STOCKER and DEHNER'S
Pediatric Pathology
FOURTH EDITION

STOCKER and DEHNER'S Pediatric Pathology

FOURTH EDITION

EDITORS

Aliya N. Husain, MD
Professor
Department of Pathology
University of Chicago
Chicago, Illinois

J. Thomas Stocker, MD
Professor of Pathology, Pediatrics, and Emerging Infectious Disease
Department of Pathology
Uniformed Services University of the Health Sciences
Bethesda, Maryland

Louis P. Dehner, MD
Professor
Division of Anatomic and Molecular Pathology
Department of Pathology and Immunology
Washington University in St. Louis
Attending Surgical Pathologist
Lauren V. Ackerman Laboratory of Surgical Pathology
Barnes-Jewish and St. Louis Children's Hospitals at the Washington University Medical Center
St. Louis, Missouri

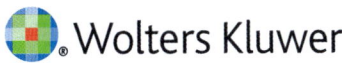

Philadelphia • Baltimore • New York • London
Buenos Aires • Hong Kong • Sydney • Tokyo

Acquisitions Editor: Ryan Shaw
Product Development Editor: Kate Marshall
Production Project Manager: David Orzechowski
Design Coordinator: Joan Wendt
Senior Manufacturing Coordinator: Beth Welsh
Marketing Manager: Dan Dressler
Prepress Vendor: SPi Global

4th edition

Copyright © 2016 Wolters Kluwer

Third Edition, Copyright © 2011 Wolters Kluwer Health / Lippincott Williams & Wilkins. Second Edition, Copyright © 2001 Lippincott Williams & Wilkins, a Wolters Kluwer business. First Edition, Copyright © 1992 by Lippincott-Raven Publishers. All rights reserved. This book is protected by copyright. No part of this book may be reproduced or transmitted in any form or by any means, including as photocopies or scanned-in or other electronic copies, or utilized by any information storage and retrieval system without written permission from the copyright owner, except for brief quotations embodied in critical articles and reviews. Materials appearing in this book prepared by individuals as part of their official duties as U.S. government employees are not covered by the above-mentioned copyright. To request permission, please contact Wolters Kluwer at Two Commerce Square, 2001 Market Street, Philadelphia, PA 19103, via email at permissions@lww.com, or via our website at lww.com (products and services).

9 8 7 6 5 4 3 2 1

Printed in China

Library of Congress Cataloging-in-Publication Data
Stocker & Dehner's pediatric pathology / editors, Aliya N. Husain, J. Thomas Stocker, Louis P. Dehner. — Fourth edition.
    p. ; cm.
Pediatric pathology
Stocker and Dehner's pediatric pathology
ISBN 978-1-4511-9373-2
 I. Husain, Aliya N., editor. II. Stocker, J. Thomas, editor. III. Dehner, Louis P., 1940-, editor. IV. Title: Pediatric pathology. V. Title: Stocker and Dehner's pediatric pathology.
   [DNLM: 1. Pathologic Processes. 2. Pediatrics. 3. Pathology—methods.   WS 200]
   RJ49
   618.92'007—dc23

2015015789

This work is provided "as is," and the publisher disclaims any and all warranties, express or implied, including any warranties as to accuracy, comprehensiveness, or currency of the content of this work.

This work is no substitute for individual patient assessment based upon healthcare professionals' examination of each patient and consideration of, among other things, age, weight, gender, current or prior medical conditions, medication history, laboratory data and other factors unique to the patient. The publisher does not provide medical advice or guidance and this work is merely a reference tool. Healthcare professionals, and not the publisher, are solely responsible for the use of this work including all medical judgments and for any resulting diagnosis and treatments.

Given continuous, rapid advances in medical science and health information, independent professional verification of medical diagnoses, indications, appropriate pharmaceutical selections and dosages, and treatment options should be made and healthcare professionals should consult a variety of sources. When prescribing medication, healthcare professionals are advised to consult the product information sheet (the manufacturer's package insert) accompanying each drug to verify, among other things, conditions of use, warnings and side effects and identify any changes in dosage schedule or contradictions, particularly if the medication to be administered is new, infrequently used or has a narrow therapeutic range. To the maximum extent permitted under applicable law, no responsibility is assumed by the publisher for any injury and/or damage to persons or property, as a matter of products liability, negligence law or otherwise, or from any reference to or use by any person of this work.

LWW.com

DEDICATION

To my mother, Khadija Omar, who has inspired me throughout my life
and in memory of my father, Zahid Omar, who saw only the
beginnings of his children's lives.
Aliya N. Husain

To my wife, Pat, the Center of my life, at 49 years together and counting,
and to our children: Rick, his wife Cathy and sons Jack and Joseph (both smarter
than I ever was); David and daughter Sydney; and Meg and her wife Melissa.
How joyful and full they make our lives.
J. Thomas Stocker

To my multigenerational family and that "other" family, my residents,
and fellows through all these rewarding years. All of you have kept me young.
Louis P. Dehner

Contributors

Hikmat A. Al-Ahmadie, MD
Assistant Attending
Department of Pathology
Memorial Sloan Kettering Cancer Center
New York, New York

Raymond G. Areaux, Jr., MD
Assistant Professor
Pediatric Ophthalmology & Strabismus
Department of Ophthalmology & Visual Neurosciences
University of Minnesota
Minneapolis, Minnesota

Jennifer Dien Bard, PhD, D(ABMM), FCCM
Director, Clinical Microbiology Laboratory
Department of Pathology and Laboratory Medicine
Children's Hospital Los Angeles
Assistant Professor
Clinical Pathology
Keck School of Medicine
University of Southern California
Los Angeles, California

Kevin E. Bove, MD
Professor
Department of Pathology
Cincinnati Children's Hospital Medical Center
Cincinnati, Ohio

Theonia K. Boyd, MD
Director, Anatomic Pathology
Department of Pathology
Boston Children's Hospital
Staff Pathologist
Division of Women's and Perinatal Pathology
Department of Pathology
Brigham and Women's Hospital
Associate Professor of Pathology
Harvard Medical School
Boston, Massachusetts

John J. Buchino, MD
Emeritus Professor
Departments of Pathology and Pediatrics
University of Louisville
Emeritus Chief
Department of Pathology
Kosair Children's Hospital
Louisville, Kentucky

Mariana M. Cajaiba, MD
Assistant Professor
Department of Pathology and Laboratory Medicine
Ann & Robert H. Lurie Children's Hospital of Chicago
Northwestern University Feinberg School of Medicine
Chicago, Illinois

J. Douglas Cameron, MD, MBA
Professor
Department of Ophthalmology and Visual Neurosciences
Director of Research
University of Minnesota
Minneapolis, Minnesota

Anthony Chang, MD
Associate Professor
Department of Pathology
University of Chicago Medical Center
Chicago, Illinois

Nicole Cipriani, MD
Assistant Professor
Department of Pathology
The University of Chicago
Chicago, Illinois

Choladda V. Curry, MD
Hematopathologist/Cytopathologist
Department of Pathology
Baylor College of Medicine/Texas Children's Hospital
Houston, Texas

Robert F. Debski, MD
Assistant Professor
Departments of Pathology and Pediatrics
University of Louisville
Chief
Department of Pathology
Kosair Children's Hospital
Louisville, Kentucky

Louis P. Dehner, MD
Professor
Division of Anatomic and Molecular Pathology
Department of Pathology and Immunology
Washington University in St. Louis
Attending Surgical Pathologist
Lauren V. Ackerman Laboratory of Surgical Pathology
Barnes-Jewish and St. Louis Children's Hospitals at the Washington University Medical Center
St. Louis, Missouri

Michelle M. Dolan, MD
Associate Professor
Department of Laboratory Medicine and Pathology
University of Minnesota Medical School
Minneapolis, Minnesota

Christopher Dunham, MD
Neuropathologist
Clinical Associate Professor
UBC Children's and Women's Health Centre of B.C.
Head
Division of Anatomic Pathology
Vancouver, British Columbia

Jonathan Eisenstat, MD
Associate Medical Examiner
Georgia Bureau of Investigation
Division of Forensic Sciences
Decatur, Georgia

Laura S. Finn, MD
Associate Pathologist
Department of Laboratories
Seattle Children's Hospital
Department of Pathology
University of Washington School of Medicine
Seattle, Washington

Michael K. Fritsch, MD, PhD
Associate Professor
Department of Pathology and Laboratory
Medicine
Ann & Robert H Lurie Children's Hospital of Chicago
Chicago, Illinois

Anjum Hassan, MD
Associate Professor
Pathology and Immunology
Director FFPE FISH in Cytogenomics and Molecular
Pathology
Washington University in St. Louis, School
of Medicine
Barnes Jewish Hospital
St. Louis, Missouri

M. John Hicks, MD, DDS, MS, PhD
Professor of Pathology
Departments of Pathology and Immunology,
and Pediatrics
Baylor College of Medicine
Texas Children's Hospital
Houston, Texas

D. Ashley Hill, MD
Chief
Division of Pathology
Children's National Medical Center
Washington, District of Columbia

Aliya N. Husain, MD
Professor
Department of Pathology
University of Chicago
Chicago, Illinois

Jason A. Jarzembowski, MD, PhD
Interim Medical Director
Pathology and Laboratory Medicine
Children's Hospital of Wisconsin
Interim Chief (Pediatric Pathology)
Associate Professor
Department of Pathology
Medical College of Wisconsin
Milwaukee, Wisconsin

Raj P. Kapur, MD, PhD
Professor
Department of Pathology
University of Washington
Seattle, Washington

Selene Koo, MD, PhD
Molecular Genetic Pathology Fellow
Department of Pathology
University of Chicago Medical Center
Chicago, Illinois

Michael Kyriakos, MD
Professor
Division of Surgical Pathology
Washington University School of Medicine
St. Louis, Missouri

Haresh Mani, MD
Pathologist
Department of Pathology
Inova Fairfax Hospital
Falls Church, Virginia

Andrea N. Marcogliese, MD
Associate Professor of Pathology & Immunology
Texas Children's Hospital
Baylor College of Medicine
Houston, Texas

Rohit Mehra, MD
Assistant Professor of Pathology
Member-Michigan Center for Translational
Pathology
MLabs Genitourinary Service Line Director
Co-Director, University of Michigan Rapid Autopsy Discovery
Program
University of Michigan Hospital and Health Systems
Ann Arbor, Michigan

Gary W. Mierau, PhD
Electron Microscopist
Pathology and Laboratory Medicine
Children's Hospital Colorado
Aurora, Colorado

Lili Miles, MD
Director, Anatomic Pathology
Department of Pathology and Laboratory Medicine
Nemours Children's Hospital
Orlando, Florida

Kamran M. Mirza, MD, PhD
Assistant Professor
Department of Pathology
Loyola University Medical Center
Maywood, Illinois

Ivan P. Moskowitz, MD, PhD
Associate Professor
Departments of Pediatrics, Pathology, and
Human Genetics
The University of Chicago
Chicago, Illinois

Rish K. Pai, MD, PhD
Associate Professor
Department of Laboratory Medicine and
Pathology
Mayo Clinic College of Medicine
Scottsdale, Arizona

David Parham, MD
Chief of Anatomic Pathology
Children's Hospital Los Angeles
Professor of Pathology
Keck School of Medicine
Los Angeles, California

Kathleen Patterson, MD
Associate Pathologist
Department of Pathology
Seattle Children's Hospital
Seattle, Washington

Arie Perry, MD
Professor of Pathology and Neurological Surgery
Director of Neuropathology and Neuropathology Fellowship
Program
University of California, San Francisco
Department of Pathology, Division of
Neuropathology
San Francisco, California

Jennifer Pogoriler, MD, PhD
Assistant Professor
Department of Pathology and Laboratory
Medicine
The Children's Hospital of Philadelphia
Philadelphia, Pennsylvania

Peter Pytel, MD
Associate Professor
Director of Neuropathology
Department of Pathology
The University of Chicago
Chicago, Illinois

Sarangarajan Ranganathan, MD
Medical Director, Anatomic Pathology
Children's Hospital of Pittsburgh of UPMC
Professor
Department of Pathology
University of Pittsburgh
Pittsburgh, Pennsylvania

Vijaya B. Reddy, MD, MBA
Professor and Associate Chair
Department of Pathology
Rush Medical College
Chicago, Illinois

Raymond W. Redline, MD
Professor of Pathology and Reproductive Biology
Case Western Reserve University School of Medicine
Section Leader: Pediatric Pathology, Gynecologic Pathology
University Hospitals Case Medical Center
Cleveland, Ohio

Robyn C. Reed, MD, PhD
Pathologist
Department of Pathology
Children's Hospitals and Clinics of Minnesota
Minneapolis, Minnesota

Pierre A. Russo, MD
Chief of Anatomic Pathology
The Children's Hospital of Philadelphia
Perelman School of Medicine at the University of
Pennsylvania
Philadelphia, Pennsylvania

Hiroyuki Shimada, MD, PhD, FRCPA
Pathologist
Department of Pathology and Laboratory Medicine
Children's Hospital Los Angeles
Professor
University of Southern California Keck School of Medicine
Los Angeles, California

Joseph R. Siebert, PhD
Professor
Departments of Pathology and Pediatrics
University of Washington
Department of Laboratories
Seattle Children's Hospital
Seattle, Washington

J. Thomas Stocker, MD
Professor of Pathology, Pediatrics and Emerging Infectious
Disease
Department of Pathology
Uniformed Services University of the Health Sciences
Bethesda, Maryland

Mariko Suchi, MD, PhD
Associate Professor
Department of Pathology
Medical College of Wisconsin
Department of Pathology and Laboratory Medicine
Children's Hospital of Wisconsin
Milwaukee, Wisconsin

Darrel Waggoner, MD
Professor
Department of Human Genetics
Department of Pediatrics
The University of Chicago
Chicago, Illinois

Eric P. Wartchow, PhD
Electron Microscopist
Pathology and Laboratory Medicine
Children's Hospital Colorado
Aurora, Colorado

Jerry T. Wong, MD, PhD
Resident
Department of Pathology
University of Chicago
Chicago, Illinois

Xiangdong Xu, MD, PhD
Assistant Professor
Department of Pathology
University of California San Diego VA
San Diego Health System
San Diego, California

Preface

Given the pace of new findings, many driven by first- and second-generation molecular studies, the only means of maintaining currency in any reference text such as this fourth edition is an online publication with weekly or monthly updates. However, any reference with succeeding editions should strive to maintain the basic information with its less mutable cove to which are added the latest findings and observations. We have encouraged our fellow authors to keep these principles in mind as they have gone through their chapters.

As we reflect on this current edition in light of the history of this text from its first edition in 1992, it remains the comprehensive volume on all major aspects of the pathologic anatomy of childhood disorders. The editors would like to thank the various experts who have shared their knowledge and insights to make the last three editions so valuable to readers.

This edition is also an opportunity to consider the future of pediatric pathology in this period of organ and system-based subspecialty pathology. Even within the confines of a children's hospital, there are the pediatric hematopathologists, pediatric-gastrointestinal pathologists, and the list goes on. The pediatric pathologist generalist is unlikely to find himself or herself in competition for the perinatal–neonatal autopsy since there is no CPT code for that important activity. From the first edition, we have been particularly attentive to those questions that are posed to us about a baby who has been denied a postnatal existence or who only experienced it for a few brief moments or days. As pediatric pathologists, we find ourselves in the unique position to provide some answers to questions in the case of a too brief life.

We see this current edition as a small light to help illuminate the large world inhabited by small people—children. We have once again been joined by a group of fellow pathologists who append "pediatric" in front of the pathologist. We have all labored for the same purpose to provide for you who will take this reference from your shelf in the hope of finding "the answer." We have done our best to at least help the reader to get started on the road to finding "the answer." After all, finding the answer is a process which is sometimes a beginning and not the end.

Preface to the First Edition

Several years ago, the editors of this volume were lamenting the fact that a third edition of Kissane's *Pathology of Infancy and Childhood* was unlikely because John Kissane had committed himself to another formidable publishing enterprise. Our British colleagues in pediatric pathology have authored two fine references (Keeling's *Fetal and Neonatal Pathology* and Berry's *Paediatric Pathology*), but it was our opinion that a comprehensive volume on all major aspects of the pathologic anatomy of childhood disorders ranging from chromosomal syndromes and neoplasms to forensic pathology was needed. At this juncture in our deliberations, we were confronted with the daunting nature of the potential task at hand given the required range of expertise necessary to cover all of these areas. Our attention turned to the reservoir of such abilities that exists in an organization of which we are privileged to be members, the Society for Pediatric Pathology, formerly known as the Pediatric Pathology Club. Many of the contributors to this volume are friends and colleagues whom we met through the Society for Pediatric Pathology.

It was Albert Einstein who acknowledged the fact that we all stand on the shoulders of giants, and certainly pediatric pathology has evolved to its present state through the seminal contributions of the "first" generation of North American pediatric pathologists. Some of these include Maude Abbott, Dorothy Andersen, James B. Arey, J. Bruce Beckwith, Jay Bernstein, William A. Blanc, Robert P. Bolande, John Craig, John R. Esterly, Sidney Farber, George Fetterman, Enid Gilbert-Barness, M. Daria Haust, John M. Kissane, Benjamin H. Landing, A. James McAdams, Harry B. Neustein, William A. Newton, Ella Oppenheimer, Eugene V. Perrin, Edith Potter, Harvey S. Rosenberg, Marie Valdes-Dapena, Gordon Vawter, and F.W. Wigglesworth, to mention only a few. Virtually all of us in the second and now third generation of pediatric pathologists can call one of these extraordinary individuals our mentor.

Because we the editors are also the coauthors of several chapters in this textbook, we appreciate firsthand the many hours that our contributors have invested in the completion of their manuscripts. The time, experience, and patience necessary to compile information into the concise prose required by a textbook of this type are greatly appreciated. This textbook belongs to all of these authors collectively, despite the connotations of the cover and title page.

We also thank our colleagues and friends at our respective institutions for their understanding and support during the prolonged gestation and difficult delivery of this textbook. At the Armed Forces Institute of Pathology, these include Robert McMeekin, MD, Robert F. Karnei, MD, Vernon Armbrustmacher, MD, Nancy Roberts, Luther Duckett, Lisa Penalver, and Venetia Valiga. At the University of Minnesota, Ellis S. Benson, MD, Dale Snover, MD, and Diane Perez, and at the Washington University Medical Center, Emil Unanue, MD, Mark R. Wick, MD, Eleanor Grob, and Patricia Dixon are recognized for their special support.

J. Thomas Stocker, MD
Louis P. Dehner, MD

Acknowledgments

Dr. Husain would like to acknowledge the strong support and academic environment provided by Dr. Thomas Krausz, Vice Chair and Director of Anatomic Pathology, and Dr. Vinay Kumar, Chairman of Pathology, University of Chicago.

Dr. Dehner would like to acknowledge the herculean efforts of Jeannie Doerr who provided encouragement throughout this process. Linda Hankins arrived at the right time so that this project could be completed. Another member of the team, Margaret Chesney, was able to bring clarity especially for the many tables in his chapters. Once again Walter Clermont provided his skills as a medical photographer par excellence to guarantee the highest quality of illustrations.

Contents

section I General Pathology

Chapter 1 Techniques in Pediatric Pathology
  Chapter 1A The Pediatric Autopsy 1
    J. Thomas Stocker

  Chapter 1B Fine-Needle Aspiration 18
    John J. Buchino and Robert F. Debski

  Chapter 1C Molecular Techniques in Pediatric Pathology 21
    Jason A. Jarzembowski and D. Ashley Hill

  Chapter 1D Electron Microscopy 51
    Gary W. Mierau, Eric P. Wartchow, and M. John Hicks

Chapter 2 First and Second Trimester Pregnancy Loss 60
  Jennifer Pogoriler and Theonia K. Boyd

Chapter 3 Chromosomal Abnormalities 77
  Robyn C. Reed, Michelle M. Dolan, Raj P. Kapur, and Joseph R. Siebert

Chapter 4 Congenital Anomalies and Malformation Syndromes 103
  Joseph R. Siebert

Chapter 5 Inborn Errors of Metabolism 135
  Peter Pytel, Selene Koo, and Darrel Waggoner

Chapter 6 Congenital and Acquired Systemic Infectious Diseases 194
  Haresh Mani, David Parham, and Jennifer Dien Bard

Chapter 7 Pediatric Forensic Pathology 260
  Jonathan Eisenstat

Chapter 8 Transplant Pathology 292
  Rish K. Pai, Anthony Chang, and Aliya N. Husain

section II Organ System Pathology

Chapter 9 The Placenta 325
  Raymond W. Redline

Chapter 10 The Nervous System 351
  Christopher Dunham and Arie Perry

Chapter 11 The Eye 410
  J. Douglas Cameron and Raymond G. Areaux, Jr.

Chapter 12 The Respiratory Tract 444
  Louis P. Dehner, J. Thomas Stocker, Haresh Mani, D. Ashley Hill, and Aliya N. Husain

Chapter 13 The Cardiovascular System 524
  Ivan P. Moskowitz, Selene Koo, Aliya N. Husain, and Kathleen Patterson

Chapter 14 The Gastrointestinal Tract 581
  Pierre A. Russo

Chapter 15 The Liver, Gallbladder, and Biliary Tract 654
  Sarangarajan Ranganathan and M. John Hicks

Chapter 16 The Pancreas 763
  Mariko Suchi

Chapter 17 The Kidney and Lower Urinary Tract 800
  Laura S. Finn and Aliya N. Husain

Chapter 18 The Female Reproductive System 865
  Michael K. Fritsch and Mariana M. Cajaiba

Chapter 19 The Male Reproductive System, Including Intersex Disorders 894
  Hikmat A. Al-Ahmadie and Rohit Mehra

Chapter 20 Breast 927
  Louis P. Dehner

Chapter 21 The Pineal, Pituitary, Parathyroid, Thyroid, and Adrenal Glands 947
  M. John Hicks, Nicole Cipriani, Peter Pytel, and Hiroyuki Shimada

Chapter 22 Oral, Maxillofacial, Head and Neck Pathology in Pediatrics 1019
  M. John Hicks

Chapter 23 The Lymph Nodes, Spleen, and Thymus 1057
  Kamran M. Mirza, Choladda V. Curry, and Andrea N. Marcogliese

Chapter 24 The Bone Marrow 1092
  Xiangdong Xu and Anjum Hassan

Chapter 25 Soft Tissue 1124
  Louis P. Dehner, D. Ashley Hill, and Jason A. Jarzembowski

Chapter 26 The Skin 1214
  Vijaya B. Reddy

Chapter 27 Neuromuscular Diseases 1256
  Kevin E. Bove and Lili Miles

Chapter 28 Skeletal System 1298
  Louis P. Dehner and Michael Kyriakos

List of Appendices 1387
Index 1435

SECTION I
General Pathology

CHAPTER 1A

The Pediatric Autopsy

J. Thomas Stocker, M.D.

As described by the Autopsy Committee of the College of American Pathologists, the autopsy is "a medical–surgical procedure by a physician for the welfare of the living through the study of those patients for whom all our current knowledge and technology were inadequate" (1). The use of the autopsy in medicine as a tool of discovery and education has declined frighteningly in the past 25 years, with some newer hospitals not even including an autopsy suite in their design. In many hospitals, including university hospitals, the autopsy incidence (autopsies compared to number of deaths) has dropped well below 20%, often reaching as low as 2% to 5%. Pediatric hospitals have historically had a higher incidence, often as high as 75% or more, but in recent years, this incidence has declined as well. In a survey in 2005 (by the author) of 15 children's hospitals, the autopsy rate for in-hospital deaths varied from 15% to 48% with an average of 32%, and that figure represented a 5% to 10% drop from the rate in 2000 at these same children's hospitals.

Many excellent textbooks and protocols have been written describing methods for performing an autopsy. The following is a technique the author has developed over the past 40 years, often incorporating many techniques from these textbooks and colleagues' experience. This type of autopsy has proven useful to the author, but is by no means the only procedure that might be used.

THE STANDARD PEDIATRIC AUTOPSY

Autopsy Permit

The first step with any autopsy is examination of the autopsy permit for its completeness. This includes a determination of the nature of the death of the patient and whether it may be under medical examiner jurisdiction (i.e., a coroner's case). It is imperative that the pathologist performing the autopsy be intimately familiar with the criteria for medical examiner jurisdiction in the community in which the patient died. The College of American Pathology maintains a state-by-state file of these criteria (www.CAP.org).

Following examination of the autopsy permit, the clinical chart of the patient should be reviewed and a call placed (if possible) to the attending physician or other members of the medical team responsible for the patient. In addition to a review of the clinical or hospital course of the patient, the medical team should be asked what questions they might have that the autopsy should address.

A variety of forms and protocols are available for the pediatric autopsy, and one of these might be used or one designed specifically to address the types of patients in a particular hospital.

Instrumentation

The instruments used in performing the pediatric autopsy are often quite different than those used in adult autopsies, both in type and size (Figure 1A-1). Pediatric autopsies, particularly those done on fetuses and neonates, require smaller and more delicate instruments than the "full-sized" instruments used on larger children or adults (Table 1A-1). In morgues where adult autopsies are also done, it is often wise to keep the instruments used for the pediatric autopsy in a separate area, even under lock and key, if necessary, to assure they are not used (and abused) doing autopsies on adults.

External Examination

The external examination of the body is one of the most important aspects of the pediatric autopsy for it offers information about the general health of the infant/child, offers

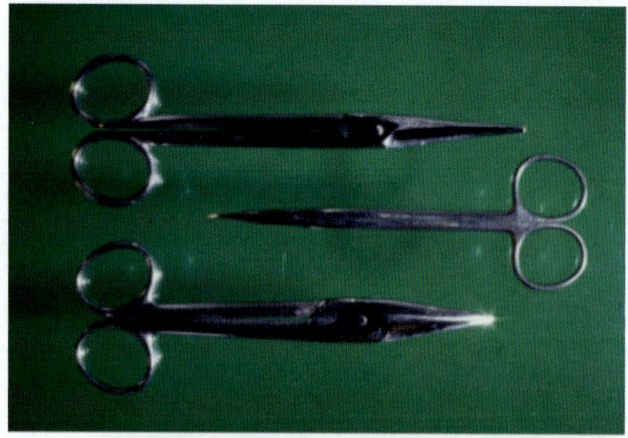

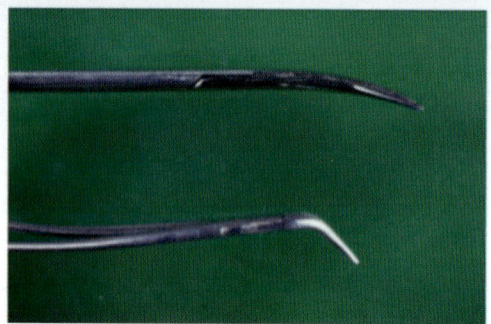

FIGURE 1A-1 • **Top:** Small instruments such as these scissors that are proportional to the size of the infant are vital to the performance of the autopsy. **Bottom:** Curved and tapered ends are helpful in dissecting and holding tissues.

as measurements, photographs, and descriptive phrases, accuracy and completeness of the examination are all the more important.

General measurements include body weight, body length (crown–heel and crown–rump [in neonates]) (Figure 1A-2), arm span from the tip of the fingers of one hand to the tip of the fingers on the other hand (which in most cases approximates the crown–heel length) (eFigure 1A-1), and head (occiput to frontal) (Figure 1A-3), chest (at level of nipples) (eFigure 1A-1), and abdominal (at level of umbilicus) circumference (eFigure 1A-2). This information can be recorded in the autopsy description or on drawings included in the final autopsy report. External markings such as needle marks, IV tubes, chest tubes, incisions, abrasions, etc. also need to be recorded and can be illustrated on standard drawings (eFigure 1A-4). These measurements are particularly important when performing a "forensic autopsy" (see Chapter 7).

FACE, EYES, EARS, MOUTH (EXTERNAL AND INTERNAL)

Examination of the *face* begins with an overall view to determine symmetry and gross abnormalities. As facial abnormalities often predict brain abnormalities, special attention should be paid to midfacial development (hypertelorism/hypotelorism, nasal bridge deformities) and hair patterns. The hair growth pattern usually consists of one or two whorls in the upper occipital/parietal area. More than two whorls or actual defects in the scalp (eFigure 1A-2) are often associated with underlying CNS abnormalities. The anterior and posterior fontanelles should be examined for their size (maximum length and width), shape, and "fullness"

evidence of therapy, and portends what might be expected when the body is opened. And since, with the exception of skin sections taken for microscopic examination, the "shell" of the patient will be documented and recorded only

TABLE 1A-1	INSTRUMENTS USED IN PERFORMING THE PEDIATRIC AUTOPSY

Scissors
 a. Thin, small, with tapered points and curved tip, used more for dissection than cutting. Limit their use to soft tissues, and organs, not for bone, cartilage, or dense tissues.
 b. Medium sized, straight, or curved for opening bowel.
 c. Large or heavier ones for opening calvarium and vertebral column.

Forceps
 a. Small and medium sized, but WITHOUT teeth (which only tears tissue)

Hemostats
 a. Small and medium sized
 b. Straight and curved

Scalpels
 a. No. 10 size curved for most routine work
 b. No. 1 size with pointed tip for delicate cutting
 c. Double edged, rectangular for sectioning organs such as the spleen, lung, liver, and kidneys

Knives
 a. Straight, of various sizes for sectioning larger organs such as the liver, brain, or organs of larger children

Balances for weighing
 a. Standard hanging balance for weighing neonates or small children
 b. Electronic balance (accurate to 0.1 g) for weighing organs

Probes of various diameters to establish patency of various openings including nares, ears, ureters, urethra, biliary tract, heart valves, patency of foramen ovale, and ductus arteriosus.

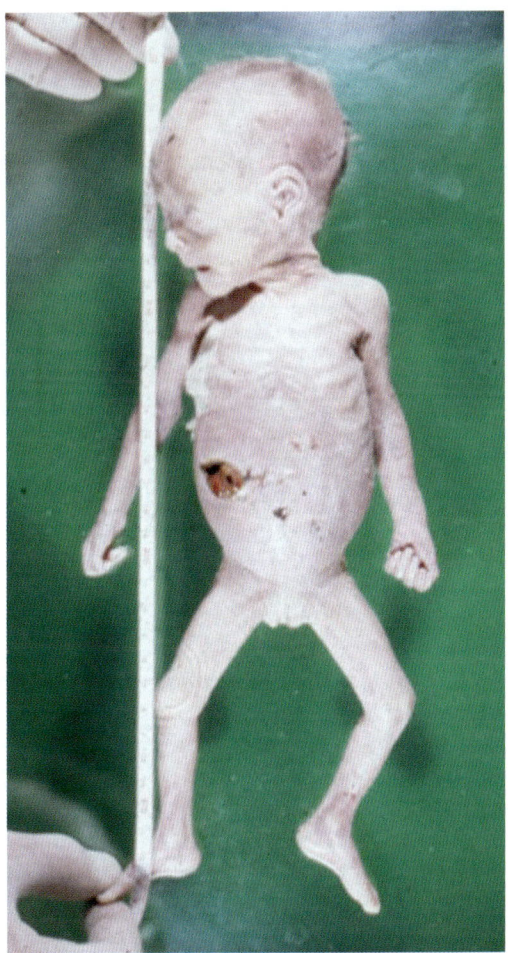

FIGURE 1A-2 • Full body view showing crown-heel measurement.

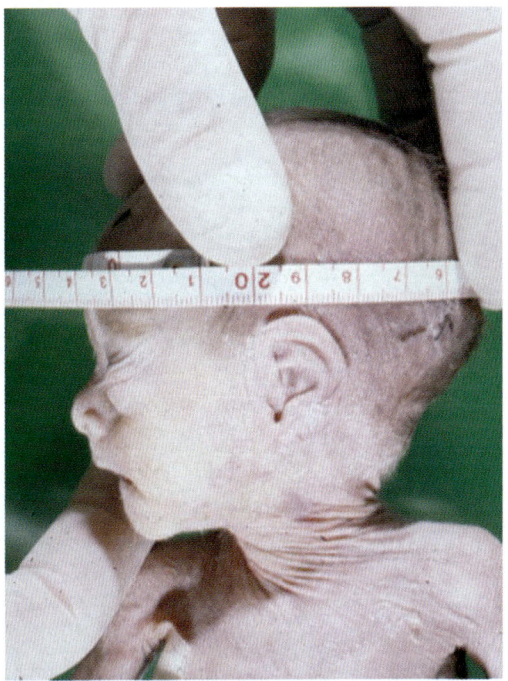

FIGURE 1A-3 • Head circumference is measured in the frontal–occipital plane.

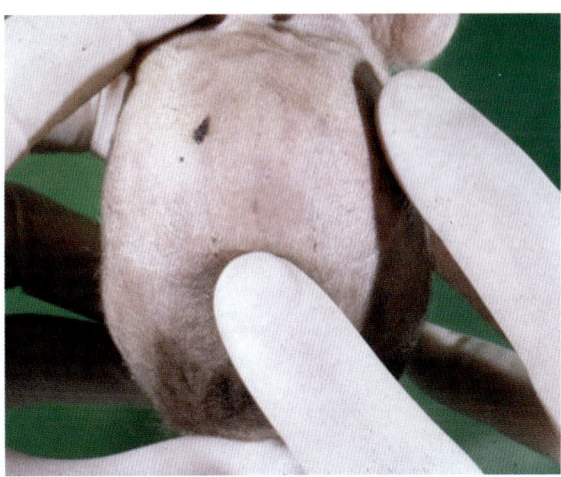

FIGURE 1A-4 • Head examination includes palpation and measurement of the anterior fontanelle.

(i.e., bulging, depressed) (Figure 1A-4). The *neck* should be flexed and extended as far as possible to determine its range of motion (Figure 1A-5A, B).

The *eyes* are examined for both size and location. The measurement of each palpebral fissure should, in a normal infant, equal the intercanthal distance (Figure 1A-6) effectively dividing the face at the level of the eyes into three equal expanses. If the fissure length exceeds the intercanthal distance, the eyes are closer together than normal (hypotelorism), and conversely, if the intercanthal distance exceeds the palpebral fissure length, the eyes are too far apart (hypertelorism).

Examination of the eye itself includes the diameter of each pupil and comparison with each other to determine if the eyes are of equal size (eFigure 1A-3). If one is smaller than the other, microphthalmia may be present. If there is a question, the eyeballs may be removed from within the cranium after the brain is removed (see CNS examination). The pupils are also examined for their symmetry and completeness (vs. aniridia) and their color (which may be difficult to determine in a premature infant).

The *nose* examination includes its position and shape (e.g., upturned, flat) with evaluation of cartilage development. A curved probe can be used to determine the patency of the choanae (posterior nasal apertures) (Figure 1A-7). The lip beneath the nose (the prolabium) should be observed and determined if longer than usual (associated with the fetal alcohol syndrome).

Examination of the *ears* begins with determining their position on the side of the head relative to the level of the palpebral fissures. In near-term and term infants, the tip of the ears should be above the level of the palpebral fissures, or they are considered to be "low set." As the ears develop *in utero*, they "move" upward as the lower face and jaw develop and expand, reaching and then rising above the palpebral fissure level in late third trimester.

The ears are also examined for patency of the external auditory canal (via small caliber probe) by pulling down

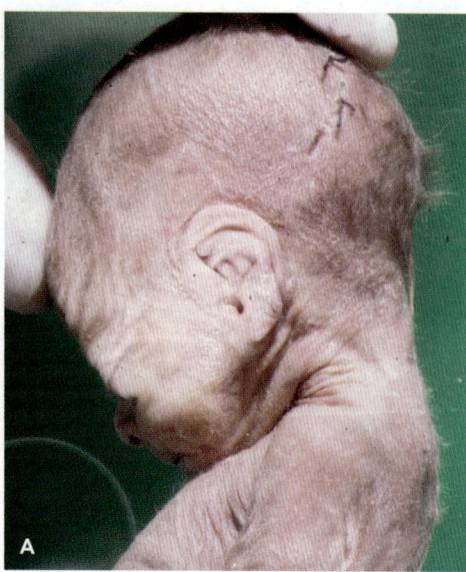
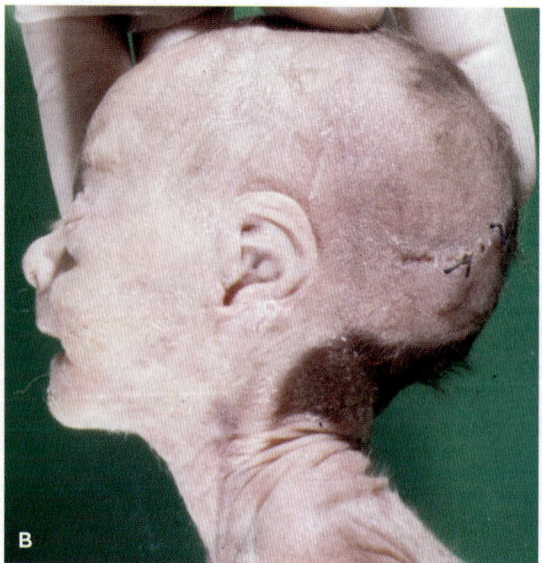

FIGURE 1A-5 • Check the mobility of the neck by flexing **(A)** and extending **(B)** it.

on the earlobe as the probe is inserted (Figure 1A-8). The external ear (pinna or auricle) should be evaluated for its shape and completeness and for the presence of cartilage.

The *mouth* should be inspected both externally and internally. A finger can be inserted into the mouth to examine the alveolar ridges of the jaw for the presence (or absence) of teeth and for determination of the shape and completeness of the palate (eFigure 1A-4). The tongue can be palpated as well but may also be removed intact after the thoracic organs have been removed (see below).

ARMS, HANDS, FINGERS

The *upper extremities* are examined for symmetry, mobility, and the presence of skin lesions. The *axilla* should be palpated for the presence of lymph nodes or other masses. The positioning and mobility of the fingers should be noted along with their length. Some chromosomal anomalies (e.g., trisomies 13 and 18) may produce an overlapping of the little finger over the fourth finger and the index finger over the third finger (eFigure 1A-5). Children with Down syndrome (trisomy 21) often display short metacarpals and phalanges and hypoplasia of the midphalanx of the fifth finger (eFigure 1A-6). Nails should be examined for the presence of hypoplasia or dysplasia. Radiographs of the extremities may be helpful in identifying skeletal abnormalities (e.g., radial hypoplasia of the VATER association) or recent or old fractures. In fact, in cases of suspected nonaccidental trauma (NAT), a full skeletal survey would be important.

The *palms of the hands* should be examined for aberrant patterning, most notably for the presence of a simian crease or a malpositioned axial triradius, common findings in Down syndrome but also seen in a wide variety of other syndromes.

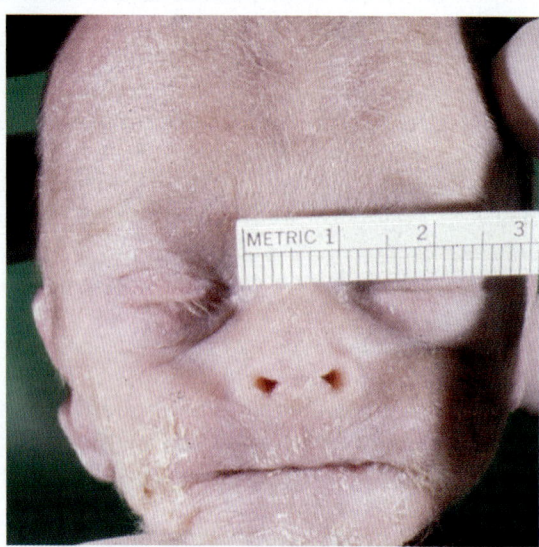

FIGURE 1A-6 • Measuring the intercanthal distance.

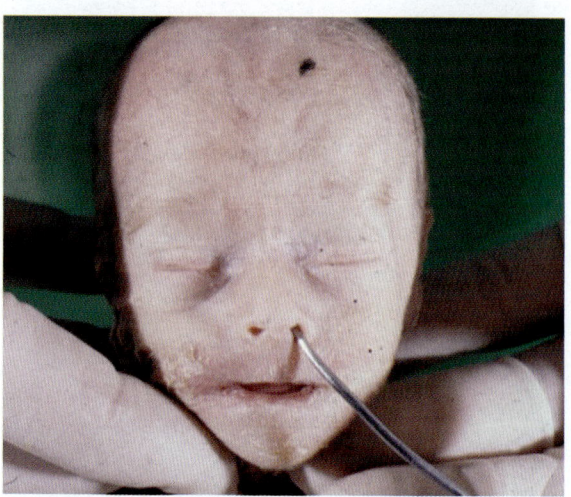

FIGURE 1A-7 • Examination of the nose includes checking for the patency of each naris into the upper pharynx with a probe or curved suturing needle.

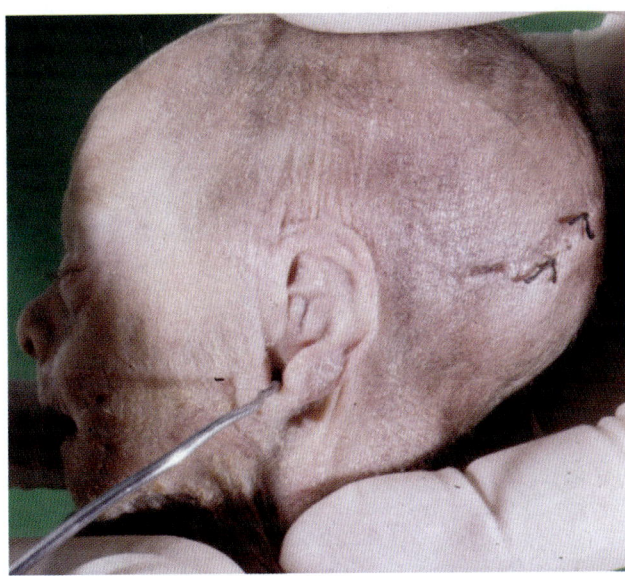

FIGURE 1A-8 • Probing the external auditory canal.

CHEST: FRONT AND BACK

Examination of the chest begins with the determination of its symmetry, position of the nipples, and length and positioning of the sternum (e.g., pectus excavatum or carinatum). The junction of the neck with the chest should be examined to note the shape and the length of the neck (short neck or webbed skin). The clavicles should be palpated for degree of development (e.g., hypoplasia) and the presence of fractures. Breast development should be determined using a system such as the Tanner stage I to V system (2).

Turning the body over or rolling it on its side allows examination of the back for symmetry (e.g., scoliosis, lordosis) and the presence of lesions. Particularly important in infants is the presence of spinal and vertebral column defects indicative of meningomyelocele and spina bifida, remembering that one form, spinal bifida occulta, may not be visible as a skin defect.

At this point, prior to the opening of the chest and abdomen, aspiration of the thorax for air, blood, and/or fluid can be performed. In young children, in particular, the presence of air or fluid in each hemithorax can be determined as well as its amount. With the body in the supine position, a 12- to 14-gauge needle on a 5- to 25-mL syringe (depending on the size of the child), can be inserted parallel to the autopsy table at the rib–sternal junction between the 4th and 5th or 5th and 6th ribs, being careful to avoid the heart (Figure 1A-9). When inserted through the parietal pleura, aspiration of air or fluid within the free space of the hemithorax can be attempted. If nothing is present as the syringe plunger is pulled back, the plunger when released will move back toward the needle. If air or fluid is present, it will be withdrawn as the plunger is pulled back until it can no longer be done. At this point, the amount of fluid/air in the syringe can be measured and, if a sterile draw has been done, the fluid may be sent for culture. If the plunger is pulled back to its maximum length, the needle and/or syringe can be removed, the amount of air/fluid can be measured and expelled from the syringe, and then the needle and/or syringe can be reinserted into the same needle hole for aspiration of as much air/fluid as is left (repeating as many times as needed). The same procedure can then be performed on the other hemithorax. This allows for an accurate measurement of the amount of pneumothorax, hemithorax, or transudate/exudate present on each side.

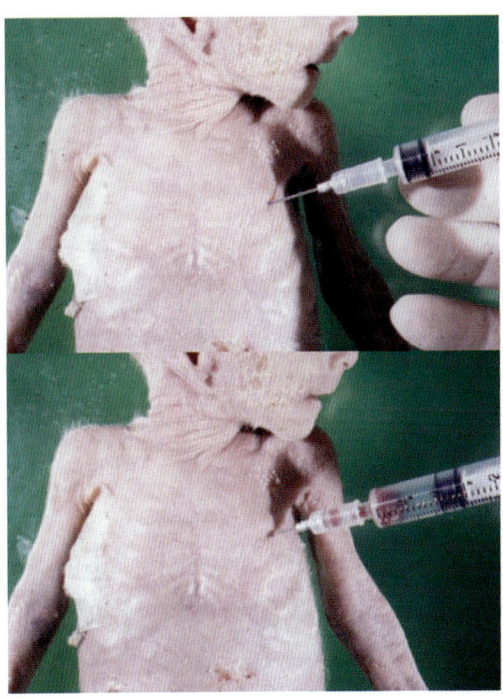

FIGURE 1A-9 • **Top**: A needle is inserted between the upper ribs at an angle parallel to the sternum. **Bottom**: If air or fluid is present in the thorax, it can be withdrawn and measured (or cultured, if appropriate cleansing is performed).

ABDOMEN: FRONT AND BACK INCLUDING ANUS/VAGINA, URETHRA

The shape of the abdomen should be evaluated looking for distension (e.g., ascites or abdominal air), depression (e.g., secondary to dehydration), and wall thickness (edema, muscular atrophy, etc.). Sterile aspiration of abdominal fluid may be performed for culture prior to incising the abdominal wall. Signs of premortem medical intervention such as needle marks or incisions should be recorded. In newborn infants, the umbilicus should be examined for evidence of inflammation or necrosis and, if present, the stump of the umbilical cord may be examined for the presence of two umbilical arteries and one umbilical vein. Discoloration of the abdominal wall may indicate underlying hemorrhage, infection, or gastrointestinal necrosis as in neonatal necrotizing enterocolitis (eFigure 1A-7).

The external genitalia can be examined for anatomic development and, in infant boys, the presence or absence of

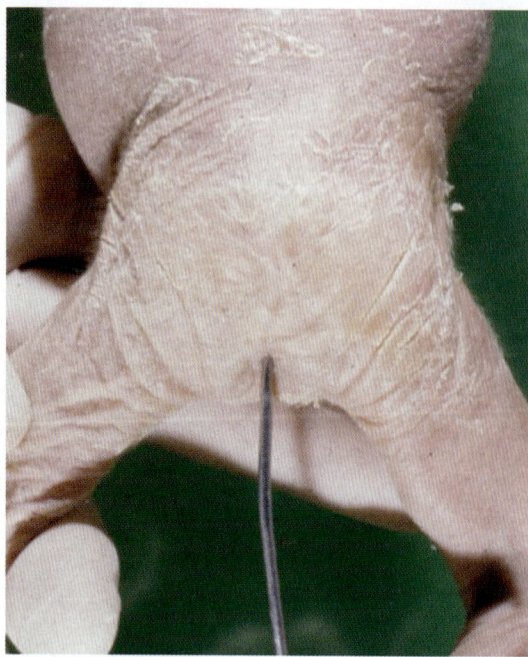

FIGURE 1A-10 • The anus (and penis or vagina) should be probed for patency.

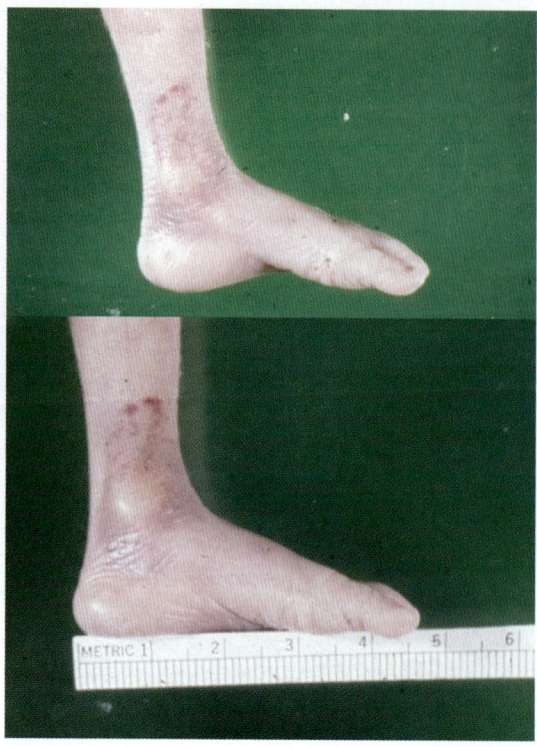

FIGURE 1A-11 • Examination of the foot includes its overall development and configuration (arched versus "rocker-bottom") (**top**) as well as its length (**bottom**), which correlates with gestational age.

testes in the scrotum should be noted along with the size and development of the penis. A staging system can be used to describe pubic hair growth in male and females. In females, the patency of the vaginal opening may be determined with a probe (eFigure 1A-8). Similarly, the anus should be probed for patency in neonates, recognizing that anal atresia may be higher than the anal opening (Figure 1A-10). The presence of meconium is a clear sign of anal patency.

LEGS, FEET, TOES

The lower extremities should be examined for symmetry and length (i.e., in proportion to trunk and arm length). In infants, the hips can be rotated to determine laxity. Feet should be examined for the presence of an arch to the sole (Figure 1A-11), versus a "rocker-bottom" configuration as may be seen with certain trisomies (eFigure 1A-9). Five toes should be present on each foot, and the spaces between toes should be of equal depth.

Special Techniques and Studies
Photography

Photography is an integral and highly important part of any autopsy, particularly images of abnormalities or gross pathology for which microscopic sections may be inadequate documentation. And with the availability of digital technology, many photographs can be taken with the "excess or unnecessary" images easily removed at no cost. While fixed photography equipment is useful, a handheld camera is more easily utilized and encourages the taking of images throughout the performance of the autopsy.

Basic images should include the external surface of the body (front and back) and anterior and lateral views of the face. Incisions and other surface marks on the face trunk and extremities may be photographed and documented particularly in cases of suspected NAT. A ruler placed at the edge of the picture helps define the dimensions of a lesion. Images of internal organs are taken as needed to document anatomic abnormalities or specific pathologic changes (e.g., necrosis, hemorrhage).

Radiography

Imaging via x-rays, MRI, or CT can be important in diagnosing and documenting skeletal abnormalities from chondrodysplasias to fractures. They may also be helpful in recording the presence of such things as pneumothorax, pneumopericardium, and pneumoperitoneum, along with documenting the extent of tumor involvement in metastatic diseases.

LABORATORY TECHNIQUES
Cultures

"Standard" cultures (aerobic and anaerobic bacterial) of blood, lung, and CSF may be taken, or appropriate cultures (fungal and/or viral) might be determined as the clinical history suggests or as the autopsy progresses and signs of infection are noted (e.g., cloudy abdominal fluid in peritonitis or aspirated fluid from an unsuspected cyst or abscess).

Unusual studies are those that extend beyond the limits of the standard autopsy as described in the autopsy permit, for example, examination of the organs of the chest and abdomen, and the brain. Removal of the eyes or long bones of the arms and legs might be needed to diagnose diseases of the eyes or to define a particular type of musculoskeletal dysplasia. (Special permission for these procedures may be needed.)

Cytogenetics

Tissue for cell culture should be taken as soon as possible after death (and having the autopsy permit signed and witnessed). Chromosome studies should be considered in embryos and fetuses when the maternal history or the appearance of the embryo/fetus suggests the presence of chromosomal abnormalities. "Large" chromosomal abnormalities such as trisomies or deletion of a major portion of a long or a short arm are often associated with significant external abnormalities such as midline defects (facial dysmorphia), hand or feet changes (syndactyly, "rocker-bottom" feet), and scalp defects (see Chapters 3 and 4).

The source of the tissue is dependent on the time after death in which the sample is obtained (see below).

Internal Examination

Chest and Abdomen

Unless the clinical history or appearance of the body suggests otherwise (e.g., a large gastroschisis or previous thoracic or abdominal surgery with sutured incisions still present), the opening of the body is most commonly done via a "Y"-shaped incision (Figure 1A-12) or some variation (e.g., "U"-shaped over chest with extension to the symphysis pubis). In either case, the incision begins in the anterior axillary line at the level of the clavicle and extends to the xiphoid just below the sternum and then up to the opposite anterior axillary line. In a neonate or infant, the chest incision can be positioned through or adjacent to the nipples to allow sampling of breast tissue while obtaining a section of skin. Subcutaneous tissue may also be measured (thickness) (eFigure 1A-10) and observed to determine the state of nutrition of the infant or the state of hydration. Edema can often be noted in the subcutaneous tissue of the chest. From the point below the xiphoid, the incision is extended toward the symphysis pubis on either side of the umbilicus. The skin of the chest and abdomen is reflected to either side after dissecting it free from the sternum and thoracic cage (eFigure 1A-11). The abdominal skin is freed along the lower rib margin.

The following measurements may be made prior to removing the chest plate (Figure 1A-13). The size of the liver is judged by measuring the distance that it extends below the rib margin (assuming no diaphragmatic hernia is present). Measurements are made in the anterior axillary lines, the midclavicular line, and the midline (eFigures 1A-12 and 1A-13). If the liver does not extend to the left anterior axillary line, the distance it does extend to the left can be recorded by measuring the distance from the midline to where it disappears beneath the rib margin (eFigure 1A-14). Other measurements include

1. The distance the spleen tip extends below (or above) the rib margin.
2. The distance the gallbladder extends above or below the margin of the liver—done primarily to see that a gallbladder is present.
3. The distance the urinary bladder extends above the symphysis pubis.

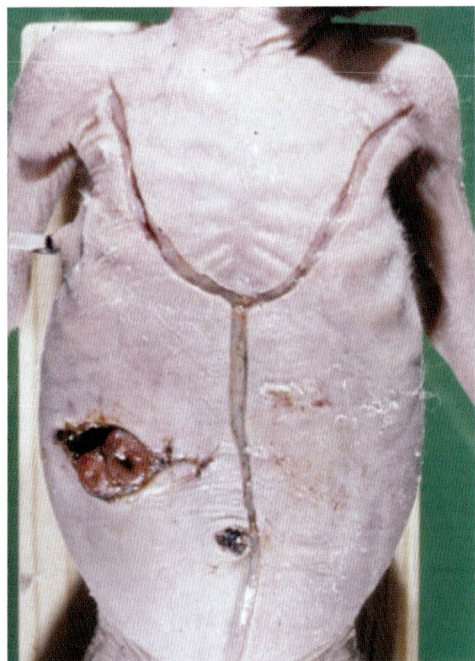

FIGURE 1A-12 • A "standard" Y-shaped incision is used to gain access to the thorax and abdomen. Note the gastronomy site in the right upper quadrant.

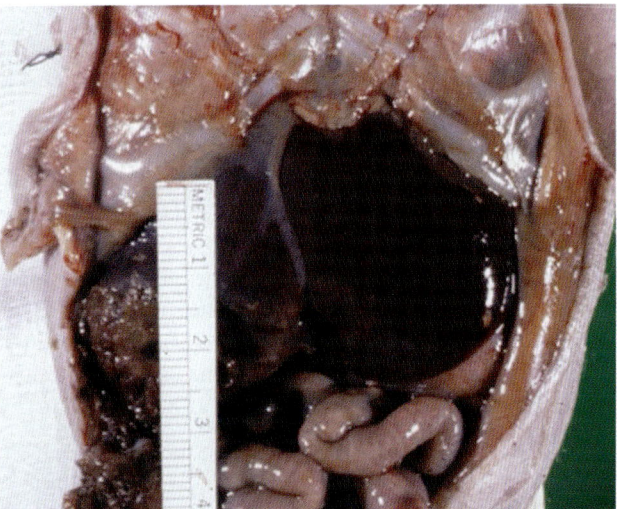

FIGURE 1A-13 • With the abdomen open, but before removal of the chest plate, the abdominal organs can be examined. Here, the size of the liver is determined by measuring its extension below the lower sternal border, in this measurement in the right midclavicular line.

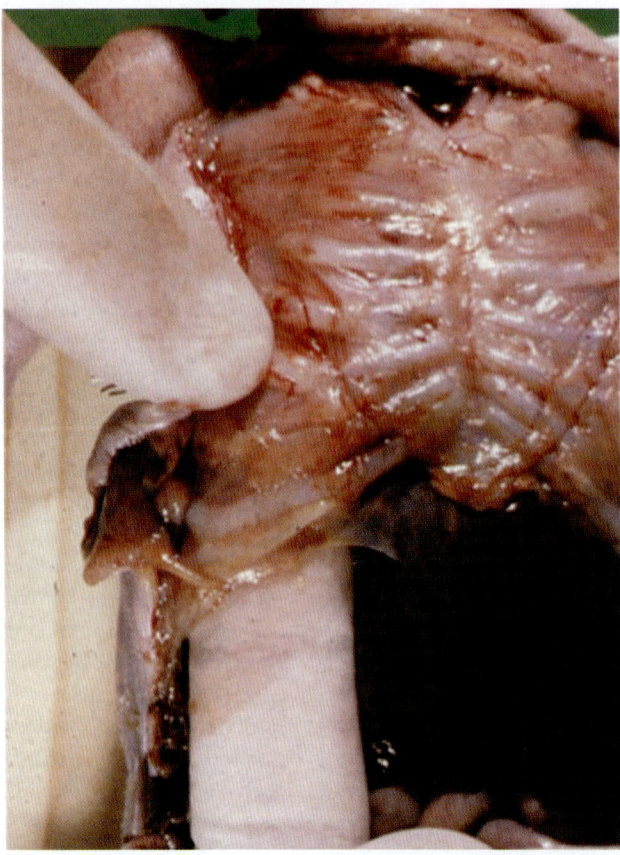

FIGURE 1A-14 • The height of the diaphragm is measured by inserting a finger up under the lower sternal border and palpating its upward extension to the highest rib or intercostal space.

4. The root and the radius of the mesentery. The root is determined by moving the bowel toward the upper right quadrant and measuring the length of its attachment to the vertebral column (eFigure 1A-15). The radius is determined by placing one end of a ruler on the vertebral column where the mesentery attaches and pulling up a segment of small bowel and measuring the distance from the vertebral column to where it attaches at the mesenteric border of the bowel (eFigure 1A-16).
5. The amount the diaphragm leaflets are pushed up into the thorax by the abdominal organs. This is done by placing a finger beneath the rib margin in the right and left midclavicular line and feeling how high the leaflets extend (Figure 1A-14). This is determined by noting where one can feel one's finger in relationship to a rib or intercostal space (e.g., 5th intercostal space or 6th rib) (eFigure 1A-17). This measurement is significant for determining whether the diaphragm leaflets are intact and whether air or fluid (e.g., blood, pus) in the thorax has forced the leaflets down.

THYMUS

The thymus in infants is often quite large and may obstruct the view of the pericardium and great vessels of the heart. It is usually helpful to dissect the thymus free from the other chest organs and weigh it before proceeding to the examination of the heart and lungs. Care must be taken to include the portion of the thymus that extends "outside" the chest into the cervical tissues of the neck.

BLOOD CULTURE

When a blood-borne infection is suspected, a blood culture may be obtained prior to dissecting the cardiovascular system. An easy approach is to open the pericardial sac and, after measuring any fluid that may be present, use a needle and syringe (after searing the surface of the right atrium with a heated spatula) (eFigure 1A-18A,B) to withdraw blood for culture (Figure 1A-15). *Caution*: if a cardiac anomaly is suspected, one may choose to sterilize and withdraw blood from the inferior vena cava just prior to its entering the heart, thus avoiding damage to the atrium by the heated spatula.

LUNG CULTURE

Lung tissue for culture may easily be obtained from the right or left lower lobe by immobilizing it with a forceps or hemostat, searing the surface with a heated spatula, and, using a sterile scalpel, excising a piece of lung tissue (eFigure 1A-19A to C).

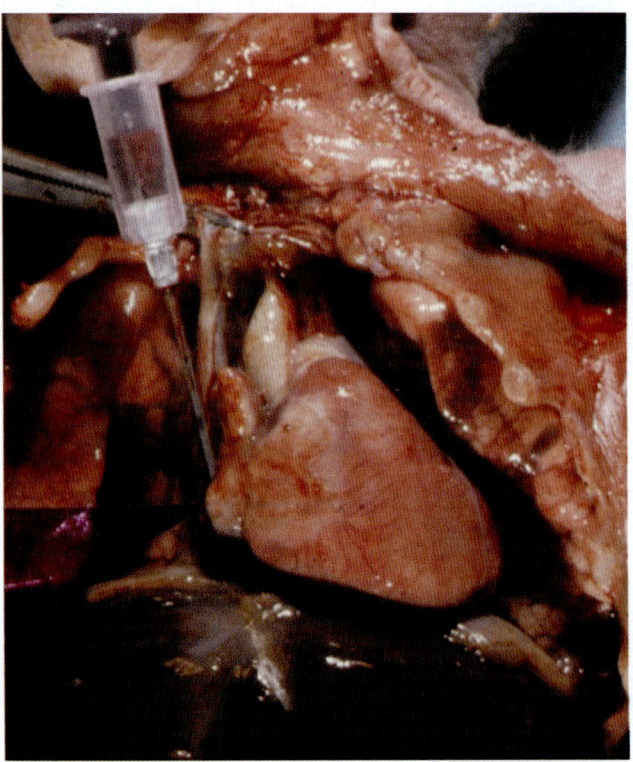

FIGURE 1A-15 • A blood culture can be taken from the inferior vena cava or the right atrium after searing the appropriate area with a heated spatula.

TISSUE FOR CYTOGENETICS

Before taking tissue for examination and culture, contact the laboratory performing the analysis and obtain appropriate media (such as RPMI) for transportation. Tissues that may be used for cell culture include the amniotic membranes of the placenta, spleen, and blood for lymphocytes and skin, fascia, pericardium, pleura, and retroperitoneal tissue for fibroblasts. The sooner this tissue can be placed in the appropriate media, the better chance for successful growth, but fibroblasts from fascia and skin may often still be successfully harvested 24 to 48 hours after death.

CARDIAC/THORACIC RATIO

Prior to removal of the organs of the chest, the width of the heart at its widest point should be measured and compared to the width of the thorax at the same point (Figure 1A-16). The ratio is helpful in detecting cardiac anomalies since a ratio of greater than 0.5 is often associated with many of these anomalies. With this initial suspicion, a "nonstandard" approach to the heart's dissection may be employed (see later).

REMOVING THE ORGANS

Organ-by-Organ Versus Rokitansky

Removal and examination of the chest and abdominal organs can be done one organ at a time or by removing the neck, chest, and abdominal organs as one unit (Rokitansky technique). The latter technique is best performed by beginning in the area of the neck and working caudally. The neck organs are dissected by working around the larynx, esophagus, and descending aorta, freeing them with blunt dissection from the soft tissues laterally and behind. Anteriorly, the left brachial artery, the left carotid artery, and the right brachiocephalic artery may be tied off and transected to allow access to them by the mortician (eFigure 1A-20). When dissection has extended behind and laterally above the larynx, the region above the epiglottis can be transected allowing the complete larynx with attached esophagus to be pulled inferiorly (eFigure 1A-21A, B). Following this, the left lung can be pulled aside to allow an incision to be made along the spinal column just behind the esophagus and aorta. When this procedure is repeated on the right side, the neck organs along with the heart/lung/esophagus can be pulled forward (eFigure 1A-22). The abdominal organs are mobilized by cutting the diaphragm (a good time to take a section for microscopic examination) along the contour of the body wall and dissecting inferiorly along the spinal column, freeing up the spleen and kidney on the left and the liver and kidney on the right. Care must be taken to avoid cutting across the ureters as they pass along the sides of the spinal column before entering the bladder. At this point, the urethra and rectum (and vagina in a female) must be transected (eFigure 1A-23A, B) and freed from the soft tissue of the pelvis allowing the entire neck, chest, and abdominal block to be removed intact.

Note: In a premature infant, it is often prudent to remove the ovaries or testes (if undescended) prior to performing the Rokitansky technique in order to not "lose" them during the dissection (eFigure 1A-24).

It may also be helpful in some cases to perform a *"modified" Rokitansky technique* and remove one or more of the organs before removing the entire block (e.g., remove the spleens in cases of polysplenia, or the bowel in cases of intestinal atresia or duplication).

TESTES/OVARIES

As noted above, it is often easier to remove the ovaries (and testes if undescended) shortly after opening the abdomen. The small size of an infant's ovaries may make locating them difficult. By finding the uterus and fallopian tubes behind the urinary bladder, one can locate the ovaries adjacent to the tubes. They can then be removed, weighed, and often submitted in toto for microscopic examination. Larger ovaries from older infants and young girls may be hemisected. These often contain small fluid-filled cysts.

Testes that are present in the scrotum may be removed by pressure on the scrotum in the direction of the inguinal canal, then inserting a forceps into the canal from the open abdomen, pulling on the vas deferens, and extracting both the vas deferens and testis. This can then be examined for the presence of a vascular malformation or a hydrocele before dissecting the testis free from the vas deferens and attached soft tissue, weighing it and submitting a section for microscopic examination.

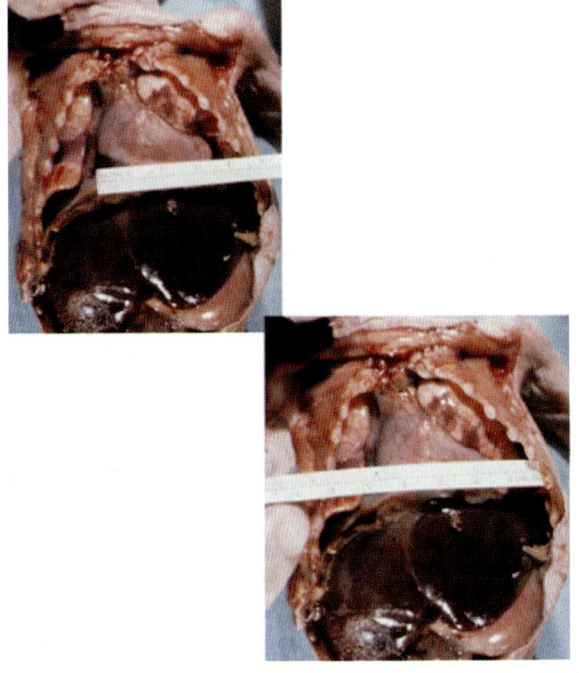

FIGURE 1A-16 • The cardiothoracic ratio is determined by measuring the width of the heart (**top**) at its widest point and the width of the thoracic cavity (**bottom**) at its widest internal point.

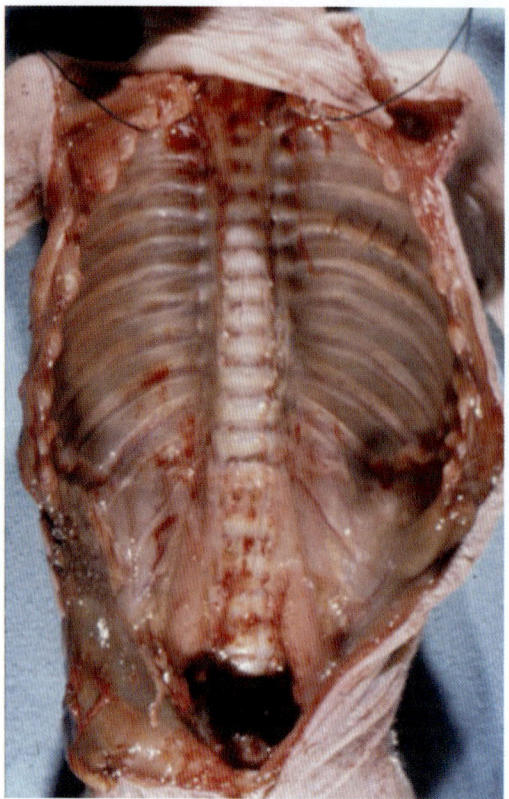

FIGURE 1A-17 • With all organs removed, the ribs and vertebral column can be examined for developmental abnormalities, and the psoas muscle can be sampled for histologic sections.

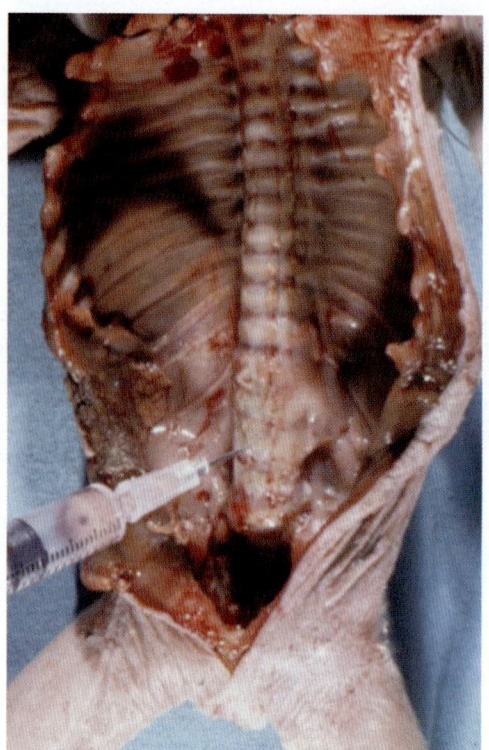

FIGURE 1A-18 • CSF can be obtained for culture and other purposes by inserting a long needle through the intervertebral disc of a lumbar vertebra after sterilizing the area.

EXAMINATION OF THE BODY CAVITY

Following removal of the chest and abdominal organs, the body cavity can be examined for abnormalities of the *ribs* and spinal cord (Figure 1A-17). *Vertebral bodies* may be noted to be irregular, for example, butterfly vertebrae in the VATER association (Vertebral or Vascular anomaly, Anal atresia, TracheoEsophageal fistula, Renal or Radial abnormality), or out of alignment, for example, scoliosis or lordosis (eFigure 1A-25). Special attention should be given to the area in which the ribs abut the spinal column as this is a region in which rib fractures, both old and recent, may be observed. A section of rib including the costochondral junction may be taken for microscopic examination of bone and bone marrow.

VERTEBRAL COLUMN/SPINAL CORD

CSF Culture

A culture of the cerebral spinal fluid is relatively easy in an infant and a young child. Once all the abdominal organs have been removed, the intervertebral disc region of one of the lumbar discs can be seared with a hot spatula (eFigure 1A-26), and a long needle (in an infant) or a spinal tap needle may be inserted through the disc into the spinal canal (Figure 1A-18). Aspiration not only supplies fluid for culture but can also be used for documenting hemorrhage (eFigure 1A-27). In a small infant, the head may need to be elevated to provide enough fluid in the spinal canal for aspiration.

Section of Psoas Muscle

The psoas muscles provide an easily accessible source of skeletal muscle and often include ganglion cells from the paraspinal ganglia (eFigure 1A-28).

Removing the Vertebral Column

While older children may require spinal cord removal similar to that of an adult, infants, particularly neonates, have vertebral columns easily removed from an abdominal approach to provide ready access to the spinal cord. This is accomplished by *making* an incision through two of the lowest intervertebral discs and then bending the pelvis backward to allow a pair of round-ended scissors into the vertebral canal to transect the pedicles on both sides of the vertebral columns (eFigure 1A-29A to D). As one moves caudally, the vertebral column can be lifted to allow the thoracic and cervical vertebral to be freed up by cutting their pedicles. To remove the vertebral column completely, the highest cervical intervertebral disc accessible can be transected. Upon removal of the vertebral column, vertebral body anomalies may again be noted, and a vertebral body may be taken for microscopic examination following fixation and decalcification.

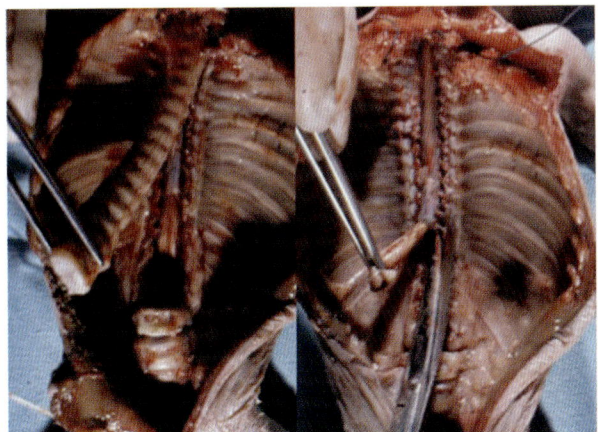

FIGURE 1A-19 • Following removal of the vertebral column (**left**), the spinal cord along with its dura can be removed from the spinal canal (**right**).

Removing the Spinal Cord

With the vertebral column removed, the spinal cord in its dura can be dissected free by cutting across the spinal nerves exiting through the dura (Figure 1A-19). The spinal cord may be dissected at this time with cross sections taken from the upper, mid, and lower levels or may be placed in fixative with the brain for dissection after fixation (eFigure 1A-30A,B).

SEPARATION AND EXAMINATION OF HEART/LUNG

Prior to separating the heart lung block from the abdominal organs, assuming the Rokitansky technique was used to remove the organs, an examination of the *esophagus* should be performed. This is done by placing the block, so its posterior surface is exposed. The entrance to the esophagus behind the larynx can then be entered with a pair of scissors and an incision made from the opening to the point the esophagus passed through the diaphragm. This posterior exposure allows examination of the internal surface of the esophagus with particular attention paid to the portion of the anterior wall of the esophagus lying adjacent to the trachea. Esophageal atresia will be easily discovered if present, and the presence of tracheoesophageal fistula, particularly of the "H" type (see Chapter 12), can be established prior to the esophagus being separated from the trachea. Following this examination, the upper portion of the esophagus is separated from the larynx and the mediastinal tissue and left intact for examination with the remainder of the gastrointestinal tract.

Section Thoracic/Abdominal Aorta and Inferior Vena Cava

With the esophagus separated from the thoracic organs, the descending aorta can be examined for abnormalities (Figure 1A-20) and, if none are present, transected beyond the arch and freed from the mediastinal tissues to be left with the abdominal organs. This leaves the chest and abdominal organs attached by only the inferior vena cava, which, when transected as near to the diaphragm/liver as possible, separates the two blocks.

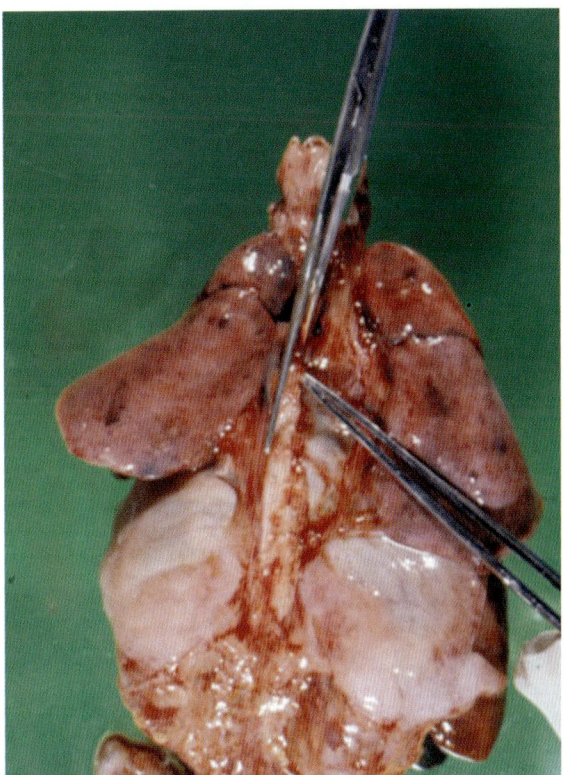

FIGURE 1A-20 • The thoracic aorta and the esophagus can be opened while the abdominal and thoracic organ block is still intact. Here, the aorta is opened along the posterior aspect of the organ block.

Examination of the Chest Block

If the clinical history suggests a cardiac malformation, if the cardiac/thoracic ratio is greater than 0.5, or if external examination of the heart is noticeably abnormal, consideration should be given to a "fixed inflation" of the heart (see below) prior to opening the atria and ventricles. If no abnormality is suspected, the heart may be opened in a standard fashion.

Standard Examination of the Heart

The heart should be separated from the lungs following identification and transection of the pulmonary arteries and veins, noting their anatomic relationships (i.e., origin and position). The heart may then be weighed and examined by opening the chambers along the line of blood flow. This is most easily accomplished by opening the right atrium between the inferior vena cava and the atrial appendage. This incision leaves intact the sinoatrial node that is located in the anterior wall of the right atrium just below the entrance of the superior vena cava. A pair of scissors can be used to cut through the lateral wall of the right atrium, through the tricuspid valve and along the lateral portion of the right ventricular wall. With the right side of the heart thus opened, the atrium can be examined for completeness of the foramen ovale and the entrance of the coronary sinus. The tricuspid can be measured (circumference) and the leaflets inspected, and the right ventricle can be measured for the thickness of the free wall.

The next incision, most easily accomplished with a pair of blunt-nosed scissors, extends up the anterior wall of the right ventricle adjacent to the septum and along the outflow tract into and then through the pulmonary valve. This allows examination of the septum for ventricular septal defects and for measurement of the pulmonary valve circumference and presence of three cusps. With the pulmonary valve opened, the right and left pulmonary artery branches can be identified as can the ductus arteriosus (for patency, circumference, and length).

The left side of the heart is examined by cutting between the openings of the pulmonary veins and then down the lateral wall of the left atrium, through the mitral valve and along the wall of the left ventricle. The mitral valve circumference can be measured and the leaflets observed for orientation and completeness. The left ventricular wall thickness is determined, and the septum is examined for defects. The systemic outflow tract is then opened with an incision through the anterior wall of the left ventricle adjacent to the septum and behind the mitral leaflet into the aorta. When opening the aorta, care must be taken to move the opened pulmonary trunk aside and continue the incision through the aortic valve. The opened valve circumference may be measured and the three cusps observed, noting the position of the origin of the coronary arteries above and behind two of the cusps (the right and left coronary sinuses). Finally, the arch of the aorta is examined for anomalies (e.g., coarctation, patent ductus, etc.). If myocardial infarction is suspected, the right and left ventricles may be "bread-loafed" remembering that the papillary muscles are often affected first in infants with myocardial damage.

Fixed Inflation and Dissection of the Heart

The study of an organ by removing, inflating, and fixing prior to its dissection is useful primarily for examining (and retaining for teaching) the heart but could also be used for other "hollow" organs such as the small or large bowel and the urinary or gallbladder (eFigures 1A-31–1A-48).

The technique for the heart involves separating the heart from the lungs by tying off (as far from the heart as possible) all the vessels including the pulmonary arteries, pulmonary veins, superior and inferior vena cavae, and arteries of the aortic arch, then attaching the heart via cannulas to the superior vena cava and a pulmonary vein, and inflating it under mild pressure (e.g., 20-cm water) with a mixture in four parts to one of 100% alcohol and 37% formalin. Following approximately 24 hours in this fixative, the heart is "opened" by transecting each of the vessels that have been tied off and opening a series of "windows" in the atria, ventricles, and pulmonary trunk and aorta above the valves.

The windows begin with a square or rectangular opening in the right atrium, and after examination of the interior of the atrium and the tricuspid valve, continue with a triangular opening in the right ventricle dictated by any anomalies that may be observed, for example, an incomplete tricuspid valve or a high ventricular septal defect. After observing the anatomy of the right ventricle, its outflow tract can be examined from the window into the right ventricle as well as from a rectangular window opening in the pulmonary trunk just above the pulmonary valve.

The left side of the heart is approached with a window in the left atrium made from incisions connecting the openings for the pulmonary veins, or, to spare the veins, a window just "inside" the locations of the pulmonary veins. With the atrium open, the upper aspect of the mitral valve can be observed and, if normal, the left ventricle can be opened with an incision from the apex of the ventricle, parallel to the ventricular septum, and upward through the anterior and posterior wall, creating a hinge-like opening through which the interior of the ventricle and the lower portion of the mitral valve can be examined. The outflow tract through the aorta can also be observed from the ventricular side and, with a rectangular window cut into the aorta above the aortic valve, from the aortic side.

The incisions involved in creating the windows also allow access to atrial and ventricular myocardial tissue, as well as aortic and pulmonary artery wall for microscopic sections.

Following dissection, the heart can be processed through various concentrations of alcohol and then xylene as is performed with other tissues submitted for processing for microscopic sections. The processing may take a day or more in each solution, and then when the xylene has cleared the heart, it is placed in a paraffin bath under a slight vacuum, which will help speed the impregnation of the tissue. When removing the heart from the heated paraffin, it should be rotated in all planes to clear the paraffin from the heart chambers and vessel openings. Doing this over Bunsen burner with a low flame allows the excess paraffin to exit more rapidly. The heart can then be cooled slowly and retained for future study or teaching purposes.

Examination of the Thymus

This includes weighing and describing it (size, shape, consistency, etc.) and submitting a representative section for microscopic examination.

Examination/Removal of Thyroid and Parathyroids

The thyroid is usually readily visible adjacent to the lower larynx and can be dissected free intact. The weight should be taken, the organ described, and a representative section submitted for microscopic examination. The parathyroid glands may only rarely be visible in an infant, and to ensure that they are available for microscopic examination (if clinical history warrants), the entire thyroid gland and adjacent soft tissue may need to be submitted for microscopic examination.

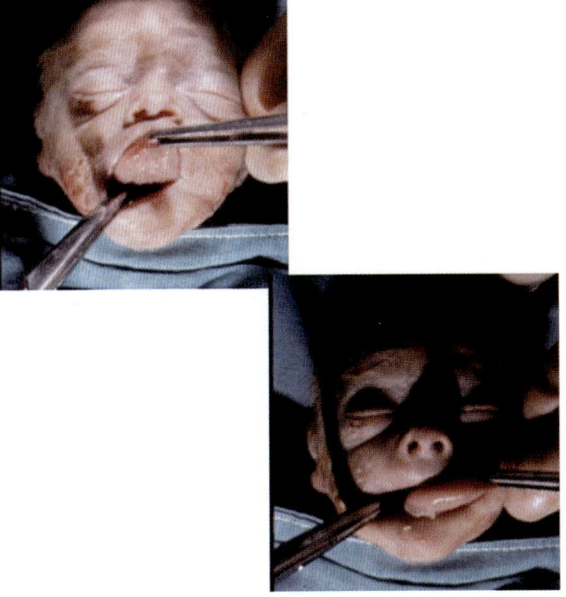

FIGURE 1A-21 • The tongue is removed by lifting it with a pair of forceps toward the top of the mouth (**top**) and then incision and separating the base and lateral surfaces of the tongue from the floor of the mouth (**bottom**).

Removal/Examination of the Tongue

While not necessary or feasible in most cases, removal of the tongue not only allows more extensive examination of the mouth and nasopharynx but also provides another specimen of skeletal muscle for microscopic examination. Once the larynx has been removed (or in continuity with the removal of the chest organs), the tongue may be freed from the mandible by cutting with a scalpel (or preferably a pair of scissors) along the inner edge of the mandible. Care must be taken to not cut the lips or outside of the mouth (Figure 1A-21). A safe way to avoid this possibility is to use a pair of scissors (rather than a scalpel) and only opening the blades after inserting the pair of scissors inside the mouth.

EXAMINATION OF THE RESPIRATORY SYSTEM

Following removal of the heart from the heart/lung block as described above, the respiratory system can be examined. The pulmonary arteries and veins should be identified and examined for the presence of clots (emboli). If present, the arteries or veins should be opened along their length into the lung to determine the extent of the vascular obstruction.

The *larynx* (with thyroid and parathyroids removed) should be separated from the trachea and then examined for patency from above and below. It may then be hemisected from anterior to posterior, allowing a view of the vocal cords and laryngeal mucosa.

The *trachea* should also be probed for patency and for the size of the lumen throughout. Externally, the cartilage plates along its circumference should be examined for the presence of complete rings. The trachea may then be resected at the carina leaving as much as possible of the right and left main stem bronchi.

Lung examination begins by weighing the right and the left lungs separately and noting the lobation of the lobes (two on the left and three on the right) and their color and consistency (eFigure 1A-31). At this point, it is often helpful to inflate one of the lungs with formalin by inserting a syringe in the mainstem bronchus and slowly injecting 10 to 50 mL of formalin depending on the size of the lungs. A hemostat may then be used to close off the bronchus and the lung placed in formalin for an hour or two (or overnight if possible) before dissecting. The other lung is examined by gently probing the bronchi and vessels and then sectioning the lung perpendicular to the hilum. This allows examination of the parenchyma for lesions (cysts, abscesses, areas of consolidation and hemorrhage). Sections should be taken from obvious areas of pathology as well as from pleural and hilar regions. While a section may be taken from each of the five lobes, in small lungs, a slice of the entire lung may fit into one cassette.

EXAMINATION OF THE ABDOMINAL ORGANS

In females, separate the *uterus and fallopian tubes* from the abdominal block (ovaries already removed and weighed).

Spleen

The spleen may have been removed earlier (see above), but if not, should now be dissected from the abdominal block with special attention paid to the areas adjacent to the spleen and liver for smaller "accessory" spleens. If none are present, the spleen can be weighed, sectioned, and described, and a sample can be taken for microscopic examination (eFigure 1A-32).

Liver

From the anterior portion of the abdominal block, the diaphragm can be removed and the liver examined. The biliary tract is difficult to dissect in a small infant, but its patency can be demonstrated by making an incision in the duodenum in the region of the ampulla of Vater. The gallbladder can then be compressed against the liver, and if the biliary tree is patent, bile can be expressed through the ampulla (Figure 1A-22). If no bile is seen, the extrahepatic biliary tree may have to be dissected along its length. Following this, the liver can be removed from the block, weighed, described, and sectioned at 1.0-cm intervals with representative tissue taken for microscopic examination.

Adrenals and Kidneys

From the rear of the abdominal block, the aorta can be opened to observe the origin and patency of the celiac axis, mesenteric arteries, and renal/adrenal arteries as well as the

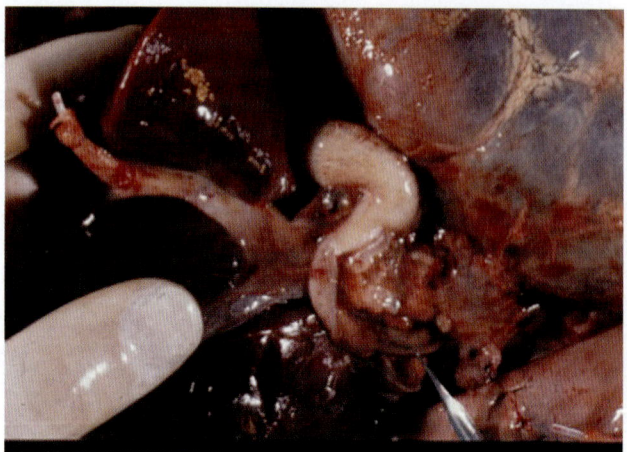

FIGURE 1A-22 • The biliary tree can be examined for patency by first opening the duodenum in the region of the ampulla of Vater and then compressing the gallbladder (note thumb over gallbladder) and observing the flow of bile from the ampulla (at tip of scissors).

iliac arteries. The renal veins can also be observed entering the inferior vena cava and their patency observed. The adrenals can be dissected from the kidneys, weighed, described, and sectioned with a cross section taken from each adrenal for microscopic examination.

The kidneys, ureters, and bladder can be dissected en bloc either with or without the renal arteries and section of the aorta (eFigure 1A-33). After identifying the origin, course, and entrance into the bladder of each ureter, each kidney can be removed, weighed, and examined by clearing off the soft tissue from the capsule (without stripping the capsule) and bisecting the kidney. The cortex and medullary thicknesses are measured and examined for lesions before sections are taken for microscopic examination. The renal pelvis should be opened and the entrance to the ureters examined, followed by opening the entire length of the ureters into the bladder. The bladder itself should be opened and the mucosa examined before a section is taken for microscopic examination. The urethra can be probed for patency and when opened in a male, the prostate can be examined and a section submitted for microscopic examination.

Note: In cases of suspected *urethral stricture or atresia*, it may be helpful to remove the urethra along with the external genitalia, most noticeably the penis in male infants. This is accomplished by separating the symphysis pubis and dissecting the penis in continuity with the bladder. It may also be helpful to fix the penis and distal portion of the bladder and then cross-section the specimen and submit it in its entirety.

Removing, Measuring, and Sectioning the Bowel

The bowel may be removed prior to removing the chest/abdomen block or when dissecting the abdominal organs. In either event, the bowel is best separated from the other organs by beginning in the area of the sigmoid/rectum and working toward the stomach, using a pair of curved scissors to cut along the mesenteric attachment as close to the bowel wall as possible, being careful to identify (and not cut across) the appendix when working near the cecum. In a small infant, the bowel may be wrapped around one's fingers as one progresses from the sigmoid to the duodenum. The bowel may be transected at the duodenum at the point it passes beneath the inferior duodenal fold. The entire bowel can then be laid out on a cutting board for measuring the length and width of the small intestine, colon, and appendix. If lesions are identified along the length of the bowel, they may be cross-sectioned and examined, or the entire length of the bowel may be opened for inspection before sectioning (eFigure 1A-34).

The most proximal part of the gastrointestinal tract (esophagus, stomach, and upper duodenum) along with the pancreas is then (if not previously done) separated from the diaphragm and liver. The incision in the previously opened esophagus (see under "Separation and Examination of Heart/Lung") can be extended through the gastroesophageal junction, along the edge of the stomach and through the pylorus into the duodenum. Gastric contents can be observed and a portion saved for further analysis if appropriate. Beyond the pylorus, the ampulla of Vater is again identified (see Liver above) and its relationship to the pancreas observed. The pancreas can then be dissected from its attachment to the duodenum, weighed, described, and sections taken from the head and tail for microscopic examination. With the entire gastrointestinal tract now opened, portions along its length (2 × 1 cm) may be taken (esophagus ×1, esophageal–gastric junction ×1, stomach ×2, small bowel ×3, appendix ×1 and colon ×2) and placed on paper (Figure 1A-23) for fixation and sectioning at a later time (overnight is best, but only 1 to 3 hours in 37% formalin is usually sufficient).

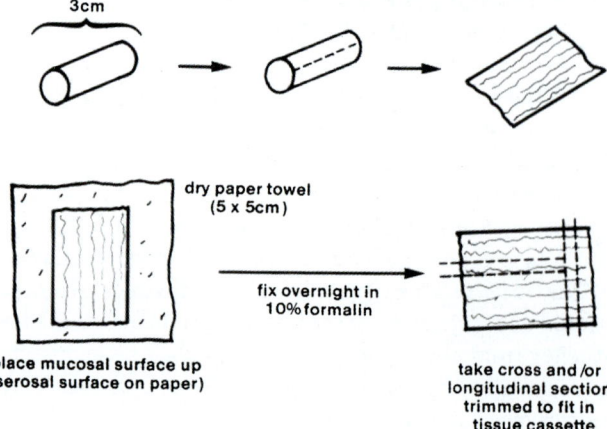

FIGURE 1A-23 • Technique for fixing thin-walled tissue on paper towels before sectioning.

Note: In situations in which the bowel is extremely fragile, particularly in cases of necrotizing enterocolitis, it may be best to leave the small bowel and colon intact with the mesentery and fix the entire specimen in formalin prior to dissection.

Central Nervous System

Examination of the Scalp

The scalp should be examined for abnormalities in the pattern of the growth of the hair, looking for two or more swirls of growth; the more swirls or defects in hair growth, the more likely there will be abnormalities in the structure of the brain. The anterior and the posterior fontanelles should be palpated in infants to check for fullness or depression.

Opening the Scalp

An intermastoid, suboccipital incision (Figure 1A-24) allows reflection of the scalp anteriorly to the level of the eyebrows and posteriorly to below the posterior fontanelle (eFigure 1A-35A, B). In young infants, pushing a finger between the scalp and the calvarium and rolling the skin forward may accomplish this. In older children, dissection of the tissue between the scalp and calvarium may require a pair of scissors or a scalpel.

Measuring the Calvarium

With the fontanelles exposed, they may again be palpated and measured (length and width) (eFigure 1A-36). The calvarium can also be examined for developmental defects, fractures, or hemorrhage.

Opening the Calvarium

In infants whose calvarium has not completely ossified, the calvarium may be opened with a scalpel and a pair of scissors along the unfused sutures. Examination of the sagittal sinus

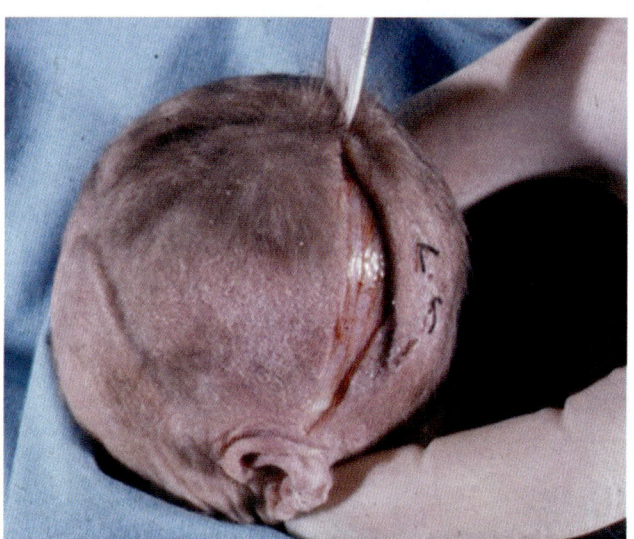

FIGURE 1A-24 • The scalp is opened with an incision between the ears at the level below (posterior to) the crown of the head, that is, an intermastoid suboccipital incision.

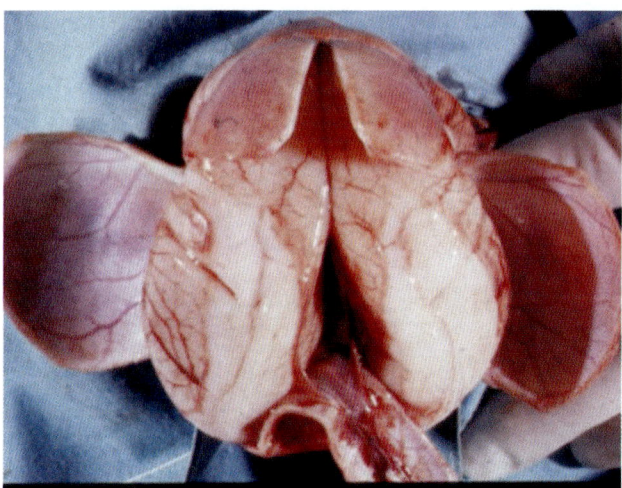

FIGURE 1A-25 • The calvarium can be opened by cutting lateral to each side of the sagittal suture and then along the sutures between the frontoparietal and parietooccipital bones. After examining the sagittal vein, the suture line is reflected posteriorly **(bottom),** and the parietal bones are reflected laterally to expose the brain.

may be done by cutting with a pair of scissors through the parietal bone from the anterior fontanelle to the posterior fontanelle about one centimeter to each side of the sagittal suture. Lifting the edge of the strip left in the middle allows a view of the intact sinus (eFigure 1A-37A to C).

Extending the incisions parallel to the sagittal suture to the anterior and the posterior portions of the calvarium and then laterally from both ends of the incision into the parietal bone (on both the right and the left sides) until they are 1 to 4 cm apart (depending on the size of the head), allow both parietal/frontal bones to be reflected laterally (Figure 1A-25, eFigure 1A-38). By cutting across the anterior extension of the sagittal suture and reflecting it posteriorly, the brain is exposed. The calvarium of older infants and children is removed as one would for an adult.

Removing the Brain

The brain of a small infant is removed from anterior to posterior by placing one's hand behind the head (with the reflected sagittal suture between the middle and the ring fingers and tilting the head backward [Figure 1A-26]). As the brain falls away from the base of the skull, the cranial nerves, pituitary stalk, and tentorium can be cut across as they come into view. Eventually, one can see into the spinal canal and insert a pair of scissors to cut across the spinal cord well below the brainstem. At this point, the brain should easily be "delivered" into the hand held beneath the head.

Examination of the Excised Brain

Following removal, the brain should be weighed and the external features examined including the basic development of the cerebral cortex related to the infant's gestational age (see Addendum). The vessels at the base of the brain may also be examined, but further manipulation of the brain

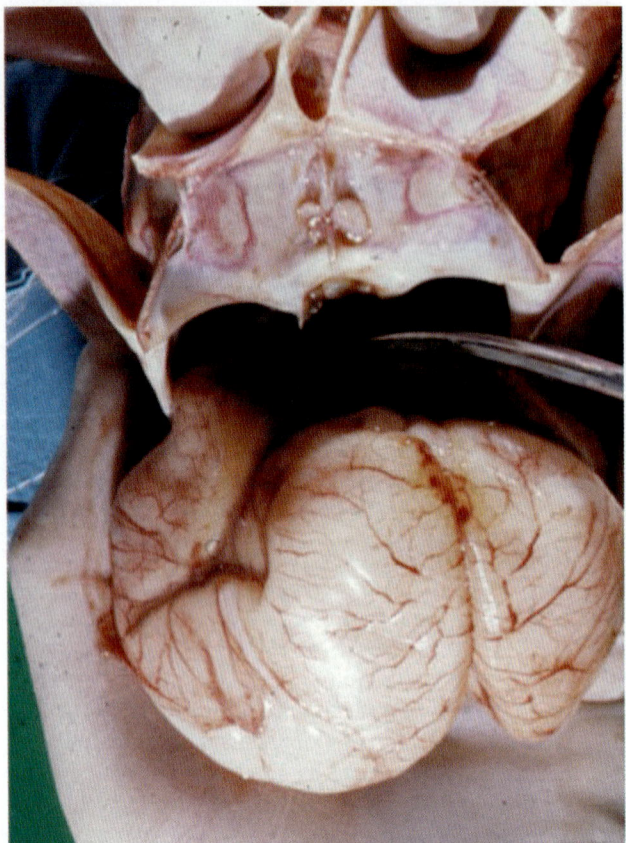

FIGURE 1A-26 • Remove the brain by tipping the head posteriorly and transecting the cranial nerves, tentorium, and spinal cord.

should be put off until it can be made more firm by fixing in formalin (10% to 37%) for 1 to 2 weeks. Placing the container with the brain near a source of low heat (e.g., a radiator or a heat vent) may hasten the fixation.

Sectioning the Brain and Spinal Cord

The spinal cord, if removed via the abdominal approach, can be fixed along with the brain. Examination consists of opening the dura along its length and then sectioning the cord at 0.5- to 1.0-cm intervals saving two or more sections for microscopic examination.

The *brain after fixation* should be examined for gross abnormalities (e.g., area of hemorrhage or necrosis, developmental anomalies such as holoprosencephaly) and a unique approach to dissection determined by the abnormalities. In most instances, however, major anomalies are not seen, and a more "standard" approach may be taken. This consists first of examining the vessels at the base of the brain after gently removing the meninges. The circle of Willis should be identified and any variations recorded. The cerebellum and brainstem can be removed from the rest of the brain by making a transverse section in the region of the cerebral peduncles (eFigure 1A-39A, B). In a small infant's brain, this cerebellar/brainstem block may be cut transversely at 0.5- to 1.0-cm intervals to view the cerebellar folia and dentate nucleus along with the lower brainstem (eFigure 1A-40A to C). In larger brains, the brainstem might be separated from the cerebellum prior to sectioning.

If significant hemorrhage is present in the cerebral hemispheres, the meningeal arteries may be followed into the cerebrum to search for a site of an aneurysm or rupture. After the exterior of the cerebral hemispheres has been examined, the brain is placed "base up" and transverse (coronal) sections made at 1.0- to 1.5-cm intervals (depending on the size of the brain) from the anterior lobe through the occipital lobe (eFigure 1A-41). If possible, these sections (often only five or six in infants but as many as 12 to 15 in older children) should include ones through the stalk of the pituitary, the mammillary bodies, the apex of the interpeduncular fossa, and the top of the cerebral peduncles. This allows close examination of the numerous nuclei of the deep gray matter.

CNS Microscopic Sections

Routine sections include, but are not limited to brainstem (pons), cerebellum including dentate nucleus, frontal (or occipital) cortex and white matter, hippocampus, internal capsule/posterior limb/thalamus, cervical, thoracic, and lumbar spinal cord and additional sections of specific lesions—for example, tumor, necrosis, and hemorrhage (Figure 1A-27).

Examination of the Inside of the Cranium

Removal of the Pituitary

The pituitary can easily be removed from the hypophyseal fossa of the sella turcica after the brain has been removed. The gland is usually quite soft and delicate, and the best approach is made by using a pair of small curved scissors to dissect around and beneath the gland.

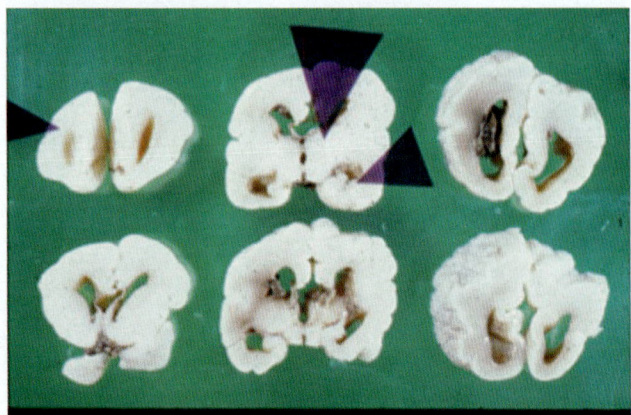

FIGURE 1A-27 • Standard histologic sections from the brain include portions of the cerebrum, hippocampus, and basal nuclei (*arrows*) along with sections of cerebellum and brain stem.

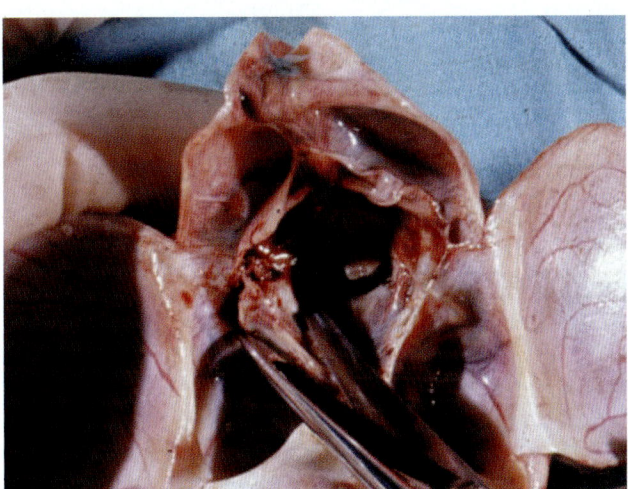

FIGURE 1A-28 • The middle ear is exposed by removing the petrous portion of the temporal bone.

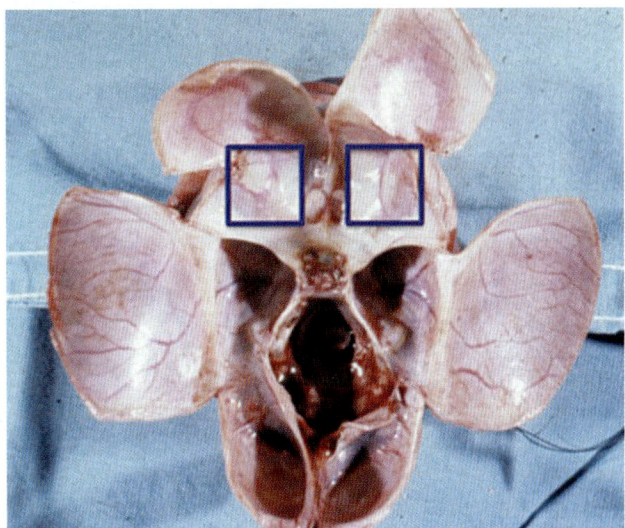

FIGURE 1A-29 • The opened calvarium provides access to the eyes through the roof of the orbits (*indicated with squares*).

Opening of Middle Ear

The middle ear can be visualized by removing the petrous portion of the temporal bone with a pair of heavy (bone) scissors or with saw cuts on either side of the petrous protrusion (Figure 1A-28). With removal of the bone, the middle ear can be examined for infection (pus or cloudy fluid) and a culture performed if indicated. The bones of the middle ear (malleus, incus, and stapes) can also be seen.

Removal of eye/s can be performed from beneath the eyelids by cutting around the orbital septum and palpebral ligaments holding the eyeball to the bones of the orbit, and then dissecting posteriorly to separate the ocular muscles and transect the optic nerve. Care must be taken to avoid damage to the eyelid and skin of the face.

A less potentially damaging approach is through the opened skull following removal of the brain. Access to the eye is made by cutting an opening in the superior surface of the orbital plate of the frontal bone (Figure 1A-29). In a newborn, this can often be done with a scalpel and a pair of scissors but may require a saw in older patients. When the opening is large enough to accommodate the size of the eyeball, the optic nerve and orbital muscles can be dissected and visualized, then transected. As the eye is moved posteriorly, the ligaments holding the eye to the orbit can be cut across (with special care taken to avoid cutting the eyelid) and the eye pulled through the opening in the orbital plate.

Preparing the Remains for Disposition

Following the completion of gross autopsy examination, all tissues NOT taken for microscopic examination, long-term storage, or teaching purposes (in accordance with the autopsy permit) should be returned to the body in a plastic bag of appropriate size. This includes the chest plate and vertebral column. The body and scalp over the calvarium can be sewn closed. Consulting with morticians as to their preference is often helpful. The outside of the body should be appropriately tagged for identification, washed, dried, and wrapped in appropriate material for transfer to the funeral home.

References

1. College of American Pathologists Pamphlet. *Autopsy: aiding the living by understanding death*. Northfield, IL.
2. Marshall WA, Tanner JM. Variations in pattern of pubertal changes in girls. *Arch Dis Child* 1969;44:291–303.

CHAPTER 1B

Fine-Needle Aspiration

John J. Buchino, M.D., and Robert F. Debski, M.D.

Fine-needle aspiration (FNA) was first reported in the early 1930s by Martin and Ellis (1) and Stewart (2), but the procedure did not gain widespread acceptance until after Zajicek published his monograph in 1974 (3). Although several studies and monographs have established the usefulness of FNA in pediatrics, many pediatric centers have been slow to adopt this invaluable technique. Those that have adopted this technique, however, have found it to be a relatively easy, low-cost diagnostic procedure that can provide a great deal of information (4). Several important advantages of FNA are listed in Table 1B-1. It is important that clinicians recognize that FNA is most applicable in discrete mass lesions, generally not in diffuse processes such as cellulitis or a pulmonary infiltrate. Typical indications for the use of FNA in children are summarized in Table 1B-2. For several reasons (given below), it is strongly recommended that a pathologist perform FNA of all palpable lesions and that a pathologist should be present to assist when a radiologist performs an image-guided FNA of deep-seated lesions, regardless of image modality (CT, MRI, ultrasound, etc). Thereupon, the pathologist is able to obtain an accurate history and observe the exact size and location of the lesion. The person performing the aspiration is best able to evaluate whether the lesion has been penetrated. As one gains experience, the texture of the lesion and consistency of the aspirated material assist in the formulation of a differential diagnosis. The pathologist is also best able to prepare the smears and triage the aspirate material for ancillary studies.

The standard equipment required for FNA is listed in Table 1B-3. If need be, the equipment and supplies can easily be carried in a phlebotomy tray to the patient's bedside or, preferably, to a treatment room. Outpatient FNA should be performed in a clinic or hospital-based setting with adequate room for the patient, parents, and assistants, as well as the pathologist. An adjacent area or an appropriate cart for rapid staining and microscopic evaluation is highly desirable. Although untoward complications are extremely rare with the aspiration of superficial lesions, the procedure room should be equipped to handle emergencies, as with any other area in which clinical procedures are carried out.

In general, relatively few complications are associated with FNA. The most common is bruising or swelling at the FNA site. Inadvertent puncture of a vessel may result in a small hematoma. Nevertheless, a history of a possible bleeding diathesis should always be obtained. A vasovagal response or light-headedness may occur in a small percentage of patients (be aware, parents may also feel faint when observing the procedure). A pneumothorax is possible when a chest wall lesion or a lesion in the supraclavicular space is aspirated. Seeding of tumor in the needle tract, while reported, is a markedly rare occurrence (5).

The FNA technique is outlined in Figure 1B-1. This is essentially the same as the technique used for adults. Of note, the use of an FNA syringe holder (i.e., "aspirator" or "aspiration gun") and the specific type (i.e., "pistol-grip" or "pencil-grip" syringe holder) are optional. In children, the standard size of needle for a superficial lesion is usually 1 inch, 23 gauge. A 23-gauge needle recovers adequate material for diagnosis in more than 90% of cases and is unlikely to cause any significant organ or vessel trauma. A 22-gauge needle may facilitate the drainage of purulent material but should not be used in regions where a major vessel may be sheared (e.g., near the carotid artery). The pathologist must also be mindful of spatial differences, such as decreased chest wall thickness in infants and small children.

When performing an FNA on an infant or child, adequate control of the patient is imperative. Nobody wants to attempt the aspiration of a moving target. Thus, a skilled assistant, such as a nurse or pathology assistant, is invaluable in this situation. Since the procedure is relatively brief, the assistant is usually able to hold and control infants less than 1 year of age in the desired position. Children older than 6 years can generally cooperate well when talked through the procedure. Children between 12 months and 6 years, however, can be difficult because of their lack of comprehension of what is happening and their strength. Sedation should be used whenever possible. Most tertiary care pediatric services now have sedation teams that are adept at sedating children for short procedures. The choice of sedatives may

TABLE 1B-1	ADVANTAGES OF FNA
Low cost	
Low risk	
Rapid diagnosis	
No general anesthesia necessary	
Outpatient setting, appropriate in most cases	
Ancillary tests, possible in most cases	
Special stains	
Immunohistochemistry	
Flow cytometry	
Electron microscopy	
Molecular studies (FISH, PCR)	
Direct interaction with the patient and family	

TABLE 1B-3	EQUIPMENT NEEDED FOR FNA
Needles (22 to 25 gauge, 1 inch)	
Syringes (10 to 20 mL)	
Local anesthetic (optional)	
Alcohol prep, Betadine	
Syringe holder ("aspiration gun") (optional)	
Gauze	
Glass slides	
Paper clips	
Fixatives (95% ethanol, CytoLyt, etc.)	
Adhesive bandage	
Gloves	
Sterile culture container/media (optional)	
Flow cytometry media (RPMI) (optional)	

vary and is somewhat dependent on the personal preference of the anesthesiologist and/or the pathologist. When sedation is used, the child must be monitored in the appropriate fashion. If sedation is not available, a papoose wrap may be employed to immobilize the child. Also, use a local anesthetic whenever possible. The only exceptions to the use of a local anesthetic are a known allergy and a lesion so small that the injected anesthetic will make it difficult to palpate and properly sample the lesion.

Prior to actually performing the FNA procedure, the pathologist and assistant should verify patient identification, the site to be aspirated, and that a consent form for the procedure has been signed. The site to be aspirated should have been marked in the presence of the patient's parents/guardians. Once the entire team is ready, the pathologist may proceed with the aspiration.

Typically, several separate aspirations are necessary to obtain adequate material for cytologic evaluation. The number of aspirates may vary somewhat depending on the amount and type of material obtained. A significant advantage to FNA is that material can be obtained for ancillary studies in addition to standard cytomorphology. Of note, ancillary studies usually require additional aspirations, which may or may not be possible.

The utility of ancillary studies has recently blossomed and enhanced the field of FNA, more than ever as pathologists are expected to "do more with less." An FNA workup may now include special stains, immunohistochemistry, flow cytometry, and molecular studies. These ancillary techniques may be applied to direct smears, cytospin centrifugations, and/or cell blocks. Cell block preparations, in particular, are processed similar to small biopsies in surgical pathology and, thus, are advantageous for certain ancillary studies, especially immunohistochemistry and molecular studies (i.e., FISH). Cytomorphology will continue to be the cornerstone of FNA, but with continued advancements, ancillary studies play an important role today and in years to come, assisting pathologists with diagnoses and guiding clinicians with therapy (6,7).

The most common condition for which children are referred for FNA is persistent lymphadenopathy. In contrast to the adult population, malignancy is present in only a very small percentage of children with enlarged lymph nodes (8). Since infections are the most common cause of enlarged lymph nodes in children, microbiology cultures and special stains can have a significant positive yield (9). Flow cytometry may play a crucial role by detecting a monoclonal or polyclonal lymphoid population.

Several articles and monographs have described various lesions encountered in the pediatric population and diagnosed by FNA (10–12). Although it is helpful to be familiar with these, the algorithmic approach offered by Howell et al. (13) serves as an excellent starting point in the evaluation of FNA smears. For those pathologists considering initiating an FNA service, practicing on fresh surgical specimens (and preparing touch preps when possible) can be helpful to gain experience with little risk.

A pathologist should be mindful of common pitfalls in the diagnosis of lesions by FNA in children. These include (a) obtaining inadequate material because of inadequate patient control; (b) attempting to aspirate an ill-defined swelling rather

TABLE 1B-2	INDICATIONS FOR FNA
Indication	Example
Mass lesion of unknown cause	Any mass ≥0.5 cm
Alternative to surgery	High-risk surgical candidate (e.g., child in respiratory distress secondary to a large anterior mediastinal mass)
Diagnosis of a non-resectable tumor	Large retroperitoneal neuroblastoma
Confirmation of a metastasis	Pulmonary lesion in a child with Wilms tumor
Support of a clinical diagnosis	Persistent lymphadenopathy
Preoperative planning	Thyroid or salivary gland lesion

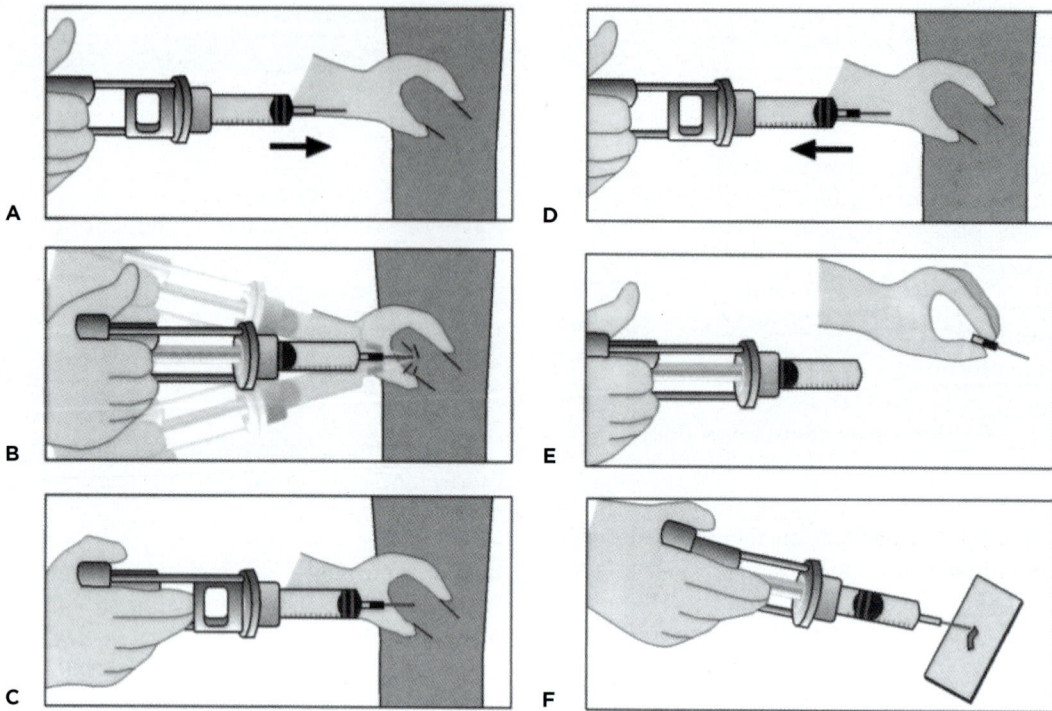

FIGURE 1B-1 • Aspiration technique. **A:** Insert the needle attached to the syringe and holder into the mass while stabilizing the mass with the other hand. **B:** Create negative pressure while moving the needle back and forth until aspirate is present on the needle hub. **C:** Release negative pressure. **D:** Remove the needle from the mass. **E:** Detach the needle from the syringe and fill the syringe with air. **F:** Attach the needle to the syringe and express the aspirate onto a slide or into medium.

than a discrete, palpable mass; and (c) lacking familiarity with the differential diagnosis of lesions in children.

The accuracy of an FNA diagnosis in pediatrics varies depending on the type of lesion aspirated and the experience of the pathologist obtaining and interpreting the specimen. In several published series of pediatric FNA, the sensitivity has been greater than 90% and the specificity greater than 95% in distinguishing benign from malignant lesions (14). The percentage of samples inadequate for diagnosis typically ranges from 5% to 10%.

Finally, essential to achieving an accurate diagnosis by FNA is clear communication between the clinician and the pathologist, both before and after the procedure. This was best stated by Dr. Fred Stewart in 1933: "Diagnosis by aspiration is as reliable as the combined intelligence of the clinician and the pathologist make it" (2).

References

1. Martin HE, Ellis EB. Biopsy by needle puncture and aspiration. *Am Surg* 1930;92:169–181.
2. Stewart FW. The diagnosis of tumors by aspiration biopsy. *Am J Pathol* 1933;9:801–812.
3. Zajicek J. *Aspiration Biopsy Cytology Part I: Cytology of Supradiaphragmatic Organs.* New York, NY: Karger; 1974.
4. Howell L. Changing role of fine-needle aspiration in the evaluation of pediatric masses. *Diagn Cytopathol* 2001;24(1):65–70.
5. Postovsky S, Elhasid R, Weyl Ben Arush M, et al. Local dissemination of hepatocellular carcinoma in a child after fine-needle aspiration (Letter to the Editor). *Med Pediatr Oncol* 2001;36:667–668.
6. Barroca H, Carvalho J, Gil da Costa M, et al. Detection of N-myc amplification in neuroblastomas using Southern blotting on fine needle aspirates. *Acta Cytol* 2001;45:169–172.
7. Buchino JJ, Lee HK. Specimen collection and preparation in fine-needle aspirations in children. *Am J Clin Pathol* 1998;109:54–58.
8. Handa U, Mohan H, Bal A. Role of fine needle aspiration cytology in evaluation of paediatric lymphadenopathy. *Cytopathology* 2003;14:66–69.
9. Buchino JJ, Jones VF. Fine-needle aspiration in the evaluation of children with lymphadenopathy. *Arch Pediatr Adolesc Med* 1994;48:1327–1330.
10. Buchino JJ. Cytopathology in pediatrics. In: Wied GL, ed. *Monographs in Clinical Cytology*, Vol. 13. Basel, Switzerland: Karger; 1991:1–7.
11. Geisinger KR, Silverman JF, Wakely PE. *Pediatric Cytopathology.* Chicago, IL: ASCP Press; 1994:4–5.
12. Vielh P, Howell LP. Techniques. In: Kline TS, ed. *Guides to Clinical Aspiration Biopsy. Pediatrics.* New York, NY: Igaku-Shoin; 1994:5–8.
13. Howell L, Russell LA, Howard PH, et al. The cytology of pediatric masses: a differential diagnostic approach. *Diagn Cytopathol* 1992;8:107–115.
14. Drut R, Drut R, Pollono D, et al. Fine-needle aspiration biopsy in pediatric oncology patients. *J Pediatr Hematol Oncol* 2005;27:370–376.

CHAPTER 1C
Molecular Techniques in Pediatric Pathology

Jason A. Jarzembowski, M.D., Ph.D., and D. Ashley Hill, M.D.

INTRODUCTION

Rapid advances in the understanding of the molecular and genetic basis of disease have led to an increasingly information-rich and complex working environment for the pediatric pathologist. In addition to providing insight into the pathology and biology of disease, these advances have led to improvements and refinements in diagnosis, risk stratification, prediction of outcome, determination of eligibility for new targeted therapies, and gene-based screening for disease risk. Molecular techniques have become the standard of care in the pathologic evaluation of hematopoietic diseases, pediatric tumors, infectious diseases, immunodeficiencies, metabolic diseases, and chromosomal/genetic disorders. Pediatricians and surgeons, armed with the latest literature on the gene expression profile of a given set of tumors or a newly described mutation associated with a congenital defect, are anxious to apply these new discoveries to their patients' specimens. With a solid understanding of disease morphology and pathogenesis coupled with access to advanced technology and tissue resources, pediatric pathologists are in an advantageous position to utilize this wealth of information in a manner that is clinically important to today's patients. Here, we discuss several molecular techniques focusing on relevance to the standard practice of a pediatric pathologist. We include a broad overview of the technical aspects of each methodology with the utility of each method illustrated by applications to specific pediatric diseases. Because detailed descriptions of all techniques and all relevant diseases are beyond the scope of this chapter, key references and helpful websites are suggested for a more in-depth discussion.

Tissue Handling

The appropriate management of complicated pediatric specimens submitted to the pathology laboratory begins well before the slides cross the microscope stage. Even before the child is in the operative suite, it is fundamental that pathologists participate in the preoperative treatment planning. Establishing an open line of communication with the referring physicians and surgeons will ensure that the pathology team is well prepared for special handling requirements. This is a good opportunity to consider the differential diagnosis and plan ahead for appropriate specimen transport; intraoperative assessment of tissue adequacy, preliminary diagnosis, and margin evaluations when necessary; and tissue requirements for potential ancillary testing and clinical trial enrollment (Table 1C-1). Debski and colleagues have written an excellent review on the approach to handling pediatric tumors that applies to other specimen types as well (Figure 1C-1) (1).

Specific Molecular Techniques

Most pathology laboratories today have a sizeable arsenal of molecular tools that can be deployed to assist in diagnosis, predict treatment efficacy, or provide other pertinent clinicopathologic information. The first group of assays described—flow cytometry, immunohistochemistry (IHC), and immunofluorescence—are all protein based and predicated on the specific recognition of antigen by antibody. Those in the second group are all nucleic acid–dependent and include traditional cytogenetics, *in situ* hybridization, polymerase chain reaction (PCR), and the continually evolving worlds of microarray technology and next-generation sequencing (NGS).

FLOW CYTOMETRY

Background

Since its inception in the 1970s, flow cytometry has gained widespread acceptance and is today considered an essential component of the diagnostic workup of hematopoietic neoplasms and immunodeficiency disorders. This methodology allows for rapid identification of cell surface molecules and their coexpression patterns, thus separating subpopulations

TABLE 1C-1 TYPICAL TISSUE REQUIREMENTS FOR COMMONLY USED MOLECULAR DIAGNOSTIC TECHNIQUES

Methodology	Tissue Amount	Fresh	Frozen	FFPE
Flow cytometry	<1 cm³	✓		
FISH/ISH	4- to 10-μm sections			✓
Immunofluorescence	4- to 10-μm sections		✓	
Immunohistochemistry	4- to 10-μm sections		Some	✓
Cytogenetics	<1 cm³	✓		
PCR	Varies	✓	✓	
Microarray	<1 cm³	✓	✓	✓

FFPE, formalin-fixed paraffin-embedded; FISH/ISH, (fluorescence) *in situ* hybridization; PCR, polymerase chain reaction.

of cells such as monocytes from lymphocytes, B from T lymphocytes, or CD4+ from CD8+ T lymphocytes. Aberrant marker profiles or absolute cell counts can also be easily determined. The diagnosis and classification of leukemias and lymphomas are thoroughly discussed elsewhere in this book. Herein, we describe the general theory and method with special attention to specimen processing and practical applications.

Method

The most common specimens submitted for flow cytometry are peripheral blood, bone marrow aspirates, cerebrospinal fluid, and lymph nodes. For peripheral blood (except for paroxysmal nocturnal hematuria [PNH] studies) and bone marrow specimens, erythrocytes are removed by lysis or differential centrifugation. A portion of the sample is spun onto a slide for assessment of cell viability and possible contaminating debris. From this, total cell counts can be estimated, which determines how many analysis tubes can be run; approximately 10^6 cells are needed for optimal results from a typical reaction tube. When testing will be applied to solid samples, the tissue should be immediately transported on saline-moistened gauze or in fresh RPMI medium to the laboratory. Touch preparations for cytologic evaluation are useful in guiding the triage of the sample for light microscopy, flow cytometry, cytogenetics, and storage in a −80°C freezer for subsequent studies. Flow cytometry requires a small (3 to 5 mm³) piece of viable tissue placed in fresh RPMI

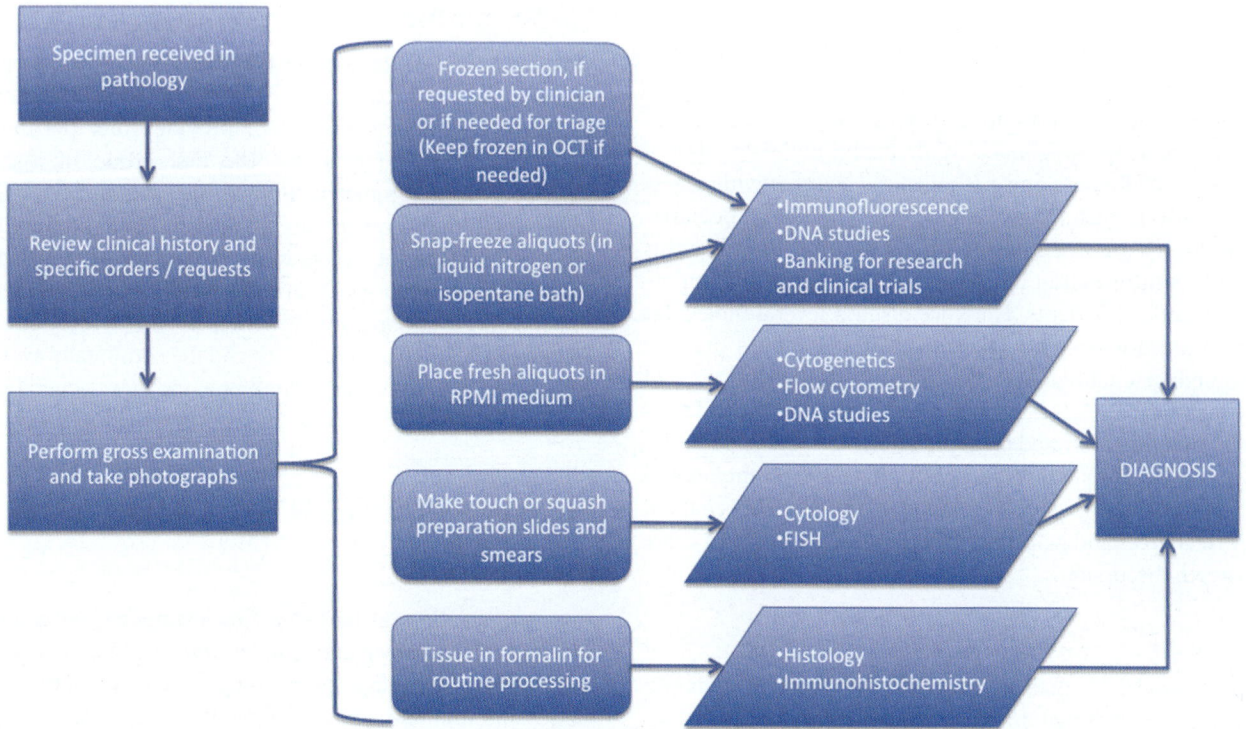

FIGURE 1C-1 • Recommended triage and sampling protocol for pediatric specimens.

or similar medium. If subsequent processing will be delayed for more than an hour or so, the tissue should be finely diced to maximize exposure to the nutritive medium and prolong viability (2). Once at the flow cytometry laboratory, the tissue is carefully teased apart and separated into a single-cell suspension (3–5).

For the next step, cell aliquots are mixed with surface antigen–specific antibodies that have been conjugated to fluorescent dyes, such as phycoerythrin (PE), fluorescein isothiocyanate (FITC), and phthalocyanines (PC5, PC7). After a short incubation to allow the conjugated antibodies to bind their target surface antigens on the cells in the aliquot, the sample is loaded into the flow cytometer (Figure 1C-2). The cell suspension flows through capillary tubing, eventually streaming single file through the detection chamber. Here, one or more lasers "interrogate" each cell, determining the forward scatter (roughly correlating with size), the side scatter (roughly correlating with cytoplasmic complexity or granularity), and a measurement of fluorescent dyes reflecting expression of a particular protein by the cell. Multiple antibodies can be combined in each tube to the extent that they each have a distinct fluorescent tag. For example, a single tube for profiling lymphocytes might contain CD3-PE, CD19-PC5, and kappa-FITC; the expression profile of these three surface markers can be quantitated separately because each has a different associated dye. Detection of each fluorescent signal requires a separate channel on the device, so that a four-channel flow cytometer can analyze four markers per tube and a five-channel machine can observe five molecules in concert. In addition to demonstrating the coexpression patterns of these markers on distinct cellular populations, multichannel technology also minimizes the necessary sample size and shortens analysis time by reducing the number of tubes needing to be run. Nonetheless, modern cytometers can analyze cells at flow rates exceeding 1000 cells/second.

The data obtained from each cell are recorded as an event, theoretically allowing the user to look at the individual profile of each cell in the specimen. By selecting populations of cells with a certain range of expression for a particular marker ("gating"), the relative frequency and coexpressed markers can be visualized (see Figure 1C-3, panel D). For example, one might initially gate on CD45+ cells (leukocytes only) and then observe the CD3+ and CD20+ cell populations to assess the relative B- and T-cell numbers. T cells might be gated into CD4+ and CD8+ groups. If the T cells coexpressed both markers, one might suspect an immature T-cell neoplasm such as pre-T-ALL and would then investigate other markers such as CD5, CD10, and TdT. In such a stepwise fashion, each cell subpopulation can be examined for abnormalities.

The interpretation of flow cytometric data is a dynamic process (6). Tabular reports that list the markers analyzed and the percentage of cells positive are unable to capture the complexity of such data. It is good clinical practice to review the expression patterns of the cells of interest, seeing where they lie on each plot and correlating the flow cytometric patterns with the microscopic appearance and results of other ancillary studies.

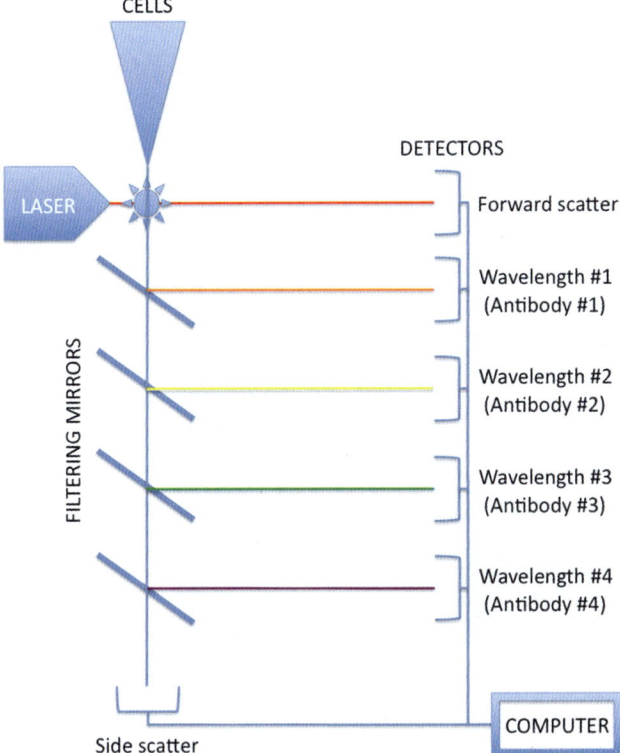

FIGURE 1C-2 • Overview of a typical four-channel flow cytometry setup. The antibody-bound cell suspension flows through the cytometer with cells passing singly through the laser beam(s). Forward scatter (**to the right**) is determined by the intensity of the light passing directly through the cell, whereas side scatter (**to the bottom**) depends on the intensity of reflected light. A series of filtering mirrors (**left**) selectively reroute light of the desired wavelength toward the detectors and allow the remainder of the beam to pass. Each antibody under investigation is conjugated to a tag that fluoresces at a different wavelength. Thus, each detector effectively measures a specific antibody and, together, four antibodies, forward scatter, and side scatter are measured simultaneously for each cell. Data are compiled by a computer processor and presented as interactive scattergrams.

Applications

Flow cytometric analysis is invaluable, not only in the diagnostic workup of leukemias and lymphomas, but in a myriad of other applications, as well. For example, in lieu of the traditional Kleihauer-Betke test, the degree of fetomaternal hemorrhage can be accurately determined using flow cytometry with antibodies directed against fetal hemoglobin (7,8). The diagnosis of PNH can be made by demonstrating an absence of GPI-linked proteins such as CD55 and CD59 (9,10). For some diseases, it is important to enumerate classes of lymphocytes such as monitoring CD4+ cell counts in HIV-infected patients, or other specific subtypes that may be

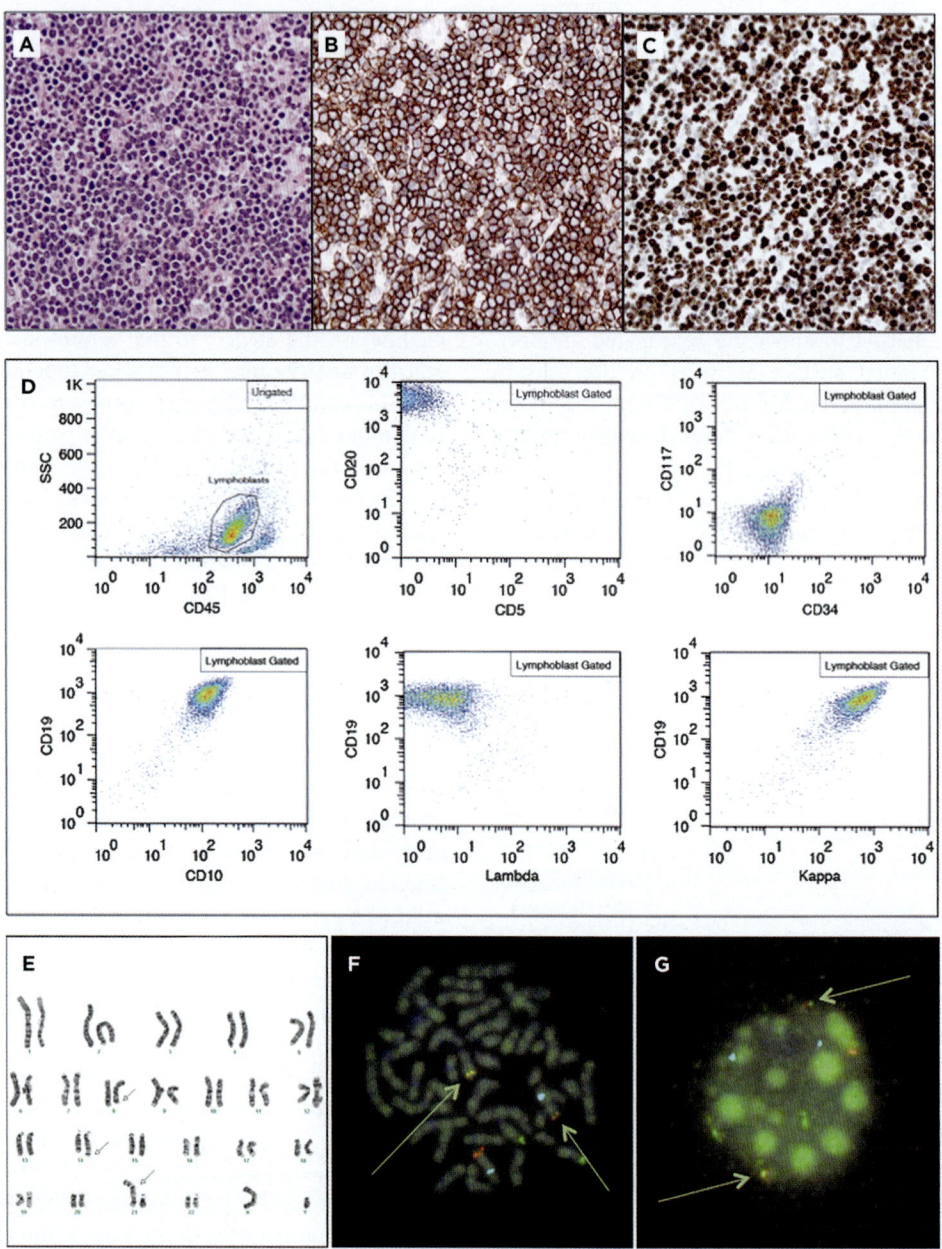

FIGURE 1C-3 • Burkitt lymphoma. Although just a small round blue cell tumor at first glance, the H&E-stained section (**A**) shows uniform cells with scant cytoplasm and a high mitotic rate along with interspersed tingible body macrophages. The lesional cells are positive for CD19 (**B**), identifying them as B lymphocytes with a near-100% proliferation rate (**C**, MIB-1 IHC). Flow cytometry (**D**) shows lymphoblasts that are negative for CD34 and CD117 (blastic and myeloblastic markers, respectively), but positive for the B-cell markers CD10 (moderate), CD19, and CD20 (bright) and kappa restricted (suggesting monoclonality). Conventional cytogenetic analysis (**E**) revealed an abnormal karyotype with a t(8;14) characteristic of Burkitt lymphoma, as well as an extra copy of 1q attached to the short arm of 21 (*arrows*). FISH was performed on both metaphase (**F**) and interphase nuclei (**G**) using *MYCC* (chr 8, *red*) and *IGH* probes (chr 14, *green*) and demonstrates several fusion genes (*in yellow*). Extra green signals indicate occasional gain of chromosome 14. (Flow cytometry plots kindly provided by Dennis W. Schauer, Clinical Immunodiagnostic and Research Laboratory, Department of Pediatrics, Medical College of Wisconsin. Karyotype and FISH analysis courtesy of Dr. Peter vanTuinen, Dynacare Clinical Cytogenetics Laboratory, Medical College of Wisconsin.)

lacking (such as in various immunodeficiencies) or present in excessive numbers (such as CD3+, CD4−, CD8−, "double-negative" T cells in autoimmune lymphoproliferative disorder) (11,12). Also, flow cytometry is being more frequently used in minimal residual disease detection—identifying small, morphologically invisible populations of leukemic or even circulating solid tumor cells, which has therapeutic and prognostic significance (13–15).

IMMUNOHISTOCHEMISTRY

Background

Over the course of the 1980's decade, IHC rapidly gained acceptance and became standard of care in most anatomic pathology laboratories. IHC boasts high sensitivity, specificity, and resiliency. Unlike immunofluorescence or many molecular techniques, IHC can be performed on formalin-fixed, paraffin-embedded tissue (FFPE). This greatly enhances its utility, especially on cases with limited material and in retrospective studies. Finally, automated stainers can easily perform IHC with minimal human hands-on time. Such machines have reduced the relative cost of IHC in many laboratories.

Method

The principle of IHC is simple enough and involves a primary antibody specific for the antigen of interest, a secondary antibody that not only binds the first antibody but is also conjugated to an enzyme, and a colorimetric indicator such as a dye that is formed or changes color via the action of the aforementioned enzyme. Thus, a molecular linkage is formed that localizes a readily discernible color (typically, brown or red) to the vicinity of the antigen of interest (Figure 1C-4) (16).

For most diagnostic and research applications of IHC, FFPE tissue is used (17,18). The application of microwave or steam heat to the tissue prior to the staining process ("antigen retrieval" or "unmasking") can improve sensitivity of the technique by reducing or reversing formalin-induced cross-linking of proteins (which modifies or blocks some epitopes required for antibody recognition). A few special antibodies have been optimized for use with frozen tissue sections, and these require the forethought to reserve a piece of the specimen for this purpose.

The primary antibody is the primary determinant of IHC reactivity. The choice of antibody is guided not only by the target antigen but also by the desired sensitivity/specificity, the reaction conditions, and the cost and reliability of product from a given manufacturer. Different antibody clones react with different portions of proteins and may yield strikingly different IHC results. Monoclonal antibodies (where all antibody molecules recognize a single epitope) are usually more specific than polyclonal sera (where the antibody molecules recognize a variety of antigenic epitopes on a single protein); however, the former are therefore more vulnerable to false-negative results when the epitope is obscured (by protein interactions or misfolding) or absent (via mutations). Perhaps the most pronounced difference between monoclonal and polyclonal antibodies is seen with carcinoembryonic antigen (CEA); fewer than 5% of all hepatocellular carcinomas stain with monoclonal CEA antibodies, whereas roughly 70% stain with polyclonal CEA antibodies in a cytoplasmic or canalicular pattern (19).

The optimal reaction conditions, such as antibody concentration and incubation time, must be determined for each new antibody, and existing protocols should be tested with each new lot of an established antibody. Excessive concentrations of antibody or prolonged incubation times may allow nonspecific binding, whereas insufficient antibody or time can yield false-negative results (20).

The choice of secondary antibody is in large part dictated by the primary antibody; the two must originate from different species so that the secondary antibody recognizes the constant portions of the primary antibody. Some manufacturers offer a secondary antibody that reacts against primary antibodies from multiple species. The variety of signaling methods and permutations thereof is too numerous to describe here. Suffice it to say, the secondary antibody is conjugated to a signal molecule—a dye, an enzyme, or a fluorescent marker—such that the location of the antibody "sandwich" can in some way be visualized.

One of the most common detection reactions involves horseradish peroxidase (HRP), which can convert a chromogen (such as TMB or DAB) into a brown-colored product. This method is susceptible to high background signal created by endogenous peroxidases found especially in erythrocytes and granulocytes; these cytoplasmic enzymes can react with the dye precursors to produce a signal indistinguishable from the intended one, except for its localization. In order to quench these enzymes and lower the background noise, pretreatment with methanol and dilute hydrogen peroxide (or other related methods) is used to denature these culprits without significantly inhibiting the subsequently used HRP. However, endogenous peroxidase activity may still hinder interpretation in enzyme-rich tissues such as spleen and bone marrow. Regardless of the specific methods employed, the end result is a color change localized to the antigenic sites of interest. A light counterstain, such as hematoxylin alone, hematoxylin and eosin, methyl green, or periodic acid–Schiff, is often employed to allow background architecture and unstained cells to be discerned.

The final step is careful interpretation. The positive control should show strong, specific staining on a section of tissue known to contain the antigen of interest. Ideally, this positive control tissue should be present on the same slide as the

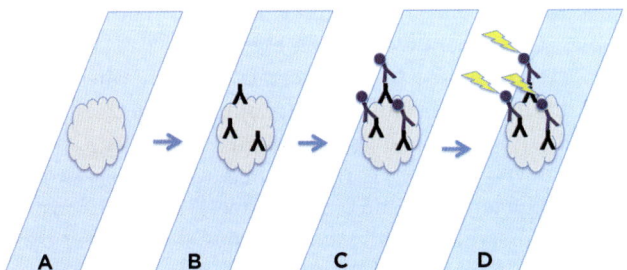

FIGURE 1C-4 • Overview of immunohistochemical staining. Tissue slides (**A**) are incubated with a primary antibody specific for the antigen of interest (**B**), to which a secondary antibody conjugated to a marker is then bound (**C**). Detection is then achieved by a colorimetric or light-producing assay (**D**).

case tissue section. Likewise, the negative control, usually performed on an additional slide of the actual case material, omits the primary antibody and should demonstrate a lack of nonspecific binding of secondary antibody, important when using a natural protein such as biotin in the antibody complex. Each case tissue section has internal controls built in, as well, in the form of blood vessels, connective tissue, or epithelium. The positive and negative staining patterns of these tissue types should be examined in addition to the staining of the areas of interest. Interpretation should include consideration of the quality, quantity, and patterns of staining. Proteins can be nuclear, cytoplasmic, and/or cytoplasmic membranous. Knowledge of the expected pattern of antibody staining in particular tissues is important for quality control.

As an ancillary diagnostic method, IHC results are usually reported as part of a more comprehensive report. Within the "Microscopic Description" or "Comment" section, the performed IHC stains should be described (in tabular or textual format) including the name of the stain, the results with lesional cells, and verification of controls. For example, "Properly controlled immunohistochemical stains demonstrate that the lesional cells are positive for a, b, and c, but negative for x, y, and z." Depending on personal and institutional preference, an explanation of these results and how they support the diagnosis may then be appended. Most laboratories automatically add a note detailing whether these stains are FDA approved for clinical use or are investigational only, which may affect the payment for these services.

Applications

The most common use for IHC is as an ancillary method in the diagnosis and detection of tumors and identification of tissue. Sometimes, its purpose is to detect or highlight a single population of cells—for example, ganglion cells (for the RET protein, in biopsies of suspected Hirschsprung disease) or endodermal sinus tumor components (by α-fetoprotein staining) of mixed germ cell tumors or teratomas (21–23). Some IHC stains lend insight into the genetic alterations in tumors like mutant-specific BRAF (24), IDH1 (25,26), and TP53 (27). EGFR and p53 expression patterns, which distinguish *de novo* pediatric and adult glioblastomas, differ between *de novo* and progressive glioblastoma in adults (28,29). The results of other IHC tests can direct and optimize treatment by confirming the presence of target molecules, for example, estrogen and progesterone receptor status for antihormonal therapy in breast carcinoma, and CD20 surface expression for rituximab in leukemia/lymphoma and autoimmune disease (30,31). As with any ancillary technique, the results of IHC alone should not determine the diagnosis or treatment but, rather, should be interpreted in the context of the morphologic appearance and clinical history.

ANTIGENS

Cytoskeleton

Three main groups constitute the cytoskeleton of human cells: thin, intermediate, and thick filaments. *Thin filaments* (5 to 6 nm) are composed of α-, β-, and γ-actins; the former are exclusively found in muscle cells and can be distinguished by antibodies such as muscle-specific actin (MSA; HHF35), smooth muscle actin (SMA), and smooth muscle myosin heavy chain (SMMS-1). For example, the IHC staining pattern differentiates between nonmuscle cells and tumors (MSA– SMA– SMMS-1–), skeletal muscle myocytes and rhabdomyosarcomas (MSA+ SMA– SMMS-1–), and smooth muscle myocytes and leiomyosarcomas (MSA+ SMA+ SMMS-1+). Myoepithelial cells and myofibroblasts also stain positively for all three markers, although to varying degrees.

Diagnostically speaking, the most useful cytoskeletal proteins are the *intermediate filaments* (10 nm). The relative composition of intermediate filaments varies by cell type and allows distinction by IHC. The major intermediate filaments include vimentin, desmin, glial fibrillary acidic protein (GFAP), and cytokeratins.

Vimentin can be found in all mesenchyme-derived cells—fibroblasts, myocytes, osteocytes, chondrocytes, Schwann cells, endothelial cells, and hematopoietic elements—often leading to its dismissal as "nonspecific." Nonetheless, a vimentin stain serves well to distinguish sarcomas and lymphomas from carcinomas. Even with the most poorly differentiated neoplasms, this distinction can usually be made. Vimentin IHC is also of great utility in confirming that tissue antigenicity has been preserved; most sections have at least focal areas of vimentin-positive cells. Necrotic tissue can be surprisingly informative, as it often maintains some degree of reactivity, often in the original pattern of distribution. In these cases, careful comparison with control tissue and nontumoral tissue in the section is necessary to ensure accurate interpretation.

Desmin shares sequence homology with vimentin and is likewise restricted to mesenchymal cells. However, unlike vimentin, desmin is only expressed at significant levels in smooth, skeletal, and cardiac myocytes. Thus, in a sense, desmin is a marker of myogenic differentiation; although the aforementioned cells contain desmin, primitive mesenchymal cells and neoplasms do not. Desmin-positive tumors include leiomyomas, leiomyosarcomas, and rhabdomyosarcomas. Of special note, desmin expression in most cardiac myocytes is limited to the intercalated discs, whereas the Purkinje fibers show diffuse cytoplasmic staining.

Glial fibrillary acidic protein (GFAP) is relatively specific for astrocytes and their corresponding neoplasms—astrocytomas, glioblastomas, and other gliomas (32). Reactive astrocytes are markedly positive and care must be taken to ensure that such a population of cells is not mistaken for the actual neoplasm (32–34). Ependymal cells and their derivative neoplasms show variable reactivity for GFAP. *Neurofilament* is actually a set of three related proteins that form fibers within the cell bodies and processes of neurons; the main diagnostic utility of a neurofilament IHC stain is to highlight neurons within tissue or tumor.

Epithelial cells are easily distinguishable by the presence of distinct *cytokeratin* profiles. Carcinomas are positive when using broad-spectrum cytokeratin antibody "cocktails" such as AE1/AE3 or CK7/CK20, which can rule out most lymphomas and sarcomas. Important exceptions include the epithelial component of synovial sarcoma (Figure 1C-5, panel C), epithelioid sarcoma, and the characteristic cytoplasmic inclusions of malignant rhabdoid tumors; the latter stain for cytokeratin, not muscle markers. More specific antibodies can help highlight organ-specific epithelium, for example, CK19 in breast or biliary tract or TTF1 in the lung and thyroid.

Thick filaments (20 to 25 nm) are composed of β-tubulin and are ubiquitous to all cell types. Thus, their diagnostic utility is limited.

Cell Surface Markers

Cell surface antigens have proven utility not only in IHC but also in flow cytometry and cell sorting. However, while flow cytometry requires fresh tissue or cell-rich fluid, the same

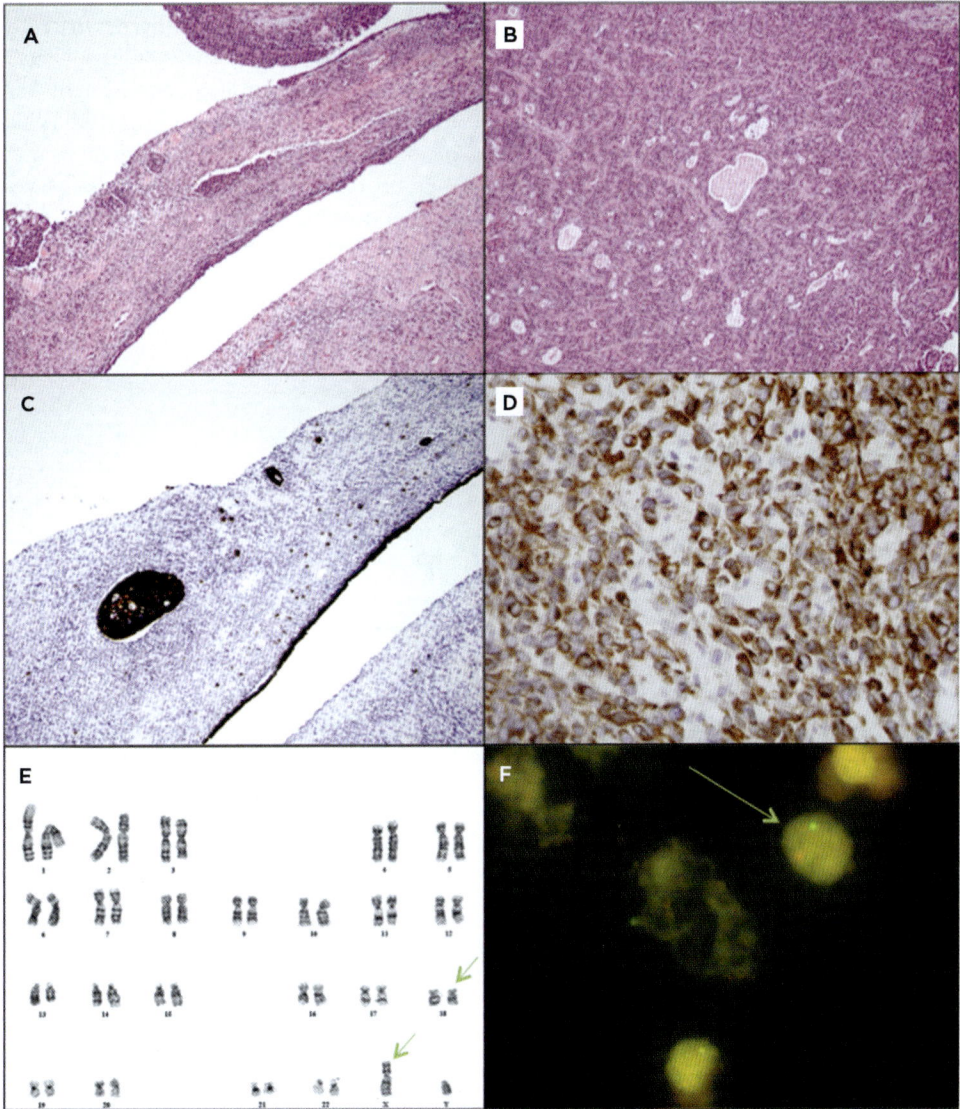

FIGURE 1C-5 • Biphasic synovial sarcoma. The H&E-stained sections (**A, B**) demonstrate a spindle cell sarcoma with areas of glandular differentiation; the latter are immunohistochemically positive for mixed cytokeratins (**C**), and the majority of the tumor cells are positive for bcl-2 (**D**). Conventional cytogenetic analysis (**E**) demonstrated t(X;18) pathognomonic for the *SYT-SSX* fusion gene of synovial sarcoma (*arrows*). Breakapart FISH probes (one red, one green from opposite ends [5′ and 3′, respectively] of the *SYT* gene) are seen separately instead of together as a single intact yellow signal (as seen in the surrounding normal cells) (**F**). (Karyotype and FISH analysis courtesy of Dr. Peter vanTuinen, Dynacare Clinical Cytogenetics Laboratory, Medical College of Wisconsin.)

markers can be evaluated on FFPE tissue by IHC. These antigens are indispensable in the diagnosis of hematopoietic neoplasms, and such use is detailed elsewhere in this book (see Chapters 22 and 23).

Many of these cell surface molecules are numerically designated as a "cluster of differentiation," or "CD." For example, the normal constituent cells of the mature immune system can be roughly grouped by their expression of these proteins: B lymphocytes (positive for CD19, CD20 [L26], CD79a; Figure 1C-3), T lymphocytes (positive for CD3, CD4, CD8), and natural killer cells (positive for CD56). Myeloblasts stain for CD34 and CD117 (c-kit), two markers also associated with other neoplasms; a CD34 stain is positive in synovial sarcoma and some vascular tumors, and CD117 positivity is an important finding in gastrointestinal stromal tumors (35).

Macrophages and histiocytes exhibit granular staining in their cytoplasm for CD68, a component of lysosomal membranes (more accurately, a *lysosomal* surface marker); CD1a is specific for Langerhans cells and T lymphoblasts (36–39). Mast cells have membrane positivity for CD138, as well as cytoplasmic positivity for a characteristic enzyme, tryptase (40). This enzyme can also be detected by histochemical methods that require frozen tissue.

Endothelial cells, both nascent and tumoral, can be marked with CD31 and CD34, although these antibodies mark some other cells, as well. GLUT-1 is a useful marker for the endothelial cells of infantile hemangiomas (41), and D2-40 (podoplanin) marks lymphatic endothelium (along with mesothelium and some other tissues) (42).

Pathogens

A wide variety of viruses can be detected by antibodies specific for well-conserved antigens, including adenovirus, cytomegalovirus (CMV), herpes simplex virus (HSV) types I and II, parvovirus B19, human herpesvirus 8 (HHV8), human papilloma virus, BK virus (via large T antigen), hepatitis B virus (via surface antigen), and Epstein-Barr virus (EBV, via the latent membrane protein [LMP]). Typically, clinical suspicion, positive serologic testing, or viral cytopathic change seen on routine H&E-stained slides serves as a trigger for further workup by IHC. Companion *in situ* hybridization tests are available for both HPV and EBV (Figure 1C-6,

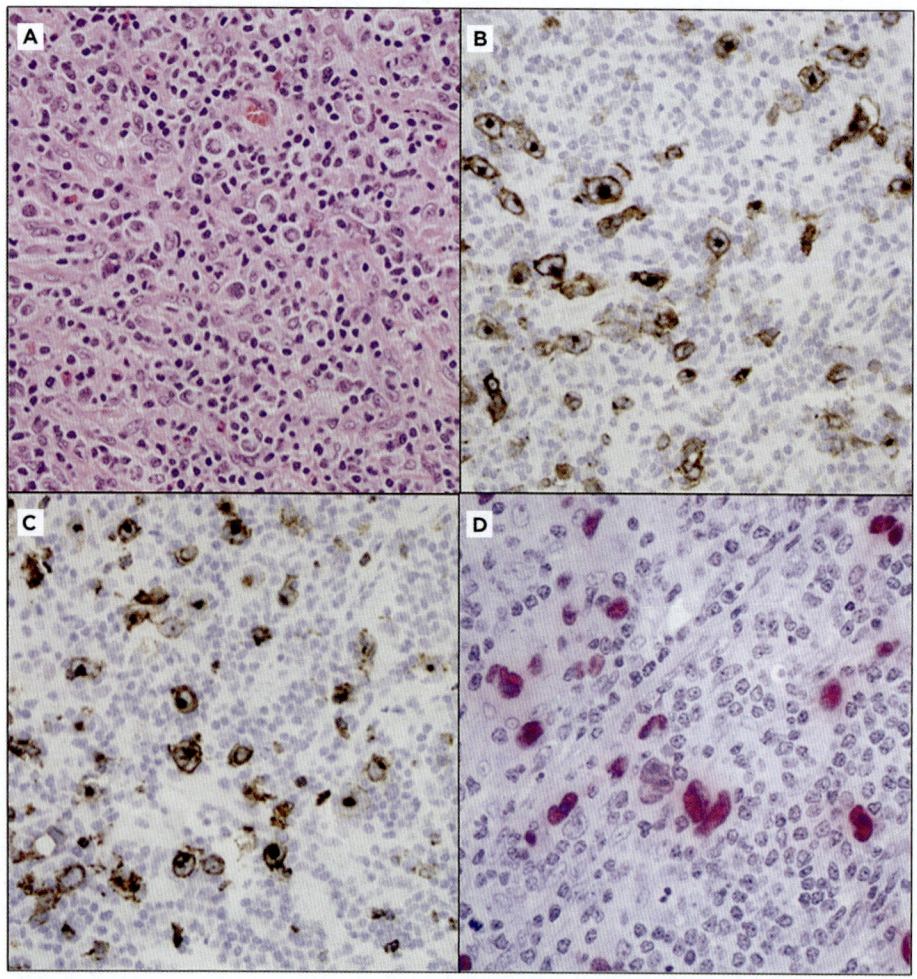

FIGURE 1C-6 • Classic Hodgkin lymphoma. The H&E-stained section (**A**) reveals scattered large cells with atypical, convoluted nuclei in a mixed inflammatory background. At lower power, fibrous bands were seen entrapping nodules of tumor. By IHC, the Hodgkin cells are positive for CD15 (**B**) and CD30 (**C**). *In situ* hybridization for EBV-encoded RNA (EBER) is positive in many of these cells (**D**, *red staining*).

panel D); these tests can identify the former as high- or low-risk subtypes. Whenever possible, viral IHC should be performed in tandem with culture and serologic testing (43).

IHC is less commonly used to identify bacteria, both because of these organisms' patchy and often sparse distribution in tissue and the greater detection sensitivity of microbiologic culture methods (43,44). However, antibodies against *Helicobacter pylori* have supplanted more traditional Steiner, Giemsa, or Alcian Yellow stains at some institutions (45,46). Also, *Pneumocystis jiroveci*, once thought to be protozoal but now formally classified as a fungus, can be easily highlighted by appropriate antibodies in IHC (47,48).

Hormones

IHC can assist in confirming the diagnosis and hormone secretion profile of many endocrine tumors. For example, pancreatic endocrine neoplasms (islet cell tumors) can be categorized as derived from alpha, beta, delta, or G cells based on immunohistochemically verifiable expression of glucagon, insulin, somatostatin, or gastrin, respectively. Likewise, VIP-producing tumors and serotonin-secreting carcinoids can be demonstrated by IHC.

In conjunction with clinical presentation, pituitary adenomas can be easily classified by IHC profiling for prolactin, adrenocorticotrophin hormone (ACTH), thyroid-stimulating hormone, growth hormone, follicle-stimulating hormone, and luteinizing hormone (49,50). This approach is especially useful with silent adenomas, which have detectable hormone(s) in the tumor cells' cytoplasm, but not in the patient's serum.

Medullary thyroid carcinoma stains positively for calcitonin, as do normal C-cells and the hyperplastic foci of multiple endocrine neoplasia syndrome. More generally, thyroid epithelial cells can be highlighted by antibodies to thyroglobulin or thyroid transcription factor-1 (TTF-1). Parathyroid hormone stains are useful in identifying parathyroid tissue, although normal, hyperplastic, and neoplastic tissues react identically.

Although less often useful in the pediatric realm, IHC for estrogen and progesterone receptors has become standard of care in the evaluation of breast cancer, serving to guide the choice of chemotherapy. Germ cell and sex cord tumors can express α-inhibin and β-human chorionic gonadotrophin (β-hCG), and the serum levels of these markers are sometimes used to monitor patients for recurrence.

Embryonal and Cancer Markers

Fetal tissues and neoplasms share expression of primitive traits, including a subset of proteins normally restricted to developmental periods. For example, α-fetoprotein can be found in fetal liver as well as hepatoblastomas, hepatomas, and endodermal sinus tumors. Placental alkaline phosphatase (PLAP) stains germ cell tumors and some carcinomas. The stem cell marker OCT4 is now replacing PLAP as a more sensitive and specific marker of germ cell neoplasms, specifically seminoma/germinoma, embryonal carcinoma, and intratubular germ cell neoplasia. Among the so-called cancer markers, CA-125 is more specific for genitourinary neoplasms, whereas CA19-9 is preferentially expressed in gastrointestinal cancers. Both these markers are also detectable in patient serum.

INI-1 (hSNF, SMARCB1, BAF47) is a particularly helpful antibody in the diagnosis of malignant rhabdoid tumor (and atypical teratoid/rhabdoid tumor), epithelioid sarcoma, and renal medullary carcinoma. Loss of nuclear INI-1 staining is predictive of INI-1 mutation or deletion that typifies this group of tumors, whereas the gene is invariably expressed in normal cells, providing a useful internal control.

Also of note is the WT1 protein, a zinc-finger transcription factor that is expressed in the course of normal urogenital development and which functions as an inactivated tumor suppressor in nephroblastoma (Wilms tumor) and other neoplasms. Wilms tumors show nuclear immunoreactivity for WT1 with most antibodies, whereas desmoplastic small round cell tumors, with canonical *EWS-WT1* gene rearrangements, are often only positive when using antibodies directed against C-terminal epitopes (51,52).

Protooncogenes

Anaplastic lymphoma kinase-1 (ALK-1) is the fusion product of a characteristic $t(2;5)$ translocation found in most anaplastic large cell lymphomas and inflammatory myofibroblastic tumors; its expression in the former is thought to portend favorable prognosis. ALK-1 is also mutated or amplified in about 20% of neuroblastomas, especially in familial variants, and may identify patients eligible for crizotinib therapy (53–55). Tyrosine kinases, such as *c-kit* (CD117), can help diagnose tumors such as gastrointestinal stromal tumors, as well as predict which lesions might respond to monoclonal antibody therapy (in this case, imatinib).

BRAF, a serine/threonine protein kinase, is often mutated in human cancers. In children, a specific V600E mutation is frequently seen in papillary thyroid carcinoma, aggressive Langerhans cell histiocytosis, and brain tumors (glioblastoma multiforme, pleomorphic xanthoastrocytomas, and gangliogliomas) (56–60). The presence of this mutation identifies tumors which might be amenable to targeted therapies.

Cell Cycle and Apoptotic Markers

The most commonly used antibody in this category is MIB-1 (Ki67), a proliferation marker frequently used to assess the proliferative activity of lesions. Although a high MIB-1 index does not define something as neoplastic, it can be used as a corroborating piece of evidence in making such a decision, or in determining the histologic grade of a tumor (Figure 1C-3, panel C). Some apoptotic markers, such as Bcl-2 and Bcl-6, have utility in identifying the lineage of hematopoietic neoplasms and other tumors (Figure 1C-5, panel D). β-catenin, a molecule involved in the Wnt signaling pathway, shows nuclear staining in desmoid tumors, Wnt pathway–related medulloblastomas, and colorectal lesions with aberrations of the APC pathway.

P53 IHC correlates with genetic *TP53* status in many pediatric tumors, including gliomas, rhabdomyosarcomas, adrenal cortical neoplasms, Wilms tumors, and pleuropulmonary blastomas (27,61–64). Aberrant p53 expression in the nucleus is usually predictive of a gene mutation; the most common deleterious mutations often interfere with protein turnover. Absent p53 expression by IHC doesn't always imply an intact p53 pathway. Nonsense mutations, deletions and chromosome 17 loss are other mechanisms by which *TP53* function can be lost.

Other

Alpha-1-antitrypsin (A1AT) is expressed in normal and neoplastic liver tissue, as well as in yolk sac tumors. Its primary diagnostic utility, however, is in identifying A1AT deficiency manifest as strong cytoplasmic positivity in the setting of hepatic or pulmonary disease; recall that the disorder affects A1AT export, not production, so the mutated protein accumulates intracellularly. A1AT is also a serine protease inhibitor (serpin), and is found in histiocytes and pancreatic and salivary duct epithelium.

Limitations

As mentioned previously, immunohistochemical stains are only useful when done properly and in a well-controlled fashion. Evaluation of appropriate controls is required every time a stain is run in order to ensure validity. Minor changes in reaction conditions or the antibody supplier can lead to major changes in results. IHC staining patterns can only be interpreted in the context of the H&E morphology, the clinical scenario, and the results of other ancillary tests. Basing a diagnosis on a single immunostain can be risky. Performing a panel of five stains that are 80% specific is bound to result in at least one stain with spurious results.

IMMUNOFLUORESCENCE

Background

Direct immunofluorescence (DIF) is a molecular technique that provides ancillary information in the diagnosis of dermatologic, renal, and transplant organ disease. DIF relies on the same antibody-antigen recognition concept as flow cytometry and IHC. The most common uses in pathology include detection of immunoglobulins, complement proteins, and fibrinogen in patient tissue sections or infectious organisms in other samples (*Pneumocystis* spp.) (65).

Method

DIF requires fresh or snap-frozen tissue as formalin and other aldehyde-derived fixatives alter the antigenicity of immunoglobulins, complement proteins, and other molecules of

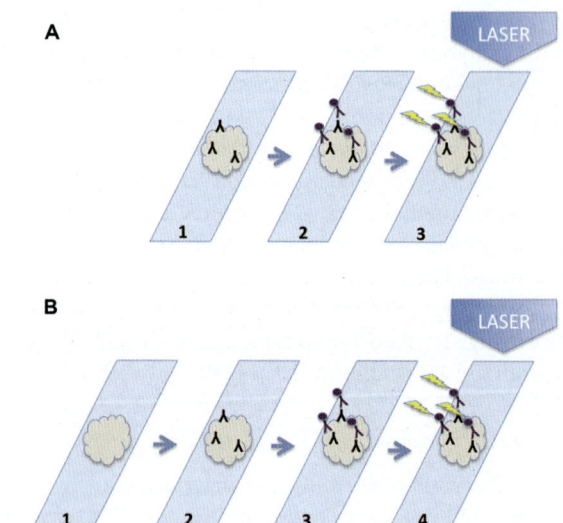

FIGURE 1C-7 • Overview of immunofluorescent staining. For DIF (**A**), slides bear tissue with native antibody of interest already bound (*1*). A secondary antibody conjugated to a fluorescent tag is then bound to the original antibodies (*2*) and then detected by laser-induced fluorescence (*3*). Indirect immunofluorescence (IIF) (**B**) is nearly identical to IHC (see Figure 1C-4), except detection requires laser excitation.

interest (66). Ammonium sulfate–based buffers that inhibit tissue proteases can be used to transport specimens from the procedure areas to the testing laboratory (67–72). Tissue is then snap frozen in OCT, sectioned in a cryostat, air dried, rehydrated, and incubated with the appropriate antibody solution. If DIF is not needed immediately, it is helpful to know that tissue antigens are stable frozen in OCT for up to 4 months at either −20°C or −70°C (65).

For most renal and skin biopsies, a typical immunofluorescence panel will include antibodies directed against IgG, IgA, IgM, C1, C3, fibrinogen, C4d (in renal transplant), properdin, and albumin—the latter as a positive control. Antibody binding and staining is similar to that for IHC but uses a fluorochrome rather than a dye for detection (Figure 1C-7). Stained slides are stored in a dark refrigerator until reading, which should occur as promptly as possible (within 24 hours) as fluorescence intensity diminishes with time.

Applications

The most common specimens that routinely involve immunofluorescence staining are for medical kidney disease and autoimmune skin disorders (Figure 1C-8). In addition to the particular stains that are positive (e.g., IgG versus IgM), the pattern (linear versus granular) and the location (basement membrane versus dermal-epidermal junction) of staining are also important in distinguishing between specific entities. (*See Chapters 17 and 26 for detailed information about DIF in kidney and skin lesions.*) Ultimately, the simultaneous consideration of all available information—clinical presentation, laboratory studies, H&E-stained sections, and DIF—is required to maximize diagnostic sensitivity and accuracy.

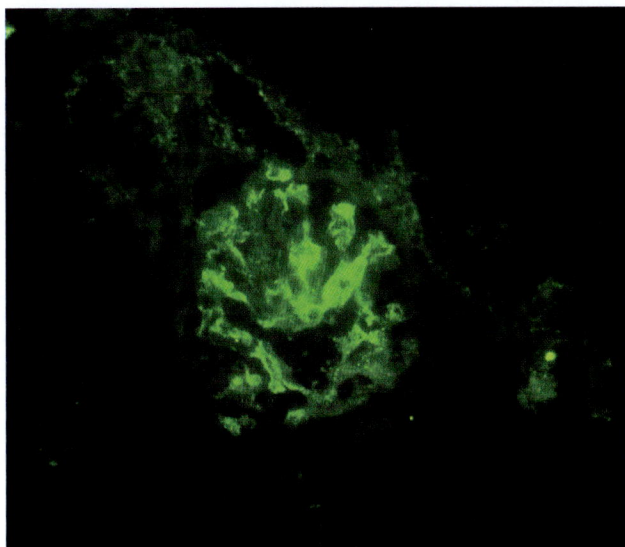

FIGURE 1C-8 • DIF for IgA in a renal core biopsy from an 11-year-old girl with gross hematuria and nephrotic-range proteinuria. Glomeruli showed diffuse IgA deposits in the mesangium and granular deposition in the capillary loops which, in conjunction with the light and electron microscopic findings, was consistent with IgA nephropathy.

FLUORESCENCE *IN SITU* HYBRIDIZATION

Background

Increasing numbers of tumors and congenital disorders are being identified as monogenic in nature, and their underlying genetic alterations are being discovered. In turn, this has yielded a large number of genetic targets that can be used in the diagnosis, prognosis, and therapeutic selection for these patients. As such, a variety of molecularly based genetic assays have been developed to investigate and analyze these targets. Instead of relying on the specificity of an antibody-antigen reaction, as in IHC and IF, fluorescence *in situ* hybridization (FISH/ISH) utilizes the base complementarity between a labeled oligonucleotide probe and a DNA or RNA sequence of interest.

One of the main advantages of FISH/ISH is its *in situ* nature—target sequences of interest are precisely localized within specific cells, the nuclear/cytoplasmic distribution can be compared, and the relative chromosomal location of two genes can be identified. This is in contrast to techniques such as PCR, microarrays, or cytogenetics, which by necessity destroy the architecture to get at the DNA, RNA, or chromosomes. Another benefit of FISH/ISH is the high specificity of nucleic acid strand interactions, which can easily distinguish between closely related gene products. Alternatively, probes can be designed against conserved sequences to detect multiple isoforms or products, for example, multiple strains of a single virus or common population variants of a polymorphous locus. Linking the probes to a fluorescent tag (in FISH) amplifies the signal and increases the sensitivity of the assay without affecting the specificity. Finally, these methods are usually suitable for use with FFPE, allowing their application in cases with limited material as well as in retrospective research or clinical studies.

Methods

The optimal tissue source for FISH/ISH assays depends on the target molecule; frozen tissue is preferable for RNA studies, whereas FFPE is suitable for DNA work as well as for some small, stable RNAs. Standard 4- to 10-μm sections are cut on a cryostat or microtome and, for FFPE, deparaffinized and rehydrated. Other potential specimen sources include touch preparations and nuclear spreads from conventional cytogenetics (Figures 1C-3, 1C-5, and 1C-9); in both instances, nuclei are fixed by alcohol- or aldehyde-based methods.

Slides are overlaid with a small amount of buffer containing the desired probe and incubated from several hours to overnight. Probes can be RNA or DNA and can be synthesized in-house from templates or purchased from a variety of commercial vendors; some of the latter sell kits with multiple probes and controls appropriately packaged together for a particular disease entity or differential diagnostic workup.

Sections are then washed to remove unbound and nonspecifically bound probe. Then, for ISH, the detection reaction is run to create a color change at the site of binding, akin to that described for IHC (Figure 1C-6, panel D). For FISH, sections are examined under a fluorescent microscope to detect the labeled probe (Figure 1C-3, panels F and G; Figure 1C-5, panel F; Figure 1C-9, panel F; and Figure 1C-10, panels B and C). Appropriate controls include probes against "housekeeping" genes, or the centromeres of uninvolved chromosomes, as well as evaluation of the analytic probes in "normal" or uninvolved cells.

Applications

FISH and ISH have wide utility in a broad range of applications. The most common may be in the detection of chromosomal translocations in solid and hematopoietic neoplasms. This analysis can be approached in two ways: looking for the fusion product, or looking for the destruction of the original gene ("breakapart"). For example, in some cases of Burkitt lymphoma (Figure 1C-3, panels F and G), the *MYCC* and *IGH* genes are involved in a *t*(8;14) translocation. In the assay pictured, the *MYCC* probe is conjugated to a red tag and the *IGH* probe to a green tag. In normal cells, two separate red signals and two separate green signals should be present. However, in Burkitt cells harboring the translocation, one set of red and green signals overlaps producing a yellow fusion signal. For the breakapart strategy, the principle is reversed: normal cells should have two intact signals, but translocation will destroy one of those signals and create two new signals. For example, in synovial sarcoma (Figure 1C-5, panel F), the central tumor cell has two separate *SYT*

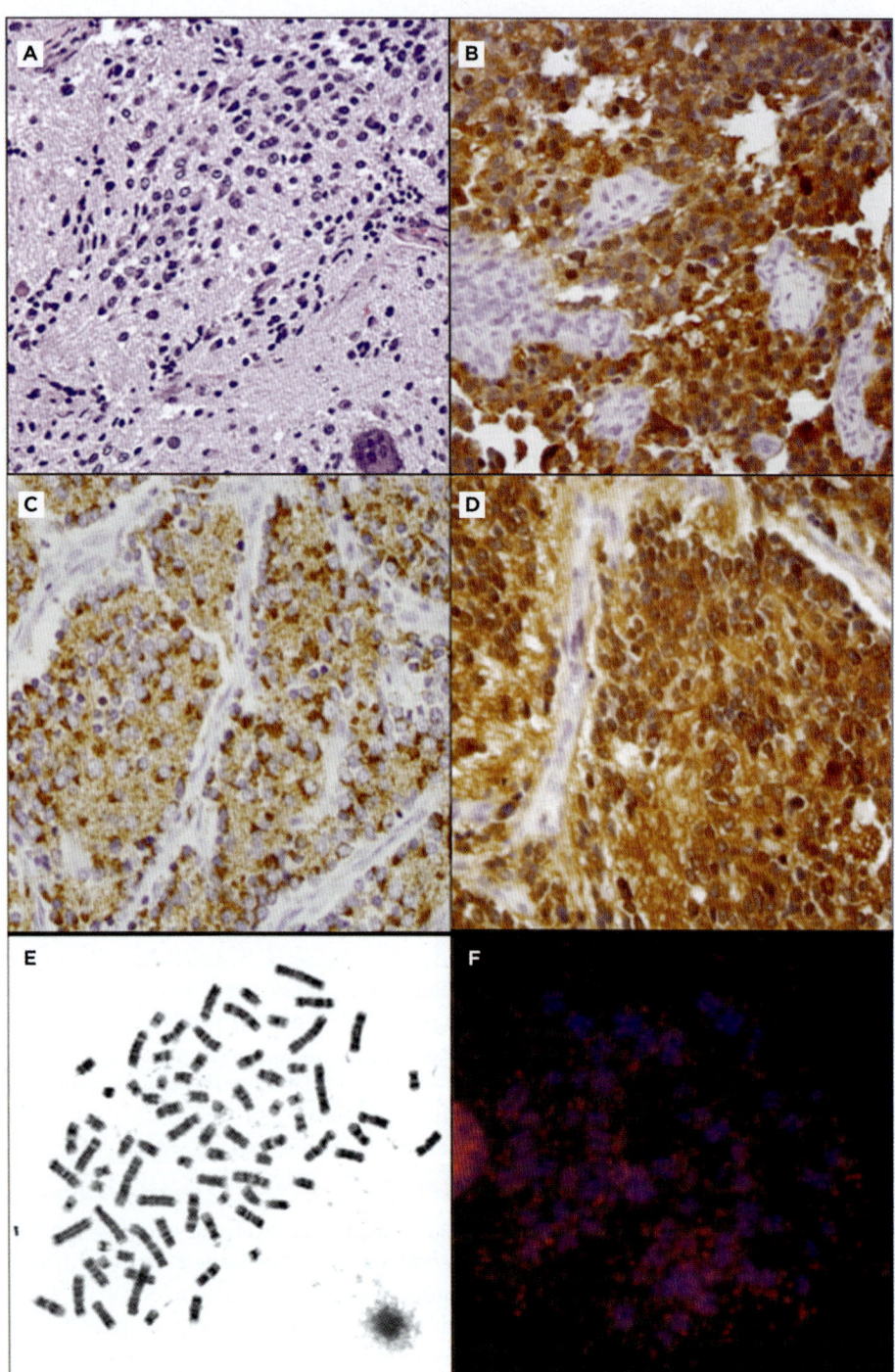

FIGURE 1C-9 • Neuroblastoma. On an H&E-stained section (**A**), small round blue cells with occasional early gangliocytoid differentiation, copious neuropil, and a low mitotic–karyorrhectic index are seen. The tumor cells are immunohistochemically positive for PGP9.5 (**B**), NB84 (**C**), and synaptophysin (**D**), confirming the diagnosis of neuroblastoma. A metaphase chromosomal spread (**E**) shows numerous double minutes in the background, which are FISH positive for *MYCN* (**F**), indicating amplification. (Chromosomal and FISH analyses courtesy of Dr. Peter vanTuinen, Dynacare Clinical Cytogenetics Laboratory, Medical College of Wisconsin.)

signals (one red and one green, from opposite ends of the gene) instead of a single intact yellow signal as seen in the surrounding normal cells.

FISH can also be used to detect copy number changes of a gene or locus, such as *MYCN* amplification in neuroblastoma (Figure 1C-9, panel F) or loss of one copy of the *hSNF5/INI1* locus in malignant rhabdoid tumor (73). In the case of *MYCN* amplification, this method is able to detect amplification whether via intrachromosomal sequence duplication or extrachromosomal double minutes (as shown). A centromeric probe should always be included in amplification assays to ensure that amplification is not merely due to whole chromosome gain (polysomy) which may have a different prognosis.

FISH is invaluable in the examination of stillbirth and intrauterine death, especially in cases of delayed delivery

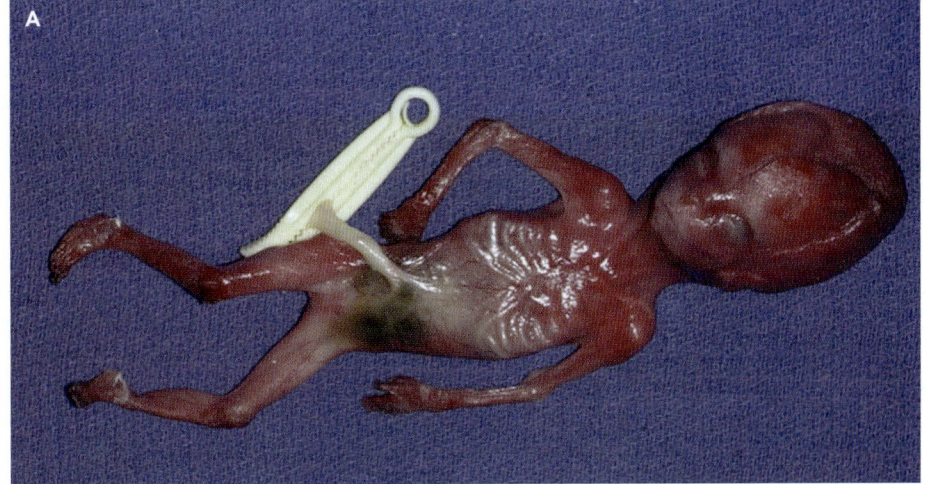
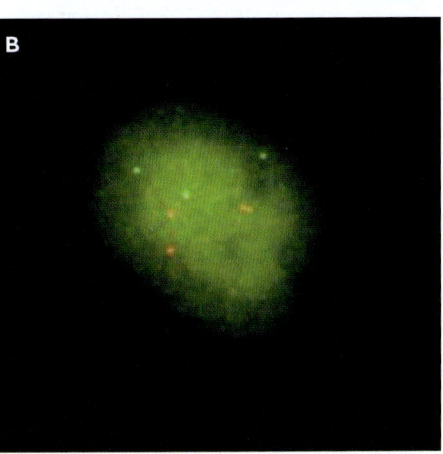
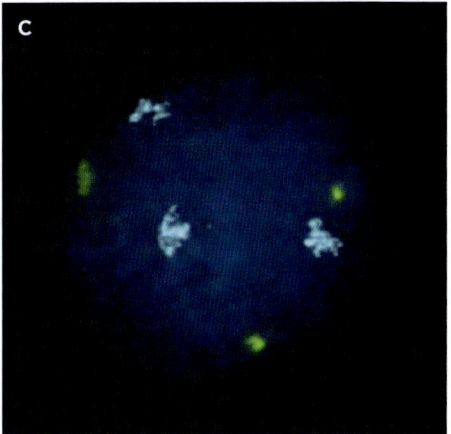

FIGURE 1C-10 • Fetal triploidy. A 29-year-old G1P0 female underwent medical pregnancy termination at 20 weeks' gestation following ultrasound diagnosis of intrauterine growth retardation, Dandy-Walker malformation, and ventricular septal heart defect (**A**) (Courtesy of Pat Rogers, Children's Hospital of Wisconsin, Audio Visual Services). Amniocentesis and FISH analysis had been performed, demonstrating triploidy (69,XXX). FISH probes in (**B**) include chromosomes 13 (*red*) and 21 (*green*) and, in (**C**), chromosomes 18 (*aqua*) and X (*green*); three copies of each chromosome are present, and no copies of the Y chromosome [*red probe* in (**C**)] are identified. (FISH analysis courtesy of Dr. Peter vanTuinen, Dynacare Clinical Cytogenetics Laboratory, Medical College of Wisconsin.)

where tissue quality is compromised. In the example case of a fetal demise with dysmorphic features (Figure 1C-10), the bottom two panels (B and C) show a standard FISH workup for common cytogenetic abnormalities in this setting—analysis of chromosomes 13, 18, 21 (most commonly implicated in stillborn trisomies), and X and Y. As shown, the fetus is triploid with three clear signals for chromosomes 13, 18, 21, and X. Not only is this study diagnostic, but essential because cells did not grow for conventional cytogenetics and karyotyping (see Chapter 3).

Nonfluorescent (colorimetric) ISH is often used as a nucleic acid version of IHC with otherwise similar techniques and applications. Most commonly, colorimetric ISH is used for detecting the abundant nucleic acids of infectious agents, such as HPV, HSV, and EBV (Figure 1C-6, panel D). ISH tends to have higher sensitivity and specificity than IHC for the companion viral proteins (74).

CYTOGENETICS

Background

Conventional cytogenetic analysis, or karyotyping, is a well-established technique that gives a broad genetic overview at a chromosomal level. It can identify constitutional disorders and demonstrate abnormalities that aid in diagnosis, often providing insight into prognosis and therapeutic effectiveness. Despite the development of increasingly sophisticated and sensitive molecular assays, cytogenetics maintains a crucial diagnostic role because of its capability to detect a wide range of abnormalities at once using a simple and cost-effective procedure.

Method

Typical specimens submitted for cytogenetic analysis include tumor or lymph node tissue, skin biopsy as a source of fibroblasts, whole blood or peripheral blood mononuclear cells, and prenatal samples from chorionic villus sampling or amniocentesis. For conventional cell culture and karyotyping, fresh viable tissue is required. For tumors and lymph nodes, a small (1 cm^3) piece of grossly viable lesional tissue usually suffices. For fetuses or neonates, a placental biopsy, taken superficially from the cleansed fetal surface, is usually an acceptable surrogate; however, care must be taken to prevent contamination of the sample with maternal cells (decidua or blood). Skin or fascia lata from autopsy cases is also usually adequate.

Samples should be immediately placed in standard tissue culture medium (such as RPMI) and kept at room temperature until transport to the cytogenetics laboratory. Often, testing can be delayed until initial workup of the case is completed—for example, with most tumors we routinely save a tissue sample in medium until the H&E-stained slides can be reviewed, and the necessity of cytogenetic testing can be evaluated. Most tissue is stable and viable for several days in culture medium at 4°C, although the risk of bacterial or fungal contamination increases over time unless antibiotics are included in the formulation of the medium. Another alternative is to submit the tissue to the cytogenetics lab for tissue culture and to make the decision about proceeding with karyotyping at a later date.

Upon receipt in the laboratory, specimens are disaggregated, and the cells are allowed to grow in culture for several days until they reach a sufficient number of actively dividing cells. At this point, a mitotic inhibitor is added that arrests the cells in metaphase with chromosomes neatly condensed and separated. Cells are cultured long enough for as many cells as possible to reach the stage of mitotic arrest, without reducing viability. The cells are then chemically treated to preserve the chromosomal integrity, fix the nuclei, and remove the cell membrane and cytoplasm. The nuclear preparation is then placed onto slides for staining and analysis.

Several different stains and procedures can be employed, but the most commonly used method is Giemsa staining (G-banding; see Figure 1C-3, panel E, and Figure 1C-5, panel E), which utilizes a limited trypsin digestion before staining with the same DNA-binding dye used elsewhere in histology, thereby producing light and dark bands across each chromosome. Other protocols utilize other chemical treatments and other dyes to specifically stain telomeres (T-banding), heterochromatin (C-banding), or AT-rich sequences (Q-banding). Each method produces a characteristic banding pattern that can be compared to known reference standards. G-banding typically yields roughly 400 bands across the genome for analysis; higher resolution banding can discriminate smaller regions but requires preparation of less condensed chromosomes, such as those in prometaphase instead of metaphase, and involves a more lengthy analysis. Standard G-banding has a detection limit of about four megabases; deletions or additions of smaller amounts of DNA may not be identified by this method.

Regarding terminology, the pattern produced by a particular method is compared to a standard reference (the Paris nomenclature) where bands are numbered according to their location on the chromosome—arm, region, band, sub-band, sub-sub-band, etc. The short arm is dubbed p (petit) and the long arm is q (queue). Bands (p11, p12, p13, …), sub-bands (p12 divided into p12.1, p12.2, p12.3, …), and sub-sub-bands (p12.2 divided into p12.21, p12.22, p12.23, …) are numbered from the centromere outward (the centromere can be considered to be both p10 and q10); p21.23 would be more telomeric than p21.22. Note that this terminology places band p3.25 between p3.1 and p3.3, as a sub-sub-band belonging to sub-band p3. A band's location is preceded by its host chromosome, such as 5q23.1, which is an area located roughly halfway out on the long arm of chromosome 5, and is properly described as "five q two three point one." Karyotypes are denoted in writing as the total diploid number of chromosomes, followed by the identities of the sex chromosomes, and then details regarding abnormalities. For example, boys and girls would usually have constitutional karyotypes of 46,XY, and 46,XX, respectively, while a female patient with Cri du chat syndrome might instead have a 46,XX,del(5p) karyotype.

Chromosomes are examined under a microscope, and their banding patterns are compared within each chromosomal pair (22 autosomal pairs and 2 sex chromosomes in each examined mitotic spread) and to the reference standards looking for aberrations in number, size, and/or composition. Standard karyotyping can detect numerical changes in chromosomes (e.g., monosomy or trisomy), duplication or loss of chromosomal material, translocations, and other disorders. Typically, the chromosomes from 20 different nuclei are examined, assuring a representative sampling in order to exclude mosaicism or a small percentage of abnormal cells, such as occasional tumor cells within a preponderance of normal cells.

Chromosomal abnormalities detectable by conventional cytogenetics are numerical or structural in nature. The former includes common constitutional disorders such as Down syndrome (trisomy 21), Edwards syndrome (trisomy 18), and Patau syndrome (trisomy 13), in all of which patients have a third, additional copy of an autosome (e.g., a girl with Down syndrome would have a 47,XX,+21 karyotype). Constitutional triploidy, three copies of all chromosomes (e.g., 69,XXX) is much less common than isolated trisomies and is almost always embryonic lethal (Figure 1C-10). Monosomies, such as Turner syndrome (45,XO), are readily detected. Again, standard analysis includes 20 cells because sporadic loss of a chromosome (or other aberration) can occur during sample preparation; an abnormality should be consistently seen in multiple cells before it is considered real. Tumors often show aneuploidy with varying numbers of each chromosome, in addition to structural aberrations.

Structural chromosomal problems occur in many different forms and appear to be the result of DNA damage and/or faulty repair. Some are balanced, in which no net material is lost, but sequences are simply rearranged; this includes translocations and inversions. Others are unbalanced, with net loss (deletions) or gain (duplications) of genetic material. These include inversions, deletions, additions, ring chromosomes, translocations with loss of one derivative chromosome, and combinations thereof.

Translocations involve swapping of material between two or more chromosomes, usually without net loss (reciprocal and balanced). However, the rearranged genes can be separated from their regulatory sequences and be aberrantly expressed or can instead be combined to produce a novel fusion protein. The former is exemplified by common translocations involving the *MYC* proto-oncogene in Burkitt lymphoma, such as t(8;14)(q24;q32), which places *MYC* under constitutive expression of the immunoglobulin heavy chain promoter, instead of its usual tightly controlled regulation (Figure 1C-3). A classic example of the latter mechanism is the Philadelphia chromosome, t(9;22)(q34;q11), seen in a subset of adult and pediatric leukemias, which juxtaposes the *BCR* and *ABL* genes to create a novel BCR-ABL fusion protein with dysregulated tyrosine kinase activity that drives oncogenesis. Note the terminology used for such events: "t" for translocation, followed by the involved chromosomes (9,22), and the regions or bands involved (q34 from chromosome 9 and q11 from chromosome 11); thus, the karyotype of a Philadelphia chromosome-positive pediatric ALL might be 46,XY,t(9;22)(q34;q11). Some balanced translocations are constitutional, but because the overall genetic content of the cells is unchanged, there is no problem detected in the carrier of a particular translocation. The problem occurs when offspring inherit only one of the abnormal parental chromosomes incurring an unbalanced genotype and, therefore, disease. A good example of this is a subset of Robertsonian translocations implicated in some cases of Down syndrome.

Applications

Probably, the most common application of conventional cytogenetics is analyzing constitutional karyotype. This usually occurs prenatally, using fetal cells obtained by chorionic villus sampling or amniocentesis, or in the neonatal period using a blood sample. Such information may guide prenatal care, anticipate difficulties in the neonatal period, portend outcomes, or guide future family planning. In instances of fetal loss or stillbirth, samples of skin or placenta should be sent for cytogenetics as part of the standard workup, especially if dysmorphic features are noted. In all cases with abnormal genetic results, and in many cases with normal karyotypes, parental referral to a genetic counselor is helpful.

Cytogenetic analysis can also provide important information in the evaluation of many neoplasms. A particular translocation may be identified that is pathognomonic for a given tumor (Figures 1C-3 and 1C-5), while other genetic aberrations may provide information on prognosis or therapeutic efficacy. For example, 95% of cases of acute promyelocytic leukemia bear a t(15;17)(q22;q12) abnormality that, besides being a diagnostic finding, can be used in molecular tests to monitor recurrence and also offers a therapeutic target—the fusion protein that results from this translocation, PML-RAR-alpha, appears to convey sensitivity to all-trans retinoic acid (75). Other prognostic genetic markers include 1p/19q loss in oligodendrogliomas, 1p/16q loss in Wilms tumor, 6q/17q loss in medulloblastoma, and 1p loss and the previously mentioned *MYCN* amplification in neuroblastoma.

Limitations

The major limitations of conventional cytogenetic analysis are threefold: the requirement for fresh, viable tissue with cells that can grow in a culture environment, the variable length of time for cells to grow and be analyzed, and the relatively low resolution of detection (four megabases). Assays such as interphase FISH and PCR can circumvent the need for growing cells and have a faster turnaround time; however, these techniques are designed for targeting precise molecular abnormalities. DNA microarrays (discussed below) provide a much higher resolution than standard karyotyping and can also detect abnormalities such as copy neutral loss of heterozygosity (LOH). Improvements in probe density, cost per sample, and software to assist in data analysis have led to chromosomal microarray assays becoming a first-line test in some laboratories. Despite continued methodologic advances in molecular pathology, karyotyping still has a major role as a simple, cost-effective method of examining the entire genome at low resolution for numerical or structural abnormalities.

POLYMERASE CHAIN REACTION

Background

The purpose of PCR is to create millions of copies of a specific segment of DNA so that it can be analyzed by its sequence, size, and complementarity to other sequences. It is used regularly in molecular diagnostics, forensic science, and research laboratories. Variations of the basic principles of PCR have led to numerous advancements in our ability to quickly and cost-effectively detect DNA sequence variants associated with specific diseases.

Methods

PCR sensitivity is best on fresh, snap frozen samples, but the technique can also be applied to formalin-fixed paraffin-embedded tissue. First, DNA is extracted from the sample of interest. If starting with RNA, total RNA is extracted and then converted into cDNA (complementary DNA) by an enzyme called *reverse transcriptase* (RT), the so-called RT-PCR. This DNA or cDNA is then mixed with free nucleotides (dNTPs), buffer, thermostable DNA polymerase, and two short, sequence-specific oligonucleotides called *primers* (Figure 1C-11). Primers are approximately 20 base pairs long and are designed so that one primer is complementary to the top strand of DNA at one end of the target segment and a second primer is complementary to the bottom strand of DNA at the other end of the target segment. Within this mixture, the target DNA or cDNA is then amplified through cycles of denaturation (at high temperatures such as 95°C), annealing (at lower temperatures defined by primer–template

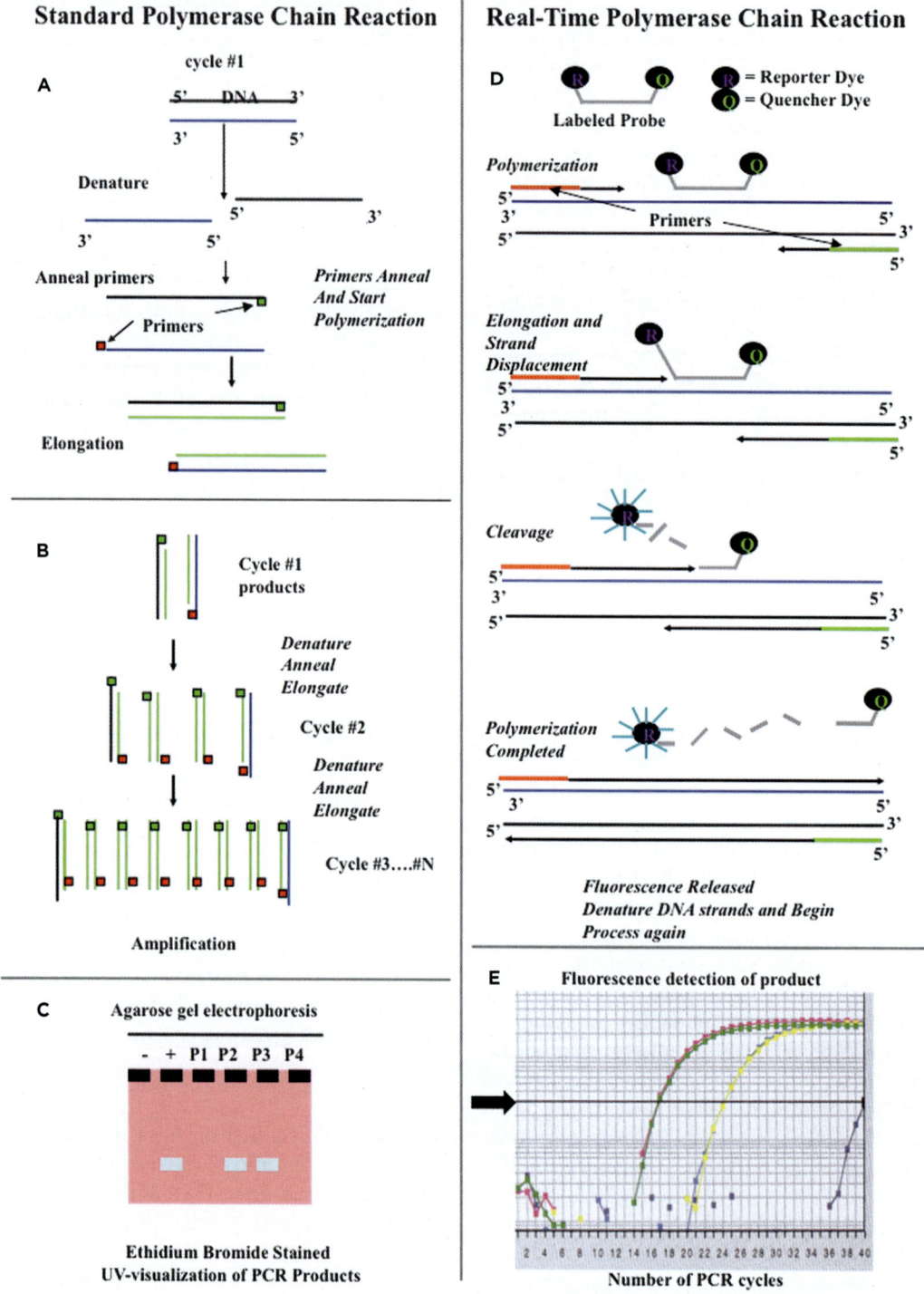

FIGURE 1C-11 • Schematic of PCR methodology. A comparison of conventional PCR (**left column**) and real-time PCR (**right column**). Conventional PCR involves denaturing of double-stranded DNA (or cDNA), annealing of primers, and elongation steps (**A, B**). The detection of amplified product typically involves agarose gel electrophoresis (**C**). **D, E**: Real-time PCR uses the same features of denaturation, annealing of primers, and elongation but adds a probe complementary to sequence in between the two end primers. This probe is labeled with both fluorescent reporter and quencher dyes that when in close proximity do not emit a signal. As the strand elongates from the 5′ primer, the probe is disrupted and cleaved, releasing the reporter dye into the solution. Once the reporter is no longer in proximity to the quencher dye, its fluorescent signal is detectable. Additional reporter dye will be released with each cycle and is proportional to the accumulated amount of amplified product. A detector measures fluorescence in real time, and the results are viewed in graphical form with quantity of signal on the y-axis and number of PCR cycles on the x-axis. The horizontal line indicates a threshold level beyond which there is exponential accumulation of signal, confirming that the specific DNA product is obtained. (**D** and **E** adapted from Applied Biosystems' TaqMan literature.)

nucleotide sequence, usually 55°C to 65°C), and elongation (70°C to 72°C). The denaturation stage separates the DNA into single strands, to which the primers can then bind during the annealing phase. During elongation, the polymerase uses the target DNA strand as a template to lengthen the primers, creating complementary double-stranded molecules; these products then serve as additional targets in the next round, allowing exponential amplification.

The amplified product is then subjected to gel electrophoresis and staining (with ethidium bromide or fluorescent analogues) where the relative size of the DNA can be determined by comparison to known standards. Confirmation that this product is the sequence of interest can be done by transferring the DNA from the gel to a nylon or nitrocellulose membrane, applying a radioactively or fluorescently labeled probe (similar to a primer, a probe is a short sequence of DNA designed to match a sequence internal to that of the primer pairs), and then placing the membrane on x-ray film. If the probe matches the sequence on the membrane, the label will expose the x-ray film at the location of the band. This process is known as *Southern blotting*. Some laboratories choose to clone and sequence PCR products for confirmation rather than blotting. Other laboratories do not perform either of these confirmatory steps; these laboratories may be at risk for reporting false positives.

Real-Time Polymerase Chain Reaction

Real-time or quantitative PCR is a variation on standard PCR that was first described by Holland et al. (76,77). It follows the same basic principles of standard RT-PCR but utilizes the 5′ exonuclease activity of the *Thermus aquaticus* (Taq) DNA polymerase coupled with fluorescence energy transfer (Figure 1C-6). First DNA is extracted from the sample of interest. If starting with RNA, the RNA is extracted and reverse transcribed into cDNA. The target cDNA or DNA is amplified in a mix containing not only a set of forward and reverse oligonucleotide primers designed to amplify sequences specific to the gene of interest but also a probe designed to match a sequence internal to that of the primer pairs. The probe is labeled with a reporter fluorescent dye at the 5′ end and a quencher fluorescent dye at the 3′ end. The quencher dye acts to decrease emission of the reporter dye as long as they are in close proximity to each other (on the ends of the same molecule). During the elongation phase of PCR, both primers and probe anneal to the target sequence if present. As the 5′ primer is extended, the 5′ exonuclease activity of the *Taq* DNA polymerase releases the fluorescent reporter dye once it reaches the 5′ end of the annealed probe; now separated from the 3′ quencher, fluorescence from the 5′ dye increases. As the specific product accumulates, additional probes anneal and then release more fluorescent signal with each PCR cycle. Rather than visualizing the PCR product after agarose gel electrophoresis and staining, the product is visualized in real time on a computer that plots the intensity of the reporter's fluorescent signal. Signal intensity is directly proportional to the amount of specific amplicon produced with each cycle of amplification. This method is capable of providing highly sensitive detection of target DNA and rapid results. Because of the elimination of postprocessing steps such as nested PCR or Southern blot confirmation, the risk of cross-contamination in association with carryover PCR product is reduced, and there is no need for radioactive materials.

Applications

PCR has numerous applications for pediatric pathologists primarily in tumor pathology, microbiologic speciation of organisms, genetic testing for mutations, and forensic identification.

Detection of Fusion Gene Transcripts

One of the first applications developed for pathology was detection of fusion gene transcripts resulting from translocations in hematopoietic and solid tumors (Table 1C-2). Although many of these translocations are also detectable by cytogenetics, the latter technique requires fresh tissue and growing cells. FISH is another method for detecting gene fusions/translocations and may perform superiorly to RT-PCR when only FFPE is available. The benefit of RT-PCR over both those techniques is that it preserves the ability to obtain sequence information from the fusion gene product. A few studies have suggested that in some tumors, the fusion type may have prognostic importance, thus designing the test to distinguish between variants may have some additional clinical utility (77,78). Also, RT-PCR can detect fusion genes in the setting of complex translocations involving small amounts of DNA (<400 kb) below the resolution of conventional chromosomal banding and karyotyping.

Molecular Microbiology

The use of PCR technology has transformed the clinical microbiology laboratory. For many microbial infections, PCR techniques have replaced standard culture or immunoassay identification (79). Real-time PCR is particularly appealing for use in microbiology for its speed over current methods (results in hours rather than days), efficacy (the ability of an organism to grow in culture is not an issue with PCR), and accuracy for speciation. Further, because real-time PCR is performed in a closed system, meaning that there is no open handling of amplified DNA products, there is a greatly decreased risk of cross-contamination. PCR-based sequencing can add additional utility to the microbiology laboratory. The sequence of 16S ribosomal RNA appears to be unique among microbial species and can be used to accurately identify organisms such

TABLE 1C-2 MOLECULAR TESTING IN PEDIATRIC DISEASES

System	Tumor	Genetic Aberration	Immunohistochemistry Pertinent Positives	Pertinent Negatives	Notes
Head and Neck	Congenital epulis	—	—	S100	S100(–) unlike other granular cell tumors
	Sinonasal papillomas	—	HPV, in a subset	—	—
	Nasopharyngeal angiofibroma	Some associated with *APC* mutations and/or FAP	β-Catenin	—	—
	Osteomas	May be associated with Gardner syndrome	—	—	—
	Teratoma	—	Varies by component	AFP to rule out yolk sac tumor component	—
	Nasopharyngeal carcinoma	HLA associations	EBV/EBER; mixed cytokeratins	Cytokeratins 7 and 20	—
	Adenoid cystic carcinoma	Some have t(6;9) (q21-24;p13-23), others have LOH at 6q.	Ductal cells: cytokeratin, EMA, and CEA. Myoepithelial cells: cytokeratin, p63, S100.	—	IHC helps identify different components.
	Pleomorphic adenoma	FLAG 1 t(3:8) (p21;q21)	Ductal cells: cytokeratin, EMA, and CEA. Myoepithelial cells: cytokeratin, p63, S100.	—	IHC helps identify different components.
	Salivary gland anlage tumor	—	Epithelial cells: cytokeratin; stromal cells: vimentin, actin, and cytokeratin	—	—
	Mucoepidermoid carcinoma	*MECT1/MAML2* translocations	Cytokeratin, including CK7	—	—
	Sialoblastoma	—	Ductal cells: cytokeratin; basaloid cells: S100 and actin	—	—
Cardiovascular	Fibroma	May be associated with Gorlin syndrome	—	—	—
	Rhabdomyoma	May be associated with tuberous sclerosis	Myoglobin, actin, desmin	S100	—
	Myxoma	May be associated with Carney syndrome	Vimentin	—	—
	Teratoma	—	Varies by component	AFP to rule out yolk sac tumor component	—

SECTION I GENERAL PATHOLOGY 39

	Tumor	Genetics	Markers	Additional markers	Notes
	Infantile hemangioma	—	GLUT1, LeY	—	—
	Kaposiform hemangioendothelioma	—	CD31, CD34, D2-40	—	—
	Epithelioid hemangioendothelioma	—	CD31, vWF; substantial fraction show cytokeratin staining	EMA	—
	Lymphangioma	—	D2-40	—	—
	Juvenile papillomatosis	—	HPV 6 and 11, cytokeratins	—	—
Respiratory	Pleuropulmonary blastoma	Germ line loss-of-function *DICER1* mutations in familial cases	Primitive stromal component similar to embryonal RMS: desmin, myogenin, MyoD1, myoglobin	—	Loss of Dicer1 staining in epithelium
	Pulmonary blastoma	—	—	—	—
	Midline poorly differentiated carcinoma	NUT translocation t(15;19) (q14;p13.1)	Cytokeratin, EMA; morule positive for CGA	—	—
	Embryonal rhabdomyosarcoma	LOH at 11p15	Muscle markers: desmin, myogenin, MyoD1, myoglobin	Rule out other SRBCTs: PGP9.5, WT1, CD99, CD45	Myogenin usually <50% (as opposed to alveolar RMS)
	Inflammatory myofibroblastic tumor	*ALK* rearrangements in some	ALK; myofibroblastic markers	—	—
	Granular cell tumor	—	S100	—	—
Gastrointestinal	Gastrointestinal stromal tumor	Mutations in *KIT* or *PDGFRA*	c-kit (CD117), vimentin, bcl-2, CD34	—	KIT staining may identify tumors suitable for monoclonal antibody therapy
	Adenocarcinoma	—	Cytokeratins, CEA, CA19.9	—	—
	Inflammatory myofibroblastic tumor	*ALK* rearrangements in some	ALK; myofibroblastic markers	—	—
	Schwannoma	—	S100, GFAP	KIT, desmin, smooth muscle actin	—
	Leiomyoma	—	Desmin, smooth muscle actin	S100, KIT	—
	Fundic gland gastric polyps	Some associated with FAP (*APC* mutations)	—	—	—
	Juvenile polyps	Cronkhite-Canada syndrome; some with *SMAD4/DPC4* mutations	—	—	—
	Peutz-Jeghers polyps	Mutations in *LKB1* gene	—	—	—
	Carcinoid tumors	—	Chromogranin, NSE, PGP 9.5, specific polypeptide hormones	—	—

(*Continued*)

TABLE 1C-2 MOLECULAR TESTING IN PEDIATRIC DISEASES (continued)

System	Tumor	Genetic Aberration	Immunohistochemistry			Notes
			Pertinent Positives	Pertinent Negatives		
Hepatobiliary	Adenoma	None known	Hep Par 1, CAM5.2, polyclonal CEA; CD34 in endothelial lining	AFP		IHC does not help distinguish adenoma from carcinoma
	Focal nodular hyperplasia	None known	Hep Par 1, CAM5.2, polyclonal CEA; CD34 in endothelial lining	—		—
	Hepatocellular carcinoma	Gains of 1q, 7q, 8q; losses of 16q	Hep Par 1, CAM5.2, polyclonal CEA; CD34 in endothelial lining	—		—
	Hepatoblastoma	Variable; some associated with BWS	AFP, hCG, Hep Par 1, polyclonal CEA	—		—
	Infantile hemangioendothelioma	—	CD31, CD34, factor VIII, GLUT1	—		—
	Mesenchymal hamartoma	Translocations involving 11, 17, and 19 t(11;19) (q11;q13.4)	Cytokeratins in ductal component; smooth muscle actin in stromal cells	—		—
	Desmoplastic small round cell tumor	t(11;22)(p13;q12) creating *EWS-WT1* fusion gene	Cytokeratin, EMA, WT1 (C-terminal epitope), CD99, NSE, PLAP	—		—
	Undifferentiated embryonal sarcoma	May have same translocation as mesenchymal hamartoma	Not much: sometimes vimentin and bcl-2	—		—
Pancreatic	Acinar cell carcinoma	—	Enzymes: lipase, trypsin, chymotrypsin	Chromogranin, synaptophysin		—
	Solid pseudopapillary tumor	Mutations in β-catenin	Vimentin, NSE, CD10, CD56, CD99, α₁-antitrypsin; nuclear β-catenin expression	Cytokeratins usually negative		—
	Pancreatoblastoma	Mutations in β-catenin/APC pathways	Enzymes: lipase, trypsin, chymotrypsin; also CEA and CA19.9	—		—
Genitourinary	Nephroblastoma (Wilms tumor)	Deletions or mutations in WT1, WT2, WT3, or WTX	WT1	—		—
	Cellular mesoblastic nephroma	t(12;15)(p13;q25) creating *ETV6-NTRK3* fusion	—	—		Same genetic aberration as congenital infantile fibrosarcoma

	Entity	Genetics	IHC Positive	IHC Negative/Other	Notes
	Ewing sarcoma/PNET	Translocations of *EWS* on 22q11; partners vary	CD99	—	—
	Clear cell sarcoma	t(10;17) and del 14q have been described	—	—	—
	Malignant rhabdoid tumor	*hSNF5* mutations/deletions (22q11)	Cytokeratin	Loss of nuclear INI1 staining, BAF47	—
	"Translocation" carcinomas	t(X;1)(p11.2;q25) and *APSL-TFE* fusion or t(6;11)(p21;q12) involving *TFEB*	Overexpression of TFE3	Cytokeratins (pan-CK and CK7), EMA	—
	Renal medullary carcinoma	Sickle cell carriers (11p15.5 mutation = HbS); possible 22q11 involvement	Cytokeratin	Loss of nuclear INI staining	—
	Angiomyolipoma	*TSC1* and *TSC2* genes—9q34 or 16p13.3 mutations	HMB45, smooth muscle actin, Melan-A	—	—
	Inflammatory myofibroblastic tumor	*ALK* rearrangements such as t(2;5)	ALK, vimentin, smooth muscle actin, desmin; variably for cytokeratin	—	—
	Embryonal rhabdomyosarcoma	LOH at 11p15	Muscle markers: desmin, myogenin, MyoD1, myoglobin	Rule out other SRBCTs: PGP9.5, WT1, CD99, CD45	Myogenin usually <50% (as opposed to alveolar RMS)
	Condyloma accuminata	—	HPV 6,11	—	—
Female Reproductive System	Clear cell adenocarcinoma	—	Cytokeratin	—	—
	Embryonal rhabdomyosarcoma	LOH at 11p15	Muscle markers: desmin, myogenin, MyoD1, myoglobin	Rule out other SRBCTs: PGP9.5, WT1, CD99, CD45	Myogenin usually <50% (as opposed to alveolar RMS)
	Dysgerminoma	I(12p)	PLAP, hCG	—	—
	Embryonal carcinoma	—	CD30, cytokeratin; less often PLAP and AFP	—	—
	Endodermal sinus tumor (yolk sac tumor)	I(12p) ±	AFP, SALL4, glypican-3	—	—
	Mature teratoma	>95% karyotypically normal	Component-specific	Rule out yolk sac tumor component: AFP	—
	Immature teratoma	60% with nonrecurrent cytogenetic abnormalities	Component-specific	Rule out yolk sac tumor component: AFP	—

(Continued)

TABLE 1C-2 MOLECULAR TESTING IN PEDIATRIC DISEASES (continued)

System	Tumor	Genetic Aberration	Immunohistochemistry Pertinent Positives	Pertinent Negatives	Notes
	Struma ovarii	—	Thyroglobulin, TTF-1	—	—
	Granulosa cell tumor	—	Inhibin, vimentin, CD99, cytokeratin	—	—
	Sertoli-Leydig cell tumor	SMARCA 4 (BRG1) inactivation mutations	CD99, WT1, inhibin, calretinin, cytokeratin	—	—
	Gonadoblastoma	Phenotypic females with 46,XY karyotype		—	—
	Small cell carcinoma		Cytokeratin, vimentin WT1	Hypercalcemia ±	—
	Complete hydatidiform mole	46,XX or 46,XY by dispermy	—	Negative for p57/KIP2 in the cytotrophoblast	Cytogenetics and p57 staining are far superior to histology for distinguishing partial versus complete moles
	Partial hydatidiform mole	Triploid: usually 69,XXY, but also 69,XXX and 69,XYY		Positive for p57/KIP2 in the cytotrophoblast	—
	Choriocarcinoma	—	hCG	Only weak hPL staining	—
	Condyloma acuminata	—	HPV 6,11	—	—
Male Reproductive System	Intratubular germ cell neoplasia	I(12p)	PLAP, OCT4, NSE, p53, ferritin, CD117, D2-40	—	—
	Embryonal rhabdomyosarcoma	LOH at 11p15	Muscle markers: desmin, myogenin, MyoD1, myoglobin	Rule out other SRBCTs: PGP9.5, WT1, CD99, CD45	Myogenin usually <50% (as opposed to alveolar RMS)
	Seminoma	I(12p)	PLAP, focal cytokeratin, vimentin, CD30, CD44	—	—
	Embryonal carcinoma	—	CD30, cytokeratin, OCT4, less often PLAP and AFP	—	—
	Endodermal sinus tumor (yolk sac tumor)	—	AFP, SALL4, glypican-3	PLAP ±	—
	Mature teratoma	>95% karyotypically normal	Component-specific	Rule out yolk sac tumor component: AFP	—

	Entity	Genetics	Immunohistochemistry	Comments
	Immature teratoma	60% with nonrecurrent cytogenetic abnormalities	Component-specific	Rule out yolk sac tumor component: AFP
	Granulosa cell tumor	—	Inhibin, vimentin, CD99, cytokeratin	—
	Sertoli cell tumor	—	Inhibin, vimentin, cytokeratin, variably for S100	PLAP, CEA
	Leydig cell tumor	—	Inhibin, melan A, vimentin, S100, chromogranin, synaptophysin; variably for cytokeratin, EMA, desmin	PLAP, CEA
Endocrine	Pituitary adenomas	—	Mono/oligoclonal hormone production	Decreased type IV collagen matrix
	Papillary thyroid carcinoma	*RET* gene mutations; also *BRAF*, *APC*, *RAS*, *TRK*	Cytokeratin, TTF-1, thyroglobulin	—
	Medullary thyroid carcinoma	*RET* mutations	Calcitonin, cytokeratin, chromogranin, TTF-1, synaptophysin, CEA	—
	Spindle epithelial tumor with thymus-like differentiation (SETTLE)	—	Cytokeratin	—
	Parathyroid adenomas/hyperplasia	*MEN1* (11q13), *RET* (10q11), or *HRPT2* (1q25)	Cytokeratin, PTH	—
	Pheochromocytoma	*RET* in MEN2-related cases; 1p losses	NSE, chromogranin, synaptophysin; S100 in sustentacular cells	Cytokeratin, EMA
	Neuroblastoma	*MYCN* amplification, *ALK* amplification or mutation	PGP9.5, NSE, synaptophysin, NB84	CD99, CD45
	Pancreatic endocrine tumors	Variable	Chromogranin, synaptophysin, NSE, specific hormones	—
Skin	Verruca vulgaris	Multiple in Cowden syndrome	HPV	—
	Tricholemmoma	Multiple in Gardner syndrome	CD34 in lesional cells	—
	Epidermoid cyst	—	—	—
	Sebaceous adenoma	Muir-Torre syndrome	—	—
	Melanocytic nevi	—	S100, Melan A, HMB4	—

(Continued)

TABLE 1C-2 MOLECULAR TESTING IN PEDIATRIC DISEASES (continued)

System	Tumor	Genetic Aberration	Immunohistochemistry		Notes
			Pertinent Positives	Pertinent Negatives	
	Cellular blue nevus	Carney complex	HMB45	S100	—
	Dermatofibroma	—	Factor XIIIa	CD34	—
	Dermatofibrosarcoma protuberans	Translocation COLIA1-PDFGB t(17;22)(q22;q13)	CD34, p53	Factor XIIIa	Same translocation as giant cell fibroblastoma
	Juvenile xanthogranuloma	—	CD68, vimentin, S100 (variable)	CD1a	—
	Langerhans cell histiocytosis	—	S100, CD1a	—	—
	Neurothekeoma	—	S100, vimentin; cellular variant positive for NKI/C3 and negative for S100	CD68	—
Soft tissue	Lipoblastoma	PLAG1 rearrangements	—	—	—
	Liposarcoma	FUS-CHOP fusion gene from t(12;16) or variant translocation	—	—	—
	Gardner fibroma	APC mutations	β-Catenin	—	—
	Desmoid fibromatosis	APC mutations	β-Catenin	—	—
	Inflammatory myofibroblastic tumor	ALK rearrangements in some	ALK; myofibroblastic markers	—	—
	Infantile fibrosarcoma	t(12;15)(p13;q25) creating ETV6-NTRK3 fusion	—	—	Same translocation as cellular mesoblastic nephroma
	Low-grade fibromyxoid sarcoma	Some with t(7;16)(q34;p11) translocation and FUS-CREB3L2 fusion	—	—	—
	Embryonal rhabdomyosarcoma	LOH at 11p15	Muscle markers: desmin, myogenin, MyoD1, myoglobin	Rule out other SRBCTs: PGP9.5, WT1, CD99, CD45	Myogenin usually <50% (as opposed to alveolar RMS)
	Alveolar rhabdomyosarcoma	t(2;13) or t(1;13) translocations fusing PAX3 or PAX7, respectively, with FOXO1	Muscle markers: desmin, myogenin, MyoD1, myoglobin	Rule out other SRBCTs: PGP9.5, WT1, CD99, CD45	Myogenin usually >50% (as opposed to embryonal RMS)
	Ossifying fibromyxoid tumor	—	S100; rarely, desmin, GFAP, and cytokeratins	—	—

Category	Tumor	Genetics/Notes	Immunohistochemistry		Other
	Soft tissue myoepithelioma	—	Cytokeratin, S100, calponin	—	—
	Synovial sarcoma	t(X;18)(p11.2;q11.2) fusing *SYT* and *SSX1* or *SSX2*	Cytokeratin and EMA in the epithelial phase	—	—
	Epithelioid sarcoma	—	Vimentin, keratin, and EMA	Loss of nuclear INI1 expression	—
	Alveolar soft part sarcoma	*TFE3-ASPL* fusion gene	—	—	—
	Clear cell sarcoma (melanoma of soft parts)	t(12;22)(q13;q13) with *EWS–ATF1* fusion	S100, HMB45	—	—
	Ewing sarcoma/PNET	Translocations of *EWS* on 22q11; partners vary	CD99	—	—
Bone	Osteochondroma	*EXT1* and *EXT2* gene mutations in multiple hereditary exostoses	—	—	—
	Chondromyxoid fibroma	6q13 rearrangements	—	—	—
	Osteomas	May be associated with Gardner syndrome	—	—	—
	Chordoma	—	S100 and epithelial markers	—	—
	Fibrous dysplasia	Seen in McCune-Albright syndrome and with *GNAS* mutations	—	—	—
Central Nervous System	Medulloblastoma	i(17q) most common, other various ones. Some cases associated with Gorlin syndrome and *PTCH* gene.	—	—	—
	Retinoblastoma	Rb loss-of-function	—	—	—
	Atypical teratoid/rhabdoid tumors	*hSNF5* gene—22q11 mutations/deletions	—	Loss of nuclear INI1 expression, BAF47	—

(*Continued*)

TABLE 1C-2 MOLECULAR TESTING IN PEDIATRIC DISEASES (continued)

System	Tumor	Genetic Aberration	Immunohistochemistry			Notes
			Pertinent Positives	Pertinent Negatives		
					Pertinent Negatives	
	Hemangioblastoma	von Hippel-Lindau syndrome	Vimentin, NSE, GFAP, inhibin A	Epithelial markers	—	—
	Dysplastic gangliocytomas	Cowden syndrome	—	—	—	—
Peripheral Nervous System	Schwannoma	Monosomy 22 or 22q loss (NF2 gene)	S100	—	—	—
	Neurofibroma	NF1	S100	—	—	—
	MPNST	Associated with NF1	Only a minority are S100 positive	—	—	—
Lymph nodes	Hodgkin lymphoma	—	CD15, CD30, EBER ISH	—	—	—
	Anaplastic large cell lymphoma	—	ALK, CD30	ALK	—	—
	Burkitt lymphoma	*MYC* translocations	CD10, CD19, near-100% MIB-1 positivity	—	—	—
	Precursor B- or T-cell lymphoblastic lymphoma/leukemia	—	TdT, lineage-specific markers (may be mixed)	—	—	—

as mycobacteria as well as to identify new pathogens (80). Further, PCR-based assessment of antimicrobial resistance genes may become more commonplace as information from microbial research laboratories makes its way to clinical application (81).

Genetic Testing for Mutations

In the last decade, hundreds of diseases have been attributed to abnormalities in the DNA sequence code. Base substitutions and insertions and deletions of coding sequences alter the production of or change the nature of proteins in a manner that is associated with particular diseases. Duchenne muscular dystrophy, cystic fibrosis, and neurofibromatosis type 1 are common examples of monogenic diseases that are amenable to PCR-based genetic testing, but there are many more in the categories of metabolic diseases, neurologic and muscular diseases, and cancer predisposition syndromes. Sequencing for commonly mutated exons (so-called mutational hot spots) in affected children or offspring of affected or carrier parents provides important information to the treating physician and parents, but full sequencing of large genes can be complex and arduous with routine PCR technology.

Forensic Identification

PCR is commonly used to amplify specific segments of DNA for forensic analysis such as for identification of victims of natural disasters, victims of crimes, and also identification of perpetrators leaving DNA evidence at a crime scene. PCR-based identification methods include analysis of sequence and length polymorphisms and mitochondrial DNA sequences. The most common method used to identify individuals is examination of 13 different loci that show variability among humans to create a "DNA fingerprint" (82).

Limitations

While PCR has become one of the most commonly used tools in molecular medicine, it is important to note its limitations. The assay is extremely sensitive and care must be taken to avoid contamination from nucleic acids in the environment, particularly in the microbiology laboratory. Laboratory technicians performing PCR testing should have adequate training and experience and understand the importance of good technique. PCR detection of sequence variants in mutation analysis is limited to base substitutions and small insertion/deletions. Detection of larger intragenic deletions currently requires other supporting methodology (83,84). PCR applications in detecting and identifying new organisms can lead to dilemmas about whether or not a newly sequenced isolate is clinically relevant. Finally, PCR testing is not "agnostic." It is not a screening test for unknown abnormalities; rather, it is applied in a target-specific manner.

ARRAY TECHNOLOGY

DNA microarrays are used as a tool to evaluate and quantify sequence information for tens of thousands to a million sequences in a single experiment. The development of microarrays required the advances of miniaturization and computer technology coupled with the knowledge of DNA sequence among multiple species. The basic methodology involves thousands/millions of small chemically generated oligonucleotide sequences representing portions of the genomic DNA sequence that are fixed to a platform such as a glass slide or silicon wafer. These sequences are "arrayed" in a manner such that the location and sequence of each probe is known and millions of probes can fit in a small area. The patient DNA (or cDNA reverse transcribed from RNA) is then labeled with a fluorescent dye and hybridized to the array. Patient DNA that has sequence identity to a probe on the array binds there and can be detected by a fluorescence detector.

There are currently three main applications of microarray technology: (a) comparative genomic hybridization (CGH), which compares the amount of patient DNA at a given locus to a reference standard, (b) single nucleotide polymorphism (SNP) detection, which assays the genotype of an individual at hundreds of thousands of sites known to be polymorphic among individuals, and (c) gene expression, which is a reflection of which genes are actively transcribed in a given sample in a relatively quantifiable manner. CGH arrays can provide information on genomic gains and losses just as in standard karyotyping albeit at a much higher resolution and without the requirement for growing cells. Karyotyping has one advantage over CGH in that karyotyping can detect balanced translocations, whereas CGH generally cannot. SNP arrays can detect SNPs or mutations that can link someone to a specific disease state, determine suitability to targeted therapy, or determine individual variations in drug metabolism. SNP arrays can also measure copy number changes including uniparental disomy. It is clear that microarray technology has transformed molecular biology and genetic research and for the same reasons, it is valuable in research, there is no shortage of potential applications in clinical molecular diagnostics.

NEXT-GENERATION SEQUENCING

For the last three decades, the Sanger method of sequencing has been the favored method of reading the base code sequence of DNA. This method uses PCR amplification of specific region(s) of interest (i.e., exons of a gene) and a capillary sequencer machine. This method is somewhat laborious but is reliable and has high fidelity. It was used to sequence the first human genome in a 13-year effort ending in 2003. Since the completion of that first human genome sequence, new powerful technology has emerged. These so-called *next-generation* sequencers can perform massively parallel DNA sequencing of clonally amplified or single DNA molecules. This technology has made sequencing entire genomes and RNA transcriptomes possible in a matter of days to weeks rather than years and has also substantially brought down the price of sequencing large areas of DNA.

NGS has replaced standard PCR-based methods for mutation detection and screening in many laboratories. Depending on the application, laboratories can design disease-specific panels for "targeted resequencing" or sequence all the coding DNA exons from all genes in the human genome that produce proteins (i.e., the exome). Each methodology has its advantages. Targeted resequencing assays generally have better sensitivity and coverage of the exons in the specific gene panel. Mutation analysis is typically faster and easier when sequencing a small number of target genes. Exome analysis has its advantages in circumstances where the targets are not known or predictable from the disease phenotype and is more often used as a discovery tool. Gene copy number can be inferred from exome sequencing data with appropriate software. On the other hand, the large amount of data generated from a human exome (8 GB text file for a single exome at 100× coverage) is still somewhat expensive to generate and also presents a challenge for storage and sharing of raw data files and sheer numbers of sequence variants to analyze. These technical issues represent a short-term problem. The more complicated aspects of using NGS in clinical diagnostics include (a) developing quality standards and proficiency testing on technology that is rapidly evolving (85,86) and (b) developing consensus interpretation guidelines for "incidental" findings of pathogenic or potentially pathogenic mutations in genes unrelated to the particular diagnostic search (e.g., BRCA1, BRCA2) (87–89).

FUTURE DIRECTIONS FOR MOLECULAR METHODS IN PEDIATRIC PATHOLOGY

Technology and its applications to medical sciences will inevitably continue to advance at an extremely rapid pace. The era of personalized medicine is coming, but that does not mean that the hematoxylin and eosin stain is no longer sufficient and cost-effective for diagnosing the vast majority of diseases. Pathologists have an important role ensuring that new methodologies are subjected to validation, quality control, and quality assurance measures just as one would naturally expect from any clinical chemistry test or immunohistochemical stain. And, pathologists and laboratory managers are especially qualified to determine the cost–benefit ratio of introducing new tests. These are very important responsibilities. Far from being at risk of replacement by technologic machinery, as pathologists we are uniquely positioned to determine which new technologies will be beneficial to the patient in terms of improving accuracy or timeliness of diagnosis, reducing costs, improving quality, or providing added benefit over currently used diagnostic methods.

Further Reading

A special issue devoted to immunohistochemistry, with individual articles devoted to various organ systems. *Arch Pathol Lab Med* 2008;132(3).

Dabbs DJ. *Diagnostic Immunohistochemistry: Theranostic and Genomic Applications.* 3rd ed. Philadelphia, PA: Saunders; 2010.

Li MM, Andersson HC. Clinical application of microarray-based molecular cytogenetics: an emerging new era of genomic medicine. *J Pediatr* 2009;155(3):311–317.

Miller MB, Tang YW. Basic concepts of microarrays and potential applications in clinical microbiology. *Clin Microbiol Rev* 2009;22(4):611–633.

Roulston D, Le Beau MM. Cytogenetic analysis of hematologic malignant disease. In: Barch MJ, Knutsen T, Spurbeck J, eds. *The AGT Cytogenetics Laboratory Manual.* 3rd ed. Philadelphia, PA: Lippincott-Raven; 1997.

Speicher M, Antonara SE, Motulsky AG, eds. *Vogel and Motulsky's Human Genetics: Problems and Approaches.* 4th ed. New York, NY: Springer; 2010.

Strachan T, Read AP. *Human Molecular Genetics.* 2nd ed. New York, NY: Wiley-Liss; 1999.

Voelkerding KV, Dames SA, Durtschi JD. Next generation sequencing: from basic research to diagnostics. *Clin Chem* 2009;55;4:1–18.

References

1. Debski R, Rutledge J, Kapur R. A plea for the masses: a gross room approach to pediatric tumors. *J Histotechnol* 2004;27:221–228.
2. Dressler LG, Visscher D. Handling, storage, and preparation of human tissues. *Curr Protoc Cytom* 2001;Chapter 5: Unit 5.2.
3. Gudgin EJ, Erber WN. Immunophenotyping of lymphoproliferative disorders: state of the art. *Pathology* 2005;37(6):457–478.
4. Haferlach T, Kern W, Schnittger S, et al. Modern diagnostics in acute leukemias. *Crit Rev Oncol Hematol* 2005;56(2):223–234.
5. Szczepanski T, van der Velden VH, van Dongen JJ. Flow-cytometric immunophenotyping of normal and malignant lymphocytes. *Clin Chem Lab Med* 2006;44(7):775–796.
6. Finn WG. Beyond gating: capturing the power of flow cytometry. *Am J Clin Pathol* 2009;131(3):313–314.
7. Davis BH, Olsen S, Bigelow NC, et al. Detection of fetal red cells in fetomaternal hemorrhage using a fetal hemoglobin monoclonal antibody by flow cytometry. *Transfusion* 1998;38(8):749–756.
8. Dziegiel MH, Nielsen LK, Berkowicz A. Detecting fetomaternal hemorrhage by flow cytometry. *Curr Opin Hematol* 2006;13(6):490–495.
9. Hall SE, Rosse WF. The use of monoclonal antibodies and flow cytometry in the diagnosis of paroxysmal nocturnal hemoglobinuria. *Blood* 1996;87(12):5332–5340.
10. Luzzatto L, Gianfaldoni G. Recent advances in biological and clinical aspects of paroxysmal nocturnal hemoglobinuria. *Int J Hematol* 2006;84(2):104–112.
11. Pattanapanyasat K, Thakar MR. CD4+ T cell count as a tool to monitor HIV progression & anti-retroviral therapy. *Indian J Med Res* 2005;121(4):539–549.
12. Sherman GG, Galpin JS, Patel JM, et al. CD4+ T cell enumeration in HIV infection with limited resources. *J Immunol Methods* 1999;222(1–2):209–217.
13. Gaipa G, Basso G, Biondi A, et al. Detection of minimal residual disease in pediatric acute lymphoblastic leukemia. *Cytometry B Clin Cytom* 2013;84(6):359–369.
14. Campana D. Minimal residual disease monitoring in childhood acute lymphoblastic leukemia. *Curr Opin Hematol* 2012;19(4):313–318.

15. Woo J, Baumann A, Arguello V. Recent advancements of flow cytometry: new applications in hematology and oncology. *Expert Rev Mol Diagn* 2014;14(1):67–81.
16. Hsu SM, Raine L, Fanger H. Use of avidin-biotin-peroxidase complex (ABC) in immunoperoxidase techniques: a comparison between ABC and unlabeled antibody (PAP) procedures. *J Histochem Cytochem* 1981;29(4):577–580.
17. Bhan AK. Immunoperoxidase. In: Colvin RB, Bhan AK, McCluskey RT, eds. *Diagnostic Immunopathology*. New York, NY: Raven Press; 1994.
18. Elias JM. *Immunohistopathology: A Practical Approach to Diagnosis*. Chicago, IL: American Society of Clinical Pathologists; 1990.
19. Kakar S, Gown AM, Goodman ZD, et al. Best practices in diagnostic immunohistochemistry: hepatocellular carcinoma versus metastatic neoplasms. *Arch Pathol Lab Med* 2007;131(11):1648–1654.
20. Fritschy JM. Is my antibody-staining specific? How to deal with pitfalls of immunohistochemistry. *Eur J Neurosci* 2008;28(12):2365–2370.
21. Nogueira AM, Barbosa AJ, Carvalho AA, et al. Usefulness of immunocytochemical demonstration of neuron-specific enolase in the diagnosis of Hirschsprung's disease. *J Pediatr Gastroenterol Nutr* 1990;11(4):496–502.
22. Perrone T, Steeper TA, Dehner LP. Alpha-fetoprotein localization in pure ovarian teratoma. An immunohistochemical study of 12 cases. *Am J Clin Pathol* 1987;88(6):713–717.
23. Robey SS, Kuhajda FP, Yardley JH. Immunoperoxidase stains of ganglion cells and abnormal mucosal nerve proliferations in Hirschsprung's disease. *Hum Pathol* 1988;19(4):432–437.
24. Long GV, Wilmott JS, Capper D, et al. Immunohistochemistry is highly sensitive and specific for the detection of V600E BRAF mutation in melanoma *Am J Surg Pathol* 2013;37(1):61–65.
25. Agarwal S, Sharma MC, Jha P, et al. Comparative study of IDH1 mutations in gliomas by immunohistochemistry and DNA sequencing. *Neuro Oncol* 2013;15(6):718–726.
26. Loussouarn D, Le Loupp AG, Frenel JS, et al. Comparison of immunohistochemistry, DNA sequencing and allele-specific PCR for the detection of IDH1mutations in gliomas. *Int J Oncol* 2012;40(6):2058–2062.
27. Pugh TJ, Yu W, Yang J, et al. Exome sequencing of pleuropulmonary blastoma reveals frequent biallelic loss of TP53 and two hits in DICER1 resulting in retention of 5p-derived miRNA hairpin loop sequences. *Oncogene* 2014;33(45):5295–5302. doi: 10.1038/onc.2014.150. Epub 2014 Jun 9.
28. Kleihues P, Ohgaki H. Primary and secondary glioblastomas: from concept to clinical diagnosis. *Neuro Oncol* 1999;1(1):44–51.
29. Sung T, Miller DC, Hayes RL, et al. Preferential inactivation of the p53 tumor suppressor pathway and lack of EGFR amplification distinguish de novo high grade pediatric astrocytomas from de novo adult astrocytomas. *Brain Pathol* 2000;10(2):249–259.
30. Smith MR. Rituximab (monoclonal anti-CD20 antibody): mechanisms of action and resistance. *Oncogene* 2003;22(47):7359–7368.
31. Teng YK, Levarht EW, Hashemi M, et al. Immunohistochemical analysis as a means to predict responsiveness to rituximab treatment. *Arthritis Rheum* 2007;56(12):3909–3918.
32. Bignami A, Schoene W. Glial fibrillary acidic protein in human brain tumors. In: DeLellis R, ed. *Diagnostic Immunohistochemistry*. New York, NY: Masson Publishing; 1981.
33. Duffy PE, Huang YY, Rapport MM, et al. Glial fibrillary acidic protein in giant cell tumors of brain and other gliomas. A possible relationship to malignancy, differentiation, and pleomorphism of glia. *Acta Neuropathol* 1980;52(1):51–57.
34. Velasco ME, Dahl D, Roessmann U, et al. Immunohistochemical localization of glial fibrillary acidic protein in human glial neoplasms. *Cancer* 1980;45(3):484–494.
35. Hasegawa T, Matsuno Y, Shimoda T, et al. Gastrointestinal stromal tumor: consistent CD117 immunostaining for diagnosis, and prognostic classification based on tumor size and MIB-1 grade. *Hum Pathol* 2002;33(6):669–676.
36. Chu T, Jaffe R. The normal Langerhans cell and the LCH cell. *Br J Cancer Suppl* 1994;23:S4–S10.
37. Gloghini A, Rizzo A, Zanette I, et al. KP1/CD68 expression in malignant neoplasms including lymphomas, sarcomas, and carcinomas. *Am J Clin Pathol* 1995;103(4):425–431.
38. Holness CL, Simmons DL. Molecular cloning of CD68, a human macrophage marker related to lysosomal glycoproteins. *Blood* 1993;81(6):1607–1613.
39. Ornvold K, Ralfkiaer E, Carstensen H. Immunohistochemical study of the abnormal cells in Langerhans cell histiocytosis (histiocytosis x). *Virchows Arch A Pathol Anat Histopathol* 1990;416(5):403–410.
40. Horny HP, Valent P. Diagnosis of mastocytosis: general histopathological aspects, morphological criteria, and immunohistochemical findings. *Leuk Res* 2001;25(7):543–551.
41. North PE, Waner M, Mizeracki A, et al. GLUT1: a newly discovered immunohistochemical marker for juvenile hemangiomas. *Hum Pathol* 2000;31(1):11–22.
42. Kalof AN, Cooper K. D2-40 immunohistochemistry—so far! *Adv Anat Pathol* 2009;16(1):62–64.
43. Woods GL, Walker DH. Detection of infection or infectious agents by use of cytologic and histologic stains. *Clin Microbiol Rev* 1996;9(3):382–404.
44. Bacchi CE, Gown AM, Bacchi MM. Detection of infectious disease agents in tissue by immunocytochemistry. *Braz J Med Biol Res* 1994;27(12):2803–2820.
45. Eshun JK, Black DD, Casteel HB, et al. Comparison of immunohistochemistry and silver stain for the diagnosis of pediatric *Helicobacter pylori* infection in urease-negative gastric biopsies. *Pediatr Dev Pathol* 2001;4(1):82–88.
46. Jonkers D, Stobberingh E, de Bruine A, et al. Evaluation of immunohistochemistry for the detection of *Helicobacter pylori* in gastric mucosal biopsies. *J Infect* 1997;35(2):149–154.
47. Linder J, Radio SJ. Immunohistochemistry of Pneumocystis carinii. *Semin Diagn Pathol* 1989;6(3):238–244.
48. Wazir JF, Macrorie SG, Coleman DV. Evaluation of the sensitivity, specificity, and predictive value of monoclonal antibody 3 F6 for the detection of Pneumocystis carinii pneumonia in bronchoalveolar lavage specimens and induced sputum. *Cytopathology* 1994;5(2):82–89.
49. Asa SL. *Tumors of the Pituitary Gland. Atlas of Tumor Pathology*, Third Series, Vol. 22. Washington, DC: Armed Forces Institute of Pathology; 1998.
50. Jarzembowski J, McKeever P. The pathologic perspective on the pituitary. *Rev Endocrinol* 2008;30–35.
51. Hill DA, Pfeifer JD, Marley EF, et al. WT1 staining reliably differentiates desmoplastic small round cell tumor from Ewing sarcoma/primitive neuroectodermal tumor. An immunohistochemical and molecular diagnostic study. *Am J Clin Pathol* 2000;114(3):345–353.
52. Murphy AJ, Bishop K, Pereira C, et al. A new molecular variant of desmoplastic small round cell tumor: significance of WT1 immunostaining in this entity. *Hum Pathol* 2008;39(12):1763–1770.
53. Janoueix-Lerosey I, Lequin D, Brugières L, et al. Somatic and germline activating mutations of the ALK kinase receptor in neuroblastoma. *Nature* 2008;455(7215):967–970.
54. Mossé YP, Laudenslager M, Longo L, et al. Identification of ALK as a major familial neuroblastoma predisposition gene. *Nature* 2008;455(7215):930–935.
55. Carpenter EL, Mossé YP. Targeting ALK in neuroblastoma–preclinical and clinical advancements. *Nat Rev Clin Oncol* 2012;9(7):391–399.
56. Fisher KE, Neill SG, Ehsani L, et al. Immunohistochemical Investigation of BRAF p.V600E mutations in thyroid carcinoma using 2 separate BRAF antibodies. *Appl Immunohistochem Mol Morphol* 2014;22(8):562–567.
57. Méhes G, Irsai G, Bedekovics J, et al. Activating BRAF V600E mutation in aggressive pediatric Langerhans cell histiocytosis: demonstration by allele-specific PCR/direct sequencing and immunohistochemistry. *Am J Surg Pathol* 2014;38(12):1644–1648.
58. Dahiya S, Haydon DH, Alvarado D, et al. BRAF(V600E) mutation is a negative prognosticator in pediatric ganglioglioma. *Acta Neuropathol* 2013;125(6):901–910.
59. Chappé C, Padovani L, Scavarda D, et al. Dysembryoplastic neuroepithelial tumors share with pleomorphic xanthoastrocytomas and

ganglogliomas BRAF(V600E) mutation and expression. *Brain Pathol* 2013;23(5):574–583.
60. Dinges HC, Capper D, Ritz O, et al. Validation of a manual protocol for BRAF V600E mutation-specific immunohistochemistry. *Appl Immunohistochem Mol Morphol* 2015 23(5):382–388.
61. Ganigi PM, Santosh V, Anandh B, et al. Expression of p53, EGFR, pRb and bcl-2 proteins in pediatric glioblastoma multiforme: a study of 54 patients. *Pediatr Neurosurg* 2005;41(6):292–299.
62. Huang J, Soffer SZ, Kim ES, et al. p53 accumulation in favorable-histology Wilms tumor is associated with angiogenesis and clinically aggressive disease. *J Pediatr Surg* 2002;37(3):523–527.
63. Leuschner I, Langhans I, Schmitz R, et al.; Kiel Pediatric Tumor Registry and the German Cooperative Soft Tissue Sarcoma Study. p53 and mdm-2 expression in Rhabdomyosarcoma of childhood and adolescence: clinicopathologic study by the Kiel Pediatric Tumor Registry and the German Cooperative Soft Tissue Sarcoma Study. *Pediatr Dev Pathol* 2003;6(2):128–136.
64. Sredni ST, Zerbini MC, Latorre MR, Alves VA. p53 as a prognostic factor in adrenocortical tumors of adults and children. *Braz J Med Biol Res* 2003;36(1):23–27.
65. Mackie RM, Young H, Campbell IA. Studies in cutaneous immunofluorescence. I. The effect of storage time on direct immunofluorescence of skin biopsies from bullous disease and lupus erythematosus. *J Cutan Pathol* 1980;7(4):236–243.
66. Holden CA, MacDonald DM. Immunoperoxidase techniques in dermatopathology. *Clin Exp Dermatol* 1983;8(5):443–457.
67. Elias J, Boss E, Kaplan AP. Studies of the cellular infiltrate of chronic idiopathic urticaria: prominence of T-lymphocytes, monocytes, and mast cells. *J Allergy Clin Immunol* 1986;78(5 Pt 1):914–918.
68. Fischer EG. To fix or not to fix: Michel's is the solution. *Int J Surg Pathol* 2006;14(1):108.
69. Michel B, Milner Y, David K. Preservation of tissue-fixed immunoglobulins in skin biopsies of patients with lupus erythematosus and bullous diseases–preliminary report. *J Invest Dermatol* 1972;59(6):449–452.
70. Mutasim DF, Pelc NJ, Supapannachart N. Established methods in the investigation of bullous diseases. *Dermatol Clin* 1993;11(3):399–418.
71. Sorelli P, Gratian MJ, Bhogal BS, et al. Immunogold electron microscopy using skin in Michel's medium intended for immunofluorescence analysis. *Clin Dermatol* 2001;19(5):638–641.
72. Vaughn Jones SA, Palmer I, Bhogal BS, et al. The use of Michel's transport medium for immunofluorescence and immunoelectron microscopy in autoimmune bullous diseases. *J Cutan Pathol* 1995;22(4):365–370.
73. Biegel JA, Rorke LB, Emanuel BS. Monosomy 22 in rhabdoid or atypical teratoid tumors of the brain. *N Engl J Med* 1989;321(13):906.
74. Fanaian NK, Cohen C, Waldrop S, et al. Epstein-Barr virus (EBV)-encoded RNA: automated in-situ hybridization (ISH) compared with manual ISH and immunohistochemistry for detection of EBV in pediatric lymphoproliferative disorders. *Pediatr Dev Pathol* 2009;12(3):195–199.
75. Licht JD. Acute promyelocytic leukemia–weapons of mass differentiation. *N Engl J Med* 2009;360(9):928–930.
76. Holland PM, Abramson RD, Watson R, et al. Detection of specific polymerase chain reaction product by utilizing the 5′—3′ exonuclease activity of Thermus aquaticus DNA polymerase. *Proc Natl Acad Sci U S A* 1991;88(16):7276–7280.
77. Sorensen PH, Lynch JC, Qualman SJ, et al. PAX3-FKHR and PAX7-FKHR gene fusions are prognostic indicators in alveolar rhabdomyosarcoma: a report from the children's oncology group. *J Clin Oncol* 2002;20(11):2672–2679.
78. Ladanyi M, Antonescu CR, Leung DH, et al. Impact of SYT-SSX fusion type on the clinical behavior of synovial sarcoma: a multi-institutional retrospective study of 243 patients. *Cancer Res* 2002;62(1):135–140.
79. Espy MJ, Uhl JR, Sloan LM, et al. Real-time PCR in clinical microbiology: applications for routine laboratory testing. *Clin Microbiol Rev* 2006;19(1):165–256.
80. Sontakke S, Cadenas MB, Maggi RG, et al. Use of broad range 16S rDNA PCR in clinical microbiology. *J Microbiol Methods* 2009;76(3):217–225.
81. Weile J, Knabbe C. Current applications and future trends of molecular diagnostics in clinical bacteriology. *Anal Bioanal Chem* 2009;394(3):731–742.
82. Project, USDHG. *DNA Forensics*. 2009 [cited 2009 11/1/2009]. Available from http://www.ornl.gov/sci/techresources/Human_Genome/elsi/forensics.shtml
83. De Lellis L, Curia MC, Catalano T, et al. Combined use of MLPA and nonfluorescent multiplex PCR analysis by high performance liquid chromatography for the detection of genomic rearrangements. *Hum Mutat* 2006;27(10):1047–1056.
84. Engert S, Wappenschmidt B, Betz B, et al. MLPA screening in the BRCA1 gene from 1,506 German hereditary breast cancer cases: novel deletions, frequent involvement of exon 17, and occurrence in single early-onset cases. *Hum Mutat* 2008;29(7):948–958.
85. Rehm HL, Bale SJ, Bayrak-Toydemir P, et al.; Working Group of the American College of Medical Genetics and Genomics Laboratory Quality Assurance Committee. ACMG clinical laboratory standards for next-generation sequencing. *Genet Med* 2013;15(9):733–747.
86. Richards CS, Palomaki GE, Lacbawan FL, et al.; CAP/ACMG Biochemical and Molecular Genetics Resource Committee. Three-year experience of a CAP/ACMG methods-based external proficiency testing program for laboratories offering DNA sequencing for rare inherited disorders. *Genet Med* 2014;16(1):25–32.
87. Evans BJ. Minimizing liability risks under the ACMG recommendations for reporting incidental findings in clinical exome and genome sequencing. *Genet Med* 2013;15(12):915–920.
88. Green RC, Berg JS, Grody WW, et al.; American College of Medical Genetics and Genomics. ACMG recommendations for reporting of incidental findings in clinical exome and genome sequencing. *Genet Med* 2013;15(7):565–574.
89. Allyse M, Michie M. Not-so-incidental findings: the ACMG recommendations on the reporting of incidental findings in clinical whole genome and whole exome sequencing. *Trends Biotechnol* 2013;31(8):439–441.

CHAPTER 1D
Electron Microscopy

Gary W. Mierau, Ph.D., Eric P. Wartchow, Ph.D.(c), and M. John Hicks, M.D., D.D.S., M.S., Ph.D.

Electron microscopy remains an essential tool for today's pediatric pathologist. Although now increasingly being used as a means to refine and guide the course of more costly and narrowly specialized diagnostic studies, the technique continues to provide for a significant number of childhood diseases the best and sometimes only means of establishing a definitive diagnosis. Offering a direct and open morphologic approach, and not being confined to hypothesis testing, it is one of the more powerful and least treacherous ancillary diagnostic techniques currently available. This having been said, it is also recognized that each special technique has its relative strengths and weaknesses in particular situations. These should be regarded as complementary tools, which are best employed using a highly selective but fully integrated approach.

We have found ancillary electron microscopic studies to be warranted in the workup of approximately five percent of surgical specimens submitted for histologic diagnosis. In contrast to the situation with adult patients, where renal specimens predominate, a very broad mix of specimens is received from pediatric patients (Figure 1D-1). Respiratory tract specimens for the evaluation of cilia morphology comprise the largest proportion of diagnostic cases, followed by liver, kidney, and muscle, and then in gradually diminishing numbers by a wide variety of other tissue types.

In addition to the more customary applications in diagnostic surgical and autopsy pathology, electron microscopy can play a valuable role in a departmental quality assurance program for example through the examination of a sampling of tumor specimens for which such studies were not initially considered necessary for diagnostic purposes. Our experience has been that this practice will lead to a reconsideration of the diagnosis in a significant number of cases.

A number of institutions are utilizing electron microscopy in the clinical laboratory as a primary means of detecting virus in diarrheal stool specimens, blood, skin vesicles, and other bodily fluids. The development of alternative technologies, such as multiplex PCR, may in time come to diminish its role in this context. Even if this does happen, this technology will remain essential for the detection of new or unusual agents.

Opportunities currently abound also for the use of electron microscopy in pathology research, in particular where integration or correlation of nonstructural with structural information is of benefit.

THE ELECTRON MICROSCOPY LABORATORY

The central element in any electron microscopy laboratory is, of course, the electron microscope itself. A basic transmission electron microscope is all that is needed for diagnostic applications (Figure 1D-2). Ease of operation, reliability, and optimal performance at low magnifications are of far greater importance in this setting than are the advanced features offered by the more expensive and more demanding "analytical" microscopes. Electron microscopes have achieved a relatively mature state of technologic development, and several manufacturers produce excellent (100 to 120 kV) instruments suitable for this application. In contrast to the situation with respect to the electron microscopes themselves, the technology associated with image capture, recording, transmission, and storage has recently undergone revolutionary changes. Digital cameras offer many advantages and have now largely replaced film cameras. Coupled with an Internet-based computerized delivery system, they enable a very significant reduction in turnaround time with relatively little compromise to quality. Other than the electron microscope, the only specialized equipment needed is an ultramicrotome. Because ultimate success with this technique depends so heavily upon the capacity to obtain quality ultrathin sections in a reliable and rapid manner, it is of greater importance to possess a modern ultramicrotome than a modern electron microscope.

A scanning electron microscope can occasionally be used to advantage (e.g., for demonstration of hair shaft abnormalities) but is not a necessity for a basic facility. Similarly, the

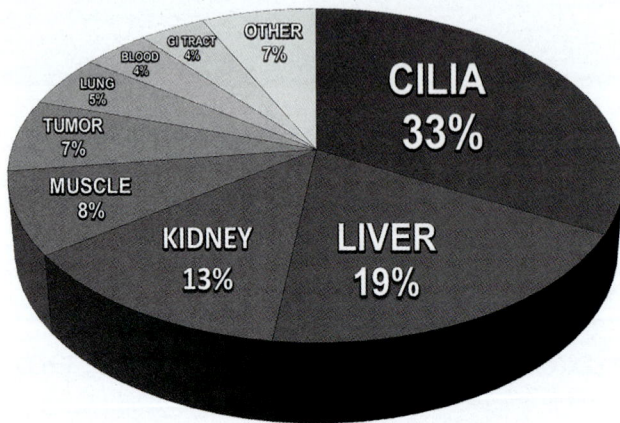

FIGURE 1D-1 • Composition of pediatric cases submitted for diagnostic ultrastructural study (Children's Hospital Colorado, 2013, n = 603).

capacity to perform elemental analysis (e.g., for heavy metal detection) or tomographic studies (e.g., for problematic cilia specimens) is a need only for larger more sophisticated referral laboratories.

Generating results within a clinically relevant time frame is crucial to a successful operation, and it is a reasonable expectation to have an interpretive report, complete with illustrations, available within two working days of specimen receipt. Even "same day" examination of specimens is possible when circumstances warrant. One dedicated technologist for every 250 specimens examined annually continues to be a reasonable guide for the staffing of a diagnostic EM facility (1). To ensure a steady and secure service, two technologists and therefore a minimum caseload of approximately 500 specimens per year are needed. Institutions with fewer specimens may be better served by outsourcing, at least the technical component of this work, to a provider that can consistently meet this standard. Overnight delivery systems and electronic data transmission mechanisms obviate any need for the EM provider to be in close proximity to the referring institution.

In providing the interpretive component of the ultrastructural studies, a number of organizational models have been shown effective. Which is best in a given situation will depend upon the particular circumstances and personnel available. In some institutions, each pathologist while on service assumes full responsibility for the submission, examination, and interpretation of their cases. In others, a designated pathologist carries the responsibility for the examination and interpretation of all cases. In the majority of laboratories, however, technical personnel (with appropriate training and guidance) do much of the examination and may even assist with the interpretation of results.

It is often assumed that the electron microscopy laboratory will be a financial liability for its parent institution. This need not be true. With attentiveness to basic business practices, and sufficient volume, an electron microscopy laboratory can be a profitable enterprise. Electron microscopy is sometimes thought of as being a very expensive and extremely slow technique, but its modern-day cost and speed is actually quite comparable to immunohistochemistry and most other ancillary diagnostic techniques. And, of course, the cost savings to be derived from utilizing the most powerful techniques available to obtain a fast and accurate diagnosis needed to minimize the length of a hospital stay should be obvious. Certainly for health care facilities already maintaining an electron microscopy laboratory, there is no economic reason not to use the technique to its fullest advantage. The major expenses associated with this endeavor are fixed rather than incremental, so its actual cost to the institution will remain virtually the same whether it is used a little or used a lot.

THE ELECTRON MICROSCOPY TECHNIQUE

While most other ancillary techniques (e.g., IHC, FISH, PCR) are restricted in application to hypothesis testing, electron microscopy can provide the right answer even when the wrong question, or no specific question,

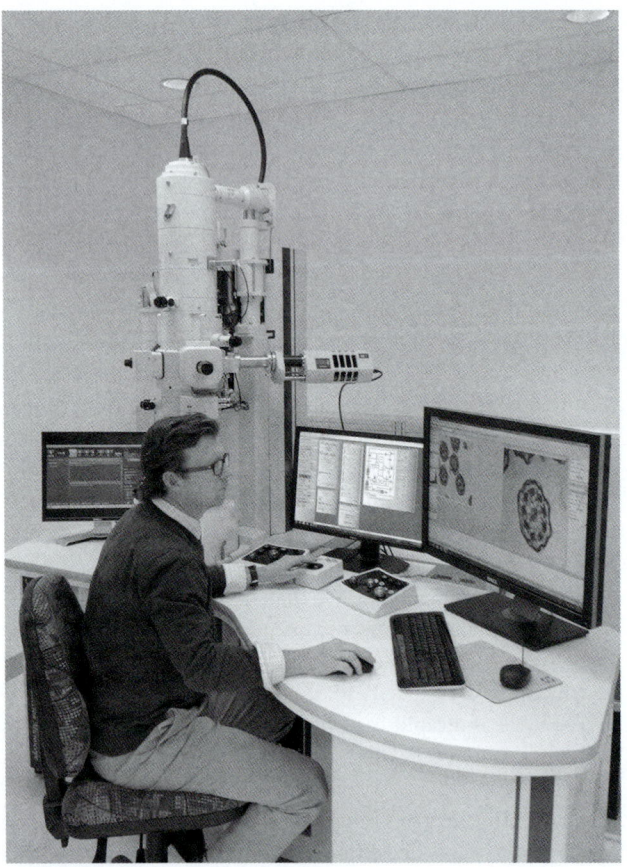

FIGURE 1D-2 • Example of transmission electron microscope suitable for diagnostic work.

is being asked. Preserving the option to perform electron microscopy is therefore an important habit to develop. Placing a bit of tissue into an appropriate fixative as a matter of routine takes little extra time and costs next to nothing—but provides excellent insurance should a diagnostic issue arise later.

Electron microscopy is not so much a different technology as a modification, and extension, of a most familiar one. Specimens for electron microscopy are handled in almost the same way as for light microscopy. Here, the standard fixative, instead of formaldehyde, is glutaraldehyde (to better preserve proteins) followed by osmium tetroxide (to better preserve lipids). Ordinary formalin preparations, if they are properly buffered (pH 7.2–7.4 range) and adjusted to moderate hypertonicity (400 to 500 mOsm), actually serve quite well as a primary fixative for electron microscopy and can be substituted when necessary. The tissues are dehydrated in a similar fashion but then are embedded in an epoxy resin to enable the cutting of thinner sections than would be possible with the softer paraffin wax used for routine histology. To cut the necessary (approximately 80 nm thick) ultrathin sections requires a similar but more refined "ultra" microtome and the use of a diamond blade. An electron beam cannot penetrate glass, so the sections are mounted on a fine-meshed screen (referred to as a grid) rather than on a glass slide. The sections are not stained in the true sense of the word (as color reactions cannot be detected with an electron microscope) but are incubated in similar fashion in heavy metal solutions (usually of uranium and lead) to selectively add contrast to various substructural components. Methodologic details for all these procedures can be found in many standard texts (2, 3). Except in its use of a beam of electrons, rather than a beam of light, the electron microscope is not very different in design or operation from that of an ordinary light microscope. It is the shorter wavelength of electrons that enables the superior point-to-point resolution and, thus, higher working magnifications offered by this instrumentation. The two techniques form a strong partnership, with the light microscope being best suited for the study of collections of cells and the electron microscope being best suited for the study of individual cells.

Under ideal conditions, specimens submitted for electron microscopy will consist of a representative sampling of appropriately sized (approximately 1 mm^3) tissue cubes placed into the most suitable fixative immediately upon removal from the patient. Real-life conditions will not always be ideal, but all is not necessarily lost if they are not. Just as an experienced automobile mechanic can still usually identify the make and model of a car after it has been involved in an accident, so can an experienced electron microscopist still usually identify the cell type and disease process involved in a partially wrecked tissue specimen. One has to be more cautious when dealing with suboptimal specimens, however, as there is a strong inverse relationship between the quality of specimen preservation and the probability of making a significant interpretive error. The safest strategy when dealing with suboptimally preserved specimens is to restrict electron microscopy to the search for some particular feature(s) predetermined to be of diagnostic relevance.

A demonstration of the deleterious effects associated with suboptimal specimen processing is presented in Figure 1D-3, which shows subsamples from the same case of Langerhans cell histiocytosis after being subjected to progressively harsher treatments. Here, it can be seen that, though the diagnosis can still be made, the degree of difficulty increases (and the degree of confidence decreases) as the quality of cellular preservation is diminished. With optimal processing (Figure 1D-3A), the richness of cytoplasmic detail almost obscures the diagnostic Birbeck granules. Substitution of formaldehyde for glutaraldehyde as the primary fixative (Figure 1D-3B) results in a significant loss of cytoplasmic detail, but, at least in this instance, this does not interfere with the identification of the critical feature. Often, it is the case that in order to perform additional specialized procedures, such as the immunohistochemical reaction for S100 protein shown here, it becomes necessary to trade off some degree of cellular preservation to maintain an adequate degree of tissue reactivity. Such applications, however, will fall mainly within the domain of research. For general purposes, when using formalin-fixed tissues for electron microscopy, it is best to refix the specimen in glutaraldehyde before proceeding with the tissue processing. As a last resort, one can retrieve paraffin-embedded tissue and reprocess it for electron microscopy. The technique is simple (4). Following removal of a carefully selected appropriately sized tissue sample from the paraffin block using a sharply pointed scalpel blade, the specimen is dewaxed overnight in xylene. Best results are obtained if, following rehydration in graded alcohols, the tissue is refixed both with glutaraldehyde and with osmium tetroxide prior to further processing. Because much of the lipid will have been extracted during the earlier processing events, one can expect poor preservation of membranes and other structures of high lipid content. Nevertheless, as shown in Figure 1D-3C, the features of key interest may still remain clearly identifiable. Structures that are composed largely of proteins (e.g., filaments, granules, intercellular junctions, immune deposits) are the most likely to remain identifiable, but sometimes, membranous structures also are preserved. It proved possible, for example, in a correlative study to demonstrate Birbeck granules in deparaffinized material from 11 of 14 cases in which they were known to exist (5). In some situations, for example, in attempting to identify a focally distributed virus, this approach may actually prove more efficacious than would an unfocused search through optimally preserved tissue. Utilization of deparaffinized tissue preserved with a nonaldehyde-type fixative (e.g., alcohol, B5, Bouin) will generally be unrewarding for, without cross-linking of proteins, nearly all substructural features are lost during processing (Figure 1D-3D).

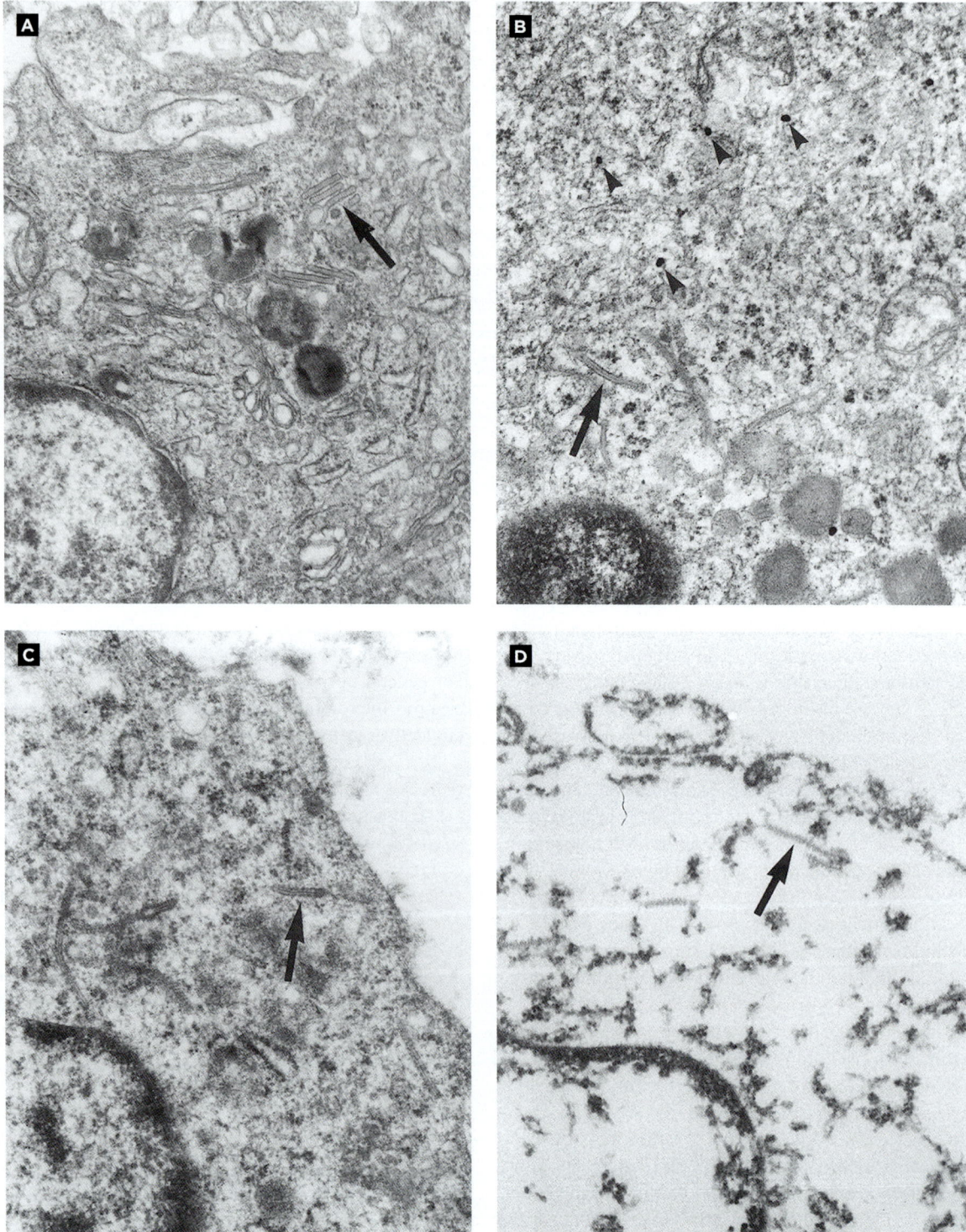

FIGURE 1D-3 • Subsamples from the same case of Langerhans cell histiocytosis subjected to variations in processing technique. **A:** Routine processing, utilizing glutaraldehyde fixation, results in optimal preservation of Birbeck granules (*arrow*) and other subcellular components. **B:** Substitution of formaldehyde for glutaraldehyde results in swelling of the mitochondria and some loss of cytoplasmic detail but has little effect on the Birbeck granules (*arrow*). The less intense fixation enables immunogold labeling of S100 protein (*arrowheads*). **C:** Birbeck granules (*arrow*) display an altered appearance but remain clearly identifiable in formalin-fixed tissue retrieved from a paraffin block. The mitochondria are reduced to smudges and most other cytoplasmic detail is lost. **D:** In B5-fixed tissue retrieved from paraffin, the Birbeck granules (*arrow*) are hardly recognizable and nearly all other components have been lost.

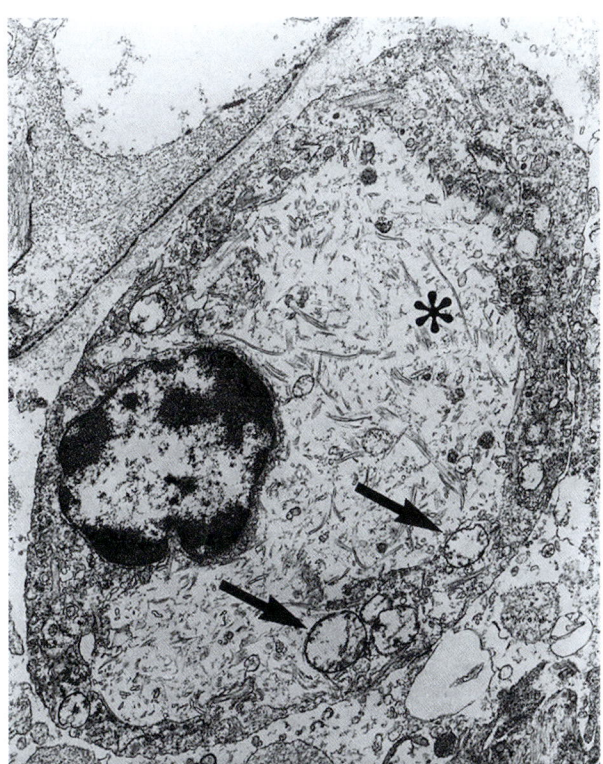

FIGURE 1D-4 • Autopsy specimen of brain showing perivascular cell with large cytoplasmic inclusion (*asterisk*). The mitochondria (*arrows*) exhibit degenerative changes, but the material within the inclusions remains well enough preserved to enable a confident diagnosis of Krabbe disease.

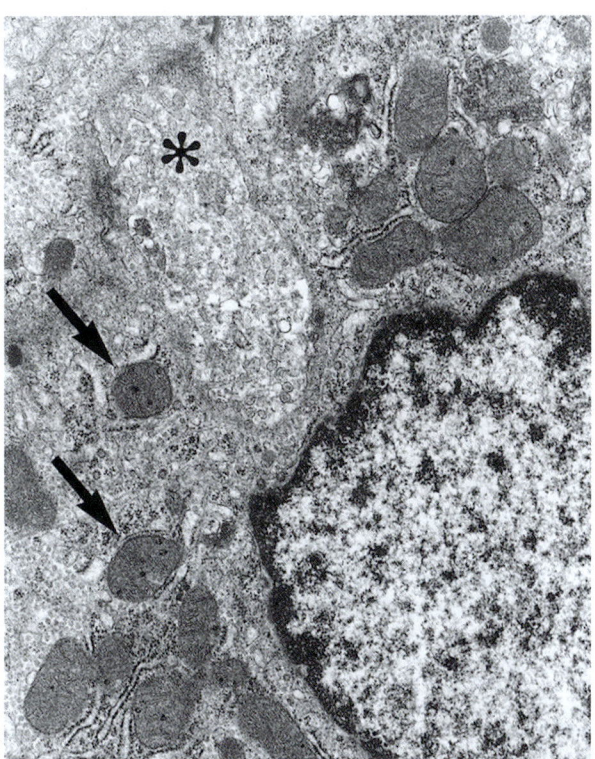

FIGURE 1D-5 • Snap frozen specimen of liver thawed in chilled glutaraldehyde shows excellent preservation of mitochondria (*arrows*) and other cellular structures and allows demonstration of the coarse granular bile (*asterisk*) characteristic of type 1 progressive familial intrahepatic cholestasis.

It is often assumed that autopsy specimens will not be suitable for electron microscopic study. This is not always the case. While some autolytic degradation is inevitable, its severity and speed of occurrence is not entirely predictable. Sometimes, as illustrated in Figure 1D-4, cellular preservation remains surprisingly good even after an extended postmortem interval. The appearance of certain organelles, such as mitochondria, is very quickly altered by anoxic conditions. One would not, therefore, want to attempt assessment of a mitochondrial disorder using autopsy material. On the other hand, many structures are quite durable and can be confidently identified even in a specimen that is very degenerated. Here again, the denser the structure, and the greater its protein content, the more likely it is to remain recognizable.

Frozen tissue as well can be used for electron microscopy. Best results are obtained when the frozen tissue is placed directly into cold glutaraldehyde and allowed to fix as it thaws. The quality of cellular preservation, particularly with respect to ice crystal damage, varies regionally within a specimen. Examination of multiple sites may therefore prove beneficial. This recovery technique is especially useful in renal pathology, in circumstances where the initial specimen submitted for electron microscopy happens not to contain any glomeruli. The technique may serve other purposes as well, as demonstrated in Figure 1D-5.

Electron microscopy is particularly well suited for the examination of fine-needle aspirate specimens (6, 7). In pediatric medicine, an electron microscopic approach to the examination of fine-needle aspirates has been found to be especially useful in the diagnosis of childhood round cell tumors (8). Since with electron microscopy it is normally the situation that relatively a relatively small number of cells are examined individually for identifying characteristics, the technique is not much compromised by the small disrupted samples produced by the aspiration procedure. Figure 1D-6A shows how a confident diagnosis can be established even with just a few neoplastic cells being present. Demonstrated in Figure 1D-6B is an ultrastructural "special stain" for glycogen that can be of particular usefulness in circumstances like these (9), as it can be applied directly to an existing ultrathin section and does not require the processing of any additional material.

With lower risk of loss during the embedding process, and within approximately the same time frame, tiny specimens of other sorts (for instance, from an endomyocardial biopsy procedure) can be embedded in epoxy resin instead of paraffin wax. More specimen detail than usual will be observed by light microscopy because of the enhanced resolution offered by the 1-μm-thick resin-embedded sections. The array of special stains utilizable with these sections is somewhat limited, but this strategy does preserve the option to use electron microscopy, which might be considered the most powerful "special stain" of all.

The introduction of flow cytometric, immunocytochemical, and molecular diagnostic techniques greatly diminished

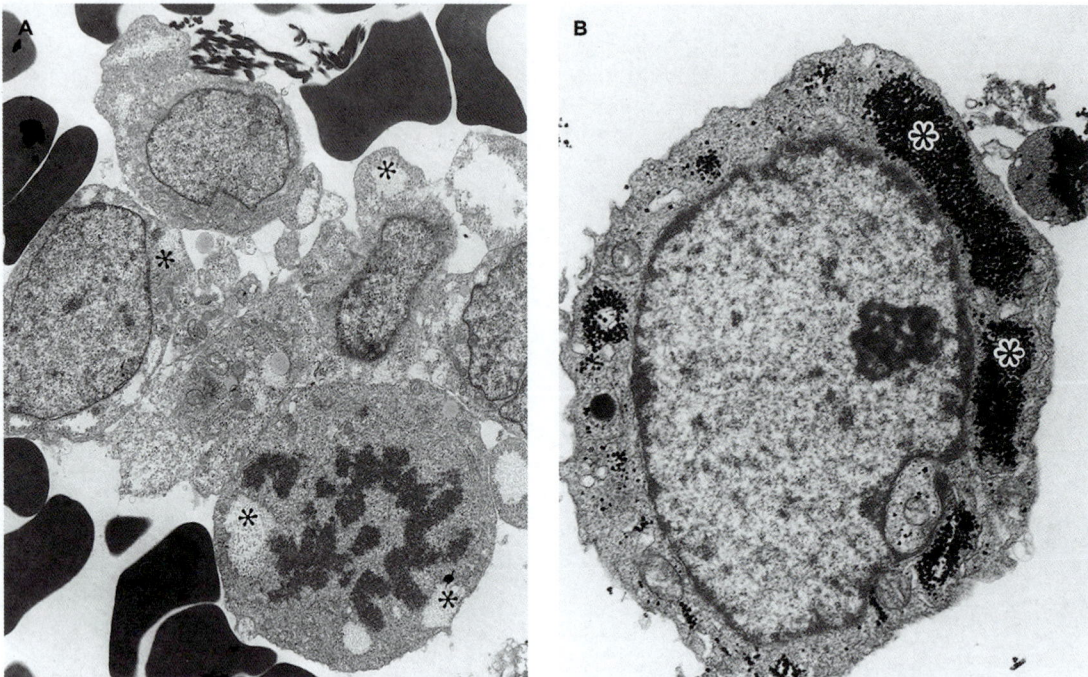

FIGURE 1D-6 • Fine-needle aspirate specimen displaying focal deposits of cytoplasmic glycogen (*asterisks*) characteristic of Ewing sarcoma. That the "moth-eaten" areas represent glycogen deposits **(A)** is easily confirmed by incubating the sections in a weak tannic acid solution prior to staining with uranyl acetate and lead citrate **(B)**.

the role for electron microscopy in the diagnosis of hematologic disorders. Nevertheless, it remains an indispensable tool for the diagnosis of certain conditions (e.g., platelet storage pool disorders). To meet the challenges presented by the minuscule specimens obtainable from some pediatric patients, droplets of blood are drawn into two or three anticoagulant-coated glass microhematocrit tubes. Immediately upon transport to the laboratory (or the next morning, in the case of late-arriving specimens), the hematocrit tubes are centrifuged and then scored and broken just below the buffy coat layer. The buffy coat samples are then gently expelled into a vial of glutaraldehyde. As the droplet settles through the fixative, it consolidates into a single small firm pellet, which can subsequently be processed with ease as a solid tissue specimen. Where larger volumes are obtainable, blood specimens are first drawn into 3-ml tubes containing sodium citrate anticoagulant and centrifuged to produce a leukocyte-enriched layer from with which the microhematocrit tubes are then filled.

In the diagnosis of peroxisomal disorders, ultrastructural studies are utilized to determine whether these organelles are normal, abnormal, reduced in number, or absent (10). Usually, this can be accomplished without the application of any special techniques. Occasionally, however, we have found it beneficial to employ the alkaline–diaminobenzidine reaction for catalase activity (11) to verify the identity of morphologically abnormally formed peroxisomes.

Another easily performed ultrastructural special stain that has upon occasion proved helpful is the uranaffin reaction. It can be used, among other things, to establish the identity of neuroendocrine granules in tumors (12) and serotonin granules in platelets (13).

Evaluation of ciliary morphology requires electron microscopy (14). Curettage specimens of nasal mucosa are especially recommended for this purpose because they produce an adequate yield of favorably oriented cilia more consistently than other biopsy methods. The brush biopsy technique, in experienced hands, also generally produces excellent results (Figure 1D-7A). Specimens from patients as young as one month of age can be successfully obtained using these techniques. We have found little need here for the use of any special fixatives or processing techniques, other than for concentrating small dispersed samples by centrifugation in an agar-based gelling agent prior to the dehydration and embedding process.

Electron microscopy, in addition to detecting viruses in solid tissue specimens, can be used for detection of viruses in body fluids and fecal specimens. The negative staining techniques used for this purpose are fast and easy to perform and need not be very elaborate. A Beckman Airfuge® ultracentrifuge can be used to help concentrate the virus onto the grid surface, but the direct technique, which requires no special equipment, works almost as well (15). The more cumbersome immunologic techniques have not performed as well for us in this regard but have occasionally proved useful in confirming the identity of a detected virus. The negative staining technique can be used with a variety of specimens (e.g., urine, blood, vesicle fluid, cerebrospinal fluid, amniotic fluid, respiratory tract secretions), but its major application in pediatrics lies in the diagnosis of acute

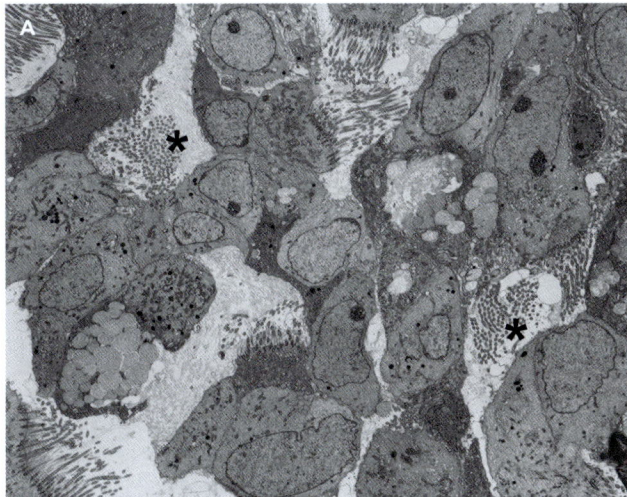
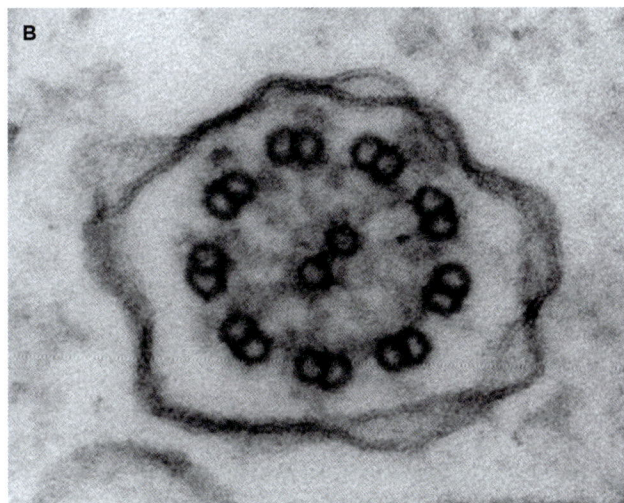

FIGURE 1D-7 • **A:** Brush biopsy specimen of nasal respiratory epithelium showing numerous favorably oriented cilia (*asterisks*). **B:** Cilium exhibiting absence of dynein arms as the cause for primary ciliary dyskinesia.

viral gastroenteritis. This very practical and cost-effective approach enables detection of all pathogens. Multiple agent infections are readily detected using this methodology (Figure 1D-8), which can be especially important when isolation procedures to stem a nosocomial outbreak are being implemented. The technique can be performed in just a matter of minutes, which may be of importance when initiation of therapy awaits establishment of a firm diagnosis or, such as in the event of a bioterrorism attack, an infectious organism requires quick identification.

ILLUSTRATIVE EXAMPLES

Electron microscopic examination can provide definitive diagnostic information in a number of situations. The most frequently requested study is for the identification of defects in ciliary structure (Figure 1D-7B). Another application in the evaluation of children with pulmonary dysfunction is for the demonstration of pulmonary interstitial glycogenosis. Electron microscopy can also be used to provide evidence of surfactant ABCA3 (Figure 1D-9A) and type B deficiencies.

When multiorgan system dysfunction is present in a neonate or infant with hepatomegaly, electron microscopic examination of a liver biopsy specimen may yield evidence of the underlying disease. Ultrastructural studies can reveal the existence of a storage disease at its earliest stages of manifestation and sometimes, such as with certain forms of glycogen storage disease, even provide a precise diagnosis. Ultrastructural studies are highly beneficial in the diagnosis of peroxisomal disorders. Electron microscopy can render a definitive diagnosis in children with significant cholestasis early in life and who may be suspected to have progressive familial intrahepatic cholestasis (Figure 1D-5), alpha-1-antitrypsin deficiency, or other diseases as a cause of their jaundice and liver dysfunction.

A substantial number of renal diseases (e.g., minimal change lesion, dense deposit disease, thin basement membrane nephropathies) can only be diagnosed with confidence using this technology. Persistent hematuria in children can be due to many different disease processes, and often, IgA nephropathy, thin basement membrane, and hereditary nephritis are considered in the differential diagnosis. In children with persistent hematuria, renal biopsy tissue is

FIGURE 1D-8 • Negative stained stool specimen from a patient infected simultaneously with rotavirus (*open arrow*), coronavirus (*curved arrow*), and a small round virus (*solid arrow*).

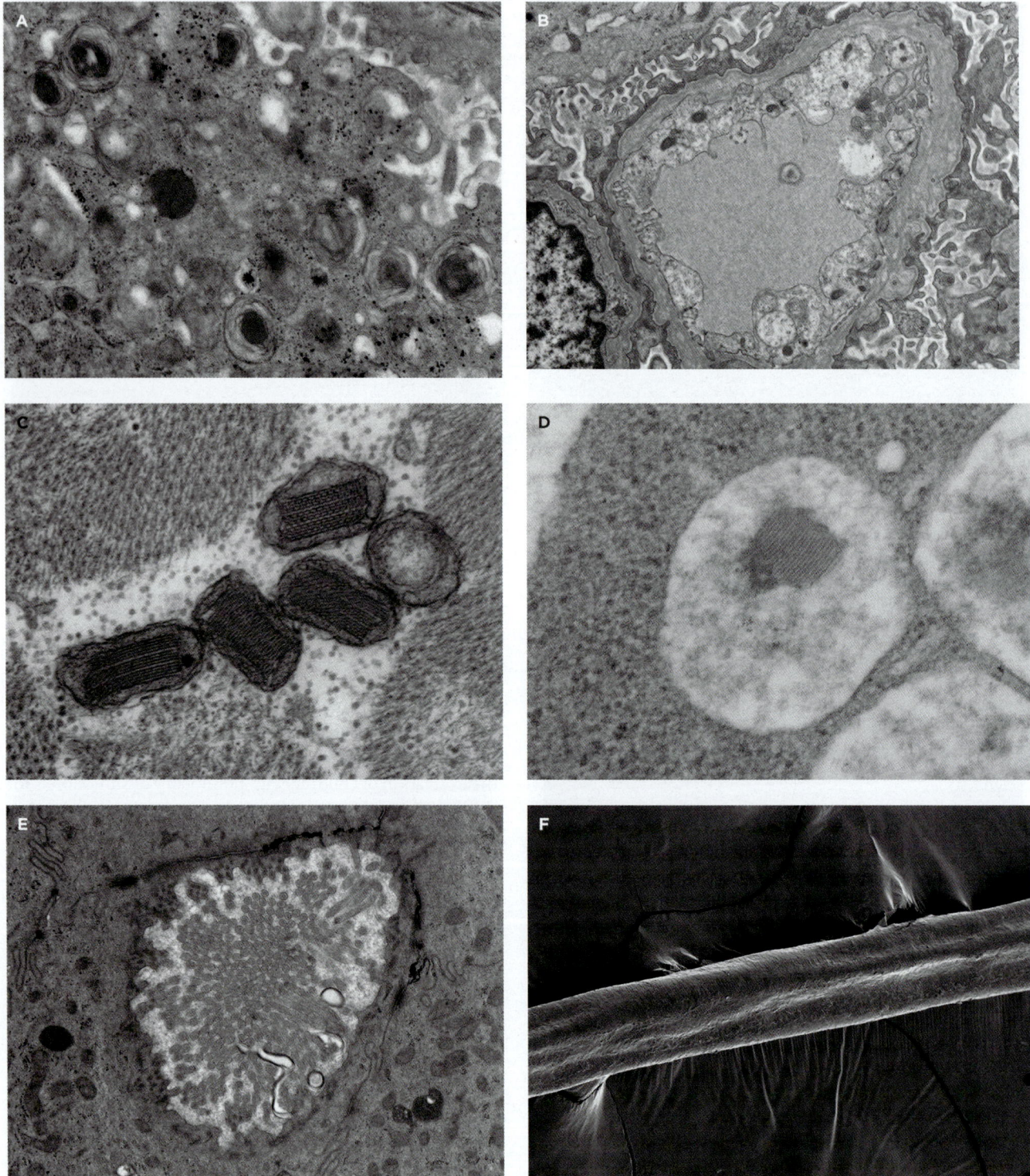

FIGURE 1D-9 • Illustrative examples of definitive diagnostic features provided by ultrastructural examination. **A:** Abnormal lamellar bodies characteristic for surfactant ABCA3 deficiency. **B:** Lamellation and basket-weave patterning of the glomerular basement membranes characteristic for hereditary nephritis. **C:** "Parking lot" inclusions within mitochondrial cristae characteristic for mitochondriopathy. **D:** "Fingerprint" inclusions within lymphocytic vacuole characteristic for juvenile-type neuronal ceroid lipofuscinosis. **E:** Intracytoplasmic lumen within enterocyte characteristic for microvillus inclusion disease. **F:** Longitudinal groove along triangular hair shaft characteristic for pili canaliculi et trianguli.

typically submitted for routine light, immunofluorescence, and electron microscopy. IgA nephropathy, for instance, is identified by immunofluorescence reactivity with IgA antibody in combination with the demonstration of paramesangial deposits by electron microscopy. Thin basement membrane disease is diagnosable only by accurate measurement of the thickness of glomerular basement membranes, which accomplished with the aid of an electron microscope. Hereditary nephritis is initially detected by electron microscopic demonstration of the characteristic lamellation and basket-weave patterning within the glomerular basement membranes (Figure 1D-9B), after which immunofluorescence studies and genetic testing more productively can be utilized to provide diagnostic confirmation.

Ultrastructural studies of muscle biopsy specimens are of particular utility in diagnosing causes of infantile hypotonia, storage diseases, and mitochondriopathies (Figure 1D-9C).

Immunohistochemical and molecular diagnostic techniques have reduced, but not eliminated, the use of electron microscopy in tumor diagnosis. Ultrastructural studies continue to be particularly helpful where immunohistochemical and/or molecular studies produce confusing or equivocal results, insufficient or aberrant neoplastic cell differentiation causes diagnostic uncertainty, an unusual or uncommon diagnosis is under consideration, or when only a limited sampling is available for study (Figure 1D-6).

Electron microscopy is often the best (i.e., fastest, cheapest, easiest, and/or only) means of screening for lysosomal storage disorders. Blood (Figure 1D-9D) is among the many types of specimens used for this purpose. Ultrastructural studies of blood are employed also for the identification of platelet storage pool disorders, the diagnosis of congenital dyserythropoietic anemia, and for the occasional problematic leukemia.

Bowel biopsies are examined, among other things, to detect furtive organisms such as microsporidia and to diagnose microvillus inclusion disease (Figure 1D-9E).

The "Other" category shown in Figure 1D-1 encompasses a wide variety of specimen types, including skin. Skin biopsy specimens are often favored for the diagnosis of storage diseases and serve as well for a variety of other purposes. Variants of epidermolysis bullosa can be placed by electron microscopy into one of four major types, after which the diagnosis may be further refined by targeted immunophenotyping and guided genetic testing. Connective tissue disorders, such as Ehlers-Danlos syndrome and cutis laxa, may be diagnosed by transmission electron microscopy. Scanning electron microscopy may be used to identify hair shaft abnormalities, such as trichorrhexis nodosa, pili torti, and pili canaliculi et trianguli (Figure 1D-9F).

To the examples and applications previously mentioned could be added a vast number of others. It is, in conclusion, emphasized that electron microscopy remains an extremely powerful, highly versatile, absolutely indispensable diagnostic technique for the current practice of pediatric pathology. Ideally, every pathologist would have an electron microscope located just down the hall and the time and expertise required to use it effectively. Fortunately, when such is not the case, modern-day transportation and communication systems allow consultative arrangements to be developed, virtually anywhere in the world, that are nearly as fast, convenient, and effectual. Barriers to the utilization of this technique are presently nonexistent.

References

1. Williams MJ. Diagnostic electron microscopy in the Veterans Administration. In: Trump BF, Jones RT, eds. *Diagnostic Electron Microscopy*. Vol. 2. New York, NY: John Wiley and Sons; 1979:1–13.
2. Bozzola JJ, Russell LD. *Electron Microscopy. Principles and Techniques for Biologists*, 2nd ed. Sudbury, MA: Jones and Bartlett Publishers; 1998.
3. Hayat MA. *Principles and Techniques of Electron Microcopy. Biological Applications*, 3rd ed. Boca Raton, FL: CRC Press; 1989.
4. Johannessen JV. Use of paraffin material for electron microscopy. *Pathol Annu* 1977;12:189–224.
5. Mierau GW, Favara BE, Brenman JM. Electron microcopy in histiocytosis X. *Ulrastruct Pathol* 1982;3:137–142.
6. Strausbauch P, Neill J, Dabbs DJ, et al. The impact of fine needle aspiration biopsy on a diagnostic electron microscopy laboratory. *Arch Pathol Lab Med* 1989;113:P1354–P1356.
7. Yazdi HM, Dardick I. Diagnostic immunocytochemistry and electron microscopy. In: Kline TS, ed. *Guides to Clinical Aspiration Biopsy. Pediatrics*. New York, NY: Igaku-Shoin; 1992:1.
8. Akhtar M, Ali MA, Sabbah R, et al. Fine-needle aspiration biopsy diagnosis of round cell malignant tumors of childhood. A combined light and electron microscopic approach. *Cancer* 1985;55:1805–1817.
9. Dingemans KP, van den Bergh Weerman MA. Rapid contrasting of extracellular elements in thin sections. *Ultrastruct Pathol* 1990;14:519–527.
10. Dimmick JE, Applegarth DA. Pathology of peroxisomal disorders. In: Landing BH, Haust MD, Bernstein J, Rosenberg HS, eds. *Genetic Metabolic Diseases*. Basel, Switzerland: Karger; 1993:45–98. (Rosenberg HS, Bernstein J, eds. Perspectives in Pediatric Pathology; vol 17.)
11. Fahimi HD. Cytochemical localization of peroxidatic activity of catalase in rat hepatic microbodies (peroxisomes). *J Cell Biol* 1969;43:275–288.
12. Payne CM, Nagle RB, Borduin VF, et al. An ultrastructural evaluation of the cell organelle specificity of the uranaffin reaction in two human endocrine neoplasms. *Submicrosc Cytol* 1983;15:833–841.
13. Payne CM. A quantitative ultrastructural evaluation of the cell organelle specificity of the uranaffin reaction in normal human platelets. *Am J Clin Pathol* 1984;81:62–70.
14. Mierau GW, Agostini R, Beals TF, et al. The role of electron microscopy in evaluating ciliary dysfunction: report of a workshop. *Ultrastruct Pathol* 1992;16:245–254.
15. Doane FW, Anderson N. *Electron Microscopy in Diagnostic Virology. A Practical Guide and Atlas*. Cambridge, UK: Cambridge University Press; 1987.

CHAPTER 2

First and Second Trimester Pregnancy Loss

Jennifer Pogoriler, M.D., Ph.D., and Theonia K. Boyd, M.D.*

Pathologic examination of the products of embryos and fetuses, both from spontaneous abortions (SAbs) and terminations of pregnancy, has become increasingly important. While such examination was once performed primarily for the purpose of furthering scientific understanding of prenatal human development, the practical medical applications of this knowledge have become clear and now form an integral part of the medical assessment and management of fertility issues (1–5). As an understanding of the factors involved in successful pregnancies has developed and as patient demand for information has increased, the role of pathologic examination has grown. Increased use of assisted fertilization techniques has heightened the interest of physicians and patients alike in understanding why pregnancies fail. This chapter will address the examination of disorders encountered in those pregnancies that end spontaneously in the first and second trimesters of gestation; the pathology of fetuses delivered after pregnancy termination after prenatal ultrasound diagnosis is beyond the scope of this chapter.

It is recognized that many conceptions do not end in live births but, rather, that there is a high rate of spontaneous loss, especially early in gestation. It is estimated that 10% to 20% of recognized pregnancies end as SAbs, with most losses occurring in the first trimester (first 12 to 14 weeks of gestation). With the demonstration of fetal cardiac activity, the miscarriage rate drops to approximately 3% to 12% (6). In a study of women with a normal prenatal visit at 6 to 11 weeks of gestational age (GA), the risk of subsequent SAb was 1.6% or less, considerably lower than for pregnancies overall (7). After the first trimester, approximately 1% to 2% of pregnancies are spontaneously aborted (8). The incidence of stillbirth at term gestation is in the order of 0.1% to 0.5%. These loss rates that persist throughout gestation, together with changing or changed societal approaches and expectations of pregnancy such as delaying childbearing until later in a woman's reproductive life and increased access to assisted reproduction methods, have led to an intense interest in understanding the cause of pregnancy loss and the implications for future reproductive success.

GA refers to the number of weeks since the last menstrual period (equivalent to menstrual dates), while developmental age (DA) or conceptual age (CA) refers to the age as determined from the time of fertilization, generally considered as approximately 2 weeks after the last menstrual period. Embryos are assessed by developmental features that correlate with age, usually given as DA. Thus, in a normal gestation, GA is DA plus 2 weeks.

The first trimester of pregnancy is the period of implantation and embryogenesis, with the completion of embryogenesis by 8 weeks of DA (10 weeks of GA). Upon completion of embryogenesis with development of all organ systems, the conceptus is referred to as a fetus. Definitions of fetus and infant vary with locale; in Canada, a fetus is considered an infant once it has reached the GA of 20 weeks or is liveborn at any GA. In the United States, by contrast, the living intrauterine conceptus is referred to as a fetus until the time of live birth. Stillbirth is defined as delivery of a deceased conceptus at or after 20 weeks of GA.

CAUSES OF EARLY SPONTANEOUS ABORTION

It is well recognized that the major causes of early SAb are lethal chromosomal abnormalities, which are usually aneuploid (any karyotype that deviates from two haploid sets of 22 autosomes and one sex chromosome, with each haploid set contributed by one parent) (9). The use of techniques such as comparative genomic hybridization (CGH) and quantitative fluorescence-polymerase chain reaction (QF-PCR) to supplement conventional cytogenetic analysis has increased the detection of chromosome abnormalities because these

---

*Based upon the prior edition chapter by Deborah E. McFadden

techniques do not require cell culture and can address the issue of maternal cell contamination. Numerous studies have shown that at least half of early SAbs are chromosomally abnormal when routine cytogenetics is performed. Array CGH may be used in cases in which tissue culture for cytogenetic analysis has failed or in which maternal cell contamination is suspected (10–12). More recent studies of preimplantation blastomeres in in vitro fertilization (IVF) patients have shown that even in young healthy couples, fewer than 10% of embryos have a normal karyotype in all blastomeres (13), although it is unclear if this is due to IVF or reflects a typical state of chromosomal instability in early embryonic life.

The distribution of chromosome abnormalities is consistent between various studies, with trisomy accounting for half of all chromosomally abnormal SAbs, polyploidies and monoploidies (primarily monosomy X) each accounting for 10% to 15%, and structural rearrangements accounting for approximately 5%. (14,15). Trisomy for two chromosomes (double trisomy) is seen in only 3% of the chromosomally abnormal early SAbs. Trisomies for chromosomes 16, 21, and 22 are most common in early SAbs. The structural abnormalities are an important subgroup because of the possibility that they have arisen from a parent who carries a rearrangement predisposing to an unbalanced karyotype in the offspring. Studies of couples who have had recurrent miscarriages show that 5% have balanced rearrangements such as reciprocal translocations (16). These individuals have an increased risk of conceiving chromosomally abnormal pregnancies as well as recurrent miscarriage (17), with the actual risk depending on the type of rearrangement and the chromosomes involved (18). Although the presence of a balanced translocation predicts a risk of increased miscarriage in future pregnancies, the risk of a liveborn infant with a translocation is extremely low, and the proposed benefit of preimplantation genetic diagnosis is to shorten the interval between pregnancies, in order to achieve a successful outcome (19) rather than to improve the overall live birth rate.

With respect to trisomic conception, the most common subset of nonviable aneuploidies, studies of parental origin have demonstrated that the largest proportion of trisomy is maternally derived. There is a strong positive correlation with maternal age, meaning that the risk of conceiving a trisomic conceptus rises with increasing maternal age (20). Hypotheses to explain this finding include abnormal chromosomal crossover, altered chromatin cohesion, and altered DNA damage checkpoints. Trisomy affects 3% of pregnancies in 25-year-old women but occurs in 35% of pregnancies in women aged 42 years (21). Most trisomies are the result of errors in meiosis I (22), although this varies for individual chromosomes. For example, trisomy 18 is more typically the result of errors in the second meiotic division, while trisomy 21 is predominantly the result of first meiotic division errors.

With the predominance of SAbs attributable to aneuploidy, it is clear that in order to ensure clinical relevance of SAb evaluations, the examination should include determination of karyotype, particularly in recurrent pregnancy loss. In the event that the examination proves normal, with normal karyotype and normal villus histology, management of persons having recurrent SAbs shifts and other etiologies for pregnancy loss must be considered (23). The investigation of those who have had chromosomally normal miscarriages with no other pathology is dependent upon the proposed nonchromosomal mechanisms of pregnancy loss. These proposed associations include exogenous environmental exposures, uterine abnormalities (24), skewed X-inactivation (25,26), disorders of endocrine function, immune disorders including conditions with autoantibodies, and thrombophilic conditions (15). The roles of these factors in miscarriage remain under investigation, and the relative significance of each has not been established with certainty. Prospective cohort studies have not shown an association between single inherited thrombophilia mutations and miscarriage, although multiple mutations may increase risk (27–30). Prophylactic anticoagulant treatment has not been shown to improve outcomes in patients with recurrent miscarriages and inherited thrombophilias, and screening for these conditions is therefore not currently recommended (31), although this practice remains controversial (30). There is less controversy about the role of antiphospholipid antibody in recurrent pregnancy loss. Antiphospholipid antibodies are found more often in women who have recurrent miscarriages (RSAb) than in other women, although the mechanism by which an antiphospholipid antibody causes pregnancy loss is not definitively known. It is speculated that it may be due to interference with trophoblast function and thus the establishment of successful implantation, mediated by early-onset inadequate decidual arteriolar perfusion, and/or due to maternal/gestational interface inflammation (32). There are no specific pathologic features identified in the first trimester SAb from women who are positive for this antibody. Later findings seen in a subset of patients are also nonspecific but include those changes seen in other causes of uteroplacental malperfusion including infarction, increased intervillous fibrin, and terminal villous hypoplasia (33–35). Current guidelines recommend screening in patients with prior venous thromboembolism, with one fetal loss or with multiple embryonic losses. Treatment with prophylactic anticoagulation may improve outcome in these patients (36). With changing reproductive patterns, such as women starting their families later in life and having fewer children, there is enhanced societal desire to diagnose and manage causes of miscarriage. Given that cytogenetic abnormalities account for the majority of first trimester abortions, it has been suggested that the evaluation of first trimester SAb with cytogenetic analysis may prove more cost effective than a standard battery of tests such as thyroid function tests, endometrial biopsy, or thrombophilia testing (37). Pathologic examination also serves to identify those conditions not associated with abnormal karyotype that may require additional investigation or treatment to increase the likelihood of successful pregnancy and to diagnose conditions in which there is a risk of neoplasia, as with molar gestations and their attendant risk of transformation to gestational trophoblastic neoplasia (GTN) (1).

FIRST TRIMESTER SPONTANEOUS ABORTION

Indication for Cytogenetic Analysis

Given that chromosome abnormality accounts for the majority of first trimester SAbs, an argument could be made for performing cytogenetic analysis on all cases. To assist in the reproductive counseling regarding cause of the SAb and risks for recurrence, karyotype is a vital piece of information. Where embryo-pathology examination was once performed only in cases of recurrent SAbs, changes in reproductive patterns and practices have altered, resulting in a broader range of cases referred for embryo-pathologic examination. Those who treat women who have had difficulty conceiving or who have had previous miscarriage(s) are anxious to know whether the pregnancy failure was the result of chromosome abnormality or if there is perhaps another etiology necessitating further investigation. Increasingly, assisted reproductive technologies (ARTs) such as IVF or intracytoplasmic sperm injection (ICSI) are utilized. There are concerns that ARTs are associated with an increased incidence of chromosome abnormalities at prenatal diagnosis and at birth, specifically for sex chromosome abnormalities in pregnancies that are the result of ICSI (38,39). However, many small studies have found a high rate of chromosomal abnormalities in both ART and naturally conceived miscarriages, and a recent meta-analysis of case-controlled studies of chromosomal abnormalities in first trimester miscarriages showed no significant differences between either IVF or ICSI and natural conception, with the risk of abnormalities increased in older women in all groups (40).

Until the natural history of ART pregnancies is delineated, the use of these technologies should be considered as an indication for cytogenetic analysis in cases of SAb. In some laboratories, the fact that the majority of first trimester SAbs are the result of chromosome abnormality is sufficient indication to perform cytogenetic analysis of *all* cases examined morphologically. In other laboratories, constraints imposed by funding structures may impose the necessity of specific clinical indication before cytogenetic studies will be funded. These other indications include a history of recurrent miscarriages (variably defined as two to three or more losses), abnormal villus morphology, abnormal or normal embryo, parental chromosome rearrangement, and maternal age 35 years or greater.

Examination

Examination of the early pregnancy loss or embryo specimen is quite different from that of a fetal specimen as the latter represents an autopsy examination of a fetus and its placenta. Examination of the products of an early pregnancy loss (spontaneous or missed abortion) is performed to identify pregnancy-related tissues (embryo and/or placental tissue) to confirm intrauterine pregnancy and to assess their morphology. This examination includes sampling of tissues for additional studies, including for cytogenetic analysis or other means of determining the chromosome complement of the conceptus. Thus, it is imperative that all specimens for embryo-pathology examination are submitted in the fresh rather than fixed state.

An assessment of the products of conception is best accomplished by examining the specimen under a dissecting microscope, ideally equipped with a camera. The presence of any embryonic or placental tissue, including implantation site, allows confirmation of intrauterine pregnancy. In the absence of pregnancy-related tissues, intrauterine pregnancy cannot be confirmed, and the report must reflect that. Decidualized endometrium may be seen in estrogen effect, including with ectopic pregnancy, and is therefore insufficient for confirmation of intrauterine pregnancy.

The morphology of the chorionic villi is characterized—their individual morphology and their distribution over the chorionic sac. Attention to whether the villi appear overly abundant and/or cystic is important because of concerns for complete or partial hydatidiform mole (CHM, PHM). Other features of embryonic development, such as amnion, yolk sac, umbilical cord, and nucleated embryofetal erythrocytes, should also be assessed.

Tissues are sampled for cytogenetic analysis and can be retained frozen for additional studies as required. In many institutions, tissue is often submitted directly to the cytogenetics laboratory by the clinicians, either from the tissue obtained at dilation and curettage or by chorionic villous sampling. Additional tissue may be retained frozen for array CGH, although this can be increasingly performed on paraffin-embedded tissue (41). Although an argument can be made to utilize array CGH in all cases of SAbs to eliminate the labor and risk of culture failure associated with conventional cytogenetic analysis, conversely, CGH will miss some anomalies seen only on karyotype (12,42–44).

The presence of embryonic tissue confirms intrauterine pregnancy and is a feature in favor of a diagnosis other than CHM, a frequent concern as edematous villi are often identified on ultrasound or at gross examination. In determining the developmental stage and thus age of the embryo, standard developmental criteria can be used (45,46). Embryos may be normally developed (Figure 2-1) according to established criteria, but this does not exclude chromosome abnormality. Most developmental tables were established without karyotype determination. Some cases do not show regularly developed embryos but rather embryos or embryonic tissues in which normal developmental features are not present, a state referred to as growth disorganization. Growth disorganization has been divided into four categories: type I growth-disorganized embryo (GD1)

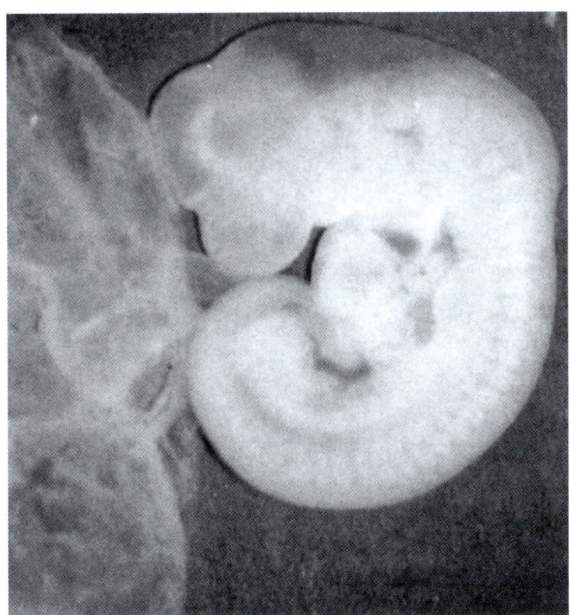

FIGURE 2-1 • Normally developed human embryo, stage 14 of development.

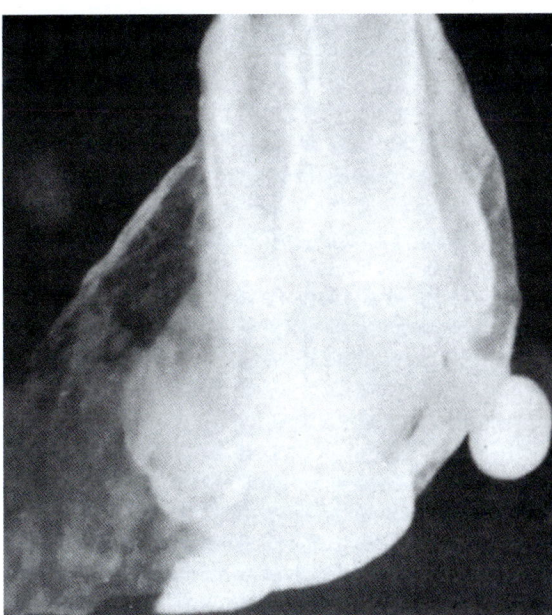

FIGURE 2-3 • Growth-disorganized embryo, GD2—1 mm nodular embryo in opened amniotic and chorionic sac.

refers to an intact empty sac (Figure 2-2), type II refers to a nodular embryo in which cranial and caudal ends cannot be distinguished (Figure 2-3), type III refers to a cylindrical embryo in which there is some cranial–caudal differentiation with retinal pigment (Figure 2-4), and type IV refers to an embryo in which there is more recognizable embryonic development but delayed growth of limbs and other developmental features (Figure 2-5). While growth disorganization is readily identified and classified, the findings are nonspecific—in all types of growth-disorganized embryos, the incidence of chromosome abnormality is similar to that encountered in SAbs in general, with the same types of chromosome abnormalities identified. Ultrasound detection of an embryo does not strictly correlate with the morphologic detection of embryonic tissue, but it has been demonstrated that the rates of abnormal karyotypes are not significantly different between SAbs in which an embryonic pole is identified on ultrasound examination and those that appear anembryonic (37,47). Approximately 60% to 70% of both anembryonic and embryonic specimens are chromosomally abnormal, although the spectrum of abnormalities may be different, with fewer monosomy X and viable autosomal trisomies in the anembryonic specimens.

Embryos may show isolated or focal abnormalities such as neural tube defects, facial clefts, or limb anomalies

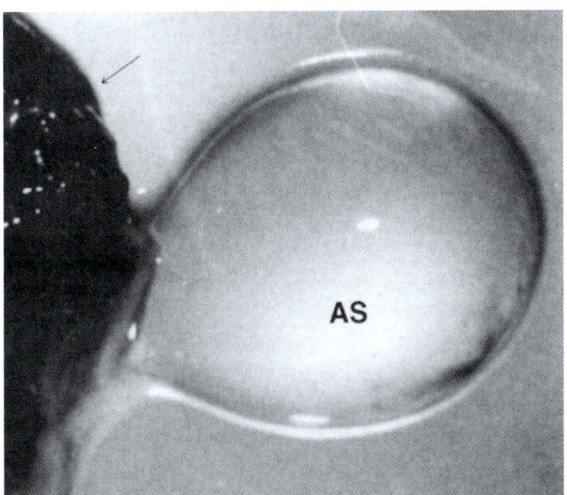

FIGURE 2-2 • Growth-disorganized embryo, GD1—intact empty amniotic sac (AS). Opened chorionic sac (*arrow*).

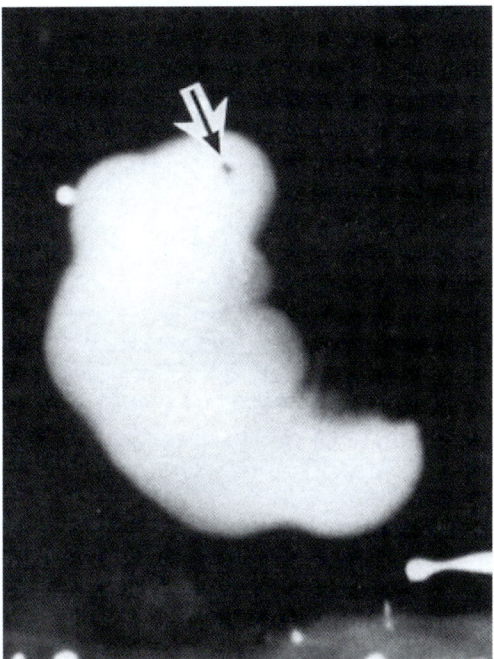

FIGURE 2-4 • Growth-disorganized embryo, GD3—cylindrical embryo with retinal pigment (*arrow*).

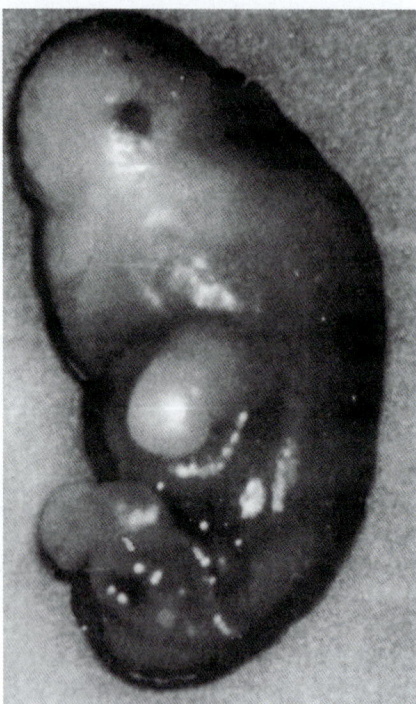

FIGURE 2-5 • Growth-disorganized embryo, GD4—delayed development of head, trunk, and limbs relative to crown-rump length.

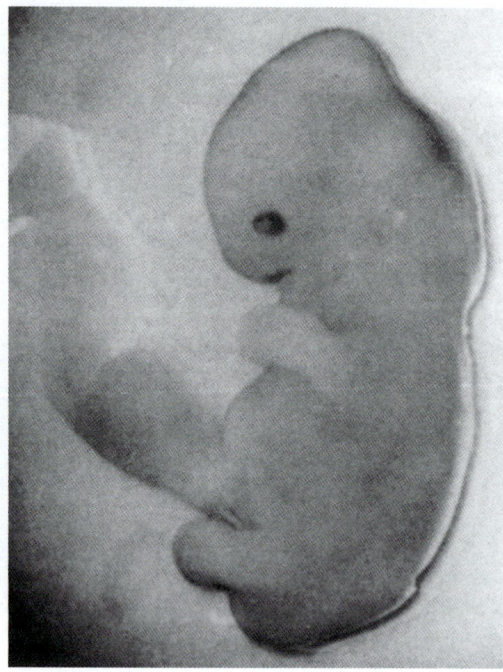

FIGURE 2-7 • Monosomy X embryo with parietal encephalocele.

(Figures 2-6 to 2-8). Many of these abnormalities, such as neural tube defects, occur in the setting of chromosome abnormality (48). In the setting of a normal karyotype, the focal defects likely have the same significance as in later gestation, and genetic counseling to discuss the findings and possible recurrence risks is indicated. Chromosomally abnormal embryos may show a number of nonspecific abnormalities, such as delay of normal limb development and various types of growth disorganizations. Embryos with trisomies more commonly encountered in later gestation and live births, such as trisomies 13, 18, and 21, may show some features in common with the phenotypes

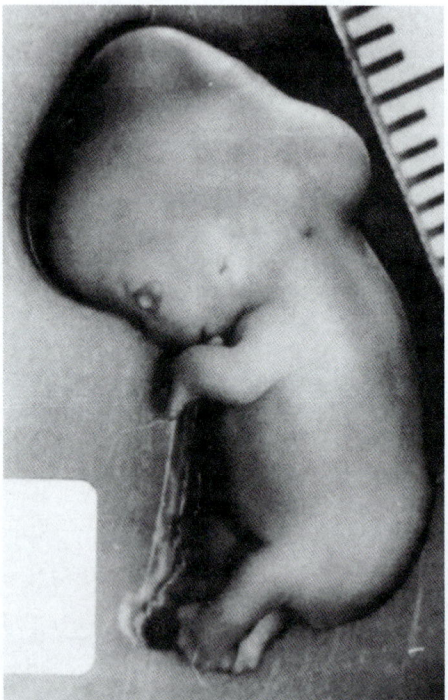

FIGURE 2-6 • Stage 20 embryo with parietal and occipital encephaloceles.

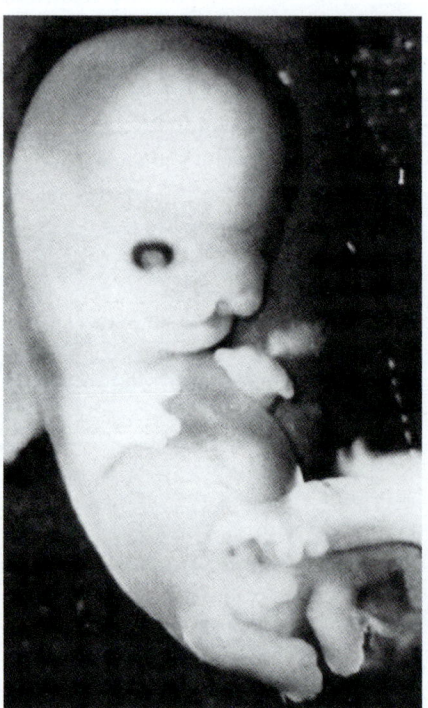

FIGURE 2-8 • Stage 18 embryo with cleft lip, absent digit in the right hand, and coloboma.

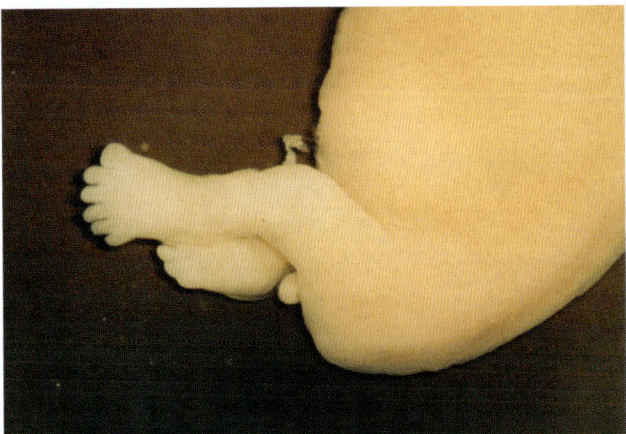

FIGURE 2-9 • Embryo with trisomy 13—postaxial polydactyly of feet.

observed in the fetal period. Most often, however, embryonic phenotypic manifestations of these trisomies are nonspecific (Figure 2-9).

Triploidy is encountered in approximately 6% of early SAbs; embryonic tissues are often identified. A phenotype thought to be characteristic of embryonic triploidy has been described and includes retarded limb development, facial dysplasia, subectodermal hemorrhage, and cystic chorionic villi (49) (Figure 2-10), but more recent series describe a wide range of phenotypic abnormalities ranging from growth-disorganized to apparently normal embryos (50). These apparently normal embryos are most often seen at approximately stage 16 of development (37 to 42 days), equivalent to

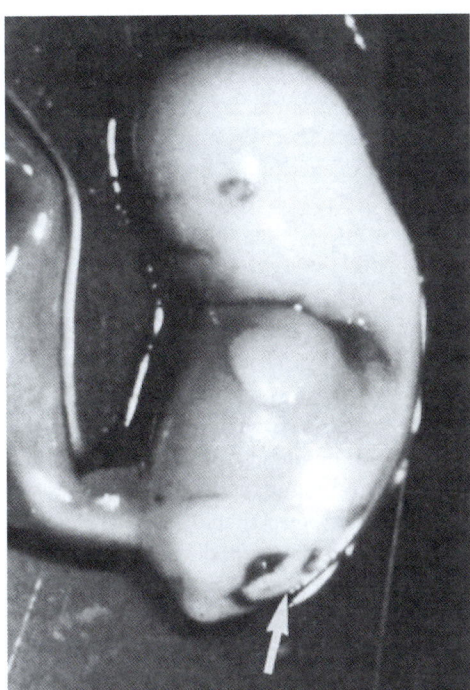

FIGURE 2-10 • Triploid embryo showing dysplastic face, delayed limb development, and defect in lumbosacral region (*arrow*).

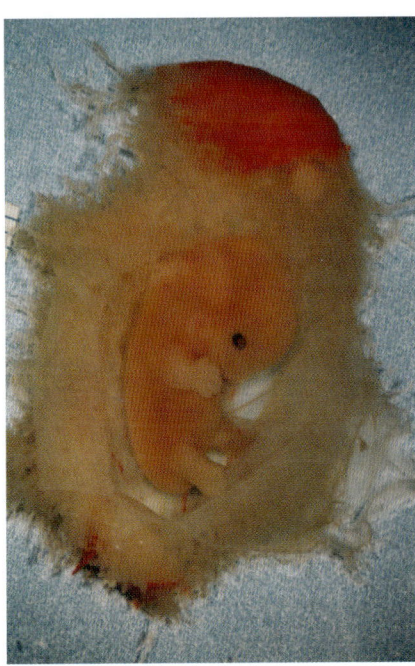

FIGURE 2-11 • Triploid embryo showing normal stage 18 phenotype, approximately 41 days DA.

approximately 7 to 8 weeks of GA (Figure 2-11). The normal and the growth-disorganized phenotypes have been seen in triploids of both maternal origin and paternal origin.

Histologic examination of placental tissues and decidua should be routinely performed in all cases. Microscopic examination of chorionic villi allows detection of many potential abnormalities including viral infections such as cytomegalovirus (CMV) and bacterial infections such as Listeriosis. In addition, other disorders such as intervillositis or conditions with increased intervillous fibrin are occasionally detected. Villous infarction is distinctly unusual and should raise concerns of maternal vascular/thrombophilic disease. Routine histologic examination of decidua allows for assessment of decidual (maternal) vasculature. In a review of the histopathology of SAbs with known karyotype, 19% of SAbs with a normal karyotype showed evidence of chronic inflammation or perivillous fibrin deposition, in contrast to 8% of those with an abnormal karyotype. The findings were even more frequent (31%) in the subset of SAbs that were chromosomally normal and occurred in a population with recurrent SAbs (51).

Chronic histiocytic intervillositis is a disorder in which there is an abnormal increase in maternal mononuclear cells, predominantly comprised of mature CD68 histiocytes, within the intervillous (maternal) space (Figure 2-12). The lesion is thought to be a maternal immune-mediated disorder; it confers a high recurrence risk in subsequent pregnancies (52–54).

Increased perivillous fibrin is another disorder in which it has been suggested that maternal immune dysregulation may play a role. Perivillous fibrin may also be increased as a degenerative change in response to prolonged intrauterine death, and distinguishing between pathologic and degenerative changes in perivillous fibrin can be difficult. When there is an obvious increase in perivillous fibrin, the lesion may be considered to account for

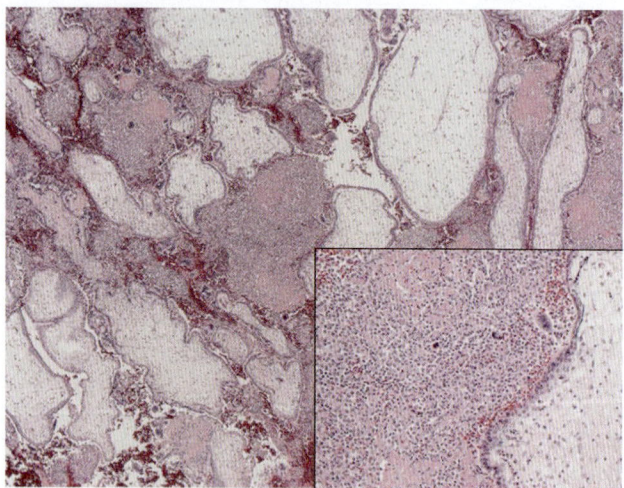

FIGURE 2-12 • Chronic (histiocytic) intervillositis in SAb at 10 weeks GA.

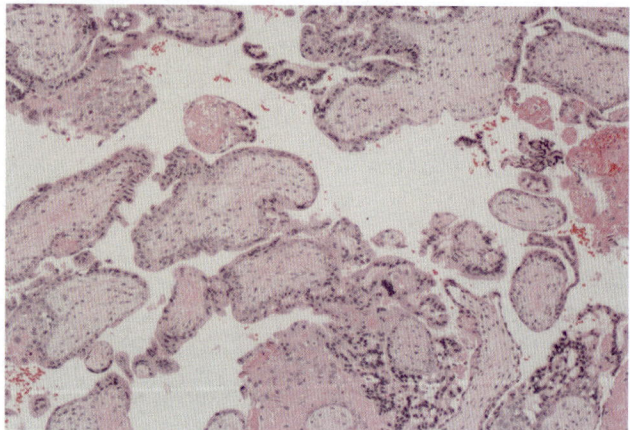

FIGURE 2-14 • Irregular ("busy") appearing trophoblastic epithelium in trisomy 22.

the loss. Some suggest that an arbitrary threshold of 50% villous involvement be used to make a pathologic diagnosis (55). Although probably etiologically heterogeneous, this entity may also recur and has been associated with recurrent SAbs.

Infection is a clear cause of pregnancy loss, with viruses, spirochetes, and bacteria all playing significant roles. Although first trimester loss may occur with syphilis, it is seen more often in losses occurring in later gestation. Listeriosis, by contrast, causes pregnancy loss throughout gestation (56). Listeriosis may occur as community outbreaks, related to improper food handling, or as a sporadic event related to ingestion of foods known to be at risk of containing Listeria, such as soft or unpasteurized cheeses. Listeriosis is characterized, histologically, by acute neutrophilic villitis with intervillous abscess formation (Figure 2-13). There is usually also an acute chorioamnionitis. Gram-positive bacilli may be demonstrated on Gram stain, although histology is usually sufficiently characteristic to allow confident diagnosis.

Excluding the small percentage of cases in which infectious, immune, or vascular causes of first trimester SAb is identified, the majority of SAbs are shown to be chromosomally abnormal. Although there are histologic features in chorionic villi that have been suggested as being more commonly observed in aneuploid pregnancies, such as irregular villous outlines, excess trophoblast inclusions, or complex invaginations, in general, these findings are nondiagnostic (57–60). Some trisomies, such as trisomy 22, may be more likely to show these features (61) (Figure 2-14).

Concern for GTN is heightened in the SAb population, as CHM and PHM may present as spontaneous or missed abortions. Historically, it has been shown that fewer than 44% of CHMs or PHMs are detected at routine first trimester ultrasound (62), providing an indication of the necessity for histologic examination of SAbs, even when a gestation appears routine at ultrasound or at the time of evacuation. The risk of GTN requiring chemotherapy has been reported to be between 15% and 28% after diagnosis of CHM (63), underscoring the importance of early diagnosis. The risk of GTN after triploid PHM is less well defined; there are case reports of choriocarcinoma occurring after triploid PHM (33,61,64,65), but others have shown that the risk of persistent GTN is rare, occurring in fewer than 5% of cases (39). Given the risks, however, some recommend that these cases be managed as would women who have had a CHM (34).

The diagnosis of early CHM and PHM can be difficult in specimens from early SAbs, perhaps more so than in the past when these pregnancies presented later in gestation. Gross examination of early hydatidiform moles may show cystic change of chorionic villi—grossly, this may be impossible to differentiate from the cystic change in partial moles and the hydropic degeneration occurring in nonmolar SAbs. Histologic diagnosis may not be possible even among experienced pathologists (66): studies have demonstrated considerable interobserver and intraobserver variability in the diagnosis of both CHM and PHM even among placental pathologists (67). A major problem that occurs in routine practice is to distinguish between hydropic abortion (degenerative change) and molar gestation. With recognition that the features in early CHM may be subtle and with the availability of karyotype determination, ploidy determination, and immunohistochemical staining for p57kip2, diagnostic accuracy is increased (68).

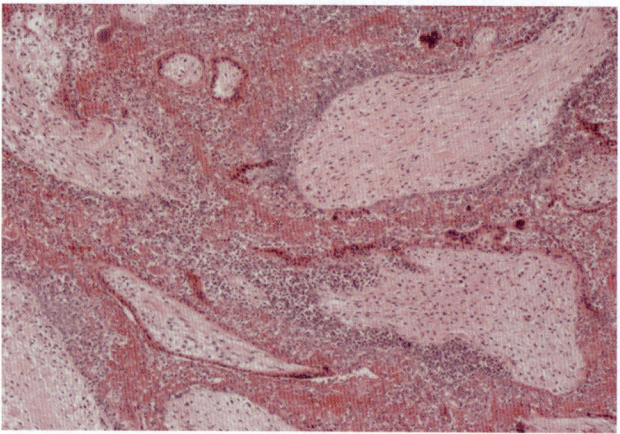

FIGURE 2-13 • Villus abscesses of Listeriosis. SAb at 14 weeks GA.

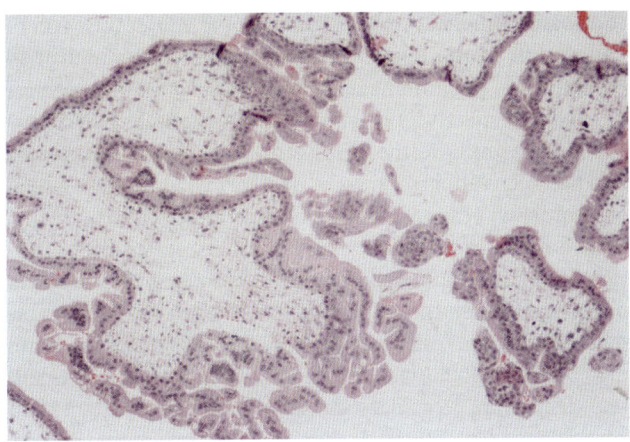

FIGURE 2-15 • Early CHM with stromal karyorrhexis.

CHMs are diploid, with both haploid complements being paternal in origin. Thus, CHMs are androgenetic, with no maternal DNA contribution present. The abnormal development in this situation is considered to be a reflection of imprinting (see Chapter 3, Table 3-17), since both maternal and paternal genetic contributions are required for normal embryonic and placental development. The classic histopathologic features of CHM are diffuse villus edema (hydropic change), cistern formation, and circumferential syncytio- and cytotrophoblast hyperplasia. Rudimentary villous vessels may be identified, but intravascular nucleated red blood cells are not seen. Stromal karyorrhexis is a feature of early CHM, thought to be related to increased stromal proliferation and apoptosis (Figure 2-15) (34). Immunohistochemical staining for p57kip2 is useful in the assessment of potential complete molar gestations because of its expression from the maternal allele only. Thus, in a CHM, by definition androgenetic, the normal p57kip2 staining of cytotrophoblast and villus stroma is absent (69,70). p57kip2 staining of triploid PHM is normal because of the maternal haploid contribution and is thus not helpful as a diagnostic aid.

Triploidy may be either paternal (diandric) or maternal (digynic) in origin. Older studies demonstrated that diandry was the predominant origin of triploidy, while more recent studies have shown that the distribution of diandric triploidy and digynic triploidy is somewhat more complex than that. In early pregnancy, the incidence of diandric triploidy is in the range of 50% to 65% (71–73). Of the two origins, it is diandric triploidy that presents as missed abortion with grossly cystic villi, with or without a final diagnosis of PHM. In the fetal and infant population, digyny clearly predominates.

PHM is characterized, classically, by two populations of villi, some with hydropic change and cistern formation and others that are small and not hydropic. The external villous contours are irregular and have been described as fjordlike. Invaginations or inclusions of trophoblast are common—so-called trophoblast pseudoinclusions—that represent complex infoldings of chorionic villi sectioned at acute angles to their longitudinal axes. There may be a lacy appearance to the syncytiotrophoblast, and circumferential trophoblast hyperplasia may be focal.

Unlike CHM, the presence of intravillous nucleated blood cells is the norm. Triploidy can be confirmed by conventional cytogenetics, flow cytometry, or molecular testing.

SECOND TRIMESTER PREGNANCY LOSS

With completion of the embryonic period, organogenesis is complete. The forces that lead to loss of pregnancy during fetal life are somewhat different than during the embryonic period. While chromosome abnormality remains a significant factor, it is considerably less prevalent than in first trimester losses (approximately 5% to 10%), and the types of chromosome abnormalities more closely resemble those seen in third trimester losses and neonates, indicating that other processes, including nonchromosomal genetic disorders, are proportionally more responsible for second trimester intrauterine demise. Nonchromosomal factors such as twinning and uteroplacental pathology assume a larger role (74), and thus, the causes of second trimester loss are more heterogeneous, with a concomitant broader range of implications for counseling and management of future pregnancies. Examination of second trimester fetal loss is similar to the investigation of intrauterine death in later gestation, requiring complete postmortem examination, including placental evaluation, with the goals of 1) identifying the cause of intrauterine demise, 2) assessing recurrence risk in future pregnancies, and 3) determining management options.

The extent of fetal postmortem examination varies between institutions, with external examination of a fresh or formalin-fixed fetus sufficing in some laboratories, while others provide complete autopsy examination. The latter is the only way of adequately assessing such specimens, and examination other than complete autopsy with examination of the placenta should be considered incomplete. As many of the cases examined in the fetal pathology service come after diagnosis of intrauterine fetal death, maceration of tissues is a problem that must be addressed. The characteristic features of various disorders are present but may be altered or obscured by the effects of maceration. Maceration is not a diagnosis and should not be considered a limitation to the examination of affected fetuses. Second trimester specimens may also come from elective terminations due to fetal structural, chromosomal, or other genetic anomalies. In these cases, both the fetus and placenta are often markedly disrupted, which may limit the ability to confirm or expand on abnormalities seen in prenatal imaging. However, an attempt to identify all possible abnormalities should be made. Comparison of ultrasound and pathologic examination of second trimester fetuses has shown that perinatal examination can identify major and minor structural abnormalities, particularly involving the face and extremities, as well as congenital heart defects that may not have been fully characterized by antemortem ultrasound evaluation (35,75).

The autopsy of fetal specimens is conducted exactly as in all other perinatal cases: a complete external examination is performed, skeletal survey is done as indicated, and internal examination with dissection of all organ systems, including central nervous system (CNS) to the extent that the methodology of termination permits, is conducted. External examination includes an assessment of all growth parameters and comparison to established normative values for determination of DA. Particular attention should be given to the detection of intrauterine growth restriction (IUGR), with consideration given to the demise-to-delivery interval of spontaneous pregnancy losses that might alter estimation of GA at demise. Sections from all identifiable organ systems are submitted for histologic examination. Cytogenetic and/or other molecular studies should be initiated in cases whereby maternal and fetal circumstances warrant investigation. Unfixed and nonmacerated fetal and placental tissues can be frozen in the event that the tissue is required for CGH or other genetic studies. When indicated, tissues can be submitted for specific molecular genetic analysis, for disorders such as hemoglobinopathies and inborn errors of metabolism. Specific infectious disease cultures, including viral cultures, can be submitted as clinically appropriate. In cases of suspected skeletal dysplasia of unknown genetic origin, fibroblast cultures can be submitted and initiated; the resultant cell line can be frozen and retained for potential future genetic testing.

It is not possible to outline all of the disorders encountered in the pathology of second trimester losses. Suffice it to say that all of the pathology encountered in later gestation, intrauterine deaths, and pregnancy losses also occurs in the second trimester, as does a proportion of chromosomal anomalies responsible for first trimester SAbs (see Chapter 4).

In general, losses occurring in the second trimester can be either intrinsic to the conceptus or a consequence of abnormalities in the intrauterine environment. In the latter setting, the fetuses are normally developed, usually well preserved, and the findings raise concerns for uterine anomalies, cervical incompetence, and/or ascending infection (76).

Uterine anomalies are present in approximately 15% of women who have recurrent miscarriages (77). Pathologic examination of the aborted fetus and placenta cannot make this diagnosis, but the finding of a nonmacerated, anatomically, and chromosomally normal fetus with no evidence of ascending infection may lead to clinical consideration of anatomic or mechanical uterine abnormalities as etiologic factors in second trimester losses/deliveries.

Ascending infection is a common cause of second trimester previable or viable preterm deliveries (3,78). Particularly in a primigravida, there may be no antecedent history or known risk factors. Postmortem examination typically shows a well-preserved, anatomically normal fetus, aside from potential contractures or deformations secondary to oligohydramnios in the event of prolonged preterm membrane rupture. Histologic examination of fetal organs may demonstrate ingestion and inspiration of infected amniotic fluid, seen as neutrophils within the gastrointestinal tract and lungs, respectively. Gross examination of the placenta may show fetal membrane and chorionic plate opacity, the histologic correlate to neutrophils in the chorion or chorioamnion. Fetal response may be present in the form of neutrophils in the fetal chorionic surface vessels and/or in the vessels of the umbilical cord (chorionic and/or umbilical vasculitis, respectively). Ascending infection has been associated with intrauterine demise in midtrimester gestations and has been reported to be more likely when there is a fetal inflammatory response to intrauterine infection (63,79).

Although a broad range of organisms is responsible for chorioamnionitis, routine culturing of the products of SAb is not performed. When there is clinical concern for specific notable diseases, such as Listeriosis or syphilis, confirmatory cultures may be indicated. Listeriosis can occur as outbreaks, and thus, knowledge of its role in gestational infection is important from an epidemiologic perspective as well as from a clinical one. Listeriosis is caused by *Listeria monocytogenes*. Infection may be caused by exposure to foods such as unpasteurized or soft cheeses as well as incompletely processed meats; outbreaks have been related to contaminated production techniques. Listeriosis may be subclinical or may be associated with gastrointestinal diseases, such as vomiting and diarrhea, or generalized malaise that includes fever and myalgia. Infection in pregnant women is associated with an increased risk of intrauterine death and SAb, including both first and second trimester SAbs.

Pathologically, Listeriosis may be suspected when external examination of a fetus shows small white lesions on the skin, which are confirmed to be cutaneous microabscesses in which organisms abound. Similar abscesses may be identified in fetal organs. Gross examination of the placenta may be normal or show characteristic gross features of ascending infection. Histologic examination usually shows chorioamnionitis that may be severe. On cut surface of the placental disk, the characteristic lesion of Listeriosis is seen as small white lesions similar to those noted on fetal postmortem examination. Microscopically, these represent acute intervillous and villous microabscesses. Gram-positive bacilli are abundant on tissue Gram stain (Figures 2-16 [skin] and 2-17 [villus micro abscess]).

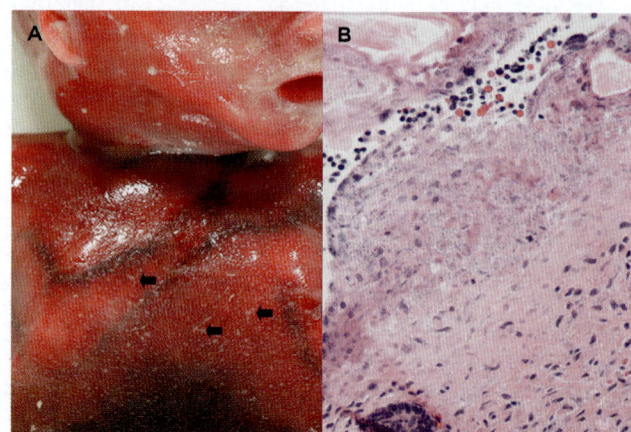

FIGURE 2-16 • Listeriosis. **A:** Gross examination shows small white nodules/plaques on the skin of second trimester fetus (*arrows*). **B:** Histologic examination shows necrosis with abundant bacteria, shown to be Gram-positive bacilli, culture positive for *Listeria monocytogenes*.

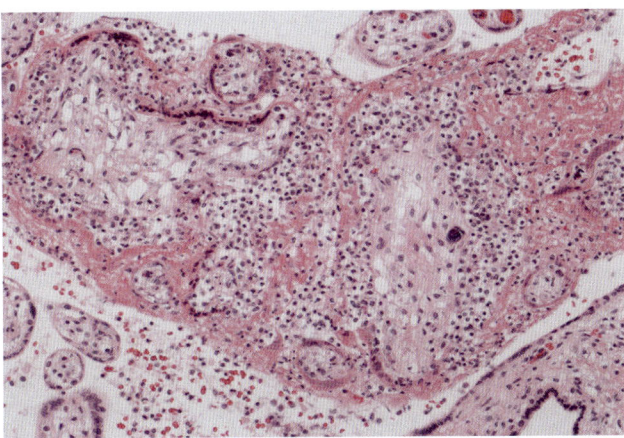

FIGURE 2-17 • Villus abscesses of Listeriosis associated with severe, acute chorioamnionitis.

Other infections, including viral infections, can account for intrauterine death in the second trimester, with CMV being the viral infection most commonly encountered in fetal death occurring in developed countries (80). Fetuses affected by CMV may appear grossly normal, aside from the effects of retention after fetal death, but may also show hepatic calcifications and CNS abnormalities. Histologic examination of fetal organs may show variably severe tissue-destructive mononuclear inflammation, and CMV inclusions may be identified by routine histology or aided by immunohistochemical staining or *in situ* hybridization. Classically, the placenta shows a "dirty" lymphoplasmacytic villitis, with villous vascular and stromal karyorrhexis and hemosiderosis. CMV inclusions are often readily identifiable on routine H&E stains (Figure 2-18), although immunohistochemistry or *in situ* hybridization can also be utilized for confirmation, as necessary. There may be a discrepancy between the severity of placental manifestations and those of the fetal organs; and in fact, it often appears that fetal organs are more likely to show inclusions and inflammation relative to the extent of placental inflammation.

Syphilis is encountered more commonly in the obstetric population of developing countries, including being responsible for fetal deaths. Spirochetes may be readily identified in fetal organs, and the placenta shows the features described elsewhere (see Chapter 9), including villitis, villus edema, and obliterative vascular changes.

Chromosomal abnormalities are encountered less often in second trimester losses than in those occurring in the first trimester, and the type of aneuploidy encountered is less varied, bearing a closer resemblance to the range observed nearer term (see Chapter 3). The trisomies encountered during life—trisomies 21, 13, and 18, as well as monosomy X and triploidy—are the most commonly identified abnormalities in the midgestational period. A minority of chromosomally abnormal fetuses survives to term; in fact, it is estimated that only 20% of trisomy 21 conceptions, 5% of trisomy 18 conceptions, and 1% of monosomy X conceptions survive to be liveborn. The mechanism allowing some of the chromosome abnormalities to survive into later gestation has been suggested as due to placental mosaicism for both an aneuploidy and normal cell line (81).

Trisomy 21

Trisomy 21 syndrome in the fetus shows the same range of developmental anomalies observed in liveborns (Chapter 3, Table 3-8), although the external facial and somatic phenotype may be less well developed. It is frequently associated with abnormalities of maternal serum markers (Chapter 3, Table 3-11). In addition, it is not unusual for midtrimester trisomy 21 to present as hydrops fetalis, with generalized subcutaneous edema and nuchal thickening that can be mistaken for a nuchal hygroma (Figure 2-19). The only

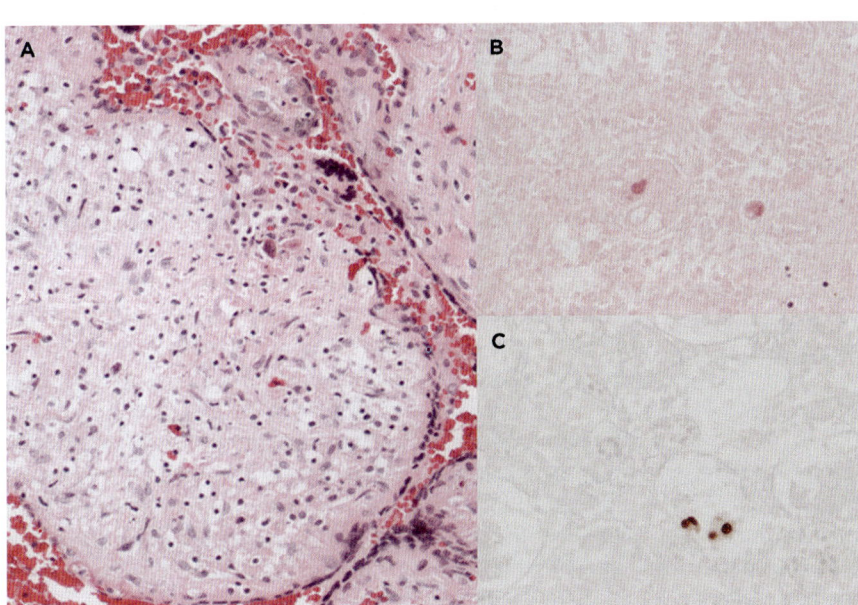

FIGURE 2-18 • CMV in macerated second trimester fetus. **A:** Villitis with viral inclusions. **B:** Viral inclusions in kidney. **C:** *In situ* hybridization for CMV highlights inclusions.

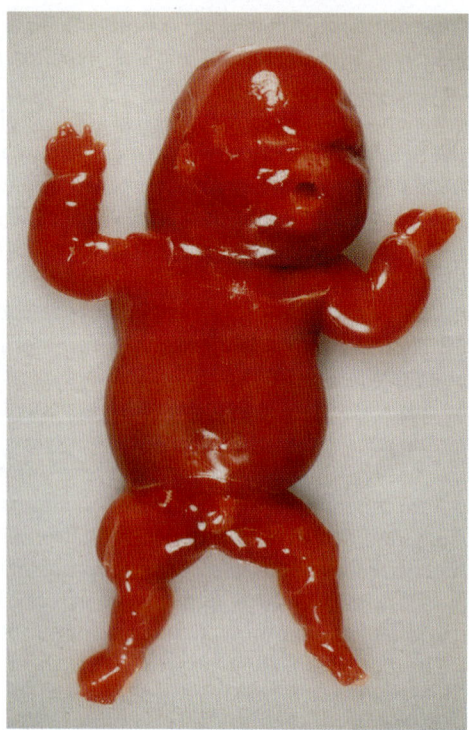

FIGURE 2-19 • Trisomy 21 syndrome. Hydropic fetus confirmed by cytogenetic analysis to have trisomy 21. No other internal anomalies.

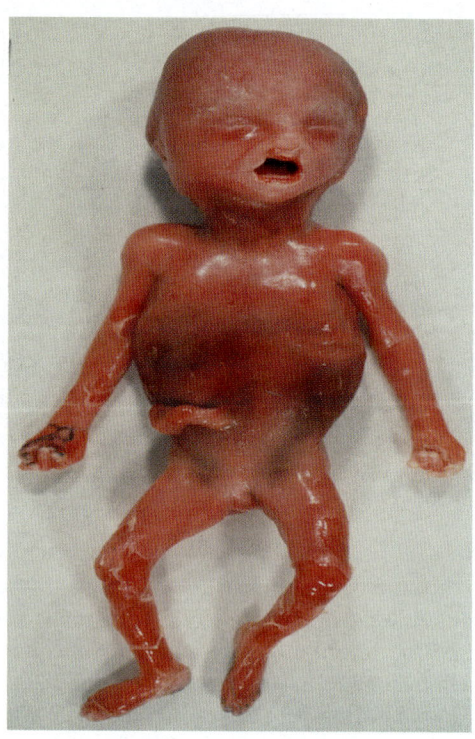

FIGURE 2-20 • Trisomy 18 syndrome. Fetus showing rounded head and rather small face with bilateral cleft lip and palate. Hands show characteristic clenched appearance. Internal examination showed horseshoe kidney, single umbilical artery, ventricular septal defect (VSD), and dysplasia of the cardiac valves.

feature observed more commonly in those trisomy 21 cases presenting as intrauterine demise as opposed to those terminated after prenatal cytogenetic diagnosis is hydrops fetalis; the other anomalies do not appear to be different between the two groups and thus do not provide an explanation to account for the survival of only some fetuses until later gestation. Although the presence of features such as atrioventricular canal-type cardiac defects, or transverse palmar creases, may suggest trisomy 21, cytogenetic analysis is required for confirmation. While cell sorting reveals an increased ratio of megakaryocytic and erythroid precursors relative to myeloid precursors in the fetal liver of second trimester trisomy 21 fetuses (82), rarely is transient myeloproliferative disorder, which predominates in the third trimester, diagnosed postnatally or postmortem (83). There is an empiric risk of recurrence of trisomy 21 on the order of 1% after an affected pregnancy (second trimester or later), whereas other chromosome abnormalities, such as monosomy X, are not associated with the increased risk of recurrence. If the trisomy 21 is the result of a Robertsonian translocation, carried in balanced form by one parent, the risk for recurrent trisomy 21 is substantially higher.

Trisomy 18

Fetuses with trisomy 18 may present as intrauterine demise without external anomalies and may be associated with abnormal maternal serum screening, including very low estriol levels. However, these fetuses typically demonstrate IUGR, which can be difficult in a case where there is maceration, as retention after fetal death may account for some of the discrepancy in fetal growth parameters. Of all the trisomic conceptuses, these fetuses display the widest range in external and internal phenotype. Having stated as much, trisomy 18 fetuses universally exhibit short sternums, with the xiphoid process present midway between the internipplary line and the umbilicus. In addition, they often exhibit a somewhat rounded appearance to the head with a small face (Figure 2-20). The hands show flexion of the fingers, with the second and fifth fingers characteristically clasped over the third and fourth, respectively. Feet may show prominent heels and may be rounded, so-called rocker bottom feet, though these features are subjective and can be overinterpreted. Internal examination may be normal or may show the internal abnormalities described in liveborns, with renal anomalies such as horseshoe kidney being one of the most commonly observed (see Chapter 3, Tables 3-9). Dysplasia of cardiac valves is encountered in most cases and has been referred to as "diaphanous dysplasia." Any number of additional anomalies may be present, including CNS defects (e.g., meningomyelocele, hydrocephalus) as well as other aberrations in phenotype (e.g., gastroschisis). Although more female than male infants are liveborn with trisomy 18, among elective terminations, the sex ratio is equal, and it has been suggested that male infants are more likely to die in utero (84–86).

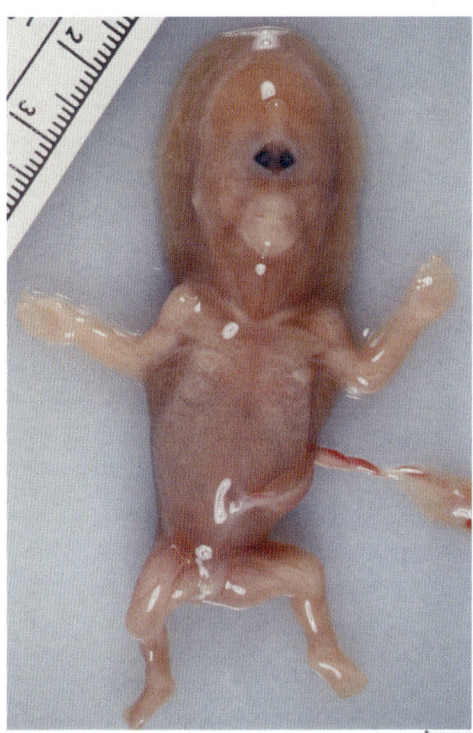

FIGURE 2-21 • Trisomy 13 syndrome. Macerated fetus showing synophthalmia with proboscis. Bilateral postaxial polydactyly of feet. Internal examination showed VSD.

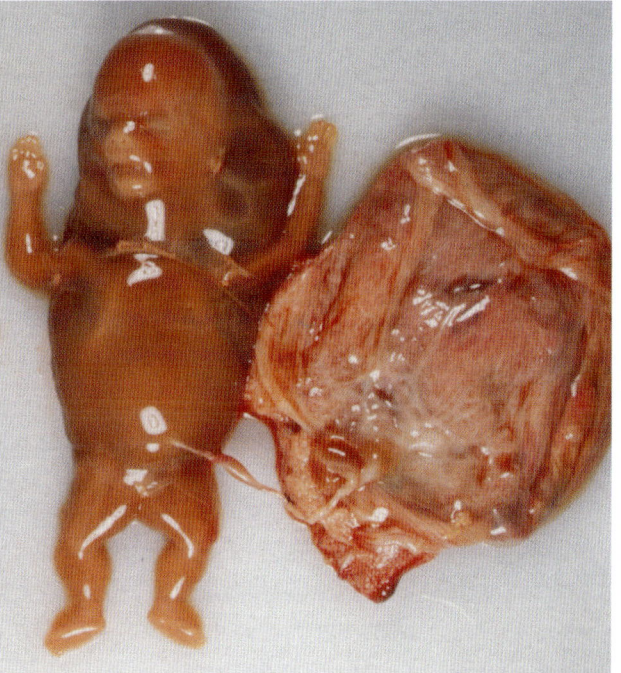

FIGURE 2-22 • Monosomy X syndrome. Macerated female fetus showing hydrops fetalis with large cystic nuchal hygroma. Internal examination showed hypoplasia of the aorta.

Trisomy 13

Trisomy 13 may also present as unanticipated fetal death, with only 5% of all trisomy 13 conceptions surviving to be liveborn. The facial anomalies are explainable by paucity of midfacial tissue, which are also reflective of brain anomalies, the most dramatic of which is holoprosencephaly. Facial anomalies include cleft lip and palate, proboscis, hypotelorism, and synophthalmia (Figure 2-21). Postaxial polydactyly of the hands and/or feet is common. There may be an omphalocele as well as internal anomalies affecting a variety of systems including the kidneys, which may be enlarged and show cystic change, and the heart, which characteristically shows tetralogy of Fallot or truncus arteriosus (see Chapter 3, Table 3–10). At gross examination, the differential diagnosis includes Meckel–Gruber and pseudotrisomy 13 syndromes.

Monosomy X

Monosomy X is also known as Turner syndrome. In the fetal period, this most commonly presents as hydrops fetalis, often with a very large cystic hygroma. Accentuation of the subcutaneous edema on the dorsal aspects of the hands and feet is characteristic but nonspecific. These fetuses are female and show normal female genitalia, internally and externally. Characteristic anomalies include left-sided cardiac anomalies such as hypoplasia of the aortic arch and/or left ventricular hypoplasia. Renal anomalies include horseshoe kidney (Figure 2-22).

Triploidy

Triploidy is the presence of an entire extra haploid set of chromosomes, which may be of maternal (digynic) or paternal (diandric) origin. Diandric triploidy has been reported in anywhere from 20% to 85% of triploid pregnancies, likely depending on the developmental stage of the pregnancy at the time of ascertainment, with diandric triploidy cases predominating in earlier abortions (50,72,87). Most but not all cases of diandric triploidy are associated with PHM (46). In the fetal period, digynic triploidy predominates (72). In general, triploidy is characterized by anomalies that affect almost every organ system and can be present in both digynic and diandric triploidies. Syndactyly of the third and fourth fingers and second and third toes is a characteristic feature of triploidy, independent of parental origin. Despite the fact that the chromosome abnormality is numerically the same, it has been proposed that imprinting leads to a fetal/placental phenotype that correlates with the parental origin of triploidy (88), although not all series have found differences based on parental origin (50). Digynic triploidy gives rise to marked asymmetric IUGR, with the head size being relatively well preserved compared to the trunk and extremities, which are markedly growth restricted (Figure 2-23). There is adrenal hypoplasia, as has been observed in other cases of severe IUGR, consistent with the concept that placental function can be operative in intrauterine adrenal growth and development. Other anomalies are varied and affect all organ systems. The placenta is abnormally small and shows no villus edema or trophoblastic hyperplasia. In diandric triploidy, growth is better preserved,

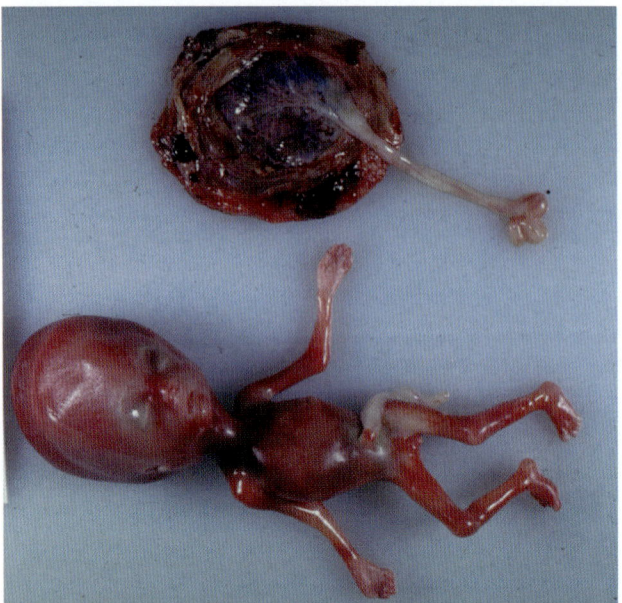

FIGURE 2-23 • Digynic triploid phenotype—the phenotype most often encountered in triploid fetuses. Asymmetric IUGR, with relative sparing of the head and thin extremities. No molar change is seen in the placenta.

but there may be symmetric IUGR (Figure 2-24). The placenta shows changes of PHM with villus edema and cistern formation; focal circumferential syncytiotrophoblast hyperplasia, which can have a lacey appearance; and trophoblast invaginations into the villus stromal core (so-called trophoblast pseudoinclusions). Fetal growth and placental differences are reflected in abnormalities observed in maternal serum screening, with digynic triploids showing markedly decreased estriol and human chorionic gonadotropin (hCG), while the diandric triploids have markedly increased levels of alpha-fetoprotein (AFP) and hCG.

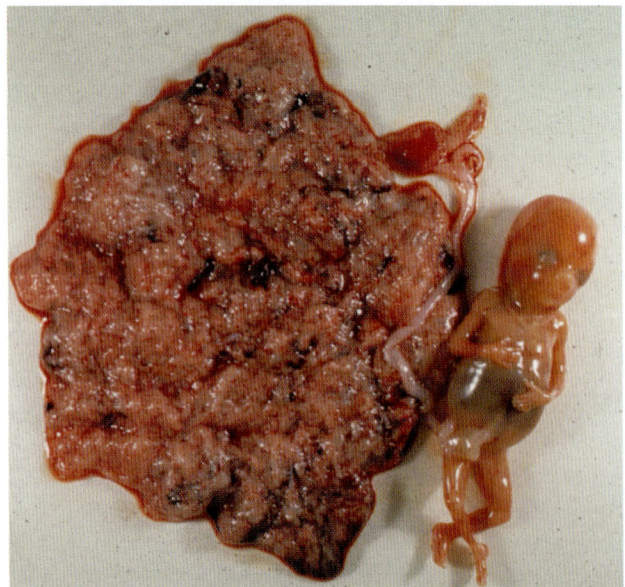

FIGURE 2-24 • Diandric triploid phenotype—the phenotype seen only rarely in triploid fetuses. Growth parameters better preserved. Large placenta shows changes of PHM.

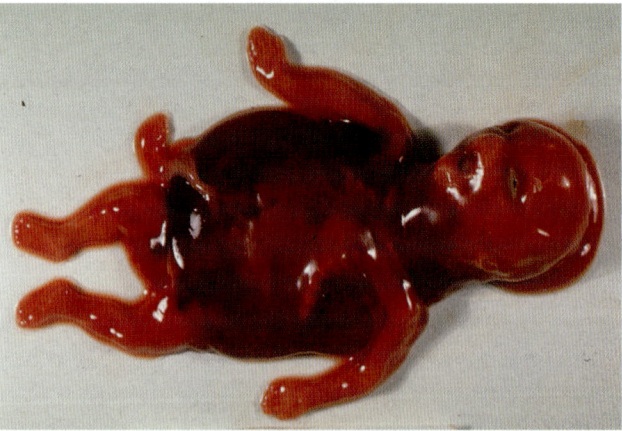

FIGURE 2-25 • Hydrops fetalis, cause not determined, after extensive investigation. Genetic counseling should include possibility of undiagnosed genetic conditions, with recurrence risks as high as 25%.

Hydrops Fetalis

Hydrops fetalis can present with second trimester fetal demise and warrants complete evaluation for diagnosis, as in those cases diagnosed as later gestational stillbirths (Figure 2-25). Although historically hydrops fetalis was often associated with Rhesus isoimmunization, with prophylactic anti-D treatment, isoimmune hydrops fetalis now accounts for less than 10% of cases. Nonimmune hydrops fetalis is much more common. The increase in extravascular fluid in these cases may be due to abnormal pathophysiology involving the heart, kidney, liver, or vessels leading to obstructed lymphatic flow, congestive heart failure with increased central venous pressure, or low plasma oncotic pressure. The differential diagnosis is extensive and includes chromosome abnormalities, infection such as CMV and parvovirus B19, hemoglobinopathies such as thalassemia, fetal arrhythmias, congenital pulmonary airway malformations, tumors (e.g., sacrococcygeal teratoma, placental chorangioma(tosis), obstructive cardiac masses), and metabolic disorders (see Chapter 4) (89,90). Accordingly, the approach to hydrops fetalis includes complete autopsy examination (91) with material reserved for cytogenetic analysis, viral cultures, PCR for parvovirus, initiation of fibroblast cultures, and retention of a variety of tissues for freezing at −70 °C in the event that additional studies such as alpha-thalassemia gene studies are required. With the exclusion of these entities, one is left with a diagnosis of hydrops fetalis of undetermined etiology. Because of the possibility of an undetected metabolic condition leading to hydrops, genetic counseling considers the risk of autosomal recessive conditions; thus, the risk of recurrence may be as high as 25% for each subsequent pregnancy.

Twinning

Monozygous twinning is associated with an increased risk of intrauterine fetal demise and may occur on the basis of placental vascular anastomoses, leading to twin–twin

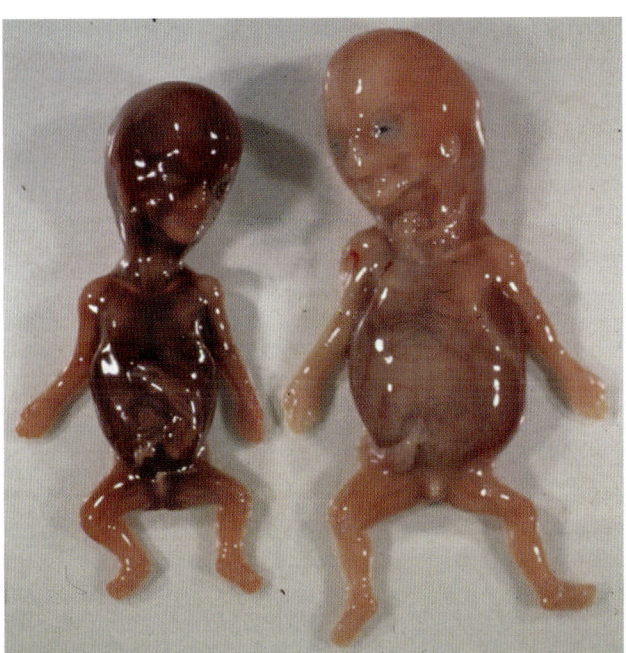

FIGURE 2-26 • Twin–twin transfusion syndrome in intrauterine death. Monochorionic twin fetuses show size difference as well as differences in the degree of congestion, consistent with circulatory imbalance.

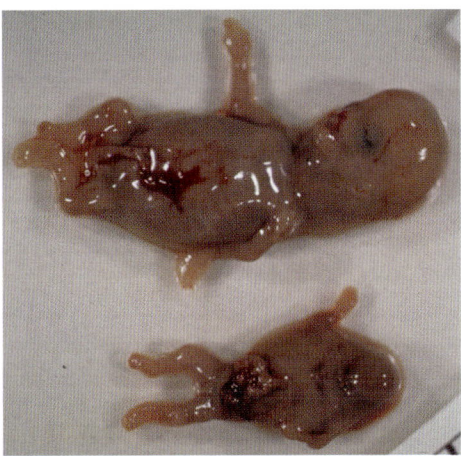

FIGURE 2-27 • TRAP sequence, with normal pump twin and acardiac recipient twin.

transfusion syndrome (Figure 2-26) or twin-reversed arterial perfusion (TRAP) sequence (92,93) in monochorionic twins. Monochorionic monoamniotic twins (MCMA) are also at risk for cord entanglement, which may lead to compromise of umbilical cord blood flow and fetal death; however, cord entanglement in this setting surprisingly does not usually affect fetal survival (94,95). Instead, MCMA twins have a higher rate of mortality than monochorionic diamniotic (MCDA) twins, primarily due to chromosomal or congenital anomalies or TRAP sequence (96). Twin–twin transfusion syndrome can be suggested in monochorionic twins if there are growth and/or perfusion discrepancies between the two fetuses (92). TRAP is a condition in which the umbilical cords of MCMA twins are implanted very close to one another, establishing large bore vascular anastomoses involving chorionic vessels. It is hypothesized that some event leads to an imbalance in the shunting of blood, resulting in reversed perfusion such that one twin receives deoxygenated blood from the other via retrograde flow through its umbilical artery. This results in hypoxia in the recipient twin with resultant aborted somatic development and organogenesis that is most severe cranially. Thus, the characteristic phenotype is an acardiac, acephalic twin (Figure 2-27). This perfusion abnormality may result in the intrauterine death of both twins, or the still-perfused acardiac twin may be delivered at term with the coexisting twin.

Umbilical Cord Compromise

Umbilical cord compromise can occur in a variety of settings and can result in fetal death (97–100). In some cases, there may be no gross fetal features to suggest the cause of death, whereas other cases show findings such as cord entanglement that could not have occurred postmortem and that thus suggest the diagnosis (Figure 2-28). Of note, there has been considerable controversy as to whether the twist at the junction of the umbilical cord with the abdominal wall, often observed in macerated fetuses, is a cause of cord blood flow compromise or a postmortem artifact. Some authors have identified placental histologic features that indicate or at least support a diagnosis of fatal umbilical cord blood flow restriction (see Chapter 9) (101,102). This underscores the importance of placental evaluation as a critical component in investigating the cause of midtrimester intrauterine demise.

Limb–Body Wall Complex

Limb–body wall complex (LBWC), a disorder within the spectrum of short cord or placental adhesion sequence, is characterized by limb anomalies, including limb aplasia or hypoplasia, associated with a large anterior body wall defect and an abnormally short umbilical cord, usually in chromosomally normal fetuses (Figure 2-29) (103,104). With routine use of detailed antenatal ultrasound examination, these

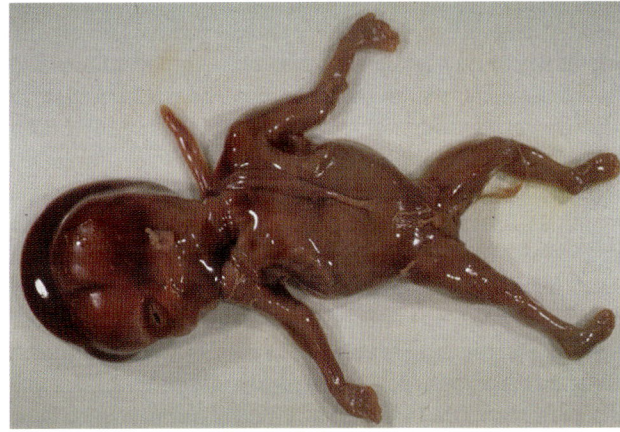

FIGURE 2-28 • Probable cord entanglement in intrauterine fetal death.

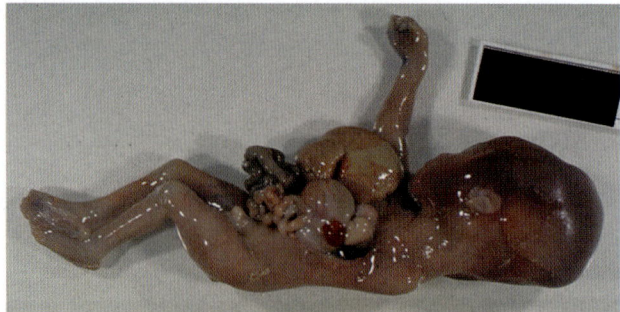

FIGURE 2-29 • BWC in intrauterine death. Large body wall defect, absence of limb, and abnormally short umbilical cord.

cases now result most commonly in pregnancy termination but may also present as early intrauterine demise, presumably due to fatally compromised umbilical cord blood flow.

Postprocedure Pregnancy Loss

Loss of pregnancy can occur after invasive prenatal procedures such as chorionic villus sampling and amniocentesis. The rate varies with institution, usually being on the order of 0.5%, although some studies show no significant increase in fetal loss in those who had amniocentesis than in those who did not (17,52). The loss can take the form of SAb or fetal death. Ascending infection and placental circulatory abnormalities are general categories that can result in postprocedural demise. For quality assurance purposes, losses occurring within a month of an invasive procedure are considered postprocedure losses. Postmortem examination should be undertaken as with any other pregnancy loss, as appropriate for the GA but to include both embryofetal and placental evaluation.

References

1. Jindal P, Regan L, Fourkala EO, et al. Placental pathology of recurrent spontaneous abortion: the role of histopathological examination of products of conception in routine clinical practice: a mini review. *Hum Reprod* 2007;22(2): 313–316.
2. Poland BJ, Lowry RB. The use of spontaneous abortuses and stillbirths in genetic counseling. *Am J Obstet Gynecol* 1974;118(3):322–326.
3. Srinivas SK, Ma Y, Sammel MD, et al. Placental inflammation and viral infection are implicated in second trimester pregnancy loss. *Am J Obstet Gynecol* 2006;195(3):797–802.
4. Szulman AE. Examination of the early conceptus. *Arch Pathol Lab Med* 1991;115(7):696–700.
5. Tasci Y, Dilbaz S, Secilmis O, et al. Routine histopathologic analysis of product of conception following first-trimester spontaneous miscarriages. *J Obstet Gynaecol Res* 2005;31(6):579–582.
6. Makrydimas G, Sebire NJ, Lolis D, et al. Fetal loss following ultrasound diagnosis of a live fetus at 6–10 weeks of gestation. *Ultrasound Obstet Gynecol* 2003;22(4):368–372.
7. Tong S, Kaur A, Walker SP, et al. Miscarriage risk for asymptomatic women after a normal first-trimester prenatal visit. *Obstet Gynecol* 2008;111(3):710–714.
8. Akolekar R, Bower S, Flack N, et al. Prediction of miscarriage and stillbirth at 11–13 weeks and the contribution of chorionic villus sampling. *Prenat Diagn* 2011;31(1):38–45.
9. Warren JE, Silver RM. Genetics of pregnancy loss. *Clin Obstet Gynecol* 2008;51(1):84–95.
10. Fritz B, Hallermann C, Olert J, et al. Cytogenetic analyses of culture failures by comparative genomic hybridisation (CGH)—re-evaluation of chromosome aberration rates in early spontaneous abortions. *Eur J Hum Genet* 2001;9(7):539–547.
11. Gao J, Liu C, Yao F, et al. Array-based comparative genomic hybridization is more informative than conventional karyotyping and fluorescence in situ hybridization in the analysis of first-trimester spontaneous abortion. *Mol Cytogenet* 2012;5(1):33.
12. Lomax B, Tang S, Separovic E, et al. Comparative genomic hybridization in combination with flow cytometry improves results of cytogenetic analysis of spontaneous abortions. *Am J Hum Genet* 2000;66(5):1516–1521.
13. Larsen EC, Christiansen OB, Kolte AM, et al. New insights into mechanisms behind miscarriage. *BMC Med* 2013;11:154.
14. Petracchi F, Colaci DS, Igarzabal L, et al. Cytogenetic analysis of first trimester pregnancy loss. *Int J Gynaecol Obstet* 2009;104(3):243–244.
15. Eiben B, Bartels I, Bahr-Porsch S, et al. Cytogenetic analysis of 750 spontaneous abortions with the direct-preparation method of chorionic villi and its implications for studying genetic causes of pregnancy wastage. *Am J Hum Genet* 1990;47(4):656–663.
16. Sugiura-Ogasawara M, Aoki K, Fujii T, et al. Subsequent pregnancy outcomes in recurrent miscarriage patients with a paternal or maternal carrier of a structural chromosome rearrangement. *J Hum Genet* 2008;53(7):622–628.
17. Ozawa N, Maruyama T, Nagashima T, et al. Pregnancy outcomes of reciprocal translocation carriers who have a history of repeated pregnancy loss. *Fertil Steril* 2008;90(4):1301–1304.
18. Stephenson MD, Sierra S. Reproductive outcomes in recurrent pregnancy loss associated with a parental carrier of a structural chromosome rearrangement. *Hum Reprod* 2006;21(4):1076–1082.
19. Keymolen K, Staessen C, Verpoest W, et al. A proposal for reproductive counselling in carriers of Robertsonian translocations: 10 years of experience with preimplantation genetic diagnosis. *Hum Reprod* 2009;24(9):2365–2371.
20. Nagaoka SI, Hassold TJ, Hunt PA. Human aneuploidy: mechanisms and new insights into an age-old problem. *Nat Rev Genet* 2012;13(7):493–504.
21. Robinson WP. *Chromosomal Genetic Disease: Numerical Aberrations. Encyclopedia of Life Sciences*. United Kingdom: Macmillan Reference Ltd; 2000.
22. Chiang T, Schultz RM, Lampson MA. Meiotic origins of maternal age-related aneuploidy. *Biol Reprod* 2012;86(1):1–7.
23. The Practice Committee of the American Society for Reproductive Medicine. Evaluation and treatment of recurrent pregnancy loss: a committee opinion. *Fertil Steril* 2012;98(5):1103–1111.
24. Salim R, Regan L, Woelfer B, et al. A comparative study of the morphology of congenital uterine anomalies in women with and without a history of recurrent first trimester miscarriage. *Hum Reprod* 2003;18(1):162–166.
25. Hogge WA, Prosen TL, Lanasa MC, et al. Recurrent spontaneous abortion and skewed X-inactivation: is there an association? *Am J Obstet Gynecol* 2007;196(4):384e1–384e6; discussion e6–e8.
26. Beever CL, Stephenson MD, Penaherrera MS, et al. Skewed X-chromosome inactivation is associated with trisomy in women ascertained on the basis of recurrent spontaneous abortion or chromosomally abnormal pregnancies. *Am J Hum Genet* 2003;72(2):399–407.
27. Said JM, Higgins JR, Moses EK, et al. Inherited thrombophilia polymorphisms and pregnancy outcomes in nulliparous women. *Obstet Gynecol* 2010;115(1):5–13.
28. Silver RM, Zhao Y, Spong CY, et al. Prothrombin gene G20210A mutation and obstetric complications. *Obstet Gynecol* 2010;115(1):14–20.
29. Dizon-Townson D, Miller C, Sibai B, et al. The relationship of the factor V Leiden mutation and pregnancy outcomes for mother and fetus. *Obstet Gynecol* 2005;106(3):517–524.
30. Davenport WB, Kutteh WH. Inherited thrombophilias and adverse pregnancy outcomes: a review of screening patterns and recommendations. *Obstet Gynecol Clin North Am* 2014;41(1):133–144.

31. ACOG Practice Bulletin No. 138: Inherited thrombophilias in pregnancy. *Obstet Gynecol* 2013;122(3):706–717.
32. Abrahams VM. Mechanisms of antiphospholipid antibody-associated pregnancy complications. *Thromb Res* 2009;124(5):521–525.
33. Medeiros F, Callahan MJ, Elvin JA, et al. Intraplacental choriocarcinoma arising in a second trimester placenta with partial hydatidiform mole. *Int J Gynecol Pathol* 2008;27(2):247–251.
34. Wells M. The pathology of gestational trophoblastic disease: recent advances. *Pathology* 2007;39(1):88–96.
35. Papp C, Szigeti Z, Joo JG, et al. The role of perinatal autopsy in the management of pregnancies with major fetal trisomies. *Pathol Res Pract* 2007;203(7):525–531.
36. Practice Bulletin No. 132: Antiphospholipid syndrome. *Obstet Gynecol* 2012;120(6):1514–1521.
37. Lathi RB, Mark SD, Westphal LM, et al. Cytogenetic testing of anembryonic pregnancies compared to embryonic missed abortions. *J Assist Reprod Genet* 2007;24(11):521–524.
38. Allen VM, Wilson RD, Cheung A. Pregnancy outcomes after assisted reproductive technology. *J Obstet Gynaecol Can* 2006;28(3):220–250.
39. Gjerris AC, Loft A, Pinborg A, et al. Prenatal testing among women pregnant after assisted reproductive techniques in Denmark 1995–2000: a national cohort study. *Hum Reprod* 2008;23(7):1545–1552.
40. Qin JZ, Pang LH, Li MQ, et al. Risk of chromosomal abnormalities in early spontaneous abortion after assisted reproductive technology: a meta-analysis. *PLoS One* 2013;8(10):e75953.
41. Kudesia R, Li M, Smith J, et al. Rescue karyotyping: a case series of array-based comparative genomic hybridization evaluation of archival conceptual tissue. *Reprod Biol Endocrinol* 2014;12:19.
42. Dhillon RK, Hillman SC, Morris RK, et al. Additional information from chromosomal microarray analysis (CMA) over conventional karyotyping when diagnosing chromosomal abnormalities in miscarriage: a systematic review and meta-analysis. *BJOG* 2014;121(1):11–21.
43. Benkhalifa M, Kasakyan S, Clement P, et al. Array comparative genomic hybridization profiling of first-trimester spontaneous abortions that fail to grow in vitro. *Prenat Diagn* 2005;25(10):894–900.
44. Schaeffer AJ, Chung J, Heretis K, et al. Comparative genomic hybridization-array analysis enhances the detection of aneuploidies and submicroscopic imbalances in spontaneous miscarriages. *Am J Hum Genet* 2004;74(6):1168–1174.
45. Harkness LM, Baird DT. Morphological and molecular characteristics of living human fetuses between Carnegie stages 7 and 23: localization of inhibin mRNA alpha and beta a subunits by in-situ hybridization. *Hum Reprod Update* 1997;3(1):59–92.
46. O'Rahilly R, Muller F. Developmental stages in human embryos: revised and new measurements. *Cells Tissues Organs* 2010;192(2):73–84.
47. Munoz M, Arigita M, Bennasar M, et al. Chromosomal anomaly spectrum in early pregnancy loss in relation to presence or absence of an embryonic pole. *Fertil Steril* 2010;94(7):2564–2568.
48. McFadden DE, Kalousek DK. Survey of neural tube defects in spontaneously aborted embryos. *Am J Med Genet* 1989;32(3):356–358.
49. Harris MJ, Poland BJ, Dill FJ. Triploidy in 40 human spontaneous abortuses: assessment of phenotype in embryos. *Obstet Gynecol* 1981;57(5):600–606.
50. Joergensen MW, Niemann I, Rasmussen AA, et al. Triploid pregnancies: genetic and clinical features of 158 cases. *Am J Obstet Gynecol* 2014;211(4):370.e1–370.e19.
51. Redline RW, Zaragoza M, Hassold T. Prevalence of developmental and inflammatory lesions in nonmolar first-trimester spontaneous abortions. *Hum Pathol* 1999;30(1):93–100.
52. Boyd TK, Redline RW. Chronic histiocytic intervillositis: a placental lesion associated with recurrent reproductive loss. *Hum Pathol* 2000;31(11):1389–1396.
53. Doss BJ, Greene MF, Hill J, et al. Massive chronic intervillositis associated with recurrent abortions. *Hum Pathol* 1995;26(11):1245–1251.
54. Marchaudon V, Devisme L, Petit S, et al. Chronic histiocytic intervillositis of unknown etiology: clinical features in a consecutive series of 69 cases. *Placenta* 2011;32(2):140–145.
55. Waters BL, Ashikaga T. Significance of perivillous fibrin/oid deposition in uterine evacuation specimens. *Am J Surg Pathol* 2006;30(6):760–765.
56. Baud D, Greub G. Intracellular bacteria and adverse pregnancy outcomes. *Clin Microbiol Infect* 2011;17(9):1312–1322.
57. van Lijnschoten G, Arends JW, De La Fuente AA, et al. Intra- and interobserver variation in the interpretation of histological features suggesting chromosomal abnormality in early abortion specimens. *Histopathology* 1993;22(1):25–29.
58. Novak R, Agamanolis D, Dasu S, et al. Histologic analysis of placental tissue in first trimester abortions. *Pediatr Pathol* 1988;8(5):477–482.
59. Minguillon C, Eiben B, Bahr-Porsch S, et al. The predictive value of chorionic villus histology for identifying chromosomally normal and abnormal spontaneous abortions. *Hum Genet* 1989;82(4):373–376.
60. Rehder H, Coerdt W, Eggers R, et al. Is there a correlation between morphological and cytogenetic findings in placental tissue from early missed abortions? *Hum Genet* 1989;82(4):377–385.
61. Cheung AN, Khoo US, Lai CY, et al. Metastatic trophoblastic disease after an initial diagnosis of partial hydatidiform mole: genotyping and chromosome in situ hybridization analysis. *Cancer* 2004;100(7):1411–1417.
62. Fowler DJ, Lindsay I, Seckl MJ, et al. Routine pre-evacuation ultrasound diagnosis of hydatidiform mole: experience of more than 1000 cases from a regional referral center. *Ultrasound Obstet Gynecol* 2006;27(1):56–60.
63. Romero R, Espinoza J, Goncalves LF, et al. The role of inflammation and infection in preterm birth. *Semin Reprod Med* 2007;25(1):21–39.
64. Matsui H, Iizuka Y, Sekiya S. Incidence of invasive mole and choriocarcinoma following partial hydatidiform mole. *Int J Gynaecol Obstet* 1996;53(1):63–64.
65. Seckl MJ, Fisher RA, Salerno G, et al. Choriocarcinoma and partial hydatidiform moles. *Lancet* 2000;356(9223):36–39.
66. Buza N, Hui P. Partial hydatidiform mole: histologic parameters in correlation with DNA genotyping. *Int J Gynecol Pathol* 2013;32(3):307–315.
67. Fukunaga M, Katabuchi H, Nagasaka T, et al. Interobserver and intraobserver variability in the diagnosis of hydatidiform mole. *Am J Surg Pathol* 2005;29(7):942–947.
68. Gupta M, Vang R, Yemelyanova AV, et al. Diagnostic reproducibility of hydatidiform moles: ancillary techniques (p57 immunohistochemistry and molecular genotyping) improve morphologic diagnosis for both recently trained and experienced gynecologic pathologists. *Am J Surg Pathol* 2012;36(12):1747–1760.
69. McConnell TG, Murphy KM, Hafez M, et al. Diagnosis and subclassification of hydatidiform moles using p57 immunohistochemistry and molecular genotyping: validation and prospective analysis in routine and consultation practice settings with development of an algorithmic approach. *Am J Surg Pathol* 2009;33(6):805–817.
70. Merchant SH, Amin MB, Viswanatha DS, et al. p57KIP2 immunohistochemistry in early molar pregnancies: emphasis on its complementary role in the differential diagnosis of hydropic abortuses. *Hum Pathol* 2005;36(2):180–186.
71. McFadden DE, Jiang R, Langlois S, et al. Dispermy—origin of diandric triploidy: brief communication. *Hum Reprod* 2002;17(12):3037–3038.
72. McFadden DE, Langlois S. Parental and meiotic origin of triploidy in the embryonic and fetal periods. *Clin Genet* 2000;58(3):192–200.
73. Zaragoza MV, Surti U, Redline RW, et al. Parental origin and phenotype of triploidy in spontaneous abortions: predominance of diandry and association with the partial hydatidiform mole. *Am J Hum Genet* 2000;66(6):1807–1820.
74. Stillbirth Collaborative Research Network Writing Group. Causes of death among stillbirths. *JAMA* 2011;306(22):2459–2468.
75. Sun CC, Grumbach K, DeCosta DT, et al. Correlation of prenatal ultrasound diagnosis and pathologic findings in fetal anomalies. *Pediatr Dev Pathol* 1999;2(2):131–142.
76. Stanek J, Biesiada J. Relation of placental diagnosis in stillbirth to fetal maceration and gestational age at delivery. *J Perinat Med* 2013;42(4):1–15.
77. Devi Wold AS, Pham N, Arici A. Anatomic factors in recurrent pregnancy loss. *Semin Reprod Med* 2006;24(1):25–32.
78. Heller DS, Moorehouse-Moore C, Skurnick J, et al. Second-trimester pregnancy loss at an urban hospital. *Infect Dis Obstet Gynecol* 2003;11(2):117–122.
79. Lahra MM, Gordon A, Jeffery HE. Chorioamnionitis and fetal response in stillbirth. *Am J Obstet Gynecol* 2007;196(3):229 e1–229 e4.

80. Al-Adnani M, Sebire NJ. The role of perinatal pathological examination in subclinical infection in obstetrics. *Best Pract Res Clin Obstet Gynaecol* 2007;21(3):505–521.
81. Kalousek DK, Barrett IJ, McGillivray BC. Placental mosaicism and intrauterine survival of trisomies 13 and 18. *Am J Hum Genet* 1989;44(3):338–343.
82. Tunstall-Pedoe O, Roy A, Karadimitris A, et al. Abnormalities in the myeloid progenitor compartment in Down syndrome fetal liver precede acquisition of GATA1 mutations. *Blood* 2008;112(12):4507–4511.
83. Heald B, Hilden JM, Zbuk K, et al. Severe TMD/AMKL with GATA1 mutation in a stillborn fetus with Down syndrome. *Nat Clin Pract Oncol* 2007;4(7):433–438.
84. Crider KS, Olney RS, Cragan JD. Trisomies 13 and 18: population prevalences, characteristics, and prenatal diagnosis, metropolitan Atlanta, 1994–2003. *Am J Med Genet A* 2008;146(7):820–826.
85. Morris JK, Savva GM. The risk of fetal loss following a prenatal diagnosis of trisomy 13 or trisomy 18. *Am J Med Genet A* 2008;146(7):827–832.
86. Cereda A, Carey JC. The trisomy 18 syndrome. *Orphanet J Rare Dis* 2012;7:81.
87. McFadden DE, Robinson WP. Phenotype of triploid embryos. *J Med Genet* 2006;43(7):609–612.
88. McFadden DE, Kalousek DK. Two different phenotypes of fetuses with chromosomal triploidy: correlation with parental origin of the extra haploid set. *Am J Med Genet* 1991;38(4):535–538.
89. Bellini C, Hennekam RC. Non-immune hydrops fetalis: a short review of etiology and pathophysiology. *Am J Med Genet A* 2012;158A(3):597–605.
90. Randenberg AL. Nonimmune hydrops fetalis part I: etiology and pathophysiology. *Neonatal Netw* 2010;29(5):281–295.
91. Rodriguez MM, Chaves F, Romaguera RL, et al. Value of autopsy in nonimmune hydrops fetalis: series of 51 stillborn fetuses. *Pediatr Dev Pathol* 2002;5(4):365–374.
92. De Paepe ME, Luks FI. What-and why-the pathologist should know about twin-to-twin transfusion syndrome. *Pediatr Dev Pathol* 2013;16(4):237–251.
93. Weber MA, Sebire NJ. Genetics and developmental pathology of twinning. *Semin Fetal Neonatal Med* 2010;15(6):313–318.
94. Rossi AC, Prefumo F. Impact of cord entanglement on perinatal outcome of monoamniotic twins: a systematic review of the literature. *Ultrasound Obstet Gynecol* 2013;41(2):131–135.
95. Dias T, Mahsud-Dornan S, Bhide A, et al. Cord entanglement and perinatal outcome in monoamniotic twin pregnancies. *Ultrasound Obstet Gynecol* 2010;35(2):201–204.
96. Dias T, Contro E, Thilaganathan B, et al. Pregnancy outcome of monochorionic twins: does amnionicity matter? *Twin Res Hum Genet* 2011;14(6):586–592.
97. Baergen RN. Cord abnormalities, structural lesions, and cord "accidents." *Semin Diagn Pathol* 2007;24(1):23–32.
98. Peng HQ, Levitin-Smith M, Rochelson B, et al. Umbilical cord stricture and overcoiling are common causes of fetal demise. *Pediatr Dev Pathol* 2006;9(1):14–19.
99. Ernst LM, Minturn L, Huang MH, et al. Gross patterns of umbilical cord coiling: correlations with placental histology and stillbirth. *Placenta* 2013;34(7):583–588.
100. Tantbirojn P, Saleemuddin A, Sirois K, et al. Gross abnormalities of the umbilical cord: related placental histology and clinical significance. *Placenta* 2009;30(12):1083–1088.
101. Ryan WD, Trivedi N, Benirschke K, et al. Placental histologic criteria for diagnosis of cord accident: sensitivity and specificity. *Pediatr Dev Pathol* 2012;15(4):275–280.
102. Parast MM, Crum CP, Boyd TK. Placental histologic criteria for umbilical blood flow restriction in unexplained stillbirth. *Hum Pathol* 2008;39(6):948–953.
103. Hunter AG, Seaver LH, Stevenson RE. Limb–body wall defect. Is there a defensible hypothesis and can it explain all the associated anomalies? *Am J Med Genet A* 2011;155A(9):2045–2059.
104. Gimenez-Scherer JA, Davies BR, Resendiz-Moran MA, et al. Abdominal wall defects: autopsy findings of distinct groups suggest different pathogenetic mechanisms. *Pediatr Dev Pathol* 2009;12(1):22–27.

CHAPTER 3

Chromosomal Abnormalities

Robyn C. Reed, M.D., Ph.D., Michelle M. Dolan, M.D., Raj P. Kapur, M.D., Ph.D., and Joseph R. Siebert, Ph.D.

Advances in genetic testing have blurred the distinction between the cytogenetic and molecular classifications of disease, and with continuing evolution of laboratory methods, "genomic" disease is becoming the preferred term. The foundational study in cytogenetics, G-banding, is still widely used, but the development of increasingly sensitive methods for investigating genomic DNA, such as fluorescence *in situ* hybridization (FISH), array-based oligonucleotide comparative genomic hybridization (a-CGH), and single nucleotide polymorphism (SNP) arrays, has expanded the scope of cytogenetic testing to include changes too small to detect by karyotype (Table 3.1, Figure 3-1). Although newer genomic technologies such as next-generation sequencing now permit screening the entire genome to the level of the nucleotide, conventional and molecular cytogenetic techniques continue to play an important role in pediatric and surgical pathology. In this chapter, we focus on constitutional abnormalities, those conditions that are present from conception or at birth and that typically have significant clinicopathologic findings. Related topics not covered in this chapter include chromosomal rearrangements associated with pediatric neoplasms, single-gene mutations, and mutations in mitochondrial DNA. Cytogenetic changes characteristic of childhood tumors are introduced as part of the discussion of specific neoplasms in other chapters and have been the subject of several excellent reviews (1–3). For information about the mitochondrial genome and related diseases, the reader is referred to the review by Schapira (4). Because knowledge about cytogenetic abnormalities and their clinicopathologic correlations is growing rapidly, the most up-to-date information about many such abnormalities can be found in online resources and current publications; several excellent resources are listed in Table 3.2.

The evolution of genomic techniques has resulted in numerous diagnostic testing options, each with advantages and disadvantages. In complex cases, a team approach to diagnosis is helpful. Cytogeneticists, molecular geneticists, clinical geneticists, and genetic counselors can provide valuable assistance to clinicians and pathologists in establishing a differential diagnosis and selecting and interpreting an appropriate sequence of tests (5). Some common indications for cytogenetic testing in pediatric pathology are listed in Table 3.3.

CYTOGENETIC TECHNIQUES

Conventional Cytogenetic Analysis (G-Banding)

G-banding is performed on metaphase (dividing) cells and permits the evaluation of the entire chromosome complement. The need for metaphase cells requires that specimens be cultured for up to several days; this is a major contributing factor to the time- and labor-intensive nature of conventional cytogenetic testing. A variety of tissue types can be cultured to yield metaphase cells for analysis, including peripheral and cord blood, chorionic villi, amniotic fluid, bone marrow, lymph nodes, and solid tumors. Technical considerations for postmortem tissue sampling are listed in Table 3.4. Analyses of peripheral and cord blood, chorionic villi, and amniotic fluid are typically performed to identify and characterize constitutional abnormalities (i.e., those present at birth and typically found in every cell), whereas analyses of bone marrow, lymph nodes, and tumors are performed to identify and characterize abnormalities associated with neoplastic disorders. Although sampling the correct area of the specimen is most critical in the case of neoplastic disorders (in which only part of the sample may be involved), it is also important in some constitutional studies. For example, placental specimens may contain cells of both fetal origin (chorionic stroma, amniocytes) and maternal origin (decidualized endometrium). Imprecise sampling may therefore result in the preferential growth of maternal cells, rather than the fetal cells of interest.

The goal of tissue culture is to optimize the conditions of cell culture media, temperature, pH, and sterility to stimulate cells to proceed through the cell cycle to mitosis. After the cells are arrested in mitosis, they are harvested, fixed, and dropped onto glass slides. The slides are then treated with a proteolytic enzyme and stained with Wright–Giemsa stain, resulting in a series of alternating light and dark bands

TABLE 3.1 CYTOGENETIC METHODS

	Karyotype	Array CGH	SNP Array	FISH	Cell-Free Fetal DNA
Appropriate samples	Chorionic villi, Amniocytes, Cord blood lymphocytes, Peripheral blood lymphocytes, Skin or soft tissue fibroblast culture	Chorionic villi, Amniocytes, Cord blood lymphocytes, Peripheral blood lymphocytes, Skin or soft tissue fibroblast culture	Chorionic villi, Amniocytes, Cord blood lymphocytes, Peripheral blood lymphocytes, Skin or soft tissue fibroblast culture	Chorionic villi, Amniocytes, Cord blood lymphocytes, Peripheral blood lymphocytes, Skin or soft tissue fibroblast culture, Formalin-fixed, paraffin-embedded tissue, Air-dried touch preps	Maternal peripheral blood
Turnaround time[a]	1–2 wk	1–2 wk	1–2 wk	1–2 d	1–2 wk
Method	Stain prophase or metaphase chromosomes, and examine banding patterns	Hybridize patient and control DNA with probes (e.g., oligonucleotides) affixed to glass slide.	Hybridize patient DNA with DNA oligomers on microarray chip.	Hybridize fluorescently labeled DNA probes to patient DNA affixed to slide	Massively parallel DNA sequencing, computer analysis
Resolution limit[b]	3–5 Mb	~50–100 kb	50–100 kb	50–400 kb	Currently, whole chromosome (21, 18, 13, X, and Y), and additional select chromosomal regions.
Notes	Requires viable, mitotically active cells. If tissue is cultured (i.e., not a direct prep), may select for biased cell subsets. Best method for detecting balanced translocations and inversions	Sensitive method for detecting small duplications and deletions. Interpretation can be complicated by copy number variants (CNV). Testing parental DNA may help determine if a CNV is benign or disease causing	Sensitive method for detecting small duplications and deletions. Can detect uniparental isodisomy	Targeted method for detecting small duplications, deletions, and translocations. Must select probes directed to specific DNA sequences.	Screening test only. Results must be confirmed with analysis of chorionic villi, amniocytes, or cord or peripheral blood. False positives can occur with CPM or maternal mosaicism (e.g., 45,X/46,XX mosaic). False negatives can occur with confined fetal mosaicism

[a] Turnaround times are approximate and dependent on a number of factors; it is critical to contact the laboratory for specific details.
[b] Limit of resolution depends on band-level resolution (G-banding) and array design and configuration (microarray).

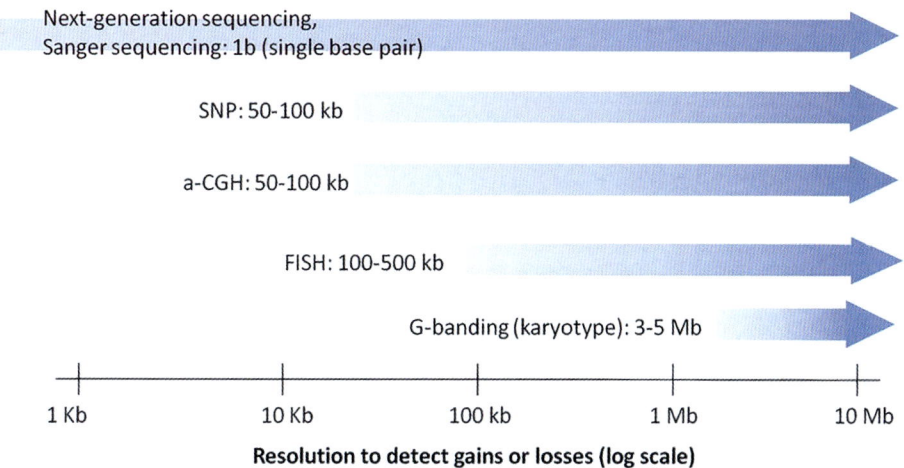

FIGURE 3-1 • Maximum resolution of cytogenetic and molecular laboratory methods. Ranges are approximate, and different laboratories may have different limits of detection and reportable ranges.

(G-bands) characteristic of each of the 22 pairs of autosomes and 2 sex chromosomes. Darkly staining (positive) G-bands are rich in adenine (A) and thymine (T) residues and have relatively few genes, in contrast with lightly staining G-bands, which are rich in guanine (G) and cytosine (C) residues and are relatively gene rich.

G-banding enables the detection across the entire genome of both numerical (gain or loss of a chromosome) and structural (e.g., translocation, deletion, inversion) abnormalities. These abnormalities are described using a specialized nomenclature provided in the International System for Human Cytogenetic Nomenclature (ISCN) (6). See Table 3-5 for a glossary of cytogenetic terms commonly encountered in the practice of pediatric pathology, including examples of commonly used ISCN nomenclature.

Molecular Cytogenetic Analysis (FISH)

Although G-banding provides a rapid way of screening the entire genome for numerical or structural chromosomal abnormalities, it is hampered by the need for dividing (metaphase) cells and by relatively low resolution (approximately 3 to 5 Mb). A major advantage to FISH is the ability to evaluate nondividing (interphase) cells, although it can also be performed on metaphase cells. Thus, FISH can be performed on specimens that cannot be cultured or that do not yield metaphase cells after culturing. FISH is a method that can be readily adapted to a variety of specimen types including cell suspensions, touch imprints, disaggregated tissues such as tumors, and paraffin-embedded tissues. Of note, it is typically not successful in specimens that have undergone decalcification. A large number of interphase cells (usually at least 200) can be rapidly evaluated by FISH, making it much faster and more sensitive than G-banding analysis.

Briefly, FISH is performed by applying fluorescently labeled probes (DNA sequences typically several hundred kb in length and complementary to known sequences) to cells that are affixed to a glass slide. The DNA of the probe and specimen are concurrently heat denatured for several minutes, and the slide is incubated at 37°C for 6 to 14 hours to allow the probe to bind to its target sequence. After washing and the addition of a nuclear counterstain such as 4′6′-diamidino-2-phenylindole (DAPI), the cells are examined under a fluorescence microscope.

Numerous different probe types are commercially available or can be developed within the laboratory. The types most frequently used to evaluate pediatric constitutional abnormalities are enumeration probes (directed against the pericentromeric region of chromosomes and used to detect chromosomal gains or losses) and locus-specific probes (directed against specific genes or loci and used to detect deletions or duplications of those regions).

Chromosomal Microarray

Array-based genomic technologies are routinely used in cytogenetic laboratories, and for the evaluation of patients with developmental delay, they are now considered the

TABLE 3.2	ONLINE RESOURCES FOR CYTOGENETICS AND MOLECULAR GENETICS

GeneReviews: genereviews.org
OMIM, Online Mendelian Inheritance in Man: omim.org
DECIPHER, Database of Chromosomal Imbalance and Phenotype in Humans Using Ensembl Resources: decipher.sanger.ac.uk
ECARUCA, European Cytogeneticists Association Register of Unbalanced Chromosome Aberrations: ecaruca.net

TABLE 3.3	INDICATIONS FOR PRENATAL GENOMIC TESTING

Structural fetal anomalies
Fetal growth restriction
Recurrent miscarriage or fetal loss
Known parental genomic abnormality

TABLE 3.4 TISSUE SAMPLING FOR CYTOGENETIC STUDIES: TECHNICAL CONSIDERATIONS

KARYOTYPE: Viable, mitotically active cells

Neonate:
- Umbilical cord blood, peripheral blood lymphocytes (if infant has not been transfused), skin fibroblasts

Recent fetal demise:
- Fibroblasts and chondrocytes remain viable the longest.
- Sample fascia, cartilage, or lung
- Use sterile blade; do not include epidermis, which may be contaminated. Avoid contacting formalin with blade.

Macerated fetus:
- Fibroblasts may still be viable. Sample fascia, tendon, or cartilage
- Chances of successful culture: ~70% within 3 days of death; case reports of success 6 days after death
- Also sample fetal surface of the placenta.

a-CGH AND SNP ARRAY: High-quality DNA
- Fresh or fresh frozen tissue when possible (liver, placenta, cord or peripheral blood, other).
- Formalin-fixed, paraffin-embedded tissue may be possible, but DNA tends to be more fragmented and may give less information.

FISH: Interphase or metaphase cells
- Air-dried touch prep slides and fresh tissue are ideal; metaphase analysis requires suspension of cultured cells.
- Formalin-fixed, paraffin-embedded tissue possible; high level of nuclear truncation due to slide preparation
- Unacceptable: frozen tissue; decalcified specimens

TABLE 3-5 GLOSSARY OF TERMS USED FREQUENTLY IN CYTOGENETICS

Aneuploidy—gain or loss of all of one or more chromosomes (e.g., trisomies, monosomies). Does not include ploidy abnormalities (e.g., haploidy, triploidy, tetraploidy). Example: 47,XX,+21—female karyotype with 47 chromosomes, including three copies of chromosome 21

Chimerism—the presence in one zygote of a cell line derived from another zygote

Deletion—loss of part of a chromosome. Example: 46,XY,del(15)(q11.2q13)—deletion within the short arm of a chromosome 15, encompassing bands 15q11.2 through 15q13

Duplication—gain of part of a chromosome. Example: 46,XX,dup(22)(q13.31q13.33)—duplication of the long arm of a chromosome 22, encompassing bands 22q13.31 through 22q13.33

Haploidy—half (23) of the normal diploid (46) chromosome complement

Insertion—intercalation of part of one chromosome into another chromosome (interchromosomal) or into a different location within the same chromosome (intrachromosomal)

Inversion—180-degree rotation of an intrachromosomal segment

Pericentric—the inverted segment includes the centromere (it involves both the short and long arms of the chromosome)

Paracentric—the inverted segment does not include the centromere (it involves only one chromosome arm).

Mosaicism—the presence of two or more cell lines derived from a single zygote

Nondisjunction—failure of homologous chromosomes or sister chromatids to segregate properly during meiosis or mitosis

Parental imprinting—differential expression of alleles based on the parent of origin

Polyploidy—one or more complete extra set of chromosomes. Examples: triploidy (69,XXX), tetraploidy (92,XXYY)

Translocation—recombination of nonhomologous parts of two chromosomes

Balanced—reciprocal translocation with no net gain or loss of chromosomal material. Example: 46,XX,t(9;22)(q34;q11.2)—translocation between the long arm of a chromosome 9 at band 9q34 and the long arm of a chromosome 22 at band 22q11.2

Unbalanced—the presence of only one of two translocation partners, resulting in net gain and loss of translocated portions of the involved chromosomes. Example: 46,XX,der(22)t(9;22)(q34;q11.2)—the presence of only the derivative (abnormal) chromosome 22 from the translocation above, resulting in net gain of material from 9q and net loss of material from 22q

Robertsonian—translocation involving fusion of the long arms of two acrocentric chromosomes (13, 14, 15, 21, or 22) with resultant loss of their short arms

Uniparental disomy—both chromosomes of a homologous pair are derived from the same parent

Heterodisomy—UPD in which the two homologues differ (due to nondisjunction in meiosis I)

Isodisomy—UPD in which the homologues are identical (due to failure of sister chromatids to separate in meiosis II)

TABLE 3-6	INCIDENCE OF ANEUPLOIDY DURING DEVELOPMENT					
Gestation (Weeks)[a]			0	6-8	20	40
	Sperm	Oocytes	Preimplantation Embryos	Spontaneous Abortions	Stillbirths	Live Births
Incidence of aneuploidy	1%-2%	~20%	~20%	35%-54%	4%-6%	0.3%-0.6%
Most common aneuploidies	Various	Various	Various	45, X, +16, +21, +22, polyploidy	45,X, +13, +18, +21, polyploidy	45, X, +13, +18, +21, XXX, XXY, XYY

[a]Data pooled from multiple references (13, 71, and two new references: Boue J, Boue A Lazar P. Retrospective and prospective epidemiological studies of 1500 karyotyped spontaneous abortuses. Teratology, 1975;12:11-26.
Menasha J, Levy B, Hirschhorn K, et al. Incidence and spectrum of chromosome abnormalities in spontaneous abortions: new insights from a 12-year study. Genet Med, 2005;7:251-63.).

first-line test (9,10). Unlike G-banding and FISH, which use metaphase and interphase cells as the substrate, microarrays evaluate DNA that has been extracted from the specimen. These assays can detect copy number gains or losses with a markedly increased resolution (typically <100 kb, depending on the array configuration). Like FISH, arrays evaluate specimen DNA with fluorescent labeled probes. However, unlike FISH, in which a single probe set is applied to patient DNA affixed to a slide, in array-based testing, the patient DNA is applied to a slide to which thousands of oligonucleotide probes are affixed. The level of resolution of these arrays is dependent on the number of these probes in the array, the distance between probes on a chromosome, and the degree to which certain chromosomal regions are "targeted" (i.e., sampled by a larger number of probes than other regions).

Two major types of arrays are in routine clinical use. a-CGH identifies regions of copy number gain or loss by hybridizing a mixture of an equal concentration of patient DNA and normal control DNA. By contrast, SNP arrays do not use a concurrent control DNA sample but rather compare the patient DNA to a well-characterized reference genome. Like a-CGH, SNP arrays can identify copy number changes but can also identify copy number neutral loss of heterozygosity, in which two copies of a chromosomal region are present, but both are derived from a single parent. Hybrid arrays containing both oligonucleotides and SNPs are also routinely used. Compared to G-banding and FISH, array-based techniques more precisely determine the size of aberrant regions as well as their gene content. A limitation of chromosomal microarrays is their ability to detect only unbalanced rearrangements leading to gain or loss of DNA; balanced rearrangements cannot be detected.

In cases where a fetal structural abnormality is identified by ultrasound, a-CGH is more sensitive than G-banding for detecting unbalanced rearrangements resulting in gain or loss of DNA (e.g., deletions, duplications). In a recent meta-analysis, a-CGH detected pathogenic abnormalities in 10% of cases with a normal karyotype (11). Similar results are found in first-trimester spontaneous abortions, where a-CGH detects abnormalities in 13% of cases with a normal karyotype (12). However, G-banding can detect some abnormalities (e.g., balanced rearrangements, polyploidy) that cannot be detected by chromosomal microarray.

CONSTITUTIONAL ABNORMALITIES

Constitutional chromosomal abnormalities are present at birth and affect all cell lines. Such abnormalities are common: for example, it is estimated that as many as 25% of conceptions are aneuploid, of which 99% are spontaneously aborted (13). The rates and types of chromosomal abnormalities detected in spontaneous abortions differ throughout gestation, with a higher rate detected in early gestation (Table 3-6). The pathology of early embryonic loss and its poor correlation with cytogenetic findings are discussed in Chapter 2.

Aneuploidy, defined as gain or loss of all of one or more chromosomes, is one of the most common types of cytogenetic abnormality found in prenatal specimens, such as chorionic villi, amniotic fluid, or spontaneous abortions (Table 3-7). The rate of aneuploidy among all liveborn infants is approximately 0.5%, although the rate in malformed infants is significantly higher (21). Most aneuploidy occurs as a result of nondisjunction, the failure of homologous chromosomes (in meiosis) or sister chromatids (in mitosis) to segregate appropriately into daughter cells (22–24). When nondisjunction occurs in meiosis, the result is an aneuploid gamete; this is the basis for most nonmosaic aneuploid conceptuses (25). Nondisjunction of autosomes (chromosomes 1 to 22), which is far more common during oogenesis than spermatogenesis, typically occurs during the first meiotic division, when homologous chromosomes segregate. In contrast, sex chromosome nondisjunction occurs more commonly during male gametogenesis in the second meiotic division, when sister chromatids separate.

TABLE 3-7	CHROMOSOMAL ANOMALIES IN SPONTANEOUS ABORTIONS
Abnormality	Reported Rate of Occurrence (%)[a]
Autosomal trisomy	50-60
Polyploidy	20-25
Monosomy X	10-20
Translocations	2-5

[a]Pooled results from references (15,16,18–20).

Mitotic nondisjunction, occurring after a zygote is formed, may result in mosaicism, that is, the presence of two distinct cell lines both derived from a single zygote. Examination of human embryos conceived by *in vitro* fertilization suggests that rates of spontaneous postzygotic nondisjunction are very high (20% to 50% of preimplantation embryos) (13,26). Although genetic or pharmacologic alterations that disrupt meiotic and mitotic checkpoints predispose to nondisjunction and aneuploidy (25), most instances of nondisjunction are sporadic. In one population-based study, spontaneous abortion due to aneuploidy was not associated with an increased risk of a similar event in subsequent pregnancies (27).

Autosomal Trisomies

Most nonmosaic autosomal trisomies arise from errors during the first meiotic division in oogenesis (28,29). Oogenesis in humans begins during fetal development. In the second trimester, oocytes arrest in late prophase of the first meiotic division and remain in a "dormant" state until one to five decades after birth. During this period of meiotic arrest, recombination between homologous chromosomes occurs (13). The physical sites of recombination, termed chiasmata, stabilize the chromosomal pairs through metaphase (30). It is believed that the prolonged meiotic arrest increases the risk of nondisjunction, possibly due to age-related loss of chiasmata.

Trisomies 13, 18, and 21 are the only autosomal trisomies compatible with survival to term. Their features are summarized in Tables 3-8, 3-9, and 3-10 and Figures 3-2, 3-3, and 3-4. Two alternative theories have been developed to explain how a trisomy results in a specific clinical phenotype (31). The "amplified developmental instability" hypothesis suggests that increased expression of hundreds of genes on the trisomic chromosome disrupts the global balance of gene expression and/or protein stoichiometry during

TABLE 3-8 MALFORMATIONS AND POSTNATAL DISORDERS ASSOCIATED WITH TRISOMY 21/DOWN SYNDROME (DS)

Malformation	% of DS[a]	Postnatal Disorder	% of DS[a]
Craniofacial[b]		**Central nervous system**	
Upslanted palpebral fissures	>50	Cognitive impairment	100
Ear anomalies	>50	Early-onset Alzheimer dementia	>50[c]
Epicanthal folds	>50	Seizures	
Flat midface	>50	**Cancer (relative risk)**	
Hypertelorism	25–50	Acute lymphoblastic leukemia (31)	
Other: brachycephaly, midline parietal hair whorl, mild microcephaly, choanal stenosis, cleft palate without cleft lip		Acute myeloid leukemia (26)	
		Lymphoma (3)	
		Colon (3)	
Cardiovascular	>50	Testicular (21)	
Atrioventricular canal	10–25	Transient abnormal myelopoiesis	5–10
Patent ductus arteriosus	10–25	**Autoimmune (relative risk)**	
Tricuspid valve defects	10–25	Crohn disease (3)	
Ventricular septal defect	5–10	Ulcerative colitis (3)	
Atrial septal defect	5–10	Celiac disease (5)	1–5
Tetralogy of Fallot	1–5	Early-onset diabetes mellitus (3)	
Other: coronary valve defects, hypoplastic right heart, hypoplastic left heart, anomalies of coronary circulation, coarctation of the aorta, other aortic anomalies, pulmonary artery stenosis, anomalies of great veins, single umbilical artery		Thyroiditis (32)	
		Autoimmune hepatitis (33)	
		Psoriasis (4)	
		Musculoskeletal	
		Hypotonia	
		Joint hyperextensibility	**>50**
		Other	>50
Digestive tract	10–25	Testicular microlithiasis	
Duodenal stenosis	5–10	Enlarged thymic Hassall corpuscles	25–50
Hirschsprung disease	1–5		
Anal atresia/stenosis	1–5	Abnormal lymphocyte subsets	10–25
Other: tracheoesophageal fistula, esophageal atresia/stenosis, nonduodenal intestinal atresia/stenosis, intestinal malrotation, ectopic anus, annular pancreas		Ocular:	10–25
		Glaucoma	10–25
		Strabismus	5–10
		Nystagmus	25–50
Respiratory		Scoliosis	
Anomalies of larynx, trachea, or bronchi		Hearing loss[d]	
Pulmonary anomalies			

TABLE 3-8 MALFORMATIONS AND POSTNATAL DISORDERS ASSOCIATED WITH TRISOMY 21/DOWN SYNDROME (DS) (continued)

Malformation	% of DS[a]	Postnatal Disorder	% of DS[a]
Genitourinary			
Obstructive defects of renal pelvis, ureter, bladder neck, or urethra	1–5		
Cryptorchidism	5–10		
Hypospadias/epispadias	1–5		
Central nervous system			
Hypoplastic superior temporal gyrus			
Flat frontal poles, retarded myelination			
Hydrocephalus			
Limb			
Clinodactyly (fifth finger)	25–50		
Single transverse palmar crease	25–50		
Syndactyly	1–5		
Other: clubfoot, polydactyly, limb reduction defects, rhizomelic shortening			
Ocular			
Brushfield spots	1–5		
Cataract	5–10		
Keratoconus	5–10		

[a]Data pooled from multiple references (34–52).
[b]Many of the craniofacial features are less distinct in fetuses than in infants or children.
[c]Onset of Alzheimer dementia is age dependent. One hundred percent have pathologic changes by age 40 years and >50% have clinical findings by age 50 years.
[d]The incidence of hearing loss varies with age and aggressive treatment of middle ear infections.

development, leading to abnormalities of development. This is supported by the presence of common features between trisomies and segmental chromosomal duplications, including craniofacial abnormalities, structural cardiac abnormalities, and cognitive impairment. The "gene dosage effect" hypothesis asserts that a small set of genes, expressed at 1.5-fold greater than normal levels, is responsible for many of the phenotypic findings. Based on phenotypic mapping studies of individuals with duplications of part of chromosome 21 and clinical features of Down syndrome, a 1.6 to 5 Mb region of the long arm of chromosome 21 has been proposed to be the "Down syndrome critical region," three copies of which are thought to account for many of the features of Down syndrome (7,65). In mice, duplication of part of chromosome 16 (homologous to human chromosome 21) results in phenotypic features similar to those in Down syndrome, including craniofacial alterations, changes in cerebellar architecture, and impaired learning and memory. Similar critical regions have been proposed for trisomy 13 (14) and trisomy 18 (66). Selective overexpression of smaller regions or single candidate genes in these homologous regions in the mouse may provide an experimental basis for understanding how trisomies influence development.

Most nonmosaic autosomal trisomies lead to early embryonic demise. Although trisomies 13, 18, and 21 are compatible with survival to term, each has a high rate of embryonic and fetal loss (Tables 3-6, 3-7, and 3-11). A retrospective examination found that 10% of fetuses with trisomy 21 and 32% with trisomy 18 diagnosed by amniocentesis subsequently died spontaneously *in utero*; deaths occurred at a constant rate throughout the second and third trimesters (76). Analysis of placentas from fetuses and infants with apparently nonmosaic trisomy 13 or 18 suggests that those surviving to term have placental mosaicism (79). It is possible that survival to term requires that at least a subset of placental cells be diploid and that nonmosaic placental trisomy 13 or 18 is always lethal. Although trisomies for each of the autosomes have been identified in spontaneous abortions, the pattern is not random; for example, trisomies 16, 21, and 22 are particularly common in the first trimester. Most trisomic abortuses manifest as highly disorganized embryos (see Chapter 2).

Prenatal diagnosis and elective termination of pregnancy also impact the rate of liveborn trisomies. Definitive prenatal diagnosis requires chorionic villus sampling, amniocentesis, or other invasive procedure to obtain tissue for genomic studies. To reduce unnecessary risks and cost associated with invasive prenatal diagnosis, noninvasive screening methods have been developed that identify pregnancies at greatest risk for aneuploidy. Sequencing of maternal plasma cell-free fetal DNA (cfDNA)

TABLE 3-9 MALFORMATIONS ASSOCIATED WITH TRISOMY 18

Malformation	% of Cases[a]
General	
Intrauterine growth restriction	25–50[b]
Fetal hydrops	5–10
Craniofacial	
Microcephaly	25–50[b]
Choroid plexus cyst	
Other: triangular facies, abnormal calvarial shape ("strawberry" skull), hydrocephalus, micrognathia, hypotelorism, cleft lip/palate, small ears, wide fontanelles, narrow nasal bridge, microstomia, short sternum	
Cardiovascular	
Ventricular septal defect	>50
Atrioventricular canal defect	25–50
Other: ectopia cordis (pentalogy of Cantrell), hypoplastic left or right heart, overriding aorta, single umbilical artery, patent ductus arteriosus, tetralogy of Fallot, double-outlet right ventricle, transposition of the great arteries, mitral valvular disease	
Digestive tract	
Omphalocele	10–25
Meckel diverticulum	>50
Other: anorectal atresia, esophageal atresia, pyloric stenosis, ectopic pancreas, abnormal liver lobation	
Respiratory	
Abnormal lung lobation, tracheal stenosis, tracheoesophageal fistula	
Genitourinary	
Abnormal genitalia, cloacal exstrophy, obstructive uropathy, horseshoe kidney, renal aplasia/hypoplasia, renal/ureteral duplication, cryptorchidism, bifid uterus	
Central nervous system	
Cerebellar and pontine hypoplasia	>50
Meningomyelocele ± Chiari malformation	10–25
Other: anencephaly, craniorachischisis, hippocampal dysplasia, agenesis of the corpus callosum, neural migration defects	
Limb	
Clenched hand with overlapping digits	>50
Radial ray defects	5–10
Rocker-bottom feet	25–50
Other: arthrogryposis, polydactyly, phocomelia, syndactyly, hypoplastic nails, ectrodactyly	
Ocular	
Coloboma, cataract, cloudy cornea, retinal hypopigmentation, microphthalmia, iridial hypoplasia	
Musculoskeletal	
Other: diaphragmatic defect, absent 12th ribs, malformed occipital bones	
Other viscera	
Hypoplasia of adrenals, thymus, thyroid, and/or gallbladder, accessory spleen	
Placenta/cord	
Umbilical cord cysts	
Small placenta	

[a]Data pooled from multiple references (15,17,53–62).
[b]Frequency as a second-trimester ultrasound finding.

is currently the most sensitive noninvasive screening method for detecting trisomy 21, with a detection rate of 98% to 100% and a false-positive rate of 0% to 0.3% (80,81). cfDNA testing is also in clinical use to detect trisomies 13 and 18; the sensitivity for detection of these aneuploidies ranges from 78% to 100%, with greater sensitivity for trisomy 18 than for trisomy 13 (80).

Because cfDNA is mostly derived from placental trophoblast cells, one potential source of false-positive and false-negative results is confined placental or fetal mosaicism, estimated to affect 1 in 1000 to 1 in 4000 pregnancies (82). Therefore, despite the high specificity, confirmatory invasive diagnostic testing (by chorionic villus sampling or amniocentesis) is required

TABLE 3-10 MALFORMATIONS ASSOCIATED WITH TRISOMY 13

Malformation	% of Cases[a]
General	
Intrauterine growth restriction	10–50[b]
Fetal hydrops	5–10
Craniofacial	
Microcephaly	10–50
Holoprosencephalic facies (cyclopia, ethmocephaly, cebocephaly, premaxillary agenesis/dysgenesis)	>50
Cleft lip/palate (midline/bilateral > unilateral)	
Hypotelorism	
Other: malformed ears, absent ear canal, aplasia cutis of scalp, choanal stenosis or atresia; hemangiomas, receding forehead, sparse curled eyelashes, natal teeth, micrognathia	
Cardiovascular	>50
Ventricular septal defect	25–50
Patent ductus arteriosus	25–50
Echogenic intracardiac foci (myocardial calcifications)	10–25
Other: dextrocardia, tetralogy of Fallot, atrial septal defect, truncus arteriosus, aortic coarctation, pulmonary atresia/stenosis, bicuspid aortic valve, single umbilical artery	
Digestive tract	
Pancreatic–splenic fusion	
Appendiceal diverticulum	
Other: omphalocele, abnormal liver lobation, intestinal atresia, Meckel diverticulum	
Respiratory	
Abnormal lung lobation	
Genitourinary	
Obstructive dysplasia	25–50
Renal/ureteral duplications	25–50
Other: cryptorchidism, double vagina, bicornuate uterus, abnormal fallopian tubes, small penis, abnormal scrotum	
Central nervous system	
Holoprosencephaly	25–50
Arhinencephaly	>50
Cerebellar malformations	25–50
Other: anencephaly, meningomyelocele, agenesis of the corpus callosum, hydrocephaly, hippocampal dysplasia, neural migratory defects, choroid plexus cyst	
Limb	
Postaxial polydactyly	~50
Other: syndactyly, rocker-bottom feet, hypoplastic nails, clubbed feet, hypoplastic nails, single transverse palmar crease, radial aplasia	
Ocular	
Microphthalmia	25–50
Coloboma of iris or retina	25–50
Other: retinal dysplasia, aniridia, anophthalmia, cataract, premature vitreous body, hypoplasia of optic nerve	
Musculoskeletal	
Dysplastic/fused lumbosacral ± thoracic vertebra, absent 12th ribs, hypoplastic sphenoid bone, diaphragmatic defect	>50
Hematologic	
Irregular neutrophil nuclei	
Increased fetal and Gower-2 hemoglobin	

[a]Data pooled from multiple references (16,55,60,61,63,64).
[b]Reported rates of IUGR appear to be higher in populations that were studied later in gestation.

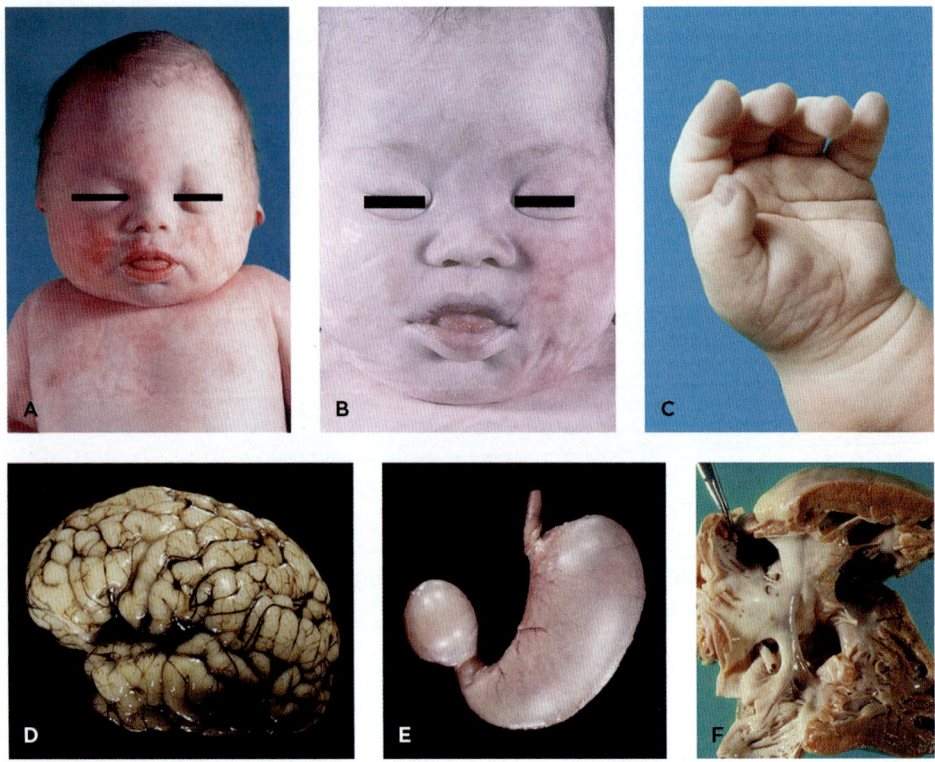

FIGURE 3-2 • Trisomy 21. **A:** 35-week fetus with typical late-gestation facies (epicanthal folds, broad nose, bulging tongue). **B:** Similar facial changes are apparent in 2-month-old infant (note increased slant of palpebral fissures). **C:** Single palmar crease. **D:** Lateral view of brain showing small superior temporal gyrus and enlarged middle temporal gyrus. **E:** Duodenal atresia. **F:** Atrioventricular canal, with large primum atrial septal defect, large ventricular septal defect in position of AV canal, and cleft septal leaflet of the tricuspid valve.

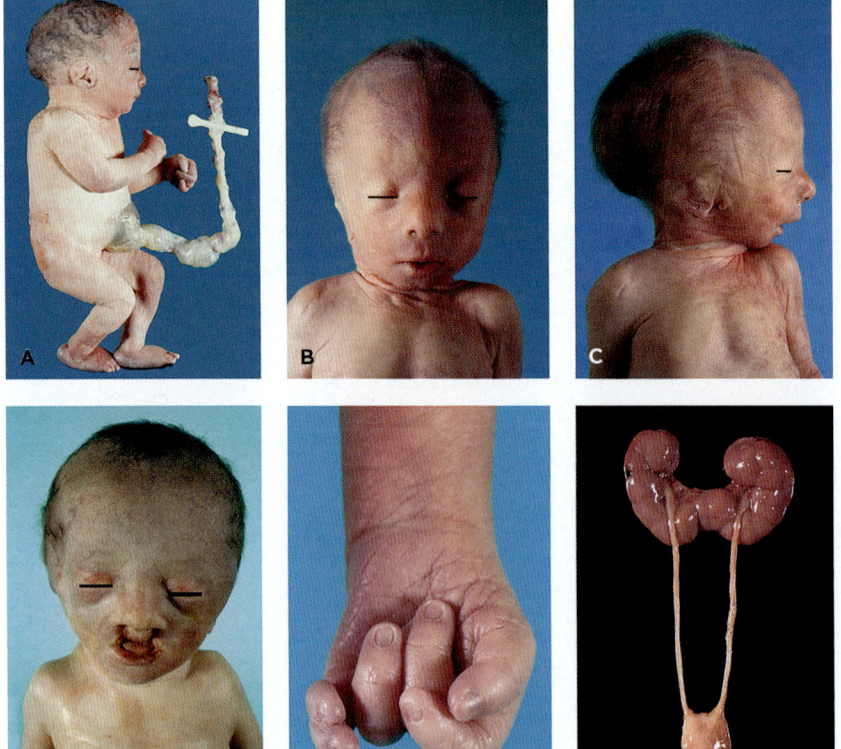

FIGURE 3-3 • Trisomy 18. **A:** Late-gestational fetus with omphalocele and rocker-bottom feet. **B:** Young infant with widely separated eyes and mild trigonocephaly. **C:** Infant shown in (**B**), with dysplastic ear and micrognathia. **D:** Infant with triangular facies, ocular hypertelorism, and bilateral cleft lip. **E:** Overlapping digits in pattern common to trisomy 18, with distal polydactyly. **F:** Horseshoe kidney (with ureters and urinary bladder).

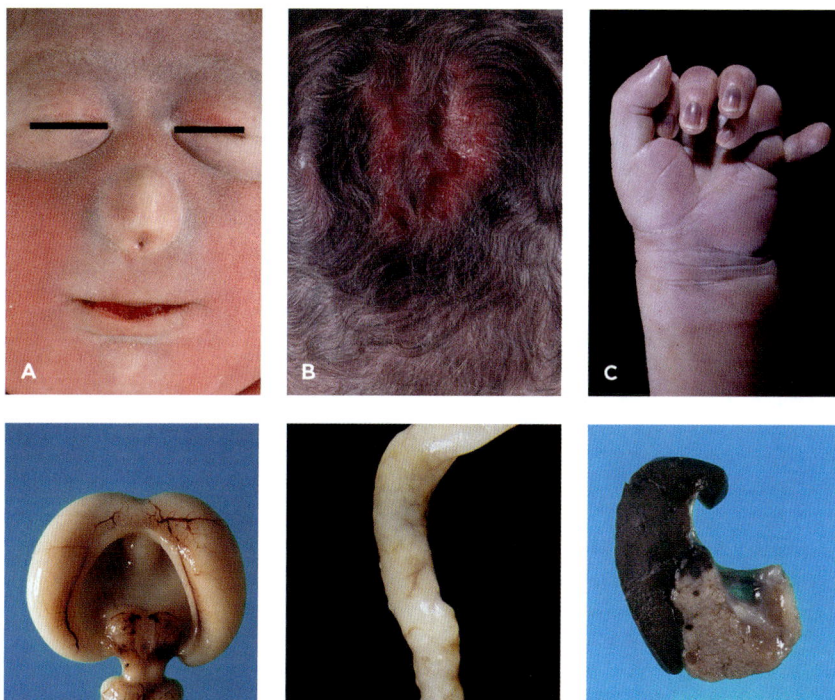

FIGURE 3-4 • Trisomy 13. **A:** Infant with cebocephaly (ocular hypotelorism and single nostril nose), one of the facial changes associated with holoprosencephaly. **B:** Aplasia cutis of the scalp. **C:** Postaxial polydactyly. **D:** Alobar holoprosencephaly. **E:** Appendiceal diverticula ("dinosaur tail") are pathognomonic for trisomy 13, although not present in every case. **F:** Fusion of spleen **(left)** and tail of pancreas (note tiny splenic islands within the pancreas).

before a decision is made to terminate the pregnancy (83). Another current testing option is an "integrated test" that includes quantitative measurement of pregnancy-associated plasma protein A, alpha-fetoprotein, unconjugated estriol, free β–human chorionic gonadotropin, and/or inhibin A in maternal serum, early second-trimester ultrasound evaluation of nuchal translucency, and maternal age (Table 3-11). This approach affords an 80% to 85% detection rate of trisomy 21, with a false-positive rate of 1% to 5% (84,85). Similar sensitivity and specificity have been reported for trisomy 18 based on a two-stage screening approach using maternal serum markers.

Approximately 50% of infants born with either trisomy 13 or trisomy 18 die within the 1st year and fewer than 5% survive to 10 years (67), with most deaths due to cardiac malformations. Surviving infants have significant neurocognitive deficits and multiple other medical complications. In contrast, the life expectancy of infants with trisomy 21 is much longer: in developed countries, more than 90% of children with Down syndrome live more than 10 years, and the current median lifespan for these individuals is approximately 60 years (68). In addition to cognitive impairment and congenital malformations, postnatal health issues often associated with trisomy 21 include hearing loss, acute leukemia, early-onset Alzheimer disease, and other conditions (Table 3-8). The most common causes of death currently are complications of congenital heart disease, pneumonia and, among patients over 40 years of age, dementia (86,87).

Autosomal Monosomies

Meiotic nondisjunction events resulting in disomic or nullisomic gametes should, in theory, result in equal percentages of trisomic and monosomic embryos. In practice, however, this is not seen because, with the exception of monosomies for chromosomes X (Turner syndrome) and in rare cases 21 (which may likely be mosaic), autosomal monosomies are lethal in embryonic life, even before implantation (88). This observation is supported by studies of embryos conceived *in vitro* (88,89). Mosaicism for cell lines with a normal karyotype and an autosomal monosomy is compatible with long-term survival, and genotype/phenotype correlations have been established for some of these cases (90,91).

Sex Chromosome Aneuploidies

At least one X chromosome is required for survival of the preimplantation embryo. Thus, 45,Y conceptuses are not observed. However, other forms of sex chromosome aneuploidy, including monosomy X or extra copies of either the X or Y chromosomes, are compatible with long-term survival and account for the majority of liveborn infants with aneuploidy.

Monosomy X (Turner Syndrome)

A 45,X karyotype is one of the most frequently encountered forms of aneuploidy in spontaneous abortions. In contrast with autosomal aneuploidies, for which maternal meiotic

TABLE 3-11	PRENATAL SCREENING MARKERS AND CLINICAL OUTCOMES FOR COMMON TRISOMIES					
	Prenatal Screening Markers		Rate of IUFD or Stillbirth[a,b]	Percentage of Liveborns Surviving to:[a]		
Trisomy	Maternal Serum Analytes	Ultrasound[c]		1 Month	1 Year	10 Years
21	↓ AFP ↓ PAPP-A ↑ fβ-HCG ↑ inhibin	1st trimester: nuchal translucency, nasal bone hypoplasia 2nd trimester: echogenic intracardiac foci, echogenic bowel, rhizomelic limb shortening, mild pyelectasis	10%–30%	>95	95	>90
18	↓ AFP ↓↓ PAPP-A ↓↓ fβ-HCG ↓ uE3	1st trimester: nuchal translucency 2nd trimester: choroid plexus cyst, clenched hands, echogenic bowel, IUGR, mild pyelectasis, mild ventriculomegaly	45%–70%	50%	5%–30%	1%
13	↓ AFP ↓↓ PAPP-A ↓↓ fβ-HCG	2nd trimester: mild pyelectasis, echogenic intracardiac foci, IUGR, mild ventriculomegaly	20%–40%	50%	15%–30%	1%

[a]References (20,67–78).
[b]After diagnosis by amniocentesis or ultrasound; does not include first-trimester losses or elective terminations of pregnancy.
[c]Nonspecific findings that significantly increase the risk for trisomy.
AFP, α-fetoprotein; PAPP-A, pregnancy-associated plasma protein A, increased inhibin A; fβ-HCG, free β-human chorionic gonadotropin; uE3, unconjugated estriol; IUGR, intrauterine growth restriction; VSD, ventricular septal defect; IUFD, intrauterine fetal demise.

nondisjunction events predominate, sex chromosome loss can involve either the maternal or paternal sex chromosome, most often during a postzygotic mitosis. Hence, mosaicism in the setting of Turner syndrome is frequent, and occult mosaicism has been speculated to exist even in those patients in whom no mosaicism is found by either G-banding or FISH (92). Turner syndrome is typically characterized by female genitalia, short stature, and a high prevalence of specific anomalies (Table 3-12, Figure 3-5) and a characteristic cognitive profile (32). The presence of mosaicism for 46,XX and/or 47,XXX cell lines may mitigate the severity of the clinical findings (100).

Only 1% of 45,X embryos survive to term. Many are lost in the first trimester, but late fetal loss is also common. Severe hydrops with massive nuchal edema is common *in utero* and usually portends a poor outcome. Extravascular fluid in the neck collects as a multiloculated cystic hygroma, a lymphatic malformation characterized by thin membranous septa and inconspicuous endothelial linings (8). Gross and microscopic studies of cystic hygroma in Turner syndrome suggest hypoplasia/agenesis of lymphatic vessels and failure of the lymphatics to connect to the venous system (33). Resolution of transient nuchal edema is proposed as the basis for the webbed neck commonly observed in Turner syndrome.

Other common malformations include aortic coarctation, hypoplastic left heart, horseshoe kidney, and streak ovaries.

Of the individuals with Turner syndrome, approximately 50% have a 45,X karyotype with no other cell line identified. The remaining cases show mosaicism for another cell line, including 46,XX, 47,XXX, 46,XY, or a variety of other structural abnormalities of the sex chromosomes, the most common of which is an isochromosome X composed of two copies of the long arm of a chromosome X joined at the centromere (100,101). Individuals with mosaicism for a cell line containing all or part of a Y chromosome exhibit a range of clinical features ranging from normal male to a Turner syndrome phenotype. Within this continuum, the gonads and external genitalia may show ambiguous differentiation. Ovotestes or other forms of gonadal dysgenesis are common and 7% to 30% of patients develop gonadoblastoma (102).

Sex Chromosome Polysomy

X chromosome inactivation is a process of epigenetic modification that silences most genes on all but one X chromosome in each cell at the blastocyst stage of development; a subset of X-linked genes normally escapes this inactivation. The process of X chromosome inactivation is

TABLE 3-12 MALFORMATIONS AND POSTNATAL ABNORMALITIES ASSOCIATED WITH MONOSOMY X/TURNER SYNDROME (TS)

Malformation	% of TS[a]	Postnatal Abnormality	% of Cases
General		**External**	
Intrauterine growth restriction	>80	Short stature	>90
Fetal hydrops (may be transient)	>80	Webbed neck	>80
Broad chest		Short neck/low hairline	>70
Widely spaced nipples		Cubitus valgus	
Inverted and/or hypoplastic nipples		Infantile external genitalia	
Craniofacial		Scant pubic/axillary hair	
Nuchal cystic hygroma		Failure to develop secondary sex characteristics	
Triangular face			
Down-slanted palpebrae		**Endocrine**	
Other: epicanthus, ptosis, high-arched narrow palate, micrognathia, hypertelorism, low-set ears, dysmorphic ears		Low estrogen and progesterone	15-30
		Elevated follicle-stimulating hormone (FSH)	
Diabetes mellitus		Autoimmune thyroiditis	
Cardiovascular	17-45	**Other**	
Coarctation of the aorta		Aortic dissection, myopia, deafness, hypertension, Crohn disease, cardiac conduction defects, chondrodysplasia of the distal radius (Madelung deformity)	
Hypoplastic left heart			
Bicuspid aortic valve			
Cystic medial necrosis of aorta			
Other: mitral valvular dysplasia, ventricular septal defect, anomalous pulmonary venous return		**Increased risk for neoplasia**	
		Melanocytic nevi, pilomatrixoma	
Genitourinary	>90	Gonadoblastoma (if portion of Y chromosome is present)	
Gonadal dysgenesis (streak gonads)		Central nervous system neoplasms	
Horseshoe kidney or other renal malformations	40		
Hypoplastic uterus			
Clitoral hypertrophy			
Central nervous system			
Mild cortical dysplasia			
Neuroglial heterotopia			
Hydrocephalus			
Limb			
Short 4th and 5th metacarpals	>50		
Other: narrow hyperconvex nails			
Ocular			
Cataracts			
Musculoskeletal			
Raised semilunar carpal bones	>60		
Inferior displacement of inner tibial growth			
Other: bone dysplasia with coarse trabeculae, scoliosis, spina bifida, vertebral fusion, cervical rib, abnormal sella turcica, dislocated hip			

[a]Data pooled from multiple references (55,93-99).

random in each cell of the inner cell mass. Therefore, each cell in a 46,XX embryo has an equal chance of inactivation of the paternally or maternally derived X chromosome. In embryos with three or more X chromosomes, most genes on all but one X chromosome are silenced. Although the dose-related effect of those genes that escape X inactivation appears to have little impact on the development of 47,XXX females, such effects are observed in males and females with gains of 3 or more X chromosomes. These individuals show cognitive impairment and mild dysmorphic features (Table 3-13). Klinefelter syndrome (47,XXY) has an incidence of approximately 1 in 1000 male births and is typically characterized in adulthood by tall stature, hypogonadism, and azoospermia. Children with Klinefelter syndrome are at increased risk for developmental delays (particularly in verbal skills including expressive language)

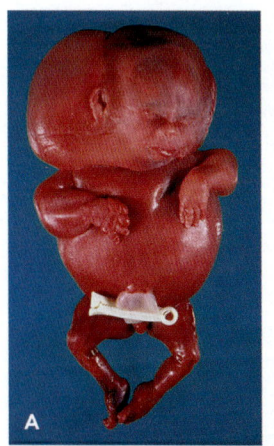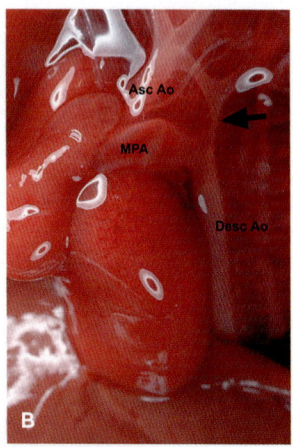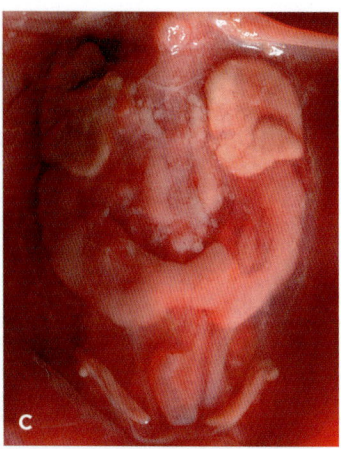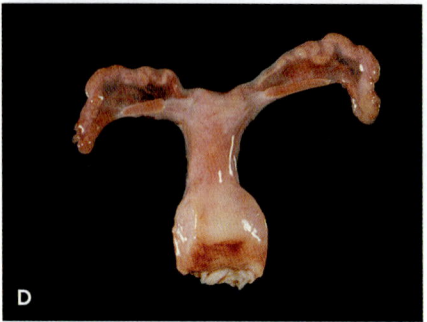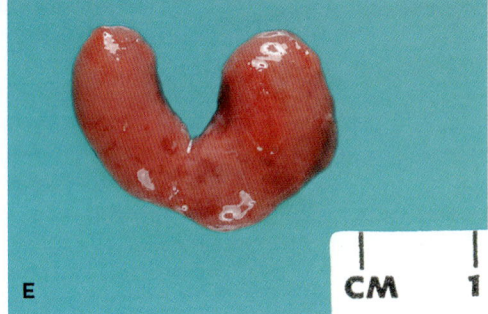

FIGURE 3-5 • 45,X. **A:** Fetus with massive cystic hygroma and hydrops. **B:** Left anterior oblique view of heart *in situ*; arrow indicates region of narrowing (coarctation) of the preductal aorta (Asc Ao, ascending aorta; MPA, main pulmonary artery; Desc Ao, descending aorta)—17 weeks. **C:** *In situ* view of low-set horseshoe kidneys and small but histologically normal ovaries—18 weeks. **D:** Streak ovaries in specimen from newborn; prominent cervix is normal for age. **E:** Small horseshoe kidney—17 weeks.

and behavioral problems (104,105), as well as other medical difficulties (106). The presence of an extra Y chromosome in males (47,XYY) confers mild language impairment, an increased incidence of autism spectrum disorders, and minor dysmorphic features (104,107,108).

Mosaicism

Mosaicism refers to the presence in an individual of more than one karyotypically distinct cell line derived from a single zygote. Usually, two cell populations are present, one with a normal chromosome complement and another with a numerical or structural abnormality. Occasionally, however, both cell lines are abnormal. The relative abundance of the two cell populations in different tissues may be highly variable within an individual. This variability may reflect the origin of a cytogenetic abnormality in a cell lineage with restricted embryologic fates and/or selective pressures that favor one of the cell lines. Because of variable tissue distributions and the possibility that the different cell lines may have different growth properties *in vitro*, cytogenetic analyses of peripheral blood lymphocytes cannot completely exclude mosaicism in other tissues. Evaluation of multiple tissues (skin, blood, placental villi, and/or amniocytes) and/or the use of more sensitive techniques such as FISH increase the likelihood of detecting mosaicism.

Mosaicism is a consequence of postzygotic mitotic errors that can occur at any stage of development. Empirical data suggest that such errors occur frequently in mitotically active cell populations (e.g., hematopoietic precursors) but that the majority of aneuploid cells are eliminated by unknown mechanisms (22). Mosaicism for a trisomic cell line can arise from a nondisjunction event occurring in a trisomic zygote ("trisomic rescue") or in a karyotypically normal zygote. Trisomic rescue, while returning a cell to diploidy, introduces the possibility of the development of uniparental disomy (UPD), in which both copies of a chromosome are inherited from a single parent (109,110). In trisomic rescue, one of the three copies of the trisomic chromosome is lost. As two of the three copies of this chromosome have come from one parent, approximately two-thirds of the time, such trisomic rescue events will result in loss of one of these two copies. In the other one-third of the time, however, the single chromosome inherited from the other parent will be lost, and both remaining copies of the chromosome will be from one parent. UPD is particularly important when the chromosome involved contains imprinted genes (genes differentially expressed based on the parent of origin), because expression of these genes will differ depending on the parental origin of the chromosome.

The phenotype of individuals with mosaicism is influenced by the percentages of each cell line in various tissues and is typically less severe than those with no evidence of mosaicism. If mosaicism arises in the cleavage-stage embryo, both aneuploid and diploid cell populations are likely to contribute to the embryonic (embryo, amnion) and extraembryonic lineages. Mitotic errors occurring later in development produce more restricted mosaicism that may be confined to either the fetus or placenta.

TABLE 3-13	SEX CHROMOSOME POLYSOMIES
Polysomy	Clinical/Pathologic Features[a]
47,XXX	Normal
47,XYY	Tall stature, hypertelorism, macroorchidism, infertility (oligospermia), mild language deficits, increased incidence of autism spectrum disorders, mild behavioral problems
47,XXY	*Klinefelter syndrome*: hypogonadism, hypogenitalism, infertility (testicular fibrosis), long limbs, gynecomastia, cognitive impairment (15%–20%), neoplasia (1%–2%) including breast cancer, leukemia/lymphoma, testicular tumors, and extragonadal germ cell tumors
48,XXXX	Cognitive impairment, mild facial anomalies, 5th finger clinodactyly
49,XXXXX	*Penta X syndrome*: microcephaly, cognitive impairment, small hands with 5th finger clinodactyly, abnormal facies, growth deficiency, patent ductus arteriosus
48,XXXY	Klinefelter syndrome with cognitive impairment, growth deficiency, radioulnar synostosis
48,XXYY	Klinefelter-like syndrome with higher incidence of cognitive impairment and behavioral abnormalities

[a]References (55,93,103).

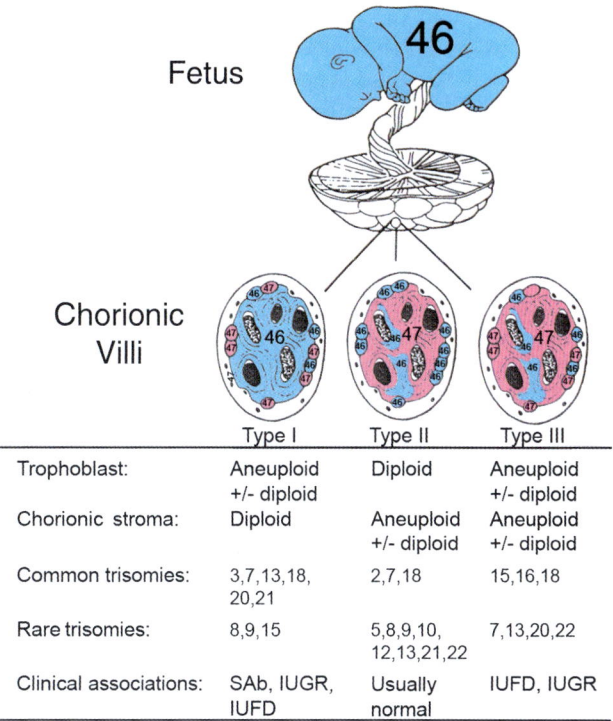

FIGURE 3-6 • Three types of CPM in which the fetus is diploid are distinguished based on whether aneuploidy cells are restricted to the trophoblast (type I), chorionic stroma (type II), or both trophoblast and chorionic stroma (type III). Trisomies commonly or rarely associated with each type and their clinical correlates are indicated in the table. (Modified from Tyson RW, Kalousek DK. Chromosomal abnormalities in stillbirth and neonatal death. In: Dimmick JE, Kalousek DK, eds. *Pathology of the Embryo and Fetus*. Philadelphia, PA: JB Lippincott; 1992, with permission.)

Confined Placental Mosaicism

Confined placental mosaicism (CPM), in which mosaicism is present in the placenta but not in the fetus, appears to be a relatively common phenomenon. Discrepant fetal and placental karyotypes have been observed in 0.5% to 2% of chorionic villus samples (9). CPM is subclassified into three types depending on whether the aneuploid population is confined to the trophoblast (type I), chorionic stroma (type II), or both cell lineages (type III) (111) (Figure 3-6). This distinction is significant because chorionic stromal cells, but not trophoblasts, replicate efficiently in cell culture. Therefore, type I CPM will not be detected by routine karyotype of cultured (indirect) preparations, although it can still be ascertained by analysis of uncultured (direct) cytotrophoblastic cells or by *in situ* methods (e.g., FISH) that evaluate specific chromosomes. Conversely, the "fetal" DNA detected in maternal serum in prenatal screening by cfDNA analysis is actually derived mainly from the trophoblast, rather than the fetus or the chorionic stroma. Hence, in type I and type III CPM, cfDNA screening may yield results that incorrectly suggest fetal aneuploidy, whereas type II CPM will not be detected by this method (82). Array-based CGH may be a more sensitive method of assessment, because it can detect all three types of CPM. Although it will not detect low-level mosaicism, it is thought that only those levels of mosaicism high enough to be detectable by a-CGH are likely to be clinically significant (112,113).

Prospective studies indicate that the vast majority of placentas with mosaicism detected by chorionic villus sampling early in gestation have no clinical significance (112). However, a small percentage of cases represent important causes of miscarriage, fetal growth restriction, intrauterine demise, and postnatal morbidity. Risks for each of these outcomes differ depending on the type of CPM (Figure 3-6). Some researchers recommend testing the placenta for CPM in cases of idiopathic fetal growth restriction (birth weight < 5th percentile) without obvious maternal, fetal, or placental causes (113).

An additional reason to test for CPM is to detect UPD, which can have significant clinical consequences depending on the chromosome involved. As noted above, UPD can arise from trisomic rescue, in which the trisomic complement is restored to a diploid complement, but both copies of the involved chromosome are derived from one parent (109,110). In CPM, the placenta retains some of the original aneuploid cell line, while the fetus has only diploid cells. The incidence of UPD in infants with CPM is low, but it may be useful to analyze placentas of idiopathic growth-restricted infants for this reason (109). SNP arrays and other specialized molecular genetic tests can be used to detect UPD, which cannot be detected by G-banding or FISH.

No specific gross or microscopic placental findings exist for CPM, although very few case series include these data. Maternal hypertension sometimes complicates CPM pregnancies and corresponding placental pathology can be present (19,109,113,114).

Polyploidy

Polyploidy refers to complete extra haploid sets of chromosomes, such as triploidy (69 chromosomes) or tetraploidy (96 chromosomes). Triploidy is common (1% of human embryos) and usually leads to spontaneous abortion between 7 and 17 weeks' gestation (115). Although the extra chromosomal set is more often of maternal (digynic) than paternal (diandric) origin, diandry may predominate in triploid early spontaneous abortions (116,117). Most, if not all, diandric triploid conceptions result from dispermic fertilization of a single oocyte (118,119). Digynic triploid conceptuses arise from errors in the first, or less often the second, meiotic division.

Most triploid embryos are spontaneously aborted (116,117,120–122) and those rare cases that do come to live birth generally die within a few hours (123). Diandric and digynic triploid conceptuses exhibit distinct phenotypes designated as type I and type II triploidy, respectively (124). Diandric fetuses that survive into the second trimester typically show growth ranging from normal to moderate symmetrical growth restriction, and partial molar transformation of their placentas, with large cystic villi and trophoblast hyperplasia (125). Survival of digynic embryos into the second and third trimesters is associated with severe asymmetrical growth restriction and small placentas that do not exhibit molar change. These phenotypic differences have been attributed to parental imprinting of genes that influence placental and fetal growth (122).

Common malformations observed in triploid fetuses include adrenal hypoplasia, syndactyly (particularly digits 3 and 4), hydrocephalus, and other defects (Table 3-14). Apart from partial mole formation, no specific malformations have been found to distinguish diandric versus digynic triploidy (125,129). Triploidy can be diagnosed by several methods, including flow cytometry, FISH, and G-banding.

Structural Chromosomal Abnormalities

The discussion thus far has focused on numerical abnormalities, that is, gain or loss of entire chromosomes. Structural abnormalities, in contrast, result in gain or loss of parts of chromosomes; common examples include deletions, duplications, and unbalanced translocations (Figure 3-7). Deletions, duplications, and inversions can arise via several mechanisms during gametogenesis, one of the most frequent of which is nonallelic homologous recombination (NAHR) (130–132). NAHR is mediated by repetitive DNA sequences, scattered throughout the genome, that are prone to recombination (133,134). Repetitive sequences on homologous chromosomes can misalign during meiosis. When crossing over events occur at these misaligned sequences, regions may be lost (deleted) from one chromosome and gained (duplicated) on its homologue (Figure 3-7). Sites in the genome that are rich in repetitive sequences are particularly prone to NAHR, leading to recurrent microdeletion and microduplication

TABLE 3-14	DIGYNIC VERSUS DIANDRIC TRIPLOIDY[a]	
	Digynic	Diandric
Fetus		
Growth	Asymmetric IUGR	Usually normal or symmetric IUGR
Craniofacial	Macrocephaly, hypertelorism, ventriculomegaly, low-set ears, microphthalmia, coloboma	Usually normal or microcephaly, ventriculomegaly
Cardiac	Normal, ventricular septal defect	Normal, ventricular septal defect
Extremities	Syndactyly between 3rd and 4th digits	Syndactyly between 3rd and 4th digits
Other	Adrenal hypoplasia, micropenis, renal malformations, pulmonary hypoplasia, Leydig cell hyperplasia	Adrenal hypoplasia, ambiguous genitalia
Placenta	Hypoplastic with no features of partial mole	Partial mole 　Edematous with cisternae in terminal villi 　Trophoblastic hyperplasia 　Scalloped villus contours
Common mechanism	Error in meiosis II	Fertilization of normal oocyte by two spermatozoa
Usual outcome	Spontaneous abortion or stillbirth	Spontaneous abortion or stillbirth

[a]References: (120,122,123,125–128).

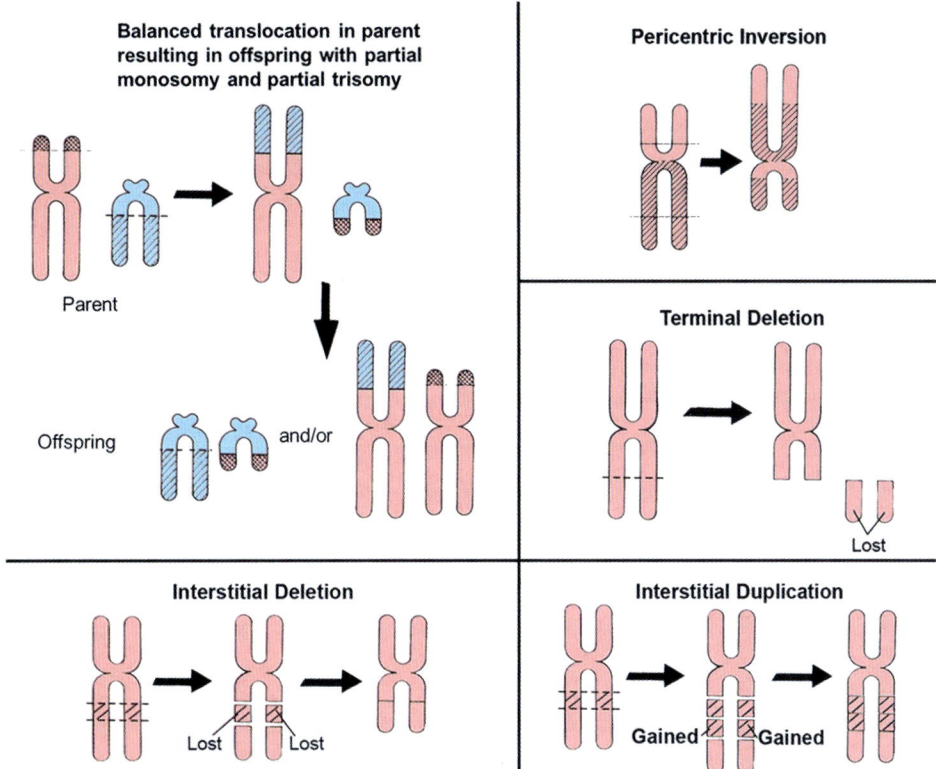

FIGURE 3-7 • Examples of chromosomal rearrangements.

syndromes, many of which have well-characterized phenotypic features (see Table 3-15). Several online databases catalog this information (see Table 3.2), and several recent review articles summarize syndromes associated with recurrent duplications and deletions (133,134). G-banding, FISH, and a-CGH findings in a representative case of a deletion are illustrated in Figure 3-8.

Translocations are another type of structural abnormality. Balanced reciprocal translocations result from an exchange of material between chromosomes with no accompanying gain or loss of genetic material. Although individuals who carry balanced translocations are not expected to manifest phenotypic findings (barring microdeletion, microduplication, or gene disruption at the translocation breakpoints), they are at increased risk for transmitting the translocation to their offspring in unbalanced form. In such cases, the offspring will inherit only one of the abnormal (derivative) chromosomes involved in the translocation and will thus have partial monosomy and partial trisomy for portions of the involved chromosomes (Figure 3-7). Therefore, when an unbalanced translocation is identified in a fetus, parental cytogenetic testing is recommended to determine whether the mother or father carries the translocation in balanced form. Such information greatly impacts genetic counseling, as there is an increased risk in future pregnancies for fetal demise or for liveborn children with congenital abnormalities.

Robertsonian translocations are a special type of translocation that result from fusion at the centromere of two acrocentric chromosomes (13, 14, 15, 21, or 22) with resultant loss of their short arms. (Because the acrocentric short arms are highly repetitive regions encoding no critical genes, loss of one or more copies is of no clinical significance). Carriers of such translocations have one normal copy of each of the acrocentric chromosomes involved, as well as the Robertsonian translocation. Because they possess two copies of each of the involved chromosomes, carriers of a Robertsonian translocation usually have a normal phenotype. However, their offspring are at risk for aneuploidy. If, during meiosis, one of the normal homologs segregates into a gamete along with the Robertsonian translocation, the resulting gamete will have two copies of that chromosome, which, after fertilization, results in trisomy.

Submicroscopic Abnormalities

Loss or gain of chromosomal material less than 3 to 5 Mb cannot be readily visualized by G-banding but can be detected by a-CGH and FISH. Several well-characterized microdeletion and microduplication syndromes relevant to fetal and pediatric medicine are listed in Table 3-15. The 22q11.2 microdeletion/microduplication syndrome, one of the most important of such disorders in pediatric pathology, is discussed in greater detail below.

Velocardiofacial/DiGeorge Syndrome

VCF/DiGeorge syndrome (also referred to as the 22q11.2 deletion syndrome) is an autosomal dominant disorder with variable penetrance and expressivity. Velocardiofacial and

TABLE 3-15 SELECTED STRUCTURAL AND SUBMICROSCOPIC CHROMOSOMAL ANOMALIES

Syndrome or Disorder	Genetic Locus (Affected Gene(s))	Clinical Findings
Velocardiofacial syndrome (VCFS)/DiGeorge	22q11.2 (*TBX1* and contiguous genes)	Conotruncal heart abnormalities, palatal insufficiency, learning difficulty, distinctive facies, hypoparathyroidism, T-cell defect
X-linked congenital adrenal hypoplasia/glycerol kinase deficiency/Duchenne myopathy	Xp21 (*DAX1, GK, DMD*)	Adrenal insufficiency, hyperglycerolemia, myopathy
Tuberous sclerosis/autosomal dominant polycystic kidney disease	16p13 (*TSC2, PKD1*)	Tuberous sclerosis, polycystic kidney disease, congenital hepatic fibrosis
Maturity-onset diabetes of the young type 5	17q12 (*TCF2*)	Glomerulocystic kidney disease, renal hypoplasia and other renal abnormalities, genital tract abnormalities, diabetes
WAGR	11p13.3 (*PAX6, D11S2163, PER, WT1*)	Wilms tumor, aniridia, genitourinary abnormalities, cognitive impairment
Smith-Magenis	17p11.2 (*RAI1*)	Failure to thrive, feeding difficulties, hypotonia, cognitive impairment, behavioral abnormalities
Rubinstein-Taybi	16p13.3 (*CBP*)	Distinctive facial features, broad thumbs and great toes, short stature, cognitive impairment
Alagille	20p12 (*JAG1*)	Cholestasis with liver bile duct paucity, pulmonary artery abnormalities, posterior embryotoxon, butterfly vertebrae, distinct facial features
Williams	7q11.23 (*ELN* + >20 contiguous genes)	Peripheral pulmonary stenosis, supravalvular aortic stenosis, connective tissue abnormalities, mild intellectual disability, growth and endocrine abnormalities
Prader-Willi/Angelman	15q11-13 (*SNURF-SNRPN* and contiguous genes)	Prader-Willi: Severe hypotonia, cognitive impairment, hyperphagia, and obesity
		Angelman: Severe cognitive impairment, ataxia, seizures
Miller-Dieker	17p13.3 (*LIS1* and contiguous genes)	Lissencephaly, seizures, severe developmental and neurologic abnormalities, distinctive facial features
Monosomy 1p36	1p36 (*KIAA1273* and contiguous genes)	Cognitive impairment, hypotonia, seizures, structural brain abnormalities, distinctive facial features
Microduplication 22q11.2	22q11.2 (same as VCFS/DiGeorge)	Variable features: normal to mildly impaired cognition, growth retardation, non-conotruncal heart defects, velopharyngeal insufficiency
Hereditary neuropathy with liability to pressure palsies (HNPP)	17p11.2 (*PMP22*; same as CMT1A)	Pressure neuropathies, usually presenting in adolescence or early adulthood
Charcot-Marie-Tooth 1A (CMT1A)	17p11.2 (*PMP22*; same as HNPP)	Slowly progressive demyelinating peripheral neuropathy with distal muscle weakness, atrophy, and sensory loss
Wolf-Hirschhorn	4p16.3 (*WHSC1, LETM1, MSX1*)	Fetal growth restriction, microcephaly, hypotonia, seizures, "Greek warrior helmet" facies
Cri du chat syndrome	5p15.2 (*CTNND2* and contiguous genes)	Fetal growth restriction, catlike cry, cognitive impairment, hypotonia, microcephaly, abnormal facies, cardiac malformation
Cat eye syndrome	tetrasomy 22q11.2	Iris coloboma, mild cognitive impairment, hypertelorism, preauricular skin tags or pits

References: (93,135–152).

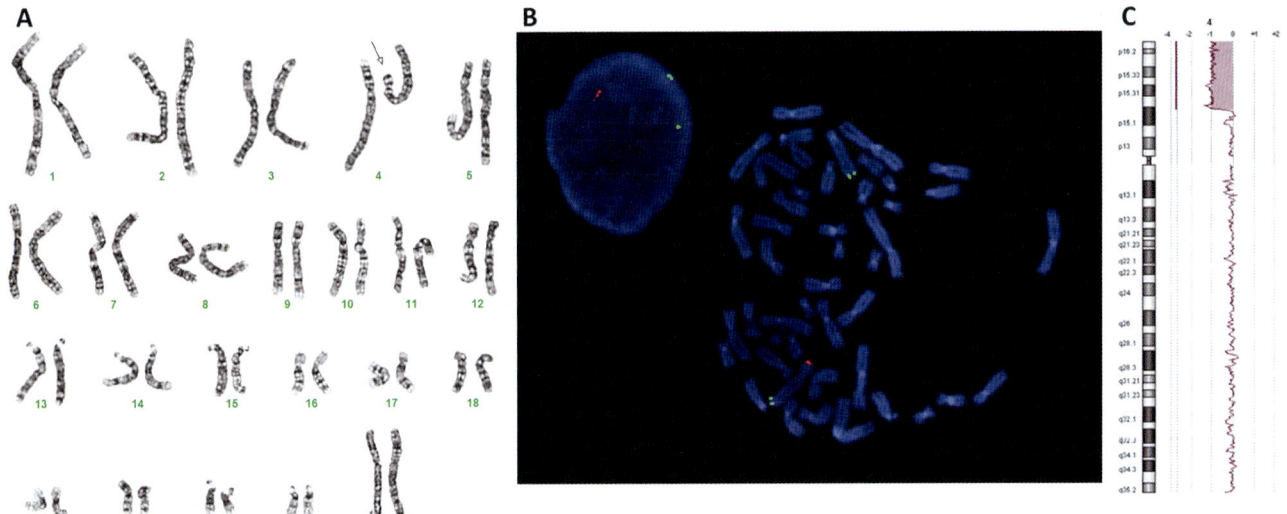

FIGURE 3-8 • Deletion of the distal short arm of a chromosome 4. **A:** The ISCN designation of this G-banded karyotype is 46,XX,del(4)(p15.1). An arrow designates the abnormal chromosome 4. **B:** FISH using a Cytocell (Cambridge, UK) probe to the Wolf-Hirschhorn syndrome critical region in 4p16.3 (*red*) and a control locus to the 4q telomere (*green*). The metaphase cell shows two copies of chromosome 4: both hybridize to the 4q telomere probe, but only one hybridizes to the 4p16.3 probe, indicating a deletion on the other #4 homolog. **C:** Oligonucleotide a-CGH showed that the deletion of 4p is approximately 29 Mb and includes over 140 genes.

DiGeorge syndromes are clinical entities that share many pathogenic and phenotypic features (153–159). Typical craniofacial abnormalities include palatal insufficiency and clefts. Cardiac malformations usually involve the conotruncal region (truncus arteriosus, tetralogy of Fallot, interrupted aortic arch, ventricular septal defect, or others); these can also be isolated findings in 22q11.2 deletion. In addition to these common elements, individuals with DiGeorge syndrome classically exhibit agenesis or hypoplasia of the thymus and parathyroid glands, resulting in T-cell defects and hypocalcemia (153).

The VCF/DiGeorge syndrome critical region (DGCR) is a 2.5-Mb segment in 22q11.2 that is deleted in 90% of patients. Due to the small size of this deletion, deletions may or may not be detectable by G-banding, but FISH using probes to the DiGeorge critical region can confirm the presence of the deletion. Additionally, because the phenotypic spectrum of this syndrome can be highly variable, the 22q11.2 deletion is often detected by microarray analysis performed as part of the genetic evaluation of the patient. The DGCR contains more than 20 genes, of which *TBX1* appears to be responsible for most of the DiGeorge phenotype (154,160). *TBX1* encodes a transcription factor that is expressed in embryonic pharyngeal arch mesoderm and the cardiac outflow tracts. A subset of patients with clinical VCF or DiGeorge syndrome and no 22q11.2 deletion detectable by FISH have *TBX1* point mutations (161), and in mouse models, disruption of the *TBX1* homologue is associated with conotruncal cardiac defects (160).

For every case of microdeletion arising via NAHR, there should be a corresponding microduplication. The widespread use of genomic techniques has identified such duplications and in some cases has identified a constellation of phenotypic findings sufficiently different than the corresponding deletion as to be considered a distinct syndrome. In other cases, however, deletions and duplications of the same region may share a number of common phenotypic findings. For example, duplication of 22q11.2 results in a variable clinical spectrum that can include velopharyngeal insufficiency, intellectual disability, mildly dysmorphic facial features, and occasional nonconotruncal congenital heart defects (162–164).

Chromosomal Instability Disorders

Several syndromes and diseases are due in part to chromosomal instability, usually resulting from defects in DNA repair. These genetic syndromes are characterized by congenital malformations, cytopenias, and/or cancer predisposition. Diagnosis has until recently required specialized laboratory techniques, including special cell culture and staining conditions with appropriate controls. However, mutational analysis of specific genes (see Table 3-16) has now replaced cytogenetic studies for many of these disorders.

Fanconi anemia (FA) is a chromosomal instability disorder characterized by pancytopenia, poor fetal and postnatal growth, and high incidence of congenital malformations (Figure 3-9) that overlap with the anomalies of the VACTERL (*v*ertebral–*a*norectal–*c*ardiac–*t*racheo*e*sophageal–*r*enal–*l*imb) association, especially radial ray abnormalities (170). Because of this phenotypic overlap, some authors have recommended testing for FA in any individual with radial ray abnormalities (171,172) or other findings in the VACTERL association (173).

Mutations in at least 15 different genes have been implicated in FA, predominantly encoding proteins that mediate

TABLE 3-16	CYTOGENETICS AND MOLECULAR GENETICS OF SELECTED CHROMOSOMAL INSTABILITY SYNDROMES			
Syndrome	Clinical Features	Cytogenetic Finding	Genetic Defect(s)	Comment
Fanconi anemia (FA)	Variable presentation, including 25%–40% of patients with no physical abnormalities. Pancytopenia, poor fetal and postnatal growth, abnormal skin pigmentation, radial ray defects, VACTERL-like malformations, increased cancer risk (AR)	Increased chromosomal breakage after exposure to a clastogenic agent	FANCA, FANCB, FANCC, BRCA2, FANCD2, FANCE, FANCF, FANCG, FANCI, BRIP1, FANCL, FANCM, RAD51C, SLX4, PALB2	Mutations in at least 15 different genes (complementation groups) can cause Fanconi anemia. Molecular genetic testing is available, but DNA breakage studies remain the most common diagnostic method. Somatic cell hybridization or gene complementation techniques can be used to target DNA testing.
Robert-SC (R-SC)	Symmetric limb reduction defects, IUGR, cleft lip/palate, other craniofacial malformations, mental retardation (AR)	Repulsion of heterochromatic regions near centromeres ("puffing") and delayed progression through metaphase ("anaphase lag")	ESCO2	
Nijmegen breakage (NB)	Characteristic facies, microcephaly, immunodeficiency, growth retardation, radiosensitivity, increased cancer risk (AR)	Increased chromosomal breakage with normal culture or after exposure to a clastogenic agent	NBS1	Nijmegen breakage syndrome is observed primarily in patients of Slavic descent due to the founder effect of a single mutation. NBS1, FANCD2, and ATM may interact with one another.
Fragile X (FRAX)	Macrocephaly, large testes, cognitive impairment (X-linked)	Chromosome breakage at Xq27.3 induced by one of several culture methods; G-banding now performed only to rule out another etiology.	FMR1	Clinical disease is associated with expansion of a trinucleotide repeat (>200 repeats) in the 5′-untranslated region of exon 1. Molecular genetic testing has replaced cytogenetic testing.
Ataxia-telangiectasia (AT)	Ataxia, telangiectasia, dysarthria, abnormal ocular movements, recurrent infections, increased cancer risk (AR)	Radiation-induced nonrandom rearrangements of chromosomes 7 and 14	ATM	AT-like disorders have been described due to mutations in other genes (e.g., MRE11).

AR, autosomal recessive; IUGR, intrauterine growth restriction; VACTERL, *v*ertebral–*a*norectal–*c*ardiac–*t*racheoesophageal–*r*enal–*l*imb malformation association.
References: (165–169).

DNA repair (Table 3-16); approximately 60% to 70% of cases are caused by mutations in the *FANCA* gene (165,174–177). Because diagnosis of FA by mutational analysis is complicated by the large number of causative genes and the possibility that the patient's disease is caused by an unidentified gene mutation, the gold standard continues to be cytogenetic analysis of patient cells that have been cultured in the presence of clastogenic agents that induce DNA breakage. Interpretation of this test is complex and requires experience with chromosomal rearrangements typical of FA, as well as robust control ranges for normal and elevated rates of chromosomal breakage.

Epigenetic Chromosomal Modifications and Associated Disorders

A large and growing number of diseases are now known to result from epigenetic chromosomal modifications, that is, changes to the DNA (e.g., methylation) or associated proteins

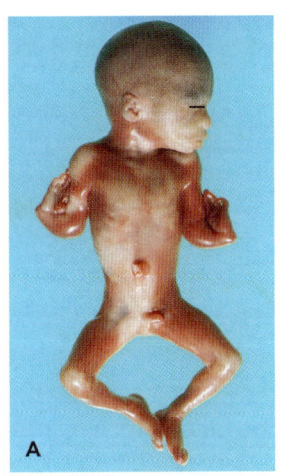 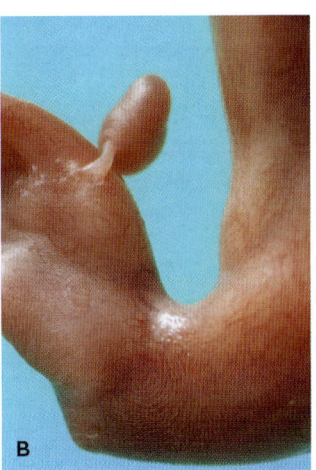 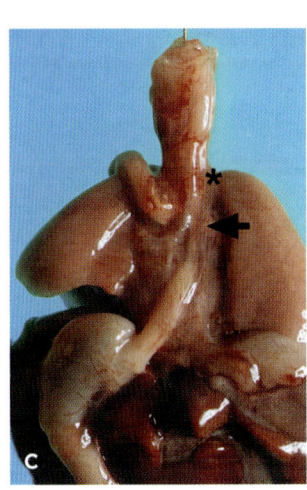

FIGURE 3-9 • Fanconi anemia. **A:** Fetus with bilateral radial aplasia. **B:** Close view of right arm and hand, showing marked deviation of wrist, secondary to radial aplasia, and tiny remnant of thumb. **C:** Posterior view of viscera, showing proximal atresia of esophagus (*asterisk*) with distal tracheoesophageal fistula (*arrow*). Thoracic aorta is reflected to left.

and RNAs that influence gene expression without altering the genetic sequence. A recent review summarizes current knowledge about mechanisms of epigenetic chromosomal modification (178). Epigenetic modifications differ among individuals, cell types, and maternally versus paternally derived chromosomes and can be influenced by environmental stimuli including circadian rhythms, nutritional status, and other factors (179,180). Because they do not change chromosomal structure or DNA sequence, epigenetic modifications cannot be detected by G-banding, FISH, or microarray, although DNA methylation can be identified using specialized laboratory methods (178). In DNA methylation, cytosine bases are covalently modified by methyl groups, a reversible process that modulates local gene expression, usually in an inhibitory way (178). X chromosome inactivation, discussed above, is an example of gene silencing, mediated by high levels of cytosine methylation. The molecular basis for X chromosome inactivation has been partially elucidated (181), but the mechanisms that regulate epigenetic modification of many autosomal genes remain poorly understood. However, a growing body of literature suggests that epigenetic modifications can be inherited and can influence risk for type 2 diabetes, cardiovascular disease, and obesity (178).

Imprinting is another mechanism of epigenetic modification. As discussed above, imprinting refers to the differential expression of genes based on their parental origin (182–188). During meiosis, imprinted regions are marked as being maternally or paternally derived. Imprinting generally involves clusters of closely spaced genes known as imprinting domains, which are regulated by discrete DNA elements termed imprinting centers. Imprinting centers are themselves regulated by differential methylation and histone modification (178). Conditions due to abnormalities of imprinting arise from altered expression of genes in the imprinted region. For example, Prader-Willi and Angelman syndromes result from differential imprinting in the same region of chromosome 15 (189–191). Prader-Willi syndrome results from absence of expression of genes normally expressed from the 15q11.2-q13 region of the paternal chromosome 15; this can be due to a microdeletion of paternal chromosome 15q11.2-13 and maternal UPD 15 or a defect in the imprinting process itself (144,192). Conversely, Angelman syndrome results from absence of expression of genes normally expressed from the same region of the maternal chromosome 15, which can be due to microdeletion of the maternal chromosome 15 or paternal UPD 15 (145,193–196).

The *IGF2/H29* locus in 11p15 is another imprinted region. Abnormal imprinting at this locus has been associated with Beckwith-Wiedemann syndrome and Russell-Silver syndrome (197–199). Paternal imprinting is associated with methylation of the *IGF2/H19* imprinting center, expression of *IGF2*, and silencing of *H19*, whereas the reverse methylation and expression patterns occur for the maternal allele. In a subset of patients with Beckwith-Wiedemann syndrome, *IGF2* is overexpressed due to either paternal UPD of 11p15 (replacement of the maternal locus by a paternal locus) or loss of imprinting (activation of the normally silent maternal locus) (200–203). In Russell-Silver syndrome, a subset of patients have hypomethylation of the paternal *IGF2/H19* imprinting center, leading to reduced expression of *IGF2* (204–207). Other pediatric disorders associated with imprinting aberrations are listed in Table 3-17.

Diseases of imprinting, particularly Beckwith-Wiedemann syndrome, appear to be more common among individuals conceived by assisted reproductive technology (ART), including ovarian stimulation, *in vitro* oocyte maturation, and *in vitro* fertilization (188,208–214). It is unclear whether this is because ART causes abnormal imprinting in the embryo or whether infertile individuals are themselves more likely to have abnormal patterns of imprinting they pass to their offspring. It is also not known if less obvious epigenetic alterations may exist at greater frequencies in individuals conceived by ART (215,216).

Future Directions

Advances in genomic technologies now permit detection of abnormalities undetectable by routine G-banding analysis. Array CGH has supplanted the G-banded karyotype as a first-line investigation for cytogenetic defects in the evaluation of patients with developmental delay (9,10) and is

TABLE 3-17 PEDIATRIC IMPRINTING DISORDERS

Disorder or Syndrome	Chromosomal Locus [Affected Gene(s)]	Phenotypic Features
Beckwith-Wiedemann	11p15.5 (*IGF2, H19, KCNQ1,* and others)	Macrosomia, large tongue, hemihypertrophy, omphalocele, ear pits, adrenocytomegaly, placental mesenchymal dysplasia, neoplasia (Wilms tumor, hepatoblastoma)
Pseudohypoparathyroidism/Albright hereditary osteodystrophy	20q13 (*GNAS*)	Developmental delay, cognitive impairment, obesity, short stature, ± hypocalcemia
Prader-Willi	15q11.2 (*MKRN3, MAGEL2, NDN,* and others)	Cognitive impairment, obesity, short stature, behavioral problems
Angelman	15q12 (*UBE3A, ATPC10C*)	Cognitive impairment, dysmorphic facies, behavioral and speech problems, ataxic gait
Transient neonatal diabetes mellitus	6q24 (*PLAGL1*)	Growth retardation, low fetal/infantile insulin levels
Russell-Silver syndrome	7p11.2 11p15.5 (*H19, IGF2*)	Short stature, asymmetric skull, triangular facies, 5th finger clinodactyly

becoming much more widely used in the evaluation of fetal loss (11,217–220). The advent of cfDNA testing now permits sensitive, noninvasive screening for cytogenetic abnormalities by a simple blood test, often obviating the need for invasive prenatal testing. When such invasive testing is performed, however, microarrays permit a higher level of resolution than currently afforded by G-banding or FISH; microarray testing in this setting is now offered in many clinical laboratories. With the development of next-generation sequencing technology, whole-exome and whole genome sequencing will likely augment or even supplant these techniques in at least some clinical situations, adding a new level of sensitivity for detecting genetic abnormalities down to single base pair alterations and further blurring the distinction between cytogenetics and molecular genetics. However, as in the past, the ability to correlate genotypic findings with phenotypic manifestations will be crucial in providing diagnostic and prognostic information to clinicians, patients, and families. Therefore, continued attention to accurate and comprehensive anatomic pathology, including pathology of the embryo and fetus, will be vital to the evolution of this field.

References

1. Braoudaki M, Tzortzatou-Stathopoulou F. Clinical cytogenetics in pediatric acute leukemia: an update. *Clin Lymphoma Myeloma Leuk* 2012;12(4):230–237.
2. Bovée JVMG, Hogendoorn PCW. Molecular pathology of sarcomas: concepts and clinical implications. *Virchows Arch* 2010;456(2):193–199. doi:10.1007/s00428-009-0828-5.
3. Romeo S, Dei Tos AP, Hogendoorn PCW. The clinical impact of molecular techniques on diagnostic pathology of soft tissue and bone tumours. *Diagn Histopathol* 2012;18(2):81–85.
4. Schapira AH V. Mitochondrial diseases. *Lancet* 2012;379(9828):1825–1834.
5. Patel P, Farley J, Impey L, et al. Evaluation of a fetomaternal-surgical clinic for prenatal counselling of surgical anomalies. *Pediatr Surg Int* 2008;24(4):391–394.
6. Shaffer L, McGowan-Jordan J, Schmid M, eds. *ISCN (2013): An International System for Human Cytogenetic Nomenclature*. Basel, Switzerland: S. Karger; 2013.
7. Park J, Oh Y, Chung KC. Two key genes closely implicated with the neuropathological characteristics in Down syndrome: DYRK1A and RCAN1. *BMB Rep* 2009;42(1):6–15.
8. Chervenak F, Isaacson G, Blakemore K. Fetal cystic hygroma. Cause and natural history. *N Engl J Med* 1983;309:822–825.
9. Miller DT, Adam MP, Aradhya S, et al. Consensus statement: chromosomal microarray is a first-tier clinical diagnostic test for individuals with developmental disabilities or congenital anomalies. *Am J Hum Genet* 2010;86(5):749–764.
10. Battaglia A, Doccini V, Bernardini L, et al. Confirmation of chromosomal microarray as a first-tier clinical diagnostic test for individuals with developmental delay, intellectual disability, autism spectrum disorders and dysmorphic features. *Eur J Paediatr Neurol* 2013;17:589–599.
11. Hillman SC, McMullan DJ, Hall G, et al. Use of prenatal chromosomal microarray: prospective cohort study and systematic review and meta-analysis. *Ultrasound Obstet Gynecol* 2013;41(6):610–620.
12. Dhillon RK, Hillman SC, Morris RK, et al. Additional information from chromosomal microarray analysis (CMA) over conventional karyotyping when diagnosing chromosomal abnormalities in miscarriage: a systematic review and meta-analysis. *BJOG* 2014;121(1):11–21.
13. Hassold T, Hunt P. To err (meiotically) is human: the genesis of human aneuploidy. *Nat Rev Genet* 2001;2:280–291.
14. Helali N, Iafolla AK, Kahler SG, et al. A case of duplication of 13q32->qter and deletion of 18p11.32->pter with mild phenotype: Patau syndrome and duplications of 13q revisited. *J Med Genet* 1996;33:600–602.
15. Bronsteen R, Lee W, Vettraino IM, et al. Second-trimester sonography and trisomy 18. *J Ultrasound Med* 2004;23(2):233–240.
16. Kjaer I, Keeling JW, Fischer Hansen B. Pattern of malformations in the axial skeleton in human trisomy 13 fetuses. *Am J Med Genet* 1997;70(4):421–426.
17. Nakamura Y, Hashimoto T, Sasaguri Y, et al. Brain anomalies found in 18 trisomy: CT scanning, morphologic and morphometric study. *Clin Neuropathol* 1986;5(2):47–52.
18. Bejjani BA, Shaffer LG. Application of array-based comparative genomic hybridization to clinical diagnostics. *J Mol Diagn* 2006;8(5):528–533.
19. Kalousek DK, Langlois S, Barrett I, et al. Uniparental disomy for chromosome 16 in humans. *Am J Hum Genet* 1993;52:8–16.
20. Machin GA, Crolla JA. Chromosome constitution of 500 infants dying during the perinatal period. With an appendix concerning other genetic

disorders among these infants. *Humangenetik* 1974;23(3):183–198.
21. Baldwin V, Kalousek D, Dimmick J. Diagnostic pathologic investigation of the malformed conceptus. *Perspect Pediatr Pathol* 1982;7:65–108.
22. Cimini D, Degrassi F. Aneuploidy: a matter of bad connections. *Trends Cell Biol* 2005;15:442–451.
23. Oliver TR, Feingold E, Yu K, et al. New insights into human nondisjunction of chromosome 21 in oocytes. *PLoS Genet* 2008;4(3):e1000033.
24. Sherman SL, Freeman SB, Allen EG, et al. Risk factors for nondisjunction of trisomy 21. *Cytogenet Genome Res* 2005;111(3–4):273–280.
25. Gardner R, Sutherland G, Shaffer L. *Chromosome Abnormalities and Genetic Counseling*. Oxford University Press: New York City, NY 4th ed.; 2012.
26. Bielanska M, Tan SL, Ao A. Chromosomal mosaicism throughout human preimplantation development in vitro: incidence, type, and relevance to embryo outcome. *Hum Reprod* 2002;17:413–419.
27. Robinson WP, Mcfadden DE, Stephenson MD. The origin of abnormalities in recurrent aneuploidy/polyploidy. *Am J Hum Genet* 2001;69: 1245–1254.
28. McFadden D, Friedman J. Chromosome abnormalities in human beings. *Mutat Res* 1997;396:129–140.
29. Nicolaidis P, Petersen M. Origin and mechanisms of non-disjunction in human autosomal trisomies. *Hum Reprod* 1998;13:313–319.
30. Roeder GS. Meiotic chromosomes: it takes two to tango. *Genes Dev* 1997;11:2600–2621.
31. Reeves RH, Baxter LL, Richtsmeier JT. Too much of a good thing: mechanisms of gene action in Down syndrome. *Trends Genet* 2001; 17(2):83–88.
32. Hong D, Kent J, Kesler S. Cognitive profile of Turner syndrome. *Dev Disabil Res Rev* 2009;15:270–278.
33. Van der Putte S. Lymphatic malformation in human fetuses. A study of fetuses with Turner's syndrome or status Bonnevie-Ullrich. *Virchows Arch A Pathol Anat Histol* 1977;376:233–246.
34. Abbag FI. Congenital heart diseases and other major anomalies in patients with Down syndrome. *Saudi Med J* 2006;27(2):219–222.
35. Douglas SD. Down syndrome: immunologic and epidemiologic associations-enigmas remain. *J Pediatr* 2005;147(6):723–725.
36. Goldacre MJ, Wotton CJ, Seagroatt V, et al. Cancers and immune related diseases associated with Down's syndrome: a record linkage study. *Arch Dis Child* 2004;89(11):1014–1017.
37. Haargaard B, Fledelius HC. Down's syndrome and early cataract. *Br J Ophthalmol* 2006;90(8):1024–1027.
38. Head E, Lott IT. Down syndrome and beta-amyloid deposition. *Curr Opin Neurol* 2004;17(2):95–100.
39. Källén B, Mastroiacovo P, Robert E. Major congenital malformations in Down syndrome. *Am J Med Genet* 1996;65(2):160–166.
40. Kava MP, Tullu MS, Muranjan MN, et al. Down syndrome: clinical profile from India. *Arch Med Res* 2004;35(1):31–35.
41. Málaga S, Pardo R, Málaga I, et al. Renal involvement in Down syndrome. *Pediatr Nephrol* 2005;20(5):614–617.
42. Massey G V, Zipursky A, Chang MN, et al. A prospective study of the natural history of transient leukemia (TL) in neonates with Down syndrome (DS): Children's Oncology Group (COG) study POG-9481. *Blood* 2006;107(12):4606–4613.
43. Milbrandt TA, Johnston CE. Down syndrome and scoliosis: a review of a 50-year experience at one institution. *Spine (Phila Pa 1976)* 2005;30(18):2051–2055.
44. Papp C, Bán Z, Szigeti Z, et al. Prenatal sonographic findings in 207 fetuses with trisomy 21. *Eur J Obstet Gynecol Reprod Biol* 2007; 133(2):186–190.
45. Schepis C, Barone C, Siragusa M, et al. An updated survey on skin conditions in Down syndrome. *Dermatology* 2002;205(3):234–238.
46. Shott SR. Down syndrome: common otolaryngologic manifestations. *Am J Med Genet C Semin Med Genet* 2006;142C(3):131–140.
47. Torfs CP, Christianson RE. Anomalies in Down syndrome individuals in a large population-based registry. *Am J Med Genet.* 1998;77(5): 431–438.
48. Uibo O, Teesalu K, Metskula K, et al. Screening for celiac disease in Down's syndrome patients revealed cases of subtotal villous atrophy without typical for celiac disease HLA-DQ and tissue transglutaminase antibodies. *World J Gastroenterol* 2006;12(9):1430–1434.
49. Vachon L, Fareau GE, Wilson MG, et al. Testicular microlithiasis in patients with Down syndrome. *J Pediatr* 2006;149(2):233–236.
50. Yokoyama T, Tamura H, Tsukamoto H, et al. Prevalence of glaucoma in adults with Down's syndrome. *Jpn J Ophthalmol* 2006;50(3):274–276.
51. Yurdakul NS, Ugurlu S, Maden A. Strabismus in Down syndrome. *J Pediatr Ophthalmol Strabismus* 2006;43(1):27–30.
52. Gilbert-Barness E, Opitz JM. Chromosome abnormalities. In: Stocker J, Dehner L, eds. *Pediatric Pathology*. Philadelphia, PA: J.B. Lippincott; 1992:41–71.
53. Chen C-P. Congenital heart defects associated with fetal trisomy 18. *Prenat Diagn* 2006;26(5):483–485.
54. Donaldson SJ, Wright CA, de Ravel TJ. Trisomy 18 with total craniorachischisis and thoraco-abdominoschisis. *Prenat Diagn* 1999;19(6): 580–582.
55. Gilbert EF, Opitz JM. Developmental and other pathologic changes in syndromes caused by chromosome abnormalities. *Perspect Pediatr Pathol* 1982;7:1–63.
56. Kinoshita M, Nakamura Y, Nakano R, et al. Thirty-one autopsy cases of trisomy 18: clinical features and pathological findings. *Pediatr Pathol* 1989;9(4):445–457.
57. Makrydimas G, Papanikolaou E, Paraskevaidis E, et al. Upper limb abnormalities as an isolated ultrasonographic finding in early detection of trisomy 18. A case report. *Fetal Diagn Ther* 2003;18(6):401–403.
58. Nyberg DA, Kramer D, Resta RG, et al. Prenatal sonographic findings of trisomy 18: review of 47 cases. *J Ultrasound Med* 1993;12(2): 103–113.
59. Shaw S-W, Cheng P-J, Chueh H-Y, et al. Ectopia cordis in a fetus with trisomy 18. *J Clin Ultrasound* 2006;34(2):95–98.
60. Siebert JR. CNS manifestations of chromosomal change. In: Golden JA, Harding BN, eds. *Developmental Neuropathology*. 1st ed. Basel, Switzerland: International Society of Neuropathology; 2004:132–141.
61. Warkany J. *Congenital Malformations*. Chicago, IL: Year Book Medical Publishers; 1974:1309.
62. Yeo L, Guzman ER, Day-Salvatore D, et al. Prenatal detection of fetal trisomy 18 through abnormal sonographic features. *J Ultrasound Med* 2003;22(6):581–590.
63. Fujinaga M, Shepard TH, Fitzsimmons J. Trisomy 13 in the fetus. *Teratology* 1990;41(2):233–238.
64. Lehman CD, Nyberg DA, Winter TC, et al. Trisomy 13 syndrome: prenatal US findings in a review of 33 cases. *Radiology* 1995;194(1): 217–222.
65. Rachidi M, Lopes C. Mental retardation in Down syndrome: from gene dosage imbalance to molecular and cellular mechanisms. *Neurosci Res* 2007;59(4):349–369.
66. Boghosian-Sell L, Mewar R, Harrison W, et al. Molecular mapping of the Edwards syndrome phenotype to two noncontiguous regions on chromosome 18. *Am J Hum Genet* 1994;55(3):476–483.
67. Baty B, Blackburn B, Carey J. Natural history of trisomy 18 and trisomy 13: I. Growth, physical assessment, medical histories, survival, and recurrence risk. *Am J Med Genet* 1994;49:175–188.
68. Bittles AH, Bower C, Hussain R, et al. The four ages of Down syndrome. *Eur J Public Health* 2007;17(2):221–225.
69. Embleton ND, Wyllie JP, Wright MJ, et al. Natural history of trisomy 18. *Arch Dis Child Fetal Neonatal Ed* 1996;75(1):F38–F41.
70. Hook EB, Topol BB, Cross PK. The natural history of cytogenetically abnormal fetuses detected at midtrimester amniocentesis which are not terminated electively: new data and estimates of the excess and relative risk of late fetal death associated with 47,+21 and some other abnormal karyotypes. *Am J Hum Genet* 1989;45(6):855–861.
71. Kalousek DK, Lau AE. Pathology of spontaneous abortion. In: Dimmick JE, Kalousek DK, eds. *Developmental Pathology of the Embryo and Fetus*. Philadelphia, PA: J.B. Lippincott; 1992:55–82.

72. Morris JK, Wald NJ, Watt HC. Fetal loss in Down syndrome pregnancies. *Prenat Diagn* 1999;19(2):142–145.
73. Oyelese Y, Vintzileos AM. Is second-trimester genetic amniocentesis for trisomy 18 ever indicated in the presence of a normal genetic sonogram? *Ultrasound Obstet Gynecol* 2005;26(7):691–694.
74. Rosen T, D'Alton ME. Down syndrome screening in the first and second trimesters: what do the data show? *Semin Perinatol* 2005;29(6):367–375.
75. Spencer K, Heath V, Flack N, et al. First trimester maternal serum AFP and total hCG in aneuploidies other than trisomy 21. *Prenat Diagn* 2000;20(8):635–639.
76. Won RH, Currier RJ, Lorey F, et al. The timing of demise in fetuses with trisomy 21 and trisomy 18. *Prenat Diagn* 2005;25:608–611.
77. Wyllie JP, Wright MJ, Burn J, et al. Natural history of trisomy 13. *Arch Dis Child* 1994;71(4):343–345.
78. Yamanaka M, Setoyama T, Igarashi Y, et al. Pregnancy outcome of fetuses with trisomy 18 identified by prenatal sonography and chromosomal analysis in a perinatal center. *Am J Med Genet A* 2006;140(11):1177–1182.
79. Kalousek DK, Barrett IJ, McGillivray BC. Placental mosaicism and intrauterine survival of trisomies 13 and 18. *Am J Hum Genet* 1989;44:338–343.
80. Langlois S, Brock J. Current status in non-invasive prenatal detection of Down syndrome, trisomy 18, and trisomy 13 using cell-free DNA in maternal plasma. *J Obstet Gynaecol Canada* 2013;2878:177–181.
81. Norwitz E, Levy B. Noninvasive prenatal testing: the future is now. *Rev Obs Gynecol* 2013;6:48–62.
82. Grati FR, Malvestiti F, Ferreira JCPB, et al. Fetoplacental mosaicism: potential implications for false-positive and false-negative noninvasive prenatal screening results. *Genet Med* 2014:1–5.
83. Benn P, Cuckle H, Pergament E. Non-invasive prenatal testing for aneuploidy: current status and future prospects. *Ultrasound Obstet Gynecol* 2013;42(1):15–33.
84. Canick JA, MacRae AR. Second trimester serum markers. *Semin Perinatol* 2005;29:203–208.
85. Wald NJ, Rodeck C, Hackshaw AK, et al. SURUSS in perspective. *Semin Perinatol* 2005;29:224–235.
86. Zhu JL, Hasle H, Correa A, et al. Survival among people with Down syndrome: a nationwide population-based study in Denmark. *Genet Med* 2013;15(1):64–69.
87. Englund A, Jonsson B, Zander CS, et al. Changes in mortality and causes of death in the Swedish Down syndrome population. *Am J Med Genet A* 2013;161A(4):642–649.
88. Munné S, Cohen J. Chromosome abnormalities in human embryos. *Hum Reprod Update* 1998;4:842–855.
89. Rubio C, Simon C, Vidal F. Chromosomal abnormalities and embryo development in recurrent miscarriage couples. *Hum Reprod* 2003;18:182–188.
90. McConnell V, Derham R, McManus D. Mosaic monosomy 14: clinical features and recognizable facies. *Clin Dysmorphol* 2004;13:155–160.
91. Pinto-Escalante D, Ceballos-Quintal JM, Castillo-Zapata I, et al. Full mosaic monosomy 22 in a child with DiGeorge syndrome facial appearance. *Am J Med Genet* 1998;76:150–153.
92. Uematsu A, Yorifuji T, Muroi J, et al. Parental origin of normal X chromosomes in Turner syndrome patients with various karyotypes: implications for the mechanism leading to generation of a 45,X karyotype. *Am J Med Genet* 2002;111:134–139.
93. Jones KL. *Smith's Recognizable Patterns of Human Malformation*. Philadelphia, PA: W.B. Saunders; 2006:778.
94. Mazzanti L, Cacciari E. Congenital heart disease in patients with Turner's syndrome. Italian Study Group for Turner Syndrome (ISGTS). *J Pediatr* 1998;133(5):688–692.
95. Sybert VP. Cardiovascular malformations and complications in Turner syndrome. *Pediatrics* 1998;101(1):E11.
96. Sybert VP, McCauley E. Turner's Syndrome. *N Engl J Med* 2004;351:1227–1238.
97. Wertelecki W, Fraumeni JF, Mulvihill JJ. Nongonadal neoplasia in Turner's syndrome. *Cancer* 1970;26(2):485–488.
98. Schoemaker MJ, Swerdlow AJ, Higgins CD, et al. Cancer incidence in women with Turner syndrome in Great Britain: a national cohort study. *Lancet Oncol* 2008;9(3):239–246.
99. Hasle H, Olsen JH, Nielsen J, et al. Occurrence of cancer in women with Turner syndrome. *Br J Cancer* 1996;73(9):1156–1159.
100. Sybert V. Phenotypic effects of mosaicism for a 47,XXX cell line in Turner syndrome. *J Med Genet* 2002;39:217–221.
101. Sybert VP, Mccauley E. Turner's syndrome. *N Engl J Med* 2004:1227–1238.
102. Gravholt CH, Fedder J, Naeraa RW. Occurrence of gonadoblastoma in females with Turner syndrome and Y chromosome material: a population study. *J Clin Endocrinol Metab* 2014;85:3199–3202.
103. Aguirre D, Nieto K, Lazos M, et al. Extragonadal germ cell tumors are often associated with Klinefelter syndrome. *Hum Pathol* 2006;37(4):477–480.
104. Ross JL, Roeltgen DP, Kushner H, et al. Behavioral and social phenotypes in boys with 47,XYY syndrome or 47,XXY Klinefelter syndrome. *Pediatrics* 2012;129(4):769–778.
105. Tartaglia N, Cordeiro L, Howell S, et al. The spectrum of the behavioral phenotype in boys and adolescents 47,XXY (Klinefelter syndrome). *Pediatr Endocrinol Rev* 2010;8 Suppl 1:151–159.
106. Aksglaede L, Link K, Giwercman A, et al. 47,XXY Klinefelter syndrome: clinical characteristics and age-specific recommendations for medical management. *Am J Med Genet C Semin Med Genet* 2013;163C:55–63.
107. Lalatta F, Folliero E, Cavallari U, et al. Early manifestations in a cohort of children prenatally diagnosed with 47,XYY. Role of multidisciplinary counseling for parental guidance and prevention of aggressive behavior. *Ital J Pediatr* 2012;38(1):52.
108. Bardsley MZ, Kowal K, Levy C, et al. 47,XYY syndrome: clinical phenotype and timing of ascertainment. *J Pediatr* 2013;163(4):1085–1094.
109. Van Opstal D, van den Berg C, Deelen W. Prospective prenatal investigations on potential uniparental disomy in cases of confined placental trisomy. *Prenat Diagn* 1998;18:35–44.
110. Shaffer LG, Agan N, Goldberg JD, et al. American College of Medical Genetics statement of diagnostic testing for uniparental disomy. *Genet Med* 2001;3(3):206–211.
111. Kalousek D, Vekemans M. Confined placental mosaicism and genomic imprinting. *Baillieres Best Pr Res Clin Obs Gynaecol* 2000;14:723–730.
112. Stetten G, Escallon CS, South ST, et al. Reevaluating confined placental mosaicism. *Am J Med Genet A* 2004;131:232–239.
113. Lestou VS, Kalousek DK. Confined placental mosaicism and intrauterine fetal growth. *Arch Dis Child Fetal Neonatal Ed* 1998;79:F223–F226.
114. Yong PJ, Langlois S, von Dadelszen P, et al. The association between preeclampsia and placental trisomy 16 mosaicism. *Prenat Diagn* 2006;26:956–961.
115. Dietzsch E, Ramsay M, Christianson A. Maternal origin of extra haploid set of chromosomes in third trimester triploid fetuses. *Am J Med Genet* 1995;58:360–364.
116. Baumer A, Balmer D, Binkert F, et al. Parental origin and mechanisms of formation of triploidy: a study of 25 cases. *Eur J Hum Genet* 2000;8(12):911–917.
117. Lindor N, Ney J, Gaffey T, et al. A genetic review of complete and partial hydatidiform moles and nonmolar triploidy. *Mayo Clin Proc* 1992;67:791–799.
118. McFadden DE, Jiang R, Langlois S, et al. Dispermy—origin of diandric triploidy. *Hum Reprod* 2002;17:3037–3038.
119. Uchida I, Freeman V. Triploidy and chromosomes. *Am J Obs Gynecol* 1985;151:65–69.
120. Zaragoza M V, Surti U, Redline RW, et al. Parental origin and phenotype of triploidy in spontaneous abortions: predominance of diandry and association with the partial hydatidiform mole. *Am J Hum Genet* 2000;66:1807–1820.
121. Genest D. Partial hydatidiform mole: clinicopathological features, differential diagnosis, ploidy and molecular studies, and gold standards for diagnosis. *Int J Gynecol Pathol* 2001;20:315–322.

122. Devriendt K. Hydatidiform mole and triploidy: the role of genomic imprinting in placental development. *Hum Reprod Update* 2005;11(2): 137–142.
123. Doshi N, Surti U, Szulman A. Morphologic anomalies in triploid liveborn fetuses. *Hum Pathol* 1983;14:716–723.
124. McFadden D, Kalousek D. Two different phenotypes of fetuses with chromosomal triploidy: correlation with parental origin of the extra haploid set. *Am J Med Genet* 1991;38:535–538.
125. Daniel A, Wu Z, Bennetts B, et al. Karyotype, phenotype and parental origin in 19 cases of triploidy. *Prenat Diagn* 2001;21:1034–1048.
126. Hassold T, Hunt P. To err (meiotically) is human: the genesis of human aneuploidy. *Nat Rev Genet* 2001:280–291.
127. Jacobs PA, Szulman AE, Funkhouser J, et al. Human triploidy: relationship between parental origin of the additional haploid complement and development of partial hydatidiform mole. *Ann Hum Genet* 1982;46(Pt 3):223–231.
128. Uchida I, Freeman V. Triploidy and chromosomes. *Am J Obstet Gynecol* 1985;151:65–69.
129. McFadden DE, Robinson WP. Phenotype of triploid embryos. *J Med Genet* 2006;43:609–612.
130. Emanuel BS. Molecular mechanisms and diagnosis of chromosome 22q11.2 rearrangements. *Dev Disabil Res Rev* 2008;14(1):11–18. doi:10. 1002/ddrr.3.Molecular.
131. Ade C, Roy-Engel A, Deininger P. Alu elements: an intrinsic source of human genome instability. *Curr Opin Virol* 2013;3:639–645.
132. Robberecht C, Voet T, Zamani Esteki M, et al. Nonallelic homologous recombination between retrotransposable elements is a driver of de novo unbalanced translocations. *Genome Res* 2013;23:411–418.
133. Watson CT, Marques-Bonet T, Sharp AJ, et al. The genetics of microdeletion and microduplication syndromes: an update. *Annu Rev Genomics Hum Genet* 2014;15:6.1–6.30.
134. Deak KL, Horn SR, Rehder CW. The evolving picture of microdeletion/microduplication syndromes in the age of microarray analysis: variable expressivity and genomic complexity. *Clin Lab Med* 2011;31(4): 543–564, viii.
135. McDonald-McGinn D, Emanuel B, Zackai E. 22q11.2 deletion syndrome. In: Pagon R, Adam M, Ardinger H, et al., eds. *Gene Reviews [Internet]*; Seattle, WA: University of Washington, Seattle; 2014.
136. Cole DE, Clarke LA, Riddell DC, et al. Congenital adrenal hypoplasia, Duchene muscular dystrophy, and glycerol kinase deficiency: importance of laboratory investigations in delineating a contiguous gene deletion syndrome. *Clin Chem* 1994;40(11 Pt 1):2099–2103.
137. Lim CC, Tan H, Thangaraju S, et al. End-stage renal disease in tuberous sclerosis complex-polycystic kidney disease contiguous gene syndrome: epidemiology, clinical manifestations and implications for transplantation. *Int Urol Nephrol* 2014;46:1869–1870.
138. Ellard S, Thomas K, Edghill EL, et al. Partial and whole gene deletion mutations of the GCK and HNF1A genes in maturity-onset diabetes of the young. *Diabetologia* 2007;50(11):2313–2317.
139. Hingorani M, Moore A. Aniridia. In: Pagon R, Adam M, Ardinger H, et al., eds. *Gene Reviews [Internet]*. Seattle, WA: University of Washington, Seattle; 2013.
140. Smith ACM, Boyd LE, Elsea SH, et al. Smith-Magenis syndrome. In: Pagon R, Adam M, Ardinger H, et al., eds. *Gene Reviews [Internet]*. Seattle, WA: University of Washington, Seattle; 2013.
141. Stevens CA. Rubinstein-Taybi syndrome. In: Pagon R, Adam M, Ardinger H, et al., eds. *Gene Reviews [Internet]*. Seattle, WA: University of Washington, Seattle; 2013.
142. Spinner NB, Leonard LD, Krantz ID. Alagille syndrome. In: Pagon R, Adam M, Ardinger H, et al., eds. *Gene Reviews [Internet]*. Seattle, WA: University of Washington, Seattle; 2013.
143. Morris CA. Williams syndrome. In: Pagon R, Adam M, Ardinger H, et al., eds. *Gene Reviews [Internet]*. Seattle, WA: University of Washington, Seattle; 2013.
144. Driscoll D, Miller J, Schwartz S, et al. Prader-Willi syndrome. In: Pagon R, Adam M, Ardinger H, et al., eds. *Gene Reviews [Internet]*; Seattle, WA: University of Washington, Seattle; 2014.
145. Dagli A, Williams C. Angelman syndrome. In: Pagon R, Adam M, Ardinger H, et al., eds. *Gene Reviews [Internet]*; Seattle, WA: University of Washington, Seattle; 2014.
146. Dobyns WB. Das S. LIS1-associated lissencephaly/subcortical band heterotopia. In: Pagon R, Adam M, Ardinger H, et al., eds. *Gene Reviews [Internet]*. Seattle, WA: University of Washington, Seattle; 2013.
147. Battaglia A. 1p36 deletion syndrome. In: Pagon R, Adam M, Ardinger H, et al., eds. *Gene Reviews [Internet]*. Seattle, WA: University of Washington, Seattle; 2013.
148. Firth HV. 22q11.2 duplication. In: Pagon R, Adam M, Ardinger H, et al., eds. *Gene Reviews [Internet]*. Seattle, WA: University of Washington, Seattle; 2013.
149. Wentzel C, Fernström M, Ohrner Y, et al. Clinical variability of the 22q11.2 duplication syndrome. *Eur J Med Genet* 2008;51(6):501–510. Available at: http://www.ncbi.nlm.nih.gov/pubmed/18707033. Accessed August 1, 2014.
150. Bird TD. Hereditary neuropathy with liability to pressure palsies. In: Pagon R, Adam M, Ardinger H, et al., eds. *Gene Reviews [Internet]*. Seattle, WA: University of Washington, Seattle; 2013.
151. Dietze I, Fritz B, Huhle D, et al. Clinical, cytogenetic and molecular investigation in a fetus with Wolf-Hirschhorn syndrome with paternally derived 4p deletion. Case report and review of the literature. *Fetal Diagn Ther* 2004;19(3):251–260.
152. McDermid HE, Morrow BE. Genomic disorders on 22q11. *Am J Hum Genet* 2002;70(5):1077–1088.
153. Goldmuntz E, Clark BJ, Mitchell LE, et al. Frequency of 22q11 deletions in patients with conotruncal defects. *J Am Coll Cardiol* 1998; 32(2):492–498.
154. Klewer S, Runyan R, Erickson R. TBX1 and the DiGeorge syndrome critical region. In: Epstein C, Erickson R, Wynshaw-Boris A, eds. *Inborn Errors of Development*; 2004:699–704.
155. McDonald-McGinn D, Emanuel B, Zackai E. 22q11.2 deletion syndrome. In: Pagon R, Adam M, Ardinger H, Bird T, Dolan C, Fong C, eds. *Gene Reviews [Internet]*; Seattle, WA: University of Washington, Seattle; 2014.
156. Schwinger E, Devriendt K, Rauch A, et al. Clinical utility gene card for: DiGeorge syndrome, velocardiofacial syndrome, Shprintzen syndrome, chromosome 22q11.2 deletion syndrome (22q11.2, TBX1). *Eur J Hum Genet* 2010;18(9):1–3.
157. Prasad SE, Howley S, Murphy KC. Candidate genes and the behavioral phenotype in 22q11.2 deletion syndrome. *Dev Disabil Res Rev* 2008;14(1):26–34. doi:10.1002/ddrr.5.
158. Papangeli I, Scambler P. The 22q11 deletion: DiGeorge and velocardiofacial syndromes and the role of TBX1. *Wiley Interdiscip Rev Dev Biol* 2013;2(3):393–403.
159. Michaelovsky E, Frisch A, Carmel M, et al. Genotype-phenotype correlation in 22q11 deletion syndrome. *BMC Med Genet* 2012;13:122.
160. Gao S, Li X, Amendt BA. Understanding the role of Tbx1 as a candidate gene for 22q11.2 deletion syndrome. *Curr Allergy Asthma Rep* 2013;13(6):613–621.
161. Yagi H, Furutani Y, Hamada H, et al. Role of TBX1 in human del22q11.2 syndrome. *Lancet* 2003;362:1366–1373.
162. Portnoï M-F. Microduplication 22q11.2: a new chromosomal syndrome. *Eur J Med Genet* 2009;52(2-3):88–93.
163. Portnoï M-F, Lebas F, Gruchy N, et al. 22q11.2 duplication syndrome: two new familial cases with some overlapping features with DiGeorge/velocardiofacial syndromes. *Am J Med Genet A* 2005;137(1):47–51.
164. Van Campenhout S, Devriendt K, Breckpot J, et al. Microduplication 22q11.2: a description of the clinical, developmental and behavioral characteristics during childhood. *Genet Couns* 2012;23:135–148.
165. Alter B, Kupfer G. Fanconi anemia. In: Pagon R, Adam M, Ardinger H, et al., eds. *Gene Reviews [Internet]*. Seattle, WA: University of Washington, Seattle; 2013.
166. Gordillo M, Vega H, Jabs EW. Roberts syndrome. In: Pagon R, Adam M, Ardinger H, et al., eds. *Gene Reviews [Internet]*. Seattle, WA: University of Washington, Seattle; 2013.
167. Varon R, Demuth I, Digweed M. Nijmegen breakage syndrome. In: Pagon R, Adam M, Ardinger H, et al., eds. *Gene Reviews [Internet]*. Seattle, WA: University of Washington, Seattle; 2013.

168. Saul RA, Tarleton JC. FMR1-related disorders. In: Pagon R, Adam M, Ardinger H, et al., eds. *Gene Reviews [Internet]*. Seattle, WA: University of Washington, Seattle; 2013.
169. Gatti R. Ataxia-Telangiectasia. In: Pagon R, Adam M, Ardinger H, et al., eds. *Gene Reviews [Internet]*. Seattle, WA: University of Washington, Seattle; 2013.
170. Giampietro PF, Davis JG, Adler-brecher B, et al. The need for more accurate and timely diagnosis in Fanconi anemia: a report from the international Fanconi anemia Registry. *Pediatrics* 1993;91(6):1116–1120.
171. Esmer C, Sánchez S, Ramos S, et al. DEB test for Fanconi anemia detection in patients with atypical phenotypes. *Am J Med Genet A* 2004;124A(1):35–39.
172. Webb ML, Rosen H, Taghinia A, et al. Incidence of Fanconi anemia in children with congenital thumb anomalies referred for diepoxybutane testing. *J Hand Surg Am* 2011;36(6):1052–1057.
173. Faivre L, Portnoi MF, Pals G, et al. Should chromosome breakage studies be performed in patients with VACTERL association? *Am J Med Genet* 2005;137A:55–58.
174. Mathew C. Fanconi anaemia genes and susceptibility to cancer. *Oncogene* 2006;25:5875–5884.
175. Kottemann MC, Smogorzewska A. Fanconi anaemia and the repair of Watson and Crick DNA crosslinks. *Nature* 2013;493(7432):356–363.
176. Smith A, Wagner J. Current clinical management of Fanconi anemia. *Expert Rev Hematol* 2012;5:513–522.
177. Kee Y, Andrea ADD. Molecular pathogenesis and clinical management of Fanconi anemia. *J Clin Invest* 2012;122(11):3799–3806.
178. Inbar-Feigenberg M, Choufani S, Butcher DT, et al. Basic concepts of epigenetics. *Fertil Steril* 2013;99(3):607–615.
179. Masri S, Sassone-Corsi P. The circadian clock: a framework linking metabolism, epigenetics and neuronal function. *Nat Rev Neurosci* 2013;14(1):69–75.
180. Osborne-Majnik A, Fu Q, Lane RH. Epigenetic mechanisms in fetal origins of health and disease. *Clin Obstet Gynecol* 2013;56(3):622–632.
181. Lee JT, Bartolomei MS. X-inactivation, imprinting, and long noncoding RNAs in health and disease. *Cell* 2013;152(6):1308–1323.
182. Biliya S, Bulla LA. Minireview. Genomic imprinting: the influence of differential methylation. *Exp Biol Med* 2010;235:139–147.
183. Lim D, Maher E. Human imprinting syndromes. *Epigenomics* 2009;1:347.
184. Tomizawa S, Sasaki H. Genomic imprinting and its relevance to congenital disease, infertility, molar pregnancy and induced pluripotent stem cell. *J Hum Genet* 2012;57:84–91.
185. Abramowitz LK, Bartolomei MS. Genomic imprinting: recognition and marking of imprinted loci. *Curr Opin Genet Dev* 2012;22(2):72–78.
186. Barlow DP. Genomic imprinting: a mammalian epigenetic discovery model. *Annu Rev Genet* 2011;45:379–403.
187. Piedrahita JA. The role of imprinted genes in fetal growth abnormalities. *Birth Defects Res A Clin Mol Teratol* 2011;91:682–692.
188. Ishida M, Moore G. The role of imprinted genes in humans. *Mol Aspects Med* 2013;34:826.
189. Gurrieri F, Accadia M. Genetic imprinting: the paradigm of Prader-Willi and Angelman syndromes. *Endocr Dev* 2009;14:20–28.
190. Buiting K. Prader-Willi syndrome and Angelman syndrome. *Am J Med Genet C Semin Med Genet* 2010;154C(3):365–376.
191. Horsthemke B, Wagstaff J. Mechanisms of imprinting of the Prader-Willi/Angelman region. *Am J Med Genet A* 2008;146A(16):2041–2052.
192. Cassidy SB, Schwartz S, Miller JL, et al. Prader-Willi syndrome. *Genet Med* 2012;14(1):10–26.
193. Kyllerman M. Angelman syndrome. In: Dulac O, Lassonde M, Sarnat H, eds. *Handbook of Clinical Neurology*. Vol. 111. 1st ed. Elsevier B.V.; 2013:287–290.
194. Mabb AM, Judson MC, Zylka MJ, et al. Angelman syndrome: insights into genomic imprinting and neurodevelopmental phenotypes. *Trends Neurosci* 2011;34(6):293–303.
195. Williams CA, Driscoll DJ, Dagli AI. Clinical and genetic aspects of Angelman syndrome. *Genet Med* 2010;12(7):385–395.
196. Van Buggenhout G, Fryns J-P. Angelman syndrome (AS, MIM 105830). *Eur J Hum Genet* 2009;17(11):1367–1373.
197. Eggermann T. Silver-Russell and Beckwith-Wiedemann syndromes: opposite (epi)mutations in 11p15 result in opposite clinical pictures. *Horm Res* 2009;71(Suppl 2):30–35.
198. Jacob KJ, Robinson WP, Lefebvre L. Beckwith-Wiedemann and Silver-Russell syndromes: opposite developmental imbalances in imprinted regulators of placental function and embryonic growth. *Clin Genet* 2013;84(4):326–334.
199. Demars J, Gicquel C. Epigenetic and genetic disturbance of the imprinted 11p15 region in Beckwith-Wiedemann and Silver-Russell syndromes. *Clin Genet* 2012;81(4):350–361.
200. Choufani S, Shuman C, Weksberg R. Molecular findings in Beckwith-Wiedemann syndrome. *Am J Med Genet C Semin Med Genet* 2013;163C(2):131–140.
201. Shuman C, Beckwith J, Smith A, et al. Beckwith-Wiedemann syndrome. In: Pagon R, Adam M, Ardinger H, et al., eds. *Gene Reviews [Internet]*; Seattle, WA: University of Washington, Seattle; 2014.
202. Weksberg R, Shuman C, Beckwith JB. Beckwith-Wiedemann syndrome. *Eur J Hum Genet* 2010;18(1):8–14.
203. Saal H. Beckwith-Wiedemann syndrome. In: Pagon R, Adam M, Ardinger H, Bird T, Dolan C, Fong C, eds. *Gene Reviews [Internet]*; Seattle, WA: University of Washington, Seattle; 2014
204. Wakeling EL. Silver-Russell syndrome. *Arch Dis Child* 2011;96(12):1156–1161.
205. Eggermann T, Begemann M, Spengler S, et al. Genetic and epigenetic findings in Silver-Russell syndrome. *Pediatr Endocrinol Rev* 2010;8:86–93.
206. Eggermann T, Spengler S, Gogiel M, et al. Epigenetic and genetic diagnosis of Silver-Russell syndrome. *Expert Rev Mol Diagn* 2012;12:459–471.
207. Eggermann T. Russell-Silver syndrome. *Am J Med Genet C Semin Med Genet* 2010;154C(3):355–364.
208. Amor DJ, Halliday J. A review of known imprinting syndromes and their association with assisted reproduction technologies. *Hum Reprod* 2008;23(12):2826–2834.
209. Kochanski A, Merritt T, Gadzinowski J, et al. The impact of assisted reproductive technologies on the genome and epigenome of the newborn. *J Neonatal Perinatal Med* 2013;6:101–108.
210. Eroglu A, Layman L. Role of ART in imprinting disorders. *Semin Reprod Med* 2012;30:92–104.
211. Soejima H, Higashimoto K. Epigenetic and genetic alterations of the imprinting disorder Beckwith-Wiedemann syndrome and related disorders. *J Hum Genet* 2013;58(7):402–409.
212. Denomme MM, Mann MRW. Genomic imprints as a model for the analysis of epigenetic stability during assisted reproductive technologies. *Reproduction* 2012;144(4):393–409.
213. Talaulikar V, Arulkumaran S. Reproductive outcomes after assisted conception. *Obstet Gynecol Surv* 2012;67:566–583.
214. Chiba H, Hiura H, Okae H, et al. DNA methylation errors in imprinting disorders and assisted reproductive technology. *Pediatr Int* 2013;55(5):542–549.
215. El Hajj N, Haaf T. Epigenetic disturbances in in vitro cultured gametes and embryos: implications for human assisted reproduction. *Fertil Steril* 2013;99(3):632–641.
216. Shufaro Y, Laufer N. Epigenetic concerns in assisted reproduction: update and critical review of the current literature. *Fertil Steril* 2013;99(3):605–606.
217. Kang JU, Koo SH. Clinical implementation of chromosomal microarray technology in prenatal diagnosis (Review). *Mol Med Rep* 2012;6(6):1219–1222.
218. Hui L, Bianchi DW. Recent advances in the prenatal interrogation of the human fetal genome. *Trends Genet* 2013;29(2):84–91.
219. Evangelidou P, Alexandrou A, Moutafi M, et al. Implementation of high resolution whole genome array CGH in the prenatal clinical setting: advantages, challenges, and review of the literature. *Biomed Res Int* 2013;2013:346762.
220. Hillman SC, McMullan DJ, Williams D, et al. Microarray comparative genomic hybridization in prenatal diagnosis: a review. *Ultrasound Obstet Gynecol* 2012;40(4):385–391.

CHAPTER 4

Congenital Anomalies and Malformation Syndromes

Joseph R. Siebert, Ph.D.

The study of congenital anomalies continues to be hampered by misunderstandings at a number of levels. In many circles, for example, the statement that "the baby was born with a genetic deformity" is often heard. In fact, this is often not the case, for many congenital anomalies are neither genetic in origin nor do they constitute a physical deformation per se. Another common, but erroneous, opinion is that hundreds or even thousands of substances in the environment cause birth defects. In fact, only 30 to 40 exogenous substances (i.e., teratogens) have been proven to have this potential. But if these issues continue to hamper our dealings professionally, they also tug at the souls of grieving parents who ask "What caused my baby's problem?" or "How did this happen?" or "Will it happen again?" These questions take on added complexity when multiple anomalies are encountered in a single patient. It can fall to the pathologist, as well as clinical specialists, to help explain these findings. The purpose of this chapter, then, is to provide a broad context for understanding the basic *patterns* of anomalies. As such, descriptions will emphasize gross features over microscopic appearances or discussions of intricate pathologic processes. For help with these latter matters, the reader is referred to chapters that cover specific organ systems.

ETIOLOGY AND PATHOGENESIS

The question of causation—etiology—is not at all simple, for etiology may be heterogeneous, that is, multiple factors may bring about a given defect. Holoprosencephaly is a powerful example, for it arises sporadically or is associated with several gene mutations, aneuploidies (e.g., trisomy 13), diseases such as maternal diabetes mellitus, and teratogens (e.g., ethyl alcohol). Robin sequence (micrognathia, cleft palate, glossoptosis) is another example, in which causes may be chromosomal, teratogenic, monogenic, disruptive (i.e., amniotic bands), or unknown.

The mechanism—or pathogenesis—responsible for a defect may be varied as well. In Robin sequence, for example, deformations may occur secondary to intrauterine constraint produced by oligohydramnios. However, reduced amniotic fluid volume may occur from premature rupture of membranes (particularly chronic leakage), renal anomalies, or placental or maternal factors.

CONCEPTS AND TERMS OF MORPHOGENESIS

In 1982, a set of standardized terms for describing human developmental abnormalities was established (1). The definitions are essential for pediatric pathologists, pediatricians, medical geneticists, and others dealing with congenital anomalies. Several additional discussions of the terminologic, historic, diagnostic, nosologic, and morphologic aspects of congenital anomalies in humans are available (2,3).

Hypoplasia refers to underdevelopment and *hyperplasia* to overdevelopment of an organism, organ, or tissue and result from a change in cell number. *Hypotrophy* and *hypertrophy* refer to a decrease and increase, respectively, in the size of an organ, tissue, or cells. *Agenesis* is the absence of a part of the body caused by a presumed absence of the anlage, or primordium. *Aplasia* refers to absence of a rudimentary structure caused by failure of the anlage to develop completely. Aplasia can be regarded as an extreme degree of hypoplasia. *Atrophy* describes the shrinkage of a previously normally developed tissue mass or organ because of a decrease in cell size or cell number.

A *developmental field* is the portion of the embryo that reacts as a coordinated unit to inductive effects with differentiation and growth (4). Developmental fields represent, then, the major branches on the morphogenetic tree. It has been suggested that the embryo itself constitutes the *primary developmental field* (5) and that other more constricted ones are operational at later stages of development. A *monotopic field defect* represents a defect in organogenesis and includes contiguous anomalies (e.g., cyclopia and holoprosencephaly; cleft lip and cleft palate). Such alterations are more likely to arise late in gestation and produce more confined defects (6). By contrast, a *polytopic field defect* is thought to result from an earlier defect during blastogenesis—the first 4 weeks of development—and occurs if abnormal inductive processes produce more distantly located and diverse defects (6,7).

The midline also acts as a developmental field (8). It represents the normal plane of cleavage in monozygotic twinning and the plane around which symmetry of visceral position is determined. It is an especially vulnerable site in terms of developmental anomalies. Morphogenetic events involving the midline include fusions, segmentation, programmed cell death with morphogenetic "necroses" or resorptions, rotations, and other developmental movements. In some anomalies involving the midline, the incidence of monozygotic twinning may be increased (e.g., sirenomelia, cloacal anomalies). Other examples of midline anomalies include the holoprosencephaly complex, agenesis of the corpus callosum, cleft lip, cleft palate, midface cleft complex, spina bifida, omphalocele, congenital heart defects, hypospadias, and imperforate anus.

A *malformation* is "a morphologic defect of an organ, part of an organ, or larger region of the body resulting from an intrinsically abnormal developmental process" (1).

A *disruption*, or secondary malformation, is "a morphologic defect of an organ, part of an organ, or a larger region of the body, resulting from the extrinsic breakdown of, or interference with, an originally normal developmental process" (1). Disruptions are causally heterogeneous and may bear close resemblance to malformations anatomically. In a given case, the distinction between a disruption and a malformation may be made on the basis of the associated malformations or the history of gestational exposure to a teratogenic agent or event. The general prevalence of birth defects is given as 3% to 5%.

A *deformation* is "an abnormal form, shape, or position of a part of the body caused by mechanical forces." It may be extrinsic, due to intrauterine constraint (e.g., lack of amniotic fluid), or intrinsic, due to a defect of the nervous system that causes hypomobility (1). Examples of deformities are talipes equinovarus and arthrogryposis. About 1% to 2% of newborn infants have deformations of some sort.

Dysplasia represents "an abnormal organization of cells into tissue(s) and its morphologic result(s)" (1). Dysplasia is therefore a process and the consequence of *dyshistogenesis*, an abnormal differentiation of tissue structure. This is in contrast to a malformation, which is a defect in morphogenesis of the organ structure. Dysplasias may or may not be metabolically induced, may involve one or several germ layers, and may be generalized or localized; they often demonstrate a sporadic pattern of occurrence (1).

Mild dysplasias, common in the normal population, include freckling, capillary hemangioma over the glabella and metopic suture area of the forehead, café au lait spots, moles, and nevi. If they are mendelian traits, they usually represent autosomal dominant mutations. Dysplasias are components of every aneuploidy syndrome and probably are one reason for the increased incidence of associated cancers. Dysplasias can be induced environmentally by radiation, viruses, and carcinogens.

Anomalies sometimes occur as groups of defects, which require additional classification. The terms described below help in categorizing anomalies but are only aids. Placing a name on a cluster of anomalies helps in organizing thoughts about a given condition but does not identify cause or mechanism or suggest recurrence risk (9).

That being said, a *syndrome* is "a pattern of multiple anomalies thought to be pathogenetically related and not known to represent a single sequence or a polytopic field defect" (1). No structural anomaly of any malformation syndrome is obligatory, and no one component is pathognomonic of any syndrome.

A *sequence* is a "pattern of multiple anomalies derived from a single known or presumed prior anomaly or mechanical factor" (1). In the Potter sequence, the pathogenetic event is oligohydramnios arising from a genetic or nongenetic cause; the causal event represents a malformation (e.g., renal agenesis or dysplasia, as in polycystic kidney) or a mechanical factor (e.g., amniotic fluid leakage). Lack of amniotic fluid restricts fetal movement and causes fetal compression, producing the typical changes of Potter sequence (Figure 4-1).

A *malformation complex* consists of "those groups of heterogeneous disorders with overlapping characteristics that are difficult to separate into specific conditions," for example, facio-auriculo-vertebral spectrum and hypoglossia–hypodactylia.

An *association* consists of "a nonrandom occurrence in two or more individuals of multiple anomalies not known to be a polytopic field defect, sequence, or syndrome" (1). Associations have also been defined as the results of "disruptive events acting on developmental fields" (10). However, the diversity of findings in associations highlights how much remains unknown about possible developmental fields. The term "association" is a temporary category that should change as conditions become better understood. An example is CHARGE syndrome, which for many years was classified as an association, until mutations in the *CHD7* gene were identified in numerous patients (11).

Jones has offered a valuable policy for naming patterns of malformations (12):

1. When the etiology is known and easily remembered, the appropriate term should be used to designate the disorder.
2. Time-honored designations should be continued unless there is good reason to change.
3. In the absence of a reasonably descriptive designation, eponyms, some of them multiple, may be used until the basic defect for the disorder is recognized. However, use of an eponym should thereafter be limited to one proper name.
4. The use of the possessive form of an eponym should be discontinued, because the author neither had nor owned the disorder.

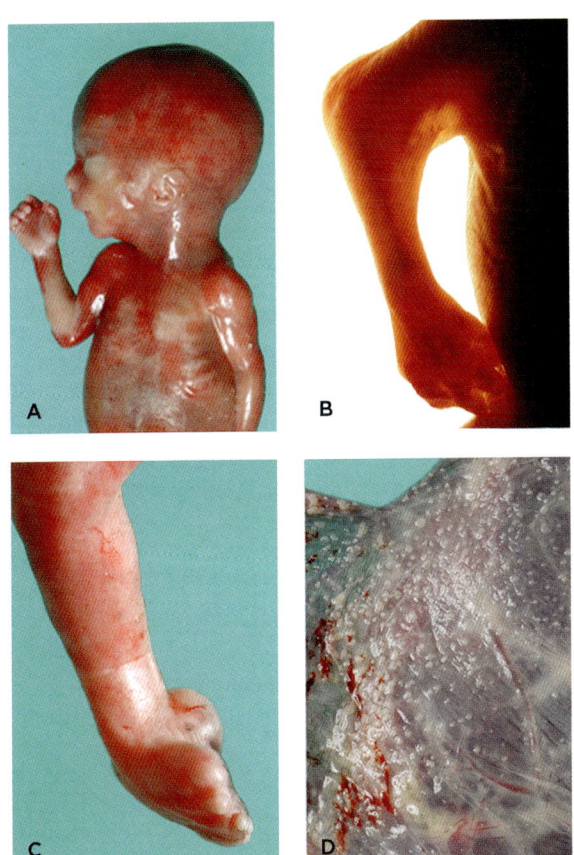

FIGURE 4-1 • Potter sequence. **A:** A 22-week fetus with a history of severe oligohydramnios (renal system normal; no history of premature rupture of membranes). Note the blunt nose, small mandible, and flattened ear. **B:** Marked skin webbing (pterygium) of right elbow developed secondary to prolonged immobilization of joint. **C:** Medial rotation of foot at ankle joint (talipes equinovarus) resulted from intrauterine constraint. **D:** Fetal surface of placenta shows amnion nodosum, a finding common in cases of oligohydramnios.

5. Designation of a disorder by one or more of its manifestations does not necessarily imply that they are either specific or consistent components of that disorder.
6. Names that may have an unpleasant connotation for the affected individual or family should be avoided.
7. The syndrome should not be designated by the initials of the originally described patients.
8. Names that are too general for a specific syndrome should be avoided.
9. Unless acronyms are extremely pertinent or appropriate, they should be avoided.

DEFORMATIONS

Amniotic Fluid Volume

Oligohydramnios, or anhydramnios, is an ominous sign, as it effectively reduces the space available to the fetus and is associated with a wide variety of fetal deformations involving the limbs and craniofacial complex. With reduced inhalation

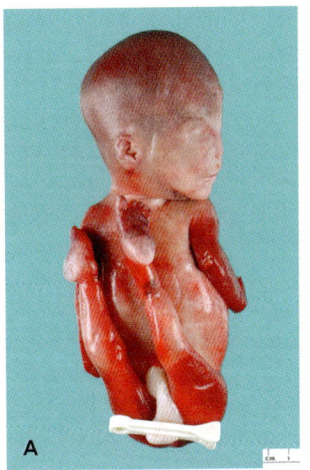 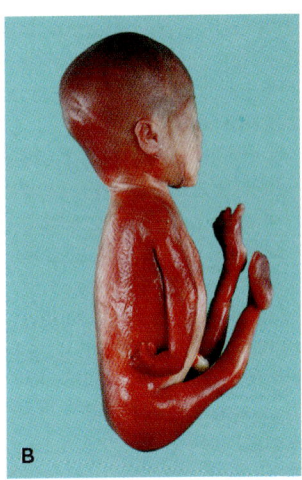

FIGURE 4-2 • Severe arthrogryposis in a 23-week fetus. Extraordinary flexion and contracture deformities and marked flattening of the face are apparent. Autopsy revealed no other fetal anomalies (karyotype 46,XX). Etiology is heterogeneous in this condition. **A:** Frontal view. **B:** Lateral view.

of fluid comes pulmonary hypoplasia, which is lethal when severe. Reduced fluid volume comes about primarily from leakage (e.g., premature rupture of membranes) or renal anomalies with reduced production of fetal urine. Placental abnormalities, with decreased fetal blood flow, can cause "prerenal" oligohydramnios.

Abnormalities of Uterus and Placental Implantation

A bicornuate uterus may cause fetal compression and constraint, resulting in a deformed fetus. Uterine malformations may also predispose the fetus to malformations arising from abnormalities in implantation, placentation, body stalk formation, and late fetal cord compression or torsion. With these occurrences comes an increased risk of stillbirth (see Chapter 18).

Neurogenic, Skeletal, and Other Causes of Deformations

Central nervous system (CNS) and skeletal muscle defects (e.g., amyoplasia) may result in deformations. The most common congenital limb deformities are tibial bowing, mild metatarsus varus, talipes equinovalgus and varus, and the flexural contractures of arthrogryposis (Figure 4-2). Skeletal dysplasias may be associated with deformities of prenatal or postnatal onset. Twins and multiple fetuses may interfere with each other's physical development and manifest deformities.

DISRUPTIONS

Ionizing Radiation

Studies of radiation exposure to pregnant women during medical treatments or warfare have provided valuable information regarding radiation-induced anomalies. It is commonly held that pregnant women should avoid all unnecessary radiation exposure. However, data regarding exact doses of radiation are often unavailable, and so actions based upon those fears (i.e., elective abortion after an exposure or suspected exposure) may be unwarranted. Counselors must use extreme caution when dealing with questions regarding radiation exposure.

Guidelines are available for this purpose (13). During pregnancy, the acceptable cumulative dose of ionizing radiation during pregnancy is 5 rads. With few exceptions, diagnostic studies produce dosages less than this level. A two-view radiograph of mother's chest, for example, exposes the fetus to just 0.00007 rads. Therefore, a mother would need the equivalent of 500 chest examinations before the fetus would be exposed to a harmful level of radiation. Because 8 to 25 weeks, and especially 10 to 17 weeks, of gestation is a highly sensitive period for CNS teratogenesis, unnecessary exposures directly to the fetus should be avoided during this time. Prenatal radiation exposure may produce a slight increase in the risk of childhood leukemia or small change in the frequency of gene mutations, but these are quite rare and not an indication for pregnancy termination.

When maternal radiation occurs at higher than diagnostic levels, the exposed fetus may exhibit generalized growth retardation, microcephaly, skull defects, eye anomalies, spina bifida, cleft palate, micromelia, clubfoot, and genital and other anomalies (14). Altered cognitive status, ranging from reduced intelligence quotient (IQ) to frank mental retardation and seizures, is recognized; MRI examinations in these patients are suggestive of neuronal migration defects (15).

Teratogenic Disruptions

A list of teratogenic agents in humans is shown in Table 4-1. Additional resources on this topic are available (16,17). While some viruses are responsible for malformations, a number of others cause congenital/neonatal or maternal disease, but not malformations per se. These include adenovirus, echovirus, hepatitis B and C virus, influenza, and West Nile virus, and are excluded from Table 4-1. Teratogens exert their influence during especially vulnerable times ("critical periods"), when specific tissues are undergoing development (Table 4-2).

Thalidomide Embryopathy

Thalidomide, a drug once used in the treatment of morning sickness, was first recognized as a teratogen by Lenz and McBride in separate reports in 1961. Exposure to thalidomide during the critical period (days 23 to 28 of gestation) results in a number of defects, the most notable of which are limb defects ranging from triphalangeal thumb to tetra-amelia or phocomelia of the upper and lower limbs, at times with preaxial polydactyly of six or seven toes per foot. Congenital heart defects, urinary tract anomalies, genital defects, gastrointestinal anomalies, eye defects, ear malformations, and dental anomalies may also occur. The drug is also used in the treatment of leprosy (i.e., erythema nodosum leprosum), certain autoimmune disorders, and cancer. For this reason, cases of thalidomide embryopathy still occur, especially in countries with a high prevalence

TABLE 4-1 TERATOGENIC AGENTS IN HUMANS

Radiation
  Atomic weapons
  Radioiodine
  Greater than therapeutic levels

Infectious Agents
  Cytomegalovirus
  Herpes simplex virus 1 and 2
  Lymphocytic choriomeningitis virus (LCMV)
  Parvovirus B-19 (erythema infectiosum)
  Rubella virus
  Syphilis
  Toxoplasmosis
  Varicella virus
  Venezuelan equine encephalitis virus

Maternal and Metabolic Imbalance
  Alcohol abuse
  Amniocentesis, early
  Chorionic villus sampling (before day 60)[a]
  Cretinism, endemic
  Diabetes mellitus
  Folic acid deficiency
  Hyperthermia
  Myasthenia gravis
  Phenylketonuria
  Rheumatic disease and congenital heart block
  Sjögren syndrome
  Virilizing tumors

Drugs and Environmental Chemicals
  Aminopterin, methylaminopterin
  Androgenic hormones
  Captopril (renal failure)
  Carbamazepine[a]
  Chlorobiphenyls
  Cocaine
  Corticosteroids[a]
  Coumarin and other anticoagulants
  Cyclophosphamide
  Diethylstilbestrol
  Diphenylhydantoin
  Enalapril (renal failure)
  Etretinate and other retinoic acid compounds
  Fluconazole (high dose)
  Iodides
  Lithium[a]
  Mercury (organic forms)
  Methimazole (scalp defects, choanal atresia)[a]
  Methylene blue (by intra-amniotic injection)
  Misoprostol[a]
  Nicotine (smoking, passive exposure, nicotine patch)
  Penicillamine
  Phenobarbitol[a]
  Sartans
  Tetracycline
  Thalidomide
  Toluene abuse
  Trimethadione
  Valproic acid

[a]Agents produce <10 defects per 1000 exposures.
Modified from Shepard TH, Lemire RJ. *Catalog of Teratogenic Agents*, 13th ed. Baltimore, MD: The Johns Hopkins University Press; 2007.

TABLE 4-2	CRITICAL PERIODS IN HUMAN TERATOGENICITY	
Teratogen	Gestational Age (Days)	Malformation
Rubella virus	0–60	Cataract; heart defect
	0–120+	Hearing deficit
Thalidomide	21–40	Limb reduction defects
Hyperthermia	18–30	Anencephaly
Male hormones in females (androgens, exogenous drugs, tumors)	Prior to 90	Clitoral hypertrophy; labial fusion
	After 90	Clitoral hypertrophy
Anticoagulants	Prior to 100	Hypoplasia of nose; stippling of epiphyses
	After 100	Possible mental retardation
Diethylstilbestrol	After 14	Vaginal adenosis (50%)
	After 98	Vaginal adenosis (30%)
	After 126	Vaginal adenosis (10%)
Radioiodine therapy	After 65–70	Atrophy ("thyroidectomy") of fetal thyroid gland
Goitrogens, iodides	After 180	Fetal goiter
Tetracycline	After 120	Staining of enamel of primary teeth
	After 250	Staining of crowns of permanent teeth

Modified from Shepard TH. Proven and suspected human teratogens-How can we sort them out? In: Crichton JU, ed. *Safe Drugs for Canadian Children—Report of the Third Canadian Ross Conference on Pediatric Research*. Montreal, Canada: Ross Laboratories; 1978:9–25 (Ref. 18).

of leprosy and access to the drug. The mechanism of action continues to be studied. The drug has anti-inflammatory properties, and some have suggested that defective angiogenesis in developing limb buds may also be operational (19).

Folic Acid Deficiency

Deficiency of folic acid results in up to 70% of neural tube deficits (NTDs), particularly anencephaly. Preconceptional intake of 0.4-mg folic acid daily reduces the incidence of NTDs by up to 90% and congenital heart defects by approximately 40% (20). The fortification of wheat flour with folic acid in the United States has resulted in a decrease in the incidence of NTDs; a similar success might also be expected with similar fortification and surveillance worldwide (21,22). In addition to aiding in the prevention of NTDs, prenatal supplementation with folic acid prevents pregnancy-induced megaloblastic anemia (23).

Folic Acid Antagonists and Derivatives

Aminopterin and methotrexate, its methyl derivative, are folic acid antagonists that have several applications and may cause a variety of anomalies. Aminopterin is used as a pesticide; both drugs are used to treat certain cancers or to end an unwanted or ectopic pregnancy, making exposure during early pregnancy possible. Craniofacial anomalies include severe hypoplasia of frontal, parietal, temporal, or occipital bones; wide fontanelles; upsweep of frontal scalp hair; broad nasal bridge; shallow supraorbital ridges; prominent eyes; cleft palate; apparently low-set ears; micrognathia; maxillary hypoplasia; and epicanthal folds. The limbs are relatively short, and dislocation of hips, short thumbs, partial syndactyly of third and fourth fingers, dextroposition of the heart, and hypotonia may occur (24).

Fetal Iodine Deficiency

The pregnant woman and her developing fetus both have an increased need for iodine. The woman deficient in dietary intake of iodine therefore puts both herself and her fetus at risk (25). The use of iodized salt has done much to reduce the risk of associated mental retardation worldwide, but is of little help to women who do not have access to this food or those who must reduce their salt intake during pregnancy.

Iodine deficiency has been called the single greatest preventable cause of intellectual disability (26). Deficiency in the fetus results in mental retardation, spastic diplegia, deafness, and strabismus (27,28) and develops from severe maternal iodine deficiency (<20 µg/day) during the first half of gestation. This is especially prevalent in regions with reduced iodine content in the soil, particularly certain European countries and mountainous areas, such as New Guinea, the Himalayas, and the Andes (29). The World Health Organization recommends a daily iodine intake of between 150 and 300 µg (30).

Trimethadione Syndrome

Trimethadione is a drug used in the treatment of seizures. A large percentage of cases are associated with pregnancy loss or abnormalities in offspring, which include delayed growth and mental development, and craniofacial (e.g., malformed ears, cleft palate), skeletal, cardiac, gastrointestinal, or genitourinary anomalies (31,32).

Valproic Acid Embryopathy

The teratogenicity of valproic acid has been well documented (16). Although valuable as an antiepileptic and mood-altering drug, valproic acid administration during pregnancy is associated with a host of anomalies, including microcephaly, trigonocephaly, porencephaly, spina bifida, other CNS defects, facial anomalies, cardiac defects, limb reduction anomalies, and genitourinary defects (33). Dosages associated with malformations have generally been 750 to 1,000 mg/day (although low-dose effects are also suspected) and exposures verified during the first trimester.

Warfarin Embryopathy

Although the contraindications of warfarin usage during pregnancy are well recognized, women, for example those with prosthetic heart valves, may take the drug during the first trimester, before pregnancy is recognized. Such exposure can result in intrauterine death or an embryopathy characterized by restricted growth, hypoplastic nose, limb defects (shortening, brachydactyly, nail hypoplasia), gastroschisis, cardiac defects, and stippled epiphyses or chondrodysplasia punctata (34,35). If exposure occurs later in gestation, CNS hemorrhage, with subsequent brain damage and mental retardation, may occur.

Synthetic Progestin Embryopathy

Exposure to synthetic progestins (e.g., 17-α-ethinyl-19-nortestosterone) early in gestation can induce enlargement of the clitoris or labioscrotal fusion in female fetuses and hypospadias in males (36). The incidence of ectopic pregnancy is increased in women who experience contraception failure from either oral progestins or implants (37). Diethylstilbestrol may cause vaginal adenosis, clear cell adenocarcinoma of the vagina or cervix, or breast cancer in prenatally exposed females and reproductive anomalies in exposed males (38,39). The use of a variety of exogenous sex hormones is not associated with increased risk of major malformations, with the exception of esophageal atresia, which carries a risk ratio of 2.87, or approximately 6 per 10,000 live births (40).

Mercury Embryopathy

Exposure of the developing human to mercury compounds has serious effects, most notably an increased incidence of growth restriction, microcephaly, and CNS damage, with consequent deficits that include blindness, hypotonia or spasticity, deafness, dysarthria, chorea, athetosis, and strabismus. In one study of maternal exposure to inorganic mercury, the prevalence of miscarriage and stillbirth was not increased (41). Both maternal ingestion and occupational exposure are recognized routes of exposure. The classic condition is Minamata disease, an epidemic that affected women living on the island of Minamata, Japan, who ingested shellfish contaminated with methylmercury (42). Pregnant women continue to be exposed, especially those living in areas of heavy industrial pollution or downstream of gold mines, where contamination of soil and water occurs (43), or those ingesting contaminated marine food (44).

Isotretinoin Embryopathy

Isotretinoin (i.e., Accutane) is a synthetic vitamin A analog, 13-*cis*-retinoic acid. Because it inhibits sebaceous gland function, the drug is valuable in the treatment of cystic acne. Administration to pregnant women is associated with a variety of serious anomalies. Miscarriage, perinatal mortality, and premature birth are reported, and survivors may have a variety of malformations or decreased mental status. Ear anomalies are common, including dysplastic, hypoplastic, or absent ears; agenesis of the external ear canal is variable. CNS abnormalities (microcephaly, hydrocephalus, porencephaly, Dandy-Walker malformation, neuronal migration defects) and conotruncal congenital heart defects are recognized (45).

Alcohol Embryopathy

Alcohol is a common and important teratogen in humans, but its influence was not fully appreciated until 1968 (46). In 1973, Jones and Smith named the condition "fetal alcohol syndrome" (FAS) (47). Effects include structural, behavioral, and neurocognitive deficits, and so a number of other designations have been used, including the earlier "fetal alcohol effect" and current "fetal alcohol spectrum disorders" (48). In a sense, the term "fetal alcohol syndrome" is unfortunate, for, although popular, it implies that alcohol exerts its primary influence on the fetus; in fact, teratogenic damage to the embryo is far more significant, hence the more accurate term "alcohol embryopathy."

A maternal history of alcohol consumption is often difficult to ascertain, but nevertheless, clinical criteria for making the diagnosis are available. Major characteristics of affected infants and children include distinctive facies (epicanthal folds, short palpebral fissures, midface hypoplasia, thin vermilion border of the upper lip, absent to indistinct philtrum, and short, upturned nose), growth restriction, malformations, and psychomotor abnormalities (49). Patients generally present with prenatal and postnatal growth retardation and CNS dysfunction, including mental retardation, hyperactivity, sleep disorders, spastic tetraplegia, seizures, and behavioral difficulties (Table 4-3). Additional disabilities may include academic or legal difficulties, inappropriate sexual behavior, and other problems related to alcohol or other drug use. Joint, limb, and conotruncal cardiac anomalies are often present; limb defects include shortness of the metatarsals and metacarpals or severe ectrodactyly (52). The unusual hirsutism that is present at birth may disappear with age. Structural brain malformations, chiefly hypoplasia or agenesis of the corpus callosum, lissencephaly, and holoprosencephaly, as well as ocular abnormalities, have been described (50,53). Recently, an abnormally angled corpus callosum, diagnosed by transfontanellar ultrasound, has been noted in a large percentage of affected infants (54). Cystic hygromas are found in patients with FAS, but also with a number of other conditions (Table 4-4). FAS has been reported in both monozygotic and dizygotic twins; the higher incidence in the

TABLE 4-3	CHARACTERISTICS OF FAS

Somatic and Cutaneous Findings
   Prenatal and postnatal growth retardation, with diminished adipose tissue content
   Hirsutism
   Cutaneous hemangiomas
Central Nervous System
   Micrencephaly
   Neuronal migration defects (heterotopia)
   Absent or hypoplastic corpus callosum
   Ventriculomegaly
   Holoprosencephaly
   Hypoplastic cerebellum
   Dysplastic brainstem
   Lissencephaly
Craniofacial
   Microcephaly
   Ocular hypertelorism
   Short palpebral fissures, sometimes downslanting or with epicanthal folds
   Microphthalmia, other eye anomalies
   Posteriorly rotated ears, with hypoplastic concha
   Low nasal bridge
   Hypoplastic midface, with hypoplastic maxillae
   Retro- or micrognathia
   Cleft lip and/or palate
   Smooth vermillion border
   Long, indistinct philtrum
   Small teeth
Cardiovascular
   Congenital heart disease, often conotruncal (e.g., tetralogy of Fallot)
   Atrial and/or ventricular septal defects
Gastrointestinal Tract
   Esophageal, duodenal, or anal atresia
   Tracheoesophageal fistula
   Pyloric stenosis
Urogenital System
   Hypospadias
   Hypoplastic labia
   Small rotated kidneys
   Hydronephrosis
Musculoskeletal Systems
   Abnormal palmar creases
   Hypoplastic nails
   Reduction defects of limbs and digits
   Pectus excavatum or carinatum
   Scoliosis
   Klippel-Feil anomaly
   Diaphragmatic hernia
   Umbilical hernia
Behavioral
   Developmental delay, mental retardation
   Irritability (in infancy)
   Hyperactivity (in childhood)
   Hypotonia, reduced coordination

Modified from Clarren SK, Smith DW. The fetal alcohol syndrome. *N Engl J Med* 1978;298:1063–1067; Clarren SK, Alvord EC, Sumi SM, et al. Brain malformations related to prenatal exposure to ethanol. *J Pediatr* 1978;92:64–67; Potter BJ, Hetzel BS. Fetal alcohol syndrome. In: Hetzel BS, Smith RM, eds. *Fetal Brain Disorders: Recent Approaches to the Problem of Mental Deficiency*. New York, NY: Elsevier North Holland; 1981 (Refs. 49–51).

TABLE 4-4	DISORDERS ASSOCIATED WITH NUCHAL CYSTIC HYGROMA

Single Gene Disorders
   Familial webbing of neck
   Lymphedema distichiasis syndrome
   Roberts syndrome
   Bieber syndrome
   Lethal multiple pterygium syndrome
   Noonan syndrome
Chromosome Disorders
   45 X (Ulrich-Turner syndrome or monosomy X)
   X-chromosome polysomy
   13q–
   18p–
   Trisomy 18
   Trisomy 21
   Trisomy 22 mosaicism
Teratogenic Disorders
   Alcohol embryopathy
   Fetal amethopterin syndrome
   Fetal trimethadione syndrome

Modified from Gilbert-Barness EF, Opitz JM. Congenital anomalies and malformation syndromes. In: Wigglesworth JS, Singer DB, eds. *Textbook of Fetal and Perinatal Pathology*. Oxford, UK: Blackwell Scientific Publications; 1991 (Ref. 55).

former has suggested a genetic influence (56). Despite small head circumference and initially slow psychomotor maturation, some infants with FAS may progress and develop intelligence within the normal range. Endocrine investigations usually show normal or near-normal levels of growth hormone, cortisol, and gonadotropins (see Chapter 21) (57). FAS is also a carcinogenic syndrome and is associated with tumors virtually identical to those seen in the fetal diphenylhydantoin (Dilantin) syndrome (see below).

Nicotine

Prenatal nicotine exposure, originating most often from maternal smoking, passive exposure to smoke, or use of nicotine-containing agents, is associated with abnormal placentation, abruption, reduced fetal growth and length of gestation, and stillbirth or neonatal mortality (58). These effects are substantial. If women did not smoke during pregnancy, it has been estimated that the prevalence of small-for-gestation babies could be reduced by 30%, abnormal placentas by 10%, premature deliveries (<37 weeks) by 30%, and premature or perinatal deaths by 15% (59). Prenatal exposure to cigarette smoke is associated with both congenital and long-term effects, including cryptorchidism, limb deficiencies, neurocognitive deficits, and decreased reproductive success in males; exposure is a recognized risk factor for increased respiratory disorders and infection, obesity, anxiety disorders, and sudden infant death syndrome.

Diphenylhydantoin Embryopathy

The antiseizure drug diphenylhydantoin and derivatives (phenytoin, Dilantin) causes a syndrome of intrauterine growth restriction, microcephaly and mental retardation, cleft palate, congenital heart defect, digital hypoplasia, and characteristic facial appearance consisting of wide-set eyes, epicanthal folds, broad sunken nasal bridge, upturned nose, and widened lips (60,61). Intellectual development may be delayed as well. Human exposure during the 5th to 6th week results in cleft lip and maxillary hypoplasia (62). The teratogenic mechanism(s) remains unclear despite abundant research.

Fetal exposure to diphenylhydantoin is also known to be carcinogenic. Neuroblastoma, ganglioneuroblastoma, extrarenal Wilms tumor, and malignant mesenchymoma have been observed in individuals exposed to diphenylhydantoin *in utero* (63).

Metabolic Disruptions

Phenylketonuria

Unmanaged maternal phenylketonuria (PKU) leads to intrauterine and postnatal growth restriction, microcephaly and mental retardation, cardiovascular defects, dislocated hips, and other more minor anomalies. The incidence of fetal defects is greatly decreased in mothers whose PKU is well controlled during pregnancy. It has been suggested that impaired accretion of two fatty acids, arachidonic and docosahexaenoic acids (structural components of the CNS), contributes to the small head, reduced vision, and mental retardation (64). In severe forms, the accumulation of phenylalanine results in the formation of CNS fibrils that resemble amyloid, suggesting that the disease may be one of abnormal protein folding (65,66). Infants of phenylketonuric mothers are heterozygous, and because phenylketonuric heterozygotes are generally normal, the defect in the fetus must be attributed to the maternal metabolic disturbance.

Diabetes Mellitus

A large number of pregnancy complications are recognized in women suffering from diabetes mellitus. Stillbirth and perinatal mortality in insulin-dependent women occur at five times the background rate; neonatal mortality is increased 15 times and infant mortality three times over the general population (67). Macrosomia complicates vaginal delivery. Type I maternal diabetes is also associated with an increased incidence of preeclampsia and pregnancy-induced hypertension (68). The effects of gestational diabetes are the subject of continuing study, but in general tend to be fewer and less severe than those arising from pregestational diabetes.

Maternal diabetes mellitus is also associated with a number of fetal anomalies, with an incidence variably estimated at two to eleven times that of the normal population (69). Defects may involve virtually every organ system, prominent examples being anencephaly, holoprosencephaly, arhinencephaly, or myelomeningocele, congenital heart defects, caudal

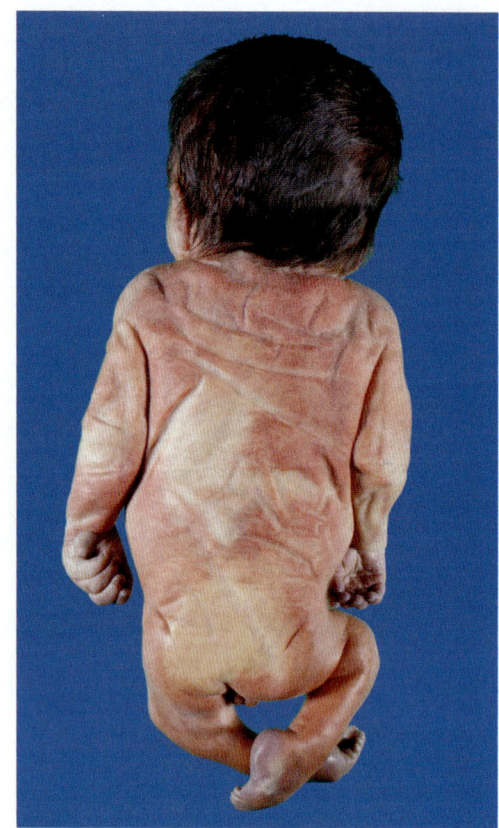

FIGURE 4-3 • Infant of diabetic mother. Pelvic girdle is reduced noticeably in this 31-week-old male with absent lumbosacral spine and malformed pelvis, indicative of caudal dysgenesis (formerly caudal regression syndrome).

dysgenesis (formerly "caudal regression")/sirenomelia, imperforate anus, radial aplasia, and renal abnormalities, including renal agenesis and dysplasia (Figure 4-3). Malformations (Table 4-5) are the most important cause of mortality in infants of diabetic mothers.

The exact role of glucose metabolism in diabetic embryopathy is highly complex and beyond the scope of this review. Current studies are centered on metabolic derangements, including oxidative stress, that inhibit regulatory genes, resulting in apoptosis of progenitor cells and malformations (70,71).

Infectious Disruptions

Infections, particularly toxoplasmosis, rubella, cytomegalovirus (CMV), herpes simplex, varicella, syphilis, and others (TORCHS), may cause fetal disruptions (see Chapter 6). The earlier in pregnancy the infection occurs, the greater is the likelihood of embryonic death or development of anomalies. The most frequent fetal abnormalities are intrauterine growth restriction, microcephaly and mental retardation, deafness, cataracts, retinopathy, microphthalmia, glaucoma, myopia, and congenital heart defects.

Periventricular calcifications and chorioretinitis are frequent in toxoplasmosis. Other organisms that may be implicated in human congenital anomalies are herpes hominis type 2, which is associated with a severe congenital brain

TABLE 4-5 CONGENITAL ANOMALIES ASSOCIATED WITH MATERNAL DIABETES MELLITUS

Central Nervous System
 Anencephaly
 Holoprosencephaly
 Arhinencephaly
 Occipital encephalocele
 Myelomeningocele

Cardiovascular System
 Atrial, ventricular septal defect
 Transposition of the great vessels
 Single ventricle, hypoplastic left heart
 Ebstein anomaly of tricuspid valve
 Pulmonic stenosis, mitral atresia
 Hypertrophic cardiomyopathy

Musculoskeletal System
 Amelia of upper limbs
 Caudal dysgenesis (regression)/sirenomelia
 Costovertebral segmentation defects

Urogenital System
 Renal adysplasia
 Unilateral renal agenesis

Craniofacial Complex
 Bilateral auricular atresia
 Cleft lip/palate
 Bifid tongue
 Microtia/anotia
 Hemifacial microstomia

Other Abnormalities
 Hypoplastic lungs
 Thymic aplasia
 Omphalocele
 Anorectal stenosis/atresia

Modified from Castori M. Diabetic embryopathy: a developmental perspective from fertilization to adulthood. *Mol Syndromol* 2013;4:74–86.

defect, varicella, Venezuelan equine encephalitis, Coxsackie virus, and syphilis. Acquired immune deficiency syndrome (AIDS) is acquired by transplacental means or during labor, delivery, or breast feeding and constitutes an enormous problem worldwide (72). In 2005 in the United States, 92% of cases of children with AIDS were attributed to maternal transmission of the human immunodeficiency virus (HIV); the incidence of neonatal HIV infection has fallen substantially in the United States with the implementation of prenatal testing, antiretroviral therapy, C-section, and avoidance of breast feeding (73).

Amnion Rupture Disruption Sequence

Early amnion rupture (or ADAM complex) may result in severe defects of the fetus, including asymmetric clefts, body wall defects, often with extrusion of viscera, and highly variable amputations (Figure 4-4). When amnion adheres to the head, marked distortions of craniofacial structures are found, with widely separated eyes, displacement of the nose onto the forehead, and exencephaloceles; swallowing of amniotic bands may produce bizarre orofacial clefts that often follow a linear pattern. Marked deformations, growth deficiency, and a short umbilical cord are also observed in this condition (74). The fetus may also be adherent to the placenta, making diagnosis straightforward. However, when strands of amnion are not identified, diagnosis is hampered, although the pattern of defects may still imply this mode of pathogenesis. In the macerated fetus, strands of tissue resembling sloughed epidermis may be identified as amnion by microscopy. Amnion may also be absent from the fetal surface of the placenta, or free membranes. The least severe form of amniotic band disruption is a constriction groove ("Streeter band") on a limb. The temporal relationship of abnormalities in early amnion rupture sequence is shown in Table 4-6.

Amnion rupture is thought to be rather common, affecting perhaps 1 of every 1,200 liveborn and stillborn fetuses. If this is the case, many occurrences apparently have few or no sequelae. Rare families with amniotic bands in relatives have been reported, but the recurrence risk appears to be negligible (76). Causes for premature rupture are not understood. The forces of uterine contraction have been implicated, but recent studies have suggested that a process of programmed weakening of membranes may operate prior to delivery (77). This observation could help explain familial recurrences (see Chapter 9 for additional details).

Chorion and Yolk Sac Rupture Sequence

While rupture of the amnion is well recognized, some have hypothesized that similar defects might arise from rupture of the chorion or yolk sac. Rupture during the 3rd week of gestation and subsequent mechanical compression of the fetus could interfere with normal cardiac descent, resulting in cleft sternum, ectopia cordis, and thoracic and pulmonary hypoplasia (78). Such cases reflect the complex nature of embryogenesis in the region. Another published example involved an infant with rudimentary occipital meningocele and transverse defects of the hands, who, by microscopy, had intestinal mucosa adherent to the scalp (79). Possible explanations included a genetic defect similar to disorganization in the rodent; homeotic transformation; abnormal juxtaposition of epidermis and yolk sac remnant (or omphaloenteric duct); or adhesion of endoderm and ectoderm to the embryo.

Ischemic and Vascular Disruptions

Interference with blood supply may result in ischemic disruptions. Cutis marmorata telangiectatica congenita is a vascular disruption characterized by atypical capillaries, venules, and veins in different cutaneous layers. Clinically, the lesions manifest as telangiectasia, capillary hemangiomata, cutis marmorata, venous hemangiomata, and varicose veins, depending on the type of vessels involved and

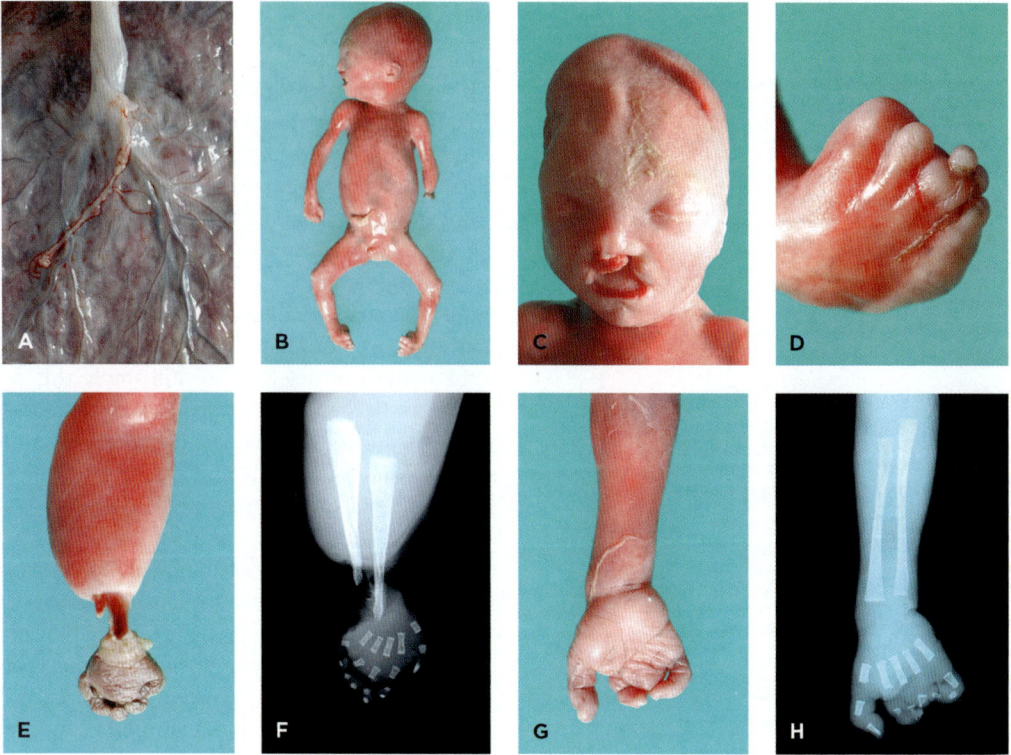

FIGURE 4-4 • Amnion rupture sequence. **A:** Close-up view of fetal surface of placenta shows tiny remnant of amnion. **B:** A 22-week male fetus with multiple amputation defects. **C:** Face with unilateral cleft lip. **D:** Right foot with syndactyly and multiple amputations of the digits. **E:** Exposed radius and ulna and necrosis of hand reflect the evolution of a band-induced amputation. **F:** Radiograph corresponding to (E). **G:** Right hand with multiple amputation defects. **H:** Radiograph corresponding to (G).

TABLE 4-6 TIMING OF ANOMALIES ASSOCIATED WITH EARLY AMNION RUPTURE

Age at Occurrence	Craniofacial Defect	Limb Defect	Other Abnormality
3–4 weeks	Anencephaly Encephalocele Meningocele Facial deformation Unusual, often linear clefting Proboscis Orbital/eye defect	Complete absence of limb	Placenta adherent to head or abdomen; short umbilical cord
5–6 weeks	Cleft lip Choanal atresia	Limb deficiency Polydactyly Syndactyly	Abdominal wall defect Thoracic wall defect Scoliosis
7 or more weeks	Cleft palate Micrognathia Ear deformity Craniosynostosis	Amniotic bands Amputation Hypoplasia Pseudosyndactyly Foot deformity Dislocation of hip Distal lymphedema	Omphalocele Short umbilical cord Ambiguous genitalia
Second, third trimester	Oligohydramnios deformation sequence, with flattened ears, blunt nose, small mandible	Pena-Shokeir phenotype Constriction bands, with lymphedema distal to site of constriction and possible autoamputation	Pulmonary hypoplasia Constriction of umbilical cord by bands may cause death when severe Altered dermal or hair pattern

Modified from Gilbert-Barness EF, Opitz JM. Congenital anomalies and malformation syndromes. In: Wigglesworth JS, Singer DB, eds. *Textbook of Fetal and Perinatal Pathology*. Oxford, UK: Blackwell Scientific Publications; 1991; Higginbottom MC, Jones KL, Hall BD, et al. The amniotic band disruption complex: timing of amniotic rupture and variable spectra of consequent defects. *J Pediatr* 1979;95:544–549 (Refs. 55,75).

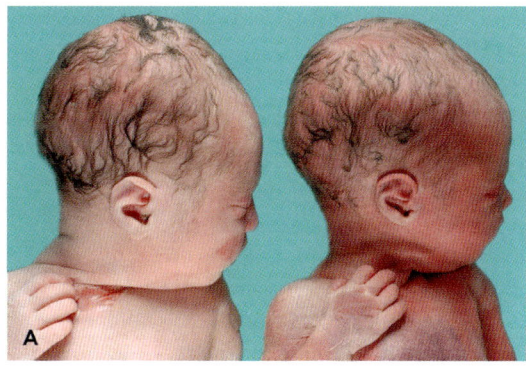
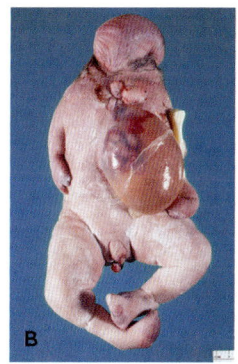

FIGURE 4-5 • Complications of monochorionic twinning. **A:** Pale, donor twin (**left**) and congested, recipient cotwin (**right**) in twin–twin transfusion syndrome. **B:** Acardiac cotwin in TRAP. Note the absence or malformation of structures of the upper body, omphalocele, and more normal lower extremities (but with anomalies of numerous digits).

the layer of skin affected. Secondary thrombosis with subsequent localized atrophy and ulceration may occur. Cutis marmorata telangiectatica congenita occurs sporadically, with female preponderance and occasional minor manifestations in close relatives.

In the Klippel-Trenaunay-Weber syndrome (see below), which usually occurs sporadically, dysplasia and capillary or cavernous hemangiomatosis and phlebectasia and varicosities with oligodactyly, syndactyly, and gigantism of digits have been observed. Congenital or postnatal hypertrophy of one or more limbs is frequent. Visceral hemangiomata may occur.

In addition to the well-recognized difficulties that arise in singletons, twins or other multiple gestations are especially at risk. Cord entanglement occurs in twins and may disrupt blood flow. Because of the variability in distance between cord insertion sites, more complications are observed in monochorionic monoamniotic than in monochorionic diamniotic placentas (21). Two additional examples of vascular disruption involve monochorionic twinning, namely twin–twin transfusion syndrome and twin reversed arterial perfusion (TRAP).

Twin–Twin Transfusion Syndrome

Twinning within the context of a shared placental disc is complicated by the presence of intraplacental vascular anastomoses. These may be small and mild or quite large, allowing significant sharing of blood between fetuses. Problems arise when blood flow is unbalanced and unidirectional, creating "pump" and "recipient" twins (Figure 4-5A). In such circumstances, the pump twin is pale and anemic, while the recipient or perfused twin is congested, possibly hydropic, and polycythemic. Differences in amniotic fluid volume can create the "stuck twin" phenomenon, with oligohydramnios in one amniotic sac (with consequent fetal deformation) and polyhydramnios in the other. The death of one twin quickly affects the well-being of the other, resulting in death or embolization of decay products, resulting in disseminated intravascular coagulation or visceral infarcts (80).

Twin Reversed Arterial Perfusion

Artery-to-artery anastomoses have a particularly striking effect when flow in one umbilical artery and aorta is reversed, a phenomenon that can be diagnosed *in utero* by Doppler flow studies. In such a circumstance, the lower body is perfused, but upper regions are not (Figure 4-5B). The heart may fail to develop (acardia); absence of the head (acardius–acephalus), upper limbs, or other viscera (e.g., lungs) often occurs.

Dysplastic Disruptions

Dysplastic disruptions include the presacral teratoma that may be associated with anencephaly, spina bifida, meningocele, or imperforate anus; duplication of the lower intestinal tract, uterus, vagina, and ureter/renal pelvis; patent urachus; cleft palate; and esophageal and duodenal atresia. Imperforate anus and sacral defects may be inherited on an autosomal dominant basis.

Hyperthermia as a Disruption

Smith and colleagues were the first to make a systematic study of the effects of hyperthermia caused by infections or sauna bathing during pregnancy (81). Hyperthermia is an antimitotic teratogen that interferes mostly with CNS development, producing NTDs, microcephaly, micrencephaly, microphthalmia, and neurogenic contractures (82). Other anomalies associated with hyperthermia include neuronal heterotopia, polymicrogyria, small midface, micrognathia, cleft lip and palate, ear, cardiac, and limb defects (e.g., arthrogryposis and syndactyly). Severe mental deficiency and seizures in infancy have also been described (81).

The presence and severity of anomalies depend upon the duration of hyperthermic episode, maximum temperature reached, and stage of development (82). Both mild temperature elevation during the preimplantation period and more significant elevations during embryonic and fetal development may manifest as anomalies. At weeks 7 to 16 of gestation, hyperthermia may be associated with hypotonia, neurogenic arthrogryposis, or CNS dysgenesis.

NONMETABOLIC DYSPLASIA SYNDROMES

The most common dysplasia syndromes are the autosomal dominant conditions: neurofibromatosis 1, von Hippel-Lindau disease, Marfan syndrome, and the osteochondrodysplasias, most of the lethal forms of which are autosomal recessive traits. These conditions are discussed in various chapters including Chapters 10, 25, and 28.

Beckwith-Wiedemann Syndrome

Two prominent overgrowth conditions are Beckwith-Wiedemann and Perlman syndromes. In the early 1960s, Beckwith and Wiedemann reported several patients with exomphalos (i.e., omphalocele), macroglossia, and gigantism. In one review, Beckwith-Wiedemann syndrome (BWS) accounted for nearly 12% of all cases of omphalocele. Craniofacial abnormalities (Figure 4-6) include microcephaly, macroglossia (which may interfere with respiration or swallowing), prominent eyes with relative infraorbital hypoplasia, capillary nevus flammeus of the central forehead and eyelids, metopic ridge in the central forehead, large fontanelles, prominent occiput, and malocclusion, with a tendency toward mandibular prognathism. A marker for the syndrome is the unusual linear fissures or pits in the lobule of the external ear and semilunar indentations of the posterior rim of the helix. Hemihypertrophy, clitoromegaly, large ovaries, hyperplastic uterus and bladder, bicornuate uterus, hypospadias, and immunodeficiency are prominent.

Interstitial cell hyperplasia of the testis, pituitary hyperplasia, neonatal polycythemia, diastasis recti, posterior diaphragmatic eventration, and cryptorchidism may also occur. Manifestations of BWS also include neonatal hypoglycemia, more generalized organomegaly, and cytomegaly of the adrenal cortex and islet cells of the pancreas. The placenta in BWS may exhibit mesenchymal dysplasia, a rare change that may be mistaken for partial hydatidiform mole. In one study, over 20% of placentas with this change were from patients with BWS (83).

The predisposition to the development of malignant tumors such as Wilms tumor, adrenocortical carcinoma, hepatoblastoma, gonadoblastoma, and brain stem glioma is widely recognized. Wilms tumor may be bilateral when it is associated with this syndrome (see Chapter 17). Even when free of tumor, the kidneys may be strikingly enlarged, and their surfaces traversed by numerous, irregularly disposed, shallow fissures that markedly increase the number of lobulations. The parenchyma is disorganized; minute lobulations crowd one another, each with a distinctly demarcated cortex and medulla. Other renal changes include persistent glomerulogenesis, medullary dysplasia, diffuse bilateral nephroblastomatosis, metanephric hamartomas, hydronephrosis and hydroureters, and duplications.

The incidence of polyhydramnios and prematurity is relatively high in BWS. Most cases are sporadic, but familial cases are recognized; dominant inheritance (with variable expressivity) is suspected in a number of cases. In the majority of cases, BWS is caused by disruption of genomic imprinting within the 11p15 region (84). This mechanism has been exhibited in dramatic fashion by the increased incidence of BWS in families utilizing assisted reproductive technologies, namely *in vitro* fertilization and intracytoplasmic sperm injection (85). The region contains several genes (e.g., *CDKN1C*, *H19*, *IGF2*, *LIT1*, *KCNQ1OT1*) responsible for normal growth. In some 10% to 20% of cases, paternal uniparental disomy is the responsible mechanism; in smaller numbers of cases, mutations, translocations, inversions, or duplications of these genes may occur.

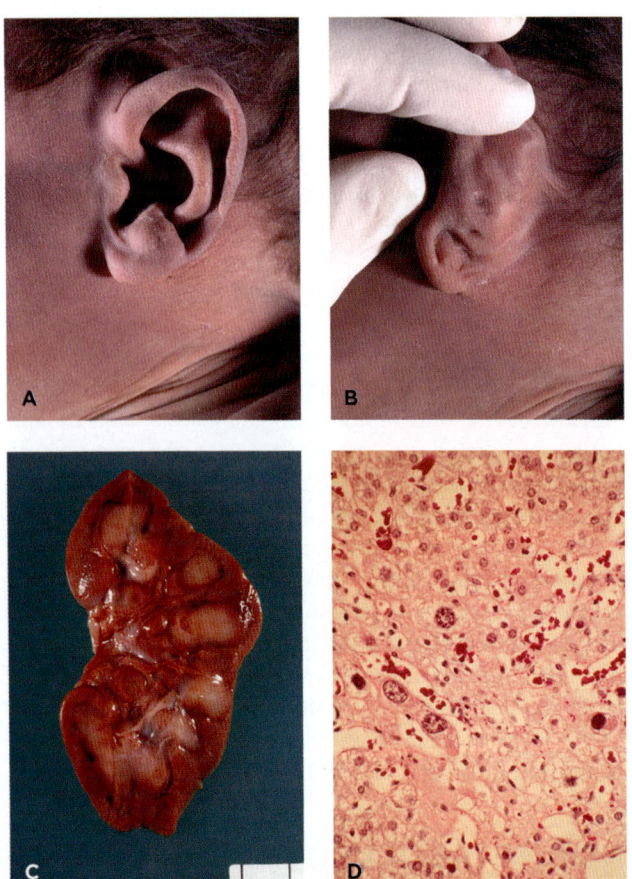

FIGURE 4-6 • Beckwith-Wiedemann syndrome. **A, B:** Ear pits were identified in this 9-month-old infant, who had a large omphalocele excised shortly after birth (46,XY, no deletion recognized). **C:** Note the distorted architecture in this dysplastic kidney. **D:** Microscopic view of adrenal gland, showing marked cytomegaly.

Perlman Syndrome

Perlman syndrome is an autosomal recessive disorder composed of macrosomia, nephromegaly with renal dysplasia (persistent fetal lobation, nephrogenic rests, immature glomeruli, sclerotic glomeruli, primitive tubular structures, and medullary hamartomatous dysplasia), Wilms tumor, hyperplasia of the endocrine pancreas with resultant hypoglycemia, cryptorchidism, multiple congenital anomalies (mostly infrequent and nonspecific ones, such as facial dysmorphia [depressed nasal bridge, anteverted upper lip], cleft lip, and cardiac anomalies), and mental retardation. The frequent occurrence of Wilms tumor has led to the speculation that persistent foci of renal dysplasia, blastema, or nephroblastomatosis constitute predisposing lesions (86). The condition resembles BWS but is distinguished on the basis of inheritance (BWS is autosomal dominant), differences in specific anomalies or facial appearance, and different natural histories and associated malformations. Death by 1 year of age is common.

METABOLIC DYSPLASIA SYNDROMES

Williams Syndrome

Williams (or Williams-Beuren) syndrome is an autosomal dominant disorder manifest by characteristic facial features, supravalvular and aortic stenosis, infantile hypercalcemia (which may be comparatively mild and transient or severe and life-threatening), and behavioral and neurologic abnormalities. Specific characteristics include growth and mental retardation, microcephaly, congenital hypotonia, and elfin face with short palpebral fissures, depressed nasal bridge, epicanthal folds, and anteverted nares. Cardiovascular defects include supravalvular aortic stenosis, peripheral pulmonary artery stenosis, pulmonary valvular stenosis, and ventricular and atrial septal defect. Renal artery stenosis with hypertension, hypoplasia of the aorta, and other arterial anomalies have been reported. Genitourinary anomalies are varied but occur in one-half to three-quarters of patients (87). Many neonates exhibit irritability, with failure to thrive. Recent investigations have focused on deletions or mutations within the Williams-Beuren critical region (7q11.23) and resulting errors in development, vitamin D catabolism, and intestinal absorption of calcium. Genes in this region include *ELN* (cardiovascular development), *RFC2* (DNA replication, general growth and development), *LIMK1* (cognition), and others.

Zellweger Syndrome

Zellweger syndrome (cerebrohepatorenal syndrome) belongs to a group of peroxisomal disorders. Genetic diseases involving peroxisomes (single membrane–bound organelles involved in multiple metabolic processes) include those in which only a single peroxisomal function is impaired—acatalasemia, X-linked adrenoleukodystrophy, and the adult form of Refsum disease—and those with impaired peroxisome biogenesis—the so-called Zellweger spectrum (consisting of Zellweger syndrome, infantile Refsum disease, and neonatal adrenoleukodystrophy) and rhizomelic chondrodysplasia punctata (88).

Zellweger syndrome develops on an autosomal recessive basis, from mutations in one of the 16 *PEX* genes (most commonly *PEX1* and *PEX6*). These encode for peroxins, proteins integral to the assembly of peroxisomes. With peroxisomal dysfunction comes the accumulation of very long chain fatty acids, which damage a number of tissues during development. Diagnosis can be complex, involving several biochemical abnormalities; a cell line, established by skin biopsy during infancy, provides fibroblasts for additional diagnostic purposes (89). The syndrome is dominated clinically by severe CNS dysfunction. Affected infants are usually born at term and do not manifest intrauterine growth restriction. Other clinical manifestations (see Table 4-7) include a pear- or light bulb-shaped head, large fontanelles, flat occiput, high forehead with shallow supraorbital ridges, a flat face, minor ear anomalies, inner epicanthal folds, Brushfield spots, mild micrognathia, and redundant neck skin.

Infants with Zellweger syndrome are severely hypotonic, with an inability to suck, reduced deep tendon reflexes, and lack of psychomotor development. The degree of hypotonia

TABLE 4-7 CLINICAL FINDINGS IN ZELLWEGER SYNDROME

Craniofacial
  Macrocephaly; high forehead and hairline; dolichocephaly
  Large anterior fontanel; open metopic suture
  Mongoloid slant of palpebral fissures, with epicanthal folds; hypertelorism; shallow supraorbital ridges
  High-arched palate; posterior cleft of palate
  Small mandible
  Minor anomalies of ears
  Redundant skin folds of neck

Limbs
  Talipes equinovarus
  Camptodactyly
  Contractures

Central Nervous System
  Hypotonia, rarely hypertonia
  Severe mental retardation
  Seizures
  Nystagmus; oculogyric fits
  Absent neonatal reflexes

Eyes
  Cataract; corneal clouding
  Glaucoma; nystagmus
  Brushfield spots
  Pigmentary retinopathy
  Optic nerve "dysplasia" or hypoplasia

Skeletal System
  Chondrodysplasia calcificans, especially involving the patella
  Delayed skeletal maturation
  Bell-shaped thorax
  Talipes equinovarus deformity

Other Findings
  Cardiac defect
  Jaundice with hepatomegaly
  Hypospadias, cryptorchidism; clitoromegaly
  Single palmar crease

Modified from Gilbert-Barness EF, Opitz JM. Congenital anomalies and malformation syndromes. In: Wigglesworth JS, Singer DB, eds. *Textbook of Fetal and Perinatal Pathology*. Oxford, UK: Blackwell Scientific Publications; 1991; Lee PR, Raymond GV. Child neurology: Zellweger syndrome. *Neurology* 2013;80:e207–e210 (Ref. 55,89).

and physical appearance can be suggestive of Down syndrome. Other manifestations include congenital heart defects (e.g., anomalies of the aortic arch, patent ductus arteriosus, ventricular septal defect), stippled calcification of the epiphyses, and hepatomegaly with signs of hepatic dysfunction and occasional jaundice. Life expectancy ranges from a few months to 2 years; death usually occurs from respiratory complications or infection.

Autopsy findings of patients with Zellweger syndrome are listed in Table 4-8. Brain abnormalities include focal lissencephaly and other cerebral gyral abnormalities, heterotopic cerebral cortex, olivary nuclear dysplasia, defects of the corpus callosum, numerous lipid-laden macrophages and histiocytes in cortical and periventricular areas, and dysmyelination. The liver is characterized by hepatic lobular disarray, or micronodular cirrhosis, biliary dysgenesis, and siderosis. The kidneys show persistent fetal lobulations with cortical cysts. Albuminuria and aminoaciduria may be observed. Other abnormalities include hypoglycemia, elevated serum iron, siderosis, hyperpipecolic acidemia, hepatic and cerebral glycogen storage, elevated very long chain fatty acids, abnormal bile acids, dicarboxylic aciduria, and hypocarnitinemia. Renal cysts have been a consistent finding and may be a pathologic marker for this condition. They are often macroscopic and both glomerular and tubular by microscopy. Occasionally, cysts appear to connect directly to terminal ends of collecting tubules without an intervening tubular segment, suggesting focally deficient metanephric differentiation. More classic cystic dysplastic changes, horseshoe kidneys, and ureteral duplication have been noted. Immunodeficiency may develop, and some patients have been diagnosed mistakenly with DiGeorge syndrome. Patients with atypical Zellweger syndrome (Versmold variant) have hypertonia and may live longer (see Chapter 5.)

SEQUENCES

Robin Sequence

The defects in Robin sequence include retro- or micrognathia, glossoptosis, and cleft soft palate. Hypoplasia of the mandible before week 9 of gestation causes the tongue to be posteriorly located, presumably preventing closure of the posterior palatal shelves. Hypoplasia may also be a result of early mechanical constraint *in utero*, limiting growth before palatine closure. Infants may have failure to thrive and feeding difficulties, requiring tracheostomy or orofacial surgery. Isolated and syndromic forms are recognized. The latter may have a genetic basis, with dysregulation of *SOX9* and *KCNJ2* postulated in a subset of cases. Associations with Stickler syndrome (see below) and blindness due to high myopia have been identified.

Prune Belly Sequence

Prune belly sequence occurs as a triad of absent or hypoplastic abdominal muscles, urinary tract defects, and cryptorchidism. The umbilicus may be displaced cephalad, with flaring of rib margins, Harrison groove, and pectus deformities, all apparently secondary to the muscle defect. Nearly three-quarters of patients have additional defects of the cardiac, pulmonary, gastrointestinal, or musculoskeletal systems (90). Most cases are sporadic, but some familial cases have been autosomal recessive.

Renal anomalies are a critical part of the spectrum. With urethral or bladder neck obstruction, more proximal segments of the urinary tract become dilated, resulting in megacystis, hydroureter, and hydronephrosis, the latter with consequent renal dysplasia. Urinary ascites may occur from overdistention and prenatal rupture of the bladder. The abdomen tends to be tense and glassy in the fetus, and, after collapse of the bladder and/or absorption of abdominal fluid, lax and wrinkled in the newborn (Figure 4-7). Neonatal death occurs in 20% of infants, usually from pulmonary

TABLE 4-8 PATHOLOGIC FINDINGS IN ZELLWEGER SYNDROME

Brain
  Abnormal cerebral gyral pattern (microgyria, pachygyria, partial lissencephaly)
  Hypoplasia or agenesis of corpus callosum
  Cerebral, cerebellar heterotopias
  Cerebellar, olivary hypoplasia
  Ventriculomegaly
  Hypoplasia/dysgenesis of optic nerve
  Leukoencephalomyelopathy
  Gliosis

Heart
  Ventricular septal defect
  Patent ductus arteriosus
  Patent foramen ovale

Liver
  Biliary dysgenesis
  Cirrhosis
  Siderosis
  Absent peroxisomes
  Abnormal mitochondria
  Diminished smooth endoplasmic reticulum

Kidney
  Cortical microcysts
  Glomerular and tubular cystic dysplasia
  Hydronephrosis
  Horseshoe kidney

Pancreas
  Islet cell hyperplasia

Thymus
  Hypoplasia/aplasia

Modified from Gilbert-Barness EF, Opitz JM. Congenital anomalies and malformation syndromes. In: Wigglesworth JS, Singer DB, eds. *Textbook of Fetal and Perinatal Pathology*. Oxford, UK: Blackwell Scientific Publications; 1991.; Lee PR, Raymond GV. Child neurology: Zellweger syndrome. *Neurology* 2013;80:e207–e210.

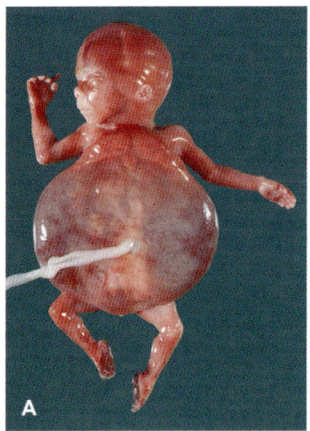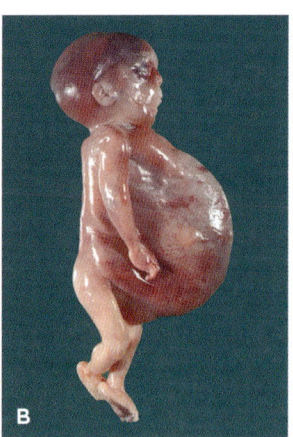

FIGURE 4-7 • Prune belly sequence. **A:** Anterior view of an 18-week male fetus with marked distention of the abdomen secondary to megacystis, bladder outlet obstruction, and severe ascites. Note talipes deformity of feet, a result of intrauterine constraint. **B:** Lateral view of a second 18-week male fetus, showing marked distention of fluid-filled abdomen. Abdominal skin takes on a wrinkled appearance when/if fluid is resorbed. The rib cage of each fetus is markedly expanded.

hypoplasia, a sequel of oligohydramnios or abdominal pressure on the diaphragm. However, long-term survival is possible, especially in patients with mild or no changes of the abdominal musculature or urinary tract. Additional complications in survivors include decreased spermatogenesis/absence of spermatogonia and salt-wasting nephritis.

Pathogenesis continues to receive attention. One hypothesis is that an early and primary insult to mesenchymal precursors of both abdominal musculature and kidney is responsible. A different view is that urethral obstruction, with massive distention of the urinary bladder and secondary stretching and thinning of abdominal skeletal muscles, occurs. Modes of urethral obstruction (posterior urethral valves, obstructing urethral diaphragm, urethral stenosis or atresia, physical kinking) continue to be studied (91). The prostate gland is generally hypoplastic or absent, but it remains unclear whether this change is primary or secondary.

ASSOCIATIONS

Because of shared molecular determinants, spatial contiguity, or close timing of morphogenetic events during early embryonic development, malformations may sometimes appear as complexes that involve several diverse tissues. When these occur repeatedly (i.e., nonrandomly) and without recognized etiology or pathogenesis, the disorders are termed associations. As the understanding of these conditions increases, the designation may change (e.g., CHARGE association is now known as CHARGE syndrome). Diagnosis can be difficult, given the degree of phenotypic overlap among associations. For example, VATER, VACTERL, CHARGE, MURCS, Fanconi syndrome, and other conditions share a number of features. That is apparent in the associations described below.

VATER Association

The acronym VATER reflects the association of vertebral defects, anal atresia, tracheoesophageal fistula with esophageal atresia, and radial and renal abnormalities (Figure 4-8) (92). Genitourinary defects include renal dysplasia or agenesis, renal ectopia, persistent urachus, hypospadias, and caudally displaced, hypoplastic penis. Prenatal growth deficiency, ear anomalies, large fontanels, cleft palate, cloacal exstrophy, and rib anomalies are also recognized. This pattern of malformations occurs sporadically.

The phenotypic variability of VATER association complicates both diagnosis and classification. VACTERL is an expansion of VATER that includes cardiac and limb defects. The overlap with müllerian duct, renal, and cervicothoracic somite malformations (MURCS) with tracheal agenesis, hemifacial microsomia, and other facial asymmetry syndromes is recognized. The VATER phenotype also overlaps with Fanconi syndrome and to a lesser degree with sirenomelia. Chromosomal breakage studies are therefore recommended for patients with features of both VATER association and Fanconi syndrome.

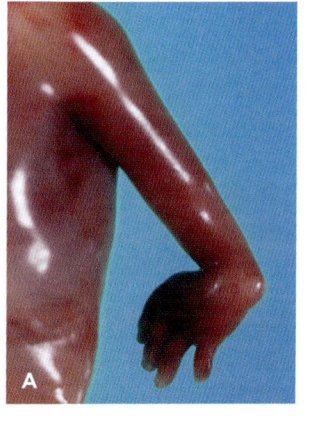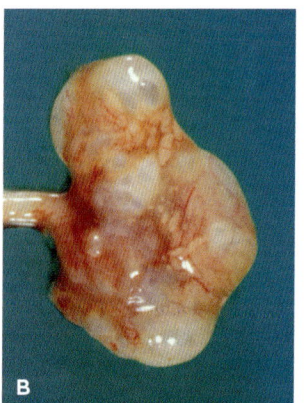
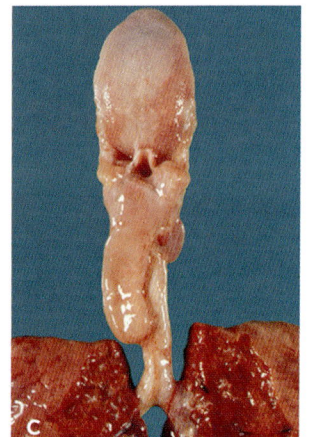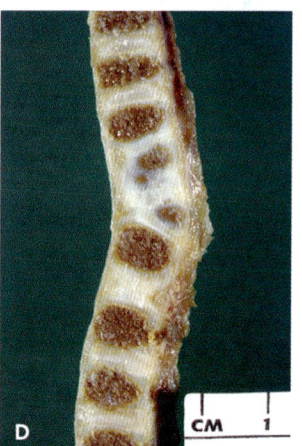

FIGURE 4-8 • VATER/VACTERL association. **A:** Marked deviation of wrist and hand; thumb and radius are absent. **B:** Cystic renal dysplasia. **C:** Esophageal atresia (without tracheoesophageal fistula) from infant with VACTERL association. **D:** Excised segment of vertebral column with hemivertebrae.

The etiology and pathogenesis of VATER association remain unknown. It has been hypothesized that anomalies derive from a common pathogenetic mechanism, namely a defect of blastogenesis prior to day 35 of gestation. Evidence comes from the fact that several critical tissues develop before 35 days, including the septa that divide rectum/anus and trachea/esophagus, radial limb bud, and mesoderm that forms the vertebral bodies. The Adriamycin animal model may contribute to future understanding of these issues (see Chapters 12, 17, and 28 for additional details).

MURCS Association

MURCS is an acronym for müllerian duct aplasia, renal aplasia, and cervicothoracic somite malformations, the latter of which are manifest as cervicothoracic vertebral defects, especially C5 to T1. The condition, also known as Mayer-Rokitansky-Küster-Hauser syndrome type II, is largely sporadic; a variety of duplications and deletions have been reported, but as yet they do not suggest a unified pattern of pathogenesis. Maternal diabetes is present in a subset of cases. Absence of the vagina, absence or hypoplasia of the uterus, and renal abnormalities occur in up to 40% of patients. Additional anomalies, including those involving the craniofacial, skeletal, and cardiac systems, complicate diagnosis (93). A male form of MURCS has been postulated; findings are azoospermia, renal anomalies, and cervicothoracic spinal abnormalities (94).

Schisis Association and Variants

Midline defects such as NTDs (e.g., anencephaly, encephalocele, meningomyelocele), oral clefts, omphalocele, and diaphragmatic hernia occur more frequently than expected (95). This so-called schisis association is frequently lethal. It occurs more often in girls, in twins (4.6%), and in breech presentations (13.7%), and is associated with lower mean birth weight and shortened gestation. Congenital cardiac defects, limb deficiencies, and defects of the urinary tract, mainly renal agenesis, have a high association. Schisis-type abnormalities appear to occur in a nonrandom fashion and have been postulated to arise during blastogenesis (96).

AUTOSOMAL DOMINANT CONDITIONS

CHARGE Syndrome

This syndrome, known originally as CHARGE association, is a dominant condition characterized by coloboma, heart disease, atresia of choanae, retarded growth, and genital and ear anomalies (97). Additional anomalies are varied and may include mild facial dysmorphia, facial palsy, cleft palate, thymic hypoplasia and mild or severe anomalies of the CNS (arhinencephaly, holoprosencephaly). Mutations in the *CHD7* gene, located at 8q12, are recognized in 65% to 70% of patients; a small number of cases may arise from mutations in *SEMA3E*, germ-line mosaicism, or on an X-linked basis. Phenotypic variability is pronounced, and diagnosis is based upon the presence of four major or three major and three minor anomalies.

Nail–Patella Syndrome

In nail–patella syndrome, or hereditary onycho-osteodysplasia, fingers and toes, especially thumbs and great toes, show onychodysplasia, hypoplasia, longitudinal ridging, and hemiatrophy. The patellae are small, absent, or dislocated; the elbows are dysplastic; small osseous spurs or horns on the iliac bones are prominent. Radial heads may be dislocated, and femoral condyles enlarged, causing valgus deformities of the knees. Glaucoma may develop or progress after birth and a peculiar heterochromia may be seen in the iris. Subtle impairment of hearing and peripheral neurologic symptoms such as sensory dysfunction are also recognized. A nephropathy is more frequent in females and varies from proteinuria, which may be transient and asymptomatic, to fibrosis and renal failure (98). Thickening of the glomerular basement membrane, with focal collections of collagen fibers and mesangial thickening, is observed. Immunofluorescence shows a nonspecific focal distribution of IgM or complement (additional details are found in Chapters 17 and 28).

One gene identified to date, *LMX1B*, on chromosome 9q34.1, is a transcription factor important to limb, renal, ocular, and brain development. However, the interfamilial and intrafamilial variability in phenotypes is highly suggestive of additional genetic involvement (99). In fact, the tuberous sclerosis complex gene (*TSC1*) is also located on chromosome 9q3, and both disorders have been recognized in the same kindred; one family member has both conditions (100).

Orofaciodigital Syndrome Type I

Orofaciodigital syndrome type I (OFD1) is an extremely variable constellation of congenital disorders and as such has engendered both attention and debate. At least 13 types have been described. Because most appear to have an autosomal recessive form of inheritance, they are not described in this section. The one additional exception is type VII (Whelan syndrome), which exhibits facial asymmetry and hydronephrosis and is thought to be autosomal dominant or X-linked dominant. Major changes in the OFD complex include hypertrophic frenula, lingual hamartomas, cleft lip or palate, ocular hypertelorism, brachydactyly, polydactyly, and syndactyly. Other organ systems, most notably the CNS and urinary tract, are affected as well. OFD1 is an X-linked dominant trait, lethal in hemizygous males prenatally and characterized by webbing between the buccal mucous membrane and alveolar ridge, partial clefts in the mid-upper lip, hypoplasia of nasal cartilages, absent lateral incisors, asymetric shortening of the digits with clinodactyly, bifid hallux with or without syndactyly, and variable mental deficiency. Mutations in the *OFD1* gene affect primary cilia, altering diverse signaling pathways. This accounts for the phenotypic variability and overlap with other ciliopathies such as Joubert and Meckel-Gruber syndromes. Patients with OFD syndrome may exhibit polycystic kidneys, biliary and ductal cysts of the liver and pancreas, and CNS anomalies (including occipital encephalocele and cerebellar dysgenesis) that are also observed in these two syndromes.

Branchio-Oto-Renal Syndrome

The branchio-oto-renal (BOR) syndrome is an autosomal dominant disorder characterized by branchial arch anomalies (i.e., preauricular pits, branchial fistulas, anomalies of the external ear), hearing loss, and renal hypoplasia and dysplasia. The syndrome is one of the more prevalent among congenital disorders that exhibit hearing loss. A preauricular pit at birth is a marker for this syndrome and suggests further workup. The renal anomalies range from minor defects to marked hypoplasia with renal failure. Mutations have been identified in *EYA1*, *SIX1*, and *SIX5* genes; other genes (*SHARPIN*, *FGF3*, and *HOXA*) may be involved as well (101).

Townes-Brocks Syndrome

Townes-Brocks syndrome is an autosomal dominant disorder with variable expressivity. Major changes include thumb anomalies (i.e., triphalangeal thumb), preaxial polydactyly, auricular anomalies, imperforate anus, cardiac defects, and anomalies of other internal organs, including renal hypoplasia and cysts. Mental retardation has been reported in a minority of patients. Endocrine abnormalities include congenital hypothyroidism and growth hormone deficiency. Additional clinical complications may include obstructive apnea and dysphagia. Anomalies overlap with the VATER/VACTERL association, hemifacial microsomia, cat eye, Baller-Gerold, and other syndromes. Diagnosis, while challenging, is important, for some of these conditions are sporadic. Towns-Brocks syndrome, by contrast, is caused by mutations in the *SALL1* gene.

Holt-Oram Syndrome

This syndrome is characterized by certain skeletal and cardiovascular abnormalities and appears as an autosomal dominant trait with variable expressivity. Skeletal abnormalities in the upper limbs range from thumb hypoplasia to phocomelia and have a preponderance of left-sided involvement. Hypoplasia or absence of the first metacarpal and radius, and defects of the ulna, humerus, clavicle, scapula, and sternum may be present. The most frequently described cardiac anomaly is a secundum-type atrial septal defect. However, a variety of other cardiac defects and anomalies of the coronary arteries have been recognized. To date, nearly 40 mutations of the gene responsible for Holt-Oram syndrome, *TBX5*, have been identified (102); missense mutations are associated with distinct phenotypes. Variability within affected families suggests that the genetic background, environmental or stochastic modifiers, or modifier genes may be important. In addition, *TBX5* is a T-box transcription factor gene that, when mutated, upregulates tumor cell proliferation and metastasis. Several older patients with Holt-Oram syndrome have been reported with malignancies. These occurrences could be coincidental, of course, although experimental support for this association is available.

Mandibulofacial Dysostosis

Mandibulofacial dysostosis, also known as Treacher Collins or Franceschetti-Klein-Zwahlen syndrome, is viewed as a nonspecific developmental field defect that may be inherited as an autosomal dominant condition. The main characteristics of this disorder are malar hypoplasia with downslanting palpebral fissures, defects of the lower lid, mandibular hypoplasia, and malformations of the external ear. Other abnormalities include partial to total absence of the lower eyelashes, external ear canal defects, conductive deafness, cleft palate, incompetent soft palate, and a projection of scalp hair onto the lateral cheek. Pharyngeal hypoplasia, microphthalmia, macrostomia or microstomia, choanal atresia, blind fistulas and skin tags between the auricle and the angle of the mouth, absence of the parotid gland, congenital heart defects, and cryptorchidism are occasionally reported. Because the majority (over 60%) of cases arise *de novo* and expression is highly variable, with different phenotypes occurring both within and between families, diagnosis and counseling can be challenging. Mutations in *TCOF1* are the most common genetic change (approximately 80%). Over 50 mutations in the gene, which encodes the protein "treacle," have been identified, and the Treacher Collins locus mapped to chromosome 5q31.3-32 (103). Mutations in *POLR1C* and *POLR1D* are observed infrequently (2%) and are autosomal recessive. In experimental models, mutations in *Tcof1* lead to increased neural crest cell death and associated craniofacial defects.

Opitz-Frias Syndrome

A rare, heterogenous condition, Opitz-Frias syndrome, also known as hypertelorism–hypospadias or G/BBB syndrome, was described and named using the initials of the surnames of the three families. Because of the overlap between G and BBB syndrome manifestations, some investigators have suggested that they are the same entity and should be called Opitz or Opitz-Frias syndrome. Affected males may exhibit cranial asymmetry, ocular hypertelorism, prominent forehead sometimes with widow's peak, broad nasal bridge, anteverted nostrils, and hypospadias or other genitourinary anomalies. Female carriers generally have only hypertelorism. Cleft lip or palate, other defects involving the upper airway, cardiac anomalies, strabismus, and downslanting palpebral fissures may be present; imperforate anus, agenesis or hypoplasia of the corpus callosum, and Dandy Walker malformation are recognized in a subset of patients. About one-half of individuals have developmental and cognitive delay. Patients may have difficulty swallowing (104). Neonatally, infants can be recognized by their hypertelorism, hypospadias, and other anomalies, such as cleft lip or palate and congenital heart defects. The syndrome is genetically heterogeneous, with both X-linked and autosomal dominant forms recognized. The former maps to Xp22 and is designated type I; the latter maps to 22q11 and is designated type II. Mutations in the *MID1* gene have been demonstrated in X-linked cases. The two forms are not easily differentiated by phenotypic means.

ACROCEPHALOSYNDACTYLY SYNDROMES

Acrocephalosyndactyly syndromes are caused by autosomal dominant mutations. The numeric designations of these entities derive from earlier classifications, and syndromes are more commonly known by their proper names. The abnormalities that occur in representative syndromes are listed in Table 4-9.

Apert Syndrome

Apert syndrome, or acrocephalosyndactyly type I, was formerly called acrocephalosyndactyly type II, Vogt cephalodactyly, or Apert-Crouzon disease. The condition can be diagnosed at birth or even prenatally and is characterized by irregular craniosynostosis (especially of coronal sutures), midface hypoplasia, syndactyly, and a broad distal phalanx of the thumb and hallux. Patients may have normal or reduced intellectual abilities. Specific craniofacial anomalies include short anteroposterior skull diameter with a high, full forehead and flat occiput, flat face, supraorbital horizontal groove, shallow orbits, ocular hypertelorism, downslanting palpebral fissures, small nose, and maxillary hypoplasia. Fusion of cervical vertebrae is variable, with involvement of C5-6 most common. This may help differentiate Apert from Crouzon syndrome, where fusion of C2-3 predominates. Cutaneous syndactyly of all toes occurs with or without osseous syndactyly. Synostosis of the radius and humerus, pyloric stenosis, ectopic anus, pulmonary aplasia, anomalous tracheal cartilages, pulmonary stenosis, cardiac malformations, cystic kidneys, hydronephrosis, and bicornuate uterus may occur. The possibility has been raised that infants with Apert syndrome with polydactyly, especially of the toes, represent a nosologically different entity. Most cases arise from *de novo*

TABLE 4-9 MAJOR FEATURES OF REPRESENTATIVE ACROCEPHALOSYNDACTYLY SYNDROMES

Apert Syndrome (Type I)	Saethre-Chotzen Syndrome (Type III)	Pfeiffer Syndrome (Type V)
Mental retardation or normal intelligence	Mental deficiency[a]	Cloverleaf skull[a]
Short anteroposterior skull diameter, with high forehead and flat occiput	Brachycephaly; high forehead	Coronal and sagittal craniosynostosis
Supraorbital horizontal groove	Coronal craniosynostosis; large fontanelles	Ocular hypertelorism
Shallow orbits	Shallow orbits	Antimongoloid palpebral fissures
Ocular hypertelorism	Ocular hypertelorism	Small nose
Downslanted palpebral fissures	Ptosis	Radiohumeral synostosis[a]
Flat face	Facial asymmetry	Broad distal phalanges of thumb, great toe
Maxillary hypoplasia	Maxillary hypoplasia	Partial syndactyly of fingers, toes
Small nose	Small ears	
Cutaneous syndactyly of all toes, with or without syndactyly	Cutaneous syndactyly	
Synostosis of radius, humerus	Single palmar crease	
Irregular thumb, toe	Broad thumbs, great toes	
Pyloric stenosis	Small stature[a]	
Ectopic anus	Hearing deficit[a]	
Pulmonary aplasia	Vertebral anomaly[a]	
Anomalous tracheal cartilage	Cryptorchidism[a]	
Pulmonic stenosis, other cardiac malformations	Renal anomalies[a]	
Cystic kidney		
Hydronephrosis		
Bicornuate uterus		

[a]Occasional abnormality.
Modified from Gilbert-Barness EF, Opitz JM. Congenital anomalies and malformation syndromes. In: Wigglesworth JS, Singer DB, eds. *Textbook of Fetal and Perinatal Pathology*. Oxford, UK: Blackwell Scientific Publications; 1991.

mutations in the fibroblast growth factor receptor 2 gene (*FGFR2*). (See Chapter 28 for additional details.)

Pfeiffer Syndrome

Pfeiffer syndrome, also known as acrocephalosyndactyly type V, arises on an autosomal dominant basis, with most cases representing new mutations. The disorder is genetically heterogeneous, with mutations in both *FGFR1* and *FGFR2* occurring. Three types of Pfeiffer syndrome are recognized. In type I, findings include craniosynostosis of coronal or sagittal sutures, ocular hypertelorism, downward slant of palpebral fissures, small nose, short fingers with broad distal phalanges of the thumbs and big toes, and partial syndactyly of fingers and toes. In type II, cloverleaf skull (kleeblattschädel) and ankylosis of the elbow (radiohumeral synostosis) are seen; type III resembles type II but manifests visceral anomalies without cloverleaf skull. Early death characterizes the latter two types, while in type I, craniofacial abnormalities tend to improve with age, and intelligence is usually normal (see Chapter 28 for additional details).

Other Related Conditions

Crouzon Craniofacial Dysostosis

Inherited as an autosomal dominant trait, Crouzon craniofacial dysostosis occurs from a *FGFR2* mutation. Most cases arise *de novo*, but several family histories have provided evidence for germ-line mosaicism. Findings in Crouzon syndrome are variable but generally include craniofacial anomalies with shallow orbits and ocular proptosis, hypertelorism, strabismus, frontal bossing, curved parrot-like nose, maxillary hypoplasia (with relative mandibular prognathism), and short upper lip. Craniosynostosis may involve coronal, lambdoid, and sagittal sutures. Associated hydrocephalus, if severe, can lead to cerebellar tonsillar herniation. The teeth are peg-shaped and widely spaced, and associated with a large tongue, deviated nasal septum, atretic auditory meatus, and deafness. Facial operations may be required to correct extreme midface hypoplasia and proptosis. A variant, Crouzon syndrome with acanthosis nigricans, is due to a mutation in *FGFR3*.

Robinow Syndrome

Robinow syndrome, or "fetal face" syndrome, is heterogeneous, with both autosomal dominant and recessive forms recognized. Some dominant forms are caused by mutations in the *WNT5A* gene, located on 3p14.3; the gene for the recessive form is *ROR2* and located on chromosome 9q22. Abnormalities include macrocephaly, large anterior fontanelle, frontal bossing, hypertelorism, large nasal bridge with small upturned nose, small mouth, gingival hyperplasia with crowded teeth, and micrognathia. The latter findings resemble a fetal face. The forearms are short ("mesomelic dwarfism") with brachydactyly; pectus excavatum, rib anomalies, hemivertebrae (sometimes with scoliosis), inguinal hernia, and cardiac anomalies may occur, along with a small, 'buried,' or absent penis, cryptorchidism, or shawl scrotum in boys and small clitoris and labia majora in girls. Many defects overlap between the two forms. However, vertebral, rib, and craniofacial anomalies appear to be more common in the recessive form, while orodental changes appear more often in the dominant form (105). *WNT5A* and *ROR2* appear to interact, but molecular details remain unclear.

Stickler Syndrome

Stickler syndrome, or hereditary arthroophthalmopathy, is phenotypically variable and genetically heterogenous (106). It is recognized in five forms. Three are autosomal dominant: types I (mutations in *COL2A1*), II (*COL11A1*), and III (*COL11A2*); two are recessive: IV (*COL9A1*) and V (*COL9A2*). The syndrome is characterized by depressed nasal bridge, epicanthal folds, midface hypoplasia, cleft of hard palate, micrognathia, deafness, and myopia complicated by frequent retinal detachment or cataracts. Hypotonia, marfanoid habitus, prominence of large joints, and spondyloepiphyseal dysplasia are also present in Stickler syndrome. Fifty percent of girls and 40% of boys have mitral valve prolapse. The syndrome should be considered in infants with Robin sequence—in one study, one-third of patients with Robin sequence were diagnosed subsequently with Sticker syndrome (107).

Noonan Syndrome

Webbing of the neck, pectus excavatum, cryptorchidism, and pulmonic stenosis (or other forms of congenital heart disease, especially hypertrophic cardiomyopathy) characterize this syndrome. Short stature, epicanthal folds, ptosis of eyelids, ocular hypertelorism, myopia, low-set or abnormal ears, anomalous vertebrae, and mental retardation are common. Edema of the dorsum of the hands and feet in the newborn may simulate that seen in the infant with Ullrich-Turner (45X) syndrome. The condition is genetically heterogeneous, with mutations in the gene *PTPN11* identified in approximately 40% of patients (108). Eight subtypes of Noonan syndrome are associated with gene mutations in *KRAS*, *SOS1*, *RAF1*, *NRAS*, *BRAF*, and *RIT1*. Patients may suffer from other conditions as well—somatic *PTPN11* mutations are also found in several childhood malignancies, including juvenile myelomonocytic, acute myeloid, and acute lymphoblastic leukemias (109). Neurofibromatosis type I has been reported in two patients with Noonan syndrome; in each patient, the mutation responsible for one disorder was inherited while the other arose *de novo*.

Brachmann-de Lange Syndrome

Cornelia de Lange, or Brachmann-de Lange syndrome (BDLS), has as major manifestations growth deficiency, profound mental retardation, synophrys, hirsutism, and thin, downturned vermilion borders (Figure 4-9). Other common anomalies are microcephaly, micrognathia, limb anomalies, dental abnormalities, such as late eruption of widely spaced teeth, and male genital abnormalities, such as cryptorchidism and hypospadias. Less common anomalies involve the eye (myopia, microcornea, astigmatism, optic atrophy, coloboma of the optic nerve, strabismus, and proptosis), choanal

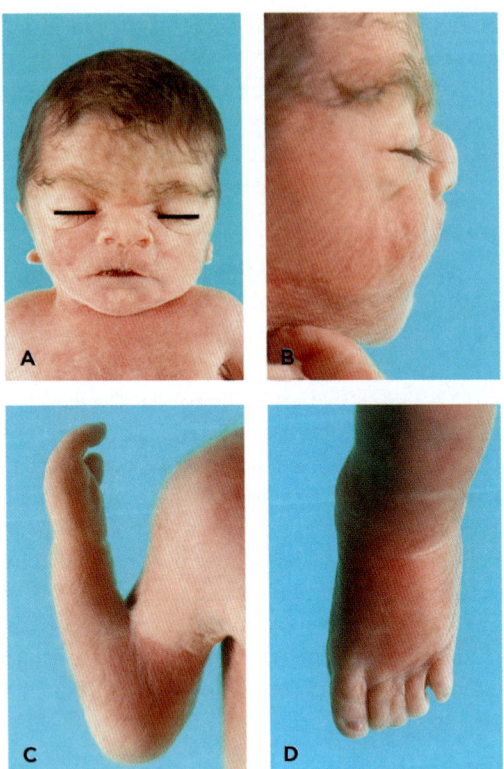

FIGURE 4-9 • Brachmann-de Lange syndrome. This 30-week fetus was born spontaneously and lived several hours, dying of respiratory failure secondary to congenital diaphragmatic hernia. **A:** Characteristic facies, with hirsutism, synophrys, ocular hypertelorism, and elongated philtrum. **B:** Lateral view showing elongated eyelashes, blunt nose, and small mandible. **C:** Severe reduction anomaly of right arm (absent ulna, third, fourth, and fifth fingers), with pterygium at elbow. **D:** Syndactyly of second and third toes.

atresia, low-set ears, cleft palate, congenital heart defects (most commonly a ventricular septal defect), hiatus hernia, gastrointestinal anomalies (e.g., duplication of the gut, malrotation of the colon, short esophagus, and pyloric stenosis), inguinal hernia, small labia majora, and absent second to third interdigital triradius. BDLS, dup(3q), and FAS show some phenotypic overlap but are distinguishable.

Both dominant and X-linked forms are recognized, although most cases develop from spontaneous mutations. Dominant cases are associated with mutations in *NIPBL*, *SMC3*, or *RAD21*. To date, about 50% to 60% of patients with BDLS have had heterozygous mutations in the *NIPBL* gene (110). X-linked BDLS arises from *SMC1A* or *HDAC8* mutations (111), which together account for at least 5% of cases.

AUTOSOMAL RECESSIVE CONDITIONS

Meckel Syndrome

Meckel first described this syndrome in 1822, and in 1934, Gruber coined the term *dysencephalia splanchnocystica*. Meckel, or Meckel-Gruber, syndrome is recessively inherited and generally leads to death in the perinatal period or early infancy from respiratory or renal failure; survival beyond this is rare. The classic diagnostic triad is occipital encephalocele, cystic kidneys, and polydactyly (Figure 4-10). However, some place more emphasis on hepatic changes than polydactyly (see below), and in fact bilateral multicystic kidneys, fibrotic changes in the liver, and occipital encephalocele or other CNS malformation have been offered as minimum diagnostic criteria (112).

Prenatal diagnosis is possible with ultrasonography, often before the 11th to 12th week; maternal serum alpha-fetoprotein levels may be elevated due to the encephalocele. Clinical and genetic heterogeneity are pronounced, and to date, 11 forms are associated with 40 gene mutations. Meckel syndrome is one of a growing number of ciliopathies, disorders characterized by aberrations in primary cilia, surface organelles that monitor the extracellular environment and effect transmembrane signaling (113). Because these processes are so fundamental to development, phenotypic changes can be widespread, varied, and overlap with other syndromes. For example, mutational analysis has shown that both Meckel and Joubert syndromes can be caused by mutations in the same gene, *MKS3*, thus accounting for the features shared by the two conditions.

Cranial rachischisis, Chiari malformation, hydrocephalus, Dandy-Walker malformation, polymicrogyria, ocular anomalies, cleft palate, congenital heart defects, hypoplasia of the adrenal glands, pseudohermaphroditism in males, and other malformations are additional findings. Excessively large, cystic, dysplastic kidneys cause marked abdominal distension. The cysts are spherical, with absent glomeruli and pronounced interstitial fibrosis; cysts display an orderly, progressive increment in size from capsule to calyx. Other genitourinary anomalies include agenesis, atresia, hypoplasia, and duplication of the ureters and absence or hypoplasia of the urinary bladder (see Chapter 17). Cysts of the liver and pancreas are encountered; hepatic fibrosis and proliferation

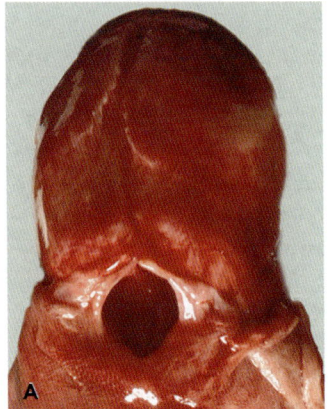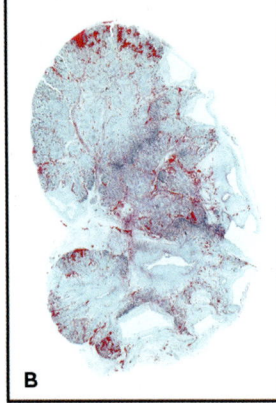

FIGURE 4-10 • Meckel-Gruber syndrome. **A:** Occipital defect marks location of encephalocele, absent at autopsy (secondary to autolysis) but identified by prenatal ultrasound. **B:** Microscopic view of cystic renal dysplasia, associated with atretic ureter; large cysts are mostly collecting tubules; other changes include tubular loss and peritubular and medullary fibrosis.

of the bile ducts (i.e., ductal plate malformation) are seen in portal tracts, and the pancreas may exhibit fibrosis as well. Severe hypoplasia of male genitalia with cryptorchidism, epididymal cysts, and ductal dilatation are common.

Smith-Lemli-Opitz Syndrome

This autosomal recessive disorder was the first true malformation complex to be associated with a metabolic derangement and the first associated with abnormal synthesis of cholesterol. Deficient cholesterol levels result from reduced activity of the final enzyme in the synthetic pathway, 7-dehydrocholesterol reductase (DHCR7). As a result, plasma concentrations of intermediate products are elevated (e.g., 7-dehydrocholesterol).

The phenotype varies from mild to severe. A distinctive craniofacial appearance with microcephaly, anteverted nostrils, ptosis of eyelids, inner epicanthal folds, strabismus, micrognathia, syndactyly of second and third toes, hypospadias, cryptorchidism, growth retardation, and mental deficiency are the main characteristics of Smith-Lemli-Opitz syndrome (114). Defects in brain morphogenesis include micrencephaly, holoprosencephaly, Dandy Walker variant, Chiari malformation type I, abnormal septi pellucidi or corpus callosum, hypoplasia of the frontal lobes, hypoplasia of cerebellum and brain stem, dilated ventricles, and irregular gyral patterns and neuronal organization (115).

Less frequent anomalies are rudimentary postaxial hexadactyly, congenital heart defect, and defects of renal and spinal cord development. Cystic renal disease, hypoplasia, hydronephrosis, and abnormalities of the ureters are frequent. Rarely, severe perineoscrotal hypospadias may be seen. The reported higher frequency of affected boys than girls may be related to a bias in ascertaining the genital anomaly. A large number of mutations have been identified in the delta-7-dehydrocholesterol reductase gene (*DHCR7*), which is localized to 11q13.4.

Leprechaunism

Leprechaunism is an autosomal recessive congenital disorder of extreme insulin resistance. Individuals with the condition, also known as Donohue or Donohue-Uchida syndrome, have a strikingly characteristic ("elflike") facial appearance with prominent ears, hirsutism, excessive skin folding with decreased subcutaneous fat, acanthosis nigricans, skeletal involvement (large hands and feet), enlarged genitalia secondary to hyperandrogenism, and hyperinsulinemia. Intrauterine growth restriction and failure to thrive, with postnatal growth and mental retardation, are recognized; additional findings may include hypertrophic cardiomyopathy and, by microscopy, cystic changes in the gonads and marked hyperplasia of pancreatic islet cells. Death from deficient energy metabolism and loss of glucose homeostasis is common in infancy and often occurs in the first year (116). Mutations in the insulin receptor gene (*INSR*), located at 19p13.2, are the cause of this condition. Prenatal diagnosis is thus possible.

Cockayne and Related Syndromes

Cockayne syndrome is an autosomal recessive disorder that manifests as two forms, type A (CSA) and type B (CSB). Mutations in the excision repair cross-complementing gene, *ERCC8*, at 5q12.1, are responsible for CSA; mutations in several genes account for CSB, chiefly *ERCC6*, at 10q11, although others in the xeroderma pigmentosum gene family (*XPB* or *ERCC3*, *XPD* or *ERCC4*, and *XPG* or *ERCC5*) are recognized (117). CSA is the classic form and characterized by retarded growth and development, short stature, premature aging, neurologic impairment (e.g., ataxia, spasticity, dementia), hearing loss, chorioretinitis, dental abnormalities, and photosensitivity (118). It generally becomes apparent in early infancy and leads to death from intercurrent infections or development of hypertension and atherosclerosis before adulthood. CNS abnormalities include microcephaly, hydrocephalus, patchy irregular loss of myelin, axons in a tigroid pattern, focal calcification (especially in basal ganglia), cerebellar atrophy, peripheral neuropathy, bizarre astrocytosis, and oligodendroglial dysplasia. CSB is a more severe, early-onset form that progresses rapidly, leading to death at 6 or 7 years.

Although understood incompletely, pathogenesis is focused on selective defects in the capacity of cells to excise damaged DNA (119). The growth of patient fibroblasts is decreased markedly following ultraviolet (UV) irradiation. Subsequent DNA synthesis is normal, but cells fail to recover RNA synthesis postirradiation. Because of these traits, prenatal diagnosis can be made on the basis of the reactivity of amniocytes to UV light.

Other conditions resemble Cockayne syndrome and may in fact constitute a Cockayne spectrum. CAMFAK syndrome (congenital cataracts, microcephaly, failure to thrive, kyphoscoliosis) is an autosomal recessive disease with central and peripheral demyelination that is similar to that seen in CS (120). A less severe variety, without failure to thrive, is termed CAMAK. MICRO syndrome, also autosomal recessive, is characterized by microcephaly, cataracts, and microcornea and should be distinguished from Cockayne and CAMFAK syndromes, but also cerebro–oculo–facial–skeletal (COFS) syndrome (121). Cultured cells from patients with COFS and Cockayne syndromes manifest hypersensitivity to UV light (in contrast to those with CAMFAK, CAMAK, or MICRO syndromes), and mutations in *CSB* and *ERCC6* have been reported in patients diagnosed with COFS (122). UV-sensitive syndrome (UVSS) is another recessive condition of faulty DNA repair and is associated with mutations in *ERCC6*, *ERCC8*, or the *UVSSA* gene.

Seckel Syndrome

Seckel syndrome (primordial or "bird-headed" dwarfism) is inherited as an autosomal recessive trait. It is associated with severe prenatal growth and mental deficiency with microcephaly and premature synostosis, narrow face with hypoplastic maxillae, prominent "beak-like" nose, malformed ears, sparse hair, clinodactyly of fifth finger, hypoplasia of proximal radius, dislocation of hip and hypoplasia of proximal fibula,

11 pairs of ribs, and cryptorchidism in boys. Numerous dental anomalies are recognized, especially hypodontia, enamel hypoplasia, crowding, and malocclusion. Cardiac anomalies are possible, among them tetralogy of Fallot and ventricular septal defect. Hematopoietic disease most often manifests as anemia, but myelodysplasia and AML have been observed as well. Schizencephaly has been reported in one patient and malignant hypertension associated with rupture of a cerebral aneurysm in another. Genes (or loci) responsible for other forms of the syndrome are recognized: SCKL1 (caused by mutations in the gene *ATR*), SCKL2 (*RBBP8*), SCKL3 (SCKL3 locus), SCKL4 (*CENPJ*), SCKL5 (*CEP152*), SCKL6 (*CEP63*), and SCKL7 (*NIN*). Mechanisms continue to be elucidated—chromosomal breakage has been documented in some cases, while others have defective DNA repair.

Dubowitz Syndrome

Dubowitz syndrome is an autosomal recessive, but possibly heterogeneous, disorder characterized by an unusual facial appearance, infantile eczema, small stature, and mild microcephaly (123). Infants with this syndrome are usually small for their gestational age and demonstrate retarded osseous maturation. The clinical manifestations include mild mental deficiency, mild microcephaly, small face, shallow supraorbital ridges, ocular hypertelorism, blepharophimosis, ptosis, rounded tip of nose, and micrognathia. In this regard, facial characteristics may resemble those of FAS. Other abnormalities include high-pitched voice, submucous cleft palate, pes planus, metatarsus adductus, hypospadias, cryptorchidism, clinodactyly of the fifth finger, and pilonidal dimple (124). A number of behavioral changes have been described, including hyperactivity and shyness; some patients like music, rhythm, and the vibrations produced by music; others dislike crowds (125). Increased chromosome breakage and susceptibility to neoplasia are complications. Mutations in the DNA Ligase IV gene and *NSUN2* have been described in subsets of patients.

Orofaciodigital Syndrome Type II (Mohr Syndrome)

Dominant forms of this condition have been reviewed earlier in the chapter. Of the 13 recognized types of OFD, most are recessive. The orofaciodigital syndrome type II is characterized by shortness of stature, conductive deafness, midline partial cleft lip, midline cleft of the tongue, hypoplasia of the maxilla and mandible, relatively short hands, partial duplication of the hallux and first metatarsal, cuneiform and cuboid bones, and normal intelligence (126).

Pena-Shokeir Phenotype

Pena-Shokeir Type I Sequence (Fetal Akinesia Deformation Sequence)

In 1974, Pena and Shokeir first described early lethal neurogenic arthrogryposis and pulmonary hypoplasia (Pena-Shokeir I syndrome or fetal akinesia deformation). Phenotypic changes appear to be nonspecific and caused by decreased or absent *in utero* movements, resulting in a series of deformations. Genetic heterogeneity is recognized. One-half of the cases are sporadic, and one-half are familial and autosomal recessive or X-linked. Hall proposed the term Pena-Shokeir "phenotype," because the condition is not a specific syndrome, but rather a physical change produced by lack of movement *in utero* (127).

Infants are small for their gestational age; approximately 30% are stillborn. Most die from the complications of pulmonary hypoplasia within days to weeks. Facial abnormalities include prominent eyes, hypertelorism, telecanthus, epicanthal folds, malformed ears, depressed tip of the nose, small mouth, high arched palate, and micrognathia (128). Small placenta and relatively short umbilical cord, the latter presumably arising from lack of fetal movement, are frequent findings. Polyhydramnios occurs due to failure of normal deglutition. Neuromuscular deficiency in the function of the diaphragm and intercostal muscles, with failure of normal excursion of amniotic fluid, causes pulmonary hypoplasia. Multiple ankyloses at elbows, knees, hips, and ankles; rocker-bottom feet; talipes equinovarus; and camptodactyly are present. Absence of the flexion creases on the fingers and palms, and sparse dermatoglyphic ridges are frequent. The phenotype may resemble that of trisomy 18, from which it should be distinguished.

Neuropathologic findings include thin cerebral and cerebellar cortices, polymicrogyria, and multiple foci of encephalomalacia, with loss of neurons and gliosis. The spinal cord is usually involved, with reduction in anterior motor horn cells. Skeletal muscles show diffuse and group atrophy consistent with neurogenic atrophy.

Prenatal diagnosis is possible, especially with prior occurrence and a high index of suspicion. Pterygium formation is one of the manifestations of the Pena-Shokeir phenotype. The lethal form of recessive multiple pterygium syndrome may represent a severe form of the Pena-Shokeir phenotype (see Chapter 28 for additional discussion).

Pena-Shokeir Type II Sequence (Cerebro-Oculo-Facio-Skeletal Syndrome)

COFS syndrome is a rare autosomal recessive disorder characterized by prenatal and postnatal growth and psychomotor retardation, scoliosis, hip dysplasia or dislocation, narrow pelvis, joint contractures and wasting, and microcephaly with abnormal facies (large ears, broad nasal bridge, overhanging upper lip, micrognathia), with death in infancy or early childhood. Defects in the CNS involve the eyes (optic atrophy, microcornea, retinal degeneration, cataracts, blepharophimosis) and degeneration of the brain and spinal cord, with calcification in white matter and basal ganglia. Changes are usually manifest at birth. Progressive cortical atrophy, with reduced white matter of the brain, is associated with generalized hypotonia and hyporeflexia or areflexia. The usual postnatal course is characterized by progressive psychomotor deterioration and death before 5 years of age.

Mutations have been identified in the CSB or xeroderma pigmentosum genes (see previous discussion), hence the syndrome's inclusion in the spectrum of defective nucleotide excision repairs (129).

Roberts Syndrome

Roberts syndrome has been described under the names pseudothalidomide or SC syndrome, SC-phocomelia syndrome, total phocomelia, hypomelia–hypotrichosis–facial hemangioma syndrome, and others. Prominent features of this malformation syndrome include nearly symmetric phocomelia-like limb deficiency, often with radial defects, prenatal and postnatal growth retardation, microbrachycephaly, eye abnormalities (i.e., shallow orbits, prominent globes, and cloudy corneas), cleft lip with or without cleft palate, and prominent premaxilla (Figure 4-11). The upper limbs may be affected more severely than the lower ones, the latter sometimes being altered by absent or hypoplastic fibulae (130). Minor craniofacial abnormalities include sparse, silver-blond hair, extensive hemangiomas, micrognathia, hypoplastic nasal cartilages, and malformed ears with hypoplastic lobules; some patients may have nuchal cystic hygroma. Autopsy studies have shown cystic dysplastic kidneys, horseshoe kidney, and ureteral stenosis with hydronephrosis. The condition is inherited as an autosomal recessive trait. Infants are stillborn or die in early infancy. Traditionally, the diagnosis has been confirmed by identifying premature centromere separation with puffing and splitting and heterochromatin repulsion. It is now known that mutations in the *ESCO2* gene are responsible for the syndrome, and for SC phocomelia, a milder variant. The gene product is required for chromatid cohesion, hence the classification of Roberts syndrome with other cohesinopathies (131).

Familial Agnathia/Holoprosencephaly

Agnathia may occur alone or with other anomalies. The association with holoprosencephaly is common and has been described in siblings, suggesting autosomal recessive inheritance; other cases are due to unbalanced translocations or appear to occur sporadically. The disorder may include inferior midline fusion of the ears (agnathia–otocephaly complex, or AGOTC) and is caused by mutations in the *PRRX1* or *OTX2* genes (132). Associations of agnathia with situs inversus, renal agenesis, ectopia cordis, and rib or vertebral anomalies have been reported, as have occurrences with tetramelia and anal atresia/situs inversus. Polyhydramnios may be a presenting feature, and the condition is almost always lethal in the fetal or neonatal period (133).

Thrombocytopenia and Absent Radius Syndrome

The thrombocytopenia absent radius (TAR) syndrome is inherited as an autosomal recessive trait; almost half of patients die during early infancy. Microdeletions in 1q21.1 have been identified in many patients (134). Limb defects

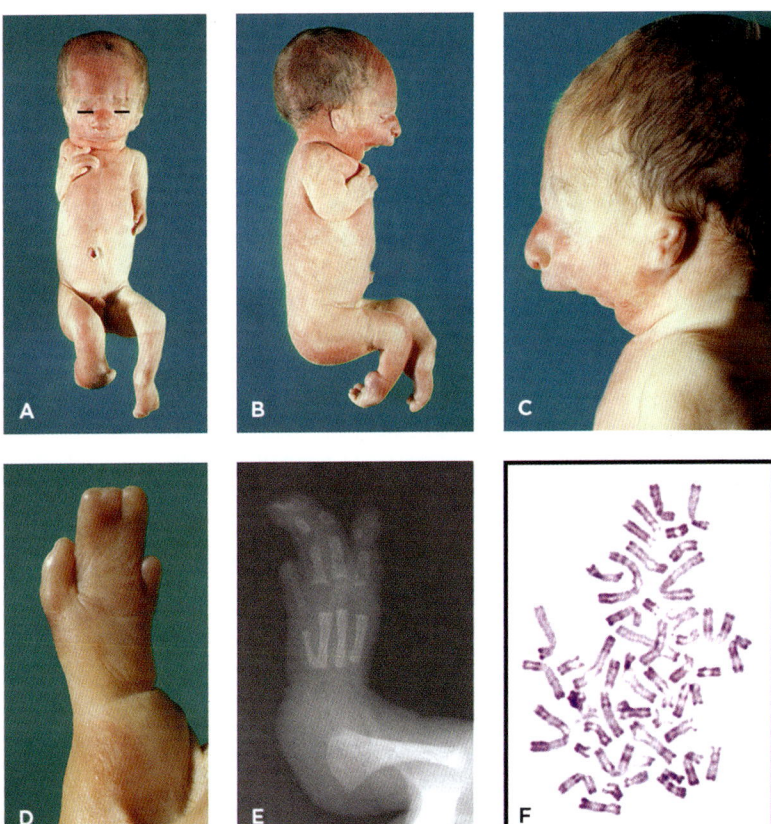

FIGURE 4-11 • Robert (pseudothalidomide) syndrome. **A:** Fetus with multiple limb malformations. **B:** Lateral view. **C:** Agnathia and severely hypoplastic ear. **D:** Phocomelia and syndactyly of upper limb. **E:** Radiograph of foot. **F:** Metaphase spread, showing prominent centromeres.

include absence or hypoplasia of the radius, despite the presence of thumbs. These defects are usually bilateral and occur with associated ulnar hypoplasia and defects of the hands, legs, and feet. Other abnormalities include congenital heart defect, spina bifida, brachycephaly, strabismus, micrognathia, syndactyly, short humerus, and dislocation of the hips. A host of additional anomalies are recognized, including lower limb, renal, and cardiac anomalies, capillary hemangiomas of the face, intracranial vascular malformations, sensorineural hearing loss, and scoliosis (135). Mental retardation occurs in 7% of patients. Prenatal diagnosis can be suggested by ultrasonography when defects of the upper limbs are recognized. Thrombocytopenia with absence or hypoplasia of megakaryocytes, leukemoid granulocytosis, eosinophilia, and anemia constitute the major hematologic abnormalities. A pronounced intolerance to cow's milk is probably related to disturbances in eosinophils. Leukemoid granulocytosis is present in over half of the patients, particularly during bleeding episodes. The development of acute myeloid leukemia has been described in an adult patient (136).

Hydrolethalus Syndrome

Hydrolethalus syndrome is characterized by hydrocephalus, midline defects of the brain (e.g., absent or hypoplastic corpus callosum, absent pituitary gland), other CNS abnormalities (hypothalamic hamartoma, fused thalami and basal ganglia, temporal and occipital lobe hypoplasia), micrognathia, limb anomalies including polydactyly, abnormal lobation of the lungs, microphthalmia, cleft lip or palate, small or absent tongue, wide or bifid nose, and low-set, malformed ears. The occipital bone is often altered by a keyhole-shaped defect at the posterior margin of the foramen magnum. Bilateral pulmonary agenesis and renal anomalies including unilateral agenesis and hypoplasia or tubular cysts are associated manifestations (137). The syndrome is autosomal recessive and tends to be lethal in the fetal or newborn period. Mutations in *HYLS1* have been identified in numerous patients (138).

A closely associated disorder is acrocallosal syndrome, which also manifests abnormalities of the corpus callosum, craniofacial complex, and digits (e.g., duplication of hallux and postaxial polydactyly). Mutations in *KIF7* have been identified in patients with both conditions. Because the gene plays an important role in the function of primary cilia, the syndromes represent new additions to the growing list of ciliopathies (139).

HETEROGENOUS AUTOSOMAL DOMINANT AND RECESSIVE DYSPLASIAS

Osteochondrodysplasias and Other Skeletal Dysplasias

Spranger et al. (140) identified three basic constitutional errors of bone development: dysostoses ("malformations of single bones, alone or in combination"), disruptions ("secondary malformations of bones"), and skeletal dysplasias ("developmental disorders of chondro-osseous tissue"). Pathologic diagnosis of these conditions requires both radiographic and histologic techniques. The latter should involve samples of affected bone and cartilage and generally includes rib (to include costochondral junction), vertebral body, and proximal and distal ends of major long bones (including osteochondral junctions).

Dysostoses may arise from defects in signaling factors, expressed only temporarily during development. Examples include those described elsewhere in this chapter, that is, Holt-Oram and Smith-Lemli-Opitz syndromes, as well as the brachydactylies, Greig polysyndactyly, and Pallister-Hall syndrome. Lesions may be asymmetric and in general do not lead to dwarfism unless the axial bones are involved.

Disruptions may arise from the action of teratogens or infectious agents. Thalidomide and warfarin embryopathies are examples presented in this chapter.

Dysplasias constitute a larger group of disorders and may be subcategorized as "primary dysplasias," which result from mutated genes that are expressed in cartilage or bone, or "secondary dysplasias," abnormalities arising from hormonal disease (e.g., hypothyroidism) or metabolic errors (e.g., hypophosphatasia). In these conditions, effects are widespread and sufficiently severe to cause dwarfism.

The osteochondrodysplasias, in order of increasing lethality, include osteogenesis imperfecta, thanatophoric dysplasia, achondrogenesis, and the short rib polydactyly syndromes (Figure 4-12). Even combined, these disorders are encountered infrequently, on the order of 16 per 100,000 births (140). However, because of the often striking changes in bones, the conditions are rather easily recognized by prenatal ultrasound, undergo therapeutic termination of pregnancy, and are seen with some frequency by fetal pathologists.

Chondrodysplasias

These are defects of collagen synthesis, principally type 2 collagen. The classification of chondrodysplasias has been approached in somewhat different manners by various authors: early clinical manifestations (lethal versus nonlethal), gross phenotype (short trunk versus normally proportioned trunk with platyspondyly versus short rib polydactyly), and predominant site of bone involvement (epiphysis, metaphysis, or spine) (140). The chondrodysplasias are associated with short stature; the major cause of death among lethal forms is pulmonary hypoplasia, resulting from rib anomalies and reduced intrathoracic volume.

Those chondrodysplasias with predominant metaphyseal involvement of tubular bones, and in some cases the spine, also include many of the same disorders that cause death *in utero* or shortly after birth (141). The physis, which is composed of resting and proliferating cartilage, enlarged chondrocytes, and calcified regions within the zone of enchondral ossification, is the site of the major histologic abnormalities. Deficiency of chondroid matrix, disorganization of chondrocytes, deviations in individual chondrocytic cytology,

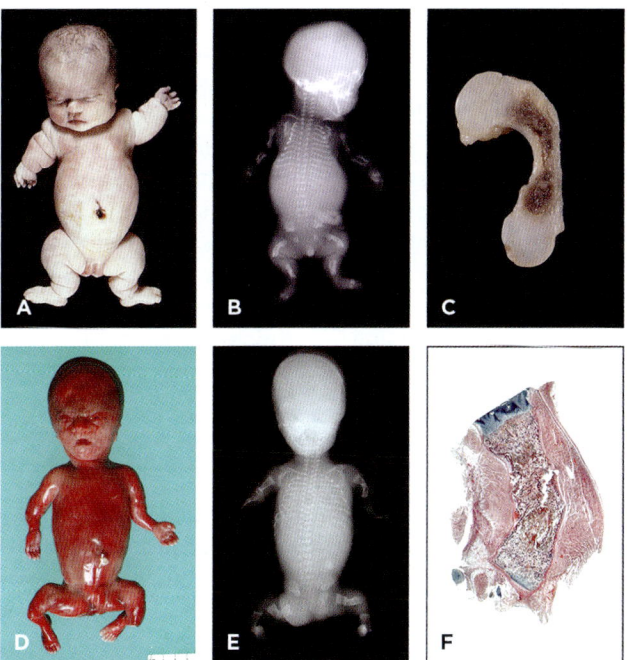

FIGURE 4-12 • Skeletal dysplasia. **A:** Full-term infant with thanatophoric dwarfism type I. **B:** Radiograph of 24-week male fetus with the same condition. Note short limbs, flat vertebral bodies, short ribs, and curved long bones, especially humeri and femora. **C:** Excised "telephone-receiver" femur is characteristic of thanatophoric dwarfism type I. **D:** A 22-week male fetus with osteogenesis imperfecta, type 2. **E:** Radiograph of same fetus. Note multiple telescoping fractures of long bones, multiple rib fractures, and poorly mineralized calvaria. **F:** Microscopic section of femur, showing multiple compression fractures.

absence of proliferating chondrocytes, degeneration of matrix, and absence or alteration of chondrocytic columnation are some of the specific microscopic features that, in differing combinations, represent the principal histopathologic findings among the various types of short trunk and non–short trunk chondrodysplasias. Nodules of immature mesenchymal tissue are interposed at the disorganized and attenuated physeal growth zone in thanatophoric dysplasia (see Chapter 28 for discussion of specific conditions).

Other Osteochondrodysplasias

Except for some very general phenotypic similarities, the nonchondrodysplasias constitute a heterogeneous group of conditions due to defects in collagen. Osteogenesis imperfecta represents a group of inherited connective tissue disorders associated with fragile bones and a number of other nonosseous abnormalities of connective tissues. The most severe form of osteogenesis imperfecta is type II, which is typically lethal in the perinatal period.

Osteopetrosis is heterogenous and either an autosomal recessive or dominant condition that is characterized by a generalized increase in bone density, especially affecting the pelvis and skull. A defect in osteoclast function has been demonstrated, particularly in the "malignant" or autosomal recessive form, with death occurring in the first decade of life. The histologic findings are diagnostic in most cases.

X-LINKED SYNDROMES

Lowe Syndrome

Hypotonia, congenital cataract, renal tubular dysfunction, and mental retardation manifest as Lowe syndrome (or, oculocerebrorenal syndrome of Lowe). The renal tubular defect causes limited ammonium production, hyperchloremic acidosis, phosphaturia, hypophosphatemia, generalized aminoaciduria, albuminuria, osteoporosis, sometimes rickets, and organic aciduria (142). Death is usually due to renal failure. The condition is monogenic, X-linked, and caused by mutations in *OCRL1* (mapped to Xq24-q26). Females are affected rarely, by a mechanism(s) that is understood incompletely.

Menkes Syndrome

Menkes, or Menkes kinky hair, syndrome is characterized by progressive cerebral deterioration with seizures, twisted and fractured hair (pili torti), and systemic copper deficiency. Affected infants have pudgy cheeks and sparse, coarse, and lightly pigmented hair that, when magnified, shows pronounced twisting and breakage. Hair changes are thought to be due to defective disulfide bonds in keratin (which are copper dependent). Nervous system findings include reduced numbers of noradrenergic fibers in the forebrain and peculiar torpedo-like swellings of catecholamine-containing axons in peripheral nerve tracts, which may relate to vascular disturbances, deterioration of the viscera, and eventual death (143). Skeletal changes in Menkes syndrome include wormian bones, metaphyseal widening, particularly of ribs and femora, and lateral spurs. Arteriograms show widespread arterial elongation and tortuosity due to reduced copper-dependent cross-linking in the internal elastic membrane of vessel walls. The condition is X-linked recessive, and caused by mutations in the *ATP7A* gene, the protein of which is involved in copper delivery and export. Survival of affected males averages 3 years or less; female carriers may have subtle changes (144). First-trimester prenatal diagnosis is possible by DNA probe.

Lesch-Nyhan Syndrome

Lesch-Nyhan syndrome is an X-linked recessive condition manifest by a deficiency of the enzyme involved in purine synthesis—hypoxanthine guanine phosphoribosyltransferase (HPRT). Patients produce excessive amounts of uric acid and suffer from profound mental retardation, characteristic self-mutilation, and motor disability. The latter stems from a severe action dystonia overlying a baseline hypotonia (145), which, with developmental delay, becomes apparent in the first few months of life; most patients never walk. Mental and behavioral changes are evident by the second to third year. The disorder is caused by mutations in the *HPRT1* gene, mapped to Xq26. The rare involvement of females may be due to uniparental disomy or lyonization. Because HPRT enzyme activity is variable, the disorder exhibits differing levels of severity. Patients with a neurologic variant of the syndrome have normal or near-normal intelligence and no self-injurious behavior. Another variant, Kelley-Seegmiller syndrome, shows excessive purine production. Prenatal diagnosis is possible by molecular genetic testing or enzyme analysis using cultured amniocytes or chorionic villi.

Opitz-Kaveggia (FG or FG-1) Syndrome

This X-linked syndrome comprises mental retardation, hypotonia, and anal malformation, sometimes with constipation. Other prominent findings are macrocephaly with megalencephaly, other craniofacial changes (hypertelorism, downslanting palpebral features, frontal bossing with upsweeping hair), hearing loss, variable agenesis of the corpus callosum, midline fusion of the mammillary bodies, heterotopia of cranial nerve nuclei, and pachygyria or other dysgenetic changes of the cerebral cortex. The condition results from mutations in the *MED12* gene, located at Xq13. X inactivation has been reported but not correlated with specific loci (146). Affected patients have lived up to 18 years of age.

Pallister Syndrome

This condition is characterized by mental retardation and anomalies of the craniofacial complex (frontal prominence, anterior cowlick, ocular hypertelorism, antimongoloid slant, broad, flat nasal bridge, midline notch of the upper lip, submucosal cleft of the hard palate, prominent mandible, and reduced number of upper central incisors). Additional changes include elbow subluxation, camptodactyly, and pes cavus (147). Patients may have grand mal seizures, strabismus, and spasticity (148). In Pallister's cases, the mother and a sister were mildly afflicted, consistent with an X-linked trait. The sister is known to have had an affected boy.

SPORADIC ABNORMALITIES

Klippel-Trenaunay-Weber (Klippel-Trenaunay) Syndrome

Features of this malformation complex include limb hypertrophy, hemangiomas that may be capillary, cavernous phlebectasias, and varicosities. The legs, buttocks, abdomen, and lower trunk are the usual sites of vascular lesions. Less common abnormalities include arteriovenous fistulas, lymphangiomas, macrodactyly, syndactyly, polydactyly, hyperpigmented nevi, and telangiectasia. Craniofacial abnormalities include asymmetric facial hypertrophy, hemangiomas, and eye abnormalities. Visceromegaly and hemangiomas of the intestinal tract, urinary system, and mesentery may be present. Anomalies of the CNS are recognized: asymmetry (hemihypertrophy) of the cerebrum and cerebellum, hydrocephalus, heterotopia, cerebral calcification or atrophy, and vascular defects such as aneurysms, arteriovenous malformation, and cavernomas. Mental deficiency and seizures may occur with facial hemangiomatosis. The overlap with Sturge-Weber syndrome is recognized (see below). Cases have been largely sporadic. Mutations in several genes (e.g., *VG5Q*, *PIK3CA*, *RASA1*) have been identified in patients with vascular malformations, but none follow a pattern that yet accounts for all the syndromic features. However, the familial occurrence of vascular nevi, hemangiomas, or other clinical signs suggests that the syndrome can be inherited on an autosomal dominant or perhaps paradominant basis. Limb hypertrophy, subcutaneous cystic spaces, and early congestive heart failure may be discernible by prenatal ultrasonography.

Sturge-Weber Dysplasia

This syndrome is characterized by hemangiomas in the facial skin, eyes (at times accompanied by glaucoma or buphthalmos), and leptomeninges (149). Cutaneous hemangiomas may occur in the trigeminal distribution, but this is not obligatory; meningeal hemangiomas may present in parietal and occipital areas. Intellectual and progressive neurologic deficits are complicated by seizures and presumably develop from impaired cerebral perfusion and perhaps localized metabolic deficits. Additional pathologic findings include cerebral cortical atrophy, sclerosis, laminar necrosis, and calcification. Somatic mosaic mutations in *GNAQ*, located at 9q21.2, are responsible for the syndrome.

Hallermann-Streiff Syndrome

Oculomandibulodyscephaly with hypotrichosis was first reported by Audry in 1893; Hallermann and Streiff described three cases independently in 1948 and 1950. The syndrome is rare, with less than 200 cases reported, and characterized by microphthalmia, a small, pinched, birdlike nose, and hypotrichosis (150). Infants have proportionately small stature, brachycephaly with frontal and parietal bossing, thin calvaria, malar hypoplasia, micrognathia, and anterior displacement of the temporomandibular joint. Hair is sparse, and skin is thin and atrophic, most prominently over the nose and suture areas of the scalp. Other craniofacial anomalies are microstomia, high, narrow, arched palate, and dental anomalies. Ocular manifestations include spherophakia, blue sclerae, nystagmus, strabismus, colobomata, glaucoma, and various chorioretinal pigment alterations; cataracts may resorb spontaneously. Nasal and mandibular anomalies may compromise respiration and feeding, requiring rhinoplasty, facial augmentation, or mandibular surgery (151). To date, most cases have been sporadic. Reported karyotypes have been normal, and inheritance patterns uncertain, with both autosomal dominant and recessive forms suggested in a few case reports.

Hypomelanosis of Ito

Hypomelanosis of Ito (systematized achromic nevus or incontinentia pigmenti achromians) appears to be a manifestation of mosaicism rather than a distinct entity, most likely involving a number of chromosomes that disrupts pigmentary genes (152). Thus, the condition has been termed "pigmentary mosaicism" and consists of a triad of scattered, streaked, whorled, or mottled areas of cutaneous hypopigmentation that fluoresce; mental deficiency; and severe intractable seizures present from birth (153). Skin manifestations bear a resemblance to those of incontinentia pigmenti and the ash leaf macule of tuberous sclerosis. Pathologic changes in the brain are variable and include cortical dysplasias, heterotopias, and hamartomas. Recognition of the cutaneous changes may alert clinicians to defects in other organ systems.

Rubinstein-Taybi Syndrome

Rubinstein-Taybi syndrome is a rare condition characterized by mental retardation and a number of physical anomalies, among which are broad thumbs and toes, bulbous fingers, slanted palpebral fissures, and hypoplastic maxilla. Other abnormalities include short stature and small cranium, seizure activity, beaked nose with nasal septum extending below nasal alae, epicanthal folds, ptosis of eyelids, long eyelashes and hypertrichosis, strabismus, low-set or malformed auricles, excess dermal ridge patterning in the thenar and first interdigital areas of the palm, cryptorchidism, and cardiac defects (particularly ventricular septal defect and patent ductus arteriosus). Cataract, colobomata, polydactyly, simian crease, and orodental and renal anomalies have been described. A large number of mutations are recognized in *CREBBP* and *EP300*, genes encoding histone acetyltransferases, coactivators important to several signaling pathways (154).

ABNORMALITIES OF UNCERTAIN ORIGIN

Short-Cord Syndrome

The length of the normal umbilical cord varies with gestational age, averaging 60 ± 13 cm at term. Cord length is static during the third trimester, presumably because the fetus is constrained in this period. This observation supports the notion that cord length is determined in part by fetal activity and the tension placed on the cord during growth. Both short and long cords are associated with an increased risk of complications during labor and delivery. The former may complicate delivery, while the latter is more easily obstructed or prolapsed (155). Factors that retard fetal movement (e.g., intrauterine compression, uterine anomaly, amniotic bands, CNS or musculoskeletal anomaly, other fetal malformation) are associated with a short umbilical cord. Such cords are associated with a variety of severe fetal anomalies, especially limb–body wall complex. This supports the additional concept that, while some cases of short cord may be due to reduced fetal motion, others may develop as part of an early defect involving the body stalk or the cord itself (156).

Nonimmune Hydrops Fetalis

Fetal hydrops is the generalized increase in fluid accumulation in serous cavities and soft tissues of the fetus (Figure 4-13). At birth, the affected infant shows gross edema and may be difficult to resuscitate because of pleural effusions, ascites, and associated lung hypoplasia. Fetal hydrops is divided into immune and nonimmune types. The most common cause of immune hydrops was once Rh isoimmunization. Since the advent of anti-D globulin (i.e., RhoGAM), most cases of fetal hydrops are nonimmune in nature (Table 4-10). The incidence of nonimmune hydrops is thought to be between 1 in 2,500 and 1 in 3,500 newborns. The pathogenetic mechanisms leading to fetal hydrops are increased intracapillary hydrostatic pressure, decreased intracapillary osmotic pressure, and damage to the peripheral capillary or vascular integrity. Extensive reviews of the differential diagnosis, pathogenesis, and etiology are available (157,158).

Chronic and severe anemia leading to hydrops may be caused by a variety of conditions, most commonly homozygous alpha-thalassemia, twin-to-twin transfusion, chronic fetomaternal transfusion, or infection by parvovirus B19. Severe, progressive anemia leads to congestive heart failure. Fetomaternal transfusion is thought to occur in at least half of all pregnancies, but the quantity of transfused blood is usually small. A Kleihauer-Betke acid elution test of the mother's blood is used to demonstrate the presence of fetal erythrocytes. The presence of fetal cells indicates bleeding from the

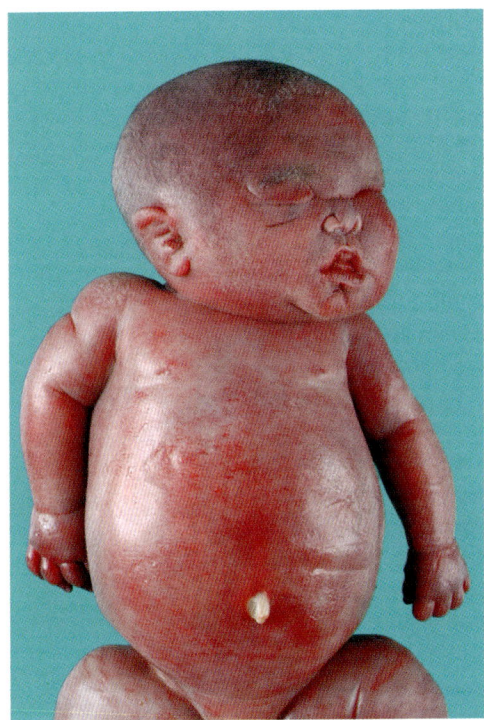

FIGURE 4-13 • Nonimmune hydrops fetalis. This 25-week female fetus suffered intrauterine fetal demise. The heart was enlarged and showed biventricular endocardial fibroelastosis. The cause of fetal hydrops was not ascertained but may have been related to maternal antiphospholipid antibody syndrome.

TABLE 4-10 CONDITIONS ASSOCIATED WITH NONIMMUNE HYDROPS FETALIS

ETIOLOGIC FACTOR
Fetal Conditions
    Severe chronic anemia *in utero*
    Fetomaternal transfusion
    Twin-to-twin transfusion
    Homozygous thalassemia
    Acardiac twinning
    Atrioventricular shunts
    Hemorrhage or thrombosis
    Maternal drugs
Placental Conditions
    Chorionic vein thrombosis
    Umbilical vein thrombosis
    Angiomyxoma of umbilical cord
    Aneurysm of umbilical cord
    Chorioangioma of placenta
Maternal Conditions
    Maternal diabetes mellitus
    Maternal nephritis
CONGENITAL ANOMALY
Cardiovascular System
    Severe congenital heart disease
    Large arteriovenous malformation
    Premature closure of foramen ovale
    Atresia or premature closure of ductus venosus
    Hypoplastic right heart
    Hypoplastic left heart
    Cardiopulmonary hypoplasia with bilateral hydrothorax
    Premature closure of ductus arteriosus, with pulmonary hypoplasia
    Fetal arrhythmia
    Cardiomyopathy
    Myocarditis
    Cardiac tumors (e.g., rhabdomyoma)
Pulmonary System
    Congenital pulmonary airway malformation
    Pulmonary hypoplasia
    Pulmonary lymphangiectasia
    Intrathoracic mass
    Diaphragmatic hernia
Gastrointestinal System
    Bowel atresia
    Duplications of the gut
    Peritonitis
Liver
    Congenital hepatitis
Kidney
    Urinary tract malformation
    Congenital nephrosis
    Renal vein thrombosis
ASSOCIATED CONDITIONS
Developmental or Genetic Disorders
    Ullrich-Turner syndrome (45X)
    Trisomy 18
    Meckel syndrome
    Pena-Shokeir phenotype
    Noonan syndrome
    Neu-Laxova syndrome
    Lethal multiple pterygium syndrome
    Skeletal dysplasia (e.g., lethal congenital short limb dysplasia)
    Multiple congenital abnormalities
Intrauterine Infection
    Syphilis
    Toxoplasmosis
    Cytomegalovirus
    Coxsackie B virus (pancarditis)
    Chagas disease
    Leptospirosis
    Parvovirus B19
Storage Disease
    Lysosomal storage disease
    Mucopolysaccharidosis
    Gaucher disease
    Gangliosidosis
    Sialidosis
Other Conditions
    Tuberous sclerosis
    Dysmaturity
    Amniotic band syndrome
    Fetal tumor (teratoma, neuroblastoma, hemangioendothelioma, angioma)

Modified from Machin GA. Hydrops revisited: literature review of 11,414 cases published in the 1980s. *Am J Med Genet* 1989;34:366–390; Bellini C, Hennekam RCM, Fulcheri E, et al. Etiology of nonimmune hydrops fetalis: a systematic review. *Am J Med Genet A* 2009;149A(5); McGillivray BC, Hall JG. Nonimmune hydrops fetalis. *Pediatr Rev* 1987;9:197–202 (Ref. 157-159).

fetal circulation into maternal circulation; by knowing the percentage of fetal cells in the maternal circulation, one can estimate the amount of blood lost by the fetus. If this quantity reaches significant proportions, it can cause fetal death. In twin-to-twin transfusion, nonimmune hydrops may be seen in the donor twin secondary to anemia (where it leads to congestive heart failure), but more often the condition occurs in the recipient twin, secondary to volume overload.

Several cardiovascular causes of hydrops are recognized. Persistent fetal arrhythmia leads to fluid accumulation and congestive failure. Congenital heart block with bradycardia suggests a diagnosis of maternal autoimmune disease (especially systemic lupus erythematosus). A number of cardiovascular anomalies can lead to intrauterine congestive heart failure, including septal defects, premature closure of the foramen ovale, premature closure of the ductus arteriosus, agenesis of the ductus venosus, and hypoplastic left ventricle.

Pulmonary causes of fetal hydrops include diaphragmatic hernia, pulmonary lymphangiectasis, and congenital airway malformation. With mediastinal shift, obstruction of the lymphatic duct and major blood vessels occurs, producing excess accumulation of fluid. Gastrointestinal atresias, midgut volvulus, and duplication are thought to cause hydrops because of decreased intravascular colloid osmotic pressure. Obstruction of the fetal urinary tract at the ureteropelvic junction or bladder outlet or renal abnormalities causing nephrosis may also be associated with fetal hydrops. In this latter case, hypoalbuminemia develops, with subsequent fluid accumulation and cardiac failure.

Chromosomal defects may be associated with cystic hygroma and often with generalized hydrops fetalis. This is commonly seen with Ullrich-Turner (45X) syndrome. Bieber syndrome manifests as a familial cystic hygroma simulating an encephalocele. Incomplete formation of the lymphatic system delays drainage into the thoracic duct. The cause of nuchal cysts and hydrops is not clear, but the condition is relatively common, and its associated conditions have been reported.

Placental abnormalities, including chorioangioma, torsion of the cord, or umbilical vein thrombosis, may also be a cause of fetal hydrops. Intrauterine infection, particularly the TORCH syndrome, may also have associated hydrops. The likely mechanism for ascites and more extreme fluid collections is usually severe hepatic injury caused by infection and consequent hypoalbuminemia and portal hypertension.

The lethal chondrodysplasias may be associated with hydrops. Conditions involving absent or abnormal fetal movement, including syndromes exhibiting the Pena-Shokeir phenotype, may manifest fetal hydrops. The mechanism leading to fluid collection is unknown. Transient *in utero* hydrops early in the second trimester is characteristic of Noonan syndrome. Lysosomal storage diseases, including Gaucher disease, GM1 gangliosidosis, mucopolysaccharidoses, disorders of sialic acid, and others have been described with fetal hydrops. Hypoproteinemia and sinusoidal obstruction of the liver by Kupffer cells swollen with storage material have been suggested as causes for the accumulation of fluid.

References

1. Spranger J, Benirschke K, Hall JG, et al. Errors of morphogenesis: concepts and terms. Recommendations of an International Working Group. *J Pediatr* 1982;100:160–165.
2. Cohen MMJ. *The Child with Multiple Birth Defects*, 2nd ed. Oxford, UK: Oxford University Press; 1997:267.
3. Opitz JM, Herrmann J, Pettersen JC, et al. Terminological, diagnostic, nosological, and anatomical-developmental aspects of developmental defects in man. *Adv Hum Genet* 1979;9:71–164.
4. Opitz JM. The developmental field concept in pediatrics. *J Pediatr* 1982;101:805–809.
5. Opitz JM. Blastogenesis and the "primary field" in human development. *Birth Defects Orig Art Ser* 1993;29:3–37.
6. Martinez-Frias ML, Frias JL. Primary developmental field III: clinical and epidemiological study of blastogenetic anomalies and their relationship to different MCA patterns. *Am J Med Genet* 1997;70:11–15.
7. Martinez-Frias ML, Frias JL, Opitz JM. Errors of morphogenesis and developmental field theory. *Am J Med Genet* 1998;76:291–296.
8. Opitz JM, Gilbert EF. CNS anomalies and the midline as a "developmental field." *Am J Med Genet* 1982;12:443–455.
9. Khoury MJ, Moore CA, Evans JA. On the use of the term "syndrome" in clinical genetics and birth defects epidemiology. *Am J Med Genet* 1994;49:26–28.
10. Lubinsky M. VATER and other associations: historical perspectives and modern interpretations. *Am J Med Genet* 1986;2:9–16.
11. Vissers LELM, van Ravenswaaij CMA, Admiraal R, et al. Mutations in a new member of the chromodomain gene family cause CHARGE syndrome. *Nat Genet* 2004;36:955–957.
12. Jones KL. *Smith's Recognizable Patterns of Human Malformation*, 6th ed. Philadelphia, PA: Elsevier Saunders; 2006.
13. American College of Obstetricians and Gynecologists (ACOG). *Guidelines for Diagnostic Imaging During Pregnancy*. Washington, D.C.: ACOG; 1995.
14. De Santis M, Di Gianantonio E, Straface G, et al. Ionizing radiations in pregnancy and teratogenesis: a review of literature. *Reprod Toxicol* 2005;20:323–329.
15. Otake M, Schull WJ. Radiation-related brain damage and growth retardation among the prenatally exposed atomic bomb survivors. *Int J Radiat Biol* 1998;74:159–171.
16. Friedman JM, Polifka JE. *Teratogenic Effects of Drugs: A Resource for Clinicians*, 2nd ed. Baltimore, MD: The Johns Hopkins University Press; 2000.
17. Shepard TH, Lemire RJ. *Catalog of Teratogenic Agents*, 13th ed. Baltimore, MD: The Johns Hopkins University Press; 2007.
18. Shepard TH. Proven and suspected human teratogens-How can we sort them out? In: Crichton JU, ed. *Safe Drugs for Canadian Children—Report of the Third Canadian Ross Conference on Pediatric Research*. Montreal, Canada: Ross Laboratories; 1978:9–25.
19. Stevens TD, Bunde CJ, Fillmore BJ. Mechanism of action in thalidomide teratogenesis. *Biochem Pharmacol* 2000;59:1489–1499.
20. Czeizel AE, Dudas I, Vereczkey A, et al. Folate deficiency and folic acid supplementation: the prevention of neural-tube defects and congenital heart defects. *Nutrients* 2013;5:4760–4765.
21. Anonymous. Spina bifida and anencephaly before and after folic acid mandate-United States, 1995–1996 and 1999–2000. *MMWR* 2004;53:362–365.
22. Bell KN, Oakley GPJ. Tracking the prevention of folic acid-preventable spina bifida and anencephaly. *Birth Defects Res A Clin Mol Teratol* 2006;76:654–657.
23. Tamura T, Picciano MF. Folate and human reproduction. *Am J Clin Nutr* 2006;83:993–1016.
24. Warkany J. Teratogenicity of folic acid antagonists. *Cancer Bull* 1981;33:76–77.
25. Glinoer D. Feto-maternal repercussions of iodine deficiency during pregnancy. An update. *Ann Endocrinol (Paris)* 2003;64:37–44.
26. Brent R. The role of the pediatrician in preventing congenital malformations. *Pediatr Rev* 2011;32:411–421.
27. Hetzel BS, Hay ID. Thyroid function, iodine nutrition, and fetal brain development. *Clin Endocrinol* 1979;11:445–460.
28. Connolly KJ, Pharoah POD, Hetzel BS. Fetal iodine deficiency and motor performance during childhood. *Lancet* 1979;2:1149–1151.
29. Murdoch DR, Harding EG, Dunn JT. Persistence of iodine deficiency 25 years after initial correction efforts in the Khumbu region of Nepal. *N Z Med J* 1999;112:266–268.
30. Anonymous. Goitre and iodine deficiency in Europe. Report of the Subcommittee for the Study of Endemic Goitre and Iodine Deficiency of the European Thyroid Association. *Lancet* 1985;1:1289–1293.
31. Feldman GL, Weaver DD, Lovrien EW. The fetal trimethadione syndrome: report of an additional family and further delineation of this syndrome. *Am J Dis Child* 1977;131:1389–1392.
32. Zackai EH, Mellman WJ, Neiderer B. The fetal trimethadione syndrome. *J Pediatr* 1975;87:280–284.
33. Ozkan M, Cetinkaya M, Koksal N, et al. Severe fetal valproate syndrome: combination of complex cardiac defect, multicystic dysplastic kidney, and trigonocephaly. *J Matern Fetal Neonatal Med* 2011;24:521–524.

34. Bates SM, Ginsberg JS. Anticoagulants in pregnancy: fetal effects. *Baillieres Clin Obstet Gynaecol* 1997;11:479–488.
35. Chan KY, Gilbert-Barness E, Tiller G. Warfarin embryopathy. *Pediatr Pathol Mol Med* 2003;22:277–283.
36. Carmichael SL, Shaw GM, Laurent C, et al. Maternal progestin intake and risk of hypospadias. *Arch Pediatr Adolesc Med* 2005;159:957–962.
37. Garcia CA, McGarry PA, Voirol M, et al. Neurological involvement in the Smith-Lemli-Opitz syndrome. *Dev Med Child Neurol* 1973;15:48–55.
38. Heinonen OP. Diethylstilbestrol in pregnancy. Frequency of exposure and usage patterns. *Cancer* 1973;31:573–577.
39. Whitehead ED, Leiter E. Genital abnormalities and abnormal semen analysis in male patients exposed to diethylstilbestrol in utero. *J Urol* 1981;125:47–50.
40. Lammer EJ, Cordero JF. Exogenous sex hormone exposure and the risk for major malformations. *JAMA* 1986;255:3128–3132.
41. Eighany NA, Stopford W, Bunn WB, et al. Occupational exposure to inorganic mercury vapour and reproductive outcomes. *Occup Med* 1997;47:333–336.
42. Matsumoto H, Koya G, Takeuchi T. Fetal Minamata disease: a neuropathological study of two cases of intrauterine intoxication by a methyl mercury compound. *J Neuropathol Exp Neurol* 1965;24:563–574.
43. Matsuyama A, Yasuda Y, Yasutake A, et al. Detailed pollution map of an area highly contaminated by mercury containing wastewater from an organic chemical factory in People's Republic of China. *Bull Environ Contam Toxicol* 2006;77:82–87.
44. Hansen JC, Gilman AP. Exposure of Arctic populations to methylmercury from consumption of marine food: an updated risk-benefit assessment. *Int J Circumpolar Health* 2005;64:121–136.
45. Lammer EJ, Chen DT, Hoar RM, et al. Retinoic acid embryopathy. *N Engl J Med* 1985;313:837–841.
46. Lemoine P, Harousseau H, Borteyru JP, et al. Les enfants de parents alcoholiques: anomalies observees. *Quest Med* 1968;25:476–482.
47. Jones KL, Smith DW. Recognition of the fetal alcohol syndrome in early infancy. *Lancet* 1973;2:999–1001.
48. Calhoun F, Attilia ML, Spagnolo PA, et al. National Institute on Alcohol Abuse and Alcoholism and the study of fetal alcohol spectrum disorders. The International Consortium. *Ann Ist Super Sanita* 2006;42:4–7.
49. Clarren SK, Smith DW. The fetal alcohol syndrome. *N Engl J Med* 1978;298:1063–1067.
50. Clarren SK, Alvord EC, Sumi SM, et al. Brain malformations related to prenatal exposure to ethanol. *J Pediatr* 1978;92:64–67.
51. Potter BJ, Hetzel BS. Fetal alcohol syndrome. In: Hetzel BS, Smith RM, eds. *Fetal Brain Disorders: Recent Approaches to the Problem of Mental Deficiency*. New York, NY: Elsevier North Holland; 1981.
52. Herrmann J, Pallister PD, Opitz JM. Tetraectrodactyly and other skeletal manifestations in the fetal alcohol syndrome. *Eur J Pediatr* 1980;133:221–226.
53. Stromland K, Pinazo-Duran MD. Ophthalmic involvement in the fetal alcohol syndrome: clinical and animal model studies. *Alcohol Alcohol* 2002;37:2–8.
54. Bookstein FL, Connor PD, Huggins JE, et al. Many infants prenatally exposed to high levels of alcohol show one particular anomaly of the corpus callosum. *Alcohol Clin Exp Res* 2007;31:868–879.
55. Gilbert-Barness EF, Opitz JM. Congenital anomalies and malformation syndromes. In: Wigglesworth JS, Singer DB, eds. *Textbook of Fetal and Perinatal Pathology*. Oxford, UK: Blackwell Scientific Publications; 1991.
56. Streissguth AP, Dehaene P. Fetal alcohol syndrome in twins of alcoholic mothers: concordance of diagnosis and IQ. *Am J Med Genet* 1993;47:857–861.
57. Hellstrom A, Jansson C, Boguszewski M, et al. Growth hormone status in six children with fetal alcohol syndrome. *Acta Paediatr* 1996;85:1456–1462.
58. Mund M, Louwen F, Klingelhoefer D, et al. Smoking and pregnancy—a review on the first major environmental risk factor of the unborn. *Int J Environ Res Public Health* 2013;10:6485–6499.
59. Werler MM. Teratogen update: smoking and reproductive outcomes. *Teratology* 1997;55:382–388.
60. Hanson JW, Smith DW. The fetal hydantoin syndrome. *J Pediatr* 1975;87:285–290.
61. Wlodarczyk BJ, Palacios AM, George TM, et al. Antiepileptic drugs and pregnancy outcomes. *Am J Med Genet A* 2012;158A:2071–2090.
62. Webster WS, Howe AM, Abela D, et al. The relationship between cleft lip, maxillary hypoplasia, hypoxia and phenytoin. *Curr Pharm Des* 2006;12:1431–1448.
63. Gilbert-Barness EF, Opitz JM. Congenital anomalies and malformation syndromes. In: Stocker JT, Dehner LP, eds. *Pediatric Pathology*. Philadelphia, PA: Lippincott Williams & Wilkins; 2001.
64. Infante JP, Huszagh VA. Impaired arachidonic (20:4n-6) and docosahexaenoic (22:6n-3) acid synthesis by phenylalanine metabolites as etiological factors in the neuropathology of phenylketonuria. *Mol Genet Metab* 2001;72:185–198.
65. Adler-Abramovich L, Vaks L, Carny O, et al. Phenylalanine assembly into toxic fibrils suggests amyloid etiology in phenylketonuria. *Nat Chem Biol* 2012;8:701–706.
66. Leandro J, Simonsen N, Saraste J, et al. Phenylketonuria as a protein misfolding disease: the mutation pG46S in phenylalanine hydroxylase promotes self-association and fibril formation. *Biochim Biophys Acta* 2011;1812:106–120.
67. Siddiqui F, James D. Fetal monitoring in type I diabetic pregnancies. *Early Hum Dev* 2003;72:1–13.
68. Leguizamon GF, Zeff NP, Fernandez A. Hypertension and the pregnancy complicated by diabetes. *Curr Diab Rep* 2006;6:297–304.
69. Dunne F, Brydon P, Smith K, et al. Pregnancy in women with type 2 diabetes: 12 years outcome data 1990–2002. *Diabet Med* 2003;20:734–738.
70. Castori M. Diabetic embryopathy: a developmental perspective from fertilization to adulthood. *Mol Syndromol* 2013;4:74–86.
71. Zabihi S, Loeken MR. Understanding diabetic teratogenesis: where are we now and where are we going? *Birth Defects Res A Clin Mol Teratol* 2010;88:779–790.
72. Merchant RH, Lala MM. Prevention of mother-to-child transmission of HIV-an overview. *Indian J Med Res* 2005;121:489–501.
73. Centers for Disease Control and prevention (CDC). Achievements in public health. Reduction in perinatal transmission of HIV infection. *MMWR* 2006;55:592–597.
74. Miller ME, Graham JM, Higginbottom MC, et al. Compression-related defects from early amnion rupture: evidence for mechanical teratogenesis. *J Pediatr* 1981;98:292–297.
75. Higginbottom MC, Jones KL, Hall BD, et al. The amniotic band disruption complex: timing of amniotic rupture and variable spectra of consequent defects. *J Pediatr* 1979;95:544–549.
76. Lubinsky M, Sujansky E, Sanger W, et al. Familial amniotic bands. *Am J Med Genet* 1983;14:81–87.
77. Moore RM, Mansour JM, Redline RW, et al. The physiology of fetal membrane rupture: insight gained from the determination of physical properties. *Placenta* 2006;27:1037–1051.
78. Kaplan LC, Matsuoka R, Gilbert EF, et al. Ectopia cordis and cleft sternum: evidence for mechanical teratogenesis following rupture of the chorion or yolk sac. *Am J Med Genet* 1985;21:187–202.
79. ten Donkelaar HJ, Hamel BC, Hartman E, et al. Intestinal mucosa on top of a rudimentary occipital meningocele in amniotic rupture sequence: disorganization-like syndrome, homeotic transformation, abnormal surface encounter or endoectodermal adhesion? *Clin Dysmorphol* 2002;11:9–13.
80. McCulloch K. Neonatal problems in twins. *Clin Perinatol* 1988;15:141–158.
81. Smith DW, Clarren SK, Harvey MA. Hyperthermia as a possible teratogenic agent. *J Pediatr* 1978;92:878–883.
82. Edwards MJ. Apoptosis, the heat shock response, hyperthermia, birth defects, disease and cancer. Where are the common links? *Cell Stress Chaperones* 1998;3:213–220.
83. Pham T, Steele J, Stayboldt C, et al. Placental mesenchymal dysplasia is associated with high rates of intrauterine growth restriction and fetal demise: a report of 11 new cases and a review of the literature. *Am J Clin Pathol* 2006;126:67–78.

84. Arnaud P, Feil R. Epigenetic deregulation of genomic imprinting in human disorders and following assisted reproduction. *Birth Defects Res C Embryo Today* 2005;75:81–97.
85. Allen C, Reardon, W. Assisted reproduction technology and defects of genomic imprinting. *BJOG* 2005;112:1589–1594.
86. Henneveld HT, van Lingen RA, Hamel BC, et al. Perlman syndrome: four additional cases and review. *Am J Med Genet* 1999;86:439–446.
87. Sammour Z, Gomes C, de Bessa J Jr, et al. Congenital genitourinary abnormalities in children with Williams-Beuren syndrome. *J Pediatr Urol* 2014;10(5):804–809.
88. Wanders RJ, Waterham HR. Peroxisomal disorders I: biochemistry and genetics of peroxisome biogenesis disorders. *Clin Genet* 2005;67:107–133.
89. Lee PR, Raymond GV. Child neurology: Zellweger syndrome. *Neurology* 2013;80:e207–e210.
90. Siebert JR, Kapur RP. Back and perineum. In: Gilbert-Barness EF, et al., eds. *Potter's Pathology of the Fetus, Infant, and Child*. Edinburgh, UK: Elsevier; 2007.
91. Siebert JR, Smith KJ, Cox LL, et al. Microtomographic analysis of lower urinary tract obstruction. *Pediatr Dev Pathol* 2014;16:405–414.
92. Quan L, Smith DW. The VATER association: vertebral defects, anal atresia, tracheoesophageal fistula with esophageal atresia, radial dysplasia. *Birth Defects Orig Art Ser* 1972;8:75–78.
93. Pittock ST, Babovic-Vuksanovic D, Lteif A. Mayer-Rokitansky-Kuster-Hauser anomaly and its associated malformations. *Am J Med Genet* 2005;135:314–316.
94. McGaughran J. MURCS in a male: a further case. *Clin Dysmorphol* 1999;8:77.
95. Czeizel A. Schisis-association. *Am J Med Genet* 1981;10:25–35.
96. Hersh JH, Angle B, Fox TL, et al. Developmental field defects: coming together of associations and sequences during blastogenesis. *Am J Med Genet* 2002;110:320–323.
97. Pagon RA, Graham JM Jr, Zonana J, et al. Coloboma, congenital heart disease, and choanal atresia with multiple anomalies: CHARGE association. *J Pediatr* 1981;99:223–227.
98. Bongers EM, Huysmans FT, Levtchenko E, et al. Genotype-phenotype studies in nail-patella syndrome show that LMX1B mutation location is involved in the risk of developing nephropathy. *Eur J Hum Genet* 2005;13:935–946.
99. Marini M, Giacopelli F, Seri M, et al. Interaction of the *LMX1B* and *PAX2* gene products suggests possible molecular basis of differential phenotypes in Nail-Patella syndrome. *Eur J Hum Genet* 2005;13:789–792.
100. Khalifa O, Al-Sakati N, Al-Mane K, et al. Combined *TSC1* and *LMX1B* mutations in a single patient. *Clin Dysmorphol* 2014;23:47–51.
101. Brophy P, Alasti F, Darbro B, et al. Genome-wide copy number variation analysis of the Branchio-oto-renal syndrome cohort identifies a recombination hotspot and implicates new candidate genes. *Hum Genet* 2013;132:1339–1350.
102. Huang T. Current advances in Holt-Oram syndrome. *Curr Opin Pediatr* 2002;14:691–695.
103. Marszalek B, Wojcicki P, Kobus K, et al. Clinical features, treatment and genetic background of Treacher Collins syndrome. *J Appl Genet* 2002;43:223–233.
104. Huning I, Kutsche K, Rajaei S, et al. Exon 2 duplication of the MID1 gene in a patient with a mild phenotype of Opitz G/BBB syndrome. *Eur J Med Genet* 2013;56:188–191.
105. Beiraghi S, Leon-Salazar V, Larson BE, et al. Craniofacial and intraoral phenotype of Robinow syndrome forms. *Clin Genet* 2011;80:15–24.
106. Stickler GB, Hughes W, Houchin P. Clinical features of hereditary progressive arthroophthalmopathy (Stickler syndrome): a survey. *Genet Med* 2001;3:192–196.
107. van den Elzen AP, Semmekrot BA, Bongers EM, et al. Diagnosis and treatment of the Pierre Robin sequence: results of a retrospective clinical study and review of the literature. *Eur J Pediatr* 2001;160:47–53.
108. Ogata T, Yoshida R. PTPN11 mutations and genotype–phenotype correlations in Noonan and LEOPARD syndromes. *Pediatr Endocrinol Rev* 2005;2:669–674.
109. Tartaglia M, Gelb BD. Noonan syndrome and related disorders: genetics and pathogenesis. *Annu Rev Genomics Hum Genet* 2005;6:45–68.
110. Schoumans J, Wincent J, Barbaro M, et al. Comprehensive mutational analysis of a cohort of Swedish Cornelia de Lange syndrome patients. *Eur J Hum Genet* 2007;15:143–149.
111. Musio A, Selicorni A, Focarelli ML, et al. X-linked Cornelia de Lange syndrome owing to SMC1L1 mutations. *Nature Genet* 2006;38:528–530.
112. Alexiev BA, Lin X, Sun CC, et al. Meckel-Gruber syndrome: pathologic manifestations, minimal diagnostic criteria, and differential diagnosis. *Arch Pathol Lab Med* 2006;130:1236–1238.
113. Barker AR, Thomas R, Dawe HR. Meckel-Gruber syndrome and the role of primary cilia in kidney, skeleton, and central nervous system development. *Organogenesis* 2014;10(1):96–107.
114. Smith DW, Lemli L, Opitz JM. A newly recognized syndrome of multiple congenital anomalies. *J Pediatr* 1964;64:210–217.
115. Lee R, Conley S, Gropman A, et al. Brain magnetic resonance imaging findings in Smith-Lemli-Opitz syndrome. *Am J Med Genet A* 2013;161:2407–2419.
116. Planchenault D, Martin-Coignard D, Rugemintwaza D, et al. Donohue syndrome or leprechaunism. *Arch Pediatr* 2014;21:206–210.
117. Lehmann AR. DNA repair-deficient diseases, xeroderma pigmentosum, Cockayne syndrome and trichothiodystrophy. *Biochimie* 2003;85:1101–1111.
118. Arenas-Sordo Mde L, Hernandez-Zamora E, Montoya-Perez LA, et al. Cockayne's syndrome: a case report. Literature review. *Med Oral Patol Oral Cir Bucal* 2006;11:E236–E238.
119. Hoeijmakers J. DNA damage, aging, and cancer. *N Engl J Med* 2009;361:1475–1485.
120. Talwar D, Smith SA. CAMFAK syndrome: a demyelinating inherited disease similar to Cockayne syndrome. *Am J Med Genet* 1989;34:194–198.
121. Graham JMJ, Hennekam R, Dobyns WB, et al. MICRO syndrome: an entity distinct from COFS syndrome. *Am J Med Genet A* 2004;128:235–245.
122. Graham JMJ, Anyane-Yeboa K, Raams A, et al. Cerebro-oculo-facio-skeletal syndrome with a nucleotide excision-repair defect and a mutated *XPD* gene, with prenatal diagnosis in a triplet pregnancy. *Am J Hum Genet* 2001;69(2):291–300.
123. Dubowitz V. Familial low birth weight dwarfism with an unusual facies and a skin eruption. *J Med Genet* 1965;2:12–17.
124. Wilroy RS, Tipton RE, Summitt RL. The Dubowitz syndrome. *Am J Med Genet* 1978;2:275–284.
125. Tsukahara M, Opitz JM. Dubowitz syndrome: review of 141 cases including 36 previously unreported patients. *Am J Med Genet* 1996;63:277–289.
126. Toriello HV. Oral-facial-digital syndromes. *Clin Dysmorphol* 1992;2:95–105.
127. Hall JG. Analysis of Pena Shokeir phenotype (invited editorial comment). *Am J Med Genet* 1986;25:99–117.
128. Pena SDJ, Shokeir MHK. Syndrome of camptodactyly, multiple ankyloses, facial anomalies and pulmonary hypoplasia: a lethal condition. *J Pediatr* 1974;85:373–375.
129. Suzumura H, Arisaka O. Cerebro-oculo-facio-skeletal syndrome. *Adv Exp Med Biol* 2010;685:210–214.
130. Temtamy SA, Ismail S, Helmy NA. Roberts syndrome: study of 4 new Egyptian cases with comparison of clinical and cytogenetic findings. *Genet Couns* 2006;17:1–13.
131. Ball ARJ, Chen YY, Yokomori K. Mechanisms of cohesion-mediated gene regulation and lessons learned from cohesinopathies. *Biochim Biophys Acta* 2014;1839:191–202.
132. Patat O, van Ravenswaaij-Arts CM, Tantau J, et al. Otocephaly-dysgnathia complex: description of four cases and confirmation of the role of OTX2. *Mol Syndromol* 2013;4:302–305.
133. Faye-Petersen OM, David E, Rangwala N, et al. Otocephaly: report of five new cases and a literature review. *Fetal Pediatr Pathol* 2006;25:277–296.
134. Albers CA, Newbury-Ecob R, Ouwehand WH, et al. New insights into the genetic basis of TAR (thrombocytopenia-absent radii) syndrome. *Curr Opin Genet Dev* 2013;23:316–323.

135. Greenhalgh KL, Howell RT, Bottani A, et al. Thrombocytopenia-absent radius syndrome: a clinical genetic study. *J Med Genet* 2002;39:876–881.
136. Go RS, Johnston KL. Acute myelogenous leukemia in an adult with thrombocytopenia with absent radii syndrome. *Eur J Haematol* 2003;70:246–248.
137. Salonen R, Herva R, Norio R. The hydrolethalus syndrome: delineation of a "new" lethal malformation syndrome based on 28 patients. *Clin Genet* 1981;19:321–330.
138. Paetau A, Honkala H, Salonen R, et al. Hydrolethalus syndrome: neuropathology of 21 cases confirmed by *HLYS1* gene mutation analysis. *J Neuropathol Exp Neurol* 2008;67:750–762.
139. Walsh DM, Shalev SA, Simpson MA, et al. Acrocallosal syndrome: identification of a novel KIF7 mutation and evidence for oligogenic inheritance. *Eur J Med Genet* 2013;56:39–42.
140. Spranger JW, Brill PW, Poznanski AK. *Bone Dysplasias: An Atlas of Genetic Disorders of Skeletal Development.* Oxford, UK: Oxford University Press; 2002.
141. Spranger JM, Maroteaux P. The lethal osteochondrodysplasias. *Adv Hum Genet* 1990;19:1–103.
142. Richards W, Donnell GN, Wilson WA, et al. The oculo-cerebro-renal syndrome of Lowe. *Am J Dis Child* 1965;109:185–203.
143. Uno H, Arya S, Laxova R, et al. Menkes syndrome with vascular and adrenergic nerve abnormalities. *Arch Pathol Lab Med* 1983;107:286–289.
144. Tumer Z. An overview and update of ATP7A mutations leading to Menkes disease and occipital horn syndrome. *Hum Mutat* 2013;34: 417–429.
145. Jinnah HA, Visser JE, Harris JC, et al. Delineation of the motor disorder of Lesch-Nyhan disease. *Brain* 2006;129:1201–1217.
146. Raynaud M, Dessay S, Ronce N, et al. Skewed X chromosome inactivation in carriers is not a constant finding in FG syndrome. *Eur J Hum Genet* 2003;11:352–356.
147. Pallister PD, Herrmann J, Spranger JW, et al. The W syndrome. *Birth Defects Orig Art Ser* 1974;10:51–60.
148. Goizet C, Bonneau D, Lacombe D. W syndrome: report of three cases and review. *Am J Med Genet* 1999;87:446–449.
149. Thomas-Sohl K, Vaslow D, Maria B. Sturge-Weber syndrome: a review. *Pediatr Neurol* 2004;30:303–310.
150. Mirshekari A, Safar F. Hallermann-streiff syndrome: a case review. *Clin Exp Dermatol* 2004;29:477–479.
151. David LR, Finlon M, Genecov D, et al. Hallermann-Streiff syndrome: experience with 15 patients and review of the literature. *J Craniofac Surg* 1999;10:160–168.
152. Taibjee SM, Bennett DC, Moss C. Abnormal pigmentation in hypomelanosis of Ito and pigmentary mosaicism: the role of pigmentary genes. *Br J Dermatol* 2004;151:269–282.
153. Quigg M, Rust RS, Miller JQ. Clinical findings of the phakomatoses: hypomelanosis of Ito. *Neurology* 2006;66:E45.
154. Negri G, Milani D, Colapietro P, et al. Clinical and molecular characterization of Rubinstein-Taybi syndrome patients carrying distinct novel mutations of the *EP300* gene. *Clin Genet* 2014;87(2) [Epub ahead of print].
155. Balkawade NU, Shinde MA. Study of length of umbilical cord and fetal outcome: a study of 1,000 deliveries. *J Obstet Gynaecol India* 2012;62:520–525.
156. Daskalakis G, Pilalis A, Papadopoulos D, et al. Body stalk anomaly diagnosed in the 2nd trimester. *Fetal Diagn Ther* 2003;18:342–344.
157. Machin GA. Hydrops revisited: literature review of 11,414 cases published in the 1980s. *Am J Med Genet* 1989;34:366–390.
158. Bellini C, Hennekam RCM, Fulcheri E, et al. Etiology of nonimmune hydrops fetalis: a systematic review. *Am J Med Genet A* 2009;149A(5): 844–851.
159. McGillivray BC, Hall JG. Nonimmune hydrops fetalis. *Pediatr Rev* 1987;9:197–202.

CHAPTER 5

Inborn Errors of Metabolism

Peter Pytel, M.D., Selene Koo, M.D., Ph.D., and Darrel Waggoner, M.D.

INTRODUCTION

Over 100 years ago, in 1908, Archibald Garrod delivered his four Croonian Lectures during which he first introduced the expression of "inborn errors of metabolism" (1). He proposed that these result from enzymatic defects in catabolic pathways. Since that time, our understanding of inborn errors of metabolism (IEM) has increased dramatically. Along with improved technology especially in molecular sequencing–based techniques, this has resulted in refinement in diagnosis and classification of IEM. Early diagnosis is increasingly important as treatments, such as dietary management and enzyme replacement, are becoming available for some patients. Although individually rare, the collective incidence of IEM is approximately 1/1500 persons.

Online genetic/metabolic disease databases such as OMIM (Online Mendelian Inheritance in Man, http://www.ncbi.nlm.nih.gov/entrez/query.fcgi?db=OMIM), MetaGene (http://www.metagene.de/index.html), GeneTests (http://www.genetests.org/), GTR (Genetic Testing Registry) (http://www.ncbi.nlm.nih.gov/gtr/) that includes a link to GeneReviews, and NORD (http://www.rarediseases.org/) are ideal sources for current information on the rapidly evolving field of IEM.

CLINICAL PRESENTATION OF INBORN ERRORS OF METABOLISM

Most metabolic diseases are autosomal recessive disorders, some are X linked, and a few are inherited as dominant traits. Carriers of recessive traits are usually asymptomatic, but female carriers of X-linked traits do sometimes show disease manifestations that vary in severity. IEM may present at any age and in a variety of ways even within the same disease entity and within the same family. IEM can lead to organ dysfunction, neurologic and medical complications, skeletal dysplasia, and dysmorphic features (Table 5-1). Symptoms may begin before birth (e.g., with hydrops fetalis or fetal ascites), at birth, with sudden death in infancy, with deterioration after a symptom-free interval, or later in life with milder symptoms and progression. On the one hand, symptoms may sometimes be confused with sepsis, delaying the diagnosis, while on the other hand, infection can lead to decompensation in IEM, becoming the trigger that leads to the first presentation.

DIAGNOSIS OF INBORN ERRORS OF METABOLISM

IEM may be diagnosed by biochemical assays, tissue histology and, more recently, molecular techniques, specifically DNA sequencing. All play an important role depending on the specific disease in question, but molecular testing has grown quickly and may soon be the best, easiest, and fastest method to make a diagnosis. Sometimes, the diagnosis is made based on newborn screening (NBS) as discussed in detail below.

Biochemical studies may allow definitive diagnosis. Routine studies include evaluation of blood glucose, lactate, ammonia, and ketones, urine organic acids, blood and urine amino acids, fatty acids, and carnitine metabolites. Biochemical assays on skin fibroblasts and lymphocytes of specific enzymes can be done for some metabolic pathways.

Morphology of tissues, including liver, muscle, skin, conjunctiva, or placenta (Table 5-2), may show characteristic findings by light microscopy (LM). Brain, lymph nodes, spleen, kidney, and heart often also show findings in IEM, but biopsies of these sites are not performed as commonly. Transmission electron microscopy (EM) of the skin, conjunctiva, mucosal ganglion cells, liver, peripheral nerve, muscle, bone marrow, or peripheral blood leukocytes is important in evaluation of some IEM (Table 5-3). Particularly for lysosomal storage diseases, ultrastructural study of these sites is a sensitive screen that can provide valuable information about stored material.

Many IEM affect the liver (2,3); in some cases (cystinosis, metachromatic leukodystrophy, Fabry disease),

TABLE 5-1	CLINICAL SYMPTOMS IN PATIENTS WITH INBORN ERRORS OF METABOLISM

Nonimmune hydrops fetalis, fetal ascites

Sudden unexpected death in infancy

Acute or episodic presentation of symptoms mimicking sepsis (lethargy, vomiting, tachypnea, shock, coma)

Failure to thrive

Macrocephaly or microcephaly

Medical complications: cardiomyopathy and arrhythmias, acute or chronic liver disease/cirrhosis, organomegaly, deafness

Neurologic complications: hypotonia/hypertonia, seizures, loss of cognitive milestones or motor skills, exercise intolerance, cramps, fatigue, and rhabdomyolysis

Ophthalmologic signs: corneal clouding, macular and retinal changes

Skeletal abnormalities including dysostosis multiplex

Dysmorphic features: coarse facial features, macroglossia

morphologic alterations have no apparent clinical consequence. In other disorders—such as tyrosinemia and glycogen storage disease (GSD) IV—progressive liver disease is common. A variety of histologic alterations—including hepatitis, steatosis, cirrhosis, cholestasis, ductopenia, ductular proliferation, neoplasia, and storage—can be seen in IEM, and many IEM cause similar morphologic alterations (see Chapter 15).

Skeletal muscle biopsy is useful for evaluation of mitochondrial myopathies, glycogen storage diseases, and some lysosomal storage diseases. Increased mitochondria with "ragged red fibers," subsarcolemmal mitochondria collections, and structurally abnormal mitochondria occur in mitochondrial myopathies. Increased muscle fiber glycogen, sometimes in vacuoles, may be present in the GSDs. Increased lipid occurs with abnormal fatty acid metabolism and with mitochondrial dysfunction (see Chapter 27).

NEWBORN SCREENING

Newborn screening (NBS) began in the 1960s with testing for phenylketonuria, and additional tests have been added since then. With the development of new technology, specifically tandem mass spectrometry (MS/MS) for NBS, it has become possible to detect many more metabolic disorders via a rapid-throughput methodology. As of January 2013, 47 states in the United States have added expanded NBS using MS/MS and screen for the majority of the recommended core conditions. Information on each state's NBS program is available through Genes-R-Us (http://genes-r-us.uthscsa.edu). The Discretionary Advisory Committee on Heritable Disorders in Newborns and Children (DACHDNC) was established under the Public Health Service Act and fulfills the functions previously undertaken by the Secretary's Advisory Committee on Heritable Disorders in Newborns and Children (SACHDNC). The committee recommends

TABLE 5-2 PLACENTAL FINDINGS IN LYSOSOMAL STORAGE DISEASES

Lysosomal Storage Disease	Affected Cells	Hydrops Fetalis
Sialidosis (mucolipidosis type I)	Syncytiotrophoblasts, Hofbauer and stromal cells	Yes
Mucolipidosis II (I-cell disease)	Syncytiotrophoblasts, Hofbauer and stromal, X cells	Yes
Mucolipidosis IV	Hofbauer and stromal cells	Yes
Sialic acid storage disease	Syncytiotrophoblasts, Hofbauer cells, endothelium, amniocytes	Yes
Galactosialidosis	Syncytiotrophoblasts	Yes
MPS I (Hurler)	Villous stromal cells	Yes
MPS III (Sanfilippo)	Syncytiotrophoblasts, Hofbauer cells, and stromal cells	Yes
MPS IVA (Morquio A)	Villous stromal cells	Yes
MPS VII (Sly)	Villous stromal cells	Yes
GM1 gangliosidosis	Syncytiotrophoblasts, Hofbauer cells	Yes
GM2 gangliosidosis (Tay-Sachs)	Syncytiotrophoblasts	
Cholesterol ester storage disease	Syncytiotrophoblasts	
Wolman disease	Syncytiotrophoblasts	Yes
GSD II	Amniocytes, endothelial cells, stromal cells	
GSD IV	Amniocytes	
Niemann-Pick A	Syncytiotrophoblasts, Hofbauer cells, fibrocytes in the cord	Yes
Gaucher disease type 2	Vessels	Yes
Fabry disease	Endothelial cells, perithelial cells, vascular smooth muscle cells	Yes

TABLE 5-3 ULTRASTRUCTURAL APPEARANCE OF LYSOSOMAL STORAGE DISEASES IN SKIN AND CONJUNCTIVAL BIOPSIES

Disorder	Ultrastructural Appearance of Predominant Storage	Stored Material	Cells Affected
Disorders with ultrastructurally characteristic storage			
Pompe disease	Electron-dense glycogen granules	Glycogen	Lymphocytes, endothelium, fibroblasts, epithelium, nerves
Cholesterol ester storage disease, Wolman disease	Cholesterol, lipids	Cholesterol ester	Fibroblasts
Infantile ceroid lipofuscinosis	Granular osmiophilic material	Saposin A, D	Perithelial and endothelial cells, smooth muscle, sweat gland epithelial cells, lymphocytes
Late infantile ceroid lipofuscinosis	Curvilinear profiles	Mitochondrial subunit c of ATPase synthase	Perithelial and endothelial cells, smooth muscle, sweat gland epithelial cells, lymphocytes
Juvenile ceroid lipofuscinosis	Curvilinear and fingerprint profiles	Mitochondrial subunit c of ATPase synthase	Perithelial and endothelial cells, smooth muscle, sweat gland epithelial cells, lymphocytes
Cystinosis	Rectangular, rhomboid, polymorphic crystals	Cystine	Fibroblasts
Metachromatic leukodystrophy	Tuffstone or herringbone bodies	Sulfatide, cholesterol, phosphatides	Peripheral nerve Schwann cells, histiocytes
Krabbe disease (globoid leukodystrophy)	Crystals with sharp corners	Galactosylceramide	Peripheral nerve Schwann cells
Fabry disease	Pleomorphic leaflets, lamellae, tubular structures	Globotriaosylceramide-containing substrates	Epithelium, fibroblasts, endothelium, lymphocytes
Disorders with ultrastructurally nonspecific storage			
Mucopolysaccharidoses (MPS) Mucolipidoses Aspartylglycosaminuria Alpha-mannosidosis Beta-mannosidosis, GM1 Gangliosidosis, I-cell disease	Lucent or fine fibrillogranular material	Oligosaccharides, glycosaminoglycans	Eccrine gland epithelium, endothelial cells (may be spared in MPS), fibroblasts, lymphocytes, macrophages, pericytes, Schwann cells, smooth muscle cells. Mucolipidosis III affects primarily fibroblasts with normal lymphocytes.
Fucosidosis, GM1 and GM2 gangliosidosis, galactosialidosis, MPS, mucolipidosis IV, and sialidosis	Fine lamellated membranous cytoplasmic bodies, zebra bodies	Gangliosides and glycolipids	Peripheral nerve Schwann cells, endothelial cells, pericytes, smooth muscle cells in Fabry disease. In Niemann-Pick and ML IV lymphocytes have storage

that every NBS program includes a uniform screening panel (Table 5-4) and advises on the addition of new tests to the screening panel (http://www.hrsa.gov/advisorycommittees/mchbadvisory/heritabledisorders/). The Web site has a list of conditions that have been nominated and are under current review.

Molecular testing for DNA mutations has been incorporated into NBS for several disorders, and this will likely increase over time. There has been discussion about the use of whole genome sequencing in NBS, which is controversial, but there is little doubt that molecular techniques will play a larger role in NBS in the future (4). Cystic fibrosis screening

TABLE 5-4 RECOMMENDED UNIFORM SCREENING PANEL FOR ALL STATES

Metabolic Disorders

Organic acid disorders

- **Core Conditions:** Propionic acidemia; methylmalonic acidemia; isovaleric acidemia; 3-methylcrotonyl-CoA carboxylase deficiency; 3-hydroxy-3-methylglutaric aciduria; holocarboxylase synthase deficiency; β-ketothiolase deficiency; glutaric aciduria
- **Secondary Conditions:** Methylmalonic acidemia with homocystinuria; malonic acidemia; isobutyrylglycinuria; 2-methylbutyrylglycinuria; 2-methylglutaconic aciduria; 2-methyl-3-hydroxybutyric aciduria

Fatty acid oxidation disorders

- **Core Conditions:** Carnitine uptake defect/carnitine transport defect; medium-chain acyl-CoA dehydrogenase deficiency; very long-chain acyl-CoA dehydrogenase deficiency; long-chain L-3 hydroxyacyl-CoA dehydrogenase deficiency; trifunctional protein deficiency
- **Secondary Conditions:** Short-chain acyl-CoA dehydrogenase deficiency; medium-/short-chain L-3 hydroxyacyl-CoA dehydrogenase deficiency; glutaric acidemia type II; medium-chain ketoacyl-CoA thiolase deficiency; carnitine palmitoyltransferase type I and II deficiencies; carnitine–acylcarnitine translocase deficiency

Amino acid disorders

- **Core Conditions:** Argininosuccinic aciduria; citrullinemia; maple syrup urine disease; homocystinuria; phenylketonuria; tyrosinemia, type I
- **Secondary Conditions:** Argininemia; hypermethioninemia; tyrosinemia types II and III

Endocrine Disorder

Congenital adrenal hyperplasia
Primary congenital hypothyroidism

Hemoglobin Disorder

S, S disease (sickle cell anemia)
S, beta-thalassemia
S, C disease

Other Disorders

Biotinidase deficiency
Critical congenital heart disease
Cystic fibrosis
Classic galactosemia
Hearing loss
Severe combined immunodeficiencies

---

includes the use of molecular techniques to detect a panel of common mutations. The initial screen is done by measurement of immunoreactive trypsinogen and then followed by molecular genetic testing of the *CFTR* gene and sweat testing. The genetic testing involves determination of a panel of common mutations, and a diagnosis is made based on a combination of sweat test results and genetic testing (5).

Several states have recently implemented screening for lysosomal storage disorders including Krabbe, Gaucher, Pompe, Fabry, and Niemann-Pick diseases and mucopolysaccharidoses I and II. Molecular testing is an important component for the follow-up of screen-positive individuals and can be used in predicting problems such as severity of disease (Gaucher) (6) and pseudodeficiency (Hurler) (7). Krabbe testing utilizes full gene sequencing in addition to enzyme determination as part of the NBS process. Detection of specific mutations associated with the severe infantile presentation of Krabbe disease is used when recommending treatment and follow-up protocols (8).

The genetic basis for most IEM is known, and Sanger sequencing has been utilized to define the mutations in affected individuals and has typically been done after biochemical or enzyme testing established the diagnosis. Although this has been a powerful tool for diagnosis, molecular techniques have been sparingly used for primary diagnosis as the technology limits how many genes can reasonably be sequenced in a single individual, and hence the need to know which gene to sequence. Next-generation sequencing (NGS) is the newest technology that utilizes massive parallel sequencing to generate large-scale sequence data, which can be used to sequence the entire exome or genome. NGS is also used to offer panel testing where many genes related to a common phenotype can be sequenced at one time. This is useful in the diagnosis of IEM and has resulted in NGS panels becoming a more common primary diagnostic technique. Three examples are reviewed below, but many diseases could illustrate this approach.

Glycogen storage disorders (GSDs) are a group of disorders of glycogen metabolism that primarily affect the liver and muscle. GSDs are classified on the basis of specific enzyme defects in glycogen production or breakdown and the various disorders lead to overlapping features of hypoglycemia, hepatomegaly, and muscle symptoms. The diagnosis of GSD once relied on invasive liver or muscle biopsies and biochemical assays to determine the specific subtype important for counseling and treatment (8). *Congenital disorders of glycosylation* (CDG) are a group of over 60 different disorders in glycosylation of proteins. CDG is characterized by multiorgan dysfunction with significant morbidity and mortality. Biochemical testing of serum transferrin is a useful screening tool for CDG but cannot diagnose the specific form of the disease (9). *Disorders of mitochondrial dysfunction* show clinical and genetic heterogeneity and are difficult to diagnose due to extreme locus and allelic heterogeneity. These diseases develop as a result of dysfunction of more than 900 genes in the nuclear and mitochondrial genome (10). NGS of a panel of genes implicated in GSDs, CDG, and mitochondrial dysfunction is now available and can be used successfully to diagnose these disorders (8–10).

LYSOSOMAL STORAGE DISEASES

The first lysosomal storage disease described was Pompe disease (11). Historically, lysosomal storage diseases were defined by the storage product, clinical features, histomorphology, and biochemical abnormalities. Nowadays, there is a shift to a molecular classification of these diseases. In this chapter, lysosomal storage diseases are defined broadly to also include diseases like neuronal ceroid lipofuscinoses (12). As such, lysosomal storage diseases are currently a group of some 50 to 70 genetic disorders with a combined incidence of approximately 1/5000 (13,14). There is an overrepresentation of some populations including Ashkenazi Jews and those of Finnish ancestry (14,15). As a group, lysosomal storage diseases are among the most commonly diagnosed metabolic disorders. Most are monogenic diseases that are inherited as autosomal recessive disorders except for three X-linked disorders (Fabry, Danon, and Hunter diseases). Many of the mutations affect lysosomal enzymes, but others disrupt lysosomal function in different ways as discussed in detail below. Table 5-5 summarizes important lysosomal storage diseases and groups them based on the function of the mutated gene. The next passages describe common themes in disease phenotype, pathophysiology, diagnosis, and treatment in this large group of diseases. Individual entities will subsequently be described following the overall order of Table 5-5.

Disease Phenotype

Lysosomal storage diseases can present at virtually any age but are most commonly encountered as pediatric diseases. Many affected patients present in early childhood. At one end of the spectrum, these diseases are a cause of nonimmune hydrops fetalis accounting overall for some 6% to 15% of such cases (16,17). On the other end of the spectrum are adult-onset presentations that may mimic other myopathies or psychiatric diseases and are therefore easily misdiagnosed.

TABLE 5-5 MASON CATEGORIES OF LYSOSOMAL STORAGE DISORDERS

Diseases caused by mutations disrupting enzyme function

(1) Sphingolipidoses
- Gaucher (types I, II, III), GBA gene encoding acid beta-glycosidase
- Fabry, GLA gene encoding alpha-galactosidase A
- Gangliosidosis GM1, GLB1 gene encoding beta-galactosidase (allelic with MPS IV; see above)
- Gangliosidosis GM2, Tay-Sachs variant, HEXA gene encoding beta-hexosaminidase A
- Gangliosidosis GM2, Sandhoff variant, HEXB gene encoding beta-hexosaminidase B
- Niemann-Pick (types A and B), SMDP1 gene encoding acid sphingomyelinase
- Metachromatic leukodystrophy, ARSA gene encoding arylsulfatase A
- Krabbe, GALC gene encoding galactosylceramidase
- Farber, ASAH1 gene encoding acid ceramidase

(2) Disorders of glycoprotein degradation (oligosaccharidoses/glycoproteinoses)
- Alpha-mannosidosis, MAN2B1 gene encoding alpha-mannosidase
- Beta-mannosidosis, MANBA gene encoding beta-mannosidase
- Fucosidosis, FUCA1 gene encoding alpha-l-fucosidase
- Sialidosis, NEU1 gene encoding neuraminidase 1
- Aspartylglucosaminuria, AGA gene encoding aspartylglucosaminidase

(3) Glycogen storage diseases—Pompe disease/adult-onset acid maltase disease

(4) Mucopolysaccharidoses
- MPS I—Hurler, Scheie, Hurler-Scheie, IDUA gene encoding alpha-l-iduronidase
- MPS II—Hunter, IDS gene encoding iduronate-2-sulfatase

(Continued)

TABLE 5-5 MASON CATEGORIES OF LYSOSOMAL STORAGE DISORDERS (Continued)

    MPS IIIA—Sanfilippo A, SGSH gene encoding sulfamidase
    MPS IIIB—Sanfilippo B, NAGLU gene encoding alpha-N-acetylglucosaminidase
    MPS IIIC—Sanfilippo C, HGSNAT gene encoding heparan-alpha-glucosaminide N-acetyltransferase
    MPS IIID—Sanfilippo D, GNS gene encoding N-acetylglucosamine-6-sulfatase
    MPS IV—Morquio A, GALNS gene encoding N-acetylgalacosamine-6-sulfatase
    MPSIV—Morquio B, GLB1 gene encoding beta-galactosidase (allelic with GM1 gangliosidosis; causative genes disrupt breakdown of keratin sulfate without affecting degradation of GM1 gangliosides)
    MPS VI—Maroteaux-Lamy, ARSB gene encoding arylsulfatase B
    MPS VII—Sly, GUSB gene encoding beta-glucuronidase
    MPS IX—Natowicz, HYAL2 gene encoding hyaluronoglucosaminidase 1
(5) Lipidosis–Wolman disease and cholesterol ester storage disease (CESD)

Nonenzymatic protein deficiencies—defects affecting, for example, trafficking, membrane proteins, lysosomal enzyme protection, or structural proteins

    Mucolipidosis II alpha/beta, III alpha/beta; GNPTAB gene encoding the alpha- and beta-subunits for GlcNAc-1-phosphotransferase
    Mucolipidosis III gamma; GNPTG, the gamma subunit for GlcNAc-1-phosphotransferase
    Mucolipidosis IV, MCOLN1 encoding mucolipin-1
    Cystinosis, CTNS gene encoding cystinosin
    Danon, LAMP2 encoding lysosomal-associated membrane protein-2
    Gaucher, atypical; PSAP gene encoding saposin C
    Gangliosidosis GM2, AB variant; GM2A gene encoding GM2 ganglioside activator protein
    Niemann-Pick type C1, NPC2 gene encoding NPC1 protein
    Niemann-Pick type C2, NPC2 gene encoding NPC2 protein
    Krabbe, atypical; PSAP gene encoding saposin A
    Metachromatic leukodystrophy, atypical; PSAP gene encoding saposin B

Ceroid lipofuscinoses

    CLN1—Haltia-Santavouri; CLN1 gene encoding PPT-1
    CLN2—Jansky-Bielschowsky; CLN2 gene encoding TPP-1
    CLN3—Spielmeyer-Sjöegren; CLN3 gene encoding CLN3 protein (battenin)
    CLN4—Parry; CLN4 (DNAJC5) gene encoding DnaJ homologue subfamily C member 5
    CLN5; CLN5 gene encoding CLN5
    CLN6; CLN6 gene encoding CLN6
    CLN7; CLN7 (MFSD8) gene encoding motility factor superfamily domain containing protein 8
    CLN8; CLN8 gene encoding CLN8
    CLN10; CLN10 (CTSD) gene encoding cathepsin D
    CLN11; CLN11 (PRN) gene encoding progranulin
    CLN12; CLN12 gene encoding CLN12/ATPase
    CLN13; CLN13 (CTSF) gene encoding cathepsin F
    CLN14; CLN14 (KCTD7) gene encoding potassium channel tetramerization domain containing protein 7

The pattern of organ involvement in a specific lysosomal storage disease depends on the nature of the accumulating substrate, its anatomic distribution, and the cell turnover rate in individual organs. Three recurring themes among these patterns of organ involvement are nervous system, liver, and skeletal involvement.

- The central and peripheral nervous systems are particularly vulnerable to lysosomal storage diseases and therefore often affected. Neurologic manifestations include developmental delay, dementia, speech impairment, deafness, visual loss, ophthalmoplegia, leukodystrophy, seizures, ataxia, peripheral neuropathy, and macrocephaly (15).

- Hepatosplenomegaly is a feature of many of these diseases including Gaucher disease, Niemann-Pick disease, and mucopolysaccharidosis (MPS). To what extent Kupffer cells or hepatocytes are affected varies depending on the disease process.
- Deposition of storage material like glycosaminoglycans in growth plates and cartilage disrupts normal development and maturation of the skeleton. As a result, these patients often have coarse, dysmorphic facial features. "Dysostosis multiplex" is a term that is often used for the skeletal manifestations that include coarse, dysmorphic facial features, short stature, as well as bone and joint abnormalities.

Beyond these three organ systems, there is a plethora of other organ manifestations as illustrated by the following examples: In Gaucher disease, involvement of the reticuloendothelial system may lead to hypersplenism causing anemia. Cardiac involvement with deposition of glycosaminoglycans in the heart valves and connective tissue is a feature of mucopolysaccharidoses (esp. MPS VI) and may be associated with valvular disease, conduction defects, and cardiomyopathy. Deposition of glycosaminoglycans in the dura and ligaments can cause spinal cord compression symptoms or carpal tunnel syndrome. Involvement of adenoids, tonsils, and epiglottis can contribute to upper airway obstruction. Deposition in the cornea can cause cataracts.

Pathophysiology

Morphologic studies illustrating accumulation of storage products have led to the name of lysosomal storage diseases. This nomenclature may, however, fall short of truly summarizing the pathogenesis of these diseases (13). In some instances, storage material may not even be lysosomal—MPS IIIB is associated with defective transfer from the Golgi to the lysosome and accumulation of storage material in disrupted Golgi. Other processes may contribute to the pathogenesis beyond accumulation of storage material:

- Toxic effect: At least in some cases, cellular and neuronal dysfunction is independent of neuronal storage. In Krabbe disease, secondary increase of the lysosphingolipid psychosine is thought to have toxic effects (12).
- Vesicle function and trafficking: Lysosomes are connected to many key vesicle and cell trafficking systems, including autophagy and exocytosis. Lysosomal storage diseases lead to disruption of pH gradients in the endomembrane system that can disrupt function of many proteins (18). Autophagy and exocytosis may be disrupted (18).
- Lipid composition: Changes in the composition of lipids in cell membranes can alter membrane fluidity and affect receptor signaling. This is, for example, observed in Niemann-Pick disease type C.
- Signaling and activation of apoptosis: Some of the accumulating storage products can act as ligands for cellular receptors. Examples include galactoceramide in Krabbe and glycosaminoglycans in mucopolysaccharidoses. These disruptions in cell signaling can lead to activation of proapoptotic pathways (12). Activation of the unfolded protein response resulting from disrupted function of the endoplasmic reticulum can also be a pathway leading to apoptosis.
- Inflammation: Niemann-Pick disease (types A, B, C) and Gaucher disease as diseases associated with prominent involvement of the reticuloendothelial system can lead to release of inflammatory cytokines from cells like microglial cells.
- Calcium homeostasis: Storage products can disrupt calcium handling in the endoplasmic reticulum affecting cellular calcium homeostasis.

Diagnosis of Lysosomal Storage Diseases

The diagnosis and classification of lysosomal storage diseases have evolved and changed. Historically, morphologic studies and biochemical documentation of enzyme deficiency in leukocytes, fibroblasts, or amniocytes were key components of the diagnostic workup. In that setting, the ultrastructural evaluation of storage material often could add valuable insight into the disease process. Histomorphologic and ultrastructural confirmation of storage material may be performed on the skin, conjunctiva, peripheral blood lymphocytes, liver, bone marrow, skeletal muscle, rectal suction biopsies sampling mucosal ganglion cells, or placenta, depending on the suspected clinical diagnosis (17,19–24). Some of the storage material may require special handling of the tissue since it may be soluble in solutions used for routine processing. The appropriate triage of a specimen may therefore include setting aside tissue for alcohol fixation (e.g., for cysteine crystals or glycogen), formalin fixation, glutaraldehyde fixation for electron microscopy, and freezing. Stored lipids can be visualized by oil red O or Sudan black–stained sections on frozen tissue or on Epon-embedded sections. The Schultz adaptation of the Liebermann-Burchard reaction has been used to stain cholesterol (25). The sugar moieties of glycosylated storage material or accumulated carbohydrates can be highlighted by PAS staining with and without diastase. Colloidal iron or Alcian blue can be utilized to stain glycosaminoglycan accumulation as seen with mucopolysaccharidoses.

Nowadays, however, our understanding of and our approach toward lysosomal storage diseases have changed dramatically with the advent of new molecular techniques (13). Genetic testing has rapidly become the main diagnostic tool. Targeted treatment options have changed the role and importance of an accurate classification from a purely prognostic aspect to a crucial step in patient management. An understanding of the morphologic manifestations of these diseases is therefore less critical for daily diagnostic practice than in the past. But studying the morphologic changes of these diseases still conveys important insights into the underlying pathophysiologic concepts. And in some unexpected cases, the diagnostic workup may start with the specimen that ends up on the workbench or under the microscope of a pathologist who will then still have to recognize the key morphologic features.

Treatment

Patients with lysosomal storage diseases are typically managed in a multidisciplinary team, and a number of general supportive care measures may be considered. Physical therapy and pulmonary assistance (BiPAP/CPAP) may be beneficial in patients with mucopolysaccharidoses. Seizure control is an important and challenging aspect of managing affected patients. Splenectomy has been performed in patients with Gaucher disease to manage hypersplenism (26). But beyond these general supportive care measures, there is a rapidly evolving field of targeted treatments that involve enzyme replacement therapies, substrate reduction therapies, pharmacologic chaperones, and bone marrow transplantation. Because of the blood–brain barrier, a commonly encountered problem is the treatment of central nervous system involvement (12). These therapeutic approaches may include the following:

- Enzyme replacement therapies are approved and used for Pompe disease, adult-onset acid maltase deficiency, non-neuropathic type I Gaucher disease, Fabry disease, MPS I S, MPS I S/H, MPS II, and MPS VI. Replacement therapies for alpha-mannosidosis, GM1 gangliosidosis, Wolman disease, and MPS IV A are in clinical trials. Studies with intrathecal administration and with combination therapies are ongoing (12,18,27,28).
- Substrate reduction therapies aim to reduce the upstream synthesis of accumulating storage products. Miglustat (*N*-butyl-deoxygalactonojirimycin) is a competitive inhibitor of ceramide glucosyltransferase and is of potential use in the treatment of Gaucher I and III as well as Niemann-Pick disease type C (27).
- Pharmacologic chaperones stabilize a protein during the transport and processing in the endoplasmic reticulum, preventing mutant protein from being sent for early degradation and allowing for the expression of mutant proteins with residual activity. Miglustat has shown beneficial effects in mouse models of Fabry disease (27).
- Bone marrow transplantation has been shown to benefit patients with Krabbe disease and Hurler disease and some patients with late-onset metachromatic leukodystrophy if performed before onset of symptoms. Skeletal dysplasia in Hurler disease is, however, not fully corrected, and treated children with Krabbe disease may still develop manifestations such as motor difficulty (15,29). Gene therapy is also being studied as another approach to treatment (30).

Lysosomal Storage Diseases Linked to Defects in Specific Enzymes

Sphingolipidoses

Gaucher Disease
Gaucher disease is the most common lysosomal storage disease (31). There are three allelic types that represent mutations in the beta-glucocerebrosidase gene (32). Type 1 Gaucher disease is the most common form and is particularly frequent in individuals of Ashkenazi Jewish heritage (33). Type 1 is nonneuronopathic and causes hepatosplenomegaly, hypersplenism, lung disease, and bony involvement. This is in contrast to types 2 and 3 that are known as neuronopathic forms because they additionally result in seizures and brain injury. Type 2 typically presents as life-threatening disease in infancy while type 3 is milder.

The enzyme defect in beta-glucocerebrosidase leads to failure of cleavage of glucose from ceramide. Glucocerebrosides are derived from glycolipids in white and red cell membranes and accumulate mainly in lysosomes of cells of the reticuloendothelial system. Characteristic Gaucher cells are large eosinophilic phagocytes with wrinkled or striated cytoplasm (Figure 5-1A–C) that are found in the liver, bone marrow, spleen, lymph nodes, tonsils, thymus, Peyer patches, alveolar septae, and Virchow-Robin space (28,31,34). Gaucher cells are capable of erythrophagocytosis and are acid phosphatase positive and label with antibody to CD68. The striations can be highlighted with Masson trichrome, aldehyde fuchsin, and PAS after diastase. Electron microscopy shows lysosomal rod-shaped or tubular lipid bilayer stacks (Figure 5-1D, E).

The liver is enlarged in all three types with accumulation of storage material in the Kupffer cells, especially in zone 3, but not the hepatocytes (34). Fibrosis may progress to cirrhosis. The spleen is enlarged, weighing as much as 10 kg, and may be uniformly pale or mottled due to storage accumulation. In the bone marrow, infiltrating Gaucher cells lead to osteopenia, sclerosis, necrosis, and pathologic fractures (35). Erlenmeyer flask deformity of the distal femur is considered diagnostic of Gaucher disease (35). No neuronal storage material is seen in the brain, but there are phagocytic cells in the Virchow-Robin spaces (28). The neuronal loss observed in patients with type 2 and 3 diseases is thought to result from lipids that are toxic to neurons. The placenta may be involved with Gaucher cells in villous vessels (17).

Diagnosis is based on quantitating beta-glucocerebrosidase activity in leukocytes or fibroblasts or by DNA analysis. There is some genotype–phenotype correlation with specific mutations associated with certain patterns of presentation. Splenectomy is performed to reduce thrombocytopenia and anemia (26). Enzyme replacement therapy effectively treats the pancytopenia and hepatosplenomegaly in type 1 patients, but the bone disease responds slowly, if at all (13,26,28).

Fabry Disease (Angiokeratoma Corporis Diffusum Universale)
Fabry disease is the result of alpha-galactosidase A (ceramide trihexosidase) deficiency leading to disordered glycosphingolipid metabolism with accumulation of globotriaosylceramide (ceramide trihexoside, ceramide digalactoside, blood group B glycolipid) containing substrates (36). Fabry disease is X linked, and 1:40,000 to 1:60,000 males are affected (37). Over 150 mutations have been identified. Clinical manifestations include extremity pain and paresthesias (acroparesthesias), hearing loss, skin and mucous membrane angiokeratomas, and corneal opacities (36). Renal impairment leads to end-stage renal disease by 20 to 40 years of age. Early death may result from renal failure,

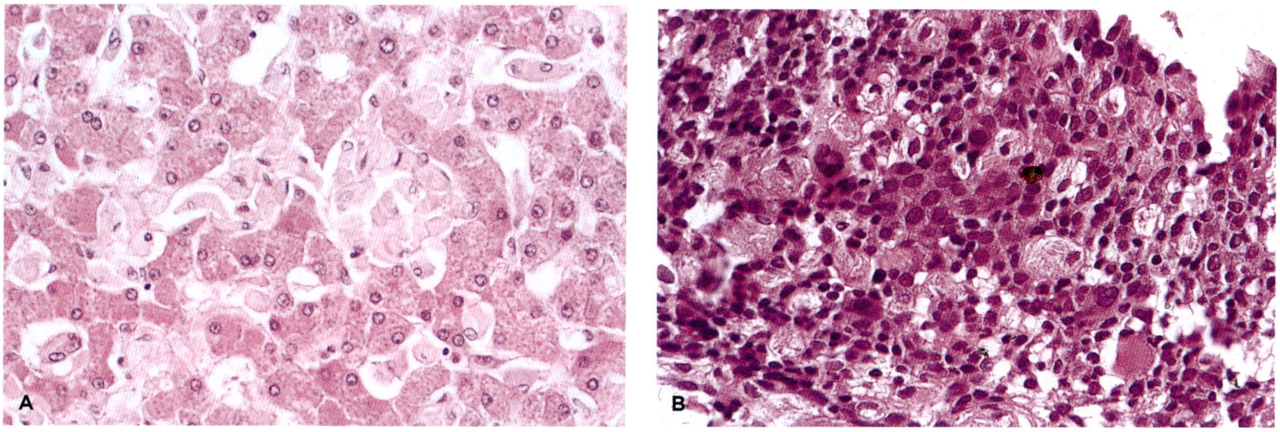

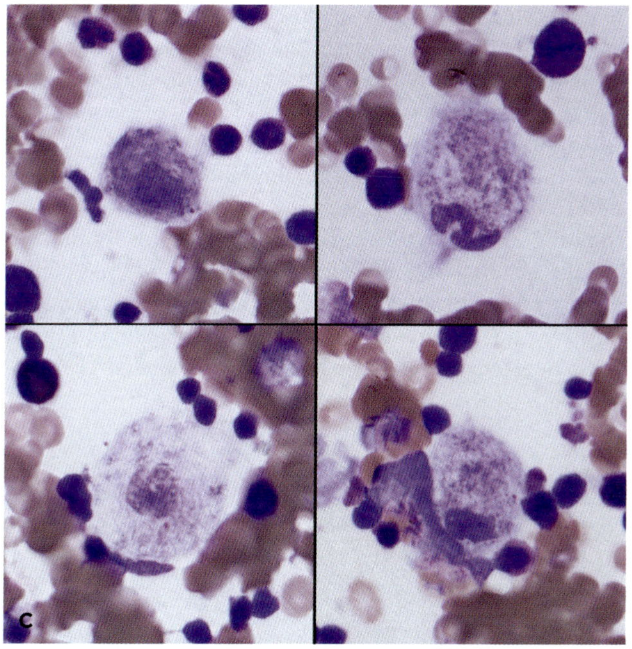

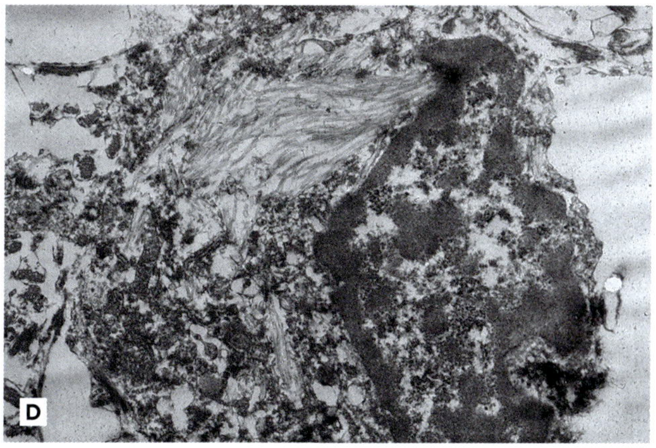

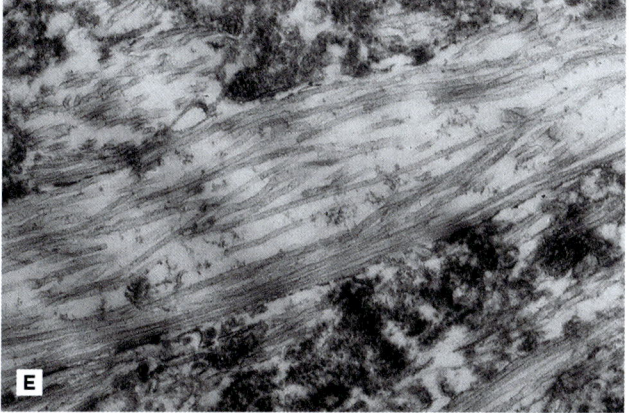

FIGURE 5-1 • Gaucher disease. **A:** The liver of a patient with Gaucher disease has prominent Kupffer cells due to pale eosinophilic expansion of the cytoplasm by lysosomal glucocerebroside storage material (H&E). **B:** Enlarged phagocytes in the spleen have a "wrinkled tissue paper" appearance of their cytoplasm because of the glucocerebroside storage (H&E). **C:** Wright-stained bone marrow aspirate from a patient with Gaucher disease showing "Gaucher cells" with a "wrinkled tissue paper" appearance of cytoplasm due to glucocerebroside storage (Wright). **D:** Ultrastructural appearance of Gaucher cell from the spleen, obtained at autopsy, showing cytoplasmic storage in upper middle and lower middle of the image, to the left of the nucleus (Uranyl acetate, lead citrate). **E:** Ultrastructurally, glucocerebroside storage material in Gaucher disease comprises rod-shaped or tubular lipid bilayer stacks with a diameter of up to 4 μm (Uranyl acetate, lead citrate).

cardiac disease, or cerebrovascular disease (38). Late-onset manifestations with cardiac disease with or without renal involvement can be seen even into the 6th decade, and the above cited incidence may underestimate the overall disease burden (37,39). In contrast to other X-linked diseases, the phenotype in female heterozygotes is variable, but can be associated with significant medical problems mimicking those of the classic disease seen in males (40). Hemizygotes and heterozygotes with B or AB blood type are more severely affected due to the additional accumulation of B-specific glycolipid.

PAS-positive glycolipid and cholesterol accumulate in lysosomes of endothelial cells, reticuloendothelial cells, and macrophages. By EM, osmiophilic lamellated leaflets and tubules are seen in endothelial, perithelial, and smooth muscle cells (41,42). Glomerular podocytes, endothelial, mesangial, interstitial, and tubular epithelial cells all contain storage material. Podocyte storage causes cellular injury, followed by glomerular capillary wall thickening, progressive mesangial matrix expansion, glomerulosclerosis, and, eventually, end-stage renal disease (Figure 5-2A to C). Some patients develop hypertrophic obstructive cardiomyopathy. Storage material in arteries can lead to luminal obstruction and ischemic lesions that may, for example, be found in the brain. There is typically no clinically significant liver involvement, but morphologic studies may show Kupffer cells that have a tan appearance in H&E sections and storage that is birefringent and crystalline in frozen sections stained with the Schultz method.

Diagnosis is based on identifying decreased alpha-galactosidase A in leukocytes or fibroblasts or by DNA analysis for the mutation. Enzyme activity is not a reliable diagnostic tool for female carriers. Their diagnosis requires mutational analysis. Enzyme replacement therapy may have benefit in Fabry patients (13,38).

Gangliosidoses

These autosomal recessive disorders all show lysosomal accumulation of glycosphingolipids (gangliosides).

GM1 Gangliosidosis

GM1 gangliosidosis and mucopolysaccharidosis IVB both are the result of mutation in the *GLB1* gene encoding beta-galactosidase (43,44). The former is associated with CNS involvement, while the latter is characterized by skeletal involvement, cardiac valvular disease, and corneal clouding but normal intellect. CNS disease is the manifestation of ganglioside accumulation, while systemic manifestations result from galactosyl oligosaccharides and keratan sulfate storage. Differences in the mutation may spare the ability of the enzyme to break down gangliosides in MPS IVB. The phenotype of patients with GM1 gangliosidosis resembles that of MPS by showing coarse facies, dysostosis multiplex, and hepatosplenomegaly, but these patients also develop rapid neurologic deterioration and seizures. Infants may have hydrops fetalis, and most patients die by the age of 2 years. A late-onset form of infantile/juvenile GM1 gangliosidosis that presents at 1 year of age is clinically similar to the early-onset form but with milder dysostosis and death by 5 years of age.

In the nervous system, sudanophilic gangliosides accumulate in the neurons causing cellular ballooning and resulting in neuronal loss, gliosis, and atrophy. By EM, the storage material includes membranous cytoplasmic bodies. Peripheral nerves are also affected. In systemic organs, PAS-positive GAG accumulation causes vacuolization of Kupffer cells, hepatocytes, glomerular visceral epithelial cells and

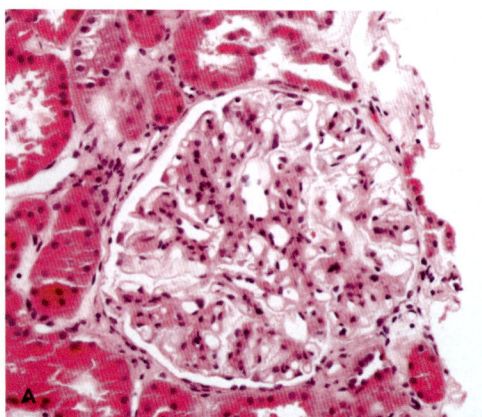
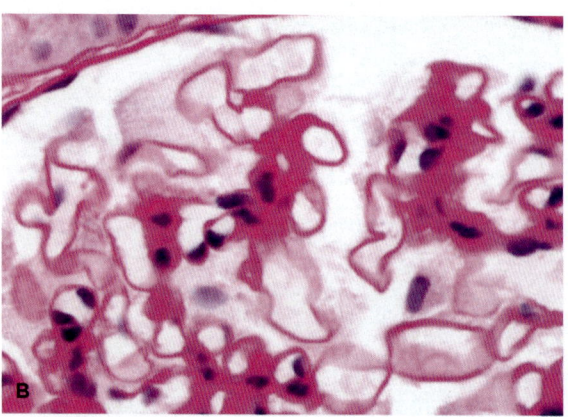
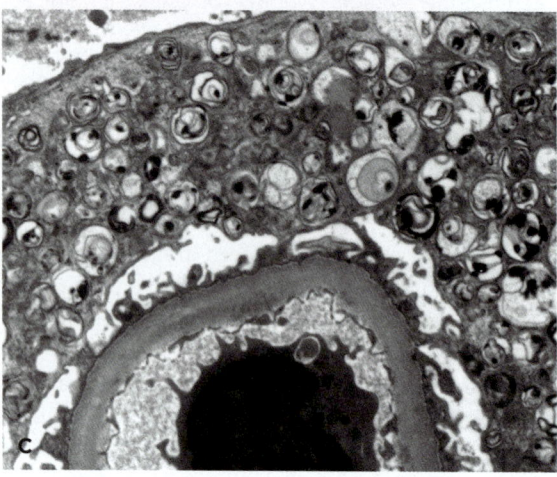

FIGURE 5-2 • Fabry disease. **A:** By LM, glomeruli in Fabry disease show mesangial expansion with prominence of pale-staining visceral epithelial cells (podocytes) (H&E). **B:** At higher magnification, podocyte cytoplasm is markedly expanded by PAS-positive storage material (PAS). **C:** Ultrastructurally, visceral epithelial cell cytoplasm is expanded by osmiophilic, lamellated leaflets and tubules, representing glycolipid and cholesterol storage (Uranyl acetate, lead citrate). (Images courtesy of Helen Liapis, M.D., Nephropath, Little Rock, AR.)

endothelial cells, placental syncytiotrophoblasts, marrow histiocytes, lymphocytes, lymph nodes, thymus, lung, intestine, pancreas, pituitary, thyroid, salivary gland, skin (including sweat glands), and conjunctiva (45,46). Visceral storage material is fibrillogranular (45,46). Definitive diagnosis rests on demonstrating beta-galactosidase deficiency in leukocytes, fibroblasts, or amniocytes or on DNA analysis.

GM2 Gangliosidosis
These gangliosidoses are due to autosomal recessive defects in lysosomal hexosaminidase with resultant accumulation of GM2 gangliosides mainly in neurons. Hexosaminidase A is a heterodimer composed of an alpha and a beta subunit. Hexosaminidase B is a homodimer composed of two beta subunits. Only hexosaminidase A can hydrolyze GM2 gangliosides.

GM2 gangliosidosis type 1 (Tay-Sachs disease, B variant): This form of GM2 gangliosidosis is due to hexosaminidase A deficiency caused by mutations in the gene encoding the alpha subunit (43,47). Hexosaminidase B is expressed. GM2-containing gangliosides accumulate particularly in the CNS. The incidence is increased in Ashkenazi Jewish populations. Psychomotor deterioration, seizures, blindness, and death by 3 to 5 years of age characterize most patients, although milder juvenile and adult forms are recognized (48). The brain is atrophic with neuronal loss and secondary gliosis; cholesterol, phospholipid, and GM2 ganglioside accumulate as sudanophilic storage in essentially all neurons. The stored material is PAS positive in frozen but not in paraffin sections. By EM, stored material in the CNS is concentrically lamellated, membranous, and granular (45,49). More pleomorphic inclusions are present in the glia. The liver appears normal by LM, but, by EM, there is granular and zebra body storage. Diagnosis is based on hexosaminidase A (decreased) and B (normal) assay in serum, leukocytes, or fibroblasts. Alternatively, DNA analysis by whole genome sequencing or targeted testing for common mutations can confirm the diagnosis.

GM2 gangliosidosis type 2 (Sandhoff disease, O variant): Patients have a mutation in the beta subunit of hexosaminidase shared by A and B, resulting in deficiency of both enzymes (hence "O" variant) (43). Clinically affected patients are indistinguishable from Tay-Sachs disease patients. The cerebral cortex is atrophic and yellowed by accumulated asialoganglioside. PAS-positive sphingolipids and glycoprotein accumulate in hepatocytes, Kupffer cells, lymphocytes, pancreatic acinar cells and histiocytes of the spleen, lymph nodes, as well as bone marrow. By EM, storage material similar to that of Tay-Sachs disease is found with prominent membranous cytoplasmic bodies in brain and heterogeneous material in viscera (45). Diagnosis can be determined by enzyme assay or DNA analysis.

GM2 activator protein deficiency (AB variant) results from mutations in the *GM2A* gene that encodes the GM2 activator protein, which acts as a substrate-specific cofactor for hexosaminidase A (43,50). The designation as "AB variant" stems from the normal expression levels of hexosaminidase A and B, which are not functional because of the defective activator protein. Clinically and pathologically, the AB variant resembles infantile Tay-Sachs and Sandhoff diseases (50,51). Visceral organs are not involved. Zebra and membranous cytoplasmic bodies accumulate (Figure 5-3A,B), and heterogeneous storage affects glial cells. Diagnosis is based on reduced activator protein level in fibroblasts and DNA analysis.

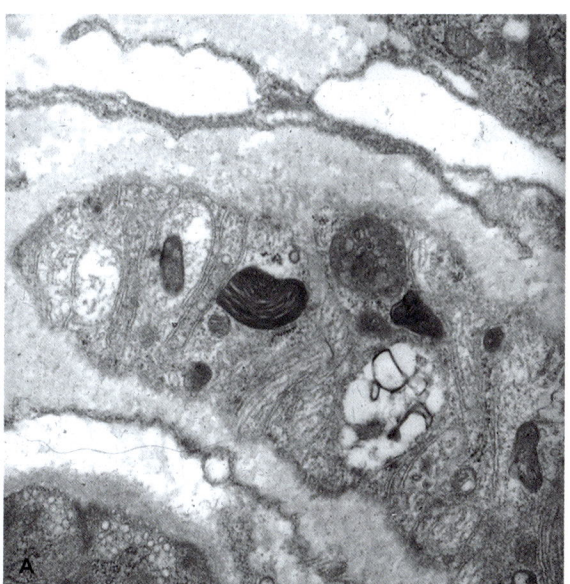 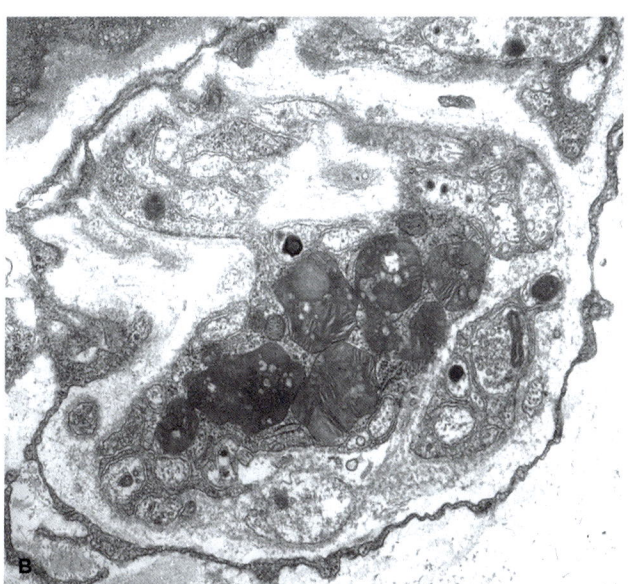

FIGURE 5-3 • Gangliosidosis. **A, B:** Membranous cytoplasmic bodies in GM2 (AB variant) gangliosidosis are heterogeneous and can show concentric or parallel structure, here in peripheral nerve axons. Though the morphology of the stored gangliosides is often not helpful in distinguishing the gangliosidoses, location of the storage material can be helpful (Uranyl acetate, lead citrate). (Image **B** from Vogler C, Rosenberg HS, Williams JC, et al. Electron microscopy in the diagnosis of lysosomal storage diseases. *Am J Med Genet Suppl* 1987;3:243–255, with permission.)

Niemann-Pick Disease (Sphingolipidoses, Sphingomyelin Lipidosis, Sphingomyelin-Cholesterol Lipidosis, NPD)

Two basic variants of Niemann-Pick disease that are discussed further below are those with acid sphingomyelinase deficiency and those with mutations in *NPC1* or *NPC2* (52). All of these are autosomal recessive. NPD A and B are the result of sphingomyelinase deficiency and are distinguished by phenotype severity and CNS involvement. Niemann-Pick disease type C with *NPC1* or *NPC2* mutation is not the result of a specific enzyme deficiency but is caused by more general impairment of intracellular lipid trafficking and membrane lipid composition (53).

Niemann-Pick disease (NPD) type A and B: Both of these variants are caused by mutations in the *SMPD1* gene that encodes sphingomyelin phosphodiesterase 1. Type A is the more common (85% of cases) and most severe, infantile, neuronopathic form of NPD (54,55). Hydrops fetalis, failure to thrive, hepatosplenomegaly, hypotonia, and progressive neurologic deterioration end with death by 3 to 4 years of age. The disease incidence is higher in the Ashkenazi Jewish populations, among which the carrier frequency is 1:80. Type B is phenotypically variable, more chronic, and non-neuronopathic. This disease variant presents in older infants or later with hepatosplenomegaly. Progressive pulmonary disease may become a major complication.

The pathologic hallmark of NPD is the *Niemann-Pick (NP) cell* (Figure 5-4A), though NP cells may be infrequent in very young children. These foamy lipid-laden histiocytes have pale yellow or tan cytoplasmic pigmentation on the H&E stain, the result of lipofuscin, sphingomyelin, ganglioside, and cholesterol storage. The vacuoles are birefringent with polarized light and stain with Sudan black B, oil red O (ORO), and Schultz reaction but stain poorly with PAS and for acid phosphatase (56). The blue green cytoplasm of histiocytes with storage stained with Wright-Giemsa stain led to the term *sea-blue histiocytes* (57).

Kupffer cells (Figure 5-4B) (and, in some cases, hepatocytes) have progressive increase in foamy cytoplasm. Portal fibrosis and cholestasis are observed, but cirrhosis is rare. Infants with NPD A may have cholestasis, bile duct paucity, pseudoglandular formation, and giant cell transformation with a neonatal hepatitis pattern. The spleen may be as much as ten times normal size with extensive infiltrate and replacement of red pulp by NP cells, some of which show erythrophagocytosis. The brain is atrophic with neuron loss, gliosis, and demyelination. Vacuolated neurons have sudanophilic, ORO-positive, and Luxol fast blue–positive storage, and foam cells and lipid-laden glia are in brain parenchyma and Virchow-Robin space (58). Ultrastructural studies can demonstrate storage of lipid with membranous lamellar or concentrically laminated myelin-like features and lipofuscin storage in many tissues including the liver, spleen, lung, bone marrow, kidney, and lymph node (Figure 5-4C to F) (56).

Diagnosis rests with identifying sphingomyelinase deficiency in leukocytes or fibroblasts. In families with a known molecular lesion, heterozygote status can be determined by DNA analysis.

Niemann-Pick disease type C: NPD C is the result of a defect of cholesterol esterification and intracellular trafficking that leads to lysosomal accumulation of sphingomyelin and unesterified cholesterol as well as secondary reduction in sphingomyelinase activity. NPD C is due to mutations in the *NPC-1* gene or less commonly the *NPC-2* gene. A type D form has been described ("NPD D") in cases from Nova Scotia with neurologic disease developing in childhood (59,60). On a genetic basis, NPD D is a variant of NPD C occurring in people of that particular heritage. The protein product of *NPC-1* is thought to facilitate the egress of cholesterol and other lipids from the late endosomes and lysosomes to other cellular compartments (53). Protean manifestations can begin any time from intrauterine life to adulthood (61,62). Patients may present with fetal ascites or with transient neonatal jaundice and hepatitis (63). Hepatosplenomegaly can occur in some patients but usually regresses over time and, in general, is less severe than that seen with NPD A or B. Neurologic disease is progressive with spasticity and seizures.

Neurovisceral storage is prominent with vacuolated cells in viscera and storage in neurons and glia. Vacuolated cells stain with Luxol fast blue, PAS, and Sudan black B and are positive for cholesterol with the Schultz reaction and for acid phosphatase. EM identifies membrane-bound whorled and dense osmiophilic lysosomal storage in skin and conjunctival cells, endothelial and perithelial cells, keratinocytes, retinal ganglion cells, retinal pigment epithelium, Schwann cells, smooth muscle cells, and fibroblasts (64). In the central nervous system, accumulation of storage material can be associated with the development of Tau-positive neurofibrillary tangles, the formation of meganeurites, and the presence of axonal spheroids.

NPD C may cause a neonatal hepatitis-like histology with giant cell transformation, fibrosis, or cirrhosis (63,65). The pathogenesis of this injury is unknown. Storage in liver is inconspicuous and easily overlooked, particularly in the setting of hepatitis. With time, whorled and irregular lamellar inclusions, clefts, and lipid storage accumulate in macrophages and Kupffer cells and to a lesser extent in hepatocytes (66). A screening test involves staining cultivated cells with filipin to detect free cholesterol. Diagnosis is based on measurement of cholesterol esterification in fibroblasts during LDL uptake and molecular analysis of the *NPC-1* or *NPC-2* genes.

Metachromatic Leukodystrophy (Sulfatide Lipidosis, MLD)

This is an autosomal recessive disease caused by mutations in the *ARSA* gene resulting in deficiency of arylsulfatase A, an enzyme that hydrolyzes galactocerebroside sulfate to galactocerebroside (67,68). The enzyme deficiency leads to accumulation of sulfated glycolipids primarily in the CNS but also in extraneural sites. The sulfated glycolipids are responsible for the phenomenon of metachromasia observed with certain

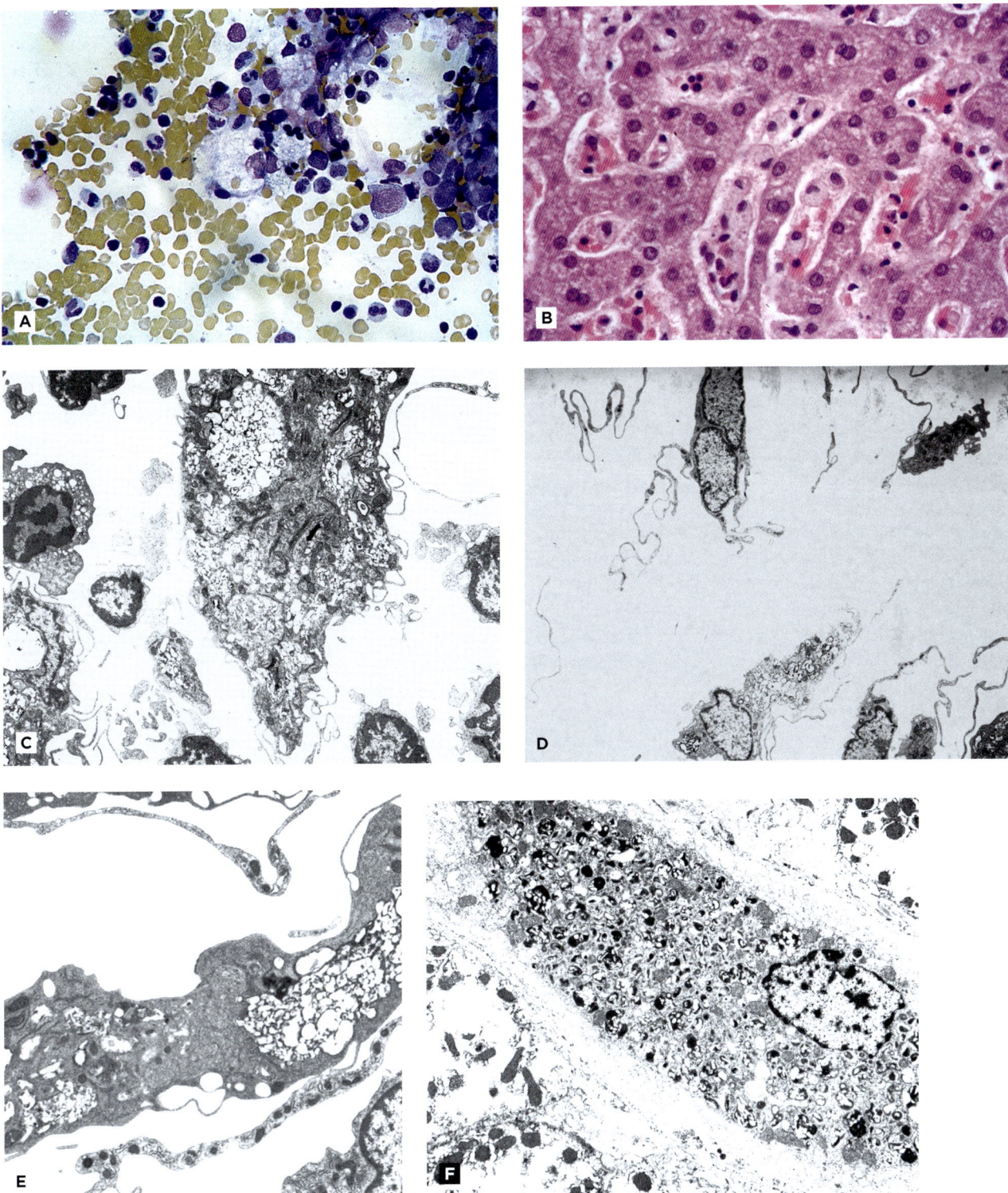

FIGURE 5-4 • Niemann-Pick disease. **A:** Several vacuolated "Niemann-Pick" cells, the pathologic hallmark of types A and B Niemann-Pick disease, are present and show "sea blue" coloration by Wright-Giemsa stain in this smear of a bone marrow aspirate. Niemann-Pick cells are capable of erythrophagocytosis and emperipolesis. **B:** Enlarged, foamy Kupffer cells in Niemann-Pick disease, as shown here, may be absent in very young children but become more prominent with time (H&E). **C–F:** Ultrastructurally, storage material in Niemann-Pick disease is a heterogeneous mix of membranous lamellar material, concentrically lamellated myelin-like material, and lipofuscin (**C–F**: Uranyl acetate, lead citrate).

aniline dyes that gave rise to the historical naming of this entity. An atypical form is caused by mutations in the cofactor saposin B (69). Different mutations have been described, and patients have a variable course with progressive neurologic disease resulting in several clinical forms with infantile, juvenile, and adult types. The central and peripheral nervous systems show demyelination, and the cerebellum is atrophic with Purkinje and granular cell loss. Spherical aggregates of metachromatic material that are 15 to 20 μm in diameter occur in oligodendrocytes, in macrophages within Virchow-Robin spaces, and in Schwann cells. This material comprises sulfatide, cholesterol, and phosphatides. In frozen sections, it stains positive with PAS, Alcian blue, and colloidal iron, and it is brown metachromatic (with 1% cresyl violet at low pH) and stains purple with toluidine blue. On electron microscopic studies, the storage material in oligodendrocytes, astrocytes, and Schwann cells is composed of closely packed, lamellar, amorphous, or prismatic material with alternating leaflets and tubules giving it a "herringbone" or "tuffstone" pattern (Figure 5-5A,B).

The gallbladder may be small and fibrotic with multiple mucosal papillomas and radiolucent choleliths; lamina propria macrophages, gallbladder epithelial cells, and intrahepatic bile ducts have storage. However, patients only rarely present with cholecystitis or pancreatitis. Liver macrophages, Kupffer cells, hepatocytes, and renal tubular epithelial cells also contain metachromatic storage.

Diagnosis is based on measuring arylsulfatase A activity. However, a low level does not prove MLD nor does a normal level exclude the diagnosis. A deficiency of the sphingolipid activator protein saposin B can result in a normal or heterozygous range arylsulfatase A level in an affected patient. Pseudoarylsulfatase A deficiency occurs when an abnormal allele that encodes only 5% to 15% of residual activity leads to low arylsulfatase A activity in a person who does not have MLD. Excessive urine sulfatides can confirm the diagnosis of MLD; a sulfatide-loading test allows distinction between patients homozygous for the pseudodeficiency allele and MLD patients.

Krabbe Disease (Galactosylceramide Lipidosis, Globoid Cell Leukodystrophy)

Autosomal recessive deficiency of galactocerebroside beta-galactosidase activity results in rapidly progressive neurologic deterioration in affected infants (67,70). An atypical variant is the result of a mutation in the cofactor saposin A. The pathology is limited largely to the nervous system. Grossly, the brain shows atrophy and discoloration of the white matter. Histologically, there is myelin loss, neuronal degeneration, and gliosis. The distinctive *globoid cells* are derived from monocyte–macrophage bone marrow stem cells and represent cells distended by PAS-positive and acid phosphatase–positive undigested psychosine (galactosylsphingosine) and galactosylceramide. The globoid cells accumulate in white matter and perivascular spaces. Psychosine accumulation causes oligodendroglia destruction and is an example of a lysosomal storage disease in which accumulated metabolites have distinct toxic effects (12). On electron microscopic studies, the storage material is composed of electron-dense, straight or curved, hollow tubular profiles in longitudinal section with crystalloid profiles in cross section (Figure 5-6A,B). Peripheral nerves have endoneural fibrosis, demyelination, and infiltration of PAS-positive macrophages, similar to the globoid cells seen in the CNS. Storage material also occurs in sweat gland epithelium. Diagnosis is based on DNA analysis or on identifying galactocerebroside beta-galactosidase deficiency in leukocytes, fibroblasts, amniotic, or chorionic cells. Specific mutations are associated with the infantile-onset form and are used in predicting outcome and therapeutic decisions about stem cell transplantation.

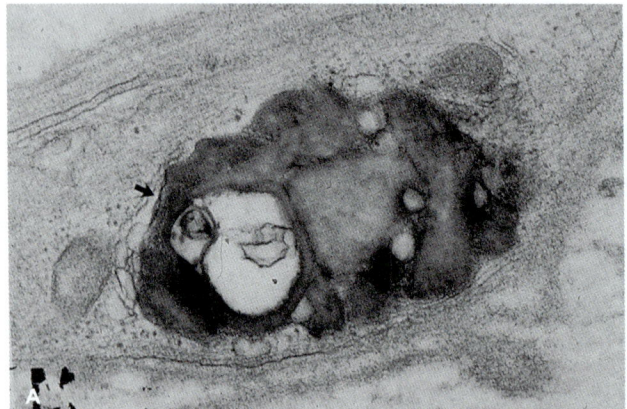
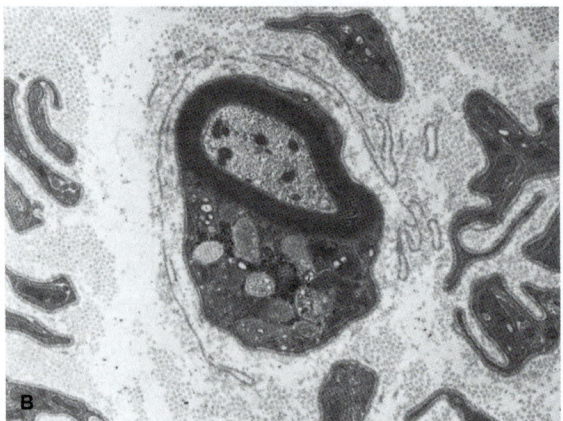

FIGURE 5-5 • Metachromatic leukodystrophy. **A:** This unmyelinated nerve from a conjunctival biopsy contains an inclusion of variable electron density. In some foci (*arrow*), closely approximated osmiophilic lamellae contribute to a subtle herringbone pattern. **B:** Myelinated nerve with pleomorphic lysosomes of variable density, "tuffstone" inclusions from a sural nerve of a patient with metachromatic leukodystrophy. (**A, B**: Uranyl acetate, lead citrate, **A:** Used from Vogler C, Rosenberg HS, Williams JC, et al. Electron microscopy in the diagnosis of lysosomal storage diseases. *Am J Med Genet Suppl* 1987;3:243–255, with permission.)

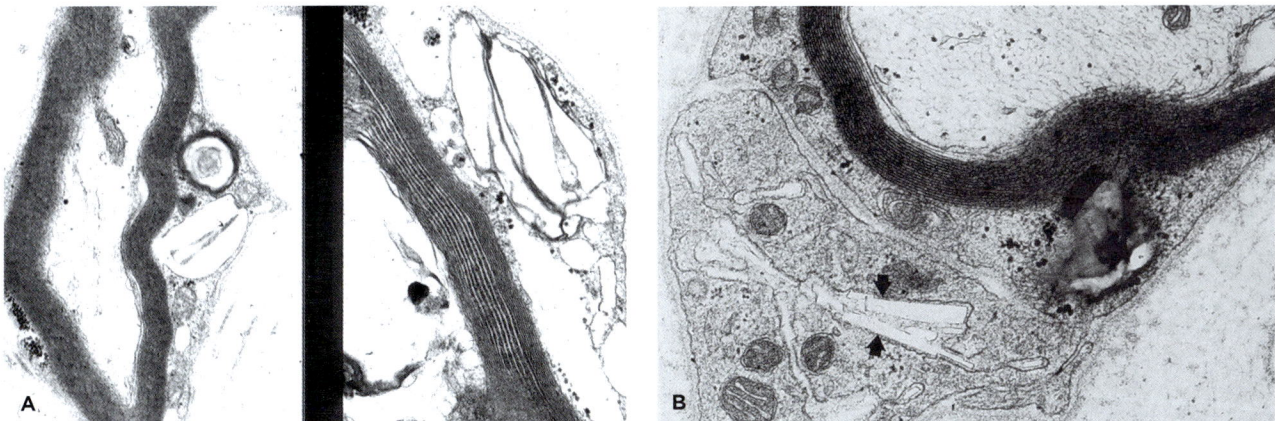

FIGURE 5-6 • Krabbe disease. **A, B:** Electron-lucent, angulated, and needle-shaped inclusions in conjunctival myelinated nerve Schwann cells, characteristic of Krabbe disease. (**A, B**: Uranyl acetate, lead citrate; **B**: Used from Vogler C, Rosenberg HS, Williams JC, et al. Electron microscopy in the diagnosis of lysosomal storage diseases. *Am J Med Genet Suppl* 1987;3:243–255, with permission.)

Farber Disease (Disseminated or Farber Lipogranulomatosis)

This rare autosomal recessive deficiency of acid ceramidase leads to accumulation of ceramide, which is formed from turnover of sphingolipids in lymph nodes, liver, kidney, and lung. Mucopolysaccharides and gangliosides also accumulate (71). Symptoms begin in infancy and include failure to thrive, vomiting, painful and progressively deformed joints, subcutaneous nodules that are especially prominent near joints, and laryngeal involvement with hoarseness and respiratory insufficiency. Clinically, histiocytosis is often in the differential diagnosis. Farber disease may present *in utero* with hydrops fetalis.

Lymph nodes, lung, larynx, spleen, liver, heart, subcutaneous, and periarticular tissues show nodular lipogranulomas containing PAS-positive storage in foam cells and multinucleated giant cells. Storage is also present in endothelial cells, pericytes, Schwann cells, hepatocytes, renal tubular epithelium, and glomerular visceral epithelial cells. Neurons are distended with PAS-positive ceramides and gangliosides. By electron microscopy, storage material consists of membrane-bound, comma-shaped curvilinear tubular profiles, termed *banana bodies* or *Farber bodies*, along with concentric lamellar, zebra body, and fibrillogranular material (72). Diagnosis is confirmed by demonstration of decreased acid ceramidase activity in leukocytes, fibroblasts, or amniocytes.

Disorders of Glycoprotein Degradation (Oligosaccharidoses/Glycoproteinoses)

These autosomal recessive disorders are due to deficiency of a lysosomal enzyme that degrades glycoprotein oligosaccharide side chains of glycoproteins (73). Defective function in lysosomal exopeptidases involved in the stepwise breakdown of glycoproteins can result in blockage of the entire pathway. Tissues accumulate glycoproteins and oligosaccharides, resulting in a phenotype that resembles that of mucopolysaccharidoses.

Alpha-Mannosidosis

Affected patients have deficient alpha-mannosidase and increased plasma levels as well as excretion of small mannose-rich oligosaccharides (73). The phenotype is variable, but in principle, this disease presents with immune deficiency manifested by recurrent infections, skeletal abnormalities, hearing impairment, speech problems, gradual impairment of cognitive function, and neuromuscular abnormalities with weakness and psychosis (74). Hepatocytes have granular or foamy cytoplasm, and Kupffer cells and hepatocytes contain reticulogranular, amorphous, or membranous storage by EM. In the brain, neurons have marked and widespread ballooning with membrane-bound vacuoles containing reticulogranular material. Diagnosis can be based on ultrastructural morphology of the skin, conjunctiva, or peripheral blood lymphocytes; demonstration of oligosacchariuria; and measurement of tissue alpha-mannosidase activity and gene testing (74).

Beta-Mannosidosis

The clinical phenotype associated with deficiency of beta-mannosidase is variable (73). Cognitive impairment is the most common presentation, but patients may also have deafness, speech problems, susceptibility to infections, hypotonia, epilepsy, peripheral neuropathy, facial dysmorphism, skeletal abnormalities, and angiokeratoma corporis diffusum (75,76). Cytoplasmic vacuoles are described in skin and bone marrow in isolated patients. The diagnosis rests on measurement of beta-mannosidase in leukocytes or fibroblasts and genetic testing.

Fucosidosis

This lysosomal storage disease, due to deficient alpha-l-fucosidase, causes accumulation of fucoside moiety–containing glycolipids, glycoproteins, and oligosaccharides (73,77). Most patients are of Italian or Spanish descent or from the southwestern United States. The presentation includes progressive

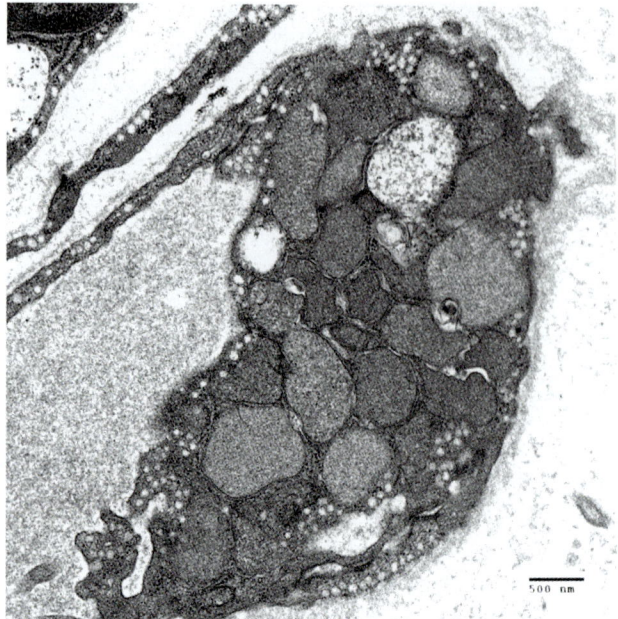

FIGURE 5-7 • Fucosidosis. Granular storage material distends the cytoplasm of this endomysial endothelial cell from a muscle biopsy of a 2-year-old girl with fucosidosis (Uranyl acetate, lead citrate).

mental retardation, seizures, recurrent infections, coarse facies, dysostosis multiplex and growth retardation, angiokeratoma corporis diffusum, and visceromegaly (73,77). The clinical course is variable. Most patients reach the second decade of life. The CNS, conjunctiva, muscle, skin and sweat gland epithelium, and peripheral blood lymphocytes all show granular lysosomal storage by EM (Figure 5-7). Diagnosis is based on demonstrating deficient alpha-l-fucosidase in leukocytes and fibroblasts. Some clinically normal individuals have low alpha-l-fucosidase levels in plasma.

Sialidosis

Sialidosis Types I and II are distinguished based on phenotype severity, but both result from mutations in the *NEU1* gene encoding lysosomal sialidase (78,79). Milder forms are associated with visual defects, cherry-red macular spots, ataxia, hyperreflexia, and seizures. More severe cases have dysostosis multiplex, cognitive impairment, hepatosplenomegaly, and Hurler-like phenotype. Definitive diagnosis is based on measurement of neuraminidase activity in cultivated fibroblasts or leukocytes.

Aspartylglycosaminuria

This autosomal recessive glycoprotein degradation defect occurs predominantly in Finland and is due to lack of aspartylglucosaminidase (80,81). Decreased cognitive function and facial and skeletal manifestations are most notable. The progression of disease is often slow with many patients living into their 30s, 40s, and 50s. Enlarged lysosomes contain aspartylglucosamine that appears as fibrillogranular storage in skin, conjunctiva, rectal mucosa, peripheral blood lymphocytes, neurons, hepatocytes, and Kupffer cells. In the CNS, delayed myelination, white matter gliosis, and gray matter atrophy are seen. Storage material may be evident in the liver, kidney, skin, and placenta as early as by the 20th week of gestation. Diagnosis is based on enzyme assay or DNA molecular analysis.

Glycogen Storage Disease: Pompe Disease (Glycogen Storage Disease Type II, GSD-II) and Adult Acid Maltase Deficiency

This glycogen storage disease is the result of mutations in the *GAA* gene encoding the lysosomal enzyme alpha-1,4-glucosidase (acid maltase) (82–85). A range of phenotypes occurs in GSD II patients, reflecting the variety of residual enzyme activity and tissue-specific isoenzymes. All are autosomal recessive. Patients with severe disease have hypotonia and cardiomegaly. These infants with classical Pompe disease die of cardiac or respiratory failure in the first few years of life. Adult-onset skeletal muscle disease is seen in late-onset cases without solid organ involvement and often results in muscle weakness in a distinct truncal distribution pattern that includes respiratory muscle weakness (86).

PAS-positive, diastase-digestible glycogen lysosomal storage is generalized but most severe in the skeletal muscle, heart, liver, and brain. Increased acid phosphatase activity indicates lysosomal distention and secondary elevation of other lysosomal enzymes (Figure 5-8A). A vacuolar myopathy with disruption of cytoplasmic structure affects skeletal, cardiac, and smooth muscle (Figure 5-8B,C). Cardiac involvement includes cardiac hypertrophy (Figure 5-8D), endocardial fibroelastosis, and arrhythmia from changes in the conduction system.

Glycogen is increased in Schwann cells, anterior horn cells, brainstem motor nuclei and spinal ganglia, myenteric plexus, astrocytes, oligodendroglia, endothelial cells, and pericytes with relative sparing of cortical neurons. Hepatocytes are only slightly enlarged with delicate glycogen-containing vacuoles. Liver lacks the mosaic pattern and nuclear glycogenation seen in other GSD (Figure 5-8E). In the kidney, glycogen accumulates in the epithelium of loops of Henle and collecting tubules, and the adrenal zona fasciculata has prominent storage.

Skin, conjunctiva, liver, muscle, lymphocytes, and placenta can show diagnostic lysosomal glycogen accumulation by EM (Figure 5-8F) (83). Glycogen in muscle is both lysosomal and cytoplasmic. Diagnosis is confirmed by demonstrating absent enzyme in dried blood spots, leukocytes, muscle, liver, or fibroblasts. In addition, DNA analysis can be utilized, which is also useful in defining patients with pseudodeficiency. Enzyme replacement therapy is available (84).

Mucopolysaccharidoses

The mucopolysaccharidoses (MPSs) are systemic diseases due to deficiency of one of the enzymes required for catabolism of glycosaminoglycans (GAG) including dermatan, heparan, chondroitin, and keratan sulfate, with resultant storage of undegraded GAG in lysosomes in a variety of cell types (12). The clinical presentation is variable but may include facial dysmorphism (Figure 5-9A,B), bone/joint dysplasia (Figure 5-9C), hepatosplenomegaly, neurologic impairment, developmental regression, and short life span to mild clinical phenotype with normal life expectancy (Table 5-6) (87,88). All MPS are autosomal recessive except X-linked Hunter syndrome. Hurler (type I) and Hunter (type II) syndromes are the most common types. Scheie and Hurler-Scheie syndromes are subtypes of MPS I with a milder disease. Some infants, particularly with MPS VII, present with hydrops (Table 5-2).

The stored GAG can be highlighted with colloidal iron and Alcian blue stains and is digested by hyaluronidase. Adding 10% cetyltrimethylammonium bromide to formalin may help preserve tissue GAG. By EM, visceral lysosomal storage is fine fibrillogranular material (Figure 5-9D).

In MPS, many organs and tissue types have lysosomal storage. The liver is typically enlarged and firm. Vacuolization is more prominent in Kupffer cells than hepatocytes. Fibrosis of the space of Disse occurs late in the disease; rarely, more severe fibrosis can develop in older patients. Coarse facial features, short stature, and bone and joint abnormalities (dysostosis multiplex) are the result of skeletal involvement. The corneas may show cloudiness. Airway obstruction and

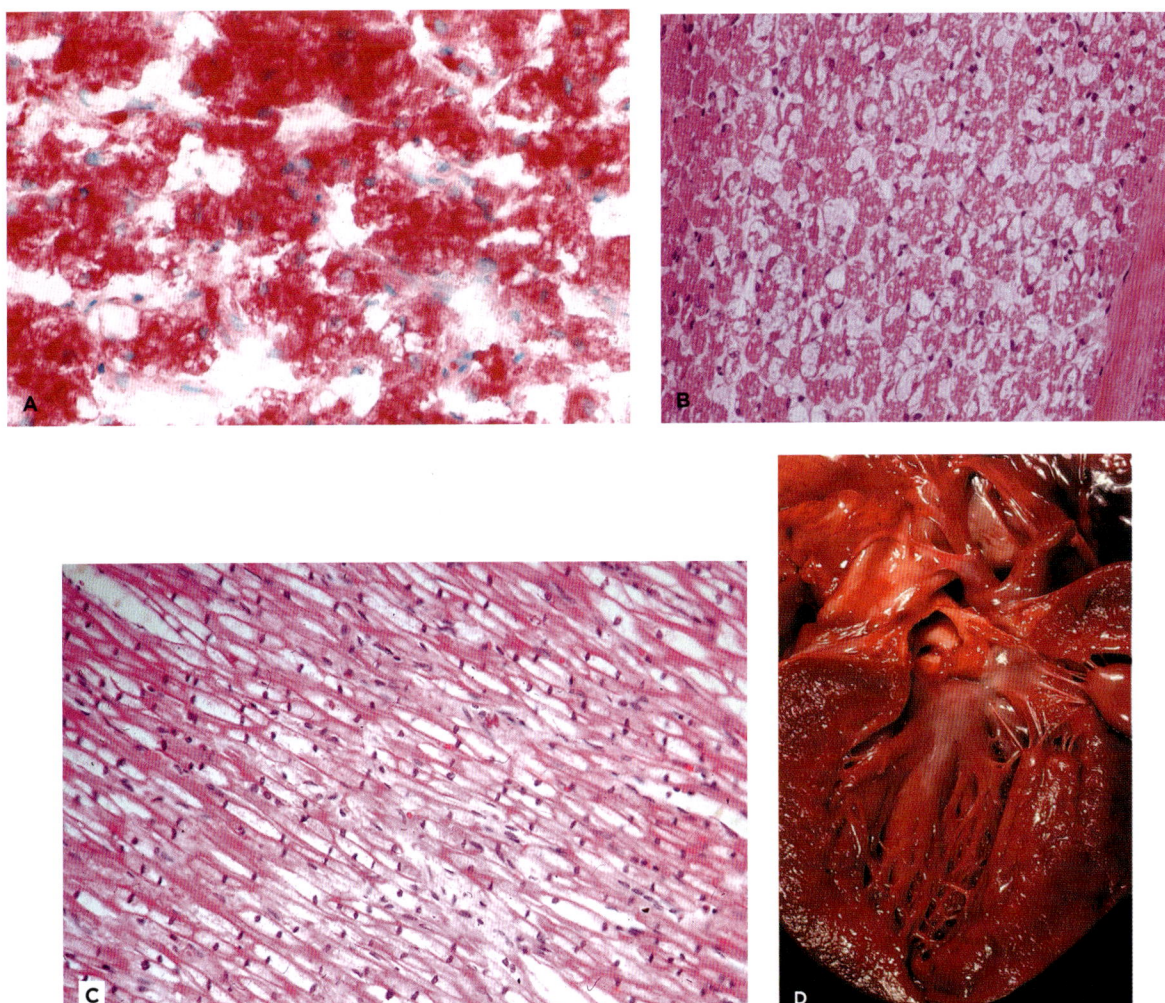

FIGURE 5-8 • Pompe disease (type II glycogen storage disease). **A:** Glycogen storage in Pompe disease is lysosomal (in contrast to glycogen storage in the other types of glycogen storage disease). The distended lysosomes also contain abundant acid phosphatase activity, which can be demonstrated histochemically, here in skeletal muscle by acid phosphatase staining (acid phosphatase stain). **B:** Vacuolar myopathy, though not specific for Pompe disease, is nonetheless characteristic and often striking in this LSD. The pale vacuoles in skeletal muscle fibers (representing glycogen storage) seen with H&E stain can be highlighted by PAS stain (not shown) (H&E). **C:** Histologically, cardiac myocytes are enlarged due to sarcoplasmic expansion by pale, often vacuolar material (H&E). **D:** Cardiac myocyte enlargement can lead to a hypertrophic gross appearance of myocardium, as seen in this image of the left ventricle from an infant who died with Pompe disease.

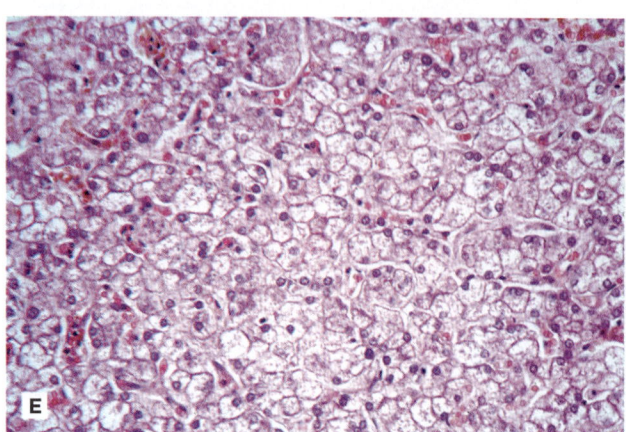
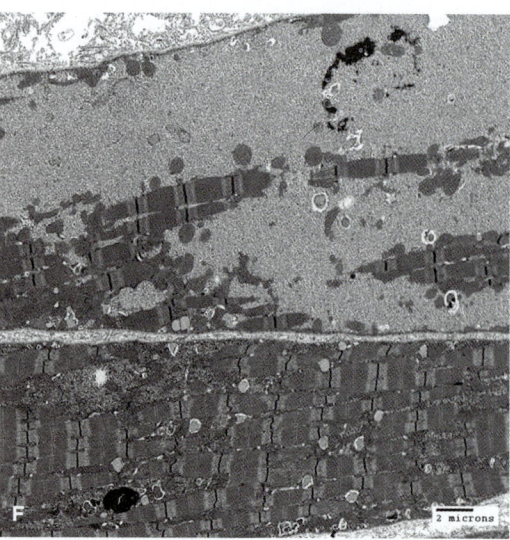

FIGURE 5-8 • *(Continued)* **E:** The histologic appearance of hepatocytes in Pompe disease is usually less striking than that of skeletal muscle. Hepatocytes are slightly enlarged with somewhat rarefied, vacuolar cytoplasm. Note the absence of glycogenated nuclei, which are typically not seen in the liver in Pompe disease but are observed in several other types of glycogen storage disease (H&E). **F:** Even though the primary defect in Pompe disease is lysosomal (in contrast to other glycogen storage diseases), glycogen accumulation is seen by ultrastructural analysis of skeletal muscle in the cytoplasm as well as within membrane-bound structures representing lysosomes.

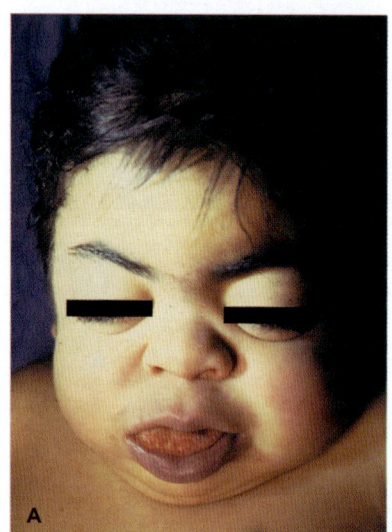
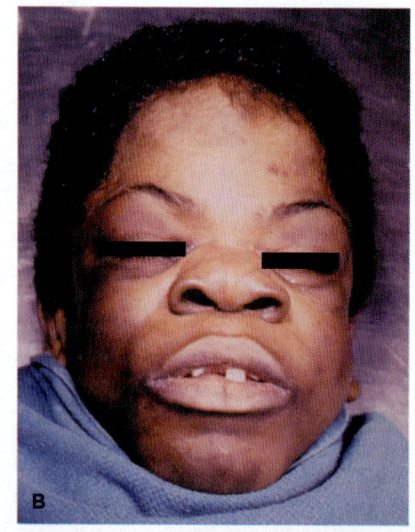
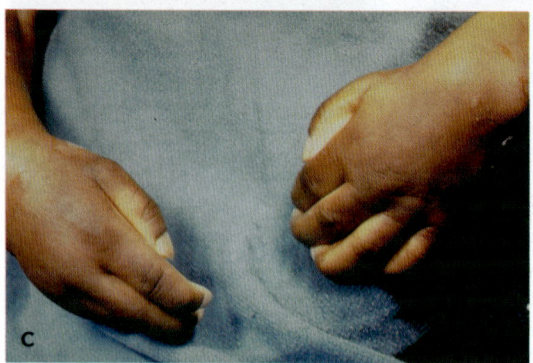
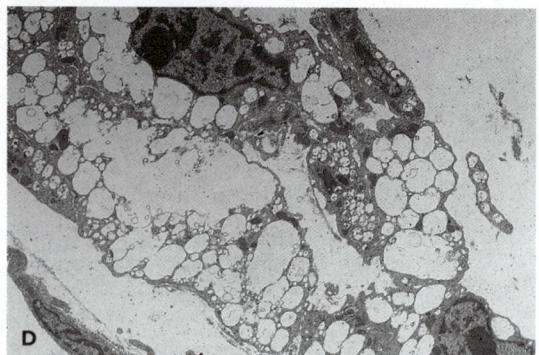

FIGURE 5-9 • Mucopolysaccharidosis. **A, B:** MPS patients have a characteristic facial appearance with coarse facial appearance, thick doughy skin, coarse hair, flattened midface, wide nasal bridge, and macroglossia, here seen in two children who died with MPS. **C:** The hands in MPS patients have joint stiffness and are held in a flexed position, a function of periarticular altered connective tissue and altered bone formation. **D:** In mucopolysaccharidosis, stored GAGs (previously called *mucopolysaccharides*) have the ultrastructural appearance of fine fibrillogranular material and clear membrane-bound vacuoles. Distinguishing different types of mucopolysaccharidosis based on ultrastructural morphologic characteristics is not possible.

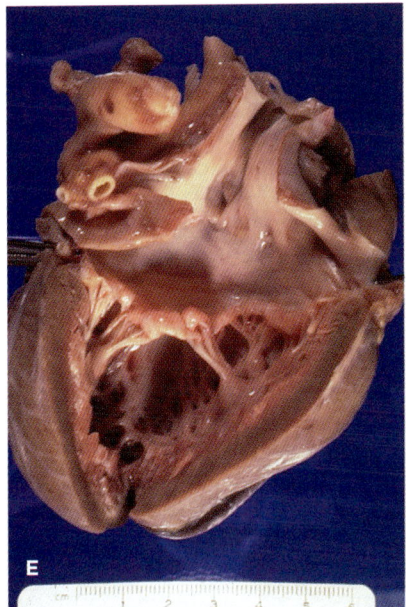
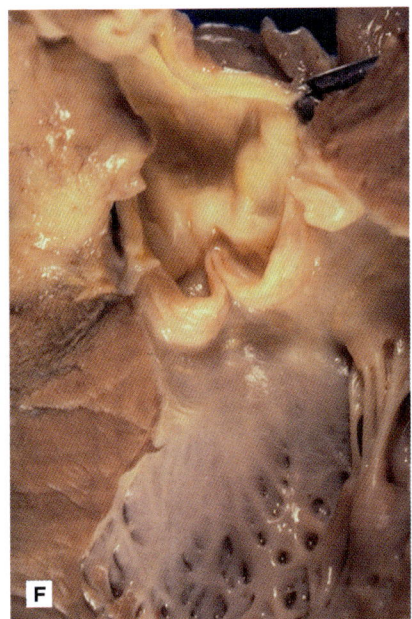
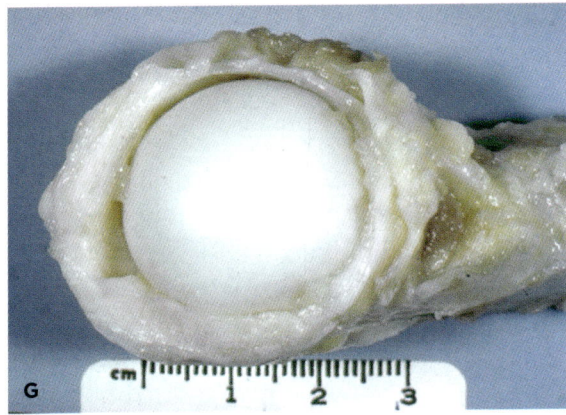
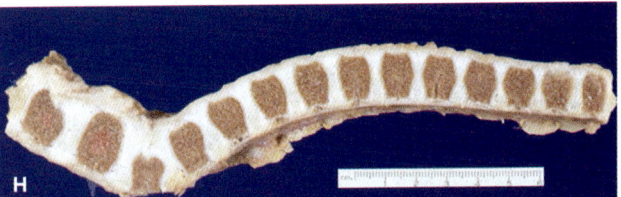
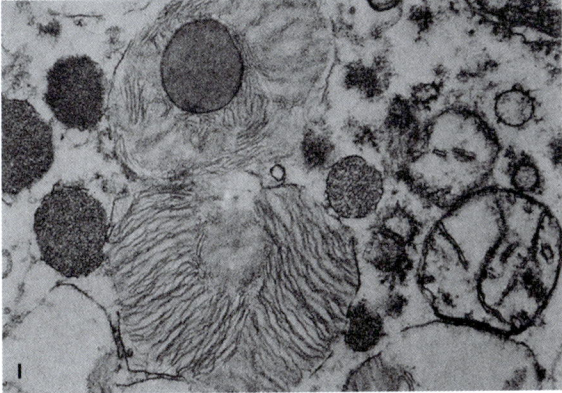

FIGURE 5-9 • *(Continued)* **E, F:** The heart in patients with MPS typically has thickened sclerotic valves, due to GAG storage in heart valve stromal cells and altered extracellular connective tissue in the valve. Endocardial thickening is also frequent. **G, H:** The femoral head of a patient from MPS shows articular synechiae and thick, poorly pliable periarticular connective tissue. These joint changes cause marked joint stiffness and make normal movement impossible. The vertebral column from an MPS patient shows characteristic anterior inferior breaking of the lower thoracic and upper lumbar areas caused by hypoplasia of the anterior superior aspect. This change results in the dorsal kyphosis or gibbus deformation often seen in MPS patients, and it is part of the widespread dysostosis multiplex. **I:** Though storage material in neurons can resemble that seen in other organs, it can also take the form of "zebra bodies," as shown in this case of Hurler syndrome (**D, I**: Uranyl acetate, lead citrate).

nerve or cord compression can be manifestations of soft tissue involvement (Figure 5-9C, G, and H) (Table 5-6) (89). Vessel walls and heart valves are often affected with storage with resultant sclerosis (Figure 5-9E,F), and endocardial fibroelastosis may occur. Neurons store both GAG and gangliosides leading to formation of membranous cytoplasmic bodies, zebra bodies, and fibrillogranular storage material (Figure 5-9I). Neuronal loss and gliosis are seen in some patients, and meningeal storage may contribute to hydrocephalus.

Diagnosis is suggested by increased urine GAG, the presence of vacuoles, and metachromatic Alder-Reilly granules in peripheral blood leukocytes. EM of the skin, conjunctiva, buffy coat, or liver can show characteristic fibrillogranular

TABLE 5-6 MUCOPOLYSACCHARIDOSES

MPS	Eponym	Enzyme Deficiency (Chromosome locus)	Stored Material	Clinical and Pathologic Findings
I	Hurler, Scheie, Hurler-Scheie	Alpha-l-iduronidase (4p16.3)	Dermatan sulfate, Heparan sulfate	Corneal clouding, dysostosis multiplex, hepatosplenomegaly, cardiac valve sclerosis, cognitive impairment, premature death (Scheie has milder phenotype without cognitive impairment), rarely hydrops fetalis
II	Hunter	Iduronate sulfatase (Xq28)	Dermatan sulfate, Heparan sulfate	Dysostosis multiplex, hepatosplenomegaly, cardiac valve sclerosis, cognitive impairment, X linked
IIIA	Sanfilippo A	Heparan N-sulfatase (sulfamidase) (17q25.3)	Heparan sulfate	cognitive impairment, mild somatic disease
IIIB	Sanfilippo B	N-acetyl-alpha-d-glucosaminidase (17q21.2)	Heparan sulfate	Similar to IIIA
IIIC	Sanfilippo C	Acetyl-CoA–alpha-glucosaminide N-acetyltransferase (8p11.21)	Heparan sulfate	Similar to IIIA
IIID	Sanfilippo D	N-acetylglucosamine-6-sulfatase (12q14.3)	Heparan sulfate	Similar to IIIA
IVA	Morquio A	Galactosamine-6-sulfatase (16q24.3)	Keratan sulfate, Chondroitin-6-sulfate	Skeletal abnormalities, corneal clouding, odontoid hypoplasia, hydrops fetalis
IVB	Morquio B	Beta galactosidase (3p21.33)	Keratan sulfate	Similar to IVA
VI	Maroteaux-Lamy	N-acetylgalactosamine-4-sulfatase (arylsulfatase B) (5q14.1)	Dermatan sulfate	Dysostosis multiplex, corneal clouding, normal intelligence
VII	Sly	Beta glucuronidase (7q11.21)	Dermatan sulfate, Heparan sulfate, Chondroitin-4,6-sulfates	Dysostosis multiplex, hepatosplenomegaly, cognitive impairment, hydrops fetalis
IX		Hyaluronidase (3p21.2–21.3)	Hyaluronan	Periarticular soft tissue masses (nodular histiocyte aggregates), short stature

lysosomal storage. LM of thick sections of tissue prepared for EM is useful for identifying the multiple clear cytoplasmic vacuoles indicative of lysosomal storage. Enzyme assay of serum, leukocytes, or fibroblast culture provides definitive diagnosis, and carrier testing using DNA analysis is practical. Enzyme replacement therapy is now available for some forms (87,88).

Lipidoses: Wolman Disease and Cholesterol Ester Storage Disease (CESD)

These are phenotypical variants of autosomal recessive mutations in the *LIPA* gene encoding lysosomal acid lipase and resulting in the accumulation of cholesterol esters and triglyceride (90–92). Severe deficiency leads to the phenotype described as Wolman disease that is characterized by failure to thrive, hepatosplenomegaly, and early death. Milder deficiencies are associated with dyslipidemia, hepatic fibrosis, and early atherosclerosis.

The enlarged liver is a distinctive bright orange-yellow with a greasy consistency. Bile duct proliferation and cholestasis are described, and periportal fibrosis with portal bridging may progress to cirrhosis. In viscera—including liver, spleen, adrenal, lymph nodes, lymphocytes, bone marrow, and intestine—cholesterol esters and triglycerides accumulate as cholesterol crystals in foamy histiocytes (Figure 5-10A,B). This storage can be identified by viewing sections of unfixed frozen tissue with polarized light (Figure 5-10C).

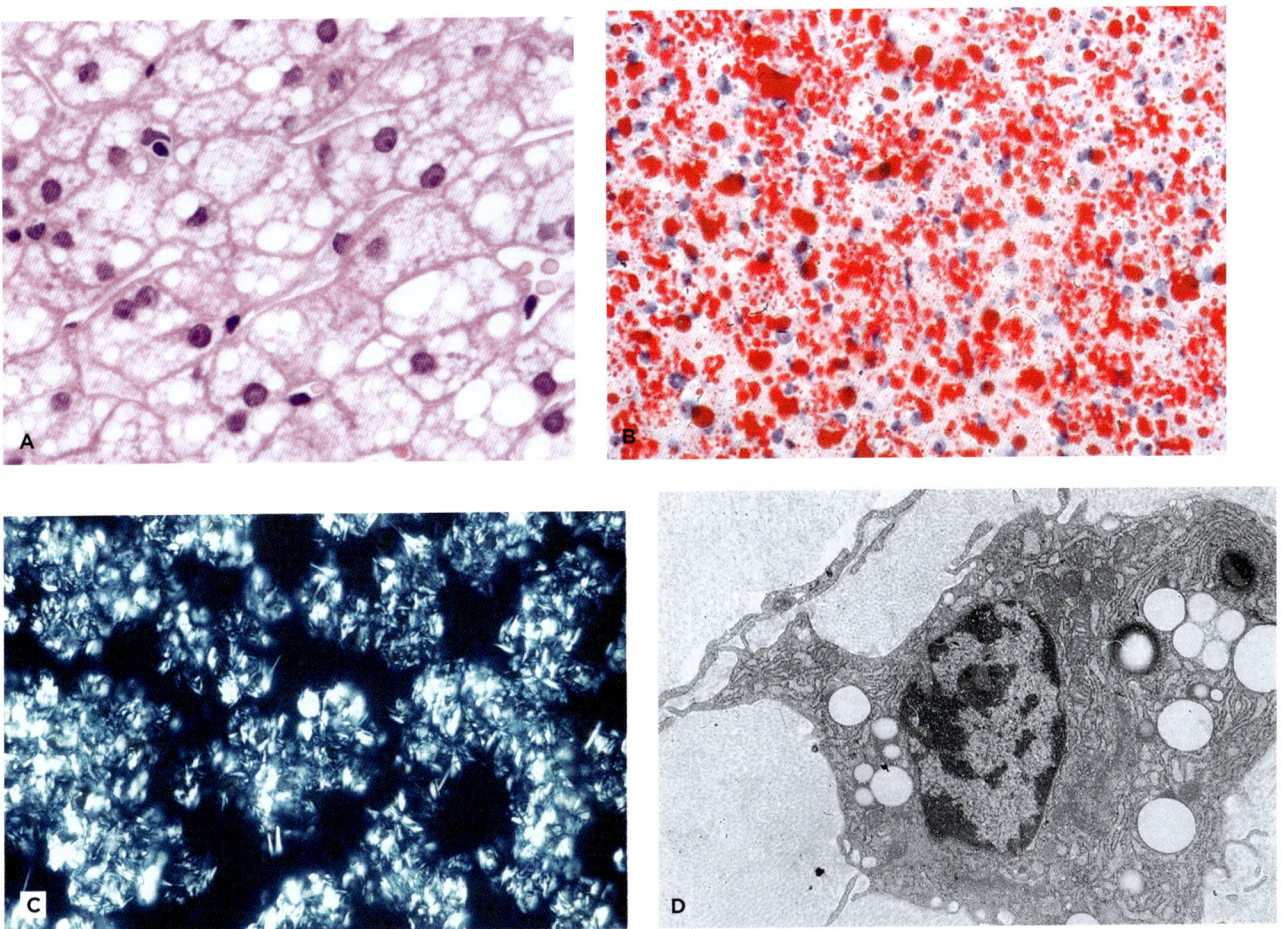

FIGURE 5-10 • Cholesterol ester storage disease. **A:** In cholesterol ester storage disease, there is widespread vacuolization of hepatocytes (H&E). **B:** Widespread cytoplasmic lipid can be demonstrated in frozen section analysis of liver tissue in cholesterol storage disease, here stained with oil red O. **C:** Hepatocellular cholesterol ester crystals are birefringent in frozen sections when viewed with polarized light. **D:** This conjunctival macrophage does not show needle-shaped clefts but does show many sharply demarcated electron-lucent vacuoles, some of which have peripheral osmiophilia, characteristic of lipid following fixation. (**D**: Uranyl acetate, lead citrate, Used from Vogler C, Rosenberg HS, Williams JC, et al. Electron microscopy in the diagnosis of lysosomal storage diseases. *Am J Med Genet Suppl* 1987;3:243–255, with permission.)

Cholesterol and triglycerides in these cells can also be highlighted histochemically with the Schultz modification of the Lieberman-Burchard reaction. EM shows lipid droplets and membrane-bound angular cholesterol clefts in hepatocytes, Kupffer cells, fibroblasts, and macrophages (Figure 5-10D). The mucosa of the small intestine, particularly duodenum and ileum, is velvety yellow due to lamina propria storage. Adrenal glands are large, hard, and bright yellow, with dystrophic calcification and necrosis of the inner fasciculata and residual fetal cortex. Oligodendroglia, some neurons of the CNS, and Schwann cells of the peripheral nervous system contain lipid. Placental syncytiotrophoblasts may be affected. Demonstration of acid lipase deficiency in tissue, cultivated fibroblasts, or leukocytes confirms the diagnosis.

Lysosomal Storage Diseases Linked to Nonenzymatic Protein Deficiencies

Some of these diseases are variants of historically and clinically discussed entities mentioned in previous sections and are therefore omitted here (AB variant of GM2 gangliosidosis, or the Niemann-Pick type C variants caused by NPC1 or NPC2 mutations).

Mucolipidoses

I-cell disease (ML II) and pseudo-Hurler polydystrophy (ML III) are autosomal recessive diseases that result from mutations that disrupt the hexameric complex of GlcNAc-1-phosphotransferase, which is composed of 2 alpha, 2 beta, and 2 gamma units (93). This enzyme complex tags newly synthesized lysosomal hydrolases for their appropriate targeting toward lysosomes by adding mannose-6-phosphate as a signal in the Golgi network (93). Phosphotransferase deficiency results in abnormal lysosomal enzyme transport. As a result, newly synthesized enzymes are secreted out of the cell instead of being transferred to lysosomes. This results in elevated plasma levels of lysosomal enzymes. The *GNPTAB* gene affected in ML II encodes the alpha- and beta-subunits of the hexameric enzyme complex, and the *GNPTG* gene affected in ML III encodes the gamma subunit.

Affected patients have features of both MPS and sphingolipidoses, hence the designation *mucolipidoses*. Clinical and radiologic findings (coarse facial features, psychomotor retardation, failure to thrive, hepatomegaly, dysostosis multiplex) are similar to those seen in MPS I, but earlier onset, a more rapid course, marked gingival hyperplasia, and absence of mucopolysacchariduria help distinguish ML II and III clinically from MPS I (94,95).

The term *I-cell disease* was coined because cultured fibroblasts from affected patients contain dense inclusions. PAS-positive and Hale colloidal iron–positive vacuoles are prominent in endothelial cells and fibroblasts and occur in lymphocytes, Kupffer cells, glomerular visceral epithelial cells, satellite cells in the muscle, myocardium, and pancreatic acinar cells (96). Storage in stromal fibroblasts of the heart is associated with valve thickening. Granulomas with finely vacuolated histiocytes may occur in lung and portal areas. Hepatocytes are normal or only mildly altered and contain triglyceride droplets.

The CNS may be normal morphologically, except for lamellar bodies in spinal ganglia neurons and anterior horn cells, or may have cerebral cortical atrophy with neuronal loss. Storage may be apparent in affected fetuses and their placentas. I-cell disease can present as nonimmune hydrops (see Table 5-1). By EM, the storage material is electron lucent or fibrillogranular and includes oligosaccharides, mucopolysaccharides, and lipids (96). EM of skin or conjunctiva can be used for diagnostic evaluation (Figure 5-11). Increased serum levels of lysosomal enzymes and decreased levels of *N*-acetylglucosamine-1-phosphotransferase provide biochemical confirmation.

ML III (pseudo-Hurler polydystrophy) symptoms are similar to ML II but milder with growth restriction, coarse facial features, cardiac valve disease, dysostosis multiplex, and corneal clouding (94,95). The pathology of ML III is not as well documented as that of ML II. Storage is identified in skin fibroblasts, but lymphocytes are normal.

Mucolipidosis type IV (ML IV, sialolipidosis, ganglioside–sialidase deficiency) results from mutations in the gene *MCOLN1*, which codes for the TRP family ion membrane channel, mucolipin 1. This putative lysosomal ion channel is thought to be involved in Fe^{2+}, Ca^{2+}, and Zn^{2+} transport and with that critical for still poorly understood aspects of lysosomal function (97). As a result, there is abnormal intracellular membrane trafficking. This disorder is classified as a mucolipidosis because of the storage of both lipids and mucopolysaccharides. Although panethnic, ML IV is more common among Ashkenazi Jews (98). Patients have severe psychomotor retardation, ophthalmologic abnormalities with corneal clouding, retinal degeneration, and optic nerve atrophy, but they do not have dysostosis multiplex seen in MPS. The overall incidence may be underestimated because of milder cases that can have a presentation mimicking cerebral palsy (98).

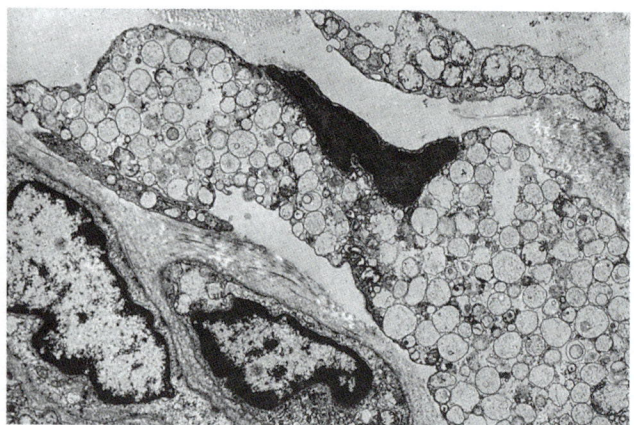

FIGURE 5-11 • I-cell disease. In I-cell disease, fibroblast cytoplasm is expanded by numerous membrane-bound vacuoles containing electron lucent to fibrillogranular material (Uranyl acetate, lead citrate).

Widespread storage affects the brain and viscera including the liver, pancreas, kidney, marrow, conjunctiva, cornea, skin, muscle, peripheral nerve, rectum, and placenta (Figure 5-12A,B). In neurons and glia, ganglioside, phospholipid, and GAG accumulation is variably PAS positive and sudanophilic and is associated with neuronal loss and astrocytosis. By EM, lysosomes contain heterogeneous material with fibrillogranular and concentric membranous bodies (Figure 5-12C).

Hypergastrinemia and achlorhydria are described (99). Chronic atrophic gastritis and enterochromaffin-like cell hyperplasia are seen along with cytoplasmic vacuolization of parietal cells due to lysosomal storage. Confirmatory diagnosis of ML IV should include screening for mutations in *MCOLN1*.

Cystinosis

In cystinosis, cystine accumulates because of defective transport of cystine out of lysosomes into the cytoplasm (100,101). This transport defect is due to an autosomal recessively inherited deficiency of cystinosin, a lysosomal membrane protein. Of the several forms of cystinosis, the most severe, nephropathic cystinosis, presents in the first year of life with Fanconi syndrome, rickets, photophobia, and short stature.

Rectangular, rhomboid, or polymorphic cystine crystals accumulate in lysosomes in most tissues, particularly in the fixed tissue macrophage system in the marrow, kidney, liver, lung, pancreas, intestine, appendix, spleen, conjunctiva,

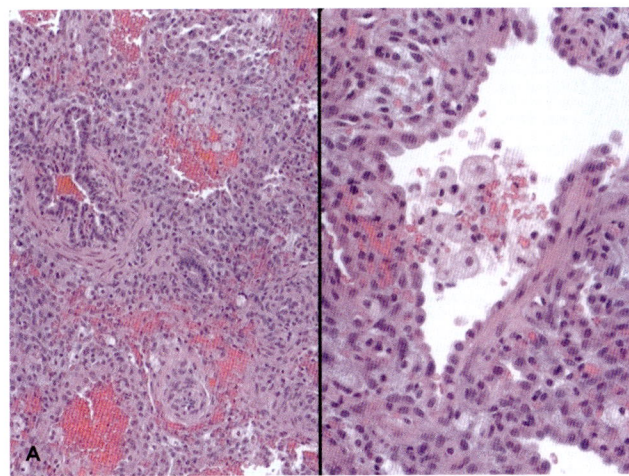
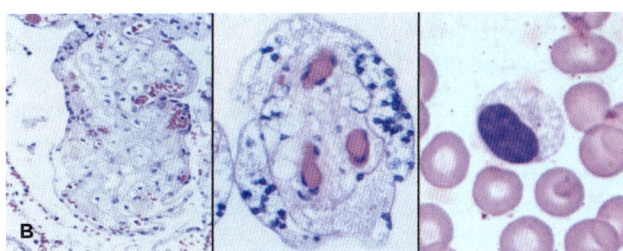
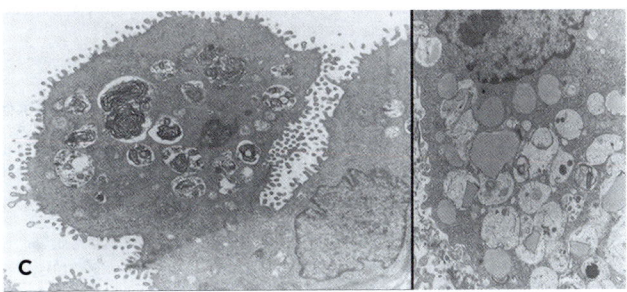

FIGURE 5-12 • Mucolipidosis IV. **A:** Foamy macrophages in lung tissue are present in this case of sialidosis (H&E). **B:** Cells of the reticuloendothelial system in sialidosis are vacuolated, as seen in chorionic villi (**left and middle images**) and a peripheral blood monocyte (**right image**) (H&E and Wright's). **C:** Ultrastructurally, storage material in sialidosis can manifest as lamellar inclusions (**left image**) or fibrillogranular material (**right image**) (Uranyl acetate, lead citrate).

cornea, retina, lymph nodes, thyroid, thymus, muscle, brain, gingiva, and placenta (Figure 5-13). The crystals are apparent in unfixed frozen or alcohol-fixed tissue examined with polarized light, which gives them a brilliant silvery birefringence. The kidney is the most severely affected organ, and cystine crystals may be present in interstitial, glomerular, and tubular cells. A "swan neck" deformity with atrophy of proximal tubule segments adjacent to cystine-containing interstitial cells is seen early in the disease. Progressive interstitial fibrosis and inflammation with tubular atrophy are associated with end-stage renal failure. Other organs are also affected, particularly after renal transplantation. Hepatomegaly is not associated with significant liver dysfunction. Perivenular Kupffer cells accumulate refractile crystals in clusters, and spaces left by crystals can be seen by EM. Pancreatic endocrine and exocrine insufficiency is due to long-standing cystine accumulation. Skeletal muscle fiber atrophy, ring fibers, and cystine crystals in endomysial cells lead to a myopathy. CNS involvement may cause nonobstructive hydrocephalus, demyelination, and cystic necrosis with calcification and spongy change. Diagnosis is based on the ophthalmologic demonstration of cystine crystals; identification of cystine crystals in bone marrow, cornea, fixed tissue macrophages, or amniocytes; and measurement of leukocyte or fibroblast cystine content. Cystinosis is an example of a lysosomal storage disease for which treatment including renal transplantation and cysteine depleting medical therapy has significantly impacted disease outcome (100).

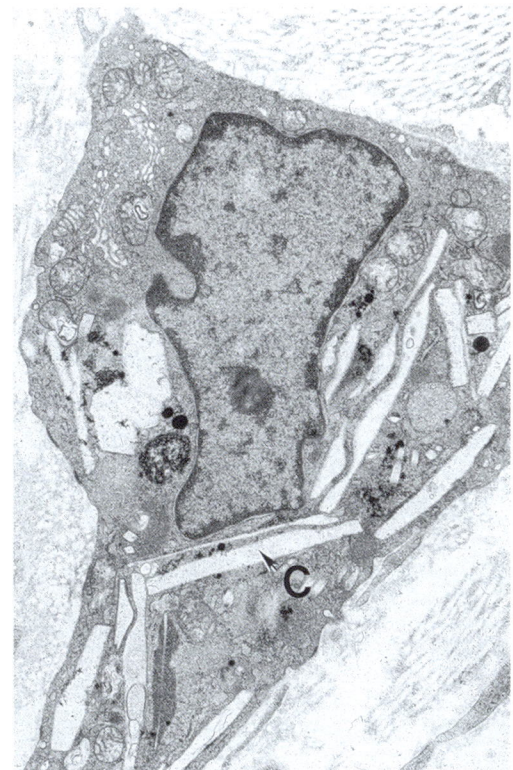

FIGURE 5-13 • Cystinosis. Electron-lucent, pleomorphic, polygonal, and rectilinear cystine crystals (C) in dermal macrophage from a 22-year-old with cystinosis. (Uranyl acetate, lead citrate; Used from Vogler C, Rosenberg HS, Williams JC, et al. Electron microscopy in the diagnosis of lysosomal storage diseases. *Am J Med Genet Suppl* 1987;3:243–255, with permission.)

Danon Disease, X-Linked Vacuolar Cardiomyopathy and Myopathy

X-linked dominant mutations in the *LAMP-2* gene encoding lysosome-associated membrane protein-2 lead to failure of fusion of endosome and lysosome (102). In males, this disorder is characterized by cognitive impairment, hypertrophic cardiomyopathy, skeletal muscle weakness, and death due to heart failure (103) in the third decade of life unless treated with heart transplantation (104). First symptoms are noted on average at an age of 12 years. Women are affected later than men, on average by about 15 years, but also develop similar disease manifestations (104).

Skeletal muscle shows the features of a vacuolar myopathy with myofiber degeneration, myofiber regeneration, and cytoplasmic vacuoles that contain PAS-positive vacuoles autophagic material. Internal cytoplasmic staining of membranous structures for proteins of the dystrophin glycoprotein complex is observed. LAMP-2 is not identifiable immunohistochemically in leukocytes, skeletal muscle, and myocardium in affected patients, and definitive diagnosis is based on DNA testing for the mutation (103).

Neuronal Ceroid Lipofuscinoses (NCL or CLN)

These were first described by Frederick Batten and are sometimes referred to as Batten disease. In other settings, the term Batten disease is used more specifically to refer to CLN3. These progressive encephalopathies affect patients at any age causing seizures, blindness, psychomotor deterioration, and premature death (105,106). The incidence is 1/10,000, and carrier frequency is approximately 1%. Collectively, CLNs are the most common inherited progressive encephalopathies of childhood. Traditionally, these were subdivided based on age of onset, disease course, and ultrastructural appearance of storage material. Currently at least 13 different forms are now defined by the underlying genetics (106a). The two most common are the classic juvenile form, CLN3, and the classic late infantile form, CLN2 (Table 5-7). The different mutations that cause CLN are not part of a single common pathway but affect different functions: CLN1 results from mutations disrupting a glycoprotein, palmitoyl-protein thiotransferase, which catabolizes proteins in the lysosome by removing thioester-linked fatty acyl groups from cysteine residues. With that, these mutations are thought to lead to ER stress and apoptosis. The gene mutated in CLN2 encodes a lysosomal exopeptidase. The gene mutated in CLN3 encodes a protein of still incompletely understood function. CLN11 interestingly is linked to mutations in the *GRN* gene that encodes progranulin. Progranulin has recently been linked to some neurodegenerative diseases.

Autofluorescent PAS-positive glycolipid accumulates in lysosomes in lymphocytes, cells in skin (particularly pericytes, endothelial, smooth muscle, and sweat gland epithelial cells), conjunctiva, skeletal muscle, and rectal mucosal neurons. As many as 10% to 20% of lymphocytes may have storage in late infantile CLN, but these cells are generally normal in adult CLN. There are differences in the ultrastructural appearance of the stored lipopigment observed in different types of CLN. CLN1 is found to have granular osmiophilic deposits and CLN2 and CLN3 with membranous patterns described as curvilinear and fingerprint bodies. Others may show a mixture of the mentioned patterns. Overall correlation between genotype and EM findings is poor because of morphologic overlap (Figure 5-14A to G) (24). The heart can show myocardial, valvular, and conduction system storage (107). Diagnosis can be made using DNA analysis, and panels of gene testing including all the associated genes are available.

TABLE 5-7 THE MORE COMMON NEURONAL CEROID LIPOFUSCINOSES

Type	Eponym	Age at Presentation	Predominant Storage[a]	Protein Defect
Infantile (INCL, CLN1)	Santavuori-Haltia	6–12 mo	Granular osmiophilic (GROD), saposin A, D	Palmitoyl-protein thioesterase 1 (PPT 1), cathepsin D
Late infantile (LICL, LINCL, CLN2)	Jansky-Bielschowsky	2–3 y	Curvilinear (in some cases also fingerprint), mitochondrial subunit c of ATP synthase	Tripeptidyl peptidase 1 (TPP1)
Juvenile (JNCL, CLN3)	Batten-Spielmeyer-Vogt	4–9 y	Fingerprint, mitochondrial subunit c of ATP synthase	Battenin (a lysosomal transmembrane protein)
Adult (ANCL, CLN4)	Kufs, Parry	30 y	Granular osmiophilic, fingerprint bodies,[b] mitochondrial subunit c of ATP synthase	Unknown

[a]There is overlap in character of storage among these disorders.
[b]Storage may be sparse outside the CNS.

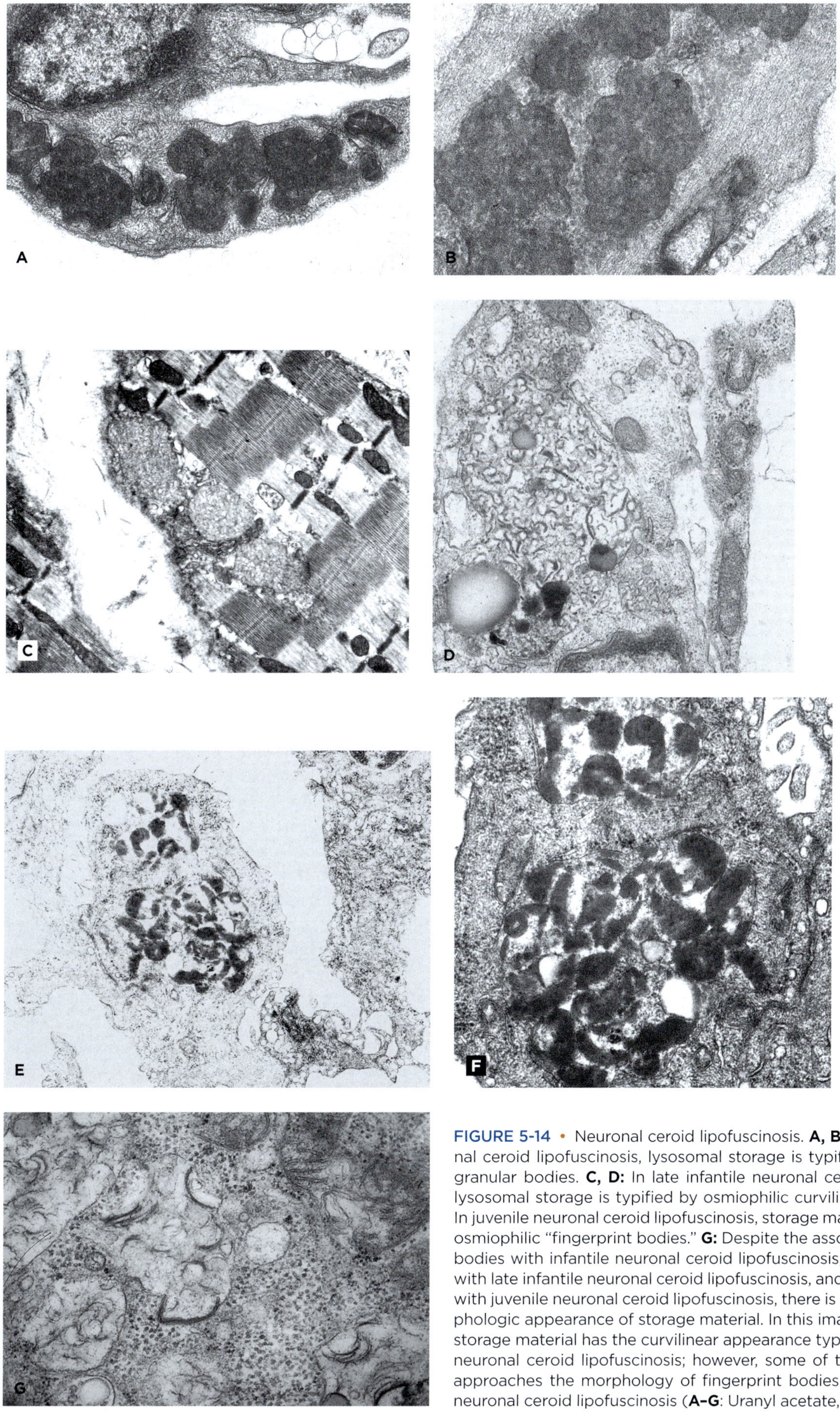

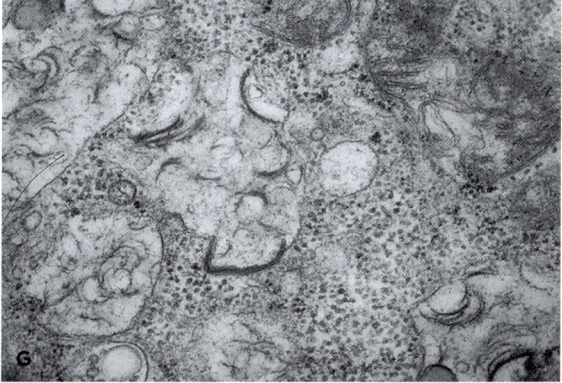

FIGURE 5-14 • Neuronal ceroid lipofuscinosis. **A, B:** In infantile neuronal ceroid lipofuscinosis, lysosomal storage is typified by osmiophilic granular bodies. **C, D:** In late infantile neuronal ceroid lipofuscinosis, lysosomal storage is typified by osmiophilic curvilinear material. **E, F:** In juvenile neuronal ceroid lipofuscinosis, storage material is typified by osmiophilic "fingerprint bodies." **G:** Despite the association of granular bodies with infantile neuronal ceroid lipofuscinosis, curvilinear bodies with late infantile neuronal ceroid lipofuscinosis, and fingerprint bodies with juvenile neuronal ceroid lipofuscinosis, there is overlap in the morphologic appearance of storage material. In this image, the bulk of the storage material has the curvilinear appearance typical of late infantile neuronal ceroid lipofuscinosis; however, some of the darker material approaches the morphology of fingerprint bodies typical of juvenile neuronal ceroid lipofuscinosis (**A–G**: Uranyl acetate, lead citrate).

AMINOACIDOPATHIES

In these disorders, amino acid catabolism is blocked because of an enzyme deficiency, with resultant accumulation of a specific amino acid.

Phenylketonuria (PKU, Hyperphenylalaninemia)

PKU is an autosomal recessive condition classically caused by mutations in the gene encoding for hepatic phenylalanine hydroxylase (PAH), which converts phenylalanine to tyrosine (108,109). In the United States, it has an incidence of about one case per 15,000 live births. Both deficient PAH and exposure to dietary phenylalanine are necessary for expression of the phenotype. The biochemical consequence is accumulation of phenylalanine and its metabolites and a relative deficiency of tyrosine, which becomes an essential amino acid in PKU patients (110). Clinical features are the result of tyrosine deficiency and elevated phenylalanine (111). The main clinical effect is in the brain with microcephaly, severe cognitive impairment, seizures, and progressive motor dysfunction. The brain injury in untreated PKU patients is secondary to phenylalanine accumulation in the blood (which increases brain phenylalanine), combined with deficiency of other large neutral amino acids (especially tyrosine and methionine). This results in abnormal brain protein synthesis, myelin turnover, and biogenic amine neurotransmission (112). Untreated patients have variable white matter alterations with spongiosis, delayed myelination or demyelination, focal myelin pallor, or breakdown with deposition of neutral fat, gliosis, and neuronal loss. In addition, affected patients have a mousy odor, eczema, and light skin and hair due to deficiency of tyrosine, a precursor of melanin.

Diagnosis is based on blood phenylalanine level. Classically, this was done using a bacterial inhibition assay (Guthrie method). Tandem mass spectrometry has recently become the main method of screening for PKU (113). A strictly reduced phenylalanine diet begun in infancy can prevent severe neurologic damage, although treated patients may have a lower IQ, psychiatric or neurologic abnormalities, and abnormal cerebral white matter; adults who relax their diet may have motor or cognitive decline (108,110). Some patients respond to treatment with BH_4, the cofactor for PAH, with reduction of phenylalanine levels, allowing a less restricted diet.

PKU variants are caused by deficiency of the PAH cofactor tetrahydrobiopterin (BH_4), due to one of several defects in the biosynthesis or recycling of BH_4 (114). Because BH_4 is also a cofactor for tyrosine and tryptophan hydroxylases and nitric oxide synthase, its deficiency also results in catecholamine and serotonin deficiencies. Deficiencies of GTP cyclohydrolase I (GTPCH), 6-pyruvoyl-tetrahydropterin synthase (PTPS), dihydropteridine reductase (DHPR), and pterin-4a-carbinolamine dehydratase (PCD) have been described (115). GTPCH and PTPS are involved in synthesis of BH_4 from GTP, and DHPR and PCD are involved in recycling BH_4. These patients respond to oral BH_4 treatment with normalization of serum phenylalanine. In addition to therapy with BH_4, these patients may also require treatment for their CNS dopamine and serotonin deficiencies, with l-dopa and 5-hydroxytryptophan, respectively, as well as carbidopa. Patients with DHPR deficiency also need folinic acid supplementation. All newborns with hyperphenylalaninemia should be screened for these less common disorders by testing for abnormal urine pterins and DHPR enzyme activity on a dried blood spot.

Pregnant women with PKU must keep phenylalanine concentrations low to prevent toxic embryopathy/fetopathy. Microcephaly, callosal hypoplasia, cognitive impairment, growth restriction, and heart malformations (aortic coarctation with hypoplastic left heart syndrome, tetralogy of Fallot, patent ductus arteriosus) are seen in heterozygous infants of PKU mothers with hyperphenylalaninemia during pregnancy.

Some patients with hyperphenylalaninemia have a milder form of PKU with residual PAH activity; they may not require dietary therapy or may only need general protein restriction. However, even women with mild PKU need to keep phenylalanine levels in a safe range for the fetus during pregnancy.

Tyrosinemia Type I (Hepatorenal Tyrosinemia)

This autosomal recessive condition is caused by deficient or defective fumarylacetoacetate hydrolase (FAH), the last enzyme in the pathway for tyrosine degradation, as a result of a number of mutations at 15q23-q25. Tyrosine degradation by FAH normally primarily occurs in hepatocytes and renal tubular epithelium (116). Tyrosinemia type I has an incidence of approximately 1 in 100,000, with an increased prevalence in French Canadians. Symptoms vary, but, in general, earlier presentation correlates with worse prognosis (117). Patients may have failure to thrive, a distinctive boiled cabbage or fishy odor, hepatomegaly, acute liver failure, cirrhosis, renal Fanconi syndrome, proteinuria, rickets, and peripheral neuropathy. In the chronic form of tyrosinemia type I, symptoms develop later and are less severe but include cognitive impairment, rickets, and hepatocellular carcinoma. Liver, kidney, and peripheral nerve damage result from accumulation of the tyrosine degradation products fumarylacetoacetate, maleylacetoacetate, and succinylacetone; these molecules may act as alkylating agents, disrupt sulfhydryl metabolism, impair DNA repair, and inhibit transport function (118).

Liver lesions can begin *in utero*. The liver is generally enlarged with sharply demarcated regenerative nodules with variegated colors, ranging from yellow to deep green. Microscopically, zones of hepatocellular collapse, cirrhosis, steatosis, intracanalicular and ductal cholestasis, cholangiolar proliferation, pseudoacinar transformation, and giant cell change are seen (119,120). Sinusoidal collagen deposition is often present. Alpha-fetoprotein is demonstrable in

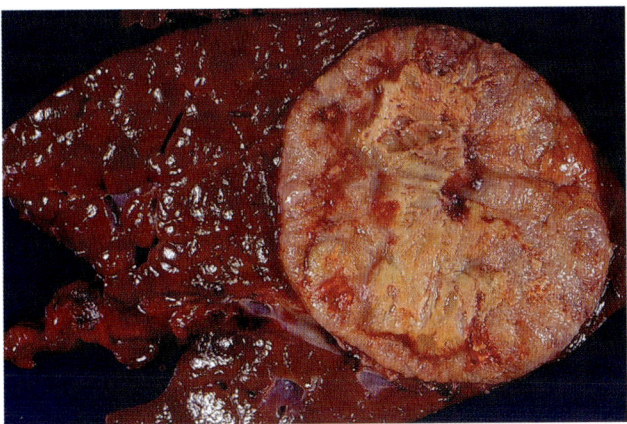

FIGURE 5-15 • Tyrosinemia. Hepatocellular carcinoma in the liver from a young child with tyrosinemia.

hepatocytes in cirrhotic areas. Dysplasia, adenomas, and hepatocellular carcinoma can be seen (Figure 5-15) (119–121). Hepatocellular carcinoma occurs in a third of patients who survive beyond 2 years of age, may occur as early as the first year of life, and may be accompanied by normal or increased alpha-fetoprotein level. Kidneys are enlarged, with cortical tubular ectasia, tubular calcification, glomerulosclerosis, interstitial nephritis, and fibrosis. Half of affected patients have hyperplasia of the islets of Langerhans, but hypoglycemia is unusual. Hypertrophic obstructive cardiomyopathy has been described (122). Axonal degeneration with demyelination similar to that seen in porphyrias occurs, and patients may have cerebral white matter spongiosis (123).

Diagnosis is based on increased levels of succinylacetone or tyrosine in dried blood samples, plasma, or urine (117). FAH activity can be assayed in lymphocytes, fibroblasts, or liver. Demonstration of two mutant alleles known to cause FAH deficiency confirms the diagnosis.

Treatment includes phenylalanine and tyrosine dietary restriction and liver transplantation. Treatment with the herbicide 2-(2-nitro-4-trifluoromethylbenzoyl)-1,3-cyclohexanedione (NTBC), which blocks the tyrosine degradation pathway and prevents accumulation of maleylacetoacetate and fumarylacetoacetate, may improve liver and renal function and reduce mortality from liver failure. It appears to reduce but not prevent the risk of developing hepatocellular carcinoma (124); patients who initiate NTBC treatment late are especially at risk for hepatocellular carcinoma.

Tyrosinemia Type II (Oculocutaneous Tyrosinemia, Richner-Hanhart Syndrome)

Oculocutaneous tyrosinemia is a rare autosomal recessive condition caused by a deficiency in cytoplasmic tyrosine aminotransferase (117,125), the first enzyme in the breakdown of tyrosine, leading to extremely high levels of plasma tyrosine. Patients have palmoplantar keratosis, corneal erosions, photophobia, and variable cognitive impairment, but no liver dysfunction. Their skin exhibits hyperkeratosis, acanthosis, and parakeratosis. Conjunctival and skin biopsies may have large lipid-like inclusion bodies with filaments and myelin-like figures in epithelium, fibroblasts, and endothelium (125).

Homocystinuria

Classical homocystinuria is an autosomal recessive disorder caused by cystathionine beta-synthetase (CBS) deficiency. Patients present in the first to second decade of life with optic lens dislocations, cognitive impairment, skeletal abnormalities, and thromboembolic disease (126,127). Patients typically present with thromboemboli approximately 10 years after initial presentation (127). Approximately 50% of untreated patients die as young adults, often due to a thromboembolic event (128). Dislocation of the optic lens and bony abnormalities appear to result from protein destabilization due to elevated homocysteine levels. Mechanisms for developing neurologic complications and thromboembolic disease are less well understood.

Affected patients have increased urine and serum homocysteine, homocystine, and methionine. NBS by tandem mass spectrometry for hypermethioninemia is useful in identifying patients with CBS deficiency (129). Some patients with homocystinuria are responsive to treatment with pyridoxal phosphate (vitamin B_6), a cofactor for CBS; nonresponders are placed on a methionine-restricted diet.

Nonketotic Hyperglycinemia (NKH, Glycine Encephalopathy)

This autosomal recessive disease is caused by mutations in the intramitochondrial glycine cleavage enzyme complex, resulting in elevated glycine levels (130). Affected children have a broad range of phenotypes. Severely affected patients develop hypotonia, lethargy, apnea, cognitive impairment, seizures, and death in the first 6 months of life. Atypical forms of the disorder are phenotypically heterogeneous (131), while patients with a transient form experience spontaneous normalization or improvement of plasma and cerebrospinal fluid glycine levels and neurologic symptoms (132). Unlike disorders of branched amino acid metabolism such as methylmalonic acidemia or propionic acidemia that also cause hyperglycinemia, there is no ketosis or organic acid excretion. Glycine accumulates in all body fluids and all tissues, including the brain; it is preferentially elevated in the cerebrospinal fluid (133).

In the CNS, abnormal myelination, callosal agenesis or thinning, cerebellar hypoplasia, gyral defects, and spongiform myelopathy (particularly of corticospinal and optic tracts and cerebellar white matter) are described (134,135). These CNS abnormalities are thought to reflect glycine function as an inhibitory neurotransmitter in the spinal cord and brain stem and as an excitatory neurotransmitter in the cortex (130). The liver may be steatotic, and skeletal muscle may have intranuclear filamentous inclusions and abnormal mitochondria (134).

The diagnosis is suggested by a cerebrospinal fluid/plasma glycine concentration ratio of greater than 0.08 and confirmed with measurement of glycine cleavage system activity in a liver biopsy (136). The normal hyperglycinuria in newborns makes measurement of the urine glycine not useful for diagnosis.

Patients are treated with substances that reduce glycine concentration (e.g., sodium benzoate or a low-protein diet) and N-methyl-d-aspartate (NMDA) receptor antagonists to prevent excitotoxicity in the cortex from excess glycine. Treatment response is variable (130).

Maple Syrup Urine Disease (MSUD, Branched-Chain Ketoaciduria)

This autosomal recessive disorder is due to a mutation in a gene encoding any subunit of the alpha-ketoacid dehydrogenase complex (137), which catalyzes the breakdown of branched-chain amino acids (leucine, isoleucine, and valine). MSUD is the most common IEM among Mennonites; in some communities, MSUD occurs in approximately 1 in 358 newborns. In non-Mennonites, the incidence is approximately 1 in 200,000 (137,138). In the classical phenotype, neonates present in the first week of life with poor feeding, alternating hyper- and hypotonia, ketoacidosis, seizures, and sudden unexpected death. Less severe, later-onset forms also occur.

The characteristic maple syrup, burnt sugar, or fenugreek odor of patients' urine, sweat, and saliva is imparted by sotolone (139). Brain abnormalities include edema, astrocytosis, and delayed myelination without myelin destruction (140). Gray matter is unaffected. Evaluation of plasma branched-chain amino acids or urine branched-chain ketoacids with tandem mass spectrometry and leukocyte or fibroblast branched-chain ketoacid decarboxylase measurement can provide the diagnosis. Traditionally, patients are placed on a restrictive diet; liver transplantation has also been found to be effective (137).

CARBOHYDRATE METABOLISM ABNORMALITIES

Galactosemia

Galactose is a simple sugar that is present in small amounts in many foods and is a part of lactose found in dairy products and baby formula. Three enzymes are critical for the sequential steps necessary for galactose metabolism: galactokinase encoded by *GALK1*, galactose-1-phosphate uridyl transferase encoded by *GALT*, and uridine diphosphate galactose-4-epimerase encoded by *GALE*. Mutations in any of these three genes can disrupt normal galactose metabolism resulting in galactosemia characterized by toxic accumulation of galactose, galactose-1-phosphate, and galactitol. These metabolites damage liver, kidneys, and lungs. All three variants of galactosemia follow an autosomal recessive inheritance pattern. The overall incidence is about 1 in 35,000. Mutations in *GALT* are described as type I and represent the most common form, while mutations in *GALK1* and *GALE* are described as types II and III, respectively (141,142). A milder variant of *GALT* mutations are described as the Duarte variant.

Severe disease clinically mimics hereditary fructose intolerance (HFI) but follows galactose feeding, usually after milk exposure, and is characterized by feeding intolerance, failure to thrive, vomiting, diarrhea, lethargy, hypotonia, hepatocellular insufficiency, jaundice, and hypoglycemia. Other complications include sepsis (often with *E. coli*) due to depressed neutrophil function and with disease progression renal failure, cataracts, cognitive impairment, hypergonadotropic hypogonadism, and ovarian failure with amenorrhea (143). Mild cases may suffer from cataracts, low bone density, ataxia, depression, and anxiety (144). Extensive liver damage may be prevented or reversed by a galactose-free diet, but CNS complications may not be avoided by dietary restriction (145).

In infants with galactosemia, the liver is enlarged and yellow with panlobular macrovesicular steatosis, followed by periportal ductular reaction with bile-plugged cholangioles surrounded by acute inflammation. The early liver lesions resemble those of HFI. By 1 to 1½ months of age, pseudoacinar transformation of hepatic plates occurs, and hepatocytes surround dilated canaliculi that may contain bile. Extramedullary hematopoiesis and iron deposition may be prominent. Fibrosis, apparent as early as 2 weeks of age, progresses to cirrhosis by 3 to 6 months. In some cases, giant cell transformation and regenerative or dysplastic nodules occur. The most severe hepatic abnormalities occur during episodes of sepsis; endotoxins may contribute to liver injury. Pancreatic islets are hyperplastic, and vacuolization of renal tubular epithelium (similar to that seen in HFI and tyrosinemia) is accompanied by tubular dilatation and necrosis. Ovarian histology in ovarian failure is variable; oocytes may be absent or reduced in number.

Diagnosis may be suspected if non–glucose-reducing substances are present in urine, although this test is neither sensitive nor specific (69). Diagnosis of classical galactosemia is based on red cell GALT assay (65) and can only be done if red cells have not been transfused in the last 3 months. GALK and GALE deficiencies can be identified by NBS if galactose is measured on a blood spot, and specific enzyme assays then confirm the diagnosis (146). Mutational analysis is commonly used to identify common variants associated with decreased enzyme activity but not requiring treatment.

Hereditary Fructose Intolerance (HFI)

Deficiency of fructose-1-phosphate aldolase (fructoaldolase B), inherited as an autosomal recessive disorder, is the result of *ALDOB* mutations and leads to fructose-1-phosphate accumulation (147,148). This toxic substrate damages the liver, kidney, and brain and inhibits glycogenolysis and gluconeogenesis, resulting in hypoglycemia, phosphate sequestration, and ATP depletion (149). It has been proposed that acute lesions in HFI are due to ATP depletion and osmotic effects of fructose-1-phosphate accumulation. Fructose-1,6-diphosphatase deficiency can cause a similar inhibition of gluconeogenesis with fructose- and fasting-induced hypoglycemia.

Symptoms develop when fructose in fruits and some vegetables or sucrose in candy is introduced into the diet, and clinical improvement occurs if fructose, sorbitol, and sucrose are withdrawn from the diet. Older children with HFI may avoid sweet foods. Liver, kidney, and intestine are affected; symptoms vary but include failure to thrive, vomiting, hepatomegaly, coagulopathy, and renal failure with renal tubular acidosis, aminoaciduria, and proteinuria. Acute liver failure may occur if fructose or sucrose is ingested in the newborn period.

Liver lesions resemble those of neonatal hepatitis and galactosemia with giant cell transformation, steatosis, ductular proliferation, cholestasis, and portal fibrosis. Acute hepatic necrosis with little inflammation may be seen in the acute phase. Progression to cirrhosis with portal hypertension, ascites, and splenomegaly occurs but is rare. Older infants may have less severe liver damage with variable steatosis and portal fibrosis. By EM, characteristic but not pathognomonic changes include "fructose holes" in hepatocytes: lucent spaces with sparse glycogen and membranous arrays surrounded by a single membrane. These lesions may result from dilated degranulated rough endoplasmic reticulum and relate to intracellular accumulation of enzyme substrate or ATP depletion. Pancreatic islet hyperplasia is seen, and, in the kidney, proximal tubule epithelium is granular and vacuolated with slight tubule dilatation.

Hypophosphatemia, metabolic acidosis, and elevated transaminases are typical but not diagnostic. Fructose tolerance test is not recommended for diagnosis because of potential danger to the patient. Analysis of leukocyte DNA for the aldolase B gene is generally performed first, and, if DNA is normal, measurement of aldolase B activity in liver or intestinal tissue can be done.

Glycogen Storage Diseases

Glycogen catabolism is an important energy source. The main glycogen storage diseases are assigned Roman numerals, but subtypes are also distinguished (150–152). The underlying enzyme defect can be in glycogen synthesis or breakdown (Table 5-8). The diseases are generally associated

TABLE 5-8   GLYCOGEN STORAGE DISEASES

Type	Eponym	Clinical	Tissues Affected	Enzyme Deficient
0		Fasting ketotic hypoglycemia, short stature, osteopenia, without hepatomegaly or weakness	Liver	Glycogen synthase
I	von Gierke 1a and 1b (non-a)	1a: most severe of GSD, recurrent hypoglycemia, hepatomegaly, nephromegaly, proteinuria, muscle atrophy, failure to thrive, xanthomas 1b also has recurrent bacterial infections	Liver, hepatic adenoma, hepatocellular carcinoma, kidney (1b: neutropenia, inflammatory bowel disease)	1a: glucose-6-phosphatase 1b: glucose-6-phosphatase translocase
II	Pompe	Hypotonia, cardiomyopathy, hepatomegaly	Muscle, heart, CNS, lymphocytes, liver, kidney, adrenal	Alpha-1,4-glucosidase (acid maltase)
III	Forbes, Cori, limit dextrinosis	Hypotonia, hypoglycemia, ketosis, growth failure, infections, hepatosplenomegaly, cardiomyopathy	Muscle, heart, liver, WBC	Amylo-1,6-glucosidase, 4-alpha-glucanotransferase (debrancher enzyme)
IV	Amylopectinosis, Andersen	Hepatosplenomegaly, cirrhosis, muscle wasting, gastroenteritis, osteoporosis, cardiomyopathy, hydrops	Liver, heart, muscle, CNS, PNS	Amylo (1,4 → 1,6) transglucosidase (brancher enzyme)
V	McArdle	Exercise intolerance, cramps, fatigue, myoglobinuria	Muscle	Muscle myophosphorylase
VI	Hers	Growth retardation, hepatomegaly, hypoglycemia	Liver	Hepatic phosphorylase
VII	Tarui	Exercise intolerance, cramps, fatigue, myoglobinuria	Muscle, hemolytic anemia	Phosphofructokinase
IX		Exercise intolerance, stiffness, weakness, includes GSD VIII and X	Liver, heart, blood cells, muscle	Phosphorylase kinase complex
XI	Fanconi-Bickel	Hepatorenal glycogen accumulation	Liver and kidney	Glucose transporter 2 (GLUT2)

CNS, central nervous system; PNS, peripheral nervous system; WBC, white blood cell.

with glycogen accumulation. Many organs are affected by glycogen storage diseases, including the liver, heart, skeletal muscle, kidney, erythrocytes, and intestine. The clinical presentation may include muscle fatigue, cramps, progressive weakness, rhabdomyolysis, hypoglycemia, acidosis, failure to thrive, or hepatomegaly. Overall incidence is approximately 1/20,000. The various GSD have specific treatments, so early identification of an enzyme defect is important.

Subtle differences in liver morphology in GSD have been described, but, in general, pathologic features are clearly distinctive in only a few GSDs, such as the light microscopic findings in GSD IV and the ultrastructural appearance of hepatocytes in GSD II and IV. In general, hepatocytes are enlarged with clear or vacuolated cytoplasm and resemble plant cells in that cell membranes appear thick, due to peripheral displacement of organelles by glycogen. Cytoplasm is PAS positive and diastase digestible. Some glycogen is lost with formalin fixation due to its water solubility; optimal glycogen preservation can be achieved by alcohol fixation or by using fresh frozen tissue. Nuclei may be glycogenated, particularly in types I and III; types VI and IX typically do not have glycogenated nuclei. Increased collagen in Disse space occurs in GSD I, III, IV, VI, and IX. By EM, cytoplasmic glycogen pools in hepatocytes, and variably sized lipid droplets occur in most GSDs but are particularly abundant in GSD I, II, and VI.

GSD 0 is not truly a GSD but is an autosomal recessive deficiency of glycogen synthase that results in ketotic hypoglycemia without hepatomegaly or muscle symptoms (153). Steatosis and a slight decrease in liver glycogen content with normal glycogen structure are seen.

GSD I (von Gierke disease). In classical GSD I, GSD Ia, the glucose-6-phosphatase enzyme complex in endoplasmic reticulum is defective. The diagnosis is based on glycogen quantitation and glucose-6-phosphatase analysis (151,154,155). In GSD Ib, glucose-6-phosphatase is normal, but a defect in glucose-6-phosphatase translocase transporter protein results in failure of enzyme transport. Both of these forms are inherited in an autosomal recessive pattern. Patients with GSD Ia present in infancy with hepatomegaly, recurrent ketotic hypoglycemia with acidosis, hyperuricemia, hyperlipidemia, seizures, liver failure, and failure to thrive (156,157). Truncal obesity, short stature, aminoaciduria, phosphaturia, muscle atrophy, and a bleeding tendency due to hypoglycemia-induced platelet dysfunction are also described. Patients with type 1b additionally have neutropenia and impaired neutrophil function, with recurrent bacterial infections and oral and intestinal mucosal ulcerations indistinguishable from Crohn disease.

In GSD Ia, liver involvement is prominent with uniformly increased hepatocellular glycogen, nuclear glycogenation, and steatosis with small- and medium-sized lipid droplets (Figure 5-16A to D). In the liver of GSD 1b patients, minimal or no nuclear glycogenation is seen, unlike in GSD Ia. Sinusoids are compressed by distended hepatocytes. Mallory bodies and zone 3 and periportal fibrosis have been reported (Figure 5-16C). Focal nodular hyperplasia, adenomas (often multiple with atypical cytologic features), dysplasia, and hepatocellular adenocarcinoma may occur in patients with GSD 1a, particularly with the G727T mutation (Figure 5-16E,F) (156). Adenomas may arise because of glucagon stimulation and can regress if hypoglycemia is reduced with diet. They are more common in boys than girls and are seen as early as 3 years of age. Hepatoblastomas have also been described in GSD I.

Nephromegaly, increased glycogen in tubular epithelium, focal segmental glomerulosclerosis, and interstitial fibrosis occur in GSD 1. Nephrocalcinosis relates to hypercalciuria due to tubular acidosis. Xanthomas and chronic pancreatitis may reflect hyperlipidemia.

GSD II (Pompe disease and adult-onset acid maltase deficiency) is included above in the section on LSD.

GSD III (Cori-Forbes disease, Forbes disease, limit dextrinosis) patients have amylo-1,6-glucosidase, 4-alpha-glucanotransferase (debrancher enzyme) deficiency, which can be measured in the liver, fibroblasts, skin, or lymphocytes. This clinically and genetically heterogeneous disorder has symptoms similar but less severe than those seen in GSD I (152,158). Progressive skeletal weakness may be a predominant feature in adults, and cardiomyopathy occurs in some patients. Hepatomegaly and hypoglycemia are seen (157). Liver failure can occur, but liver function tends to improve with age. Of the subtypes, GSD IIIa has liver and muscle involvement, GSD IIIb has liver involvement only, and GSD IIIc is an isolated muscle disease.

If restricted to muscle, enzyme assay of the muscle is required for diagnosis. Muscle biopsy may show slight fiber size variation with little vacuolization or increased glycogen. Some patients have vacuolar myopathy with glycogen accumulation at the periphery of fibers. Liver has delicate reticular septal fibrosis or, less commonly, micronodular or mixed cirrhosis, and glycogenated nuclei can occur. Hepatic adenomas occur in GSD III patients (159), and hepatocellular carcinoma can sometimes develop in a background of cirrhosis (160).

GSD IV (Andersen disease, branching enzyme deficiency, amylopectinosis). Amylo (1,4 → 1,6) transglucosidase (brancher enzyme) deficiency can be identified in the liver, muscle, leukocytes, and fibroblasts (161). GSD IV is autosomal recessive, and there are multiple mutations in the *GBE1* gene that cause enzyme deficiency. Abnormally long, relatively insoluble amylopectin-like glycogen chains with reduced branch points accumulate in all tissues, particularly the liver, skeletal muscle, and heart (152). The phenotype of the disease is variable within and between families with a spectrum that is between severe neonatal disease (162) and adult polyglucosan body disease (163). Infants with the fatal perinatal neuromuscular subtype present with severe hypotonia and cardiomyopathy, leading to early death. Infants with the classic hepatic subtype develop failure to thrive with liver dysfunction and cirrhosis but also cardiomyopathy and hypotonia. Other children have a nonprogressive

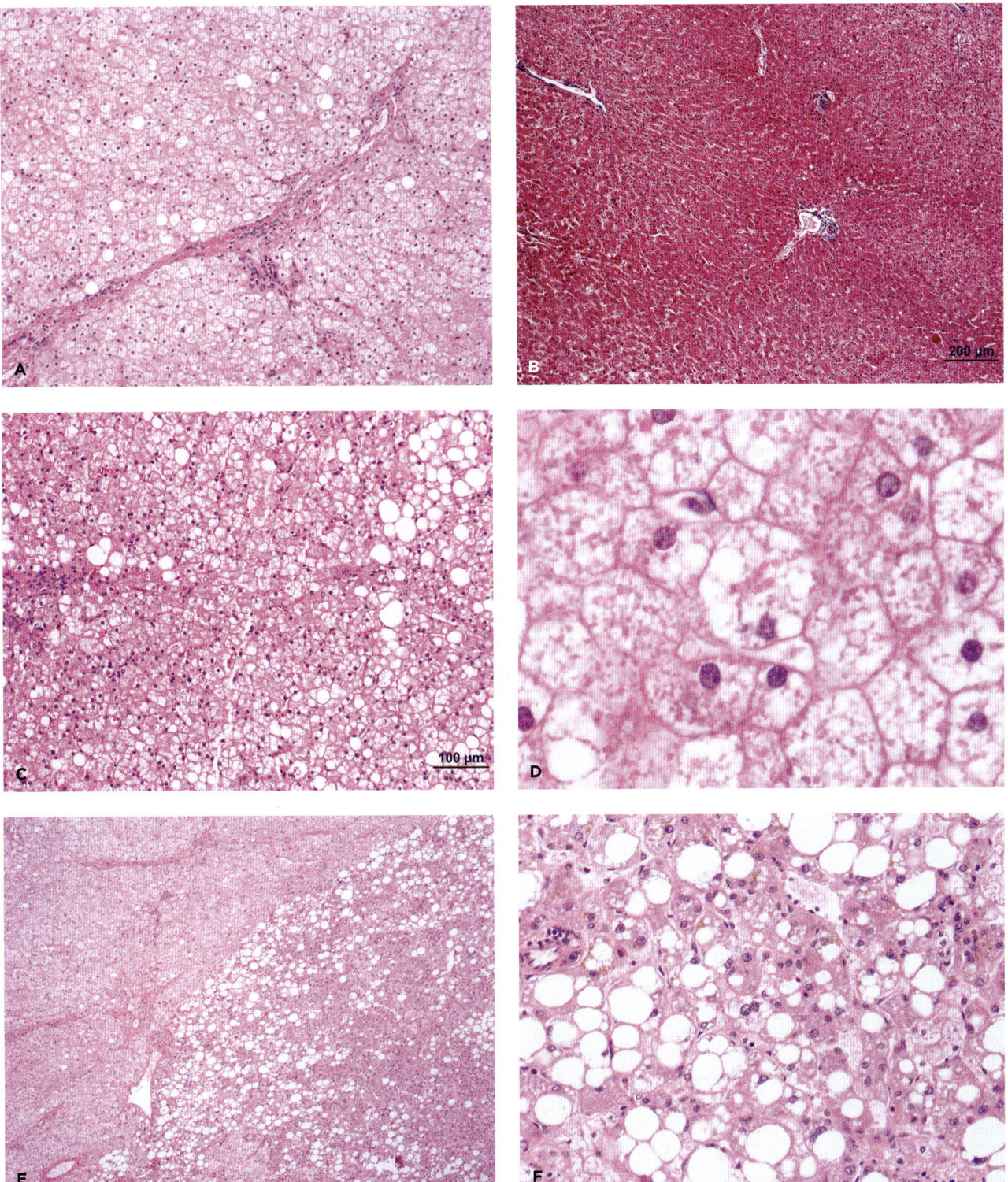

FIGURE 5-16 • Glycogen storage disease, type I. **A:** The liver in type I glycogen storage disease shows diffuse steatosis with hepatocyte distension obscuring sinusoids (H&E). **B:** Despite diffuse hepatocellular involvement, the liver in type I disease shows little (if any) fibrosis (trichrome). **C, D:** In type Ia disease, the liver shows steatosis (**C**) and hepatocellular Mallory hyaline (**D**); note the presence of glycogenated nuclei (**C**), typical of type Ia disease (H&E). **E, F:** Patients with type I GSD are at increased risk for the development of hepatocellular adenoma (with varying degrees of dysplasia), which can evolve into hepatocellular carcinoma. In (**E**), the interface between the hepatocellular adenoma (**lower right**) and nonneoplastic liver (**upper left**) is shown; in (**F**), the cells of the adenoma show dysplastic cytologic features (H&E).

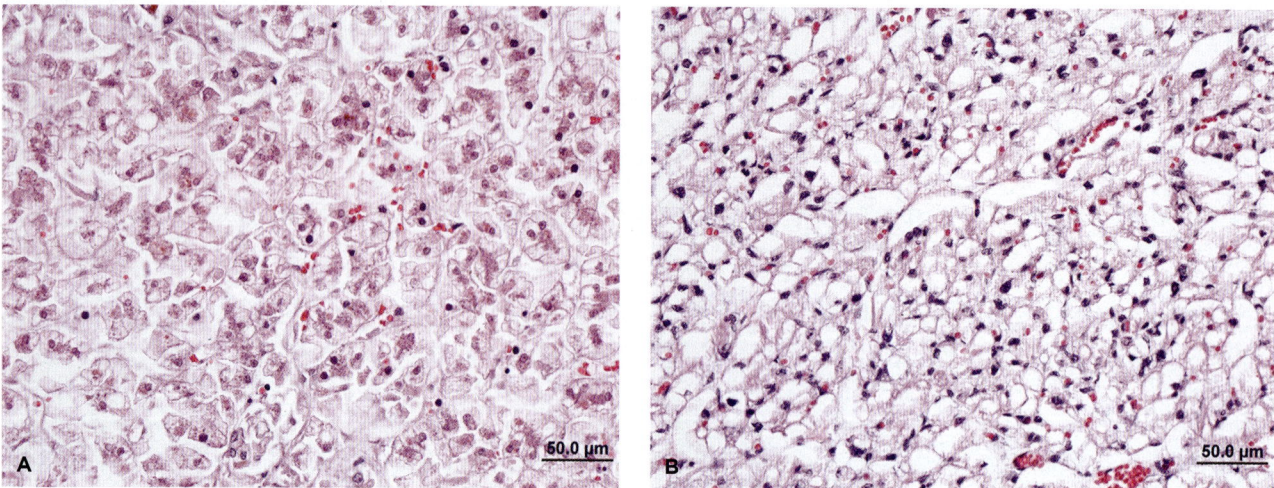

FIGURE 5-17 • Glycogen storage disease, type IV. **A:** In type IV disease, hepatocytes are enlarged with ground-glass cytoplasmic inclusions (H&E). **B:** Skeletal muscle involvement in type IV disease, with rarefaction of myofibers due to non–membrane-bound glycogen accumulation (H&E).

hepatic subtype that is not progressive in the same fashion but associated with hepatomegaly, myopathy, and hypotonia. Late-onset cases include adults presenting with adult polyglucosan body disease.

The liver is tan with a waxy or a tough leathery consistency and tiny nodules that may aggregate into larger nodules. The liver resembles that seen in Lafora disease but with progression to fibrosis and cirrhosis. Only rarely do hepatic neoplasms occur with GSD IV. Pericellular fibrosis encircles clusters of hepatocytes with round or oval ground-glass intracytoplasmic inclusions primarily in periportal hepatocytes (Figure 5-17A). These PAS-positive, diastase-resistant inclusions stain green with colloidal iron. They stain brown, blue, or not at all with Lugol iodine, and they are removed by pectinase or alpha-amylase. They often have an artifactual space around them. By EM, inclusions are non–membrane bound with undulating random delicate fibrils up to 5 nm in diameter surrounded by glycogen rosettes. Similar inclusions are seen in the heart, skeletal muscle, skin, CNS neurons, and lymph node macrophages (Figure 5-17B).

GSD V (McArdle disease) is due to autosomal recessive inherited myophosphorylase deficiency. Children with GSD V typically have exercise intolerance, but rarely this disease presents with respiratory failure in infancy (164). Patients have no rise in lactic acid after ischemic exercise. By LM, skeletal muscle may appear normal or may have mild alterations, with occasional degenerating fibers and subsarcolemmal glycogen-containing vacuoles. EM highlights subsarcolemmal and sarcoplasmic glycogen. Enzyme histochemistry and biochemical testing can show absent myophosphorylase activity.

GSD VI (Hers disease) due to hepatic phosphorylase deficiency is a relatively benign autosomal recessive disorder that causes hypoglycemia and growth failure (165). The disease improves with age: hepatomegaly decreases after puberty, and adults are typically asymptomatic. A nonuniform mosaic pattern of distended hepatocytes without nuclear glycogenation is accompanied by mild fibrosis and steatosis. Heart and skeletal muscle are not altered.

GSD VII (Tarui disease) is characterized by absent phosphofructokinase activity, easy fatigability, and exercise intolerance in children (166,167). Severe infantile cases with respiratory failure also occur. Patients have hemolytic anemia due to absence of a muscle isoenzyme in red blood cells, hyperuricemia, and myoglobinuria. Muscle has extensive subsarcolemmal and sarcoplasmic glycogen, and a few fibers contain hyaline, PAS-positive, diastase-resistant inclusions with a filamentous fine structure resembling amylopectin. Histochemical staining suggests that these are an insoluble form of glycogen.

GSD IX. Phosphorylase kinase, or phosphorylase b kinase, is composed of four separately encoded subunits, alpha, beta, gamma, and delta (168). The disease affects the liver and/or skeletal muscle. Mutations in the *PHKA2* gene are the most common and cause X-linked hepatic disease. Mutations in the *PHKA1* gene cause a rare X-linked skeletal muscle form of the disease, *PHKB* mutations are linked to autosomal recessive disease affecting the muscle and liver, and *PHKG2* mutations are linked to autosomal recessive liver disease.

GSD XI (Fanconi-Bickel syndrome) disease has hepatorenal glycogen accumulation resulting in hepatomegaly and nephromegaly, proximal tubular nephropathy, rickets, failure to thrive, glucosuria, and aminoaciduria (169,170). The disease results from mutations in the *GLUT2* gene. The severity of the clinical phenotype is variable.

FATTY ACID OXIDATION DEFECTS

A number of enzymes and transporters are involved in intramitochondrial fatty acid oxidation (FAO), and defects in these pathways lead to a heterogeneous group of disorders

TABLE 5-9	FATTY ACID OXIDATION DEFECTS

Acyl-CoA dehydrogenase deficiencies
   Medium-chain acyl-CoA dehydrogenase deficiency (MCADD, MCAD)
   Short-chain acyl-CoA dehydrogenase deficiency (SCAD)
   Long-chain 3-hydroxyacyl-CoA dehydrogenase deficiency (LCHAD)/trifunctional protein (MTP) deficiency
   Very long-chain acyl-CoA dehydrogenase deficiency (VLCAD)
   Glutaric acidemia type II (multiple acyl-CoA dehydrogenase deficiency, MADD)
Substrate transport defects
   Carnitine palmitoyltransferase (CPT) deficiency CPT I and CPT II deficiencies
   Primary systemic carnitine deficiency (carnitine transporter deficiency)
   Carnitine-acylcarnitine translocase deficiency

TABLE 5-10	METABOLIC CAUSES OF SUDDEN UNEXPECTED DEATH IN INFANCY

Inherited defects of fatty acid oxidation (FAO)
   Medium-chain acyl-CoA dehydrogenase deficiency (MCAD)
   Very long-chain acyl-CoA dehydrogenase deficiency (VLCAD)
   Long-chain 3-hydroxyacyl-CoA dehydrogenase deficiency (LCHAD)/trifunctional protein deficiency
   Glutaric acidemia type 2 (multiple acyl-CoA dehydrogenase deficiency (MADD))
   Carnitine palmitoyltransferase II deficiency (CPT II)
   Primary carnitine deficiency (carnitine transporter deficiency)
   Carnitine–acylcarnitine translocase (CAT) deficiency
Hyperammonemia/urea cycle disorders
   Ornithine transcarbamylase (OTC) deficiency
   Carbamoyl phosphate synthetase deficiency
   Argininosuccinate synthetase deficiency (citrullinemia)
   Argininosuccinate lyase deficiency (argininosuccinic aciduria)
   Lysinuric protein intolerance
Organic acidemias
   Methylmalonic acidemia
   Propionic acidemia
   Isovaleric acidemia
   Glutaric acidemia type 1
   3-Hydroxy-3-methyl-glutaryl-CoA lyase deficiency
   3-Methylcrotonyl-CoA carboxylase deficiency
Congenital lactic acidosis
   Pyruvate dehydrogenase deficiency
   Pyruvate carboxylase deficiency
   Phosphoenolpyruvate carboxykinase (PEPCK) deficiency
Amino acid disorders
   Maple syrup urine disease
   Tyrosinemia type 1
Carbohydrate disorders
   Galactosemia
   Glycogen storage disease type I
   Hereditary fructose intolerance
   Fructose-1,6-bisphosphate deficiency

(Table 5-9) (171). Inherited disorders of fatty acid transport and oxidation can present with acute liver failure and sudden unexpected death in children.

Acyl-CoA Dehydrogenase Deficiencies

Before beta-oxidation of fatty acids occurs, fatty acids must first be converted to their coenzyme A (CoA) thioesters. This conversion is catalyzed by acyl-CoA dehydrogenases, of which there are at least four types—classified based on chain lengths as short-, medium-, long-, and very long-chain dehydrogenases (171,172). Any of these four forms of acyl-CoA dehydrogenases can be deficient. Where known, inheritance is autosomal recessive.

In general, patients with acyl-CoA dehydrogenase deficiency have hypoketotic hypoglycemia, liver and skeletal muscle abnormalities, cardiomyopathy, and sudden unexpected death in childhood (Table 5-10) (173). Patients with short-chain defects may have ketotic hypoglycemia (174). Patients develop panlobular microvesicular or macrovesicular steatosis in the liver (175) and fat accumulation in the myocardium and skeletal muscle (176,177). Establishing a diagnosis may allow for successful treatment with carnitine and avoidance of prolonged fasting (173). These disorders are included in NBS programs (Table 5-4) (178).

Short-Chain Acyl-CoA Dehydrogenase Deficiency (SCADD, SCAD)

There are two clinical forms: (a) a myopathic form limited to muscle, clinically presenting with progressive weakness and exercise-induced pain in middle-aged patients, and (b) a systemic form with neonatal onset of vomiting, lethargy, acidosis, ketotic hypoglycemia, hepatomegaly, hypotonia, seizures, and microcephaly. However, the vast majority of patients with short-chain acyl-CoA dehydrogenase (SCAD) deficiency detected through NBS do not demonstrate any symptoms (179). At least 35 different inactivating mutations in the SCAD gene have been described (174); however, there is no consistent correlation between genotype and phenotype. Patients exhibit cerebral edema and fatty changes in the liver (173).

Medium-Chain Acyl-CoA Dehydrogenase Deficiency (MCADD, MCAD)

This is one of the most common IEM, with an incidence of up to 1 in 9000 to 10,000 in northern Europe (180). Homozygosity for the A985G mutation is found in 80% of affected patients (181). Patients present between 6 and 24 months of age with hypoketotic hypoglycemia after fasting, lethargy, vomiting, and sudden unexpected death (173). Fatal cases may resemble SIDS or Reye syndrome. They can also present in later life with exercise-induced muscle pain and rhabdomyolysis (182), and there is marked clinical variability even in the same family (183). The liver may be normal grossly or have minimal steatosis (184), and the heart may show lipid accumulation (180). Mitochondria may be enlarged with crystals, increased matrix density, and dilated cristae (185). Encephalopathy and cerebral edema are due to accumulation of fatty acids in the CNS (180). Octanoylcarnitine is elevated on plasma acylcarnitine analysis, and further confirmatory testing may include urine acylglycine analysis and molecular testing (186).

Long-Chain 3-Hydroxyacyl-CoA Dehydrogenase Deficiency (LCHADD, LCHAD) and Trifunctional Protein Deficiency

Long-chain 3-hydroxyacyl-CoA dehydrogenase (LCHAD) is a functional part of mitochondrial trifunctional protein (MTP), comprising LCHAD, long-chain enoyl-CoA hydratase, and long-chain thiolase activities (187). Most patients have isolated LCHAD deficiency, but some also lack activity of the other two enzymes and have generalized MTP deficiency. Similar clinical and biochemical manifestations occur in affected individuals.

Nearly all LCHAD-deficient patients have at least one G-to-C mutation at nucleotide position 1528 (G1528C) of the gene for the alpha-subunit of MTP on both chromosomes, resulting in an E474Q change in the protein. Most of these patients are homozygous for the G1528C mutation, while about 25% are compound heterozygotes for G1528C on one allele and a different LCHAD mutation on the other allele (188).

LCHAD-deficient patients typically present before 3 years of age with episodic nonketotic hypoglycemia, cardiomyopathy, and hepatomegaly (189). Infants can present shortly after birth with severe cardiomyopathy; a later-onset form presents with exercise-induced muscle pain, rhabdomyolysis, myoglobinuria, peripheral neuropathy, and retinopathy (187). Patients with MTP deficiency appear to have a similar clinical presentation (173). Elevation of 16- and 18-carbon acylcarnitines in the plasma is diagnostic; lymphocyte or fibroblast MTP activity or molecular testing is confirmatory (173).

The HELLP syndrome (hemolysis, elevated liver enzymes, and low platelet count), pre-eclampsia, and acute fatty liver of pregnancy occur in approximately one-third of mothers of fetuses with LCHAD deficiency (187). The mechanism for this association is unknown. MTP deficiency is also associated with maternal HELLP syndrome.

The liver in LCHAD-deficient patients shows steatosis, fibrosis, and cirrhosis. Fat accumulates in the skeletal and cardiac muscle and renal tubules (189).

Very-Long-Chain Acyl-CoA Dehydrogenase Deficiency (VLCADD, VLCAD)

Very-long-chain acyl-CoA dehydrogenase (VLCAD) catalyzes the first step in the beta-oxidation of fatty acids. Multiple mutations in VLCAD give rise to VLCAD deficiency, and clinical presentation is highly heterogeneous. Affected patients most commonly present with a severe neonatal form with dilated or hypertrophic cardiomyopathy, hepatomegaly, and sudden death (176). Less commonly, patients present in early childhood with hypoketotic hypoglycemia or in late childhood and early adulthood with episodic myopathy and rhabdomyolysis. Histologically, lipid accumulates in the skeletal and cardiac muscle. The liver may exhibit microvesicular and macrovesicular steatosis, cholestasis, and fibrosis.

Glutaric Acidemia Type II (Glutaric Aciduria Type II, Multiple Acyl-CoA Dehydrogenase Deficiency, MADD)

Glutaric acidemia type II is caused by deficiency of one of two proteins that transfer electrons from acyl-CoA dehydrogenases in the electron transport chain, the electron-accepting protein electron transfer flavoprotein (ETF) or ETF-ubiquinone oxidoreductase (ETF-QO). This deficiency leads to abnormal fatty acid, amino acid, and choline metabolism. Patients may present in early infancy with hypotonia, hepatomegaly, sweaty feet odor, metabolic acidosis, and nonketotic hypoglycemia; death may occur in the first few months of life in the most severe form. Congenital anomalies include cerebral cortical dysgenesis, facial dysmorphism, external genital defects, and renal cystic dysplasia (Figure 5-18A) (190). Patients exhibit lipid accumulation in the liver (Figure 5-18B), kidney, heart, and skeletal muscle (190). The liver may also have periportal hepatic fibrosis and hypoplastic biliary ducts (191). In some patients, there is gliosis of the cerebral white matter and spinal cord.

Milder forms of the disease present in infants, children, or adults as acidosis, hypoglycemia, or lipid storage myopathy (192). Some patients are responsive to riboflavin supplementation (193).

Substrate Transport Defects

Carnitine Palmitoyltransferase (CPT) Deficiency

CPT is an enzyme that catalyzes the reaction of carnitine with long-chain fatty acyl groups for transport into the mitochondria. There are two forms of this enzyme, CPT-I and CPT-II, which are associated with the outer and inner mitochondrial membranes, respectively. CPT-I exists as multiple isoforms that are specific to the liver (CPT-IA), skeletal muscle (CPT-IB), and brain (CPT-IC) (194). Deficiencies in CPT-IA and CPT-II have been described. CPT-IA deficiency affects males and females equally. Most patients with CPT-II deficiency are males, although the CPT-II gene is on an autosome.

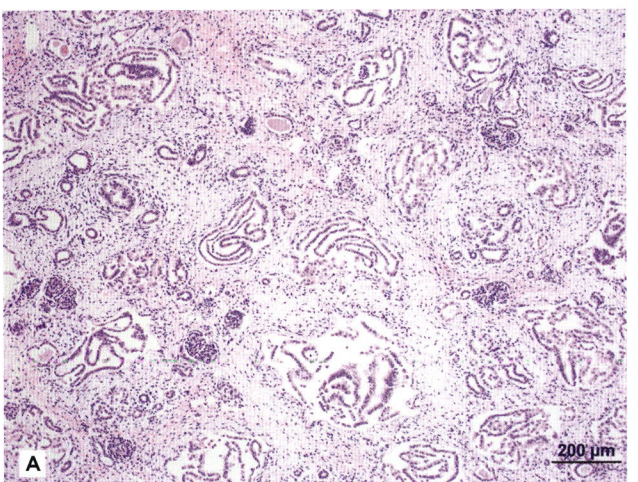 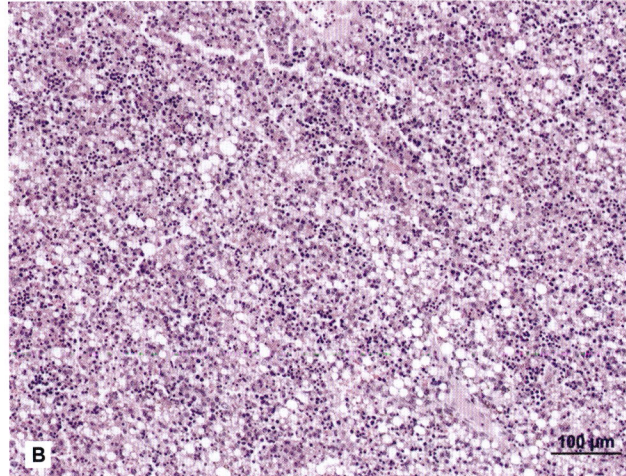

FIGURE 5-18 • Glutaric acidemia, type II. **A:** Renal dysplasia in an infant with glutaric acidemia, type II (H&E). **B:** Hepatic steatosis in glutaric acidemia, type II (as well as widespread extramedullary hematopoiesis, reflective of the patient's neonatal state) (H&E).

Patients with CPT-IA deficiency present within the first 18 months of life with attacks of hypoketotic hypoglycemia, hepatomegaly, and hypoglycemia and typically lack cardiac manifestations. Patients with CPT-II deficiency usually present between 6 and 20 years of age with recurrent myalgia and muscle stiffness after prolonged exercise or fasting and are clinically normal between attacks. They may develop acute renal failure as a result of myoglobinuria, respiratory insufficiency due to respiratory muscle involvement, and paroxysmal cardiac manifestations. Less commonly, patients may present at less than 2 years of age (infantile form) with more severe disease, with attacks of acute liver failure leading to coma, seizures, and cardiac involvement. Patients may also present within the first few days of life (neonatal form) with sudden death, dysmorphic features, cystic renal dysplasia, and neuronal migration defects, similar to ETF-QO deficiency. Patients are treated with glucose during attacks and dietary therapy with frequent meals and avoidance of long-chain fatty acids.

In patients with CPT-II deficiency, a muscle biopsy obtained when the patient is asymptomatic may be normal or have mild lipid accumulation. Biopsies obtained after an episode of myoglobinuria may exhibit fiber necrosis or atrophy. At autopsy, patients with the neonatal form of CPT-II deficiency exhibit fatty infiltration of the myocardium, liver, kidneys, adrenal glands, and skeletal muscle and polymicrogyria and glial heterotopia in the brain (195).

Carnitine Deficiency

Carnitine is an essential cofactor for transport of medium- and long-chain fatty acids across the inner mitochondrial membrane into the mitochondrial matrix, where they undergo beta-oxidation (196). Carnitine is derived either from the diet or via biosynthesis; it is made in the liver, brain, and kidneys and transported to other tissues, including muscle, which has the highest concentration of free carnitine, followed by the liver and heart (196,197).

Primary carnitine deficiency occurs in two biochemically and clinically distinct syndromes (197). Primary systemic carnitine deficiency, or carnitine uptake defect, is an autosomal recessive disorder caused by a defect in the sodium-dependent transporter protein OCTN2, which is encoded by the gene *SLC22A5*. This disease has a frequency of approximately 1 in 40,000 newborns (198). In primary systemic carnitine deficiency, liver, muscle, and plasma carnitine concentrations are all reduced. Before the age of 2 years, affected patients present with hypoketotic hypoglycemia, hepatomegaly, hyperammonemia, coma, and sudden unexpected death. Older patients typically present with cardiomyopathy. Histologically, there is lipid accumulation in skeletal and cardiac muscle and liver (199,200). In some patients, there is cardiomegaly and endocardial fibroelastosis. This disorder responds very well to treatment with carnitine supplementation (198).

Myopathic carnitine deficiency is an autosomal recessive disorder that presents as progressive weakness beginning in childhood (197). Carnitine levels are decreased in muscle but are normal or only slightly decreased in serum and liver. Lipid storage myopathy is seen, primarily in type I fibers. In many cases, no definite biochemical defect has been identified.

MITOCHONDRIAL DISORDERS

Mitochondria are the result of endosymbiosis that occurred some two billion years ago (201). Their main function is the generation of energy in the form of ATP through the respiratory chain. The steps of the respiratory chain take place at the five protein complexes, I through V. Mitochondrial diseases are a very heterogeneous group of disorders that are complex on many different levels (201–203). (a) They are associated with complex genetics that result from the interplay between mitochondrial DNA and nuclear DNA (nDNA). (b) Different biologic processes can lead to mitochondrial dysfunction.

(c) They may come to presentation at any time from infancy to adulthood. (d) They can have a myriad of different disease manifestations. (e) The classification of mitochondrial disease is therefore complex, and genotype–phenotype correlations are often difficult. But certain recurring patterns can be recognized.

(1) The genetics of mitochondrial diseases

The genetics of mitochondrial diseases are complex because two different genomes contribute to normal mitochondrial function, the mitochondrial genome and the nuclear genome (203). The mitochondrial genome (mtDNA) exists as a 16.5-kb double-stranded circular genome that contains 37 genes encoding 27 transfer RNAs (tRNAs), two ribosomal RNAs (rRNAs), and 13 structural proteins that are part of the respiratory chain subunits. Three big groups of mitochondrial diseases distinguished based on genetics are (1) cases with mtDNA defects in the form of point mutations or a single uniform deletion, (2) cases with nDNA defects, and (3) nDNA defects that disrupt normal mtDNA maintenance (Table 5-11).

Two key concepts in the genetics of mtDNA are maternal inheritance and heteroplasmy. The mitochondrial genome of an individual is all derived from the ovum and thus inherited from the mother. Only daughters therefore transmit mutations to their offspring. Heteroplasmy refers to the heterogeneous composition and distribution of mtDNA. Nuclear autosomal DNA exists in exactly two copies per cell. In contrast, each cell contains many mitochondria, and each mitochondrion has several copies of mtDNA. Some of the hundreds of copies of mtDNA in a cell may contain mutations. As many as 1/200 infants may harbor mtDNA mutations (204). Within an organism, the mtDNA carrying mutations may be unevenly distributed in different tissue types (203). Wild-type and mutant mtDNA copies may also replicate at different rates in a tissue-dependent manner. At least conceptually, clinical disease manifestations may only arise if the number of mutant copies in a given tissue reaches a certain threshold (204). Homoplasmic mutations associated with disease are however also described.

Nuclear mutations are inherited in Mendelian patterns and often present in early infancy. These either can directly affect a component of one of the five complexes of the respiratory chain often resulting in a Leigh disease–type presentation or they indirectly affect mitochondrial function by disrupting the assembly of the respiratory chain complexes, membrane composition, or mtRNA translation. Mutations of nDNA affecting mtDNA maintenance can cause defects in the replicative machinery or in enzymes controlling the pool of dNTPs necessary for mtDNA replication.

(2) Aspects of mitochondrial biology disrupted by mutations

Some mutations in nDNA or mtDNA disrupt subunits of the respiratory chain complexes. Both genomes contribute to complexes I, III, IV, and V, but complex II is exclusively encoded by nDNA. Many of the point mutations in the mtDNA affect tRNAs. These are thought to possibly affect mitochondrial function by a reduction in or impaired efficiency of mitochondrial protein synthesis. Some nDNA mutations disrupt mitochondrial function in other ways including (a) alteration of the lipid milieu of the inner nuclear membrane; (b) defects in mitochondrial RNA translation, which requires the function of many nuclear encoded proteins; (c) defects of mitochondrial dynamics that disrupt movement of mitochondria within the cell or the way they fuse and divide; and (d) mutations that disrupt mtDNA maintenance.

(3) Age of onset of mitochondrial diseases

Mitochondrial diseases can present at any age. Early childhood manifestations are often the result of mutations in nDNA, while later presentation more often results from mutations in mtDNA or from mutations causing mtDNA deletions and depletion.

(4) Clinical presentations of mitochondrial diseases

Mitochondrial diseases can present with many different clinical manifestations, none of which is specific for the diagnosis. These include cardiac involvement, neurologic manifestations including seizures and migraines, auditory loss, visual problems, endocrinopathy with diabetes or hypoparathyroidism, renal disease, gastrointestinal symptoms, and skeletal muscle involvement that often includes external eye muscle weakness resulting in ptosis (203,205).

(5) Classification of mitochondrial diseases

It is usually the clustering of manifestations and the family history that may give clues to the correct diagnosis. Some of the distinct named syndromes include MELAS (mitochondrial encephalomyopathy, lactic acidosis, and stroke-like episodes), MERRF (myoclonus epilepsy with ragged red fibers), LHON (Leber hereditary optic neuropathy), NARP (neuropathy, ataxia, retinitis pigmentosa), KSS (Kearns-Sayre syndrome), Leigh disease, and CPEO (chronic progressive external ophthalmoplegia). Some of these tend to be associated with certain mtDNA mutations and some with nDNA mutations. KSS, for example, results from large-scale deletions, MELAS from point mutations, and Leigh disease often from nDNA mutations. But genotype–phenotype correlation is not always reliable (204).

MELAS (mitochondrial encephalomyopathy, lactic acidosis, and stroke-like episodes) results from point mutations in mtDNA that affect tRNAs (most frequently m.3271T>C and m.3291T>C), but rare cases linked to DNA polymerase subunit gamma 1 subunit are described. Patients have sudden onset of stroke-like episodes, usually in adulthood, along with myopathy, ataxia, headaches, deafness, cardiomyopathy, and diabetes mellitus.

MERRF (myoclonus epilepsy with ragged red fibers) is also usually linked to point mutations in mtDNA, most often m.8344A>G. Patients have myoclonic epilepsy, cerebellar ataxia, dementia, myopathy, deafness, short stature, and increased lactate and pyruvate levels. Ragged red fibers are present in muscle biopsy along with numerous COX-negative fibers.

TABLE 5-11 MITOCHONDRIAL DEFECTS (MITOCHONDRIOPATHIES)

Primary Mitochondrial	DNA Disorders	Clinical Features	Inheritance Pattern
Rearrangements (large-scale partial deletions and duplications)	Chronic progressive external ophthalmoplegia (CPEO)	External ophthalmoplegia Ptosis	Sporadic or mitochondrial
	Kearns-Sayre syndrome (KSS)	PEO before age 20 y Pigmentary retinopathy Heart block Cerebellar ataxia Deafness Myopathy Dysphagia Diabetes mellitus Hypoparathyroidism Dementia	Sporadic or mitochondrial
	Pearson marrow pancreas syndrome	Sideroblastic anemia Exocrine pancreatic dysfunction Neonatal or infantile onset Survivors may develop KSS symptoms later in life.	Sporadic or mitochondrial
Point mutations	Diabetes mellitus and deafness		Sporadic
	Genes encoding structural proteins		
	Leber hereditary optic neuropathy LHON (G11778A, T14484C, G3460A)	Sudden loss of vision, usually bilateral, onset 18 to 30 y	Mitochondrial
	NARP (T8993G/C)(ATPase6 gene)	Males:females 4:1 Neuropathy, late childhood or adult onset Ataxia Retinitis pigmentosa	Mitochondrial
	Leigh syndrome (T8993G/C) (ATPase6 gene)	Onset of symptoms in 1st year of life Hypotonia and motor retardation Seizures Lactic acidosis Pigmentary retinopathy Necrotizing encephalomyelopathy	Mitochondrial
	Genes encoding transfer RNAs MELAS (A3243G, T3271C, A3251G)	Seizures and/or dementia Lactic acidosis Stroke-like events Ragged red fiber myopathy	Mitochondrial
	MERRF (A8344G, T8356C)	Myoclonic epilepsy Ragged red fiber myopathy	Mitochondrial
	CPEO (A3243G, T4274C)	Chronic progressive external ophthalmoplegia	Mitochondrial

(Continued)

TABLE 5-11 MITOCHONDRIAL DEFECTS (MITOCHONDRIOPATHIES) (Continued)

Primary Mitochondrial	DNA Disorders	Clinical Features	Inheritance Pattern
	Genes encoding transfer RNAs		
	Myopathy (T14709C, A12320G)		Mitochondrial
	Hypertrophic cardiomyopathy (A3243G, A4269G, A4300G)		Mitochondrial
	Diabetes and deafness (A3243G, C12258A)		Mitochondrial
	Encephalomyopathy (G1606A, T10010C)		Mitochondrial
	Genes encoding ribosomal RNAs		
	Nonsyndromic sensorineural deafness (A7445G)		Mitochondrial
	Aminoglycoside-induced non-syndromic deafness (A1555G)		Mitochondrial
Nuclear Gene Disorders			
Disorders of mtDNA maintenance	Autosomal dominant progressive external ophthalmoplegia		
	Mutations in adenine nucleotide translocator (*ANT1*)	PEO, muscle weakness, bipolar disease	AD
	Mutations in DNA polymerase (*POLG1*)	PEO, muscle weakness, psychiatric disease, neuropathy, ataxia	AD or AR
	Mutations in Twinkle helicase (*C10ORF2*)	PEO, myalgia, exercise intolerance, peripheral neuropathy, psychiatric disease	AD
	Mitochondrial neurogastrointestinal encephalomyopathy (MNGIE) (2° multiple mtDNA deletions): mutations in thymidine phosphorylase (*ECGF1*)	Onset in infant to adult ages Gastrointestinal dysmotility (pseudoobstruction) Leukoencephalopathy Neuropathy Ophthalmoplegia Myopathy	AR
	Myopathy with mtDNA depletion: mutations in thymidine kinase (*TK2*)		AR
	Encephalopathy with liver failure and mitochondrial DNA depletion: mutations in deoxyguanosine kinase (*DGUOK*), *MPV17* or *POLG1*	Neonatal or infantile onset Progressive liver disease	AR
	Mitochondrial DNA depletion due to ATP-forming beta-subunit of the Krebs cycle enzyme succinyl-CoA ligase (*SLUCA2*)	Hypotonia Muscle atrophy Hyperkinesia Severe hearing impairment Postnatal growth retardation Methylmalonic acidemia	AR

TABLE 5-11	MITOCHONDRIAL DEFECTS (MITOCHONDRIOPATHIES) (Continued)		
Primary Mitochondrial	DNA Disorders	Clinical Features	Inheritance Pattern
Primary disorders of the respiratory chain	Leigh syndrome (subacute necrotizing encephalomyopathy)		
	Complex I deficiency—mutations in complex I subunits (NDUFS2, NDUFS4, NDUFS7, NDUFS8, and NDUFV1)		AR
	Complex II deficiency—mutations in complex II flavoprotein subunit (SDHA)		AR
	Leukodystrophy and myoclonic epilepsy: complex I deficiency—mutations in complex I subunit (NDUFV1)		AR
	Cardioencephalomyopathy: complex I deficiency—mutations in complex I subunit (NDUFS2)		AR
	Optic atrophy and ataxia: complex II deficiency—mutations in complex II flavoprotein subunit (SDHA)		AD
Disorders of mitochondrial protein import	Dystonia-deafness: mutations in deafness-dystonia protein DDP1 (TIMM8)		XLR
Disorders of assembly of the respiratory chain	Leigh syndrome (subacute necrotizing encephalomyopathy)		
	Complex IV deficiency—mutations in COX assembly protein (SURF1)	Most common cause of Leigh syndrome	AR
	Complex IV deficiency—mutations in COX assembly protein (COX10)		AR
	Cardioencephalomyopathy: complex IV deficiency—mutations in COX assembly protein (SCO2)		AR
	Hepatic failure and encephalopathy:		
	Complex IV deficiency—mutations in COX assembly protein (SCO1)		AR
	Complex IV deficiency—mutations in protein affecting COX mRNA stability (leucine-rich pentatricopeptide repeat cassette, LRPPRC)		AR
	Tubulopathy, encephalopathy, and liver failure: complex III deficiency—mutations in complex III assembly (BSC1L)		AR
	Encephalopathy: complex I deficiency—mutations in the complex I assembly protein (B17.2L)		AR

(Continued)

TABLE 5-11 MITOCHONDRIAL DEFECTS (MITOCHONDRIOPATHIES) (Continued)

Primary Mitochondrial	DNA Disorders	Clinical Features	Inheritance Pattern
Disorders of RNA metabolism	Leigh syndrome (subacute necrotizing encephalomyopathy)		
	Complex IV deficiency (*LRPPRC*)		AR
	Multiple complex defects with mutations in mitochondrial elongation factor G1 (*EFG1*)		AR
Disorders of the lipid membrane	Coenzyme Q10 deficiency (*COQ2*)	Ataxia, seizures, encephalomyopathy	AR
		Cerebellar atrophy	
		Renal dysfunction	
		Treatable with coenzyme Q10	
	Barth syndrome (Tafazzin)	Cardiomyopathy	XLR
		Noncompaction of the left ventricle	
		Neutropenia	
		3-Methylglutaconic aciduria	
		Skeletal muscle myopathy	

PEO, progressive external ophthalmoplegia; AD, autosomal dominant; AR, autosomal recessive; XLR, X-linked recessive.

Kearns-Sayre syndrome (KSS) is typically associated with external ophthalmoplegia, pigmentary retinopathy, and heart block and usually presents before 20 years of age. Ptosis, cerebellar involvement, ataxia, and endocrinopathies (diabetes mellitus, hypoparathyroidism, growth hormone deficiency, Addison disease, and hypogonadism) also occur. The brain may have basal ganglia calcification. Skeletal muscle biopsy shows numerous or infrequent ragged red fibers and COX-negative fibers. Structurally abnormal mitochondria are apparent by EM. KSS is usually the result of a single deletion, most often with loss of a 4977-bp fragment. These are almost always sporadic and not maternally inherited.

Chronic progressive external ophthalmoplegia (CPEO) with ragged red fibers is generally a benign disorder with slowly progressive ophthalmoplegia, ptosis, and proximal limb weakness beginning in adolescence. Most cases are sporadic and have deletions or duplications of mtDNA. Muscle biopsy shows ragged red and cytochrome oxidase (COX)-negative fibers.

Leigh disease typically goes along with multifocal often symmetric gray matter lesions that can involve many gray matter areas but often affect the basal ganglia system. Leigh disease can result from mtDNA point mutations, especially in patients with high mutational load. In other patients, Leigh disease is the result of nDNA mutations.

Leber hereditary optic neuropathy (LHON) presents with painless acute or subacute visual loss. Often, the disease presents early in life. Optic nerve pathology with ganglion cell loss and retinal nerve fiber atrophy may be seen, but ragged red fibers are not present. In some patients, the disease results from an m11778G>A point mutation and in others from mutations in genes encoding subunits in complex I.

Multiple mitochondrial DNA deletions. Mutations in adenine nucleotide translocator-1 (*ANT-1*) and the mitochondrial helicase Twinkle (*C10ORF2*) can lead to autosomal dominant or recessive progressive ophthalmoplegia and, in some cases, multisystemic symptoms.

Mitochondrial neurogastrointestinal encephalomyopathy (MNGIE) disease. This autosomal recessive condition usually presents before age 20 years and is characterized by severe gastrointestinal dysmotility (pseudoobstruction), poor weight gain, gastroesophageal reflux, vomiting, diarrhea, abdominal pain, and abdominal distension. Patients may also have hearing loss, ptosis, external ophthalmoplegia, sensorimotor neuropathy, and leukoencephalopathy on brain MRI scan. Demyelinating peripheral neuropathy is associated with paresthesias and distal limb weakness. The gene encoding thymidine phosphorylase, *ECGF1*, is the only known gene associated with MNGIE disease. Both mitochondrial DNA depletion and multiple mitochondrial DNA deletions are found in patients with MNGIE disease.

Muscle biopsy shows ragged red fibers; eosinophilic cytoplasmic inclusions, representing enlarged mitochondria, occur in rectal submucosal ganglia and smooth muscle cells.

The duodenum may demonstrate focal atrophy or absence of the muscularis propria with increased number of nerves and focal loss of Auerbach plexus with fibrosis.

Diagnosis may be made by demonstrating elevated plasma thymidine and deoxyuridine or by demonstrating less than 10% of the control mean thymidine phosphorylase activity in buffy coat leukocytes. Respiratory chain enzyme assays on tissues demonstrate defects in single or multiple complexes. The most common defect is in cytochrome c oxidase (complex IV). Molecular genetic testing of the *ECGF1* gene detects essentially 100% of affected individuals.

Mitochondrial DNA depletion syndrome patients have disease onset in the early months of life with progressive liver failure and encephalopathy. Three nuclear-encoded mitochondrial genes associated with hepatocerebral syndrome have been identified: deoxyguanosine kinase (*DGUOK*), *MPV17*, and DNA polymerase gamma (*POLG1*).

Mutations in the *POLG1* gene have been associated with autosomal recessive Alpers syndrome characterized by progressive encephalopathy, ataxia, and liver failure; intractable seizures may be the predominant clinical feature. Liver histopathology in patients with *POLG1* mutations is variable, ranging from steatosis and mild fibrosis to marked fibrosis and cirrhosis, hepatocyte degeneration, and bile duct proliferation. Muscle biopsy shows COX-deficient fibers and ragged red fibers. Liver failure is the major presenting symptom in patients with *DGUOK* or *MPV17* mutations, although there is overlap in these defects. In DGUOK deficiency, progressive liver disease leads to steatosis, siderosis, canalicular and hepatocellular cholestasis, multinucleated giant cells, cirrhosis, and, in some patients, hepatocellular carcinoma; fatal infantile liver disease may occur with or without encephalopathy. By EM, there is accumulation of mitochondria with reduced cristae. Mutations in *MPV17*, encoding an inner mitochondrial membrane protein, have been reported in patients with infantile hepatic mtDNA depletion.

Diagnosis may be made by demonstration of depletion of mitochondrial DNA by real-time PCR analysis on liver or muscle tissue. Also, DNA analysis of the *POLG1*, *DGUOK*, and *MPV17* genes is available.

Coenzyme Q_{10} (CoQ_{10}, ubiquinone) deficiency. CoQ_{10} is a lipid-soluble component is found in all cell membranes and functions as an electron and proton carrier. CoQ_{10} deficiency is caused by mutations in the *COQ2* gene and is inherited as an autosomal recessive disorder. CoQ_{10} deficiency can present in infancy with encephalomyopathy and renal dysfunction and later in life as a myopathic form with myoglobinuria, exercise intolerance, and weakness or may be associated with cerebellar atrophy, ataxia, and seizures. It is treatable with CoQ_{10} supplementation. Muscle biopsy shows increased lipid and ragged red fibers.

Barth syndrome is due to defects in the *TAZ* gene that encodes the protein tafazzin, which influences incorporation of cardiolipin, an essential part of the inner mitochondrial membrane. This X-linked disorder causes mitochondrial myopathy with ragged red fibers, dilated cardiomyopathy with abnormal left ventricular compaction, and neutropenia.

Diagnosis of Mitochondrial Diseases

The diagnosis of mitochondrial diseases can be difficult because of the complex underlying genetics (203). In some cases, the disease presentation is suggestive of mtDNA- or nDNA-related diseases as outlined above. Mitochondrial diseases affecting skeletal muscle may be diagnosed on a muscle biopsy (204). Key diagnostic features are the following (Figure 5-19): (1) the presence of cytochrome oxidase negative fibers seen by the appropriate enzyme histochemical studies; (2) the presence of ragged red fibers in which abnormal mitochondria are seen as often subsarcolemmal aggregates that stain on the modified Gomori trichrome stain and are visualized on the SDH reaction; (3) strong succinate dehydrogenase positive blood vessels (SSVs) in m.3243A>G associated cases of MELAS; and (4) numerical increase in mitochondria and morphologically abnormal mitochondria including those containing pseudocrystalline inclusions. Biochemical testing for respiratory chain enzymes is technically difficult but can be helpful. Mutations in mtDNA may be difficult to confirm because of heteroplasmy and different percentages of mutated mtDNA in different tissues. Some tissues with high cell turnover like hematopoietic cells may select out mutant mtDNA and may therefore represent a poor specimen (205). Testing for mtDNA mutations on affected tissue like skeletal muscle can be helpful. The presence of nuclear mutations can be identified by genetic testing.

Therapy of Mitochondrial Diseases

Specific therapies for mitochondrial diseases are not yet available (202,205). The only exception is the rare case caused by coenzyme Q_{10} (CoQ_{10}, ubiquinone) deficiency, which responds to CoQ_{10} supplementation. The management of cases with mitochondrial diseases or suspected mitochondrial diseases should however include testing to diagnose disease manifestations in organ systems that may have gone undiagnosed but affect treatment. Such examples include cardiac workup to diagnose and treat arrhythmias, endocrine studies, and swallowing studies to assess for possible dysphagia.

HYPERAMMONEMIAS/UREA CYCLE DISORDERS

The urea cycle converts toxic nitrogenous waste into water-soluble urea in the liver (206,207). Defects in this pathway initially present with nonspecific symptoms (lethargy, vomiting, irritability) and progress to hyperammonemia with neurotoxicity and cerebral edema. Most untreated patients die, often with cerebral or pulmonary hemorrhage. Alternatively, children or adults with urea cycle defects can present when fasting or infection precipitates symptoms (207).

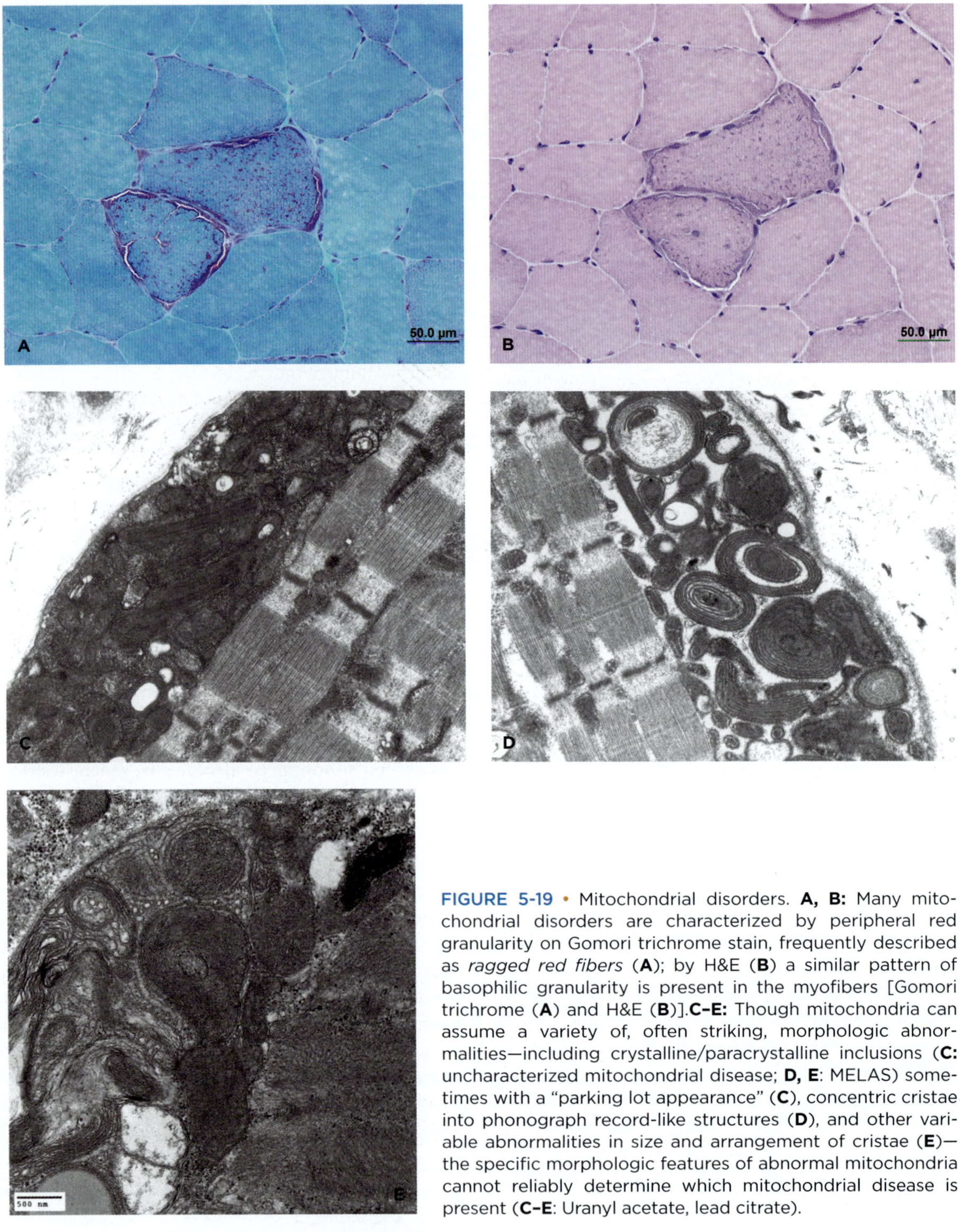

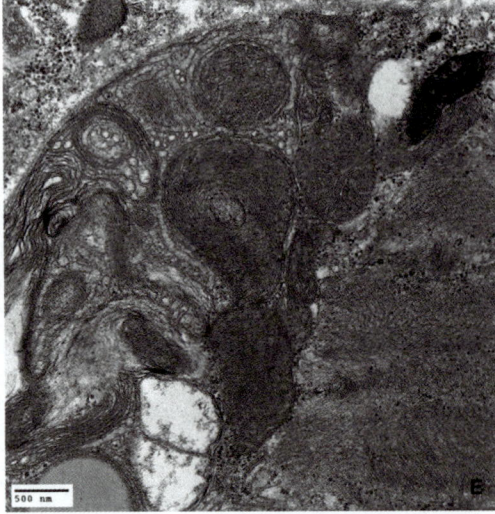

FIGURE 5-19 • Mitochondrial disorders. **A, B:** Many mitochondrial disorders are characterized by peripheral red granularity on Gomori trichrome stain, frequently described as *ragged red fibers* (**A**); by H&E (**B**) a similar pattern of basophilic granularity is present in the myofibers [Gomori trichrome (**A**) and H&E (**B**)]. **C–E:** Though mitochondria can assume a variety of, often striking, morphologic abnormalities—including crystalline/paracrystalline inclusions (**C**: uncharacterized mitochondrial disease; **D, E**: MELAS) sometimes with a "parking lot appearance" (**C**), concentric cristae into phonograph record-like structures (**D**), and other variable abnormalities in size and arrangement of cristae (**E**)—the specific morphologic features of abnormal mitochondria cannot reliably determine which mitochondrial disease is present (**C–E**: Uranyl acetate, lead citrate).

Brains of patients with urea cycle defects demonstrate extensive neuronal loss, gliosis, and Alzheimer type II astrocytes (206). Liver biopsy may be normal or show mild steatosis, glycogen accumulation, focal necrosis, interface hepatitis, or mild portal or bridging fibrosis (208). Mitochondria may be normal or have nonspecific pleomorphism and swollen or shortened cristae. Diagnosis is based on plasma or urine amino acid analysis (128).

Carbamoyl Phosphate Synthetase I (CPS I) Deficiency

Carbamoyl phosphate synthetase is a mitochondrial enzyme that catalyzes the formation of carbamoyl phosphate, the first rate-limiting step of the urea cycle (209). CPS I deficiency is a rare autosomal recessive disorder with a lethal neonatal-onset form and a milder delayed-onset form with episodic hyperammonemia (210). The liver is normal or exhibits mild-to-moderate steatosis with focal necrosis, portal fibrosis, and glycogen accumulation (208). By electron microscopy, mitochondria may be normal or dilated with increased matrix density and fragmentation of cristae (211). The brain shows patchy spongiosis and Alzheimer type II astrocytosis.

Ornithine Transcarbamylase (OTC) Deficiency

This X-linked disease is the most common urea cycle disorder (212). A large number of mutations of the OTC gene, located at Xp21, have been described. In the neonatal form, patients have emesis, hyperammonemia, progressive encephalopathy, and focal neurologic defects. Hemizygous boys typically present in the first days of life, but heterozygous girls may be intermittently symptomatic. All patients with OTC deficiency are vulnerable to valproate-associated hepatotoxicity due to inhibition of the urea cycle, and OTC-deficient heterozygote mothers may have postpartum hyperammonemic encephalopathy (213).

Histologically, the liver may be normal even in fatal disease or exhibit steatosis, mild piecemeal necrosis, nodularity and portal fibrosis with enlarged pale hepatocytes, and glycogen accumulation (208). The brain exhibits severe cerebral atrophy with ulegyria, delayed myelination, cystic degeneration most commonly in the territory of the anterior and middle cerebral arteries, neuronal loss, and Alzheimer type II astrocytosis. The cerebellar granular cell layer may be atrophic.

Diagnosis is confirmed by mutation analysis, urine amino acid analyses to identify increased orotic acid, and low leukocyte, fibroblast, or liver OTC. Patients with hyperammonemia are treated with sodium benzoate and phenylbutyrate and placed on a low-protein diet with supplemental arginine. Liver transplant may be considered in patients with life-threatening symptoms and a confirmed diagnosis of OTC deficiency (212).

Citrullinemia Type 1

This autosomal recessive disease is caused by mutations in argininosuccinate synthetase, which converts citrulline to argininosuccinate (214). It has a frequency of 1 in 40,000 to 200,000. Clinical presentation is heterogeneous. The classic neonatal-onset form presents early in life with hyperammonemic encephalopathy, failure to thrive, and death. Milder forms present with intermittent hyperammonemia during childhood and adulthood or hepatic dysfunction and neuropsychiatric symptoms during pregnancy or postpartum. Histologically, the liver exhibits diffuse hepatocyte swelling, variable fibrosis, focal necrosis, and cholestasis (208). By electron microscopy, enlarged mitochondria with increased matrix density and paracrystalline and electron-dense bodies may be seen (215).

Argininosuccinic Aciduria

This autosomal recessive disease is the second most common urea cycle defect and is caused by a defect in argininosuccinate lyase (216), which catalyzes the formation of arginine from argininosuccinate. The severe neonatal form presents within the first few days of life with hyperammonemia, tachypnea, hypothermia, seizures, and lethargy. A late-onset form presents with episodic hyperammonemia, neurocognitive disabilities, cirrhosis, systemic hypertension, and trichorrhexis nodosa (brittle hair due to arginine deficiency). The liver exhibits periportal and bridging fibrosis, micronodular cirrhosis, steatosis, and glycogen accumulation (208). Ultrastructural mitochondrial abnormalities are not seen. Diagnosis is based on a newborn screen with elevated citrulline by tandem mass spectrometry and confirmed with elevation of citrulline and argininosuccinic acid in the plasma.

Argininemia (Hyperargininemia, Arginase Deficiency)

This rare autosomal recessive disease is caused by a deficiency in arginase I, the final enzyme in the urea cycle. Patients present during childhood, later in life than other urea cycle disorders, with spastic paraplegia, cognitive defects, and epilepsy (217). Hyperammonemia is seen in a minority of patients. Rarely, liver manifestations, including hepatomegaly with steatosis and periportal fibrosis but with normal mitochondria, may be seen (218). Patients are treated with a low-protein diet.

Hyperornithinemia–Hyperammonemia–Homocitrullinuria (HHH) Syndrome

This rare autosomal recessive disorder is caused by impaired ornithine transport from the cytoplasm into mitochondria due to mutations in the *SLC25A15* gene, which encodes the ornithine transporter (219). Ornithine is produced with urea in the last step of the urea cycle. Patients present with growth retardation, seizures, and spasticity and have increased plasma ornithine concentration, elevated homo-citrulline in the urine, and episodic hyperammonemia. Electron microscopy may demonstrate increased mitochondrial number and giant pleomorphic hepatocyte mitochondria, glycogen accumulation, and increased smooth endoplasmic reticulum (220).

Lysinuric Protein Intolerance (LPI)

This autosomal recessive disorder is caused by mutations in the gene *SLC7A7*, which encodes for the light chain of a heterodimeric cationic amino acid transporter (221). The mutation results in lack of normal intestinal absorption and excessive renal loss of the cationic amino acids lysine, ornithine, and arginine, with resultant low plasma levels of these amino acids and increased urine lysine. This disease has a higher incidence in Finland, where 1 in 60,000 births is affected. Affected patients may have failure to thrive, feeding difficulty, recurrent episodes of vomiting and diarrhea, hepatomegaly, cognitive impairment, sparse hair, osteoporosis, hypotonia, and, in some cases, sudden unexpected death in infancy (222). Episodic hyperammonemia develops after protein-rich meals.

Pathologic alterations in the lungs include pneumonia with lipid deposits in the interstitium, alveolar spaces, and alveolar macrophages; interstitial lung disease; and pulmonary alveolar proteinosis (223). In the kidneys, progressive immune complex–mediated IgA mesangial proliferative or membranous glomerulonephritis is seen (224). In the liver, microvesicular steatosis, bile duct proliferation, periportal nuclear glycogen accumulation, portal fibrosis, and micronodular cirrhosis are described (224). Pancreatic acinar atrophy and fibrosis (223) and hemophagocytic lymphohistiocytosis with macrophage activation (221) can also occur. Patients are treated with a protein-restricted diet, supplementation with l-citrulline, and nitrogen-scavenging drugs (221).

ORGANIC ACIDEMIAS

In these disorders, catabolism of amino acids, carbohydrates, or fatty acids is blocked due to an enzyme or cofactor deficiency, with resultant accumulation of organic acids, which can be identified by mass spectrometry of the urine (129). Clinically, the organic acidemias are characterized by severe progressive encephalopathy with coma, seizures, and death (Table 5-12).

Propionic Acidemia

Propionic acidemia is an autosomal recessive disease caused by defects in the biotin-dependent enzyme propionyl-CoA carboxylase, which converts propionyl-CoA to methylmalonyl-CoA during branched-chain amino acid and odd-chain fatty acid metabolism. The defect leads to tissue propionic acid accumulation. Infants are symptom-free for the first few hours or weeks after birth and subsequently present with nonspecific gastrointestinal symptoms or rapidly progressive encephalopathy with hypotonia, seizures, and myoclonus progressing to coma and early death. Later-onset forms may present as acute encephalopathy, anorexia, failure to thrive, and developmental delay. Laboratory results show ketotic hyperglycemia, leukopenia, thrombocytopenia, anemia, and hyperammonemia. Decreased free carnitine, increased propionyl carnitine, and increased urine excretion of propionylglycine and methylcitrate characterize this disorder. Patients are treated with a low-protein diet, carnitine supplementation, metronidazole, and vitamin B12. Liver transplantation may partially correct the enzymatic defect but is not curative.

In early-onset forms, the brain exhibits spongy degeneration of the white matter, particularly at the gray–white matter junction in the temporal cortex and in the midbrain, pons, and medulla (225). In later-onset patients,

TABLE 5-12 ORGANIC ACIDEMIAS

Name	Common Clinical Presentation	Enzyme Deficiency	Substrate Accumulation	Laboratory Evaluation	Pathologic Findings
Propionic acidemia	Neonate: vomiting, respiratory distress, hypotonia, seizures, death	Biotin-dependent propionyl-CoA carboxylase	Propionic acid (U, B) Methylcitrate (U) Tiglylglycine (U) 3-Hydroxypropionate (U)	Ketoacidosis, hyperammonemia, hyperglycemia Neutropenia Thrombocytopenia	Brain: spongy white matter degeneration, particularly of globus pallidus
Methylmalonic acidemia	Similar to propionic acidemia	Methylmalonyl-CoA mutase	Methylmalonic acid (U, B) Methylcitrate (U) Tiglylglycine (U) 3-Hydroxypropionate (U)	Ketoacidosis, hyperammonemia, hyperglycemia Neutropenia Thrombocytopenia	Brain: spongy white matter degeneration Kidneys: interstitial fibrosis, tubular atrophy
Isovaleric acidemia	Similar to propionic acidemia May have later age of onset	Isovaleryl-CoA dehydrogenase	Isovaleric acid (B) Isovalerylglycine (U)	Acidosis Sweaty feet odor Pancytopenia	Brain: spongy white matter degeneration Liver: steatosis
Glutaric acidemia type 1	Developmental delay Macrocephaly Choreoathetosis Dystonia	Glutaryl-CoA dehydrogenase	Glutaric acid (U) 3-OH-glutaric acid (U)	Acidosis	Brain: frontotemporal atrophy, striatal degeneration, white matter spongiosis, subdural hematoma

U, urine; B, blood.

there may be degeneration of the basal ganglia and hypoxic changes with Purkinje cell and granular layer dropout in the cerebellum and Alzheimer type II astrocytes in the basal ganglia.

Methylmalonic Acidemia

Methylmalonic acidemia is an autosomal recessive disorder resulting in the accumulation of methylmalonic acid in body fluids and urine due to actual or functional deficiency of methylmalonyl-CoA mutase activity (226). This enzyme catalyzes the isomerization of methylmalonyl-CoA to succinyl-CoA, a Krebs cycle intermediate. The coenzyme adenosylcobalamin, derived from vitamin B12, is required for enzymatic activity. Mutations in the methylmalonyl-CoA mutase gene or in genes (*MMAA* and *MMAB*) encoding proteins required for the synthesis of adenosylcobalamin can give rise to this condition. Clinically, patients present similarly to those with propionic acidemia, and the pathology is nonspecific. In addition to brain changes similar to those seen with propionic acidemia, the kidneys show interstitial fibrosis, tubular atrophy, and chronic inflammation, with formation of enlarged, pale mitochondria with disrupted cristae (227). Nearly all patients with mutations in *MMAA* respond to treatment with vitamin B12, while patients with mutations in methylmalonyl-CoA mutase rarely respond to vitamin B12 therapy (226).

Isovaleric Acidemia

Isovaleric acidemia is an autosomal recessive disorder of leucine metabolism caused by a deficiency of isovaleryl-CoA dehydrogenase. Patients present either in the neonatal period or in early childhood with anion gap metabolic acidosis and a sweaty feet odor and may progress to coma and death due to cerebral edema or hemorrhage (228). Patients may have pancytopenia, acute pancreatitis, Fanconi syndrome, and cardiac arrhythmias. A diagnosis is suggested on detection of elevated C5 acylcarnitine by tandem mass spectrometry on newborn screen and confirmed with detection of isovalerylcarnitine in the plasma and isovalerylglycine in the urine. In addition to dietary restriction, patients are treated with glycine, which is enzymatically conjugated to the excess isovaleryl-CoA.

Glutaric Acidemia Type I

Glutaric acidemia type 1 is an autosomal recessive disease caused by glutaryl-CoA dehydrogenase (GCDH) deficiency. GCDH catalyzes the formation of crotonyl-CoA from glutaryl-CoA in the metabolism of the amino acids lysine, hydroxylysine, and tryptophan. Patients present with macrocephaly with an underdeveloped neocortex and CSF space expansion (micrencephalic macrocephaly) at or shortly after birth (229). The CSF space expansion can lead to stretching of veins that may rupture, giving rise to subdural hematomas and bilateral retinal hemorrhages that mimic shaken baby syndrome. Between 6 and 18 months of age, patients typically experience acute neurologic deterioration with a severe dystonic–dyskinetic syndrome following a triggering event. The central nervous system is remarkable for dilatation of the Sylvian fissures, frontotemporal atrophy, striatal degeneration, and white matter spongiosis. Diagnosis is based on increased glutaric and hydroxyglutaric acid in the urine and decreased GCDH in fibroblasts (129); molecular diagnosis is possible. Patients are treated with a low-lysine diet and carnitine supplementation.

CONGENITAL LACTIC ACIDOSIS

Increased lactate can be due to nongenetic disease (including tissue necrosis and sepsis), but there are also primary genetic disorders that lead to lactate accumulation. The normal lactate:pyruvate ratio in human plasma is 10:1 to 25:1. This ratio is typically elevated when the Krebs cycle is impaired (e.g., hypoxia), but normal or low when the defect is upstream of the Krebs cycle (e.g., pyruvate dehydrogenase deficiency) (113).

Pyruvate Dehydrogenase (PDH) Deficiency

The clinical spectrum of PDH deficiency ranges from fatal lactic acidosis in the newborn to chronic neurologic dysfunction with structural abnormalities of the brain progressing to profound cognitive impairment, microcephaly, and blindness, without systemic acidosis (230). There may be a characteristic dysmorphic appearance with a narrow head, frontal bossing, wide nasal bridge, long philtrum, and flared nostrils. The most common defect is X-linked, due to mutations in the E1 alpha-subunit of the PDH complex. Males typically present with severe neonatal lactic acidosis, while females most commonly present with neurologic symptoms. Affected males may have a thin corpus callosum or callosal agenesis and Leigh encephalopathy (symmetric cystic lesions and gliosis in the brain stem and basal ganglia) (230,231). Female heterozygotes may have as severe a presentation as affected males (Figure 5-20A–C) or may be normal. Neurodegenerative changes including cerebral atrophy, ventricular dilatation, polymicrogyria, and callosal hypoplasia may be seen (232). The E1 beta-, E2 beta-, and E3 beta-subunits of the pyruvate dehydrogenase complex are encoded by autosomal genes, and deficiencies are inherited as autosomal recessive traits. If low PDH activity is found in leukocytes or fibroblasts, the activities of the individual PDH components—E1, E2, and E3—can be assayed for further classification, and DNA analysis is available for the E1 alpha gene (230).

Pyruvate Carboxylase Deficiency

Pyruvate carboxylase, which catalyzes the conversion of pyruvate to oxaloacetate, is important in gluconeogenesis and replenishment of the Krebs cycle (233). Deficiency of pyruvate carboxylase is an autosomal recessive disorder

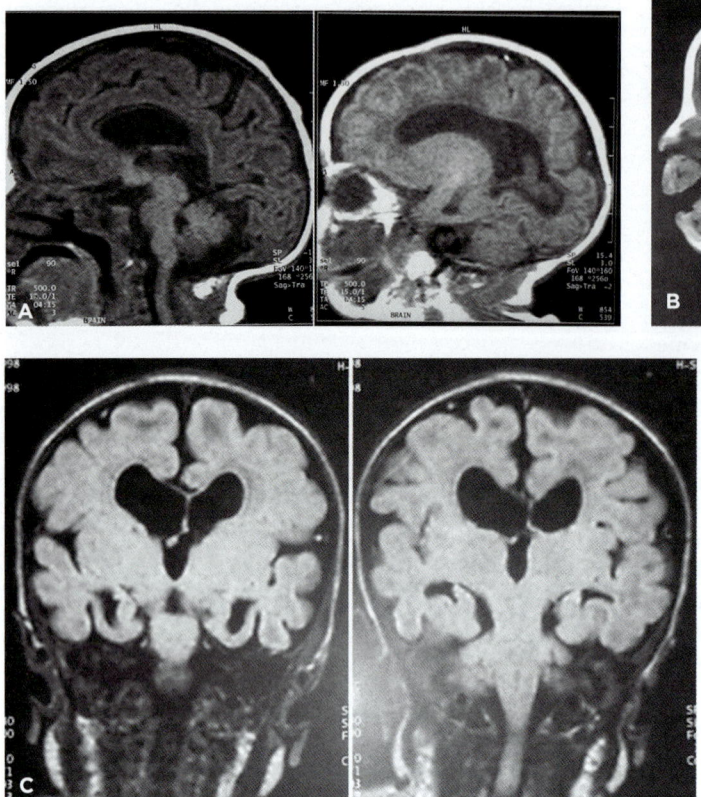
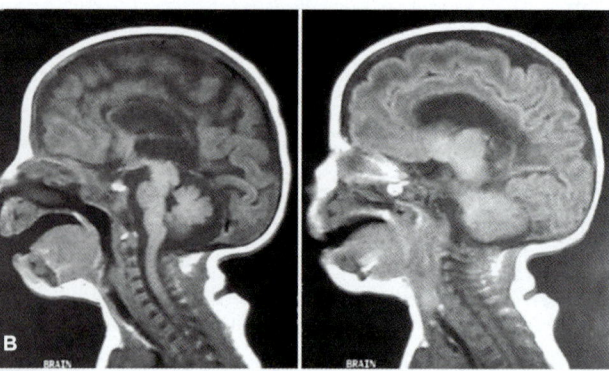

FIGURE 5-20 • Pyruvate dehydrogenase deficiency. A-C: Magnetic resonance imaging of a girl who was heterozygous for pyruvate dehydrogenase deficiency. Note atrophy, abnormal gyral formation, and absence of the corpus callosum.

with different clinical presentations, including a neonatal form with severe biotin-unresponsive lactic acidosis and death within the first few months of life, an infantile form with moderately elevated lactate, and a benign form with few sequelae. Patients may also have hepatomegaly with portal fibrosis and steatosis. Other clinical features can include cognitive impairment, developmental delay, hypotonia, high-amplitude tremors, nystagmus, and seizures. Brain findings include ischemia-like changes and cystic periventricular leukomalacia and hemorrhage.

PEROXISOMAL DISORDERS

Peroxisomes are organelles bound by a single membrane that contain a protein-rich matrix. They are spherical with a diameter of 0.1 to 1 μm, and they are larger and more abundant in the liver and kidney than in other tissues. Their number adjusts to metabolic requirement. Peroxisomes are important for alpha oxidation of branched-chain fatty acids and beta-oxidation of very long-chain fatty acids (VLCFA) but also the biosynthesis of ether phospholipids as well as bile acids. In general, peroxisomal disorders can be identified by increased tissue and body fluid levels of VLCFA, decreased plasmalogen, and increased phytanic acid levels. EM may be useful in defining the number and size of peroxisomes and in identifying trilaminate inclusions that are thought to be related to VLCFA deposition.

Peroxisomal disorders can be divided into two groups, those that result from general defects in peroxisomal biogenesis and those caused by a single enzyme deficiency (Table 5-13).

TABLE 5-13 PEROXISOMAL DISORDERS

Peroxisomal biogenesis disorders
  Zellweger syndrome spectrum (ZSS)
  Zellweger syndrome (cerebrohepatorenal syndrome)
  Neonatal adrenoleukodystrophy
  Infantile Refsum disease
  Rhizomelic chondrodysplasia punctata type 1

Single peroxisomal enzyme deficiencies
  X-linked adrenoleukodystrophy
  Acyl-CoA oxidase deficiency (pseudoneonatal adrenoleukodystrophy)
  Rhizomelic chondrodysplasia punctata type 2
  Rhizomelic chondrodysplasia punctata type 3
  D-Bifunctional protein deficiency
  2-Methylacyl-CoA racemase deficiency
  Sterol carrier protein X deficiency
  Refsum disease
  Hyperoxaluria type I (oxalosis 1)

Peroxisomal Biogenesis Disorders

Disorders of peroxisomal biogenesis are characterized by defective and/or reduced number of peroxisomes and defects in multiple peroxisomal enzymes. Genetic phenotype complementation studies and database searches have helped to define a family of genes that are key for peroxisomal function, the *PEX* genes that encode peroxins (234,235). At least 14 different *PEX* genes are recognized, and mutations in at least 13 of these have been linked to a disease phenotype. These disorders have similar biochemical findings: The Zellweger syndrome spectrum is caused by defects in any of the *PEX* genes required for normal peroxisome assembly and includes the first three diseases listed below (235,236). This spectrum includes presentations that have traditionally been described as distinct entities, Zellweger syndrome, neonatal adrenoleukodystrophy, and infantile Refsum disease. The clinical classification into these categories is primarily a reflection of disease severity and not of the gene affected.

Zellweger (cerebrohepatorenal) syndrome is the most severe of the biogenesis disorders. An autosomal recessive disease, it presents in neonates with metabolic abnormalities; distinctive facial dysmorphology; severe hypotonia; failure to thrive; mental retardation; seizures; ocular, genital, and cardiovascular malformations; renal glomerular cysts; and calcific stippling of the patellae.

In the brain, premature arrest of migrating neuroblasts during development results in site-specific cerebral microgyria and pachygyria with neuronal heterotopia, an abnormal convolution pattern and olivary dysplasia. The liver initially shows a hepatitic pattern, with hepatocellular unrest, focal necrosis, steatosis, and canalicular and cytoplasmic cholestasis with pseudoacinar and giant cell transformation. Lymphocytes and macrophages accumulate in sinusoids and portal spaces. Intrahepatic bile ducts may be normal, decreased, or hyperplastic. With time, the liver becomes firm and fibrotic with micronodular cirrhosis (2,3). By EM, peroxisomes are absent or rare in the liver and kidney. The pathogenesis of the liver injury is unknown but may relate to injury by abnormal bile acids.

Neonatal adrenoleukodystrophy is an autosomal recessive disorder that is less severe than Zellweger syndrome and is characterized by hypotonia, craniofacial dysmorphism, adrenocortical atrophy, and psychomotor deterioration. The brain shows progressive dysmyelination/demyelination of cerebral and cerebellar white matter and polymicrogyria. Hepatic peroxisomes are reduced in number and size. PAS-positive macrophages with angulate lysosomes are present in viscera and brain.

Infantile Refsum disease patients resemble those with Zellweger syndrome with hypotonia, seizures, mental retardation, hearing loss, and dysmorphic facies. Their course is milder than seen in Zellweger syndrome or neonatal adrenoleukodystrophy. Hepatomegaly with fibrosis and portal-to-portal bridging is seen, and, by EM, peroxisomes are deficient or very small (2,3). Lysosomal PAS-positive trilaminate inclusions with two dense outer and an inner lucent lamellae and an outer thickness of 6 to 14 nm accumulate first in macrophages and then in hepatocytes and suggest VLCFA storage. An elevated phytanic acid, trihydroxycoprostanoic acid, pipecolic acid, and VLCFA and decreased phytanic acid oxidase are laboratory abnormalities.

Rhizomelic chondrodysplasia punctata type 1 is a peroxisomal disorder that is genetically and biochemically distinct from Zellweger syndrome. It is due to a defect in a peroxisomal targeting gene that affects import of enzymes into peroxisomes, *PEX7*. Patients have impaired plasmalogen synthesis and phytanic acid oxidation, severe proximal limb shortening, calcific stippling in hyaline cartilage, cataracts, renal dysfunction, facial dysmorphism, ichthyosis, and death in childhood. Hepatocytes may have absent or large irregularly shaped peroxisomes. Plasma phytanic acid is increased, and RBC and tissue plasmalogen are decreased (see Chapter 28).

Single Peroxisomal Enzyme Deficiency

X-linked adrenoleukodystrophy. Affected patients have a mutation in the *ABCD1* gene that encodes ALDP (237). ALDP is thought to transport VLCFA into the peroxisome for beta-oxidation. A defect of the transport of C24:0 and C26:0 fatty acids into the peroxisome increases their level in the cytosol and increases the availability of substrate for the elongase ELOVL1 for further elongation. Elevated levels of plasma VLCFA is still a useful diagnostic test. The two basic pathologically distinct presentations are adrenomyeloneuropathy (AMN), which is associated with a noninflammatory axonal neuropathy, and the cerebral demyelinating form of X-ALD that usually causes rapidly progressive inflammatory demyelination in the brain (237). The latter results in progressive behavioral, cognitive, and neurologic deterioration and has an incidence of 1/21,000 boys. Adrenal glands are small, and zona fasciculata cells contain cytoplasmic lipid inclusions with a lamellar pattern. Lipid accumulation in CNS causes demyelination with a perivascular lymphocytic infiltrate that resembles that seen in multiple sclerosis.

Acyl-CoA oxidase deficiency (pseudoneonatal adrenoleukodystrophy) presents clinically with hypotonia, psychomotor retardation, sensory deafness, hepatomegaly, and retinopathy, with or without mild craniofacial dysmorphism. Atrophy of skeletal muscle, brainstem ganglia, and cranial nerves along with hepatic fibrosis and large PAS-positive, sudanophilic adrenal macrophages and brain astrocytes are described in this disorder. Hepatic peroxisomes are heterogeneous in size and increased in number.

Rhizomelic chondrodysplasia punctata type 2, due to dihydroxyacetonephosphate acyltransferase deficiency, presents with craniofacial abnormalities, hypotonia, cataracts, cognitive impairment, eczema, cerebral atrophy, and dwarfism with rhizomelic shortening of the upper arms but no stippled patellar calcifications.

Rhizomelic chondrodysplasia punctata type 3, due to alkyl dihydroxyacetonephosphate synthase deficiency, is clinically similar to rhizomelic chondrodysplasia punctata type 1.

d-Bifunctional protein deficiency presents with neonatal hypotonia, seizures, failure to thrive, visual abnormalities, psychomotor delay, and dysmorphism that resembles that seen in Zellweger syndrome.

2-Methylacyl-CoA racemase deficiency has a variable clinical course, with adult-onset sensorimotor neuropathy and fulminant liver disease described.

Sterol carrier protein X (SCPx) deficiency. Dystonic tremor, hypergonadotropic hypogonadism, and sensory motor neuropathy are seen in this rare disorder.

Refsum disease is due to autosomal recessively inherited phytanoyl-CoA hydroxylase deficiency that is required for alpha oxidation of the branched-chain fatty acid phytanic acid (238). Patients have deterioration of night vision, retinitis pigmentosa, anosmia, deafness, ataxia, and arrhythmias.

Hyperoxaluria type I (oxalosis 1). This rare autosomal recessive disease results from mutations in the *AGXT* gene encoding the hepatic peroxisomal alanine–glyoxylate aminotransferase (239,240). High urine oxalate, progressive oxalate nephrocalcinosis, and oxalate urolithiasis are seen, and calcium oxalates deposit in many sites including bone, soft tissue, eye, and cardiac conduction system. Patients may have renal failure, recurrent fractures, and cardiac arrhythmias and die before 20 years of age. The liver is grossly normal, but oxalate crystals may be present in the hepatic arterioles and gallbladder. The crystals have a rosette pattern with radial striations and a starburst appearance seen with polarized light.

CONGENITAL DISORDERS OF GLYCOSYLATION (CDG), FORMERLY KNOWN AS CARBOHYDRATE-DEFICIENT GLYCOPROTEIN SYNDROMES

Together with glycogen storage disease type I (discussed above) and alpha-1-antitrypsin deficiency (discussed in Chapter 15), these form a group of conditions that can all be grouped together as disorders of endoplasmic reticulum.

Congenital disorders of glycosylation (CDG) are a heterogeneous group of multisystem disorders linked to abnormal synthesis of glycan moieties of glycoproteins or glycolipid (241,242). This group of diseases has grown to include at least 45 members. This large number is reflective of the complex process involved in the process of glycosylation. N-linked glycosylation includes the following steps: (a) assembly of $Man_5GlcNAc_2$ in the cytoplasm, (b) translocation into the ER, (c) further assembly in the ER to $Glc_3Man_9GlcNAc_2$ and transfer to asparagine residues on nascent proteins, and (d) processing in the Golgi by trimming and addition of further residues. O-linked glycosylation only involves assembly in the Golgi through addition of glycans to the hydroxyl groups of threonine or serine of proteins. With the increase in entities, the classification system has changed. The most common diseases are the ones affecting N-glycosylation. These were traditionally classified as defects of assembly (group I) and processing (type II). A new proposed classification system names these according to the name of the affected gene and ending of "-CDG," for example, PMM2-CDG for cases linked to mutations in *PMM2* (241,242). All known CDGs are inherited as autosomal recessive traits except EXT1-/EXT2-CDG leading to an autosomal dominant presentation with multiple exostoses, and MAGT1-CDG, which is X-linked. Because of the abnormal assembly or processing of carbohydrate moieties of glycoconjugates, there is abnormal glycosylation of glycoproteins. Diagnosis is usually made by analyzing the glycosylation status of transferrin and apolipoprotein C-III, most commonly by isoelectric focusing, chromatography, or capillary electrophoresis. Not all cases, however, are associated with diagnostic abnormalities on these tests. Newer methodology using mass spectrometry is likely to be more informative. Subsequent confirmatory testing by enzyme assay, DNA analysis, glycan analysis on fibroblasts, or complementation assays is required if the screening test is abnormal.

CDG-I patients have a defect in assembly of *N*-glycan moieties in the cytosol and endoplasmic reticulum. CDG-Ia is the most common CDG and is caused by deficient phosphomannomutase (PMM2-CDG according to the proposed new classification) (241). Patients have a variable phenotype with eye movement abnormalities, developmental delay, hypotonia, ataxia, stroke-like episodes, seizures, and facial dysmorphism (Table 5-14). Nonimmune hydrops has also been described in CDG-Ia. CDG-Ib (MPI-CDG) is the one CDG with relative neurologic sparing. The liver is primarily affected, and patients may have cyclic vomiting, hypoglycemia, failure to thrive, liver fibrosis, and protein-losing enteropathy (Table 5-14). This form responds to oral mannose supplementation and is the one CDG with an established treatment option.

CDG-II patients have a defect in processing of *N*-glycan moieties of glycoconjugate in the Golgi. Clinical findings are variable depending upon the type and include dysmorphism, microcephaly, liver dysfunction, hypotonia, severe cognitive impairment, seizures, lipodystrophy, hypertrophic cardiomyopathy, peripheral neuropathy, and hydrops fetalis (Table 5-14).

In CDG patients, there is often severe neonatal-onset olivopontocerebellar atrophy with Purkinje and granule cell depletion; atrophy of cerebellar white matter; and loss of pontine nuclei, inferior olives, and middle and inferior cerebellar peduncles with relative sparing of dentate neurons. Outside the CNS, pleural and pericardial effusions, hypertrophic obstructive cardiomyopathy, cystic dilatation of renal tubules and collecting ducts, steatosis, ductal plate abnormalities, portal fibrosis, cirrhosis, and retinal dystrophy with pigment epithelium degeneration are seen. Many

TABLE 5-14 CARBOHYDRATE-DEFICIENT GLYCOPROTEIN DISORDERS

CDG Subtype	Gene	Protein	Major Clinical Features	Comments
CDG-Ia	PMM2	Phosphomannomutase II	Cognitive impairment (CI) Seizures Hypotonia Strabismus Abnormal fat distribution Inverted nipples Coagulopathy Cerebellar hypoplasia/atrophy Ataxia	Most common form of CDG Incidence may be 1:20,000. Enzyme and mutation analysis clinically available No treatment available Occasionally normal transferrin electrophoresis
CDG-Ib	MPI	Phosphomannose isomerase	Hepatic fibrosis Coagulopathy Protein-losing enteropathy Hypoglycemia Cyclic vomiting	Treatment with oral mannose resolves symptoms. No brain involvement; normal development
CDG-Ic	ALG6	Glucosyltransferase I Dol-p-Glc: Man(9) GlcNAc(2)-PP-dolichyl glucosyltransferase	CI	Second most common form of CDG Seizures Hypotonia Strabismus
CDG-Id	ALG3	Dolichyl-P-Man:Man(5) GlcNAc(2)-PP-dolichyl mannosyltransferase	Severe CI seizures; hypsarrhythmia Optic nerve atrophy Iris colobomas	
CDG-Ie	DPM1	Dolichol-phosphate mannose synthetase I	Severe CI Seizures Hypotonia Coagulopathy	
CDG-If	MPDU1	Mannose-P-dolichol utilization defect 1/Lec 35	CI Pigmentary retinopathy Short stature Ichthyosis	Episodes of hypertonia
CDG-Ig	ALG12	Dolichyl-P-Man:Man(7) GlcNAc(2)-PP-dolichyl mannosyltransferase	CI Hypotonia Microcephaly Frequent infections	
CDG-Ih	ALG8	Glucosyltransferase II dolichyl-P-Glc:Glc(1)Man(9)GlcNAc(2)-P-P-Dol glucosyltransferase	Hepatomegaly Protein-losing enteropathy Coagulopathy Renal failure	
CDG-Ii	ALG2	Mannosyltransferase II GDP-Man:Man(1) GlcNAc(2)-P-P-Dol mannosyltransferase	CI Severe seizures Coloboma of the eye Coagulopathy	
CDG-Ij	DPAGT1	UDP-GlcNAc: dolichol phosphate N-acetylglucosamine-1-phosphate transferase	Severe CI Seizures Hypotonia Microcephaly	

(Continued)

TABLE 5-14 CARBOHYDRATE-DEFICIENT GLYCOPROTEIN DISORDERS (Continued)

CDG Subtype	Gene	Protein	Major Clinical Features	Comments
CDG-Ik	ALG1	Mannosyltransferase I GDP-Man: GlcNAc(2)-PP-Dol mannosyltransferase	Severe CI Hypotonia Microcephaly Coagulopathy Nephrotic syndrome	
CDG-Il	ALG9	Mannosyltransferase Dol-P-Man:Man(6)- and Man(8)-GlcNAc(2)-P-P-Dol mannosyltransferase	Severe microcephaly Seizures Hypotonia Hepatomegaly	
CDG-IIa	MGAT2	GlcNAc transferase II	CI Seizures Dysmorphic facies	Normal cerebellum
CDG-IIb	GCS1	Glucosidase I	Hepatomegaly; hepatic fibrosis Seizures Hypotonia Dysmorphic facies	Normal transferrin on isoelectric focusing
CDG-IIc	SLC35C1	GDP-fucose transporter 1	CI Hypotonia Microcephaly Frequent infections; persistently elevated peripheral leukocyte count	Normal transferrin on isoelectric focusing May be treatable with fucose supplementation
CDG-IId	B4GALT1	Beta-1,4-galactosyltransferase 1	Hypotonia due to myopathy Spontaneous hemorrhage Dandy-Walker malformation with hydrocephalus	
CDG-IIe	COG7	Conserved oligomeric Golgi complex subunit 7	Severe seizures Hepatomegaly Progressive jaundice Frequent infections Cardiac failure Dysmorphic facies	Fatal in infancy
CDG-IIf	SLC35A1	CMP-sialic acid transporter	Thrombocytopenia Abnormal platelet glycoproteins	Normal transferrin on isoelectric focusing No neurologic abnormality

patients have a coagulopathy due to low levels of clotting factors, although it is usually not clinically significant except during surgery or following trauma.

LIPID METABOLISM DISORDERS

Smith-Lemli-Opitz Syndrome

This autosomal recessive disorder of cholesterol biosynthesis is due to deficiency in 7-dehydrocholesterol reductase encoded by the *DHCR7* gene (243–246). The enzyme defect leads to low levels of cholesterol and high levels of 7-dehydrocholesterol. Cholesterol levels may have an effect on normal development through different mechanisms including an effect on the sonic hedgehog signaling pathway. The variable disease phenotypes include microcephaly, holoprosencephaly, limb malformations, cognitive impairment, behavioral disorders, hypotonia, dysmorphic facies, cleft palate, ambiguous genitalia, and congenital heart disease. Plasma cholesterol is reduced; patients with very low cholesterol levels have a more severe phenotype, and cholesterol deficiency may have a role in dysmorphogenesis.

Morphologic findings include reduced myelination of the cerebral hemispheres and cranial and peripheral nerves, absent corpus callosum, cerebellar hypoplasia, abnormal gyral pattern, and altered neuronal migration. There is pancreatic enlargement and islet cell nuclear hyperchromasia, and liver has nonspecific changes (Figure 5-21A,B) with cholestasis.

Conradi-Hunermann Syndrome (CDPX2)

This X-linked dominant disorder of sterol metabolism is caused by a deficiency of sterol-Δ^8-isomerase, also known as emopamil binding protein (245–247). The enzyme encoded by the *EBP* gene converts 8-dehydrocholesterol to 7-dehydrocholesterol, one step before the enzymatic step that is abnormal in Smith-Lemli-Opitz syndrome. Typical features include chondrodysplasia punctata, cataracts, bilateral and asymmetrical limb anomalies, joint contractures, ichthyosiform skin lesions following Blaschko lines, patchy alopecia, and short stature. The skin lesions are most severe at birth and histologically show hyperkeratosis, parakeratosis, and marked acanthosis. Lesions improve with age, leaving behind follicular atrophoderma ("orange peel" lesions) and hypopigmented streaks that follow Blaschko lines. It was originally thought that this defect would be lethal in males; however, there have been two affected male patients reported (one of whom was a somatic mosaic for the genetic defect and the other of whom had a very severe phenotype). Plasma sterol analysis shows elevated 8-dehydrocholesterol and 8(9)-cholestenol. Blood cholesterol levels are typically normal (see Chapter 28).

CHILD Syndrome (Congenital Hemidysplasia with Ichthyosiform Erythroderma and Limb Defects)

This is a rare X-linked dominant disorder of sterol metabolism linked to mutations of the *NSDHL* gene, which encodes the 3β-hydroxysteroid dehydrogenase component of the

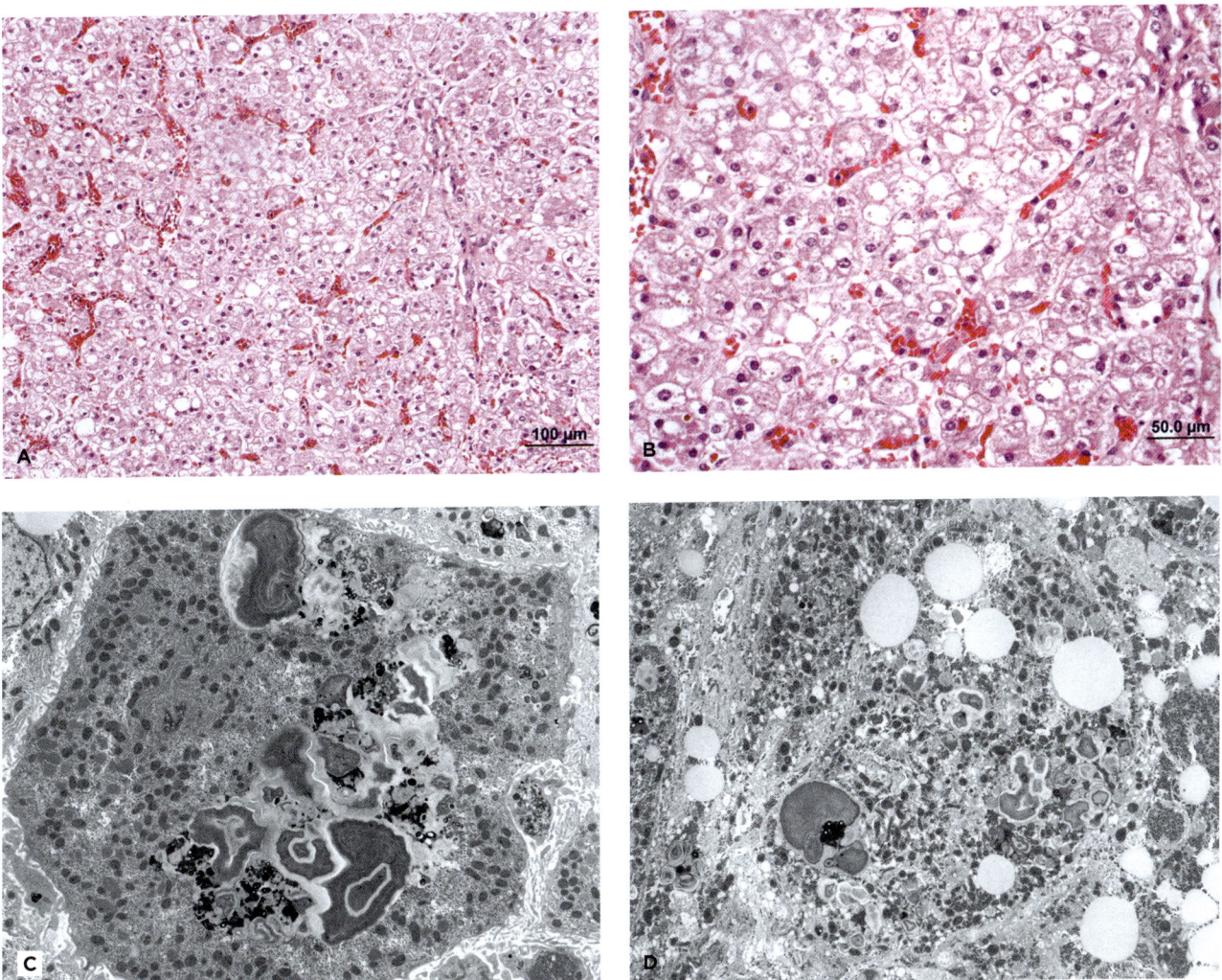

FIGURE 5-21 • Smith-Lemli-Opitz syndrome. **A, B:** Hepatocellular disarray in Smith-Lemli-Opitz syndrome (H&E). **C, D:** Hepatocytes with multiple cytoplasmic whorled structures, lamellar structures, lipid droplets, and lipofuscin in Smith-Lemli-Opitz syndrome (**C, D:** Uranyl acetate, lead citrate).

sterol-4-demethylase protein. It is characterized by unilateral ichthyosiform skin lesions, often sharply demarcated at the midline of the trunk; limb deficiencies; and punctate calcifications of the epiphyses and other cartilaginous structures (245,246,248). In addition, ipsilateral visceral anomalies can be present, including brain, renal, lung, and cardiac defects. While some of the skin lesions follow Blaschko lines, many patients have more extensive patches of abnormal skin. It is generally presumed to be lethal in males. A few patients with the CHILD phenotype have been found to have a defect in sterol-Δ^8-isomerase as in CDPX2.

The skin abnormality in the *NSDHL* defect is typically a persistent scaly, raised, and sometimes verrucous lesion. Skin biopsy of the *NSDHL* defect shows marked ichthyosiform epidermal hyperplasia, inflammation, and sometimes foamy histiocytes within the dermal papillae (referred to as *verruciform xanthoma*). The lesions may regress with age. Sterol analysis of plasma, lymphocytes, and fibroblasts shows abnormally increased levels of 4-methylsterols.

SUDDEN INFANT DEATH AND AUTOPSIES IN THE SETTING OF INBORN ERRORS OF METABOLISM

Sudden Death in Infants with Inborn Errors of Metabolism

Sudden unexpected death in infancy (SUDI) is defined as sudden unexpected death occurring before the age of 12 months and has a reported incidence of approximately 1/3000 (249). Many metabolic disorders can cause SUDI or acute metabolic crisis in infants, in some cases without preceding clinical symptoms (Table 5-15) (250,251). A key feature of the clinical history that could suggest an IEM in a young infant is deterioration in the clinical status after a symptom-free interval of hours to days. Findings that may indicate an IEM include family history of a similar sudden death, particularly in a sibling; dysmorphic features; enlarged liver, spleen, or heart; fatty or pale liver, heart, muscle, or kidney; or cerebral edema.

Inherited defects of FAO have been shown to cause 2% to 5% of SUDI cases, and these are the most common disorders presenting as SUDI (249,252). Of these, medium-chain acyl-CoA dehydrogenase deficiency (MCAD) is the most common IEM that causes SUDI. As many as a third of affected infants die during the initial presentation, often without previous clinical evidence of a FAO defect. Hypoglycemia following birth or hypoketotic hypoglycemia suggests the diagnostic possibility of MCAD.

Autopsy of Children with Suspected Inborn Errors of Metabolism

The autopsy may include photography, radiography, histology, histochemistry, ultrastructural examination, fibroblast culture, biochemical analysis, and DNA analysis (253,254).

TABLE 5-15 INBORN ERRORS OF METABOLISM THAT CAUSE HYDROPS FETALIS

Lysosomal storage disease
   Mucopolysaccharidosis types I, IVA, and VII
   I-cell disease (mucolipidosis II)
   Mucolipidosis IV
   GM1 gangliosidosis
   Wolman disease
   Fabry disease
   Farber disease
   Gaucher disease type II
   Sialidosis
   Galactosialidosis
   Niemann-Pick disease types A, C
Glycogen storage disease type IV
Long-chain hydroxyacyl-CoA dehydrogenase deficiency
Primary carnitine deficiency
Pearson marrow-pancreas syndrome
Congenital disorders of glycosylation (CDG)
Neonatal hemochromatosis

It is important to do the autopsy as soon as possible after death, preferably within 2 hours. Photographs and whole body radiographs will document dysmorphology that can be seen in a number of IEM. Hydrops suggests another group of disorders (Tables 5-2 and 5-15). There are several suggested protocols for sample collection in cases of unexpected metabolic death (255,256).

Biochemical studies will be directed based on the autopsy findings, but it is important to collect tissue and fluids that may be useful for further evaluation (Table 5-16). Since sepsis and intoxication can mimic IEM, cultures and toxicology may be necessary. Urine should be collected by catheterization or suprapubic tap, placed in a preservative-free container, and frozen at -20°C for amino and organic acid analysis. Blood, serum, and plasma are useful for whole blood acylcarnitine analysis by MS/MS, which is compared to postmortem sample reference ranges (252,256). Spotting a few drops of whole blood obtained by cardiac puncture onto filter paper (i.e., Guthrie card) is the most efficient collection method and suitable for many analyses. If more blood is available, collect heparinized blood, separate, and store plasma at -20°C. Red blood cells can be stored at +4°C (256).

If DNA is to be analyzed, collect whole blood in EDTA and keep at room temperature or +4°C until DNA can be extracted. Genomic DNA (25 to 60 μg) can be obtained from 1 to 2 mL of blood.

CSF can be obtained by cisternal puncture by hyperflexing the neck and inserting a needle between the atlas and the axis vertebrae. CSF may only provide reliable information if collected before death, but it is useful in certain circumstances, especially for mitochondrial respiratory chain diseases and organic acid and acylcarnitine analyses (256). Collect two

TABLE 5-16	SPECIMENS TO BE TAKEN IN AUTOPSY OF AN INFANT WITH POSSIBLE INBORN ERROR IN METABOLISM
Specimen	Storage
Urine	−20°C
CSF	−70°C
Whole blood in EDTA for DNA	Room temperature or +4°C
Serum	−20°C
Vitreous	−20°C
Erythrocytes	+4°C
Bile	−20°C
Skin for fibroblast culture	Room temperature or +4°C
Brain, heart, kidney, liver, skeletal muscle, adrenal	−70°C
Brain, heart, kidney, liver, skeletal muscle	In 2% glutaraldehyde

Sources: Byard RW. Sudden Death in Infancy, Childhood and Adolescence. Cambridge, UK: Cambridge University Press; 2004; Fitzpatrick D. Genetic metabolic disease. In: Keeling JW, ed. Fetal and Neonatal Pathology. London, UK/New York: Springer; 2001:153–174.

1-mL samples, one in a plain tube and one in fluoride oxalate, and store at -70°C (256). Vitreous humor can be collected into a fluoride tube and stored at -20°C for glucose and electrolyte analysis.

Bile may be the only analyzable fluid in cases where the interval between death and autopsy is long. In all cases where there is a possibility of underlying metabolic disease, a sample of bile should be obtained (256). Bile can be collected on filter paper or a Guthrie card for acylcarnitine testing or collected in a plain tube for storage at -20°C.

Tissues must be taken promptly if accurate results are to be obtained. One cubic centimeter of tissue from the brain, kidney, muscle, liver, and other viscera can be snap frozen in liquid nitrogen, wrapped in foil, and stored at -70°C. Liver and skeletal muscle can be obtained at the bedside after death (256). Fresh frozen muscle is the tissue of choice for the diagnosis of mitochondrial respiratory chain disorders. Complexes I, II, III, and IV of the respiratory chain can be measured (256). Some enzymes of intermediary metabolism are more stable, and tissue analysis may provide essential diagnostic information, even when obtained at the time of a routine autopsy. Both MCAD and LCAD in the liver may be stable up to 100 hours after death if the body is refrigerated and for 5 years if tissue is kept at -70°C.

Fibroblast culture is essential for the evaluation of many IEM, and obtaining skin for fibroblasts should be part of any autopsy on an infant or child who dies from unknown cause; this may be the only tissue on which a suspected diagnosis can be confirmed (256). Fibroblasts can be used for studies of DNA, enzymes, and metabolites and for karyotype and can be saved for future studies (257,258). Achilles tendon, kidney, pericardium, and fascia may also be used as a source of fibroblasts. Skin is not a good choice for cell culture for a macerated fetus; in that case, placental villi, kidney, lung, or heart could be used for culture. Take two pieces of tissue from different sites, using sterile technique, and place in separate sterile vials containing culture transport medium (HamF10, Eagle MEM, Dulbecco medium, or sterile normal saline if the only solution available). Taking samples at the beginning of the autopsy is recommended because of the lower risk of bacterial contamination (256). Skin fibroblasts remain viable for up to 9 days after death, but they should be obtained as soon as possible as this increases chance of successful culture. Store specimen at 4°C (not below 0°C) until it can be delivered to the cell culture lab. Cultivated fibroblasts can be cryopreserved for an indefinite period for future studies.

Histologic, histochemical, and ultrastructural findings can be a guide to diagnosis but are unfortunately often nonspecific. Liver and kidney frozen sections can be used to look for lipid. Although not specific for and not always present in FAO defects, steatosis can occur in SUDI due to these disorders. Increased glycogen suggests altered glycogen metabolism. If membrane bound, it suggests GSD type II.

Unless tissue is obtained minutes after death, ultrastructure is seldom well preserved; however, abnormal storage may remain identifiable even in autolyzed tissue. EM requires sectioning tissues into 1-mm^3 pieces and fixation in 2% glutaraldehyde. LM and histochemistry can be performed on skeletal muscle up to 24 hours after death in children using a 1 to 2 mm in diameter, 1-cm long strip of muscle frozen in liquid nitrogen-cooled isopentane (-170°C). An infant with unexplained nonimmune hydrops may show characteristic lysosomal material suggesting a storage disease in viscera, brain, placental villi, or amnion cells.

ACKNOWLEDGMENTS

The contributions of Drs. Carole A. Vogler, David S. Brink, and Dorothy K. Grange to the 3rd edition of this book, which the current chapter is based on, are gratefully acknowledged.

References

1. Rosenberg LE. Legacies of Garrod's brilliance. One hundred years—and counting. *J Inherit Metab Dis* 2008;31:574–579, doi:10.1007/s10545-008-0985-8.
2. Jevon GP, Dimmick JE. Histopathologic approach to metabolic liver disease: Part 2. *Pediatr Dev Pathol* 1998;1:261–269.
3. Jevon GP, Dimmick JE. Histopathologic approach to metabolic liver disease: Part 1. *Pediatr Dev Pathol* 1998;1:179–199.
4. Landau YE, Lichter-Konecki U, Levy HL. Genomics in newborn screening. *J Pediatr* 2014;164:14–19, doi:10.1016/j.jpeds.2013.07.028.
5. Wilcken B, Wiley V. Newborn screening methods for cystic fibrosis. *Paediatr Respir Rev* 2003;4:272–277.
6. Koprivica V, et al. Analysis and classification of 304 mutant alleles in patients with type 1 and type 3 Gaucher disease. *Am J Hum Genet* 2000;66:1777–1786, doi:10.1086/302925.
7. Aronovich EL, Pan D, Whitley CB. Molecular genetic defect underlying alpha-l-iduronidase pseudodeficiency. *Am J Hum Genet* 1996;58:75–85.

8. Wang J, et al. Clinical application of massively parallel sequencing in the molecular diagnosis of glycogen storage diseases of genetically heterogeneous origin. *Genet Med* 2013;15:106–114, doi:10.1038/gim.2012.104.
9. Jones MA, et al. Molecular diagnostic testing for congenital disorders of glycosylation (CDG): detection rate for single gene testing and next generation sequencing panel testing. *Mol Genet Metab* 2013;110:78–85, doi:10.1016/j.ymgme.2013.05.012.
10. Dinwiddie DL, et al. Diagnosis of mitochondrial disorders by concomitant next-generation sequencing of the exome and mitochondrial genome. *Genomics* 2013;102:148–156, doi:10.1016/j.ygeno.2013.04.013.
11. Hers HG. Inborn lysosomal diseases. *Gastroenterology* 1965;48:625–633.
12. Boustany RM. Lysosomal storage diseases—the horizon expands. *Nat Rev Neurol* 2013;9:583–598, doi:10.1038/nrneurol.2013.163.
13. Platt FM. Sphingolipid lysosomal storage disorders. *Nature* 2014;510:68–75, doi:10.1038/nature13476.
14. Kadali S, Kolusu A, Gummadi MR, et al. The relative frequency of lysosomal storage disorders: a medical genetics referral laboratory's experience from India. *J Child Neurol* 2014;29:1377–1382. doi:10.1177/0883073813515075.
15. Pastores GM, Maegawa GH. Clinical neurogenetics: neuropathic lysosomal storage disorders. *Neurol Clin* 2013;31:1051–1071, doi:10.1016/j.ncl.2013.04.007.
16. Bonduelle M, et al. Lysosomal storage diseases presenting as transient or persistent hydrops fetalis. *Genet Couns* 1991;2:227–232.
17. Soma H, et al. Identification of Gaucher cells in the chorionic villi associated with recurrent hydrops fetalis. *Placenta* 2000;21:412–416, doi:10.1053/plac.1999.0483.
18. Schultz ML, Tecedor L, Chang M, et al. Clarifying lysosomal storage diseases. *Trends Neurosci* 2011;34:401–410, doi:10.1016/j.tins.2011.05.006.
19. Alroy J, Ucci AA. Skin biopsy: a useful tool in the diagnosis of lysosomal storage diseases. *Ultrastruct Pathol* 2006;30:489–503, doi:10.1080/01913120500520986.
20. Ceuterick-de Groote C, Martin JJ. Extracerebral biopsy in lysosomal and peroxisomal disorders. Ultrastructural findings. *Brain Pathol* 1998;8:121–132.
21. Libert J. Diagnosis of lysosomal storage diseases by the ultrastructural study of conjunctival biopsies. *Pathol Annu* 1980;15:37–66.
22. Prasad A, Kaye EM, Alroy J. Electron microscopic examination of skin biopsy as a cost-effective tool in the diagnosis of lysosomal storage diseases. *J Child Neurol* 1996;11:301–308.
23. Vogler C, Rosenberg HS, Williams JC, et al. Electron microscopy in the diagnosis of lysosomal storage diseases. *Am J Med Genet Suppl* 1987;3:243–255.
24. Anderson GW, Goebel HH, Simonati A. Human pathology in NCL. *Biochim Biophys Acta* 2013;1832:1807–1826, doi:10.1016/j.bbadis.2012.11.014.
25. Weber AF, Phillips MG, Bell JT Jr. An improved method for the Schultz cholesterol test. *J Histochem Cytochem* 1956;4:308–309.
26. Kim SU. Lysosomal storage diseases: stem cell-based cell- and gene-therapy. *Cell Transplant* 2014. doi:10.3727/096368914X681946.
27. Hollak CE, Wijburg FA. Treatment of lysosomal storage disorders: successes and challenges. *J Inherit Metab Dis* 2014;37:587–598. doi:10.1007/s10545-014-9718-3.
28. Takahashi T, et al. Enzyme therapy in Gaucher disease type 2: an autopsy case. *Tohoku J Exp Med* 1998;186:143–149.
29. Lund TC. Hematopoietic stem cell transplant for lysosomal storage diseases. *Pediatr Endocrinol Rev* 2013;11(Suppl 1):91–98.
30. Sondhi D, et al. Partial correction of the CNS lysosomal storage defect in a mouse model of juvenile neuronal ceroid lipofuscinosis by neonatal CNS administration of an adeno-associated virus serotype rh.10 vector expressing the human CLN3 gene. *Hum Gene Ther* 2014;25:223–239, doi:10.1089/hum.2012.253.
31. Chen M, Wang J. Gaucher disease: review of the literature. *Arch Pathol Lab Med* 2008;132:851–853. doi:10.1043/1543-2165(2008)132[851:GDROTL]2.0.CO;2.
32. Jmoudiak M, Futerman AH. Gaucher disease: pathological mechanisms and modern management. *Br J Haematol* 2005;129:178–188. doi:10.1111/j.1365-2141.2004.05351.x.
33. Diaz GA, et al. Gaucher disease: the origins of the Ashkenazi Jewish N370S and 84GG acid beta-glucosidase mutations. *Am J Hum Genet* 2000;66:1821–1832, doi:10.1086/302946
34. Murray GJ, Oliver KL, Jin FS, et al. Studies on the turnover of exogenous mannose-terminal glucocerebrosidase in rat liver lysosomes. *J Cell Biochem* 1995;57:208–217. doi:10.1002/jcb.240570205
35. Wenstrup RJ, Roca-Espiau M, Weinreb NJ, et al. Skeletal aspects of Gaucher disease: a review. *Br J Radiol* 2002;75(Suppl 1):A2–A12.
36. Schiffmann R. Fabry disease. *Pharmacol Ther* 2009;122:65–77. doi:10.1016/j.pharmthera.2009.01.003
37. Clarke JT. Narrative review: Fabry disease. *Ann Intern Med* 2007;146:425–433.
38. Germain DP, et al. Analysis of left ventricular mass in untreated men and in men treated with agalsidase-beta: data from the Fabry Registry. *Genet Med* 2013;15:958–965. doi:10.1038/gim.2013.53.
39. Nakao S, et al. Fabry disease: detection of undiagnosed hemodialysis patients and identification of a "renal variant" phenotype. *Kidney Int* 2003;64:801–807, doi:10.1046/j.1523-1755.2003.00160.x.
40. Wang RY, Lelis A, Mirocha J, et al. Heterozygous Fabry women are not just carriers, but have a significant burden of disease and impaired quality of life. *Genet Med* 2007;9:34–45. doi:10.1097GIM.0b013e31802d8321.
41. Bradshaw SE. Electron microscopy illuminates the pathology of Fabry nephropathy. *Nat Rev Nephrol* 2011;7:126.
42. Fischer EG, Moore MJ, Lager DJ. Fabry disease: a morphologic study of 11 cases. *Mod Pathol* 2006;19:1295–1301. doi:10.1038/modpathol.3800634.
43. Patterson MC. Gangliosidoses. *Handb Clin Neurol* 2013;113:1707–1708. doi:10.1016/B978-0-444-59565-2.00039-3.
44. Regier DS, Tifft CJ. In: Pagon RA, ed. GeneReviews(R); 1993 Seattle (WA): University of Washington, Seattle; 1993-2015. Available from: http://www.ncbi.nlm.nih.gov/books/NBK164500/.
45. Itoh H, Tanaka J, Morihana Y, et al. The fine structure of cytoplasmic inclusions in brain and other visceral organs in Sandhoff disease. *Brain Dev* 1984;6:467–474.
46. Petrelli M, Blair JD. The liver in GM1 gangliosidosis types 1 and 2. A light and electron microscopical study. *Arch Pathol* 1975;99:111–116.
47. Neufeld EF. Natural history and inherited disorders of a lysosomal enzyme, beta-hexosaminidase. *J Biol Chem* 1989;264:10927–10930.
48. Rucker JC, et al. Neuro-ophthalmology of late-onset Tay-Sachs disease (LOTS). *Neurology* 2004;63:1918–1926.
49. von Specht BU, et al. Enzyme replacement in Tay-Sachs disease. *Neurology* 1979;29:848–854.
50. Mahuran DJ. Biochemical consequences of mutations causing the GM2 gangliosidoses. *Biochim Biophys Acta* 1999;1455:105–138.
51. Schepers U, et al. Molecular analysis of a GM2-activator deficiency in two patients with GM2-gangliosidosis AB variant. *Am J Hum Genet* 1996;59:1048–1056.
52. Vanier MT. Niemann-Pick diseases. *Handb Clin Neurol* 2013;113:1717–1721. doi:10.1016/B978-0-444-59565-2.00041-1.
53. Peake KB, Vance JE. Defective cholesterol trafficking in Niemann-Pick C-deficient cells. *FEBS Lett* 2010;584:2731–2739. doi:10.1016/j.febslet.2010.04.047.
54. McGovern MM, Aron A, Brodie SE, et al. Natural history of Type A Niemann-Pick disease: possible endpoints for therapeutic trials. *Neurology* 2006;66:228–232. doi:10.1212/01.wnl.0000194208.08904.0c.
55. Schuchman EH. The pathogenesis and treatment of acid sphingomyelinase-deficient Niemann-Pick disease. *J Inherit Metab Dis* 2007;30:654–663. doi:10.1007/s10545-007-0632-9.
56. Narita T, Nakazawa H, Hizawa Y, et al. Glycogen storage disease associated with Niemann-Pick disease: histochemical, enzymatic, and lipid analyses. *Mod Pathol* 1994;7:416–421.
57. Dawson PJ, Dawson G. Adult Niemann-Pick disease with sea-blue histiocytes in the spleen. *Hum Pathol* 1982;13:1115–1120.
58. Ledesma MD, Prinetti A, Sonnino S, et al. Brain pathology in Niemann Pick disease type A: insights from the acid sphingomyelinase knockout mice. *J Neurochem* 2011;116:779–788. doi:10.1111/j.1471-4159.2010.07034.x.

59. Greer WL, et al. The Nova Scotia (type D) form of Niemann-Pick disease is caused by a G3097-->T transversion in NPC1. *Am J Hum Genet* 1998;63:52–54. doi:10.1086/301931.
60. Jan MM, Camfield PR. Nova Scotia Niemann-Pick disease (type D): clinical study of 20 cases. *J Child Neurol* 1998;13:75–78.
61. Patterson MC, et al. Recommendations for the diagnosis and management of Niemann-Pick disease type C: an update. *Mol Genet Metab* 2012;106:330–344. doi:10.1016/j.ymgme.2012.03.012.
62. Rosenbaum AI, Maxfield FR. Niemann-Pick type C disease: molecular mechanisms and potential therapeutic approaches. *J Neurochem* 2011;116:789–795. doi:10.1111/j.1471-4159.2010.06976.x.
63. Spiegel R, et al. The clinical spectrum of fetal Niemann-Pick type C. *Am J Med Genet A* 2009;149A:446–450. doi:10.1002/ajmg.a.32642.
64. Hahn AF, et al. Nerve biopsy findings in Niemann-Pick type II (NPC). *Acta Neuropathol* 1994;87:149–154.
65. Semeraro LA, Riely CA, Kolodny EH, et al. Niemann-Pick variant lipidosis presenting as "neonatal hepatitis." *J Pediatr Gastroenterol Nutr* 1986;5:492–500.
66. Elleder M, et al. Liver findings in Niemann-Pick disease type C. *Histochem J* 1984;16:1147–1170.
67. Kohlschutter A. Lysosomal leukodystrophies: Krabbe disease and metachromatic leukodystrophy. *Handb Clin Neurol* 2013;113:1611–1618. doi:10.1016/B978-0-444-59565-2.00029-0.
68. Renaud DL. Lysosomal disorders associated with leukoencephalopathy. *Semin Neurol* 2012;32:51–54. doi:10.1055/s-0032-1306386.
69. Henseler M, et al. Analysis of a splice-site mutation in the sap-precursor gene of a patient with metachromatic leukodystrophy. *Am J Hum Genet* 1996;58:65–74.
70. Sakai N. Pathogenesis of leukodystrophy for Krabbe disease: molecular mechanism and clinical treatment. *Brain Dev* 2009;31:485–487. doi:10.1016/j.braindev.2009.03.001.
71. Park JH, Schuchman EH. Acid ceramidase and human disease. *Biochim Biophys Acta* 2006;1758:2133–2138. doi:10.1016/j.bbamem.2006.08.019.
72. Zappatini-Tommasi L, Dumontel C, Guibaud P, et al. Farber disease: an ultrastructural study. Report of a case and review of the literature. *Virchows Arch A Pathol Anat Histopathol* 1992;420:281–290.
73. Michalski JC, Klein A. Glycoprotein lysosomal storage disorders: alpha- and beta-mannosidosis, fucosidosis and alpha-N-acetylgalactosaminidase deficiency. *Biochim Biophys Acta* 1999;1455:69–84.
74. Malm D, Nilssen O. Alpha-mannosidosis. *Orphanet J Rare Dis* 2008;3:21. doi:10.1186/1750-1172-3-21.
75. Bedilu R, et al. Variable clinical presentation of lysosomal beta-mannosidosis in patients with null mutations. *Mol Genet Metab* 2002;77:282–290.
76. Molho-Pessach V, et al. Angiokeratoma corporis diffusum in human beta-mannosidosis: report of a new case and a novel mutation. *J Am Acad Dermatol* 2007;57:407–412. doi:10.1016/j.jaad.2007.01.037.
77. Willems PJ, et al. Fucosidosis revisited: a review of 77 patients. *Am J Med Genet* 1991;38:111–131. doi:10.1002/ajmg.1320380125.
78. Caciotti A, et al. Type II sialidosis: review of the clinical spectrum and identification of a new splicing defect with chitotriosidase assessment in two patients. *J Neurol* 2009;256:1911–1915. doi:10.1007/s00415-009-5213-4.
79. Seyrantepe V, et al. Molecular pathology of NEU1 gene in sialidosis. *Hum Mutat* 2003;22:343–352. doi:10.1002/humu.10268.
80. Aronson NN Jr. Aspartylglycosaminuria: biochemistry and molecular biology. *Biochim Biophys Acta* 1999;1455:139–154.
81. Arvio P, Arvio M, Marttinen E, et al. Excessive infantile growth and early pubertal growth spurt: typical features in patients with aspartylglycosaminuria. *J Pediatr* 1999;134:761–763.
82. Banugaria SG, et al. The impact of antibodies on clinical outcomes in diseases treated with therapeutic protein: lessons learned from infantile Pompe disease. *Genet Med* 2011;13:729–736. doi:10.1097/GIM.0b013e3182174703.
83. Bembi B, et al. Diagnosis of glycogenosis type II. *Neurology* 2008;71:S4–S11. doi:10.1212/WNL.0b013e31818da91e.
84. Bembi B, et al. Management and treatment of glycogenosis type II. *Neurology* 2008;71:S12–S36. doi:10.1212/WNL.0b013e31818da93f.
85. Prater SN, et al. The emerging phenotype of long-term survivors with infantile Pompe disease. *Genet Med* 2012;14:800–810. doi:10.1038/gim.2012.44.
86. Laforet P, et al. Juvenile and adult-onset acid maltase deficiency in France: genotype-phenotype correlation. *Neurology* 2000;55:1122–1128.
87. Lampe C, Bellettato CM, Karabul N, et al. Mucopolysaccharidoses and other lysosomal storage diseases. *Rheum Dis Clin N Am* 2013;39:431–455. doi:10.1016/j.rdc.2013.03.004.
88. Wraith JE. Mucopolysaccharidoses and mucolipidoses. *Handb Clin Neurol* 2013;113:1723–1729. doi:10.1016/B978-0-444-59565-2.00042-3.
89. Stevenson DA, Steiner RD. Skeletal abnormalities in lysosomal storage diseases. *Pediatr Endocrinol Rev* 2013;10(Suppl 2):406–416.
90. Bernstein DL, Hulkova H, Bialer MG, et al. Cholesteryl ester storage disease: review of the findings in 135 reported patients with an underdiagnosed disease. *J Hepatol* 2013;58:1230–1243. doi:10.1016/j.jhep.2013.02.014.
91. Reynolds T. Cholesteryl ester storage disease: a rare and possibly treatable cause of premature vascular disease and cirrhosis. *J Clin Pathol* 2013;66:918–923. doi:10.1136/jclinpath-2012-201302.
92. Zhang B, Porto AF. Cholesteryl ester storage disease: protean presentations of lysosomal acid lipase deficiency. *J Pediatr Gastroenterol Nutr* 2013;56:682–685. doi:10.1097/MPG.0b013e31828b36ac (2013).
93. Kornfeld S. Trafficking of lysosomal enzymes in normal and disease states. *J Clin Invest* 1986;77:1–6. doi:10.1172/JCI112262.
94. Bargal R, et al. When Mucolipidosis III meets Mucolipidosis II: GNPTA gene mutations in 24 patients. *Mol Genet Metab* 2006;88:359–363. doi:10.1016/j.ymgme.2006.03.003.
95. Otomo T, et al. Mucolipidosis II and III alpha/beta: mutation analysis of 40 Japanese patients showed genotype-phenotype correlation. *J Hum Genet* 2009;54:145–151. doi:10.1038/jhg.2009.3.
96. Koga M, et al. Histochemical and ultrastructural studies of inclusion bodies found in tissues from three siblings with I-cell disease. *Pathol Int* 1994;44:223–229.
97. Kiselyov K, et al. TRPML: transporters of metals in lysosomes essential for cell survival? *Cell Calcium* 2011;50:288–294. doi:10.1016/j.ceca.2011.04.009.
98. Wakabayashi K, Gustafson AM, Sidransky E, et al. Mucolipidosis type IV: an update. *Mol Genet Metab* 2011;104:206–213. doi:10.1016/j.ymgme.2011.06.006.
99. Schiffmann R, et al. Constitutive achlorhydria in mucolipidosis type IV. *Proc Natl Acad Sci U S A* 1998;95:1207–1212.
100. Nesterova G, Gahl WA. Cystinosis: the evolution of a treatable disease. *Pediatr Nephrol* 2013;28:51–59. doi:10.1007/s00467-012-2242-5.
101. Wilmer MJ, Schoeber JP, van den Heuvel LP, et al. Cystinosis: practical tools for diagnosis and treatment. *Pediatr Nephrol* 2011;26:205–215. doi:10.1007/s00467-010-1627-6.
102. Nishino I, et al. Primary LAMP-2 deficiency causes X-linked vacuolar cardiomyopathy and myopathy (Danon disease). *Nature* 2000;406:906–910. doi:10.1038/35022604.
103. Charron P, et al. Danon's disease as a cause of hypertrophic cardiomyopathy: a systematic survey. *Heart* 2004;90:842–846. doi:10.1136/hrt.2003.029504.
104. Boucek D, Jirikowic J, Taylor M. Natural history of Danon disease. *Genet Med* 2011;13:563–568. doi:10.1097/GIM.0b013e31820ad795.
105. Cenik B, Sephton CF, Kutluk Cenik B, et al. Progranulin: a proteolytically processed protein at the crossroads of inflammation and neurodegeneration. *J Biol Chem* 2012;287:32298–32306. doi:10.1074/jbc.R112.399170.
106. Hawkins-Salsbury JA, Cooper JD, Sands MS. Pathogenesis and therapies for infantile neuronal ceroid lipofuscinosis (infantile CLN1 disease). *Biochim Biophys Acta* 2013;1832:1906–1909. doi:10.1016/j.bbadis.2013.05.026.
106a. Carcel-Trullols J, Kovacs AD, Pearce DA. Cell biology of the NCL proteins: What they do and don't do. Biochim Biophys Acta [epub ahead of print]. doi:10.1016/j.bbadis.2015.04.027.
107. Hofman IL, van der Wal AC, Dingemans KP, et al. Cardiac pathology in neuronal ceroid lipofuscinoses—a clinicopathologic correlation in three patients. *Eur J Paediatr Neurol* 2001;5(Suppl A):213–217.

108. Blau N, van Spronsen FJ, Levy HL. Phenylketonuria. *Lancet* 2010;376:1417–1427. doi:10.1016/S0140-6736(10)60961-0.
109. Scriver CR. The PAH gene, phenylketonuria, and a paradigm shift. *Hum Mutat* 2007;28:831–845. doi:10.1002/humu.20526.
110. Phenylketonuria due to phenylalanine hydroxylase deficiency: an unfolding story. Medical Research Council Working Party on Phenylketonuria. *BMJ* 1993;306:115–119.
111. Paine RS. The variability in manifestations of untreated patients with phenylketonuria (phenylpyruvic aciduria). *Pediatrics* 1957;20:290–302.
112. Kölker S, et al. Pathogenesis of CNS involvement in disorders of amino and organic acid metabolism. *J Inherit Metab Dis* 2008;31:194–204. doi:10.1007/s10545-008-0823-z.
113. Debray F-G, et al. Diagnostic accuracy of blood lactate-to-pyruvate molar ratio in the differential diagnosis of congenital lactic acidosis. *Clin Chem* 2007;53:916–921. doi:10.1373/clinchem.2006.081166.
114. Dudesek A, et al. Molecular analysis and long-term follow-up of patients with different forms of 6-pyruvoyl-tetrahydropterin synthase deficiency. *Eur J Pediatr* 2001;160:267–276.
115. Opladen T, Hoffmann GF, Blau N. An international survey of patients with tetrahydrobiopterin deficiencies presenting with hyperphenylalaninaemia. *J Inherit Metab Dis* 2012;35:963–973. doi:10.1007/s10545-012-9506-x.
116. Tanguay RM, et al. Different molecular basis for fumarylacetoacetate hydrolase deficiency in the two clinical forms of hereditary tyrosinemia (type I). *Am J Hum Genet* 1990;47:308–316.
117. Scott CR. The genetic tyrosinemias. *Am J Med Genet C Semin Med Genet* 2006;142C:121–126. doi:10.1002/ajmg.c.30092.
118. van Dyk E, Steenkamp A, Koekemoer G, et al. Hereditary tyrosinemia type 1 metabolites impair DNA excision repair pathways. *Biochem Biophys Res Commun* 2010;401:32–36. doi:10.1016/j.bbrc.2010.09.002.
119. Dehner LP, et al. Hereditary tyrosinemia type I (chronic form): pathologic findings in the liver. *Hum Pathol* 1989;20:149–158.
120. Russo P, O'Regan S. Visceral pathology of hereditary tyrosinemia type I. *Am J Hum Genet* 1990;47:317–324.
121. Seda Neto J, et al. HCC prevalence and histopathological findings in liver explants of patients with hereditary tyrosinemia type 1. *Pediatr Blood Cancer* 2014;61:1584–1589. doi:10.1002/pbc.25094.
122. Lindblad B, et al. Cardiomyopathy in fumarylacetoacetase deficiency (hereditary tyrosinaemia): a new feature of the disease. *J Inherit Metab Dis* 1987;10:319–322. doi:10.1007/BF01811439.
123. Russo PA, Mitchell GA, Tanguay RM. Tyrosinemia: a review. *Pediatr Dev Pathol* 2001;4:212–221. doi:10.1007/s100240010146.
124. Masurel-Paulet A, et al. NTBC treatment in tyrosinaemia type I: long-term outcome in French patients. *J Inherit Metab Dis* 2008;31:81–87. doi:10.1007/s10545-008-0793-1.
125. Goldsmith LA. Molecular biology and molecular pathology of a newly described molecular disease—tyrosinemia II (the Richner-Hanhart syndrome). *Pathobiology* 1978;46:96–113. doi:10.1159/000162885.
126. Mudd SH. Hypermethioninemias of genetic and non-genetic origin: a review. *Am J Med Genet C Semin Med Genet* 2011;157C:3–32. doi:10.1002/ajmg.c.30293.
127. Mudd SH, et al. The natural history of homocystinuria due to cystathionine beta-synthase deficiency. *Am J Hum Genet* 1985;37:1–31.
128. Testai FD, Gorelick PB. Inherited metabolic disorders and stroke. Part 2: Homocystinuria, organic acidurias, and urea cycle disorders. *Arch Neurol* 2010;67:148–153. doi:10.1001/archneurol.2009.333.
129. Ozben T. Expanded newborn screening and confirmatory follow-up testing for inborn errors of metabolism detected by tandem mass spectrometry. *Clin Chem Lab Med* 2013;51:157–176. doi:10.1515/cclm-2012-0472.
130. Veríssimo C, et al. Nonketotic hyperglycinemia: a cause of encephalopathy in children. *J Child Neurol* 2013;28:251–254. doi:10.1177/0883073812441063.
131. Dinopoulos A, Matsubara Y, Kure S. Atypical variants of nonketotic hyperglycinemia. *Mol Genet Metab* 2005;86:61–69. doi:10.1016/j.ymgme.2005.07.016.
132. Applegarth DA, Toone JR. *J Inherit Metab Dis* 2004;27:417–422.
133. Perry TL, et al. Nonketotic hyperglycinemia. *N Engl J Med* 1975;292:1269–1273. doi:10.1056/NEJM197506122922404.
134. Agamanolis DP, Potter JL, Herrick MK, et al. The neuropathology of glycine encephalopathy. *Neurology* 1982;32:975–985.
135. Agamanolis DP, Potter JL, Lundgren DW. Neonatal glycine encephalopathy: biochemical and neuropathologic findings. *Pediatr Neurol* 1993;9:140–143. doi:10.1016/0887-8994(93)90051-D.
136. Applegarth DA, Toone JR. Nonketotic hyperglycinemia (glycine encephalopathy): laboratory diagnosis. *Mol Genet Metab* 2001;74:139–146. doi:10.1006/mgme.2001.3224.
137. Burrage LC, Nagamani SCS, Campeau PM, et al. Branched-chain amino acid metabolism: from rare Mendelian diseases to more common disorders. *Hum Mol Genet* 2014;23:R1–R8. doi:10.1093/hmg/ddu123.
138. Puffenberger EG. Genetic heritage of the Old Order Mennonites of southeastern Pennsylvania. *Am J Med Genet C Semin Med Genet* 2003;121C:18–31. doi:10.1002/ajmg.c.20003.
139. Podebrad F, et al. 4,5-Dimethyl-3-hydroxy-2 [5h]-furanone (sotolone)—the odour of maple syrup urine disease. *J Inherit Metab Dis* 1999;22:107–114.
140. Martin JJ, Schlote W. Central nervous system lesions in disorders of amino-acid metabolism. *J Neurol Sci* 1972;15:49–76. doi:10.1016/0022-510X(72)90121-9.
141. McCorvie TJ, Timson DJ. Structural and molecular biology of type I galactosemia: disease-associated mutations. *IUBMB Life* 2011;63:949–954. doi:10.1002/iub.510.
142. McCorvie TJ, Timson DJ. The structural and molecular biology of type I galactosemia: enzymology of galactose 1-phosphate uridylyltransferase. *IUBMB Life* 2011;63:694–700. doi:10.1002/iub.511.
143. Ridel KR, Leslie ND, Gilbert DL. An updated review of the long-term neurological effects of galactosemia. *Pediatr Neurol* 2005;33:153–161. doi:10.1016/j.pediatrneurol.2005.02.015.
144. Waisbren SE, et al. The adult galactosemic phenotype. *J Inherit Metab Dis* 2012;35:279–286. doi:10.1007/s10545-011-9372-y.
145. Karadag N, et al. Literature review and outcome of classic galactosemia diagnosed in the neonatal period. *Clin Lab* 2013;59:1139–1146.
146. Berry GT. Galactosemia: when is it a newborn screening emergency? *Mol Genet Metab* 2012;106:7–11. doi:10.1016/j.ymgme.2012.03.007.
147. Davit-Spraul A, et al. Hereditary fructose intolerance: frequency and spectrum mutations of the aldolase B gene in a large patients cohort from France—identification of eight new mutations. *Mol Genet Metab* 2008;94:443–447. doi:10.1016/j.ymgme.2008.05.003.
148. Santer R, et al. The spectrum of aldolase B (ALDOB) mutations and the prevalence of hereditary fructose intolerance in Central Europe. *Hum Mutat* 2005;25:594. doi:10.1002/humu.9343.
149. Bouteldja N, Timson DJ. The biochemical basis of hereditary fructose intolerance. *J Inherit Metab Dis* 2010;33:105–112. doi:10.1007/s10545-010-9053-2.
150. Roach PJ, Depaoli-Roach AA, Hurley TD, et al. Glycogen and its metabolism: some new developments and old themes. *Biochem J* 2012;441:763–787. doi:10.1042/BJ20111416.
151. Shin YS. Glycogen storage disease: clinical, biochemical, and molecular heterogeneity. *Semin Pediatr Neurol* 2006;13:115–120. doi:10.1016/j.spen.2006.06.007.
152. Oldfors A, DiMauro S. New insights in the field of muscle glycogenoses. *Curr Opin Neurol* 2013;26:544–553. doi:10.1097/WCO.0b013e328364dbdc.
153. Weinstein DA, Correia CE, Saunders AC, et al. Hepatic glycogen synthase deficiency: an infrequently recognized cause of ketotic hypoglycemia. *Mol Genet Metab* 2006;87:284–288. doi:10.1016/j.ymgme.2005.10.006.
154. Chou JY, Jun HS, Mansfield BC. Glycogen storage disease type I and G6Pase-beta deficiency: etiology and therapy. *Nat Rev Endocrinol* 2010;6:676–688. doi:10.1038/nrendo.2010.189.
155. Chou JY. The molecular basis of type 1 glycogen storage diseases. *Curr Mol Med* 2001;1:25–44.
156. Froissart R, et al. Glucose-6-phosphatase deficiency. *Orphanet J Rare Dis* 2011;6:27. doi:10.1186/1750-1172-6-27.

157. Mayatepek E, Hoffmann B, Meissner T. Inborn errors of carbohydrate metabolism. *Best Pract Res Clin Gastroenterol* 2010;24:607–618. doi:10.1016/j.bpg.2010.07.012.
158. Hershkovitz E, et al. Glycogen storage disease type III in Israel: presentation and long-term outcome. *Pediatr Endocrinol Rev* 2014;11:318–323.
159. Franchi-Abella S, Branchereau S. Benign hepatocellular tumors in children: focal nodular hyperplasia and hepatocellular adenoma. *Int J Hepatol* 2013;2013:215064. doi:10.1155/2013/215064.
160. Demo E, et al. Glycogen storage disease type III-hepatocellular carcinoma a long-term complication? *J Hepatol* 2007;46:492–498. doi:10.1016/j.jhep.2006.09.022.
161. Magoulas PL, El-Hattab AW. In: Pagon RA, et al., eds. *GeneReviews(R)*; Seattle (WA): University of Washington, Seattle; 1993-2015. Available from: http://www.ncbi.nlm.nih.gov/books/NBK115333/.
162. Escobar LF, Wagner S, Tucker M, et al. Neonatal presentation of lethal neuromuscular glycogen storage disease type IV. *J Perinatol* 2012;32:810–813. doi:10.1038/jp.2011.178.
163. Paradas C, et al. Branching enzyme deficiency: expanding the clinical spectrum. *JAMA Neurol* 2014;71:41–47. doi:10.1001/jamaneurol.2013.4888.
164. Lucia A, et al. McArdle disease: another systemic low-inflammation disorder? *Neurosci Lett* 2008;431:106–111. doi:10.1016/j.neulet.2007.11.028.
165. Burwinkel B, et al. Mutations in the liver glycogen phosphorylase gene (PYGL) underlying glycogenosis type VI. *Am J Hum Genet* 1998;62:785–791.
166. Bruser A, Kirchberger J, Schoneberg T. Altered allosteric regulation of muscle 6-phosphofructokinase causes Tarui disease. *Biochem Biophys Res Commun* 2012;427:133–137. doi:10.1016/j.bbrc.2012.09.024.
167. Toscano A, Musumeci O. Tarui disease and distal glycogenoses: clinical and genetic update. *Acta Myol* 2007;26:105–107.
168. Goldstein J, Austin S, Kishnani P, et al. In: Pagon RA, et al., eds. *GeneReviews(R)*; Seattle (WA): University of Washington, Seattle; 1993-2015. Available from: http://www.ncbi.nlm.nih.gov/books/NBK55061/.
169. Al-Haggar M. Fanconi-Bickel syndrome as an example of marked allelic heterogeneity. *World J Nephrol* 2012;1:63–68. doi:10.5527/wjn.v1.i3.63.
170. Grunert SC, Schwab KO, Pohl M, et al. Fanconi-Bickel syndrome: GLUT2 mutations associated with a mild phenotype. *Mol Genet Metab* 2012;105:433–437. doi:10.1016/j.ymgme.2011.11.200.
171. Gregersen N, Bross P, Andresen BS. Genetic defects in fatty acid beta-oxidation and acyl-CoA dehydrogenases. Molecular pathogenesis and genotype-phenotype relationships. *Eur J Biochem* 2004;271:470–482. doi:10.1046/j.1432-1033.2003.03949.x.
172. Bartlett, K. & Eaton, S. Mitochondrial beta-oxidation. *Eur J Biochem* 2004;271:462–469. doi:10.1046/j.1432-1033.2003.03947.x.
173. Wanders R, et al. Disorders of mitochondrial fatty acyl-CoA β-oxidation. *J Inherit Metab Dis* 1999;22:442–487.
174. Jethva R, Bennett MJ, Vockley J. Short-chain acyl-coenzyme A dehydrogenase deficiency. *Mol Genet Metab* 2008;95:195–200. doi:10.1016/j.ymgme.2008.09.007.
175. Yang Z, Lantz PE, Ibdah JA. Post-mortem analysis for two prevalent beta-oxidation mutations in sudden infant death. *Pediatr Int* 2007;49:883–887. doi:10.1111/j.1442-200X.2007.02478.x.
176. Aliefendioğlu D, et al. A newborn with VLCAD deficiency. Clinical, biochemical, and histopathological findings. *Eur J Pediatr* 2007;166:1077–1080. doi:10.1007/s00431-006-0350-6.
177. Singla M, Guzman G, Griffin AJ, et al. Cardiomyopathy in multiple Acyl-CoA dehydrogenase deficiency: a clinico-pathological correlation and review of literature. *Pediatr Cardiol* 2008;29:446–451. doi:10.1007/s00246-007-9119-6.
178. Kaye CI, et al. Newborn screening fact sheets. *Pediatrics* 2006;118:e934–e963, doi:10.1542/peds.2006-1783.
179. van Maldegem BT, Wanders RJA, Wijburg FA. Clinical aspects of short-chain acyl-CoA dehydrogenase deficiency. *J Inherit Metab Dis* 2010;33:507–511. doi:10.1007/s10545-010-9080-z.
180. Schatz UA, Ensenauer R. The clinical manifestation of MCAD deficiency: challenges towards adulthood in the screened population. *J Inherit Metab Dis* 2010;33:513–520. doi:10.1007/s10545-010-9115-5.
181. Wilcken B. Fatty acid oxidation disorders: outcome and long-term prognosis. *J Inherit Metab Dis* 2010;33:501–506. doi:10.1007/s10545-009-9001-1.
182. Ruitenbeek W, et al. Rhabdomyolysis and acute encephalopathy in late onset medium chain acyl-CoA dehydrogenase deficiency. *J Neurol Neurosurg Psychiatr* 1995;58:209–214.
183. Korman SH, et al. Homozygosity for a severe novel medium-chain acyl-CoA dehydrogenase (MCAD) mutation IVS3-1G>C that leads to introduction of a premature termination codon by complete missplicing of the MCAD mRNA and is associated with phenotypic diversity ranging from sudden neonatal death to asymptomatic status. *Mol Genet Metab* 2004;82:121–129. doi:10.1016/j.ymgme.2004.03.002.
184. Treem WR, et al. Medium-chain and long-chain acyl CoA dehydrogenase deficiency: clinical, pathologic and ultrastructural differentiation from Reye's syndrome. *Hepatology* 1986;6:1270–1278.
185. Santer R, Schmidt-Sommerfeld E, Leung YK, et al. Medium-chain acyl CoA dehydrogenase deficiency: electron microscopic differentiation from Reye syndrome. *Eur J Pediatr* 1990;150:111–114.
186. Sim KG, Hammond J, Wilcken B. Strategies for the diagnosis of mitochondrial fatty acid β-oxidation disorders. *Clin Chim Acta* 2002;323:37–58. doi:10.1016/S0009 8981(02)00182-1.
187. Rakheja D, Bennett MJ, Rogers BB. Long-chain L-3-hydroxyacyl-coenzyme a dehydrogenase deficiency: a molecular and biochemical review. *Lab Invest* 2002;82:815–824. doi:10.1097/01.LAB.0000021175.50201.46.
188. IJlst L, Ruiter JP, Hoovers JM, et al. Common missense mutation G1528C in long-chain 3-hydroxyacyl-CoA dehydrogenase deficiency. Characterization and expression of the mutant protein, mutation analysis on genomic DNA and chromosomal localization of the mitochondrial trifunctional protein alpha subunit gene. *J Clin Invest* 1996;98:1028–1033. doi:10.1172/JCI118863.
189. Tyni T, Pihko H. Long-chain 3-hydroxyacyl-CoA dehydrogenase deficiency. *Acta Paediat* 1999;88:237–245.
190. Slukvin II, Salamat MS, Chandra S. Morphologic studies of the placenta and autopsy findings in neonatal-onset glutaric acidemia type II. *Pediatr Dev Pathol* 2002;5:315–321. doi:10.1007/s10024-001-0213-0.
191. Wilson GN, et al. Glutaric aciduria type II: review of the phenotype and report of an unusual glomerulopathy. *Am J Med Genet A* 1989;32:395–401. doi:10.1002/ajmg.1320320326.
192. Angle B, Burton BK Risk of sudden death and acute life-threatening events in patients with glutaric acidemia type II. *Mol Genet Metab* 2008;93:36–39. doi:10.1016/j.ymgme.2007.09.015.
193. Spiekerkoetter U. Mitochondrial fatty acid oxidation disorders: clinical presentation of long-chain fatty acid oxidation defects before and after newborn screening. *J Inherit Metab Dis* 2010;33:527–532. doi:10.1007/s10545-010-9090-x.
194. Bonnefont J-P, et al. Carnitine palmitoyltransferases 1 and 2: biochemical, molecular and medical aspects. *Mol Aspects Med* 2004;25:495–520. doi:10.1016/j.mam.2004.06.004.
195. Meir K, et al. Severe infantile carnitine palmitoyltransferase II deficiency in 19-week fetal sibs. *Pediatr Dev Pathol* 2009;12:481–486. doi:10.2350/08-10-0548.1.
196. Stanley CA. Carnitine deficiency disorders in children. *Ann N Y Acad Sci* 2004;1033:42–51. doi:10.1196/annals.1320.004.
197. Kerner J, Hoppel C. Genetic disorders of carnitine metabolism and their nutritional management. *Annu Rev Nutr* 1998;18:179–206. doi:10.1146/annurev.nutr.18.1.179.
198. Longo N, Amat di San Filippo C, Pasquali M. Disorders of carnitine transport and the carnitine cycle. *Am J Med Genet C Semin Med Genet* 2006;142C:77–85. doi:10.1002/ajmg.c.30087.
199. Bennett MJ, Hale DE, Pollitt RJ, et al. Endocardial fibroelastosis and primary carnitine deficiency due to a defect in the plasma membrane carnitine transporter. *Clin Cardiol* 1996;19:243–246.
200. Tripp ME, et al. Systemic carnitine deficiency presenting as familial endocardial fibroelastosis: a treatable cardiomyopathy. *N Engl J Med* 1981;305:385–390. doi:10.1056/NEJM198108133050707.

201. DiMauro S, Schon EA, Carelli V, et al. The clinical maze of mitochondrial neurology. *Nat Rev Neurol* 2013;9:429–444. doi:10.1038/nrneurol.2013.126.
202. Farrar GJ, Chadderton N, Kenna PF, et al. Mitochondrial disorders: aetiologies, models systems, and candidate therapies. *Trends Genet* 2013;29:488–497. doi:10.1016/j.tig.2013.05.005.
203. Davis RL, Sue CM. The genetics of mitochondrial disease. *Semin Neurol* 2011;31:519–530. doi:10.1055/s-0031-1299790.
204. Elliott HR, Samuels DC, Eden JA, et al. Pathogenic mitochondrial DNA mutations are common in the general population. *Am J Hum Genet* 2008;83:254–260. doi:10.1016/j.ajhg.2008.07.004.
205. Pfeffer G, Chinnery PF. Diagnosis and treatment of mitochondrial myopathies. *Ann Med* 2013;45:4–16. doi:10.3109/07853890.2011.605389.
206. Braissant O. Current concepts in the pathogenesis of urea cycle disorders. *Mol Genet Metab* 2010;100(Suppl 1):S3–S12. doi:10.1016/j.ymgme.2010.02.010.
207. Häberle J. Clinical and biochemical aspects of primary and secondary hyperammonemic disorders. *Arch Biochem Biophys* 2013;536:101–108. doi:10.1016/j.abb.2013.04.009.
208. Yaplito-Lee J, Chow C-W, Boneh A. Histopathological findings in livers of patients with urea cycle disorders. *Mol Genet Metab* 2013;108:161–165. doi:10.1016/j.ymgme.2013.01.006.
209. Martínez AI, Pérez-Arellano I, Pekkala S, et al. Genetic, structural and biochemical basis of carbamoyl phosphate synthetase 1 deficiency. *Mol Genet Metab* 2010;101:311–323. doi:10.1016/j.ymgme.2010.08.002.
210. Häberle J, et al. Molecular defects in human carbamoyl phosphate synthetase I: mutational spectrum, diagnostic and protein structure considerations. *Hum Mutat* 2011;32:579–589. doi:10.1002/humu.21406.
211. Zimmermann A, Bachmann C, Colombo JP. Ultrastructural pathology in congenital defects of the urea cycle: Ornithine transcarbamylase and carbamoyl phosphate synthetase deficiency. *Virchows Arch* 1981;393:321–331. doi:10.1007/BF00430832.
212. Gordon N. Ornithine transcarbamylase deficiency: a urea cycle defect. *Eur J Paediatr Neurol* 2003;7:115–121.
213. Cordero DR, Baker J, Dorinzi D, et al. Ornithine transcarbamylase deficiency in pregnancy. *J Inherit Metab Dis* 2005;28:237–240. doi:10.1007/s10545-005-5514-4.
214. Woo HI, Park H-D, Lee Y-W. Molecular genetics of citrullinemia types I and II. *Clin Chim Acta* 2014;431:1–8. doi:10.1016/j.cca.2014.01.032.
215. Zamora SA, Pinto A, Scott RB, et al. Mitochondrial abnormalities of liver in two children with citrullinaemia. *J Inherit Metab Dis* 1997;20:509–516.
216. Erez A, Nagamani SCS, Lee B. Argininosuccinate lyase deficiency—argininosuccinic aciduria and beyond. *Am J Med Genet C Semin Med Genet* 2011;157C:45–53.
217. Carvalho DR, et al. Clinical features and neurologic progression of hyperargininemia. *Pediatr Neurol* 2012;46:369–374. doi:10.1016/j.pediatrneurol.2012.03.016.
218. Braga AC, Vilarinho L, Ferreira E, et al. Hyperargininemia presenting as persistent neonatal jaundice and hepatic cirrhosis. *J Pediatr Gastroenterol Nutr* 1997;24:218.
219. Camacho JA, et al. Hyperornithinaemia-hyperammonaemia-homocitrullinuria syndrome is caused by mutations in a gene encoding a mitochondrial ornithine transporter. *Nat Genet* 1999;22:151–158. doi:10.1038/9658.
220. Nakajima M, et al. Clinical, biochemical and ultrastructural study on the pathogenesis of hyperornithinemia-hyperammonemia-homocitrullinuria syndrome. *Brain Dev* 1988;10:181–185. doi:10.1016/S0387-7604(88)80025-1.
221. Ogier de Baulny H, Schiff M, Dionisi-Vici C. Lysinuric protein intolerance (LPI): a multi organ disease by far more complex than a classic urea cycle disorder. *Mol Genet Metab* 2012;106:12–17. doi:10.1016/j.ymgme.2012.02.010.
222. de Klerk JB, Duran M, Huijmans JG, et al. Sudden infant death and lysinuric protein intolerance. *Eur J Pediatr* 1996;155:256–257.
223. Parto K, Kallajoki M, Aho H, et al. Pulmonary alveolar proteinosis and glomerulonephritis in lysinuric protein intolerance: case reports and autopsy findings of four pediatric patients. *Hum Pathol* 1994;25:400–407.
224. McManus DT, et al. Necropsy findings in lysinuric protein intolerance. *J Clin Pathol* 1996;49:345–347.
225. Feliz B, Witt DR, Harris BT. Propionic acidemia: a neuropathology case report and review of prior cases. *Arch Pathol Lab Med* 2003;127:e325–e328. doi:10.1043/1543-2165(2003)127<e325:PAANCR>2.0.CO;2.
226. Tanpaiboon P. IEM digest. *Mol Genet Metab* 2005;85:2–6. doi:10.1016/j.ymgme.2005.03.008.
227. Zsengellér ZK, et al. Methylmalonic acidemia: a megamitochondrial disorder affecting the kidney. *Pediatr Nephrol* 2014;29:2139–2146. doi:10.1007/s00467-014-2847-y.
228. Vockley J, Ensenauer R. Isovaleric acidemia: new aspects of genetic and phenotypic heterogeneity. *Am J Med Genet A* 2006;142C:95–103. doi:10.1002/ajmg.c.30089.
229. Strauss KA, Puffenberger EG, Robinson DL, et al. Type I glutaric aciduria: Part 1. Natural history of 77 patients. *Am J Med Genet A* 2003;121C:38–52. doi:10.1002/ajmg.c.20007.
230. Brown GK, Otero LJ, LeGris M, et al. Pyruvate dehydrogenase deficiency. *J Med Genet* 1994;31:875.
231. Brown GK. Pyruvate dehydrogenase E1α deficiency. *J Inherit Metab Dis* 1992;15:625–633. doi:10.1007/BF01799619.
232. Brown G. Pyruvate dehydrogenase deficiency and the brain. *Dev Med Child Neurol* 2012;54:395–396.
233. García-Cazorla A, et al. Pyruvate carboxylase deficiency: metabolic characteristics and new neurological aspects. *Ann Neurol* 2005;59:121–127. doi:10.1002/ana.20709.
234. Fujiki Y, Yagita Y, Matsuzaki T. Peroxisome biogenesis disorders: molecular basis for impaired peroxisomal membrane assembly: in metabolic functions and biogenesis of peroxisomes in health and disease. *Biochim Biophys Acta* 2012;1822:1337–1342. doi:10.1016/j.bbadis.2012.06.004.
235. Waterham HR, Ebberink MS. Genetics and molecular basis of human peroxisome biogenesis disorders. *Biochim Biophys Acta* 2012;1822:1430–1441. doi:10.1016/j.bbadis.2012.04.006.
236. Poll-The BT, Engelen M. Peroxisomal leukoencephalopathy. *Semin Neurol* 2012;32:42–50. doi:10.1055/s-0032-1306385.
237. Kemp S, Berger J, Aubourg, P. X-linked adrenoleukodystrophy: clinical, metabolic, genetic and pathophysiological aspects. *Biochim Biophys Acta* 2012;1822:1465–1474. doi:10.1016/j.bbadis.2012.03.012.
238. Wanders RJ, Komen J, Ferdinandusse S. Phytanic acid metabolism in health and disease. *Biochim Biophys Acta* 2011;1811:498–507. doi:10.1016/j.bbalip.2011.06.006.
239. Cochat P, Groothoff J. Primary hyperoxaluria type 1: practical and ethical issues. *Pediatr Nephrol* 2013;28:2273–2281. doi:10.1007/s00467-013-2444-5.
240. Hoppe, B. An update on primary hyperoxaluria. *Nat Rev Nephrol* 2012;8:467–475. doi:10.1038/nrneph.2012.113.
241. Jaeken J. Congenital disorders of glycosylation. *Ann N Y Acad Sci* 2010;1214:190–198. doi:10.1111/j.1749-6632.2010.05840.x.
242. Jaeken J. Congenital disorders of glycosylation (CDG): it's (nearly) all in it! *J Inherit Metab Dis* 2011;34:853–858. doi:10.1007/s10545-011-9299-3.
243. DeBarber AE, Eroglu Y, Merkens LS, et al. Smith-Lemli-Opitz syndrome. *Expert Rev Mol Med* 2011;13:e24. doi:10.1017/S146239941100189X.
244. Nowaczyk MJ, Irons MB. Smith-Lemli-Opitz syndrome: phenotype, natural history, and epidemiology. *Am J Med Genet C Semin Med Genet* 2012;160C:250–262. doi:10.1002/ajmg.c.31343.
245. Kelley, RI, Herman, GE. Inborn errors of sterol biosynthesis. *Annu Rev Genom Hum Genet* 2001;2:299–341. doi:10.1146/annurev.genom.2.1.299.
246. Kanungo S, Soares N, He M, et al. Sterol metabolism disorders and neurodevelopment—an update. *Dev Disabil Res Rev* 2013;17:197–210. doi:10.1002/ddrr.1114.

247. Canueto J, Giros M, Gonzalez-Sarmiento R. The role of the abnormalities in the distal pathway of cholesterol biosynthesis in the Conradi-Hunermann-Happle syndrome. *Biochim Biophys Acta* 2014;1841:336–344. doi:10.1016/j.bbalip.2013.09.002.
248. Seeger MA, Paller AS. The role of abnormalities in the distal pathway of cholesterol synthesis in the Congenital Hemidysplasia with Ichthyosiform erythroderma and Limb Defects (CHILD) syndrome. *Biochim Biophys Acta* 2014;1841:345–352. doi:10.1016/j.bbalip.2013.09.006.
249. Loughrey CM, Preece MA, Green A. Sudden unexpected death in infancy (SUDI). *J Clin Pathol* 2005;58:20–21. doi:10.1136/jcp.2004.020677.
250. Lovera C, et al. Sudden unexpected infant death (SUDI) in a newborn due to medium chain acyl CoA dehydrogenase (MCAD) deficiency with an unusual severe genotype. *Ital J Pediatr* 2012;38:59. doi:10.1186/1824-7288-38-59.
251. Opdal SH, Rognum TO. The sudden infant death syndrome gene: does it exist? *Pediatrics* 2004;114:e506–e512. doi:10.1542/peds.2004-0683.
252. Pryce JW, Weber MA, Heales S, et al. Tandem mass spectrometry findings at autopsy for detection of metabolic disease in infant deaths: postmortem changes and confounding factors. *J Clin Pathol* 2011;64:1005–1009. doi:10.1136/jclinpath-2011-200218.
253. Ernst LM, Sondheimer N, Deardorff MA, et al. The value of the metabolic autopsy in the pediatric hospital setting. *J Pediatr* 2006;148:779–783. doi:10.1016/j.jpeds.2006.01.040.
254. Pinar H. Postmortem findings in term neonates. *Semin Neonatol* 2004;9:289–302. doi:10.1016/j.siny.2003.11.003.
255. Leonard JV, Morris AA. Inborn errors of metabolism around time of birth. *Lancet* 2000;356:583–587.
256. Olpin SE. The metabolic investigation of sudden infant death. *Ann Clin Biochem* 2004;41:282–293. doi:10.1258/0004563041201473.
257. Bliss LA, et al. Use of postmortem human dura mater and scalp for deriving human fibroblast cultures. *PLoS One* 2012;7:e45282. doi:10.1371/journal.pone.0045282.
258. Meske V, Albert F, Wehser R, et al. Culture of autopsy-derived fibroblasts as a tool to study systemic alterations in human neurodegenerative disorders such as Alzheimer's disease—methodological investigations. *J Neural Transm* 1999;106:537–548.

CHAPTER 6

Congenital and Acquired Systemic Infectious Diseases

Haresh Mani, M.D., David Parham, M.D., and Jennifer Dien Bard, Ph.D., D(ABMM), F.C.C.M.

As it takes two to make a quarrel, so it takes two to make a disease, the microbe and its host.—Charles V. Chapin, 1856–1941

Infections are the leading global cause of death in the pediatric population. The optimism that accompanied the advent of antibiotics in the mid-20th century was premature, and even advances such as immunization and improved sanitation have not stopped microbial reemergence. The importance of infectious diseases is underscored by ever-increasing antimicrobial resistance and resurgence of infections such as tuberculosis (TB), malaria, and syphilis, once thought eradicated from developed countries. International travel has removed boundaries from the spread of infection, as exemplified by the rapid spread of infections such as severe acute respiratory syndrome (SARS) across countries. In this chapter, we aim to provide an overview of systemic infections that the pediatric pathologist is likely to encounter. Infections that are predominantly confined to a single organ system (e.g., poliomyelitis, hepatitis) are not considered in this chapter, even though they may occasionally cause systemic manifestations. The reader is directed to chapters dealing with specific organ systems for information on such infections. Further, since it is impossible to comprehensively detail all facets of various systemic infections in a single chapter, we have generously referenced resources for the reader with specific interests. Detailed information is also available in standard textbooks including Feigin and Cherry's *Textbook of Pediatric Infectious Diseases* (1), Connor and Chandler's *Pathology of Infectious Diseases* (2), and the *American Academy of Pediatrics Red Book* (www.aapredbook.com).

THE PATHOGENESIS OF INFECTIOUS DISEASES

An infection is the result of an encounter between an infectious agent and a susceptible host. The microorganism is the *sine qua non*, but the occurrence of the disease, its pathophysiology, and its outcome are determined by host and environmental factors. A discussion of microbial virulence factors is beyond the scope of this chapter; various reviews cover the topic in considerable depth (3,4).

HOST FACTORS

Host genetic factors, immune status, age, and geographic location determine the likelihood and severity of infection. The heritability of infectious disease susceptibility is a complex factor modified by developmental and maturational changes in host defense, from embryo through adolescence, with resultant differences in response to infection (5,6). Polymorphisms in genes coding for proteins that recognize bacterial pathogens [such as Toll-like receptor 4, CD14, Fc(gamma)RIIa, and mannose-binding lectin] and the response to bacterial pathogens [with elaboration of cytokines such as tumor necrosis factor-α, interleukin (IL)-1α, IL-1β, IL-1 receptor agonist, IL-6, IL-10, heat shock proteins, angiotensin I–converting enzyme, plasminogen activator inhibitor-1] can influence response to bacterial stimuli (7).

Immunologic maturity and immunodeficiencies (quantitative and qualitative) also determine infection susceptibility. Since they have developmentally immature immune systems, neonates and infants are at a relative immunologic disadvantage. The immaturity of the fetal immune system helps prevent "premature rejection" by the host (the mother). Paradoxically, this potential benefit also increases the risk of infections for the fetus and the prematurely born neonate. Term newborns have a higher frequency of microbial infections than older children and adults; extremely premature newborns (<28 weeks of gestation) have a 5- to 10-fold higher frequency than term newborns. Immunologic immaturity also obscures clinical symptoms in neonatal sepsis. Recent advancements in developmental immunology provide a framework for understanding the mechanisms underlying the propensity of infections in the preterm, near-term, and term newborn (8). The immune environment during early life favors innate over acquired immunity. Innate immunity against pathogens represents the critical first-line barrier of host defenses, as newborns have a naïve adaptive immune system. However, innate immune mechanisms are also relatively impaired in neonates as compared to older children and adults, thereby increasing neonatal susceptibility to infections (9). Further, the neonate is unable to produce antibody to thymus-independent antigens such as bacterial polysaccharides, although transplacentally acquired maternal antibodies confer some protection for the first few months of life. Neonatal B-cells have an immature phenotype, and the neonatal spleen has a different cellular composition; unlike adults, neonatal accessory cells, that is, macrophages and dendritic cells, appear to produce less stimulatory cytokines and an overabundance of inhibitory cytokines (10).

Children with immunodeficiencies (primary or acquired) have an increased risk of infections (Tables 6-1 and 6-2). Impaired splenic function (due to asplenia, disease, or splenectomy) significantly increases the risk of life-threatening bacterial sepsis, especially with capsulated organisms, necessitating pneumococcal and meningococcal immunizations. Secondary factors such as comorbidities (Table 6-3), medications, and nutritional status also dictate clinical course. Most organisms causing disease in a setting of immunodeficiency are "opportunists" and are ubiquitous in the internal or external environment where they ordinarily do no harm. Systemic or repeated local infections may be the first manifestation of unsuspected primary immunodeficiency. A family history of unusual infections, age at presentation, specific type of infection (e.g., *Aspergillus* in chronic granulomatous disease, *Pneumocystis* in severe combined immunodeficiency), recurrent otitis media, need for IV antibiotics, and lymphopenia are additional warning signs (11).

ENVIRONMENTAL FACTORS

Over 50 years ago, Haldane proposed that the prevalence of thalassemia in malaria-endemic areas was due to the heterozygotic advantage it conferred against malaria, despite its otherwise deleterious effects. Table 6-4 outlines examples of the influence of geographic, political, and socioeconomic factors on infectious diseases that account for a major part of the world's infant morbidity and mortality. Infectious disease risks associated with international travel are diverse and depend on the destination, planned activities, and baseline medical history. Common infections associated with travel to developing countries include malaria, diarrhea, respiratory infections, and cutaneous larva migrans (12). Children have special needs and vulnerabilities that should be addressed when preparing for travel abroad (13). Natural disasters also exacerbate the risk of infections due to changes in the environment, in human conditions, and in the vulnerability to existing pathogens and are associated with many infectious diseases including diarrheal diseases, acute respiratory infections, malaria, leptospirosis, measles, dengue fever, viral hepatitis, typhoid fever, meningitis, tetanus, and cutaneous mucormycosis (14).

On a less global scale, certain local environments must frequently be considered as contributors to disease. Such

TABLE 6-1 INFECTIONS ASSOCIATED WITH PRIMARY IMMUNODEFICIENCIES

Infection	Host Factor
General associations	
Recurrent respiratory and pyogenic infections by extracellular bacteria: *Streptococcus pneumoniae*, *Haemophilus influenzae*, *Staphylococcus aureus*	Antibody deficiencies
Chronic or severe infections with intracellular pathogens: viruses, mycobacteria, *Pneumocystis carinii*, *Toxoplasma gondii*, and others	Deficiencies of T lymphocytes
Specific associations	
Chronic viral encephalitis	X-linked agammaglobulinemia
Echovirus dermatomyositis	
Polio vaccine–induced paralysis	
Severe parainfluenza infection	Severe combined immunodeficiency
Severe varicella	Cartilage–hair hypoplasia
Severe Epstein-Barr virus infection	X-linked lymphoproliferative syndrome
Recurrent meningococcal sepsis	Complement deficiencies
Disseminated gonococcal infection	
Staphylococcal skin infections	Neutrophil abnormalities
Mucosal and periodontal infections	
Infections with *Aspergillus* sp., *S. aureus*, *Pseudomonas cepacia*, *Chromobacterium violaceum*	Chronic granulomatous disease
BCGosis and atypical mycobacteria	NF-γ and IL-12 deficiencies
Persistent mucocutaneous candidiasis	Chronic mucocutaneous candidiasis
Chronic/recurrent giardiasis	IgA deficiency

BCG, Bacille Calmette-Guérin; INF, interferon; IL, interleukin; IgA, immunoglobulin A.

TABLE 6-2 CONGENITAL IMMUNODEFICIENCIES WITH AN INCREASED RISK OF SEPSIS[a]

Immunodeficiency	Characteristic Susceptibility[b]	Estimated Sepsis Occurrence, %[c]
Innate immune defects		
Complement deficiency	*Neisseria*	28
Mannose-binding lectin	*Neisseria, S. pneumoniae, H. influenzae*	
NEMO deficiency	*Klebsiella, S. pneumoniae*, mycobacteria	86
IRAK4 deficiency	Gram-positive bacteria	75
TLR-4	Gram-negative bacteria	
Caspase-12 defect		
CGD	*S. aureus, Salmonella, Burkholderia, Candida, Aspergillus, Nocardia*	21 (X-linked) 10 (autosomal)
Leukocyte adhesion deficiency	*Pseudomonas aeruginosa*	28
Specific granule deficiency		
Severe chronic neutropenia		3[d]
Type 1 cytokine axis defects	Mycobacteria, *Salmonella*	
Chediak-Higashi syndrome	*S. aureus*	
Adaptive immune defects		
SCID	Usual opportunistic infections and severe viral infections (RSV, VZV, HSV, CMV)	5[e]
Agammaglobulinemia	HiB, *S. pneumoniae*, enteric infections, *Pseudomonas*	10[f]
Hyper-IgM	Severe sinopulmonary infections, *Pneumocystis, Pseudomonas, Escherichia, Giardia, Cryptosporidium*	13
Hyper-IgE	Recurrent pneumonias (*S. aureus, S. pneumoniae, HiB*), eczema	
CVID	Respiratory infections (HiB, *S. pneumoniae*), GI infections (*C. jejuni, Salmonella, Giardia*)	1[g]
Transient hypogammaglobulinemia of infancy		
IgG subclass deficiency		
Ataxia-telangiectasia	Gram-positive bacteria, severe sinopulmonary infections	5
IPEX	Enteric bacteria	
Wiskott-Aldrich syndrome		36
NK-cell deficiency	Severe viral infections (CMV, HSV, VZV) beyond infancy	

[a]Sepsis, caused by bacteremia, fungemia, or viremia.
[b]Characteristic infectious susceptibility that can be useful in considering a particular diagnosis.
[c]Occurrence of sepsis within a particular population.
[d]Bacteremia in additional 15%.
[e]As high as 30% in reticular dysgenesis and 16% in Omenn syndrome.
[f]As a presenting manifestation before immunoglobulin replacement therapy.
[g]Higher in the Good syndrome variant (16%).

NEMO, nuclear factor-B; TLR, toll-like receptor; CGD, chronic granulomatous disease; SCID, severe combined immunodeficiency; Ig, immunoglobulin; CVID, common variable immunodeficiency; IPEX, immunodysregulation, polyendocrinopathy, enteropathy, X-linked.

Sources: Orange JS. Congenital immunodeficiencies and sepsis. *Pediatr Crit Care Med* 2005;6(3 Suppl):S99–S107.; Randolph AG, McCulloh RJ. Pediatric sepsis: important considerations for diagnosing and managing severe infections in infants, children, and adolescents. *Virulence* 2014;5(1):179-189.

TABLE 6-3. PRIMARILY NONIMMUNE DISORDERS INFLUENCING INCIDENCE AND SEVERITY OF INFECTION

	Site	Predominant Organisms	Proposed Mechanism
Metabolic disorders			
Diabetes mellitus	Skin, GU tract	*S. aureus*, *E. coli*, yeasts, *Zygomycetes*	Impaired phagocytosis, neutrophilic chemotaxis, and opsonization
Galactosemia	Bacteremia, meningitis	*E. coli*, Viridans group streptococci	Impaired phagocytosis due to hypoglycemia
Uremia	Pneumonia, septicemia	Unspecified	Impaired macrophage function
Iron deficiency	Unspecified	Unspecified	Impaired bacterial killing
Nephrotic syndrome	Peritonitis	*S. pneumoniae*, enteric bacilli	Unknown, protein loss (?)
Intravenous lipid	Pulmonary arteritis, fungemia	*Malassezia furfur*	Lipophilic organism
Circulatory alterations			
Congenital/rheumatic heart disease	Endocarditis, pericarditis	Viridans group streptococci, *S. aureus*	Endocardial damage due to jet effects, turbulence
Sickle cell disease	Meningitis, systemic osteomyelitis	*S. pneumoniae*, *Salmonella* spp.	Ischemia, functional asplenia, defective opsonization
Exudative enteropathy	Pneumonia, gastroenteritis	*S. pneumoniae*, enteric bacilli, *Giardia*	Intestinal loss of immunoglobulins and lymphocytes
Cystic fibrosis	Bronchitis, bronchiectasis, pneumonia	*S. aureus*, *Pseudomonas*	Defective ciliary movement, mechanical obstruction due to hyperviscosity of mucus
Immobile cilia syndromes	Otitis, sinusitis, bronchitis, bronchiectasis	*H. influenzae*, *Neisseria*, staphylococci, streptococci, *Pseudomonas*	Defective ciliary motility
GU obstruction/malfunction	Pyelonephritis, cystitis	*E. coli*, *Proteus*, *Enterobacteria*	Urinary stasis, instrumentation, trauma
Barrier defects			
Eczema, exfoliative dermatitis	Impetigo, sepsis	Staphylococci, β-hemolytic streptococci	Mechanical loss of skin barrier
Burns	Skin, sepsis	*Pseudomonas*, *S. aureus*, *S. epidermidis*, fungi, VZV, HSV	Changes in flora, physiochemical properties of the skin
Skull fractures	Meningitis	*S. pneumoniae*	Direct access to CSF via respiratory passages and sinuses
Neural tube defects	Meningitis	*S. pneumoniae*, enteric bacteria, staphylococci	Direct access to CSF from skin
Foreign bodies			
Arterial and venous catheters	Phlebitis, omphalitis, endocarditis, arteritis, liver abscess	*S. epidermidis*, *Pseudomonas*, yeasts	Barrier bypass, nidus for infection
CSF shunts	Meningitis, peritonitis, septicemia, endocarditis, phlebitis	*S. epidermidis*, *S. aureus*, enteric organisms	Barrier bypass, nidus for infection
Prostheses	Endocarditis	*S. aureus*, *S. epidermidis*	Nidus for infection
Aspiration	Pneumonia, lung abscess	Anaerobes	Aspiration of infected material, bronchial obstruction by foreign bodies, necrosis of airway epithelium
Splenectomy	Fulminant septicemia	*S. pneumoniae*, *Salmonella*	
Malnutrition	Pneumonia	Measles, HSV, staphylococci, enteric bacteria, *Pneumocystis*	Depression of complement, cell-mediated immunity, and phagocytosis

CSF, cerebrospinal fluid; GU, genitourinary.
? = Pathogenesis suspected, but largely unknown at present.

TABLE 6-4 INFLUENCE OF ENVIRONMENTAL FACTORS ON INFECTIOUS DISEASES

	Example	Comment
Geographic		
Climate	Malaria	Requires summer average over 21°C
Geologic characteristics	Onchocerciasis	Insect vector develops in fast-flowing rivers
Animal reservoirs	Toxoplasmosis	Oocysts produced in cats
Vector availability	Chagas disease	Transmitted by triatomid insects
Political and economic		
Population density/overcrowding	Tuberculosis	Complex relationship, including ease of droplet transmission, malnutrition, presence of other chronic diseases
Political structure and stability	Measles, polio	Can be eradicated by effective and sustained public health and immunization programs
War, refugee status	Malaria	Refugee-borne global spread of disease
Socioeconomic status	Tetanus	Most common cause of neonatal death in countries with lowest per capita income
Cultural/behavioral patterns	AIDS	Sexual and parenteral transmission of disease in homosexuals and drug addicts
Nosocomial sources of infection		
Pediatric ICU	*S. aureus, E. coli, Klebsiella, Enterobacter, Serratia*	Pediatric ICU–acquired infections less common than adult ICU–acquired
Neonatal ICU	Staphylococci, *E. coli*	Susceptibility increased because of absence of normal flora
Day care	Diarrheal illnesses, hepatitis A, *H. influenzae*, upper respiratory viruses	Close person-to-person contact in a highly susceptible population with behavior patterns facilitating transmission
Contaminated ventilatory equipment	*Pseudomonas, Serratia*	Aerosols and nebulizers are reservoirs; cystic fibrosis patients especially affected
Contaminated IV fluids	*E. coli, Erwinia, Pseudomonas*	Contamination of containers
Contaminated water/air supplies	*Legionella*	Reservoirs in drinking water supply and air conditioning equipment. Rarely seen in normal children

ICU, intensive care unit; IV, intravenous.

nosocomial environments as intensive care units, neonatal nurseries, day care centers, schools, and summer camps play a role either by serving as reservoirs for pathogenic microbes or by facilitating their spread in a susceptible population. Biofilm formation may also be important in bacterial pathogenesis (15). Hospitalized or chronically ill children are exposed additionally to equipment and pharmaceutical agents that may be the source of iatrogenic infections. Lack of personal hygiene and exposure to pets, soil, and natural environments are additional factors to consider in children.

Infections and Teratogenesis

In order to act as a teratogen, an agent must be capable of crossing the placenta at an early stage of embryogenesis or organogenesis and either inhibit cell growth and differentiation or produce cell destruction. The spectrum of resulting defects depends on both the timing and the severity of the insult. Dysmorphogenetic syndromes produced by fetal infection are remarkable in their clinical and morphologic variability. Of the large number of agents causing fetal infection, only rubella, cytomegalovirus (CMV), varicella-zoster virus (VZV), herpes simplex virus (HSV), toxoplasma, and syphilis are firmly established as human teratogens. Teratogenic effects of human immunodeficiency virus (HIV) infection, independent of drug abuse or concomitant opportunistic infection, have not been confirmed. Evidence linking coxsackieviruses and mumps to congenital heart defects and endocardial fibroelastosis, respectively, is also inconclusive.

In utero infections can result in a variety of adverse fetal outcomes. Microorganisms damage fetal cells or tissues by elaborating toxic substances, interrupting cell division or migration, and/or evoking (or depressing) host inflammatory and repair responses. Depending on the organism and the timing of the insult, intrauterine infection may result in a variety of lesions with variable severity. Prenatal congenital infections caused by *Toxoplasma gondii*, rubella, CMV, HSV, VZV, and *Treponema* account for approximately 5% to 15% of IUGR cases (16). Table 6-5 lists various viral infections associated with adverse fetal outcomes (17).

Intrapartum or neonatal infections are more limited in scope than those occurring *in utero* because of the more

TABLE 6-5 VIRAL INFECTIONS ASSOCIATED WITH ADVERSE FETAL OUTCOMES

	Transmission						
Virus	*In Utero*	During Delivery	Breast Milk	Incidence per 1000 Live Births	Present in AF/Fetus in Unaffected Cases	Clinical Consequences at Birth	Postnatal
HSV	+	+++	++	0.04	Yes	IUGR, death, multiorgan disease	Recurrence
CMV	+++	+++	+++	5–22	Yes	IUGR, CNS disease, CID	Developmental delay, deafness
Adenovirus	+++	–	++	Unknown	Yes	IUGR, fetal hydrops	Unknown
AAV	+	+	++	Unknown	Unknown	Prematurity	—
EV	+	–	+++	Unknown	Unknown	Myocarditis	Neurodevelopmental delay, diabetes
HHV6	+	+	+	Unknown	Yes	Encephalitis	Unknown
LCMV	+	–	+	Unknown	Unknown	CNS disease, eye disease, death	Blindness
Parvovirus	++	+	+	Unknown	Unknown	Fetal hydrops	Anemia
Rubella	++	–	+	0.01	Unknown	CNS disease, eye disease	Deafness, exanthem
VZV	+	++	++	0.01	Yes	Limb disease, CNS disease	Disseminated VZV

+, rare; ++, frequent; +++, common.

AAV, adenovirus associated virus; AF, amniotic fluid; CID, chronic inflammatory disease; CMV, cytomegalovirus; CNS, central nervous system; EV, enterovirus; HHV, human herpes virus; HSV, herpes simplex virus; IUGR, intrauterine growth restriction; LCMV, lymphocytic choriomeningitis virus; VZV, varicella-zoster virus.

Modified from: Rawlinson WD, Hall B, Jones CA, et al. Viruses and other infections in stillbirth: what is the evidence and what should we be doing? *Pathology* 2008;40:149–60. Ref. (17).

advanced developmental state of the infant. Nonetheless, they produce acute and possibly fatal disease (e.g., neonatal herpes virus infection), persistent tissue or organ dysfunction (e.g., postnatal CMV infection), or late complications (e.g., obstructive hydrocephalus resulting from neonatal meningitis).

TRANSMISSION

Maternal–fetal transmission is specific to the pediatric population, and it may occur *in utero* ("vertical transmission") or during breast-feeding. Other routes of transmission including inhalation, ingestion, and inoculation are similar in adults and children. Routes of fetal and neonatal infection have been thoroughly reviewed by Blanc (18). These are illustrated in Figure 6-1 and summarized in Table 6-6.

VERTICAL TRANSMISSION

Pathways of vertical transmission include those occurring *in utero* (transplacental and ascending), intrapartum (in the birth canal, from maternal genital and gastrointestinal tracts), and immediately postnatal (although, strictly speaking, this is not vertical transmission). Although *in utero* infection can occur during any trimester, its timing significantly affects clinical course. Organisms may ascend from the maternal genital tract along the cervix to the amniotic sac through either intact or ruptured membranes. This ascending route is the preferred one for HSV, most

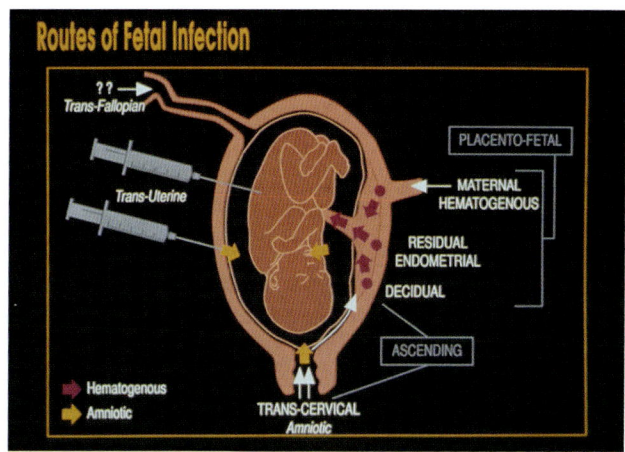

FIGURE 6-1 • Routes of fetal infection.

TABLE 6-6 PREDOMINANT PATHWAYS OF THE MAJOR FETAL AND NEONATAL INFECTION

Transplacental	Ascending	Postpartum
Bacteria		
Listeria[a]	Group B streptococci	*Staphylococci*[a]
Treponema pallidum	Enteric bacilli[b]	*Pseudomonas*[a]
Mycobacterium tuberculosis	*Haemophilus influenzae*	Nongroup B streptococci[b]
Borrelia	*Neisseria gonorrhea*	
Campylobacter fetus (?)	Anaerobes	
	Actinomyces	
	Fusobacteria	
Viruses		
Cytomegalovirus[c]	Herpes simplex[c]	Respiratory syncytial virus
Human immunodeficiency virus		Coxsackie B[a]
Rubella		
Mumps		
Measles		
Variola		
Vaccinia		
Poliovirus		
ECHO		
Hepatitis B[c]		
Western equine encephalitis		
Human parvovirus		
Varicella-zoster[a]		
Epstein-Barr virus		
Protozoa		
Toxoplasma		
Plasmodium		
Trypanosoma		
Babesia		
Fungi		
Coccidioides	*Candida*[c]	
	Aspergillus	
	Torulopsis	
Mycoplasmas		
	Mycoplasma hominis	
	Ureaplasma urealyticum	

[a]Also utilize ascending route.
[b]Also utilize hematogenous route.
[c]Also acquired postnatally.

bacteria, and *Candida*. Hematogenous spread of maternal blood-borne organisms across the placenta is the pathway used by most viruses and protozoa such as plasmodia and toxoplasma.

Perinatal infections commonly occur from exposure to maternal blood, body fluids, stool, or urine. The likelihood of infection varies significantly with the specific organism and various host factors (e.g., passively acquired antibody levels in the infant) and the IgG nadir in serum. Intrapartum transmission is more likely in a setting of prolonged labor combined with an infected maternal birth canal. Premature fetal inspiration results in perinatal pneumonia with high mortality. Postnatally acquired infections are transmitted most commonly through contact with caregivers (parents, relatives, visitors, and health care providers), the environment (medical equipment, other fomites), or breast milk (19). In most perinatal infections due to maternal transmission, the infant is exposed before illness is diagnosed in the mother and frequently occurs even before the mother becomes ill. Examples include maternally derived measles, enteroviral infection, chicken pox, and hepatitis.

BREAST MILK TRANSMISSION

Human milk protects against both specific pathogens and many illnesses (e.g., necrotizing enterocolitis, bacteremia, meningitis, respiratory tract illness, diarrheal disease, and otitis media). Breast milk enhances nonpathogenic flora, decreases colonization with enteropathogens, aids development of the respiratory and intestinal mucosal barriers, provides secretory IgA and functioning immune cells (neutrophils, macrophages, T and B lymphocytes), and prevents gut inflammation and immunomodulation (20). Breast milk–associated infections include HIV-1, human T-lymphotropic virus-1 (HTLV-1), CMV, measles virus, and streptococci (21). Bacterial infections are rarely, if ever, transmitted to infants through breast milk. Although infections associated with breast milk are more commonly transmitted through other mechanisms, at least temporary cessation of breast-feeding has been recommended in certain maternal bacterial infections associated with *Neisseria gonorrhoeae*, *Haemophilus influenzae*, group B streptococci (GBS; *Streptococcus agalactiae*), staphylococci, *Borrelia burgdorferi*, *Treponema pallidum*, and *Mycobacterium tuberculosis*.

EVALUATION OF SUSPECTED FETAL INFECTION

Given the incredibly wide spectrum of fetal infections, pathologists must properly evaluate fetal and neonatal deaths. Infection should be suspected in newborns exhibiting any or all of the following: intrauterine growth restriction, failure to thrive, hydrops, jaundice, hepatosplenomegaly, skin rashes, hydrocephalus, microcephaly, eye lesions such as microphthalmia, chorioretinitis, and cataract. Wigglesworth has outlined a procedure for evaluating these infants by using serologic studies, radiology, bacteriologic studies including dark-field examination, and viral diagnostic studies including culture and electron microscopy (22). Nucleic acid amplification techniques have enabled the identification of infectious agents hitherto difficult or impossible to detect (23). It cannot be overemphasized that histopathologic examination constitutes only one facet of adequate autopsy examination in suspected prenatal or perinatal infection.

VIRAL INFECTIONS

Most significant viral infections in neonates or infants occur through transplacental or intrapartum transmission. The risk of transmission depends on whether the maternal infection is primary (e.g., HSV, HIV-1), secondary reactivation (e.g., HSV, CMV), or chronic (e.g., hepatitis B, HIV-1, HTLV-1). Fetal and neonatal viral infections are multifaceted. Many agents are teratogens and can affect the fetus or infant at any stage, leading to fetal death, malformation, self-limited or ongoing infection, and late sequelae. Table 6-7 summarizes the main features of fetal and neonatal viral infections, while Table 6-8 outlines the major pathologic features of commonly seen viral infections in infants and older children. Of the more commonly encountered viral illnesses in children, many exclusively involve the nervous system (e.g., poliomyelitis, rabies) and are discussed in *Chapter 10*. Respiratory tract pathogens are included in *Chapter 12*, and the hepatitis viruses in *Chapter 15*. Of the remainder, relatively few are encountered by the pathologist; many are opportunists in immunocompromised children. In general, these disseminated opportunistic viral infections resemble their perinatal infectious counterparts. For comprehensive information, the reader is referred to Feigin and Cherry's textbook (1); only selected infections will be discussed here.

CYTOMEGALOVIRUS

CMV, the largest member of the family Herpesviridae, is encountered in all populations. A ubiquitous pathogen, CMV seroprevalence in adult populations ranges from 50% to 90%. It is the most common cause of congenital infection in the United States, with frequencies ranging from 0.2% to 2.2% of liveborn babies in the United States. Unlike congenital rubella and toxoplasmosis, intrauterine CMV transmission occurs in some women who are CMV seroimmune before pregnancy, at a much lower frequency than primary intrauterine infections. Approximately 1% of all congenitally infected infants excrete CMV in their urine within 3 weeks after birth; about 5% manifest perinatal disease at birth, and 15% develop late sequelae (24). More children may be affected by congenital CMV than by other perinatal diseases such as Down syndrome, fetal alcohol syndrome, and spina bifida. CMV is, therefore, one of the most common causes of birth defects and childhood disability.

Transmission

CMV infection may be transplacental, perinatal, or postnatal. Early, hematogenous gestational infections are the most devastating. Rarely, congenital CMV infection recurs in subsequent pregnancies. Primary CMV infection may rarely occur in the mother during delivery or lactation, and the lack of maternal antibody protection in these cases increases the risk for illness in the infant, although infections are rarely associated with clinical illness in full-term infants (25,26). Congenital and perinatal CMV immunity is complex; fetal protection cannot be assured with maternal immunity, since reinfection with a novel strain can occur (27). Infants who are susceptible (e.g., due to prematurity, seronegative mothers, or immunodeficiency) can have severe disease. CMV is also commonly reactivated in a setting of congenital or acquired immunodeficiency. Childcare centers also significantly transmit CMV, propagated by frequent mouthing of hands and toys. Approximately 20% to 40% of toddlers in day care shed the virus for years. These children function as an important infectious source for other children, parents, and daycare workers. After puberty, CMV infection is mainly sexually

TABLE 6-7 VIRAL INFECTION IN THE FETUS AND NEONATE

	Abortion	Stillbirth	Intrauterine Growth Restriction	Congenital Defects	Acute Perinatal Infection	Late Effects
Rubella	+	+	+	Cataract, retinopathy, sensorineural deafness, patent ductus arteriosus, pulmonary stenosis, VSD, microcephaly, cognitive impairment	Interstitial pneumonitis, cholestatic hepatitis with giant cell transformation, anemia, thrombocytopenia, myocarditis, immunopathy, osteoporosis, pancreatitis	Interstitial pulmonary fibrosis, hepatic fibrosis/cirrhosis, biliary atresia, arteriopathy with infarction, diabetes mellitus, chronic lymphocytic thyroiditis, panencephalitis, autism (?)
Cytomegalovirus	?	+	+	Microcephaly, hydrocephaly, microphthalmia	Necrotizing meningoencephalitis with arterial and periventricular calcification, hepatitis with giant cell transformation, cholangitis, inclusions in lung, renal tubules, rare pneumonitis and interstitial nephritis	Deafness, neurologic deficits, optic atrophy, noncirrhotic portal hypertension, and vascular and periventricular calcifications (brain) Hypoganglionosis of bowel (see *Pediatr Pathol* 1984;2:85-102)
Herpes simplex	+	+	+	Microcephaly, hydranencephaly, microphthalmia	Hepatoadrenal necrosis, vesicular skin rash, vesicular/ulcerated stomatitis, esophagitis, necrotizing pneumonitis, chorioretinitis	Psychomotor retardation
Varicella-zoster	?	?	+	Limb hypoplasia, rudimentary digits, cutaneous scars in dermatome distribution, chorioretinitis, microphthalmia	Typical varicella, acute disseminated varicella with necrotizing cutaneous and visceral lesions	Blindness, psychomotor retardation

	Abortion	Stillbirth	Intrauterine Growth Restriction	Congenital Defects	Acute Perinatal Infection	Late Effects
HIV	+	+	+	None	See Table 6-9A	See Table 6-9B
Parvovirus	+	+	−	Ocular defects	Anemia, hydrops, hepatic fibrosis, siderosis	?
Hepatitis B	−	−	−	−	Acute hepatitis, giant cell transformation, chronic active hepatitis, fulminant hepatitis	Cirrhosis, carrier state hepatocellular carcinoma
Hepatitis A	+	−	+	−	Rare	−
Mumps	+	+	−	Not proved	Perinatal parotitis (extremely rare)	Endocardial fibroelastosis (?)
Influenza	+	+	−	Unlikely	Rare influenza pneumonia, apnea	−
Vaccinia	+	+	+	−	Generalized vaccinia	−
Variola	+	+	?	?	Smallpox	−
Measles	+	+	−	?	Measles pneumonia	−
Polio	+	+	+	−	Paralytic polio	Paralysis
Echo	−	−	−	−	Meningitis, DIC	−
Coxsackie B	?	?	−	−	Disseminated disease, meningoencephalitis, myocarditis	−
Adenovirus	−	−	−	−	Pneumonia	−
RSV	−	−	−	−	Apnea, bronchiolitis, pneumonia	Asthma (?), COPD

DIC, disseminated intravascular coagulation; VSD, ventricular septal defect. +, occurs; −, does not occur.

TABLE 6-8 COMMON SYSTEMIC VIRAL INFECTIONS IN INFANTS AND CHILDREN

Virus	Localized or Self-Limited Disease	Disseminated or Serious Disease	Specific Inclusions	Comments
Adenoviruses	Acute respiratory illness (types 1, 2, 3, 4, 7, 21) Laryngotracheitis, pneumonia	Types 1, 2, 4, 5, 7, 11 Hepatitis, massive hepatic necrosis Pneumonia, hemorrhagic cystitis, gastroenteritis, meningoencephalitis	1. Large basophilic indistinctly demarcated intranuclear inclusion (smudge cells) 2. Smaller eosinophilic intranuclear with incomplete halo	Easily confused with disseminated HSV infection
Cytomegalovirus	Mononucleosis	Interstitial pneumonia Gastroenteritis Retinitis, encephalitis, glomerulonephritis	1. Large amphophilic or basophilic nuclear inclusions with distinct halo. 2. Smaller basophilic PAS-positive indistinct cytoplasmic inclusions	Disease in immunocompromised host is similar to neonatal pattern.
Herpes simplex	Localized oral, skin, or genital vesicular or ulcerated eruption, may be extensive	Hepatitis, hepatoadrenal necrosis, stomatitis, esophagitis, encephalitis, pneumonia	1. Type A eosinophilic nuclear inclusions with halo 2. Type B basophilic or amphophilic nuclear inclusions filling nucleus with peripheral chromatin rim, often multinucleate cells	Either type I or type II may disseminate: disseminated form resembles neonatal disease.
Varicella-zoster	Localized herpes zoster, acute varicella, generalized vesicular eruption	Disseminated zoster Progressive disseminated varicella, pneumonia, meningoencephalitis, hepatitis	Multinuclear or mononuclear cells with nuclear type A inclusions, indistinguishable from HSV inclusions	Associated with Reye syndrome
Epstein-Barr virus	Mononucleosis	Fatal mononucleosis, hepatitis, myocarditis, immunodeficiency various hematologic phenotypes in X-linked lymphoproliferative syndrome	None	Implicated in oncogenesis, especially in X-linked lymphoproliferative syndrome, posttransplant lymphoproliferative syndrome
Rubeola	Uncomplicated primary measles, skin, conjunctiva, respiratory tract	Progressive measles	Cytoplasmic and nuclear inclusions in epithelial and Warthin-Finkeldey giant cells	Subacute sclerosing panencephalitis, late
Mumps	Parotitis	Orchitis/oophoritis Meningitis, pancreatitis Mastitis, nephritis, arthritis	None	Late sequelae include deafness and diabetes mellitus.

TABLE 6-8 COMMON SYSTEMIC VIRAL INFECTIONS IN INFANTS AND CHILDREN (Continued)

Virus	Localized or Self-Limited Disease	Disseminated or Serious Disease	Specific Inclusions	Comments
Coxsackievirus	Coxsackieviruses A; benign, self-limited febrile illness with respiratory disease	Coxsackieviruses B, myocarditis, meningoencephalitis	None	
Echoviruses	Mild nonspecific febrile illness with respiratory disease	Hepatitis, hepatic necrosis, meningitis, adrenal and renal hemorrhage	None	
Variola (smallpox)	Disease declared eradicated by WHO in 1980		Cytoplasmic Guarnieri bodies. Nuclear changes inconsistent	
Vaccinia	Eczema vaccinatum	Disseminated vaccinia	Indistinguishable from smallpox	
Hantavirus	?	Hantavirus pulmonary syndrome in adolescents	None	Noncarcinogenic pulmonary edema

HSV, herpes simplex virus; PAS, periodic acid–Schiff; WHO, World Health Organization.

transmitted. Virus is present in urine; oropharyngeal, cervical, and vaginal secretions; breast milk; semen; and tears and can be shed intermittently for years.

Clinical Features

Transplacental transmission can result in congenital infection and neurologic sequelae. Perinatal and postnatal transmission usually fails to produce clinical disease except in extremely preterm infants (28). Around approximately 90% of infants born with congenital CMV infection do not exhibit clinical abnormalities at birth (so-called asymptomatic congenital CMV infection). Of the 40,000 children annually born with congenital CMV infection, approximately 10% to 15% exhibit clinical signs or symptoms. Infection involves multiple organ systems, particularly the reticuloendothelial and central nervous systems (CNS). Commonly observed physical signs in these infants include petechiae, jaundice, and hepatosplenomegaly (Figure 6-2). Neurologic abnormalities such as microcephaly and lethargy affect a significant proportion. Other physical signs include intrauterine growth restriction, chorioretinitis, optic atrophy, and seizures. Postnatally acquired infection results in neonatal sepsis with apnea, bradycardia, hepatitis, leukopenia, and prolonged thrombocytopenia. Older children with severe infection are typically immunodeficient. Disseminated CMV infection produces fever, leukopenia, thrombocytopenia, pneumonia, hepatitis, chorioretinitis, adrenalitis, and encephalitis. Infected infants may have the characteristic "blueberry muffin" lesions, a hemorrhagic purpura with mobile gray–blue skin papules that contain dermal extramedullary hematopoiesis. CNS lesions are irreversible and affect prognosis. Symptomatic liver disease commonly occurs, ranging from mild inclusion body cholangitis to severe cholestatic hepatitis (Figure 6-2). Noncirrhotic portal fibrosis with portal hypertension is rare but results in potentially lethal late sequela. Glomerulonephritis, ascites, and pulmonary hypoplasia are also described. A syndrome of hepatosplenomegaly, respiratory distress, a peculiar gray pallor, and atypical lymphocytosis occurs in multiple transfused low-birth-weight infants in this setting. Interstitial inclusion body pneumonitis (Figure 6-2) likely causes the high (24%) mortality rate.

Pathology

Morphologic hallmarks of CMV infection comprise cytomegaly with extremely large (25 to 40 μm) inclusion-bearing cells and both nuclear and cytoplasmic inclusions; often, the nucleolus is retained within the inclusion, appearing as an "accessory body" (29). A clear zone around the inclusion with chromatin margination renders an "owl's eye" appearance. Inclusions vary from eosinophilic to deeply basophilic, depending on developmental stage. The inclusions are periodic acid–Schiff (PAS) and GMS positive, although immunostains are commonly used to specifically identify the virus. They are also CD15-positive, creating potential confusion with Hodgkin lymphoma. Potential virocytes include endothelial cells, epithelial cells (notably the biliary tree, pneumocytes, many exocrine cells, and renal tubular cells), fibroblasts, and histiocytes. Patchy, focal necrosis with mononuclear cells, occasionally neutrophils, and vascular and parenchymal calcifications characterizes the infection. Calcifications most commonly affect the developing brain. Giant cell transformation of hepatocytes is not a frequent feature.

Congenital neurologic and hematologic damage and developmental defects are evident at birth in 10% of

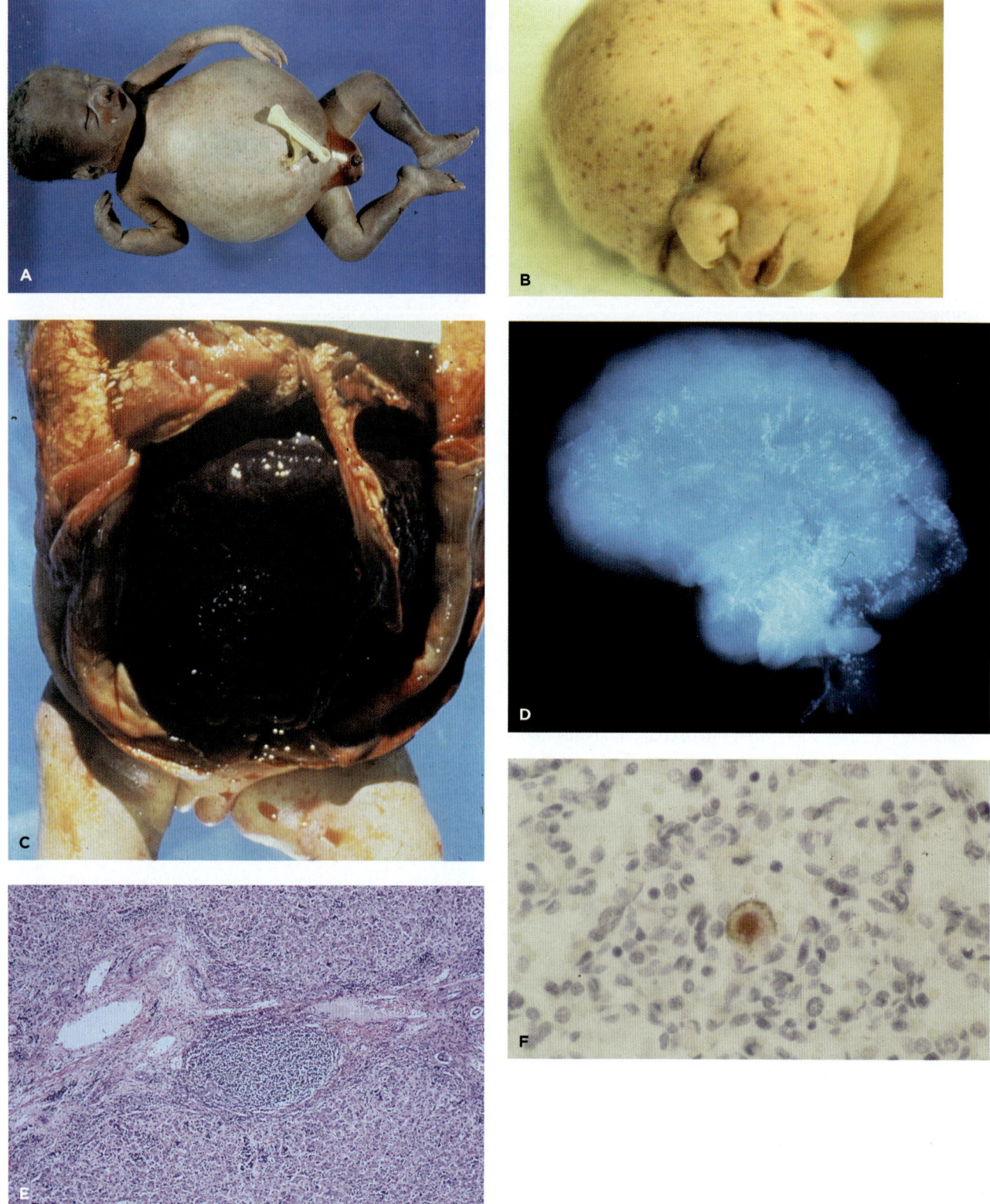

FIGURE 6-2 • Congenital CMV infection. **A:** Body with marked ascites. **B:** Face with petechiae as well as elsewhere. **C:** Abdominal cavity at autopsy showing hepatosplenomegaly. **D:** Skull x-ray with diffuse calcification secondary to necrosis. (See Malinger G, Lev D, Zahalka N, et al. *Am J Neuroradiol* 2003;24:28–32.) **E:** CMV hepatitis with inflammation around a bile duct and within the lobules. **F:** Lung: CMV immunostain with large nuclear inclusion.

CMV-infected babies. During infancy, sequelae such as sensorineural deafness, psychomotor retardation, and cerebral palsy may develop even in infants lacking symptoms at birth. About 20% of all infected neonates suffer sequelae of a congenital CMV infection (30).

Laboratory Diagnosis

When large inclusion-bearing cells are present, morphologic diagnosis is straightforward. Sensitivity of histopathologic methods can be improved with immunocytochemical and molecular virologic techniques. The reference method for diagnosing congenital CMV infection involves isolating the virus in cell culture from urine collected within 3 weeks of birth, but a positive result after the third week may result from vaginal secretions, breast-feeding, or untested transfusions (30). Detection of CMV in the saliva and urine of infants is accomplished easily because newborns with congenital CMV shed large amounts of virus into these body fluids. Blood is also a useful specimen to detect viral DNA or pp65 antigen in peripheral blood leukocytes, but these methods have not been evaluated for diagnosing congenital CMV infection. Viral DNA can be detected in neonatal blood dried on paper (DBS). The DBS test is simpler, faster, and less costly than viral isolation. The samples can be safely stored for extended periods, so diagnosis can be made even after several years. The DBS method is reported to have high sensitivity (71% to 100%) and specificity (99% to 100%) (31).

Laboratory findings in 50% of symptomatic CMV-infected neonates include conjugated hyperbilirubinemia, thrombocytopenia, and elevations of hepatic transaminases reflecting the involvement of the hepatobiliary and reticuloendothelial systems (28). Viral culture of amniotic fluid can identify fetal infection, but a false negative is common. Polymerase chain reaction (PCR) assays on amniotic fluid may have better sensitivity and specificity but require the presence of viremia in the peripheral blood and may not identify every congenital CMV infection.

Prognosis and Outcome

Mortality rate among symptomatic children is now less than 5%. Of the symptomatic children who survive infancy, most will suffer mild to severe psychomotor and perceptual handicaps, and approximately one half will develop sensorineural hearing loss, cognitive impairment, and microcephaly (28). Predictors of adverse neurologic outcome include microcephaly, chorioretinitis, presence of other neonatal or neurologic abnormalities, and cranial abnormalities on CT scans. Petechiae and intrauterine growth restriction independently predict hearing loss. Children asymptomatic at birth have a better long-term prognosis, but approximately 10% develop sensorineural hearing loss, often bilateral. Neurologic complications occur in asymptomatic congenital CMV infection less frequently than in symptomatic infection. This inability to predict outcome in infants at risk for the development of hearing loss and other sequelae necessitates monitoring and follow-up of all children with congenital CMV infection (32).

HERPES SIMPLEX VIRUS (HSV)

First described as hepatoadrenal necrosis by Haas in 1935 (33), HSV types 1 and 2 cause severe perinatal infections and, less frequently, prenatal and postnatal infections. HSV-2 predominates, and about 20% of infections are caused by HSV-1 (34). The risk to the infant is highest at the time of delivery in mothers with primary genital herpes, but fetal infection may occur in the absence of visible maternal lesions.

Transmission

Most HSV infections in infants are acquired during passage through an infected birth canal. Maternal skin infections and even nipple lesions, as well as paternal disease, pose a threat to the infant. Severe fetal intrauterine infection can also occur as a consequence of either primary or recurrent maternal infection. HSV antigen in endometrium, decidua, and placenta suggests possible transplacental passage. Case reports demonstrate HSV infections in infants caused by maternal HSV-positive breast lesions, and conversely, virus from primary infantile gingivostomatitis may infect the mother's breast.

Clinical Features

Neonatal infections manifest in the first week of life. Although the neonatal form of the disease may be relatively benign, the majority of cases result in death from disseminated disease with meningoencephalitis (50%) or serious neurologic impairment (30%). The clinical presentation is variable and diagnosis may be extremely difficult; seizures, cyanosis, shock, and bleeding diatheses are common manifestations. Since no specific sign or symptom is diagnostic, the diagnosis should be strongly considered in the presence of HSV risk factors, atypical sepsis, unexplained acute hepatitis, or focal seizure activity. Neonatal HSV infection may be either disseminated or relatively localized. In general, the younger the patient at presentation, the more disseminated the lesions. Infants with subclinical encephalitis usually have skin and mucous membrane lesions (Figure 6-3A). Conversely, at least one-third of newborns with disseminated HSV do not have detectable skin or mucous membrane lesions at the time of presentation (34). In older infants and children, clinical presentations include orolabial and genital herpes, herpes gladiatorum, herpetic whitlow, eczema herpeticum, and ocular herpes. Herpes encephalitis in older children is an emergency that requires a high index of suspicion to diagnose (35).

Pathology

The pathologic hallmark of disseminated HSV are patchy and focal well-demarcated punctate areas of yellow-tan to hemorrhagic coagulative necrosis with little cellular inflammatory reaction at the periphery of irregular zones of necrosis (Figure 6-3B, C) (34). There are two types of inclusions (Figure 6-3D). Early infectious inclusions (Cowdry type B) stain variably (usually amphophilic, sometimes basophilic), are homogeneous and glassy, occupy the entire nucleus, and

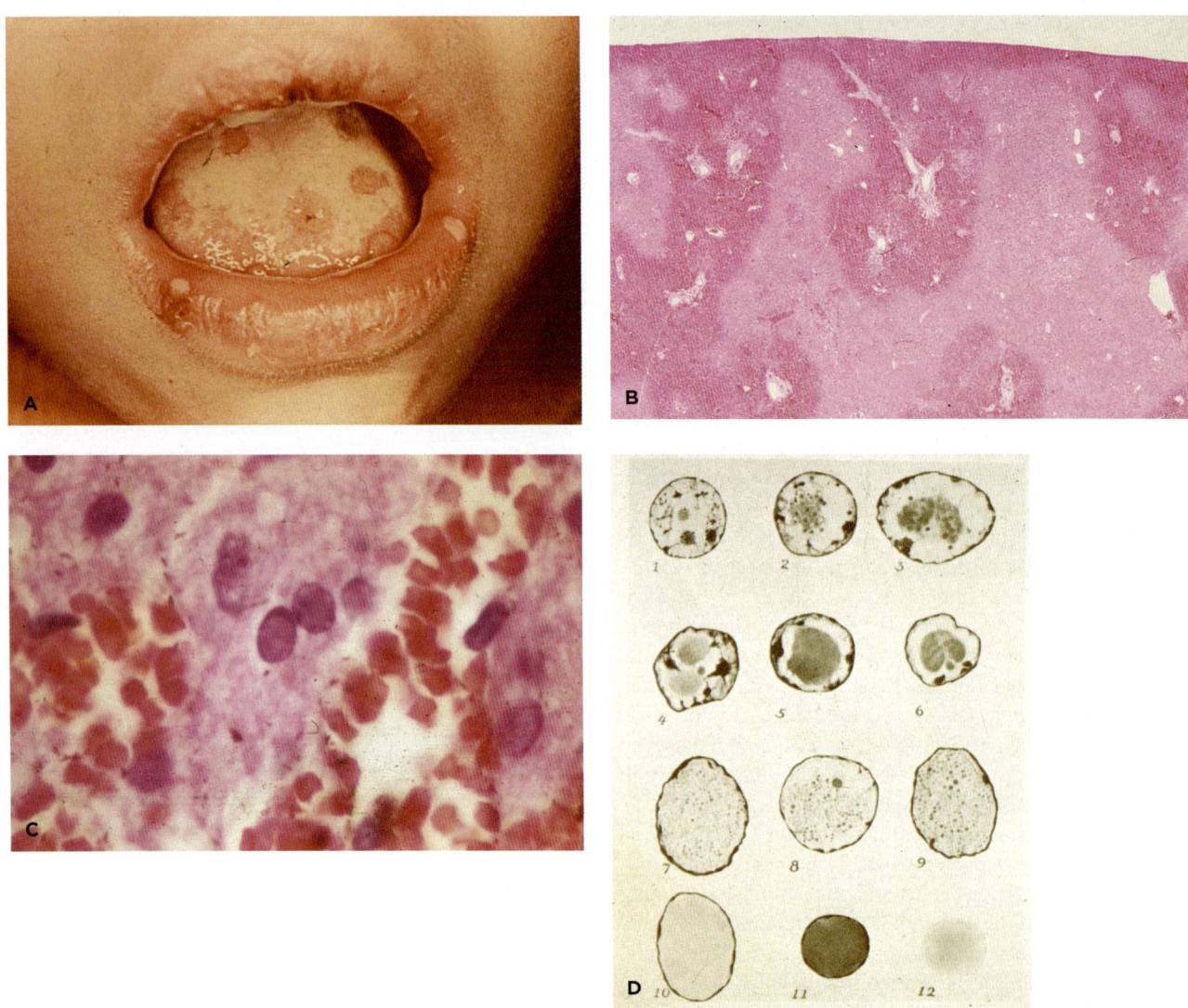

FIGURE 6-3 • Herpes simplex infection. **A:** Herpetic stomatitis. **B:** Liver (low power) with multifocal areas of coagulative necrosis. **C:** Liver (high power) with smooth nuclear inclusions usually at the interface between the necrotic and viable parenchyma. **D:** Pictorial representation of inclusions—camera lucida drawings by *E. Piotti*; each nucleus corresponds to the types of inclusions seen in the first reported case of HSV infection. (With permission from Singer DB. Pathology of neonatal Herpes simplex virus infection. *Perspect Pediatr Pathol* 1981;6:243–278.)

push the chromatin to the nuclear membrane. The later inclusions (Cowdry type A) are smaller, deeply eosinophilic, round, or polygonal and separated from the nuclear membrane by a clear halo. Multinucleated cells are more likely to contain Cowdry type B inclusions. Type A inclusions reflect excess viral capsid material following extrusion of encapsidated viral DNA. Seventy-five to eighty percent of cases of disseminated HSV involve liver (Figure 6-3B, C) and adrenal glands. Lesions may also be seen in the lung, brain, spleen, bone marrow, and GIT. Care must be exercised in the evaluation of necrotizing and ulcerated skin or mucous membrane lesions; HSV inclusions can usually be found at the periphery of such lesions, as secondary bacterial or yeast infection may obscure the underlying viral lesion.

Laboratory Diagnosis

If vesicular or ulcerated lesions are present, a firm diagnosis is usually possible using smears of vesical fluid or scrapings of the base of the lesional. In properly stained smears, identification of the characteristic, often multiple inclusions is straightforward; epithelial cells contain one or more large intranuclear inclusions, described with three Ms: Multinucleation of cells, Molding of nuclei, and Margination of chromatin (Figure 6-3D). Morphologic distinction from varicella-zoster inclusions is not possible, but in the usual clinical setting, this is not a problem. Both immunohistochemical and molecular biologic techniques can be used in distinguishing HSV from other viruses. Resistance testing of antivirals to HSV-1 can be done by phenotypic and genotypic methods. Phenotypic methods are cumbersome but allow clear interpretation of results, whereas genotypic methods are faster but may be diagnostically less conclusive (36).

Prognosis and Outcome

Neonatal herpes is a potentially devastating illness, with 80% mortality without treatment. Even with therapy, the mortality rate for disseminated disease remains very high (50%). About 25% of survivors may have neurologic defects and/or blindness. Maternal therapy or prophylactic infant treatment, in certain situations, may decrease shedding, hasten clinical resolution, and protect the patient.

The consequences of neonatal HSV infection can be severe (37). Disease may be localized to skin, eye, and mouth (SEM disease), involve the CNS, or disseminate to multiple organs. Most survivors in the latter two categories have neurologic sequelae. Neonatal herpes may occur in the absence of skin lesions; if infection is suspected, swabs of the oropharynx, conjunctiva, rectum, skin lesions, mucosal lesions, urine, and cerebrospinal fluid (CSF) should be promptly submitted for laboratory studies (38).

HUMAN PARVOVIRUS INFECTION

Parvovirus B19, better known as a cause of erythema infectiosum (fifth disease), is a single-stranded DNA virus of the *Erythrovirus* genus that primarily targets erythroid precursors in the bone marrow. Because the erythrocyte P antigen is the cellular receptor for the virus, individuals lacking this antigen are resistant to infection.

Transmission

Transmission occurs through contact with respiratory droplets, saliva, and, less commonly, blood and urine. Seroprevalence data show that peak parvovirus infections occur in school-age children. Modes of entry into bloodstream and placenta are not clearly known.

Clinical Features

Intrauterine infection (39) results in fetal anemia, a pronounced leukoerythroblastic reaction, and hepatitis with excessive iron deposition. Parvovirus is a major cause of disease and possibly accounts for up to 16% of cases of "idiopathic" nonimmune hydrops (40). In Anand's series (39), two of six affected pregnancies resulted in fetal hydrops and death, whereas the other four infants were normal. Fetal and perinatal presentations other than hydrops have been described. Ocular lesions include microphthalmia, aphakia, and dysplasia of sclera, anterior segment, and retina. Liveborn infants can present with a lethal constellation of anemia, petechial rash, purpuric "blueberry muffin" lesions, and severe liver disease with hepatic fibrosis and siderosis that mimic the syndrome of neonatal hemochromatosis (41).

Although postnatal infection is frequently asymptomatic, the best known clinical illness is immune-mediated erythema infectiosum or fifth disease. Fifth disease is a highly contagious pediatric illness with a slapped cheek appearance and lacy erythematous exanthem on the face, trunk, and proximal limbs in children. Adults manifest arthralgias and arthritis. Severe consequences occur most often in individuals with hemoglobinopathy, red blood cell abnormalities, or immunodeficiency. Erythroid abnormalities include pure red cell aplasia and aplastic anemia (especially aplastic crisis in a setting of chronic hemolytic anemia). Vasculitis and hemophagocytic syndrome can also occur. In some series, parvovirus has been the agent most frequently associated with myocarditis, but the significance of this finding has been questioned in an autopsy study.

Pathology

The bone marrow shows variable degrees of erythroid hypoplasia. Morphologic abnormalities in red cell precursors include giant pronormoblasts with vacuoles and multiple nucleoli. Distinctive eosinophilic intranuclear inclusions occur in erythroid lineage cells. By DNA hybridization and electron microscopy, inclusions contain B19 virus (39), and the virus is readily detected in tissue with immunohistochemical and PCR techniques (40). Histologic studies on very young fetuses show ocular malformations and generalized intense inflammatory reactions. The first clue to the infection may be infected red cells in the fetal capillaries of the placenta.

RUBELLA

Rubella is caused by a single-stranded RNA virus. Originally described by Gregg as a classic triad of cataracts, deafness, and congenital heart disease (42), the "expanded rubella syndrome" is rare in countries where rubella vaccination is the norm. However, congenital rubella syndrome (CRS) is unfortunately not just a subject of historical interest. Existence of both a nonimmune population of women of childbearing age and the many survivors of the 1964 to 1965 epidemic attest to the continued importance of this disease. Investigation of adult individuals enables delineation of late effects of congenital infection (43).

Transmission

Rubella virus is capable of infecting the fetus at any time during gestation. Virus reaches the fetus in emboli of necrotic placental tissue and then affects the fetus by at least three mechanisms: (a) inhibition of cell growth, (b) cytolysis, and (c) compromise of blood supply (43). These factors consequently incite necrosis, inflammation, and scarring in virtually limitless combinations and permutations. Unlike CMV, maternal antibodies to rubella virus protect the fetus from infection. Postnatal and childhood infections are transmitted through inhalation of droplets of nasopharyngeal secretions. Per the CDC, endemic rubella and CRS have been eliminated from the United States through 2011, but international importation continues (44).

Clinical Features

The incidence and pattern of fetal rubella vary strikingly with gestational age at the time of maternal viremia. Congenital heart defects result from infection in the first trimester of gestation, deafness and neurologic deficits follow infection through the 4th gestational month, and retinopathy ensues through the 5th gestational month. Infection late in gestation more likely produces inflammatory and destructive lesions, without evidence of malformation. The probability of the fetus suffering significant damage decreases from 80% to 90% in first trimester to near 0% beyond 20 weeks. In either case, the virus is recoverable for months to years after birth. With the possible exception of microcephaly, most CNS abnormalities result from meningoencephalitis and/or necrosis. Necrosis, presumably ischemic, is related to the vascular lesions seen in a majority of cases. True developmental malformation is rare (43). A late-onset chronic progressive panencephalitis with neuropathologic changes similar to subacute sclerosing panencephalitis (SSPE) occurs in the second decade of life in some survivors of CRS. These changes include meningeal and perivascular infiltrates of lymphocytes and plasma cells with glial nodules, predominantly in the white matter. Rubella virus has been recovered from these late lesions. Deafness in CRS is related both to CNS damage causing central auditory imperception and to inflammation and scarring in the cochlea. CRS and Down syndrome are considered to be the main causes of combined deafness and blindness in patients over 18 years of age, whereas CHARGE syndrome is the main cause in children (45). Disseminated sequelae may relate to vascular spread and cytopathic effects on endothelial cells. Deafness, cardiovascular and neurologic damage, and retinopathy are rare if infection occurs beyond the second trimester, suggesting a protective role of maternal antibodies (46).

Postnatal rubella presents as a prodrome followed by a characteristic postauricular lymphadenopathy. Fine maculopapular rash appears 1 to 5 days later, starting in the face and spreading to limbs and trunk and lasting about 3 days. Complications are infrequent but include immune manifestations such as arthritis, encephalitis, Guillain-Barré syndrome, and thrombocytopenia. Surveillance of postnatal and congenital infection is an essential component of CRS prevention, since rubella is difficult to diagnose on clinical grounds alone. Laboratory differentiation of rubella from other exanthems, such as measles, parvovirus B19, human herpes virus 6, enteroviruses, and various endemic arboviruses, is essential. Current testing includes RT-PCR and sequencing for diagnosis and epidemiologic surveillance, and oral fluid tests for detection of rubella-specific IgG and IgM salivary antibody responses (47).

Pathology

A wide spectrum of cardiovascular disease is seen in CRS. In addition to the characteristic patent ductus arteriosus, lesions most commonly include pulmonary artery branch stenosis, myocarditis, and systemic arterial hypoplasia and stenosis. Valvular sclerosis has been frequent in some series (43). The arterial lesion of CRS is distinctive and possibly unique: fibromuscular intimal proliferation, devoid of inflammatory change, leads to patchy and focal vascular stenosis. The media and adventitia are usually not disrupted, and there is no calcification (except in the brain). Chronic meningeal inflammation, perivascular lymphocytic infiltrates, gliosis, and mineralization of cerebral arterioles may occur. Transient bone lesions consist of focal osteopenia and growth inhibition. Metaphyseal changes reminiscent of syphilis, that is, longitudinal radiologic striations, occur in one-half of the patients. Interstitial pneumonitis is seen in up to 75% of CRS infants and may persist for up to a year after birth. Alterations of the lymphoreticular system are variable; both precocious germinal centers (from viral antigenic stimulus) and lymphoid depletion are encountered. Histiocytic proliferation and erythrophagocytosis may be seen. Hepatic changes include cholestatic hepatitis, giant cell transformation, necrosis, extramedullary hematopoiesis, and fibrosis; cirrhosis may ensue. On occasion, bile duct proliferation mimics extrahepatic biliary atresia; true biliary atresia has been reported anecdotally. Eye changes include cataracts, lens necrosis, ciliary body inflammation, iridocyclitis, and retinitis. Interstitial nephritis and chronic lymphocytic thyroiditis have also been described. The placenta may show villitis, villous stromal necrosis and sclerosis, and vascular endothelial lesions (48). Due to its short and benign course, no specific histopathologic features characterize postnatal rubella infection.

Laboratory Diagnosis

Serologic testing for IgM antibodies is the primary diagnostic test to confirm acute rubella infection. Additional diagnostic tests include paired IgG serology, molecular testing, and rubella IgG avidity testing.

Prognosis and Outcome

Characteristically, CRS sequelae affect the eyes (cataracts or retinopathy) and hearing (sensorineural deafness). Multiorgan involvement may include myocarditis, hepatitis, cytopenia, meningoencephalitis, and visceromegaly. Cardiac teratogenic effects include patent ductus arteriosus, pulmonary artery stenosis, and supra-aortic stenosis. Long-term effects of intrauterine rubella infection include an increase in the prevalence of diabetes, thyroid disorders, early menopause, and osteoporosis (49). HLA haplotypes that are associated with autoimmune disorders occur in increased frequency. Approximately 20% of CRS survivors develop diabetes mellitus, usually in the second or third decade. Persistent viral infection has been implicated as the virus may be recovered from the pancreas and lymphocytic infiltration of the pancreas may be seen at postmortem exam. Postnatal growth retardation probably results from active virus, as evidenced by its prolonged shedding in nasopharyngeal secretions.

VARICELLA ZOSTER VIRUS

VZV (human herpes virus 3) is a double-stranded DNA virus. The existence of a fetal varicella syndrome was suggested in 1974, although the first case had been reported years earlier. Several studies describe the defects associated with fetal varicella infection, and a specific neonatal syndrome is associated with maternal varicella (but not by maternal zoster) occurring during the first half of pregnancy (50).

Transmission

Congenital VZV infections are transmitted transplacentally. The risk of embryopathy with maternal infection in the first 20 weeks of gestation is estimated at 0.4% to 2%. Intrauterine insult occurring between 8 and 20 weeks of gestation results in a fetal disease with distinctive herpes zoster-like dermatome distribution. Although the virus has not been isolated from affected fetuses or newborns, virus specific IgM has been demonstrated in affected fetus and VZV DNA sequences have been recovered from the placenta. Neonatal varicella infection follows *in utero* near-term exposure or postnatal contact with the mother or others (household or nursery). Infants delivered of mothers who were infected more than 5 days before delivery fared best, presumably because there was time for production and transfer of maternal antibody. Perinatal infection can be severe when the mother presents with chicken pox exanthem from 5 days before to 2 days after delivery, since maternal transplacental viremia occurs without sufficient time for maternal–fetal antibody transfer. Postnatal transmission occurs via respiratory droplets and contact or aerosolization of virus from varicella or zoster skin lesions. Infection peaks in winter and spring.

Clinical Features

Fetal varicella results in multiple defects of skin, limbs, eyes, and brain, giving an impression of a sudden devastating, but self-limited, herpes zoster–like in utero illness (50). All patients exhibit cicatricial skin lesions corresponding to the affected dermatome. There is frequent associated hypoplasia of the underlying bone and soft tissue. Hypoplastic limbs, many seriously deformed by scarring, occur in 80% of cases. Occasional calcification of the liver suggests dissemination, and viral-like inclusions can be seen in the lung. CNS involvement may take the form of necrotizing encephalitis with calcification. Microphthalmia, severe chorioretinitis with scarring, and cataract lead to blindness. Neurologic abnormalities frequently correspond anatomically to the afflicted dermatome and include limb paresis, microcephaly, Horner syndrome, cranial nerve palsies, and cortical atrophy.

Neonatal varicella in the newborn may be limited to the skin (Figure 6-4) or disseminate widely; disseminated disease carries a very high mortality rate, largely due to varicella pneumonia. Older children develop a prodrome for 2 to 3 days, followed by a transient scarlatiniform rash that may precede or accompany the characteristic varicelliform rash, which appears on the trunk and spreads out as crops of 1- to 4-mm maculopapular lesions. These progress to clear fluid-filled vesicles ("dew drop on a rose petal") and pustules, with accompanying distressing pruritus. Lesions of various stages are seen in a given patient, and the patient remains infectious until all the lesions have crusted. Excoriation may leave shallow pink depressions that lead to scars when complicated by secondary bacterial infection. Vesicles may also develop on mucous membranes and leave multiple small ulcers. Rarely, there may be septic shock, hemolytic–uremic

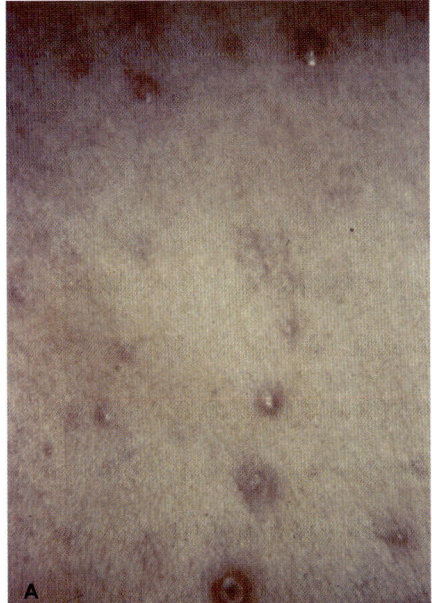 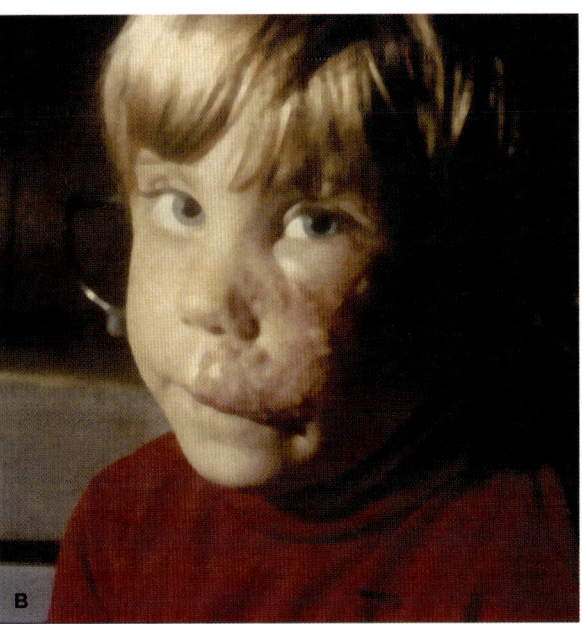

FIGURE 6-4 • Varicella-zoster virus infection. **A:** Neonatal varicella with skin lesions. **B:** Herpes zoster in an older child.

syndrome, necrotizing pneumonia, encephalitis, hepatitis, and/or Reye syndrome (51).

VZV infects sensory nerves, migrates to sensory ganglia during acute infections, and remains latent there, to cause later herpes zoster (Figure 6-4). Involvement of nonneuronal satellite cells, which interface with multiple neurons, may allow the virus to involve large geographic areas (e.g., an entire dermatome) during reactivation. A prodrome of pain, itching, burning, and paresthesia may precede the characteristic zosteriform eruption by 4 to 5 days, as may constitutional symptoms such as headache, fever, and malaise. Lesions may continue to develop within the dermatome over a week and last for 2 to 3 weeks but may last longer in debilitated and immunodeficient patients. Ulcers, scaling, hyperpigmentation, and secondary bacterial infection with resultant scarring may complicate the clinical picture. Herpes zoster is uncommon in childhood.

Pathology

Chicken pox is a clinical diagnosis. However, Tzanck smears of vesicular or pustular fluid (of varicella or zoster) allows rapid identification of VSZ-infected cells by demonstrating intranuclear inclusions and giant cells similar to those seen in HSV infection. Skin biopsies also show features similar to HSV, that is, ballooning degeneration progressing to acantholytic intraepidermal vesicle sometimes involving adnexa. Unlike HSV infection, dermal leukocytoclastic vasculitis with occasional hemorrhage may occur. Inclusions begin as faint basophilic intranuclear bodies with peripheral chromatin condensation, later becoming eosinophilic with a surrounding halo. An immunostain is available for specific identification. Disseminated VZV may induce hemorrhagic necrosis in a variety of organs, with little or no inflammation or eosinophilic intranuclear inclusions. Pulmonary lesions consist of an interstitial mononuclear infiltrate, edema, hemorrhage, and hyaline membranes, all apparent within focal, sharply defined centrilobular areas of necrosis (51).

Laboratory Diagnosis

Culture, direct fluorescent antibody assay (DFA), and PCR assays are available for diagnosis of VZV-induced disease. Serologic tests are available but not recommended for diagnosis.

Prognosis and Outcome

Chicken pox is almost always self-limited. Death from chicken pox is distinctly unusual (12 deaths/100,000 cases), except in immunodeficient patients in whom pneumonia, meningoencephalitis, and hepatitis may develop (52). Less frequently, other systemic manifestations may occur, including nephritis, myocarditis, arthritis, myositis, uveitis, orchitis, and idiopathic thrombocytopenic purpura (53). Reye syndrome has been described following treatment with salicylates, and aspirin is contraindicated in patients with chicken pox.

HUMAN IMMUNODEFICIENCY VIRUS (HIV)

The first cases of pediatric acquired immunodeficiency syndrome (AIDS) were reported in 1982–1983, soon after recognition of adult disease. Over 90% of cases of childhood HIV infection are acquired by vertical transmission. HIV/AIDS in children resembles adult disease in both its primary viral cytopathic effect on the lymphoid and nervous systems and its secondary immunodeficiency effects including opportunistic infections and neoplasia. Adult and pediatric HIV infection also differs with respect to diagnostic methods, effects on the response capability of the developing immune system, etiologies of secondary infections, and type and distribution of pathologic lesions. HIV-2 causes clinical disease similar to HIV-1 but with a significantly slower progression to immune suppression. In West African infants, there is infrequent HIV-2 vertical transmission and no cases of late postnatal seroconversion (54). HIV-2 transmission through breast milk occurs less commonly than for HIV-1, but the risk and possible factors contributing to transmission have not been adequately quantified. Recent volumes have detailed the epidemiology, immunopathogenesis, molecular biology, and clinicopathologic aspects of pediatric AIDS (55–57). The CDC surveillance case definitions for HIV and AIDS are shown in Tables 6-9A, 6-9B, and 6-10 (58).

Transmission

Vertical transmission is the most common mode of acquisition of pediatric HIV. Transmission of virus by breast-feeding, sexual abuse, and heterosexual or homosexual relationships accounts for most of the remainder. The risk of transmission through transfusion of blood or blood products has been almost eliminated. Vertical transmission can take place *in utero*, intrapartum, or postpartum, through breast-feeding. To some extent, the resultant infections can be distinguished on the basis of culturable virus or HIV genome in cord and infant blood. The best predictor of transmission risk is maternal viral burden, as measured by maternal plasma HIV-1 RNA level. Levels under 500 copies per milliliter imply minimal risk of perinatal transmission (59). Treatment of HIV-infected mothers with effective antiviral agents has significantly decreased the rate of vertical transmission. Obstetric interventions such as caesarian section or shortening of postrupture transmembrane exposure may also decrease the rate of perinatal infection (60). Coinfections appear to increase the risk of mother-to-child HIV transmission such as chorioamnionitis, maternal genital infection (e.g., HSV), systemic infections (e.g., hepatitis B), mastitis, and infant infections (e.g., periodontitis, oral candidiasis, and diarrhea) (61). Despite their immature immune system and prolonged repetitive exposure to breast milk, most infants born to HIV-infected women escape infection. In infected infants, the course and response to treatment depend upon the timing (*in utero*, intrapartum, or during breast-feeding) and potentially the route of infection, probably

TABLE 6-9A	2008 SURVEILLANCE CASE DEFINITION FOR HIV INFECTION AMONG CHILDREN AGED <18 MONTHS[a]

Criteria for definitive or presumptive HIV infection

Child born to an HIV-infected mother and laboratory criterion or at least one other criteria met

Laboratory criterion for definitive HIV infection

Positive results on two separate specimens (not including cord blood) using HIV virologic (nonantibody) tests (HIV nucleic acid detection is method of choice)

Laboratory criterion for presumptive HIV infection

Criterion for definitively HIV infected not met, and

Positive result on one specimen (not including cord blood) using HIV virologic tests AND no subsequent negative results from HIV virologic or antibody tests

Other criteria (for cases that do not meet above laboratory criteria)

HIV infection diagnosed by a physician or qualified medical care provider based on the laboratory criteria and documented in a medical record. Oral reports of prior laboratory test results are not acceptable.

or

When test results regarding HIV infection status are not available, documentation of a condition that meets the criteria in the 1987 pediatric surveillance case definition for AIDS

Criteria for uninfected with HIV, definitive or presumptive

Child born to an HIV-infected mother is either definitively or presumptively uninfected with HIV if (1) the criteria for definitive or presumptive HIV infection are not met and (2) at least one of the following laboratory criteria or other criteria are met.

Laboratory criteria for uninfected with HIV, definitive

At least two negative HIV DNA or RNA virologic tests from separate specimens, both of which were obtained at age ≥1 mo and one of which was obtained at age ≥4 mo

or

At least two negative HIV antibody tests from separate specimens obtained at age ≥6 mo

and

No other laboratory or clinical evidence of HIV infection[b]

Laboratory criteria for uninfected with HIV, presumptive

Two negative RNA or DNA virologic tests, from separate specimens, both of which were obtained at age ≥2 wk and one of which was obtained at age ≥4 weeks

or

One negative RNA or a DNA virologic test from a specimen obtained at age ≥8 weeks

or

One negative HIV antibody test from a specimen obtained at age ≥6 mo

or

One positive HIV virologic test followed by at least two negative tests from separate specimens, one of which is a virologic test from a specimen obtained at age ≥8 wk or an HIV antibody test from a specimen obtained at age ≥6 mo

and

No other laboratory or clinical evidence of HIV infection[b]

Other criteria (for cases that do not meet above laboratory criteria)

Determination of uninfected with HIV by a physician or qualified medical care provider based on the laboratory criteria and who has noted the HIV diagnostic test results in the medical record. Oral reports of prior laboratory test results are not acceptable

and

No other laboratory or clinical evidence of HIV infection[b]

Criteria for indeterminate HIV infection

Child born to an HIV-infected mother if the criteria for infected with HIV and uninfected with HIV are not met

[a]These guidelines are intended for public health surveillance only and are not a guide for clinical diagnosis.

[b]No positive results from virologic tests (if tests were performed) and no AIDS-defining condition for which no other underlying condition indicative of immunosuppression exists (see Table 6-10).

Modified from Schneider E, Whitmore S, Glynn KM, et al.; Centers for Disease Control and Prevention. Revised surveillance case definitions for HIV infection among adults, adolescents, and children aged <18 mo and for HIV infection and AIDS among children aged 18 mo to <13 years—United States, 2008. *MMWR* 2008;57(RR-10):1–12.

TABLE 6-9B 2008 SURVEILLANCE CASE DEFINITION FOR HIV INFECTION AMONG CHILDREN AGED 18 MONTHS TO <13 YEARS[a]

Criteria for HIV infection

At least one of laboratory criteria or the other criterion should be met.

Laboratory criteria

Positive result from a screening test for HIV antibody (e.g., reactive EIA), confirmed by a positive result from a supplemental test for HIV antibody (e.g., Western blot or indirect immunofluorescence assay)

or

Positive result or a detectable quantity by an HIV virologic (nonantibody) tests[b]

Other criterion (for cases that do not meet laboratory criteria)

HIV infection diagnosed by a physician or qualified medical care provider based on the laboratory criteria and documented in a medical record. Oral reports of prior laboratory test results are not acceptable.

Criteria for AIDS

Children aged 18 mo to <13 y are categorized for surveillance purposes as having AIDS if the criteria for HIV infection are met and at least one of the AIDS-defining conditions has been documented.

[a]These guidelines are intended for public health surveillance only and are not a guide for clinical diagnosis. The 2008 laboratory criteria for reportable HIV infection among persons aged 18 mo to <13 y exclude confirmation of HIV infection through the diagnosis of AIDS-defining conditions alone (see Table 6-10). Laboratory-confirmed evidence of HIV infection is now required for all reported cases of HIV infection among children aged 18 mo to <13 y.

[b]For HIV screening among children aged 18 mo to <13 y infected through exposure other than perinatal exposure, HIV virologic (nonantibody) tests should not be used in lieu of approved HIV antibody screening tests. A negative result (i.e., undetectable or nonreactive) by an HIV virologic test (e.g., viral RNA nucleic acid test) does not rule out the diagnosis of HIV infection.

TABLE 6-10 AIDS-DEFINING ILLNESSES IN THE PEDIATRIC AGE GROUP

Bacterial infections, multiple or recurrent[a]
Candidiasis of bronchi, trachea, or lungs
Candidiasis of esophagus[b]
Cervical cancer, invasive[c]
Coccidioidomycosis, disseminated or extrapulmonary
Cryptococcosis, extrapulmonary
Cryptosporidiosis, chronic intestinal (>1-month duration)
Cytomegalovirus disease (other than liver, spleen, or nodes), onset at age >1 mo
Cytomegalovirus retinitis (with loss of vision)[b]
Encephalopathy, HIV related
Herpes simplex: chronic ulcers (>1-month duration) or bronchitis, pneumonitis, or esophagitis (onset at age >1 mo)
Histoplasmosis, disseminated or extrapulmonary
Isosporiasis, chronic intestinal (>1-month duration)
Kaposi sarcoma[b]
Lymphoid interstitial pneumonia or pulmonary lymphoid hyperplasia complex[a,b]
Lymphoma, Burkitt (or equivalent term)
Lymphoma, immunoblastic (or equivalent term)
Lymphoma, primary, of brain
Mycobacterium avium complex or *M. kansasii*, disseminated or extrapulmonary[b]
M. tuberculosis of any site, pulmonary,[b,c] disseminated,[b] or extrapulmonary[b]
Mycobacterium, other species or unidentified species, disseminated[b] or extrapulmonary[b]
Pneumocystis jiroveci pneumonia[b]
Pneumonia, recurrent[b,c]
Progressive multifocal leukoencephalopathy
Salmonella septicemia, recurrent
Toxoplasmosis of brain, onset at age >1 mo[b]
Wasting syndrome attributed to HIV

[a]Only among children aged <13 y. (CDC. 1994 Revised classification system for human immunodeficiency virus infection in children <13 years of age. *MMWR* 1994;43[No. RR-12].)

[b]Condition that might be diagnosed presumptively.

[c]Only among adults and adolescents aged ≥13 y. (CDC. 1993 Revised classification system for HIV infection and expanded surveillance case definition for AIDS among adolescents and adults. *MMWR* 1992;41[No. RR-17].)

Source: Schneider E, Whitmore S, Glynn KM, et al.; Centers for Disease Control and Prevention. Revised surveillance case definitions for HIV infection among adults, adolescents, and children aged <18 mo and for HIV infection and AIDS among children aged 18 mo to <13 years—United States, 2008. *MMWR* 2008;57(RR-10):1–12.

due to immunologic factors. Immune factors may be responsible for the adverse effects even in infants who escape actual infection (62).

Breast-feeding by an HIV-1–positive mother increases transmission risk by 4% to 22% over the risk for prior prenatal and perinatal transmission. However, the lack of acceptable, feasible, affordable, sustainable, and safe (AFASS) water for breast milk alternatives complicates infant feeding practices in less developed nations. Unless AFASS criteria are satisfied, current WHO/UNICEF guidelines recommend exclusive breast-feeding for all infants for at least the first 6 months because of reduced infant mortality among exclusively breast-fed, HIV-exposed infants (63). Conversely, the avoidance of breast-feeding in maternal HIV-1 infection is an important component of preventing mother-to-child transmission in the United States and other developed countries. Issues related to breast milk HIV-1 transmission include the increased risk of primary maternal HIV-1 infection during lactation, the health of the HIV-1–infected mother, the presence of virus, potentially immunologically protective factors and factors that enhance HIV-1 transmission in breast milk, and possible interventions that prevent or limit HIV-1 transmission through breast milk (64). These interventions include early weaning, education, and support to decrease the occurrence of mastitis or nipple lesions, antiretroviral therapy for the mother or infant, treating the human milk to decrease the viral burden (ultraviolet light, freezing, and thawing), and stimulating the infant's immune defenses with active or passive immunization.

Clinical Features

Clinical manifestations include hepatosplenomegaly, lymphadenopathy, failure to thrive, fever of unknown origin (FUO), chronic diarrhea, various infections, parotitis, chronic otitis media, lymphoid interstitial pneumonitis (LIP), HIV nephropathy, HIV encephalopathy, HIV cardiomyopathy, idiopathic thrombocytopenia purpura, and lymphoma. Age-specific data suggest that HIV manifestation changes with the child's age, and these may further vary based on geographic location (65–67). HIV encephalopathy, HIV cardiomyopathy, idiopathic thrombocytopenia purpura, and lymphoma may occur later than other manifestations.

There is great variation in rapidity of onset, age of onset, and rate of progression in pediatric AIDS. In perinatally infected infants, the onset of symptomatic disease occurs at 6 to 8 months of age, as compared with a mean of about 18 months in transfusion-acquired pediatric AIDS (and years in adults). This extremely rapid progression undoubtedly reflects early disruption of differentiation in the developing cellular immune system that results from HIV-induced destruction of CD4 lymphocytes before the establishment of a fully developed immunologic response. There is also marked variation in the rate of progression of HIV in pediatric patients once they are symptomatic. Some perinatally infected children have onset of disease in the first year of life characteristically with *Pneumocystis jiroveci* pneumonia (PJP; formerly *Pneumocystis carinii* pneumonia, PCP), HIV encephalopathy, and recurrent severe bacterial infections. Another group is characterized by onset after the first year and a more indolent and chronic course of mucosal candidiasis, LIP, and cardiovascular disease. The reason(s) for these differences are, as yet, unclear. Children with AIDS do not show the marked degree of lymphopenia seen in adults but are more likely to have hyperglobulinemia. Cutaneous anergy is seen in infants. Severe bacterial infections are extremely common in pediatric AIDS, occurring in over 80% of affected children. Among pediatric opportunistic infections, candidiasis is the most frequent (Figure 6-5), beginning as oral thrush and affecting the entire GIT; PJP is the most frequent fatal infection in infancy (Figure 6-5). Other common opportunistic pathogens, depending on geographic distribution and/or population, include CMV (Figure 6-5), *Mycobacterium avium/intracellulare*, tuberculosis (TB), aspergillosis, cryptococcosis, cryptosporidiosis, histoplasmosis, HSV, adenoviral pneumonia, measles, and respiratory syncytial virus (RSV). About 25% of children with AIDS develop a lymphoproliferative syndrome with generalized lymphadenopathy and splenomegaly.

Children with HIV demonstrate lower motor, cognitive, and adaptive functioning compared to uninfected children. Risk factors that may negatively affect the development of infected children include neurologic abnormalities, progression of the disease, and poor environmental factors (68). Anemia, also a very common complication of pediatric HIV infection, is associated with a poor prognosis. Failure of erythropoiesis may be the most important mechanism for anemia (69). Survival in children with AIDS is in general shorter than survival in HIV-infected adults.

Clinical manifestations in children living with HIV/AIDS differ from those in adults, due to a poorly developed immunity that allows greater dissemination throughout various organs. In developing countries, HIV-infected children have an increased frequency of malnutrition and common childhood infections such as otitis, pneumonia, gastroenteritis, and TB. Symptoms common to many treatable conditions, such as recurrent fever, diarrhea, and generalized dermatitis, tend to be more persistent and severe and often do not respond as well to treatment (70).

Pathology

All of the pathologic lesions that occur in adults with HIV infection are seen in children, but there are significant differences in frequency and distribution (71). Pathologies identified more frequently in children include thymic lesions, pulmonary lymphoid and lymphoproliferative disorders (LPDs), and arteriopathy. Polyclonal B-cell lymphoproliferative disorders (PBLD) and malignant lymphoma, especially of brain, are the common neoplasms in children; Kaposi sarcoma is rarely encountered. Table 6-11 outlines the systemic pathology of pediatric HIV infection. Systemic mycoses that are more frequent in HIV-positive patients include cryptococcosis, histoplasmosis, coccidioidomycosis, blastomycosis, paracoccidioidomycosis, sporotrichosis, penicilliosis,

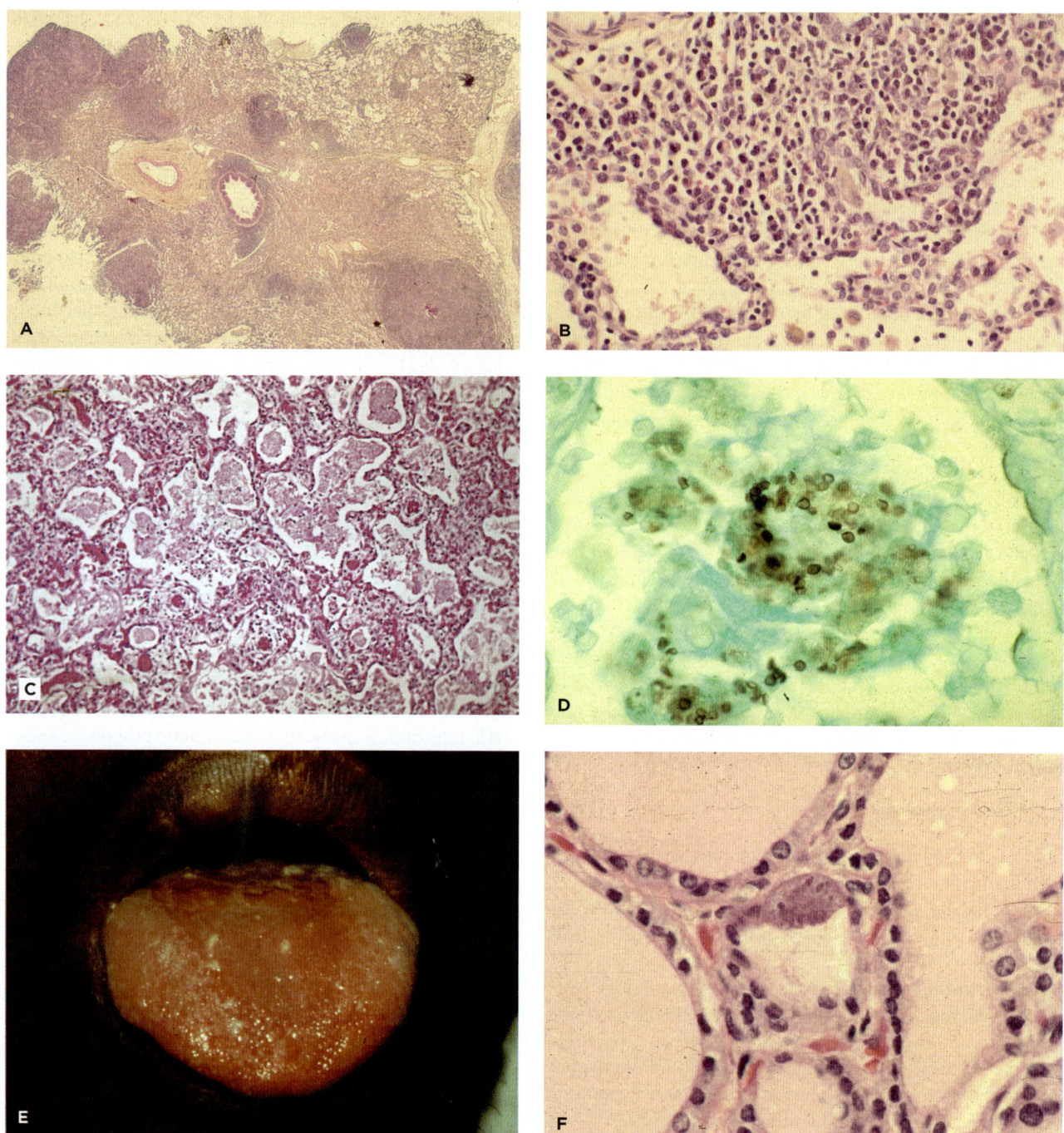

FIGURE 6-5 • HIV infection. **A, B:** Lymphoid interstitial pneumonia (low power and high power) with follicular bronchiolitis and diffuse interstitial lymphoplasmacytic inflammation. **C, D:** *Pneumocystis jiroveci* pneumonia—foamy alveolar material with saucer- or cup-shaped organisms that stain heavily with silver (GMS stain). **E:** Oral thrush (candidal glossitis). **F:** Incidental HSV inclusions in thyroid follicular cells.

and aspergillosis (72). Among parasitic infections, *Cryptosporidium parvum* and *Isospora belli* are the two most important enteric pathogens, and leishmaniasis, strongyloidiasis, and toxoplasmosis are the three main opportunistic systemic infections. These infections are also seen in association with the immune reconstitution inflammatory syndrome following highly active anti-retroviral therapy (HAART) (73).

Lymphoid Organs

The thymic lesions of childhood HIV infection include precocious or marked involution, marked reduction or absence of Hassall corpuscles, and thymitis. Thymitis may take the form of follicular, mononuclear, or plasma cell infiltrates. Thymic dysfunction and thymic involution occur during HIV disease and have been associated with rapid progression

TABLE 6-11 SYSTEMIC PATHOLOGY OF PEDIATRIC HIV INFECTION

Organ/System

Placenta
- Increased weight
- Chorioamnionitis
- Funisitis/fetal vasculitis
- Villitis

Growth and development
- Increased fetal wastage, intrauterine demise
- Failure to thrive/wasting
- No increase in malformations

Thymus
- Small size, cortical atrophy
- Lymphoid depletion
- Warthin-Finkeldey–type giant cells
- Accelerated involution
- Fibrosis, plasmacytosis
- Calcified, cystic, or small Hassall corpuscles

Spleen
- Splenomegaly
- Immunoblastic proliferation
- Lymphoid depletion
- Histiocytosis
- Hemophagocytosis
- Opportunistic infection
- "Kaposiform" spindle cell proliferation

Lymph nodes
- Follicular hyperplasia, histiocytosis
- Plasmacytosis
- Multinucleate giant cells
- Hemophagocytosis
- Lymphoid depletion, fibrosis
- Lymphoproliferative disorders
- "Kaposiform" spindle cell proliferation
- Opportunistic infection

Bone marrow
- Hypoplasia or hyperplasia
- Myelodysplasia
- Plasmacytosis, histiocytosis
- Eosinophilia, lymphoid aggregates
- Hemosiderosis, fibrosis, granulomas
- Serous fat atrophy

Cardiovascular system
- Dilated cardiomyopathy
- Myocarditis, pericarditis
- Vasculitis, vascular calcification
- Coronary and cerebral aneurysm
- Inflammation and fibrosis of conducting system

Lung
- Opportunistic infection, especially PCP, CMV, RSV
- Lymphoproliferative disorders (PLH, LIP, PBLD)
- Malignant lymphoma
- Giant cell pneumonia
- Smooth muscle neoplasms

Organ/System

Gastrointestinal tract
- Opportunistic infection, especially *Candida*, CMV, MAIC, Cryptosporidium, Isospora, Salmonella, Shigella
- Lymphoid depletion of MALT
- Lymphoproliferative disorders
- Neoplasms (lymphoma, smooth muscle tumors, Kaposi sarcoma)
- Ulcers of undetermined etiology
- Pneumatosis, pseudomembranous enteritis

Liver
- Chronic active hepatitis, including HBV and HCV, giant cell hepatitis
- Opportunistic infection, especially CMV, adenovirus, MAI

Pancreas
- Acute and chronic pancreatitis, some associated with pentamidine or dideoxyinosine
- Opportunistic infection (CMV, MAIC, *Candida*)
- Steatonecrosis
- Islet hypertrophy and fibrosis
- Dilatation of ducts and acini
- Nodular lymphoid infiltrates

Kidney
- HIV-associated nephropathy: focal and segmental glomerulosclerosis, mesangial hyperplasia, immune complex glomerulonephritis, and minimal change disease
- Opportunistic infection (CMV, *Candida*, MAIC)
- Nephromegaly
- Nephrocalcinosis

Skin
- Opportunistic infection (*Candida*, HSV, VZ, HPV)
- Molluscum contagiosum
- Scabies
- Seborrheic dermatitis
- Kaposi sarcoma

Nervous system
- Cerebral atrophy, multinucleate giant cells, microglial nodules, vascular mineralization
- Lymphoma
- Opportunistic infection (*Candida*, CMV, MAIC, progressive multifocal leukoencephalopathy)
- Nonspecific white matter pallor or gliosis

in infants perinatally infected with HIV. Perivascular sclerosis is common. Thymic involvement may be due to direct infection or may represent an autoimmune process. Thymic recovery may be achieved in some patients as a result of potent antiretroviral therapy. Extensive thymic damage may, however, hamper immune reconstitution, particularly in pediatric patients (74).

Although splenomegaly is commonly seen in HIV-infected children, there is lymphoid depletion, architectural disarray, increased macrophages, and functional hyposplenia. Cytologically, lymphoid organs show many large lymphocytes, immunoblasts, and also giant cells (polykaryocytes). Progression to lymphoma and Castleman disease may occur in nodal and extranodal sites. Quijano has detailed histopathologic findings in lymph nodes (75).

Lungs

HIV-related pulmonary lymphoid and lymphoproliferative lesions including pulmonary lymphoid hyperplasia (PLH), lymphocytic interstitial pneumonia (LIP), and PBLD (71) are more common in children than in adults. PLH is a peribronchial infiltrate of benign lymphoid follicles, often with germinal centers. LIP is characterized by a significant infiltrate of lymphocytes, plasmacytoid cells, plasma cells, and the occasional large immunoblastic cell that expand the interstitial septa (Figure 6-5). There is much overlap between PLH and LIP; they often coexist, hence the designation PLH-LIP complex. These disorders constitute a spectrum of disease related to Epstein-Barr virus (EBV) infection and may eventuate in PBLD or in malignant lymphoma

Central Nervous System

Neurologic manifestations are frequent in children with AIDS (76); HIV-related encephalopathy is characterized by low IQ, loss of developmental milestones, microcephaly, progressive weakness, and seizures. Morphologic features include gross brain atrophy, hydrocephalus, diffuse gliosis, multinucleated giant cells, microglial nodules, basal ganglia mineralization, HIV encephalitis, corticospinal tract degeneration, and siderocalcinosis of blood vessels. Common lesions not directly related to HIV infection are lymphomas and cerebrovascular accidents. Opportunistic CNS infections are relatively uncommon, limited predominantly to monilial and cytomegaloviral encephalitides. CNS lymphoma, although less common in children than in adults, is the most common malignancy in pediatric AIDS and is usually EBV-associated. Myelin abnormalities occur both in the brain and the spinal cord and are attributed to delayed myelination, myelin injury, and/or wallerian degeneration. Progressive multifocal leukoencephalopathy (PML) is rare in children. It has been suggested that most of the CNS effects of HIV infection cannot be attributed to detectable levels of viral antigen but may be due to circulating cytokines and other soluble factors. The prevalence of HIV encephalopathy has not decreased despite use of HAART; as patients live longer, the prevalence of CNS manifestations may actually increase.

Other Viscera

Liver disease manifests as hepatomegaly with altered enzymes, cholestasis, and/or hepatitis. Cholestatic hepatitis may be the first clue to a pediatric HIV infection. Giant cell transformation of hepatocytes is associated with poor outcomes in these children and is often associated with inflammation and diffuse fibrosis. Viral hepatitis and HAART-induced toxicity may contribute to liver injury (77–79). Morphologically, these may show chronic hepatitis with varying activity and/or cholestatic hepatitis. GI manifestations are similar to that in adults, the pathology including HIV enteropathy, opportunistic infections, and EBV-associated smooth muscle tumors (79). Renal lesions include focal segmental glomerulosclerosis, mesangial hypercellularity, microcystic transformation of renal tubules, immune complex glomerulonephritis, minimal change disease, and nephromegaly (due to glomerulomegaly, tubular dilatation, and interstitial inflammation) (80,81). Secondary changes include drug-related nephrotoxicity and opportunistic infections. Salivary glands are often affected early giving an appearance of chronic mumps. In HIV-associated arteriopathy, small- and medium-sized vessels in many organs (heart, lung, spleen, kidney, intestine, and brain) show fibrous intimal thickening, fragmentation or loss of elastica, and calcification. This results in luminal narrowing, aneurysmal dilatation, and distal ischemic lesions. HIV infects the fetus through the placenta. Although chorioamnionitis, cytotrophoblastic hyperplasia, and other lesions have been identified in placentas of HIV-infected women, no lesion is specific for HIV infection (82). HIV antigens have been found in placental Hofbauer cells, trophoblasts, and villous endothelial cells. Infected placental macrophages may infect fetal circulating cells or fetal endothelial cells.

Laboratory Diagnosis

As in adults, HIV-1 causes the majority of cases of childhood AIDS, but the diagnosis is more difficult in infants. In infants under the age of 18 months, HIV antibody tests such as the enzyme-linked immunosorbent assay (ELISA), Western blot, and rapid tests are not used, since maternal HIV antibodies may persist in the child until 6 to 18 months. In this age group, definitive diagnosis of HIV infection requires two positive viral detection assays on separate specimens or documentation of an AIDS-defining illness (58,83). For children aged 18 months to 13 years, laboratory-confirmed evidence of HIV infection is required in addition to the presence of one or more AIDS-defining conditions, to meet the surveillance case definition for AIDS (58). The salient differences between the 2007 World Health Organization (WHO) and 2008 CDC revised surveillance definitions are outlined in Table 6-12 (58).

MEASLES

The causative agent of measles (rubeola) is a single-stranded RNA paramyxovirus virus of the genus *Morbillivirus*. Although global deaths from measles have decreased notably

TABLE 6-12 COMPARISON OF WHO AND CDC STAGES OF HIV INFECTION[a]

WHO Stage[b]	WHO T-lymphocyte count and percentage[c]	CDC Stage[d]	CDC T-lymphocyte Count and Percentage
Stage 1 (HIV infection)	CD4+ T-lymphocyte count of ≥500 cells/μL	Stage 1 (HIV infection)	CD4+ T-lymphocyte count of ≥500 cells/μL or CD4+ T-lymphocyte percentage of ≥29
Stage 2 (HIV infection)	CD4+ T-lymphocyte count of 350–499 cells/μL	Stage 2 (HIV infection)	CD4+ T-lymphocyte count of 200–499 cells/μL or CD4+ T-lymphocyte percentage of 14–28
Stage 3 (advanced HIV disease [AHD])	CD4+ T-lymphocyte count of 200–349 cells/μL	Stage 2 (HIV infection)	CD4+ T-lymphocyte count of 200–499 cells/μL or CD4+ T-lymphocyte percentage of 14–28
Stage 4 (acquired immunodeficiency syndrome [AIDS])	CD4+ T-lymphocyte count of <200 cells/μL or CD4+ T-lymphocyte percentage of <15	Stage 3 (AIDS)	CD4+ T-lymphocyte count of <200 cells/μL or CD4+ T-lymphocyte percentage of <14

[a]For reporting purposes only.
[b]Among adults and children aged ≥5 y.
[c]Percentage applicable for stage 4 only.
[d]Among adults and adolescents (aged ≥13 y). CDC also includes a fourth stage, stage unknown: laboratory confirmation of HIV infection but no information on CD4+ T-lymphocyte count or percentage *and* no information on AIDS-defining conditions.

From Schneider E, Whitmore S, Glynn KM, et al.; Centers for Disease Control and Prevention. Revised surveillance case definitions for HIV infection among adults, adolescents, and children aged <18 mo and for HIV infection and AIDS among children aged 18 mo to <13 years—United States, 2008. *MMWR* 2008;57(RR-10):1–12.

in past decades, due to both increases in immunization rates and decreases in measles case fatality ratios (CFRs), the values for measles CFR remain imprecise, resulting in continued uncertainty about the actual toll that measles exacts (84,85). Recent resurgent measles outbreaks in sub-Saharan Africa, Europe, and the United States show the ease with which measles virus can re-enter communities if high levels of population immunity are not sustained (86).

Transmission

Measles is highly contagious and is spread by aerosols and droplets of respiratory secretions. The viral receptor is CD46 for viral H and F glycoproteins, and viremia is mediated through infection of lymphoid and endothelial cells. Host innate immune responses are effective in promptly eliminating the virus (87).

Clinical Features

After a 1- to 2-week incubation period, there is a prodrome (of fever, cough, rhinorrhea, and/or conjunctivitis) with the development of Koplik spots characteristically seen in the oral mucosa. This is followed by an erythematous maculopapular (morbilliform) rash that begins on the face, spreads to the trunks and limbs (Figure 6-6A), and fades about 6 days later in the same order in which it had appeared.

Complications are a result of progressive viral replication, secondary bacterial or viral infections, and/or an abnormal host–immune response. The most common complications are bacterial pneumonia or otitis media, the former being the most frequent cause of death. Other complications are febrile convulsions, encephalitis, chronic diarrhea, and liver function abnormalities. Pulmonary complications (secondary pneumonia, giant cell pneumonia, and atypical measles pneumonia) are the most feared. Prophylactic antibiotics may help prevent respiratory complications (88), although this has been refuted.

While rare, the measles virus can infect the CNS and trigger fatal CNS disease (89). CNS complications can occur from days to years after acute infection and include acute postinfectious allergic encephalitis, acute progressive measles (inclusion body) encephalitis, pseudotumor cerebri, and subacute sclerosing panencephalitis (SSPE). SSPE has an average 6-year latent period after infection/vaccination and is manifested as progressive cognitive impairment, motor dysfunction, seizures, coma, and death in 1 to 2 years.

Pathology

The pathology of measles infection is characterized by two types of multinucleated giant cells. Warthin-Finkeldey giant cells are seen in lymphoid tissues throughout the body during the incubation period, while epithelial giant cells occur in the epithelia of all major organs (Figure 6-6B,C). The giant cells may contain nuclear and/or cytoplasmic inclusions. Interstitial pneumonitis is characteristic, with or without a granulomatous response. Allergic phenomena (atypical measles pneumonia and postinfectious encephalitis) are

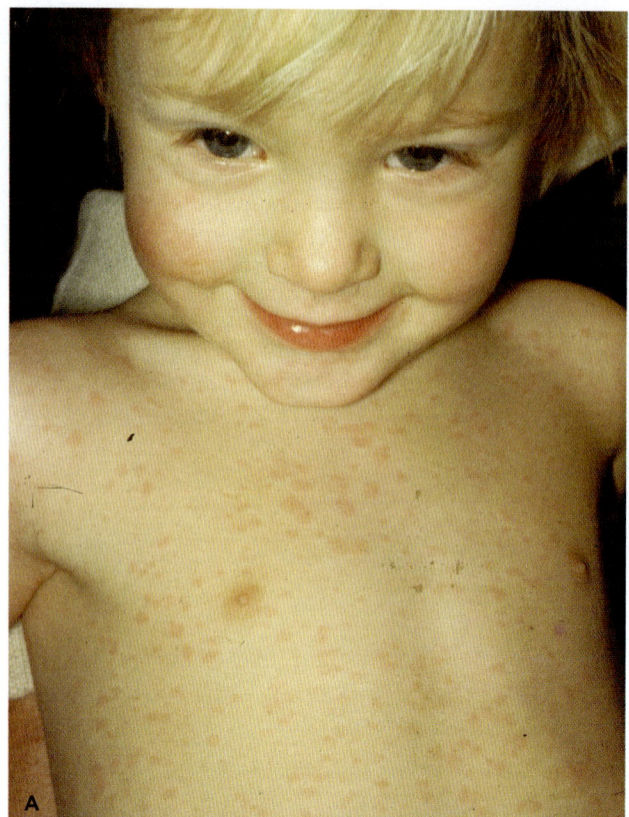
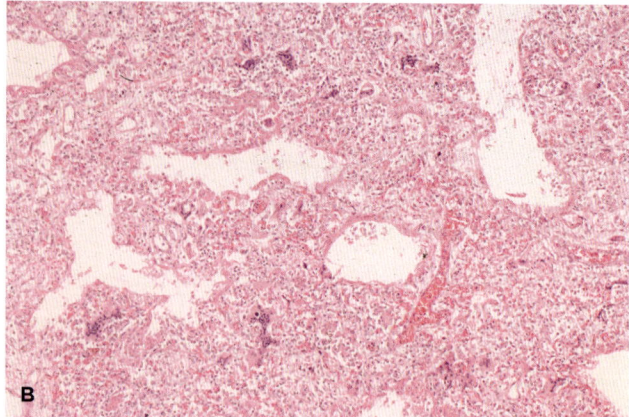
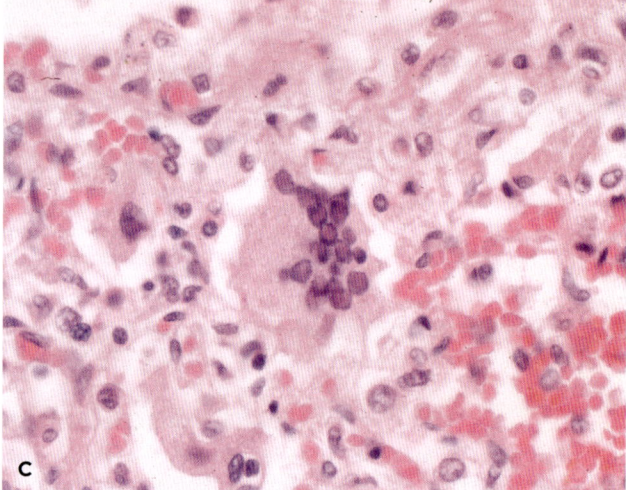

FIGURE 6-6 • Measles. **A:** Clinical feature of morbilliform rash on the chest. **B:** Measles pneumonia showing scattered giant cells (low power). **C:** Warthin-Finkeldey giant cells in measles pneumonia.

characterized by vascular injury and necrosis. SSPE may occur as sequelae, following infection of neurons and glial cells; histopathologically, there is lymphocytic vascular cuffing, gliosis, and demyelination. Both immunohistochemical and *in situ* hybridization techniques are available to demonstrate the virus in tissues; this helps differentiation from RSV, VZV, and parainfluenza, since all these agents can cause giant cell pneumonia with a granulomatous response. Although laboratory tests are rarely required to diagnose measles, laboratory confirmation is an important component of disease surveillance in all settings. The CDC has recommended serum-based diagnostics as the "gold standard" for this purpose, although alternative specimens such as dried blood spots and oral fluid samples are viable alternatives for surveillance (90).

EPSTEIN-BARR VIRUS

EBV is a gamma–human herpes virus that infects B-lymphocytes and epithelial cells of the pharyngeal mucosa, salivary gland ducts, and uterine cervix. The diverse clinical disease spectrum includes infectious mononucleosis (IM), LPDs, lymphoepithelioma-like (nasopharyngeal) carcinomas, and rare smooth muscle neoplasms. Infection of epithelial cells is lytic (productive), with resultant full cycle of viral replication and release of infectious viral particles into secretions. On the other hand, infection of B-lymphocytes is predominantly latent (nonproductive), with the potential for immortalization and activation of infected cells. Only a limited set of genes are expressed during latent cycle infection [EBV nuclear antigens (EBNAs) and three latent membrane proteins (LMPs)]; these define different latency patterns (91).

EBV is ubiquitous and transmitted primarily by saliva, although transmission by blood transfusion and allogeneic bone marrow transplantation is also documented. Sexual transmission has also been proposed as a route of infection (92). Very little is known about the risk of congenital EBV infections, with only one well-documented case in the literature. Since most adult women have become seropositive during childhood, primary EBV infection during pregnancy is rare, whereas reactivation of a latent EBV infection seems to occur more often in seropositive pregnant women as compared to control subjects. However, only primary infection (and not reactivation) may be harmful to the embryo or fetus. Worldwide, primary subclinical infection occurs within the first few years of life, and symptomatic IM occurs when infection is delayed to adolescence or beyond.

Infectious Mononucleosis

IM is a self-limiting lymphoproliferative disease with a benign course. The highest rates of IM occur between 10 and 19 years of age (6 to 8 cases per 1000 persons per year), although mild infections in younger children may often be undiagnosed. Rates of infection are highest in closeted populations of young adults such as active-duty military personnel and college students (11 to 48 cases per 1000 persons per year) (93).

Most clinical symptoms are due to the host's immune response. The incubation period is estimated to be 5 to 7 weeks, followed by a prodrome of 3 to 5 days (with headache, malaise, and fever) and the characteristic triad of fever, sore throat, and extensive cervical lymphadenopathy/tonsillar enlargement. Pharyngeal inflammation and transient palatal petechiae are also common. Other frequent clinical manifestations include splenomegaly (identified in all patients by ultrasonography) and hepatomegaly with transient hepatic dysfunction. EBV infection must be considered in children with FUO. Younger children may show less typical and less severe clinical disease. Atypical lymphocytes appear in circulation from 1 to 4 weeks after disease onset. These atypical cells are mainly activated oligoclonal CD8-positive cytotoxic T-cells, with only a small proportion representing EBV-infected B cells; in fact, the CD8 proliferation may result in a reduction of the CD4/CD8 ratio. Uncomplicated illness usually lasts for 2 to 4 weeks. Complications of IM involve the hematopoietic system (anemia, thrombocytopenia, neutropenia), heart (pericarditis, myocarditis), nervous system (meningoencephalitis, cerebellitis, Guillain-Barré syndrome, Bell palsy, transverse myelitis, autoimmune neuropathies, psychiatric diseases), skin (ampicillin-associated rash, Gianotti-Crosti syndrome), kidneys (nephritis, glomerulopathies), and immune system (hypo- and hypergammaglobulinemia, autoantibodies) (94). Although most patients are advised to avoid contact sports to prevent potentially serious splenic rupture, this is a rare complication (approximately 0.1%). "Virus-associated hemophagocytic syndrome" is an unusual consequence of unknown pathogenesis, characterized by a benign generalized histiocytic proliferation with marked hemophagocytosis in bone marrow and lymph nodes. Usually, IM is an acute, self-limiting disease that occurs only once in the host's lifetime. However, some patients suffer from recurrent fever, persistent hepatosplenomegaly, hematologic abnormalities, neuromyasthenia, and the so-called chronic fatigue syndrome. Many of these patients reveal immunologic abnormalities such as deficient natural killer (NK) cell activity and abnormal antibody responses to the different EBV antigens. Prolonged illness after IM may be due to altered immunity rather than increased viral load.

Differential diagnoses for suspected IM include streptococcal pharyngitis, toxoplasmosis, CMV pharyngitis, acute HIV infection, and other viral pharyngitis (95). The presence of splenomegaly, posterior cervical adenopathy, axillary adenopathy, and inguinal adenopathy is most useful in considering the possibility of IM, while the absence of cervical adenopathy and fatigue is most helpful in dismissing the diagnosis. Hoagland's criteria for the diagnosis of IM are widely cited: at least 50% lymphocytes and at least 10% atypical lymphocytes in the presence of fever, pharyngitis, and adenopathy, with confirmation by a positive serologic test. Although specific, these criteria are not highly sensitive; only about one-half of symptomatic patients with a positive heterophile antibody test meet all the criteria.

Diagnosis rests on viral serology and the detection of the EBV genome, viral antigens, or infectious virus in saliva or lymphoid tissues. The accidental discovery of elevated heterophile antibody by Paul and Bunnell in 1932 forms the basis for the heterophile agglutination reaction. Although they are relatively specific, IgM heterophile antibody tests are somewhat insensitive, particularly in the first weeks of illness. Heterophile antibody tests are less sensitive in patients younger than 12 years, detecting only 25% to 50% of infections in this group, compared with 71% to 91% in older patients. Antibodies to viral capsid antigen (i.e., VCA-IgG and VCA-IgM) are produced slightly earlier than the heterophile antibody and are more specific for EBV infection; in acute infection, IgM anti-VCA antibodies are present and anti-EBNA antibodies are absent. The VCA-IgG antibody persists past the stage of acute infection and signals the development of immunity. A past infection is identified by the absence of IgM antibodies and the presence of IgG antibodies against VCA and EBNA. However, anti-EBNA antibodies may not be detected in immunodeficient children. Patients with latent infection have elevated antibodies against early antigen (EA). Although no evidence-based or consensus guidelines have been proposed to guide the evaluation of patients with suspected IM, Ebell has proposed an algorithmic approach based on the percentage of atypical lymphocytes and absence of streptococcal pharyngitis (95). At present, nucleic acid hybridization (by Southern blot, *in situ* hybridization, or PCR) is the most specific method for the detection of EBV in clinical material. The laboratory diagnosis of IM has been recently reviewed (96).

Histologically, enlarged lymph nodes show a predominant paracortical expansion (Figure 6-7A–C), with atypical cells that are predominantly cytotoxic T-cells (CD8 and TIA-1 positive). EBV-infected cells are best identified by *in situ* hybridization for EBV-encoded small RNA (EBER) (Figure 6-7D). Histologic findings of EBV-associated hepatitis include minimal swelling and vacuolization of the hepatocytes, and a peculiar sinusoidal infiltration of T-cells in a "bead of strings" pattern (Figure 6-7E), in addition to periportal inflammation.

EBV-Associated Neoplasms

Neoplasms associated with latent EBV infection include lymphomas, nasopharyngeal carcinoma, lymphoepithelial carcinomas in various viscera, smooth muscle tumors, and inflammatory pseudotumor-like follicular dendritic cell

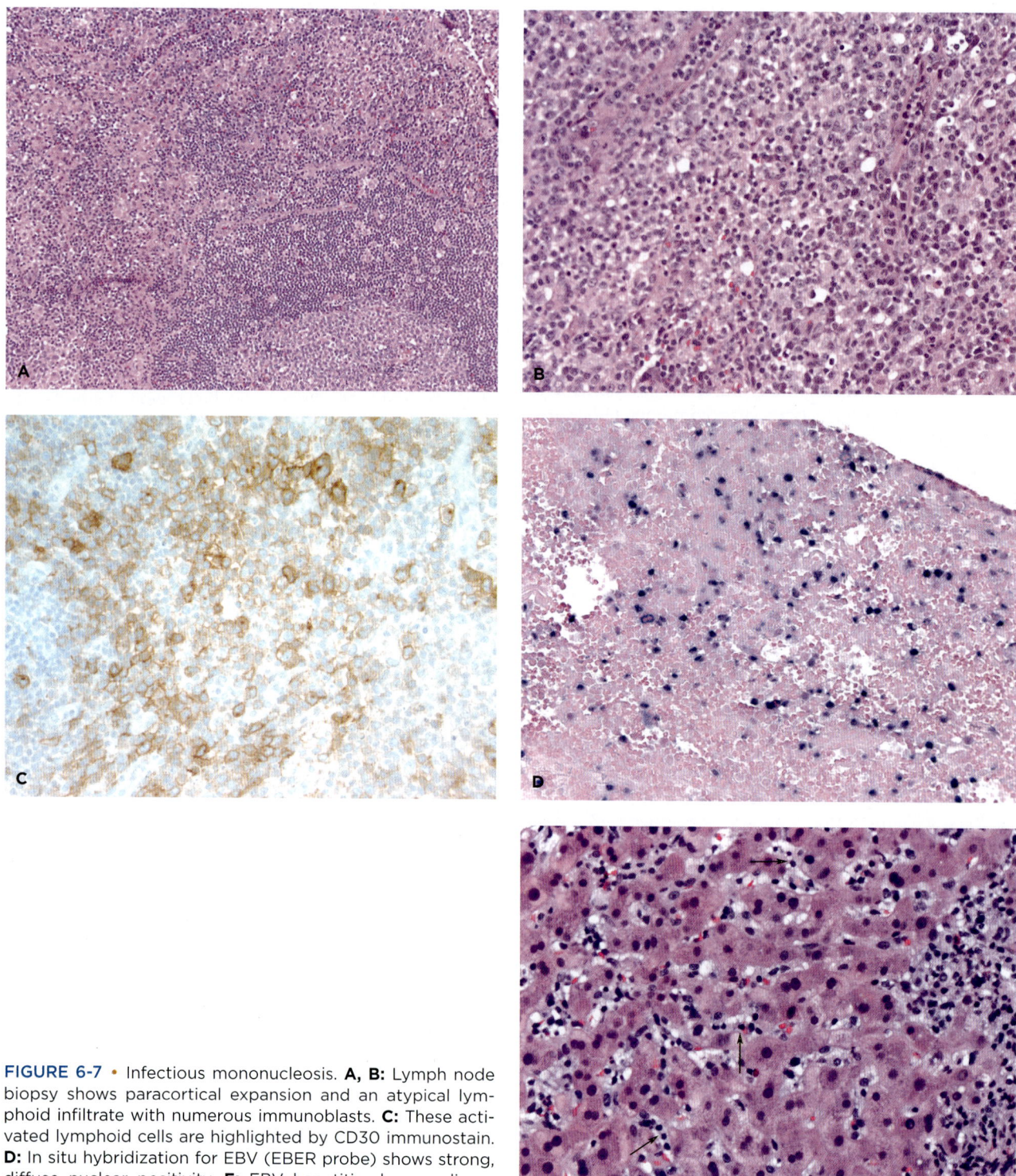

FIGURE 6-7 • Infectious mononucleosis. **A, B:** Lymph node biopsy shows paracortical expansion and an atypical lymphoid infiltrate with numerous immunoblasts. **C:** These activated lymphoid cells are highlighted by CD30 immunostain. **D:** In situ hybridization for EBV (EBER probe) shows strong, diffuse nuclear positivity. **E:** EBV hepatitis shows a linear T-cell infiltrate in liver sinusoids

tumor (91,97–99). Different latency patterns are associated with different neoplasms (e.g., type I with Burkitt lymphoma, type II with Hodgkin lymphoma and nasopharyngeal carcinoma, and type III with posttransplant LPDs), with type III latency expressing more EBV proteins and being more immunogenic and type I being the least immunogenic (91). In lymphomagenesis, EBV plays either a direct role (such as in posttransplant LPDs and HIV-associated immunoblastic lymphoma occurring in immunodeficient individuals) or as a cofactor (such as in Burkitt lymphoma and some T-/NK-cell malignancies occurring in immunocompetent individuals). EBV-associated T-/NK-cell LPD (EBV-T/NK LPD) of children and young adults is generally referred to with the blanket nosologic term of severe chronic active EBV infection (CAEBV) and overlaps with a unique disease previously described as infantile fulminant EBV-associated T-LPD. This disease is rare, is associated with high morbidity and mortality, and appears to be more prevalent in East Asian countries. The major signs and symptoms include fever, hepatomegaly, splenomegaly, liver dysfunction, thrombocytopenia, anemia, lymphadenopathy, hypersensitivity to mosquito bites, skin rash, hydroa vacciniforme, diarrhea, and uveitis. A classification system for EBV-T/NK LPD of children and young adults has been proposed based on morphology (polymorphic or monomorphic) and clonality (polyclonal or monoclonal NK or cytotoxic T-cells) (100).

VIRAL HEMORRHAGIC FEVERS

The combination of fever and hemorrhage can be caused by viruses, rickettsiae, bacteria, protozoa, and fungi. However, conventionally, the term "hemorrhagic fever" refers to fever and hemorrhage caused by viruses transmitted by arthropods ("arboviruses") and rodents. Viruses implicated in this syndrome are diverse and include arenaviridae (e.g., lassa virus), bunyaviridae (e.g., Hanta virus, Rift Valley fever), flaviviridae (e.g., yellow fever, dengue), chikungunya, and filoviridae (e.g. Ebola, Marburg) (101,102). The detailed description of each of these conditions is beyond the scope of this chapter. Certain general features common to these syndromes will be outlined, using dengue as a prototype (103). The clinical differential diagnoses include leptospirosis, rickettsial fevers (e.g., typhus), complicated malaria, and disseminated intravascular coagulopathy (DIC) following severe sepsis of any etiology. Viral hemorrhagic fevers have become a major concern in the recent past. Agents such as dengue virus have caused many recent epidemics; more than 1.2 million cases of dengue fever and dengue hemorrhagic fever (DHF) were reported to the WHO from 56 countries in the 1998 pandemic (104).

Transmission

Many of these arboviral fevers are transmitted to humans by mosquito bites (dengue is transmitted by the female Aedes mosquito). Several ecologic factors have contributed to a significant increase in the incidence of dengue fever and the emergence of DHF as a major public health problem in America and Asia. Prenatal or perinatal transmission has been reported in rare instances. There is no evidence for transmission of dengue virus in breast milk, nor more severe disease in breast-fed infants compared with formula-fed infants. There has been no documented person-to-person transmission of dengue virus without a mosquito vector.

Clinical Features

Dengue viruses cause dengue fever, DHF, and dengue shock syndrome (DSS) in infants less than 1 year of age, but rarely in those younger than 3 months. The disease spectrum ranges from a mild flu-like illness to life-threatening manifestations with severe hypotension (due to vascular dysregulation), vascular abnormalities (manifested as conjunctival suffusion, flushing, and exanthem), capillary instability (manifested as edema), and hemorrhage (due to a combination of thrombocytopenia and microvascular damage with DIC). Visceral involvement manifests variably as renal, pulmonary, hepatic, and neurologic dysfunction and as a result of lymphoid necrosis and depletion. Infection of mononuclear cells leads to cytokine activation and plays a central role in the pathogenesis of DHF. Antibody-dependent enhancement due to preexisting antidengue IgG against the infecting strain causes more severe disease.

Infants and young children with dengue usually have only a nonspecific febrile illness, with a rash that is difficult to distinguish from other viral illnesses. The more severe cases usually occur in older children and adults, characterized by a rapidly rising temperature and severe headache, myalgia, and arthralgia that last for 5 to 6 days. Many patients have an initial macular to maculopapular rash that later becomes diffusely erythematous. Minor hemorrhagic manifestations such as petechiae, epistaxis, and gingival bleeding occur. Although dengue fever may be incapacitating, its prognosis is favorable and most patients generally recover after 7 to 10 days of illness. DHF, on the other hand, is an acute febrile illness with hemorrhagic manifestations, thrombocytopenia, and evidence of increased vascular permeability resulting in loss of plasma from the vascular compartment. Hypoproteinemia, an elevated hematocrit, and serous effusion are indicators of plasma leakage, which may progress to circulatory failure, so-called Dengue shock syndrome (DSS). The patient may die within 24 hours or may recover quickly following appropriate volume replacement and supportive therapy. Neurologic manifestations may occur in the absence of shock (105). Complications such as hepatic dysfunction and fluid overload are more commonly found in infants, and the case fatality rate is also higher in this age group (106).

Pathology

Morphologically, there is variably prominent capillary dilatation, endothelial swelling, edema, and/or vasculitis with fibrin thrombi. Target organs are different in different syndromes; for example, in hantavirus syndromes, the major target organ may be the lung or the kidney with brain, liver, and spleen being secondary target organs. Each involved organ may show features of severe injury such as diffuse alveolar damage, renal tubular necrosis, and medullary hemorrhage, and features of DIC may be present.

OTHER SYSTEMIC VIRAL INFECTIONS

Disseminated *adenoviral* disease usually occurs in immunocompromised hosts, posttransplantation, or in neonates and manifests with clinically significant destructive hepatitis. Rarely, infection may occur in healthy children. The hepatitis is characterized by variable necrosis with intranuclear amphophilic or basophilic viral inclusions with peri-inclusional clearing or, in late stages, smudge cells. Adenovirus may also cause enterocolitis and pneumonia and has been associated with intussusception. Respiratory and disseminated infections are associated with significant morbidity and mortality in neonates (107).

Enteroviral infections include poliomyelitis, EV 71 neurologic disease, neonatal EV disease, coxsackievirus, and echovirus (108). *Echovirus* can cause flu-like symptoms in any age group. However, fatal and severe infections are almost exclusively reported in neonates and infants. The spectrum of illness includes encephalitis, meningitis, hepatitis, and other unusual manifestations such as myocarditis, orchitis, postviral fatigue syndrome, and transient erythroblastopenia of childhood. *Coxsackieviruses* are implicated in hand, foot, and mouth disease (Figure 6-8), myocarditis, and aseptic meningitis.

HTLV infection is endemic in southwest Japan, the Caribbean, South America, and sub-Saharan Africa (109). Transmission is through sexual contact, intravenous drug abuse, infected blood and blood products, and breast milk. The frequency of transmission and the contributing factors to sexual and mother-to-child transmission remain uncertain. HTLV transmission is more frequent in breast-fed than formula-fed infants. Duration of breast-feeding correlates with transmission rate. Transmission is also associated with higher maternal provirus levels and HTLV-1 antibody titers (110). The median time of transmission has been estimated at 11 to 12 months of age. Complete avoidance of breastfeeding is reportedly effective in preventing mother-to-child transmission. HTLV-1 causes adult T-cell leukemia/lymphoma (ATLL), a chronic, progressive neuropathy called HTLV-1-associated myelopathy, and tropical spastic paraparesis associated with various other chronic conditions (uveitis, arthritis, Sjögren syndrome, infective dermatitis, and a persistent lymphadenitis in children). Early life infection carries the greatest risk for later development of ATLL. In areas of low prevalence, the likelihood of a false-positive HTLV-1 test is high; therefore, repeat testing is often indicated. In a pregnant woman, antibody titer testing and proviral load quantification are appropriate to estimate the risk for transmission to the infant. HTLV-2 causes at least two forms of chronic ataxia (spastic or tropical).

Mumps has been reported to be resurgent in the United States; over 2,500 cases were reported in 2006 alone (Figure 6-9). The majority of these cases occurred in college students aged 18 to 25 years, even though most had been vaccinated with two doses of measles, mumps, and rubella-containing vaccines. Kancherla has reviewed mumps and discussed potential mechanisms for vaccine failure (111). Detection of serum IgM is reportedly better at 3 days or more following symptom onset, although virologic assays are more sensitive in the first 2 days. Thus, selection of testing methods and timing of sample collection are important factors in the ability to confirm infection among vaccinated persons (112).

"NEW" VIRAL INFECTIONS

Better detection techniques and faster spread of information have allowed identification of new pathogens and early detection of pandemics in the past decade. The H1N1 influenza virus, first reported in 2009 (113–115), can cause severe pediatric disease (116). The influenza virus remains an important challenge, given its ability to mutate at a very high level. Although the common circulating influenza virus strains (H1N1 and H3N2) are not virulent enough to cause mortality, mutated strains may be lethal, especially in children (117).

Severe acute respiratory syndrome (SARS) is caused by a coronavirus (HCoV-NL63), identified in 2004 and transmitted primarily by respiratory droplets. In the pediatric cases reported in the literature, children had mild respiratory illness, although the severity of the disease in adolescents seemed more similar to that in adults (118,119). Infants born to mothers with confirmed SARS were born prematurely, presumably because of maternal illness. Two of the five infants described developed severe abdominal disease (coronavirus has been linked to necrotizing enterocolitis), although coronavirus was not identified in any of the infants (120). The Middle East respiratory syndrome is also caused by a coronavirus (121). Most affected children are reportedly asymptomatic. *West Nile virus* (WNV) infection leads to approximately one case of severe neurologic disease per every 20 cases of nonspecific febrile illness and every 150 to 300 cases of asymptomatic infection (seroconversion). Clinical illness is rare in infants and children (122). Transmission occurs primarily through the bite of Culex mosquitoes, but it may also occur during pregnancy (123), through organ transplants, following percutaneous exposure in laboratory workers, and possibly via transfusion of blood products. One case of possible WNV transmission through breast-feeding has been reported (124). However, the absence of illness in this infant (and most infants/children), the transient nature of maternal viremia with WNV infection, and the rarity of such a transmission event suggest that there is no reason to avoid breast-feeding or breast milk when a mother is infected with WNV (21).

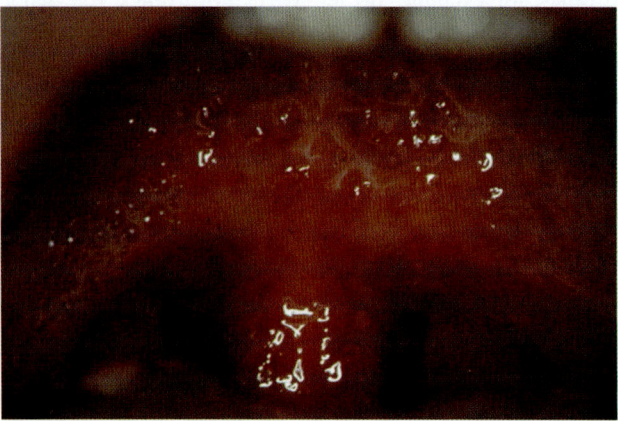

FIGURE 6-8 • Coxsackie infection with vesicular oral mucosal lesions.

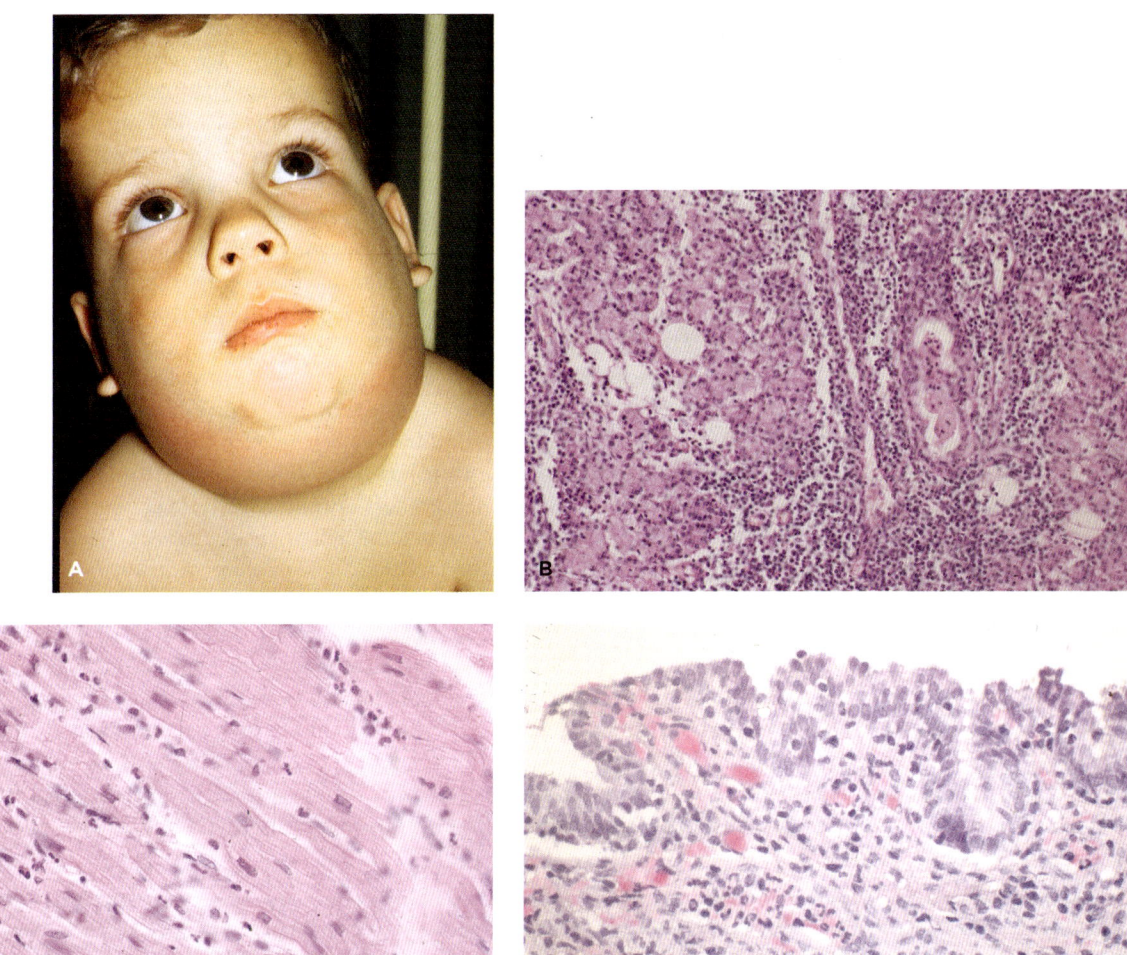

FIGURE 6-9 • Mumps. **A:** Bilateral parotitis is seen in this clinical photograph. **B:** Histologic appearance of parotitis is shown with a diffuse lymphocytic infiltrate. **C:** Mumps myocarditis is characterized by the presence of a lymphocytic infiltrate and focal myonecrosis. **D:** Acute epididymo-orchitis in mumps is seen as an active lymphocytic infiltrate in the interstitium (see Chapter 12).

Human metapneumovirus (HMPV), discovered in 2001, is an important cause of respiratory syncytial virus (RSV)-negative respiratory tract infections, typically affecting children between 2 and 3 years of age (125). It is most frequently detected soon after the RSV season. HMPV was classified as the first human member of the *Metapneumovirus* genus, of the family *Paramyxoviridae*. At least two genetic lineages of HMPV are circulating in humans, with two sublineages each. Antibody responses are elicited against the highly conserved F protein of HMPV, and may provide protection against infection (126) (see Chapter 12).

The human bocavirus (HBoV), discovered in 2005, is famous for being the first virus identified by "molecular virus screening" of nasopharyngeal samples (127). HBoV has been detected worldwide in mainly respiratory and stool samples and is most common in young children aged 6 to 24 months with respiratory tract infections or gastroenteritis. Details such as transmission routes, clear causality, presentation modes, and clinical relevance of HBoV are still unclear (128).

BACTERIAL INFECTIONS

We will give an overview of neonatal sepsis followed by a discussion of the more common infections caused by individual groups of bacteria.

NEONATAL SEPSIS

Sepsis is a leading cause of death in infants and children, with over 42,000 cases of severe sepsis reported annually in the United States and millions worldwide. Sepsis is especially devastating in the neonatal population. Neonates significantly differ from adults in multiple respects including their naïve immune system, pathophysiologic response to sepsis, and response to treatment (129). One half of the children with severe sepsis in the United States are infants, and one half of these are low- or very low-birth-weight babies. Incidence and mortality rates vary by age and the presence of underlying disease, if any. Attack rates for infants of colonized mothers also vary with the organisms, their serotype, and the presence or absence of maternal antibody. Sepsis neonatorum denotes fulminant bacterial sepsis occurring within the first 30 days of life, and clinically characterized by abrupt onset, rapid progression, often without demonstrable anatomic localization and very high morbidity and mortality rates even with appropriate antibiotic therapy. The clinical manifestations are protean and include hypothermia, hyperthermia, respiratory distress, and feeding disturbances. Clinical distinction from noninfectious disease, especially hyaline membrane disease, is frequently impossible, and thorough microbiologic evaluation is mandatory in all cases of neonatal death. Unfortunately, sepsis is a term that has been, and continues to be, used very loosely in clinical practice, limiting comparison of studies from around the globe. Although bacteremia, systemic inflammatory response syndrome (SIRS), and septicemia have been defined for the adult population, these cannot be directly extrapolated to the pediatric population. Definitions for the pediatric population have been agreed upon in consensus (Table 6-13) (130,131). SIRS is the body's response to an infectious or noninfectious insult. The name is only partially accurate since patients who develop SIRS have both an initial proinflammatory state (i.e., initially hyperimmune) and a later anti-inflammatory state (i.e., hypoimmune). The pathophysiology of SIRS is complex (132). One major difference in the definition of sepsis in children versus adults is the age-specific cutoffs for physiologic- and organ system-related laboratory parameters.

Based on the timing of infection, neonatal sepsis is subclassified as early onset (in the first week of life and especially within the first 24 hours), late onset (7 to 30 days of age), or very late onset (beyond 30 days). Early-onset disease is associated with obstetric complications including fever, prolonged labor, prolonged membrane rupture, and premature delivery. The predominant organisms causing early-onset infections are GBS (133) and enteric bacilli, especially *Escherichia coli*. Universal antenatal screening has significantly reduced the incidence of GBS sepsis in the United States from 1.5 to 0.3/1000 live births over the past three decades. An algorithm has been developed to manage early neonatal GBS sepsis. Less common early-onset pathogens include other streptococci, enterococci, *Listeria*, *Haemophilus influenzae*, *Streptococcus pneumoniae*, *Chlamydia*, and other organisms in the maternal genital flora. These organisms can also cause late- or very late-onset bacterial infections. Antibiotic-resistant strains of gram-negative bacilli and staphylococci are important nosocomial pathogens in hospital settings.

Positive blood cultures can establish an infectious etiology for a patient's illness and provide susceptibility testing and optimization of antimicrobial therapy. The key principles in obtaining blood cultures include choosing the best

TABLE 6-13 DEFINITIONS OF SIRS, INFECTION, SEPSIS, SEVERE SEPSIS, AND SEPTIC SHOCK

SIRS
The presence of at least two of the following four criteria, one of which must be abnormal temperature or leukocyte count:
- Core temperature of >38.5°C or <36°C
- Tachycardia, defined as a mean heart rate >2 SD above normal for age in the absence of external stimulus, chronic drugs, or painful stimuli or otherwise unexplained persistent elevation over a 0.5- to 4-h time period OR for children <1-y old; bradycardia, defined as a mean heart rate <10th percentile for age in the absence of external vagal stimulus, β-blocker drugs, or congenital heart disease or otherwise unexplained persistent depression over a 0.5-h time period.
- Mean respiratory rate >2 SD above normal for age or mechanical ventilation for an acute process not related to underlying neuromuscular disease or the receipt of general anesthesia.
- Leukocyte count elevated or depressed for age (not secondary to chemotherapy-induced leukopenia) or >10% immature neutrophils.

Infection
A suspected or proven (by positive culture, tissue stain, or polymerase chain reaction test) infection caused by any pathogen OR a clinical syndrome associated with a high probability of infection. Evidence of infection includes positive findings on clinical exam, imaging, or laboratory tests (e.g., white blood cells in a normally sterile body fluid, perforated viscus, chest radiograph consistent with pneumonia, petechial or purpuric rash, or purpura fulminans).

Sepsis
SIRS in the presence of or as a result of suspected or proven infection.

Severe sepsis
Sepsis plus one of the following: cardiovascular organ dysfunction OR acute respiratory distress syndrome OR two or more other organ dysfunctions.

Septic shock
Sepsis and cardiovascular organ dysfunction.

From Goldstein B, Giroir B, Randolph A; International Consensus Conference on Pediatric Sepsis. International pediatric sepsis consensus conference: definitions for sepsis and organ dysfunction in pediatrics. *Pediatr Crit Care Med* 2005;6(1):2–8.

available phlebotomy site, paying attention to aseptic technique, obtaining an adequate volume of blood, obtaining specimen prior to initiation of antibiotics, and providing a sufficient number of blood culture sets. Technical variables that can affect results include culture medium, the ratio of blood to broth, and additives that inactivate antimicrobial agents. Organisms requiring special considerations are mycobacteria, *Bartonella*, anaerobes, and fungi. However, blood cultures are often negative since infants may have low-level bacteremia, and the blood volume drawn is usually suboptimal compared to the patient's weight. Measures of leukocytosis, acute-phase proteins, procalcitonin, cytokines, cell surface antigens, inter-alpha inhibitor proteins, and bacterial genomes have been used in combination to improve diagnosis of neonatal sepsis, but not as stand-alone test (134). Real-time PCR methods that simultaneously detect the 25 most important bacterial and fungal species, causing approximately 90% of all bloodstream infections, have been proposed for routine assessment of neonatal sepsis (135).

Regardless of the agent, pathologic changes in infants with neonatal sepsis vary little. Since the organism is commonly acquired from the mother's genital tract, the main pathologic finding in early-onset disease is widespread pneumonia. The lungs are heavy, red, and airless. Histologically, there is a widespread, relatively uniformly distributed, intra-alveolar polymorphonuclear exudate. In infants dying within the first few hours of life, there may be little polymorphonuclear infiltrate, with collapse and congestion predominating. Hyaline membranes may be present and often contain large numbers of bacteria. Interstitial infiltrates may be prominent in GBS sepsis. Pulmonary hemorrhage is frequently seen. Systemic lesions are decidedly uncommon; splenitis is seen in 30% of cases, and meningitis is rare.

Late-onset neonatal sepsis, in contrast, has no association with obstetric complications. In a study on 6215 infants admitted to National Institute of Child Health and Human Development (NICHD) Neonatal Research Network (NRN) centers, 70% of first episode late-onset infections were caused by gram-positive organisms, and coagulase-negative staphylococci (CoNS) accounted for 48% (136). Gram-negative bacilli, *Candida albicans*, and GBS also cause late-onset neonatal sepsis. The route of acquisition is uncertain. Vertical transmission can be documented in most GBS disease (most commonly subtype III) and in some cases of *E. coli* infections. Horizontal transmission from home or nursery contacts presumably accounts for the remainder. The onset is either insidious or fulminant, and mortality is less than that seen in early-onset disease. Bacteremia results in meningeal seeding in virtually all case. Ventriculitis is the rule and, together with arachnoidal fibrosis, accounts for the high incidence of hydrocephalus in survivors. Various scoring systems are available to estimate the severity of illness and organ dysfunction (137).

Sepsis may have distinct characteristics in patients with congenital immunodeficiencies, such as a paradoxically milder course due to an incomplete inflammatory response or a more severe course due to a lack of regulatory responses and a higher pathogen burden. Preterm infants are especially susceptible to late-onset sepsis, often due to gram-positive bacterial infections, causing substantial morbidity and mortality. Newborns suffer innate immune weaknesses including diminished skin integrity, impaired Th1-polarizing responses, low complement levels, and diminished expression of plasma antimicrobial proteins and peptides (138). An association is seen between types of immunodeficiencies and the class of infecting organisms (Tables 6-1 and 6-2) (139).

STAPHYLOCOCCAL INFECTIONS

Staphylococcus aureus and coagulase-negative staphylococci (CoNS) are frequently encountered pathogens in the young. Staphylococcal infection usually occurs in late neonatal life; 40% to 90% of nursery infants at 5 days of age are colonized by *S. aureus*, predominately on the skin and nares. The morphologic hallmark of CoNS infection is suppurative inflammation with necrosis (Figure 6-10), with or without systemic inflammation; any organ or organ system may be involved. Cutaneous and subcutaneous infections can progress to necrotizing fasciitis, which may become fulminant. Methicillin-resistant *S. aureus* (MRSA) changed the epidemiology, clinical manifestations, laboratory approach, antibiotic management, and prevention of pediatric staphylococcal infections (140). Spread of MRSA occurs in school and day care settings. Community-acquired MRSA causes nosocomial infections in neonatal intensive care units. Nursery outbreaks of *S. aureus* infections have been traced to postnatal contact with mothers, health care workers, and contaminated, unpasteurized, banked breast milk. Differentiating between isolates that have the *pvl* genes and those that are negative for *pvl* has major therapeutic implications.

The most common bloodstream infection encountered in neonatal and pediatric intensive care units is by CoNS (141). CoNS infections are almost always associated with intravenous catheters or invasive procedures. The organism is a normal skin commensal, so that differentiating infection from colonization and contamination can be difficult. CoNS infections have high mortality rates and are frequently methicillin resistant. Colonization rates are as high as 60% to 90% for infants hospitalized at 2 weeks of age.

Staphylococci also cause diseases due to elaboration of soluble toxins, including food poisoning, staphylococcal scalded skin syndrome (SSSS), and toxic shock syndrome (TSS). SSSS is caused by an epidermolytic exotoxin produced by phage group II *Staphylococcus*, resulting in large intraepidermal bullae with rupture and exfoliation (Figure 6-10). Fluid loss and/or secondary infection may be fatal. TSS is rare under age 10 and peaks in teenagers. Predisposing factors include tampon use, surgical procedures, skin infections, and abortions. TSS toxin I causes massive intravascular fluid loss that leads to edema, diarrhea, and hypotensive shock. Signs include red, edematous mucous membranes and erythema,

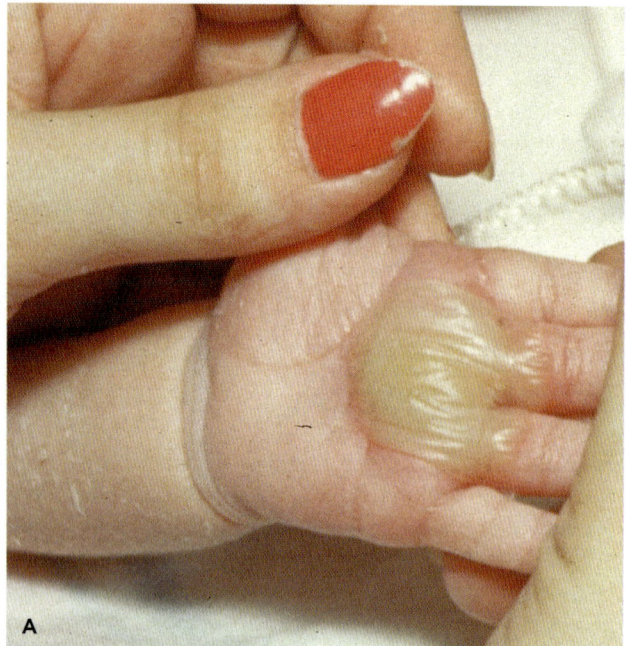
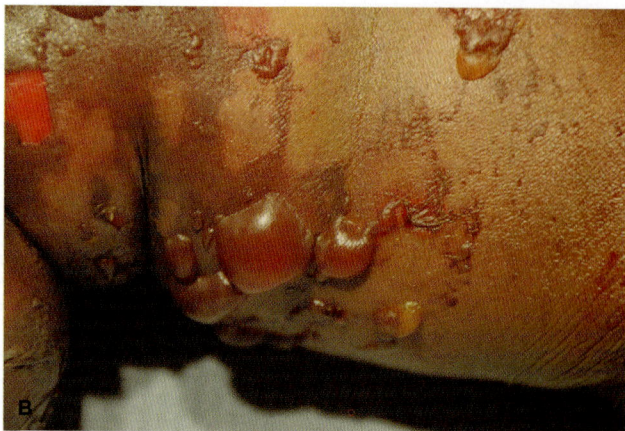
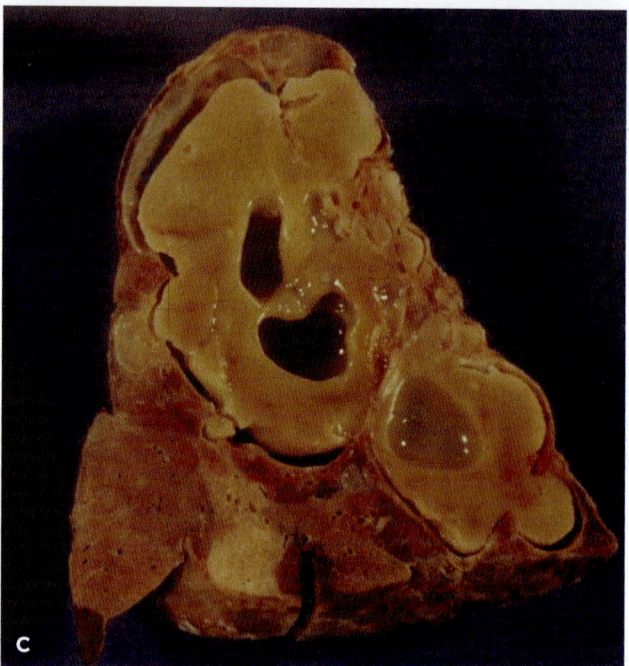

FIGURE 6-10 • Staphylococcal infections. **A:** Impetigo with bullous features. **B:** Staphylococcal scalded skin syndrome (toxic epidermal necrolysis) following MRSA infection. **C:** Partially "healed" or resolving staphylococcal lung abscess.

edema, and ulceration that involves the cervix, vagina, and perineum. Autopsies reveal few specific findings, as there is no evidence of bacterial invasion of tissues, and inflammatory reaction is negligible. Reported findings include genitourinary tract ulceration, mild lymphoid depletion, SSSS-like skin lesions, and mild and nonspecific inflammation in kidney, liver, heart, and muscle.

STREPTOCOCCAL INFECTIONS

Pathogenic group A streptococci (GAS; *Streptococcus pyogenes*) are comprised of a number of serotypes based on the M protein. GAS produces disease by at least three mechanisms: (a) direct tissue invasion of skin and upper airways (impetigo, erysipelas, cellulitis, pharyngitis, tonsillitis, necrotizing fasciitis, necrotizing pneumonia), (b) toxin elaboration (scarlet fever), and (c) immune-mediated mechanisms (acute glomerulonephritis and rheumatic fever) (Figure 6-11). The prevalence of invasive GAS disease with resultant bacteremia and/or streptococcal TSS is on the rise (142). Nonsuppurative immunologic complications can occur even in the neonate. Maternal carriage is an important factor in neonatal GAS disease. Early-onset disease is associated with concurrent maternal infection that manifests as respiratory distress, pneumonia, and toxic shock–like syndrome, while late-onset disease causes soft tissue infections and meningitis.

Non-GAS infections are mainly encountered in the newborn. *Streptococcus pneumoniae* is a common cause of pneumonia, meningitis, and otitis media (143). In asplenic patients, it is the single most common cause of sepsis, accounting for almost 50% of cases. *Streptococcus pneumoniae* has also been recognized as a cause of invasive soft tissue disease and a toxic shock–like syndrome in previously healthy children. GBS is transmitted primarily *in utero* and during delivery and is an important cause of early-onset neonatal sepsis, meningitis, and pneumonia (144). Several variables are used to identify increased GBS infection risk in

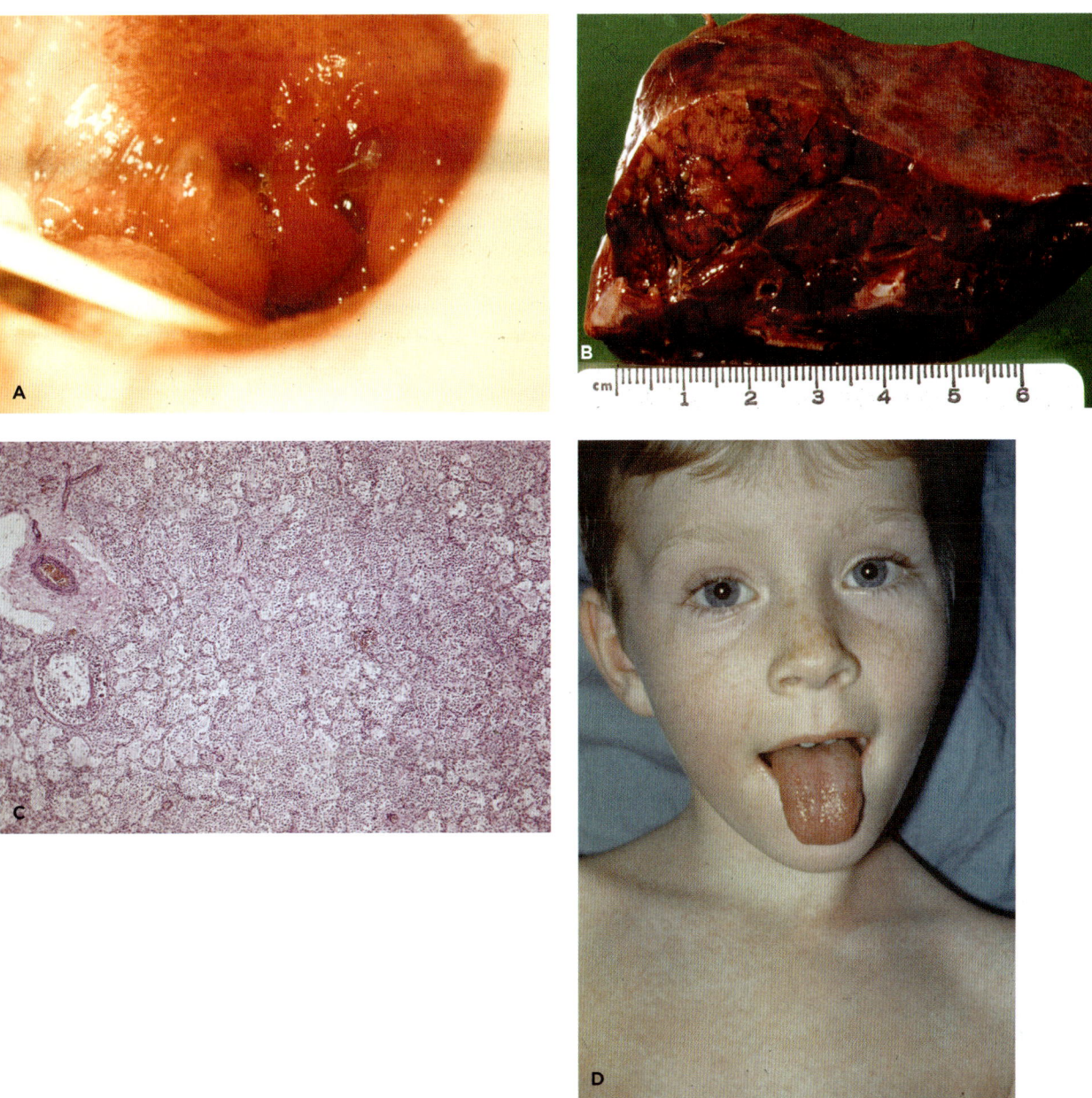

FIGURE 6-11 • Streptococcal infections. **A:** Streptococcal pharyngitis with erythematous, congested mucosa. **B:** Congenital streptococcal pneumonia with diffuse involvement. **C:** Diffuse alveolar exudates of neutrophils and fibrin in congenital streptococcal pneumonia. **D:** Scarlet fever with erythematous mucous membranes and tongue.

the neonate and to recommend intrapartum antimicrobial prophylaxis for infants at high risk (145). Other streptococcal infections, although much less common than GBS, are occasionally encountered (146–149). Viridans group streptococci (VGS) are of particular concern in neutropenic children, with septic shock and mortality of 10%. VGS infection may be accompanied by neurologic complications, myocarditis, and acute respiratory distress syndrome. Their incidence and severity have increased during the past 15 years, and antibiotic resistance is commonplace. VGS infection may cause amniotic fluid infection in midgestation with resultant fetal–neonatal sepsis.

ENTEROCOCCI

Enterococci are among the top four causes of nosocomial bacteremia in the United States (150) as they can survive on hands and inanimate surfaces. Risk factors for enterococcal bacteremia include prolonged hospital stay, exposure to antibiotics, central venous catheter use, and necrotizing enterocolitis. They cause urinary tract infections, bloodstream infections (including neonatal sepsis and infections in older children), catheter-associated bacteremia, endocarditis, intra-abdominal infection, and meningitis. Enterococci are normal inhabitants of the human GIT. Virulence is dictated by genes that cluster in distinct regions termed pathogenicity islands (PAIs), and transfer and deletion of these are frequent. The management of patients with enterococcal infections requires identifying the susceptibility of the isolate and the site of infection, both of which are key factors in providing optimal therapy. Vancomycin-resistant enterococci (VRE) are increasing in prevalence and guidelines have been released for their control (151).

NEISSERIA INFECTIONS

Neisseria gonorrhoeae can be transmitted *in utero*, intrapartum, or postpartum. Gonococcal conjunctivitis is the most frequent clinical manifestation of neonatal infection (Figure 6-12), but septicemia and arthritis can also develop (152). Increasingly common gonococcal infections outside of the perinatal period are associated with sexual abuse/sexual activity in children and adolescents; their clinical and pathologic features are similar to those in adults.

Neisseria meningitidis is a major cause of childhood morbidity and mortality (153), the spectrum of disease including bacteremia, fulminant sepsis (meningococcemia), meningitis, and pneumonia. Human disease is caused by five serogroups (A, B, C, Y, and W135), with serogroup B being commonly implicated in children less than 2 years of age. Fulminant meningococcemia ("purpura fulminans"), the form most likely to be encountered by the pathologist, is a catastrophic condition with hemorrhagic skin lesions that progress to gangrene (Figure 6-13A). Lethargy or irritability, petechiae, and purpura are followed by circulatory collapse, shock, and death. The time from first symptom to death may be only a few hours. The combination of circulatory collapse, purpura, and bilateral adrenal cortical hemorrhage constitutes the Waterhouse-Friderichsen syndrome. The petechial skin lesions consist of extravasated red cells from small vessels, absence of vasculitis, fibrin thrombi, and organisms identified within endothelial cells or in smears from the lesions. Purpuric lesions show hemorrhagic infarction of skin and subcutis with vascular thrombi. The pathogenesis of these lesions and their extremely variable clinical course are not well understood. Reminiscent of generalized Schwartzman reaction, the pathologic picture implicates an endotoxin-mediated process. Adrenal hemorrhage (Figure 6-13B, C), although striking, is unlikely to cause acute adrenal insufficiency and, by itself, does not cause death, given the great reserves of the adrenal. Acquired deficiencies of proteins C and S are probably more important players in fulminant meningococcemia. The propensity for severe disease in infants and very young children may be due to the fact that the protein C system is incompletely developed at this age. Early specific diagnosis, essential for optimal management, is based on CSF microscopy, culture, latex agglutination, and molecular techniques. Latex agglutination allows serotyping, while molecular methods are rapid and helpful in patients who have already received antibiotics. Traditional clinical prognostic signs include duration of petechiae, hypotension, presence of meningitis, leukopenia, and lack of elevation of erythrocyte sedimentation rate. The clinical syndrome of purpura fulminans may also be caused by infections with other bacteria (e.g., *E. coli*, *S. pneumoniae*, *P. mirabilis*) and viruses (varicella, rubella).

ENTEROBACTERIACEAE

Except in the neonate, the enteric bacilli are either gastrointestinal pathogens or systemic opportunists in the compromised host. Depending on the nature of the underlying disease, they cause pneumonia, septicemia, and localized suppurative reactions (Figure 6-14). The cellular reaction, when present, is entirely nonspecific, but it must be emphasized that profoundly leukocytopenic patients show inflammatory reactions that may consist solely of edema, vascular engorgement, hemorrhage, and fibrin deposition, with little or no cellular reaction. Enteric, usually food-borne, infections with verotoxin-producing strains of *E. coli* (O5l7: H7) are responsible for hemolytic uremic syndrome.

SALMONELLA INFECTION (TYPHOID)

These gram-negative bacilli can cause localized infection (e.g., gastroenteritis by *S. enterica* serovar Typhimurium) or systemic infection (e.g., typhoid by *S. enterica* serovar Typhi). Typhoid and paratyphoid fever are relatively

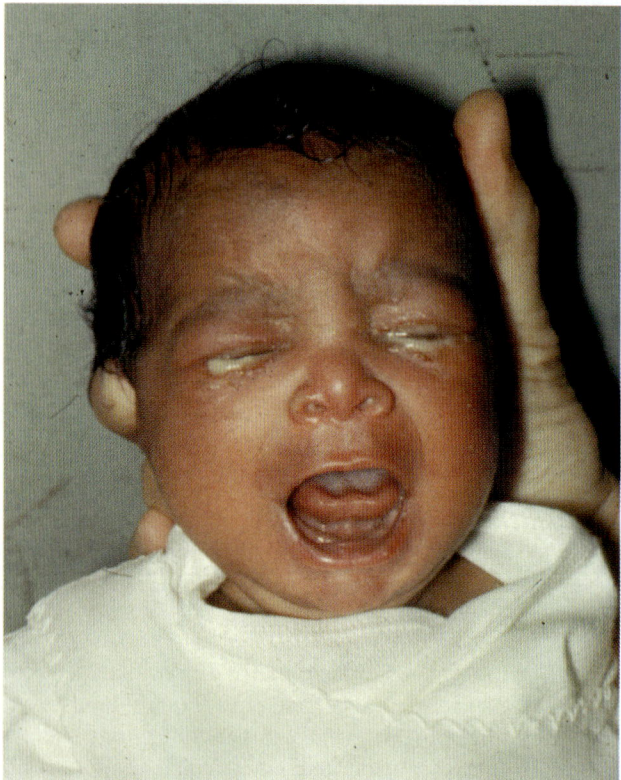

FIGURE 6-12 • Severe purulent gonococcal conjunctivitis is present in this infant.

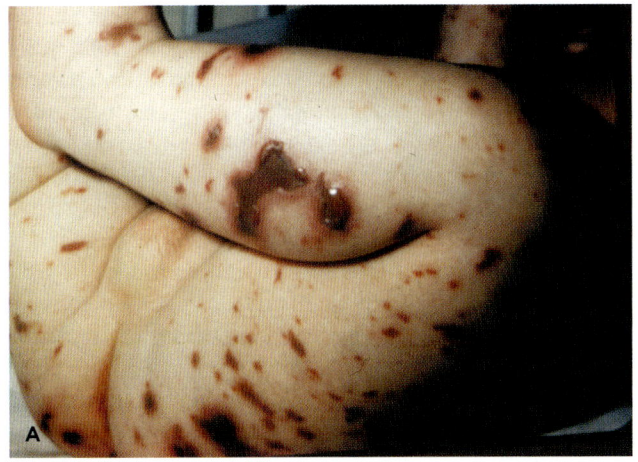
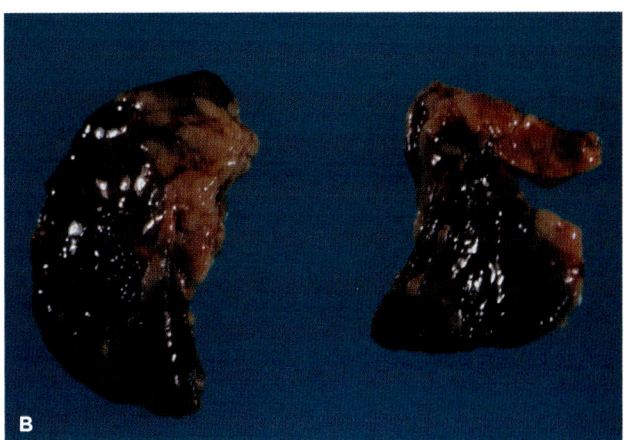
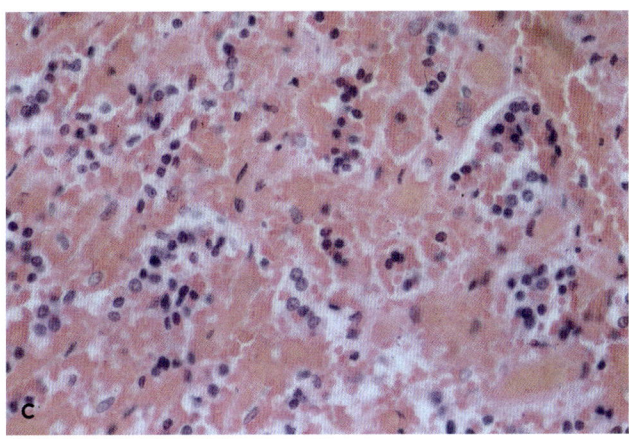

FIGURE 6-13 • Fulminant meningococcemia. **A:** Numerous petechial and ecchymotic foci with features of purpura fulminans of a consumptive coagulopathy. **B:** Bilateral adrenal hemorrhages of the Waterhouse-Friderichsen syndrome. **C:** The adrenal shows the presence of hemorrhagic necrosis.

common in developing countries, with a worldwide estimated 13.5 million episodes in 2010 (interquartile range 9.1 to 17.8 million) (154). Transmission is fecal–oral and results from poor sanitation and fecal contamination of water and dairy products. After an incubation period of 5 to 30 days, a febrile phase develops with stepwise daily elevations in temperature sometimes associated with rose spots on the trunk, bradycardia, and leukopenia. Fever can be high grade and continuous, last for 3 weeks, and presage decline and convalescence. In the present antibiotic era, patients may present with fever, diarrhea, abdominal pain, and hepatosplenomegaly. Specific symptoms and signs may be inapparent in children. The bacteria gain access to the bowel wall and disseminate via lymphatics to lymph nodes, spleen, and liver. *Salmonella* proliferate in bile-amplified enterohepatic circulation. Intestinal typhoid ulcers result from necrosis of hyperplastic Peyer patches and therefore array along the long axis of the small bowel. Histology reveals numerous

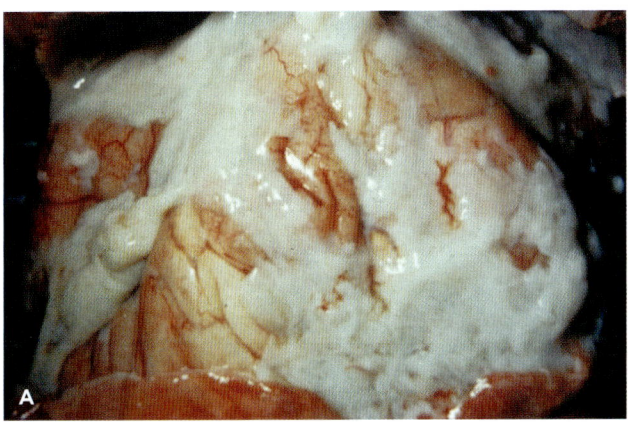
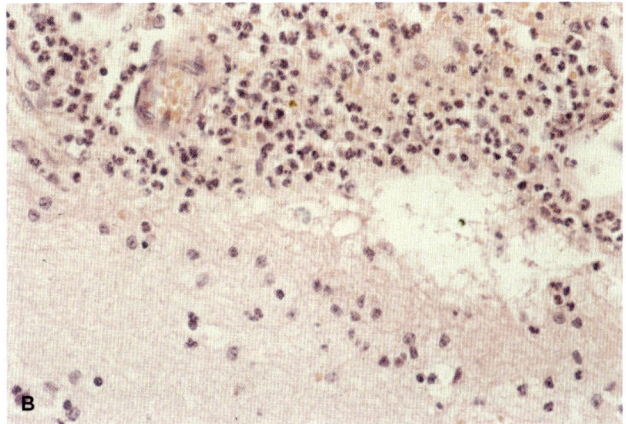

FIGURE 6-14 • **A:** Acute *E. coli* meningitis with purulent exudate covering convexities. **B:** Neutrophils filling the subarachnoid space.

macrophages (so-called typhoid cells or Mallory cells) forming "soft granulomas" with erythro- and lymphophagocytosis, plasma cells, and activated lymphocytes. Macrophage aggregates (so-called typhoid nodules) may be seen in the spleen, liver, bone marrow, kidneys, salivary glands, and testes. A fibrinous exudate may be seen on the splenic capsule that later becomes organized to produce the "sugar-coated" ("zuckergleiss") spleen. Laboratory diagnosis is by culture (*S. typhi* isolates are positive from blood or bone marrow by the first week and stool by the third week), serology (Widal test), and more specific assays (155). Complications include ileus, acute renal failure, cardiac arrhythmia (with sudden death), massive intestinal hemorrhage (following Peyer patch necrosis), pancreatic dysfunction, intestinal perforation, peritonitis, Zenker degeneration of abdominal skeletal muscles, liver necrosis, splenic rupture, and DIC (156). Atypical manifestations include pneumonitis, pericarditis, osteomyelitis (especially in sickle cell anemia patients), dactylitis, pericarditis, arthritis, meningitis, cerebellar ataxia, myelonecrosis, and a generalized hemophagocytic syndrome (157). When a carrier stage develops, patients excrete bacteria in their stool and urine, posing a health hazard to society, as exemplified by the infamous Typhoid Mary.

HAEMOPHILUS INFLUENZAE

This small gram-negative coccobacillus is a commensal of the upper respiratory tract and a major cause of morbidity and mortality in infants and young children. Colonization by capsular *H. influenzae* type B (HiB) is uncommon in a healthy individual, but it can cause severe disease in patients with respiratory compromise or immunodeficiency. Transmission is through direct contact and by respiratory droplets. There is no evidence for its transmission through breast milk, which actually limits oropharyngeal colonization. Most invasive disease outside the neonatal age group results from infection by HiB. Infections range from mild (e.g., conjunctivitis and otitis media) to life-threatening (epiglottitis, meningitis, pericarditis, pneumonia, septic arthritis, and facial cellulitis). Until recently, HiB was the major cause of meningitis in infants accounting for 80% of cases under the age of 2 years and for at least one-third of infantile bacterial pneumonia. This has decreased significantly in countries where the use of the HiB conjugate vaccines is the norm (158). In the upper airway, *H. influenzae* causes life-threatening acute epiglottitis (Figure 6-15). The larynx and especially the epiglottis are the site of marked congestion, edema, and leukocytic infiltration, which may completely occlude the small infant airway. The cherry red appearance is helpful in distinguishing this condition from severe viral laryngotracheitis (croup), which is occasionally severe enough to cause airway obstruction in this age group. Nontypeable strains commonly cause lower respiratory infections but can also cause invasive disease. In children, they are also the most common cause of bacterial conjunctivitis and the second most common cause (after *S. pneumoniae*) of otitis media. *H. influenzae* also causes acute chorioamnionitis. Histopathologic features of *H. influenzae* infection do not differ from other bacterial illness.

DIPHTHERIA

Diphtheria is caused by a toxin produced by *Corynebacterium diphtheriae* carrying a particular lysogenic bacteriophage; all of the gross and microscopic features of the disease can be

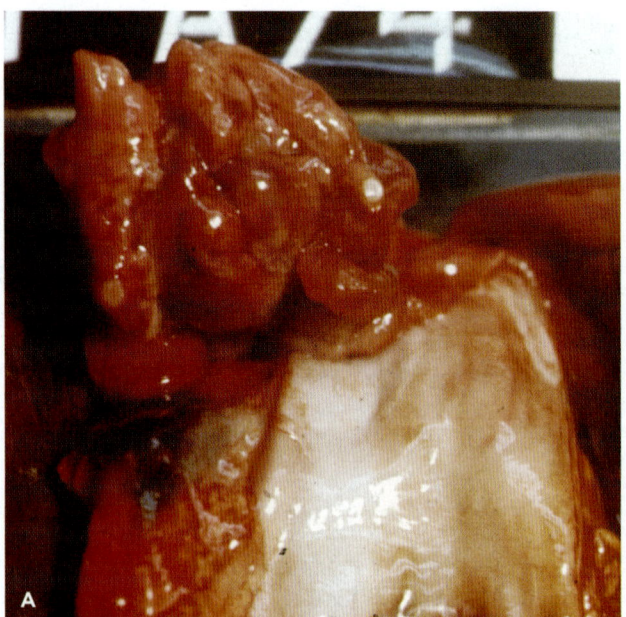
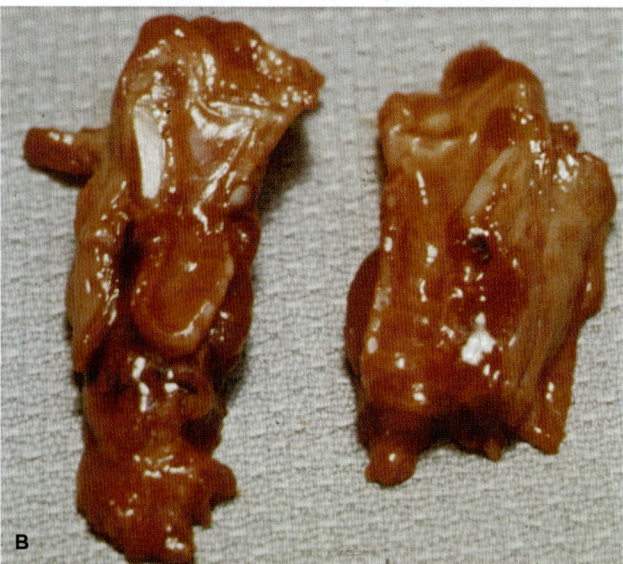

FIGURE 6-15 • *Haemophilus influenzae* epiglottitis. **A:** Marked induration and enlargement of the epiglottis are features in this autopsy case. **B:** Involvement of the entire epiglottis and larynx by *H. influenzae* results in these gross findings.

produced by purified toxin. The toxin can affect all cells of the body but is most damaging to nerves, kidneys, and heart, and it halts addition of amino acids to elongating polypeptide chains. Humans are the only identified reservoirs and symptom-free carriers. The major sources of infection are fomites and secretions from patients in the incubation stage of disease. Initial toxin-induced necrosis of upper airway epithelium with abundant fibrin exudation leads to the typical fibrinous pseudomembrane overlying mildly inflamed submucosa, accompanied by tremendous edema of the soft tissues of the neck. Death is related to airway obstruction, toxin-mediated cardiomyopathy/myocarditis, and diphtheritic peripheral and cranial neuropathy.

Despite large-scale immunization, rare cases of diphtheria continue to occur in nonimmunized children and unprotected young adults. Although universal immunization has significantly reduced its incidence, toxigenic strains remain in circulation, posing a constant threat to people with low levels of seroprotection.

Corynebacterium ulcerans has been increasingly implicated as an emerging zoonotic agent of diphtheria from animals such as cats or dogs (159).

PERTUSSIS

Pertussis is an acute respiratory tract infection, generally two weeks in duration, manifested by a paroxysmal cough, posttussive emesis, or inspiratory whoop (160). The term whooping cough derives from the high-pitched gasp occurring after a paroxysm of coughing and usually seen in young children over 6 months of age (161). Clinically, pertussis progresses through three stages: a nonspecific catarrhal stage lasting one to two weeks, a paroxysmal stage sometimes persisting many weeks, and a convalescent stage. The paroxysmal coughing, an attempt to clear thick mucus from the tracheobronchial tree, can cause distension of neck veins, bulging of eyes, lacrimation, and posttussive emesis. In recent years, there has been resurgence in pertussis. Adults are considered the main reservoir, and booster vaccination in adult life may be beneficial as a community preventive measure (see Chapter 12).

Most cases of pertussis are caused by *Bordetella pertussis*, but other species (*Bordetella parapertussis*, *Bordetella bronchiseptica*, and *Bordetella holmesii*) have also been implicated. Unlike *B. pertussis*, which is a respiratory pathogen, *B. holmesii* can also cause bacteremia (162). *Bordetella* species have tropism for respiratory ciliated cells and are typically noninvasive. Histologically, the infection is characterized by acute bronchitis and bronchiolitis with epithelial denudation (Figure 6-16). The test of choice for diagnosis is culture of nasopharyngeal aspirates or posterior nasopharyngeal swabs. Although highly specific, *Bordetella* is difficult to culture, with low sensitivity. Yield is greatest within the first two weeks of symptom onset, when the infection may not be clinically suspected. The use of PCR-based tests is well accepted and increases detection of pertussis by 19% compared with culture alone (161). Other tests, including DFA and serology, are not as useful (163).

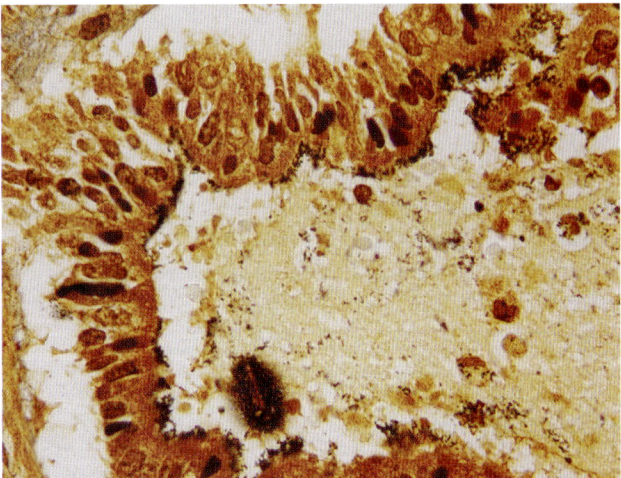

FIGURE 6-16 • Pertussis infection. Bronchial lumen filled with mucus and short coccobacilli (Bordetella) (Modified Warthin-Starry stain). Section courtesy of Dr. Cynthia Trevenen, Alberta Children's Hospital, Calgary.

INFECTIONS BY OTHER GRAM-NEGATIVE BACILLI

Ubiquitous in soil and water, *Pseudomonas aeruginosa* infection occurs almost exclusively as an opportunistic pathogen, frequently associated with cystic fibrosis. It also causes gangrenous lesions in the skin (pyoderma gangrenosum) and GIT of patients with malignancy. Primarily a nosocomial infection, *Pseudomonas* sepsis occurs as a late-onset disease in very low-birth-weight infants and carries a 50% mortality rate. Occasional cases may be associated with chorioamnionitis. *Pseudomonas* sepsis is characterized by necrotizing vasculitis, involving both arteries and veins. The vessel wall is replaced by collections of organisms, often with very little cellular infiltrate, and hemorrhagic infarction results at the affected site. Particularly affected are the skin and mucous membranes (especially of the intestinal tract), manifesting as deep red or violaceous raised plaques, which rapidly undergo necrosis. Patients may also have a hemorrhagic necrotizing bronchopneumonia (Figure 6-17).

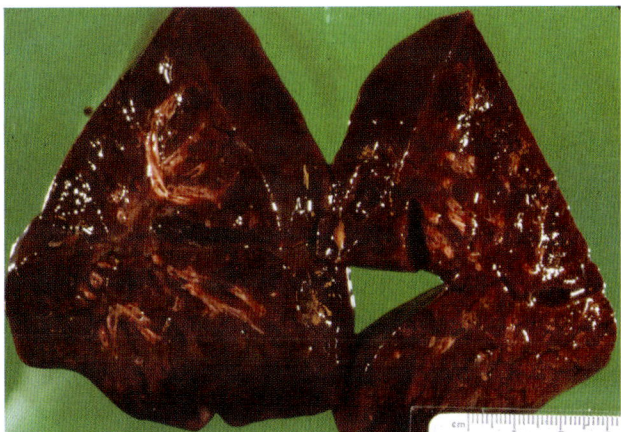

FIGURE 6-17 • Necrotizing hemorrhagic pneumonia caused by *Pseudomonas aeruginosa*.

Serratia marcescens, an infrequent pathogen in the newborn, is usually nosocomially acquired through foreign bodies and instrumentation. *Serratia* sepsis is a late-onset disease with severe meningitis and a high mortality rate.

Citrobacter species are an increasingly recognized cause of neonatal sepsis, meningitis, hemorrhagic encephalitis, and brain abscess. The majority of cases present in the first 10 days of life. Most cases are apparently nosocomial, following surgical manipulation of umbilical cord stumps, but early-onset sepsis suggests that vertical transmission may also occur.

LISTERIOSIS

Listeria monocytogenes is a small, gram-positive bacillus that acts as a facultative intracellular parasite. The organism is a common intestinal and vaginal commensal. Human listeriosis presents as one of three clinical forms including febrile gastroenteritis, maternal–fetal/neonatal listeriosis, or bacteremia with or without CNS involvement. Infections are uncommon, and the estimated incidence of listeriosis during pregnancy is 12 cases per 10^5 (164). Listeriosis during pregnancy is associated with second trimester abortion and infrequently causes premature delivery or stillbirth. Up to two-thirds of viable neonates develop overt infection due to either transplacental or intrapartum transmission (164). Perinatal infection is an uncommon cause of severe disease in the neonate.

Neonatal listeriosis is classified as either early (occurring in the first 5 to 7 postnatal days) or late infection. Early-onset infection is due to types Ia, Ib, and IVb, while type IVb predominates in late-onset infection. Early disease is associated with maternal infection, often overt at the time of delivery, and with meconium staining of the amniotic fluid. Clinical presentations include neonatal sepsis with pneumonia, bacteremia, and/or meningitis (164). In some neonates, the infection manifests as "granulomatosis infantiseptica" with salmon pink rash mucosal nodules, and widespread microabscesses and granulomas especially in the liver, spleen, and lungs (Figure 6-18). In contrast, late-onset infection usually occurs in full-term neonates delivered from uncomplicated pregnancies and presents as meningitis between the second and eighth week of life (165). Late-onset infection is presumed to be acquired from the maternal vaginal tract at the time of delivery. Listerial meningoencephalitis cannot be distinguished from other systemic bacterial or viral infections. Most frequently involved organs include the adrenals, liver, GIT, skin, and tracheobronchial tree. Mortality of untreated early-onset infection is 100%; survivors have CNS sequelae including hydrocephalus and cognitive impairment. Factors determining *L. monocytogenes* virulence have been reviewed (166).

Systemic infection is marked by bacterial replication in mononuclear cells in the liver, spleen, and bone marrow. Parasitized monocytes play an important role in CNS invasion (167). The histopathologic features depend largely on the duration of the disease. Inflammatory foci may consist solely of necrosis with little cellular reaction (although fibrin thrombi and hemorrhage may be prominent) or miliary abscesses may be seen, particularly in liver and adrenal glands. Gram, Warthin-Starry, and immunohistochemical stains help identify organisms in tissues. The lesions after several days in patients who mount a specific immune response assume a granulomatous appearance as mononuclear cells replace polymorphonuclear leukocytes in the abscesses. Irrespective of route (transplacental or ascending) of infection, placental infection is common, causing intervillous and intravillous microabscesses with necrotizing villitis and chorioamnionitis. A definitive diagnosis of listeriosis is made by culturing *L. monocytogenes*. Blood and CSF are the most useful specimens; serologic assays are not useful.

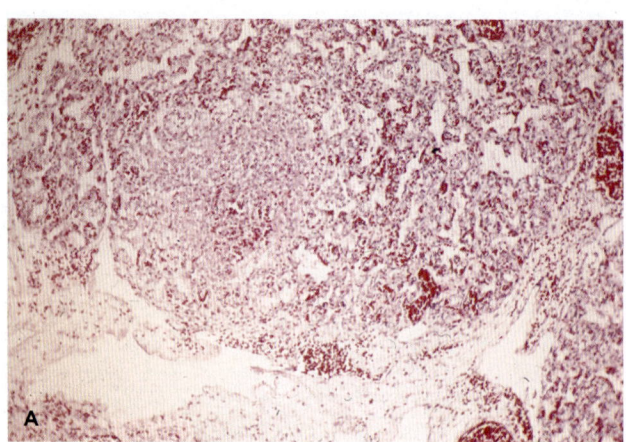
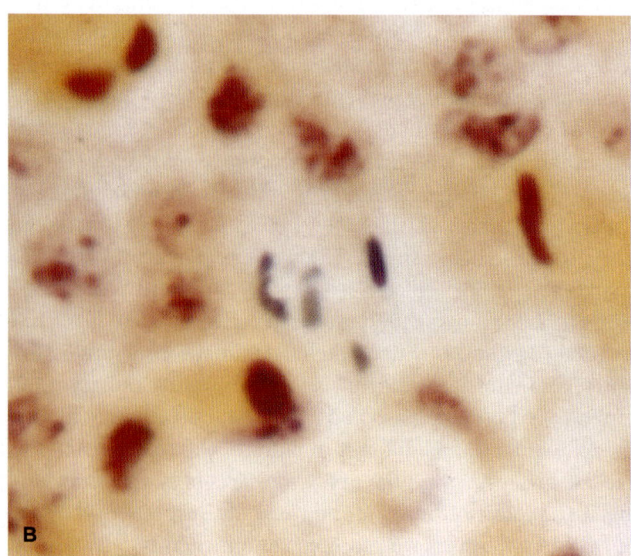

FIGURE 6-18 • Listeriosis. **A:** Lung abscess is seen in this infant with numerous such lesions with minimal inflammation. **B:** Brown-Hopps stain highlights the rod-shaped bacteria.

SYPHILIS

Treponemes are microaerophilic spiral gram-negative bacteria that are 6 to 20 µm long and 0.1 to 0.5 µm in diameter. Without Warthin-Starry stains, this thickness is less than the resolution limits of conventional light microscopy, but it can be visualized by darkfield or phase contrast microscopy. Similar to Lyme disease, *T. pallidum* causes multisystem disease in stages. Humans are the sole natural host of *T. pallidum*. The WHO estimates that maternal syphilis leads to 460,000 abortions/stillbirths and 270,000 liveborn infants with congenital syphilis yearly. The frequency of congenital syphilis in a specific locale is determined ultimately by the prevalence of syphilis among adults and the effectiveness of prenatal screening and treatment. HIV-infected pregnant women are at high risk for having active syphilis. Pediatric syphilis has been the subject of many reviews (168,169).

Transmission

Transmission of syphilis occurs through contact via sex, open lesions, or secretions from the lesions in the skin and mucous membranes. Congenital syphilis occurs in the fetus through placentitis, whereas perinatal infection occurs by contact with the spirochete during passage through the birth canal. As early as 9 to 10 weeks of gestation, *T. pallidum* can cross the placenta and infect the developing fetus throughout pregnancy. Vertical transmission during pregnancy occurs more frequently with primary or secondary syphilis than with latent maternal disease. Fetal infection is most efficient during the early stages of maternal infection; at this time, the transmission rate approaches 100%. The risk of transmission diminishes after 4 years of infection, even when the mother is untreated. Postnatal infection can occur in the infant through contact with open lesions or secretions in the infected mother or another adult. If syphilitic lesions involve the breast or nipples, then breast-feeding or expressed breast milk should be avoided until the mother has completed treatment and the lesions have healed. There is no evidence for transmission of *T. pallidum* in breast milk of mothers without a breast or nipple lesion.

Clinical Features

Fetal infection can result in spontaneous abortion, stillbirth, early congenital syphilis, and late congenital syphilis (Figure 6-19). Congenital syphilis does not have a primary stage and may result in perinatal death in more than 40% of affected, untreated pregnancies. Manifestations in surviving infants traditionally have been divided into early- and late-onset types. Early manifestations appear in the first 2 years of life, when secondary syphilis-like lesions result from transplacental spirochetemia. Late-onset disease is seen in children older than 2 years and is not considered contagious.

Many features are nonspecific, but certain lesions are pathognomonic, and the disease can be recognized in severely macerated stillborns in one-third to one-half of congenital syphilis cases. Infection occurring prior to the 5th month

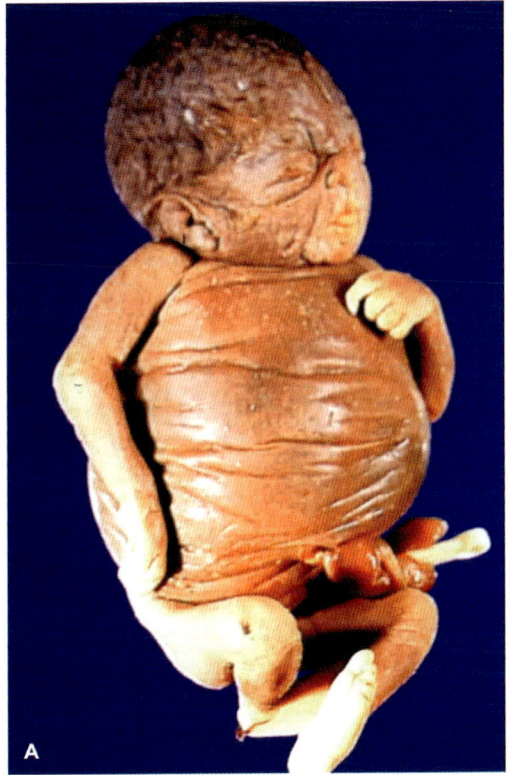
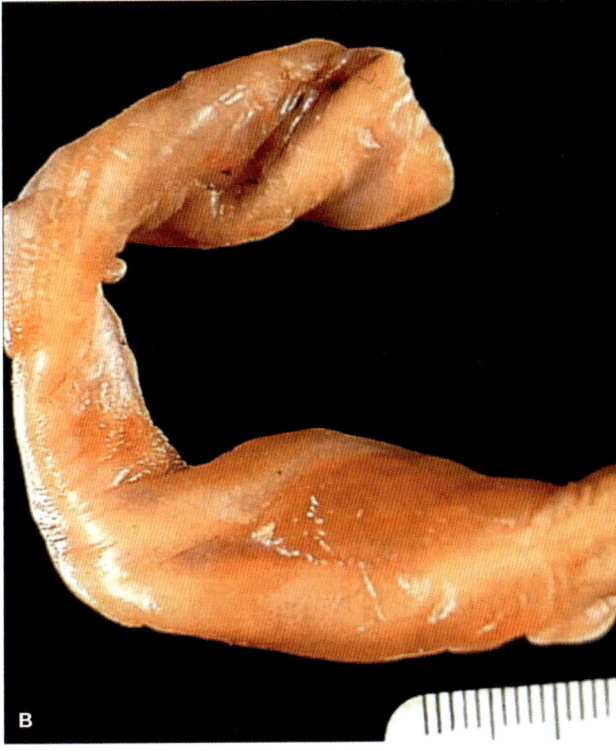

FIGURE 6-19 • Congenital syphilis with its various features. **A:** Congenital syphilis with hydrops fetalis. **B:** Congenital syphilis with "barber pole" funisitis.

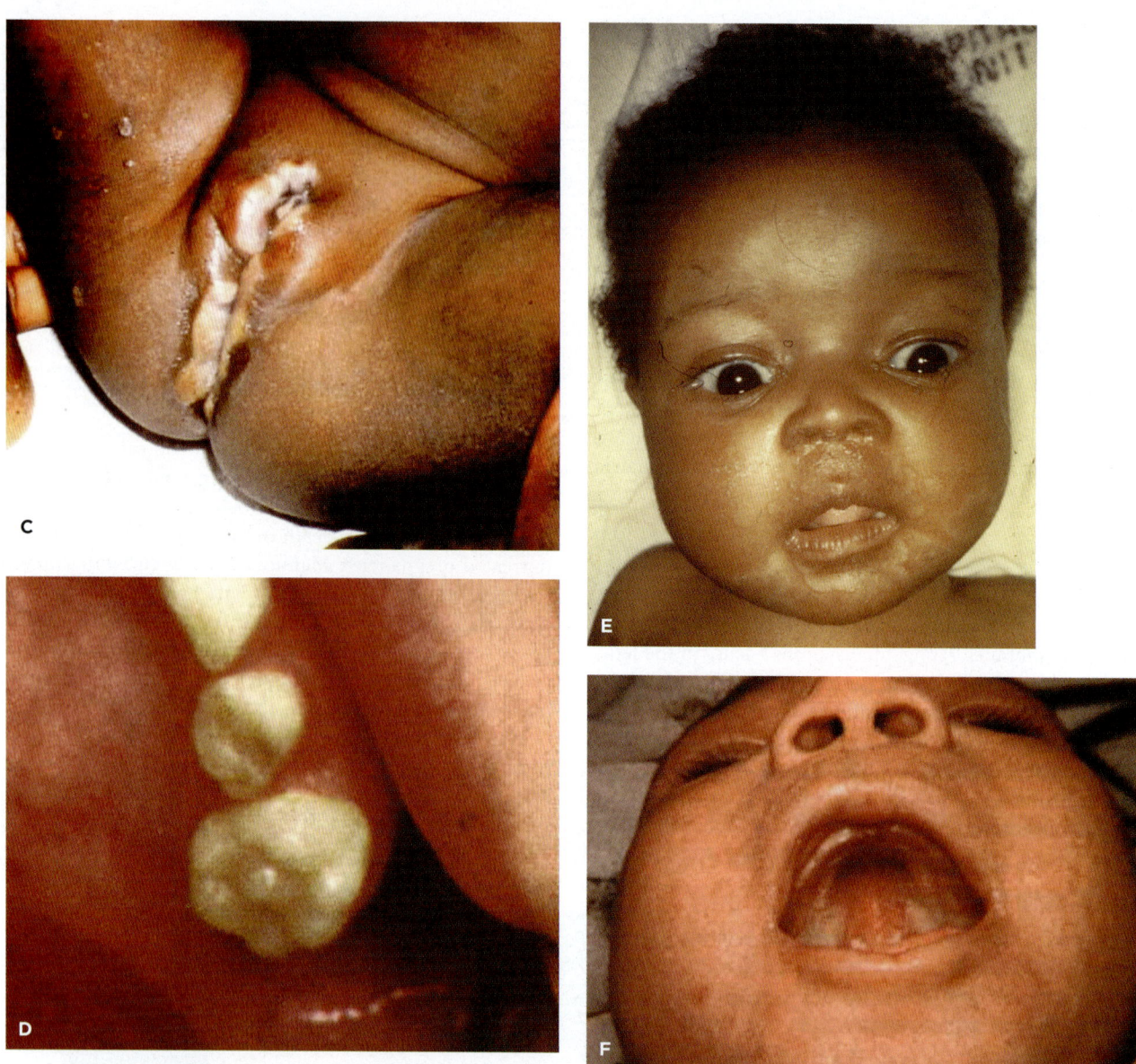

FIGURE 6-19 • (*Continued*) **C:** Labial lesions in neonatal syphilis forming condylomata lata. **D:** Bifid molar as a malformative manifestation in tooth development. **E:** Snuffles as a nasal discharge secondary to obstructive nasopharyngitis. The mucopurulent discharge contains viable organisms. **F:** Mucous patches representing an ulcerative mucositis.

of intrauterine life does not cause destructive changes and organogenesis is unaffected. Hepatomegaly and/or hydrops may be the only gross evidence of disease in the macerated second and third trimester stillborn infant (Figure 6-19A); however, organisms are abundant in all organs, even after extensive autolysis. Congenital syphilis can clinically mimic a number of neonatal conditions, including other congenital infections (CMV, HSV, rubella, and toxoplasma), bacterial sepsis, and blood group incompatibility. A negative Coombs test with hydrops may suggest congenital syphilis, as well as parvovirus infection. Asymptomatic at birth, most early-onset congenital syphilis cases are identified only by routine prenatal screening. If untreated, symptoms develop within weeks or months. Stillborns and highly symptomatic premature newborns exhibit an enlarged liver and spleen, skeletal involvement, and often pneumonia and bullous skin lesions. In less severe infections, the early signs of congenital syphilis include poor feeding and snuffles (syphilitic rhinitis; Figure 6-19E). Early manifestations of congenital infection vary and involve multiple organ systems. Hepatomegaly occurs almost universally, with biochemical evidence of liver dysfunction. The most striking lesions affect the mucocutaneous tissues and bones. Mucous patches, rhinitis, and condylomatous lesions characterize mucous membrane involvement in congenital syphilis (Figure 6-19F). Nasal fluid is highly infectious. Snuffles are quickly followed by a diffuse maculopapular desquamative rash with extensive sloughing of the epithelium, particularly on palms, soles, and perioral and perianal regions. A vesicular rash and bullae may develop, weep, and desquamate. These lesions teem with spirochetes and are highly infectious. Bone involvement with multiple symmetric periostitis and joint osteochondritis occurs in 60% to 80% of untreated early congenital infections. Bone involvement can be very painful, causing immobility (pseudoparalysis of Parrot). Tibial metaphyseal demineralization (Wimberger sign) is seen radiologically. Bone involvement usually resolves spontaneously within 6 months. Neurosyphilis may be present even with normal CSF findings. Alternatively, in the first 6 months, it may present as acute meningitis or a chronic meningovascular neurosyphilis at the end of the first year of life, with progressive hydrocephalus, cranial nerve palsies, seizures, and neurodevelopmental regression. Cerebral infarction from syphilitic endarteritis may occur in the second year of life. Anemia, thrombocytopenia, leukopenia, and leukocytosis are common. The late manifestations of congenital syphilis are a consequence of scarring from the early systemic disease and involve teeth (Figure 6-19D), bones, eyes, the eighth cranial nerve, and CNS.

In older children and adolescents, syphilis is sexually transmitted and may be the result of sexual abuse. Manifestations and diagnosis are similar to that in adults. Neurosyphilis occurs in approximately 30% of patients with secondary syphilis; CSF pleocytosis and proteinosis are typical findings. Neurosyphilis may be clinically silent or present with meningeal, cranial nerve, or spinal nerve involvement. In addition to mucocutaneous involvement, secondary syphilis can also manifest with iritis, anterior uveitis, arthritis, and nephrotic syndrome, probably caused by deposition of immune complexes composed of treponemal antigens, fibronectin, antibodies, and complement. Secondary syphilitic lesions resolve without treatment in 1 to 2 months. The infection then enters a latent period, without overt evidence of disease. The signs of secondary syphilis can recur during the first year (early latency) but not thereafter (late latency). Relative immunity to reinfection exists during latency, and approximately 60% of untreated patients will not progress from latency to tertiary syphilis. The remaining patients progress after latent periods of 3 to 10 years. This time frame renders acquired tertiary syphilis a very rare occurrence during childhood and adolescence.

Pathology

Silverstein suggested that histopathologic changes of syphilis require development of fetal immune competence. Humoral immunity is insufficient to control the infection, and cell-mediated immunity is suppressed during the primary and secondary stages. Ultimate eradication occurs when T-cells infiltrate syphilitic lesions. *T. pallidum* may escape immune surveillance by antigenic variation. Although primary syphilis elicits a Th1 immune response, progression to the secondary stage is accompanied by a shift to a Th2 response, allowing for incomplete clearance of the pathogen. In pregnancy, fetal infection induces intense inflammatory responses and prostaglandins that may be responsible for the various manifestations of congenital syphilis (170).

The main pathologic changes of syphilis occur in pancreas, liver, GIT, bones, and nasal mucosa as inflammation, scarring, and developmental delay. The liver shows diffuse inflammation and fibrosis with formation of coarse nodules (hepar lobatum). Osteochondritis and periostitis of joints, long bones, palate, and nasal cartilage lead to skeletal deformities. Lung involvement leads to pale airless, heavy, and fibrotic lungs (pneumonia alba). The viscera in general appears immature for gestational age with prominent extramedullary hematopoiesis, persistence of fetal adrenal cortex, active glomerulogenesis, and persistence of fetal stroma in many organs, notably the pancreas and the pulmonary interstitium. The inflammatory response is mainly mononuclear and may be difficult to distinguish from extramedullary hematopoiesis. Polymorphonuclear leukocytes occur in response to tissue necrosis, producing the typical Dubois abscess. Gummata are rare in newborns. Oppenheimer and Dahms provide a complete description of the pathologic changes of congenital syphilis and describe a pathognomonic triad comprised of interstitial inflammation, pressure atrophy, and fibrosis of the pancreas with pressure atrophy of the parenchyma, pneumonia alba, and thickening of the bowel wall by submucosal infiltrates and fibrosis. An obliterative endarteritis, consisting of concentric endothelial and fibroblastic proliferative thickening with plasma cell infiltration, should suggest syphilis. This endarteritis is also found in all stages of acquired syphilis (in the primary chancre, polymorphonuclear leukocytes, and macrophages often can be seen ingesting treponemes).

Placental examination in suspected cases allows early diagnosis. Grossly, the placenta is large and heavy. Syphilitic placentitis is histologically characterized by histiocytic-predominant villitis, proliferative endovasculitis of the stem villi (perivasculitis with concentric mural vascular sclerosis), and necrotizing umbilical periphlebitis. The umbilical periphlebitis is pathognomonic and comprises of abscess-like necrotic foci in the Wharton jelly, with eosinophilic perivenous precipitates. Other histopathologic findings include villous dysmaturity, hypercellular villi with variable acute and chronic inflammation, numerous Hofbauer cells, endarteritis, perivascular fibrosis, numerous intravascular nucleated red cells, proliferative fetal vascular changes, chorioamnionitis, necrotizing funisitis, and/or plasma cell deciduitis. Spirochetes may be difficult to demonstrate in the placenta, and their absence does not exclude the diagnosis. Spirochetes are easier to demonstrate in the umbilical cord (171).

Laboratory Diagnosis

Definitive diagnosis requires demonstration of the spirochete; *T. pallidum* is a long (15-μm) slender organism optimally identified by darkfield examination. If fresh preparations are not available, Levaditi, Dieterle, Steiner, or Warthin-Starry stains are helpful. An immunohistochemical procedure has been described, and PCR diagnosis has been useful in selected cases. In the appropriate clinical setting, a diagnosis may also be made if serum quantitative antibody titer is at least four times greater than the maternal titer. The CSF Venereal disease research laboratory (VDRL) test is reactive, and/or the IgM FTA-ABS is positive.

Prognosis and Outcome

If the newborn survives, progressive inflammation and fibrosis lead to the stigmata of late congenital syphilis: gummatous facial deformities (perforated palate and saddle nose), skeletal defects [frontal bossing, short maxillae, mandibular protuberance, high palatal arch, scaphoid scapulae, saber shins, Clutton joints, sternoclavicular thickening (Higoumenakis sign)], dental abnormalities (Hutchinson incisors, mulberry molars), rhagades, meningovasculitis leading to eighth nerve damage and optic atrophy, interstitial keratitis, and neurosyphilis.

LEPTOSPIROSIS

Leptospirosis is a zoonotic disease caused by a single nontreponemal spirochete species (*Leptospira interrogans*) with several subgroups. An emerging global disease, the disease occurs in seasonal epidemic forms in tropical countries, especially South and Southeast Asia. Although primarily a zoonosis, humans are infected by exposure to water or soil contaminated with animal urine or by the bite of a rat flea. Transplacental infection and fetal death have been documented. The majority of leptospiral infections are either subclinical or mild, but some patients develop complications due to multiorgan system involvement, with fatality rates over 40% (172). After an incubation period of 2 to 30 days, a flu-like septicemic phase ensues, followed by an immune phase involving kidneys, liver, meninges, eyes, skin, pancreas, heart, spleen, and lymph nodes. Clinical presentation depends upon the predominant organs involved. Because of its protean manifestations, leptospirosis is often misdiagnosed and underreported. The more severe form (Weil disease) is characterized by jaundice, coagulopathy, and hematuria (hence the term "icterohemorrhagica"). When fatal, death is usually due to renal failure (173), although pulmonary involvement can also be a serious life threat (174). Identification methods include direct (darkfield) microscopy, culture, and the most widely used reference standard method—the microscopic agglutination test (175). In the first week, blood and CSF cultures are positive, while in the immune phase, leptospires may be recoverable only from the urine. Pathology reflects organ dysfunction and features of coagulopathy. Mortality is high in fulminant cases. Antibiotic therapy may cause a Jarisch-Herxheimer–type reaction with clinical worsening.

LYME DISEASE

Lyme disease is the most common tick-borne infection in both North America and Europe. In the United States, Lyme disease is caused by the spirochete *Borrelia burgdorferi*, transmitted by the bite of the deer tick species *Ixodes scapularis* and *I. pacificus*.

Transmission

Transplacental spread to the fetus is reported; first trimester infection may be followed by premature delivery with demonstrable spirochetes in many viscera and severe congenital cardiovascular abnormalities, including hypoplasia of the aorta and endocardial fibroelastosis. However, whether or not *B. burgdorferi* directly causes fetal illness or abnormality is debated. Prenatal transmission is uncommon, even in endemic areas. The case against congenital infection is strong as no inflammation is seen in the placentas or tissues from children where spirochetes have been identified. Further, longitudinal population studies and serosurveys have not shown any consistent evidence of adverse fetal effects of Lyme disease during pregnancy (176), even when the placenta is infected. Although *B. burgdorferi* DNA has been found in breast milk, there is no evidence for lactiferous transmission (177).

Clinical Features

Lyme disease is characterized by multiorgan system involvement (skin, heart, joints, and nervous system) that occurs in three stages: early localized, early disseminated, and late. Following tick bite, an acute phase is characterized by the erythema migrans rash with or without systemic manifestations such as fever, headache, photophobia, myalgias, generalized lymphadenopathy, and severe fatigue, without localizing signs. Erythema migrans is a round or oval, expanding erythematous skin lesion that develops at the site of deposition of *B. burgdorferi* and typically become apparent approximately 7 to 14 days after tick detachment. It should be at least 5 cm in largest diameter for secure diagnosis. The nonscaly and nonpruritic lesions may vary from erythematous to targetoid to vesicular. Secondary skin lesions may arise by hematogenous dissemination from the site of primary infection. A tick bite hypersensitivity reaction is favored over erythema migrans if an urticarial erythematous skin lesion appears during *Ixodes* attachment, develops within 48 hours of detachment, measures less than 5 cm, and reduces in size over the 24 to 48 hours following its appearance. Early Lyme disease manifestations also include neurologic symptoms (cranial neuropathy, especially Bell palsy, meningoradiculitis, and encephalitis), carditis (heart block or myopericarditis), and Borrelial lymphocytoma. Late manifestations include recurrent large joint (typically knee) arthritis, late neurologic disease (encephalopathy, encephalomyelitis, and peripheral neuropathy), and acrodermatitis chronica atrophicans (178). Acrodermatitis chronica atrophicans starts as a doughy bluish-red swelling on the extensor surfaces of the hands and feet and resolves over months to years with atrophy ("cigarette paper skin"). Most clinical features are immune mediated by elaboration of various cytokines. There is no well-accepted definition of post-Lyme disease syndrome. Erythema migrans, seen in nearly 90% of children with Lyme disease, is the only manifestation of Lyme disease in the United States that is clinically diagnostic in the absence of laboratory confirmation. In a community-based prospective study of 201 children with Lyme disease, the initial manifestations were single erythema migrans (66%), multiple erythema migrans (23%), arthritis (7%), facial palsy (3%), aseptic meningitis (1%), and carditis (0.5%) (177).

Pathology

Histopathologically, Lyme disease manifests a perivascular and interstitial infiltration of lymphocytes, plasma cells, and histiocytes in involved organs. Borrelia may be demonstrated in the acute hemorrhagic lesions of erythema migrans. Inflammatory changes are minimal to absent in neonates and, for that reason, spirochetes may be more numerous. Placental changes range from none to a chorionic villitis with histiocytes, plasma cells, increased Hofbauer cells, and intervillous and intravillous spirochetes. Borrelial lymphocytoma, a rare cutaneous manifestation of Lyme disease, presents as a solitary bluish-red swelling with a diameter of up to a few centimeters, most commonly on the earlobe in children and the breast, on or near the nipple, in adults. It may be the only sign of Lyme disease and persist for months. It contains a dense lymphoid infiltrate with or without germinal centers in the cutis and subcutis that may suggest the diagnosis of a lymphoma to the unaware; however, the infiltrate is polyclonal. Lesions of acrodermatitis chronica atrophicans show a pronounced lymphoplasmacellular infiltration of the skin and sometimes the subcutis, with or without atrophy (179).

Laboratory Diagnosis

Diagnosis of Lyme disease is based on serology, and careful quality control procedures are required (178). First-tier testing most often uses polyvalent ELISA. If the first-tier assay result is positive or equivocal, then the same serum specimen is retested by separate IgM and IgG immunoblots. For patients with symptoms in excess of 4 weeks, reactivity must be present on the IgG immunoblot for the patient to be considered seropositive. In areas with high endemicity, seropositivity rates may exceed 4%. False-positive results may be due to cross-reaction with viruses, autoimmune diseases, and other spirochetes. Although useful for research studies, culture of *Borrelia* species from skin or blood or identification of *B. burgdorferi* DNA by PCR is not recommended for diagnosis in routine clinical care (178).

Prognosis and Outcomes

Long-term prognosis is excellent following treatment, irrespective of whether the children present with erythema migrans alone, early disseminated disease, or late Lyme disease. Recurrence of arthritis may occur among patients with HLA-DR2, HLA-DR3, or HLA-DR4 phenotypes. Children with Lyme neuroborreliosis have been reported to have persistent facial nerve palsy (180). It has been suggested that therapy of pregnant women with syphilis and Lyme borreliosis should follow the same strategy, since both diseases have similar etiologic, clinical, and epidemiologic characteristics (181).

Coinfections Associated with Lyme Disease

I. scapularis, the vector for *B. burgdorferi*, may also transmit *Anaplasma phagocytophilum* (previously referred to as *Ehrlichia phagocytophila*) and/or *Babesia microti*, the primary cause of babesiosis. Thus, a bite from an *I. scapularis* tick may lead to the development of Lyme disease, human granulocytic anaplasmosis (HGA, formerly known as human granulocytic ehrlichiosis), or babesiosis as a single infection or, less frequently, as a coinfection (178). Coinfection should be considered in patients who present with more severe initial symptoms than are commonly observed with Lyme disease alone, especially in those who have unexplained leukopenia, thrombocytopenia, or anemia and high-grade fever for over 48 hours despite receiving antibiotic therapy appropriate for Lyme disease. Coinfection may also be indicated by persistence of systemic viremic symptoms after resolution of erythema migrans. Endemic to coastal New England, babesiosis is an erythrocyte parasitic infection that causes a mild hemolytic disease with fever and perinatal transplacental babesiosis has been reported. On peripheral smears, babesial organisms may be mistaken for malarial parasites. HGA is discussed under "Ehrlichiosis."

Tick-Borne Lymphadenopathy

Tick-borne lymphadenopathy is an infection probably caused by *Rickettsia conorii* and *R. slovaca* and transmitted by the tick *Dermacentor marginatus* (182). The tick bite is usually on the scalp, where a necrotic eschar forms, surrounded by a perilesional erythematous halo. As the name suggests, there is painful regional lymphadenopathy.

OTHER SPIROCHETAL INFECTIONS

Nonvenereal treponematoses (and their causative agents) include yaws (*T. pertenue*), pinta (*T. carateum*), and bejel (*T. endemicum*) (183). They are restricted to the tropics and subtropics, affect children and young adults, and are transmitted by direct personal contact, fomites (bejel), or arthropod vectors (yaws and pinta). Spirochetes multiply at site of primary infection and disseminate to regional lymph nodes. Although bejel and yaws have a systemic spirochetemia with tertiary lesions in bones and joints, unlike syphilis transplacental infection aortic and neurologic involvements do not usually occur. Yaws affects the skin as fissured, verrucous, or oozing lesions; bejel causes mucocutaneous lesions of the mouth and nasopharynx; and pinta occurs as serpiginous plaques on the foot, hand, or arm.

Abramowsky et al. have described a novel nontreponemal spirochetosis eliciting a pronounced lymphoplasmacytic response in fetal intestine, lung, and meninges in second trimester fetuses and associated with chorioamnionitis and villitis. The organism is morphologically distinct from those causing syphilis, leptospirosis, and borreliosis (184).

CLOSTRIDIAL INFECTIONS

Clostridia are ubiquitous, gram-positive, anaerobic, spore-forming bacillus present in the environment, soil, and the gastrointestinal tracts of humans, animals, and insects. Most clostridial syndromes are caused by toxins elaborated by the bacteria and include botulism, tetanus, myonecrosis (gas gangrene), and pseudomembranous colitis. Clostridial toxins are strongly antigenic and can be neutralized by antisera, a fact that is often used in therapy.

Botulism, an acute neuromuscular paralysis, is an acute systemic toxemia, not strictly an infection (185). It is caused by absorption of preformed botulinum toxin produced by *Clostridium botulinum*, usually from the GIT, although the toxin may rarely also be absorbed from infected wounds. The most common sources of food-borne botulism are home-canned fruits, vegetables, fish, honey, corn syrup, and the skin of fresh fruits such as grapes. It presents as a descending paralysis (cranial nerves, limbs, and trunk) about 12 to 36 hours after ingestion of toxin. Infant botulism presents with constipation, difficulty in feeding, weak cry, hypotonia, and drooling, progressing to cranial neuropathy and ventilatory failure. There are no specific morphologic findings. An association with sudden infant death syndrome has been postulated, but the data are inconclusive. Botulism most frequently occurs between 6 weeks and 6 months of age, with the youngest reported patient being 6 days of age. Breast milk may protect against botulism by causing more acid stools and increasing the presence of *Bifidobacterium* species, thereby limiting the intestinal presence of *C. botulinum* or its spores.

Tetanus, caused by the toxin tetanospasmin produced by *C. tetani*, is a major cause of neonatal–infant mortality in many developing countries. Neonatal tetanus follows contamination of the umbilical stump due to poor hygiene and certain traditional practices, especially when mothers are not adequately immunized. Tetanus neonatorum presents as generalized weakness and failure to nurse and progresses to muscular rigidity, spasms, and death in over 90% of affected infants. There are no characteristic morphologic features. Older nonimmunized children can develop tetanus following trauma; often, the colonized wound may be trivial.

Gas gangrene or clostridial myonecrosis caused by clostridial exotoxins (especially lecithinase) follows penetrating or crush injuries contaminated with soil or feces. Infection may also be nontraumatic in patients with reduced resistance to infections, following an insult to the intestines permitting transmucosal migration of intestinal clostridia into the blood. The myonecrosis is characterized by severe tissue damage associated with gas- and fluid-filled bullae in necrotic skeletal muscle and surrounding soft tissues. Inflammation in the gangrenous muscle is scant to absent. *C. perfringens* causes about 80% of these infections, followed by *C. septicum* and other clostridia. Infection progresses very rapidly in the absence of prompt diagnosis and treatment. Higher mortality rates are seen with *C. septicum* infections. Neutrophil dysfunction (e.g., malignancies), bowel ischemia (e.g., hemolytic uremic syndrome), and trauma predispose to *C. septicum* infection in children (186).

Pseudomembranous colitis is a toxin-mediated condition produced by overgrowth of *C. difficile* in the large intestine.

ZOONOSES

Space does not permit discussion of this large group of bacterial diseases that exist largely in domestic and wild animals and are secondarily acquired by humans. Examples include brucellosis, anthrax, tularemia, and plague. Although the clinical and epidemiologic aspects of these conditions may be distinctive in the pediatric age group, their pathologic manifestations do not differ from those in adults. Comprehensive reviews are available (187–190). Anthrax, plague, and tularemia, potential agents of bioterrorism, are discussed in a later section. Brucellosis is briefly outlined below.

Brucellosis

Humans are accidental hosts to brucellosis. We acquire the disease by directly contacting infected animals (cattle, pigs, or sheep) or by ingesting contaminated milk/milk products. *Brucella* species gain entry through skin abrasions, gastrointestinal tract, respiratory tract, or conjunctiva and then localize in the reticuloendothelial system (lymph node, spleen, liver, and bone marrow). After an incubation period of 3 to 4 weeks, the patient has nonspecific symptoms including fever, chills, profuse sweats, body aches, mental inattention, and depression. Pathologic changes in involved organs include nonspecific inflammation, lymphoid hyperplasia, and (non-necrotizing or necrotizing) granulomas. *Brucella* species can be cultured from such specimens as blood or bone marrow. The organism is a potential bioagent for terrorism ("select agent"), and limited laboratory workup should be performed due to the low infectious dose required for infection. A presumptive diagnosis is made by demonstrating rising antibody titers in the serum. Complications include sacroiliitis, osteomyelitis (especially vertebral), neurobrucellosis (meningitis, encephalitis, radiculopathy, myelitis, and peripheral neuropathy), infective endocarditis, and mycotic aneurysms (191).

TUBERCULOSIS

Mycobacterial disease in children is encountered by the pathologist in three clinical forms: pulmonary TB, disseminated HIV-associated *M. avium* infection, and infections with lymphadenopathy caused by atypical mycobacteria (usually *Mycobacterium fortuitum*, *M. scrofulaceum*, or *M. avium-intracellulare*).

An estimated one-third of the world's population (2 billion people) is infected with the tubercle bacillus. The WHO estimates that more than 8 million new cases of TB occur each year, with 3 million persons dying from the disease. Childhood TB, defined as TB in patients less than 15 years of age, accounts for 2% to 40% of all cases (192). The current WHO practice of reporting only acid-fast bacillus (AFB) smear–positive cases underestimates global incidence and prevalence, since 95% of infected children may be AFB smear–negative (193). Difficulties in diagnosis stem from the low yield of mycobacteriologic cultures and the reliance on clinical case definitions (194). The epidemiology of pediatric TB continues to be shaped by risk factors such as age, race, immigration, poverty, overcrowding, and HIV/AIDS because primary disease and its complications are more common in children. The pathogenesis of disease differs from that in adults, leading to differences in clinical and radiographic manifestations in pediatric TB. In some regions, TB accounts for 10% to 15% of all pediatric deaths.

Transmission

Pediatric TB occurs in congenital- and postnatal-acquired forms; congenital TB is rare. Infection of the fetus may be transplacental (50% of cases) or by aspiration or ingestion of infected amniotic fluid (in maternal tuberculous endometritis or villitis). Transplacental infection leads to primary complex formation in the liver or lungs, whereas amniotic infection leads to primary disease in the lungs or gastrointestinal tract (195). Radiologic (CT scan) findings and the time course of the development of lesions may distinguish the two modes of transmission. Perinatal TB is acquired from postnatal transmission from the mother, adult caregiver, health care worker, or other infectious source (e.g., *M. bovis* in cow's milk).

Acquired TB is transmitted by inhalation of infective airborne mucous droplets generated by an infected individual or produced by therapeutic manipulation (aerosol treatments, sputum induction, and through manipulation of lesions). The bacteria may also gain access via the skin, mucous membranes, conjunctiva, or ingestion. The risk of acquiring disease is greatest shortly after the initial infection develops, and it is associated inversely with age, from birth to 8 years of age. For unknown reasons, a second disease peak occurs during late adolescence and early adult life (192). Pediatric patients with TB are usually not infectious. They lack cavities with a large number of bacilli, and the relatively weak cough of young children is not conducive to airborne transmission.

Clinical Features

Congenital TB presents with nonspecific symptoms during the second or third week of life (poor feeding, poor weight gain, cough, lethargy, irritability, fever) and may mimic other congenital infections such as syphilis, CMV, or neonatal sepsis. To make a diagnosis of congenital TB, the infant should have proven lesions, postnatal transmission should be excluded by thorough contact investigation of close contacts including health care workers, and there should be at least one of the following: papular or petechial lesions in the first week of life, documentation of TB infection of the placenta or the maternal genital tract, or a primary complex in the liver (caseating hepatic granulomas) (195). Hepatosplenomegaly, respiratory distress, fever, lymphadenopathy, and abdominal distension are the most common signs and symptoms (196). Most infants have abnormal chest radiographs, usually showing a miliary pattern, hilar and mediastinal lymphadenopathy, or parenchymal infiltrates and, less commonly, multiple rim-enhancing pulmonary nodules with central hypodense areas. Fetal involvement is much less common than placental TB (197). The primary focus may be either in the liver or in the lung, depending on the route of access, and widespread miliary disease ensues. Perinatal TB presents at a later time than congenital TB; however, clinical manifestations may be similar to those of congenital TB.

Clinical features of acquired TB depend on the evolution of disease. In contrast to adults and older adolescents, the clinical manifestations of TB in children are usually related to primary TB. Inhaled bacilli induce a localized pneumonia at a terminal airway (the Ghon focus); with resultant local tuberculous lymphangitis and hilar adenopathy, this forms the primary complex. An occult lymphohematogenous spread may disseminate bacilli to a variety of target organs, where the bacilli may survive for decades. Most children do not develop further disease but instead develop "latent tubercular infection" (LTBI) with a positive tuberculin skin test result and no clinical or radiographic evidence of TB. Others (especially younger children) develop progressive primary TB, In these cases, the primary focus continues to grow even after the development of cellular immunity, and they may caseate centrally, liquefy, and empty into the bronchi resulting in further spread (Figure 6-20). Pleural involvement results from hematogenous spread or direct spread from a subpleural parenchymal or lymph node focus and may present as pleural effusions or tuberculous empyema. Pleural TB is uncommon in children younger than 6 years and extremely rare before 2 years of age. Bloodstream dissemination can cause extrapulmonary disease, including cervical lymphadenopathy (scrofula) and meningitis. Less common forms of extrathoracic disease include osteoarticular, abdominal, GI, genitourinary, and/or cutaneous lesions. Extrapulmonary TB must be considered when evaluating children with a history of persistent fevers. Meningitis develops when caseating lesions in the cerebral cortex invade the meninges and disseminate into the subarachnoid space. Children less than 2 years of age are likely to experience a rapid progression of meningitis to hydrocephalus, seizures, and cerebral edema, whereas older children have a basal meningitis that slowly progresses over weeks (198). A less frequent manifestation of CNS disease, tuberculomas form when caseous foci within the brain enlarge and become encapsulated. Miliary TB occurs when large numbers of bacilli disseminate through the bloodstream and cause simultaneous disease in two or more organs, typically with millet-sized lesions (Figure 6-20A). Miliary disease frequently has an insidious presentation with

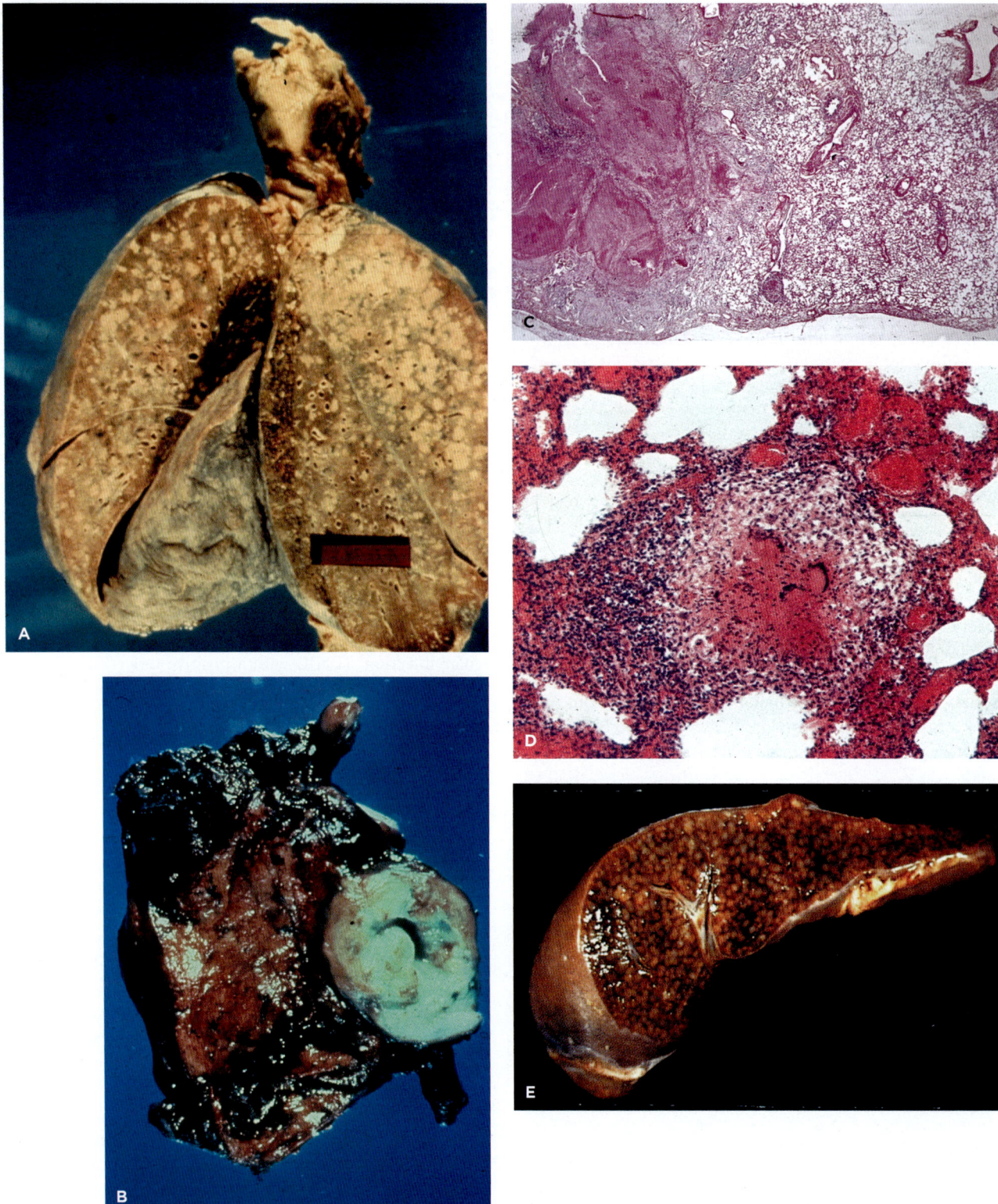

FIGURE 6-20 • Tuberculosis. **A:** Miliary pulmonary disease. **B:** Fibrocaseous cavitary lesion of secondary/progressive tuberculosis. **C:** Caseating granulomas in the lung (low power). **D:** Tuberculous granuloma, lung with central necrosis, and Langhans-type giant cells. **E:** Spleen with military tuberculosis.

fever, lymphadenopathy, and hepatosplenomegaly developing before radiographic abnormalities. As many as 50% of children with military TB have a negative tuberculin skin test at presentation. Extrapulmonary TB occurs in 9% to 23% of pediatric cases (199–201).

Infected children have a comparatively higher risk of progression to active disease than adults: 43% of infants, 24% of 1- to 5-year-olds, and 15% of 11- to 15-year-olds develop disease if not treated for latent TB. In immunocompetent children, the risk of developing clinical TB is highly age dependent; young children have the greatest risk of severe manifestations. After reaching the age of 10 years, children are much more likely to manifest primarily pulmonary adult-type disease. Factors that increase the risk of progression from infection to disease include anergy, immunosuppressive therapy, HIV coinfection, malnutrition, other medical conditions (e.g., renal and liver failure, diabetes mellitus, or cancer), and intercurrent viral infections (e.g. measles). In contrast to adults, children have a relative deficiency of macrophage and dendritic cell function and tend to develop Th2-type T-cell responses to mycobacterial infection characterized by lack of CD8-positive cell response and production of CD4-positive cells, IL-4 and IL-5 (202). Although BCG vaccination may not prevent infection, it reduces the hematogenous complications of primary infection (203) and is reportedly efficacious in preventing tuberculous meningitis.

Pathology

The histopathologic features of TB are similar in children and adults. The classic morphologic feature of TB is the caseating granuloma (Figure 6-20B-E). Immunocompromised children may have lesions that teem with intra- and extracellular acid-fast bacilli, without granuloma formation.

Laboratory Diagnosis

Because children have less specific signs and symptoms of disease, they tend to have paucibacillary disease and fewer positive mycobacterial cultures and have increased risk for progression to disseminated disease, diagnosis can be challenging (194). Microscopy (acid-fast stains, auramine–rhodamine fluorescence) and culture techniques (solid, liquid, radiometric, and nonradiometric systems) still remain the mainstay of diagnosis. Molecular amplification systems (PCR, NASBA, TMA, and LCR) can identify *M. tuberculosis*, nontuberculous mycobacteria, and rifampin (rpoB gene)/isoniazid (katG gene) resistance. Although molecular assays have high sensitivity and specificity in smear-positive sputum, test sensitivity varies in smear-negative sputum and extrapulmonary specimens (204). Unfortunately, congenital and perinatal TB often eludes diagnosis until autopsy. In some series, tuberculous sepsis is the most common clinically unrecognized fatal infection found at autopsy, particularly in anergic children with a negative skin test.

RICKETTSIAL INFECTIONS

Rickettsiae are arthropod-borne intracellular coccobacilli that cause spotted fevers, typhus, and scrub typhus. A related organism, *Coxiella burnetii*, causes Q fever. The clinical and pathologic spectrum of rickettsial disease is discussed thoroughly by Walker et al. (205). Their epidemiologic features are listed in Table 6-14. Rickettsial disease is characterized by fever, headache, and (except for Q fever) rash. The pathologic substrate is inflammation of small blood vessels. Although it is reported from every state, Rocky Mountain spotted fever (RMSF) is endemic in the southeastern and south-central United States and coastal New England.

TABLE 6-14 RICKETTSIAL DISEASES

Disease	Agent	Transmission	Geographic Distribution
Spotted fever group			
Rocky Mountain spotted fever	*R. rickettsii*	Tick bite	Western hemisphere
Rickettsial pox	*R. akari*	Tick bite	USA, Russia, Korea
Boutonneuse fever	*R. conorii*	Tick bite	Mediterranean, Africa, India
Tick typhus	Several	Tick bite	Asia, Australia, central Europe
Typhus group			
Epidemic typhus	*R. prowazekii*	Louse feces	Worldwide
Brill-Zinsser disease	*R. prowazekii*	Recrudescent form of epidemic typhus	Worldwide
Murine typhus	*R. mooseri (R. typin)*	Rat flea feces	Worldwide
Scrub typhus	*R. tsutsugamushi*	Mite bite	Japan, Southeast Asia, Pacific
Q fever	*Coxiella burnetii*	Aerosol	Worldwide
Ehrlichiosis			
Sennetsu fever	*E. sennetsu*	Tick bite	Japan, Malaysia
Monocytic ehrlichiosis	*E. chaffeensis*	Tick bite	United States, Portugal, Mali
Granulocytic ehrlichiosis	Unnamed species	Tick bite	United States: Midwest, northeast

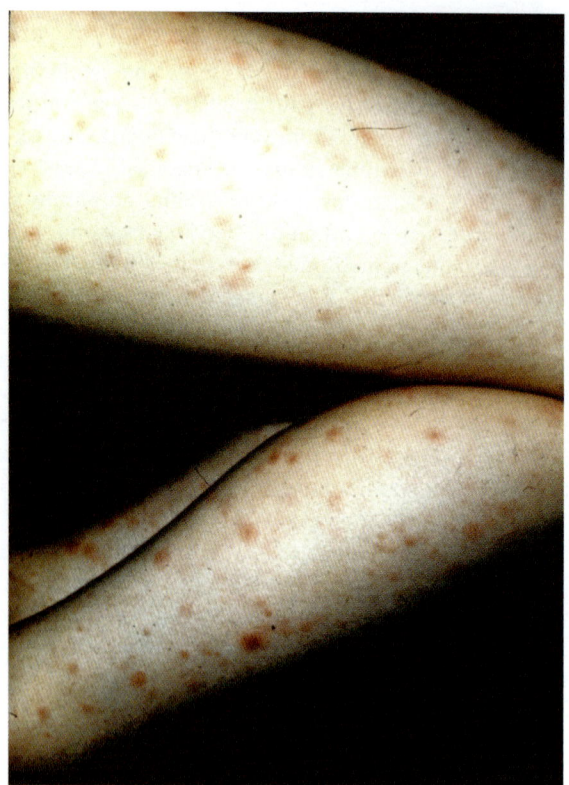

FIGURE 6-21 • Rocky Mountain spotted fever—lesions on the legs.

Rickettsiae enter the blood during a tick bite and penetrate blood vessels. They multiply in endothelial cells and vascular smooth muscle, resulting in a systemic vasculitis, the basis for rash (Figure 6-21), interstitial pneumonia, myocarditis, hepatic portal triaditis, meningoencephalomyelitis, and interstitial nephritis. Leakage of fluid from the injured vessels leads to edema and hypovolemia, and vascular necrosis and inflammation initiate consumption coagulopathy. The vasculitis of RMSF involves capillaries, venules, and arterioles; the cellular inflammatory reaction comprised of mainly macrophages and lymphocytes, with few polymorphonuclear leukocytes. Eccentric microthrombosis and microinfarction frequently result. Rickettsial organisms are visible, albeit very small (<2 μm), and may be demonstrated with difficulty using Giemsa or immunostains. Diagnosis, however, is serologically accomplished by the Weil-Felix test or by specific complement fixation. PCR-based methods are also available.

Ehrlichiosis

Ehrlichiae are small pleomorphic coccobacilli in the family Anaplasmataceae. They are tick-borne obligate intracellular parasites currently grouped with the rickettsiae. Human ehrlichiosis is reportable and is on the rise. Ehrlichiae infect macrophages, monocytes, and neutrophils. The three species causing infections include *E. chaffeensis*, causing human monocytic ehrlichiosis (HME); *A. phagocytophilum*, causing human granulocytic ehrlichiosis (HGA); and *Ehrlichiosis ewingii*, causing human ewingii ehrlichiosis (206). Patients present with fever and myalgias, with or without rash and other systemic manifestations. Lab findings include leukopenia, thrombocytopenia, and elevated transaminases. Although uncommon, complications include meningitis, pneumonitis, renal failure, and septic shock. Ehrlichiosis is diagnosed by blood smear examination or PCR in the first week of infection and by serology beyond 2 weeks (206). Cultures are available in specialized centers. A high index of suspicion is required for diagnosis, especially in tick-endemic regions. The peripheral blood contains intracytoplasmic morulae. The bone marrow is usually panhypercellular, with increased histiocytes, granulomas, ring granulomas, erythrophagocytosis, plasmacytosis, and lymphoid aggregates. The liver contains sinusoidal and portal lymphohistiocytic infiltrates and hepatocyte necrosis, and the spleen shows focal necrosis on a background of mild histiocytosis. Interstitial pneumonitis and pulmonary hemorrhage have also been reported. Other organs may show nonspecific perivascular lymphohistiocytic infiltrates. Immunohistochemical stains are available for diagnosis. Most of the literature pertains to adult infections, and the incidence and the natural course in children are unclear (207).

HGA, as the name suggests, is a rickettsial infection of neutrophils, rarely seen in children. Clinical manifestations are nonspecific and may include fever, chills, headache, and myalgias. The incubation period is 5 to 21 days. In most cases, HGA is a mild, self-limited illness, even without antibiotic therapy. However, serious manifestations, including fatal outcome, have been reported in immunocompromised patients. Chronic infection due to *A. phagocytophilum* has not been described in humans. Laboratory features may include leukopenia, lymphopenia, thrombocytopenia, and mild elevation of liver enzyme levels. HGA can be detected in blood samples by smear examination, PCR, or HL60 cell culture. Identification of characteristic intragranulocytic inclusions on blood smear is the most rapid diagnostic method, but such inclusions are often scant in number or sometimes absent. Overlying platelets or other types of inclusions unrelated to HGA can be misinterpreted by inexperienced observers. The most sensitive diagnostic method is paired (acute-phase and convalescent-phase) serologic testing using an indirect fluorescent antibody assay; acute-phase testing alone is not sufficiently sensitive. Serologic testing is often the only way to diagnose a patient who has already begun to receive antibiotic treatment. Perinatal transmission from mother to child, possibly transplacental, has been reported.

MYCOPLASMA INFECTIONS

Mycoplasma and *Ureaplasma* are the smallest free living microorganisms, lacking cell wall peptidoglycans. *Mycoplasma hominis* and *Ureaplasma urealyticum* are frequent inhabitants of the maternal genital tract. They are associated with placental and perinatal pathology including chorioamnionitis (208), funisitis (209), diffuse decidual leukocytoclastic necrosis (210), fetal vasculitis (211), fetal demise, prematurity (210), premature rupture of membranes, cerebral white

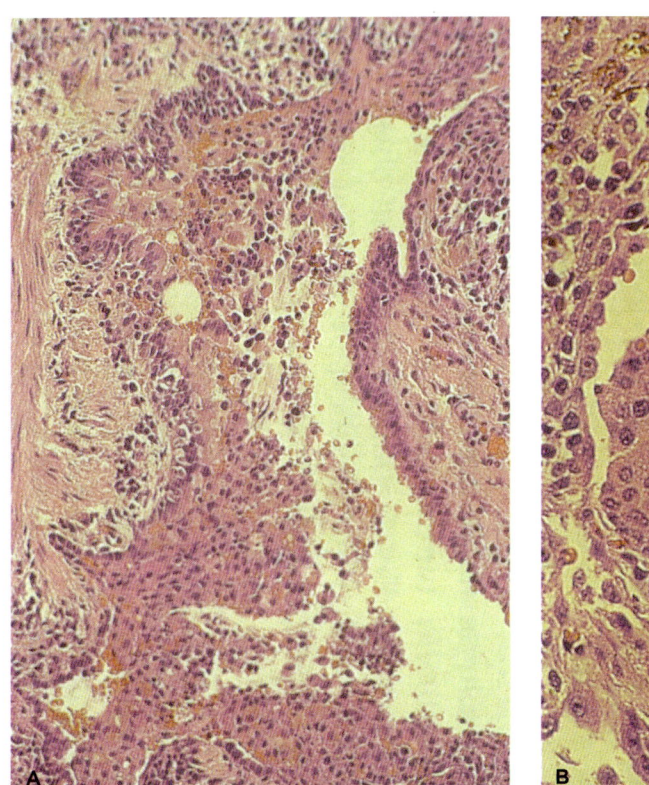 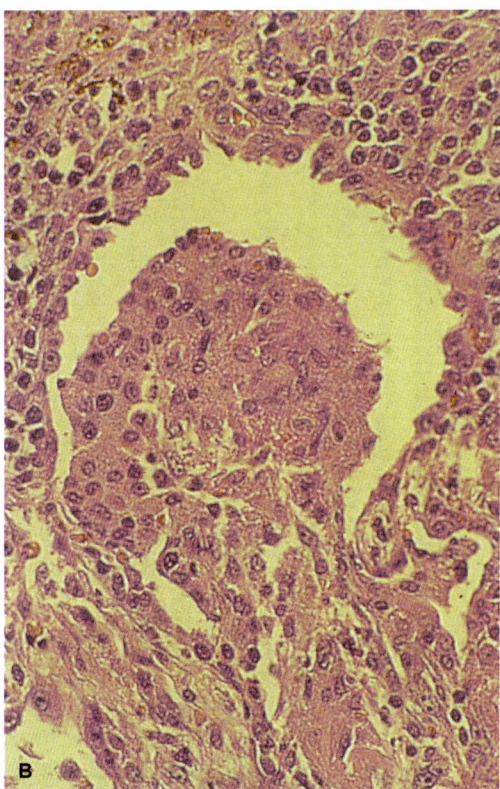

FIGURE 6-22 • Mycoplasma pneumonia. **A:** Inflamed bronchiole with epithelial hyperplasia and surface necrosis. **B:** Partial occlusion of bronchiole.

matter echolucency (211), and chronic lung disease of the newborn (212). However, because both these organisms may be recovered from perfectly normal infants, establishing a causal relationship to disease may be difficult and requires vigorous exclusion of other pathogens. Histopathology of infected tissues varies from no pathologic changes to necrosis, with or without an associated inflammatory reaction.

While the most typical syndrome is tracheobronchitis, pneumonia may be the most severe type of *Mycoplasma pneumoniae* infection in older children (213). The pneumonia is insidious in onset. Chest radiographs show bronchopneumonia (often involving a single lower lobe), plate-like atelectasis, nodular infiltration, and hilar adenopathy. As many as 25% of persons infected with *M. pneumoniae* experience extrapulmonary complications at variable time periods or even in the absence of respiratory illness (214–216). Extrapulmonary pathology may be due to infection of other organs and/or host immune response to infection. These include neurologic (meningoencephalitis, encephalomyelitis, aseptic meningitis, cerebellar ataxia, isolated abducens palsy, ocular myasthenia, syndromatic inappropriate antidiuretic hormone (SIADH), transverse myelopathy, and Guillain-Barré syndrome) (217), dermatologic (maculopapular eruptions, erythema nodosum, erythema multiforme, and Stevens-Johnson syndrome), musculoskeletal (myalgias, arthritis, and rhabdomyolysis), gastrointestinal (diarrhea, pancreatitis, cholestatic hepatitis), hematologic (hemolysis, DIC, thrombocytopenia, thrombocytosis) (218), cardiovascular (vasculitis, pericarditis, and myocarditis), renal (glomerulonephritis, renal failure, interstitial nephritis, and IgA nephropathy) (214), and lower genital tract (219) manifestations. Histopathologic findings include bronchial epithelial ulceration with peribronchial and interstitial inflammation (Figure 6-22). Bronchiolitis obliterans, type II pneumocyte hyperplasia, diffuse alveolar damage, lung abscess, and fibrinous pleuritis have also been reported, as have long-term sequelae including pleural scarring, bronchiectasis, and pulmonary fibrosis. Active lymphocytic myocarditis may occur. The infection is routinely diagnosed by serologic methods, although PCR and culture-based techniques are also available. Serology is more likely to be positive in children with pneumonia rather than upper respiratory tract infection or bronchitis (218).

CHLAMYDIAL INFECTIONS

Chlamydiae are obligate intracellular pathogens; *Chlamydia trachomatis* and *C. pneumoniae* are important human pathogens, while *C. psittaci* is an important cause of zoonosis. Chlamydial infections in children have been comprehensively reviewed (220,221). *C. psittaci* and *C. trachomatis*, consisting of many subtypes, cause several distinct conditions in children (Table 6-15).

Chlamydia pneumoniae infects children of all ages. It is a common human respiratory pathogen with asymptomatic nasopharyngeal carriage occurring in up to 5% of the

TABLE 6-15	CHLAMYDIAL DISEASE IN CHILDHOOD		
Organism	Disease	Pathologic Features	Transmission
C. psittaci	Ornithosis (Psittacosis)	Interstitial lobular or lobar pneumonia	Aerosol from infected birds
C. trachomatis			
Types A, B, C	Trachoma	Chronic progressive conjunctivitis with scarring leading to blindness. Cytoplasmic inclusions in early stage	Contact
Types D-M	Inclusion conjunctivitis	Acute follicular conjunctivitis with cytoplasmic inclusions	Contact
	Nongonococcal urethritis, proctitis, salpingitis, cervicitis	Nonspecific, but prominent plasma cells and lymphoid nodules	Venereal; rare in prepubertal children and suggest sexual abuse
	Neonatal pneumonia and conjunctivitis	Interstitial pneumonitis with rare inclusions	Transit through birth canal
Types L_1, L_2, L_3	Lymphogranuloma venereum	Cutaneous ulcer, granulomatous lymphadenitis with stellate abscesses	Venereal

population. The nasopharynx is probably the most frequent site of perinatally acquired chlamydial infection, with approximately 70% of infected infants having positive cultures at that site. Most infections are asymptomatic and may persist for over 2 years. The clinical presentation ranges from mild atypical pneumonia similar to Mycoplasma infection to severe disease. The role of *Chlamydia* in upper respiratory, sinus, and middle ear infections is unclear. Infants with chlamydial pneumonia will usually be symptomatic before the 8th week of life, with the insidious development of nasal obstruction and/or discharge, tachypnea, and a repetitive, staccato cough. In very young infants, infection may be more severe and be associated with apnea. Possible laboratory findings include a distinctive peripheral eosinophilia, mild arterial hypoxemia, and elevated serum immunoglobulins. Untreated disease can linger or recur. Pulmonary disease takes the form of an interstitial pneumonitis or rarely necrotizing bronchiolitis and consolidation. Because the pneumonia is rarely fatal, pathologic descriptions are few, and no characteristic features have been described. Definitive diagnosis is by cell culture, but this technique is labor-intensive and requires special media for collection and transportation. Although serology is commonly used for diagnosis, infection may occur without seroconversion (222). PCR methods also allow for definitive diagnosis.

Chlamydia trachomatis infection is arguably the most prevalent sexually transmitted infection in the United States, with prevalence rates exceeding 10% among sexually active adolescents. Infection tends to be asymptomatic and of long duration. The rectum and vagina may also be infected at birth, but in older children, organisms in these sites may indicate sexual abuse. If a pregnant woman has active infection, the infant may acquire the infection during vaginal delivery and develop inclusion body conjunctivitis or pneumonitis. All pregnant women should be tested during their first prenatal visit and again during the third trimester if they are at high risk (25 years of age or other risk factors such as new or multiple sexual partners). The evidence linking *C. trachomatis* to premature delivery and fetal loss is inconclusive. Transmission of the organism in nurseries or neonatal intensive care units has not been reported, so that there is no indication that infants with chlamydial infections should be isolated.

During vaginal delivery, up to 50% of infants exposed to chlamydiae develop conjunctivitis (221). The incubation period for chlamydial conjunctivitis is 5 to 14 days after delivery or earlier if membranes have prematurely ruptured. The severity ranges from mild injection to purulent discharge with pseudomembrane formation. Clinical differentiation from gonococcal ophthalmia may be difficult. Inclusion conjunctivitis is characterized by clearly defined cytoplasmic microcolonies or inclusions in conjunctival epithelial cells. These contain large amounts of glycogen that is readily demonstrated with iodine or PAS stains. Regardless of treatment, the conjunctivitis mostly resolves spontaneously during the first few months. However, inflammation persists in occasional infants, who develop a micropannus (neovascularization of the cornea) and scarring trachoma. Approximately 70% of infants with perinatal chlamydial infection develop asymptomatic nasopharyngeal infection; about 30% of these develop pneumonia (221). The latter present between 4 and 12 weeks of age with cough and tachypnea, but no fever. Radiographs do not show any consolidation. Laboratory tests reveal eosinophilia and elevated immunoglobulin levels. As in adults, infected adolescents may develop urethritis, epididymitis, bartholinitis, endometritis, subclinical salpingitis, and perihepatitis (Fitz-Hugh-Curtis syndrome).

Except for inclusion body conjunctivitis, early trachoma, and neonatal inclusion body pneumonia, the clinical and pathologic features of chlamydial infections are not specific. Although cell culture techniques are the gold standard for laboratory diagnosis, enzyme immunoassays, direct fluorescent antibody assays, nucleic acid amplification tests, and microimmunofluorescence serology are more commonly used. However, nonculture techniques may yield false-positive results (221,222).

ACTINOMYCOTIC INFECTIONS

Actinomycosis is a chronic suppurative inflammatory process caused primarily by *Actinomyces* species, particularly *Actinomyces israelii*, usually acting in concert with other bacteria. The organism is a part of the normal flora of the mouth. In the absence of underlying risk factors, actinomycosis is rare in children (223). The cervicofacial form of the disease is more likely to be encountered than abdominal and thoracopulmonary disease, and it may be seen following trauma, surgery, or even tooth extraction (especially in a setting of caries). Diagnosis requires a high degree of suspicion. In all locations, the lesion is an indolent, burrowing suppurative process with large aggregates of organisms forming "sulfur granules" with distinctive peripheral clubbing. The organism is rather pleomorphic, and diagnosis should ideally be confirmed by culture. Colonization of the tonsillar crypts is a common event, but it typically occurs with bilateral enlargement and obstructive sleep apnea, rather that true infection.

Nocardiosis is mostly caused by two branching gram-positive coccobacilli species, *Nocardia asteroides* and *N. brasiliensis*. Both obligate aerobes are weakly acid fast, which helps to distinguish them from *Actinomyces* species. They are soil inhabitants that mostly act as opportunistic pathogens. Primary infection takes many forms including pulmonary abscesses (often multiple and coalescent), pneumonia, or coin lesions. Extrapulmonary spread occurs most often to brain and kidney. In any location, the histologic hallmark is liquefaction necrosis and suppuration. The organisms, although small, are readily identifiable on Gram, acid fast, or silver methenamine stains. In the absence of immunosuppression, nocardiosis is unusual in children.

FUNGAL INFECTIONS

Of *in utero* fungal infections, only candidiasis occurs with any frequency. *Candida glabrata* and *Aspergillus* have been shown to reach the fetus by the ascending transcervical route, while *Coccidioides* spreads by a hematogenous route (18).

Candidiasis ascends from the maternal genital tract and causes chorioamnionitis, from where it can gain access to the fetal skin and upper respiratory and intestinal tracts. Thus, it causes a generalized cutaneous rash, aspiration pneumonia (Figure 6-23), and intestinal mucositis (224). Affected infants are frequently growth restricted, and many are stillborn or abortuses. In recent years, candidiasis has been recognized as a complication of the intensive care of low-birth-weight infants. Risk factors include parenteral nutrition, central arterial or venous catheters, and a history of broad-spectrum antibiotic therapy. These infants are older than the true congenital cases and tend to have more visceral dissemination with nephritis, carditis, endophthalmitis, arthritis, osteomyelitis, and meningitis. Large aggregates of pseudohyphae may form endocardial vegetations and urinary tract fungus balls. The lesions grossly resemble the miliary abscesses of listeriosis on occasion and may be confused with HSV. The cellular reaction to candidiasis is suppurative and budding yeast and pseudohyphae are easily demonstrated in the lesions with routine PAS, methenamine silver, or even Gram stains. *C. glabrata* is an occasional cause of neonatal sepsis in premature infants. *Candida* infections in later childhood range from relatively mundane cutaneous and mucous membrane infections (diaper rash, thrush, glossitis) to fatal septicemic illness with widespread miliary abscesses (225), particularly in immunocompromised children. Chronic mucocutaneous candidiasis is a particular form of cellular immunodeficiency with defective T-cell response to *Candida* antigens. In the immunodeficient or multiple antibiotic-treated patients, *Candida* organisms enter through intestinal or respiratory tract mucosa, producing local ulceration, necrosis, and hematogenous spread. The usual suppurative reaction may be blunted in the leukopenic host. The usual tissue form of candidiasis is a small unencapsulated budding yeast with occasional blastospores having elongated germ tubes. Confusion with *Aspergillus* arises when serially budding organisms are attached end to end to form pseudohyphae. A slight "pinching in" of *Candida*, resembling sausage links at the site of attachment, is a helpful diagnostic feature. *C. glabrata* does not form pseudohyphae. Further confusion

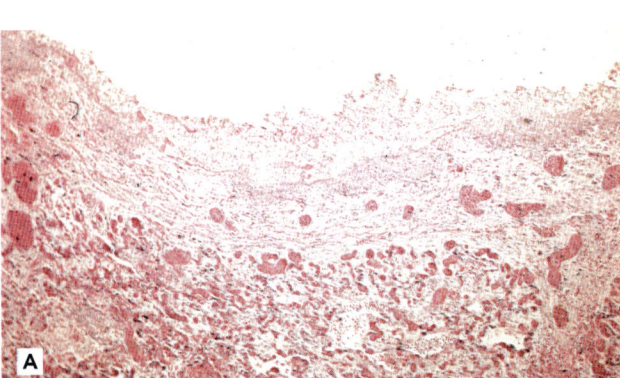
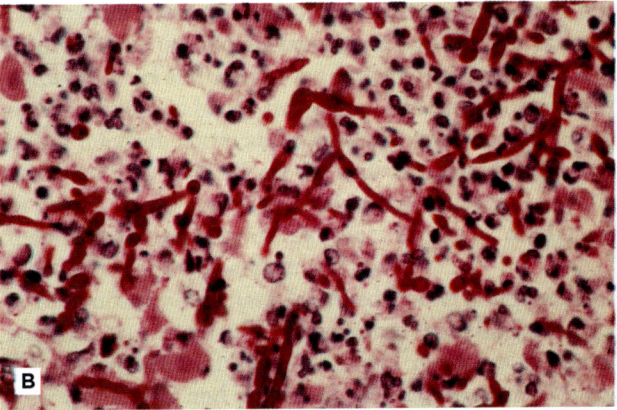

FIGURE 6-23 • **A:** Candidal pleuritis. **B:** Candidal pneumonia with yeast and pseudohyphal phase organisms (PAS stain).

with *Aspergillus* arises when masses of pseudohyphae cause vascular occlusion, thrombosis, and infarction.

Other fungi are occasionally encountered in the neonatal age group, chiefly as complications of intensive measures in seriously compromised infants. *Malassezia furfur* colonization and sepsis in neonates are related to indwelling Broviac catheters and long-term parenteral alimentation using lipid emulsion. It is a lipophilic yeast that localizes in pulmonary vessels, the site of parenteral lipid deposits administration. The organism is a tiny (2- to 4-µm) budding yeast with a distinctive "heel and sole" outline well seen on silver stains. Rare cases of gastrointestinal zygomycosis clinically mimic necrotizing enterocolitis and show diffuse invasion of bowel wall, with necrosis and fungal invasion of vessels.

Fungal diseases of older infants and children fall into two categories: the endemic mycoses, characterized by sharply defined geographic boundaries and occurrence in normal (nonimmunosuppressed) hosts, and the opportunistic mycoses, ubiquitous in the environment but not ordinarily causing disease in healthy persons (225).

In North America, the endemic mycoses include blastomycosis, endemic in the eastern states, histoplasmosis in the Mississippi and Ohio River valleys, and coccidioidomycosis in the southwest. They have several features in common:

1. The organisms are dimorphic fungi; with rare exception, the yeast form is the one seen in tissue.
2. All three are primarily pulmonary diseases with clinical and morphologic features similar to TB.
3. Disseminated disease is the exception and tends to occur in very young children or immunocompromised patients.
4. All evoke a host response that is primarily granulomatous or mixed granulomatous and suppurative.
5. All are likely to be misdiagnosed, especially when encountered outside of their usual locale or clinical setting.

Blastomycosis in children ranges from asymptomatic to disseminated forms and is a rare cause of osteomyelitis. Most symptomatic disease consists of pneumonic infiltration or consolidation with or without cavitation (226). Microscopically, there is a mixed granulomatous and suppurative reaction. *Blastomyces dermatitidis* is a large, thick-walled yeast easily visible in sections or smears. Characteristic broad-based budding is a distinguishing feature of this mold. Delayed diagnosis may result in dissemination even in immunocompetent hosts.

Histoplasmosis is asymptomatic in the majority of infected children. Acute pulmonary or disseminated disease may be seen in young infants or immunocompromised children (227). Dissemination occurs in pediatric HIV-infected patients. In the lung, histoplasmosis provokes a caseating, granulomatous reaction indistinguishable from TB; likewise, organisms may be very few (Figure 6-24). In the disseminated form of histoplasmosis, the organisms are found within macrophages, particularly in the reticuloendothelial system. Sclerosing mediastinitis is a rare manifestation. In endemic areas, histoplasmosis is a common cause of hepatic granulomas. *Histoplasma capsulatum* is a tiny, budding yeast best demonstrated with silver stains. An immunoperoxidase method has been described, and PCR techniques are useful in archival tissues.

Coccidioides immitis is a soil inhabitant that causes self-limited, often asymptomatic pulmonary disease in well children. Dissemination is unusual and seems to occur in the very young or immunocompromised. The pulmonary disease shows many clinical and morphologic similarities to histoplasmosis, but *C. immitis* exists in tissues as large double-walled spherules (sporangia), 20 to 100 m in diameter, containing myriads of tiny endospores that are released by rupture of the spherule (Figure 6-25).

The main opportunists are four fungi: two yeasts (*Candida* and *Cryptococcus*) and two mycelial forms (*Aspergillus* and Zygomycetes). They all have an ability to cause invasive and life-threatening infections in immunosuppressed or patients on antibiotic therapy.

Cryptococcus neoformans infection is rarely encountered in immunocompetent children. Meningitis, pneumonia,

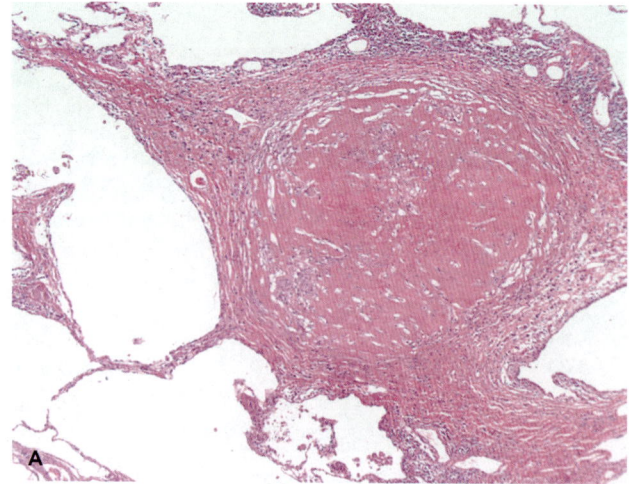
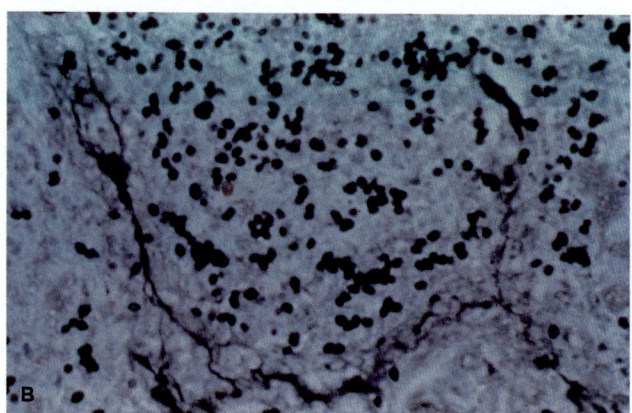

FIGURE 6-24 • **A:** Histoplasma nodule, lung. **B:** Organisms highlighted by a GMS stain.

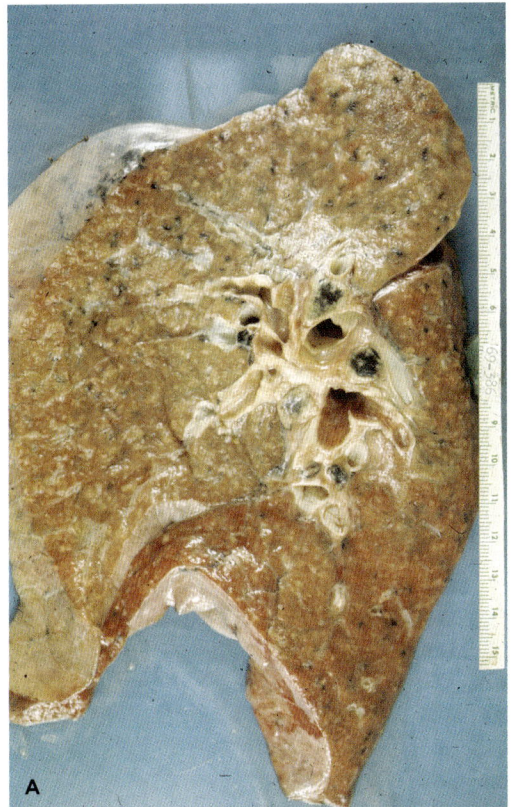
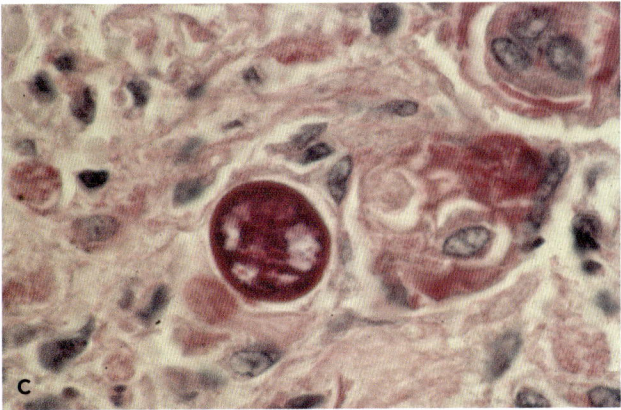
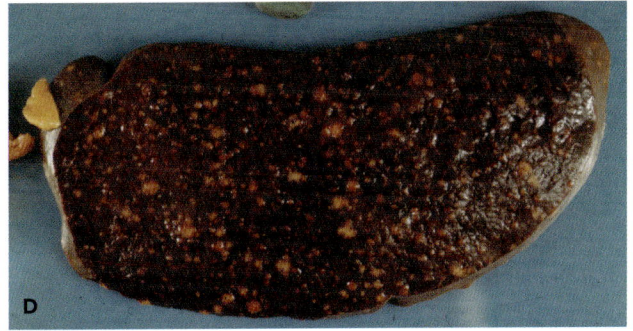
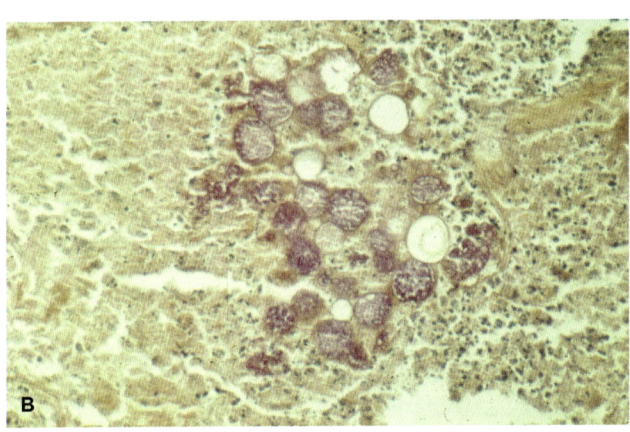

FIGURE 6-25 • Coccidioidomycosis. **A:** Cross-section of lung with disseminated disease. **B:** Focal necrosis in the lung with the thick capsules of the sporangia staining red. **C:** Endospores in large sporangium. **D:** Spleen in a case of disseminated infection.

cutaneous lesions, and disseminated disease have been reported, usually in the immunocompromised host (particularly secondary to HIV). Two forms of inflammatory reaction are recognized: granulomatous inflammation and a gelatinous mass. The latter is composed of large numbers of organisms almost devoid of cellular reaction. The organism is a multiple budding yeast with a thick mucoid capsule that typically appears as a clear space; however, some strains have a thin capsule. The capsule may be visualized with mucicarmine stain and sometimes shows radial striations.

Aspergillosis is caused by several species, *Aspergillus fumigatus* being the most common. Four types of disease occur in children: hypersensitivity pneumonitis, saprophytic colonization of pre-existing pulmonary cavities ("aspergilloma"), invasive pulmonary aspergillosis, and disseminated aspergillosis (225). Invasive pulmonary and disseminated aspergilloses occur almost exclusively in immunocompromised children. Aspergillosis is presumptively diagnosed in tissues by identifying dichotomously branching septate hyphae uniformly 7 to 8 microns in diameter. However, rare opportunistic fungi (e.g., *Fusarium, Pseudallescheria*, pheohypomycosis, and others) share these features. Partially treated or long-standing lesions may show broader septae, morphologically overlapping with Zygomycetes. Only the fruiting heads, comprised of vesicles with phialides and *conidia,* are absolutely diagnostic, but these only occur in aerated tissues. Radial or sunburst arrangement and a wavelike configuration are characteristic. The inflammatory reaction is suppurative and necrotizing. *Aspergillus* shares with Zygomycetes (and to a lesser extent, *Candida*), a propensity for vascular invasion leading to infarction. *Aspergillus* is present in the sputum in a minority of patients, and the diagnosis is frequently established by lung biopsy; areas of infarction and necrosis distal to a fungal thrombus may not contain demonstrable fungi.

Zygomycosis (or mucormycosis) is caused by several fungi (*Rhizopus* species, *Mucor* species, and *Absidia* species). All are indistinguishable from each other in tissues. These organisms are opportunists and are rarely, if ever, seen in normal children. Rhinocerebral and endobronchial zygomycosis occur almost invariably in diabetic children. Pulmonary, gastrointestinal, and disseminated diseases are seen in children with malignancy. The typical pattern of tissue involvement includes granulomatous or suppurative inflammation, vascular invasion and thrombosis, and infarction. These fungi show coenocytic hyphae of rather variable diameter (5 to 20 μm) that branch at right angles. Folds and wrinkles may mimic septation.

Although histopathology is a major diagnostic tool in diagnosing fungal infections, diagnostic errors may result from morphologic mimics, use of inappropriate terminology, and incomplete knowledge of mycology (228). Template diagnosis formats have been suggested to minimize errors; further species identification requires microbiology cultures or molecular techniques.

PARASITIC DISEASES

Common protozoal and helminthic diseases are listed in Tables 6-16 and 6-17. Although parasitic infections have become more frequent even in the developed world, space does not permit a detailed review of each entity. Many of these organisms cause disease more or less confined to one organ system, and these are discussed in the appropriate sections. Valuable sources for further details include *Pathology of Infectious Diseases* by Connor et al. (2), *Atlas of Human Parasitology* by Ash and Orihel (229), and Feigin and Cherry's encyclopedic *Textbook of Pediatric Infectious Diseases* (1). Protozoal infections of the fetus and neonate will be briefly discussed below.

TOXOPLASMOSIS

Toxoplasma gondii is a protozoan of the family Coccidia. The organism is a parasite of worldwide distribution; its definitive host is the cat. Clinical, epidemiologic, and pathologic features are the subject of excellent reviews (230,231). Congenital toxoplasmosis, with very rare exceptions, occurs

TABLE 6-16 PROTOZOAL INFECTIONS

Category	Organism	Disease	Transmission
Intestinal protozoa			
Amebae	*Entamoeba histolytica*	Amebiasis, liver abscess	Fecal-oral
Flagellates	*Giardia lamblia*	Giardiasis	Fecal-oral
Ciliates	*Balantidium coli*	Ciliary dysentery	Fecal-oral
Coccidia	*Cryptosporidium*	Gastroenteritis	Meat, fecal-oral
Extraintestinal protozoa			
Amebae	*Naegleria fowleri*	Meningoencephalitis	Warm water
	Acanthamoeba culbertsoni	Meningoencephalitis	Warm water
Flagellates	*Trichomonas vaginalis*	Genitourinary infections	Venereal
Coccidia	*Toxoplasma gondii*	Mononucleosis-like syndrome, lymphadenitis, disseminated	Infected meat oocysts in soil, sand, cat litter
Sporozoa	*Pneumocystis jiroveci*	Pneumonia, rarely disseminated	Droplet
Blood-borne protozoa			
Sporozoa	*Plasmodium vivax*	Malaria	Arthropod born (mosquito)
	P. ovale	Malaria	Mosquito
	P. malariae	Malaria	Mosquito
	P. falciparum	Malaria	Mosquito
	Babesia microti	Babesiosis	Tick bite
Flagellates	*Leishmania tropica*	Cutaneous leishmaniasis	Arthropod borne (sand flies)
	L. mexicana	Cutaneous leishmaniasis	Sand flies
	L. braziliensis	Mucocutaneous leishmaniasis	Sand flies
	L. donovani	Visceral leishmaniasis (kala-azar)	Sand flies
	Trypanosoma cruzi	Chagas disease	Triatomine (reduviid) bugs
	T. gambiense	African sleeping sickness	Tsetse flies (360)
	T. rhodesiense	African sleeping sickness	Tsetse flies

TABLE 6-17 HELMINTHIC DISEASES

Category	Organisms	Disease	Transmission
Nematodes			
Intestinal	Ascaris lumbricoides	Ascariasis	Egg ingestion
	Enterobius vermicularis	Pinworm	Egg ingestion
	Ancylostoma duodenale	Old world hookworm	Skin penetration
	Necator americanus	New world hookworm	Skin penetration
	Strongyloides stercoralis	Intestinal and disseminated strongyloidiasis	Skin penetration
	Trichuris trichiura	Whip worm	Egg ingestion
Tissue	Trichinella spiralis	Trichinosis	Ingestion of larvae
	Toxocara canis, T. cati	Visceral larva migrans	Egg ingestion
	Ancylostoma braziliense A. caninum	Cutaneous larva migrans	Skin penetration
Filarial worms	Wuchereria bancrofti	Lymphangitis, elephantiasis	Mosquitos
	Brugia malayi	Lymphangitis, elephantiasis	Mosquitos
	Loa loa	Subcutaneous nodules, conjunctivitis	Chrysops flies
	Onchocerca volvulus	River blindness, subcutaneous nodules, dermatitis	Black flies
	Dirofilaria immitis	Pulmonary disease (coin lesions)	Mosquitos
Cestodes			
Intestinal	Diphyllobothrium latum	Fish tapeworms	Ingestion of raw fish
	Hymenolepis nana	Dwarf tapeworms	Fecal-oral egg ingestion
	Taenia solium	Pork tapeworm	Ingestion of rare pork
	Taenia saginata	Beef tapeworm	Ingestion of rare beef
Larval	Taenia solium	Cysticercosis	Fecal-oral
	Echinococcus	Hydatid disease	Egg ingestion
	Diphyllobothrium sp.	Sparganosis	Copepod ingestion
Trematodes			
Intestinal	Fasciolopsis buski	Giant intestinal fluke	Larva ingestion (aquatic plants)
Liver and lung	Opisthorchis sinensis	Oriental liver fluke	Ingestion of raw or undercooked fish
	Fasciola hepatica	Sheep liver fluke	Larva ingestion (aquatic plants)
	Paragonimus westermani	Lung fluke	Larva ingestion (undercooked crabs and crayfish)
Blood	Schistosoma mansoni	Schistosomiasis (intestinal)	Skin penetration
	S. haematobium	Schistosomiasis (urinary tract)	Skin penetration
	S. japonicum	Schistosomiasis (intestinal)	Skin penetration

only with primary maternal infection. The exact route of transmission to the fetus is unknown, but clearly, the placenta is involved. About 5 per 1000 nonimmune pregnant women may acquire toxoplasma infection, with a 10% to 100% risk of transmission to the baby, with more efficient transmission later in pregnancy. However, the risk of infection causing harm to the fetus is greater in early pregnancy. Prenatal diagnosis is now feasible, and maternal therapy during gestation appears to lessen the ill effects on the fetus (232). Among congenital infections, there is a wide spectrum of severity; most are asymptomatic, but 10% to 12% have severe morbidity, and a few infants die. The characteristic clinical picture consists of fever, hydrocephalus or microcephaly, hepatosplenomegaly, jaundice, chorioretinitis, seizures, cerebral calcifications, and CSF pleocytosis. Newborns that die from toxoplasmosis generally have disseminated disease, even when clinical signs are confined to brain and eyes. Organisms may be identified in brain, eye, middle ear, blood vessels, heart, testes, adrenal, lung, kidney, muscle, and, occasionally, liver, spleen, and lymph nodes (Figure 6-26). The organisms appear in tissues both encysted and free. The cysts are round or oval bodies 10 to 30 m in diameter with a thick wall that is certainly visible on hematoxylin and eosin sections but better demonstrated with PAS, silver, or immunoperoxidase stains. Within the cyst are densely packed tiny trophozoites, 2 µm in diameter. The intact cysts are either intracellular or extracellular and rarely excite an inflammatory response. They rupture to liberate free trophozoites into the tissues. The host reaction is quite heterogenous and depends somewhat on the stage of disease. Acute lesions are characterized

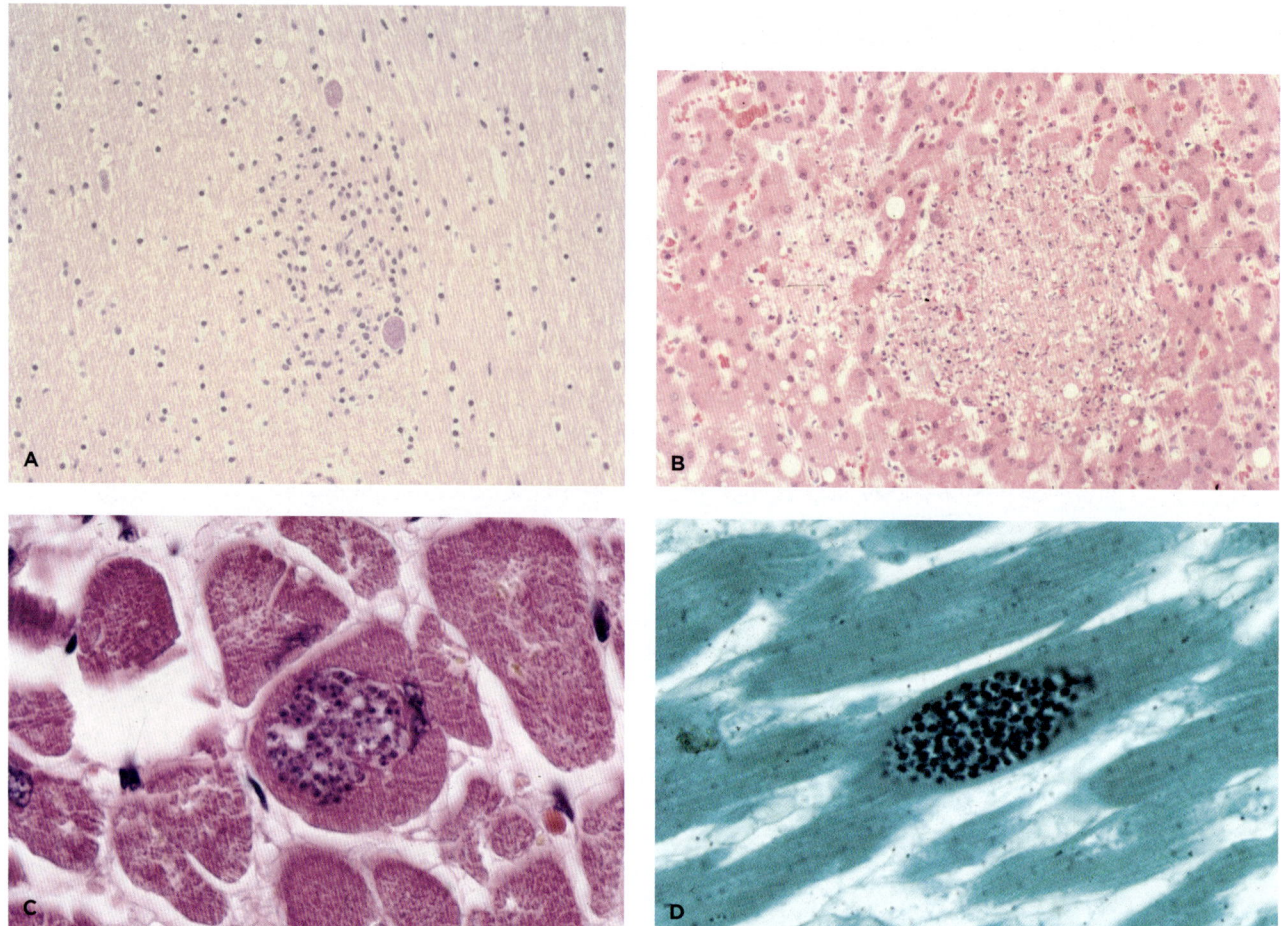

FIGURE 6-26 • Toxoplasmosis. **A:** Brain with microglial nodule and encysted organisms. **B:** Toxoplasmosis involving the liver with a granuloma-like lesion. **C:** Myocarditis with cyst forms within the muscle cells. **D:** Organisms highlighted by GMS stain.

by suppurative reaction, some eosinophilic infiltrates, and liquefactive necrosis, which may be extensive and confluent in the brain. Dystrophic calcification is most conspicuous in the brain. Trophozoites are numerous in these lesions. At a later stage, suppuration gives way to a nonnecrotizing, granulomatous disease. Cysts are less common but are more frequently encountered in and around granulomas. Healing stages are highly variable in morphology, with granulation tissue, gliosis, and fibrosis. Encysted organisms may persist in many tissues.

OTHER PROTOZOAL INFECTIONS

In endemic areas, malaria and trypanosomiasis constitute a threat to the fetus during episodes of maternal parasitemia. Congenital malaria, however, appears to be relatively rare; any *Plasmodium* species may be encountered. Affected infants develop fever, irritability, jaundice, and hepatosplenomegaly; the disease is usually not suspected, and the diagnosis is almost invariably made by peripheral blood smear. Most reported fetal deaths due to malaria are associated with maternal falciparum malaria. It is not clear whether maternal anemia or fetal infection plays the more important role in fetal demise, but parasites and malarial pigment may be identified in affected fetuses.

In Central and South America and Mexico, congenital Chagas disease results from transplacental spread of *Trypanosoma cruzi* to the fetus (233). In endemic areas, *T. cruzi* is a major cause of abortion and prematurity. Approximately 1% to 10% of pregnancies in women with chronic *T. cruzi* infection result in infants born with congenital infection (234). Most infected newborns are asymptomatic or have nonspecific findings such as low birth weight, prematurity, or low Apgar scores. Other signs include hepatosplenomegaly, anemia, and thrombocytopenia. When the disease follows an acute form in the neonate, organisms are found in many organs. The acute lesions are mixed granulomatous and suppurative. Amastigotes of *T. cruzi* are found within histiocytes and are indistinguishable from those of *Leishmania* species. Meningoencephalitis, myocarditis, and respiratory distress have a high association with mortality (234).

Entamoeba histolytica is an important cause of morbidity in developing countries and causes amoebic colitis, hepatitis, liver abscess (Figure 6-27), and related complications.

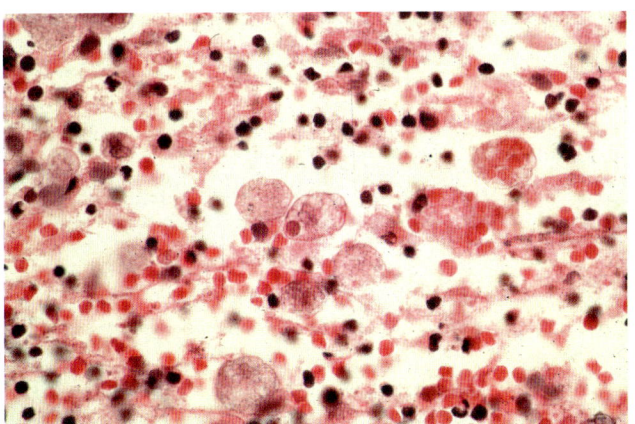

FIGURE 6-27 • *E. histolytica*—organisms showing erythrophagocytosis.

Leishmania species can cause cutaneous (Figure 6-28) or systemic disease, with significant morbidity.

SYSTEMIC INFECTIOUS AGENTS WITH BIOTERRORISM POTENTIAL

Fears of bioterrorism have exaggerated the importance of various infectious agents, to the point of being considered in the routine differential diagnosis of many human illnesses. These agents have been categorized based, among other things, on their ease of dissemination or transmission, high mortality, degree of social disruption, and need for special preparation (235). Although any or all of the highest-risk biologic agents (including inhalation anthrax, pneumonic plague, smallpox, tularemia, botulism, and viral hemorrhagic fevers) can be seen in the pediatric patient, several agents might closely resemble some of the more common childhood illnesses (Table 6-18) (53,236). Selected infections are briefly outlined hereunder:

Smallpox is a highly contagious infection, caused by the variola virus, which is a strict human pathogen with no carrier state. Although smallpox was the first human epidemic disease to be eradicated, its high infectivity, ease of person-to-person transmission, high mortality, and lack of specific chemotherapeutic agents make it an important biologic weapon, especially since the majority of the world population would be susceptible to infection. Following aerial transmission, the virus spreads and multiplies in the reticuloendothelial system during the incubation period. A second phase of viremia ensues, associated with prodromal nonspecific symptoms, followed by the characteristic skin lesions. The differential diagnosis of smallpox includes infection by VZV, HSV, measles, vaccinia, impetigo from *S. aureus*, and epidermolysis bullosa (53). Unlike chicken pox, however, fever precedes the rash by 2 to 3 days, the palms and soles are commonly involved, and the vesicles are all in the same stage. Histologically, in smallpox, the papillary dermis shows signs of inflammation and capillary endothelial swelling, followed by reticulating degeneration of the overlying epidermis with the presence of basophilic inclusions (Guarneri bodies), unlike HSV or VZV. Lysis of the infected cells leads to vesiculation; after 4 to 7 days, the clear vesicles become filled with neutrophils. The pustular fluid is usually bacteriologically sterile, unless secondarily infected. The umbilication characteristic of the mature smallpox vesicle is due to persistent septa and fixed dermal adnexa. Once the host immune response controls the infection, the vesicular fluid is resorbed and a scab is formed 10 to 15 days after the appearance of the rash. The scabs fall off by 3 weeks once the basal epithelium is replaced, leaving scars proportional to the depth of dermal involvement. Mucosal lesions are similar, except that they are covered by slough. The road to smallpox eradication, the weapon potential of the variola virus, and possible remedies have been reviewed by Raghunath (237). The Advisory Committee on Immunization Practices recommends not vaccinating pregnant or breast-feeding women or children less than 18 years old in pre-event smallpox vaccination programs (238). Secondary contact vaccinia from smallpox vaccine is rare (Figure 6-29), estimated to occur at a rate of 5 to 7 cases per 100,000 vaccines.

Anthrax, caused by *Bacillus anthracis*, is a worldwide zoonotic disease. Transmission in humans occurs through contact with animals or animal products (e.g., wool) and

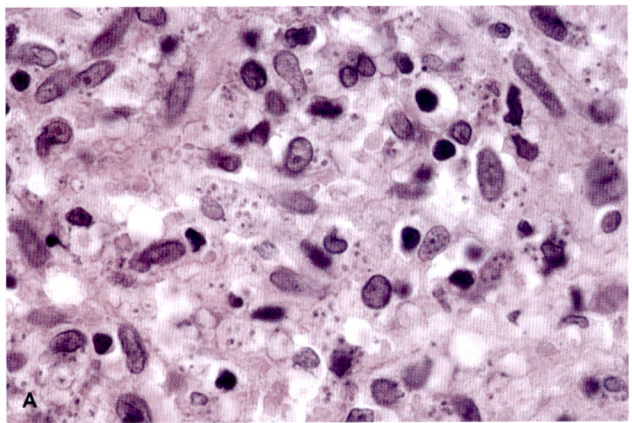
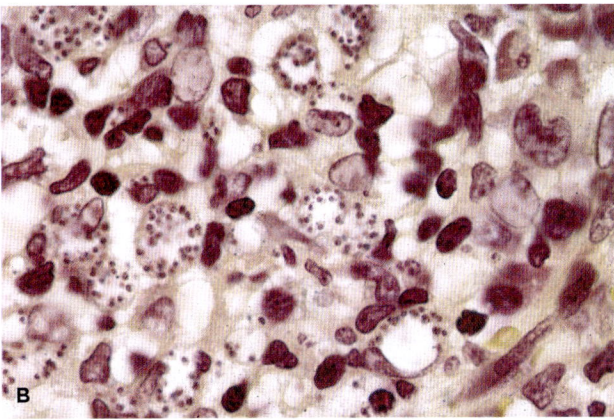

FIGURE 6-28 • Cutaneous leishmaniasis. **A:** Intracellular organisms (within histiocytes) (H&E). **B:** Brown-Hopps stain highlights organisms with their nucleus and kinetoplast.

TABLE 6-18 DIFFERENTIAL DIAGNOSIS OF INFECTIONS BY AGENTS WITH BIOTERRORISM POTENTIAL

Agent	Differential Diagnosis
Smallpox: variola major	Chicken pox–herpes zoster Herpes Measles Mumps Vaccinia Epidermolysis bullosa Impetigo from *Staphylococcus aureus*, coagulase positive, group 2
Anthrax: *Bacillus anthracis*	Inhalation type: respiratory syncytial virus–"flu/cold" Cutaneous type: insect bites, cat scratch disease Gastrointestinal type: rotavirus, Norwalk virus
Plague: *Yersinia pestis*	Cat scratch disease: *Bartonella henselae* Insect bites Necrotizing fasciitis: peripheral infarction Toxic shock syndrome Stevens-Johnson syndrome
Tularemia: *Francisella tularensis*	"Flu cold" *Haemophilus influenzae* Primary pulmonary hemosiderosis Inhalation toxin with adult respiratory distress syndrome
Botulism: *Clostridium botulinum*	Viral gastroenteritis Inflammatory bowel disease Autoimmune disorder: dysarthria, generalized weakness Drug reaction Polio: paralysis Myasthenia gravis

Source: Stocker JT. Clinical and pathologic differential diagnosis of selected potential bioterrorism agents of interest to pediatric health care providers. *Clin Lab Med* 2006;26:329–344.

from person to person by way of cutaneous lesions. Anthrax occurs in three forms: cutaneous, gastrointestinal, and inhalational. The cutaneous form accounts for nearly 95% of cases in children and adults. Pulmonary and gastrointestinal infections may be complicated by sepsis and meningitis. In the initial stages, the cutaneous form mimics insect bites or cat scratch disease, the gastrointestinal form mimics viral gastroenteritis, and the pulmonary form resembles RSV or similar infections, leading to delay in instituting specific therapy (53). The hallmark lesions are edema and hemorrhage, including hemorrhagic thoracic lymphadenitis, hemorrhagic mediastinitis with radiographic mediastinal space expansion, meningeal hemorrhage/edema (so-called cardinal's cap) (in over 90% cases), and hemorrhagic mesenteric lymphadenitis (in 20% cases) (239,240). The causative gram-positive bacilli may be identified in smear preparations of lymph node, spleen, or blood. After presumed exposure, antimicrobial prophylaxis is recommended for up to 60 days. Adverse effects of prolonged antimicrobial use may cause added pathology, although little information is available on effects of such prolonged use.

Plague is a bacterial zoonosis caused by *Yersinia pestis*, acquired through infected flea bites, and manifested as bubonic, septicemic, or pneumonic forms (241). Most commonly, the bubonic form presents with one or more enlarged, tender, regional lymph nodes, so-called bubo, as a result of migration of bacteria from the bite site to the regional lymph nodes. A local skin lesion (papule, vesicle, ulcer, or eschar) may be seen at the bite site. There is marked neutrophilia (40,000 to 100,000 cells/μL), blood cultures are often positive (50%), and the organism may be identified readily in aspirates of the buboes. Morphologically, lymph nodes show congestion and edema progressing to extranodal hemorrhage and necrosis. The bacteria resist phagocytosis causing lymph node necrosis and may be seen as extracellular aggregates within necrotic foci. Ulceration and cutaneous fistulae may occur. The bacteria may be recognized in sections and smears by their bipolar "safety pin" morphology or by the identification of monoclonal antibodies to the F1 antigen of *Y. pestis*. Destruction of the lymph nodes is followed by bacteremia, septicemia, and endotoxemia. Pneumonic plague causes dyspnea, chest pain, cough, and hemoptysis, while patients with septicemic plague often have prominent gastrointestinal symptoms and abdominal pain. Gangrene of the fingers, toes, or the tip of the nose, caused by small-vessel thrombosis, is referred to as "black death." All three forms may have systemic manifestations of gram-negative sepsis. Septicemic and pneumonic plague progress rapidly and are usually fatal without prompt treatment; bubonic plague has a mortality rate of 50% to 60%.

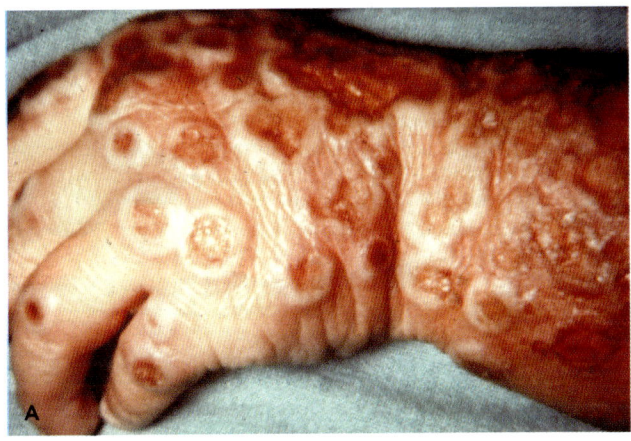
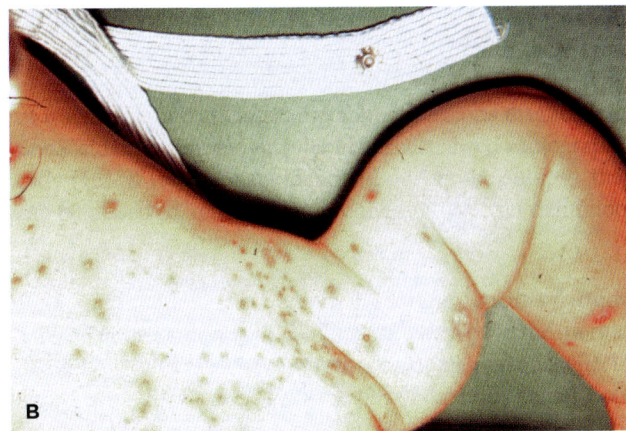

FIGURE 6-29 • Vaccinia. **A:** Well-developed lesions on the hand. **B:** Disseminated early lesions.

ACKNOWLEDGMENT

The authors acknowledge their keen appreciation and gratitude for the services of Ms. Rossana Desrochers, who ably assisted in the editing of this chapter.

References

1. Cherry JD, Demmler-Harrison GJ, Kaplan SL, eds. *Feigin and Cherry's Textbook of Pediatric Infectious Diseases*, 7th ed. Philadelphia, PA: Saunders; 2014.
2. Connor D, Chandler FW, Manz H, et al., eds. *Pathology of Infectious Diseases*. Standford, CT: Appleton and Lange; 1997.
3. Nizet V. Understanding how leading bacterial pathogens subvert innate immunity to reveal novel therapeutic targets. *J Allergy Clin Immunol* 2007;120:13–22.
4. van der Poll T, Opal SM. Host–pathogen interactions in sepsis. *Lancet Infect Dis* 2008;8(1):32–43.
5. Cooke GS, Hill AV. Genetics of susceptibility to human infectious disease. *Nat Rev Genet* 2001;2(12):967–977.
6. Strunk T, Burgner D. Genetic susceptibility to neonatal infection. *Curr Opin Infect Dis* 2006;19:259–263.
7. Dahmer MK, Randolph A, Vitali S, et al. Genetic polymorphisms in sepsis. *Pediatr Crit Care Med* 2005;6(3 suppl):S61–S73.
8. Clapp DW. Developmental regulation of the immune system. *Semin Perinatol* 2006;30(2):69–72.
9. Kenzel S, Henneke P. The innate immune system and its relevance to neonatal sepsis. *Curr Opin Infect Dis* 2006;19:264–270.
10. Landers CD, Chelvarajan RL, Bondada S. The role of B cells and accessory cells in the neonatal response to TI-2 antigens. *Immunol Res* 2005;31:25–36.
11. Cant A, Battersby A. When to think of immunodeficiency? *Adv Exp Med Biol* 2013;764:167–177.
12. Fox TG, Manaloor JJ, Christenson JC. Travel-related infections in children. *Pediatr Clin North Am* 2013;60:507–527.
13. Maloney SA, Weinberg M. Prevention of infectious diseases among international pediatric travelers: considerations for clinicians. *Semin Pediatr Infect Dis* 2004;15(3):137–149.
14. Kouadio IK, Aljunid S, Kamigaki T, et al. Infectious diseases following natural disasters: prevention and control measures. *Expert Rev Anti Infect Ther* 2012;10:95–104.
15. Joo HS, Otto M. Molecular basis of in vivo biofilm formation by bacterial pathogens. *Chem Biol* 2012;19:1503–1513.
16. Longo S, Borghesi A, Tzialla C, et al. IUGR and infections *Early Hum Dev* 2014;90S1:S42–S44.
17. Rawlinson WD, Hall B, Jones CA, et al. Viruses and other infections in stillbirth: what is the evidence and what should we be doing? *Pathology* 2008;40:149–160.
18. Blanc WA. Pathology of the placenta, membranes, and umbilical cord in bacterial, fungal, and viral infections in man. *Monogr Pathol* 1981;(22):67–132.
19. Klein JO, Baker CJ, Remington JS, et al. Current concepts of infections of the fetus and newborn infant. In: Remington JS, Klein JO (eds): *Infectious Diseases of the Fetus and New Born Infant*, 5th ed. Philadelphia, PA: WB Saunders; 2006:3–25.
20. Goldman AS. The immune system of human milk: antimicrobial, antiinflammatory and immunomodulating properties. *Pediatr Infect Dis J* 1993;12:664–671.
21. Lawrence RM, Lawrence RA. Breast milk and infection. *Clin Perinatol* 2004;31:501–528.
22. Wigglesworth JS. Quality of the perinatal autopsy. *Br J Obstet Gynaecol* 1991;98:617–619.
23. Garcia-de-Lomas J, Navarro D. New directions in diagnostics. *Pediatr Infect Dis J* 1997;16:S43–S48.
24. Pass R. Cytomegalovirus infection. *Pediatr Rev* 2002;23:163–170.
25. Schleiss MR. Acquisition of human cytomegalovirus infection in infants via breast milk: natural immunization or cause for concern? *Rev Med Virol* 2006;16(2):73–82.
26. Hamprecht K, Maschmann J, Vochem M, et al. Epidemiology of transmission of cytomegalovirus from mother to preterm infant by breastfeeding. *Lancet* 2001;357:513–518.
27. Schleiss MR. Cytomegalovirus in the neonate: immune correlates of infection and protection. *Clin Dev Immunol* 2013;2013:501801.
28. Ross SA, Boppana SB. Congenital cytomegalovirus infection: outcome and diagnosis. *Semin Pediatr Infect Dis* 2005;16(1):44–49.
29. Becroft DM. Prenatal cytomegalovirus infection: epidemiology, pathology and pathogenesis. *Perspect Pediatr Pathol* 1981;6:203–241.
30. Demmler GJ, Infectious Diseases Society of America and Centers for Disease Control. Summary of a workshop on surveillance for congenital cytomegalovirus disease. *Rev Infect Dis* 1991;13(2):315–329.
31. Barbi M, Binda S, Caroppo S. Diagnosis of congenital CMV infection via dried blood spots. *Rev Med Virol* 2006;16:385–392.
32. Rivera LB, Boppana SB, Fowler KB, et al. Predictors of hearing loss in children with symptomatic congenital cytomegalovirus infection. *Pediatrics* 2002;110:762–767.
33. Hass GM. Hepato-adrenal necrosis with intranuclear inclusion bodies: report of a case. *Am J Pathol* 1935;11:127–142.
34. Singer DB. Pathology of neonatal herpes simplex virus infection. *Perspect Pediatr Pathol* 1981;6:243–278.
35. Sanders JE, Garcia SE. Pediatric herpes simplex virus infections: an evidence-based approach to treatment. *Pediatr Emerg Med Pract* 2014;11(1):1–19.
36. Sauerbrei A, Bohn K. Phenotypic and genotypic testing of HSV-1 resistance to antivirals. *Methods Mol Biol* 2014;1144:149–165.
37. Kimberlin D. Herpes simplex virus, meningitis and encephalitis in neonates. *Herpes* 2004;11(Suppl 2):65A–76A.
38. Kimberlin DW. Neonatal herpes simplex infection. *Clin Microbiol Rev* 2004;17:1–13.

39. Anand A, Gray ES, Brown T, et al. Human parvovirus infection in pregnancy and hydrops fetalis. *N Engl J Med* 1987;316:183–186.
40. Essary LR, Vnencak-Jones CL, Manning SS, et al. Frequency of parvovirus B19 infection in nonimmune hydrops fetalis and utility of three diagnostic methods. *Hum Pathol* 1998;29:696–701.
41. Vogel H, Kornman M, Ledet SC, et al. Congenital parvovirus infection. *Pediatr Pathol Lab Med* 1997;17:903–912.
42. Gregg NM. Congenital defects associated with maternal rubella. *Aust Hosp* 1947;14(11):7–9.
43. Rosenberg HS, Oppenheimer EH, Esterly JR. Congenital rubella syndrome: the late effects and their relation to early lesions. *Perspect Pediatr Pathol* 1981;6:183–202.
44. Papania MJ, Wallace GS, Rota PA, et al. Elimination of endemic measles, rubella, and congenital rubella syndrome from the Western hemisphere: the US experience. *JAMA Pediatr* 2014;168:148–15.
45. Abou-Elhamd KA, ElToukhy HM, Al-Wadaani FA. Syndromes of hearing loss associated with visual loss. *Eur Arch Otorhinolaryngol* 2014;271:635–646.
46. Webster WS. Teratogen update: congenital rubella. *Teratology* 1998;58:13–23.
47. Banatvala JE, Brown DWG. Rubella. *Lancet* 2004;363(9415):1127–1137.
48. Kaplan C. The placenta and viral infections. *Semin Diagn Pathol* 1993;10:232–250.
49. Forrest JM, Turnbull FM, Sholler GF, et al. Gregg's congenital rubella patients 60 years later. *Med J Aust* 2002;177:664–667.
50. Alkalay AL, Pomerance JJ, Rimoin DL. Fetal varicella syndrome. *J Pediatr* 1987;111:320–323.
51. Fleisher G, Henry W, McSorley M, et al. Life-threatening complications of varicella. *Am J Dis Child* 1981;135:896–899.
52. Pfeiffer H, Varchmin-Schultheiss K, Brinkmann B. Sudden death in childhood due to varicella pneumonia: a forensic case report with clinical implications. *Int J Legal Med* 2006;120:33–35.
53. Stocker JT. Clinical and pathologic differential diagnosis of selected potential bioterrorism agents of interest to pediatric health care providers. *Clin Lab Med* 2006;26:329–344.
54. Ekpini ER, Wiktor SZ, Satten GA, et al. Late postnatal mother-to-child transmission of HIV-1 in Abidjan, Cote d'Ivoire. *Lancet* 1997;349:1054–1059.
55. Joshi VV. *Pathology of AIDS and Other Manifestations of HIV Infection.* New York, NY: Igaku-Shoin; 1990:384.
56. Moran CMF, ed. *Systemic Pathology of HIV infection and AIDS in Children.* Armed Forces Institute of Pathology. Washington, D.C.: ARP Press; 1997:325.
57. Ortiz AM, Silvestri G. Immunopathogenesis of AIDS. *Curr Infect Dis Rep* 2009;11:239–245.
58. Schneider E, Whitmore S, Glynn KM, et al.; Centers for Disease Control and Prevention. Revised surveillance case definitions for HIV infection among adults, adolescents, and children aged <18 months and for HIV infection and AIDS among children aged 18 months to <13 years—United States, 2008. *MMWR Recomm Rep* 2008;57(RR-10):1–12
59. Mofenson LM, Lambert JS, Stiehm ER, et al. Risk factors for perinatal transmission of human immunodeficiency virus type 1 in women treated with zidovudine. Pediatric AIDS Clinical Trials Group Study 185 Team. *N Engl J Med* 1999;341:385–393.
60. Landesman SH, Kalish LA, Burns DN, et al. Obstetrical factors and the transmission of human immunodeficiency virus type 1 from mother to child. The Women and Infants Transmission Study. *N Engl J Med* 1996;334:1617–1623.
61. King CC, Ellington SR, Kourtis AP. The role of co-infections in mother-to-child transmission of HIV. *Curr HIV Res* 2013;11:10–23.
62. Tobin NH, Aldrovandi GM. Immunology of pediatric HIV infection. *Immunol Rev* 2013;254:143–169.
63. World Health Organization *HIV and Infant Feeding Technical Consultation—Consensus Statement.* Geneva, Switzerland: World Health Organization; 2007:1–5.
64. Read JS, American Academy of Pediatrics Committee on Pediatric AIDS. Human milk, breastfeeding, and transmission of human immunodeficiency virus type 1 in the United States. *Pediatrics* 2003;112:1196–1205.
65. Laufer MK, van Oosterhout JJ, Perez MA, et al. Observational cohort study of HIV-infected African children. *Pediatr Infect Dis J* 2006;25:623–627.
66. Shah I. Age related clinical manifestations of HIV infection in Indian children. *J Trop Pediatr* 2005;51(5):300–303.
67. Singh HK, Gupta A, Siberry GK, et al. The Indian pediatric HIV epidemic: a systematic review. *Curr HIV Res* 2008;6:419–432.
68. Burns S, Hernandez-Reif M, Jessee P. A review of pediatric HIV effects on neurocognitive development. *Issues Compr Pediatr Nurs* 2008;31(3):107–121.
69. Calis JC, van Hensbroek MB, de Haan RJ, et al. HIV-associated anemia in children: a systematic review from a global perspective. *AIDS* 2008;22:1099–1112.
70. Merchant RH, Lala MM. Common clinical problems in children living with HIV/AIDS: systemic approach. *Indian J Pediatr* 2012;79:1506–1513.
71. Joshi VV, Oleske JM. Pulmonary lesions in children with the acquired immunodeficiency syndrome: a reappraisal based on data in additional cases and follow-up study of previously reported cases. *Hum Pathol* 1986;17:641–642.
72. Ramos-e-Silva M, Lima CM, Schechtman RC, et al. Systemic mycoses in immunodepressed patients (AIDS). *Clin Dermatol* 2012;30:616–627.
73. Nissapatorn V, Sawangjaroen N. Parasitic infections in HIV infected individuals: diagnostic & therapeutic challenges. *Indian J Med Res* 2011;134:878–897.
74. Ye P, Kirschner DE, Kourtis AP. The thymus during HIV disease: role in pathogenesis and in immune recovery. *Curr HIV Res* 2004;2:177–183.
75. Quijano G, Siminovich M, Drut R. Histopathologic findings in the lymphoid and reticuloendothelial system in pediatric HIV infection: a postmortem study. *Pediatr Pathol Lab Med* 1997;17:845–856.
76. Dickson DW, Llena JF, Nelson SJ, et al. Central nervous system pathology in pediatric AIDS. *Ann N Y Acad Sci* 1993;693:93–106.
77. Gil AC, Lorenzetti R, Mendes GB, et al. Hepatotoxicity in HIV-infected children and adolescents on antiretroviral therapy. *Sao Paulo Med J* 2007;125:205–209.
78. Schuval S, Van Dyke RB, Lindsey JC, et al.; Pediatric ACTGPST. Hepatitis C prevalence in children with perinatal human immunodeficiency virus infection enrolled in a long-term follow-up protocol. *Arch Pediatr Adolesc Med* 2004;158(10):1007–1013.
79. Velasco-Benitez CA. Digestive, hepatic, and nutritional manifestations in Latin American children with HIV/AIDS. *J Pediatr Gastroenterol Nutr* 2008;47(Suppl 1):S24–S26.
80. McCulloch MI, Ray PE. Kidney disease in HIV-positive children. *Semin Nephrol* 2008;28:585–594.
81. Ray PE. Taking a hard look at the pathogenesis of childhood HIV-associated nephropathy. *Pediatr Nephrol* 2009;24:2109–2119.
82. D'Costa G F, Khadke K, Patil YV. Pathology of placenta in HIV infection. *Indian J Pathol Microbiol* 2007;50(3):515–519.
83. Read JS, Committee on Pediatric AIDS. Diagnosis of HIV-1 infection in children younger than 18 months in the United States. *Pediatrics* 2007;120:e1547–e1562.
84. Moss WJ, Griffin DE. Global measles elimination. *Nat Rev Microbiol* 2006;4:900–908.
85. Wolfson LJ, Grais RF, Luquero FJ, et al. Estimates of measles case fatality ratios: a comprehensive review of community-based studies. *Int J Epidemiol* 2009;38:192–205.
86. Moss WJ, Griffin DE. Measles. *Lancet* 2012;379:153–164.
87. Hahm B. Hostile communication of measles virus with host innate immunity and dendritic cells. *Curr Top Microbiol Immunol* 2009;330:271–287.
88. Kabra SK, Lodha R. Antibiotics for preventing complications in children with measles. *Cochrane Database Syst Rev* 2008;(3):CD001477.
89. Young VA, Rall GF. Making it to the synapse: measles virus spread in and among neurons. *Curr Top Microbiol Immunol* 2009;330:3–30.
90. Centers for Disease Control & Prevention. Recommendations from an ad hoc Meeting of the WHO Measles and Rubella Laboratory Network (LabNet) on use of alternative diagnostic samples for measles and rubella surveillance. *MMWR* 2008;57:657–660.

91. Cohen JI, Kimura H, Nakamura S, et al. Epstein-Barr virus-associated lymphoproliferative disease in non-immunocompromised hosts: a status report and summary of an international meeting, 8–9 September 2008. *Ann Oncol* 2009;20:1472–1482.
92. Higgins CD, Swerdlow AJ, Macsween KF, et al. A study of risk factors for acquisition of Epstein-Barr virus and its subtypes. *J Infect Dis* 2007;195(4):474–482.
93. Candy B, Chalder T, Cleare AJ, et al. Recovery from infectious mononucleosis: a case for more than symptomatic therapy? A systematic review. *Br J Gen Pract* 2002;52:844–851.
94. Jenson HB. Acute complications of Epstein-Barr virus infectious mononucleosis. *Curr Opin Pediatr* 2000;12:263–268.
95. Ebell M. Epstein-Barr virus infectious mononucleosis. *Am Fam Physician* 2004;70:1279–1287.
96. Gulley ML, Tang W. Laboratory assays for Epstein-Barr virus-related disease. *J Mol Diagn* 2008;10:279–292.
97. Delecluse HJ, Feederle R, O'Sullivan B, et al. Epstein Barr virus-associated tumours: an update for the attention of the working pathologist. *J Clin Pathol* 2007;60:1358–1364.
98. Deyrup AT. Epstein-Barr virus-associated epithelial and mesenchymal neoplasms. *Hum Pathol* 2008;39:473–483.
99. Rezk SA, Weiss LM. Epstein-Barr virus-associated lymphoproliferative disorders. *Hum Pathol* 2007;38:1293–1304.
100. Ohshima K, Kimura H, Yoshino T, et al. Proposed categorization of pathological states of EBV-associated T/natural killer-cell lymphoproliferative disorder (LPD) in children and young adults: overlap with chronic active EBV infection and infantile fulminant EBV T-LPD. *Pathol Int* 2008;58:209–217.
101. Carneiro SC, Cestari T, Allen SH, et al. Viral exanthems in the tropics. *Clin Dermatol* 2007;25:212–220.
102. Gould EA, Solomon T. Pathogenic Flaviviruses. *Lancet* 2008;371:500–509.
103. Potts JA, Rothman AL. Clinical and laboratory features that distinguish dengue from other febrile illnesses in endemic populations. *Trop Med Int Health* 2008;13:1328–1340.
104. Ligon BL. Dengue fever and dengue hemorrhagic fever: a review of the history, transmission, treatment, and prevention. *Semin Pediatr Infect Dis* 2005;16(1):60–65.
105. Kamath SR, Ranjit S. Clinical features, complications and atypical manifestations of children with severe forms of dengue hemorrhagic fever in South India. *Indian J Pediatr* 2006;73:889–895.
106. Kalayanarooj S, Nimmannitya S. Clinical presentations of dengue hemorrhagic fever in infants compared to children. *J Med Assoc Thai* 2003;86(Suppl 3):S673–S680.
107. Ronchi A, Doern C, Brock E, et al. Neonatal adenoviral infection: a seventeen year experience and review of the literature. *J Pediatr* 2014;164:529–535e1–4.
108. Abzug MJ. The enteroviruses: problems in need of treatments. *J Infect* 2014;68(Suppl 1):S108–S114.
109. Gotuzzo E, Moody J, Verdonck K, et al. Frequent HTLV-1 infection in the offspring of Peruvian women with HTLV-1-associated myelopathy/tropical spastic paraparesis or strongyloidiasis. *Rev Panam Salud Publica* 2007;22:223–230.
110. Hisada M, Maloney EM, Sawada T, et al. Virus markers associated with vertical transmission of human T lymphotropic virus type 1 in Jamaica. *Clin Infect Dis* 2002;34:1551–1557.
111. Kancherla VS, Hanson IC. Mumps resurgence in the United States. *J Allergy Clin Immunol* 2006;118:938–941.
112. Rota JS, Rosen JB, Doll MK, et al. Comparison of the sensitivity of laboratory diagnostic methods from a well-characterized outbreak of mumps in New York City in 2009. *Clin Vaccine Immunol* 2013;20:391–396.
113. Jain R, Goldman RD. Novel influenza A(H1N1): clinical presentation, diagnosis, and management. *Pediatr Emerg Care* 2009;25(11):791–796.
114. Neumann G, Noda T, Kawaoka Y. Emergence and pandemic potential of swine-origin H1N1 influenza virus. *Nature* 2009;459:931–939.
115. Stein RA. Lessons from outbreaks of H1N1 influenza. *Ann Intern Med* 2009;151(1):59–62.
116. Kwan-Gett TS, Baer A, Duchin JS. Spring 2009 H1N1 influenza outbreak in King County, Washington Disaster. *Med Public Health Prep* 2009;3(Suppl 2):S109–S116.
117. Khanna M, Kumar P, Choudhary K, et al. Emerging influenza virus: a global threat. *J Biosci* 2008;33:475–482.
118. Bitnun A, Allen U, Heurter H, et al.; Other Members of the Hospital for Sick Children SIT Children hospitalized with severe acute respiratory syndrome-related illness in Toronto. *Pediatrics* 2003;112:e261.
119. Hon KL, Leung CW, Cheng WT, et al. Clinical presentations and outcome of severe acute respiratory syndrome in children. *Lancet* 2003;361:1701–1703.
120. Shek CC, Ng PC, Fung GP, et al. Infants born to mothers with severe acute respiratory syndrome. *Pediatrics* 2003;112:e254.
121. Memish ZA, Al-Tawfiq JA, Assiri A, et al. Middle East respiratory syndrome coronavirus disease in children. *Pediatr Infect Dis J* 2014;33(9):904–906.
122. Petersen LR, Marfin AA. West Nile virus: a primer for the clinician. *Ann Intern Med* 2002;137:173–179.
123. Centers for Disease Control and Prevention. Intrauterine West Nile virus infection—New York, 2002. *MMWR* 2002;51:1135–1136.
124. Petersen LR, Roehrig JT, Hughes JM. West Nile virus encephalitis. *N Engl J Med* 2002;347:1225–1226.
125. Baer G, Schaad UB, Heininger U. Clinical findings and unusual epidemiologic characteristics of human metapneumovirus infections in children in the region of Basel, Switzerland. *Eur J Pediatr* 2008;167:63–69.
126. Cox RG, Erickson JJ, Hastings AK, et al. Human metapneumovirus virus-like particles induce protective B and T cell responses in a mouse model. *J Virol* 2014;88(11):6368–6379.
127. Allander T, Tammi MT, Eriksson M, et al. Cloning of a human parvovirus by molecular screening of respiratory tract samples. *Proc Natl Acad Sci USA* 2005;102:12891–12896.
128. Jartti T, Hedman K, Jartti L, et al. Human bocavirus-the first 5 years. *Rev Med Virol* 2012;22:46–64.
129. Luce WA, Hoffman TM, Bauer JA. Bench-to-bedside review: developmental influences on the mechanisms, treatment and outcomes of cardiovascular dysfunction in neonatal versus adult sepsis. *Crit Care* 2007;11:228.
130. Goldstein B, Giroir B, Randolph A; International Consensus Conference on Pediatric Sepsis. International pediatric sepsis consensus conference: definitions for sepsis and organ dysfunction in pediatrics. *Pediatr Crit Care Med* 2005;6(1):2–8.
131. See LL. Bloodstream infection in children. *Pediatr Crit Care Med* 2005;6(3 Suppl):S42–S44.
132. Robertson CM, Coopersmith CM. The systemic inflammatory response syndrome. *Microbes Infect* 2006;2006:5.
133. Oh W. Early onset neonatal group B streptococcal sepsis. *Am J Perinatol* 2013;30:143–147.
134. Shah BA, Padbury JF. Neonatal sepsis: an old problem with new insights. *Virulence* 2014;5:170–178.
135. Mussap M, Molinari MP, Senno E, et al. New diagnostic tools for neonatal sepsis: the role of a real-time polymerase chain reaction for the early detection and identification of bacterial and fungal species in blood samples. *J Chemother* 2007;19(Suppl 2):31–34.
136. Stoll BJ, Hansen N, Fanaroff AA, et al. Late-onset sepsis in very low birth weight neonates: the experience of the NICHD Neonatal Research Network. *Pediatrics* 2002;110:285–291.
137. Lacroix J, Cotting J; Pediatric Acute Lung Injury; Sepsis Investigators (PALISI) Network. Severity of illness and organ dysfunction scoring in children. *Pediatr Crit Care Med* 2005;6(3 Suppl):S126–S134.
138. Power Coombs MR, Kronforst K, Levy O. Neonatal host defense against Staphylococcal infections. *Clin Dev Immunol* 2013;2013:826303.
139. Orange JS. Congenital immunodeficiencies and sepsis. *Pediatr Crit Care Med* 2005;6(3 Suppl):S99–S107.
140. Kaplan SL. Community-acquired methicillin-resistant Staphylococcus aureus infections in children. *Semin Pediatr Infect Dis* 2006;17(3):113–119.
141. Venkatesh MP, Placencia F, Weisman LE. Coagulase-negative staphylococcal infections in the neonate and child: an update. *Semin Pediatr Infect Dis* 2006;17(3):120–127.

142. Martin JM, Green M. Group A streptococcus. Semin Pediatr Infect Dis 2006;17(3):140–148.
143. Hoffman JA, Mason EO, Schutze GE, et al. Streptococcus pneumoniae infections in the neonate. Pediatrics 2003;112:1095–1102.
144. Centers for Disease Control and Prevention. Trends in perinatal group B streptococcal disease—United States, 2000–2006. MMWR Morb Mortal Wkly Rep 2009;58:109–112.
145. American Academy of Pediatrics Committee on Infectious Diseases and Committee on Fetus and Newborn. Revised guidelines for prevention of early-onset group B streptococcal (GBS) infection. Pediatrics 1997;99:489–496.
146. Dyson AE, Read SE. Group G streptococcal colonization and sepsis in neonates. J Pediatr 1981;99:944–947.
147. Jeffery H, Mitchison R, Wigglesworth JS, et al. Early neonatal bacteraemia. Comparison of group B streptococcal, other Gram-positive and Gram-negative infections. Arch Dis Child 1977;52(9):683–686.
148. Siegel JD, McCracken GH Jr. Group D streptococcal infections. J Pediatr 1978;93:542–543.
149. Siegel JD, McCracken GH Jr. Sepsis neonatorum. N Engl J Med 1981;304:642–647.
150. Butler KM. Enterococcal infection in children. Semin Pediatr Infect Dis 2006;17:128–139.
151. Recommendations of the Hospital Infection Control Practices Advisory Committee (HICPAC). Recommendations for preventing the spread of vancomycin resistance. MMWR 1995;44:1–13.
152. Ingram DL. Neisseria gonorrhoeae in children. Pediatr Ann 1994;23:341–345.
153. Rouphael NG, Stephens DS. Neisseria meningitidis: biology, microbiology, and epidemiology. Methods Mol Biol 2012;799:1–20.
154. Buckle GC, Walker CL, Black RE. Typhoid fever and paratyphoid fever: systematic review to estimate global morbidity and mortality for 2010. J Glob Health 2012;2:010401.
155. Darton TC, Blohmke CJ, Pollard AJ. Typhoid epidemiology, diagnostics and the human challenge model. Curr Opin Gastroenterol 2014;30:7–17.
156. Connor BA, Schwartz E. Typhoid and paratyphoid fever in travellers. Lancet Infect Dis 2005;5(10):623–628.
157. Hoffner RJ, Slaven E, Perez J, et al. Emergency department presentations of typhoid fever. J Emerg Med 2000;19(4):317–321.
158. Bisgard KM, Kao A, Leake J, et al. Haemophilus influenzae invasive disease in the United States, 1994–1995: near disappearance of a vaccine-preventable childhood disease. Emerg Infect Dis 1998;4(2):229–237.
159. Zakikhany K, Efstratiou A. Diphtheria in Europe: current problems and new challenges. Future Microbiol 2012;7:595–607.
160. Faulkner A, Skoff T, Martin S, et al. Pertussis. In: Roush SW and Baldy LM (eds): *Manual for the Surveillance of Vaccine-Preventable Diseases*. Atlanta, GA: Centers for Disease Control and Prevention; 2008: 10.1–10.12.
161. Kline JM, Lewis WD, Smith EA, et al. Pertussis: a reemerging infection. Am Fam Physician 2013;88:507–514.
162. Pittet LF, Emonet S, Schrenzel J, et al. Bordetella holmesii: an under-recognised Bordetella species. Lancet Infect Dis 2014;14:510–519.
163. Zouari A, Smaoui H, Kechrid A. The diagnosis of pertussis: which method to choose? Crit Rev Microbiol 2012;38:111–121.
164. Mylonakis E, Paliou M, Hohmann EL, et al. Listeriosis during pregnancy: a case series and review of 222 cases. Medicine (Baltimore) 2002;81:260–269.
165. Mylonakis E, Hohmann EL, Calderwood SB. Central nervous system infection with Listeria monocytogenes. 33 years' experience at a general hospital and review of 776 episodes from the literature. *Medicine (Baltimore)* 1998;77:313–336.
166. Dussurget O. New insights into determinants of Listeria monocytogenes virulence. Int Rev Cell Mol Biol 2008;270:1–38.
167. Drevets DA, Bronze MS. Listeria monocytogenes: epidemiology, human disease, and mechanisms of brain invasion. FEMS Immunol Med Microbiol 2008;53(2):151–165.
168. Hollier LM, Harstad TW, Sanchez PJ, et al Fetal syphilis: clinical and laboratory characteristics. Obstet Gynecol 2001;97(6):947–953.
169. Woods CR. Syphilis in children: congenital and acquired. Semin Pediatr Infect Dis 2005;16(4):245–257.
170. Peeling RW, Hook EW III. The pathogenesis of syphilis: the Great Mimicker, revisited. J Pathol 2006;208:224–232.
171. Sheffield JS, Sanchez PJ, Wendel GD Jr, et al. Placental histopathology of congenital syphilis. Obstet Gynecol 2002;100:126–133.
172. Vijayachari P, Sugunan AP, Shriram AN. Leptospirosis: an emerging global public health problem. J Biosci 2008;33:557–569.
173. Cerqueira TB, Athanazio DA, Spichler AS, et al. Renal involvement in leptospirosis—new insights into pathophysiology and treatment. Braz J Infect Dis 2008;12:248–252.
174. Dolhnikoff M, Mauad T, Bethlem EP, et al. Pathology and pathophysiology of pulmonary manifestations in leptospirosis. Braz J Infect Dis 2007;11:142–148.
175. Ahmad SN, Shah S, Ahmad FM. Laboratory diagnosis of leptospirosis. J Postgrad Med 2005;51(3):195–200.
176. Strobino BA, Williams CL, Abid S, et al. Lyme disease and pregnancy outcome: a prospective study of two thousand prenatal patients. Am J Obstet Gynecol 1993;169:367–374.
177. Shapiro ED. Lyme disease in children. Am J Med 1995;98:69S–73S.
178. Wormser GP, Dattwyler RJ, Shapiro ED, et al. The clinical assessment, treatment, and prevention of lyme disease, human granulocytic anaplasmosis, and babesiosis: clinical practice guidelines by the Infectious Diseases Society of America. Clin Infect Dis 2006;43:1089–1134.
179. Mullegger RR. Dermatological manifestations of Lyme borreliosis. Eur J Dermatol 2004;14:296–309.
180. Skogman BH, Croner S, Nordwall M, et al. Lyme neuroborreliosis in children: a prospective study of clinical features, prognosis, and outcome. Pediatr Infect Dis J 2008;27:1089–1094.
181. Hercogova J, Vanousova D. Syphilis and borreliosis during pregnancy. Dermatol Ther 2008;21(3):205–209.
182. Porta FS, Nieto EA, Creus BF, et al. Tick-borne lymphadenopathy: a new infectious disease in children. Pediatr Infect Dis J 2008;27: 618–622.
183. Parish JL. Treponemal infections in the pediatric population. Clin Dermatol 2000;18:687–700.
184. Abramowsky C, Beyer-Patterson P, Cortinas E. Nonsyphilitic spirochetosis in second-trimester fetuses. Pediatr Pathol 1991;11(6):827–838.
185. Ferrari ND III, Weiss ME. Botulism. Adv Pediatr Infect Dis 1995;10:81–91.
186. Smith-Slatas CL, Bourque M, Salazar JC. Clostridium septicum infections in children: a case report and review of the literature. Pediatrics 2006;117:e796–e805.
187. Chomel BB. Zoonoses of house pets other than dogs, cats and birds. Pediatr Infect Dis J 1992;11:479–487.
188. Morrison G. Zoonotic infections from pets: understanding the risk and treatment. Postgrad Med 2001;110(1):24–26, 29–30, 35–36.
189. Nicoll A. Children, avian influenza H5N1 and preparing for the next pandemic. Arch Dis Child 2008;93(5):433–438.
190. Stirling J, Griffith M, Dooley JS, et al. Zoonoses associated with petting farms and open zoos. Vector Borne Zoonotic Dis 2008;8(1):85–92.
191. Franco MP, Mulder M, Gilman RH, et al. Human brucellosis. Lancet Infect Dis 2007;7(12):775–786.
192. Mandalakas AM, Starke JR. Current concepts of childhood tuberculosis. Semin Pediatr Infect Dis 2005;16(2):93–104.
193. Nelson LJ, Wells CD. Global epidemiology of childhood tuberculosis. Int J Tuberc Lung Dis 2004;8:636–647.
194. Feja K, Salman L. Tuberculosis in children. *Clin Chest Med* 2005;26(2):295–312.
195. Cantwell MF, Shehab ZM, Costello AM, et al. Brief report: congenital tuberculosis. *N Engl J Med* 1994;330:1051–1054.
196. Adhikari M, Pillay T, Pillay DG. Tuberculosis in the newborn: an emerging disease. Pediatr Infect Dis J 1997;16:1108–1112.
197. Ormerod P. Tuberculosis in pregnancy and the puerperium. Thorax 2001;56:494–499.

198. Diagnostic Standards and Classification of Tuberculosis in Adults and Children. This official statement of the American Thoracic Society and the Centers for Disease Control and Prevention was adopted by the ATS Board of Directors, July 1999. This statement was endorsed by the Council of the Infectious Disease Society of America, September 1999. Am J Respir Crit Care Med 2000;161(4 Pt 1):1376–1395.
199. Maltezou HC, Spyridis P, Kafetzis DA. Extra-pulmonary tuberculosis in children. Arch Dis Child 2000;83(4):342–346.
200. Nelson LJ, Schneider E, Wells CD, et al. Epidemiology of childhood tuberculosis in the United States, 1993–2001: the need for continued vigilance. Pediatrics 2004;114:333–341.
201. Marais BJ, Gie RP, Schaaf HS, et al. The natural history of childhood intra-thoracic tuberculosis: a critical review of literature from the pre-chemotherapy era. Int J Tuberc Lung Dis 2004;8:392–402.
202. Lewinsohn DA, Gennaro ML, Scholvinck L, et al. Tuberculosis immunology in children: diagnostic and therapeutic challenges and opportunities. Int J Tuberc Lung Dis 2004;8:658–674.
203. Udani PM. BCG vaccination in India and tuberculosis in children: newer facets. Indian J Pediatr 1994;61:451–462.
204. Pearce EC, Woodward JF, Nyandiko WM, et al. A systematic review of clinical diagnosis systems used in the diagnosis of tuberculosis in children. AIDS Res Treat 2012;2012(2012):401896.
205. Walker DH, Paddock CD, Dumler JS. Emerging and re-emerging tick-transmitted rickettsial and ehrlichial infections. Med Clin North Am 2008;92:1345–1361.
206. Dumler JS, Madigan JE, Pusterla N, et al. Ehrlichioses in humans: epidemiology, clinical presentation, diagnosis, and treatment. Clin Infect Dis 2007;45(Suppl 1):S45–S51.
207. Schutze GE BS, Buckingham SC, Marshall GS, et al.; Tick-borne Infections in Children Study (TICS) Group. Human monocytic ehrlichiosis in children. Pediatr Infect Dis J 2007;26:475–479.
208. Hecht JL, Onderdonk A, Delaney M, et al.; ELGAN Study Investigators. Characterization of chorioamnionitis in 2nd-trimester C-section placentas and correlation with microorganism recovery from subamniotic tissues. Pediatr Dev Pathol 2008;11(1):15–22.
209. Egawa T, Morioka I, Morisawa T, et al. Ureaplasma urealyticum and Mycoplasma hominis presence in umbilical cord is associated with pathogenesis of funisitis. Kobe J Med Sci 2007;53:241–249.
210. Goldenberg RL, Faye-Petersen O, Andrews WW, et al. The Alabama Preterm Birth Study: diffuse decidual leukocytoclastic necrosis of the decidua basalis, a placental lesion associated with preeclampsia, indicated preterm birth and decreased fetal growth. J Matern Fetal Neonatal Med 2007;20:391–395.
211. Dammann O, Allred EN, Genest DR, et al. Antenatal mycoplasma infection, the fetal inflammatory response and cerebral white matter damage in very-low-birth weight infants. Paediatr Perinat Epidemiol 2003;17(1):49–57.
212. Honma Y, Yada Y, Takahashi N, et al. Certain type of chronic lung disease of newborns is associated with Ureaplasma urealyticum infection in utero. Pediatr Int 2007;49:479–484.
213. Esposito S, Cavagna R, Bosis S, et al. Emerging role of Mycoplasma pneumoniae in children with acute pharyngitis. Eur J Clin Microbiol Infect Dis 2002;21:607–610.
214. Sanchez-Vargas FM, Gomez-Duarte OG. Mycoplasma pneumoniae—an emerging extra-pulmonary pathogen. Clin Microbiol Infect 2008;14:105–117.
215. Timitilli A, Di Rocco M, Nattero G, et al. Unusual manifestations of infections due to Mycoplasma pneumoniae in children. Infez Med 2004;12:113–117.
216. Waites KB, Talkington DF. Mycoplasma pneumoniae and its role as a human pathogen. Clin Microbiol Rev 2004;17:697–728.
217. Yis U, Kurul SH, Cakmakci H, et al. Mycoplasma pneumoniae: nervous system complications in childhood and review of the literature. Eur J Pediatr 2008;167:973–978.
218. Othman N, Isaacs D, Daley AJ, et al. Mycoplasma pneumoniae infection in a clinical setting. Pediatr Int 2008;50:662–666.
219. Deligeoroglou E, Salakos N, Makrakis E, et al. Infections of the lower female genital tract during childhood and adolescence. Clin Exp Obstet Gynecol 2004;31(3):175–178.
220. Darville T. Chlamydia trachomatis infections in neonates and young children. Semin Pediatr Infect Dis 2005;16(4):235–244.
221. Hammerschlag MR. Chlamydia trachomatis and Chlamydia pneumoniae infections in children and adolescents. Pediatr Rev 2004;25:43–51.
222. Dowell SF, Peeling RW, Boman J, et al; C. pneumoniae Workshop Participants. Standardizing Chlamydia pneumoniae assays: recommendations from the Centers for Disease Control and Prevention (USA) and the Laboratory Centre for Disease Control (Canada). Clin Infect Dis 2001;33:492–503.
223. Bartlett AH, Rivera AL, Krishnamurthy R, et al. Thoracic actinomycosis in children: case report and review of the literature. Pediatr Infect Dis J 2008;27:165–169.
224. Darmstadt GL, Dinulos JG, Miller Z. Congenital cutaneous candidiasis: clinical presentation, pathogenesis, and management guidelines. Pediatrics 2000;105:438–444.
225. Walsh TJ, Gonzalez C, Lyman CA, et al. Invasive fungal infections in children: recent advances in diagnosis and treatment. Adv Pediatr Infect Dis 1996;11:187–290.
226. Schutze GE, Hickerson SL, Fortin EM, et al. Blastomycosis in children. Clin Infect Dis 1996;22:496–502.
227. Butler JC, Heller R, Wright PF. Histoplasmosis during childhood. South Med J 1994;87(4):476–480.
228. Sangoi AR, Rogers WM, Longacre TA, et al. Challenges and pitfalls of morphologic identification of fungal infections in histologic and cytologic specimens: a ten-year retrospective review at a single institution. Am J Clin Pathol 2009;131:364–375.
229. Ash LR, Orihel TC. Atlas of Human Parasitology., 5th ed. Chicago, IL, ASCP Press; 2007.
230. Beazley DM, Egerman RS. Toxoplasmosis. Semin Perinatol 1998;22:332–338.
231. Montoya JG, Liesenfeld O. Toxoplasmosis. Lancet 2004;363:1965–1976.
232. Naessens A, Jenum PA, Pollak A, et al. Diagnosis of congenital toxoplasmosis in the neonatal period: a multicenter evaluation. J Pediatr 1999;135:714–719.
233. Bern C, Montgomery SP, Herwaldt BL, et al. Evaluation and treatment of chagas disease in the United States: a systematic review. JAMA 2007;298:2171–2181.
234. Torrico F, Alonso-Vega C, Suarez E, et al. Maternal Trypanosoma cruzi infection, pregnancy outcome, morbidity, and mortality of congenitally infected and non-infected newborns in Bolivia. Am J Trop Med Hyg 2004;70:201–209.
235. Ferguson NE, Steele L, Crawford CY, et al. Bioterrorism web site resources for infectious disease clinicians and epidemiologists. Clin Infect Dis 2003;36:1458–1473.
236. Patt HA, Feigin RD. Diagnosis and management of suspected cases of bioterrorism: a pediatric perspective. Pediatrics 2002;109:685–692.
237. Raghunath D. Smallpox revisited. Curr Sci 2002;83:566–576.
238. Wharton M, Strikas RA, Harpaz R, et al. Recommendations for using smallpox vaccine in a pre-event vaccination program. Supplemental recommendations of the Advisory Committee on Immunization Practices (ACIP) and the Healthcare Infection Control Practices Advisory Committee (HICPAC). MMWR Recomm Rep 2003;52:1–16.
239. Guarner J, Jernigan JA, Shieh WJ, et al.; Inhalational Anthrax Pathology Working Group. Pathology and pathogenesis of bioterrorism-related inhalational anthrax. Am J Pathol 2003;163:701–709.
240. Meyer MA. Neurologic complications of anthrax: a review of the literature. Arch Neurol 2003;60(4):483–488.
241. Koirala J. Plague: disease, management, and recognition of act of terrorism. Infect Dis Clin North Am 2006;20:273–287.

CHAPTER 7
Pediatric Forensic Pathology

Jonathan Eisenstat, M.D.

INTRODUCTION

Forensic pathology is the field of medicine that deals with the investigation of death utilizing the scientific method as it pertains to the court of law. It is the study and investigation of bodily disease, injury, and death. Forensic pathologists are medical doctors who have completed at least an anatomic pathology residency and a forensic pathology fellowship. There are only approximately 500 board-certified forensic pathologists in the United States. Most often, the forensic pathologist is asked to determine the cause and manner of an individual's death, although consults on live patients for wound interpretation do occasionally occur. The *cause of death* is essentially why the person died. The *underlying cause of death* is the etiologically specific disease or injury that, unbroken by any sufficient intervening cause, initiated the lethal sequence of events that led to the individual's death. For example, if a child sustained a traumatic brain injury at the age of 1 year and survived for a period of time on a ventilator, subsequently developing pneumonia, and eventually succumbed to the pneumonia, the incident that started this chain of events was the head injury, and thus, it is considered the underlying cause of death. The immediate cause of death in this case would be the pneumonia. The *manner of death* reflects the circumstances under which the individual died. It is divided into five categories (six in some jurisdictions). According to the National Association of Medical Examiners Guide for Manner of Death Classification (1), the following are the accepted categories of manner of death: natural—due solely to a natural disease process or as a result of aging; accident—when an injury or poisoning causes death, without evidence of intent to harm; suicide—as a result of an intentional self-inflicted act; homicide—as a result of a volitional act committed by another person; and undetermined—when the manner could not be determined after a thorough investigation; and some have suggested a sixth manner as therapeutic complication/misadventure—this manner of death is utilized when an individual dies as a result of a known complication of a medical procedure (2). For instance, if a femoral line is placed in a patient and the patient develops a retroperitoneal hemorrhage resulting in death, this is a known complication of this procedure and should be classified as such. Deeming a manner of death to be a therapeutic complication/misadventure is a nonjudgmental determination that takes the burden away from the pathologist of having to decide if this should be called a natural death or an accident. It is not synonymous with negligence or malpractice. Pediatric deaths can fall into any of these categories. As of 2010, the National Vital Statistics System of the CDC (3) showed that the most common manner of death in children less than 1 year old was natural, mostly due to congenital anomalies. If congenital anomalies and short gestation, which mainly cause death in the first month of life, were to be removed, sudden infant death syndrome (SIDS) would be the most prevalent cause of death in the first year of life. Unintentional injuries were the leading cause of death between the ages of 1 and 44 years. These accidental deaths include motor vehicle accidents, drug intoxications, and asphyxial deaths such as drowning or choking, to mention a few. Suicides and homicides become more prevalent with increasing age.

The medicolegal death investigation system varies throughout the United States. Some states are strictly medical examiner systems, some are coroner systems, and others are a combination of coroner and medical examiner. As described above, medical examiners are medical doctors trained in the investigation of death. Coroners may be physicians but are usually lay individuals who are locally elected officials. They can have varying levels of medical knowledge and education, from a high school degree to a doctorate. They most often are elected by the citizens of a particular county and are responsible for receiving death calls, responding to certain scenes and pronouncing death in certain circumstances. They are also the individuals who sign the death certificates of unattended or traumatic deaths that occur in their jurisdiction. The coroner often consults with the medical examiner concerning the cause and manner of a person's death. The weakest link of the coronial system is the potential difference between what the medical examiner determines the cause and manner of death to be and what the coroner decides (4). The majority of forensic pathologists practicing in the United States do so in a medical examiner setting, whether or not the overall system is a coroner system. Sixty-five percent of the 3145 county-equivalent jurisdictions in the United States have coroners as their chief medicolegal officers (5).

Different jurisdictions have different laws concerning what types of cases fall under the purview of the medical examiner. In general, any death of a non–terminally ill child, where there is a traumatic injury or the death is unwitnessed, should at a minimum be referred to the medical examiner and/or coroner. The medical examiner office will then decide if the case warrants an examination by the forensic pathologist. All homicides, no matter how delayed the death is, warrants an exam by the medical examiner office. Other traumatic cases may be taken on a case-by-case basis depending on the level of suspicion and concern by law enforcement, the prosecutor's office, and other public officials. If a child has a natural disease where the death is expected, depending on the circumstances surrounding the death, the medical examiner may decline jurisdiction.

Child fatality review committees meet on a regular basis to review child death cases. They are composed of representatives from different agencies. Child advocates, pediatricians, law enforcement, district attorneys, and medical examiners partake in these meetings. The aim of the child fatality review is to identify possible deficiencies within the system and attempt to correct them as well as identify any trends that may be occurring.

FORENSIC AUTOPSY

The forensic autopsy, as with the hospital autopsy, is performed to determine the child's cause of death. In the hospital setting, the natural disease process is the main focus of the examination. In the forensic setting, any natural disease should be documented, but there are a number of other questions that need to be answered and specimens that should be procured. These include interpretation of injuries, determining the manner of the child's death, collection of biologic specimens for a multitude of ancillary studies, collection of trace evidence (hair and fibers), and sometimes identifying the child. The questions that need to be answered are not only medical but also of a legal nature.

External Examination

The autopsy begins with an external examination. The first external procedure that should be performed is the taking of photographs of the body as it is received in the morgue, prior to any manipulation of the body. This will allow for documentation of any articles of clothing, personal effects, injuries, and medical intervention. The clothing, personal effects, and therapeutic devices should then be removed, and the body should be photographed naked. All clothing and personal effects received with the body should be documented and, if deemed necessary, retained as evidence. Clothing is usually retained only in homicide cases. A head-to-toe evaluation should then take place with documentation of all natural and traumatic findings. This includes looking in the oral cavity, ears, female external genitalia, and anus. If the child is an uncircumcised male, the foreskin should be retracted and examined. The standard measurements (crown–heel, crown–rump, head circumference, chest circumference, abdominal circumference, foot length) should be taken and compared to standard growth charts. As the external examination is proceeding, any finding with potential evidentiary value should be retained, including trace evidence such as fibers and hairs that appear to be other than those from the child. When child abuse is suspected, scalp hair from the child should be taken and retained. This can become important if the scene reveals an impact site on a wall or other surface, where hair may be present. The decedent's hair that was pulled at autopsy can be compared with that found at the scene. All of this needs to be done maintaining appropriate chain of custody and documentation. When documenting a significant injury, the location on the body should be described in relation to a standard anatomical landmark. The most common landmarks used are the head, feet, shoulder, and midline of the torso. For example, an injury may be located 12 cm below the top of the head and 1 cm left of the midline. This may be important when different scenarios are given in an attempt to explain the causation of the injury. Correlation between the different scenarios and the location of the injuries on the child's body may prove or disprove one or all of the histories presented. Diagrams should be available and used if necessary as they may become extremely valuable in trying to convey your findings to a family or jury.

When examining a body, both at the scene and in the autopsy suite, documentation of postmortem changes is important. These changes should be conveyed through pictures as they may have progressed from the time the body is examined at the place of death to the time of autopsy. The standard postmortem changes that are usually documented (rigor mortis, livor mortis, algor mortis, and decomposition) have been studied in adults; thus, in children, the timing of these changes may be different than is stated below. We know that children have a lower muscle mass than do adults and lose heat at a quicker rate, both of which play a role in the rate of postmortem change. *Rigor mortis* is the stiffening of the body. It is the result of cross-linking of actin and myosin to form actinomyosin as the level of ATP decreases. In general, this process begins within 2 to 6 hours after death and starts in the smaller muscle groups first (6). By 12 hours, rigor is usually fully formed and stays as such for another 12 hours before it begins to fade. *Livor mortis* is the settling of the blood via gravity after circulation ceases. Lividity appears within 30 minutes after death and will become "fixed" after about 12 hours. Prior to becoming fixed, the blood will move with gravity as the body is moved. Once fixed, no matter how the body is moved, lividity will not follow gravitational pull and will remain in the same anatomic location. This is why photographs of the child at the scene are extremely important; it may be the only time you can see the true lividity pattern, which correlates with the position of the child when found (Figure 7-1). *Algor mortis* is the change

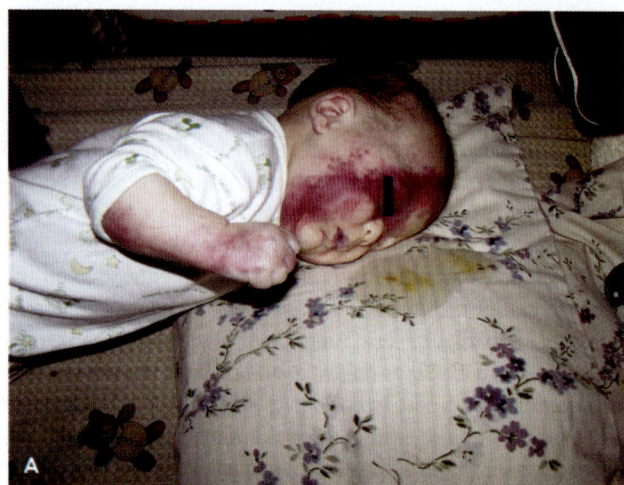
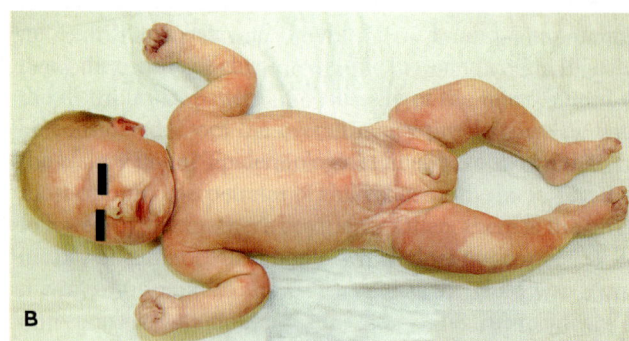

FIGURE 7-1 • **A:** Photograph at scene showing lividity on the anterior surface of the body. **B:** Photograph at autopsy showing the lividity on the face much less recognizable.

in body temperature after death. Variables that need to be considered when evaluating algor mortis are the decedent's antemortem temperature (did he or she have a fever?) and the temperature and humidity of the environment where the body was found. Certain drugs may increase an individual's temperature as well, such as cocaine and methamphetamine. Once the individual dies, the body temperature will start to equilibrate with the ambient temperature. Algor mortis is not a very reliable marker for determining the time since death. *Decomposition* consists of autolysis, putrefaction, and mummification. *Autolysis* is the result of internal cell breakdown due to the body's innate enzymes, commonly seen in the pancreas. *Putrefaction* is the result of bacteria and fungi spreading throughout the body. These organisms degrade the tissues resulting in gaseous by-products that lead to the foul odor associated with decomposition, softening of the organs, and microscopic bubbles seen on histologic analysis. *Mummification* is the drying out of the tissues secondary to an arid environment. If a stillborn fetus is being evaluated, the postmortem changes are the result of maceration. *Maceration* is due to the fetus floating in a pool of amniotic fluid with resultant skin changes such as erythema and sloughing, brown-red discoloration starting at the umbilical stump, liquefaction of internal organs, and microscopic loss of nuclear basophilia of the tubular cells of the renal cortex (Figure 7-2). Nonfetal bodies that are found in environments containing moisture can result in adipocere, a waxy substance produced by hydrolysis and hydrogenation of body fat, usually as a result of *Clostridium perfringens*. Other postmortem changes that may occur and should be documented include insect activity and animal predation. In certain cases, evaluation of the insects can be performed by an entomologist, and an opinion can be rendered concerning how long the child has been dead.

After the initial assessment, photographs, and external examination have been completed, any injuries, or suspected injuries, should be thoroughly documented. They should be described, measured, and photographed with a ruler and case identifier. If the injury is suggestive of a bite mark, an L-shaped ruler should be used in the photograph. After all of the injuries have been documented, punch biopsies can be taken and processed for histologic analysis. More specific details of various injuries are described below.

The internal examination starts with a "Y"-shaped incision. Documentation of any subcutaneous soft tissue injuries should be documented and photographed. If there is any abnormal fluid accumulation in any of the cavities, it should be measured and described. The chest plate will then be removed after documenting any fractures that may be present. The internal organs should be examined *in situ* to assess for any injury, malformation, or natural disease process. Internal body fluids, such as blood (if unable to be obtained externally) and urine, should be collected at this time and placed into the correct tube to be sent for analysis. Bile and blood should be collected and placed on specifically designed cards for metabolic and biologic studies. In infants, it is recommended to remove all of the organs en bloc as this allows for a better evaluation of the interconnections

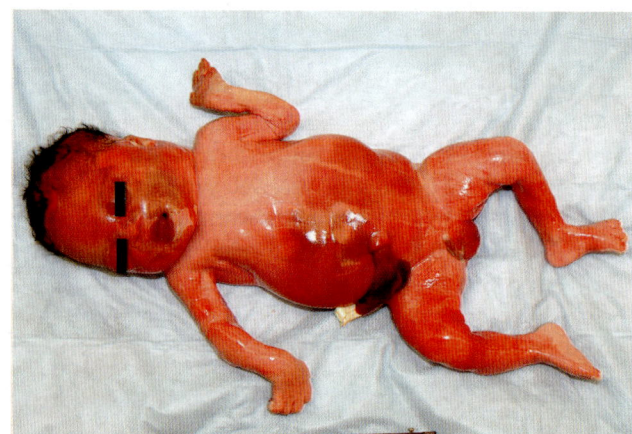

FIGURE 7-2 • Macerated fetus showing erythema and skin sloughing. This is indicative of a death *in utero*, thus ruling out a live birth.

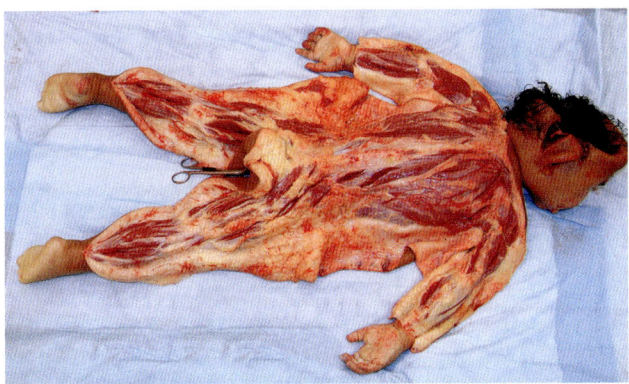

FIGURE 7-3 • Posterior dissection of an infant to evaluate for trauma. The posterior neck, back, and all four extremities are dissected into the soft tissues to look for hemorrhage.

between the organs and vasculature. The pleura should be stripped to allow for direct visualization of the ribs, and if any abnormality is identified, that portion of the rib should be removed. A radiograph of that specimen can be taken prior to decalcification, dissection, and histologic evaluation. If injuries are identified, or there is the suspicion of abuse, a posterior dissection of the neck, back, and all four extremities should be performed (Figure 7-3). This allows for evaluation of the soft tissues as well as direct visualization of the posterior aspect of the vertebrae and the long bones of the extremities. All of these steps need to be performed because skeletal injuries in children are often beyond the scope of the standard autopsy and radiology (7–9). In 2009, Love and Sanchez introduced a new technique, the pediatric skeletal examination (PSE) (10), to evaluate fractures in suspected child abuse cases. This is a fairly labor-intensive and time-consuming procedure that involves dissection down to the bone to allow for direct visualization of fractures. Love et al. (11) reviewed 94 cases of suspected inflicted trauma, half of which utilized the PSE and half of which did not. They showed that more fractures were identified with the PSE than without and determined that it was a valuable tool.

The autopsy is only one of the many tools utilized by the forensic pathologist in formulating his or her conclusions. Some of the other methodologies available to the forensic pathologist include radiology, photography (both antemortem and postmortem), metabolic analysis, toxicology, vitreous chemical analysis, microbiology, odontology, anthropology, trace evidence, ballistics, and biology (DNA). Depending on the case, any combination of the above ancillary studies may be utilized; in addition to investigation, which should be performed in every case.

Radiology

Every infant who presents for autopsy, as well as any child or adolescent with penetrating injury or suspected abuse, should undergo skeletal radiography. In infants, the entire skeleton should be x-rayed, whether it be a digital skeletal survey, computed tomography, magnetic resonance imaging, or multiple individual films that reveal the entire skeleton. A single plain film "babygram" is discouraged as the most common of inflicted skeletal injuries are often missed with these types of films. Radiology is extremely important as certain types of fractures, such as classic metaphyseal lesions diagnostic of nonaccidental trauma, may be better visualized radiographically (12). If fractures are identified during the autopsy, they can be dissected, removed, and reimaged for better definition.

Photography

Photography is an extremely important ancillary study. Overall photographs of the body as it is received in the morgue should be taken prior to removal of clothing, personal effects, and therapeutic devices. Photographs of the body naked, both front and back, should then be taken. All injuries should be photographically documented. Sometimes, photographs of the child in life can be compared to postmortem photographs to highlight similarities or differences. These photographs may be used in a court of law to portray injuries or a lack thereof.

Metabolic Analysis

Metabolic studies can be requested on either blood or bile stain cards to test for the more common metabolic disorders. The CDC, Office of the Chief Medical Examiner in Virginia, and a private laboratory conducted a population-based study of all child deaths under 3 years of age from 1996 to 2001 and revealed that 1% of these children had a positive metabolic screen using tandem mass spectrometry. Not only does this help identify the cause of the child's death but also it may prevent a false determination of child maltreatment as well as help prevent a subsequent death of one of the child's siblings (13).

Toxicology

Toxicology should be performed on all cases. This is to rule out both accidental and intentional intoxications. Certain drugs can be found in breast milk, while other drugs can be transferred to the child via transdermal patches. Some parents have been known to hide drugs in their child's diapers, while some children have found their way into their parent's prescription and/or illicit drugs. Gray top tubes contain potassium oxalate, which is an anticoagulant, and sodium fluoride, a cholinesterase inhibitor. These tubes should be used when submitting blood for toxicologic analysis as they will help prevent degradation of certain drugs (14).

Chemistry

Vitreous humor is the best postmortem biologic specimen to use for the analysis of electrolytes and glucose. It should be aspirated only after a negative internal evaluation of the retrobulbar soft tissues and perioptic nerve sheaths. Dehydration patterns and diabetes mellitus can be diagnosed using this specimen. The procedure of withdrawing vitreous humor involves inserting a 20-gauge needle attached to a 6- or 10-mL syringe into the globe just anterior to the lateral canthus. After puncturing the globe, slight pressure should be used to aspirate the gelatinous fluid, being careful not to go too deep or use too much force, as the retina may be damaged making analysis unreliable. Only clear fluid should be sent for testing as the contamination by blood or tissue will alter the results.

Cultures

Infectious diseases are one of the most important public health concerns; thus, cultures should be considered in all autopsies. However, there are many who believe that postmortem cultures are of minimal or no value. Issues that arise when considering the value of postmortem cultures include contamination and postmortem spread of organisms. Essentially, bacteria in deceased individuals are similar to those in a laboratory culture as they can spread without any resistance from antibodies. Most contaminated specimens grow multiple organisms, whereas a single organism should arouse suspicion of a true infection. Even with a "positive" culture, it is of vital importance to perform microscopic analysis of the tissues in an attempt to determine if these positive cultures are the result of a true infection or the result of postmortem overgrowth. If organisms are seen microscopically, the presence or absence of inflammation will help make the determination if the bacteria are due to postmortem overgrowth or a true antemortem infection. Once the body is opened, there is rapid contamination of the surfaces of the internal organs from fluids that have now been exposed to external organisms; thus, a sterile technique is needed. When procuring a culture of an internal organ, the prosector must first sear the surface of that organ to sterilize it. This can be accomplished by taking a scalpel blade or spatula, heating it with a flame, and touching the surface of the organ until it is dried and black or white from the burn. Utilizing a sterile blade, a puncture of that organ should be performed through the burned surface and a culture swab placed through that opening. If any bodily fluid enters that site, it is deemed contaminated. This should all be done before removal of any organ. Another factor in deciding if blood cultures should be performed relies on the circumstances of the case. Cultures in the majority of postmortem examinations rarely reveal significant new information; thus, it may be difficult to justify the cost of the test (15). In addition, the amount of blood that is often obtained at postmortem examination in children is minimal, and decisions must be made how that blood is best utilized (cultures, toxicology, metabolic analysis, etc.). The procedure to aspirate cerebrospinal fluid for viral and/or microbiologic studies should be performed in the same fashion as a clinical spinal tap would be done. Swab the skin with alcohol or Betadine, use a sterile needle to enter the interspinous space, and aspirate. As multiple attempts may be necessary, it is recommended to start caudally with each reattempt moving cranially. This is to prevent migration of blood into the specimen. Other options are aspirating CSF through the foramen magnum or ventricles (15).

Odontology and Anthropology

Odontology and anthropology consultation can be used on an "as-needed" basis. Odontology can be used for identification purposes via comparison with antenatal dental films, which is rare in infants but may become more prevalent in the teenage years. Dental cavities and fillings can be used for comparison as well. Evaluating the eruption pattern of the teeth may assist in aging of the individual. Anthropology is a valuable resource for a number of reasons. A forensic anthropologist can help with the identification of a person, as well as perform trauma analysis on skeletal remains. They can measure certain bones and compare them to a standardized chart as well as inspect ossification zones to estimate the age the child was when he/she died.

Scene Investigation

Scene investigation is an extremely important component of death investigation, and in certain cases, it may be the most critical. It may be performed in the presence of, or by, law enforcement, the coroner, and/or the medical examiner. Photographs should be taken of every scene as it may be the only time you will be able to see the site of the incident and/or death undisturbed, as it was when the individual died. Photographs should include the overall view of the scene and continue progressively closer until the exact location of death is found. The child should be photographed where found, both front and back, as progression of postmortem changes may occur between the time of the scene investigation and the time of the autopsy. This is well known with lividity, which may appear on the posterior aspect of the child's body by the time of autopsy but was anteriorly distributed at the scene, indicating a prone position and possible asphyxia. Interviews should be performed at the initial scene visit. These interviews should be taken from the caregivers, others in the residence at the time of the death, and neighbors. These individuals should be interviewed separately to see if all of their stories coincide. Interviews may be performed a second time, if necessary. The overall surroundings should be assessed, that is, cleanliness of the residence, appearance of other children, food in the refrigerator, appropriateness of toys for the child's age, animals, infestation, weapons, medications/drugs, and child's sleeping environment, to name a few. A doll reenactment (in the case of an infant sleep-related death) can aid in the assessment of the child's position when laid down to sleep and when found, including the surroundings, and in injury related deaths to allow the caregiver to show his/her version of how the injury may have occurred. If available, a buckwheat doll without any specific anatomical features should be used. An "F" can be written on the front and a "B" can be written on the back (Figure 7-4). The doll should be given to the individual who found the child, and he or she should be asked to show exactly what position the child was in when found. This should be photographed and/or videotaped. Any potential evidence should be procured and brought with the body to the autopsy. Many times, the body has been removed from the scene, either by emergency medical personnel or by personal vehicle. This does not negate the importance of a scene investigation. An investigator should be sent to the location where the child was found to perform a thorough investigation despite the fact that the scene may have been altered. The body should be photographed in the hospital, if that is where the child

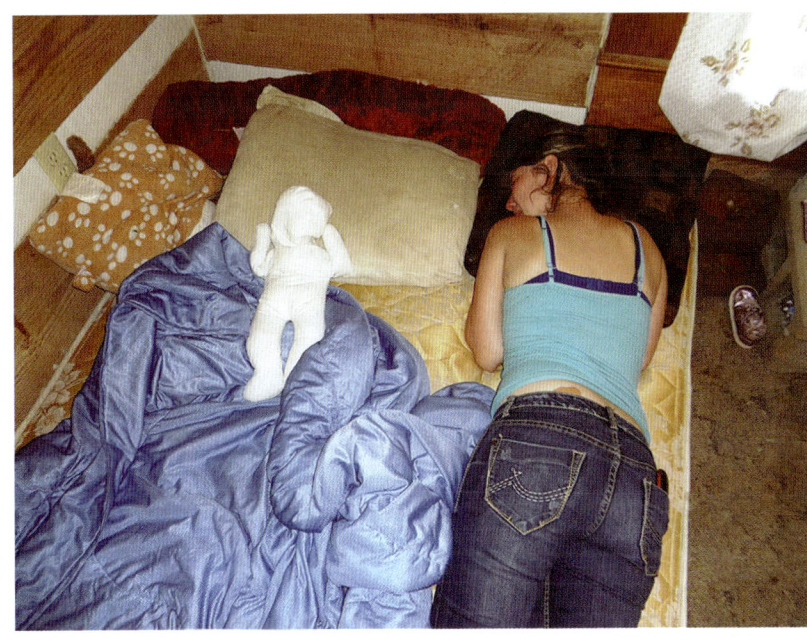

FIGURE 7-4 • Buckwheat doll used for a reenactment of the child's position when found. An "F" can be written on the doll to indicate the child's front, and a "B" can be written on the doll to indicate the child's back.

was taken. If there are patterned injuries to the body, look throughout the residence for implements that may have been used, and submit those to the medical examiner office for evaluation. All of the information that has been gleaned from the scene investigation will be evaluated in conjunction with the autopsy findings to determine the cause and manner of death.

Medical devices used in resuscitation should be left in place and documented to prevent any misinterpretation of findings at autopsy. As in any hospital autopsy, the medical history is of great importance. Medical records, including, but not limited to, birth records, pediatrician records, reports of emergency medical services, and records from the emergency department from the final admission, should be requested and reviewed. It is important to remember that just because a child has a significant medical history, it does not mean that he or she can't die an unnatural death.

An important topic that the forensic pathologist is confronted with is organ donation. In most jurisdictions, the organ procurement agency consults with the medical examiner before proceeding with harvesting on cases that fall under the medical examiner's jurisdiction. In addition to solid organ donation, the eyes, skin, long bones, and heart for heart valves may be procured. This is a very important and potentially lifesaving procedure that needs to be approached in a delicate manner. One needs to carefully weigh the potential benefits of donation to live patients while not disrupting any evidence that may affect the determination of cause and manner of death and possible litigation. Child abuse deaths are the cases that are most often denied donation due to the potential for disrupting evidence on the skin and within the body cavities. A major concern is the alteration of rib fractures, whether acute or remote, and the possibility of causing a posterior rib fracture as a result of a thoracotomy for harvesting the heart or lungs. One method for harvesting of the heart and/or lungs that has been proposed is a modified thoracotomy technique where an autopsy-type incision is made into the skin and the chest is opened through serial incisions of the anterior cartilaginous segments of the ribs. This prevents any strain being placed on the ribs that may result in alterations of fractures (16). Rarely, organ procurement will proceed despite objection from the medical examiner. This may result in an undetermined cause and manner of death as well as animosity between agencies (17). The best way to prevent a situation such as this is to have open and good communication with your local organ donation group. Part of the communication necessary to maintain a good working relationship between the autopsy pathologist and the organ procurement organizations includes the sharing of findings from the procuring institution, autopsy findings, and laboratory results. Photographs can be taken prior to, and during, the procurement. The organ and tissue procurement agencies are required to perform a number of tests to make sure that what they are transplanting is safe for the recipient. The results of these tests can and should be shared with the medical examiner and may aid in determining the cause and manner of the child's death. One must remember that you have a responsibility not only to those requiring organs but also to the families of the deceased individual as well as the deceased himself/herself.

SUDDEN DEATH

In the pediatric forensic setting, the most common presentation of death will be that of a sudden unexplained death, most often in infancy. Approximately 4000 infants die suddenly and unexpectedly each year in the United States without any prior medical history (18). These deaths are most often determined to be due to SIDS, sudden unexplained infant death (SUID, a.k.a. sudden unexplained death in infancy, SUDI), or asphyxia. Epidemiologically, SUID and

SUDI are all coded with the same ICD code as SIDS deaths. The basic difference between these three categories includes sleep environment and evidence, or lack thereof, of asphyxia at the scene and/or autopsy. An analysis of 3136 sleep-related sudden unexpected infant deaths revealed that 24% were sleeping in a crib or on their back when found, 70% were on a sleep surface other than a recommended crib or bassinet, 64% were found on their side or stomach, and 49% were sleeping with an adult (19). The differences in certification of these types of deaths are discussed below. The Centers for Disease Control and Prevention has issued a standardized SUID investigation checklist available to any agency wishing to utilize it for child death investigation (20).

Sturner outlined common errors in forensic pediatric pathology that highlight the necessity of much of what has been described above (21). The ten categories of errors that he highlighted include an incomplete or absent scene investigation, including the "bed of death" and environmental analysis such as temperature; inadequate or insufficient photography, including the position of the child when found and videography if necessary; improper postmortem interval assessment, such as forgetting that rigidity can become complete within a few hours and body temperature equilibrates within its surroundings quickly, especially in children; inadequate or incomplete medical records, including birth records; incomplete preautopsy study, such as body measurements; inadequate gross autopsy examination, such as forgetting to evaluate the gastrointestinal tract; incomplete microscopic examination, forgetting to examine all organs under the microscope; incomplete laboratory studies, such as toxicology and metabolic analysis; failure to differentiate and document artifacts, such as distinguishing antemortem from postmortem changes; and failure to give appropriate importance and significance to findings, such as how much alveolar acute inflammation constitutes a significant pneumonia (21).

Sudden Infant Death Syndrome (SIDS)

The term SIDS was initially coined in 1969 to define any unexpected death of an infant or young child that remained unexplained after a thorough investigation, including autopsy. It is essentially a diagnosis of exclusion. Currently, to determine that a death is due to SIDS, one has to adhere to a strict guideline, which includes a child between the age of 1 month and 1 year, without any pre-existing conditions including prematurity, and being found supine on an appropriate sleep surface without anything that could compromise the child's ability to breathe. The diagnosis cannot be made until a complete autopsy has been performed, including toxicology, histology, metabolic analysis, review of medical records, and a thorough scene investigation. If no other potential or actual etiologically specific pathology is found, the cause of death can be deemed SIDS. The rate of SIDS has decreased dramatically over the years. The reason for the decreased incidence is twofold: (a) the back to sleep campaign, and (b) the change in the definition of SIDS. In 1994, the National Institute of Child Health and Development initiated the Back to Sleep campaign. Over the following 10 years, the rate of SIDS deaths decreased by greater than 50%, decreasing from 1.34 per 1000 live births to 0.64 per 1000 births (22). A number of risk factors for SIDS have been identified such as male sex, black race, and winter months. Most cases of SIDS occur before 6 months of age, usually between 2 and 4 months of age. A meta-analysis of 35 case control studies revealed that both prenatal and postnatal maternal smoking was associated with an increased risk of SIDS (23). This was dose dependent and suggested that maternal cessation of smoking may be protective against SIDS. Another meta-analysis, this time on 18 studies, showed that breastfeeding of any extent and duration was protective against SIDS, possibly as a result of its immunologic benefits (24,25). There is a divide between medical examiners as to the manner of death in SIDS cases, whether it be natural or undetermined. Many believe that all external factors have been ruled out and thus it is a natural death, whereas others believe that we still do not know why the child died and thus it deserves an undetermined manner. The autopsy in these cases is essentially negative, thus ruling out any obvious natural disease or traumatic injury. A common finding at autopsy is the presence of petechiae on the serosal surfaces of the thymus, lungs, and heart. These are nonspecific findings, which can be seen in other causes, such as asphyxia. Microscopically, these petechiae may be seen, as well as pulmonary edema, congestion, and slight hemorrhage. Recent research has focused on morphologic differences in the brainstems of children who have died of SIDS suggesting that these cases may be due to immature development of the centers responsible for arousal, cardiovascular, and respiratory functions. When these children are faced with an environmental stressor, they are vulnerable to sudden death. This has led to the triple risk model: underlying vulnerability, critical stage of development (peak between 2 and 4 months of postnatal life), and an exogenous stressor (26,27). Intrinsic and extrinsic risk factors have been identified. The intrinsic risk factors include African American race, male gender, prematurity, and prenatal maternal smoking or alcohol use, whereas extrinsic risk factors include any physical stressor present around the time of death such as prone or side sleep, bed sharing, over bundling, soft bedding, or the child's face being covered (26). Ninety-nine percent of SIDS infants had at least 1 intrinsic or extrinsic risk factor, and 75% had at least 1 of each (26). As will be described below, a diagnostic shift has taken a number of these extrinsic factors and changed the terminology from SIDS to SUID (sudden unexplained infant death) (27). There is an adage that the first unexpected death of a child in a family may be SIDS, a subsequent death may be deemed undetermined, and a third death is a homicide until proven otherwise.

Recent studies have highlighted the prevalence of cardiac channelopathies in sudden infant deaths. Some of the more well-known disorders that are identified in sudden death in young individuals are long QT syndrome, Brugada syndrome, short QT syndrome, and catecholaminergic polymorphic ventricular tachycardia. Long QT syndrome has a prevalence of 1 in 2500 and is currently known to involve over 700 mutations in 12 genes (28). Mutations in repolarizing cardiac potassium channels KCNQ1/Kv7.1 (LQT1) and hERG1/Kv11.1 (LQT2) are the most common and predispose the individual to ventricular arrhythmias, syncope, and sudden cardiac death (29). Schwartz et al. identified that 50% of a cohort of SIDS deaths had a prolongation of the corrected QT interval and that if there was the presence of a prolonged corrected QT interval in the first week of life, it imparted a 41.6 times increased risk of SIDS (30). The other disorders mentioned have varying mutations and lethality but usually present with the same symptoms. The above-mentioned known channelopathies are seen in SIDS cases but research on children who have died of SIDS shows that the majority of the channelopathies in these deaths are related to mutations in the sodium channels (29). The importance of identifying a channelopathy as the cause of death is not only to help the family come to an understanding of why their child died but to alert the family to the possibility of a sibling having the same mutation and to refer him or her for evaluation. Other genetic abnormalities have been found in infants who die suddenly and unexpectedly, such as medium-chain acyl-CoA dehydrogenase (MCAD) deficiency, which is the most common inherited disorder of fatty acid metabolism, which presents in early childhood with a potentially fatal episode of hypoketotic hypoglycemic crisis (28).

An apparent life-threatening event (ALTE), which used to be termed "near miss SIDS," is defined as "an episode that is frightening to the observer, since it is characterized by some combination of apnea (centrally or occasionally obstructive), color change (usually cyanotic or pallid, but occasionally erythematosus or plethoric), and marked change in muscle tone (usually marked limpness), choking or gagging" (31). In approximately half of these cases, an underlying etiology such as episodic gastroesophageal reflux, respiratory infection, and seizure disorder is found. The other half are termed idiopathic (32). Current research has focused on polymorphisms in genes that regulate brainstem neurotransmitters. The medullary serotonin or 5-hydroxytryptamine (5-HT) system with the serotonin transporter gene (5-HTT) regulates multiple autonomic homeostatic functions such as ventilation, thermoregulation, and arousal (28). Abnormalities in the genes that regulate these functions can have serious consequences and thus are thought to possibly play a role in sudden infant deaths. Serotonin seems to play a role in these deaths and may be a valuable tracer for the risk of SIDS in a child with idiopathic ALTE (32). There have been varying reports as to the number of infants who have experienced an ALTE prior to a lethal episode.

Sudden Unexplained Infant Death (SUID)

SUID utilizes the findings in SIDS but adds in one or a number of the above-mentioned risk factors. The most common investigative findings that result in a death being deemed an SUID instead of an SIDS is bed sharing with an adult in an adult-sized bed (Figure 7-5). Bed sharing is a controversial subject with many believing it is an unsafe sleep environment and others believing it to be safe and promote bonding between the caregiver and child. A nationwide telephone survey revealed that 19.4% of mothers shared a bed with their infant more than 50% of the time, 27.6% bed shared sometimes, and 52.7% never bed shared (33). Another study in Oregon, which represented a greater diversity in its study population, revealed that 35.2% of mothers frequently bed shared, 41.4% sometimes bed shared, and 23.4% never did (34). This, or any of the other risk factors of an unsafe sleep environment, raises the possibility of an asphyxial death, but there is no way to prove it without a confession from the caregiver that the caregiver, or another individual in the bed, was lying on top of the child when he/she was found (see following section for asphyxial deaths) or that the face was

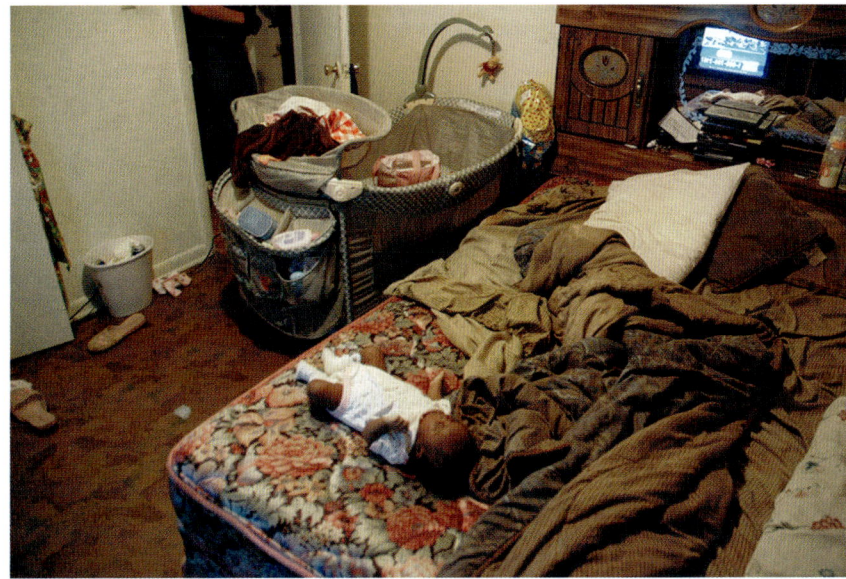

FIGURE 7-5 • "Unsafe sleep environment." The child was found bed sharing with adults in the adult-sized bed that contained soft bedding and pillows. Notice the bassinet that was not being used for sleep.

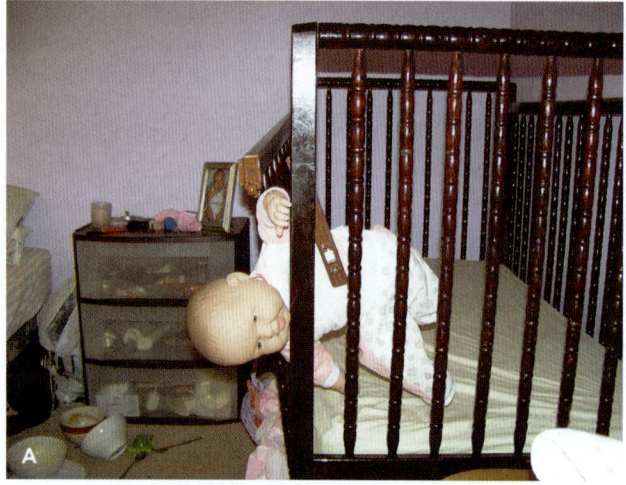 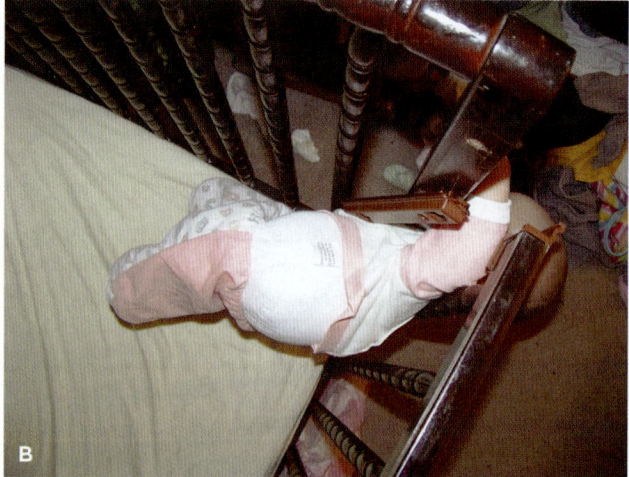

FIGURE 7-6 • Wedging. Doll reenactment of a child who was found wedged between the slats of a crib. **A:** View from the side. **B:** View from above. Autopsy revealed a demarcation line at the level of the wedging.

covered in some manner. The weakness of the infant neck muscles makes the infant more prone to asphyxia as a result of rebreathing carbon dioxide and decreased oxygen intake. The autopsies in these cases are most often also essentially negative, but the history or scene investigation shows an unsafe environment.

Asphyxia

The autopsy of a child who died of asphyxia is also quite often completely negative. For this reason, the investigation may hold the key to determining the cause of death to be asphyxia. This may be elucidated by a doll re-enactment with photographs, documentation of the postmortem changes at the scene, and witness accounts. The autopsy in these cases may show pallor over the nose and mouth, indicating pressure over these areas, or a line of demarcation in lividity suggestive of compression (Figure 7-6). Asphyxial deaths can result from wedging (the child wedged between two surfaces such as a mattress and wall), overlaying (an individual found lying on top of the child), or obstruction of the face (such as by a blanket or pillow). Overlaying is most often seen in children less than 5 months of age but has been found in children up until 2 years of age (35). As the number of bed sharers increases so does the risk of overlaying. The bed sharers do not need to be adults. There have been documented cases of other children, often siblings, found lying on top of one another where the child located beneath the other child was dead. Parental intoxication increases the risk of overlaying, and some states have even considered criminal charges against these parents. The child may not be able to cry out as the mouth and nose may be covered and the thorax compressed. If the history conveyed by the caregiver suggests the possibility of overlaying but external examination reveals multiple cutaneous or oral injuries, inflicted trauma should be strongly considered. Homicidal asphyxia, such as smothering, can be very difficult to diagnose at autopsy as these examinations may be completely unremarkable as well. In these cases, the pathologist should pay specific attention to the oral region. One may see abrasions of the lips or nose and lacerations of the mucosal surface of the lips or frenula (Figure 7-7). There has been the suggestion by some that severe pulmonary hemorrhage and/or a marked number of intra-alveolar siderophages is consistent with an asphyxial death. Krous *et al.* looked at 444 cases of infant deaths that were determined to die of SIDS, accidental suffocation, or inflicted suffocation (36). They reviewed the files and microscopic slides to evaluate for intrathoracic petechiae, pulmonary hemorrhage, and siderophages. They

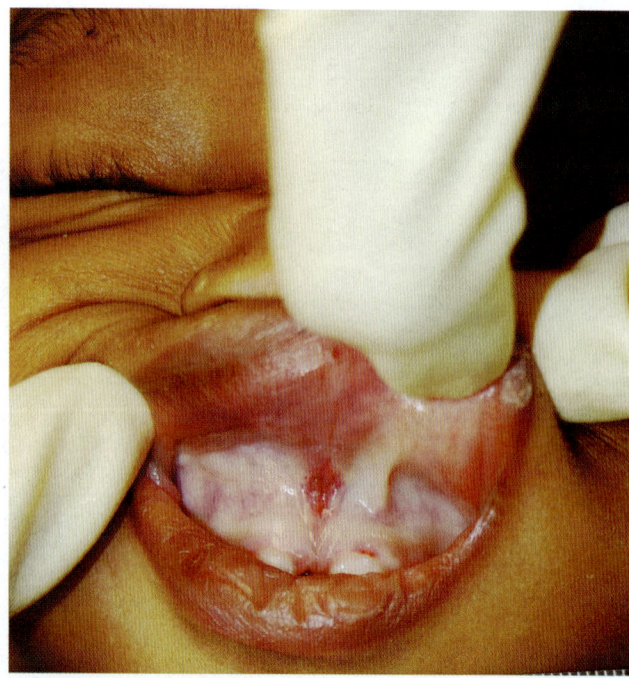

FIGURE 7-7 • Laceration of the upper frenulum in a case of homicidal asphyxia (smothering).

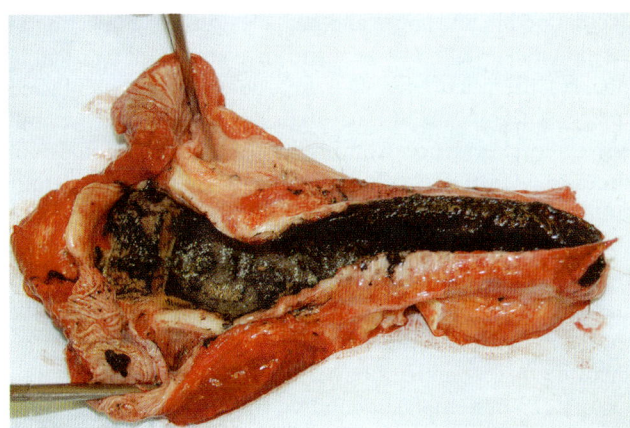

FIGURE 7-8 • Dark black soot within the tracheobronchial tree of an individual who died in a house fire. This, in conjunction with a positive carboxyhemoglobin saturation above 10%, indicates that the child was alive prior to the fire.

determined that any of these findings in isolation cannot confidently be used to distinguish between a diagnosis of SIDS or suffocation, but if there is significant pulmonary hemorrhage, a thorough inspection of the body for signs of trauma should be considered. In addition, when the number of intra-alveolar siderophages is prominent, the diagnosis of idiopathic pulmonary hemosiderosis should be considered (37). This is a rare disease with a possible hereditary component and a clinical history of cough and hemoptysis. In the acute setting, acute pulmonary hemorrhage is its usual presentation.

Special subtypes of asphyxia include drowning and smoke inhalation. In drowning deaths, a full autopsy examination should be performed in an attempt to identify any natural disease or traumatic event that may have led to the drowning. In infants, drowning often occurs in the bathtub, especially if they are not attended to appropriately, whereas toddlers drown in pools more often as they may wander and enter the pool without the ability to swim. Once adolescence is reached, the risks change to include open bodies of water. Toxicologic analysis should be performed in these cases as often there is the combination of alcohol and swimming that contribute to the death of these adolescents. Young children are considered a high-risk group for deaths due to smoke inhalation, the most common scenario occurring as a result of a house fire. Autopsy examination of these children should be performed not only to test for a carboxyhemoglobin level but also to rule out other injuries. Carboxyhemoglobin saturation is one test used to identify if the child may have been alive prior to the start of the fire, which will be displayed by a carboxyhemoglobin level of 10% or more. Indicators that suggest carbon monoxide exposure include cherry-red lividity and cherry-red discoloration of the viscera. Black soot may be found focally or throughout the tracheobronchial tree (Figure 7-8).

Accidental strangulation is another form of asphyxia that used to be seen more often but has decreased in incidence due to the acts of the Consumer Product Safety Commission, public awareness, and manufacturing changes. Common household items that have led to accidental strangulation include pull strings on window blinds and pacifier strings. Ligature hanging can be seen in the teenage years as a result of suicidal intent or accidentally due to autoerotic asphyxia or "pass out games." Just the weight of the head is needed to cause death via hanging; thus, it is not uncommon to find the individual sitting, kneeling, or with the feet touching the ground (Figure 7-9A). These cases deserve the attention of the medical examiner due to the sensitive nature of these deaths. Determining the cause and manner of death in these cases may elicit strong emotional responses from families. External examination of the neck in any form of hanging may reveal a ligature furrow around the neck. This is usually composed of an area of depression with abrasion or dried yellow skin. The furrow usually has a horizontal orientation on the anterior neck and angles upward and backward behind both ears in suicidal hangings but may have a different configuration

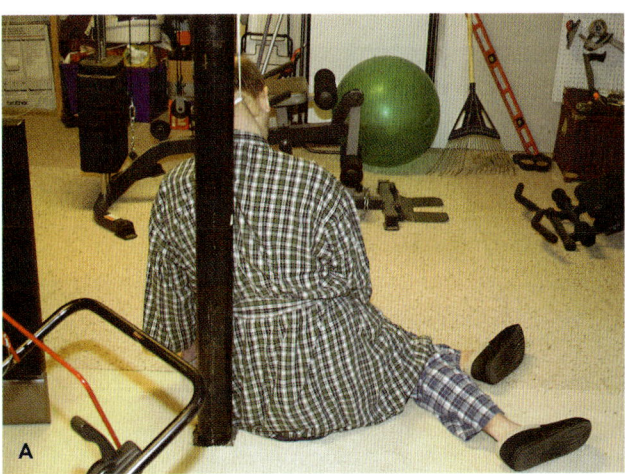
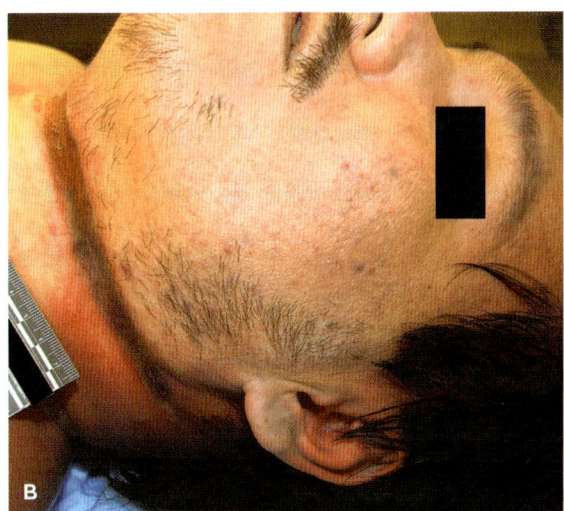

FIGURE 7-9 • Suicidal hanging. **A:** Note that the body is not fully suspended. Only the weight of the head is necessary to cause death. **B:** Ligature furrow on the neck after removal of the ligature.

in other types of hangings, depending on the position of the body (Figure 7-9B). The furrow findings will be present if the individual was hanging for at least a number of minutes to hours. Internal examination of the neck should reveal the lack of intramuscular hemorrhage in the strap muscles, and there should not be any fracture of the hyoid bone or thyroid cartilage. The same is true in the case of autoerotic asphyxia, except that the ligature furrow may have varying configurations depending on the apparatus that was used. Autoerotic asphyxia describes an act performed by an individual seeking to heighten orgasm by restricting oxygen to the brain. This is usually done by placing a ligature around the neck, which is attached to an escape mechanism that allows the person to release the tension on the neck prior to passing out. Essentially, these deaths are due to the failure to utilize the escape mechanism in a timely manner, most likely due to the individual losing consciousness. Once again, scene investigation may be the most important aspect of the investigation. Suicidal hangings may have a "note of intent" at the scene, or messages may be found on the individual's phone or social media account that sheds light on his or her mental state. In autoerotic asphyxia cases, the scene has often been altered prior to law enforcement or emergency medical services arrival due to the social stigma that may accompany this type of death. At the scene of an autoerotic asphyxial death, look for any sort of pornography, clothing of the opposite sex, and any information on the deceased's computer that may indicate the possibility of experimentation. The manner of death in autoerotic asphyxia cases is accident. The mechanism of death in any of these cases is usually one of vascular occlusion and not as a result of airway occlusion. Depending on the width of the ligature used, pressure will be placed on the jugular veins first and carotid arteries next. Petechiae can be seen on the conjunctivae, oral mucosa, and face when the drainage of blood from the brain is halted due to occlusion of the veins with continuation of blood supply to the brain through the carotid arteries. Asphyxial games (a.k.a. the choking game, Space Monkey, Funky Chicken, etc.) are becoming more prevalent in the teenage population. Autopsy findings include florid facial petechiae, but often, there is absence of conjunctival petechiae. These games are often performed in isolation, as opposed to historically being done in groups. The mechanism of death is similar to those of autoerotic asphyxia, but there is no elaborate setup and no sexual connection. If the right questions are asked, the investigator may be able to elicit a history of playing this game with a continuous attempt to prolong the length of time of asphyxia (38). Cervical spine fracture, "hangman's fracture," is not seen in any of the above described cases as they occur in judicial hangings or the rare instance where an individual jumps from a height with a noose around the neck. There needs to be a drop from a height with rapid deceleration to cause this type of fracture.

Injuries, Nonaccidental and Accidental

Injuries to a child may be accidental or nonaccidental. Children who present with injuries should be examined by a physician who specializes in the evaluation of these types of injuries. This is of vital importance in order to avoid a false accusation of child abuse and possible criminal conviction of an individual who is innocent and vice versa. It is important to note that the lack of external trauma does not rule out inflicted injury as significant internal injuries can be found without any external evidence. Conversely, external trauma does not necessarily correlate with internal injuries and is not definitively diagnostic of child abuse. When documenting injuries, the distribution, pattern, and severity of the injuries need to be considered. Does the overall injury profile correlate with the history given? Epidemiologic studies have shown that the most common perpetrator of child abuse is the biologic father followed by the mother's boyfriend. Often, there is the given history of a minor fall at home, which does not correlate with the injuries found to the child, or that the child was found unresponsive with no traumatic history. The true incidence of inflicted head injury is not known as the child may present with nonspecific signs that resolve, and a false diagnosis, such as a viral syndrome, may be given. The most common form of abusive injury is that of head trauma with abdominal trauma being the second most common form of inflicted trauma. Hospitalization rates for abused children aged 0 to 3 years have remained relatively stable at 2.36 per 10,000 over the last 14 years, the most prevalent group being those under 1 year old. If there is a previous report from child protective services concerning a specific child, there is a 3 times higher risk of that child suffering a sudden unexplained death (39).

Blunt Force Injuries

The most common form of injury found in child death investigation is that of blunt force. The cutaneous manifestations are usually in the form of contusions, abrasions, or lacerations. A contusion (bruise) is the result of a blunt impact that tears the subcutaneous vessels leading to bleeding beneath the skin (Figure 7-10). Of note, a contusion should not be aged on gross examination; thus, punch biopsies of identified contusions should be processed for microscopic examination. Many variables may affect the color and size of a contusion, including the individual's skin color, coagulation disorders,

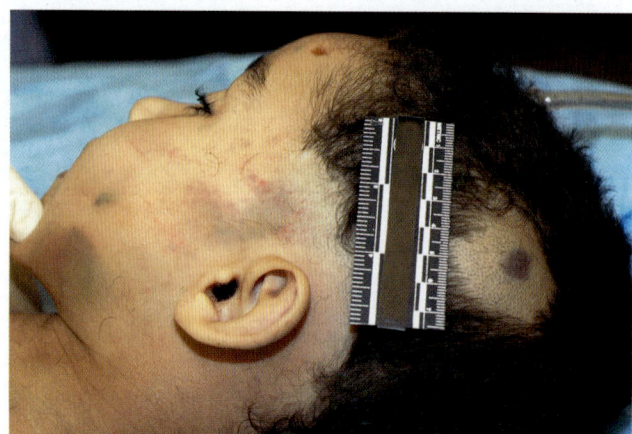

FIGURE 7-10 • Multiple contusions (bruises) of varying colors along the entirety of the left side of the child's face as a result of a blunt force trauma.

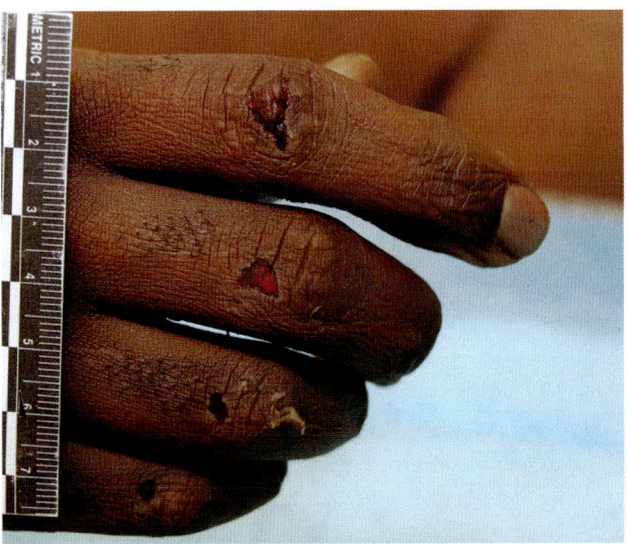

FIGURE 7-11 • Abrasions (scrapes) as a result of blunt force trauma.

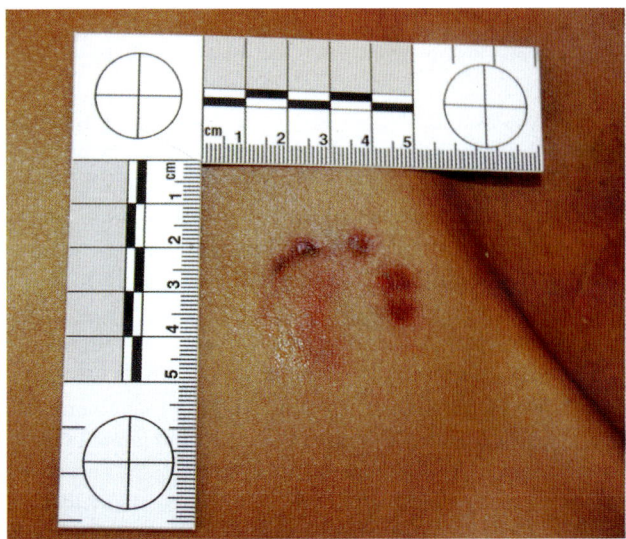

FIGURE 7-13 • Bite mark. Notice the combination of abrasion and contusion in a unique pattern. An L-shaped ruler should be used in the photograph.

inflammatory disorders, hormonal abnormalities, depth of the bleeding, location on the body, amount of blood, and the light in which the injury is evaluated. Studies of bruising in adults showed development of a bruise within 30 minutes of a traumatic insult. The size of the contusion varied but generally decreased over time (40). The one color change that may be utilized is that yellow discoloration indicates at least 18 hours since the onset of the injury due to the presence of hemosiderin. Histology may be helpful in the determination of aging a contusion but is still an estimation and not specific. In general, perivascular polymorphonuclear leukocytes may be visible around 4 hours after injury, with a peripheral infiltration by around 12 hours. Macrophages peak around 16 to 24 hours and may contain hemosiderin by 72 hours. Fibroblasts may appear at 2 to 4 days (41). An abrasion (scrape) is the result of shearing off of the superficial layers of the epidermis (Figure 7-11). A laceration is a splitting of the skin due to a

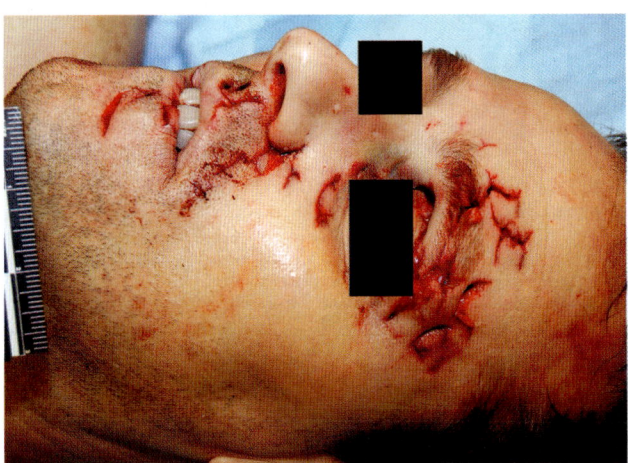

FIGURE 7-12 • Multiple lacerations (splitting of the skin) as a result of blunt force trauma. If the edges were pulled apart, "bridging" of the subcutaneous nerves and vessels would be present.

blunt impact. Examining the depths of a laceration may reveal strands of vessels and nerves "bridging" one side of the wound to the other (Figure 7-12). This helps in distinguishing a laceration from a stab wound, which will cut across all of the deep tissues, including the vessels and nerves.

A unique type of blunt force injury is the bite mark. It can comprise all of the above three blunt force trauma characteristics but often has a distinct ovoid shape (Figure 7-13). If you suspect a wound to be a bite mark, it should be immediately swabbed with a sterile cotton tip applicator that has been moistened with sterile saline or water. The swab should then be placed in a sterile container and submitted to serology to evaluate for the presence of saliva and subsequently for DNA if so desired. A control swab should be taken from a different part of the child's body. If a bite mark is identified, the pathologist should strongly consider collecting a sexual assault kit. At a minimum, this should include oral, genital, and anal swabs. Depending on the physical maturity level of the child, fingernail clippings, scalp hair, and pubic hair combings may be obtained as well. A forensic odontologist can aid in the evaluation of a potential bite mark and render an opinion as to the likelihood that the impressions on the skin were caused by the teeth of a specific individual.

Children of different ages have distinct usual patterns of accidental injuries that coincide with their physical developmental stage. Infants are relatively immobile and thus should not have contusions to any part of their body. As the child begins to "cruise," contusions may be seen on the forehead and cheeks. Toddlers often have injuries to the knees, shins, elbows, and forearms. All of these injuries should be evaluated on an individual case basis. Certain areas of the body are relatively protected and should increase the suspicion that an injury is inflicted, not accidental. These include the buttocks, lower back, midline of the abdomen, philtrum, and submental space. A reevaluation of these injuries can be performed the following day, after refrigeration, as they may become more prominent and more easily identified. Physically abused children have significantly more bruises and more areas on the body injured than do non–physically abused children. Inflicted contusions are often linear, petechial, clustered, or patterned. They are much more likely to have bruises on the buttocks, genitalia, cheeks, neck, trunk, head, anterior thighs, and arms, whereas bruises on the forehead, nose, mouth, and chin are common in both inflicted and accidental scenarios (42).

A patterned injury is one that has characteristics suggestive of an object that may have caused the injury. These can range from a surface onto which the child fell to an implement that was used to inflict the injury. Common implements used by perpetrators include hands, belts, fly swatters, and other household objects. The resultant injury to the skin will vary depending on the amount of force used and what part of the child's body was impacted. If the skin is struck with enough velocity, such as a slap, the pressure will push the blood to the periphery resulting in maximal distortion at the periphery. This will cause rupture of the peripheral vessels resulting in either petechiae or contusion outlining the shape of the implement and leaving a relatively pale area of unremarkable skin underlying the point of contact (Figure 7-14). As the amount of force increases, the vessels at the point of contact will be damaged as well, resulting in bruising over the entire area of contact. If the force remains high but the velocity is decreased, the contusion will be displayed at the point of contact, but the periphery may be spared and thus a direct image of the implement may be present. These patterns can be fairly unique and suggestive of certain objects. Once a patterned injury is identified, the investigator should be contacted and asked to visit the scene in an attempt to locate any

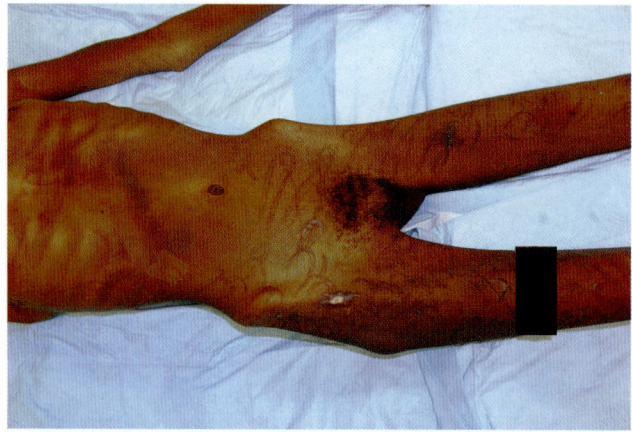

FIGURE 7-15 • Patterned injury caused by a looped electrical cord. Note how the injury conforms to the dimensions of the body.

suspicious objects. Another important finding to consider is if the injury is planar or if it conforms to the dimensions of the body. For instance, does the injury on the thigh stay in one plane or does it conform to the angulation of the body such as starting on the lateral thigh and continuing uninterrupted over the anterior and medial aspect of the thigh. If it does conform to the dimensions of the body, the implement is malleable, such as an electrical cord or belt (Figure 7-15), and investigators should be informed to collect these items from the scene. A vertical gluteal cleft injury occurs when a child is beaten over the buttocks; the convex surface flattens, and the regions immediately lateral to the vertical gluteal cleft, which are the interface between impacted and nonimpacted tissue, are subjected to shearing injury. The resulting pattern consists of vertically oriented, parallel linear contusions located on either side of the midline (Figure 7-16).

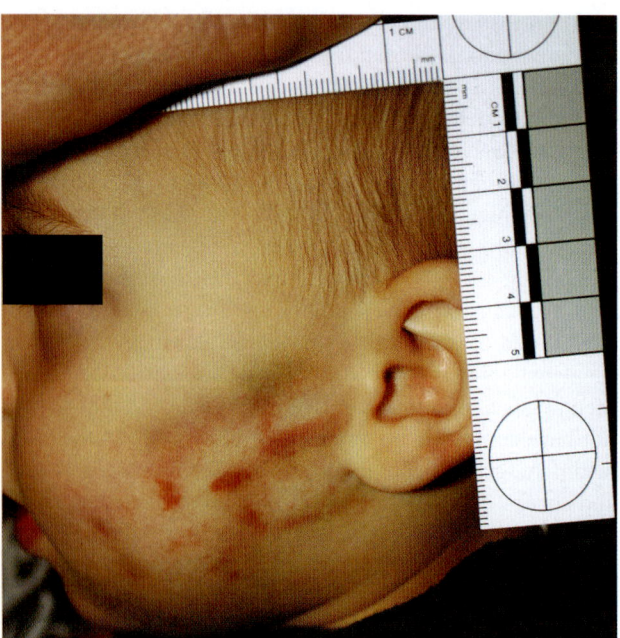

FIGURE 7-14 • Patterned contusion as the result of an open hand slap to the face.

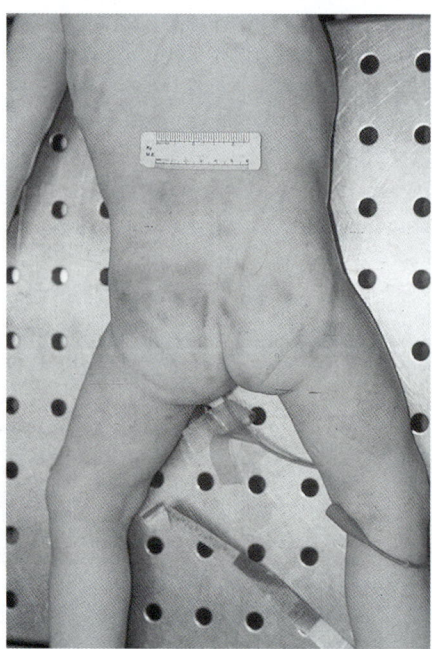

FIGURE 7-16 • Vertical gluteal cleft contusions.

A rim of petechiae may develop along the apex of the ear following direct blunt impact for the same reason. In these two examples, the pattern is dictated by the shape of the body and the anatomic lines of stress rather than by the shape of the object (43). When an injury over a joint is examined, it is helpful to move the joint into various positions. An injury viewed as irregular in the anatomic position may emerge as a pattern injury as the extremity is flexed or rotated. A "brush or burn abrasion" occurs when there is tangential contact of the skin with a solid surface, such as when a pedestrian is struck by a vehicle and subsequently strikes the pavement resulting in "road rash" (Figure 7-17).

Blunt impact injuries of the head may be focal or diffuse with scalp contusions, skull fractures, intracranial hemorrhage, and/or parenchymal injuries. Externally, abrasions, contusions, or lacerations may be seen. As stated earlier, the presence or absence of external trauma does not necessarily correlate with the internal findings. Upon reflection of the scalp, any hemorrhage in the soft tissues or galea should be documented prior to removal of the skull (Figure 7-18). The skull should then be evaluated prior to its removal and after it has been removed. Skull fractures in accidental falls are most often linear and nondisplaced and involve only one bone, usually a parietal bone. There is rarely an underlying intracranial injury. If there are multiple fractures, or the fracture crosses a suture line, the injury is more often inflicted (Figure 7-19). If significant pressure is placed on the head, there can be crushing injuries with multiple skull fractures resulting in deformity of the head. This is seen in cases such as automobiles that roll over a child. Focal internal injuries, such as an epidural hemorrhage, are consistent with an accidental mechanism, such as an object "toppling over" onto the child causing a focal impact and tearing of the middle meningeal artery.

Another important component of blunt impact injury evaluation is that of fractures involving sites other than the skull. If fractures are suggested on preautopsy radiology

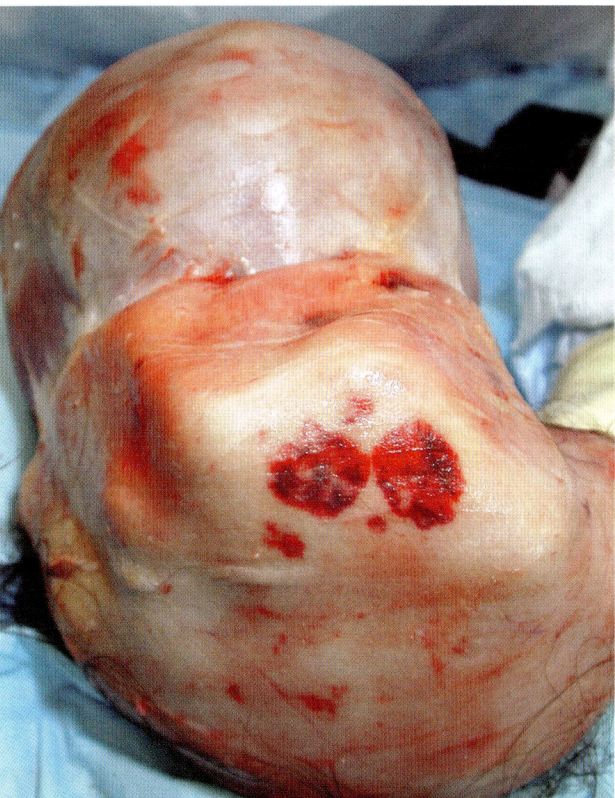

FIGURE 7-18 • Subscalpular soft tissue hemorrhage indicative of a blunt impact injury of the head.

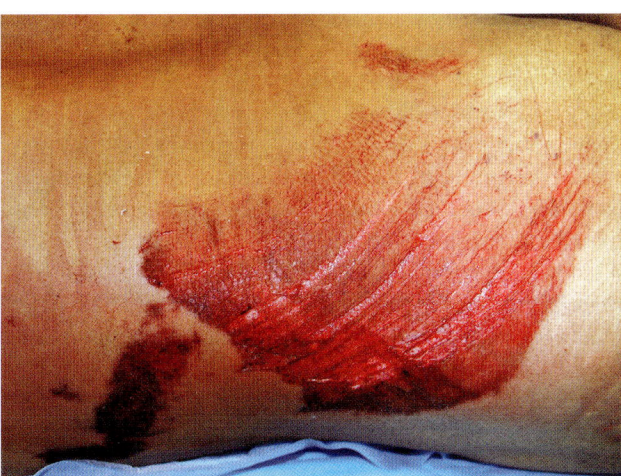

FIGURE 7-17 • Brush abrasion from a tangential impact with the ground in an individual who was ejected in a motor vehicle accident.

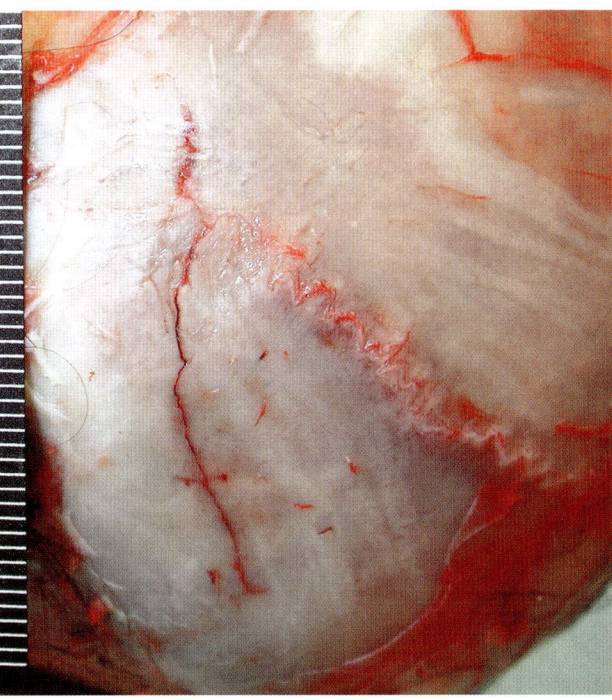

FIGURE 7-19 • Skull fracture that crosses the suture line. This is more consistent with an inflicted injury.

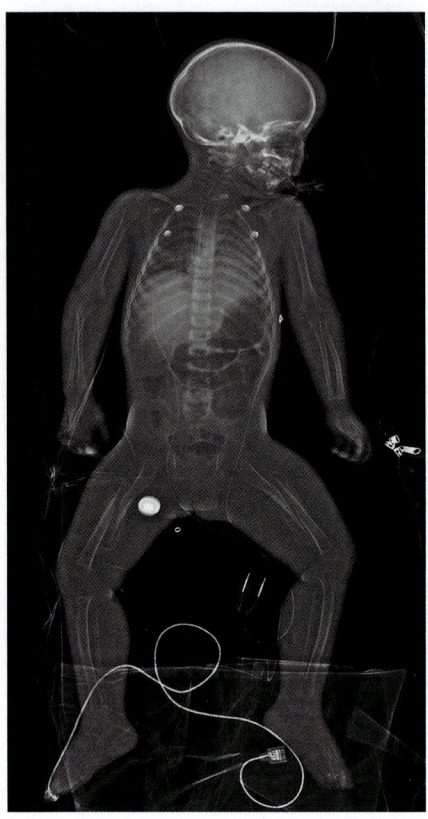

FIGURE 7-20 • Digital radiograph showing bilateral femur fractures. These bones should be dissected out for further studies.

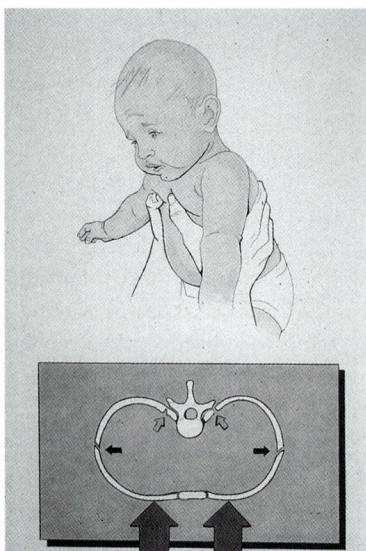

FIGURE 7-21 • Schematic representation of the production of abusive rib fractures. Anteroposterior squeezing results in posterior or lateral rib fractures.

studies (Figure 7-20), the particular bone seen as suspicious on radiology should be dissected and removed. All other bony areas should at a minimum be evaluated *in situ*. Not only will the prosector be able to evaluate the surrounding soft tissues and bony structures but, if necessary, can excise other bones for further radiographic and histologic examination. If access to a pediatric radiologist is available, it would be beneficial to review the films with him/her as certain fractures can be subtle. Kleinman has grouped skeletal injuries according to their relative specificity for abuse (44). Those with a high specificity for abuse, particularly in infants, include classic metaphyseal lesions, posterior rib fractures, scapular fractures, spinous process fractures, and sternal fractures. Classic metaphyseal lesions of the long bones are fairly specific for inflicted trauma. As the soft tissues are dissected away, hemorrhage and surrounding tissue reaction can be inconspicuous or abundant. This variation is a direct result of the difference in healing patterns between adults and children. The primary lesion consists of a planar disruption through the primary spongiosa. The distal femur and proximal tibia are the most common sites of these fractures, which are often bilateral. The lesions are thought to be produced by torsional and tractional forces generated when the infant is twisted or pulled by an extremity or when the extremities are subjected to shear strains during violent shaking. Although extremely telling of abuse, these lesions are difficult to date because the usual markers, such as subperiosteal formation of new bone, are often lacking (44,45). Fractures of the shaft of a long bone are four times more frequent than are epiphyseal–metaphyseal injuries and are the most common fracture seen in child abuse (46–49). However, these fractures are of low specificity in ambulatory children (50,51). Indeed, nondisplaced oblique or spiral fractures of the tibia are so frequently caused by accidental falls in ambulating youngsters that they are referred to as "toddler's fractures" (44,52). The specificity for abuse increases as the age of the child decreases; spiral diaphyseal fractures of nonambulatory infants are highly suspect. Rib fractures, especially those that are posterior, are highly suspect for abuse. The ribs of young children are much more pliable than are those of an adult, and fractures are much less common. The method by which these fractures occur is via anterior–posterior pressure, usually by an adult squeezing the thorax (Figure 7-21), causing levering of the ribs over the transverse process of the spine (53). Findings suggestive of rib fractures being caused by inflicted anterior–posterior compression include fingertip abrasions and contusions on the torso, vertical crushing of the internal surface of the rib with a lack of fracture on the external surface, and severity of the injury inconsistent with the proposed mechanism, which often includes forceful CPR (54). Less frequent are fractures of the lateral aspect of the ribs, which, when attributed to nonaccidental trauma, are most often fractured on the inner cortex (54,55). These fractures may be difficult to identify both radiographically and at autopsy. Hemorrhage over the ribs may alert the prosector to the possibility of a fracture and closer examination may reveal a linear fracture line (Figure 7-22). Older fractures may show callus formation, which will be visible radiologically and easily seen at autopsy. The fractured ribs should be removed, decalcified,

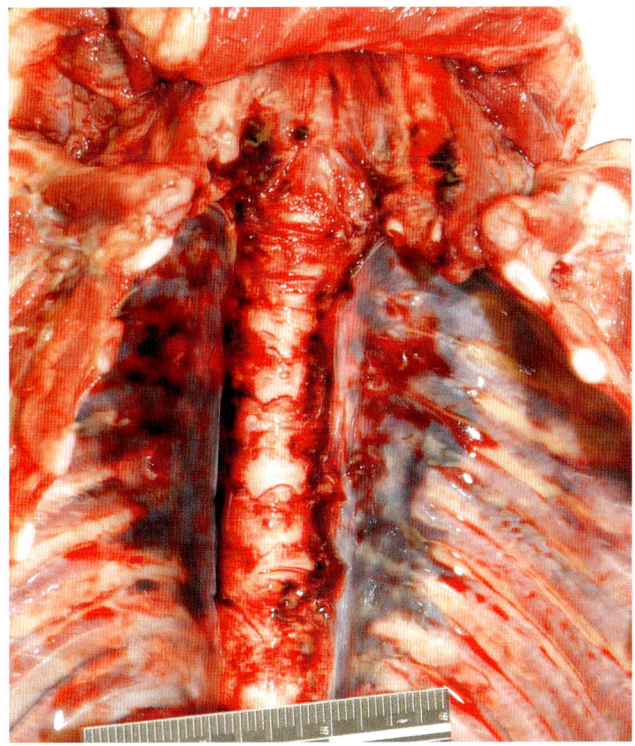

FIGURE 7-22 • Subpleural hemorrhage of the posterior rib cage. The pleura was removed to reveal acute fractures.

and submitted for histologic analysis (Figure 7-23). If necessary, forensic anthropology consultation can be extremely helpful, not only in aging the fractures but in determining the direction of the fractures and the stress needed to develop specific fractures (54). They can be x-rayed again after removal for better definition. Histology may reveal varying ages of healing reflecting a repetitive pattern of injury. Attempting to specifically age a fracture can be difficult as healing rates vary by the child's age. Younger infants form calluses faster than do older infants. A child's body may be discarded in an attempt to conceal a birth or a crime only to be found later when it is already skeletonized. In these types of cases, a forensic anthropologist should be consulted to help in determination of age, race, stature, and trauma analysis.

The internal organs of the chest and abdomen are also susceptible to blunt force injuries, with abdominal blunt trauma being the second leading cause of death in child abuse. This usually involves a large amount of force over a small surface area; that is, a punch, kick, or stomp. These forces can result in an internal organ being compressed between the site where the force is being applied and the relatively immobile spine. Lacerations of the internal organs can occur and lead to internal bleeding or spillage of intestinal contents. There does not have to be cutaneous evidence of injury to have internal trauma, but sometimes, a patterned injury on the skin can be helpful in determining what caused the injury, such as the tread of a shoe (Figure 7-24). The most commonly affected hollow viscus in blunt abdominal trauma includes the duodenum and jejunum, while the most commonly injured solid organs are the liver and pancreas (Figure 7-25). The mortality rate in victims with abusive hollow viscus perforations is very high [71% in a study by Ledbetter (56)], and they often present for medical care in extremis or are dead at the scene. Historical information usually reveals that the child has been ill, with nausea and vomiting, for a time period ranging from hours to days. Histologic evaluation of the injured viscus can aid in aging the injury. The mechanism of death in liver laceration is exsanguination. A pancreatic laceration is supportive evidence of significant blunt force trauma to the abdomen and if survived may lead to pancreatitis and pancreatic pseudocyst formation. The rib cage acts as protection for the underlying thoracic organs; thus, there are relatively fewer injuries to the heart and lungs; however, when there is rapid forceful anteroposterior pressure placed on the thorax, such as in a stomping, a rupture of the heart,

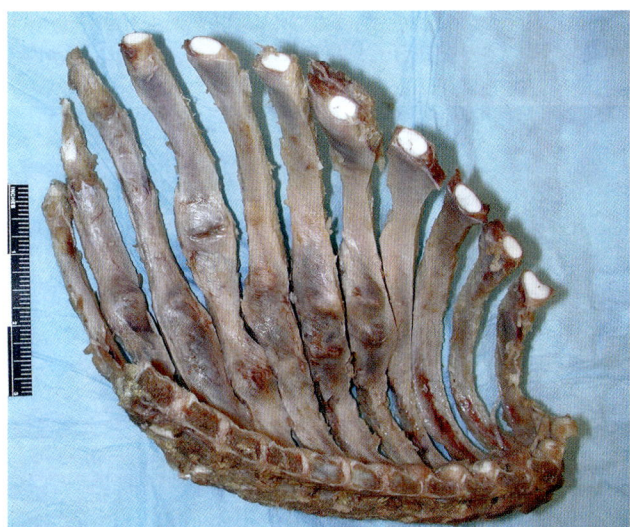

FIGURE 7-23 • Partial rib cage, after formalin fixation, removed for further examination due to multiple fractures of varying ages.

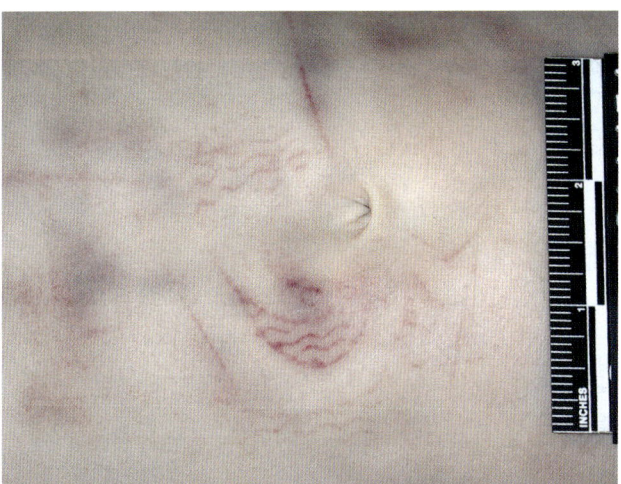

FIGURE 7-24 • Contusion on the abdomen with impression of the tread of a shoe. Internal injuries included lacerations of the liver and pancreas (see Figure 7-25).

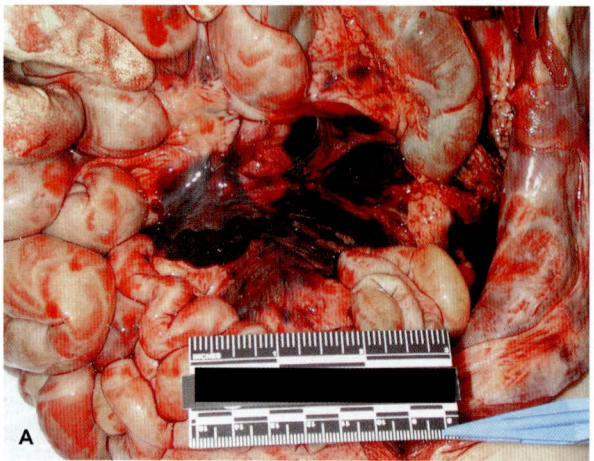 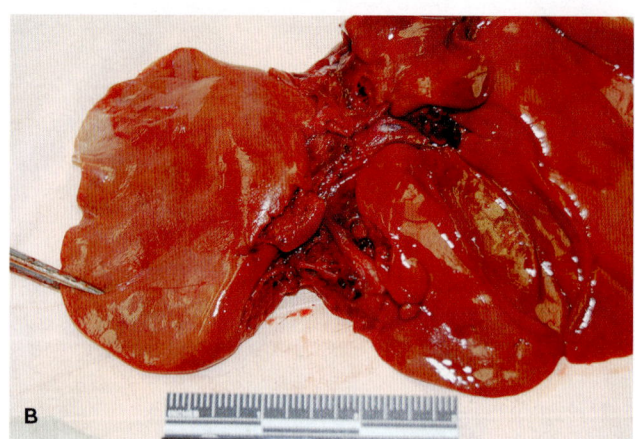

FIGURE 7-25 • Internal injuries of the blunt abdominal trauma from Figure 7-24. **A:** Mesenteric hemorrhage. **B:** The liver was lacerated with resultant hemoperitoneum.

most often at the junction of the right atrium with the venae cavae, has been documented. This leads to cardiac tamponade and death (Figure 7-26).

MIMICS

There are a number of natural disease processes that can "mimic" inflicted injuries. It is important to have knowledge of these as they are often used in legal proceedings as a defense for nonaccidental trauma. The following are a few of the disorders to consider:

"Mongolian spots" (Figure 7-27), also known as congenital dermal melanocytosis, are gray-blue patches that are usually on the lower back/buttocks but can be anywhere on the body. They are present at birth and usually disappear within the first few years but may persist for life. They can be confused with contusions, but a small incision into the skin will reveal the lack of any underlying hemorrhage. Microscopic evaluation shows dermal proliferation of melanocytes.

Impetigo contagiosa is an infectious disease usually caused by *Staphylococcus aureus* or group A streptococcus and is most often seen in preschool-age children. The lesions, which usually occur in exposed areas, begin as relatively circular vesicopustules that rupture quickly and can be mistaken for cigarette burns (Figure 7-28). After rupture, the lesions become covered with a thick yellow crust. Histologically, the vesicopustule is located in the upper layers of the epidermis and contains numerous neutrophils. It also may contain Gram-positive cocci.

Staphylococcal scalded skin syndrome is characterized by large, flaccid bullae caused by a toxin produced by staphylococcus that rupture almost immediately. It usually presents in an extracutaneous fashion, such as with pharyngitis or conjunctivitis. These lesions may be mistaken for scald burns.

Ehlers-Danlos syndrome is an inherited connective tissue disorder currently with ten different subtypes. Some subtypes are characterized by poor wound healing with extremely thin skin, prolonged bleeding, and subsequent scarring (57). Due to the fact that these patients may present with a severe injury that is associated with a history of minor trauma, such lesions have been confused with abusive injuries. A number

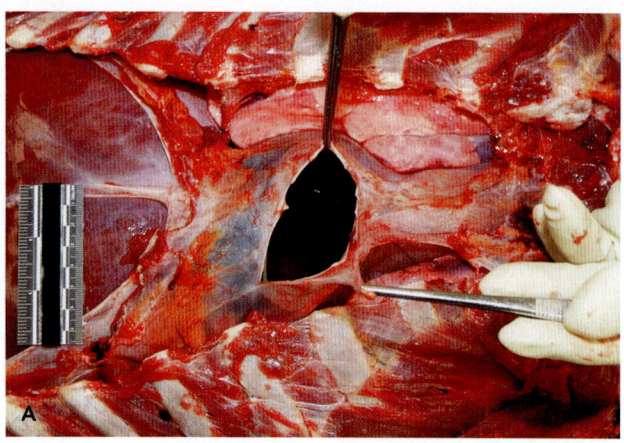 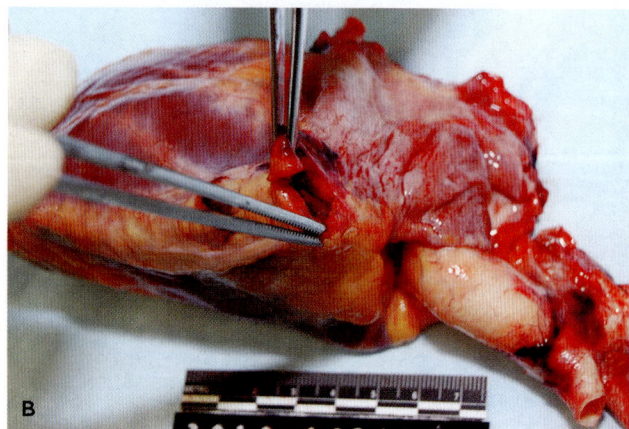

FIGURE 7-26 • **(A)** Cardiac tamponade as a result of a stomp to the chest, with **(B)** laceration of the right atrium.

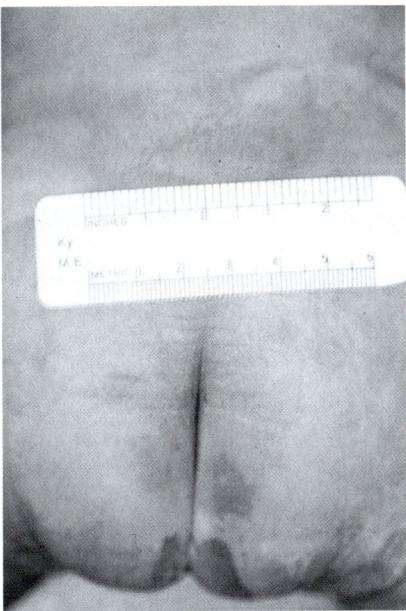

FIGURE 7-27 • "Mongolian spot." Dissection into the skin and soft tissues will fail to reveal any hemorrhage.

of hematologic disorders can lead to easy bruising and may be confused with nonaccidental trauma as well.

Various cultural healing methods may be mistaken as abuse if the pathologist is not aware of them. Two of the more common of these practices are coining and cupping. Cao gio (coining) involves rubbing coins along certain distributions to alleviate ailments. The same therapeutic intention is seen with cupping.

Osteogenesis imperfect (OI) is a rare disorder of type I collagen that results in abnormal bone fragility. Type I collagen is the major structural protein of the extracellular matrix of bone, skin, dentin, sclera, and tendon (58,59). OI is a phenotypically and genotypically heterogenous group of inherited disorders involving mutations in the genes that encode for type I collagen (59). Four main types of OI are known. Type I is the most common. It is characterized by abnormal fragility with osteoporosis, blue sclerae, defective dentition (dentinogenesis imperfecta), and

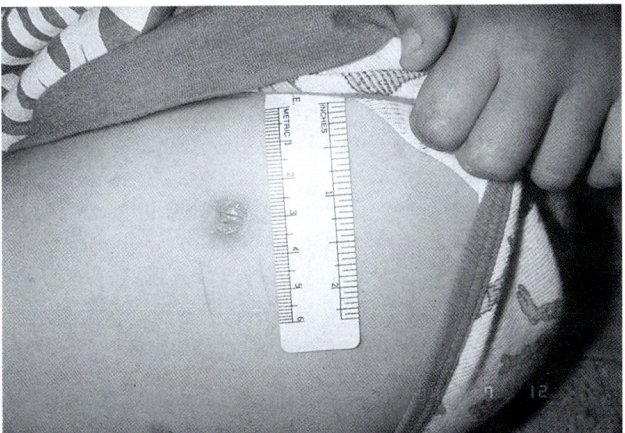

FIGURE 7-28 • Impetigo contagiosa, initially alleged to be a cigarette burn.

presenile hearing impairment. Other features common in OI type I include wormian bones of the skull and short stature. OI type I accounts for approximately 80% of all cases of OI. It is inherited in an autosomal dominant fashion. The family history is extremely useful in evaluating children for OI type I. OI type II is known as the fetal or perinatal form. Severe osteopenia is generally apparent at birth, and intrauterine growth retardation is present. The majority of children with OI type II succumb within the first few weeks of life. These infants display deep blue-black sclerae, a characteristic facies, severe skeletal deformities, and multiple fractures and osteopenia at birth. Because of the obvious bony deformities, this form is unlikely to be mistaken for child abuse (60). Type III is thought to be caused by a sporadic mutation. The majority of patients with type III OI display characteristic triangular faces. These infants may have fractures at birth. The color of the sclerae may appear normal. Children with type III often display shortening, bowing, and angulation of the long bones in addition to growth retardation. Type IV, the rarest form, is most often confused with abuse. Osteopenia and deformity are present but may be mild. Type IV children usually have wormian bones and abnormal dentition is common. Metaphyseal fractures in OI are different from the metaphyseal corner fractures and bucket-handle fractures seen classically in child abuse (61). Although the potential for misdiagnosis exists, the probability is very small given the relative prevalences of type IV OI and abusive fractures (62). Microscopically, the osseous tissue of a child with OI demonstrates a relative abundance of osteocytes. The extracellular matrix is reduced; thus, the cells are much closer together than is normal (63). The diagnosis of OI remains a clinical one, based on the patient and family history and on the findings of diagnostic imaging and physical examination. A skin biopsy for collagen analysis or blood for DNA analysis may be used as a confirmatory test (59). Of importance, one must remember that there are spontaneous mutations without any family history of OI and blue sclera can be present in infants up to 4 months of age (59). There has been the suggestion by a few of a disorder known as temporary brittle bone disease. The presumption is that there is a temporary fragility of collagen due to deficiencies in trace elements such as copper. Children with this presumed disorder have a transient predisposition to sustaining fractures with normal handling (64). The majority of experts do not accept temporary brittle bone disease as a true diagnosis (see Chapter 28).

Rickets (vitamin D deficiency) can lead to multiple pathologies in various organ systems, including the skeleton. Skeletal findings in rickets include softening of the skull (craniotabes), pseudodiastasis of the cranial sutures, transverse lucencies of the forearms and ribs, compression fractures of the vertebrae, and lower extremity long bone fractures. The metaphyses show changes, such as fractures, which are most commonly symmetric and medial and occur in the fastest growing long bones first. An interesting finding is that these fractures are often asymptomatic and heal rather rapidly without the usual stages of healing once treatment begins. Aging of these fractures is not possible due to the abnormal healing pattern (65). Other features that have been described include loss of cortical distinction, subperiosteal new bone formation in the long bone diaphysis, insufficiency fractures and Looser zones (pseudofractures) of the ribs and forearms. As breastfeeding becomes more prevalent and babies are breastfed longer, the number of children with vitamin D deficiency has increased.

Short falls are often given as an explanation for head injury. Review of the literature concerning witnessed, corroborated falls reveals that children generally tolerate such forces well, even better than adults. This has been explained by factors that are unique to children, such as a smaller mass, which reduces the deceleration force on impact, and a higher proportion of cartilage and subcutaneous fat (66). Several authors have documented series of children sustaining minor household falls. In 1977, Helfer et al. reviewed a series of 246 children with a history of falling out of bed; 85 of the children were hospitalized at the time of their fall (67). No child in the study sustained central nervous system damage. The benign nature of falling out of bed was confirmed by two additional studies of falls in hospitals, one involving 76 children and another involving 207 children falling from beds, cribs, or chairs (68,69). No serious injuries occurred in either study. Stairway falls have also been examined and characterized as an initial "moderate impact" fall, followed by a series of minor impacts. Joffe and Ludwig documented 363 cases of falls down stairs seen in a pediatric emergency department (70). The majority of the children had only superficial injuries, and no child sustained life-threatening injuries or required intensive care (70). Several series of witnessed, corroborated free falls in children have also been published. Barlow and colleagues examined 61 children during a 10-year period who were admitted to the hospital after falling from a height of one or more stories (71). Of the children who fell three stories or less, 100% survived. Mortality in those falling from the fifth and sixth floors was 50%. In one study of 106 witnessed, corroborated free falls in children less than 3 years old, only one death occurred, which was a child who fell from 60 feet. The author concluded that falls of less than 10 feet are unlikely to produce serious or life-threatening injury (72). In yet another series, 70 children with a mean age of 5 years fell from heights ranging from one to 17 stories, and all survived (73). A study of fatal head injury with a history of a fall revealed only three fatalities from witnessed falls—all from heights greater than 10 feet and none with evidence of retinal hemorrhage or axonal injury. And yet in this same study, 19 fatalities occurred in children whose initial history was of a fall of 5 to 6 feet or less, but subsequent investigation revealed that most of these cases were actually inflicted trauma with an initially false history (74). A study of 317 children brought to a children's trauma center with a history of a fall revealed only one death in 117 children falling from 10 to 45 feet, and seven deaths in children allegedly falling 4 feet or less. In all seven of the fatalities after a short fall, other factors suggested a false history (75). Compiling the multiple available studies, Chadwick concludes, "Death from a fall is now considered very unlikely when the fall is less than 20 feet" (76).

Cardiopulmonary resuscitation is also often used as an attempt to explain inflicted injuries. The anatomical areas affected by CPR include the head, neck, and torso due to assisted ventilation and chest compressions. There can be perinasal and perioral contusion and abrasion, but there should not be any injury to the frenula. CPR does not cause retinal hemorrhages, but aggressive ventilation may lead to pneumothorax and rupture of the stomach. Review of the emergency medical services trip sheet and interviews with the first responders can shed light on any injuries that were present prior to their resuscitative efforts, what type of resuscitation they performed, and what injuries they may have caused. The mask used for resuscitation can be requested and retained to allow comparison with the injuries found at examination. Medications given to the child during resuscitation and intubation should be reviewed to assure that any drugs found in postmortem toxicology was given by medical personnel and not prior to medical intervention. In children, unlike adults, rib and sternal fractures rarely, if ever, occur as a result of CPR; this has even proven true in children with an underlying bone disease (54,77–83). Ribs in children are flexible and more resilient against fracture. In the absence of radiographic evidence of bone disease, unexplained rib fractures are highly suggestive of abuse. Often, such rib fractures are associated with other signs of abuse and/or different stages of rib healing. Recent radiographic studies have examined subtle CPR-related rib fractures (84). When present, these rib fractures are not usually associated with hemorrhage and are extremely difficult to notice without removal of the parietal pleura. A study of 923 children up to 14 years of age without underlying bone disease who underwent external CPR revealed that only three of these children sustained rib fractures and that all of the fractures were anteriorly distributed (80). These children were resuscitated by a mixture of medical personnel and bystanders for a length of time from 1 to 150 minutes.

Inherited metabolic conditions may cause signs and symptoms that can be confused with abuse (85–87). Methylmalonic aciduria may present as failure to thrive (57). Glutaric aciduria type I is an inherited metabolic disorder that can be confused initially with head trauma. Children with glutaric aciduria type I may present at age 6 to 18 months with encephalopathic crisis following a minor illness. This encephalopathic crisis may lead to destruction of the basal ganglia. Children with glutaric aciduria type I characteristically display a head circumference above the 95th percentile at birth. Continued rapid growth of the head circumference after birth leads to macrocephaly with frontal bossing (88). Glutaric aciduria type I may be diagnosed by a metabolic screen performed on blood (see Chapter 5).

Accidental blunt impact injuries that are often evaluated in the medical examiner office include those that occur in a number of accidental situations. These range from motor vehicle accidents to household accidents, such as objects falling on the child. From a public safety standpoint, these cases are important so as to document any defect in a certain product. This may prevent future unnecessary deaths. In the case of motor vehicle accidents, the type of child restraint, if one was used, should be evaluated to see if it was defective and if it was installed appropriately.

Shaken Baby Syndrome, Shaken Impact Syndrome, Abusive Head Trauma

Shaken baby syndrome is an extremely controversial topic. It was initially described in 1971 by Guthkelch and later in 1974 by Caffey, who termed it as "whiplash shaken infant syndrome" (89,90). The name has undergone numerous iterations including shaken baby syndrome, shaken blunt impact, and abusive head trauma. The classic triad has been described as subdural hemorrhage most often a thin layer, retinal hemorrhage and cerebral edema or anoxic encephalopathy. The debate has centered around the question: is shaking alone adequate enough to cause these injuries? There have been perpetrator confessions where the only mechanism was shaking and the child had the above constellation of findings. Much more commonly, a site of impact is identified, not necessarily on the skin surface, but within the subscalpular soft tissues. Infants and young children have unique characteristics that come into play in central nervous system trauma. The skull is pliable and unilaminar, with unfused sutures, open fontanels, and a flat shallow base. The brain constitutes a significantly larger percentage of the total body weight in children than in adults (up to 30% in children versus 2% to 3% in adults) (91), and this large, heavy head rests on a relatively weak neck. The infant's brain is less myelinated, has smaller axons, and has higher water content. The biomechanics of "shaken baby syndrome" have been argued by numerous experts over many years. Many believe that rotational injury causes shearing of the subdural bridging veins and intraparenchymal axons (Figure 7-29), while others believe that these are secondary findings as a result of other intracranial pathologies. Tearing of the subdural bridging veins can lead to subdural hemorrhage, which usually presents with a thin film of hemorrhage in the subfalcine region or over the convexities, but is rarely large enough to form a space-occupying lesion (Figure 7-30). There are those who believe that the subdural hemorrhage is a secondary phenomenon due to a number of physiologic changes such as anoxic/ischemic encephalopathy or following intradural hemorrhage (92). Matshes et al. suggest that the subdural hemorrhage is secondary to anoxic/ischemic encephalopathy due to hyperextension/hyperflexion injury to the cervical spinal cord during violent shaking, blunt impact, or both. The most common spinal regions injured are the nerve roots of C3 to C5 resulting in damaged innervation to the diaphragm and thus respiratory compromise (93). This is due to the fact that the relatively heavy head is weakly supported to the remainder of

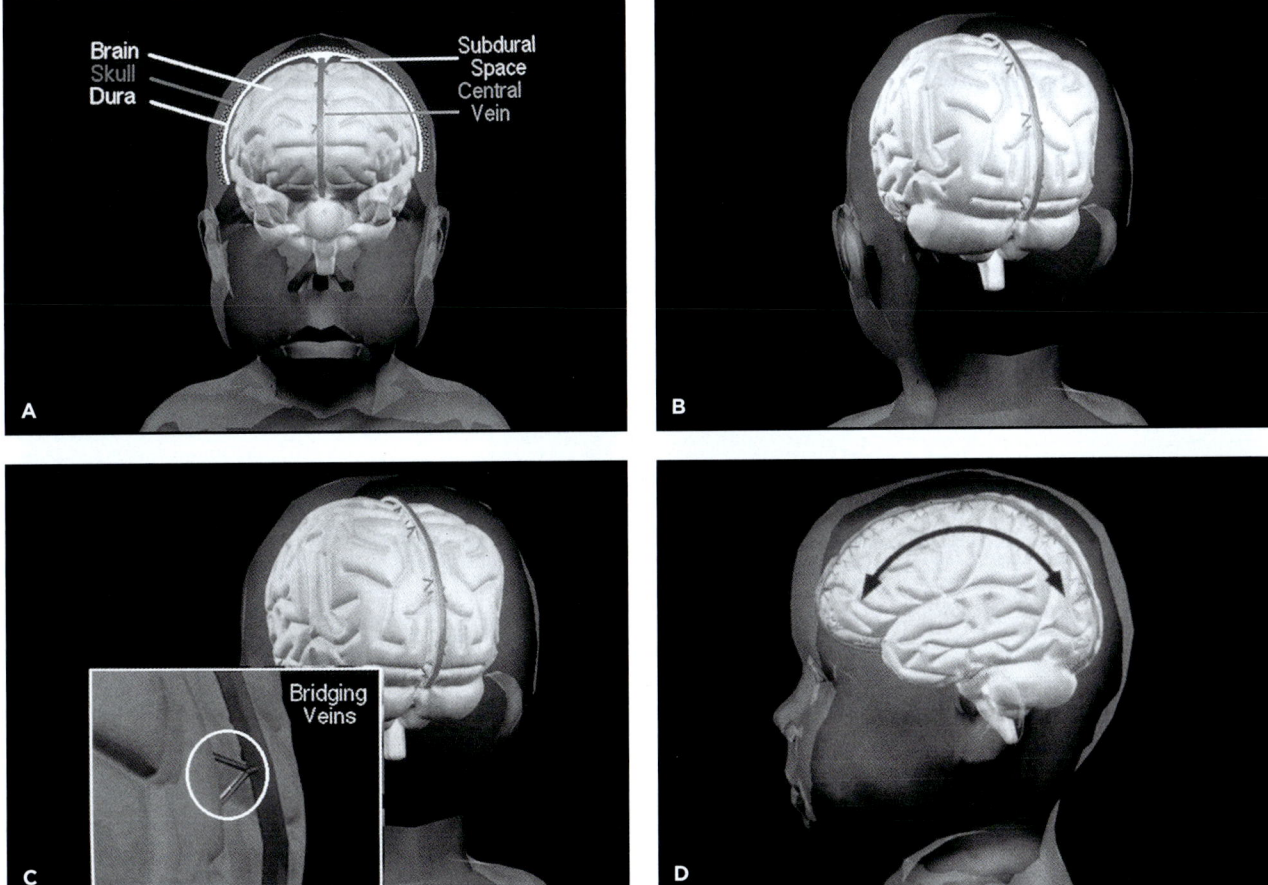

FIGURE 7-29 • Schematic representation of abusive head trauma. **A:** The various structures are defined. **B:** The central vein in the sagittal midline. **C:** Small bridging veins traversing the subdural space. **D:** Rotation of the central nervous system in angular acceleration.

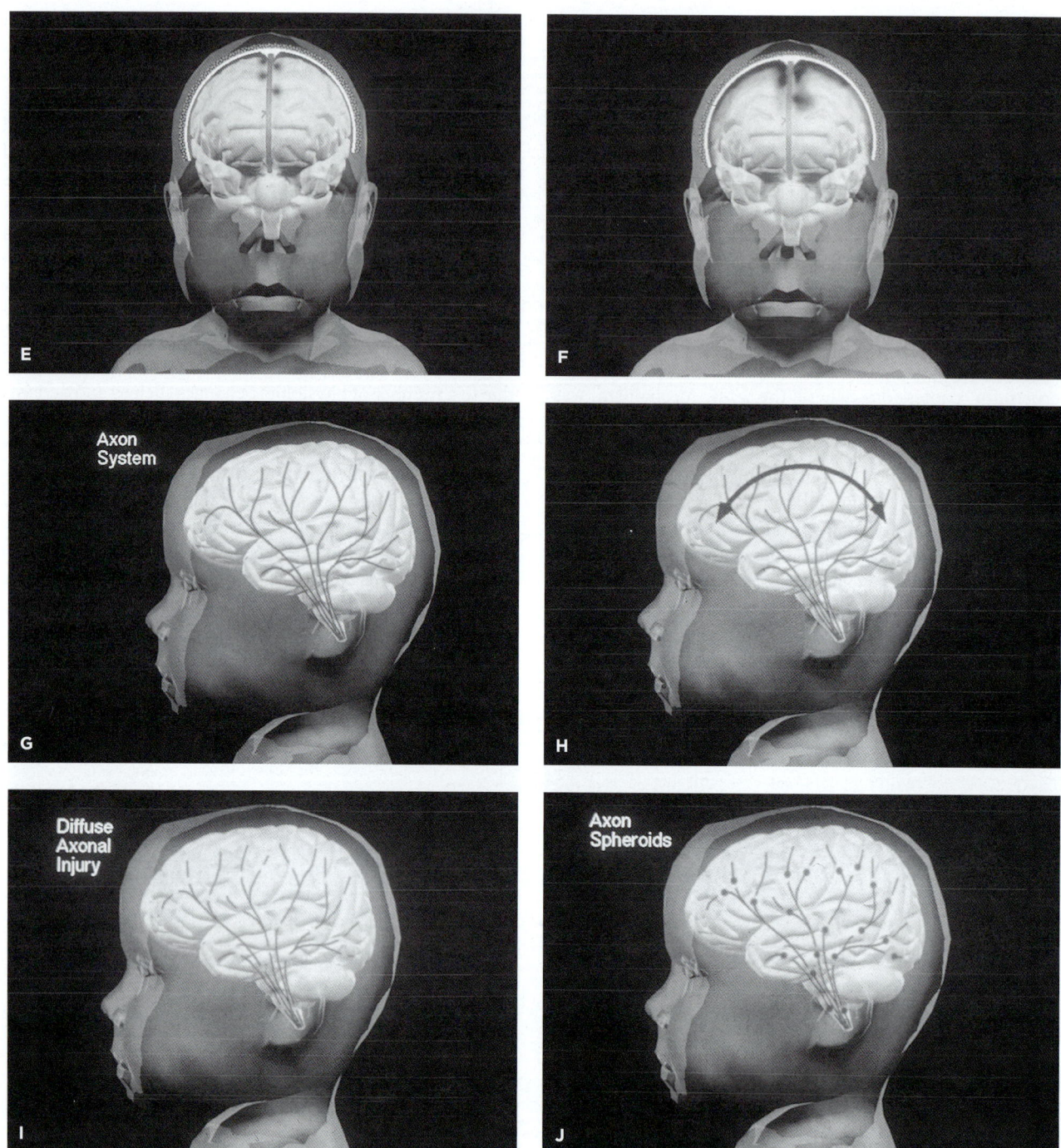

FIGURE 7-29 • *(Continued)* **E:** Parafalcine subdural hemorrhage. **F:** Subdural hemorrhage over the convexities. **G:** Depiction of the axon system. **H:** Rotation of the central nervous system with shearing. **I:** Resultant diffuse axonal injury. **J:** Eventual appearance of axon spheroids (Courtesy of Dan Davis, M.D., Hennepin County Medical Examiner's Office, Minneapolis, Minnesota).

the body by underdeveloped muscles. In addition, the cervical vertebrae are incompletely ossified; thus, they can stretch beyond the normal limits of ligamentous injury and subluxation (91), resulting in cervical spinal cord injuries under distraction, hyperflexion, and hyperextension forces. As the child is shaken, the head undergoes sheer and tensile forces and the neck undergoes compressive forces (91). Just as the bridging veins can be damaged due to shearing forces so can the axons within the parenchyma of the brain and brainstem (Figure 7-31). Diffuse axonal injury is seen grossly as focal hemorrhages in the corpus callosum, fornix, corona radiata, and rostrolateral brainstem. Microscopic evaluation shows axonal bulbs and beta-amyloid precursor protein (β-APP) positivity. These gross and microscopic findings take time

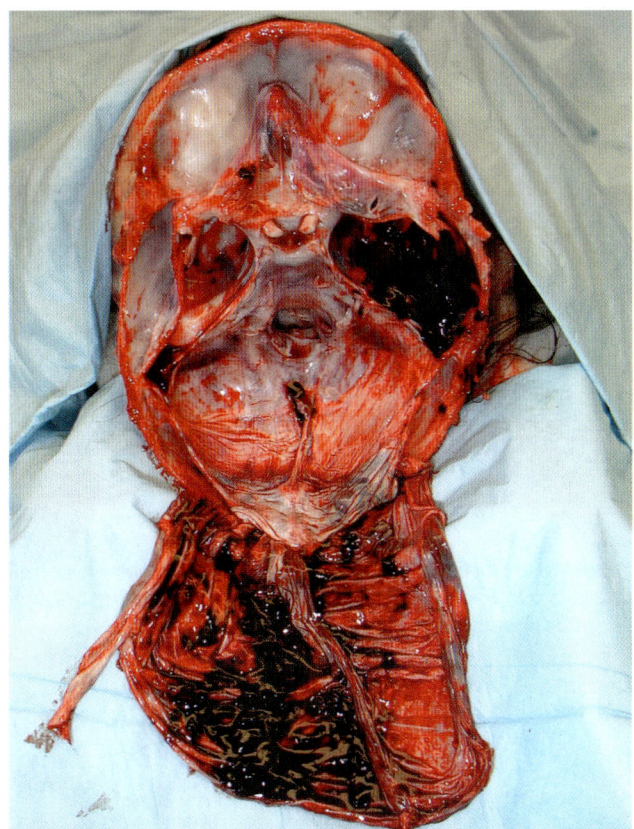

FIGURE 7-30 • Abusive head trauma with a thin layer of subdural hemorrhage.

to form, on the order of a few hours; thus, they may not all be seen if the child dies quickly. β-APP accumulates at or near the location of axonal injury. It can be a difficult stain to interpret, especially if the child survives long enough to form cerebral infarcts as staining will be positive in both of these situations, but the distribution of positivity may aid in distinguishing traumatic axonal injury from ischemic injury.

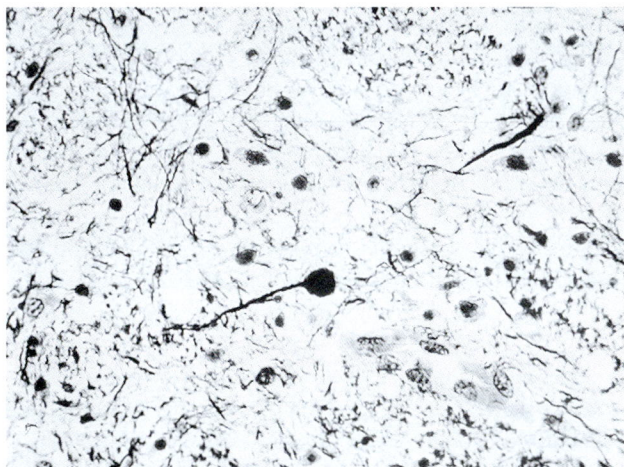

FIGURE 7-31 • An axon spheroid visualized with a silver stain. B-APP may be used to highlight axonal injury (Silver stain, ×250; courtesy of Mitch Moray, M.D., Hennepin County Medical Examiner's Office, Minneapolis, Minnesota).

If the child is maintained on a ventilator and is pronounced dead after several weeks, microglial nodules may be seen. Clinically, a rotational injury with axonal injury will present with immediate alteration in neurologic status, such as lethargy and failure to attach to the breast or bottle.

"Tin ear syndrome" is a term used to denote a subset of rotational acceleration injuries that results in unilateral ear bruising, ipsilateral subdural hemorrhage with cerebral edema, and hemorrhagic retinopathy. All patients in a series of children with these findings were toddlers between 2 and 3 years of age with thin subdural hemorrhages over the convexities and uncal herniation. These children presented to the emergency department with a Glasgow Coma Scale of 8 or less, and all of them died within 72 hours of admission. The forces required to produce this triad of findings would need to be strong enough and directed at the ear so as to preclude an accidental manner (94).

Retinal hemorrhage is another finding that has become controversial as, despite the fact that it is more often seen in abusive head trauma, there are other conditions in which it may be present. The retina is multilayered and extends from the optic nerve to the ora serrata at the periphery. Hemorrhage can occur within and in between the different layers as well as be focal or extensive. In abusive head trauma cases associated with retinal hemorrhage, the majority have multifocal hemorrhage with approximately 2/3 having too numerous to count retinal hemorrhages, which extend to the periphery (95). These hemorrhages have a predilection for forming at sites of vitreoretinal attachments, such as the periphery, perivascular regions, and posterior pole (95). Other situations where retinal hemorrhages can be seen include sepsis, coagulopathy, increased intracranial pressure, and after vaginal delivery. Hemorrhages associated with vaginal delivery are usually resolved by the end of the first month of life. The retinal hemorrhages in these cases are more focal and unilayered, whereas in abusive head trauma, they are usually bilateral, more numerous, multilayered and extend to the ora serrata (Figure 7-32). If the forces are great enough, there may be hemorrhage within the vitreous

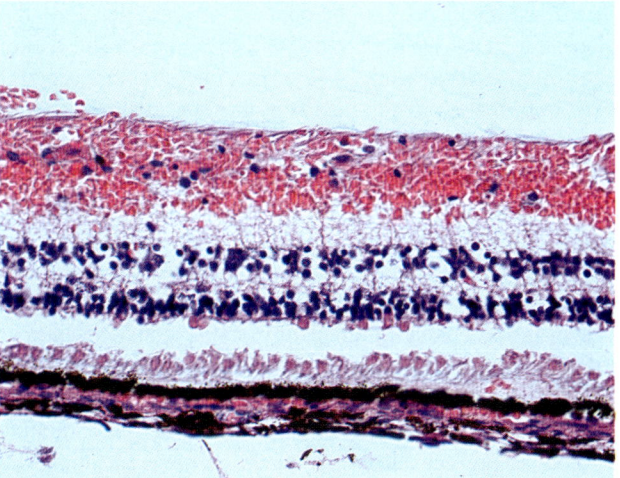

FIGURE 7-32 • Microscopic view of retinal hemorrhages.

humor. Retinoschisis, which is splitting of the retinal layers, may also occur. Blood will accumulate in the space formed by the splitting, most often between the internal limiting membrane and the nerve fiber layer (95). Purtscher retinopathy is another distinct pattern of retinal hemorrhage seen following traumatic chest compression asphyxia. It is characterized by large white patches on the retina in the macular and peripupillary areas (96,97). It has been reported in association with battered child syndrome (98). It is known that retinal hemorrhage can occur secondary to increased intracranial pressure via concomitant increased intraocular pressure (IOP). As the IOP increases, capillary perfusion decreases, and thus, oxygenation decreases. The more capillaries that fail, the greater the hemorrhage that may be seen (92). This may all be true, but the overall distribution of the hemorrhages and a thorough investigation of the circumstances surrounding the child's death and autopsy findings should help elucidate the true nature of the retinal hemorrhages. As retinal hemorrhages can resolve within 24 hours as well as develop while in the hospital due to secondary effect, prompt evaluation by an ophthalmologist is important. Superficial hemorrhages are most often resolved by 3 days (up to 1 week) and deeper hemorrhages are usually gone by 1 month (up to 6 weeks). When a child presents with retinal hemorrhage in the first month and a half of life, birth-related retinal hemorrhage should be considered (95). Dating retinal hemorrhages is not precise, but the presence of hemosiderin suggests injury of at least 18 hours. Vitreous humor should never be drawn prior to evaluating the retrobulbar soft tissues and perioptic nerve sheaths for hemorrhage. The drawing of vitreous humor may introduce hemorrhage into the vitreous itself or within the layers of the retina and possibly even cause retinoschisis.

Procedurally, once the brain is removed, the dura should be stripped to allow for visualization of the base of the skull. After documenting any fractures, the middle ears should be examined after removing the petrous ridges. Any hemorrhage should be noted and any pus should be cultured. The eyes and optic nerves should then be examined after removing the orbital plates. This involves dissection of the extraocular muscles and removal of the optic nerve from within the sphenoid bone. A careful dissection needs to be done so as to not penetrate the globe. If hemorrhage is identified in the retrobulbar soft tissues or perioptic nerve sheaths, both eyes should be removed and fixed in formalin prior to further evaluation. Attention should be focused on which portion of the perioptic nerve sheath has hemorrhage, as different etiologies may be associated with hemorrhage in just the intracranial portion versus the portion within the bone. After fixation, the eyes and optic nerves should be sectioned and submitted for histologic evaluation (Figure 7-33). A posterior neck dissection will allow visualization of the soft tissues, musculature, and spinous processes of the spine. The spine should be unroofed to expose the underlying spinal cord, and some suggest removing the entirety of the cervical spine and spinal cord intact as one unit. Whole mounts of cross sections at different levels of the spine, including the nerve roots, can be processed for histologic analysis. Most spinal

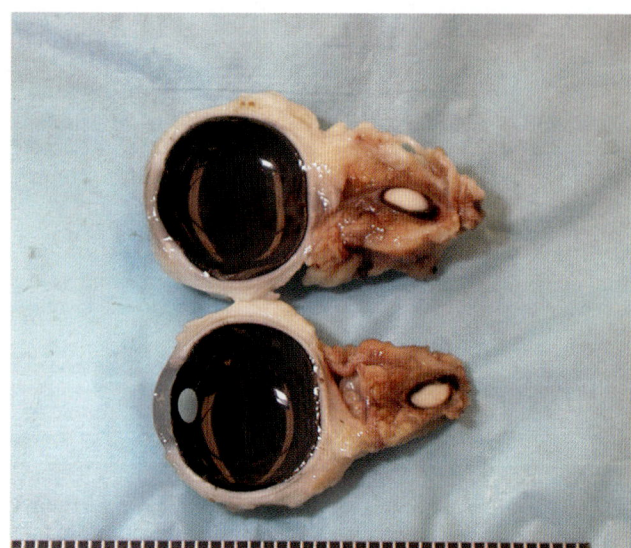

FIGURE 7-33 • Dissection of the eyes and optic nerves after formalin fixation. Notice the retinal hemorrhages and perioptic nerve sheath hemorrhage.

cord injuries identified in cases of abuse are incidental findings, either radiographically or at autopsy (99).

Neglect

Neglect is essentially the omission of the basic needs of a child, whether it be food, medicine, clothing, shelter, education, emotional support, or safety needs. Neglect is the most common type of childhood maltreatment but is a rare cause of pediatric mortality (86). It may manifest in many ways and can be extremely difficult to identify. Lack of parental, or caregiver, oversight can lead to toxic ingestions of illicit drugs or prescription medicine, drowning, environmental exposure, and malnutrition; to list a few. The majority of these children are less than 3 years old as this is the age when children are less able to seek out food or assistance from others. Malnutrition and dehydration as a manifestation of neglect are most prevalent in young children, especially infants with an average age of 6 months, as they are unable to feed themselves or obtain food. These children also have a large energy requirement as a result of rapid growth. Dehydration may be suggested by poor skin turgor; which is evidenced by a slow return to normal after the skin is pinched into a tent like configuration. If dehydration is considered, vitreous humor should be submitted to the chemistry lab for electrolyte analysis. Postmortem electrolyte analysis should be performed on vitreous humor, not blood, as blood undergoes rather rapid alterations in the electrolytes, whereas in vitreous, it is more stable. Dehydration can be found in three main forms: hypotonic, isotonic, and hypertonic. Hypotonic dehydration, with low sodium, chloride, and potassium, is the result of a number of underlying etiologies, including cystic fibrosis, adrenal insufficiency, and bacillary dysentery. Isotonic dehydration is usually the result of diarrhea due to viral gastroenteritis. In this situation, water is lost in diarrhea and sodium is lost at a similar rate. This is the most common form of dehydration in children.

Hypertonic dehydration, with elevated sodium, is seen with increased salt intake, diabetes mellitus, diabetes insipidus, hyperthermia, and decreased water intake. Sodium, potassium, and urea nitrogen will be elevated. This type is what is usually seen with neglect and is associated with the highest mortality rate (86). The mechanism of death is usually a cardiac arrhythmia. Vitreous analysis is also helpful in looking for hyperglycemia. It may reveal an initial presentation of diabetes mellitus. A low vitreous glucose should not be used to diagnose hypoglycemia as glucose decreases postmortem, even within the vitreous fluid. Neglect can result in minimal morbidity if it is reversed quickly but can result in death if it is allowed to continue. The most severe form of neglect usually involves starvation. This is seen more often in children in the early years before they have the ability to seek out food and water for themselves. A review of the child's medical records, if the child has ever been to a doctor, may shed light on the overall health of the child. Attention should be placed on the child's growth charts for any evidence of a time when the child's weight began to drop off the curve. The child's feeding schedule should be evaluated and any bottle or formula should be retained. The contents of the bottle can be evaluated and compared to the recommended preparation. There are instances where the formula has been mixed with too much water resulting in malnourishment and water intoxication. Radiology may reveal demineralization and evidence of other deficiencies. At autopsy, the overall loss of adipose tissue leads to an emaciated look (Figure 7-34). The head may appear enlarged with a prominent occiput relative to the torso due to decreased neck fat, the eyes may be sunken due to loss of orbital fat, and the cheeks may be sunken due to atrophy of the buccal fat pad. The outline of the ribs may be visualized through the skin, the iliac crests may be prominent, and the abdomen may be scaphoid. There may be prominent atrophy of the extremities. Posteriorly, the spinous processes of the vertebrae may appear prominent. The skin may appear wrinkled due to the loss of subcutaneous fat, and these children have a predisposition to forming decubitus ulcers. The anterior fontanel may appear depressed, which will be obvious after reflection of the scalp. Upon opening of the body, the lack of adipose tissue is obvious both beneath the skin and throughout the cavities. The fat that does remain is usually brown fat, which can be confirmed microscopically. The weight of the child may be below the 5th or 3rd percentile. The internal organ weights may be low. The entirety of the gastrointestinal tract should be evaluated both on its serosal surface and within the lumen. Any intestinal contents should be documented and possibly retained. The lack of intestinal contents should be described as well. There may be firm fecaliths as a result of dehydration. Protein deficiency may be manifest via hepatic microvesicular steatosis. Other microscopic changes may include calcified involution of the thymus with a "starry sky" appearance and adrenal gland atrophy with depletion of lipid. When a child is starved, the body will utilize its glycogen stores from liver and muscle in the first few days leading to gluconeogenesis from amino acids over the next week and a half to two weeks. This results in a decrease in muscle mass. Subsequently, energy is produced by fatty acid metabolism with ketone formation and eventually protein catabolism (100). Neglected children are prone to multiple complications as a result of their compromised immune systems and protein status (86). The most common of these are infectious, such as bronchopneumonia and urinary tract infection. There is a common recurring history relayed by the individual responsible for caring for the neglected child that minimizes the duration or effects of the neglect and/or is inconsistent with the findings at autopsy (86). When investigating these deaths, a complete feeding history should be obtained, including how often the child was fed, what the child was fed (breast milk, formula, cereal, etc.), and what ratio of water to formula was used. Scene investigation should not only document the overall surroundings but should focus on the presence or absence of food throughout the residence. It is not rare to find a fully stocked kitchen, while at the same time food has obviously been withheld from the child. Review of the child's medical history is important to track the child's weight from birth until death and document any medical diagnosis the child may hold.

Before a death is deemed to be the result of neglect, which carries with it a manner of homicide, one must rule out an underlying organic cause for the emaciated appearance. Such organic diseases include partial cleft palate, other oral motor abnormalities, intestinal malabsorption, cystic fibrosis, protein-losing enteropathies, abetalipoproteinemia, pyloric stenosis, celiac disease, malignancies, and congenital metabolic disorders (e.g., congenital adrenal hyperplasia and glycogen storage diseases). In these cases, absorption of the nutrients and calories necessary for development and the expenditure of energy are inadequate. Even if an underlying organic disease is identified, one must ask why the child was not taken for medical treatment, as the emaciated appearance is quite obvious. Diseases such as cystic fibrosis, MCAD, diabetes mellitus, cognitive impairment/chromosomal abnormalities, congenital adrenal hyperplasia, and viral gastroenteritis can cause dehydration. Mentally impaired children are at increased risk for dehydration because their intake may be inadequate as a result of swallowing difficulties associated with neuromuscular incoordination. Other conditions associated with such findings include congenital heart disease, cerebral palsy, and

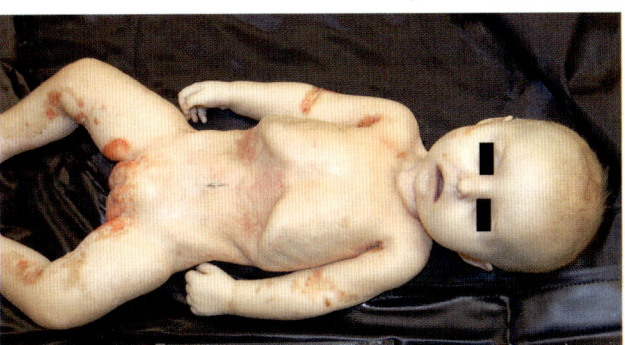

FIGURE 7-34 • Neglect. Notice the emaciated appearance with visualization of the bony structures through the skin.

chromosomal abnormalities. Metabolic and/or genetic screening can be important to rule out a number of these mimics of neglect.

Every now and then, a child will die of hyperthermia due to the surrounding environment. The two most common scenarios in which these deaths occur are when a child is left in a vehicle on a hot day and when a child is sleeping, at which time the child is either swaddled or wrapped too tightly in too many blankets. Autopsy findings in these cases are nonspecific and include petechiae of the conjunctivae, skin, and thoracic cavity as well as pulmonary and cerebral edema. If the child survived for a longer period of time, muscle necrosis, visceral cellular degeneration, gastrointestinal hemorrhage, focal myocardial necrosis, renal tubular necrosis, rhabdomyolysis, and disseminated intravascular coagulation may occur (101). Clinically, these children will become disoriented and delirious, possibly have seizures, and eventually become comatose. Children are at greater risk for serious complications and even death due to hyperthermia as they have a larger body surface area compared to their weight, higher basal metabolic rate, reduced ability to lose heat through sweating, and decreased ability to remove themselves from a dangerous situation. These are predisposing factors to increasing core body temperature and dehydration. Studies have shown that the temperature within most vehicles can reach at least 123°F within 15 minutes with the temperatures reaching 75% of their maximum within 5 minutes. The symptoms described above are reached within 20 minutes of the child being enclosed within the vehicle (102). Investigation of these deaths revolves around documentation of the ambient temperature outside the vehicle, temperature within the vehicle, duration the child was left unattended in the vehicle, and the body temperature of the child as close to when he/she was found as possible. Sometimes, the only history concerning the body temperature will be that the child's skin felt hot.

Fetal/Neonatal Deaths

These cases often initially come to medical attention when the mother presents to the hospital with vaginal bleeding and the doctor notices that the mother was recently pregnant. Different states have varying definitions as to what constitutes a viable fetus. Seri et al. (103) summarized the current literature well by showing that infants born at less than or equal to 23 weeks' gestational age and/or with a birth weight $\leq$ 500 g have virtually no chance for survival whereas those neonates born at $\geq$ 25 weeks gestation and/or weighing $\geq$ 600 g have a 60% to 70% survival rate with approximately 50% showing no neurologic deficit. The gray zone between these gestational ages and weights is one where there is a debate as to how to approach these newborns. On occasion, the medical examiner is asked to perform an examination on a "fetus." These may be fetuses/newborns found in a nonhospital setting, where there is suspicion for a nonnatural death, an unattended delivery, the suspicion of trauma or toxin, or an abandoned fetus (104). The main questions posed usually include the following: Was the baby born alive or was it stillborn? Is there any antemortem trauma? What caused the child's death? In all of these cases, the placenta should be requested for examination. Fetal death is defined as death prior to complete expulsion from the mother, irrespective of the gestational age or cause of death. A neonatal death is defined as a death occurring after complete expulsion from the mother, indicative of a live birth. The etiology of fetal demise has changed somewhat over the years, but intrauterine infections, lethal malformations, fetal growth restriction, and placental abruption continue to be the more common causes of fetal death (104). When evaluating whether the child was born dead or alive, the prosector must look for maceration, gastric contents, and if there is air in the lungs. Maceration is consistent with death prior to rupture of the membranes as a result of floating in the amniotic fluid without circulation throughout the fetus. Evaluation of the contents of the stomach may reveal the presence of material not consistent with amniotic fluid, such as toilet water, which would be consistent with inhalation/aspiration if delivered in a toilet. The "float test" is a controversial method of determining if the child was born alive or dead. Procedurally, the distal trachea is tied off and the lungs are placed in water or formalin to see if they will float or not. If they float, it indicates the presence of air in the lungs suggesting the child had taken a breath. Microscopic analysis should be performed to evaluate for air in the alveolar spaces and within the pulmonary interstitium. Putrefaction with gas formation must be ruled out as the reason for a positive "float" test. If the baby died before taking a breath, the lungs may be red, rubbery, and airless. The lungs will not be inflated with air; thus, the pleural cavities will not be filled with the lungs, giving the appearance that they are collapsed. A child can die during labor, usually as a result of asphyxia or trauma. Wisser et al. examined 59 newborns delivered vaginally for the presence of caput succedaneum and facial petechiae. They found that caput succedaneum and facial petechiae are not uncommon after vaginal delivery but that caput succedaneum usually resolves within the first few days of life and the petechiae were never extensive (105). The remainder of the examination should use the same protocol as if this was an infant death, except that the placenta should be examined if it is available. Examination of the end of the umbilical cord may reveal vascular abnormalities, multiple sharp force injuries due to cutting of the cord after delivery, and evidence of a vital reaction upon microscopic examination. If it has been determined that the death did not occur in utero, a full investigation into the cause and manner of the postpartum death must be undertaken. All of the previously defined manners of death are possible, including sequelae of a natural disease, environmental exposure to the elements resulting in hypo- or hyperthermia, and inflicted injury.

Investigation may shed light on the mother's state of mind before, during, and after the pregnancy, that is, if she and/or others knew she was pregnant. There are "striking similarities in features of mothers committing infanticide," such as average intelligence, living at home with parents at time of delivery, attempted concealment of pregnancy, statements on questioning that the child was born dead, lack of plans for delivery or for care of the infant thereafter, delivery alone in a high-risk location or circumstance, concealment of the delivery, and concealment of the infant and placenta.

Burns

There are a number of different types of burns. The most common burns seen in the pediatric setting include scald, contact, and thermal. When evaluating burns, degree of the burn, distribution on the body, and pattern are of the utmost importance.

The most common history received when a child presents with scald burns includes the pulling of a pot of boiling water on itself or getting into a bathtub where the water is too hot. The developmental stage of the child needs to be considered in these situations. Is the child capable of reaching up and pulling down a pot of hot water or climbing over the side of a bathtub? The pattern of the burn on the body is critical. When a pot of hot water is pulled down onto oneself, the water will strike the upper extremities and the top front of the head and splash down to involve the anterior neck and torso. These are often asymmetric and of varying degrees. Clothing may alter the appearance and distribution of the burns. Immersion into hot water as a form of punishment/abuse most often manifests as burns with distinct demarcation lines. If the child is held by the upper body and dipped into hot water, stocking-like demarcation of the burn may be present. If the child is cradled and immersed into hot water, the burns will display a distribution consistent with the child retracting away from the water (Figure 7-35). These will be seen as burns on the body with sparing of the areas of flexion, such as the popliteal fossa, inguinal region and antecubital fossae. These burns are usually of similar severity (Figure 7-36). Deaths due to scald burns are not immediately fatal. They usually cause death by their delayed complications of electrolyte disturbances or infectious processes. If the perpetrator's contention is that it was a tap water scald burn, the water heater should be examined and the temperature setting documented. If the location where the injury occurred (i.e., bathtub) still contains water, the temperature may be measured. Unfortunately, the investigation usually takes place too long after the fact for the water temperature to give a reading that accurately reflects the temperature at the time of the incident. The American Academy of Pediatrics recommends a "safe setting" of hot water heaters at 125°F or less. At 125°F, contact with water for 2 minutes is required to produce a full-thickness burn. At 130°F and higher, full-thickness burns can result with exposure times of 30 seconds or less (106,107).

Contact burns are a well-known form of abuse. These occur when a heated surface is placed on the child's body. Common items used to inflict these injuries include cigarettes, curling irons, and clothing irons (Figure 7-37). The pattern of these injuries, whether acute, healing, or already scarred, can be useful in identifying the item that was used to cause the burn. Burns in varying stages of healing may indicate a pattern of repetitive abuse. As stated earlier, impetigo may be confused with contact burns.

Thermal injuries are most often the result of a house fire where the child was unable to escape. Examination of these children may reveal burns ranging from first degree to complete charring (Figure 7-38). Radiographs and a complete autopsy should be performed to rule out any trauma the child may have sustained prior to the fire. Artifacts associated with thermal injuries include splitting of the skin, fractures of bones, and epidural hemorrhage. A trained forensic pathologist should be able to differentiate these from true antemortem trauma.

Factitious Disorder Imposed on Another (Munchausen Syndrome by Proxy)

The term *Munchausen syndrome by proxy* (MSBP) was coined in 1977 by Meadow to describe illnesses in children produced by their caregivers (107). The syndrome was named as an extension of the disorder known as Munchausen syndrome, in which a patient "creates" an illness to obtain the attention afforded persons playing a "sick role." The name of the disorder has undergone numerous iterations, with the Diagnostic and Statistical Manual of Mental Disorders (DSM-5) in 2013 giving it the name "factitious disorder imposed on another." Originally, MSBP was defined as a cluster of four elements:

1. A child's illness is simulated (faked) or produced by a parent or someone who is in loco parentis.
2. The child is presented for medical assessment and care, usually persistently, and medical procedures are often performed.
3. The perpetrator denies knowledge of the cause of the child's illness.
4. Acute symptoms and signs of the illness abate when the child is separated from the perpetrator (108).

It must be stressed that the above definition excludes physical abuse only, sexual abuse only, and nonorganic failure to thrive only. In this particular disorder, the perpetrator (most often the mother) creates or feigns illness in the child to gain

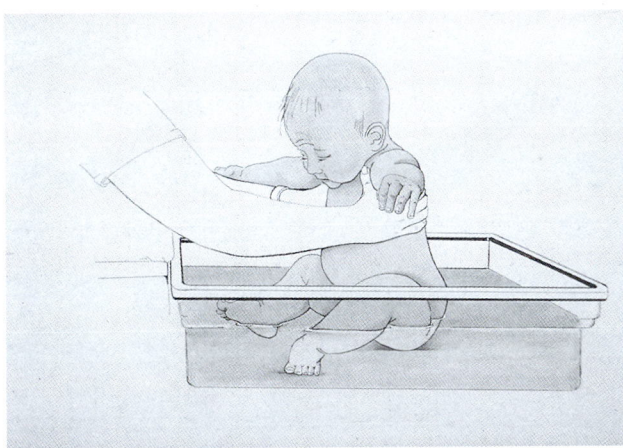

FIGURE 7-35 • Immersion into hot water pattern.

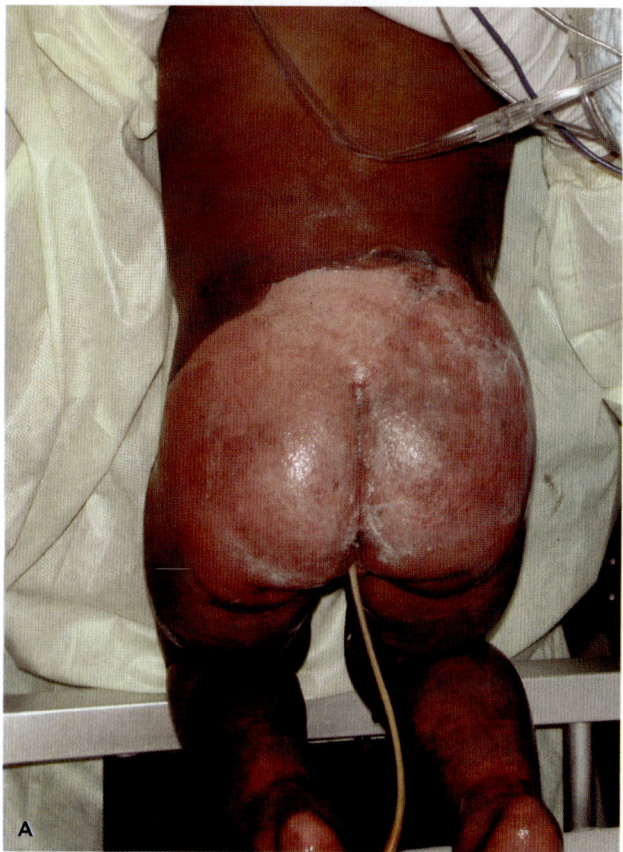
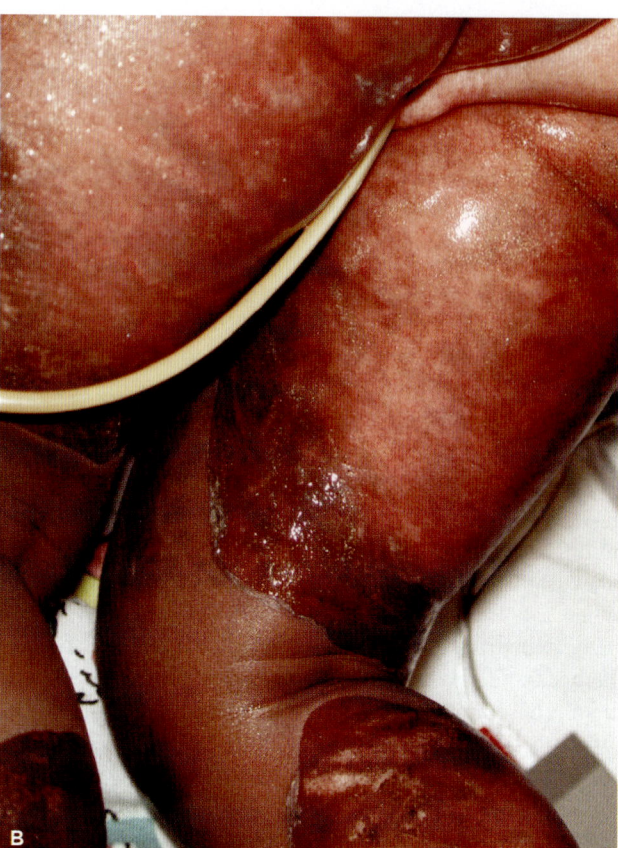

FIGURE 7-36 • **A:** Immersion burns on a child dipped into scalding hot water. **B:** There is sparing of the knees and popliteal fossae.

attention from the medical community. The methods by which disorders are created in the victims are often elaborate and almost beyond belief. In the series of 117 cases, common presentations included bleeding, seizures, central nervous system depression, apnea, diarrhea, vomiting, fever, and rash (108,109). Methods of production of various illnesses include forced oral ingestion of drugs or other substances (including salt), intentional manual suffocation, and intentional injection of nonprescribed substances and bacteria (110).

More recently, because of widespread inappropriate application of the term, Meadow (111) has suggested further specifications for its use. These include the following actions by and characteristics of the perpetrator:

1. A person intentionally produces or feigns physical or psychological signs or symptoms in someone under his or her care.

FIGURE 7-37 • Contact burn with a space heater. These burns were found on multiple anatomical locations in this infant consistent with nonaccidental trauma.

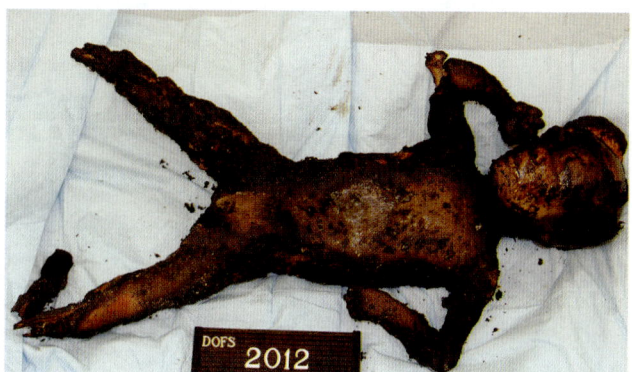

FIGURE 7-38 • Charred body of a child that died in a house fire.

2. The motivation for the perpetrator's behavior is to assume the sick role by proxy.
3. External incentives for the behavior (such as economic gain) are absent.
4. The behavior is not better accounted for by another mental disorder.

Meadow stresses that the key discriminator in the above criteria is the second one—"in relation to the children, the mother would be harming the child (making the child ill) in order herself to assume the sick role and all its benefits" (111). The more recent definition in the DSM-5 includes the addition of deception by the perpetrator as an essential criterion (109). It should be stressed that this disorder is not merely a "game" or an act of histrionics on the part of the mother. It constitutes true physical abuse and may be fatal if not detected by the medical community. Indeed, Rosenberg's series displayed a mortality rate of 9% (108). All the children who died were under the age of 3 years; the most common symptoms in these children were apnea and decreased levels of consciousness (108).

In recent years, covert video surveillance in the rooms of suspected victims in these cases has proved useful in detecting and documenting this form of abuse. In such a procedure, the patient is admitted to a hospital room equipped with a hidden video monitor. Close by is an observation area where designated persons (law enforcement officers, hospital personnel) monitor the parental activities in the child's room. It is important that observation be continuous in these cases, so that intervention occurs in a timely fashion if the child is abused or assaulted. In a series published by Southall et al. in 1997, the use of covert video monitoring led to the identification and documentation of abuse in 33 of 39 suspected cases (112). Although vocal critics of such surveillance have emerged, it is certain that many of the cases presented in the article would not have been confirmed without such evidence, and the children would have remained "in harm's way" with the abusive caregiver.

When a case of possible factitious disorder imposed on another is evaluated, all records should be completely and thoroughly reviewed. It is important to check multiple sources, including health insurance companies, to make sure that all medical evaluations have been discovered. It is helpful to construct a time line, as these are usually complicated, protracted cases. Such a time line is helpful in "keeping the facts straight" and is useful in explaining the condition and history to law enforcement officers, attorneys, and other laypersons. Information gleaned from extensive review of the often voluminous medical records should include documentation of admissions, outpatient and emergency department visits, calls to the physician, consultations, invasive procedures, and prescribed medications. An issue that should be considered during a review of medical records is the number of times visits were initiated by the caregiver, as opposed to the number of visits representing physician-ordered rechecks and specialty consultations. When a suspected victim of factitious disorder imposed on another presents to the emergency department, blood and urine should be obtained for toxicologic analysis because multiple cases of forced ingestion of medication have been documented in these cases (108,113). When this diagnosis is considered, one should always keep in mind that the most common reason why a parent persistently seeks medical attention for a child is genuine illness of the child.

Sharp Force Injuries

Sharp force injuries consist of two main types of injuries, stab wounds and incised wounds (Figure 7-39). The basic difference between the two has to do with measurements. A stab wound is deeper into the body than it is long on the surface of the skin. An incised wound is longer on the surface of the skin than it is deep into the body. Both of these can be caused by the same instrument, such as a knife, scissors, or sharp glass. Sharp force injuries, in contrast to blunt force injuries,

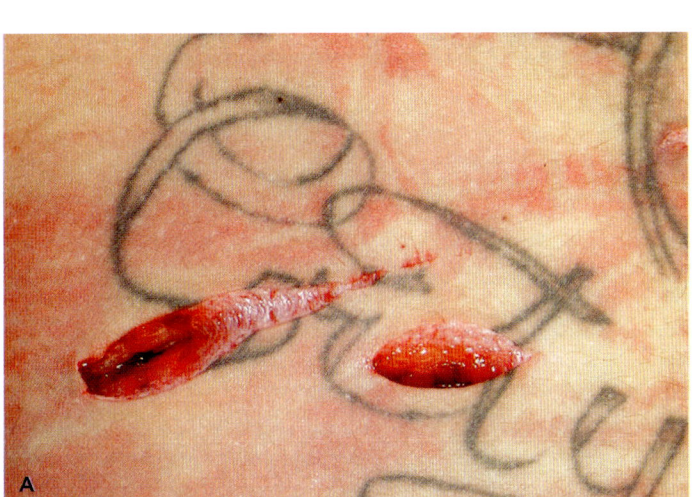
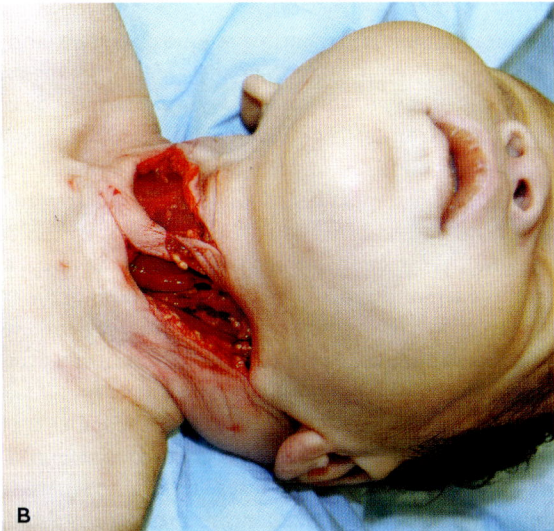

FIGURE 7-39 • **A:** Stab wound. It penetrates deeper into the body than it is long on the surface of the skin. The margins are sharp, and there is no tissue bridging. **B:** Incised wound. It is longer on the surface of the skin than it is deep into the body.

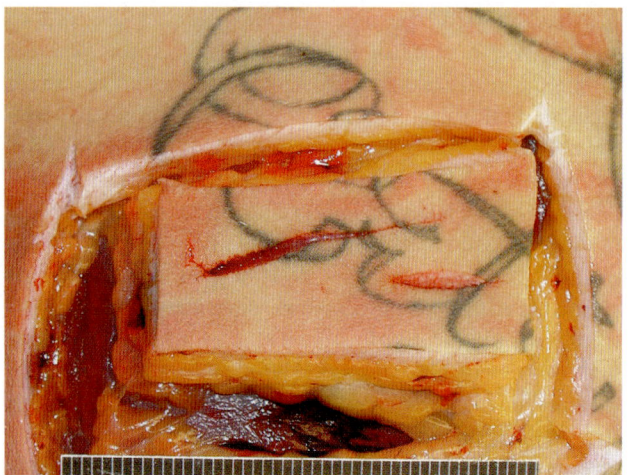

FIGURE 7-40 • Stab wound. Same stab wound as in Figure 7-39A but after removal of normal skin tension. The true dimensions of the injury are seen, and the characteristics of the confluences can be identified (blunt versus sharp edge).

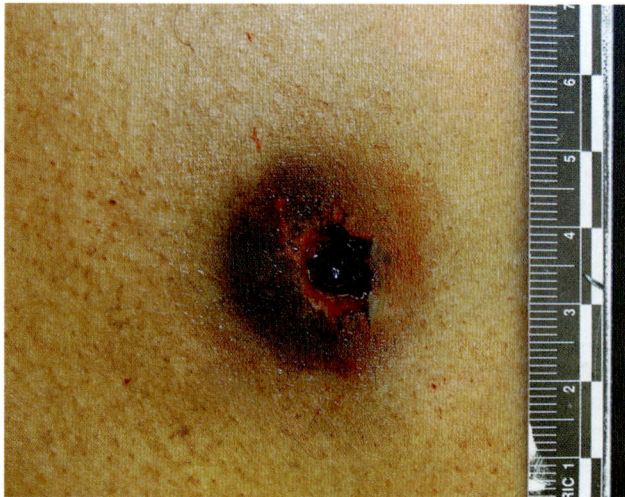

FIGURE 7-41 • Close range gunshot wound. There is dark soot around the entrance wound but no stippling.

usually have sharp margins without associated abrasion or tissue bridging within the depth of the wound. When measuring the dimensions of these wounds, you must keep in mind that the skin has lines of tension (Langer lines) that can alter the appearance of these wounds. To get an accurate measurement, the tension must be released, either by pushing the edges of the wound together with your hand or by cutting into the dermis around the wound (Figure 7-40). This will not only allow you to measure the true length of the wound but also evaluate the confluences for their sharpness or bluntness. This may be important in helping identify a suspected weapon. In addition, the location on the body, total number of injuries, distribution of the wounds, and severity of the injuries may help in distinguishing accidental, suicidal, and homicidal manners.

Gunshot Wounds

In younger children, gunshot wounds are rare and most often are the result of accidental incidents. In the teenage years, suicides and homicides become the more predominant manner of death due to gunshot wounds. A common scenario encountered in early childhood is one in which a child finds a gun, picks it up, looks down the barrel, and fires. Important questions to ask in cases such as these include the range of fire, directionality of the bullet and the physical ability of the child to actually hold the gun and pull the trigger. The range of fire should be close if it is truly self-inflicted, the direction should be from the front to the back, and the child should have the ability to squeeze the trigger on his/her own (Figure 7-41). When a weapon is fired, the bullet is pushed out of the barrel by the forces produced by ignition of gunpowder resulting in heated gases. The bullet emerges from the end of the barrel followed by the heated gases and burned gunpowder. Unburned particles of gunpowder follow shortly thereafter. Depending on the distance between the end of the barrel and the individual's body, certain characteristics may be seen that helps in determining the range of fire. The range of fire is divided into four general categories: contact range is when the barrel of the weapon is in contact with the skin or overlying clothing and may result in searing (burning) of the skin, deposition of burned gunpowder around the entrance wound and within the wound itself, abrasions or lacerations around the entrance wound, and pink discoloration of the underlying musculature as a result of the emitted gases. If the contact wound is over a bony structure, most often the skull, the gases may become trapped between the skin and skull, resulting in a stellate laceration radiating from around the entrance wound as well as the formation of an imprint from the end of the weapon on the skin (Figure 7-42). Close range is when the end of the weapon is so close to the skin

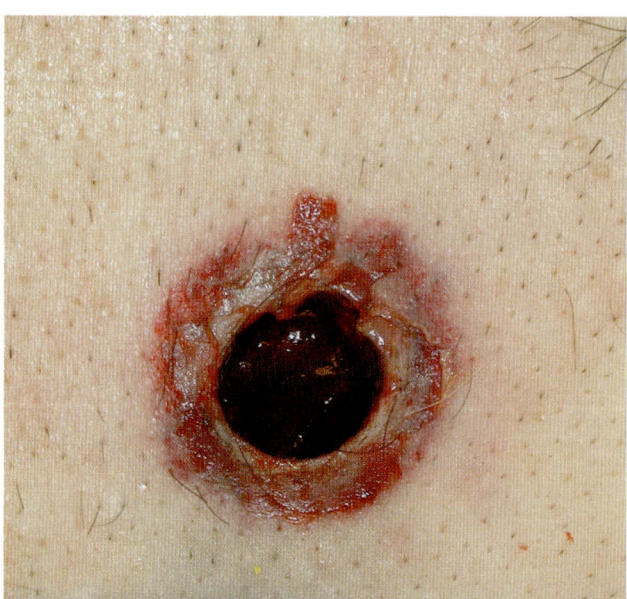

FIGURE 7-42 • Contact range gunshot wound. Searing (burning) and abrasion around the margins of the entrance wound and a rectangular shaped abrasion at the 12:00 position suggestive of the sight of a weapon.

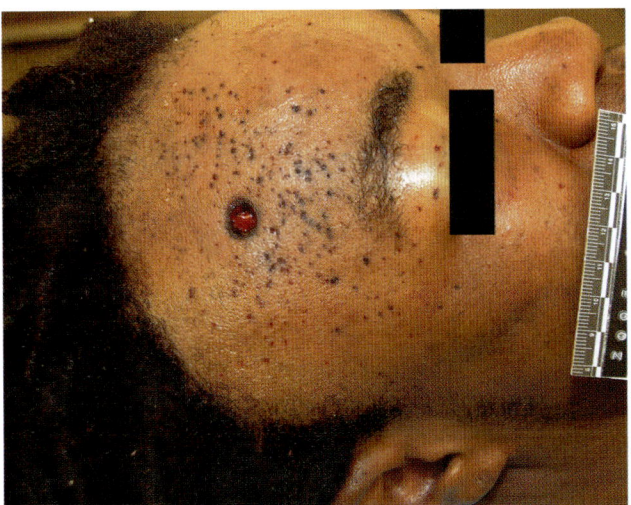

FIGURE 7-43 • Intermediate range gunshot wound. Stippling (small punctate abrasions) are seen around the entrance wound. These are due to unburned particles of gunpowder striking the skin.

that only the powder soot and some searing is seen around the entrance wound. Intermediate range is when unburned gunpowder, which is manifest as stippling or tattooing seen as reddish-brown punctate abrasions with possible fragments of gunpowder embedded within them, are around the entrance wound (Figure 7-43). As the distance from the skin increases, the zone of stippling increases until it is no longer present. Indeterminate range is when there are no distinguishing findings around the entrance wound other than a marginal abrasion caused by the bullet scraping the skin as it enters the body. The exact distance from which the weapon was from the body when it was fired in any of the above ranges vary depending on the weapon, projectile, and type of powder the projectile was loaded with. Exit gunshot wounds are most often slitlike or stellate perforations and have edges that easily reapproximate. The pathway of the projectile through the body can be of importance as it may corroborate or disprove a scenario that has been presented to law enforcement. The pathway should be described in three planes: anterior–posterior, superior–inferior, and lateral. The anatomy that is either penetrated (the bullet enters and stays within) or perforated (the bullet enters and exits) should be described as this may become important when asked about survivability and pain and suffering. Usual anatomic landmarks used when describing gunshot wounds on the skin include the top of the head (distance below), sole of the foot (distance above), midline of the body (distance left or right of), and anterior (ventral) surface of the body (distance posterior to).

CONCLUSION

The approach to the investigation of childhood deaths involves multiple disciplines and may have significant public health, personal, and legal ramifications. Consulting other professionals, such as radiologists, ophthalmologists, law enforcement, department of family and child services, and geneticists can be crucial in determining the cause and manner of death in these difficult cases. Many jurisdictions utilize a child fatality review system where individuals from different disciplines meet and discuss childhood deaths. These committees often include representatives from the medical examiner office, department of family and child services, law enforcement, district attorney, and public health. This may help identify deficiencies across all professions as well as identify emerging trends that may be of public concern. It is important to remember that forensic pathologists do not work in a vacuum. The child's medical history, social history, and investigative information as well as collaboration with multiple other experts and agencies are all imperative in coming to the correct conclusion.

References

1. Hanzlick R, Hunsacker JC, Davis GJ. *A Guide for Manner of Death Classification*. Atlanta, GA: National Association of Medical Examiners; 2002:29.
2. Gill JR, Goldfeder LB, Hirsch CS. Use of "therapeutic complication as a manner of death. *J Forensic Sci* 2006;51(5):1127–1133.
3. Center for Disease Control and Prevention. 10 Leading Causes of Death by Age Group, United States 2011. 2014. http://www.cdc.gov/injury/wisqars/pdf/leading_causes_of_death_by_age_group_2011-a.pdf Accessed July 22, 2014.
4. Hanzlick RL, Fudenberg J. Coroner versus medical examiner systems: can we end the debate? *Acad Forensic Pathol* 2014;4(1):10–17.
5. Hanzlick RL. A perspective on medicolegal death investigation in the United states: 2013. *Acad Forensic Pathol* 2014;4(1): 2–9.
6. Chakravarthy M. "Rigor mortis" in a live patient. *Am J Forensic Med Pathol* 2010;31(1):87–88.
7. Kleinman PK, Marks SC, Blackbourne B. The metaphyseal lesion in abused infants: a radiologic-histopathologic study. *AJR Am J Roentgenol* 1986;146(5):895–905.
8. Kleinman PK, Marks SC, Adams VI, et al. Factors affecting visualization of posterior rib fractures in abused infants. *AJR Am J Roentgenol* 1988;150(3):635–638.
9. Kleinman PK, Nimkin K, Spevak MR, et al. Follow-up skeletal surveys in suspected child abuse. *AJR Am J Roentgenol* 1996;167(4):893–896.
10. Love JC, Sanchez LA. Recognition of skeletal fractures in infants: an autopsy technique. *J Forensic Sci* 2009;54(6):1443–1446.
11. Love JC, Wiersema JM, Derrick SM, et al. The value of the pediatric skeletal examination in the autopsy of children. *Acad Forensic Pathol* 2014;4(1):100–108.
12. Laskey AL, Haberkorn KL, Applegate KE, et al. Postmortem skeletal survey practice in pediatric forensic autopsies: a national survey. *J Forensic Sci* 2009;54(1):189–191.
13. Centers for Disease Control and Prevention. Contribution of selected metabolic diseases to early childhood deaths—Virginia, 1996–2001. *MMWR Morb Mortal Wkly Rep* 2003;52(29):677–679.
14. Toennes SW, Kauert GF. Importance of vacutainer selection in forensic toxicological analysis of drugs of abuse. *J Anal Toxicol* 2001;25(5):339–343.
15. Roberts FJ. Procurement, interpretation, and value of postmortem cultures. *Eur J Clin Microbiol Infect Dis* 1998;17(12):821–827.
16. Wolf DA, Derrick SM, Wood RP. Preservation of evidence during pediatric organ donation: a modified thoracotomy procedure designed to increase consent in medical examiner cases. *Prog Transplant* 2011;21(1):67–70; quiz 71.
17. Wolf DA, Derrick SM. Undetermined cause and manner of death after organ/tissue donation. *Am J Forensic Med Pathol* 2010;31(2):113–116.

18. Centers for Disease Control and Prevention. Sudden Unexpected Infant Death (SUID). Available at http://www.cdc.gov/sids/aboutsuidandsids.htm. Accessed May 19, 2014.
19. Schnitzer PG, Covington TM, Dykstra HK. Sudden unexpected infant deaths: sleep environment and circumstances. *Am J Public Health* 2012;102(6):1204–1212.
20. U.S. Department of Health and Human Services, Center for Disease Control and Prevention, Division of Reproductive Health. Sudden Unexplained Infant Death Investigation (SUIDI) Reporting Form. http://www.cdc.gov/sids/pdf/suidi-form2-1-2010.pdf
21. Sturner WQ. Common errors in forensic pediatric pathology. *Am J Forensic Med Pathol* 1998;19(4):317–320.
22. Task Force on Sudden Infant Death Syndrome. The changing concept of sudden infant death syndrome: diagnostic coding shifts, controversies regarding the sleep environment, and new variables to consider in reducing risk. *Pediatrics* 2005;116(5):1245–1255.
23. Zhang K, Wang X. Maternal smoking and increased risk of sudden infant death syndrome: a meta-analysis. *Leg Med (Tokyo)* 2013;15(3):115–121.
24. Hauck FR, Thompson JM, Tanabe KO, et al. Breastfeeding and reduced risk of sudden infant death syndrome: a meta-analysis. *Pediatrics* 2011;128(1):103–110.
25. Young J, Watson K, Ellis L, et al. Responding to evidence: breastfeed baby if you can—the sixth public health recommendation to reduce the risk of sudden and unexpected death in infancy. *Breastfeed Rev* 2012;20(1):7–15.
26. Trachtenberg FL, Haas EA, Kinney HC, et al. Risk factor changes for sudden infant death syndrome after initiation of Back-to-Sleep campaign. *Pediatrics* 2012;129(4):630–638.
27. Bechtel K. Sudden unexpected infant death: differentiating natural from abusive causes in the emergency department. *Pediatr Emerg Care* 2012;28(10):1085–1089; quiz 90–91.
28. Courts C, Madea B. Genetics of the sudden infant death syndrome. *Forensic Sci Int* 2010;203(1–3):25–33.
29. Tfelt-Hansen J, Winkel BG, Grunnet M, et al. Cardiac channelopathies and sudden infant death syndrome. *Cardiology* 2011;119(1):21–33.
30. Schwartz PJ, Stramba-Badiale M, Segantini A, et al. Prolongation of the QT interval and the sudden infant death syndrome. *N Engl J Med* 1998;338(24):1709–1714.
31. National Institutes of Health Consensus Development Conference on Infantile Apnea and Home Monitoring, Sept 29 to Oct 1, 1986. *Pediatrics* 1987;79(2):292–299.
32. Filonzi L, Magnani C, Nosetti L, et al. Serotonin transporter role in identifying similarities between SIDS and idiopathic ALTE. *Pediatrics* 2012;130(1):e138–e144.
33. Willinger M, Ko CW, Hoffman HJ, et al. Trends in infant bed sharing in the United States, 1993–2000: the National Infant Sleep Position study. *Arch Pediatr Adolesc Med* 2003;157(1):43–49.
34. Lahr MB, Rosenberg KD, Lapidus JA. Bedsharing and maternal smoking in a population-based survey of new mothers. *Pediatrics* 2005;116(4):e530–e542.
35. Collins KA. Death by overlaying and wedging: a 15-year retrospective study. *Am J Forensic Med Pathol* 2001;22(2): 155–159.
36. Krous HF, Chadwick AE, Haas EA, et al. Pulmonary intra-alveolar hemorrhage in SIDS and suffocation. *J Forensic Leg Med* 2007;14(8):461–470.
37. Masoumi H, Chadwick AE, Haas EA, et al. Unclassified sudden infant death associated with pulmonary intra-alveolar hemosiderosis and hemorrhage. *J Forensic Leg Med* 2007;14(8):471–474.
38. Andrew TA, Fallon KK. Asphyxial games in children and adolescents. *Am J Forensic Med Pathol* 2007;28(4):303–307.
39. Schwartz KA, Preer G, McKeag H, et al. Child maltreatment: a review of key literature in 2013. *Curr Opin Pediatr* 2014;26(3):396–404.
40. Scafide KR, Sheridan DJ, Campbell J, et al. Evaluating change in bruise colorimetry and the effect of subject characteristics over time. *Forensic Sci Med Pathol* 2013;9(3):367–376.
41. Perper JA. Microscopic forensic pathology. In: Spitz W, ed. *Medicolegal Investigation of Death*. Springfield, IL: Charles C Thomas Publisher; 1993:660–661.
42. Kemp AM, Maguire SA, Nuttall D, et al. Bruising in children who are assessed for suspected physical abuse. *Arch Dis Child* 2014;99(2):108–113.
43. Feldman KW. Patterned abusive bruises of the buttocks and the pinnae. *Pediatrics* 1992;90(4):633–636.
44. Kleinman PK. Skeletal trauma: general considerations. In: Kleinman PK, ed. *Diagnostic Imaging of Child Abuse*, 2nd ed. St. Louis, MO: Mosby; 1998:12–22.
45. Kleinman PK, Spevak MR. Variations in acromial ossification simulating infant abuse in victims of sudden infant death syndrome. *Radiology* 1991;180(1):185–187.
46. Kerr MA, Black MM, Krishnakumar A. Failure-to-thrive, maltreatment and the behavior and development of 6-year-old children from low-income, urban families: a cumulative risk model. *Child Abuse Negl* 2000;24(5):587–598.
47. Leonidas JC. Skeletal trauma in the child abuse syndrome. *Pediatr Ann* 1983;12(12):875–881.
48. Leventhal JM, Thomas SA, Rosenfeld NS, et al. Fractures in young children. Distinguishing child abuse from unintentional injuries. *Am J Dis Child* 1993;147(1):87–92.
49. Loder RT, Bookout C. Fracture patterns in battered children. *J Orthop Trauma* 1991;5(4): 428–433.
50. Blakemore LC, Loder RT, Hensinger RN. Role of intentional abuse in children 1 to 5 years old with isolated femoral shaft fractures. *J Pediatr Orthop* 1996;16(5):585–588.
51. Merten DF, Carpenter BL. Radiologic imaging of inflicted injury in the child abuse syndrome. *Pediatr Clin North Am* 1990;37(4):815–837.
52. Dunbar JS, Owen HF, Nogrady MB, et al. Obscure tibial fracture of infants—the Toddler's fracture. *J Can Assoc Radiol* 1964;15:136–144.
53. Kleinman PK, Schlesinger AE. Mechanical factors associated with posterior rib fractures: laboratory and case studies. *Pediatr Radiol* 1997;27(1):87–91.
54. Gunther WM, Symes SA, Berryman HE. Characteristics of child abuse by anteroposterior manual compression versus cardiopulmonary resuscitation: case reports. *Am J Forensic Med Pathol* 2000;21(1):5–10.
55. Kleinman PK, Marks SC Jr, Nimkin K, et al. Rib fractures in 31 abused infants: postmortem radiologic-histopathologic study. *Radiology* 1996;200(3):807–810.
56. Ledbetter DJ, Hatch EI Jr, Feldman KW, et al. Diagnostic and surgical implications of child abuse. *Arch Surg* 1988;123(9):1101–1105.
57. Wardinsky TD. Genetic and congenital defect conditions that mimic child abuse. *J Fam Pract* 1995;41(4):377–383.
58. Marini JC, Gerber NL. Osteogenesis imperfecta. Rehabilitation and prospects for gene therapy. *JAMA* 1997;277(9):746–750.
59. Singh Kocher M, Dichtel L. Osteogenesis imperfecta misdiagnosed as child abuse. *J Pediatr Orthop B* 2011;20(6):440–443.
60. Gahagan S, Rimsza ME. Child abuse or osteogenesis imperfecta: how can we tell? *Pediatrics* 1991;88(5):987–992.
61. Ablin DS, Greenspan A, Reinhart M, et al. Differentiation of child abuse from osteogenesis imperfecta. *AJR Am J Roentgenol* 1990;154(5):1035–1046.
62. Kleinman PK. Diagnostic imaging in infant abuse. *AJR Am J Roentgenol* 1990;155(4):703–712.
63. Bullough PG, Davidson DD, Lorenzo JC. The morbid anatomy of the skeleton in osteogenesis imperfecta. *Clin Orthop Relat Res* 1981(159): 42–57.
64. Sprigg A. Temporary brittle bone disease versus suspected non-accidental skeletal injury. *Arch Dis Child* 2011;96(5):411–413.
65. Keller KA, Barnes PD. Rickets vs abuse: a national and international epidemic. *Pediatr Radiol* 2008;38(11):1210–1216.
66. Warner KG, Demling RH. The pathophysiology of free-fall injury. *Ann Emerg Med* 1986;15(9):1088–1093.
67. Helfer RE, Slovis TL, Black M. Injuries resulting when small children fall out of bed. *Pediatrics* 1977;60(4):533–535.
68. Lyons TJ, Oates RK. Falling out of bed: a relatively benign occurrence. *Pediatric* 1993;92(1):125–127.
69. Nimityongskul P, Anderson LD. The likelihood of injuries when children fall out of bed. *J Pediatr Orthop* 1987;7(2):184–186.

70. Joffee M, Ludwig S. Stairway injuries in children. *Pediatrics* 1988;82(3 Pt 2):457–461.
71. Barlow B, Niemirska M, Gandhi RP, et al. Ten years of experience with falls from a height in children. *J Pediatr Surg* 1983;18(4):509–511.
72. Williams RA. Injuries in infants and small children resulting from witnessed and corroborated free falls. *J Trauma* 1991;31(10):1350–1352.
73. Musemeche CA, Barthel M, Cosentino C, et al. Pediatric falls from heights. *J Trauma* 1991;31(10):1347–1349.
74. Reiber GD. Fatal falls in childhood. How far must children fall to sustain fatal head injury? Report of cases and review of the literature. *Am J Forensic Med Pathol* 1993;14(3):201–207.
75. Chadwick DL. Falls and childhood deaths: sorting real falls from inflicted injuries. *APSAC Advis* 1994;7:24–25.
76. Chadwick DL, Chin S, Salerno C, et al. Deaths from falls in children: how far is fatal? *J Trauma* 1991;31(10):1353–1355.
77. Hashimoto Y, Moriya F, Furumiya J. Forensic aspects of complications resulting from cardiopulmonary resuscitation. *Leg Med (Tokyo)* 2007; 9(2):94–99.
78. Hoke RS, Chamberlain D. Skeletal chest injuries secondary to cardiopulmonary resuscitation. *Resuscitation* 2004;63(3):327–338.
79. Krischer JP, Fine EG, Davis JH, et al. Complications of cardiac resuscitation. *Chest* 1987;92(2):287–291.
80. Maguire S, Mann M, John N, et al. Does cardiopulmonary resuscitation cause rib fractures in children? A systematic review. *Child Abuse Negl* 2006;30(7):739–751.
81. Sewell RD, Steinberg MA. Chest compressions in an infant with osteogenesis imperfecta type II: no new rib fractures. *Pediatrics* 2000;106(5):E71.
82. Wininger KL. Chest compressions: biomechanics and injury. *Radiol Technol* 2007;78(4):269–274.
83. Worn MJ, Jones MD. Rib fractures in infancy: establishing the mechanisms of cause from the injuries—a literature review. *Med Sci Law* 2007;47(3):200–212.
84. Dolinak D. Rib fractures in infants due to cardiopulmonary resuscitation efforts. *Am J Forensic Med Pathol* 2007;28(2):107–110.
85. Collins KA, Nichols CA. A decade of pediatric homicide: a retrospective study at the Medical University of South Carolina. *Am J Forensic Med Pathol* 1999;20(2):169–172.
86. Knight LD, Collins KA. A 25-year retrospective review of deaths due to pediatric neglect. *Am J Forensic Med Pathol* 2005;26(3):221–228.
87. Marcus BJ, Collins KA. Childhood panhypopituitarism presenting as child abuse: a case report and review of the literature. *Am J Forensic Med Pathol* 2004;25(3):265–269.
88. Baric I, Zschocke J, Christensen E, et al. Diagnosis and management of glutaric aciduria type I. *J Inherit Metab Dis* 1998;21(4):326–340.
89. Guthkelch AN. Infantile subdural haematoma and its relationship to whiplash injuries. *Br Med J* 1971;2(5759):430–431.
90. Caffey J. The whiplash shaken infant syndrome: manual shaking by the extremities with whiplash-induced intracranial and intraocular bleedings, linked with residual permanent brain damage and mental retardation. *Pediatrics* 1974;54(4):396–403.
91. Bandak FA. Shaken baby syndrome: a biomechanics analysis of injury mechanisms. *Forensic Sci Int* 2005;151(1):71–79.
92. Gabaeff SC. Challenging the pathophysiologic connection between subdural hematoma, retinal hemorrhage and shaken baby syndrome. *West J Emerg Med* 2011;12(2):144–158.
93. Matshes EW, Evans RM, Pinckard JK, et al. Shaken infants die of neck trauma, not brain trauma. *Acad Forensic Pathol* 2011;1(1):82–91.
94. Hanigan WC, Peterson RA, Njus G. Tin ear syndrome: rotational acceleration in pediatric head injuries. *Pediatrics* 1987;80(5):618–622.
95. Levin AV. Retinal hemorrhage in abusive head trauma. *Pediatrics* 2010;126(5):961–970.
96. Billmire ME, Myers PA. Serious head injury in infants: accident or abuse? *Pediatrics* 1985;75(2):340–342.
97. Buys YM, Levin AV, Enzenauer RW, et al. Retinal findings after head trauma in infants and young children. *Ophthalmology* 1992;99(11): 1718–1723.
98. Tomasi LG, Rosman NP. Purtscher retinopathy in the battered child syndrome. *Am J Dis Child* 1975;129(11):1335–1337.
99. Rooks VJ, Sisler C, Burton B. Cervical spine injury in child abuse: report of two cases. *Pediatr Radiol* 1998;28(3):193–195.
100. Gill JR. Pediatric starvation by neglect. *Acad Forensic Pathol* 2013;3(1): 46–53.
101. Hiss J, Kahana T, Kugel C, et al. Fatal classic and exertional heat stroke—report of four cases. *Med Sci Law* 1994;34(4):339–343.
102. Krous HF, Nadeau JM, Fukumoto RI, et al. Environmental hyperthermic infant and early childhood death: circumstances, pathologic changes, and manner of death. *Am J Forensic Med Pathol* 2001;22(4): 374–382.
103. Seri I, Evans J. Limits of viability: definition of the gray zone. *J Perinatol* 2008;28(Suppl 1):S4–S8.
104. Sims MA, Collins KA. Fetal death. A 10-year retrospective study. *Am J Forensic Med Pathol* 2001;22(3):261–265.
105. Wisser M, Rothschild MA, Schmolling JC, et al. Caput succedaneum and facial petechiae-birth-associated injuries in healthy newborns under forensic aspects. *Int J Legal Med* 2012;126(3):385–390.
106. Moritz AR, Henriques FC. Studies of thermal injury: II. The relative importance of time and surface temperature in the causation of cutaneous burns. *Am J Pathol* 1947;23(5):695–720.
107. DiMaio DJ, DiMaio VJM. *Forensic Pathology*. Boca Raton, FL: CRC Press; 1993:314.
108. Rosenberg DA. Web of deceit: a literature review of Munchausen syndrome by proxy. *Child Abuse Negl* 1987;11(4):547–563.
109. Bass C, Glaser D. Early recognition and management of fabricated or induced illness in children. *Lancet* 2014;383(9926):1412–1421.
110. Reece RM. Unusual manifestations of child abuse. *Pediatr Clin North Am* 1990;37(4):905–921.
111. Meadow R. What is, and what is not, 'Münchhausen syndrome by proxy'? *Arch Dis Child* 1995;72(6):534–539.
112. Southall DP, Plunkett MC, Banks MW, et al. Covert video recordings of life-threatening child abuse: lessons for child protection. *Pediatrics* 1997;100(5):735–760.
113. Feldman KW, Christopher DM, Opheim KB. Münchausen syndrome/bulimia by proxy: ipecac as a toxin in child abuse. *Child Abuse Negl* 1989;13(2):257–261.

CHAPTER 8

Transplant Pathology

Rish K. Pai, M.D., Ph.D., Anthony Chang, M.D., and Aliya N. Husain, M.D.

Solid organ transplantation is the optimal mode of therapy for a variety of end-stage diseases, with somewhat variable long-term outcome depending on the organ, as is discussed in this chapter (small bowel, liver, pancreas, kidney, heart, and lung). Kidney and liver transplants are relatively more common; thus, these are presented in greater detail. Although there are many organ-specific features in posttransplantation pathology, there are also many similarities. Postsurgical complications have markedly decreased due to better techniques and donor and recipient management. Immunosuppressive regimens, including multiple drug combinations, are standard of care. Antibody-mediated rejection (AMR) is uncommon, while acute cellular rejection occurs in a majority of recipients and can usually be treated effectively. Chronic rejection is a fibrosing process that continues to be the major limiting factor to long-term survival, and is more frequent in lung and kidney than in heart or liver allografts. These immunocompromised patients are susceptible to both the usual bacterial as well as opportunistic infections, which often involve the lung. Posttransplant lymphoproliferative disease (PTLD), reported to occur in 3% to 5% of recipients, appears to be decreasing even further. It can involve the transplanted organ (rare in heart) as well as extranodal sites such as the gastrointestinal tract.

TRANSPLANT IMMUNOLOGY

Overview

The success of transplantation depends, in large part, on the immune response of the recipient to the donor tissue. The phenomenon of graft rejection was first identified by Peter Medawar in the early 1940s. Medawar and others demonstrated that allogeneic skin grafts (graft from a genetically distinct individual of the same species) would undergo rapid necrosis; however, syngeneic skin grafts (graft from a genetically identical individual) would survive. As almost all solid organ transplants occur between two genetically different individuals (allogeneic graft), many potential foreign or nonself molecules (alloantigens) are available to elicit an immune response and lead to graft failure. Most of these alloantigens are derived from polymorphic genes inherited from both parents and expressed codominantly. One of the most important alloantigens responsible for rejection is encoded by the major histocompatibility complex (MHC). There are three different histopathologic categories of rejection: antibody-mediated (including hyperacute) rejection, acute rejection, and chronic rejection, each of which can also be characterized by immunologic effector mechanisms (humoral versus cell mediated). As transplant immunology is a complex field, only a limited discussion of this broad topic is presented here, and interested readers are referred to many excellent reviews for further reading (1,2).

Antibody-Mediated Rejection

The most severe form of AMR is hyperacute rejection, which is characterized by thrombotic occlusion of the graft vasculature that begins within minutes to hours after blood vessel anastomosis. The mechanism involves preformed antibodies present in the recipient that bind to donor endothelial cells and elicit an immune response characterized by complement activation. Complement proteins are powerful serum proteins that are able to damage cells through either cell lysis or recruitment of inflammatory cells such as neutrophils and macrophages. Classical complement activation occurs when an antibody of the IgM or IgG subclass binds to its cognate antigen and activates C1q. Activation of complement leads to the destruction of donor endothelial cells, resulting in thrombosis. The IgM antibodies responsible for hyperacute rejection are mainly those against the carbohydrate ABO blood group antigen expressed primarily on red blood cells but also on vascular endothelial cells. As most donors and recipients are matched with respect to their ABO subtypes, hyperacute rejection due to anti-ABO antibodies is rare. Although a few centers are successful in performing ABO-incompatible transplantation, it is done only occasionally.

Most forms of AMR occur due to the patient acquiring donor-specific antibodies sometime during the posttransplant period. The incidence is variable depending on the transplanted organ, as detailed in each of the specific sections below.

Acute Allograft Rejection

Acute allograft rejection is commonly encountered in solid organ transplants and has been an area of extensive research. Classically, acute rejection is characterized by the presence of infiltrating lymphocytes that mediate direct killing, macrophage activation, and tissue damage. The lymphocytes involved in this process include $CD4^+$ T-cells, $CD8^+$ T-cells, natural killer (NK) cells, and B cells. Much of transplant immunology has been focused on the role of T cells in rejection, as they are the principal mediators of acute rejection. Indeed, much of the immunosuppressive therapies in use today are directed toward interfering with T-cell function. The mechanism underlying T-cell activation is complex and involves direct presentation of alloantigens (non–self-MHC molecules) to recipient T-cells by donor-derived leukocytes and indirect presentation of alloantigens to recipient T-cells by recipient leukocytes. The process by which recipient T-cells can be directly activated by non–self-MHC molecules on donor cells is still a mystery to most immunologists. During T-cell development in the thymus, those cells, with T-cell receptors, with high affinity for self-MHC molecules are deleted and only those with low affinity for self-MHC survive, thus preventing nonspecific T-cell activation (negative selection) (3). However, in the transplant setting, recipient peripheral T-cells are exposed to *non–self*-MHC. Immunologists hypothesize that since T-cells with high affinity for these MHC molecules were not deleted by negative selection, there will be a significant proportion (up to 1%) of circulating recipient T-cells with high affinity for non–self-MHC (4). These T-cells could become activated and mediate allograft rejection. The subsequent secretion of cytokines leads to macrophage, neutrophil, and NK cell recruitment (through chemokine and adhesion molecule expression) and tissue destruction (through reactive oxygen species, arachidonic acid metabolites, thrombosis, etc.). In addition, through direct allorecognition, donor $CD8^+$ T-cells can mediate killing. Direct allorecognition is thought to be the principle mechanism by which cellular rejection is mediated.

Indirect recognition of alloantigens is much better understood immunologically as it mirrors what occurs during infections. In this pathway, recipient antigen-presenting cells (dendritic cells and macrophages) phagocytose donor antigens and process them into peptides for presentation on class I and class II MHC. T-cells specific for these peptide: MHC complexes then can become activated and mediate rejection. The proportion of T-cells that would be activated in such a manner is much smaller than in direct allorecognition, and for many years, the significance of this pathway of T-cell activation has been unclear. Recently, indirect presentation has gained the interest of transplant immunologists as it can on its own mediate rejection (5). Moreover, indirect presentation is essential in producing highly specific antidonor antibodies (6). The donor-specific antibodies are mainly directed against donor MHC, both class I and class II. Once formed, these antibodies can bind to donor leukocytes and activated endothelial cells (anti-MHC class II) or all donor cells (anti-MHC class I) resulting in tissue damage through activation of complement and recruitment of inflammatory cells. Indeed, the use of C4d, a product of the complement cascade, as a surrogate of antibody-mediated complement activation has helped pathologists recognize acute humoral rejection (7,8).

Chronic Allograft Rejection

Histologically, chronic rejection in most organs is characterized by fibrosis and vascular damage, and immunologically, this process most likely represents repeated bouts of acute rejection (sometimes subclinical). Thus, both cell-mediated and humoral mechanisms most likely contribute to chronic rejection. Upon activation, some T cells can differentiate into effector cells that produce fibrosing cytokines (9) resulting in collagen deposition and parenchymal extinction. In addition, other cytokines such as platelet-derived growth factor and basic fibroblast growth factor can induce proliferation of smooth muscle cells leading to narrowing of the graft vessels. Moreover, antidonor antibodies have been shown to activate endothelial proliferation and vascular remodeling in animal models (6). The resulting ischemia further leads to parenchymal loss and graft dysfunction. Other causes of late graft dysfunction might not necessarily be related to immune-mediated rejection. Indeed, systemic disease such as diabetes, hyperlipidemia, viral infections, etc. can all contribute to late graft dysfunction and should be differentiated from chronic rejection.

Allograft Tolerance

Understanding the immunologic mechanisms of allograft rejection has been essential in developing new therapies as well as defining new histopathologic entities (acute humoral rejection); however, many questions remain. One of the most active fields in transplant immunology is uncovering the mechanisms behind allograft tolerance. The goal of such research is to determine which patients can be removed from immunosuppressive therapy due to tolerance toward the donor allograft. This is particularly important in the pediatric population as immunosuppressive therapy is a major cause of morbidity and mortality. To date, no serologic or histopathologic data can accurately predict graft survival upon withdrawal of medications; however, evidence points to a role of donor-derived leukocytes in mediating allograft tolerance. It is hypothesized that patients who become microchimeras are more likely to become tolerant to their allografts (10). This finding is supported by the early observations that solid organ allografts are accepted to a great extent in individuals who are also receiving partial bone marrow transplants (11). In addition, the greater acceptance of liver allografts is thought to be due to the large number of donor-derived leukocytes present in this organ, some of which may be pluripotent stem cells that can migrate to recipient bone marrow and persist. The recent appreciation of regulatory T cells has also shed light on allograft tolerance. Regulatory T cells have been shown to suppress the function of effector T cells, and active research is underway to enhance the activity of regulatory T cells in order to achieve allograft tolerance (12).

TRANSPLANT PATHOLOGY OF THE INTESTINE

Overview

The introduction of improved immunosuppression has led to a rise in small intestinal transplantation that is of particular importance to the pediatric pathologist as many of the disorders requiring transplantation occur in children: intestinal atresia, necrotizing enterocolitis, intestinal volvulus, Crohn disease, gastroschisis, massive resections, Hirschsprung disease, neuronal intestinal dysplasia, neuropathic and myopathic pseudoobstruction, protein-losing enteropathy, and microvillus inclusion disease (13–15). When the liver disease is mild, the intestine can be transplanted in isolation. Signs of portal hypertension and cirrhosis mandate intestinal transplantation in combination with the liver or as part of a multivisceral organ transplant. Indeed, patients receiving combined intestinal/liver transplantation or a multivisceral organ transplant experience fewer episodes of acute rejection and improved overall survival at 5 years (16). Currently, the major obstacle to intestinal transplantation is the availability of appropriate grafts. In particular, size matching is of extreme importance as many pediatric patients have contracted abdominal cavities as a result of previous surgeries.

The pathologist's role in intestinal transplantation is to evaluate mucosal biopsies in patients with graft dysfunction or as part of a surveillance program. Most institutions routinely take protocol biopsies for the first few months and when clinically indicated thereafter. In evaluating mucosal biopsies, the pathologist must correlate histologic findings with the clinical and endoscopic findings. As with most transplant specimens, a systematic approach evaluating the overall architecture, surface and crypt epithelium, inflammatory infiltrate, and vasculature can prevent pitfalls in diagnosis.

Preservation Injury and Hyperacute Rejection

Due to the intestinal villous circulation, the regenerative compartment of the epithelium is protected from ischemia; thus, preservation injury is less worrisome than in other solid organs. Biopsies taken prior to transplantation demonstrate lamina propria edema and separation of the epithelium from the basement membrane. Shortly after reperfusion, numerous mitoses can be seen within the regenerative compartment along with capillary congestion, villous blunting, and a mild neutrophilic infiltrate (17). Biopsies taken a week after transplantation usually show normal histology even when earlier epithelial damage was quite severe. Hyperacute (antibody-mediated) rejection in small bowel transplants has recently been described, and there is some overlap with preservation injury; however, distinction between the two is usually not difficult. In instances of hyperacute rejection, there is a positive cross-match indicating preformed donor-specific antibodies. These antibodies damage the endothelium leading to fibrin thrombi within the lamina propria vasculature resulting in severe congestion and focal hemorrhage. Neutrophils can be seen marginating within the congested vessels. The presence of fibrin thrombi and severe congestion distinguishes hyperacute rejection from preservation injury (18).

Acute Rejection

Unlike liver allografts, acute rejection is common and remains a major cause of intestinal graft failure. Acute rejection is clinically characterized by nonspecific symptoms such as fever, nausea, vomiting, increased stomal output, abdominal pain, and distention. In severe acute rejection, hemodynamic instability may occur, leading to shock. Endoscopically, acute rejection is characterized by granularity, diminished peristalsis, and, in some cases, mucosal ulceration. Acute rejection can occur at any time in the post-transplant period; however, the first episode of rejection usually occurs within 100 days (14,15). The landmark paper by Lee et al. (17) analyzed the first 62 intestinal transplants performed at the University of Pittsburgh and was the first study to develop histologic criteria for the diagnosis of acute rejection. Subsequent modifications have led to a well-developed histologic grading system for acute rejection that provides a reliable assessment of severity (19).

The histologic manifestations of acute rejection include crypt apoptosis, increased lamina propria inflammatory cell infiltrate, and crypt architectural distortion. During most episodes of acute rejection, all biopsies taken from multiple sites will show histologic features of rejection; however, in approximately 20% of cases, only the ileum will be involved. Crypt apoptosis is the earliest histologic sign of rejection, and apoptotic counts should be routinely performed on mucosal biopsy specimens. Rejection is characterized by greater than six apoptotic bodies per ten consecutive crypts, and in mild acute rejection, crypt apoptosis is the dominant histologic feature (Figure 8-1). In addition, mild localized collections of inflammatory cells (predominately activated/blastic lymphocytes with lesser numbers of eosinophils and neutrophils) are present around small venules and capillaries in the deep mucosa. Peyer patches become enlarged and contain large numbers of activated lymphocytes. The crypt epithelium commonly shows features of regeneration including mucin depletion, nuclear enlargement, and hyperchromasia. A mild increase in intraepithelial lymphocytes and occasional neutrophils is typically seen. The villi are shortened, and the crypts may be distorted due to lamina propria expansion.

Moderate rejection is characterized by increased crypt apoptotic bodies and a diffuse inflammatory cell infiltrate characterized by activated lymphocytes. Crypt apoptotic bodies begin to appear in the midportions of the crypt and

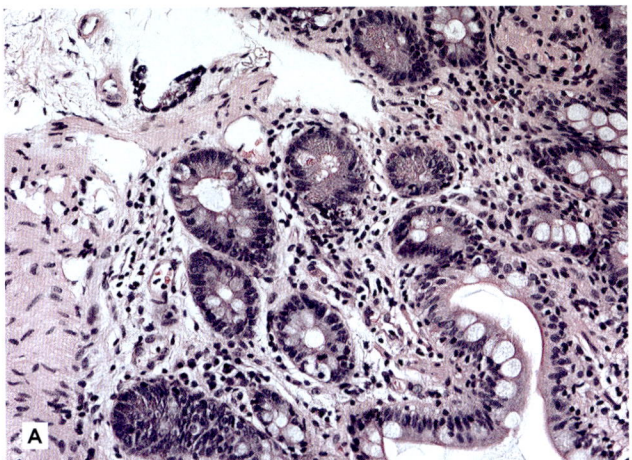
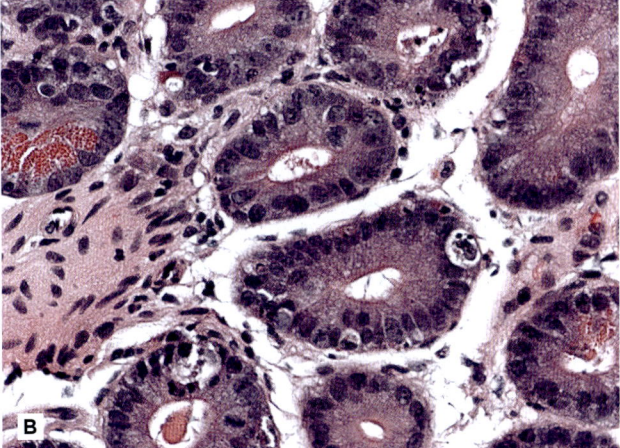

FIGURE 8-1 • Mild acute rejection of small bowel allografts. **A:** The villous architecture is usually preserved, and there is only a mild increase in lamina propria inflammation. **B:** Prominent apoptotic bodies are the most evident feature (Photos courtesy of Dr. Reetesh Pai, Stanford University).

confluent apoptosis in a single crypt may be seen. The villi are flattened to a greater extent; however, extensive ulceration is not common. In severe acute rejection, crypt apoptotic body counts are further increased (up to 20) (Figure 8-2). Mucosal ulcerations are common and, in its place, are fibrinous neutrophilic exudates mimicking pseudomembranous colitis. Care should be taken when evaluating biopsies for acute rejection 100 days post transplant as the inflammatory infiltrate is generally mild and crypt apoptosis is the only dominant histologic feature (17).

Chronic Rejection

Chronic rejection in the intestine is less common than in heart, kidney, and lung (20). Patients with chronic rejection have persistent diarrhea despite increased immunosuppressive therapy. Endoscopic and radiographic findings of chronic rejection include loss of mucosal folds, mural thickening, focal ulcers, and decreased arborization of the mesenteric vasculature. Clinically, chronic rejection is encountered late in the posttransplant period, with most cases occurring months after transplantation. There are many factors associated with the development of chronic rejection. Those individuals with acute rejection within 30 days of transplantation and those with severe acute rejection are more likely to develop chronic rejection. Other risk factors include prolonged cold ischemic time, old donor age, and episodes of cytomegalovirus (CMV) infection (20). Simultaneous liver transplantation greatly protects from chronic rejection most likely by decreasing the number of acute rejection episodes. The pathologic process that results in chronic rejection involves arterial obliteration; however, arteries are rarely sampled in endoscopic biopsies. Thus, on mucosal biopsies, one can only suggest possible chronic rejection based on downstream features of chronic ischemia. Early histologic changes that suggest possible

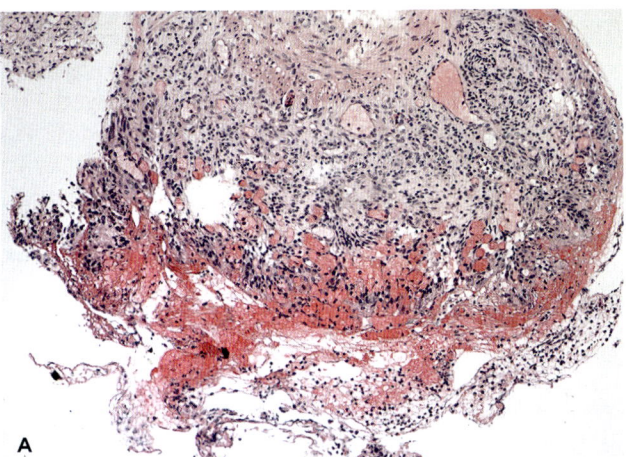
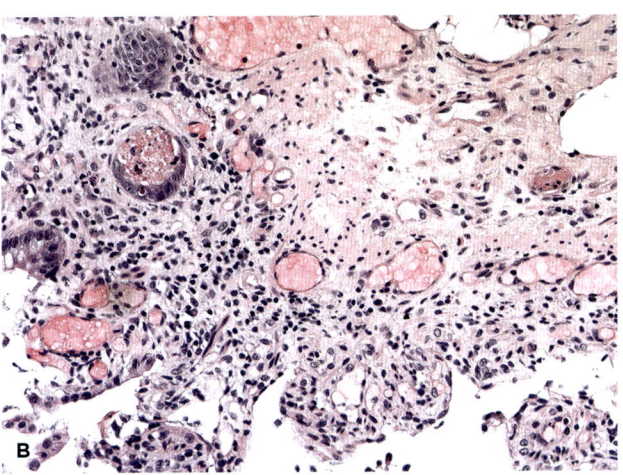

FIGURE 8-2 • Severe acute rejection of small bowel allografts. **A:** Surface ulceration with a prominent lymphocytic infiltrate is common. **B:** Crypts are typically lost, and the surviving crypts are severely damaged. This differential diagnosis includes ischemia and infection (Photos courtesy of Dr. Reetesh Pai, Stanford University).

chronic rejection include patchy mild fibrosis and focal crypt loss. These nonspecific changes can persist for months. With worsening ischemia due to progression of chronic rejection, there is extensive loss of the intestinal crypts, villous atrophy, mucosal ulceration, and increased lamina propria inflammation and fibrosis. The surviving crypts show evidence of chronic damage including pyloric gland metaplasia (17,20). Once chronic rejection proceeds to the severe stage, the graft is very likely to fail. At resection, the vasculature should be adequately sampled to find the characteristic changes of chronic rejection. In addition, extensive neural hyperplasia is a common finding at resection (21).

Complications of Transplantation

Infection remains a very common complication of transplantation, whether in the postoperative setting or due to immunosuppressive therapies. The majority of infections are bacterial infections although fungal infections are also encountered (15). Of more importance to the pathologist is recognizing viral infections, in particular CMV, Epstein-Barr virus (EBV), and adenovirus. CMV infection is encountered in 5% to 29% of intestinal allograft specimens and can clinically mimic acute rejection (15). Negative CMV serology in the pediatric recipient is associated with increased CMV infection when transplanted with a serologic positive donor (22). In the majority of specimens, a moderate neutrophilic and mononuclear cell infiltrate is seen in the lamina propria as well as in the crypts. Ulceration with abundant granulation tissue can be seen in severe cases. In severely immunocompromised individuals, inflammation may be mild. In addition, crypt atrophy, cell dropout, and apoptotic bodies may be present, mimicking rejection. The characteristic CMV inclusions are mainly confined to the endothelial and stromal cells (Figure 8-3); however, epithelial cells can be infected in severe cases.

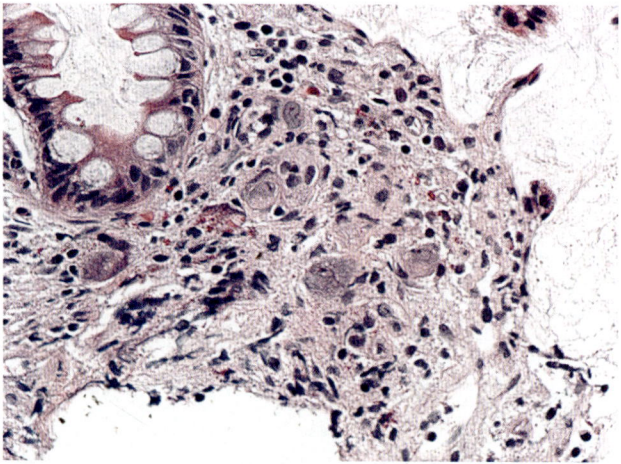

FIGURE 8-3 • CMV infection of small bowel allograft. In CMV infection, an inflammatory infiltrate with ulceration, crypt atrophy, and apoptotic bodies can be seen; however, the characteristic cytoplasmic and nuclear inclusions are key in differentiating CMV infection from rejection (Photo courtesy of Dr. Reetesh Pai, Stanford University).

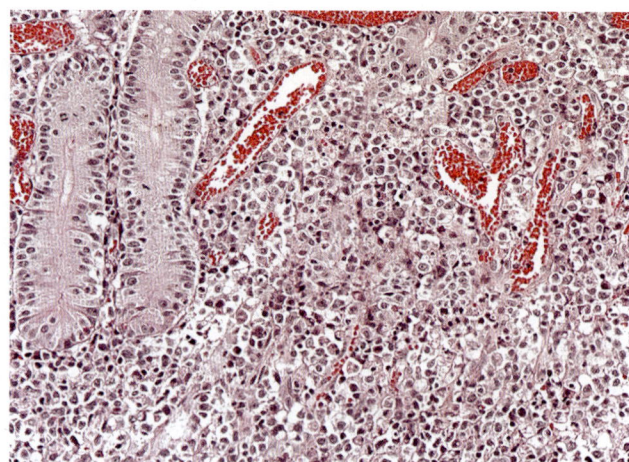

FIGURE 8-4 • Posttransplant lymphoproliferative disorder of small bowel allografts. PTLD is commonly characterized by an atypical inflammatory infiltrate, which can be mixed (polymorphous) as in this case or monomorphic. In situ hybridization for EBER can be helpful in confirming the diagnosis (Photo courtesy of Dr. Reetesh Pai, Stanford University).

Adenovirus is a very common cause of pediatric gastroenteritis; however, until recently, infection of allografts has not been routinely recognized. Pinchoff et al. (23) found a high prevalence of adenoviral infection in pediatric small bowel allografts. Adenoviral enteritis most commonly affects the ileum and is characterized by smudgy epithelial cell nuclear inclusions, epithelial hyperplasia with disarray, and a prominent lymphoplasmacytic infiltrate.

EBV infection is another serious complication in the posttransplant period as it can lead to PTLD (24). EBV infection is associated with a wide histologic spectrum, from simple lymphoid hyperplasia to non-Hodgkin lymphoma. When evaluating a specimen, particular attention should be paid to the type of lymphoid infiltrate (Figure 8-4). If small lymphocytes predominate, one can be reassured; however, the presence of large atypical lymphoid cells should prompt concern for PTLD and in situ hybridization for EBV early RNA (EBER) should be performed. A large number of EBER-positive cells (>15 per high-power field) with a heterogeneous population of lymphoid cells, including immunoblasts, plasma cells, and large cleaved cells, are characteristic of polymorphous PTLD (Figure 8-4) (24). If the lymphoid population is homogenous, the designation of monomorphic PTLD is made, and further classification is made according to established criteria (24). The vast majority of monomorphic PTLDs are B cell in origin; however, T-cell PTLDs have been described.

The Gastrointestinal Tract in Graft Versus Host Disease

The intestinal tract is one of the three major target organs in graft versus host disease (GVHD) (25,26). The skin and the liver are the other two organs affected when donor lymphoid cells are transfused into immunosuppressed host. GVHD usually occurs in the setting of bone marrow transplantation but may also rarely occur following the transfusion of nonirradiated blood into patients with primary or secondary immunodeficiency disorders (27). Conceptually, GVHD mirrors allograft rejection as donor leukocytes recognize recipient tissues as "foreign" and attempt to "reject" them. Thus, the immunologic effector mechanisms are similar.

The gastrointestinal tract is affected in at least half of patients with acute GVHD and classically occurs within the first 100 days posttransplantation; however, persistent, recurrent, or late-onset acute GVHD is a well-recognized phenomenon (25). Intestinal GVHD is usually heralded by profuse watery diarrhea, which indicates involvement of the small intestine and colon. Occasionally, the upper gastrointestinal tract will be involved first or exclusively; the symptoms are nausea, vomiting, and anorexia. Acute intestinal GVHD is usually diagnosed by colonoscopic biopsy or endoscopic biopsy of the upper gastrointestinal tract. The earliest histologic changes occur deep in the crypts (the regenerative compartment) with epithelial infiltration by lymphocytes and subsequent apoptosis of individual glandular cells (28,29) (Figure 8-5). The minimum necessary criteria to diagnose acute GVHD are variable across institutions. At a minimum, more than one apoptotic body per biopsy fragment is necessary to consider a diagnosis of acute GVHD (30). However, in the setting of cytomegaloviral infection, recent chemotherapy, and features suspicious for medication injury, it may not be possible to definitively diagnosis GVHD. If appropriate therapy is not instituted, glandular destruction and ulceration are seen. Complete crypt loss, villous atrophy, and extensive mucosal denudation occur in advanced acute GVHD. In the esophagus, vacuolization and inflammation of the epithelial basal layer with apoptosis of squamous epithelial cells and eventual desquamation and ulceration are seen (31).

Chronic GVHD is a more insidious process that primarily affects the skin and liver. The intestinal tract is largely spared; however, features of chronic injury can be seen (32). In the esophagus, a scleroderma-like fibrosis and dysmotility may develop (33). In the evaluation of all the phases of intestinal GVHD, opportunistic infections must be ruled out (31). Interestingly, mycophenolate mofetil, a commonly used immunosuppressive drug in solid organ transplantation, can give rise to histologic findings similar to acute GVHD (34).

TRANSPLANT PATHOLOGY OF THE LIVER

Overview

In the United States, approximately 10% of the total number of liver transplants occur in the pediatric population (35). The indications for liver transplant are diverse (Table 8-1) (35); the most common continues to be extrahepatic biliary atresia.

TABLE 8-1 INDICATIONS FOR PEDIATRIC LIVER TRANSPLANTATION

Noncholestatic cirrhosis
    Autoimmune hepatitis
    Chronic viral hepatitis
Cholestatic liver disease/cirrhosis
    Caroli disease
    Choledochol cyst
    Primary sclerosing cholangitis
Biliary atresia
    Extrahepatic
    Alagille syndrome
    Hypoplasia
Acute hepatic necrosis
    Acute viral hepatitis
    Drugs
Metabolic diseases
    Alpha-1-antitrypsin deficiency
    Wilson disease
    Hemochromatosis
    Tyrosinemia
    Primary oxalosis
    Glycogen storage disease types Ia, Ib, III, and IV
    Hyperlipidemia
    Urea cycle disorders
    Crigler-Najjar syndrome
Malignant neoplasms
    Hepatoblastoma
    Hepatocellular carcinoma
Other
    Cystic fibrosis
    Budd-Chiari syndrome
    Congenital hepatic fibrosis
    TPN/hyperalimentation
    Familial cholestasis
    Hepatic adenomatosis

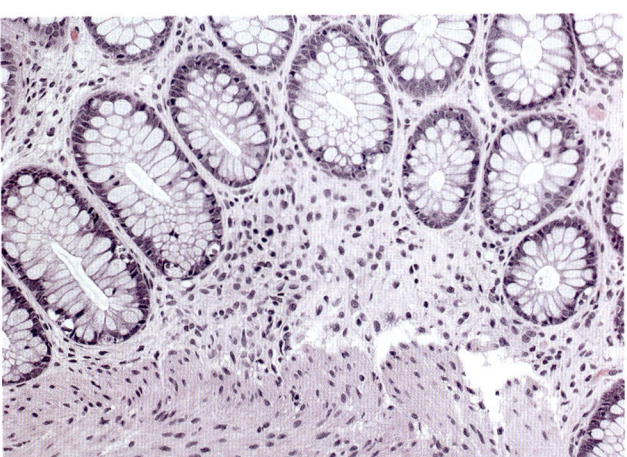

FIGURE 8-5 • GVHD of the small bowel. GVHD is characterized by apoptosis of individual epithelial cells lining the crypts similar to acute rejection seen in small bowel transplants. If severe, complete villous loss and surface ulceration can be seen.

Early in pediatric transplantation, the survival rates were dismal as only 30% of patients survived greater than 1 year (13). With improved surgical techniques, patient screening, and immunosuppression, the current 1-year patient survival is 90% and the 5-year survival is 80%. Graft survival is 85% at 1 year and 67% at 5 years (35). The early days of pediatric liver transplantation were also complicated by a shortage of appropriate-sized liver allografts. With the advent of reduced-sized liver transplantation, living-related transplantation, and, most importantly, split-liver transplantation, the shortage of pediatric liver allografts has been somewhat alleviated (13,36,37). In split-liver transplants, the whole adult cadaveric liver is divided into two functional segments: one for adults (right trisegment) and one for children (left lateral segment). Recent studies have shown that split-liver recipients have comparable survival to whole liver recipients (38,39). Despite these improvements, surgical complications continue to be more common when compared with adults (13,36,40). In particular, the use of partial liver allografts predisposes to biliary complications (41). In addition, hepatic artery thrombosis (HAT) is more common in pediatric patients owing to the technically difficult surgery. However, the improvement in surgical techniques and postoperative management has improved, allowing many of these grafts to be saved. Portal vein thrombosis is occasionally encountered, which, in most cases, resolves without need for intervention (40). Hepatic vein thrombosis is rarely encountered except in patients undergoing liver transplantation for Budd-Chiari syndrome. Bowel perforation is common in the pediatric population as most of these patients have had previous abdominal surgery and suffer from poor nutrition. Other complications of liver transplant can be roughly grouped into the time periods in which they are most likely to occur (Table 8-2) (42).

The initial outcome of the liver allograft depends on the health of the donor liver, the amount of ischemic time the allograft suffered, the presence of preformed antiallograft antibodies, and complications encountered during surgery and the perioperative period. Acute rejection and viral infections tend to occur between 1 week and 2 months post transplantation, whereas chronic rejection and recurrent disease are late manifestations. However, the timing can vary significantly (e.g., late-onset acute rejection), and biopsy interpretation remains essential.

Preservation Injury

Preservation (harvesting) injury results from donor and tissue procurement factors that contribute to poor allograft function in the perioperative period. In order to diagnose preservation injury, one must exclude injury due to surgical complications, immunologic reactions, and drug toxicity. Warm and cold ischemia preferentially damages hepatocytes and endothelial cells, respectively. Endothelial cell damage leads to interference with vascular blood flow and subsequent allograft injury. Many donor factors can increase the susceptibility of the allograft to ischemic time. One of the most studied is the presence of donor macrovesicular steatosis. Transplantation of liver allografts with greater than 50% macrovesicular steatosis, on frozen section analysis, may result in poor graft function as steatotic hepatocytes are sensitive to ischemic damage. Other donor factors that influence graft function include fibrosis, chronic liver disease,

TABLE 8-2 APPROXIMATE TIMELINE OF BIOPSY FINDINGS IN LIVER TRANSPLANTATION

Posttransplant Interval	Complications	Histologic Features
Early (0-7 d)	Preservation/harvesting injury	Centrilobular pallor, ballooning degeneration, cholestasis
	Humoral rejection	Extensive necrosis and perivenular hemorrhage; positive C4d
	Early hepatic artery thrombosis	Zonal hepatocyte and bile duct necrosis
Middle (7-30 d)	Acute cellular rejection	Mixed portal infiltrate, bile duct damage, and endothelialitis
	CMV hepatitis	Microabscesses and viral inclusions
Late (>30 d)	Recurrent disease	Features of original disease
	Chronic rejection	Bile duct and arteriolar loss, foam cell arteriopathy
	Late-onset acute rejection	Perivenular inflammation, interface and lobular activity, less endothelialitis and portal inflammation than classic acute rejection
	PTLD	Atypical lymphoid infiltrate, EBER+
	Late hepatic artery thrombosis	Centrilobular hepatocyte dropout, biliary obstruction
	De novo autoimmune hepatitis	Lymphoplasmacytic infiltrate with interface activity

hemodynamic instability, infections, donor atherosclerosis, and donor age (43,44).

Clinically, preservation injury is characterized by poor bile production and persistent elevations of serum ALT and AST. The histologic features of preservation injury are usually apparent within 1 to 2 days after revascularization. In mild preservation injury, mild centrilobular hepatocyte ballooning and canalicular cholestasis are commonly seen. Occasionally, neutrophils may be present. On low-power microscopic evaluation, preservation injury can be suggested by pallor in the centrilobular areas. The hepatocyte injury is rapidly reversible; however, the cholestasis may persist for several weeks (Figure 8-6). In more severe injury, zonal necrosis and severe neutrophilia may be seen. In these biopsies, bile ductular proliferation as well as cholestasis may be prominent. In patients receiving a steatotic liver, reperfusion results in lysis of the steatotic hepatocytes with formation of sinusoidal fat droplets that disrupt hepatic blood flow. The extracellular fat may persist for weeks after initial injury. Resolution of hepatic injury is the hallmark of preservation injury, but if severe, the allograft may fail resulting in primary nonfunction. If hepatocyte injury persists beyond 1 week, other diagnoses such as rejection and obstructive cholangitis should be considered.

It is our practice to report the percentage of macrovesicular steatotic hepatocytes, the amount of fibrosis, and the presence of perivenular necrosis (45) to our transplant surgeons who ultimately determine allograft use.

Hepatic Artery Thrombosis

As previously mentioned, HAT remains a significant problem in pediatric liver transplantation and is a complication in 5% to 10% of pediatric liver allografts (40). The incidence of HAT increases with decreasing age due to the smaller size of the arterial anastomosis. As the hepatic artery is the sole blood supply to the biliary tree, HAT should be sought whenever a biliary leak is found. HAT can occur early in the posttransplant period or late (occurring >30 days post transplant). Early HAT is associated with severe graft dysfunction and high mortality rate. In early HAT, rapid diagnosis and repair of the vascular tree are essential in reversing biliary damage and prevention of allograft failure. Even with aggressive treatment, retransplantation may be necessary; however, in one study, 40% of children with HAT survived without retransplantation (46).

In late HAT, the allograft is less susceptible to damage as collaterals have formed. Indeed, many patients are asymptomatic. Symptomatic patients commonly present with recurrent cholangitis, biliary tract strictures (due to prolonged ischemic damage), abscess, and fever. Biopsy findings in HAT are nonspecific, variable, and irregularly distributed within the graft (42). The earliest histologic features of arterial insufficiency include scattered apoptotic hepatocytes and increase mitotic activity (30). If ischemia persists, coagulative necrosis of the centrilobular hepatocytes is frequently encountered along with bile duct necrosis. In late HAT, features of biliary obstruction are encountered, including canalicular cholestasis, cholate stasis, and bile ductular proliferation. In addition, centrilobular hepatocyte ballooning and dropout are commonly seen. Although these findings suggest HAT, definitive diagnosis requires clinical correlation.

Biliary Complications

In children, biliary tract complications are more numerous due to surgical difficulties and the use of split-liver allografts (36,40,47). Clinically, biliary complications should be suspected when preferential increases in alkaline phosphatase and gamma-glutamyl transferase occur. Minor strictures may be asymptomatic with only minor elevations in biliary enzymes, whereas complete obstruction, cholangitic abscess, and ascending cholangitis result in fever, jaundice, right upper quadrant pain, and bacteremia. In the acute phase, liver biopsies show portal edema, ductular reaction, canalicular cholestasis, and a portal inflammatory cell infiltrate rich in neutrophils that is intimately associated with the proliferating ductules. Chronic obstruction leads to cholate stasis, chronic portal inflammation, focal bile duct loss, and portal fibrosis. Progression to biliary cirrhosis can occur if the obstruction is not relieved. Biliary–vascular fistula is a serious complication that warrants prompt surgical correction. Histologically, bile is found in blood vessels often with a giant cell reaction, and red blood cells are found within bile ducts.

Antibody-Mediated (Humoral) Rejection

The liver is relatively resistant to injury by antidonor antibodies for multiple reasons including clearance of antibodies by resident Kupffer cells, dual blood supply, and large sinusoidal surface area, which facilitates absorption of antibodies (48).

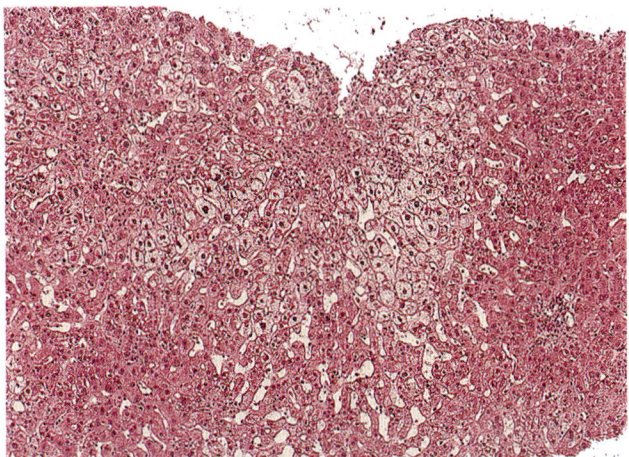

FIGURE 8-6 • Preservation injury of liver allografts. Pallor in the centrilobular areas with hepatocyte ballooning occurring shortly after transplantation is characteristic of mild preservation injury. Hepatocyte and canalicular cholestasis can also be quite prominent in some cases.

Antidonor antibodies may be preformed or develop *de novo*. Preformed antibodies against ABO blood group antigens can give rise to hyperacute AMR; however, the significance of preformed and *de novo* antibodies against other antigens, particularly HLA, is less clear.

Hyperacute AMR is suspected first in the operating room when the liver becomes swollen and hard and bile is not produced, soon after revascularization. Hemostasis may be difficult to achieve in these patients. Histologically, hyperacute rejection may be difficult to distinguish from primary nonfunction. In severe cases (mostly those due to ABO incompatibility), there tend to be large areas of infarction, portal vein thrombi, and necrotizing arteritis. With appropriate clinical history, such as positive cross-match and short ischemic time, hyperacute rejection may be suggested.

There is much conflicting literature regarding the significance of donor-specific antibodies in ABO-compatible livers. In this setting, the donor-specific antibodies are often against the HLA complex. Some patients with high levels of donor-specific antibodies may develop liver injury that is characterized by centrilobular hepatocyte ballooning, canalicular cholestasis, scattered acidophil bodies, and bile ductular proliferation. These features may be indistinguishable from preservation injury and biliary outflow impairment. Some biopsies also show features of acute cellular rejection, and these cases may be less responsive to conventional immunosuppression. Unlike cardiac and renal allograft biopsies, immunohistochemistry for C4d has limited diagnostic utility. However, in the setting of donor-specific antibodies, clinical evidence of graft dysfunction, and histologic evidence of graft injury, the presence of diffuse stromal staining for C4d in greater than 50% of portal tracts supports the diagnosis of AMR (49).

Acute Cellular Rejection

Acute rejection is fairly common in pediatric liver allografts. Most episodes occur within the first few months after transplantation and can easily be controlled by traditional immunosuppressive therapy. However, a somewhat distinct form of acute rejection can occur late in the posttransplant period, aptly termed late acute rejection. These rejection episodes tend to be more resistant to standard immunosuppressive therapy and have unique histologic features. Most cases of late acute rejection in children are due to inadequate immunosuppression (50). Clinically, acute rejection can be asymptomatic when mild. More severe cases present with fever, decreased bile flow, and elevations in liver chemistry tests. The gold standard for confirming the diagnosis remains liver biopsy; however, communication between the pathologists and clinician is essential in determining which patients with rejection require increased immunosuppression.

In 1997, the Banff working group convened to develop histologic criteria outlining three core histologic features: (a) portal inflammation, (b) subendothelial inflammation, and (c) bile duct damage (51) (Figure 8-7). The portal inflammation is mixed. Activated (blastic) lymphocytes and small mononuclear cells tend to predominate; however, eosinophils, macrophages, and neutrophils can be prominent. PTLD should be kept in mind when a monotonous portal infiltrate consisting of blastic lymphocytes is present without other features of rejection. The presence of mononuclear inflammatory cells between the endothelial cells of the portal or central vein and the underlying basement membrane, referred to as endothelialitis, is another common feature of rejection. Occasionally, central vein endothelialitis and/or perivenulitis may be the only prominent feature of acute rejection. Bile duct damage is manifested by the presence of mononuclear cells inside the basement membrane and between cholangiocytes. In addition, the bile duct epithelium shows loss of apical cytoplasm (increased nuclear/cytoplasmic ratio), paranuclear vacuolization, nucleoli, nuclear overlap, mitosis, apoptotic bodies, and cytoplasmic eosinophilia. To make a diagnosis of acute rejection, two of three of the above histologic features must be present. The diagnosis is further strengthened if greater than 50% of bile ducts are damaged or if unequivocal endothelialitis is present.

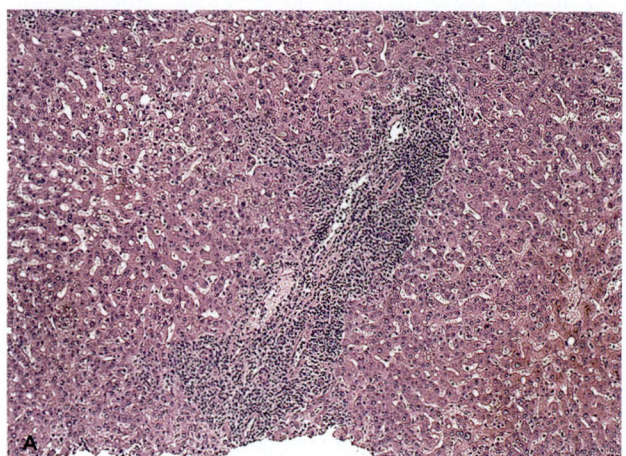 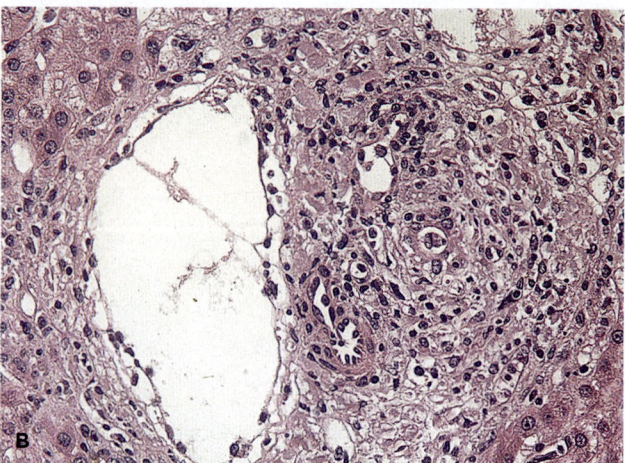

FIGURE 8-7 • Acute rejection of liver allografts. **A:** The portal tracts in acute rejection are expanded by a dense mixed inflammatory infiltrate. **B:** Definitive evidence of endothelialitis along with bile duct damage confirms the diagnosis.

Once the diagnosis of acute rejection is made based on the above criteria, an indication of the global severity should be given. In mild acute rejection, portal inflammation is mild. In moderate rejection, most or all of the portal tracts are expanded by an inflammatory infiltrate. In severe rejection, there is spillover into the hepatic parenchyma with hepatocyte necrosis, both periportal and perivenular. A rejection activity index has been developed to further characterize the severity of rejection and is routinely reported at some institutions (51,52).

As mentioned, late-onset acute rejection has some unique morphologic features when compared with acute rejection occurring early in the posttransplant period (50,53). Late acute rejection tends to have less portal inflammation, increased interface activity, less endothelialitis, and more lobular activity; however, traditional features of acute rejection should still be present. In some cases, only centrilobular pathology exists with perivenular inflammation and zone 3 hepatocyte dropout (isolated central perivenulitis).

Chronic Rejection

Chronic rejection has become relatively rare with current immunosuppressive therapy. Some studies report almost no cases of chronic rejection in pediatric patients (54); however, chronic rejection does occur and is an important cause of late graft failure. Factors associated with chronic rejection include a primary diagnosis of autoimmune liver disease, late-onset acute rejection, nonwhite race, baseline immunosuppression, certain tumor necrosis factor-2 alleles, and CMV infection (controversial) (55–57). Despite the name, many cases of chronic rejection occur within months of transplant (2 to 6 months) and lead to graft failure within 2 years. Indeed, unlike other solid organ allografts, chronic rejection in the liver decreases with time, except for a small group of patients with late-onset chronic rejection.

The classic presentation of chronic rejection is that of a patient with multiple episodes of acute rejection who develops progressive cholestasis and elevations in alkaline phosphatase, bilirubin, and gamma-glutamyl transferase and is unresponsive to immunosuppressive therapy. Rarely, patients present with chronic rejection in the absence of any documented history of acute rejection.

As chronic rejection most commonly results from repeated bouts of acute rejection, there will be a period of overlap. Conceptually, acute rejection refers to reversible and active lesions in which there is hepatocyte apoptosis and blastic portal inflammation, whereas chronic rejection is generally nonreversible and refers to loss of key structures. If both features are present, both acute and chronic rejection should be diagnosed based on their respective criteria. Late clinical findings of chronic rejection include hepatic infarction and loss of synthetic function. Clinically and pathologically, chronic rejection can resemble biliary obstruction and ischemic cholangiopathy.

Like acute rejection, there are three histopathologic features of chronic rejection: (a) bile duct atrophy, (b) foam cell arteriopathy, and (c) bile duct loss, at least one of which should be present (52,58). The diagnosis of chronic rejection mainly depends upon bile duct features as the characteristic foam cell arterial changes are rarely encountered on routine liver biopsies. Thus, it is important to exclude other causes of duct injury or loss such as HAT, obstructive biliary disease, recurrent chronic hepatitis, drug reactions, and CMV infections. The bile duct damage is thought to be ischemic in nature due to damage to the peribiliary arterial plexus. The earliest manifestations of bile duct injury include eosinophilic transformation of the biliary cytoplasm, uneven nuclear spacing, syncytial formation, nuclear enlargement and hyperchromasia, and ducts with focal epithelial cell loss (Figure 8-8A). At this early stage of chronic rejection, it is thought that these changes may be reversible with

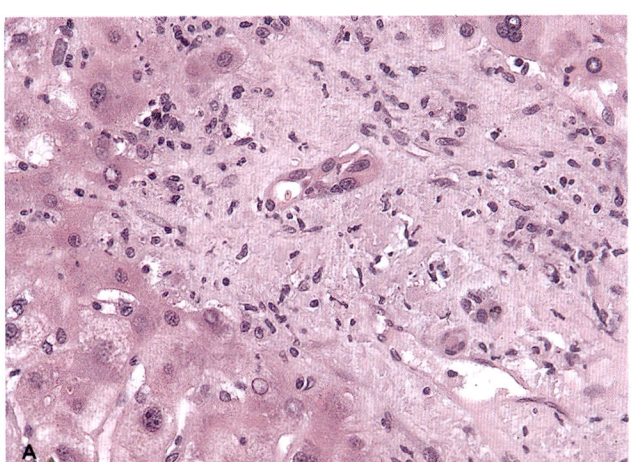
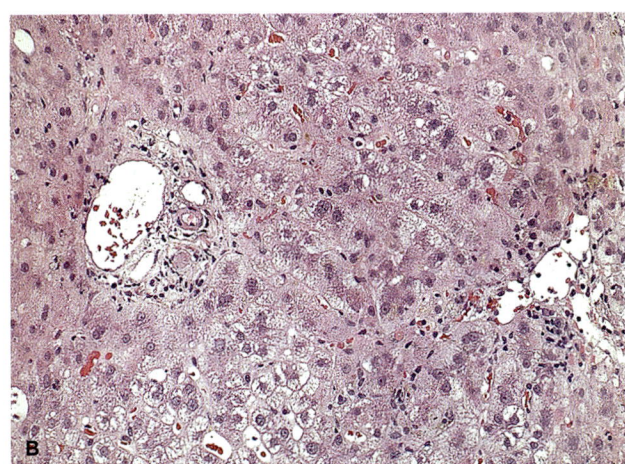

FIGURE 8-8 • Chronic rejection of liver allografts. **A:** In early chronic rejection, the biliary nuclear/cytoplasmic ratio is increased, and the cytoplasm shows prominent eosinophilia. **B:** In late chronic rejection, the bile ducts are lost, and only portal veins and, to a lesser extent, terminal hepatic arterioles remain to identify portal tracts. There is an "empty" appearance to the often diminutive portal tracts.

immunosuppression. In late chronic rejection, bile ducts and, to a lesser extent, terminal hepatic arterioles are lost (Figure 8-8B). When quantifying bile duct and arterial loss, it is essential to remember that in a normal liver, not all portal tracts contain these structures. In fact, between 5% and 10% of portal tracts do not contain bile ducts or hepatic artery branches (59). Thus, bile duct loss is only significant if greater than 20% of the portal tracts do not have bile ducts. However, quantification of bile duct and arterial loss can be complicated in late chronic rejection as portal tracts can be difficult to visualize. In these cases, portal tracts should be inferred from location within the lobule, presence of hepatic arteries, and shape. Additionally, inflammatory cells may obscure bile ducts. In such cases, immunohistochemistry for cytokeratin 7 may be useful in determining bile duct number; however, care must be taken to count only true bile ducts and not ductules (60).

Foam cell arteriopathy is another hallmark of chronic rejection; however, it is best appreciated in large-sized and medium-sized hepatic artery branches that can only be sampled on hepatectomy specimens. Early chronic rejection is characterized by accumulation of foam cells within the intima without luminal compromise. In late rejection, foam cell accumulation with luminal compromise predominates. Changes in large bile ducts can also be appreciated in hepatectomy specimens, including fibrosis of the wall, epithelial sloughing, and papillary hyperplasia. In most cases of chronic rejection, both bile duct loss and foam cell arterial changes coexist; however, up to 15% of cases may have only one feature.

Centrilobular changes can also be seen in chronic rejection and may be a prominent feature. In early chronic rejection, perivenular mononuclear inflammation, hepatocyte dropout, acidophil bodies, pigmented macrophages, and mild fibrosis are commonly seen. Late chronic rejection is characterized by perivenular fibrosis that can be extensive, resulting in bridging fibrosis. Vascular damage due to chronic rejection may be a cause of these centrilobular changes; however, immunologic factors may also contribute to these findings. Centrilobular cholestasis can also be prominent, especially when bile duct loss becomes severe. Many factors not related to chronic rejection may also lead to similar centrilobular changes such as viral hepatitis, venous outflow obstruction, and HAT. Thus, definitive diagnosis of chronic rejection must rely on bile duct and arterial changes.

De Novo and Recurrent Autoimmune Hepatitis

Patients who are transplanted due to autoimmune hepatitis (AIH) can develop recurrent disease (30% by 5 years); however, some patients without any prior history develop a syndrome remarkably similar to classic AIH termed *de novo* AIH, plasma cell hepatitis, or immune-mediated hepatitis. The diagnosis of *de novo* or recurrent AIH requires the presence of autoantibodies, lymphoplasmacytic portal inflammation with prominent interface and lobular activity, serologic evidence of liver injury, hypergammaglobulinemia, and no evidence of viral hepatitis, drug-related hepatitis, or rejection (Figure 8-9) (53).

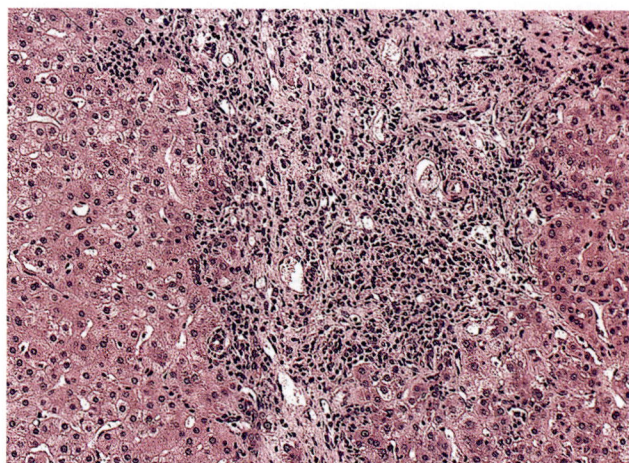

FIGURE 8-9 • *De novo* autoimmune hepatitis. The portal tract is expanded by a dense lymphoplasmacytic infiltrate with prominent interface and lobular activity. Along with elevated ANA titers, these findings are consistent with a *de novo* autoimmune hepatitis.

Other Recurrent Diseases

In children, recurrent hepatitis C or B is generally not routinely encountered as chronic viral hepatitis is an uncommon indication of pediatric liver transplantation. In addition, intrinsic metabolic or synthetic liver disease does not recur in the allograft. However, metabolic diseases that secondarily affect the liver can recur in the allograft. These diseases include Niemann-Pick disease, Gaucher disease, cystinosis, and erythropoietic protoporphyria (61).

Recent evidence has confirmed that primary sclerosing cholangitis (PSC) can recur in approximately 5% to 20% of patients with most recurrences diagnosed more than 1 year post transplant (62). Moreover, PSC patients are at a higher risk of developing rejection and worsening inflammatory bowel disease after transplantation. Because in the posttransplant setting there are many causes of biliary disease, the diagnosis of recurrent PSC is often difficult, and no gold standard exists. Thus, close clinical, radiologic, and histopathologic correlation is required to make this diagnosis. The presence of nonanastomotic biliary strictures is suggestive of recurrent PSC but only if occurring late in the posttransplant period. In addition, other causes of late-onset biliary strictures, such as chronic rejection, arterial insufficiency, and biliary infections must be excluded. Early stricturing is more likely due to complications of preservation injury and HAT. Biopsies showing characteristic "onion-skinning" cholangitis or fibro-obliterative changes have been shown to occur only in allografts from PSC patients, but these features are seen only in a small percentage of patients. Thus while specific absence of these features does not rule out recurrent PSC. Features of biliary obstruction are more commonly seen in recurrent PSC; however, these features are nonspecific.

Currently, guidelines suggest that recurrent PSC should be suggested in cases with a confirmed diagnosis of PSC before transplant; if there is cholangiographic evidence of extrahepatic biliary obstruction, beading, and irregularities at least greater than 90 days after transplantation; or if there is histologic evidence of fibrous cholangitis and/or fibro-obliterative lesions with or without ductopenia, biliary fibrosis, or biliary cirrhosis.

Idiopathic Posttransplantation Chronic Hepatitis

Recently, a group of patients without any previous history or serologic evidence of viral hepatitis or drug reaction has been shown to develop a picture resembling chronic hepatitis late in the posttransplant period (63). Remarkably, in one pediatric study, 64% of allograft biopsies at 10 years post transplant had histopathologic features of chronic hepatitis including portal inflammation, necroinflammatory activity, and fibrosis. Less than 5% of these cases met the criteria of *de novo* AIH; only 2 of 113 were positive for hepatitis C, whereas no cause was found in the vast majority of cases. Although only a subset met the criteria for *de novo* AIH, many patients had increased ANA and SMA titers, some above 1:100. It is possible that these clinical and histopathologic abnormalities represent a subclinical form of *de novo* AIH or atypical chronic rejection. These authors suggest that reinstitution of steroid therapy may be beneficial to these patients. As most institutions do not routinely obtain protocol liver biopsies late in the posttransplant course, these findings have yet to be corroborated at other institutions.

Posttransplant Opportunistic Infections

As the pediatric transplant recipient may be naïve for many viral infections and many would not have completed their vaccinations, viral infections of the allograft tend to be more severe. Indeed, even live attenuated viral vaccines are contraindicated in transplant patients due to the possibility of graft infections. Viral infections occur most commonly 1 week to 2 months after transplantation and tend to follow episodes of acute rejection due to increased immunosuppression (42). Thus, distinction between ongoing acute rejection and new-onset viral infection may be difficult clinically and histologically. The most common viral infections leading to graft dysfunction are CMV and EBV. However, other, rarer viral infections such as adenovirus, varicella virus, and herpes simplex virus can lead to graft failure.

CMV hepatitis is fairly common in pediatric liver transplantation, affecting up to 10% of allografts. However, with the advent of prophylactic CMV therapy, the incidence and severity of disease have been reduced. Close monitoring of patients receiving an allograft from a CMV positive donor, is essential as CMV hepatitis tends to be more common and more severe. CMV infection of the allograft can lead to a variety of histologic manifestations, some of which overlap with acute rejection. As classic eosinophilic nuclear inclusions are rare and may be absent, reliance on multiple histologic features is necessary. Mild-to-moderate lymphocytic portal inflammation is found in almost all cases of CMV hepatitis. In addition, one of the most sensitive, but not specific, findings in CMV hepatitis is the presence of scattered clusters of necrotic hepatocytes surrounded by a neutrophilic infiltrate forming microabscesses (Figure 8-10A). However, microabscesses can be found in a wide variety of conditions such as biliary obstruction, ischemia, other infections, and sepsis (64), and therefore, CMV immunohistochemistry is indicated when microabscesses are present. Kupffer cell hyperplasia, hepatocyte ballooning, and parenchymal inflammation are other common findings. Slight lymphocytic cholangitis may be seen and should not be mistaken for acute rejection.

Pediatric transplant recipients commonly develop manifestations of EBV infection that can ultimately lead to PTLD. Naïve recipients of EBV-positive allografts are at a much higher risk of developing infection in the posttransplant period. Interestingly, transplantation for Langerhans cell histiocytosis also predisposes to EBV-associated PTLD (41). Clinically, EBV infection first manifests as fever, pharyngitis, lymphadenitis, and jaundice. Liver enzymes are typically elevated. EBV infection results in a wide variety of histologic manifestations in the liver allograft. Nonspecific findings such as portal inflammation and sinusoidal mononuclear infiltrates, often forming linear aggregates, are common. Scattered acidophil bodies, hepatocyte ballooning, and mild lobular disarray with pseudoacinar formation and plate hypertrophy are commonly seen. If EBV infection is not controlled, progression to PTLD may occur. Early lesions consist of atypical lymphocytes in the portal inflammatory cell infiltrate. Endothelialitis may be present, closely mimicking acute rejection. Differentiation relies on the presence of a monotonous portal infiltrate with few atypical lymphocytes rather than the mixed infiltrate seen in acute rejection (Figure 8-10C). Frank PTLD can range from diffuse large B-cell lymphoma to Hodgkin-like lymphoma. Extrahepatic involvement is common. *In situ* hybridization for EBER as well as immunohistochemistry for CD20, kappa, and lambda is useful to confirm the diagnosis (Figure 8-10D).

Adenovirus, though rare, is more common in pediatric transplant recipients than in adults who are more likely to have protective immunity (65). Clinically, patients present with fever, difficulty breathing, diarrhea, and liver dysfunction. Usually, infection occurs in the first 3 months, and serotype 5 is the most common. Random geographic areas of necrosis are characteristic of adenoviral hepatitis (Figure 8-10B). Smudgy and granular viral nuclear inclusions can be found at the edge of the necrotic zones and can be documented by immunohistochemistry. HSV and VZ are other rare causes of posttransplant viral hepatitis and can lead to fulminant hepatic failure if infection goes unrecognized. Once again, infection is more common and more severe in pediatric patients as they are more likely to lack protective immunity. HSV and VZ cause similar histopathologic findings, and because it is difficult to separate these two infections based on H&E alone,

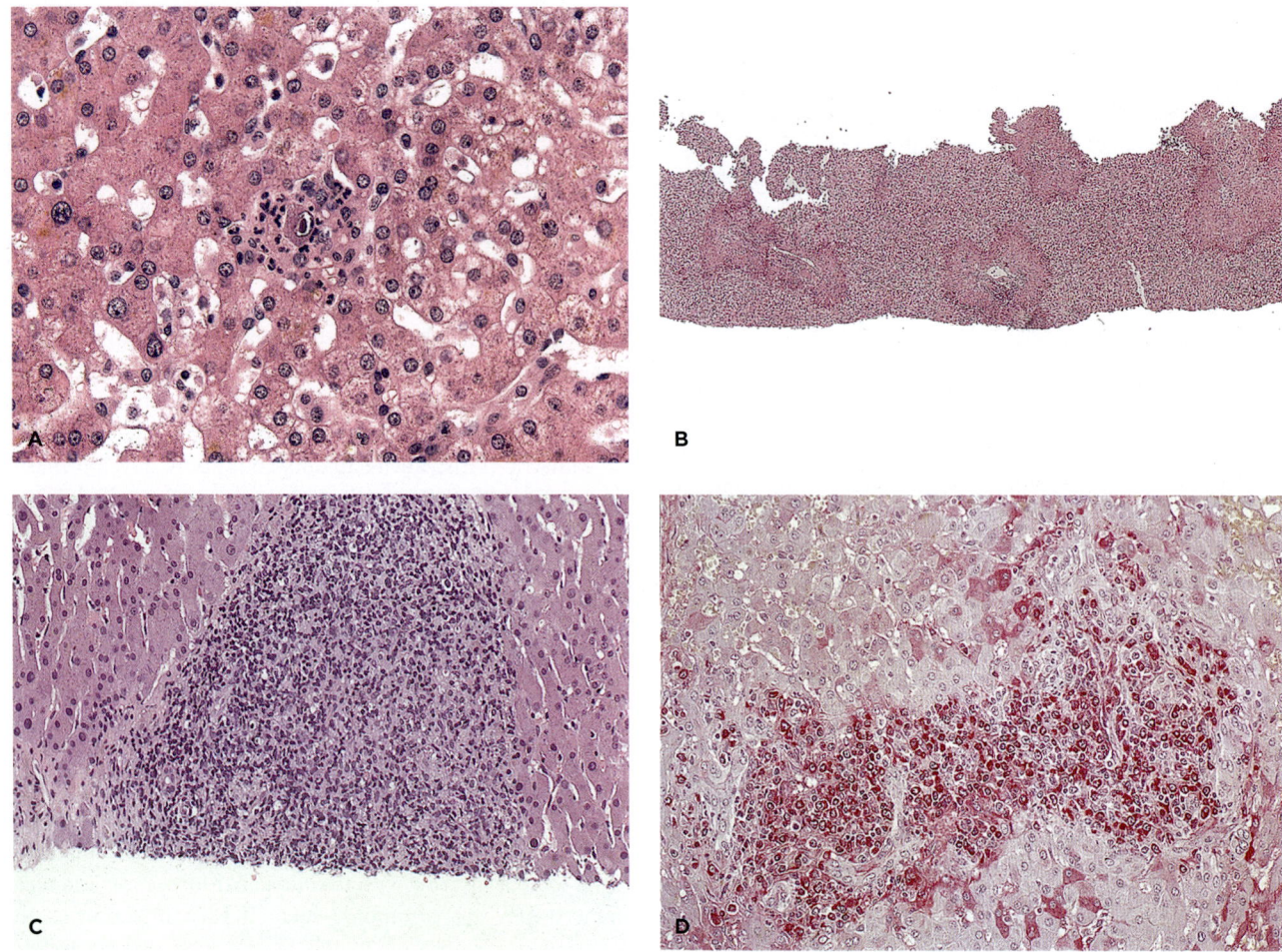

FIGURE 8-10 • Posttransplant infections of the liver allograft. **A:** CMV is a common infection in the posttransplant setting. Characteristic findings include microabscesses near infected cells. **B:** Adenovirus infection, although rare, is a serious complication in the pediatric setting. Zonal necrosis along with smudgy nuclear inclusions is characteristic. **C:** The histologic findings in PTLD are varied. In severe cases, the portal tracts are greatly expanded by a dense, atypical lymphoid infiltrate. **D:** *In situ* hybridization for EBER may be essential in confirming the diagnosis of PTLD.

immunohistochemistry is required. As in adenoviral hepatitis, random confluent areas of coagulative-type necrosis are common. In the center of the necrotic areas, ghost hepatocytes and neutrophils are seen. At the edge of these zones, virally infected hepatocytes with characteristic ground-glass intranuclear inclusions may be present. Multinucleated infected hepatocytes are sometimes seen. If VZ or HSV is suspected, rapid communication to the clinicians is essential. Immediate antiviral therapy and cessation of immunosuppression may reduce graft dysfunction and prevent graft failure.

The Liver in Bone Marrow Transplantation

Bone marrow transplantation is used in the management of a wide variety of diseases, including aplastic anemia, leukemia, and immune disorders (26). Hepatic changes seen in these patients may be related to chemotherapy and total-body irradiation in preparation for transplantation, GVHD, or the infections to which these immunocompromised individuals are susceptible. Veno-occlusive disease (VOD) or sinusoidal occlusive syndrome (SOS) is a complication of chemotherapy (particularly cyclophosphamide-based regimens) and may be mild, with full recovery, or severe and lead to death (66). VOD usually occurs within the first 30 days after transplantation; however, late-onset VOD has been reported with newer chemotherapeutic regimens (67). Chemotherapeutic agents damage the sinusoidal endothelial cell layer, resulting in deposition of extracellular matrix in the sinusoids and terminal hepatic veins occluding blood flow. This results in ascites, weight gain, painful hepatomegaly, and jaundice. In the early phase, centrilobular hemorrhage is associated with damaged venules and sinusoids (Figure 8-11). There is narrowing of the lumina and widening of the subendothelial zone, which may contain collagen fibers, siderophages, and cell fragments. Progression is manifested by partial to complete occlusion of the venules and sinusoids and centrizonal hepatocellular atrophy. The reticulin stain is particularly helpful in identifying the occlusive sinusoidal and venular lesions (Figure 8-11).

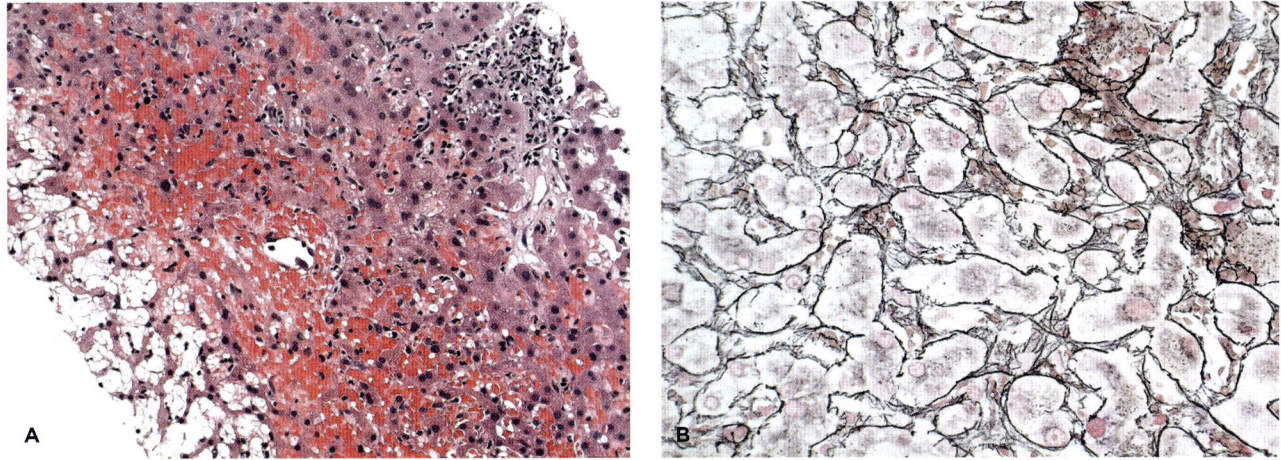

FIGURE 8-11 • Veno-occlusive syndrome/sinusoidal obstructive syndrome. **A:** VOD/SOS is characterized by centrilobular hemorrhage and necrosis. **B:** A reticulin stain is helpful in highlighting the sinusoidal and venular deposition of extracellular matrix.

Cholestasis and distortion of the lobular architecture may occur (68). Mild disease is followed by recovery by day 20, but death from fulminant hepatic failure occurs in some cases.

Immunologic mechanisms of rejection in liver allograft recipients and GVHD in bone marrow transplant patients are similar. They manifest many of the same histopathologic changes in the liver. Both are characterized by portal inflammation and bile duct injury in the acute phase and severe duct damage and duct loss in the chronic stages (69). The acute form of GVHD manifests 3 to 4 weeks after transplantation with a skin rash, diarrhea, and jaundice. The early changes consist of mild, nonspecific lobular hepatitis. Liver biopsy specimens evaluated 1 to 2 weeks after the onset of the disease show characteristic bile duct abnormalities. The bile ducts show epithelial degeneration and necrosis and lymphocytic infiltration (Figure 8-12A). Destruction of ducts and ductular proliferation occurs with progressive disease. There is a lymphocytic portal inflammation, but spillover is usually minimal. Mild hepatocellular changes, occasional acidophil bodies, and cholestasis are seen in the lobule. Endothelialitis of the portal and central veins may be seen (70).

Chronic GVHD affects 30% of long-term survivors. It may be preceded by acute GVHD or develop in patients without prior episodes of disease. Chronic liver disease is seen in most patients with chronic GVHD with multisystem involvement or as a limited disorder with cutaneous and hepatic involvement, which has a more favorable prognosis. Although cirrhosis and its complications are unusual, micronodular cirrhosis leading to death from hepatic failure has been reported (25,26). The liver in chronic GVHD may show a histologic appearance of chronic hepatitis with portal infiltration by mononuclear cells. Long-standing GVHD results in bile duct loss (Figure 8-12B). Additional findings include portal infiltration by plasma cells and cholestasis with pseudoxanthomatous changes. Endothelialitis is not a feature of chronic GVHD (70).

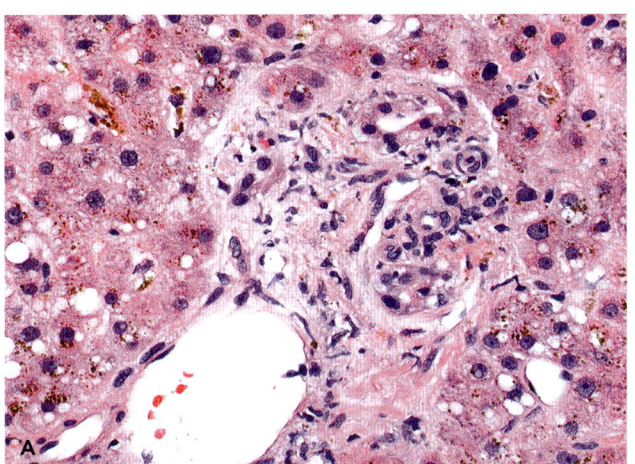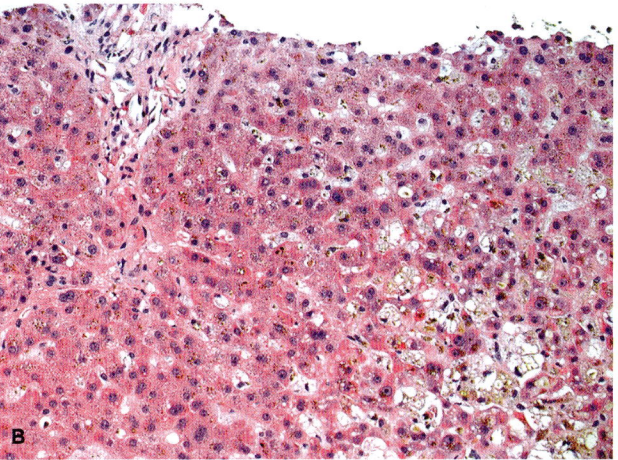

FIGURE 8-12 • GVHD of the liver. **A:** GVHD is characterized by destruction of the bile ducts with lymphocytic infiltration. Extensive iron deposition is commonly seen in these bone marrow transplant patients. **B:** In chronic GVHD, bile ducts are lost and cholestasis is evident (Photos courtesy of Dr. John Hart, University of Chicago).

TRANSPLANT PATHOLOGY OF THE PANCREAS

Overview and the Role of Histopathology

Pancreatic transplantation is becoming increasingly utilized for type I diabetes mellitus and is most commonly performed in conjunction with a kidney allograft due to end-stage renal failure. As end-stage renal failure in type I diabetes occurs mainly in adulthood, the pediatric pathologist is rarely asked to evaluate pancreatic biopsies in this setting. Moreover, histopathologic evaluation of pancreatic graft biopsies is rarely indicated in current practice for a variety of reasons. First, the pancreas is a very active exocrine and endocrine organ; thus, levels of synthetic products produced by the pancreas can accurately gauge graft function. Second, biopsies from the kidney have proven to be a fairly accurate surrogate in evaluating pancreatic rejection in patients who receive kidney/pancreas transplants (71). Third, in some instances, biopsies can be difficult to obtain and could cause severe injury to the pancreatic duct and vessels. Despite these caveats, biopsies obtained from the pancreatic grafts can occasionally provide useful information to the clinician, and at some large centers, biopsies are routinely performed (72).

Histopathology of Acute and Chronic Rejection

In 1997, a histologic grading scheme was proposed for acute rejection that divided acute rejection into six grades based on the degree of septal, acinar, ductal, and vascular inflammation (73). Inflammation in the islets of Langerhans is rarely encountered and is not a feature of acute rejection. This grading scheme showed good reproducibility, prognostic significance, correlation with laboratory data, and response to immunosuppressive treatment. Chronic rejection is characterized by fibrous expansion of the septal areas and loss of acinar parenchyma. Islets initially are not affected; however, extensive fibrosis can lead to loss of glycemic control. The vascular changes are similar to those seen in other solid organs with intimal and medial fibrosis and narrowing of the lumen. Critical to the evaluation of allograft pancreatic biopsies is assessment for other causes of graft dysfunction such as bacterial, fungal, or viral infections, especially CMV infection (74). Clinically and histologically, CMV pancreatitis can mimic acute rejection; however, the presence of the characteristic nuclear inclusions in endothelial or stromal cells is diagnostic.

RENAL TRANSPLANT PATHOLOGY

Overview

From 2007 to 2011, over 6800 pediatric patients suffered from end-stage renal disease (ESRD) in the United States (75). Of these, 38% received a kidney transplant and 4% died within the first year. The most common pediatric causes of ESRD are aplastic/hypoplastic/dysplastic kidneys (15.9% of total), obstructive uropathy (15.6%), and focal segmental glomerulosclerosis (FSGS) (11.7%).

Approximately 750 renal transplants are performed annually for patients less than 18 years old in the United States and approximately 300 were living donor (LD) allografts with the vast majority of these from a parent (76). Native nephrectomy for polyuria, severe proteinuria (including hyperlipidemia and thrombophilia), recurrent pyelonephritis, and refractory hypertension will be considered for a minority of pediatric patients (77). One-year allograft survival improved from 91% in 1987 to 1995 to 94% in 1996 to 2000 for LD and 81% to 93% for deceased donor (DD), and the projected allograft half-life (the time at which one-half of allografts will be lost) improved from 15.4 (LD) and 9.5 (DD) years in the 1987 to 1989 cohort to 25.4 and 16.4 years, respectively, for the 1996 to 1998 cohort (78).

Important morbidities in pediatric renal transplant recipients are growth failure, cardiovascular disease, and infectious diseases (79), and infectious diseases now exceed rejection as the most common reason for hospitalization in these patients (80).

Pediatric renal allograft biopsies may be either indication (i.e., graft dysfunction) or protocol biopsies. Interpretation of transplant biopsies is challenging due to the numerous injuries that can simultaneously harm the allograft, which include donor disease, surgical complications, allograft rejection, drug toxicities, opportunistic infections, recurrent or de novo renal diseases, and PTLD. The widely used Banff classification of renal allograft pathology defines a "minimal" sample for interpretation as seven glomeruli and one artery and an "adequate" sample as at least ten glomeruli and two arteries and recommends that there be two cores or at least two separate cortical areas (81,82). Multiple levels should be examined with hematoxylin and eosin (H&E), periodic acid–Schiff (PAS), Jones methenamine silver stains, and trichrome; and immunofluorescence or immunohistochemical studies for C4d should be performed. Additional studies to be performed include immunofluorescence microscopy for other immunoglobulin and complement components to establish recurrent or *de novo* disease, immunohistochemical studies for T- and B-lymphocytes, and *in situ* hybridization for EBV to exclude PTLD when these conditions are suspected clinically or pathologically.

Hyperacute and Accelerated Acute Rejection and Delayed Graft Function

Hyperacute and accelerated rejections primarily represent variants of acute antibody–mediated (humoral) rejection due to preformed antidonor antibodies, but this has become exceedingly rare with the advancement of cross-matching techniques. Rare T-cell–mediated cases of hyperacute rejection have been reported. Hyperacute rejection is characterized by graft swelling and tenderness and anuria almost immediately or within the first few days after transplantation. Arterioles and glomerular capillaries are distended by thrombi that contain platelets and erythrocytes, which lead to necrosis of glomerular endothelium and tubular epithelium. Neutrophils marginate in small vessels and peritubular capillaries. C4d deposition along peritubular capillaries similar to that seen in acute and chronic antibody-mediated rejection (cAMR), as discussed below, is often seen in hyperacute rejection (83). The disease formerly known as accelerated acute rejection is also caused by preformed antibodies that may not be detectable until the plasma cell clone has been stimulated by the graft. It typically occurs 1 to 12 weeks after transplantation and is manifested by necrotizing arteritis or a thrombotic microangiopathy (TMA). Severe vascular occlusion due to sickle cell trait can mimic hyperacute rejection (84). Delayed graft function may be caused by a variety of donor factors, peritransplant ischemic injury, or drug toxicity. Typical histologic findings are reminiscent of acute tubular necrosis and include dilation of tubular lumens, loss of the proximal tubular brush border, epithelial cell necrosis and apoptosis, and cellular casts (85). Of note, biopsies performed at the time of kidney transplantation can demonstrate increased numbers of neutrophils within glomerular and peritubular capillaries, which is likely due to ischemia–reperfusion injury and mimics AMR.

Acute Rejection

Historically, renal allografts in children had higher rates with earlier and more refractory episodes of acute rejection than allografts in adults (79), but with improved immunosuppressive therapy, the 12-month probability of acute rejection in children in the NAPRTCS series decreased from 54% to 13% in LD allografts and 69% to 16% in DD recipients between 1987–1990 and 2003–2005, respectively. 53% of LD allografts and 47% of DD allografts achieved complete reversal of rejection (return to baseline creatinine values), and only 4% and 6%, respectively, lost their grafts or died as a result of acute rejection (76). For LD allografts, the relative risk of developing acute rejection is increased in African Americans, history of prior transplant or more than five blood transfusions, HLA mismatch, lack of induction therapy, and female gender; and for DD recipients, additional risk factors include recipient age less than 1 year, prior dialysis, and cold ischemic time greater than 24 hours (76). Tables 8-3 and 8-4 summarize the criteria for the scoring of lesions and classification of patterns of rejection in the Banff classification of renal allograft pathology.

Acute T-Cell–Mediated Rejection

The two criteria for acute T-cell–mediated rejection (TCMR) in the Banff classification (type I) are the following: (a) mononuclear cell infiltrates involving more than 25% of the parenchyma (≥i2; see Table 8-3); (b) at least two foci with five to ten intraepithelial mononuclear cells ("tubulitis") for type IA in a tubular cross-section or greater than 10 mononuclear cells for type IB in a tubular cross-section (approximately 10 tubular epithelial cells) (Figure 8-13A). Interstitial inflammation alone without tubulitis is not diagnostic of acute (type I) rejection, but the presence of interstitial inflammation between well-preserved tubules is abnormal. In this scenario, polyomavirus nephropathy (PVN) may not always exhibit characteristic viral cytopathic changes, especially for JC virus, and this diagnosis should be excluded using SV40 immunohistochemistry. Sufficient interstitial inflammation (>25%) without tubulitis containing at least 5 lymphocytes or any degree of tubulitis with less than 25% interstitial inflammation are considered borderline or "suspicious" for acute rejection. In the latter situation, the administration of immunosuppressive therapy prior to biopsy may very quickly reduce the interstitial inflammatory response while tubulitis can persist, but this clinical information may not be provided at the time of biopsy evaluation and, in that context, i1t2 (or 10% to 25% interstitial inflammation and 5 to 10 lymphocytes per tubular cross-section; see Table 8-3) lesions may indicate rejection (82). Interstitial inflammation is not graded in areas of interstitial fibrosis/tubular atrophy, the immediate subcapsular cortex, and the adventitia around large veins, but this is being reevaluated (86). The interstitial infiltrate in acute rejection is often mixed, but the presence of prominent aggregates of eosinophils, especially if the inflammation is centered around the medulla, may suggest a drug-induced acute interstitial nephritis. The presence of numerous intratubular aggregates of neutrophils or neutrophilic tubulitis raises the diagnostic consideration of pyelonephritis. The presence of numerous plasma cells can be observed in rejection (particularly antibody mediated), PVN, or PTLD. Similarly, while tubulitis should be assessed in the most severely involved area, there should be more than one focus with the highest grade of involvement, and since tubulitis in atrophic tubules may be seen in the absence of rejection, it should not be graded in tubules that show a 50% or greater reduction in caliber. Most of the infiltrating lymphocytes in acute rejection will be T cells, and a predominantly B-cell infiltrate raises the question of a PTLD (82), while nodular aggregates of B-cell aggregates in a predominantly T-cell infiltrate may identify allografts that will be refractory to standard antirejection therapy but responsive to anti–B-cell immunotherapy (87).

Intimal arteritis (or endarteritis), seen as lymphocytic infiltration beneath the endothelium of arteries (Figure 8-13B), is the defining criterion for acute (type II) rejection, which has always been considered to represent TCMR. However, recent data suggests that some of these may represent AMR (88). Type IIA shows mild-to-moderate endarteritis in at least one arterial cross-section (v1), and type IIB shows severe intimal arteritis with at least a 25% reduction of the luminal area in at least one arterial cross-section (v2) (82). Because of the potential for sampling error, the most severely involved artery should be graded. Lymphocytes in venous walls or lymphocytes attached to (but not beneath) the arterial endothelium do not satisfy the diagnostic criterion for type II rejection, but these findings should trigger examination of deeper tissue sections, as intimal arteritis can be focal. Transmural arteritis or fibrinoid necrosis with

TABLE 8-3 BANFF CLASSIFICATION OF RENAL ALLOGRAFT PATHOLOGY (82,126)—I. LESION SCORING[a]

Lesion	Code	Grade 0	Grade 1	Grade 2	Grade 3	Comment
Findings associated with T-cell–mediated rejection						
Tubulitis	t	None	≥2 foci with 1–4 intraepithelial lymphocytes per tubular cross-section or per 10 epithelial cells	≥2 foci with 5–10 intraepithelial lymphocytes per tubular cross-section or per 10 epithelial cells	≥2 foci with >10 intraepithelial lymphocytes per tubular cross-section or per 10 epithelial cells OR ≥2 areas of tubular basement membrane destruction with i2/i3 inflammation and t2 tubulitis elsewhere	Do not count atrophic tubules <50% normal size.
Interstitial inflammation	i	<10% of unscarred parenchyma	10%–25% of unscarred parenchyma	26%–50% of unscarred parenchyma	>50% of unscarred parenchyma	Indicate >5%–10% eosinophils, neutrophils, or plasma cells and B-cell nodules with an asterisk (*).
Total interstitial inflammation[b]	ti	<10% of total parenchyma	10%–25% of total parenchyma	26%–50% of total parenchyma	>50% of total parenchyma	
Arteritis	v	No intimal arteritis	≥1 artery with intimal arteritis and <25% luminal occlusion	≥1 artery with intimal arteritis and ≥25% luminal occlusion	≥1 artery with fibrinoid change and transmural arteritis with medial smooth muscle necrosis	Indicate infarction and/or interstitial hemorrhage with an asterisk (*).
Findings associated with antibody-mediated rejection						
C4d staining	C4d	Negative (0%)	Minimal (1–9% of area with ≥2+ linear staining along peritubular capillaries)	Focal positive (10–50% of area with ≥2+ linear staining along peritubular capillaries)	Diffuse positive (>50% of area with ≥2+ linear staining along peritubular capillaries)	Immunohistochemistry may be one grade less sensitive than immunofluorescence.
Glomerulitis	g	None	Glomerulitis in a minority of glomeruli	Segmental or global glomerulitis in 25–75% of glomeruli	Glomerulitis (mostly global) in all or almost all glomeruli	Specify types of inflammatory cells.
Peritubular capillaritis	ptc	No luminal inflammatory cells in cortical peritubular capillaries	≥10% cortical peritubular capillaries with at most 3–4 luminal inflammatory cells	≥10% cortical peritubular capillaries with at most 5–10 luminal inflammatory cells	≥10% cortical peritubular capillaries with a maximum of >10 luminal inflammatory cells	Specify type(s) of luminal cells (mononuclear cell versus neutrophil) and extent (focal versus diffuse).

TABLE 8-3	BANFF CLASSIFICATION OF RENAL ALLOGRAFT PATHOLOGY (82,126)—I. LESION SCORING[a] (Continued)					
Lesion	Code	Grade 0	Grade 1	Grade 2	Grade 3	Comment
Glomerular double contour	cg	Double contours in <10% of peripheral capillary loops in most severely affected nonsclerotic glomerulus	Double contours in 10–25% of peripheral capillary loops in the most severely affected nonsclerotic glomerulus	Double contours in 26–50% of capillary loops in the most severely affected nonsclerotic glomerulus	Double contours in >50% of peripheral capillary loops in the most severely affected nonsclerotic glomerulus	
Chronic changes						
Tubular atrophy	ct	No tubular atrophy	≤25% of cortical tubules	26–50% of cortical tubules	>50% of cortical tubules	
Interstitial fibrosis	ci	≤5% of cortical area	6–25% of cortical area	26–50% of cortical area	>50% of cortical area	Do not score subcapsular fibrosis. Elastica breaks, inflammatory cells in fibrosis suggest chronic rejection.
Subintimal fibrosis in arteries	cv	No chronic vascular changes	≤25% luminal narrowing by fibrointimal thickening	26–50% luminal narrowing	>50% luminal narrowing	
Findings associated with calcineurin inhibitor toxicity						
Arteriolar hyalinization	ah	No PAS-positive hyaline thickening	Mild-to-moderate PAS-positive hyaline thickening in at least one arteriole	Moderate-to-severe PAS-positive hyaline thickening in more than one arteriole	Severe PAS-positive hyaline thickening in many arterioles	
Alternate arteriolar hyalinization[b]	aah	No typical lesions of CNI arteriolopathy	Nodular hyaline deposits in only one arteriole and no circumferential involvement	Nodular hyaline deposits in more than one arteriole, but no circumferential involvement	Circumferential hyaline involvement; independent of the number of arterioles involved	

[a]Note the number of glomeruli and arteries present and number of sclerotic glomeruli.
[b]Total interstitial inflammation and alternate arteriolar hyalinization are undergoing evaluation and have not been officially incorporated into the Banff classification.

lymphocytic inflammation is the criterion by which type III acute rejection is defined. Interstitial hemorrhage and infarction are not sufficient for a diagnosis of type III rejection but are designated with an asterisk after the "v" score (82) and examination of deeper tissue sections should be performed to avoid overlooking either type II or III rejection, which can be focal lesions.

Acute Antibody-Mediated Rejection

Demonstration of diffuse linear C4d deposition along peritubular capillaries (C4d3) (Figure 8-13C) has become the hallmark of AMR (82) and is seen in 20% to 30% of biopsies for acute rejection. C4d is an inactive fragment of complement component C4 that binds covalently to endothelial cells, thereby avoiding the modulation that makes the immunoglobulins responsible for initiating the attack undetectable. In normal kidneys, immunofluorescent staining for C4d is found in mesangial regions and at the vascular pole of glomeruli, presumably a consequence of the physiologic turnover of immune complexes, but peritubular capillary staining is characteristic of AMR (89). Other histopathologic features of AMR include neutrophils in peritubular and glomerular capillaries, but the Banff classification has categories of AMR in which there is C4d staining without these features, alone, and with changes consistent with acute tubular necrosis (Table 8-4). AMR typically has its onset 1 to 3 weeks after transplantation but may arise after several months or years, especially if immunosuppression is decreased. There is no correlation with HLA match, ischemic time, or donor age. During episodes of rejection, C4d-positive cases show higher

TABLE 8-4	BANFF CLASSIFICATION OF RENAL ALLOGRAFT PATHOLOGY (126)—II. DIAGNOSTIC CATEGORIES
T-cell–mediated rejection	
Suspicious/borderline changes	(v0 and (i0/i1 and t1, t2, or t3)) OR (v0 and (i2/i3 AND t1))
IA	v0 and (i2/i3 and t2)
IB	v0 and (i2/i3 and t3)
IIA	v1
IIB	v2
III	v3
Chronic active	cv > 0 with mononuclear cells in subintimal fibrosis
Antibody-mediated rejection	
C4d+	C4d*, antidonor antibody detected, and no morphologic evidence of acute or chronic rejection
I	C4d*, antidonor antibody detected, and ATN-like change with minimal interstitial inflammation
II	C4d*, antidonor antibody detected, and (ptc > 0 and/or g > 0 and/or thromboses)
III	C4d*, antidonor antibody detected, and v3
Chronic active	C4d*, antidonor antibody detected, (cg > 0 and/or ct > 0 and/or ci > 0 and or cv > 0)
Interstitial fibrosis and tubular atrophy without evidence of any specific etiology	
I	ct1 and ci0 or 1
II	ct2 and ci2
III	ct3 and ci3

*C4d grade 2 or 3 by IF on frozen or C4d > 0 by IHC.

serum creatinine levels and are less responsive to steroid and anti–T-cell immunotherapy compared to C4d-negative cases (8), and long-term graft survival is significantly reduced (90). Most patients with positive C4d staining have HLA class I or II donor-specific antibodies, but ABO and non-HLA antiendothelial antibodies have been demonstrated in a few patients (8). As our recognition of AMR improves, the 2013 Banff classification now recognizes C4d-negative AMR, given that donor-specific antibody titers can wax and wane and detection of C4d may be dependent on the immunolocalization technique as immunohistochemistry (IHC) is generally less sensitive than immunofluorescence (IF) microscopy.

Chronic Rejection

Chronic T-Cell–Mediated Rejection

The presence of foam cells or foamy macrophages in the arterial intima may be the only specific pathologic feature of chronic type II rejection. All other pathologic features of chronic glomerular or tubulointerstitial injury are not specific for allograft rejection. Therefore, establishing a diagnosis of chronic rejection can only be made with sequential biopsies, and even in that scenario, the contribution of other concurrent injuries, such as chronic ischemia, calcineurin inhibitor (CNI) toxicity, infection, and others, cannot be excluded. As a result, chronic allograft nephropathy (CAN) was a term that was created to acknowledge these limitations. However, CAN as a term has fallen out of favor and was specifically removed from the Banff classification in 2005. Interstitial fibrosis and tubular atrophy is the preferred description with an emphasis on the underlying etiology, if known. Although some nephropathologists still prefer to use CAN to describe the constellation of chronic allograft changes, it is essential to understand that CAN is a "wastebasket" term that encompasses many different injuries and does not represent a single mechanism of injury.

Chronic Antibody-Mediated Rejection

Chronic transplant glomerulopathy frequently manifests with proteinuria and represents a chronic phase of AMR. Injury of the glomerular endothelial cells causes detachment from the original glomerular basement membranes, but over time, the endothelial cell continues to produce a matrix that forms a second layer, which results in duplication or occasionally multilayering of the GBM (Figure 8-13D). Immunofluorescent microscopy of chronic transplant glomerulopathy may show nonspecific segmental granular deposits of IgG or IgM and C3 in the capillary wall and mesangium, and electron microscopy shows widening of the subendothelial space due to accumulation of electron lucent flocculent material, but no electron-dense deposits, which contrasts with recurrent or *de novo* membranoproliferative glomerulonephritis (MPGN). A similar injury involving the peritubular capillary basement membranes can also be observed (Figure 8-13E). Electron microscopy is the most sensitive method to observe these alterations, but when severe, these changes also can be seen by light microscopy; C4d peritubular capillary deposition can be present but is more likely to be absent in cAMR. Of note, a small subset of patients with AMR may develop *de novo* membranous nephropathy (dnMN) of which approximately 50% also manifest with chronic transplant glomerulopathy. Truong et al. found a close association between acute rejection and dnMN, and an autopsy of one patient revealed that the membranous glomerular changes were limited to the allograft and not the native kidneys (91). Therefore, dnMN may represent an unusual manifestation of AMR, but this pathogenic mechanism is not understood. dnMN was reported in initial allografts of seven children, four of whom developed MN in subsequent allografts (92). Some initial data suggested that the subepithelial immune complexes of dnMN consisted of IgG1, which contrasted with idiopathic or recurrent MN due to phospholipase A2 receptor that consisted primarily of IgG4. However, more recent data precludes the use of IgG subclass identification to distinguish *de novo* from recurrent

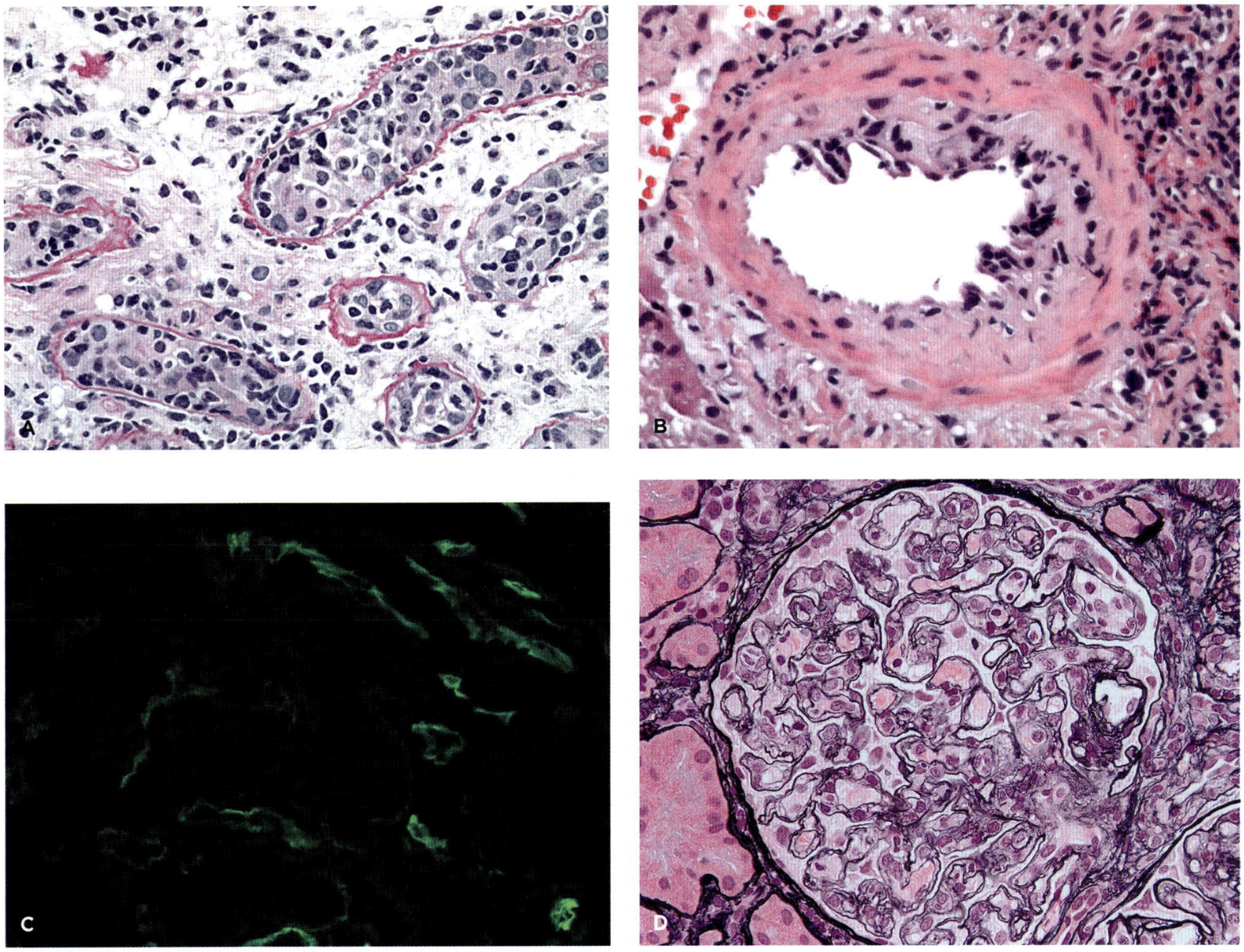

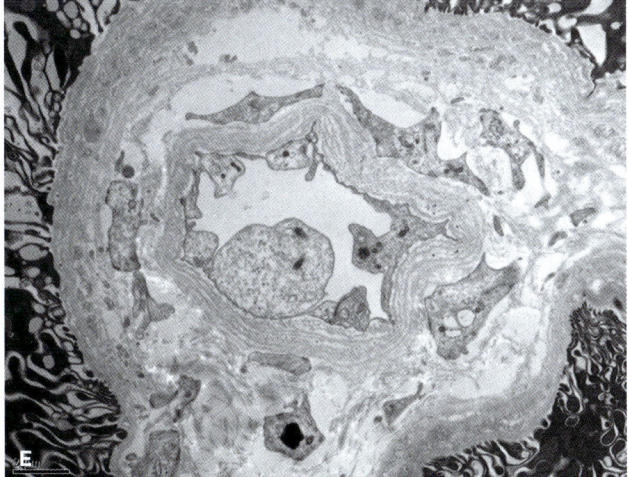

FIGURE 8-13 • Acute and chronic rejection. **A:** Tubulitis is a feature of acute T-cell–mediated rejection, and the greater than 10 intraepithelial lymphocytes per 10 epithelial cells in nonatrophic or only partially atrophic tubules seen here is a t3 lesion (PAS). **B:** Intimal arteritis is indicative of grade II acute rejection, and the 25% to 30% luminal narrowing seen here is a borderline v2 lesion (H&E). **C:** Bright C4d deposition along peritubular capillaries between tubules is the hallmark of active antibody-mediated rejection. **D:** Double contours along glomerular capillary loops are a sign of chronic antibody-mediated rejection (Jones methenamine silver). **E:** Multilayering of the peritubular capillary basement membrane is another sign of chronic antibody-mediated rejection.

MN (93). Fibrointimal thickening with reduplication of the internal elastica (cv) and arteriolar hyaline change (ah) may be related to hypertension; peripheral hyaline nodules in arterioles suggest chronic calcineurin inhibitor (cyclosporine, tacrolimus) toxicity as discussed below; marked tubular ectasia with Tamm-Horsfall casts raises the question of chronic obstruction; and intratubular neutrophils, lymphoid follicles, and viral inclusions are seen in infections (94).

Polyomavirus Nephropathy

Over the past 15 years, PVN has become the most important infection in kidney transplant patients. The human polyomavirus family consists of BK, JC, and SV40 viruses. BK and, to a much lesser degree, JC viruses (both named after the initials of the patients from which they were first isolated) are the primary causes of PVN, which develops in

2% to 9% of renal transplant recipients, and one-half of these patients lose graft function. Up to 90% of the population worldwide is BKV seropositive, and the virus is known to persist in renal allografts (95). Histologically, confirmed BKV nephropathy developed in six of 173 (3.5%) pediatric renal transplant recipients 4 to 47 months after transplant (median 15 months), which led to reduced long-term graft function, and BKV nephropathy was significantly associated with recipient seronegativity (96). PVN is characterized by enlarged nuclei with basophilic nuclear inclusions in tubular epithelial cells (Figure 8-14) that may impart a "ground-glass" appearance, while central pale inclusions surrounded by dark chromatin and vesicular nuclei have also been described. Immunohistochemistry for the large T antigen of SV40 confirms the presence of active viral replication, and one single positive nucleus is diagnostic of PVN. In early stages of viral replication, SV40 immunohistochemistry may be positive in normal-appearing nuclei, which more commonly are found in the distal nephron segments in the renal medulla (97). As the PVN progresses, proximal tubules and even glomerular epithelial cells can demonstrate viral replication, and the prominence of glomerular epithelial cells can even mimic a cellular crescent (98). In late stages of PVN, inclusion-bearing cells may be negative (83). Interstitial inflammation and tubulitis are characteristic findings for PVN, which can mimic the diagnosis of acute (type I) rejection. Establishing the diagnosis of concurrent TCMR and PVN is challenging, but the finding of prominent interstitial inflammation with only rare SV40 tubular epithelial cell nuclear positivity by immunohistochemistry would support this possibility. TCMR may preferentially involve the renal cortex, while early PVN should be limited to the renal medulla. SV40 immunohistochemistry should be performed on any "borderline" inflammatory infiltrates that are suspicious for acute TCMR. A three-stage schema for PVN is based on the degree of IF/TA, which correlates with allograft survival (99). Inclusion-bearing cells, known as "decoy" cells, can be identified in the urine, and in a prospective study of 78 adult renal allograft recipients, decoy cell shedding was seen in 30%, viremia assessed by nested PCR in 13%, and biopsy-proven nephropathy in 8%. With biopsy as the diagnostic standard, decoy cells had a sensitivity of 100% and specificity of 71%, and BKV viremia had a sensitivity of 100% and specificity of 88%, but the viral load in patients with BKV nephropathy was significantly higher than in those without nephropathy (95). Adenovirus nephritis is rare and should be considered in the differential diagnosis when there is tubular necrosis, interstitial hemorrhage, and granulomatous inflammation surrounding infected tubules.

Immunosuppressive Drug Toxicity

Of the immunosuppressive agents currently used in solid organ transplantation, the CNI, cyclosporine and tacrolimus, have the most significant renal toxicity. The monoclonal and polyclonal antibodies that deplete the T-cell pool (OKT3 and antilymphocyte and antithymocyte globulins [ATG]) or inhibit interleukin-2 (basiliximab and daclizumab) rarely cause renal disease (100). However, there have been case reports of glomerular and larger renal vessel thrombosis with OKT3 (83). Steroids and antiproliferative agents have numerous adverse effects but generally do not cause renal lesions. However, sirolimus has been reported to delay recovery from acute renal failure in cultured mouse proximal tubular epithelium (101) and to result in delayed graft function, which resulted in myoglobin casts when sirolimus was used in combination with tacrolimus (102), possibly because these two drugs are metabolized by the same pathway (85). Sirolimus has also been reported to rarely cause reversible proteinuria and TMA (83).

CNI can cause characteristic lesions in glomeruli, tubules, the interstitium, and vessels. Glomerular TMA and isometric vacuolization of proximal tubular epithelial cells indicate acute or ongoing toxic injury, while chronic toxicity results in hyaline changes in arterioles and interstitial fibrosis/tubular atrophy in a "striped" distribution (94). The differential diagnosis of glomerular TMA includes AMR, but CNI-induced TMA does not show C4d staining along peritubular capillaries. The cytoplasmic vacuoles in CNI tubulopathy are small and uniform, in contrast to the large irregular vacuoles seen with ischemic tubular injury, and they do not stain with H&E or PAS stains. The differential diagnosis includes an osmotic nephrosis due to agents such as mannitol and intravenous immunoglobulin. Arteriolar lesions include ballooning of smooth muscle cells, probably an early and reversible lesion like isometric vacuolization in tubules, and PAS-positive mural hyaline nodules along the adventitial aspect of the vessel (Figure 8-15). The differential diagnosis of the hyalinosis includes diabetes mellitus and hypertension, but the subadventitial nodules are relatively specific for CNI toxicity (83).

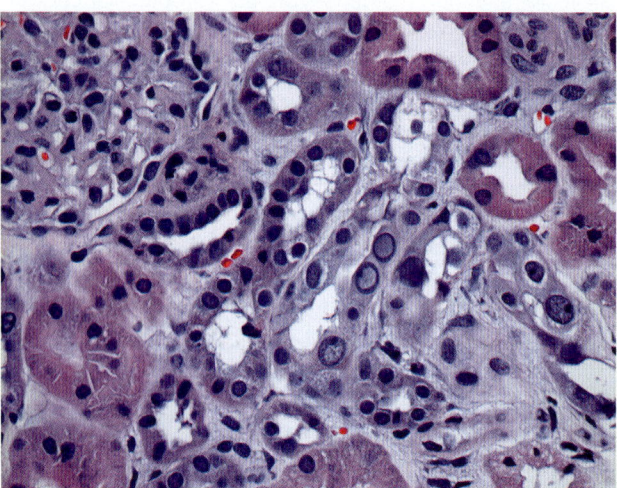

FIGURE 8-14 • Enlarged nuclei with intranuclear inclusions in infected tubular epithelial cells are characteristic of polyomavirus nephropathy (H&E).

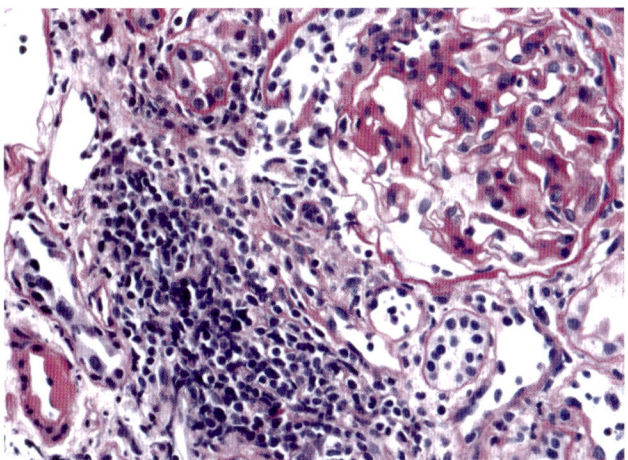

FIGURE 8-15 • The PAS-positive nodules in the wall of the arteriole at the lower left are seen in calcineurin inhibitor toxicity (PAS).

Recurrent Disease

Recurrence of the original disease that necessitated renal transplantation accounts for 7.9% of allograft loss in children (76). In addition, any acquired renal disease may develop *de novo* in renal allografts. The most common recurrent disease in pediatric renal allograft recipients is FSGS, which accounts for 12% of ESRD leading to transplantation in all children and adolescents in the United States and 23% among African American patients and recurs in the allograft in 20% to 50% of patients. Rapid progression from onset to ESRD, younger age, white race, mesangial proliferation on biopsy, and recurrent disease in one allograft are associated with a higher risk of recurrence (79). Autosomal recessive FSGS due to NPHS2 mutations appears to have a much lower risk of recurrence after transplantation (103). Recurrences occur early, 78% within the first posttransplant month (103), and patients with primary FSGS also experience twice the rate of early graft nonfunction/acute tubular necrosis, requiring dialysis compared to all other groups, raising the question of subclinical recurrence (79).

MPGN type I accounts for 2.1% of ESRD leading to transplantation in children (76) and recurs in 30% to 77% of allografts, resulting in loss of the graft in approximately one-fourth to one-third of patients with recurrent disease (103). Dense deposit disease (formerly MPGN type II) accounts for 0.9% of pediatric renal transplants (76) and recurs in nearly all allografts (103). Lupus nephritis accounts for 1.6% of ESRD leading to transplantation in children (76) and may recur in 30% of allografts, but the incidence of graft failure due to recurrent disease is low (103). IgA nephropathy accounts for 1.3% of pediatric renal transplants (76) and has been reported to recur in 65% of adults who had a graft biopsy for any reason (104). However, graft loss from recurrence was only 7% in one pediatric series and 3% in adults (103). Henoch-Schönlein purpura nephritis accounts for 1.4% of ESRD leading to transplantation in children (76), and recurrence has been reported in 53% of allografts, all from living-related donors, and 22% of grafts were lost (103). Congenital nephrotic syndrome (CNF) accounts for 2.6% of pediatric renal transplants (76), and though proteinuria recurs in 25% of patients with the Finnish type of CNF who receive transplants, these patients do not appear to have recurrent CNF (105). MGN accounts for 0.5% of ESRD leading to transplantation in children (76), and recurrence has been reported in adults but not in children. Familial nephritis accounts for 2.2% of pediatric renal transplants (76), but half of males with X-linked Alport syndrome will require transplantation by age 25. This genetic disease does not recur in the allograft, but crescentic glomerulonephritis due to antiglomerular basement membrane antibodies develops in 3% to 5% of transplanted Alport males and nearly 90% of these grafts fail (106).

Hemolytic uremic syndrome (HUS) is the most common cause of acute renal failure in children in developed countries and accounts for 2.7% of pediatric renal transplants (76). HUS rarely recurs in transplanted children with classic postdiarrheal HUS, but the recurrence rate of atypical HUS (aHUS) due to either factor H or factor I deficiency is 80% to 90%. Of note, both complement regulatory proteins are synthesized by the liver, but aHUS due to membrane cofactor only has a 20% recurrence rate as the kidney allograft may be able to provide sufficient quantities of the missing protein. Recombinant antibody targeting complement component C5 (eculizumab) is a promising therapeutic agent that inhibits the formation of C5a and the subsequent proinflammatory and prothrombotic events. A TMA indistinguishable from HUS may develop in transplants as a result of AMR, drug toxicity (oral contraceptives, cyclosporine, and, rarely, OKT3), pregnancy, or other infection.

Cystinosis accounts for 2.1% of ESRD leading to transplantation in children (76), and cystine deposits commonly occur in renal allografts of patients with cystinosis. This does not appear to affect graft function, but neither does the renal allograft prevent the systemic complications of cystinosis. In contrast, recurrence of oxalate deposits in oxalosis, which accounts for 0.5% of pediatric renal transplants (76), does impair graft function, and combined liver and kidney transplantation is the preferred treatment. Graft survival in children transplanted for ESRD due to urologic abnormalities is comparable to children with normal urinary tracts if the abnormalities can be corrected and careful attention is paid to possible sources of infection (107). Wilms tumor (WT) and Denys-Drash syndrome (DDS) each account for 0.5% of pediatric renal transplants (76), and transplantation should be delayed for 1 to 2 years after completion of chemotherapy.

Posttransplant Lymphoproliferative Disorders

According to the Organ Procurement and Transplantation Network, PTLDs occur in 2% of pediatric renal transplant recipients, which is substantially greater than the 0.5% incidence in adults (108). Seronegativity for EBV in recipients imparts greater than a fourfold increased risk for PTLD. There is also a continuum of pathologic lesions ranging from benign lymphoid hyperplasia to polymorphic PTLD to monomorphic PTLD, and tissue from suspected cases should be handled in the same manner as a suspected non-Hodgkin lymphoma, with samples sequestered for possible flow cytometry, immunohistochemical studies for T cells and B cells, *in situ* hybridization for EBV, and B-cell gene rearrangement studies. Typically, the interstitial infiltrate is very dense and either is monomorphic or contains a range of lymphoid cells, but neutrophils, eosinophils, tubulitis, and endarteritis are usually absent. Since most PTLDs are B-cell proliferations, in contrast to the predominantly T-cell proliferation in acute TCMR, and more than 90% harbor the EBV genome, a combination of immunohistochemistry for T cells and B cells and *in situ* hybridization for EBV-encoded nuclear RNAs (EBERs) can establish the diagnosis (109).

PATHOLOGY OF HEART TRANSPLANTATION

Overview

In 1967, the first successful human heart transplant was achieved, but survival was limited by infection, graft failure/hemodynamic collapse, and rejection. Important milestones include introduction of biopsy forceps for percutaneous endomyocardial biopsies in 1973, the development of CNI and the introduction of cyclosporine A in the heart transplant population in 1980, and the introduction of ATG in 1990 for both induction and treatment of rejection.

Volumes and Indications

The total number of pediatric heart transplant procedures reported to the Registry of the International Society of Heart and Lung Transplantation (ISHLT) has been gradually increasing from 400 in the year 2000 to 565 in 2011 (110). The first year of life is the single most common year for a heart transplant procedure in patients aged 18 years and younger. The indications for transplantation include congenital cardiac malformations in the infant [most often after surgery(ies), but this has been decreasing], and in the older child cardiomyopathy (dilated) (which has been increasing over the years), congenital malformation [also after surgery(ies)], endocardial fibroelastosis, Adriamycin toxicity, and retransplantation for chronic rejection. Dilated cardiomyopathy does not recur in the transplanted heart. The patient is at higher risk for developing chronic rejection again after retransplantation for it.

Surgical Complications

In the current setting, surgical complications are exceedingly rare and include hemorrhage and wound infections.

Rejection

Endomyocardial biopsy (EMB) remains the gold standard for rejection surveillance. It has a high sensitivity and specificity for the diagnosis of acute cellular rejection. There are currently no cardiac imaging modalities or serum markers that can replace it. Typically, surveillance biopsies are performed once weekly for the first month, every 2 weeks for the 2nd month, and every 6 to 8 weeks between the 3rd and 12th months. After the first year, the frequency can be decreased to quarterly, biannually, or annually. The current working formulation suggests a minimum of three step levels for microscopic examination. No special stains are routinely required. Unstained slides can be saved for immunohistochemical staining if needed. One to two pieces of biopsy should be obtained in addition and frozen for immunofluorescence staining, if clinically indicated (111).

Hyperacute rejection is graft injury triggered by preformed antibodies and occurs rapidly after implantation of the graft, usually within minutes to hours. This type of rejection is now extremely rare.

Acute cellular rejection consists of an inflammatory infiltrate that is predominantly a T-cell–mediated response directed against the cardiac allograft. A substantial increase in activated B-lymphocytes and NK cells is seen in moderate rejection, suggesting their important role as promoters and effectors of cellular rejection. Eosinophils and neutrophils are also present in severe rejection. The grading system for acute cellular rejection has been revised by the ISHLT such that the old system can easily be translated into the new one, which is simpler and more reproducible (Table 8-5; Figures 8-16 to 8-21; eFigures 8-1 and 8-2) (112). In most transplant centers, mild as well as focal moderate rejection (grades 1A, 1B, 2/1R) is not treated if patient is asymptomatic, and there is no clinical indication of rejection. However, other centers do treat focal moderate

TABLE 8-5 OLD AND REVISED GRADING SYSTEMS OF THE ISHLT FOR ACUTE CELLULAR CARDIAC REJECTION

1990	2005
No rejection (grade 0)	No rejection (grade 0R)
Focal, mild acute rejection (grade 1A)	Mild, low-grade rejection: interstitial and/or perivascular cellular infiltrate with up to one focus of myocyte damage (grade 1R)
Diffuse, mild acute rejection (grade 1B)	
Focal, moderate acute rejection (grade 2)	
Multifocal moderate rejection (grade 3A)	Moderate, intermediate-grade rejection: two or more foci of cellular infiltrate with associated myocyte damage (grade 2R)
Diffuse, moderate rejection (grade 3B)	Severe, high-grade rejection: diffuse cellular infiltrate with multifocal myocyte damage ± edema, ± hemorrhage ± vasculitis (grade 3R)
Severe acute rejection (grade 4)	

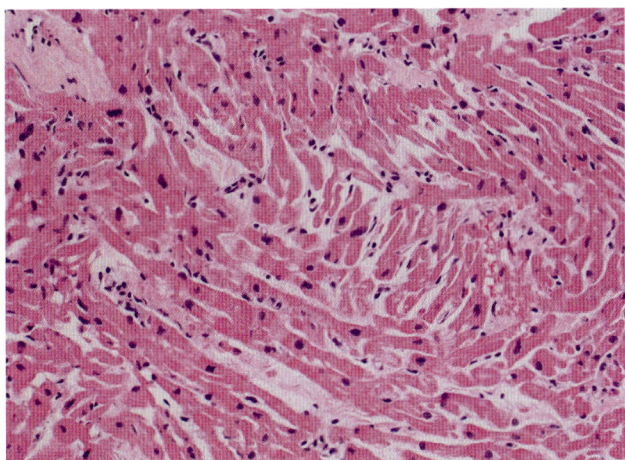

FIGURE 8-16 • Negative for acute cellular rejection (grade 0/0R). Pediatric heart biopsies appear more cellular than adults do since the myocytes are smaller. Also, capillary endothelium can be quite prominent in posttransplant biopsies (H&E, 200×).

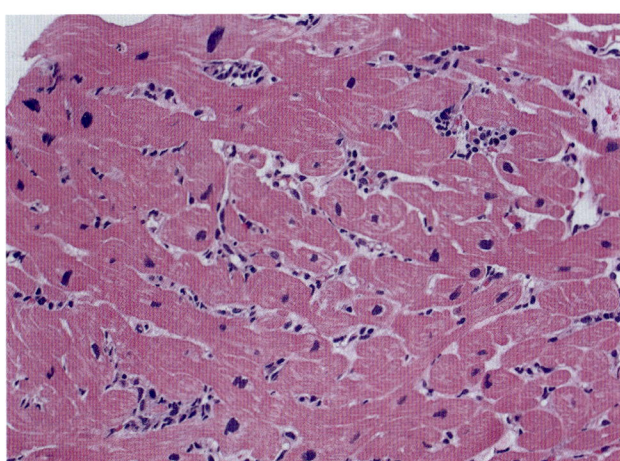

FIGURE 8-18 • Mild acute cellular rejection (grade 1B/1R). There is a sparse but diffuse lymphocytic infiltrate between myocytes, without any myocyte damage (H&E, 200×).

rejection; thus, pathologists are expected to report both the old and the revised grades.

Antibody-Mediated Rejection

AMR is an immunopathologic process associated with the production of antidonor-reactive antibodies in which injury to the graft is, in part, the result of activation of the complement system. It occurs in about 10% to 15% of cardiac recipients. It is poorly responsive to conventional immunosuppression, which targets the cellular arm of the immune response. Risk factors for developing AMR include blood transfusions, previous transplantation, use of ventricular assist devices, presence of positive B-cell flow cytometry cross-match, and elevated panel-reactive and donor-specific antibodies. AMR has been associated with the development of cardiac allograft vasculopathy (CAV) and decreased survival (113).

Histologic features are capillary endothelial changes (swelling or denudation with congestion), macrophages and neutrophils in capillaries, interstitial edema, and/or hemorrhage and fibrin in vessels. However, these are relatively nonspecific findings and often absent in early AMR. C4d deposition (strong diffuse endothelial staining) can be detected by immunofluorescence on frozen sections (Figure 8-22) or paraffin immunohistochemistry (Figure 8-23) (114). One should be aware that there is significant background staining, which should be disregarded. The ISHLT recommends grading pathologic AMR as pAMR 0 (negative), pAMR 1(H+) (histopathologic AMR alone), pAMR 1(I+) (immunopathologic AMR alone), pAMR 2 (histopathologic and immunopathologic findings are both present), and pAMR3 (severe pathologic AMR with interstitial hemorrhage, capillary fragmentation, mixed inflammatory infiltrates, endothelial cell pyknosis, and/or karyorrhexis and marked edema and immunopathologic findings are present) (115).

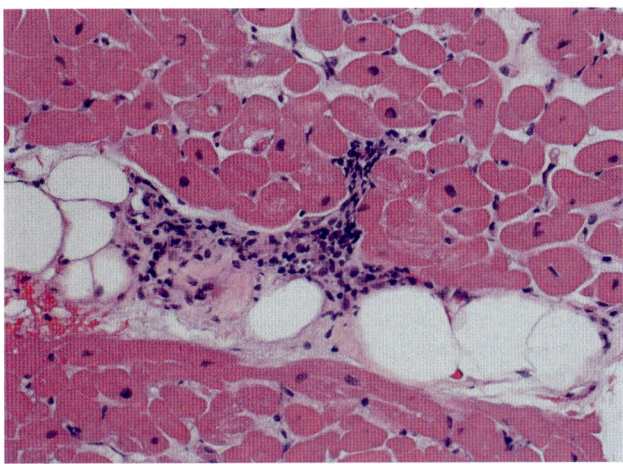

FIGURE 8-17 • Focal mild acute cellular rejection (grade 1A/1R). There is a focal infiltrate of lymphocytes between the myocytes and involving fat, which is often present in posttransplant biopsies (H&E, 200×).

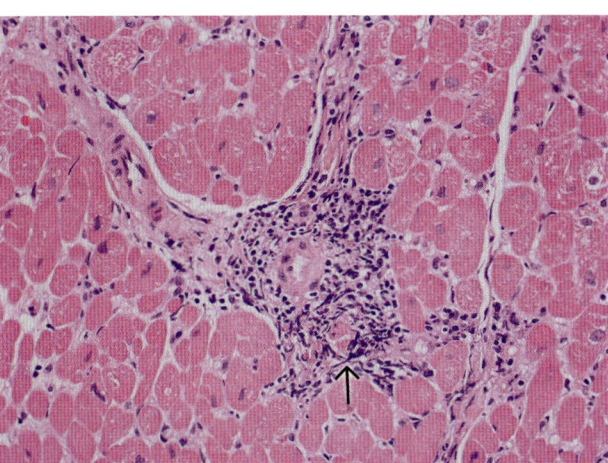

FIGURE 8-19 • Focal moderate acute cellular rejection (grade 2/1R). There is one focus of activated lymphocytes associated with myocyte damage (arrow) (H&E, 200×).

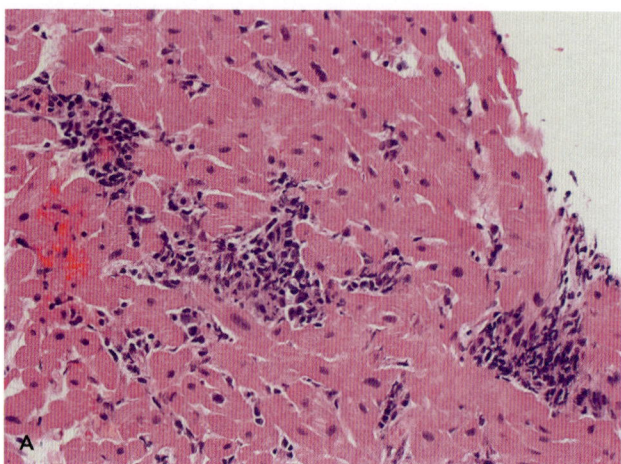

FIGURE 8-20 • Multifocal moderate acute cellular rejection (grade 3A/2R). The biopsy has two separate foci of moderate rejection seen in **(A)** and **(B)** (H&E, 200×).

Chronic rejection (CAV) involves both epicardial and intramural coronary arteries. The whole length of the coronary vessels is usually affected. There is diffuse concentric narrowing with luminal stenosis due to intimal fibrosis (eFigures 8-3 and 8-4) with long-term lesions resembling conventional atherosclerosis (Figure 8-24). The incidence of CAV in children increases over time (only 53% are free of CAV at 14 years post transplant) (110). Infant recipients and children 1 to 5 years of age had the lowest risk of CAV, likely due to their lower incidence of acute cellular rejection.

Infection

These chronically immunosuppressed patients are prone to bacterial and opportunistic infections mostly in the lungs, GI tract, skin, and nervous system. Infection of the heart itself is rare; toxoplasmosis and CMV are seen most often.

The incidence of PTLD seems to be decreasing from the 3% to 5% reported in the past, perhaps due to better immunosuppressive regimens. The proliferation is EBV driven and can be polyclonal lymphoplasmacytoid or monoclonal. It most often involves extracardiac sites such as lymph nodes, gastrointestinal tract, lung, and skin.

Other Complications

Hypertension is reported in 47% at 1 year, 63% at 5 years, and 72% of pediatric recipients at 10 years after transplantation. Hyperlipidemia also increases steadily to 38% at 10 years after pediatric transplantation (116). 5% of patients required renal replacement therapy in the form of dialysis or renal transplant by 11 years post transplant. 18% of patients developed a malignancy by 15 years post transplant, the vast majority being lymphoma (110).

Other Biopsy Findings

Quilty Lesion

This is an endocardial lymphocytic lesion composed of mature lymphocytes with a central dendritic cell network upon which the B- and T cells are organized (neolymphogenesis)

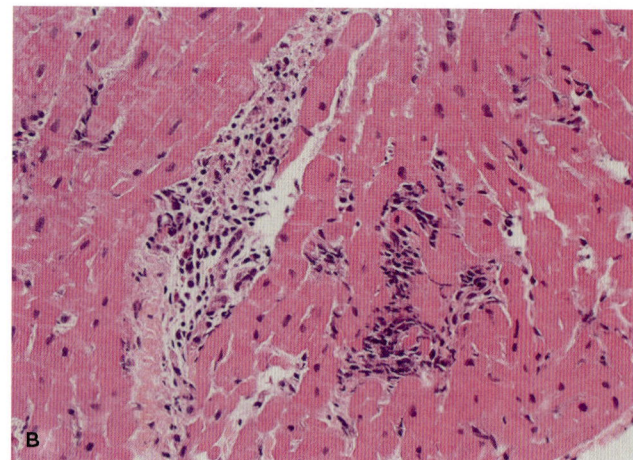

FIGURE 8-21 • Diffuse moderate acute cellular rejection (grade 3B/3R). There is a marked infiltrate associated with myocyte damage and few eosinophils and neutrophils (H&E, 200×).

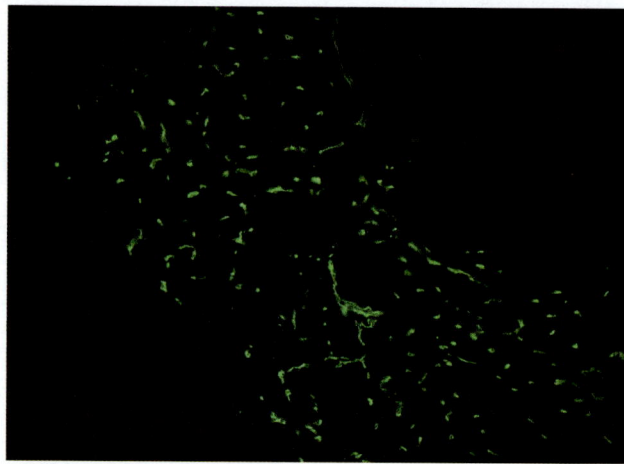

FIGURE 8-22 • Positive C4d staining is seen in all the vessels in this heart biopsy (Courtesy of Dr. Anthony Chang, University of Chicago Medical Center, indirect immunofluorescence, 40×).

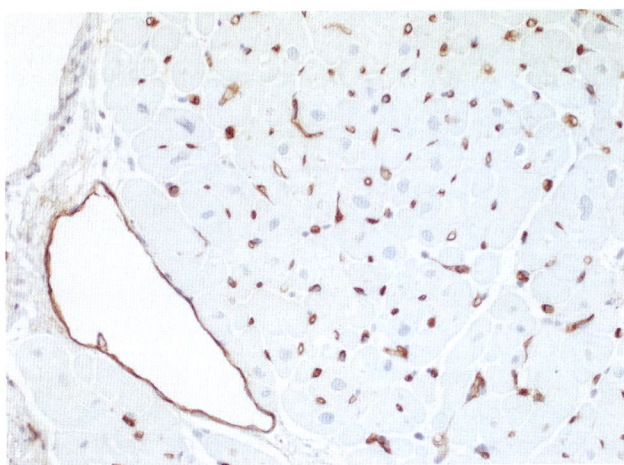

FIGURE 8-23 • Positive C4d staining is seen in all the vessels in this heart biopsy with strong endothelial staining (immunohistochemical stain, 200×).

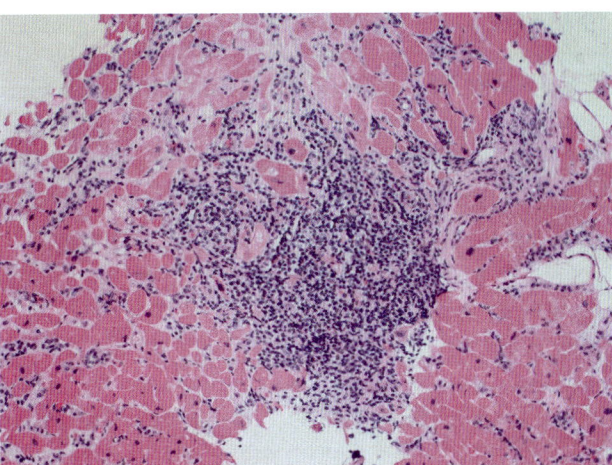

FIGURE 8-25 • Quilty lesion. This EMB shows a large infiltrate between myocytes, composed of mature lymphocytes with multiple capillaries (H&E, 100×).

(117). The infiltrate often extends into the underlying myocardium where it may be associated with myocyte damage and fibrosis (Figure 8-25). It is not known to be related to acute or chronic rejection, infection, ischemic time, or poor outcome. The main issue is to differentiate it from cellular rejection and avoid overtreatment (eFigures 8-5 to 8-8)

Adipose Tissue

Over time, more and more fat accumulates in the transplanted heart and can be seen in the endomyocardial biopsies (eFigure 8-9). Only when epicardial mesothelium is identified should one alert the cardiologist as to the possibility of perforation.

Site of Previous Biopsy

Due to the structure of the heart, the bioptome tends to be guided to the same location for each biopsy. Thus, it is very common to see organizing biopsy site with fibrin, mild inflammation, granulation tissue, and fibrosis (eFigure 8-10).

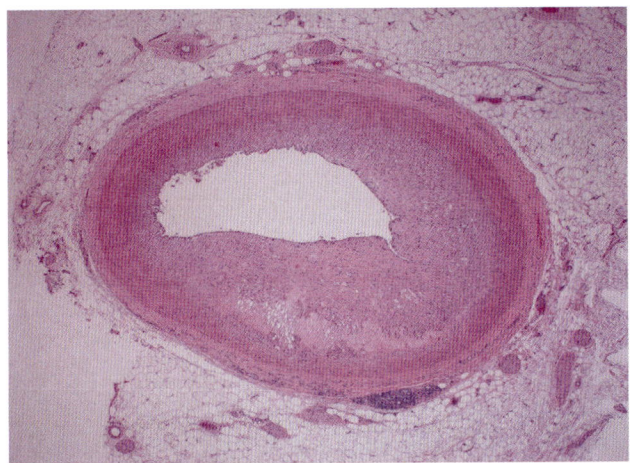

FIGURE 8-24 • Chronic rejection (CAV) is seen in this epicardial coronary artery, which has eccentric intimal fibrosis (H&E, 20×).

Calcifications

Occasionally, dystrophic microcalcifications are seen on biopsy. These can be located in the myocyte or in areas of scarring.

Fibrosis

Focal fibrosis is often seen on biopsy, especially after the first year post transplantation. It may represent old biopsy site, healed infarct, or drug-induced fibrosis.

Outcome

For recipients surviving the first year post transplant, the median conditional survival was greater than 21 years for those who received a transplant in the first year of life, 20.6 years for those whose transplant occurred between 1 and 5 years of age, 16.7 years for recipients between 6 and 10 years of age, and 16.1 years for adolescents (110).

PATHOLOGY OF LUNG TRANSPLANTATION

Lung transplantation, single, bilateral, or, less often, heart–lung, has been an accepted mode of therapy for a variety of end-stage lung diseases for over 30 years. Methods of evaluation of allograft dysfunction are variable and, depending on the clinical differential diagnosis, can include transbronchial biopsy (TBB), bronchoalveolar lavage (BAL) with culture, endobronchial biopsy (EBB), and, least often, wedge biopsy and fine needle aspiration biopsy (FNAB).

Volumes and Indications

Since 2005, the number of procedures worldwide that are reported to the ISHLT have been fairly constant, with 107 lung transplants in 2011. The majority of recipients are between 12 and 17 years of age with less than five procedures per year in infants (118). The most common indications for children are cystic fibrosis (CF) and primary pulmonary arterial hypertension (PPAH), in contrast to adults who are transplanted for emphysema, CF, idiopathic pulmonary fibrosis, and PPAH. Heritable surfactant deficiency and alveolar capillary dysplasia are indications in neonates. There is no recurrence of original disease in children except for the rare patient who gets retransplanted for chronic rejection and is at higher risk for developing chronic rejection again.

Vascular Complications

Postsurgical obstruction/thrombosis of the arterial or venous anastomosis, although rare, is a surgical emergency. Inflammatory cells, endothelial disruption, and recent thrombus are seen in the early posttransplant period, while organizing/organized thrombus, stenosis, and fibrosis with foreign body giant cells are present in the intermediate to late period.

Airway Anastomotic Complications

The anastomosis heals by formation of granulation tissue, the surface of which reepithelializes in a few days. Occasionally, exuberant polypoid granulation tissue forms, which may need to be removed. Varying degrees of ischemic injury, manifested as coagulative necrosis of airway wall components, are commonly present. Superimposed infection may interrupt and complicate the healing process. Common organisms found on culture, EBB, and special stains include fungi (*Candida* and *Aspergillus* sp.) and bacteria. Fungi tend to invade necrotic cartilage. Dehiscence of the anastomosis can allow infection to spread into the mediastinum. Healing may result in fibrosis and stenosis of the airway, treatment for which includes stent placement.

Primary Graft Dysfunction

Primary graft dysfunction occurs in 22% of pediatric lung recipients (similar to adults) in the first 30 days after transplantation due to some combination of ischemia, reperfusion, surgical trauma, denervation, and interruption of lymphatics, resulting in endothelial injury and pulmonary edema with or without diffuse alveolar damage (DAD). Recovery occurs in the majority of patients in a few days to weeks with supportive therapy, although the mortality and morbidity rates are high (119).

Rejection

Definite diagnosis and grading of rejection (especially acute rejection) are based on light microscopic examination of tissue obtained by TBB, which may be performed based on the clinical symptoms or based on a surveillance protocol. Since rejection is a patchy process, it is recommended that five fragments of alveolated lung tissue be examined at three different levels stained with H&E. A working formulation for the grading of pulmonary allograft rejection, initially developed in 1990 and revised in 1996 (Table 8-6) and 2007, is widely used (120).

TABLE 8-6 WORKING FORMULATION FOR THE CLASSIFICATION AND GRADING OF PULMONARY ALLOGRAFT REJECTION

A. Acute rejection (perivascular)
   Grade 0—none
   Grade 1—minimal
   Grade 2—mild
   Grade 3—moderate
   Grade 4—severe
B. Airway inflammation—lymphocytic bronchitis/bronchiolitis
   Grade 0—none
   Grade 1—minimal
   Grade 2—mild
   Grade 3—moderate
   Grade 4—severe
C. Chronic airway rejection—bronchiolitis obliterans
   Ca. Active
   Cb. Inactive
D. Chronic vascular rejection—accelerated graft vascular sclerosis

Modified from Yousem SA, Berry GJ, Cagle PT, et al. Revision of the 1990 working formulation for the classification of pulmonary allograft rejection. Lung Rejection Study Group. *J Heart Lung Transplant* 1996;15:1–15.

Antibody-Mediated Rejection

Only a few well-documented cases of AMR (formerly referred to as hyperacute rejection) of the lung (all in adults) have been reported in the literature (121). Preformed antibodies bind to the endothelium and epithelium of the donor lung and activate inflammatory, complement, and coagulation cascades. Within minutes to hours after transplantation, there is progressive respiratory failure, pulmonary edema, and pleural effusion, with complete opacification of the allograft seen on radiologic examination. The histologic features of AMR include DAD, alveolar hemorrhage, interstitial neutrophilia, fibrin thrombi, and vasculitis. There is deposition of IgG and complement in the alveolar septa. Complement fragments C3d and C4d may also be detected. If fresh frozen tissue is not available for immunofluorescence studies, C4d deposition can be demonstrated in the vascular endothelium by IHC. Only strong endothelial staining without background should be interpreted as positive. A few cases of AMR have also been described in the first year after transplantation, all in adults (122).

Acute Rejection

Acute rejection is a cell-mediated process during which there is progressive infiltration of the graft by host mononuclear cells. Immune cell activation causes release of inflammatory chemokines and upregulation of adhesion molecules. Major cellular targets include endothelial and epithelial cells. With current immunosuppressive therapy, it is rare for a lung transplant recipient to die of acute cellular rejection.

Although acute rejection can develop as early as 3 days to many years post transplant, most patients experience some rejection commonly around 3 months, with most episodes occurring between 2 and 9 months (123). Noncompliance with immunosuppressive medications is a significant cause of late episodes of acute rejection.

Acute rejection is characterized by a predominantly lymphocytic infiltrate with scattered eosinophils, neutrophils, and plasma cells. The infiltrate is located in the perivascular areas and/or the submucosa of airways. In minimal acute rejection (grade A1/B1), there are scattered infrequent perivascular and airway mononuclear infiltrates forming two to three layers that are not obvious at low magnification (Figure 8-26). Mild acute rejection (grade A2/B2) consists of greater than three layers of activated lymphocytes, eosinophils, and neutrophils around small blood vessels (Figure 8-27) or a band-like infiltrate in the airway submucosa (eFigure 8-11). Moderate acute rejection (A3/B3) is characterized by an extension of the inflammation into alveolar septa with or without vasculitis or a band-like infiltrate in the submucosa extending into the airway epithelium with focal epithelial necrosis. In severe acute rejection (grade A4/B4), diffuse perivascular, interstitial, and airspace infiltrates associated with pneumocyte damage, macrophages, hyaline membranes, hemorrhage, and neutrophils or epithelial ulceration with fibrinopurulent exudates are seen.

In the 2007 revision, the grading of perivascular and interstitial infiltrates remains the same (i.e., A0 to A4); however, the airway inflammation is changed to B0 (none), B1R (low grade, 1996 B1 and B2), grade B2R (high grade, 1996 B3 and B4) (120). The latter poses a problem for those centers that treat grade B2 rejection in a manner similar to grade A2. Asymptomatic minimal rejection is clinically insignificant and not treated. Mild (grade A2/B2) and higher grades are treated irrespective of symptoms.

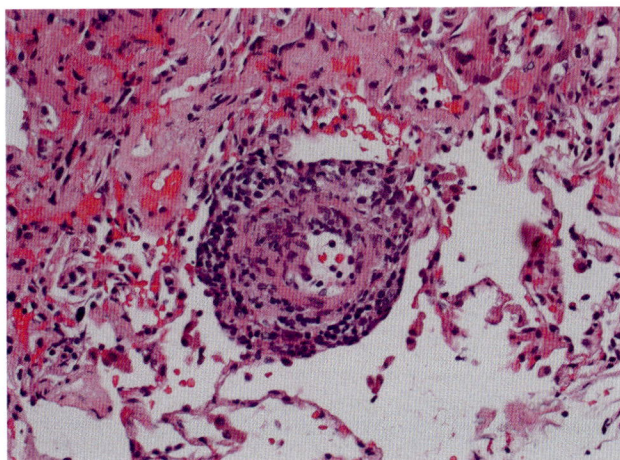

FIGURE 8-27 • Mild acute cellular rejection of the lung (A2). There is a complete perivascular cuff, more than three layers thick, which is readily apparent at low power (H&E, 40×).

The main differential diagnosis is infection, and microbiologic cultures and TBB are most useful to distinguish this (eFigure 8-12). Aspiration is a common event, which is gaining more significance since it may trigger episodes of acute rejection and increase the risk of patients to develop chronic rejection (eFigures 8-13 to 8-15). Bronchial-associated lymphoid tissue (BALT) is often prominent in lung transplant recipients, and care should be taken not to overcall it as rejection (eFigure 8-16).

Chronic Rejection

In the lung, chronic rejection is primarily manifested as bronchiolitis obliterans (BO). Despite improved baseline immunosuppression and treatment of acute rejection, BO remains the most important cause of late graft failure. Although its etiology and pathogenesis are still not completely understood, acute rejection is certainly one of the most important risk factors. In general, the process of chronic rejection is believed to occur in stages. The initial wave of antibody-mediated response is paralleled by a cellular infiltrate in which the monocyte/macrophage compartment plays a central role as the critical effector cells. The high antigenicity of airway epithelial cells through the up-regulated expression of MHC, adhesion and costimulatory molecules, together with the abundance of antigen-presenting cells and circulating lymphocytes, provide an increased propensity to damage of these structures, similar to epithelial-lined conduits in other solid allografts (e.g., bile ducts, pancreatic ducts, and renal tubules). The production of inflammatory mediators and growth factors contribute to the fibroproliferative response of the damaged graft leading to BO.

Although the term chronic implies a late temporal process, BO can be seen as early as 3 to 6 weeks after transplantation but primarily occurs 1 or more years later. The onset of chronic rejection is insidious with vague general symptoms and nonproductive cough. There is progressive dyspnea on exertion and irreversible decline in pulmonary function

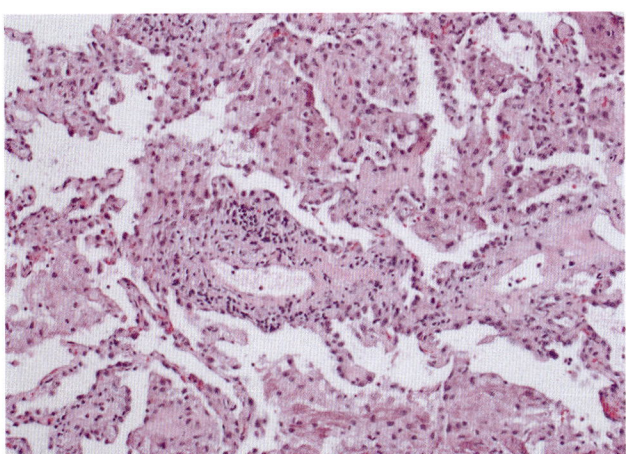

FIGURE 8-26 • Minimal acute cellular rejection of lung (A1). There is an incomplete perivascular cuff of lymphocytes (H&E, 100×).

tests, not explained by other causes such as infection. When the decline is greater than 10% of baseline, a clinical diagnosis of bronchiolitis obliterans syndrome (BOS) is made, which does not need pathologic confirmation. BOS is graded from 1 to 3 based on the degree of loss of lung function (124). When the clinical diagnosis is not clear, a wedge biopsy is often needed since BO is a patchy process and diagnostic yield of TBB is low.

BO is patchy both in distribution and severity in individual lobes and in the same airway. There is submucosal fibrosis, which either bulges asymmetrically into the lumen and causes partial obstruction or is concentric and causes total obstruction (Figure 8-28; eFigures 8-17 to 8-20). Chronic vascular rejection occurs much less frequently and is histologically similar to the transplant vasculopathy seen in other solid organ allografts (intimal fibrosis and vascular thickening); however, in the lung, it does not usually cause significant allograft dysfunction.

The main histologic differential diagnosis is organizing pneumonia (formerly known as bronchiolitis obliterans organizing pneumonia or BOOP), which is a healing response to various forms of lung injury and manifests as loose fibromyxoid plugs of connective tissue within alveoli and bronchioles. On the other hand, BO is a dense scar tissue (mature collagen) within small airways.

Once there has been a decrease in lung function due to BO, it cannot be reversed, but aggressive immunosuppression can stabilize the disease for variable periods of time. Some patients can live with BO for a few years, but others have progressive dysfunction and complications and die unless retransplanted.

Infections

Like any immunocompromised patient, lung transplant recipients are at high risk of developing infections, which can be bacterial, viral, or fungal, and may cause tracheobronchitis, localized infection of the airway anastomosis, or pneumonia. Most bacterial infections occur in the first posttransplant month, whereas viral and fungal infections tend to be seen in the 3- to 6-month period since they are on immunosuppressive drugs. Lung transplant patients remain susceptible to infections for the rest of their lives especially in that substantial population of children transplanted because of CF (50% of cases in most pediatric lung transplant programs).

Microscopic findings depend on the etiology of the infection and the host response, which may be minimal. Bacterial infections usually elicit neutrophilic infiltration of airway, interstitium, and alveolar spaces. Occasionally, there is only bacterial growth and infarction with no inflammation. The most common viral infection is caused by CMV, which often infects endothelial cells. This may lead to bleeding complications after diagnostic TBB. CMV is diagnosed by finding the classical single intranuclear and multiple small cytoplasmic inclusions in an enlarged cell (eFigure 8-21). Treated patients often have smudged, eosinophilic inclusions, which may be difficult to identify as CMV (Figure 8-29). Adenovirus infection is more common in children, and scattered adult and pediatric patients develop serious pneumonias due to the other respiratory viruses (respiratory syncytial virus, parainfluenza, influenza). Fungal infections are often caused by *Aspergillus* or *Candida* sp. especially in children with CF. Pneumocystis pneumonia is rare due to routine prophylaxis.

In the very early stage of CMV infection, IHC staining against immediate-early antigen may demonstrate nuclear positivity in cells lacking diagnostic cytopathic changes (Figure 8-30). IHC is also very useful for confirming the diagnosis in patients already on treatment for CMV.

The main differential diagnosis is from acute rejection, since the symptoms are similar. Infection may precipitate rejection and vice versa. Infections can be very difficult to treat, with new resistant strains emerging in some patients. Prophylaxis plays an important role in preventing pneumocystis and CMV pneumonia.

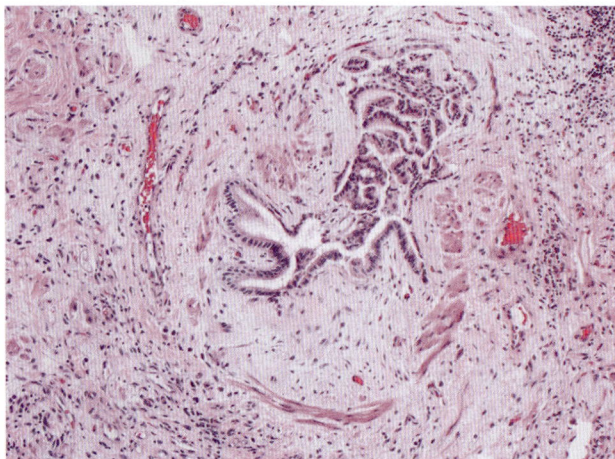

FIGURE 8-28 • Chronic rejection (bronchiolitis obliterans). Eccentric submucosal fibrosis partially occludes the lumen of this bronchiole (H&E, 100×).

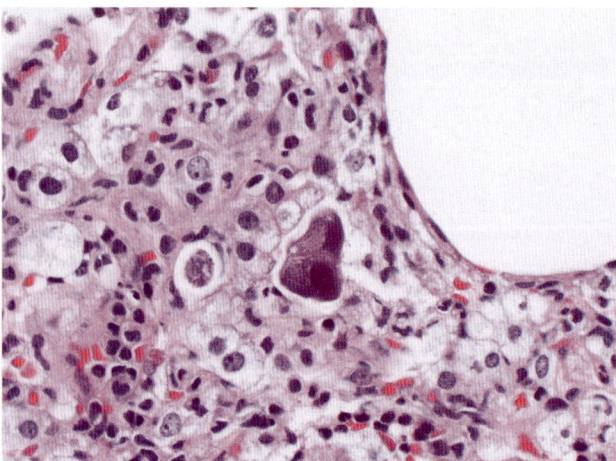

FIGURE 8-29 • Treated CMV. Soon after treatment, CMV inclusions become eosinophilic and smudged as seen in this photomicrograph (H&E, 200×).

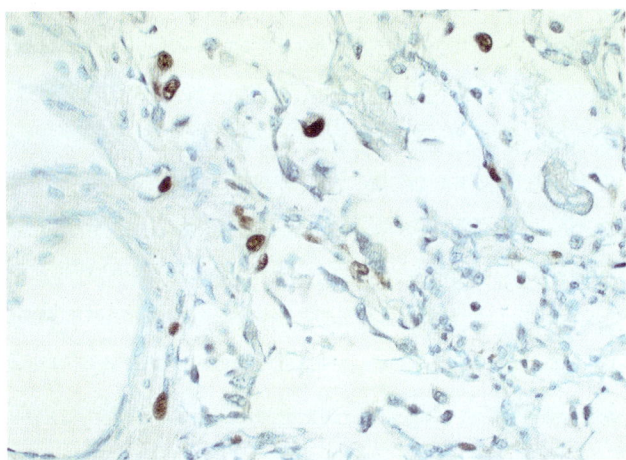

FIGURE 8-30 • Early CMV pneumonitis. In the lung transplant recipient, detection of any nuclear stain even without classic intranuclear inclusions is indicative of CMV infection (immunohistochemical stain, 200×).

OTHER FORMS OF LUNG INJURY

DAD, organizing pneumonia, acute interstitial pneumonia, and interstitial fibrosis may all be seen as nonspecific responses to lung injury in the posttransplant patient. The etiology of these responses is diverse and is not specifically related to either acute or chronic rejection.

Posttransplant Lymphoproliferative Disorder

PTLD occurs in 3% to 5% of lung transplant recipients with frequent involvement of the allograft, often as one or multiple nodules. A high index of suspicion should be maintained, and the diagnosis can be suggested on FNAB and TBB. Particularly with low-grade lesions, the need to obtain adequate tissue for complete workup may require a wedge biopsy. The histologic and molecular features are similar to those seen in any other transplant patient (Chapter 22).

Outcome

Advances in donor management, surgical techniques, and immunosuppressive drugs have led to improvement in the short-term survival of patients. However, in contrast to other solid organ transplants, over half of the lung transplant recipients (pediatric and adult) continue to suffer and die of chronic rejection (BO) 3 to 10 years post transplantation (118).

Pulmonary Complications After Hematopoietic Stem Cell Transplant

With the use of effective infection prophylaxis, noninfectious causes of pulmonary dysfunction after stem cell transplant are the major pulmonary causes of morbidity and mortality. These include acute and chronic graft versus host disease, idiopathic pneumonia syndrome, diffuse alveolar hemorrhage, pulmonary VOD, and organizing pneumonia (125).

References

1. Chinen J, Buckley RH. Transplantation immunology: solid organ and bone marrow. *J Allergy Clin Immunol* 2010;125(2 Suppl 2):S324–S335. doi: 10.1016/j.jaci.2009.11.014
2. Heeger PS, Dinavahi R. Transplant immunology for non-immunologist. *Mt Sinai J Med* 2012;79(3):376–387. doi: 10.1002/msj.21314
3. Starr TK, Jameson SC, Hogquist KA. Positive and negative selection of T cells. *Annu Rev Immunol* 2003;21:139–176.
4. Pietra BA. Transplantation immunology 2003: simplified approach. *Pediatr Clin North Am* 2003;50(6):1233–1259.
5. Gould DS, Auchincloss H Jr. Direct and indirect recognition: the role of MHC antigens in graft rejection. *Immunol Today* 1999;20(2):77–82.
6. Colvin RB, Smith RN. Antibody-mediated organ-allograft rejection. *Nat Rev Immunol* 2005;5(10):807–817.
7. Collins AB, Schneeberger EE, Pascual MA, et al. Complement activation in acute humoral renal allograft rejection: diagnostic significance of C4d deposits in peritubular capillaries. *J Am Soc Nephrol* 1999;10(10):2208–2214.
8. Mauiyyedi S, Colvin RB. Humoral rejection in kidney transplantation: new concepts in diagnosis and treatment. *Curr Opin Nephrol Hypertens* 2002;11(6):609–618.
9. Mannon RB. Therapeutic targets in the treatment of allograft fibrosis. *Am J Transplant* 2006;6(5 Pt 1):867–875.
10. Wekerle T, Sykes M. Mixed chimerism and transplantation tolerance. *Annu Rev Med* 2001;52:353–370.
11. Main JM, Prehn RT. Successful skin homografts after the administration of high dosage X radiation and homologous bone marrow. *J Natl Cancer Inst* 1955;15(4):1023–1029.
12. Waldmann H, Chen TC, Graca L, et al. Regulatory T cells in transplantation. *Semin Immunol* 2006;18(2):111–119.
13. Ghobrial RM, Farmer DG, Amersi F, et al. Advances in pediatric liver and intestinal transplantation. *Am J Surg* 2000;180(5):328–334.
14. Kato T, Tzakis AG, Selvaggi G, et al. Intestinal and multivisceral transplantation in children. *Ann Surg* 2006;243(6):756–764; discussion 764–756.
15. Reyes J, Bueno J, Kocoshis S, et al. Current status of intestinal transplantation in children. *J Pediatr Surg* 1998;33(2):243–254.
16. Jugie M, Canioni D, Le Bihan C, et al. Study of the impact of liver transplantation on the outcome of intestinal grafts in children. *Transplantation* 2006;81(7):992–997.
17. Lee RG, Nakamura K, Tsamandas AC, et al. Pathology of human intestinal transplantation. *Gastroenterology* 1996;110(6):1820–1834.
18. Wu T, Abu-Elmagd K, Bond G, et al. A clinicopathologic study of isolated intestinal allografts with preformed IgG lymphocytotoxic antibodies. *Hum Pathol* 2004;35(11):1332–1339.
19. Wu T, Abu-Elmagd K, Bond G, et al. A schema for histologic grading of small intestine allograft acute rejection. *Transplantation* 2003;75(8):1241–1248.
20. Parizhskaya M, Redondo C, Demetris A, et al. Chronic rejection of small bowel grafts: pediatric and adult study of risk factors and morphologic progression. *Pediatr Dev Pathol* 2003;6(3):240–250.
21. Noguchi Si S, Reyes J, Mazariegos GV, et al. Pediatric intestinal transplantation: the resected allograft. *Pediatr Dev Pathol* 2002;5(1):3–21.
22. Manez R, Kusne S, Green M, et al. Incidence and risk factors associated with the development of cytomegalovirus disease after intestinal transplantation. *Transplantation* 1995;59(7):1010–1014.
23. Pinchoff RJ, Kaufman SS, Magid MS, et al. Adenovirus infection in pediatric small bowel transplantation recipients. *Transplantation* 2003;76(1):183–189.
24. Finn L, Reyes J, Bueno J, et al. Epstein-Barr virus infections in children after transplantation of the small intestine. *Am J Surg Pathol* 1998;22(3):299–309.
25. McDonald GB, Shulman HM, Sullivan KM, et al. Intestinal and hepatic complications of human bone marrow transplantation. Part I. *Gastroenterology* 1986;90(2):460–477.

26. McDonald GB, Shulman HM, Sullivan KM, et al. Intestinal and hepatic complications of human bone marrow transplantation. Part II. *Gastroenterology* 1986;90(3):770–784.
27. Moroff G, Luban NL. The irradiation of blood and blood components to prevent graft-versus-host disease: technical issues and guidelines. *Transfus Med Rev* 1997;11(1):15–26.
28. Snover DC, Weisdorf SA, Vercellotti GM, et al. A histopathologic study of gastric and small intestinal graft-versus-host disease following allogeneic bone marrow transplantation. *Hum Pathol* 1985;16(4):387–392.
29. Washington K, Bentley RC, Green A, et al. Gastric graft-versus-host disease: a blinded histologic study. *Am J Surg Pathol* 1997;21(9):1037–1046.
30. Shulman HM, Kleiner D, Lee SJ, et al. Histopathologic diagnosis of chronic graft-versus-host disease: National Institutes of Health Consensus Development Project on Criteria for Clinical Trials in Chronic Graft-versus-Host Disease: II. Pathology Working Group Report. *Biol Blood Marrow Transplant* 2006;12(1):31–47.
31. Snover DC. Graft-versus-host disease of the gastrointestinal tract. *Am J Surg Pathol* 1990;14(Suppl 1):101–108.
32. Asplund S, Gramlich TL. Chronic mucosal changes of the colon in graft-versus-host disease. *Mod Pathol* 1998;11(6):513–515.
33. Mekori YA, Claman HN. Is graft-versus-host disease a reliable model for scleroderma? *Ric Clin Lab* 1986;16(4):509–513.
34. Papadimitriou JC, Cangro CB, Lustberg A, et al. Histologic features of mycophenolate mofetil-related colitis: a graft-versus-host disease-like pattern. *Int J Surg Pathol* 2003;11(4):295–302.
35. The Organ Procurement and Transplantation Network. [Internet] 2007 [cited]; Available from: http://www.optn.org
36. Hendrickson RJ, Karrer FM, Wachs ME, et al. Pediatric liver transplantation. *Curr Opin Pediatr* 2004;16(3):309–313.
37. Kulkarni S, Malago M, Cronin DC II. Living donor liver transplantation for pediatric and adult recipients. *Nat Clin Pract Gastroenterol Hepatol* 2006;3(3):149–157.
38. Azoulay D, Astarcioglu I, Bismuth H, et al. Split-liver transplantation. The Paul Brousse policy. *Ann Surg* 1996;224(6):737–746; discussion 746–738.
39. Kalayoglu M, D'Alessandro AM, Knechtle SJ, et al. Preliminary experience with split liver transplantation. *J Am Coll Surg* 1996;182(5):381–387.
40. McDiarmid SV. Management of the pediatric liver transplant patient. *Liver Transpl* 2001;7(11 Suppl 1):S77–S86.
41. Sieders E, Peeters PM, TenVergert EM, et al. Analysis of survival and morbidity after pediatric liver transplantation with full-size and technical-variant grafts. *Transplantation* 1999;68(4):540–545.
42. Washington K. Update on post-liver transplantation infections, malignancies, and surgical complications. *Adv Anat Pathol* 2005;12(4):221–226.
43. Ploeg RJ, D'Alessandro AM, Knechtle SJ, et al. Risk factors for primary dysfunction after liver Transplantation—a multivariate analysis. *Transplantation* 1993;55(4):807–813.
44. Rull R, Vidal O, Momblan D, et al. Evaluation of potential liver donors: limits imposed by donor variables in liver transplantation. *Liver Transpl* 2003;9(4):389–393.
45. Gaffey MJ, Boyd JC, Traweek ST, et al. Predictive value of intraoperative biopsies and liver function tests for preservation injury in orthotopic liver transplantation. *Hepatology* 1997;25(1):184–189.
46. Stringer MD, Marshall MM, Muiesan P, et al. Survival and outcome after hepatic artery thrombosis complicating pediatric liver transplantation. *J Pediatr Surg* 2001;36(6):888–891.
47. McDiarmid SV. Current status of liver transplantation in children. *Pediatr Clin North Am* 2003;50(6):1335–1374.
48. Demetris AJ, Markus BH. Immunopathology of liver transplantation. *Crit Rev Immunol* 1989;9(2):67–92.
49. Hübscher SG. Antibody-mediated rejection in the liver allograft. *Curr Opin Organ Transplant* 2012;17(3):280–286. doi: 10.1097/MOT.0b013e328353584c
50. D'Antiga L, Dhawan A, Portmann B, et al. Late cellular rejection in paediatric liver transplantation: aetiology and outcome. *Transplantation* 2002;73(1):80–84.
51. Demetris AJ, Batts KP, Dhillon AP, et al. Banff schema for grading liver allograft rejection: an international consensus document. *Hepatology* 1997;25(3):658–663.
52. Lefkowitch JH. Diagnostic issues in liver transplantation pathology. *Clin Liver Dis* 2002;6(2):555–570.
53. Demetris AJ, Adeyi O, Bellamy CO, et al. Liver biopsy interpretation for causes of late liver allograft dysfunction. *Hepatology* 2006;44(2):489–501.
54. Jain A, Mazariegos G, Pokharna R, et al. Almost total absence of chronic rejection in primary pediatric liver transplantation under tacrolimus. *Transplant Proc* 2002;34(5):1968–1969.
55. Evans PC, Smith S, Hirschfield G, et al. Recipient HLA-DR3, tumour necrosis factor-alpha promoter allele-2 (tumour necrosis factor-2) and cytomegalovirus infection are interrelated risk factors for chronic rejection of liver grafts. *J Hepatol* 2001;34(5):711–715.
56. Gupta P, Hart J, Cronin D, et al. Risk factors for chronic rejection after pediatric liver transplantation. *Transplantation* 2001;72(6):1098–1102.
57. van den Berg AP, Klompmaker IJ, Hepkema BG, et al. Cytomegalovirus infection does not increase the risk of vanishing bile duct syndrome after liver transplantation. *Transpl Int* 1996;9(Suppl 1):S171–S173.
58. Demetris A, Adams D, Bellamy C, et al. Update of the International Banff Schema for Liver Allograft Rejection: working recommendations for the histopathologic staging and reporting of chronic rejection. An International Panel. *Hepatology* 2000;31(3):792–799.
59. Crawford AR, Lin XZ, Crawford JM. The normal adult human liver biopsy: a quantitative reference standard. *Hepatology* 1998;28(2):323–331.
60. Harrison RF, Patsiaoura K, Hubscher SG. Cytokeratin immunostaining for detection of biliary epithelium: its use in counting bile ducts in cases of liver allograft rejection. *J Clin Pathol* 1994;47(4):303–308.
61. Jaffe R. Liver transplant pathology in pediatric metabolic disorders. *Pediatr Dev Pathol* 1998;1(2):102–117.
62. Graziadei IW. Recurrence of primary sclerosing cholangitis after liver transplantation. *Liver Transpl* 2002;8(7):575–581.
63. Evans HM, Kelly DA, McKiernan PJ, et al. Progressive histological damage in liver allografts following pediatric liver transplantation. *Hepatology* 2006;43(5):1109–1117.
64. Lamps LW, Pinson CW, Raiford DS, et al. The significance of microabscesses in liver transplant biopsies: a clinicopathological study. *Hepatology* 1998;28(6):1532–1537.
65. Hoffman JA. Adenoviral disease in pediatric solid organ transplant recipients. *Pediatr Transplant* 2006;10(1):17–25.
66. Wadleigh M, Ho V, Momtaz P, et al. Hepatic veno-occlusive disease: pathogenesis, diagnosis and treatment. *Curr Opin Hematol* 2003;10(6):451–462.
67. Pai RK, van Besien KH, Hart J, et al. Clinicopathologic features of late-onset veno-occlusive disease/sinusoidal obstruction syndrome after high dose intravenous busulfan and hematopoietic cell transplant. *Leuk Lymphoma* 2012;53(8):1552–1557. doi: 10.3109/10428194.2012.661052
68. Shulman HM, Fisher LB, Schoch HG, et al. Veno-occlusive disease of the liver after marrow transplantation: histological correlates of clinical signs and symptoms. *Hepatology* 1994;19(5):1171–1181.
69. Starzl TE, Demetris AJ. Transplantation milestones. Viewed with one- and two-way paradigms of tolerance. *JAMA* 1995;273(11):876–879.
70. Snover DC, Weisdorf SA, Ramsay NK, et al. Hepatic graft versus host disease: a study of the predictive value of liver biopsy in diagnosis. *Hepatology* 1984;4(1):123–130.
71. Randhawa P. Allograft biopsies in management of pancreas transplant recipients. *J Postgrad Med* 2002;48(1):56–63.
72. Klassen DK, Weir MR, Cangro CB, et al. Pancreas allograft biopsy: safety of percutaneous biopsy-results of a large experience. *Transplantation* 2002;73(4):553–555.
73. Drachenberg CB, Papadimitriou JC, Klassen DK, et al. Evaluation of pancreas transplant needle biopsy: reproducibility and revision of histologic grading system. *Transplantation* 1997;63(11):1579–1586.
74. Klassen DK, Drachenberg CB, Papadimitriou JC, et al. CMV allograft pancreatitis: diagnosis, treatment, and histological features. *Transplantation* 2000;69(9):1968–1971.

75. Pediatric ESRD. *Am J Kidney Dis* 2014;63(1):e295–e306.
76. Smith JM, Stablein DM, Munoz R, et al. Contributions of the Transplant Registry: The 2006 Annual Report of the North American Pediatric Renal Trials and Collaborative Studies (NAPRTCS). *Pediatr Transplant* 2007;11(4):366–373.
77. Sharbaf FG, Bitzan M, Szymanski KM, et al. Native nephrectomy prior to pediatric kidney transplantation: biological and clinical aspects. *Pediatr Nephrol* 2012;27:1179–1188
78. Benfield MR, McDonald RA, Bartosh S, et al. Changing trends in pediatric transplantation: 2001 Annual Report of the North American Pediatric Renal Transplant Cooperative Study. *Pediatr Transplant* 2003;7(4):321–335.
79. Benfield MR. Current status of kidney transplant: update 2003. *Pediatr Clin North Am* 2003;50(6):1301–1334.
80. Puliyanda DP, Stablein DM, Dharnidharka VR. Younger age and antibody induction increase the risk for infection in pediatric renal transplantation: a NAPRTCS report. *Am J Transplant* 2007;7(3):662–666.
81. Haas M, Sis B, Racusen LC, et al.; Banff Meeting Report Writing Committee. Banff 2013 meeting report: inclusion of c4d-negative antibody-mediated rejection and antibody-associated arterial lesions. *Am J Transplant* 2014;14(2):272–283.
82. Racusen LC, Solez K, Colvin RB, et al. The Banff 97 working classification of renal allograft pathology. *Kidney Int* 1999;55(2):713–723.
83. Colvin RB, Nickeleit V. Renal transplant pathology (Chapter 28). In: Jennette JC, Olson JL, Schwartz MM, et al., eds. *Heptinstall's Pathology of the Kidney*, 6th ed. Philadelphia, PA: Lippincott Williams & Wilkins; 2007;1349–1447.
84. Kim L, Garfinkel MR, Chang A, et al. Intragraft vascular occlusive sickle crisis with early renal allograft loss in occult sickle cell trait. *Hum Pathol* 2011;42(7):1027–1033.
85. Smith KD, Wrenshall LE, Nicosia RF, et al. Delayed graft function and cast nephropathy associated with tacrolimus plus rapamycin use. *J Am Soc Nephrol* 2003;14(4):1037–1045.
86. Mengel M, Reeve J, Bunnag S, et al. Scoring total inflammation is superior to the current Banff inflammation score in predicting outcome and the degree of molecular disturbance in renal allografts. *Am J Transplant* 2009;9(8):1859–1867.
87. Lehnhardt A, Mengel M, Pape L, et al. Nodular B-cell aggregates associated with treatment refractory renal transplant rejection resolved by rituximab. *Am J Transplant* 2006;6(4):847–851.
88. Lefaucheur C, Loupy A, Vernerey D, et al. Antibody-mediated vascular rejection of kidney allografts: a population-based study. *Lancet* 2013;381(9863):313–319.
89. Feucht HE. Complement C4d in graft capillaries—the missing link in the recognition of humoral alloreactivity. *Am J Transplant* 2003;3(6):646–652.
90. Herzenberg AM, Gill JS, Djurdjev O, et al. C4d deposition in acute rejection: an independent long-term prognostic factor. *J Am Soc Nephrol* 2002;13(1):234–241.
91. Truong L, Gelfand J, D'Agati V, et al. De novo membranous glomerulonephropathy in renal allografts: a report of ten cases and review of the literature. *Am J Kidney Dis* 1989;14(2):131–144.
92. Heidet L, Gagnadoux ME, Beziau A, et al. Recurrence of de novo membranous glomerulonephritis on renal grafts. *Clin Nephrol* 1994;41(5):314–318.
93. Huang CC, Lehman A, Albawardi A, et al. IgG subclass staining in renal biopsies with membranous glomerulonephritis indicates subclass switch during disease progression. *Mod Pathol* 2013;26(6):799–805.
94. Solez K, Colvin RB, Racusen LC, et al. Banff '05 Meeting Report: differential diagnosis of chronic allograft injury and elimination of chronic allograft nephropathy ('CAN'). *Am J Transplant* 2007;7(3):518–526.
95. Hirsch HH, Knowles W, Dickenmann M, et al. Prospective study of polyomavirus type BK replication and nephropathy in renal-transplant recipients. *N Engl J Med* 2002;347(7):488–496.
96. Smith JM, McDonald RA, Finn LS, et al. Polyomavirus nephropathy in pediatric kidney transplant recipients. *Am J Transplant* 2004;4(12):2109–2117.
97. Meehan SM, Kraus MD, Kadambi PV, et al. Nephron segment localization of polyoma virus large T antigen in renal allografts. *Hum Pathol* 2006;37(11):1400–1406.
98. Celik B, Randhawa PS. Glomerular changes in BK virus nephropathy. *Hum Pathol* 2004;35(3):367–370.
99. Masutani K, Shapiro R, Basu A, et al. The Banff 2009 Working Proposal for polyomavirus nephropathy: a critical evaluation of its utility as a determinant of clinical outcome. *Am J Transplant* 2012;12(4):907–918.
100. Smith JM, Nemeth TL, McDonald RA. Current immunosuppressive agents: efficacy, side effects, and utilization. *Pediatr Clin North Am* 2003;50(6):1283–1300.
101. Lieberthal W, Fuhro R, Andry CC, et al. Rapamycin impairs recovery from acute renal failure: role of cell-cycle arrest and apoptosis of tubular cells. *Am J Physiol Renal Physiol* 2001;281(4):F693–F706.
102. Pelletier R, Nadasdy T, Nadasdy G, et al. Acute renal failure following kidney transplantation associated with myoglobinuria in patients treated with rapamycin. *Transplantation* 2006;82(5):645–650.
103. Seikaly MG. Recurrence of primary disease in children after renal transplantation: an evidence-based update. *Pediatr Transplant* 2004;8(2):113–119.
104. Ponticelli C, Traversi L, Banfi G. Renal transplantation in patients with IgA mesangial glomerulonephritis. *Pediatr Transplant* 2004;8(4):334–338.
105. Laine J, Jalanko H, Holthofer H, et al. Post-transplantation nephrosis in congenital nephrotic syndrome of the Finnish type. *Kidney Int* 1993;44(4):867–874.
106. Kashtan CE. Renal transplantation in patients with Alport syndrome. *Pediatr Transplant* 2006;10(6):651–657.
107. Bereket G, Fine RN. Pediatric renal transplantation. *Pediatr Clin North Am* 1995;42(6):1603–1628.
108. *2012 Annual Report of the U.S. Organ Procurement and Transplantation Network and Scientific Registry of Transplant Recipients: Transplant Data 2002–2012*. Rockville, MD; Richmond, VA; Ann Arbor, MI: Department of Health and Human Services, Health Resources and Services Administration, Healthcare Systems Bureau, Division of Transplantation; United Network for Organ Sharing; University Renal Research and Education Association.
109. Trpkov K, Marcussen N, Rayner D, et al. Kidney allograft with a lymphocytic infiltrate: acute rejection, posttransplantation lymphoproliferative disorder, neither, or both entities? *Am J Kidney Dis* 1997;30(3):449–454.
110. Dipchand AI, Kirk R, Edwards LB, et al; International Society for Heart and Lung Transplantation. The Registry of the International Society for Heart and Lung Transplantation: sixteenth official pediatric heart transplantation report—2013; focus theme: age. *J Heart Lung Transplant* 2013;32(10):979–988. doi: 10.1016/j.healun.2013.08.005. PubMed PMID: 24054806.
111. Tan CD, Baldwin WM III, Rodriguez ER. Update on cardiac transplantation pathology. *Arch Pathol Lab Med* 2007;131(8):1169–1191.
112. Stewart S, Winters GL, Fishbein MC, et al. Revision of the 1990 working formulation for the standardization of nomenclature in the diagnosis of heart rejection. *J Heart Lung Transplant* 2005;24(11):1710–1720.
113. Everitt MD, Hammond ME, Snow GL, et al. Biopsy-diagnosed antibody-mediated rejection based on the proposed International Society for Heart and Lung Transplantation working formulation is associated with adverse cardiovascular outcomes after pediatric heart transplant. *J Heart Lung Transplant* 2012;31(7):686–693. doi: 10.1016/j.healun.2012.03.009. Epub 2012 May 1, PubMed PMID: 22551931.
114. Fedson SE, Daniel SS, Husain AN. Immunohistochemistry staining of C4d to diagnose antibody-mediated rejection in cardiac transplantation. *J Heart Lung Transplant* 2008;27(4):372–379.
115. Berry GJ, Burke MM, Andersen C, et al. The 2013 International Society for Heart and Lung Transplantation Working Formulation for the standardization of nomenclature in the pathologic diagnosis of antibody-mediated rejection in heart transplantation. *J Heart Lung Transplant* 2013;32(12):1147–1162. doi: 10.1016/j.healun.2013.08.011. PubMed PMID: 24263017.

116. Boucek MM, Aurora P, Edwards LB, et al. Registry of the International Society for Heart and Lung Transplantation: tenth official pediatric heart transplantation report—2007. *J Heart Lung Transplant* 2007;26(8):796–807.
117. Sattar HA, Husain AN, Kim AY, et al. The presence of a CD21+ follicular dendritic cell network distinguishes invasive Quilty lesions from cardiac acute cellular rejection. *Am J Surg Pathol* 2006;30(8):1008–1013.
118. Benden C, Edwards LB, Kucheryavaya AY, et al.; International Society for Heart and Lung Transplantation. The Registry of the International Society for Heart and Lung Transplantation: sixteenth official pediatric lung and heart-lung transplantation report—2013; focus theme: age. *J Heart Lung Transplant* 2013;32(10):989–997. doi: 10.1016/j.healun.2013.08.008. PubMed PMID: 24054807.
119. Meyers BF, de la Morena M, Sweet SC, et al. Primary graft dysfunction and other selected complications of lung transplantation: a single-center experience of 983 patients. *J Thorac Cardiovasc Surg* 2005;129(6):1421–1429.
120. Stewart S, Fishbein MC, Snell GI, et al. Revision of the 1996 working formulation for the standardization of nomenclature in the diagnosis of lung rejection. *J Heart Lung Transplant* 2007;26(12):1229–1242.
121. Camargo JJP, Camargo SM, Schio SM, et al. Hyperacute rejection after single lung transplantation: a case report. *Transplant Proc* 2008;40(3):867–869.
122. Witt CA, Gaut JP, Yusen RD, et al. Acute antibody-mediated rejection after lung transplantation. *J Heart Lung Transplant* 2013;32(10):1034–1040. doi: 10.1016/j.healun.2013.07.004. Epub 2013 Aug 13. PubMed PMID: 23953920; PubMed Central PMCID: PMC 3822761.
123. Husain AN. Transplantation related lung pathology (Chapter 24). In: Zander DS, Farver C, eds. *Pulmonary Pathology*. Philadelphia, PA: Elsevier; 2008.
124. Rosen JB, Smith EO, Schecter MG, et al. Decline in 25% to 75% forced expiratory flow as an early predictor of chronic airway rejection in pediatric lung transplant recipients. *J Heart Lung Transplant* 2012;31(12):1288–1292. doi: 10.1016/j.healun.2012.09.010. Epub 2012 Oct 25. PubMed PMID: 23102913.
125. Haddad IY. Stem cell transplantation and lung dysfunction. *Curr Opin Pediatr* 2013;25(3):350–356. doi: 10.1097/MOP.0b013e328360c317. Review. PubMed PMID: 23652684.

SECTION II
Organ System Pathology

CHAPTER 9
The Placenta

Raymond W. Redline, M.D.

INTRODUCTION

Perinatal pathology, the subdiscipline of pediatric pathology devoted to the study of abnormal pregnancy outcomes, is a dynamic specialty interfacing with obstetrician–gynecologists, neonatologists, and clinical geneticists. A central tenet of this field is that analysis of adverse pregnancy outcome begins with study of the placenta and its adnexa. The fetus is entirely dependent on the placenta for sustenance and protection throughout gestation. Indeed, the placenta has been called a "diary of intrauterine life." Artificial barriers are often placed between the study of so-called products of conception resulting from early pregnancy loss and placentas submitted to pathology following complications of later pregnancy. Such a separation has no anatomic or functional basis and has probably hindered a complete and holistic understanding of the underlying biologic factors responsible for adverse outcomes in couples with sporadic or recurrent pregnancy loss. The first part of this chapter briefly summarizes key stages of placental development as a basis for understanding the problems of the first and early second trimester. The second part will outline the structure of the mature placenta to provide an anatomic framework for disease processes occurring in the late second and third trimester of pregnancy.

EARLY PREGNANCY

Development

The fertilized zygote undergoes a series of cleavage divisions to form a solid 16 cell morula by 5 days following ovulation (1). Between 5 and 8 days, a number of important events occur; the loose aggregate of cells become compacted, cells at the periphery develop tight junctions and begin transporting fluid into the center of the morula (blastocyst formation), and the surrounding zona pellucida is shed as the blastocyst attaches to, crosses, and invades the endometrium (Figure 9-1). The formation of tight cell–cell junctions at the periphery of the blastocyst marks the emergence of the trophectoderm lineage (trophoblast), which is the principal component of the placenta. Transport of fluid into the blastocyst and invasion of the gestational endometrium (decidua) foreshadow the two most important functions of trophoblast throughout gestation: transport of maternal substrates to the fetus and tissue remodeling of the uterus to ensure adequate delivery of these substrates. Cells within the blastocyst (inner cell mass) separate into two lineages: epiblast, which gives rise to the epithelium surrounding the amnionic cavity (day 8) and the embryonic germ layers (days 15 to 28), and hypoblast, which forms the connective tissue of the placenta (extraembryonic mesoderm) and the primary yolk sac.

Development of the maternal and fetal placental circulations occurs in parallel. The maternal circulation begins when uterine capillaries are eroded by the outer layer of primitive syncytial trophoblasts at the periphery of the blastocyst allowing blood to flow into lacunar spaces that form within the trophoblast. These lacunae gradually enlarge to form the intervillous space. Trophoblasts also migrate against flow into the arterial circulation forming cellular plugs that limit perfusion of the intervillous space (Figure 9-2A) (2). During this period, the walls of the spiral arteries are remodeled in a series of events that includes dissolution of the muscular media, dilatation of the lumen, and reconstitution of the vessel wall by extracellular matrix; all mediated by trophoblasts within the vessel lumen. By the time the trophoblastic plugs disappear at approximately 10 weeks of gestation, the structural integrity of the developing placenta is sufficient to withstand the high

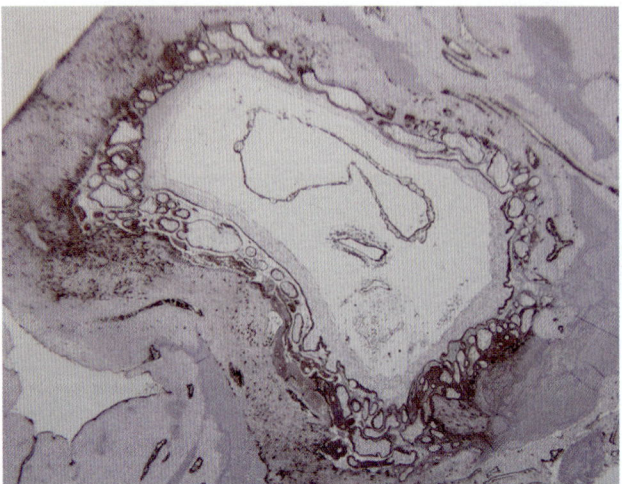

FIGURE 9-1 • Early implanting gestational sac (cytokeratin stain): portions of embryo and unattached amnionic sac are surrounded by circumferential primary villi anchored in the peripheral cytotrophoblast shell with early intermediate trophoblasts infiltrating the adjacent endometrium.

oxygen tension and pressures of arterial blood flow. Extension of the remodeling process to the deeper arteries in the inner third of the myometrium occurs between 10 and 18 weeks of pregnancy. During this period and beyond, the placenta also expands laterally by attachment to and cooptation of large veins at its margins (so-called marginal sinus formation) (3). By the end of pregnancy, approximately 80 and 100 spiral arteries open into the intervillous space.

The fetal circulation of the placenta develops in two phases (4). Extraembryonic mesoderm migrates out into the trophectoderm between the lacunar spaces to form so-called "primary villi." A villous capillary plexus then develops within the extraembryonic mesoderm via local inductive interactions with trophoblasts (Figure 9-2B). This plexus eventually becomes connected to the embryonic circulation via anastomoses with large vessels growing out from the fetus into the extraembryonic connective tissue covering the trophoblastic portion of the placenta (chorionic plate). These fetal vessels reach the placenta via the body stalk, later to become the umbilical cord (UC). Paired arteries within the body stalk develop alongside the allantoic duct, and a vein develops alongside the omphalomesenteric duct. Vascularized extraembryonic mesoderm in the primary villi subsequently expands to form villous trees, largely driven by branching angiogenesis. As these trees increase in complexity and the placenta enlarges, the more proximal fetoplacental vessels develop a muscular media and form stem villous arteries and veins.

The final stage of early placental development is formation of the membranes. The first event occurring at about 9 to 11 weeks of gestation is disappearance of the extraembryonic coelom and primitive yolk sac resulting in attachment of the amnionic sac surrounding the fetus to the chorionic connective tissue covering the trophoblastic portion of the placenta. This is followed at 11 to 17 weeks by the gradual atrophy and collapse of the intervillous space in portions of the placenta away from the implantation site. It has been suggested that higher oxygen tension due to the lack of endovascular trophoblast plugs in arteries away from the implantation site triggers this pattern of peripheral atrophy (5). Finally, at about 17 to 20 weeks, the enlarging gestational sac makes contact with and fuses with the opposite side of the uterus forming the mature multilayered placental membrane composed of vascularized decidua vera, avascular decidua capsularis, chorionic trophoblasts (chorion laeve) and connective tissue, and amnionic connective tissue and epithelium.

Multiple Pregnancies

Background

Twins (and higher-order multiple pregnancies) develop following either fertilization of multiple eggs (dizygotic twins) or fission of a single fertilized egg (monozygotic twins). The incidence of dizygotic twinning is variable in different

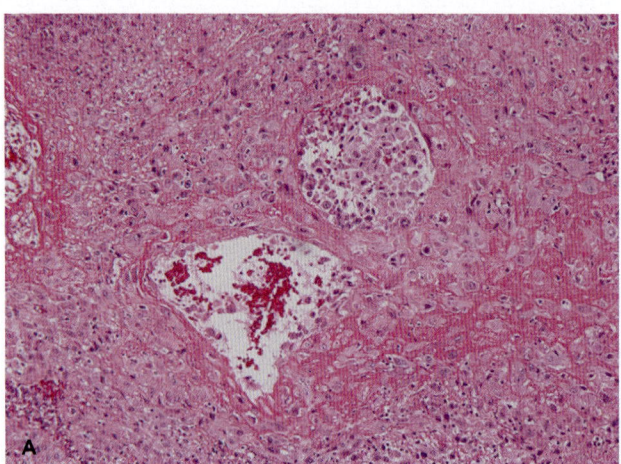 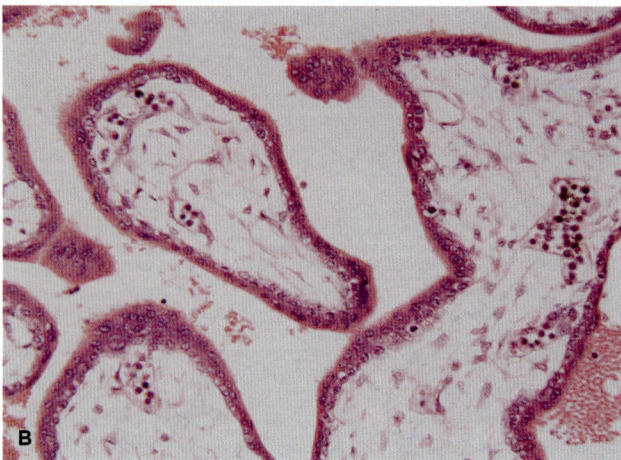

FIGURE 9-2 • Early pregnancy vascular development: **(A)** spiral arteries surrounded by intermediate trophoblasts with luminal plugs of endovascular trophoblasts and remodeling of the vessel wall and **(B)** fetal capillaries arising from pluripotent villous stromal cells induced by villous trophoblasts.

populations and depends on the frequency of polyovulation, either naturally occurring due to higher endogenous FSH levels or induced by drugs used in association with assisted reproductive technology. Monozygotic twinning occurs at a constant rate in most populations and can be associated with a variety of different placental types (Figure 9-3). The classic explanation for the differences in placental morphology in monozygotic twin placentas is temporal: separation prior to blastocyst formation leads to separate placentas (dichorionic diamnionic), separation between blastocyst formation and amniogenesis to a single placenta with separate amnionic sacs (monochorionic diamnionic), and separation after amniogenesis to a single placenta with one amnionic sac (monochorionic monoamnionic). A new theory posits that monozygotic twinning is always an early postfertilization event and that placental monochorionicity and monoamnionicity depend on proximity and fusion of membrane layers rather than embryo splitting (6). This concept is supported by a recent report that on rare occasions dizygotic twins can fuse to form a monochorionic placenta (7). Secondary fusion due to proximity has also been proposed as an explanation for conjoined twins (8).

Essentially, all monochorionic twin placentas have vascular connections. Most are surface anastomoses involving chorionic arteries or veins (artery to artery and vein to vein) that lead to sharing of blood (chimerism) but do not cause circulatory imbalance (9). One unusual exception is when large arteries with closely apposed UC insertion sites are connected. In this situation, an artery from one twin may develop sufficient pressure to reverse the circulatory flow in the second twin (twin reversed arterial perfusion {TRAP} sequence) leading to secondary atrophy of the heart and other rostral structures and resulting in the development of an acardiac fetus (10). A second more common exception occurs during the period when the villous circulation connects with the embryonic circulation. Crossed intertwin connections at that time can lead to shared zones that are perfused by the arterial circulation of one twin and drained by the venous system of the other (deep arteriovenous anastomoses).

Pathology

The main task for the pathologist in multiple pregnancies is to determine the number of chorions and amnions in each placenta, usually by direct inspection followed by confirmatory histologic sections from the dividing membrane. This examination is not required when the placental discs are completely separate. If a single placenta is noted and the dividing membrane is opaque, then two amnions flanking a fused central chorion is most likely (dichorionic diamnionic placentas). This is confirmed at gross examination by peeling the three layers, and the placentas should be separated for weighing and further examination. If the dividing membrane is translucent, only two amnions are most likely (monochorionic diamnionic placenta). The chorionic layer is absent because it surrounds, but does not divide, the two fetal sacs. This anatomy can again be confirmed by peeling only two layers. A monochorionic placenta is, as the name suggests, a single organ that should be weighed without further separation. Inspection of the chorionic plate for surface anastomoses should then be performed followed by injection studies to look for deep arteriovenous anastomoses. Air injection studies are a quick and easy method for demonstrating clinically significant connections (1). More complete injection studies using colored or radio-opaque dyes are usually only conducted in a research context. Discordant twin growth, usually defined as a greater than 25% difference in body weights, is a significant complication of both dichorionic and monochorionic gestations. Pathologic lesions other than transfusion syndrome (see below) that are significantly associated with discordant growth include peripheral cord insertion, avascular villi, and indicators of maternal vascular malperfusion (11,12).

Clinical Correlation

Twin gestations of all types are at increased risk for premature delivery, intrauterine growth restriction (IUGR), preeclampsia, and cerebral palsy. Many of these complications are more frequent in the smaller and/or the nonpresenting (second) twin. Twin-to-twin transfusion syndrome (TTTS),

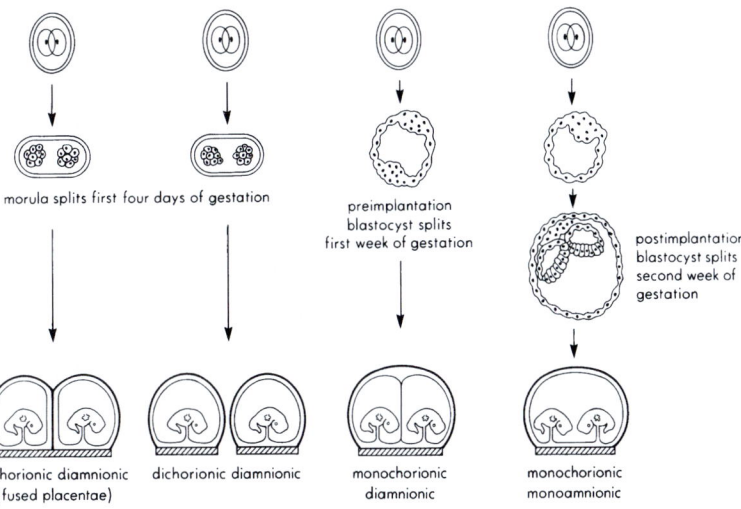

FIGURE 9-3 • Diagrammatic representation of placentation in monochorionic twinning. (From Gersell DJ, Kraus FT. Diseases of the placenta. In: Kurman RJ, ed. *Blausteins Pathology of the Female Genital Tract*. New York: Springer Verlag, 1998:986, with permission.)

affecting monochorionic twins, is a specific form of discordant twin growth caused by large deep arteriovenous anastomoses without accompanying superficial arterial anastomoses (9). TTTS is characterized by growth restriction and oligohydramnios in the donor twin and macrosomia, congestive heart failure, and polyhydramnios in the recipient. Twin anemia polycythemia sequence (TAPS) is another clinical syndrome characterized by differences in hemoglobin concentrations in twins developing secondary to chronic net transfusion across smaller arteriovenous anastomoses. Finally, acute antenatal or intrapartum transfusion occurs when previously balanced anastomoses become unbalanced due to changes in fetal blood pressures or secondary occlusion of bridging fetal vessels. The most dramatic example of acute transfusion occurs after fetal demise of one twin. In this case, sudden shifts of blood from the survivor to the decedent result in a very high risk of perinatal brain damage.

Gestational Trophoblastic Disease
Background

Trophoblast may be separated into two major subtypes, villous and extravillous (13). Neoplasia involving villous trophoblast leads to choriocarcinoma while that of extravillous trophoblasts results in either placental site trophoblastic tumor (PSTT) or epithelioid trophoblastic tumor (ETT) (14). More than half of choriocarcinomas are preceded by molar pregnancies (complete or partial hydatidiform moles). All molar pregnancies have an overrepresentation of paternal chromosomes. Complete moles form after fertilization of an empty ovum and contain only paternal chromosomes while partial moles usually follow double fertilization of a single egg and thus have a 2:1 ratio of paternal to maternal chromosomes. Studies in mice have shown that trophoblast proliferation is largely driven by growth-promoting factors that are transcribed exclusively from paternally inherited genes while antiproliferative genes are often expressed only from maternal alleles (15). An increased frequency of molar pregnancies explains the increased incidence of choriocarcinoma in Asian populations. Although occasionally developing after molar pregnancy, PSTT and ETT most commonly follow term pregnancies, often years after delivery. It is well documented that some extravillous trophoblast is left behind after delivery and can persist for many years. Although not proven, these persistent rests of trophoblasts, known as placental site nodules, might be precursors for these rare tumors.

Pathology

Molar pregnancies are characterized by villous edema and trophoblastic hyperplasia (16). Edema is often extreme leading to cavitation of the villous stroma. In complete moles, the edema and hyperplasia affect the entire conceptus while in partial moles, they affect only a subgroup of villi (Figure 9-4A). Partial moles also show irregularly shaped

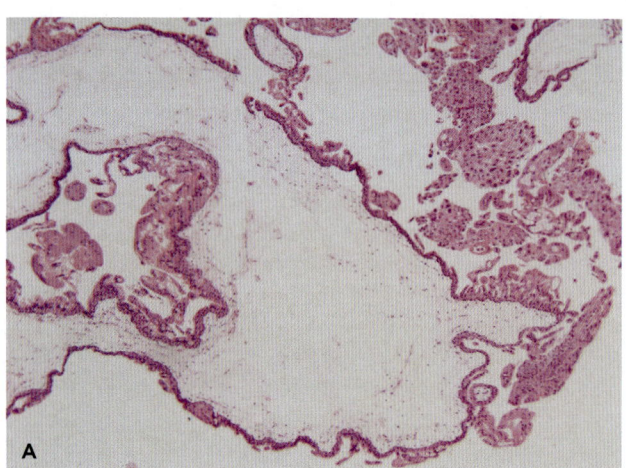
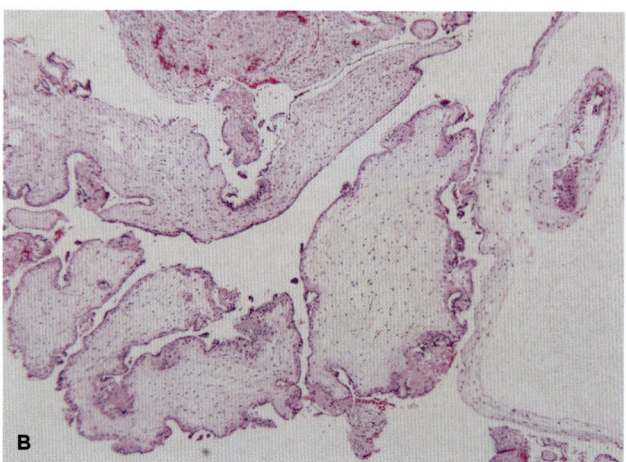
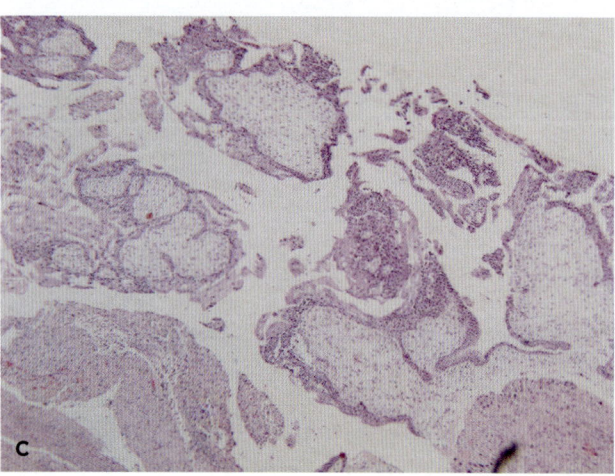

FIGURE 9-4 • Molar pregnancy: **(A)** complete hydatidiform mole—uniformly hydropic villi with central cisterns and circumferential trophoblastic hyperplasia, **(B)** partial hydatidiform mole—molar villi (*left*) and irregularly shaped fibrotic villi (*right*) showing mild circumferential syncytiotrophoblast hyperplasia, and **(C)** early complete hydatidiform mole—bulbous villous branching, densely cellular myxoid stroma, and trophoblastic hyperplasia.

dysmorphic villi (Figure 9-4B). The classic complete mole is easily diagnosed based on clusters of fluid-filled vesicles (hydatidiform or "grape-like" change) and marked trophoblastic hyperplasia. However, with the current use of early ultrasound approximately one-third of complete moles are evacuated at a stage before the development of edema or diffuse trophoblastic hyperplasia. These early complete moles can be difficult to recognize but manifest a number of helpful diagnostic features including a cauliflower-like growth pattern, densely cellular myxoid villous stroma, focal trophoblastic hyperplasia, and atypia of implantation site trophoblasts (Figure 9-4C). Occasionally, early pregnancy specimens show nonspecific trophoblastic hyperplasia in the absence of molar villi. Cytogenetic study of these specimens has shown a high prevalence of the two relatively uncommon karyotypes, trisomies 7 and 15 (17). Whether these cases have an increased risk of later choriocarcinoma is not known.

Choriocarcinomas often present with large areas of uterine hemorrhage and necrosis. The cellular areas show a typical pattern characterized by clusters of 10 to 50 mononuclear cytotrophoblasts surrounded by a wreath-like garland of syncytial trophoblasts (Figure 9-5A). The mononuclear cytotrophoblastic cells show mild-to-moderate nuclear atypia with prominent nucleoli and a watery clear cytoplasm. The multinucleate syncytial trophoblastic cells have enlarged hyperchromatic nuclei and a deeply eosinophilic-purple cytoplasm. Syncytial trophoblasts stains intensely for human chorionic gonadotropin (hCG), human placental lactogen (hPL), and inhibin, while the cytotrophoblasts lacks these hormones but expresses p63. Both cell types are cytokeratin positive (13,14).

PSTT is derived from mature extravillous trophoblasts and are characterized by large mononuclear cells with significant nuclear atypia and abundant intensely eosinophilic cytoplasm (Figure 9-5B). Binucleation is occasionally seen, but larger numbers of nuclei, as seen in syncytial trophoblasts, are rare. Unlike normal intermediate trophoblasts, tumor cells invade in large cohesive sheets and are associated with tissue necrosis. Tumor cells stain positively for cytokeratin, inhibin, and hPL, but are only weakly or focally positive for hCG and p63 (13,14).

ETT are derived from so-called transitional extravillous trophoblasts and are composed of nests of vacuolated or eosinophilic cells often in a hyaline matrix, bearing a striking resemblance by both light microscopy and immunostaining to the cells of the membranous chorion laeve (Figure 9-5C). They tend to grow in a nodular expansile pattern in the lower uterine segment or cervix where they can mimic squamous carcinomas. Their immunohistochemical profile includes diffuse expression of cytokeratin and p63 plus focal/variable expression of inhibin, hCG, and hPL (13,14).

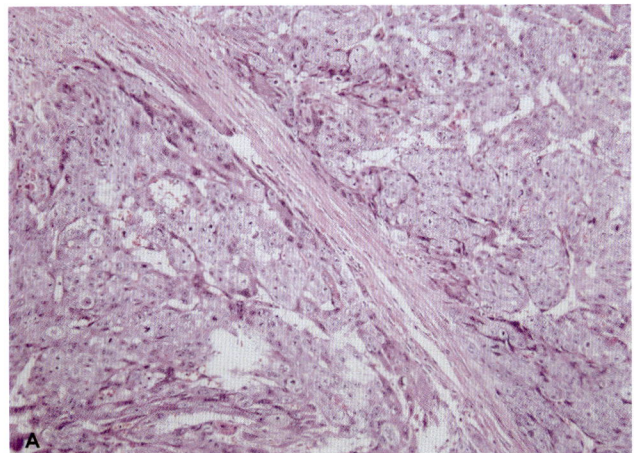
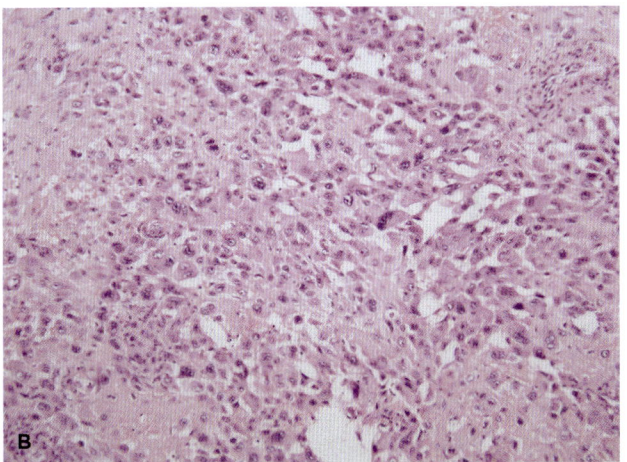
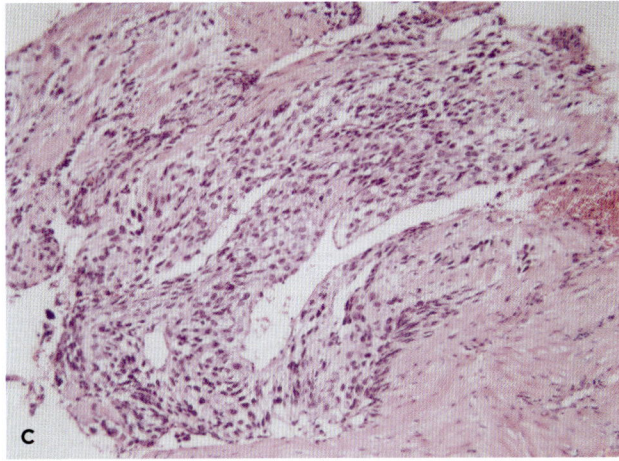

FIGURE 9-5 • Trophoblastic tumors: **(A)** choriocarcinoma—clusters of mononuclear cytotrophoblasts surrounded by a wreath-like garland of poorly differentiated syncytial trophoblasts, **(B)** placental site trophoblastic tumor—loosely cohesive sheets of atypical intermediate trophoblasts with strongly eosinophilic cytoplasm, and **(C)** epithelioid trophoblastic tumor—sheets of vacuolated extravillous trophoblast invading myometrium.

Clinical Correlation

All preneoplastic and neoplastic lesions of trophoblasts are combined under the rubric gestational trophoblastic disease. While molar pregnancies are usually confirmed by tissue diagnosis, postmolar choriocarcinomas are often managed based solely on serum monitoring of the tumor marker, hCG, and radiographic imaging. Persistence or elevation of hCG levels after evacuation of a molar pregnancy is treated empirically with single agent chemotherapy. Tumors with extremely high hCG levels or metastasis to organs other than the lung are treated with multiple agent chemotherapy. Bulky uterine disease may necessitate hysterectomy. PSTT and ETT usually present with vaginal bleeding. Curettage is suspicious for a neoplasm, and hCG levels are usually positive, but often at low levels. Radiographic studies confirm a mass lesion, and hysterectomy is performed. Unlike choriocarcinoma, PSTT and ETT are relatively indolent and only rarely metastasize. However, they respond poorly to chemotherapy, so local control is paramount. Clinical management of early pregnancy specimens suspicious for, but not diagnostic of, gestational trophoblastic disease (avillous trophoblasts or villi with nonspecific trophoblastic hyperplasia) should include at least one follow-up hCG titer to ensure return to baseline.

Missed Abortion/Anembryonic Pregnancy

Background

The term missed abortion refers to a pregnancy in which a nonviable chorionic sac is retained in the uterus requiring curettage for evacuation. Early gestational sacs lacking sonographic and/or histologic evidence of embryonic development (anembryonic pregnancy) are most common. A large percentage of such specimens have embryonic lethal chromosomal abnormalities (18). Chromosomally normal anembryonic pregnancies probably represent major disruptions of early embryogenesis due to teratogens, sporadic mutations in major developmental genes, or random errors in morphogenesis (see chapter 3).

Pathology

Anembryonic pregnancies show a typical histopathologic profile. Typical features include a relatively thin chorionic membrane, and uniformly edematous (hydropic) villi (Figure 9-6A). Amnion, yolk sac, UC, and embryonic tissue are usually absent, and no fetal blood vessels are apparent. The uniformly hydropic nature of the villi is caused by continuing trophoblast transport of fluid into villi without egress to a fetal circulation. With prolonged retention, the hydropic villi may undergo secondary fibrosis (hyalinization). Gestational endometrium and implantation site in these cases usually lack hemorrhagic/ischemic degeneration or other abnormalities.

Clinical Correlation

The management of women with early pregnancy losses, particularly when recurrent, is highly dependent on the nature of the loss. A careful pathologic examination can often guide clinical management in cases where cytogenetic analysis either has not been obtained or is unsuccessful (18). Recognition of anembryonic gestation (sometimes referred to as "blighted ovum" or hydropic abortus) by early ultrasound or pathologic examination is clinically useful in that it identifies a cohort with a high rate of aneuploidy and hence a low recurrence rate. Early and late missed abortions with normally vascularized villi, thromboinflammatory lesions, or endometrial pathology are much more likely to recur in subsequent pregnancies.

Miscarriages (Threatened, Incomplete, and Complete Abortions)

Background

The term miscarriage refers to an early pregnancy in varying stages of being spontaneously expelled from the mother (threatened, incomplete, and complete abortions). Many occur following previous fetal demise. These cases represent a heterogenous mixture of chromosomally normal and abnormal gestations, some with fetal malformations, deformations, or disruptions. An uncommon, but clinically important, subgroup is miscarriage with evidence of an underlying thromboinflammatory process. These processes are more frequent in patients with recurrent miscarriages and may represent aberrant maternal responses to pregnancy (18). One specific maternal condition, antiphospholipid antibody syndrome, has been associated with vascular thrombosis, hemorrhage, and complement-mediated damage to maternal endothelial cells and/or trophoblasts.

Pathology

The most common phenotype in spontaneous miscarriage is a well-developed chorionic sac with an adherent amnion, hyalinized villi with partially involuted fetal vasculature, and a combination of hemorrhage and necrosis in the implantation site and gestational endometrium (Figure 9-6B). Another common subtype contains a normally formed, viable or recently deceased embryo or fetus plus a large amount of fresh intervillous hemorrhage (so-called Breus mole). In addition to intervillous hemorrhage, these specimens show normally vascularized chorionic villi with early stromal–vascular karyorrhexis and, in some cases, thrombosis or congestion of spiral arteries with an absence of endovascular trophoblastic plugs (Figure 9-6C, D). Specimens with evidence for a thromboinflammatory process are much less common. Three variants have been described: (a) maternal floor infarction/massive perivillous fibrin deposition (discussed later), (b) chronic histiocytic intervillositis, characterized by extensive infiltration of the intervillous space by a

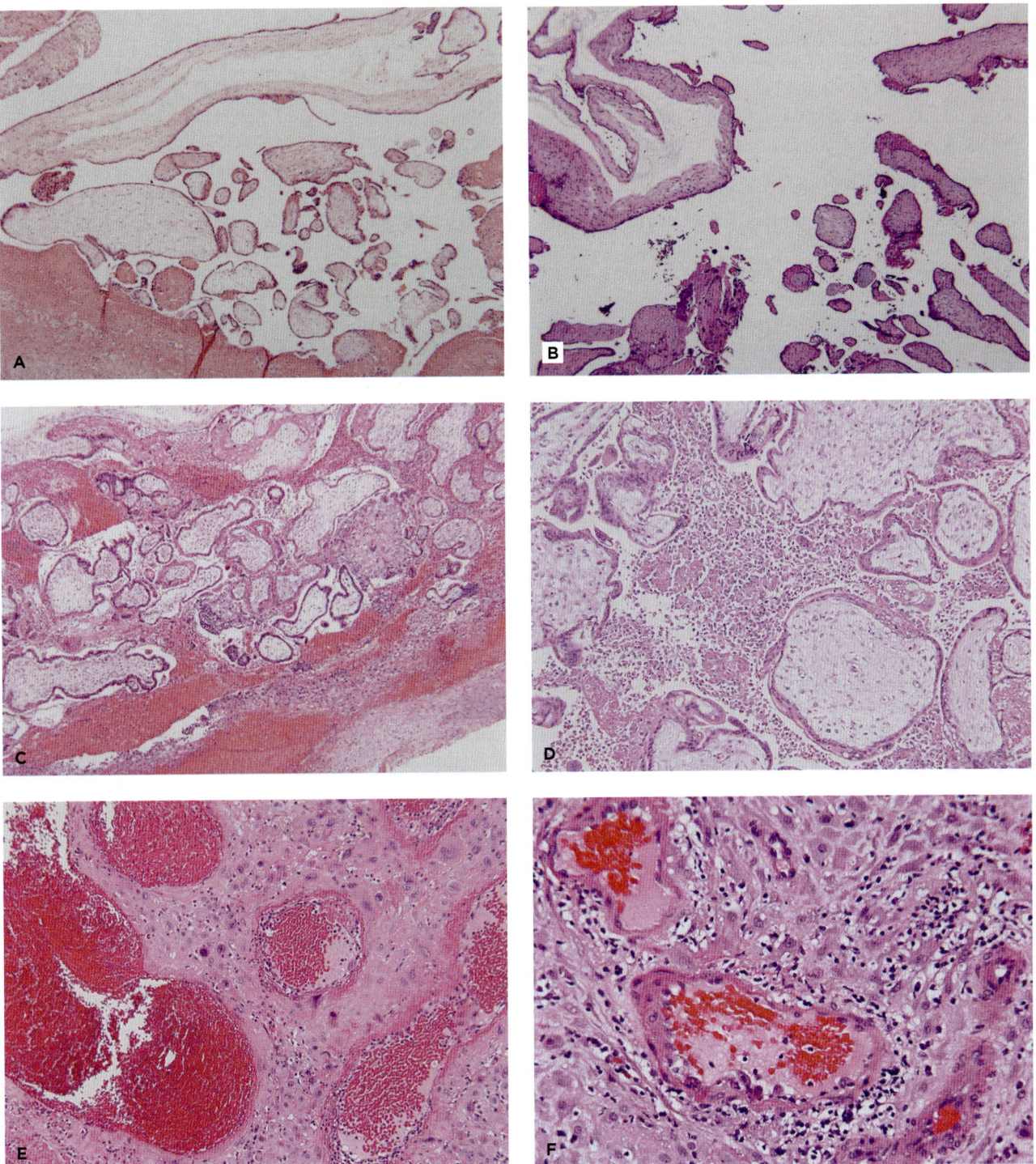

FIGURE 9-6 • Early pregnancy losses: **(A)** anembryonic pregnancy—uniformly hydropic villi adjacent to chorion without an adherent amnion, **(B)** hyalinized villi with adjacent fused chorioamnion, consistent with remote fetal death, **(C)** Breus mole—well-preserved villi with marked intervillous hemorrhage, **(D)** pathologic congested spiral arteries lacking endovascular trophoblastic plugs, **(E)** chronic histiocytic intervillositis—early chorionic villi surrounded by sheets of immature monocyte–macrophages **(F)** spiral arterioles with marked chronic perivasculitis in maternal autoimmune disease.

monomorphic infiltrate of monocyte–macrophages (Figure 9-6E), and (c) decidual arteriopathy, often accompanying antiphospholipid syndrome or other autoimmune diseases, and characterized by vasculitis, mural hypertrophy, perivascular decidual fibrin deposition, and/or plasma cell infiltration (Figure 9-6F) (18,19).

Clinical Correlation

Patients with recurrent, chromosomally normal miscarriages, particularly in association with thromboinflammatory lesions and/or the antiphospholipid antibody syndrome, are often treated with low-dose heparin and/or aspirin. Less commonly, more aggressive anticoagulation, intravenous gamma globulin, or corticosteroids have been utilized. Previous therapeutic options that have largely been abandoned include other types of immunosuppressive drugs, diethyl stilbestrol, progesterone, and immunization with paternal leukocytes.

Congenital Infections

Background

Although ascending infections involving organisms from the cervicovaginal tract do occur in the first half of pregnancy (discussed later), the majority of early infections are acquired hematogenously (1,20). Most occur after primary maternal infections, since previous exposure generally elicits protective antibodies. Organisms infecting both placenta and fetus include spirochetes (*Treponema pallidum*), parasites (*Toxoplasma gondii, Trypanosoma cruzi*), and viruses (cytomegalovirus, varicella zoster virus, herpes simplex virus, rubella virus, poxviruses). Those that usually infect only the placenta include *Plasmodium falciparum, Borrelia burgdorferi*, and *Schistosoma hematobium*. Other organisms cross the placenta to infect the fetus without eliciting placental inflammation including Parvovirus B19, HIV, hepatitis B, and the enteroviruses. The majority of congenital infections begin in the second trimester. First-trimester infections are less common, but more severe, and those occurring in the earliest stages of pregnancy often spare the products of conception entirely.

Pathology

Organisms restricted to the placenta usually involve either the decidua or the intervillous space. Histologic findings include local accumulations of fibrin and a mixed acute and chronic inflammatory infiltrate. Infections involving both fetus and placenta generally cause a diffuse placentitis with chronic inflammation of the chorion, decidua, and villous stroma. Two overlapping patterns are seen. The first, characterized by edematous villi with increased Hofbauer cells, is typical of syphilis (Figure 9-7A). The second, characterized by fibrotic villi with evidence of remote hemorrhage and villous plasma cells, is typical of CMV (Figure 9-7B). Some infections have unique features allowing a specific histopathologic diagnosis. These include the presence of organisms or viral inclusions in the villous stroma (CMV, herpes simplex virus, varicella zoster virus, *T. cruzi*), UC (*T. pallidum, T. gondii*), or intervillous space (*P. falciparum, S. hematobium*).

Clinical Correlation

A common clinical mnemonic for congenital infection is the acronym TORCH, standing for Toxoplasma, Other agents, Rubella virus, Cytomegalovirus, and Herpes simplex virus. In the United States, CMV and syphilis account for more than 90% of cases. Infants with any TORCH infection share common features including IUGR, pancytopenia, hepatosplenomegaly, and coagulopathy. Each infection also has specific features, a description of which is beyond the scope of this chapter. A standard serologic screen known as the "TORCH titer" tests for maternal IgG specific for the common TORCH agents and is part of the routine workup for IUGR or suspected antenatal maternal infection. Specific testing for IgM is required to distinguish recent from remote infection. Many infections are diagnosed by PCR testing of fetal blood or amniotic fluid obtained by amniocentesis.

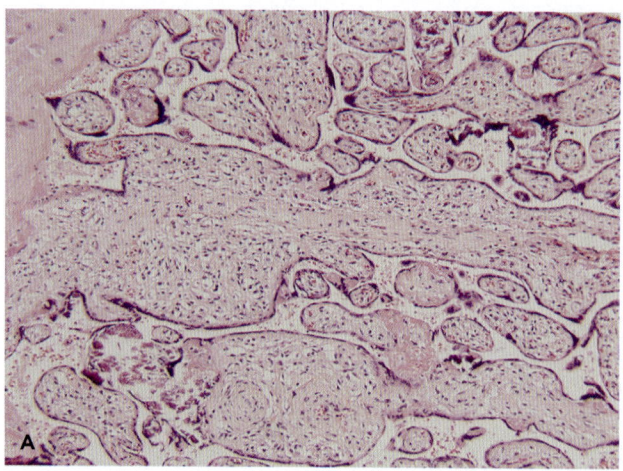 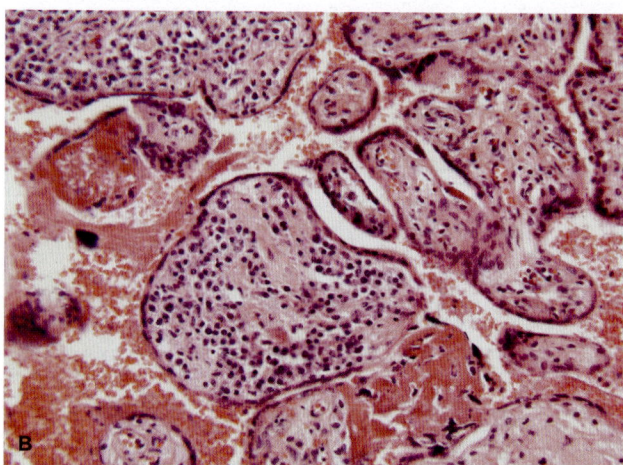

FIGURE 9-7 • TORCH infections: **(A)** syphilis—histiocytic villitis with villous edema and **(B)** CMV-plasma cell villitis with villous fibrosis.

LATE PREGNANCY

Anatomy

The mature placenta is composed of four distinct compartments of structure–function:

1. Fetoplacental vasculature: UC, chorionic plate and vascularized villous stroma
2. Interhemal membrane: villous trophoblasts and adjacent maternal intervillous space
3. Basal plate: anchoring villi, decidua, and underlying maternal uterine vasculature
4. Placental membranes: amnion, chorion, and adjacent maternal decidua.

The fetoplacental vasculature begins at the UC, a squamous epithelial-covered conduit usually measuring between 40 and 70 cm in length at term that conducts fetal blood from the umbilicus to some location on the chorionic plate (or occasionally the adjacent placental membranes). The UC contains paired arteries that spiral around a central vein; all surrounded by a hyaluronate-rich matrix (Wharton jelly), which provides considerable protection from external compression. The two arteries are connected at or just before their insertion site into the chorionic plate by an anastomosis (Hyrtl's anastomosis). The chorionic plate (also known as the fetal surface) is composed of fibroconnective tissue supporting large muscular arteries and veins that distribute fetal blood flow from the UC to a family of 20 and 30 large villous trees (4). These villous trees protrude from the underside of the chorionic plate, branch several times, and conduct fetal blood through a succession of ever smaller arteries and veins, terminating in capillaries that interface with the trophoblastic interhemal membrane. The larger (proximal) villi are separated into stem and intermediate villi with the latter representing the arteriolar level at which blood flow into the gas exchanging terminal (distal) villi is regulated. Maturation of the villous tree with advancing gestational age in the third trimester is characterized by an increase in the number of distal relative to proximal villi, decreased distal villous connective tissue, peripheralization of villous capillaries, and the formation of specialized vasculosyncytial membranes that optimize gas exchange. There is, however, considerable regional variation in maturity such that well-perfused villi overlying the opening of the maternal spiral artery at the center of a cotyledon may appear considerably less mature than those at the "watershed" between spiral arteries at the periphery of the cotyledon (Figure 9-8A, B). The two critical anatomic features to be maintained in this compartment are patency of large proximal villous vessels and a short diffusion distance between fetal capillaries and distal villous trophoblasts.

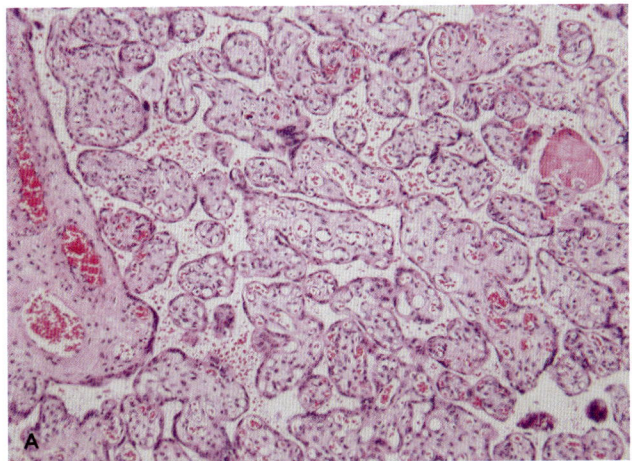
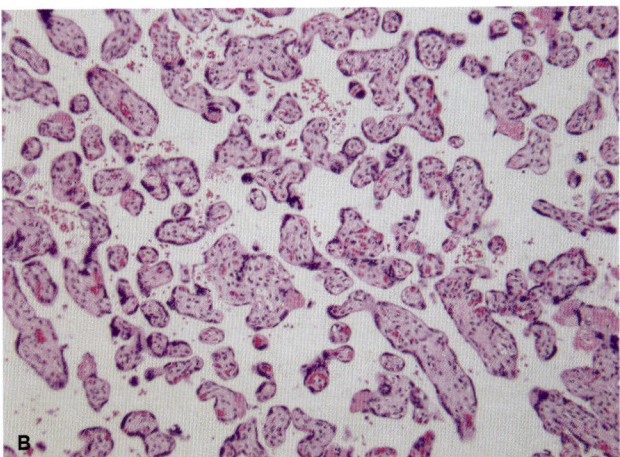
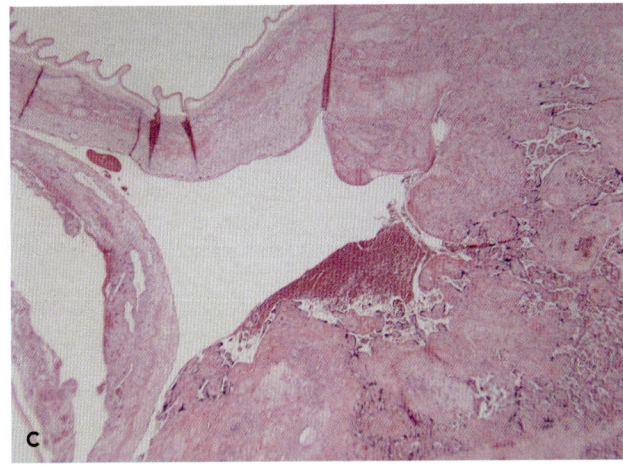

FIGURE 9-8 • Normal placental anatomy at term: **(A)** central lobule—distal villi are enlarged with abundant stroma, numerous capillaries, and uniform layer of villous trophoblasts, **(B)** peripheral lobule—distal villi are much smaller with scant peripheral capillaries and prominent syncytial knots, and **(C)** margin/membrane—peripheral villi extend into a large venous space within the basal plate that is covered by fused amniochorion and decidua.

The interhemal membrane consists of multinucleate syncytiotrophoblastic cells, a few scattered, basally located cytotrophoblastic stem cells, and an underlying basement membrane. Each cytotrophoblastic stem cell is the progenitor for 80 to 100 differentiated syncytiotrophoblastic cells that fuse into large syncytial sheets forming a mosaic covering the entire villous tree (21). Turnover of syncytiotrophoblasts occur via clustering of nuclei into syncytial knots that are later shed into the maternal circulation (22). Critical features at the interhemal membrane are cellular viability; appropriate maturation in terms of endocrine, transport, anticoagulant, and immunoprotective function; and accessibility to maternal blood flow—meaning absence of adherent fibrin or inflammatory exudate in the intervillous space.

The basal plate consists of so-called anchoring villi embedded in maternal endometrium, ectatic maternal spiral arteries, and tangentially oriented maternal veins. Extravillous trophoblasts, differentiating from villous cytotrophoblastic stem cells on the underside of the anchoring villi diffusely, infiltrate the maternal endometrium and elaborate large amounts of a fibronectin-rich extracellular matrix forming the Nitabuch layer, which provides structural integrity and unites the diverse components of the basal plate into a coherent anatomic structure. Basal plate arteries normally lack a smooth muscle layer, having been remodeled by endovascular extravillous trophoblasts. Adequate arterial remodeling is a critical feature of mature placentas allowing adequate blood flow into the intervillous space. Lateral villous trees grow into maternal veins at the periphery of the placenta resulting in the formation of large sinusoidally dilated veins that surround the disc (Figure 9-8C) (3). These structures were previously misinterpreted as a continuous marginal venous sinus.

The placental membranes appear to be a distinct structure, but this appearance is deceptive. Membranes form by secondary involution of early placental tissue not included in the final placental disc, and their basic anatomic architecture is the same. The amnion and chorionic connective tissue overly a trophoblastic region containing scattered involuted chorionic villi. This trophoblast coalesces as the intervillous space is obliterated to form a distinct zone known as the chorion leave, composed largely of transitional extravillous trophoblast) (13). The chorion laeve is supported by the underlying maternal decidua. Critical features in this compartment are maintenance of integrity and contiguity of all layers. In particular, chorionic prostaglandin dehydrogenase in chorion laeve trophoblasts must be functionally active and spatially positioned to inactivate labor-inducing prostaglandins elaborated by the amnion, decidua, and myometrium. Inflammatory or ischemic damage to these cells can result in the premature onset of labor (23).

Chronic Disease Processes

Disease processes affecting the placenta in late pregnancy can be classified in a variety of ways including anatomic location, mechanism of injury, or clinical presentation. One way that is particularly useful for understanding the causal sequence of events leading to adverse pregnancy outcomes is time of onset. The rationale for such a separation is that earlier placental lesions can significantly decrease placental reserve lowering the threshold for fetal injury and resulting in an enhanced effect of comparatively minor stressors at the time of parturition (preconditioning). In the following scheme, the term chronic refers to lesions evolving over weeks, subacute to those evolving over many hours to days, and acute to those evolving over just a few hours.

Maternal Vascular Malperfusion

Background

Chronic maternal vascular malperfusion of the intervillous space can result from a variety of causes including underlying cardiac insufficiency, failure to expand intravascular volume during pregnancy, or abnormalities in uteroplacental arteries. It is currently believed that the major process leading to malperfusion is failure of extravillous trophoblasts to appropriately invade and remodel the uterine spiral arteries. While the exact mechanism remains uncertain, a likely sequence of events appears to be early hypoxia at the implantation site leading to dysregulation of renin–angiotensin, vascular endothelial growth factor, integrin, and tissue protease expression and resulting in impaired trophoblasts differentiation and inadequate tissue invasion (24,25). In the absence of normal arterial remodeling, the placenta is inadequately perfused leading to decreased fetoplacental growth and, in some cases, the release of vasoactive mediators that cause the clinical syndrome known as preeclampsia. Several of these mediators have been identified including soluble VEGF receptor 1 (sflt-1), soluble endoglin, and circulating AT1 receptor antibodies (24,26).

Pathology

Placentas affected by maternal malperfusion generally show two or more of a constellation of pathologic abnormalities (27). Important and sometimes overlooked features include decreased weight for gestational age and decreased placental weight relative to that of the infant (increased fetoplacental weight ratio). These features correlate with impairment of placental growth (distal villous hypoplasia) as the fetus sacrifices placental reserve (estimated at up to 30% of weight) in order to supply critical vascular beds such as the central nervous and cardiovascular systems (Figure 9-9A). Complete obstruction to villous blood flow secondary to spiral artery thrombosis leads to villous infarction (Figure 9-9B). Partial obstruction leads to stasis with intervillous fibrin deposition (Figure 9-9C), hypoxia with accelerated syncytiotrophoblast turnover and increased syncytial knots (Figure 9-9D), and localized ischemia with villous agglutination (Figure 9-9E). This process is now referred to as accelerated villous maturation. A quantitative approach to the diagnosis of increased syncytial knotting has been described (28). Particularly, useful for diagnosis is an alternating pattern of villous crowding with knots, fibrin, and agglutination with intervening areas of villous paucity (hypoplasia) that can easily be recognized at scanning magnification (Figure 9-9F). Three other site-specific abnormalities may also be present: (a) Persistent muscularization of spiral arteries and aggregation of placental site giant cells in the basal plate correlating with superficial implantation. (b) Decidual arteriopathy, either medial hypertrophy (Figure 9-9G) or fibrinoid necrosis (acute atherosis) (Figure 9-9H), linked to either underlying vascular disease or the pregnancy-specific vasoactive mediators discussed above. It is most frequently detected in small arterioles in the placental membranes near the disc margin, and (c) a thin UC (<8 mm diameter) reflecting fetal extracellular volume depletion and decreased hydration of Wharton jelly.

Clinical Correlation

Placental malperfusion is associated with a variety of adverse outcomes including IUGR, spontaneous preterm birth preceded by either premature labor or premature rupture of membranes, and an increased risk for the development of preeclampsia (29,30). Clinical conditions predisposing to malperfusion include essential hypertension, diabetes mellitus, connective tissue disease, chronic renal insufficiency, and underlying maternal coagulopathies including thrombophilic mutations and antiphospholipid syndrome. Many patients have one or more components of the metabolic syndrome, characterized by obesity, abnormal serum lipid levels, enhanced production of acute phase inflammatory mediators, and a predisposition to vascular damage related to oxidative stress. Patients with placental malperfusion and metabolic syndrome are also at risk for

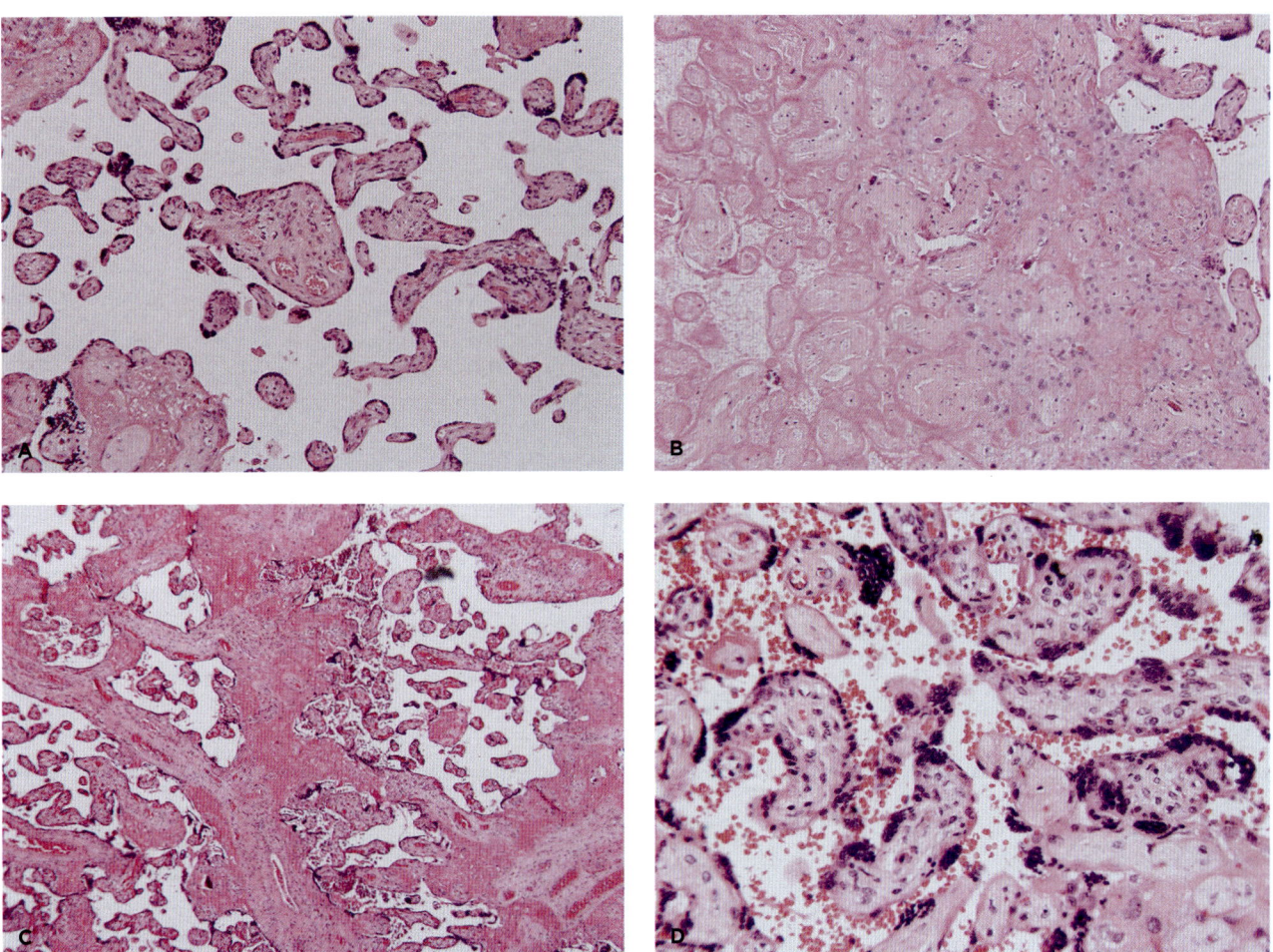

FIGURE 9-9 • Maternal vascular malperfusion: **(A)** distal villous hypoplasia—decreased number of long thin poorly branching distal villi, **(B)** villous infarction—large aggregate of nonviable villi with collapse of the intervillous space and remote ischemic necrosis of the villous trophoblasts, **(C)** increased intervillous fibrin—irregular aggregates of fibrin-coating large proximal villi and protruding from denuded portions of the distal villous tree, **(D)** increased syncytial knots—numerous aggregates of large numbers of syncytiotrophoblastic nuclei within the villous trophoblast layer,

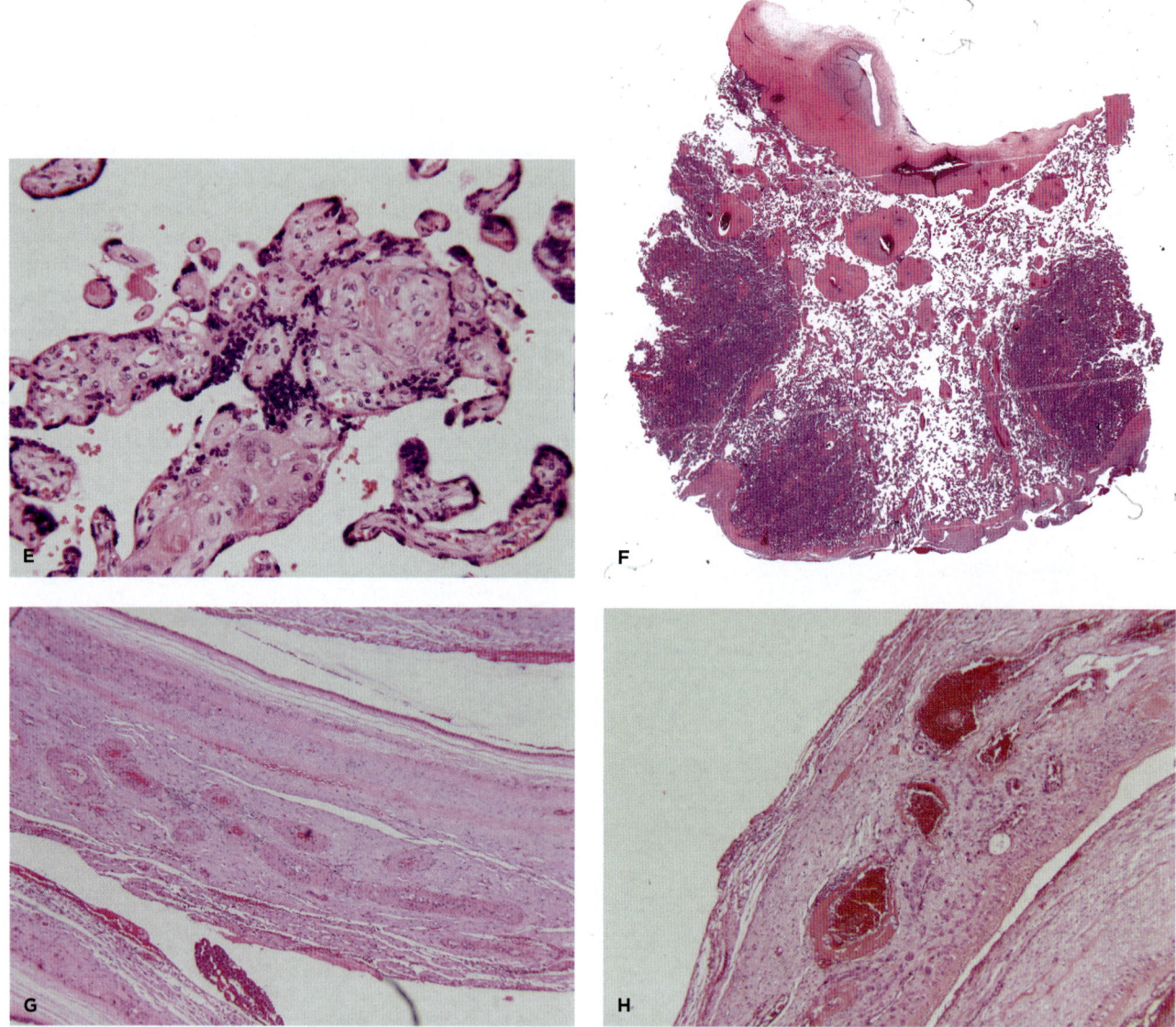

FIGURE 9-9 • (*Continued*) **(E)** villous agglutination—small areas of aggregated villi with syncytial knots and intervillous fibrin (microinfarct), **(F)** whole slide image showing alternating areas of villous crowding (knots, fibrin, and agglutination) and paucity (distal villous hypoplasia), **(G)** mural hypertrophy of decidual arterioles—hypertrophy of the vascular smooth muscle wall (arteriolosclerosis), and **(H)** acute atherosis of decidual arterioles—fibrinoid necrosis of the vascular smooth muscle wall with scattered aggregates of embedded lipid laden macrophages.

developing cardiovascular disease, type II diabetes, and sleep-disordered breathing in later life.

Fetal Vascular Malperfusion

Background
There are two distinct types of fetal vascular malperfusion, each causing a distinct pattern of placental injury (31). The first, *chronic partial or intermittent UC compression*, is often associated with a clinical history of UC entanglement or a predisposing UC lesion (excessive length, hypercoiling, membranous insertion, cord tethering) leading to compression of the umbilical vein, increased placental venous pressure, and global reduction in perfusion of the distal-most portions of the villous tree (32,33). The second, *fetal thrombotic vasculopathy* (FTV), is caused by thrombosis of large fetal placental vessels leading to with segmental degeneration of all dependent downstream villi. Potential causes of FTV are best summarized by Virchow classic triad of risk factors; stasis, loss of endothelial resistance to coagulation, and circulating hypercoagulability. Stasis due to UC obstruction is the major risk factor for FTV. Other causes of stasis include fetal cardiovascular insufficiency, sometimes associated with congenital heart malformations, and polycythemia, often associated with hemoconcentration. Loss of endothelial resistance to coagulation may occur with severe fetal inflammation, antiphospholipid syndrome, and other forms of vessel wall damage. Hypercoagulability can be associated with maternal platelet disorders or diabetes and

fetal thrombophilic mutations involving protein C, protein S, antithrombin II, factor V, prothrombin 2010, and methyltetrahydrofolate reductase (34,35). Interaction between risk factors is probably an important factor in many cases of FTV.

Pathology
Histologic findings consistent with global fetal malperfusion (chronic partial/ intermittent UC obstruction) include pressure-related intramural fibrin deposition (intimal fibrin cushions) within the walls of large placental veins (Figure 9-10A), relative immaturity and patchy edema of villous parenchyma, and scattered small foci (<10 villi per focus) of avascular villi. Histologic findings consistent with total segmental fetal vascular occlusion (FTV) include organizing thrombi within large chorionic or stem villous vessels (seen in approximately 1/3 of cases) (Figure 9-10B), obliteration of the lumen of medium-sized vessels by proliferating smooth muscle cells and subendothelial fibroblasts (fibromuscular

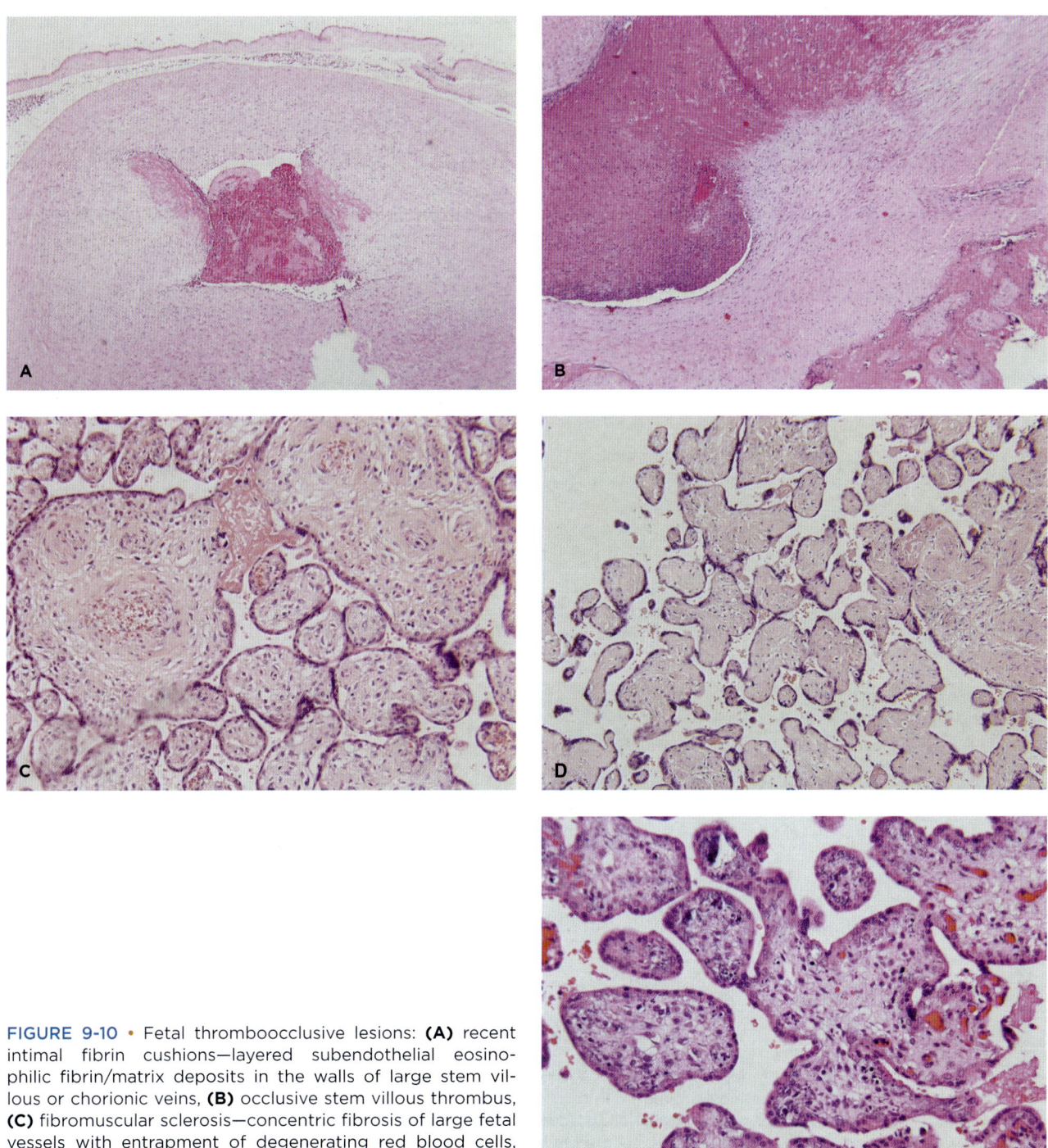

FIGURE 9-10 • Fetal thromboocclusive lesions: **(A)** recent intimal fibrin cushions—layered subendothelial eosinophilic fibrin/matrix deposits in the walls of large stem villous or chorionic veins, **(B)** occlusive stem villous thrombus, **(C)** fibromuscular sclerosis—concentric fibrosis of large fetal vessels with entrapment of degenerating red blood cells, **(D)** extensive hyalinized avascular distal villi, and **(E)** distal villi with degenerative stromal–vascular karyorrhexis.

sclerosis) (Figure 9-10C), and large contiguous foci of distal villi with degenerative changes (>10 villi per focus). Longstanding thrombosis leads to hyalinized avascular villi (Figure 9-10D). More recent occlusion leads to villous stromal–vascular karyorrhexis (also known as hemorrhagic endovasculitis) characterized by fragmentation of red blood cells, endothelial cells, and villous stromal fibroblasts (Figure 9-10E). The segmental nature of the villous changes in FTV distinguishes it from similar, but more uniform, degenerative changes seen throughout the placentas of stillbirths (36). One diagnostic threshold for FTV has been set at an average of greater than 15 affected villi/ slide (31). Smaller numbers of avascular villi should also be reported.

Clinical Correlation

Both FTV and chronic partial UC obstruction are significant risk factors for IUFD and cerebral palsy (37,38). FTV may also be associated with thromboembolic disease in the fetus (39,40). The finding of any substantial number of avascular villi has been correlated with IUGR, chronic monitoring abnormalities, and discordant twin growth (12,41).

Villitis of Unknown Etiology

Background

Localized lymphohistiocytic villous stromal inflammation is common, being seen in approximately 9% to 10% of term pregnancies (42,43). While localized infiltrates could reflect unrecognized infections, extensive investigation over many years has failed to reveal organisms, and neither mothers nor infants have shown any consistent clinical or laboratory evidence of an infectious process. These villous infiltrates are largely composed of CD8-positive maternal T lymphocytes, many of which coexpress CD25 (44). It is currently believed that this lesion, known by convention as villitis of unknown etiology (VUE), is the result of maternofetal cell trafficking causing a localized host-versus-graft reaction in the villous tree.

Pathology

Most cases of VUE are characterized by small groups of less than 10 affected villi in either a random or predominantly basal distribution, low-grade VUE (Figure 9-11A), and basal villitis (Figure 9-11B), respectively. Less commonly,

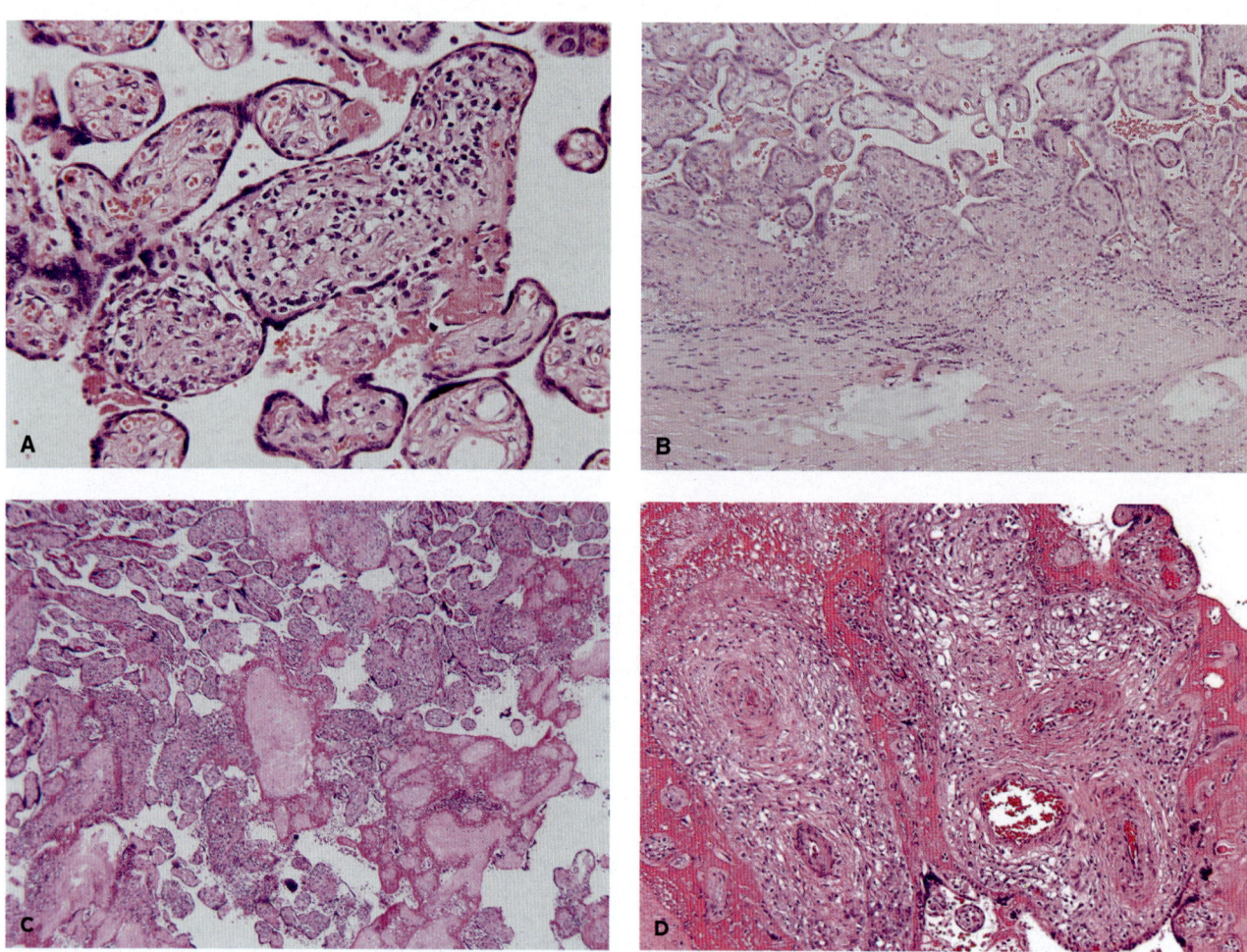

FIGURE 9-11 • Chronic villitis (VUE): **(A)** focal VUE—clusters of less than 10 villi with a nonuniform lymphohistiocytic infiltrate in the villous stroma, **(B)** basal VUE—lymphohistiocytic infiltrate involving anchoring stem and adjacent villi accompanied by a lymphoplasmacytic infiltrate in the decidua basalis, **(C)** patchy/diffuse VUE—aggregates of 10 or more chronically inflamed villi, and **(D)** VUE with obliterative fetal vasculopathy—marked perivascular chronic inflammation involving stem villi leading to vascular occlusion.

larger groups of villi are involved (patchy or diffuse VUE) (Figure 9-11C). These cases are classified as high-grade VUE. Stem villous vasculitis with luminal obliteration represents a special subcategory of high-grade VUE where lymphocytic infiltration extends to the proximal villi or even the chorionic plate (Figure 9-11D) (31). This pattern is often associated with extensive downstream avascular villi and has been termed obliterative fetal vasculopathy. VUE of all types is often accompanied by a lymphoplasmacytic infiltrate in the basal plate (chronic deciduitis). Diffuse perivillous fibrin deposition and intervillositis with a polymorphous inflammatory infiltrate including neutrophils (active chronic villitis) are other associated features, most commonly seen with high-grade VUE. The presence of neutrophils or plasma cells increases the possibility of an underlying infection. Histiocytic giant cells, on the other hand, are common and do not suggest an infectious etiology.

Clinical Correlation
Low-grade VUE is generally not associated with adverse outcomes (43). Predominantly, basal villitis is increased with underlying uterine abnormalities such as previous curettage, chronic endometritis, low implantation, and adherent placentas (45). High-grade VUE is associated with IUGR and stillbirth (41,46). Obliterative fetal vasculopathy is a risk factor for cerebral palsy and other forms of neurologic impairment (47). Recurrence of VUE occurs in approximately 10% to 25% of cases and is more common with high-grade histology (45). Also of interest is the association of VUE with ovum donation pregnancies where the fetus shares no antigens with the mother (48).

Villous Stromal–Vascular Maldevelopment

Background
Normal third-trimester villous development is dominated by nonbranching angiogenesis, which drives elongation of the distal villous tree (4). Vascular growth normally exceeds stromal growth leading to the formation of terminal villi characterized by minimal amounts of villous stroma and close apposition of fetal capillary loops to attenuated areas of overlying syncytiotrophoblasts known as vasculosyncytial membranes. Processes that uncouple the normal balance between vascular and stromal growth lead to either excessive stroma or abnormal vascular patterning. These disorders can be separated into three groups: distal villous immaturity (maturation defect), villous capillary lesions (diffuse chorangiosis, multifocal chorangiomatosis, and chorangioma), and less specific dysmorphic patterns including at the most extreme end of the spectrum, mesenchymal dysplasia (49–51). Possible etiologies include elevated levels of insulin and insulin-like growth factors, hypoxia-related angiogenic factors such as vascular endothelial growth factor and the angiopoietins, pressure-related vascular remodeling, and genetic or epigenetically altered developmental gene expression.

Pathology
Delayed villous maturatioin (distal villous immaturity) is defined by a constellation of abnormalities including decreased fetoplacental weight ratio, placentomegaly, excessive distal villous stroma (fibroblasts, macrophages, and/or extracellular fluid), predominantly central villous capillaries, a thick cellular layer of villous trophoblasts, and decreased vasculosyncytial membranes (Figure 9-12A). *Villous capillary lesions* are separated into three subgroups. Villous chorangiosis is confined to distal villi, and the vessels are lined by endothelium alone. This lesion is defined by an increase in the number of capillary cross sections in otherwise normal villi (more than 10 per villus in at least 10 villi in several H&E-stained sections with at least some villi showing 15 to 20 capillary cross-sections) (Figure 9-12B). Placental chorangiomas are expansile tumor-like lesions usually arising from major stem villi beneath the chorionic plate or at the placental margins (Figure 9-12C). Histologically, they resemble capillary hemangiomas and are composed of a mixture of endothelial cells, pericytes, and fibroblasts. Multifocal chorangiomatosis arises in the loose reticular connective tissue of immature intermediate villi and is characterized by proliferating small vessels composed of both endothelial cells and pericytes surrounding an intact central villous core (Figure 9-12D). Rather than expanding eccentrically to form a mass as in chorangioma, the vessels in chorangiomatosis extend proximally and distally to form large zones of vascular proliferation. "Dysmorphic villi" is a general term used to describe a variety of different global derangements in placental structure. The most dramatic example is mesenchymal dysplasia characterized by gross expansion of stem villi including a combination of vascular proliferation, stromal overgrowth, and formation of villous cisterns resembling those in complete hydatidiform mole (Figure 9-12E) (16,51). Other dysmorphic patterns include irregular villous contour, excessive numbers of trophoblast inclusions, abnormal vascular patterning, and parenchymal disproportion with an exaggeration of proximal relative to distal villi (18,52,53).

Clinical Correlation
Delayed villous maturation is common in diabetic pregnancies and may also be increased in placentas with chronic UC obstruction (49). It is seen in some otherwise unexplained stillbirths and a subset of growth-restricted fetuses (54). Villous chorangiosis is also increased with maternal diabetes and can accompany a variety of other chronic and subacute pathologic lesions (55). Notably, it is increased in placentas associated with high altitude, smoking, air pollution, and maternal anemia and may represent a compensatory physiologic adaptation to reduced oxygen tension in the absence of malperfusion (56). Placental chorangiomas are most frequent at sites, such as the placental margin, and in scenarios such as preeclampsia and multiple gestation that are also associated with relative hypoxia (50). In rare cases, they may be disseminated throughout the placenta causing stillbirth

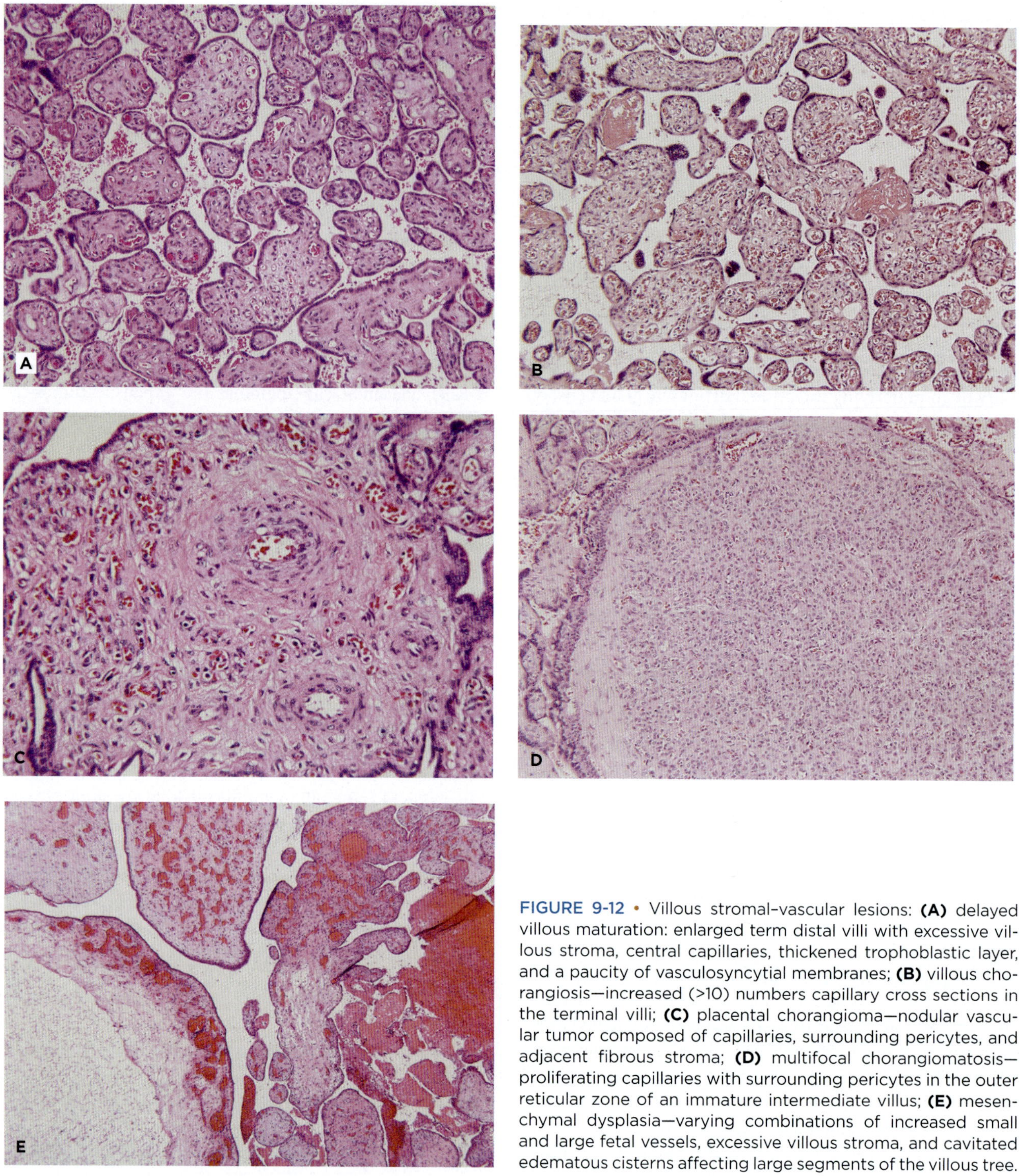

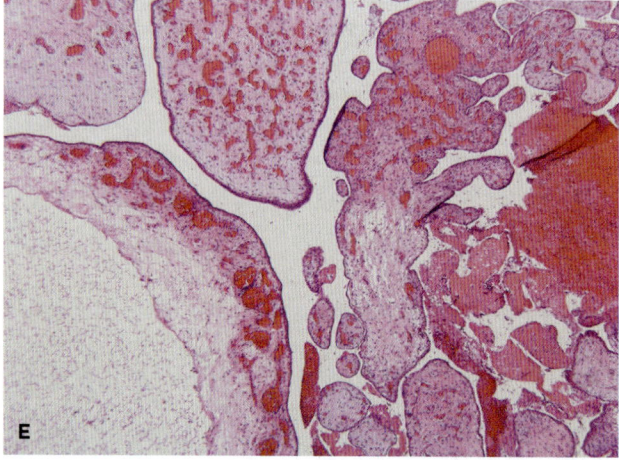

FIGURE 9-12 • Villous stromal-vascular lesions: **(A)** delayed villous maturation: enlarged term distal villi with excessive villous stroma, central capillaries, thickened trophoblastic layer, and a paucity of vasculosyncytial membranes; **(B)** villous chorangiosis—increased (>10) numbers capillary cross sections in the terminal villi; **(C)** placental chorangioma—nodular vascular tumor composed of capillaries, surrounding pericytes, and adjacent fibrous stroma; **(D)** multifocal chorangiomatosis—proliferating capillaries with surrounding pericytes in the outer reticular zone of an immature intermediate villus; **(E)** mesenchymal dysplasia—varying combinations of increased small and large fetal vessels, excessive villous stroma, and cavitated edematous cisterns affecting large segments of the villous tree.

and sometimes recurring in subsequent pregnancies. They are occasionally associated with hemangiomas in the fetus (57). Large chorangiomas can sometimes trap platelets leading to fetal consumptive coagulopathy or act as arteriovenous shunts leading to heart failure and hydrops fetalis. Multifocal chorangiomatosis is more common in preterm placentas and has been associated with IUGR and fetal malformations (50). Dysmorphic villi may be seen in aneuploid gestations, confined placental mosaicism, Beckwith-Wiedemann syndrome, and a subgroup of preterm infants with IUGR and normal pulsed flow Doppler testing (18,53,58,59).

Chronic Marginal Abruption

Background
As discussed above, lateral growth of the placenta involves remodeling of large uterine veins (3). These large obliquely

oriented structures are prone to disruption with changes in uterine conformation (rupture of membranes, premature cervical dilatation), lack of support by the surrounding endometrium (severe inflammation, defective implantation), or elevated intramural pressure (compression of larger upstream maternal veins) (60,61). Unlike arterial rupture, which tends to be central and forceful, and results in abruptio placenta (see below), venous hemorrhages tend to be marginal and occur at relatively low pressure (62). If not associated with immediate delivery, they can present clinically with threatened abortion, recurrent vaginal bleeding, or subchorionic hematomas on ultrasound. Factors associated with chronic marginal abruption include chorioamnionitis, multiparity, smoking, and oligohydramnios (63).

Pathology

Chronic marginal abruption is associated with a constellation of placental findings including old marginal blood clot, circumvallate membrane insertion, chorioamnionic hemosiderin deposition, and green (biliverdin) staining of the fetal surface (63,64). Circumvallation that is due to chronic marginal abruption develops as a consequence of blood accumulating in the space between the decidua and chorion leading to undermining or folding of the marginal chorionic plate and should be associated with adjacent hemosiderin deposition (Figure 9-13A, B). Hemosiderin usually stains blue by iron stain but in some cases may be iron negative due to encrustation by glycoproteins. Any pigment seen in a premature placenta favors chronic marginal abruption, as opposed to meconium that is uncommon before 37 weeks.

Clinical Correlation

Chronic marginal abruption is often associated with oligohydramnios, a clinical presentation known as chronic abruption–oligohydramnios sequence (65). Hemorrhages can be detected by early ultrasound as so-called subchorionic hematomas, and serial sonography has documented the development of placental circumvallation following repeated episodes of vaginal bleeding and subchorionic hemorrhage (66). Chronic marginal abruption is an important cause of preterm delivery and has been associated with an atypical form of neonatal lung disease (64,67). Finally, acute marginal abruption resulting in immediate delivery is an important cause of preterm delivery and must be distinguished from abruptio placenta by pathologic evaluation (62).

Perivillous Fibrin/Fibrinoid Deposition

Background

Maternal floor infarction/massive perivillous fibrin deposition (MFI/PVF) is characterized by the accumulation of excessive amounts of fibrin and extracellular matrix-rich fibrinoid around gas exchanging distal villi in the lower two-thirds of the placenta (68). It must be distinguished from perivillous fibrin plaques that have a similar histologic pattern, but a more localized distribution (69), and increased intervillous fibrin that adheres to but does not surround groups of proximal and distal villi in cases of maternal malperfusion (discussed above). MFI/PVF is an idiopathic lesion. Among other possibilities, it could represent a primary abnormality, an aberrant secondary response to trophoblastic injury, or an exaggerated reaction to local circulatory stasis. Associations with maternal autoimmune disease and thrombophilia suggest extrinsic maternal causation, while reports of weight discordance in twins and an association with long-chain 3-hydroxyacyl-CoA dehydrogenase (LCHAD) deficiency are more consistent with intrinsic fetal susceptibility (70–73). The pathogenesis of localized perivillous fibrin plaques is also not well understood.

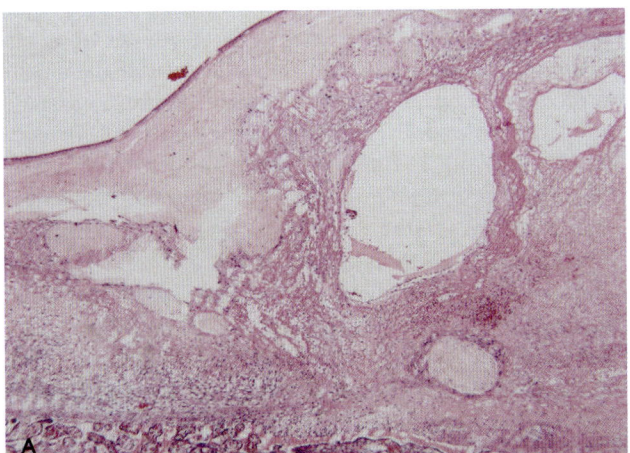
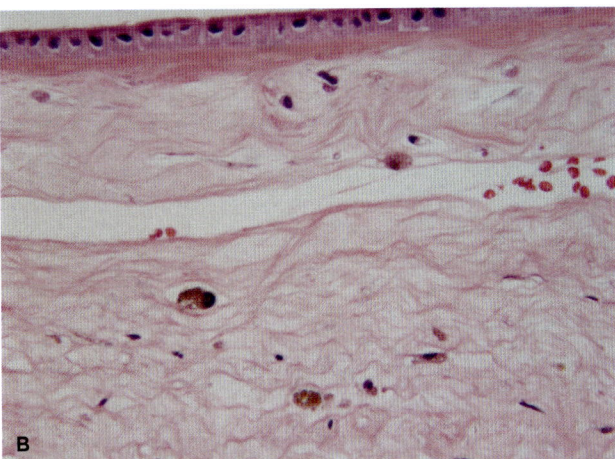

FIGURE 9-13 • Chronic abruption: **(A)** circumvallation—nonperipheral membrane insertion with underlying organizing blood clot and **(B)** membrane hemosiderin—cytoplasmic golden-brown refractile pigment within macrophages in the chorioamnion.

Pathology

MFI/PVF can present with a variety of patterns ranging from basal–predominant with a rind-like gross thickening of the basal plate to diffuse with fine lacy strands of fibrin marbling the entire cut surface of the placenta (so-called "Gitterinfarkt"). In some cases, degenerative changes such as eosinophilia or karyorrhexis of villous trophoblasts and stroma may be seen. The features that distinguish it from increased intervillous fibrin are circumferential encasement of distal villi and extravillous trophoblasts within the fibrinoid matrix (Figure 9-14). Localized plaques of perivillous fibrin can be seen at all gestational ages. In some cases, these plaques may be multifocal or focally complex, but they never occupy a significant proportion of the total villous parenchyma. They are of little clinical significance and must not be misdiagnosed as MFI/PVF (69). Reexamination of the gross placental specimen to assess overall extent of involvement is often useful in making the distinction. Both lesions can be distinguished from villous infarction by maintenance of normal villous spacing (absence of collapse of the intervillous space) and the lack of acute or chronic ischemic changes (trophoblastic eosinophilia and necrotic cellular debris).

Clinical Correlation

MFI/PVF is a rare, but important, placental lesion associated with high rates of spontaneous abortion, stillbirth, severe IUGR, and neurologic impairment (68,74). Furthermore, it is a recognized cause of recurrent reproductive failure with an overall recurrence risk of 50% or higher (75). MFI/PVF most commonly presents in the second or early third trimester and can progress quite rapidly (72). Arrest of fetal growth, decreased pulsed flow Doppler studies, and abnormal biophysical profile are common, and delivery at the earliest possible opportunity has been recommended (76). No controlled trials of therapy have been conducted, but heparin and/or aspirin have been used in some cases (71).

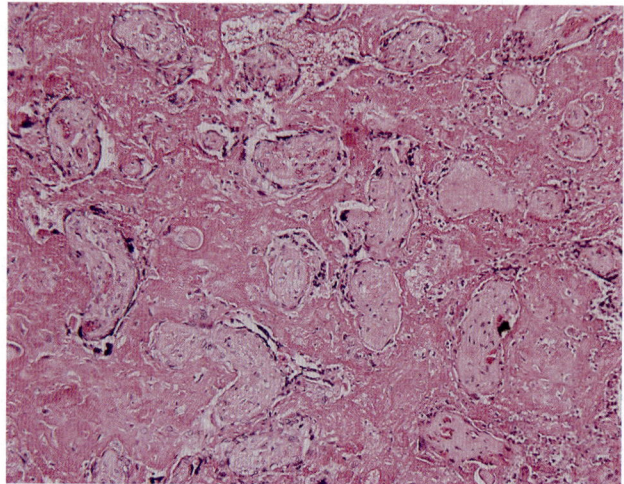

FIGURE 9-14 • Massive perivillous fibrin deposition/maternal floor infarction: eosinophilic fibrin/matrix material with embedded intermediate trophoblasts completely surrounding large portions of the distal villous tree.

SUBACUTE DISEASE PROCESSES

Amniotic Fluid Infection/Chorioamnionitis

Background

The products of conception develop in a normally sterile uterine cavity. However, parturition necessitates communication with the external environment, and the pathway for egress, the cervicovaginal tract, like most other body orifices, has a rich and complex microbial flora including aerobic and anaerobic bacteria, mycoplasma, and fungi. This site can also harbor organisms with a particular capacity to infect the products of conception, such as group B streptococci and *Listeria monocytogenes*. Direct connection between the gestational sac and the cervicovaginal tract does not occur until about 18 to 19 weeks when the membranes fuse to the uterocervical lining (77). After that time, the cervical mucus plug, placental membranes, and, most importantly, the closed cervical os protect the fetoplacental unit from ascending infection. Failure of these mechanisms allows organisms to enter the endometrial cavity and amniotic fluid where local immunosuppression and fetal immaturity inhibit an effective response. The inflammatory response to microorganisms in the amniotic fluid is comprised of maternal neutrophils emanating from both the intervillous circulation and small venules in the membranous decidua. The maternal response is supplemented by a fetal response comprised of neutrophils emanating from large vessels of the UC and chorionic plate. The term chorioamnionitis indicates the placental layers (chorion and amnion) through which maternal and fetal neutrophils traverse to reach the site of infection. While the majority of amniotic fluid infections occur via the ascending route, other pathways exist including hematogenous seeding from distant sites, contiguous spread from other pelvic organs, and direct inoculation of organisms during diagnostic procedures such as amniocentesis.

Pathology

Any pathologic description of chorioamnionitis must distinguish its two components, the maternal and fetal inflammatory responses. Each of these in turn should be subcategorized in terms of spatiotemporal progression (stage) and severity (grade) (78). The stages of maternal infection are (a) acute subchorionitis (neutrophils restricted to subchorionic fibrin and/or the membranous decidual–chorionic interface) (Figure 9-15A), (b) acute chorioamnionitis (neutrophils in chorion and amnion), and (c) necrotizing chorioamnionitis (amnionic epithelial necrosis). Significant necrosis is defined by karyorrhexis of neutrophils, desquamation of amnionic epithelial cells, and intense eosinophilia of the amnionic basement membrane (Figure 9-15B). The stages of fetal infection are (a) neutrophils in chorionic vessels (chorionic vasculitis) and/or umbilical vein (umbilical phlebitis), (b) neutrophils in one or both umbilical arteries (umbilical arteritis), and (c) neutrophils and neutrophilic debris forming arcs around umbilical vessels in the Wharton jelly (necrotizing funisitis) (Figure 9-15C). Severe

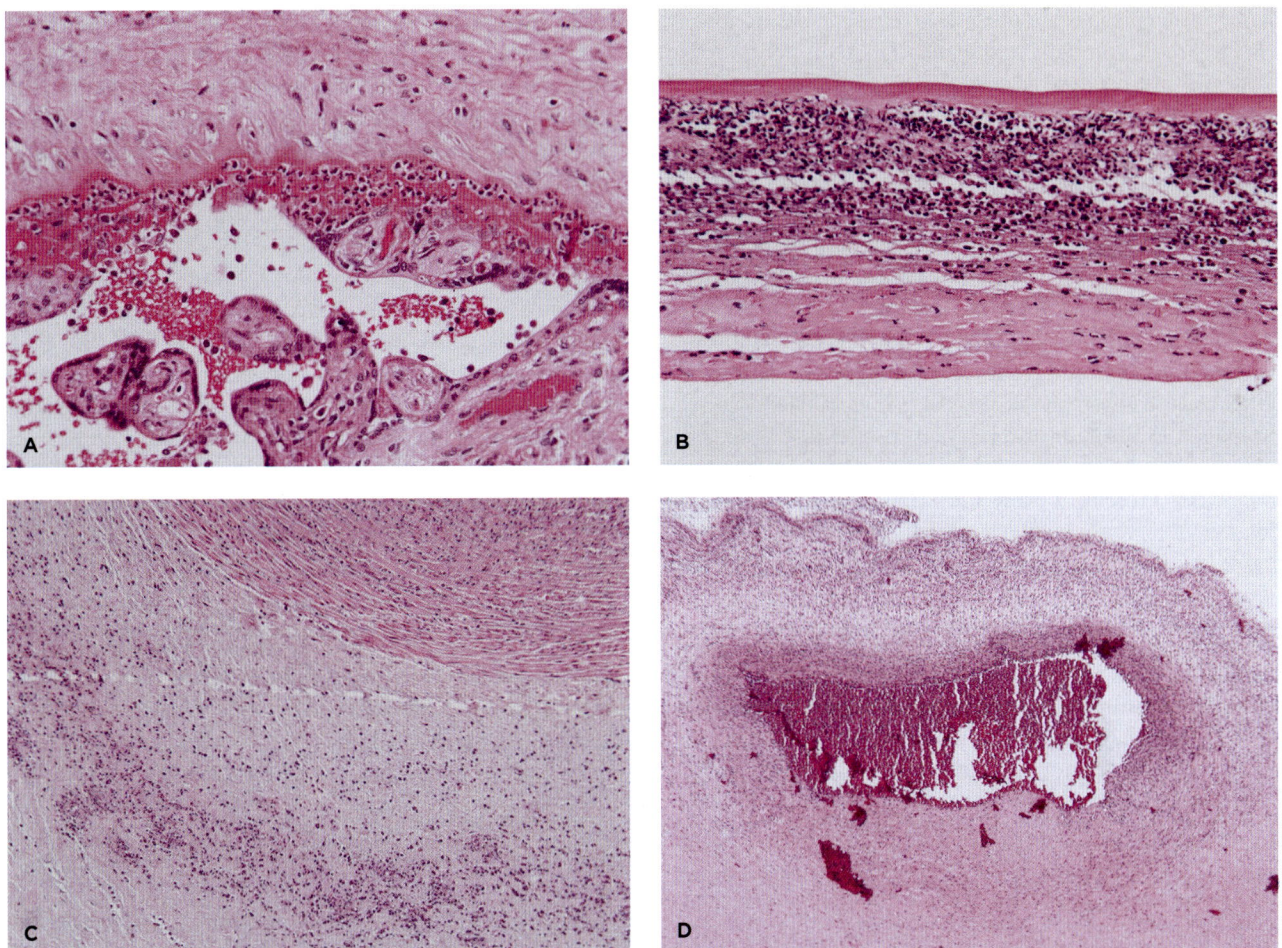

FIGURE 9-15 • Chorioamnionitis: **(A)** early subchorionitis—diffuse neutrophilic infiltration of the subchorionic fibrin, **(B)** necrotizing chorioamnionitis—necrosis and sloughing of amniocytes combined with a thickened eosinophilic basement membrane and karyorrhexis of adjacent neutrophils, **(C)** necrotizing funisitis—loosely organized perivascular arcs of eosinophilic precipitate and degenerating neutrophilic debris in the umbilical Wharton jelly, and **(D)** intense chorionic vasculitis—near confluent neutrophilic infiltration of the amnionic side of major chorionic vessels accompanied by myocyte disarray and/or endothelial activation.

maternal responses are defined by large accumulations of neutrophils (microabscesses) under the chorion and severe fetal responses by near-confluent neutrophilic infiltration, attenuation, and degenerative changes within the amnionic aspect of the chorionic vessel wall (intense chorionic vasculitis) (Figure 9-15D). Severe fetal responses can, in some cases, promote the formation of mural vascular thrombi that can sometimes embolize to the fetus.

Clinical Correlation

The prevalence of histologic chorioamnionitis is inversely proportional to gestational age reaching over 50% below 28 weeks, and placental infection is the leading cause of premature delivery at less than 32 weeks (79). Premature cervical dilatation is the most important risk factor for infection. Chorioamnionitis is usually preceded by either membrane rupture or labor. In general, the ability to effectively eradicate chorioamnionitis using antibiotics is limited, and delivery cannot usually be forestalled. Spread of organisms from the infected placenta to the fetus (early onset sepsis) is uncommon, and chorioamnionitis is only rarely a direct cause of stillbirth. Exceptions include group B streptococcus, Listeria, and coliform bacilli. Recently, the fetal response to amniotic fluid infection has received special attention (fetal inflammatory response syndrome). Some evidence suggests that various aspects of this response including circulating cytokines, bacterial toxins, and activation of the coagulation cascade predispose to CNS injury and other types of neonatal morbidity (80).

Meconium-Related Changes

Background

Transient episodes of acute hypoxia can trigger redistribution of antenatal blood flow resulting in the release of fetal stool (meconium) into the amniotic fluid. This vagally mediated reflex is believed to be an adaptation preserving adequate perfusion to more critical vascular beds such as the central nervous and cardiovascular systems. In most cases, the hypoxic episodes are caused by transient UC occlusion, which is most common postterm as the fetus continues to grow and move in the face of decreases in the amount of protective amniotic fluid and UC Wharton jelly. Meconium is composed of large amounts of bile acid and phospholipases, substances that can have caustic effects on fetal and placental tissues. Particularly, susceptible are large umbilical and chorionic blood vessels (81). The amount of meconium passed and the volume of amniotic fluid available to suspend it are important variables in determining both its effects on the placenta and the fetal lungs. Since meconium diffuses relatively slowly through tissue, duration of exposure is the critical factor in terms of toxic effects on fetal blood vessels. Prolonged exposure is also relevant insofar as it is an indicator of hypoxic episodes occurring remote from the time of delivery. Prolonged exposure to meconium and the fetal inflammatory component of chorioamnionitis may also synergize to cause more severe forms of chorionic vessel wall injury (37,47).

Pathology
The pathologist's role is not to diagnose meconium passage but rather to estimate duration of exposure and any secondary effects. Meconium is a fine particulate red-brown pigment generally found in vacuolated tissue macrophages.

Other membrane pigments such as hemosiderin and lipofuscin have a different appearance, are not associated with a clinical history of meconium-stained fluid, and do not cause degenerative changes in the amnion such as dehiscence from the chorion, necrosis of amniocytes, and connective tissue edema (Figure 9-16A). Based on *in vitro* experiments, it is believed that meconium pigment–laden macrophages appear in amnion approximately 1 hour after release and in the membranous decidua at about 3 hours (82). Significant accumulations of pigment-laden macrophages in the deeper layers of the chorionic plate and Wharton jelly and green staining of the UC probably take at least 6 to 12 hours (Figure 9-16B). A rare, but clinically significant, lesion associated with prolonged meconium exposure is meconium-associated vascular necrosis (81). This lesion is characterized by apoptosis of peripheral myocytes in the umbilical and chorionic vessels (Figure 9-16C).

Clinical Correlation
Meconium passage occurs in approximately 14% of all deliveries, but rarely before 34 weeks of gestation. While statistically associated with obstetric and neonatal complications, it is neither a specific nor sensitive indicator for them. Meconium aspiration syndrome, defined as respiratory distress requiring oxygen therapy associated with

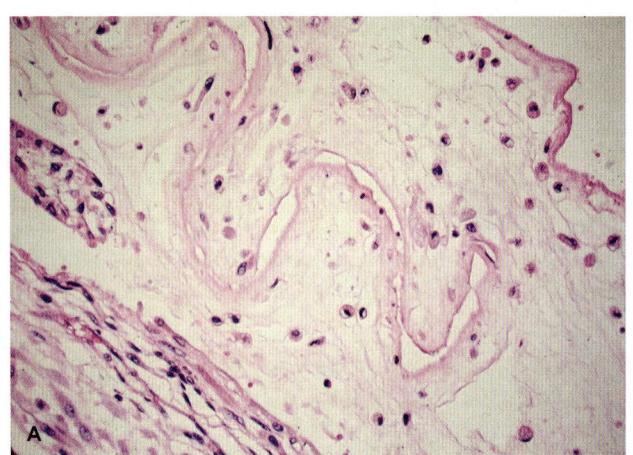

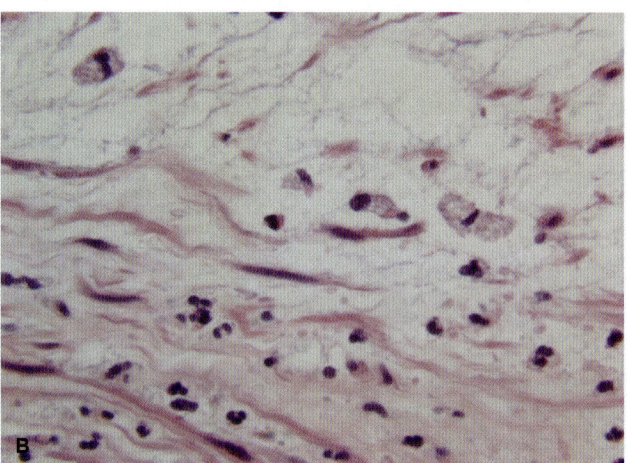

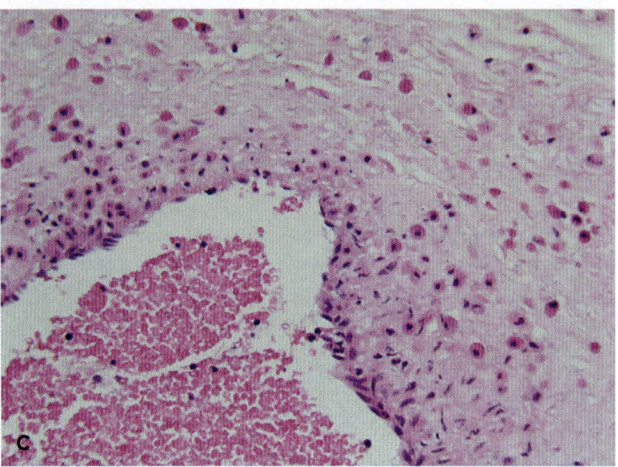

FIGURE 9-16 • Meconium-related changes: **(A)** numerous vacuolated pigment-laden macrophages and amnionic edema with necrosis of amniocytes, **(B)** numerous vacuolated pigment-laden macrophages deep in the connective tissue of the chorionic plate, and **(C)** meconium-associated vascular necrosis—diffuse eosinophilic cytoplasmic degeneration and nuclear pyknosis (apoptosis) of peripheral vascular smooth muscle cells in the vessels of the chorionic plate and/or umbilical cord.

meconium release and an abnormal chest x-ray, is associated with serious respiratory and neurologic complications and a significant mortality rate. Autopsy cases often reveal deep inspiration of meconium leading to plugging of airways and chemical damage to the pulmonary parenchyma. Meconium-associated vascular necrosis has been strongly associated with adverse neurologic outcomes (47).

Increased Circulating Fetal Nucleated Red Blood Cells

Background
Prolonged and/or repetitive periods of antenatal fetal hypoxemia are well-documented causes of central nervous damage in experimental pregnancy models (83). While an underlying placental cause for hypoxia is sometimes indicated by one or more of the pathologic lesions, in other cases, there is no recognizable pattern of injury. One useful indicator of sustained and/or severe fetal hypoxemia is an increased number of circulating fetal nucleated red blood cells (NRBC) in the placental circulation (84). This physiologic response is the result of both premature release of red blood cell precursors into the systemic circulation and increased fetal erythropoiesis. It is, at least in part, mediated by hypoxia-inducible elements in the promoter regions of erythropoietin.

Pathology
The identification of increased NRBCs in the placental circulation is particularly useful in cases such as stillbirth where neonatal blood counts are not available. While erythroblastosis is easily recognized (Figure 9-17A), the detection of lesser numbers of circulating normoblasts requires systematic examination of distal villi at high magnification (Figure 9-17B). A simple semiquantitative method for recognizing increased NRBCs in the placenta has been described (85). The finding of 10 or more NRBC in 10 high-power (40×) microscopic fields correlates with a neonatal NRBC count of greater than 2500/mm^3 within the first 2 hours of life.

Clinical Correlation
Increased circulating NRBCs signifies decreased oxygen availability in the fetal hematopoietic microenvironment. This can result from maternal hypoxemia, decreased placental oxygen transfer, or insufficient fetal oxygen-carrying capacity (anemia). Accumulation of red blood cell precursors in fetal hematopoietic tissues and large scale release into the circulation requires a time interval measured in hours. Estimates of the time required to see significant numbers of NRBCs vary and are controversial. Pathologic data and available animal studies suggest that a significant elevation of NRBCs in a previously normal host probably requires at least 6 to 12 hours to develop (84–87). Persistence of elevated NRBC for several days postnatally generally indicates a longer period of antenatal hypoxia. Significantly elevated placental NRBCs have been associated with fetal anemia, IUGR, CNS lesions, and IUFD (37,88,89).

Fetomaternal Hemorrhage

Background
Fetomaternal hemorrhage (FMH) represents disruption of villous capillaries with bleeding into the intervillous space and is an inevitable complication of the close proximity of maternal and fetal circulations in the human placenta. Small amounts of FMH occur in at least 50% of pregnancies (90). More substantial hemorrhages of up to 40 mL occur in 8% of pregnancies and hemorrhages greater than 40 mL in 0.3% to 1%. Diagnosis of FMH requires either flow cytometry or the Kleihauer-Betke testing. These tests are performed on a peripheral blood sample from the mother, and the volume of hemorrhage is calculated from the percentage of fetal cells relative to the maternal blood volume.

Pathology
Definitive diagnosis of massive FMH is only confirmed by direct measurement of fetal red blood cells in the maternal circulation, and appropriate testing should be performed in all cases of stillbirth and unexplained adverse outcomes.

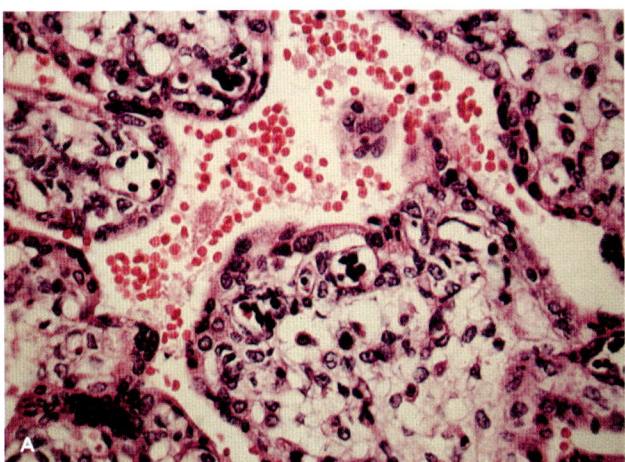
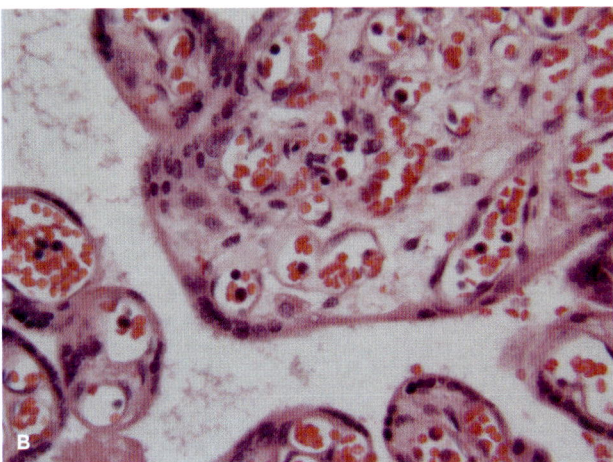

FIGURE 9-17 • Increased circulating fetal NRBC: **(A)** marked increase in circulating NRBC—clusters of immature NRBC including erythroblasts in villous capillaries and **(B)** mild-to-moderate increase in circulating NRBC—scattered normoblasts in terminal villous capillaries.

Placental findings that suggest the diagnosis in the proper clinical context are intervillous thrombi, markedly increased circulating NRBCs, and/or placental signs of hydrops fetalis (placentomegaly, villous immaturity, diffuse villous edema) (Figure 9-18A). Intervillous thrombi are spherical collections of clotted blood that are completely surrounded by villous tissue (Figure 9-18B). They have been shown to represent sites of villous disruption with fetal bleeding (91), However, these lesions are very common and are not useful indicators of significant FMH unless multiple or large (92). One characteristic finding in cases of massive FMH is marked constriction of arterioles and dilatation of venules in large stem villi.

Clinical Correlation
Predisposing factors for significant FMH include severe maternal malperfusion, placental edema, and tissue disruption associated with abruptio placenta, amniocentesis, maternal trauma, or external cephalic version. Most cases have none of these factors (90). Typical antenatal findings include decreased fetal movements and nonreactive fetal monitoring, sometimes with a distinct sinusoidal fetal heart rate pattern. Affected fetuses and neonates are at risk for circulatory failure, CNS damage, hydrops fetalis, and/or stillbirth due to a combination of hypovolemia and chronic high-output congestive heart failure related to fetal anemia.

Acute Disease Processes
Maternal Arterial Hemorrhages
Background
Acute maternal arterial hemorrhage due to the sudden separation of a significant portion of the placenta from its underlying maternal blood supply is an important cause of acute hypoxic injury. Three major factors predispose to arterial rupture: (a) an abnormal arterial wall (e.g., acute atherosis in preeclampsia), (b) physical force (e.g., trauma or tissue disruption), and (c) ischemia–reperfusion injury (e.g., vasospasm associated with vasoactive mediators such as cocaine or nicotine). The most common clinical cause of arterial hemorrhage is abruption placenta, often accompanied by preeclampsia and often occurring before the onset of labor. Other causes, generally occurring during labor, are rupture of a complete placenta previa and rupture of the uterus with attempted vaginal delivery following a previous C-section. Placental findings in these latter two conditions are relatively nonspecific and will not be discussed further.

Pathology
Correlation between the clinical and pathologic diagnosis of abruptio placenta is only fair, and the only gold standard for diagnosis is direct visualization of a large hematoma at the time of C-section. Nevertheless, most affected placentas show one or more of a constellation of findings that allow a pathologic diagnosis to be made with some confidence. The best pathologic evidence is a retroplacental hematoma with either placental indentation or intraplacental extension (Figure 9-19A). Other supportive findings include a compression crater in the basal plate, microscopic evidence of interstitial hemorrhage within decidual tissues, diffuse retromembranous hemorrhage, very early villous infarction (Figure 9-19B), and recent villous stromal hemorrhage (Figure 9-19C) (93). Finally, lesions associated with chronic maternal malperfusion, as listed above, are often seen with abruptio placenta and strengthen the diagnosis.

Clinical Correlation
The classical clinical signs of abruptio placenta are vaginal bleeding, abdominal pain, and uterine rigidity. Hypertension, maternal substance abuse, advanced maternal age, low pregnancy weight gain, grand multiparity, and strenuous physical labor are known predisposing risk factors. Abruptio placenta and other causes of significant acute maternal arterial hemorrhage are associated with a variety of adverse outcomes including preterm delivery, IUGR, stillbirth, and hypoxic ischemic encephalopathy.

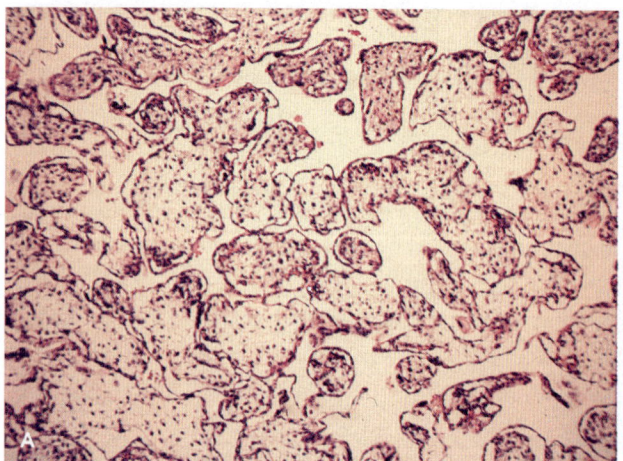
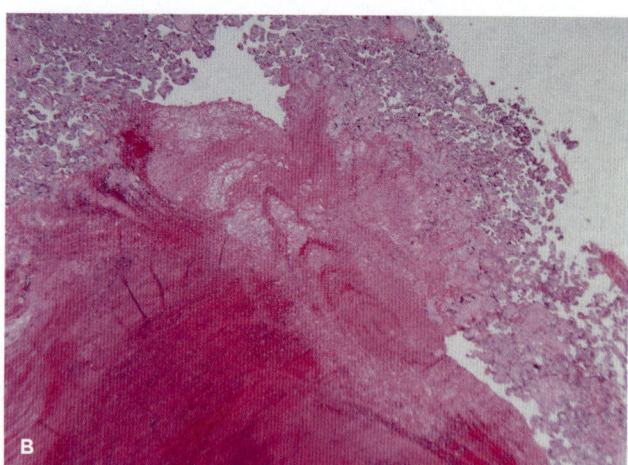

FIGURE 9-18 • Fetomaternal hemorrhage: **(A)** villous hydrops-marked stromal edema with artifactual dehiscence of the villous trophoblast layer and **(B)** intervillous thrombus—fresh laminated hematoma completely surrounded by distal villi.

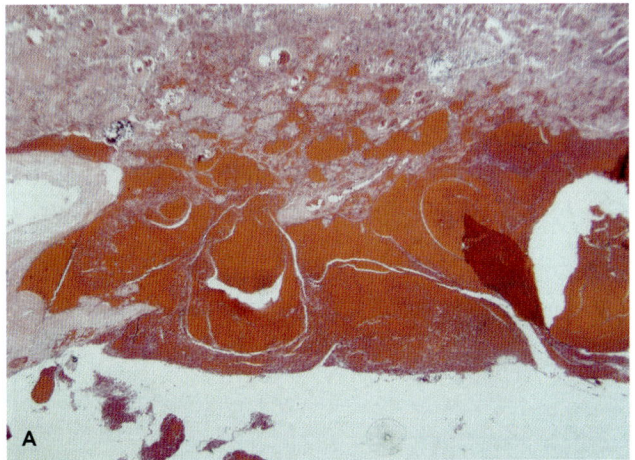
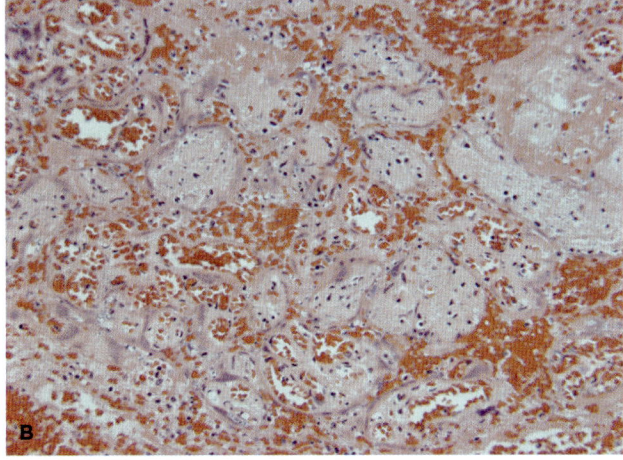
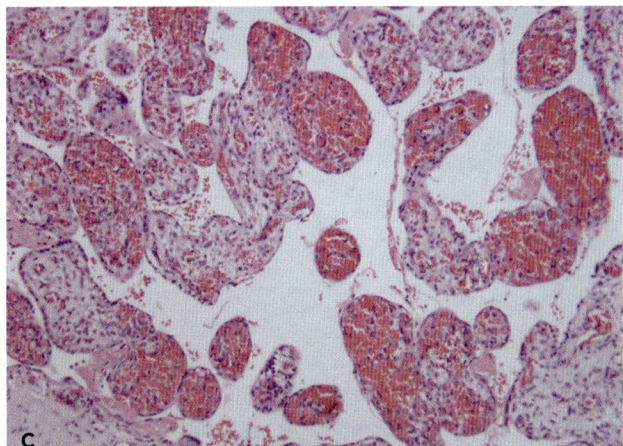

FIGURE 9-19 • Abruptio placenta: **(A)** laminated blood clot spreading within, indenting, and focally perforating the basal plate, **(B)** recent villous infarction—eosinophilic degeneration and karyorrhexis of villous trophoblasts with partial collapse of the intervillous space, and **(C)** villous stromal hemorrhage—diffuse fresh hemorrhage filling the stroma of immature distal villi.

Umbilical Cord Accident

Background

A second cause of acute hypoxic injury is complete obstruction of umbilical blood flow. Obstruction to flow can occur via a variety of mechanisms including compression of the UC between the fetus and the bony pelvis (UC prolapse), tight UC knots, and UC entanglements around fetal body parts (94). Scenarios increasing the risk of UC accident include an excessively long UC, decreased amniotic fluid volume, and sudden changes in fetal position. The umbilical vein is the more easily compressed structure by virtue of its thin wall.

Pathology

While, the UC may show a distinct abnormality such as a tight overhand knot (Figure 9-20A), often the only clue suggesting obstruction is a difference in diameter and/or color on opposite sides of a putative site of obstruction (Figure 9-20B). Recently, the degree of dilatation in chorionic and large stem villous veins has been used to help make the diagnosis of cord obstruction (Figure 9-20C) (95). Specifically, dilatation of chorionic and/or major stem villous veins relative to adjacent arteries of at least 4:1 in sections taken the UC insertion site was shown to be indicative of UC accident as the cause of death in a significant fraction of term and near-term stillborns. Pathologic abnormalities that may predispose to UC obstruction include excessive length, hypercoiling, decreased Wharton jelly, membranous insertion, and tethering to the chorionic surface by an amniotic web (Figure 9-20D).

Clinical Correlation

The overall correlation between clinical UC entanglements and adverse outcomes is weak and controversial. This reflects the fact that the severity and duration of cord occlusion are poorly estimated by the observed state of the UC at the time of delivery. However, UC accidents in general are well-recognized causes of stillbirth. UC prolapse, in particular, is an important cause of intrapartum fetal demise in preterm and/or breech deliveries (95). Transient UC occlusion is correlated with meconium release and the fetal heart rate pattern known as variable decelerations. Variable decelerations can develop a "late" component, a pattern indicative of acidosis and suggestive of more prolonged and severe occlusion. Significant obstruction to umbilical venous flow prevents oxygenated placental venous blood from returning to the fetus and therefore can be associated with dramatic differences between umbilical arterial and venous pH and base excess values (96).

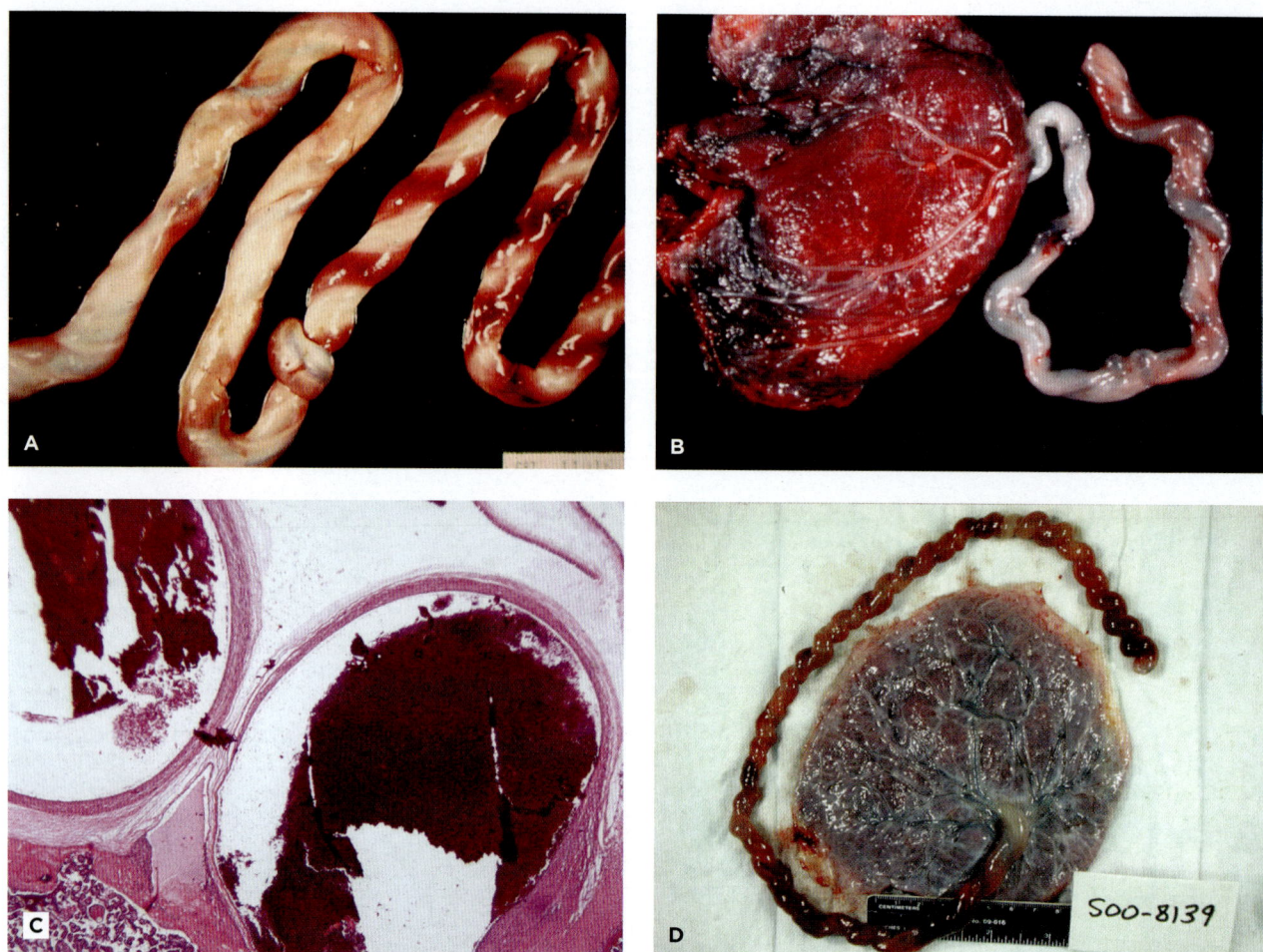

FIGURE 9-20 • Umbilical cord accidents: **(A)** tight overhand umbilical cord knot with marked morphologic changes in vessels on one side of the obstruction, **(B)** acute cord prolapse—transverse indentation of the umbilical cord with congestion on the fetal side, **(C)** markedly dilated chorionic plate veins, and **(D)** excessive long, diffusely hypercoiled, and macerated umbilical cord associated with an intrauterine fetal demise.

Fetal Hemorrhage

Background

Finally, the least common mechanism of acute hypoxic injury is fetal hemorrhage, most notably secondary to ruptured vasa previa. Ruptured vasa previa represents tearing of chorionic vessels traversing the placental membranes and is most commonly related to membranous insertion of the UC. Other varieties of acute fetal hemorrhage include massive intrapartum FMH (see above), iatrogenic rupture of umbilical or chorionic vessels as the result of an invasive procedure, and sequestration of extravasated blood in the placenta (subamnionic or subchorionic hemorrhage), UC (umbilical hematomas), or fetus (most commonly involving the liver, lung, or central nervous system).

Pathology and Clinical Correlation

Fetal hemorrhages in the placenta should always be carefully correlated with adjacent structural changes and the clinical history. Fetal vessels in the fetal membranes are common with peripheral UC insertions, and these vessels often tear during the third stage of labor after delivery of the infant. Tears showing significant amounts of adjacent hemorrhage, distortion of neighboring tissues, or an organized hematoma may in some cases be significant. Likewise, subamnionic and intraumbilical hemorrhages commonly occur with traction on the UC after delivery. In all circumstances, a diagnosis of fetal hemorrhage should be made with extreme caution in the absence of significant fetal distress or a history of neonatal anemia or signs of hypovolemia.

References

1. Kraus FT, Redline R, Gersell DJ, et al. *Placental Pathology*. Washington, DC: American Registry of Pathology; 2004.
2. Jauniaux E, Gulbis B, Burton GJ. The first trimester gestational sac limits rather than facilitates oxygen transfer to the foetus—a review. *Placenta* 2003;24(Suppl A):S86–S93.
3. Craven CM, Zhao L, Ward K. Lateral placental growth occurs by trophoblast cell invasion of decidual veins. *Placenta* 2000;21(2–3):160–169.
4. Demir R, Kaufmann P, Castellucci M, et al. Fetal vasculogenesis and angiogenesis in human placental villi. *Acta Anat* 1989;136(3):190–203.
5. Jauniaux E, Hempstock J, Greenwold N, et al. Trophoblastic oxidative stress in relation to temporal and regional differences in maternal

placental blood flow in normal and abnormal early pregnancies. *Am J Pathol* 2003;162(1):115–125.
6. Herranz G. The timing of monozygotic twinning: a criticism of the common model. *Zygote* 2013;5:1–14.
7. Souter VL, Kapur RP, Nyholt DR, et al. A report of dizygous monochorionic twins. *N Engl J Med* 2003;349(2):154–158.
8. Spencer R. Conjoined twins: theoretical embryologic basis. *Teratology* 1992;45(6):591–602.
9. Lewi L, Deprest J, Hecher K. The vascular anastomoses in monochorionic twin pregnancies and their clinical consequences. *Am J Obstet Gynecol* 2013;208(1):19–30.
10. Benson CB, Bieber FR, Genest DR, et al. Doppler demonstration of reversed umbilical blood flow in an acardiac twin. *J Clin Ultrasound* 1989;17(4):291–295.
11. Hanley ML, Shen-Schwartz S, Anath CV, et al. Birthweight discordancy in twin gestation—is it related to discordancy of placental mass or histopathologic lesions. *Am J Obstet Gynecol* 2000;178:S83.
12. Redline RW, Shah D, Sakar H, et al. Placental lesions associated with abnormal growth in twins. *Pediatr Dev Pathol* 2001;4(5):473–481.
13. Lee Y, Kim KR, McKeon F, et al. A unifying concept of trophoblastic differentiation and malignancy defined by biomarker expression. *Hum Pathol* 2007;38(7):1003–1013.
14. Shih IM, Kurman RJ. p63 expression is useful in the distinction of epithelioid trophoblastic and placental site trophoblastic tumors by profiling trophoblastic subpopulations. *Am J Surg Pathol* 2004;28(9):1177–1183.
15. Barton SC, Surani MA, Norris ML. Role of paternal and maternal genomes in mouse development. *Nature* 1984;311(5984):374–376.
16. Banet N, Descipio C, Murphy KM, et al. Characteristics of hydatidiform moles: analysis of a prospective series with p57 immunohistochemistry and molecular genotyping. *Mod Pathol* 2013;27(2):238–254.
17. Redline RW, Hassold T, Zaragoza MV. Determinants of trophoblast hyperplasia in spontaneous abortions. *Mod Pathol* 1998;11:762–768.
18. Redline RW, Zaragoza MV, Hassold T. Prevalence of developmental and inflammatory lesions in non-molar first trimester spontaneous abortions. *Hum Pathol* 1999;30:93–100.
19. Nayar R, Lage JM. Placental changes in a first trimester missed abortion in maternal systemic lupus erythematosus with antiphospholipid syndrome: a case report and review of the literature. *Hum Pathol* 1996;27:201–206.
20. Bittencourt AL, Garcia AG. The placenta in hematogenous infections. *Pediatr Pathol Mol Med* 2002;21(4):401–432.
21. Simpson RA, Mayhew TM, Barnes PR. From 13 weeks to term, the trophoblast of human placenta grows by the continuous recruitment of new proliferative units: a study of nuclear number using the dissector. *Placenta* 1992;13(5):501–512.
22. Mayhew TM, Barker BL. Villous trophoblast: morphometric perspectives on growth, differentiation, turnover and deposition of fibrin-type fibrinoid during gestation. *Placenta* 2001;22(7):628–638.
23. van Meir CA, Matthews SG, Keirse MJ, et al. 19-Hydroxyprostaglandin dehydrogenase: implications in preterm labor with and without ascending infection. *J Clin Endocrinol Metab* 1997;82(3):969–976.
24. Irani RA, Xia Y. The functional role of the Renin-Angiotensin system in pregnancy and preeclampsia. *Placenta* 2008;29(9):763–771.
25. Caniggia I, Winter J, Lye SJ, et al. Oxygen and placental development during the first trimester: implications for the pathophysiology of preeclampsia. *Placenta* 2000;21(Suppl A):S29–S30.
26. Levine RJ, Lam C, Qian C, et al. Soluble endoglin and other circulating antiangiogenic factors in preeclampsia. *N Engl J Med* 2006;355(10):992–1005.
27. Redline RW, Boyd T, Campbell V, et al. Maternal vascular underperfusion: nosology and reproducibility of placental reaction patterns. *Pediatr Dev Pathol* 2004;7:237–249.
28. Loukeris K, Sela R, Baergen RN. Syncytial knots as a reflection of placental maturity: reference values for 20 to 40 weeks' gestational age. *Pediatr Dev Pathol* 2010;13(4):305–309.
29. Arias F, Victorio A, Cho K, et al. Placental histology and clinical characteristics of patients with preterm premature rupture of membranes. *Obstet Gynecol* 1997;89:265–271.
30. De Wolf F, Brosens I, Renaer M. Fetal growth retardation and the maternal arterial supply of the human placenta in the absence of sustained hypertension. *Br J Obstet Gynaecol* 1980;87:678–684.
31. Redline RW, Ariel I, Baergen RN, et al. Fetal vascular obstructive lesions: nosology and reproducibility of placental reaction patterns. *Pediatr Dev Pathol* 2004;7:443–452.
32. Baergen RN, Malicki D, Behling C, et al. Morbidity, mortality, and placental pathology in excessively long umbilical cords: retrospective study. *Pediatr Dev Pathol* 2001;4(2):144–153.
33. Machin GA, Ackerman J, Gilbert-Barness E. Abnormal umbilical cord coiling is associated with adverse perinatal outcomes. *Pediatr Dev Pathol* 2000;3(5):462–471.
34. Oppenheimer EH, Esterly JR. Thrombosis in the newborn: comparison between infants of diabetic and nondiabetic mothers. *J Pediatr* 1965;67(4):549–556.
35. Vern TZ, Alles AJ, KowalVern A, et al. Frequency of factor V-Leiden and prothrombin G20210A in placentas and their relationship with placental lesions. *Hum Pathol* 2000;31(9):1036–1043.
36. Genest DR. Estimating the time of death in stillborn fetuses. 2. Histologic evaluation of the placenta—a study of 71 stillborns. *Obstet Gynecol* 1992;80(4):585–592.
37. Redline RW. Cerebral palsy in term infants: a clinicopathologic analysis of 158 medicolegal case reviews. *Pediatr Dev Pathol* 2008;11(6):456–464.
38. Saleemuddin A, Tantbirojn P, Sirois K, et al. Obstetric and perinatal complications in placentas with fetal thrombotic vasculopathy. *Pediatr Dev Pathol* 2010;13(6):459–464.
39. Dahms BB, Boyd T, Redline RW. Severe perinatal liver disease associated with fetal thrombotic vasculopathy. *Pediatr Dev Pathol* 2002;5(1):80–85.
40. Leistra-Leistra MJ, Timmer A, van Spronsen FJ, et al. Fetal thrombotic vasculopathy in the placenta: a thrombophilic connection between pregnancy complications and neonatal thrombosis? *Placenta* 2004;25(Suppl A):S102–S105.
41. Redline RW, Patterson P. Patterns of placental injury: correlations with gestational age, placental weight, and clinical diagnosis. *Arch Pathol Lab Med* 1994;118:698–701.
42. Knox WF, Fox H. Villitis of unknown aetiology: its incidence and significance in placentae from a British population. *Placenta* 1984;5:395–402.
43. Redline RW. Villitis of unknown etiology: noninfectious chronic villitis in the placenta. *Hum Pathol* 2007;38(10):1439–1446.
44. Katzman PJ, Murphy SP, Oble DA. Immunohistochemical analysis reveals an influx of regulatory T cells and focal trophoblastic STAT-1 phosphorylation in chronic villitis of unknown etiology. *Pediatr Dev Pathol* 2011;14(4):284–293.
45. Redline RW, Abramowsky CR. Clinical and pathologic aspects of recurrent placental villitis. *Hum Pathol* 1985;16:727–731.
46. Derricott H, Jones RL, Heazell AE. Investigating the association of villitis of unknown etiology with stillbirth and fetal growth restriction—a systematic review. *Placenta* 2013;34(10):856–862.
47. Redline RW. Severe fetal placental vascular lesions in term infants with neurologic impairment. *Am J Obstet Gynecol* 2005;192:452–457.
48. Styer AK, Parker HJ, Roberts DJ, et al. Placental villitis of unclear etiology during ovum donor in vitro fertilization pregnancy. *Am J Obstet Gynecol* 2003;189(4):1184–1186.
49. Redline R. Distal villous immaturity. *Diagn Histopathol* 2012;18(5):189–194.
50. Ogino S, Redline RW. Villous capillary lesions of the placenta: distinctions between chorangioma, chorangiomatosis, and chorangiosis. *Hum Pathol* 2000;31:945–954.
51. Pham T, Steele J, Stayboldt C, et al. Placental mesenchymal dysplasia is associated with high rates of intrauterine growth restriction and fetal demise: a report of 11 new cases and a review of the literature. *Am J Clin Pathol* 2006;126(1):67–78.
52. Kliman HJ, Segel L. The placenta may predict the baby. *J Theor Biol* 2003;225(1):143–145.
53. Dicke JM, Huettner P, Yan S, et al. Umbilical artery Doppler indices in small for gestational age fetuses: correlation with adverse outcomes and placental abnormalities. *J Ultrasound Med* 2009;28(12):1603–1610.

54. Stallmach T, Hebisch G, Meier K, et al. Rescue by birth: defective placental maturation and late fetal mortality. *Obstet Gynecol* 2001;97(4):505–509.
55. Altshuler G. Chorangiosis: an important placental sign of neonatal morbidity and mortality. *Arch Pathol Lab Med* 1984;108:71–74.
56. Soma H, Watanabe Y, Hata T. Chorangiosis and chorangioma in three cohorts of placentas from Nepal, Tibet and Japan. *Reprod Fertil Dev* 1996;7:1533–1538.
57. Benirschke K. Recent trends in chorangiomas, especially those of multiple and recurrent chorangiomas. *Pediatr Dev Pathol* 1999;2:264–269.
58. Goodfellow LR, Batra G, Hall V, et al. A case of confined placental mosaicism with double trisomy associated with stillbirth. *Placenta* 2011;32(9):699–703.
59. McCowan LM, Becroft DM. Beckwith-Wiedemann syndrome, placental abnormalities, and gestational proteinuric hypertension. *Obstet Gynecol* 1994;83(5 Pt 2):813–817.
60. Craven CM, Chedwick LR, Ward K. Placental basal plate formation is associated with fibrin deposition in decidual veins at sites of trophoblast cell invasion. *Am J Obstet Gynecol* 2002;186(2):291–296.
61. Pritchard JA, Mason R, Corley M, et al. Genesis of severe placental abruption. *Am J Obstet Gynecol* 1970;108:22–27.
62. Harris BA. Peripheral placental separation: a review. *Obstet Gynecol Surv* 1988;43:577–581.
63. Naftolin F, Khudr G, Benirschke K, et al. The syndrome of chronic abruptio placentae, hydrorrhea, and circumvallate placenta. *Am J Obstet Gynecol* 1973;116:347–350.
64. Redline RW, Wilson-Costello D. Chronic peripheral separation of placenta. The significance of diffuse chorioamnionic hemosiderosis. *Am J Clin Pathol* 1999;111(6):804–810.
65. Elliott JP, Gilpin B, Strong TH, Jr., et al. Chronic abruption-oligohydramnios sequence. *J Reprod Med* 1998;43(5):418–422.
66. Bey M, Dott A, Miller JM. The sonographic diagnosis of circumvallate placenta. *Obstet Gynecol* 1991;78:515–517.
67. Yoshida S, Kikuchi A, Sunagawa S, et al. Pregnancy complicated by diffuse chorioamniotic hemosiderosis: obstetric features and influence on respiratory diseases of the infant. *J Obstet Gynaecol Res* 2007;33(6):788–792.
68. Andres RL, Kuyper W, Resnik R, et al. The association of maternal floor infarction of the placenta with adverse perinatal outcome. *Am J Obstet Gynecol* 1990;163:935–938.
69. Becroft DM, Thompson JM, Mitchell EA. Placental infarcts, intervillous fibrin plaques, and intervillous thrombi: incidences, co-occurrences, and epidemiological associations. *Pediatr Dev Pathol* 2004;7(1):26–34.
70. Bendon RW, Hommel AB. Maternal floor infarction in autoimmune disease: two cases. *Pediatr Pathol Lab Med* 1996;16(2):293–297.
71. Katz VL, DiTomasso J, Farmer R, et al. Activated protein C resistance associated with maternal floor infarction treated with low-molecular-weight heparin. *Am J Perinatol* 2002;19(5):273–277.
72. Redline RW, Jiang JG, Shah D. Discordancy for maternal floor infarction in dizygotic twin placentas. *Hum Pathol* 2003;34(8):822–824.
73. Griffin AC, Strauss AW, Bennett MJ, et al. Mutations in long-chain 3-hydroxyacyl coenzyme a dehydrogenase are associated with placental maternal floor infarction/massive perivillous fibrin deposition. *Pediatr Dev Pathol* 2012;15(5):368–374.
74. Adams-Chapman I, Vaucher YE, Bejar RF, et al. Maternal floor infarction of the placenta: association with central nervous system injury and adverse neurodevelopmental outcome. *J Perinatol* 2002;22(3):236–241.
75. Bane AL, Gillan JE. Massive perivillous fibrinoid causing recurrent placental failure. *BJOG* 2003;110(3):292–295.
76. Mandsager NT, Bendon RW, Mostello D, et al. Maternal floor infarction of placenta: prenatal diagnosis and clinical significance. *Obstet Gynecol* 1994;83:750–754.
77. Goldenberg R, Hauth J, Andrews W. Intrauterine infection and preterm delivery. *N Engl J Med* 2000;342:1500–1507.
78. Redline RW, Faye-Petersen O, Heller D, et al. Amniotic infection syndrome: nosology and reproducibility of placental reaction patterns. *Pediatr Dev Pathol* 2003;6:435–448.
79. Mueller-Heubach E, Rubinstein DN, Schwarz SS. Histologic chorioamnionitis and preterm delivery in different patient populations. *Obstet Gynecol* 1990;75(4):622–626.
80. Gomez B, Romero R, Ghezzi F, et al. The fetal inflammatory response syndrome. *Am J Obstet Gynecol* 1998;179:194–202.
81. Altshuler G, Arizawa M, Molnar-Nadasdy G. Meconium-induced umbilical cord vascular necrosis and ulceration: a potential link between the placenta and poor pregnancy outcome. *Obstet Gynecol* 1992;79:760–766.
82. Miller PW, Coen RW, Benirschke K. Dating the time interval from meconium passage to birth. *Obstet Gynecol* 1985;66:459–462.
83. Myers RE. Four patterns of perinatal brain damage and their conditions of occurrence in primates. *Adv Neurol* 1975;10:223–234.
84. Naeye RL, Lin HM. Determination of the timing of fetal brain damage from hypoxemia-ischemia. *Am J Obstet Gynecol* 2001;184(2):217–224.
85. Redline RW. Elevated circulating fetal nucleated red blood cells and placental pathology in term infants who develop cerebral palsy. *Hum Pathol* 2008;39(9):1378–1384.
86. Blackwell SC, Hallak M, Hotra JW, et al. Timing of fetal nucleated red blood cell count elevation in response to acute hypoxia. *Biol Neonate* 2004;85(4):217–220.
87. Minior V, Levine B, Guller S, et al. Antenatal fetal hypoxemia gradually increases fetal nucleated red blood cells in a rat model. *Am J Obstet Gynecol* 2004;191:S168.
88. Soothill PW, Nicolaides KH, Campbell S. Prenatal asphyxia, hyperlacticaemia, hypoglycaemia, and erythroblastosis in growth retarded fetuses. *Br Med J* 1987;294:1051–1053.
89. Cohen MC, Peres LC, Al-Adnani M, et al. Increased number of fetal nucleated red blood cells in the placentas of term or near-term stillborn and neonates correlates with the presence of diffuse intradural hemorrhage in the perinatal period. *Pediatr Dev Pathol* 2014;17(1):1–9.
90. Faxelius G, Raye J, Gutberlet R, et al. Red cell volume measurements and acute blood loss in high-risk newborn infants. *J Pediatr* 1977;90(2):273–281.
91. Kaplan C, Blanc WA, Elias J. Identification of erythrocytes in intervillous thrombi: a study using immunoperoxidase identification of hemoglobins. *Hum Pathol* 1982;13:554–557.
92. Devi B, Jennison RF, Langley FA. Significance of placental pathology in transplacental haemorrhage. *J Clin Pathol* 1968;21(3):322–331.
93. Mooney EE, al Shunnar A, O'Regan M, et al. Chorionic villous haemorrhage is associated with retroplacental haemorrhage. *Br J Obstet Gynaecol* 1994;101(11):965–969.
94. Spellacy WN, Graven H, Fisch RO. The umbilical cord complications of true knots, nuchal coils and cords around the body. *Am J Obstet Gynecol* 1966;94:1136–1142.
95. Parast MM, Crum CP, Boyd TK. Placental histologic criteria for umbilical blood flow restriction in unexplained stillbirth. *Hum Pathol* 2008;39(6):948–953.
96. Martin GC, Green RS, Holzman IR. Acidosis in newborns with nuchal cords and normal Apgar scores. *J Perinatol* 2005;25(3):162–165.

CHAPTER 10
The Nervous System

Christopher Dunham, M.D., and Arie Perry, M.D.

GENERAL NEUROPATHOLOGIC PROCESSES AND PRINCIPLES

The practice of neuropathology demands an extensive knowledge of normal central nervous system (CNS) cytology and architecture, in addition to common artifacts. During development, the CNS (from fetal life and beyond) changes dramatically, especially in terms of histology, making pathologic assessments even more challenging. A full discussion of normal CNS histology and common artifacts is beyond the scope of this text. Some of the more common neuropathologic changes and pathophysiologic processes are introduced below.

The CNS contains a variety of neurons, which vary in size from the small neocortical granular (stellate) neurons (<15 μm) to the large neocortical pyramidal neurons (measuring from 10 to 100 μm for the Betz cells of the primary motor cortex). Pyramidal neurons are often considered the morphologic prototype that bears ample lightly basophilic cytoplasm, darker clumpy Nissl substance, a large central nucleus, a prominent nucleolus (the "owl's eye"), and coarse cytoplasmic processes. Neocortical neurons exhibit a prominent apical dendrite oriented perpendicular to the cortical surface. Neurons may display several different cytologic abnormalities, some of which are specific, but others may be nonspecific and thus requiring interpretation in the correct clinicopathologic context. *Acutely necrotic neurons* (i.e., "dead") are a form of nonspecific change that contain two essential components: (a) shrunken pyknotic angular nuclei and (b) cytoplasmic eosinophilia ("red is dead") (Figure 10-1A). Although commonly caused by ischemia (and hence often referred to as ischemic neurons), any process that causes acute neuronal death may lead to the formation of such neurons (e.g., hypoxia, hypoglycemia, carbon monoxide, epilepsy, herpes simplex virus [HSV] encephalitis). Acute neuronal death is much more difficult to appreciate in fetal brains that contain a predominance of primitive neurons (small dark nuclei with little cytoplasm); in such cases, nuclear fragmentation or karyorrhexis (at times in keeping with apoptosis) can be appreciated on high magnification (Figure 10-1B). A large variety of *neuronal inclusions* may be seen, including both intranuclear and intracytoplasmic types. These inclusions vary tremendously in color, size, and shape, from essentially rounded and eosinophilic/basophilic to more fibrillar (e.g., neurofibrillary tangle). These inclusions are commonly seen in viral and neurodegenerative/metabolic diseases. Abnormal vacuolization of the cytoplasm can be seen and may correlate with swelling of ultrastructural elements (e.g., mitochondria). Vacuolization that seemingly occurs within the neuropil (the meshwork of neuronal processes among which all the cell bodies of the neocortex reside) may be a result of neuronal loss, edema, or the expansion of neuronal processes (which occurs with the prion diseases or "spongiform" encephalopathies) or may be artifactual in nature. Some damaged neurons, for instance, those near infarction, may undergo mineralization (i.e., ferruginization). Damage to the axon can also lead to several cytologic alterations. Disruption of the axon may result in chromatolytic changes that include swelling of the soma, dispersion of the Nissl substance, eccentric displacement of the nucleus, and accumulation of cytoskeletal filaments. This latter event results in axonal spheroids (i.e., swellings) that can be highlighted with immunohistochemical (IHC) stains (e.g., β-amyloid precursor protein [β-APP]) (Figure 10-2). The distally transected portion of the axon degenerates and initially forms ovoids that are later taken up by macrophages, which serve to localize areas of degeneration (1). Somewhat more fusiform axonal spheroids known as "torpedoes" are commonly found in the upper cerebellar cortex and reflect Purkinje cell damage.

Normal astrocytes are situated throughout the gray (protoplasmic astrocytes) and white (fibrillary astrocytes) matter. For the most part, these astrocytes partake in their physiologic functions rather inconspicuously. However, in response to almost any insult, these cells undergo proliferation (i.e., hyperplasia) and enlargement (i.e., hypertrophy) termed reactive *astrocytosis or gliosis*, which has been equated to the "scar tissue" of the CNS (notably, the few perivascular and meningeal fibroblasts in the CNS only rarely participate to form true collagen-rich scars as seen elsewhere in the body; e.g., organizing CNS abscesses). The normally inapparent cytoplasmic processes of astrocytes (by routine H&E staining)

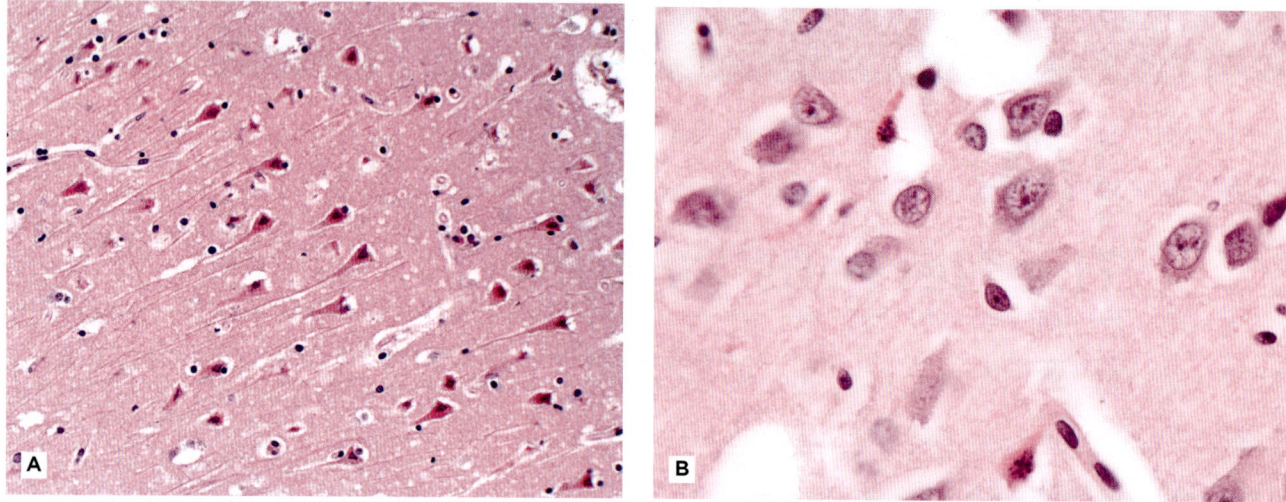

FIGURE 10-1 • Acutely "necrotic" or dead neurons. **A:** Adult. **B:** Premature infant. Note the nuclear fragmentation (i.e., karyorrhexis) and eosinophilic cytoplasm in two shrunken subicular neurons.

accumulate intermediate glial fibrillary acid protein (GFAP) filaments after stimulation and thus take on a starburst-like pattern (Figure 10-3). In contrast to astrocytic neoplasms, these reactive astrocytes are typically distributed evenly throughout the parenchyma. *Myelination glia* (an oligodendrocyte precursor) are a notable pitfall to the determination of gliosis in the newborn; these glia also display relatively abundant eosinophilic cytoplasm, but they are a normal finding in the actively myelinating nervous system. Although their distinction from gliosis is often difficult, myelination glia often display hyperchromatic small round nuclei associated with cytoplasm that is shaped like a comet (2). In the more chronic stages of gliosis, the cytoplasmic processes of astrocytes retract and become less obvious on routine staining, although their nuclei remain in increased number and continue to mark areas of prior damage. Gliosis occurring in the cerebellar cortex in response to Purkinje cell loss is termed *Bergmann gliosis*, which is characterized by parallel fibrillary processes radiating through the molecular layer toward the pial surface and the accumulation of astrocytic nuclei within the Purkinje layer. The somewhat nonspecific form of gliosis that occurs immediately under the neocortical pia mater is called *Chaslin gliosis*, a reaction that is often attributed to previous seizure activity. Occasionally found within these areas of long-standing gliosis are the brightly eosinophilic corkscrew-shaped structures termed *Rosenthal fibers* (RFs) and less often *eosinophilic granular bodies* (EGBs); however, these structures are also seen in a variety of neoplastic (e.g., pilocytic astrocytoma [PA]) and nonneoplastic (i.e., Alexander disease) conditions (Figure 10-4). RFs have a characteristic ultrastructural appearance, manifesting as an electron-dense core surrounded by fibrillary material. An entirely nonspecific but characteristic astrocytic reaction occurs in abnormal physiologic states often associated with hyperammonemia; under these conditions, *Alzheimer-type II astrocytes* (of no relation to Alzheimer disease) accumulate,

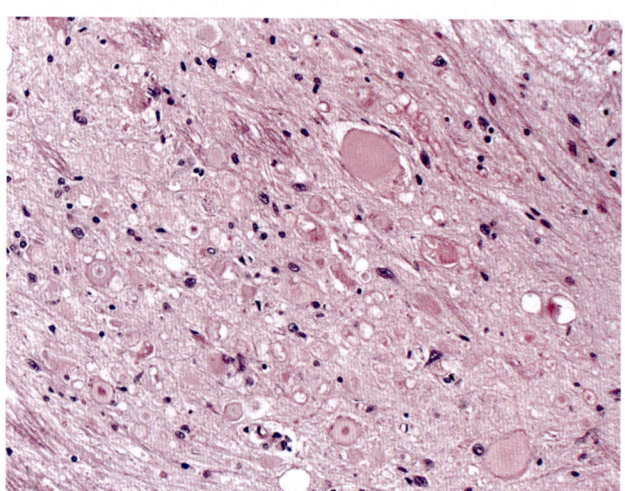

FIGURE 10-2 • Axonal spheroids from a case of infantile neuroaxonal dystrophy (i.e., Seitelberger disease).

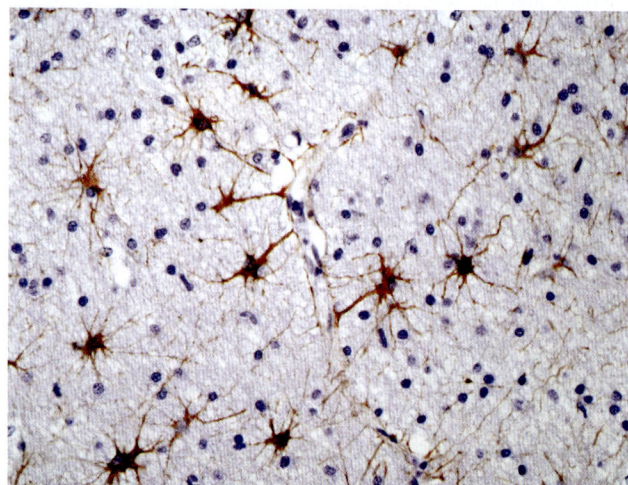

FIGURE 10-3 • Reactive gliosis (Glial fibrillary acidic protein immunohistochemistry (IHC)).

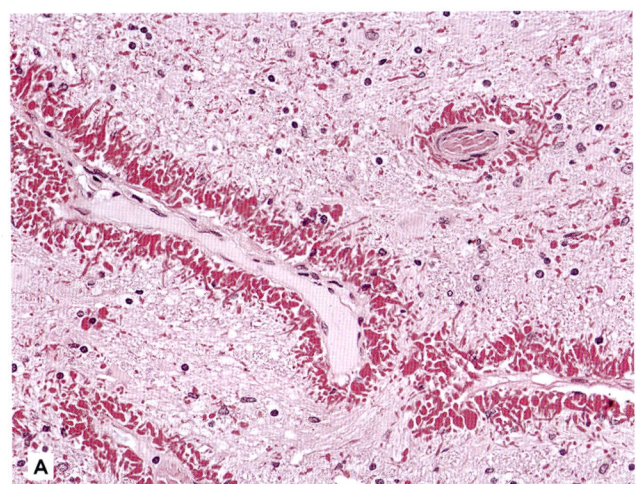 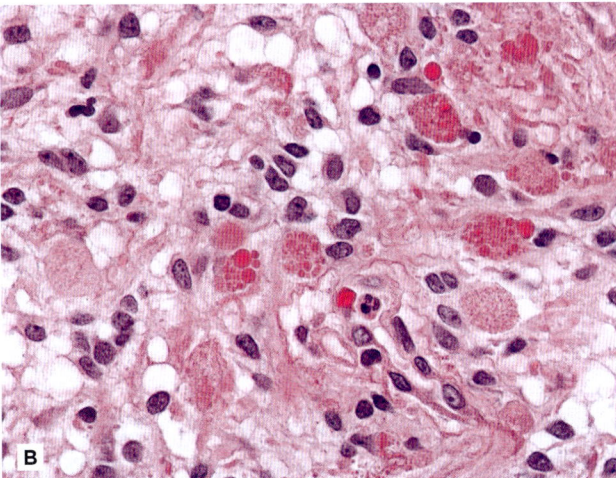

FIGURE 10-4 • Rosenthal fibers and eosinophilic granular bodies are nonspecific eosinophilic structures that are most commonly seen in the context of long-standing gliosis or within low-grade primary brain neoplasms. **A:** Perivascular accumulation of RFs in this case of Alexander disease. **B:** EGBs within the microcystic component of a pilocytic astrocytoma.

particularly in the basal ganglia and deep layers of the neocortex. These astrocytes, often seen in pairs, exhibit inconspicuous cytoplasm, enlarged pale nuclei, and occasionally a prominent nucleolus. Astrocytes may bear inclusions, both cytoplasmic and nuclear, although these are often difficult to appreciate on routine stains, necessitating the use of special stains and IHC for their detection.

Normal oligodendroglia inconspicuously fulfill their metabolic roles (most importantly myelination) from a histologic point of view. As opposed to astrocytes, the spectrum of pathology occurring in oligodendroglia is much more restricted. By routine staining, the delicate processes of normal oligodendroglia are inconspicuous, while their hyperchromatic, round regular nuclei are sometimes surrounded by small clear haloes representing a retraction artifact of formalin fixation. As may be predicted, insults affecting oligodendroglia result in demyelination (i.e., myelin loss), which can be elucidated with myelin special stains (e.g., Luxol fast blue [LFB]). Usually, there is concomitant oligodendroglial dropout and astrocytic gliosis. Some pathologic processes cause myelin to separate between its layers, resulting in intramyelinic splitting, which manifests as vacuolar change in the white matter on light microscopy. Like astrocytes, oligodendroglia may bear abnormal nuclear (e.g., progressive multifocal leukoencephalopathy [PML]) or cytoplasmic (e.g., multiple system atrophy [MSA]) inclusions, the latter of which usually require special/IHC stains for their detection. The normally subtle cytoplasm of oligodendroglia may become more conspicuous when they suffer cytotoxic insults (e.g., ischemia).

Pathologic reactions of the ventricular lining cells, or ependyma, are generally very limited and nonspecific. These normally columnar to cuboidal cells form a simple (i.e., single layered) epithelium. With hydrocephalus (HCP) or cerebral atrophy, the epithelium stretches and becomes atrophic, or even discontinuous. Soon after acute injury, subependymal astrocytes proliferate and produce nodular excrescences that protrude into the ventricular cavity. Although previously termed *granular ependymitis*, this nonspecific pathologic reaction is not always related to an underlying inflammatory process; as such, the terms subventricular gliosis or ependymal granulations are preferable. If exuberant, this gliosis may entrap portions of ependyma resulting in subependymal rosettes/tubules. As with the other cellular elements of the CNS, residual ependymal cells may bear inclusions, usually of viral etiology (e.g. cytomegalovirus [CMV]).

Microglial reactions are unique to the CNS. *Microglia* are inflammatory and antigen-presenting cells derived from bone marrow monocytes. The nuclei and cytoplasmic processes of these parenchymal cells often blend imperceptibly into the normal CNS tissue. Generally, they are of two types: (a) *resident microglia* are those that reside within the neuropil (and also the perivascular space) and do not undergo significant turnover with hematogenous monocytes and (b) *perivascular microglia*, whose population is continually renewed via hematogenous monocytes (2). Activated microglia have also been termed *rod cells* since, after parenchymal insult, their presence is heralded by a proliferation of small elongate naked-appearing nuclei. After CNS damage, perivascular microglia phagocytose necrotic debris and accordingly accumulate lipid material, which distends their cytoplasm yielding a foamy appearance. In contrast, resident microglia are stimulated by smaller degrees of parenchymal damage (e.g., individual neuronal necrosis), with two basic pathologic patterns seen. First, there may be a diffuse microglial activation, wherein rod cells are evenly distributed throughout the diseased tissue; some have termed this uniquely CNS reaction "neuroinflammation" (3) (Figure 10-5A). Second, and often associated with viral encephalitides, are *microglial nodules*, which are roughly spherical aggregates of microglia (Figure 10-5B). Microglia may also surround and digest dying neurons, a process termed *neuronophagia*.

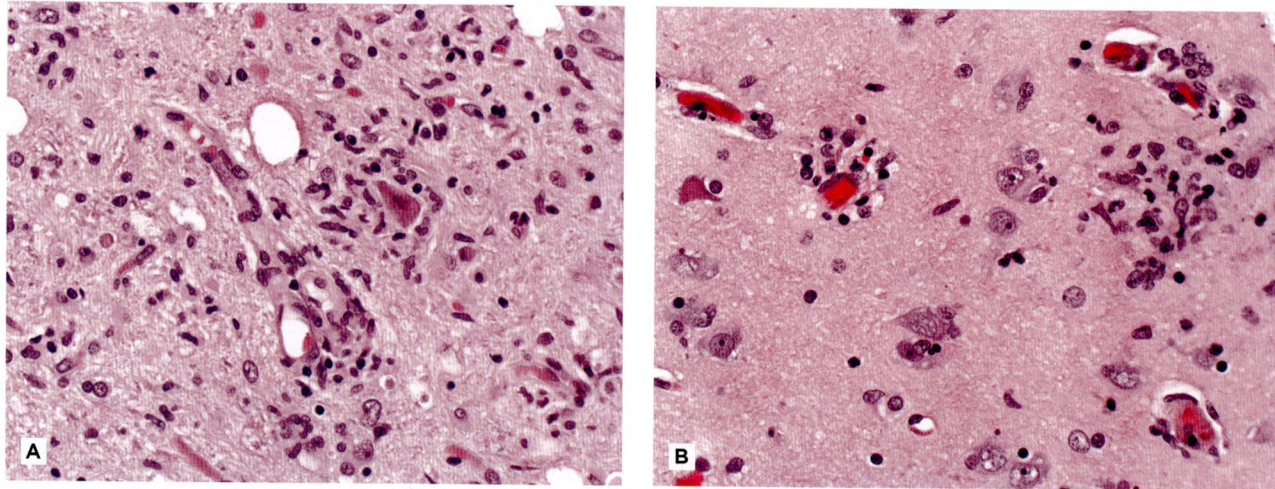

FIGURE 10-5 • Activated microglia. **A:** Neuronophagia is seen within this diffuse microgliosis. **B:** In addition to some perivascular lymphocytes, a microglial nodule is seen toward the right side of the figure.

Increased Intracranial Pressure, Edema, and Hydrocephalus

Once the cranial sutures fuse early in postnatal life, the skull essentially acts as a rigid closed box, the contents of which include brain parenchyma, blood, and cerebrospinal fluid (CSF). A mature brain (approximately 1400 g) contains 75 mL each of blood and CSF (*Note*: a term brain weighs approximately 300 to 350 g). This CSF results in a normal intracranial pressure (ICP) of 15 mm Hg. The cerebral perfusion pressure (CPP) equals the mean arterial pressure minus the ICP. Cerebral blood flow (CBF), which for the brain is normally 50 mL/100 g/min, is calculated by dividing CPP by resistance (i.e., the vasculature). Through *autoregulation*, the CBF is kept constant despite changes in the systemic blood pressure. Notably, the autoregulatory capabilities of the prenatal cerebral vasculature are poor, making the brain vulnerable to fluctuations in blood pressure. When a mass-forming disease process increases the intracranial contents and elevates ICP (e.g., brain tumor), the brain compensates by expelling contents from the "closed box" so as to maintain the CBF at near normal levels. CSF leaves the cranial cavity first, and once autoregulatory mechanisms fail, blood is expelled (i.e., global ischemia), and then finally brain tissue (i.e., cerebral herniation). Several dural folds exist in the cranial cavity (e.g., cerebral falx, tentorium) and effectively serve to compartmentalize the brain. However, these extremely tough pieces of connective tissue are unyielding in the setting of increased ICP. In response to a mass lesion, brain tissue will shift or herniate from one compartment to the next, resulting in tissue damage (including contusion). Subfalcine, transtentorial (i.e., uncal), and tonsillar herniations are the most important forms, with the latter often being fatal due to compression of nearby cardiorespiratory centers in the medulla (1).

Cerebral edema is a local or generalized accumulation of fluid within the brain parenchyma that can result in increased ICP. If severe, cerebral edema may result in herniation. There are three main types of cerebral edema: (a) vasogenic, (b) cytotoxic, and (c) hydrocephalic. The *blood–brain barrier* (BBB) results from the specialized properties of the endothelial cells, their intercellular junctions, and a relative lack of vesicular transport (4). Breakdown of the BBB results in *vasogenic* cerebral edema. This type of cerebral edema is often seen in the context of CNS neoplasia and is responsive to steroid therapy. *Cytotoxic* cerebral edema refers to the intracellular swelling that occurs in neurons, glia, and endothelial cells. It results from failure of the ATP-dependent Na^+/K^+ pump and subsequent osmotic accumulation of intracellular fluids. Cytotoxic cerebral edema occurs after hypoxia, or more commonly with global ischemia due to cardiac arrest. *Hydrocephalic* cerebral edema is the result of transependymal CSF accumulation. Both vasogenic and hydrocephalic cerebral edema are elucidated by hyperintense signals seen on T2-weighted MRI and fluid-attenuated inversion recovery (FLAIR) sequences. Notably, these forms of cerebral edema are not mutually exclusive and often occur simultaneously. Grossly, the edematous brain exhibits congestion, with flattening of gyri and narrowing of sulci. There may be evidence of cerebral herniation (see above) manifesting as areas of necrosis and hemorrhage. Certain types of herniation routinely cause compression of large arteries and hence infarction (e.g., uncal herniation with posterior cerebral artery compression and primary occipital lobe infarction). On coronal sectioning, the ventricles are collapsed from surrounding pressure and appear slit like. By histology, the parenchyma is pale and vacuolated.

Hydrocephalus (HCP) refers to the accumulation of excess CSF and concurrent expansion of the cerebral ventricles (Figure 10-6). CSF can accumulate under normal ICP, usually in the context of cerebral atrophy; this is called HCP *ex vacuo*. Conventional HCP occurs under the pressure of excess CSF, usually resulting from a paucity of CSF absorption but also more uncommonly from abnormal CSF production (e.g., from a choroid plexus papilloma [CPP]).

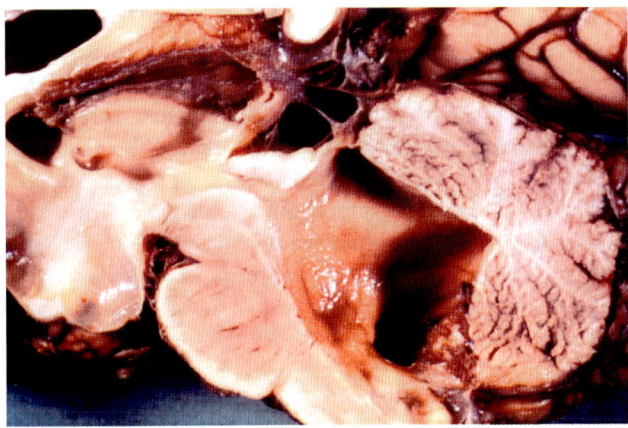

FIGURE 10-6 • Hydrocephalus. There is marked dilatation proximal to and including the fourth ventricle in this sagittally sectioned autopsy of the brain, which also exhibited evidence of meningitis.

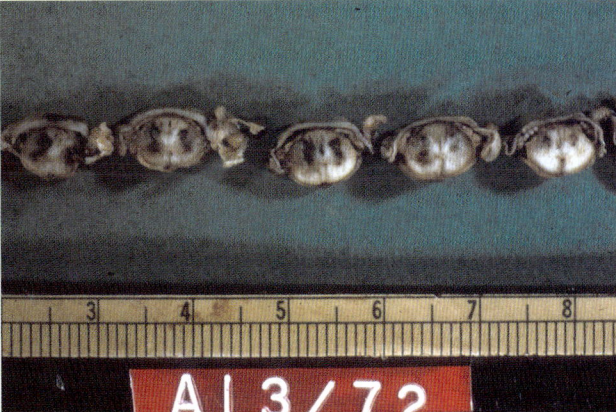

FIGURE 10-7 • Laceration and intraparenchymal hemorrhage within the spinal cord secondary to a complicated breech delivery seen here in cross sections of the spinal cord.

HCP due to impaired resorption can be *communicating* or *noncommunicating*, with the former resulting from a lack of arachnoid granulation–mediated CSF uptake, and the latter being caused by an obstruction in the ventricular system. Communicating HCP is often a result of meningitis or subarachnoid hemorrhage (SAH), while more rare causes include arachnoid villi aplasia or dural venous sinus obstruction. Noncommunicating HCP may be primary (i.e., congenital) or secondary (i.e., acquired). Primary causes include aqueductal stenosis (e.g., related to gliosis, atresia/forking, or an obstructing septum) and X-linked HCP (caused by mutations in the *L1CAM* gene on Xq28). Secondary causes include tumor, hemorrhage, or infection. Several structural CNS abnormalities may exhibit concurrent HCP (e.g., holoprosencephaly [HPE]) of unknown pathogenesis, and some suggest that the nonspecific term ventriculomegaly may be more appropriate in these cases.

TRAUMA

Birth

Various craniospinal injuries may be mechanically incurred at birth. A number of extracranial hemorrhages may occur within the scalp whose layers can be remembered via the mnemonic "scalp" (*s*kin, *c*onnective tissue, *a*poneurosis epicranialis or galea, *l*oose connective tissue, *p*eriosteum). Hemorrhage into the subcutaneous connective tissue is called *caput succedaneum*. There may be subgaleal bleeding and subperiosteal hemorrhage (i.e., *cephalhematoma*) that often occur over the parietal bone, which may be attributable to forceps delivery. Usually, these hemorrhages resolve after a few weeks or months. Perinatal skull fractures are also frequently parietal in location and often linear in quality. Depressed skull fractures tend to be more common in children over 2 years of age. Separation of the squamous and lateral aspects of the occipital bone is called *occipital osteodiastasis*, and this may result in contusion of the cerebellum and posterior fossa subdural hemorrhage (SDH) (5). Epidural hemorrhage is less common than SDH and SAH. A cerebral contusion with subsequent evolution to intracerebral/intraventricular hemorrhage (ICH/IVH) is rare. However, white matter tears that are potentially hemorrhagic (i.e., gliding or internal contusions) may be seen in young infants and are thought to arise from shearing forces between the gray and white matter.

The spinal cord may absorb tractional or rotational forces at the time of birth. Breech and cephalic deliveries typically result in upper thoracic/low cervical and midcervical damage, respectively. Large forces can result in laceration (i.e., tearing) of the parenchyma (Figure 10-7). Petechial hemorrhages and axonal spheroids may be seen microscopically. Clinical outcome is variable; there may be acute respiratory failure and death or, in those survivors who are initially hypotonic, spasticity. The brachial plexus may be injured via tractional forces at the time of delivery. Damage to the C5-6 roots results in shoulder deficits (i.e., Erb paralysis), whereas the wrist and digits are affected with C8-T1 insult (Klumpke paralysis). Simplistically, surgical repair involves resection of the resultant traumatic neuroma with anastomosis of more normal proximal and distal nerve stumps; frozen section assessment of the degree of nerve stump viability may be requested intraoperatively.

Infancy and Childhood

Pediatric patients may suffer from both accidental and nonaccidental (i.e., inflicted or abusive) injury. Motor vehicle accidents (MVAs), falls, and assaults are the leading causes of pediatric neurotrauma. The neuropathology of severe or fatal head injury in children older than 1 year is very similar to that seen in adults (1). Infants less than 1 year old suffer a different pattern of injuries, which is thought to be related to the unique and immature anatomic features seen at this age (6). These include a highly deformable skull, unfused cranial sutures, a high head-to-body ratio, an elastic spinal column with immature joints, reduced neck muscle tone, and a relatively unmyelinated brain. Accordingly, the cause of death in fatal infant craniospinal injury is often related to cerebral edema, secondary to hypoxia–ischemia. The craniocervical junction is particularly vulnerable and damage to vital brainstem cardiorespiratory centers may account for the frequent clinical presentation of apnea (6). SDH may be seen and is typically thin and bilateral (see below).

Inflicted Injury in Infants

The pathogenesis of fatally inflicted CNS injury among infants is controversial. Several terms have been used to describe the classic pattern injuries and circumstances, the most common of which is likely "shaken baby syndrome." Many disfavor the use of this term since it implies knowledge of the mechanisms surrounding injury; hence, the term "inflicted injury" or "nonaccidental injury" is preferred. Infants suffering from inflicted injury often present clinically in a moribund state with respiratory distress or apnea. There may be lethargy, irritation, poor feeding, vomiting, and seizures. Fundoscopy may reveal retinal hemorrhages, and CT/MRI often reveals cerebral swelling and a diffuse thin layer of subarachnoid blood. In addition to inflicted mechanisms, this clinical feature may be mimicked by other etiologic entities, including MVAs, vasculopathies/coagulopathies, infection, dehydration, and metabolic abnormalities; hence, a thorough forensic-based investigation of these cases may be required (see Chapter 7).

Autopsy of an infant with inflicted injury needs to be meticulous since many findings may be subtle. Extracranial injuries may include rib and long bone fractures, which may be more conspicuous in older children. A variety of cranial fractures and hemorrhages is somewhat characteristic but nevertheless nonspecific in isolation. Skull fractures are relatively common in infants despite the inherent deformability of these bones at this age. Fractures tend to be linear and may result in dural tears and resultant CSF leaks (e.g., rhinorrhea, otorrhea). *Growing fractures* occur when a portion of the leptomeninges herniates through the dural defect and intercede between the two sides of a bony interruption; with time, CSF accumulates in a cyst-like space and erodes bone, thus preventing proper healing. In general, skull fractures are most often parieto-occipital. Several different types of hemorrhage may also be incurred. *Epidural hemorrhage* occurs between the outer surface of the dura and the adjacent skull. It is uncommon in infants, possibly because the dura is tightly adherent to the skull, and since the middle meningeal artery is more easily displaced than torn (6). *SDH* is common yet different than the space-occupying variety seen in older children and adults. They are thin and bilateral and are often described as "trivial." Accordingly, infant SDHs are not thought to be due to the tearing of bridging veins, and they tend to be accompanied by retinal hemorrhages (which are somewhat nonspecific). SAH and IVHs are generally negligible. *Cerebral contusions* are essentially "brain bruises," which manifest as areas of parenchymal hemorrhage and necrosis among the crests of gyri. Acutely, the hemorrhage of contusions is perivascular and oriented perpendicular to the cortical surface. Although they may be seen beneath skull fractures, contusions are generally uncommon. Cerebral edema is often the immediate cause of death and is related to global hypoxic–ischemic injury. As mentioned above, the craniocervical junction is particularly susceptible to injury, especially that which is related to stretch. Careful dissection of the cervical paraspinal muscles may reveal soft tissue hemorrhage. Spinal epidural hemorrhage may be seen but must be cautiously interpreted since this can be artifactually induced. When the craniocervical region suffers from severe hyperextension injury, *pontomedullary rents* (or tears) may be identified. If the injured infant survives but dies later on, signs of cerebral atrophy in keeping with hypoxic–ischemic encephalopathy (HIE) may be seen.

Although *diffuse axonal injury* (DAI) was previously purported to be the underlying neuropathology in infant-inflicted injury, it is only identified in rare cases As opposed to DAI, the axonal damage in infant-inflicted injury is localized often to the lower pons and upper medulla and particularly to descending corticospinal tracts (7). In addition, axonal damage may be apparent in the cervical and other spinal roots (8). Axonal spheroids can be seen on routine stains about 24 hours after injury, but IHC staining for β-APP can highlight microscopic axonal damage 2 hours or less after injury (9). The lysosomal marker, CD68, is often used to label microglia and may be used to highlight the acute and more remote cellular reactions to axonal damage. HIE is frequent and is seen more diffusely throughout the brain; usually, HIE is the most prominent finding in cases of infant-inflicted injury. Early features include acute neuronal necrosis, parenchymal vacuolation, microglial activation, and myelin pallor, whereas in chronic stages, parenchymal rarefaction predominates with neuronal loss and gliosis.

SUDDEN INFANT DEATH SYNDROME

Sudden infant death syndrome (SIDS) is a complex multifactorial disorder. SIDS is generally defined as the sudden unexpected death of an infant (<1 year in age) that often occurs during sleep and for which no cause of death is identified despite thorough history, death scene investigation, and autopsy. Numerous factors are associated with SIDS, but the role to which each impacts this disorder remains elusive. Many of these factors are hypothesized in terms of their effect on the infant's innate autonomic physiologic response to normal homeostatic stressors (e.g., apnea, hypercarbia/blood pH, hypotension). These infant responses are largely mediated by brainstem nuclei. Maternal factors increasing the risk of SIDS include low socioeconomic status, low maternal education, cigarette smoking, and alcohol consumption. These maternal factors may play a role in predisposing the embryo/infant to hypoxic–ischemic damage (e.g., periventricular leukomalacia [PVL]) or brainstem abnormalities, which can be seen pathologically in a subset of SIDS cases (10); notably, the histopathologic changes seen in SIDS cases are often inconspicuous. Cerebellar and more so medullary abnormalities have been hypothesized. Derivatives of the rhombic lip (e.g., external granule layer [EGL] of the cerebellum, the inferior olive, and the arcuate nucleus) have also been implicated in SIDS. More recently, focus has been directed toward possible abnormalities in the medullary serotonergic (5HT) nuclei, as championed by Hannah Kinney and colleagues (11,12). These nuclei have been suggested to normally modulate and integrate autonomic, respiratory, and somatomotor responses to homeostatic stressors; in particular, lowered 5HT receptor binding has been demonstrated in the arcuate nucleus (13). Susceptibility genes have been proposed, as evidenced by the detection of polymorphisms in the promoter regions/coding sequences; candidate genes include the 5HT transporter, IL-10, and heat shock protein 60 (6). Rare SIDS-like cases have even been associated with cardiac sodium channel mutations (causing arrhythmias) and inborn errors of metabolism (especially medium chain acetyl-CoA dehydrogenase deficiency). In addition to its association with sleep, death in SIDS is often associated with the prone position. Integration and synthesis of these factors have led to the *triple-risk model* of SIDS (14). This model proposes that there are three key factors leading to infant death when present simultaneously: (a) a vulnerable infant (i.e., those with pathophysiologic abnormalities), (b) a critical period of development (the peak incidence of SIDS cases occurs at 2 to 4 months and may be related to brain maturation), and (c) an exogenous stressor (e.g., prone sleeping). As researchers continue to unravel the mysteries of this disorder, management and minimization of these recognizable risk factors are the best means of preventing this devastating syndrome (see Chapter 7).

STRUCTURAL MALFORMATIONS OF THE CNS

Neural Tube Defects, Axial Mesodermal Defects, and Tail Bud Defects

Classic embryology describes three primitive germ layers: endoderm, mesoderm, and ectoderm. Near 16 days postovulation, the mesodermally derived notochord induces the development of CNS tissue from the overlying ectoderm; the signaling molecule sonic hedgehog (Shh) is important to this process. This newly formed neuroectoderm first thickens into the neural plate. A longitudinal neural groove then develops, and subsequently at 18 to 20 days postovulation, neural folds arise from the lateral aspects of the plate. The neural crest (the forerunner of the spinal, cranial nerve and autonomic ganglia, leptomeninges, Schwann cells, melanocytes, and other tissues) originates from the apices of these folds, which eventually meet at distinct closure sites in the midline to form the neural tube. In humans, two initial closure sites are well recognized, one (site 1) at the cervical–occipital boundary (on day 22 postfertilization) and a second (site 2) at the extreme rostral end of the neural plate. A third closure site at the forebrain–midbrain boundary may also exist. Fusion of the neural fold proceeds bidirectionally from site 1 and caudally from site 2. Fusion of the cranial portion of the neural tube is completed at the anterior neuropore (24 days postfertilization), which subsequently develops into the lamina terminalis. The caudal aspect of the neural tube finishes closure at the posterior neuropore (28 days postfertilization). In general, the process of neural tube formation is called neurulation and is divided into two aspects: (a) primary neurulation describes the fusion of neural folds, which form the rostral aspects of the CNS, and (b) secondary neurulation describes the formation of the caudal-most neural tube (i.e., lumbosacral spinal cord) that occurs through canalization of a solid mass of cells. Primary and secondary neurulated tissues eventually join to form the complete neural tube. After neural tube formation, the axial skeleton begins its development and eventually encases the maturing CNS. The skull has a dual origin: the cranial vault and occiput develop from axial mesoderm (endochondral bone formation), while the skull base and facial bones arise from the cranial neural crest (membranous bone). The vertebrae also arise from the axial mesoderm.

Neural Tube Defects

Neural tube defects (NTDs) are the result of defective neural tube closure during the 3rd to 4th week of gestational age (GA). The true incidence of NTD is difficult to determine since severe forms lead to spontaneous abortion. Birth prevalence has been estimated to be between 3/1000 and 7/1000 depending on several factors, including geography (e.g., high prevalence in Northern Ireland) (15). There is a spectrum of CNS involvement, from widespread (e.g., complete craniorachischisis) to more focal (e.g., lumbosacral myelomeningocele). Patients with focal spinal forms may survive with motor and sensory deficits below the level of nonclosure, which include rectal and urinary sphincter involvement (e.g., incontinence, urinary tract infections). Additional problems may include HCP, Chiari II malformation, and kyphosis. Although the use of folic acid supplements has reduced the frequency of NTDs, the therapeutic mechanism remains unclear. *Craniorachischisis* is the most severe form of NTD wherein there is complete failure of neural tube closure such that the brain and spinal cord are exposed to the amniotic fluid. There may be some forebrain development rostrally, but neural tube closure is usually deficient distal to the midbrain. In *anencephaly*, which is now usually encountered near midgestation after termination of pregnancy, the defective neural tube is generally limited to the cranial and cervical regions (Figure 10-8A). The skull vault is absent, the skull base is malformed (thick and flat anomalous sphenoid bones), and the orbits are shallow. The majority of the brain (minus portions of the anterior pituitary, cranial nerves, medulla, and some cerebellar folia) is replaced by the *area cerebrovasculosa*. This CSF-filled cystic angiomatous area contains neuroglial-derived tissues (including ependyma, neurons, neuroblasts, and choroid plexus) and numerous thin-walled, closely packed, and congested blood vessels. Contrary to most descriptions

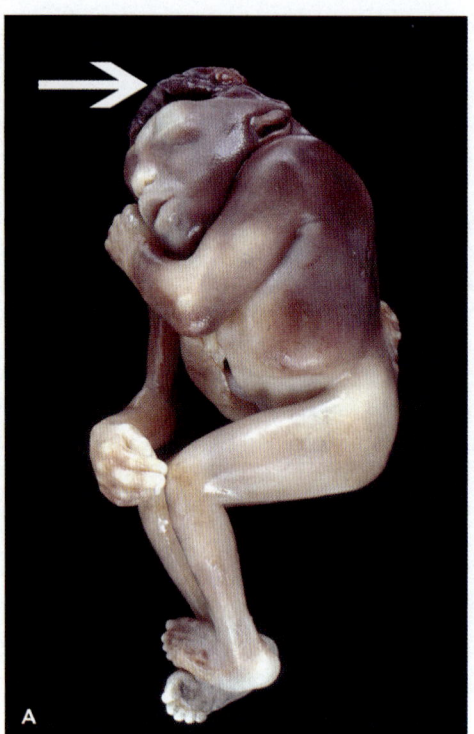
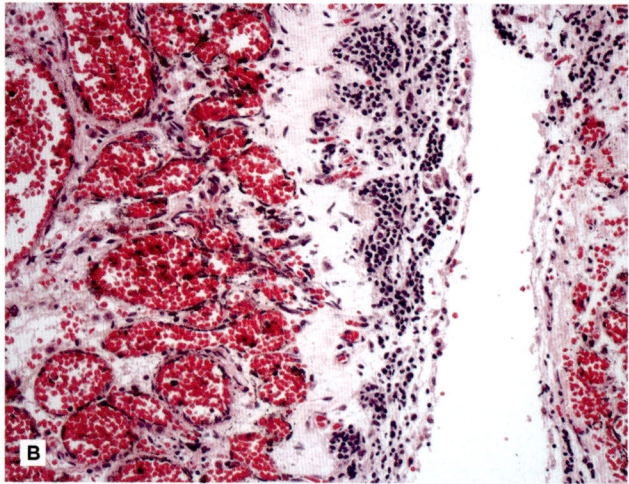

FIGURE 10-8 • Anencephaly. **A:** Because of the absent calvarium (or "skull cap"), malformed vascularized neuroglial tissue (i.e., area cerebrovasculosa) can be directly visualized (see *arrow*). **B:** Microscopically, the area cerebrovasculosa usually displays a very organized layered architecture, with a superficial primitive neural layer and a subjacent vascular layer (H&E, 200×).

that describe disorganization, the neuroglial and vascular components of the area cerebrovasculosa are usually quite organized across cases and produce a laminar structure; the neuroglial tissue, which often has a nodular substructure, forms a layer that is usually more superficially situated than the vascular layer (Figure 10-8B). Occasionally, a third layer composed of macrophages is seen actively breaking down the primitive neural tissue. Atrophic, keratinizing, squamous epithelium that is continuous with normal skin covers the defect. Due to the deficiency of cerebral tissue, there is a paucity of descending spinal cord tracts. Overlying spinal leptomeninges are vascular and may contain glioneuronal heterotopias (6). Associated non-CNS abnormalities include hypoplastic adrenals and lungs, plus an enlarged thymus (16). *Myelomeningoceles* can occur throughout the spinal cord, but those affecting the lumbosacral region are the most frequent (Figure 10-9). An association with the Chiari II malformation is frequently appreciated in those cases with lumbosacral myelomeningoceles, prenatal surgical closure of which has been shown to mitigate clinical sequelae (17). The spinal cord may be "closed" (i.e., no NTD *per se*) or "open" posteriorly as a flattened lesion. Closed lesions are cystic and covered by a delicate membrane/skin that contains a hydromyelic cord. Open lesions contain a vascularized mass of disorganized neuroglial tissue called the *area medullovasculosa* that is covered by atrophic cutaneous tissue. In either case, the spinal cord and meninges herniate through an associated vertebral

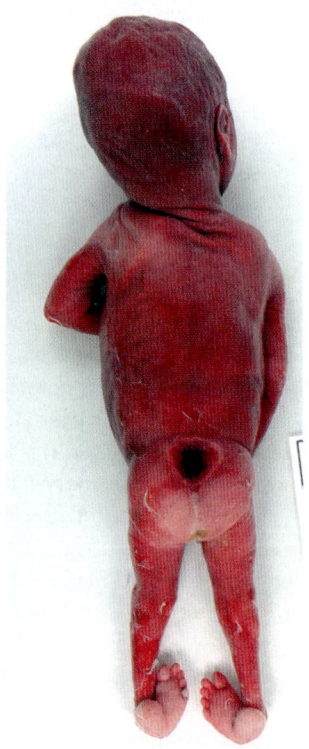

FIGURE 10-9 • Lumbosacral myelomeningocele, 23 weeks gestational age. This NTD was associated with Chiari II type changes in the brain. In passing, note the clubbed foot deformity.

defect. There may be additional spinal cord abnormalities above the NTD (e.g., hydromyelia, syringomyelia, and diplomyelia).

Herniation Through Axial Mesodermal Defects

Portions of CNS tissue (with proper neural tube closure) may herniate through axial mesodermal (i.e., bony) defects. These include encephaloceles and meningoceles. *Encephaloceles* may be anteriorly located (frontoethmoidal cases are common in Southeast Asia), but occipital cases are the most frequent (Figure 10-10). Occipital encephaloceles can involve the foramen magnum and include portions of the cerebellum, brainstem, and occipital lobe (e.g., Chiari III malformation). *Meckel-Gruber syndrome* is a lethal autosomal recessive disorder that is characterized by the triad of CNS malformations (especially occipital encephalocele), cystic dysplasia of the kidneys, and ductal plate malformations of the liver (18). It can be detected by ultrasound prior to 14 weeks' gestation. There is genetic linkage to three loci: 17q21-24 (*MKS1*), 11q13 (*MKS2*), and 8q24 (*MKS3*). *Meningoceles* are typically lumbosacral in location. All three layers of meninges herniate through the bony vertebral defect, while the spinal cord remains in a normal position. Accompanying spinal cord defects may be seen and include hydromyelia, syringomyelia, diastematomyelia, and cord tethering.

Tail Bud Defects

Tail bud defects are thought to involve abnormalities of secondary neurulation. Cord abnormalities are lumbosacral and include hydromyelia (dilatation of the central canal), diastematomyelia (splitting of the cord into hemisections, often due to a bony spur), diplomyelia (duplication of the spinal cord), and cord tethering. The *tethered cord syndrome* per se involves lower limb motor and sensory deficits, pain, and neuropathic bladder, all of which presumably result from traction on distal cord elements. There may be a thickened filum terminale, low or dilated conus medullaris, spinal lipoma, or other abnormalities in the lumbosacral cord or sacral region in general (6). Detethering frequently leads to clinical improvement. Surgical specimens often reveal an increase in dense collagenous tissue and foci of fat cells, the latter of which is not a normal constituent of the filum terminale (19).

Disorders of Forebrain Development

The early development of the forebrain and midline structures, as it pertains to the neuropathology of structural malformations, is described in greater elsewhere (1,20). In brief, three primary brain vesicles are present by the 4th week of GA: (a) prosencephalon (forebrain), (b) mesencephalon (midbrain), and (c) rhombencephalon (hindbrain). Forebrain induction is thought to be governed by the prechordal plate, the ventralizing molecule Shh, and the dorsalizing molecule bone morphogenic protein 7. By constraining growth in the ventral midline of the forebrain primordium, the relatively rapid dorsolateral growth leads to the formation of paired telencephalic secondary vesicles by the 6th week GA. There are five secondary brain vesicles: (a) the telencephalon (cerebral hemispheres and basal ganglia) and (b) diencephalon (thalamic substructures), both arising from the prosencephalon; (c) the mesencephalon; (d) the metencephalon (pons and cerebellum) and (e) myelencephalon (medulla), both arising from the rhombencephalon. Shh also induces the optic primordium to divide and grow out from the diencephalon at 4 to 5 weeks GA. The paired olfactory vesicles are induced by the olfactory placodes and their ingrowing olfactory nerves at 6 weeks GA. The anterior commissure begins its development at 10 weeks GA, arising from or adjacent to the lamina terminalis. At this same time, the fornices and hippocampal primordia arise nearby and grow in a reverse C-shaped manner en route to their destination in the temporal lobe. The corpus callosum arises at 12 weeks

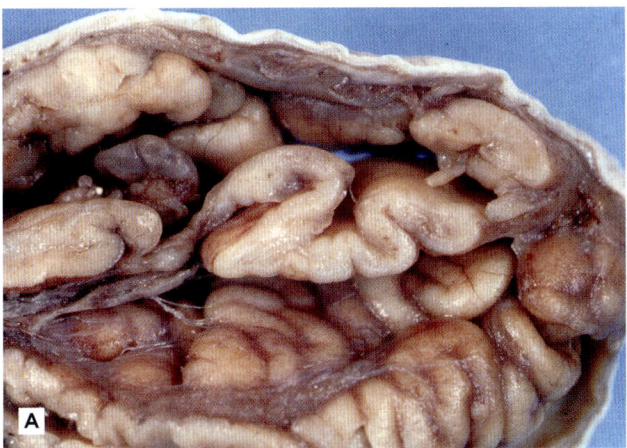
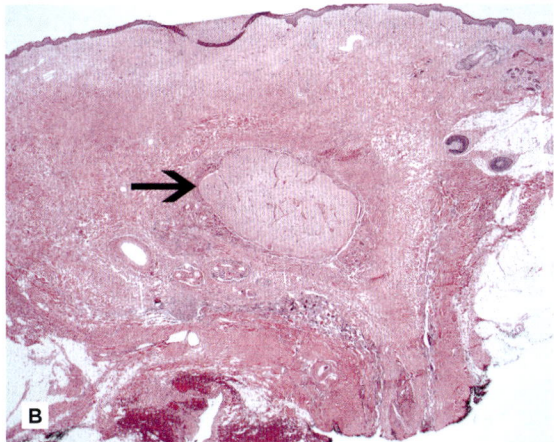

FIGURE 10-10 • Encephalocele. **A:** Atrophic cutaneous tissue overlies brain parenchyma in this surgical specimen. (Image courtesy of Dr. Beth Levy, St. Louis University.) **B:** Histologically, neuroglial tissue (*arrow*) is embedded within the deep subcutaneous connective tissue from a more subtly involved example.

GA from the massa commissuralis, which is slightly rostral and superior to the anterior commissure. It grows in a rostrocaudal manner and in doing so results in the formation of the septum pellucidum at 20 weeks GA.

Holoprosencephaly and Agenesis of the Corpus Callosum

HPE is a disorder of induction and patterning of the rostral neural tube occurring at 4 to 5 weeks GA. This may be the result of a faulty prechordal plate (21). The majority of cases are sporadic, and the incidence is approximately 5/100,000 to 9/100,000 live births. Risk factors for HPE include maternal diabetes and possibly alcohol consumption. Chromosomal abnormalities are commonly seen, the most frequent of which is trisomy 13 (Patau syndrome). Molecular genetic investigations have revealed several genes that are potentially mutated in HPE, including *SIX3* (HPE2), *SHH* (HPE3), *TGIF* (HPE4), *ZIC2* (HPE5), and *PTCH* (HPE7). Mutation of the sonic hedgehog gene (SHH) is most commonly seen, a finding that is especially intriguing in light of its normal role in neuroectodermal induction. HPE may be seen in the context of a well-recognized syndrome, such as Smith-Lemli-Opitz syndrome (due to a defect in cholesterol biosynthesis). Notably, the Shh molecule must undergo autoproteolytic cleavage for proper functioning, which in turn is dependent on cholesterol attachment to its carboxy-terminus. HPE has a variable clinical picture; severe forms result in death early in life or midgestational termination, while more mild forms allow survival into adulthood. Craniofacial and ocular abnormalities that can be present have been hypothesized to be a result of defective mesencephalic neural crest (22) (Figure 10-11A). Microcephaly (i.e., small head) is common; brains are correspondingly micrencephalic (i.e., low weight) and often less than 100 g at term. There may be hypotonia, seizures, developmental delay, and cognitive impairment. Hypofunctioning of the pituitary gland results in pan-endocrinopathies.

There are three main clinicopathologic categories of HPE that together likely represent a spectrum of disease severity. Lobar, semilobar, and alobar forms correspond to increasingly severe structural and clinical diseases, which is generally defined by the extent of the midline longitudinal fissure. In less severe forms, the fissure can be seen "cleaving" the cerebrum into two cerebral hemispheres more caudally. In *alobar HPE*, the most commonly encountered form on the pediatric neuropathology service, the longitudinal fissure is absent and results in a single cerebral mass or "holosphere." The Sylvian fissure, the gyrus rectus, and the olfactory structures are also absent. This anomalous gyral pattern prohibits the delineation of cerebral lobes. The holosphere is horseshoe shaped and contains a single ventricle that opens posterodorsally (Figure 10-11B). The opening of this ventricle is covered by a delicate membranous roof that attaches to the tentorium; this membrane may balloon to form a dorsal cyst. The lateral aspects of this membrane are

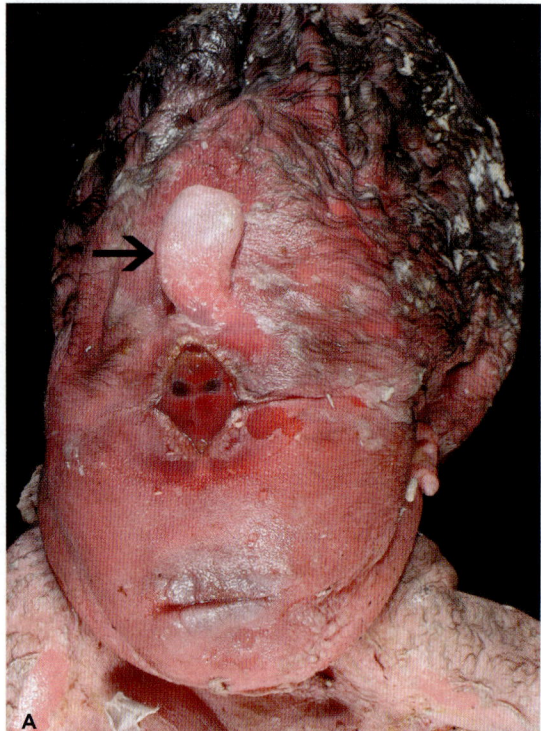
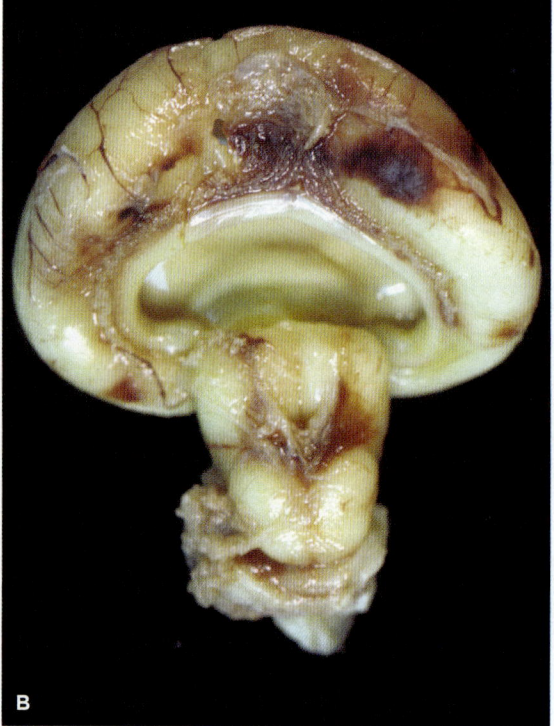

FIGURE 10-11 • Alobar holoprosencephaly. **A:** Examination of the face reveals a proboscis (*arrow*), which is superior to a single orbit bearing two fused globes. **B:** Superior and caudal views of the brain reveal the horseshoe-shaped holosphere containing a single ventricle that opens posterodorsally. (Images courtesy of Dr. Robert Schmidt, Department of Pathology and Immunology, Washington University School of Medicine, St. Louis, MO.)

bounded by a single, arch-shaped hippocampus. The floor of the single ventricle is formed by the fused deep gray nuclei. Although the corpus callosum is absent, there is no bundle of Probst (see below). The anterior commissure and the septum pellucidum are also absent. Both the brain stem and the cerebellum are grossly normal (with the exception of hypoplastic corticospinal tracts). The skull base is malformed. The anterior aspects of the circle of Willis are anomalous, and both the anterior and middle cerebral arteries are replaced by a disorganized collection of vessels called the *rete mirabile*. Microscopically, the cortical gray matter is occasionally dysplastic (1,16,23). In affected cases, it is excessively thick and dyslaminated and may demonstrate a progressively abnormal lateromedial gradient of architectural disturbance (22). The sparsely cellular external layer is segmented and arranged into irregular clusters, which may form thick cords of neurons that can traverse the entire pallium (i.e., developing cortical gray matter). There may be acellular deep zones or "glomeruli." The deeper neocortical neurons are often maloriented. Norman et al. suggest that the abnormal cortex seen in the context of HPE is unique to this disorder (16). The leptomeninges of the holosphere can be laden with glioneuronal rests and form a superficial "crust" over the brain, reminiscent of leptomeningeal neuroglial heterotopia. The architecture of the hippocampi, deep gray nuclei, and cerebellum is also often abnormal, with the latter exhibiting dysplasia, heterotopia, and an association with trisomy 13. The least severe *lobar* form of HPE, despite its resemblance to a normal brain, still contains the cerebral cortex that is continuous across the midline (at the frontal pole, in the orbital region or above the corpus callosum causing *cingulosynapsis*) (Figure 10-12). Portions of the olfactory structures and posterior corpus callosum may be present. *Semilobar* HPE is intermediate in appearance. In the recently described *middle hemispheric variant* of HPE, portions of the deep gray nuclei and frontoparietal lobe are fused across the midline, with relative rostral, caudal, and ventral brain sparing.

Agenesis of the corpus callosum (ACC) may be isolated or seen in combination with other CNS abnormalities. These associations (e.g., a neuronal migration disorder [NMD]) make it difficult to assess the clinical impact of ACC *per se*. However, isolated ACC is most often asymptomatic and found incidentally on imaging. Potential signs and symptoms may include seizures, cognitive impairment, subtle perceptual deficits, or a disconnection-like syndrome. ACC may be associated with a well-recognized syndrome (e.g., Aicardi) or an inborn error of metabolism (e.g., nonketotic hyperglycinemia). Pathologically, the characteristic findings of ACC are seen grossly on coronal sectioning of the brain (24). Agenesis may be complete or partial, with latter forms being found more caudally (i.e., splenium) in keeping with the rostrocaudal embryologic development of the corpus callosum. Laterally situated and longitudinally orientated bundles of white matter are usually identified immediately superior to the lateral ventricles; these are called *the bundles of Probst* and are thought to represent misdirected callosal fibers (Figure 10-13). The normal dorsolateral angles of the lateral ventricles take on an abnormal superior orientation (i.e., "batwing ventricles"). The distended membranous roof of the 3rd ventricle displaces the fornices and leaves of the septum pellucidum laterally. The cingulate gyrus is replaced by several short radiating gyri and the anterior commissure may also be absent; these features are best appreciated on medial inspection of the brain prior to coronal sectioning of the cerebral hemispheres. Other structural abnormalities that may accompany ACC include HCP (in this context, often occurring in the posterior cerebral hemispheres and termed *colpocephaly*), olfactory hypoplasia, and NMDs (see below).

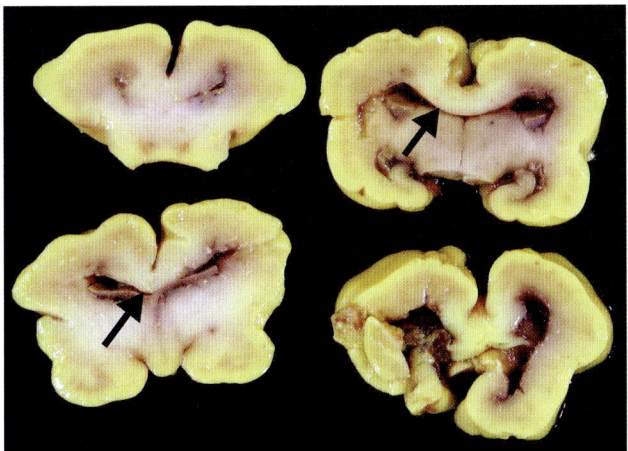

FIGURE 10-12 • Cingulosynapsis. This 24- to 25-week gestational aged fetus with semilobar holoprosencephaly displays midline fusion of the rostral most aspect of the cerebral hemispheres (**top right**). In addition, grey matter (*arrows*) located in a region consistent with the cingulate gyrus is seen abnormally crossing the midline (i.e., cingulosynapsis); note that the corpus callosum, which is normally well demarcated from the overriding cingulate gyrus, is ill defined.

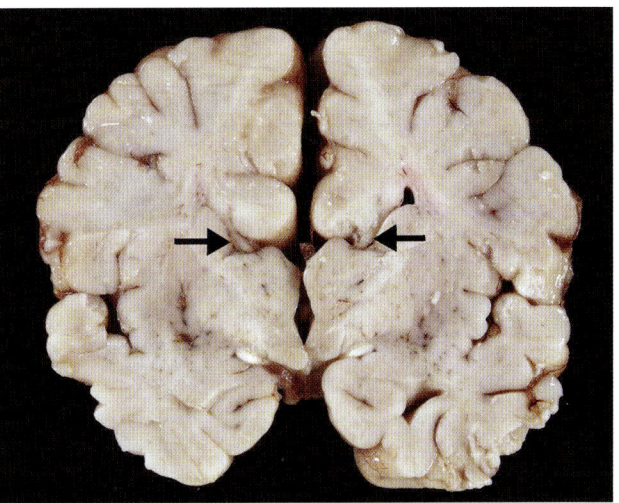

FIGURE 10-13 • Agenesis of the corpus callosum. A 2-month-old infant male. History of sudden unexpected death and cosleeping. Coronal sections of the brain do not reveal a normal corpus callosum; in its absence, dorsolaterally directed "bundles of Probst" (*arrows*) are noted.

A subset of ACC may be the result of mechanically impeding mass lesion (e.g., lipoma), but the pathogenesis of most other cases is unclear. Some have speculated that abnormalities in the "glial sling," which normally guides commissural fibers across the midline, may be a potential cause of ACC (25).

Other disorders of forebrain induction include olfactory aplasia, atelencephaly, aprosencephaly, and abnormalities involving the septum pellucidum (1,2). Just as the development of the cingulate gyrus and that of the corpus callosum are linked, so are those of the olfactory bulbs and the gyrus rectus; true olfactory aplasia is usually accompanied by the absence of the gyrus rectus.

Cell Migration and Specification Disorders

The embryology of early neocortical development is reviewed in greater detail by Golden and others (6,20). The wall of the early neural tube is composed of a pseudostratified neuroepithelial layer. By 4 weeks GA, the outer preplate zone has emerged from the inner ventricular zone of neuroepithelium. The preplate is composed of two layers: an outer layer of *Cajal-Retzius cells* (CRCs) (i.e., neurons) and an inner layer of *subplate neurons*. These transient subplate neurons play an important role in the early organization of neocortical connectivity. CRCs secrete *reelin*, an important extracellular matrix protein that assists migrating neuroblasts in finding their correct neocortical laminar destination. By 6 weeks GA, *radial glia* processes have essentially spanned the cortical mantle and aligned themselves perpendicular to the brain surface. These radial glia processes serve as physical guides for the migrating neuroblasts, which will form the cortical plate and eventual neocortex. The process of *radial migration* is complex and involves numerous molecules, including neuregulin, ErbB4, cell adhesion molecules, astrotactin, extracellular matrix molecules, and their receptors (6,20). A two-part physical barrier to overmigration lies in the marginal zone (i.e., laminae I) of the pallium and is composed of (a) the glia limitans, which is formed by the expanded end feet of the radial glia and the basal lamina of pial blood vessels, and (b) the horizontal processes and synapses of CRCs. Neuroblasts leave the ventricular zone to populate the cortical plate, "split the preplate," and form the future neocortical laminae in an inside-to-outside sequence, with the deepest layers forming prior to more superficial layers (i.e., laminae VI prior to V). These neuroblasts migrate in waves between 6 and 20 weeks GA. Despite this migration, histologic evidence of lamination in the neocortex is essentially absent at midgestation (save for the molecular layer) and the neocortex forms a very cell-dense and well-delimited band. Over the subsequent 10 weeks, neocortical lamination gradually emerges, and the 6-layer appearance is often appreciated by 30 weeks' gestation. In addition to radial migration, there is also *tangential migration* to the developing neocortex. In tangential migration, migrating neuroblasts are guided by neuronal processes to their destination; this form of migration is utilized by the future inhibitory interneurons of the neocortex that arise from the medial and lateral ganglionic eminences (i.e., the germinal matrix) and travel along axonal processes that run parallel to the cortical surface. Initially, the primitive neocortex is overpopulated by neurons, and their numbers are normally culled by apoptosis, the latter of which is usually difficult to identify with any significant frequency in fetal autopsy brains. The remaining neurons terminally differentiate and establish the connectivity pattern indicative of the developed neocortex.

Lissencephaly, Types I and II

Lissencephaly type I (i.e., classical type) is a diffuse and abnormally "smooth" (i.e., agyric) cerebral surface, whereas pachygyria represents a more focal agyric abnormality among more normally gyrated cortex. Lissencephaly type I is caused by disrupted neocortical cell migration. A number of additional CNS malformations may be associated with lissencephaly type I, and imaging that reveals such features can guide genetic testing. Four main genes have been linked to lissencephaly type I and some appear associated with distinct histopathology (6). *LIS1* (17p13.3) encodes the LIS1 protein [aka platelet-activating factor acetyl hydrolase 1 subunit β1 (PAFAH1β1)] that is involved in a complex cellular cascade, which influences dynein (and hence cell movement) and possibly cell proliferation. LIS1 is associated with Miller-Dieker syndrome. *XLIS* (or *DCX*; Xq22.3-23) encodes doublecortin, which is a microtubule-associated protein; while affected males have lissencephaly type I, females exhibit *subcortical band heterotopia* (SBH; see "Cerebral Heterotopia" below). The reelin protein (encoded by the *RELN* gene; 7q22) is the extracellular ligand that influences intracellular downstream targets (e.g., LIS1 protein). Clinically, *RELN* mutation causes lissencephaly type I associated with cerebellar malformations. Finally, *ARX* (Xp21) encodes a transcription factor important in CNS/PNS development; mutations result in lissencephaly type I and ambiguous genitalia. The general clinical features of lissencephaly type I include developmental delay, cognitive impairment, seizures (including infantile spasms), and microcephaly.

Pathologically, lissencephaly type I is characterized by thickened neocortical gray matter and a paucity of white matter (Figure 10-14). The agyric cortex may be preferentially seen more rostrally (*XLIS* or *RELN* mutation) or caudally (*LIS1* mutation). Foci of pachygyria tend to have an ill-defined border with more normal brain. Heterotopic gray matter may be seen in the periventricular and deep white matter, and if associated with an *XLIS* mutation, a subcortical band of gray matter may be seen. There may be HCP. The cerebellum is typically hypoplastic in cases associated with *RELN* mutations. The inferior olives may be dysplastic, and the corticospinal tracts may be abnormal. Classically, the histology of lissencephaly type I is described as a malformed four-layer cortex: (a) the outer first layer (i.e., molecular layer) is fairly normal and contains CRCs, (b) the second layer contains large maloriented pyramidal neurons, (c) the cell poor third layer may be myelinated in older children,

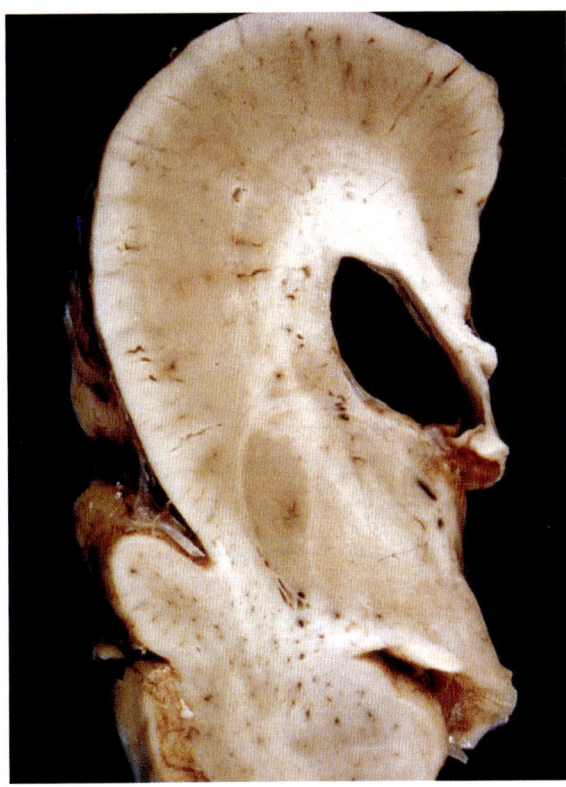

FIGURE 10-14 • Lissencephaly type I. The markedly thickened cerebral gray matter displays an absence of gyration. There is a concomitant paucity of cerebral white matter (coronal section). (Image courtesy of Dr. Beth Levy, St. Louis University.)

and (d) the fourth layer is thick and contains disorganized small to medium pyramidal and granular neurons. This classic four-layer pattern corresponds to the *LIS1* mutation and is more prominent in posterior cerebral aspects. Recent investigations have suggested additional histologic variants, including four-layer anteriorly predominant (*DCX* mutation), three-layer (*ARX* mutation), and two-layer forms (26).

The cell migratory defect in *lissencephaly type II* (i.e., cobblestone type) appears to be one of overmigration. A defective glia limitans allows radial glial processes to extend beyond the normal limits of the neocortex, facilitating the excessive migration of neuroglial precursors. Lissencephaly type II shares a thickened neocortical gray ribbon and at times an agyric surface with lissencephaly type I. However, the five main autosomal recessive syndromes associated with lissencephaly type II exhibit a characteristic triad of cerebral, ocular, and muscle diseases that are not seen in type I disease. These syndromes include *Walker-Warburg syndrome, Fukuyama congenital muscular dystrophy (FCMD), muscle–eye–brain disease, congenital muscular dystrophy type 1D (MDC-1D),* and *MDC-1C*, a disorder associated with fukutin-related protein (*FKRP*) mutations. FCMD is the most common (incidence of 3/100,000/year) and characteristically occurs in Japan. The abnormalities in these syndromes (and hence lissencephaly type II) are thought to be due to defective glycosylation, in particular O-mannosylation. Glycosylation is a common posttranslational protein modification and, in general, is important to normal development. *O-glycosylation of α-dystroglycan* appears particularly important to the etiology of these conditions (27). Pathologically, these micrencephalic brains have a lissencephalic cortex that may have a "bumpy" quality (i.e., cobblestone). The gray–white junction tends to be distinct below the thickened gray matter. The white matter is deficient and there may be HCP. The brain stem is small, in part due to hypoplastic corticospinal tracts. The cerebellum in these cases is characteristically small, especially in the vermal region, and cases of Walker-Warburg syndrome may exhibit features of a Dandy-Walker malformation (DWM) and an occipital encephalocele. Microscopically, the cortex is very disorganized and unlaminated. Superficial aspects tend to be more abnormal and may resemble polymicrogyria. The gray–white junction may exhibit a nodular appearance. The deep and superficial areas are separated by large internalized and hyalinized blood vessels that likely represent the original, and overrun, leptomeningeal vasculature. Less severely affected areas may contain a leptomeningeal "crust" of glioneuronal heterotopia. The cerebellum is disorganized, and although the internal granular and Purkinje neurons retain their somewhat normal relations, the normal architecture is disrupted. Bands of white matter are seen over the cerebellar surface. The overall appearance of the cerebellum may also resemble polymicrogyria.

Polymicrogyria

Polymicrogyria is a cortical malformation where the neocortical gray matter ribbon may seem grossly thickened but microscopically is actually thin, excessively folded, and fused. Intrinsic and acquired origins for this lesion have been proposed (6). The risk factors for polymicrogyria include (a) intrauterine infection (e.g., "TORCH"), (b) intrauterine ischemia, (c) metabolic diseases (e.g., Zellweger syndrome), and (d) a family history. Polymicrogyria may also be associated with well-recognized syndromes. Karyotypic abnormalities have been noted (e.g., −1p36, −22q11), but with the exception of *FGFR3* mutations in thanatophoric dwarfism, specific mutational information is limited (28). Clinically, localized polymicrogyria may be asymptomatic, but more often, it is associated with developmental delay, psychomotor retardation, spastic diplegia, pseudobulbar palsy, and epilepsy. MRI highlights this abnormal cortex and may reveal additional structural abnormalities (e.g., decreased white matter or other white matter changes, calcification, schizencephaly, porencephaly). Grossly, the cerebral surface in polymicrogyria is irregular and bumpy. Coronal sections reveal thickened neocortical gray matter composed of serpiginous, heaped-up thin layers. Polymicrogyria may be widespread and symmetric or focal and asymmetric. Cingulate and striate cortices are often spared. Polymicrogyria may be seen in the relatively spared temporal lobe of hydranencephaly or adjacent to porencephalic defects. Microscopically, the cortex is composed of numerous attenuated, excessively folded, and fused layers (Figure 10-15). Fusion of adjacent molecular

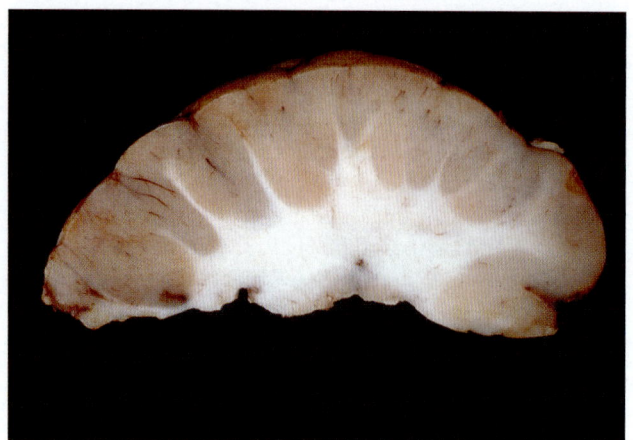

FIGURE 10-15 • Polymicrogyria. Transverse sectioning of this surgical brain specimen reveals abnormal undulation of the cortical ribbon.

layers results in a branching pattern of paucicellular tissue, which often bears a central blood vessel. The cortex is usually unlayered but may be four layered (similar to lissencephaly type I). However, Judkins et al. suggested that categorization of polymicrogyria by lamina is artificial since the neocortical laminae are normally formed but neuronally depleted; as such, this group suggested that polymicrogyria is not a cell migratory disorder, but rather a postmigrational malformation of cortical development (29). In passing, leptomeningeal glioneuronal and nodular heterotopias may also be seen alongside polymicrogyria.

Cerebral Heterotopia

Cerebral heterotopia refers to malformative lesions wherein groups of cytologically normal brain cells (i.e., neurons and glia) do not reach their neocortical destination. Three main categories are discussed here: leptomeningeal heterotopia (LH), periventricular heterotopia (PH), and SBH. LH and PH are often associated with other CNS malformations, while SBH is usually seen in isolation. LH is likely the most common of these three forms and is usually focal. Genetic and epigenetic risk factors are associated with each form of cerebral heterotopia. Genetic syndromes linked to LH include trisomy 13, HPE, and lissencephaly type II. The genetics of PH are complex, but one X-linked form involves mutations of *FLNA* (Xq28) (30). SBH is usually due to mutations in the *XLIS* gene (i.e., doublecortin, *DCX*) (see above). Epigenetic risk factors likely represent the most common mechanisms underlying LH/PH and include HIE, PVL, and germinal matrix/subpial hemorrhage. Damage to the glia limitans and radial glia likely underlies the pathogenesis of LH and PH, respectively. It is difficult to assess the clinical impact of these heterotopias since LH and PH are frequently associated with other CNS malformations. However, cognitive impairment and seizures often accompany all three forms of cerebral heterotopia. Grossly, LH is often inapparent unless seen in the context of lissencephaly type II. SBH appears as a band of gray matter (outside of the intragyral white matter) that is flanked on either side by white matter. On close inspection, the gray matter of the SBH may be broken up into nodules, which are split by white matter bundles. PH may also be confluent (i.e., band-like) or nodular, the latter being more common. Like LH, PH is associated with abnormal adjacent neocortex (cortical dysplasia with LH and polymicrogyria with PH). Microscopically, all three forms of cerebral heterotopia appear similar. Pyramidal and granular neurons are associated with glia and other normal neocortical elements, but there is no lamination and the neurons are maloriented. In LH, there is usually some connection to the underlying cortex.

"Malformations of Cortical Development," Including Focal Cortical Dysplasia

This group of epileptogenic CNS malformations regrettably has been plagued by a plethora of confusing terminology. *Malformations of cortical development* (MCD) are now the preferred umbrella term that encompasses several entities including the NMDs (see above), focal cortical dysplasia (FCD), and microdysgenesis. Previously, the term "cortical dysplasia" was often used nonspecifically to describe many different abnormal cortical histologies. "Microdysgenesis" has similarly been utilized in the past to describe milder abnormalities in cortical architecture (e.g., excess white matter neurons, excess perivascular oligodendroglia in the white matter, "glioneuronal hamartia," abnormal neuronal clustering, dyslamination, cortical columnarization) (31); however, the term *mild MCD* is now favored over microdysgenesis (see below). At the time of publication of the previous edition of this textbook, the 2004 classification of Palmini et al. was considered most apt (32). Under that system, FCD was divided into two tiers and included 4 entities: FCD Ia, Ib, IIa, and IIb. The most recent 2011 consensus on the classification of FCD has created a new third tier (FCD IIIa-d) to recognize those cases where dysplastic cortex is seen in combination with a presumed primary lesion (see below) (33).

FCDs are relatively common in surgical specimens, especially in centers with multidisciplinary epilepsy programs. The seizures associated with FCD usually manifest in the first decade. A variety of genetic predispositions and environmental insults have been hypothesized to play a role in the pathogenesis of FCD. At what time FCD arise during development is unclear (i.e., insult occurring before, during, or after neuroglial migration). Genetic studies have suggested general roles for the PI3K/mTOR and reelin pathways. In addition, polymorphisms of the *TSC1* gene have been associated with FCD type IIb, while polymorphisms of the *TSC2* gene have been seen with ganglioglioma (GG) and FCD type IIa. Identification of these lesions has been facilitated by MRI (34), and although a number of relatively nonspecific changes can be seen, the "transmantle sign" (involving T2/flair signal hyperintensities trailing down from the abnormal cortex and through the white matter toward the ventricular surface) is a fairly specific feature of FCD.

Pathologically, FCD may be grossly inapparent or seen as a focal thickening of gray matter with blurring of the underlying gray–white matter junction. According to the newest 2011 consensus paper regarding classification, FCD I is primarily categorized by abnormalities of radial migration (i.e., excessive column formation), FCD Ia, and/or tangential (i.e., dyslamination), FCD Ib, organization or a combination of both, FCD Ic. Microcolumns of FCD Ia are defined by the presence of at least 8 vertically oriented small diameter neurons that are arranged perpendicular to the cortical surface. In FCD Ib, the normal hexalaminar appearance of the neocortex is disturbed, either transcortically or focally (e.g., laminae II or IV can be missing or are significantly deplete of neurons). In both FCD Ia and Ib, (a) the gray white junction can be blurred by heterotopic neurons, (b) immature small diameter neurons can be present, and (c) hypertrophic neurons can be identified outside of layer V. The hallmark of FCD II is the *dysmorphic neuron*. Dysmorphic neurons are maloriented and/or abnormally large neurons with atypical coarse Nissl substance and thick dendritic processes. Cytoplasmic vacuolation can be seen. These neurons are highlighted by nonphosphorylated neurofilament protein (NFP) IHC or by Bielschowsky silver staining. *Balloon cells* have abundant glassy eosinophilic "astrocyte-like" cytoplasm and eccentrically placed "neuron-like" vesicular nuclei, often with prominent nucleoli; larger than gemistocytes, these cells may demonstrate neuronal, glial, or hybrid features by routine staining and by IHC (e.g., coexpressing GFAP and neuronal markers). Balloon cells, which are at times multinucleate and clustered, can be seen throughout the neocortical gray matter but most often aggregate in the subcortical white matter resulting in blurring of the gray–white junction (Figure 10-16). Dysmorphic neurons are seen in both FCD IIa and IIb, but balloon cells are restricted to FCD IIb (i.e., "Taylor's type" FCD). The dyslamination of FCD II is different from FCD I; in FCD II, all neocortical lamina are obscured with the exception of layer I. However, both may have heterotopic neurons in layer I or the white matter, the latter resulting in blurring of the gray–white junction. Other changes may be numerous but often include gliosis, hypomyelinated zones, an abnormally myelinated layer I, and calcification (6).

FCD type IIb is often indistinguishable from the tubers of tuberous sclerosis (TS) and as such may represent a form fruste of this condition, a hypothesis that is somewhat strengthened by genetic studies (see above). The histologic changes of FCD may also be seen in hemimegalencephaly, an epileptogenic disorder that describes the syndromic or isolated occurrence of an enlarged abnormal hemisphere associated with hemiparesis and developmental delay (6). However, the scarcely reported histology of fetal hemimegalencephaly seems more subtle and typified by accelerated cortical differentiation.

Antenatal Disruptive Lesions

Although in some sense, this group of lesions could be considered malformative; they are generally considered to result from a hypoxic–ischemic insult to the developing brain. These insults are acquired *in utero* and intrauterine infections may play a role in the etiology of some. *Hydranencephaly* is the severe and diffuse necrosis of the cerebral mantle and deep gray (with concomitant HCP *ex vacuo*) due to perfusion failure of the internal carotid territory at 15 to 16 weeks' gestation. The residual mantle is markedly thinned, and there is evidence of secondary brainstem and spinal cord atrophy. There may be sparing of parenchyma supplied by the posterior cerebral artery. *Porencephaly* describes the focal transmantle necrosis of the cerebrum (most often in the middle cerebral artery territory) wherein the ventricle communicates with the subarachnoid space. Polymicrogyria, gliosis, and calcification often rim the porencephalic defect. If there is bilateral middle cerebral artery damage that spares the cingulate gyri (i.e., leaving a "handle"), the resulting defect is called *basket brain*. *Schizencephaly* describes a nontransmantle cleft in the cerebrum. *Multicystic encephalopathy* (MCE) is the result of a diffuse white/gray matter insult to the cerebrum, causing multifocal necrosis and cystic change (Figure 10-17). The insult in MCE is presumed to occur late in gestation since the general architecture of the brain is maintained, but some cases have been described in newborns.

Microcephaly and Micrencephaly

Microcephaly refers to a small head, whereas *micrencephaly* refers to a small brain. Some authors have used the term "microcephaly" interchangeably to refer to both. If one excludes brains with hypoplasia/atrophy due to other entities (e.g., HPE, antenatal disruptive lesions), the possibility of a rarely encountered *primary* micrencephaly should be considered.

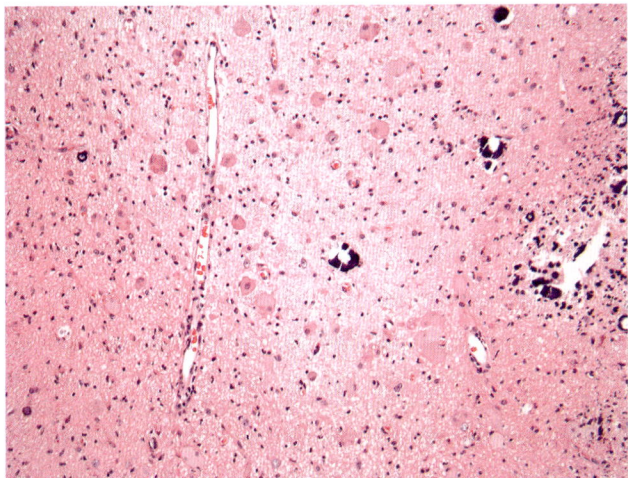

FIGURE 10-16 • FCD type IIb. Balloon cells are seen within the gliotic and calcified white matter immediately subjacent to malformed cortical gray matter.

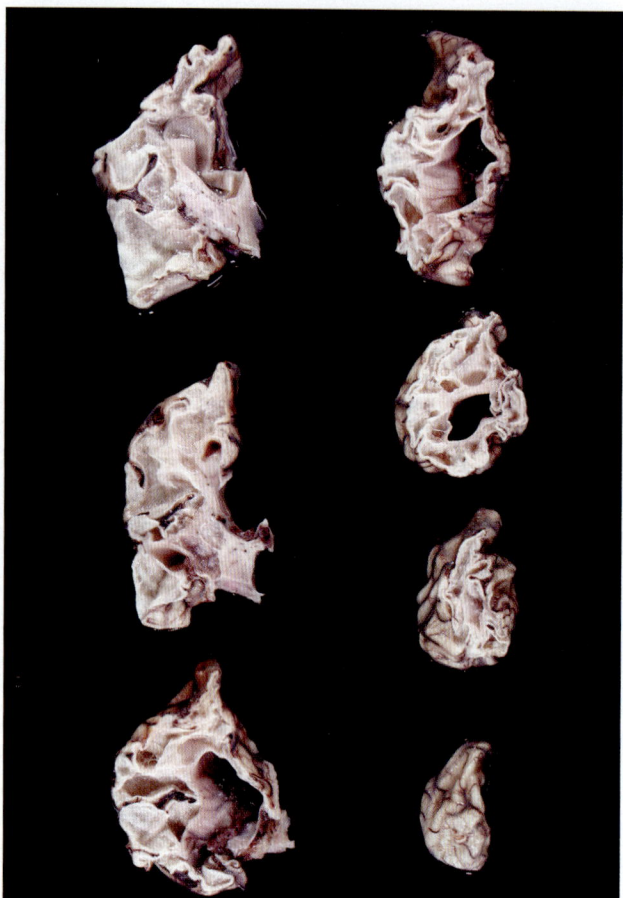

FIGURE 10-17 • Microcystic encephalopathy (MCE). Coronal sections of the left cerebral hemisphere from this 2-month-old female reveal prominent pathology in keeping MCE. PCR testing of formalin-fixed paraffin-embedded tissues revealed the presence of HSV-2.

Hindbrain Malformations

As described above, by the 6th week of GA, the secondary brain vesicles that give rise to the cerebellum and pons (metencephalon), in addition to the medulla (myelencephalon), have begun their development. There are similarities in the development of the hindbrain and the spinal cord. The alar and basal plates give rise to the dorsal sensory and ventral motor spinal cord horns, respectively. With respect to the hindbrain, its dorsal aspect is essentially splayed out such that the motor basal plates lie medially, while the sensory alar plates lie laterally. The metencephalic alar plates fuse and give rise to the cerebellum. The Purkinje and deep gray neurons of the cerebellum arise from the ventricular zone of the alar plate, while the eventual internal granule neurons arise from the upper aspect of an alar plate derivative called the *upper rhombic lip* (35). A lateral to medial outward migration of granule neuron precursors has populated the EGL by 14 weeks and persists until 1 year of age. Neurons from the EGL migrate inward to their eventual destination in the internal granule layer. The flocculonodular, anterior, and posterior lobes are already identifiable by 12 weeks GA. Cerebellar folia can be seen by 20 weeks.

The precerebellar nuclei (i.e., pontine, inferior olivary, and arcuate nuclei) arise from the *lower rhombic lip*.

Chiari and Dandy-Walker Malformations

Although the Chiari malformations are discussed in the context of the hindbrain, their actual pathogenesis is unclear (see below). Three forms are well recognized. *Chiari I* malformations are characterized by the caudal displacement (not true herniation) of the cerebellar tonsils through the foramen magnum and into the upper cervical spinal canal. Chiari I malformations are often associated with syringomyelia. The clinical picture includes neck pain and signs/symptoms associated with syringomyelia (i.e., "cape-like" or "hanging" dissociated sensory loss in the shoulders and arms) that develops in older teenagers and young adults. Pathologically, surgical resection specimens reveal leptomeningeal sclerosis and gliosis with neuronal loss in the cerebellar cortex of the affected tonsillar tissue. Pathogenesis of the Chiari I malformation is unclear. *Chiari II* malformations (previously known as the Arnold-Chiari malformation) occur in young children and describe the caudal displacement of cerebellar vermis into the upper cervical spinal canal plus added hindbrain abnormalities. Ninety-five percent of Chiari II malformations are associated with a lumbosacral myelomeningocele (6). Maternal vitamin A deficiency is a risk factor for Chiari II. The clinical picture of Chiari II is dominated by HCP and the myelomeningocele. Pathologically, the fourth ventricle, midbrain, pons, and medulla are all elongated and caudally displaced. There may be "tectal beaking" and an S-shaped "kinking" of the medulla onto the dorsal spinal cord (Figure 10-18). Moreover, careful dissection of fetuses with Chiari II invariably demonstrates kinking of the medulla without cerebellar herniation upon midgestational termination, suggesting that medullary kinking precedes cerebellar herniation in the natural history of this disorder. With respect to the skull, the posterior fossa is small and there are often abnormally rostrally coursing cranial nerves. Additional CNS malformations may include PH, polymicrogyria, and pachygyria. Pathogenesis of the Chiari II malformation is unknown. Hypotheses include (a) hydrodynamic (related to mechanic pressure from HCP or excess CSF egress from the myelomeningocele), (b) cord tethering, (c) a defect in neurulation, or (d) a defect in the posterior fossa mesenchyme leading to restricted cerebellar growth. Since myelomeningoceles invariably accompany Chiari II, some have suggested that the NTD causes the brain findings characteristic of Chiari II due to egress of CSF through the NTD. To the latter, recent studies from Children's Hospital of Philadelphia (CHOP) have demonstrated that fetal surgery to close the associated NTD helps ameliorate later clinical symptomatology (17). *Chiari III* malformations are rare and are defined by an occipitocervical encephalocele (which includes cerebellar tissue) that is accompanied by a distorted brain stem and abnormal local anatomy. The clinical picture is similar to Chiari II but is more severe and the prognosis is

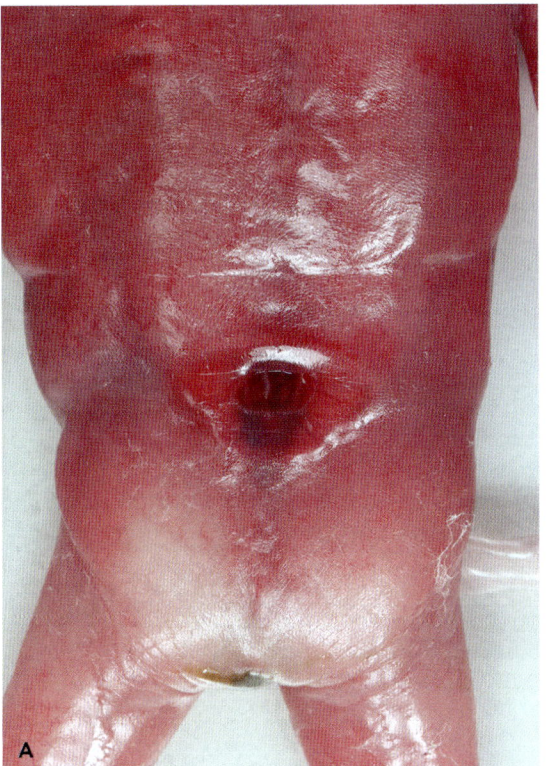 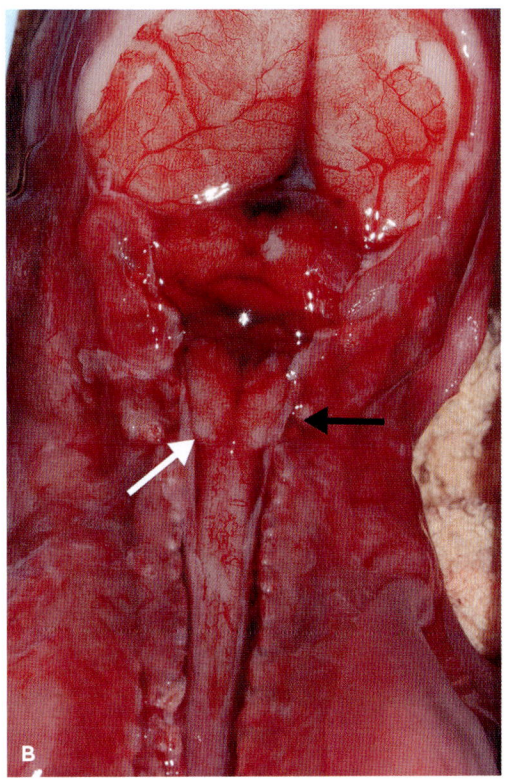

FIGURE 10-18 • Chiari II malformation and related lumbosacral neural tube defect in a 20- to 21-week gestational aged female fetus. **A:** Gross examination confirms the presence of a neural tube defect, which upon further sampling for microscopy confirmed the presence of an intact spinal cord, suggesting the presence of a meningocele. **B:** As is typical of this gestational age, herniating cerebellar vermis is not detected in this posterior dissection; rather, a kinked medulla (*white arrow*) is appreciated herniating through the foramen magnum and past the C1 vertebra (the latter is dissected away and its stump is indicated by the *black arrow*).

poor. Pathologic changes may include cerebellar dysplasia. Pathogenesis is also unclear but is likely related to defective neurulation.

The *Dandy Walker Malformation* (DWM) typically presents sporadically in infancy as an isolated finding or in association with other CNS malformations. Common clinical features of DWM include HCP and increased ICP. Surprisingly, cerebellar signs/symptoms are less common, but there may be concomitant cognitive impairment. DWM is characterized by five main pathologic features. First, there is cystic dilatation of the fourth ventricle. Second, the cerebellar vermis is hypoplastic or absent. Third, DWM is characterized by a large posterior fossa. Fourth, and likely related to the large posterior fossa, is the elevation of the tentorium and related dural sinuses. Finally, there is HCP. The Dandy-Walker variant has only some of the features of the DWM, which includes an anteriorly rotated vermis with or without fourth ventricular dilatation. The pathogenesis of the DWM is unknown, but maldevelopment of the fourth ventricular roof and its outlet foramina (especially Magendie) is thought to be important. Maternal isoretinoin use is a risk factor. Pathologically, the main findings are those seen grossly (see above). The fourth ventricular cyst wall is composed of an outer pial and inner ependymal layers, with residual cerebellar parenchymal in between.

A variety of additional cerebellar malformations has been characterized. Cerebellar heterotopia and dysplasia are reviewed by Golden (6). Rare malformations include cerebellar agenesis, Joubert syndrome, pontoneocerebellar hypoplasia, and granular cell aplasia. *Blake pouch cyst* is an emerging entity causing HCP and occasionally delayed neurologic development. All ages can be affected. Etiologically, it is thought to be due to nonperforation of the foramen of Magendie (36). Grossly, a Blake pouch cyst results in an enlarged 4th ventricle and possibly a degree of vermal hypoplasia or anterior rotation and displacement. Histologically, the wall of a Blake pouch cyst is characterized by leptomeninges, ependyma, and choroid plexus.

Malformations of the brain stem are numerous but rare. Some are described elsewhere in this chapter (i.e., Moebius syndrome, X-linked HCP with congenital absence of the pyramids). Olivary heterotopia and dysplasias of the dentate nucleus and inferior olive may occur in association with a number of different CNS malformations or syndromes, and in light of their origin from the metencephalic alar plate, it is not surprising that these may occur in conjunction with cerebellar abnormalities. *Dentato-olivary dysplasia* (DOD) can be seen in many clinical contexts and takes on a variety of pathologic forms. Of note, DOD can be seen in the context of "intractable epilepsy in infancy,"

TABLE 10-1	CNS CYSTS	
Cyst Type	Common Sites	Pathology
Neurenteric (i.e., endodermal)	Intradural, extramedullary, and ventral to the cervical spinal cord	Cuboidal to columnar respiratory-type or GI-type epithelium covering a connective tissue stroma. Possible goblet cells and cilia. Immunohistochemistry[a] (IHC)
Colloid	Anterosuperior third ventricle near the Foramen of Monroe	Simple columnar epithelium. Possible cilia. Cyst contents PAS positive. IHC[a]
Rathke cleft	Sella	Similar to neurenteric. Degenerate forms with atrophic epithelium and xanthogranulomatous inflammation. IHC[a]
Dermoid	Midline: fontanelle, fourth ventricle, cauda equina	Stratified squamous epithelium with dermal adnexal appendages. Cyst contents (grossly "cheesy"): degenerate keratinocytes, sebaceous material, hair, etc.
Epidermoid	Cerebellopontine angle (CPA), parasellar, diploe of skull	Similar to dermoid epithelium but without dermal appendages. Keratinizing epithelium. Cyst contents: "dry" keratin. Gross "pearly" appearance
Ependymal	Intraventricular, leptomeningeal, intraparenchymal	Columnar epithelium similar to ependyma. Possible cilia. No goblet cells. IHC: GFAP positive and S100 protein positive
Choroid plexus	Lateral ventricles	Simple cuboidal to columnar epithelium. Cytokeratin positive and S100 positive
Pineal	Pineal parenchyma	Three layers: (a) internal fibrillar layer with RFs. IHC: GFAP positive. (b) Pineal parenchymal "middle" layer. IHC: synaptophysin positive. (c) Outer connective tissue layer
Blake pouch	Posterior fossa	Cyst wall composed of leptomeninges, ependyma, and choroid plexus
Arachnoid	CPA, Sylvian fissure	CSF filled. Inner arachnoid (EMA positive) and outer connective tissue layers

[a]Cytokeratin and EMA positive, with collagen IV immunoreactive subepithelial basement membrane. Usually CK7 positive, CK20 negative.

where pathologically it takes on a distinctive appearance characterized by a primitive C-shaped inferior olive and globular dentate nucleus (37).

Cystic Lesions of the CNS

"Cysts" within the CNS are biologically benign and nonneoplastic. Their characteristic sites and pathology are summarized in Table 10-1. During embryologic development, ectopic placement of germ layer tissue may account for the formation of many of these lesions.

METABOLIC, NEURODEGENERATIVE, AND MISCELLANEOUS DISORDERS

Lysosomal Storage Disorders

Lysosomes are the digestive organelles of the cell. They contain numerous hydrolytic enzymes (e.g., phosphatases, nucleases, glycosidases, proteases, sulfatases, phospholipases) that assist in normal cellular metabolism. These enzymes are often directed to cleave off the sugar chains from larger macromolecules. A deficiency in one or more of the glycoprotein enzymes results in a *lysosomal storage disorder* (LSD). The LSDs are uncommon disorders that often result in progressive and multisystemic diseases that are fatal in childhood. LSD can be subdivided into categories, which are roughly based on the class of macromolecule that is not correctly metabolized; these include (a) sphingolipidoses (lipids), (b) mucopolysaccharidoses (MPS) (disaccharide molecules of glycosaminoglycans [GAGs]), (c) glycoproteinoses (glycoproteins), and (d) a number of miscellaneous LSDs, which include the neuronal ceroid lipofuscinoses (NCL) and Pompe disease (type II glycogenosis) (38).

The LSDs are generally autosomal recessive disorders that are usually the result of a mutation in the gene that encodes a particular lysosomal enzyme. There is extensive clinicopathologic overlap among the LSDs as a whole, many of which are individually indistinguishable without ancillary biochemical and genetic testing (see Chapters 5 and 28).

Conceptually, the LSDs can be divided into four basic clinicopathologic phenotypes: (a) neuronal lipidoses, (b) leukodystrophies, (c) storage histiocytoses, and (d) MPS (or the Hurler phenotype) (38). Most LSD storage products are water soluble and thus are washed out during routine histologic processing, whose residual feature is clear, vacuolated, and

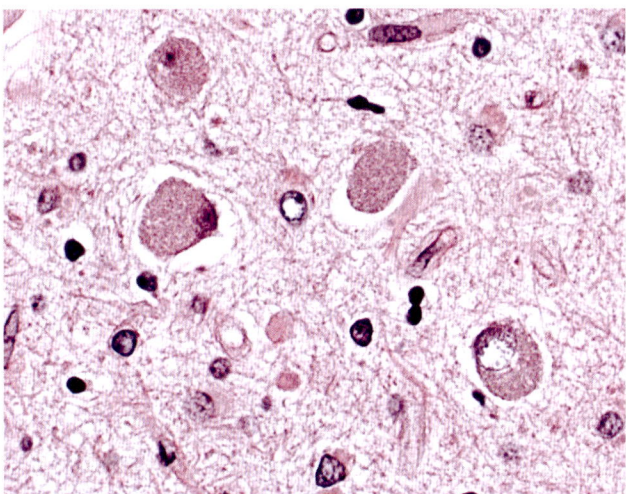

FIGURE 10-19 • Neuronal lipidosis (NL). The cytoplasm of these neurons is markedly distended by lipofuscin-like storage products in this example of neuronal ceroid lipofuscinosis (NCL).

distended cytoplasm of involved cells. This accumulated material mechanically disrupts cellular processes and eventually leads to cell death. The *neuronal lipidoses* are characterized by substrate storage in cytoplasm of neurons, leading to the gross finding of megalencephaly early in the disease course (Figure 10-19). Subsequent neuronal death and gliosis eventually result in cerebral atrophy. Involvement of the retina may lead to the characteristic "cherry-red spot," while other clinical manifestations of the neuronal lipidosis (NL) phenotype include psychomotor impairment and dementia, loss of acquired motor and perceptual skills, epilepsy, and myoclonus. The *leukodystrophies*, which are part of the LSDs (e.g., metachromatic leukodystrophy [MLD] and Krabbe leukodystrophy [KLD]), are the result of substrate accumulation in oligodendrocytes and Schwann cells, causing loss of myelin and myelinating cells. Clinical manifestations include psychomotor retardation, spasticity, ataxia, visual abnormalities, and a demyelinating peripheral neuropathy. Substrate accumulation in mesenchymal and epithelial cells, in addition to the extracellular matrix, results in the *Hurler phenotype*. Clinically, these patients have core features, which include coarse facies, skeletal and joint abnormalities (i.e., dysostosis multiplex and arthropathies), organomegaly, cloudy corneas, cardiovascular disease, and CNS disease (entrapment neuropathies, HCP, and NL). Finally, substrate storage in monocytes/macrophages causes the *storage histiocytosis* (SH) phenotype, which clinically manifests in hepatosplenomegaly, and hematologic and skeletal abnormalities. Table 10-2 lists a subset of the LSD, their specific enzymatic defects, and some of their characteristic clinicopathologic features (note: MLD and KLD are further described below) (see Chapter 5).

Leukodystrophies

The *leukodystrophies* are a group of genetically based progressive disorders that share common abnormalities in myelin formation and metabolism. These disorders have hence been referred to as *dysmyelinating*, to distinguish them from acquired demyelinating disorders (e.g., multiple sclerosis) where myelin is thought to form normally but is later destroyed. Pathogenetically, the leukodystrophies are a heterogeneous group of disorders, which, for example, include some of the lysosomal and peroxisomal storage disorders. These disorders often have onset during childhood, but adults can also be affected. Clinically, they can affect numerous neurologic modalities and hence result in a myriad of signs and symptoms, which may include psychomotor impairment and dementia; pyramidal and extrapyramidal manifestations including spastic paraparesis, ataxia, and visual and hearing abnormalities; as well as signs of bulbar involvement. Characteristic clinical manifestations (i.e., age of onset, signs/symptoms) may accompany specific forms of leukodystrophy. The white matter of not only the CNS but also the PNS [e.g., MLD, KLD, and, less so, adrenoleukodystrophy (ALD)] may be affected. Some leukodystrophies are more systemic in nature and thus bear extra-CNS/PNS disease manifestations (e.g., adrenal and testicular involvement with ALD; biliary and renal involvement with MLD). Genetically, many of these disorders are inherited in an autosomal recessive manner; however, some follow an X-linked or sporadic pattern.

Pathologically, the leukodystrophies characteristically cause bilaterally symmetric white matter–predominant disease that can involve the cerebrum, brain stem, cerebellum, and even the spinal cord. Usually, subcortical U-fibers are spared from myelin destruction (Figure 10-20A). There may be a rostral (Alexander disease, MLD) or caudal (ALD; KLD) predominance of cerebral white matter disease. In general, early stages of disease are characterized by widespread myelin destruction with relative axonal preservation; macrophages are often present and distended by bubbly periodic acid-Schiff (PAS)-positive cytoplasmic material. Later stages often demonstrate axonal and oligodendrocyte destruction plus reactive gliosis. Characteristic pathologic changes often accompany individual leukodystrophies and hence assist in diagnosis (Table 10-3; Figure 10-20B). A subset of leukodystrophies are considered "sudanophilic" since macrophages and other cells that accumulate indigestible substrates stain positive with Sudan B or Oil Red O fat stains. Included in these sudanophilic leukodystrophies are ALD, Pelizaeus-Merzbacher disease (PMD), and a host of less well-described entities that may contain characteristic histopathology including calcification, pigmentation, meningeal angiomatosis, and cavitation with oligodendrocyte proliferation (e.g., vanishing white matter disease), the latter of which recently has been linked to mutations in any of the genes encoding subunits of the eukaryotic translation factor eIF2B (39,40).

Peroxisomal Disorders

Peroxisomes are cellular organelles that have a single membrane enclosing a matrix wherein biochemical reactions take place. Peroxisomes generate hydrogen peroxide (H_2O_2), a molecule that assists in oxidizing several cellular toxins. However, H_2O_2 can itself be toxic; hence, peroxisomes contain

TABLE 10-2 LYSOSOMAL STORAGE DISEASES

LSD	Enzymatic/Protein Deficiency	Stored Material	Characteristic Clinicopathologic Features
GM1 gangliosidosis	β-Galactosidase	GM1 ganglioside, keratan sulfate	NL, MPS, cherry-red spot[a]
GM2 gangliosidosis (Tay-Sachs and Sandhoff)	Hexosaminidase A and/or B	GM2 gangliosides	NL, SH (Sandhoff), cherry-red spot[a]
Niemann-Pick A/B	Sphingomyelinase	Sphingomyelin	NL, SH (Niemann-Pick cells), cherry-red spot[a]
Niemann-Pick C	ER membrane protein with role in intracellular cholesterol transport	Phospholipids and glycolipids	NL, SH (Niemann-Pick cells), axonal swellings, and neurofibrillary tangles[a]
Gaucher disease	Glucocerebrosidase	Glucocerebroside	SH with Gaucher cells ("wrinkled tissue paper")[a]
Fabry disease	α-Galactosidase	Trihexosylceramide	Painful peripheral neuropathy; ischemic CNS and heart disease; bathing trunk telangiectasias, renal, and eye disease[a]
Farber granulomatosis	Ceramidase	Ceramide	NL, LD, cherry-red spot; painful arthropathy, subcutaneous nodules, and hoarseness related to lipid granulomas[a]
MPS type I: Hurler disease	α-L-Iduronidase	Dermatan and heparan sulfate	MPS, mental retardation, dysostosis multiplex, cloudy corneas, heart disease. EM: reticulogranular inclusions
NCL 1–4	Palmitoyl protein thioesterase (NCL1), tripeptidyl peptidase (NCL2)	Saposin A&D (NCL1), SCMAS (subunit C of mitochondrial ATPase synthase), (NCL2–4)	NL. EM: granular osmiophilic deposit (NCL1), curvilinear bodies (NCL2), fingerprint bodies (NCL3), or "mixed" with lipofuscin-like (NCL4)
Pompe disease (glycogenosis type 2)	α-Glucosidase (acid maltase)	Glycogen (membrane bound and free by EM)	Vacuolar myopathy, cardiomegaly, macroglossia

EM: in general, many of these disorders contain membranous cytoplasmic or zebra body inclusions within lysosomes; GM1 may contain added reticulogranular material; Gaucher disease exhibits tubular inclusions; Farber granulomatosis features "banana bodies."

[a]Sphingolipidoses.

LSD, lysosomal storage disease; NL, neuronal lipidosis; MPS, mucopolysaccharidosis; SH, storage histiocytosis; ER, endoplasmic reticulum; NCL, neuronal ceroid lipofuscinosis.

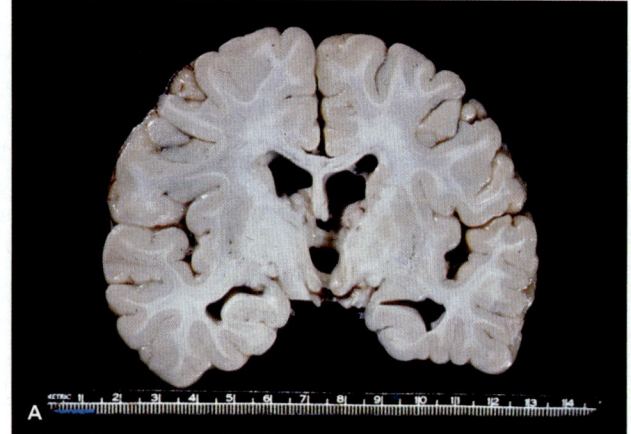
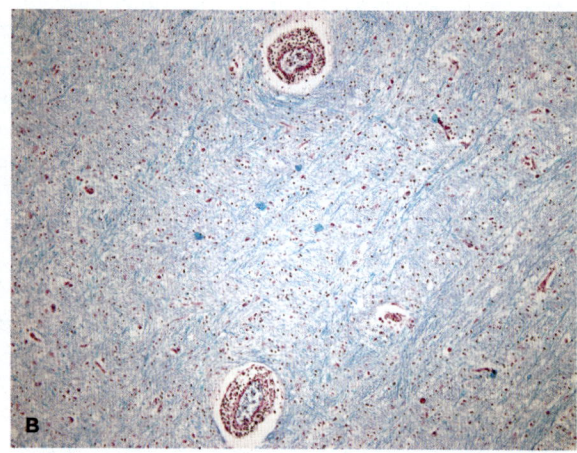

FIGURE 10-20 • Leukodystrophy. **A:** Coronally sectioned case of Krabbe disease demonstrates symmetric dysmyelination of cerebral white matter with relative sparing of the subcortical U-fibers. (Image courtesy of Dr. Barry Rewcastle.) **B:** LFB–PAS-stained case of ALD demonstrates pale white matter and characteristic perivascular lymphocytic cuffing.

TABLE 10-3 THE LEUKODYSTROPHIES

Leukodystrophy	Biochemical/Genetic Abnormality (Chromosomal Locus)	Characteristic Pathology
Adrenoleukodystrophy (ALD)	Deficiency of a peroxisomal ATP-binding cassette transporter, resulting in accumulation of VLCFAs. X-linked (Xq28)	Perivascular lymphocytic inflammation. EM: trilaminar inclusions. Striated lamellar cytoplasm inclusions in CNS and select systemic organs
Metachromatic leukodystrophy (MLD)	Aryl-sulfatase A deficiency. Accumulate sulfatide (22q13)	Metachromatic material (using acidic cresyl violet or toluidine blue) in the brain (macrophages), PNS (Schwann cells), and viscera (biliary epithelium and renal tubules). EM: herringbone, prismatic, and tuft stone inclusions
Krabbe leukodystrophy (KLD)	Galactocerebroside b-galactosidase deficiency. Accumulate psychosine (14q25-31)	Globoid cells, often perivascular. PNS: hypertrophic neuropathy with fibrosis and "onion bulbs." EM: tubular inclusions
Alexander disease	Sporadic mutation of the GFAP gene (17q21)	RF accumulation, especially in perivascular and subpial locations. Grossly cavitated white matter. EM: amorphous electron-dense material surrounded by 10-nm intermediate filaments
Canavan disease	Aspartoacylase deficiency. Accumulate N-acetylaspartate (17p13-ter)	More central aspects of central myelin lost with relative oligodendroglial and axonal sparing. Vacuolation at neocortical gray–white junction. No macrophages and little gliosis (versus other LSDs). EM: myelin splitting at intraperiod line plus elongate mitochondrial with "ladderlike" cristae
Pelizaeus-Merzbacher disease (PMD)	Deficiency of normal proteolipid protein (PLP). Accumulate abnormally folded PLP in the ER. X-linked (Xq22)	Perivascular patchy dysmyelination (i.e., tigroid)

catalase, an enzyme that serves to break down H_2O_2 into water and oxygen. Peroxisomes also play an important role in the β-oxidation of very-long-chain fatty acids (VLCFAs), plasmalogen biosynthesis (an important cell membrane and myelin component), cholesterol biosynthesis, and the metabolism of amino acids, bile acids, and purine nucleotides. Knowledge of these basic biologic functions is clinically useful since the routine laboratory workup of the peroxisomal disorders often involves initial assessment of VLCFAs, hepatic peroxisomes, and red blood cell plasmalogens.

There are two main categories of peroxisomal disorders: (a) *peroxisomal biogenesis disorders* (e.g., Zellweger spectrum, and rhizomelic chondrodysplasia punctata type 1) and the (b) *single peroxisome enzyme–protein deficiencies* (e.g., X-ALD, D-bifunctional protein deficiency, and adult Refsum disease) (38). In general, these disorders are neuropathologically characterized by NMD, leukodystrophy-like white matter abnormalities, CNS lipid deposition, and systemic abnormalities (including the adrenal cortex and liver). Both the biogenesis disorders and the single enzymes deficiencies are inherited in an autosomal recessive fashion, with the exception of X-lined ALD. The biogenesis disorders involve mutations in the PEX genes, which encode the peroxin proteins that are important to peroxisomal functioning. *Zellweger spectrum* includes three disorders, which are considered to form a spectrum of diseases related to mutations in a number of genes, including *PEX1*. These include (from most to least severe) the following: Zellweger syndrome, neonatal ALD, and infantile Refsum disease. *Zellweger syndrome* (a.k.a. cerebrohepatorenal syndrome) is a systemic disorder primarily affecting the liver (cirrhosis) and brain. Patients have dysmorphic facies and neurologic manifestations that include psychomotor impairment, hypotonia, depressed deep tendon and Moro reflexes, seizures, and nystagmus. These infants die within the first year of life. Neuropathologic findings include NMDs (e.g., pachygyria, polymicrogyria), leukodystrophy-like white matter abnormalities, abnormalities of rhombic lip–derived structures (dentate nucleus/inferior olivary dysplasias, cerebellar heterotopias), and prominent deposition of sudanophilic lipid in the CNS (primarily within macrophages and showing trilaminar appearance on EM) (Chapters 5 and 15).

Mitochondrial Disorders

The mitochondria are the "powerhouse" of the cell. They produce the energy needed for life in the form of ATP via aerobic respiration. The final stages of aerobic respiration are mediated by the electron transport chain, which comprises five protein complexes that are embedded within the inner mitochondrial membrane. Each of these five complexes is composed of multiple protein subunits (86 in total), most of which are encoded by nuclear DNA. The mtDNA genome is circular and double stranded and includes 16,569 base pairs. Up to ten copies of the mtDNA genome may be seen within a cell. This genome encodes for 22 tRNAs, 2 rRNAs, and 13 subunits of the electron transport chain. Genetically induced defects in the assembly or formation of the electron transport chain, or in the maintenance of the mitochondrial DNA, result in mitochondrial disorders. Dysfunction of the electron transport chain presumably results in cell death via numerous mechanisms, including energy deprivation, free radical toxicity, and apoptosis. Since electron transport chain functioning relies on proteins encoded by both mitochondrial and nuclear DNA, mitochondrial disorders may be inherited via either maternal or classic Mendelian patterns.

Mitochondrial disorders, as with the LSDs, may display significant clinicopathologic overlap. Many of these disorders, when viewed in isolation, may be caused by more than one mutation, and in turn, any given mutation may lead to more than one phenotype. This biologic complexity makes the diagnosis of mitochondrial disorders challenging. These disorders are often described as encephalomyopathies, since muscle (cardiac and skeletal) and brain tissues are usually affected due to their heavy reliance on mitochondrial energy production. Clinically, the presence of a mitochondrial disorder may be suspected via characteristic lab abnormalities, which often include an elevation in blood/CSF lactate and the lactate-to-pyruvate ratio. *Ragged red fibers* (RRF) are a common manifestation of muscle disease and represent a localized proliferation of abnormal mitochondria. RRFs are detected histochemically on frozen sections via modified Gomori trichrome (dark red) or succinic dehydrogenase (dark blue) stains (Figure 10-21A). The cytochrome oxidase C (COX) stain often fails to stain such affected fibers (i.e., "pale fibers"). By EM, the abnormal mitochondria of RRFs may take several unusual configurations including concentric spirals and rectangular paracrystalline arrays that resemble "parking lots" (Figure 10-21B). It is important to note that RRFs are not entirely specific for the mitochondrial disorders and that not all mitochondrial disorders bear RRFs. Other common neuropathologic findings seen among the mitochondrial disorders include hypoxic–ischemic-like and infarct-like changes, intramyelinic edema/spongy myelinopathy, tract/system degenerations, and vascular mineralization (deep gray and adjacent white matter, dentate nucleus, and the brain stem). As our knowledge of mitochondrial disorders has evolved, so too has the number of better recognized individual entities (38). Below, only a few of the more common mitochondrial disorders are briefly discussed.

Mitochondrial encephalopathy with lactic acidosis and strokes (MELAS) is a maternally inherited disorder that most often results from an adenine to guanine point mutation at nucleotide 3243 of mtDNA. This mutation is within the gene that encodes the tRNA for leucine. Those afflicted are usually young, although both the age of onset and initial presentation may be quite variable. Sudden focal neurologic signs (e.g., hemiplegia, hemianopsia, seizures), migraine-like attacks, or more nonspecific symptoms (such as vomiting or a change in mental status) may be seen. Myopathic features include proximal limb weakness, fatigability, and deficits in eye movements. Episodes of such neurologic dysfunction tend to be recurrent. Pathologically, foci of necrotic brain

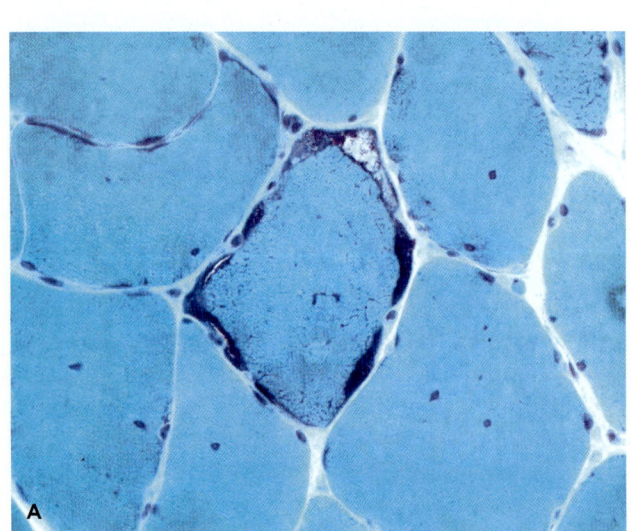
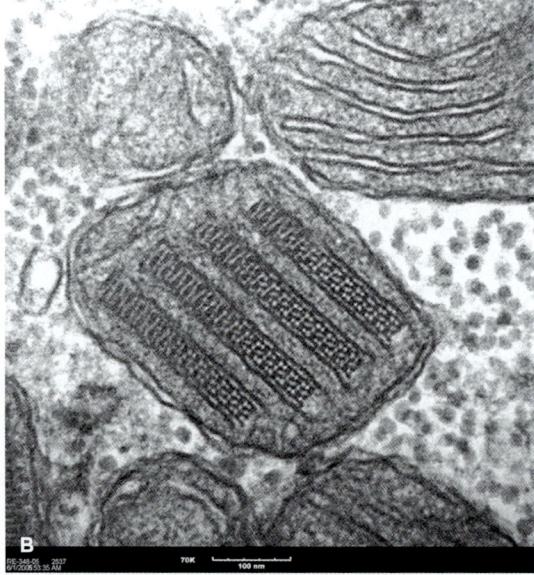

FIGURE 10-21 • Mitochondrial myopathy. **A:** Ragged rough fiber. (Modified Gomori trichrome.) **B:** EM reveals abnormal mitochondria with paracrystalline ("parking lot") inclusions.

damage resemble true infarcts; however, these lesions do not follow standard vascular distributions. The occipital lobes, deep gray matter (which also may demonstrate vascular mineralization), and cerebellum are often affected. RRFs are present.

Myoclonic epilepsy with ragged red fibers (MERRF) is another maternally inherited disorder. MERRF most often results from an adenine to guanine point mutation at nucleotide 8344 of mtDNA. This mutation is within the gene that encodes the tRNA for lysine. Like MELAS, those afflicted are often young. Clinical features include a proximal myopathy, myoclonic epilepsy, sensorineural hearing loss, cognitive deficits, short stature, and ataxia. Pathologic changes involve neuronal loss and gliosis among the dentatorubroolivary system, substantia nigra, dorsal column nuclei (gracile and cuneate), and Clarke's column. Vascular mineralization may be noted in the deep gray matter, and muscle pathology includes RRFs.

Leigh disease (subacute necrotizing encephalopathy) is most frequently caused by germ line rather than mitochondrial mutations and, hence, usually inherited in an autosomal recessive pattern. Genes encoding subunits of the electron transport chain complexes I, II, IV, and V may be mutated, or alternatively, there may be a deficiency of pyruvate dehydrogenase. Disease onset often manifests prior to 2 years of age and includes weight loss, vomiting, psychomotor impairment, and weakness. Movement disorders, ataxia, eye abnormalities (optic atrophy, ophthalmoplegia, nystagmus), respiratory difficulties, hypotonia, and epilepsy are also often characteristic. Pathologically, the deep gray and brainstem are primarily affected by vasculonecrotic lesions. The brainstem tegmentum, inferior colliculi, and substantia nigra are characteristically affected. Grossly, these lesions are atrophic, soft, and symmetrically distributed. Microscopically, the findings resemble those seen in Wernicke-Korsakoff syndrome (although hemorrhagic features are absent and the mamillary bodies are normal). Typical lesions bear rarefaction of the neuropil with spongiosis and relative neuron preservation, foamy macrophages, and gliosis and an increased density of capillaries that is thought to result from vascular proliferation and/or neuropil collapse.

Kearns-Sayre syndrome (KSS) is a sporadic disorder that is most frequently due to a deletion in the mtDNA genome (approximately 5 kb). KSS is usually of pediatric onset and is neurologically characterized by eye findings (ophthalmoplegia, ptosis, retinitis pigmentosa, and vision loss), hearing deficits, weakness, ataxia, proximal myopathy, cognitive impairment, and seizures. Extra-CNS abnormalities include short stature, often fatal cardiac pathology (cardiomyopathy and conduction problems), and plus additional GI, renal, and endocrine perturbations. Chronic progressive external ophthalmoplegia (CPEO) may be seen as a component of KSS or alternatively can be the sole manifestation of a mitochondrial disorder. Neuropathologic abnormalities classically include RRFs on muscle biopsy and a diffuse spongy myelinopathy. This white matter pathology is not accompanied by prominent gliosis or macrophagic infiltrates. As can be seen in many of the disorders characterized by spongy myelinopathy, splitting of myelin lamellae at the intraperiod line results in vacuole formation. Like many mitochondrial diseases, deep gray matter may bear vascular mineralization. Correlating with clinical ataxia, cerebellar pathology includes Purkinje neuron dendritic deformities plus eventual neuronal dropout.

Amino Acid Disorders

Amino acid disorders are rare inherited (mostly autosomal recessive) deficits in the enzymatic degradation of amino acids. This group includes the urea cycle disorders, phenylketonuria (PKU), nonketotic hyperglycinemia, homocystinuria, maple syrup urine disease (MSUD), and some of the organic acidemias (e.g., propionic and methylmalonic acidemia). Although some of these diseases have an insidious onset and pursue a chronic course, most follow a severe and fatal clinical picture in early childhood. Encephalopathy/psychomotor impairment, seizures, and motor findings (spasticity, tetraplegia) are seen. Neurologic dysfunction is thought to be related to a combination of toxic biochemical accumulations (e.g., amino acid intermediaries, hyperammonemia), deficits in the biosynthesis of key metabolic compounds, and energy dysfunction. Neuropathologic alterations commonly include a spongy myelinopathy (like that seen in KSS) that tends to affect infratentorial structures, Alzheimer-type II astrocytes (see below), and neocortical/deep gray hypoxic–ischemic lesions. Vascular pathology (i.e., infarction) is characteristic of homocystinuria (see Chapter 5).

Congenital Disorders of Glycosylation

The *congenital disorders of glycosylation* (CDGs) are an uncommon but evolving group of relatively recently described inborn errors of metabolism. *N*- and *O*-linked glycan synthesis/processing are affected and ultimately result in hypoglycosylated glycoproteins; hence, these disorders are often multisystemic in nature. These disorders are inherited in an autosomal recessive manner, and the genetic basis underlying many of the CDGs is a missense mutation. Isoelectric focusing of transferrin is the common test used in the diagnosis of CDGs. CDG type Ia is the most common and best described entity. The R141H missense mutation in the *PMM2* gene on 16p13.3-13.2 is the most frequent mutation in CDG Ia. Infants are affected in the early stages by prominent psychomotor impairment, ataxia, and alternating strabismus. This early phase of disease is often fatal. If the patient survives, later neurologic manifestations include retinitis pigmentosa, seizures, and stroke-like episodes. Other clinical aspects of CDG Ia may include hypotonia, feeding problems, liver disease (fatty infiltration and cirrhosis, leading to coagulopathies), pericardial effusions, dysmorphic features (inverted nipples, subcutaneous buttock fat pads, and contractures), and musculoskeletal abnormalities. Neuropathologic features are dominated by olivopontocerebellar atrophy (OPCA); EM may reveal myelin-like lysosomal inclusions.

Acquired Metabolic Disorders and Vitamin Deficiencies

Acquired metabolic diseases affecting the nervous system are numerous. They are encountered more frequently in adults, although pediatric examples are clinically and pathologically similar. Some of these include hypoglycemia, electrolyte disorders (e.g., central pontine myelinolysis [CPM], disorders of calcium hemostasis), hepatic encephalopathy, porphyria, uremic, and dialysis-related encephalopathy. Several vitamin deficiencies may also characteristically lead to neurologic disease. These include thiamine (B1) and Wernicke-Korsakoff syndrome, pyridoxine (B6), B12 (subacute combined degeneration), nicotinic acid (pellagra), folic acid, vitamin A (intoxication also possible), and vitamin E.

Neurodegenerative and Miscellaneous Disorders

There are a number of neurodegenerative and more nondescript neurologic disorders that characteristically affect the pediatric population. A subset of these entities is discussed below.

Alpers-Huttenlocher syndrome (progressive neurodegeneration of childhood [PNDC]) is now considered by many to reside among the mitochondrial disorders (41). This disease manifests in infancy and is characterized by the acute onset of intractable seizures, developmental delay, hypotonia, ataxia, cortical blindness, failure to thrive, and liver disease (which pathologically reveals bile duct proliferation and cirrhosis). Death frequently occurs by 3 years of age. Molecular genetic studies have revealed mtDNA depletion and mutations in the polymerase gamma *(POLG)* gene. Genetic transmission has been suggested to be autosomal recessive. Gross pathologic findings reveal a patchy neocortical atrophy that has a predilection for the visual cortex. Along with thalamic and focal hippocampal atrophy, there may be concomitant HCP *ex vacuo*. Microscopically, the neocortex is especially affected by a spongy rarefaction, with superimposed neuronal loss and gliosis; severe cases are transcortical, while less involved cortex shows these abnormalities more superficially. These spongy changes are reminiscent of those seen in Creutzfeldt-Jakob disease (CJD). Neuronal loss is often prominent in the inferior olives. Neutral fat deposition in diseased parenchyma is highlighted with Oil Red O staining.

Axonal spheroids are a microscopic accompaniment of many diseases that affect the nervous system. When numerous, these axonal spheroids may signify the presence of a *neuroaxonal dystrophy (NAD)*. Axonal spheroids are rounded eosinophilic structures ranging in size from 20 to 120 μm. They are highlighted with silver stains or by various IHC stains (e.g., NFP and ubiquitin). EM reveals mitochondrial, membrane-bound electron-dense granule, and tubulomembranous structures, all among an amorphous matrix; intermediate filaments are surprisingly sparse but if seen are often displaced toward the periphery. Two NADs are discussed further: infantile neuroaxonal dystrophy (INAD, or Seitelberger disease) and neurodegeneration with brain iron accumulation type 1 (NBIA; pantothenate kinase–associated neurodegeneration [PANK] or Hallervorden-Spatz disease). Both are rare progressive neurologic diseases.

INAD typically has an onset just after 1 year of age. Sporadic and familial forms (with an autosomal recessive inheritance pattern) may be seen. A definitive pathogenesis has not been defined. Normal development may be seen early on, but psychomotor impairment eventually develops. Weakness, hypotonia, depressed deep tendon reflexes, visual difficulties, and cerebellar deficits (ataxia, pendular nystagmus) may also be seen clinically. Terminal stages of disease (between 6 and 15 years of age) include tetraplegia/spasticity with decerebrate posturing, bulbar palsies, and bowel/bladder incontinence. Gross pathologic examination reveals cerebral and cerebellar atrophy with HCP *ex vacuo*. Optic nerves may be atrophic as well. The globus pallidus is large and pale early on but later takes on a rusty discoloration. Microscopically, the deep gray matter, brain stem (including the substantia nigra), cerebellar cortex, and spinal cord are especially affected; abnormalities include axonal spheroids (central, peripheral, and in the autonomic nervous systems), spongy degeneration, gliosis, and lipid/iron pigment accumulation (especially within the globus pallidus and the substantia nigra reticulata). These regions, as well as a few white matter tracts (e.g., corticospinal, spinobulbar, optic, olfactory), may display demyelination-like pathology.

NBIA occurs in both sporadic and familial (autosomal recessive) forms and may have an onset at any age. Infantile (<1-year old), late infantile (2- to 5-year old), juvenile ("classic") 7- to 15-year old), and rarely adult-onset cases have been described. Infantile/late infantile cases are often fatal before 10 years of age and are more often associated with mutations in the *PANK2* gene. An insidious gait disorder with hypotonia often heralds the onset of disease, although psychomotor deficits may predate such manifestations. Hyperkinetic movement disorders are a key clinical feature and are seen in approximately 50%; these include choreoathetosis, dystonia, and tremors, which may result in dysarthria, dysphagia, and abnormal extraocular movements. Additional neurologic deficits include ataxia and nystagmus, visual abnormalities, hyperreflexia with a Babinski response, and leg amyotrophy. Cognitive impairment leads to dementia. *HARP syndrome* (hypo-β-lipoproteinemia, acanthocytosis, retinitis pigmentosa, and pallidal degeneration) is considered to reside within the NBIA clinicopathologic spectrum (42). MRI findings characteristically reveal the "eye of the tiger" sign where a ringlike region of T2 hypointensity is seen in the globus pallidus externa and the substantia nigra, while T2 hyperintensity is seen in the globus pallidus interna. Gross pathology reveals atrophy within the cerebrum and cerebellum; this atrophy has a rusty hue in the globus pallidus interna and substantia nigra (Figure 10-22). Microscopically, the pallidonigral system is characteristically affected by iron pigment deposition, neuronal loss, gliosis, and spheroid formation. Granular pigment containing iron, lipofuscin, and

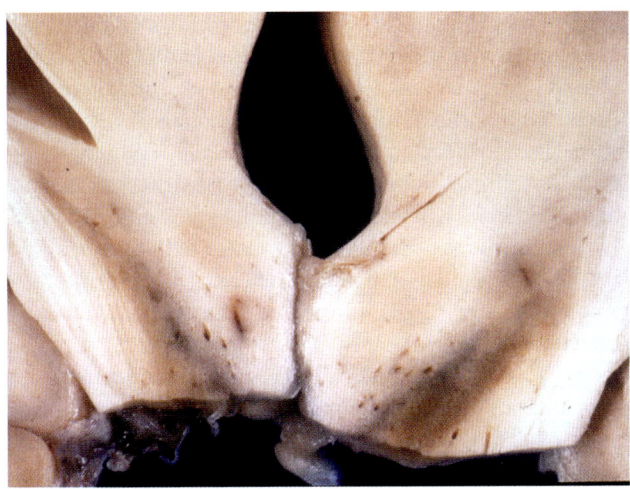

FIGURE 10-22 • NIBA (PANK or HSD). This coronal brain section reveals a rusty discoloration of the substantia nigra.

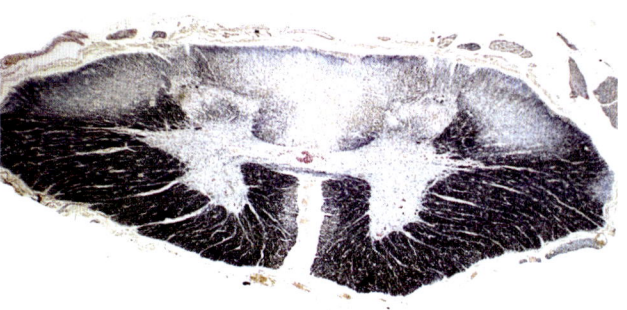

FIGURE 10-23 • Friedreich ataxia (FA). In this myelin-stained histologic preparation of the spinal cord in transverse section, there is a symmetric lack of staining in the dorsal columns, corticospinal tracts, and less so in the spinocerebellar tracts.

neuromelanin may be intracellular (neuronal somata and axons, astrocytes, and microglia) or extracellular. Spheroids may also be seen in other deep gray nuclei, as well as the neocortex, the brainstem tegmentum, and the spinal cord. Notably, the peripheral nervous system is not affected.

Neurodegenerative disorders that prominently affect the cerebellum are numerous but uncommon. Secondary forms of cerebellar disease (i.e., paraneoplastic, toxic/nutritional, vascular, infectious/inflammatory, prion related, and metabolic) will not be discussed here. Primary forms of cerebellar disease may be inherited or sporadic (e.g., MSA, idiopathic degeneration) in nature. Familial cerebellar ataxia may follow an autosomal recessive or dominant pattern of inheritance. Some of the more common forms of autosomal recessive (Friedreich ataxia [FA]; ataxia telangiectasia [AT]) and autosomal dominant diseases (the "spinocerebellar ataxias"; dentatorubropallidoluysian atrophy [DRPLA]; and the episodic ataxias [EA1 and EA2]) are discussed below.

FA is a progressive multisystem disorder that typically has an onset prior to 15 years of age and results in death by the end of the fourth decade. This disorder involves an abnormally expanded intronic GAA trinucleotide repeat within the frataxin (*FXN*) gene located on 9q13-21.1. The product of this gene encodes for a mitochondrial protein involved in iron transport; protein dysfunction is thought to lead to iron accumulation and oxidative neuronal damage. Ataxia (of gait, limb and voice, or dysarthria) is the result of cerebellar and sensory degeneration. There is a loss of position and vibratory sense, along with areflexia. A pyramidal pattern of leg weakness is accompanied by a Babinski response. Extra-CNS manifestations include pes cavus, scoliosis, cardiomyopathy, and diabetes mellitus. Gross pathologic CNS findings are generally limited to atrophic dorsal roots of the spinal cord; ischemic CNS disease may be seen and may be attributed to cardiac disease. Microscopic changes are prominent within the spinal cord and include tract degenerations (spinocerebellar, corticospinal, and dorsal columns) plus degeneration of Clarke's columns (Figure 10-23). The dorsal root ganglia show neuronal depletion with associated nodules of Nageotte (proliferation of satellite cells that normally rim sensory neurons of the dorsal root ganglia). Large myelinated sensory fibers are lost in peripheral nerves. Neuronal loss in the accessory cuneate and gracile nuclei reflects transsynaptic degeneration. Neuronal loss and gliosis are seen in the vestibular, cochlear, and superior olivary nuclei. Cerebellar abnormalities include white matter gliosis plus neuronal loss in the dentate nuclei with concomitant superior cerebellar peduncle atrophy. Hypoxic–ischemic changes may be seen in the cerebellum and neocortex.

Strictly speaking, *spinocerebellar atrophy* (SCA) is a heterogeneous group of autosomal dominant neurodegenerative disorders affecting the cerebellum and additional CNS structures. The reciprocal circuitry between the cerebellar cortex, dentate nucleus, and the inferior olive (the "cerebellar module") is thought to be particularly important to the pathogenesis of ataxia (43). The number of disorders included under the rubric of SCA continues to grow at a rapid pace, and types 1 to 36 have recently been described (note: there is no SCA 33 or 34) (1,44). Many of the SCAs are trinucleotide repeat disorders, of which six forms (SCA 1 to 3, 6, 7, and 17) bear expanded CAG coding repeats along with clinical evidence of "genetic anticipation," wherein the repeat becomes progressively longer, and disease onset is progressively earlier with increasing disease severity for each subsequent generation of patients. SCA 10 and 31 are exceptional in that they exhibit pentanucleotide repeats of ATTCT and TGGAA, respectively. Despite their recognition, the mechanism by which these repeats cause disease is unclear.

Although the typical age of onset is usually after the fifth decade, pediatric forms of SCA may be seen. The spectrum of neurologic deficits includes cerebellar dysfunction (truncal and limb ataxia, dysarthria, nystagmus), abnormal gait, spasticity, weakness, parkinsonism and other extrapyramidal movement disorders, pyramidal signs, autonomic dysfunction, sensory abnormalities (including visual difficulties), and cognitive impairment. Some SCAs cause a multitude of neurologic deficits, while others are considered "purely" cerebellar. SCA 3 (or Machado-Joseph disease) is the most common form among this group of diseases. Pathologic descriptions are available for only a subset of these disorders. SCA 2 affects many neurologic systems. The gross brain weight is reduced, and there is OPCA. Although there may be gross cerebellar atrophy in SCA 6, one of the "purely" cerebellar forms, such atrophy is not conspicuous in SCA 3. Microscopically, both SCA 2 and SCA 6 demonstrate cerebellar cortical atrophy with Purkinje cell dropout, while the cerebellar disease in SCA 3 targets the dentate nucleus (with neuron loss and "grumose degeneration"). SCA 2 demonstrates neuronal dropout from the basis pontis and inferior olive. The spinal cord is abnormal in both SCA 2 and 3; while both demonstrate fiber loss in the posterior columns and neuronal loss in Clarke's nucleus, SCA 3 exhibits additional lateral column degeneration reminiscent of FA (but without dorsal spinal root involvement). IHC may reveal diagnostically useful intranuclear inclusions or more diffuse staining in the SCAs with expanded CAG repeats (SCA 6 bears abnormal cytoplasmic staining only). These inclusions may stain with antibodies targeting the abnormal gene product involved, expanded polyglutamine residues (e.g., IC2), ubiquitin, or against other "chaperone" proteins.

Spinal muscular atrophy (SMA) is an autosomal recessive neuromuscular disorder resulting from the homozygous mutation or deletion of the *SMN1* gene on 5q13. Three forms are generally recognized. *SMA 1* (or Werdnig-Hoffmann disease) has an onset in infancy. Proximal extremity muscle weakness progresses to involve the axial and diaphragmatic muscles; there may be bulbar involvement with respiratory insufficiency related to intercurrent infection and aspiration. Death is often seen prior to 1 year of age. In *SMA 2*, early motor development may be normal, but weakness prevails by 3 months of age. There may be lingual atrophy and hand tremor. Fasciculations and depressed deep tendon reflexes are also seen. Eventually, contractures and kyphoscoliosis develop. Most die by 25 years of age. *SMA 3* is a more chronic and insidious form but still may have a young onset. A functional motor deficit is appreciated and includes clinical weakness. Knee jerk reflexes are depressed and there may also be hand tremor. This subtype does not affect respiratory musculature or lead to shortened life span. Pathologically, SMA 3 exhibits an adult pattern of muscle denervation with angulated fibers, whereas SMA 1 and 2 show grouped atrophy with small rounded fibers intermixed with hypertrophic type I fibers, the latter possibly reflecting a compensatory response (Figure 10-24). In the end stage, endomysial connective tissue and fat replacement may mimic a muscular dystrophy. Within the CNS, all forms of disease demonstrate gross anterior spinal root atrophy, with anterior horn lower motor neuron loss and concomitant gliosis microscopically. Earlier stages may feature neuronophagia and chromatolytic neurons. The latter may also be seen in the thalamus and can be a useful diagnostic feature. Bulbar motor neurons may also be affected.

Autism

Autism is an enigmatic and increasingly common neurologic disorder characterized by three key features: impaired social interaction, communication deficits (both verbal and nonverbal), and restricted/stereotyped behavior. Onset is before 3 years of age, and there is a 4:1 male-to-female sex distribution. Prevalence has most recently been estimated at 1/150 live births. The term autism spectrum disorders (ASD) is also often used to reflect the widely held notion that there are likely multiple overlapping forms rather than a single disorder, including Asperger disorder with enhanced language fluency and higher-level functioning. Genetic factors are critical, but rather than a simple Mendelian pattern of inheritance, multiple genes are likely to be involved in predisposition. In particular, duplication of chromosome 15q11-q13 is observed in a subset, and there appears to be a strong linkage between this GABA β3 subunit–encoding locus and the clinical feature of "insistence on sameness" (45).

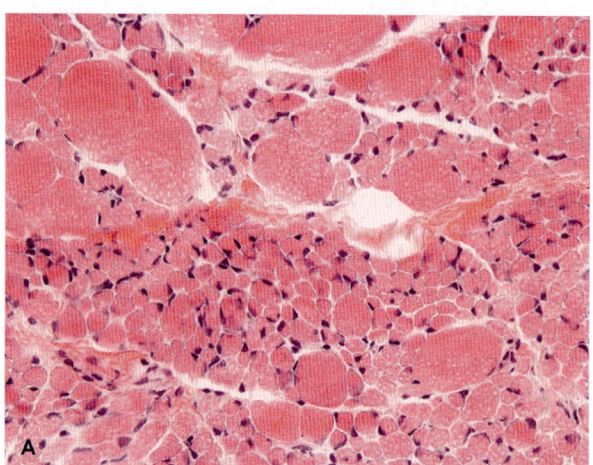 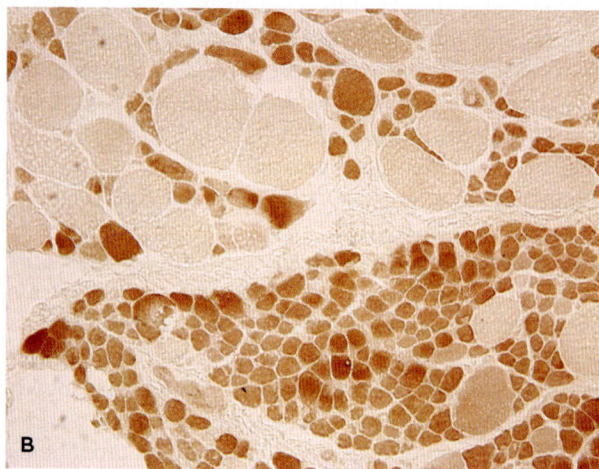

FIGURE 10-24 • Spinal muscular atrophy (SMA). **A:** H&E-stained frozen section of skeletal muscle reveals the typical distribution of rounded atrophic and enlarged fibers. **B:** Many of the latter prove to be type I (ATPase pH 9.4).

Neurotransmitter studies have suggested deficits in GABA-A receptors (hippocampal formation), ACh receptors (frontal and parietal lobes plus the cerebellar cortex), and decreased 5HT synthesis (dentatothalamocortical pathway) (46–48). Although the prevalence of autism is clearly higher in monozygotic (60% to 90% concordance) versus dizygotic (5% to 10% concordance) twins, environmental factors likely play a significant etiologic role as well. Neuropathologic descriptions remain limited, although the most common gross finding, especially in young patients, is a nonspecific megalencephaly. A recent review by Blatt summarizes the widespread, yet highly variable neuropathologic abnormalities reported in autism, including neocortical, limbic, and olivocerebellar changes (49). Purkinje cell dropout is common in some series, but not others. Limbic structures (including the amygdala, hippocampus, and entorhinal cortex) exhibit small and closely packed neurons. Neocortical malformations may be seen and include a thickened neocortex, focal increased neuronal density, dyslamination, pyramidal neuronal malorientation, an increase in white matter, and molecular layer neurons. Cortical microcolumns, thought to be the smallest functional unit of the neocortex, have also been studied and found to be abnormally developed (50). Several brain regions, including the vertical limb of the nucleus of the diagonal band of Broca, the dentate nucleus, and the inferior olive, demonstrate neuronomegaly in younger patients with autism, followed by atrophy in older patients; there may be superimposed neuronal loss in some of these regions.

Epilepsy

Epilepsy may be a manifestation of a number of different disorders that cause dysfunctioning of the neocortex. Vascular, infectious, traumatic, autoimmune, neoplastic, metabolic, malformative, and neurodegenerative are some of the etiologic classes that may be involved in the pathogenesis of epilepsy. Epilepsy in the context of "malformations of cortical development" (in particular, *focal cortical dysplasia*) is discussed in detail above. Epileptogenic lesions of wide ranging etiology are frequently resected and encountered on the surgical pathology service. In reviewing their surgical pathology experience, Pasquier et al. (51) reviewed 327 cases of drug-resistant epilepsy and highlighted the spectrum of disease that may be seen in this context. Included within these specimens was a large number displaying a common form of idiopathic pathology to which we will limit our discussion here: *mesial temporal sclerosis* (MTS). MTS (also known as Ammon horn sclerosis or hippocampal sclerosis) is not usually associated with a clear genetic abnormality and does not have a clear pathogenesis. However, some cases are associated with a history of prolonged febrile seizures during infancy, and moreover, the pathology is similar if not identical to that seen within the context of hypoxic–ischemic injury. MTS may be seen in isolation or in conjunction with a second form of temporal lobe pathology (e.g., neoplasm, vascular formation, cortical dysplasia). Gross pathology reveals atrophy of the hippocampal formation with concomitant dilatation of the adjacent inferior temporal horn of the lateral ventricle (Figure 10-25A). Microscopically, neuronal loss and gliosis are most striking in the CA1 and CA4 (i.e., endfolium) hippocampal subregions (Figure 10-25B). Neuronal loss, dispersion, and/or duplication may also be seen within the dentate granular layer. Dysmorphic neurons may occasionally be seen in the endfolium and, like some of the dentate granule neuron alterations, may be a reactive, rather than primary component of MTS. A microscopically similar type of neurodegenerative pathology, often termed "hippocampal sclerosis," is occasionally seen in the elderly population, but unlike MTS, it is associated with TDP-43 immunopositive inclusions on microscopy (52).

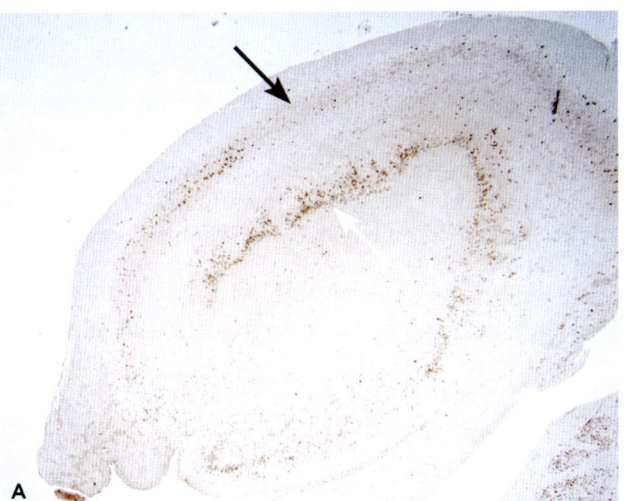
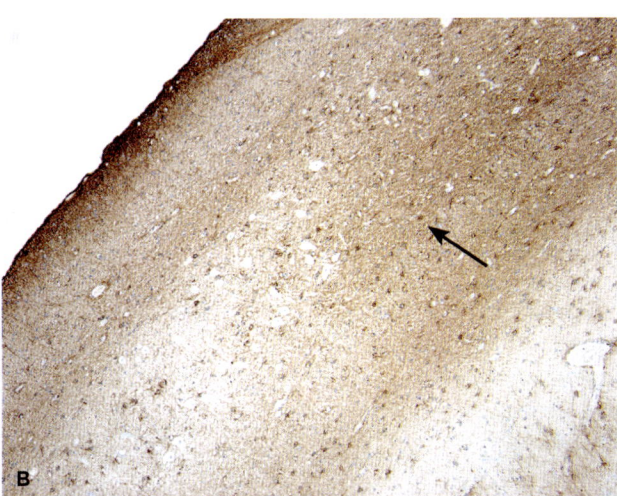

FIGURE 10-25 • Mesial temporal sclerosis (MTS). **A:** Using NeuN immunohistochemistry, this low-power magnification image reveals a dropout of neurons in the hippocampal CA1 subregion (*black arrow*), as well as neuronal dispersion within the dentate granule layer of the hippocampal formation (*white arrow*). **B:** GFAP-stained section reveals marked gliosis of CA1. Note: unstained neurons (**left**) taper off into a region of more intense gliosis (*arrow*).

Neoplasia

Primary CNS tumors are common in pediatrics and only superseded by lymphoid–hematopoietic neoplasia in terms of frequency (53). Although adults and children may incur similar tumors, their relative frequencies vary significantly with age. In children, PAs are the most frequent, followed by medulloblastoma and ependymoma (Table 10-4). With respect to infants (i.e., <1-year-old), low-grade astrocytomas (including PAs and pilomyxoid astrocytoma [PMA]) are also most common; however, the most common malignancy may now be "atypical teratoid rhabdoid tumor" (ATRT) rather than medulloblastoma, given widespread use of INI1 IHC

TABLE 10-4 THE MAIN HISTOLOGIC TYPES OF PRIMARY CNS TUMORS IN CHILDREN AND THEIR RELATIVE FREQUENCIES

Tumor Type, WHO Grade	Percentage
Pilocytic astrocytoma (PA), I	23.5
Diffuse astrocytoma, II	5
Anaplastic astrocytoma, III	7.2
Glioblastoma (GBM), IV	7.2
Pleomorphic xanthoastrocytoma (PXA), II–III[a]	1.9
Subependymal giant cell astrocytoma (SEGA), I	2.5
Medulloblastoma, IV	16.3
Ependymoma, II–III[a]	10.1
Craniopharyngioma (CPG), I	5.6
Germ cell tumors	2.5
Ganglioglioma (GG), I–III[a]	2.5
Meningioma, I–III[a]	2.5
Supratentorial primitive neuroectodermal tumor (sPNET), IV	1.9
Pineal parenchymal tumors (PPTs) (pineocytoma; pineoblastoma), II–IV	1.9
Atypical teratoid rhabdoid tumor (ATRT), IV	1.3
Choroid plexus tumors (CPTs) (papilloma; carcinoma), I and III	0.9
Desmoplastic infantile ganglioglioma (DIG)/astrocytoma (DIA), I	0.6
Dysembryoplastic neuroepithelial tumor (DNT), I	0.6
Pituitary adenoma	0.9
Schwannoma	1.3
Neurofibroma	0.3
Langerhans cell histiocytosis	0.6

[a]Tumors where a range of grades are listed, the highest grade is generally called "anaplastic."
Data from Rickert CH, Paulus W. Epidemiology of central nervous system tumors in childhood and adolescence based on the new WHO classification. *Childs Nerv Syst* 2001;17(9):503-11.

(54). For daily practice, the WHO Classification of Tumors of the Nervous System (2007) is currently considered the standard diagnostic scheme (Table 10-5) (56). Nonetheless, despite continued advances in our knowledge of neoplasia, several pediatric tumors remain difficult to classify and even those that otherwise resemble their adult counterparts are biologically and genetically unique.

Clinical Considerations

The presenting signs and symptoms of pediatric brain tumors are largely similar to those described in adults (Table 10-6). However, tumors occurring in infancy often display more insidious features (e.g., failure to thrive, irritability) that often mislead initial clinical workup. As such, neuroradiologic studies are an important tool, often serving as a surrogate for gross pathology, particularly in small biopsies. Therefore, such studies should optimally be reviewed prior to intraoperative consultation. CT and MR images (including T1 +/− gadolinium enhancement, T2, flair, diffusion-weighted imaging, and susceptibility-weighted imaging/gradient echo sequences) greatly assist in refining the differential diagnosis by revealing locations and diagnostically useful patterns (e.g., cystic lesions with a mural nodule).

Treatment strategies generally involve surgery, radiotherapy, and chemotherapy. Radiotherapy and chemotherapy are often reserved for high-grade/malignant neoplasms, although commonly used in lower-grade tumors as well when complete resection is not possible. While radiotherapy can be highly effective, it is often avoided in children under 3 years of age due to its damaging effects on the developing nervous system. In such cases, many oncologists opt for high-dose chemotherapy-only options (e.g., the Head Start regimen). A more thorough assessment of therapeutic neurooncology is available elsewhere (57).

General Pathologic Considerations

The workup of pediatric CNS tumors often employs both routine and ancillary pathologic studies. As classification schemes are regularly updated, it is important to review prior surgical specimens at the time of recurrence or progression, as previous diagnoses occasionally need revision. Initial tumor evaluation often begins at the time of intraoperative consultation, with cytologic smear/touch preparations and frozen sections frequently undertaken to guide surgical management. The *frozen section* provides a preliminary diagnosis and enables tissue allocation algorithms, the latter of which are increasingly being utilized for tumor banking, local research, ancillary molecular testing, and participation in clinical protocols. However, diagnostic accuracy ultimately remains most critical, and therefore, first priority should always be given to allocating tissue to optimally preserved permanent sections. Retention and processing of cavitronic ultrasound aspirator (CUSA) material may be somewhat less preserved than resected tissue due to partial autolysis and other artifacts but can nonetheless be essential to the final diagnosis, especially in the

TABLE 10-5 WHO CLASSIFICATION OF TUMORS OF THE NERVOUS SYSTEM

Tumors of neuroepithelial tissue
Astrocytic tumors
    Pilocytic astrocytoma (PA)
    Pilomyxoid astrocytoma
    Subependymal giant cell astrocytoma (SEGA)
    Pleomorphic xanthoastrocytoma (PXA)
    Diffuse astrocytoma
    Fibrillary astrocytoma
    Protoplasmic astrocytoma
    Gemistocytic astrocytoma
    Anaplastic astrocytoma
    Glioblastoma (GBM)
    Giant cell GBM
    Gliosarcoma
    Gliomatosis cerebri
Oligodendroglial tumors
    Oligodendroglioma
    Anaplastic oligodendroglioma
Oligoastrocytic tumors
    Oligoastrocytoma
    Anaplastic oligoastrocytoma
Ependymal tumors
    Subependymoma
    Myxopapillary ependymoma
    Ependymoma
        Cellular
        Papillary
        Clear cell
        Tanycytic
    Anaplastic ependymoma
Choroid plexus tumors (CPTs)
    Choroid plexus papilloma (CPP)
    Atypical CPP
    Choroid plexus carcinoma (CPC)
Other neuroepithelial tumors
    Astroblastoma
    Chordoid glioma of the third ventricle
    Angiocentric glioma
Neuronal and mixed glioneuronal tumors
    Dysplastic gangliocytoma of cerebellum (Lhermitte-Duclos)
    Desmoplastic infantile astrocytoma/ ganglioglioma
    Dysembryoplastic neuroepithelial tumor (DNT)
    Gangliocytoma
    Ganglioglioma (GG)
    Anaplastic ganglioglioma
    Papillary glioneuronal tumor
    Rosette-forming glioneuronal tumor of the fourth ventricle
    Central neurocytoma
    Extraventricular neurocytoma
    Cerebellar liponeurocytoma
    Paraganglioma of the filum terminale
Tumors of the pineal region
    Pineal parenchymal tumors (PPTs)
    Pineocytoma
    PPT of intermediate differentiation
    Pineoblastoma
    Papillary tumor of the pineal region
Embryonal tumors
    Medulloblastoma
    Desmoplastic–nodular medulloblastoma
    Medulloblastoma with extensive nodularity
    Anaplastic medulloblastoma
    Large cell medulloblastoma
    CNS primitive neuroectodermal tumors (PNETs)
    CNS PNET, NOS
    CNS neuroblastoma
    CNS ganglioneuroblastoma
    Medulloepithelioma
    Ependymoblastoma
    Atypical teratoid/rhabdoid tumor

Tumors of cranial and paraspinal nerves
Schwannoma (neurilemmoma, neurinoma)
    Cellular
    Plexiform
    Melanotic
Neurofibroma
    Plexiform
Perineurioma
    Intraneural perineurioma
    Soft tissue perineurioma
Malignant peripheral nerve sheath tumor (MPNST)
    Epithelioid
    MPNST with divergent mesenchymal and/or epithelial differentiation
    Melanotic

(Continued)

TABLE 10-5 WHO CLASSIFICATION OF TUMORS OF THE NERVOUS SYSTEM (continued)

Tumors of the meninges	Epithelioid hemangioendothelioma
Tumors of meningothelial cells	Hemangiopericytoma
Meningioma	Angiosarcoma
Meningothelial	Kaposi sarcoma
Fibrous (fibroblastic)	Primary melanocytic lesions
Transitional (mixed)	Diffuse melanocytosis
Psammomatous	Melanocytoma
Angiomatous	Malignant melanoma
Microcystic	Meningeal melanomatosis
Secretory	Other neoplasms related to the meninges
Lymphoplasmacyte rich	Hemangioblastoma
Metaplastic	**Lymphomas and hematopoietic neoplasms**
Chordoid	Malignant lymphomas
Clear cell	Plasmacytoma
Atypical	Granulocytic sarcoma
Papillary	**Germ cell tumors**
Rhabdoid	Germinoma
Anaplastic (malignant)	Embryonal carcinoma
Mesenchymal tumors	Yolk sac tumor
Lipoma	Choriocarcinoma
Angiolipoma	Teratoma
Hibernoma	Mature
Liposarcoma (intracranial)	Immature
Solitary fibrous tumor	Teratoma with malignant transformation
Fibrosarcoma	Mixed germ cell tumors
Malignant fibrous histiocytoma	**Tumors of the sellar region**
Leiomyoma	Craniopharyngioma (CPG)
Leiomyosarcoma	Adamantinomatous
Rhabdomyoma	Papillary
Rhabdomyosarcoma	Granular cell tumor
Chondroma	Pituicytoma
Chondrosarcoma	Spindle cell oncocytoma of the adenohypophysis
Osteoma	**Metastatic tumors**
Osteosarcoma	
Osteochondroma	
Hemangioma	

Modified from the WHO 2007 classification scheme (55).

context of small tumors. Fixing a small portion of the tumor (i.e., 1 mm³) in glutaraldehyde for ultrastructural analysis is recommended when the initial diagnosis is in question. If sufficient tissue is provided, a fragment should also be snap frozen and stored for future studies. If only a small portion of tumor remains for formalin-fixed paraffin-embedded (FFPE) tissue, requesting a number of unstained sections upfront will reduce the risk of sectioning through the entire specimen.

Evaluation of the FFPE material allows the first precise characterization of tumor. Primary CNS tumors may simplistically be considered as either "well circumscribed" or "diffusely infiltrating," and this dichotomization often assists in narrowing the differential diagnosis. Glial, neuronal, embryonal, and a number of other cytologic features can usually be appreciated on routine stains. Detail should be directed at the nuclear features since these are often key to many diagnoses (especially gliomas). *Degenerative-type atypia*

TABLE 10-6 PRESENTING SIGNS AND SYMPTOMS OF PEDIATRIC BRAIN TUMORS

Symptom/Sign Category	Specific Feature
General illness	Irritability, listlessness, failure to thrive, loss of developmental milestones, behavioral disturbance, poor feeding
Increased ICP or HCP	Headache, nausea, vomiting, macrocephaly, "sun-setting eyes," papilledema
Focal neurologic disturbances ("focality")	Seizures
	Motor deficits (e.g., weakness)
	Visual field loss/deficit (e.g., Parinaud)
	Neuroendocrine dysfunction
	Cranial neuropathies
	Cerebellar dysfunction (nystagmus, ataxia, Romberg sign, abnormal tone, tremor, vertigo, etc.)
	Long tract signs (paraparesis, hyperreflexia, Babinski sign)

(large hyperchromatic nuclei, often bearing cytoplasmic pseudoinclusions) is a common feature to many low-grade primary brain tumors and should not be overinterpreted as a concerning finding in the absence of other malignant features. *Mitotic activity* is critical to the grading of many CNS primary tumors, and specific cutoff numbers [generally expressed as #/10 high-powered fields (HPF)] exist for some tumor types; however, since most of the tumor-specific cutoff numbers were established in adult cohorts, their relevancy to the pediatric population could be questioned since pediatric tumors tend to have greater levels of proliferation in general, especially in infancy (56). *Grading* is generally based not on the entirety of the specimen but on the most malignant portion identified (i.e., "one rotten apple spoils the bunch"). *Microvascular proliferation* (MVP), also referred to as endothelial proliferation or endothelial hyperplasia, represents foci of multilayering in small blood vessels; several cellular elements (including smooth muscle cells, pericytes, and endothelial cells) are identified in these hyperplastic walls despite the focus on endothelia in the name. It is an important finding in the diffuse gliomas, as is *necrosis* (which may be pseudopalisading), where both of these features raise the WHO grade in diffuse gliomas, but not in PA. The latter scenario draws importance to one cardinal rule in brain tumor pathology: tumor classification always precedes grading. EGBs and RFs, while nonspecific, usually imply the presence of a slow-growing neoplasm, as do other features including hyalinization of small blood vessels and calcification.

IHC plays an important ancillary role in the diagnosis of brain tumors. The more commonly utilized stains are listed in Table 10-7. Special histochemical stains and ultrastructural modalities have largely been supplanted by IHC, but the former still have great utility in some scenarios. The *reticulin* histochemical stain is frequently used to identify extracellular matrix deposition in several tumors (e.g., PXA, gliosarcoma, GG, desmoplastic–nodular medulloblastoma) and in some tumors may stain in a pericellular pattern (e.g., schwannoma), indicative of basal lamina (although the immunostain collagen IV is a more specific marker). PAS and PAS-with-diastase stains confirm the presence of glycogen within the cytoplasm of tumor cells (diastase sensitive), while the latter also highlights EGBs and other lysosome-rich processes. A *trichrome* stain highlights RFs in addition to collagen and fibrin. The *Bielschowsky* silver stain labels axons (similar to phosphorylated NFP IHC) and often the ganglion cell component of glioneuronal tumors. LFB, counterstained with H&E or PAS, can be used to stain myelin and, hence, highlight tumor infiltration of white matter, or active demyelination (note: myelin breakdown products within macrophages is first blue, then changes to magenta or PAS positive with time and concomitant degradation), as seen in tumefactive (or tumor-like) multiple sclerosis. Ultrastructural analysis remains the gold standard for a few tumor types, such as ependymoma. The cilia, basal bodies, and intercellular "zipper-like" junctions of ependymoma are often well preserved and may even be identified in FFPE tissue. Electron microscopy can also help support the presence of neuronal differentiation when dense-core granules, clear vesicles, microtubule-filled processes, and synapse formation are seen.

Genetic studies are becoming more frequent in the daily practice of neuropathology. *Karyotyping* remains an excellent method of globally screening rare pediatric brain tumors for cytogenetic abnormalities. Several pediatric brain tumors are amenable to testing, and some may exhibit signature molecular alterations. However, karyotyping is gradually being supplanted by *chromosomal microarrays* (a.k.a. array comparative genomic hybridization) and other genome or methylome screening modalities, given higher sensitivities and broader coverage. *Fluorescence in situ hybridization* (FISH) is occasionally used in the workup of several tumor types, including astrocytomas, oligodendrogliomas, medulloblastomas, ATRTs, and meningiomas. Polymerase chain reaction (PCR)–based *loss of heterozygosity* (LOH) analysis is also used by some, as is *chromogenic in situ hybridization* (CISH). Although not routinely performed, many research protocols involve *whole-genome* and/or *whole-exome sequencing* to identify mutations that can aid in tumor diagnosis and therapy (58,59). As such, high-throughput techniques, elucidating the underpinnings of pediatric brain tumors, are anticipated to become routinely employed for diagnostic, prognostic, and predictive evaluation of affected patients in the future.

TABLE 10-7 IHC STAINS COMMONLY USED IN THE INVESTIGATION OF PEDIATRIC CNS TUMORS

Stain	Utility
GFAP	Glial differentiation, primarily in gliomas, reactive gliosis
S-100 protein	Nonspecific neuroectodermal marker, gliomas, DNT (OLCs), CPT, nerve sheath tumors, melanocytic tumors, histiocytic tumors
Neuronal markers[a]	Facilitate identification of a "neuronal component" in a tumor. Synaptophysin and chromogranin also for neuroendocrine differentiation; NFP labels normal axons and hence infiltration.
Cytokeratin[b]	Epithelial differentiation in CPTs, ATRT, metastatic carcinoma
EMA	Ependymoma[c], meningioma, ATRT, metastatic carcinoma
CD34	Epileptogenic tumors: GG and PXA
INI1/BAF47	ATRT[d]
c-kit	Germinomatous differentiation in germ cell tumors
Ki-67	Proliferative marker
CD68	Lysosomal marker; used to identify reactive elements, including macrophages and microglia; histiocytic tumors
p53	Labels many tumors including astrocytic tumors, high-grade CPTs and MPNSTs. Particularly useful to identify "naked nuclei" of an infiltrating astrocytoma when strongly positive
HMB-45 and Melan-A	Melanocytic markers
CD45, CD20 and CD79a, CD3	Markers of white blood cells (CD45 is general, CD20 and CD79a for B-cells, and CD3 for T-cells) in reactive conditions and lymphoma
IDH1	Detects the R132H mutation in the IDH1 gene, which is common in diffusely infiltrating astrocytomas that progress over time to glioblastoma, GBM (i.e., secondary GBM); however, such mutation, and corresponding immunohistochemical positivity, is generally limited in the pediatric population to those older than 14 y of age (see text for details).
Beta-catenin	Nuclear positivity is a strong and sensitive marker of the WNT molecular group of medulloblastomas and in turn is a favorable prognostic marker. Adamantinomatous craniopharyngiomas, which frequently bear a CTNNB1 mutation, are also correspondingly positive.
GAB1	Marker of the SHH molecular group of medulloblastomas
Collagen IV	Marker of basal lamina
BRAF V600E	Detects the V600E mutation in the BRAF oncogene
Muscle markers[e]	Muscle type differentiation in rhabdomyosarcoma, ATRT, medullomyoblastoma

[a]Neuronal markers: synaptophysin, NeuN, NFP, MAP-2, chromogranin.
[b]CAM 5.2 (low molecular weight cytokeratin most commonly used).
[c]Ependymomas also stain with CD99 in a membranous and dot-like pattern.
[d]For ATRT, a triad of vimentin, EMA and SMA positivity also useful.
[e]Includes SMA, MSA, desmin, myogenin, myoglobin, and caldesmon.
DNT, dysembryoplastic neuroepithelial tumor; OLC, oligodendroglial-like cells; CPTs, choroid plexus tumors; NFP, neurofilament; ATRT, atypical teratoid rhabdoid tumor; GG, ganglioglioma; PXA, pleomorphic xanthoastrocytoma; MPNST, malignant peripheral nerve sheath tumor.

What follows here is a brief account of the pertinent pathologic and molecular genetics of the most common pediatric brain neoplasms. More complete descriptions are presented elsewhere (56,60–62).

Gliomas

Pilocytic Astrocytomas

PAs, WHO grade I, are slowly growing tumors that most commonly occur in the cerebellum, hypothalamus, and in relation to the optic pathway (especially in relation to NF1), although cerebral, brain stem, and spinal cord cases also occur. Imaging often reveals a cystic lesion bearing an enhancing mural nodule.

Histologically, PAs are fairly discrete GFAP-positive tumors that exhibit only limited infiltration of adjacent native parenchyma. They are classically described as *biphasic* with (a) compact areas that contain spindled cells with long thin fibrillary processes (i.e., "piloid" or hairlike) emanating from opposite ends of the cell (i.e., bipolar) and (b) more loosely textured microcystic areas populated by small cells

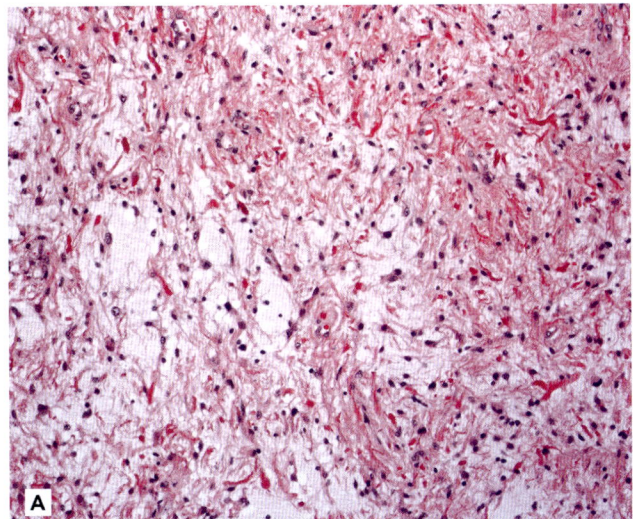 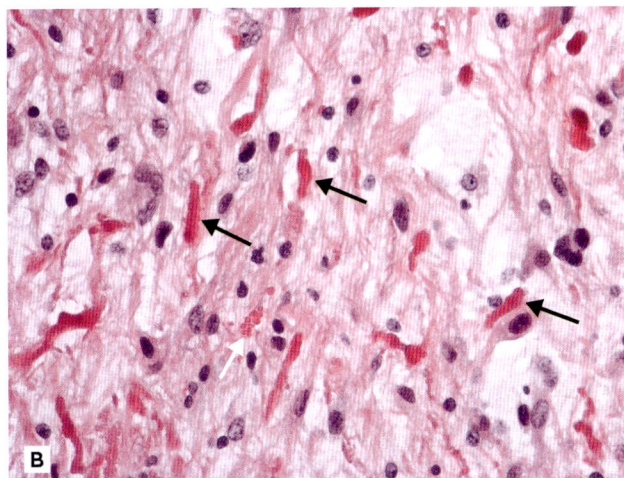

FIGURE 10-26 • Pilocytic astrocytoma (PA). **A:** Medium-power magnification demonstrating the typical biphasic architecture including solid and microcystic areas. **B:** High-power magnification demonstrating bland oval tumor nuclei beset in a fibrillary background composed of long, thin, and delicate cytoplasmic (i.e., piloid) processes. Numerous Rosenthal fibers (*black arrows*) are seen, as is one eosinophilic granular body (EGB; *white arrow*).

with round-oval nuclei bearing short cytoplasmic processes (Figure 10-26A, B); typically, RFs are seen in the former areas, while EGBs are seen in the latter. Degenerative atypia (see above) and vascular hyalinization are both common. Several histologic features, taken out of context, can raise suspicion of a more ominous neoplasm, in particular a diffusely infiltrating type glioma. Areas of a PA may closely resemble diffusely infiltrating astrocytoma (DA) or oligodendroglioma. MVP, often termed "glomeruloid type," can closely mimic that found in high-grade gliomas and may be accompanied by bland "infarct-like" necrosis. Occasionally, the MVP in PA forms linear arrays. Mitotic activity can be seen but is generally low. Extension into the adjacent subarachnoid space is fairly common, but does not adversely impact prognosis. Cases of *anaplastic PA* (WHO grade III), which secondarily develop the typical features of a high-grade DA (see below), have been reported but are exceedingly rare (63). *Pilomyxoid astrocytomas* (PMA) are considered by some to be an infantile variant of PA, since some cases of PMA have been shown to histologically evolve into PA (55). Moreover, Johnson et al. demonstrated that PMA and PA reside along a histologic spectrum (64). Typically, PMAs occur in the hypothalamus and are characterized by a monotonous population of small oval-to-elongate cells; these cells are embedded in mucoid background and form occasional perivascular pseudorosettes similar to those seen in ependymoma along with mitoses, necrosis, and variable infiltration. This proposed variant has been suggested to recur and seed the CSF spaces more frequently than typical PA (65). Accordingly, PMA has been considered a more aggressive variant and designated as WHO grade II in the 2007 WHO classification scheme. With the exceptions of anaplastic and pilomyxoid variants, however, most PAs are WHO grade I and behave in a favorable manner.

Several recent studies have significantly unraveled the molecular genetic features of PA. The vast majority demonstrate abnormalities of the MAPK pathway. Tandem duplication and fusion of KIAA1549 and the *BRAF* oncogene (a.k.a. the "BK" fusion) is the most commonly encountered mutation and is seen in approximately 3/4s of all cerebellar PAs (66,67). Similar *BRAF* alterations were also noted in the so-called "diffuse pilocytic astrocytomas" of the cerebellum studied by Ida and colleagues, supporting the notion that most pediatric astrocytomas of the cerebellum are prognostically favorable despite occasional cases with concerning histologic features (68). Whole-genome sequencing has additionally uncovered somatic mutations in both FGFR1 and NTRK2 in PA, which in turn has highlighted additional therapeutic targets for this very common pediatric brain tumor (59).

Diffusely Infiltrating Astrocytomas

DAs, WHO grades II to IV, are much less common than PAs in the pediatric population, as opposed to adults. Nonetheless, DAs remain an important group of tumors as these are essentially incurable with current therapeutic techniques. They may affect all aspects of the neuraxis, but they have an obvious predilection for white matter, and a much greater proclivity for both the thalamus and the basis pontis than adult counterparts (the latter is referred to as *diffuse intrinsic pontine glioma*, DIPG). DAs are grossly gray-tan-to-gelatinous tumors that obscure the native gray–white boundaries; higher-grade examples often contain additional hemorrhage and necrosis. Microscopically, tumor cells invade adjacent brain structures in a single cell manner and have a tendency to aggregate around or next to pre-existing structural elements such as neurons, blood vessels, and pia;

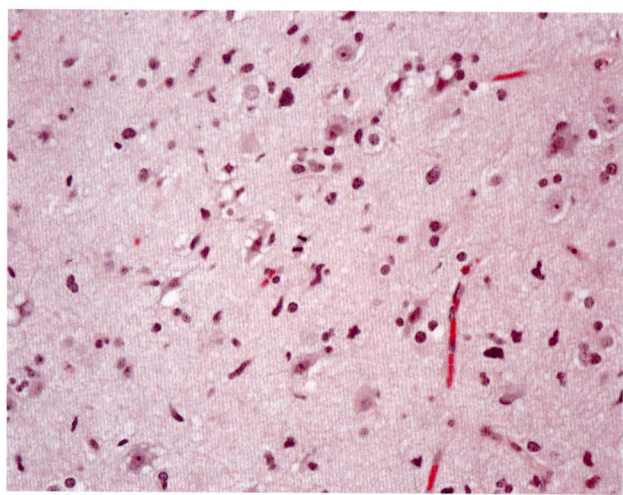

FIGURE 10-27 • Anaplastic astrocytoma, WHO grade III. Enlarged, hyperchromatic, and irregular tumor nuclei are associated with little cytoplasm and are seen diffusely invading neocortical gray matter.

these are called *secondary structures of Scherer*. Infiltration of the white matter can be highlighted via IHC for phosphorylated NFP wherein native axons are seen among the tumor cells. Irregularly arranged, the morphology of infiltrating astrocytic tumor cells ranges from uniform, and minimally atypical, to highly pleomorphic in terms of both their cytoplasmic and nuclear features (Figure 10-27). Eosinophilic cytoplasm is often seen in fibrillary (elongate) and gemistocytic (eccentric "belly-like") forms, with GFAP-positive processes often being few in number and coarse. In contrast, reactive astrocytes are evenly spaced and have a "starburst" appearance with several thin processes radiating in all directions. "Naked nuclei" (i.e., nuclei without discernible cytoplasm on routine staining) are common or predominant in fibrillary astrocytomas, making their identification difficult in cases with only mild hypercellularity and atypia. Nuclear features often reflect tumor grade. In general, the lowest grade tumors (i.e., WHO II) display less pleomorphism; they are moderately hyperchromatic and oval to angulated and bear indistinct nuclear membranes/nucleoli. In higher-grade examples (i.e., WHO III to IV), nuclei often become increasingly pleomorphic and hyperchromatic.

DA *grading criteria* are currently fairly well defined. The four key features are encompassed by the mnemonic "AMEN": nuclear atypia, mitoses, endothelial proliferation, and necrosis. WHO grade II tumors show nuclear atypia alone. One mitotic figure is generally not considered sufficient to warrant an anaplastic designation, especially in large resections (69). WHO grade III tumors (i.e., *anaplastic astrocytoma*) generally exhibit mitotic activity (at least two to three mitoses within the entire surgical material, although specific cutoffs required have not been universally accepted, particularly in the youngest patients). Suspicion of a higher-grade neoplasm is also often deduced from radiologic enhancement, which often (but not always) correlates with the presence of MVP. Either MVP or necrosis (in particular pseudopalisading necrosis, wherein tumor cells cluster or palisade around an area of central necrosis) elevates the grade to IV [i.e., *glioblastoma* (GBM)].

The inherently infiltrative nature of diffuse astrocytomas precludes surgical resection, and recurrences are inevitable. Although some studies suggest better outcomes for childhood versus adult DAs, the prognosis remains poor (70). A recent epidemiologic study of 987 children and adults estimated the median survival times for grades II, III, and IV DAs at 5.6, 1.6, and 0.4 years, respectively (71).

The traditional *EGFR* amplifications (seen in primary or de novo GBM) versus *TP53* and *IDH* mutations (secondary GBMs developing from a lower-grade precursor) molecular pathogenic dichotomy, which characterizes adult DAs, are not applicable to pediatric DAs, with the general exception of a small subset of teenagers harboring "adult-type" gliomas (72,73). However, phosphatase and tensin homolog (PTEN) mutations, which characterize both primary and secondary adult GBMs, may also be seen in children and appear to portend a poor prognosis (72). Over the past several years, IDH1 mutations have been uncovered in secondary GBMs, lower-grade astrocytomas, and oligodendrogliomas, but with respect to children, Pollack et al. demonstrated that this mutation is primarily confined to those patients over 14 years of age (74); as such, standard IDH1 IHC, which identifies the R132H mutation, largely does not play a significant role in pediatric neuropathology, except in older children. To better define the differences between pediatric and adult high-grade astrocytomas, Paugh et al. conducted high-resolution analysis of genomic imbalances using single nucleotide polymorphism microarrays and gene expression microarrays. This study found that the *PDGFRA* gene was the predominant target of focal amplification in pediatric high-grade astrocytomas; in addition, pediatric cases demonstrated more frequent gains of 1q, less frequent gains of chromosome 7, and less frequent loss of 10q versus adult cases (75). More recent studies of WHO grade II DAs have revealed mutations in the transcription factor gene *MYBL1* and the related gene *MYB*, as well as abnormalities in the tyrosine kinase gene *FGFR1* (76). With respect to pediatric high-grade astrocytomas, current research has now focused attention upon epigenetic alterations and has identified recurrent driver mutations in histone and chromatin remodeling genes, including *H3F3A* (which encodes for histone H3.3), *SETD2*, and *ATRX* (76). DIPGs most commonly harbor histone H3.3 or H3.1 K27M mutations, in addition to recently identified recurrent activating mutations in the activin receptor gene *ACVR1* (58). The former are also commonly found in other highly aggressive midline astrocytomas involving the thalamus and spinal cord. In contrast, mutations at the G34 site of the same gene are associated with high-grade cerebral hemispheric gliomas of intermediate prognosis and older age of onset (mostly adolescents and young adults) (77).

Ependymomas

Ependymomas, WHO grades II to III, are discrete radiologically enhancing gliomas, which in children most often occur in relation to the fourth ventricle. Supratentorial and spinal cord cases also occur, the latter of which are more common in adults. Of several microscopic variants (classic, cellular, papillary, clear cell, tanycytic, and myxopapillary), the classic and cellular types are the most common. The microscopic interface with the adjacent brain is often sharp. Tumor cells are more often fibrillar, but epithelial morphologies can be seen. Fibrillarity is often most characteristic within the GFAP-positive nuclear-free zones of perivascular pseudorosettes, whereas the cells lining the less common true ependymal rosettes and canals typically appear epithelioid and label with epithelial membrane antigen (EMA) (Figure 10-28A, B). The epithelial quality of many ependymomas is further reflected by cytoplasmic dot-like positivity upon IHC staining for EMA and CD99. Although not routinely used to make the diagnosis of ependymoma in current clinical practice, electron microscopy can facilitate the diagnosis, especially in challenging cases, by demonstrating long zipper-like intercellular junctions, microvilli, cilia, and intracytoplasmic lumina.

Numerous grading criteria have been proposed to distinguish usual WHO grade II ependymomas from their WHO grade III "anaplastic" counterpart. Although the WHO clearly recognizes anaplastic ependymomas, the criteria by which they are distinguished are regrettably vague and lack quantitative parameters (i.e., "increased cellularity," "brisk mitoses") (56). Adding to the confusion, several past studies attempted to define anaplastic criteria, but no consensus has been achieved. Ho et al. suggested that two of the following four criteria were indicative of anaplasia: mitoses ≥4/10 HPF, hypercellularity, MVP, and necrosis (78). Other studies have found atypia, hypercellularity, and MVP to be reliable prognosticators (79,80). Kurt el al. suggested that indicators of cellular proliferation, in particular cell density–adjusted mitotic rates and Ki-67 labeling indices, to be especially important (81), while Tabori et al. demonstrated that telomerase activity is reflective of anaplasia, typified by IHC positivity for h-TERT (82). Some researchers have also suggested that grading might need to be location specific (i.e., supratentorial versus posterior fossa). Tihan et al. studied 96 pediatric posterior fossa ependymomas and demonstrated that by their well-defined criteria ("anaplasia" was defined by 2 or more of the following criteria: MVP, palisading necrosis, hypercellularity with nuclear pleomorphism/hyperchromasia, and mitoses >10/10 hpf), anaplastic ependymomas incurred a shorter event-free survival (83).

Ependymomas are usually treated with surgery and, in many cases, radiation. Unfortunately, chemotherapy has not been demonstrated to be consistently effective in treatment. With respect to prognosis, "gross total resection" has been the sole consistent favorable indicator. Radiotherapy is often withheld in children under 3 years of age because of the heightened risk of CNS damage in this cohort. Five-year progression-free survival (PFS) and overall survival (OS) rates for grade II and grade III ependymomas were 90% and 93% versus 27% and 61%, respectively (79).

To date, no single genetic feature characterizes the majority of pediatric ependymomas. While loss of chromosome 22q is the most commonly seen abnormality overall, this usually occurs in the context of adult spinal cases and in NF2 patients. Loss of the tumor suppressor gene *4.1B* (DAL-1 on 18p11.3) has been noted to be more common in intracranial examples (especially in the "clear cell variant"), and abnormalities of the *4.1R* gene (on 1p32-33) may also be important (84,85). Various comparative genomic hybridization studies on pediatric intracranial ependymoma have revealed gain on 1q (spinal cases may show gain of chromosome 7) and losses on chromosomes 6q, 9, 13, and 17p in subsets of tumors (86). Poorer clinical outcomes have been suggested in cases with (a) partial chromosomal losses (or structural alterations) and gain of 1q (87) and (b) elevated ErbB2/4 receptor coexpression levels, which is especially predictive when combined with the Ki67 labeling index and extent of resection (88). In addition, microarray and quantitative PCR data have suggested several potential genes of interest in the pathogenesis of pediatric ependymoma (89), with patterns supporting a possible histogenetic link to radial glia (90).

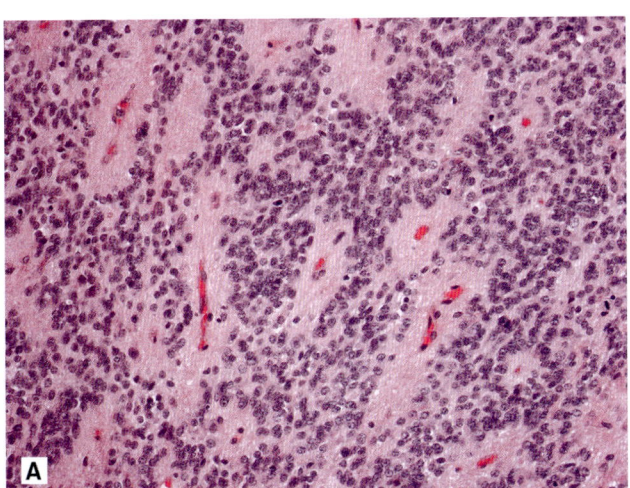 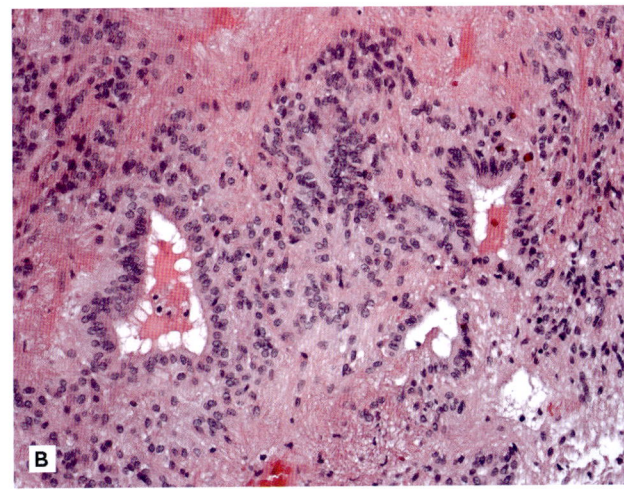

FIGURE 10-28 • Posterior fossa ependymoma, WHO grade II; medium to high magnification. **A:** Perivascular pseudorosettes. **B:** True rosettes.

With respect to posterior fossa ependymomas, recent transcriptional profiling by Witt and colleagues suggested the presence of two distinct clinicopathologic groups, so-called A and B (91). Group A was characterized by younger age, lateral tumor location, a balanced genome, and increased risks of recurrence, metastases (at recurrence), and death. Groups A and B were further defined by via LAMA2 and NELL2 IHC, respectively, with only 16% of all cases being either double positive or double negative for these markers. This molecular dichotomy likely underpins the well-recognized association between extent of surgical resection and clinical outcome and as such suggests that molecular profiling might provide a more accurate prognostic tool. Although further data is required, the delineation of two prognostically different groups of ependymoma may set the stage for tailored therapy wherein some patients could be potentially spared from the harmful effects of radiotherapy.

Less Common Gliomas

Additional relatively discrete and generally low-grade gliomas include pleomorphic xanthoastrocytomas (PXA), subependymal giant cell astrocytomas (SEGA), and desmoplastic infantile astrocytomas/gangliogliomas (DIAs/DIG) (56). These neoplasms are usually associated with a favorable prognosis post resection and are briefly discussed below. *Astroblastoma*s are a rare discrete form of glioma that contain mostly epithelioid and variably GFAP-positive cells arranged in distinctive astroblastic rosettes (i.e., perivascular pseudorosettes containing broad-based cellular processes). Vascular hyalinization is characteristic and often marked in lower-grade examples. Both high- and low-grade forms of astroblastoma have been proposed (56). Like ependymoma, dot-like cytoplasmic EMA expression may be seen, but the tumor generally lacks the fibrillarity seen in ependymoma. *Gliomatosis cerebri* is another rare but well-recognized form of diffuse glioma defined by widespread infiltration involving more than two lobes and potentially infratentorial structures (56). Types I and II are recognized, with the latter being associated with a distinct mass. It is likely that this simply represents an exaggerated form of conventional diffuse gliomas, although prognosis is poor for these patients even when the histologic grade otherwise appears low grade, with the majority of patients dying within 12 months (56). Histologically, gliomatosis cerebri usually demonstrates astrocytic, or more rarely oligodendroglial cytology. *Angiocentric glioma* is a recently described benign (WHO grade I), cortically based, epileptogenic primary neoplasm that displays ependymal-like IHC and ultrastructural features, but elongate astrocytoma-like cytology and a perivascular/subpial infiltrative growth pattern (56,92).

In comparison with adults, *oligodendrogliomas* (WHO grades II and III) are much less common in children. These tumors, as largely defined in adults, are generally white matter–based lesions of the cerebrum that have a tropism for the neocortical gray matter. Secondary structures of Scherer and calcification tend to be more prominent in oligodendrogliomas as opposed to DAs. The typical "fried-egg" appearance of tumor cells is a helpful, although not entirely consistent, tissue-processing artifact wherein round/regular tumor nuclei are surrounded by a clear halo of cytoplasm. Delicate chicken-wire–type vasculature courses between the tumor cells. Scattered mitotic activity is tolerated within grade II forms. In general, mitotic activity greater than 6/10 hpf and/or MVP is necessary for a designation of anaplastic oligodendroglioma (WHO grade III) (93). Oligodendrogliomas are probably best known for their favorable prognosis and chemotherapeutic responsiveness when accompanied by codeletion of the 1p and 19q chromosomal arms (94). Unfortunately, this genetic signature is more commonly encountered in adult oligodendrogliomas and is only rarely encountered in pediatric cases (84,95). Given this lack of a molecular signature in this age group and the fact that oligodendroglioma-like mimics are more common in children than true oligodendrogliomas, one should carefully exclude tumors such as PA, clear cell ependymoma, dysembryoplastic neuroepithelial tumor (DNT), and neurocytic tumors, among others before diagnosing a "pediatric oligodendroglioma."

Pleomorphic xanthoastrocytomas, PXA, WHO grades II and III, are commonly epileptogenic and superficially located in the neocortex of the temporal lobe. Histologic features are quite characteristic, but prior to its recognition as a distinct entity, PXA was commonly misdiagnosed as a GBM. Large pleomorphic cells are variably GFAP positive and often contain substantial eosinophilic to lipidized clear vacuolated cytoplasm. Spindle-shaped cells are arranged in interweaving fascicles that often engender a mesenchymal quality, which is accompanied by pericellular reticulin deposition. EGBs and perivascular lymphocytes are typical. Both subarachnoid space involvement and a limited infiltrative component can be seen. Grading criteria have been proposed to mark a subset of PXAs that are associated with a poor prognosis; five or more mitoses/10 hpf and necrosis have been suggested as criteria for "anaplastic PXA" (56). Previous comparative genomic hybridization work has demonstrated homozygous 9p21.3 mutations involving the *CDKN2A/p14ARF/CDKN2B* loci in a subset of cases. Additionally, a more recent study has shown that PXA commonly harbors a *BRAF V600E* mutation (57/87; 66% of cases) (96). The latter raises the possibility of BRAF inhibitor chemotherapy, and an early trial investigating the utility of vemurafenib in four patients with PXA suggested some beneficial effect on the tumors of three patients in the context of only minimal toxicity (97).

SEGA, WHO grade I, is almost entirely restricted to patients with TS (see later discussion). They usually occur near the foramen of Monro and accordingly result in obstructive HCP. Whether this entity is neoplastic or hamartomatous remains unclear. Imaging reveals contrast enhancement and often calcification. Tumor cells contain abundant glassy eosinophilic cytoplasm and, despite the name, are more aptly considered large than truly "giant" (giant cells of a giant cell GBM are much larger, more bizarre, and often multinucleate). Both spindled and epithelioid to gemistocyte-like cells are seen, typically forming sweeping fascicles and occasional perivascular pseudorosettes. Nuclei often bear prominent nucleoli, resulting in comparisons to ganglion-like cells. These hybrid astrocytic/neuronal features are reiterated in the immunoprofile that sometimes reveals coexpression of GFAP and neuronal markers. Accordingly, some experts have favored the alternative term "subependymal giant cell tumor." Mitoses, MVP, and necrosis are usually absent.

Embryonal Tumors

Embryonal tumors comprise approximately 20% of pediatric CNS tumors. Histologically, they are united by their so-called "small round blue cell" morphology that is characterized by primitive appearing cells exhibiting a high nuclear-to-cytoplasmic ratio, hyperchromatic nuclei, and often high mitotic–karyorrhectic indices. All are cell dense and malignant and carry a WHO grade IV designation. Embryonal tumors include medulloblastoma, the umbrella category "central nervous system primitive neuroectodermal tumor" (CNS PNET), and ATRT. Pineoblastomas are also a form of embryonal tumor but are discussed later, along with other pineal parenchymal tumors (PPT).

Medulloblastoma

Medulloblastomas are the most common embryonal tumor. These infiltrative tumors of the cerebellum most commonly arise in the vermis but can originate in the cerebellar hemispheres. Although characterized by a multilineage potential, medulloblastomas most often manifest at least limited evidence of neuronal differentiation morphologically (e.g., Homer Wright rosettes, neuropil formation, neurocytic differentiation) or immunohistochemically, but occasionally outright ganglioid/ganglionic maturation is appreciated. Less commonly, medulloblastomas may exhibit glial, skeletal muscle, and/or melanocytic types of differentiation.

Radiographically, medulloblastomas are contrast-enhancing tumors that may contain necrosis. Medulloblastomas have a proclivity to escape the confines of the cerebellar parenchyma and invade the subarachnoid space; in doing so, they elicit extra-axial deposition of reticulin fibers (i.e., desmoplastic reaction). As such, it is not surprising that some medulloblastomas may further seed CSF pathways, leading to the formation of "drop metastases" to the spinal cord. Distant metastases may also rarely occur (most frequently bone and lymph nodes).

Numerous histologic subtypes of medulloblastoma exist, the most common of which include *classic*, *desmoplastic–nodular* (DN), *medulloblastoma with extensive nodularity* (MBEN), and *large cell anaplastic* (LCA) (56). Classic medulloblastomas contain patternless sheets of "small round blue cells," with or without *Homer Wright rosettes* (a.k.a. neuroblastic rosettes); the latter are constituted by primitive tumor cells that surround a central island of delicate fibrillar neuropil (Figure 10-29A).

LCA medulloblastomas are characterized by two types of tumor cells, either of which may predominate: (a) *large cells* are rounded and contain enlarged vesicular nuclei, prominent nucleoli, and variable amounts of cytoplasm, and (b) *anaplastic cells* are similarly enlarged but show significant nuclear atypia and hyperchromasia. Both often display cell wrapping, apoptotic lakes, and increased proliferation (Figure 10-30). Attempts at grading medulloblastomas, which essentially amounts to assessing the degree and extent of cytologic anaplasia, have concluded that greater degrees of anaplasia are associated with worse clinical outcomes (98,99). Whereas some advocate separating large cell and anaplastic variants, others have advocated lumping them together since both features are often seen in the same case, both frequently harbor *MYC* gene amplifications, and prognostic/therapeutic implications for each subtype are essentially the same.

DN medulloblastomas have a characteristic low-power appearance of rounded pale islands (i.e., nodules) of tumor,

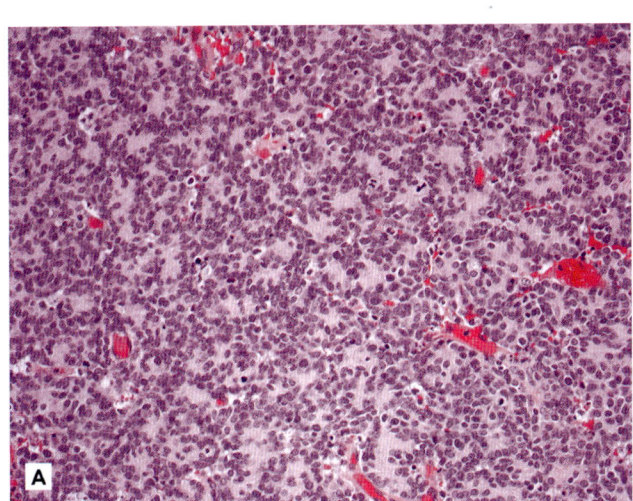 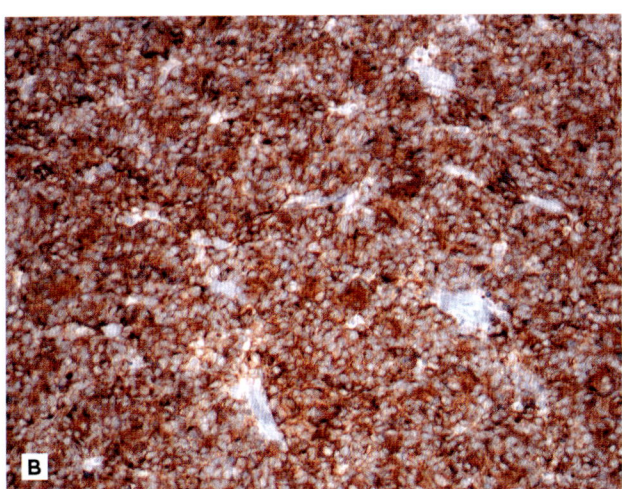

FIGURE 10-29 • Medulloblastoma, "classic" subtype, medium to high magnification. **A:** Numerous Homer Wright rosettes and scattered mitoses are seen. **B:** Strong synaptophysin immunohistochemistry is seen, particularly in the fibrillar cores of the Homer Wright rosettes.

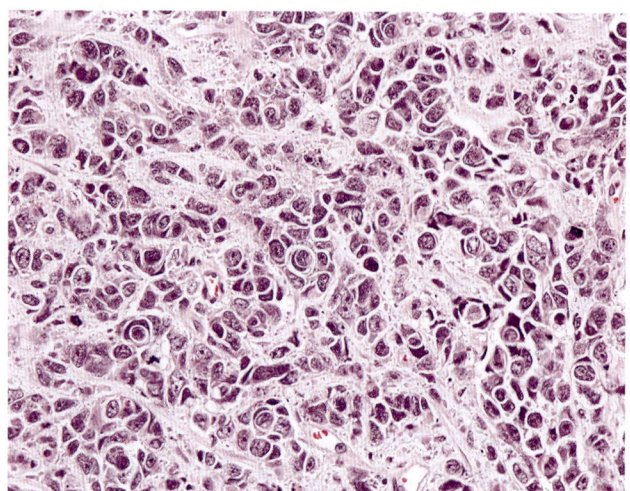

FIGURE 10-30 • Large cell–anaplastic medulloblastoma. "Cell wrapping" is prominent in this example.

separated by darker internodular tumor. The *pale islands* are less cellular and composed of more mature neurocyte-like cells with uniform round-oval, less mitotically active nuclei embedded within neuropil-rich, reticulin-poor background. The *internodular tumor* is more cellular and primitive appearing, with mitotically active cells embedded within reticulin-rich matrix. Sometimes, parallel rows of single tumor cells are identified (i.e., cellular streaming). Tumors bearing a predominance (i.e., >95%) of large irregular pale islands (which are often grossly or radiologically visible) with minimal internodular primitive areas have been termed *MBENs* (formerly known as "cerebellar neuroblastoma"); these rare medulloblastomas seen primarily in infants are considered to form a prognostically more favorable subgroup (56).

IHC confirmation of medulloblastoma is achieved in most cases by demonstrating synaptophysin positivity. The latter ranges from strong and diffuse (Figure 10-29B) to weak and patchy. Lack of synaptophysin staining should lead to consideration of other diagnostic entities, although rare examples of medulloblastoma may be negative. While most medulloblastomas display at least focal GFAP positivity, some of the staining may be attributed to nonneoplastic astrocytes embedded within the tumor that display long and thin processes. Tumor cell fractions with true GFAP positivity are minor in most, though rare examples with greater glial differentiation invoke differentials that may include high-grade astrocytomas and ependymomas. Neuronal differentiation can further be demonstrated in subset of cases with NeuN IHC. The Ki67 proliferative index is generally high but noticeably lower within the nodules of the DN variant. Additionally useful immunostains include beta-catenin (to identify the prognostically favorable WNT molecular subgroup [see below]), GAB1 (to identify the Shh subtype), and p53 (strong and diffuse staining correlated with poor prognosis).

Several biologic pathways have been implicated in medulloblastoma pathogenesis. *Sonic hedgehog* (SHH) is important to cerebellar granular cell development, and mutations in the SHH signaling pathway (most notably the *PTCH* gene associated with Gorlin syndrome) have been linked to the DN variant histologically and potential therapeutic targeting clinically (100). Cytoplasmic expression of GAB1 by IHC serves as a useful surrogate for identifying this molecular subtype and is typically expressed in the internodular cells of the DN variant but is also seen in some classic medulloblastomas (101). In 2010, the current molecular landscape of medulloblastoma was more clearly established by Northcott et al. based upon gene expression profiles. They were able to demonstrate 4 distinct molecular groups of medulloblastoma: *WNT, SHH, group C, and group D* (102), the latter two groups now referred to as *groups 3 and 4* (103). Attempts to find surrogate IHC markers for each of these subsets have met with partial success. However, in an attempt to circumvent interlaboratory variations in IHC staining techniques, Northcott et al. utilized a novel technique developed by NanoString Technologies called the nCounter Analysis System (nCAS). This technique utilizes specific oligonucleotide probes linked to specific fluorescence barcodes to identify particular mRNA molecules and in turn assess the degree of gene transcription. By using nCAS, Northcott et al. were able to demonstrate economical, rapid, reliable, and reproducible molecular group assignment by interrogating the activity of only 22 select genes; unfortunately, this technique is not widely available or certified for clinical use currently.

Approximately 15% of sporadic medulloblastomas involve mutations in the *WNT pathway*, which includes contributions from APC (related to Turcot syndrome), axin, GSK-3beta, beta-catenin, and the transcription factor complex TCF/LEF (104). This subtype is often identified by the presence of monosomy 6 by FISH, although nuclear immunoreactivity for beta-catenin (as opposed to nonspecific cytoplasmic expression) is a particularly practical way to identify this subtype (101). Unfortunately, there are currently no reliable methods for distinguishing the other two major molecular subtypes (groups 3 and 4) from one another immunohistochemically (discussed below). As such, cases that are negative for GAB1 and nuclear beta-catenin expression may be classified as "non-WNT/non-SHH," currently representing the largest group encountered clinically.

When considering the entire group of medulloblastomas, overexpression of the ERBB2 receptor has been associated with poor clinical outcome, while elevated Trk-C expression and DN medulloblastoma histology have been linked to more favorable behavior (73,105). The most common cytogenetic alteration in medulloblastomas involves loss of chromosome 17p, most often resulting from the formation of an *isochromosome 17q* [i(17q)] with an associated duplication of the long arm; i17q is encountered in about 30% of cases (86), most of which fall into molecular groups 3 and 4 (102). Isolated losses of 17p have been associated with aggressive behavior, as have amplifications in the MYC oncogenes, either *MYCC* (mostly in group 3) or *MYCN* (mostly in group 4); such amplifications are seen in approximately 10% of cases (73,104).

Five-year survival rates for medulloblastomas have continually improved over the last 25 years, rising from 36% in 1980 to the current standard of 70% to 80%. However, this has come with a significant price in terms of long-term side effects, since craniospinal radiation is particularly toxic to the developing CNS, especially in those children less than 5 years old. In turn, high-dose chemotherapy-only approaches have been developed and have demonstrated encouraging short- and long-term results (106).

Central Nervous System Primitive Neuroectodermal Tumors

The CNS PNET category of embryonal tumor subsumes the older term "supratentorial primitive neuroectodermal tumor" (sPNET) in order to reflect that rare cases may occur in the brain stem or spinal cord (i.e., CNS PNET, not otherwise specified), as well as the rare variants such as central neuroblastoma, ganglioneuroblastoma, medulloepithelioma, and ependymoblastoma (56). Recent work has suggested a close relationship between ependymoblastoma, medulloepithelioma, and a relative diagnostic newcomer termed "embryonal tumor with abundant neuropil and true rosettes" (ETANTR) (see below and Table 10-8).

CNS PNETs are contrast enhancing and may exhibit calcification, hemorrhage, and/or necrosis. Histologically, these tumors are composed of undifferentiated/poorly differentiated neuroepithelial cells. Superficially, they are reminiscent of classic medulloblastomas, although they often exhibit a greater degree of divergent differentiation, both on routine staining (e.g., Homer Wright rosettes, perivascular pseudorosettes, ependymal canals, pigmented cells, neurons) and IHC (positivity seen with neuronal markers including synaptophysin, GFAP, muscle markers, and epithelial markers).

A previously held conceptualization suggested that all CNS embryonal neoplasms were of a similar origin. In particular, CNS PNET was originally considered to simply represent the supratentorial form of medulloblastoma. However, prognosis for CNS PNET has been demonstrated to be significantly worse than for medulloblastoma. Moreover, gene expression profiling and CGH data support their separation (100,107). In particular, comparative genomic hybridization has revealed that CNS PNETs, as compared to medulloblastoma, do not demonstrate i(17q) or –10q, but rather exhibit +1q, –16p, and –19p (107). With respect to CNS PNET, Li et al. suggested a role for the pRB/Ink4/p53 and DNA repair pathways in their development (108). Others found *MYC* (especially *MYCN*) gene amplifications and anaplastic/large cell histology to be common (109). Given considerable biologic and genetic differences, CNS PNET and medulloblastoma are currently considered separate entities.

Medulloepithelioma is a rare variant that displays histology reminiscent of the embryonic neural tube (56). Neuroepithelium arranged in papillary, tubular, and/or trabecular arrangements are seen. The neuroepithelium exhibits an external limiting membrane, and often, multiple lines of differentiation including neural, glial, and mesenchymal are found. In addition, sheets of "small round blue cells" can be appreciated. Ependymoblastic rosettes (see below) may also be seen.

In *ependymoblastomas*, the background of "small round blue cells" is interrupted by the formation of distinctive multilayered true rosettes called "ependymoblastic rosettes" (56). The presence of additional neoplastic neuropil distinguishes the former from a more recently identified tumor called *ETANTR* (110). However, recent genetic studies have further established a close link between ependymoblastomas, medulloepitheliomas, and ETANTR. Among 41 tumors (20 ETANTR and 21 ependymoblastoma), Korshunov et al. found FISH evidence for amplification of 19q13.42 in 37 of 41 cases (111). Rare examples of medulloepithelioma have similarly shown this signature amplicon (112). In turn, the unifying term "embryonal tumors with multilayered rosettes" (ETMR) was coined. Additional work by Korshunov et al. has identified LIN28A as a potent diagnostic marker of ETMR (113).

In a recent study of 142 CNS PNETs examining transcriptional and copy number profiles, Picard et al. (114) identified three main molecular groups: (a) primitive neural, (b) oligoneural, and (c) mesenchymal. The primitive neural group was characterized clinically by a higher proportion of females, younger age, and poor survival. The mesenchymal group had the highest incidence of metastases at diagnosis. LIN28 and OLIG2 were suggested to be promising diagnostic and prognostic markers of the primitive neural and oligoneural groups, respectively; given the work of Korshunov (see above), it seems likely that the primitive neural molecular group of Picard et al. is characterized by histologic features of ETMR.

Atypical Teratoid/Rhabdoid Tumor

ATRT is a highly malignant tumor seen almost exclusively in infants. These tumors are often large, cystic, hemorrhagic, and enhancing. ATRTs can be seen anywhere along the neuraxis; in the posterior fossa, they have a proclivity for the cerebellopontine angle. Routine and IHC stains yield a polyphenotypic pattern (i.e., presence of multiple lineage-associated markers that are usually not coexpressed). Characteristic to ATRT are rhabdoid cells, which exhibit eccentrically placed vesicular nuclei, prominent nucleoli, and a globular or fibrillar eosinophilic paranuclear inclusion (Figure 10-31A), corresponding to whorled bundles of intermediate filaments ultrastructurally. Areas of both mesenchymal and epithelial differentiation may be noted. Primitive appearing cells may predominate in some cases and cause diagnostic confusion with CNS PNET or medulloblastoma (115,116). The IHC profile is highly variable but typically includes a triad of positivity for EMA, smooth muscle actin (SMA), and vimentin.

ATRTs usually result from biallelic inactivation of the *INI1/BAF47/hSNF5/SMARCB1* gene tumor suppressor gene (located at 22q11) via either large-scale deletion (which may be identified with FISH) or smaller single-base-pair mutations (detected through gene sequencing). Although initially

TABLE 10-8 CANCER PREDISPOSITION (NEUROCUTANEOUS) SYNDROMES

Syndrome	Gene (Locus)	Nervous System Pathology	Extraneural Manifestations
Neurofibromatosis type 1	NF1 (17q11)	Neurofibromas (diffuse, nodular, plexiform); MPNSTs; optic/hypothalamic gliomas; diffuse astrocytomas; "UBOs"	Skin (café au lait spots, axillary freckling); Lisch nodules; pheochromocytoma; carcinoid tumors; rhabdomyosarcoma; CML; bone lesions
Neurofibromatosis type 2	NF2 (22q12)	Bilateral vestibular schwannomas; schwannosis; multiple meningiomas; MA; spinal cord ependymomas; glial microhamartoma	Minimal skin stigmata (rare plexiform schwannomas); cataracts.
Ataxia telangiectasia (AT)	ATM (11q22-23)	Cerebellar degeneration; intracranial hemorrhage; cytomegaly and nuclear atypia (CNS and extra-CNS tissues)	Mucocutaneous and conjunctival telangiectasias; immunodeficiency and related respiratory infections; tumor predilection and radiation sensitivity
Neurocutaneous melanosis syndrome	sporadic	Diffuse melanocytosis, melanocytoma, or primary malignant melanoma of the leptomeninges	Cutaneous nevi (giant and or multiple, including the congenital nevus of Ota)
Nevoid basal cell carcinoma (Gorlin) syndrome	PTCH (9q22.3)	Medulloblastoma with extensive nodularity; meningioma; CNS malformations (agenesis of the corpus callosum, cerebral falcine calcifications; HCP)	Odontogenic keratocysts; palmar/plantar dyskeratoses; skeletal malformations; ovarian fibromas; melanoma; leukemia/lymphoma; breast/lung carcinoma
Von Hippel-Lindau (VHL)	VHL (3p25-26)	Hemangioblastomas (cerebellum, retina); papillary endolymphatic sac tumor (PELST)	Renal cell carcinoma; pheochromocytoma; pancreatic tumors; polycythemia
Cowden	PTEN/MMA C1 (10q23)	DGCC (Lhermitte-Duclos disease)	Verrucous skin; cobblestone oral papules; trichilemmomas; colonic polyps; thyroid nodules; breast carcinoma
Li-Fraumeni	TP53 (17p13.3)	Gliomas (astrocytoma, ependymoma; ± multicentric); cerebral PNETs; CPTs; meningioma; schwannoma	Bone and soft tissue sarcomas; leukemia; adrenocortical/breast carcinoma; visceral epithelial malignancies
Turcot	Type 1: hMLH1 (3p21); hMSH2 (2p22-21); hPMS2 (7p22) Type 2: APC (5q21)	Type 1: GBM (younger onset versus sporadic) Type 2: medulloblastoma	Type 1: ±hereditary nonpolyposis colorectal carcinoma Type 2: familial adenomatous polyposis
Familial retinoblastoma	RB (13q14)	Retinoblastoma; pineoblastoma	Osteosarcoma

CML, chronic myeloid leukemia; MPNST, malignant peripheral nerve sheath tumor; UBOs, unidentified bright object on T2 weighted or FLAIR MR images; MA, meningioangiomatosis.

it was thought that only 75% of ATRTs demonstrated abnormalities in *SMARCB1*, Jackson et al. showed that nearly 100% of cases bear biallelic alteration in this gene (117). From the initial work of Judkins et al. (118), a highly sensitive and specific IHC stain (usually referred to as "INI1") for this gene's protein product has become commercially available; nonneoplastic nuclei retain nuclear staining of this ubiquitously expressed protein, whereas there is loss of expression in tumor nuclei (Figure 10-31B). These extremely aggressive tumors often cause death within 1 year. Rare examples of ATRT resulting from inactivation of other SWI/SNF chromatin remodeling genes besides *SMARCB1* have

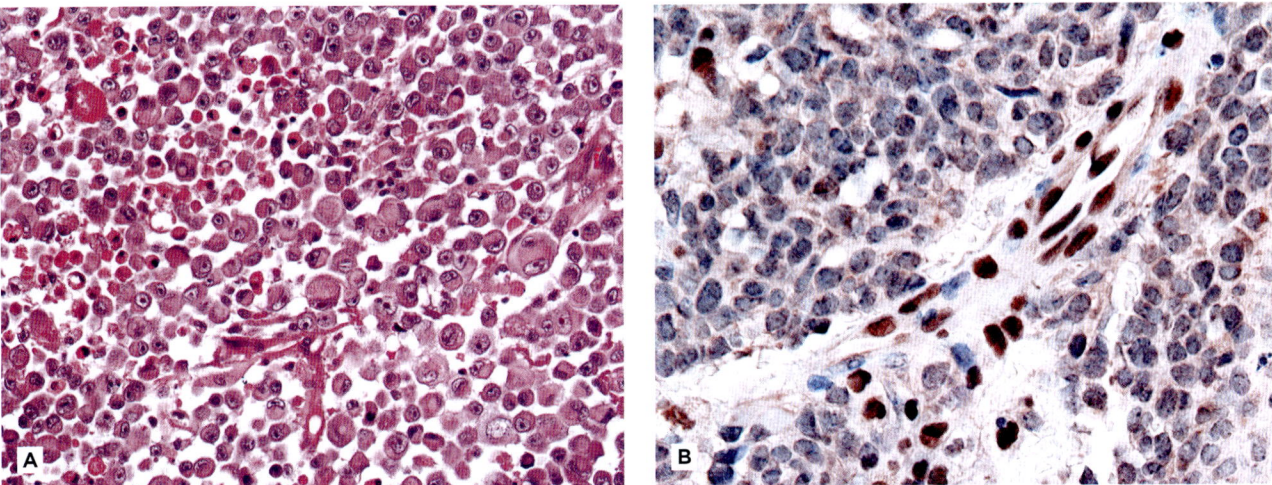

FIGURE 10-31 • Atypical teratoid rhabdoid tumor (ATRT). **A:** Rhabdoid cells. **B:** INI1/BAF-47 immunohistochemistry demonstrating a lack of staining in tumor nuclei, while nonneoplastic lymphocytes and endothelial cells retain nuclear positivity.

been reported, including the *SMARCA4* gene encoding the BRG1 protein (119).

More recently, Hasselblatt's group and others have identified a second pediatric INI1 immunonegative primary CNS tumor that surprisingly appears to carry a favorable prognosis. *Cribriform neuroepithelial tumors* (i.e., CRINET) usually emanate from the 3rd/4th ventricle and are contrast enhancing (120). Histologically, these nonrhabdoid tumors are populated by fairly primitive cells that form cribriform strands, trabeculae, and cystic spaces, as well as more solid areas. The surfaces that the tumor cells create are characteristically EMA positive. In line with INI1 immunonegativity, Hasselblatt et al. demonstrated 4 base pair duplication in exon 4 of *SMARCB1*. A Vancouver family was recently encountered with several family members afflicted with similar posterior fossa tumors, and preliminary genetic data demonstrated a germline duplication involving exon 6 of *SMARCB1* (54).

Tumors Related to the Third Ventricle/Suprasellar Space

Craniopharyngiomas (CPGs), WHO grade I, are squamous epithelial neoplasms that are thought to be derived from remnants of Rathke pouch. They are typically suprasellar and result in dysfunction of the hypothalamic–pituitary axis, visual difficulties, obstructive HCP, and increased ICP. These contrast-enhancing, cystic and calcified tumors contain a characteristic thick dark fluid similar to "machinery oil," which may result in chemical meningitis when spilled *in vivo*. Wet mount specimens of the latter, when viewed under polarized light, reveal eye-catching cholesterol crystals. Since the *papillary* histologic variant primarily affects adults almost exclusively, the discussion below focuses upon the adamantinomatous variant, which is most commonly seen in children.

Adamantinomatous CPGs are typically present in children, although there is also a second smaller peak in adults.

Epithelial cells are arranged in sheets, whorls, trabeculae, and lining cystic spaces. Solid foci bear orderly islands of epithelia with (a) peripheral or basal palisades, (b) adjacent polygonal cells, and (c) a loose meshwork of epithelial cells termed *stellate reticulum* resulting from intercellular fluid accumulation (Figure 10-32). Cellular outlines (or "ghosts") of squamoid tumor cells with brightly eosinophilic cytoplasm and indistinct nuclei constitute *wet keratin*, a diagnostic feature even in the absence of viable epithelium. A xanthogranulomatous inflammatory reaction is typical and accompanied by needle-shaped clear cholesterol clefts and necrosis. The ragged interface with adjacent brain is typified by dense piloid gliosis (including RFs), which may resemble PA in the absence of adjacent epithelium. IHC is positive for cytokeratins and EMA. The outcome is dependent on the extent of surgical resection and tumor size, with 10-year survivals ranging from 64% to 96% (56). Mutational and

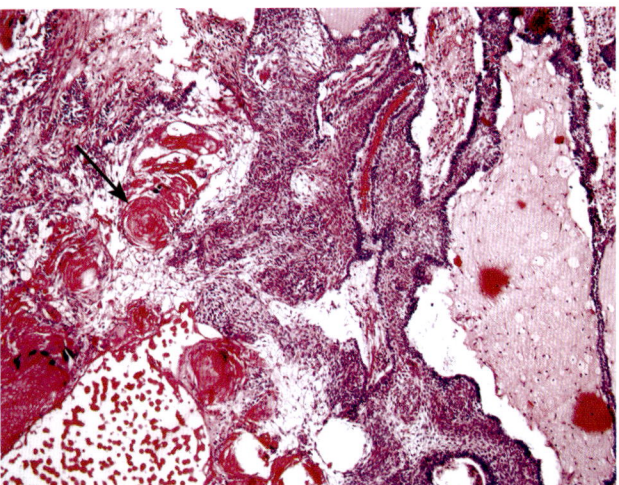

FIGURE 10-32 • Adamantinomatous CPG. In addition to its characteristic epithelium, "wet keratin" (*arrow*) can be seen and often bears "ghosts" of degenerate tumor cells.

IHC analyses have suggested a role for aberrant WNT pathway signaling in adamantinomatous CPGs; in one study, exon 3 of beta-catenin was mutated in 77% of these tumors, with corresponding nuclear accumulation of beta-catenin in 94% (121).

Germ cell tumors are thought to be derived from ectopically placed germ cells during gestation and epidemiologically are very common in eastern Asia. Included in this group are germinoma, yolk sac tumor, choriocarcinoma, embryonal carcinoma, teratoma (mature and immature variants), and mixed neoplasms (comprised of two or more of the preceding types). Pineal and suprasellar regions are especially favored; at times, "synchronous" (and separate) lesions may be detected in each of these two areas. Suprasellar lesions typically result in dysfunction of the hypothalamic–pituitary axis and abnormal vision, whereas pineal lesions result in Parinaud syndrome and HCP. Occasionally, large germ cell tumors affect the fetal brain; these often take the form of immature teratoma. Clinical outcomes correlate with certain subtypes and segregate into favorable (e.g., germinoma, teratoma) and unfavorable groups (e.g., yolk sac tumor, choriocarcinoma, embryonal carcinoma), the latter of which are often suspected via imaging/gross features of necrosis and hemorrhage. Histologic features of CNS germ cell tumors are essentially identical to their extra-CNS counterparts (nongerminomatous examples are discussed in Chapters 18 and 19). Especially when considering a differential diagnosis of a "mixed" germ cell tumor, a battery of IHC stains should be employed to confirm impressions on routine staining; such a battery typically includes CD117 (c-kit)/placental alkaline phosphatase (PLAP), beta-hCG, CD30, OCT3/4, CAM 5.2, and AFP (56).

CNS *germinomas* have characteristic histology composed of two cell types. The neoplastic component has large round-to-oval epithelioid cells that are glycogen-rich and have a clear-to-eosinophilic cytoplasm; the associated nucleus is large, vesicular and bears a prominent nucleolus (Figure 10-33A). The second cell type comprises a variably prominent reactive lymphocytic infiltrate, which is dispersed within an architectural lobularity created by delicate fibrovascular septae. This inflammation can also be granulomatous and may overshadow the tumor cells, occasionally leading to a misdiagnosis of inflammatory disorders; this pitfall is particularly important to consider when dealing with small biopsy specimens. Immunohistochemically, the large tumor cells stain positively for PLAP and c-kit (CD117) in a membranous pattern, of which the latter is now preferred (122) (Figure 10-33B). Occasionally when attempting to confirm the presence of CNS germinoma, it is necessary to resort to immunostaining with OCT3/4, which, on a cautionary note, stains the tumor nuclei of both germinoma and embryonal carcinoma. Genetic studies have demonstrated similar cytogenetic alterations within CNS and extra-CNS germinomas: *isochromosome 12p* [i(12p)]. Germinomas are extremely radiosensitive and chemosensitive and are therefore among the prognostically favorable group of CNS germ cell tumors, with 5-year survival rates varying from 80% to 96% (61).

PPTs are thought to be derived from the native pineocyte, a neuron-like cell with photoreceptor and neuroendocrine characteristics. These contrast-enhancing tumors obstruct CSF flow and compress adjacent structures, classically resulting in Parinaud syndrome. Three main PPTs are recognized: pineoblastoma, pineocytoma, and PPT of intermediate grade (PPTIG). Pineoblastoma, WHO grade IV, primarily affects children, while pineocytoma, WHO grade II, usually occurs in adults. PPTIG is, as its name implies, "intermediate" in terms of grade and clinical features and is considered WHO grade II or III. Jouvet et al. have proposed an alternative four-tier grading scheme for PPTs, where pineocytomas are grade I, PPTIG are split into grade II and III categories, and pineoblastomas are grade IV; the degrees of mitotic activity and NFP staining in tandem serve to differentiate these groups into prognostically meaningful categories (123). *Pineoblastomas* can be poorly demarcated and may contain

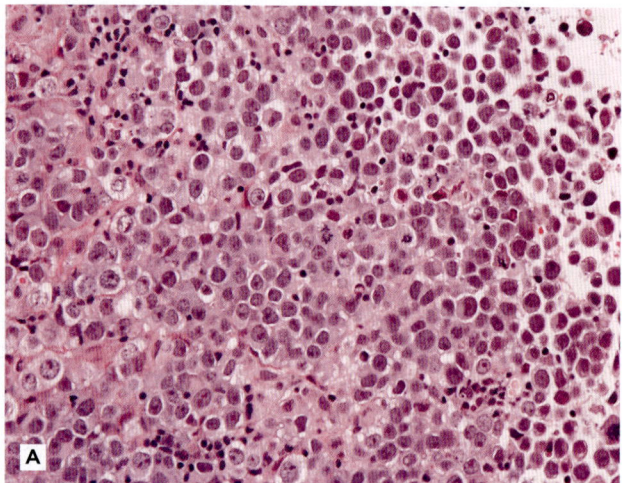
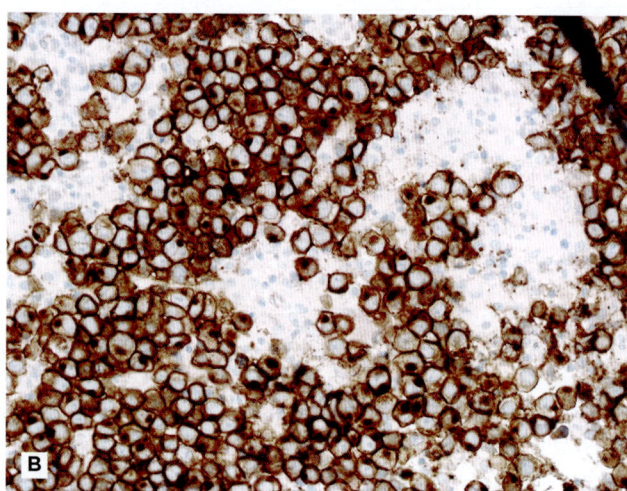

FIGURE 10-33 • Intracranial germinoma. **A:** Typical biphasic histology including large mitotically active cells and reactive lymphocytes. **B:** CD117 (c-kit) immunohistochemistry demonstrating membranous positivity in the large tumor cells.

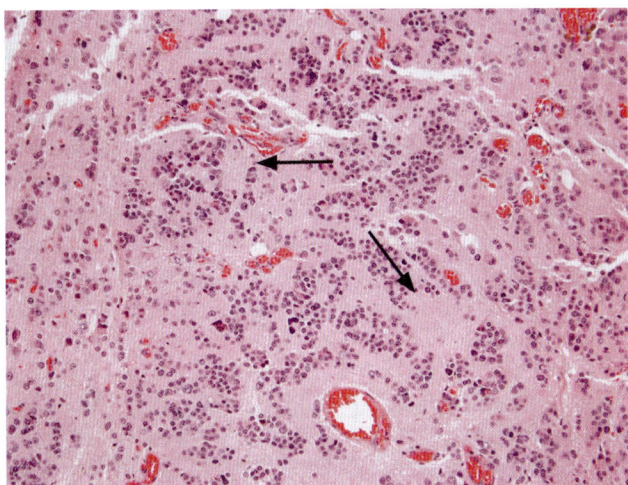

FIGURE 10-34 • Pineocytoma. Pineocytic rosettes (*arrows*), which are larger than Homer Wright rosettes, and are scattered throughout this example.

hemorrhage and or necrosis. Histologically, these embryonal tumors are populated by primitive mitotically active cells similar to those of medulloblastoma and CNS PNET. They may contain Homer Wright and/or Flexner-Wintersteiner rosettes, but not the pineocytic rosettes that are characteristic of pineocytoma. *Pineocytomas* bear uniform small mature cells with round-oval bland nuclei and moderate amounts of eosinophilic cytoplasm. These cells closely resemble the neurocytes encountered in central neurocytoma. Mitoses and necrosis are infrequent. Pineocytic rosettes resemble Homer Wright rosettes but are larger and more irregular, being formed by mature rather than primitive cells (Figure 10-34). Degenerative atypia can be striking and ganglionic differentiation may also be seen. IHC reveals staining for neuronal markers, especially synaptophysin, but also for the more nonspecific neural/neuroendocrine marker, neuron-specific enolase (NSE). In general, the grading of PPTs integrates cytology, mitotic activity, the presence or absence of necrosis, pineocytic/Homer Wright/Flexner-Wintersteiner rosettes, and extent of NFP staining (61) (see also above). Five-year survival rates for pineocytoma and pineoblastoma have been estimated at 86% and 58%, respectively (56). The genetics of pineoblastoma are reviewed elsewhere (108,124).

Neuronal and Mixed Glioneuronal Tumors
Ganglioglioma

Gangliogliomas (GG) (usually WHO grade I) are epileptogenic tumors that preferentially occur in the temporal lobe. The defining feature is presence of *dysmorphic neurons*. Their morphology deviates from normal neurons (large vesicular nucleus, prominent nucleolus, basophilic cytoplasm bearing Nissl substance) in exhibiting binucleation or multinucleation, vacuolated cytoplasm, and clumpy irregularly formed Nissl substance (Figure 10-35A). Coarse irregular processes and Alzheimer-type degenerative changes (including neurofibrillary tangles and granulovacuolar degeneration) may be seen. Architecturally, the ganglion cells are often clumped or haphazardly arranged in comparison to the laminar, well-ordered arrangement of normal cortex. However, in areas where the glial component predominates, GGs may resemble DA, oligodendroglioma, and even PA. *Gangliocytomas* are essentially GGs without the glial component; in cases where a glial component is more equivocal, a diagnosis of "ganglion cell tumor" may be more appropriate. Connective tissue–rich areas and calcification may be present. Although generally considered noninfiltrating neoplasms, neuropil-like areas (including axons) indistinguishable from native parenchyma are frequent and make the designation of infiltration versus neoplastic neuropil difficult. Additionally, like PAs, there is nearly always at least some infiltration found microscopically. EGBs and perivascular lymphocytes are common. Features characteristic of high-grade gliomas (mitoses and necrosis) are usually absent, although MVP is fairly common.

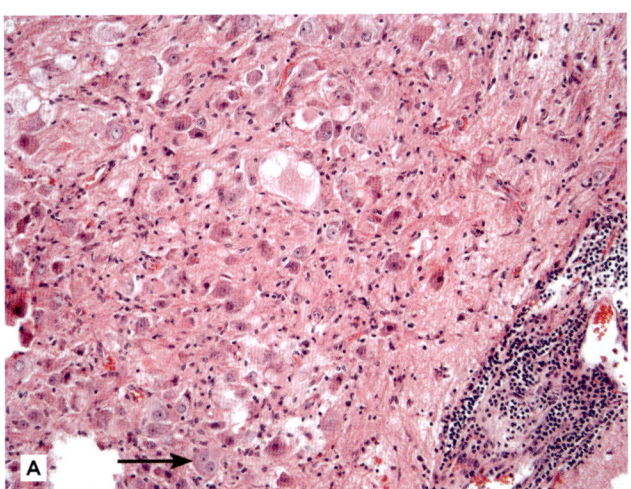
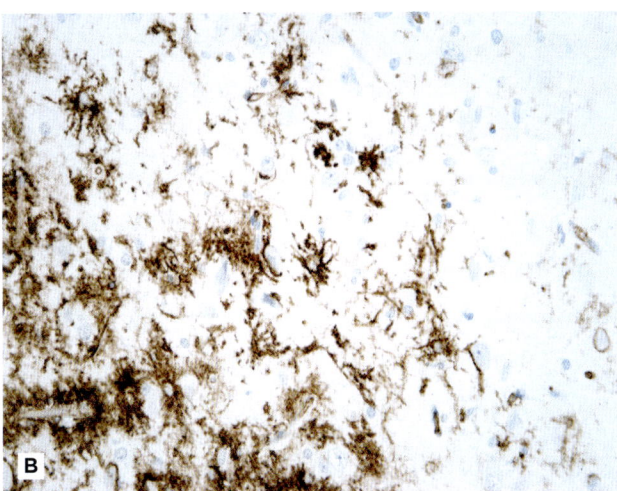

FIGURE 10-35 • Ganglioglioma (GG). **A:** H&E section reveals numerous neoplastic neurons, including vacuolated and binucleate (*arrow*) forms. **B:** CD34 immunohistochemistry highlights tumor cells with highly ramifying cytoplasmic processes.

High-grade glial transformation (i.e., anaplastic GG, WHO grade III) is exceedingly rare and difficult to define (61). The glial and neuronal components can be highlighted immunohistochemically with GFAP and neuronal markers (most commonly synaptophysin), respectively. Additionally, scattered CD34 positivity has been suggested to be characteristic of GG, both within tumor cells and in the adjacent dysplastic cortex (125) (Figure 10-35B). Electron microscopy can also be used to support the finding of neuronal differentiation. As described above, recent genetic studies have shown that, similar to PXA, a significant number of GG exhibit the *BRAF V600E* mutation, suggesting a potential link between these tumors (96), as well as DNTs (see below) (126). Prognosis is favorable with surgical resection.

Dysembryoplastic Neuroepithelial Tumor

DNT, WHO grade I, is a controversial lesion that was first described in 1988 by Daumas-Duport (127). Although currently considered a mixed glioneuronal tumor by the WHO, some consider it a hamartomatous mass (56). These epileptogenic lesions are cortically based (rare exceptions involve the septum pellucidum, basal ganglia, thalamus, or other sites) and have a marked predilection for the temporal lobe. Imaging may reveal calcifications, cyst-like nodules, and contrast enhancement, including a rim-enhancing pattern. The histologic hallmark of classic DNT is the *specific glioneuronal element*, which is composed of columns of bundled axons/capillaries (arranged perpendicular to the cortical surface) that are lined by oligodendroglial-like cells (OLC). The exact histogenesis of the OLC is debated; most are strongly S-100 and OLIG2 positive, but negative for both GFAP and neuronal markers, similar to mature oligodendrocytes. However, rare NeuN staining has been seen suggesting at least limited overlap with neurocytic cells. The patterned intracortical nodules and the specific glioneuronal elements are rich in pale basophilic mucin, within which are often nondysmorphic *floating neurons* (Figure 10-36A, B). Stellate astrocytes may be seen among the specific glioneuronal element. Complex and simple forms of DNT are the most commonly recognized. *Complex* DNTs feature additional glial nodules that may resemble PA or less often, DA. In some recurrent examples, only a glial nodule is evident (128). Additionally, this component may exhibit rare mitoses, nuclear atypia, necrosis, and even MVP, but these features are not common and do not imply a poor prognosis. Similarly, nodules resembling GG can be seen, warranting a diagnosis of composite GG/DNT. Foci of cortical dysplasia may be seen in the adjacent nonneoplastic brain (i.e., FCD type IIIb; see prior discussion). Even more controversial is the proposed *nonspecific* variant of DNT, a diagnosis that is not widely accepted (129). DNTs have a favorable prognosis, even after subtotal resection. Genetic studies of DNT are rare, but unlike their most common adult histologic mimic, oligodendrogliomas, they lack 1p and 19q codeletions (56,61,130,131). Additionally, a subset harbors the *BRAF V600E* mutation commonly seen in PXA and GG (126).

Other Neuronal/Glioneuronal Tumors

Desmoplastic infantile ganglioglioma/desmoplastic infantile astrocytoma (DIG/DIA), WHO grade I, is a distinctive tumor usually occurring in the first year of life. These large superficial lesions often have dural attachment, cyst formation, and contrast enhancement. Macrocephaly and increased ICP herald its presence. Histologically, reticulin-rich desmoplastic areas contain spindled cells with a fascicular or storiform arrangement; these areas often obscure the astrocytic component that often requires GFAP IHC to fully appreciate. The latter resemble slender fibrillary astrocytes embedded within the densely desmoplastic stroma; scattered small gemistocytes may also be seen. Neurons, typically smaller than those seen in GG, can likewise be inconspicuous and may only be appreciated with IHC or electron microscopy; if present, the term "DIG" applies, but if absent the designation DIA is more appropriate. Alternatively, some neuro-

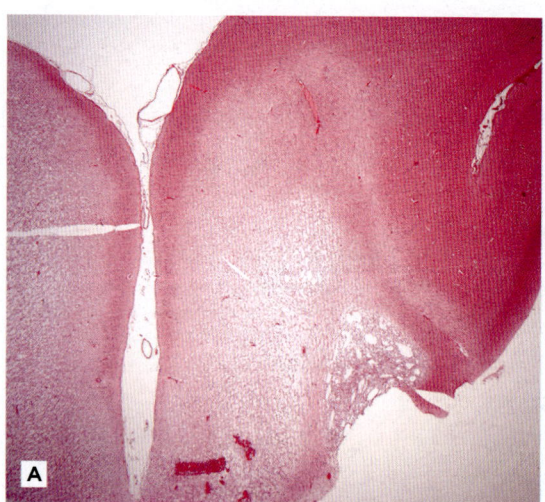
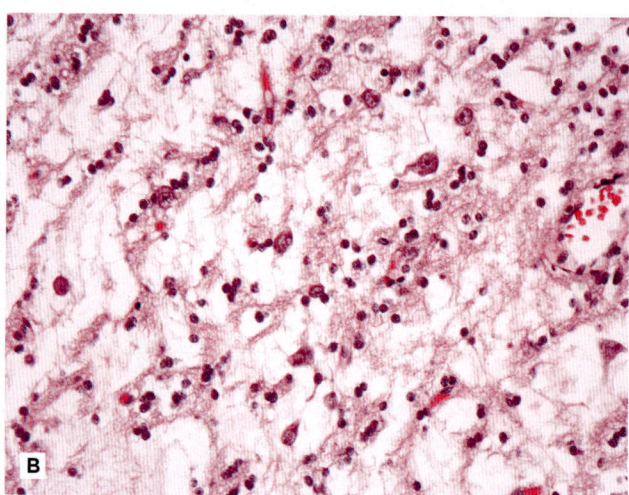

FIGURE 10-36 • Dysembryoplastic neuroepithelial tumor (DNT). **A:** Low-power microscopy reveals a cortically based neoplasm. **B:** High-power microscopy demonstrates "floating neurons" and "oligodendroglial-like cells."

pathologists have favored the umbrella term "desmoplastic tumor of infancy" to encompass all cases regardless of the presence or absence of a neuronal component. Less commonly, more classic GG-like foci, complete with EGBs, may be present. Worrisome and mitotically active PNET-like foci bearing MVP and necrosis may be seen but fortunately do not impact prognosis, since these patients usually enjoy favorable outcomes after surgery. Whether true "malignant" forms of DIG/DIA exist is unclear (132).

Dysplastic gangliocytoma of the cerebellum (Lhermitte-Duclos disease) (DGCC), WHO grade I, is a unique cerebellar neoplasm nearly invariably associated with Cowden syndrome in adults, but much less often in children (133). Predictably, these patients present with signs and symptoms of cerebellar dysfunction and CSF obstruction. These solid tumors are characteristically striped on T2-weighted MRI due in part to thickened folia. Microscopically, a distinctive abnormal architecture is seen and has been likened to cortex "flipped inside-out." More normal cerebellar cortex is progressively replaced by two layers. The outer layer consists of parallel arrays of myelinated axons, whereas the inner layer is composed of abnormal smaller and larger neurons (ganglioid and ganglion-like, respectively), which replace the internal granular cells. These ganglion cells may resemble Purkinje cells but are far too numerous, disordered, and pleomorphic. Abnormal vascular proliferation may be noted in the subarachnoid space and white matter, which in turn may be vacuolated. Since patients with Cowden syndrome bear germline mutations in the PTEN tumor suppressor gene on chromosome 10q23, genetic studies (including sporadic cases) have investigated the PTEN/Akt/mTOR pathway. IHC and mutational analyses have confirmed frequent PTEN mutations and secondary activation of mTOR (133,134). A workup for other features of Cowden syndrome may also be warranted since such patients are at risk for numerous systemic manifestations, including breast and gastrointestinal carcinomas, although again this association is much less common in cases of childhood onset DGCC.

Choroid Plexus Tumors

Choroid plexus tumors (CPTs) are intraventricular papillary epithelial tumors that are derived from the choroid plexus (56). They are intensely contrast-enhancing lesions that often present with increased ICP and HCP. Although CPTs may affect any site where native choroid plexus resides, the lateral ventricle is the most frequent location noted in affected children.

CPP, WHO grade I, closely resembles normal choroid plexus in that papillae contain a fibrovascular core, a simple to cuboidal epithelium with minimal to mild atypia, and little mitotic activity. However, this neoplastic epithelium differs from normal choroid plexus in being more cell dense and lacking the normal surface hobnail (i.e., bumpy) architecture (Figure 10-37A). Mesenchymal type metaplasia, pigmented epithelium, and focal ependymal differentiation are rare, except for the latter that usually manifests with GFAP immunoreactivity.

Choroid plexus carcinoma (CPC), WHO grade III, is a rare tumor that usually presents before 3 years of age. The papillary architecture characteristic of CPP is variably replaced by areas of solid tumor growth (Figure 10-37B). The epithelium is clearly anaplastic in most examples, although transitions with better-differentiated areas are occasionally seen and may suggest a role for progressive malignant transformation in some. A hypercellular pseudostratified epithelium is formed by tumor cells with high nuclear-to-cytoplasmic ratios. Nuclei are hyperchromatic and mitotic activity is generally prominent (>5 per 10 HPF). Foci of necrosis are characteristic, and MVP may be seen. CPCs often invade the adjacent brain parenchyma.

Atypical CPP is considered an intermediate WHO grade II variant, which has been defined by a minimum of two mitoses per 10 HPF, often containing at least two of the following as well: hypercellularity, pleomorphism, foci of solid growth, and necrosis (135).

In general, CPT IHC reveals positivity for cytokeratins and S-100 protein, with the latter often being more limited in CPCs. Unlike most carcinomas, EMA is usually negative and

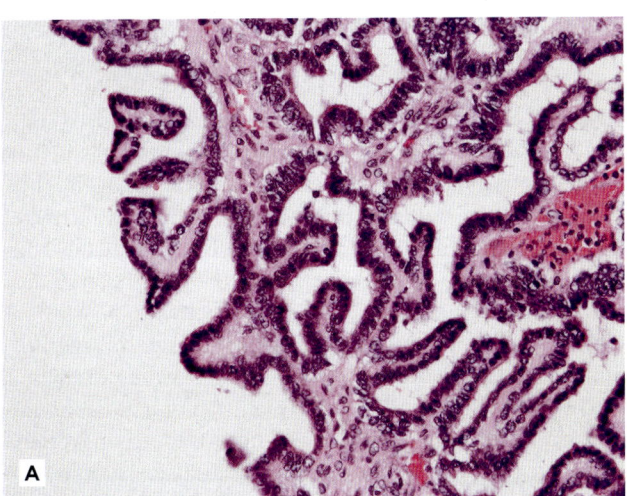
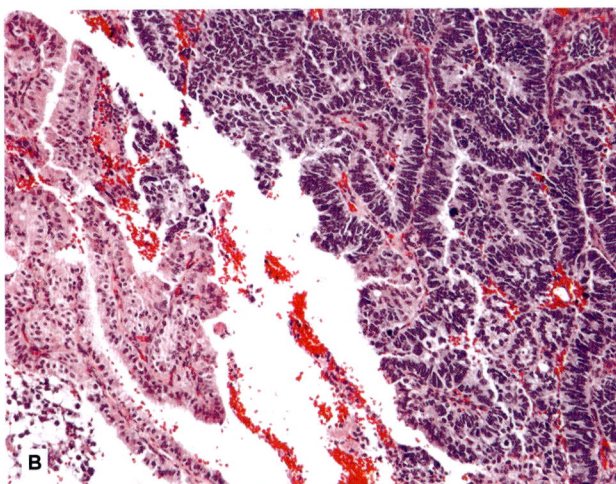

FIGURE 10-37 • Choroid plexus tumors (CPTs). **A:** Choroid plexus papilloma (CPP). **B:** CPC; note the better-differentiated area, left, versus the more poorly differentiated tumor, right.

focal GFAP expression is relatively common. Transthyretin and synaptophysin staining have been touted as markers of CPTs, but these are generally unreliable due to low specificities.

The genetics of CPTs are reviewed by Kamaly-Asl et al. (136). *TP53* mutations may be frequent in CPC (especially those related to Li-Fraumeni syndrome) but are rare in CPP. Kamaly et al. further suggest that rare cases of CPC with *SMARCB1* mutations are truly ATRT, an important differential diagnostic consideration, since this tumor afflicts the same age group, can be intraventricular, and may show papillary features. CPP is often cured with surgery (5-year survival 100%), while CPC often grows rapidly and has an unfavorable prognosis (5-year survival 40%) (56).

Miscellaneous CNS Tumors

A variety of less common CNS tumors arise in pediatric patients. As opposed to adults, meningeal-based tumors, in particular meningioma, are uncommon (137). Pituitary adenoma is also much more common in adults. Nerve sheath tumors (including schwannoma and neurofibroma) are covered in the soft tissue chapter (Chapter 25), whereas bony skull–based tumors (including chordoma, Langerhans cell histiocytosis) are covered in the chapter on the skeletal system (Chapter 28). Primary melanocytic lesions (melanomas, melanocytoma) are rare and thought to be derived from leptomeningeal melanocytes, hence their typical extra-axial location; they are morphologically and genetically analogous to cutaneous blue nevi, ocular melanocytomas, and the melanomas that arise from them (138), although they can sometimes be difficult to distinguish from pigmented schwannomas that arise from nearby nerve roots. Vascular tumors are similarly rare, with hemangioblastomas being common only in adults. Their presence in children strongly raises the possibility of von Hippel-Lindau (VHL) disease.

Cancer Predisposition Syndromes

The most common syndromes encountered in a pediatric practice are summarized in Table 10-8. The multisystemic nature of these syndromes is evidenced by the fact that patients incur both neoplastic and nonneoplastic forms of pathology. While many of these syndromes are inherited in an autosomal dominant pattern, some (e.g., AT) are autosomal recessive, while others (e.g., neurocutaneous melanosis syndrome) appear sporadically. The specific clinical diagnostic criteria for each of these syndromes are not given here; for such, the reader is directed to other texts (38,56,62).

INFECTIOUS DISEASE

Bacterial Infections
Acute Meningitis

Neonatal acute bacterial meningitis is most frequently due to group B streptococcus (*Streptococcus agalactiae*) and *Escherichia coli*. Several other Gram-positive (*Listeria monocytogenes* and *Staphylococcus aureus*) and Gram-negative (*Citrobacter*, *Klebsiella*, *Enterobacter*, *Proteus*, *Salmonella* species, and *Pseudomonas aeruginosa*) bacteria may also be causative. Infants and young children are affected primarily by *S. pneumoniae*, *Neisseria meningitidis*, and *Haemophilus influenzae* type b (Hib), while children older than 5 years (like adults) are infected most frequently with the former two pathogens. Notably, immunization with the Haemophilus, pneumococcal, and meningococcal conjugate vaccines has significantly reduced the incidence of previously devastating infections (139).

Bacteria reach the CNS via hematogenous spread, often from an upper respiratory focus, or direct spread from a contiguous site of disease (i.e., mastoids, inner ear, nasal sinus, mouth). Neonates often acquire organisms via passage through an infected birth canal. Once arriving at the CNS, breech of the BBB is facilitated by bacterial surface proteins, although most enter the CSF at sites without an intact BBB such as the choroid plexus, after which craniospinal dissemination can occur rapidly. Although host immune defenses and antimicrobial therapy may effectively neutralize the pathogen, bacterial products can persist in stimulating the inflammatory response (139).

Focal neurologic deficits, changes in mental status, fever, rash, seizures, and signs of meningeal irritation herald the presence of acute meningitis. Nonspecific changes such as irritability, lethargy, poor feeding, apneic spells, and a bulging fontanelle may be seen in infants. CSF examination is key to the diagnosis, and findings include granulocytic pleocytosis, elevated protein, decreased CSF to serum glucose ratio, and identification of organisms on Gram stain. Definitive diagnosis is made with culture, organism-specific PCR, and latex agglutination tests.

Gross examination of the brain affected by meningitis reveals diffuse edema and possibly cerebral herniation. The surface vasculature is congested. A light-colored thick leptomeningeal exudate may be seen grossly (Figure 10-38A) but may be less prominent in partially treated cases and those that die in the early stages of disease. Focal areas of parenchymal softening are suggestive of infarction. Microscopic sections reveal a neutrophil-predominant exudate (Figure 10-38B) (lymphocytes and macrophages are seen in later stages) that often extends along intracortical Virchow-Robin spaces. This inflammation can result in a vasculitis with secondary thrombosis (and hence infarction). Choroid plexitis and ventriculitis may also be seen. Organisms are highlighted with the Gram stain but may be difficult to find in treated examples. Complications among survivors predictably follow the areas of pathologic damage. Cortical infarcts lead to focal neurologic deficits (e.g., spasticity, dysphasia) and seizures and, when widespread, may result in cognitive impairment (or when less pronounced, learning disabilities and behavioral disturbances). Resolution of leptomeningeal inflammation with concomitant fibrosis overlying cranial nerves may result in cranial nerve palsies (e.g., hearing loss). Scarring (i.e., parenchymal gliosis, ependymal granulations, and meningeal fibrosis) can obstruct the flow of CSF causing HCP (see Chapter 6).

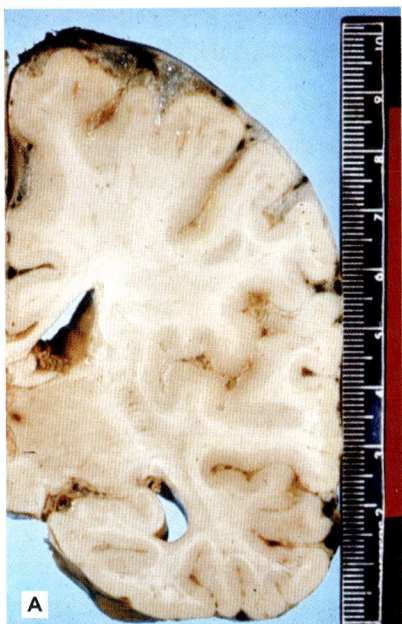
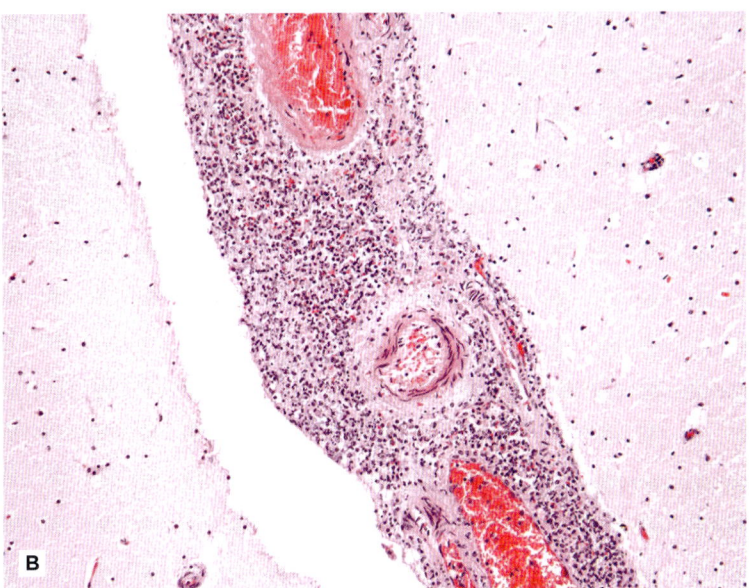

FIGURE 10-38 • Acute bacterial meningitis. **A:** Coronal section of the cerebrum reveals abundant purulent material within the leptomeninges. **B:** Microscopy highlights a neutrophil-rich leptomeningeal infiltrate.

Cerebral Abscess

Bacteria, which cause abscesses, like those causing meningitis, also arrive at the CNS via hematogenous or direct contiguous spread. Children with congenital heart disease are particularly predisposed to hematogenous dissemination of bacteria, resulting in abscesses within brain regions receiving a high blood flow (e.g., middle cerebral artery territory). Dental infections (i.e., abscesses), mastoiditis, paranasal sinusitis, or otitis media may traverse local anatomic boundaries and lead to abscess formation in adjacent brain parenchyma.

The spectrum of microorganisms causing abscesses has changed with time (140). While the incidence of *S. aureus* has been decreasing, the identification of anaerobes has increased. *Streptococcus milleri* and *S. viridans* are frequently associated with direct brain inoculation and hematogenous spread, respectively, and as a group, aerobic and anaerobic forms of streptococcus cause 60% to 70% of cerebral abscesses (1). Other causative aerobic and microaerophilic bacteria may include *Haemophilus*, Gram-negative enteric bacilli, and *Pseudomonas aeruginosa*. Common anaerobes include Bacteroides, Peptostreptococcus, Fusobacterium, Propionibacterium, Prevotella, and Actinomyces. Penetrating head injuries, neurosurgical procedures, and immunocompromised states all predispose to abscess formation, with the latter invoking less common bacterial (e.g., *Nocardia*, *Listeria*, *Mycobacterial* species), fungal (e.g., *Candida*, *Aspergillus*, *Cryptococcus*, *Histoplasma*, *Coccidioides*, and *Mucor*), and parasitic (e.g., *Toxoplasmosis*) pathogens. MR imaging most often reveals a mass with a thin smooth rim of enhancement, the latter raising a differential diagnosis with GBM or other neoplasms. The resulting gross and microscopic appearance of cerebral abscesses evolves through stages. Early stages (<4 days) begin with a *cerebritis* that grossly appears as an ill-defined area of hyperemia and edema; microscopically, endothelial swelling is accompanied by perivascular and parenchymal neutrophils. After roughly 4 days, areas of confluent necrosis emerge, as both macrophage and mononuclear infiltrates become more conspicuous. An early granulation tissue reaction at the margin of necrosis heralds the initiation of *capsule formation* at approximately 10 days; chronic inflammatory cells are noted within the capsule, which is in turn surrounded by edema and reactive astrocytosis in the adjacent brain. A well-formed reticulin-rich capsule is noted at 2 weeks, at which time the classic multilayered abscess wall is best appreciated. Organisms (most highlighted with special stains) are seen at all stages of evolution, particularly at the capsule-necrosis boundary.

Subdural empyema and epidural abscesses are uncommon and not discussed further here.

Chronic Bacterial Infections

Mycobacteria uncommonly cause infection in North American children. Most cases are seen in immunocompromised patients (in particular, those with AIDS) and those in the developing world. *Mycobacterium tuberculosis* (TB) causes meningitis (the most common form of disease), tuberculous masses (i.e., tuberculomas), and spinal epidural abscesses. Initial infection results from inhalation of bacteria-laden droplets; subsequent CNS spread is related to hematogenous dissemination. Reactivation of a focus of latent CNS infection (i.e., a "tubercle" or "Rich focus") is also a source of active disease. Symptoms in children are subacute (occur over 2 to 3 weeks) and may include fever, meningismus, signs of increased ICP (headache, nausea, and vomiting), seizures, cranial nerve palsies, and epilepsy, with subsequent changes in mental status. Examination may reveal a 6th cranial nerve palsy. Diagnosis may be made on CSF specimens via culture (often slow growing), PCR, or direct visualization using Ziehl-Neelsen or auramine rhodamine fluorescence staining (see below).

Gross pathologic findings include a gelatinous and, at times, nodular leptomeningeal exudate that is often most prominent along the Sylvian fissure and base of the brain. The choroid plexus and ventricular lining may be similarly affected and result in HCP. Areas of parenchymal softening are suggestive of superimposed infarcts related to *endarteritis obliterans* with vascular thrombosis. Necrotizing granulomas are typical but are often less well formed or replaced by a diffuse histiocytic infiltrate in immunocompromised hosts. Chronic type inflammatory cells, variable fibrosis, and multinucleated (Langhans type) giant cells may be accompanied, albeit rarely in most cases, by acid-fast bacilli on Ziehl-Neelsen staining (i.e., "red snappers"). Inflammation may spill over into the adjacent brain, causing microglial activation and gliosis. Tubercles are the nodular macroscopic confluence of these granulomas, while the histologically similar tuberculomas are grossly "mass forming."

Other bacteria causing chronic CNS disease are uncommon but include Lyme disease (*Borrelia burgdorferi*) and syphilis (*Treponema pallidum*).

Viral Infections

Viral meningitis is defined as a febrile illness associated with clinical signs of meningeal irritation but lacking neurologic dysfunction and positive cultures. These often banal cases occur with seasonal and geographic variations; rarely do they come to the attention of the neuropathologist. The most common causative entities include the enteroviruses (echoviruses, Coxsackie A and B, and enterovirus *per se*) and HSV-2 (i.e., Mollaret meningitis). Histology reveals, at best, a scanty lymphocytic predominant perivascular and leptomeningeal infiltrate, which may affect the choroid plexus and creep into the superficial aspects of the brain parenchyma.

Viral encephalitis also causes fever but is additionally characterized by brain parenchymal dysfunction manifesting as an altered state of consciousness and/or objective signs of neurologic dysfunction (i.e., seizures, focal neurologic deficits); the equivalent pathologic process occurring in the spinal cord is called *myelitis*. Mixed forms (i.e., meningoencephalitis or encephalomyelitis) also occur. Each of these main pathologic processes can result in either acute or chronic disease depending on the particular type of viral pathogen involved. The clinical severity of diseases induced by these viruses ranges from minimal to fatal. Antivirals exist for some pathogens (e.g., HSV and acyclovir), but care is limited to supportive therapy for others. Diagnoses are made by serology, culture (in the past from CNS biopsy specimens), and PCR-based assays (especially of CSF), which uncover specific viral nucleic acids.

Herpes simplex virus (HSV) is one of the most common members of the Herpesviridae family, a group of generally necrotizing double-stranded DNA viruses that also include varicella-zoster virus (VZV), CMV, and Epstein-Barr virus (EBV). Viral DNA is enclosed in a nucleocapsid and surrounded by a viral envelope. Neonatal disease is most often caused by HSV type 2, while the less frequent childhood form of infection is caused by HSV type 1. Neonatal disease is usually acquired in the perinatal period from an infected mother bearing recurrent but often asymptomatic genital disease (141). Neonates present within the first 4 weeks of life with one of three main forms of disease: (a) localized skin, eyes, or mouth (SEM) disease including vesicles and/or keratoconjunctivitis; (b) encephalitis ± SEM; or (3) diffuse or disseminated HSV with SEM, encephalitis, and multiple visceral organ disease. These affected infants may be lethargic and irritable, feed poorly, and suffer from seizures. Pathology reveals a diffusely swollen and congested brain. Hemorrhagic and necrotic lesions of the gray and white matter are accompanied by macrophages and lymphocytes. Intranuclear viral inclusions may be seen within neurons, glia, and/or endothelia. Survivors are left with a parenchymal loss and gliosis, which, when widespread and severe, can be labeled as *multicystic encephalomalacia* (142) (Figure 10-17).

Childhood disease is much less common and presents in a similar fashion to that in adults. Primary HSV infection is often asymptomatic, although some may develop oropharyngeal ulcers. Once the virus is absorbed, it replicates and subsequently travels in a retrograde fashion along sensory axons (e.g., olfactory or trigeminal) toward the respective ganglion where a latent infection ensues. Reactivation of viral disease is accompanied by replication and anterograde travel down sensory axons toward the periphery whereupon mucocutaneous vesicles erupt. *HSV encephalitis* is thought to arise either with primary infection or after reactivation of latent trigeminal ganglia disease. Common clinical presenting features include fever, headache, altered mental status, and seizures. The classic distribution of disease (see below) may be seen via imaging, and definitive diagnosis using PCR to find viral DNA in the CSF has largely supplanted brain biopsy. Swelling, congestion, hemorrhage, and necrosis are typically localized initially (often asymmetrically) to the posterior orbitofrontal cortex, temporal lobes, cingulate gyrus, and insulae (Figure 10-39A). Acutely necrotic (i.e., "red") neurons are accompanied by parenchymal lymphocytes and macrophages, plus the nonspecific but characteristic viral encephalitic features of perivascular lymphocytes, microglial activation, microglial nodule formation, and neuronophagia. Neuronal, glial, and/or endothelial intranuclear viral inclusions (Figure 10-39B) may be difficult to appreciate in some cases, wherein IHC staining for HSV can be very helpful. Endothelial and hence vascular involvement may result in thrombosis and infarction. A necrotizing myelopathy may be seen but is rare. In survivors, the extensive residual damage usually manifests in the form of cystic encephalomalacia.

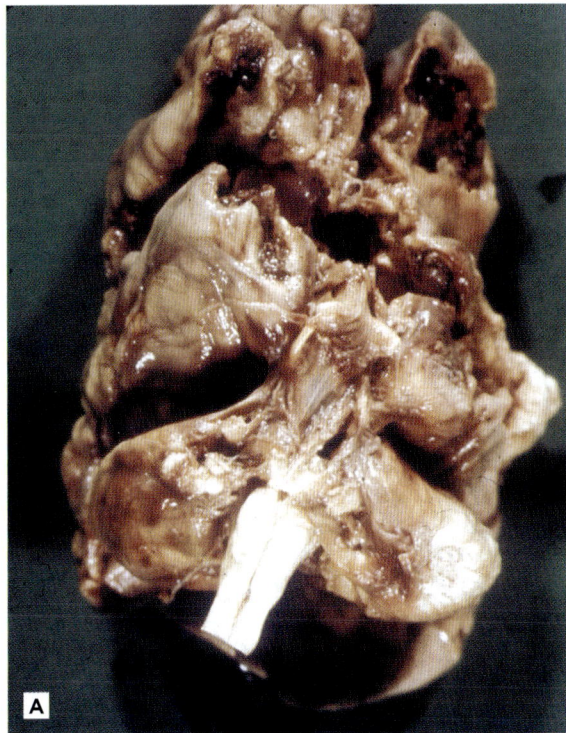
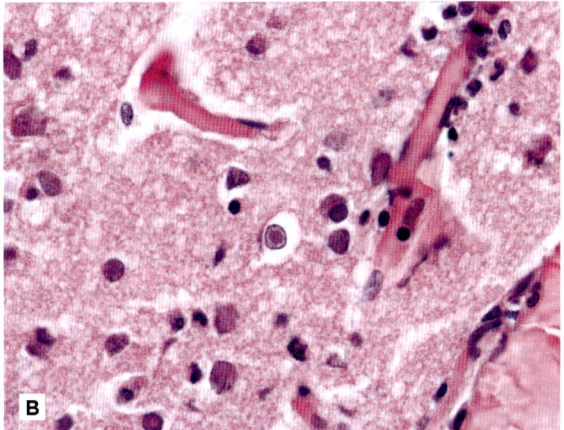

FIGURE 10-39 • Herpes simplex encephalitis. **A:** Ventral view of the brain demonstrating marked hemorrhagic necrosis in a congenital case caused by HSV 2 (image courtesy of Dr. Barry Rewcastle). **B:** High-power histology showing an eosinophilic intranuclear inclusion, likely within a glial cell.

CMV is the most common intrauterine viral infection. Congenital CMV is usually acquired transplacentally from a newly infected mother, and while acquisition is most successful in third trimester gestations, first-trimester infections lead to the most severe (often systemic and fatal) disease. Survivors are left with sequelae that include hearing loss, language disorders, microcephaly (the most common neurologic presentation), cognitive impairment, seizures, chorioretinitis, and motor deficits. Imaging reveals micrencephaly, cerebral microcalcifications (often periventricular), HCP, and gyral abnormalities. Diagnosis of fetal infection can be made via viral culture or PCR of amniotic fluid, or by fetal IgM serology. Gross pathology confirms the imaging impressions and may reveal porencephaly and polymicrogyria. Microscopy reveals a necrotizing ventriculoencephalitis, with areas of calcification and gliosis. Perivascular lymphocytes are accompanied by macrophages and activated microglia (± nodules). Cytomegalic cells bear a single haloed intranuclear inclusion (i.e., Cowdry A) associated with abundant cytoplasm also containing multiple small inclusions (Figure 10-40); IHC often highlights more widespread involvement than is appreciated by routine stains. Subependymal gliosis may result in HCP. CMV infections are less common in older children and are largely restricted to immunosuppressed patients (e.g., those with HIV) with systemic disease, which may be related to reactivation of latent bone marrow virus. Symptoms may include changes in mental status, nystagmus, and cranial nerve palsies, all of which are often indicative of a poor prognosis. Pathologically, several forms of disease may be seen including encephalitis of varying severity, ventriculitis, and lumbosacral myeloradiculitis (see Chapter 6).

Primary infection with *VZV* results in chicken pox (varicella), whereas reactivation of latent sensory ganglia disease causes shingles (zoster). Either form of VZV may result in CNS disease, which is typically necrotizing and accompanied by intranuclear inclusions. Varicella may cause an embryopathy, transient cerebellitis, meningoencephalitis (which can resemble *acute disseminated encephalomyelitis* [ADEM]) and has been associated with *Reye syndrome* (an

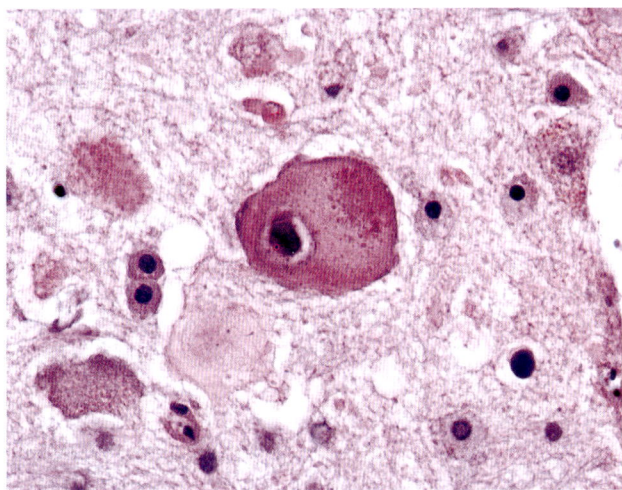

FIGURE 10-40 • CMV encephalitis. Cytomegalic cell containing a large intranuclear inclusion.

encephalopathic illness that has been correlated with salicylate ingestion). Zoster has been associated with encephalitis, myeloradiculitis, and a vasculopathy/vasculitis. *Varicella embryopathy* is acquired transplacentally and results in the most severe disease when acquired in the first half of gestation. Cutaneous scarring, limb hypoplasia, chorioretinitis, cataracts, and cognitive impairment are seen. Pathologically, scarring and gliosis are seen within the meninges and parenchyma, respectively, with the latter showing evidence of degeneration, but rarely an active necrotizing infection with demonstrable virus. A chronic inflammatory infiltrate is accompanied by microglial activation. There may be neuronal loss and degeneration within the dorsal root ganglia, anterior horns, and posterior/lateral funiculi, along with denervation muscular atrophy. Vasculitis (±granulomatous) with infarction is seen in AIDS patients. The recent development of a live attenuated vaccine will likely decrease the future incidence of VZV-related CNS disease.

The *arboviruses* are a group of mostly single-stranded RNA viruses that are usually transmitted to humans via mosquitos. Infections are seasonally distributed and generally occur in the summer and fall. While West Nile virus has garnered much of the spotlight over the last decade or so, it only rarely results in symptomatic CNS disease in pediatric patients. More common in children, yet still rare, are Western and Eastern equine encephalitides and La Crosse encephalitis (143). Incubation periods are less than 3 weeks and presenting symptoms include fever, malaise, and myalgias. Neurologic disease is diverse and includes aseptic meningitis, increased ICP, altered level of consciousness (which can lead to coma), motor deficits, and seizures. Diagnosis is made via serology or via PCR-specific RNA assay of the CSF. Gross pathology may reveal swelling, congestion, hemorrhage, and, if severe, necrosis. Some arboviruses tend to affect certain areas of the brain and spinal cord, but despite these predilections, the microscopic features are nonspecific (1). Chronic leptomeningeal inflammation is accompanied by the typical features of encephalitis (microglial activation, microglial nodules, perivascular lymphocytes) and occasionally perivascular hemorrhage/myelin destruction. Vessels may be thrombosed, but only rare and severe cases demonstrate significant necrosis. Notably, although viral inclusions are absent on routine staining, IHC staining (available for some arboviruses) can help to highlight neuronal and glial infection.

Although more commonly associated with meningitis, the *enteroviruses* (see above) may rarely cause a poliomyelitis. These small single-stranded RNA viruses (including the formerly more common poliovirus) cause a lytic infection of motor neurons in the anterior horn of the spinal cord and in the brain stem. Initial infection is via the fecal–oral route, and after hematogenous dissemination, the virus enters the CNS. Roughly 10 days after the resolution of a nonspecific flu-like illness, a prodrome of fever, headache, vomiting, meningismus, irritability, and myalgia ensues. Paralytic encephalomyelitis follows this prodrome and is often asymmetric and lower extremity predominant. Gross pathologic findings are uncommon, but severe cases include congestion, hemorrhage, and necrosis of motor nuclei within the brain stem and spinal cord anterior gray matter. Microscopically, affected areas are intensely inflamed. Parenchyma and leptomeninges first contain neutrophils and later lymphocytes plus activated microglia (with microglial nodules and neuronophagia). Chronic forms of disease manifest as areas of neuronal loss, gliosis, and scanty inflammatory infiltrates.

The *measles virus* is a single-stranded RNA pathogen from the Paramyxoviridae family. Measles is a highly contagious virus that is acquired through inhalation. Primary infection is systemic and results in fever, a maculopapular rash, and rarely CNS disease, which can include aseptic meningitis or ADEM. Measles mediates two less common chronic CNS diseases that are rare in areas that have consistently provided the MMR vaccine: *measles inclusion body encephalitis* (MIBE) (which occurs in the immunocompromised patients a few months after primary infection) and *subacute sclerosing panencephalitis* (SSPE). Re-emergence of measles has recently been seen in relation to a lack of immunization over concerns the latter causes autism, despite lack of evidence to support this notion. SSPE results in CNS disease approximately 5 to 10 years after primary infection, with rare examples occurring after vaccination. In SSPE, the viral genome is mutated such that the virus is unable to assemble or bud from infected cells. Clinical disease progresses through the early stages of cognitive and behavioral dysfunction, through motor deficits, seizures, and ataxia, followed by autonomic dysfunction, altered mental status, and finally death. Median survival is less than 2 years. Diagnosis can be made via antibody titers or PCR of fresh frozen brain. Pathologically, the gross brain may show signs of atrophy and leukodystrophy-like changes. A meningoencephalitis is seen microscopically, with lymphocytic infiltrates (including perivascular) and parenchymal microglial activation. The neocortex and deep cerebral gray and white matter regions are especially involved. There may be neuronal loss, and Alzheimer-like neurofibrillary tangles may be identified in residual neurons. Extensive white matter gliosis (i.e., "sclerosing") may be accompanied by demyelinated patches. Intranuclear eosinophilic and haloed viral inclusions may be seen in neurons and oligodendroglia, but these are often sparse, necessitating IHC for their detection.

Human immunodeficiency virus (HIV) is a single-stranded RNA retrovirus that causes AIDS. HIV infection is acquired by numerous routes, including sexual, hematologic, iatrogenic (e.g., contaminated instruments), and perinatal. This latter mode of infection is the most common in children. Primary infection may result in aseptic meningitis, after which a reservoir of virus is established in CD4-positive T-cells, macrophages, and microglia. With viral-mediated destruction, CD4-positive T-cells plummet to numbers less than 200/µL; thereafter, the systemic and CNS features of AIDS ensue. CNS disease related to AIDS includes (a) direct HIV infection, (b) opportunistic infections, (c) nonspecific

CNS damage (related to ischemia, metabolic insults), and (d) treatment-related disease (e.g., AZT myopathy). *Highly active antiretroviral therapy* (HAART) appears to have significantly impacted the patterns (i.e., incidence, prevalence) of AIDS-related disease in developed nations, especially in terms of reducing opportunistic infections (144). However, these opportunistic infections are much less common in children as compared to adults regardless of therapy. Moreover, socioeconomic barriers have impeded the implementation of HAART therapy in many developing nations. *HIV encephalitis/encephalopathy* (HIVE) and *vacuolar myelopathy* are disorders that are thought to be directly related to CNS HIV infection. Almost 40% of HIV-positive children develop HIVE, which is the most frequent HIV-specific disease and tends to occur in the later stages of immune suppression (145). Clinically, HIVE is characterized by developmental delay, apathy, seizures, and spastic quadriparesis (6). Grossly, HIVE brains may be atrophic, although the degree of pathology is often underwhelming compared to the severity of clinical manifestations. Microscopically, the *multinucleated giant cell* is characteristic; it is thought to be of phagocytic lineage, expresses HIV antigens, and harbors virus (146). Loosely aggregated microglia and glial cells (similar to microglial nodules) and perivascular (at times vasculitic) inflammatory infiltrates may be seen and predominate in the deep cerebral white matter, basal ganglia, and brain stem. Leukoencephalopathic features can be present and include white matter myelin pallor and gliosis; there also may be degeneration of the corticospinal tracts. Somewhat characteristic of pediatric AIDS brains are the angiocentric calcifications seen within basal ganglia and frontal white matter.

Fungal Infections

Fungal infections are most common in pediatric patients who are immunocompromised. Typically, these pathogens gain access to the CNS by hematogenous dissemination, often via lung infection. CNS invasion may be accompanied by only a sparse inflammatory reaction, which in part may be related to the patient's immunosuppression and innate mechanisms of immune evasion by various fungi. The clinicopathologic features of the most commonly encountered fungal pathogens are summarized in Table 10-9. Other CNS fungal infections include Mucormycosis, Coccidiomycosis, Blastomycosis, Histoplasmosis, and Chromoblastomycosis.

Parasitic Infections

Parasitic infections of the pediatric CNS are uncommon. Two of the most common, toxoplasmosis and neurocysticercosis (NCC), are briefly described below. Other parasitic infections include cerebral malaria, amoebic infections (e.g., *Entamoeba histolytica*, *Naegleria fowleri*, *Acanthamoeba* species), neuroschistosomiasis, trypanosomiasis, and helminthic infections (e.g., *Echinococcus granulosus*).

Toxoplasmosis is caused by *Toxoplasma gondii*, an obligate intracellular protozoan. Cats are the definitive host, and human infection is acquired via inadvertent ingestion of parasitic oocysts passed through feline feces. Primary infection is essentially asymptomatic in the immunocompetent individual; although the immune system may prevent the development of disease, the parasite is not eradicated and lies dormant in muscle/brain cysts. Of particular interest is CNS toxoplasmosis in congenital form or in the immunosuppressed patient. *Congenital toxoplasmosis* results from transplacental spread of organisms primarily during initial maternal infection and parasitemia. Like CMV, transmission of disease is most efficient during late gestation but more severe earlier on (highest risk for severe disease is 10 to 24 weeks). Following birth, affected infants classically present with the *Sabin tetrad*, which includes seizures, chorioretinitis, cerebral calcifications, and HCP. The pathology of congenital toxoplasmosis differs from the disease seen in older immunosuppressed individuals. Parasites proliferate in ependymal and periventricular regions, disseminating widely from there. Ependymal destruction and gliosis result

TABLE 10-9 SUMMARY OF COMMON FUNGAL INFECTIONS

Organism	Fungal Morphology	Source	Clinical Presentation	Pathology
Cryptococcus neoformans	Narrow budding yeast; polysaccharide capsule	Pigeon excreta Inhaled	Subacute to chronic meningitis	Thick gelatinous meninges and soap bubble deep gray matter lesions. Perivascular yeast accumulation. PAS positive and mucicarmine positive
Candida albicans	Pseudohyphae and yeast	Endogenous (e.g., GI, GU, skin)	Low-grade meningitis	Cerebritis and microabscesses in an ACA/MCA distribution. PAS and Grocott methenamine silver (GMS) positive
Aspergillus species (*fumigatus* and *flavus*)	Acutely branching septated hyphae	Soil Inhaled	Hemorrhagic infarction and abscess formation	Hyphal angioinvasion ± granulomatous reaction. PAS positive and GMS positive

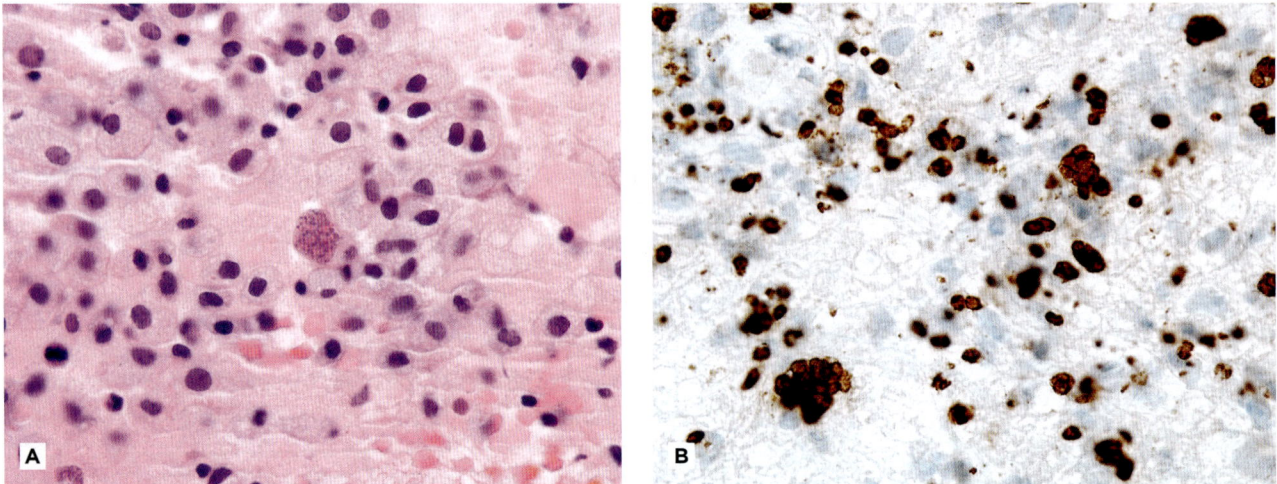

FIGURE 10-41 • Toxoplasmosis. **A:** An encysted organism (bradyzoites) is accompanied by foamy macrophages and coagulative necrosis. **B:** Immunohistochemistry against toxoplasmosis helps to highlight free-living tachyzoite forms that mimic karyorrhectic debris on routine staining.

in obstructive HCP. There is leptomeningeal, parenchymal, and perivascular inflammation, in addition to vascular thrombosis with secondary coagulative necrosis with mineralization. Inflammation is chronic, and there is often microglial activation. Encysted *bradyzoites* are more easily appreciated, whereas extracellular *tachyzoites* may be difficult to distinguish from karyorrhectic nuclear debris; in these cases, IHC stains and electron microscopy help to highlight the parasites (Figure 10-41). Toxoplasmosis disease related to immunosuppression is associated with reactivation of a dormant infection. Clinical presentation is variable but can include changes in mental status, features of increased ICP, and focal neurologic deficits. Imaging usually reveals multiple ring-enhancing lesions. Pathologically, areas of hemorrhage and necrosis are often centered upon the basal ganglia. Microscopically, foci of *coagulative necrosis* are surrounded by mononuclear and neutrophilic inflammation plus granulation tissue, gliosis, encephalitis, and/or vasculitis. These pathologic changes depend in part on the immune status of the host: greater degrees of suppression are associated with less inflammation and scarring. Vascular damage with superimposed thrombosis is often present. Older lesions can become cystic.

NCC is likely the most common parasitic CNS infection worldwide. Humans are the definitive host in the non-CNS form of disease wherein larval forms residing in poorly cooked pork are ingested; thereafter, the larvae mature into the adult tapeworms (*Taenia solium*), which reside in the GI tract. CNS disease occurs when humans become the intermediate host after eating food contaminated with tapeworm eggs (or oocytes). Once ingested, the eggs develop into larvae, which burrow through the GI tract wall and disseminate hematogenously throughout the body (including the CNS and muscle). Numerous larval cysts may develop within the brain and often remain asymptomatic for years. However, if the larvae are in eloquent brain or die, an intense inflammatory reaction may occur and herald the parasites' presence via new onset seizures or a myriad of location-dependent specific neurologic signs and symptoms. Imaging reveals one or more 1 to 2 cm ring-enhancing cystic lesions that may bear a calcified parasitic *scolex*. Microscopically, the larval cyst wall contains three layers: outer/cuticular, middle/cellular, and inner/reticular/fibrillary components. Favorable sections of the scolex may reveal parts of the four muscular suckers and or the double row of 22 to 32 hooklets (i.e., teeth) (Figure 10-42). Once the larvae dies and begins to degenerate, a chronic inflammatory response (including multinucleate giant cells, eosinophils, and neutrophils) ensues and a zone of granulation tissue may eventually wall off the deceased larva, which in turn undergoes fibrosis and mineralization.

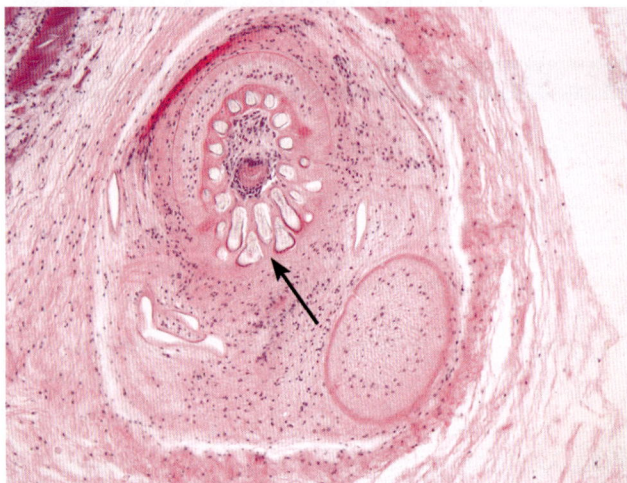

FIGURE 10-42 • Neurocysticercosis (NCC). This viable larval form has been favorably sectioned and reveals the characteristic hooklets of the scolex (*arrow*).

VASCULAR DISORDERS

Several pediatric CNS disorders fall under the rubric of vascular pathology. These include both congenital and acquired disorders, and they may affect all pediatric age groups. In general, these cause an interruption of blood supply (either global or localized), which results in ischemia and/or hemorrhage. The incidence of pediatric CNS vascular disorders varies considerably; likely, the most commonly encountered entities are those affecting premature infants (e.g., HIE and germinal matrix hemorrhage [GMH]). The gray or white matter may be preferential targets of damage.

Hypoxic-ischemic encephalopathy (HIE) is a common form of injury, especially in premature infants. HIE causes a global insult (e.g., with septic shock or cardiac arrest). The clinical impact may be minimal or may lead to profound neurologic impairment and even death. The areas of the brain that are susceptible to damage are age dependent; premature infants suffer damage primarily in the periventricular white matter (i.e., PVL and perinatal telencephalic leukoencephalopathy), deep gray matter (i.e., basal ganglia and thalamus), hippocampal subiculum, cerebellum, and basis pontis, while term infants and older children exhibit hippocampal CA1 and neocortical damage preferentially. However, these general patterns are only guidelines and damage can be more widespread in all ages. Regional factors associated with increased vulnerability include (a) high metabolic activity; (b) vascular watershed zones; and (c) specific neurotransmitter receptor distributions (especially glutaminergic). These factors contribute to the general concept of *selective vulnerability*, which dictates that certain areas of the CNS are preferentially susceptible to certain injurious processes, such as hypoxia and ischemia. Grossly, there may be cerebral swelling, dusky gray matter, white matter infarcts, and loss of normal gray–white junctions that eventually result in cerebral atrophy.

The microscopic CNS pathologic changes of HIE are age and region dependent. Neocortical damage may occur in a variety of patterns. As with any HIE, the initial phase is one of cerebral swelling and edema that manifests as parenchymal pallor and vacuolation. *Acute neuronal death* (i.e., "red neurons") occurs within the first 24 hours. If mature neurons contain ample cytoplasm (i.e., large pyramidal neurons), the latter will become brightly eosinophilic (Figure 10-1A). The neuronal nucleus becomes pyknotic and angulated. However, if cells are small and immature (i.e., little cytoplasm), evidence of HIE will be limited to nuclear fragmentation (i.e., karyorrhexis) (Figure 10-1B). If the nucleus fragments into multiple rounded bodies, cell death may be considered *apoptotic* rather than necrotic. *Apoptotic neurons* can be seen throughout the neocortical laminae, but they are often preferentially seen in the external granular layer. Microglial activation (highlighted by the use of CD68 IHC) is a common early occurrence, while foamy macrophages appear after a few days; this phagocytic activity is often marked by the presence of mitoses after the onset of HIE and is confirmed by increased Ki67 labeling in the damaged area. Vascular changes include early swelling of endothelia, while capillary proliferation occurs after a week. Reactive gliosis is generally not apparent until 1 week after injury. Some have suggested that the premature brain cannot demonstrate gliosis in the first half of gestational development, which would facilitate the rough dating of an *in utero* insult; however, exceptions to this rule clearly exist (147). Mineralization within neurons and macrophages may be seen after 10 to 14 days. Notably, these changes are very similar to those of frank infarction, although the latter typically involves all cell types within a vascular region, rather than individual neurons. For example, vascular watershed zones are particularly susceptible to HIE, resulting in selective neuronal necrosis, but if injury is more severe, complete parenchymal involvement occurs (i.e., watershed infarction). Near-term infants may display a peri-Rolandic or rarely a columnar distribution of cortical damage. The sulcal cortical depths are particularly susceptible to HIE, leading over time to deep sulcal atrophy and superficial sparing; grossly, this pathology is termed *ulegyria* because of the "mushroomlike" appearance of the affected gyrus.

The hippocampus is somewhat more resistant to the effects of HIE in premature infants, as compared to its more classic involvement in older children and adult patients. After the first few months of age, HIE damage in the hippocampus typically manifests as acute necrosis in Sommer sector (CA1) and the end folium (i.e., CA4), while CA2 (the "dorsal resistant zone") is largely spared. Later stages are characterized by neuronal loss and gliosis (i.e., hippocampal sclerosis). However, in term and particularly premature infants, the pattern and cytology of hippocampal damage differs; the *subiculum* is more commonly affected and neuronal death manifests as apoptosis, and when accompanied by similar changes in the basis pontis the misnomer *pontosubicular necrosis* can be applied (the more apt term would be "pontosubicular apoptosis") (148). On a cautionary note, the CA1 subregion typically contains smaller premature neurons until 2 years of age, and as such, this should not be overinterpreted as neuronal shrinkage in the context of acute neuronal necrosis (149).

HIE may preferentially affect the deep gray nuclei (including the basal ganglia and thalami), primarily in preterm but also term infants. These nuclei display a high metabolic activity near term, which might underlie their susceptibility to insult (150). Histologic changes are similar to those in the neocortex. While acute damage usually results in neuronal necrosis in older infants, apoptotic neurons can be seen in the basal ganglia of premature infants/fetuses suffering HIE. As a response to injury, the deep gray nuclei may also display abnormal myelination, wherein oligodendroglia mistakenly invest reactive astrocytic, rather than axonal processes. Grossly, these deep gray nuclei adopt a marbled appearance called *status marmoratus*. Survivors with this type of damage may suffer clinically from cerebral palsy.

The cerebellum is also commonly affected by HIE. Both the cortex and dentate nuclei are often damaged. While Purkinje and dentate neurons die via necrosis, internal granule neurons are lost by apoptosis (6).

Overall, the brain stem is uncommonly affected by HIE (with the exception of the aforementioned pontosubicular necrosis). The inferior olives and more laterally situated medullary tegmental neurons may incur necrosis, but other changes are generally rare. Severe HIE may result in bilaterally symmetric dorsal lower brainstem necrosis, which may explain the pathogenesis behind a subset of *Moebius syndrome* cases (facial diplegia and bilateral abducens palsies) (151). Only severe cases of HIE tend to affect the entirety of the brain stem and for that matter the spinal cord.

If HIE occurs during prenatal life, the pathways and cytoarchitecture of the developing brain may be significantly disturbed. Accordingly, this may lead to secondary malformations (i.e., acquired and not congenital). The type of malformation that results is GA dependent. It would be predicted that earlier insults result in more profound malformations. *Polymicrogyria*, *schizencephaly*, and *porencephaly* (see earlier discussions) are thought to result from early damage, while some forms of cortical dysplasia and hippocampal sclerosis are considered to be of late onset (6).

The white matter may be preferentially damaged in premature (and less so term) infants. The most common type of pathology is PVL. PVL is now less frequently encountered in its classic and striking "cystic form" than it was in the past, likely because of advances in prenatal care. Nonetheless, noncystic forms are still frequently observed at autopsy. Premature infants between the GAs of 24 and 35 weeks (peak age is 28 weeks) are most frequently affected. Besides age, two of the most important risk factors include fetomaternal cardiorespiratory instability (e.g., fetal cerebral hypoperfusion and immature cerebral autoregulatory mechanisms) and intrauterine infection (e.g., chorioamnionitis). These two factors may act synergistically to trigger an inflammatory response (in part mediated by reactive astrocytes and activated microglia) that primarily targets the premyelinating oligodendrocytes of the fetal brain via excitotoxic amino acid–based mechanisms, oxidative stress, and cytokine cascades (152). Clinically, these premature infants are generally "sick" (i.e., septic with unstable cardiac and respiratory function), and neurologically, they may have weak legs and seizures. The more uncommonly affected term infant often suffers from congestive heart disease or a congenital diaphragmatic hernia. Long-term sequelae include cerebral palsy, cognitive deficits (mental retardation, learning deficits), behavioral abnormalities, and epilepsy. Twenty-five percent of SIDS cases display evidence of PVL at autopsy. Unfortunately, the genetic features of PVL are still not well understood.

Pathologically, PVL is defined by two features: (a) *periventricular necrosis* that may be cystic and mineralized (Figure 10-43) and (b) evidence for a more *diffuse white matter gliosis*, sometimes referred to as "perinatal telencephalic leukoencephalopathy." Some have conceptualized these two lesional components as the vascular "core" and the "penumbra," respectively. Adding further to the vascular hypothesis is the suggestion that the periventricular areas of predilec-

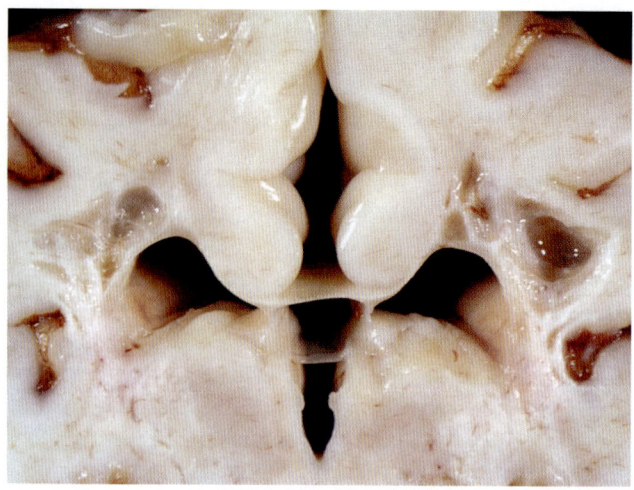

FIGURE 10-43 • Periventricular leukomalacia (PVL). Coronal section of the brain demonstrating cystic abnormalities in the white matter; note the markedly thinned corpus callosum.

tion likely represent a region of vascular watershed during this age (1). Microscopically, periventricular white matter damage begins with the development of coagulative necrosis of all cell types within the first 24 hours of the insult (all cells develop nuclear pyknosis and eosinophilic cytoplasm). Axonal spheroids are seen on routine staining but can be further highlighted with β-APP IHC. Activated microglia, elucidated with CD68 IHC, are prominent in early stages. Within the first week, macrophages infiltrate the areas of necrosis and are surrounded by early reactive gliosis. Gross cavitation and mineralization (of axons) can be seen after a few weeks. Cystic spaces collapse to form glial scars or areas of encephalomalacia. Small areas of necrosis, the type of lesion more commonly seen in current pediatric neuropathologic practices, do not result in residual cystic degeneration over time but rather lead to the formation of glial scars. Destruction of axons during this process undoubtedly affects the development of the overlying neocortical gray matter and likely accounts for subsequent cytoarchitectural abnormalities. Surrounding these areas of periventricular necrosis is a more subtle penumbra of diffuse white matter gliosis that is relatively devoid of axonal pathology. Moreover, diffuse gliosis without a necrotic component may be seen as a manifestation of PVL (6). Prominent loss of premyelinating oligodendrocytes from these areas leads to delayed and impaired myelination. Since premature infants are mainly at risk, it is not uncommon to see coexistent GMH (see below) and HIE.

GMH is also characteristic of premature infants. Given subependymal origin of hemorrhages, IVH is regularly present as well. Although in rare examples, term infants may also experience GMH and IVH, the latter is more often a result of choroid plexus hemorrhage, possibly related to congenital vascular malformation (see below). Age is the most important risk factor, with the incidence of GMH being inversely proportional to GA. Those infants less than 28 weeks GA are at the greatest risk for severe GMH (153). Other risk factors may include respiratory compromise (which is interrelated with age), intrauterine growth restriction (IUGR), fetomaternal sepsis (e.g., related to chorioamnionitis), hypothermia, intubation, and transportation between hospitals. Although the large veins of the germinal matrix are the likely source of the hemorrhage, the exact pathogenesis of GMH remains unclear. The germinal matrix is a major source of neuroglial precursors and persists until 34 weeks' gestation (involution occurs by 38 to 40 weeks' gestation). Enhanced fibrinolytic activity is characteristic of the involuting matrix making it susceptible to hemorrhage, in part due to the lack of sufficient parenchymal support of the matrix vasculature and poor hemostasis. Hypoxic–ischemic injury of the germinal matrix may further impair the already primitive autoregulatory capabilities of these vessels, making them vulnerable to fluctuations in CPP.

Clinically, GMH usually presents within the first 24 to 48 hours after birth. There may be a decreased level of consciousness or irritability, a tense fontanelle, and seizure activity. Severe GMH is often fatal (153). Occult cases of GMH are presumably of less clinical severity. Grading the GMH has been widely applied to ultrasonography. Grade I is confined to the germinal matrix; grade II additionally includes IVH that in grade III causes HCP; and finally, grade IV adds intraparenchymal "extension" of hemorrhage beyond the germinal matrix. This "extension" in grade IV cases may not be purely direct; in fact, many experts suggest that hemorrhage extending beyond the confines of the germinal matrix and into the adjacent brain is more likely to be related to *venous infarction*. Clinically speaking, higher grades of GMH correlate with greater degrees of long-term neurologic disability (6). Grossly, the appearance of GMH is in keeping with the aforementioned grading scheme (Figure 10-44). Extension of ventricular blood through the foramina of the fourth ventricle into the basal cisterns yields a subarachnoid component that likely plays a role in chronic HCP. Areas of parenchyma adjacent to GMH may be necrotic (with microscopic mineralization) and often show concomitant PVL. Microscopically, there are relatively few reactive changes in the parenchyma, especially in cases dying acutely.

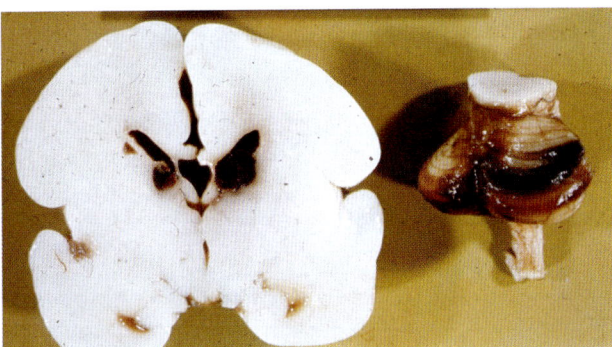

FIGURE 10-44 • Bilateral GMH. Hemorrhage on the left side has extended into the adjacent ventricular system and out into the subarachnoid space (cisterna magna) overlying the cerebellum through the foramina of the fourth ventricle (coronal section). (Image courtesy of Dr. Barry Rewcastle.)

A variety of acquired vascular disorders may be seen in children, many of which are rarely encountered by the neuropathologist. Essentially, all of these disorders result in "stroke" (i.e., infarction). Risk factors for pediatric stroke include diabetes, cardiac abnormalities (e.g., congenital and rheumatic heart disease, arrhythmias), thrombophilias, hyperhomocysteinemia, hematologic conditions, trauma, drug use (e.g., smoking, amphetamines), hypertension, obesity, and oral contraceptive use. Meningitis often leads to infarction via inflammation, damage, and thrombosis of leptomeningeal vessels (i.e., secondary vasculitis). Clinically, pediatric and adult stroke may present similarly (i.e., focal signs/symptoms and or more global neurologic impairment). Angiography and diffusion-/perfusion-weighted MRI studies are frequently used in the patient's workup. Microscopically, edema and congestion precede acute neuronal cell death that is most readily visible by 24 hours. At 1 to 2 days, there is infiltration of neutrophils (PMNs) and endothelial swelling. Within the first week, PMNs make way for macrophages. Angiogenesis and reactive gliosis are seen by 2 weeks. Later stages are characterized by neuronal loss, gliosis, and cystic degeneration. Well-recognized clinicopathologic entities that have a relative predilection for the CNS vasculature include Moyamoya disease, fibromuscular dysplasia, venous sinus thrombosis, arterial dissection, vasculitides (e.g., Takayasu arteritis, primary angiitis of the CNS), and vasculopathies (e.g., HIV vasculopathy). Many systemic disorders characteristically affect the large and small blood vessels of the CNS including systemic lupus erythematosus, other collagen vascular disorders, sickle cell disease, antiphospholipid antibody syndrome, fat emboli, thrombotic thrombocytopenic purpura, and hemolytic uremic syndrome.

Many of the congenital CNS vascular anomalies are also uncommonly seen. *Berry (i.e., saccular) aneurysms* are extremely rare in young children. A defective internal elastic lamina may predispose to their formation over time and thus accounts for the low prevalence in this population. These often present with massive and fatal SAH. The key to their discovery is a careful dissection of blood and the circle of Willis in the fresh state when structures are more manipulatable. Microscopically, the aneurysm wall is focally attenuated; the internal elastic lamina and media are replaced by fibrous connective tissue, and possibly atherosclerosis plus hemosiderin.

Vascular malformations include arteriovenous malformations (AVMs), cavernous hemangiomas (i.e., cavernous angiomas or "cavernomas"), venous angiomas, and capillary telangiectasias, the former two of which are more commonly symptomatic. *AVMs* may present with hemorrhage or with ischemic signs and symptoms that relate to arteriovenous shunting and vascular steal. Arterial feeders and draining veins are usually well appreciated angiographically. Microscopically, there are arteries, veins, and "arterialized veins" of varying mural thickness and caliber, often with entrapped fragments of gliotic brain between these abnormal vessels. Hybrid vessels appear partly arterial and partly venous in favorable histologic sections. Staining of the internal elastic lamina (e.g., Musto Movat, Verhoeff van Gieson) assists in highlighting the arterial components. Recent and remote hemorrhage may be seen in the abnormal vessels, as well as gliotic brain. Evidence of embolization may be seen in the form of foreign material within the vascular lumina of the malformation. *Cavernous angiomas* are essentially venous structures that present as mass lesions, which may cause hemorrhage, focal neurologic deficits, or seizures. Gradient echo and susceptibility-weighted MRI sequences highlight these malformations. Microscopically, hyalinized veins of various calibers are packed together in a back-to-back fashion, generally excluding intervening parenchyma in most examples. Gliosis and signs of prior hemorrhage surround these abnormal blood vessels.

Vein of Galen aneurysms are actually arteriovenous fistulas that are associated with aneurysmal dilatation of the vein of Galen. These are thought to arise early in gestation (between 6 and 11 weeks) (6). The posterior cerebral artery is a frequent "feeder artery." The most common clinical presentation is high-output congestive heart failure in a young child. Vascular steal may lead to atrophy and parenchymal necrosis (with dystrophic calcification). Microscopically, feeder vessels are dilated and hypertrophic, while the "aneurysmal" vein similarly displays a thickened wall. Vessels in the adjacent brain parenchyma may also be hyperplastic in response to high-pressure shunting.

Meningioangiomatosis (MA) is a form of meningovascular malformation or hamartoma occurring either in the setting of NF2 or sporadically (154). The former is typically asymptomatic, whereas the latter usually presents before adulthood with seizures and/or headache. MA often features plaque-like meningothelial, smooth muscle, and fibroblast-like spindle cell proliferations that extend down the Virchow-Robin perivascular spaces into the cortex (Figure 10-45). The surrounding brain is gliotic and often displays dysmorphic neurons, dystrophic calcification, and fibrosis. In contrast to pure MA, cases associated with an overlying meningioma likely represent an unusual mimic with perivascular tumoral spread, rather than an underlying malformation. Other CNS vascular anomalies include Fowler syndrome, meningocerebral angiodysplasia/renal agenesis, and Sturge-Weber-Dimitri disease (i.e., encephalotrigeminal angiomatosis) (6).

References

1. Ellison D. *Neuropathology: A Reference Text of CNS Pathology*, 3rd ed. Edinburgh, UK; New York, NY: Mosby, 2013:xiii, 879.
2. Ellison D, Love S. *Neuropathology: A Reference Text of CNS Pathology*, 2nd ed. Edinburgh, UK; New York, NY: Mosby; 2004:xii, 755.
3. Dickson D. *Neurodegeneration: The Molecular Pathology of Dementia and Movement Disorders*, 2nd ed. Chichester, West Sussex: Wiley-Blackwell, 2011.
4. Kandel ER. *Principles of Neural Science*, 5th ed. New York, NY: McGraw-Hill; 2013:1–1709.
5. Currarino G. Occipital osteodiastasis: presentation of four cases and review of the literature. *Pediatr Radiol* 2000;30(12):823–829.
6. Golden JA, Harding BN; International Society of Neuropathology. *Developmental Neuropathology*. Basel, Switzerland: International Society of Neuropathology, 2013:386.
7. Geddes JF, Hackshaw AK, Vowles GH, et al. Neuropathology of inflicted head injury in children. I Patterns of brain damage. *Brain* 2001;124(Pt 7):1290–1298.
8. Shannon P, Smith CR, Deck J, et al. Axonal injury and the neuropathology of shaken baby syndrome. *Acta Neuropathol* 1998;95(6):625–631.
9. Geddes JF, Whitwell HL, Graham DI. Traumatic axonal injury: practical issues for diagnosis in medicolegal cases. *Neuropathol Appl Neurobiol* 2000;26(2):105–116.
10. Matturri L, Ottaviani G, Lavezzi AM. Maternal smoking and sudden infant death syndrome: epidemiological study related to pathology. *Virchows Arch* 2006;449(6):697–706.
11. Kinney HC, Thach BT. The sudden infant death syndrome. *N Engl J Med* 2009;361(8):795–805.
12. Paterson DS, Trachtenberg FL, Thompson EG, et al. Multiple serotonergic brainstem abnormalities in sudden infant death syndrome. *JAMA* 2006;296(17):2124–2132.
13. Kinney HC, Randall LL, Sleeper LA, et al. Serotonergic brainstem abnormalities in Northern Plains Indians with the sudden infant death syndrome. *J Neuropathol Exp Neurol* 2003;62(11):1178–1191.
14. Filiano JJ, Kinney HC. A perspective on neuropathologic findings in victims of the sudden infant death syndrome: the triple-risk model. *Biol Neonate* 1994;65(3–4):194–197.
15. Frey L, Hauser WA. Epidemiology of neural tube defects. *Epilepsia* 2003;44(Suppl 3):4–13.
16. Norman MG. *Congenital Malformations of the Brain: Pathologic, Embryologic, Clinical, Radiologic, and Genetic Aspects*. New York, NY: Oxford University Press, 1995:xii, 452.
17. Adzick NS, Thom EA, Spong CY, et al. A randomized trial of prenatal versus postnatal repair of myelomeningocele. *N Engl J Med* 2011;364(11):993–1004.
18. Alexiev BA, Lin X, Sun CC, et al. Meckel-Gruber syndrome: pathologic manifestations, minimal diagnostic criteria, and differential diagnosis. *Arch Pathol Lab Med* 2006;130(8):1236–1238.
19. Tehli O, Hodaj I, Kural C, et al. A comparative study of histopathological analysis of filum terminale in patients with tethered cord syndrome and in normal human fetuses. *Pediatr Neurosurg* 2011;47(6):412–416.
20. Donkelaar HJt, Lammens M, Hori A, et al. *Clinical Neuroembryology: Development and Developmental Disorders of the Human Central Nervous System*. Berlin, Germany; New York, NY: Springer, 2006:xi, 536.

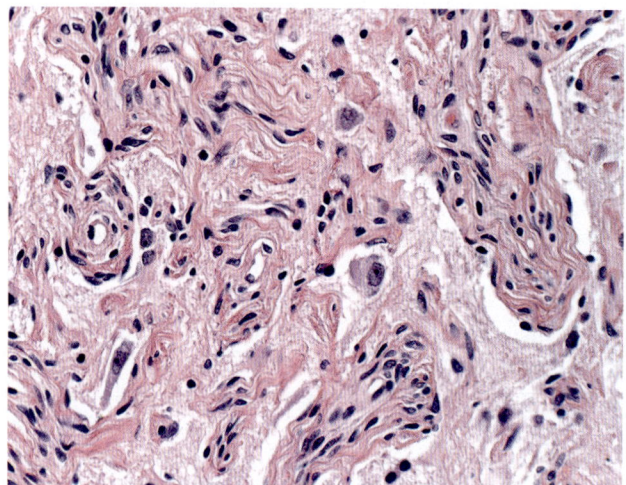

FIGURE 10-45 • MA characterized by a variably hyalinized, fibroblast-like perivascular spindle cell proliferation, adjacent to normal-appearing or mildly dysmorphic cortical neurons.

21. Dale JK, Vesque C, Lints TJ, et al. Cooperation of BMP7 and SHH in the induction of forebrain ventral midline cells by prechordal mesoderm. *Cell* 1997;90(2):257–269.
22. Sarnat HB, Flores-Sarnat L. Neuropathologic research strategies in holoprosencephaly. *J Child Neurol* 2001;16(12):918–931.
23. Sarnat HB. *Cerebral Dysgenesis: Embryology and Clinical Expression.* New York, NY: Oxford University Press, 1992:x, 473.
24. Loeser JD, Alvord EC Jr. Agenesis of the corpus callosum. *Brain* 1968;91(3):553–570.
25. Davila-Gutierrez G. Agenesis and dysgenesis of the corpus callosum. *Semin Pediatr Neurol* 2002;9(4):292–301.
26. Forman MS, Squier W, Dobyns WB, et al. Genotypically defined lissencephalies show distinct pathologies. *J Neuropathol Exp Neurol* 2005;64(10):847–857.
27. Martin-Rendon E, Blake DJ. Protein glycosylation in disease: new insights into the congenital muscular dystrophies. *Trends Pharmacol Sci* 2003;24(4):178–183.
28. Hevner RF. The cerebral cortex malformation in thanatophoric dysplasia: neuropathology and pathogenesis. *Acta Neuropathol* 2005;110(3):208–221.
29. Judkins AR, Martinez D, Ferreira P, et al. Polymicrogyria includes fusion of the molecular layer and decreased neuronal populations but normal cortical laminar organization. *J Neuropathol Exp Neurol* 2011;70(6):438–443.
30. Sheen VL, Dixon PH, Fox JW, et al. Mutations in the X-linked filamin 1 gene cause periventricular nodular heterotopia in males as well as in females. *Hum Mol Genet* 2001;10(17):1775–1783.
31. Kasper BS, Stefan H, Buchfelder M, et al. Temporal lobe microdysgenesis in epilepsy versus control brains. *J Neuropathol Exp Neurol* 1999;58(1):22–28.
32. Palmini A, Najm I, Avanzini G, et al. Terminology and classification of the cortical dysplasias. *Neurology* 2004;62(6 Suppl 3):S2–S8.
33. Blumcke I, Thom M, Aronica E, et al. The clinicopathologic spectrum of focal cortical dysplasias: a consensus classification proposed by an ad hoc Task Force of the ILAE Diagnostic Methods Commission. *Epilepsia* 2011;52(1):158–174.
34. Ruggieri PM, Najm I, Bronen R, et al. Neuroimaging of the cortical dysplasias. *Neurology* 2004;62(6 Suppl 3):S27–S29.
35. ten Donkelaar HJ, Lammens M, Wesseling P, et al. Development and developmental disorders of the human cerebellum. *J Neurol* 2003;250(9):1025–1036.
36. Cornips EM, Overvliet GM, Weber JW, et al. The clinical spectrum of Blake's pouch cyst: report of six illustrative cases. *Childs Nerv Syst* 2010;26(8):1057–1064.
37. Harding BN, Boyd SG. Intractable seizures from infancy can be associated with dentato-olivary dysplasia. *J Neurol Sci* 1991;104(2):157–165.
38. Prayson RA. *Neuropathology*, 2nd ed. Philadelphia, PA: Elsevier/Saunders, 2012:1. Online resource (xv, 630 p.).
39. Rodriguez D, Gelot A, della Gaspera B, et al. Increased density of oligodendrocytes in childhood ataxia with diffuse central hypomyelination (CACH) syndrome: neuropathological and biochemical study of two cases. *Acta Neuropathol* 1999;97(5):469–480.
40. van der Knaap MS, Leegwater PA, Konst AA, et al. Mutations in each of the five subunits of translation initiation factor eIF2B can cause leukoencephalopathy with vanishing white matter. *Ann Neurol* 2002;51(2):264–270.
41. Gordon N. Alpers syndrome: progressive neuronal degeneration of children with liver disease. *Dev Med Child Neurol* 2006;48(12):1001–1003.
42. Ching KH, Westaway SK, Gitschier J, et al. HARP syndrome is allelic with pantothenate kinase-associated neurodegeneration. *Neurology* 2002;58(11):1673–1674.
43. Koeppen AH. The pathogenesis of spinocerebellar ataxia. *Cerebellum* 2005;4(1):62–73.
44. van de Warrenburg BP, Sinke RJ, Kremer B. Recent advances in hereditary spinocerebellar ataxias. *J Neuropathol Exp Neurol* 2005;64(3):171–180.
45. Shao Y, Cuccaro ML, Hauser ER, et al. Fine mapping of autistic disorder to chromosome 15q11-q13 by use of phenotypic subtypes. *Am J Hum Genet* 2003;72(3):539–548.
46. Blatt GJ, Fitzgerald CM, Guptill JT, et al. Density and distribution of hippocampal neurotransmitter receptors in autism: an autoradiographic study. *J Autism Dev Disord* 2001;31(6):537–543.
47. Chugani DC, Muzik O, Rothermel R, et al. Altered serotonin synthesis in the dentatothalamocortical pathway in autistic boys. *Ann Neurol* 1997;42(4):666–669.
48. Perry EK, Lee ML, Martin-Ruiz CM, et al. Cholinergic activity in autism: abnormalities in the cerebral cortex and basal forebrain. *Am J Psychiatry* 2001;158(7):1058–1066.
49. Blatt GJ. The neuropathology of autism. *Scientifica (Cairo)* 2012;2012:703675.
50. Casanova MF, Buxhoeveden DP, Switala AE, et al. Minicolumnar pathology in autism. *Neurology* 2002;58(3):428–432.
51. Pasquier B, Peoc HM, Fabre-Bocquentin B, et al. Surgical pathology of drug-resistant partial epilepsy. A 10-year-experience with a series of 327 consecutive resections. *Epileptic Disord* 2002;4(2):99–119.
52. Nelson PT, Schmitt FA, Lin Y, et al. Hippocampal sclerosis in advanced age: clinical and pathological features. *Brain* 2011;134(Pt 5):1506–1518.
53. Rickert CH, Paulus W. Epidemiology of central nervous system tumors in childhood and adolescence based on the new WHO classification. *Childs Nerv Syst* 2001;17(9):503–511.
54. Dunham C, Pillai S, Steinbok P. Infant brain tumors: a neuropathologic population-based institutional reappraisal. *Hum Pathol* 2012;43(10):1668–1676.
55. Ceppa EP, Bouffet E, Griebel R, et al. The pilomyxoid astrocytoma and its relationship to pilocytic astrocytoma: report of a case and a critical review of the entity. *J Neurooncol* 2007;81(2):191–196.
56. Louis DN, Ohgaki H, Wiestler OD, et al. *WHO Classification of Tumours of the Central Nervous System*, 4th ed. Lyon, France: IARC, 2007:312.
57. Ullrich NJ, Pomeroy SL. Pediatric brain tumors. *Neurol Clin* 2003;21(4):897–913.
58. Buczkowicz P, Hoeman C, Rakopoulos P, et al. Genomic analysis of diffuse intrinsic pontine gliomas identifies three molecular subgroups and recurrent activating ACVR1 mutations. *Nat Genet* 2014;46(5):451–456.
59. Jones DT, Hutter B, Jager N, et al. Recurrent somatic alterations of FGFR1 and NTRK2 in pilocytic astrocytoma. *Nat Genet* 2013;45(8):927–932.
60. Burger PC. *Smears and Frozen Sections in Surgical Neuropathology: A Manual*. Baltimore, MD: PB Medical Pub, 2009:xii, 678.
61. Burger PC, Scheithauer BW, Vogel FS. *Surgical Pathology of the Nervous System and its Coverings*, 4th ed. New York, NY: Churchill Livingstone, 2002:xii, 657.
62. Perry A, Brat DJ. *Practical Surgical Neuropathology: A Diagnostic Approach*. Philadelphia, PA: Churchill Livingstone/Elsevier, 2010:xxxiii, 620.
63. Rodriguez FJ, Scheithauer BW, Burger PC, et al. Anaplasia in pilocytic astrocytoma predicts aggressive behavior. *Am J Surg Pathol* 2010;34(2):147–160.
64. Johnson MW, Eberhart CG, Perry A, et al. Spectrum of pilomyxoid astrocytomas: intermediate pilomyxoid tumors. *Am J Surg Pathol* 2010;34(12):1783–1791.
65. Tihan T, Fisher PG, Kepner JL, et al. Pediatric astrocytomas with monomorphous pilomyxoid features and a less favorable outcome. *J Neuropathol Exp Neurol* 1999;58(10):1061–1068.
66. Forshew T, Tatevossian RG, Lawson AR, et al. Activation of the ERK/MAPK pathway: a signature genetic defect in posterior fossa pilocytic astrocytomas. *J Pathol* 2009;218(2):172–181.
67. Horbinski C. To BRAF or not to BRAF: is that even a question anymore? *J Neuropathol Exp Neurol* 2013;72(1):2–7.
68. Ida CM, Lambert SR, Rodriguez FJ, et al. BRAF alterations are frequent in cerebellar low-grade astrocytomas with diffuse growth pattern. *J Neuropathol Exp Neurol* 2012;71(7):631–639.

69. Giannini C, Scheithauer BW, Burger PC, et al. Cellular proliferation in pilocytic and diffuse astrocytomas. *J Neuropathol Exp Neurol* 1999;58(1):46–53.
70. Broniscer A, Gajjar A. Supratentorial high-grade astrocytoma and diffuse brainstem glioma: two challenges for the pediatric oncologist. *Oncologist* 2004;9(2):197–206.
71. Ohgaki H, Kleihues P. Population-based studies on incidence, survival rates, and genetic alterations in astrocytic and oligodendroglial gliomas. *J Neuropathol Exp Neurol* 2005;64(6):479–489.
72. Raffel C, Frederick L, O'Fallon JR, et al. Analysis of oncogene and tumor suppressor gene alterations in pediatric malignant astrocytomas reveals reduced survival for patients with PTEN mutations. *Clin Cancer Res* 1999;5(12):4085–4090.
73. Ullrich NJ, Pomeroy SL. Molecular genetics of pediatric central nervous system tumors. *Curr Oncol Rep* 2006;8(6):423–429.
74. Pollack IF, Hamilton RL, Sobol RW, et al. IDH1 mutations are common in malignant gliomas arising in adolescents: a report from the Children's Oncology Group. *Childs Nerv Syst* 2011;27(1):87–94.
75. Paugh BS, Qu C, Jones C, et al. Integrated molecular genetic profiling of pediatric high-grade gliomas reveals key differences with the adult disease. *J Clin Oncol* 2010;28(18):3061–3068.
76. Fontebasso AM, Bechet D, Jabado N. Molecular biomarkers in pediatric glial tumors: a needed wind of change. *Curr Opin Oncol* 2013;25(6):665–673.
77. Sturm D, Witt H, Hovestadt V, et al. Hotspot mutations in H3F3A and IDH1 define distinct epigenetic and biological subgroups of glioblastoma. *Cancer Cell* 2012;22(4):425–437.
78. Ho DM, Hsu CY, Wong TT, et al. A clinicopathologic study of 81 patients with ependymomas and proposal of diagnostic criteria for anaplastic ependymoma. *J Neurooncol* 2001;54(1):77–85.
79. Korshunov A, Golanov A, Sycheva R, et al. The histologic grade is a main prognostic factor for patients with intracranial ependymomas treated in the microneurosurgical era: an analysis of 258 patients. *Cancer* 2004;100(6):1230–1237.
80. Merchant TE, Jenkins JJ, Burger PC, et al. Influence of tumor grade on time to progression after irradiation for localized ependymoma in children. *Int J Radiat Oncol Biol Phys* 2002;53(1):52–57.
81. Kurt E, Zheng PP, Hop WC, et al. Identification of relevant prognostic histopathologic features in 69 intracranial ependymomas, excluding myxopapillary ependymomas and subependymomas. *Cancer* 2006;106(2):388–395.
82. Tabori U, Ma J, Carter M, et al. Human telomere reverse transcriptase expression predicts progression and survival in pediatric intracranial ependymoma. *J Clin Oncol* 2006;24(10):1522–1528.
83. Tihan T, Zhou T, Holmes E, et al. The prognostic value of histological grading of posterior fossa ependymomas in children: a Children's Oncology Group study and a review of prognostic factors. *Mod Pathol* 2008;21(2):165–177.
84. Rajaram V, Gutmann DH, Prasad SK, et al. Alterations of protein 4.1 family members in ependymomas: a study of 84 cases. *Mod Pathol* 2005;18(7):991–997.
85. Singh PK, Gutmann DH, Fuller CE, et al. Differential involvement of protein 4.1 family members DAL-1 and NF2 in intracranial and intraspinal ependymomas. *Mod Pathol* 2002;15(5):526–531.
86. Pfeifer JD. *Molecular Genetic Testing in Surgical Pathology*. Philadelphia, PA: Lippincott, Williams & Wilkins, 2006:474.
87. Dyer S, Prebble E, Davison V, et al. Genomic imbalances in pediatric intracranial ependymomas define clinically relevant groups. *Am J Pathol* 2002;161(6):2133–2241.
88. Gilbertson RJ, Bentley L, Hernan R, et al. ERBB receptor signaling promotes ependymoma cell proliferation and represents a potential novel therapeutic target for this disease. *Clin Cancer Res* 2002;8(10):3054–3064.
89. Suarez-Merino B, Hubank M, Revesz T, et al. Microarray analysis of pediatric ependymoma identifies a cluster of 112 candidate genes including four transcripts at 22q12.1-q13.3. *Neuro Oncol* 2005;7(1):20–31.
90. Taylor MD, Poppleton H, Fuller C, et al. Radial glia cells are candidate stem cells of ependymoma. *Cancer Cell* 2005;8(4):323–335.
91. Witt H, Mack SC, Ryzhova M, et al. Delineation of two clinically and molecularly distinct subgroups of posterior fossa ependymoma. *Cancer Cell* 2011;20(2):143–57.
92. Wang M, Tihan T, Rojiani AM, et al. Monomorphous angiocentric glioma: a distinctive epileptogenic neoplasm with features of infiltrating astrocytoma and ependymoma. *J Neuropathol Exp Neurol* 2005;64(10):875–881.
93. Giannini C, Scheithauer BW, Weaver AL, et al. Oligodendrogliomas: reproducibility and prognostic value of histologic diagnosis and grading. *J Neuropathol Exp Neurol* 2001;60(3):248–262.
94. Cairncross JG, Ueki K, Zlatescu MC, et al. Specific genetic predictors of chemotherapeutic response and survival in patients with anaplastic oligodendrogliomas. *J Natl Cancer Inst* 1998;90(19):1473–1479.
95. Kreiger PA, Okada Y, Simon S, et al. Losses of chromosomes 1p and 19q are rare in pediatric oligodendrogliomas. *Acta Neuropathol* 2005;109(4):387–392.
96. Schindler G, Capper D, Meyer J, et al. Analysis of BRAF V600E mutation in 1,320 nervous system tumors reveals high mutation frequencies in pleomorphic xanthoastrocytoma, ganglioglioma and extra-cerebellar pilocytic astrocytoma. *Acta Neuropathol* 2011;121(3):397–405.
97. Chamberlain MC. Salvage therapy with BRAF inhibitors for recurrent pleomorphic xanthoastrocytoma: a retrospective case series. *J Neurooncol* 2013;114:237–240.
98. Eberhart CG, Kepner JL, Goldthwaite PT, et al. Histopathologic grading of medulloblastomas: a Pediatric Oncology Group study. *Cancer* 2002;94(2):552–560.
99. Giangaspero F, Wellek S, Masuoka J, et al. Stratification of medulloblastoma on the basis of histopathological grading. *Acta Neuropathol* 2006;112(1):5–12.
100. Pomeroy SL, Tamayo P, Gaasenbeek M, et al. Prediction of central nervous system embryonal tumour outcome based on gene expression. *Nature* 2002;415(6870):436–442.
101. Ellison DW, Dalton J, Kocak M, et al. Medulloblastoma: clinicopathological correlates of SHH, WNT, and non-SHH/WNT molecular subgroups. *Acta Neuropathol* 2011;121(3):381–396.
102. Northcott PA, Korshunov A, Witt H, et al. Medulloblastoma comprises four distinct molecular variants. *J Clin Oncol* 2010;29(11):1408–1414.
103. Taylor MD, Northcott PA, Korshunov A, et al. Molecular subgroups of medulloblastoma: the current consensus. *Acta Neuropathol* 2011;123(4):465–472.
104. Tamber MS, Bansal K, Liang ML, et al. Current concepts in the molecular genetics of pediatric brain tumors: implications for emerging therapies. *Childs Nerv Syst* 2006;22(11):1379–1394.
105. Grotzer MA, Janss AJ, Phillips PC, et al. Neurotrophin receptor TrkC predicts good clinical outcome in medulloblastoma and other primitive neuroectodermal brain tumors. *Klin Padiatr* 2000;212(4):196–199.
106. Dhall G, Grodman H, Ji L, et al. Outcome of children less than three years old at diagnosis with non-metastatic medulloblastoma treated with chemotherapy on the "Head Start" I and II protocols. *Pediatr Blood Cancer* 2008;50(6):1169–1175.
107. Inda MM, Perot C, Guillaud-Bataille M, et al. Genetic heterogeneity in supratentorial and infratentorial primitive neuroectodermal tumours of the central nervous system. *Histopathology* 2005;47(6):631–637.
108. Li MH, Bouffet E, Hawkins CE, et al. Molecular genetics of supratentorial primitive neuroectodermal tumors and pineoblastoma. *Neurosurg Focus* 2005;19(5):E3.
109. Behdad A, Perry A. Central nervous system primitive neuroectodermal tumors: a clinicopathologic and genetic study of 33 cases. *Brain Pathol* 2010;20(2):441–450.
110. Dunham C, Sugo E, Tobias V, et al. Embryonal tumor with abundant neuropil and true rosettes (ETANTR): report of a case with prominent neurocytic differentiation. *J Neurooncol* 2007;84(1):91–98.
111. Korshunov A, Remke M, Gessi M, et al. Focal genomic amplification at 19q13.42 comprises a powerful diagnostic marker for embryonal tumors with ependymoblastic rosettes. *Acta Neuropathol* 2010;120(2):253–260.
112. Nobusawa S, Yokoo H, Hirato J, et al. Analysis of chromosome 19q13.42 amplification in embryonal brain tumors with ependymoblastic multilayered rosettes. *Brain Pathol* 2012;22(5):689–697.

113. Korshunov A, Ryzhova M, Jones DT, et al. LIN28A immunoreactivity is a potent diagnostic marker of embryonal tumor with multilayered rosettes (ETMR). *Acta Neuropathol* 2012;124(6):875–881.
114. Picard D, Miller S, Hawkins CE, et al. Markers of survival and metastatic potential in childhood CNS primitive neuro-ectodermal brain tumours: an integrative genomic analysis. *Lancet Oncol* 2012;13(8):838–848.
115. Haberler C, Laggner U, Slavc I, et al. Immunohistochemical analysis of INI1 protein in malignant pediatric CNS tumors: lack of INI1 in atypical teratoid/rhabdoid tumors and in a fraction of primitive neuroectodermal tumors without rhabdoid phenotype. *Am J Surg Pathol* 2006;30(11):1462–1468.
116. Fleming AJ, Hukin J, Rassekh R, et al. Atypical teratoid rhabdoid tumors (ATRTs): the British Columbia's Children's Hospital's experience, 1986–2006. *Brain Pathol* 2012;22(5):625–635.
117. Jackson EM, Sievert AJ, Gai X, et al. Genomic analysis using high-density single nucleotide polymorphism-based oligonucleotide arrays and multiplex ligation-dependent probe amplification provides a comprehensive analysis of INI1/SMARCB1 in malignant rhabdoid tumors. *Clin Cancer Res* 2009;15(6):1923–1930.
118. Judkins AR, Mauger J, Ht A, et al. Immunohistochemical analysis of hSNF5/INI1 in pediatric CNS neoplasms. *Am J Surg Pathol* 2004;28(5):644–650.
119. Hasselblatt M, Gesk S, Oyen F, et al. Nonsense mutation and inactivation of SMARCA4 (BRG1) in an atypical teratoid/rhabdoid tumor showing retained SMARCB1 (INI1) expression. *Am J Surg Pathol* 2011;35(6):933–935.
120. Hasselblatt M, Oyen F, Gesk S, et al. Cribriform neuroepithelial tumor (CRINET): a nonrhabdoid ventricular tumor with INI1 loss and relatively favorable prognosis. *J Neuropathol Exp Neurol* 2009;68(12):1249–1255.
121. Buslei R, Nolde M, Hofmann B, et al. Common mutations of beta-catenin in adamantinomatous craniopharyngiomas but not in other tumours originating from the sellar region. *Acta Neuropathol* 2005;109(6):589–597.
122. Kamakura Y, Hasegawa M, Minamoto T, et al. C-kit gene mutation: common and widely distributed in intracranial germinomas. *J Neurosurg* 2006;104(3 Suppl):173–180.
123. Jouvet A, Saint-Pierre G, Fauchon F, et al. Pineal parenchymal tumors: a correlation of histological features with prognosis in 66 cases. *Brain Pathol* 2000;10(1):49–60.
124. Miller S, Rogers HA, Lyon P, et al. Genome-wide molecular characterization of central nervous system primitive neuroectodermal tumor and pineoblastoma. *Neuro Oncol* 2011;13(8):866–879.
125. Blumcke I, Wiestler OD. Gangliogliomas: an intriguing tumor entity associated with focal epilepsies. *J Neuropathol Exp Neurol* 2002;61(7):575–584.
126. Chappe C, Padovani L, Scavarda D, et al. Dysembryoplastic neuroepithelial tumors share with pleomorphic xanthoastrocytomas and gangliogliomas BRAF(V600E) mutation and expression. *Brain Pathol* 2013;23(5):574–583.
127. Daumas-Duport C, Scheithauer BW, Chodkiewicz JP, et al. Dysembryoplastic neuroepithelial tumor: a surgically curable tumor of young patients with intractable partial seizures. Report of thirty-nine cases. *Neurosurgery* 1988;23(5):545–556.
128. Ray WZ, Blackburn SL, Casavilca-Zambrano S, et al. Clinicopathologic features of recurrent dysembryoplastic neuroepithelial tumor and rare malignant transformation: a report of 5 cases and review of the literature. *J Neurooncol* 2009;94(2):283–292.
129. Daumas-Duport C, Varlet P, Bacha S, et al. Dysembryoplastic neuroepithelial tumors: nonspecific histological forms—a study of 40 cases. *J Neurooncol* 1999;41(3):267–280.
130. Fujisawa H, Marukawa K, Hasegawa M, et al. Genetic differences between neurocytoma and dysembryoplastic neuroepithelial tumor and oligodendroglial tumors. *J Neurosurg* 2002;97(6):1350–1355.
131. Perry A, Fuller CE, Banerjee R, et al. Ancillary FISH analysis for 1p and 19q status: preliminary observations in 287 gliomas and oligodendroglioma mimics. *Front Biosci* 2003;8:a1–a9.
132. Al-Kharazi K, Gillis C, Steinbok P, et al. Malignant desmoplastic infantile astrocytoma? A case report and review of the literature. *Clin Neuropathol* 2013;32(2):100–106.
133. Zhou XP, Marsh DJ, Morrison CD, et al. Germline inactivation of PTEN and dysregulation of the phosphoinositol-3-kinase/Akt pathway cause human Lhermitte-Duclos disease in adults. *Am J Hum Genet* 2003;73(5):1191–1198.
134. Abel TW, Baker SJ, Fraser MM, et al. Lhermitte-Duclos disease: a report of 31 cases with immunohistochemical analysis of the PTEN/AKT/mTOR pathway. *J Neuropathol Exp Neurol* 2005;64(4):341–349.
135. Jeibmann A, Hasselblatt M, Gerss J, et al. Prognostic implications of atypical histologic features in choroid plexus papilloma. *J Neuropathol Exp Neurol* 2006;65(11):1069–1073.
136. Kamaly-Asl ID, Shams N, Taylor MD. Genetics of choroid plexus tumors. *Neurosurg Focus* 2006;20(1):E10.
137. Perry A, Dehner LP. Meningeal tumors of childhood and infancy. An update and literature review. *Brain Pathol* 2003;13(3):386–408.
138. Kusters-Vandevelde HV, van Engen-van Grunsven IA, Kusters B, et al. Improved discrimination of melanotic schwannoma from melanocytic lesions by combined morphological and GNAQ mutational analysis. *Acta Neuropathol* 2010; 120(6): 755–764.
139. Chavez-Bueno S, McCracken GH Jr. Bacterial meningitis in children. *Pediatr Clin North Am* 2005;52(3):795–810, vii.
140. Saez-Llorens X. Brain abscess in children. *Semin Pediatr Infect Dis* 2003;14(2):108–114.
141. Kimberlin DW. Herpes simplex virus infections of the central nervous system. *Semin Pediatr Infect Dis* 2003;14(2):83–89.
142. Schutz PW, Fauth CT, Al-Rawahi GN, et al. Granulomatous herpes simplex encephalitis in an infant with multicystic encephalopathy: a distinct clinicopathologic entity? *Pediatr Neurol* 2014;50(4):392–396.
143. Romero JR, Newland JG. Viral meningitis and encephalitis: traditional and emerging viral agents. *Semin Pediatr Infect Dis* 2003;14(2):72–82.
144. Gray F, Chretien F, Vallat-Decouvelaere AV, et al. The changing pattern of HIV neuropathology in the HAART era. *J Neuropathol Exp Neurol* 2003;62(5):429–440.
145. Bell JE, Lowrie S, Koffi K, et al. The neuropathology of HIV-infected African children in Abidjan, Cote d'Ivoire. *J Neuropathol Exp Neurol* 1997;56(6):686–692.
146. Sharer LR. Pathology of HIV-1 infection of the central nervous system. A review. *J Neuropathol Exp Neurol* 1992;51(1):3–11.
147. Squier M, Chamberlain P, Zaiwalla Z, et al. Five cases of brain injury following amniocentesis in mid-term pregnancy. *Dev Med Child Neurol* 2000;42(8):554–560.
148. Rossiter JP, Anderson LL, Yang F, et al. Caspase-3 activation and caspase-like proteolytic activity in human perinatal hypoxic-ischemic brain injury. *Acta Neuropathol* 2002;103(1):66–73.
149. Friede RL. *Developmental Neuropathology*, 2nd rev. and expanded edn. Berlin; New York, NY: Springer-Verlag; 1989:xvi, 577.
150. Thorngren-Jerneck K, Ohlsson T, Sandell A, et al. Cerebral glucose metabolism measured by positron emission tomography in term newborn infants with hypoxic ischemic encephalopathy. *Pediatr Res* 2001;49(4):495–501.
151. Sarnat HB. Watershed infarcts in the fetal and neonatal brainstem. An aetiology of central hypoventilation, dysphagia, Moibius syndrome and micrognathia. *Eur J Paediatr Neurol* 2004;8(2):71–87.
152. Volpe JJ. Cerebral white matter injury of the premature infant-more common than you think. *Pediatrics* 2003;112(1 Pt 1):176–180.
153. Gleissner M, Jorch G, Avenarius S. Risk factors for intraventricular hemorrhage in a birth cohort of 3721 premature infants. *J Perinat Med* 2000;28(2):104–110.
154. Perry A, Kurtkaya-Yapicier O, Scheithauer BW, et al. Insights into meningioangiomatosis with and without meningioma: a clinicopathologic and genetic series of 24 cases with review of the literature. *Brain Pathol* 2005;15(1):55–65.

CHAPTER 11
The Eye

J. Douglas Cameron, M.D., MBA, and Raymond G. Areaux, Jr., M.D.

INTRODUCTION

The observations and opinions of surgical pathologists are critical in managing many pediatric ocular conditions including potentially fatal entities such as retinoblastoma and suspected nonaccidental trauma.

Because pediatric ophthalmic surgical specimens tend to be infrequent, this chapter includes a discussion of pertinent ocular anatomy and pivotal events in embryologic development of the eye; the intention is to provide a context for pathologic features. In addition, the type of surgical procedure used to obtain the tissue specimen is described to assist in understanding the origin of the specimen and orientation of gross specimens.

This chapter is organized by the types of tissue most frequently received in the laboratory: eyelid tissue, conjunctiva, cornea, vitreous, orbital soft tissues, whole globes removed surgically, and globes removed at autopsy. Crystalline lens tissue removed because of congenital cataracts and extraocular muscle tissues removed during some types of strabismus procedures are infrequently processed because histologic observations of this type of specimen are not relevant to management of the ocular abnormality.

THE EYELID

Structure of the Eyelid

The eyelid is covered by stratified squamous epithelium associated with a thin keratin layer. The surface merges with the mucous membrane at the mucocutaneous junction located on the eyelid margin (Figure 11-1). The epidermis is associated with pilosebaceous units, eccrine glands, and apocrine glands. The apocrine glands have no recognized function in the eyelid tissues. The cilia are the product of a modified pilosebaceous unit in that there are no associated piloerector muscles and there is a prominent sebaceous component (glands of Zeis). The tarsal plate is a dense collagenous structure that supports the delicate eyelid and houses a large volume of sebaceous glands (the meibomian glands). No cartilage is present in the eyelid. The holocrine secretion of the meibomian gland is applied to the tear film surface from pores located along the eyelid margin anterior to the mucocutaneous junction and posterior to the eyelid cilia (1,2).

Vascular Abnormalities of the Eyelid

Infantile hemangioma is a benign proliferation of blood vessels of the soft tissue of the face that may involve both eyelids and the orbit. The proliferation does not usually involve the contents of the globe. The cutaneous lesions are red and lobulated and may markedly distort the contours of the face (Figure 11-2). The lesions are rarely biopsied for risk of hemorrhage but occasionally may be surgically debulked. Initially, there is capillary lesion in a lobular pattern characterized by proliferation of endothelial cells around a small-caliber vascular channel. The lesion is not encapsulated, and lobules of the hemangioma extend into the surrounding soft tissue. With time, the endothelial profile flattens and the lumen becomes more prominent as interstitial tissue develops. The lesions appear clinically within the first month of life and may enlarge over several years before spontaneously involuting by approximately age 7 years. In the interim, obstruction of vision by mechanical eyelid ptosis or secondary astigmatism from mechanical distortion of the cornea may interfere with normal visual development resulting in *amblyopia* (developmental arrest of visual function, which may become permanent without treatment, "lazy eye") (3).

Surgical treatment of these lesions in children requires extreme precision. Steroids injected into the lesion may be seen as amorphous material in the vascular lumen or in the interstitial space (4). Central retinal artery occlusion has been reported with intralesional injections (5). Since 2008, beta-blockers have become the most common treatment for inducing regression of hemangiomas (6). Superficial lesions may be treated topically without surgical intervention (7).

Nevus flammeus is a congenital vascular lesion in the distribution of the first and second divisions of the trigeminal nerve. The vascular abnormality is present at birth and does not progress or regress. The cutaneous lesion may be treated with laser but is generally not biopsied (8). Nevus flammeus is clinically important because this vascular mal-

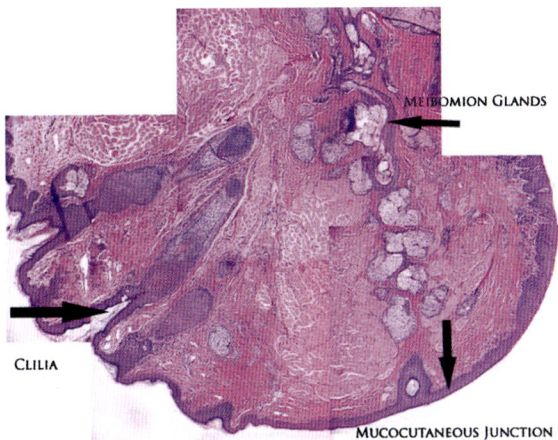

FIGURE 11-1 • Structure of the eyelid: the anterior surface of the eyelid is composed of stratified squamous epithelium with a thin keratin layer. The keratinized surface merges with mucous membrane lining the posterior surface of the eyelid at the mucocutaneous junction (*arrow*). Large pilosebaceous units represent the eyelashes that lack a piloerector muscle. Meibomian gland secretion covers the surface of the tear film at the mucocutaneous junction (hematoxylin–eosin stain, original magnification ×40).

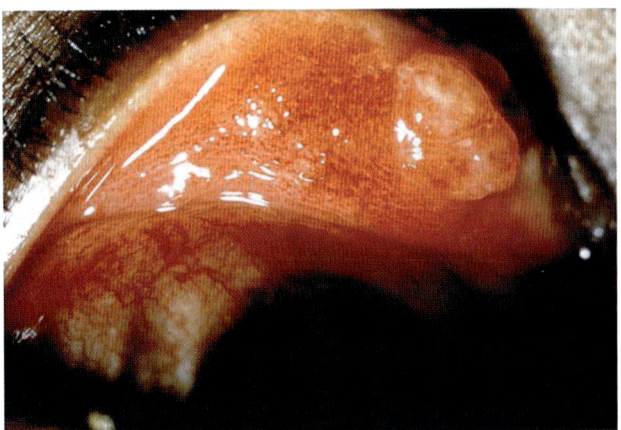

FIGURE 11-3 • Pyogenic granuloma is a clinical term used by ophthalmologists to refer to a transient fibrovascular response in a mucous membrane (the conjunctiva). With remodeling normally found in the repair process, the lesion will spontaneously diminish over time. The lesion is occasionally removed if it causes symptoms related to eyelid dysfunction.

formation is frequently associated with ipsilateral glaucoma and ipsilateral choroidal hemangioma. Glaucoma results from ipsilateral elevation of episcleral venous pressure. The choroidal component is difficult to treat and may progress to serious retinal detachment, a potential cause of loss of vision (9).

Inflammatory Abnormalities of the Eyelid

Pyogenic granuloma refers to a polypoid lobular capillary hemangioma of the skin in the discipline of dermatopathology. This term is used by clinical ophthalmologists to describe a granulation tissue reaction usually located in the tarsal conjunctiva, which is a response to mechanical trauma or to the presence of a chalazion (Figure 11-3). Pyogenic granuloma is an impaired wound healing process (10). A reddish lobulated mass develops on the conjunctival surface that may be large enough to protrude through the interpalpebral fissure. The overlying mucous membrane may show effects of drying and reactive squamous proliferation. In the subepithelial tissue, there are acute and chronic inflammatory reactions associated with multiple delicate vascular channels and an edematous stroma (granulation tissue). Conjunctival pyogenic granuloma will usually spontaneously involute over days to weeks. Topical steroids may be prescribed in the acute inflammatory phase to encourage involution. The area may be excised later if the mass interferes with surface lubrication of the eye or results in malpositioning of the eyelid margin or unacceptable appearance.

Chalazion is a granulomatous reaction to sebaceous products of the meibomian gland of the eyelid. This condition is often misinterpreted as a "sty," which is an abscess of a pilosebaceous unit. The meibomian gland duct becomes occluded, and sebaceous gland content ruptures into the surrounding soft tissue. The affected area is initially tender but evolves into a firm nontender nodule. The tissue is usually friable amorphous gray tissue composed of a lipogranulomatous reaction with foreign body and occasional Langhans-type giant cells (Figure 11-4). The surrounding normal tissue is usually not represented in the specimen; however, infiltration among the fibers of the orbicularis muscle may be observed occasionally.

Generally, the nodule resolves over weeks or months and responds to warm compresses and scrubbing of the eyelid margin. In some individuals, there may be multiple episodes in different locations in the eyelid. In adults, multiple chalazia occurring in the same location is a risk factor for sebaceous carcinoma. In children, chalazia may mechanically induce refractive error or ptosis or contribute to progressive ptosis. Thus, incision and curettage may be performed if there is risk of amblyopia (11).

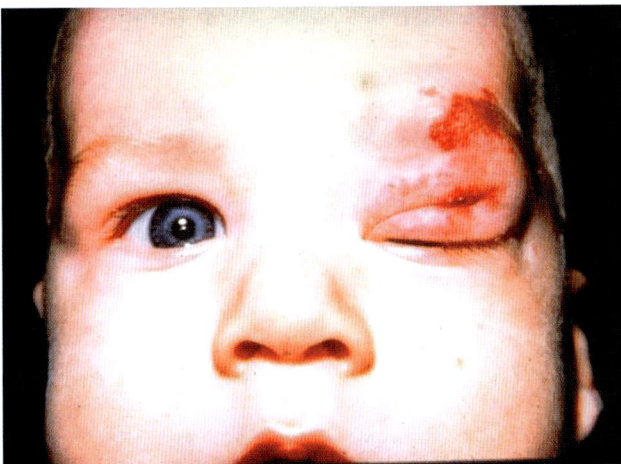

FIGURE 11-2 • Infantile hemangiomas in the periorbital soft tissue of the face cause dysfunction of the eyelid because of mechanical ptosis. If the eye is not stimulated by formed images, the retinal function will not develop (amblyopia).

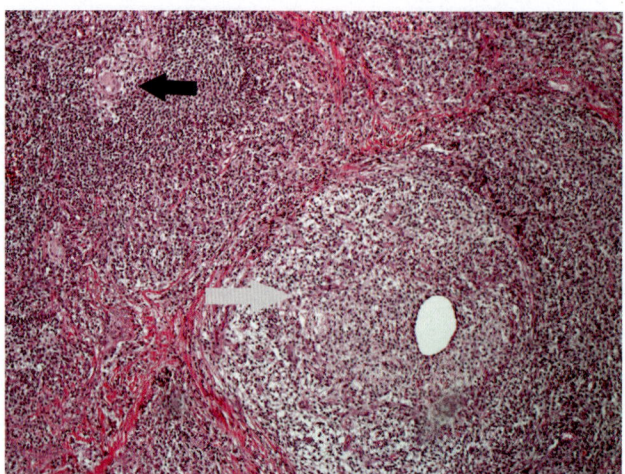

FIGURE 11-4 • Chalazion is a lipogranulomatous reaction to a lipid globule (*white arrow*) representing sebaceous secretion from a ruptured meibomian gland of the eyelid (*black arrow*). The rupture is thought to be the result of blockage of the outlet mechanism of the gland. The tissue submitted will often be limited to the contents of the chalazion (hematoxylin–eosin stain, original magnification ×100).

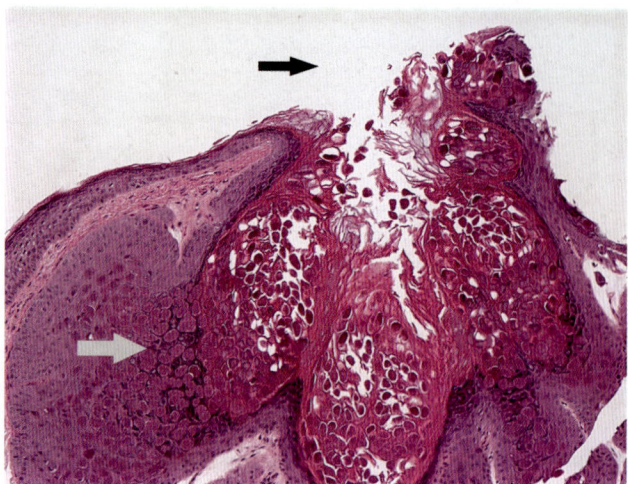

FIGURE 11-5 • Molluscum contagiosum consists of virus-infected cells (*white arrow*) of the eyelid margin that may cause regional conjunctivitis because of exfoliation of infected cells and debris (*black arrow*) (hematoxylin-eosin stain, original magnification ×20).

Juvenile xanthogranuloma (nevoxanthoendothelioma) is a non–Langerhans cell histiocytosis (LCH) but shares a common CD34 precursor cell with LCH and may occur in adults as well (12). Well-defined purple to red nodules appear on the skin and anterior surface of the eye (13). The reaction may also appear in the orbit and in the uveal tract. Lesions in the iris may cause spontaneous hyphema, which may be bilateral. The cutaneous lesions are characterized by mononuclear lipidized or nonlipidized cells and Touton giant cells. The lesions tend to involute spontaneously and may respond to topical or periocular steroids. Occasionally, intraocular lesions cause intractable glaucoma requiring enucleation. The mononuclear cells are usually limited to the uveal tract but may involve adjacent structures as well (see chapter 25).

Molluscum contagiosum is a poxvirus infection of the epithelium of the skin in children aged 1 to 4 years with risk factors of swimming and eczema (14). Multiple, well-demarcated, elevated, umbilicated, nontender nodules develop on the skin. Shedding of viral particles from infected epithelial cells near the lid margin may produce a localized, persistent, follicular conjunctivitis, which brings the patient to clinical attention. This infection is often associated with immune deficiency. The lesion consists of acanthotic stratified squamous epithelial cells with prominent intracytoplasmic inclusions (Figure 11-5). The contents of infected cells desquamate into the environment from the umbilicated region. Conjunctival follicular reaction from molluscum contagiosum is difficult to treat medically. Lid margin lesions often require surgical excision.

A *sty* or *hordeolum* is an abscess of one of the adnexal units of the eyelid skin. This condition is very infrequent and is generally not biopsied. An external hordeolum is superficial, and an internal hordeolum is located deeper in the eyelid skin. In most cases, a lesion described clinically as a sty may actually be a chalazion (see above).

The orbital septum is a fibrous diaphragm extending from the periosteum of the orbital rim to the eyelid margin. Its major function is to compartmentalize and protect orbital fat from external influences. *Preseptal cellulitis* is a bacterial infection of the subcutaneous tissue of the eyelid anterior to the orbital septum that may present with a dramatic increase in preseptal and facial soft tissue volume and even abscess. In contradistinction, infection posterior to the orbital septum (*orbital cellulitis*) causes minimal facial swelling but marked swelling of the intraorbital tissues forcing the globe to move anteriorly (proptosis or exophthalmos). The malposition of the globe as well as direct inflammation of extraocular muscles may limit ocular motility (*ophthalmoparesis*) resulting in double vision (*diplopia*). Orbital cellulitis most commonly results from secondary spread of sinusitis across the lamina papyracea of the medial orbital wall, bacterial seeding from trauma that violates the orbital septum or orbital walls, or more rarely from hematogenous spread (15). The orbital septum is a profound barrier to inflammation; it is extremely rare for a preseptal cellulitis to seed the postseptal space without a traumatic bridge in an immunocompetent host. The infected tissue is rarely biopsied, although fine needle aspirations may be used for culturing microorganisms. The most common organisms found are *Haemophilus influenzae* and *Streptococcus* species. Treatment is with intravenous systemic antibiotics and close inpatient monitoring. Functional compromise of the globe (e.g., worsening vision, an afferent pupillary defect, markedly elevated intraocular pressure) is evidence of a sight-threatening compartment syndrome that requires urgent surgical decompression.

Neoplastic Lesions of the Eyelid

Melanocytic nevus is a proliferation of abnormal melanocytes at the dermal–epidermal junction. Clinically, the lesions appear as hyperpigmented areas of the skin that vary in degree and extent of pigmentation (see Chapter 26). Children are infrequently affected; however, the distinction from melanoma by histologic criteria is difficult (16).

Spindle cell and epithelioid nevus (Spitz nevus) is a proliferation of melanocytes that has many histologic features of melanoma even though the clinical course is usually benign. The lesion may present as a rapidly enlarging, well-demarcated nodule of the eyelid skin (17). Histologic patterns include spindle and epithelioid cell as well as mixed types. The mitotic rate is usually low, and actively dividing cells are generally located near the superficial dermis. The size of the melanocytes usually diminishes toward the base of the lesion. Regional lymph node metastasis has been reported; however, even in those cases, the long-term course remains favorable. Cutaneous malignant melanoma of the skin may arise in childhood (18) (see Chapter 26).

Oculodermal melanocytosis is congenital hyperpigmentation of the skin associated with involvement of the ipsilateral episcleral tissue located deep to the conjunctiva. Hyperpigmentation is present at birth and generally remains stationary in intensity and extent throughout the life of the individual. The lesions may become more prominent during puberty (19). An increased concentration of typical melanocytes is located at the dermal–epidermal junction and in the episcleral tissue. There is minimal risk of malignant transformation of cutaneous and episcleral melanocytes. There is an increased risk for ipsilateral uveal melanoma, particularly for Caucasians. Malignant transformation may also occur in the nevus itself as well as orbit, optic nerve, and brain (20).

Xeroderma pigmentosum is an autosomal recessive defect in the DNA repair systems of the body. Exposure to ultraviolet light induces the formation of basal cell carcinoma, squamous cell carcinoma, and malignant melanoma in the facial skin of even young children (21). The number of lesions is characteristically large. Children may also develop squamous cell carcinoma of the conjunctiva as well as pterygia. Ocular surface scarring from these lesions may significantly affect visual function (22). There is no treatment to replace the deficient DNAse that normally repairs ultraviolet-damaged DNA. Treatment of individual lesions is accomplished by standard surgical therapy. Prevention is attempted by limiting exposure of the facial skin to sunlight.

Basal cell nevus syndrome (Gorlin-Goltz) is an autosomal dominant condition associated with the development of basal cell carcinoma at multiple sites (22). Basal cell carcinoma of the eyelid has been observed in a 16-year-old. The eyelid lesions tend to be aggressive and may involve the orbit (23). In addition to cutaneous malignancies, there are associated skeletal abnormalities such as odontogenic cysts of the jaw and bifid ribs. Palmar and plantar pits as well as cognitive impairment and intracranial calcifications may be present. As with other ectodermal dysplasia syndromes, the ocular surface may be abnormal due to ocular surface abnormalities. Degenerative pannus (scarring between corneal epithelium and Bowman membrane) may be associated with loss of vision.

Neurofibromatosis type I (NF-1) is an autosomal dominant condition in which various types of abnormally produced cytokines lead to the development of neoplasia of various types. The syndrome is recognized by the presence of hyperpigmented cutaneous regions with a smooth contour (café au lait) spots and proliferation of elements of peripheral nerve (neurofibroma) within the eyelid skin. The neurofibromas are acquired and consist of nodular or plexiform patterns. The nodular form generally does not affect eyelid function. The plexiform variety may produce massive enlargement of the soft tissues of the face including the eyelid, causing major deformations of the eyelid margin (ptosis, ectropion, or entropion), which can result in amblyopia via visual axis occlusion, induction of astigmatism, or corneal scarring. Surgical debulking of lesions is occasionally performed to improve eyelid function, which is often only partially successful. The lesion consists of proliferation of all cellular elements of the peripheral nerve including axons, Schwann cells, and perineural cells. Occasionally, the native peripheral nerve trunk can be identified. The lesions of plexiform deformity are often progressive. In this tissue as well as elsewhere, there is a risk of developing malignant peripheral nerve sheath tumors (see chapter 25).

Optic pathway glioma may be found in 15% to 20% of individuals with NF-1 and may account for significant morbidity in young children. Symptoms include vision loss, proptosis, and precocious puberty (24). Proptosis and glaucoma have been reported on the ipsilateral side of orbitofacial NF-1 (25). The association of NF-1 and uveal melanoma appears to be coincidental (26) (see Chapter 10).

Surgical Procedures of the Eyelid

An eyelid biopsy may be a simple removal of an ellipse of skin because of the suspicion of cutaneous neoplasm. These specimens are handled as are cutaneous biopsies elsewhere. When a lesion involves the eyelid margin, particularly near the punctum, the surgery becomes more complicated because scarring in the region of a punctum may cause lacrimal drainage abnormalities (chronic tearing, epiphora) and because scarring of the eyelid margin may damage the cornea. Some type of superficial lamellar dissection in the region of the punctum may be done to spare punctal function. For lid margin lesions, a full-thickness wedge of eyelid is removed because restoration of lid margin function is facilitated. A lid-splitting procedure removes the tissue either anterior or posterior to the anterior border of the tarsal plate. Full-thickness and partial-thickness lid margin specimens are generally oriented perpendicular to the lid margin (or row of cilia) with nasal and lateral surgical margins. During pediatric ptosis repair surgery, the levator palpebrae superioris and underlying Muller's muscles may be partially resected to elevate the eyelid. Submitted specimens from patients with congenital ptosis are remarkable for fibrofatty infiltration of the levator muscle tissue.

THE EYE

Structure of the Eye

The eye (globus oculi) is an extension of the brain that collects and transmits images gathered from the environment.

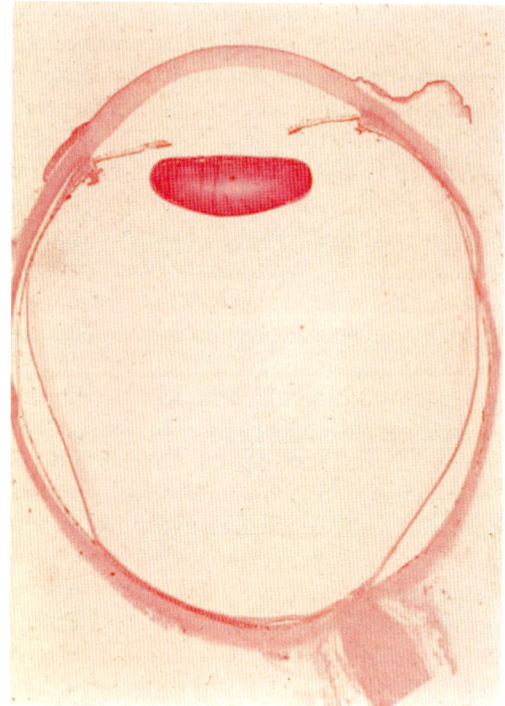

FIGURE 11-6 • The normal eye. The anterior segment is composed of the cornea, anterior chamber and the posterior chamber, and crystalline lens. The posterior segment is composed of the vitreous, retina, choroid, and optic nerve.

These structures convert energy from a restricted portion of the electromagnetic spectrum via a photochemical process into impulses that can be integrated with the electrochemical processes of the brain (1,2).

THE CONJUNCTIVA

Structure of the Conjunctiva

The conjunctiva extends from the eyelid margin to the junction of the cornea and sclera (the limbus). The conjunctiva is a mucous membrane with many specialized regions. Along the internal lining of the eyelid (the tarsal conjunctiva), the surface is tightly adherent to the tarsal plate. There is redundant conjunctiva at the forniceal regions of the eyelid to allow full mobility of the globe. The conjunctiva over the globe (bulbar conjunctiva) is loosely applied. The associated accessory lacrimal tissue is regional and clinically inconspicuous. There is associated nonnodal lymphoid tissue in the subepithelial space, particularly in the region of the fornix. The conjunctival surface is composed of stratified, nonkeratinizing epithelium containing a variable number of intraepithelial goblet cells found most prominently in the bulbar conjunctiva (Figure 11-7). Dendritic melanocytes and antigen-processing cells (Langerhans cells) are present throughout the surface epithelium. The underlying tissue is nonspecific, delicate fibrovascular tissue (substantia propria). The substantia propria of the conjunctiva fuses with the fibrovascular tissue of the globe (episcleral tissue and Tenon capsule) at the limbus but is otherwise distinct and separate. Lymphatic channels are present throughout the substantia propria of the conjunctiva to the limbus where they form arcades. The limbus is one of the locations of stem cells and is a common site for the development of both squamous cell carcinoma and malignant melanoma. Lymphatic channels of the conjunctiva drain to the preauricular, parotid, and submental nodes (1,2).

Two elements are essential: a method of focusing light (the anterior segment) and method of detecting and transferring images from the external environment to the brain (posterior segment). The anterior segment is composed of the cornea, the anterior chamber, the iris, the posterior chamber, and the crystalline lens (Figure 11-6). These structures transmit and refract light by reorienting parallel rays of light to a focal point. The posterior segment is composed of the vitreous, the retina, the optic disc, the uveal tract, and the sclera.

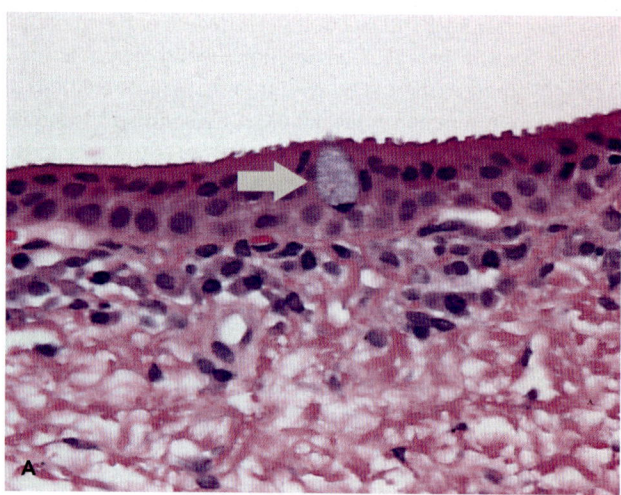
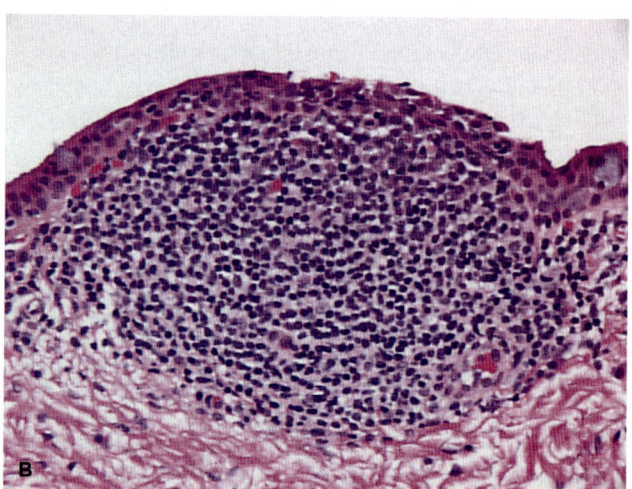

FIGURE 11-7 • **A:** The normal conjunctiva is composed of nonkeratinizing squamous epithelium containing goblet cells (*arrow*). Goblet cells are concentrated in the bulbar conjunctiva (hematoxylin–eosin stain, original magnification ×100). **B:** There is normally a nonnodal collection of lymphocytes within the stroma of the conjunctiva, particularly in the far periphery (conjunctival fornix) (hematoxylin–eosin stain, original magnification ×100).

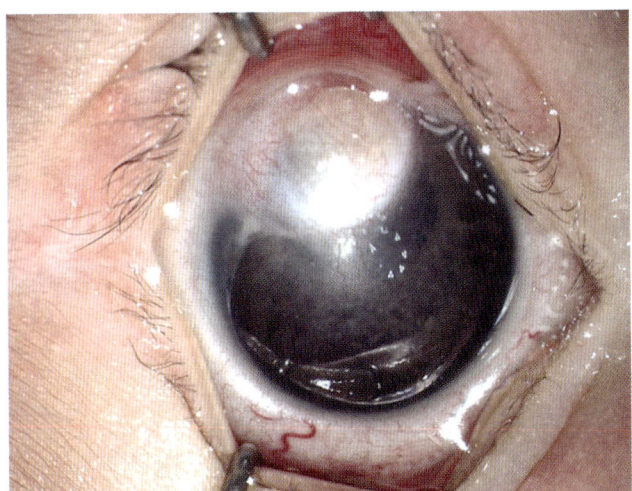

FIGURE 11-8 • Limbal dermoid. The dense opacity is located at the limbus (junction of cornea and sclera) and involves both structures as well as the iris and lens in this severe case. The radius of curvature of the clinically uninvolved cornea may be markedly distorted (irregular astigmatism) and may seriously limit visual function. The condition is not progressive but does not involute spontaneously.

Developmental Abnormalities of the Conjunctiva

Developmental abnormalities of the conjunctiva are infrequent. Occasionally, redundant, tortuous, dilated lymphatic vessels (lymphangiectasia) are present that may lead to symptoms because of dryness of elevated portions of the tissue or because of hemorrhage into the lymphatic spaces.

Episcleral osseous choristoma is due to embryonic rests of bone in the episcleral tissue, which may present as a stationary nodule often in the upper temporal quadrant of the conjunctiva or of the lower eyelid (27). The lesion generally consists of mature bone surrounded by mature fibrous tissue.

Limbal dermoid of the conjunctiva is a choristomatous nodule of dermal tissue, usually located at the limbus (Figure 11-8). The nodule may also be situated on the central corneal surface with only a minimal connection with the vascular system of the conjunctiva. The mass may obstruct the visual axis or alter the contour of the cornea and thereby cause amblyopia. The surface is nonkeratinizing squamous epithelium overlying dermal elements including mature fat. The lesion may involve the full thickness of the cornea and sclera but usually does not involve intraocular structures (Figure 11-9) (28). The lesion is usually solid without cystic elements as are found in cystic dermoid of the orbit (see below). Surgical removal may not result in normalization of corneal curvature.

Neuronal ceroid lipofuscinosis is a group of neurodegenerative diseases inherited in an autosomal recessive pattern that results in accumulation of lipopigments within cells and consequent disruption of cellular function (29). The conjunctiva is considered a convenient site for diagnostic biopsy. Intracellular "curvilinear bodies and fingerprint bodies" are found by examination with transmission electron microscopy (Figure 11-10) (see Chapters 5 and 10).

Inflammatory Conditions of the Conjunctiva

Microbial infections of the conjunctiva due to bacteria, viruses, and fungi occur commonly but are rarely biopsied. Trachoma remains a worldwide cause of significant blindness that results from infection with *Chlamydia trachomatis*. Early stages of the disease are characterized by an indolent follicular conjunctivitis. Late in the evolution of the disease, superficial scarring of the tarsal conjunctiva causes

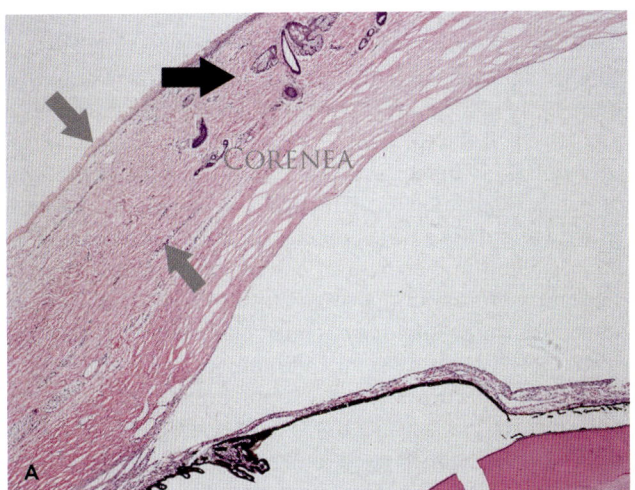
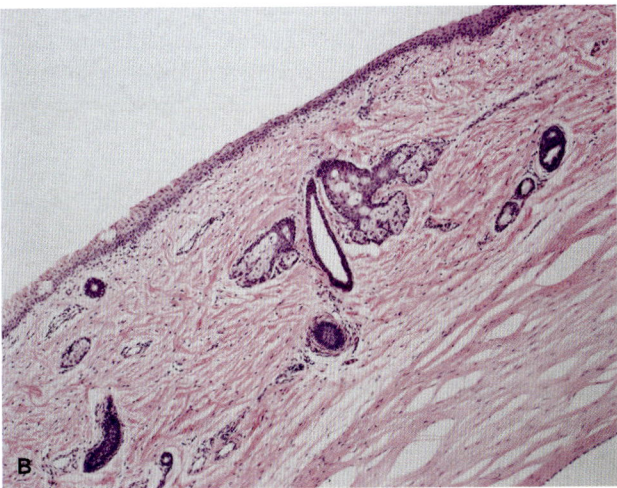

FIGURE 11-9 • Limbal dermoid, light micrograph. **A:** Solid dermoid is present at the limbus (junction of cornea and sclera) involving the eye of a child, which was enucleated for other reasons. The conjunctiva is markedly thickened (between two *gray arrows*) (hematoxylin–eosin stain, original magnification ×20). **B:** Mature pilosebaceous units as well as eccrine and apocrine glands are present. The lesion tends to remain stationary in size and location. If the opacity involves the central visual axis, retinal function may not develop in a normal manner (amblyopia) (hematoxylin–eosin stain, ×40 original magnification).

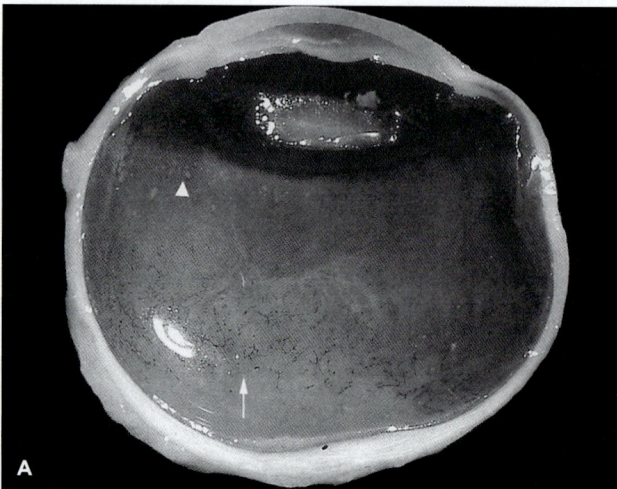 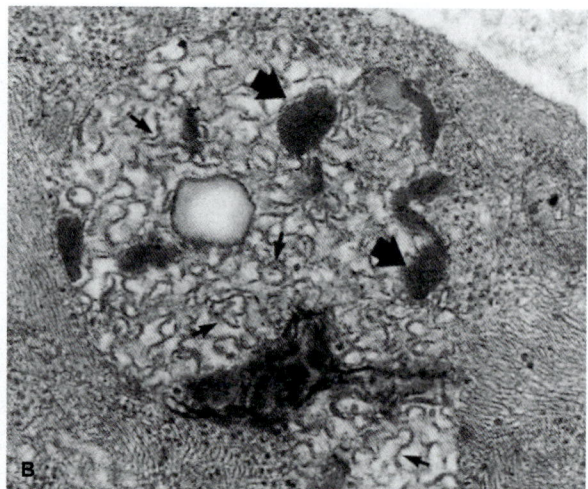

FIGURE 11-10 • **A:** Neuronal lipofuscinosis is a neurodegenerative disease resulting in pigment degeneration of the retina (*arrow* and *arrowhead*). **B:** The conjunctiva may be used as a biopsy site to confirm the diagnosis by transmission electron microscopy. Within affected cells, curvilinear and fingerprint bodies are recognized (*arrows*).

contraction (entropion), forcing eyelashes (cilia) to contact and damage the superficial cornea. Blindness results from secondary corneal scarring and not from the conjunctival infection. Treatment of these advanced cases is surgical.

Ligneous conjunctivitis is an accumulation of fibrin in the subepithelial space of mucous membranes throughout the body, caused by a systemic reduction in the levels of plasminogen (30). The condition usually presents in young females due to conjunctival symptoms (itching, burning, decreased vision) because of the presence of subconjunctival nodules composed of a woody-like accumulation of fibrin (31). The overlying epithelium is usually unremarkable, although signs of drying (epithelial thinning, reactive keratinization) may be present. Amorphous fibrin sometimes associated with an acute or chronic nongranulomatous inflammatory infiltrate may be present. Topical plasminogen concentrate has been used for treatment (32). Ligneous conjunctivitis may be associated with congenital occlusive hydrocephalus and juvenile colloid milium (31).

Melanocytic Abnormalities of the Conjunctiva

Melanosis of the conjunctiva is recognized clinically as hyperpigmentation of the conjunctiva without alteration of the surface contour of the conjunctiva. The lesion is present at birth or develops in early childhood as a yellow-brown to brownish black discoloration. There is a larger than average number of typical melanocytes and a higher than average accumulation of melanin in the conjunctival epithelium basal layers. This lesion is not a precursor for melanoma.

Melanosis of the episclera and scleral tissue is visible melanosis of the tissues deep to the conjunctiva, although the normal, transparent conjunctiva is visible as an area of slate gray discoloration. Heterochromia iridis and hyperpigmentation of the uveal tract may be present. Hyperpigmentation may extend to the meninges of the optic nerve and the brain. The contour of the overlying conjunctiva is not altered. The lesion may also present at birth and is generally stationary. A larger than average number of melanocytes is present as individual cells or small clusters interspersed in connective tissue. There is an increase in the number of melanocytes in the uveal tract; these melanocytes are larger than the indigenous melanocytes. The melanocytes are relatively hyperpigmented (Figure 11-11). This lesion is a risk factor for melanoma, which arises in the ipsilateral uveal tract or deep orbital tissues but not in the conjunctiva.

Nevus of Ota is a risk factor for ipsilateral uveal and orbital melanoma, particularly in Caucasians. In addition to hyperpigmentation of the eye (melanosis oculi) and orbit, there is hyperpigmentation of the eyelid and periorbital facial skin. Meningeal melanocytoma has also been associated with the nevus of Ota (33).

Melanocytic nevus of the conjunctiva is an accumulation of abnormal nevus cells in the region of the conjunctival epithelium. Early in life, in the junctional nevus stage, the nevus is a relatively well-demarcated area of the conjunctiva, which may not alter the surface contour and may be amelanotic or lightly pigmented. Conjunctival nevi are often associated with an anomalous development of the conjunctival epithelium, where the conjunctival epithelium is drawn into the substantia propria of the conjunctiva to form solid nests of squamous epithelium or cysts lined by squamous epithelium (Figure 11-12). The cysts may alter the surface contour of the conjunctiva, particularly if the cystic lining contains goblet cells or accessory lacrimal tissue that secretes into the lumen of the cysts. The melanocytes may be extensively pleomorphic, ranging from spindle-shaped cells to epithelioid cells. These atypical melanocytes may occur in the epithelium of the inclusion cysts giving the false impression of lymphatic spread of a melanoma. Clusters of melanocytic nevus cells may indent the lining of lymphatic channels also giving the appearance of lymphatic invasion.

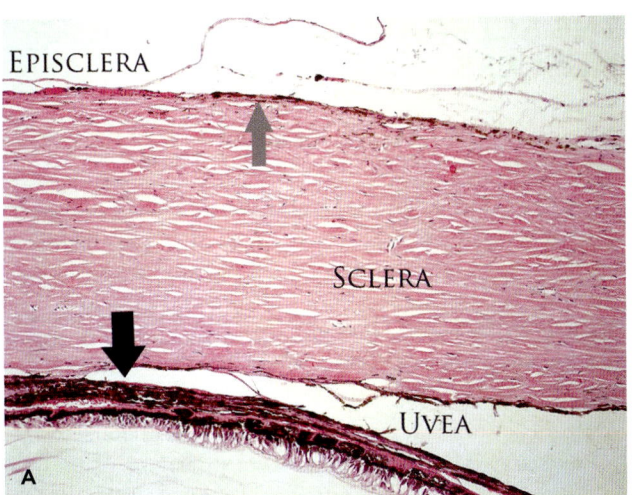
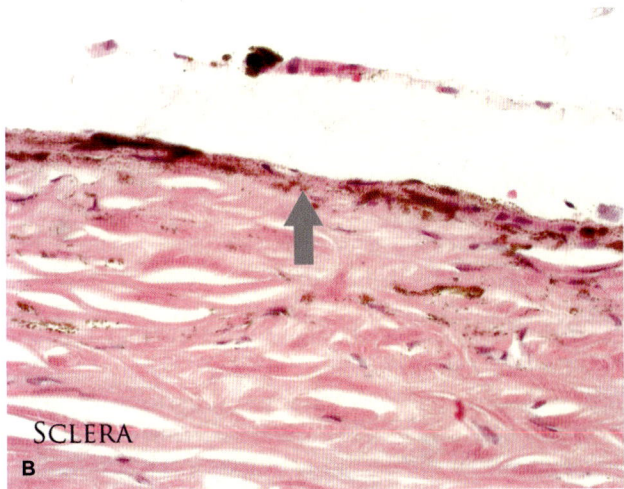

FIGURE 11-11 • **A:** Melanosis oculi may be associated with hyperpigmentation of the uveal tract (*black arrow*) as well the episcleral surface (*gray arrow*). The uveal pigmentation is a clinical risk factor for the development of uveal melanoma (hematoxylin–eosin A ×40 original magnification). **B:** The hyperpigmentation of the episcleral fibrous tissue is clearly visible clinically but subtle histopathologically (*gray arrow*) (hematoxylin–eosin stain, original magnification ×200).

Later in the natural history of a conjunctival melanocytic nevus, a dermal component develops (compound nevus). At puberty, there may be proliferation of melanocytes and increased density of pigmentation creating concern about the presence of a conjunctival melanoma. The nevus may appear to enlarge because of simultaneous proliferation of the squamous epithelial component of the inclusion cysts and increasing volume of the contents of the cyst (34). Irritation from drying of the elevated surface of the conjunctiva may also add to the impression of growth due to reactive inflammation and vascularization (35).

Melanoma of the conjunctiva may arise from a preexisting nevus or *de novo* even though primary acquired melanosis (PAM) with atypia does not generally occur in the pediatric age group but may be on the increase (18). A review of the international literature by Taban found 28 reported cases of conjunctival melanoma in individuals under the age of 15 years (36,37).

A conjunctival melanoma is an atypical proliferation of conjunctival melanocytes that has the potential of widespread metastasis and death. In the presence of a preexisting nevus or in the absence of histologic signs of a pre-existing

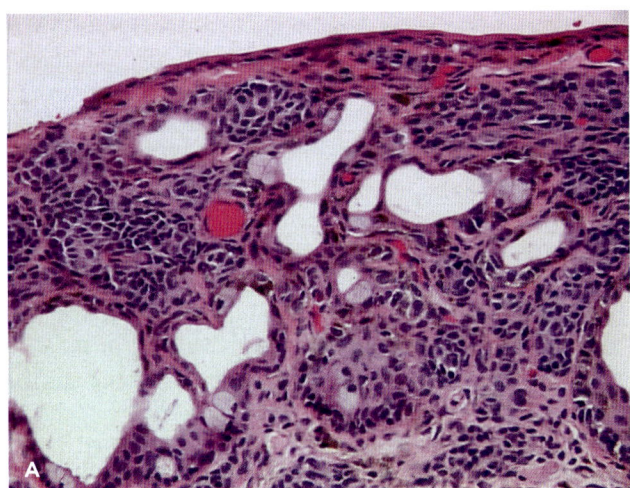
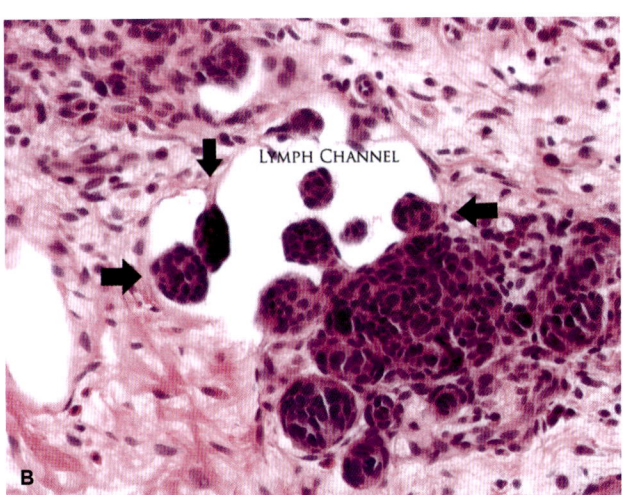

FIGURE 11-12 • **A:** Conjunctival nevus. The surface stratified squamous cells are somewhat flattened. Multiple cysts lined by squamous epithelial cells are located among nests of nevus cells in the subepithelial tissue. Material accumulating in the cystic spaces may simulate growth by clinical appearance (hematoxylin–eosin stain, original magnification ×100). **B:** Aggregates of melanocytic nevus cells may indent the lining of lymphocytic channels in the conjunctival stroma suggesting lymphatic. The appearance of the cells is bland and the aggregates are covered by lymphatic endothelial cells (hematoxylin–eosin, original magnification ×400).

nevus, there is invasion of the substantia propria of the conjunctiva by malignant melanocytes. Features of malignancy include the presence of mitotic figures, atypical melanocytes in clusters, lack of the expected maturation with depth, and infiltrative growth at the deep margin. Cytologic features such as a spindle-shaped appearance of the cells is of no prognostic significance.

Squamous carcinoma of the conjunctiva rarely involves the pediatric age group, though it may be seen in xeroderma pigmentosum (38). The lesion may present as a papilloma, a gelatinous lesion, or as a leukoplakic mass of the conjunctiva. The initial histopathologic findings are atypia progressing to carcinoma *in situ*. The lesions are invasive if the underlying basement membrane is breached. Squamous cell carcinoma of the conjunctiva is usually indolent but may spread to regional nodes. Spindle cell and mucoepidermoid variants tend to be more aggressive and may invade the eye itself.

Surgical Procedures of the Conjunctiva

The repair process of the conjunctiva results in scarring that may restrict movement of the globe and may result in a cosmetically unacceptable appearance. Therefore, biopsies of the conjunctiva are generally limited in extent even in the presence of a suspected malignancy. Most biopsy sites of the conjunctiva are described in reference to the limbus (e.g., the specimen is from the 3 o'clock position of the right eye and extended nasally). Biopsies for the diagnosis of systemic disease (e.g., sarcoidosis) are often performed in the inferior fornix where there is a normal high density of resting lymphocytes. Surgical access to the eye (limbal incision, orbital biopsy) and for strabismus procedures is through the conjunctiva. Inclusion cysts may arise at a suture line if the wound margins are not precisely apposed. Inclusion cysts may be removed by a second procedure to improve cosmetic appearance. Conjunctival tissue is essentially a nonrenewable resource, making the surgeon hesitant to remove any more tissue than is absolutely necessary. When there is not enough conjunctiva to close a defect, amniotic membrane transplant tissue is often used to improve healing.

Histopathologic interpretation of a conjunctival biopsy is often difficult because this tissue, which may harbor potentially serious disease (melanoma, lymphoma, rhabdomyosarcoma), is delicate and can be easily crushed with the forceps; furthermore, the samples are usually small. Adding to the processing problem is the tendency of the conjunctival tissue to curl or deform, if immersion fixed in formalin. The optimal method of submission is to fix the conjunctiva after the tissue has been flattened on support media such as filter paper. Many tumors of significance arise at the limbus (the junction of cornea and sclera). Therefore, the tissue sections are usually oriented perpendicular to the limbus. Close communication with the surgeon is necessary to establish tissue margins of significance.

THE SCLERA AND EXTRAOCULAR MUSCLES

Structure of the Sclera and Extraocular Muscles

The sclera is formed by randomly oriented collagenous fibers that are more hydrated than the cornea and are therefore opaque. The sclera contains elastin fibers to accommodate changes in intravascular blood volume during systole and diastole. There are seven extraocular muscles that course through each orbit with various actions. The horizontal and cyclovertical muscles are responsible for ocular motility while the levator is responsible for eyelid excursion.

The sclera is relatively thin at the insertions of the four rectus muscles and the insertion of the superior oblique. The insertion of the inferior oblique is muscular rather than tendinous; therefore, there is no compensatory thinning. The sclera is breached by multiple ostia for the short and long posterior ciliary arteries posteriorly, the vortex veins near the equator, sensory nerves anteriorly, and multiple emissary channels carrying aqueous to the venous system near the limbus. Blood vessels supplying the anterior segment of the eye are located within the rectus muscle belly. There are two vessels in each rectus muscle, except the lateral rectus, which contains only one vessel. Disruption of more than four of these arteries during strabismus surgery can result in anterior segment ischemia.

THE CORNEA

Structure of the Cornea

The cornea is the dominant element of the optical system of the eye, providing up to 80% of its refracting power. The power of the cornea is determined by its curvature, a feature that is highly conserved throughout life. The cornea is composed primarily of extracellular matrix (the corneal stroma). The principal component of the corneal stroma is uniform type I collagen bundles separated at a precise distance by highly specialized and uniform proteoglycans. The interfiber distance is determined by the degree of hydration of the proteoglycans (Figure 11-13). The anterior surface of the cornea is composed of extraordinarily homogeneous nonkeratinizing squamous epithelium. The corneal epithelium does not contain goblet cells or antigen-processing cells. The normal basement membrane of the corneal epithelium is not visible by light microscopy. It rests on an acellular band of dense type I collagen (Bowman membrane) that is found only in primates and birds. Bowman membrane probably functions in maintaining corneal curvature, does not thicken with age, and is not restored if damaged by pathologic processes (Figure 11-14). The corneal endothelium is derived from neural crest and not mesoderm and, therefore, is not stained by vascular endothelial markers (e.g., factor VIII); rather, it is S100 positive. The corneal endothelium produces a thick basement

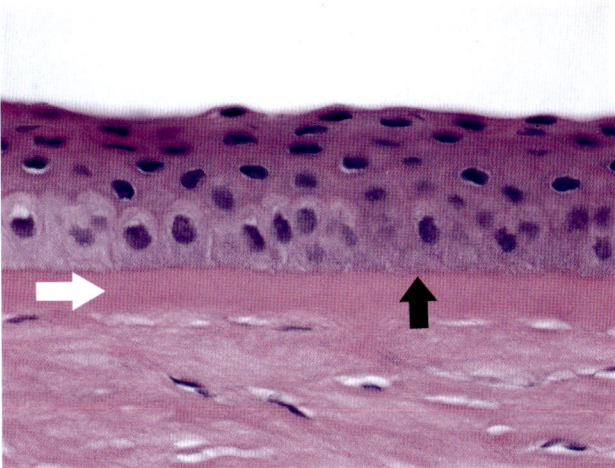

FIGURE 11-14 • Normal corneal anterior surface. The corneal surface is nonkeratinized and is composed of uniform cells. The epithelial basement membrane is not visible by light microscopy when the epithelium is normal (*black arrow*). Bowman layer is acellular type I collagen that is not replaced if damaged (*white arrow*) (periodic acid/Schiff stain, original magnification ×200).

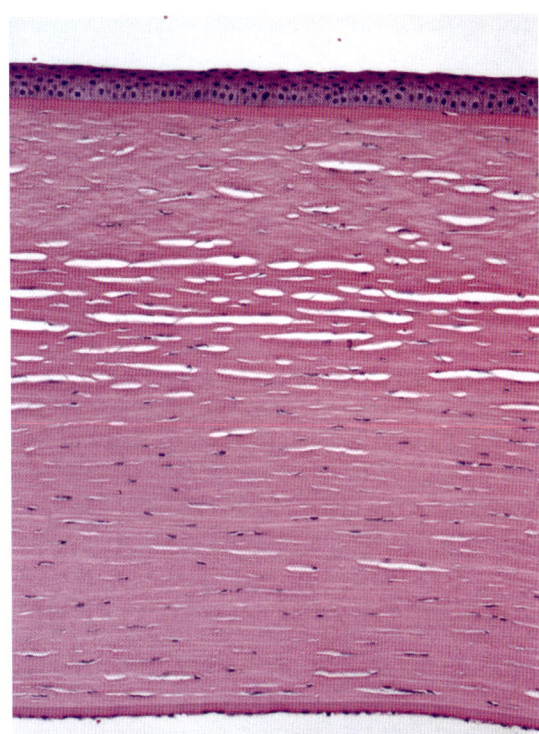

FIGURE 11-13 • Normal cornea. The surface epithelium is stratified, nonkeratinized squamous epithelium that does not contain goblet cells. The epithelial basement membrane is not visible by light microscopy when the epithelium is normal. The corneal stroma is composed of uniform collagenous fibers regularly separated by proteoglycans. The splitting artifact of the stroma between collagenous lamellae is a normal finding. Lack of the splitting artifact correlates with clinical corneal edema. Descemet membrane continues to thicken throughout life. There are no firm architectural attachments between Descemet membrane and corneal stroma and Descemet membrane and corneal endothelial cells. Corneal endothelial cells are similar to mesothelial cells of the pleura and maintain corneal hydration (periodic acid/Schiff stain, original magnifications ×20).

membrane (Descemet membrane) that is not physically attached to the corneal stroma and thickens continuously throughout life (1,2).

Developmental Abnormalities of the Cornea

There is a small range of tolerance of corneal diameter in which the normal optical properties of the cornea function. Similarly, the radius of curvature must be precise in order to focus light on the retina.

Microcornea is a condition in which the cornea is less than 9 mm in diameter (horizontal limbus to limbus) at 1 year of age. Other anatomic abnormalities such as microphthalmos with cyst or persistent hyperplastic primary vitreous (PHPV) often coexist. Even nonsyndromic-associated abnormalities of the trabecular meshwork are likely to cause glaucoma. The cornea tissue generally has a normal histologic appearance except in the case of Peters anomaly (see following).

Megalocornea is a condition in which the cornea is greater than 11.5 mm in diameter (horizontal limbus to limbus) at 1 year of age. Developmental abnormalities are generally stationary and tend to be bilateral. Megalocornea may be associated with dislocated crystalline lens (ectopia lentis) and other abnormalities of the anterior segment. The structure of the cornea in megalocornea is generally normal.

Peters anomaly most likely results from failure of separation of the cornea from the crystalline lens during embryonic development. In most cases the central posterior corneal stroma, Descemet membrane, and central corneal endothelium are absent. Rupture of Descemet membrane during forceps delivery or with corneal enlargement from glaucoma (buphthalmos with Haab striae) may appear similar histologically.

Herpes Simplex Keratitis

The herpes simplex virus initially affects the body as a systemic infectious disease with the cutaneous expression being a vesicular dermatitis. Live virus is retained in the gasserian ganglion and, for undetermined reasons, will periodically travel via sensory peripheral nerve to infect the corneal epithelium. Cytopathologic effects of the infected cells are seen as a linear, branching ulcer of the corneal epithelium (dendritic figure). With repeated episodes of infection, the corneal stroma becomes involved, not with direct viral infection but with lymphocytic infiltration, peripheral vascularization, and proteolysis of the extracellular matrix (discoid herpes keratitis, metaherpetic keratitis). The cornea can thin to the point of rupture. There may or may not be an intact epithelial covering. Bowman membrane ulcerates and Descemet membrane ruptures resulting in perforation of the cornea. A foreign body granulomatous response to the severed ends of either or both Bowman membrane and Descemet membrane is a unique response in herpes simplex keratitis. There may be an extensive lymphocytic infiltrate in the keratoplasty specimen that may not be appreciated clinically. The degree of vascularization of the cornea is a risk factor for immunologic corneal rejection (39) (see Chapter 6).

Acanthamoeba Keratitis

Acanthamoeba is a protozoa commonly found in soil and water. The organism can gain access to the cornea via microabrasions often associated with wearing contact lenses (40). The organism is neurotropic accounting for the extreme pain associated with infection. Organisms can be identified clinically by using confocal microscopy (41). The trophozoite form is motile and is able to spread extensively throughout the corneal stroma creating necrotizing keratitis and scarring. The encysted form can be identified throughout the cornea with most commonly used stains (Figure 11-15). There may be a limited inflammatory response because of treatment with anti-inflammatory drugs. *Acanthamoeba* is resistant to most forms of therapy (42). Occasionally, biopsy for diagnosis or penetrating keratoplasty for advanced stages of the infection is performed.

Dystrophic Conditions of the Cornea

Corneal dystrophies are metabolic abnormalities of the cornea that cause clinically detectable opacities. The prevalence of corneal dystrophy is extremely low. Most dystrophies are inherited in an autosomal dominant pattern (except macular corneal dystrophy, congenital hereditary endothelial dystrophy type 2 (CHED 2), lattice type 3, and gelatinous dystrophy, which are autosomal recessive), bilateral, symmetric, and progressive (at markedly variable rates) and recur in corneal grafted tissue. Even though the conditions are inherited, they generally do not progress sufficiently to be treated with

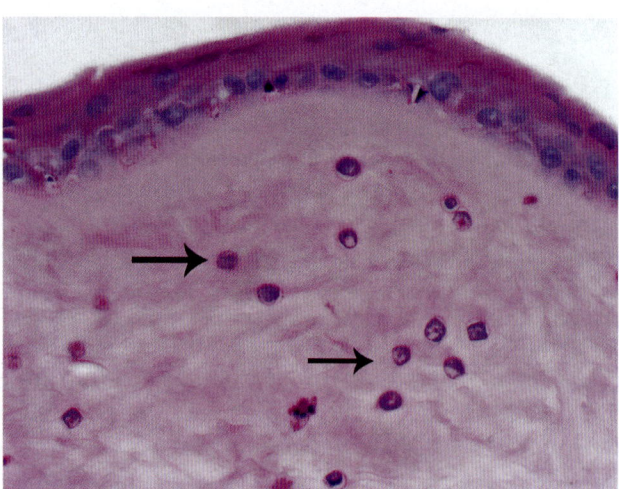

FIGURE 11-15 • *Acanthamoeba* keratitis. Multiple encysted *Acanthamoeba* organisms are present throughout the corneal stroma (periodic acid/Schiff stain, original magnification ×200).

penetrating keratoplasty in the pediatric age group except for CHED.

CHED is a congenital structural abnormality of the corneal stroma and endothelium that is inherited in both autosomal recessive (43,44) and autosomal dominant forms (45). The two forms are genetically distinct but both involve a region of chromosome 20 (46) with the recessive form mapping to 20p13 (47). Both corneas of an affected individual become thickened and opaque. An affected corneal collagen fiber diameter is nearly twice the normal diameter and is haphazardly arranged in a manner that limits transmission of light. Descemet membrane is often thin and the endothelium is abnormal. Treatment has traditionally been surgical.

Recently, multiple corneal dystrophies that were thought to be distinct clinically have been found to have a common genetic defect in the BIGH-3 gene (TGF-βI h3 gene located at 5q31) (48,49). This discovery has totally changed the classification of the affected corneal stromal dystrophies: Reis-Bücklers, lattice types I and III, granular, Avellino, and Thiel-Behnke corneal dystrophy (50).

Dystrophies of Bowman membrane (Reis-Bücklers and Thiel-Behnke dystrophies) occur very rarely. There is destruction of Bowman membrane possibly due to a protease produced in the corneal epithelium. *Granular corneal dystrophy* is an abnormality of protein metabolism of the corneal epithelial cells. Well-demarcated deposits occur initially in the anterior corneal stroma and progress to accumulate in deeper stromal layers. The intervening collagen is normal. *Lattice corneal dystrophy* type I is an accumulation of amyloid in the corneal stroma often in a linear pattern associated with the genetic abnormality at 5q31. Other subgroups of lattice corneal dystrophy involve other processes leading to amyloid deposition and are also rare. *Avellino corneal dystrophy* presents initially with features of granular corneal dystrophy and then progresses to develop features of lattice corneal dystrophy ("dystrophy" is an essential part of the name JDC). Studying affected patients living in Avellino, Italy, with this mixed clinical picture led to the discovery of the common genetic defect at 5q31 which is associated with multiple phenotypic expressions (51).

Map-dot-fingerprint (MDF) dystrophy, also known as anterior basement membrane dystrophy, is one of the most commonly occurring "dystrophies." MDF dystrophy is characterized by excessive production of basement membrane material by the corneal epithelial cells (52). The epithelium is loosely adherent because of abnormal adhesive properties of the redundant basement membrane. Corneal abrasions tend to occur more frequently (recurrent erosion) (Figure 11-16). Secondary reactive degeneration of the Bowman membrane and anterior corneal stroma may occur if the abrasions are extensive, leading to superficial corneal opacification that is permanent. The condition rarely affects the pediatric age group and is treated with lubrication.

Macular corneal dystrophy is an abnormality of mucopolysaccharide production by corneal keratocytes (53). The condition is inherited in an autosomal recessive pattern and

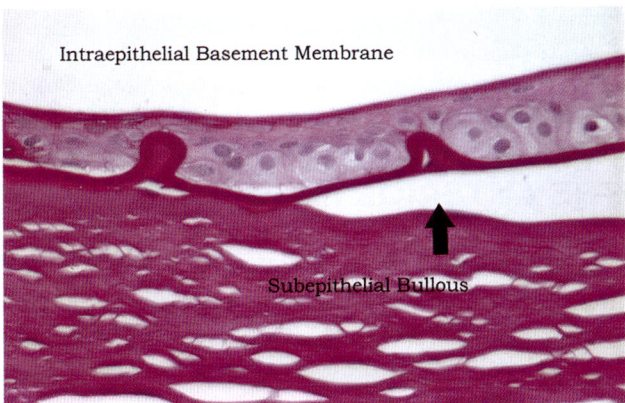

FIGURE 11-16 • Map-dot-fingerprint dystrophy. Epithelial cells have produced a defective basement membrane with abnormal adhesive characteristics. The epithelium has separated from the Bowman membrane to form a subepithelial bulla. The bullae are fragile and may rupture causing exposure of nerve endings and pain. The absence of epithelial cover is a risk factor for corneal infection (periodic acid/Schiff stain, original magnification ×100).

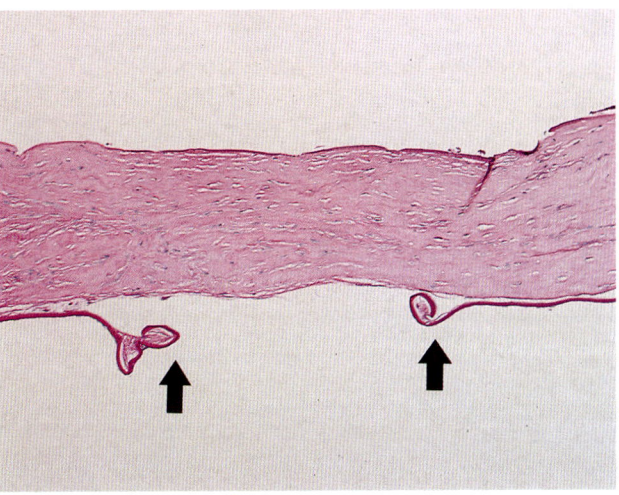

FIGURE 11-18 • Corneal hydrops. The lack of tensile strength of the cornea has progressed to the point of rupture of Descemet membrane, exposing the relatively dehydrated corneal stroma to be exposed to aqueous humor (arrows). Hydration of the corneal stroma results in opacity in the region of rupture. With time, the posterior cornea may repair causing at least partial clearing of the stroma and improved vision (periodic acid/Schiff stain, original magnification ×40).

most cases are caused by mutations in CHST6 gene. Unlike the other corneal dystrophies, there is a systemic abnormality in a subset of those with macular corneal dystrophy.

Keratoconus is an acquired localized stromal thinning of the cornea, usually located in the inferior nasal quadrant (Figure 11-17). The thin area is displaced anteriorly by normal levels of intraocular pressure altering the anterior corneal curvature. Keratoconus is not considered to be a corneal dystrophy. Its etiology has not been established but appears to relate to abnormal activity of the matrix metalloproteinases normally produced by corneal keratocytes. The natural history is one of progressive myopia and irregular astigmatism that can be corrected initially with contact lenses. In time, some cases progress to corneal stromal scarring in the region of the cone (the area of maximal distortion). The stroma becomes thin to the point where corneal rupture is possible. Rupture of Descemet membrane in the region of the cone may allow aqueous from the anterior chamber to instantaneously hydrate the normally dehydrated corneal stroma (corneal hydrops). There is sudden appearance of corneal opacity that may slowly clear over weeks or months as the corneal endothelium repairs. Complete clarity is rarely accomplished. Distinct, focal breaks of Bowman membrane characterize keratoconus. Scarring of variable degrees is associated with the breaks in Bowman membrane. In the event of corneal hydrops, there is rupture of Descemet membrane. The severed ends of Descemet membrane generally curl inward. Endothelial cells may migrate over exposed posterior corneal stroma to establish a new, but considerably thinner Descemet membrane (Figure 11-18). Keratoconus is still one of the most common indications for penetrating keratoplasty in children (54). However, clinical trials of corneal collagen cross-linking via ultraviolet radiation are being evaluated as a nonsurgical option.

Degenerations of the Cornea

Band keratopathy is a degeneration of the anterior cornea often associated with chronic anterior uveitis or chronic keratitis. It appears as superficial opacification of the anterior cornea with focal oval well-demarcated areas of translucency that causes marked loss of vision. Calcium is deposited in Bowman membrane and corneal stroma by dystrophic calcification (Figure 11-19). The calcified Bowman membrane is as fragile as an eggshell and may fracture and extrude onto the anterior corneal surface. Chelation of calcium deposits with ethylenediamine-tetraacetic acid (EDTA) may debulk the lesions and improve vision.

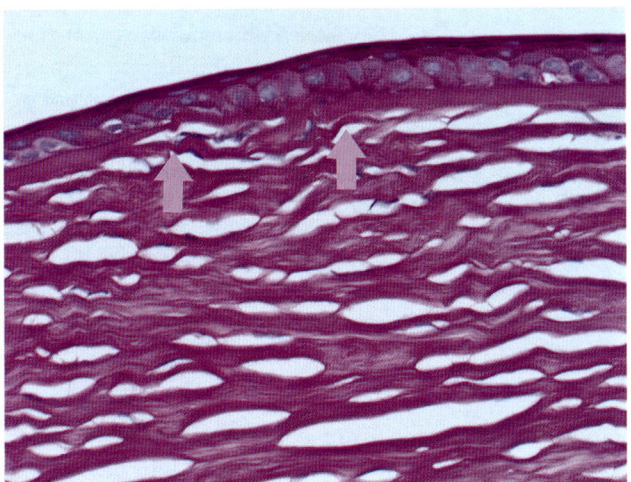

FIGURE 11-17 • Keratoconus. There is a break in the Bowman membrane (arrows) that is associated with alteration of the anterior contour of the cornea (formation of a "cone") (periodic acid/Schiff stain, original magnification ×200).

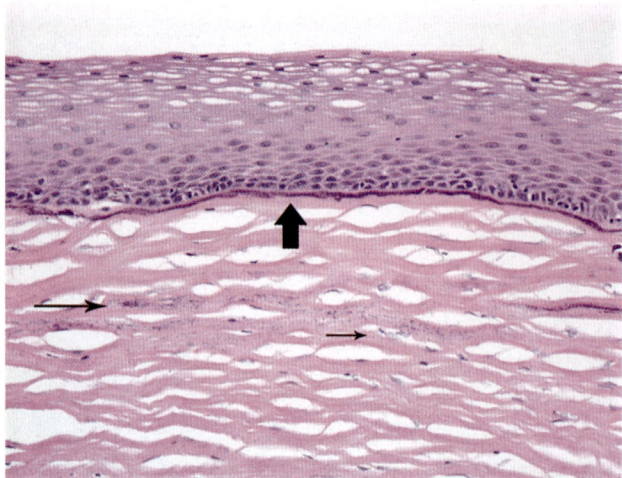

FIGURE 11-19 • Band keratopathy is dystrophic calcification of the Bowman membrane (*large arrow*) and corneal stroma (*small arrows*) following chronic keratitis or uveitis. In advanced cases, the calcified Bowman membrane may fracture and be displaced onto the corneal surface causing a foreign body sensation (hematoxylin-eosin stain, original magnification ×40).

Surgical Procedures of the Cornea

Biopsy of the cornea is performed infrequently except in the case of infection (fungus and *Acanthamoeba*) that is resistant to therapy. Repair processes of the cornea result in loss of transparency, and therefore, biopsies are extremely small and originate as far away from the visual axis (center of the cornea) as possible. Most of the biopsy specimens, in the case of suspected fungus, will be submitted for culture; however, histopathologic evaluation in cases of suspected *Acanthamoeba* is more likely to be diagnostic than microbiologic studies.

Classically, full-thickness penetrating keratoplasty has been the most common method of treating disease-damaged corneas. A trephine, usually 7.5 mm in diameter, is used to create an incision through the cornea. The entire specimen is submitted only after the donor graft is in place and secured. Drying artifacts of the host cornea may accumulate during the interval. The most common indications for penetrating keratoplasty in the pediatric age group are congenital corneal opacities, keratoconus, and opacity from corneal trauma. Newer surgical techniques have been developed in which only the specific layer (lamella) of the cornea that has been altered by disease is removed. Currently, the most common deep lamellar procedure in children is removal and replacement of Descemet membrane, often with part of the posterior corneal stroma (Descemet stripping endothelial keratoplasty, DSEK), which may be used for CHED. Surface damage of the cornea may be treated with anterior lamellar keratoplasty or keratectomy, often with placement of an amniotic membrane graft.

Corneal refractive surgery changes the optical qualities of the cornea by altering its thickness and curvature. Currently, the two most common procedures are photorefractive keratectomy (PRK) and laser *in situ* keratomileusis (LASIK). Because the optical system of the eye is not stable until age 18 to 22 years, these procedures are generally not performed on children.

THE ANTERIOR SEGMENT

Structure of the Anterior Segment

The anterior segment is divided into anterior and posterior chambers by the plane of the iris. The anterior chamber is bordered anteriorly by the cornea, peripherally by the anterior chamber aqueous filtering apparatus (the trabecular meshwork), and posteriorly by the iris stroma and the anterior crystalline lens capsule at the pupil. Aqueous is produced by the nonpigmented epithelium of the ciliary processes and flows through the pupil into the anterior chamber. The aqueous nourishes the anterior hemisphere of the crystalline lens and all of the tissues bordering the anterior chamber. Spent aqueous is filtered into the systemic vascular system, at the periphery of the anterior chamber initially, through a porous trabecular meshwork, and then through a protein membrane (the juxtacanalicular connective tissue [JXT]). Beyond the JXT, the aqueous is discharged through the canal of Schlemm, through emissary veins, and finally into veins of the general circulatory system. Abnormalities of drainage (glaucoma) usually occur in the JXT. Tumor cells in the anterior chamber may exit the eye via the aqueous drainage channels.

The trabecular meshwork collagen cores are covered by an endothelium contiguous with the corneal epithelium. There is no epithelial or endothelial lining of the anterior surface of the iris. The iris stroma is variably pigmented by dendritic melanocytes allowing for iris "color." The degree of iris epithelial pigmentation is uniformly dense despite the degree of iris stromal pigmentation. The vessels of the iris stroma are unique because of a very thick adventitial lining. The blood column cannot be seen during clinical evaluation. The thick adventitia is probably necessary because of the continuous movement of the iris associated with changes in pupil diameter. The sphincter muscle at the pupil is located in the iris stroma. The dilator muscle fibers are located in the cytoplasm of the anterior iris pigment epithelium.

The posterior chamber is bordered by the posterior surface of the iris, the equatorial crystalline lens, the ciliary body, and the anterior border of the vitreous (the vitreous face). The posterior chamber contains aqueous. The lens zonules extend through the posterior chamber from posterior ciliary body to the lens equator and are freely mobile in that space.

Glaucoma

Glaucoma is an imbalance between intraocular production of aqueous and drainage of aqueous into the systemic circulation, which results in increased intraocular pressure and progressive optic neuropathy by a variety of proposed mechanisms. Any developmental abnormality of the anterior segment may lead to glaucoma; the more extensive the architectural abnormality, the more likely is glaucoma to develop. In the vast majority of cases, the imbalance is caused by abnormalities of filtration rather than overproduction of aqueous. Increased intraocular pressure will not decrease aqueous production until the intraocular pressure is in the range of the diastolic blood pressure.

Congenital Glaucoma

In the pediatric age group, the tissues of the eye remain pliable to the point where increased intraocular pressure may actually expand the dimensions of the eye leading to enlargement of the cornea and anterior–posterior dimensions of the globe (buphthalmos). The expansion is not uniform enlargement of the globe; rather, it is stretching of the thinnest portion of the eye wall at the junction of the cornea and sclera (the intercalary zone). In advanced cases of glaucoma from any cause, the anterior chamber may collapse allowing the anterior surface of the iris to come in contact with the posterior surface of the cornea (total anterior synechiae), further limiting the ability of aqueous to exit the eye. The front of the eye may bulge forward (ectasia) and the ectatic area may become lined by iris (anterior staphyloma).

In many cases of congenital glaucoma, there is no histologic sign of architectural abnormality of the anterior chamber angle including the delicate trabecular meshwork. However, developmental anatomic abnormalities range from total immaturity of the draining structures to regional minimal structural changes. Except in extreme cases, the intraocular pressure cannot be predicted from the nature of the architectural changes.

In the pediatric age group, one of the most common forms of secondary glaucoma is neovascular glaucoma. In this situation, ischemia of the retina induces formation of local angiogenic factors (e.g., vascular endothelial growth factor [VEGF]). The process stimulates angiogenesis of the anterior surface of the iris. This fibrovascular growth flattens the contour of the anterior iris (clearly seen by light microscopy) and also causes adhesions between the anterior surface of the iris and the posterior surface of the peripheral cornea (peripheral anterior synechia [PAS]). The PAS limit aqueous access to the trabecular meshwork and cause increased intraocular pressure. This mechanism is found in retinopathy of prematurity, advanced retinoblastoma, and uncontrolled diabetic retinopathy, among others.

Sustained increased intraocular pressure causes degeneration of the ganglion cell and nerve fiber layer of the retina. The exact cause for internal retinal atrophy has not been definitely determined for all types of glaucoma. In addition, there is retrodisplacement of the structural support of the optic disc (the lamina cribrosa), which is a finding unique to increased intraocular pressure. In other forms of atrophic optic neuropathy, the position of the lamina cribrosa relative to the surrounding sclera is not affected. Progressive loss of retinal ganglion cell axons progressively increases the cup-to-disc ratio to the point of "total cupping" of the optic disc. This clinical finding can be confirmed by anterior–posterior histologic sections of the eye if the plane of section is through the optic disc. Total optic cupping correlates with total loss of optic nerve axons, widening of pial septa, and enlargement of the subretinal space. The character of the dura is not changed by increased intraocular pressure.

Surgical Treatment of Glaucoma

Generally, the aim of glaucoma surgery is to re-establish aqueous filtration (goniotomy or trabeculotomy) or to bypass the usual pathway with a subconjunctival fistula (trabeculectomy) or shunt (tube-shunting procedure). In a goniotomy and trabeculotomy, a needle or microscopic blade is used to penetrate the trabecular meshwork. The trabeculectomy procedure produces a permanent fistula between the anterior chamber and the episcleral surface. In shunting procedures, a silicone tube is placed in the anterior chamber to route aqueous posteriorly to a filtration chamber placed at the equator of the eye and covered by conjunctiva and Tenon's capsule.

THE CRYSTALLINE LENS

Structure of the Crystalline Lens

The crystalline biconvex lens is located in the visual axis posterior to the iris diaphragm and contributes about 30% of the refractive power of the eye. Until approximately age 40 years, the lens is pliable enough to allow variable focus from distance to near. After age 40, the lens loses its pliability and bifocals or reading spectacles are necessary for near tasks.

The crystalline lens is surrounded by a dense type IV collagen capsule that is variable in thickness. The thickest portion of the capsule is at the point of insertion of the supportive lens zonule system of fibers and is thinnest at the posterior pole, adjacent to the vitreous in the visual axis. The lens cortex and nucleus are initially entirely cellular. In the anterior hemisphere, there is a single layer of cuboidal "epithelial cells" that terminate at the lens equator by forming a curvilinear "lens bow" (the stem cells of the lens). The remainder of the lens cells lose their nuclei and become anucleate lens fibers. The lens fibers have a very regular structure associated with few organelles but have an intricate system of ball-and-socket connections between lens fibers. Lens fibers are continuously added to the surface of the cortex beneath the lens. The older fibers are compacted in the central lens and tend to become opaque (nuclear cataract). Lens zonules originate from the surface cells of the pars plana, anterior to the vitreous base, and extend through the posterior chamber to the equator of the lens. Zonules are composed of fibrillin, maintain lens position, and change lens shape (and optical power) during accommodation (1,2).

Developmental Abnormalities of the Crystalline Lens

The crystalline lens develops from an invagination of the surface ectoderm to form the lens vesicle. The developing lens interacts with the retina derived from the neuroectoderm to form the functional aspects of the eye. Neural crest cells form the supportive tissue of the eye and orbit. Fibers of the lens cortex form a visible suture in the shape of an inverted Y anteriorly and an inverted Y posteriorly. Subtle changes in lens biochemistry may lead to opacification of lens fibers as punctate or diffuse opacities or opacification of the Y sutures. A rich, temporary, vascular plexus (tunica vasculosa lentis) supports the lens during embryonic development, which will undergo apoptosis approximately at birth. At that time, nutritional support for the lens changes to the aqueous produced by the cilia epithelium. The tunica vasculosa lentis may be retained in various degrees to form fibrovascular membranes in the papillary space (persistent fetal vasculature.) The lens is supported by a system of zonules composed primarily of fibrillin. Variations in zonular structure may allow various degrees of lens dislocation (55).

Primary aphakia is an exceedingly rare event because of the contribution of the lens to ocular development; if the lens is not present, the remainder of the globe is unable to develop.

Microphakia may occur in generalized ocular abnormalities such as *PHPV*. In this situation, abnormalities of the vitreous will limit development of the lens. Eyes affected by PHPV are usually small with limited visual potential. Many complex factors determine lens size, most of which are not yet fully characterized. The microphakic lens is usually also spherical. The abnormal shape may be caused by deficiencies in the quality or quantity of lens zonules (56,57).

A *pyramidal cataract* is a dense elevation on the anterior surface of the lens usually in the visual axis. In addition, there may be absence of axial posterior corneal stroma and Descemet membrane and endothelium (Peters syndrome).

Phakomatous choristoma is the presence of ectopic lens tissue in the cutaneous structures of the anterior orbital soft tissue, usually in the inferior nasal quadrant. The abnormal lens is characterized by basement membrane–producing epithelial cells and primitive lens fibers. The condition is usually stationary and not associated with other ocular abnormalities (58,59).

Congenital Lens Opacities

Congenital cataracts are the final expression of many types of developmental and metabolic defects and are relatively rare (60). Autosomal dominant transmission with high penetrance is most common, but autosomal recessive and X-linked transmissions also occur. It is not surprising that several cataract types have been linked to regions that regulate crystalline genes, the major proteins of the lens fibers (61). The pathologic features of congenital cataracts are classified by geographic localization of the clinical opacity.

Anterior polar cataracts arise in the papillary space as an elevated plaque that may be the result of faulty separation of the lens vesicle from the surface ectoderm or may be the result of a momentary toxic environment (e.g., inflammation) during gestation. *Posterior polar cataracts* are more likely related to failure of involution of components of the tunica vasculosa lentis (*Mittendorf dot*). Opacification in the region of the Y sutures is common and is estimated to occur in at least 20% of the population. Congenital cataract may affect any region of the lens with markedly variable degrees and patterns of relative opacity. A *cerulean cataract* is a club-shaped opacity with a blue tinge. A *zonular congenital cataract* has opacification in zones around a clear nucleus. In contrast, the fetal nucleus may be translucent or totally opaque as found in the *rubella syndrome*. There is potential risk indicated by cataract as there is intracellular sequestration of live virus within the central fiber cells of the lens, which may persist long after birth and may cause viral endophthalmitis if released during cataract surgery.

Lens Opacities in Genetic Diseases

There are dozens of other syndromes of known or suspected genetic cause in which some form of cataract has been described; however, seldom are the clinical characteristics of the lens opacity specific for that syndrome. The most common lens opacity in these often autosomal dominant diseases is the posterior subcapsular cataract (PSC). What may be difficult to determine is whether the cataract is directly due to the genetic defect or is a secondary effect of the disease process.

In *galactosemia*, polysaccharides may accumulate in the lens, changing the state of hydration and the clarity of the lens. If the biochemical abnormality is corrected through dietary measures early in the course of the disease, the lens may return to its normal state of transparency. If the condition persists, secondary structural changes in the lens will cause permanent opacity (see Chapter 5).

Environmental Lens Opacities

The developing lens is extremely sensitive to changes in its biochemical microenvironment. Even transient changes may lead to localized opacities in specific regions of the lens cortex. The closer the opacity to the epicenter of the lens, the more likely the event was early in development. Lens opacities formed in this manner generally do not progress after birth and may not affect visual function.

Rubella

The rubella virus may gain access to the developing lens and infect the cells of the lens cortex during pregnancy. Infection in this manner produces a dense white (pearl-like) cataract that may be limited to the embryonic nucleus. The cataract is distinguished by retention of lens cells with nuclei in the center of the lens, which, in normal development, would have involuted and disappeared except at the equatorial lens bow (Figure 11-20). Rubella virus remains viable in the lens for years after birth (57). Early surgical procedures designed to remove congenital cataracts piecemeal may have contributed to virus release into the eye and subsequent viral panophthalmitis.

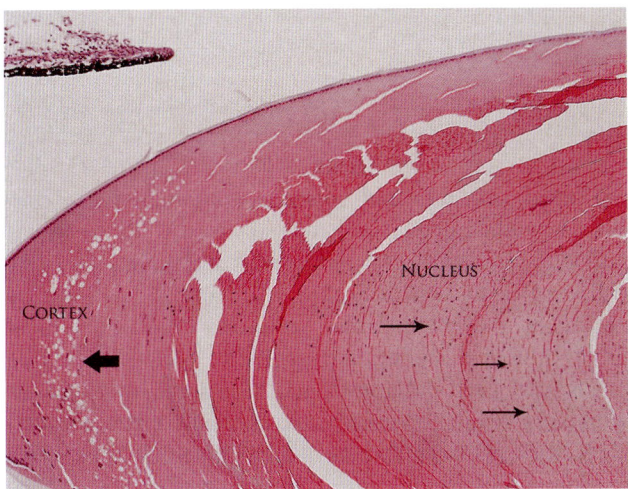

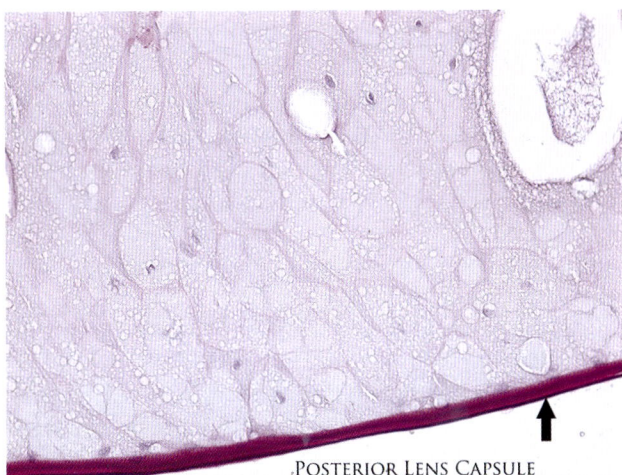

FIGURE 11-20 • Rubella cataract. Normally, there are no nucleated crystalline lens cells in the center of the lens, the lens nucleus. With rubella infection early in gestation, the central lens cells are infected with the rubella virus, retain their nuclei (*small arrows*), and are densely opaque. There is also some degeneration of the lens cortex (*large arrow*), which also causes peripheral translucent opacity (hematoxylin–eosin stain, original magnification ×20).

FIGURE 11-22 • Posterior subcapsular cataract (PSC). Lens epithelial cells have migrated from the lens equator to the posterior cortex of the lens in the visual axis. The cells have retained their nuclei and are irregular in shape and size manifesting as a "ground-glass" appearance of the posterior lens cortex clinically (periodic acid/Schiff stain, original magnification ×40).

Toxic Cataract

With chronic damage from anterior uveitis, the anterior lens epithelial cells will be stimulated to undergo fibrous metaplasia resulting in dense anterior subcapsular cataract (Figure 11-21). Following trauma, intraocular inflammation, or vitrectomy, crystalline lens cells may migrate from the lens equator to the posterior pole of the lens to create a "ground-glass" opacification of the posterior lens cortex. The migrating cells retain their nuclei but are very polymorphic. The PSC cells are said to resemble urothelial cells of the bladder and have been called "bladder cells" (Figure 11-22) (55).

Traumatic Cataract

The crystalline lens will instantly become opaque if the lens capsule is disrupted allowing fluid to disturb the homogeneity of the lens cortex as in a penetrating injury of the cornea or sclera. A shock wave associated with blunt trauma may also cause the formation of a cataract; however, the clinical onset of the opacity may be days or years following the injury. This type of cataract may be characterized by posterior migration of the lens epithelium from the equator along the internal surface of the posterior capsule to the posterior pole of the lens. This type of PSC is also associated with advanced diabetes mellitus, with chronic treatment with corticosteroids, and with inflammation (62).

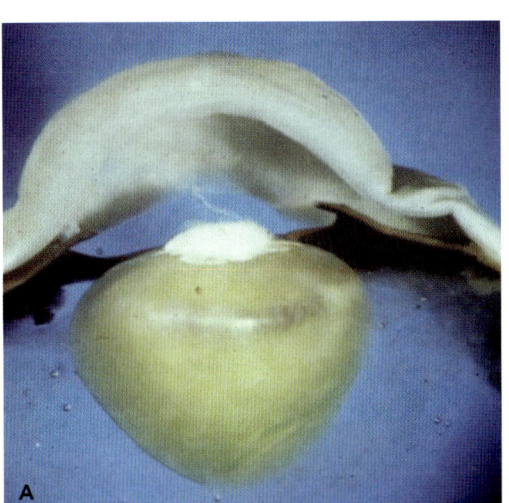

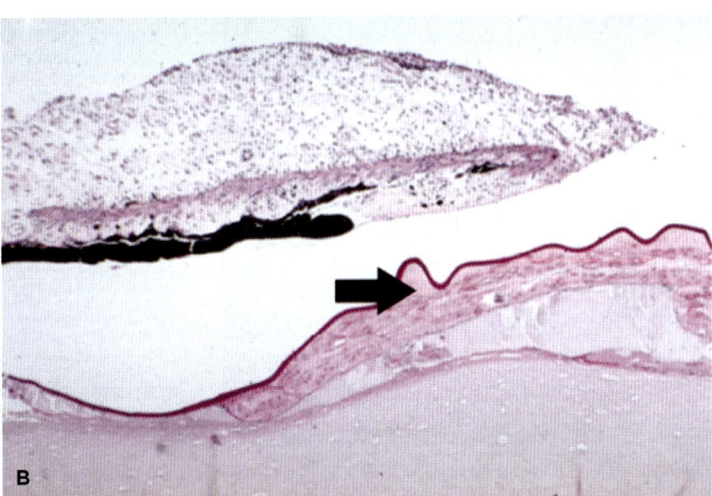

FIGURE 11-21 • Anterior subcapsular cataract. **A:** The cornea is opaque from long-standing anterior uveitis and keratitis creating a toxic environment in the anterior chamber. **B:** Crystalline lens repair processes have caused a dense anterior subcapsular cataract (*arrow*) by fibrous metaplasia of the crystalline lens epithelium. The lens capsule undulates because of contracture of the fibrous scar (periodic acid/Schiff stain, original magnification ×40).

The Zonular Apparatus and Lens Dislocation (Ectopia Lentis)

The lens zonules are composed of a cystine-rich glycoprotein fibrillin, which is encoded on chromosome 15q21.1 (63). A lens is *luxated* when it is completely dislocated from its normal position and the zonular support is nearly or completely absent. *Subluxated* lenses are partially removed from their normal position with variable degrees of zonular support remaining (Figure 11-23).

The most common cause of lens subluxation–luxation in most large series has been trauma. It usually follows penetrating injury or severe contusive injury and is often associated with cataract and rhegmatogenous retinal detachment.

Marfan syndrome is the most common heritable cause of crystalline lens dislocation; it is caused by mutations in the fibrillin-1 gene (*FBN1*) on chromosome 15q21.1. The most important systemic abnormality of Marfan syndrome is the high risk of dissecting aneurysm of the aorta. Lens subluxation may be present at birth or may appear after birth and may be stationary or progressive. The zonules can be easily seen stretching from the periphery of the lens across the peripheral pupillary space. The subluxated lens may be normal in size or small, with a flatter curvature of the lower half and a posterior bulge as a result of weakness or absence of the inferior zonules. The zonular bundles may be thin, thick, or of normal caliber but in most cases show thin and poorly aggregated zonules (see Chapter 13).

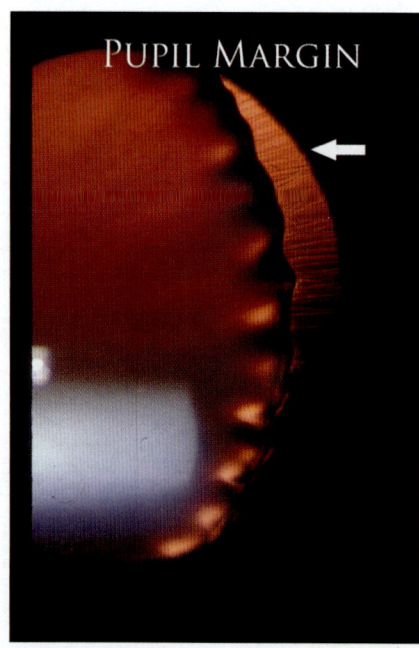

FIGURE 11-23 • Crystalline lens dislocation. The center of the lens is displaced (subluxated) from the pupillary margin (*white arrow*) but is not completely dislocated (luxated). Stretched zonules can be seen extending from the margin of the lens posteriorly to their insertion. The majority of lens zonules attached to the elevated portions of the lens margin.

Surgical Procedures of the Crystalline Lens

Whereas cataract extraction is one of the most common surgical procedures performed in the United States on the elderly, cataract surgery is infrequently performed in the pediatric age group with the most common indications being congenital or inflammation-related cataracts (e.g., uveitis associated with juvenile rheumatoid arthritis and trauma). Surgery is usually performed through a small corneal incision. The opaque material of the lens is removed by mechanical aspiration through a sophisticated auger-like device. In children over 1 year of age, the cataract may be replaced by a synthetic intraocular lens (IOL) constructed of various types of biostable (usually plastic) polymers. In infancy, an IOL is generally not used initially but is implanted secondarily later in childhood. Even with an IOL implant, children require glasses for near tasks because modern monofocal IOLs correct only for distance, and multifocal lenses are not indicated for children.

The cataractous lens is almost always removed in small degraded components and not submitted for histopathologic examination. The central anterior lens capsule is always removed to allow access to the crystalline lens intraoperatively (except in rare cases of intact total lensectomy). In children, the posterior lens capsule and anterior hyaloid face of the vitreous body are also removed because they invariably opacify due to the child's robust immune response (whereas posterior capsular opacification is only clinically significant in about 10% of adults after cataract surgery). The resultant fibrous cyclitic membranes may be treated with a laser procedure (YAG capsulotomy) or surgical excision.

THE VITREOUS

Structure of the Vitreous

The vitreous is composed of a type II collagen matrix containing hyaluronic acid. The majority of the vitreous is composed of water and may attain a volume of 4 mL weighing 4 g. The vitreous is formed near the junction adherent to the internal surface of the retina at the optic disc, in the region of the peripheral macula, along the course of retinal blood vessels, and at the posterior surface of the crystalline lens. The matrix of the vitreous degenerates over time (usually beyond the pediatric age) and separates from the surface of the posterior retina forming "floaters," which cast a symptomatic shadow on the retina. The vitreous is a biochemical sink and also functions in maintaining retinal attachment (1,2).

Surgical Procedures of the Vitreous

The entire vitreous can be surgically removed (vitrectomy) without immediate effect on the structure of the eye. In most cases, a cataract will develop due to subtle biochemical alteration. Vitrectomy is most often used to remove acquired mechanical factors affecting the retina (e.g., epiretinal membrane formation associated with macular hole and subretinal neovascularization from a variety of causes). Vitrectomy is also used to correct fibrovascular membranes (traction retinal detachment) that are found in advanced stages of diabetic retinopathy. Occasionally, vitrectomy is used in pediatric cases for diagnostic purposes (diffuse infiltrating retinoblastoma, medulloepithelioma). The specimen often contains only a small number of cells, as is found in fine needle aspirations used at other sites. Usually, the histopathologic diagnosis is established by examining a cellblock. Fine needle aspiration is rarely done intraocularly because the mechanical forces generated during aspiration are much more difficult to control than the aspiration forces generated by the highly sophisticated vitrectomy instrument.

Intermediate uveitis or pars planitis is a localized inflammation probably of autoimmune origin that involves the vitreous base and peripheral retina. Children and young adults are primarily affected. The majority of affected patients are asymptomatic and become symptomatic only with secondary changes such as cystoid macular edema (reactive swelling of the retina), cataract, or glaucoma. In the region of the peripheral retina, there is phlebitis and retinal edema. The vitreous structure collapses and becomes opaque over the area of proliferation of the nonpigmented epithelium of the ciliary body. Granulomatous inflammation is present in the region of reactive proliferation. Medulloepithelioma of the ciliary body and diffuse infiltrating retinoblastoma may present in a similar manner.

Familial exudative vitreoretinopathy is a congenital abnormality of the peripheral retinal circulation resulting in secondary extracellular matrix abnormalities throughout the vitreous in the form of organized membranes and focal opacities (snowflake-like) (64). Autosomal dominant, recessive, and X-linked inheritance patterns have been identified. At least five mutations associated with familial exudative vitreoretinopathy have been identified on the long arm of chromosome 11. Along with the basic vascular abnormality, the membranes are responsible for causing retinal detachment, displacement of the macula, cataract, and anterior chamber angle closure (64).

THE RETINA AND UVEAL TRACT

Structure of the Retina and Uveal Tract

The retina is a highly organized construct of neuroglial elements that serve to transduce light into an electrical signal, which is then transmitted via the ganglion cells through the optic nerve to the visual cortex. The uveal tract is the underlying metabolic engine and heat-sink of the eye.

The main architectural structure of the retina is provided by the Muller cells. Incident light travels through the full thickness of the retina before it is absorbed by visual pigments in the photoreceptor outer segments and is converted into electrical signals for the brain. The outer limiting membrane of the retina is not a true retina but a series of attachments between Muller cells and photoreceptors. The visual pigments of the rods are embedded in the plasma membrane of separate disc-shaped structures of the photoreceptor outer segments. The visual pigments of the cones are located in a folded but continuous plasma membrane of the outer segments. In both the rods and cones, the signal is transported from the photoreceptor outer segments via cilia to the photoreceptor inner segments. The photoreceptor inner segments contain abundant mitochondria. The visual signal is then passed to the horizontal, bipolar, and amacrine signal-processing cells in the middle retina across connections in the outer plexiform layer. A series of synapses in this layer forms the middle limiting membrane. The modified signal is then passed to the ganglion cells across connections of the inner plexiform layer and passed to the lateral geniculate via long axonal processes that make up the optic nerve (Figure 11-24).

Muller cells, modified astrocytes, support the retina by extending from the internal limiting membrane (a true basement membrane that it produces) across the full thickness of the neurosensory retina to the external limiting membrane that is actually a series of connections between the apical portion of the Muller cell and the photoreceptor cells. The nuclei of the Muller cells are located in the same region as the nuclei of the photoreceptors. The retina also contains microglia and oligodendroglia. The central retinal artery supplies the internal retina to the level of the middle limiting membrane. There are three layers of capillaries posteriorly and two layers in the equatorial retina. Beyond the equator, there is a single capillary layer, and at the periphery, the retina is solely supplied by external sources in the uveal tract.

The retinal pigment epithelium (RPE) is derived from neuroectodermal cells of the outer layer of the optic cup. The RPE cell is among the first in the body to produce melanin, a molecule that is necessary for the development of the neurosensory retina. The retina does not fully develop in

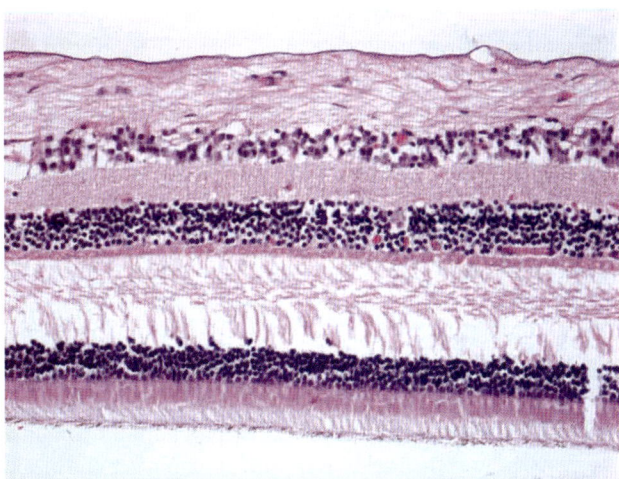

FIGURE 11-24 • The normal retina: the retina contains photoreception system, an image processing system, and image transmission system. The retina is rarely biopsied (hematoxylin–eosin stain, original magnification ×20).

ocular albinism. The melanin granules, which are large and oval, are easily distinguished as individual granules by light microscopy. Collections of extracellular RPE melanin in the vitreous may be mistaken for bacteria. In contrast, individual melanin granules in the dendritic melanocytes of the uveal tract have a small diameter that is not easily resolvable by light microscopy. The RPE is a monolayer of cells residing on its basement membrane with an undulating basal surface and long apical processes. The apical processes interdigitate among the photoreceptor outer segments and help to physically isolate individual photoreceptor outer segments. Interphotoreceptor mucoid substance is also present among the photoreceptor outer segments. Among the functions of the RPE is metabolism of spent photoreceptor outer segment lipoproteins and visual pigment molecules. The RPE has no physical connection with the overlying neurosensory retina but is held in place by physiologic forces generated between the vitreous and the choroid. If these factors are altered, or if the physical integrity of the neurosensory retina is violated by the formation of a physical hole, the retina will detach from the RPE (retinal detachment).

The fovea centralis is the most highly specialized region of the retina. It is a thin area of the retina located directly in the visual axis in the center of a portion of the retina designated as the macula. The macula is a region of the retina generally lying between the temporal inferior and superior vascular arcades. All factors that might interfere with the transmission of light are eliminated. The internal limiting membrane is thin; the internal retina including ganglion cells and nerve fiber layer are absent; the internal retinal circulation is absent; and the external plexiform layer is oriented obliquely to reach peripherally located ganglion cells. Only cones are present and are in such a high concentration that their profiles are cylindrical rather than cone-shaped. The RPE is thicker in this region and there is a higher concentration of melanin granules. In the center, there is an avascular zone of 500 mm diameter where nutrition is solely supplied by the uveal tract vessels (choriocapillaris). There is compensatory thickening of the ganglion cell and nerve fiber layer in the retina immediately peripheral to the fovea centralis.

The uveal tract receives its blood supply from the short and long posterior ciliary system. The larger vessels are located external and progressively diminish in caliber to finally form the choriocapillaris, which is a large-volume chamber lined by fenestrated vascular endothelial cells. The basement membrane of the vascular endothelium, a layer of extracellular matrix containing elastin, and the basement membrane of the RPE cells together make up Bruch membrane. In the region between lumens of the choriocapillaris vessels, Bruch membrane is composed of only two layers. Venous blood is drained via vortex veins located in each quadrant through a long intrascleral channel to mix with systemic venous blood on the episcleral surface. Among the vascular channels, there is a dense concentration of dendritic melanocytes characterized by retention of intracellular small-caliber melanin granules. The uveal tract also contains the long posterior ciliary nerve, a branch of the trigeminal, and may contain collections of peripheral nervous system ganglion cells.

The retina is protected from vascular insults by a blood–retinal barrier similar in function and form to the blood–brain barrier. The vessels of the choriocapillaris are porous but any extravascular fluid is blocked from retinal penetration by intercellular tight junctions near the apical portions of the RPE cells. Similarly, the vascular endothelial cells of the intraretinal vascular system are connected by tight junctions to form the intraretinal portion of the blood–retinal barrier. This barrier may be breached by either inflammation or degeneration.

Tumors of the Retina and Uveal Tract

Retinoblastoma is a malignant tumor of the retina, resulting from an uncontrolled proliferation of retinoblasts, which are pluripotential neuroectodermal cells that differentiate into the various components of normal mature retina. The malignancy is capable of widespread metastases leading to death. The tumor initially proliferates in the plane of the retina but is capable of involving all structures within the eye. The tumor may spread to the central nervous system via the optic nerve and through lymphatics and blood vessels to tissues at distant sites.

This tumor has become a model for heritable malignant tumors based on a genetic deletion of the Rb (retinoblastoma) gene. The genetic defect at chromosome 13q14 is associated with retinoblastoma in early childhood. The Knudson two-hit hypothesis states that retinoblastoma arises as a result of two mutational events (65). If one or both chromosomal 13q14 regions are normal, no retinoblastoma develops. If both chromosomes 13 have a 13q14 deletion or functional abnormality, retinoblastoma results. When both mutations occur in the same somatic postzygotic cell, a single unilateral retinoblastoma results. Because the mutations occur in a somatic cell, this condition is, therefore, not inherited. In the hereditary form, the first mutation occurs in a germinal prezygotic cell, which means that this mutation is present in all resulting somatic cells, and a second mutation occurs in the somatic postzygotic cells, resulting in multiple retinal tumors as well as nonretinal tumors in other sites at different times of life, such as sarcomas. In the inherited form with a germ-line mutation (i.e., a carrier of the retinoblastoma genetic abnormality), the probability of developing the tumor is 95 in 100 (66).

The tumor arises when the retinoblastoma gene is absent (point deletion) or nonfunctional in affected cells. The protein produced by the gene (RB1) is a phosphoprotein that inhibits progression through the cell cycle by binding to DNA. The RB1 protein functions as a tumor suppressor in the retina by inhibiting proliferation and promoting differentiation of retinal progenitor cells. In the absence of this protein, there is an accumulation of proliferating embryonic retinal cells. In the eye, the tumor arises in differentiated retina, may arise in multiple sites of the same eye, and may develop in both eyes.

Retinoblastoma is inherited in an autosomal dominant pattern with incomplete penetrance even though at a cellular level the disease is autosomal recessive. In heritable retinoblastoma, all of the 200 million cells of the developing retina of an individual are susceptible to acquiring a second mutation. Even though the probability of any one cell being damaged is low, the chance of one hit in 200 million is high.

Small subsets of cases of retinoblastoma arise in children with extensive deletions in chromosome 13. In addition, these children may exhibit holoprosencephaly, midface dysmorphism including cleft lip and palate, and mental and growth retardation. This is the least frequent form of retinoblastoma (67).

Retinoblastoma is the most common intraocular neoplasm in children with a frequency of 1 in 16,000 to 1 in 20,000 live births in the United States. The incidence of retinoblastoma decreases with age. There is no significant sex or race predilection, and 20% to 35% of the cases are bilateral (resulting from germ-line mutations), although only 5% of all children with retinoblastomas have a family history of retinoblastoma. The tumor occurs in both sexes and is found in all cultures and all geographic areas. The incidence of heritable retinoblastoma appears stable. There is a recent suggestion that the incidence of nonheritable, unilateral retinoblastoma is increasing in certain groups due to environmental influences (nutritional deficiencies and human papillomavirus infection).

The heritable form is likely when another family member has been identified with retinoblastoma. Approximately 40% of cases of retinoblastoma are heritable. This form is generally diagnosed before age 12 months, much earlier than the nonheritable form. In 80% of cases of heritable retinoblastoma, retinal tumors are multiple in each eye and are found in both eyes. An associated intracranial pinealoblastoma (primitive neuroectodermal tumor or trilateral retinoblastoma) is found in 2% to 3% of cases. The RB gene defect at chromosome 13q14 is associated with other malignant tumors, so the children who survive heritable retinoblastoma are at risk of developing osteosarcoma, soft tissue sarcoma, and other mesenchymal tumors during the first two decades of life or later. In adulthood, there is a significant risk of developing malignant melanoma and central nervous system tumors. In the elderly, there is an increased incidence of cancer of the bladder. The 30-year cumulative incidence rate for second, nonocular, primary tumors is approximately 26%. The risk may be increased with radiation and chemotherapy (68).

The nonheritable form arises spontaneously and comprises about 60% of cases. The average age at presentation is 24 months. There is generally a single tumor in one eye. There is no detectable chromosomal abnormality and, therefore, a lower risk of developing retinoblastoma in succeeding generations. These children have the same risk for second primary tumors as the general population.

Historically, untreated retinoblastoma has presented as a fungating mass emanating from a ruptured globe. There was often associated facial soft tissue invasion and involvement

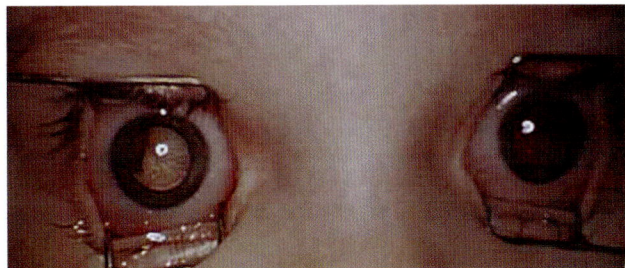

FIGURE 11-25 • Retinoblastoma. The right pupil appears white (leukocoria) because of light reflecting off a large intraocular tumor (retinoblastoma) through a clear lens and cornea. Cataract and corneal opacification are features of only an advanced retinoblastoma that fills the entire eye.

of the central nervous system. Death usually followed in the subsequent weeks or months.

Currently, retinoblastoma is often discovered by parents or relatives who notice a difference between the quality of the light reflex in one eye relative to the other either in person or on viewing family photographs (Figure 11-25). At this relatively early stage, usually at age less than 3 years, the eye does not appear to be inflamed and the child does not appear to be aware of loss of vision. The tumor, whether limited to the posterior retina, in the vitreous or in the subretinal space associated with retinal detachment, will reflect the light that is normally absorbed by blood pigments and melanin in the RPE and choroid. Children with retinoblastoma may also present with strabismus (misalignment of the visual axes of the two eyes), iris neovascularization (response to retinal ischemia leading to heterochromia, dilated fixed pupil, secondary glaucoma), or tumor accumulation in the anterior chamber (neoplastic hypopyon). More advanced cases may present with signs of intraocular inflammation (panophthalmitis), or ruptured globe with orbital extension. In some cases of regressed retinoblastoma, the sole clinical sign may be a small calcified tumor in the plane of the retina with surrounding RPE scarring.

Leukocoria (white pupil) is not an exclusive sign of retinoblastoma. Any condition that changes absorption of ambient light to reflection of that light through the pupil may cause this sign. Some of the more common nonretinoblastoma conditions presenting with leukocoria include PHPV (a developmental anomaly of the vitreous resulting in intraocular fibrosis and retinal detachment), Coats disease (a developmental vascular malformation of the retina leading to retinal detachment), and presumed ocular toxocariasis (a parasitic intraocular infection leading to intraocular scarring and retinal detachment).

Clinical findings may be unilateral or bilateral. Bilateral cases are often asymmetric. Retinoblastoma appears initially as an isolated or multicentric translucent-to-opaque thickening or globular expansion of the retina in any quadrant of the eye (Figure 11-26). Larger tumors become vascularized with a feeding artery and a draining vein. Focal opacities within larger masses correspond to areas of dystrophic calcification. The mass progressively enlarges and expands into the vitreous where it may simulate vitreous inflammation or into the

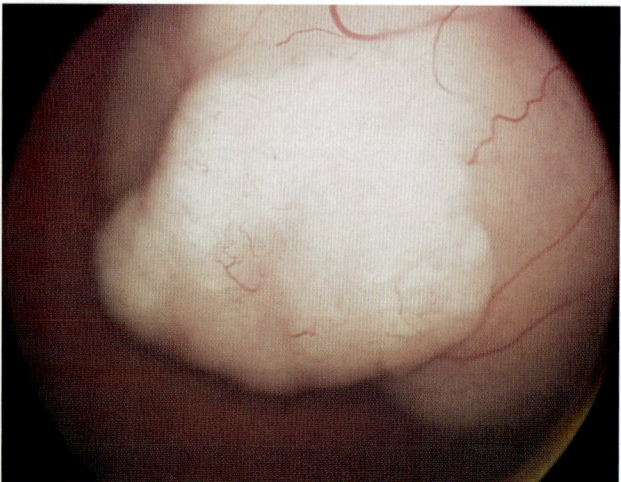

FIGURE 11-26 • Retinoblastoma. The intraocular tumor causing the leukocoria in Figure 11-25 extends into the vitreous space from the retina. Areas of calcification and irregular vascularization are evident.

subretinal space causing a serous retinal detachment. The mass continues to enlarge to fill the entire posterior compartment and displaces the lens–iris diaphragm anteriorly (Figure 11-27). Retinal ischemia associated with tumor growth will promote neovascularization of the anterior iris surface. The anterior contour of the iris flattens and the pupil may become distorted, enlarged, and nonreactive. The delicate neovascular vessels may hemorrhage and deposit hemosiderin within the iris stroma that darkens the iris color (heterochromia iridis). Neovascularization of the trabecular meshwork interferes with the egress of aqueous and causes the intraocular pressure to rise (neovascular glaucoma). The sclera of a child is pliable and may markedly expand in an anterior–posterior dimension resulting in a large eye (buphthalmos). Increased intraocular pressure also causes corneal decompensation, opacification, and scarring. With additional tumor growth, the tumor will seek sites of weakness in the eye wall (cornea and sclera). The largest opening is the scleral canal containing the optic nerve, the most likely and earliest site of extraocular extension. The tumor may also extend through any of the numerous scleral ostia; however, this stage in the evolution of the tumor is not visible clinically. When extraocular, the tumor may extend through the lymphatics of the conjunctiva and infiltrate the soft preseptal tissues of the orbit and facial lymph nodes. Direct expansion to the posterior septal orbital tissues is usually across the posterior sclera, presenting as proptosis. The cornea is the most likely site of frank rupture of the eye when the tumor completely fills the eye. Choroidal invasion allows extension through the blood vessels and spread to distant sites.

Fluorescein angiography of the retinoblastoma is characterized by early filling and late hyperfluorescence associated with leakage of fluorescein into the vitreous. Echographic features of retinoblastoma include general low internal reflectivity alternating with intense hyperreflectivity in regions of dystrophic calcification. There is a shadow effect posterior to thick areas of the tumor.

Standard radiography has been important in identifying intraocular opacities (dystrophic calcification) and outlining signs of extraocular extension. Dystrophic calcification, however, can occur in nonneoplastic conditions, particularly those associated with degeneration (e.g., following trauma). Computed tomography (CT) and magnetic resonance imaging (MRI) allow more precise recognition of extraocular extension. CT scans are avoided as much as possible in children with retinoblastoma as the additional radiation poses a significant increased risk for secondary malignancy in these patients predisposed by their tumor-suppressor gene defect. Furthermore, CT was often used to look for calcifications within the lesion to lend diagnostic support for retinoblastoma, but several other diseases that may masquerade as retinoblastoma may display calcification. MRI is particularly important in the detection of mass lesions in the pineal and suprasellar regions of the brain (trilateral retinoblastoma). By CT imaging, retinoblastoma has approximately the same density as brain. By MRI T1-weighted imaging, the tumor is hyperdense relative to the vitreous, and by T2-weighted imaging, the tumor is hypodense relative to the vitreous. There is minimal to marked enhancement on contrast-enhanced T1-weighted images with fat suppression techniques.

In most cases of retinoblastoma, the external dimensions of the eye are normal for the patient's age. The exceptions

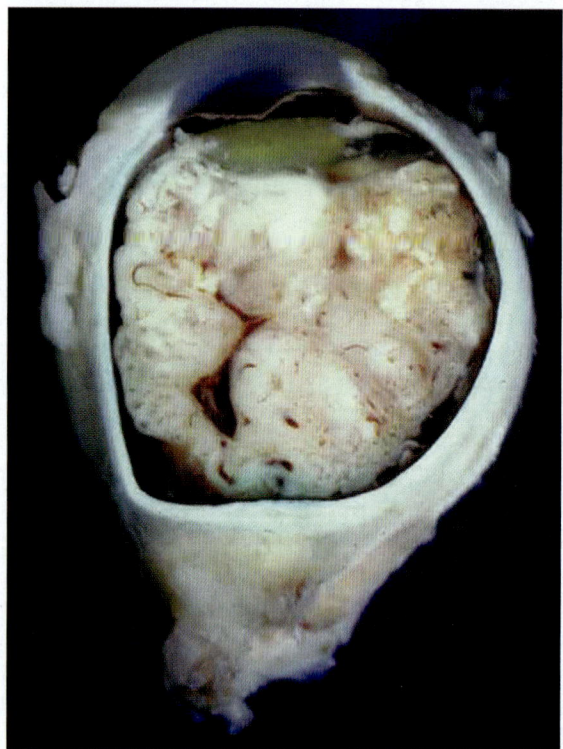

FIGURE 11-27 • Retinoblastoma. The tumor has filled the entire volume of the posterior segment and is displacing the lens–iris diaphragm anteriorly. The cut surface of the tumor has a "brain-like" quality. Multiple calcific highlights are present.

are rare and are associated with developmental abnormalities affecting the size of the globe (e.g., microphthalmos) and advanced cases with buphthalmos or frank rupture of the globe. On gross sectioning, the tumor has a brain-like consistency associated with focal areas of dystrophic calcification. The tumor may arise in any region of the retina. The location of greatest clinical significance is near the optic disc.

There are several growth patterns. The tumor may remain confined to the plane of the retina usually at the retinal periphery in a rare variant of retinoblastoma, diffuse infiltrating retinoblastoma. The usual tumor is densely white or gray with an irregular outline that is sharply demarcated from surrounding differentiated, uninvolved retina. In most cases, the tumor invades the vitreous (endophytic growth pattern), into the subretinal space (exophytic growth pattern), or both. Tumor within the vitreous is poorly supported by blood vessels and develops extensive areas of necrosis giving it a friable character that appears similar to inflammation within the vitreous. This form of tumor extension may also be associated with metastatic seeding to the surface of the retina or optic disc making the distinction between multiple primary sites and multiple metastatic sites difficult. The posterior chamber, the anterior chamber, and the surface of the optic disc may similarly be seeded by tumor from the vitreous. Tumor in the subretinal space is associated with serous fluid accumulating in the subretinal space and detaching the overlying retina. Advanced tumors may invade the choroidal tissues (69).

The final growth pattern is regression. Retinoblastoma may progress in one eye and regress in the other. The remaining tumor tissue is often extensively calcified and surrounded by RPE reaction for a variable distance from the main tumor.

The cross-sectional diameter of the optic disc in most patients is 1.5 mm. Immediately posterior to the lamina cribrosa, the ganglion cell axons acquire a myelin coat increasing the cross-sectional diameter of the optic nerve (dural sheaths and neural axis) to 3.0 mm. Any optic nerve cross-sectional diameter greater than 3.0 mm harbors extraocular retinoblastoma until proven otherwise. The desired length of the optic nerve specimen is a minimum of 10 mm. Removal of 20 mm of optic nerve is technically possible, even in a child. A short optic nerve specimen is a poor prognostic risk factor.

It is unusual for a cataract to form, except in the most advanced tumors characterized by extensive necrosis. In these cases, iris neovascularization and anterior chamber hemorrhage (hyphema) may be a presenting clinical feature.

The majority of the tumor cells are characterized by large vesicular nuclei with homogeneously dispersed chromatin of variable shape and size without a nucleolus. There is only a small amount of visible cytoplasm. Retinoblastoma cells are positive with S100 but are usually negative with glial fibrillary acidic protein (GFAP). Ultrastructurally, the cells contain few internal organelles. In some regions, there may be triplication of the nuclear membrane. Numerous mitotic figures are present throughout the tumor. There may be some background cells with features of glial cells; however, it is difficult to distinguish neoplastic glial cells from reactive glial cells originating in surrounding normally differentiated retina. Outside the confines of the retina (e.g., in the subretinal space), retinoblastoma cells tend to adhere to each other in small clusters. Multiple bizarre cells may be present. Inflammatory cells and macrophages may be present in vitreous samples.

There are several types of more differentiated cells generally grouping in the form of rosettes. Rosettes are composed of one or two layers of nuclei encircling a central space. Mitotic figures may be seen in the cells making up the rosettes. Some rosettes are incompletely formed and blend with the surrounding undifferentiated cells. Rosettes are usually found in random areas of greater differentiation rather than within areas of totally undifferentiated retinoblasts.

The most primitive and least specific of the forms is the Homer-Wright rosette. It is composed of poorly differentiated cells with distinct neuroblastoma-like features. The central portion of the rosette does not form a definitive lumen but contains neurofibrillary processes and is thought to be composed of cells with ganglion cell characteristics. This type of configuration is found in neuroblastoma of the adrenal gland and cerebellar medulloblastoma among others. The Homer-Wright rosette appears much less frequently in retinoblastoma than the Flexner-Wintersteiner rosette.

The Flexner-Wintersteiner rosette is more differentiated and more specific for retinoblastoma as compared with the Homer-Wright rosette (Figure 11-28). The layer of cuboidal cells is taller and has a more definite epithelial-like character. The apical portion of the cell forms an inner limiting structure of terminal bars, delimiting the cells from a central lumen. The central lumen contains acid mucopolysaccharide that is similar to the acid mucopolysaccharide found in the interphotoreceptor mucoid substance. Some cells may have characteristics of inner photoreceptor elements such as abundant nuclei, cytoplasmic microtubules, and 9 + 0 cilia. Occasionally, laminated membranous structures resembling the discs of rod outer segments have been identified.

The fleurette is the most differentiated and is the most specific for retinoblastoma but is identified in only 6% of cases of retinoblastoma. This type of rosette is more linear

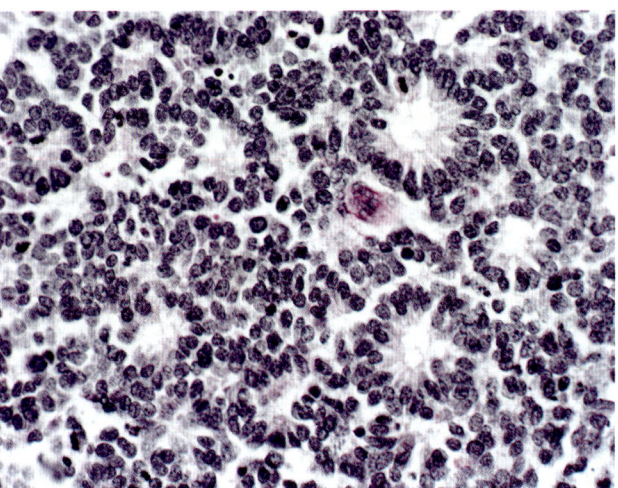

FIGURE 11-28 • Retinoblastoma. Flexner-Wintersteiner rosettes are an indication of tumor differentiation.

than round and is composed of more differentiated cells with small, less basophilic nuclei and prominent eosinophilic cytoplasm. Cytoplasmic processes extend through a fenestrated membrane in a cluster-like configuration suggesting a bouquet of flowers (i.e., a "fleurette"). There may be associated areas of deposited calcium, but mitotic figures are rare in fleurettes and there is no necrosis. The cells have ultrastructural characteristics of cone photoreceptors.

Tumor cells spread initially in the plane of the retina. There does not seem to be any architectural resistance of either the inner or outer retina to the advance of the tumor cells. The tumor spreads across the inner limiting membrane into the substance of the vitreous. In the vitreous, proliferation of blood vessels appears to be limited. Tumor cells are arranged in sleeves around dilated blood vessels originating in the retina. Approximately 50 to 200 cells are seen surrounding the lumen of blood vessels in contrast with the one to two cell layers that make up a true rosette. The thickness of the sleeve depends on the metabolic activity of the cells of the tumor. Twenty to one hundred and ten micrometers from the vessel lumen, there is ischemic necrosis and dystrophic calcification but little or no inflammatory infiltrate. Extensive cellular necrosis leads to liberation of substantial amounts of DNA that can deposit and be identified by light microscopy along the internal limiting membrane of the retina, along blood vessel walls, and along the posterior crystalline lens capsule.

The mode of spread for retinoblastoma includes local extension, extension into the optic nerve and intracranial spread, and hematogenous distant metastases. Spherules of tumor cells separate from the primary tumor in the vitreous and deposit on the inner limiting membrane and secondarily reinvade the retina at a site distant from the original tumor. Spherules also gain access to the posterior chamber where aqueous convection currents carry the cells to the iris surface and trabecular meshwork of the anterior chamber (Figure 11-29). Aqueous seeding may simulate a hypopyon (a layer of inflammatory cells in the inferior anterior chamber).

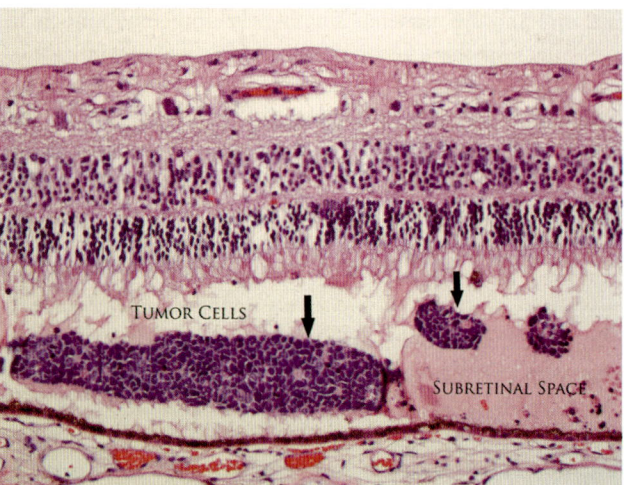

FIGURE 11-30 • Tumor cells (*arrows*) have extended from the plane of the retina into the subretinal space (hematoxylin–eosin stain, original magnification ×20).

Tumor cells readily cross the external limiting membrane of the retina and enter into the subretinal space (Figure 11-30). Disturbance of RPE function due to the presence of tumor cells breaks down the blood retinal barrier and allows fluid to accumulate in the subretinal space (serous retinal detachment). There is no secondary neovascularization to support tumor cells in the subretinal space. Nutrition appears to be derived from the serous fluid itself. Tumor cells become configured into spherules as in the vitreous cavity; however, the inner most cells of the spherules tend to be necrotic rather than the externally situated cells in the vitreous. Cells may obtain access to the space under the RPE and across Bruch membrane and choriocapillaris to the vessel-rich choroidal layer.

Retinoblastoma spreads in the plane of the retina, to the optic disc, through the lamina cribrosa into the substance of the optic nerve (Figure 11-31). Once beyond the lamina cribrosa, extraocular extension has occurred (Figure 11-32).

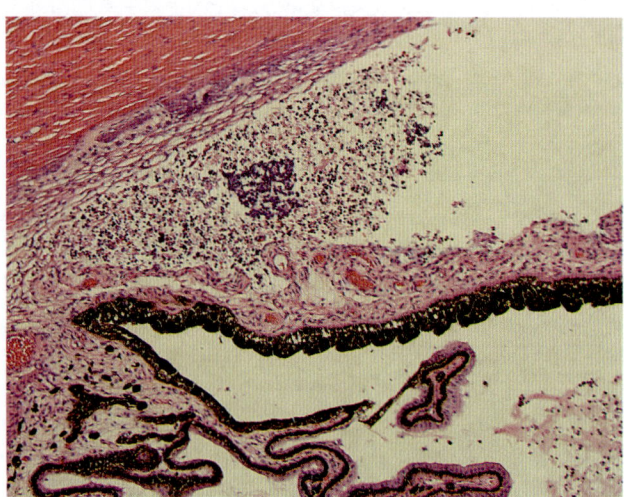

FIGURE 11-29 • Retinoblastoma. Both viable and necrotic tumors have extended into the anterior chamber in a case of advanced retinoblastoma (hematoxylin–eosin stain, original magnification ×40).

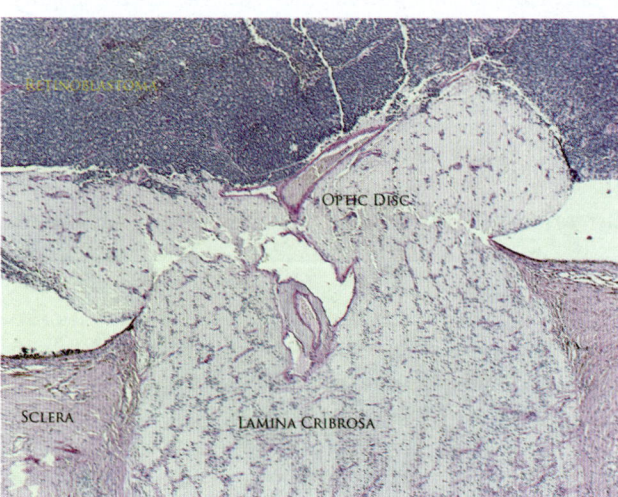

FIGURE 11-31 • Retinoblastoma. The intraocular retinoblastoma has extended to the superficial tissues of the optic disc but not through the lamina cribrosa (hematoxylin–eosin stain, original magnification ×20).

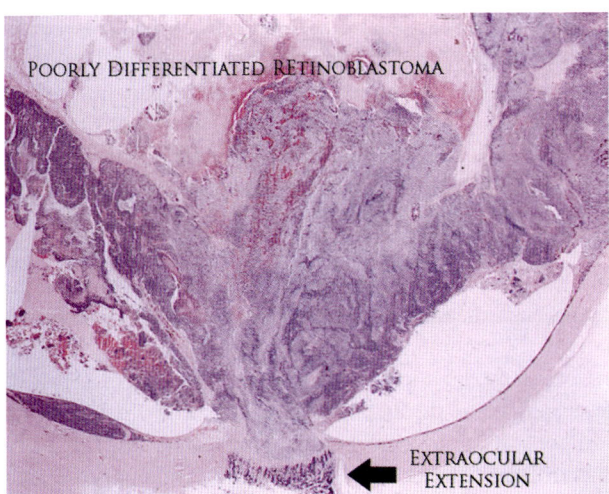

FIGURE 11-32 • Retinoblastoma. The tumor has spread beyond the lamina cribrosa to the optic nerve (hematoxylin–eosin stain, original magnification ×20).

The tumor in the optic nerve axis has access to the subarachnoid space through which it is able to spread throughout the central nervous system (Figure 11-33).

In the uveal tract, tumor cells have access to the intravascular compartment and may spread extensively to the liver, bones, and lungs. Massive choroidal invasion is defined as a mass of retinoblastoma cells measuring 3 mm or more and not reaching the sclera (Figures 11-34 and 11-35) (70). In the anterior chamber, tumor cells may traverse the trabecular meshwork to gain access to episcleral tissue including the lymphatics of the conjunctival stroma. The lymphatic channels collect at the preauricular nodes and submental nodes of the soft tissues of the face.

Tumor cells may escape the eye along surgical wounds in those unfortunate cases where retinoblastoma has been mis-

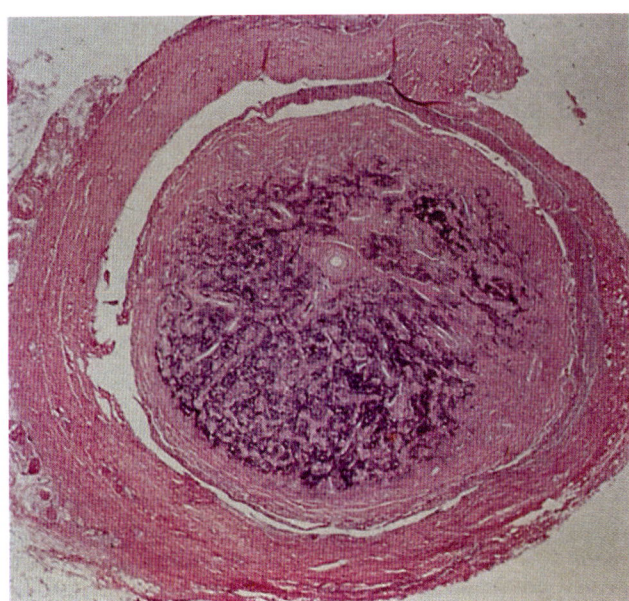

FIGURE 11-33 • Retinoblastoma tumor cells have completely replaced the axons of the optic nerve (hematoxylin–eosin stain, original magnification ×20).

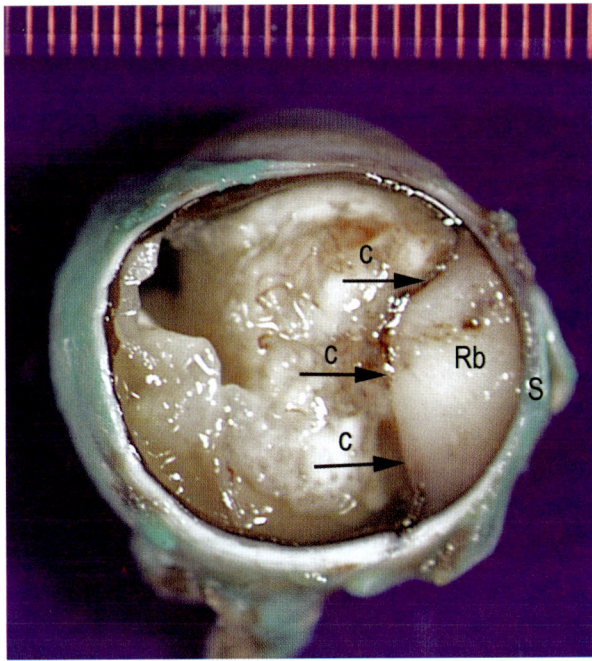

FIGURE 11-34 • Retinoblastoma. Massive invasion of the choroid has occurred. The main tumor has extended across the choroid [C] into the uveal tract (Rb). The tumor extends across the full thickness of the choroid and comes in contact with the sclera (S). The degree of involvement greatly exceeds 3 mm in dimension (actual measurement 18 × 10 × 10 mm) is a definite risk factor of extraocular extension.

interpreted as a congenital cataract and the cataract has been surgically removed.

In terms of prognostic factors, besides tumor size and location, a differentiated tumor with abundant Flexner-Wintersteiner rosettes has a better prognosis than one without rosettes. Similarly, a tumor composed entirely of fleurettes (retinocytoma) has a much better prognosis. Although many

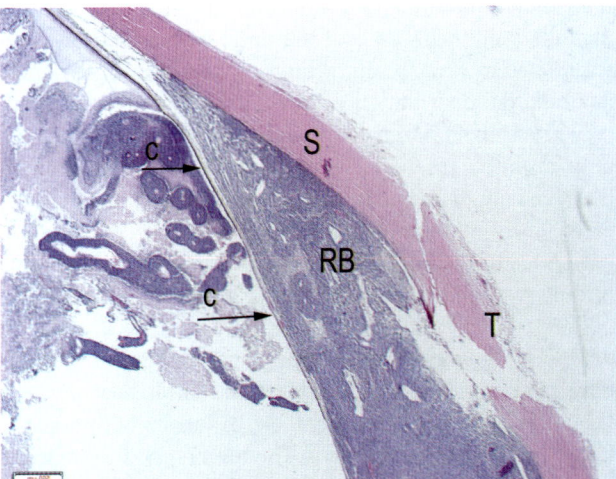

FIGURE 11-35 • Retinoblastoma. Choroidal invasion of the retinoblastoma (RB) occupies the extensive area of suprachoroidal space (between the choroid [C] and the sclera [S]). The hiatus in the sclera (T) is the site of postenucleation tumor tissue sampling for genetic studies. Access is with a 6.0-mm trephine (hematoxylin–eosin, original magnification ×02).

factors affect the prognosis, the most important is the extent of invasion by the retinoblastoma, with extension into the optic nerve and choroid being the two most important predictors of outcome and extraocular invasion being the most important predictor of death. Massive choroidal invasion and extension into the sclera are associated with a high incidence of systemic metastases. With respect to assessing extraocular extension, it is important to note that isolated episcleral "free-floating" tumor cells may sometimes represent artifact of dislodged tumor cells during opening of the globe. Subretinal pigment epithelial or superficial choroidal extension is frequent and is not very significant. Uveal inflammation in the presence of choroidal invasion is associated with a poor prognosis. Full-thickness choroidal involvement is associated with 60% mortality. Thus, massive choroidal involvement, deep choroidal involvement with emissarial extension short of the surface of the eye, concomitant choroidal inflammation, and a large tumor are associated with an adverse outcome. With respect to invasion of the optic nerve, invasion up to but not beyond the lamina cribrosa has relatively little prognostic significance, but invasion up to the line of transection is a poor prognostic sign. Tumor beyond the lamina cribrosa and involving the pia arachnoid also is associated with a poor prognosis. Presence of iris neovascularization is a poor prognostic sign and may relate to the quantitative volume of tumor and to significant choroidal invasion. Besides local extension and intracranial involvement, distant metastases may involve long bones and skull, viscera (most often the liver), and lymph nodes (71,72).

Treatment of retinoblastoma is case specific and includes argon laser photocoagulation, cryoablation, intravitreal chemotherapy, intra-arterial (ophthalmic artery) chemotherapy, and enucleation. The prognosis for retinoblastoma has improved in Western countries from high mortality to high survivability. In regions where accessibility to medical care is limited, the mortality remains high.

Medulloepithelioma is a rare tumor originating from the medullary epithelial cells of the optic vesicle that have differentiated toward the epithelium of the ciliary body. There is a bimodal distribution of tumors presenting as congenital lesions in children and acquired lesions in adults. In both instances, the clinical and histopathologic distinction between benign and malignant lesions may be difficult in the early stages of tumor progression. The single best differentiating feature is invasion of adjacent tissues and even that finding can be found in tumors with an indolent course.

Congenital medulloepitheliomas tend to arise in the first decade of life presenting with pain, decreased vision, a sectoral cataract (leukocoria), or increased intraocular pressure (73). The tumors are not heritable. A ciliary body mass is found by clinical examination. The tumors tend to be white or gray with an irregular, sometimes cystic surface. The cystic components of the tumor may separate from the primary mass and may float freely in the anterior chamber or even in the vitreous. Infrequently, the tumor may arise in the plane of the RPE or along the course of the optic nerve. The tumor is composed of primitive neuroblastic cells arranged in chords or sheets of cells associated with an extracellular matrix containing hyaluronic acid. Flexner-Wintersteiner (photoreceptor differentiation) and Homer-Wright rosettes (ganglion cell differentiation) lined by a single layer of cells may be present. In addition, primitive rosettes (ciliary epithelial differentiation) may be present; however, this type of rosette is lined by several layers of undifferentiated neuroepithelial cells. Reactive proliferation and formation of a cellular membrane may also occur and extend across the vitreous face. Because there is often an inconsistent degree of pleomorphism and variable mitotic activity, the natural history may be difficult to predict by cytologic features. Invasion of adjacent uveal structures, especially extension to and through the sclera, is a distinct risk factor for additional local invasion, although the tumor only rarely produces distant metastasis. Tumors significantly affecting ocular function are often treated with enucleation because of the uncertainty of the natural history of any individual tumor and the difficulty in determining the significance of involvement of adjacent structures, particularly the vitreous.

A subgroup of medulloepitheliomas (*teratoid medulloepithelioma*) contain heterotopic elements, particularly cartilage; however, brain and muscle tissue may also be present. Again, histologic clues to a malignant course are not distinctive enough for certain categorization. Tumors with heterotopic elements tend to have a more aggressive course. Treatment criteria for the two groups are similar because the heterotopic elements cannot be distinguished clinically with any degree of certainty. The overall mortality in one series was reported in the range of 10%.

Benign and malignant acquired medulloepitheliomas also occur but arise most often in adults. Again, the distinction between benign and malignant lesions may be difficult. Treatment is usually surgical depending on symptoms and volume of tumor (74). It is recognized that ocular medulloepithelium may occur in the DICER1-related disorders (74a).

THE OPTIC NERVE

Structure of the Optic Nerve

The optic disc is formed by the confluence of ganglion cell axons exiting through a canal in the posterior medial portion of the sclera to form the optic nerve. The hydraulic integrity of the globe at this point is maintained by a sieve-like structure, the lamina cribrosa, that interdigitates with the axons as they pass through the sclera. The majority of the fibers exit via large pores in the superior and inferior lamina. The exiting fibers form a central concavity, the optic cup, which is not covered by the internal limiting membrane of the retina but does contain glial tissue. The region is not supplied by the central retinal artery but by end arteries of the short posterior ciliary system, which is a branch of the ophthalmic artery.

Just beyond the lamina cribrosa, oligodendroglia form a myelin sheath around each axon. This addition increases the diameter of the optic nerve from 1.5 mm at the scleral canal to 3.0 mm in the myelinated portion. The axons of the optic nerve are supplied by branches of the ophthalmic artery in the arachnoid, extending across the subarachnoid space to the pia. The central retinal artery crosses the dura and arachnoid 12 mm posterior to the lamina to assume a central position in the proximal optic nerve but does not supply the optic nerve itself. The dura of the optic nerve is contiguous with the periosteum of the orbital apex and with the sclera. The subdural space is truncated or closed through the optic canal of the sphenoid bone. The subarachnoid space of the optic nerve is contiguous with the subarachnoid space of the central nervous system (1,2).

Surgical Procedures of the Optic Nerve

The optic nerve is a large structure, but is surgically inaccessible because of its position in the posterior orbit. The surgical approach often involves removal of a portion of the orbital rim or direct access via a crainiotomy. Fistulization of the meninges (optic nerve fenestration) has been attempted in certain limited medical conditions that do not usually affect the pediatric age group.

Optic nerve gliomas are juvenile pilocytic astrocytomas that cause fusiform enlargement of the optic nerve. In many cases, the tumor limits visual potential but is not a threat to the life of the child. Approximately 20% of persons with NF-1 will have optic nerve gliomas, but most children diagnosed with an optic pathway glioma have NF-1. These tumors may undergo malignant transformation (75,76). Only rarely will an optic nerve glioma extend into the eye. Two cytologic patterns are found in pilocytic astrocytomas: areas of fibrillar matrix with oval to round nuclei and a more mucoid matrix that may contain microcysts. Rosenthal fibers (intracellular electron-dense material surrounded by glial elements), eosinophilic granular bodies (membrane-bound intracellular osmophilic material), and microcalcifications also characterize the lesion. Neither Rosenthal fibers nor granular bodies are unique to pilocytic astrocytoma. Chemotherapy is the mainstay of treatment for cases with progressive loss of vision, though surgical resection of the optic nerve or enucleation may be necessary if there is sufficient proptosis to cause degeneration of the cornea or abnormal development of the orbit. The primary risk factor for a poor outcome is involvement of the optic chiasm (see Chapter 10) (77).

Meningioma of the optic nerve may arise in the arachnoid sheath of the optic nerve (primary optic nerve meningioma) or may involve the orbit from an intracranial meningioma, usually one situated along the sphenoid ridge. Optic nerve meningioma is uncommon. Most are of the transitional and meningotheliomatous types. They usually do not invade the eye itself but may cause proptosis and ophthalmoplegia due to mass effect of the tumor. Treatment is usually surgical. Treatment with external beam radiation is being evaluated (78).

THE ORBIT

Structure of the Orbit

The globe is housed in a 30-mL orbit bordered by bone that provides physical protection for the globe, primarily by the presence of the orbital rim. The interior orbit is separated from the soft tissues of the face by the orbital septum, a fibrous membrane that originates from the periosteum of the facial bones at the orbital rim. The rectus and oblique muscles have their origin at the periosteum of the orbital apex and function to align the two globes, allowing the brain to receive two slightly dissimilar images providing for perception of depth. The veins traversing the orbit have no valves. Direction of blood flow is determined by differential pressure gradients between the internal and external carotid systems. The only epithelial structure in the orbit is the lacrimal gland, a portion of which is located anterior to the orbital septum (the palpebral lobe) and a portion is posterior to the septum (the orbital lobe). The ducts from the orbital lobe extend through the palpebral lobe to reach ostia in forniceal region of the conjunctiva. There are no lymphatic channels or lymph nodes in the orbit except the lymphoid tissue associated directly with the lacrimal gland. The only cartilaginous structure in the orbit is the trochlea in the superior nasal orbit that serves as a pulley to direct orientation of the superior oblique tendon. Orbital soft tissue is divided into multiple intercommunicating compartments by delicate fibrous septa. The area between the rectus muscles has been referred to as the intraconal space, but that space has no unique functional or prognostic significance for tumors. Preseptal soft tissue forms the eyelids, the conjunctiva, and the lacrimal drainage apparatus. The eyelids protect the eye from the external environment and close when stimulated by visual threats, movement of the eyelashes, or disturbance of corneal sensation. The orbicularis oculi closes the eyelids, and the levator palpebrae open the eyelids. The eyelid is also responsible for forming and maintaining the tear film. The tear film has at least three functional layers: an aqueous portion that contains oxygen and other nutrients, a mucous portion that allows smooth layering of the aqueous portion, and a lipid portion that retards evaporation of the aqueous portion. The major volume of aqueous is not formed by the lacrimal gland in the orbit but is formed by accessory lacrimal gland acini located in the upper eyelid, the upper conjunctival fold (the fornix), and the conjunctiva directly covering the globe (bulbar conjunctiva). The lacrimal gland itself plays only a minor reflex role of tear film function. Tear film components exit via puncta located at the superior and inferior nasal eyelid margins. Tears and surface debris flow through the canaliculus to the nasal lacrimal duct and finally to the lateral wall of the nasal mucosa under the inferior turbinate. A pumping mechanism for aqueous is thought to function via contraction of the orbicularis oculi. The caruncle is a sequestered portion of the lower eyelid margin and contains all of the dermal elements of the eyelid but is covered by mucous membrane contiguous with the conjunctiva (1,2).

Tumors and Surgical Procedures of the Orbit

As indicated with the optic nerve, surgical approaches to the orbit are technically difficult and undertaken only with strong clinical indications. Lacrimal gland tissue is usually removed anteriorly through the skin and orbital septum. Particularly, when adenoid cystic carcinoma is encountered, bone in the region of the lacrimal fossa is often removed. Because of the evolution of treatment of rhabdomyosarcoma, only a biopsy sampling of the tumor is required prior to chemotherapy and radiation (although debulking procedures may be performed). In the past, the entire contents of the orbit including all eyelid tissue to the orbital rim (exenteration) were required. Tumors located in the posterior orbit are best approached via a frontal craniotomy. Occasionally, expanded orbital contents are decompressed into an adjacent sinus cavity such as in aggressive Graves disease. Release of trapped orbital contents in an orbital floor fracture is indicated only if the entrapped tissue causes major abnormalities of movement of the globe.

A *dermoid cyst* of orbital tissue is a cystic choristoma usually containing benign dermal elements that tend to progressively enlarge because of internal desquamation of the surface epithelium and adnexal units. The cyst arises from embryonic rests of mesenchyme that tend to be adjacent to membranous bones particularly in the region of facial fusion lines (79). A classification by location has been proposed. Juxtasutural cysts are often found along the orbital rim and are attached to bone by fibrous septa that do not distort the bone. Sutural dermoid cysts (including giant dermoid cysts) originate in the synostosis of orbital bones and may extend within cancellous bone or may extend either into the orbital cavity or into the intracranial cavity. This type of cyst is associated with defects of bone and may develop the appearance of a draining sinus. A soft tissue dermoid cyst develops within soft tissue and is not associated with bone.

Orbital dermoid cysts may develop either anterior or posterior to the orbital septum. Cysts present anterior to the orbital septum tend to occur at an earlier age (usually before age 5 years) and are often found at orbital rim suture lines. The cyst is usually a smooth, firm, nontender, oval mass along the superior orbital rim and is less than 2 cm in diameter. Cysts posterior to the orbital septum tend to be associated with intraorbital suture lines and present at a later age. Anteriorly positioned cysts may herniate through the orbital septum. Posterior lesions may extend through the superior orbital fissure or into the temporal fossa. Medial lesions generally do not extend into the ethmoid air cells, but superior cysts may extend into the frontal sinus. Most lesions present in the first two decades, although presentation in advanced age is also possible. There is no gender specificity.

There has been a distinction between epidermoid cysts that do not contain adnexal elements and dermoid cysts that do contain adnexal elements. However, the histologic distinction does not guide management and the general term dermoid cyst is most often used. The lining of the cyst is stratified, keratinizing squamous epithelium with or without adnexal units. When adnexal units are present, the cyst wall is usually more robust than in those lesions without adnexal units. The cyst may contain desquamated squamous epithelium, cholesterol, hemorrhage (hemosiderin), hair, or calcium. The contents may subdivide into various fluid levels. In regions were the cyst wall has ruptured, there is granulomatous foreign body reaction and fibrous reaction that may be extensive.

Generally, there is progressive enlargement of the lesion because of expanding volume of the intraluminal contents. Continuous pressure may cause erosion through bone into contiguous tissues and spaces. There is no malignant transformation. Treatment is surgical excision with care to remove the cyst intact as ruptured contents are highly proinflammatory and rupture increases the likelihood of incomplete excision of the cyst wall and recurrence. Lesions that are fixed to bone, in an atypical location, or occur in the clinical setting of craniofacial dysostosis may extend intracranially and should be imaged prior to excision to define their extent.

Langerhans cell histiocytosis (LCH) is a clonal proliferative disorder with multiple clinically distinct forms (Hand-Schüller-Christian disease, Letterer-Siwe disease, and eosinophilic granuloma). The pathophysiology of LCH is not fully understood; however, there is no evidence of metabolic abnormality or infection (80). Recurrent mutation in the BRAF gene has been demonstrated in 57% of cases (81) The Langerhans cell is an immune-processing cell of the monocyte–macrophage system found among the squamous epithelial cells in the skin, in bone marrow, and in the paracortical region of lymph nodes as well as multiple other sites. Despite the clinical dissimilarity, all these diseases have a histologic pattern that suggests a granulomatous inflammatory infiltrate containing pathologic Langerhans cells. The normal Langerhans cell has dendritic processes, an eccentric folded nucleus, small nucleolus, and a cytoplasmic structure, the Birbeck granules that have central striation and a "tennis racket" profile. The function of the Birbeck granule is unknown, but it appears to be composed of plasma membrane components.

The light microscopic pattern of LCH is that of chronic granulomatous inflammation characterized by an infiltrate of histiocytes, lymphocytes, giant cells, and eosinophils. The presence of eosinophils is not essential for the diagnosis of LCH. Pathologic Langerhans cells lack dendritic processes but retain Birbeck granules. S100 positivity differentiates Langerhans cells from other macrophages. Birbeck granules can be detected only by transmission electron microscopy and are found in only 20% of the cases studied. Langerhans cells can be identified by CD1a and Langerin stains. The number of CD1a-stained cells generally decreases as the lesion matures or regresses.

The prevalence of LCH in children under age 15 years ranges between 4.6 and 8.9 per 100,000 (82,83). There have been no reported instances of familial, time, or geographic location clustering (80). There appears to be no gender specificity. LCH may present as a single system disease with a lesion in a single tissue type or a multisystem disease including disseminated forms. Orbital involvement most often presents as a single system disease of orbital bone. The onset of proptosis is acute, and there are associated signs of inflammation.

The degree of involvement is highly variable. When the lesion is located in orbital bones, there has been concern that there would be progression to central nervous system involvement and such lesions have been treated with chemotherapy with conflicting opinions about long-term benefit. Extraocular lesions of sufficient size may cause intraocular findings of compression (choroidal folds, optic disc swelling) and compressive optic neuropathy. Rarely, LCH may present as uveitis where a vitreous biopsy could be interpreted as containing only macrophages and other benign inflammatory cells (unless stained for CD1a). Secondary glaucoma may develop if the trabecular meshwork is affected. The eyelid skin is unusually not involved. Late recurrences have been reported (see Chapters 22 and 27). Single system disease survival is nearly 100%. Multisystem disease survival is associated with an 80% survival. Age at presentation of less than 1 year is a risk factor for a poor prognosis. LCH itself is a risk factor for secondary malignancy including Hodgkin lymphoma and acute leukemia. Treatment includes surgical debulking, chemotherapy, and simple observation.

Lymphangioma is a developmental abnormality of lymphatic vessels and their precursor cells and lymphoid tissue in the soft issue of the orbit. Normally, no lymphatic channels or populations of lymphocytes are found in the orbit; thus, this lesion is a choristoma and presents at birth, although the condition may not present clinically until advanced age. One clinical classification is by the character of hemodynamics in the lesion (no flow, venous flow, or arterial flow) that guides surgical and other means of therapy (84). There is no gender specificity with the majority of lesions presenting in the first decade.

Lesions of various sizes and degrees of functional significance may be found in the eyelid, the conjunctiva, anterior (preseptal) orbital soft tissue, and posterior (postseptal) orbital soft tissue. The eye itself is not involved. Noncontinuous vascular lesions may be present in patients with intracranial vascular lesions. The size of the lymphangioma may vary with posture, straining, or inflammation of the upper respiratory tract. There is usually less effect during indolent periods on the optical system than that found with hemangioma of similar volume. There is minimal pain unless acute hemorrhage suddenly expands the volume of the lesion. In this circumstance, there may be various degrees of loss of vision, development of an afferent pupillary defect, choroidal folds, optic disc swelling, and compressive optic neuropathy (potentially to the point of complete and permanent loss of vision). Hemorrhage may be spontaneous or associated with trauma and is more likely to occur in a child or adolescent than in older persons. This event is also more likely in the postoperative period after debulking procedures. Long-standing lesions beginning in childhood may result in expansion of the orbital contours.

The gross appearance is that of diffuse lesion with no external capsule. The cut surface is composed of vascular channels of various sizes that may contain translucent fluid or hemorrhage or both. The vascular channels are separated by fibrous septa that also may contain areas of fresh to old brownish hemorrhage. The vascular channels are lined by low-profile vascular endothelial cells with little apparent support by pericytes or extracellular matrix. Within the fibrous septa, there are variable amounts of lymphoid tissue, some of which may contain germinal centers. By transmission electron microscopy, endothelial cell gaps and fragmented basement membrane may be seen.

Treatment is limited to embolization and surgical debulking. Multiple procedures are often necessary. In extreme cases, due to corneal exposure and ulceration, enucleation of the eye may be necessary (85).

Idiopathic inflammatory disease of the orbit (also known as inflammatory pseudotumor of the orbit) is a syndrome of inflammation of the soft tissues of the orbit of undetermined cause. The condition may arise at any age (range 2 to 89 years) with no gender predilection. Approximately 5% of cases arise in the 2 to 18 years age group. The usual presentation is orbital pain. The onset is often explosive and may be either unilateral or bilateral. The bilateral cases may be simultaneous or sequential. The presentation tends to be bilateral in children (44%). Other common findings are ophthalmoparesis, proptosis, and a palpable mass. Cerebrospinal fluid pleocytosis may be present in cases of extraorbital inflammation. Imaging findings include thickening of extraocular muscles including the tendon insertion to the sclera (in contrast with thyroid ophthalmopathy where the tendon is spared), lacrimal gland enlargement, contrast enhancement of the sclera, and inflammation of orbital fat. Histologic findings include pleomorphic inflammation, fibrovascular tissue proliferation, and fat necrosis (granulomatous inflammation to fat necrosis). There is no clonal restriction. The plasma cells may be IgG4 positive (6). Early in the course of the disease, there is a fine collagenous stroma and a rich cellular infiltrate consisting of plasma cells, eosinophils, and lymphocytes. Later in the course of disease, there is often a dense deposition of extracellular matrix and a granulomatous pattern in the region of fat necrosis. The rate of progression and response to treatment is variable. Bilaterality is a risk factor for poor therapeutic response. The histologic character of the lesion may not be predictive of therapeutic success. Treatment is high-dose systemic prednisone or periocular steroid injections in localized cases. Radiation and other immunomodulatory drugs are reserved for refractory cases (86).

Rhabdomyosarcoma is the most common sarcoma in children as a proliferation of primitive rhabdomyoblasts. There are two distinct clinical presentations. The most characteristic is the sudden, unexplained onset of signs of inflammation in a child suggestive of preseptal or orbital cellulitis, except that there is no response to conventional treatment, indicating that a biopsy is necessary. In the embryonal variant, there may be marked pleomorphism of cells, which are often spindled, with prominent nucleoli and a variable degree of cytoplasmic eosinophilia. Rarely, actin and myosin filaments may be identified by PTAH staining. Myosin filaments and sarcomeric units with Z-banding are evident in the tumor cells by transmission electron microscopy. The immunohistochemical profile is positive for desmin, smooth muscle actin, and focally for myogenin. A rare subtype is the botryoid rhabdomyosarcoma that may present in the subconjunctival space or anterior orbital soft tissues, suggestive of a lymphoma. It is most often seen in older children and its prognosis is more favorable than with other types of rhabdomyosarcoma.

In older children, the alveolar variant may present in paraorbital sinuses and secondarily may involve the tissues of the orbit. Clinical signs are those of a soft tissue mass in the orbit or more likely in the ethmoid sinuses with temporal displacement of the globe. The tumor is composed of aggregation of primitive round cells with an acellular center vaguely suggestive of alveoli of a normal lung. Positive immunohistochemical markers include those for muscle with strong reactivity for myogenin (also see Chapter 25).

Treatment of orbital rhabdomyosarcoma is no longer surgical (orbital exenteration) but a combination of chemotherapy and radiation after diagnostic fine needle aspiration or biopsy (87). Mutation-associated sarcomas have a worse prognosis.

Tumors of the lacrimal gland, which is the only epithelial structure of the orbit, most often tend to be the result of inflammation or lymphoma, generally in the adult age groups. The most common epithelial tumor of the lacrimal gland is pleomorphic adenoma (benign mixed tumor), which is generally found in adults. The most common malignant tumor of the lacrimal gland is *adenoid cystic carcinoma*, which can occur in the pediatric age group. Early clinical signs and tumefaction of this neoplasm may be subtle. The most common histologic pattern is that of proliferation of small cells with hyperchromatic nuclei in a "Swiss cheese" pattern. Solid, basaloid, and sclerosis patterns are also possible. The tumor tends to spread early due to its propensity to involve perineural spaces, to adjacent orbital bone. Evaluation of surgical margins in this situation is at best problematic. The long-term outcome for all cases is generally poor (88).

OCULAR TRAUMA

The most common indication for the surgical removal of an eye in the pediatric age group is trauma. Loss of visual function of the eye is usually due to a combination of hemorrhage, inflammation, and ultimately glaucoma.

Accidental trauma to the eye is categorized into nonpenetrating or penetrating trauma. The distinction is important in guiding the initial therapy of the injured eye. Generally, a nonpenetrating injury does not require surgical repair, although the degree of injury in many cases exceeds that found in penetrating injury. Surgical repair is usually necessary in cases of penetrating trauma (open globe injury).

In most cases of severe trauma treated with enucleation, there is a rupture or laceration of the corneal–scleral coat, the "eye wall." Most ruptures are found in the region of the corneal–scleral limbus, which is a normally thin region of the eye wall. Lacerations are also most commonly found in the anterior eye wall but may also be located posteriorly. By the time of enucleation, there usually has been fibrovascular repair of the eye wall wound that can be identified by discontinuity of the collagen pattern, rupture of Bowman or Descemet membrane, or interruption of one of the pigmented coats of the eye. The anterior chamber is usually disorganized and PAS are present. The lens may be totally absent, be represented by crystalline lens remnants (best identified by periodic acid/Schiff staining), or show changes of anterior or posterior fibrous metaplasia of the crystalline lens epithelial cells. The retina is most often detached with blood or serous fluid in the subretinal space. The surface of the retina may undulate due to the formation of a contracted membrane on its surface (epiretinal membrane). The vitreous may be contracted and filled with inflammatory cells or with proliferating fibrovascular tissue (proliferative vitreoretinopathy). There may be hemorrhage within, superficial to, or deep to any of the coats of the eye. The choroid may be infiltrated by nongranulomatous or granulomatous inflammatory cells either diffusely (see below) or focally. The optic nerve frequently has signs of early or advanced atrophy (62).

The eye may be collapsed if there has been loss of intraocular contents, including the lens, vitreous, and retina. Intraocular foreign material may be present, depending on the nature of the original injury. Identifying foreign material is aided by the use of polarized light.

The eye is removed within 2 weeks, if there is no clinical indication of retention of useful vision (no light perception) in order to reduce the risk of losing vision in the contralateral eye because of sympathetic ophthalmia.

Sympathetic ophthalmia is a bilateral granulomatous inflammation of the uveal tract appearing 5 days to many years following trauma to one of the two eyes. The inflammation is thought to be due to an autoimmune response to an unknown type of antigen that is expressed during trauma. The first clinical indication of the presence of sympathetic ophthalmia is a loss of the ability to focus at near objects (accommodation) followed by a generalized uveitis. Untreated, the uveitis in the initially uninvolved eye may be more severe than in the injured eye. The major histologic sign is a granulomatous inflammatory response in any portion of the uveal tract characterized by epithelioid histiocytes and giant cells. The giant cells may contain melanin pigment, but this finding is not specific to sympathetic ophthalmia. There is generally an intense infiltrate of lymphocytes but not plasma cells or eosinophils in the surrounding tissue. Epithelioid histiocytes also accumulate between the RPE and Bruch membrane (Dalen-Fuchs nodules) (Figure 11-36). Dalen-Fuchs nodules may also be found in sarcoid uveitis. There may be some sparing of the choriocapillaris in the noninjured (sympathizing) eye, but the finding is not specific for sympathetic ophthalmia. An inflammatory reaction to exposed lens protein (lens-induced uveitis or phacoanaphylactic endophthalmitis) is also found in some cases. All of the histologic findings are nonspecific. To establish the

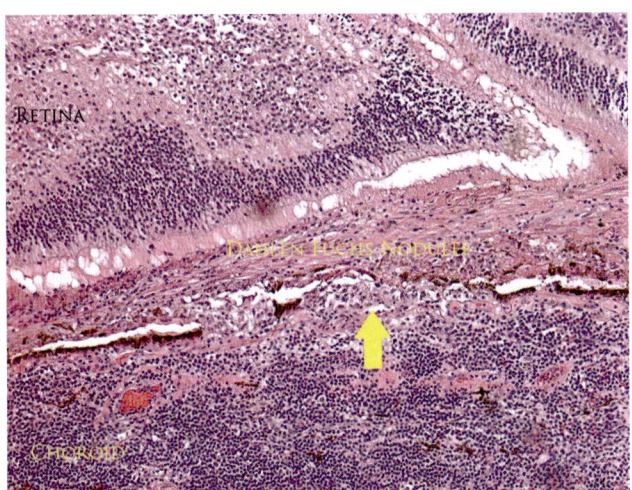

FIGURE 11-36 • Sympathetic ophthalmia. There is a massive chronic granulomatous inflammatory infiltration of the uveal tract. Epithelioid histiocytes have accumulated between the RPE and Bruch membrane (*arrow*). The features of the retina are distorted by trauma, inflammation, and sectioning artifacts (hematoxylin–eosin stain, original magnification ×40).

diagnosis of sympathetic ophthalmia, there must be a history of some type of ocular trauma, which may include such surgical procedures such as cyclocryotherapy (freezing of the ciliary body to treat intractable glaucoma) or pars plana vitrectomy (see above).

Eyes removed within the 2-week risk period for sympathetic ophthalmia may still have suture material at sites of penetration of the sclera and may also have surgical appliances used in retinal detachment repair (scleral buckles) and treatment of glaucoma (glaucoma filtration devices) on the episcleral surface. There may be considerable fibrosis from the episcleral tissue at sites of injury and at surgical sites even a few days after the original injury.

Eyes removed months or years following trauma are generally small and shrunken and have assumed a cuboidal shape (phthisis) (Figure 11-37). The ocular degeneration may be so advanced as to make identification of laterality difficult. The most reliable landmarks are the insertion of the superior and inferior oblique muscles. On sectioning, there may be extreme resistance because of dystrophic calcification both in the remaining lens tissue and in the plane of the RPE. Decalcification for several days is often necessary. Histologically, there is often scarring and vascularization of the cornea, complete fibrosis of the anterior chamber, atrophy of the iris, cataract (portions of which may be calcified), total retinal detachment with atrophy and gliosis, fibrosis of the vitreous, and, most often, profound optic atrophy. The most important observations are those of the uveal tract to determine the presence or absence of sympathetic ophthalmia. In adults, it is also important to determine if this "blind painful eye" has been harboring a neoplasm such as malignant melanoma (62).

Orbital and Ocular Surgery After Trauma

In cases of intraocular tumor or advanced degeneration of the eye from trauma or other insults (atrophia bulbi, phthisis bulbi), the entire eye is removed (enucleation). The volume of the eye is replaced with a spherical implant (e.g., acrylic, porous polyethylene, hydroxyapatite, or dermis fat graft) to which the rectus muscles are ideally reattached and covered with conjunctiva. A contact lens–like prosthesis ("glass eye") is then placed behind the eyelids but anterior to the conjunctiva. The prosthesis should be removed and cleaned similar to cleaning a contact lens. In some circumstances, particularly with advanced endophthalmitis, and when there is no evidence of intraocular malignancy, the cornea and ocular contents are removed leaving the rectus muscles attached to the sclera, which is left in place (evisceration). Processed coral material (hydroxyapatite) is placed in the scleral shell. Fibrous tissue will grow into and stabilize the coral relative to the sclera. A prosthesis is attached to the coral by a peg, which extends through a fistula in the conjunctiva. Increased mobility of the prosthesis is the clinical advantage to evisceration versus enucleation.

AUTOPSY SPECIMENS OF THE EYE

Removing the eyes of a child at autopsy is a very uncommon event, except when there is suspicion of child abuse homicide. Globes may be removed via an anterior approach as with surgical enucleation or may be removed through a window created in orbital roof. Whichever approach is used, it is important to obtain as much optic nerve as possible and to obtain a sample of orbital fat.

In most cases of death due to shaking or simple blunt force injury in which death occurred shortly following the injury, there is little external sign of trauma. There is also usually no abnormality of the cornea, anterior chamber, or external surface of the globe. It is important to note any signs of scleral thinning indicated by a blue tinge of the sclera, which may be found in very young infants or in individuals affected by

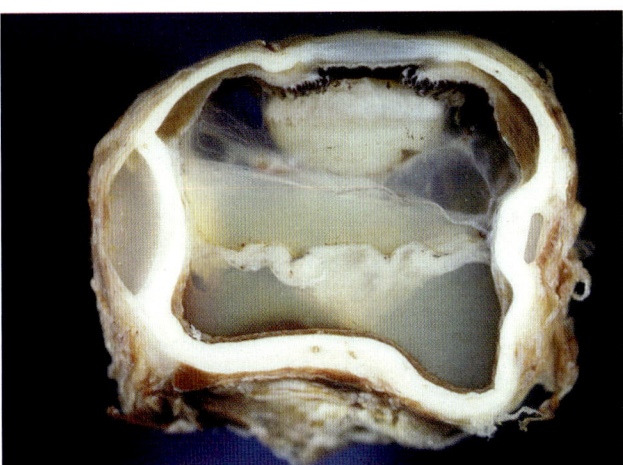

FIGURE 11-37 • Phthisis. This eye has degenerated following surgical repair for a detached retina. The eye is small and cuboidal in shape.

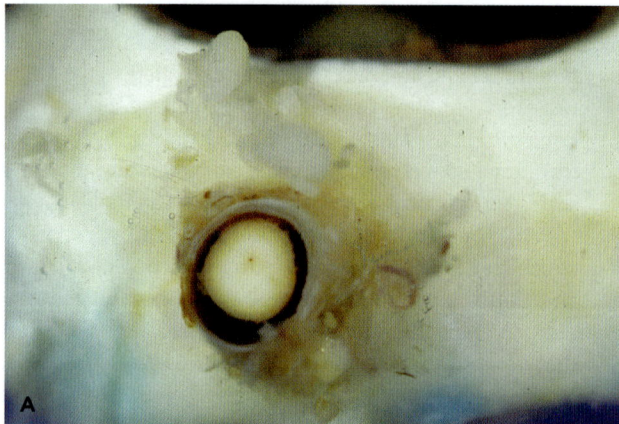
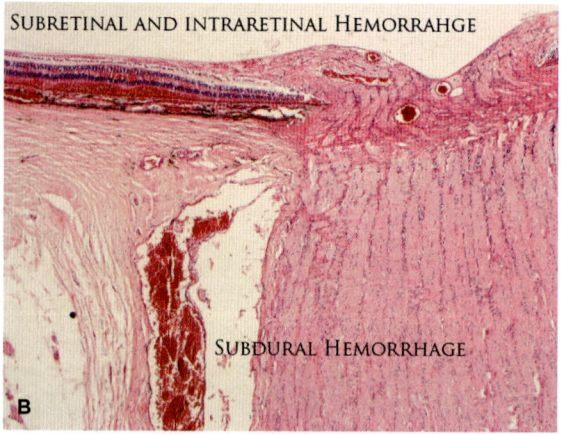

FIGURE 11-38 • Nonaccidental trauma. **A:** The cross section of the optic nerve is normal at 3.0 mm. There is extensive hemorrhage in the subdural and subarachnoid spaces. **B:** Subdural and subretinal hemorrhages are present in this low-magnification view.

osteogenesis imperfecta. Subdural and subarachnoid hemorrhage of the optic nerve is indicated also by a blue-to-gray discoloration of the dura. Cross sections of the optic nerve itself are normal in diameter and character; however, there may be marked expansion of the dural and subdural spaces by hemorrhage (Figure 11-38). On sectioning of the eye, the cornea, lens, and anterior chamber generally are normal. Retinal hemorrhages may be present. The location and extent of the intraretinal hemorrhage, particularly if the hemorrhage extends to the ora serrata, is an important observation (Figure 11-39). The retina in the region of the macula may also be elevated. Hemorrhage may extend into the vitreous itself. Histologically, the hemorrhages may be located completely within the architecture of the retina (intraretinal), between the neurosensory retina and the RPE (subretinal), between the retina and the cortex of the vitreous (subhyaloid), or within the vitreous (intravitreal). There may also be signs of disruption of the internal limiting membrane in the region of the macula. Hemorrhage may also be noted in the sclera at the insertion of the dura of the optic nerve (the circle of Zinn-Haller). Hemorrhage may be found in the surrounding orbital fat (see Chapter 7).

In cases where the child died after a longer interval from abuse, the hemorrhages may be less apparent. There may be atrophy and gliosis in the region of resolved retinal hemorrhage. There may or may not be hemosiderin staining in the area of suspected former hemorrhage. There may be considerable optic atrophy (89).

SUMMARY

The most common eyelid specimens in the pediatric age group usually consist of inflammatory lesions: molluscum contagiosum and chalazion. Most important lesions would be those of metastatic neuroblastoma in very young children and rhabdomyosarcoma in slightly older children. There is a variant of rhabdomyosarcoma with a subconjunctival presentation, the botryoid variant. Basal cell carcinoma and squamous cell carcinoma can occur with xeroderma pigmentosum but are otherwise uncommon. Sebaceous cell carcinoma can occur but again is extremely rare.

Conjunctival nevus may be an important clinical problem in the pediatric age group. Malignant melanoma can occur in

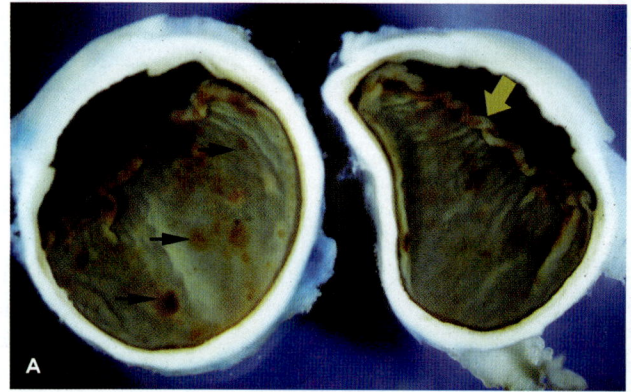
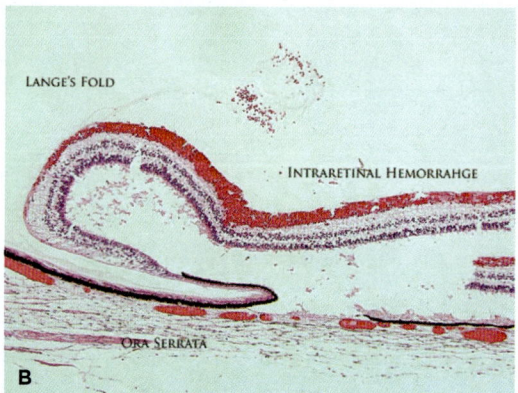

FIGURE 11-39 • Nonaccidental trauma. **A:** Hemorrhages are found throughout the retina (*black arrows*) and extend as far anteriorly as the ora serrata (*yellow arrow*). **B:** Intraretinal hemorrhage is shown extending to the ora serrata.

very young children, but most of the pigmented lesions will be nevi. Concern is generated because of enlarging size due to expansion of subepithelial squamous cysts, increased pigmentation found during adolescence, and inflammation of the nevus from a combination of factors. Pterygium and squamous cell carcinoma are found generally in a much older age group.

Corneal tissue is most often evaluated because of surgical treatment of keratoconus. Confirmatory findings include focal ruptures of Bowman membrane and occasionally rupture of Descemet membrane (corneal hydrops). Other corneal specimens will be submitted following accidental trauma and will show evidence of repair with fibrous proliferation. Corneal dystrophies, except for CHED in some restricted geographic areas, are not commonly treated with surgery in this age group. An important biopsy evaluation would be for *Acanthamoeba* keratitis, particularly if there is a history of correction of refractive error with soft contact lenses.

Cataracts in this age group are treated surgically, but the tissue is generally not examined histologically.

Retina, vitreous, and uveal tract are very infrequently evaluated by fine needle aspiration biopsy. The major exception would be anterior chamber paracentesis for diffuse infiltrating retinoblastoma as a differential diagnosis in the evaluation of protracted intermediate uveitis, both found in the older child–younger teenage group. Congenital melanoma of the uveal tract has been reported, but uveal melanoma generally occurs in the fifth to sixth decade.

The most common orbital lesions in children include ruptured dermoid cyst and various vascular developmental abnormalities such as lymphangioma. Idiopathic orbital inflammation (orbital inflammatory pseudotumor) can occur in children where the presentation is often bilateral and the progression more aggressive. Rhabdomyosarcoma has a predilection for orbital tissue in children. Surgical treatment for rhabdomyosarcoma is now not as common as formerly, being replaced currently by combinations of chemotherapy and occasionally radiation. The biopsy of orbital tumor tissue is often essential in managing treatment strategies for rhabdomyosarcoma. Adenoid cystic carcinoma of the lacrimal gland can occur in children. Its treatment at any age is difficult as the outcome tends to be poor.

The treatment of retinoblastoma is in rapid evolution. Enucleation, once the standard of care for all cases of retinoblastoma, is now done selectively and often after prior treatment with chemotherapy, cryotherapy, photocoagulation, transpupillary thermotherapy, and, occasionally, radiation. All therapeutic efforts will change the histologic appearance of the primary tumor. Definite histologically defined risk factors, especially optic nerve involvement by the retinoblastoma tumor, continue to guide therapy when enucleation is performed. The most important part of gross examination of a retinoblastoma eye is extremely careful evaluation of the surgical margin at the site of transection of the optic nerve. Sections of the retinoblastoma eye must include levels through the optic disc.

Most eyes enucleated in children are the result of irreparable trauma to the eye. The most important histologic observations include those for diffuse granulomatous inflammation of the uveal tract with or without signs of Dalen-Fuchs nodules (i.e., sympathetic ophthalmia). Sarcoidosis and other inflammatory lesions may have exactly the same histologic appearance as sympathetic ophthalmia. Correlation of histopathologic findings of the pathologist with clinical findings of the ophthalmologist is essential in establishing the diagnosis of sympathetic ophthalmia. Eyes removed many years following the original trauma may even become small externally and distorted internally (phthisis bulbi). The evaluation for sympathetic ophthalmia remains an important function of the pathologist even if the interval between the injury and enucleation has been decades.

Autopsy eye specimens are usually collected for assessment of ocular developmental abnormalities as part of evaluation for congenital syndromes (e.g., trisomy 13 or 18) or as a part of a homicide investigation for child abuse. In cases of suspected nonaccidental injury, important observations include external signs of ocular injury; the apparent thinness of the sclera (osteogenesis imperfecta); sign of cataract formation; the presence, location, and extent of retinal hemorrhage; the presence and extent of vitreous hemorrhage; the presence and extent of subretinal hemorrhage; signs of traction retinal detachment; signs of intrascleral hemorrhage at the scleral insertion of the dura of the optic nerve (circle of Zinn-Haller); the presence of hemorrhage in the soft tissues of the orbit; presence and extent of subdural and subarachnoid hemorrhage; and finally the presence and degree of optic atrophy.

References

1. Hogan MJ, Alvarado JA, Weddell JE. *Histology of the Human Eye*. Philadelphia, PA: W.B. Saunders Company; 1971.
2. Fine B, Yanoff M. *Ocular Histology. A Text and Atlas*, 2nd ed. New York: Harper and Row; 1979.
3. Levi M, Schwartz S, Blei F, et al. Surgical treatment of capillary hemangiomas causing amblyopia. *J AAPOS* 2007;11(3):230–234.
4. Verity DH, Restori M, Rose GE. Natural history of periocular capillary haemangiomas: changes in internal blood velocity and lesion volume. *Eye* 2006;20(10):1228–1237.
5. Egbert JE, Schwartz GS, Walsh AW. Diagnosis and treatment of an ophthalmic artery occlusion during an intralesional injection of corticosteroid into an eyelid capillary hemangioma. *Am J Ophthalmol* 1996;121(6):638–642.
6. Jakobiec FA, Stacy RC, Mehta M, et al. IgG4-positive dacryoadenitis and Kuttner submandibular sclerosing inflammatory tumor. *Arch Ophthalmol* 2010;128(7):942–944.
7. Chambers CB, Katowitz WR, Katowitz JA, et al. A controlled study of topical 0.25% timolol maleate gel for the treatment of cutaneous infantile capillary hemangiomas. *Ophthal Plast Reconstr Surg* 2012;28(2):103–106.
8. Shirley MD, Tang H, Gallione CJ, et al. Sturge-Weber syndrome and port-wine stains caused by somatic mutation in GNAQ. *N Engl J Med* 2013;368(21):1971–1979.
9. Paulus YM, Jain A, Moshfeghi DM. Resolution of persistent exudative retinal detachment in a case of Sturge-Weber syndrome with anti-VEGF administration. *Ocul Immunol Inflamm* 2009;17(4):292–294.

10. Godfraind C, Calicchio ML, Kozakewich H. Pyogenic granuloma, an impaired wound healing process, linked to vascular growth driven by FLT4 and the nitric oxide pathway. *Mod Pathol* 2013;26(2):247–255.
11. Bagheri A, Hasani HR, Karimian F, et al. Effect of chalazion excision on refractive error and corneal topography. *Eur J Ophthalmol* 2009;19(4):521–526.
12. Bains A, Parham DM. Langerhans cell histiocytosis preceding the development of juvenile xanthogranuloma: a case and review of recent developments. *Pediatr Dev Pathol* 2011;14(6):480–484.
13. Shields CL, Thaler AS, Lally SE, et al. Massive macronodular juvenile xanthogranuloma of the eyelid in a newborn. *J AAPOS* 2014;18(2):195–197.
14. Olsen JR, Gallacher J, Piguet V, et al. Epidemiology of molluscum contagiosum in children: a systematic review. *Fam Pract* 2014;31(2):130–136.
15. Georgakopoulos CD, Eliopoulou MI, Stasinos S, et al. Periorbital and orbital cellulitis: a 10-year review of hospitalized children. *Eur J Ophthalmol* 2010;20(6):1066–1072.
16. Plaza JA, De Stefano D, Suster S, et al. Intradermal spitz nevi: a rare subtype of spitz nevi analyzed in a clinicopathologic study of 74 cases. *Am J Dermatopathol* 2014;36(4):283–294; quiz 295–287.
17. Hiscott P, Seitz B, Naumann GO. Epithelioid cell Spitz nevus of the eyelid. *Am J Ophthalmol* 1998;126(5):735–737.
18. Slade AD, Austin MT. Childhood melanoma: an increasingly important health problem in the USA. *Curr Opin Pediatr* 2014;26(3):356–361.
19. Sinha S, Cohen PJ, Schwartz RA. Nevus of Ota in children. *Cutis* 2008;82(1):25–29.
20. Munoz-Hidalgo L, Lopez-Gines C, Navarro L, et al. BRAF V600E mutation in two distinct meningeal melanocytomas associated with a nevus of ota. *J Clin Oncol* 2014;32(20):e72–e75.
21. Radhadevi CV, Charles KS, Lathika VK. Orbital malignant melanoma associated with nevus of ota. *Indian J Ophthalmol* 2013;61(6):306–309.
22. Chaurasia S, Mulay K, Ramappa M, et al. Corneal changes in xeroderma pigmentosum: a clinicopathologic report. *Am J Ophthalmol* 2014;157(2):495–500 e492.
23. Honavar SG, Shields JA, Shields CL, et al. Basal cell carcinoma of the eyelid associated with Gorlin-Goltz syndrome. *Ophthalmology* 2001;108(6):1115–1123.
24. Hutt-Cabezas M, Karajannis MA, Zagzag D, et al. Activation of mTORC1/mTORC2 signaling in pediatric low-grade glioma and pilocytic astrocytoma reveals mTOR as a therapeutic target. *Neuro Oncol* 2013;15(12):1604–1614.
25. Morales J, Chaudhry IA, Bosley TM. Glaucoma and globe enlargement associated with neurofibromatosis type 1. *Ophthalmology* 2009;116(9):1725–1730.
26. Honavar SG, Singh AD, Shields CL, et al. Iris melanoma in a patient with neurofibromatosis. *Surv Ophthalmol* 2000;45(3):231–236.
27. Gayre GS, Proia AD, Dutton JJ. Epibulbar osseous choristoma: case report and review of the literature. *Ophthalmic Surg Lasers* 2002;33(5):410–415.
28. Mohammad AE, Kroosh SS. Huge corneal dermoid in a well-formed eye: a case report and review of the literature. *Orbit* 2002;21(4):295–299.
29. Rakheja D, Narayan SB, Bennett MJ. Juvenile neuronal ceroid-lipofuscinosis (Batten disease): a brief review and update. *Curr Mol Med* 2007;7(6):603–608.
30. Yohe SL, Reyes M, Johnson DA, et al. Plasminogen deficiency as a rare cause of conjunctivitis and lymphadenopathy. *Am J Surg Pathol* 2009;33(2):313–319.
31. Schuster V, Seregard S. Ligneous conjunctivitis. *Surv Ophthalmol* 2003;48(4):369–388.
32. Mehta R, Shapiro AD. Plasminogen activator inhibitor type 1 deficiency. *Haemophilia* 2008;14(6):1255–1260.
33. Rahimi-Movaghar V, Karimi M. Meningeal melanocytoma of the brain and oculodermal melanocytosis (nevus of ota): case report and literature review. *Surg Neurol* 2003;59(3):200–210.
34. Zamir E, Mechoulam H, Micera A, et al. Inflamed juvenile conjunctival naevus: clinicopathological characterisation. *Br J Ophthalmol* 2002;86(1):28–30.
35. Maly A, Epstein D, Meir K, et al. Histological criteria for grading of atypia in melanocytic conjunctival lesions. *Pathology* 2008;40(7):676–681.
36. Taban M, Traboulsi EI. Malignant melanoma of the conjunctiva in children: a review of the international literature 1965–2006. *J Pediatr Ophthalmol Strabismus* 2007;44(5):277–282; quiz 298–279.
37. Shields CL, Markowitz JS, Belinsky I, et al. Conjunctival melanoma: outcomes based on tumor origin in 382 consecutive cases. *Ophthalmology* 2011;118(2):389–395 e381–e382.
38. Shao L, Newell B, Quintanilla N. Atypical fibroxanthoma and squamous cell carcinoma of the conjunctiva in xeroderma pigmentosum. *Pediatr Dev Pathol* 2007;10(2):149–152.
39. Shtein RM, Elner VM. Herpes simplex virus keratitis: histopathology and corneal allograft outcomes. *Expert Rev Ophthalmol* 2010;5(2):129–134.
40. Carvalho FR, Foronda AS, Mannis MJ, et al. Twenty years of Acanthamoeba keratitis. *Cornea* 2009;28(5):516–519.
41. Erie JC, McLaren JW, Patel SV. Confocal microscopy in ophthalmology. *Am J Ophthalmol* 2009;148(5):639–646.
42. Dart JK, Saw VP, Kilvington S. Acanthamoeba keratitis: diagnosis and treatment update 2009. *Am J Ophthalmol* 2009;148(4):487–499 e482.
43. Aldahmesh MA, Khan AO, Meyer BF, et al. Mutational spectrum of SLC4A11 in autosomal recessive CHED in Saudi Arabia. *Invest Ophthalmol Vis Sci* 2009;50(9):4142–4145.
44. Shah SS, Al-Rajhi A, Brandt JD, et al. Mutation in the SLC4A11 gene associated with autosomal recessive congenital hereditary endothelial dystrophy in a large Saudi family. *Ophthalmic Genet* 2008;29(1):41–45.
45. Aldave AJ, Han J, Frausto RF. Genetics of the corneal endothelial dystrophies: an evidence-based review. *Clin Genet* 2013;84(2):109–119.
46. Callaghan M, Hand CK, Kennedy SM, et al. Homozygosity mapping and linkage analysis demonstrate that autosomal recessive congenital hereditary endothelial dystrophy (CHED) and autosomal dominant CHED are genetically distinct. *Br J Ophthalmol* 1999;83(1):115–119.
47. Mohamed MD, McKibbin M, Jafri H, et al. A new pedigree with recessive mapping to CHED2 locus on 20p13. *Br J Ophthalmol* 2001;85(6):758–759.
48. Holland EJ, Daya SM, Stone EM, et al. Avellino corneal dystrophy. Clinical manifestations and natural history. *Ophthalmology* 1992;99(10):1564–1568.
49. Stone EM, Mathers WD, Rosenwasser GO, et al. Three autosomal dominant corneal dystrophies map to chromosome 5q. *Nat Genet* 1994;6(1):47–51.
50. Yang J, Han X, Huang D, et al. Analysis of TGFBI gene mutations in Chinese patients with corneal dystrophies and review of the literature. *Mol Vis* 2010;16:1186–1193.
51. Folberg R, Stone EM, Sheffield VC, et al. The relationship between granular, lattice type 1, and Avellino corneal dystrophies. A histopathologic study. *Arch Ophthalmol* 1994;112(8):1080–1085.
52. Ramamurthi S, Rahman MQ, Dutton GN, et al. Pathogenesis, clinical features and management of recurrent corneal erosions. *Eye* 2006;20(6):635–644.
53. Abbruzzese C, Kuhn U, Molina F, et al. Novel mutations in the CHST6 gene causing macular corneal dystrophy. *Clin Genet* 2004;65(2):120–125.
54. Feder RS, Kshettry P. Noninflammatory ectatic disorders. In: Krachmer JH, Mannis MJ, Holland EJ, eds. *Cornea*. Philadelphia, PA: Elsevier Mosby; 2005.
55. Cameron JD, Streeten BW. Pathology of the lens. In: Albert DM, Miller JW, Azar DT, Blodi BA, eds. *Albert and Jakobiec's Principles and Practice of Ophthalmology*. Vol. 4. Philadelphia, PA: Saunders Elsevier; 2008:3653–3678.
56. Ceron O, Lou PL, Kroll AJ, et al. The vitreo-retinal manifestations of persistent hyperplasic primary vitreous (PHPV) and their management. *Int Ophthalmol Clin*. 2008;48(2):53–62.
57. de Visser L, Braakenburg A, Rothova A, et al. Rubella virus-associated uveitis: clinical manifestations and visual prognosis. *Am J Ophthalmol* 2008;146(2):292–297.
58. McMahon RT, Font RL, McLean IW. Phakomatous choristoma of eyelid: electron microscopical confirmation of lenticular derivation. *Arch Ophthalmol* 1976;94(10):1778–1781.
59. Zimmerman LE. Phakomatous choristoma of the eyelid. A tumor of lenticular anlage. *Am J Ophthalmol* 1971;71(1 Pt 2):169–177.
60. Graw J. Congenital hereditary cataracts. *Int J Dev Biol* 2004;48(8–9):1031–1044.

61. Deng H, Yuan L. Molecular genetics of congenital nuclear cataract. *Eur J Med Genet* 2014;57(2-3):113-122.
62. Cameron JD. Ocular Trauma. In: Klintworth GK, Garner A, eds. *Garner and Klintworth's Pathobiology of Ocular Disease*. Vol. 3. New York: Informa Healthcare, 2008:333-360.
63. Nemet AY, Assia EI, Apple DJ, et al. Current concepts of ocular manifestations in Marfan syndrome. *Surv Ophthalmol* 2006;51(6):561-575.
64. Benson WE. Familial exudative vitreoretinopathy. *Trans Am Ophthalmol Soc* 1995;93:473-521.
65. Knudson A. Retinoblastoma: teacher of cancer biology and medicine. *PLoS Med* 2005;2(10):e349.
66. Dyer MA, Harbour JW. Cellular and genetic events in retinoblastoma tumorigenesis. In: Singh AD, Damato BE, Pe'er J, et al. eds. *Clinical Ophthalmic Oncology*. Vol. 3. Philadelphia, PA: Saunders Elsevier; 2007: 405409.
67. Seidman DJ, Shields JA, Augsburger JJ, et al. Early diagnosis of retinoblastoma based on dysmorphic features and karyotype analysis. *Ophthalmology* 1987;94(6):663-666.
68. Murphree AL, Singh AD. Heritable retinoblastoma: the RB1 cancer predisposition syndrome. In: Singh AD, Damato BE, Pe'er J, et al. eds. *Clinical Ophthalmic Oncology*. Saunders Elsevier, 2007:428-433.
69. Chevez-Barrios P, Eagle RC Jr, Marbach P. Histologic features and prognostic factors. In: Singh AD, Damato BE, Pe'er J, et al., eds. *Clinical Ophthalmic Oncology*. Philadelphia, PA: Saunders Elsevier; 2007:468-483.
70. Sastre X, Chantada GL, Doz F, et al. Proceedings of the consensus meetings from the International Retinoblastoma Staging Working Group on the pathology guidelines for the examination of enucleated eyes and evaluation of prognostic risk factors in retinoblastoma. *Arch Pathol Lab Med* 2009;133(8):1199-1202.
71. Eagle RC Jr. High-risk features and tumor differentiation in retinoblastoma: a retrospective histopathologic study. *Arch Pathol Lab Med* 2009;133(8):1203-1209.
72. Kaliki S, Shields CL, Rojanaporn D, et al. High-risk retinoblastoma based on international classification of retinoblastoma: analysis of 519 enucleated eyes. *Ophthalmology* 2013;120(5):997-1003.
73. Broughton WL, Zimmerman LE. A clinicopathologic study of 56 cases of intraocular medulloepitheliomas. *Am J Ophthalmol* 1978;85(3):407-418.
74. Saunders T, Margo CE. Intraocular medulloepithelioma. *Arch Pathol Lab Med* 2012;136(2):212-216.
74a. Priest JR, Williams GM, Manera R, et al. Ciliary body medulloepithelioma: four cases associated with pleuropulmonary blastoma—a report from the International Pleuropulmonary Blastoma Registry. *Br J Ophthalmol* 2011;95(7):1001-1005.
75. Lewis RA, Gerson LP, Axelson KA, et al. von Recklinghausen neurofibromatosis II Incidence of optic gliomata. *Ophthalmology* 1984;91(8):929-935.
76. Liu GT, Katowitz JA, Rorke-Adams LB, et al. Optic pathway gliomas: neoplasms, not hamartomas. *JAMA Ophthalmol* 2013;131(5): 646-650.
77. Nair AG, Pathak RS, Iyer VR, et al. Optic nerve glioma: an update. *Int Ophthalmol* 2014;34:999-1005.
78. Harold Lee HB, Garrity JA, Cameron JD, et al. Primary optic nerve sheath meningioma in children. *Surv Ophthalmol* 2008;53(6): 543-558.
79. Garrity JA, Henderson JW, Cameron JD. Cysts and celes. In: Garrity JA, Henderson JW, Cameron JD, eds. *Henderson's Orbital Tumors*, 4th ed. Philadelphia, PA: Lippincott Williams & Wilkins, 2007:33-61.
80. Margo CE, Goldman DR. Langerhans cell histiocytosis. *Surv Ophthalmol* 2008;53(4):332-358.
81. Badalian-Very G, Vergilio J-A, Degar BA, et al. Recurrent BRAF mutations in Langerhans cell histiocytosis. *Blood* 2010;116(11): 1919-1923. doi: 10.1182/blood-2010-04-279083. PMC 3173987. PMID 20519626).
82. Stalemark H, Laurencikas E, Karis J, et al. Incidence of Langerhans cell histiocytosis in children: a population-based study. *Pediatr Blood Cancer* 2008;51(1):76-81.
83. Guyot-Goubin A, Donadieu J, Barkaoui M, et al. Descriptive epidemiology of childhood Langerhans cell histiocytosis in France, 2000-2004. *Pediatr Blood Cancer* 2008;51(1):71-75.
84. Garrity JA, Henderson JW, Cameron JD. Vascular Hamartomas, hyperplasia, and neoplasms. In: Garrity JA, Henderson JW, Cameron JD, eds. *Henderson's Orbital Tumors*, 4th ed. Philadelphia, PA: Lippincott Williams & Wilkins, 2007:210-215.
85. Couch SM, Garrity JA, Cameron JD, et al. Embolization of orbital varices with N-butyl cyanoacrylate as an aid in surgical excision: results of 4 cases with histopathologic examination. *Am J Ophthalmol* 2009;148(4):614-618 e611.
86. Garrity JA, Henderson JW, Cameron JD. Inflammatory orbital pseudotumors. In: Garrity JA, Henderson JW, Cameron JD, eds. *Henderson's Orbital Tumors*, 4th ed. Philadelphia, PA: Lippincott Williams & Wilkins, 2007:343-351.
87. Chen B, Perry JD. Rhabdomyosarcoma. In: Singh AD, Damato BE, Pe'er J, et al., eds. *Clinical Ophthalmic Oncology*. Saunders Elsevier; 2007:581-585.
88. Shields JA, Shields CL. *Lacrimal Gland Primary Epithelial Tumors. An Atlas and Textbook. Eyelid, Conjunctival and Orbital Tumors*. Philadelphia, PA: Wolters Kluwer/Lippincott Williams & Wilkins, 2009:699-726.
89. Cameron JD, Emerson MV. Ophthalmic pathologic findings in infantile traumatic brain injury. In: Troncoso JC, Rubio A, Fowler DR, eds. *Essential Forensic Neuropathology*. Philadelphia, PA: Wolters Kluwer/Lippincott Williams & Wilkins, 2010:203-217.

CHAPTER 12
The Respiratory Tract

Louis P. Dehner, M.D., J. Thomas Stocker, M.D., Haresh Mani, M.D., D. Ashley Hill, M.D., and Aliya N. Husain, M.D.

DEVELOPMENT OF THE LUNG

The lung begins as a pouch or groove originating from the primitive foregut in week 3 of embryologic development, when the embryo is 3 mm long. As the groove enlarges caudally, a tubular lung bud is formed; the upper portion develops into the epithelium of the larynx and the caudal portion into the epithelium of the tracheobronchial tree (1).

The embryonic period of lung development (Table 12-1) begins in week 4 of gestation as the single lung bud from the foregut divides into two primary bronchial buds, the forerunners of the right and left lungs (Figure 12-1A to C). During week 5 of gestation, the primary bronchi divide. Each forms three lobar buds that, by the end of week 6 of gestation, divide again to form 10 segmental bronchi on the right and 8 to 9 on the left. These potential airways consist of a central core of epithelial cells surrounded by loose primitive mesenchyme that contains widely separated capillaries. The primitive pulmonary arteries begin to form from the sixth aortic arch, near the end of the embryonic period. The pulmonary veins begin as evaginations of the left atrium during week 4 of gestation and coalesce with the mesenchymal capillary plexus early in week 5. These early events with the branching morphogenesis and alveolarization are accompanied by microvascularization of the small airspaces for postnatal gas exchange (2). There are several important signaling pathways involved in early lung development (3–5). Lung has been discussed by Correia-Pinto and associates (6). MicroRNAs (miRNA) are important in the regulation of lung development at the levels of proliferation, apoptosis, differentiation, and morphogenesis (7). DICER1 is an RNase III enzyme that performs the final step in generating immature miRNAs (5). The loss of DICER1 in lung epithelium early in development results in loss of branching and the formation of lung cysts (8).

The pseudoglandular period (weeks 6 to 16 of gestation) begins with the completion of the proximal airways and encompasses the development of the conducting airway system to the level of the terminal bronchioles (Figure 12-2A, B).

The pseudostratified columnar epithelium of the proximal airway displays cilia at week 10 of gestation. The appearance of cilia extends to the epithelial cells of the peripheral airways by week 13. Goblet cells appear in the bronchial epithelium at weeks 13 to 14 of gestation, and submucosal glands begin as solid buds originating from the basal layers of the epithelium by weeks 15 to 16. Smooth muscle cells develop around airways by the end of gestational week 7 and organize to form an identifiable wall to the larger bronchi by week 12. Lymphatics appear first in the hilar region of the lung in gestational week 8 and in the lung itself by week 10. Cartilage is first seen in week 4 of gestation and forms distinct rings along the trachea and main bronchi by the end of week 10.

TABLE 12-1 PHASES OF INTRAUTERINE LUNG DEVELOPMENT

Phase	Gestation Period	Major Event
Embryonic	26 days to 6 weeks	Development of major airways
Pseudoglandular	6–16 weeks	Development of airways to terminal bronchioles
Acinar or canalicular	16–28 weeks	Development of acinus and its vascularization
Saccular	28–34 weeks	Subdivision of saccules by secondary crests to term
Alveolar	34 weeks (and beyond)	Alveolar acquisition

Adapted from Langston C. Prenatal lung growth and pulmonary hypoplasia. In: Stocker JT, ed. *Pediatric Pulmonary Disease*. Washington, DC: Hemisphere, 1989:2, with permission.

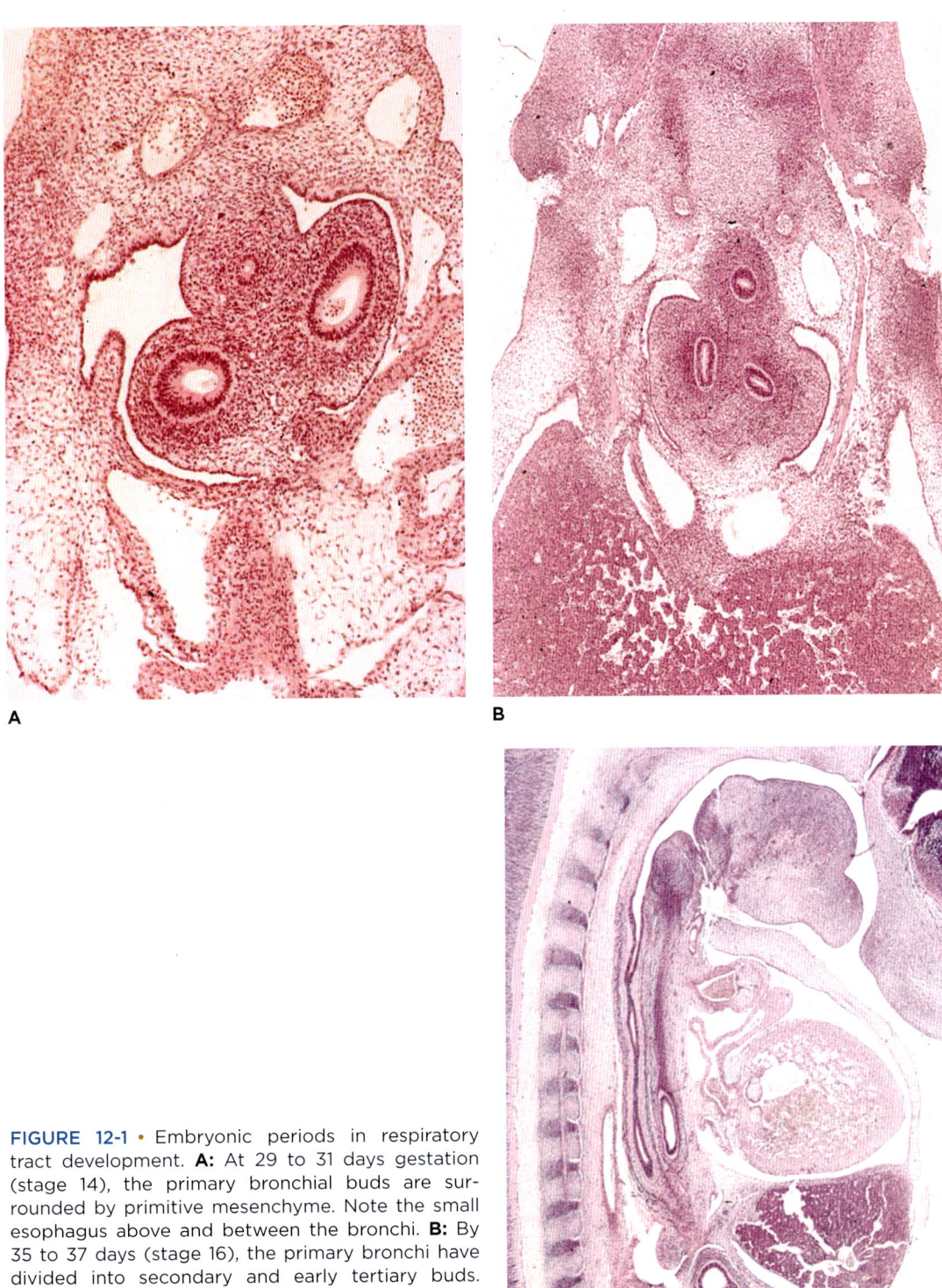

FIGURE 12-1 • Embryonic periods in respiratory tract development. **A:** At 29 to 31 days gestation (stage 14), the primary bronchial buds are surrounded by primitive mesenchyme. Note the small esophagus above and between the bronchi. **B:** By 35 to 37 days (stage 16), the primary bronchi have divided into secondary and early tertiary buds. Note the centrally located esophagus and the large amount of hepatic parenchyma (lower half). **C:** In a sagittal plane of a 37- to 40-day (stage 17) embryo, the relationship between the esophagus (nearest vertebral column) and trachea (between esophagus and heart) can be seen. The heart and liver are ventral to the foregut structures.

The acinar or canalicular period extends from weeks 17 to 28 of gestation and is characterized by the development of the basic structure of the gas-exchanging portion of the lung (Figure 12-3A, B). Smooth-walled respiratory bronchioles, lined by cuboidal epithelium, subdivide into multiple, irregular alveolar ducts. By week 20 of gestation, the cells lining the ducts develop into type II pneumocytes with lamellar and multivesicular bodies associated with surfactant synthesis.

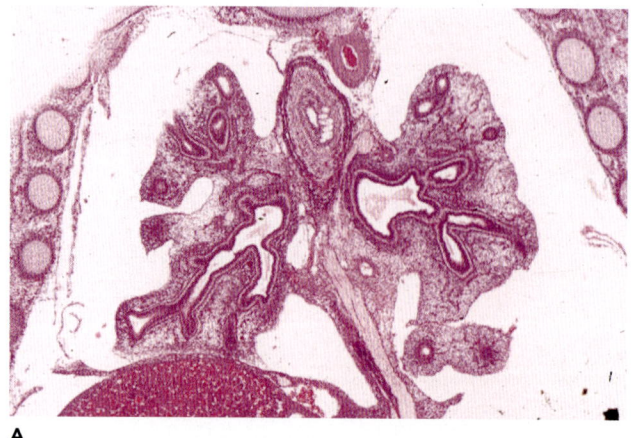
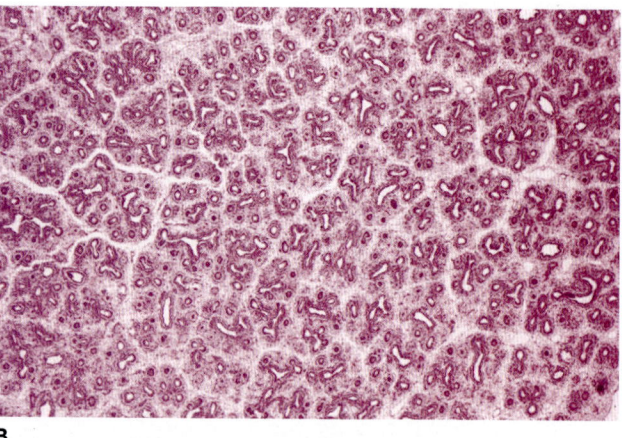

FIGURE 12-2 • Pseudoglandular period. **A:** At 9 weeks of gestation, the proximal airways are present throughout the right and left lobes. **B:** By 13 weeks, bronchiolar development is well under way, and early division into lobules and clusters of acini is apparent.

Type I pneumocytes then differentiate from type II cells to form the thin air–blood interface required for gas exchange. As the interstitium thins in the latter portion of the acinar period, the capillaries of the interstitium proliferate and come to lie beneath the type I cells. Submucosal glands in the trachea and bronchi progress from tubules to mucus-containing acini. By week 24, the cartilage has extended to the most distal bronchi.

The saccular period begins at week 28 of gestation with the development of secondary crests, which are formed as distal airspaces divide into smaller units (Figure 12-4A, B). With an accompanying marked decrease in the interstitial tissue and further increase in the capillary bed, a complex, interwoven capillary network develops in the wall of the saccules. This provides for effective gas exchange as alveoli begin to develop at the end of the period (32 to 36 weeks of gestation).

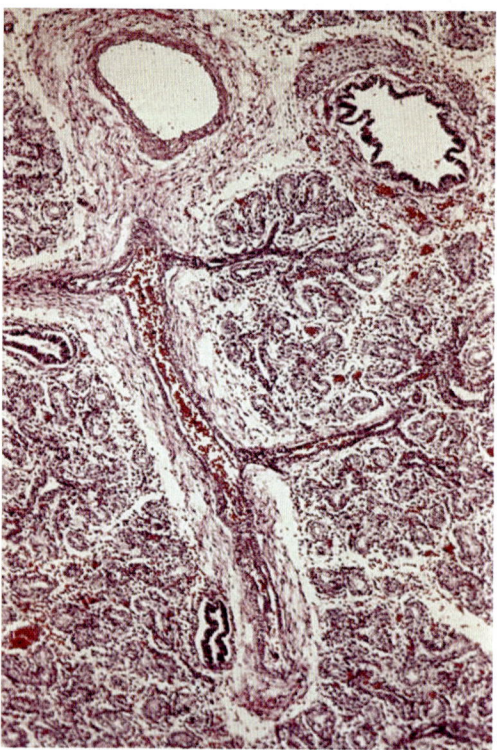
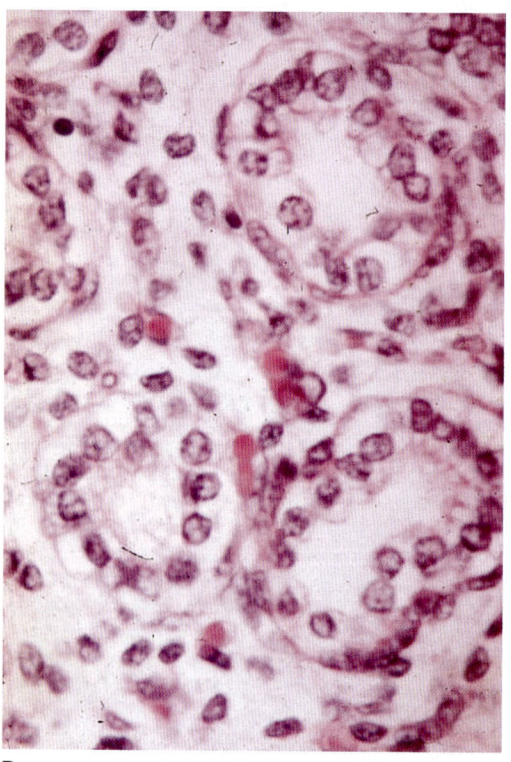

FIGURE 12-3 • Acinar period. **A:** In a 370-g fetus, acinar development is characterized by pulmonary arteries and proximal bronchioles surrounded by alveolar ducts still widely separated by mesenchymal tissue. **B:** The alveolar duct structures are lined by cuboidal epithelium (early type II cells), and blood-filled capillaries are present just beneath the cells.

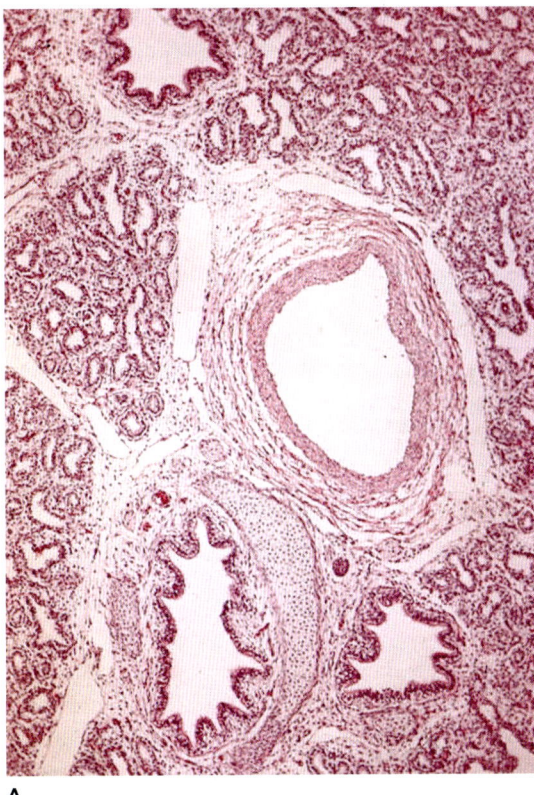
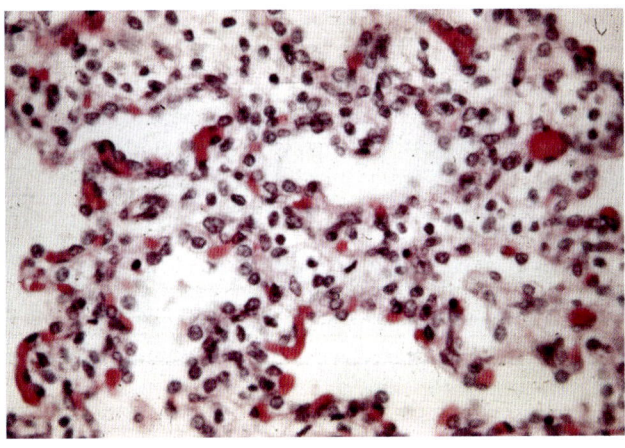

FIGURE 12-4 • Saccular period. **A:** In a 650-g fetus, discrete acini are identifiable within a lobule. **B:** Secondary crests are covered by thinning type I cells, which expose capillary beds immediately beneath the cells.

The final period of development, the alveolar period, begins *in utero* at 32 to 36 weeks of gestation and extends until 18 to 24 months after birth. Alveoli develop as flask-shaped structures with thin walls whose double capillary network meshes to appear as a single capillary bed (Figure 12-5). At term, type I pneumocytes are extremely thin, resulting in an air–blood barrier of only 0.2 mm including the type I cell, the underlying basement membrane, and the cytoplasm of the capillary endothelial cell. Lymphatic channels are distributed around pulmonary arteries, bronchi, and bronchioles and extend along interlobular septa to anastomose with a plexus beneath the pleura. Lymphatic spaces do not exist between alveoli.

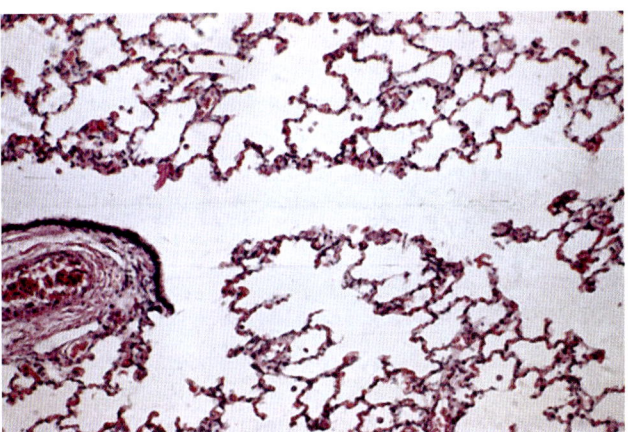

FIGURE 12-5 • Alveolar period. At 2 months of age, a respiratory bronchiole (**left**) gives rise to alveolar ducts, alveolar saccules, and thin-walled alveoli.

The vascular supply of the lungs changes appreciably in late gestation and infancy. The bronchial arterial circulation, originating from the aortic arch, supplies the bronchi, bronchioles, and interlobular septa in older children and adults; however, the bronchial artery contributes substantially to the circulation of the alveolar ducts and alveoli in the central portions of the lungs through bronchopulmonary artery anastomoses *in utero* and in early infancy.

At birth, the surface area of the lung is about 4 m^2, with the number of alveoli ranging from 10 to 150 million (mean of 53 million). Alveoli increase in number after birth, reaching the adult range of 300 to 600 million alveoli by 2 years of age. Thereafter, lung growth occurs in terms of volume and alveolar size, with no further increase in the number of small air spaces (alveoli).

NASOPHARYNX

Choanal Atresia

Choanal atresia occurs in about 1 in 5–8000 live births and consists of unilateral or bilateral occlusion of the airway between the posterior nasal passage and the nasopharynx (9). The entity has been seen in monozygotic twins and has also been noted following radiotherapy for nasopharyngeal carcinoma. The septum blocking the airway is usually composed of bone or cartilage, but in as many as 20% to 50% of cases, it may be composed of a mucous membrane alone (10). Choanal atresia may exist as an isolated sporadic lesion, in an autosomal dominant form, or possibly in an autosomal recessive form. It has been associated with palatal defects, tracheoesophageal fistula (TEF), congenital heart malformations, trisomy 6, Pfeiffer syndrome, Treacher Collins syndrome, the fetal carbimazole syndrome, and the CHARGE (Coloboma, Heart defect, choanal Atresia, Retardation, Genital, Ear anomaly) association (CHD7 mutation on 8q12.2) of which it is a major component.

Cleft Lip and/or Palate

Cleft lip, with or without unilateral and bilateral involvement of the hard palate, the soft palate, or both, is the most common malformation of the respiratory tract. It occurs once in 750 live births as an isolated anomaly or as part of a wide variety of chromosomal, inherited, and noninherited syndromes, of which over 250 have been described (11). Cleft palate is associated with other anomalies in 47% of cases, cleft lip and palate in 37%, and cleft lip alone in 14%. Anomalies most frequently seen are those in the central nervous system (CNS) and skeletal system, followed by urogenital and cardiovascular anomalies. Maternal cigarette smoking and alcohol use are associated with a 1.6- to 2.0-fold increase in isolated cleft lip, cleft palate, or both (12). The incidence of cleft lip and palate is dose related, increasing with increased cigarette smoking.

Laryngocele

A laryngocele is an abnormal dilation of the laryngeal saccule that extends upward within the false vocal fold and is in communication with the laryngeal lumen. It is filled with air, although mucoid or purulent contents may be seen following obstruction and infection, respectively. Laryngoceles occur rarely in childhood but may present as airway obstruction or as a neck mass in a neonate or an older child (13,14). The lesion, seen predominantly in boys and containing air or fluid or both, may be within the larynx behind the thyroid cartilage (33%), external to the larynx (25%), or involving both locations (15). Currently, laryngoceles are classified as either internal (confined medial to the thyrohyoid membrane) or combined (when it extends further laterally), since the existence of a purely external laryngocele has been refuted (16). Etiologic factors include congenital increased laryngeal pressure, or mechanical obstruction (such as by tumors including laryngeal papillomas). Since they are outpouchings of the laryngeal wall, they are lined by either respiratory or squamous epithelium. Infection of the lesion may occur (pyolaryngocele), leading to acute respiratory distress.

Laryngomalacia

Stridor and feeding difficulties in the newborn may be caused by laryngomalacia due to flaccidity of a long epiglottis, short arytenoepiglottic folds, or bulky arytenoid swellings, resulting in partial obstruction of the larynx. Kay and Goldsmith (17) have developed a classification based on the underlying pathophysiologic processes, with type 1 characterized by a foreshortened or tight aryepiglottic fold, type 2 defined by the presence of redundant soft tissue in the supraglottis, and type 3 applying to cases caused by other etiologies. Potentially serious complications of the obstruction include pulmonary hypertension and cor pulmonale, sudden death during respiratory tract infections, failure to thrive, and possible impaired intellectual development secondary to episodes of hypoxia and hypercapnia. Twenty percent of these infants have severe neurologic compromise or multiple congenital anomalies. Surgical procedures including supraglottoplasty have been used in severe cases (about 10% to 15% of cases) and have been successful in relieving respiratory symptoms in 80% of those cases (18). Laryngomalacia-induced stridor has been reported in patients with Pierre Robin, acrocallosal, Marshall-Smith, cri du chat, fetal warfarin, Down, Freeman-Sheldon, and Mohr syndromes. A familial form of laryngomalacia has also been described.

Laryngeal Stenosis and Atresia

Supraglottic, glottic, and subglottic developmental webs may produce varying degrees of laryngeal stenosis and have been described in families with an autosomal dominant inheritance pattern. Fraser syndrome is associated with congenital stenosis or atresia in 30% of cases, along with other anomalies (19).

Subglottic stenosis, as an acquired lesion, has been seen secondary to short-term and long-term intubation in the neonatal intensive care unit (NICU) with increased incidence when the infant is intubated for longer periods (20). With acquired stenosis, dense submucosal fibrous connective tissue is present circumferentially in the subglottic area and may narrow the lumen significantly. Submucosal glands are usually absent, and the cricoid cartilage may display evidence of erosion.

Congenital laryngeal atresia occurs in three patterns (21):

1. Type 1, atresia of both supraglottic and infraglottic portions of the larynx
2. Type 2, atresia of the infraglottic region (Figure 12-6A, B)
3. Type 3, glottic atresia

Associated conditions include esophageal atresia (EA), TEF, "total sequestration" of the lungs in the absence of TEF, anal anomalies, urinary tract malformations, skeletal anomalies, and heart malformations. Many of the conditions are part of the vertebral, anal atresia, cardiac, TEF, renal, and limb (VATER or VACTERL) association. Other associations include partial diaphragmatic obliteration, Fraser syndrome, DiGeorge developmental field defect, and partial trisomy 9. Pulmonary hyperplasia has been noted in infants who have laryngeal atresia, with lung weights ranging from 150% to 300% of normal.

Laryngotracheoesophageal Cleft

Failure in formation of the tracheoesophageal septum, normally complete by day 35 of gestation, leads to the development of one of four forms of laryngotracheoesophageal cleft (22) (Figure 12-7A to D):

1. Supraglottic interarytenoid cleft (50% of cases)
2. Partial cricoid cleft

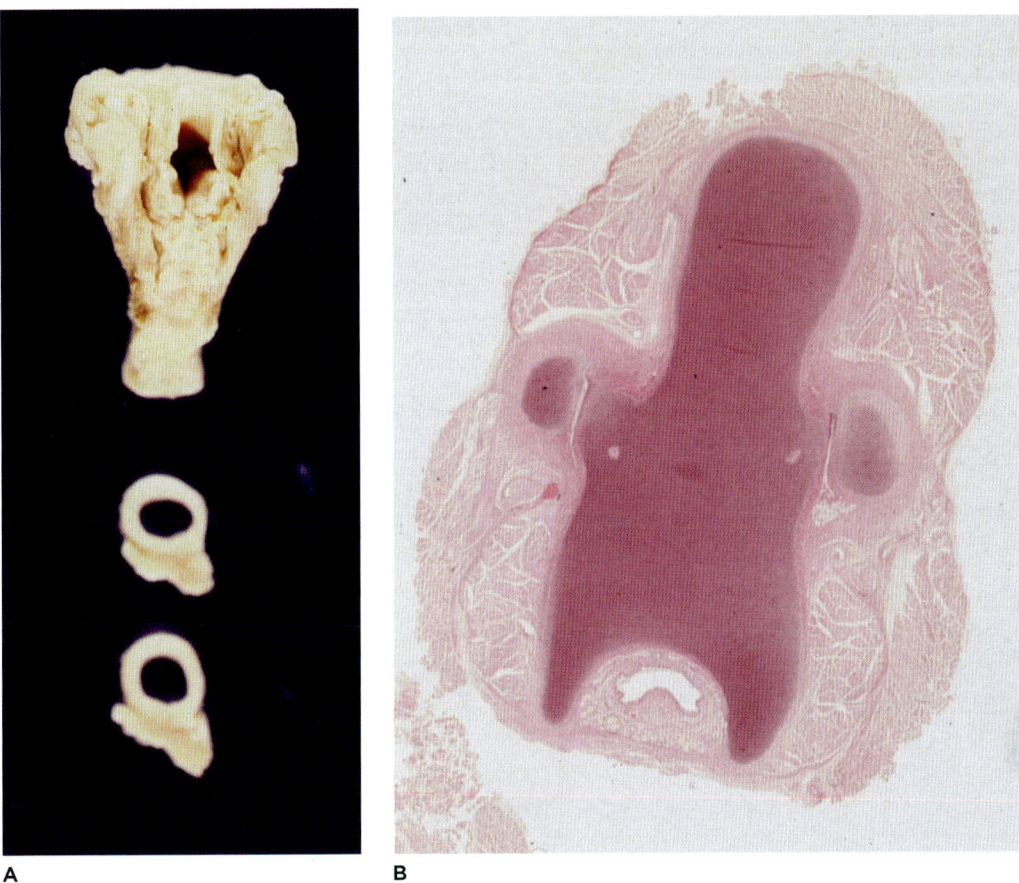

FIGURE 12-6 • Laryngeal atresia. **A:** The larynx reveals a patent upper opening (**upper piece**) and a patent trachea (**lower two cross sections**). **B:** A histologic section from the area in the region of the cricoid cartilage reveals only a pinpoint lumen (**bottom center**).

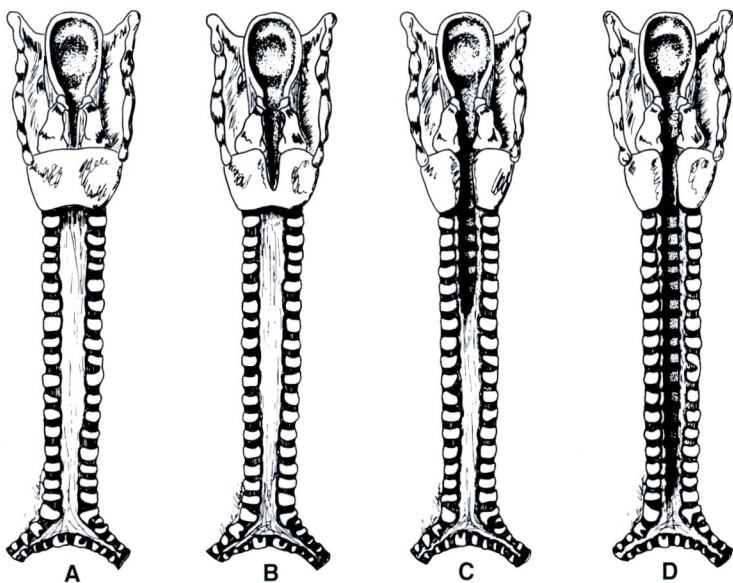

FIGURE 12-7 • Types of laryngotracheoesophageal cleft. **A:** Supraglottic interarytenoid cleft. **B:** Partial cricoid cleft. **C:** Total cricoid cleft. **D:** Complete cleft to level of carina.

3. Total cricoid cleft
4. Complete cleft of the trachea to the level of the carina

Maternal polyhydramnios is seen in many cases, and a familial occurrence has been reported with relative frequency. Associated conditions include TEF and other elements of the VATER association, pulmonary hypoplasia, exstrophy of the bladder, polysplenia, double outlet right ventricle, and the G syndrome.

TRACHEA

Tracheal Agenesis

Tracheal agenesis is a rarely occurring, uniformly fatal malformation that is usually associated with tracheoesophageal or bronchoesophageal fistula. Various classifications divide the entity into three to seven types (Figure 12-8A to G);

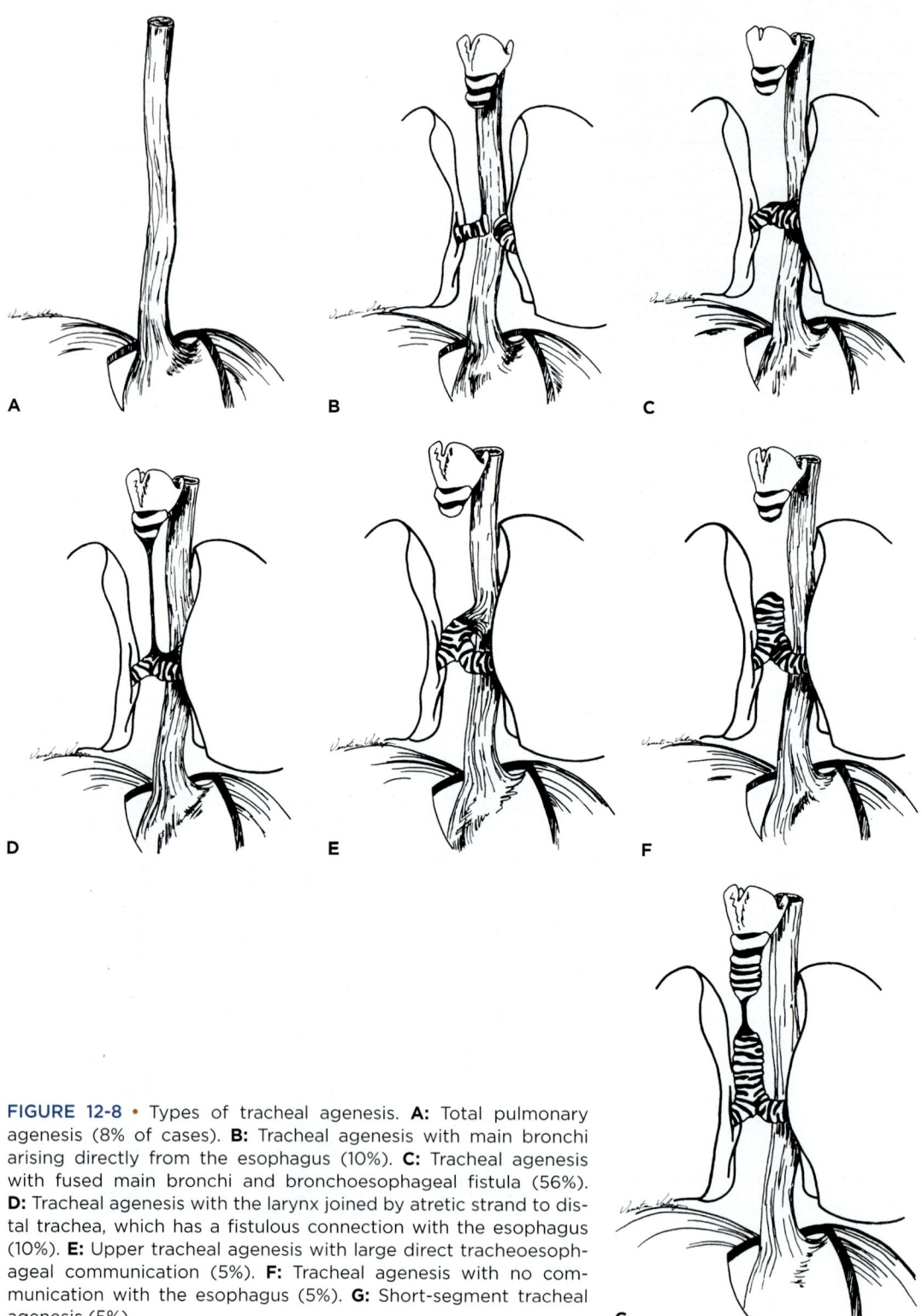

FIGURE 12-8 • Types of tracheal agenesis. **A:** Total pulmonary agenesis (8% of cases). **B:** Tracheal agenesis with main bronchi arising directly from the esophagus (10%). **C:** Tracheal agenesis with fused main bronchi and bronchoesophageal fistula (56%). **D:** Tracheal agenesis with the larynx joined by atretic strand to distal trachea, which has a fistulous connection with the esophagus (10%). **E:** Upper tracheal agenesis with large direct tracheoesophageal communication (5%). **F:** Tracheal agenesis with no communication with the esophagus (5%). **G:** Short-segment tracheal agenesis (5%).

however, nearly 70% of cases consist of agenesis of the entire trachea with a small fistulous connection between the esophagus and the carina (Figure 12-8C to E) (23,24). The lungs may be normally developed or totally absent (pulmonary agenesis). In the rare cases of tracheal agenesis with no fistulous connection to the esophagus (i.e., total sequestration of the lungs), the lungs are uniformly distended, histologically resembling extralobar sequestration (25). There is a male predominance of approximately 2:1 and an association with maternal polyhydramnios in tracheal agenesis. In addition to the anomalies of the VATER association, tracheal agenesis has been seen in association with duodenal atresia, annular pancreas, syndactyly, and CNS malformations. Evans et al. (24) describe four groups based on the type of anomalies associated with the tracheal agenesis: group 1, anomalies restricted to the trachea, larynx, and cardiovascular system; group 2, severe cardiovascular anomalies and abnormal lung lobulation; group 3, a caudal component in addition to thoracic abnormalities, with anal and renal anomalies being common; and group 4, multisystem involvement with a high incidence of aberrant vessels, complex cardiac malformations, lung lobation defects, and anomalies of other foregut derivatives.

Tracheal Bronchus

This rare anomaly, also known as bronchus suis, is defined by a bronchus to the right upper lobe arising at the junction of the mid and distal one-third of the right lateral trachea (26).

Tracheal Stenosis

Laryngeal or tracheal stenosis is usually seen as an acquired lesion related to intubation or to the presence of a foreign body; congenital stenosis of the trachea is rare (27). Congenital stenosis may be diffuse, funnel-like, or segmental. Diffuse, generalized hypoplasia accounts for about 30% of cases, funnel-shaped or "carrot-shaped" stenosis for 20%, and segmental stenosis for the remaining 50%. Segmental stenosis may be due to complete tracheal cartilage rings, "napkin-ring" stenosis, or too small but normally shaped rings with a narrow pars membranosa (Figure 12-9) (28). Associated anomalies include anomalous bronchi, TEF, unilateral pulmonary agenesis, Crouzon syndrome, Larsen syndrome, Down syndrome, Alagille syndrome, and ventricular septal defect.

Tracheal stenosis, or narrowing, may also be produced by extrinsic pressure, most commonly by abnormally placed or abnormally large blood vessels including

- Vascular ring due to double aortic arch
- Vascular ring due to right aortic arch
- Aberrant right subclavian artery
- Anomalous innominate artery
- Anomalous left carotid artery—aneurysmal left and right pulmonary arteries
- "Sling" retrotracheal left pulmonary artery

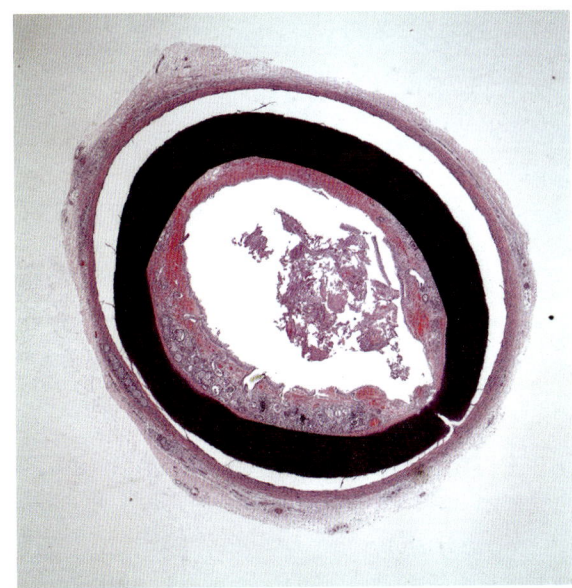

FIGURE 12-9 • Tracheal stenosis. A cross section from the mid trachea shows a complete cartilage ring beneath the mucosa, significantly narrowing the tracheal lumen.

Advances in surgical management of congenital tracheal stenosis have improved survival, especially since the advent of extracorporeal membrane oxygenation (ECMO) (29).

Tracheomalacia

Congenital tracheomalacia (i.e., soft or collapsing trachea) is exceedingly rare and overlaps with tracheal stenosis secondary to cartilage plate deficiency (30). Isolated cases have, however, been reported in association with Down syndrome, EA, CHARGE association, Larsen syndrome, pulmonary vascular sling, polychondritis, and various chondrodystrophies including Ellis–van Creveld syndrome, Langer-type mesomelic dwarfism, and diastrophic dysplasia. Aortopexy has been successfully employed in the treatment of tracheomalacia in infants. Acquired tracheomalacia may be seen in infants and young children who have been intubated for prolonged periods or as a result of trauma, radiation, or a neoplasm (31).

Tracheobronchiomegaly

Tracheobronchiomegaly, or the Mounier-Kuhn syndrome, usually involves men 20 to 40 years of age but has been reported in children of both sexes and has a familial occurrence, suggesting an autosomal recessive type of inheritance (32). The tracheal diameter exceeds the normal by three standard deviations. Saccular bulging of the intercartilaginous membranes is frequent. The disorder has been noted in a child with cutis laxa and in adults with Ehlers-Danlos syndrome.

Tracheoesophageal Fistula and Esophageal Atresia

EA, with or without TEF, occurs sporadically with an incidence of 1 in 3500 live births (33). Maternal polyhydramnios

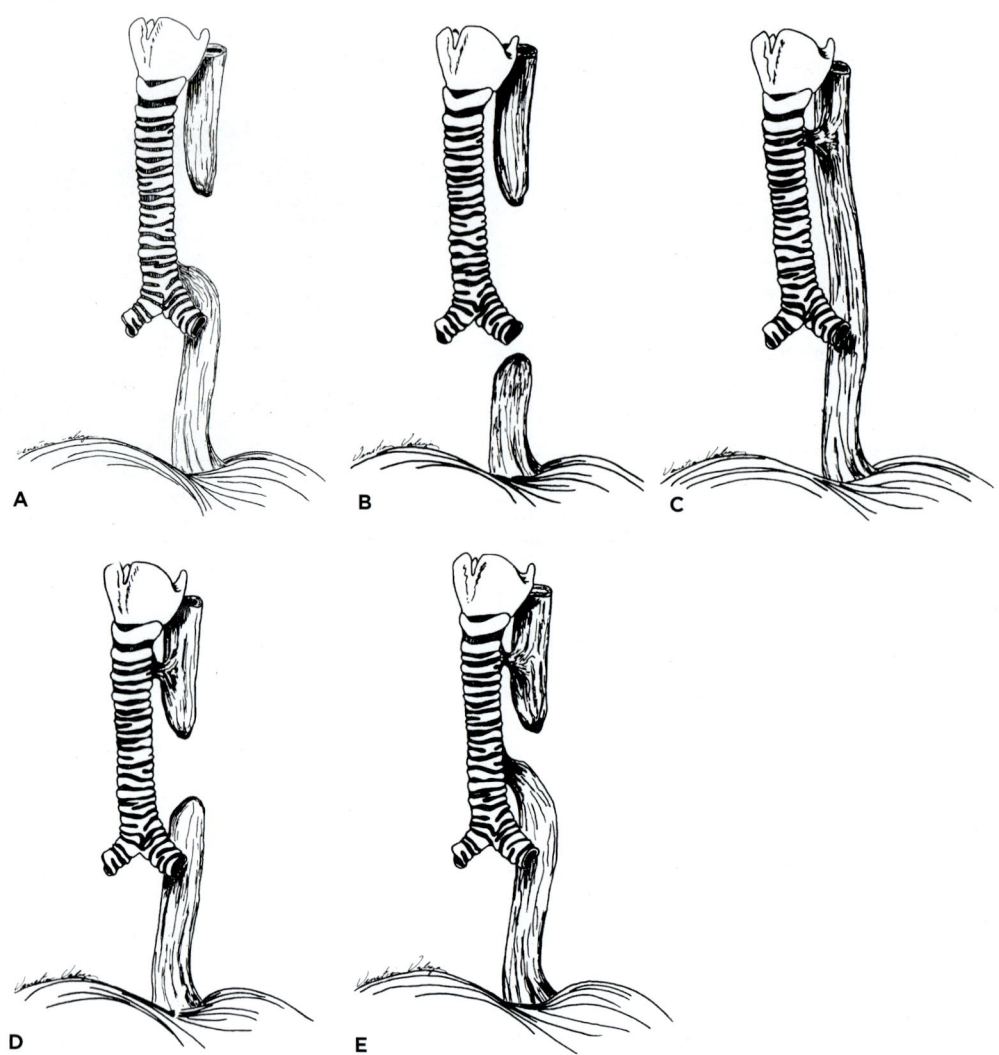

FIGURE 12-10 • Types of tracheoesophageal fistula (TEF) and esophageal atresia (EA). **A:** EA with TEF to the distal esophageal segment (>85% of cases in various series). **B:** EA without TEF (8%). **C:** TEF without EA (4%). **D:** EA with TEF to the proximal esophageal segment (1%). **E:** EA with TEF to both proximal and distal esophageal segments (1%).

is present in more than 30% of cases, and nearly 35% of the infants are premature. The anomaly can be divided into five (or more) types (Figure 12-10A to E). More than 95% of the patients have EA with the clinical findings of excessive oral and pharyngeal secretions or choking, cyanosis, or coughing during first attempts at feeding. While 98% are sporadic, the remaining have separate genetic factors (34).

TEF and EA can be most easily demonstrated at autopsy by removing the esophagus and trachea en bloc (see Chapter 1) and then opening the esophagus lengthwise along its posterior or dorsal margin. EA is readily apparent as a blind pouch (Figure 12-11A, B), but a small fistula between the anterior or ventral portion of the esophagus and the trachea can also be visualized, as can the rare esophagobronchial fistula. Histologically, squamous metaplasia of the trachea and bronchi may be seen in 80% of patients, primarily along the posterior wall of the trachea but frequently extending around the entire internal surface of the trachea and into the bronchi. The segment of esophagus may show tracheobronchial remnants in the form of abnormal mucous glands and ducts, abnormal mucin secretion, the presence of cartilage, and a disorganized muscle coat (31). Aspiration of gastric contents may be present in the lung, producing pneumonia with foreign body giant cell reaction.

Associated anomalies are seen in 49% to 72% of infants with EA and TEF, with multiple anomalies frequently present (Table 12-2) (35). A nonrandom association of TEF with other malformations has been recognized in about 45% of cases and given the acronyms of VATER, VACTER, or VACTERL (vertebral, anal, cardiac, tracheoesophageal, renal, or radial and limb anomalies) (33). Other less frequently associated anomalies include congenital pulmonary airway malformation (CPAM), diaphragmatic hernia, duodenal atresia, biliary atresia, sirenomelia, trisomy 18,

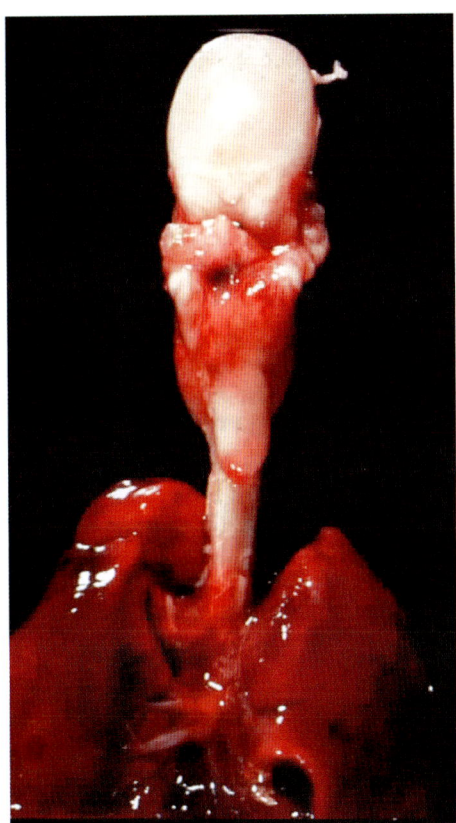 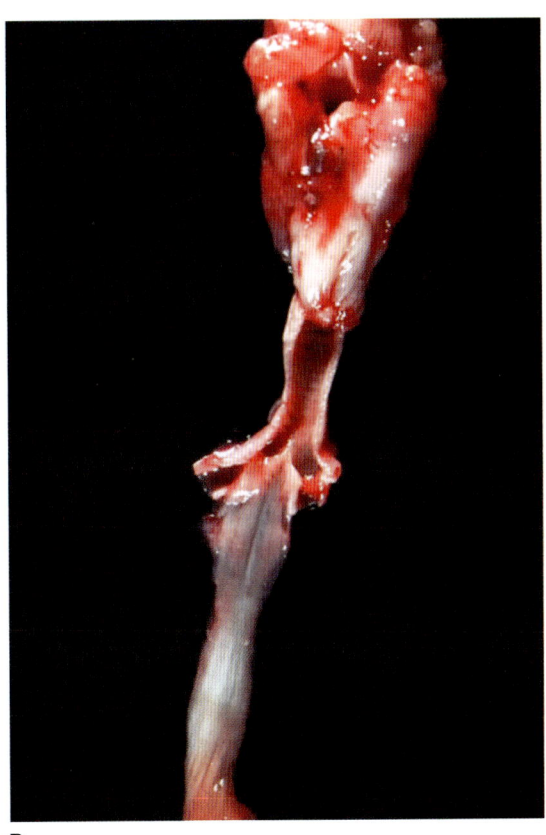

FIGURE 12-11 • TEF and EA. **A:** In a posterior view of the tongue **(top)**, trachea, and lung, the esophagus is seen to end in a blind pouch **(center)**. **B:** With the trachea and esophagus open posteriorly, a fistula can be seen connecting the carina with the distal end of the esophagus.

and intracardiac epithelial cyst. TEFs may develop in burn patients, with foreign body impaction such as a disc battery (36), and following radiation and chemotherapy for mediastinal malignancies, including lymphoma (37).

Postsurgical survival of patients with EA and TEF has increased steadily over the last 50 years, presently ranging from 75% to over 90% (38). The highest mortality rate occurs in infants with low birth weight or with coexisting cardiac malformations. TEF may recur after surgical repair in nearly 10% of cases (39). Tracheal narrowing may persist for years in nearly one-third of the patients, along with respiratory infections and gastroesophageal reflux. Histologically, esophageal inflammation may be seen in 51% of cases, Barrett esophagus in 6%, and Helicobacter pylori infection in 21% of cases (40). An increased incidence of esophageal adenocarcinoma in adulthood in patients with TEF has been suggested (41).

TABLE 12-2 ANOMALIES ASSOCIATED WITH ESOPHAGEAL ATRESIA AND TRACHEOESOPHAGEAL FISTULA

Organ System	Incidence (%)	Most Frequent Examples
Musculoskeletal	15–24	Vertebral defects, rib defects, radial amelia, caudal dysgenesis
Cardiovascular	11–49	Ventricular septal defect, patent ductus arteriosus, right aortic arch
Gastrointestinal	20	Imperforate anus, malrotation, duodenal atresia
Genitourinary agenesis	12–50	Renal malposition, renal cysts or hypospadias, horseshoe kidney
Craniofacial	10	Choanal stenosis, ear malformations, micrognathia
Central nervous system	7	Hydrocephalus
Pulmonary	2	CPAM, pulmonary hypoplasia

Adapted from Stocker JT. Congenital and developmental diseases. In: Dail DH, Hammer SP, eds. *Pulmonary Pathology*. 2nd ed. Heidelberg, Germany: Springer-Verlag, 1994:163, with permission.

BRONCHUS

Bronchial Atresia

Bronchial atresia is an entity seen almost exclusively in infants and is thought by some to be the underlying cause in the entire spectrum of parenchymal malformations from infantile (congenital) lobar emphysema (ILE), CPAMs to sequestration in almost 80% of cases (38). Cases of bronchial atresia with mild emphysema, however, have been reported in children from 1 day to 13 years of age (median, 4 years) with symptoms of chronic cough and fever in nearly all of the cases, often related to the recurrent pneumonia noted in more than 90% of cases (42). The atretic bronchus is connected to the right lower lobe, left upper lobe, and right upper lobe in decreasing order of frequency. Histologically, the affected bronchus may be obstructed by circumferential or eccentric luminal fibrosis with or without abnormalities of the cartilage plates and filled with mucin to create a "mucocele." The fibrosis may be the result of *in utero* inflammation in the neonate or possibly postpartum inflammation in the case of children and adults.

Bronchial stenosis may also be associated with ILO. The lumen of the bronchus may be intrinsically narrowed by postinflammatory fibrosis or by an intraluminal mass such as aspirated meconium or other foreign material, bronchial adenoma, ectopic thyroid tissue, or bronchial mucosal web. Extrinsic causes of bronchial stenosis include parabronchial masses such as teratoma and bronchogenic cyst, enlarged or abnormally located pulmonary arteries, and cardiac or left atrial enlargement. Bronchial stenosis has also been associated with EA and TEF. More recently, studies have also suggested that bronchial stenosis and/or atresia are common features of CPAM, extralobar sequestration, intralobar sequestration (ILS), EA, and TEF (38,43). It is often difficult to demonstrate bronchial atresia and/or stenosis unless a dissecting microscope is used and the lesion is looked for carefully. The presence of an intrabronchial mucocele is helpful.

Bronchomalacia

Bronchomalacia and tracheobronchomalacia are seen most frequently in premature infants treated for prolonged periods with mechanical ventilation (39). Congenital bronchomalacia is rare and occurs when there is abnormal development of bronchial cartilage, leading to collapse of the lumen and possible development of secondary pneumonia. Bronchomalacia has also been suggested as a cause of sudden death in infancy and early childhood. Deficiency of subsegmental bronchial cartilage with bronchial collapse is also a feature of Williams-Campbell syndrome and has been noted in children with Larsen syndrome. Children with Down syndrome have a high incidence (up to 50%) of laryngomalacia, tracheomalacia, and bronchomalacia (44).

Histologically, the affected bronchus is decreased in size, with the usual cartilage plates replaced by scattered small islands of immature-appearing cartilage. The lung distal to the collapsed bronchus may show pneumonia or is distended in a pattern typical of ILO. Bronchial stents are used in the treatment of this abnormality but have been associated with complications including an aortobronchial fistula (39).

Bronchial Isomerism Syndromes

Bronchial isomerism results in "mirror–image" lungs (i.e., bilateral right or left lung) and is associated with five types of "polysplenia/asplenia" or heterotaxy syndromes (36).

Type 1, Ivemark asplenia syndrome, is a nonfamilial malformation complex involving bilateral right-sidedness, including absence of the spleen, intestinal malrotation, symmetric liver, and bilateral three-lobed "right" lungs with bronchi for both lungs. A variety of cardiac malformations are also associated with this type, including right aortic arch, symmetric venae cavae, transposition of the great vessels, and total anomalous pulmonary venous return.

Type 2, M-anisosplenia, involves boys who have one or more larger and one or more smaller spleens, along with congenital heart malformations, bilateral three-lobed "right" lungs, and relatively normal visceral situs.

Type 3, the polysplenia syndrome, is characterized by a bilateral two-lobed "left" lung bronchial pattern with intestinal malrotation, symmetric liver, congenital heart malformations, and 4 to 14 uniform small spleens.

Type 4, F-anisosplenia, involves females who have bilateral two-lobed "left" lungs, congenital heart malformation (usually double outlet right ventricle), and anisosplenia.

Type 5, O-anisosplenia, is characterized by bilateral two-lobed "left" lungs, an approximately 50% incidence of intestinal malrotation, multiple spleens, an equal sex ratio, and congenital heart malformations, particularly double-outlet right ventricle, ostium atrioventriculare commune, or both (see Chapter 13).

Abnormal Bronchial Branching and Origin

Abnormal branching patterns, mostly minor anomalies such as double stem superior segments of lower lobe bronchi and trifurcation of the left upper lobe bronchus, are seen in nearly 10% of bronchograms (45). However, major anomalies are also seen, including double right lobe bronchus, accessory cardiac bronchus, tracheal origin of the right upper lobe bronchus (also called preparterial bronchus), and bridging bronchus (46).

McLaughlin et al. (47) noted a tracheal origin of a bronchus in 2% of 412 symptomatic patients younger than 5 years of age who were undergoing bronchoscopy. The various forms of tracheal bronchus (Figure 12-12) may lead to recurrent episodes of pneumonia requiring resection of the bronchus and lobe. Other anomalies are noted in more than 75% of patients with tracheal bronchus. Wells et al. (48) suggest that in patients with sling left pulmonary artery, the tracheal bronchus often associated with the right upper lobe may represent the "normal" origin of the bronchus,

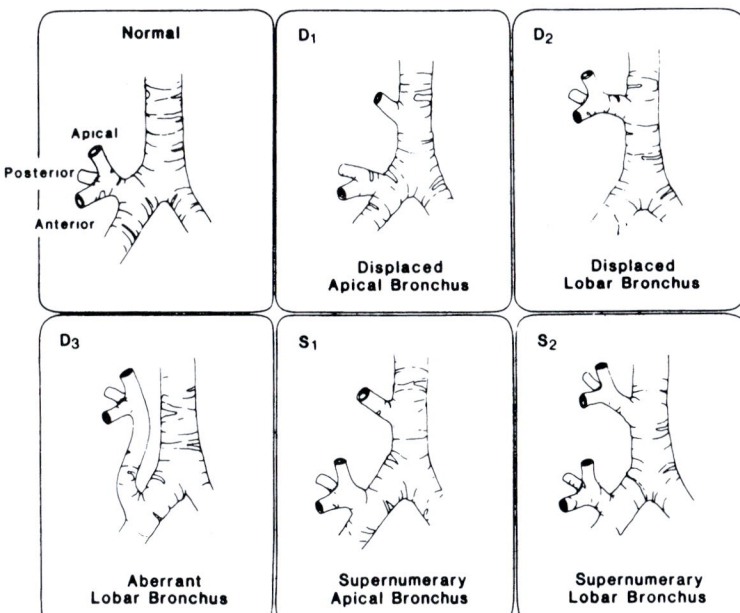

FIGURE 12-12 • Anatomic variations of right upper lobe bronchus. (From McLaughlin FJ, Strieder DJ, Harris GB, et al. Tracheal bronchus: association with respiratory morbidity in childhood. *J Pediatr* 1985;106:751, with permission.)

and the bronchi supplying the right middle and lower lobes are branches of the left main bronchus that are crossing or "bridging" the mediastinum (Figure 12-13). They note that the origin of the tracheal bronchus is at the normal level of tracheal bifurcation (T4-5), and the bifurcation of the bronchi supplying the left lung and right middle and lower lobes is at the T6-7 level.

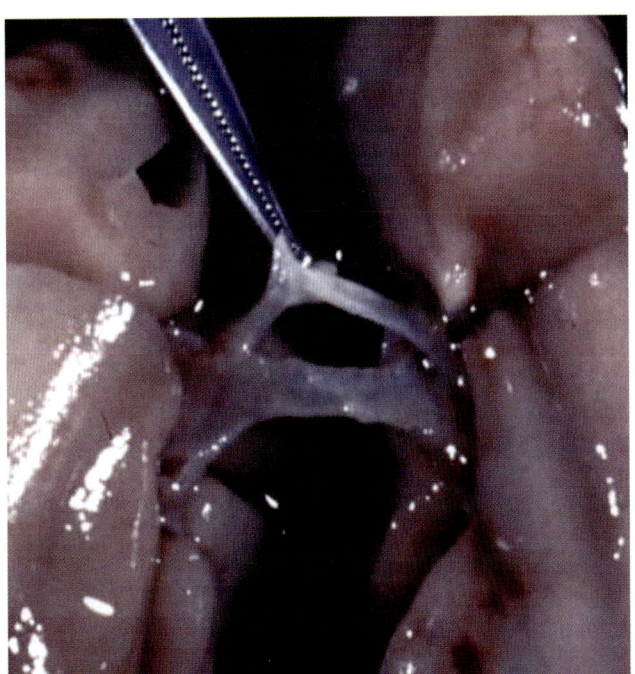

FIGURE 12-13 • A bronchus "bridges" the mediastinum in the case of tracheal agenesis.

Bronchobiliary and Bronchoesophageal Fistulae

Bronchoesophageal fistula probably represents a variation of TEF but may also be seen with infectious diseases such as tuberculosis and has been reported in association with Crohn disease.

Congenital bronchobiliary fistula rarely occurs; however, when it does, it is usually located between the right mainstem bronchus and the left hepatic duct (49). The bronchobiliary fistula is thought to represent a duplication of the upper gastrointestinal tract from its junction with the airway to the level of the ampulla of Vater. The fistula arises from the proximal portion of the right main bronchus, accompanies the esophagus through the diaphragm, and joins the biliary tree at the left hepatic duct. In its proximal portion, the tract resembles a bronchus with cartilage rings and respiratory epithelium, and in its distal portion, the tract resembles a bile duct or esophagus. Bronchobiliary fistulas may be seen in older children and adults and has been described secondary to biliary obstruction, liver infections (such as echinococcosis), and liver tumors (such as undifferentiated embryonal sarcoma).

Bronchogenic Cyst

The bronchogenic cyst is a discrete, extrapulmonary fluid-filled mass. It is most frequent in the hilar or middle-mediastinal area but may be present in a midline location from the subcutaneous region of the suprasternal area to beneath the diaphragm (1,50,51). They need to be differentiated from esophageal and enteric duplication cysts and pericardial cysts that may also be present in the mediastinal region. Bronchogenic cysts are rarely connected to the tracheobronchial tree or involve the pulmonary parenchyma. Case

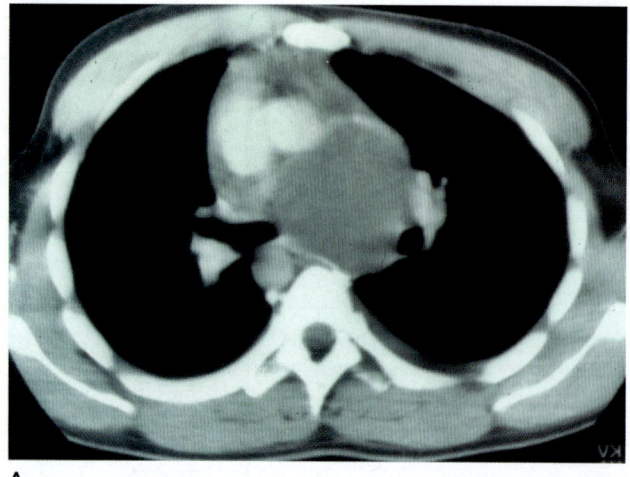
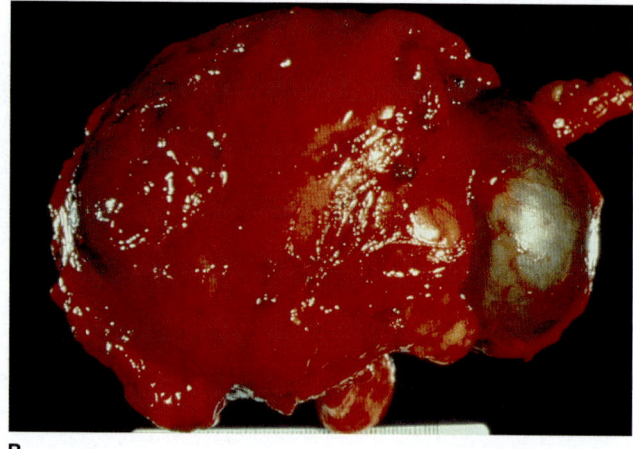
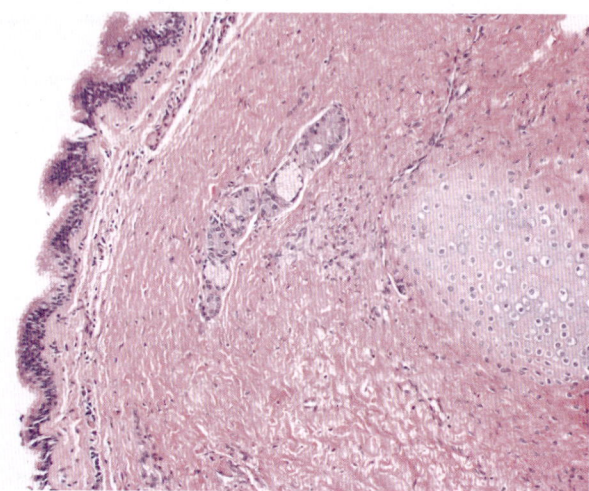

FIGURE 12-14 • Bronchogenic cyst. **A:** A CT of the chest displays a large mass in the middle mediastinum. **B:** A resected bronchogenic cyst, which was separate from the lung, is covered by connective tissue. **C:** Ciliated pseudostratified columnar epithelium overlies a wall composed of fibrous connective tissue, glands, and a cartilage plate in a bronchogenic cyst.

reports of "intrapulmonary bronchogenic cysts" probably represent instances of type 1 CPAM (52).

Bronchogenic cysts are seen most frequently in children and young adults as incidental findings on chest radiographs, at surgery, or at autopsy, but they may present with symptoms related to secondary infection of the cyst, including fever, hemorrhage, or perforation. In infants, bronchogenic cysts located near the trachea, especially the carina, may produce obstruction and respiratory distress.

In infants, the gross appearance of the cysts consists of a 1- to 4-cm, smooth-to-irregular, spheroid mass attached to, but not in communication with, the tracheobronchial tree (Figure 12-14A to C). The cysts may contain clear serous fluid, but if they are infected, the fluid may be turbid or hemorrhagic. In older patients, the cysts may reach a diameter of 8 to 10 cm and may be found throughout the mediastinum as well as in or beneath the diaphragm. Extrathoracic cysts are usually confined to the subcutaneous region in the suprasternal area (53).

Microscopically, the lining of the cyst is composed of ciliated cuboidal to pseudostratified columnar epithelium. Cartilage plates and seromucous glands are present in the wall, as is fibromuscular connective tissue (Figure 12-14C). The presence of striated muscle and stratified squamous or columnar epithelium suggests an esophageal cyst (Figure 12-15). Enteric cysts are lined by mucus-secreting columnar epithelium and contain gastric glands with parietal cells in the wall. All three types of cysts may display squamous metaplasia, mucosal ulceration, inflammation, extensive necrosis, or a combination of these, making an exact diagnosis difficult. Pericardial cysts are lined by mesothelium.

Bronchogenic cysts have been noted between the sequestration and the midline in association with extralobar sequestrations in older children. This suggests that the cysts have arisen from "rests" of bronchogenic cells along the abortive foregut tract that gave rise to the sequestration (54).

Plastic Bronchitis

Children with cardiac defects, especially in those requiring a Fontan procedure (1% to 2% of cases) or an underlying pulmonary disease (asthma or allergic disease), may develop obstructive bronchial cast (55,56). There are two types of casts: type I, cellular casts made up of inflammatory cells with fibrin, and type II, acellular casts composed mainly

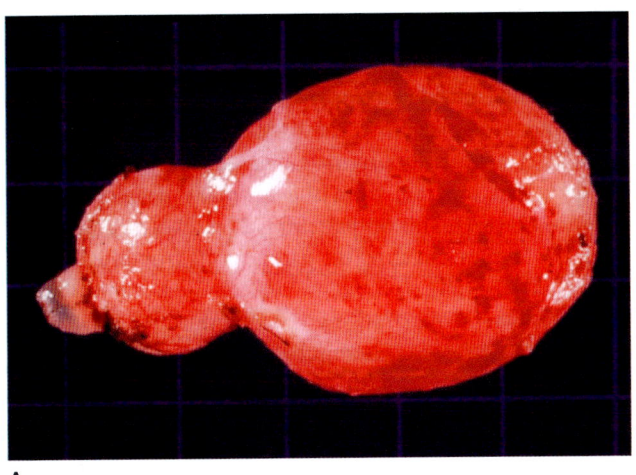
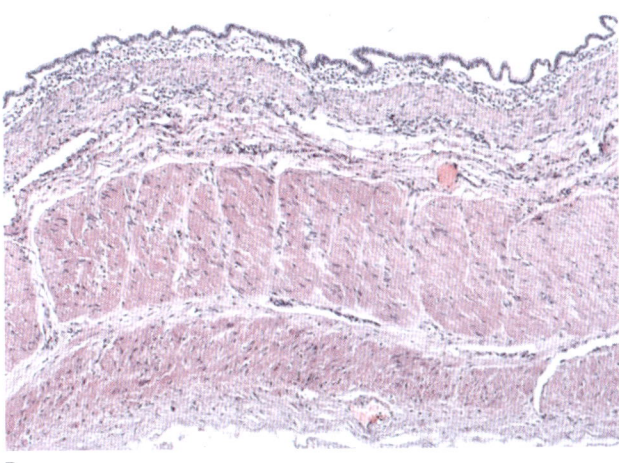

FIGURE 12-15 • Esophageal cyst. **A:** A cystic structure was resected from the middle mediastinum adjacent to the esophagus. **B:** Columnar epithelium overlies a wall composed of thick muscular bands in this esophageal cyst from the mediastinum.

of mucin. Other underlying causes include cystic fibrosis (CF), neoplasia, alpha-thalassemia, beta-thalassemia, and acute chest syndrome of sickle cell disease. Secretory hyperresponsiveness with excess mucin secretion is regarded as the basis for the disorder (57).

Grossly, the cast is a partial or complete mold of the bronchial tree with either tube-like features or partially or completely solid cores. Those composed of acellular mucin may be partially clear to opaque. Microscopically, the cast has a mucofibrinous appearance with or without inflammatory cells and cellular debris. In the case of hypersensitivity airway disease or asthma, the cast contains eosinophils and Charcot-Leyden crystals.

LUNG

Pulmonary Agenesis

Complete absence of both lungs is extremely unusual and incompatible with life. However, unilateral agenesis, involving one or more lobes, has been seen in 1 in 10,000 to 20,000 autopsies and, in the absence of other severe anomalies, is compatible with long-term survival (58). There is a 1.3:1 female predominance with unilateral agenesis; the right and left lungs are absent with equal frequency. Associated anomalies are noted in about 75% of cases and include, in decreasing order of frequency, cardiovascular, gastrointestinal, skeletal, and urogenital systems (59). Cardiovascular malformations include dextrocardia, septal defects, patent ductus arteriosus, and total anomalous pulmonary venous return. Skeletal anomalies include hemivertebrae and a high frequency of thumb malformations, especially triphalangeal thumb (Mardini-Nyhan association) (60). Along with the radial and vertebral anomalies, imperforate anus and TEF have been described, suggesting an association of pulmonary agenesis with the VATER or VACTERL association (61). There are also some phenotypic similarities to the syndrome associated with inactivation of ERK/MAP kinase genes MEK1 and MEK2 (62).

The larynx and upper trachea are usually well-formed in unilateral pulmonary agenesis, although with bilateral agenesis the total trachea may be absent. The lower trachea in unilateral agenesis may continue directly into the existing lung as a tracheobronchus or bifurcate at the carina, giving rise to a rudimentary blind-ending bronchus on the side of the agenesis. The pulmonary artery and vein to the side of the agenesis are absent or hypoplastic and may have an unusual course to the lung, often forming a pulmonary sling (63). Shift of the mediastinum to the side of the agenesis is usually present, often giving the appearance of dextrocardia in right-sided agenesis. Studies in older infants have demonstrated an absolute increase in the number of alveoli in the existing lung despite a reduced number of bronchial generations and pulmonary artery branches.

Abnormal Lobation, Location, and Shape

Abnormalities of lobation of the lung are usually of little clinical significance unless they are associated with other anomalies such as the asplenia or polysplenia syndrome (discussed earlier in chapter). Lobes may be fused to give the appearance of a single lobe on the right or left, or pleural fissures may produce the appearance of multiple lobes. The appearance of multiple lobes may be seen in infants with long-standing healed bronchopulmonary dysplasia (64). Fusion of the lungs in the midline behind the heart produces a conjoined, or "horseshoe," lung analogous to the horseshoe kidney. Additional anomalies are often present in association with horseshoe lung, including those of the VATER association and the PAGOD syndrome (pulmonary hypoplasia, agonadism, omphalocele, dextrocardia, and diaphragmatic defect), among others (65). Bronchial supply to both lungs may be anatomically normal, but there is usually an anomalous pulmonary artery supply and venous drainage resembling that seen in scimitar syndrome.

Herniation of the lung across the mediastinum into the opposite hemithorax, associated with ILO, CPAM, extralobar sequestration, and other conditions, occurs relatively frequently (1). The lung can also herniate outside the thoracic cavity, usually into the neck. Cervical herniation or "protrusion" is most frequently reported as a "normal variant" in some infants and children. It may also be seen, however, as a result of trauma or surgery, and in association with iniencephalus, the Klippel-Feil syndrome, and the cri du chat syndrome. A familial occurrence has been noted, and the condition is thought to be an autosomal dominant hereditary disease. Herniation through the diaphragm and intercostal spaces may also occur.

Pulmonary Sequestration

Sequestration is defined by a segment of lung parenchyma with its own systemic arterial blood supply independent of the normal lung. There are two basic types of sequestrations: extralobar (ELS) and intralobar (ILS) (1).

Extralobar Sequestration

Extralobar sequestrations of the lung are distinctly different from ILSs in that they are discrete masses of pulmonary parenchyma outside the normal pleural investment of the lung and are not connected to the tracheobronchial tree (25). They apparently originate from an outpouching of the foregut, and separate from the normally developing lung (Figure 12-16A). This outpouching then loses its connection with the foregut, isolating the parenchyma from the tracheobronchial tree (54).

Extralobar sequestrations are diagnosed prenatally in about 25% of cases, and about 60% of these patients present by 3 months of age (67). Presenting symptoms, often noted on the first day of life, include cyanosis, dyspnea, and difficulty in feeding. Approximately 10% of patients are asymptomatic. Fetal nonimmune hydrops, anasarca, pleural effusion, or localized edema may be present along with maternal polyhydramnios. Extralobar sequestrations may be seen in older children, occasionally in association with a bronchogenic cyst, and they have been reported in adults as old as 81 years of age. There is a slight female predominance.

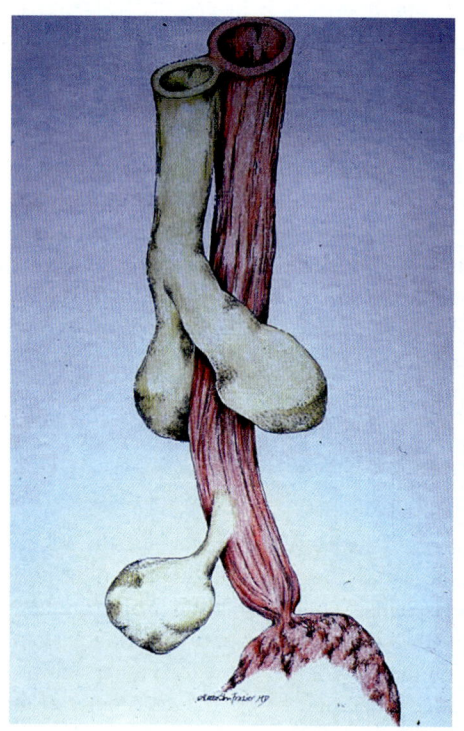
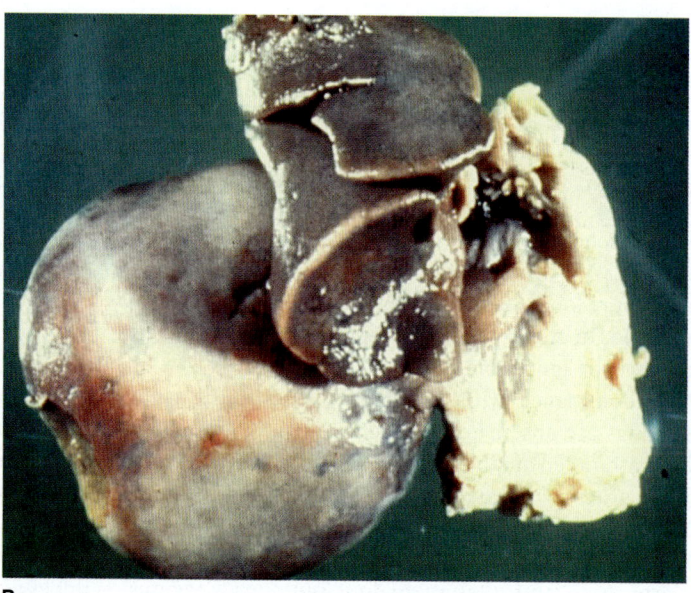

FIGURE 12-16 • Extralobar sequestration. **A:** The normal lung develops as an evagination from the foregut (**top half**). A second evagination (**bottom**) from the foregut gives rise to lung tissue not attached to the normally developing lung. **B:** A large right-sided thoracic mass is attached to the mediastinum by a thin vascular pedicle. Note the hypoplasia of the right lung.

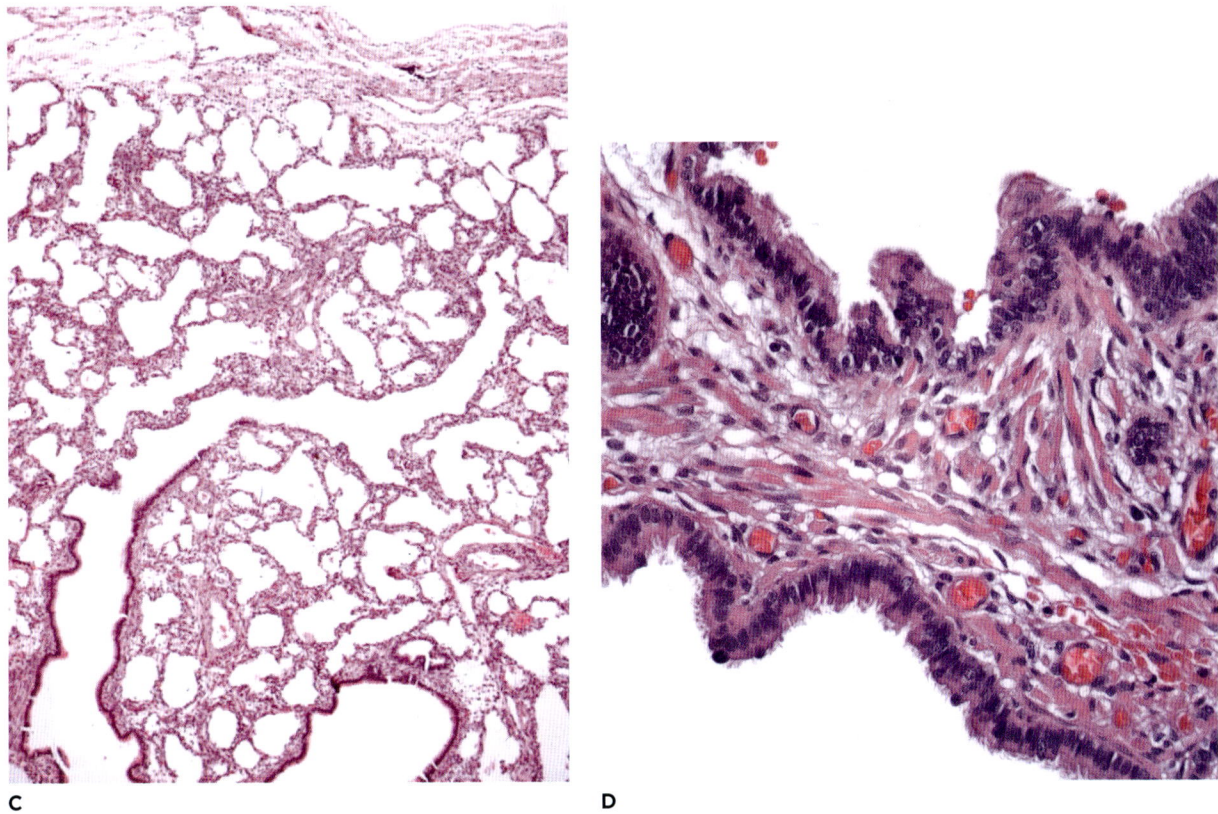

FIGURE 12-16 • (Continued) C: The pulmonary parenchyma is uniformly dilated from the bronchioles to the most distal alveoli. D: Back-to-back bronchiole-like structures typical of CPAM type 2 are seen in 50% of extralobar sequestrations. Note also the rhabdomyomatous dysplasia.

Associated anomalies are present in more than 65% of cases of extralobar sequestration, with 50% of lesions containing CPAM type 2 within the sequestration or, less frequently, in a lobe of the "normal" lung. The ELS/CPAM cases are seen more frequently in the first 3 months of life and on the left side (67). Other anomalies include bronchogenic cyst, cardiovascular malformations, bronchopulmonary foregut connection, pectus excavatum, absence of pericardium, and diaphragmatic hernia with concomitant pulmonary hypoplasia. High levels of CA19–19 have been reported in a few cases of extralobar sequestration.

Extralobar sequestration is usually a single round to ovoid lesion ranging from 0.5 to 15 cm in diameter (Figure 12-16B). In a report of 50 cases, 48% of the lesions were located in the left hemithorax, 20% in the right hemithorax, 8% in the anterior mediastinum, 6% in the posterior mediastinum, and 18% beneath the diaphragm (67). The blood supply to the extralobar sequestration is through a direct branch of the thoracic or abdominal aorta in over 75% of cases. The remaining receive their blood supply from smaller systemic arteries, the pulmonary artery, or rarely, from a systemic artery (25). Venous drainage is through the systemic circulation in over 80% of cases; the remaining 20% of cases are drained either partially or completely by the pulmonary veins, or, rarely, by the portal vein (68).

Grossly, the lesion is covered by a smooth to wrinkled pleura overlying a fine, reticular network of lymphatics. These lymphatics may be prominent in 30% or more of cases. Cut sections of the lesion display homogenous, pink-to-tan tissue resembling normal pulmonary parenchyma, or clusters of small cysts. Prominent subpleural lymphatics may also be seen.

Microscopically, extralobar sequestrations consist of uniformly dilated bronchioles, alveolar ducts, and alveoli in a normal acinar pattern (Figure 12-16C). Bronchioles are usually tortuous with undulating cuboidal to columnar epithelium. In 50% of cases, the lesion may consist partially or entirely of back-to-back, dilated, bronchiole-like structures typical of CPAM type 2 (Figure 12-16D). Lymphatics are unremarkable in the majority of cases but may be dilated and increased in number beneath the pleura and around bronchovascular bundles, occasionally resembling congenital pulmonary lymphangiectasia (CPL) (Figure 12-16C). Although they are rare, infarction, arteritis, and inflammation may be present in an extralobar sequestration. In the absence of severe anomalies, survival is good, although with large intrathoracic lesions, the associated pulmonary hypoplasia may be severe enough to cause death. Rhabdomyomatous dysplasia is seen in 25% to 30% of cases (Figure 12-16D).

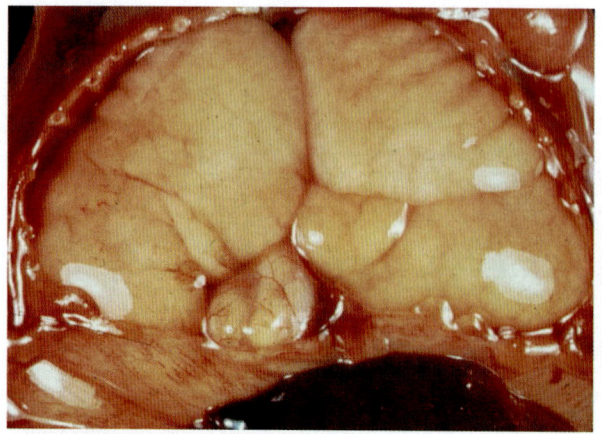

FIGURE 12-17 • Hyperplastic lungs in the case of laryngeal atresia are massively enlarged, displaying the markings of the ribs on their surface.

"Total" Sequestration with Pulmonary Hyperplasia

Infants with laryngeal or tracheal atresia without TEF have, in effect, "total" sequestration of the lungs and display a histologic appearance virtually identical with that seen in extralobar sequestration. The lungs are often two to four times the expected weight and crowd the chest cavity, flattening the diaphragm and leaving an impression of the ribs on the visceral pleural surface (Figure 12-17) (25). Similar pulmonary changes may be seen with *in utero* hyperextension of the neck that appears to compress and obstruct the larynx. Scurry et al. (69) have noted normal sized or hyperplastic lungs in infants with varying degrees of upper airway obstruction despite the presence of renal dysgenesis and oligohydramnios, conditions more frequently associated with pulmonary hypoplasia. Lymphatics are unremarkable. Atresia or obstruction of a single bronchus to a lobe may lead to hyperplasia of that lobe and the development of one form of ILE (see below) (66).

Intralobar sequestration

Intralobar sequestration (ILS), by definition, consists of a portion of lung within the normal pleural investment that is isolated (sequestered) from the tracheobronchial tree and is supplied by a systemic artery (Figure 12-18) (25,70). Although a small percentage of ILSs are clearly congenital in origin and might more correctly be called arteriovenous malformations (71), the vast majority of ILSs are probably acquired lesions formed through

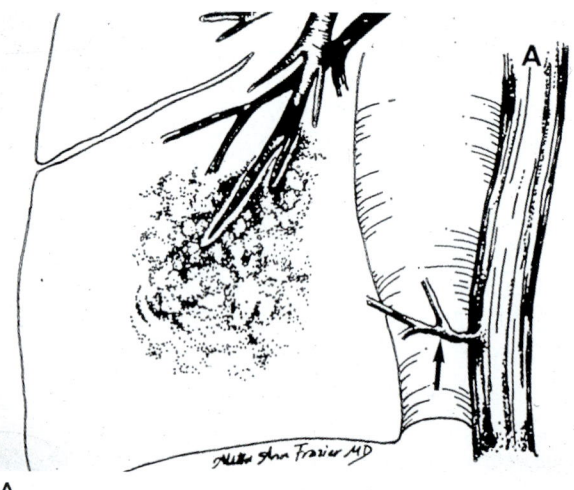
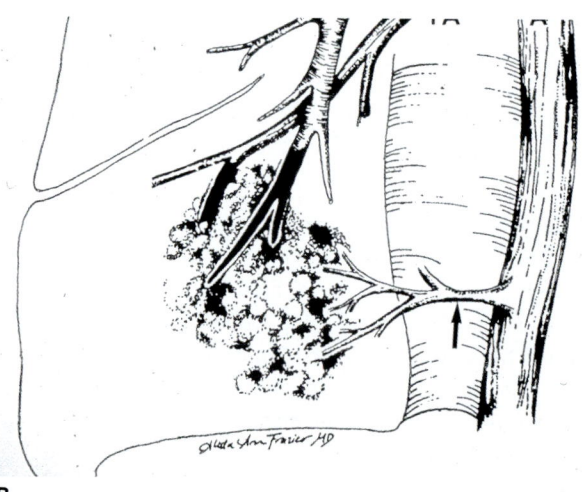
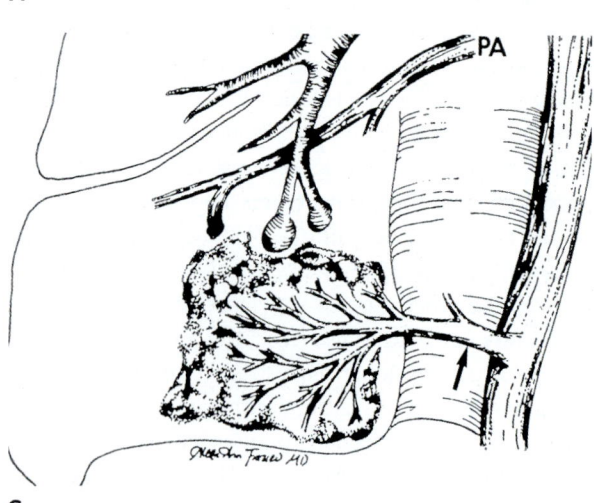

FIGURE 12-18 • Sequence of events in the formation of intralobar pulmonary sequestration. **A:** Occlusion of a bronchial branch by means such as aspirated material or inflammatory debris can lead to the development of pneumonia distal to the occlusion. **B:** As the pneumonia persists or progresses, the lung seeks oxygenated blood to aid in resolution and repair. If pulmonary artery flow is inadequate, systemic blood supplying pleural granulation tissue through the pulmonary ligament arteries may be "parasitized." **C:** As the pneumonia resolves (or progresses or recurs), the major arterial supply to the sequestered portion of lung is derived from the hypertrophied pulmonary ligament artery (or arteries). (From Stocker JT, Malczak HT. A study of pulmonary ligament arteries: relationship to intralobar pulmonary sequestration. *Chest* 1984;86:611, with permission.)

repeated episodes of pneumonia. During the course of these episodes, normal pulmonary ligament arteries become hypertrophic to provide the systemic artery supply (Figure 12-18A to C) (70,72). Some examples of ILS may develop within a previously existing malformation (e.g., CPAM). The following evidence suggests the acquired nature of ILS (66,73):

- ILS is rarely seen in the newborn (<15 cases described in children younger than 5 years of age).
- ILS is infrequently associated with other congenital malformations.
- ILS is limited to the lower lobes in 98% of cases, allowing access to normally occurring pulmonary ligament arteries.
- ILS-affected patients have a frequent history of repeated pulmonary infections.
- ILS presents with a clinical picture of chronic or recurrent pneumonia (e.g., cough, sputum production) in over 85% of cases.

ILSs involve the lower lobe in 98% of cases with this probably reflecting the availability, within pleural granulation tissues, of branches of normally occurring pulmonary ligament arteries or arteries within the diaphragm that are parasitized for access to oxygen-rich systemic blood. The pulmonary ligament arteries originate from the thoracic aorta and extend through the pulmonary ligament between the mediastinum and the lower lobes of the lung (70). No comparable arteries except the bronchial arteries are present for potential use by the upper lobes in cases of chronic or recurrent pneumonia.

Radiographic findings include cystic areas, some with fluid levels, along with homogeneous and inhomogeneous shadows (74). Lack of communication with the tracheobronchial tree is demonstrable by bronchography in about 85% of cases; the other 15% of cases show some communication between the bronchial tree and the sequestration. Arteriography demonstrates single (84%) or multiple (10%) systemic arteries (Figure 12-19A, B). The majority of the arteries (73%) originate from the thoracic aorta, but about 21% originate from the abdominal aorta or celiac axis and another 4% from the intercostal arteries. In rare instances, arteries may originate from the coronary, subclavian, innominate, internal thoracic, or pericardiophrenic arteries. Venous drainage occurs through the pulmonary veins in 95% of cases, and the remaining 5% of cases drain into the systemic circulation. Increased serum levels of CA19-19 and CA125 have been noted in patients with ILS (75).

ILS is located on the left side in 55% of cases and on the right in 45% of cases; bilateral involvement is rare. Grossly, the sequestered segment of lung displays variable pleural thickening with adhesions between mediastinal structures, the diaphragm, and the parietal pleura. Variably sized (1 mm to 5.0 cm) cysts filled with thin to viscid fluid are noted amid a dense fibrous parenchyma on cut section (Figure 12-19).

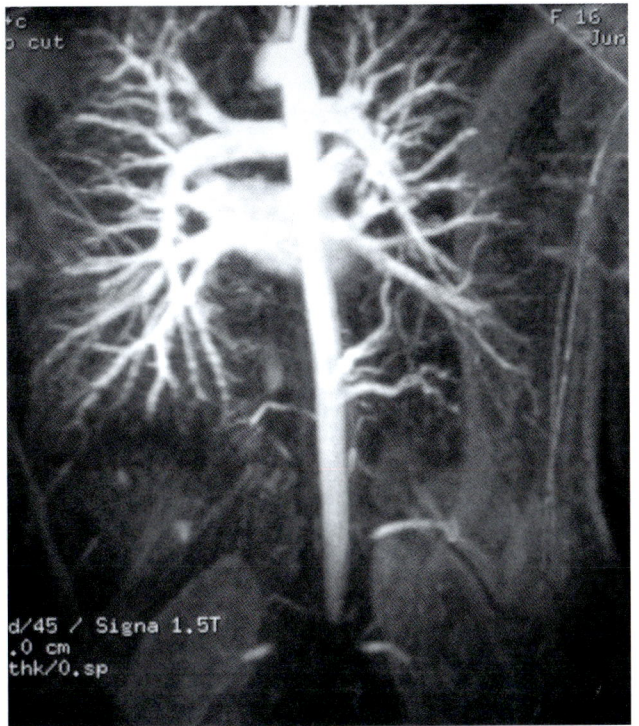

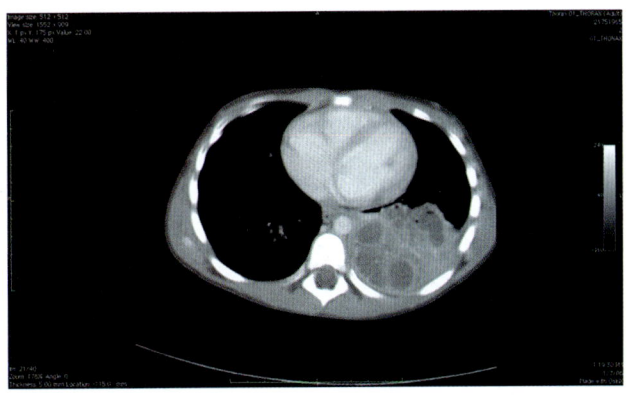

FIGURE 12-19 • Intralobar sequestration. **A:** An arteriogram demonstrates arteries arising from the descending aorta (**mid right**) supplying a portion of pulmonary parenchyma. **B:** A CT demonstrates a mass in the posterior area of the right hemithorax.

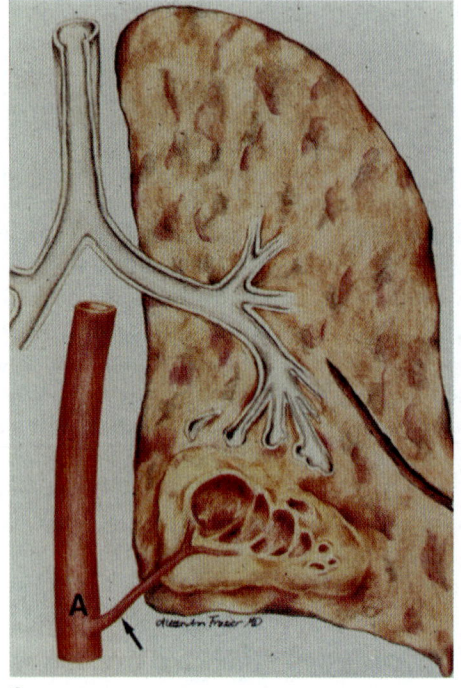 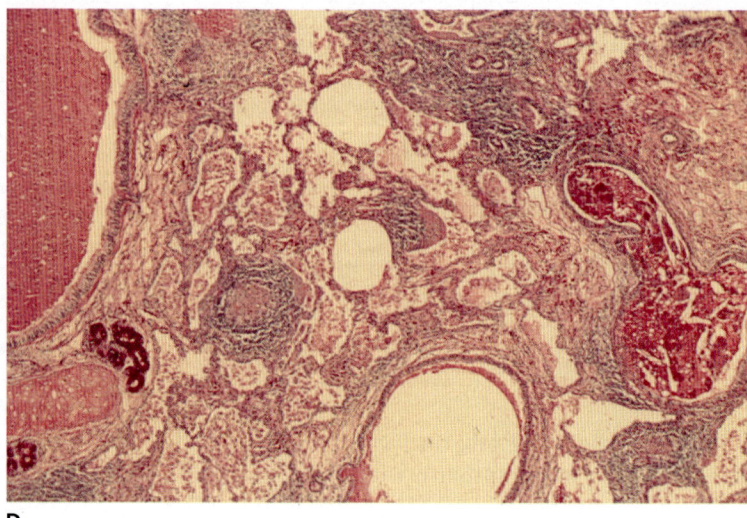

C   D

FIGURE 12-19 • (Continued) **C:** An artery arising from the descending aorta and passing through the pulmonary ligament supplies a cystic portion of the lung in the left lower lobe. **D:** Dense fibrous connective tissue containing lymphoid aggregates surrounds irregular cysts filled with debris and macrophages.

Microscopically, the pulmonary parenchyma is distorted by chronic inflammation and fibrosis (Figure 12-19D). The cysts are lined with cuboidal or columnar epithelium and are filled with amorphous eosinophilic material, foamy macrophages, or both. Elastic and muscular arteries are present within the interstitium and may show medial hypertrophy, thrombosis, and arteritis (76).

Pulmonary Hypoplasia

Pulmonary hypoplasia is the incomplete or defective development of the lung resulting in overall reduced size due to reduced numbers or size of acini (Figure 12-20A). Lung weight and lung weight–to–body weight ratio are the simplest means of determining whether hypoplasia exists. The normal lung weight–to–body weight ratio for term and near-term infants is 0.022 (range 0.012 to 0.025) (77). Emery and Mithal (78) describe a radial alveolar count using a line intersect method in which a line is drawn from a terminal bronchiole perpendicular to the nearest septal division or pleura surface (Figure 12-20B). The number of alveoli intersected by the line determines the count with the mean for term infants of 4.4 ± 0.9 (79). Alveolar counting and lung volume measurements may also be used to define hypoplasia (80). Two-dimensional or three-dimensional ultrasound and MRI have also been used in determining whether the lungs of an *in utero* fetus or newborn infant may be hypoplastic. However, secondary changes such as bronchopneumonia or pulmonary hemorrhage which increase the weight of the lungs create difficulties in the assessment for the presence of hypoplasia on basis of lung weight alone. One simple but less precise observation is the distance of a terminal bronchiole from the pleural surface.

Pulmonary hypoplasia is noted in more than 10% of neonatal autopsies and occurs in association with another malformation (or malformations) in more than 85% of cases (81). The most frequently occurring anomalies are diaphragmatic defects and renal malformations (Table 12-3), but a wide variety of anomalies have been described (1). The common feature of most of these anomalies is that they directly or indirectly compromise the thoracic space available for lung growth. The cause of the decreased thoracic space may be intrathoracic (e.g., abdominal contents herniated through a defect in the diaphragm) or extrathoracic (e.g., enlarged cystic kidneys). The thorax itself may be abnormal as in Jeune asphyxiating thoracic dystrophy, spondyloepiphyseal dysplasia congenita, and achondroplasia (82). *In utero* accumulation of fluid within the thorax as pleural effusion or chylothorax has also been implicated in the production of pulmonary hypoplasia.

Pulmonary hypoplasia may also occur in the absence of other anomalies or in cases of prolonged preterm premature rupture of amniotic membranes leading to oligohydramnios, loss of fetal cushioning, and lack of amniotic fluid pressure and growth factors which would normally be inhaled into

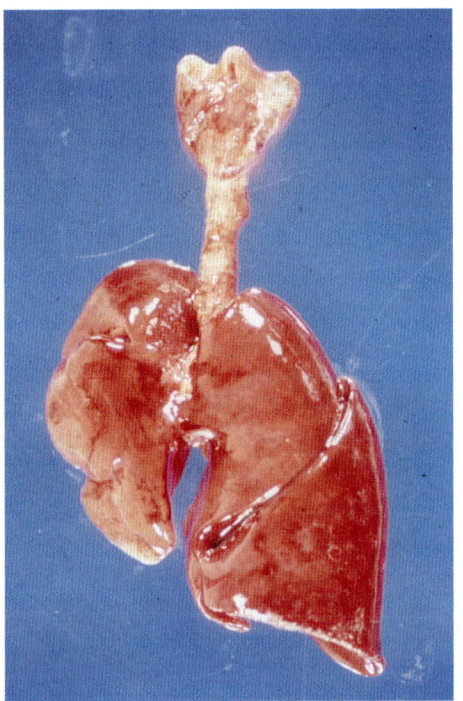 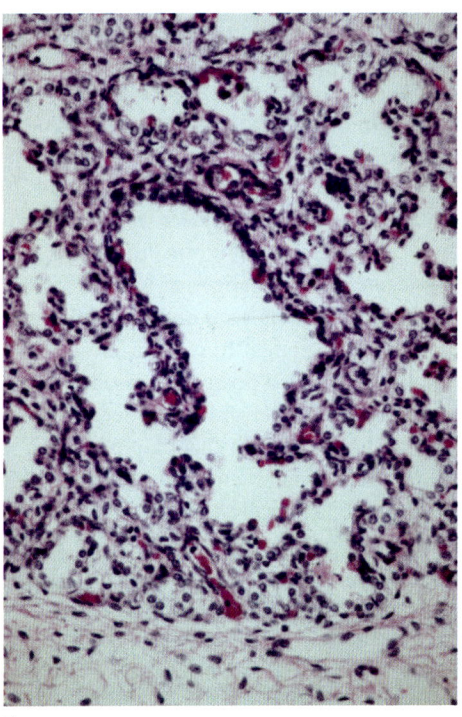

FIGURE 12-20 • Pulmonary hypoplasia. **A:** The right lung is markedly diminished in size, secondary to herniated abdominal organs through a right-sided diaphragmatic hernia. By weight, the left lung is also hypoplastic. **B:** At the periphery of an acinus in this hypoplastic lung, a radial alveolar count (RAC) is far below the normal of 4 to 6 for a term infant, confirming the diagnosis of hypoplasia.

TABLE 12-3 ANOMALIES ASSOCIATED WITH PULMONARY HYPOPLASIA

Common
- Diaphragmatic hernia
- Renal agenesis, bilateral
- Renal dysgenesis, bilateral
- Obstructive uropathy
- Polycystic renal disease (autosomal recessive)
- Large abdominal wall defects

Infrequent
- Diaphragmatic hypoplasia or eventration
- Anophthalmia/microphthalmia—usually in association with diaphragmatic hernia
- Hemolytic disease of the newborn
- Pleural effusion, as with nonimmune fetal hydrops
- Musculoskeletal abnormalities, such as thoracic dystrophies
- Anencephaly
- Scimitar syndrome
- Chromosomal anomalies, including trisomy 13, 18, and 21

Rare
- Abdominal pregnancy
- Ascites secondary to congenital cytomegalovirus infection
- Cloacal dysgenesis
- Congenital hydropericardium
- Down syndrome (probably postnatal "hypoplasia")
- Eagle-Barrett syndrome
- Giant cervical teratoma
- Glutaric acidemia, type II
- Homozygous β-thalassemia
- Horseshoe lung
- Hypoplasia of the arcuate nucleus
- Laryngotracheoesophageal cleft
- Neonatal hypophosphatasia
- Pena-Shokeir syndrome, type I
- Phrenic nerve agenesis
- Right-sided cardiovascular malformation, as with hypoplastic right side of the heart and pulmonary valve or artery atresia
- Rhabdomyoma in tuberous sclerosis
- Thoracic neuroblastoma
- Upper cervical spinal cord
- Extralobar sequestration

the lung (81). As with infants with hypoplasia secondary to other anomalies, these infants present with respiratory distress, are difficult to ventilate, and frequently have episodes of pneumothorax (PT) and interstitial pulmonary emphysema (IPE). Potter sequence with sloping forehead, flattened face and nose, receding chin, large ears, broad spade-like hands, and deformations of the limbs secondary to compression by the uterus in the absence of adequate amniotic fluid is a consistent finding in cases associated with oligohydramnios from any cause. Pulmonary hypoplasia has been noted in children with Down syndrome, but it is thought to result from failure of the lung to develop properly in the postnatal period (83).

At autopsy, the lungs may be either uniformly reduced in size or markedly asymmetric (e.g., with diaphragmatic hernia). In cases in which the pulmonary hypoplasia is the direct cause of death, the lung weight usually is less than 40% of expected and is often as low as 20% to 30%. Histologically, the acini are small for the infant's gestational age, but alveolar and capillary development is usually consistent with the gestational age.

Infantile (Congenital) Lobar Emphysema (Overinflation)

ILO is the overinflation or hyperplasia of a pulmonary lobe as the result of a partial or complete obstruction of the bronchus to the lobe by intrinsic or extrinsic factors (66) (Table 12-4). More recently, it is being recognized that not all cases involve the whole lobe; rather a segment is involved, especially on the left side where the upper segments are involved, sparing the lingula. This is especially important to recognize, since these patients may be cured by segmentectomy (84). Boys are more frequently affected than girls (1.5:1). ILO presents in the first week of life in about 50% of cases (with about 40% presenting in the first day of life) and in the first 6 months of life in over 80%, but ILO can occasionally be seen in children and young adults from 7 months to 20 years of age. Symptoms are those of mild respiratory distress increasing over a period of hours to days to weeks; cyanosis, respiratory infections, vomiting, choking, and feeding difficulties may also be seen. Rarely, the lesion may present as a sudden PT (66). Imaging studies reveal, in the classic form (see below), a characteristic hyperlucent, overdistended lobe producing mediastinal shift and compression of the uninvolved lobes (85) (Figure 12-21A). In the polyalveolar lobe form (see below), imaging may display a lobe of normal lucency but one that occupies a disproportionate part of the hemithorax with mediastinal shift. Less frequently, retained lung fluid may be seen in the involved hyperexpanded lobe (usually the polyalveolar lobe type) on initial examination but which may clear over subsequent days. Associated anomalies are present in 5% to 40% of patients, and 70% of these anomalies are cardiovascular (86). The upper lobes are involved in over 95% of cases—the left slightly more often than the right. Multiple lobe involvement occurs in about 15% of cases, usually with at least one lobe being an upper lobe. Bilateral involvement has been reported in one case involving the left upper and right middle lobes. Lower lobe involvement is rarely seen except in the "acquired" form of ILO, as in premature infants receiving mechanical ventilation who develop granulation tissue obstruction of a lower lobe bronchus, probably as a result of endotracheal tube suctioning (87).

Grossly, the lobe *in vivo* and after resection is hyperexpanded with individual alveoli, which may be readily visualized (Figure 12-21B). Microscopically, two patterns (classic and polyalveolar) are identified. Nearly, 70% (the classic pattern) display a uniform overdistension of apparently normally developed acini with alveolar saccules and alveoli three to ten times the normal size but with radial alveolar counts (RAC) similar to those of age-matched controls (Figure 12-21C) (66). There may be focal disruption of alveolar walls. The other 30% (the polyalveolar pattern) show only little overdistension of what appear to be "complex" acini of the type seen in polyalveolar lobes and hyperplastic lungs (Figure 12-21D), and these have RACs that are two standard deviations beyond the mean of age-matched controls. Seventy-five percent of these infants with polyalveolar lobe present clinically within the first day or two of life and are likely to show radiologic features of retained lung fluid (88,89). Examination of the bronchus to the lobe may reveal stenosis, atresia, or intrinsic obstruction, or the bronchus may be unremarkable if extrinsic compression was present. Cartilage abnormalities of the bronchial wall have been described, but special techniques must be employed to demonstrate these changes convincingly.

TABLE 12-4 CAUSES OF INFANTILE LOBAR OVEREXPANSION

Bronchial abnormality
  Bronchial stenosis
  Bronchial atresia
  Abnormal origin of bronchus
Extrinsic obstruction of bronchus
  Vascular anomaly
    Pulmonary artery sling
    Anomalous pulmonary venous return
    Left-to-right shunting with dilated pulmonary arteries
  External mass
    Bronchogenic cyst
Intrinsic obstruction of bronchus
  Aspirated meconium
  Mucous plug
  Granulation tissue
  Bronchial mucosal folds
  Torsion of bronchus
  Foreign body

Adapted from Stocker JT. Congenital and developmental diseases. In: Dail DH, Hammer SP, eds. *Pulmonary Pathology*. Heidelberg, Germany: Springer-Verlag, 1989:55, with permission.

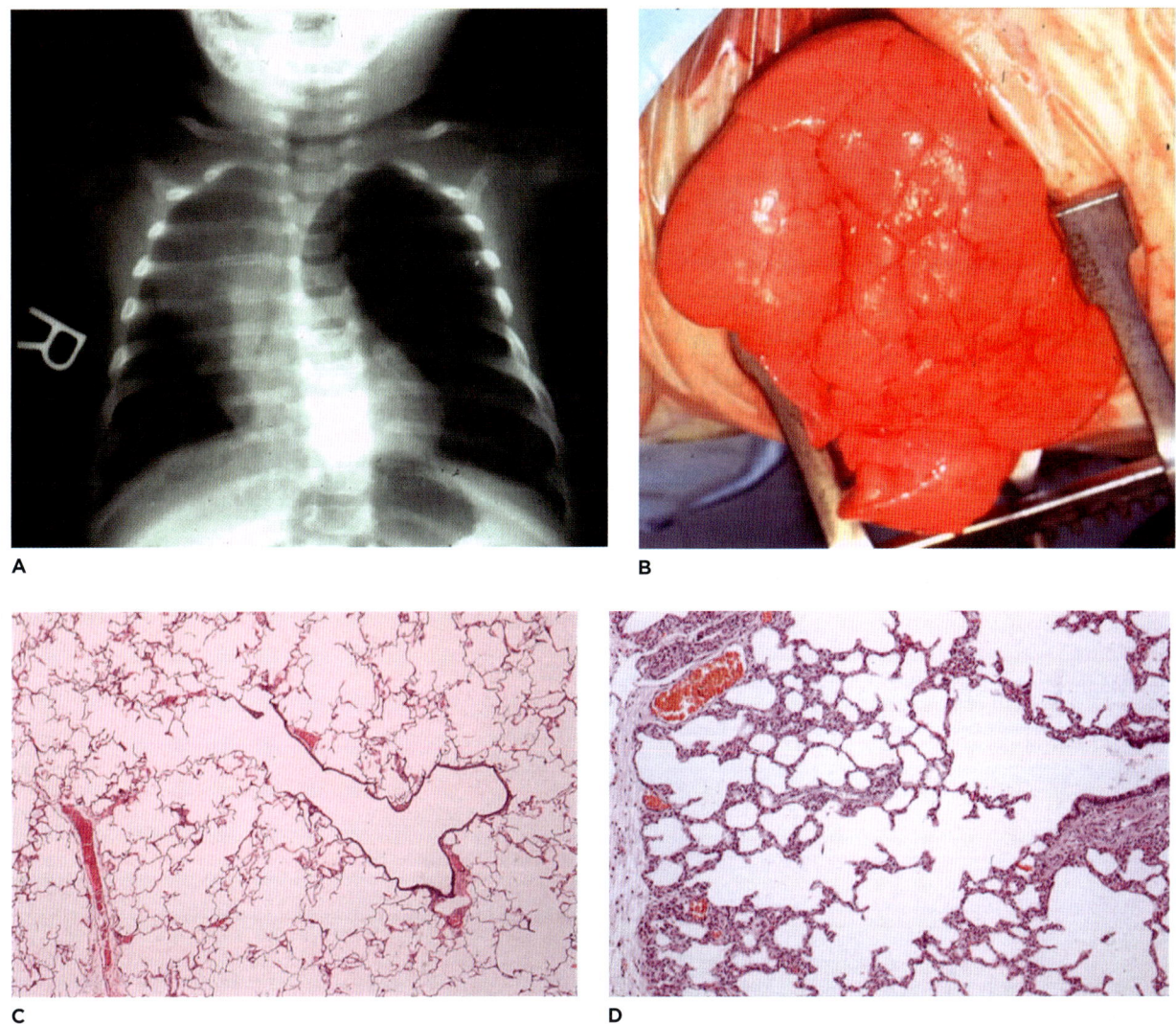

FIGURE 12-21 • Infantile lobar overinflation. **A:** A hyperinflated left lung shifts the mediastinum to the right. **B:** At surgery, the hyperinflated lung bulges from the opening in the thorax. **C:** "Classic" form of ILO. The alveolar duct and alveoli are dilated to 3 to 10 times the normal size but are otherwise unremarkable. **D:** "Hyperplastic" form of ILO. While not overinflated, this lung displays a complex acinar formation with a larger number of alveoli (and consequently a large radial alveolar count) than would be expected at this age.

Surgical resection of the involved lobe is curative, although nonsurgical management has been successful in unusual cases (85).

Congenital Pulmonary Lymphangiectasis

CPL is a rare, usually fatal disorder that presents in the first hours to days of life (90); 5% to 10% of affected infants are stillborn. It is characterized by the presence of dilated thin-walled to thick-walled lymphatics within the interlobular septa and beneath the pleura of the lung. CPL may be seen as a primary disorder or as secondary to obstructive cardiovascular lesions, particularly total anomalous pulmonary venous return, but it may occur as part of a generalized lymphangiectasis or as an isolated pulmonary lesion (91). There is a distinct male predominance of over 2.5:1. Symptoms include cyanosis and acute respiratory distress. Fluid abnormalities including chylothorax, pleural effusion, fetal hydrops, and maternal polyhydramnios have been described *in utero* and postpartum (92). In addition to the 60% of cases with cardiovascular anomalies, CPL is associated with renal malformations, generalized lymphangiectasis, and other anomalies, in another 20% of cases (1). The diagnosis of CPL in the absence of cardiovascular or other anomalies, should be strongly suspect.

The lungs in CPL are bulky, firm, noncompressible, and covered by a milky network of dilated subpleural lymphatics (Figure 12-22A). Rarely, a single lobe is involved by this process (93). On cut section, the lymphatics are fluid-filled and extend from the interconnecting subpleural network into the interlobular septa and around the bronchovascular bundles (Figure 12-22B). Microscopically, the lymphatics are diffusely

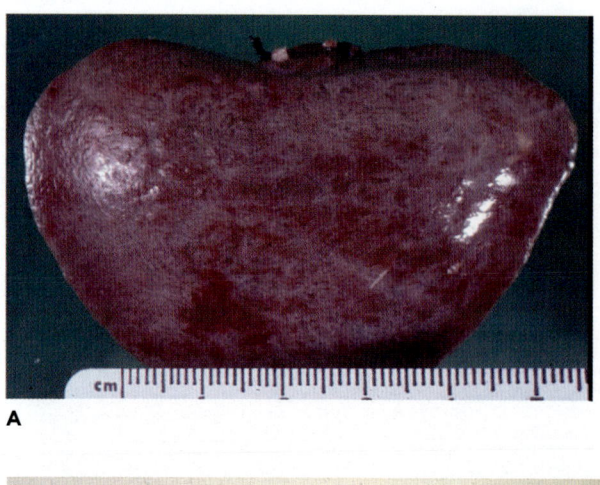
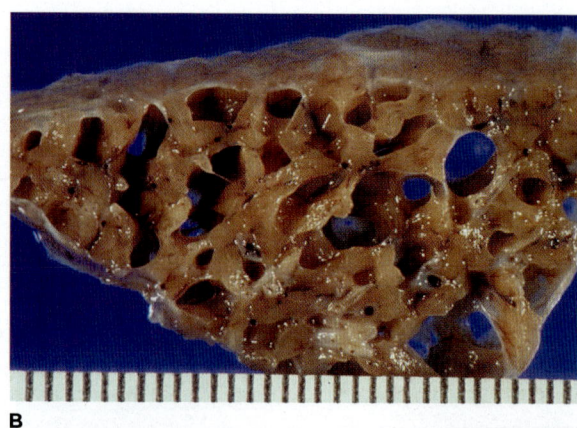
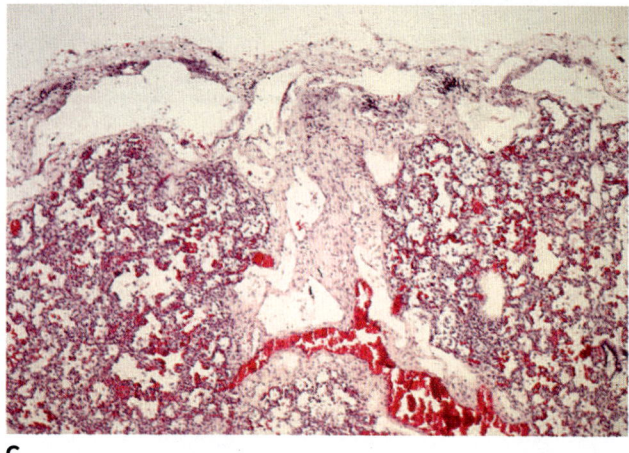
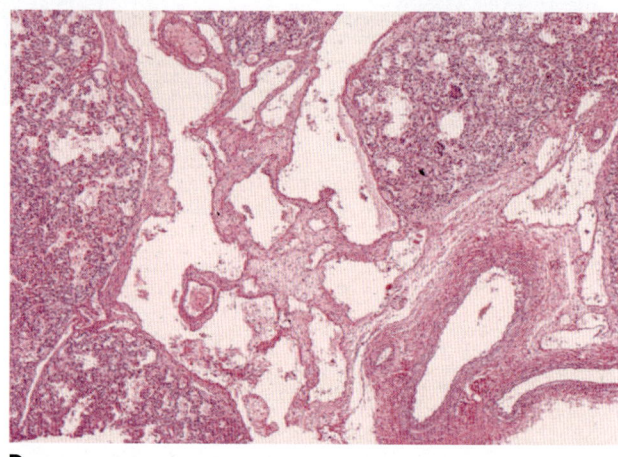

FIGURE 12-22 • Congenital pulmonary lymphangiectasis. **A:** A fine network of dilated lymphatics is present beneath the pleura, most notably where interlobular septa intersect the pleura. **B:** Cut section of the lung from an infant total anomalous pulmonary venous return reveals enormously dilated lymphatics. **C:** Dilated lymphatics extend laterally beneath the pleura (**top**) and centrally along an interlobular septum (**center**). Note the slight increase in connective tissue between the channels. **D:** Numerous dilated lymphatics extend along interlobular septa surrounding bronchovascular bundles.

and uniformly dilated and may appear to be increased in number. Identification of lymphatics can be aided by CD31 and D2-40 immunohistochemistry and can help differentiate the lesion from IPE. These small, irregular cysts are lined with a thin layer of endothelial cells and surrounded by a loose myxoid to occasionally dense connective tissue that often contains foci of extramedullary hematopoiesis. Clusters of lymphatics surround bronchovascular bundles within the interlobular septa and may separate acini beneath the pleura (Figure 12-22C, D). This is in contrast to the air-filled, larger, "unlined" cysts of IPE that are limited to the interlobular septa and do not extend laterally beneath the pleura.

Congenital Pulmonary Airway Malformation

CPAM is a developmental anomaly of the lung, with an incidence of about 1 in 5000 live births, that can be separated into four major types based on clinical and pathologic features (Figure 12-23) (94). The former designation "CCAM" was changed to "CPAM" to reflect the fact that the lesions as described below are "cystic" in only two of the four types and "adenomatoid" in only one type (type 3). CPAM more accurately encompasses three types in this classification. CPAMs are the most common surgically resected pulmonary malformation in children. CPAM is a unilateral lesion in about 95% of cases and involves a single lobe in 80% to 90% of cases. The right and left sides of the lung are nearly equally involved, with the lower lobes affected in about 60% of cases.

CPAM, type 0, also known as acinar dysplasia or agenesis, is a rarely occurring, infrequently described malformation that is largely incompatible with life (95). It may be regarded as the most extreme form of pulmonary hypoplasia. It is seen in term and premature infants who are cyanotic at birth and survive only a few hours and is associated with cardiovascular abnormalities and dermal hypoplasia. Grossly, the lungs are small and firm and have a diffusely granular

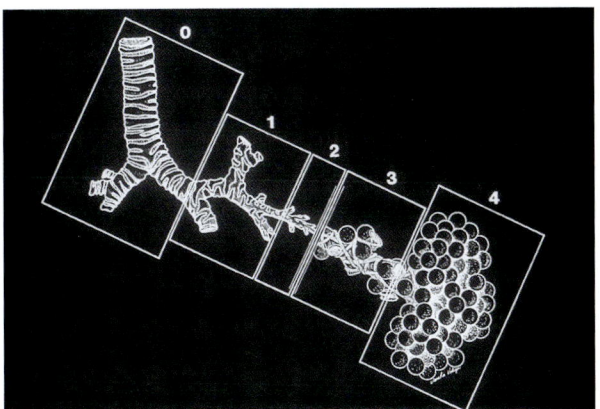

FIGURE 12-23 • Classification of CPAM. The classification is based on the similarity in appearance of the hamartomatous components of the lesion with the various areas of the normal tracheobronchial tree. Type 0, composed of bronchus-like structures, appears to be a malformation of the most proximal tracheobronchial tree. Type 1, containing bronchus-like and proximal bronchiole-like structures, mimics the distal bronchial tree and proximal acinus. Type 2, composed of bronchiole-like structures, resembles the bronchiolar segment of the acinus. Type 3, composed of bronchiole-like structures and alveolar ducts and saccules lined by cuboidal epithelium, resembles the midacinar region. Type 4, with thin-walled structures lined by type 1 alveolar lining cells, should be diagnosed correctly as PPB type 1. (From Stocker JT. Congenital and developmental diseases. In: Dail HD, Hammer SP, eds. *Pulmonary pathology*. 2nd ed. New York: Springer-Verlag, 1994:182, with permission.)

surface (Figure 12-24A). Microscopically, tissue consists of bronchus-like structures with muscle, glands, and numerous cartilage plates (Figure 12-24B). Prominent mesenchymal tissue separates these structures and contains extramedullary hematopoiesis, large thin-walled vascular channels, and collections of amorphic basophilic debris. Rarely, structures resembling proximal bronchioles are present, along with a few scattered acini at the periphery of the lesion.

CPAM, type 1, the large or predominant cyst type, presents primarily within the first week to month of life but can be seen in older children and even young adults (Figure 12-25A). It accounts for nearly 65% of cases and is usually readily amenable to surgery with a good prognosis. Grossly, the type 1 lesion is characterized by single or multiple large cysts (3 to 10 cm in diameter) surrounded by smaller cysts and compressed normal parenchyma (Figure 12-25B, C). Microscopically, the larger cysts are lined with ciliated, pseudostratified columnar epithelium and the smaller ones by cuboidal to columnar epithelium (Figure 12-25D, E). More than 45% of the cases display segments of mucus-producing cells among the epithelial lining of the larger cysts or in bronchioles and alveolar duct-like structures adjacent to the larger cysts (Figure 12-25F). These mucous cells are recognized to be precursors for adenocarcinomas (Figure 12-26) (see below—Tumors) that have been described in association with type 1 CPAM (96,97). The walls of the CPAM, type 1 cysts are composed of elastic tissue overlying fibromuscular connective tissue, and in 5% to 10% of cases, cartilage plates.

CPAM, type 2, the medium cyst type, accounts for 10% to 15% of cases, is seen exclusively within the first year of life and has a poorer outcome owing to its more frequent association with other anomalies, some of which are incompatible with life (e.g., renal agenesis). The type 2 lesion is composed of cysts 0.5 to 2.0 cm in diameter (rarely larger) that are evenly distributed and blend with the adjacent normal parenchyma (Figure 12-27A). The cysts occasionally surround normal appearing bronchi. The typical back-to-back bronchiole-like structures are lined by cuboidal to columnar epithelial cells with a thin underlying fibromuscular layer (Figure 12-27B).

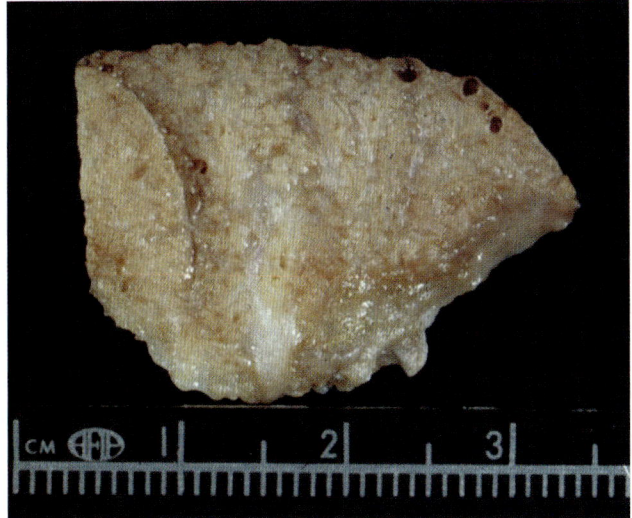

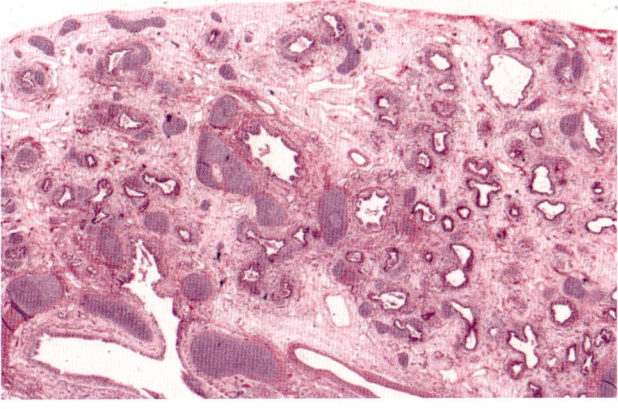

FIGURE 12-24 • CPAM, type 1 (congenital acinar dysplasia). **A:** A small nodular mass representing the right lung is largely devoid of air. A similar lung was present on the left side. **B:** Bronchial-like structures are surrounded by irregular cartilage plates and loose mesenchyme-containing thin-walled vascular structures.

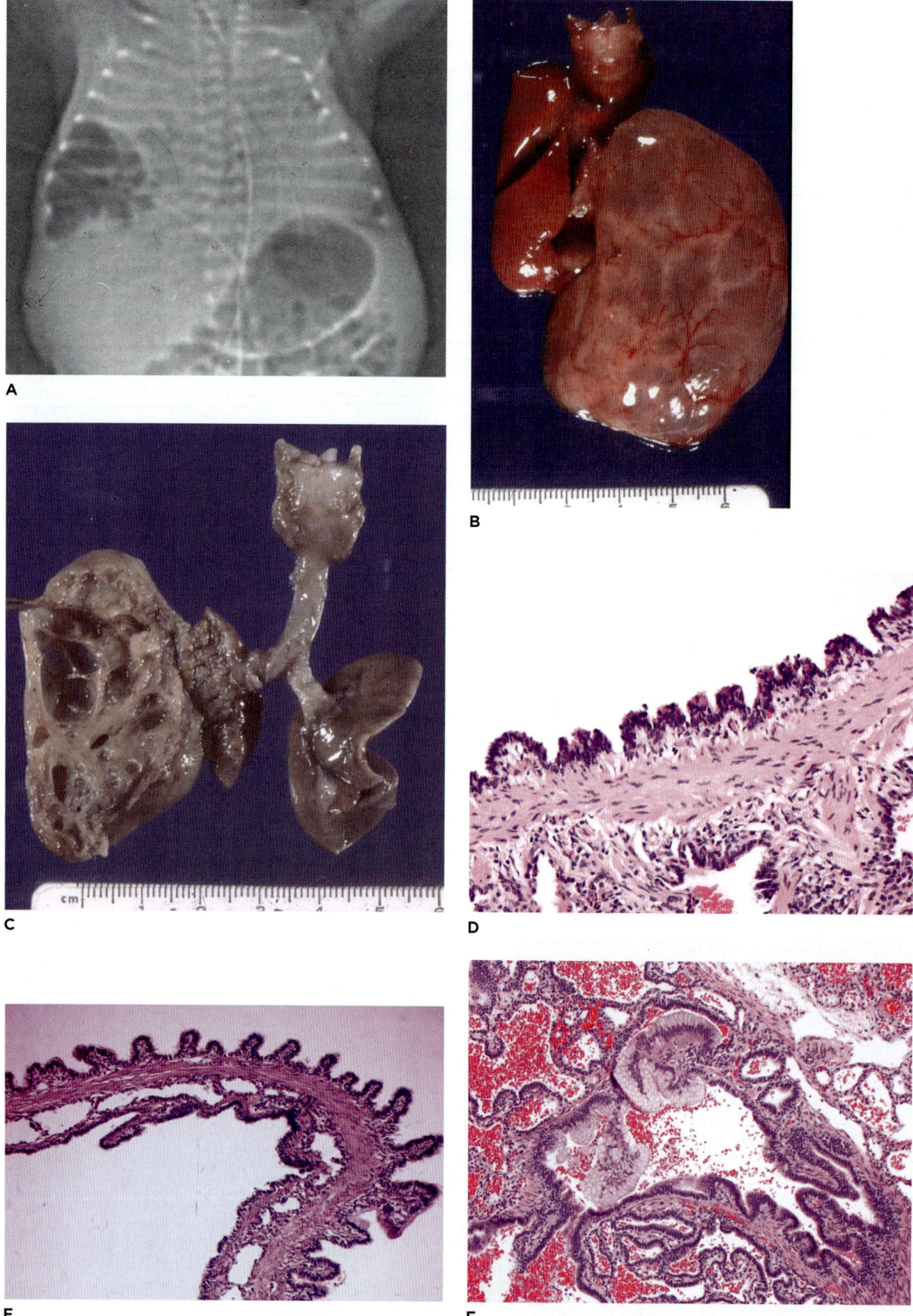

FIGURE 12-25 • CPAM, type 1. **A:** A cystic mass is present in the lower right hemithorax in a newborn with respiratory distress. **B:** Multiple large, fluid-filled cysts distend the left lobe from a fetus in the second trimester. **C:** When opened, the mass consists of intercommunication cysts. **D:** Cysts of type 1 CPAM are characteristically lined by ciliated intercommunicating in a sawtooth configuration with underlying fibromuscular connective tissue. **E:** A larger cyst wall (**top**) is covered by columnar epithelium in a papillary configuration. Note the columnar epithelial lining of the smaller cysts as well. **F:** Clusters of mucogenic cells are present along the cyst lining.

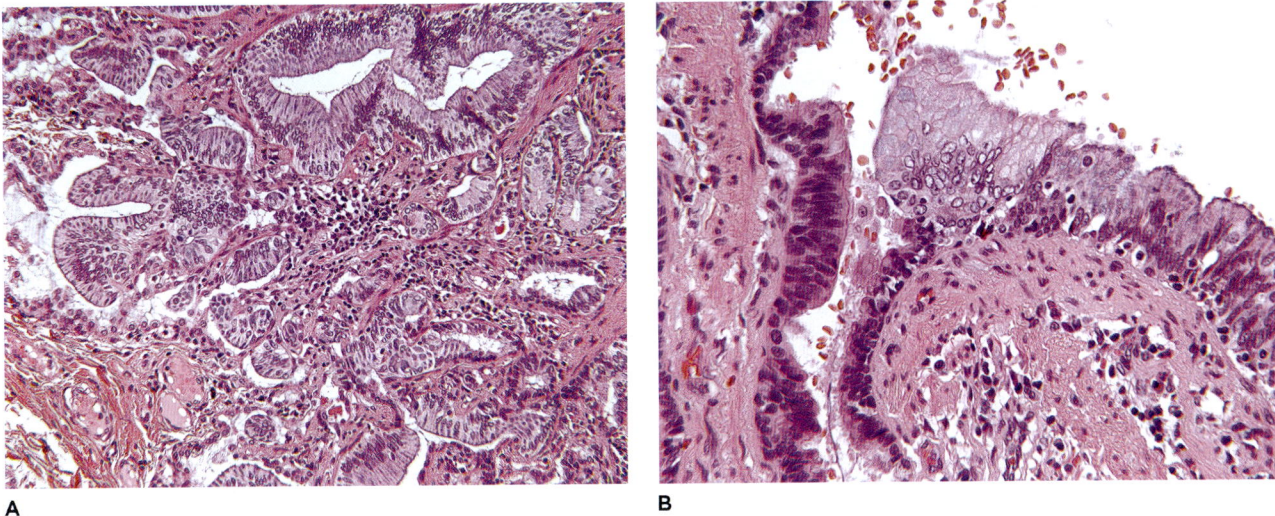

FIGURE 12-26 • CPAM type I. **A:** Mucinous metaplasia in the lung of an 18-year old who presented with a right middle lobe cyst. **B:** The mucinous epithelium has low-grade cytologic features, but it is thought that the changes are a precursor to mucinous adenocarcinoma.

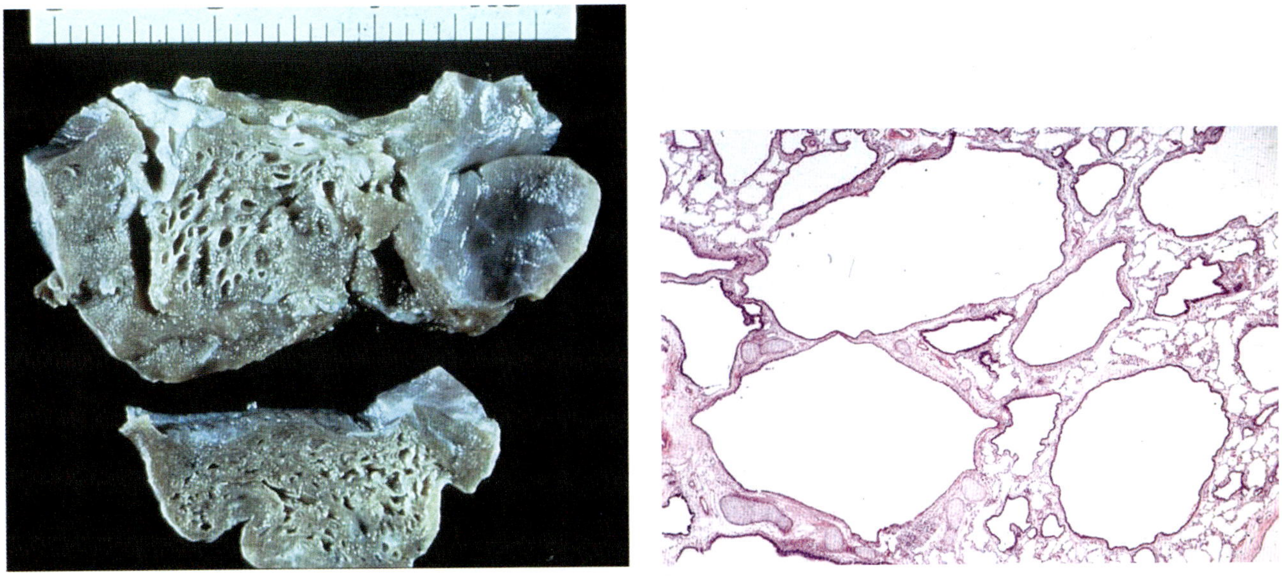

FIGURE 12-27 • CPAM, type 2. **A:** Small cysts (0.2 to 0.5 cm) are scattered throughout the lobe and blend with normal parenchyma. **B:** The back-to-back bronchiole-like structures are separated by structures resembling alveolar ducts. **C:** In a variant of type 2, striated muscle fibers are present in the connective tissue between and around cysts.

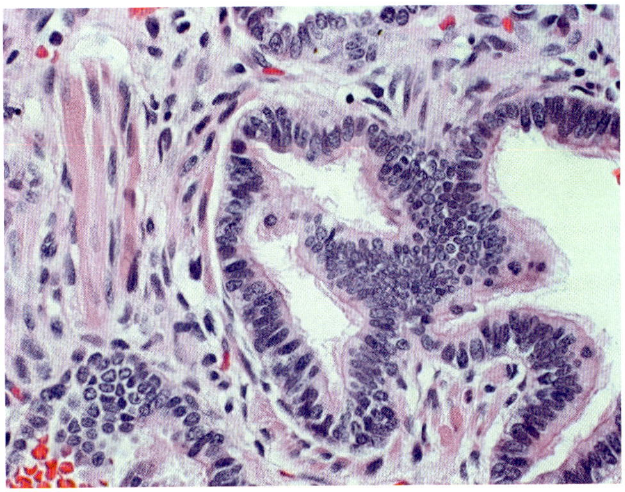

Mucous cells and cartilage plates are absent except as components of "entrapped" normal bronchi. A variant or subgroup of the type 2 lesion, termed rhabdomyomatous dysplasia, contains ribbons of striated muscle fibers throughout the lesion, both in association with the cysts and between alveolar ducts and around blood vessels (Figure 12-27C). The cysts of this rhabdomyomatous variant may be less prominent than other type 2 lesions. Rhabdomyosarcoma has been reported to originate from CPAM, but this likely represents a primary pleuropulmonary blastoma (PPB) rather than being secondary to CPAM. CPAM, type 2-like features are present in 50% of extralobar sequestrations (67).

CPAM, type 3, the small cystic or solid type, occurs infrequently (5% of cases), is seen exclusively in the first days to month of life, has a notable male predominance, and owing to its large size and association with maternal polyhydramnios and fetal anasarca, has a high mortality rate. Increased maternal levels of serum alpha-fetoprotein have been anecdotally noted in the second trimester in association with CPAM type 3. CPAM, type 3, the original lesion described by Ch'in and Tang (98), consists of a large, bulky, parenchymal mass involving an entire lobe or even an entire lung (Figure 12-28A, B). The mass effect of the lesion consistently produces mediastinal shift and often results in hypoplasia of the uninvolved lung. Cysts are rarely larger than 0.2 cm in diameter, with the exception of scattered larger bronchiole-like structures. Microscopically, the lesion resembles an immature lung devoid of bronchi. Irregular, stellate-shaped, bronchiole-like structures lined with cuboidal epithelial cells are surrounded by alveolar ductules and saccules that are also lined by cuboidal cells, imparting the "adenomatoid" appearance for which this lesion was originally named (Figure 12-28C). Mucous cells, cartilage, and rhabdomyomatous cells are not present, and there is a paucity of vessels within the lesion.

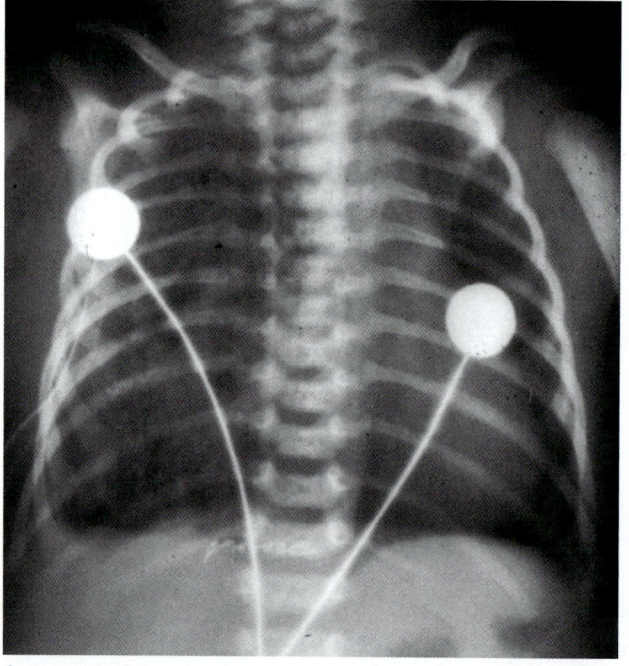

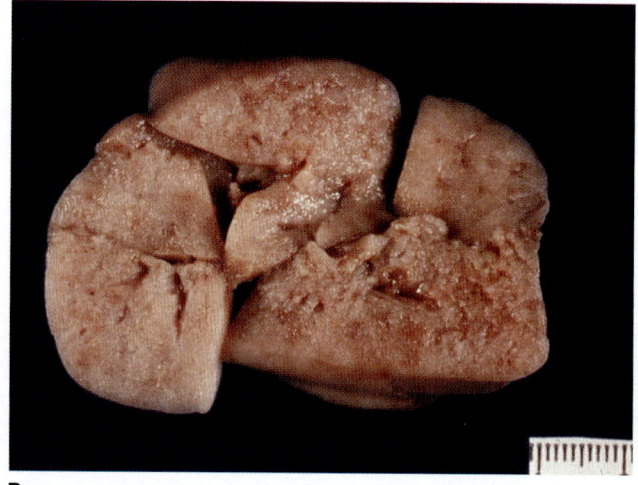

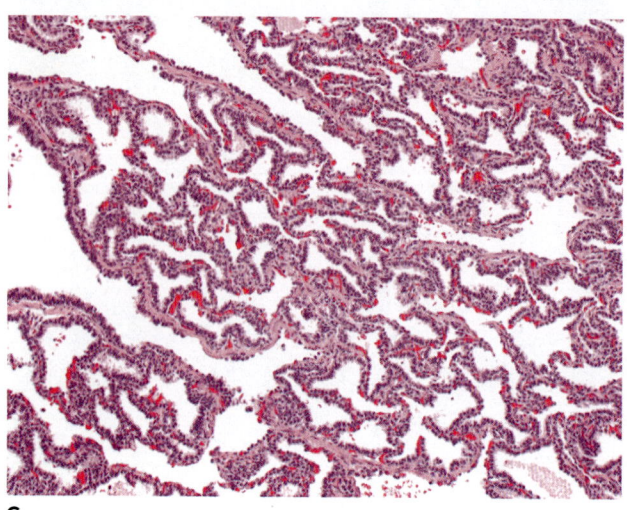

FIGURE 12-28 • CPAM, type 3. **A:** A large air-containing mass in the right hemithorax pushes the mediastinum to the left. **B:** The resected lesion is nearly solid with only a few slit-like openings. **C:** Randomly distributed irregular bronchiole-like structures are separated by dilated alveolus-like structures all of which are lined by cuboidal epithelial cells, imparting an adenomatoid (or gland-like) appearance.

CPAM, type 4, the peripheral acinar cyst type, is composed of large cysts lined by pneumocytes and it is very important to recognize it as the purely cystic pleuropulmonary blastoma (type 1 PPB). It is recommended that all children should be tested for DICER 1 mutation which is the first hit (of two-hits, see below) and is present in 70% of PPBs including those that are nonrecurring. Complete resection and close long-term follow-up are necessary (97). Once type 1 PPB has been excluded, CPAM type 4 is indeed rare if it exists at all. It is seen equally in boys and girls, with an age range of newborn to 4 years and accounts for 10% to 15% of cases. Before the recognition of type 1 PPB, most of these cases were included in the CPAM type 1 category. Clinically, the type 4 lesions may present with mild respiratory distress, sudden respiratory distress from tension PT, pneumonia, or on occasion, as an incidental finding with no symptoms (94). Radiographically, the lesion displays large air-filled cysts with mediastinal shift. The lesion involves a single lobe in about 80% of cases and rarely may be bilateral. Grossly, large thin-walled cysts are present at the "periphery" of the lobe and appear to be lined by a smooth membrane (Figure 12-29A). Microscopically, the cysts are lined by flattened

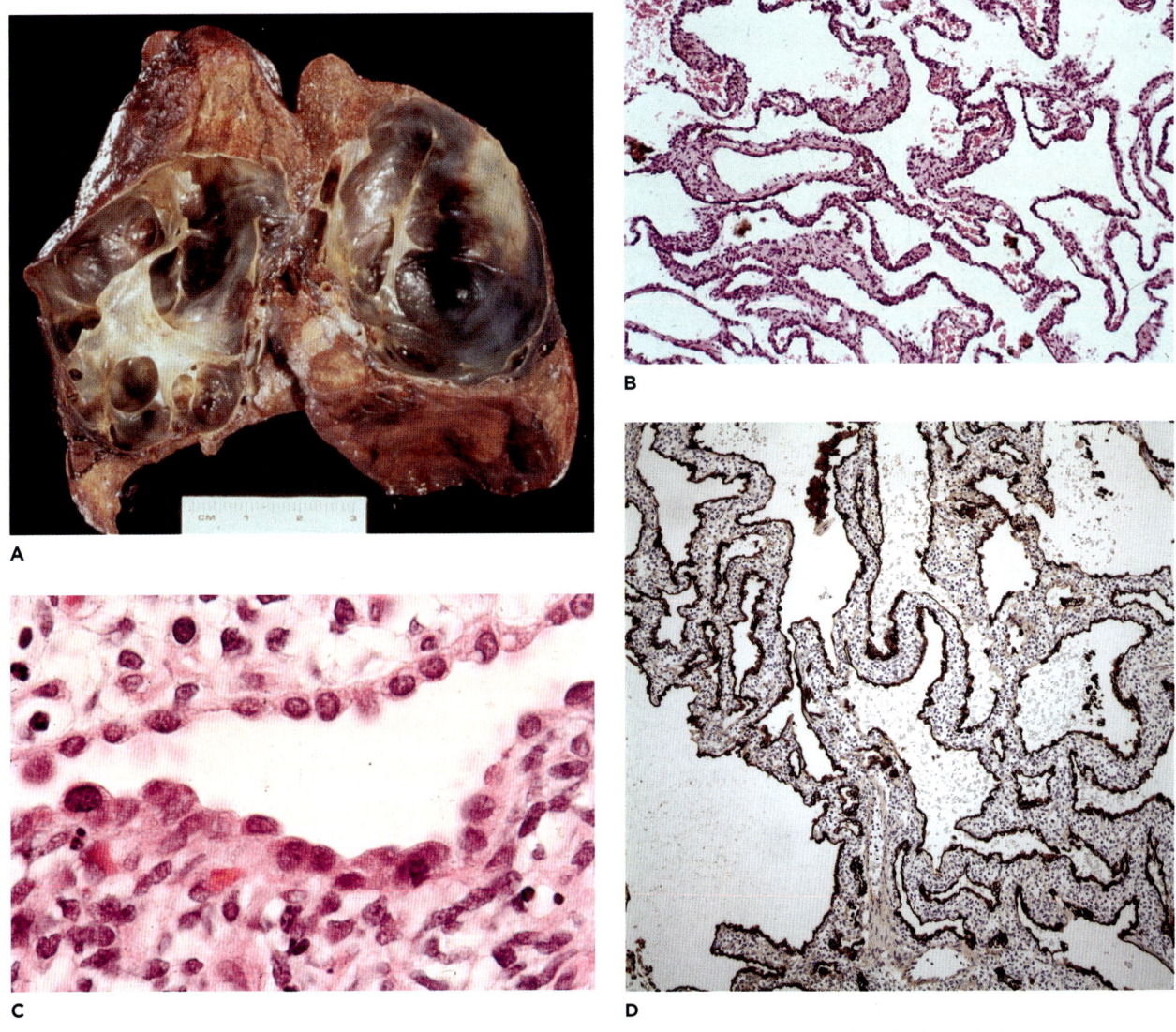

FIGURE 12-29 • PPB, type 1 (in the past diagnosed as CPAM type 4). **A:** The lung is distended by thin, almost translucent cyst walls. **B:** The walls of the cysts are composed of loose mesenchyme covered by an indistinct epithelial lining not apparent at this magnification (hematoxylin and eosin stain, original magnification ×25). **C:** The cyst walls are variously covered by an attenuated epithelium of alveolar lining cells (hematoxylin and eosin stain, original magnification ×150). **D:** The epithelium stains positively for cytokeratin (H&E, ×50). Note: Because of the similarities between PPB type 1 and CPAM type 4, it is best to consider these lesions as having the potential to progress to PPB types 2 and 3. All patients with such cystic lesions must have complete surgical excision with clear margins. If any doubt exists as to the correct diagnosis, the case should be referred to the International PPB Registry to ensure correct follow-up and management of the patient.

epithelial cells (type I and II pneumocytes), with occasional low cuboidal epithelium seen (Figure 12-29B to D). The wall of the cyst is composed of loose mesenchymal tissue with prominent arteries and arterioles. It must be emphasized that PPB type 1 and CPAM, type 4 are one in the same and should be viewed and managed as PPB.

Ultrasonography has been demonstrated to be a highly useful modality in the *in utero* diagnosis of CPAM. *In utero* serial sonography has demonstrated the gradual reduction in the size of CPAM, type 1 and 2, with subsequent normal development of the uninvolved lung (99,100). Anomalies are noted in 15% to 20% of all cases of CPAM, particularly in association with the type 2 lesion (94,101) including bilateral renal agenesis/dysgenesis, extralobar pulmonary sequestration, cardiovascular malformation, diaphragmatic hernia, hydrocephalus and macrocephaly, myelomeningocele, jejunal atresia, prune belly syndrome, sirenomelia, bilateral nephromegaly, Pierre Robin syndrome, pulmonary hypoplasia, skeletal malformation, bile duct hypoplasia, left heart hypoplasia, polycytosis of a solitary medial kidney, and congenital nephrotic syndrome (diffuse mesangial sclerosis).

Congenital Alveolar Capillary Dysplasia

Congenital alveolar capillary dysplasia with or without misalignment of pulmonary veins (ACD/MPV) is a uniformly fatal rare entity that presents as respiratory distress, progressive hypoxemia, and pulmonary hypertension in the newborn (102). Familial occurrence has been noted (103); most cases are sporadic, with familial cases showing paternal imprinting (Table 12-5). Many cases have been reported to harbor microdeletions in the *FOX* gene cluster on 16q24.1 and mutations in the *FOXF1* gene, a transcription factor that is involved in organogenesis (104). It is characterized by the failure of formation and ingrowth of alveolar capillaries. Broad alveolar septa with large alveolar capillaries within the septal wall are the hallmark of this disorder (Figure 12-30A to D) (105). Capillaries are centrally placed well beneath the basement membrane of the alveolar lining cells and surrounded by loose mesenchyme (Figure 12-30C). Ectatic veins are present within bronchovascular bundles, occasionally within the adventitia of the pulmonary arteries, and may form an intermittent ring around the bronchiole (Figure 12-30B). Small muscularized arteries are also present within the acini, extending to the precapillary area (Figure 12-30D). Other changes include paucity of alveolar capillaries and abnormal capillary size and location, seen as centrally located thin-walled dilated and congested alveolar wall vessels. Special stains including Movat pentachrome, trichrome, elastic, CK7 (for pulmonary epithelium), CD31 (for microvasculature), and SMA (for vascular smooth muscle) may be used to highlight the constellation of histologic changes. High capillary apposition and density may correlate with survival beyond the neonatal period. About a third of the patients with ACD/MPV also have pulmonary lymphangiectasis (106,107) and about 80% have anomalies of other organ systems (108). Treatment with inhaled nitric oxide and ECMO has prolonged life but has been uniformly unsuccessful in changing the fatal outcome of this disorder without lung transplantation.

Peripheral Cysts of the Lung

Peripheral, air-containing cysts of the lung can be seen in neonates, infants, and young children; it occurs in association with Down syndrome, as a result of pulmonary infarction, or in association with idiopathic spontaneous PT (109). Occlusion of the pulmonary artery in infants can result in peripheral infarction of the lung, which, with necrosis and organization, can produce subpleural cysts of varying size. Gonzalez et al. (110) reported peripheral cysts in 18 of 98 patients with Down syndrome and suggested that the cysts are an intrinsic feature of the disease that may result from reduced postnatal production of peripheral small air passages and alveoli. The 0.2- to 1.0-cm air-filled cysts are located beneath the pleura and are formed of vascular fibrous connective tissue walls lined by alveolar lining cells (Figure 12-31A, B). The cysts communicate with more centrally located bronchioles and alveolar ducts. The cysts resemble those seen in the upper lobes of adult males with idiopathic spontaneous PT and have also been noted in a case of ILE (66).

Acute Lung Injury and Respiratory Distress Syndrome

Acute lung injury is a pattern of diffuse alveolar damage (DAD) seen in association with clinical acute respiratory distress syndrome (RDS). Previously referred to as hyaline membrane disease (HMD), acute lung injury is characterized by firm, atelectatic lungs with an uneven air expansion pattern, focal hemorrhage, edema fluid in alveoli, and hyaline

TABLE 12-5 ANOMALIES ASSOCIATED WITH CONGENITAL CAPILLARY ALVEOLAR DYSPLASIA

Anophthalmia and distinct eyebrows
Familiary microphthalmia
Degeneration of the anterior segment of the eye
Atrioventricular septal defect and quadricuspid pulmonary valve
Down syndrome
Gastrointestinal
Duodenal atresia and anorectal anomaly
Intestinal malrotation
Total colonic Hirschsprung disease
Duodenal atresia
Left-right asymmetry
Arteriovenous malformation of the liver
Bilateral ureteropelvic junction obstruction
Atrioseptal defect
Abnormally lobulated lungs
Hydronephrosis
Urethral atresia
Atrioventricular canal

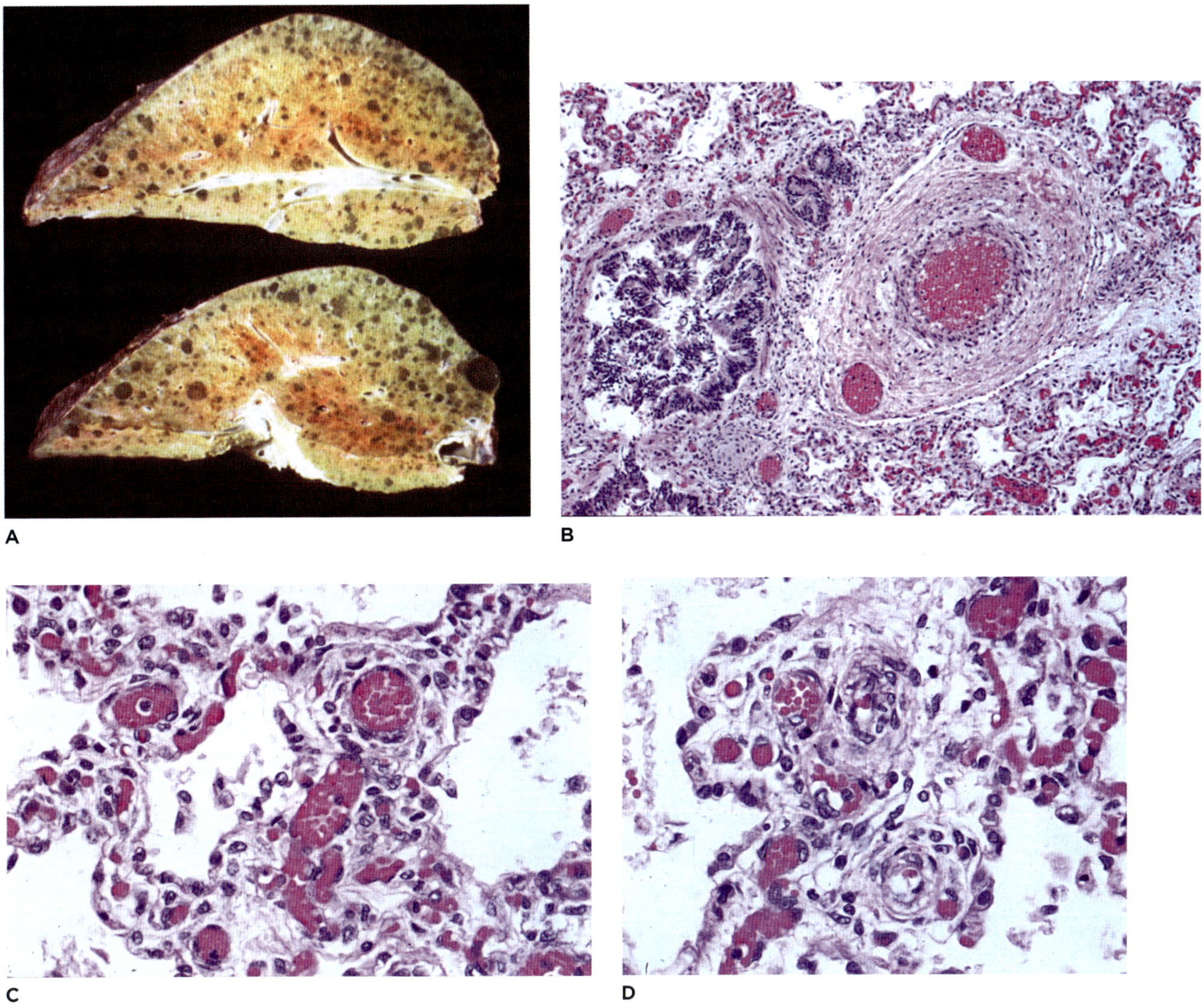

FIGURE 12-30 • Congenital alveolar capillary dysplasia. **A:** Bulky stiff lungs display focal hemorrhage and prominent interlobular septa. **B:** Dilated veins are present adjacent to and within the adventitia of a pulmonary artery (**center-right**). **C:** Broad alveolar septa contain many centrally located capillaries with only a few of them approaching the alveolar epithelium. **D:** Muscularized arteries are present within alveolar septa well away from bronchioles.

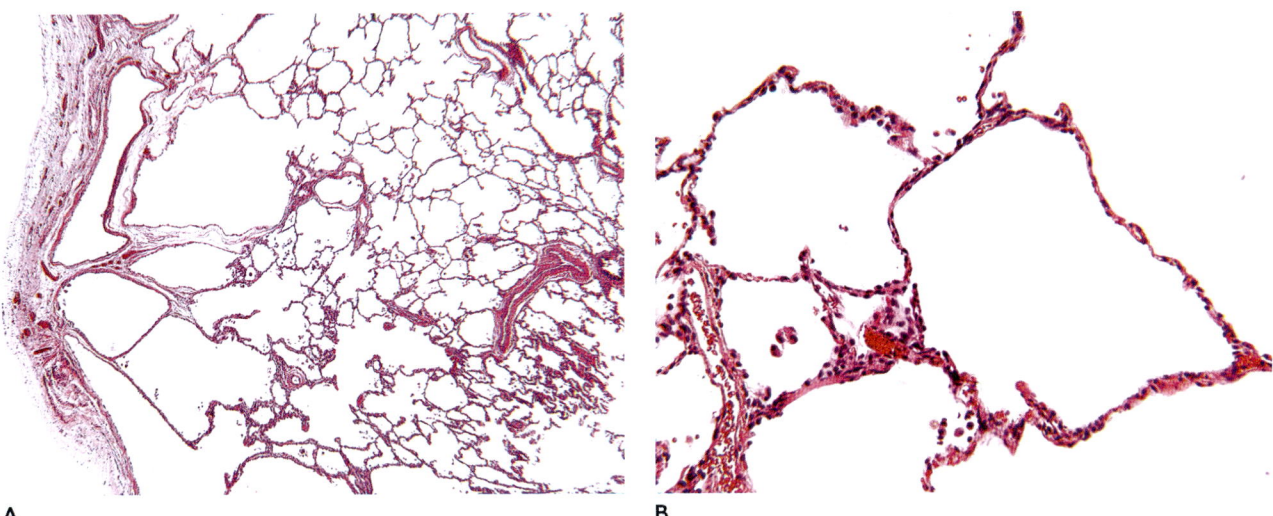

FIGURE 12-31 • Peripheral lung cysts in a 4-year-old male with trisomy 21. **A:** This lung biopsy demonstrates the presence of multiple pulmonary cysts residing beneath the pleural surface. **B:** These cysts represent a growth abnormality in the formation of small airspaces.

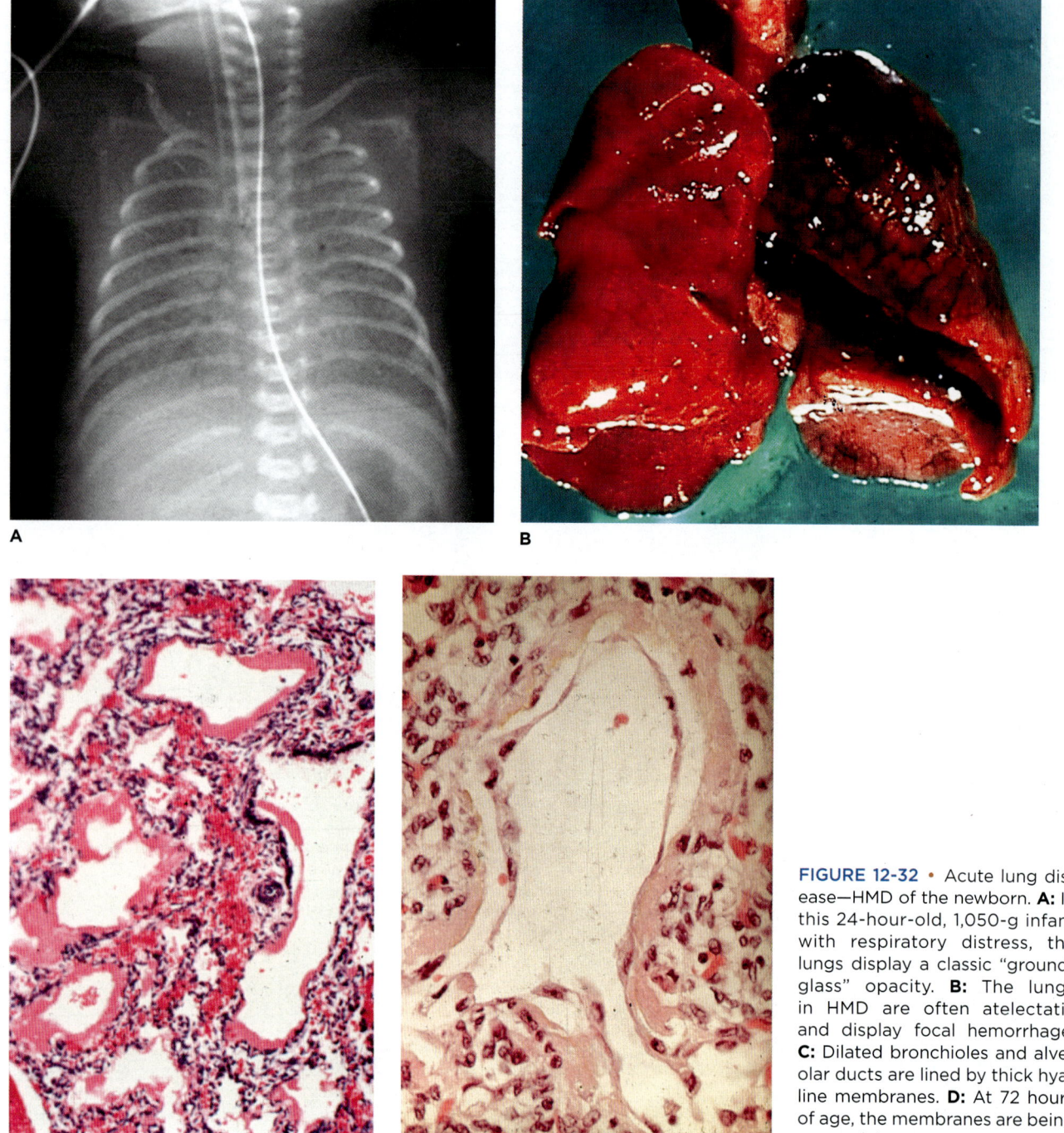

FIGURE 12-32 • Acute lung disease—HMD of the newborn. **A:** In this 24-hour-old, 1,050-g infant with respiratory distress, the lungs display a classic "ground-glass" opacity. **B:** The lungs in HMD are often atelectatic and display focal hemorrhage. **C:** Dilated bronchioles and alveolar ducts are lined by thick hyaline membranes. **D:** At 72 hours of age, the membranes are being covered by regenerating alveolar lining cells.

membranes along terminal and respiratory bronchioles and alveolar ducts. In the pediatric age group, DAD has been typically described in neonates with surfactant deficiency, although other causes include infections, inhalational injury, sepsis, and systemic shock. Breathing difficulty is common in the early neonatal period, occurring in up to 7% of newborn infants, and is not synonymous with RDS. Other common causes of breathing difficulty in term newborn infants include transient tachypnea of the newborn, pneumonia, meconium aspiration syndrome (MAS), persistent pulmonary hypertension of the neonate, and PT (111).

Infants present with tachypnea, intercostal retractions, and hypoxemia and display a typical x-ray image of ground-glass alterations of the lungs with an air bronchogram and diffusely scattered reticulogranular opacities (Figure 12-32A) (1). Grossly, the lungs are firm and resemble the liver more than the lung. Microscopically, there is an uneven air expansion pattern with atelectatic acini and dilated bronchioles and alveolar ducts (Figure 12-32B). Scattered foci of alveolar hemorrhage and edema are present, but most striking is the presence of smooth, homogeneous, pink membranes lining terminal and respiratory bronchioles and alveolar ducts, particularly at points of division or branching (Figure 12-32C). These hyaline membranes are composed of necrotic alveolar lining cells, plasma transudate, inhaled amniotic fluid including squames and fibrin. Hemorrhage is often present. Hyaline membranes may be seen in infants who die as early as 3 to 4 hours after birth and are uniformly present as well-formed structures by 12 to 24 hours in infants with RDS. In the absence of severe disease requiring high oxygen tensions and ventilatory pressures, at 36 to 48 hours, the membranes begin to organize and separate from the underlying wall to be replaced by alveolar lining cells or bronchiolar cuboidal or columnar epithelium (Figure 12-32D). Bacteria may alter the appearance of the membranes by producing fragmented, faintly basophilic structures, with organisms often readily demonstrable by Gram stain on or within the membranes. Conditions associated with hyperbilirubinemia (e.g., kernicterus, intraventricular hemorrhage, intrahepatic bile stasis, disseminated intravascular coagulation) may produce, in infants surviving 3 or more days, yellow hyaline membranes as a result of the presence of unconjugated bilirubin.

Surfactant replacement therapy, although radically decreasing the incidence of acute lung injury in premature infants and its morbidity and mortality in these infants, does not appear to alter the pathologic features of DAD in infants dying of RDS. However, treated children may show a slightly higher incidence of pulmonary hemorrhage and a lower incidence of IPE and PT (112). Surfactant therapy appears to accelerate the rate of epithelial cell regeneration (113).

The pathophysiology of acute RDS in the neonate has been divided into eight categories: alveolar fluid transport, surfactant, innate immunity, apoptosis, coagulation, direct alveolar epithelial injury by bacterial products, ventilator-associated lung injury, and repair. The biological baseline network of genes and protein expression is reportedly different in children with RDS, as compared to adults (114). Beyond the neonatal period, causes of RDS are similar to those in adults. In a prospective, multicenter, observational study covering 21 pediatric intensive care units, pneumonia and sepsis were the most common causes of acute RDS; the authors found a lower acute RDS incidence and mortality in children than those reported for adults (115). In a masked, randomized, placebo-controlled trial in 24 children's hospitals in six different countries, surfactant did not improve outcomes relative to placebo in children with direct lung injury/acute RDS (116).

Bronchopulmonary Dysplasia (Chronic Lung Disease of Prematurity)

Bronchopulmonary dysplasia was first described in 1967 by Northway et al. (117). In a retrospective study, they described the clinical and pathologic features of 19 infants dying following mechanical ventilation with high concentrations of oxygen for severe HMD (RDS). The pathology was correlated with clinical and radiographic findings and included a 2- to 3-day period of acute RDS, followed by a weeklong period of "regeneration," another 10-day period of transition to chronic disease, and a final period of chronic disease extending beyond 1 month of life. The pathologic features in the first stage included the typical findings of HMD (e.g., atelectasis, uneven air expansion pattern, hemorrhage, and hyaline membranes). During the second stage, there was necrosis of bronchiolar and alveolar epithelium with persistence of hyaline membranes (Figure 12-32A to C). In the transition to chronic disease, injury to alveolar epithelium continued, along with widespread bronchial and bronchiolar mucosal metaplasia and marked mucus secretion. Clusters of hyperexpanded alveoli alternated with areas of atelectasis. In the chronic stage, bronchioles displayed marked peribronchiolar smooth muscle hypertrophy associated with clusters of "emphysematous alveoli." The birth weights of the 19 infants dying of bronchopulmonary dysplasia varied from 900 to 2466 g, with two-thirds of them weighing more than 1300 g. Bonikos et al. (118) suggested that bronchopulmonary dysplasia was due to the toxic effects of oxygen, poor bronchial drainage, and the effects of mechanical ventilation.

In the 10 years following that initial brief description of the pathology of BPD, a number of other studies described in more detail the pathologic features including the changes noted in alveoli, airways, lymphatics, vessels, and connective tissue as criteria for the staging of bronchopulmonary dysplasia. In 1976, Bonikos et al. (119) described a severe necrotizing bronchiolitis in the acute stages of BPD and implicated prolonged exposure to high levels of oxygen as a major feature in the cause of bronchiolitis. Since that time, a number of additional factors, including infection, inflammation, poor nutrition, dehydration, and others, have been implicated in the pathogenesis of BPD (120). In addition to the bronchiolitis, there is a prominent alveolar septal fibrosis in the healed stages along with an increased incidence of cardiac hypertrophy.

The sequelae of this necrotizing bronchiolitis were described by Stocker in 1986 in a series of 28 patients with long-standing "healed" bronchopulmonary dysplasia, who died at 3 to 40 months of age (64). Noting the presence of deep pleural fissures and acini with varying degrees of alveolar septal fibrosis (Figure 12-33), it was suggested that the necrotizing bronchiolitis seen in the acute phases, while prohibiting adequate ventilation, often served to "protect" acini from damage by mechanical ventilation or high levels of oxygen (Figure 12-34A to C). Stocker also suggested that the alveolar fissures might represent areas of complete loss of acini corresponding to the marked decrease in internal surface area and number of alveoli noted by Sobonya et al. (121). The 6- to 10-fold reduction in number of alveoli suggested not only an absolute loss of some acini but a generalized reduction in lung growth. In 1991, Margraf et al. (122) confirmed the reduction in lung volume and small airway density noted by Sobonya.

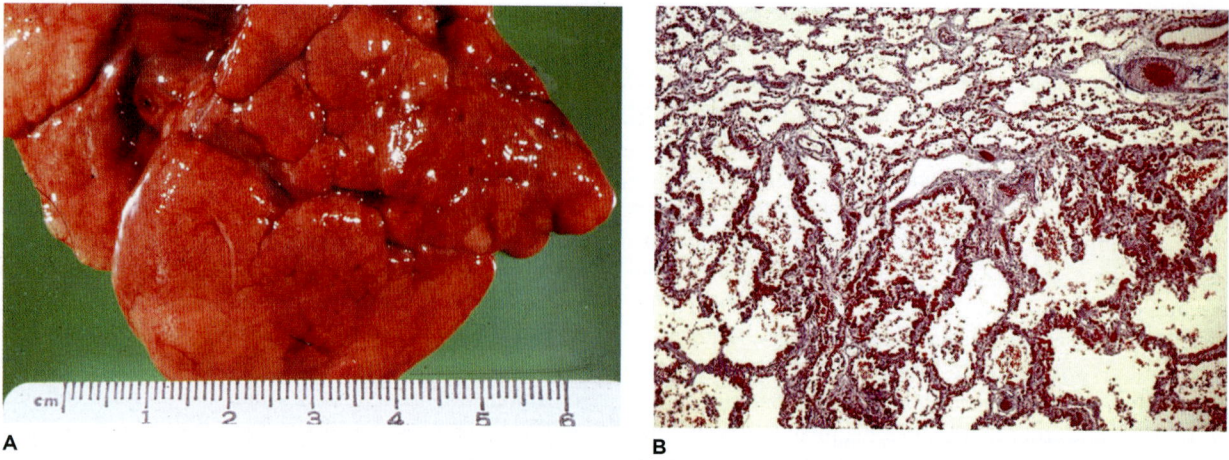

FIGURE 12-33 • Long-standing healed bronchopulmonary dysplasia. **A:** Irregular clefting and fissuring of pulmonary lobes probably represent the loss of acini during the acute phases of BPD. **B:** The acinus at top represents the one "protected" by occluded bronchioles from the damage of barotrauma and high oxygen pressures. At the bottom, this acinus displays the diffuse alveolar septal fibrosis caused by previous exposure to barotrauma and high oxygen pressures (Masson trichrome, x25).

In recent years, with the advent of surfactant replacement therapy and increased sophistication in the use of mechanical ventilation (including high frequency jet ventilation) and oxygen supplementation, another stage in the evolution of the pathology of bronchopulmonary dysplasia has been seen. Although the occasional case of "classic" acute bronchopulmonary dysplasia with necrotizing bronchiolitis, alveolar cell hyperplasia, and peribronchiolar and alveolar septal fibroplasia is still seen along with focal alveolar septal fibrosis in the older patient (Figure 12-35A to D), the few infants who now die from bronchopulmonary dysplasia display what might best be described as "acinar simplification." These simplified acini are characterized by uniformly dilated alveoli whose walls consist of thin alveolar septa with little or no interstitial fibrosis (123).

The bronchioles are similarly unremarkable, with only an occasional mild increase in peribronchiolar musculature. These changes seem to represent an "arrest" of development of the acini, with a resulting markedly decreased number of alveoli within each acinus (Figure 12-36A to C). As a result, the surface area of the lung is significantly decreased even in the absence of significant pathology (e.g., alveolar septal fibrosis).

Although high concentrations of oxygen over prolonged periods of time are known to cause alveolar cell hyperplasia and necrotizing bronchiolitis with resulting alveolar septal fibrosis,

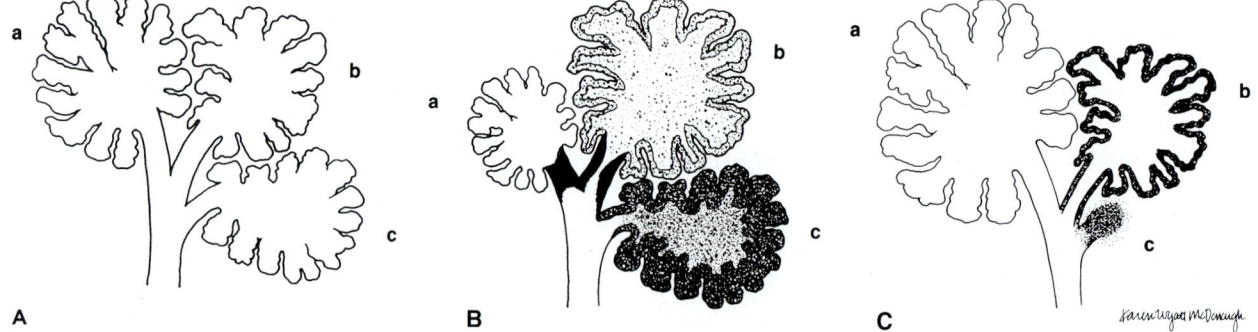

FIGURE 12-34 • Bronchopulmonary dysplasia (BPD) before the advent of surfactant replacement therapy. **A:** Schematic representation of three uniformly distended acini (*a* to *c*) with associated bronchiole, alveolar ducts, and alveoli. **B:** In the early stages of BPD, hyaline membranes or necrotic debris may totally occlude a bronchiole (*a*) protecting the distal acinus. Bronchioles that remain partially or completely open (*b*, *c*) allow the distal acinus to be exposed to varying degrees of injury from barotrauma and high oxygen tension. **C:** In the healed stages of BPD with resolution of the bronchiolar obstruction in (**A**), the "protected" distal acinus expands and continues to develop new alveoli. Depending on the degree of injury, acini may atrophy and disappear (*c*), producing pleural fissures (see Figure 12-33A), or display varying degrees of alveolar septal fibrosis (*b*) and be inhibited from further alveolar development. (From Stocker JT. Pathologic features of long-standing "healed" bronchopulmonary dysplasia: a study of 28 3- to 40-month-old infants. *Hum Pathol* 1986;17:943, with permission.)

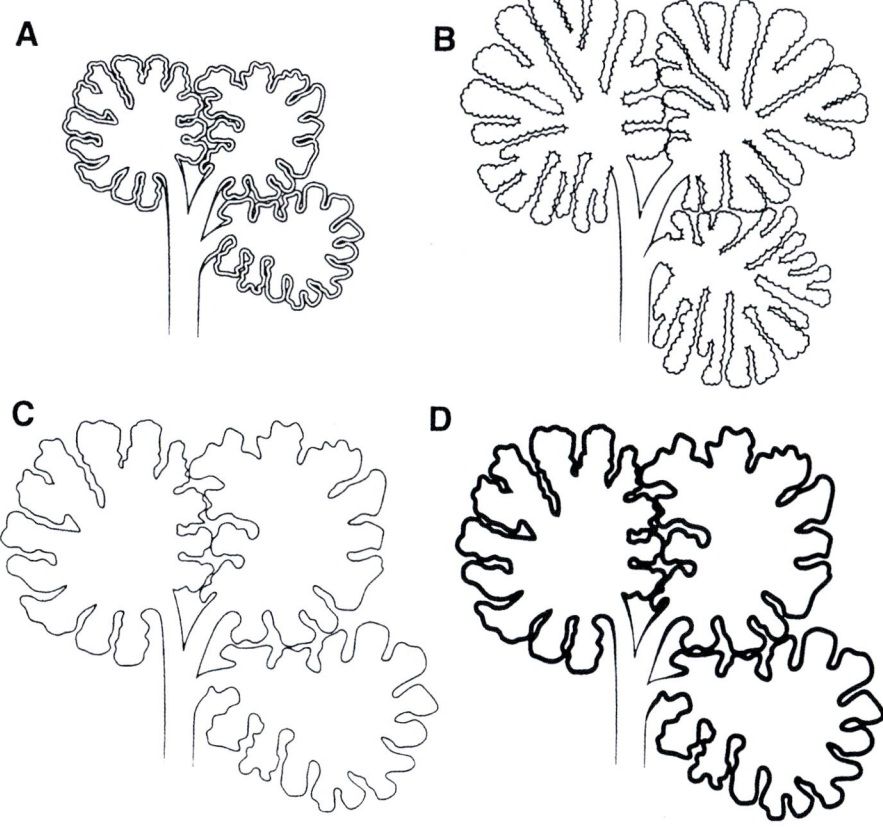

FIGURE 12-35 • Chronic lung disease of the premature (CLDP) since the advent of surfactant replacement therapy. **A:** Schematic representation of three normally expanded and aerated pulmonary acini in an immature infant. Note the appropriately thick septa of the developing lung. **B:** With normal lung growth and development, the acini not only increase in size [relative to (A)] but also in complexity with the appearance of "new" alveolar saccules and alveoli. **C and D:** In infants receiving surfactant replacement therapy who develop moderate-to-severe CLDP, the acini increase in size [relative to (A)] but show little, if any, increase in the number of alveolar saccules or alveoli. The alveolar septa in (**C**) appear normal in thickness compared with the less-injured or uninjured lung (**B**), or they may display a uniform mild alveolar septal fibrosis as in (**D**).

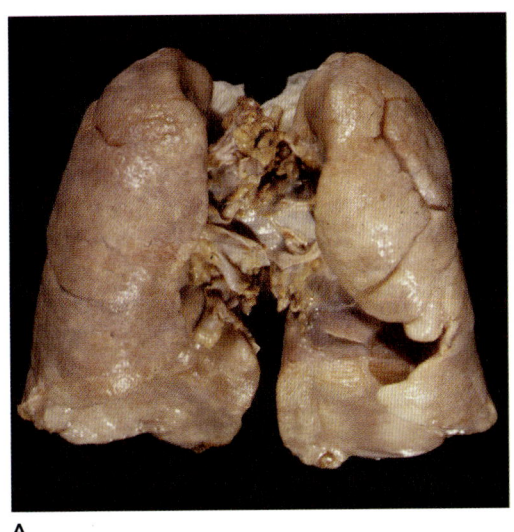

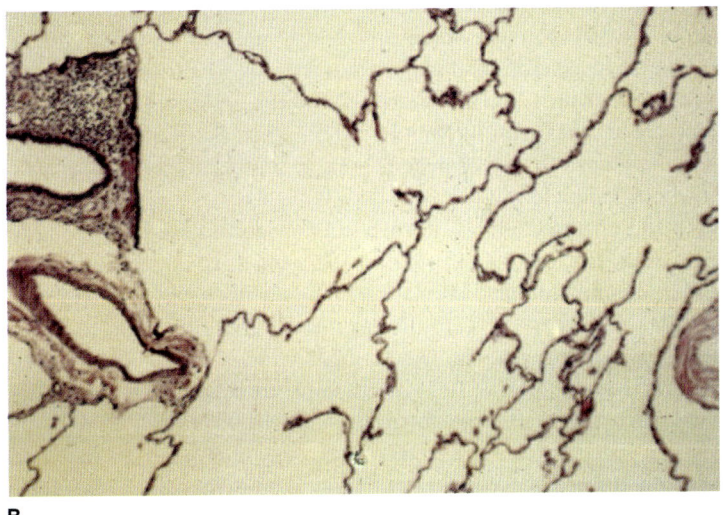

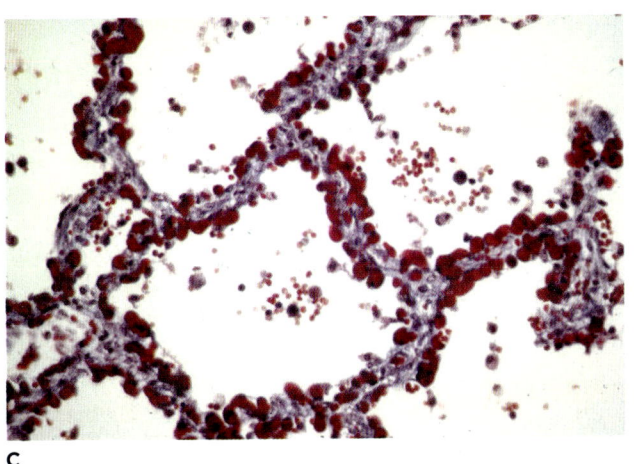

FIGURE 12-36 • Chronic lung disease of the premature. **A:** The lung appears largely unremarkable with an evenly aerated parenchyma. **B:** In this section of lung from a 4-month-old infant born at 26 weeks gestation who developed moderate respiratory distress and clinical BPD, the acini are simplified with dilated alveolar ducts and saccules and with very few alveoli arising from them. **C:** In this section of lung from a 2-month-old infant born at 28 weeks gestation who developed severe prolonged respiratory distress and clinical BPD, the alveolar septa of all acini show mild though uniform interstitial fibrous thickening.

it is possible that low levels of oxygen (25% to 35%), while not producing significant alteration in the epithelial lining of the lung or not causing damage sufficient to cause septal fibrosis, may, in very immature infants, inhibit growth of the lung, that is, the development of new alveolar ducts and alveoli. Although the lung appears to "mature" and alveolar septa appear to thin and expand to resemble the septa of term infants, there is no accompanying significant increase in the surface area of the lung through an increase in number of alveoli. Thus, although recent advances in mechanical ventilation have limited the amount of injury to the bronchiole (i.e., no necrotizing bronchiolitis), the continued patency of all bronchioles throughout the course of therapy allows equal injury or inhibition of growth to all acini from even low levels of oxygen therapy.

Husain et al. (123) examined the lungs at autopsy of 22 patients with BPD, of whom 14 had received surfactant therapy, and compared them with 15 age-matched controls. Using readily available morphometric techniques [RAC and mean linear intercept (MLI)], they displayed a virtual arrest of alveolar development in both the surfactant-treated and nonsurfactant-treated infants whether or not the typical feature of long-standing healed BPD (i.e., alveolar septal fibrosis) was present. Incidentally, septal fibrosis was infrequently seen in surfactant-treated BPD patients even though their disease was severe enough to contribute significantly to their death. The RAC/MLI ratio (an indicator of the number of alveoli) in the BPD patients who lived weeks to months was virtually unchanged from that expected at the infant's birth weight. In other words, an infant born at 28 weeks' gestation, who developed HMD and BPD and lived for 12 weeks, had the same number of alveoli as the one born at 28 weeks' gestation who died in a few days.

As a result of surfactant replacement therapy and sophisticated methods of ventilation, we now see a much smaller percentage of immature and premature infants with chronic lung disease, and when this chronic lung disease does occur, it does not at all resemble the BPD described in the 1970s and 1980s. The classic features of BPD (necrotizing bronchiolitis, epithelial cell hyperplasia, bronchiolar muscular hyperplasia, and alveolar septal fibrosis) are, in fact, rarely seen today. The chronic lung disease of prematurity of today is an extremely subtle disease (at least from a pathologic perspective) that manifests itself primarily as an inhibited or arrested growth and development of the lung. The etiology of this type of failure of development is unclear. Long-term sequelae of BPD include late sudden unexpected death, lobar overinflation, and right, left, or biventricular myocardial hypertrophy (124).

Surfactant Dysfunction Disorders

Surfactants are a mixture of lipids and proteins that are required to reduce alveolar surface tension, and their deficiency is the primary cause of neonatal RDS. There are three different proteins with important roles in surfactant function and metabolism: surfactant protein B (SP-B), surfactant protein C (SP-C), and an ATP-binding cassette family of transports member A3 (ABCA3) (Table 12-6). Mutations in any of the genes encoding for the three different proteins can result in significant lung disease (125). Infants with an inability to produce SP-B typically develop significant respiratory distress and radiographic evidence of diffuse lung disease soon after birth. Chorionic villous sampling can be used to identify the homozygous state *in utero* (126).

Lung disease is rapidly progressive over the next several months requiring lung transplantation, although infants with milder mutations may have some surfactant production and may not require transplantation. Patients with SP-C mutations have a variable clinical course and may even be discovered in adulthood, depending on the specific mutation (125). In infants with SP-C mutations, clinical improvement has been reported even years after mechanical ventilation. Patients with ABCA3 deficiency also have a highly variable clinical course (127). ABCA3 deficiency has an autosomal recessive inheritance pattern, and the most common mutation, E292V, is associated with milder disease. Thyroid transcription factor-1 (TTF-1), also known as Nkx2.1 or TITF1, is one of a number of transcription factors important for the expression of several genes involved in surfactant production and function, SP-A, SP-B, SP-C, and ABCA3 (125). Mutations or deletions in TTF-1 result in the so-called brain–thyroid–lung phenotype since TTF-1 is important in the development of these organs. A high index of suspicion is required in patients who present with any combination of hypothyroidism, neurologic symptoms, and respiratory disease. Respiratory presentation may range from life-threatening respiratory distress in the newborn to chronic lung disease and patterns of recurrent pulmonary infections. No single common mutation is currently recognized. Although not related to surfactants, mutations in the α-chains (*CSF2RA*) and affinity-enhancing β-chains (*CSF2RB*) of the granulocyte–macrophage colony-stimulating factor receptor leading to pulmonary alveolar proteinosis (PAP) have also been identified in children (128).

Grossly, the lungs in surfactant dysfunction disorders are heavy and appear consolidated. Microscopically, in the early stages, alveoli are lined by a continuous layer of cuboidal alveolar lining cells (Figure 12-37A). As the disease progresses, alveoli may be filled with eosinophilic granular material admixed with desquamated alveolar cells and macrophages resembling congenital alveolar proteinosis (Figure 12-37B). In the later stages, alveolar septa are widened by fibroblasts producing alveolar septal fibrosis, although the alveolar cell hyperplasia persists (Figure 12-37C). Immunohistochemical stains of the typical SP-B–deficient lung demonstrate decreased to absent SP-B and normal-to-increased amounts of A and C in alveolar lining cells (Figure 12-37D, E). Electron microscopy displays alveolar type II cells with irregular electron-dense bodies, which also may be present in alveolar spaces and macrophages (Figure 12-37F) (129). Treatment may include oxygen, nutritional supplementation, mechanical ventilation, and courses of oral or pulse glucocorticoid therapy, with lung transplantation being the only hope for patients with persistent respiratory failure and end-stage lung disease.

TABLE 12-6 CLINICAL, GENETIC, AND PATHOLOGIC FEATURES OF CONGENITAL SURFACTANT DEFICIENCIES[a]

Surfactant deficiencies	Onset age	Disease severity	Outcome	Histology	Gene mutation	SP-type expression	EM properties
Surfactant protein-B	Term infants	Respiratory distress, progressive respiratory failure	Death at 3-6 months, some patients with milder phenotype and prolonged survival	Widened interstitium, interstitial fibrosis, arrested acinar development, type II epithelial hyperplasia, features of alveolar proteinosis	SFlPB gene 65% frameshift codon 121 mutation, autosomal recessive	SP-A +, Pro-SP-B –, SP-B –, Pro-SP-C +, SP-C –	Composite irregular membranovesicular lamellar bodies
Surfactant protein-C	Variable, early infancy to 6th decade of life	Variable phenotype	Variable phenotype, asymptomatic adults	Interstitial fibroplasias, hyperplasia of type II pneumocytes, mild interstitial inflammation, granular alveolar proteinaceous deposits	SFTPC gene autosomal dominant/dominant negative/incomplete penetrance, heterozygous mutations	SP-A +, Pro-SB +, SP-B +, SP-C +/–, alveolar accumulation of aberrantly processed pro-SP-C	Vesicular lamellar bodies with dense cores, homo- or heteromeric Pro SP-C aggregates in severely affected infants
ABCA3	Term infants, some patients <1 year, some patients 5-7 years	Moderate-to-severe respiratory distress, progressive respiratory failure	Death within 3 months, protracted course in some older patients with milder phenotype	Alveolar-type II cell hyperplasia, interstitial thickening, alveolar macrophage accumulation, alveolar proteinaceous deposits, pulmonary fibrosis in fatal disease	ABCA3 gene, homo- and heterozygous mutations	SP-A +, Pro-SP-B +, SP-B +/reduced, Pro-SP-C +/–, SP-C –	"Fried egg" inclusions with tightly packed concentric membranes and electron dense aggregates in type II pneumocytes and alveolar macrophages

SP, surfactant protein.

From Bruder E, et al. Ultrastructural and molecular analysis in fatal neonatal interstitial pneumonia caused by a novel ABCA3 mutation. *Mod Pathol* 2007;20:1009-1018, with permission.

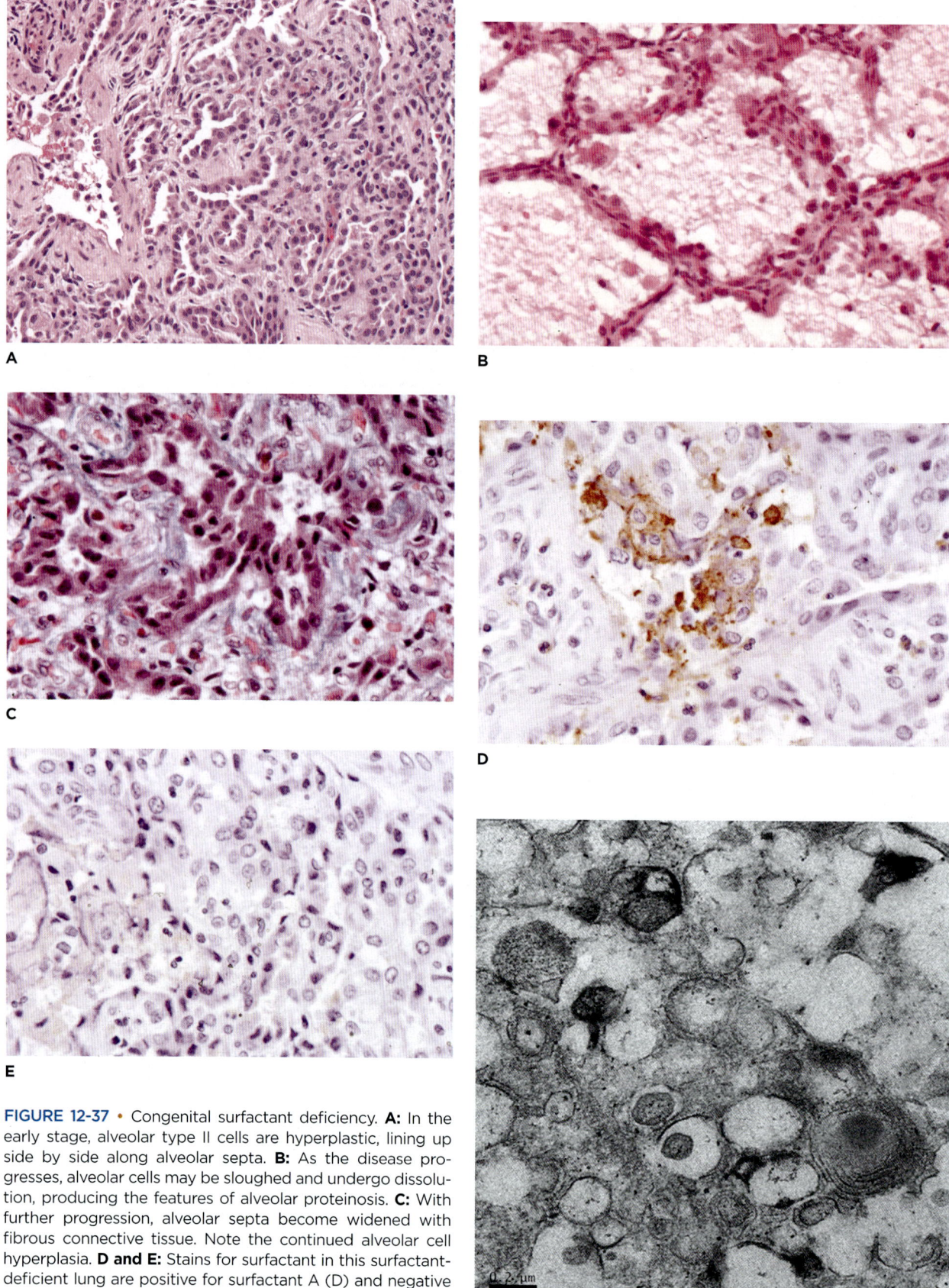

FIGURE 12-37 • Congenital surfactant deficiency. **A:** In the early stage, alveolar type II cells are hyperplastic, lining up side by side along alveolar septa. **B:** As the disease progresses, alveolar cells may be sloughed and undergo dissolution, producing the features of alveolar proteinosis. **C:** With further progression, alveolar septa become widened with fibrous connective tissue. Note the continued alveolar cell hyperplasia. **D and E:** Stains for surfactant in this surfactant-deficient lung are positive for surfactant A (D) and negative for surfactant B (E). **F:** The characteristic ultrastructural finding is the presence of so-called fried egg type lamellar bodies.

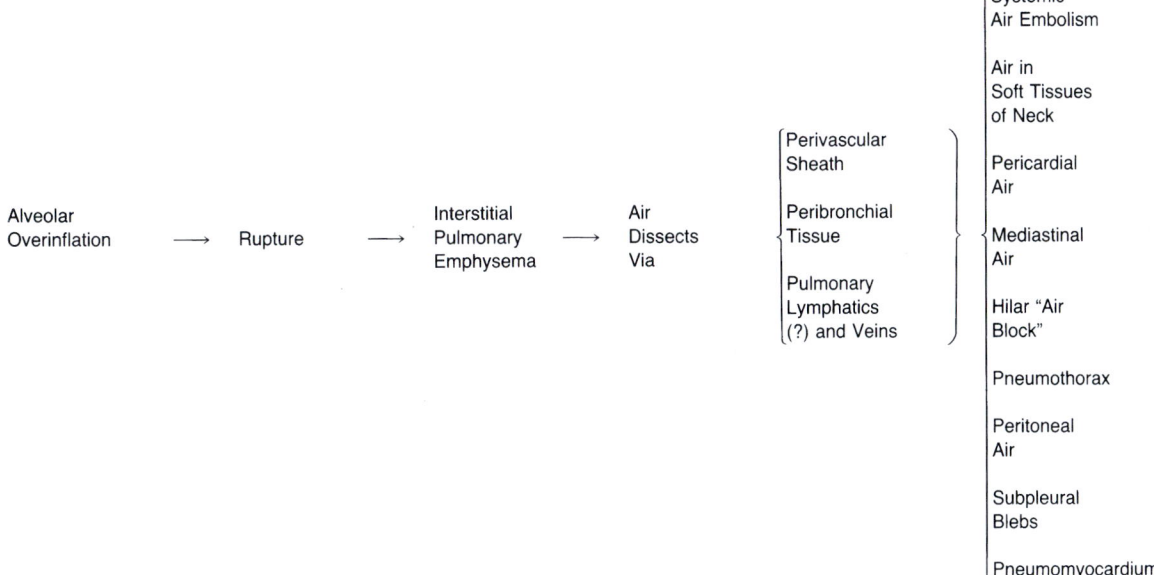

FIGURE 12-38 • Potential complications related to mechanical ventilation and pulmonary interstitial air. (From Askin FB. Pulmonary interstitial air and pneumothorax in the neonate. In: Stocker JT, ed. *Pediatric Pulmonary Disease*. Washington, DC: Hemisphere, 1989:166, with permission.)

Interstitial Pulmonary Emphysema

IPE is the dissection by air around bronchovascular bundles and along interlobular septa as the result of rupture of alveoli, usually in association with mechanical ventilation (Figure 12-38). Dissection of air peripherally through the pleura produces PT, whereas medial dissection can lead to pneumomediastinum, pneumopericardium, and, rarely, pneumomyocardium (Figure 12-39A to C) (1). Although these air leaks can occasionally be observed in normal infants and may spontaneously occur in about 5% of infants with RDS, the highest incidence is seen in infants with RDS who are receiving mechanical ventilation. Although the incidence of IPE and its complications in NICUs was as high as 40% or

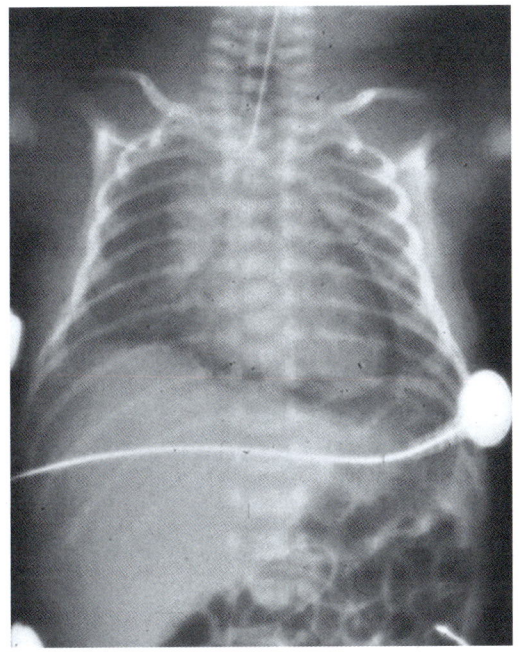
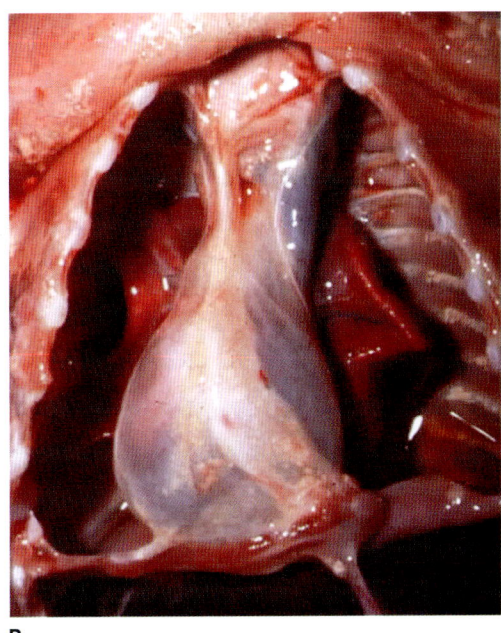

FIGURE 12-39 • Pneumopericardium, PT, and pneumomediastinum. **A:** In this chest x-ray, air can be seen within the pericardial sac surrounding the heart (pneumopericardium), and in the right hemithorax (PT). **B:** At autopsy, the air distended the pericardial sac.

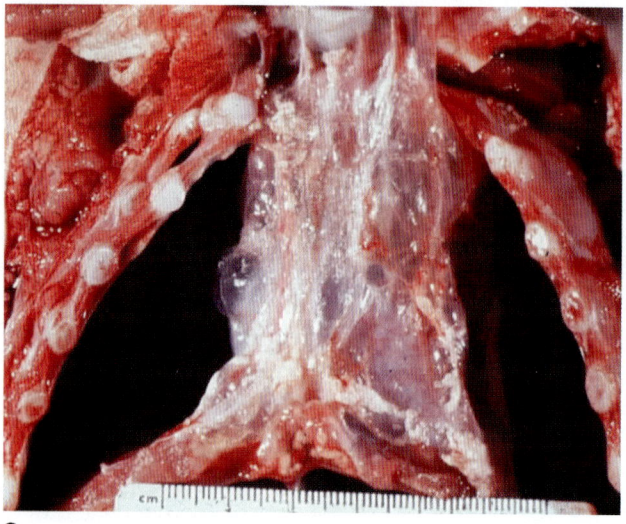

FIGURE 12-39 • (continued) **C:** Blebs of air dissect the tissues of the mediastinum (pneumomediastinum).

more among all NICU patients 30 years ago, early administration of surfactant and increasingly sophisticated means of ventilation have reduced the incidence to 20% to 35% in only the sickest infants. Those particularly at risk include infants with lower 1- and 5-minute APGAR scores, increased surfactant utilization, and higher inspired oxygen concentration. IPE has also been reported in 20% of patients dying of acute asthma, as a result of cardiopulmonary resuscitation, and in association with a variety of infectious diseases (130).

IPE can be acute (<7 days' duration) or persistent and may be localized to a single lobe or distributed diffusely through all lobes (131). Acute IPE (AIPE) presents grossly as 0.1- to 0.5-cm air blebs located beneath the pleura along junctions between the interlobular septa and the pleura (Figure 12-40A). On cut section, round to oval air spaces may be seen around bronchovascular bundles and along the interlobular septa (Figure 12-40B). Only rarely do the air-filled cysts dissect laterally from the septa beneath the pleura, which aids in the differentiation of IPE from CPL. Microscopically, the cysts of AIPE are confined to the interlobular septal and peribronchial region, compressing the adjacent blood vessels and acini (Figure 12-40C). The walls consist primarily of loose connective tissue and compressed parenchyma. AIPE may incorporate some of the lymphatics of the interlobular septa, but the vast majority of cysts appear to be formed from air-dissected connective tissue. Subpleural lymphatics are rarely involved and appear unremarkable.

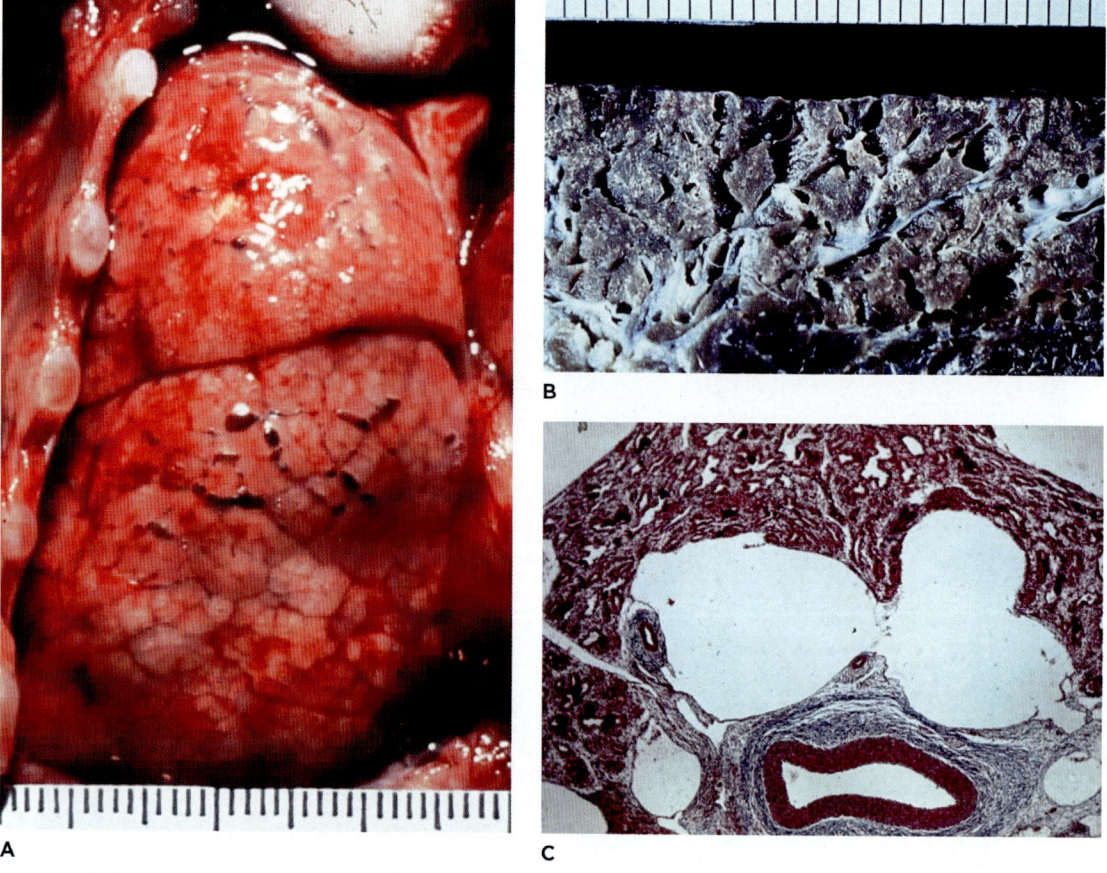

FIGURE 12-40 • Acute interstitial pulmonary emphysema. **A:** Air can be seen beneath the pleura at the junction of interlobular septa and pleura. **B:** Round to oval air-containing cysts are present within interlobular septa. The cysts extend radially from the hilum to the pleura. **C:** The pulmonary artery (**bottom**) is surrounded and partially compressed by air-filled spaces.

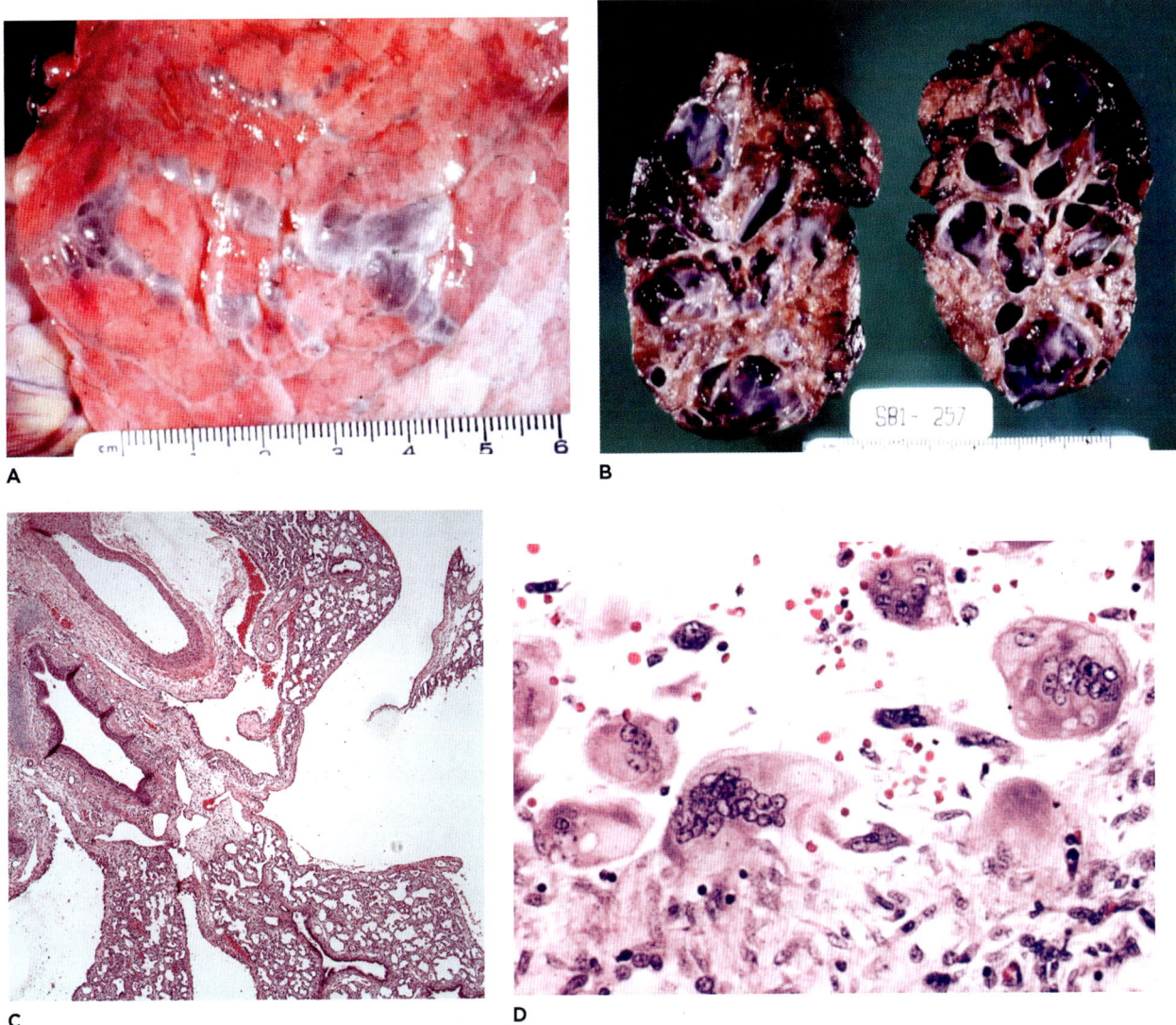

FIGURE 12-41 • Persistent interstitial pulmonary emphysema. **A:** Air blebs are noted beneath a partially "clouded" pleura. **B:** Intercommunicating, irregular, air-filled cysts lined by a smooth membrane compress the pulmonary parenchyma. **C:** The irregular cysts extend along interlobular septa. The cyst walls are composed of fibrous connective tissue of varying thickness, irregularly covered by foreign body giant cells. Note the bronchus (**left**). **D:** The foreign body giant cells contain multiple, eccentrically placed nuclei amid a smooth to granular cytoplasm.

Persistent interstitial pulmonary emphysema (PIPE) occurs in infants with AIPE that lasts more than 1 week. The cysts of PIPE may be localized to a single lobe or, when seen in association with BPD, diffusely radiate throughout most or all of the lobes. PIPE is grossly characterized by multiple 0.1- to 0.3-cm cysts localized to the interlobular septa and extending radially from the hilum to the pleura (Figure 12-41A, B). Cysts in the localized form of PIPE tend to be larger than those in lungs that are diffusely involved, occasionally as large as 5 cm. The intercommunicating, irregularly shaped cysts are air-filled and lined with a smooth glistening membrane. A communication between the airway system and the interstitium may be demonstrable. Microscopically, the cysts are composed of a thin to thick fibrous connective tissue wall intermittently "lined" with multinucleated foreign body giant cells, the pathognomonic feature of PIPE (Figure 12-41C, D). The adjacent parenchyma is usually compressed and, in the diffuse form, frequently displays the features of BPD. Treatment of localized PIPE consists of surgical resection or a variety of forms of selective intubation, mechanical ventilation, or both (132).

Aspiration

Aspiration of material into the tracheobronchial tree can occur *in utero*, during delivery, or in the neonate or young child (Table 12-7). The material aspirated may obstruct the major airways and produce sudden respiratory distress and even death (e.g., tracheal obstruction from aspiration of a peanut), or the distribution of the material may be more diffuse, leading to a "chemical" pneumonitis (e.g., aspiration of meconium or gastric contents). Aspiration of amniotic fluid

TABLE 12-7	SOURCES OF ASPIRATED MATERIAL

Amniotic debris
Meconium
Blood
Milk
Gastric contents
Foreign bodies
    Plants
    Pins
    Pieces of toys
    Small batteries
Toxic fluids
    Kerosene
    Furniture polish
    Mineral oil

in utero is a normal physiologic process, and a few sloughed squamous epithelial cells ("squames") can be seen in the lungs of virtually every term or near-term infant, but massive aspiration of amniotic debris may be seen in postterm infants or in infants with oligohydramnios.

Grossly, the lungs are expanded and firm. Microscopically, squames distend alveolar ducts and alveoli. As noted above, however, small number of squames can be seen in the lungs of virtually all infants born after 34 to 36 weeks of gestation.

Meconium staining of amniotic fluid is seen in up to 29% of all pregnancies and was noted in 12.15% of 176,790 neonates reported by Wiswell et al. (133). Approximately, 5.5% of meconium-stained neonates (0.66% of all neonates) develop the MAS. Boys are more frequently affected than girls. MAS may cause death in approximately 4% of affected neonates.

Meconium aspiration syndrome (MAS) presents as respiratory distress in the meconium-stained neonate and requires mechanical ventilation in about 30% of cases. Pneumothoraces are noted in more than 11% of MAS infants. ECMO and surfactant lavage have contributed to the increasing survival of neonates with MAS.

Meconium, the residual of gastrointestinal secretions accumulated in the lower gastrointestinal tract of the fetus, can, when aspirated, obstruct the trachea, bronchi, and bronchioles. The tenacious green-yellow material can frequently be seen grossly as plugs within bronchi and bronchioles on cut section of the lung. Microscopically, the material is composed of amorphous, acellular, faintly basophilic debris (Figure 12-42A). In infants surviving more than a few hours, a chemical pneumonitis develops with alveoli filled with neutrophils and basophilic debris. Meconium has been shown to induce an inflammatory response via complement and CD14 (134). Chronic intrauterine meconium aspiration may cause pulmonary infarction, rupture, and meconium embolism.

Aspiration of maternal blood during delivery may produce clinical features that mimic pulmonary hemorrhage. In infants, milk may be aspirated during feeding or regurgitation. Older infants with esophageal reflux or neurologic disorders (e.g., cerebral palsy) are also prone to aspiration. Gastric contents may obstruct bronchi or bronchioles and produce a chemical pneumonitis in which meat and vegetable fibers may be identified in association with granulomata and foreign body giant cells (Figure 12-42B to D).

Aspirated foreign bodies are responsible for about 2000 deaths a year in children, usually lodge in the upper airway or bronchi, and include virtually any object that will pass through the glottis into the larynx (135). Bronchial obstruction may lead to acute or chronic pneumonia including the development of an ILS (25).

Aspirated fluid such as kerosene, mineral oil, and furniture polish may result in severe pulmonary damage including DAD, lipoid pneumonia, and diffuse necrosis. ECMO has been helpful in treating these patients, as well as patients with meconium aspiration (see below).

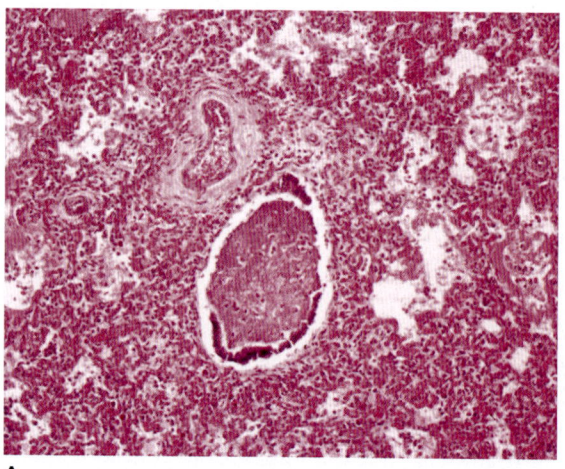 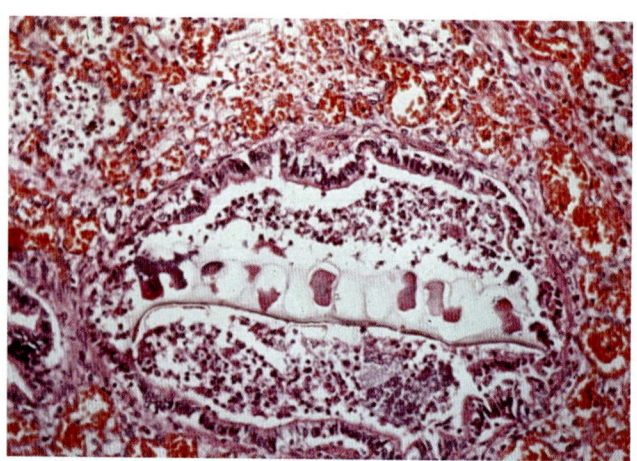

FIGURE 12-42 • Aspiration. **A:** Meconium. Amorphous debris containing scattered neutrophils occludes a bronchiole in this term infant who was intensely meconium stained. **B:** Vegetable fibers are accompanied by acute bronchiolitis.

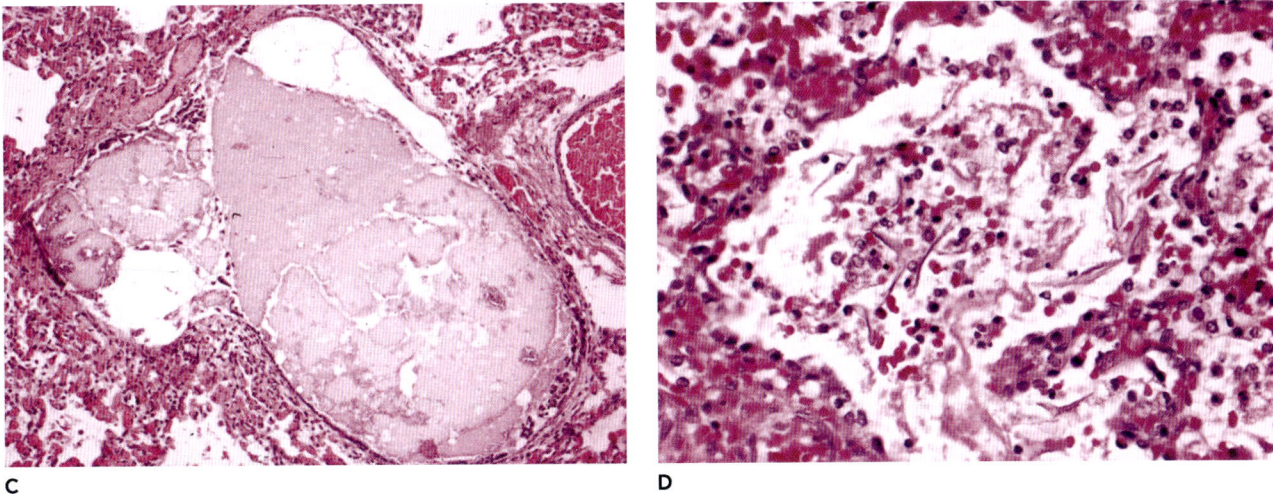

FIGURE 21-42 • (continued) **C:** Gastric contents—milk. **D:** Amniotic debris.

Extracorporeal Membrane Oxygenation

The development of ECMO and its use in the treatment of meconium aspiration, alveolar capillary dysplasia, diaphragmatic hernia (among other causes of pulmonary hypoplasia), *Listeria monocytogenes* infection, and congenital heart malformations have produced a variety of pathologic changes involving the lung and other organs (129).

Chou et al. (136) have described the autopsy findings in 23 infants receiving ECMO therapy and noted the presence of interstitial and intra-alveolar hemorrhage along with hyaline membrane formation during the first few days of therapy. They described the hyperplasia of type II pneumocytes and bronchial epithelial cells after 2 days of ECMO therapy in some patients and, by 7 days, in all patients. Interstitial fibrosis was also noted beginning at 7 days. After 15 days of treatment, there was replacement of the terminal airways and alveoli by tall columnar and mucin-producing epithelium (Figure 12-43). Squamous metaplasia of bronchial epithelium was also seen in the majority of patients, and one patient developed mucinous metaplasia as well. Clusters of calcified material were present in the alveoli of 7 of 23 cases. Long-term survivors of ECMO show a high frequency of hyperinflation and airway obstruction (137). Among children who did not survive while on ECMO and were autopsied, over 50% had a major pathologic finding which was not identified during life; the most common finding at autopsy in these children was myocardial infarction in the presence of the most common primary diagnosis of congenital heart disease in 60% of cases (138). Extrapulmonary changes include ischemic neuronal necrosis, focal cerebral infarcts, intracerebral hemorrhages, periventricular leukomalacia, pericardial hemorrhage, carotid artery injury, and retinal vasculopathy.

Bronchiectasis

Bronchiectasis is defined pathologically by dilatation of the bronchi due to a chronic inflammatory process leading to intrinsic injury to the airway and the surrounding supportive tissues. In terms of the clinical settings in children, bronchiectasis is either associated with CF or a number of other conditions ranging from immunodeficiencies of primary or secondary types, metabolic disorders like α-1-antitrypsin deficiency, and ciliary dyskinesia disorders. These various underlying disorders come to clinical attention because of recurrent lower respiratory tract infections leading to the recognition of bronchiectasis, which in turn is evaluated to determine whether the latter is a manifestation of CF or other underlying non-CF condition (139).

CF-associated bronchiectasis with chronic respiratory failure is the most common clinical-pathologic setting of bronchiectasis in the first two decades of life in our institutional experience and is reflected by the pediatric lung transplantation service (St. Louis Children's Hospital) in which 50% of transplants are performed for CF. In the developed world, CF accounts for 50% or more of cases of bronchiectasis in children, but in the developing world tuberculosis, pertussis and other recurrent lung infections remain important in the etiopathogenesis (140).

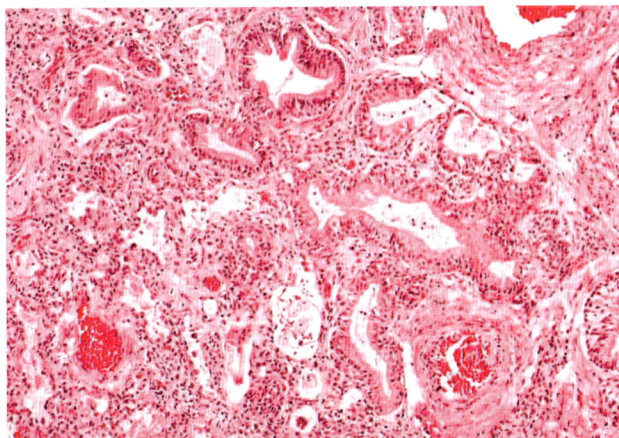

FIGURE 12-43 • Extracorporeal membrane oxygenation. This term infant with a large left-sided diaphragmatic hernia and severe pulmonary hypoplasia was on ECMO for 16 days before dying. Note the alveolar septal fibrosis and the replacement of the terminal airways and alveoli (**right**) by cuboidal to columnar epithelium.

CF is one of a group of inherited disorders known as "channelopathies" which are characterized by a dysfunction of ion channels in the cell membrane (141). In the case of CF, an autosomal recessive disorder, there are loss of function mutations in the CF transmembrane conductance regulator (CFTR) gene, a member of the ATP-binding cassette family of membrane proteins, which affects the physical properties of mucus in the various mucin-producing organs including the lung, intestinal tract, and pancreas (142–144). Some 2000 mutations have been identified in the CFTR gene, and Phe508del is one of the most prevalent mutations (145). Newborn screening for CF in the United States is an established practice. Bronchiectasis eventually develops in excess of 80% to 85% of those with CF and is observed in its early stages in the first year of life in 8% to 10% of children and in 35% to 40% by 4 years of age (146). The mucoid variant of *Pseudomonas aeruginosa* promotes and accelerates the progression of bronchiectasis (147–149). However, the airway in CF is the site of a polymicrobial biome of pathogens including nontuberculosis mycobacteria, Aspergillus, and viruses (150). Lungs as explant specimens are hypervoluminous in some as a result of air trapping and in many cases, the parenchyma is often strikingly unremarkable for a distance from the airway, but in the immediate vicinity of the ectatic airways, there is often chronic inflammation and fibrosis (Figure 12-44A, B). Mucus plugs or thickened mucus is present in the dilated airways which often extend to the periphery of the cut surface of the lungs. Cartilage may or may not be apparent grossly but is usually identified in the larger, more central bronchi (Figure 12-44A, B). Acute inflammation is a characteristic microscopic finding despite the chronicity of the process clinically (Figure 12-44C). Despite the number of neutrophils, these cells are dysfunctional and have a role in disease progression (151,152). The epithelial lining of the

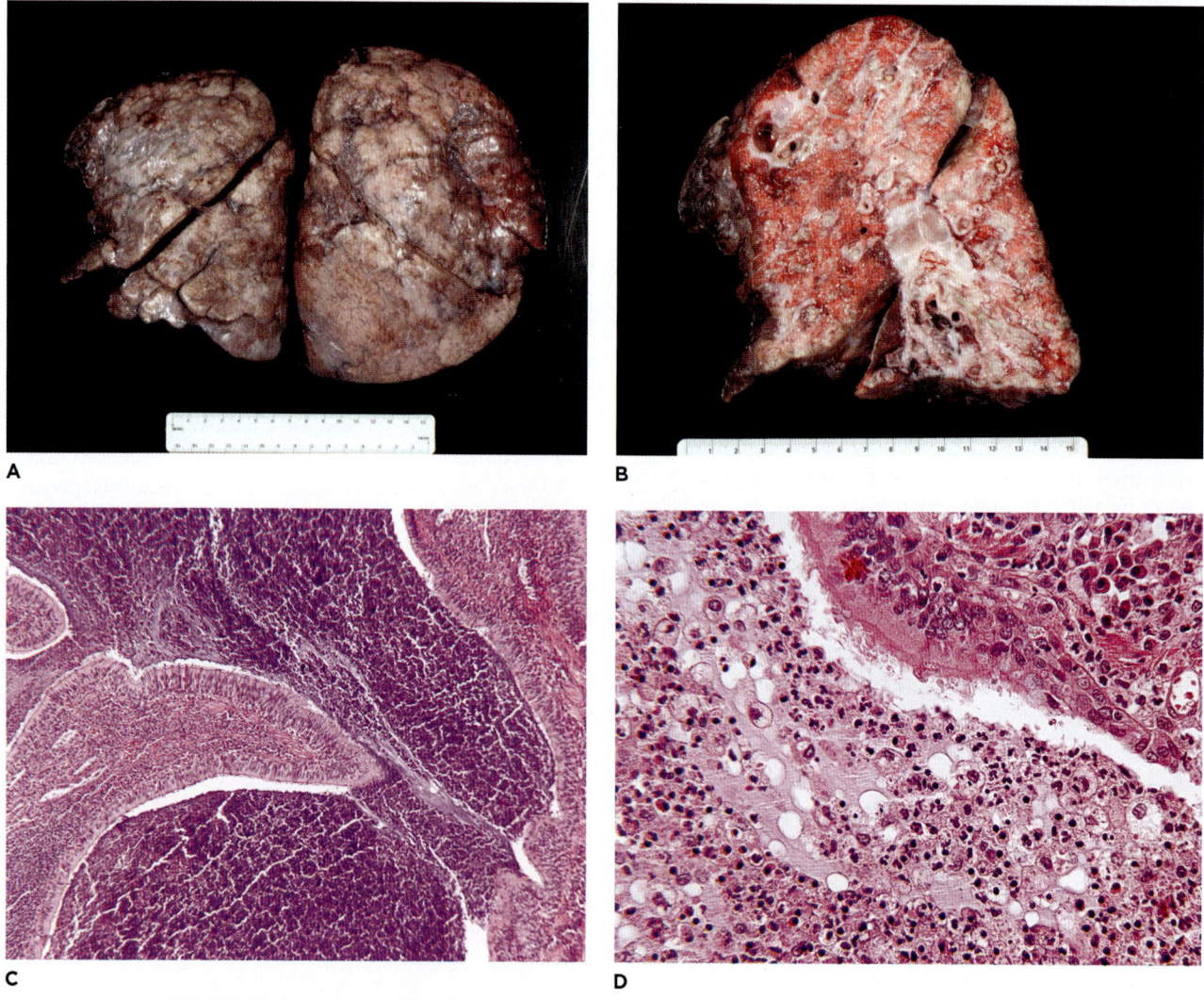

FIGURE 12-44 • Cystic fibrosis—associated bronchiectasis. **A:** The explanted lungs from a 14-year-old female showing hypervoluminous appearance from the exterior. **B:** The cut surface reveals the ectatic bronchi filled with dense tenacious secretions. **C:** Low power fields demonstrating the impacted mucin with its basophilic appearance reflecting the heavy bacterial content. **D:** Despite the chronicity of the airway inflammation, neutrophils are a prominent component of the inflammation response.

airway may be retained with abundant cytoplasmic mucin and/or squamous metaplasia (Figure 12-44D). Eosinophils in the inspissated mucin may indicate the presence of coincidental allergic bronchopulmonary aspergillosis (153). Despite the intensity of the inflammation in the airways, the small airspaces may only show the presence of pulmonary macrophages secondary to the proximal obstruction, but otherwise minimal abnormalities (154). Pulmonary hypertensive vascular changes are present in some cases.

Non-CF bronchiectasis in children living in the developed world is relatively uncommon (155). There are a number of clinical associations such as postinfectious complication in immune competent or deficient children, congenital disease as in the primary ciliary dyskinesia (PCD) or Williams-Campbell syndrome (absence of cartilage in subsegmental bronchi) and chronic aspiration syndrome (impaired neurodevelopmental disorders) (156,157). Approximately 50% to 60% of cases are either postpneumonic in immunocompetent children or in children with a primary or secondary immunodeficiency (155,158). Recurrent pneumonia is the typical clinical presentation, and oftentimes, a viral etiology is responsible for an exacerbation (159). An underlying etiology for the bronchiectasis and recurrent pneumonia may not be apparent even after a thorough diagnostic evaluation, but primary ciliary disorder (PCD) and immunodeficiency disorders are two occult conditions (160–162).

PCD is a group of autosomal recessive disorders (incidence between 1:10,000 and 40,000, more common in ethnic Asians) whose pathogenesis is on the basis of structural abnormalities in cilia and whose clinical consequences are recurrent rhinosinusitis, chronic otitis media, pneumonia, and male infertility. It is estimated that 1.5% to 15% of cases of non-CF bronchiectasis are due to PCD (158). These children may experience respiratory distress and situs inversus totalis (Kartagener syndrome) in 50% of cases (163,164). A number of mutations responsible for the various components of axonemal structure have been identified; these are detected morphologically by electron microscopy, usually performed on a nasal biopsy (165,166). This latter category of PCDs constitutes the so-called motor ciliopathy, whereas there are a number of sensory ciliopathies to include autosomal recessive polycystic kidney disease and Meckel-Gruber syndrome as two examples (164).

The Williams-Campbell syndrome, or familial congenital bronchiectasis, is a disorder characterized by a deficiency of bronchial cartilage distal to the main segmental bronchi, usually of the fourth to sixth order (167). Cartilage is absent, markedly diminished, or soft. The syndrome usually is seen in the neonatal period or early infancy, and familial cases have been reported. The disease may proceed rapidly or have a more benign course compatible with prolonged survival. Lung transplantation may be unsuccessful because of cartilage problems in the recipients' residual right and left mainstem bronchi.

Pulmonary Abscess

Pulmonary abscess or abscesses are observed at autopsy in children over a broad range of conditions from acute bronchopneumonia with microabscesses in premature infants with underlying complications developing in the setting of BPD or those older children with a hematologic disorder (168). An abscess in the right lower lobe is more likely on the basis of aspiration. Oral anaerobes, *Staphylococcus aureus*, streptococcal species, and *Klebsiella pneumoniae* are more common in primary abscesses, and gram-negative pathogens are the hallmark of a secondary lung abscess (169).

Pulmonary Hemorrhage

Hemorrhage into the alveoli and/or interstitium of the lung is a frequent finding in tissue removed at surgery at all ages and in most cases is procedure-related. However, pulmonary hemorrhage in neonatal lungs is frequently associated with acute RDS but may also occur in association with patent ductus arteriosus, erythroblastosis, congestive heart failure, disseminated intravascular coagulation, congenital malformations, acute pneumonia, systemic lupus erythematosus, Goodpasture syndrome, and rarely, as an isolated finding (Table 12-8) (170,171). The incidence of neonatal massive pulmonary hemorrhage, defined as hemorrhage involving more than two-thirds of the lung, is seen in up to 40% of neonatal autopsies. The appearance of hemorrhage may also be produced by the intrapartum aspiration of maternal blood, which mimics both the clinical and pathologic features of intrinsic massive pulmonary hemorrhage; identification of the maternal versus fetal origin of alveolar erythrocytes permits this distinction to be made. Diffuse pulmonary hemorrhage is also a manifestation of idiopathic pulmonary hemosiderosis (IPH) and pulmonary capillaritis (small vessel vasculitis) with antineutrophilic cytoplasmic autoantibodies (ANCAs) in the clinical setting of granulomatosis with polyangiitis (proteinase 3-ANCA), microscopic polyangiitis (myeloperoxidase–ANCA) and Churg-Strauss syndrome (MPO-ANCA) (172). In one series, 50% of children with pulmonary capillaritis were ANCA positive (173). MPO-ANCA with transplacental transfer to the baby and neonatal lupus erythematosus are two other associations with pulmonary capillaritis (174,175). A biopsy shows variably prominent alveolar hemorrhage, and the septa may appear congested. Fibrin and hemosiderin-laden macrophages are often accompanying findings. Neutrophils and karyorrhectic fragments are found in capillary-sized vessels. A similar reaction may be found in the alveolar septa. Henoch-Schönlein purpura may present with pulmonary hemorrhage and leukocytoclastic vasculitis (176). Both Goodpasture syndrome (anti-GBM disease) and celiac disease do not display small vessel vasculitis in the presence of alveolar hemorrhage except in those cases with a positive ANCA (177,178). Some viral infections, hematopoietic stem cell transplantation and pulmonary veno-occlusive disease are accompanied by lung hemorrhage.

TABLE 12-8 DISORDERS ASSOCIATED WITH DIFFUSE PULMONARY HEMORRHAGE AND HEMOSIDEROSIS IN INFANCY AND CHILDHOOD

Idiopathic pulmonary hemosiderosis (isolated)
Pulmonary hemosiderosis associated with sensitivity to cow's milk
Pulmonary hemosiderosis and glomerulonephritis
    With antibodies to GBM (Goodpasture syndrome)
    Without antibodies to GBM (usually immune-complex glomerulonephritis)
Pulmonary hemosiderosis associated with collagen vascular or purpuric disease
    Systemic lupus erythematosus
    Wegener granulomatosis
    Polyarteritis nodosa
    Rheumatoid arthritis
    Schönlein-Henoch purpura
    Idiopathic thrombocytopenic purpura
Pulmonary hemosiderosis secondary to cardiac disease
    Intrapulmonary vascular lesions or malformations
    Chronic left-sided or right-sided heart failure (e.g., mitral stenosis)
    Pulmonary hypertension
    Pulmonary veno-occlusive disease
    Pulmonary lymphangiomyomatosis
    Arteriovenous fistulas and other congenital vascular malformations
    Vascular thrombosis with infarction

GBM, glomerular basement membrane.
From Cutz E. Idiopathic pulmonary hemosiderosis and related disorders in infancy and childhood. *Perspect Pediatr Pathol* 1987;11:49, with permission.

Pulmonary Veno-Occlusive Disease

Pulmonary venous obstruction may be secondary to congenital cardiac malformations such as mitral stenosis or cor triatriatum, or it may be due to an intrinsic disease of the pulmonary veins, that is, pulmonary veno-occlusive disease (PVOD). PVOD, often clinically misdiagnosed as primary pulmonary hypertension, mainly affects children and young adults (179). Patients with PVOD present with symptoms of right-sided heart failure. Radiologic examination shows prominent pulmonary arteries with Kerley B lines, interlobular septal thickening, and pleural effusion. CT scans confirm pulmonary artery enlargement, smoothly thickened interlobular septae, and ground glass opacities. Microscopically, pulmonary veins and venules show eccentric intimal fibrosis that narrows and occludes pulmonary veins of all calibers and sizes. Partially recanalized veins can be highlighted by trichrome and elastic stains. A variety of secondary changes are seen including "venous infarcts" adjacent to occluded veins, lymphatic dilatation, and hypertrophied arterioles and small arteries. Evidence of pulmonary hemorrhage and chronic passive congestion includes presence of alveolar siderophages and iron encrustation of vascular and interstitial elastic fibers ("endogenous pneumoconiosis").

Its cause is unknown, although viral infections (including HIV), antiphospholipid antibody, and drugs have been implicated. PVOD has also been seen to develop in patients following bone marrow transplantation and as a component of pulmonary capillary hemangiomatosis (PCH). No effective treatment is available, and prognosis is poor; lung transplantation has been tried.

Pulmonary Alveolar Proteinosis

PAP is now defined as a macrophage dysfunction disorder and is identified pathologically by the uniform accumulation of surfactant lipids and protein in the small airspaces (180,181). Most cases are examples of auto-immune PAP which is caused by autoantibodies to granulocyte–macrophage colony-stimulating factor (GM-CSF) (182). Congenital PAP is due to mutation of GM-CSF receptor. Congenital surfactant deficiencies (dysfunction disorders) are discussed above. Cases of PAP presenting in later infancy and childhood are associated with lysinuric protein intolerance, B- or T-cell immune deficiency, or a hematologic disorder. Nocardia, mycobacteria, and fungi should be ruled out in a biopsy with PAP.

Pulmonary Alveolar Microlithiasis

Pulmonary alveolar microlithiasis is a rare and unusual disorder reported worldwide as single cases or in siblings or other family members (183). Patients often are asymptomatic with a diffuse miliary pattern concentrated along bronchovascular bundles, interlobular septa, and beneath the pleura on routine chest x-ray study (184). Diagnosis is made by demonstrating calcium phosphate microconcretions on bronchoalveolar lavage or lung biopsy. An autosomal recessive inheritance pattern has been proposed, and one case has been associated with the Waardenburg anophthalmia syndrome. The disease progresses with eventual pulmonary hypertension, cor pulmonale, and respiratory failure.

Pulmonary Hemosiderosis

Hemosiderin in the lung usually indicates previous hemorrhage or aspiration of blood and is thus relatively nonspecific (Table 12-8). Macrophages containing hemosiderin can be found in alveolar or interstitial regions in association with conditions such as infection, blood dyscrasia, chronic heart failure, pulmonary hypertension, and neoplasia. There exists a group of rare disorders that are characterized by single or repeated episodes of bleeding that can lead to massive hemorrhage or progress to chronic pulmonary disease. Based on the clinical, laboratory, and immunopathologic findings, they are divided into two categories:

1. IPH, with pulmonary hemorrhage as an isolated process
2. Secondary pulmonary hemorrhage associated with immunologically mediated renal or vascular disease.

Idiopathic Pulmonary Hemosiderosis

IPH presents with iron deficiency anemia, hypoxemia (85%), dyspnea, and hemoptysis (65%). It occurs primarily in children 3 to 6 years of age but can be seen in children as young as 4 to 6 months of age. Consanguinity and environmental factors may be involved in the development of IPH (185). Sex incidence is equal, and 15% to 20% of cases occur in adolescents and young adults. Less specific nonpulmonary symptoms include fever (in as many as 79% of cases), lymphadenopathy, hepatomegaly, and splenomegaly. Radiographically, early stages are characterized by patchy or diffuse pulmonary infiltrates or massive confluent shadows that may rapidly clear. In later stages of the disease, there is a perihilar reticulation or a pattern of diffuse interstitial disease. The clinical triad of hemoptysis, iron deficiency anemia, and diffuse parenchymal infiltrates is strongly suggestive of IPH (185). The presence of hemosiderin-laden macrophages on bronchoalveolar lavage is also highly correlated with IPH, with the presence of 35% or more hemosiderin-laden macrophages associated with a sensitivity of 100% and a specificity of 96% (186).

Hypochromic microcytic anemia is seen in virtually all cases of IPH, and eosinophilia is present in 12% to 15% of patients (187). Bone marrow examination shows reactive erythroid hyperplasia and depleted iron stores. Levels of serum iron are low, and total iron binding capacity is increased. Most patients with IPH have normal renal function without circulating autoantibodies (compare with Goodpasture syndrome; see Chapter 17). An association with celiac disease has also been reported and, rarely, juvenile dermatomyositis. Although some children with IPH may die of massive hemorrhage shortly after presentation, other patients have a history of progressive respiratory insufficiency leading to death 2 to 5 years after diagnosis. Immunosuppressants have been empirically used in therapy, and a 5-year survival of 86% was reported in 17 patients receiving corticosteroids (188,189).

Lung biopsy and autopsy specimens show varied involvement. Focal areas of consolidation are common owing to massive accumulations of hemosiderin-laden macrophages, which obliterate alveolar spaces and are associated with interstitial fibrosis (190). Stainable iron is present in alveolar and tissue macrophages, free in connective tissues, and encrusting elastic fibers of small blood vessels and alveolar septa (Figure 12-45A to C). There is mild-to-moderate alveolar cell hyperplasia, peribronchial lymphoid hyperplasia, and

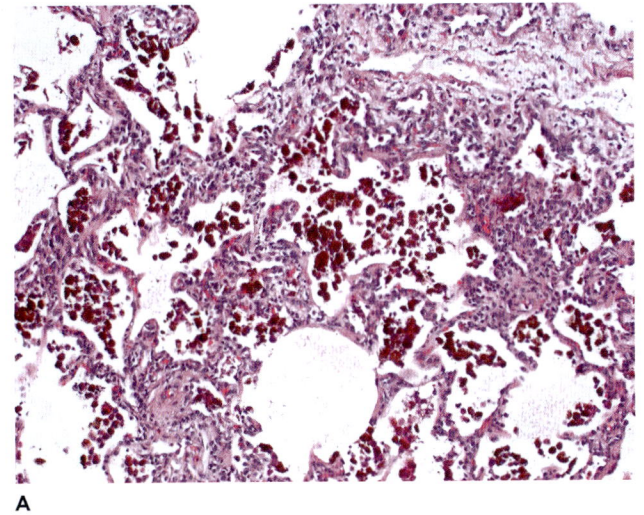

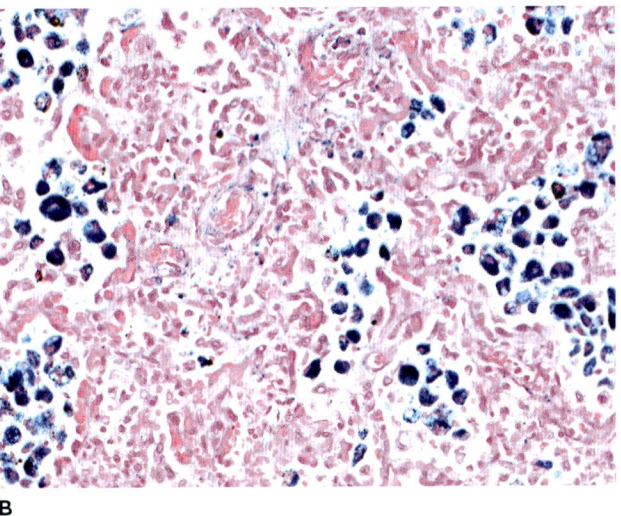

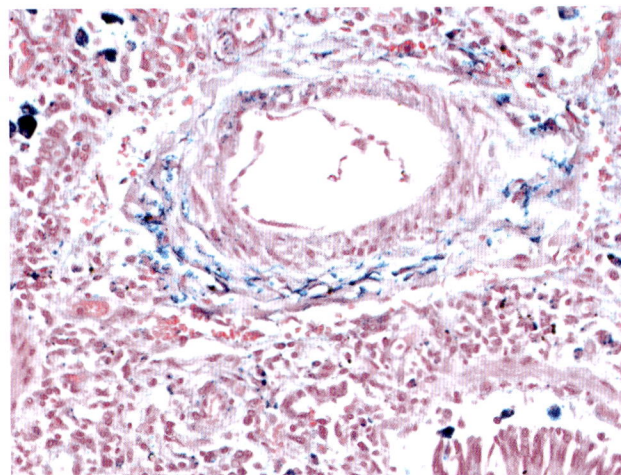

FIGURE 12-45 • Idiopathic pulmonary hemosiderosis. **A:** Hemosiderin is present in clusters of alveolar and septal macrophages. **B:** An iron stain demonstrates masses of iron in alveolar macrophages and in connective tissue. **C:** Iron is also present in the media as well as encrusting elastic fibers adjacent to a pulmonary artery.

alveolar septal mastocytosis. Immunofluorescence is negative for immunoglobulin, complement and antibasement membrane antibodies (191).

Infectious Diseases

Infectious diseases are described in detail in Chapter 6. Certain organisms specifically or primarily affecting the lungs bear special mention.

Respiratory Syncytial Virus

Respiratory syncytial virus (RSV) is an important respiratory pathogen of infancy and childhood, responsible for sizeable outbreaks of infection each year. An RNA virus, RSV occurs in regularly recurring epidemics in midwinter and early spring. It has been identified as causing 5% to 40% of pneumonias (50% of viral pneumonias), from 50% to 90% of cases of bronchiolitis, and from 10% to 30% of cases of persistent bronchitis in young children (192).

RSV presents clinically with fever, cough, rhinitis, pharyngitis, and dyspnea and can produce severe enough bronchiolitis to require hospitalization in 1% to 2% of cases, primarily in children 2 to 5 months of age, accounting for 90,000 hospital admissions annually in the United States. The mortality rate in these hospitalized patients is 1% to 3%, causing 4500 deaths in infants and children in the United States annually. RSV may, however, be associated with a higher mortality rate in children infected with pathogens such as adenovirus, pneumococcus, cytomegalovirus, and *Pneumocystis jiroveci*. Of patients with RSV requiring mechanical ventilation, the majority have at least one additional risk factor for a severe course of infection (prematurity 50%, chronic lung disease 20%, congenital heart disease 35%, immunodeficiency 20%) (193). Of those dying of RSV, Thorburn noted one of the following preexisting medical conditions in every patient–chromosomal abnormalities 29%, cardiac lesions 27%, neuromuscular disorder 15%, chronic lung disease 12%, large airway abnormality 9%, and immunodeficiency 9% (194).

In fatal cases, RSV produces extensive alveolar and terminal bronchiolar plugging by granular eosinophilic debris accompanied by peribronchiolar lymphocytic inflammation and edema.

Eosinophils may be an integral part of the inflammatory process. In less severely involved areas, bronchiolar epithelium displays uneven proliferation with a polypoid appearance, squamous metaplasia, and desquamation. Syncytial giant cells may be present along alveolar walls and may contain granular, mildly basophilic cytoplasmic inclusions, which may also be seen in bronchial, bronchiolar, and alveolar epithelia (Figure 12-46A to C). Dense cytoplasmic

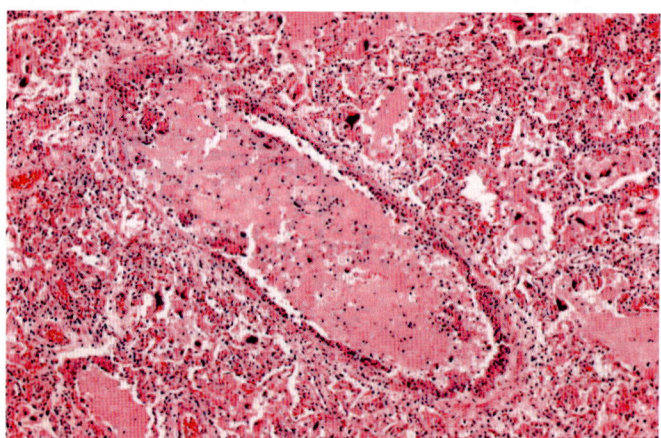

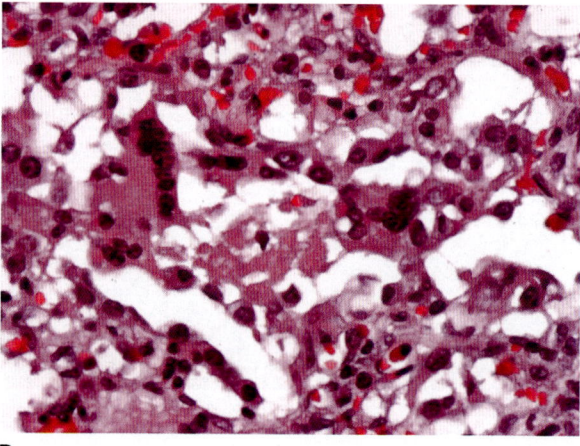

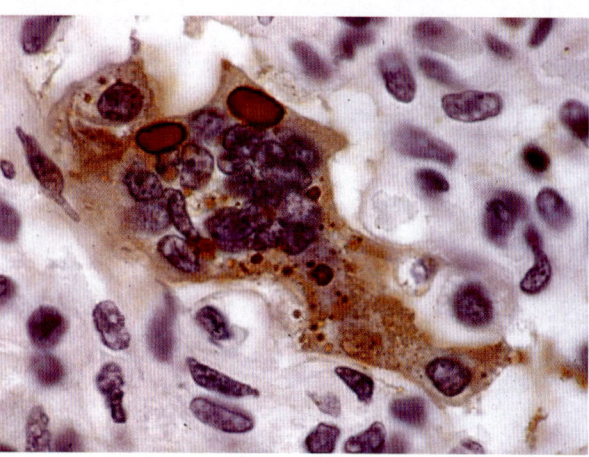

FIGURE 12-46 • Respiratory syncytial virus. **A:** Amorphous inflammatory debris fills a bronchiole and surrounding alveoli. Note the syncytial giant cells throughout the section. **B:** Hyperplastic alveolar cells line the surface of this alveolus, which contains numerous syncytial giant cells. **C:** The cytoplasmic viral inclusions stain intensely positive for RSV.

inclusions can be demonstrated by electron microscopy (192). RSV antigen can be demonstrated in formalin-fixed, paraffin-embedded autopsy tissue by immunohistochemical techniques (Figure 12-46C).

Human Metapneumovirus

Human metapneumovirus (HMPV) is in the Paramyxoviridae family and accounts for nearly 10% of community-acquired alveolar pneumonia. When compared with infants with RSV pneumonia, children with HMPV are older and have a more common history of acute otitis media requiring tympanocentesis, wheezing and gastrointestinal symptoms, and a lower hospitalization rate. HMPV is also seen more frequently than RSV in children with congenital abnormalities, particularly those with cardiopulmonary problems and when associated with an increased ventilatory requirement (195). Vargas et al. (196) have described the pathology of HMPV infections. Bronchoalveolar lavage shows epithelial degenerative changes and eosinophilic cytoplasmic inclusions within epithelial cells, multinucleate giant cells, and histiocytes. Lung biopsy additionally shows chronic airway inflammation and intra-alveolar foamy and hemosiderin-laden macrophages. Several other "new" viruses have been identified as etiologic agents in acute respiratory illnesses with similarities to RSV and hMPV; these organisms include human bocavirus, coronaviruses NL63 and HKU1 and enteroviruses, in particular EV-D68 which has also been associated with polio-like manifestations (197–200).

Adenovirus

Adenovirus, a DNA virus, is frequently associated with gastroenteritis in infants and young children but also accounts for 5% to 11% of cases of bronchitis, 2% to 10% of bronchiolitis, and 4% to 10% of pneumonia in children (201). Adenovirus infections are seen most frequently in children younger than 5 years of age who spend portions of their days in child care centers or other closed environments. Infections are also common in grade and junior high school children during winter, spring, and early summer.

Severe cases of pneumonia are most common in children 3 to 18 months of age and are associated with adenovirus types 3, 7, and 21. To this list, human ADV-14 has been added as an emerging infection (202). The onset is acute, and the child presents with high fever, persistent cough, lethargy, diarrhea, vomiting, and pharyngitis. Adenovirus infection with or without interstitial pneumonia has been implicated in up to 25% of sudden deaths in infants. Extrapulmonary complications (e.g., meningitis, myocarditis) are common, and serious pulmonary sequelae (e.g., bronchiectasis, bronchiolitis obliterans [BO], unilateral hyperlucent lung) are seen in 14% to 60% of cases with documented lower respiratory tract disease (203).

The pneumonia is characterized by severe necrotizing bronchitis, bronchiolitis, and alveolitis. Adjacent to areas of necrosis, the alveolar and bronchiolar epithelial cells are enlarged and contain small eosinophilic and larger basophilic intranuclear inclusions. These inclusions have a characteristic amphophilic (smudged) appearance and can be confirmed by immunohistochemistry. When viewed by electron microscopy, it can be seen that these inclusions contain viral particles that measure 70 to 80 nm and are arrayed in a tight periodic pattern along diagonals, which create hexagonal unit groups.

Legionella Pneumonia

Legionella pneumonia is infrequent in infants and children but may be one of the many infections seen in immunocompromised patients.

Chlamydia Pneumoniae

Chlamydia pneumoniae, an obligate intracellular bacterial parasite, is a well-known oculogenital pathogen that can also produce pneumonia in infants (204). Respiratory distress is noted in premature infants, and a progressive staccato cough is seen in older infants. The disease is readily treatable with antibiotics, and the mortality rate is low, unless complicated by other infections or DAD. Lung biopsy specimens display interstitial and intra-alveolar infiltrates of lymphocytes, plasma cells, histiocytes, eosinophils, and neutrophils. Necrotizing bronchiolitis may be present, along with emphysema, airway plugging, and atelectasis. Intracytoplasmic *Chlamydia* inclusions are only rarely seen in the lung.

Pertussis

Pertussis (whooping cough), an infection caused by the bacterial organism, *Bordetella pertussis*, and less commonly by three related types, was in decline through the 1970s, but the incidence has steadily increased over the past 30 years as more children have not had the benefit of vaccination (205). In children, the highest rates of infection are found in infants 6 months of age or less (206). The clinical manifestations are largely indistinguishable from the other infectious causes of acute respiratory illnesses. In infants, pertussis may be mistaken for sudden infant death syndrome. The diagnosis is generally established by serology and/or molecular detection. The pathologic findings range from acute bronchopneumonia, necrotizing bronchitis and bronchiolitis, and DAD (Figure 12-47A, B).

Eosinophilic Pneumonia

Acute eosinophilic pneumonia (AEP), while rare in the pediatric age group, can be seen in older children and is characterized by acute onset respiratory distress, eosinophilic infiltration in the lung, resolution of symptoms with corticosteroids, and the absence of relapse (207). An increase in peripheral blood hypersegmented eosinophils may precede the onset of symptoms. Bronchoalveolar lavage also demonstrates the presence of many eosinophils. Although the etiology of AEP is often unknown, it has been associated with a wide variety of drugs, parasites, and other infectious agents. The lungs are consolidated with alveoli filled with eosinophils and macrophages, accompanied in about

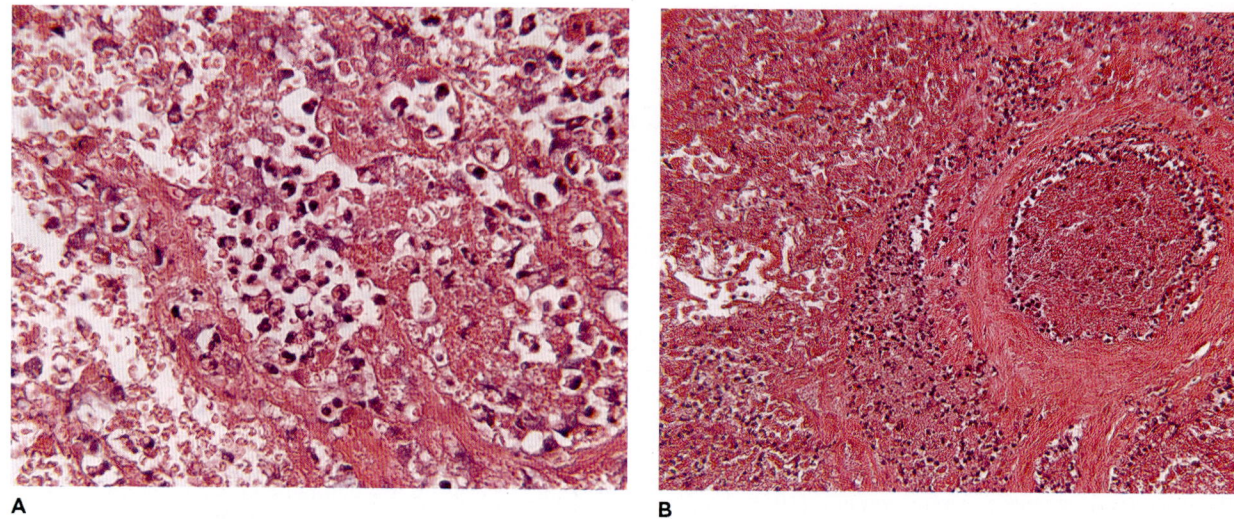

FIGURE 12-47 • Pertussis. **A:** The lungs at autopsy in this 3-month-old male with PCR proven pertussis pneumonia show the presence of necrotizing bronchopneumonia. **B:** Extensive hemorrhage and hyaline membranes are noted elsewhere in the lungs.

50% of the cases with an eosinophilic proteinaceous exudate. The interstitium may be widened by a mixture of inflammatory cells rich in eosinophils but also containing plasma cells and lymphocytes. Alveolar cells may be hyperplastic. Chronic eosinophilic pneumonia is rarely seen in children.

Interstitial Lung Diseases

As the name implies, these are diseases that primarily affect the interstitium (alveolar walls, interlobular septae, and connective tissue surrounding bronchovascular bundles) of the lung. They are bilateral with multilobar involvement. Terminology and definitions of acute and chronic interstitial lung diseases (ILDs) have evolved over the last few years, both in children and adults (208). Use of uniform criteria has helped characterize clinicopathological entities whose course, response to treatment, and prognosis are better understood, although there are still many patients whose diseases cannot be classified. It has also become evident that responses to lung injuries occur in certain pathologic patterns that can be recognized on light microscopy, such as organizing pneumonia, which point to a differential diagnosis but are not specific for a disease.

The spectrum of diseases seen in the pediatric population is almost completely different from that in adults. Idiopathic pulmonary fibrosis/usual interstitial pneumonia and smoking-related disorders are never seen in children. A nonspecific interstitial pneumonia (NSIP) pattern may be seen in children with collagen vascular disease and in certain surfactant dysfunction mutations (SP-C and ABCA3). In the *International Classification of Diseases, Ninth Revision* (ICD-9), codes have been added for several of the so-called ChILD (children's ILD) disorders as subheadings under the general heading of "Other alveolar and parietoalveolar pneumonopathy" (ICD-9 code heading 516.395). Acute interstitial pneumonia (ICD 516.33) is rare in children but is a rapid idiopathic progression of diffuse interstitial disease that histologically resembles DAD (see the section on Acute Lung Injury above). Lymphocytic interstitial pneumonia (ICD 516.35) in children is most commonly associated with immunocompromised status seen with HIV and immunodeficiency and lymphoproliferative disease in children. Cryptogenic organizing pneumonia (ICD 516.36), formerly known as BO with organizing pneumonia, may be seen in association with infection, autoimmune disease, posttransplantation (lung and bone marrow), drug reaction, and chemotherapy treatments. A desquamative interstitial pneumonia (DIP) pattern (ICD 516.37) should raise a possibility of surfactant dysfunction mutations (209).

The efforts of the Committee on Childhood Interstitial Lung Disease (ChILD) have proposed standard clinical and pathologic criteria for ILD in children 2 years old or less at presentation (210). These groups are listed below; the first four categories of disorders are seen predominantly in infants.

1. Diffuse developmental disorders
    a. Acinar dysplasia (CPAM, type 0)
    b. Congenital alveolar dysplasia
    c. Alveolar capillary dysplasia with misalignment of pulmonary veins
2. Growth abnormalities reflecting deficient alveolarization
    a. Pulmonary hypoplasia
    b. Chronic neonatal lung disease
    c. Related to chromosomal disorders
    d. Related to congenital heart disease
3. Specific conditions of undefined etiology
    a. Neuroendocrine cell hyperplasia of infancy (NEHI)
    b. Pulmonary interstitial glycogenosis (PIG)
4. Surfactant dysfunction disorders
    a. Surfactant protein B mutations
    b. Surfactant protein C mutations
    c. ABCA3 mutations
    d. Histology consistent with surfactant dysfunction disorder

    i. Pulmonary alveolar proteinosis
    ii. Chronic pneumonitis of infancy
    iii. Desquamative interstitial pneumonia
    iv. Nonspecific interstitial pneumonia
5. Disorders related to systemic disease processes
   a. Immune-mediated collagen vascular disorders
   b. Storage disease
   c. Sarcoidosis
   d. Langerhans cell histiocytosis (LCH)
   e. Malignant infiltrates
6. Disorders of the normal host-presumed immune intact
   a. Infectious/postinfectious processes
   b. Related to environmental agents
    i. Hypersensitivity pneumonitis
    ii. Toxic inhalation
   c. Aspiration syndrome
   d. Eosinophilic pneumonia
7. Disorders of the immunocompromised host
   a. Opportunistic infections
   b. Related to therapeutic interventions
   c. Related to transplantation and rejection
   d. Diffuse alveolar damage, unknown etiology
8. Disorders masquerading as ILD
   a. Arterial hypertensive vasculopathy
   b. Congestive changes related to cardiac dysfunction
   c. Veno-occlusive disease
   d. Lymphatic disorders

As evident from the above groups, these include all diffuse lung diseases including developmental disorders, not just interstitial diseases. However, this is a workable framework in which to develop a differential diagnosis when looking at a lung biopsy. Many of these conditions are discussed in other sections of this chapter.

Chronic Lung Disease of Infancy

After excluding known causes of ILDs, such as surfactant disorders and complications of prematurity (bronchopulmonary dysplasia), there remains a group of infants who were born at term or near term and developed slowly progressive respiratory insufficiency several days or weeks after birth. On biopsy, there is a mild chronic interstitial inflammation with minimal-to-mild fibrosis, reactive type 2 pneumocytes, and some simplification of alveolar architecture. Possible etiologies are postinfectious changes, nutritional deficiencies, and circulatory imbalances such as edema.

Neuroendocrine Cell Hyperplasia of Infancy

NEHI, previously referred to as persistent tachypnea of infancy, is a respiratory disorder of unknown cause, typically presenting in the first year of life with significant tachypnea, hypoxemia, and failure to thrive. High-resolution CT scan typically shows ground-glass opacities most commonly occurring in the right middle lobe and lingula, with air trapping in the lower lobes. Infant pulmonary function testing reveals air trapping and airway obstruction. The diagnostic gold standard of NEHI is a lung biopsy showing increased numbers of bombesin-immunopositive pulmonary neuroendocrine cells within bronchioles and alveolar ducts without evidence of other abnormalities, and limited or absent inflammation (211,212). BAL evaluation does not show high numbers of inflammatory cells or cytokines. Treatment is supportive, with oxygen supplementation and steroid use during wheezing episodes. All patients in the initial series improved and survived for a mean of 5 years (213). Outcomes are excellent, although some patients may remain symptomatic into early adulthood.

Pulmonary Interstitial Glycogenosis

This entity was first described in infants who presented with tachypnea, hypoxemia, and diffuse interstitial infiltrates with overinflated lungs on chest radiographs in the first month of life (214). Lung biopsies from all cases showed expansion of the interstitium by spindle-shaped and polygonal cells containing periodic acid–Schiff-positive, diastase-labile material consistent with glycogen (Figure 12-48A, B).

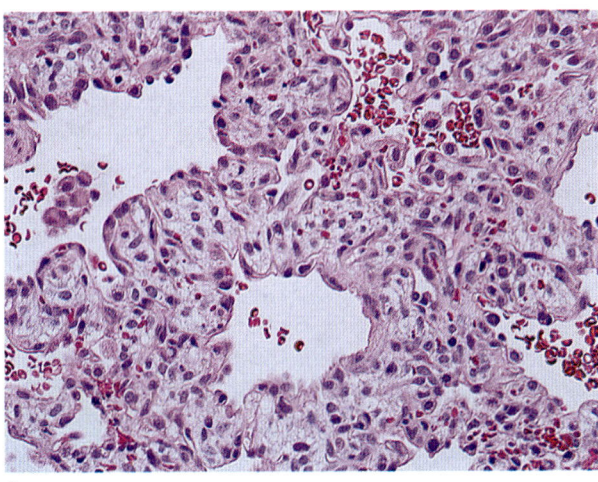
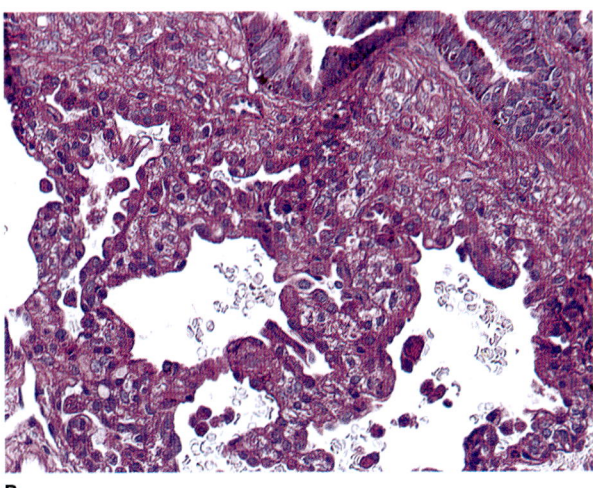

FIGURE 12-48 • Pulmonary interstitial glycogenosis. **A:** The widened interstitium is the result of the apparent persistence of uncommitted stromal cells with abundant clear cytoplasm. **B:** This PAS stain shows strong positivity in the cytoplasm of the stromal cells.

On immunohistochemistry, these cells are vimentin-positive but negative for leukocyte common antigen, lysozyme, and other macrophage markers, thereby confirming their mesenchymal origin. The hallmark finding on electron microscopy is the presence of primitive interstitial mesenchymal cells with abundant monoparticulate glycogen and few other cytoplasmic organelles. Alveolar lining cells show minimal or no glycogen. On lung biopsy, two characteristic patterns of PIG have been observed: diffuse interstitial PIG without other abnormalities, and so-called patchy PIG involvement in preterm patients with alveolar growth abnormalities (215). The latter is characterized by alveolar simplification, characterized by enlarged and poorly septated airspaces at low power (so-called alveolar simplification), as well as variable interstitial widening. In most cases, this is a relatively benign disease with resolution of signs and symptoms over the course of a few months, with or without treatment. However, deaths have been reported when there is coexistent cardiovascular disease or other alveolar growth abnormalities (216).

Bronchiolitis Obliterans

BO is differentiated from cryptogenic organizing pneumonitis since the latter is principally centered in small airspaces and is the resolving stage of active pneumonitis. In contrast, BO represents a process that is bronchiole or small airway centered with irreversible injury to the airways in most cases. There are a number of etiologies; it can be a sequel of severe lower respiratory tract infection, especially adenovirus and *Mycoplasma pneumonia* (217,218). It is a leading cause of death 1-year postlung transplantation in children (219). The sequence of events begins with peribronchiolar and endobronchial lymphocyte infiltrates and eventual destruction of smooth muscle with fibromyxoid reaction in the airway. There is progressive fibrosis, obliteration, and eventual loss of any remnants of small airways (220).

LUNG TUMORS

Compared to the experience in the adult population, primary pulmonary neoplasms in children are distinctly uncommon. Most malignant disease in the lungs of children is metastatic in nature; many of the more common primary solid malignancies of childhood are known for their spread to the lungs including Wilms tumor, rhabdomyosarcoma, Ewing sarcoma, and osteosarcoma. One institutional review revealed that 80% of all lung tumors in children were secondary or metastatic lesions and accounted for 90% or more of all malignant disease in the lungs of children (221).

Amini et al. (222) have reviewed the role of multidetector CT in the management of pediatric lung neoplasms.

Metastatic Disease

Murrell et al. (223) analyzed factors that most accurately predict the diagnosis of a malignancy in a radiologically detected lung nodule in the pediatric oncology patient; they concluded that peripherally located lesions measuring between 5 and 10 mm in children with a history of a solid malignancy were most likely malignant.

Osteosarcomas is the most common of these various malignancies to be seen as a surgical specimen since metastatectomy has been one approach in the management of these patients (224). The individual nodule may be composed of viable osteosarcoma or osteoid or bone without apparent tumor cells. In the case of *Ewing sarcoma* and *synovial sarcoma*, these tumors are also known to occur in the lung as primary neoplasms, but a prior history and/or presence of multiple nodules establish the metastatic nature of the tumor (225). *Neuroblastoma* is one of the more common malignancies of childhood but is infrequent as a source of lung metastasis (226). Granulomas and organizing pneumonitis are lesions that produce pseudometastasis (223). *Wilms tumor*, *hepatoblastoma*, and *rhabdomyosarcoma* are other childhood malignancies that are encountered most frequently as one or multiple nodules in the lungs (227,228).

Primary Neoplasms

Primary neoplasms of the lung and airway in children and adolescents in aggregate constitute a small, but important set of tumors. As some measure of the validity of the latter comment, a total of 40 primary lung tumors in patients between the ages of 3 months to 19 years were identified over a 90-year period at Children's Hospital, Boston (229).

Bronchial carcinoid (low-grade neuroendocrine tumor [NET]) and inflammatory myofibroblastic tumor (IMT) together accounted for 38% of the 40 cases, and an additional six cases (15%) were examples of PPB. With the initial report of the latter neoplasm in 1988, both the carcinoid and IMT have been displaced by the PPB as the most frequent primary neoplasm of the lung in childhood (221).

Neville et al. (230) analyzed the SEER registry data from 1973 to 2004 and found that the age-adjusted incidence of tumors of the lung and bronchus in children had remained stable at 0.049 per 100,000 persons. In their analysis, 160 patients were identified, with a median age of 16 years at diagnosis. The most common tumor type was an endocrine tumor (52%), likely a bronchial carcinoid or well-differentiated NET in most instances, followed by sarcoma (11%) and mucoepidermoid carcinoma (MEC) (9%). Overall survival was greater than 381 months with a 15-year survival of 65%. Males had better survival than females (381 versus 288 months), and those with endocrine neoplasms and MECs had the best survival. Small cell carcinoma had the worst median survival (<5 months). Surgery improved the 10-year survival from 32% to 75%. Multivariate analysis demonstrated nonsurgical treatment and nonendocrine tumor histology to be independent prognostic factors for tumor-related deaths.

Nonepithelial Mesenchymal Neoplasms

Pleuropulmonary Blastoma

PPB constitutes approximately 50% of all primary malignant tumors of the lung in children and between 25% and 30% of all benign and malignant pulmonary neoplasms in the first two decades of life (221). Even smaller series of lung tumors in children reflect the primacy of PPB (231). However, those studies antedating the initial report of PPB in 1988 obviously do not directly acknowledge this neoplasm; it is probably represented in the diagnostic categories of rhabdomyosarcoma or mesenchymal sarcoma arising in a congenital lung cyst or possibly pulmonary blastoma (PB) (Table 12-9).

The behavior of PPB, a tumor presenting clinically in one of its three basic pathologic types, has been documented recently in a series of 350 cases from the International PPB Registry (232). The age at clinical presentation is correlated with type I through type III PPB morphology, reflecting tumor progression, as it evolves from the purely multicystic lesion (type I) with a median age at diagnosis of 8 months, the intermediate cystic and solid stage (type II) with a median age of 35 months, and the purely solid (type III) with a median age of 41 months. The 5-year disease-free survival for types I, II, and III is 80%, 60%, and 37%, respectively (232). Almost two-thirds of children with a PPB have a heterozygous germline mutation in DICER1 (233). In addition to PPB, extrapulmonary manifestations of the DICER1-PPB familial tumor predisposition syndrome include cystic nephroma of the kidney, nasal chondromesenchymal hamartoma, Sertoli-Leydig tumor of the ovary, embryonal rhabdomyosarcoma of the cervix and other sites, intestinal hamartomatous polyps, ciliary body medulloepithelioma, hyperplasia and differentiated carcinomas of the thyroid, pituitary blastoma, and pineoblastoma (233).

Type I PPB is arguably the most important pathologic expression of this neoplastic process because of its clinical and imaging resemblance to other congenital lung cysts in the first year of life (234,235). Failure to recognize and manage the type I or cystic PPB at this stage in its evolution may

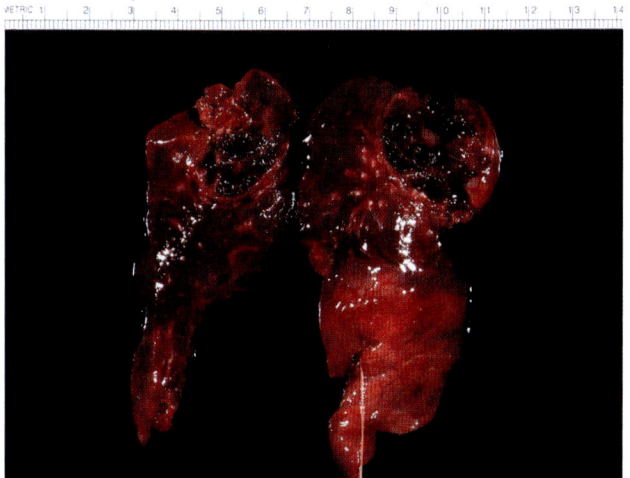

FIGURE 12-49 • Pleuropulmonary blastoma, type I in a 3-month-old female. A lobectomy was performed showing the presence of a circumscribed hemorrhagic multiseptated cyst.

be followed by the less favorable type II or unfavorable type III PPB. At this point in our understanding of PPB, it is difficult to ascertain the proportion of type I lesions that will progress to a type II or III PPB. It is this conundrum with the inability to differentiate type I PPB from CPAM that has generated discussion in the pediatric surgical literature in regard to congenital lung cysts (236,237). However, the cystic or type I PPB should be considered in the differential diagnosis of any congenital lung cyst and even more so when there is more than one pulmonary cyst since CPAM rarely presents as multifocal lesions.

Pathologically, the type I lesion is located in the periphery of the lung beneath the pleura as a delicately septated multicystic structure whose appearance is optimally demonstrated in a resected segment of lung or with the suspension of the collapsed cyst in fluid (Figure 12-49). If a mass is identified grossly in this multicystic lesion, the specimen likely represents a type II PPB with the cystic component of a type I PPB which has progressed to a solid primitive multipatterned sarcoma whose features are shared with the type III PPB.

If a portion of lung accompanies the type I PPB, a zone of transition from normal peripheral airspaces to the formation of the cysts is often appreciated, but normal lung parenchyma is not intermixed with the multicystic structures in type I PPB unlike CPAM. The septa forming the cysts are generally lined by a low cuboidal epithelium rather than the ciliated bronchiolar-type epithelium of the CPAM. Immediately beneath the epithelium, there are continuous or discontinuous compact zones of small primitive round cells with or without rhabdomyoblastic differentiation (Figure 12-50A to D). The presence of the small primitive cells beneath the surface may be readily appreciated throughout the multicystic structure or exquisitely localized in one or multiple foci. It is for this reason that the entire specimen should be examined microscopically. This population of small cells has the potential to

TABLE 12-9	PRIMARY PULMONARY TUMORS IN CHILDREN
Benign	**62 Total**
Inflammatory pseudotumor	52
Chondromatous hamartoma	3
Granular cell myoblastoma	3
Leiomyoma	2
Bronchial chondroma	1
Teratoma	1
Malignant	**81 Total**
Bronchial adenoma	
Carcinoid	35
Mucoepidermoid	9
Adenoid cystic	2
Bronchogenic carcinoma	
Adenocarcinoma	14
Squamous cell carcinoma	7
Small cell carcinoma	3
Large cell carcinoma	3
Sarcoma	
Fibrosarcoma	8

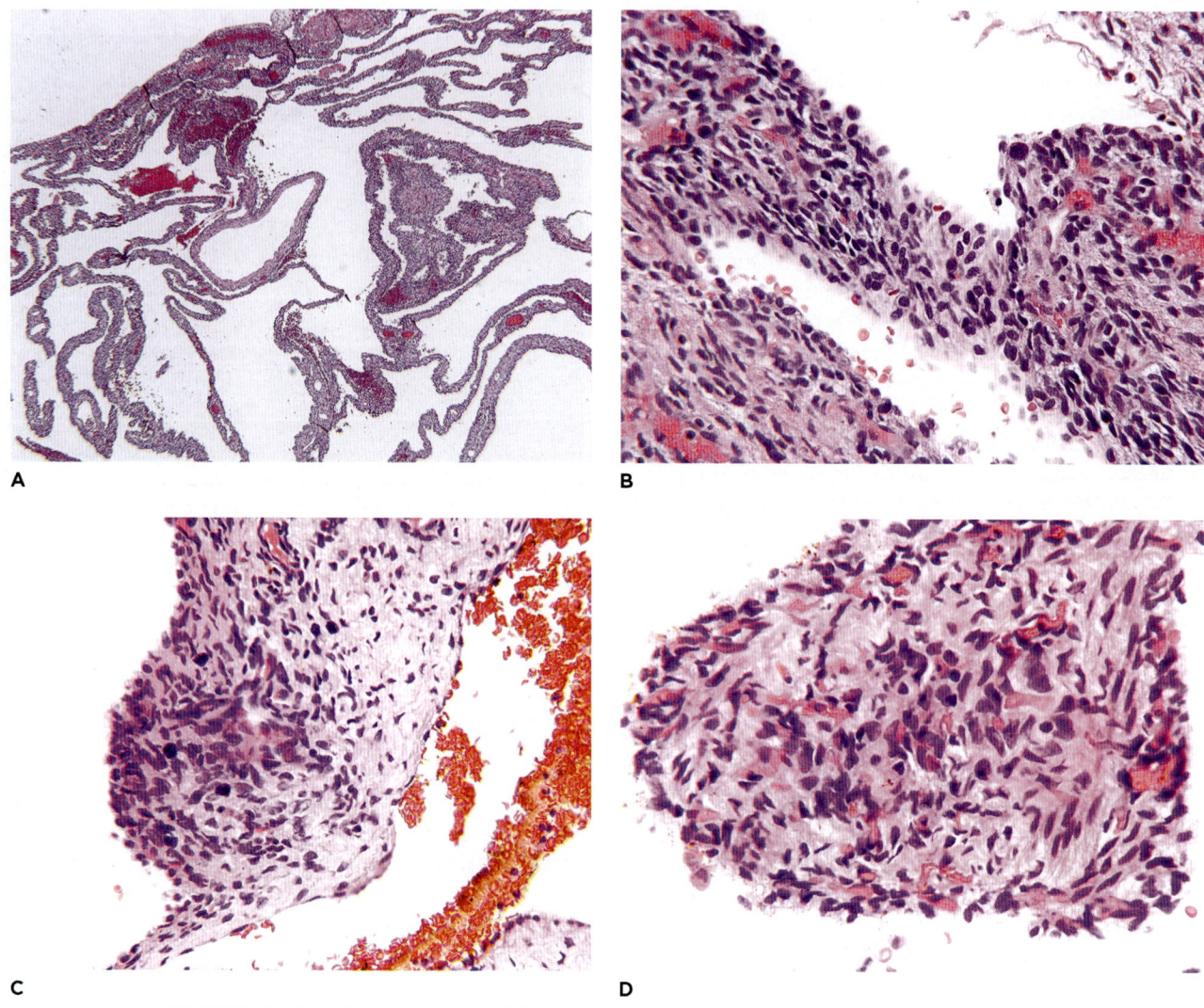

FIGURE 12-50 • Pleuropulmonary blastoma, type I. **A:** Low power overview of multicystic architecture and uniform septal thickness. **B:** The septum in this field has been widened by the proliferation of immature spindled and primitive round cells. **C:** This field displays adjacent widened septa and condensation of rhabdomyoblasts beneath the surface epithelium as an area of cellular density. **D:** Rhabdomyoblasts scattered in a background of primitive small round and spindle-shaped cells.

proliferate and differentiate along rhabdomyoblastic lines; this process is often accompanied by expanded and hypercellular septal areas that are regarded as features of tumor progression of a type I to a type II or III PPB. Another feature of type I PPB is the presence of small subepithelial nodules of immature chondrocytes resembling fetal cartilage; these nodules are not present or identified in all cases.

The location at the periphery of the lung and the multicystic architecture are characteristic in themselves to qualify as a type I PPB since primitive small cells, rhabdomyoblasts, or nodules of immature cartilage may not be present in the septa, but rather a fibrous or fibrovascular stroma. These latter findings are the features of the "type Ir PPB" which is regarded as a PPB that has failed to progress to the next pathologic stage of a type II or type III PPB. Unlike the type I PPB which is diagnosed in the first year of life, type Ir PPB is recognized well into later childhood and even young adulthood (232).

Type II and type III PPBs differ morphologically in that there are no identifiable cystic or type I foci in the latter (Figure 12-51A to C). Type III PPB is purely solid tumor that is often hemorrhagic, necrotic, and friable and can measure in excess of 10 cm in most cases (Figure 12-52 A–D). Several histologic patterns are recognizable in those resected specimens without prior adjuvant chemotherapy. Blastemal, rhabdomyoblastic, spindled, cartilaginous, and anaplastic foci are the five basic histologic patterns, but each tumor has its own unique combinations of these several patterns; almost all PPBs with a solid component have anaplastic, blastemal, and rhabdomyoblastic components. Immunohistochemical evaluation of the solid areas of PPB types II and III demonstrate a rhabdomyoblastic pheno-

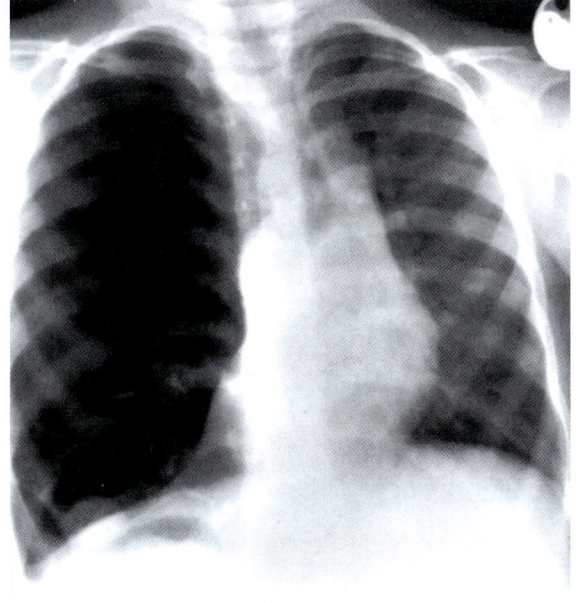
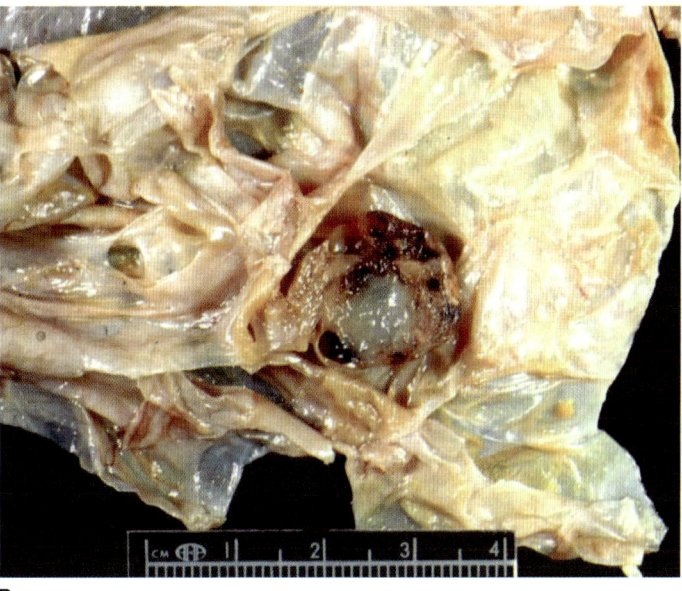
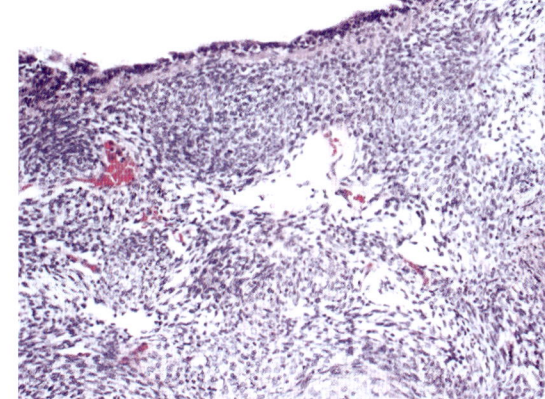

FIGURE 12-51 • PPB, type II, cystic/solid. **A:** A large cystic lesion occupies the entire right hemithorax. Note the opacity just above the right leaflet of the diaphragm. **B:** The opened resected specimen is composed of multiple cysts and a small, irregular, partially solid nodule. **C:** The nodule is covered by cuboidal epithelium and is composed of rhabdomyosarcoma, chondrosarcoma, and other areas of undifferentiated sarcoma.

type in part and p53 expression. A minority of cases are composed of chondrosarcoma and/or high-grade spindle cell sarcoma with some resemblance to dedifferentiated chondrosarcoma.

A small biopsy of a type II or III PPB with its limited sampling of a large mass shows one of the several patterns, often embryonal rhabdomyosarcoma or spindle cell sarcoma. These biopsies are a prelude to adjuvant chemotherapy so that it is important to correlate the pathologic findings in these small specimens with the imaging if possible. If a child less than 6 years old has a large solid or solid and cystic mass occupying the thoracic cavity, PPB is the likely diagnosis in most cases but not exclusively so. The examination of the postchemotherapy resection specimen is important since it provides an opportunity to determine whether the PPB is type II or III since there is a correlation with outcome (232).

Inflammatory Myofibroblastic Tumor

IMT, formerly called inflammatory pseudotumor or plasma cell granuloma (both terms no longer recommended), is a specific clinicopathologic entity which is associated with a translocation of the ALK gene (2p23) with different fusion partners or with pericentric inversions; approximately 40% to 50% of IMTs of the lung are ALK positive by immunohistochemistry (238–240). It is generally acknowledged that the pathologic diagnosis of IMT, regardless of the primary site (bladder, mesentery, small intestine), is based upon the morphologic features without the requirement for ALK expression assuming that other similar appearing

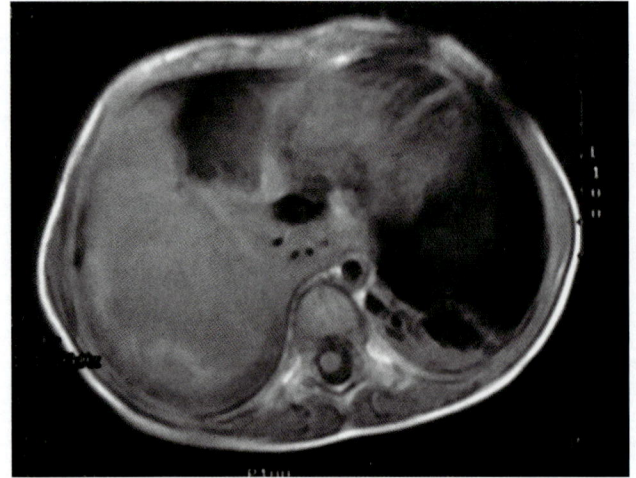
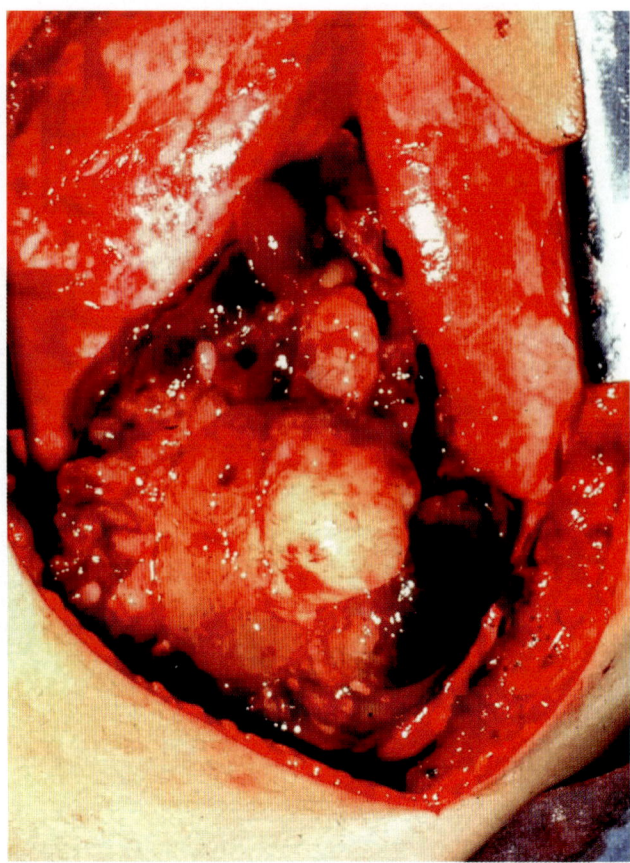
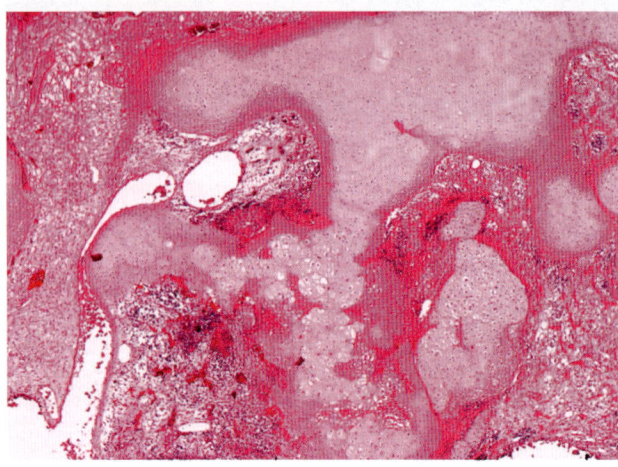
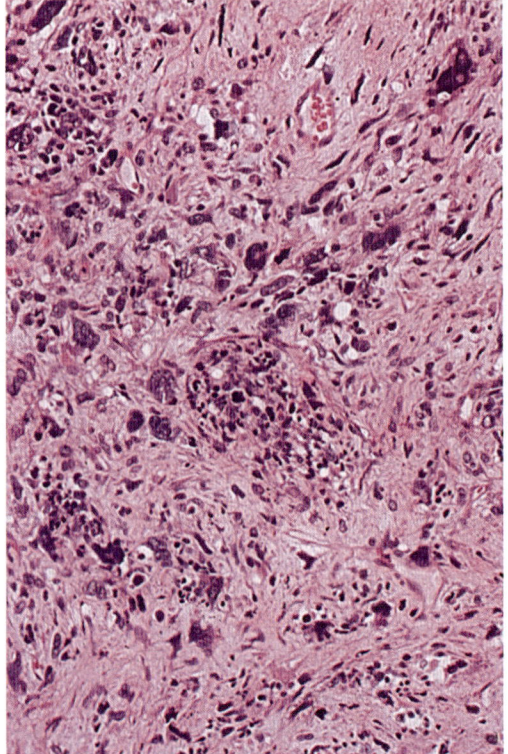

FIGURE 12-52 • PPB, type III, solid. **A:** A large mass fills the anterior portion of the right hemithorax of a 1-year-old boy. **B:** A multilobulated mass of hemorrhagic and focally necrotic tissue is seen *in situ* attached to the pleura. **C:** Immature cartilage blends with blastemal and mesenchymal components. **D:** Clusters of anaplastic blastemal cells displaying marked mitotic activity are separated by fibrovascular septa.

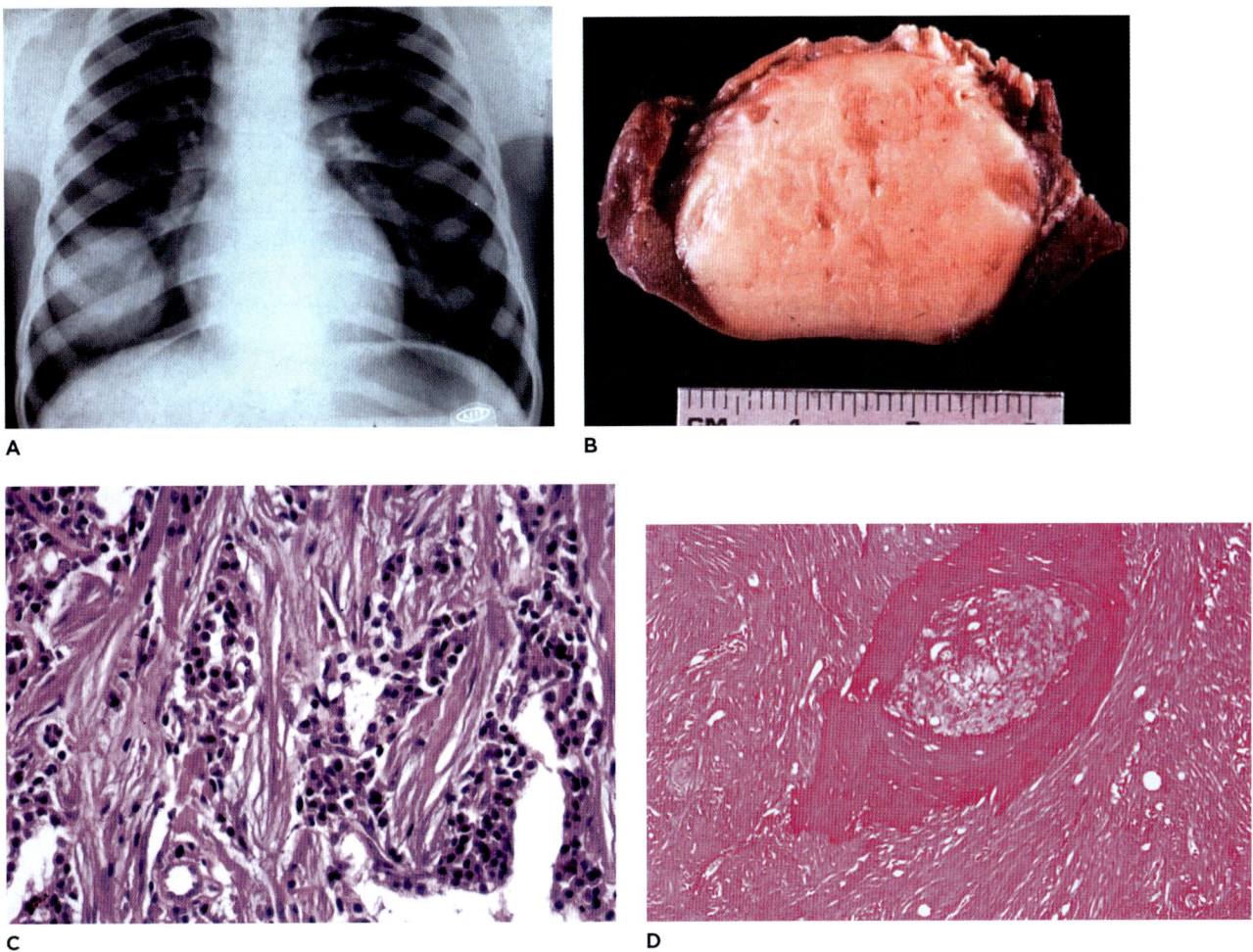

FIGURE 12-53 • Inflammatory myofibroblastic tumor. **A:** A discrete round mass is present in the right lower lobe of this 4-year-old boy. **B:** A circumscribed nodule bulges from the cut surface of a resected section of the lung. **C:** Interlacing fascicles of myofibroblasts are separated by an infiltrate of lymphocytes and plasma cells. **D:** A densely sclerotic area contains a focus of osteoid-like stroma.

fibroinflammatory processes have been excluded from the differential diagnosis.

An asymptomatic mass in the lung is the most common presentation of an IMT, usually in a child between 8 and 15 years; 25% or fewer patients have fever, anemia, and/or weight loss (Figure 12-53A). In some of the symptomatic cases, elevated levels of IL-6 are thought to be responsible for the constitutional manifestations that often resolve after resection. Though the majority of children only have pulmonary involvement, there are infrequent cases of multicentric or "metastatic" IMTs. Surgical resection is the treatment of choice, usually a lobectomy, and is curative in 90% or more of cases. However, this neoplasm can locally recur in an aggressive manner. There is a low potential for metastatic behavior, but the problem is distinguishing a metastasis from multicentric disease.

The pathologic findings are those of a well circumscribed, firm mass with grey-white to tan appearance, measuring 3 to 10 cm in diameter. Dystrophic calcifications are noted either by imaging or gross examination in 25% to 35% of cases (Figure 12-53B). The presence of hemorrhage and/or necrosis should suggest an alternative interpretation to IMT such as an infectious process or even a high-grade malignant neoplasm; the latter scenario is very uncommon in children. The microscopic features vary from a compact spindle cell proliferation with a variably prominent population of mature plasma cells to a densely collagenized background with a paucicellular appearance (Figure 12-53C, D). Spindle cells with an intermixture of foamy histiocytes yield a fibrohistiocytic pattern. Foci of epithelioid cells have been correlated with aggressive clinical behavior (241). Mitotic activity is variable, and the presence of marked pleomorphism and anaplasia should suggest another diagnosis.

The spindle cells commonly express smooth muscle actin by immunohistochemistry but are nonreactive for desmin and h-caldesmon in most cases. There is an association between the pattern of ALK immunostaining and the fusion partner. The plasma cells are polyclonal; there are some putative cases of IMT with a dominant IgG4 population, but there is a sense that the IgG4-sclerosing disorders and IMT are separate

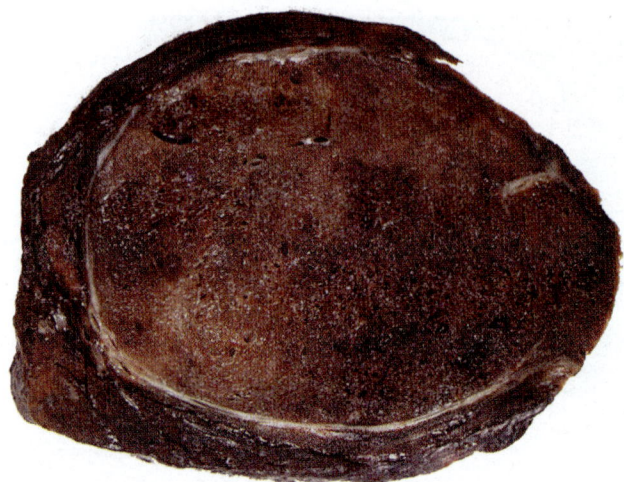

FIGURE 12-54 • Fetal lung interstitial tumor. This tumor was discovered shortly after birth as a solid mass which on gross examination was a spongy rather than a firm texture and is sharply demarcated from the adjacent lung.

entities (242). The trachea or bronchus is another site of IMT in children where it presents as an endobronchial mass (243).

Fetal Lung Interstitial Tumor

Fetal lung interstitial tumor (FLIT) is an entity that was identified among "lung tumors" in neonates and infants with the question of type I PPB (244). However, these lesions presented as a mass rather than as a cyst and may be accompanied by fetal hydrops (245). A spongy, well circumscribed mass whose microscopic appearance has a microscopic resemblance to fetal lung at 20 to 24 weeks of gestation (Figure 12-54). The interstitium is occupied by uniform, immature stromal cells with clear, glycogen-rich cytoplasm (Figure 12-55A, B). Solid foci of spindle cells have the immunophenotype of myofibroblasts or smooth muscle. An A2M-ALK translocation has been identified in one case (246). To date, there have been no known recurrences after lobectomy.

Congenital Peribronchial Myofibroblastic Tumor

Congenital peribronchial myofibroblastic tumor (CPMT) is an extremely rare but well-characterized spindle cell tumor that is detectable by prenatal ultrasonography (247,248). Nonimmune fetal hydrops is yet another clinical manifestation (249). A solitary lobar-based mass in association with a major airway has a glistening, tan-white trabeculated surface on sectioning. These tumors measure 3 to 6 cm in greatest dimension in most cases. The two histologic components of the CPMT include fascicles of spindle cells with and without a compact pattern on the basis of extracellular material in the background (Figure 12-56A to D). Mitotic figures are easily identified but no atypical forms in most cases. Lobules and irregular islands of immature spindle cells are interspersed in the background. Though the gross appearance conveys the impression of a well-demarcated tumor, involvement of the adjacent parenchyma occurs along and into the airspace septa. The immunophenotype is generally restricted to vimentin and equivocal positivity for smooth muscle actin in some cases (Figure 12-56D). CPMT has some resemblance to congenital mesoblastic nephroma and chest wall hamartoma, two other lesions occurring in infancy.

Myofibroma

Myofibroma (myofibromatosis) is one of the more common fibrous tumors of childhood typically presenting in the skin or soft tissues. When there is visceral involvement, it is usually in the context of generalized or multifocal disease with the lung as one of the affected sites (250,251). In these cases, there are several nodules in the lungs. Few examples of solitary myofibroma of the lung are reported (252,253). The pathologic features are identical to the counterpart in the soft

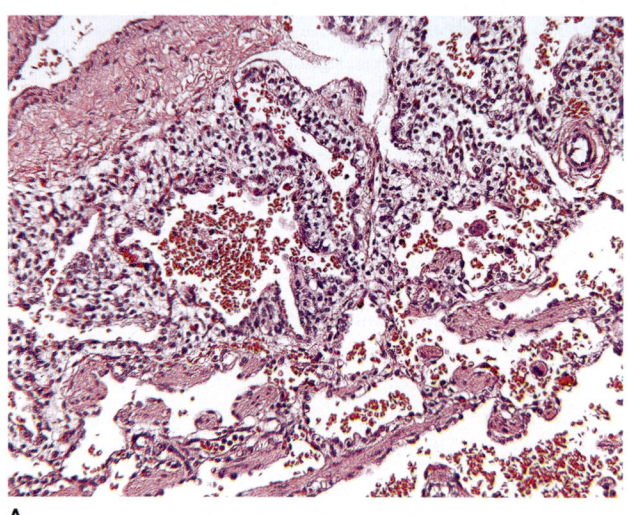
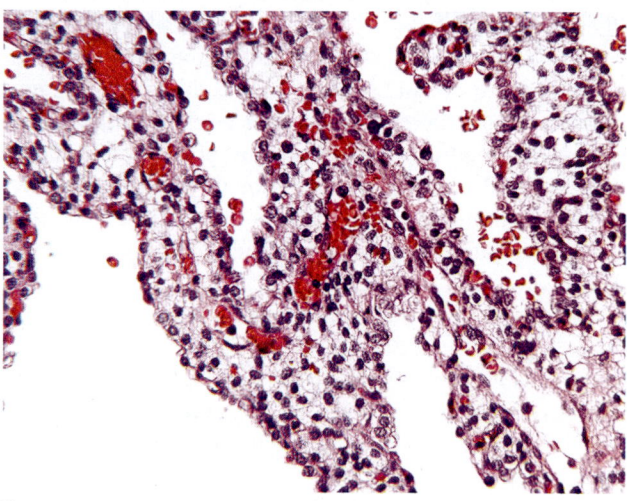

FIGURE 12-55 • Fetal lung interstitial tumor. A: A portion of thin fibrous capsule and a microcystic architecture of uniform septa that are occupied by interstitial cells. B: Here, the septal cells are seen as polygonal cells with abundant clear cytoplasm. These interstitial cells do not form a cambium layer-like formation like the cystic PPB.

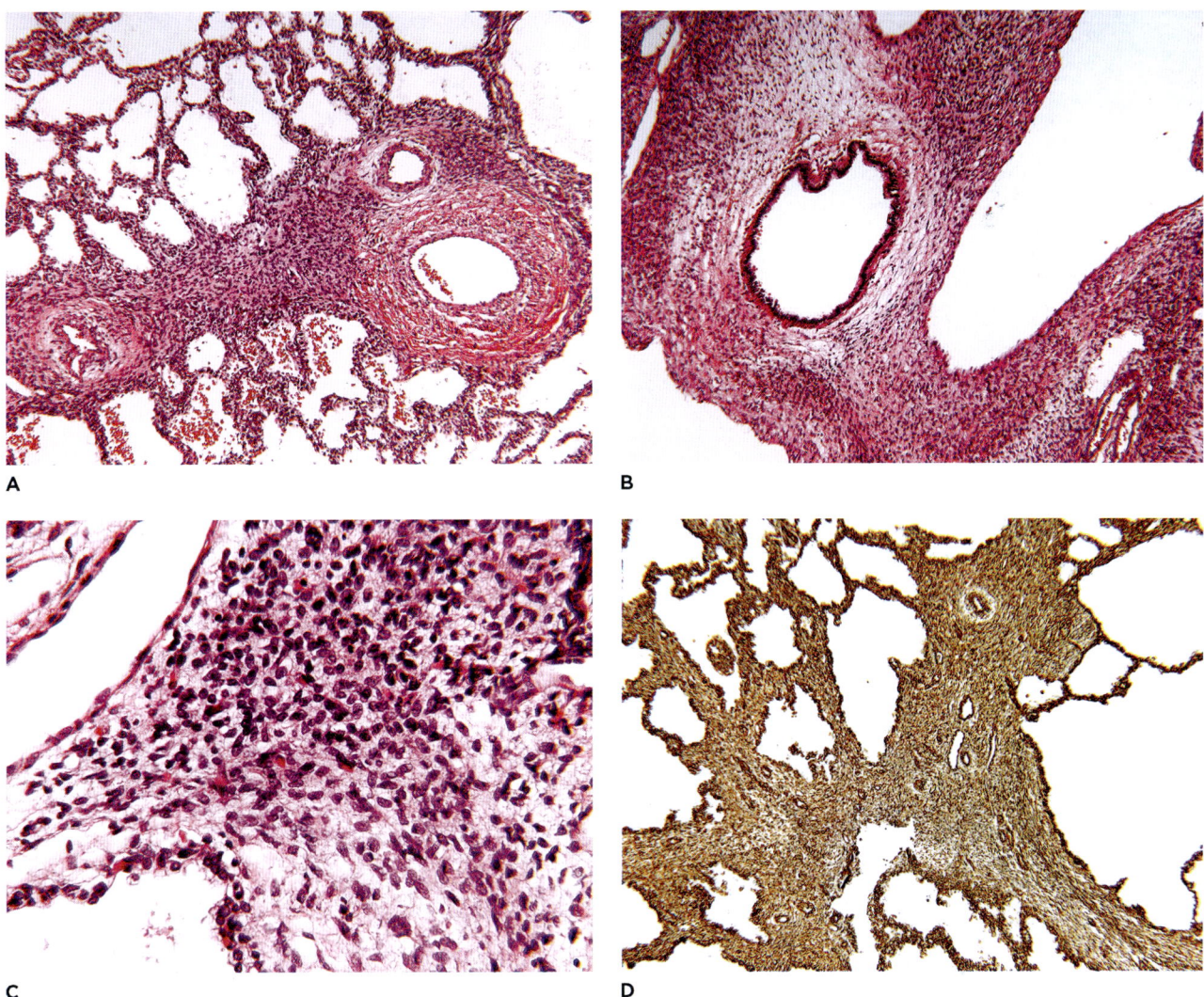

FIGURE 12-56 • Congenital peribronchial myofibroblastic tumor. **A:** This tumor presented as a suspected CPAM in a newborn. The proliferation of spindle cells shows a peribronchial and interstitial pattern. **B:** An airway is surrounded by a concentric proliferation of spindle cells with a limited pattern of involvement of the adjacent lung parenchyma. **C:** Immature-appearing spindle cells have a resemblance to CIF. **D:** The immunophenotype of the spindle cells is limited to vimentin.

tissues. Angiocentric lesions are optimally identified at the periphery of the mass as it abuts the lung parenchyma.

Other examples of spindle cell, fibrous tumors of the lung, and/or pleura have been documented mainly as single case studies whose importance resides in the awareness that solitary fibrous tumor, calcifying fibrous pseudotumor, and desmoid fibromatosis occur as intrapulmonary or pleural masses in children (254–256).

Chondroid Neoplasms

Pure chondroid neoplasms or those tumors with a cartilaginous component are represented by a heterogeneous group of lesions. Chondroma of the airway as one or more nodules in the lungs of a female child or adolescent should raise the possibly of the Carney triad of gastrointestinal stromal tumors and paragangliomas (257). The chondroma is composed of cellular hyaline cartilage. Microscopic nodules of fetal-appearing cartilage are found in type I PPB and sarcomatous nodules of cartilage are present in the solid areas of type II and type III PPBs. Metastatic germ cell neoplasms to the lungs can be composed in part of nonsarcomatous appearing cartilage. Salivary gland–type neoplasms of the lung, typically in a pleomorphic adenoma-like category, may have a cartilaginous component. Chondromatous hamartoma presenting as a solitary lesion in the periphery of the lung or rarely as multiple lesions is extremely uncommon in children despite its presumed maldevelopmental nature. Lobules of mature or immature cartilage are accompanied by small glands or tubules at the periphery of the chondroid nodules (Figure 12-57). A endobronchial lesion has been reported in an 8-month-old male (258).

Vascular Tumors

Vascular tumors or tumor-like lesions of the lung are infrequent in children despite the fact that this category of vascular anomalies is common in the skin and soft tissues of children. One airway hemangioma was found among

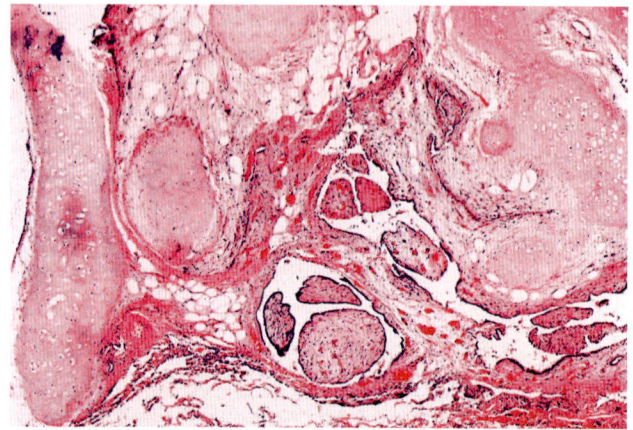

FIGURE 12-57 • Chondromatous hamartoma. Irregular lobules of cartilage are separated by vascular adipose tissue and fibrous connective tissue (H&E ×30).

20 benign respiratory tract tumors in one series; in another series of 40 tumors, five different vascular lesions, including nine cases of vascular malformations and hemangioma-hemangiomatosis (23%), were identified (221,229). *Infantile hemangioma* is known to present in the glottis, subglottic region, or trachea with a preference for the subglottic region (259). Like its counterpart elsewhere, these tumors have a lobulated pattern of capillary-like vascular spaces that are immunopositive for GLUT-1 (Figure 12-58A to C).

Pulmonary capillary hemangiomatosis (PCH) is a rare disorder which is characterized by a multifocal, nodular proliferation of small vascular spaces within the interstitium and with abrupt transition to normal lung (260–262). There is also extension into lymphatics and veins. Subintimal proliferation occurs in both small arteries and veins as well as muscular hypertrophy. Pulmonary hypertension with cor pulmonale is the major complication. It is thought that PCH and PVOD are related disorders. A mutation in the EIF2AK4 gene has been detected in affected brothers (263). Similar vascular lesions in the lung have been reported in association with congenital cardiac defects and trisomy 21 (264).

Epithelioid hemangioendothelioma (EHE), a low-grade malignant vascular neoplasm, presents in the liver and/or lungs, often in patients less than 40 years old. These tumors have a recurrent t(1;3)(p36;q25) translocation (WWTR1-CAMTA1 fusion gene) (265). A second translocation in EHE has been identified involving the fusion transcript, YAP1-TFE3 (266). Pulmonary infiltrates and/or nodules are the presenting features (267). The tumor is composed of round

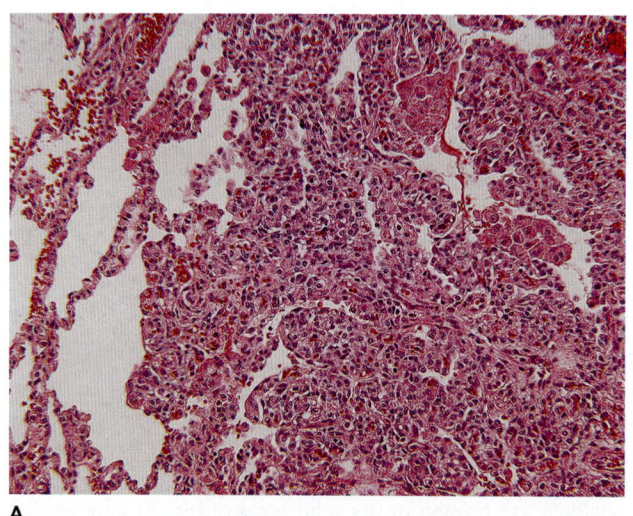

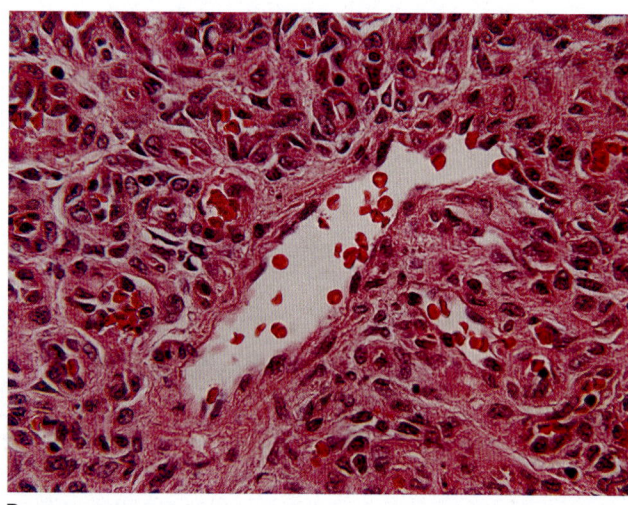

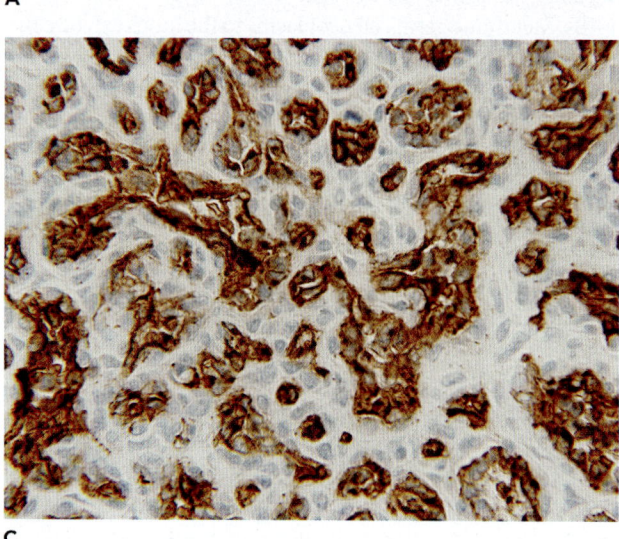

FIGURE 12-58 • Infantile hemangioma. **A:** One of multiple nodules in this biopsy reveals an interstitial process with encroachment on the small airspaces. **B:** This field shows the presence of small vascular spaces. **C:** GLUT-1 immunopositivity identifies the vessels as characteristic of infantile hemangioma.

or polygonal cells with cytoplasmic vacuoles present within a pale to hyaline myxoid stroma.

Kaposi sarcoma with pulmonary involvement is reported in HIV-infected children and in those who have received human stem cell transplantation (268–270). Reticulonodular infiltrates in both lung fields are accompanied by other visceral sites of disease. Compact spindle cells are accompanied by interposed erythrocytes and zonal eosinophilic bodies. Nuclear positivity for HHV-8 confirms the diagnosis.

Other vascular lesions include several whose pathogenesis is likely that of a malformation and others of less certain pathogenesis and even histogenesis. Sclerosing hemangioma (so-called) or pneumocytoma typically presents as a solitary, peripheral lesion, but rarely as multiple nodules. This well-circumscribed lesion occurs infrequently in older children and adolescents in whom there is also a female predilection (271,272). Though this tumor behaves in a benign fashion, there are examples of spread to regional lymph nodes including a case in a 10-year-old girl (273). A solid to papillary tumor is composed of epithelioid cells with or without a sclerotic stroma. Blood-filled spaces may be present. Histiocytes and plasma cells are prominent in some cases (274). The combination of epithelioid cells and stroma can lead to a diagnosis of EHE. Because of the expression of TTF-1 and napsin A, a primitive respiratory epithelial cell is a favored histogenetic proposal (275).

Lymphangiomatosis and lymphangiomyomatosis (LAM) are similar in respect to their appearance as cystic lesions of the lung but are pathogenetically distinct entities. The former disorder is a malformation of lymphatics (276,277). It may be difficult to differentiate the dilated interstitial lymphatic spaces in lymphangiomatosis from lymphangiectasia (278). However, pulmonary lymphangiomatosis is accompanied by other extrapulmonary manifestations including involvement of the pleura, mediastinum, chest wall, and bone (Gorham-Stout disease). LAM is a member of the perivascular epithelioid cell tumor (PEComa) family of neoplasms that are characterized immunophenotypically by HMB-45, melan-A, and smooth muscle actin expression (279). Females are overwhelmingly affected with early manifestations in the late second and third decades of life (280,281). LAM occurs in the setting of tuberous sclerosis complex (TSC1 on 9q34 or TSC2 on 16p13) or sporadically with an inactivating somatic mutation in the TSC2 gene. Microscopically, the lung biopsy shows the presence of cysts and nodules of immature smooth muscle and clear cells (LAM cells) unlike the more mature smooth muscle which accompanies the lymphatics in lymphangiomatosis. LAM cells are not only in the walls of lymphatics but also around other vascular structures and small airways (282). In addition to the previously noted immunophenotype, LAM cells are positive for β-catenin (283). An argument has been made that LAM is a low-grade metastasizing neoplasm (284). Another related neoplasm in the lung is the clear cell "sugar" tumor which is very rare and even more so in childhood (285,286).

Vascular malformations of the lung likely include some "cavernous" hemangiomas, but the most representative process is the arteriovenous malformation (287,288). Hereditary hemorrhagic telangiectasia (HHT, Rendu-Osler-Weber disease) is an autosomal dominant disorder with four mutations in genes critical for normal angiogenesis: type 1, endoglin (ENG, HHT1); type 2, ACVRL1 (previously ALK1, HHT2); type 3, SMAD4 (HHT with juvenile polyps); and type 4, GbF2 (HHT 5). Most cases of HHT are type 1 (53%) or type 2 (47%) (289,290). Common symptomatic organs are the brain, liver, and lungs. Pulmonary AVMs were discovered in 35% of children with HHT in one study and in 45% in another (291,292). The pathologic findings can range from numerous dilated small vessels within the interlobar septa with a hemangiomatous or telangiectatic appearance to a racemose of grouped thick- and thin-walled vessels in a background of fibrosis, chronic inflammation, and hemosiderin-laden macrophages. Without the benefit of special stains, it may be difficult to differentiate between arteries and veins. There are also the intravascular changes associated with embolization.

Hematolymphoid and Histiocytic Disorders

Infiltrative disorders are composed of lymphocytes, Langerhans cells, and dendritic cells. Lymphoproliferative disorders (LPDs) include a spectrum of reactive, infectious, and neoplastic processes (293). The reactive types of LPD in children are follicular peribronchitis/peribronchiolitis and lymphocytic interstitial pneumonitis (LIP). In both forms, the question of a primary or secondary immunodeficiency disorder should be considered and answered in those children who are infants or young children. Nodules of lymphocytes with reactive germinal centers especially prominent around small airways are features of follicular peribronchiolitis. Similar findings may be seen in the presence of airway obstruction. LIP is a manifestation of a perturbation in the immune system whether hypersensitivity, autoimmune, or immunodeficiency in nature. If the lymphocytic infiltrates are accompanied by small epithelioid granulomas, then hypersensitivity pneumonitis in the category of bird fancier's lung is a likely possibility (294). Similar-appearing poorly organized granulomas or those resembling the "naked" granulomas of sarcoid may represent so-called granulomatous LIP which is seen in common variable immunodeficiency (295,296). It has been recognized that HIV-AIDS in children is complicated by LIP with interstitial and small airspace infiltrates of small CD8 and CD20 lymphocytes (297). Epstein-Barr virus (EBV) appears to have a role together with HIV-1 (EBV/p24 carrying cells) in the pathogenesis of LIP in these children (298). Posttransplant lymphoproliferative disorder (PTLD) is an EBV associated complication that occurs in both children and adults who are solid organ or bone marrow transplant recipients (see Chapters 8 and 23).

Leukemic infiltration of the lung in children may be found at autopsy and rarely may be the initial clinical presentation with acute respiratory failure in the case of juvenile myelomonocytic leukemia (299–301).

Histiocytic disorders involving the lungs in descending order of importance in children and adolescents are LCH, juvenile xanthogranuloma (JXG), and hemophagocytic lymphohistiocytosis (HLH) (302). Pulmonary LCH is rare in children as the only site of involvement, whereas the lungs are involved in 20% to 50% of children with multisystem disease (303). In the latter setting, lung involvement has been regarded as an unfavorable prognostic variable but that has been challenged recently (304). A distinction should be made between LCH in children and primary pulmonary LCH in young adults who present with interstitial reticulonodular infiltrates and cystic lesions (305). The imaging findings are similar in children and young adults with LCH of the lung (306). BRAF V600E–activating mutations have been detected in 30% to 50% of cases of LCH, presenting in the lung or in extrapulmonary sites (307). MAP2K1 mutations are found in those cases of LCH without BRAF mutations (308). Aggregates of Langerhans cells are present within a background of lymphocytes and a variable population of eosinophils whose density obscures the parenchyma in the background. The destruction of the parenchyma results in the cystic and interstitial fibrotic changes. JXG with involvement in children likewise is found most often in infants with multisystem disease (309). Unlike pulmonary LCH, discrete nodules rather than infiltrates is the typical feature of JXG in the lung. Mononuclear cells with or without accompanying eosinophils and rare Touton giant cells are the histologic findings. CD1a and factor XIIIa discriminate LCH from JXG, respectively. Both Rosai-Dorfman disease and HLH rarely have pulmonary manifestations (310–312).

Epithelial Neoplasms

The topic of epithelial neoplasms of the respiratory tract is one by most measures that should be brief. However, there are several entities such as juvenile laryngeal papillomatosis, NUT-midline carcinoma (NMC), and adenocarcinoma arising in CPAM that have an especial resonance in children. Among 14 primary malignant neoplasms of the lung in children in one series, four cases (29%) were epithelial including two carcinoids (low-grade NET) and one each of MEC and squamous cell carcinoma (SCC). In the same series, squamous papillomas accounted for eight (40%) of 20 benign tumors. Our experience with primary malignant epithelial neoplasms is summarized in Table 12-10.

Juvenile Laryngotracheal Papillomatosis

Juvenile laryngotracheal papillomatosis (JLP) is a HPV-directed infection of the squamous mucosa of the upper airway with the ability to spread into the lower respiratory tract to involve the tracheobronchial tree. Almost 2% of children have HPV DNA detected in the oral cavity or oropharynx (313). The larynx is the most common and often only site of the papillary or papillomatous proliferation of the infected squamous mucosa with an estimated frequency of 1:1500–2000 or 4.5 per 100,000 infants and children in the United States per year with some variation among different countries (314). There are approximately 2000–2300 newly diagnosed cases of JLP in children per year (315). Most cases of JLP in childhood are diagnosed at or before 5 years of age, but there are cases whose diagnosis is delayed into later childhood. Though there are more than 150 HPV subtypes, virtually all cases are due to HPV6 or HPV11 or infrequently both subtypes (316). There is considerable variation from one series to another in the ratio of HPV 6 to HPV11 cases; however, HPV11 is detected with greater frequency in the more aggressive, frequently recurring lesions as well as in those cases with spread along the trachea (requiring tracheostomy) and into the bronchi and lungs (317). More aggressive disease is seen in those children whose symptoms have their onset before 3 years of age. Within the larynx and trachea, the growth has a papillary or sessile architecture with replacement of the normal squamous mucosa over the mucosal surface and shows the morphology of a benign squamous papilloma with orderly stratified squamous epithelium covering a vascular connective tissue core or stalk (318). Those frequently recurring lesions often are associated with cytologic atypia, frequent mitotic figures, and fewer koilocytes that may cause concern about squamous intraepithelial neoplasia. Nuclear hyperchromatism and atypical mitotic figures are absent in most cases. Tracheobronchial involvement is seen in 1% to 3% of cases with such spread (Figure 12-59A to D) (318). Solid and cavitary lesions are composed of papillae and nodules of squamous epithelium (Figure 12-59B to D) (319). The incidence of lung involvement in recurrent papillomatosis has been estimated at

TABLE 12-10 PRIMARY MALIGNANT EPITHELIAL NEOPLASMS OF THE LUNG IN THE FIRST TWO DECADES OF LIFE

Type	No (%)	Age (Range Yr., Mean)	Sex (M/F)
Well-differentiated neuroendocrine neoplasm (carcinoid)	10 (35)	(10–19, 18)	7/3
Squamous cell carcinoma	6 (21)	(7 m/o – 19, 11)	6/0
Poorly differentiated carcinoma	5 (17)	(1–20, 14)	2/3
Mucoepidermoid carcinoma	3 (10)	(6–17, 13)	1/2
Salivary gland analogue carcinoma	3 (10)	3–15, 10	3/10
Neuroendocrine carcinoma	2 (6)	(5, 20-)	1/1

From the files of the Lauren V. Ackerman Laboratory of Surgical Pathology, St. Louis Children's Hospital, Washington University Medical Center, St. Louis, MO.

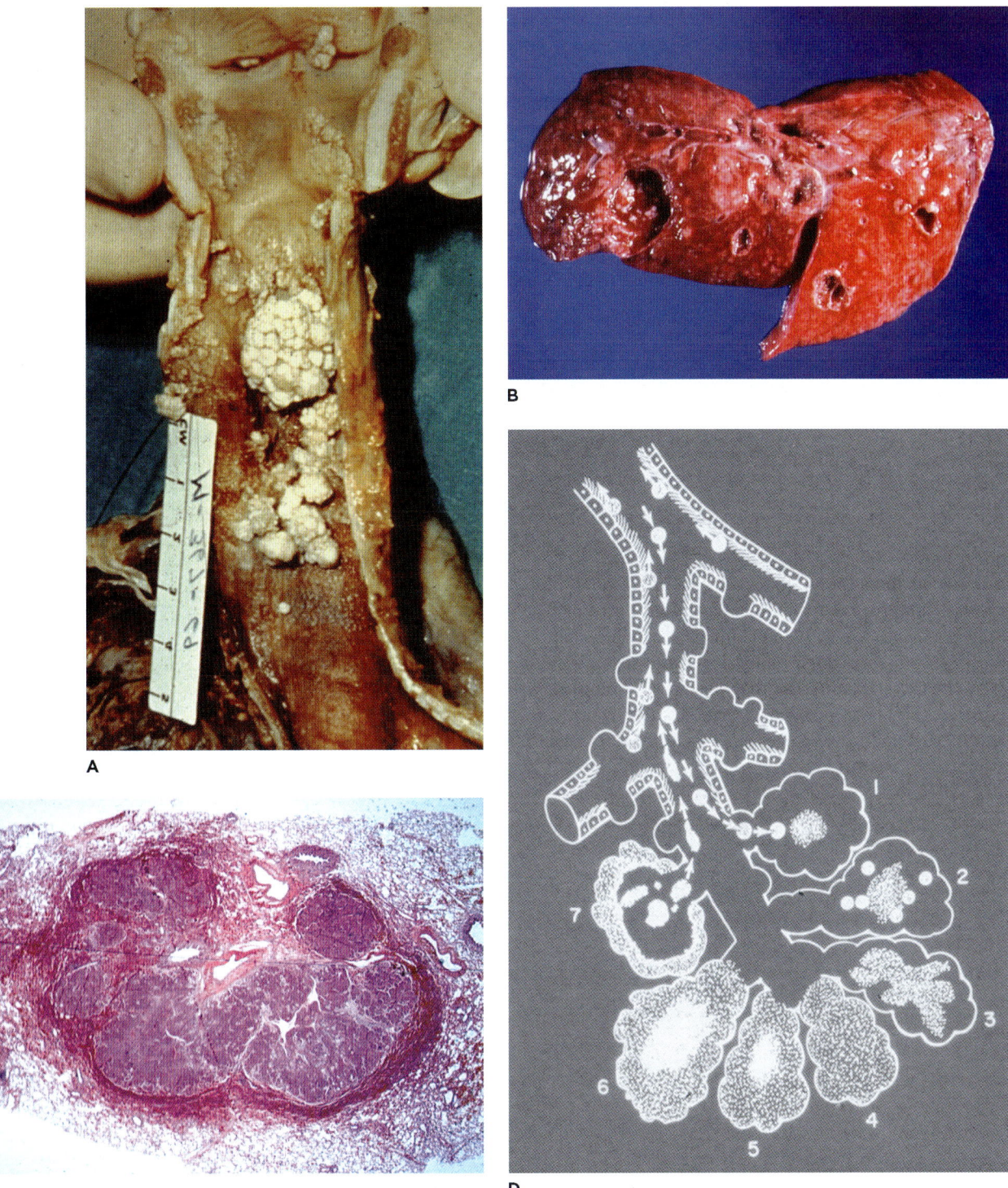

FIGURE 12-59 • Juvenile laryngotracheal papillomatosis. **A:** The larynx and trachea are covered by papillary growths of firm, tan tissue. **B:** The lung contains cystic areas where fragments of tissue broken off from the trachea and larynx have settled into the distal airways. **C:** Fragments of squamous papillomas that disseminated to the lung have proliferated to fill alveoli. **D:** Fragments of papillomas from the larynx and trachea can move down the trachea to lodge in alveolar ducts and alveoli (*1, 2*), where they can proliferate and extend throughout adjacent acini. Central cavitation of large lesions may take place (*5 to 7*) with further spread of the tissue fragments. (From Kramer SS, Wehunt WD, Stocker JT, et al. Pulmonary manifestations of juvenile laryngotracheal papillomatosis. *AJR Am J Roentgenol* 1985;144:687, with permission.)

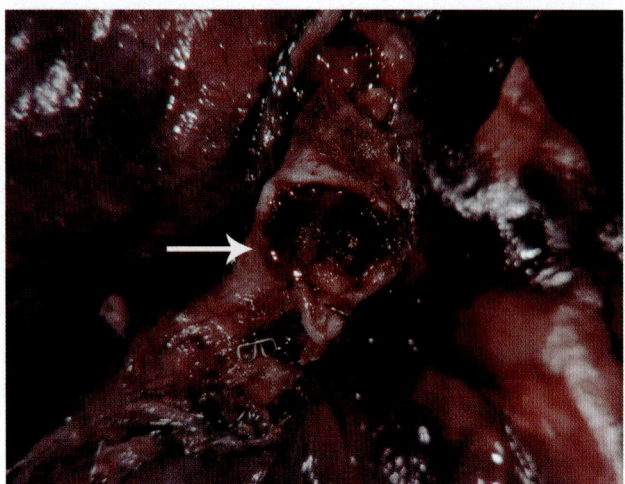

FIGURE 12-60 • Well-differentiated NET. The lumen of the bronchus is obstructed by a hemorrhagic and grayish-tan mass (arrow) in this 16-year-old male.

3.3% (317). Dissemination and subsequent growth of the benign squamous epithelium may be extensive enough to produce respiratory insufficiency and, rarely, death. SCC of the lung has been reported in patients with recurrent JLP with an incidence of almost 15% in those cases with pulmonary involvement (317,320,321).

Neuroendocrine Tumors

NET (classic carcinoid or low-grade NET) of the lung is the most common extraappendiceal primary site for this category of neoplasms in the first two decades of life (322). Our own numbers reflected a similar experience (Table 12-10). Approximately 30% of all NETs in children present in the lung once appendiceal NETs are excluded (323). Although regarded as a malignant neoplasm, the prognosis is excellent in most cases. Greater than 50% of primary malignant epithelial neoplasms in children are low-grade NETs or carcinoids. It is unusual for a carcinoid to present before 10 years of age though exceptions exist. Because of the endobronchial locations in most cases, recurrent respiratory infections are commonly documented in the medical history. An endobronchial mass with a smooth, polypoid appearance with an intact mucosa is the gross appearance (Figure 12-60). The tumor commonly surrounds, infiltrates, and replaces the subairway tissues with focal invasion of the lung parenchyma. The individual tumor cells are monotonous with slightly eccentric to central nuclei whose chromatin has a finely granular quality. An amphophilic to eosinophilic cytoplasm is apparent. Mitotic figures are generally sparse which is reflected in a Ki-67 index of less than 5% (324). Several patterns of tumor cells may be encountered including trabecula, cords, nests, and ribbons in variable proportions or dominated by one of these patterns (Figure 12-61A, B). A spindled pattern is more typical of the peripheral low-grade NET. Osseous metaplasia is seen on occasion. Immunohistochemistry is usually not necessary in most cases, but CAM 5.2, synaptophysin, and chromogranin are consistently expressed, and cytokeratin AE1/AE3 may be nonreactive. Resection is curative in most cases. Micrometastasis may be present in a regional lymph node in 10% to 25% of cases without appreciably altering the favorable outcome. The indolent clinical behavior is similar to the incidentally discovered appendiceal carcinoid in a child. Atypical carcinoid, high-grade large cell neuroendocrine carcinoma, and small cell carcinoma are rarely seen before 20 years of age (Figure 12-62A to D).

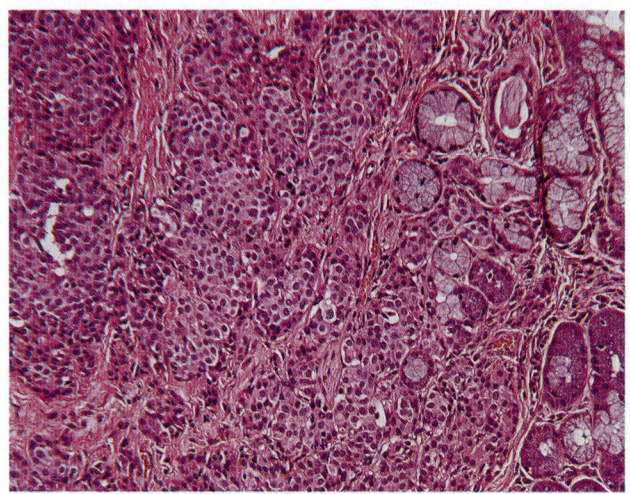
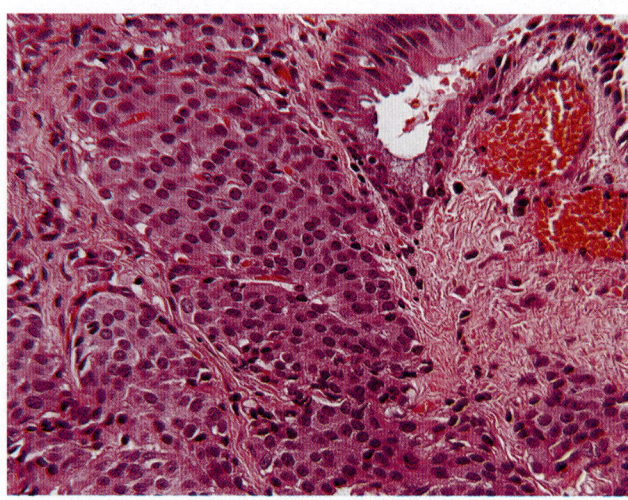

FIGURE 12-61 • Well-differentiated NET (carcinoid). **A:** Nests of tumor infiltrate through the wall of the bronchus. **B:** Nests of tumor are composed of uniform tumor cells with low-grade nuclear features and minimal mitotic activity.

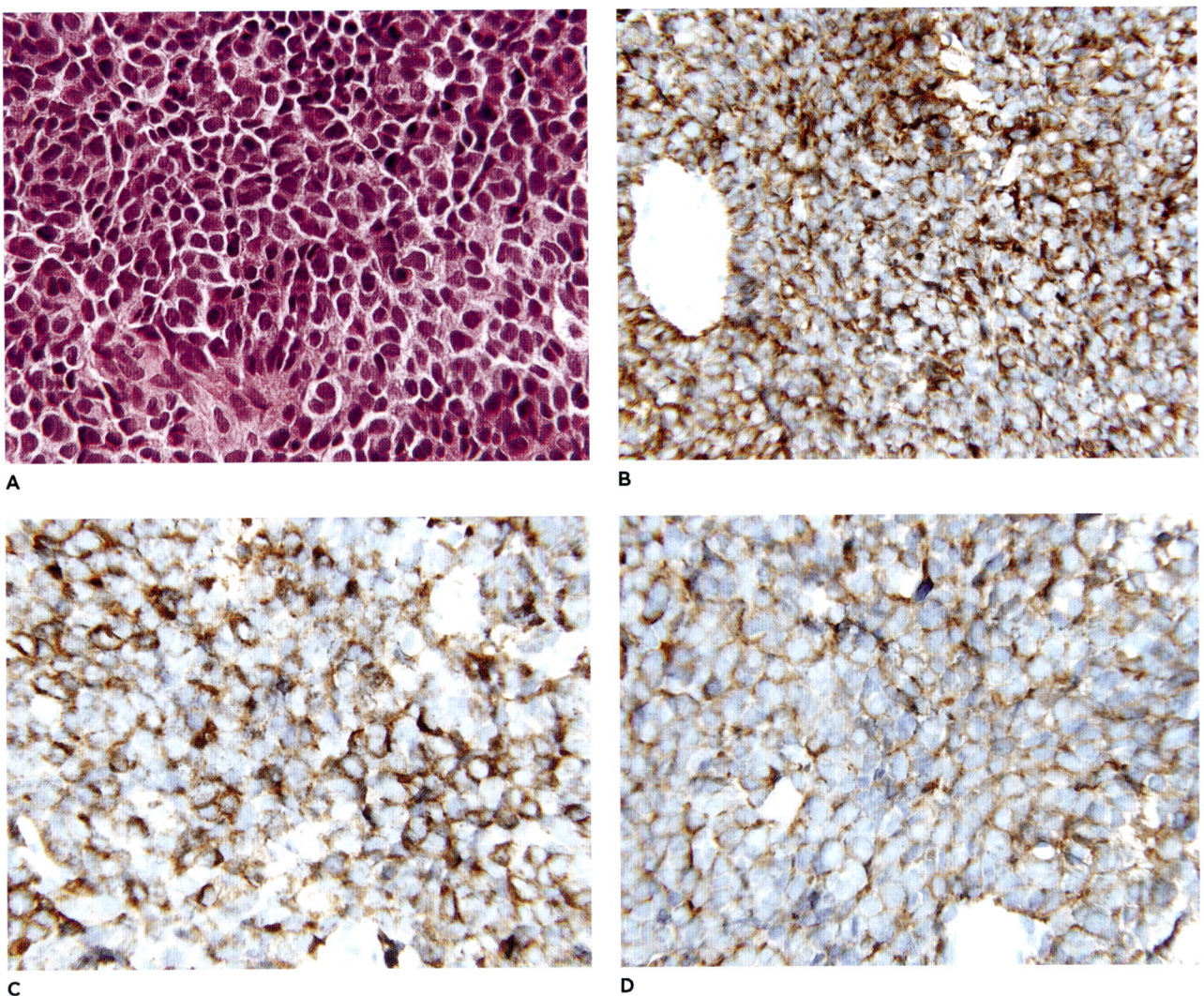

FIGURE 12-62 • High-grade neuroendocrine carcinoma. **A:** This biopsy from a 15-year-old male presented with several months of chest pain and a 7.5-cm mass in the right upper lobe. The tumor is composed of intermediate-sized malignant cells with hyperchromatic nuclei. **B:** The tumor cells are diffusely positive for cytokeratin CAM 5.2, but nonreactive for vimentin. **C:** Diffuse positivity for chromogranin. **D:** Synaptophysin positivity with diffuse pattern, but CD99 is nonreactive.

Primary Carcinomas

Carcinomas of the lung in children can be grouped into several categories: salivary gland type including MEC, adenoid cystic carcinoma (ACC) and myoepithelial-pleomorphic adenoma-like carcinoma, SCC arising in tracheobronchial papillomatosis, NMC, and adenocarcinoma arising in CPAM type I (325–327).

Mucoepidermoid Carcinoma

MEC accounts for up to 20% of bronchial tumors and about 10% of all primary pulmonary malignant tumors (328). Because of the origin in a main stem bronchus, obstructive manifestations are similar to the low-grade NET. An obstructing, soft, polypoid mass has a solid and cystic pattern with an admixture of mucus-secreting, intermediate, and squamous cells arranged in sheets and glands (Figure 12-63) and may have an accompanying dense lymphoplasmacytic infiltrate (329). Those MECs with a substantial squamous component are higher grade and higher stage, and have worse outcomes (330). Translocation $t(11;19)$ has been reported in the pulmonary MEC as in other sites, and the MECT1-MAML2 fusion transcript may be associated with better prognosis in these tumors (331,332). Neither TTF-1 nor napsin A is expressed by bronchial MECs.

Adenoid Cystic Carcinoma

ACC accounts for less than 5% of tracheal or bronchial tumors in children (326). Groups of basaloid cells arranged in cribriform cords or nested profiles are the histologic features. Accumulation of extracellular mucoid or hyaline material within the clusters imparts the characteristic cribriform

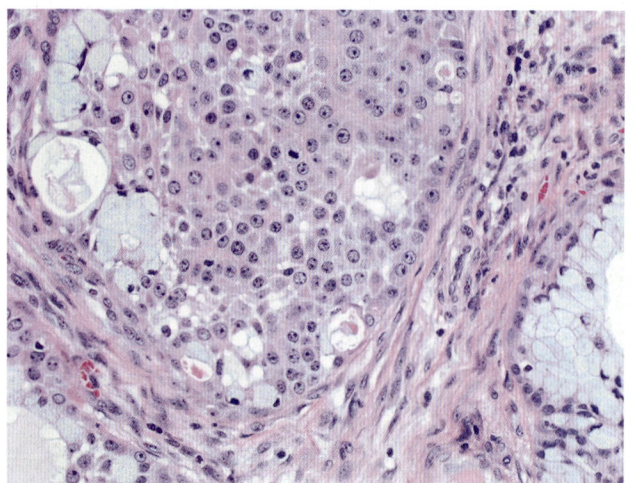

FIGURE 12-63 • Bronchial MEC. Epidermoid and intermediate cells are admixed with mucinous cells in the same tumor cluster (H&E, ×200).

pattern. Treatment is by resection, and although metastases may occur, prognosis is relatively favorable (333).

Other salivary gland–type malignancies are rare in children, with only anecdotal reports of acinic cell carcinoma of the bronchus (334,335) and epithelial–myoepithelial carcinoma. One of these neoplasms had the features of pleomorphic adenoma, but with metastases in regional lymph nodes (336).

Squamous Cell Carcinoma

SCC of the lung arising in the background of tracheobronchial papillomatosis is well-to-moderately differentiated and is recognized as small infiltrating nests in a desmoplastic stroma in association with adjacent foci of papillomatosis (Figure 12-64A,B). This rare complication is present in those cases of HPV 11–associated laryngotracheobronchial papillomatosis with E6 and E7 expression (337–339).

NUT-Midline Carcinoma

NMC is a poorly differentiated carcinoma that may express p16, but there is no association with HPV (340). This highly aggressive neoplasm has a predilection for the lung and thymus as well as other less common sites (341). Most cases present in adolescents or young adults, but there is at least one congenital case (342). A fusion transcript involving the NUT gene (15q14) and BRD4 gene—$t(15;19)$ (q13;p13.1) or BRD4-NUT is present in most cases. Microscopically, keratinizing nests of tumor abruptly transition to primitive-appearing tumor cells at the periphery or alternatively the tumor is poorly differentiated to the point that its epithelial nature may be difficult to appreciate without immunohistochemistry (Figure 12-65). These tumors are immunoreactive for CK7, p63, CD34, and focally for CK20 (343). There is overexpression of nuclear NUT by immunohistochemistry (344). NUT rearrangement has been detected in small cell carcinomas in children (345).

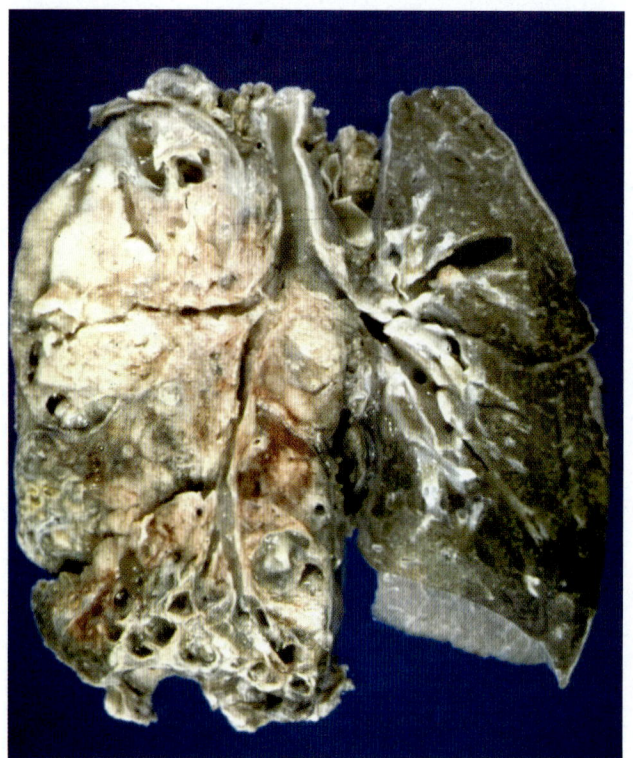

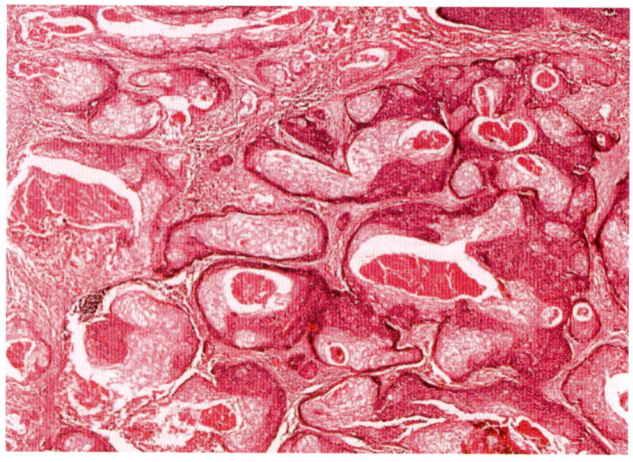

FIGURE 12-64 • Squamous cell carcinoma. **A:** The entire right lung of this 10-year-old boy is infiltrated by dense tan-white tumor. **B:** Clusters of well-differentiated stratified squamous epithelial cells invade the parenchyma (H&E, ×30).

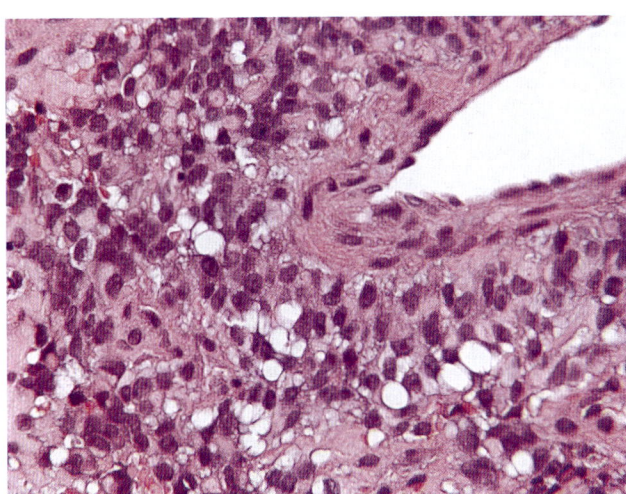

FIGURE 12-65 • NUT-midline carcinoma. This biopsy from the left mainstem bronchus of a 19-year-old female shows a poorly differentiated carcinoma with a vague nesting pattern and NUT-nuclear positivity (Contributed by Omar Hameed, MD, Nashville, TN).

Adenocarcinoma

Adenocarcinoma was seen in 2 (5%) of 40 primary lung neoplasms in children in one series (229). Adenocarcinoma in situ (formerly bronchioloalveolar carcinoma) (AIS) arising in association with type 1 CPAM has been documented in several case studies (Figure 12-66A, B). It is proposed that the adenocarcinoma is tumor progression from mucinous or goblet cell metaplasia/hyperplasia which is present in some 30% to 35% of type 1 CPAMs (346–348). Most mucinous AISs are diagnosed in older children or young adults, but there is one putative case in a neonate (349). EGFR and KRAS mutations have been detected in these neoplasms as in other examples of adenocarcinomas of the lung in adults (350–352). Another clinical setting for adenocarcinoma of the lung in children is carcinoma occurring as a second malignant neoplasm in a survivor of a first malignancy in childhood (353). Well-circumscribed fetal adenocarcinoma is discussed in the next section on pulmonary blastoma.

Pulmonary Blastoma

PB is a biphasic malignant neoplasm of lung that occurs predominantly in adults and was a poor candidate as the pulmonary counterpart of the other solid embryonic neoplasm of childhood. There is no histogenetic relationship between PB and PPB (354). The latter is a complex multi-patterned sarcoma, whereas PB is a type of sarcomatoid carcinoma of the lung (354). Well-differentiated fetal adenocarcinoma (WDFA) is regarded as a monophasic PB and like PB expresses nuclear β-catenin. (355). There is a report of WDFA in a 16-year-old individual with a germ-line mutation in DICER1 (356).

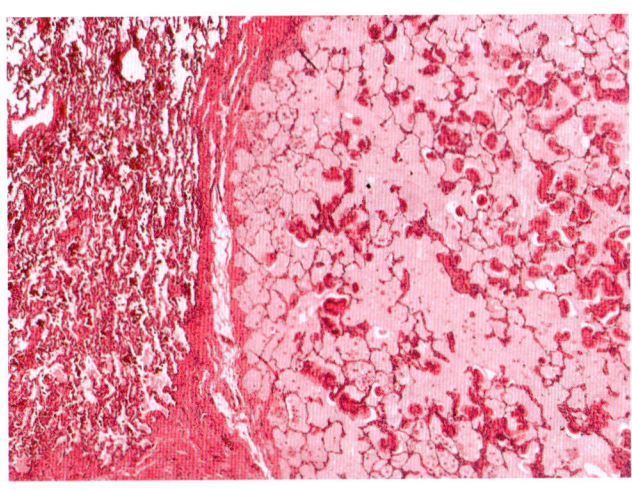
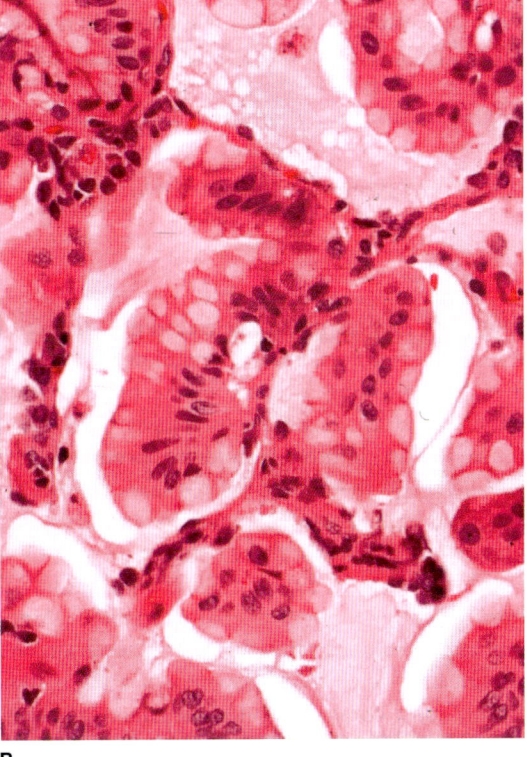

FIGURE 12-66 • Adenocarcinoma. **A:** A large, peripherally placed tumor nodule is composed of dilated alveoli filled with mucin and clusters of tumor cells (H&E, ×30). **B:** Alveolar septa are lined by papillary growths of columnar epithelial cells with irregular basal nuclei and apical mucin. Note the mucin lying free in the alveoli (H&E, ×300).

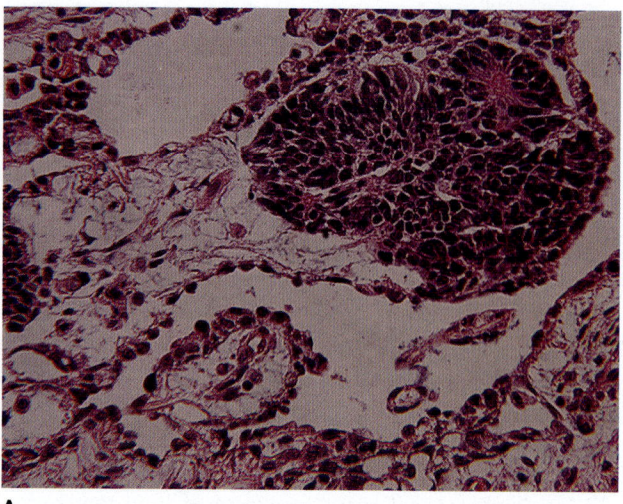 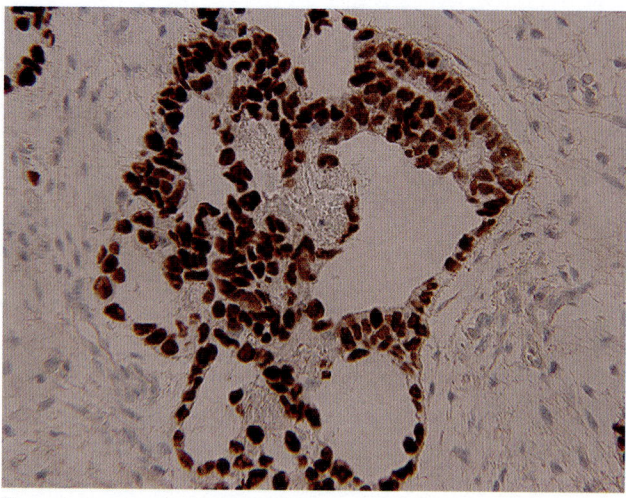

FIGURE 12-67 • Yolk sac tumor. **A:** A 6-month-old male presented with a mass in the right lower lobe. Glandular profiles with papillary unfoldings (Schiller-Duval body) are accompanied by other immature teratomatous elements including neuroepithelium. **B:** SALL4 nuclear immunostaining highlights the yolk sac tumor.

Germ Cell Neoplasms

Germ cell neoplasms in children are generally thought in terms of the sacrococcygeal region or the gonads, and the lung as a site of metastatic spread. However, there are several examples of intrapulmonary teratomas, but like the more common mediastinal teratomas, these tumors are also seen in adults in the third and fourth decades of life (357–359). One of the youngest examples is a mature teratoma in the lung of a 2-year-old male (359). There are eight cases of malignant teratoma of the lung; some of these tumors occurred in individuals 20 years old or less at diagnosis (360). Yolk sac tumor was present in one of these tumors, similar to that seen in a case in a 6-month-old male (Figure 12-67).

Miscellaneous Other Disorders of Lung

Sarcoidosis

Sarcoidosis is a chronic multisystem disorder characterized by the formation of noncaseating granulomata in the skin, lymph nodes, and lung as some of the more commonly affected sites that are accessible for biopsy. In a pediatric database of ILD in children, sarcoidosis accounted for 10% of cases (361). Less than 5% of sarcoid cases present before 20 years of age. There are two distinct age-dependent clinical presentations in childhood: those between 13 and 15 years of age with multisystem disease resembling the adult cases and those other children 4 years old or less with skin, eye, and joint manifestations (362–364). Childhood sarcoidosis is seen with near-equal frequency in boys and girls and is significantly more common in African-Americans (55% to 80% of cases) and Native Americans (5%), where cases tend to be clustered in the southeastern United Sates (362).

Older children frequently present with respiratory symptoms, weight loss, adenopathy, and headache; 50% of children have restrictive lung disease which is documented in clinical and imaging studies (364). Nearly all have bilateral hilar lymphadenopathy, which is frequently associated with bilateral paratracheal adenopathy (Figure 12-68A). Extrapulmonary manifestations are seen in 10% to 15% of childhood cases. Angiotensin-converting enzyme is elevated in approximately 50% of childhood cases, and although not specific for sarcoidosis, its presence does correlate with disease activity (362).

Pulmonary involvement is observed in less than 25% of children younger than 4 years of age but 50% or more of older children have restrictive ILD (365). It begins as alveolitis consisting of inflammatory cells and immune effector cells in the interstitium and airspaces. As the alveolitis progresses, epithelioid cells develop, and the typical small noncaseating granulomas are formed. Some necrosis is seen in granulomas, but it has more necrobiotic features than caseation. Extensive central necrosis may be an infectious process or the rare necrotizing sarcoid granulomatosis (366,367). The noncaseating granulomas are sharply circumscribed and composed of a focal collection of radially arranged epithelioid cells and multinucleated giant cells surrounded by a rim of lymphocytes (Figure 12-68B, C). The large epithelioid cells have pale, eosinophilic cytoplasm with round or oval nuclei. The giant cells, 150 to 300 nm in diameter, are of the Langhans cellular type formed from the coalescence of epithelioid cells. These cells may contain large, nonspecific, concentrically laminated, basophilic inclusion bodies (Schaumann bodies), or small star-shaped inclusion bodies with a central core of multiple radiating curved spines (asteroid bodies) (368). The granulomata contain fibroblasts and varying amounts of amorphous hyaline or reticular material, which increases with the age and maturation of the granulomata. The granulomas are found in the interstitium of the lung as well as in the subepithelial or perivascular stroma (368).

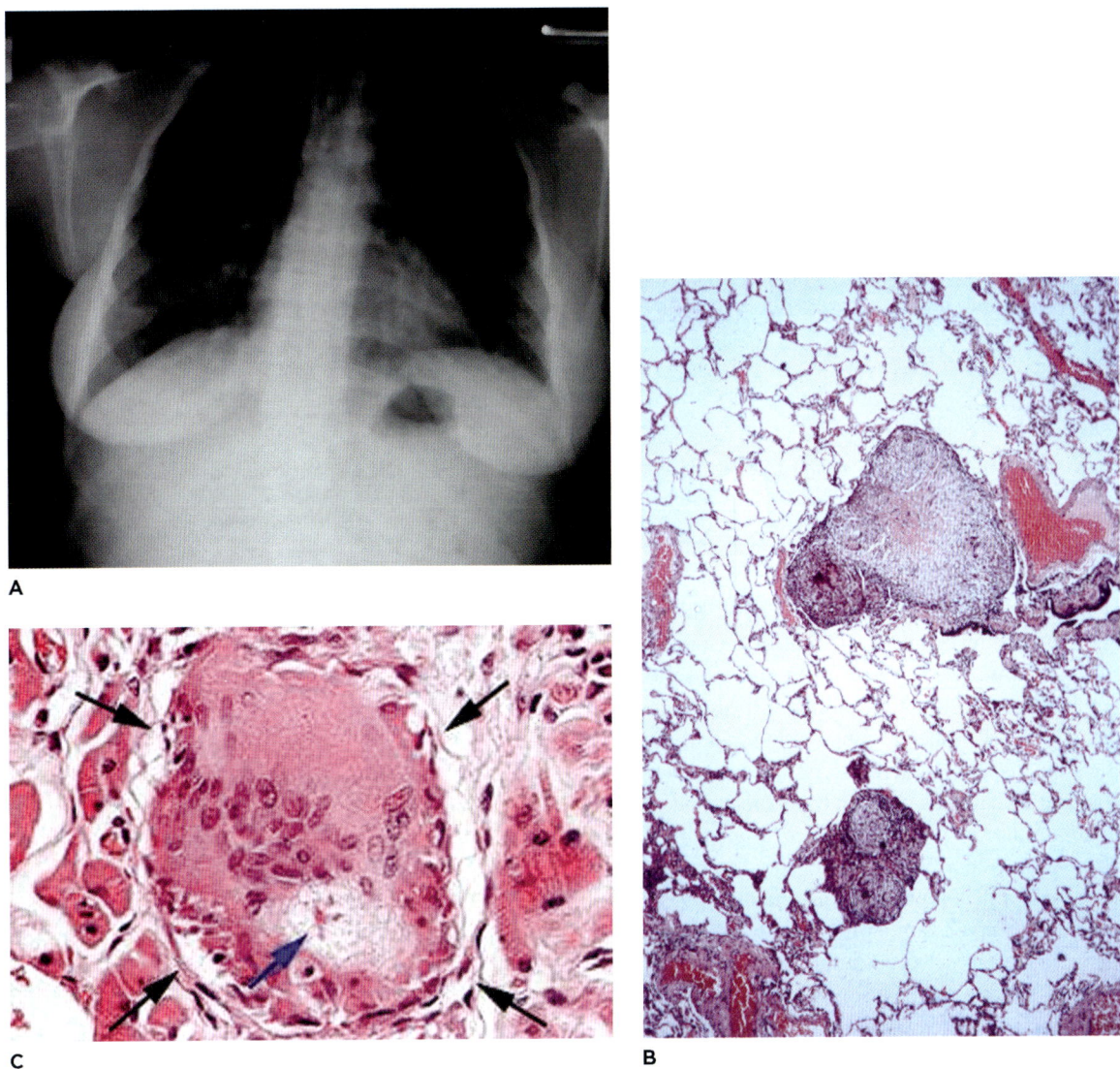

FIGURE 12-68 • Sarcoidosis. **A:** Bilateral hilar lymphadenopathy is present in this 14-year-old African American female. **B:** Several noncaseating granulomas are present in a random distribution in the lung. **C:** A granuloma showing a multinucleated giant cell (*black arrow*) with asteroid body (*blue arrow*).

Granulomata may completely resolve to leave normal lung parenchyma or, with hyalinization and fibrosis, give rise to nonspecific interstitial pulmonary fibrosis and, rarely in children, end-stage honeycomb lung. Involvement of the upper airway is unusual.

Infectious granulomas and sarcoid are the two commonest causes of pulmonary granulomas (369). However, noninfectious granulomas are seen in children with Crohn disease and common variable immunodeficiency (370–372).

Asthma

Asthma or reactive airway disease is the most common chronic disease of childhood (373). There are numerous variables that are involved in the increased risk for development of asthma in childhood, ranging from genetic predisposition to various environmental factors including tobacco smoke exposure *in utero* and second-hand exposure in infancy, urban versus nonurban residence, exposure to mold and domestic insects such as cockroaches, and respiratory viral infections to highlight some of the associations (373,374). Infants who are born prematurely also have an increased risk for asthma (375). Bacterial pathogens, in particular *Moraxella catarrhalis* and *Streptococcus pneumoniae* contribute to initiation of exacerbation of asthma (376). Immunologic mediators include CD4 (+) variants. On the basis of sputum examination, there is eosinophilic and non-eosinophilic (neutrophilic) asthma. The latter group predominates in severe refractory asthma (377). The magnitude of the problem of childhood asthma is documented by the fact that 9.6% of U.S. children have asthma (378). Only 0.02% of children requiring hospitalization have a fatal course. There has been a decrease in the mortality rate from asthma over the past decade (379). At autopsy, the lungs are often hypervoluminous with foci of atelectasis. Mucus plugs composed of soft, gelatinous, or rubbery grey materials fill medium-to-small bronchi. The smooth muscle of bronchi is markedly thickened, often

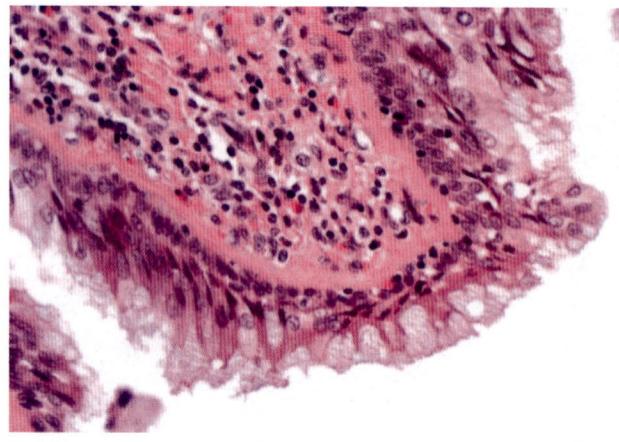 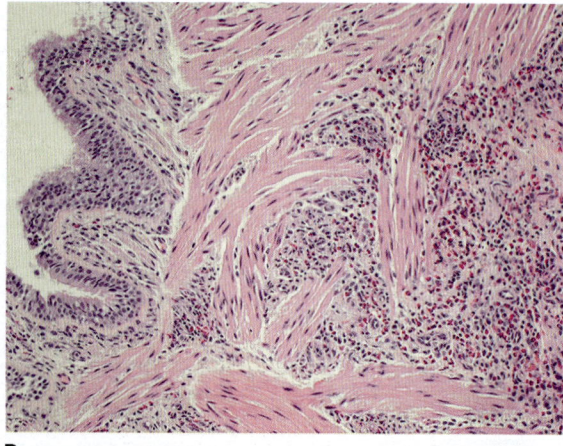

FIGURE 12-69 • Asthma. **A:** A markedly thickened undulating basement membrane separates the lumen of a bronchus from the muscular wall that is heavily infiltrated with eosinophils, lymphocytes, and plasma cells (H&E, ×100). **B:** The wall of the bronchus displays markedly thickened muscle layers (H&E, ×20).

2.5-fold or more than normal (Figure 12-69A, B). There is also a prominent thickening of the basal lamina of the mucosa, and the submucosa shows edema, vessel dilatation, and an inflammatory infiltrates of eosinophils, plasma cells, lymphocytes, and neutrophils. The bronchial mucosal lining and the submucosal glands display an increased number of goblet cells. Microscopically, the mucus plugs in bronchioles and smaller bronchi may contain small linear whorled strands of material that are twisted in a common direction with a central highly refractile densely coiled or braided coil, called a Curschmann spiral. Inflammatory cells are admixed with the material in the lumen, and degranulated eosinophils may form crystals, called Charcot-Leyden crystals. Sloughed segments of respiratory epithelium may also be present as Creola bodies. These structures—Curschmann spirals, Charcot-Leyden crystals, and Creola bodies—may also be found in sputum specimens of asthmatic patients. Similar findings are seen in allergic bronchopulmonary aspergillosis. Neutrophils may be more in evidence in those cases of severe, refractory asthma.

DIAPHRAGM

Abnormalities of the diaphragm can be both congenital and acquired. Developmental anomalies include accessory diaphragm (AD), agenesis of one or both leaflets, defective formation with herniation, and aplasia or hypoplasia of muscle with eventration. Acquired diseases such as traumatic rupture, denervation, and muscular atrophy are also noted.

The diaphragm develops from the septum transversum, pleuroperitoneal membranes, and dorsal mesentery during weeks 4 to 8 of gestation when the pleuroperitoneal folds and septum transversum converge and fuse (380–382). This embryologic event is complex as evidenced by the presence of other congenital anomalies in 40% to 50% of infants with congenital diaphragmatic hernia (CDH) (Table 12-11) (383–386).

TABLE 12-11 ANOMALIES ASSOCIATED WITH CONGENITAL DIAPHRAGMATIC HERNIA

Respiratory Tract
- Hypoplasia
- Extralobar sequestration
- Tracheoesophageal fistula
- Congenital pulmonary airway malformation

Cardiovascular System
- Tetralogy of Fallot
- Endocardial cushion defect
- Atrial and ventricular septal defects
- Ectopia cordis
- Coarctation of the aorta
- Pulmonic stenosis

Gastrointestinal Tract
- Imperforate anus
- Omphalocele
- Pyloric stenosis
- Stomach duplication
- Malrotation of bowel

Genitourinary Tract
- Hydronephrosis
- Multicystic kidney
- Duplicated collecting system

Chromosomal Anomalies
- Trisomy 18 and 21

Other Conditions
- Arthrogryposis
- Cleft lip and palate
- Meningomyelocele
- Hemivertebrae
- Fetal alcohol syndrome
- Cornelia de Lange syndrome
- Syndactyly
- Ullrich-Turner syndrome

Modified from Stocker JT. Congenital and developmental diseases. In: Dail DH, Hammer SP, eds. *Pulmonary Pathology*. Heidelberg, Germany: Springer-Verlag, 1994, with permission.

Congenital Diaphragmatic Eventration

Congenital diaphragmatic eventration (CDE) accounts for 5% of abnormalities in the formation of the diaphragm (383). Unlike CDH, the diaphragm is anatomically intact, but there is complete or incomplete muscularization of the membranous diaphragm (Figure 12-70A–C). Like CDH, there is compression of the thoracic space by abdominal organs to the lung itself, but there is no direct access by these organs. Various other anomalies are found in association with CDE (387,388). There is a report of CDE which presented with fetal hydrops (389).

Accessory Diaphragm

AD or more appropriately accessory hemidiaphragm is rare and even less common than CDE (390). There is a right-sided preference where a septum attaches anteromedial to the diaphragm and pericardium and posterior to the 5th, 6th, or 7th ribs (380). This anomaly may go undetected if asymptomatic. A fibrous structure with or without skeletal muscle is the principal histologic finding, and in this respect, it resembles CDE. When the lung is entrapped, there is hypoplasia. Cardiovascular anomalies may be present as well. Complete absence of the diaphragm and agenesis of the hemidiaphragm are other very uncommon defects (385).

Congenital Diaphragmatic Hernia

CDH is an important major anomaly accounting for 8% of all birth defects, occurs in 1:3000–5000 births and is responsible for 1% to 2% of infant deaths (382,391–393). Most cases are sporadic, and 50% to 60% of cases are not accompanied

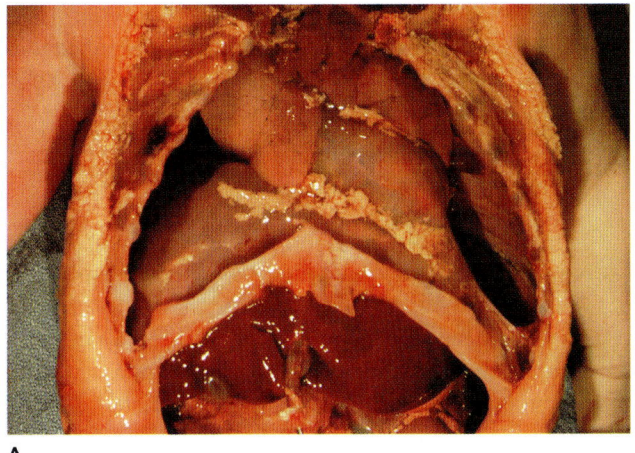

A

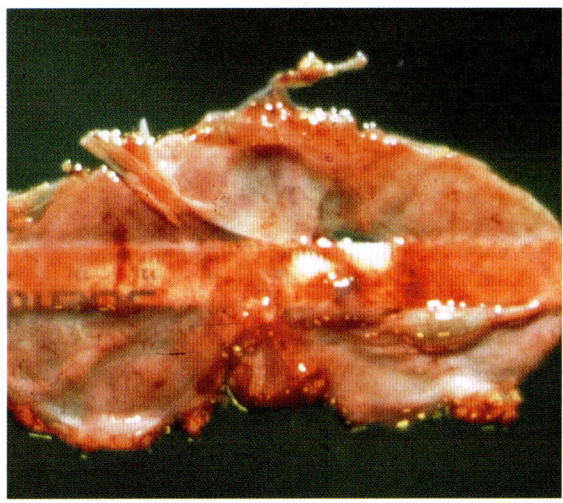

B

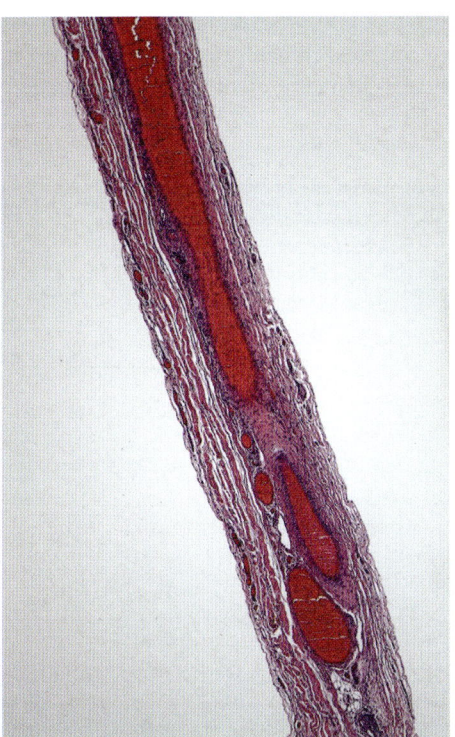

C

FIGURE 12-70 • Diaphragmatic eventration. **A:** The thorax in this newborn is markedly reduced in size by the elevation of the diaphragm and protrusion upward of the abdominal organs. **B:** At autopsy, the diaphragm consisted only of a thin and largely translucent membrane. **C:** A section of the diaphragm displays only vessels and a few strands of muscle between the thoracic and abdominal membranes (H&E, ×50).

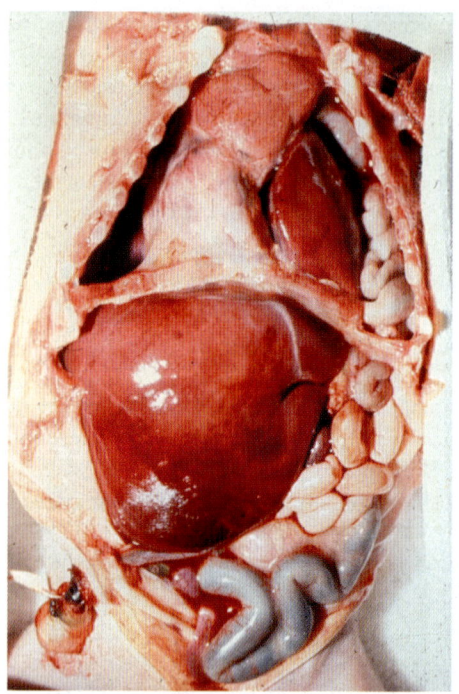 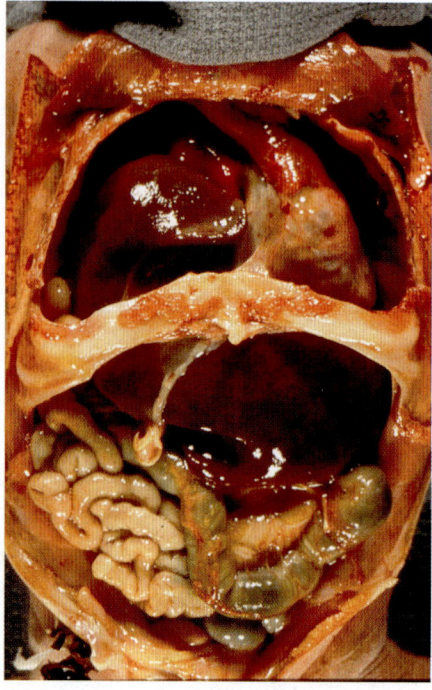

FIGURE 12-71 • Diaphragmatic hernia. **A:** A large defect in the left leaflet of the diaphragm allows herniation of the liver and portions of gastrointestinal tract into the left hemithorax. **B:** A similar defect of the right leaflet allowed the liver to herniate and shifted the mediastinum to the left side. When the liver is returned through the diaphragm to the abdomen at the time of autopsy, the profound hypoplasia of the right lung can be seen.

by additional anomalies. Those cases of complex CDH with other malformations are more likely a manifestation of a single gene disorder or chromosomal abnormality which is present in 6% to 40% of cases (382,383). Fryns syndrome is the most common autosomal recessive disorder associated with CDH and is found in 1% of all cases (394). The posterolateral aspect of the diaphragm on the left at the foramen of Bochdalek is the site of the hernia in 80% to 90% of cases (Figure 12-71) (388). A rim of skeletal muscle may or may not be present in the posterolateral location. Into this defect, stomach (rarely complicated by a volvulus), intestine, liver, and spleen are displaced into the left thoracic space. Approximately 10% of hernias are located on the right and 5% are bilateral (388). When the hernia is right sided, the defect is often partially or completely occluded by the liver, and the consequences to the right lung are considerably reduced when compared to the morbidity of the left lung. The diagnosis of CDH may be delayed when it occurs on the right side. Defects in the anterior and central portion of the diaphragm include the Morgagni hernia which is either in the retro- or parasternal region; central tendinous defect and anterior hernia are associated with the pentalogy of Cantrell with thoracoabdominal wall defect, lower sternal cleft, deficient diaphragmatic pericardium with or without ectopia cordis and cardiac anomalies (395,396). There are several sources of morbidity associated with CDH and none more important than the effects on the growth of the lung, especially the left lung (397–399). The pulmonary hypoplasia associated with CDH appears to be more consequential than that seen in other conditions with pulmonary hypoplasia (384). The growth abnormality may be more complex than simply insufficient space within the left thoracic space as suggested by some laboratory studies (400). Persistent pulmonary hypertension is another source of morbidity that generally resolves, but if not, contributes to an unfavorable clinical outcome (401–404). There has been a steady, incremental improvement in the survival of infants with CDH over the past 20 years which is approximately 70% (405). Adverse prognostic variables from the CDH Study Group are summarized in Table 12-12 (405). Pulmonary hypoplasia is life threatening when lung weights are less than 30% to 40% of expected weight. One difficulty with weight alone is the frequent secondary changes present in the lungs at autopsy.

TABLE 12-12 FACTORS ADVERSELY EFFECTING OUTCOME IN CONGENITAL DIAPHRAGMATIC HERNIA[a]

Fryns syndrome-associated CDH
Congenital cardiac defect (solitary ventricle)
Early clinical presentation (<30 days)
Large size defect with agenesis
Pulmonary hypoplasia requiring extracorporeal membrane oxygenation
Presence of other congenital anomalies, especially but not limited to EA
Prematurity with bronchopulmonary dysplasia
Persistent pulmonary hypertension

[a]From Congenital Diaphragmatic Hernia Study Group. From Harting MT, Lally KP. The congenital diaphragmatic hernia study group registry update. *Semin Fetal Neonatal Med* 2014;19:370–375.

References

1. Stocker JT. Congenital and developmental diseases. In: Dail DH, Hammer SP, eds. *Pulmonary Pathology*, 2nd ed. New York: Springer-Verlag, 1994:155–190.
2. Kimura J, Deutsch GH. Key mechanisms of early lung development. *Pediatr Dev Pathol* 2007;10(5):335–347.
3. Ornitz DM, Yin Y. Signaling networks regulating development of the lower respiratory tract. *Cold Spring Harb Perspect Biol* 2012;4(5).
4. Cardoso WV, Lu J. Regulation of early lung morphogenesis: questions, facts and controversies. *Development* 2006;133(9):1611–1624.
5. Herriges M, Morrisey EE. Lung development: orchestrating the generation and regeneration of a complex organ. *Development* 2014;141(3):502–513.
6. Correia-Pinto J, Gonzaga S, Huang Y, et al. Congenital lung lesions—underlying molecular mechanisms. *Semin Pediatr Surg* 2010;19(3):171–179.
7. Cushing L, Jiang Z, Kuang P, et al. The roles of microRNAs and protein components of the miRNA pathway in lung development and diseases. *Am J Respir Cell Mol Biol* 2015;52:397–408.
8. Wagh PK, Gardner MA, Ma X, et al. Cell and developmental stage-specific Dicer1 ablation in the lung epithelium models cystic pleuropulmonary blastoma. *J Pathol* 2015;236:41–52.
9. da Fontoura Rey Bergonse G, Carneiro AF, Vassoler TM. Choanal atresia: analysis of 16 cases–the experience of HRAC-USP from 2000 to 2004. *Rev Bras Otorrinolaringol (Engl Ed)* 2005;71(6):730–733.
10. Hsu CY, Li YW, Hsu JC. Congenital choanal atresia: computed tomographic and clinical findings. *Chung Hua Min Kuo Hsiao Erh Ko I Hsueh Hui Tsa Chih* 1999;40(1):13–17.
11. Warrington A, Vieira AR, Christensen K, et al. Genetic evidence for the role of loci at 19q13 in cleft lip and palate. *J Med Genet* 2006;43(6):e26.
12. Lorente C, Cordier S, Goujard J, et al. Tobacco and alcohol use during pregnancy and risk of oral clefts. Occupational Exposure and Congenital Malformation Working Group. *Am J Public Health* 2000;90(3):415–419.
13. Pennings RJ, van den Hoogen FJ, Marres HA. Giant laryngoceles: a cause of upper airway obstruction. *Eur Arch Otorhinolaryngol* 2001;258(3):137–140.
14. Chu L, Gussack GS, Orr JB, et al. Neonatal laryngoceles. a cause for airway obstruction. *Arch Otolaryngol Head Neck Surg* 1994;120(4):454–458.
15. Chen JL, Messner AH, Chang KW. Familial laryngomalacia in two siblings with syndromic features. *Int J Pediatr Otorhinolaryngol* 2006;70(9):1651–1655.
16. Zelenik K, Stanikova L, Smatanova K, et al. Treatment of laryngoceles: what is the progress over the last two decades? *Biomed Res Int* 2014;819:453.
17. Kay DJ, Goldsmith AJ. Laryngomalacia: a classification system and surgical treatment strategy. *Ear Nose Throat J* 2006;85(5):328–331, 336.
18. Olney DR, Greinwald JH, Jr, Smith RJ, et al. Laryngomalacia and its treatment. *Laryngoscope* 1999;109(11):1770–1775.
19. Eskander BS, Shehata BM. Fraser syndrome: a new case report with review of the literature. *Fetal Pediatr Pathol* 2008;27(2):99–104.
20. Choi SS, Zalzal GH. Changing trends in neonatal subglottic stenosis. *Otolaryngol Head Neck Surg* 2000;122(1):61–63.
21. Gatti WM, MacDonald E, Orfei E. Congenital laryngeal atresia. *Laryngoscope* 1987;97(8 Pt 1):966–969.
22. Leboulanger N, Garabedian EN. Laryngo-tracheo-oesophageal clefts. *Orphanet J Rare Dis* 2011;7:81.
23. Heimann K, Bartz C, Naami A, et al. Three new cases of congenital agenesis of the trachea. *Eur J Pediatr* 2007;166(1):79–82.
24. Evans JA, Greenberg CR, Erdile L. Tracheal agenesis revisited: analysis of associated anomalies. *Am J Med Genet* 1999;82(5):415–422.
25. Stocker JT. Sequestrations of the lung. *Semin Diagn Pathol* 1986;3(2):106–121.
26. Doolittle AM, Mair EA. Tracheal bronchus: classification, endoscopic analysis, and airway management. *Otolaryngol Head Neck Surg* 2002;126(3):240–243.
27. Tsugawa J, Satoh S, Nishijima E, et al. Development of acquired tracheal stenosis in premature infants due to prolonged endotracheal ventilation: etiological considerations and surgical management. *Pediatr Surg Int* 2006;22(11):887–890.
28. Faust RA, Stroh B, Rimell F. The near complete tracheal ring deformity. *Int J Pediatr Otorhinolaryngol* 1998;45(2):171–176.
29. Cordovilla Zurdo G, Cabo Salvador J, Sanz Galeote E, et al. Congenital heart defects with tracheal and bronchial stenoses: surgical treatment with extracorporeal circulation. *An Esp Pediatr* 1999;51(2):149–153.
30. Berrocal T, Madrid C, Novo S, et al. Congenital anomalies of the tracheobronchial tree, lung, and mediastinum: embryology, radiology, and pathology. *Radiographics* 2004;24(1):e17.
31. Dutta HK, Mathur M, Bhatnagar V. A histopathological study of esophageal atresia and tracheoesophageal fistula. *J Pediatr Surg* 2000;35(3):438–441.
32. Sane AC, Effmann EL, Brown SD. Tracheobronchiomegaly. The Mounier-Kuhn syndrome in a patient with the Kenny-Caffey syndrome. *Chest* 1992;102(2):618–619.
33. Shaw-Smith C. Oesophageal atresia, tracheo-oesophageal fistula, and the VACTERL association: review of genetics and epidemiology. *J Med Genet* 2006;43(7):545–554.
34. Pinheiro Paulo, Silva Ana, Pereira Regina. Current knowledge on esophageal atresia. *World J Gastroenterol* 2012;18(28):3662–3672.
35. La Placa S, Giuffre M, Gangemi A, et al. Esophageal atresia in newborns: a wide spectrum from the isolated forms to a full VACTERL phenotype? *Ital J Pediatr* 2013;39:45.
36. Landing BH. Five syndromes (malformation complexes) of pulmonary symmetry, congenital heart disease, and multiple spleens. *Pediatr Pathol* 1984;2(2):148–151.
37. Birman C, Beckenham E. Acquired tracheo-esophageal fistula in the pediatric population. *Int J Pediatr Otorhinolaryngol* 1998;44(2):109–113.
38. Kunisaki SM, Fauza DO, Nemes LP, et al. Bronchial atresia: the hidden pathology within a spectrum of prenatally diagnosed lung masses. *J Pediatr Surg* 2006;41(1):61–65.
39. Pillai JB, Smith J, Hasan A, et al. Review of pediatric airway malacia and its management, with emphasis on stenting. *Eur J Cardiothorac Surg* 2005;27(1):35–44.
40. Rintala RJ, Pakarinen MP. Long-term outcome of esophageal anastomosis. *Eur J Pediatr Surg* 2013;23(3):219–225.
41. Schneider A, Michaud L, Gottrand F. Esophageal atresia: metaplasia, *Barrett Dis Esophagus* 2013;26(4):425–427.
42. Landing B, Wells T. Tracheobronchial anomalies in children. *Perspect Pediatr Pathol* 1973;1:1–32.
43. Riedlinger WF, Vargas SO, Jennings RW, et al. Bronchial atresia is common to extralobar sequestration, intralobar sequestration, congenital cystic adenomatoid malformation, and lobar emphysema. *Pediatr Dev Pathol* 2006;9(5):361–373.
44. Bertrand P, Navarro H, Caussade S, et al. Airway anomalies in children with Down syndrome: endoscopic findings. *Pediatr Pulmonol* 2003;36(2):137–141.
45. Atwell SW. Major anomalies of the tracheobronchial tree: with a list of the minor anomalies. *Dis Chest* 1967;52(5):611–615.
46. Stokes JR, Heatley DG, Lusk RP, et al. The bridging bronchus. Successful diagnosis and repair. *Arch Otolaryngol Head Neck Surg* 1997;123(12):1344–1347.
47. McLaughlin FJ, Strieder DJ, Harris GB, et al. Tracheal bronchus: association with respiratory morbidity in childhood. *J Pediatr* 1985;106(5):751–755.
48. Wells TR, Takahashi M, Landing BH, et al. Branching patterns of right pulmonary artery in cardiovascular anomalies. *Pediatr Pathol* 1993;13(2):213–223.
49. Wang CR, Tiu CM, Chou YH, et al. Congenital bronchoesophageal fistula in childhood. Case report and review of the literature. *Pediatr Radiol* 1993;23(2):158–159.
50. Sauvat F, Fusaro F, Jaubert F, et al. Paraesophageal bronchogenic cyst: first case reports in pediatric. *Pediatr Surg Int* 2006;22(10):849–851.

51. Mehta RP, Faquin WC, Cunningham MJ. Cervical bronchogenic cysts: a consideration in the differential diagnosis of pediatric cervical cystic masses. *Int J Pediatr Otorhinolaryngol* 2004;68(5):563–568.
52. Tireli GA, Ozbey H, Temiz A, et al. Bronchogenic cysts: a rare congenital cystic malformation of the lung. *Surg Today* 2004;34(7):573–576.
53. Zvulunov A, Amichai B, Grunwald MH, et al. Cutaneous bronchogenic cyst: delineation of a poorly recognized lesion. *Pediatr Dermatol* 1998;15(4):277–281.
54. Stocker JT, Kagan-Hallet K. Extralobar pulmonary sequestration: analysis of 15 cases. *Am J Clin Pathol* 1979;72(6):917–925.
55. Tanase D, Ewert P, Eicken A. Plastic bronchitis: symptomatic improvement after pulmonary arterial stenting in four patients with Fontan circulation. *Cardiol Young* 2013;25:1–3.
56. Brogan TV, Finn LS, Pyskaty DJ, Jr, et al. Plastic bronchitis in children: a case series and review of the medical literature. *Pediatr Pulmonol* 2002;34(6):482–487.
57. Rubin BK, Priftis KN, Schmidt HJ, et al. Secretory hyperresponsiveness and pulmonary mucus hypersecretion. *Chest* 2014;146(2):496–507.
58. Hasegawa T, Oshima Y, Maruo A, et al. Pediatric cardiothoracic surgery in patients with unilateral pulmonary agenesis or aplasia. *Ann Thorac Surg* 2014;97(5):1652–1658.
59. Osborne J, Masel J, McCredie J. A spectrum of skeletal anomalies associated with pulmonary agenesis: possible neural crest injuries. *Pediatr Radiol* 1989;19(6–7):425–432.
60. Hastings R, Harding D, Donaldson A, et al. Mardini-Nyhan association (lung agenesis, congenital heart, and thumb anomalies): three new cases and possible recurrence in a sib-is there a distinct recessive syndrome? *Am J Med Genet A* 2009;149A(12):2838–2842.
61. Knowles S, Thomas RM, Lindenbaum RH, et al. Pulmonary agenesis as part of the VACTERL sequence. *Arch Dis Child* 1988;63(7 Spec No):723–726.
62. Boucherat O, Nadeau V, Berube-Simard FA, et al. Crucial requirement of ERK/MAPK signaling in respiratory tract development. *Development* 2014;141(16):3197–3211
63. Lin JH, Chen SJ, Wu MH, et al. Right lung agenesis with left pulmonary artery sling. *Pediatr Pulmonol* 2000;29(3):239–241.
64. Stocker JT. Pathologic features of long-standing "healed" bronchopulmonary dysplasia: a study of 28 3- to 40-month-old infants. *Hum Pathol* 1986;17(9):943–961.
65. Kim JB, Park JJ, Ko JK, et al. A case of PAGOD syndrome with hypoplastic left heart syndrome. *Int J Cardiol* 2007;114(2):270–271.
66. Mani H, Suarez E, Stocker JT. The morphologic spectrum of infantile lobar emphysema: a study of 33 cases. *Paediatr Respir Rev* 2004;5(Suppl A): S313–S320.
67. Conran RM, Stocker JT. Extralobar sequestration with frequently associated congenital cystic adenomatoid malformation, type 2: report of 50 cases. *Pediatr Dev Pathol* 1999;2(5):454–463.
68. Kamata S, Sawai T, Nose K, et al. Extralobar pulmonary sequestration with venous drainage to the portal vein: a case report. *Pediatr Radiol* 2000;30(7):492–494.
69. Scurry JP, Adamson TM, Cussen LJ. Fetal lung growth in laryngeal atresia and tracheal agenesis. *Aust Paediatr J* 1989;25(1):47–51.
70. Stocker JT, Malczak HT. A study of pulmonary ligament arteries. Relationship to intralobar pulmonary sequestration. *Chest* 1984;86(4):611–615.
71. Walford N, Htun K, Chen J, et al. Intralobar sequestration of the lung is a congenital anomaly: anatomopathological analysis of four cases diagnosed in fetal life. *Pediatr Dev Pathol* 2003;6(4):314–321.
72. Stocker JT, Dehner LP. Acquired neonatal and pediatric diseases. In: Dail DH, Hammer SP, eds. *Pulmonary Pathology*, 2nd ed. New York: Springer-Verlag, 1994:191–254.
73. Shanmugam G, MacArthur K, et al. Congenital lung malformations–antenatal and postnatal evaluation and management. *Eur J Cardiothorac Surg* 2005;27(1):45–52
74. Frazier AA, Rosado de Christenson ML, Stocker JT, et al. Intralobar sequestration: radiologic-pathologic correlation. *Radiographics* 1997;17(3):725–745.
75. Komatsu H, Mizuguchi S, Izumi N, et al. Pulmonary sequestration presenting elevated CA19-9 and CA125 with ovarian cysts. *Ann Thorac Cardiovasc Surg* 2014;20:686–688.
76. Wei Y, Li F. Pulmonary sequestration: a retrospective analysis of 2625 cases in China. *Eur J Cardiothorac Surg* 2011;40(1):e39–e42.
77. De Paepe ME, Friedman RM, Gundogan F, et al. Postmortem lung weight/body weight standards for term and preterm infants. *Pediatr Pulmonol.* 2005;40(5):445–448
78. Emery JL, Mithal A. The number of alveoli in the terminal respiratory unit of man during late intrauterine life and childhood. *Arch Dis Child* 1960;35:544–549.
79. Askenazi SS, Perlman M. Pulmonary hypoplasia: lung weight and radial alveolar count as criteria of diagnosis. *Arch Dis Child* 1979;54(8):614–618.
80. Husain AN, Hessel RG. Neonatal pulmonary hypoplasia: an autopsy study of 25 cases. *Pediatr Pathol.* 1993;13(4):475–484.
81. Page DV, Stocker JT. Anomalies associated with pulmonary hypoplasia. *Am Rev Respir Dis* 1982;125(2):216–221.
82. Weaver KN, Johnson J, Kline-Fath B, et al. Predictive value of fetal lung volume in prenatally diagnosed skeletal dysplasia. *Prenat Diagn* 2014;34(13):1326–1331.
83. McDowell KM, Craven DI. Pulmonary complications of Down syndrome during childhood. *J Pediatr* 2011;158(2):319–325.
84. Krivchenya DU, Rudenko EO, Dubrovin AG. Congenital emphysema in children: segmental lung resection as an alternative to lobectomy. *J Pediatr Surg.* 2013;48(2):309–314. doi: 10.1016/j.jpedsurg.2012.11.009.
85. Karnak I, Senocak ME, Ciftci AO, et al. Congenital lobar emphysema: diagnostic and therapeutic considerations. *J Pediatr Surg* 1999;34(9):1347–1351.
86. Ozcelik U, Gocmen A, Kiper N, et al. Congenital lobar emphysema: evaluation and long-term follow-up of thirty cases at a single center. *Pediatr Pulmonol* 2003;35(5):384–391.
87. Miller KE, Edwards DK, Hilton S, et al. Acquired lobar emphysema in premature infants with bronchopulmonary dysplasia: an iatrogenic disease? *Radiology* 1981;138(3):589–592.
88. Giudici R, Leao LE, Moura LA, et al. Polyalveolosis: pathogenesis of congenital lobar emphysema?. *Rev Assoc Med Bras* 1998;44(2):99–105.
89. Cleveland RH, Weber B. Retained fetal lung liquid in congenital lobar emphysema: a possible predictor of polyalveolar lobe. *Pediatr Radiol* 1993;23(4):291–295.
90. Bellini C, Boccardo F, Campisi C, et al. Congenital pulmonary lymphangiectasia. *Orphanet J Rare Dis* 2006;1:43.
91. Nobre LF, Muller NL, de Souza Junior AS, et al. Congenital pulmonary lymphangiectasia: CT and pathologic findings. *J Thorac Imaging* 2004;19(1):56–59.
92. Dempsey EM, Sant'Anna GM, Williams RL, et al. Congenital pulmonary lymphangiectasia presenting as nonimmune fetal hydrops and severe respiratory distress at birth: not uniformly fatal. *Pediatr Pulmonol* 2005;40(3):270–274.
93. Rettwitz-Volk W, Schlosser R, Ahrens P, et al. Congenital unilobar pulmonary lymphangiectasis. *Pediatr Pulmonol* 1999;27(4):290–292.
94. Stocker JT. Congenital pulmonary airway malformation—a new name for and an expanded classification of congenital cystic adenomatoid malformation of the lung. *Histopathology* 2002;41(suppl. 2):424–430
95. Rutledge JC, Jensen P. Acinar dysplasia: a new form of pulmonary maldevelopment. *Hum Pathol* 1986;17(12):1290–1293.
96. Mani H, Shilo K, Galvin JR, et al. Spectrum of precursor and invasive neoplastic lesions in type 1 congenital pulmonary airway malformation: case report and review of the literature. *Histopathology* 2007;51(4):561–565.
97. Priest JR, Williams GM, Hill DA, et al. Pulmonary cysts in early childhood and the risk of malignancy. *Pediatr Pulmonol* 2009;44(1):14–30.
98. Ch'in KY, Tang MY. Congenital adenomatoid malformation of one lobe of a lung with general anasarca. *Arch Pathol* 1949;48:221–225.
99. Azizkhan RG, Crombleholme TM. Congenital cystic lung disease: contemporary antenatal and postnatal management. *Pediatr Surg Int* 2008;24(6):643–657.

100. Fine C, Adzick NS, Doubilet PM. Decreasing size of a congenital cystic adenomatoid malformation in utero. *J Ultrasound Med* 1988; 7(7):405–408.
101. Stocker JT, Madewell JE, Drake RM. Congenital cystic adenomatoid malformation of the lung. Classification and morphologic spectrum. *Hum Pathol* 1977;8(2):155–171.
102. Janney CG, Askin FB, Kuhn C, III. Congenital alveolar capillary dysplasia—an unusual cause of respiratory distress in the newborn. *Am J Clin Pathol* 1981;76(5):722–727.
103. Langenstroer M, Carlan SJ, Fanaian N, et al. Congenital acinar dysplasia: report of a case and review of the literature. *AJP Rep* 2013;3(1):9–12.
104. Sen P, Yang Y, Navarro C, et al. Novel FOXF1 mutations in sporadic and familial cases of alveolar capillary dysplasia with misaligned pulmonary veins imply a role for its DNA binding domain. *Hum Mutat* 2013;34(6):801–811.
105. Pucci A, Zanini C, Ferrero F, et al. Misalignment of lung vessels: diagnostic role of conventional histology and immunohistochemistry. *Virchows Arch* 2003;442(6):597–600.
106. Melly L, Sebire NJ, Malone M, et al. Capillary apposition and density in the diagnosis of alveolar capillary dysplasia. *Histopathology* 2008;53(4):450–457.
107. Langston C. Misalignment of pulmonary veins and alveolar capillary dysplasia. *Pediatr Pathol* 1991;11:163–170.
108. Sen P, Thakur N, Stockton DW, et al. Expanding the phenotype of alveolar capillary dysplasia (ACD). *J Pediatr* 2004;145(5):646–651.
109. Stocker JT, McGill LC, Orsini EN. Post-infarction peripheral cysts of the lung in pediatric patients: a possible cause of idiopathic spontaneous pneumothorax. *Pediatr Pulmonol* 1985;1(1):7–18.
110. Gonzalez OR, Gomez IG, Recalde AL, et al. Postnatal development of the cystic lung lesion of Down syndrome: suggestion that the cause is reduced formation of peripheral air spaces. *Pediatr Pathol* 1991; 11(4):623–633.
111. Edwards MO, Kotecha SJ, Kotecha S. Respiratory distress of the term newborn infant. *Paediatr Respir Rev* 2013;14(1):29–36.
112. Toti P, Buonocore G, Rinaldi G, et al. Pulmonary pathology in surfactant-treated preterm infants with respiratory distress syndrome: an autopsy study. *Biol Neonate* 1996;70(1):21–28.
113. Gonda TA, Hutchins GM. Surfactant treatment may accelerate epithelial cell regeneration in hyaline membrane disease of the newborn. *Am J Perinatol* 1998;15(9):539–544.
114. Smith LS, Zimmerman JJ, Martin TR. Mechanisms of acute respiratory distress syndrome in children and adults: a review and suggestions for future research. *Pediatr Crit Care Med* 2013;14(6):631–643.
115. Lopez-Fernandez Y, Azalra AM, de la Olivia P, et al. Pediatric acute lung injury epidemiology and natural history (PED-ALIEN) network. Pediatric acute lung injury epidemiology and natural history study: Incidence and outcome of the acute respiratory distress syndrome in children. *Crit Care Med* 2012;40(12):3238–3245.
116. Willson DF, Thomas NJ, Tamburro R, et al. Pediatric acute lung and sepsis investigators network. Pediatric calfactant in acute respiratory distress syndrome trial. *Pediatr Crit Care Med* 2013;14(7):657–665.
117. Northway WH, Jr., Rosan RC, Porter DY. Pulmonary disease following respirator therapy of hyaline-membrane disease. bronchopulmonary dysplasia. *N Engl J Med* 1967;276(7):357–368.
118. Bonikos DS, Bensch KG, Northway WH, Jr, et al. Bronchopulmonary dysplasia: the pulmonary pathologic sequel of necrotizing bronchiolitis and pulmonary fibrosis. *Hum Pathol* 1976;7(6):643–666.
119. Bonikos D, Bensch K, Northway WJ. Oxygen toxicity in the newborn. The effect of chronic continuous 100 percent oxygen exposure on the lungs of newborn mice. *Am J Pathol* 1976;85:623–650.
120. Bancalari E, Claure N, Sosenko IR. Bronchopulmonary dysplasia: changes in pathogenesis, epidemiology and definition. *Semin Neonatol* 2003;8(1):63–71.
121. Sobonya RE, Logvinoff MM, Taussig LM, et al. Morphometric analysis of the lung in prolonged bronchopulmonary dysplasia. *Pediatr Res* 1982;16(11):969–972.
122. Margraf LR, Tomashefski JF, Jr, Bruce MC, et al. Morphometric analysis of the lung in bronchopulmonary dysplasia. *Am Rev Respir Dis* 1991; 143(2):391–400.
123. Husain AN, Siddiqui NH, Stocker JT. Pathology of arrested acinar development in postsurfactant bronchopulmonary dysplasia. *Hum Pathol* 1998;29(7):710–717.
124. Walsh MC, Yao Q, Horbar JD, et al. Changes in the use of postnatal steroids for bronchopulmonary dysplasia in 3 large neonatal networks. *Pediatrics* 2006;118(5):e1328–e1335.
125. Nogee LM. Genetic basis of children's interstitial lung disease. *Pediatr Allergy Immunol Pulmonol* 2010;23(1):15–24.
126. Stuhrmann M, Bohnhorst B, Peters U, et al. Prenatal diagnosis of congenital alveolar proteinosis (surfactant protein B deficiency). *Prenat Diagn* 1998;18(9):953–955.
127. Bullard JE, Nogee LM. Heterozygosity for ABCA mutations modifies the severity of lung disease associated with a surfactant protein C gene (SFTPC) mutation. *Pediatr Res* 2007;62(2):176–179.
128. Suzuki T, Maranda B, Sakagami T, et al. Hereditary pulmonary alveolar proteinosis caused by recessive CSF2RB mutations. *Eur Respir J* 2011;37(1):201–204.
129. Bruder E, Hofmeister J, Aslanidis C, et al. Ultrastructural and molecular analysis in fatal neonatal interstitial pneumonia caused by a novel ABCA3 mutation. *Mod Pathol* 2007;20(10):1009–1018.
130. McAdams RM. Risk factors and clinical outcomes of pulmonary interstitial emphysema in extremely low birth weight infants. *J Perinatol* 2006;26(8):521–522; author reply 522–523.
131. Stocker JT, Madewell JE. Persistent interstitial pulmonary emphysema: another complication of the respiratory distress syndrome. *Pediatrics* 1977;59(6):847–857.
132. Chalak LF, Kaiser JR, Arrington RW. Resolution of pulmonary interstitial emphysema following selective left main stem intubation in a premature newborn: an old procedure revisited. *Paediatr Anaesth* 2007; 17(2):183–186.
133. Wiswell TE, Tuggle JM, Turner BS. Meconium aspiration syndrome: have we made a difference? *Pediatrics* 1990;85(5):715–721.
134. Salvesen B, Fung M, Saugstad OD, et al. role of complement and CD14 in meconium-induced cytokine formation. *Pediatrics* 2008;131(3):e496–e505.
135. Baharloo F, Veyckemans F, Francis C, et al. Tracheobronchial foreign bodies: presentation and management in children and adults. *Chest* 1999;115(5):1357–1362.
136. Chou P, Blei ED, Shen-Schwarz S, et al. Pulmonary changes following extracorporeal membrane oxygenation: autopsy study of 23 cases. *Hum Pathol* 1993;24(4):405–412.
137. Hamutcu R, Nield TA, Garg M, et al. Long-term pulmonary sequelae in children who were treated with extracorporeal membrane oxygenation for neonatal respiratory failure. *Pediatrics* 2004;114(5):1292–1296.
138. Blanco C, Steigman C, Probst N, et al. Discrepancies between autopsy and clinical findings among patients requiring extracorporeal membrane oxygenator support. *ASAIO J* 2014;60(2):207–210.
139. Patria MF, Esposito S. Recurrent lower respiratory tract infections in children: a practical approach to diagnosis. *Paediatr Respir Rev* 2013; 14(1):53–60.
140. Redding GJ, Byrnes CA. Chronic respiratory symptoms and diseases among indigenous children. *Pediatr Clin North Am* 2009;56(6): 1323–1342.
141. Kim JB. Channelopathies. *Korean J Pediatr* 2014;57(1):1–18.
142. Kreda SM, Davis CW, Rose MC. CFTR, mucins, and mucus obstruction in cystic fibrosis. *Cold Spring Harb Perspect Med* 2012;2(9):a009589.
143. Ehre C, Ridley C, Thornton DJ. Cystic fibrosis: an inherited disease affecting mucin-producing organs. *Int J Biochem Cell Biol* 2014; 52:136–145.
144. Cant N, Pollock N, Ford RC. CFTR structure and cystic fibrosis. *Int J Biochem Cell Biol* 2014;52:15–25.
145. Rowe SM, Verkman AS. Cystic fibrosis transmembrane regulator correctors and potentiators. *Cold Spring Harb Perspect Med* 2013; 3(7):a009761.

146. Stick SM, Brennan S, Murray C, et al. Bronchiectasis in infants and preschool children diagnosed with cystic fibrosis after newborn screening. *J Pediatr* 2009;155(5):623–628.
147. Kosorok MR, Zeng L, West SE, et al. Acceleration of lung disease in children with cystic fibrosis after *Pseudomonas aeruginosa* acquisition. *Pediatr Pulmonol* 2001;32(4):277–287.
148. West SE, Zeng L, Lee BL, et al. Respiratory infections with Pseudomonas aeruginosa in children with cystic fibrosis: early detection by serology and assessment of risk factors. *JAMA* 2002;287(22):2958–2967.
149. Farrell PM, Collins J, Broderick LS, et al. Association between mucoid Pseudomonas infection and bronchiectasis in children with cystic fibrosis. *Radiology* 2009;252(2):534–543.
150. Pattison SH, Rogers GB, Crockard M, et al. Molecular detection of CF lung pathogens: current status and future potential. *J Cyst Fibros* 2013;12(3):194–205.
151. Gifford AM, Chalmers JD. The role of neutrophils in cystic fibrosis. *Curr Opin Hematol* 2014;21(1):16–22.
152. Dhooghe B, Noel S, Huaux F, et al. Lung inflammation in cystic fibrosis: pathogenesis and novel therapies. *Clin Biochem* 2014;47(7–8):539–546.
153. de Almeida MB, Bussamra MH, Rodrigues JC. Allergic bronchopulmonary aspergillosis in paediatric cystic fibrosis patients. *Paediatr Respir Rev* 2006;7(1):67–72.
154. Southern KW. Cystic fibrosis and forms frustes of CFTR-related disease. *Respiration* 2007;74(3):241–251.
155. Fall A, Spencer D. Paediatric bronchiectasis in Europe: what now and where next? *Paediatr Respir Rev* 2006;7(4):268–274.
156. Dagli E. Non cystic fibrosis bronchiectasis. *Paediatr Respir Rev* 2000;1(1):64–70.
157. Noriega Aldave AP, William Saliski D. The clinical manifestations, diagnosis and management of Williams-Campbell Syndrome. *N Am J Med Sci* 2014;6(9):429–432.
158. Stafler P, Carr SB. Non-cystic fibrosis bronchiectasis: its diagnosis and management. *Arch Dis Child Educ Pract Ed* 2010;95(3):73–82.
159. Kapur N, Mackay IM, Sloots TP, et al. Respiratory viruses in exacerbations of non-cystic fibrosis bronchiectasis in children. *Arch Dis Child* 2014;99(8):749–753.
160. Ogershok PR, Hogan MB, Welch JE, et al. Spectrum of illness in pediatric common variable immunodeficiency. *Ann Allergy Asthma Immunol* 2006;97(5):653–656.
161. Hoving MF, Brand PL. Causes of recurrent pneumonia in children in a general hospital. *J Paediatr Child Health* 2013;49(3):E208–E212.
162. Jesenak M, Banovcin P, Jesenakova B, et al. Pulmonary manifestations of primary immunodeficiency disorders in children. *Front Pediatr* 2014;2:77.
163. Busquets RM, Caballero-Rabasco MA, Velasco M. Primary ciliary dyskinesia: clinical criteria indicating ultrastructural studies. *Arch Bronconeumol* 2013;49(3):99–104.
164. Ferkol TW, Leigh MW. Ciliopathies: the central role of cilia in a spectrum of pediatric disorders. *J Pediatr* 2012;160(3):366–371.
165. Leigh MW, Pittman JE, Carson JL, et al. Clinical and genetic aspects of primary ciliary dyskinesia/Kartagener syndrome. *Genet Med* 2009;11(7):473–487.
166. Pifferi M, Di Cicco M, Piras M, et al. Up to date on primary ciliary dyskinesia in children. *Early Hum Dev* 2013;89(Suppl 3):S45–S48.
167. George J, Jain R, Tariq SM. CT bronchoscopy in the diagnosis of Williams-Campbell syndrome. *Respirology* 2006;11(1):117–119.
168. Chan PC, Huang LM, Wu PS, et al. Clinical management and outcome of childhood lung abscess: a 16-year experience. *J Microbiol Immunol Infect* 2005;38(3):183–188.
169. Patradoon-Ho P, Fitzgerald DA. Lung abscess in children. *Paediatr Respir Rev* 2007;8(1):77–84.
170. Godfrey S. Pulmonary hemorrhage/hemoptysis in children. *Pediatr Pulmonol* 2004;37(6):476–484.
171. Coffin CM, Schechtman K, Cole FS, et al. Neonatal and infantile pulmonary hemorrhage: an autopsy study with clinical correlation. *Pediatr Pathol* 1993;13(5):583–589.
172. Ameur SB, Niaudet P, Baudouin V, et al. Lung manifestations in MPO-ANCA associated vasculities in children. *Pediatr Pulmonol* 2014;49(3):285–290.
173. Fullmer JJ, Langston C, Dishop MK, et al. Pulmonary capillaritis in children: a review of eight cases with comparison to other alveolar hemorrhage syndromes. *J Pediatr* 2005;146(3):376–381.
174. Bansal PJ, Tobin MD. Neonatal microscopic polyangiitis secondary to transfer of maternal myeloperoxidase-antineutrophil cytoplasmic antibody resulting in neonatal pulmonary hemorrhage and renal involvement. *Ann Allergy Asthma Immunol* 2004;93(4):398–401.
175. Morton RL, Moore C, Coventry S, et al. Pulmonary capillaritis and hemorrhage in neonatal lupus erythematosus (NLE). *J Clin Rheumatol* 2004;10(3):130–133.
176. Rajagopala S, Shobha V, Devaraj U, et al. Pulmonary Hemorrhage in Henoch-Schonlein purpura: a case report and systematic review of the English literature. *Semin Arthritis Rheum* 2013;42(4):391–400.
177. Bogdanovic R, Minic P, Markovic-Lipkovski J, et al. Pulmonary renal syndrome in a child with coexistence of anti-neutrophil cytoplasmic antibodies and anti-glomerular basement membrane disease: case report and literature review. *BMC Nephrol* 2013;14:66.
178. Testa ME, Maffey A, Colom A, et al. Pulmonary hemorrhage associated with celiac disease. *Arch Argent Pediatr* 2012;110(4):e72–e76.
179. Frazier AA, Franks TJ, Mohammed TL, et al. From the Archives of the AFIP: pulmonary veno-occlusive disease and pulmonary capillary hemangiomatosis. *Radiographics* 2007;27(3):867–882.
180. Wang T, Lazar CA, Fisbein MC, et al. Pulmonary alveolar proteinosis. *Semin Respir Crit Care Med* 2012;33(5):498–508.
181. Ben-Dov I, Segel MJ. Autoimmune pulmonary alveolar proteinosis: clinical course and diagnostic criteria. *Autoimmun Rev* 2014;13(4–5):513–517.
182. Carey B, Trapnell BC. The molecular basis of pulmonary alveolar proteinosis. *Clin Immunol* 2010;135(2):223–235.
183. Al-Alawi AS. Familial occurrence of pulmonary alveolar microlithiasis in 3 siblings. *Saudi Med J* 2006;27(2):238–240.
184. Marchiori E, Goncalves CM, Escuissato DL, et al. Pulmonary alveolar microlithiasis: high-resolution computed tomography findings in 10 patients. *J Bras Pneumol* 2007;33(5):552–557.
185. Kiper N, Gocmen A, Ozcelik U, et al. Long-term clinical course of patients with idiopathic pulmonary hemosiderosis (1979–1994): prolonged survival with low-dose corticosteroid therapy. *Pediatr Pulmonol* 1999;27(3):180–184.
186. Salih ZN, Akhter A, Akhter J. Specificity and sensitivity of hemosiderin-laden macrophages in routine bronchoalveolar lavage in children. *Arch Pathol Lab Med* 2006;130(11):1684–1686.
187. Cohen S. Idiopathic pulmonary hemosiderosis. *Am J Med Sci* 1999;317(1):67–74.
188. Saeed MM, Woo MS, MacLaughlin EF, et al. Prognosis in pediatric idiopathic pulmonary hemosiderosis. *Chest* 1999;116(3):721–725.
189. Milman N, Pedersen FM. Idiopathic pulmonary haemosiderosis. Epidemiology, pathogenic aspects and diagnosis. *Respir Med* 1998;92(7):902–907.
190. Corrin B, Jagusch M, Dewar A, et al. Fine structural changes in idiopathic pulmonary haemosiderosis. *J Pathol* 1987;153(3):249–256.
191. Cutz E. Idiopathic pulmonary hemosiderosis and related disorders in infancy and childhood. *Perspect Pediatr Pathol* 1987;11:47–81.
192. Stocker JT, Conran RM, Fishback N. Respiratory syncytial virus. In: Conner DH, Chandler FW, eds. *Pathology of Infectious Diseases*, vol 1. Stanford, CT: Appleton & Lange, 1997:287–295.
193. von Renesse A, Schildgen O, Klinkenberg D, et al. Respiratory syncytial virus infection in children admitted to hospital but ventilated mechanically for other reasons. *J Med Virol* 2009;81(1):160–166.
194. Thorburn K. Pre-existing disease is associated with a significantly higher risk of death in severe respiratory syncytial virus infection. *Arch Dis Child* 2009;94(2):99–103.
195. Zhang SX, Tellier R, Zafar R, et al. Comparison of human metapneumovirus infection with respiratory syncytial virus infection in children. *Pediatr Infect Dis J* 2009;28(11):1022–1024.

196. Vargas SO, Kozakewich HP, Perez-Atayde AR, et al. Pathology of human metapneumovirus infection: insights into the pathogenesis of a newly identified respiratory virus. *Pediatr Dev Pathol* 2004;7(5):478–486.
197. Renois F, Bouin A, Andreoletti L. Enterovirus 68 in pediatric patients hospitalized for acute airway diseases. *J Clin Microbiol* 2013;51(2):640–643.
198. Debiaggi M, Canducci F, Ceresola ER, et al. The role of infections and coinfections with newly identified and emerging respiratory viruses in children. *Virol J* 2012;9:247.
199. Brodzinski H, Ruddy RM. Review of new and newly discovered respiratory tract viruses in children. *Pediatr Emerg Care* 2009;25(5):352–360.
200. Stephenson J. CDC tracking enterovirus D-68 outbreak causing severe respiratory illness in children in the Midwest. *JAMA* 2014;312(13):1290.
201. Cherry JD, Nauifuram S. Adenoviruses. In: Cherry J, Dennler-Harrison GJ, Kaplan SL, et al. eds. *Feigin and Cherry Textbook of Pediatric Infectious Diseases*, 7th ed. Philadelphia, PA: WB Saunders 2014,1888–1911.
202. Gautret P, Gray GC, Charrel RN, et al. Emerging viral respiratory tract infections-environmental risk factors and transmission. *Lancet Infect Dis* 2014;14:1113–1122.
203. Murtagh P, Kajon A. Chronic pulmonary sequelae of adenovirus infection. *Pediatr Pulmonol Suppl* 1997;16:150–151.
204. Chandran L, Boykan R. Chlamydial infections in children and adolescents. *Pediatr Rev* 2009;30(7):243–250.
205. Theofiles AG, Cunningham SA, Chia N, et al. Pertussis outbreak, southeastern Minnesota, 2012. *Mayo Clin Proc* 2014;89(10):1378–1388.
206. Wood N, McIntyre P. Pertussis: review of epidemiology, diagnosis, management and prevention. *Paediatr Respir Rev* 2008;9(3):201–211.
207. Jeong YJ, Kim KI, Seo IJ, et al. Eosinophilic lung diseases: a clinical, radiologic and pathologic overview. *Radiographics* 2007;27(3):617–637.
208. Churg A, Muller NL. *ATLAS of Interstitial Lung Disease Pathology*. Philadelphia, PA: Lippincott Williams & Wilkins, 2014;127–137.
209. Cazzato S, di Palmo E, Ragazzo V, et al. Interstitial lung disease in children. *Early Hum Dev* 2013;89(Suppl 3):539–543.
210. Kurland G, Deterding RR, Hagood JS, et al. An official American Thoracic Society clinical practice guideline: classification, evaluation, and management of childhood interstitial lung disease in infancy. *Am J Respir Crit Care Med* 2013;188(3):376–394.
211. Dishop MK. Diagnostic pathology of diffuse lung disease in children. *Pediatr Allergy Immunol Pulmonol* 2010;23(1):69–85.
212. Young LR, Brody AS, Inge TH, et al. Neuroendocrine cell distribution and frequency distinguish neuroendocrine cell hyperplasia of infancy from other pulmonary disorders. *Chest* 2011;139(5):1060–1071.
213. Deterding RR, Pye C, Fan LL, et al. Persistent tachypnea of infancy is associated with neuroendocrine cell hyperplasia. *Pediatr Pulmonol* 2005;40(2):157–165.
214. Canakis AM, Cutz E, Manson D, et al. Pulmonary interstitial glycogenosis: a new variant of neonatal interstitial lung disease. *Am J Respir Crit Care Med* 2002;165(11):1557–1565.
215. Deutsch GH, Young LR. Histologic resolution of pulmonary interstitial glycogenosis. *Pediatr Dev Pathol* 2009;12(6):475–480.
216. Deterding RR. Infants and young children with children's interstitial lung disease. *Pediatr Allergy Immunol Pulmonol* 2010;23(1):25–31.
217. Moonnumakal S, Fan LL. Bronchiolitis obliterans in children. *Curr Opin Pediatr* 2008;20:272–278.
218. Li YN, Liu L, Qiao HM, et al. Post-infectious bronchiolitis obliterans in children: a review of 42 cases. *BMC Pediatr* 2014;14:238.
219. Kapila A, Baz MA, Valentine VG, et al. Reliability of diagnostic criteria for bronchiolitis obliterans syndrome after lung transplantation: a survey. *J Heart Lung Transplant* 2015;34(1):65–74.
220. Barker AF, Bergeron A, Rom WN, et al. Obliterative bronchiolitis. *N Engl J Med* 2014;370:1820–1828.
221. Dishop MK, Kuruvilla S. Primary and metastatic lung tumors in the pediatric population: a review and 25-year experience at a large children's hospital. *Arch Pathol Lab Med* 2008;132(7):1079–1103.
222. Amini B, Huang SY, Tsai J, et al. Primary lung and large airway neoplasms in children: current imaging evaluation with multidetector computed tomography. *Radiol Clin North Am.* 2013;51(4):637–657.
223. Murrell Z, Dickie B, Dasgupta R. Lung nodues in pediatric oncology patients: a prediction rule for when to biopsy. *J Pediatr Surg* 2011;46(5):833–837.
224. Harting MT, Blakely ML, Jaffe N, et al. Long-term survival after aggressive resection of pulmonary metastases among children and adolescents with osteosarcoma. *J Pediatr Surg* 2006;41(1):194–199.
225. Stanelle EJ, Christison-Lagay ER, Wolden SL, et al. Pulmonary metastasectomy in pediatric/adolescent patients with synovial sarcoma: an institutional review. *J Pediatr Surg* 2013;48(4):757–763.
226. Tokmak H, Kebudi R, Gumus T, et al. Pulmonary metastasis in neuroblastoma at initial diagnosis. *J Pediatr Hematol Oncol* 2012;34(7):581–582.
227. Murrell Z, Dasgupta R. What predicts the risk of recurrent lung metastases? *J Pediatr Surg* 2013;48(5):1020–1024.
228. Dantonello TM, Winkler P, Boelling T, et al. Embryonal rhabdomyosarcoma with metastases confined to the lungs: report from the CWS Study Group. *Pediatr Blood Cancer* 2011;56(5):725–732.
229. Yu DC, Grabowski MJ, Kozakewich HP, et al. Primary lung tumors in children and adolescents: a 90-year experience. *J Pediatr Surg* 2010;45(6):1090–1095.
230. Neville HL, Hogan AR, Zhuge Y, et al. Incidence and outcomes of malignant pediatric lung neoplasms. *J Surg Res* 2009;156(2):224–230.
231. Demir HA, Yalcin B, Ciftci AO, et al. Primary pleuropulmonary neoplasms in childhood: fourteen cases from a single center. *Asian Pac J Cancer Prev* 2011;12(2):543–547.
232. Messinger YH, Stewart DR, Priest JR, et al. Pleuropulmonary blastoma: a report on 350 central pathology-confirmed pleuropulmonary blastoma cases by the International Pleuropulmonary Blastoma Registry. *Cancer* 2015;121(2):276–285.
233. Doros LA, Schultz KA, Stewart DR, et al. Dicer1-related disorders. 2014. In: Pagan RA, Adam MP, Aroinger HH, et al., eds. *Gene Reviews [Internet]*. Seattle, WA: University of Washington, Seattle, 1993–2014.
234. Bondioni MP, Gatta D, Lougaris V, et al. Congenital cystic lung disease: prenatal ultrasound and postnatal multidetector computer tomography evaluation. Correlation with surgical and pathological data. *Radiol Med* 2014;119(11):842–851.
235. Fitzgerald DA. Congenital cyst adenomatoid malformations: resect some and observe all? *Paediatr Respir Rev* 2007;8:67–76.
236. Nasr A, Himidan S, Pastor AC, et al. Is congenital cystic adenomatoid malformation a premalignant lesion for pleuropulmonary blastoma? *J Pediatr Surg* 2010;45(6):1086–1089
237. Muller CO, Berrebi D, Kheniche A, et al. Is radical lobectomy required in congenital cystic adenomatoid malformation? *J Pediatr Surg* 2012;47(4):642–645.
238. Farris AB 3rd, Mark EJ, Kradin RL. Pulmonary "inflammatory myofibroblastic" tumors: a critical examination of the diagnostic category based on quantitative immunohistochemical analysis. *Virchows Arch* 2007;450(5):585–590.
239. Mano H. ALKoma: a cancer subtype with a hared target. *Cancer Discov* 2012;2(6):495–502.
240. Minoo P, Wang HY. ALK-immunoreactive neoplasms. *Int J Clin Exp Pathol* 2012;5(5):397–410.
241. Marino-Enriquez A, Wang WL, Roy A, et al. Epithelioid inflammatory myofibroblastic sarcoma: an aggressive intra-abdominal variant of inflammatory myofibroblastic tumor with nuclear membrane or perinuclear ALK. *Am J Surg Pathol* 2011;35(1):135–144.
242. Bhagat P, Bal A, Das A, et al. Pulmonary inflammatory myofibroblastic tumor and IgG4-related inflammatory pseudotumor: a diagnostic dilemma. *Virchows Arch* 2013;463(6):743–747.
243. Fujino H, Park YD, Uemura S, et al. An endobronchial inflammatory myofibroblastic tumor in a 10-yr-old child after allogeneic hematopoietic cell transplantation. *Pediatr Transplant* 2014;18(5):E165–E168.
244. Dishop MK, McKay Em, Kreiger PA, et al. Fetal lung interstitial tumor (FLIT): A proposed newly recognized lung tumor of infancy to be differentiated from cystic pleuropulmonary blastoma and other developmental pulmonary lesions. *Am J Surg Pathol* 2010;34(12):1762–1772.

245. Lazar DA, Cass DL, Dishop MK, et al. Fetal lung interstitial tumor: a cause of late gestation fetal hydrops. *J Pediatr Surg* 2011;46(6):1263–1266.
246. Onoda T, Kanno M, Sato H, et al. Identification of novel ALK rearrangement A2M-ALK in a neonate with fetal lung interstitial tumor. *Genes Chromosomes Cancer* 2014;53(10):865–874.
247. Huppmann AR, Coffin CM, Hoot AC, et al. Congenital peribronchial myofibroblastic tumor: comparison of fetal and postnatal morphology. *Pediatr Dev Pathol* 2011;14(2):124–129.
248. de Noronha L, Cecilio WA, da Silva TF, et al. Congenital peribronchial myofibroblastic tumor: a case report. *Pediatr Dev Pathol* 2010;13(3):243–246.
249. Calvo-Garcia MA, Lim FY, Stanek J, et al. Congenital peribronchial myofibroblastic tumor: prenatal imaging clues to differentiate from other fetal chest lesions. *Pediatr Radiol* 2014;44(4):479–483.
250. Coffin CM, Neilson KA, Ingles S, et al. Congenital generalized myofibromatosis: a disseminated angiocentric myofibromatosis. *Pediatr Pathol Lab Med* 1995;15(4):571–587.
251. Pelluard-Nehme F, Coatleven F, Carles D, et al. Multicentric infantile myofibromatosis: two perinatal cases. *Eur J Pediatr* 2007;166(10):997–1001.
252. Yeniel AO, Ergenoglu AM, Zeybek B, et al. Prenatal diagnosis of infantile myofibromatosis of the lung: a case report and review of the literature. *J Clin Ultrasound* 2013;41:38–41.
253. Okuda KV, Fitze G, Pablik J, et al. Infantile myofibromatosis as an unusual cause for unilateral atelectasis in an infant. *Pediatr Blood Cancer* 2014;61(7):1158–1159.
254. Geramizadeh B, Banani A, Moradi A, et al. Intrapulmonary solitary fibrous tumor with bronchial involvement: a rare case report in a child. *J Pediatr Surg* 2010;45(1):249–251.
255. Soyer T, Ciftci AO, Gucer S, et al. Calcifying fibrous pseudotumor of lung: a previously unreported entity. *J Pediatr Surg* 2004;39(11):1729–1730.
256. Krause LM, Schey WL, Bassuk A, et al. Intrathoracic desmoid tumor in a child. *Pediatr Radiol* 1985;15(2):131–133.
257. Carney JA. Carney triad. *Front Horm Res* 2014;41:92–110.
258. Abdulhamid I, Rabah R. Endobronchial chondromatous hamartoma in an infant. *Pediatr Pulmonol* 2003;35(1):67–69.
259. Saetti R, Silvestrini M, Cutrone C, et al. Treatment of congenital subglottic hemangiomas: our experience compared with reports in the literature. *Arch Otolaryngol Head Neck Surg* 2008;134(8):848–851.
260. Oviedo A, Abramson LP, Worthington R, et al. Congenital pulmonary capillary hemangiomatosis: report of two cases and review of the literature. *Pediatr Pulmonol* 2003;36(3):253–256.
261. Almagro P, Julia J, Sanjaume M, et al. Pulmonary capillary hemangiomatosis associated with primary pulmonary hypertension: report of 2 new cases and review of 35 cases from the literature. *Medicine (Baltimore)* 2002;81(6):417–424.
262. Lantuejoul S, Sheppard MN, Corrin B, et al. Pulmonary veno-occlusive disease and pulmonary capillary hemangiomatosis: a clinicopathologic study of 35 cases. *Am J Surg Pathol* 2006;30(7):850–857.
263. Best DH, Sumner KL, Austin ED, et al. EIF2AK4 mutations in pulmonary capillary hemangiomatosis. *Chest* 2014;145(2):231–236.
264. Aiello VD, Thomaz AM, Pozzan G, et al. Capillary hemangiomatosis like-lesions in lung biopsies from children with congenital heart defects. *Pediatr Pulmonol* 2014;49(3):E82–E85.
265. Mucientes P, Gomez-Arellano L, Rao N. Malignant pleuropulmonary epithelioid hemangioendothelioma—Unusual presentation of an aggressive angiogenic neoplasm. *Pathol Res Pract* 2014;210(9):613–618.
266. Antonescu CR, Le Loarer F, Mosquera JM, et al. Novel YAP1-TFE3 fusion defines a distinct subset of epithelioid hemangioendothelioma. *Genes Chromosomes Cancer* 2013;52(8):775–784.
267. Reich S, Ringe H, Uhlenberg B, et al. Epithelioid hemangioendothelioma of the lung presenting with pneumonia and heart rhythm disturbances in a teenage girl. *J Pediatr Hematol Oncol* 2010;32(4):274–276.
268. Abbas AA, Jastaniah WA. Extensive gingival and respiratory tract Kaposi sarcoma in a child after allogenic hematopoietic stem cell transplantation. *J Pediatr Hematol Oncol* 2012;34(2):e53–e55.
269. Theron S, Andronikou S, Du Plessis J, et al. Pulmonary Kaposi sarcoma in six children. *Pediatr Radiol* 2007;37(12):1224–1229.
270. Sala I, Faraci M, Magnano GM, et al. HHV-8-related visceral Kaposi's sarcoma following allogeneic HSCT: report of a pediatric case and literature review. *Pediatr Transplant* 2011;15(1):E8–E11.
271. Devouassoux-Shisheboran M, Hayashi T, Linnoila RI, et al. A clinicopathologic study of 100 cases of pulmonary sclerosing hemangioma with immunohistochemical studies: TTF-1 is expressed in both round and surface cells, suggesting an origin from primitive respiratory epithelium. *Am J Surg Pathol* 2000;24(7):906–916.
272. Keylock JB, Galvin JR, Franks TJ. Sclerosing hemangioma of the lung. *Arch Pathol Lab Med* 2009;133(5):820–825.
273. Miyagawa-Hayashino A, Tazelaar HD, Langel DJ, et al. Pulmonary sclerosing hemangioma with lymph node metastases: report of 4 cases. *Arch Pathol Lab Med* 2003;127(3):321–325.
274. Kalhor N, Staerkel GA, Moran CA. So-called sclerosing hemangioma of lung: current concept. *Ann Diagn Pathol* 2010;14(1):60–67.
275. Schmidt LA, Myers JL, McHugh JB. Napsin A is differentially expressed in sclerosing hemangiomas of the lung. *Arch Pathol Lab Med* 2012;136:1580–1584.
276. Alvarez OA, Kjellin I, Zuppan CW. Thoracic lymphangiomatosis in a child. *J Pediatr Hematol Oncol* 2004;26(2):136–141.
277. Satria MN, Pacheco-Rodriguez G, Moss J. Pulmonary lymphangiomatosis. *Lymphat Res Biol* 2011;9(4):191–193.
278. Reiterer F, Grossauer K, Morris N, et al. Congenital pulmonary lymphangiectasis. *Paediatr Respir Rev* 2014;15(3):275–280.
279. Martignoni G, Pea M, Reghellin D, et al. Molecular pathology of lymphangioleiomyomatosis and other perivascular epithelioid cell tumors. *Arch Pathol Lab Med* 2010;134(1):33–40.
280. Urban T, Lazor R, Lacronique J, et al. Pulmonary lymphangioleiomyomatosis. A study of 69 patients. Groupe d'Etudes et de Recherche sur les Maladies "Orphelines" Pulmonaires (GERM"O"P). *Medicine (Baltimore)* 1999;78(5):321–337.
281. Wataya-Kaneda M, Tanaka M, Hamasaki T, et al. Trends in the prevalence of tuberous sclerosis complex manifestations: an epidemiological study of 166 Japanese patients. *PLoS One* 2013;8(5):e63910.
282. Clarke BE. Cystic lung disease. *J Clin Pathol* 2013;66(10):904–908.
283. Flavin RJ, Cook J, Fiorentino M, et al. β-catenin is a useful adjunct immunohistochemical marker for the diagnosis of pulmonary lymphangioleiomyomatosis. *Am J Clin Pathol* 2011;135(5):776–782.
284. McCormack FX, Travis WD, Colby TV, et al. Lymphangioleiomyomatosis: calling it what it is: a low-grade, destructive, metastasizing neoplasm. *Am J Respir Crit Care Med* 2012;186(12):1210–1212.
285. Gora-Gebka M, Liberek A, Bako W, et al. The "sugar" clear cell tumor of the lung-clinical presentation and diagnostic difficulties of an unusual lung tumor in youth. *J Pediatr Surg* 2006;41(6):e27–e29.
286. Nehra D, Vagefi PA, Chang H, et al. Clear cell sugar tumor of the lung masquerading as tuberculosis in a pediatric patient. *J Thorac Cardiovasc Surg* 2010;139(5):e109–e109.
287. Papla B, Bialas M, Urbanczyk K, et al. Pulmonary arteriovenous malformations in children and young adults. *Pol J Pathol* 2012;63(3):184–188.
288. Webber ED, Rescorla FJ. Hemopneumothorax caused by vascularized bullae and a pulmonary hemangioma in an adolescent boy. *J Pediatr Surg* 2012;47(4)e23–e25.
289. McDonald J, Pyeritz RE. Hereditary hemorrhagic telangiectasia. In: Pagon RA, Adam MP, Ardinger HH, et al. eds. GeneReview [Internet]. Seattle, WA: University of Washington, Seattle, 2000 June 26 [updated 2014 Jul 24].
290. Mei-Zahav M, Letarte M, Faughnan ME, et al. Symptomatic children with hereditary hemorrhagic telangiectasia: a pediatric center experience. *Arch Pediatr Adolesc Med* 2006;160(6):596–601.
291. Latino GA, Al-Saleh S, Alharbi N, et al. Prevalence of pulmonary arteriovenous malformations in children versus adults with hereditary hemorrhagic telangiectasia. *J Pediatr* 2013;163(1):282–284.
292. Giordano P, Lenato GM, Suppressa P, et al. Hereditary hemorrhagic telangiectasia: arteriovenous malformations in children. *J Pediatr* 2013;163(1):179–186.

293. Guinee D. Update on pulmonary and pleural lymphoproliferative disorders. *Diagn Histopathol* 2008;14:474–498.
294. Chan AL, Juarez MM, Leslie KO, et al. Bird fancier's lung: a state-of-the-art review. *Clin Rev Allergy Immunol* 2012;43(1–2):69–83.
295. Adeleye A, Kelly M, Write NA, et al. Granulomatous lymphocytic interstitial lung disease in infancy. *Can Respir J* 2014;21(1):20–22.
296. Prasse A, Kayser G, Warnatz K. Common variable immunodeficiency-associated granulomatous and interstitial lung disease. *Curr Opin Pulm Med* 2013;19(5):503–509.
297. Toro AA, Altemani AM, da Silva MT, et al. Epstein-Barr virus (EBV) gene expression in interstitial pneumonitis in Brazilian human immunodeficiency virus-1-infected children: is EBV associated or not? *Pediatr Dev Pathol* 2010;13(3):184–191.
298. Bhoopat L, Rangkakulnuwat S, Ya-In C, et al. Relationship of cell bearing EBER and p24 antigens in biopsy-proven lymphocytic interstitial pneumonia in HIV-1 subtype E infected children. *Appl Immunohistochem Mol Morphol* 2011;19(6):547–551.
299. Ross JS, Ellman L. Leukemic infiltration of the lungs in the chemotherapeutic era. *Am J Clin Pathol* 1974;61(2):235–241.
300. Winer-Muram HT, Rubin SA, Fletcher BD, et al. Childhood leukemia: diagnostic accuracy of bedside chest radiography for severe pulmonary complications. *Radiology* 1994;193(1):127–133.
301. Gustafsson B, Hellebostad M, Ifversen M, et al. Acute respiratory failure in 3 children with juvenile myelomonocytic leukemia. *J Pediatr Hematol Oncol* 2011;33(8):e363–e367.
302. Nagarjun Rao R, Moran CA, Suster S. Histiocytic disorders of the lung. *Adv Anat Pathol* 2010;17(1):12–22.
303. Odame I, Li P, Lau L, et al. Pulmonary Langerhans cell histiocytosis: a variable disease in childhood. *Pediatr Blood Cancer* 2006;47(7):889–893.
304. Ronceray L, Potschger U, Janka G, et al. Pulmonary involvement in pediatric-onset multisystem Langerhans cell histiocytosis: effect on course and outcome. *J Pediatr* 2012;161(1):129–133.
305. Suri HS, Yi ES, Nowakowski GS, et al. Pulmonary Langerhans cell histiocytosis. *Orphanet J Rare Dis* 2012;19(7):16.
306. Bano S, Chaudhary V, Narula MK, et al. Pulmonary Langerhans cell histiocytosis in children: a spectrum of radiologic findings. *Eur J Radiol* 2014;83(1):47–56.
307. Roden AC, Hu X, Kip S, et al. BRAF V600E expression in Langerhans cell histiocytosis: clinical and immunohistochemical study on 25 pulmonary and 54 extrapulmonary cases. *Am J Surg Pathol* 2014;38(4):548–551.
308. Brown NA, Furtado LV, Betz BL, et al. High prevalence of somatic MAP2K1 mutations in BRAF V600E-negative Langerhans cell histiocytosis. *Blood* 2014;124(10):1655–1658.
309. Fan R, Sun J. Neonatal systemic juvenile xanthogranuloma with an ominous presentation and successful treatment. *Clin Med Insights Oncol* 2011;5:157–161.
310. Freeman HR, Ramanan AV. Review of haemophagocytic lymphohistiocytosis. *Arch Dis Child* 2011;96(7):688–693.
311. Natu SA, Keskar US, Behera MK, et al. Haemophagocytic lymphohistiocytosis with lung cavity and lytic bone lesion in a 45 day infant. *J Clin Diagn Res* 2014;8(3):156–157.
312. Shulman S, Katzenstein H, Abramowsky C, et al. Unusual presentation of Rosai-Dorfman disease (RDD) in the bone in adolescents. *Fetal Pediatr Pathol* 2011;30(6):442–447.
313. Smith EM, Swarnavel S, Ritchie JM, et al. Prevalence of human papillomavirus in the oral cavity/oropharynx in a large population of children and adolescents. *Pediatr Infect Dis J* 2007;26(9):836–840.
314. Larson DA, Derkay CS. Epidemiology of recurrent respiratory papillomatosis. *APMIS* 2010;118(6–7):450–454.
315. Wiatrak BJ, Wiatrak DW, Broker TR, et al. Recurrent respiratory papillomatosis: a longitudinal study comparing severity associated with human papilloma viral types 6 and 11 and other risk factors in a large pediatric population. *Laryngoscope* 2004;114(11 Pt 2 Suppl 104):1–23.
316. Donne AJ, Hampson L, Homer JJ, et al. The role of HPV type in recurrent respiratory papillomatosis. *Int J Pediatr Otorhinolaryngol* 2010;74(1):7–14.
317. Gelinas JF, Manoukian J, Cote A. Lung involvement in juvenile onset recurrent respiratory papillomatosis: a systematic review of the literature. *Int J Pediatr Otorhinolaryngol* 2008;72(4):433–452.
318. Somers GR, Tabrizi SN, Borg AJ, et al. Juvenile laryngeal papillomatosis in a pediatric population: a clinicopathologic study. *Pediatr Pathol Lab Med* 1997;17(1):53–64.
319. Kramer SS, Wehunt WD, Stocker JT, et al. Pulmonary manifestations of juvenile laryngotracheal papillomatosis. *AJR Am J Roentgenol* 1985;144(4):687–694.
320. Lie ES, Engh V, Boysen M, et al. Squamous cell carcinoma of the respiratory tract following laryngeal papillomatosis. *Acta Otolaryngol* 1994;114(2):209–212.
321. Simma B, Burger R, Uehlinger J, et al. Squamous-cell carcinoma arising in a non-irradiated child with recurrent respiratory papillomatosis. *Eur J Pediatr* 1993;152(9):776–778.
322. Broaddus RR, Herzog CE, Hicks MJ. Neuroendocrine tumors (carcinoid and neuroendocrine carcinoma) presenting at extra-appendiceal sites in childhood and adolescence. *Arch Pathol Lab Med* 2003;127(9):1200–1203.
323. Redlich A, Wedhsung K, Boxberger N, et al. Extra-appendiceal neuroendocrine neoplasms in children—data from the GPOH-MET 97 study. *Klin Padiatr* 2013;225:315–319.
324. Liu SZ, Staats PN, Goicochea L, et al. Automated quantification of Ki-67 proliferative index of excised neuroendocrine tumors of the lung. *Diagn Pathol* 2014;16:9 doi: 10.1186/s13000-014-0174z.
325. Molina JR, Aubry MC, Lewis JE, et al. Primary salivary gland-type lung cancer: spectrum of clinical presentation, histopathologic and prognostic factors. *Cancer* 2007;110(10):2253–2259
326. Roby BB, Drehner D, Sidman JD. Pediatric tracheal and endobronchial tumors: an institutional experience. *Arch Otolaryngol Head Neck Surg* 2011;137(9):925–929
327. Lal DR, Clark I, Shalkow J, et al. Primary epithelial lung malignancies in the pediatric population. *Pediatr Blood Cancer* 2005;45(5):683–686.
328. Qian X, Sun Z, Pan W, et al. Childhood bronchial mucoepidermoid tumors: a case report and literature review. *Oncol LCH* 2013;6(5):1409–1414.
329. Shilo K, Foss RD, Franks TJ, et al. Pulmonary mucoepidermoid carcinoma with prominent tumor-associated lymphoid proliferation. *Am J Surg Pathol* 2005;29(3):407–411.
330. Chin CH, Huang CC, Lin MC, et al. Prognostic factors of tracheobronchial mucoepidermoid carcinoma—15 years experience. *Respirology* 2008;13(2):275–280.
331. Serra A, Schackert HK, Mohr B, et al. t(11;19)(q21;p12 p13.11) and MECT1-MAML2 fusion transcript expression as a prognostic marker in infantile lung mucoepidermoid carcinoma. *J Pediatr Surg* 2007;42(7):E23–E29
332. Roden AC, Garcia JJ, Wehrs RN, et al. Histopathologic, immunophenotypic and cytogenetic features of pulmonary mucoepidermoid carcinoma. *Mod Pathol* 2014;27(11):1479–1488.
333. Hartman GE, Schochat SJ. Primary pulmonary neoplasms of childhood: a review. *Ann Thorac Surg* 1983;1983:108
334. Katz DR, Bubis JJ. Acinic cell tumor of the bronchus. *Cancer* 1976;38(2):830–832.
335. Sabaratnam R, Anunathan R, Govender D. Acinic cell carcinoma: an unusual case of bronchial obstruction in an child. *Pediatr Dev Pathol* 2004;7:521–526.
336. Rosenfeld A, Schwartz D, Garzon S, et al. Epithelial-myoepithelial carcinoma of the lung: a case report and review of the literature. *J Pediatr Hematol Oncol* 2009;31(3):206–208.
337. Cook JR, Hill DA, Humphrey PA, et al. Squamous cell carcinoma arising in recurrent respiratory papillomatosis with pulmonary

involvement: emerging common pattern of clinical features and human papillomavirus serotype association. *Mod Pathol* 2000;12(8):914–918.
338. Saumet L, Damay A, Jeziorski E, et al. Bronchopulmonary squamous cell carcinoma associated with HPV 11 in a 15-year-old girl with a history of severe recurrent respiratory papillomatosis: a case report. *Arch Pediatr* 2011;18(7):754–757.
339. Shehata BM, Otto KJ, Sobol SE, et al. E6 and E7 oncogene expression by human papilloma virus (HPV) and the aggressive behavior of recurrent laryngeal papillomatosis (RLP). *Pediatr Dev Pathol* 2008;11(2):118–121.
340. Salles PG, Moura Rde D, Menezes LM, et al. Expression of P16 in NUT carcinomas with no association with human papillomavirus (HPV). *Appl Immunohistochem Mol Morphol* 2014;22(4):262–265.
341. Bauer DE, Mitchell CM, Strait KM, et al. Clinicopathologic features and long-term outcomes of NUT midline carcinoma. *Clin Cancer Res* 2012;18(20):5773–5779.
342. Shehata BM, Steelman CK, Abramowsky CR, et al. NUT midline carcinoma in a newborn with multiorgan disseminated tumor and a 2-year-old with a pancreatic/hepatic primary. *Pediatr Dev Pathol* 2010;13(6):481–485.
343. Shah AA, Jeffus SK, Stelow EB. Squamous cell carcinoma variants of the upper aerodigestive tract: a comprehensive review with a focus on genetic alterations. *Arch Pathol Lab Med* 2014;138(6):731–744.
344. Bair RJ, Chick JF, Chauhan NR, et al. Demystifying NUT midline carcinoma: radiologic and pathologic correlations of an aggressive malignancy. *AJR Am J Roentgenol* 2014;203(4):W391–W399.
345. Taniyama TK, Nokihara H, Tsuta K, et al. Clinicopathological features in young patients treated for small-cell lung cancer: significance of immunohistological and molecular analyses. *Clin Lung Cancer* 2014;15(3):244–247.
346. MacSweeney F, Papagiannopoulos K, Goldstraw P, et al. An assessment of the expanded classification of congenital cystic adenomatoid malformations and their relationship to malignant transformation. *Am J Surg Pathol* 2003;27(8):1139–1146.
347. Stacher E, Ullmann R, Halbwedl I, et al. Atypical goblet cell hyperplasia in congenital cystic adenomatoid malformation as a possible preneoplasia for pulmonary adenocarcinoma in childhood: A genetic analysis. *Hum Pathol* 2004;35(5):565–570.
348. Lantuejoul S, Nicholson AG, Sartori G, et al. Mucinous cells in type 1 pulmonary congenital cystic adenomatoid malformations as mucinous bronchioloalveolar carcinoma precursors. *Am J Surg Pathol* 2007;31(6):961–969.
349. Li J, Chen GS, Zhang X, et al. Congenital cystic adenomatoid malformations with associated mucinous bronchioloalveolar carcinoma in a neonate. *Fetal Pediatr Pathol* 2014;33(1):29–34.
350. Ishida M, Igarashi T, Teramoto K, et al. Mucinous bronchioloalveolar carcinoma with K-ras mutation arising in type 1 congenital cystic adenomatoid malformation: a case report with review of the literature. *Int J Clin Exp Pathol* 2013;6(11):2597–2602.
351. Hasegawa M, Sakai F, Arimura K, et al. EGFR mutation of adenocarcinoma in congenital cystic adenomatoid malformation/congenital pulmonary airway malformation: a case report. *Jpn J Clin Oncol* 2014;44(3):278–281.
352. Salomao M, Levy B, Nahum O, et al. Genomic alterations in pulmonary adenocarcinoma in situ in an adolescent patient. *Arch Pathol Lab Med* 2014;138:559–563.
353. Kayton ML, He M, Zakowski MF, et al. Primary lung adenocarcinomas in children and adolescents treated for pediatric malignancies. *J Thorac Oncol* 2010;5(11):1764–1771.
354. Weissferdt A, Moran C. Malignant biphasic tumors of the lungs. *Adv Anat Pathol* 2011;18:179–189.
355. Luo C, Yeung S, Liu Z, et al. Pulmonary well-differentiated fetal adenocarcinoma with platelet-derived growth factor receptor (PDGFR)α expression. *Cancer Biol Ther* 2012;13(14):1384–1389.
356. Wu Y, Chen D, Bian L, et al. DICER1 mutations in a patient with an ovarian sertoli-Leydig tumor, well-differentiated fetal adenocarcinoma of the lung, and familial multinodular goiter. *Eur J Med Genet* 2014;57:621–625.
357. Mondal K, Dasgupta S. Mature cystic teratoma of the lung. *Singapore Med J* 2012; 53:e237–e239.
358. Sawant A, Kandra A, Narra S. Intrapulmonary cystic teratoma mimicking malignant pulmonary neoplasm. *BMJ Case Rep* 2012;2012 pii: bcr0220125770.
359. Dar R, Mushtaque M, Wani S, et al. Giant intrapulmonary teratoma: a rare case. *Case Rep Pulmonol* 2011;2011:298653.
360. Giunchi F, Segura J. Primary malignant teratoma of lung: report of a case and review of the literature. *Int J Surg Pathol* 2012;20:523–527.
361. Nathan N, Taam RA, Epaud R, et al. A national internet-linked based database for pediatric interstitial lung diseases: the French network. *Orphanet J Rare Dis* 2012;7:40.
362. Shetty AK, Gedalia A. Childhood sarcoidosis: a rare but fascinating disorder. *Pediatr Rheumatol* 2008;6:16.
363. Fretzayas A, Moustaki M, Vougiouka O. The puzzling clinical spectrum and course of juvenile sarcoidosis. *World J Pediatr* 2011;7:103–110.
364. Sileo C, Epaud R, Mahloul M, et al. Sarcoidosis in children: HRCT findings and correlation with pulmonary function tests. *Pediatr Pulmonol* 2014;49:1223–1233.
365. Deverriere G, Flamans-Klein A, Firmin D, et al. Early onset pediatric sarcoidosis, diagnostic problems. *Arch Pediatr* 2012;19:707–710.
366. Yeboah J, Afkhami M, Lee C, et al. Necrotizing sarcoid granulomatosis. *Curr Opin Pulm Med* 2012;18:493–498.
367. Panigada S, Ullmann N, Sacco O, et al. Necrotizing sarcoid granulomatosis of the lung in a 12-year-old boy with an atypical clinical course. *Pediatr Pulmonol* 2012;47:831–835.
368. Ma Y, Gal A, Koss MN. The pathology of pulmonary sarcoidosis: update. *Semin Diagn Pathol* 2007;24:150–161.
369. Mukhopadhyay S, Farver CF, Vaszar LT, et al. Causes of pulmonary granulomas: a retrospective study of 500 cases from seven countries. *J Clin Pathol* 2012;65:51–57.
370. Damen GM, van Kriekin JH, Hoppenreijs E, et al. Overlap, common features and essential differences in pediatric granulomatous inflammatory bowel disease. *J Pediatr Gastroenterol Nutr* 2010;51:690–697.
371. Vadlamudi NB, Navaneethan U, Thame KA, et al. Crohn's disease with pulmonary manifestations in children: 2 case reports and review of the literature. *J Crohns Colitis* 2013;7:e85–e92.
372. Artac H, Bozkurt B, Talim B, et al. Sarcoid-like granulomas in common variable immunodeficiency. *Rheumatol Int* 2009;30:109–112.
373. Gold Dr, Wright R. Population disparities in asthma. *Annu Rev Public Health* 2005;26:89–113.
374. Dick S, Friend A, Dynes K, et al. A systematic review of associations between environmental exposures and development of asthma in children aaged up to 9 years. *BMJ Open* 2014;4(11):e006554.
375. Been JV, Lugtenberg MJ, Smets E, et al. Preterm birth and childhood wheezing disorders: a systematic review and meta-analysis. *PLoS Med* 2014;11(1):e1001596.
376. Szefler SJ. Advances in pediatric asthma in 2014: moving toward a population health perspective. *J Allergy Clin Immunol* 2015;135:644–652.
377. Chung KF. Defining phenotypes in asthma: a step towards personalized medicine. *Curr Opin* 2014;74:719–728.
378. Hasegawa K, Tsugawa Y, Brown DF, et al. Childhood asthma hospitalizations in the United Sates, 2000–2009. *J Pediatr* 2013;163:1127–1133.
379. Moorman JE, Akinbami LJ, Bailey CM, et al. National surveillance of asthma: United States, 2001–2010. *Vital Health Stat 3* 2012;35:1–67.
380. Mayer S, Metzger R, Kluth D. The embryology of the diaphragm. *Semin Pediatr Surg* 2014;20:161–169.
381. Chavhan GB, Babyn PS, Cohen RA, et al. Multimodality imaging of the pediatric diaphragm: anatomy and pathologic conditions. *Radiographics* 2010;30:1797–1817.
382. Wynn J, Yu L, Chung WK. Genetic causes of congenital diaphragmatic hernia. *Semin Fetal Neonatal Med* 2014;19:324–330.
383. Kantarci S, Donahoe PK. Congenital diaphragmatic hernia (CDH) etiology as revealed by pathway genetics. *Am J Med Genet C Semin Med Genet* 2007;15:217–226.

384. Hidaka N, Ishii K, Mabuchi A, et al. Associated anomalies in congenital diaphragmatic hernia: perinatal characteristics and impact on postnatal survival. *J Perinat Med* 2015;43:245–252.
385. Slavotinek AM. The genetics of common disorders—congenital diaphragmatic hernia. *Eur J Med Genet* 2014;57:418–423.
386. Slavotinek AM. Single gene disorders associated with congenital diaphragmatic hernia. *Semin Med Gen* 2007;145C:172–183.
387. Singal AK, Srinivas M, Bhatnagar V. Bronchopulmonary foregut malformation in association with diaphragmatic eventration. *J Pediatr Surg* 2006;41:1329–1331.
388. Kuo HC, Chang CY, Leung JH. Pulmonary sequestration and diaphragmatic eventration in a 6-month-old infant. *Pediatr Neonatal* 2012; 53:63–67.
389. Iskender C, Tarim E, Yalcinkaya C. Prenatal diagnosis of right diaphragmatic eventration associated with fetal hydrops. *J Obstet Gynacol Res* 2012;38:858–862.
390. Radhakrishnan J, Bean J, Piazza DJ, et al. Accessory hemi-diaphragm. *J Pediatr Surg* 2014;49:1326–1331.
391. McGivern MR, Best KE, Rankin J, et al. Epidemiology of congenital diaphragmatic hernia in Europe: a register-based study. *Arch Dis Child Fetal Neonatal Ed* 2014;0:F1-F8.
392. Robinson PD, Fitzgerald DA. Congenital diaphragmatic hernia. *Paediatr Respir Rev* 2007;8:323–335.
393. Pagon RA, Adam MP, Ardinger HH, et al. Congenital diaphragmatic hernia overview. *GeneReviews [Internet]*. Seattle, WA: University of Washington, Seattle, 1993–2014. 2006 Feb 1 [updated 2010 Mar 16].
394. Pagon RA, Adam MP, Ardinger HH, et al. Fryns syndrome. *GeneReviews [Internet]*. Seattle, WA: University of Washington, Seattle, 1993–2015. 2007 Apr 18 [updated 2015 Jan 29].
395. Jagtap SV, Dhirajkumar BS, Jain A, et al. Complete pentalogy of Cantrell (POC) with phocomelia and other associated rare anomalies. *J Clin Diagn Res* 2014;8:FD04–FD05.
396. Engum SA. Embryology, sternal clefts, ectopia cordis, and Cantrells's pentalogy. *Semin Pediatr Surg* 2008;17:154–160.
397. Jesudason EC, Connell MG, Fernig DG, et al. Early lung malformations in congenital diaphragmatic hernia. *J Pediatr Surg* 2000;35:124–128.
398. Akinkuotu AC, Sheikh F, Cass DL, et al. Are all pulmonary hypoplasias the same? A comparison of pulmonary outcomes in neonates with congenital diaphragmatic hernia, omphalocele and congenital lung malformation. *J Pediatr Surg* 2015;50:55–59.
399. Peetsold MG, Heij HA, Kneepkens CM, et al. The long-term follow-up of patients with a congenital diaphragmatic hernia: a broad spectrum of morbidity. *Pediatr Surg Int* 2009;25:1–17.
400. Kool H, Mous D, Tibboel D, et al. Pulmonary vascular development goes awry in congenital lung abnormalities. *Birth Defects Res C Embryo Today* 2014;102:343–358.
401. Muratore CS, Kharasch V, Lund DP, et al. Pulmonary morbidity in 100 survivors of congenital diaphragmatic hernia monitored in a multidisciplinary clinic. *J Pediatr Surg* 2001;36:133–140.
402. Lusk LA, Wai KC, Moon-Grady AJ, et al. Persistence of pulmonary hypertension by echocardiography predicts short-term outcomes in congenital diaphragmatic hernia. *J Pediatr* 2015;166(2):251–256.
403. Sluiter I, Reiss I, Kraemer U, et al. Vascular abnormalities in human newborns with pulmonary hypertension. *Expert Rev Respir Med* 2011;5:245–256.
404. Acker SN, Mandell EW, Sims-Lucas S, et al. Histologic identification of prominent intrapulmonary anastomotic vessels in severe congenital diaphragmatic hernia. *J Pediatr* 2015;166:178–183.
405. Harting MT, Lally KP. The congenital diaphragmatic hernia study group registry update. *Semin Fetal Neonatal Med* 2014;19:370–375.

CHAPTER 13

The Cardiovascular System

Ivan P. Moskowitz, M.D., Ph.D., Selene Koo, M.D., Ph.D., Aliya N. Husain, M.D., and Kathleen Patterson, M.D.

CONGENITAL MALFORMATIONS OF THE CARDIOVASCULAR SYSTEM

Incidence

The heart, first recognizable at 15 days of gestation, develops from a single tube into a four-chambered structure via an extraordinary series of loopings and septations (1). Given the complexity of cardiac development, it is not surprising that congenital cardiac defects account for the vast majority of cases of cardiac disease in childhood. The reported incidence of congenital heart disease (CHD) varies widely, ranging from 2.4/1000 to 8.8/1000 live births (2). The incidence statistics vary depending on the age of the patient population, the criteria used for diagnosis and inclusion in a study, and the length of study group follow-up. However, inclusion of defects that present later in life but that originate during fetal heart development, and are therefore congenital, such as bicuspid aortic valve, increases the incidence to 3% of live births (3).

Etiology

The etiology of congenital heart malformations has been historically thought to be multifactorial, with both genetic and environmental factors playing a role (4). However, no published epidemiologic work rules out a genetic etiology for the majority of CHD. Recent genetic advances suggest that the genetic basis of CHD is complex, potentially involving interactions between many genes (3). From 15% to 45% of patients with CHD have additional developmental anomalies, including chromosomal and nonchromosomal syndromes, malformation associations or sequences, and teratogen-associated defects (5). Genetic factors have long been recognized as a major player; historically, 10% of patients with CHD exhibit a trisomy, monosomy, duplication, or deletion on routine cytogenetic study, with trisomy 21 being the most common, whereas improved genetic techniques have allowed microdeletions and mutations of single genes to be identified in many of the developmental syndromes that include CHD as a major factor, with the 22q11 deletion, characteristic of the DiGeorge/velocardiofacial syndrome, being the most prevalent (4,6,7). The ever-increasing number of identified chromosomal abnormalities linked with heart malformations unfortunately does not mean that genetic screening can predict a specific form of CHD. Instead, it has become clear that mutations at multiple genetic loci can cause the same cardiac malformation and that mutations at a single locus can cause multiple different malformations. Meanwhile, molecular and biochemical analysis of normal gene products from many of these CHD-associated genes is leading to increased understanding of the developmental mechanisms in the heart (1). The advent of novel genetic techniques such as next-generation sequencing portends a rapid increase in our understanding of the genetic basis of CHD. Rather than providing a list of genes currently associated with CHD that will be quickly out of date, the reader is referred to recent reviews on the subject (e.g., 3).

CHD is fundamentally a defect of cardiovascular development, and increased understanding of cardiovascular development will help explain the etiology of the defects observed in human CHD. Cardiovascular development proceeds rapidly during early embryonic life through a series of well-defined steps (1). These include the generation of bilaterally paired groups of cardiac progenitor cells from lateral plate mesoderm, coalescing into the cardiac crescent, the migration of cardiac progenitors to the midline and the generation of the linear heart tube, the rapid growth and stereotyped rightward (D-looped) looping of the heart tube, the rapid growth of the cardiac chambers, and septation of the atria, ventricles, and outflow tract to form the final four-chambered heart with the capacity for distinct pulmonary and systemic blood flow. Cardiac development relies on both extrinsic developmental processes, such as left–right determination, and intrinsic developmental processes, such as cardiac septation. In the former, the proper establishment of the left–right axis of the body plan during gastrulation allows correct D-looping of the heart tube and appropriate development of each of the chambers with appropriate situs, or right- versus left-sided characteristics. Correct D-looping of the heart tube in turn establishes a necessary scaffold for successful completion of the following steps in cardiovascular development. Appropriate pathologic evaluation of CHD specimens will independently evaluate the situs and other structural components of the specimen (see Classification section below).

Pathophysiology

The fetal human heart approximates the structure of the mature human heart by 8 weeks of gestational age, the earliest organ to undergo morphologic development. Tremendous growth of the fetal heart occurs between 8 weeks gestational age and birth; however, the major morphologic decisions are complete by 8 weeks of gestational age. The majority of structural cardiac abnormalities observed in human CHD are therefore present very early during fetal life. Although some developmental defects will affect the ability of the fetal heart to perform its fetal circulatory function, such lesions would cause fetal lethality, not CHD (present at "birth," by definition). Such lesions are observed in fetal autopsies, a large percentage of which are affected by abnormal hearts. However, because CHD lesions are structurally present early in fetal life but not clinically disclosed until after birth, CHD lesions must be clinically silent to fetal circulation but clinically apparent to postnatal circulation. The fetal to neonatal circulatory transition (including closure of the ductus arteriosus and foramen ovale) can be considered a selective switch, clinically unveiling the cardiac defects observed in human CHD. The requirement that CHD lesions be silent to fetal circulation and unveiled by the perinatal circulatory transition places significant structural constraints on the specific types of structural abnormalities that are observed in human CHD. Three major classes, (a) shunts, (b) obstruction to flow, and (c) routing abnormalities of the great vessels comprise the vast majority of structural abnormalities observed in CHD. In the normal heart, the pulmonary and systemic vascular circuits are completely separate, functioning as two parallel circuits. Loss of this separation results in shunting of blood between the two circuits. The size and the predominant direction of the shunt (i.e., right to left or left to right) are dynamic and determined by a variety of factors, including the relative resistance to flow in the two circuits and the presence or the absence of an associated obstructive lesion. Shunting lesions, often not apparent at birth when resistance in the two circuits is similar, become clinically evident over time with the normal decrease in pulmonary vascular resistance (PVR). In general, right-to-left shunts are associated with cyanosis, and left-to-right shunts with increased pulmonary blood flow, congestive heart failure, and a risk for the development of pulmonary artery hypertension.

Obstructive lesions can occur at almost any site in either of the circuits, with the cardiac chambers proximal to the site of obstruction showing hypertrophy in response to the increased workload. In general, right-sided obstruction produces decreased pulmonary blood flow and cyanosis; left-sided obstruction results in decreased systemic blood flow. In cases of severe obstruction, the obstructed circuit is often dependent on blood flow across the ductus arteriosus (i.e., ductus-dependent lesions), and symptoms characteristically appear at the time of ductus closure in the first days of life.

The great arterial attachments to the ventricular mass complete a normally separate systemic and pulmonary circuit. Normally, the pulmonary artery receives blood only from the right ventricle and aorta blood only from the left ventricle. Observed abnormalities of great arterial attachment include each of the possible alternate combinations of ventricular–great arterial attachment, including transposition of the great arteries, in which the pulmonary artery receives flow from the left ventricle and aorta from the right ventricle; double-outlet right ventricle (DORV), in which both great arteries are attached to the right ventricle; and, rarely, double-outlet left ventricle (DOLV), in which both great arteries are attached to the left ventricle. A summary of the clinicopathologic features in some of the more common congenital cardiac defects is presented in Table 13-1.

TABLE 13-1 CONGENITAL HEART DEFECTS: MAJOR CLINICAL FINDINGS

	SHUNT		PBF				
	L→R	R→L	INC	DEC	Cyanosis	Ductus Dependent	Complications
ASD	X	—	X	—	—	—	PVOD
ECD	X	—	X	—	—	—	PVOD
VSD	X	—	X	—	—	—	PVOD
TGV	—	—	X	—	X	X	PVOD
TRUN	X	—	X	—	—	—	PVOD
EBS	—	X	—	X	X	—	Arrhythmia
TOF	—	X	—	X	X	—	Polycythemia
HRHS	—	X	—	X	X	X	—
HLHS	—	—	—	—	—	X	Shock
PDA	X	—	X	—	—	—	PVOD

PBF, pulmonary blood flow; L→R, left to right; R→L, right to left; INC, increased; DEC, decreased; ASD, atrial septal defect; ECD, endocardial cushion defect; VSD, ventricular septal defect; TGV, transposition of the great vessels; TRUN, truncus arteriosus; EBS, Ebstein malformation; TOF, tetralogy of Fallot; HRHS, hypoplastic right heart syndrome; HLHS, hypoplastic left heart syndrome; PDA, patent ductus arteriosus; PVOD, pulmonary vascular obstructive disease.

Classification

An accurate classification of congenital heart malformations requires knowledge of the normal anatomy of the heart and a careful systematic approach to the examination. Normal values for heart weight relative to age and body size are readily available; normal values for the ventricular wall thickness and valve sizes have been reported for fetuses and newborns by Oyer et al. (8) and for infants and children by Rowlatt et al. (9) and Scholz et al. (10).

Cardiac Situs

Following a careful external examination of the shape and the position of the heart, the situs of the chambers of the heart is evaluated. With the relationships of the great vessels and venous drainage pattern, a sequential evaluation of the three segments of the heart (atria, ventricles, and great vessels) is undertaken. The connections of the segments, the relationship between the chambers within a segment, and the morphology of the segments are all assessed (11–13) (Table 13-2). When this segmental approach is used for classification, normal connections, relationships, and morphology are not incorporated into the diagnosis. In the majority of cases of CHD, a single defect is present (e.g., a ventricular septal defect [VSD]), and the heart is classified on the basis of that solitary anomaly. In more complex cases, situs relationships lead the diagnosis, and are followed by morphologic defects, in order of severity (13).

Situs refers to the position of a body part relative to other body parts. Because the human body has left–right differences, which develop either normally or abnormally, normal or abnormal situs can be determined. The morphologic features of the right (right atrium, liver) can be distinguished from those of the left (left atrium, stomach, spleen). There are three types of situs: (a) situs solitus, or normal situs; (b) situs inversus, the mirror image of situs solitus; and (c) situs ambiguus. Situs ambiguus is a general term for uncertain situs, characteristic of heterotaxy syndrome. This can include cases in which both sides of the body develop with "right" characteristics (asplenia syndrome) or "left" characteristics (polysplenia syndrome). The situs patterns of the atria and visceral organs are almost always the same. Normal situs allows normal cardiac/ventricular looping (D-loop). Inverted situs results in mirror-image looping (L-loop). Ambiguous situs will often cause abnormal looping, which in turn may cause structural abnormalities such as septal or conotruncal abnormalities (13).

TABLE 13-2 SEQUENTIAL EXAMINATION OF HEART SEGMENTS

Atrial situs: determined by position of morphologic RA
   Situs solitus: RA on right; LA on left
   Situs inversus: RA on left; LA on right
   Situs ambiguus: indeterminate atrial situs
     Bilateral right-sided atria
     Bilateral left-sided atria
Atrioventricular connections
   Atrioventricular concordance: RA→RV; LA→LV
   Atrioventricular discordance: RA→LV; LA→RV
   Ambiguous (indeterminate) connection
     Double-inlet ventricle: RA + LA→one ventricle
   Absence of one atrioventricular connection
Ventricular organization
   Normal or D-looped: morphologic RV to the right of the morphologic LV
   Inverted or L-looped: morphologic RV to the left of the morphologic LV
Ventricular morphology
   Three normal components: inlet, trabecular, and outlet
     Trabecular component determines morphologic right and left ventricles.
   Rudimentary chamber: absent inlet portion
Ventriculoarterial connections
   Ventriculoarterial concordance: RV→ PA; LV→Ao
   Ventriculoarterial discordance: RV→Ao; LV→PA
   Double-outlet ventricle: one ventricle→PA + Ao
   Single outlet of heart: includes truncus, pulmonary atresia, aortic atresia

RA, right atrium; RV, right ventricle; LA, left atrium; LV, left ventricle; PA, pulmonary artery; Ao, aorta.

Dextrocardia

Dextrocardia, in which the heart is located in the right side of the chest with a right-sided apex, occurs with situs inversus, situs ambiguus, and as an isolated finding (14). Except when occurring with situs inversus, the incidence of associated intracardiac and extracardiac anomalies is high (2). Dextrocardia should be distinguished from dextroposition, in which the heart is displaced to the right side of the chest with a left-sided apex (14).

Situs Ambiguus

Situs ambiguus (heterotaxia) occurs when the usual markers of situs are disorganized or missing as a result of disruption of the left–right axis determination early in development (15–17). The two best-described forms of situs ambiguus are asplenia (bilateral right sidedness) and polysplenia (bilateral left sidedness). The "sidedness" of the heart is determined by the atrial appendage morphology (16). The heterotaxic syndromes are frequently associated with complex congenital heart and venous malformations and a variety of extracardiac defects (15). Molecular studies have identified a variety of genes involved in left–right patterning during development (17).

Juxtaposition of Atrial Appendages

Juxtaposition of the atrial appendages, diagnosed when both atrial appendages reside partially or completely on the same side of the great vessels, is a harbinger of underlying heart malformations (16,18). Left-sided juxtaposition accounts for 86% of cases, with tricuspid atresia and transposition of the

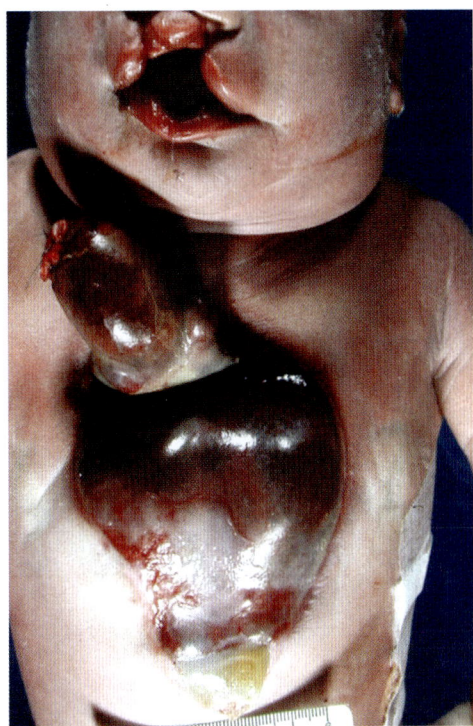

FIGURE 13-1 • Infant with multiple congenital anomalies including cleft lip seen at the top of the photograph and an anterior defect in the chest and abdomen through which the heart and liver protrude.

great vessels the most common associated malformations. On the flip side, 11% of hearts with tricuspid atresia and 3% of hearts with D-transposition exhibit left-sided juxtaposition of the atrial appendages (18).

Ectopia Cordis

Ectopia cordis, a rare anomaly in which the heart is partially or totally outside the chest (Figure 13-1), is subclassified according to the location of the defect (14,19). Thoracic ectopia cordis, the most common type, is the result of a sternal cleft. The heart is usually located on the anterior surface of the chest without skin or a pericardial covering. Thoracoabdominal (abdominal) ectopia cordis is associated with a defect in the lower sternum, diaphragm, and abdominal wall; the heart is usually located with the abdominal viscera in a common omphalocele sac. Intracardiac defects occur frequently but are not inevitable (19).

Malformations of the Venous System

Systemic Venous Anomalies

Systemic venous blood returns to the heart via five sources: superior vena cava, coronary veins, hepatic veins, inferior vena cava, and azygos veins. With normally lateralized situs (situs solitus or situs inversus), anomalies of the systemic venous system are not uncommon but usually of little clinical significance. With situs ambiguus, complex systemic venous malformations are the rule.

Persistent Left Superior Vena Cava (LSVC)
A persistent LSVC is present in 0.3% to 0.5% of the general population and up to 10% of patients with other cardiovascular anomalies (14,20). Absence of the innominate vein serves as a clue to the presence of a persistent LSVC in approximately 40% of cases (14). The LSVC traverses the posterior surface of the left atrium to enter the coronary sinus in the AV sulcus. The wall between the coronary sinus and the left atrium becomes unroofed in approximately 8% of cases, resulting in drainage of the LSVC into the left atrium (20). This latter morphology occurs most frequently in the setting of the heterotaxy syndromes (21).

Coronary Sinus Ostium Atresia
With atresia of the coronary sinus ostium, a rare anomaly, cardiac venous drainage relies on a persistent LSVC with a patent innominate vein or other left-to-right connection. The obstructed coronary sinus ostium by itself creates few clinical problems, but ligation of the persistent LSVC should be avoided during heart surgery (21).

Interruption of the Inferior Vena Cava with Azygos Continuation
Anomalies of the inferior vena cava are much less common. Infrahepatic interruption of the inferior vena cava with azygos continuation results in an absence of the inferior vena cava between the renal and hepatic veins (14,20). The inferior vena cava below the renal veins drains via an enlarged azygos vein, which enters the thorax through the aortic hiatus and joins the superior vena cava just superior to its junction with the right atrium. This anomaly is usually associated with other cardiovascular malformations and is frequently present in the polysplenia syndrome (14,15).

Pulmonary Venous Anomalies

Pulmonary venous anomalies are listed in Table 13-3.

Partial Anomalous Pulmonary Venous Connection
Anomalous pulmonary venous connection refers to a group of conditions in which the pulmonary venous drainage is routed partially or totally to the right atrium.

TABLE 13-3	PULMONARY VENOUS MALFORMATIONS
Partial anomalous pulmonary venous connection	
Sinus venosus ASD	
Scimitar syndrome	
Total anomalous pulmonary venous connection	
Supradiaphragmatic	
Supracardiac	
Intracardiac	
Infradiaphragmatic	
Pulmonary vein atresia	
Cor triatriatum	

In the more common anomaly, partial anomalous pulmonary venous connection, blood from one or more, but not all, of the pulmonary veins drains into a systemic vein or right atrium. This anomalous drainage is right sided in more than 80% of cases and most frequently enters the superior vena cava or the right atrium (14,22). More than 80% of cases occur in the setting of sinus venosus atrial septal defects (ASDs) as described earlier. The scimitar syndrome represents a variant of partial anomalous pulmonary venous connection characterized by anomalous pulmonary venous drainage into the inferior vena cava with a variety of associated cardiopulmonary anomalies. The most frequent associations include right lung hypoplasia, dextrocardia, systemic arterial supply to the lung, and abnormal bronchial anatomy (23).

Total Anomalous Pulmonary Venous Connection

Total anomalous pulmonary venous connection, in which all the pulmonary veins drain to the systemic circuit, is subclassified according to the route of the abnormal venous drainage and the presence or absence of obstruction to that drainage (24,25) (Table 13-4). The most common route of drainage is through a vertical vein that arises from a confluence of the pulmonary veins posterior to the left atrium, traverses superiorly along the left side of the mediastinum, and drains into the innominate vein at its junction with the left subclavian vein (14,25). Less frequently, the common trunk drains into the superior vena cava, right atrium, coronary sinus, or subdiaphragmatic portal venous system (Figure 13-2). In up to 10% of cases, the pulmonary veins drain to multiple different sites (25,26). Drainage is obstructed in approximately 60% of cases of total anomalous pulmonary venous connection, with the cardiac sites having the lowest risk and the infracardiac the highest risk for obstruction (25,26) (Table 13-4). The venous drainage can be obstructed by intrinsically small vessels, external compression, or interposition of a capillary bed (14,25). The pulmonary venous obstruction leads to early and often severe pulmonary hypertensive changes, manifested as medial hypertrophy of the pulmonary arteries

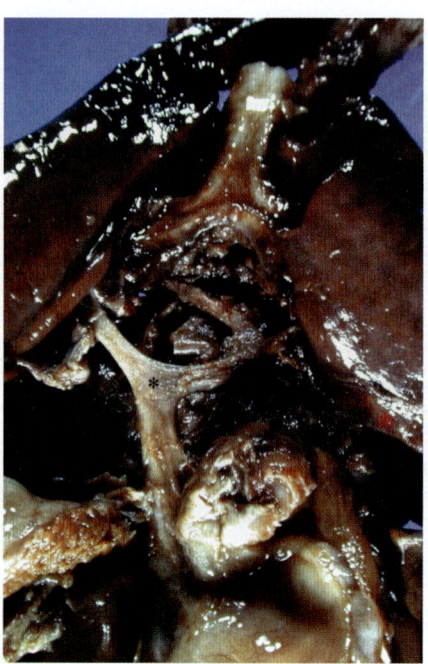

FIGURE 13-2 • Total anomalous pulmonary venous connection, infradiaphragmatic type, seen from the posterior view. A confluence of the pulmonary veins (*asterisk*) is isolated from the left atrium and drains into a vertical vein. This vein traverses the diaphragm to enter the portal venous system of the liver.

and veins combined with intimal proliferation and eventually arterialization in the pulmonary veins (25). Total anomalous pulmonary venous connection is associated with other cardiac anomalies in approximately one-third of cases, particularly with the heterotaxy syndromes (14,25). The clinical manifestations of total anomalous pulmonary venous connection vary with the degree of obstruction and the resultant PVR. With significant obstruction and high levels of resistance, cyanosis, heart failure, and death occur in the first months of life. With low resistance, infants may be asymptomatic at birth, and right-sided heart failure is the predominant manifestation (24). Surgical correction in the modern era yields more than 90% short-term survival with only rare late deaths, usually caused by pulmonary venous stenosis (24–26). In large series, risk factors for death include young age at surgery, cardiac or infracardiac connection sites, and preoperative pulmonary venous obstruction (26).

Pulmonary Vein Atresia/Stenosis

In pulmonary vein atresia, the entire pulmonary venous system drains into a common chamber from which there is no site for egress (14,24). In pulmonary vein stenosis, which is less severe, luminal narrowing occurs at the venoatrial junction of one or more of the pulmonary veins.

Cor Triatriatum

In cor triatriatum, the left atrium is partitioned by a fibromuscular shelf separating the pulmonary venous compartment from the atrial appendage and the mitral valve orifice compartment (14,24). The dividing membrane contains

TABLE 13-4	TOTAL ANOMALOUS PULMONARY VENOUS CONNECTION: CLASSIFICATION	
Site of Connection	% Total	% Obstructed
Supracardiac	45%	45%
Left innominate vein	25%–35%	
Right SVC	10%–15%	
Cardiac	25%	0%–20%
Coronary sinus	15%–20%	
Right atrium	5%–15%	
Infracardiac	25%	80%–90%
Portal vein	15%–25%	
Mixed	5%–10%	35%–60%

a variably sized opening, which results in most instances in pulmonary venous obstruction. The foramen ovale may open into either compartment; when the opening is proximal to the obstruction, it can function as an escape valve for the pulmonary venous obstruction (14,27).

Septal Malformations

Malformations of the Atrial Septum

The atrial septum forms from three distinct embryonic structures: the septum primum, endocardial cushions, and septum secundum (28). In the fetus, blood flows freely between the right and the left atria via the foramen ovale, bordered by the superior right-sided septum secundum (limbus of fossa ovalis) and the inferior left-sided septum primum (valve of fossa ovalis). This opening normally fuses during the first year of life. However, in 25% to 30% of people, this fusion never occurs, leaving a "probe-patent" or "valvular-competent" foramen ovale (29).

Atrial Septal Defect
ASD can occur in one or more of four sites (Figure 13-3; Table 13-5). A secundum ASD, the most common type, manifests as multiple perforations of, a deficiency in, or absence of the fossa ovalis flap valve (14,30). In patients with a probe-patent fossa ovalis, a secondary functional secundum ASD may appear following atrial dilatation. An isolated secundum ASD usually remains asymptomatic through childhood with 80% to 90% closing spontaneously, especially when of a small size (<4 mm diameter) (31). Defects greater than 8 mm, on the other hand, rarely close spontaneously, requiring surgical closure (31).

Primum defects, a form of AV septal defect, are discussed later. Sinus venosus defects result from a deficiency of the posterior superior aspect of the atrial wall that normally separates the right pulmonary veins from the superior vena cava/right atrium junction. A defect in this area therefore

TABLE 13-5	TYPES OF ATRIAL SEPTAL MALFORMATION
Septal defects	
Secundum ASD	
Primum ASD	
Sinus venosus ASD	
Coronary sinus ASD	
Single atrium (cor triloculare biventriculare)	
Premature closure of foramen ovale	

almost always occurs in conjunction with partial anomalous pulmonary venous return (32). Coronary sinus defects result from an unroofing or a fenestration of the coronary sinus on the posterior aspect of the left atrium and occur most often in association with a persistent left superior vena cava (LSVC) (21). Although most isolated ASDs occur sporadically, they can be inherited as an autosomal dominant anomaly with or without associated conduction system abnormalities (33,34).

Single Atrium
Complete absence of the atrial septum, a rare anomaly, results in a single atrial cavity, also termed *common atrium* or *cor triloculare biventriculare*. The single atrium usually accompanies other severe cardiac anomalies and is often associated with situs ambiguus (14).

Premature Closure of the Foramen Ovale
Premature closure of the foramen ovale manifests as a normally positioned but imperforate foramen ovale, an unidentifiable fossa ovalis, or an aneurysmal pouch bulging into the left atrium. The restricted mixing *in utero* can be complicated by hydrops fetalis and the hypoplastic left heart syndrome (14).

Malformations of the Ventricular Septum

The ventricular septum is a complex structure that can be divided into four components: inlet, trabecular, outlet, and membranous. From the right ventricular aspect, the inlet septum lies superiorly and posteriorly behind the septal tricuspid valve, the trabecular septum occupies the apex, the outlet septum sits between the crista supraventricularis and the pulmonary valve, and the membranous septum lies at the anteroseptal tricuspid commissure, where the tricuspid, mitral, and aortic valves converge (Figure 13-4). From the left ventricular aspect, the inlet septum lies posteriorly adjacent to the mitral valve, the trabecular septum occupies the apical region, the outlet septum sits beneath the right cusp of the aortic valve, and the membranous septum lies below the right and posterior aortic valve commissure (Figure 13-4).

VSDs, the most common type of congenital heart defect, can occur anywhere in the ventricular septum (35). VSDs are subclassified according to the nature of the defect rim and its anatomic position in the septum (Table 13-6).

Perimembranous (membranous, infracristal) defects account for up to 80% of VSDs (35). These defects are most easily seen from the left side, where they lie in the left

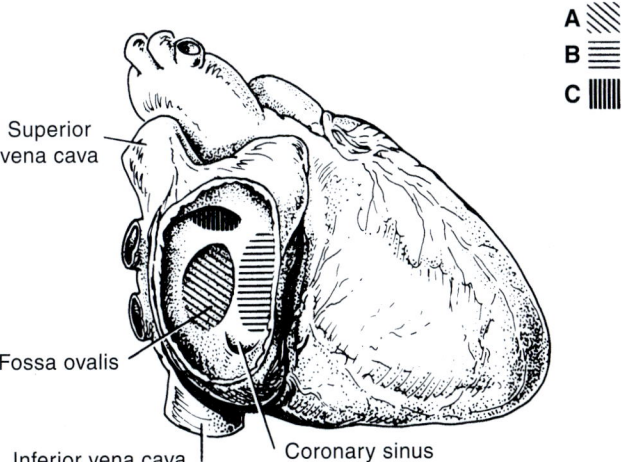

FIGURE 13-3 • The positions of various ASDs from the perspective of the right atrium, which has been opened laterally. **A:** Secundum defect. **B:** Primum defect. **C:** Sinus venosus defect.

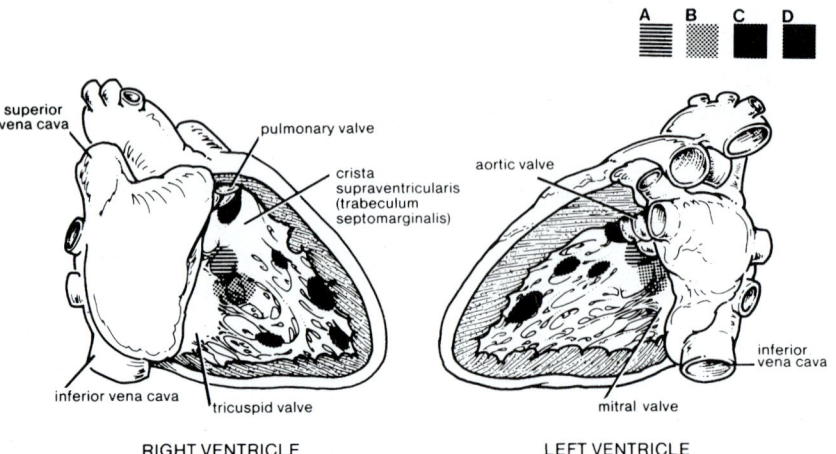

FIGURE 13-4 • The positions of the ventricular septal components and the corresponding VSTs from the lateral perspectives of the opened right and left ventricles. **A:** Membranous septum and perimembranous defect. **B:** Inlet septum and defect. **C:** Trabecular septum and trabecular muscular defects. **D:** Outlet septum and defect.

ventricular outflow tract just beneath the aortic valve (Figure 13-5). In the right ventricle, they reside beneath the crista supraventricularis and behind the papillary muscle of the conus, partially obscured by the septal leaflet of the tricuspid valve (36) (Figure 13-6).

Outlet (infundibular) defects account for 5% to 7% of VSDs in the Western world but nearly 30% of VSDs in Japan and the East Asia. These defects are often roofed by pulmonary and aortic valve tissue (i.e., doubly committed subarterial) (35,36) and can be complicated by prolapse of the right coronary cusp of the aortic valve into the defect or by aortic regurgitation. Outlet and occasionally perimembranous trabecular defects may be associated with malalignment between the outlet and the trabecular portions of the ventricular septum. Anterior malalignment results in aortic override and posterior malalignment results in pulmonic override. Either can be complicated by subaortic stenosis, often with associated arch anomalies (37).

Inlet defects, which account for 5% to 8% of VSDs, reside beneath the septal leaflet of the tricuspid valve, but posterior and inferior to the position of perimembranous trabecular defects. Although inlet defects are similar in location to the VSD component of AV septal defects, hearts with isolated inlet defects do not show the other characteristic features of AV septal defects (35).

Muscular trabecular defects, representing 5% to 20% of VSDs, can range in size from minuscule to physiologically significant and often occur as multiples (35).

Clinical manifestations of a VSD usually first appear at the age of 2 to 6 weeks, when the normal drop in PVR results in the onset of a harsh holosystolic murmur at the left sternal border. The size of the defect and the state of the PVR rather than the anatomic location of the defect determine the nature of the symptoms (Table 13-7). In VSDs with large shunts, congestive heart failure may be resistant to therapy, and the risk for pulmonary vascular obstructive disease is substantial (38).

TABLE 13-6	VENTRICULAR SEPTAL DEFECTS: CLASSIFICATION	
Defect Rim	Defect Location	Historical
Perimembranous	Inlet	Posterior AV canal
	Outlet	Supracristal Infundibular
	Trabecular	Membranous Infracristal
Muscular	Inlet	AV canal
	Outlet	Infundibular Subpulmonic Supracristal
	Central trabecular	Infracristal
	Remote trabecular	Muscular
Doubly committed subarterial	Outlet	Infundibular Supracristal

AV, atrioventricular.

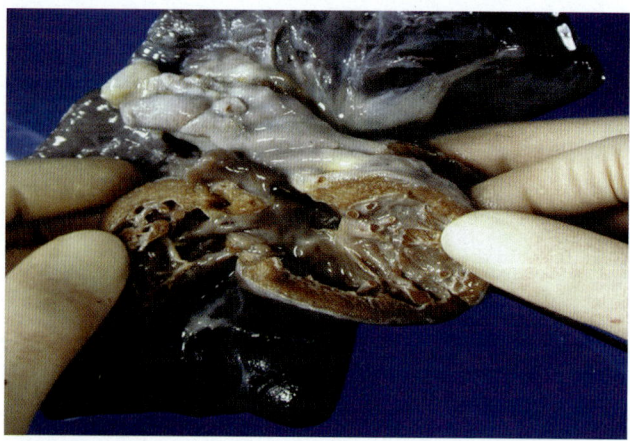

FIGURE 13-5 • Ventricular septal defect. An opened left ventricle with the free wall reflected laterally contains a perimembranous defect, visible in the outflow tract inferior to the aortic valve. The probe visible in the right ventricle in Figure 13-6 traverses the defect opening.

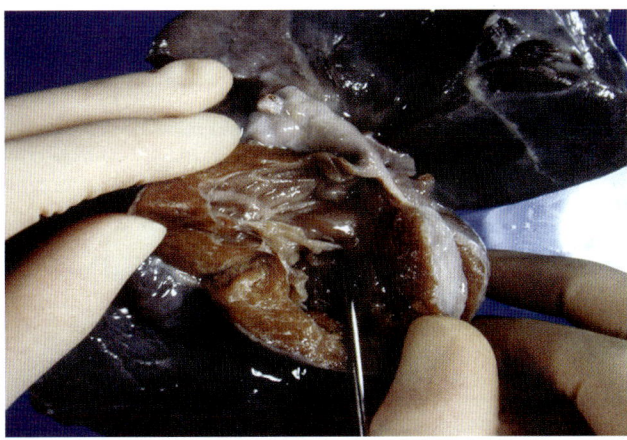

FIGURE 13-6 • Ventricular septal defect. An opened right ventricle with the free wall reflected superiorly contains a perimembranous defect hiding beneath the septal leaflet of the tricuspid valve. The probe traversing the defect is visible from the left ventricular aspect in Figure 13-5.

Spontaneous closure occurs in 25% to 40% of all VSDs and in up to 85% if the defect is small (38,39). Closure of membranous VSDs by overgrowth of fibrous connective tissue or adherence of the tricuspid valve septal leaflet can result in the formation of a ventricular septal "aneurysm." Ventricular septal aneurysms, with or without complete defect closure, are common in patients with VSD, usually appearing after 2 years of age (40).

The penetrating and branching bundles of the conduction system traverse the membranous portion of the ventricular septum (36,41). This relationship is of particular concern during the surgical repair of perimembranous and inlet defects. Anomalies in the conduction system or an ill-placed suture can result in postoperative bundle branch block or, rarely, sudden death (36).

Malformations of the Atrioventricular Septum

The AV septum is a structure at the crux of the heart that comprises the lower atrial septum and upper ventricular septum, including the atrioventricular valves (42). In the embryo, the AV septum forms at the site of fusion of the four endocardial cushions (43). The spectrum of lesions resulting from defects of the AV septum has been traditionally called *endocardial cushion defects* (Figure 13-7). AV septal defect displays the following features (42):

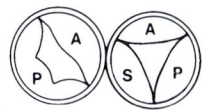
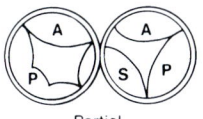
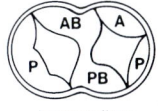
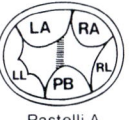
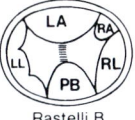
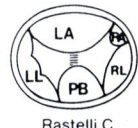

FIGURE 13-7 • Diagrammatic representation of the atrioventricular valves as viewed from the atria in a normal heart and with various atrioventricular septal defects. A, anterior leaflet; P, posterior leaflet; S, septal leaflet; AB, anterior bridging leaflet; PB, posterior bridging leaflet; LA, left anterior leaflet; RA, right anterior leaflet; RL, right lateral leaflet; LL, left lateral leaflet.

1. A decrement of tissue at the crest of the ventricular inlet, lending the inlet septum a "scooped out" appearance
2. Elongation of the left ventricular outflow tract, which creates the "gooseneck" deformity
3. Abnormal formation of the AV valves, with a characteristic "cleft" in the left-sided anterior leaflet

AV septal defects are subdivided into partial and complete forms, depending on the morphology of the AV valve leaflets.

Partial Atrioventricular Septal Defect
Partial AV septal defect is defined by the presence of two discrete AV valve annuli. Partial AV septal defects account for approximately one-third of cases (44). Most hearts in this group contain an ostium primum ASD (Figure 13-8) in conjunction with a cleft in the anterior mitral valve leaflet (42,44). The cleft mitral leaflet inserts, commissure-like, on the ventricular septum. The septal leaflet of the tricuspid valve displays variable degrees of deficiency. When both the mitral and the tricuspid valves are cleft, the

TABLE 13-7 VENTRICULAR SEPTAL DEFECTS: CLINICAL GROUPS

Group	Defect Size	Shunt	PVR	Complications	Prognosis/Therapy
1	Small	L→R	Nl	SBE	Spontaneous closure 75%–83%
2	Moderate	L→R	Nl	SBE CHF	Surgical closure required 15%–20%
3	Large	L→R	Nl Inc	SBE CHF	Surgical closure <2 years
4	Large	R→L	Inc	CHF Cyanosis	Inoperable

PVR, pulmonary vascular resistance; L→R, left to right; R→L, right to left; Nl, normal; Inc, increased; SBE, subacute bacterial endocarditis; CHF, congestive heart failure.

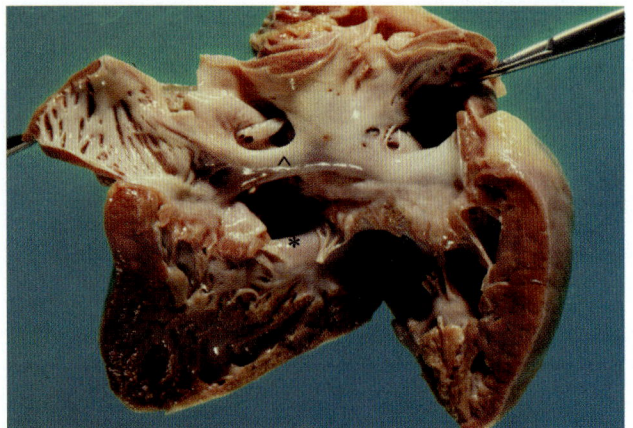

FIGURE 13-8 • Complete atrioventricular septal defect. A complete atrioventricular septal defect is readily visible centrally in this opened left atrium and ventricle. At the upper rim of the defect, a band of atrial septal tissue marked by the ^ separates the upper secundum ASD from the lower ostium primum ASD. The lower rim of the defect marked by the * represents the upper rim of the ventricular septum. The anterior and the posterior bridging leaflets of the common AV valve extend over the defect without chordal insertion.

Complete Atrioventricular Septal Defect

In the complete AV septal defect (*complete AV canal*) (Figure 13-8), the single AV orifice is guarded by five valve leaflets: posterior (inferior) bridging, right lateral, left lateral, right anterior, and left anterior (superior, bridging) (44). The complete AV septal defect is further subclassified according to the extent of septal bridging of the left anterior leaflet and the site of medial insertion:

Rastelli A: minimal bridging, attachment to right rim of septum or medial papillary muscle
Rastelli B: moderate bridging, attachment to an aberrant right apical papillary muscle
Rastelli C: marked bridging, attachment to the anterolateral papillary muscle of the right ventricle

Rastelli types A and C account for the vast majority of cases.

Additional cardiovascular anomalies occur in up to 50% of hearts with either partial or complete AV septal defects (45). The commonly associated anomalies vary in the different subtypes of AV septal defect, as outlined in Table 13-8. At least 50% of patients have trisomy 21 with a variety of other syndromes in another 25% including the heterotaxy syndromes in particular. The ventricles are "unbalanced" in approximately 10% of AV septal defects, with dominant right and dominant left ventricles occurring in nearly equal numbers (44). Clinically, the large left-to-right shunt precipitates severe congestive heart failure. Pulmonary hypertensive vascular changes can appear in the first year of life, further complicating the clinical picture (46). Early surgical repair, usually in the first year of life, is recommended.

valves insert, commissure-like, onto the rim of the ventricular septum; a connecting tongue of valve tissue covers the ventricular septum and closes the ring. The size of the defect in the ventricular septum also varies in these hearts, and in some cases, the valve leaflets may be less firmly adherent to the ventricular septum so that some interventricular shunting occurs (44).

TABLE 13-8 ATRIOVENTRICULAR SEPTAL DEFECTS: ASSOCIATED CARDIAC ANOMALIES AND SYNDROMES

Type AVSD	Relative Incidence (% of Total)[a]	Associated Syndrome[b]	Associated CV Anomalies[c]
Partial	35%	33% with trisomy 21	All AVSD:
Complete[d]	65%	48% with trisomy 21	Subaortic stenosis
			Coarctation of the aorta
			Patent ductus arteriosus
			Double-orifice mitral valve
			Parachute mitral valve
			Tetralogy of Fallot
			Double outlet right ventricle
			Common atrium
Rastelli A	55%–70%	Trisomy 21	Subaortic stenosis
Rastelli B	<10%	—	Valvular aortic stenosis
			Coarctation of aorta
			Hypoplastic left ventricle
Rastelli C	25%–40%	Heterotaxy	Tetralogy of Fallot
			Double-outlet right ventricle
			Common atrium

[a]See references (44,45,261–264).
[b]See references (44,261,263).
[c]See references (265–269).
[d]See references (45,265,270).
AVSD, atrioventricular septal defect; CV, cardiovascular.

TABLE 13-9	TYPES OF CONOTRUNCAL MALFORMATIONS

Transposition of the great vessels
    Complete transposition (D-transposition)
    Corrected transposition (L-transposition)
Double-outlet ventricles
    Double-outlet right ventricle
    Double-outlet left ventricle
Persistent truncus arteriosus
Aortopulmonary window (aortopulmonary septal defect)

D, dextro; L, levo.

Malformations of the Conus and Truncus

The conotruncal structures of the heart arise embryologically from the distal aspect of the heart tube and represent the outflow region of the developing heart. Embryologic research demonstrates the importance of cells derived from the neural crest in normal conotruncal development (47). This finding is reflected in humans by the close association between conotruncal malformations and the DiGeorge/velocardiofacial syndrome and its associated 22q11.2 chromosomal deletion (48). Table 13-9 outlines the spectrum of malformations that occur in the conotruncal region.

Transposition of the Great Vessels

In transposition of the great vessels, the aorta arises from the right ventricle and the pulmonary artery from the left ventricle (i.e., discordant ventriculoarterial connections). The transposed aorta thus originates in an anterior position, to either the right (dextrotransposition, or D-transposition) or the left (levotransposition, or L-transposition) of the pulmonary artery. Hearts with transposition are further classified according to their AV connection, as depicted in Figure 13-9.

Complete Transposition

Complete transposition, the most common form, accounts for 2.5% to 6.5% of all congenital heart malformations (see Table 13-16), with a 2:1 male predominance (49). The D-transposed aorta ascends parallel and to the right of the pulmonary artery rather than following its normal, twisted course (Figure 13-10). Internal examination reveals AV concordance with ventriculoarterial discordance (50). The aorta originates from the normally positioned morphologic right ventricle, with a muscular band separating the aortic and the tricuspid valves; the pulmonary artery arises posteriorly from the normally positioned morphologic left ventricle and is in fibrous continuity with the anterior mitral valve leaflet. The coronary arteries originate from one or both of the "facing sinuses" of the aorta (i.e., the sinuses adjacent to the pulmonary artery) (15,50). The anatomic course traversed by the coronary arteries varies considerably, a feature of significance when arterial switch surgery is planned (51,52).

A VSD accompanies the complete transposition in approximately 40% of cases, with 40% to 60% of the VSDs showing septal malalignment. Anterior (rightward) malalignment, present in 20% to 25% of cases with VSD, results in subaortic (right ventricular outflow tract) obstruction, often with associated coarctation (53). Pulmonary (left ventricular outflow tract) obstruction occurs in 25% to 30% of hearts with or without VSD, secondary to a malaligned VSD or subvalvular fibrous or fibromuscular tissue bundles (49,52,53).

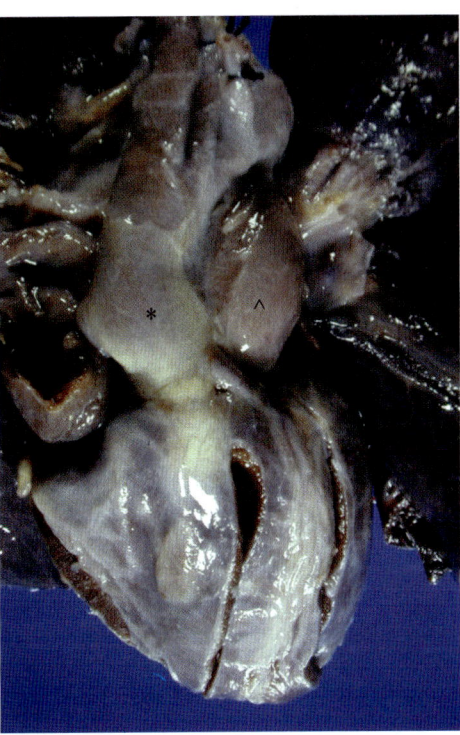

FIGURE 13-10 • Complete transposition of the great vessels from the anterior aspect of the heart. The aorta, marked with *, is situated to the right and slightly anterior to the pulmonary artery, marked with ^. The two vessels ascend in a parallel course.

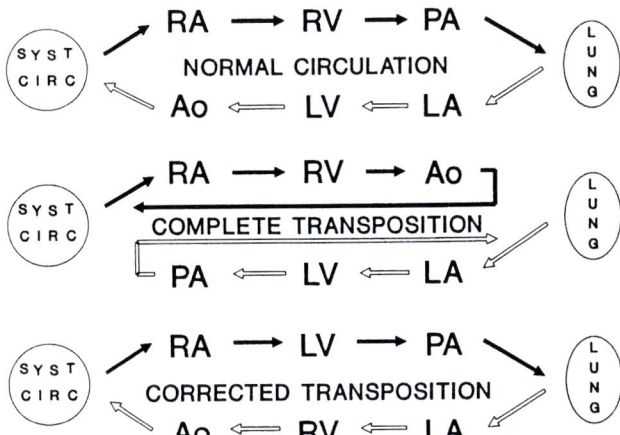

FIGURE 13-9 • Diagrammatic representation of normal blood flow (**top**), blood flow through complete transposition (**middle**), and blood flow through "corrected" transposition (**bottom**). Syst circ, systemic circulation; RA, right atrium; RV, right ventricle; PA, pulmonary artery; LA, left atrium; LV, left ventricle; Ao, aorta.

Corrected Transposition

In the much less common corrected transposition, also known as L-*transposition* or *ventricular inversion*, an L-transposed aorta ascends parallel to and to the left of the pulmonary artery. Internally, both AV and ventriculoarterial discordance are present. The right atrium is in continuity with a right-sided morphologic left ventricle from which the pulmonary artery arises; the left atrium is in continuity with a left-sided morphologic right ventricle from which the aorta originates; and blood flow is thus anatomically "corrected" (54) (Figure 13-9). The defect is frequently associated with other congenital anomalies, including tricuspid valve dysplasia, pulmonary outflow tract obstruction, and VSDs (54). AV discordance can occur with other types of ventriculoarterial connections, including DORV and ventriculoarterial concordance (55).

Double-Outlet Ventricle

Double-Outlet Right Ventricle

Of the two forms of double-outlet ventricle (Table 13-9), DORV is the more common, accounting for 1% to 1.5% of congenital heart defects (2). The term *DORV* denotes a heart in which both great vessels originate from the right ventricle. The strictest criterion requires that both great arteries arise exclusively from the right ventricle, with no fibrous continuity between the mitral and the outflow valves (56,57). A somewhat less strict criterion requires only that both great vessels arise exclusively from the right ventricle; 50% to 60% of such hearts display at least focal fibrous continuity between the mitral and

TABLE 13-10	DOUBLE-OUTLET RIGHT VENTRICLE: RELATIONSHIP OF GREAT ARTERIES	
Root of Ao Relative to Root of PA	Descriptive Terms	Ascending Ao and PA
Posterior and right	Normal or dextroposition	Spiral
Parallel and right	Side by side	Parallel
Anterior and right	D-malposition	Parallel
Anterior and left	L-malposition	Parallel

Ao, aorta; PA, pulmonary artery; D, dextro; L, levo.

the outflow valves (58,59). A VSD almost always accompanies the DORV, serving as the only site for left ventricular outflow. The variable location of the VSD relative to the pulmonary and aortic valves serves to define pathologic subcategories (56,57,60) (Figure 13-11). The anatomic relationship between the great arteries also varies, as outlined in Table 13-10. In earlier reports, the side-by-side relationship of the great arteries was described as the most frequent one, but more recent series describe the posterior normal pattern as the most common (56,58). The wide varieties of coronary artery anomalies that are associated with side-by-side or malposed great arteries affect surgical repair options and procedures (57,61).

The Taussig-Bing malformation, first described in 1949 (62), is an uncommon variant of DORV in which the VSD is subpulmonic and no pulmonary stenosis is present. When strict criteria are used, fewer than 10% of DORV are of the Taussig-Bing variant (56). When broader criteria are used ("a spectrum of anomalies unified by a juxtapulmonary VSD with malalignment of the infundibular septum"), some hearts can be classified both as the Taussig-Bing variant and as transposition of the great vessels with a malaligned VSD (59,62).

Various other cardiac malformations accompany many DORVs. Pulmonary infundibular stenosis with or without valvular stenosis occurs in 40% to 70% of hearts (56,58). ASDs are not uncommon; complete AV septal defects are less common (24). Left-sided inflow and outflow obstructive lesions may be accompanied by left ventricular hypoplasia (58).

The clinical presentation of DORV depends on the location of the VSD and the presence of associated malformations, particularly pulmonary stenosis (Table 13-11). Surgical correction varies depending on the anatomic configuration of the heart (57,61) (Table 13-11).

Double-Outlet Left Ventricle

DOLV is a rare malformation in which both great vessels arise predominantly from the morphologic left ventricle; a VSD accompanies the vast majority (63,64). Similar to DORV, the DOLV is classified by the location of the VSD relative to the great vessels (63). The DOLV with subaortic VSD is frequently complicated by pulmonary outflow tract

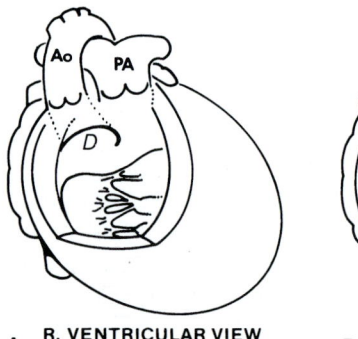
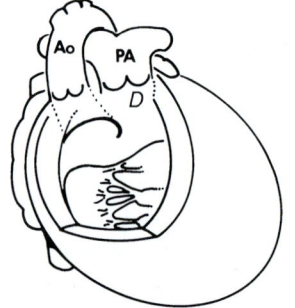
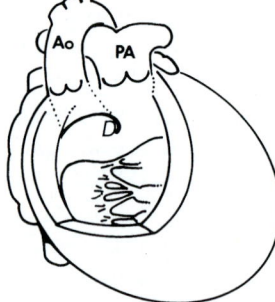
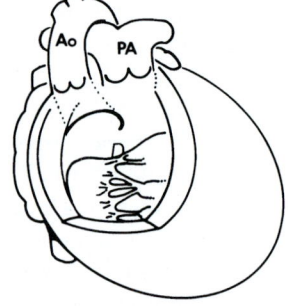

FIGURE 13-11 • The sites, D, of the VSDs in a DORV. **A:** Subaortic (60% to 65% of total cases). **B:** Subpulmonic (25% to 30%). **C:** Doubly committed (5% to 15%). **D:** Remote (10% to 15%). Ao, aorta; PA, pulmonary artery.

TABLE 13-11 DOUBLE-OUTLET RIGHT VENTRICLE: CLINICOPATHOLOGIC CATEGORIES

Clinical Type	VSD Location	RVOTO	LVOTO	Surgical Repair
VSD	Subaortic Doubly committed	Absent	Absent	Intraventricular tunnel
TOF	Subaortic Doubly committed	Present	Absent	TOF type
TGV	Subpulmonic (Taussig-Bing)	Absent	Often present	Arterial switch + VSD closure Intraventricular tunnel Damus-Kaye-Stansel
Remote VSD	Noncommitted	Absent	Often present	Intraventricular tunnel Single ventricle repair

VSD, ventricular septal defect; TOF, tetralogy of Fallot; TGV, transposition of the great vessels; RVOTO, right ventricular outflow tract obstruction; LVOTO, left ventricular outflow tract obstruction.

obstruction and DOLV with subpulmonic VSD by aortic outflow tract obstruction (63,64).

Persistent Truncus Arteriosus

Persistent truncus arteriosus is defined as a single arterial trunk that originates from a single semilunar valve and supplies the aorta, one or both pulmonary arteries, and the coronary arteries (Figure 13-12). The truncal valve is tricuspid in 50% to 70% of cases, quadricuspid in 25%, and bicuspid in most of the rest. The truncal vessel overlies and usually overrides an infundibular VSD, although occasionally, it is predominantly committed to one ventricular chamber. The truncal valve is always in fibrous continuity with the mitral valve; fibrous continuity may also be present between the truncal and tricuspid valves. The truncal valve leaflets are frequently thickened and myxomatous, with valvular insufficiency present in approximately 15% to 30%. The coronary arteries originate from the sinuses of the truncal valve in a variable pattern, with a single coronary artery present in 15% to 20% (65).

A classification devised by van Praagh creates a separate subtype for this latter finding and also acknowledges the rare case in which there is no VSD (66). The classification was subsequently revised by van Praagh to simplify the scheme in a surgically meaningful fashion (67) (Table 13-12).

Associated anomalies most frequently involve the aortic arch and include absent ductus arteriosus (>50%), right-sided aortic arch (20% to 35%), and interrupted aortic arch type B (10%) (65). Extracardiac anomalies, especially those related to DiGeorge syndrome, occur in 20% to 30%, and the DiGeorge syndrome–associated chromosome 22q11 deletion can be detected by fluorescence *in situ* hybridization (FISH) in 35% to 50% of infants with persistent truncus arteriosus (68,69).

The early clinical manifestation of congestive heart failure results from intracardiac shunting and markedly excessive pulmonary blood flow. The excessive pulmonary blood flow also produces rapidly progressive pulmonary hypertensive vascular disease; early surgical repair is therefore recommended.

Aortopulmonary Window

Aortopulmonary window, or *aortopulmonary septal defect*, is a rare malformation characterized by a defect in the vessel wall between the ascending aorta and the main pulmonary artery. The defect may lie proximally (just above the aortic and the pulmonary valves), distally (in the upper ascending aorta adjacent to the right pulmonary artery), or as a combined opening that involves the majority of the ascending aorta (14). Associated anomalies, present in more than 50% of cases, commonly include a VSD, interrupted aortic arch type A, and anomalous origin of one pulmonary artery from the ascending aorta (70). Although aortopulmonary window occurs in

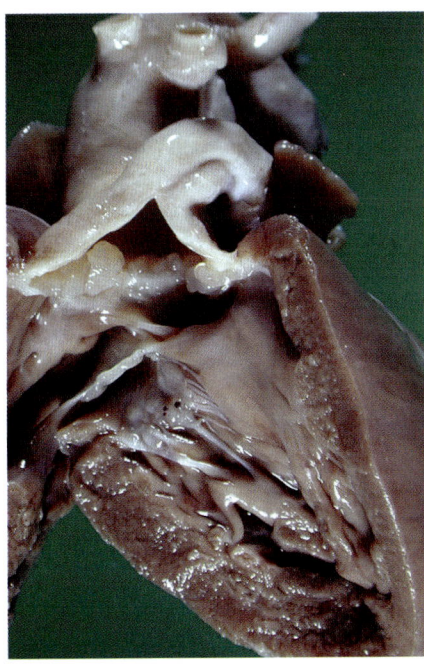

FIGURE 13-12 • Truncus arteriosus. The left ventricle free wall has been lifted to uncover the smooth-surfaced left ventricular outflow tract with a VSD opening at the top. Above the VSD lies a somewhat nodular truncus arteriosus valve. The main pulmonary artery almost immediately branches to the left from the common trunk; the aorta continues ascending posteriorly.

TABLE 13-12 TRUNCUS ARTERIOSUS CLASSIFICATION

Collett and Edwards	van Praagh	Modified van Praagh
Type 1 PAs arise as a single main artery and then divide.	*Type 1* PAs arise as a single main artery and then divide.	*Large aorta type* TA with confluent or near confluent PAs
Type 2 PAs arise separately but next to each other.	*Type 2* PAs arise separately.	
Type 3 PAs arise widely separated.		
	Type 3 One PA branch "absent" Arises from ductus or aorta	TA (large aorta type) with absence of one PA
	Type 4 Aortic arch hypoplastic or interrupted	*Large pulmonary artery type* TA with IAA or severe COTA
	Type A = VSD present	
	Type B = VSD absent	

PA, pulmonary artery; VSD, ventricular septal defect; TA, truncus arteriosus; IAA, interrupted aortic arch; COTA, coarctation of the aorta.

the same general region as persistent truncus arteriosus, it is not seen in the chromosome 22q11 deletion syndromes (70).

Malformations of the Ventricular Inflow Tracts

Tricuspid Valve Malformations

Tricuspid Atresia

Tricuspid atresia, in which the only outlet to the right atrium is via a patent fossa ovalis or an ASD, accounts for 1% to 1.5% of congenital heart malformations (5). The markedly hypoplastic right ventricle, positioned along the right anterosuperior border of the heart, has no inlet segment. The markedly dilated right atrium contains no grossly identifiable valvular tissue in more than 85% of cases (18,71). A dimple in the muscular atrial floor, presumably marking the site of the missing valve, may have a fibrous attachment to the right ventricle but often is instead in continuity with the left ventricle by transillumination and pinprick studies (18). The remaining 5% to 15% of hearts display a tricuspid valve remnant in the form of an imperforate fibrous membrane. A muscular VSD, termed the *outlet foramen*, allows communication between the dominant left ventricular chamber and the rudimentary right ventricle; however, the VSD or the infundibular outflow tract may be restrictive (71).

Tricuspid atresia is subclassified according to the size of the VSD, concordance or discordance of the great vessels, and the presence or absence of pulmonary stenosis/atresia (Table 13-13). The clinical symptoms depend on these anatomic variables; more than 50% of cases present with cyanosis and murmur in the newborn period (72). In the vast majority of hearts, the right ventricle is too small to function adequately as a pumping chamber, and univentricular repair is required.

Ebstein Malformation

Ebstein malformation accounts for less than 1% of all cases of CHD but is the most common cause of isolated tricuspid stenosis or insufficiency (2,73). It is characterized by adherence of variable portions of the septal and posterior tricuspid valve leaflets to the right ventricular wall, with "atrialization" (i.e., downward displacement of the functional annulus) of a portion of the right ventricle (Figure 13-13) (73,74). The anterior valve annulus insertion is normally positioned, with a large, redundant, and often muscularized leaflet. The margin of the leaflet may be attached to the posteroinferior right ventricular wall and produce obstruction and in some cases complete occlusion of the AV orifice (Figure 13-14) (74). Tricuspid regurgitation occurs across the dilated AV junction (true annulus). Right-to-left shunting across a patent fossa ovalis or ASD and supraventricular arrhythmias due to accessory conduction pathways frequently complicate Ebstein malformation. A variety of

TABLE 13-13 TRICUSPID ATRESIA: CLINICAL CLASSIFICATION

I. Normally related great vessels (60%–70%)
   A. Intact ventricular septum with pulmonary atresia
   B. Small VSD with pulmonary stenosis
   C. Large VSD without pulmonary stenosis
II. D-transposition of the great arteries (25%–30%)
   A. VSD with pulmonary atresia
   B. VSD with pulmonary stenosis
   C. VSD without pulmonary stenosis
II. Malposition other than D-transposition of the great arteries (5%)

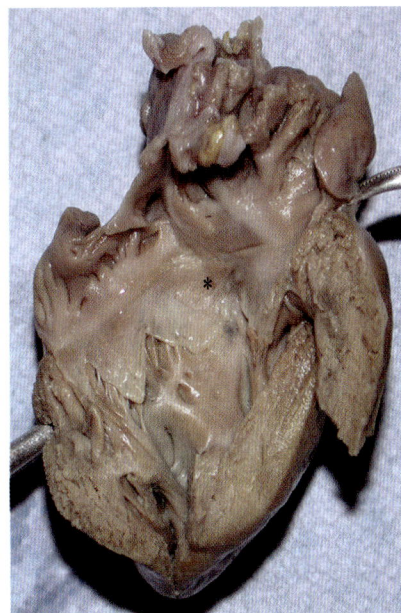

FIGURE 13-13 • Mild form of Ebstein anomaly. The opened right atrium and right ventricle display a markedly thickened ventricular wall. The septal (*asterisk*) and posterior leaflets of the tricuspid valve are fixed to the underlying ventricular wall.

other associated cardiovascular defects, most commonly pulmonary valvular stenosis, pulmonary atresia, or a VSD, occur in 30% to 40% of cases (73,75).

Given the broad range of anatomic alterations encompassed by Ebstein malformation, it is not surprising to find a broad range of clinical manifestations for the disorder. One-third to one-half of patients present in the newborn period with cyanosis and a murmur; the mortality rate among such infants is high, particularly when the malformation is associated with additional cardiac anomalies (73). In many patients, however, the diagnosis is delayed until the second decade of life or later, when arrhythmias often represent the major clinical problem (73,75).

Mitral Valve Malformations

Mitral Stenosis

The normal mitral valve apparatus is a complex structure with four primary components: annulus, anterior and posterior valve leaflets, chordae tendineae, and anterolateral and posteromedial papillary muscles. A variety of malformations affecting any or all of the valve components result in congenital mitral stenosis and insufficiency (76) (Table 13-14). A supramitral ring, a ridge of connective tissue at the atrial surface of the mitral leaflets, usually occurs with deformities of the mitral valve apparatus (77). Valve hypoplasia, in which the valve components are small but otherwise normally formed, is most commonly associated with left ventricle hypoplasia, VSDs, and coarctation of the aorta (COTA) (14,77). The "typical" mitral stenosis manifests as lesions at both the valvular and the subvalvular areas including valve dysplasia with commissure fusion, obliteration of the intrachordal spaces, and shortening of the chordae tendineae and papillary muscles. Associated malformations include tetralogy of Fallot (TOF), COTA, and subaortic stenosis with a near-normal–sized left ventricle (14,77). The double-orifice mitral valve results when excessive valve tissue bridges between the anterior and posterior valve leaflets to create two, usually unequally sized, orifices, both supported by chordal attachments that insert into often abnormally positioned papillary muscle. The double-orifice valve almost always occurs in company with other cardiac malformations, especially AV septal defects (approximately 50% of cases) or left-sided obstructive lesions (40%) (78). Two forms of cleft mitral valve without associated primum ASD or VSD have been described (78):

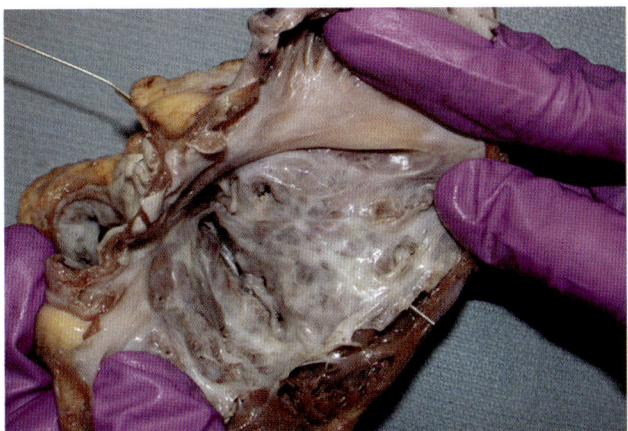

FIGURE 13-14 • Severe form of Ebstein anomaly. The opened right atrium uncovers a markedly enlarged and dysplastic anterior tricuspid leaflet attached to the apical myocardium by tiny chordae. A probe placed in the pulmonary artery traverses the remaining right ventricular cavity and appears at the base of this dysplastic valve, illustrating the severe obstruction to pulmonary inflow and outflow created by this defect.

TABLE 13-14 MITRAL VALVE MALFORMATIONS

Supravalvular lesions
  Supramitral ring
Valvular lesions
  Valve hypoplasia
  Valve dysplasia
    Commissural fusion
    Valve leaflet excess or agenesis
  Double-orifice valve
  Cleft mitral valve
Subvalvular lesions
  Parachute deformity (single papillary muscle)
  Funnel deformity (shortened fused chordae)
  Arcade deformity (papillary muscle fused with valve)
Mixed
  Shone syndrome

1. Associated with normally related great vessels and a shortened inlet septum (i.e., forme fruste of an AV septal defect)
2. Associated with TGA or DORV and a normal inlet septum

Parachute deformity of the mitral valve, defined as insertion of all the chordae into a single papillary muscle group, also usually occurs with other malformations of the heart, particularly VSDs and obstructive lesions of the aortic valve and arch (14,77,79). The eponym *Shone syndrome* denotes the association of a parachute mitral valve with a supramitral ring, subaortic stenosis, and COTA (79,80).

Mitral Atresia
Mitral atresia, defined as the absence of a left AV connection, is marked on the left atrial aspect by muscular atrial floor with or without a visible dimple or, less commonly, by an imperforate membrane (14,81,82). The microscopic examination of hearts with no grossly obvious membrane between the left atrium and the left ventricle uniformly reveals a fibrous connection at the presumed site of the absent valve (81). The outlet for pulmonary venous return is by way of a patent fossa ovalis or less commonly an ASD (14). Rarely, the fossa ovalis is prematurely closed, and pulmonary venous return is shunted to the right side of the heart by anomalous venous connections (14,83). When the great vessels are normally related, mitral atresia is most commonly associated with aortic atresia and, as such, is included in the hypoplastic left heart syndrome. The left ventricle exists as a diminutive chamber lined by translucent endocardium, which in some cases is evident only on microscopic examination of the posterosuperior aspect of the hypertrophic right ventricle (14,82). Less often, a VSD is present and a patent aortic valve arises from either the right (DORV) or the left ventricular chamber (14,82).

Floppy Mitral Valve
Floppy mitral valve represents the central defect in the floppy mitral valve (FMV)/mitral valve prolapse (MVP)/mitral valve regurgitation (MVR) triad. The primary defect in the "floppy" valve is deposition of acid mucopolysaccharides and dissolution of the collagen in the pars spongiosa and fibrosa of the valve (84). The accumulation of myxoid material leads to thickened and enlarged valve leaflets often with increased chordal insertions on the ventricular surface, elongation of the chordae tendineae, and dilatation of the valve annulus (84). With prolapse, the valve becomes "hooded," defined as the presence of ballooning to a height of at least 4 mm and involving at least one-half of the anterior or two-thirds of the posterior mitral leaflets (85). The myxomatous degeneration in the valve leaflets is without inflammation and does not lead to fusion of the valve commissures, distinguishing these valvular changes from those of rheumatic fever (RF). Similar myxomatous changes occur elsewhere in the heart, including the conduction system, a feature that likely explains the associated arrhythmias and the conduction defects.

The reported incidence of FMV/MVP/MVR varies considerably, with less than 1% to 5% of children exhibiting clinical or echocardiographic features of MVP (86). In the pediatric population, the incidence increases with age; MVP is extremely rare before 2 years of age. Most children are asymptomatic, presenting with the characteristic late systolic "click" on auscultation; an occasional child presents with chest pain of unclear etiology (86). Skeletal anomalies, especially pectus excavatum, are common (87). The 2:1 female predominance described in adults is also observed in some but not all groups of children studied (86). Progressive MVR, a major problem in adults with FMV, occurs rarely during childhood. Other complications, including infectious endocarditis, thromboembolism, arrhythmias, and even sudden death, do occur occasionally in the pediatric population (86).

Univentricular Atrioventricular Connection

The term *univentricular AV connection* denotes the connection of the AV valves to a single ventricular cavity (82). Table 13-15 lists at least some of the terms previously used for this condition and outlines the range of anomalies encompassed. The anatomy of such hearts can be highly complex and variable, so that sequential segmental analysis is an essential tool for accurate classification (82).

Double-Inlet Ventricle
In double-inlet left ventricle, the most common of the double-inlet malformations, both the left and right AV valves open into a dominant left ventricular cavity (88). The rudimentary right ventricle occupies the right anterosuperior border of a normally related, D-looped left ventricle or the left anterosuperior border of an inverted, L-looped left ventricle. The rudimentary right ventricle communicates with the dominant left ventricle via a variably sized VSD. The great vessels are

TABLE 13-15 UNIVENTRICULAR ATRIOVENTRICULAR CONNECTION

Common synonyms
  Single ventricle
  Common ventricle
  Holmes heart
  Univentricular heart
  Cor triloculare biatriatum
  Primitive ventricle
Anatomic subtypes
  Double-inlet ventricle
    Double-inlet left ventricle
    Double-inlet right ventricle
    Double-inlet ventricle of mixed morphology (absent ventricular septum)
    Double-inlet ventricle of indeterminate morphology
  Single-inlet ventricle
    Mitral atresia
    Tricuspid atresia
  Common-inlet ventricle
  Overriding atrioventricular valves

transposed in the vast majority of cases but may be normally related, atretic, or in a double-outlet configuration.

Common-Inlet Ventricle

In common-inlet ventricle, both atria communicate with a single ventricle via a common AV valve (88). Many of these hearts represent the extreme form of unbalanced AV septal defect and thus include a dominant right or left ventricular cavity and a rudimentary second ventricle. Less often, the common AV valve communicates with a single ventricular chamber of indeterminate type without an identifiable rudimentary ventricle. These hearts frequently have abnormal ventriculoarterial connections as well.

Straddling and Overriding Atrioventricular Valves

An AV valve annulus may override, or its chordal insertion may straddle, the ventricular septum (88,89). In hearts with valve annulus override, the AV connection is assigned to the ventricle to which more than 50% of the valve annulus is attached. Straddling of the chordae without valve annulus override does not change the AV connection designation.

Malformations of the Ventricular Outflow Tracts

Pulmonary Outflow Tract and Valve Malformations

Tetralogy of Fallot

TOF accounts for 3.5% to 10.5% of all CHD and represents the most common cyanotic CHD. In approximately 33% of cases, four components comprise the TOF: infundibular pulmonic stenosis, VSD, aortic valve dextroposition, and right ventricular hypertrophy (Figure 13-15). All of these anatomic components are a consequence of a single embryologic abnormality, anterosuperior malalignment of the outlet septum (Figures 13-15 and 13-16). The morphologic detail surrounding these four components can vary considerably (14,90,91). Infundibular pulmonic stenosis leads to decreased pulmonary blood flow with an associated small pulmonary artery (Figure 13-16). Over time, the stenosis becomes exacerbated by hypertrophy of the infundibular septum or cristal structures (91). The invariably large and nonrestrictive VSD is perimembranous in 75% of cases, located in the muscular outlet in 20%, and subarterial only rarely (90,91). The degree of aortic override varies from 15% to 95%. In the extreme situation, the differentiation of TOF from DORV depends on the presence of the characteristic infundibular stenosis and fibrous continuity between the aortic and mitral valves; some investigators classify hearts with more than 50% aortic override as TOF with DORV (59).

The pulmonary valve is abnormal in 66% to 75% of cases. It is most often bicuspid but may be unicuspid or stenotic by virtue of thickened dysplastic valve leaflets (14,90,91). The 20% to 25% of cases with an imperforate pulmonary valve orifice are classified as pulmonary atresia with VSD, discussed in more detail later. The pulmonary arteries show a range of accompanying abnormalities that include localized stenosis at the origin of the pulmonary artery branches, central pulmonary

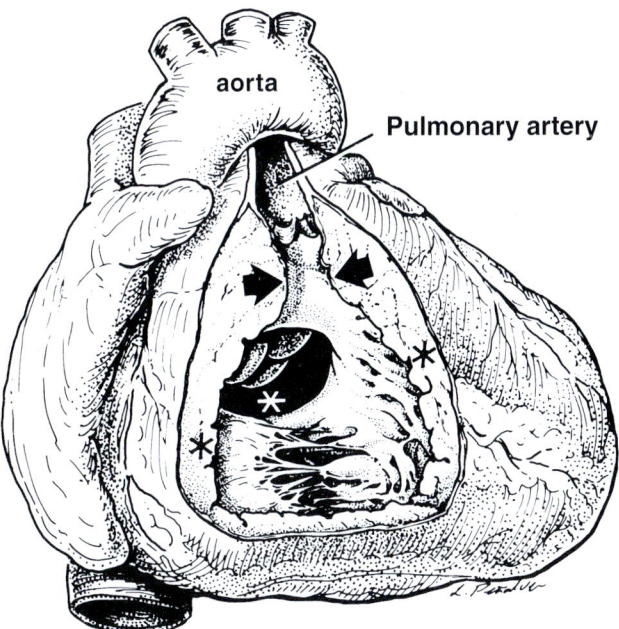

FIGURE 13-15 • An opened anterior right ventricle illustrates the four primary features of TOF: marked narrowing of the pulmonary infundibulum (between *arrows*); a large perimembranous VSD (*white asterisk*); dextroposed overriding aorta, visible through the VSD; and hypertrophy of the right ventricular myocardium (*black asterisk*).

artery discontinuity, absent left pulmonary artery branch, and pulmonary hilar artery hypoplasia (91,92). When the pulmonary artery stenosis is severe, pulmonary artery hypertension may develop after surgical repair of the TOF (93). In 3% to 6% of cases, the pulmonary valve is absent and the pulmonary arteries are dilated; this dilatation may be significant.

A variety of other cardiovascular defects occur with TOF. TOF occurs as part of a recognizable syndrome, most commonly DiGeorge syndrome or trisomy 21 (92). Commonly associated anomalies include right-sided aortic arch (20% to 30%) and absent ductus arteriosus (20% to 25%) (92). Although a patent fossa ovalis occurs commonly in infants with TOF, a true ASD is present in only 20% to 25%.

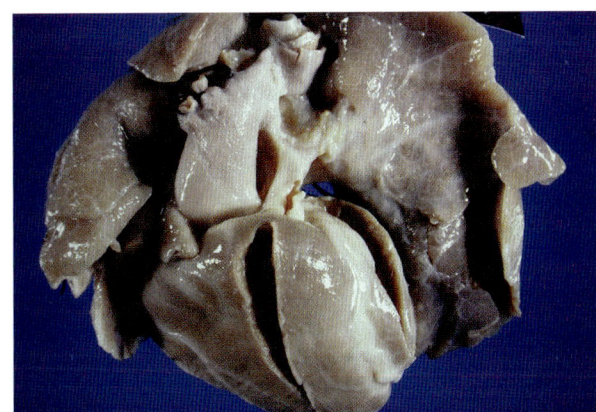

FIGURE 13-16 • Heart and lungs removed at autopsy with an unrepaired TOF. An incision through the anterior right ventricle ends at the base of a small pulmonary artery. The markedly enlarged aorta arises behind and to the right of the pulmonary artery.

A complete AV septal defect accompanies TOF in 1% to 2% of cases, most often in children with trisomy 21.

Hypoxia and cyanosis are the principal symptoms of TOF, their severity varying with the degree of pulmonary obstruction (92). In the presence of marked stenosis or atresia, cyanosis is evident in the neonatal period. More commonly, cyanosis appears in the first 6 months of life, associated with increasing infundibular stenosis.

Pulmonary Atresia with Ventricular Septal Defect
Although the designation pulmonary atresia (PA) with VSD (PA/VSD) is frequently used as a synonym for TOF with PA, not all hearts with PA/VSD display the hypoplastic right ventricular infundibulum characteristic of TOF (94). Most commonly, a dimple (more rarely recognizable fused bicuspid valve cusps) marks the site of the pulmonary valve. Abnormalities of the pulmonary arteries include a connection of confluent, bilateral pulmonary arteries to the right ventricle by an atretic cord, absence of the left pulmonary artery, and absence of all intrapericardial pulmonary arteries (95). This latter group was classified as truncus arteriosus type IV in the past. The ductus arteriosus supplies blood to one or both of the pulmonary arteries in 40% to 65% of cases. The lungs also receive blood via collateral arteries that originate from the descending aorta and supply the pulmonary arteries via intrapulmonary, hilar, or extrapulmonary anastomoses (95). Chromosome 22q11 deletion increases the likelihood of an absent ductus arteriosus and a major aortopulmonary collateral artery supply. With a major aortopulmonary collateral artery supply, hypoplasia and arborization of the pulmonary arteries make surgical management problematic (96).

Absent Pulmonary Valve
Absent pulmonary valve is a rare anomaly usually associated with TOF (97). At the site of the expected valve, a narrow valve annulus is rimmed by rudimentary, nodular, gelatinous tissue with massive poststenotic dilatation (97). More complex pulmonary artery anomalies, including discontinuity of the main pulmonary arteries, anomalous origin of the pulmonary arteries, and absence of the left pulmonary artery, occur less often (97,98). The ductus arteriosus is frequently absent (50). Dilated pulmonary arteries can compress the adjacent bronchi and cause respiratory compromise; abnormalities of the intrapulmonary arteries and bronchi may exacerbate these pulmonary problems (98).

Pulmonary Stenosis with Intact Ventricular Septum
Pulmonary stenosis with intact ventricular septum (IVS) accounts for 2.5% to 9.0% of all cases of CHD (Table 13-16). The obstruction is usually valvular, with secondary right ventricular hypertrophy and poststenotic dilatation of the pulmonary trunk. The valve is most often dome-shaped with fused cusps and a single central orifice, but it may be unicuspid, bicuspid, or tricuspid with partially fused commissures (99,100). Thickened dysplastic valve leaflets with nonfused cusps occur sporadically and as one form of pulmonary

TABLE 13-16 PREVALENCE OF CONGENITAL HEART DEFECTS

Type	Range (%)[a]	M:F
VSD	30–52	1:1
PDA	2.5–8.5	1:2
TOF	3.5–10.5	1:1
COTA	4.5–6.5	3:2
TGA	2.5–6.5	2:1
ASD	6.0–8.0	1:2
PS-IVS	2.5–9.0	1:1
AVSD	1.5–9.5	2:3
HLHS	2.0–5.0	3:2
AS	3.0–6.0	2:1

[a]Percentage of total for ten most common defects; see references (39,271–278).

VSD, ventricular septal defect; PDA, patent ductus arteriosus; TOF, tetralogy of Fallot; COTA, coarctation of the aorta; TGA, transposition of the great arteries; ASD, atrial septal defect; PS-IVS, pulmonary stenosis with intact ventricular septum; AVSD, atrioventricular septal defect; HLHS, hypoplastic left heart syndrome; AS, aortic stenosis.

stenosis in Noonan syndrome. The pulmonary artery trunk usually exhibits poststenotic dilatation; pulmonary artery hypoplasia is rare even with critical stenosis. Symptoms depend on the severity of the stenosis. Critical stenosis, presenting as cyanosis in infancy, requires early intervention (100). More commonly, infants are asymptomatic; stenosis develops and worsens in early childhood in approximately 15%, and many remain asymptomatic into adulthood. Secondary infundibular stenosis due to right ventricular hypertrophy can further complicate the course over time (101).

Subvalvular Stenosis
Pulmonary subvalvular or infundibular stenosis, which accounts for fewer than 10% of cases of pulmonary stenosis with IVS, occurs when fibrous thickening at the junction of the trabecular and outlet segments divides the right ventricle into two chambers; it may also be caused by tubular hypoplasia of the infundibulum (14). Double-chamber right ventricle is a closely related anomaly in which hypertrophied muscle bands cross the right ventricular cavity just proximal to the infundibulum and divide a high-pressure proximal chamber from a low-pressure infundibular chamber. The majority of hearts with double-chamber right ventricle exhibit other anomalies, most often (65% to 75%) a VSD (102).

Supravalvular and Peripheral Pulmonary Artery Stenosis
Supravalvular or pulmonary artery stenosis occurs as a localized area of narrowing in the pulmonary trunk or branch or as multiple areas of narrowing throughout the pulmonary artery tree (103,104). The stenosis is subclassified into four types, based on the site of the obstruction, with type III accounting

TABLE 13-17	SUPRAVALVULAR AND PERIPHERAL PULMONARY ARTERY STENOSIS

Type I Single central stenosis of:
  A Main pulmonary artery
  B Right main pulmonary artery
  C Left main pulmonary artery
Type II Bifurcation stenosis
  A Short, localized stenosis
  B Long, narrow segments of stenosis
Type III Multiple stenoses of peripheral segmental arteries
Type IV Multiple stenoses of peripheral and central arteries

for approximately one-third of cases (104) (Table 13-17). Associated cardiac malformations, present in approximately 66% of cases, include VSD, ASD, valvular pulmonary stenosis, and TOF (104,105). A variety of malformation syndromes include pulmonary artery stenosis (Table 13-18).

Pulmonary Atresia with Intact Ventricular Septum
PA with IVS accounts for 1% to 3% of all cases of CHD. The atresia is usually valvular, with a fibrous membrane containing commissural lines present at the expected site of the valve (14,106). The pulmonary artery is funnel-shaped and usually only mildly to moderately hypoplastic (14,106). The right ventricular myocardium is hypertrophied and the cavity of variable size, with the size of the tricuspid valve directly related to the size of the right ventricle. The right ventricle and tricuspid valve are usually small, often with associated pulmonary infundibular stenosis or atresia (106,107). Right ventricle–coronary artery fistulas develop in more than 50% of hearts with small ventricular cavities; in a subgroup of these hearts, the volume of flow through the fistula results in right ventricle–dependent coronary blood flow. Accompanying coronary artery luminal stenosis and vessel atrophy proximal to the fistula site can result in myocardial ischemia and sudden death (108). At the opposite extreme, the right ventricular cavity may be dilated, with the tricuspid valve showing dysplasia and often Ebsteinization (106,107).

TABLE 13-18	PULMONARY ARTERY STENOSIS–ASSOCIATED MALFORMATION SYNDROMES	
Syndrome	Location of Stenosis	References
Rubella	Peripheral pulmonary arteries	(279)
Williams	Peripheral pulmonary arteries	(267,280)
Alagille	Peripheral pulmonary arteries	(281)
Noonan	Main pulmonary artery	(282)

PA with IVS is a severe form of CHD in which pulmonary blood flow depends on a patent ductus arteriosus. The definitive surgical management varies according to the degree of right ventricular hypoplasia, the presence and severity of coronary artery fistula, and the status of the tricuspid valve with options including a variety of outflow tract ("biventricular") repairs, univentricular repair, or transplantation (106,109).

Aortic Outflow Tract and Valve Malformations

Aortic Valvular Stenosis
The left ventricular outflow tract may be obstructed at any level, but the most common form of obstruction is aortic valvular stenosis. The spectrum of abnormal valvular morphology is similar to that in pulmonary valvular stenosis, but a bicuspid valve is the most common form (14,110). Bicuspid aortic valves are not congenitally stenotic and many remain asymptomatic throughout childhood, with a significant subset progressing quickly to significant stenosis requiring intervention. Unicommissural and the less common tricuspid dysplastic and dome-shaped valves are stenotic from birth and therefore more likely to be symptomatic in early childhood. With congenitally stenotic valves, the left ventricle may be dilated, normal in size, or hypoplastic. In infants with severe stenosis, endocardial fibroelastosis (EFE) and subendocardial ischemic damage often further complicate the picture (110). COTA commonly accompanies a congenitally malformed aortic valve in two clinical settings: critical aortic stenosis (110) and bicuspid valves related to Turner syndrome.

Subvalvular Aortic Stenosis
Discrete subvalvular aortic stenosis most frequently takes the form of a fibroelastic diaphragm just beneath the base of the aortic valve; less common forms include a thickened diaphragm with a muscular base or a tunnellike narrowing of the outflow tract (14,111). Commonly associated heart defects, present in 50% to 75% of cases, include a malaligned VSD, aortic valvular stenosis or regurgitation, aortic coarctation, and AV septal defects (110,111). These subaortic lesions rarely present in infancy, and current theories consider them to be acquired progressively, perhaps on the framework of an underlying subtle deformation of the outflow tract (111,112).

Supravalvular Aortic Stenosis
Supravalvular aortic stenosis occurs in three forms (113,114):

1. An hourglass deformity caused by a constrictive annular ridge at the superior margin of the sinuses of Valsalva (66%)
2. A discrete fibromuscular membrane with a central opening in the lumen of the aorta (12%)
3. A diffuse hypoplasia of the ascending aorta with involvement of the arch and the branches (23%)

The coronary arteries may also be involved in the process, with ostial stenosis or luminal narrowing resulting in myocardial ischemia or even sudden death (113). Supravalvular aortic stenosis occurs sporadically but may also be familial or part of the Williams syndrome (115).

Aortic Atresia

Aortic atresia, the most common defect seen in the hypoplastic left heart syndrome (116), shows a 2:1 to 3:1 male predominance (14,116,117). In isolated aortic atresia, the mitral valve and the left ventricular cavity are hypoplastic, with secondary left ventricular EFE and myocardial hypertrophy (116). In the 30% to 50% of cases with associated mitral atresia, the left ventricle is diminutively (Figure 13-17) visible only on serial sections or definitively identified only on microscopic examination (116,117). VSDs, present in fewer than 10% of cases, may on the other hand be associated with a more normally sized ventricular cavity, with or without EFE (14,117). The site of the aortic valve may be invisible, or the valve may be represented by an imperforate membrane (116). The ascending aorta is represented by a narrow vessel functioning as a conduit to the coronary arteries, which arise normally. In 60% to 80% of cases, a discrete COTA is present (117). The descending aorta may then appear to arise from the ductus arteriosus, which is widely patent in most cases (117). Coronary artery changes and ventricle–coronary artery connections, similar to those complicating PA, have been described in the left coronary artery and ventricle of hearts with aortic atresia and mitral stenosis.

Hypoplastic Left Heart Syndrome

Hypoplastic left heart syndrome is a clinicopathologic condition in which underdevelopment of the left side of the heart and the ascending aorta results in obstruction to the pulmonary venous outflow and dependence on a patent ductus arteriosus for adequate systemic blood flow. Without surgical intervention, severe congestive heart failure and death invariably ensue, usually in the first 2 months of life (2). The uniform right atrial and ventricular enlargement combined with the small left ventricle, ascending aorta, and aortic arch gives these hearts a characteristic external appearance (116) (Figure 13-18). Pulmonary venous outflow depends on a left-to-right shunt across the atrial septum, usually via a patent fossa ovalis or secundum ASD (14). However, hypoplastic left heart syndrome is associated with and possibly caused by premature closure of the foramen ovale in 5% to 10% of cases; in this situation, the pulmonary venous return must be shunted to the right side of the heart via anomalous venous connections or intramyocardial sinusoids (83,117). The closed fossa ovalis worsens the already present pulmonary venous obstruction and predisposes an infant to significant pulmonary hypertension early in life. Stenotic or atretic mitral and aortic valves, with or without COTA, are the usual malformations resulting in hypoplastic left heart syndrome (116). Staged surgical correction of the hypoplastic left heart syndrome (Table 13-19) and neonatal cardiac transplantation have dramatically improved the outlook for infants with this otherwise uniformly fatal disorder (118).

Malformations of the Aortic Arch System

Ductus Arteriosus

The ductus arteriosus differs from the aorta and pulmonary arteries in that its media is formed predominantly of smooth muscle layers (119,120). Control of ductus patency during

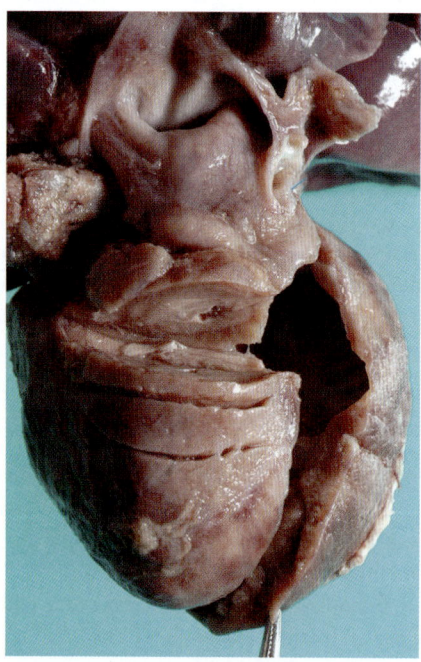

FIGURE 13-17 • Posterior view of a heart removed at autopsy with mitral atresia and a hypoplastic left ventricle. At the left, an incision opens into the large dilated right ventricle. Serial transverse sections across the thick posterior wall of the right atrium reveal a tiny opening just beneath an atretic mitral valve that represents the residuum of the left ventricle.

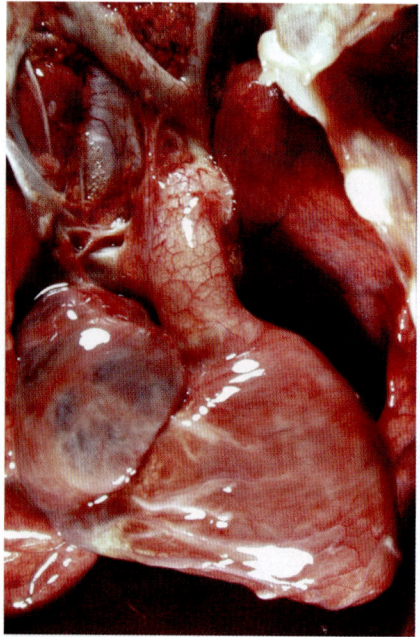

FIGURE 13-18 • External view of a heart with hypoplastic left heart syndrome, as seen from the anterior aspect. A dilated right atrial appendage hugs the large pulmonary artery and atrioventricular groove. A large right ventricle occupies the entire anterior ventricular surface.

TABLE 13-19	HYPOPLASTIC LEFT HEART: MULTISTAGE "NORWOOD" REPAIR
Stage 1: Initial palliative surgery at age 1–3 weeks	
Purpose	Establish unobstructed systemic blood supply
	Limit pulmonary blood flow and pressure to normal levels
Procedures	Transect proximal main pulmonary artery
	Allograft reconstruction of ascending aorta (i.e., neoaorta)
	Pulmonary root–neoaorta anastomosis
	Atrial septectomy
	Blalock-Taussig shunt
Stage 2: Intermediate palliation at age 4–6 months	
Purpose	Decrease right ventricular load
Procedure	Superior vena cava–right pulmonary artery anastomosis (i.e., bidirectional Glenn procedure)
Stage 3: Definitive repair at age 18 months–2 years	
Purpose	Complete separation of pulmonary and systemic venous blood
Procedure	Tunnel anastomosis between inferior vena cava and right pulmonary artery (i.e., Fontan variant procedure)

fetal life relies on many factors, including relatively low oxygen tension and high circulating prostaglandins (119). In normal full-term infants, the rapidly rising oxygen and the falling prostaglandin levels result in functional ductus closure within 15 hours of birth. In premature infants, the immature state of the ductal response combined with relative hypoxia and prostaglandin excess leads to persistent ductal patency in 40% of infants weighing less than 2000 g and up to 80% of infants weighing less than 1200 g (120).

Patent Ductus Arteriosus
A persistently patent ductus arteriosus beyond the first 2 or 3 weeks of life accounts for 2.5% to 8.5% of cases of CHD with a 2:1 female predominance (Table 13-16). In these older infants, the persistence of ductal patency is probably caused by an inherent structural abnormality, and prostaglandin inhibitors rarely induce closure (120). Grossly, the patent ductus is usually thin-walled with a smooth intima, in contrast to the thick-walled irregular appearance of the normally closing ductus (14). Occasionally, the communication between the pulmonary artery and the aorta is in the form of a window at the expected site of the ductus (14). Microscopically, the internal elastic lamina is intact rather than fragmented, and a paucity of the intimal cushions present in the normal ductus can be seen.

In children outside the newborn period, a patent ductus arteriosus without other structural heart defects raises the possibility of an underlying infectious or genetic disorder. Patent ductus arteriosus is a frequent manifestation of the congenital rubella syndrome (14). Familial recurrence has been documented in approximately 3% of cases, and abnormal neural crest development may play a role (121,122).

The clinical manifestations of patent ductus arteriosus relate to the size of the left-to-right shunt. Children with a small shunt are usually asymptomatic, coming to medical attention because of the characteristic continuous murmur. With increasing shunt size, congestive heart failure develops. Like patients with other right-to-left shunting lesions, these patients are at risk for the development of pulmonary obstructive vascular disease (14,119).

Obstructive Anomalies of the Aortic Arch

The aortic arch can be divided into three segments: proximal transverse, distal transverse, and isthmus (123) (Table 13-20). Obstructive arch anomalies occur in any of the segments with varying frequency, depending on the type of obstruction.

Coarctation of the Aorta
COTA, defined as a discrete area of narrowing in the descending aorta, accounts for 4.5% to 6.5% of congenital heart defects (Table 13-16). In the vast majority of instances, the coarctation is located in the upper thoracic aorta opposite the ductus arteriosus insertion site, and the previously used "preductal" and "postductal" designations have been replaced in the newer literature with the broader "juxtaductal" designation (14). The site of narrowing is formed by a shelf of fibroelastic tissue and smooth muscle that is in continuity with similar tissue in the ductus (14).

TABLE 13-20	AORTIC ARCH SEGMENTS	
Arch Segment	Anatomic Location	Diameter[a]
A. Isthmus	Between L subclavian and ductus	≥40%
B. Distal transverse	Between L carotid and L subclavian	≥50%
C. Proximal transverse	Between R innominate and L carotid	≥60%

[a]% of diameter compared with ascending aorta.
L, left; R, right

Associated cardiovascular anomalies, present in 50% to 60% of cases, include bicuspid aortic valve (40% to 50%), VSD (40% to 50%), and a variety of complex obstructive lesions of the left side of the heart (24%) (124). The associated VSDs show malalignment and abnormalities of the left outflow tract that could reduce aortic arch blood flow in utero. Decreased arch flow is postulated to play a role in the pathogenesis of the obstructive aortic arch lesions.

Clinical symptoms of coarctation are related to the severity of the obstruction. In infancy, coarctation presents with heart failure; these infants often have associated tubular hypoplasia (14,125). Children less than 1 year old at diagnosis are usually asymptomatic and present with upper extremity hypertension and decreased pulse and blood pressure. Surgical repair can be accomplished by resection of the coarctation ridge and end-to-end anastomosis of the aorta.

Tubular Hypoplasia

The term *tubular hypoplasia* denotes an elongated (>5 mm) and hypoplastic segment of aortic arch, usually with an associated discrete coarctation site (14,125). In normal infants, the diameter of the aortic arch is smaller than that of the ascending aorta (123). The normal values used to determine whether true arch hypoplasia is present are outlined in Table 13-20. In the vast majority of instances, tubular hypoplasia is associated with other complex heart malformations, most often left ventricular hypoplasia or DOLV (123). Amato et al. (126) have proposed a classification system for coarctation that incorporates many of these anatomic variables (Table 13-21).

Interruption of the Aortic Arch

Complete obstruction of the aortic arch is subdivided into two lesions. In aortic arch atresia, an imperforate membrane or cord occludes the arch isthmus (14). Interruption of the aortic arch refers to a complete loss of aortic arch continuity, which is subclassified according to the interruption site (127) (Table 13-22). Blood flow to the lower body depends on a patent ductus arteriosus; most hearts also contain a VSD (127). In a smaller number (one-third to two-third), additional anomalies accompany the interrupted arch (127). DiGeorge syndrome and its associated chromosome 22q11 deletion are identified in approximately 30% of cases, with 90% of the cases of deletion occurring with the type B interruption (127).

TABLE 13-22 INTERRUPTED AORTIC ARCH SUBCLASSIFICATION

Type	Interruption Site	Relative Incidence
A	Isthmus	15%–30%
B	Distal transverse arch	70%–85%
C	Proximal transverse arch	0%–8%

Aortic Arch-Branching Anomalies

The normal aortic arch, ductus arteriosus, and main pulmonary arteries develop from a sequence of six paired vessels, which then persist or disappear (128). The most significant of the myriad of anomalies that can result will be discussed briefly here.

Left Aortic Arch with Aberrant Right Subclavian Artery

The aberrant right subclavian artery originates distal to the left subclavian artery as a fourth branch of a left aortic arch, coursing behind the esophagus to the right arm. It occurs as an asymptomatic and usually isolated anomaly in 0.5% of the general population (129). It also accompanies other anomalies, appearing in 0.9% of children undergoing cardiac catheterization for other heart disease (129). During its retroesophageal course, the aberrant artery compresses the esophagus; it rarely causes symptoms, but the anomaly is visible on barium swallow. Rarely, a right-sided ductus arteriosus attaches to the anomalous right subclavian artery to form a vascular ring (128,129).

Right-Sided Aortic Arch

A right-sided aortic arch, defined by a rightward sweep of the aorta as it arches into the posterior mediastinum, may display mirror-image branching or may be accompanied by a variety of additional branching anomalies (129). A right aortic arch with mirror-image branching, the most common arch anomaly, is by itself of no clinical significance but almost always accompanies other cardiac malformations, especially TOF, which is present in 50% of cases (129). Hearts with mirror-image branching usually retain a left-sided ductus.

An aberrant left subclavian artery originating distal to the right subclavian artery as a fourth arch branch is the most frequent right-sided arch-branching anomaly. The aberrant subclavian artery follows a retroesophageal course to enter the left side of the chest, where it usually attaches to a left-sided ductus arteriosus or ligamentum arteriosum to form a vascular ring. The origin of the aberrant subclavian artery from the aortic arch frequently appears dilated—hence the designation of *Kommerell diverticulum* (128,129). Additional cardiac malformations accompany the right-sided arch with aberrant left subclavian artery in less than 20% of cases (128,129).

TABLE 13-21 COARCTATION OF THE AORTA: SURGICAL CLASSIFICATION[a]

Type I Primary coarctation
  A. With ventricular septal defect
  B. With other major cardiac defects
Type II Coarctation with isthmus hypoplasia
  A. With ventricular septal defect
  B. With other major cardiac defects
Type III Coarctation with tubular hypoplasia of isthmus and transverse arch
  A. With ventricular septal defect
  B. With other major cardiac defects

[a]All types with or without patent ductus arteriosus.

Vascular Rings

Vascular rings are malformations of the aortic arch structures that encircle and compress the trachea and the esophagus, causing respiratory symptoms and dysphagia. The most common vascular rings are formed by a double aortic arch, a right aortic arch with aberrant left subclavian artery and left ductus, or an anomalous left pulmonary artery (pulmonary sling). The most common of these, the double aortic arch, occurs with associated cardiac anomalies in less than 20% of cases (128). The anomalous left pulmonary artery (pulmonary sling) originates from the right pulmonary artery anterior to the right main bronchus and then passes between the trachea and the esophagus to enter the hilum of the left lung. A variety of tracheobronchial and cardiovascular anomalies occur in at least 50% of these infants, with tracheal cartilaginous rings or tracheal stenosis being the most common (130).

Malformations of the Coronary Arteries
Anomalous Origin of the Left Coronary Artery

A coronary artery anomaly of clinical significance is anomalous origin of the left coronary artery from the pulmonary trunk, a rare malformation (131). Beyond the newborn period, blood from the low-pressure pulmonary artery inadequately perfuses the high-pressure left ventricular myocardium. The resulting myocardial ischemia manifests clinically as congestive heart failure and pathologically as extensive subendocardial fibrosis or fibroelastosis and anterolateral wall infarction (131,132). The clinical course depends largely on the adequacy of the collateral flow that develops during the first weeks of life (132). Most infants become symptomatic in the first months of life, and 65% to 85% die in early childhood if the anomaly is not corrected by surgery (14,131). An anomalous origin of the right coronary artery is usually inconsequential because the low-pressure right ventricle is adequately perfused by blood from the low-pressure pulmonary artery (14,131).

HEREDITARY AND NONHEREDITARY FUNCTIONAL CARDIOVASCULAR DISEASES

Myocardial Disease
Cardiomyopathies

The designation *cardiomyopathy* (CMP) encompasses a heterogeneous group of diseases with dysfunction of the myocardium, unaccompanied by structural malformations, as the defining pathophysiologic abnormality. The American Heart Association (AHA) classification scheme is outlined in Table 13-23 (133). CMP occurs rarely in children, with 0.74 to 1.24 cases per 100,000 children in a year (134). In the pediatric population, dilated CMP (DCMP) accounts for 50% to 60% of cases and hypertrophic CMP (HCMP) another 25% to 40%

TABLE 13-23 CARDIOMYOPATHY: CLASSIFICATION

WHO 1980	WHO 1995	AHA 2006 (133)	
Cardiomyopathy	Cardiomyopathy	Primary cardiomyopathy	
Dilated	Dilated	Genetic	
Hypertrophic	Hypertrophic	Hypertrophic	
Restrictive	Restrictive	Arrhythmogenic RVC/D	
Unclassified	Arrhythmogenic RV	LV noncompaction	
Endocardial fibroelastosis	Unclassified	Conduction system disease	
Histiocytoid	Fibroelastosis	Ion channelopathies	
Fiedler myocarditis	Non compacted myocardium	Mixed (genetic and nongenetic)	
Specific heart muscle disease	Mildly DCMP	Dilated	
Infective	Mitochondrial CMP	Primary restrictive nonhypertrophied	
Metabolic	Specific cardiomyopathy	Acquired	
General system disease	Ischemic CMP	Myocarditis (inflammatory CMP)	
Heredofamilial	Valvular CMP	Stress (Takotsubo) CMP	
Sensitivity and toxic reaction	Hypertensive CMP	Others	
	Inflammatory CMP	Secondary cardiomyopathy	
	Metabolic CMP	Infiltrative	Storage
	Others	Endomyocardial	Toxicity
		Endocrine	Cardiofacial
		Inflammatory (granulomatous)	
		Neuromuscular/neurologic	
		Nutritional deficiencies	
		Autoimmune/collagen	
		Electrolyte imbalance	
		Consequence of cancer therapy	

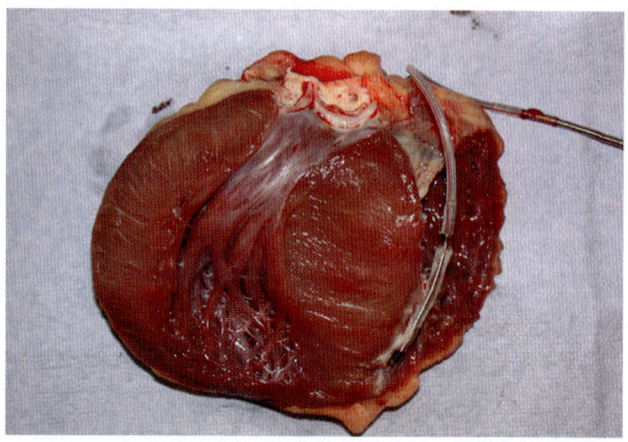

FIGURE 13-19 • Coronal section through an explanted heart with hypertrophic cardiomyopathy as viewed from behind. A catheter marks the right atrium and right ventricle. Two cusps of the aortic valve are visible above the markedly thick-walled left ventricle. The hypertrophic interventricular septum narrows and distorts the left ventricular outflow tract.

(134). The clinical approach to a child presenting with CMP has been nicely summarized by Schwartz et al. (135).

Primary Cardiomyopathies

Hypertrophic Cardiomyopathy. HCMP is characterized by left ventricular hypertrophy, either symmetric or asymmetric, with a small ventricular cavity in a structurally normal heart (Figure 13-19). Idiopathic hypertrophic subaortic stenosis, hypertrophic obstructive CMP, and muscular subaortic stenosis are among the more than 50 synonyms used in the past (136).

At explant or autopsy, the heart is massively enlarged, weighing as much as two to three times the normal weight. The thickening of the left ventricular free wall and the interventricular septum may be either symmetric (concentric) or asymmetric. With asymmetric hypertrophy, which accounts for approximately two-thirds of cases, the thickness of the interventricular septum at its base measures greater than 1.3 times the thickness at the posterior left ventricular free wall (S/P ratio) (137). This asymmetric hypertrophy is often accompanied by an enlarged elongated mitral valve (136,137). The resulting abnormal mitral valve movement contributes to left ventricular outflow tract obstruction. This physiologic state may be marked by a fibrous imprint of the mitral valve septal leaflet on the opposing septal endocardium (137).

At the microscopic level, HCMP manifests a triad of features: myocyte hypertrophy, interstitial fibrosis, and myofiber disarray defined by whorled and intertwined clusters of myocytes surrounding a central fibrotic core (136,137). At the ultrastructural level, the myofilaments also display "disarray." Myofiber disarray is unfortunately not pathognomonic of HCMP but can occur in secondary hypertrophy. The intramyocardial arteries in HCMP often display dysplastic changes similar to those seen in fibromuscular dysplasia (136,137). This small vessel disease may contribute to the myocardial ischemia, interstitial fibrosis, and development of a dilated phase late in the course of the disease (138).

It should be noted that the S/P ratio of greater than 1.3 is not an appropriate criterion in stillborn or newborn infants. In the developing heart, the ventricular septum is disproportionately thick and an S/P ratio greater than 1.3 occurs in greater than 90% of embryos and young fetuses, in 65% of older fetuses, and in 25% of normal-term newborns (139).

Primary HCMP represents a common autosomal dominant disorder with an estimated incidence of 1:500 in the general population (136). Causative mutations in at least ten different genes encoding sarcomere proteins have been identified in families with HCMP, with mutations in the myosin-binding protein C or β-myosin heavy chains accounting for 80% of cases (136,140). Mutations can also be identified in up to 60% of adults with sporadic HCMP (140). In children under 10 years of age, underlying metabolic or syndromic causes, including Noonan syndrome in particular, account for 20% to 35% of cases of HCMP (136). The spectrum of diseases that can present with HCMP is broad, as outlined in Table 13-24.

In primary HCMP, the symptoms of hypertrophy most commonly develop only after adolescent growth has been completed (136). However, up to one-third of cases can present in infancy. In infants, the hypertrophy tends to cause restriction of right ventricular outflow in addition to obstruction of left ventricular outflow (136). When this occurs, HCMP may masquerade clinically as pulmonary valvular stenosis, congenital mitral insufficiency, VSD, EFE, or myocarditis. Sudden death may occur in 1% to 2% of affected children, whether they are symptomatic or not (136).

Arrhythmogenic Right Ventricular Dysplasia. Arrhythmogenic right ventricular dysplasia (ARVD) or arrhythmogenic right ventricular cardiomyopathy (ARVC) is characterized by partial or massive transmural fibrofatty replacement of the right ventricular myocardium with associated ventricular arrhythmias (142,143).

Hearts removed at transplant or autopsy are large with the right ventricle appearing yellow or white. The fatty replacement occurs initially in the anterior free wall of the right ventricle adjacent to the septum, with progressive involvement extending to the lateral ventricular wall (142,143) (Figure 13-20). In the most severe cases, the entire right ventricle may be involved. In areas of thinning, the ventricle wall may display focal aneurysm formation (142,143). At microscopic examination, fat mixed with variable amounts of fibrous tissue and inflammatory cells replaces the normal myocardium (142,143). The extension of fat and fibrosis into the conduction pathways correlates the histopathology with the clinical course (142). The left ventricle may be thickened in 15% of cases and shows histologic features of patchy fibrosis with or without subepicardial fat infiltration in up to 50% of cases (142,143). Distinguishing the normal fatty infiltration of the right ventricle, which occurs with increasing age and obesity, from ARVD can be difficult. Suggested criteria include the association of fat with disorganized myocardium and presence of fibrosis with the fat (144).

TABLE 13-24　HYPERTROPHIC CARDIOMYOPATHY

Autosomal dominant inheritance

	Gene	Locus
Familial HCMP		
Defect in cardiac myosin-binding protein C	MYBPC3	11p11.2
Defect in cardiac β-myosin heavy chain	MYH7	14q12
Defect in cardiac troponin T	TNNT2	1q32
Defect in cardiac troponin I	TNNI3	19q13.4
Defect in myosin light chain 2	MYL2	12q23-q24.3
Defect in myosin light chain 3	MYL3	3p
Defects in α-tropomyosin	TPM1	15q22.1
Defect in cardiac α-actin	ACTC1	15q14
Defect in titin	TTN	2q31
HCMP with Wolff-Parkinson-White syndrome	PRKAG2	7q36

  Noncompaction of the left ventricle[a]
  Syndromic disorders
    Noonan syndrome
    Friedreich ataxia
    Myotonic dystrophy
    Cardiofaciocutaneous syndrome
    Leopard syndrome/lentiginosis/multiple lentigines
    Neurofibromatosis
    Beckwith-Wiedemann syndrome
    Telecanthus, multiple congenital anomalies
    Deaf mutism
    Rubinstein-Taybi syndrome

Autosomal recessive inheritance
  Total lipodystrophy, insulin resistance, leprechaunism
  Costello syndrome

Sporadic
  Infant of diabetic mother[a]

Infiltrative (storage) disorders
  Disorders of glycogen metabolism
    Glycogen storage disease type II (Pompe disease: acid maltase deficiency)
    Glycogen storage disease type IIb (Danon disease: lysosome-associated membrane protein-2)
    Glycogen storage disease type III (Cori disease: debranching enzyme)
    Glycogen storage disease type IX (cardiac phosphorylase kinase deficiency)
  Disorders of mucopolysaccharide degradation
    Mucopolysaccharidosis type I (Hurler syndrome)[a]
    Mucopolysaccharidosis type II (Hunter syndrome)
    Mucopolysaccharidosis type III (Sanfilippo syndrome)
    Mucopolysaccharidosis type IV (Morquio syndrome)
    Mucopolysaccharidosis type VII (Sly syndrome)
  Disorder of glycosphingolipid degradation (Fabry disease)
  Disorder of glycosylceramide degradation (Gaucher disease)
  Disorder of N-glycosylation
  Disorder of phytanic acid oxidation (Refsum disease)[a]
  Disorders of combined ganglioside/mucopolysaccharide and oligosaccharide degradation
    GM1 gangliosidosis[a]
    GM2 gangliosidosis (Sandhoff disease)[a]

Diminished energy production (mitochondrial disorders)
  Disorders of pyruvate metabolism
    Pyruvate dehydrogenase complex deficiency (Leigh disease)
  Disorders of oxidative phosphorylation
    Complex I deficiency
    Complex III deficiency (histiocytoid CMP)

(Continued)

TABLE 13-24 HYPERTROPHIC CARDIOMYOPATHY (continued)

Complex IV deficiency (muscle and Leigh disease forms)
Complex V deficiency
Mitochondrial transfer RNA mutation
    MERRF syndrome[a]
    MELAS syndrome
Mitochondrial DNA deletions and duplications
    Kearns-Sayre syndrome
    Barth syndrome (3-methylglucuronic aciduria type II)[a]
    Sengers syndrome

Disorders of fatty acid metabolism
    Primary carnitine deficiency[a]
    Very-long-chain acyl-CoA dehydrogenase deficiency
    Long-chain acyl-CoA dehydrogenase deficiency
    Long-chain 3-hydroxyacyl-CoA dehydrogenase deficiency[a]
    Multiple acyl-CoA dehydrogenase deficiency (glutaric acidemia type II)

Toxic intermediary metabolite
    Disorders of amino acid or organic acid metabolism
    Tyrosinemia

[a]Causes both HCMP and DCMP.
DCMP, dilated cardiomyopathy; HCMP, hypertrophic cardiomyopathy; AR, autosomal recessive; CMP, cardiomyopathy.
Modified from reference (135).
See also Callis TE, Jensen BC, Weck KE, et al. *Expert Rev Mol Diagn* 2010;10:329–351.

ARVD clinically presents with an arrhythmia or sudden death in young adults, especially males (M:F, 2.7:1), and has been reported in children as young as 5 years (142,144). ARVD presents as a familial disease in 50% of cases with both autosomal dominant and autosomal recessive (Naxos disease) inheritance patterns (142,144). The overall disease prevalence is estimated at 1:5,000 with certain regions (e.g., Greek island of Naxos) having an increased prevalence (144). ARVD accounts for up to 5% of sudden unexpected deaths in young adults. Patients with known disease experience an annual mortality rate of approximately 2% due to arrhythmia or right heart failure (144). Therefore, treatment often requires aggressive measures such as radiofrequency ablation, implantable defibrillators, or transplantation (144).

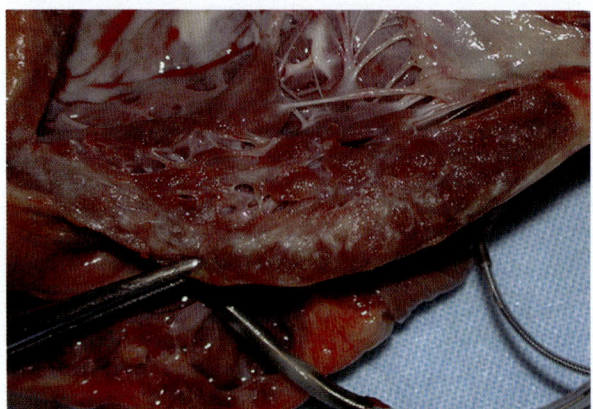

FIGURE 13-20 • In this case of arrhythmogenic right ventricular dysplasia, a close-up view of the right ventricular wall cut surface shows near complete replacement of the normally deep red myocardium by pale yellow fibrofatty tissue.

Noncompaction of the Ventricular Myocardium. Noncompaction of the ventricular myocardium (NCVM), also called *persistence of spongy myocardium*, refers to a luminal meshwork of interlacing endomyocardial trabeculae intersected by irregular endocardial-lined sinusoids that communicate with the ventricular lumen (145,146). A similar pattern of spongy myocardium occurs in the very early stages of heart embryogenesis (145,146). During normal development, as the coronary arteries and veins develop, the sinusoids involute and the surrounding myocardium becomes compacted, proceeding from the epicardium to endocardium and base to apex (146). The earliest description of noncompaction included hearts both with and without associated complex malformations (146). The noncompacted sinusoids in hearts with severe malformations, PA with IVS in particular, connect with the subepicardial coronary arteries, whereas the sinusoids in hearts with isolated noncompaction communicate with the ventricular lumen (145). Isolated noncompaction, recognized with increasing frequency in recent years, occurs at all ages (145,146). In recent studies, it accounts for up to 10% of heart lesions presenting to pediatric cardiology clinics (145).

The clinical diagnosis of NCVM hinges on echocardiographic findings with the diagnostic criteria varying between institutions (145,147). The echocardiographic features of dilated, restrictive, or hypertrophic CMP may accompany the noncompaction (145,147). These echocardiographic findings correlate with the pathologic changes described in hearts examined at autopsy or following transplant (145,147). The left ventricular cavity contains poorly defined papillary muscles as an initial clue to the diagnosis. The excess trabeculation may or may not be grossly visible on the luminal surface.

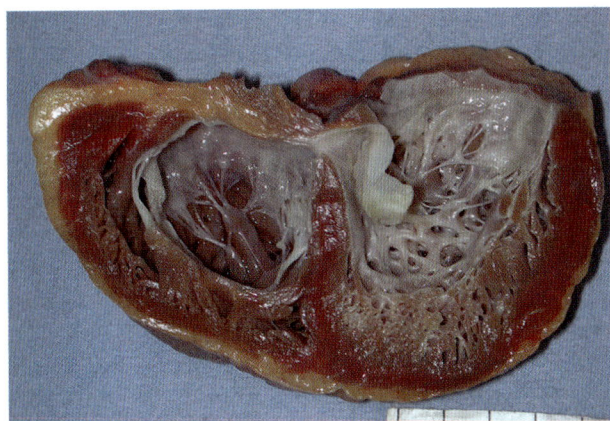

FIGURE 13-21 • Coronal section through an explanted heart with noncompaction as viewed from the front. Both the right and left ventricles of this globular heart appear thick-walled and dilated. The endocardium appears whitened due to EFE, particularly in the left ventricle. At the apex of the left ventricle, only the external 25% of the wall has the appearance of normal deep red compact myocardium. The fine trabeculations characteristic of noncompaction occupy the majority of the wall.

Full-thickness sections from the ventricular apex and/or free wall will, however, yield the histologic picture of deep invaginations of endocardial-lined spaces with variable degrees of associated fibroelastosis. The normal luminal trabeculae are of variable thickness and a definitive pathologic diagnosis of noncompaction requires that the trabeculae and intervening sinusoids account for at least 50% of the myocardial wall thickness (Figure 13-21) (147). Although left ventricular involvement represents the hallmark of this disease, the right ventricle is also involved in approximately 40% of cases (146).

Dilated Cardiomyopathy. DCMP represents a spectrum of disorders in which a dilated, poorly contracting, failing heart exhibits systolic and diastolic dysfunction. DCMP represents the common endpoint for multiple underlying conditions (Table 13-25).

The gross appearance of a heart with DCMP is the same regardless of the cause (148). The key feature is biventricular dilatation (Figure 13-22), and often, all four cardiac chambers are dilated. The enlarged heart may weigh 25% to 50% more than normal and has a globular appearance. The dilated flabby, pale left ventricular wall is of normal thickness or appears thinned despite hypertrophy of the myofibers. Stasis in the large end-diastolic atrial and ventricular cavities results in the formation of mural thrombi. Interstitial myocardial fibrosis is the histologic feature common to all cases of DCMP, whatever the cause (148). Because these histologic features are generally nonspecific, the diagnosis of DCMP based on biopsy material is difficult.

In childhood, an underlying etiology can be identified in 33% to 60% of cases of DCMP with lymphocytic myocarditis accounting for 15% to 45% (149,150). Biopsy early in the course of disease leads to a higher number of myocarditis diagnoses (150). Under the new classification scheme, these cases would be termed *inflammatory CMP* and are discussed further later.

TABLE 13-25 DILATED CARDIOMYOPATHY

Nongenetic conditions
  Infectious or postinfectious conditions
    Enteroviruses
    Mumps
    Corynebacterium diphtheriae
  Endocrine/vitamin/mineral disorders
    Thyrotoxicosis
    Hypothyroidism
    Vitamin E and selenium deficiency
    Infants of diabetic mothers[a]
  Cellular toxicity
    Anthracycline toxicity
    Hemochromatosis
    Alcohol
    Cyclophosphamide

Genetic/familial conditions
  Infiltrative (storage) disorders
    Glycogen storage disease type IV
      (Andersen disease: branching enzyme deficiency)
    Mucopolysaccharidosis type I (Hurler syndrome)[a]
    Mucopolysaccharidosis type VI (Maroteaux-Lamy syndrome)
  Disorders of oxidative phosphorylation
    Complex I deficiency
    Mitochondrial transfer RNA mutations
      MERRF syndrome[a]
    Mitochondrial DNA deletions and duplications
    Barth syndrome (3-methylglucuronic aciduria type II)[a]
  Disorders of fatty acid metabolism
    Primary or systemic carnitine uptake deficiency[a]
    Long-chain 3-hydroxyacyl-CoA dehydrogenase deficiency[a]
  Toxic intermediary metabolite disorders
    Propionic acidemia
    Ketothiolase deficiency
  Familial and neuromuscular conditions
    Familial DCMP
    Familial DCMP with conduction defects
    Isolated ventricular noncompaction[a]
    Muscular dystrophies
      Duchenne and Becker muscular dystrophy
      Emery-Dreifuss muscular dystrophy
      Myotonic dystrophy[a]
      Limb-girdle muscular dystrophy
      Congenital muscular dystrophy
    Congenital myopathies
      Centronuclear (myotubular) myopathy

(Continued)

TABLE 13-25	DILATED CARDIOMYOPATHY (continued)
Congenital myopathies (continued)	
Nemaline rod myopathy[a]	
Minicore–multicore myopathy	
Friedreich ataxia[a]	
Refsum disease[a]	

[a]Cause both DCMP and HCMP
DCMP, dilated cardiomyopathy; HCMP, hypertrophic cardiomyopathy.
Modified from reference (135).

Familial DCMP accounts for 10% to 45% of cases depending on the study methods used (149,150). Familial forms of DCMP cover a broad spectrum of disease processes (Table 13-25). The most common familial diseases are neuromuscular, with the majority having a known underlying muscular dystrophy. In a small subgroup of patients, however, the CMP represents the presenting feature of the underlying neuromuscular disorder. The identification of clinical features such as weakness, elevated creatine kinase, lactic acidosis, ptosis, granulocytopenia, and conduction abnormalities can help focus the search for the underlying genetic defect (135).

In a large combined prospective and retrospective review of DCMP in childhood, the majority of children (>70%) presented in congestive heart failure with the median age at diagnosis of 1.5 years; 42% were under 1 year. There was an M:F ratio of 3:2 and a 2 to 3× increased incidence in the black versus white populations (149). Fifty percent of children in this study died or required heart transplant.

Restrictive Cardiomyopathy. Restrictive CMP (RCMP) represents a heart in which the ventricular diastolic volume is decreased with near-normal systolic function and wall thickness. This wall "stiffness" results from infiltrative or fibrotic disorders that may be primary in the heart or secondary to a systemic disorder. RCMP occurs rarely in childhood accounting for less than 5% of all cardiomyopathies, with the majority of cases being familial isolated CMP (151).

Hearts from patients with the echocardiographic features of RCMP include three pathologic forms (151). The "pure" restrictive form manifests a normal weight with small ventricular size and no hypertrophy; the hypertensive restrictive form manifests increased weight, with free wall and septal hypertrophy; the dilated restrictive form manifests increased weight without hypertrophy and with mild ventricular dilatation. Microscopic examination similarly displays overlapping features including fibrosis, hypertrophy, and even myofiber disarray (151). With the restricted ventricular filling, atrial dilatation is often striking (152). The increased left ventricular filling pressure leads to pulmonary hypertension and associated right ventricular hypertrophy.

In children, RCMP most often occurs as a primary myocardial disease rather than secondary to infiltrative processes (152). Although the majority of primary and familial RCMP cases are idiopathic, some have now been linked to some of the same genetic mutations found in HCMP (153). CMP associated with underlying genetic disorders, such as Noonan syndrome, can also present as RCMP rather than HCMP.

Although children with RCMP can present at any age, in most series, the mean age is under 5 years (152). Symptoms at presentation often reflect the increased PVR. The long-term prognosis in these children is poor, with up to 60% dying within 5 years of diagnosis (152).

Endocardial Fibroelastosis. EFE is a focal or a diffuse proliferation of fibroelastic tissue beneath the endocardium of any chamber of the heart, but predominantly the left ventricle. EFE occurs in both structurally normal and structurally malformed hearts. In the past, EFE in a structurally normal heart was considered a form of primary CMP. In recent years, with the overall improved understanding of the cardiomyopathies, EFE is no longer considered a primary form of CMP and has instead been relegated to the status "associated finding" in a wide variety of cardiomyopathic processes.

EFE gives the normally thin translucent endocardium a white opaque appearance (Figure 13-23). Microscopic examination reveals subendocardial layers of dense collagen and elastic fibers that extend into all the crevices of the chamber walls and even into the myocardium to surround vessels and groups of myocytes. Focal dystrophic calcification and necrosis may also occur. The elastic fibers in EFE often appear larger, more darkly staining, and more uniformly oriented than those found in the subendocardial fibrosis that follows ischemic heart disease.

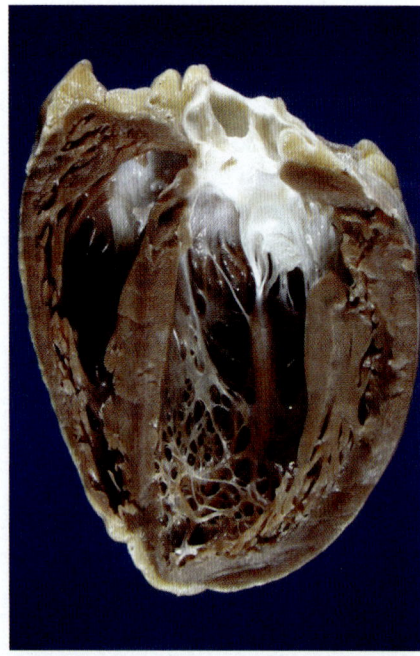

FIGURE 13-22 • Coronal section through an explanted heart with dilated cardiomyopathy. Both ventricles appear dilated with minimally thickened myocardium.

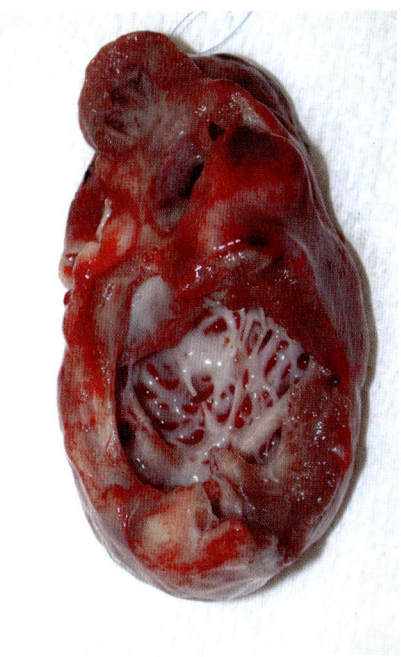

FIGURE 13-23 • Posterior view of an infant heart with windows opened into the left atrium and the left ventricle. The left ventricle endocardium appears white due to the diffuse EFE.

Myocarditis (Inflammatory Cardiomyopathy). Although the term *myocarditis* denotes inflammation of the myocardium, experienced physicians and pathologists recognize that the clinical and morphologic diagnosis of myocarditis can be exceedingly difficult. The current widely accepted criteria for a morphologic diagnosis of myocarditis require the presence of an inflammatory infiltrate directly associated with myocyte damage that occurs in the absence of ischemic changes associated with vascular disease (Figure 13-24) (154).

The macroscopic appearance of the heart, clinically or at autopsy, depends on the age of the patient, causative agent, time course of the infection, and associated complications. In acute fulminant myocarditis, the myocardium is often flabby; it may have a gray and glassy cast and be studded with

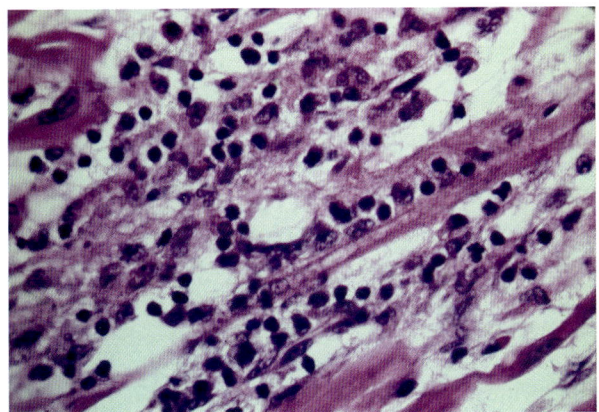

FIGURE 13-24 • Acute myocarditis. Mononuclear cells infiltrate frayed and damaged cardiac myocytes. (Hematoxylin and eosin stain, original magnification 400x.)

scattered hemorrhagic foci. Although their overall shape may not be altered, the ventricular walls are usually much softer than expected (155). With more long-standing disease, multifocal fibrosis of the ventricular wall and septum and endocardial thickening are common.

Microscopic features include inflammation and myocyte damage. Myocyte damage, best seen in longitudinal section, consists of necrosis and myocyte debris, degenerative changes and altered staining characteristics (especially with Masson trichrome), and vacuolization, which causes a ragged, frayed appearance of the myocyte margins and cellular disruption with infiltration of inflammatory cells. The nature of the inflammatory infiltrate varies with the time course and underlying etiology; infiltrates may be diffuse or focal and may include neutrophils, lymphocytes, macrophages, plasma cells, eosinophils, and/or giant cells (GCs) (154). The histologic appearance of the inflammatory infiltrate, coupled with the type and extent of the myocyte damage, may offer clues to the cause of myocarditis (155).

Endomyocardial biopsy currently serves as the major tool for diagnosing myocarditis based on the Dallas criteria (Table 13-26). However, these criteria are fraught with problems of sampling and interobserver variability. In an attempt to address biopsy interpretation difficulties, among other things, a new set of diagnostic criteria has been advanced by the World Health Organization (156).

Myocarditis presents clinically in one of three patterns: sudden unexpected death, acute heart failure, and more insidious heart disease that can mimic DCMP. In one large autopsy series, myocarditis accounted for 7% of sudden deaths. Luckily, myocarditis presents more commonly as acute heart failure, manifesting as a wide spectrum of clinical symptoms. Diagnosis relies on ECG and echocardiographic features, with identification of the underlying organisms usually requiring serologic studies. The incidence of acute myocarditis is best estimated from a large prospective study of myocarditis in Finnish military conscripts with a mean age of 20 years that yielded an incidence of 0.17/1000 person-years. With aggressive clinical support, the death rate in this group is less than 10% and the vast majority recovers normal heart function. Young age of onset renders the best long-term prognosis. The one exception to this overall good outlook is idiopathic GC myocarditis, discussed later.

Myocarditis has been linked to most human pathogens and also to a variety of noninfectious conditions (141,157) (Table 13-27).

Bacterial myocarditis occurs rarely, usually as a complication of septicemia. Streptococci, Staphylococci, and *Neisseria* cause suppurative myocarditis (14); in rickettsial infections, organisms directly invade the endothelium of myocardial vessels. Bacterial exotoxins have been implicated as the causative mechanism in diphtheria-related myocarditis (14,157). The suggestion that a bacterial infection could elicit myocarditis through antigenic mimicry has received support from studies of *Chlamydia spp.* infections and heart disease.

Protozoal myocardial infections, rare in North America and Europe, lead to significant diseases in many parts of

| TABLE 13-26 | MYOCARDITIS |

Dallas Criteria
Myocarditis: requires both inflammation and myocyte damage
Borderline myocarditis: inflammation without myocyte damage
Inflammation: lymphocytes ± neutrophils ± giant cells ± eosinophils
Myocyte damage: Frank fiber necrosis and/or intracellular lymphocytes and/or fiber vacuolization or disruption
First biopsy
   Myocarditis with/without fibrosis
   Borderline myocarditis
   No myocarditis
Subsequent biopsies (requires myocarditis diagnosis on first biopsy)
   Ongoing (persistent) myocarditis with/without fibrosis
   Resolving (healing) myocarditis with/without fibrosis
      Inflammation still present; no myofiber necrosis; reparative changes present
   Resolved (healed) myocarditis with/without fibrosis
      No inflammation in myocardium (may be in center of scar)

WHO Criteria
Myocarditis: ≥14 leukocytes/mm^2 or clusters of ≥3 T cells in myocardium; leukocytes quantitated using IHC
First biopsy
   Acute (active) myocarditis: ≥14 leukocytes/mm^2 + myocyte damage ± fibrosis
   Chronic myocarditis: ≥14 leukocytes/mm^2 without myocyte damage ± fibrosis
Subsequent biopsies
   Ongoing (persistent) myocarditis: may be acute or chronic
   Resolving (healing) myocarditis: acute or chronic but "sparser" than first biopsy
   Resolved (healed) myocarditis: no inflammation in myocardium

the world. Chagas disease (*Trypanosoma cruzi*), an endemic infection in South and Central America, represents the most common form of myocarditis worldwide (141). Acute disseminated infection occurs predominantly in children following a focal lesion. Chronic Chagas disease is a leading cause of cardiac failure and sudden death in endemic areas (14). Toxoplasmosis (*Toxoplasma gondii*) is widespread and may be acquired or occur *in utero*, but isolated myocardial disease is uncommon. Necrotizing inflammation with edema, lymphocytes, histiocytes, and plasma cells is typical. Occasionally, pseudocysts or sporozoites are seen. *Toxocara canis* causes severe granulomatous inflammation with an occasionally intense eosinophilic infiltrate (157). *Trichinella spiralis* infection may lead to cardiac failure with focal or diffuse infiltration by lymphocytes and eosinophils; the parasites are rarely found in the sites of myocardial injury, having been either destroyed or passed directly into the circulation (14). Echinococcal heart disease is rare in North America but is common in countries with large sheep-grazing programs.

Viral infections account for most cases of infectious myocarditis, with many implicated agents (Table 13-27). Coxsackievirus B is the most commonly recognized cause in infants and children. Although polymorphonuclear leukocytes may predominate initially, lymphocytes, plasma cells, and eosinophils soon replace them, followed by fibroblasts attempting repair (14).

The diagnosis of viral myocarditis can be established by (a) isolation and identification through cytopathic effects in culture, (b) identification of pathognomonic tissue changes with light or electron microscopy, (c) tissue identification of specific viral antigens with monoclonal antibodies, (d) recognition of a fourfold rise in specific antibodies in acute and convalescent serum samples, and (e) specific identification with molecular methods (157). Most acute cases are identified by serologic study. In recent years, molecular methods, in particular PCR, have become widely used to test for viral genomes in inflamed myocardial tissue. Using these techniques, viral genomes can be detected in up to 46% of cases.

The role viral infection plays in biopsy-proven chronic myocarditis remains unclear. Using PCR, viral nucleic acid can be detected in biopsy material from 10% to 60% of patients presenting with DCMP. In infants with primary EFE, mumps virus and adenovirus have been identified by PCR, suggesting *in utero* viral infection as an etiology for this disorder. Early studies suggested that treatment with steroids and other immunoregulatory drugs improved the clinical outcome; more recent studies call this into question.

Idiopathic GC myocarditis represents a distinct clinical entity with a rapidly progressive course leading to death or cardiac transplant in 89% of patients (158). The pathologic features include three phases of disease, which may all be present simultaneously within the same heart (159). The acute phase includes extensive zones of myocardial necrosis with an associated mixed inflammatory infiltrate including CD8-positive T lymphocytes, eosinophils, and macrophages including multinucleated GCs. Despite the GCs, granulomas are not seen, distinguishing this disorder from infectious and sarcoid-related GC disease. In the healing phase, granulation tissue containing inflammatory GCs mixed with myocardial GCs replaces the necrotic regions. Healed areas contain fibrous scar tissue without GCs. Although predominantly an adult disease, GC myocarditis does occur in the pediatric age range, predominantly in the second decade. A variety of features have led to the speculation that GC myocarditis represents an autoimmune disorder: (a) about 20% of patients have an underlying autoimmune disease, especially inflammatory bowel disease (158); (b) GC myocarditis occurred in a child with common variable immunodeficiency, a disorder prone to the development of autoimmune disorders; and (c) recurrent disease occurs in approximately 25% of transplanted hearts (158).

TABLE 13-27 AGENTS AND CONDITIONS ASSOCIATED WITH MYOCARDITIS

I. Infections
  A. Viruses
    Enterovirus

Coxsackie A	Coxsackie B	Echovirus	Poliovirus

    Adenovirus
    Herpes virus

Cytomegalovirus	Herpes simplex	Varicella	Epstein-Barr

    Influenza A or B
    Paramyxovirus

Respiratory syncytial virus	Measles	Mumps	

    Parvovirus

Human immunodeficiency virus	Hepatitis B	Hepatitis C	
Rubella	Dengue virus	Yellow fever virus	

  B. Bacteria
    Gram positive

Streptococcus	*Staphylococcus*	*Corynebacterium diphtheriae*	*Clostridium*

    Gram negative

Neisseria	*Brucella*	*Salmonella*	*Haemophilus influenzae*
Serratia marcescens			

    Acid-fast
      Mycobacterium tuberculosis
    Spirochetes

Leptospira	*Treponema pallidum*	*Borrelia*	

    Rickettsiae

Rickettsia rickettsii	*Rickettsia prowazekii*		

    Other

Chlamydia	*Mycoplasma pneumoniae*	*Coxiella burnetii*	
Actinomycetes	Nocardia		

  C. Fungi

Candida	*Histoplasma*	*Aspergillus*	*Coccidioides*
Cryptococcus	*Blastomyces*	Zygomycetes (mucormycosis)	

  D. Parasites

Trypanosoma cruzi	*Toxoplasma gondii*	*Entamoeba histolytica*	
Toxocara canis	*Schistosoma*	Visceral larva migrans	
Trichinella	*Echinococcus*	Cysticercosis	

II. Noninfectious
  A. Connective tissue disease

Rheumatic heart disease		Systemic lupus erythematosus	
Rheumatoid heart disease		Mixed connective tissue disease	
Ulcerative colitis		Scleroderma	

  B. Drugs and toxins

Anthracyclines	Acetazolamide	Antibiotics	
Cyclophosphamide	Amphotericin B	Indomethacin	
Phenytoin	Heavy metals	Cocaine	

  C. Other

Giant cell myocarditis	Sarcoidosis	Kawasaki disease	Thyrotoxicosis

Secondary Cardiomyopathies

Glycogen Storage Disorders. The glycogen storage diseases (GSDs) are predominantly autosomal recessive conditions characterized by a deficiency in one of the enzymes involved in the synthesis or degradation of glycogen. Significant cardiac involvement occurs in GSD types IIa (Pompe disease) and IIb (Danon disease).

Pompe disease (GSD type IIa) results from a deficiency in α-1,4-glucosidase (acid maltase), leading to accumulation of lysosomal glycogen in the heart and skeletal muscle. The disease manifests as infantile and late (adult-onset) forms, depending on the severity of the enzyme deficiency. With complete loss of the enzyme (infantile Pompe), glycogen accumulates in the heart at a rapid rate, leading to onset of disease in the first month or two of life and death in the first year. Involved infants invariably display cardiomegaly on chest X-ray and a hypertrophic left ventricle by ECG and echocardiogram. At autopsy, the heart weighs three to ten times the expected weight for age and the walls of all the chambers appear thickened, giving the heart a globular appearance. Mild degrees of EFE may be present. On microscopic examination, the cardiac myocytes appear markedly distended by vacuolated and lacy cytoplasm due to the accumulation of PAS-positive digestible glycogen displacing the myofibrils (160). Ultrastructural exam shows the glycogen to be at least partially membrane-bound, a feature that distinguishes Pompe disease from other forms of GSD. The deficiency of α-1,4-glucosidase (acid maltase) can be readily proved in muscle, fibroblasts, lymphocytes, or urine (see Chapter 5).

Danon disease (GSD type IIb) is an X-linked dominant disorder caused by primary deficiency of lysosome-associated membrane protein-2 (LAMP-2). Affected males present during childhood with muscle weakness, HCMP, and frequently (70%) mental retardation, with death from cardiac failure in the second or the third decade (161). Affected females also almost invariably manifest disease, but at an older age. At the time of diagnosis, ECG displays features of both left ventricular hypertrophy and rhythm disturbance including Wolff-Parkinson-White (WPW) syndrome and bundle branch block. The pathologic changes are best described in skeletal muscle biopsies (161). Muscle fibers contain PAS- and acid phosphatase–positive inclusions that exhibit dystrophin and sarcoglycan staining of their membranes. Ultrastructural study shows the intracytoplasmic membrane-bound vacuoles to contain glycogen mixed with cytoplasmic debris.

Mucopolysaccharidoses. *Mucopolysaccharidoses* (MPS) represent a group of lysosomal storage disorders caused by defects in the intralysosomal degradation of acid mucopolysaccharides (glycosaminoglycans). Seven forms of MPS have been identified, all but one of which are transmitted in an autosomal recessive fashion (see Chapter 5). Cardiovascular abnormalities occur in most forms of MPS, with the degree of involvement varying between forms

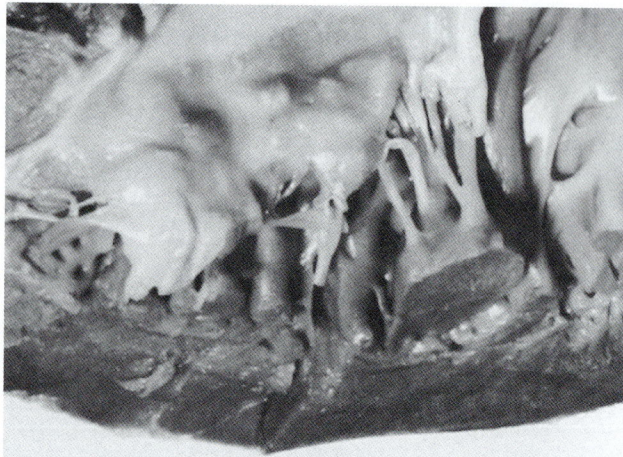

FIGURE 13-25 • Mucopolysaccharidosis type IV. A thickened, nodular mitral valve is characteristic of most MPS.

and over time for any one form (162). During life, valvular insufficiency due to thickening of the mitral—or less often aortic—valve represents the most significant cardiovascular complication (162). At autopsy, more extensive involvement can be identified. These cardiovascular changes are best described in MPS I (Hurler syndrome) (163). The valves and the endocardium of all four cardiac chambers are thickened, the mitral valve especially so, with irregular nodules along its free margin (Figure 13-25). The coronary arteries appear thickened with luminal narrowing; the aorta and systemic vessels exhibit substantial intimal plaque formation. Subendocardial fibrosis may be severe, especially in the left ventricle, with occasional patients presenting as newborns with EFE. Histologically, the thickened connective tissues of the cardiovascular system and other sites are populated by vacuolated "Hurler" cells containing large vesicles of soluble acid mucopolysaccharides and glycolipids. Ultrastructurally, membrane-bound vacuoles contain concentric and parallel lamellae (163) (see Chapter 5).

Mucolipidoses. Mucolipidosis II alpha/beta (I-cell disease) (gene locus 12q23.2) is an autosomal recessive disorder caused by mutations in the gene encoding for N-acetylglucosamine-1-phosphate transferase (*GNPTAB*), leading to defective targeting of multiple lysosomal hydrolases that degrade lipids and mucopolysaccharides. This disease has a Hurler-like clinical presentation. Fibroblasts accumulate storage material, leading to thickened and nodular valvular leaflets and abnormal chordae (164). The coronary artery intima may contain foam cells. Progressive left ventricular hypertrophy can contribute to the risk for sudden death in some patients.

Gangliosidoses. The gangliosidoses are autosomal recessive enzymatic defects of glycosphingolipid metabolism. Although manifesting predominantly as disorders of neuronal tissues, accumulation of storage material in the myocardium mimicking that seen in MPS may cause significant disease in at least two of these disorders (see Chapters 5 and 10).

GM1 gangliosidosis, resulting from a deficiency in acid β-galactosidase, causes storage of GM1 ganglioside material in neuronal tissue and glycosaminoglycans and glycopeptides in visceral organs (165). Cardiac involvement occurs in a subgroup of infants, manifesting as CMP or valve insufficiency. Foamy histiocytes containing PAS and Alcian blue–positive storage material accumulate in the heart valves, subendocardial regions, and vessel adventitia (165).

GM2 gangliosidosis type II (Sandhoff disease) results from deficiency of the hexosaminidase β-subunit. Storage material consisting of membrane-bound bodies containing laminated lipid and granular material is found in connective tissue cells throughout the heart (166). The resulting cardiac disease manifests clinically as HCMP and valvular insufficiency.

Fabry Disease. Fabry (Anderson-Fabry) disease, an X-linked recessive inborn error of glycosphingolipid metabolism (gene locus Xq22.1), results from a deficiency of lysosomal α-galactosidase A (ceramide trihexosidase). The disease occurs with an incidence of 1 in 40,000 to 117,000 male live births and accounts for 3% to 4% of unexplained LVH in young adult males (167). Although commonly considered an adult disease, symptoms begin in childhood. The majority of patients manifest neurologic pain and/or skin angiokeratomas, and nearly 40% have cardiac manifestations in the second decade. Cardiac disease manifests most commonly as left ventricular hypertrophy and less commonly with clinically significant valve and conduction system alterations. Neutral glycosphingolipids deposit in lysosomes of cells throughout the body, with the renal, cardiovascular, and peripheral nervous systems taking the largest "hit" (167). In cardiac muscle cells, the deposits are perinuclear and displace contractile elements toward the periphery. In frozen tissue, the storage material is PAS-positive and birefringent. At electron microscopic study, the deposits form intralysosomal aggregates of concentric or parallel lamellae (167).

N-Glycosylation Disorders. *N*-glycosylation disorders are a group of multisystemic diseases caused by at least 12 different defects in the attachment of *N*-linked oligosaccharide chains to glycoproteins. Hypertrophic or dilated CMP complicates at least a small subgroup of these patients (168). Cardiac manifestations including pericardial effusions and HCMP may be the presenting symptoms in some patients. Endomyocardial biopsy in one patient with DCMP revealed nonspecific findings of myocyte hypertrophy and interstitial fibrosis without inflammation (168).

Fatty Acid Oxidation Defects. Fatty acid oxidation is a complex metabolic pathway that can go awry at a variety of points, leading to cardiac dysfunction (Table 13-28) (169). The majority of these enzyme defects present in infancy, with abnormal free carnitine levels and acylcarnitine profiles serving as diagnostic clues. Primary carnitine deficiency presents with hypoglycemia and CMP (170). The CMP may be either dilated or hypertrophic; there is often associated EFE. In both biopsy and autopsy material, the cytoplasm of skeletal muscle and cardiac myocytes contains accumulations of neutral lipid vacuoles with associated large aggregates of mitochondria (171). Carnitine palmitoyltransferase 2 and carnitine-acylcarnitine translocase deficiencies often present with an arrhythmia with or without associated CMP (see Chapter 5).

Mitochondrial Electron Transport Chain Disorders. Mitochondria are the site of energy production via oxidative phosphorylation in the cell. The electron transport chain pathways involved in oxidative phosphorylation include five enzyme complexes, each including multiple proteins encoded by a mix of mitochondrial DNA (mtDNA) and nuclear DNA (nDNA). Mitochondrial enzyme deficiencies can be derived from either mtDNA or nDNA mutations. This fact, combined with the ability of mitochondria to divide independent of cell division (heteroplasmy), results in an exuberant array of phenotypic variations for the electron transport chain deficiencies. A group of mitochondrial enzyme deficiency syndromes have been identified, some of which include cardiac manifestations, especially hypertrophic or dilated CMP and conduction defects, as an important element. Up to 40% of patients with mitochondrial cytopathy manifest cardiac disease, with approximately 10% of patients presenting as an isolated CMP (172). Patients with a mitochondrial disorder including CMP follow a more severe clinical course compared with patients without CMP (172,173) (see Chapter 5).

The pathologic features of mitochondrial disease in cardiac muscle include replacement of the cardiac myofibers by pools of mitochondria that ultrastructurally may contain closely compacted stacks or circular arrays of cristae (173). In a subgroup of patients, negative COX staining of frozen tissue serves as a clue to the diagnosis. Making a definitive diagnosis of a mitochondrial cytopathy is, however, not

TABLE 13-28 FATTY ACID OXIDATION DISORDERS WITH CARDIOMYOPATHY

Enzyme	Gene
Carnitine transporter	OCTN2
Carnitine-acylcarnitine translocase	CACT
Carnitine palmitoyltransferase II	CPT2
Very-long-chain acyl-CoA dehydrogenase	VLCAD
Short-chain acyl-CoA dehydrogenase	SCAD
Mitochondrial trifunctional protein	HADHA, HADHB
Electron transfer flavoprotein dehydrogenase[a]	ETFDH
Electron transfer flavoprotein-α[a]	ETFA
Electron transfer flavoprotein-β[a]	ETFB

[a]These deficiencies are also known as glutaric acidemia type II.
CoA, coenzyme A.

straightforward, requiring not only light and electron microscopic examination of the endomyocardial biopsy material but also mtDNA and nDNA analysis of blood or tissue and frequently electron transport chain analysis of fresh/frozen skeletal muscle.

Iron Overload. The most common form of severe iron overload in childhood is transfusional siderosis, or secondary hemochromatosis, caused by repeated transfusions. The excess iron is primarily deposited in the mononuclear phagocyte system, and by itself, it does not cause significant cellular dysfunction or injury. During long-term transfusion therapy, cardiac iron deposits become readily demonstrable but usually cause no clinical problems.

The juvenile form of hereditary hemochromatosis is caused by mutations in the hemojuvelin (*HJV*, 1q21.1) or hepcidin (*HAMP*, 19q13.1) genes, rather than the *HFE* gene common in adult hemochromatosis. Clinical features are similar to those in adult disease but with earlier onset of cardiac symptoms and endocrine dysfunction. Iron accumulation begins early in life and causes clinical symptoms including arrhythmias and DCMP before the age of 30 years. The heart may be two or three times the normal weight with rusty brown discoloration (174). On microscopic exam, iron deposits, readily identified by histochemical staining, are visible in both myocardial connective tissue cells and in cardiac myocytes.

Neuromuscular Disorders. Given the similar myofibrillar structure in skeletal and cardiac muscle fibers, it is not surprising that cardiac involvement occurs as a part of many neuromuscular diseases (175). DCMP is the most common form. Conduction abnormalities and arrhythmias without apparent cardiac histopathology are also common (see Chapter 27).

Muscular Dystrophies. Both the Duchenne and the Becker forms of muscular dystrophy involve mutations in the dystrophin gene (Xp21.2-21.1). At autopsy, most patients with this X-linked recessive disorder have DCMP with epicardial and extensive interstitial fibrosis (176). Dystrophic changes may also develop in the left ventricular papillary muscles with MVP or involve the conduction system. In a small subgroup of people with a dystrophin gene mutation, DCMP may be the presenting feature of the disease.

Emery-Dreifuss muscular dystrophy is a slowly progressive form of muscular dystrophy that presents with contractures of the elbows and ankles. This phenotype occurs in both X-linked (emerin gene, Xq28) and autosomal dominant or recessive (lamin A gene, 1q22) forms (175). Cardiac involvement manifests as conduction defects, with DCMP occurring less frequently. Mutations in the lamin gene can also cause DCMP with conduction defects without skeletal muscle involvement.

Myotonic dystrophy, an autosomal dominant disorder characterized by delayed skeletal muscle relaxation (myotonia), results from an abnormal expansion of a CTG trinucleotide repeat in the 3′ untranslated region of the *DMPK* gene (19q13) (177). This disorder exhibits anticipation, with children of affected individuals exhibiting earlier disease onset and greater severity of disease in both the heart and skeletal muscle. Dystrophic changes in the heart manifest most frequently as conduction defects, although left ventricular hypertrophy, dilatation, MVP, and ventricular noncompaction can also occur (177).

Congenital Myopathies. Myofibrillar myopathies are a group of neuromuscular disorders that can be caused by mutations in several genes, including desmin. They present in the second decade of life with muscle weakness, cramps, or exercise intolerance. A DCMP frequently accompanies and may predate the myopathy in affected families. The disorder is typically transmitted in an autosomal dominant fashion with variable penetrance.

Central core disease is a slowly progressive form of congenital myopathy diagnosed by the distinctive pathologic absence of central mitochondria in skeletal muscle. Most cases can be linked to a mutation in the ryanodine receptor (*RYR1*) gene on chromosome 19 and lack an associated heart disease. However, the central core phenotype has also been identified in skeletal muscle from patients with HCMP and a mutation in the β-myosin heavy-chain (*MYH7*) gene on chromosome 14 (178). Mutations in a different region of the *MYH7* gene have been identified in myosin storage myopathy, in which myofibers contain aggregates of myosin myofilaments beneath the cell membrane.

Friedreich Ataxia. Friedreich ataxia, the most common form of inherited ataxia, results from expansion of a GAA trinucleotide repeat in the frataxin (*FXN*) gene (9q13) (179). The frataxin gene is involved with mitochondrial iron metabolism, and mitochondrial dysfunction is believed to be the mechanism behind this disorder. Cardiac disease, usually manifesting as HCMP, complicates the clinical course in 65% to 75% of patients. The severity of the cardiac manifestations correlates with the number of GAA repeats. Examination of the heart at autopsy reveals myocyte hypertrophy and fibrosis with myocyte degeneration and iron deposition.

Inflammatory/Autoimmune Disorders

Systemic Lupus Erythematosus. Most of the classic autoimmune diffuse connective tissue diseases, including systemic lupus erythematosus (SLE), rheumatoid arthritis, scleroderma, polyarteritis nodosa, and dermatomyositis, occur in children and adolescents. These diseases manifest overlapping clinical features, with heart involvement occurring as a component in many. SLE, which includes a well-studied significant cardiac component, will be the focus of the discussion here.

In the pediatric population, SLE usually occurs after the age of 9 years with a striking (3-10:1) female predominance (180). Patients present with a low-grade fever and malaise, progressing to involvement of the joints, skin, serosal membranes, and kidneys. There is a large clinical and serologic overlap between the various autoimmune connective tissue disorders, with a positive double-stranded DNA antibody helping to discriminate SLE from the other forms. A transient similar condition may occur in infants born to mothers with active SLE (see later). Cardiac disease, involving any and all portions of the heart, occurs commonly.

Pericardium. In collected autopsy series, pericarditis occurs in 62% of SLE cases (181). Clinical evidence of pericardial disease occurs in approximately 25% of patients. The pericardial effusion is typically neutrophilic with normal or low glucose, mimicking bacterial pericarditis (182). Histopathologic changes in the pericardium include mesothelial proliferation and necrosis with a fibrinous exudate and underlying inflammation and granulation tissue formation. Fibrous obliteration of the pericardial space occurs infrequently.

Myocardium. Autopsy series identify myocarditis in up to 50% of hearts, though clinical evidence of myocarditis occurs in only about 10% of patients (180,182). Echocardiographic studies identify left ventricular hypertrophy and/or abnormal wall motion in 20%. Histologic features include perivascular inflammation, interstitial inflammation with or without necrosis, and interstitial fibrosis. The demonstration of immune complex deposition in intramyocardial vessels indicates that the myocarditis can be attributed, at least in part, to the underlying autoimmune disorder. The presence of hypertension and coronary vascular narrowing in many patients suggests that at least some of the myocardial disease occurs as a secondary complication.

Endocardium and Valves. In his classic descriptions, Gross (183) described discrete vegetations of three types on the valves and endocardium in SLE: the "pyramidal ridge type," similar to that seen in RF; the "massive thrombotic type" around commissures, similar to that seen in nonbacterial endocarditis; and the "flat spreading type," which he considered the most characteristic form. These latter lesions represent the most notable gross cardiac feature in SLE, "nonbacterial verrucous" or "Libman-Sacks" endocarditis. Libman-Sacks endocarditis manifests as smooth and friable vegetations, up to about 4 mm in greatest diameter, which can be flat and granular, warty, or nodular, resembling mulberries. These vegetations, found most often on the mitral valve, are most commonly located away from the line of closure and may be difficult to identify by echocardiogram. Similar vegetations often spread along the chordae tendineae and onto the endocardium. Microscopic changes begin on the surface of the valve leaflets and include hematoxylin bodies, valvular necrosis without bacteria, widespread multinucleated eosinophilic coalescent bodies, and a characteristic valvulitis with plasma cells and thick granulation bud capillaries (183). The valve under the vegetations is minimally deformed. A second type of valve abnormality in SLE, diffuse thickening without discrete vegetations, is found predominantly in adults with long-standing disease. Valvular disease is identified at autopsy in up to 65% of patients (180) and by echocardiography in 20% to 35%. In some cases, the Libman-Sacks vegetations have been attributed to antiphospholipid antibody deposition (182).

Neonatal SLE. Neonatal SLE manifests as characteristic skin lesions and cardiac involvement, especially heart block, with other systemic organ involvement occurring only rarely. The skin rash may not be present at birth, typically appears on the face and scalp by 2 months of age, and disappears by 6 months of age. The heart disease frequently manifests *in utero*, with bradycardia frequently detectable before 30 weeks of gestation. Virtually all infants and their mothers have demonstrable 48-kD SSB/La, 52-kD SSA/Ro, and/or 60-kD SSA/Ro autoantibodies; approximately 40% of mothers lack symptoms of autoimmune disease. The antibodies apparently cross-react with fetal cardiac tissue, resulting in permanent damage to the conduction system. Histologic studies of the conduction system in these infants show the AV node and parts of the bundle branches to be replaced by fibrous scar tissue; a few lymphocytes may also be present as a residuum of prior inflammatory damage (184,185). When diagnosed *in utero*, complete heart block as a result of maternal autoantibodies leads to death in approximately 40% of cases (186), with fetal hydrops a particularly poor prognostic marker. When diagnosed in the neonatal period, morbidity is much lower (approximately 5%), but nearly all infants who survive require placement of a pacemaker. Secondary DCMP and EFE may further complicate the long-term cardiac function in these children.

Rheumatic Fever and Rheumatic Heart Disease. RF, once the leading cause of death in young people age 5 to 20, has nearly disappeared from the developed world, but it remains the leading cause of acquired heart disease in the developing world. Acute RF is characterized by (a) migratory polyarthritis of large joints; (b) carditis; (c) erythema marginatum, a striking evanescent skin rash; (d) subcutaneous nodules; and (e) Sydenham chorea, a neurologic disorder with features of involuntary, purposeless, rapid movements (187). These five features represent the major Jones diagnostic criteria for RF (Table 13-29). The presenting symptoms in an individual patient may vary greatly, making a definite diagnosis of RF difficult. Rheumatic heart disease represents the long-term cardiac sequelae of the carditis associated with RF.

RF represents a delayed autoimmune reaction to group A β-hemolytic streptococcal pharyngitis. Whether strep throat leads to RF depends on several factors, including the M-protein type of the infecting bacteria, the genetic background of the infected individual, and the socioeconomic environment surrounding the infection (187). The appropriate infecting agent evokes a T- and B-cell response against the myosin-like M-protein, which then cross-reacts with antigens in myocardium, endothelium, and neurons.

TABLE 13-29	DIAGNOSIS OF RHEUMATIC FEVER AND HEART DISEASE—2002–2004 WHO CRITERIA (BASED ON REVISED JONES CRITERIA)
Major manifestations	
• Carditis	
• Polyarthritis	
• Chorea	
• Erythema marginatum	
• Subcutaneous nodules	
Minor manifestations	
• Clinical: fever, polyarthralgia	
• Laboratory: elevated acute-phase reactants (ESR, WBC count)	
• Electrocardiogram: prolonged P–R interval	
Supporting evidence of preceding streptococcal infection within the last 45 days	
• Elevated or rising antistreptolysin-O or other streptococcal antibody, OR	
• Positive throat culture, OR	
• Rapid antigen test for group A streptococci, OR	
• Recent scarlet fever	
Diagnostic category	**Criteria**
Primary episode of RF	2 major **or** 1 major + 2 minor manifestations **Plus** Evidence of preceding group A streptococcal infection
Recurrent attack of RF in patient **without** established RHD	2 major **or** 1 major + 2 minor manifestations **Plus** Evidence of preceding group A streptococcal infection
Recurrent attack of RF in patient **with** established RHD	2 minor manifestations **Plus** Evidence of preceding group A streptococcal infection
Rheumatic chorea Insidious-onset rheumatic carditis	Other major manifestations or evidence of group A streptococcal infection not required
Chronic valve lesions of RHD (presenting with pure mitral stenosis or mixed mitral valve disease and/or aortic valve disease)	Do not require any other criteria to be diagnosed as RHD

RF, rheumatic fever; RHD, rheumatic heart disease.

The pathologic response to this autoimmune disorder results in formation of Aschoff bodies, comprising central fibrinoid necrosis surrounded by inflammatory cells (Figure 13-26). Included in the inflammation are lymphocytes, plasma cells, and a characteristic histiocytic cell with ragged edges and a vesicular nucleus containing a dense central spiculated bar of chromatin named the Anitschkow cell.

The carditis, which occurs in roughly 50% of RF patients, involves all layers of the heart. The most clinically significant disease is involvement of the heart valves. The mitral valve is involved alone in 40% to 50% of cases, the aortic and the mitral valves together in 35% to 40%, the aortic valve alone in 15% to 20%, and the mitral, aortic, and tricuspid valves together in 2% to 3%. On gross examination, the valves display a nearly continuous row of translucent verrucae near the closure margins of swollen, focally hemorrhagic valve leaflets. On the mitral and tricuspid valves, the verrucae lie on the atrial surfaces, a few millimeters from the free edges;

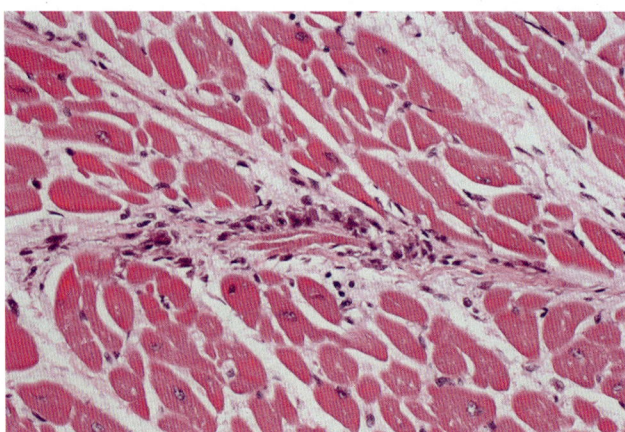

FIGURE 13-26 • Acute rheumatic carditis. A characteristic Aschoff body is seen in this section of the left ventricle. There is a central degenerating fiber surrounded by large mononuclear cells (200×).

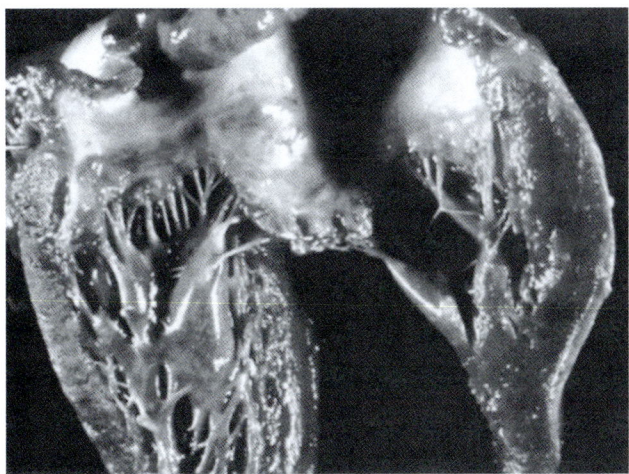

FIGURE 13-27 • Acute rheumatic carditis. Characteristic dark, nodular excrescences line the margins of closure on the mitral valve leaflets. Rarely seen today, these sites often heal as fibrous nodules with associated valvular distortion. (Courtesy of Roma Chandra, M.D., National Children's Hospital, Washington, DC.)

the attached chordae may also be involved (Figure 13-27). Verrucae on the aortic and pulmonic valves involve the ventricular surface. Microscopically, the entire leaflet is usually inflamed and edematous with focal formation of Aschoff bodies; new vessels extend from the base of the valve into the leaflet. In about half of the patients, a series of thickened subendocardial ridges, the MacCallum patch, develops in the left atrium immediately above and perpendicular to the posterior leaflet of the mitral valve (14,187). The ventricular endocardium is rarely involved. Rheumatic myocarditis results in left heart dilatation with minimal associated inflammation early in the course (187). With time, mononuclear cell infiltrates and Aschoff bodies are often found in the edematous perivascular or subendocardial interstitium of the interventricular septum and left ventricle. Rheumatic pericarditis develops only in people with valvular disease (187). Characteristically, a fibrinous exudate thickens the pericardium, binding the visceral and parietal layers together and obliterating the pericardial space. Microscopically, fibrin layers containing scattered neutrophils cover the reactive mesothelial surfaces. Beneath this layer lie infiltrates of lymphocytes, plasma cells, macrophages, and polymorphonuclear leukocytes. With resolution of the acute phase, the exudate may resolve completely or leave adhesions.

Infant of Diabetic Mother Cardiomyopathy. Maternal diabetes places an infant at significantly increased risk of heart disease at birth, including both a 5 to 10× greater relative risk of having a malformed heart and a 15% to 40% risk of HCMP in an otherwise normally formed heart (188). The HCMP remains asymptomatic in the majority of infants but may also present with congestive heart failure or even stillbirth (188,189). The HCMP is often asymmetric; occasionally, septal hypertrophy causes a transient left ventricular outflow obstruction. The ventricular hypertrophy usually resolves completely in 2 to 12 months. Given the transient and rarely fatal nature of this disorder, histologic examination of involved myocardium is limited. In the few studied cases, the myocardium appears hypertrophic with EFE in some cases (188). Myofiber disarray similar to that seen in familial HCMP is seen in some cases.

Ischemic Myocardial Necrosis. Ischemic myocardial necrosis is relatively common in the normal and malformed hearts of infants and children, especially those in which profound hypoperfusion develops for any reason. Ischemia primarily damages the papillary muscles and ventricular subendocardium of either ventricle. Thus, sampling the infant heart requires examination of all the papillary muscles, the adjacent free ventricular and atrial walls, and the ventricular septal myocardium near the membranous septum. Since the myocardial fibers of the papillary muscles and much of the subendocardium are arrayed longitudinally, sections taken along the long axis of the heart give the best sampling yield (190). Small deep red or yellow ischemic foci near the apex of a papillary muscle represent the earliest and mildest form of injury. The more severe the injury in papillary muscles, the greater the likelihood of subendocardial necrosis in the ventricular free walls (191). Longitudinal sections through the septum may expose unsuspected large infarcts near the AV ring that may involve the AV node or the bundle of His.

For the most part, the histopathology of ischemic myocardial injury in children resembles that in adult humans. However, in very young infants, the chronology of injury repair does not follow that of adults and is in fact not well defined. Using birth as the time of injury yields the following chronology of pathologic changes (191):

- 0 to 9 hours—Histopathologic evidence of ischemic injury in the myocardium may be entirely lacking; coagulative necrosis, contraction band necrosis, and wavy fibers may be seen. The ninth component of complement (C9), part of the C5-C9 membrane attack complex, has been used to identify sites of very early perinatal myocardial injury.
- 24 to 48 hours—Myocyte necrosis manifests as cytoplasmic eosinophilia and nuclear pyknosis; cross-striations may persist in necrotic fibers; marginated cells in capillaries may be the only neutrophilic response.
- 72 to 96 hours—Neutrophils infiltrate the margins of necrotic foci; mononuclear, vascular, and fibroblastic responses may be slowed by associated systemic problems.

Dystrophic calcification is common in the most frequent sites of perinatal myocardial injury, such as the papillary muscles and ventricular subendocardial myocytes. Massive myocardial calcification may occur in perinates subjected to hypoxic–ischemic injury.

Endomyocardial Biopsy and Heart Transplant

Diagnostic Biopsy

The usefulness of myocardial biopsy in the evaluation of CMP remains controversial. The initial evaluation includes history, physical examination, electrocardiography, echocardiography, and metabolic/genetic screens (135). When these studies fail to identify an underlying etiology, especially in the setting of DCMP, cardiac catheterization with endomyocardial biopsy often becomes indicated. Given the broad differential diagnoses encompassed, appropriate handling of the biopsy material requires (a) communication with the cardiologists regarding the patient's clinical picture, (b) information about specific disorders being addressed by the biopsy, and (c) adequate tissue samples.

Heart Explants

At the time of heart transplantation, examination of the explanted heart yields an opportunity to confirm, further delineate, or change the prior clinical diagnosis. Examination of cardiomyopathic hearts has yielded previously unknown diagnoses of noncompaction and arrhythmogenic right ventricular CMP.

Transplant Biopsy

Transplant biopsies play an integral role in the management of cardiac transplant patients. Findings in transplant biopsies are discussed in Chapter 8.

Conduction System Abnormalities

The conduction system represents a part of the heart that is functionally important but anatomically difficult to identify. The physiology of the conduction system and its broad range of abnormalities are beyond the scope of this chapter. However, basic understanding of conduction system anatomy is important for pathologists, especially if they examine the hearts of children at autopsy or after cardiac transplantation.

The cardiac conduction system includes the sinoatrial (SA) node, atrioventricular (AV) node, bundle of His, and bundle branches (192,193). The SA node lies in the right atrium near its junction with the superior vena cava. Electrical impulses from the SA node are transmitted via the atrial myocardium to the AV node. The AV node lies just above the septal leaflet of the tricuspid valve, within the triangle of Koch. From the AV node, the electrical impulse is transmitted via the bundle of His through the central fibrous body and membranous septum to the superior margin of the muscular interventricular septum. Here, the conduction tract divides, forming bundle branches that extend along the right and left sides of the septum. These bundle branches pass the impulse to an interweaving network of subendocardial Purkinje fibers, which transmit the signal simultaneously to the entire right and left ventricular myocardium.

Histologic examination of the AV node and its connections to the ventricular myocardium represents the key to most pathologic examinations of the conduction system (193,194). Under the microscope, the nodal tissue includes three zones: (a) an inner zone of pale-staining specialized myocardial cells containing sparse myofibrils and inconspicuous striations embedded within a fibrous stroma, (b) an outer zone of normal atrial myocardium, and (c) an intermediate zone containing transitional cells with a mixed appearance. Both the SA and AV nodes are innervated by sympathetic and parasympathetic nerve fibers.

Interfering with this normal conduction at any point along the pathway can result in arrhythmias. Arrhythmias can be divided into three basic types: supraventricular tachycardia, AV conduction disorders, and ventricular tachycardias (195) (Table 13-30).

Supraventricular tachycardias are predominantly medical disorders that rarely cause sudden death, with Wolff-Parkinson-White (WPW) syndrome being the main exception. WPW results from the presence of an accessory conduction pathway connecting atrial and ventricular muscle. This accessory pathway crosses the AV sulcus, bypassing the normal AV node (196). Pathologic evaluation for accessory pathways requires systematic study of the entire AV rim. The faster conduction through these accessory pathways leads to pre-excitation of the ventricular muscle and the diagnostic ECG findings of a short PR interval, delta wave, and widened QRS complex. Pre-excitation due to accessory pathways occurs with a prevalence of 1 to 3/1000 in the general population. Less commonly, ventricular pre-excitation result from accelerated conduction through a hypoplastic AV node. In about 10% to 20% of cases, WPW occurs in association with other congenital abnormalities, especially Ebstein malformation. An autosomal dominant form of WPW seen in association with HCMP is caused by mutations in the *PRKAG2* gene.

TABLE 13-30	ARRHYTHMIA CLASSIFICATION	
	Neonate	Child
Supraventricular tachycardia		
Primary atrial tachycardia	10%–15%	10%–15%
Sinus tachycardia		
Atrial flutter		
Atrial fibrillation		
Atrial re-entry		
AV nodal tachycardia	<5%	5%–30%
AV nodal re-entry		
Junctional ectopia		
Accessory connection mediated	>80%	>60%
Wolff-Parkinson-White[a]		
AV conduction disorders (AV block)[a]		
Congenital		
Acquired		
Ventricular tachycardia		
Scar mediated		
Cardiomyopathy related		
Long QT syndrome[a]		
Idiopathic		

[a]Disorders discussed in text.
AV, atrioventricular.

The abnormal conduction circuits can result in supraventricular tachycardia that manifests in young infants as congestive heart failure or collapse and in older children as anxiety, chest discomfort, syncope, or cardiac arrest. In symptomatic children, the lifetime risk for sudden death is estimated at 3% to 4%. However, not all individuals with pre-excitation ECG changes develop symptomatic arrhythmias. Asymptomatic adults have a very low risk of cardiac arrest/sudden death. The risk for cardiac arrest or sudden death in asymptomatic children is currently not known. In children with "high-risk" features (positive family history, multiple accessory pathways), ablation of the accessory pathways results in improved survival. The appropriate use of invasive treatment in asymptomatic children will depend on ascertaining appropriate risk stratification criteria.

AV conduction disorders (AV block), caused by interruption of impulse conduction from the atria to the ventricles, are further characterized as to the degree (first, second, and third or complete) of block. Congenital AV block (CAVB) is associated with a variety of heart malformations, in particular AV septal defects and left atrial isomerism. AV block may also occur following surgical repair of heart defects or ablation of arrhythmogenic foci (197). In the fetus, CAVB can lead to hydrops, with an associated high risk for fetal or neonatal death (186,197).

When not associated with underlying heart disease, CAVB occurs most commonly (85%) in the setting of maternal autoimmune disease with anti-SSA/Ro and/or anti-SSB/La antibodies. Fetal CAVB complicates pregnancy in only 2% of women with positive anti-SSA/Ro or SSB/La, and the risk for recurrence following a pregnancy with CAVB is less than 20%. In fetuses and infants with antibody-induced CAVB, histopathologic examination reveals fibrosis and calcification with or without inflammation in the AV node and along the conduction pathway (184,185). Antibody-induced CAVB is permanent, with 60% to 90% of children requiring pacemaker implantation (186).

Ventricular tachycardia has a broad spectrum of precipitating causes, of which the long QT syndrome (LQTS) is of particular interest. LQTS, which manifests as QT prolongation and slowed repolarization on ECG, encompasses a group of disorders affecting cardiac muscle potassium, sodium, and calcium channels (channelopathies). Currently, LQTS can be subdivided into 13 major genotypes (LQT1–LQT13) (198–200) (Table 13-31), with LQT1, LQT2, and LQT3 accounting for up to 90% of cases. Some of the genotypes also have extracardiac abnormalities. Individuals with LQTS have a significant risk of syncope and sudden death, with relative risk and event triggers (exercise, emotional stress, sleep) correlating with genotype. LQTS mutations, especially in *SCN5A*, have been identified in up to 10% of SIDS cases (201) and up to 20% of sudden cardiac deaths in older children.

Catecholaminergic polymorphic ventricular tachycardia (CPVT), a form of ventricular tachycardia with a distinctive bidirectional polymorphic pattern on ECG, leads to recurrent episodes of stress-related syncope in childhood; CPVT

TABLE 13-31 LONG QT SYNDROME

Type	Gene	Locus	Protein	Mode of inheritance	Phenotype
LQT1	KCNQ1	11p15.5	Kv7.1	AD, AR	RWS, JLNS
LQT2	KCNH2	7q35-q36	Kv11.1	AD	RWS
LQT3	SCN5A	3p21-p24	Nav1.5	AD	RWS, JLNS, Brugada syndrome
LQT4	ANK2	4q25-q27	Ankyrin B	AD	RWS
LQT5	KCNE1	21q22.1	MinK	AD	RWS, JLNS
LQT6	KCNE2	21q22.1	MiRP1	AD	RWS
LQT7	KCNJ2	17q23	Kir2.1	AD	Andersen-Tawil syndrome
LQT8	CACNA1C	12p13.3	Cav1.2	AD	Timothy syndrome
LQT9	CAV3	3p25	Caveolin 3	AD	RWS
LQT10	SCN4B	11q23.3	Nav1.5 β-4 subunit	AD	RWS
LQT11	AKAP9	7q21-q22	Yotiao	AD	RWS
LQT12	SNTA1	20q11.2	Syntrophin-α1	AD	RWS
LQT13	KCNJ5	11q24	Kir3.4	AD	RWS

AD, autosomal dominant.
AR, autosomal recessive.
RWS, Romano-Ward syndrome: ECG changes only.
Brugada syndrome: ECG changes only.
JLNS, Jervell and Lange-Nielsen syndrome: ECG changes + sensorineural hearing loss.
Andersen-Tawil syndrome: ventricular arrhythmia, periodic paralysis, dysmorphic facies, syndactyly, clinodactyly, cleft palate, scoliosis.
Timothy syndrome: ventricular arrhythmia, heart malformation, syndactyly, immunodeficiency, dysmorphic facies, autism.

type 1 is caused by mutations in the cardiac ryanodine receptor gene (*RYR2*) (201). Mutations in *RYR2* have been identified in 1.5% of sudden unexpected childhood deaths.

These molecular genetic findings in infant and childhood sudden deaths emphasize the importance of a comprehensive autopsy examination including molecular and genetic testing in cases of unexpected sudden death.

Endocardial Diseases

The major pathologic process that affects the endocardium is endocarditis, defined by the presence of inflammatory cells within the endocardium. With few exceptions, the surface of an inflamed endocardium is marked by friable or partly healed excrescences termed *vegetations*. Although heart valves are the most common sites, endocarditis also occurs on atrial walls, along the chamber trabeculae, and on the papillary muscles or chordae tendineae. Endocarditis due to microbial infection has classically been termed bacterial endocarditis and without infection nonbacterial endocarditis. With the increasing incidence of fungal endocarditis in recent years, the more general terms infective and noninfective endocarditis are replacing the classic language.

Noninfective Endocarditis

Noninfective endocarditis does not occur commonly in childhood. In a review of large published series of nonbacterial thrombotic endocarditis, only 3.2% of the reported cases occurred under 20 years of age (202). Noninfective endocarditis can be further subdivided into three groups (Table 13-32), with the rheumatic and Libman-Sacks forms discussed previously.

Nonbacterial thrombotic endocarditis is believed to occur in the setting of endothelial/endocardial injury, which serves

TABLE 13-32 FEATURES OF INFECTIVE AND NONINFECTIVE ENDOCARDITIS

Infective Endocarditis		Noninfective Endocarditis		
Bacterial	Fungal	Rheumatic	Thrombotic	Libman-Sacks
Underlying disease				
CHD	Surgically repaired CHD	Rheumatic fever	Indwelling arterial catheter	Systemic lupus erythematosus
Rheumatic heart disease	Prosthetic valve		Malignancy	
Prematurity	Immune deficit		Hypercoagulable state	
	IV drug abuse		Severe burn	
Valve before onset of endocarditis				
Normal	Normal	Normal	Normal	Normal
Abnormal	Abnormal			
	Prosthetic			
Appearance of vegetations				
Variable size	Large	Small (<4 mm)	Small, uniform size	Variable size
Tan and friable	Friable	Row near cusp margin	Friable	Ventricular surface
			Patchy along cusp margin	
Valve ulceration and perforation				
Ulceration ±	Ulceration ±	No	No	No
Perforation ±	Rare perforation			
Mural involvement				
Rare	Rare	Rare	Rare	Common
Common sites				
Septal defects	Prosthetic valve	Mitral valve	Neonates: right heart valves	Tricuspid valve
Suture lines	Suture lines	Aortic valve	Others: left heart valves	Mitral valve
Damaged valve				
Peripheral embolization				
Common	Common	Rare	Occasional	Rare
Often large				

as a nidus for platelet aggregation and thrombus formation. The associated vegetations, characterized by single or multiple, white–tan to pink, friable, verrucous projections of variable size, lie along the contact margins of the valve leaflets. Vegetations may occur as obvious warty, nodular, or sessile lesions occupying part or all of a valve leaflet, or they may be so small as to escape detection until coming to light under the microscope. They consist of fibrin strands among which lie trapped platelets, scattered erythrocytes, and occasional leukocytes. The underlying valves may appear normal or may be thickened and fibrotic (202). The actual valvular inflammatory reaction is minimal, in contrast to the pronounced reaction seen in infective endocarditis (IE). Visceral emboli are common, occurring in about 40% of cases, and resemble the parent lesions on the heart valve (202). Neonates primarily have right-sided lesions associated with intracardiac catheters, persistent fetal circulation, and disseminated intravascular coagulation. In older children and adults, the vegetations occur more often on the aortic and mitral valves and are associated with underlying malignancy, hypercoagulable states, septicemia, and extensive burns.

Infective Endocarditis

IE also occurs infrequently in children. The overall incidence of IE seems to be on the rise, and the few pediatric studies available suggest a similar trend in children. In the past, RF served as the major underlying condition. Although this remains true in much of the developing world (203), in developed countries, underlying congenital heart defects serve as the nidus for infection in the majority of pediatric patients (204). The degree of risk for developing IE varies with the type of defect; the highest risk occurs in patients with complex cyanotic heart defects, prior episodes of endocarditis, or repairs that include placement of shunt or prosthetic valve material (205). Neonates with IE do not usually have underlying congenital heart defects; risk factors include prematurity and the presence of long-term indwelling central venous catheters.

The clinical presentation for children with IE includes fever and malaise, with a new or changing heart murmur, when detectable, serving as a clue. Embolic phenomena occur in approximately 15% of patients (203,204). With long-standing disease, splenomegaly and immunologic stimulation leading to hypergammaglobulinemia, autoantibody formation, and immune complex deposition may further confuse the clinical picture. Neonates more often present with a septic picture including thrombocytopenia, disseminated intravascular coagulation, and septic emboli. Echocardiographic demonstration of vegetations aids in the diagnosis of IE, particularly in children without complex heart defects (204). Diagnosis depends on clinical or pathologic findings (Table 13-33) that include positive blood cultures and echocardiographic identification of vegetations (206).

The formation of infected vegetations begins with endothelial injury or erosion, often at a site of turbulent blood flow. The injury site serves as a nidus for fibrin clot formation. Gram-positive organisms, which account for 90% of identified organisms, have a propensity to adhere to fibronectin and

TABLE 13-33 DIAGNOSIS OF INFECTIVE ENDOCARDITIS: MODIFIED DUKE CRITERIA

Pathologic Criteria

Organisms identified in vegetation, embolized vegetation, or cardiac abscess by either culture or histology

OR

Pathologic lesions (vegetation or cardiac abscess) + histologic confirmation of endocarditis

Clinical Criteria

Two major criteria

OR

One major and three minor criteria

OR

Five minor criteria

Major Criteria

1. Positive blood culture:
   —Typical IE microorganisms from 2 separate blood cultures

   OR

   —Microorganisms consistent with IE from 2 blood cultures drawn >12 hours apart *or* All of 3 or majority of ≥4 separate blood cultures, with first and last drawn ≥1 hour apart

   OR

   —Single positive blood culture for *Coxiella burnetii* or antiphase 1 IgG antibody titer >1:800

2. Evidence of endocardial involvement:
   —Positive echocardiogram for IE:
   Oscillating intracardiac mass *or*
   Abscess *or*
   New partial dehiscence of prosthetic valve

   OR

   —New valvular regurgitation

Minor Criteria

1. Predisposing heart condition or intravenous drug use
2. Fever >38°C
3. Vascular phenomena: major artery emboli, pulmonary infarcts, intracranial hemorrhage, mycotic aneurysm, conjunctival hemorrhage, Janeway lesions
4. Immunologic phenomena: glomerulonephritis, Osler nodes, Roth spots, rheumatoid factor
5. Microbiologic evidence
   Positive blood culture not meeting major criteria *or*
   Serologic evidence of active infection with consistent organism

IE, infective endocarditis.

lamin within the clot material and activate further clot formation. In the past, viridans streptococci were the most common organisms causing IE; in more recent years, *S. aureus* has become nearly as common (204). Gram-negative, fastidious,

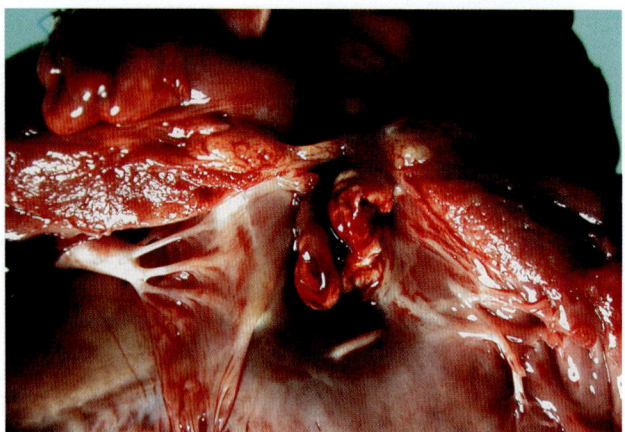

FIGURE 13-28 • Close-up view of the left ventricular outflow tract from a child with bicuspid aortic valve and *Streptococcus* endocarditis. Two large irregular vegetations obscure and partially destroy the aortic valve leaflets.

and fungal organisms are identified infrequently, occurring most often in the setting of prior heart surgery, underlying immunodeficiency, or central line placement (Figure 13-28).

The infected vegetations tend to occur on the atrial surface of the AV valves and the ventricular surface of the outflow valves (207). In neonates without underlying heart malformations, the vegetations are often right-sided. With underlying heart malformations, the vegetations may occur at the edge of VSDs or at the site of flow turbulence on the ventricular or malformed valve surface. The infective organisms elicit an acute inflammatory response leading to destruction and perforation of the valve tissue. The infection may spread into the adjacent vessel or heart tissue, leading to abscess or fistula formation. Microscopically, acute vegetations consist of granular, heaped-up layers of fibrin, platelets, necrotic material, and polymorphonuclear leukocytes. Organisms may or may not be identified. Similar neutrophil-rich infiltrates with granulation tissue formation help distinguish infected from noninfected prosthetic valve specimens. With time (and antibiotic treatment), organisms are lost and the damaged valve tissue undergoes calcification, chronic and at times granulomatous inflammation, and granulation tissue formation. Whether a native valve was initially normal or not, the subsequently damaged valve becomes a potential site for recurrent endocarditis.

Pericardial Diseases

Pericarditis

The two-layered pericardium forms a sac around the heart that normally contains less than 30 mL of serous fluid. However, when the pericardium becomes inflamed, the normally smooth mesothelium lining the sac becomes rough. A fibrinous exudate, rich in fibrinogen and other plasma proteins, accumulates as a dull-colored film over the pericardial surface. Friction between the two roughened surfaces results in the pericardial friction rub that serves as a clinical marker of pericarditis. In many instances, pericarditis also leads to increased fluid volume in the pericardial sac. The serous versus purulent versus hemorrhagic nature of this fluid varies with the underlying etiology.

Pericarditis occurs in a wide variety of clinical settings (Table 13-34) (208). When the etiology is viral or noninfectious, a lymphocyte-rich serous effusion accompanies a fibrinous exudate. Viral pericarditis typically follows a respiratory or gastrointestinal illness; enteroviruses are a common responsible viral agent (208). Noninfectious pericarditis may complicate a variety of systemic illnesses, including RF, SLE, juvenile rheumatoid arthritis, and Kawasaki disease (208,209). Postoperative pericardial effusions occur in approximately 15% to 25% of children undergoing open heart surgery (210). Approximately 25% of these postoperative effusions become symptomatic (postpericardiotomy syndrome).

Purulent pericarditis is largely caused by pyogenic bacteria, with the most common cause in North American children being *Staphylococcus aureus* (208,209). Purulent pericarditis usually results from a primary infection spreading to the pericardium either by direct extension from an adjacent purulent pneumonia, mediastinitis, or empyema or by hematogenous seeding from pyelonephritis or osteomyelitis (209). Most patients are acutely ill with fever, tachypnea, and even chest pain. A shaggy, thick, yellow or gray exudate covers the pericardial surfaces (Figure 13-29). Organisms are numerous, and large numbers of neutrophils infiltrate the pericardium and surrounding tissue.

Tuberculous pericarditis develops as a direct extension of infection from tracheobronchial lymph nodes or from hematogenous spread. The clinical onset may be insidious with fever and chest pain. Pericardiocentesis often returns bloody fluid containing numerous lymphocytes and few neutrophils. Acid-fast bacilli can be identified in fluid smears from 15% to 40% of patients, and biopsy of the thickened pericardium often reveals caseating granulomas (208).

TABLE 13-34 CAUSES OF PERICARDITIS

Infectious agents
   Viral
   Bacterial
   Fungal
   Parasitic
Immunologically mediated
   Rheumatic fever
   Systemic lupus erythematosus
   Scleroderma
   Postpericardiotomy syndrome
   Drug hypersensitivity
Other
   Uremia
   Postsurgical
   Neoplasia
   Trauma
   Radiation

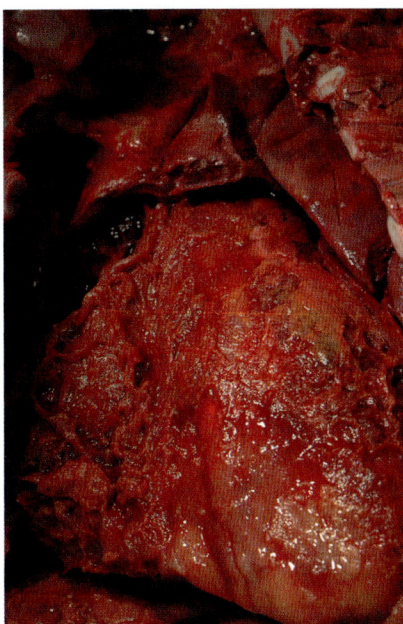

FIGURE 13-29 • The opened pericardium in an immunocompromised patient with disseminated *Aspergillus* infection. The pericardium appears thickened and shaggy due to the intense inflammatory response to the infection.

Chronic or healed pericarditis manifests in two major patterns, adhesive (obliterative) and constrictive. Adhesive pericarditis is characterized by the presence of small nodules of vascularized granulation tissue between fibrin aggregates and mesothelial cell proliferations leading eventually to partial or complete obliteration of the pericardial cavity. In the more clinically significant constrictive pericarditis, the heart becomes encased in a dense fibrous and even calcified shell, the rigidity of which may mechanically interfere with cardiac diastolic function and venous return to the atria (208).

Developmental Abnormalities

Congenital aplasia of the pericardium occurs as either complete or partial absence of the parietal pericardium. When complete, the defect is usually asymptomatic. Partial deficiency, which occurs mostly over the left side of the heart, may be complicated by herniation and strangulation of myocardium (211). Small defects may be associated with other congenital mediastinal lesions, such as bronchogenic cysts, pulmonary sequestration, or ectopia cordis. The defect is thought to result from a failure of the normal pleuropericardial foramen to close in the pleuropericardial membrane.

Pericardial cysts are thin-walled, generally unilocular structures filled with clear fluid. They tend to be benign and asymptomatic and are encountered in children only rarely at autopsy. The cysts are most often located at the costophrenic angles but may also appear higher in the mediastinum. They vary markedly in size and consist of mesothelium lining thin walls of fibrous tissue. Though believed to be developmental, the embryonic origin of these cysts remains unclear.

Extracardiac Vascular Disease

Pulmonary Hypertension

Pulmonary hypertension, defined as a mean pulmonary artery pressure at rest of greater than 25 mm Hg, represents a common pathophysiologic state arrived at from a variety of etiologic pathways. Advances in understanding the underlying vascular biology, physiology, and genetics, combined with new treatment modalities, led in 2003 to a proposed revision in the classification of these disorders. This classification was updated in 2013 in Nice (Table 13-35) (212). In pediatrics, persistent pulmonary hypertension of the newborn (PPHN) and pulmonary hypertension complicating L→R shunts represent the most common etiologies, with heritable primary (idiopathic or familial) pulmonary hypertension accounting for many of the remaining cases. Before discussing the specifics of these conditions, it seems prudent

TABLE 13-35 PULMONARY HYPERTENSION—NICE CLASSIFICATION (2013)

1. Pulmonary arterial hypertension
   1.1. Idiopathic[a]
   1.2. Heritable[a]
      1.2.1. *BMPR2*
      1.2.2. *ALK1, ENG, SMAD9, CAV1, KCNK3*
      1.2.3. Unknown
   1.3. Drug and toxin induced
   1.4. Associated with:
      1.4.1. Connective tissue disease
      1.4.2. HIV infection
      1.4.3. Portal hypertension
      1.4.4. Congenital heart disease[a]
      1.4.5. Schistosomiasis
1′. Pulmonary venoocclusive disease and/or pulmonary capillary hemangiomatosis
1″. Persistent pulmonary hypertension of the newborn[a]
2. Pulmonary hypertension due to left heart disease[a]
   2.1. Left ventricular systolic dysfunction
   2.2. Left ventricular diastolic dysfunction
   2.3. Valvular disease
   2.4. Congenital/acquired left heart inflow/outflow tract obstruction and congenital cardiomyopathies
3. Pulmonary hypertension due to lung disease and/or hypoxia
4. Chronic thromboembolic pulmonary hypertension
5. Pulmonary hypertension with unclear multifactorial mechanisms (e.g., hematologic disorders, sarcoidosis, Langerhans cell histiocytosis, lymphangioleiomyomatosis, metabolic disorders, chronic renal failure)

[a]Disorders discussed in text.

to review (a) normal pulmonary vascular development and (b) the pathologic changes associated with pulmonary artery hypertension.

Normal Pulmonary Vascular Development
The vasculature in fully developed lung includes preacinar and intra-acinar arteries. The preacinar arteries travel in parallel with the pulmonary airways and contain a well-developed muscle wall. The preacinar pulmonary arterial tree develops in synchrony with the pulmonary airways, becoming completely formed by 16 to 17 weeks of gestation (213). The intra-acinar arteries arise as a network of supernumerary vessels that supply the terminal airspaces, and in the adult carry up to 40% of the pulmonary blood flow (213). The development of the terminal airspaces and the intra-acinar arteries begins *in utero* but is incomplete at birth and continues for many months thereafter. The formation of a muscle layer around the intra-acinar arteries lags behind the development of the alveoli, and the medial muscle of these intra-acinar arteries normally extends into the alveoli only after 8 to 10 years of age (214).

The pathophysiology of the pulmonary vasculature clearly differs before and after birth. In the fetus, there is little pulmonary blood flow, with high PVR due to increased thickness of the artery walls. At birth, this high PVR rapidly falls due to release of nitric oxide and prostacyclin from the pulmonary artery endothelial cells, with resultant dilatation of the pulmonary arteries. Subsequent thinning of the muscular media requires time and is complete only at 4 months of age (213).

Pulmonary Artery Hypertensive Changes
Pulmonary artery hypertension results in a constellation of changes outlined in Table 13-36 (215). The pulmonary artery changes were traditionally graded by the Heath-Edwards grading system. However, with the advances in drug treatment modalities gained from improved understanding of the underlying pathophysiology of pulmonary hypertension, this scoring system has lost most of its value. Complex lesions are a marker of severe disease. The plexiform lesion is defined by "glomeruloid" endothelial proliferation that extends through an area of vessel wall destruction into perivascular tissue. This lesion frequently occurs adjacent to an area of concentric intimal fibrosis at an artery branch point. Plexiform lesions are not specific to primary/idiopathic pulmonary hypertension but also occur in the setting of cardiac shunting lesions. They are however not a feature of PPHN (215). The dilatation lesion refers to an area of artery wall thinning, often located distal to a plexiform lesion. These dilated areas can serve as a focal point for hemorrhage.

Persistent Pulmonary Hypertension of the Newborn
PPHN occurs when the fetal circulation fails to adapt normally at birth due to underdevelopment, maldevelopment, or maladaptation (214). The failed drop in PVR leads to right→left shunting at the foramen ovale and ductus arteriosus, with resultant central cyanosis. PPHN most often occurs as a hypoxia-related maladaptation secondary to underlying pneumonia, sepsis, or meconium aspiration. In infants with meconium aspiration, there is also abnormal extension of smooth muscle into the media of the more peripheral, normally nonmuscular intra-acinar arteries, suggesting *in utero* onset of the vascular dysfunction (214). In approximately 20% of cases, peripheral muscle extension occurs without an obvious underlying etiology, resulting in "idiopathic" PPHN (216). Epidemiologic studies suggest that nonsteroidal anti-inflammatory drugs taken by the mother may play a role in this vasculopathy. PPHN also occurs when the lungs fail to grow normally, resulting in a parallel underdevelopment of the pulmonary vasculature. This manifests most dramatically in infants with congenital diaphragmatic hernias, who often develop severe respiratory insufficiency following repair (214). In recent years, the use of vasodilators, prostacyclin, and ECMO has dramatically improved the survival of these infants.

Congenital Heart Disease with Left→Right Shunt
A left→right shunt, particularly at the posttricuspid valve level, results in increased volumes of blood flow at an increased pressure in the lungs. This stimulates smooth muscle hyperplasia along with the intimal changes of pulmonary hypertension. An additional feature seen in the left→right shunt scenario is a decrease in numbers of peripheral arteries (217). If the shunt can be repaired early enough, these pulmonary hypertensive changes are reversible. However, if the repair is delayed, the pulmonary vascular changes can become nonreversible and the pulmonary hypertension will

TABLE 13-36 PULMONARY ARTERIAL HYPERTENSION PATHOLOGIC GRADING

Pulmonary Arteriopathy	Heath and Edwards Grade
Pulmonary arteriopathy with isolated medial hypertrophy	Grade 1
Pulmonary arteriopathy with medial hypertrophy + intimal thickening (cellular or fibrotic)	
Concentric laminar intimal fibrosis	Grades 2–3
Eccentric or concentric non-laminar intimal fibrosis	
Pulmonary arteriopathy with complex lesion	Grades 4–6
Plexiform lesion	Grades 4–6
Dilatation lesion	Grades 4–6
Necrotizing arteritis	Grade 6
Pulmonary arteriopathy with isolated necrotizing arteritis	Grade 6

Adapted from reference (215).

continue to progress following surgery. Predicting in an individual patient how quickly pulmonary hypertensive changes will progress to a nonreversible stage remains problematic. Age at surgery plays a role. In one study, in infants with a variety of shunting lesions operated upon before 9 months, PVR uniformly returned to normal postoperatively, irrespective of pulmonary vascular histology. In older infants, medial wall thickening greater than 2× normal resulted in an increased risk of persistent pulmonary hypertension following surgery (217). In the worst-case scenario, pulmonary hypertension progresses to a point where PVR exceeds systemic vascular resistance and the shunt becomes right→left with resultant cyanosis (Eisenmenger syndrome).

Familial and Idiopathic Pulmonary Artery Hypertension
Primary pulmonary hypertension (PPH) occurs as a familial disease in 6% to 12% of cases, with the remainder occurring sporadically. The striking female predominance observed in adults with PPH is less obvious in children, where the M:F ratio is 1:1.3 to 1.5 (216,218). The familial disease follows an autosomal dominant inheritance pattern with incomplete penetrance and genetic anticipation (successive generations with worse disease) (218). In approximately 70% of families, a mutation in the gene encoding bone morphogenetic protein receptor-2 (*BMPR2*) can be identified; similar mutations occur in approximately 25% of sporadic cases (216,218). The involved pulmonary arteries display the range of pathologic changes described earlier. Improved understanding of the pathophysiology of pulmonary hypertension in recent years has led to significant improvements in treatment for patients with PPH. This disease, which once led to death within a year of diagnosis, can now be managed in most patients by initially using vasodilator therapy, with lung transplantation as a final option.

Pulmonary Hypertension with Obstructive Left Heart Disease
In the face of obstruction to pulmonary venous return, the vascular changes in the lungs include not only arterial but also venous thickening. With extrapulmonary venous obstruction, the pulmonary arteries develop medial hypertrophy and intimal fibroplasia without the more complex lesions. The pulmonary veins also develop medial hyperplasia with "arterialization," that is, formation of a discrete internal and external elastic lamina. These venous changes, though striking, are reversible following repair of the obstructive defect. The long-term outcome depends on the severity of the associated arterial disease.

Systemic Arterial Disease

Arteriopathy
Generalized arterial calcification of infancy (GACI) or idiopathic infantile arterial calcification (IIAC) represents a metabolic disorder of the arteries resulting in deposition of calcium hydroxyapatite in and around the internal elastic lamina and intimal fibrous proliferation. The calcification occurs in any artery, with the coronary arteries involved in greater than 75% of cases and the cerebral arteries involved only rarely. The calcification may elicit an inflammatory response including lymphocytes, eosinophils, and foreign body GCs. Ultrastructural exam identifies hydroxyapatite deposition in the elastic lamina, collagen fibers, smooth muscle, and fibroblasts. This rare condition most often presents as heart failure in early infancy but may manifest prenatally as nonimmune hydrops. The artery luminal narrowing caused by the calcification and intimal proliferation can lead to ischemic injury in involved organs, most commonly the heart, with 85% of infants dying in the first 6 months. In some families, GACI occurs in an autosomal recessive pattern with loss-of-function mutations in *ENPP1*, a gene that encodes for a protein with nucleotide pyrophosphatase activity.

Fibromuscular dysplasia represents a noninflammatory disorganization and fibrosis of large muscular arteries leading to segmental luminal narrowing, with the renal, internal carotid, coronary, celiac, hepatic, and mesenteric arteries most frequently involved. The pathologic changes can involve all layers of the vessel wall. Several forms have been described, including medial fibroplasia, perimedial fibroplasia, medial hyperplasia, and intimal fibroplasia (219). In medial fibroplasia, disorderly arrays of medial smooth muscle cells form luminal ridges that narrow the artery lumen. Between the ridges, the artery contains abnormally thin layers of otherwise normal smooth muscle cells. This alternating thick and thin luminal diameter gives an angiographic appearance of a "string of beads." Perimedial fibroplasia is characterized by layers of circumferential elastic-like tissue between the media and the adventitia. With intimal fibroplasia, the intima may be thickened and the internal elastic lamina duplicated and fragmented. Alternatively, the internal and the external elastic laminae may be disrupted and the intima and the media may merge. Fibromuscular dysplasia accounts for up to 45% of renal hypertension cases in childhood, with multifocal vascular involvement present in many. A form of severe arterial dysplasia involving the aorta, its main branches, and the coronary arteries has been described in both stillborn infants and infants with sudden death. The vessels in these infants display medial thickening due to hyperplasia of the elastic fibers.

Aneurysms
Aneurysmal vessel dilatation, rare in childhood, occurs both as a primary defect in vessel wall structure and secondary to underlying inflammatory or infectious disease (220). Inherited/genetic causes of aortic aneurysms are the focus here.

Dilatation and dissection of the ascending aorta occur most commonly in Marfan syndrome but may also complicate a spectrum of other disorders (Table 13-37) (221). In all these disorders, microscopic examination reveals cystic medial degeneration with accumulation of mucopolysaccharides in the tunica media of the involved aorta (220). At the ultrastructural level, the elastic lamella appears torn with

TABLE 13-37 AORTIC ANEURYSMS

Syndrome	Gene	Locus
Marfan	FBN1	15q21.1
Loeys-Dietz	TGFBR1	9q22
	TGFBR2	3p24
Ehlers-Danlos type IV	COL3A1	2q32
Bicuspid aortic valve	NOTCH1	9q34
Arterial tortuosity	SLC2A10	20q13
Familial thoracic aortic aneurysm and dissection (FTAAD)	MYH11 (with patent ductus arteriosus)	16p13
	ACTA2 (with livedo reticularis)	10q23
Menkes	ATP7A	Xq21.1
Turner	Not applicable	Monosomy X

loss of the connection between elastic lamella and smooth muscle cells.

Marfan syndrome is an autosomal dominant disorder of connective tissue with high penetrance but variable phenotype due to the broad spectrum of organ involvement. Marfan syndrome is caused by mutations in the fibrillin-1 gene (*FBN1*, 15q21.1), with approximately 25% of cases representing new mutations. A set of diagnostic criteria, combining clinical and genetic features, has been devised to aid in accurate diagnosis (222). To distinguish Marfan syndrome from related conditions, the revised Ghent diagnostic criteria for Marfan syndrome emphasize (a) clinical features, especially aortic root dilatation or dissection and ectopia lentis, (b) a family history of Marfan syndrome, and (c) the genetic finding of an *FBN1* mutation (222). Signs of the disease can appear at any age, but most patients are diagnosed in the second or third decade. There is a severe "neonatal" form of Marfan syndrome, associated with mutations in exons 24 to 32 of the fibrillin-1 gene (223), that presents in infancy with aortic dilatation accompanied by mitral and tricuspid regurgitation and emphysema, with death often occurring in the first 2 years.

Loeys-Dietz syndrome mimics many of the clinical features of Marfan syndrome, with craniofacial features of hypertelorism, low-set ears, and bifid uvular or cleft palate serving to distinguish the two (222,224). Loeys-Dietz syndrome is an autosomal dominant disorder caused by mutations in the genes for transforming growth factor-β receptors 1 or 2 (*TGFBR1*, *TGFBR2*). Aortic dilatation progresses to dissection at a younger age in these patients, with a mean age of death at 26 years (224).

Ascending aortic dilatation also occurs with increased frequency in Turner syndrome and in patients with a bicuspid aortic valve (221). The distribution of the aneurysms in the bicuspid aortic valve patients is somewhat different from that of Marfan syndrome. In Marfan syndrome, the dilatation occurs predominantly at the level of the aortic valve cusps, whereas in the bicuspid aortic valve group, the dilatation extends for a longer distance up the aorta. A subset of patients with bicuspid aortic valve and aneurysm formation has mutations in *NOTCH1*.

Ehlers-Danlos syndrome is a heterogeneous group of at least six generalized disorders of connective tissue synthesis, many involving different forms of collagen and their genes (225). Ehlers-Danlos syndrome type IV (vascular type) manifests as thin-walled vessels and a diffuse decrease in elastic tissue in the media, deposition of acid mucopolysaccharide material between the medial elastic lamellae, and a decrease in adventitial and medial collagen. Aortic dilatation with dissection and rupture, often intra-abdominal in location, can complicate the clinical course and even cause death (225). This form of Ehlers-Danlos syndrome is caused by a mutation in the *COL3A1* gene, which encodes collagen type III and is transmitted in an autosomal dominant fashion.

Menkes disease is an X-linked recessive disorder associated with the defective intestinal absorption of copper. Disease manifestations result from reduced activity of the numerous copper-dependent enzymes. One such enzyme, lysyl oxidase, plays a role in formation and repair of extracellular matrix material. With impaired enzyme activity, vessel wall tensile strength is diminished, leading to aneurysm formation in high-flow vessels. Arterial walls exhibit abnormalities of the internal elastic lamina at both the light and electron microscopic level (226) (see Chapter 5).

Atherosclerosis

A spectrum of inherited disorders causes congenital hypercholesterolemia; the complicating atherosclerotic cardiovascular disease occurs in childhood in a subgroup of these disorders (227) (Table 13-38). Atherosclerosis in childhood has been best described in familial hypercholesterolemia caused by a mutation in the gene encoding the receptor for low-density lipoprotein (gene locus 19p13.2). Mutations in this gene occur frequently, with heterozygotes identified at a frequency of 1 in 500 (227). About one person in a million is a homozygote; these patients have plasma cholesterol levels in excess of 650 mg/dL from infancy. Study of an involved 20-week fetus revealed lipid deposits already present in the aortic intima. Aortic atherosclerosis, although generalized, tends to be worse in the ascending aorta near the coronary arteries and in the thoracic segment, and can result in supravalvular aortic stenosis as well as stenosis of the coronary artery ostia (228). Deposits of foam cells in the aortic and mitral valves with fibrosis and cholesterol clefts also cause valvular stenosis or insufficiency. Disease is widespread throughout the coronary arteries, and death from coronary artery disease can occur as early as 3 years of age. Treatment modalities include plasmapheresis, high-dose statins, and bypass surgery to treat the coronary artery disease, as well as the possibility of liver transplantation to reverse the metabolic defect.

TABLE 13-38	INHERITED HYPERCHOLESTEROLEMIAS			
Disorder	Inheritance Pattern	Protein	Gene	Childhood CVD
Homozygous familial hypercholesterolemia	AD	Low-density lipoprotein receptor	LDLR	Yes
Heterozygous familial hypercholesterolemia	AD	Low-density lipoprotein receptor	LDLR	No
Familial defective apolipoprotein B	AD	Apolipoprotein B-100	APOB	No
Autosomal dominant hypercholesterolemia	AD	Proprotein convertase subtilisin/kexin 9	PCSK9	No
Autosomal recessive hypercholesterolemia	AR	Low-density lipoprotein receptor adaptor protein 1	LDLRAP1	Variable
Sitosterolemia	AR	ATP-binding cassette G5	ABCG5	Yes
		ATP-binding cassette G8	ABCG8	

CVD, cardiovascular disease; AD, autosomal dominant; AR, autosomal recessive.

Vasculitis

Vasculitis by definition is an inflammatory, even destructive, process involving arteries and veins that can occur as one of many manifestations in a broad spectrum of infectious and inflammatory disorders. Involvement of the heart and great vessels occurs predominantly in two of these vasculitic disorders: Kawasaki disease (KD) and Takayasu arteritis.

Kawasaki Disease (Mucocutaneous Lymph Node Syndrome). Kawasaki disease (KD), also called *mucocutaneous lymph node syndrome*, is an acute febrile exanthematous vasculitis that affects infants and young children. First reported in Japanese children in 1967, KD is now recognized worldwide. Although the initial febrile illness is self-limited, the vasculitic damage to the coronary arteries can lead to ischemic heart disease and occasionally death. In the developed world, KD now represents the most common cause of acquired heart disease in childhood.

KD occurs almost exclusively in young children, with peak incidence at 6 months to 1 year and greater than 75% of cases occurring before 5 years of life. There is a slight male predominance (M:F 1.5:1) and a prominent racial trend (Table 13-39) (229,230). This racial trend is reflected in the reported incidence of KD in Japan of 137.7 cases per 100,000 children, compared with that in the United States of 17.1 per 100,000 children.

Although the epidemiologic features of KD, including its acute febrile nature, seasonal occurrence, age of onset, and temporal and geographic clustering, point to an infectious etiology, a causal agent continues to elude detection. The possibility that it represents a response to superantigens of group A *Streptococcus* or *Staphylococcus aureus* has attracted attention but has not been proven. An alternative theory suggests an antigen-mediated immune response, with IgA plasma cells playing a central role. Epidemiologic data also suggest an underlying genetic predisposition to developing KD.

The disease typically presents as a sudden febrile illness in young children between 6 months and 5 years of life. The fever, which lasts 5 days or more, is accompanied by the development of bilateral conjunctivitis, erythematous changes of the lips and oral cavity, a nonvesicular polymorphic rash of the trunk, erythematous desquamation of the palms and soles, and cervical lymphadenopathy (229,230). This constellation of features (Table 13-40) evolves over a 10-day time period, often obscuring the diagnosis particularly in the early stages. Affected children often manifest a marked increase in acute-phase reactants, and the erythrocyte sedimentation rate is generally elevated (229). This initial febrile illness is self-limited, but in 20% to 35% of patients, the underlying vasculitis leads to coronary artery aneurysm formation (231,232). The risk of coronary artery disease is highest in young infants, a group in which the symptoms are also most likely to be

TABLE 13-39	KAWASAKI DISEASE EPIDEMIOLOGY: GENETIC FACTORS
Seasonal incidence	
Japan—biphasic winter and summer peak	
United States—winter/spring peak	
Race-specific incidence (highest to lowest)	
Asian or Pacific Islander	
African American	
Hispanic	
Caucasian	
Host factors	
Increased risk in siblings (10× population risk)	
Increased risk in twins (approximately 60× population risk)	

Compiled from references (229,230).

TABLE 13-40	CLINICAL CRITERIA FOR KAWASAKI DISEASE DIAGNOSIS

Fever persisting for ≥5 days
Presence of at least four of the following clinical features:
    Bilateral nonpurulent conjunctivitis
    Oral mucosal changes: erythema, cracked lips, strawberry tongue, or pharyngeal injection
    Polymorphous exanthematous skin rash
    Extremity changes
        Acute: desquamative erythema of palms and soles; edema of hands and feet
        Subacute: periungual peeling of digits
    Cervical lymphadenopathy (usually unilateral)
Patients with fever and less than four clinical features can be diagnosed with KD if coronary artery changes are identified with echocardiography or angiography.

Compiled from references (229,230).

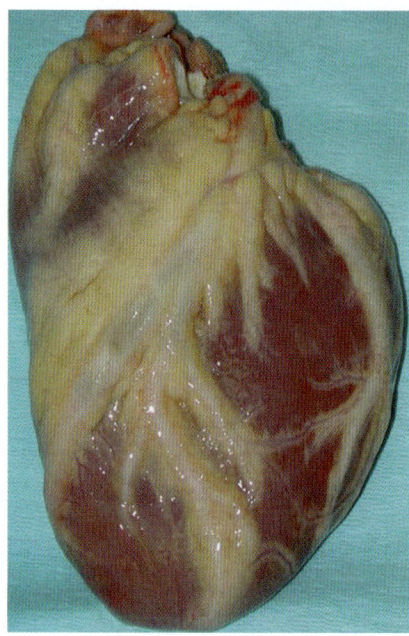

FIGURE 13-30 • Kawasaki disease. The heart from this 4-year-old is enlarged, has excessive fat deposition, and shows thick, dilated coronary arteries.

incomplete. The natural history of the aneurysms depends on their size and shape (231). Overall, 50% of the aneurysms resolve in the first 2 years; 20% become stenotic. Giant aneurysms (≥8 mm), which account for 20% of all aneurysms, do not resolve and 45% become stenotic. Although the death rate from KD overall is significantly below 1%, up to 40% of children with stenotic vessels experience myocardial infarction, with death in 18% (231). The advent of intravenous immunoglobulin therapy has dramatically reduced the incidence of coronary artery aneurysms, particularly when given within 10 days of disease onset.

The pathologic features of KD are almost entirely limited to autopsy studies and therefore represent the most severe pathologic changes. Within the first 10 days, vessel walls appear edematous (Figure 13-30) with acute inflammation in the perivascular soft tissue and vasa vasorum. Beginning and ending within 2 weeks of disease onset, there is self-limited necrotizing arteritis with accompanying neutrophilic infiltrate involving the medium-sized muscular and elastic arteries and proceeding from the endothelium to the adventitia (233). A subacute/chronic vasculitis begins within the first 2 weeks and can be seen months to years after diagnosis; histologically, predominantly small lymphocytes and clusters of plasma cells and eosinophils spread from perivascular tissue toward the lumen, in the opposite direction from the necrotizing arteritis. The subacute/chronic vasculitis can lead to aneurysm formation, thrombosis, and luminal myofibroblastic proliferation with progressive stenosis (234). In the acute phase, pericarditis, myocarditis, and endocarditis are often present with involvement of the conduction system (234). Over time, myocardial fibrosis and EFE appear. Endomyocardial biopsies from KD patients also reveal evidence of myocardial fibrosis with or without inflammation, although progression to CMP is not a described feature. In resected regressing aneurysms and coronary arteries from former KD patients dying of unrelated disease, intimal thickening with or without organizing thrombus material raises the speculation that KD may lead to early-onset coronary vascular disease.

Takayasu Arteritis. Takayasu arteritis (235) represents a form of large vessel vasculitis first described as "pulseless disease" because of subclavian artery occlusion. The vasculitis manifests in the aorta and its main branches initially as chronic granulomatous inflammation in the media and adventitia of the vessel wall. Subsequent thrombosis and intimal and wall fibrosis may lead to vessel occlusion; alternatively, the damaged vessel may be aneurysmally dilated. Symptoms of fever, malaise, arthralgias, and myalgias reflect the underlying inflammatory process. Occlusive symptoms, which vary depending on the anatomic location of the involved vessels, include seizures or stroke, renal hypertension, extremity claudication, aortic regurgitation, and pulmonary hypertension. Virtually all patients manifest multifocal bruits and/or absent pulses at presentation as a clue to the underlying disease. Takayasu arteritis predominantly affects young women and occurs most commonly in Asia, India, and Latin America (236). The underlying etiology for this rare disorder remains unknown.

CARDIAC TUMORS

Primary cardiac tumors occur rarely in both adults and children. Even among infants presenting for evaluation of

Ref. No.	Age Range (No.)	Rhabdomyoma (%)	Fibroma (%)	Teratoma (%)	Myxoma (%)	Histiocytoid (%)	Other Benign (%)	Malignant (%)
(239)	Fetal (89)	64	7	22	0	0	7	0
	Neonatal (135)	47	16	15	4	11	5	2
(240)	<1 year (35)	54	23	3	0	6	6	8
	1-15 years (56)	36	23	2	7	4	9	20
(237)	0-17 years (56) (Benign only)	79	11	2	0	0	8	—

cardiac disease, tumors account for only 0.2% to 0.4% of lesions (2,237). New imaging techniques have led to increased numbers of tumors identified during life. Fetal echocardiographic studies report cardiac tumors in 0.11% to 0.14% of referred pregnancies (238), with prenatal ultrasound identifying 21% of congenital cardiac tumors in one study (237).

The type of primary cardiac tumor present varies considerably with age (Table 13-41). In fetuses and newborn infants, rhabdomyomas account for the vast majority, followed by pericardial teratomas (238,239). During the first 2 years of life, rhabdomyomas continue to be the most common tumor, with fibromas representing the second most common (240). Myxomas, the most common tumor in adults, account for 7% of tumors in children, occurring almost exclusively in adolescents (240). In rare instances, a cardiac tumor (especially rhabdomyoma) occurs in association with a heart malformation (241). The space-occupying aspect of these tumors suggests that they in fact may play a role in inducing the associated malformation.

Benign Tumors
Rhabdomyomas

This most common cardiac tumor in infants occurs as a solitary, or more often (77% to 90%) (242,243) multiple, nodules anywhere in the heart (Figure 13-31). They are highly associated with tuberous sclerosis (TS), occurring in 40% to 60% of TS patients examined echocardiographically (241,242). Rhabdomyomas may be the first clue to the diagnosis of TS, with 70% to 80% of fetuses and infants carrying rhabdomyomas subsequently having a diagnosis of TS confirmed (242). Rhabdomyomas display a striking propensity to regress spontaneously. When identified in infancy, 50% to 70% will regress, especially when associated with TS (241). Tumors identified in older children are less likely to regress.

Clinically, many rhabdomyomas remain asymptomatic. Larger rhabdomyomas may project from the ventricular wall or septum into the cardiac cavity and obstruct cardiac flow or valvular motion (242). Disruption of the conduction system with resultant arrhythmias also frequently occurs. The tumors come to light in fetuses due to nonimmune hydrops, arrhythmias, a mass noted on routine prenatal ultrasound, or a family history of TS (238). Postnatally, tumors may present clinically with a murmur, heart failure, arrhythmia, or sudden death. When symptomatic, partial resection to relieve symptoms may be required, but more aggressive surgical intervention is contraindicated.

Grossly, rhabdomyomas appear as well-circumscribed, yellow-to-gray nodules that vary in size from microscopic to 10 cm in diameter (244). They occur with about equal frequency in either ventricle. They also may occur in the atrial walls; they have not been described in cardiac valves (243). Microscopically, the typical rhabdomyoma cells are much larger (up to 80 µm in diameter) than those of normal myocardium due to accumulation of glycogen within the cell cytoplasm, resulting in the formation of "spider cells." By electron microscopy, the "spider cells" contain abundant glycogen, few myofibrils, scattered leptofibrils, and poorly developed sarcoplasmic reticulum. Well-formed intercalated disclike intercellular junctions surround the periphery of the cells, mimicking cardiac myoblasts (243). The clinical pattern of multiple tumors that tend to regress, combined with the ultrastructural appearance of the tumor cells, supports the concept that cardiac rhabdomyomas represent a hamartomatous rather than a neoplastic process.

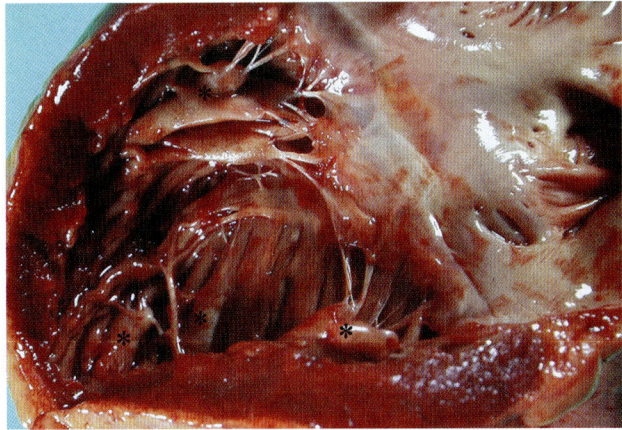

FIGURE 13-31 • Multiple small rhabdomyomas. In this opened left ventricular cavity, the trabeculae appear thickened and somewhat pale due to multiple small rhabdomyomas, highlighted by *asterisk*. These rhabdomyomas were asymptomatic in this child with tuberous sclerosis.

Cardiac Fibroma

Cardiac fibromas are the second most common tumor outside the fetal period; they present most frequently (>1/3 of cases) in the first year of life, with the remaining spread out over the following two decades (245). Fibromas characteristically arise as a single ventricular mass in an otherwise normal child, although a small subgroup occurs with Gorlin syndrome (245). Patients present with cardiomegaly, arrhythmias, and heart failure; sudden death occurs in one-third of cases, probably as the result of arrhythmias or outflow obstruction (243,245). The tumors arise most frequently in the left ventricle or interventricular septum but may also occur in the right ventricle and occasionally in the atria (244,245). They can be large, occasionally exceeding 10 cm (243). On cut surface, these firm white trabeculated tumors grossly resemble a leiomyoma (Figure 13-32). Microscopically, the tumors display a monomorphic population of bland spindled cells embedded within a variably collagenized stroma that often appears infiltrative at the periphery (243). Tumors from young infants tend to appear more cellular and mitotically active, features that do not denote more aggressive behavior (244,245). In older children, calcification and focal cystic degeneration become more prevalent. Although benign, cardiac fibromas do not regress and in fact tend to slowly increase in size (244). Surgical excision is the treatment of choice; unresectable tumors may require transplantation.

Teratomas

Teratomas are the second most common cardiac tumor in fetuses, with 50% of this rare tumor being diagnosed before or during the first month of life and two-thirds in the first year (246,247). In its more common intrapericardial location, the tumor originates from the external surface of the heart base and gives rise to an often marked pericardial effusion (246,247). Compression of the heart by the mass combined with the effusion leads to nonimmune hydrops in the fetus and cardiac tamponade in infants (239). Intrauterine pericardiocentesis is reported to effectively relieve the fetal distress. Surgical excision is curative. Rarely, teratomas occur in the interventricular septum, where they clinically mimic cardiac rhabdomyomas and fibromas (246). The pathologic features of the tumor are similar to benign teratomas occurring elsewhere in the body (239). Intrapericardial bronchogenic cysts overlap clinically with teratomas and may be included as teratomas in the older literature (246,247).

Myxomas

Myxomas are the most common (50% to 75%) cardiac tumor in adults (243) but account for only 5% of tumors in infancy and 15% to 20% of tumors in older children and adolescents (239,240,243). They arise from the endocardium, usually adjacent to the fossa ovalis, in the left (75%) or right (18%) atrium (243,248). Presenting symptoms include one or more components of a clinical triad (Table 13-42) (243,248,249). Although the vast majority of atrial myxomas occur sporadically, approximately 5% occur in families as part of Carney complex (Table 13-42) (250,251). Carney complex, an autosomal dominant disorder, results from a mutation in the *PRKAR1A* gene (locus 17q22-24) in up to 70% of cases (250,251). The syndromic form of atrial myxoma tends to occur at a younger age, in atypical locations, and with a higher frequency of multiple recurrent tumors as compared with the sporadic form (252). Atrial myxomas occurring in children and adolescents should therefore elicit a search for other manifestations of this complex in both patients and other family members.

Identical pathologic features occur in syndromic and sporadic forms of atrial myxoma (243,244,248,253). Grossly, the tumors appear gelatinous with a narrow or broad base and

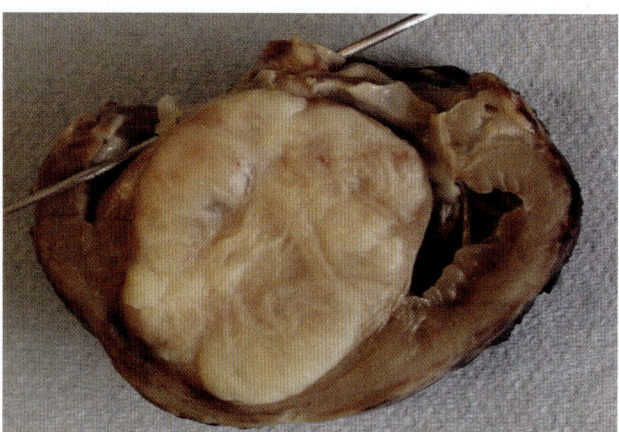

FIGURE 13-32 • Cardiac fibroma. In this transverse section of an explanted heart as viewed from the back, a white firm trabeculated mass replaces the interventricular septum and protrudes into the left and right ventricular cavities. A probe inserted into the aortic valve exits into the left ventricular chamber under the mitral valve leaflet, highlighting the obstruction to the left ventricular outflow caused by this large cardiac fibroma.

TABLE 13-42	ATRIAL MYXOMAS—CLINICAL FEATURES

Clinical Triad (248,249)
Valvular obstruction
Tumor emboli
Constitutional symptoms
    Malaise, fever, weight loss, anemia, elevated ESR, hypergammaglobulinemia
Carney Complex (250,251)
    Skin lesions: lentigines, blue nevi, other pigmented lesions
    Myxomas: cardiac, breast, skin, mucous membranes, bone
    Breast: ductal adenomas
    Psammomatous melanotic schwannomas
    Osteochondromyxomas
    Endocrine abnormalities:
        Adrenal: primary pigmented nodular adrenocortical disease (PPNAD)
        Pituitary: adenoma
        Thyroid: nodules, carcinoma
        Testicle: large-cell calcifying Sertoli cell tumor

a frond-like or smooth surface. The cut surface appears variegated with scattered gritty calcification. Microscopically, stellate or elongate cells with scant eosinophilic cytoplasm disperse singly or as small nests, trabeculae, or perivascular rings in an acid mucopolysaccharide-rich myxoid matrix. With immunohistochemical stains, the cells mark reliably with vimentin and variably with endothelial, actin, and cytokeratin markers (249,253).

Histiocytoid Cardiomyopathy

Histiocytoid cardiomyopathy is a rare myocardial disease of infancy and early childhood characterized by cardiomegaly, incessant ventricular tachycardia, and sudden death. More than 70 cases have been reported under a variety of synonyms, including isolated cardiac lipidosis, xanthomatous CMP, foamy myocardial transformation of infancy, oncocytic CMP, myocardial hamartoma, and Purkinje cell tumor (254,255). The lesion presents almost exclusively in the first 2 years of life, with a 75% predominance in girls (254). In a subgroup of these patients, both cardiac and noncardiac malformations occur, including ASDs, VSDs, EFE, hypoplastic left heart, corneal opacities, microphthalmia, cataracts, cleft palate, hydrocephalus, agenesis of the corpus callosum, and renal cysts (254).

At surgery or autopsy, the heart is often enlarged, with the left ventricular surface studded by multiple flat to round, smooth, yellow-to-tan–white nodules that may or may not be visible to the naked eye. Similar nodules may also occur on the papillary muscles, right ventricle, atria, and all four heart valves (254,256). Histologically, the nodules contain cells that differ from adjacent myocardial cells in both their larger size (20 to 40 μm diameter) and the pale foamy nature of their cytoplasm, which gives them their histiocytoid appearance (Figure 13-33). Nodules of similar cells are also often present in the conduction system, the midmyocardium, and beneath the epicardium. Immunohistochemical stains identify the cells as myocardial in origin based on positive muscle-specific actin and myosin and negative lysozyme and CD68 (257). These foamy cells contain only small amounts of glycogen and lipid; the mitochondria-rich nature of the cytoplasm becomes evident only at the ultrastructural level. By electron microscopy, these swollen abnormal myocytes contain abundant mitochondria with only rare peripherally placed myofibrils, scattered leptofibrils, no T tubules, and decreased numbers of desmosomes (256,257).

The pathogenesis for this unusual condition remains controversial. The ultrastructural features suggest a relationship with primitive Purkinje cells (256) or primitive myocardial cells and support a hamartomatous process. Comparable cellular changes may occur in other organs of infants with cardiac lesions. The finding of respiratory chain enzyme deficiencies and mtDNA mutations in a few cases raises the possibility of an underlying mitochondrial disorder (255). The possibility of an X-linked chromosomal abnormality has been suggested in a few other cases (258). Whole genome expression analysis suggests a possible role for downregulation of the IL-33/ST2 signaling pathway in the pathogenesis of this condition (259).

Unfortunately, the diagnosis of histiocytoid CMP is most often made at autopsy. When the presenting ventricular arrhythmia can be initially controlled medically, subsequent electrophysiologic mapping and surgical ablation of the lesions can lead to long-term survival. Cardiac transplantation has also been reported.

Other Benign Tumors

A variety of other benign tumors and malformations have been described in the heart (Table 13-43). Vascular tumors may occur in the setting of multiple cutaneous hemangiomas (239).

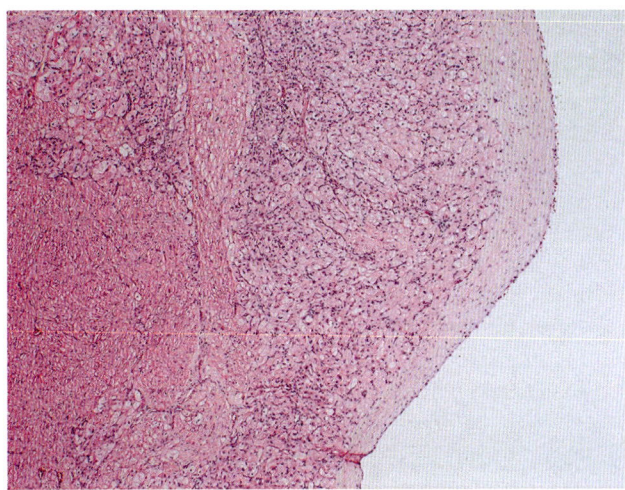

FIGURE 13-33 • Histiocytoid cardiomyopathy. Enlarged, granular-appearing, histiocytoid myocytes in the subendocardial area contrast with the normal compact myocytes on the left. (Hematoxylin and eosin stain, original magnification 100×.)

TABLE 13-43 OTHER BENIGN CARDIAC TUMORS AND MALFORMATIONS

Tumor	% of Benign Cardiac Tumors
Hemangioma and vascular malformation	4%
Mesothelioma of AV node	4%
Inflammatory myofibroblastic tumor	2%
Neurofibroma	<1%
Bronchogenic cyst	
Lipoma	
Lipoblastoma	
Multicystic hamartoma	

See references (240,243,244).

TABLE 13-44	MALIGNANT CARDIAC TUMORS

Primary (285,286)
  Rhabdomyosarcoma
  Fibrosarcoma
  Undifferentiated sarcoma
  Angiosarcoma
  Leiomyosarcoma
  Malignant peripheral nerve sheath tumor
  Synovial sarcoma
  Osteosarcoma
  Malignant germ-cell tumor
  Myeloid sarcoma
  Lymphoma
Secondary (metastatic) (260,287)
  Non-Hodgkin lymphoma
  Neuroblastoma
  Wilms tumor
  Hepatoblastoma
  Hepatoma
  Rhabdomyosarcoma
  Fibrosarcoma
  Undifferentiated sarcoma
  Osteosarcoma
  Ewing sarcoma
  Melanoma
  Adrenal carcinoma
  Malignant germ-cell tumor
  Hodgkin lymphoma
  Pleuropulmonary blastoma

Malignant Tumors

Malignant tumors account for less than 1% of the primary cardiac tumors in the fetus and newborn. In older infants and children, malignancies become more prevalent, accounting for 10% to 20% of primary cardiac tumors (240,243). In children, as in adults, metastatic tumors outnumber primary cardiac malignancies (260). Secondary malignant tumors may be distant metastases or arise from direct extension. The range of reported primary and metastatic malignant tumors is summarized in Table 13-44.

References

1. Srivastava D. Making or breaking the heart: from lineage determination to morphogenesis. *Cell* 2006;126(6):1037–1048.
2. Fyler DC, Buckley LP, Hellenbrand WE, et al. Report of the New England Regional Infant Cardiac Program. *Pediatrics* 1980;65:377–461.
3. Gelb BD, Chung WK. Complex genetics and the etiology of human congenital heart disease. *Cold Spring Harb Perspect Med* 2014;4(7):a013953. doi: 10.1101/cshperspect.a013953.
4. Brennan P, Young ID. Congenital heart malformations: aetiology and associations. *Semin Neonatol* 2001;6:17–25.
5. Pradat P, Francannet C, Harris JA, et al. The epidemiology of cardiovascular defects, part I: a study based on data from three large registries of congenital malformations. *Pediatr Cardiol* 2003;24:195–221.
6. Goldmuntz E. DiGeorge syndrome: new insights. *Clin Perinatol* 2005;32:963–978.
7. Ransom J, Srivastava D. The genetics of cardiac birth defects. *Semin Cell Dev Biol* 2007;18:132–139.
8. Oyer CE, Sung CJ, Friedman R, et al. Reference values for valve circumferences and ventricular wall thicknesses of fetal and neonatal hearts. *Pediatr Dev Pathol* 2004;7:499–505.
9. Rowlatt UF, Rimoldi HJA, Lev M. The quantitative anatomy of the normal child's heart. *Pediatr Clin North Am* 1963;10:499–588.
10. Scholz DG, Kitzman DW, Hagen PT, et al. Age-related changes in normal human hearts during the first 10 decades of life. Part I (Growth): a quantitative anatomic study of 200 specimens from subjects from birth to 19 years old. *Mayo Clin Proc* 1988;63:126–136.
11. Anderson RH. How should we optimally describe complex congenitally malformed hearts? *Ann Thorac Surg* 1996;62:710–716.
12. Devine WA, Debich DE, Anderson RH. Dissection of congenitally malformed hearts, with comments on the value of sequential segmental analysis. *Pediatr Pathol* 1991;11:235–259.
13. Van Praagh R. The segmental approach to diagnosis in congenital heart disease. *Birth Defects Orig Artic Ser* 1972;8:4–23.
14. Arey JB. *Cardiovascular Pathology in Infants and Children*. Philadelphia, PA: W.B. Saunders Company, 1984.
15. Moller JH, Nakib A, Eliot RS, et al. Congenital cardiac disease associated with polysplenia: a developmental complex of bilateral "left-sidedness". *Circulation* 1967;36:789–799.
16. Sharma S, Devine WA, Anderson RH, et al. The determination of atrial arrangement by examination of appendage morphology in 1842 heart specimens. *Br Heart J* 1988;60:227–231.
17. Belmont JW, Mohapatra B, Towbin JA, et al. Molecular genetics of heterotaxy syndromes. *Curr Opin Cardiol* 2004;19:216–220.
18. Thoele DG, Ursell PC, Ho SY. Atrial morphologic features in tricuspid atresia. *J Thorac Cardiovasc Surg* 1991;102:606–610.
19. Leca F, Thibert M, Khoury W, et al. Extrathoracic heart (ectopia cordis). Report of two cases and review of the literature. *Int J Cardiol* 1989;22:221–228.
20. Geva T, Van Praagh S. Abnormal systemic venous connections. In: Allen HD, Gutgesell HP, Clark EB, et al., eds. *Moss & Adams' Heart Disease in Infants, Children & Adolescents: Including the Fetus and Young Adults*, 6th ed. Philadelphia, PA: Lippincott Williams & Wilkins, 2001:773–798.
21. Adatia I, Gittenberger-de Groot AC. Unroofed coronary sinus and coronary sinus orifice atresia: implications for management of complex congenital heart disease. *J Am Coll Cardiol* 1995;25:948–953.
22. Gustafson RA, Warden HE, Murray GF, et al. Partial anomalous pulmonary venous connection to the right side of the heart. *J Thorac Cardiovasc Surg* 1989;98:861–868.
23. Najm HK, Williams WG, Coles JG, et al. Scimitar syndrome: twenty years' experience and results of repair. *J Thorac Cardiovasc Surg* 1996;112:1161–1169.
24. Geva T, Van Praagh S. Anomalies of the pulmonary veins. In: Allen HD, Gutgesell HP, Clark EB, et al., eds. *Moss & Adams' Heart Disease in Infants, Children & Adolescents: Including the Fetus and Young Adults*, 6th ed. Philadelphia, PA: Lippincott Williams & Wilkins, 2001:736–772.
25. Delisle G, Ando M, Calder AL, et al. Total anomalous pulmonary venous connection: report of 93 autopsied cases with emphasis on diagnostic and surgical considerations. *Am Heart J* 1976;91:99–122.
26. Karamlou T, Gurofsky R, Al Sukhni E, et al. Factors associated with mortality and reoperation in 377 children with total anomalous pulmonary venous connection. *Circulation* 2007;115:1591–1598.
27. Richardson JV, Doty DB, Siewers RD, et al. Cor triatriatum (subdivided left atrium). *J Thorac Cardiovasc Surg* 1981;81:232–238.
28. Briggs LE, Kakarla J, Wessels A. The pathogenesis of atrial and atrioventricular septal defects with special emphasis on the role of the dorsal mesenchymal protrusion. *Differentiation* 2012;84(1):117–130. doi: 10.1016/j.diff.2012.05.006.
29. Hagen PT, Scholz DG, Edwards WD. Incidence and size of patent foramen ovale during the first 10 decades of life: an autopsy study of 965 normal hearts. *Mayo Clin Proc* 1984;59:17–20.

30. Porter CJ, Feldt RH, Edwards WD, et al. Atrial septal defects. In: Allen HD, Gutgesell HP, Clark EB, et al., eds. *Moss and Adams' Heart Disease in Infants, Children & Adolescents: Including the Fetus and Young Adults*, vol. 6. Philadelphia, PA: Lippincott Williams & Wilkins, 2001:603–617.
31. Azhari N, Shihata MS, Al-Fatani A. Spontaneous closure of atrial septal defects within the oval fossa. *Cardiol Young* 2004;14:148–155.
32. al Zaghal AM, Li J, Anderson RH, et al. Anatomical criteria for the diagnosis of sinus venosus defects. *Heart* 1997;78:298–304.
33. Yi Li Q, Newbury-Ecob RA, Terrett JA, et al. Holt-Oram syndrome is caused by mutations in *TBX5*, a member of the *Brachyury (T)* gene family. *Nat Genet* 1997;15:21–29.
34. Basson CT, Bachinsky DR, Lin RC, et al. Mutations in human cause limb and cardiac malformation in Holt-Oram syndrome. *Nat Genet* 1997;15:30–35.
35. Anderson RH, Lenox CC, Zuberbuhler JR. The morphology of ventricular septal defects. *Perspect Pediatr Pathol* 1984;8:235–268.
36. Milo S, Ho SY, Wilkinson JL, et al. Surgical anatomy and atrioventricular conduction tissues of hearts with isolated ventricular septal defects. *J Thorac Cardiovasc Surg* 1980;79:244–255.
37. Zielinsky P, Rossi M, Haertel JC, et al. Subaortic fibrous ridge and ventricular septal defect: role of septal malalignment. *Circulation* 1987;75:1124–1129.
38. Hoffman JIE, Rudolph AM. The natural history of ventricular septal defects in infancy. *Am J Cardiol* 1965;16:634–653.
39. Mitchell SC, Korones SB, Berendes HW. Congenital heart disease in 56,109 births. Incidence and natural history. *Circulation* 1971;43:323–332.
40. Nugent EW, Freedom RM, Rowe RD, et al. Aneurysm of the membranous septum in ventricular septal defect. *Circulation* 1977;56:I82–I84.
41. Anderson RH, Ho SY, Becker AE. The surgical anatomy of the conduction tissues. *Thorax* 1983;38:408–420.
42. Becker AE, Anderson RH. Atrioventricular septal defects: what's in a name? *J Thorac Cardiovasc Surg* 1982;83:461–469.
43. Pierpont MEM, Markwald RR, Lin AE. Genetic aspects of atrioventricular septal defects. *Am J Med Genet* 2000;97:289–296.
44. Silverman NH, Zuberbuhler JR, Anderson RH. Atrioventricular septal defects: cross-sectional echocardiographic and morphologic comparisons. *Int J Cardiol* 1986;13:309–331.
45. Suzuki K, Ho SY, Anderson RH, et al. Morphometric analysis of atrioventricular septal defect with common valve orifice. *J Am Coll Cardiol* 1998;31:217–223.
46. Newfeld EA, Sher M, Paul MH, et al. Pulmonary vascular disease in complete atrioventricular canal defect. *Am J Cardiol* 1977;39:721–726.
47. Kirby ML, Gale TF, Stewart DE. Neural crest cells contribute to normal aorticopulmonary septation. *Science* 1983;220:1059–1061.
48. Khositseth A, Tocharoentanaphol C, Khowsathit P, et al. Chromosome 22q11 deletions in patients with conotruncal heart defects. *Pediatr Cardiol* 2005;26:570–573.
49. Wernovsky G. Transposition of the great arteries. In: Allen HD, Gutgesell HP, Clark EB, et al., eds. *Moss and Adams' Heart Disease in Infants, Children and Adolescents: Including the Fetus and Young Adults*, vol. 6. Philadelphia, PA: Lippincott Williams & Wilkins, 2001:1027–1084.
50. Anderson RH, Weinberg PM. The clinical anatomy of transposition. *Cardiol Young* 2005;15:76–87.
51. Smith A, Arnold R, Wilkinson JL. An anatomical study of the patterns of the coronary arteries and sinus nodal artery in complete transposition. *Int J Cardiol* 1986;12:295–307.
52. Mavroudis C, Backer CL. Transposition of the great arteries. In: Mavroudis C, Baker CJ, eds. *Pediatric Cardiac Surgery*, 3rd ed. Philadelphia, PA: Mosby, 2003:442–475.
53. Milanesi O, Ho SY, Thiene G, et al. The ventricular septal defect in complete transposition of the great arteries: pathologic anatomy in 57 cases with emphasis on subaortic, subpulmonary, and aortic arch obstruction. *Hum Pathol* 1987;18:392–396.
54. Van Praagh R, Papagiannis J, Grunenfelder J, et al. Pathologic anatomy of corrected transposition of the great arteries: medical and surgical implications. *Am Heart J* 1998;135:772–785.
55. de Albuquerque AT, Rigby ML, Anderson RH, et al. The spectrum of atrioventricular discordance. A clinical study. *Br Heart J* 1984;51:498–507.
56. Sridaromont S, Feldt RH, Ritter DG, et al. Double outlet right ventricle: hemodynamic and anatomic correlations. *Am J Cardiol* 1976;38:85–94.
57. Hagler DJ. Double-outlet right ventricle and double outlet left ventricle. In: Allen HD, Gutgesell HP, Clark EB, et al., eds. *Moss and Adams' Heart Disease in Infants, Children and Adolescents: Including the Fetus and Young Adults*, vol. 6. Philadelphia, PA: Lippincott Williams & Wilkins, 2001:1102–1128.
58. Lev M, Bharati S, Meng L, et al. A concept of double-outlet right ventricle. *J Thorac Cardiovasc Surg* 1972;64:271–281.
59. Ueda M, Becker AE. Classification of hearts with overriding aortic and pulmonary valves. *Int J Cardiol* 1985;9:357–369.
60. Anderson RH, Ho SY, Wilcox BR. The surgical anatomy of ventricular septal defect part IV: double outlet ventricle. *J Card Surg* 1996;11:2–11.
61. Walters HLI, Pacifico AD. Double outlet ventricles. In: Mavroudis C, Backer CL, eds. *Pediatric Cardiac Surgery*, 3rd ed. Philadelphia, PA: Mosby, 2003:408–441.
62. Taussig HB, Bing RJ. Complete transposition of the aorta and the levoposition of the pulmonary artery: clinical, physiological and pathological findings. *Am Heart J* 1949;37:551–559.
63. Tchervenkov CI, Walters HL, Chu VF. Congenital heart surgery nomenclature and database project: double outlet left ventricle. *Ann Thorac Surg* 2000;69:S264–S269.
64. Van Praagh R, Weinberg PM, Srebro JP. Double-outlet left ventricle. In: Adams FH, Emmanouilides GC, Riemenschneider TA, eds. *Heart Disease in Infants, Children, and Adolescents*, 4th ed. Baltimore, MD: Lippincott Williams & Wilkins, 1989:461–748.
65. Crupi G, Macartney FJ, Anderson RH. Persistent truncus arteriosus: a study of 66 autopsy cases with special reference to definition and morphogenesis. *Am J Cardiol* 1977;40:569–578.
66. Van Praagh R, Van Praagh S. The anatomy of common aorticopulmonary trunk (truncus arteriosus communis) and its embryologic implications. A study of 57 necropsy cases. *Am J Cardiol* 1965;16:406–425.
67. Van Praagh R. Truncus arteriosus: what is it really and how should it be classified? *Eur J Cardiothorac Surg* 1987;1:65–70.
68. Mair DD, Edwards WD, Julsrud PR, et al. Truncus arteriosus. In: Allen HD, Gutgesell HP, Clark EB, et al., eds. *Moss and Adams' Heart Disease in Infants, Children and Adolescents: Including the Fetus and Young Adults*, vol. 6. Philadelphia, PA: Lippincott Williams & Wilkins, 2001:910–923.
69. Goldmuntz E, Clark BJ, Mitchell LE, et al. Frequency of 22q11 deletions in patients with conotruncal defects. *J Am Coll Cardiol* 1998;32:492–498.
70. Kutsche LM, Van Mierop LH. Anatomy and pathogenesis of aorticopulmonary septal defect. *Am J Cardiol* 1987;59:443–447.
71. Scalia D, Russo P, Anderson RH, et al. The surgical anatomy of hearts with no direct communication between the right atrium and the ventricular mass-so-called tricuspid atresia. *J Thorac Cardiovasc Surg* 1984;87:743–755.
72. Epstein ML. Tricuspid atresia. In: Allen HD, Gutgesell HP, Clark EB, et al., eds. *Moss and Adams' Heart Disease in Infants, Children and Adolescents: Including the Fetus and Young Adults*, 6th ed. Philadelphia, PA: Lippincott Williams & Wilkins, 2001:799–809.
73. Attenhofer Jost CH, Connolly HM, Dearani JA, et al. Ebstein's anomaly. *Circulation* 2007;115:277–285.
74. Schreiber C, Cook A, Ho SY, et al. Morphologic spectrum of Ebstein's malformation: revisitation relative to surgical repair. *J Thorac Cardiovasc Surg* 1999;117:148–155.
75. Celermajer DS, Bull C, Till JA, et al. Ebstein's anomaly: presentation and outcome from fetus to adult. *J Am Coll Cardiol* 1994;23:170–176.
76. Attenhofer Jost CH, Connolly HM, O'Leary PW, et al. Left heart lesions in patients with Ebstein anomaly. *Mayo Clin Proc* 2005;80:361–368.
77. Ruckman RN, Van Praagh R. Anatomic types of congenital mitral stenosis: report of 49 autopsy cases with consideration of diagnosis and surgical implications. *Am J Cardiol* 1978;42:592–601.
78. Van Praagh S, Porras D, Oppido G, et al. Cleft mitral valve without ostium primum defect: anatomic data and surgical considerations based on 41 cases. *Ann Thorac Surg* 2003;75:1752–1762.

79. Tandon R, Moller JH, Edwards JE. Anomalies associated with the parachute mitral valve: a pathologic analysis of 52 cases. Can J Cardiol 1986;2:278–281.
80. Shone JD, Sellers RD, Anderson RC. The developmental complex of "parachute mitral valve," supravalvular ring of left atrium, subaortic stenosis and coarctation of the aorta. Am J Cardiol 1963;11:714–725.
81. Gittenberger-de Groot AC, Wenink AC. Mitral atresia: morphological details. Br Heart J 1984;51:252–258.
82. Ho SY, Zuberbuhler JR, Anderson RH. Pathology of hearts with a univentricular atrioventricular connection. Perspect Pediatr Pathol 1988;12:69–99.
83. Beckman CB, Moller JH, Edwards JE. Alternate pathways to pulmonary venous flow in left-sided obstructive anomalies. Circulation 1975;52:509–516.
84. Virmani R, Atkinson JB, Forman NB, et al. Mitral valve prolapse. Hum Pathol 1987;18:596–602.
85. Edwards JE. Floppy mitral valve syndrome. Cardiovasc Clin 1988;18:249–271.
86. Greenwood RD. Mitral valve prolapse: incidence and clinical course in a pediatric population. Clin Pediatr (Phila) 1984;23:318–320.
87. Bissett GSI, Schwartz DC, Meyer RA, et al. Clinical spectrum and long term follow-up of isolated mitral valve prolapse in 119 children. Circulation 1980;62:423–429.
88. Hagler DJ, Edwards WD. Univentricular atrioventricular connection. In: Allen HD, Gutgesell HP, Clark EB, et al., eds. Moss and Adams' Heart Disease in Infants, Children and Adolescents: Including the Fetus and Young Adults, vol. 6. Philadelphia, PA: Lippincott Williams & Wilkins, 2001:1129–1150.
89. Milo S, Ho SY, Macartney FJ, et al. Straddling and overriding atrioventricular valves: morphology and classification. Am J Cardiol 1979;44:1122–1134.
90. Anderson RH, Allwork SP, Ho SY, et al. Surgical anatomy of tetralogy of Fallot. J Thorac Cardiovasc Surg 1981;81:887–896.
91. Anderson RH, Weinberg PM. The clinical anatomy of tetralogy of Fallot. Cardiol Young 2005;15:38–47.
92. Siwik ES, Patel CR, Zahka KG, et al. Tetralogy of Fallot. In: Allen HD, Gutgesell HP, Clark BJ, et al., eds. Moss & Adams' Heart Disease in Infants, Children & Adolescents: Including the Fetus and Young Adults, 6th ed. Philadelphia, PA: Lippincott Williams & Wilkins, 2001:880–902.
93. Kinsley RH, McGoon DC, Danielson GK, et al. Pulmonary arterial hypertension after repair of tetralogy of Fallot. J Thorac Cardiovasc Surg 1974;67:111–120.
94. Tchervenkov CI, Roy N. Congenital heart surgery nomenclature and database project: pulmonary atresia–ventricular septal defect. Ann Thorac Surg 2000;69:S97–S105.
95. Hadjo A, Jimenez M, Baudet E, et al. Review of the long-term course of 52 patients with pulmonary atresia and ventricular septal defect: anatomical and surgical considerations. Eur Heart J 1995;16:1668–1674.
96. Johnson RJ, Sauer U, Buhlmeyer K, et al. Hypoplasia of the intrapulmonary arteries in children with right ventricular outflow tract obstruction, ventricular septal defect, and major aortopulmonary collateral arteries. Pediatr Cardiol 1985;6:137–143.
97. Gutgesell HP, Goldmuntz E. Congenital absence of the pulmonary valve. In: Allen HD, Gutgesell HP, Clark EB, et al., eds. Moss and Adams' Heart Disease in Infants, Children and Adolescents: Including the Fetus and Young Adults, vol. 6. Philadelphia, PA: Lippincott Williams & Wilkins, 2001:903–909.
98. Buendia A, Attie F, Ovseyevitz J, et al. Congenital absence of pulmonary valve leaflets. Br Heart J 1983;50:31–41.
99. Stamm C, Anderson RH, Ho SY. Clinical anatomy of the normal pulmonary root compared with that in isolated pulmonary valvular stenosis. J Am Coll Cardiol 1998;31:1420–1425.
100. Gikonyo BM, Lucas RV, Edwards JE. Anatomic features of congenital pulmonary valvar stenosis. Pediatr Cardiol 1987;8:109–116.
101. Gielen H, Daniels O, van Lier H. Natural history of congenital pulmonary valvar stenosis: an echo and Doppler cardiographic study. Cardiol Young 1999;9:129–135.
102. Cil E, Saraclar M, Ozkutlu S, et al. Double-chambered right ventricle: experience with 52 cases. Int J Cardiol 1995;50:19–29.
103. Franch RH, Gay BB Jr. Congenital stenosis of the pulmonary artery branches: a classification, with post mortem findings in two cases. Am J Cardiol 1963;35:512.
104. Gay BB Jr, Franch RH, Shuford WH, et al. Roentgenologic features of simple and multiple coarctations of the pulmonary artery and branches. Am J Roentgenol 1963;90:599.
105. Latson LA, Prieto LR. Pulmonary stenosis. In: Allen HD, Gutgesell HP, Clark EB, et al., eds. Moss & Adams' Heart Disease in Infants, Children & Adolescents: Including the Fetus and Young Adults, 6th ed. Philadelphia, PA: Lippincott Williams & Wilkins, 2001:820–844.
106. Zuberbuhler JR, Anderson RH. Morphological variations in pulmonary atresia with intact ventricular septum. Br Heart J 1979;41:281–288.
107. Choi YH, Seo JW, Choi JY, et al. Morphology of tricuspid valve in pulmonary atresia with intact ventricular septum. Pediatr Cardiol 1998;19:381–389.
108. Hausdorf G, Gravinghoff L, Keck EW. Effects of persisting myocardial sinusoids on left ventricular performance in pulmonary atresia with intact ventricular septum. Eur Heart J 1987;8:291–296.
109. Vricella LA, Kanani M, Cook AC, et al. Problems with the right ventricular outflow tract: a review of morphologic features and current therapeutic options. Cardiol Young 2005;14:533–549.
110. Brown JW, Stevens LS, Holly S, et al. Surgical spectrum of aortic stenosis in children: a thirty-year experience with 257 children. Ann Thorac Surg 1988;45:393–403.
111. Newfeld EA, Muster AJ, Paul MH, et al. Discrete subvalvular aortic stenosis in childhood: study of 51 patients. Am J Cardiol 1976;38:53–61.
112. Vogt J, Dische R, Rupprath G, et al. Fixed subaortic stenosis: an acquired secondary obstruction? A twenty-seven year experience with 168 patients. Thorac Cardiovasc Surg 1989;37:199–206.
113. Stamm C, Li J, Ho SY, et al. The aortic root in supravalvular aortic stenosis: the potential surgical relevance of morphologic findings. J Thorac Cardiovasc Surg 1997;114:16–24.
114. Peterson TA, Todd DB, Edwards JE. Supravalvular aortic stenosis. J Thorac Cardiovasc Surg 1965;50:734–741.
115. Zalzstein E, Moes CA, Musewe NN, et al. Spectrum of cardiovascular anomalies in Williams-Beuren syndrome. Pediatr Cardiol 1991;12:219–223.
116. Aiello VD, Ho SY, Anderson RH, et al. Morphologic features of the hypoplastic left heart syndrome—a reappraisal. Pediatr Pathol 1990;10:931–943.
117. Mahowald JM, Lucas RV Jr, Edwards JE. Aortic valvular atresia: associated cardiovascular anomalies. Pediatr Cardiol 1982;2:99–105.
118. Hagemo PS, Skarbo A-B, Rasmussen M, et al. An extensive long term follow-up of a cohort of patients with hypoplasia of the left heart. Cardiol Young 2007;17:51–55.
119. Schneider DJ, Moore JW. Patent ductus arteriosus. Circulation 2006;114:1873–1882.
120. Moore P, Brook MM, Heymann MA. Patent ductus arteriosus. In: Allen HD, Gutgesell HP, Clark EB, et al., eds. Moss and Adams' Heart Disease in Infants, Children and Adolescents: Including the Fetus and Young Adults, vol. 6. Philadelphia, PA: Lippincott Williams & Wilkins, 2001:652–669.
121. Ho SY, Anderson RH. Anatomical closure of the ductus arteriosus: a study in 35 specimens. J Anat 1979;128:829–836.
122. Satoda M, Zhao F, Diaz GA, et al. Mutations in TFAP2B cause Char syndrome, a familial form of patent ductus arteriosus. Nat Genet 2000;25:42–46.
123. Machii M, Becker AE. Hypoplastic aortic arch morphology pertinent to growth after surgical correction of aortic coarctation. Ann Thorac Surg 1997;64:516–520.
124. Beekman RH. Coarctation of the aorta. In: Allen HD, Gutgesell HP, Clark EB, et al., eds. Moss and Adams' Heart Disease in Infants, Children and Adolescents: Including the Fetus and Young Adults, vol. 6. Philadelphia, PA: Lippincott Williams & Wilkins, 2001:988–1010.

125. Pellegrino A, Deverall PB, Anderson RH, et al. Aortic coarctation in the first three months of life: an anatomopathological study with respect to treatment. *J Thorac Cardiovasc Surg* 1985;89:121–127.
126. Amato JJ, Galdieri RJ, Cotroneo JV. Role of extended aortoplasty related to the definition of coarctation of the aorta. *Ann Thorac Surg* 1991;52:615–620.
127. Loffredo CA, Ferencz C, Wilson PD, et al. Interrupted aortic arch: an epidemiologic study. *Teratology* 2000;61:368–375.
128. Kussman BD, Geva T, McGowan FX Jr. Cardiovascular causes of airway compression. *Pediatr Anesth* 2004;14:60–74.
129. Weinberg PM. Aortic arch anomalies. In: Allen HD, Gutgesell HP, Clark EB, et al., eds. *Moss & Adams' Heart Disease in Infants, Children & Adolescents: Including the Fetus and Young Adults*, 6th ed. Philadelphia, PA: Lippincott Williams & Wilkins, 2001:707–772.
130. Gikonyo BM, Jue KL, Edwards JE. Pulmonary vascular sling: report of seven cases and review of the literature. *Pediatr Cardiol* 1989;10:81–89.
131. Matherne GP. Congenital anomalies of the coronary vessels and the aortic root. In: Allen HD, Gutgesell HP, Clark EB, et al., eds. *Moss & Adams' Heart Disease in Infants, Children & Adolescents: Including the Fetus and Young Adults*, 6th ed. Philadelphia PA: Lippincott Williams & Wilkins, 2001:675–688.
132. Smith A, Arnold R, Anderson RH, et al. Anomalous origin of the left coronary artery from the pulmonary trunk. Anatomic findings in relation to pathophysiology and surgical repair. *J Thorac Cardiovasc Surg* 1989;98:16–24.
133. Maron BJ, Towbin JA, Thiene G, et al. Contemporary definitions and classification of the cardiomyopathies: an American Heart Association Scientific Statement from the Council on Clinical Cardiology, Heart Failure and Transplantation Committee; Quality of Care and Outcomes Research and Functional Genomics and Translational Biology Interdisciplinary Working Groups; and Council on Epidemiology and Prevention. *Circulation* 2006;113:1807–1816.
134. Lipshultz SE, Sleeper LA, Towbin JA, et al. The incidence of pediatric cardiomyopathy in two regions of the United States. *N Engl J Med* 2003;348:1647–1655.
135. Schwartz ML, Cox GF, Lin AE, et al. Clinical approach to genetic cardiomyopathy in children. *Circulation* 1996;94:2021–2038.
136. Maron BJ. Hypertrophic cardiomyopathy in childhood. *Pediatr Clin North Am* 2004;51:1305–1346.
137. Hughes SE. The pathology of hypertrophic cardiomyopathy. *Histopathology* 2004;44:412–427.
138. Basso C, Thiene G, Corrado D, et al. Hypertrophic cardiomyopathy and sudden death in the young: pathologic evidence of myocardial ischemia. *Hum Pathol* 2000;31:988–998.
139. Maron BJ, Verter J. Disproportionate ventricular septal thickening in the developing normal human heart. *Circulation* 1978;57:520–526.
140. Richard P, Charron P, Carrier L, et al. Hypertrophic cardiomyopathy: distribution of disease genes, spectrum of mutations, and implications for a molecular diagnosis strategy. *Circulation* 2003;107:2227–2232.
141. Feldman AM, McNamara D. Myocarditis. *N Engl J Med* 2000;343:1388–1398.
142. Tabib A, Loire R, Chalabreysse L, et al. Circumstances of death and gross and microscopic observations in a series of 200 cases of sudden death associated with arrhythmogenic right ventricular cardiomyopathy and/or dysplasia. *Circulation* 2003;108:3000–3005.
143. Thiene G, Basso C, Calabrese F, et al. Pathology and pathogenesis of arrhythmogenic right ventricular cardiomyopathy. *Herz* 2000;25:210–215.
144. Kies P, Bootsma M, Bax J, et al. Arrhythmogenic right ventricular dysplasia/cardiomyopathy: screening, diagnosis, and treatment. *Heart Rhythm* 2006;3:225–234.
145. Freedom RM, Yoo SJ, Perrin D, et al. The morphological spectrum of ventricular noncompaction. *Cardiol Young* 2005;15:345–364.
146. Weiford BC, Subbarao VD, Mulhern KM. Noncompaction of the ventricular myocardium. *Circulation* 2004;109:2965–2971.
147. Burke A, Mont E, Kutys R, et al. Left ventricular noncompaction: a pathological study of 14 cases. *Hum Pathol* 2005;36:403–411.
148. Edwards WD. Cardiomyopathies. *Hum Pathol* 1987;18:625–635.
149. Towbin JA, Lowe AM, Colan SD, et al. Incidence, causes, and outcomes of dilated cardiomyopathy in children. *JAMA* 2006;296:1867–1876.
150. Daubeney PEF, Nugent AF, Chondros P, et al. Clinical features and outcomes of childhood dilated cardiomyopathy. Results from a national population-based study. *Circulation* 2006;114:2671–2678.
151. Angelini A, Calzolari V, Thiene G, et al. Morphologic spectrum of primary restrictive cardiomyopathy. *Am J Cardiol* 1997;80:1046–1050.
152. Denfield SW, Rosenthal G, Gajarski RJ. Restrictive cardiomyopathies in childhood: etiologies and natural history. *Tex Heart Inst J* 1997;24:38–44.
153. Mogensen J, Kubo T, Duque M, et al. Idiopathic restrictive cardiomyopathy is part of the clinical expression of cardiac troponin I mutations. *J Clin Invest* 2003;111:209–216.
154. Aretz HT, Billingham ME, Edwards WD, et al. Myocarditis. A histopathologic definition and classification. *Am J Cardiovasc Pathol* 1986;1:3–14.
155. Marboe CC, Fenoglio JJ. Pathology and natural history of human myocarditis. *Pathol Immunopathol Res* 1988;7:226–239.
156. Richardson P, McKenna W, Bristow M, et al. Report of the 1995 World Health Organization/International Society and Federation of Cardiology Task Force on the Definition and Classification of Cardiomyopathies. *Circulation* 1996;93:841–842.
157. Calabrese F, Thiene G. Myocarditis and inflammatory cardiomyopathy: microbiological and molecular biological aspects. *Cardiovasc Res* 2003;60:11–25.
158. Cooper LT, Berry GJ, Shabetai R, et al. Idiopathic giant-cell myocarditis—natural history and treatment. *N Engl J Med* 1997;336:1860–1866.
159. Litvosky SH, Burke AP, Virmani R. Giant cell myocarditis: an entity distinct from sarcoidosis characterized by multiphasic myocyte destruction by cytotoxic T cells and histiocytic giant cells. *Mod Pathol* 1996;9:1126–1134.
160. Thurberg BL, Lynch Maloney C, Vaccaro C, et al. Characterization of pre- and post-treatment pathology after enzyme replacement therapy for Pompe disease. *Lab Invest* 2006;86:1208–1220.
161. Sugie K, Yamamoto A, Murayama K, et al. Clinicopathological features of genetically confirmed Danon disease. *Neurology* 2002;58:1773–1778.
162. Mohan UR, Hay AA, Cleary MA, et al. Cardiovascular changes in children with mucopolysaccharide disorders. *Acta Paediatr* 2002;91:799–804.
163. Renteria VG, Ferrans VJ, Roberts WC. The heart in the Hurler syndrome: gross, histologic and ultrastructural observations in five necropsy cases. *Am J Cardiol* 1976;38:487–501.
164. Gilbert EF, Dawson G, zu Rhein GM, et al. I-cell disease, mucolipidosis II. Pathological, histochemical, ultrastructural and biochemical observations in four cases. *Z Kinderheilkd* 1973;114:259–292.
165. Suzuki Y, Oshima A, Nanba E. β-Galactosidase deficiency (β-galactosidosis): GM1 gangliosidosis and Morquio B disease. In: Scriver CR, Beaudet AL, Sly WS, et al., eds. *The Metabolic & Molecular Bases of Inherited Disease*, 8th ed. New York: McGraw-Hill, 2001:3775–3809.
166. Blieden LC, Desnick RJ, Carter JB, et al. Cardiac involvement in Sandhoff's disease: inborn error of glycosphingolipid metabolism. *Am J Cardiol* 1974;34:83–88.
167. Linhart A, Elliott PM. The heart in Anderson-Fabry disease and other lysosomal storage disorders. *Heart* 2007;93:528–535.
168. Gehrmann J, Sohlbach K, Linnebank M, et al. Cardiomyopathy in congenital disorders of glycosylation. *Cardiol Young* 2003;13:345–351.
169. Shekhawat PS, Matem D, Strauss AW. Fetal fatty acid oxidation disorders, their effect on maternal health and neonatal outcome: impact of expanded newborn screening on their diagnosis and management. *Pediatr Res* 2005;57:78R–86R.
170. Pierpont ME, Breningstall GN, Stanley CA, et al. Familial carnitine transporter defect: a treatable cause of cardiomyopathy in children. *Am Heart J* 2000;139:s96–s106.
171. Tripp ME, Katcher ML, Peters HA, et al. Systemic carnitine deficiency presenting as familial endocardial fibroelastosis. A treatable cardiomyopathy. *N Engl J Med* 1981;305:385–390.

172. Scaglia F, Towbin JA, Craigen WJ, et al. Clinical spectrum, morbidity, and mortality in 113 pediatric patients with mitochondrial disease. *Pediatrics* 2004;114:925–931.
173. Holmgren D, Wahlander H, Eriksson BO, et al. Cardiomyopathy in children with mitochondrial disease: clinical course and cardiological findings. *Eur Heart J* 2003;24:280–288.
174. Kelly AL, Rhodes DA, Roland JM, et al. Hereditary juvenile haemochromatosis: a genetically heterogeneous life-threatening iron-storage disease. *QJMed* 1998;91:607–618.
175. Finsterer J, Stollberger C. Cardiac involvement in primary myopathies. *Cardiology* 2000;94:1–11.
176. Frankel KA, Rosser RJ. The pathology of the heart in progressive muscular dystrophy: epimyocardial fibrosis. *Hum Pathol* 1976;7:375–386.
177. Sovari AA, Bodine CK, Farokhi F. Cardiovascular manifestations of myotonic dystrophy-1. *Cardio Rev* 2007;15:191–194.
178. Fananapazir L, Dalakas MC, Cyran F, et al. Missense mutations in the beta-myosin heavy-chain gene cause central core disease in hypertrophic cardiomyopathy. *Proc Natl Acad Sci U S A* 1993;90:3993–3997.
179. Koeppen AH. Friedreich's ataxia: Pathology, pathogenesis, and molecular genetics. *J Neurol Sci* 2011;303:1–12.
180. Spencer CH, Patwardhan A, Roble SL. Inflammatory noninfectious cardiovascular diseases. In: Allen HD, Driscoll DJ, Shaddy RE, Feltes TF, eds. *Moss and Adams' Heart Disease in Infants, Children, and Adolescents Including the Fetus and Young Adult*, 8th ed. Philadelphia, PA: Lippincott Williams & Wilkins, 2012:1311–1349.
181. Miner JJ, Kim AHJ. Cardiac manifestations of systemic lupus erythematosus. *Rheum Dis Clin North Am* 2014;40:51–60.
182. Moder KG, Miller T, Tazelaar HD. Cardiac involvement in systemic lupus erythematosus. *Mayo Clin Proc* 1999;74:275–284.
183. Gross L. The cardiac lesions in Libman-Sacks disease. With a consideration of its relationship to acute diffuse lupus erythematosus. *Am J Pathol* 1940;16:375–407.
184. Ho SY, Esscher E, Anderson RH, et al. Anatomy of congenital complete heart block and relation to maternal anti-Ro antibodies. *Am J Cardiol* 1986;58:291–294.
185. Meckler KA, Kapur RP. Congenital heart block and associated cardiac pathology in neonatal lupus syndrome. *Pediatr Dev Pathol* 1998;1:136–142.
186. Jaeggi ET, Hamilton RM, Silverman ED, et al. Outcome of children with fetal, neonatal or childhood diagnosis of isolated congenital atrioventricular block: a single institution's experience of 30 years. *J Am Coll Cardiol* 2002;39:130–137.
187. Tani LY. Rheumatic fever and rheumatic heart disease. In: Allen HD, Driscoll DJ, Shaddy RE, et al, eds. *Moss & Adams' heart disease in infants, children & adolescents: including the fetus and young adults*, 8th ed. Lippincott Williams & Wilkins, 2012:1303–1330.
188. Ullmo S, Vial Y, Di Bernardo S, et al. Pathologic ventricular hypertrophy in the offspring of diabetic mothers: a retrospective study. *Eur Heart J* 2007;28:1319–1325.
189. Russell NE, Holloway P, Quinn S, et al. Cardiomyopathy and cardiomegaly in stillborn infants of diabetic mothers. *Pediatr Dev Pathol* 2008;11:10–14.
190. Donnelly WH, Hawkins H. Optimum examination of the normally formed perinatal heart. *Hum Pathol* 1987;18:55–60.
191. Donnelly WH. Ischemic myocardial necrosis and papillary muscle dysfunction in infants and children. *Am J Cardiovasc Pathol* 1987;1:173–188.
192. Anderson RH, Ho SY. The architecture of the sinus node, the atrioventricular conduction axis, and the internodal atrial myocardium. *J Cardiovasc Electrophysiol* 1998;9:1233–1248.
193. Berry GJ, Billingham ME. Normal heart. In: Mills SE, ed. *Histology for Pathologists*, 4th ed. Philadelphia, PA: Lippincott Williams & Wilkins, 2012:563–584.
194. Gulino SPM. Examination of the cardiac conduction system: forensic application in cases of sudden cardiac death. *Am J Forensic Med Pathol* 2003;24:227–238.
195. Deal BJ, Jacobs JP, Mavroudis C. Congenital Heart Surgery Nomenclature and Database Project: arrhythmias. *Ann Thorac Surg* 2000;69(4 suppl):S319–S331.
196. Anderson RH, Ho SY. Anatomy of the atrioventricular junctions with regard to ventricular preexcitation. *Pacing Clin Electrophysiol* 1997;20:2072–2076.
197. Schmidt KG, Ulmer HE, Silverman NH, et al. Perinatal outcome of fetal complete atrioventricular block: a multicenter experience. *J Am Coll Cardiol* 1991;17:1360–1366.
198. Amin AS, Pinto YM, Wilde AAM. Long QT syndrome: beyond the causal mutation. *J Physiol* 2013;591:4125–4139.
199. Cerrone M, Napolitano C, Priori SG. Genetics of ion-channel disorders. *Curr Opin Cardiol* 2012;27:242–252.
200. Abriel H, Zaklyazminskaya EV. Cardiac channelopathies: genetic and molecular mechanisms. *Gene* 2013;517:1–11.
201. Sweeting J, Semsarian C. Cardiac abnormalities and sudden infant death syndrome. *Paediatr Respir Rev* 2014;15:301–306.
202. Lopez JA, Ross RS, Fishbein MC, et al. Nonbacterial thrombotic endocarditis: a review. *Am Heart J* 1987;113:773–784.
203. Sadiq M, Nazir M, Sheikh SA. Infective endocarditis in children–incidence, pattern, diagnosis and management in a developing country. *Int J Cardiol* 2001;78:175–182.
204. Saimon L, Prince A, Gersong WM. Pediatric infective endocarditis in the modern era. *J Pediatr* 1993;122:847–853.
205. Gewitz M, Taubert KA. Infective endocarditis and prevention. In: Allen BS, Driscoll DJ, Shaddy RE, et al., eds. *Moss & Adams' Heart Disease in Infants, Children & Adolescents: Including the Fetus and Young Adult*, 8th ed. Lippincott Williams & Wilkins, 2013:1363–1376.
206. Li JS, Sexton DJ, Mick N, et al. Proposed modifications to the Duke criteria for the diagnosis of infective endocarditis. *Clin Infect Dis* 2000;30:633–638.
207. Thiene G, Basso C. Pathology and pathogenesis of infective endocarditis in native heart valves. *Cardiovasc Pathol* 2006;15:256–263.
208. Johnson JN, Cetta F. Pericardial diseases. In: Allen BS, Driscoll DJ, Shaddy RE et al., eds. *Moss & Adams' Heart Disease in Infants, Children & Adolescents: Including the Fetus and Young Adult*, 8th ed. Lippincott Williams & Wilkins, 2013:1350–1362.
209. Roodpeyma S, Sadeghian N. Acute pericarditis in childhood: a 10-year experience. *Pediatr Cardiol* 2000;21:363–367.
210. Cheung EW, Ho SA, Tang KK, et al. Pericardial effusion after open heart surgery for congenital heart disease. *Heart* 2003;89:780–783.
211. Montaudon M, Roubertie F, Bire F, et al. Congenital pericardial defect: report of two cases and literature review. *Surg Radiol Anat* 2007;29:195–200.
212. Simonneau G, Gatzoulis MA, Adatia I, et al. Updated clinical classification of pulmonary hypertension. *J Am Coll Cardiol* 2013;62(Suppl D):D34-D41.
213. Hislop AA, Pierce E. Growth of the vascular tree. *Paediatr Resp Rev* 2000;1:321–327.
214. Geggel RL, Reid LM. The structural basis of PPHN. *Clin Perinatol* 1984;2:525–549.
215. Pietra GG, Capron F, Stewart S, et al. Pathologic assessment of vasculopathies in pulmonary hypertension. *J Am Coll Cardiol* 2004;43:S25-S32.
216. Berger S, Konduri GG. Pulmonary hypertension in children: the twenty-first century. *Pediatr Clin North Am* 2006;53:961–987.
217. Rabinovitch M, Keane JF, Norwood WI, et al. Vascular structure in lung tissue obtained at biopsy correlated with pulmonary hemodynamic findings after repair of congenital heart defects. *Circulation* 1984;69:655–667.
218. Adatia I. Recent advances in pulmonary vascular disease. *Curr Opin Pediatr* 2002;14:292–297.
219. Slovut DP, Olin JW. Fibromuscular dysplasia. *N Engl J Med* 2004;350:1862–1871.
220. Sarkar R, Coran AG, Cilley RE, et al. Arterial aneurysms in children: clinicopathologic classification. *J Vasc Surg* 1991;13:47–56.
221. Jain D, Dietz HC, Oswald GL, et al. Causes and histopathology of ascending aortic disease in children and young adults. *Cardiovasc Pathol* 2011;20:15-25.
222. Loeys BL, Dietz HC, Braverman AC, et al. The revised Ghent nosology for the Marfan syndrome. *J Med Genet* 2010;47:476–485.

223. Faivre L, Collod-Beround G, Loeys BL, et al. Effect of mutation type and location on clinical outcome in 1,013 probands with Marfan syndrome or related phenotypes and *FBN1* mutations: an international study. *Am J Hum Genet* 2007;81:454–466.
224. Loeys BL, Schwarze U, Holm T, et al. Aneurysm syndromes caused by mutations in the TGF-β receptor. *N Engl J Med* 2006;355:788–798.
225. Byers PH. Disorders of collagen biosynthesis and structure. In: Scriver CR, Beaudet AL, Sly WS et al., eds. *The Metabolic & Molecular Bases of Inherited Disease*, 8th ed. New York: McGraw-Hill, 2001:5241–5285.
226. Murakami H, Kodama H, Nemoto N. Abnormality of vascular elastic fibers in the macular mouse and a patient with Menkes' disease: ultrastructural and immunohistochemical study. *Med Electron Microsc* 2002;35:24–30.
227. Rahalkar AR, Hegele RA. Monogenic pediatric dyslipidemias: classification, genetics and clinical spectrum. *Mol Genet Metab* 2008;93:282–294.
228. Kawaguchi A, Miyatake K, Yutani C, et al. Characteristic cardiovascular manifestation in homozygous and heterozygous familial hypercholesterolemia. *Am Heart J* 1999;137:410–418.
229. Satou GM, Giamelli J, Gewitz MH. Kawasaki disease: diagnosis, management, and long-term implications. *Cardio Rev* 2007;15:163–169.
230. Burns JC, Glode MP. Kawasaki syndrome. *Lancet* 2004;364:533–544.
231. Kato H, Sugimura T, Akagi T, et al. Long-term consequences of Kawasaki disease: a 10- to 21-year follow-up study of 594 patients. *Circulation* 1996;94:1379–1385.
232. Suzuki A, Kamiya T, Kuwahara N, et al. Coronary arterial lesions of Kawasaki disease: cardiac catheterization findings of 1100 cases. *Pediatr Cardiol* 1986;7:3–9.
233. Orenstein JM, Shulman ST, Fox LM, et al. Three linked vasculopathic processes characterize Kawasaki disease: A light and transmission electron microscopic study. *PLoS One* 2012;7:e38998.
234. Fujiwara H, Hamashima Y. Pathology of the heart in Kawasaki disease. *Pediatrics* 1978;61:100–107.
235. Hall S, Barr W, Lie JT, et al. Takayasu arteritis. A study of 32 North American patients. *Medicine (Baltimore)* 1985;64:89–99.
236. Parra JR and Perler BA. Takayasu's disease. *Semin Vasc Surg* 2003;16:200-208.
237. Beghetti M, Gow RM, Haney I, et al. Pediatric primary benign cardiac tumors: a 15-year review. *Am Heart J* 1997;134:1107–1114.
238. Groves AM, Fagg NL, Cook A, et al. Cardiac tumours in intrauterine life. *Arch Dis Child* 1992;67:1189–1192.
239. Isaacs H. Fetal and neonatal cardiac tumors. *Pediatr Cardiol* 2004;25:252–273.
240. Burke A, Virmani R. Classification and incidence of cardiac tumors. *Tumors of the Heart and Great Vessels*, 3rd Series. Washington, DC: Armed Forces Institute of Pathology 1996; 1–11.
241. Nir A, Tajik AJ, Freeman WK, et al. Tuberous sclerosis and cardiac rhabdomyoma. *Am J Cardiol* 1995;76:419–421.
242. Webb DW, Thomas RD, Osborne JP. Cardiac rhabdomyomas and their association with tuberous sclerosis. *Arch Dis Child* 1993;68:367–370.
243. McAllister HAJ, Hall RJ, Cooley DA. Tumors of the heart and pericardium. *Curr Probl Cardiol* 1999;24:57–116.
244. Freedom RM, Lee KJ, MacDonald C, et al. Selected aspects of cardiac tumors in infancy and childhood. *Pediatr Cardiol* 2000;21:299–316.
245. Burke A, Rosado-de-Christenson M, Templeton PA, et al. Cardiac fibroma: clinicopathologic correlates and surgical treatment. *J Thorac Cardiovasc Surg* 1994;108:862–870.
246. Marx GR, Moran AM. Cardiac tumors. In: Allen BS, Driscoll DJ, Shaddy RE et al., eds. *Moss & Adams' Heart Disease in Infants, Children & Adolescents: Including the Fetus and Young Adult*, 8th ed. Lippincott Williams & Wilkins, 2013:1549–1564.
247. Burke A, Virmani R. Heterotopias and tumors originating from ectopic tissues. In: Burke A, Virmani R, eds. *Tumors of the Heart and Great Vessels, 3rd Series*. Washington, DC: Armed Forces Institute of Pathology, 1996:111–125.
248. Burke A, Virmani R. Cardiac myxoma. *Tumors of the Heart and Great Vessels*, 3rd Series. Washington, DC: Armed Forces Institute of Pathology, 1996;21–46.
249. Reynen K. Cardiac myxomas. *N Engl J Med* 1995;333:1610–1617.
250. Boikos SA, Stratakis CA. Carney complex: the first 20 years. *Curr Opin Oncol* 2007;19:24–29.
251. Wilkes D, McDermott DA, Basson CT. Clinical phenotypes and molecular genetic mechanisms of Carney complex. *Lancet Oncol* 2005;6:501–508.
252. McCarthy PM, Piehler JM, Schaff HV, et al. The significance of multiple, recurrent, and "complex" cardiac myxomas. *J Thorac Cardiovasc Surg* 1986;91:389–396.
253. Burke AP, Virmani R. Cardiac myxoma. A clinicopathologic study. *Am J Clin Pathol* 1993;100:671–680.
254. Shehata BM, Patterson K, Thomas JE, et al. Histiocytoid cardiomyopathy: three new cases and a review of the literature. *Pediatr Dev Pathol* 1998;1:56–69.
255. Vallance HD, Jeven G, Wallace DC, et al. A case of sporadic infantile histiocytoid cardiomyopathy caused by the A8344G (MERRF) mitochondrial DNA mutation. *Pediatr Cardiol* 2004;25:538–540.
256. Kearney DL, Titus JL, Hawkins EP, et al. Pathologic features of myocardial hamartomas causing childhood tachyarrhythmias. *Circulation* 1987;75:705–710.
257. Gelb AB, Van Meter SH, Billingham ME, et al. Infantile histiocytoid cardiomyopathy—myocardial or conduction system hamartoma: what is the cell type involved? *Hum Pathol* 1993;24:1226–1231.
258. Bird LM, Krous HF, Eichenfield LF, et al. Female infant with oncocytic cardiomyopathy and microphthalmia with linear skin defects (MLS): a clue to the pathogenesis of oncocytic cardiomyopathy? *Am J Med Genet* 1994;53:141–148.
259. Shehata BM, Bouzyk M, Tang W, et al. Identification of candidate genes for histiocytoid cardiomyopathy (HC) using whole genome expression analysis: analyzing material from the HC registry. *Pediatr Dev Pathol* 2011;14:370–377.
260. Chan HSL, Sonley MJ, Moësmd CAF, et al. Primary and secondary tumors of childhood involving the heart, pericardium, and great vessels: a report of 75 cases and review of the literature. *Cancer* 1985;56:825–836.
261. Carmi R, Boughman JA, Ferencz C. Endocardial cushion defect: further studies of "isolated" versus "syndromic" occurrence. *Am J Med Genet* 1992;43:569–575.
262. Marino B, Vairo U, Corno A, et al. Atrioventricular canal in Down syndrome. Prevalence of associated cardiac malformations compared with patients without Down syndrome. *Am J Dis Child* 1990;144:1120–1122.
263. Feldt RH, Edwards WD, Porter CJ, et al. Atrioventricular septal defects. In: Allen HD, Gutgesell HP, Clark EB, et al., eds. *Moss and Adams' Heart Disease in Infants, Children and Adolescents: Including the Fetus and Young Adults*, vol. 6. Philadelphia, PA: Lippincott Williams & Wilkins, 2001:618–635.
264. Bharati S, Lev M. The spectrum of common atrioventricular orifice (canal). *Am Heart J* 1973;86:553–561.
265. Tenckhoff L, Stamm SJ. An analysis of 35 cases of the complete form of persistent common atrioventricular canal. *Circulation* 1973;48:416–427.
266. Rastelli GC, Kirklin JK, Titus JL. Anatomic observations on complete form of persistent common atrioventricular canal with special reference to atrioventricular valves. *Mayo Clin Proc* 1966;41:296–308.
267. Piccoli GP, Gerlis LM, Wilkinson JL, et al. Morphology and classification of atrioventricular defects. *Br Heart J* 1979;42:621–632.
268. Gallo P, Formigari R, Hokayem NJ, et al. Left ventricular outflow tract obstruction in atrioventricular septal defects: a pathologic and morphometric evaluation. *Clin Cardiol* 1991;14:513–521.
269. Redmond JM, Silove ED, De Giovanni JV, et al. Complete atrioventricular septal defects: the influence of associated cardiac anomalies on surgical management and outcome. *Eur J Cardiothorac Surg* 1996;10:991–995.
270. Piccoli GP, Wilkinson JL, Macartney FJ, et al. Morphology and classification of complete atrioventricular defects. *Br Heart J* 1979;42: 633–639.
271. Bound JP, Logan WF. Incidence of congenital heart disease in Blackpool 1957-1971. *Br Heart J* 1977;39:445–450.
272. Carlgren LE. Incidence and prevalence of congenital heart disease. *Acta Paediatr Scand Suppl* 1970;206:14–15.

273. Dickinson DF, Arnold R, Wilkinson JL. Congenital heart disease among 160 480 liveborn children in Liverpool 1960 to 1969. Implications for surgical treatment. *Br Heart J* 1981;46:55–62.
274. Feldt RH, Avasthey P, Yoshimasu F, et al. Incidence of congenital heart disease in children born to residents of Olmsted County, Minnesota, 1950–1969. *Mayo Clin Proc* 1971;46:794–799.
275. Ferencz C, Neill CA. Cardiovascular malformations: prevalence at livebirth. In: Freedom RM, Benson LN, Smallhorn JF, eds. *Neonatal heart disease*, 1st ed. London, UK: Springer-Verlag, 1992:20–34.
276. Perry LW, Neill CA, Ferencz C, et al. Infants with congenital heart disease: The cases. In: Ferencz C, Loffredo CA, Rubin JD, et al., eds. *Epidemiology of Congenital Heart Disease*. Mount Kisco, NY: Futura Publishing Company, Inc., 1993:33–62.
277. Tanner K, Sabrine N, Wren C. Cardiovascular malformations among preterm infants. *Pediatrics* 2005;116:e833–e838.
278. Kramer HH, Majewski F, Trampisch HJ, et al. Malformation patterns in children with congenital heart disease. *Am J Dis Child* 1987;141:789–795.
279. Rosenberg HS, Oppenheimer EH, Esterly JR. Congenital rubella syndrome: the late effects and their relation to early lesions. *Perspect Pediatr Pathol* 1981;6:183–202.
280. Kim YM, Yoo SJ, Choi JY, et al. Natural course of supravalvar aortic stenosis and peripheral pulmonary arterial stenosis in Williams' syndrome. *Cardiol Young* 1999;9:37–41.
281. Levin SE, Zarvos P, Milner S, et al. Arteriohepatic dysplasia: association of liver disease with pulmonary arterial stenosis as well as facial and skeletal abnormalities. *Pediatrics* 1980;66:879–883.
282. Burch M, Sharland M, Shinebourne E, et al. Cardiologic abnormalities in Noonan syndrome: phenotypic diagnosis and echocardiographic assessment of 118 patients. *J Am Coll Cardiol* 1993;22:1189–1192.
283. Report of the WHO/ISFC task force on the definition and classification of cardiomyopathies. *Br Heart J* 1980;44:672–673.
284. Report of the 1995 World Health Organization/International Society and Federation of Cardiology Task Force on the Definition and Classification of Cardiomyopathies. *Circulation* 1996;93:841–842.
285. Davis JS, Allan BJ, Perez EA, et al. Primary pediatric cardiac malignancies: the SEER experience. *Pediatr Surg Int* 2013;29:425–429.
286. Uzun O, Wilson DG, Vujanic GM, et al. Cardiac tumours in children. *Orphanet J Rare Dis* 2007;2:11.
287. Huh J, Noh CI, Kim YW, et al. Secondary cardiac tumor in children. *Pediatr Cardiol* 1999;20:400–403.

CHAPTER 14

The Gastrointestinal Tract

Pierre A. Russo, M.D.

EMBRYOLOGY

The gastrointestinal tract forms during the 4th week as the cephalocaudal and lateral folds of the trilaminar germ disk develop and incorporate the dorsal part of the endoderm-lined yolk sac into the body cavity to form a tubelike gut. During early embryonic life, the vitelline or omphalomesenteric duct provides an open connection between the midgut and the yolk sac (Figure 14-1). This connection becomes progressively longer and narrower as gestation proceeds and eventually forms part of the umbilical cord. By week 10, the communication between the lumen of the midgut and the umbilicus becomes obliterated and soon disappears.

The laryngotracheal diverticulum develops from the ventral foregut during week 4 of gestation (Chapter 12). Gradual formation of an esophagotracheal septum along the length of the laryngotracheal diverticulum separates the ventral respiratory and the dorsal digestive tubes (Figure 14-2). The common origin of the trachea and esophagus from the foregut results in various forms of fistulas if separation is incomplete.

During the 2nd month of embryonic life, rapid cellular proliferation within the digestive tube results in a transient partial obliteration of the duodenal lumen, the so-called solid stage of development. Recanalization occurs by week 8 of gestation. Rapid midgut growth within the relatively small body cavity results in a temporary herniation of the lengthening midgut into the umbilical stalk during weeks 6 to 11 (Figure 14-3). During this physiologic herniation, the intestinal loops rotate counterclockwise, a process that continues as the intestinal loops return to the abdominal cavity during weeks 10 and 11, so that the cecum comes to lie in the right side of the abdomen. If this orderly process fails to occur or is anomalous, the locations of the small and large intestine, mesentery, and fixation points of the intestine to the body wall will be abnormal. The hindgut, or posterior portion of the primitive digestive tube, initially ends posteriorly in the cloaca, separated from superficial ectoderm by the cloacal membrane (Figure 14-4). A transverse ridge, the urorectal septum, grows posteriorly from the umbilical stalk and gradually divides the cloaca into a ventral portion, the urogenital sinus, and a dorsal portion, the future rectum and anus. This division is normally complete at the end of week 6 of gestation. The membrane covering the anal canal disappears by week 9, so that communication between the digestive tract and the amniotic cavity is established caudally.

DISORDERS OF THE ESOPHAGUS

Congenital Abnormalities

Persistent Embryonic Epithelium

The embryonic and early fetal esophagus is lined by ciliated stratified columnar epithelium. The transformation to stratified squamous epithelium is usually complete by week 25 of gestation, but occasionally, a patch of superficial columnar epithelium persists at birth, especially in premature infants. Persistent embryonic epithelium is usually found incidentally at autopsy as microscopic foci in either the proximal or distal end of the esophagus and is of little clinical consequence. This change is limited to surface epithelium only; glandular mucosa, as in gastric heterotopia of the esophagus, is not present. Because it is not usually found after early infancy, persistent embryonic epithelium is presumed to be replaced by squamous epithelium.

Heterotopic Gastric Mucosa (Inlet Patch)

Single or multiple small patches (5 to 30 mm) of gastric cardiac- or fundic-type mucosa can sometimes be found incidentally in the cervical esophagus (eFigure 14-1). The incidence in patients undergoing esophagogastroduodenoscopy has been reported to be up to 10% (1). These patches of heterotopic gastric epithelium usually are not clinically important and are rarely biopsied since most endoscopists are familiar with them. In contrast to Barrett esophagus (BE), inlet patches occur in the upper esophagus and are surrounded by squamous mucosa; however, confusion with BE can occur if the endoscopic findings are not communicated

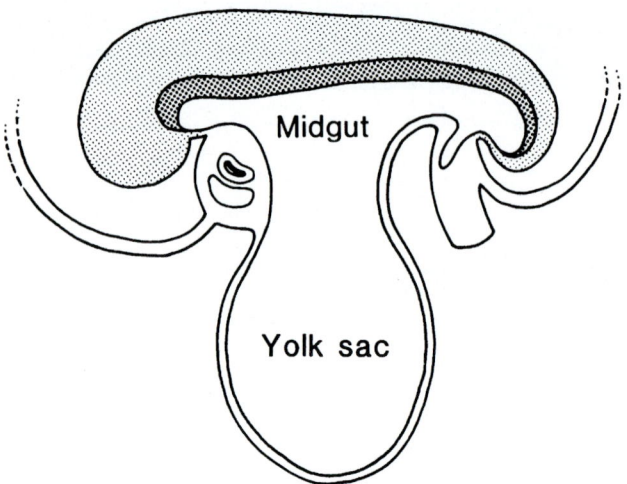

FIGURE 14-1 • During week 4 of gestation, head and tail folds of the embryo surround portions of the yolk sac. An open connection between the primitive midgut and the yolk sac exists. After this connection narrows, it is known as the vitelline or omphalomesenteric duct.

to the surgical pathologist. They can be colonized by *Helicobacter pylori* organisms (1).

Esophageal Duplication

GI duplications represent an array of lesions with a confusing terminology that includes enteric remnants, dorsal enteric cysts, neurenteric cysts, and posterior mediastinal cysts. The simple classification proposed by Dimmick and

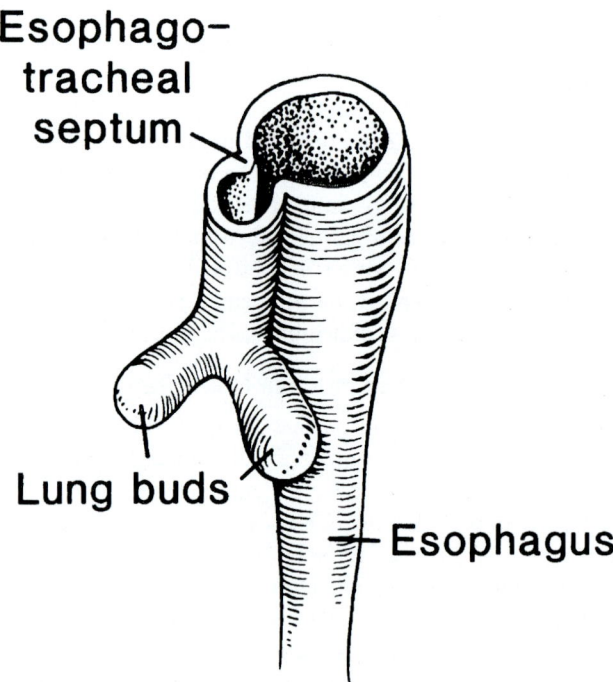

FIGURE 14-2 • Development of the respiratory system from the foregut at week 4 of gestation. The esophagotracheal septum develops from the two lateral folds that migrate toward the midline to separate the developing respiratory diverticulum from the primitive gut.

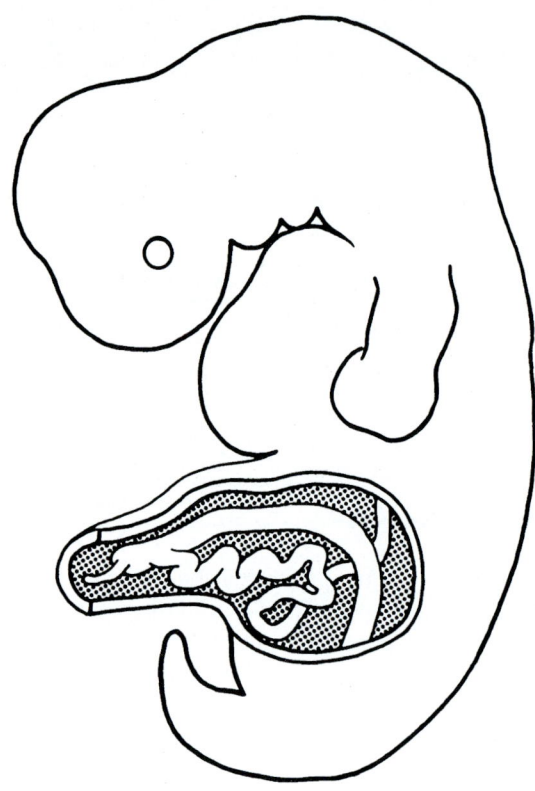

FIGURE 14-3 • Physiologic gut herniation in an embryo at week 8 of gestation. Rapid elongation of the intestine in a relatively small abdominal cavity causes the gut to herniate into the umbilical cord. This herniation resolves at the end of the 3rd month of gestation. A failure in the normal events at this stage explains the omphalocele and malrotation.

Hardwick (2), which divides these lesions into duplications and neurenteric (dorsal enteric) cysts, is preferred. Duplication of the esophagus is rare. The duplicated segment may be a separate cylindrical tube alongside part of the normal esophagus with a complete mucosa, submucosa, and two-layered muscularis externa (double esophagus). Alternatively, a spherical, intramural esophageal cyst may form and share a portion of muscularis propria with the adjacent esophageal wall. Esophageal duplication occurs most often in the thorax adjacent to the distal two-thirds of the esophagus, but it may also occur in the lateral cervical area. Esophageal duplication cysts may be asymptomatic and discovered incidentally, or they may cause tracheal or esophageal compression. The epithelium is either stratified squamous or columnar; the latter is derived from persistent embryonic esophageal ciliated columnar epithelium. Distinction between esophageal and bronchogenic cysts may be difficult because they occur at similar locations in the mediastinum and show similar ciliated columnar epithelium. The diagnosis of esophageal cyst is made if a two-layered muscularis externa is present. A bronchial origin is favored if cartilage or respiratory glands are identified. The generic designation of "foregut cyst" is used in cases in which the lining epithelium is primitive columnar without the distinguishing features cited.

of the foregut into tracheal and esophageal channels during the first month of embryonic life. Additional congenital anomalies (usually midline) occur in 50% of these infants, directly affecting the prognosis. Congenital heart diseases, especially ventricular septal defect, patent ductus arteriosus, and tetralogy of Fallot, are seen in 30% of cases of esophageal atresia, and imperforate anus occurs in approximately 10%. In babies with multiple malformations, the VATER (vertebrae, anal, tracheoesophageal, radial, and renal anomalies) association or the VACTERL (vertebrae, anal, cardiac, tracheoesophageal, renal, and limb) association should be considered. Approximately one-third of the infants with esophageal atresia are born prematurely, so that morbidity is further increased.

Variations in the anatomy of esophageal atresia and tracheoesophageal fistula are diagrammed in Figure 12-10 (see Chapter 12). Esophageal atresia without tracheoesophageal fistula occurs rarely, and tracheoesophageal fistula without esophageal atresia (H-type fistula) is even more unusual. The most common type is esophageal atresia with distal tracheoesophageal fistula, which accounts for 85% of the cases (Figure 14-5). The esophagus ends in a blind pouch in the upper chest, and the lower portion of the esophagus is connected to the trachea at or near the carina by a tracheoesophageal fistula less than 0.5 cm in diameter (see Figure 12-10). During breathing, air enters the stomach through the fistula, and as the stomach becomes distended, gastric secretions

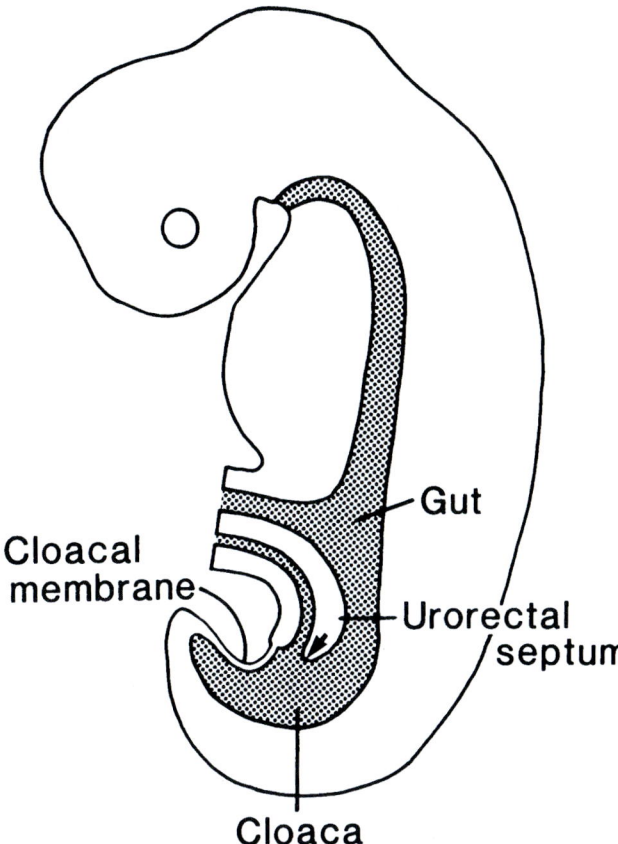

FIGURE 14-4 • Primitive hindgut region in an embryo at 6 weeks of gestation. The urorectal septum grows posteriorly to divide the cloaca into a urogenital portion separate from the intestinal portion. Note the intact cloacal membrane.

Neurenteric Cyst (Remnant) of the Mediastinum

Neurenteric remnants include diverticula, fistulas, cysts, and fibrous cords, which originate from the dorsal midline of the gastrointestinal tract and attach to or pass through the vertebral column and spinal cord cranial to their enteric origins and may continue to the skin of the dorsal midline overlying the involved vertebra. They are located at any level but are most common in the cervicothoracic and lumbosacral area. When located in the posterior mediastinum, neurenteric cysts may be confused with esophageal duplication cysts. Most are associated with vertebral anomalies, and about 25% have intraspinal anomalies (3). The walls of these remnants or cysts can be composed of all the normal layers of the gastrointestinal tract, and neuroglial tissue is found in the lesions involving the spinal cord and vertebrae. The epithelial lining is most often gastric mucosa, which can result in ulceration, perforation, and hemorrhage. Small-intestinal mucosa and primitive columnar epithelial lining have also been described.

Esophageal Atresia and Tracheoesophageal Fistula

Esophageal atresia and tracheoesophageal fistula occur together in most cases. The dual anomalies, which occur in approximately one in 3000 births, result from faulty division

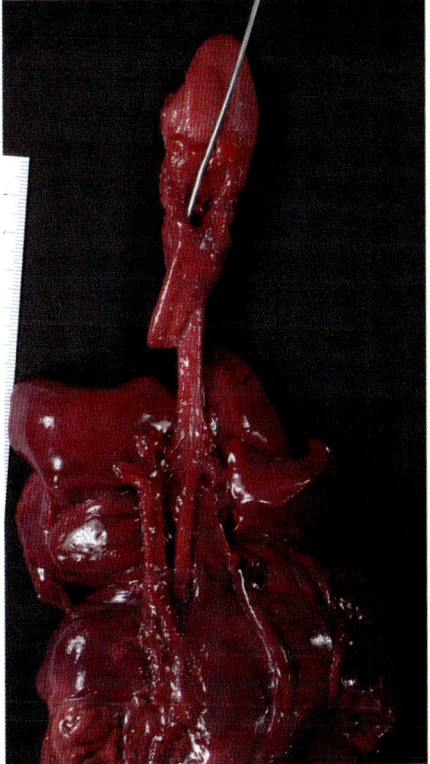

FIGURE 14-5 • Tracheoesophageal fistula at autopsy (posterior view of thoracic organ block). The probe is in the blind upper portion of the esophagus, and the tracheoesophageal fistula arises at the tracheal bifurcation.

pass through the fistula into the lungs, causing pneumonia. The infant cannot swallow oral secretions or food; attempts at feeding produce regurgitation and aspiration. The diagnosis is suggested by the inability to pass a tube from the mouth to the stomach and is confirmed by plain x-ray films of the chest and abdomen. Treatment is surgical and consists of extrapleural transection of the fistula and anastomosis of the two ends of the esophagus.

Isolated esophageal atresia without an associated fistula, found in 7% to 8% of cases, is usually characterized by blind proximal and distal esophageal pouches, often separated by a wide gap. Multiple surgical procedures are usually required for repair.

In the relatively rare cases of isolated tracheoesophageal fistula without esophageal atresia (H-type fistula), the diagnosis is often delayed beyond the newborn period. Patients with this anomaly present with coughing or choking during feeding and with recurrent pneumonia. Histologic study of the tracheoesophageal fistula often reveals foci of primitive ciliated columnar epithelium, respiratory glands, and even cartilage. These tracheobronchial elements and abnormalities in smooth muscle may extend for some distance into the distal esophagus (tracheobronchial remnant-choristoma).

Esophageal Stenosis

In most cases, esophageal stenosis is an acquired lesion caused by gastroesophageal reflux (GER) with severe peptic esophagitis. However, rare forms of congenital esophageal stenosis have been described, resulting from tracheobronchial remnants, fibromuscular hypertrophy, or membranous mucosal rings and webs (4). About half of the cases are associated with atresia. Sloughing of esophageal mucosa occurs in inherited epidermolysis bullosa, which is complicated by stenosis.

Acquired Diseases
Esophagitis Due to Gastroesophageal Reflux

GER is common during the first few months of life, as evidenced by the frequent occurrence of effortless regurgitation at this age. It is considered a physiologic process secondary to immature esophageal peristaltic and lower esophageal sphincter function and gradually improves during the first year of life. Physiologic reflux is a normal function that serves a protective role in the postprandial period (5). GER disease (GERD) refers to reflux associated with mucosal damage or with symptoms impairing quality of life. Reflux esophagitis is reported to occur in 2% to 5% of the population, and esophagitis is present in 15% to 60% of children with symptoms of reflux (5).

The symptoms of reflux esophagitis differ with the age of the patient. Infants show effortless regurgitation and sometimes forceful vomiting, excessive irritability, apnea, and failure to thrive as a consequence of caloric losses. Older children present with vomiting and poorly characterized abdominal or chest pain. Patients of any age may exhibit gastrointestinal blood loss (from esophageal ulceration), failure to thrive, and recurrent pulmonary problems (e.g., asthma, pneumonia, and night cough). Most children with reflux esophagitis are otherwise normal, but certain groups of children are predisposed, including those with neurodevelopmental problems, cystic fibrosis, and bronchopulmonary dysplasia and those who have undergone repair of esophageal atresia and tracheoesophageal fistula in infancy. Esophageal pH monitoring, esophageal manometry, and barium esophagography may be used in patient evaluation. If a patient has signs of esophagitis, such as pain, gastrointestinal blood loss, or failure to thrive, esophagoscopy and esophageal biopsy are indicated.

Histologic features in children with reflux esophagitis are similar to those widely described in adults with the same condition (Figure 14-6). Diagnostic histologic findings include intraepithelial inflammation with eosinophils, lymphocytes, and neutrophils and epithelial changes such as basal cell hyperplasia (>15% to 20% of total epithelial thickness), papillary elongation (>50% of epithelial thickness), and spongiosis. These findings may be noted even in endoscopically normal mucosa (6). Epithelial changes correlate well with pH monitoring studies and may be the only histologic features present when patients have begun treatment with antireflux agents. However, basal cell hyperplasia and papillary elongation may be difficult to assess in poorly oriented biopsies. They are also common in biopsies obtained from near the squamocolumnar junction (Z-line) in patients without reflux. Spongiosis, also a sensitive marker of epithelial cell injury, is usually best observed in the lower cell layers and can be evaluated even in poorly oriented biopsies. Intraepithelial eosinophils appear to be the earliest and most specific correlate of reflux esophagitis in infants. It should be noted that eosinophils can also be present in other conditions such as Crohn disease (CD), food impaction and infections and are particularly prominent in eosinophilic esophagitis (EoE). Lymphocytes and Langerhans cells are normally present in the esophageal squamous

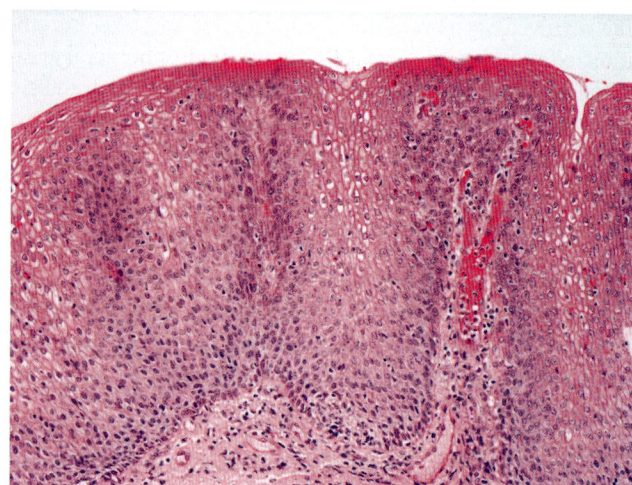

FIGURE 14-6 • Reflux esophagitis. Note the presence of basal cell hyperplasia and lengthening of the papillae. There are also scattered intraepithelial eosinophils (hematoxylin and eosin, 200×).

mucosa, so the determination of an abnormal increase in these cells is subjective. Increased intraepithelial lymphocytes (IELs) may be noted in chronic inflammatory bowel disease (IBD), in celiac disease, and in association with *H. pylori* gastritis. In a recent study in the pediatric population, a marked increase in IELs (>50/hpf) was associated with CD and found in 28% of patients with CD (7).

In otherwise healthy pediatric outpatients, occasional cases of infectious esophagitis, particularly herpes simplex esophagitis, present with signs and symptoms mimicking those of reflux esophagitis. Ingestion of caustic substances, CD, and dermatologic conditions, such as bullous pemphigoid and Stevens-Johnson syndrome, are rare possibilities, and other suggestive clinical findings are usually present. In children who are immunosuppressed or severely debilitated from another illness, infectious esophagitis is an important diagnostic consideration (Table 14-1).

The treatment of GERD consists primarily of acid suppression and enhancing gastric emptying. Acid blockade with antacids, H2 receptor antagonists, or proton pump inhibitors are the mainstay of GERD therapy. Gastroesophageal fundoplication is performed in cases refractory to medical therapy or strictures or those at risk for pulmonary complications; failure rates of 5% to 20% have been reported (5). Sequelae of GER include ulcers (usually of the distal one-third of the esophagus and often associated with blood loss), stricture, and BE.

Barrett Esophagus

BE, in which columnar epithelium replaces the normal squamous lining of the distal esophagus, is an acquired metaplastic condition caused by chronic GER. It is now established that even in children, BE is invariably found in association with severe reflux esophagitis; however, it is rare in children, occurring in only a small percentage that undergo biopsy for symptomatic GER. Usually, older children, not infants, are affected. BE cannot be predicted by the clinical presentation; the symptoms are those of the associated reflux esophagitis.

The changes in BE affect the lower portion of the esophagus (Figure 14-7A) and involvement may be either circumferential or patchy. BE is currently defined by the American College of Gastroenterology as endoscopically recognizable columnar metaplasia of the normal esophageal squamous mucosa that is histologically confirmed to have intestinal metaplasia, defined by the presence of goblet cells (Figure 14-7B) (8). The squamous mucosa proximal to the affected esophagus often shows changes of reflux esophagitis. Well-formed barrel-shaped goblet cells are usually easily recognizable with ordinary hematoxylin and eosin staining, but recognition can be enhanced and confirmed by staining with Alcian blue at pH 2.5, which imparts a blue color to intestinal-type acidic mucins. A pitfall is that Alcian blue–positive cells can be observed in the gastroesophageal junction of normal fetuses and young children, in the absence of goblet cells. In Great Britain, columnar-type mucosa without goblet cells is accepted as diagnostic of BE, provided the endoscopist is certain that the biopsies were obtained from the tubular esophagus and not the proximal stomach (9). Thus, the location of the biopsy site in relation to the lower esophageal sphincter must be known by the pathologist before BE can be diagnosed. However, because the endoscopic landmarks used to separate esophagus and stomach (primarily the upper extent of the gastric rugal folds) are not precise, particularly in the presence of a hiatal hernia, confusion between distal esophagus and gastric cardia is possible. Barrett mucosa has the potential to progress to dysplasia and, after many years, to adenocarcinoma in about 1% to 2% of cases. Patients with BE need to undergo routine, frequent monitoring, although there currently is no consensus on the frequency of surveillance in children. Adenocarcinoma in BE in children is very rare but has been reported in a patient as young as 8 years old (10).

Eosinophilic Esophagitis

EoE is a relatively recently described condition in which patients with a severe esophageal eosinophilia present with symptoms that are otherwise indistinguishable from those secondary to reflux esophagitis but fail to respond to conventional antireflux therapy or antireflux surgery. A recent set of diagnostic guidelines were developed for EoE in 2011 and include the following: (a) patients present with an isolated esophageal eosinophilia (other GI histology is normal) and symptoms of esophageal dysfunction; (b) the degree of eosinophilia in these patients is almost always greater than 15 eosinophils per high-magnification microscopic field; (c) disorders such as GERD and PPI-responsive esophageal eosinophilia need to be excluded; and (d) the symptoms and histologic abnormalities improve with either steroid or restriction diet therapy (11). The frequent association of extraintestinal allergic symptoms (asthma, eczema, and chronic rhinitis) in these patients has led to the hypothesis of an antigen- (food)/immune-mediated etiology for this type of esophagitis. It is still a matter of debate whether a damaged mucosa, say by reflux, could predispose to the development of EoE or whether changes in food processing are to blame. In young children, presenting symptoms include difficulty feeding, prolonged irritability and crying, failure to thrive,

TABLE 14-1 CAUSES OF ESOPHAGITIS IN CHILDREN

- Gastroesophageal reflux
- Allergy
- Food impaction
- Infections
- Ingestion of corrosive agents
- Prolonged retention of medication pills
- Trauma
- Repaired esophageal atresia
- Crohn disease
- Radiation
- Motility disorder

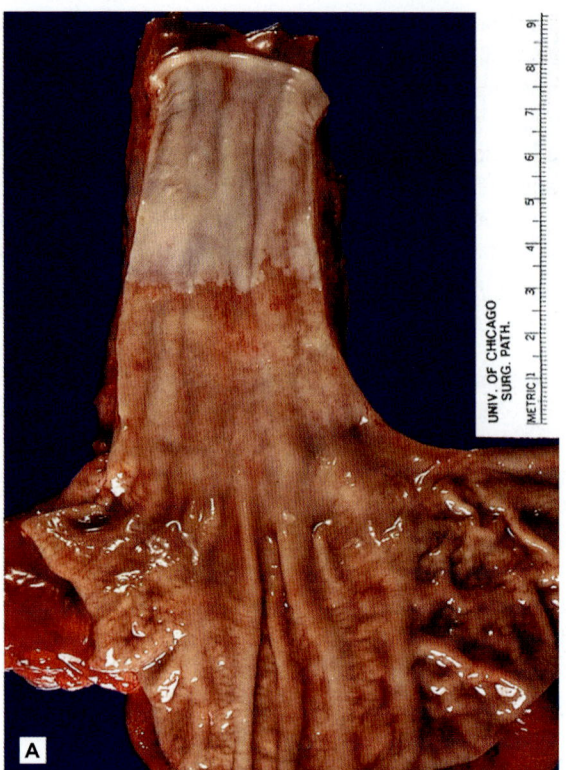
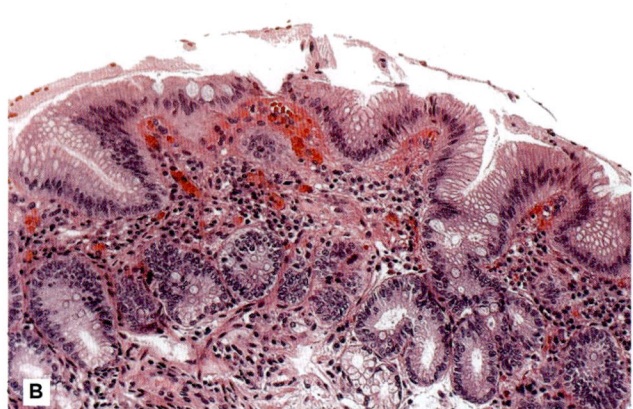

FIGURE 14-7 • Barrett esophagus. **A:** Esophagectomy specimen exhibiting a 5-cm circumferential segment of Barrett mucosa. **B:** Barrett mucosa, characterized by specialized columnar mucosa with goblet cells (hematoxylin and eosin, 200×).

and growth delay. Adolescents and adults diagnosed with this disorder often suffer from significant dysphagia and the development of esophageal strictures. Esophageal fibrosis in the deeper submucosal and muscular layers occurs in many patients with EoE, and left untreated, EoE may cause a severe narrowing of the esophagus.

Characteristic endoscopic findings include wrinkled or thickened esophageal squamous mucosa, sometimes with circumferential rings, linear furrows, or tiny vesicles. Endoscopic biopsies of the esophagus typically reveal a heavy but sometimes patchy infiltrate of eosinophils, frequently forming microabscesses near the luminal surface (Figure 14-8A to C). As previously mentioned, 15 eosinophils in any single high-power field (HPF) (400×) should be regarded as consistent with EoE in the proper clinical context (12). Other features include extracellular eosinophil granules, basal cell hyperplasia, and lamina propria fibrosis.

The presence of inflammatory changes that are equally severe in biopsies from the mid esophagus and distal esophagus is also a useful finding in making the diagnosis of EoE (since reflux changes are typically more severe distally than proximally). The presence of admixed neutrophils, on the other hand, favors the presence of reflux esophagitis, since in general, only eosinophils are present in EoE unless ulceration has occurred. Biopsies of the gastric cardia can also be useful in distinguishing between reflux esophagitis and EoE. In reflux esophagitis, the cardia is uniformly inflamed (i.e., "carditis"), while in EoE, the cardia is typically not inflamed. The presence or absence of increased eosinophils in any gastric or duodenal biopsies obtained during the endoscopy should also be mentioned in the surgical pathology report, to address the possibility of a more generalized eosinophilic gastrointestinal disorder. In some cases, it is not possible to make a firm histologic distinction between EoE and severe reflux esophagitis. Correlation with the clinical history and the endoscopic appearance is often sufficient to arrive at the proper diagnosis, but 24-hour esophageal pH monitoring may be necessary in some patients. Other causes of esophageal eosinophilia need also be considered (Table 14-2).

The current treatment for EoE includes topical swallowed corticosteroids or systemic steroids, hypoallergenic diets, or combination of each. Esophageal dilatation may be required for strictures that are unresponsive to medical therapy.

Infectious Esophagitis

Infectious esophagitis is rare except in hospitalized, immunosuppressed, and debilitated children, who are at significant risk for the development of esophagitis in association with infection by Candida species, herpes simplex virus, and cytomegalovirus (CMV). Bacterial infection is a practical consideration only as a superinfection.

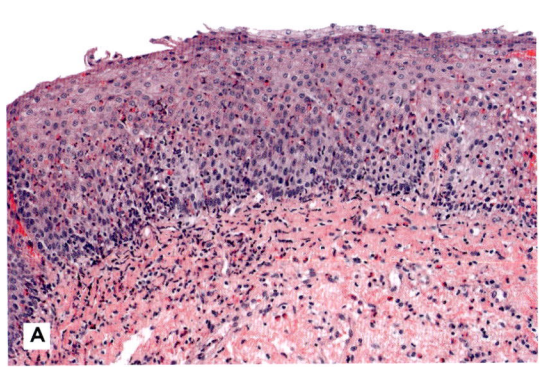
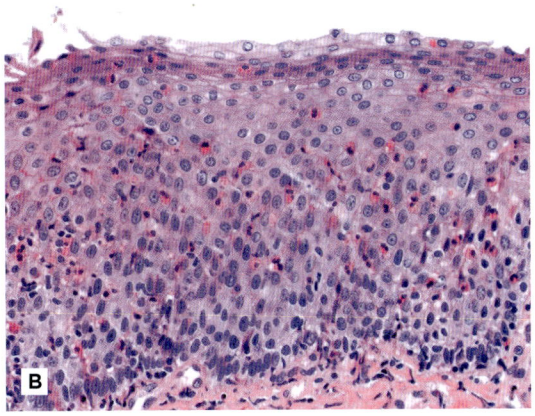
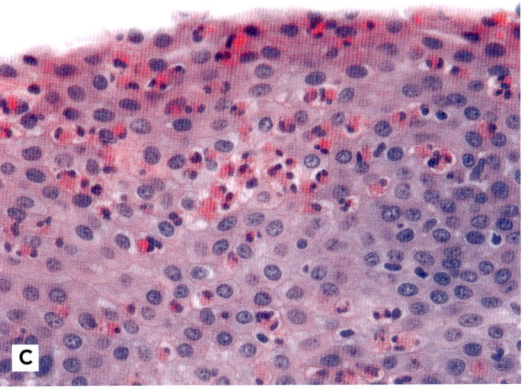

FIGURE 14-8 • Eosinophilic esophagitis. **A:** Low power showing basal cell hyperplasia. Note the fibrosis of the subepithelial stroma. **B:** There are more than 40 eosinophils per high-power field. **C:** An eosinophilic microabscess in the superficial epithelium (hematoxylin and eosin, **A:** 100×, **B:** 200×, **C:** 400×).

Herpes Simplex Esophagitis

Herpes esophagitis presents as odynophagia and is often accompanied by gingivostomatitis. Multiple small, discrete ulcers separated by normal mucosa are distributed throughout the esophagus (Figure 14-9A). In severe cases, confluent ulceration can occur. Microscopically, severe necrotizing esophagitis, abundant neutrophils, and ulceration are found. Epithelial cells at ulcer margins often demonstrate discrete eosinophilic intranuclear inclusions (Cowdry type A) or ground-glass intranuclear inclusions (Cowdry type B) (Figure 14-9B, C). Only the squamous cell can be infected by the herpes simplex virus; so if the biopsy consists only of granulation tissue and necrotic debris, no comment can be made regarding the presence or absence of this infection but IHC for HSV1 or HSV2 may be helpful. Although it occurs most often in immunosuppressed persons, herpetic esophagitis may occasionally be found in otherwise normal children.

Candida Esophagitis

Immunosuppression, premature birth, cancer chemotherapy, and AIDS are the most significant risk factors for the development of esophageal candidiasis in infants and children, although infection can also occur in patients without predisposing illnesses (13). Esophageal involvement is common in children with mucocutaneous candidiasis. In debilitated patients, esophageal infection may lead to systemic candidiasis. The gross appearance is usually a combination of white plaques and ulcerations. Histologically, the plaques consist of masses of pseudohyphae and yeast forms admixed with inflammatory debris and fibrin (eFigure 14-2A to C). Superficial collections of neutrophils should alert to the presence of organisms.

Cytomegalovirus Esophagitis

CMV esophagitis is uncommon and limited to immunosuppressed persons. It rarely occurs alone; it is usually part of a systemic CMV infection or an infection involving the whole gastrointestinal tract. In contrast to herpes simplex esophagitis, CMV cannot infect squamous epithelial cells, and the viral cytopathic effect is seen in stromal elements, endothelium, and submucosal glandular epithelium; so if the biopsy consists only of squamous epithelium, no comment can be made regarding the presence or absence of this infection.

TABLE 14-2 CAUSES OF ESOPHAGEAL EOSINOPHILIA

- Eosinophilic esophagitis
- Gastroesophageal reflux disease
- PPI-responsive esophageal eosinophilia
- Eosinophilic gastroenteritis
- Crohn disease
- Hypereosinophilic syndrome
- Achalasia
- Vasculitis, pemphigus, connective tissue disease
- Infection
- Food impaction

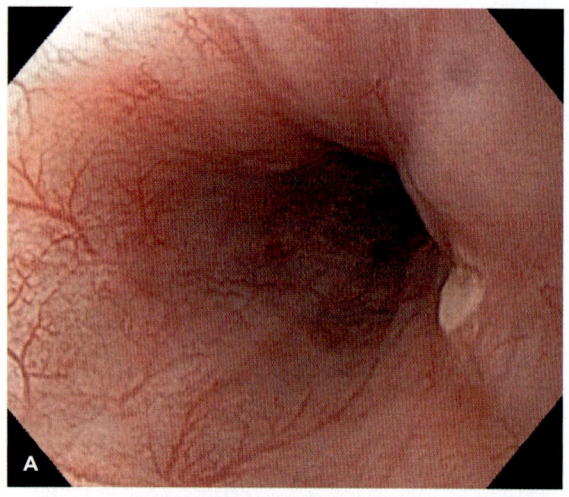
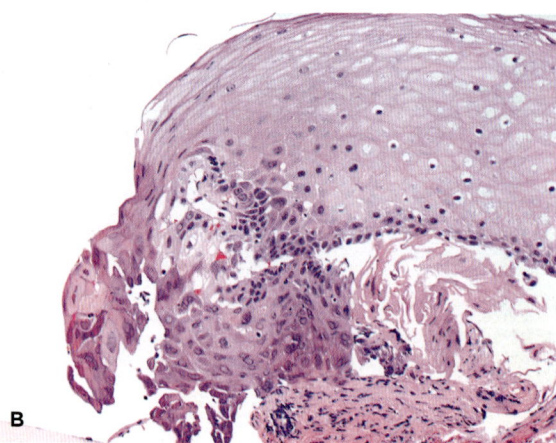
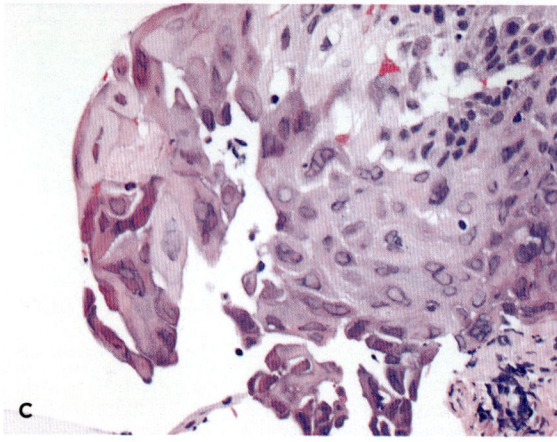

FIGURE 14-9 • Herpes simplex virus esophagitis. **A:** Endoscopic appearance of a midesophageal ulcer. **B:** Viral inclusions in squamous epithelium at the edge of the ulcer 200x. **C:** High power to demonstrate typical intranuclear inclusions and multinucleated cells 400x.

DISORDERS OF THE STOMACH

Congenital Anomalies

Hypertrophic Pyloric Stenosis

Although pyloric stenosis (PS) most likely presents between the 2nd and 4th week of life, there have been reports of PS in the newborn as well as in infants aged 4 months (14). PS is a common condition, seen in 1 of 200 infant boys. The male-to-female ratio is 5:1 or greater, and white, firstborn boys are at greatest risk. An increased concordance rate in twins and increased recurrence rate in siblings have been reported (15). Neurons supplying the circular muscle layer of the pylorus lack activity of the enzyme nitric oxide synthase. The circular muscle layer undergoes hypertrophy and elongation, and gastric outlet obstruction ensues. Progressive nonbilious vomiting, the primary manifestation, commences at 2 to 6 weeks of age in an otherwise healthy infant. The diagnosis is suggested when the hypertrophic pyloric muscle mass, approximately the size of an olive, is palpated in the right upper quadrant after a feeding. Abdominal x-ray films show marked gaseous distension of the stomach, and barium studies demonstrate a narrow and elongated pyloric channel ("string sign"). Treatment is surgical. At operation, the hypertrophic pyloric muscle appears as an elongated sphere ("olive"), approximately 2.5 cm long and 1.5 cm in diameter. A longitudinal surgical incision of the hypertrophic muscle down to the submucosa (pyloromyotomy) immediately and efficaciously relieves the obstruction. Occasional postmortem observations indicate that the circular layer of muscularis propria is hypertrophic, hyperplastic, and disorganized in appearance. The outer, longitudinal muscle layer is attenuated and of variable thickness.

Antral Web

A very unusual cause of gastric outlet obstruction in young infants is an antral web (antral diaphragm) of fibrous tissue and gastric mucosa obstructing the antrum a few centimeters proximal to the pylorus. A small, central aperture, usually no more than several millimeters in diameter, permits passage of some stomach contents; variability in the size of the opening explains the variability in age at presentation. The diagnosis is made by barium studies, and endoscopy is often difficult.

Duplication

Gastric duplication presents as a cystic mass on the greater curvature or at the pylorus and may present with bleeding, rupture, or obstruction. The pathologic features are similar to those of the more commonly encountered small-intestinal duplication. The mucosa of a gastric duplication resembles stomach mucosa in most cases, but primitive or simplified gut epithelium or intestinal mucosa is also encountered.

Pancreatic Heterotopia and Pancreatic Acinar Metaplasia

Heterotopic pancreatic tissue is most commonly noted in the stomach and proximal small bowel, although it can be seen in the liver, spleen, umbilicus, and other sites. Heterotopic pancreatic tissue also affects small-bowel stenoses, duplications, and diverticula. It is often detected incidentally on imaging studies or at autopsy. The majority of patients are asymptomatic. It usually forms a sessile mass in the antrum; a central depression may be seen, corresponding to the opening of the pancreatic duct draining the heterotopic tissue. It consists histologically of acinar and endocrine pancreas. The term *adenomyoma* has been applied to a variant characterized by a predominance of pancreatic duct structures interlaced with smooth muscle bundles but without pancreatic parenchyma. Occasionally, ulceration develops in the overlying mucosa and causes epigastric pain. More commonly in our experience, is the usually incidental histologic finding of clusters or small lobules of pancreatic acinar cells located in the deep gastric antral mucosa, which has been called *pancreatic acinar metaplasia*. This lesion is distinct from pancreatic heterotopia in that it is a histologic finding without an associated mass or recognizable endoscopic features and does not include pancreatic ducts or endocrine tissue. It has been associated with chronic gastritis in adults, whereas there are no distinct clinical or endoscopic features in children (16).

Acquired Diseases

Spontaneous Gastric Perforation in the Neonate

Spontaneous perforation of the body of the stomach is a rare but frequently fatal condition that can occur in both preterm and term infants, especially those under intensive care (17). The cause of the perforation is inapparent, although it often occurs in an area of hemorrhagic or coagulative necrosis and may be ischemic or traumatic in origin. The usual presentation is sudden abdominal distension and pneumoperitoneum.

Gastritis

A list of the types of gastritis in children is much shorter than a similar list in adults because of the absence of many of the atrophic, metaplastic, and dysplastic conditions of the adult stomach. However, it is clear that gastritis occurs with considerable frequency in children and adolescents. Numerous classification schemes exist, but for practical purposes, gastritis is categorized by etiology if apparent.

Hemorrhagic and Erosive Gastritis

The etiology of acute hemorrhagic gastritis is multifactorial, with ischemia, stress, and drug therapy playing contributory roles. Drugs known to damage the gastric mucosa include aspirin, corticosteroids, alcohol, and nonsteroidal anti-inflammatory drugs (NSAIDs), such as indomethacin. The ingestion of corrosive substances also causes a similar picture. At endoscopy, a diffusely injected and edematous mucosa, often with petechial hemorrhages and small erosions, is seen. In severe cases, which usually occur in very ill children hospitalized for sepsis, hemorrhagic shock, major surgery, burns, central nervous system disorders, or other severe illness, the changes are most severe in the gastric body and fundus.

Biopsies are usually not obtained in these severely ill patients, and therefore, this condition is usually seen at the time of autopsy. The histologic changes essentially represent a chemical injury to the gastric mucosa caused by reduced host defense against the injurious action of gastric acid and digestive enzymes. Hemorrhage and mucosal edema dominate the histologic picture. Significant inflammation is not present except directly adjacent to areas of ulceration (eFigure 14-3A, B).

Helicobacter pylori Gastritis

Since the early 1980s, it has been recognized that diffuse antral gastritis is caused by infection with *H. pylori*, a small coccoid or spirillar gram-negative bacillus. This organism, which is the pathogen responsible for the associated symptoms and pathologic changes, is not an opportunist or a commensal. Children with *H. pylori* infection usually present with nausea, vomiting, and epigastric pain. Endoscopy shows erythema, particularly in the antrum, and, in the more severe cases, erosion, antral nodularity, and thickened gastric folds. However, there is no good correlation between the endoscopic and histologic findings of gastritis. That is, in many cases where endoscopic findings of gastric mucosal erythema, granularity, or erosion are described, biopsies are entirely unremarkable. Conversely, in many cases where the gastric mucosa is described as endoscopically normal, gastritis may be evident histologically.

According to guidelines recently published by the North American and the European Societies for Pediatric Gastroenterology Hepatology and Nutrition (NASPGHAN and ESPGHAN), the initial diagnosis of *H. pylori* infection should be based on endoscopy with gastric biopsies (one each from the antrum and corpus) plus either a positive rapid urease test or a positive culture (18). The rapid urease or CLO (for *Campylobacter*-like organism) test is inexpensive and sensitive, and is based on the production of urease by the organism, which causes a change in the color of the test solution. Serologic studies are also sensitive, but positivity may persist for some time after eradication of the organism. On biopsy, the organisms are most reliably found in the antrum, although the fundus and cardia of the stomach may also be affected. The bacilli can be seen faintly on ordinary preparations stained with hematoxylin and eosin, but they are more easily seen with Giemsa, Genta, Warthin-Starry, or immunoperoxidase staining; they appear as small curved or slightly twisted rods, 4 to 5 μm in length, within the mucous coat overlying the surface or superficial foveolar epithelium (Figure 14-10). The presence of the organisms is almost invariably accompanied by neutrophils.

The antral mucosa exhibits a diffuse superficial infiltrate composed primarily of plasma cells and lymphocytes. Active foci of neutrophilic infiltration may be seen in the lamina propria or in glandular or surface epithelium. Although lymphoid aggregates are normal in the gastric mucosa, the

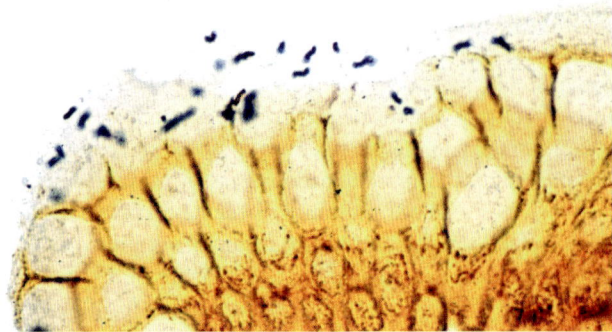

FIGURE 14-10 • *Helicobacter pylori* organisms over antral mucosa (Warthin-Starry stain, 400×).

presence of lymphoid follicles with germinal centers is highly suggestive of past or current *H. pylori* infection. In patients on a proton pump inhibitor for dyspepsia or symptoms of GER, the *H. pylori* organism may migrate to cause active gastritis of the gastric body mucosa, resulting in an inactive appearance of the antral gastritis.

Eradication of the organism is recommended for children with *H. pylori*–positive peptic ulcer disease and is based on the use of a proton pump inhibitor in combination with two antibiotics for 7 to 14 days (18). This typically results in prompt disappearance of the organisms and the neutrophilic component of the mucosal inflammatory cell infiltrates. By contrast, it may take many months for the lymphocytic and plasma cell infiltrates to disappear. Biopsies obtained during this period may be diagnosed as inactive gastritis. The diagnosis of inactive gastritis can be difficult, as there are a number of lamina propria lymphocytes and plasma cells in the gastric mucosa normally (19). As a general rule of thumb, when the density of plasma cells is such that they are clustered and touching each other, this can be regarded as indicative of inactive gastritis. In some patients with inactive antral gastritis, there may not be an antecedent diagnosis of *H. pylori* gastritis, as the infection may have been treated incidentally during antibiotic treatment of infection elsewhere (e.g., otitis media). Treatment failure is not uncommon and is usually related to antibiotic resistance, and options for these children usually include repeat EGD with culture and antibiotic susceptibility testing (18).

Even though *H. pylori* causes duodenal ulcers, the organism is not found in duodenal mucosa except in instances of gastric metaplasia of the duodenum, which is rare in children. The mechanism of duodenal ulcer formation in *H. pylori* infection is thought to involve increased acid secretion as a response to the gastric infection, as well as direct damage by the organism in the areas of duodenal gastric foveolar metaplasia.

In addition to the immediate morbidity of gastritis and ulcer disease in children and adults, infection with *H. pylori* is known to carry a risk for future adenocarcinoma of the stomach and gastric lymphoma arising in mucosa-associated lymphoid tissue (MALT).

The histologic differential diagnosis of *H. pylori* gastritis includes a small number of unusual conditions of the stomach with distinctive clinical and histologic findings, including involvement by eosinophilic gastroenteritis (EG) (Figure 14-11), CD, chronic granulomatous disease (CGD), and Henoch-Schönlein purpura (HSP). Lymphocytic gastritis, defined as greater than 25 lymphocytes for every 100 epithelial cells in the gastric mucosa (20), is most frequently associated with celiac disease in children (eFigure 14-4). It is not likely to be associated with *H. pylori* infection unless neutrophils are also present (21).

Helicobacter heilmannii (Gastrospirillum hominis) Gastritis

Helicobacter heilmannii infection of the stomach is more rare and not as serious or chronic a disease as is *H. pylori* gastritis. The clinical presentation and histologic features are similar except that *H. heilmannii* gastritis is more focal and less intense compared to *H. pylori* gastritis (22). In addition,

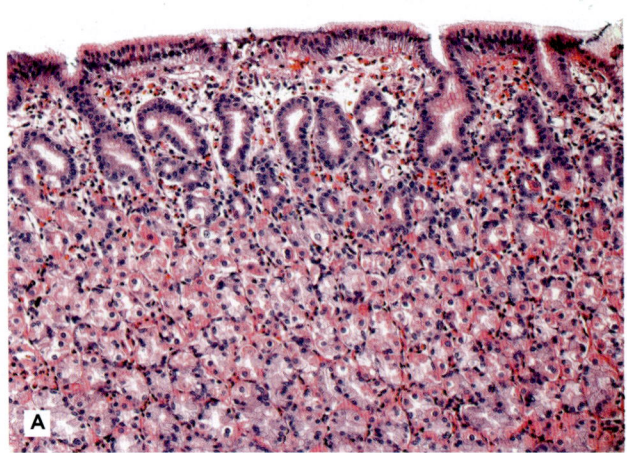
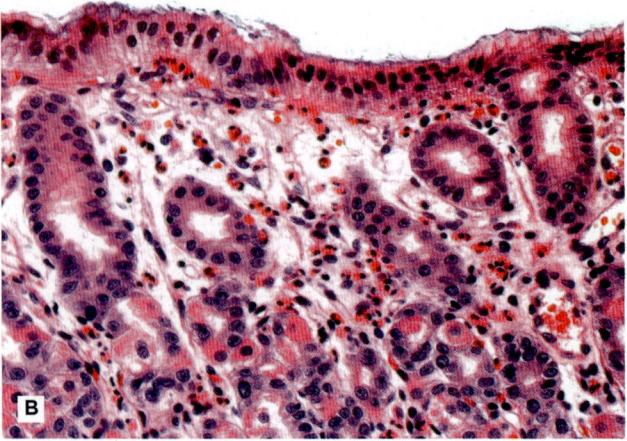

FIGURE 14-11 • Eosinophilic gastritis. **A:** A pure infiltrate of abundant eosinophils 200×. **B:** Eosinophils infiltrate the surface epithelium 400×.

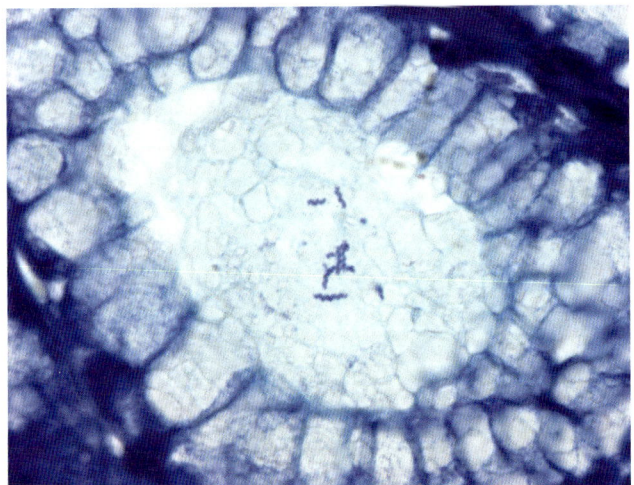

FIGURE 14-12 • *Helicobacter heilmannii* organisms over antral mucosa (Giemsa stain, 1000×).

H. heilmannii is a larger organism than *H. pylori*, more obviously spiraled, and more readily seen on sections stained with hematoxylin and eosin (Figure 14-12). *Helicobacter heilmannii* and *H. pylori* may coexist; the treatment is similar.

Peptic Ulcer Disease

Peptic ulcers are of two types: acute (stress) and chronic. They are also classified as primary and secondary, the latter associated with systemic disease. Nearly all peptic ulcers occur in the stomach and duodenum, but they may occur in any location where acid- and pepsin-secreting gastric mucosa is found, including Meckel diverticulum.

Most cases of childhood and adult chronic ulcers have been shown to be caused by infection with *H. pylori*, though it has been more recently recognized that a significant proportion of chronic duodenal ulcers (20% to 40%) are not related to *H. pylori*, drugs, or any other identifiable cause (23). Chronic (or primary) peptic ulceration in children is the same acid peptic disease that is so common in adults. This condition can develop in children as young as 4 or 5 years old, although it is more common in preadolescents and adolescents of either sex. It is most common in adolescent boys. Duodenal ulcer is more common than is gastric ulcer. Chronic abdominal pain is the most frequent presenting symptom. More than 50% of the patients have hematemesis, melena, or occult bleeding at the time of presentation. At endoscopy, chronic peptic ulcers are usually round to oval, less than 2 cm in diameter, well delineated from the surrounding mucosa by sharp margins, and covered by exudate at the base.

Microscopically, granulation tissue and scar tissue form the ulcer base, which often extends deep into the muscularis propria. The stomach invariably shows active antral gastritis, and *H. pylori* is usually identified. If the ulcer is duodenal, active duodenitis is usually present in surrounding, non-ulcerated mucosa. Chronic peptic ulcers usually heal with a medical regimen. Other causes of peptic ulcer disease in children include the Zollinger-Ellison syndrome, cystic fibrosis, short bowel syndrome, and hyperparathyroidism. The Zollinger-Ellison syndrome is rare, occurs mainly in middle-aged adults but has been reported in children, and is characterized by peptic ulceration resistant to therapy, giant gastric rugal folds, and increased serum levels of gastrin. Ulceration due to mucosal injury caused by NSAIDs or other medications is also a diagnostic consideration in older children. Among 360 children with gastritis studied by Dohil et al. (24), 55% had no detectable cause.

Ménétrier Disease

Ménétrier disease is found primarily in adults but is known to occur in children. Though similarities exist, the clinical course and etiology are different. In adults, the cause is unknown and the disease is usually severe and often requires gastrectomy. Childhood cases are often self-limited, and most are caused by CMV infection. Classic Ménétrier disease presents with epigastric or abdominal pain and weight loss. In contrast to adults, children often also present with complications of protein-losing gastropathy, such as ascites, pleural effusions, and periorbital or peripheral edema.

Unlike the adult form, Ménétrier disease in children does not spare the antrum, and hypertrophic gastric folds can be seen throughout the stomach. Histologic features include mucous cell hyperplasia, pronounced elongation and tortuosity of the usually short gastric pits (foveolae), glandular atrophy, and reversal of the usual pit-to-gland ratio. Cysts lined by superficial mucous cells are found deep in the mucosa. Inflammation is more prominent in children than in adults, reflecting the infectious etiology in most children. CMV inclusions are often evident in biopsy material in children. Gastric and urine cultures, serology, polymerase chain reaction and immunohistochemistry, and/or *in situ* hybridization may be useful ancillary tests. Other associations have included allergy, autoimmunity, and other infections, such as *Campylobacter* and herpes.

Ménétrier disease is difficult to diagnose in superficial mucosal biopsy specimens. The differential diagnosis includes other causes of large gastric folds: *H. pylori* gastritis, EG, chronic varioliform gastritis, lymphoma, lymphangiectasia, and other infectious gastritides such as tuberculosis, syphilis, and histoplasmosis.

Foveolar hyperplasia of the antrum in neonates may be caused by prostaglandin therapy administered to maintain patency of the ductus arteriosus in certain forms of congenital heart disease (25). Usually, the clinical setting, antral location, and presence of hypoalbuminemia make it possible to distinguish this group of neonates from those with Ménétrier disease.

Granulomatous Gastritis

Ectors et al. (26) presented the spectrum of causes or associations of granulomatous gastritis in 71 adults. CD constituted 52%; isolated idiopathic granulomatous gastritis, 25%; foreign body granulomas, 10%; and the remainder were related to tumors, sarcoidosis, Whipple disease, vasculitis, or unclassifiable. In our experience, CD is by far the most common cause in children followed remotely by CGD. CGD, an inherited defect of granulocytes, may lead to pyloric outlet obstruction. Endoscopically, in such patients, the antral mucosa is thickened and irregular, and surgical specimens have inflamed mucosa, submucosa, and muscularis. The infiltrate contains mononuclear inflammatory cells, multinucleate histiocytes, and eosinophils. Some have granulomas and foci of necrosis.

Crohn Disease of the Stomach

Involvement of the stomach by CD usually occurs in association with disease in the more common locations—the distal ileum and colon. In a review of 230 children with CD by Lenaerts et al. (27), 30% had lesions of the esophagus, stomach, and duodenum. On occasion, the initial presentation of CD is as a gastroduodenal process. In such cases, the antrum is usually involved, often in continuity with the proximal duodenum. Obstruction of the gastric outlet is a feature shared with EG and some cases of *H. pylori* gastritis. The histology of gastric CD is similar to that in other sites. Particularly suggestive of gastroduodenal CD is the combination of distinctly focal acute inflammation causing destruction of glandular epithelium plus spotty chronic inflammation similar to the characteristic focal involvement of the distal gastrointestinal tract in CD. This focally enhanced pattern of active gastritis in CD is usually distinct from the more diffuse, superficial and plasma cell predominant pattern of gastritis due to *H. pylori* infection. In a retrospective study of 238 children with upper gastrointestinal biopsies, focal gastritis was present in 65% of patients with CD and in 20.8% of patients with ulcerative colitis (UC), compared to 2.3% of controls without IBD and one of 39 with *H. pylori* (28). The presence of granulomas is very helpful in addition to these nonspecific inflammatory features. Pascasio reviewed 438 consecutive biopsies in children with gastritis looking for histologic markers for CD such as granulomas and focal glandulitis (29). Of 58 patients diagnosed as having CD by colonic biopsy and other standard criteria, 34 (77%) were predicted to have CD by gastric biopsy alone. Eosinophils were a significant component in many of the inflammatory foci. In their experience, none of the focal glandulitis biopsies had a history of UC.

Polyps and Tumors of the Stomach

Gastric polyps are rare in children. Juvenile polyps and Peutz-Jeghers polyps may occur in the stomach as part of a generalized polyposis syndrome. Gastric hyperplastic polyps are rare in children but can occur in the setting of *H. pylori* gastritis. Fundic gland polyps are a more common clinically insignificant consequence of chronic administration of proton pump inhibitors used to treat GERD and dyspepsia. They are usually small and often multiple and are restricted to the oxyntic mucosa of the proximal stomach. Histologically, they can be difficult to distinguish from normal gastric fundic mucosa as the histologic features can be subtle, despite the endoscopic appearance of a polypoid lesion. The diagnostic histologic features include dilatation of the fundic glands and parietal cells with cytoplasmic protrusions extending into the glandular lumina. Cytoplasmic vacuolization of parietal cells is also common. The complete absence of lamina propria inflammation and edema is a striking feature of these polyps (eFigure 14-5). The surrounding flat fundic mucosa often exhibits histologic features similar to but not as pronounced as those evident in the polyps. Fundic gland polyps also develop commonly in patients with familial polyposis coli. Thus, if a fundic gland polyp is identified in a young patient not taking a proton pump inhibitor, colonoscopy to exclude colonic polyposis may be indicated. Dysplasia does occur in fundic gland polyps associated with familial polyposis coli but is exceedingly rare in the sporadic setting (30). For this reason, it is not necessary to remove multiple sporadic fundic gland polyps.

Gastric teratomas are large, bulky multicystic masses that project into the gastric lumen or outward into the peritoneal space. Heterotopic pancreatic tissue should be considered in the differential diagnosis of gastric tumors.

Malignant tumors of the stomach are quite rare in children. MALT lymphomas associated with *H. pylori* infection and Burkitt lymphomas are the most common types of lymphoma reported (31). Adenocarcinoma of the stomach is distinctly rare but has been reported in otherwise normal children. It is also known to occur in ataxia–telangiectasia and other primary immunodeficiency disorders. Rare examples of inflammatory myofibroblastic tumor and rhabdomyosarcoma have also been reported.

Gastrointestinal Stromal Tumors

Gastrointestinal stromal tumors (GISTs) occur mainly in middle-aged and older patients, with an estimated incidence of about 5000 cases annually in the United States (32). Approximately 85% occur in the stomach, with most of the remainder occurring in the small bowel. Presentation elsewhere in the gastrointestinal tract is unusual. About 1% of GISTs present in children, either as sporadic tumors or in the setting of a syndrome. The vast majority of, but not all, GISTs in children occur in the stomach. Iron deficiency anemia is the most common presenting symptom in sporadic cases, while abdominal pain, a palpable mass, or vomiting occurs rarely (33). Two closely related syndromes feature GIST: the Carney triad and the Carney-Stratakis syndrome. Carney triad is used to describe patients with paragangliomas, pulmonary chondromas, and GIST. About 85% of patients with Carney triad are female, and the GISTs are often multifocal, which is unusual for sporadic tumors. Despite extensive molecular analysis, a specific underlying genetic defect has not been identified in patients with Carney triad (34) Carney-Stratakis syndrome designates a separate group of patients with GISTs and paragangliomas but no pulmonary chondromas. In these patients, autosomal dominant transmission has been demonstrated and germ-line mutations in any of three mitochondrial complex II succinate dehydrogenase (SDH) enzyme subunits (SDHB, SDHC, or SDHD) have been documented (35). GISTs can also develop in individuals with neurofibromatosis type 1, although usually not in childhood.

GISTs are presumed to develop from the interstitial cells of Cajal, which are thought to represent the pacemaker cells throughout the gastrointestinal tract. These cells are normally located within the myenteric plexus and the muscularis propria and have an important role in the regulation of peristalsis. In adults, approximately 90% of GISTs are associated with gain-of-function mutations of the KIT or PDGFR genes. In contrast, these mutations are only present in 15% of pediatric GISTs (32). Thus, the molecular pathogenesis of pediatric GIST is distinct from the adult counterparts, and the underlying mechanisms are currently undefined.

Pediatric GISTs can be of spindle cell or epithelioid morphology, and mixed forms are also common. Among sporadic tumors, epithelioid tumors are more common overall, but spindle cell morphology is more common in boys. The epithelioid tumors are composed of round to polygonal cells, which may have little or abundant cytoplasm. Cytoplasmic vacuolization is common in these tumors and sometimes can be so prominent as to produce a signet ring cell–like appearance (Figure 14-13A, B). The vacuoles do not stain for mucosubstances, glycogen, or fat and appear to represent an artifact of formalin fixation. The spindle cell variant of the tumor resembles smooth muscle tumors (SMT), but the cells are usually not as long and slender. Areas of hyaline fibrosis are common in both spindle cell and epithelioid variants of the tumor (see Chapter 25).

The diagnosis of GIST is confirmed by immunohistologic detection of cytoplasmic reactivity in tumor cells with the c-kit antibody. Even in pediatric tumors where 15% or less of the tumors have mutations in either the c-kit or PDGFRA genes, most of the tumors still express c-kit by immunohistochemistry. In adults, immunohistologic detection utilizing a recently developed antibody-designated DOG1 has been reported as highly sensitive and specific for the diagnosis of GISTs, including those that are nonreactive with the c-kit antibody (36). The antigen detected by the DOG1 antibody is uniformly present in Cajal cells throughout the gastrointestinal tract, but not in mast cells, unlike the c-kit protein (37). In one study, 9 of 11 pediatric GISTs were reactive with the DOG1 antibody (38).

In the pediatric population, the differential diagnosis of GIST includes leiomyoma, inflammatory myofibroblastic tumor, desmoid fibromatosis, and monophasic synovial sarcoma. In addition to the greater degree of spindle cell eosinophilia, leiomyoma can be excluded based on immunohistochemical negativity for CD117 and DOG1. Prognostic stratification for GISTs has relied primarily on tumor size and mitotic rate (mitotic figures per 50 HPFs) (39). Management recommendations for pediatric GIST depend on KIT and PDGFRA mutation status as it is presumed that pediatric GIST carrying a KIT or PDGFRA mutation will have a similar evolution and response as adult GIST. In these cases, the mainstay of treatment is imatinib mesylate, an inhibitor that binds to the intracellular portion of KIT and inhibits intracellular signaling. For the majority of children with mutation-negative tumors, the primary treatment is complete surgical resection with the goal of obtaining negative margins, which usually means either a total gastrectomy or a local wedge resection. Adjuvant imatinib is not recommended in mutation-negative GIST as it is not believed to be effective. In the St Jude experience, the incidence of local recurrence was high after primary resection (70%), and greater than 80% after re-resection, with most recurrences manifesting as small peritoneal nodules (35). Because of the usually indolent nature of GISTs in children, surveillance without therapy is recommended for asymptomatic patients with unresectable or metastatic disease.

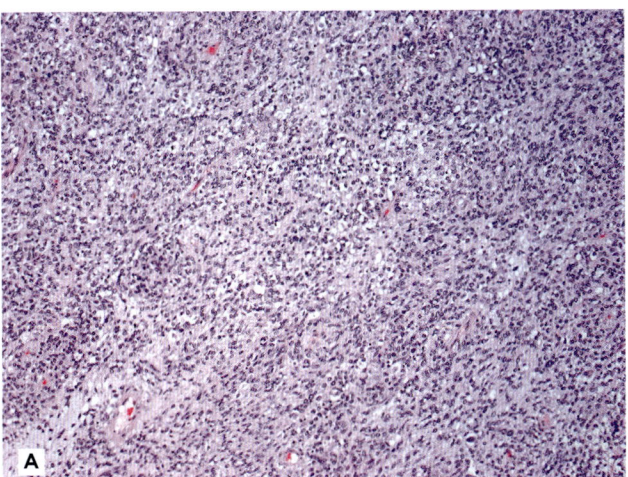
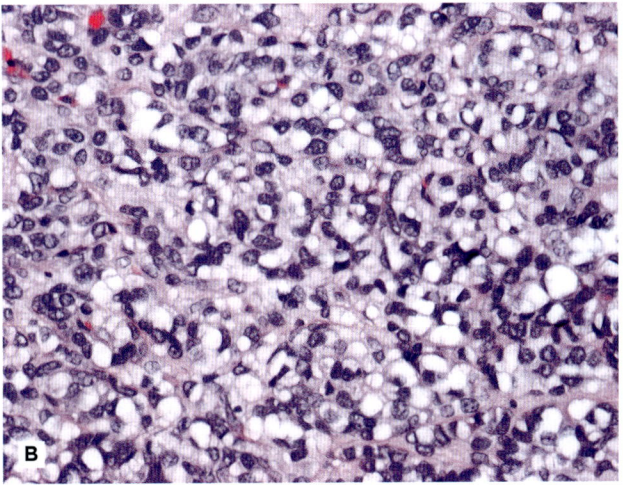

FIGURE 14-13 • Gastric gastrointestinal stromal tumor. **A:** This example demonstrates epithelioid histology, which is more common in the pediatric age group 100×. **B:** Cytoplasmic vacuoles are sometimes prominent, as seen here 200×.

DISORDERS OF THE SMALL AND LARGE INTESTINE

Congenital Abnormalities

Omphalocele

Omphalocele (exomphalos), which has an incidence of about 2 per 10,000 births (40), is a developmental defect of the anterior abdominal wall in which the abdominal musculature, fascia, and skin are absent in the midline at the point of insertion of the umbilical cord. Abdominal organs extrude anteriorly through the defect and are covered by a saclike membrane consisting of amnion externally and parietal peritoneum internally (Figure 14-14). Omphalocele results from failure of the intestine to return to the body cavity after its normal herniation into the umbilical stalk during embryonic life. Omphaloceles vary in size; the defect may be a few centimeters in diameter, or most of the anterior abdominal wall may be lacking. Depending on the size of the defect, small intestine, liver, spleen, and pancreas may be in the sac. The umbilicus usually inserts at the dome of the sac, and umbilical vessels ramify across the membrane. Intrauterine rupture of the sac may occur; exposure of the gut to amniotic fluid results in edema, bowel wall thickening, and matting of intestinal loops. Such cases must be distinguished from gastroschisis. The intestine is nearly always malrotated and shorter than normal.

Other congenital anomalies are found in at least one-third of these infants, including gastrointestinal malformations, congenital heart disease, genitourinary anomalies, imperforate anus, and central nervous system defects. The incidence of omphalocele is increased in infants with trisomy 18, trisomy 13, and trisomy 21. Omphalocele is a key feature of Beckwith-Wiedemann syndrome (gigantism, macroglossia, hemihypertrophy, visceromegaly, and hypoglycemia).

The prognosis in omphalocele is usually determined by the other anomalies and the size of the defect. Emergent operation is not necessary for intact omphaloceles, allowing workup of the neonate for concurrent abnormalities. The sac can be closed primarily if the defect is small or by staged procedures for larger defects using mesh to close the defect (40).

Gastroschisis

Gastroschisis results from a relatively small, usually right-sided paraumbilical abdominal wall defect, which is distinctly separate from the normally placed umbilicus. Loops of bowel, not covered by a membrane, extrude through the opening (Figure 14-15). Because the extruded intestine has been bathed in amniotic fluid *in utero*, it appears abnormally thickened and edematous and may be coated with fibrin. The intestine is usually not rotated and is much shorter than normal. Jejunoileal atresia is another recognized association. In contrast to omphalocele, gastroschisis is rarely associated with concurrent major congenital anomalies (41).

The condition has a prevalence of about 1 in 10,000 live births, probably higher if stillbirths and aborted fetuses are included, with a reported increase in the last 30 years (42). Its etiology is unknown; incomplete closure of the lateral folds of the abdomen during development and occlusion or disruption of the right omphalomesenteric artery have been proposed. Maternal factors such as smoking and use of certain medications may play a role (43). Treatment consists of surgical closure of the defect at birth or staged procedures with the use of prosthetic material.

Malrotation

The term malrotation includes a group of congenital positional and associated abnormalities of the intestine and mesentery resulting from nonrotation or abnormal rotation and fixation of the developing embryonic gut. During the most rapid period of growth, the embryonic intestine extends outside the abdominal cavity and initially rotates 90 degrees counterclockwise around the superior mesenteric artery (Figure 14-3). During weeks 10 and 11 of gestation, the intestine returns to the abdomen in sequential stages, with a further 180 degrees counterclockwise rotation until

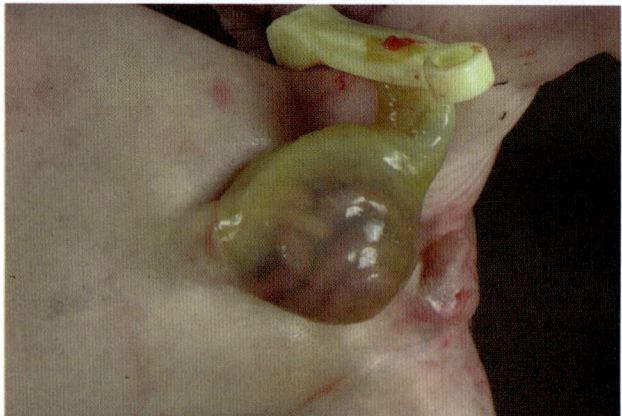

FIGURE 14-14 • Omphalocele. A translucent membrane covers the abdominal organs, which are protruding through an abdominal wall defect in this newborn. Note the insertion of the umbilicus into the center of the omphalocele sac.

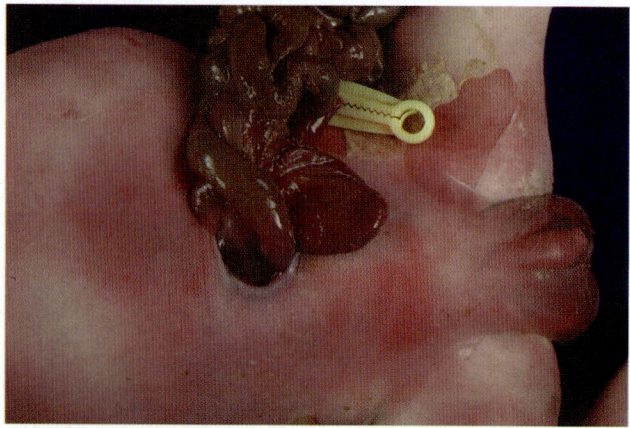

FIGURE 14-15 • Gastroschisis. Loops of intestine extrude through an abdominal wall defect located to the right of the normally placed umbilicus. The intestines are not covered by a sac.

the duodenum comes to rest in its usual position posterior to the superior mesenteric artery. The cecum and right colon, initially located in the right upper quadrant of the abdomen after the return phase, then "descend" into the right lower quadrant anterior to the superior mesenteric artery. At week 11, fixation of the gut to the abdominal wall occurs. A broad-based mesentery extending from the ligament of Treitz to the ileocecal area attaches the intestine to the posterior abdominal wall and stabilizes it. The right and left portions of the colon become fixed retroperitoneally.

Failure of this sequence to take place at all (nonrotation) or failure at any step produces a spectrum of malrotation abnormalities. Any arrest in the process of rotation also tends to interfere with the normal mesenteric fixation of the bowel and results in a narrow mesenteric base and a mobile intestine that is predisposed to volvulus. A person with an incompletely rotated bowel is likely to have abnormal mesenteric fixations and associated extrinsic intestinal obstruction and volvulus. Malrotation often occurs together with other congenital anomalies, including duodenal atresia, omphalocele, gastroschisis, jejunoileal atresia, and Meckel diverticulum.

Variations of malrotation are diagrammed in Figure 14-16. In the case of nonrotation (Figure 14-16A), the duodenum is directed inferiorly and lacks the usual sweep to the left. The distal portion of the duodenum and the ascending colon lie together in the midabdomen and are attached to the abdominal wall posteriorly by a very short mesenteric root containing the superior mesenteric artery. The descending colon is not fixed. The narrow mesenteric root and nonfixed descending colon result in midgut volvulus and duodenal obstruction (Figure 14-16C). The rapid progression of volvulus causes the most dreaded and lethal complication of malrotation, which is cessation of mesenteric artery blood flow at the base of the twisted mesentery and infarction of the entire midgut. Midgut volvulus usually presents in the first month of life with intestinal obstruction. Normal rotation of the duodenal loop with nonrotation of the colon is associated with the same potential for midgut volvulus (Figure 14-16B).

In the variation of normal colonic rotation with nonrotation of the duodenum, abnormal mesenteric bands may intermittently obstruct the duodenum. In another variation, both the duodenum and the colon rotate normally, but the ascending colon does not become fixed. Abnormal peritoneal (Ladd) bands between the hepatic flexure and the right abdominal wall may obstruct the duodenum (Figure 14-16D).

Intestinal Atresia and Stenosis

Intestinal atresia is the complete absence of a segment of the intestine or complete occlusion of the intestinal lumen. Either situation is a common cause of neonatal intestinal obstruction, with a prevalence of 2 in 10,000 live births (44). The rates of atresia in the duodenum and in the more distal jejunum and ileum are approximately equal; colonic atresia

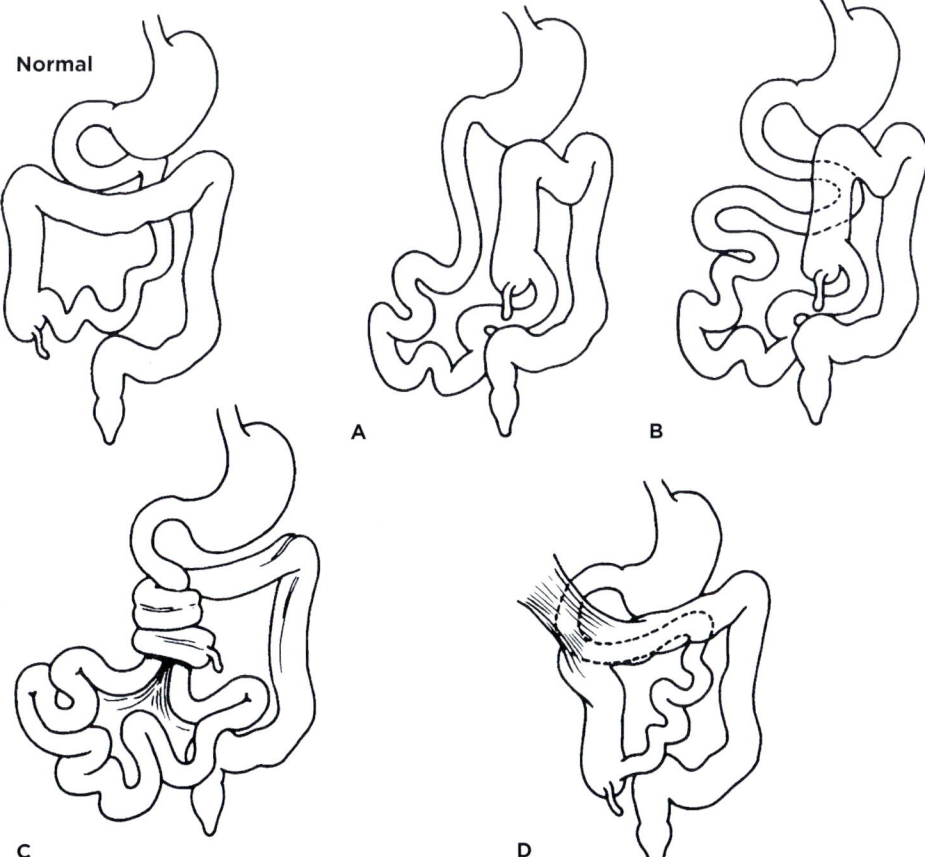

FIGURE 14-16 • Normal rotation and variations in position of stomach and intestines due to malrotation. **A:** Nonrotation of duodenum and colon. **B:** Nonrotation of colon. **C:** Midgut volvulus resulting from a narrow mesenteric root and nonfixed descending colon in malrotation. Occlusion of mesenteric blood flow leads to midgut infarction. **D:** Ladd (peritoneal) fibrous bands **(upper left)** may extend from the lateral abdominal wall to the right colon, compressing and obstructing the duodenum.

is much less frequent. Multiple jejunoileal atresias are found in approximately 10% of cases and can be associated with a number of disorders (44).

Clinical, pathologic, histologic, and experimental observations indicate that most jejunoileal atresias and stenoses are secondary malformations. The disruptions may be caused by intrauterine vascular accidents, with infarction and subsequent resorption or scarring of the affected segment. The fact that bile and squamous epithelial cells are often found distal to the obstruction suggests that the lumen was patent early in gestation. The presence of serosal fibrosis and meconium indicates previous (intrauterine) intestinal perforation and peritonitis. Experimental occlusion of portions of the mesenteric circulation in fetal animals results in identical atretic lesions. Atresias are associated with known vascular insults, such as intrauterine malrotation with volvulus, intussusception, internal hernia, and constricting gastroschisis. Familial patterns in some cases of multiple jejunoileal atresias indicate that not all cases result from vascular accidents. An inherited lethal form of multiple intestinal atresias reported mainly in French Canadians has been associated with mutations in the gene TTC7A located on chromosome 2p21 (45). Examination of the bowel showed sievelike lumina in most of these cases (46).

Approximately 75% of all intestinal stenoses and 40% of all intestinal atresias are duodenal. Intrinsic duodenal atresias and stenoses most often involve the first and second portions, the foregut portion of the duodenum, in close proximity to the entrances of the biliary and pancreatic ducts. This explains the association of duodenal atresia with hepatobiliary and pancreatic duct abnormalities. The embryologic basis of duodenal atresia also differs from that of jejunoileal and colonic atresia. Because most cases of duodenal atresia are of the membranous type, they probably result from a lack of central vacuolization during the solid cord stage of duodenal development. The rate of associated anomalies in infants with duodenal atresia is high. One-fourth of infants with duodenal atresia have Down syndrome, an association not noted with atresia at other sites. Additional congenital anomalies associated with duodenal atresia include cardiac and renal malformations, esophageal atresia, imperforate anus, and vertebral anomalies. Annular pancreas and malrotation are each found in approximately one-fourth of infants with duodenal atresia (47). Jejunoileal atresia is less likely to be associated with other anomalies, although an association has been reported with cystic fibrosis, with an estimated risk factor for cystic fibrosis 210 times higher in Caucasian infants with jejunoileal atresia than those without atresia (48).

The symptoms of intestinal atresia depend on the level of gastrointestinal tract affected. Duodenal and proximal jejunal atresia cause maternal polyhydramnios (secondary to reduced absorption of swallowed amniotic fluid), vomiting, and abdominal distension in the first 24 hours of life; these symptoms are delayed with more distal obstruction. Abdominal radiographs show gaseous distension of the stomach with duodenal atresia and, in lower intestinal atresias, air–fluid levels. Many cases of jejunoileal atresia are now detected by prenatal ultrasonography.

Intestinal atresias have been classified according to their gross appearance (49) (Figure 14-17A). Type I has an intact intestinal wall and mesentery but a septal or membranous luminal obstruction. Because the proximal segment is obstructed, its diameter greatly exceeds that of the distal segment. In type II, two intestinal segments with blind ends are separated by a fibrous cord. Histologic examination of a type II atresia usually shows a recognizable intestinal wall with muscularis layers but fibrous obliteration of the mucosa and submucosa. The frequent presence of luminal granulation tissue, fibrosis, and calcification suggests previous ischemia and healing. In type III, the most common, two blind ends are present without an intervening cord; a wedge-shaped mesenteric defect is also present. Type III may also be associated with a congenitally short small intestine. In the "apple-peel" or "Christmas tree" variety of extensive jejunal atresia, the intestine is very short and the distal ileal segment is coiled around its arterial blood supply (the ileocecal artery) (Figure 14-17B).

Intestinal segments adjacent to regions of atresia or stenosis should be examined for changes suggestive of cystic fibrosis: dilated glands with eosinophilic inspissated secretions, unusually viscid secretions in the lumen, and hyperplasia of goblet cells.

Congenital intestinal stenosis is less common than intestinal atresia; it may be solitary or multiple and may affect a short or long segment. The bowel diameter is greatly reduced, although the lumen is patent throughout. Histologic examination of the intestinal wall often shows evidence of previous ischemia and healing, including mucosal atrophy, submucosal fibrosis, and scarring of smooth muscle. As in intestinal atresia, most cases are presumed to result from an intrauterine ischemic insult, although a history of an untoward event during pregnancy is often lacking.

Duplications of the Gastrointestinal Tract

Gastrointestinal (enteric) duplications are tubular or cystic structures that lie alongside the intestinal tube. The duplication and the intestinal tube often share a muscular wall (intramural); less often, the duplication is separated from the intestine proper but in close proximity to it (extramural). Duplications may occur anywhere near the gastrointestinal tract from the neck to rectum; the single most common site is the ileum (Figure 14-18A).

Symptoms vary widely, depending on the location of the duplication. Thoracic enteric duplication cysts are usually extramural and found in the posterior mediastinum; they present with respiratory symptoms in infancy and may communicate across the diaphragm with the intra-abdominal gastrointestinal tract. Abdominal duplications may present with pain, a palpable mass, intestinal obstruction, and, if peptic ulceration occurs in ectopic gastric mucosa, intestinal bleeding.

Multiple duplications are found in 5% of patients. The usual intestinal duplication is a cystic mass located on the mesenteric border. It ranges in size from 2 to 7 cm in diameter, although much larger ones may also be found (Figure 14-18B). The cyst lumen usually does not communicate with the

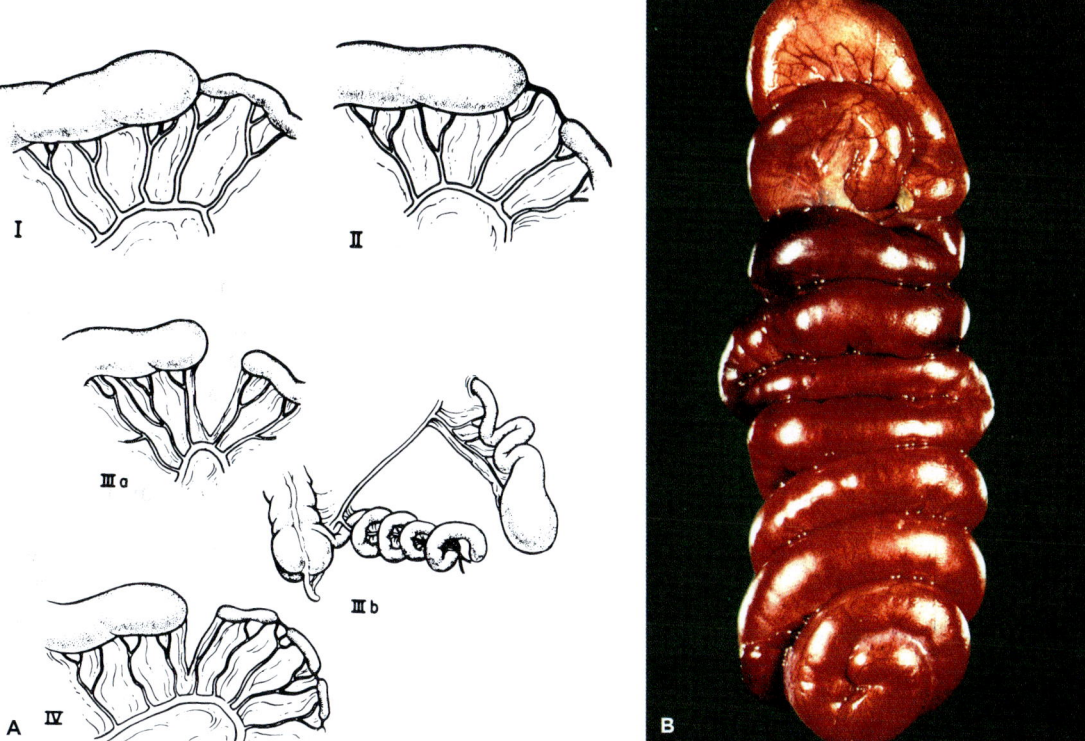

FIGURE 14-17 • **A:** Classification of intestinal atresia. I: Mucosal (membranous) atresia with intact bowel wall and mesentery; II: blind intestinal ends attached by a fibrous cord; IIIa: blind intestinal ends separated by a V-shaped mesenteric defect without an intervening cord; IIIb: "apple-peel" atresia; and IV: multiple atresia. (From Grosfeld JL. Jejunoileal atresia and stenosis. In: Welch KJ, Randolph SG, Ravich MM, et al., eds. *Pediatric Surgery*, 4th ed. Chicago, IL: Year Book; 1986:843, with permission.) **B:** Apple-peel or Christmas tree atresia.

intestinal lumen. Occasionally, tubular duplications paralleling a long segment of intestine are found, usually incidentally. Noncommunicating cysts are filled with mucoid material and histologically mimic normal gastrointestinal tract with enteric mucosa, submucosa, muscularis propria, and a myenteric plexus. Intramural duplications usually do not have a complete muscularis layer but rather share a muscularis layer with the adjacent intestine. The mucosa may resemble adjacent normal

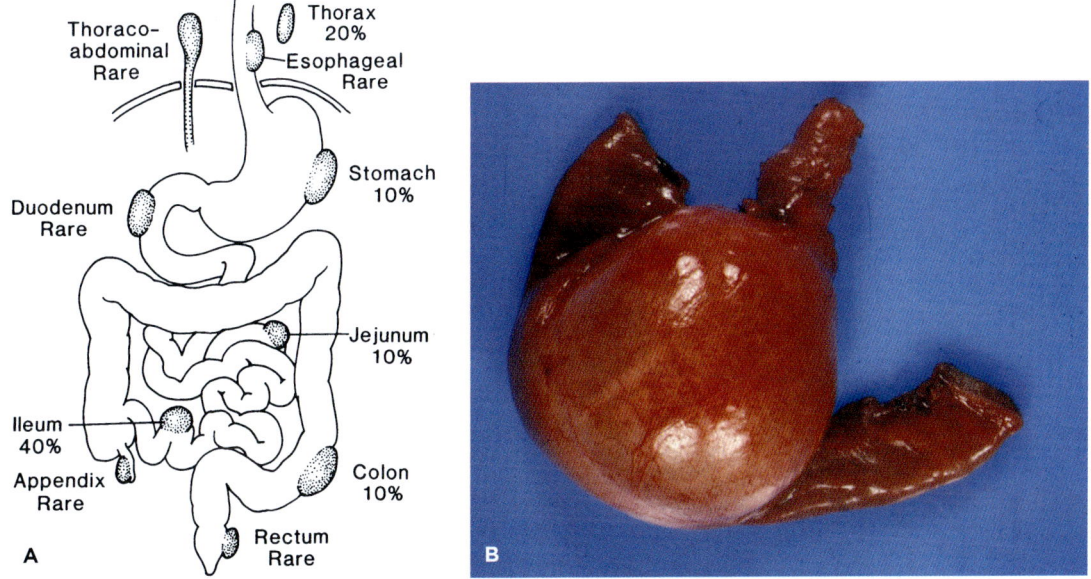

FIGURE 14-18 • **A:** Locations and incidence of gastrointestinal duplication cysts. **B:** Cystic duplication of the small intestine.

gastrointestinal mucosa, but it is often very simplified and difficult to categorize except that columnar epithelium bears a generic resemblance to intestinal surface epithelial cells. Cilia may be present, as in embryonic intestinal epithelium. Gastric mucosa is found in approximately 20% of duplications and may cause peptic ulceration in unlikely sites, such as the ileum and posterior mediastinum. Intestinal duplications in the abdomen must be distinguished from a Meckel diverticulum and other vitelline duct remnants, mesenteric cyst (which lacks intestinal wall morphology), and cystic lymphangioma.

Meckel Diverticulum and Other Vitelline Duct Anomalies

The vitelline (omphalomesenteric) duct usually becomes obliterated by week 10 of embryonic life and subsequently disappears completely. In approximately 2% of the population, however, it remains in various forms (Figure 14-19A to E). These include Meckel diverticulum or, less commonly, a fibrous cord extending from ileum to umbilicus, a cyst, or an umbilical sinus. Many of these remnants are asymptomatic, but others cause symptoms that develop most frequently in the first few years of life.

Meckel diverticulum is the most common vitelline duct remnant and also the most common congenital anomaly of the gastrointestinal tract. It results from incomplete obliteration of the vitelline duct at the ileum and appears as a 1- to 5-cm finger-like protrusion of the intestine on the antimesenteric surface of the middle ileum (Figure 14-19D). When found incidentally at autopsy or surgery, most Meckel diverticula are lined by small-intestinal epithelium. Those causing symptoms are likely to contain heterotopic gastric mucosa (Figure 14-20A, B), which secretes acid and leads to peptic ulceration of adjacent intestinal mucosa with subsequent abdominal pain, rectal bleeding, and occasionally intestinal perforation. Approximately 25% of all Meckel diverticula contain foci of gastric mucosa. Occasionally, a Meckel diverticulum may invert into the intestinal lumen and serve as the lead point of an ileal intussusception.

Other vitelline duct remnants are much less common than Meckel diverticulum. A vitelline cyst (Figure 14-19B) results from partial obliteration of the vitelline duct and presents

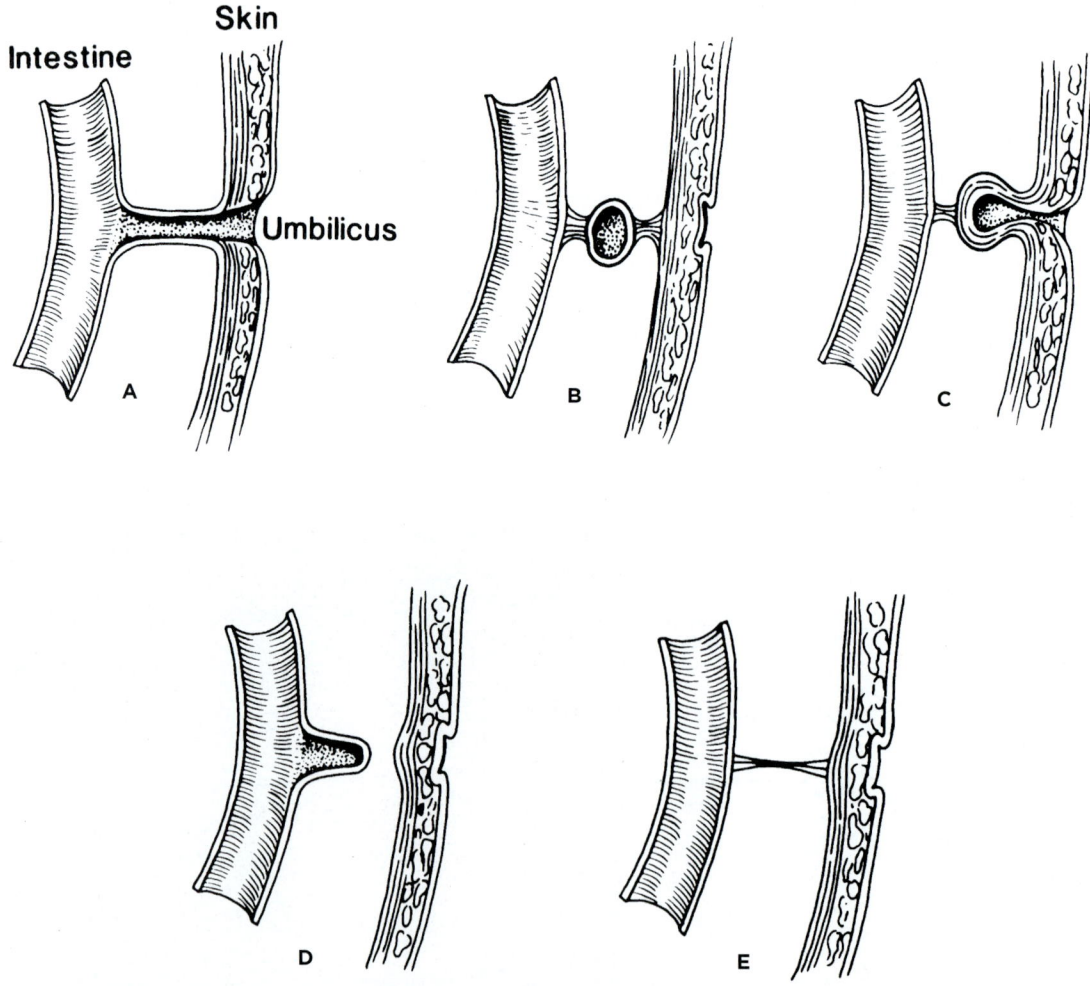

FIGURE 14-19 • Vitelline (omphalomesenteric) duct anomalies. **A:** Persistence of the entire vitelline duct from the ileum to umbilicus. **B:** Vitelline duct cyst. **C:** Vitelline duct and umbilical sinus. **D:** Meckel diverticulum. **E:** Vitelline band.

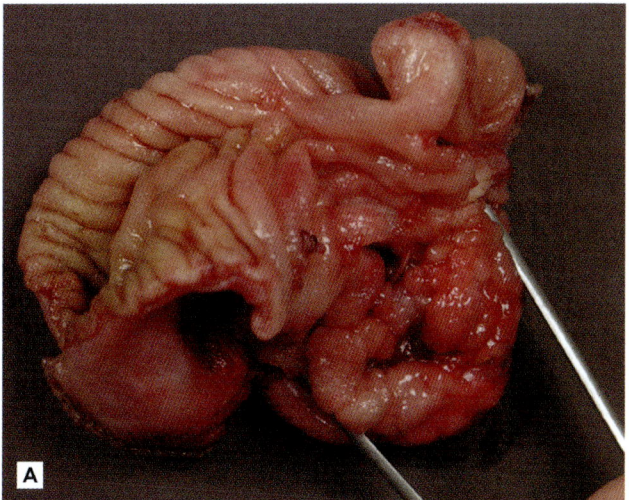
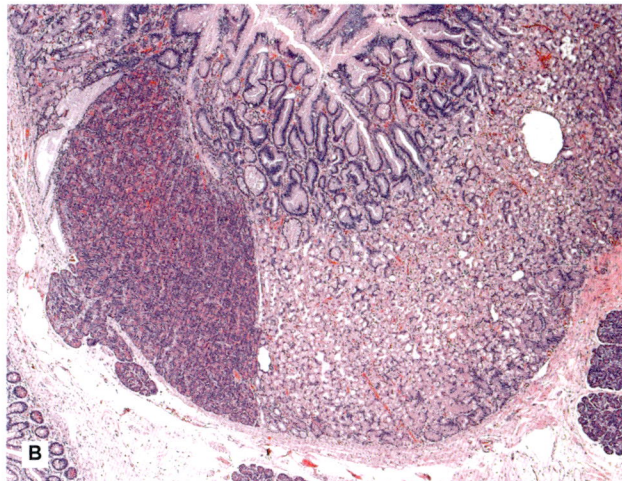

FIGURE 14-20 • Meckel diverticulum. **A:** Gastric mucosa within an opened Meckel diverticulum. **B:** Ectopic gastric fundic and pancreatic tissue in the mucosa line the diverticulum 100×.

as a mass subjacent to the umbilicus. Microscopically, the cyst wall resembles that of the intestine and is lined by mucus-secreting intestinal epithelium. A vitelline band is a fibrous cord that persists after obliteration of the vitelline duct (Figure 14-19E). These bands extend from umbilicus to ileum, a Meckel diverticulum, or a vitelline cyst and they may serve as a fulcrum for volvulus. Persistence of part of the vitelline duct at the umbilicus causes an umbilical sinus, which presents with mucous discharge from the umbilicus (Figure 14-19C). This must be distinguished from the very rare persistence of the entire vitelline duct (Figure 14-19A). Vitelline cysts and sinuses at the umbilicus are distinguished histologically from urachal remnants at the same site by the presence of intestinal or columnar epithelium. Urachal remnants have a urothelial lining.

Meconium and Meconium Abnormalities

Meconium is the dark green–to-black mucoid material that fills the neonatal colon and distal small intestine. It consists predominantly of water (75%) admixed with mucous glycoproteins, swallowed vernix caseosa, gastrointestinal secretions, bile, pancreatic enzymes, plasma proteins, minerals, and lipids. More than 90% of healthy term newborns pass a meconium stool averaging 200 mL within the first 24 hours of life, and nearly all have done so by 48 hours. Abnormalities of meconium (e.g., in cystic fibrosis) or of intestinal motility (e.g., in Hirschsprung disease) result in delayed meconium passage.

Meconium Ileus

Meconium ileus is neonatal obstruction of the ileal lumen by abnormally viscid and inspissated meconium containing an abnormally high level of albumin. Most but not all cases occur as the initial manifestation of cystic fibrosis; 10% to 15% of patients with cystic fibrosis are born with meconium ileus. Rarely, infants with congenital pancreatic or pancreatic duct abnormalities have meconium ileus without cystic fibrosis, but these account for fewer than 5% of cases. Thus, the diagnosis of cystic fibrosis should be pursued in every infant with meconium ileus. In the classic case, the distal one-third of the ileum has a nearly normal diameter, but the lumen is filled with dense gray beadlike or solid meconium having the consistency and appearance of putty. The middle one-third of the ileum, proximal to the obstructing meconium, is dilated and filled with dark gelatinous or tarlike meconium. Because the colon in meconium ileus is empty throughout the fetal life, its diameter is smaller than normal.

Microscopically, the distal ileal lumen is filled with hypereosinophilic, focally calcified meconium. Intestinal glands are dilated, often V-shaped, and plugged with hypereosinophilic secretions that are continuous with the luminal meconium. Approximately 50% of the patients with meconium ileus have meconium peritonitis or other complications of meconium ileus, which include intestinal atresia and volvulus.

The overall survival rate of infants with meconium ileus exceeds 80%, although they often have a prolonged hospital course.

Meconium Peritonitis

Intestinal perforation *in utero* causes meconium to be released into the peritoneal space. Between 33% and 50% of patients with meconium peritonitis have meconium ileus and cystic fibrosis. In the remaining patients, perforation may be the result of intrauterine intestinal obstruction resulting from atresia, vascular insufficiency, malrotation with volvulus, mesenteric hernias, or congenital bands. Meconium peritonitis is usually seen just after birth and is temporally remote from the intrauterine intestinal perforation that caused it. At gross examination, the peritonitis is usually organized, with fibrosis, calcifications, and often dense intestinal adhesions. Occasionally encountered is a meconium pseudocyst, a collection of soft meconium walled off by peritoneal fibrosis.

Microscopically, collections of squames and bile pigment in the peritoneal space, florid fibrosis, and calcifications indicate the presence of meconium. Inflammation is usually chronic, and a well-developed foreign body response to squames and calcifications may be noted. Because the fetal gut is sterile, the degree of inflammation is much less than in the usual case of postnatal peritonitis. If meconium is released into the peritoneal space during intrauterine life, when the inguinal canal to the scrotum is patent, the migration of meconium into the paratesticular area results in a condition called meconium periorchitis (50). Inguinal and even labial meconium masses may also occur, although more rarely, in girls (51).

Meconium Plug

Meconium plug is a syndrome of neonatal colonic obstruction caused by a plug of desiccated meconium, usually in the ascending colon or, in infants with a very low birth weight, the ileum or proximal colon. It is a much less serious condition than meconium ileus, but it may present with a similar clinical picture. The condition may resolve spontaneously, or the plug may pass after a contrast barium enema, and the infant has no further problems. Meconium plug syndrome has been associated with Hirschsprung disease, cystic fibrosis, and maternal tocolysis (52). However, most infants with a meconium plug have none of these conditions.

Gastrointestinal Involvement in Cystic Fibrosis

Cystic fibrosis is a lethal autosomal recessive disease involving multiple organ systems resulting from abnormalities in the gene coding for the cystic fibrosis transmembrane conductance regulator (CFTR), a membrane glycoprotein found in secretory and absorptive surfaces (Chapters 5, 12, and 15). It occurs in approximately 1 in 3500 newborns in the United States (53). Mutations in the gene that encodes CFTR result in faulty electrolyte transport across epithelial surfaces and subsequent dehydration of luminal contents, which in turn leads to obstruction of glands and ducts by thick, viscid secretions. The pancreas, intestines, and lungs are the chief organ systems affected. Gastrointestinal symptoms may be present at birth and almost invariably appear during the first few months of life (Table 14-3). Malabsorption resulting from exocrine pancreatic insufficiency is a prominent manifestation in nearly all children and adults with cystic fibrosis.

Meconium ileus is the first sign of cystic fibrosis in approximately 10% to 15% of patients (54). It usually presents as intestinal obstruction in the first hours or days of life but has also been diagnosed antenatally by obstetric ultrasonography. It should be considered a manifestation of cystic fibrosis until proven otherwise. Up to one-half of infants with meconium ileus have concurrent gastrointestinal manifestations of cystic fibrosis, including meconium peritonitis, small-intestinal atresias and stenoses, duplication, volvulus, microcolon, and mesenteric bands or adhesions.

TABLE 14-3 GASTROINTESTINAL MANIFESTATIONS OF CYSTIC FIBROSIS

Gastroesophageal reflux and Barrett esophagus
Malabsorption and pancreatic insufficiency
Meconium ileus, peritonitis, and meconium plug syndrome
Microcolon
Small-intestinal obstruction and atresia
Intussusception
Volvulus
Rectal prolapse
Brunner gland hyperplasia
Fibrosing colonopathy (due to pancreatic enzyme replacement)
Pneumatosis intestinalis
Mucocele
Gallbladder disease

Distal intestinal obstruction syndrome, formerly called *meconium ileus equivalent*, is partial or total distal intestinal obstruction by inspissated fecal material occurring in older children and adults with cystic fibrosis. It has nothing to do with meconium. Viscid intestinal contents, a change in dietary habits, dehydration, and temporary disturbances in motility are all thought to play a role. It is more frequent in adults than in children and is associated with more severe genotypes. There is no association with a history of meconium ileus (55). *Fibrosing colonopathy* is a rare distinctive noninflammatory stricturing process of the colon first described in patients with cystic fibrosis in the 1990s, when it was linked to the ingestion of new preparations of high-dose pancreatic enzyme replacement capsules (56). The condition usually presents with partial or complete intestinal obstruction, and symptoms may mimic those of distal ileal obstruction syndrome (meconium ileus equivalent) or chronic IBD. Fibrosing colonopathy usually affects a long segment of the ascending colon but may involve the entire colon. The lumen is compromised by circumferential submucosal fibrosis along the length of the strictured segment. Fibrosis of the lamina propria, mucosal ulceration, acute and chronic mucosal inflammation, and granulation tissue can also be seen. One series noted increased numbers of eosinophils in the mucosa (57) Current recommendations use lower daily doses of enzyme replacement.

HIRSCHSPRUNG DISEASE

Hirschsprung disease (HSCR, aganglionosis) is characterized by an absence of intramural parasympathetic ganglion cells in the distal gastrointestinal tract resulting in persistent contraction of the affected segment and subsequent colonic obstruction. HSCR is a congenital disorder with an incidence of one per 5000 live births. The condition results from defective craniocaudal migration of vagal neural crest cells (the progenitors of ganglion cells), which populate the entire length of the bowel by the 7th week of gestation. Mutation of one or more HSCR susceptibility genes is the major basis of the disorder (58). More than a dozen genes have been associated with HSCR, the major one being the RET gene, a protooncogene, which codes for a transmembrane receptor, which has also been identified as disease causing in MEN 2A and which maps to chromosome 10q11.2.

More than 90% of patients with Hirschsprung disease are born at full term with a normal birth weight. Presenting symptoms in neonates include delayed passage of meconium (>48 hours), vomiting, abdominal distension, and, in some cases, enterocolitis. In most cases, Hirschsprung disease is an isolated congenital anomaly (70% of patients), but associations have been noted with Down syndrome (10% of patients with Hirschsprung disease have Down syndrome) and other syndromes such as Bardet-Biedl, Mowat-Wilson, multiple endocrine neoplasia (MEN type 2A), Smith-Lemli-Opitz, Waardenburg, and central hypoventilation syndrome (Haddad or Ondine syndrome).

The aganglionic segment in Hirschsprung disease begins at the anal sphincter and extends proximally (Figure 14-21A to E). In 80% of cases, aganglionosis is limited to the rectum and distal sigmoid colon, referred to as short-segment disease. In the remaining patients, the aganglionic segment is longer (long-segment Hirschsprung disease) and extends as far proximally as the splenic flexure or transverse colon in 10% and the cecum in 5% (total colonic aganglionosis or Zuelzer-Wilson disease). In rare cases, aganglionosis extends into the small intestine and may reach as far as the proximal duodenum. Short-segment disease is 5.5 times more common in males, is less likely to recur in siblings, and has features suggestive of multifactorial inheritance. By contrast, long-segment aganglionosis shows a significantly lower male gender bias, higher recurrence rate, and genetic properties suggestive of dominant inheritance with incomplete penetrance (58). In the usual case, barium enema shows a narrow rectum and rectosigmoid colon with a proximal funneling transition to a dilated sigmoid colon. Neonates and infants with long aganglionic segments do not have this diagnostic radiologic picture. Anal manometry is another valuable diagnostic tool used in certain clinical settings. Despite the relative rarity of Hirschsprung disease, it enters into the differential diagnosis of many other conditions because of its

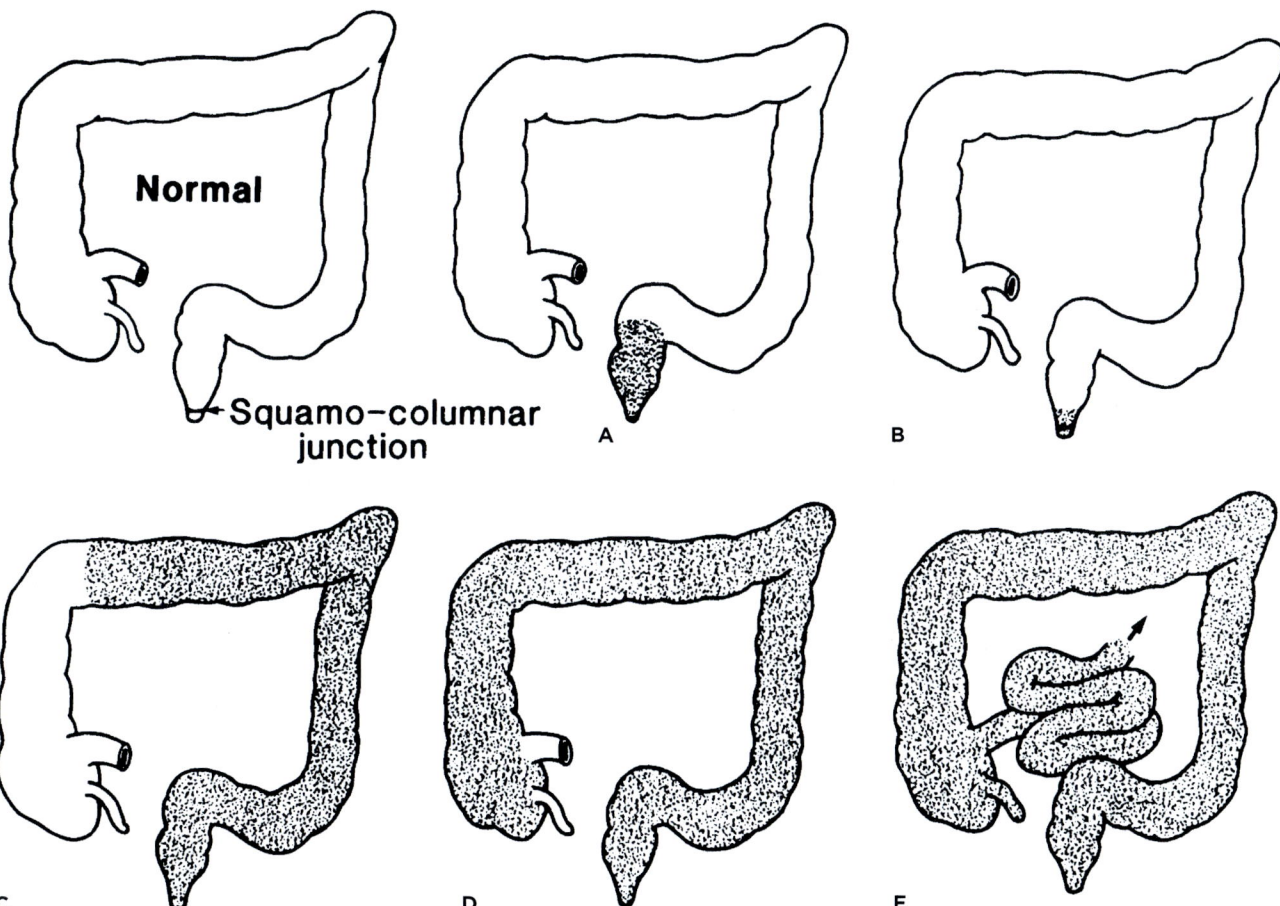

FIGURE 14-21 • Distribution of affected colon in Hirschsprung disease (stippled area). **A:** Rectosigmoid aganglionosis. **B:** Ultrashort Hirschsprung disease affected the distal rectum near the anal sphincter. **C:** Long-segment Hirschsprung disease with involvement of the hepatic flexure. **D:** Total colonic aganglionosis. **E:** Aganglionosis involving the entire colon and the distal small bowel (in exceptional cases, the distal duodenum may be involved).

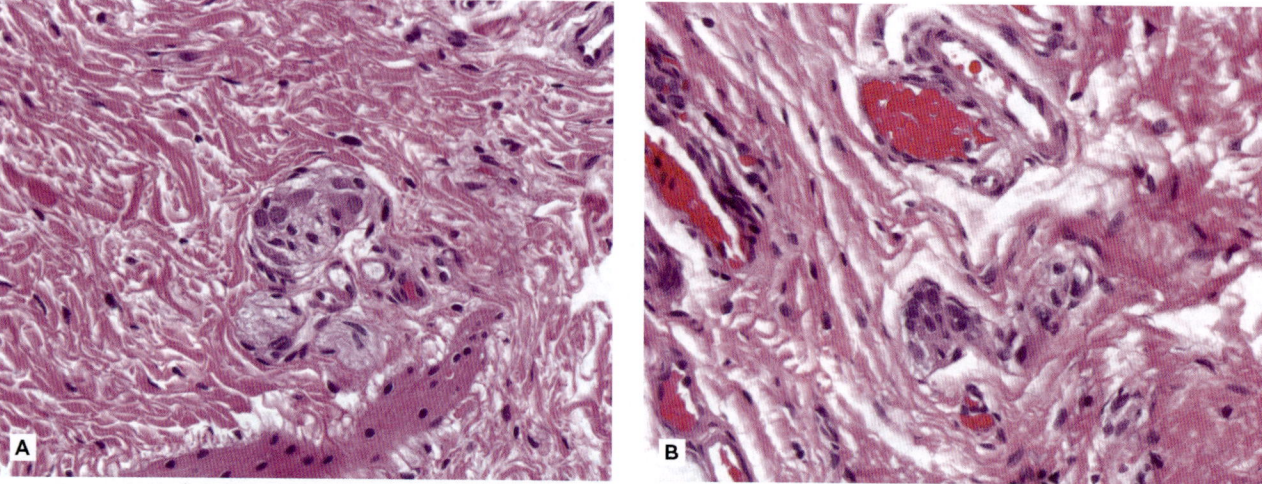

FIGURE 14-22 • Normal submucosal ganglion cells. **A:** In this 7-month-old child, ganglion cells are easy to identify 400x. **B:** In this 8-day-old infant, the ganglion cells are immature appearing and therefore more difficult to identify 400x. (Courtesy of Dr. Eduardo Ruchelli, The Children's Hospital of Philadelphia.)

varied modes of presentation and the common occurrence of functional constipation in children.

Although radiographic and manometric studies are routine diagnostic screening procedures, microscopic evaluation of rectal biopsies is the gold standard for the diagnosis of this disorder. The biopsy should be performed at least 1 to 1.5 cm above the dentate line in order to avoid the normal zone of hypoganglionic distal rectum (59). Thus, the first task of the surgical pathologist is to assess the adequacy of the biopsy material. A biopsy that contains squamous or anal transitional epithelium should be reported as inadequate and the absence of ganglion cells in such a specimen is disregarded. The biopsy must also contain an adequate thickness of submucosa in order to evaluate for loss of ganglion cells. An accepted rule of thumb is that in a well-oriented biopsy, the portion of submucosa sampled should be at least one-third the total cross-sectional area of the biopsy (58).

The absence of ganglion cells in an adequate biopsy is diagnostic of HSCR. However, careful examination of a large number of serial sections of each biopsy (75–100) is necessary before a diagnosis of Hirschsprung disease is made. As the average distance between submucosal ganglia may be up to 500 μm, a few sections 3 to 5 μm in thickness may miss the ganglia and result in a false diagnosis of aganglionosis. Further, ganglion cells in neonates can have an immature morphology that can be difficult to recognize in H&E sections, particularly in the submucosa (Meissner plexus), and confusion between endothelial cells and neuronal cells may lead to a false-negative diagnosis (Figure 14-22A, B). One useful feature present in most, but not all, patients with HSCR is the presence of multiple submucosal hypertrophic extrinsic nerve fibers; the presence of nerve fibers with a diameter greater than 40 mm is reported to be characteristic of HSCR (Figure 14-23) (60). Thick submucosal nerve fibers are reportedly less common in short-segment Hirschsprung disease and in total colonic aganglionosis.

Histochemical demonstration of acetylcholinesterase-positive cholinergic nerve fibers within the lamina propria with the presence of thick ropey fibers in the muscularis mucosa provides supportive evidence for the diagnosis of Hirschsprung disease, since they are not present in normal individuals (Figure 14-24). However, this change may not be always evident in patients under the age of 6 months, particularly in short-segment Hirschsprung disease. In addition, this technique can only be performed on frozen sections, requiring the clinician to obtain extra biopsies, and the staining procedure must be followed meticulously using freshly prepared reagents.

Immunohistochemical staining with calretinin has recently become a reliable alternate ancillary method to acetylcholinesterase staining. Calretinin is a calcium-binding protein that is expressed by a subset of submucosal and myenteric ganglion cells, some of which extend neurites into the mucosa.

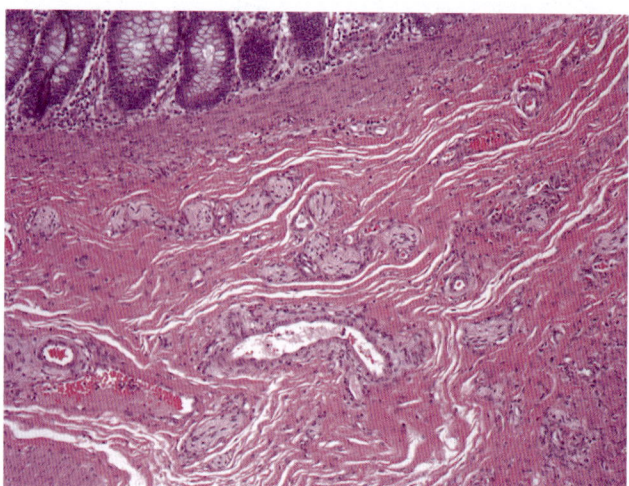

FIGURE 14-23 • Hypertrophic submucosal nerve fibers in a patient with Hirschsprung disease 100x.

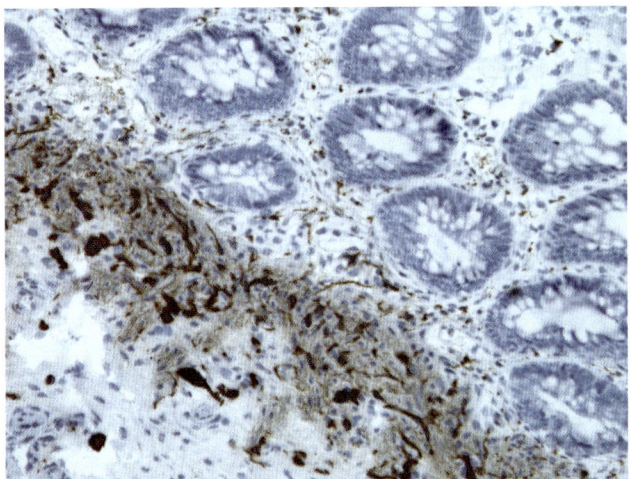

FIGURE 14-24 • Acetylcholinesterase stain of a rectal biopsy in a patient with Hirschsprung disease. Note the presence of abnormal ropey nerve fibers in the muscularis mucosae and lamina propria 400×.

A number of different histochemical stains (using lactic dehydrogenase, alpha-naphthyl esterase, and NADPH-diaphorase on frozen sections) and different antibodies (S-100, NSE, bcl-2, bone morphogenic protein 1A, and RET) to detect ganglion cells in paraffin sections have been proposed over the years but are not superior to H&E coupled with either acetylcholinesterase or calretinin and thus have not found widespread clinical use.

The definitive treatment of HSCR is surgical, and a number of different operations can be performed. The Swenson and Soave procedures involve removal of the aganglionic segment (in the case of the Soave procedure the mucosa and submucosa of the aganglionic segment are stripped) with creation of a ganglionated neorectum using normally innervated bowel, in either a one-step or two-step procedure with an intervening ostomy. On the other hand, in the Duhamel procedure, ganglionated bowel is brought down and anastomosed directly to the aganglionic segment. In either case, intraoperative seromuscular biopsies for examination of the myenteric (Auerbach) plexus are required mainly to identify normally ganglionated bowel for the anastomosis or ostomy. Seromuscular biopsies should be a minimum of 5 mm in length and require proper orientation and sectioning perpendicular to the serosa to visualize both layers of the muscularis propria to confirm the presence or absence of ganglion cells within the myenteric plexus. Ideally, the specimen should present a shrimplike or C-shaped profile. The myenteric plexus and ganglion cells within seromuscular biopsies are larger and easier to interpret than those in the submucosal plexus, provided the biopsy is adequate and there are no artifacts. In HSCR, nerves are present, usually thicker than normal, and ganglion cells are completely absent. Frozen sections performed above the grossly narrowed segment, to confirm that normal numbers of ganglion cells are present, allow the surgeon to identify the proper

The observation was made that patients with Hirschsprung disease lacked calretinin-immunoreactive submucosal nerve fibers in the aganglionic segment of the colon (61). Absence of calretinin-immunoreactive small nerves or neurites in the lamina propria and muscularis mucosae, with appropriate positive and negative control sections, has now been shown to be the equivalent of AChE histochemistry as a confirmative finding in HSCR (62,63) (Figure 14-25). A clear advantage is that calretinin immunostaining can be performed on formalin-fixed paraffin-embedded sections, obviating the need for additional biopsies or frozen sections. An important caveat that remains to be confirmed in further studies is the presence of calretinin-immunoreactive fibers extending into very short segment of aganglionic colon, complicating the diagnosis of very short segment HSCR (64).

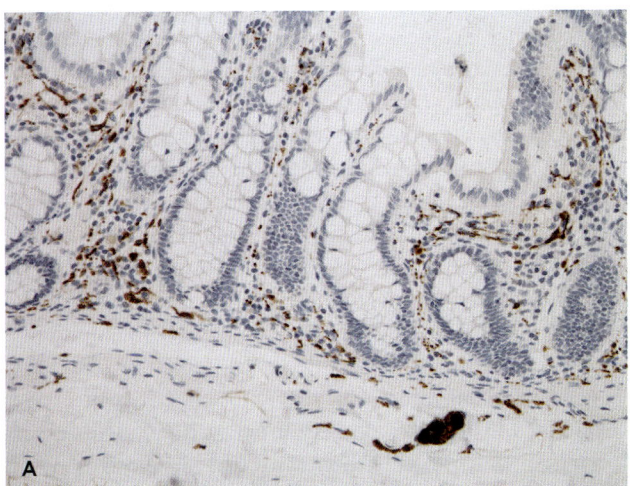 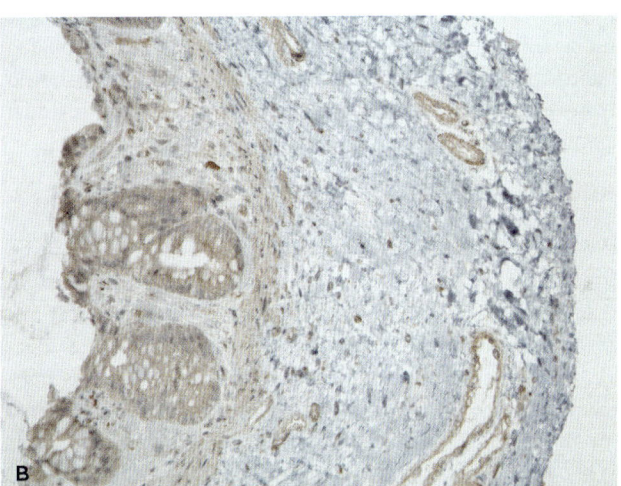

FIGURE 14-25 • Calretinin immunostains performed on sections from suction rectal biopsies. **A:** In a normal infant, calretinin reactive submucosal nerve fibers and neurites in the lamina propria are prominent 200×. **B:** In an infant with Hirschsprung disease, there is no reactivity in the submucosa or lamina propria in the aganglionic segment 200×.

level at which to transect the colon. An important point to remember when examining these frozen sections is that colonic segments from patients with HSCR usually contain a transition zone of variable length, with some degree of hypoganglionosis and hypertrophic nerves, immediately proximal to the aganglionic segment. As definitive anastomosis in this zone is associated with continuing postoperative constipation, intraoperative frozen sections must ensure that the segment of bowel used for anastomosis has a normal complement of ganglion cells and normal-caliber nerves (65).

Finally, examination of the resected bowel in HSCR is done to confirm the diagnosis of aganglionosis, determine the length of the aganglionic segment, map the transition zone, and verify the integrity of the innervation of the proximal margin. The latter is best accomplished by examining a complete full-thickness circumference of the margin.

Hirschsprung-associated enterocolitis (HAEC) is a dreaded complication of this disorder and a major cause of morbidity. It can occur before surgical treatment and from 3 weeks to 20 months after the pull-through operation (66) and can develop in aganglionic and ganglionated bowel. Several factors have been associated with an increased risk of developing HAEC: delay in diagnosis, increased length of the aganglionic segment, and trisomy 21. In one series, 45% of patients with trisomy 21 and Hirschsprung disease had enterocolitis (67).

Patients with HAEC present with abdominal distension, vomiting, fever, lethargy, and shock; abdominal radiographs reveal a distended proximal colon and absence of air in the rectosigmoid region, a useful feature, which has been termed the "cutoff" sign (66). Pathologic features can vary from a mild acute cryptitis to a full-blown mucosal ischemic necrosis; some cases may have a pseudomembranous appearance. A grading system for the histopathologic findings has been proposed (68). Neonates may present with a picture suggesting necrotizing enterocolitis (NEC) with pneumatosis intestinalis (69).

The mortality rates vary from 0% to 30%, with lower rates observed in more recent studies (70). It requires aggressive management including antibiotics (71). In cases of repeated enterocolitis, the possibility of persistent obstruction should be investigated, including rectal biopsies to rule out residual aganglionosis.

Chronic Intestinal Pseudo-Obstruction

The term intestinal pseudo-obstruction denotes greatly impaired or absent peristalsis without mechanical obstruction to luminal flow. Pseudo-obstruction is a clinical syndrome, not a pathologic diagnosis, and encompasses a wide spectrum of entities. A classification of these disorders was published recently, the major subclasses of which are neurogenic and myopathic (Table 14-4). The guidelines proposed by this working group also offer diagnostic criteria for these various entities, using both H&E and immunohistochemistry (72).

Visceral neuropathies essentially fall into two main groups: quantitative disorders, where there is an abnormality in the number of enteric neural cells (absent, as in Hirschsprung disease; hypoganglionosis; and hyperganglionosis), and qualitative disorders, where there is a cytomorphologic abnormality. The latter include acquired disorders such as inflammatory and degenerative neuropathies (Chagas disease, lymphocytic and eosinophilic ganglionitis, laxative-induced neurotoxicity) and cytologic abnormalities such as intraneuronal nuclear inclusions, an inherited disorder. The diagnosis of a quantitative abnormality such as hypoganglionosis is less easily accomplished because of a lack of robust quantitative data from normal controls (73). Values for neuronal density appear to vary with age, the region of bowel sampled, the degree of intestinal dilatation, and the methodology. **Hypoganglionosis** is encountered most frequently in the transition zone proximal to an aganglionic segment. A recent systematic review of isolated hypoganglionosis (not in association with HSCR) identified only 92 published cases, the diagnosis of which remains uncertain given the differences in methodologic workup. Most reported patients presented with some form of slow transit constipation and the outcome has been variable (74). The authors also concluded that diagnosis required

TABLE 14-4 CLINICAL CLASSIFICATION OF PEDIATRIC INTESTINAL PSEUDO-OBSTRUCTION

NEUROPATHIES
  Aganglionosis (Hirschsprung disease)
  Hypoganglionosis
    Congenital
    Acquired
  Hyperganglionosis
    Ganglioneuromatosis
    Intestinal neuronal dysplasia
  Retarded neuronal maturation
  Gliopathies
MYOPATHIES
  Muscular malformations
    Diffuse abnormal layering of small-intestinal smooth muscle
    Segmental additional smooth muscle coat
    Focal absence of smooth muscle
  Degenerative visceral myopathy
    Familial
    Sporadic
    Inflammatory
  Visceral involvement in muscular dystrophies
COMBINED
  Mitochondrial disorders
  Megacystis-microcolon-intestinal hypoperistalsis syndrome
COLONIC DESMOSIS
IDIOPATHIC (NO DIAGNOSTIC PATHOLOGY)

From Kapur R. Motor disorders. In: Russo P, Ruchelli E, Piccoli D, eds. *Pathology of Pediatric Gastrointestinal and Liver Disease.* Heidelberg, Germany: Springer Verlag; 2014a:249-317, with permission.

full-thickness biopsies. Other techniques have tried to detect abnormalities in the myenteric plexus not otherwise observable on routine H&E sections. For example, silver staining of thick sections of muscularis propria embedded flat to view the myenteric plexus have resulted in the description of a number of rare abnormalities but have not found wide application in clinical diagnosis (75,76). More modern techniques including confocal microscopy and digitalization with three-dimensional viewing of the enteric nervous system offer the possibility of a better understanding of these conditions.

Hyperganglionosis can be encountered mainly in two situations: ganglioneuromas and intestinal neuronal dysplasia (IND). Ganglioneuromas can occur anywhere in the alimentary tract but are most commonly seen in the colon and rectum. The most common form is the isolated polypoid ganglioneuroma, which occurs more frequently in children. These can be sessile or pedunculated, may be grossly indistinguishable from juvenile or hamartomatous polyps, and are usually not associated with disturbances in intestinal motility, neurofibromatosis, or MEN syndromes. On histologic examination, the lamina propria is expanded by a proliferation of ganglion cells and Schwann cells. Multiple ganglioneuromatous polyps (ganglioneuromatous polyposis) are associated with juvenile polyposis and Cowden syndrome (CS). The diffuse form of ganglioneuromatosis is characterized by a proliferation of ganglioneuromatous tissue extensively involving submucosal and myenteric plexuses, which can produce structural thickening along the bowel wall (77). The latter is associated with multiple endocrine neoplasia type 2B (MEN2B), CS, and neurofibromatosis.

IND has been described in association with Hirschsprung disease and as an isolated form. The latter is a controversial entity, with histologic diagnostic criteria that have varied since its initial description 40 years ago, and is neither well described nor widely accepted in the English medical literature. It has been divided into two forms by its proponents: IND-A, the rarest form, and IND-B. Patients with IND-A have been reported to present with constipation since early infancy. Histopathologic descriptions feature hypoplasia of the sympathetic innervation of the myenteric plexus, detected by catecholamine immunofluorescence on frozen sections, in association with hyperplasia of myenteric ganglion cells and increased acetylcholinesterase staining in the lamina propria (78). IND-B, on the other hand, is characterized by the presence of "giant" (>8 ganglion cells) submucosal ganglia (Figure 14-26). There may be associated increased acetylcholinesterase staining of the lamina propria. However, since it is now recognized that giant ganglia are more numerous in premature infants and neonates, this criterion is felt to be diagnostic only in patients older than 4 years of age. Current criteria rely on histoenzymologic stains for dehydrogenases to highlight ganglion cells on 15-μm-thick frozen sections, with "giant" ganglia involving a minimum of 20% of all submucosal ganglia (79). The applicability of these criteria to the evaluation of H&E-stained 4 μm-thick paraffin sections is uncertain. The clinical significance of these findings is equally unclear, and conservative management

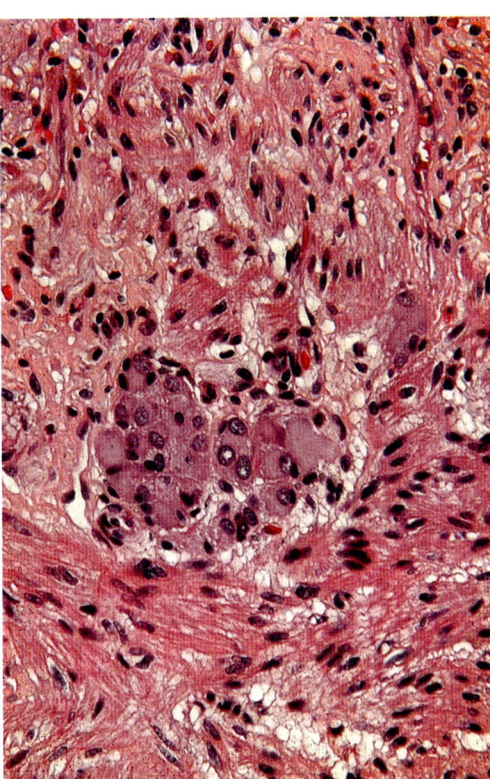

FIGURE 14-26 • Giant ganglion in a patient with intestinal neuronal dysplasia 400×.

is considered sufficient, without the need for surgical resection (79). The reproducibility of the histologic diagnosis of IND-B remains poor, and some investigators believe these features may represent a normal variant of postnatal development rather than a pathologic process (80).

Visceral myopathies can usually be appreciated by conventional microscopy, although full-thickness specimens of intestinal wall are necessary because the abnormalities are in the muscularis propria. Degeneration, atrophy, and sometimes fibrosis of intestinal smooth muscle are revealed by hematoxylin and eosin stain and enhanced by Masson trichrome stain. The outer, longitudinal layer of the muscularis propria is almost always more affected than the inner, circular layer. Most patients, except those with congenital megacystis–microcolon–intestinal hypoperistalsis syndrome (MMIHS), present later in childhood or adolescence. MMIHS is a congenital disorder with possible autosomal recessive inheritance diagnosed at birth or by prenatal ultrasonography. Affected infants present with abdominal distension, vomiting, microcolon, and markedly distended bladder and/or ureters. According to a recent review of more than 200 cases, mortality is high, with survivors maintained by parenteral nutrition or bowel transplant (81). Smooth muscle degenerative changes also occur secondarily in the muscular dystrophies, particularly Duchenne muscular dystrophy, in whom esophageal and gastric dysmotility are more common than intestinal pseudo-obstruction. Major pathologic changes include atrophy and fibrosis of the muscularis propria and muscularis mucosa, though few descriptions exist (82). Intestinal dysmotility can also be a key feature of mitochondriopathies, which include mitochondrial neurogastrointestinal encephalomyopathy (MNGIE); mitochondrial myopathy, epilepsy, lactic acidosis, and strokelike episodes (MELAS); and Alpers disease. Pathologic features include patchy atrophy of the muscularis externa and eosinophilic cytoplasmic inclusions in enteric ganglion cells (83). Diffuse abnormal layering of the intestinal smooth muscle is a relatively recently described X-linked disorder with distinctive pathologic features characterized by a trilaminar arrangement of the muscularis propria (84). Other alterations of the visceral smooth muscle include the "brown bowel syndrome," due to lipofuscin deposition in the muscularis propria resulting from vitamin E deficiency (85) and disorders such as myocyte hypertrophy with honeycomb fibrosis, alpha smooth muscle actin deficiency, and loss of the pacemaker cells of Cajal [reviewed in (58)].

Acquired Diseases
Intussusception

Intussusception, or the invagination of a portion of the intestine into itself, is a relatively common pediatric surgical problem. Infants, particularly those between 5 and 9 months of age, are most commonly affected. More than 90% of cases of childhood intussusception begin at the ileocecal valve, and the intussusceptum may reach as far as the descending colon or rectum. Progressive compression of the blood supply of the invaginated bowel causes edema, hemorrhage, and ischemic necrosis. In the classic case, severe, intermittent, colicky pain begins suddenly in an infant, followed after a few hours by vomiting and the passage of blood and mucus from the rectum. Barium enema is both diagnostic and therapeutic. The obstructing mass of invaginated bowel can be recognized, and if the congestion and edema are not too advanced, the application of hydrostatic pressure by the radiologist reduces the intussusception. Operative reduction is required if barium enema reduction fails, as happens in 20% to 30% of cases (86).

Gangrene of a portion of the intussusceptum necessitates segmental intestinal resection in approximately 10% of cases. These specimens exhibit edema, congestion, and coagulative and hemorrhagic necrosis indicative of combined ischemia and venous outflow obstruction.

In most cases, the cause is unknown. Large Peyer patches have been proposed as the possible lead point in many cases. Lymphoid hyperplasia due to adenovirus infection has been implicated in a subset of patients (Figure 14-27A to C). Use of the first commercially available oral rotavirus vaccine was associated with an increased risk of intussusception in chil-

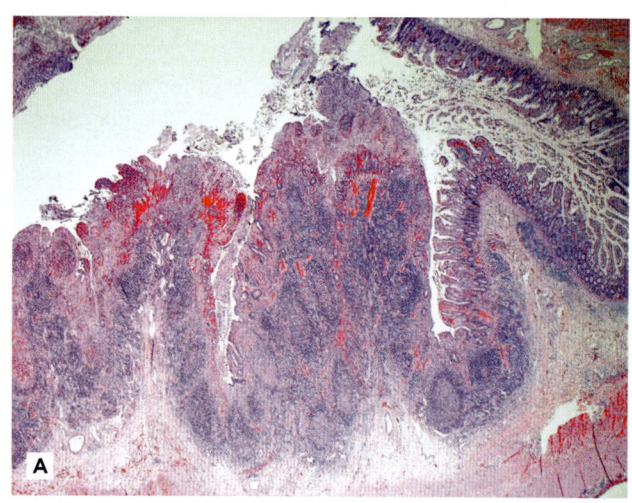
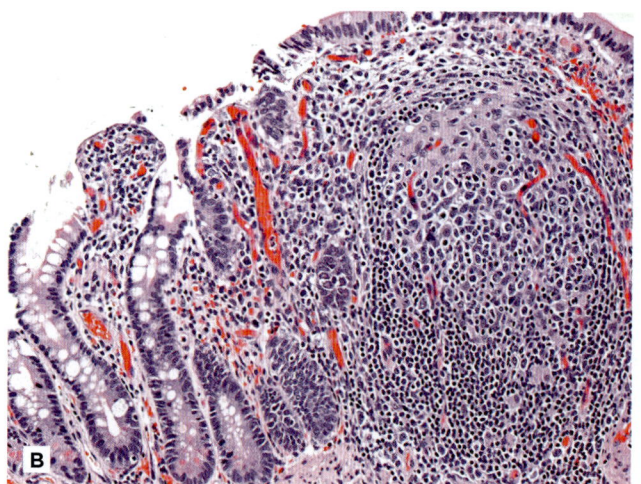
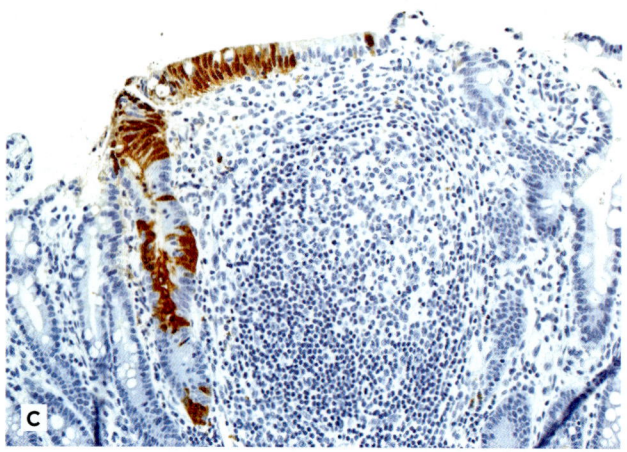

FIGURE 14-27 • Small-bowel intussusception in an infant due to adenovirus infection. **A:** Histologic section from the lead point of the intussusception demonstrating lymphoid hyperplasia 20x. **B:** High power demonstrates smudgy intranuclear inclusion within enterocytes 200x. **C:** Immunostain utilizing an adenovirus antibody confirms the diagnosis 200x.

dren, leading to withdrawal of the vaccine from the market (87). Newer-generation vaccines do not appear to have this risk (88).

Approximately 10% of cases of childhood intussusception do not conform to the typical picture. In children past infancy and in atypically located intussusceptions (i.e., those not in the ileocecal valve region), a discrete lead point is usually identified. Meckel diverticulum, Peutz-Jeghers polyps, juvenile polyps, small-intestinal duplications, and Burkitt lymphoma have been implicated.

GASTROINTESTINAL INFECTIONS

Infections of the gastrointestinal tract are the leading cause of morbidity in infants and children in all parts of the world (Table 14-5). Mortality resulting from this group of illnesses

TABLE 14-5 PEDIATRIC GASTROINTESTINAL INFECTIONS

Organism	Location	Symptom/Syndrome	Histology	Means of Diagnosis
Bacteria				
Helicobacter pylori	Stomach, especially antrum	Epigastric abdominal pain in surface	Active chronic nonspecific gastritis; organisms visible mucous coat	Histologic identification of bacilli on biopsy, culture of endoscopic biopsy
Salmonella (S. enteritidis, S. typhi, S. choleraesuis)	Distal SI, especially ileum, colon	Gastroenteritis; inflammatory, bloody, mucoid stools; enteric (typhoid) fever	Acute enteritis with exudation, hemorrhage, focal ulceration; acute infective colitis; hypertrophy, necrosis, and macrophage infiltration of Peyer patches, mesenteric LN	Stool culture, blood culture (S. typhi)
Shigella	Colon, distal SI	Bloody, mucoid stools, diarrhea, cramps, fever, convulsions	Acute infective colitis	Stool culture
Vibrio cholerae	SI	Massive watery diarrhea and dehydration	Minimal change	Stool culture
Escherichia coli				
Enteropathogenic	SI	Diarrhea	Enteritis; may show villous atrophy	Stool culture and serotyping
Enterotoxigenic	SI	Watery diarrhea, traveler's diarrhea	Minimal change	Stool culture and serotyping
Enteroinvasive	Distal SI, colon	Bloody, mucoid diarrhea	Acute infective colitis	Stool culture and serotyping
Enterohemorrhagic	Colon, distal SI	Bloody diarrhea, hemolytic uremic syndrome	Acute infective colitis	Stool culture on selective medium, serotyping, toxin assay
Campylobacter jejuni	SI, colon	Abdominal pain, diarrhea, bloody stools	Acute enteritis, acute infective colitis, acute appendicitis, mesenteric adenitis	Stool culture
Yersinia enterocolitica	Entire GI tract especially ileum, appendix, colon	Diarrhea, abdominal pain, fever	Enteritis with ulcerations and microabscesses; terminal ileitis mimicking Crohn disease; necrotizing appendicitis; acute infective colitis with aphthoid ulceration; mesenteric adenitis	Stool culture
Clostridium difficile	Colon	Pseudomembranous colitis, antibiotic-associated diarrhea	Pseudomembranous colitis, acute colitis	Toxin assay on stools
Listeria monocytogenes	SI, colon; systemic spread in immunosuppressed	Fever, gastroenteritis	ND for GI tract	Stool culture, rectal swab on selective media

(Continued)

TABLE 14-5 PEDIATRIC GASTROINTESTINAL INFECTIONS (Continued)

Organism	Location	Symptom/Syndrome	Histology	Means of Diagnosis
Aeromonas	Colon, SI	Acute watery diarrhea; dysenteric-like illness, colitis	Acute colitis	Stool culture
Mycobacterium avium complex	SI, colon	Diarrhea, abdominal pain, malabsorption in AIDS	Acid-fast bacilli in macrophages throughout lamina propria	Identification of acid-fast bacilli in macrophages in lamina propria of intestinal biopsy
Fungi				
Candida	All GI tract	Depends on location	Pseudohyphae and yeast forms with acute inflammation	Fungal stain on biopsy
Protozoa				
Giardia lamblia	Proximal SI	Diarrhea, malabsorption, failure to thrive	Proximal SI changes range from minimal change to chronic inflammation and villous atrophy. Organisms on H&E	Stool examination for cysts; mucus smears of intestinal biopsy; identification visible of trophozoites on proximal SI biopsy
Cryptosporidium	Small intestine in normal hosts; stomach, SI, and colon in AIDS patients	Watery diarrhea	Minimal change or mild, nonspecific enteritis; organisms visible on H&E	Stool examination for cysts; identification by histologic examination of proximal SI biopsy
Entamoeba histolytica	Colon	Hematochezia, diarrhea, bloody, mucoid diarrhea	Diffuse acute colitis, microulcerations, deep ulcers undermining mucosa, organism visible on H&E	Stool examination for trophozoites and cysts; identification of trophozoites on histologic examination of colonic biopsy; serology; identification of organism on biopsy
Viruses				
Rotavirus	SI	Watery diarrhea, vomiting	Enterocyte necrosis, partial villous atrophy, mononuclear inflammation	Stool ELISA
Norwalk virus	SI	Watery diarrhea, vomiting	See text	Stool ELISA, PCR on stool
Adenovirus	Colon, SI	Diarrhea	Inclusions in surface epithelium	Identification of inclusions on biopsy
Astrovirus	ND	Diarrhea	ND	ELISA on stool
Calicivirus	ND	Diarrhea	ND	
Cytomegalovirus	All parts of GI tract	GI bleeding, hemorrhagic colitis, esophagitis	Focal necrotizing colitis, esophagitis, gastritis; inclusions visible in endothelium and mesenchymal cells	Identification of inclusions on endoscopic biopsy, culture of biopsy or stool, and IHC
Herpes simplex	Esophagus, colon	Esophagitis, colitis	Small focal (aphthous) ulcerations, inclusion in epithelium	Identification of inclusions on biopsy, culture of biopsy, and IHC

GI, gastrointestinal; H&E, hematoxylin and eosin; LN, lymph node; SI, small intestine; ND, not described; ELISA, enzyme-linked immunosorbent assay; RT-PCR, reverse transcriptase polymerase chain reaction; IHC, immunohistochemistry.

is common in infants in underdeveloped countries where malnutrition contributes to the poor outcome. In developed countries, gastroenteritis and diarrhea are frequent causes of illness, but they seldom cause death because nutrition is better and medical care and intravenous fluids are available.

Viral Diarrhea

Most cases of acute infection, gastroenteritis, and diarrhea in infants and children are caused by viruses (89). Typically, the viruses localize in the small intestine and cause a noninflammatory, watery diarrhea; neutrophils and red blood cells are not found in the stool. Patients usually have nausea, vomiting, and low-grade fever. Infants are often quite ill and may become severely dehydrated.

Rotaviruses

Rotavirus is the leading cause of severe childhood gastroenteritis requiring hospital admission and, though prevalent worldwide, most deaths occur in developing countries (90). Children younger than 2 years are most susceptible; are usually ill for 4 to 7 days and are most likely to be admitted to a hospital for treatment of dehydration resulting from watery diarrhea and vomiting. Rotavirus was first identified by electron microscopy in small-intestinal epithelial cells and later in the stools of infants with diarrhea. Rotavirus infection was formerly diagnosed by the ultrastructural identification of virus particles in stools, but this method has been replaced by ELISA of stool samples. Biopsies are almost never performed during the acute illness, but several morphologic studies have shown proximal small-intestinal mucosal injury with surface enterocyte necrosis, partial villous atrophy, and chronic inflammation in the lamina propria (91). The loss of enterocytes greatly reduces the capacity of the intestine to absorb fluid and electrolytes, and the effect is compounded when damage to brush border enzymes results in malabsorption. The mucosa takes 3 to 8 weeks to recover; during this time, malabsorption may persist (91). Immunodeficient patients may take months to clear the virus and suffer a more chronic illness. Two licensed rotavirus vaccines are now available.

Norwalk Virus

Norwalk virus (also formerly known as norovirus) is the second most commonly encountered cause of viral gastroenteritis. Cases tend to occur in clusters, and epidemics are more frequent in children of school age than in infants. This is a briefer, less severe illness characterized by vomiting and watery diarrhea ("winter vomiting virus"). No method to diagnose this infection is readily available, although immunoelectron microscopy and recently developed ELISAs to detect viral antigen and antibody responses are used in reference laboratories. Only samples taken from patients during diarrhea epidemics are likely to be studied by these means. Histologic studies are sparse, but villous blunting, infiltration of mononuclear cells and neutrophils into the lamina propria, and vacuolization of enterocytes have been described (92). Villous atrophy and increased IELs mimicking celiac disease have also been observed (93).

Electron microscopic studies of stool specimens during outbreaks of gastroenteritis and diarrhea have led to the identification of other viruses, although none of these is encountered as often as rotavirus and Norwalk virus.

Enteric Adenovirus

Enteric adenoviruses are serologically distinct from respiratory adenoviruses, and for a long time, they eluded detection except by electron microscopy and difficult immunologic methods not widely available. Several outbreaks of enteric adenovirus gastroenteritis have been described in normal infants, and this infection is a common cause of pediatric viral gastroenteritis. Immunocompromised patients, particularly those with AIDS, are highly susceptible to adenovirus infection. Patients with solid organ and bone marrow transplants are also at risk.

Nonspecific watery diarrhea with vomiting, dehydration, and abdominal pain characterizes the illness. Lactose intolerance and other malabsorptive states may follow adenovirus enteritis and last for months. Adenoviral infection can result in intestinal mucosal lymphoid hyperplasia, which can form the lead point of an intussusception; in one study, adenovirus was observed in the appendix of more than one-third of specimens from children operated for ileocecal intussusception (94). Adenovirus nuclear inclusions can be identified by light microscopy within infected surface epithelial cells, but the presence of adenovirus should be confirmed by immunohistochemical stains (Figure 14-27A to C).

Cytomegalovirus

CMV infection of the GI tract occurs almost exclusively in immunocompromised individuals, especially in AIDS, and in transplanted patients, and has also been reported in chronic IBD patients treated with immunosuppression (95). Any site in the gastrointestinal tract can be affected, from esophagus to colon. In the most severe cases, the patient often has evidence of a systemic infection, with CMV pneumonia, hepatitis, and retinitis. Symptoms vary according to the affected site of the gastrointestinal tract. Particularly characteristic is a fulminant hemorrhagic colitis with multiple focal ulcerations resulting from CMV vasculitis and thrombosis; this sometimes leads to toxic megacolon, necrotizing colitis, and intestinal perforation (96). Esophageal involvement is usually distal, with ulcerations and erythema. Gastric and small-intestinal involvement is also generally manifested as erosions and ulcerations. Because it tends to affect blood vessels, CMV infection often presents with gastrointestinal bleeding. The diagnosis is made by endoscopic biopsy, with typical inclusion bodies usually seen in vascular endothelium, mesenchymal cells of the lamina propria, and more rarely in glandular epithelial cells (Figure 14-28A, B). Inclusions are not seen in squamous cells. Variable degrees of acute and chronic inflammation, vasculitis, thrombosis, and

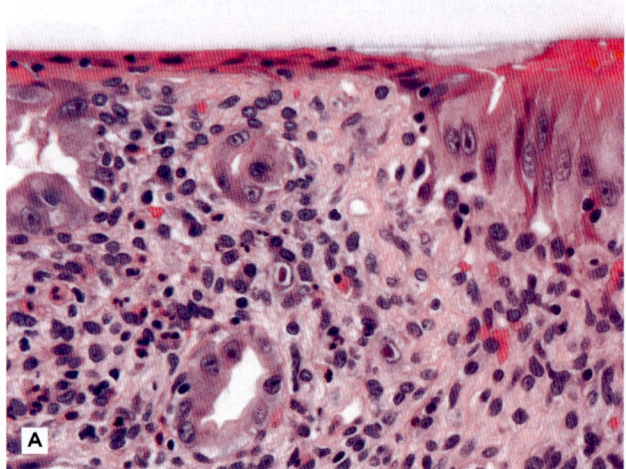 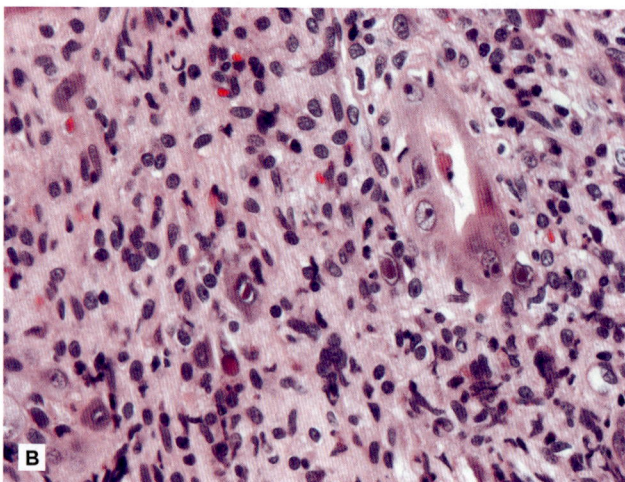

FIGURE 14-28 • CMV colitis in a child status post stem cell transplantation. **A:** Mild colitis is evident in this biopsy 400x. **B:** Several classic intranuclear viral inclusions are present 400x.

ulceration are present, depending on the extent of the infection and the degree of ulceration.

Herpes Simplex Virus

Gastrointestinal infection with this group of viruses is usually limited to immunosuppressed patients, although herpes esophagitis occasionally develops in normal children. In the gastrointestinal tract, herpesvirus most commonly causes esophagitis (see previous section) or proctocolitis. At both sites, aphthous and more extensive ulceration is characteristic. Viral cytopathic changes and inclusions are most commonly seen in squamous epithelium, but glandular epithelium and mesenchymal cells may also be involved. The accompanying inflammation commonly contains neutrophils and histiocytes.

Other Viruses

Other recently described viruses associated with gastroenteritis include astrovirus, sapovirus, and parechovirus (97).

Postenteritis enteropathy refers to infants who develop chronic diarrhea following an acute viral gastroenteritis. These children may require parenteral nutrition. Small-bowel biopsies usually reveal focal, patchy villous atrophy and mild-to-moderate inflammation. More severe cases may resemble celiac disease, though IELs are usually not increased. An associated carbohydrate intolerance may develop because of a reduction in disaccharidase activity (98).

Bacterial Diarrhea

Salmonella species, *Shigella* species, and *Campylobacter jejuni* are the most common causes of dysentery in the United States (99). Bacteria cause diarrhea through multiple pathophysiologic mechanisms, depending on the pathogen. Infectious diarrhea may manifest as acute watery diarrhea; as dysentery, with grossly bloody stools; or as persistent (>14 days) or chronic (>30 days) diarrhea. Organisms such as *C. jejuni* invade the mucosa, usually in the colon and distal small intestine, and cause epithelial necrosis and a neutrophilic response, resulting in loss of absorptive capacity. In contrast, enteropathogenic *Escherichia coli* and *Vibrio cholerae* secrete enterotoxins, which increase cyclic nucleotide-mediated secretion without penetration of the intestinal mucosa. With the latter, watery diarrhea is characteristic, and neutrophils and blood are not found in the stool. The tissue response is less pronounced and usually localized to the small intestine. *Shigella dysenteriae* and *Clostridium difficile* produce cytotoxins, which cause cell death (100). A mucosal biopsy is not usually obtained if the organism is identified by stool culture, but a biopsy may be performed in a patient with infectious colitis before the organism is cultured or if rectal bleeding persists. In such cases, the pathologist may be asked to distinguish between an infectious ("acute self-limited") colitis and early chronic IBD (see later).

Salmonella

Salmonella-induced diarrhea is a worldwide food-borne and waterborne illness. In the United States and Canada, infants and children are most often affected. In a large series of infants with diarrhea at the Hospital for Sick Children, Toronto, *Salmonella* organisms were the most common bacterial pathogens isolated. Infants may present with the acute onset of watery diarrhea, abdominal pain, and fever, but a dysenteric presentation with mucus, pus, and blood in the stools is also encountered. *Salmonella* organisms penetrate the intestinal mucosa and invade the submucosa, stimulating a neutrophilic response, epithelial necrosis with focal ulceration, hyperemia, and sometimes hemorrhage. In typhoid fever (*Salmonella typhi* infection), the organisms are carried by macrophages to intestinal lymphoid tissues, particularly Peyer patches, which become hyperplastic and necrotic. From there, bacilli enter the bloodstream. Morbidity and mortality are high (101). The more common childhood enteric infections with other strains of *Salmonella* (*S. enteritidis* and *S. typhimurium*) are usually acquired through the ingestion of contaminated eggs, poultry, and other animal products, and their course is more self-limited. The histology of the usually self-limited acute enteritis caused by *Salmonella* species is rarely observed in clinical practice. However, a colonic mucosal biopsy specimen is occasionally encountered and shows nonspecific edema, neutrophilic exudate in the lamina propria and epithelium, and crypt abscesses. Rarely does a colonic biopsy in salmonellosis show the florid crypt abscess formation, goblet cell depletion, and chronic crypt alterations characteristic of UC. Nontyphoidal Salmonella infection has become less common in AIDS patients in the developed world with the use of highly active antiretroviral therapy (HAART), while it has emerged as a major public health problem in developing countries (102).

Shigella

The *Shigellae* are a major cause of infectious diarrhea worldwide and include four species: *S. dysenteriae*, the prototype organism producing dysentery, *S. flexneri*, *S. boydii*, and *S. sonnei*. Direct invasion of the colonic epithelium and lamina propria by the organism causes cell death, ulceration, and hemorrhage. *Shigella* also produces potent toxins, known as Shiga toxins, which compound the intestinal damage. *Shigella* colitis is characterized by superficial ulceration, purulent mucosal exudate, and, in severe cases, confluent hemorrhagic necrosis of large areas of mucosa with pseudomembrane formation. The microscopic picture is that of an acute colitis with ulceration, crypt abscess formation, and goblet cell depletion (eFigure 14-6). In fulminant cases, distinction from UC can be difficult in the absence of culture results.

The potent Shiga toxins produce watery diarrhea in some cases and also have far-reaching effects throughout the body. Hemolytic uremic syndrome (HUS) occurs in about 13% of dysenteric patients with shigellosis due to *Shigella dysenteriae* infections (mostly linked to serotype SD1), affecting mainly children less than 5 years old in Africa and Asia, where it is a leading cause of death from this infection (103). Shiga toxin is an enzymatically active protein with an A to B subunit structure. The A subunit of the toxin binds to the membranes of glomerular, colonic, and endothelial cells, is endocytosed, and causes cell death by interfering with ribosomal function, whereas the B subunit binds Shiga toxin to the glycolipid globotriaosylceramide (Gb3) receptor on endothelial cells. Shiga toxin also induces endothelial cells to produce excess von Willebrand and platelet-activating factors, as well as causing platelet activation (104). *Shigellae* in addition contain a lipopolysaccharide (LPS or endotoxin), which can mediate vascular injury (103).

Vibrio cholerae

Cholera is rarely encountered in developed countries, but it is an important cause of morbidity and mortality in children worldwide. Cholera is a classic example of enterotoxigenic diarrhea, in which massive fecal fluid losses rapidly lead to dehydration in the absence of any tissue invasion by the organism, whose enterotoxin stimulates the secretion of water and electrolytes and inhibits absorption by epithelial cells. Morphologic changes are minimal. Surface epithelium of the small intestine remains intact, and at most, a mild increase in cellularity of the lamina propria and vascular congestion are observed (105).

Escherichia coli

Escherichia coli are gram-negative lactose-fermenting bacilli that consist of many strains, ranging from those that make up the normal gut flora to highly pathogenic strains. They can usually only be distinguished from each other by immunochemical or genotyping methods. The major categories of diarrhea-causing *E. coli* include *enterotoxigenic* (traveler's diarrhea), *enteroinvasive* (a major cause of dysentery), *enteropathogenic* (diarrhea in infants), *enterohemorrhagic*, and *enteroaggregative E. coli* (the latter also referred to as *enteroadherent E. coli*). Enterohemorrhagic *E. coli* include the serogroup O157:H7, the most common serogroup responsible for enterohemorrhagic colitis. Infections can be sporadic or epidemic, especially in institutional settings. Infections occur throughout the year but seem to have a predilection for warmer months. Outbreaks related to improperly cooked ground beef consumption have been highly publicized (106). Individuals at extremes of age appear most susceptible, with children younger than 4 years at greatest risk for infections and susceptibility to HUS. HUS occurs in about 12% of children with *E. coli* O157:H7 infection (107). The pathogenesis of the disorder involves adhesion to and invasion of mucosal epithelial cells with production of Shiga toxins Stx 1 and Stx 2. Stx 1 is identical to Shiga toxin of *Shigella* SD1, whereas Stx 2 is 56% homologous with Stx 1 and is the primary virulence factor for *E. coli* O157:H7.23.

The incubation period for *E. coli* O157:H7 is 3 to 4 days, and the average duration of illness is 7 days. Bloody diarrhea, vomiting, and fever usually manifest by the 3rd to 5th day of the illness (107). Nonbloody *E. coli* O157:H7 infections tend to be less severe and of shorter duration. Colonoscopic findings demonstrate nonuniform and nonspecific mucosal erythema and edema mainly in the ascending and transverse colon. Barium enema demonstrates signs of bowel edema and submucosal hemorrhage, such as thumbprinting. Stool culture is the primary means of identifying *E. coli* O157:H7, though Stx 1 and Stx 2 can be assayed in stool by ELISA (99).

Histopathologic changes include features of both ischemic and acute infectious colitis. With associated HUS, the changes predominantly affect the left colon and are dominated by hemorrhage, mucosal necrosis, and fibrin thrombi in mucosal and submucosal vessels (Figure 14-29). Severe cases requiring surgery or observed at autopsy are noted to have a swollen, hemorrhagic mucosa, frequently ulcerated and often partially covered by pseudomembranes. An acute colitis pattern with involvement primarily of the right colon is seen in those cases without associated HUS, featuring a variably intense neutrophilic infiltrate with pericryptitis, crypt microabscesses, and, less commonly, pseudomembranes.

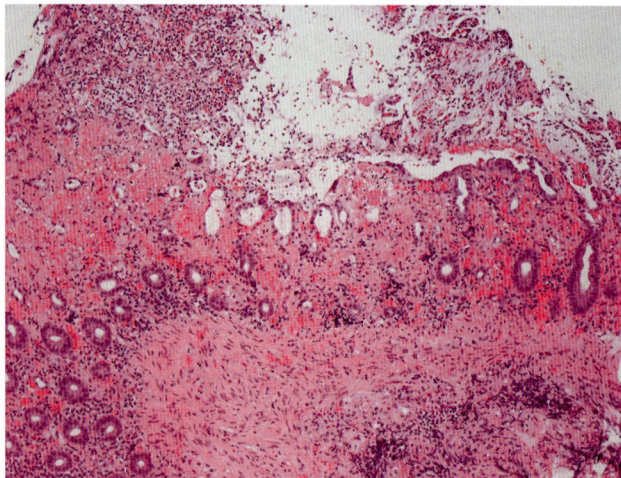

FIGURE 14-29 • Colitis due to *E. coli* O157:H7. The combination of histologic features of infectious colitis seen at each end of the biopsy and ischemic changes in the middle of the biopsy is typical of this infection 200×.

Major gastrointestinal complications of HUS include stricture, perforation, intussusception, hemoperitoneum, and pancreatitis.

Campylobacter jejuni

Campylobacter jejuni is a major cause of acute bacterial diarrhea in older infants and children in developed countries (100). Virtually unknown as recently as the early 1970s because of the unique conditions required for it to grow in culture, *C. jejuni* is now isolated as often as *Salmonella*, *Shigella*, and enteropathogenic strains of *E. coli* from children with diarrhea. Ordinary laboratory stool culture techniques are unsatisfactory to isolate this fastidious organism; a microaerophilic environment and selective media must be used. *Campylobacter* infection is acquired from animals in which the organism is a commensal, including pets and poultry, and from contaminated water or milk. The infection presents with abdominal pain, low-grade fever, and diarrhea that becomes bloody after a few days. Direct examination of the stool usually shows neutrophils. The illness is usually self-limited and lasts approximately 1 week, but it may linger for 5 or 6 weeks or relapse after initial improvement. Jejunum, ileum, colon, rectum, and appendix may all be affected. *Campylobacter* colitis may be sufficiently severe to mimic CD, with cobblestone mucosa and aphthous ulcers. Toxic megacolon has also been described. Rectal and colonic biopsy specimens show an infective proctocolitis with edema, neutrophils in the lamina propria, and crypt abscesses (eFigure 14-7).

Yersinia

Yersinia infections (yersiniosis) are caused by two pathogenic types, *Yersinia enterocolitica* (*YE*) and *Yersinia pseudotuberculosis* (*YP*). Both can cause mesenteric lymphadenitis, appendicitis, and terminal ileitis, which can mimic acute appendicitis or stricturing CD of the terminal ileum (108).

Infection with *Y. enterocolitica* is more common in colder climates and during winter; it usually causes an acute self-limited colitis (ASLC) and is an important bacterial cause of diarrhea in Scandinavian countries and Canada. Exposure to undercooked pork is a predisposing factor (109). As the organism is dependent on a rich iron source for growth, children administered frequent blood transfusions, such as those affected by thalassemia, are at increased risk (110). *Y. pseudotuberculosis* is also a food-borne pathogen that has been associated with community outbreaks. It has, in addition, been reported as a cause of acute interstitial nephritis and may result in systemic manifestations similar to Kawasaki disease (111). The anatomic pathologist may encounter relatively severe or prolonged cases of *Yersinia* infection in a variety of circumstances: acute inflammation and mucosal ulceration of the colon, necrotizing appendicitis and periappendicitis, terminal ileitis thought to be CD, or even severe mesenteric lymphadenitis mistaken for intestinal lymphoma. Severe infections with *Y. enterocolitica* can result in a florid lymphoid hyperplasia of the mucosa and submucosa of the terminal ileum and cecum, eventuating in ulceration of the overlying mucosa (eFigure 14-8A, B). Gram-negative bacilli may be observed on occasion. Granulomatous inflammation of the bowel, appendix, and mesenteric lymph nodes is characteristic of *Y. pseudotuberculosis* but may be seen with *Y. enterocolitica*. The differential diagnosis includes mycobacterium and CD. Though distinguishing between yersiniosis and CD may be difficult, evidence of chronic disease, such as crypt distortion, muscular hypertrophy, and neural hyperplasia, would favor the latter, whereas necrotizing granulomas would favor the former.

Yersinia enterocolitica is usually identified by stool culture. The organism grows on standard selective stool culture media, such as MacConkey agar, but overgrowth of normal flora makes identification difficult unless specific subculturing and other identification techniques are used.

Clostridium difficile

Clostridium difficile is a gram-positive, anaerobic bacillus pathogen that accounts for up to 25% of cases of antibiotic-associated diarrhea and most cases of antibiotic-associated pseudomembranous colitis. Though most frequently associated with *C. difficile* infection, pseudomembranous colitis can be observed with other entities, such as NEC and Hirschsprung-associated enterocolitis. Less than 1% of healthy adults are *C. difficile* carriers, although 25% of adults recently treated with antibiotics appear to be colonized (112). Host and bacterial factors, which determine *C. difficile* colitis and asymptomatic carriage, are not clear. It appears that antecedent disruption of normal colonic bacterial flora is a risk factor for *C. difficile*–induced colitis. Any antibiotic therapy is capable of producing infection by *C. difficile*; however, those antibiotics, which alter intestinal flora, appear to be most responsible. Independent of antibiotic usage, additional risk factors for *C. difficile* colitis include CD, UC, general anesthesia, chemotherapeutics, neutropenia, and cystic fibrosis. Recently, an epidemic strain, the NAP1 strain, has been associated with increased virulence and also antibiotic resistance (113). The situation in infants is more complex. *C. difficile* is harbored in 30% to 70% of healthy neonates, in whom the organism may produce toxin without causing disease. The carriage rate decreases abruptly in the first 5 months of life but does not decline to adult levels until approximately 2 years of age. However, *C. difficile* is known to cause severe disease in certain groups of young infants, particularly those with Hirschsprung disease and malignancies, in whom organisms can be demonstrated to invade colonic mucosa; the large size of the bacilli and spore formation are unique in this setting. *C. difficile* infection may present a continuum of colonic symptoms, from mild diarrhea and abdominal cramping with a lack of systemic symptoms to toxic megacolon, perforation, and peritonitis. Symptoms of *C. difficile* infection usually begin during or shortly following antibiotic therapy but may be delayed for several weeks. Diarrhea may become severe and debilitating with systemic symptoms including fever, malaise, anorexia, and dehydration. Occult or frank intestinal bleeding may be present. Endoscopic findings reveal characteristic yellow plaques, 2 to 10 mm in diameter, interspersed with normal-appearing mucosa. The earliest histologic lesions consist of foci of epithelial necrosis with a neutrophilic infiltrate and eventuate into epithelial loss and disrupted crypts. The pathognomonic volcano-like membranes consist of epithelial debris, mucus, and neutrophil-rich exudates. Late lesions consist of extensive mucosal necrosis and destruction, essentially indistinguishable from ischemic colitis or severe IBD. A demonstration of *C. difficile* toxins in the stool is the diagnostic gold standard with high sensitivity (94% to 100%) and specificity (114). Stool culture is not the method for establishing diagnosis as culture is difficult and many *C. difficile* strains are not toxicogenic. Relapse of infection following therapy and the development of vancomycin-resistant strains are emerging problems. Surgical intervention may be required in extreme cases.

Aeromonas

In the 1990s, Aeromonas species were increasingly implicated in a variety of gastrointestinal illnesses, although they are still relatively uncommon isolates in the microbiology laboratory. In young children, acute watery diarrhea or gastroenteritis is the usual presentation. More rarely, especially in adults, an acute dysenteric illness is seen, sometimes with a severe colitis mimicking chronic IBD (115).

Protozoal Infections
Giardia lamblia (Intestinalis)

Giardia lamblia is a flagellated protozoan capable of causing diarrhea and malabsorption in human hosts (Table 14-5). In some parts of the world, cyst forms of the organism can be frequently identified in the stools of asymptomatic carriers, but in developed countries, ingestion of the organism usually leads to clinically apparent illness. Toddlers and children and persons with selective IgA deficiency and other primary immunodeficiencies are more susceptible to infection. Case clusters of giardiasis have been reported in day care centers and residential institutions. Travel to foreign countries and ingestion of water from untreated sources are also risk factors.

Affected children manifest diarrhea, nausea, weight loss, malabsorption, and failure to thrive. The host ingests the cyst form of the organism. In the proximal small intestine, the cyst wall dissolves and trophozoites are released; these adhere to the brush border of epithelial cells, damaging the microvilli. In small-intestinal biopsy specimens, trophozoites are 10 to 18 μm long, have an arched or curved appearance at high levels of magnification, and are visible at the surface of enterocytes or in the mucous coat (eFigure 14-9). They do not invade tissue. The trophozoites can be highlighted with a trichrome stain.

In immunocompetent hosts, small-bowel biopsies generally show no significant reaction. The villous architecture is usually normal, but increased numbers of chronic inflammatory cells and eosinophils in the lamina propria may be seen (22). Patients with severe diarrhea and malabsorption show variable degrees of villous atrophy and more severe chronic inflammation. Patients with selective IgA deficiency or other immunodeficiency syndromes are highly susceptible to giardiasis, and villous atrophy and inflammation are usually more severe in these cases. Absence or a marked decrease in plasma cells is an important clue. Identification of Giardia in the intestine should prompt consideration of an immunodeficiency, although normal infants and children can also become infected. However, the diagnosis can be overlooked.

Metronidazole is the mainstay of treatment, and some apparent treatment failures may be due to lactose intolerance, which can persist for some time after successful eradication. The diagnosis is best accomplished by microscopic examination of stool specimens for Giardia cysts. Commercial ELISAs are available to detect Giardia antigens in stool. All too often, however, microscopic examination of a duodenal biopsy specimen will provide the first clue that a patient has giardiasis.

Cryptosporidium

Cryptosporidium was first identified as a human pathogen in 1976, as a rare cause of self-limited, watery diarrhea in immunocompetent persons (116). Clusters of diarrhea in day care centers and families have been described. In the early 1980s, Cryptosporidium was identified with increasing frequency as a cause of severe chronic diarrhea in patients with AIDS, and cryptosporidiosis is one of the opportunistic infections that often heralds the onset of AIDS. Once immunodeficient patients are infected, they are plagued with chronic diarrhea, which is often severe and difficult to eradicate. Cryptosporidium species are present in a large number of domestic and wild animals. Both zoonotic spread and person-to-person spread occur. In 1993, a widely publicized outbreak in Milwaukee, Wisconsin, was traced to contamination of the municipal water supply (117). Oocysts are

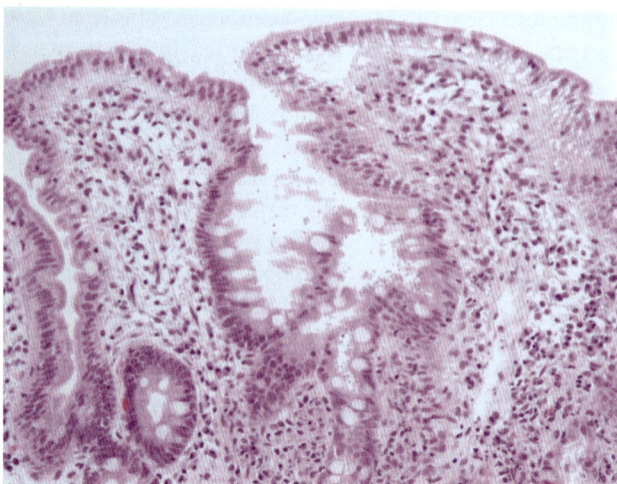

FIGURE 14-30 • Cryptosporidium infection in the small bowel. Numerous small dotlike organisms line the crypt luminal surfaces 200×.

ingested orally and progress through stages of the life cycle in the proximal small intestine where they are recognized on the surface of epithelial cells in mucosal biopsy specimens as a line of spherical basophilic structures 3 to 4 μm in diameter. They are recognizable with hematoxylin and eosin stains, but they also may be stained with Giemsa. They usually cause minimal morphologic changes in the intestine except for chronic inflammatory infiltration of the lamina propria (Figure 14-30). Electron microscopy reveals destruction of enterocyte microvilli. Diagnosis is accomplished by microscopic examination of stool specimens for oocysts with an acid-fast stain. ELISA kits are commercially available to aid in the detection of oocysts. The infection is self-limited in normal hosts. No satisfactory treatment is available for chronic infection in immunosuppressed persons.

Entamoeba histolytica

Entamoeba histolytica infection (amebiasis) is a major cause of diarrhea in third world countries. In the United States, it is diagnosed most often in southwestern states, especially in Hispanic patients and those who have recently traveled to Latin America. Infection may be asymptomatic (carrier state), or it may cause isolated hematochezia or a dysentery-like syndrome with diarrhea and blood and mucus in the stools. Infection is usually acquired through contaminated water or food and can spread by the fecal–oral route (22). The diagnosis is made by finding cysts or trophozoites in fresh stool smears or trophozoites in biopsy material. The diagnosis may also be made serologically by an elevated indirect hemagglutination titer.

In acute amebic infection, the organism invades the colon and causes a diffuse acute inflammation that may be difficult to distinguish from UC or CD, both endoscopically and pathologically. Rectal biopsy specimens often show no more than edema, scattered intraepithelial and lamina propria neutrophils, and a mild increase in lamina propria cellularity. Superficial microscopic ulcerations usually indicate invasion of the trophozoites into the lamina propria. Organisms resemble large, pale foamy histiocytes, 15 to 30 μm in diameter, with a pale nucleus and ingested red blood cells in the cytoplasm. They may be found in the surface mucous coat or in the superficial lamina propria beneath a microscopic ulceration (Figure 14-31A to D). Organisms are not found in up to 50% of rectal biopsy specimens from patients with acute-onset amebiasis (118). Examination of stool smears is a more sensitive method of diagnosis. In advanced cases, amebiasis causes multiple ulcerations, particularly in the cecum and ascending colon. Microscopically, these have a characteristic flask shape at low levels of magnification, a consequence of epithelial undermining. At this stage, abundant trophozoites are found in the intestinal wall. Sequelae include intestinal perforation, peritonitis, lymphatic and hematogenous dissemination, and systemic amebiasis.

Other Protozoal Infections

Blastocystis hominis is a protozoan that inhabits the lower intestinal tract and was believed to be a nonpathogenic commensal until relatively recent reports implicated it as a cause of diarrhea in both immunocompromised and immunocompetent individuals. Fecal microscopy using the Gomori modification of the trichrome stain has revealed the organisms in 3% to 4% of stool samples of patients with watery diarrhea and the sole observable parasite in 1% to 2% of cases (119,120). Exposure to well water or travel to foreign countries was commonly noted in infected children. Intestinal biopsies have been normal (120) or have shown a nonspecific colitis (121); intracytoplasmic basophilic bodies surrounded by a halo have been noted in crypt epithelium (121). Most patients with acute symptoms respond to a 10-day course of metronidazole, although some patients may have persistent symptoms.

Dientamoeba fragilis has been recovered in the stools of children with both acute and chronic diarrhea. The incidence appears to vary according to locale and population, this protozoan observed in 9% of samples from children in the Los Angeles area (122), but in only 0.3% of samples from patients from Montreal (123). Infection with *D. fragilis* may manifest as an eosinophilic colitis and should be included in the differential diagnosis of patients with chronic diarrhea and gut eosinophilia, especially in those who respond poorly to proper elimination diets (123). Accurate diagnosis is dependent on proper stool sample fixation and concentration methods (123). Infection with *Cyclospora*, also referred to as "cyanobacterium-like bodies," has been reported in children with prolonged diarrhea. Diagnosis rests on identification of the parasite by examination of stool samples with either d'Antoni iodine or an acid-fast stain (124,125).

Fungal Disease of the Gastrointestinal Tract

Candida is regarded as part of the normal flora in healthy persons. It becomes a pathogen only in cases of immunodeficiency, immunosuppression, debilitation, or during prolonged antibiotic therapy. Since the onset of the AIDS

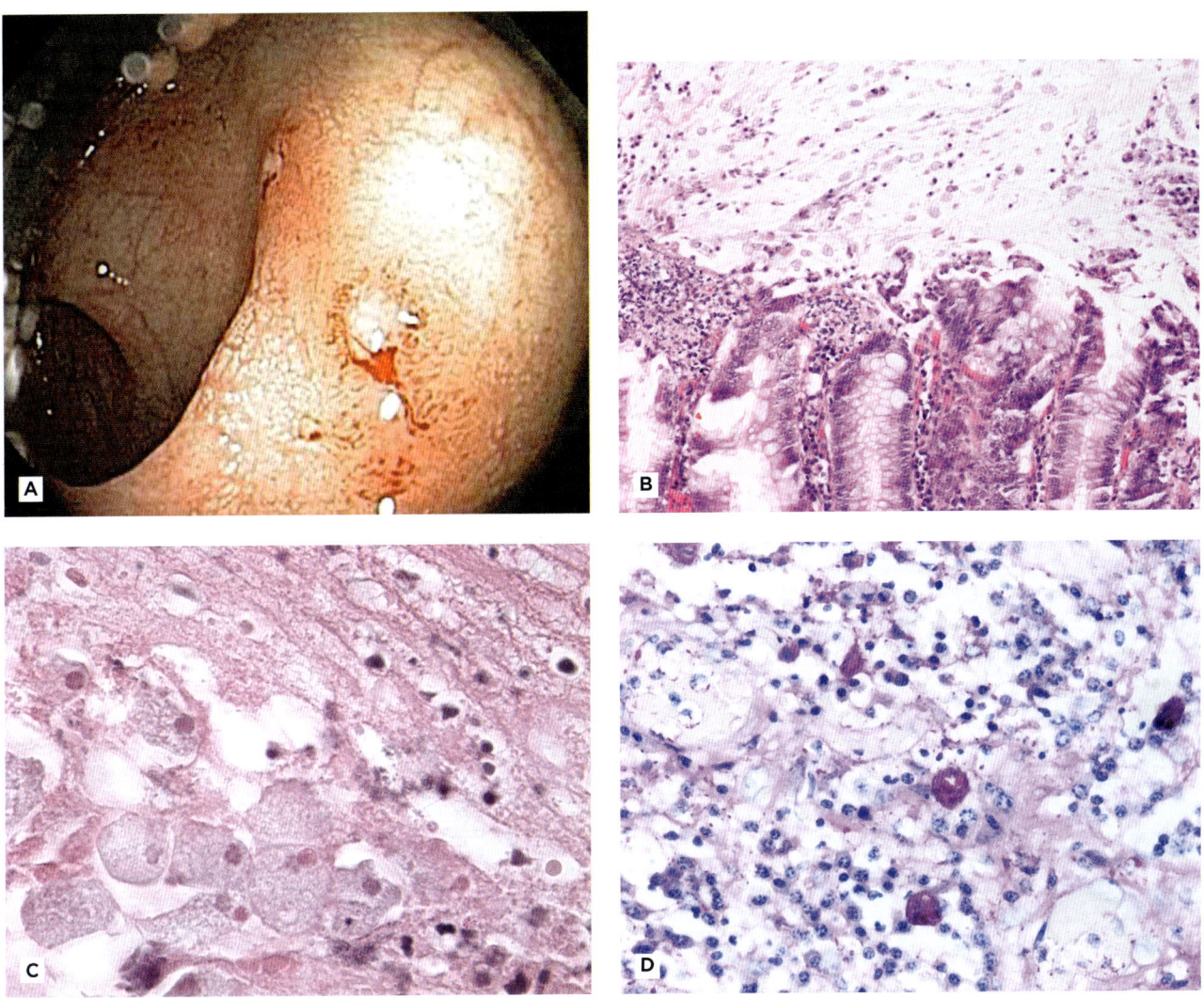

FIGURE 14-31 • *Entamoeba histolytica* colitis. **A:** Colonoscopy revealed scattered ulcers. **B:** Trophozoites can be seen within mucus and debris at the luminal surface 200×. **C:** The trophozoites are slightly larger than histiocytes and contain ingested red blood cells (oil immersion, photo courtesy of Dr Emma Furth, Hospital of the University of Pennsylvania). **D:** The organisms are highlighted in a PAS stain 400×.

epidemic, esophageal candidiasis has been recognized as an AIDS-defining condition in many patients. Candidiasis develops in most patients with AIDS sometime during their illness. Zygomycosis and *Aspergillus* infection are also usually limited to debilitated and immunosuppressed patients. The gastrointestinal tract is often the portal of entry for fungal septicemia in these people. Any portion of the gastrointestinal tract may be infected by these three groups of fungi. Multiple fungal microabscesses a few millimeters in diameter or focal ulcerations are grossly identifiable on mucosal surfaces. *Histoplasma capsulatum* may cause gastrointestinal disease in immunocompetent persons in endemic areas.

MALABSORPTION

Malabsorption in children has many causes, only some of which have anatomic correlates of concern to the pathologist viewing an abnormal biopsy specimen. Conditions associated with a failure to absorb nutrients but without diagnosable histologic abnormalities include pancreatic and liver diseases, enterocyte enzyme deficiencies, alterations of normal bacterial flora, some infections, some immunodeficiency states, and decreases in intestinal surface area. These extraintestinal, enzymatic, metabolic, and other nonstructural causes of malabsorption in children are discussed in standard textbooks and review articles.

Children with malabsorption of any cause usually present with growth failure, bulky or diarrheal stools, and anemia. Edema and hypoalbuminemia occur if inadequate protein is absorbed or if serum protein is lost through the intestine. Steatorrhea results in a failure to absorb fat-soluble vitamins, associated with a prolonged prothrombin time and manifestations of bleeding (vitamin K deficiency), rickets and hypocalcemia (vitamin D deficiency), and night blindness (vitamin A deficiency). Zinc malabsorption produces a characteristic dermatitis. Anemia results from malabsorption of iron, folate, or vitamin B_{12}. The laboratory diagnosis of malabsorption is complex but usually includes documentation of fat, carbohydrate, and protein loss in the stools. A 72-hour quantitative stool fat excretion is used to quantify steatorrhea. Carbohydrate absorption is evaluated by means of the H2 breath test, fecal pH, and D-xylose absorption. Serum proteins, immunoglobulins, calcium, carotene, folic acid, and vitamin B_{12} are all subject to intestinal loss and can be measured directly. Stool is cultured and examined for ova and parasites, especially *G. lamblia*. Because cystic fibrosis is a common cause of malabsorption in children in North America and northern Europe, a sweat test is often performed. Antitissue transglutaminase and antiendomysial antibodies are sought in serum to rule out celiac disease.

The focus of this section will be on causes of malabsorption in children that are likely to be encountered by the pathologist and are listed in Table 14-6. Of the causes of intestinal malabsorption, the most commonly encountered in developed countries are celiac disease, temporary postgastroenteritis syndrome (postenteritis enteropathy), cow's milk protein intolerance, short gut syndrome (postoperative), CD, and immunodeficiency states.

The Intestinal Biopsy in Children

Intestinal biopsies are most frequently obtained from the duodenum via forceps during endoscopic examination (EGD). Biopsies from both proximal and distal duodenum are recommended, including biopsies of endoscopically normal mucosa, as many disorders affecting the duodenum have a focal distribution. In children, for example, the lesions in gluten-sensitive enteropathy (GSE) may be patchy, and villous atrophy may coexist with normal mucosa. An adequate biopsy should have four to five well-oriented villi in a row, and observation of four normal villi in a row is generally an indication that the specimen is normal. Accurate evaluation of villous morphology requires careful attention to proper orientation of the specimen. Some laboratories have found that orientation of the specimen on filter paper prior to fixation is helpful. We have found that rapid immersion of the specimen in fixative is preferable to having the endoscopist place the biopsy on filter paper, which may result in excessive stretching or drying of the specimen. In addition to obtaining biopsies for routine histology, samples may also be snap-frozen (for disaccharidase analysis) or submitted for electron microscopy (for confirmation of microvillous inclusion disease). Histologic evaluation of the small-bowel biopsy should proceed systematically, to include (a) adequacy of the sampling, as determined by the number and site of the biopsy specimens, (b) assessment of the villous architecture with evaluation of the villus-to-crypt (V:C) ratio, (c) evaluation of the length of the crypts (hyperplasia, hypoplasia), (d) the appearance of the surface enterocytes and their brush border, (e) an evaluation of the quantity of IELs, (f) the cellularity of the lamina propria (plasma cells may be absent or decreased in some primary immunodeficiencies), and (g) the presence of microorganisms (Giardia, cryptosporidia). The normal villus height–to–crypt depth ratio in the duodenum is about 3:1 in children, and higher in the distal as compared to the proximal duodenum. More recent studies from the duodenum suggest that the normal number of IELs has an upper limit of 20 to 25/100 epithelial cells (126). The lamina propria contains a mixture of plasma cells (mostly IgA secreting), CD4+ T lymphocytes, and lesser numbers of eosinophils, histiocytes, and mast cells. Newborns usually lack plasma cells in the first week of life, gradually acquiring them during the first month of life, with IgM-containing plasma cells predominating. By 3 months of life, IgA plasma cells predominate.

Congenital Transport and Enzymatic Disorders

Except for those disorders associated with fat processing, small-intestinal biopsies in most congenital disorders of transport are generally normal or only very slightly abnormal. Therefore, a normal-appearing small-bowel mucosa from a patient with prolonged diarrhea, especially a young infant, should alert the clinician to a consideration of these entities.

The clinical feature of carbohydrate malabsorption resulting from congenital disaccharidase deficiency and glucose–galactose malabsorption is an osmotic diarrhea due to the unabsorbed solute in the ileum. The diagnosis is obtained

TABLE 14-6 CAUSES OF MALABSORPTION AND CHRONIC DIARRHEA OF INFANCY AND CHILDHOOD

Congenital transport and enzymatic disorders
    Glucose–galactose malabsorption
    Disaccharidase deficiency
    Lysinuric protein intolerance
    Abetalipoproteinemia
    Chylomicron retention disease
    Sodium chloride diarrhea
    Primary bile acid malabsorption
Congenital defects of intestinal epithelial differentiation
    Microvillus inclusion disease
    Tufting enteropathy
    Enteroendocrine cell dysgenesis
Autoimmune enteropathy
Gluten-sensitive enteropathy (celiac disease)
Postviral enteropathy and bacterial overgrowth
Bacterial infections (e.g., Mycobacterium avium–intracellulare)
Parasitic infections (Giardia and Cryptosporidium)
Eosinophilic enteritis
    Intestinal lymphangiectasia
    Crohn disease
Congenital immunodeficiencies
Cystic fibrosis
Langerhans cell histiocytosis

by the determination of disaccharidase activities in homogenates of small-bowel biopsies or by breath testing. Congenital disaccharidase and transporter deficiencies are rare, and are more often secondary, resulting from diffuse mucosal damage due to infectious gastroenteritis, GSE, or other food allergies. Severe mucosal injury may outpace expression of brush border enzymes and transporter proteins, thus worsening the diarrhea and malabsorption.

Disorders of amino acid transport rarely feature prominent gastrointestinal manifestations, except for lysinuric protein intolerance, which results from mutations in the SLCA7 gene that codes for the dibasic amino acid transporter system (127). This clinically manifests as failure to thrive with vomiting and diarrhea. Other complications include lupus, hemophagocytic lymphohistiocytosis, and sudden infant death. Intestinal biopsies in cases of congenital chloride diarrhea and congenital sodium diarrhea have been reported as normal or showing only mild partial villus atrophy. Heubi et al. (128) described a severe refractory diarrhea due to a primary disorder of bile acid absorption; intestinal biopsies were normal. It is worth noting that bile acid–related diarrheas are far more commonly secondary to chronic pancreatic insufficiency, or to loss of ileal surface due to NEC, or extensive surgical resection.

Lipid Transport Disorders

Most clinical disorders of fat malabsorption result from severe liver disease, pancreatic disease (such as cystic fibrosis), or extensive ileal resection (as in CD) with loss of the enterohepatic circulation of bile acids. Intestinal biopsies play a limited role in the diagnosis of these disorders. However, primary abnormalities of fat transport within the enterocyte, though much less frequent, can result in a characteristic vacuolization of the enterocyte in intestinal biopsies. The three main disorders of lipid trafficking are **abetalipoproteinemia**, **hypobetalipoproteinemia**, and **chylomicron retention disorder (Anderson disease)**.

Abetalipoproteinemia is an autosomal recessive disorder characterized by the absence of apo B–containing lipoproteins. The molecular basis for the defect is a mutation of the gene coding for microsomal triglyceride transfer protein (MTP), located on chromosome 4q22. MTP is responsible for assembly of lipoprotein particles, and for the proper folding of apo B, preventing its premature degradation. Fatty acids within intestinal cells thus cannot be exported as chylomicrons. Patients have diarrhea and fat malabsorption usually appearing within the first few months of life, with acanthocytosis, and deficiencies in fat-soluble vitamins resulting in retinitis pigmentosa and neurologic symptoms. There is clinical heterogeneity, however, with signs and symptoms presenting in older patients in a significant proportion of cases. Serum levels of cholesterol and triglycerides are typically low and do not rise after a fatty meal. **Hypobetalipoproteinemia** is an autosomal dominant disorder due to a mutation in the apo B gene located on chromosome 2, leading to a truncated apo B protein (129). Homozygous patients have a clinical and histologic phenotype essentially indistinguishable from abetalipoproteinemia, whereas heterozygous patients have only a mild phenotype. **Chylomicron retention (Anderson) disease** is similar to abetalipoproteinemia in its gastrointestinal manifestations and impact on growth, though acanthocytosis is usually absent and neurologic and ocular abnormalities are less severe. Also, in contrast to abetalipoproteinemia, serum fasting triglyceride levels are normal and hypocholesterolemia is less marked. The causative gene, SAR1B, codes for a GTPase associated with coat protein carriers involved in endoplasmic reticulum to Golgi transport, particularly in chylomicron and LDL transport (130).

These disorders have similar pathologic features. The duodenal mucosa has a pale appearance on endoscopy with normal esophageal and gastric mucosa. Villous morphology is preserved though some patients may demonstrate mild villous atrophy. The characteristic feature is diffuse vacuolization of the enterocytes resulting from fat accumulation, the vacuolar appearance resulting from leaching of the fat by routine histologic processing (Figure 14-32A). Lipid vacuoles fill the enterocytes on electron microscopy (Figure 14-32B), and because the enterocyte cannot export lipids, none is noted in the extracellular space or in the lacteals. Acanthocytosis resulting from abnormal lipoproteins in red blood cells is usually noted on peripheral blood smears in abetalipoproteinemia and can be an important clue to the diagnosis (Figure 14-32C).

Congenital Defects of Intestinal Epithelial Differentiation

Microvillus Inclusion Disease

Microvillus inclusion disease (MVID) is an autosomal recessive disease characterized by refractory secretory diarrhea usually occurring within the first week of life, though a late-onset form may manifest in the first few months of life. Investigation of clusters of cases within the Navajo population identified mutations in the gene MYO5B located on chromosome 18q21 (131). MYO5B codes for myosin Vb, part of a family of proteins responsible for actin-dependent organelle transport and regulation of endosome recycling. Mutations in a related gene, MYO5A, cause Griscelli syndrome, an immunodeficiency disorder characterized by abnormal transfer of melanin granules to keratinocytes (132). Patients with MVID are dependent on total parenteral nutrition (TPN), though improved survival may require small-bowel transplantation. Small-bowel biopsies are usually characterized by severe villus atrophy, mild or moderate crypt hyperplasia, and a variable degree of inflammation in the lamina propria but without crypt destruction (Figure 14-33A). The diagnosis may be strongly suspected on paraffin-embedded sections by the absence of a distinct brush border using the periodic acid–Schiff (PAS) stain and by the presence of a diffuse PAS-positive staining of the apical portion of the enterocytes (Figure 14-33B). Similar observations are noted using immunohistochemical staining for alkaline phosphatase and

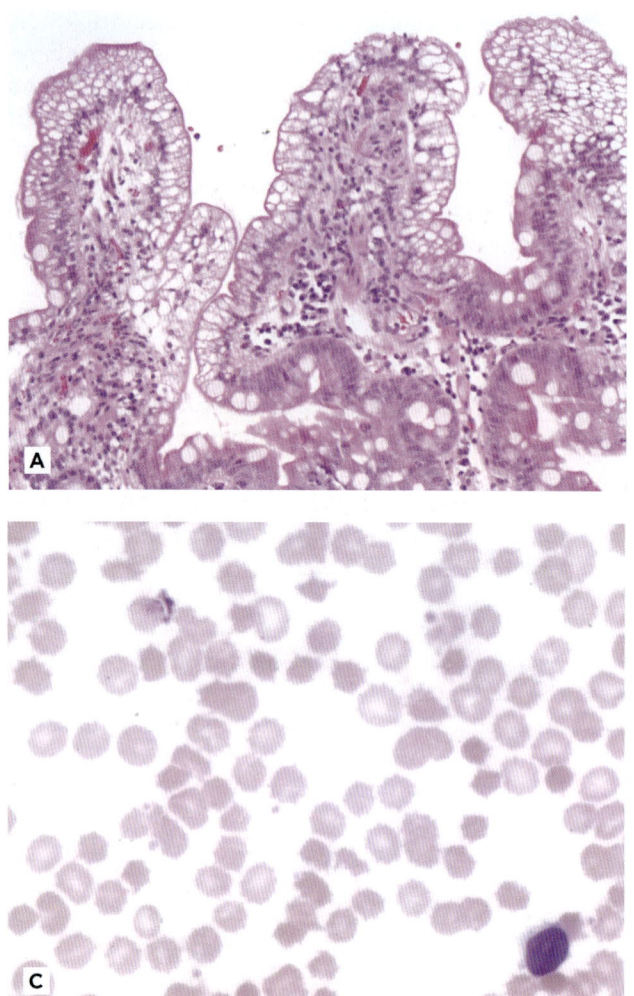
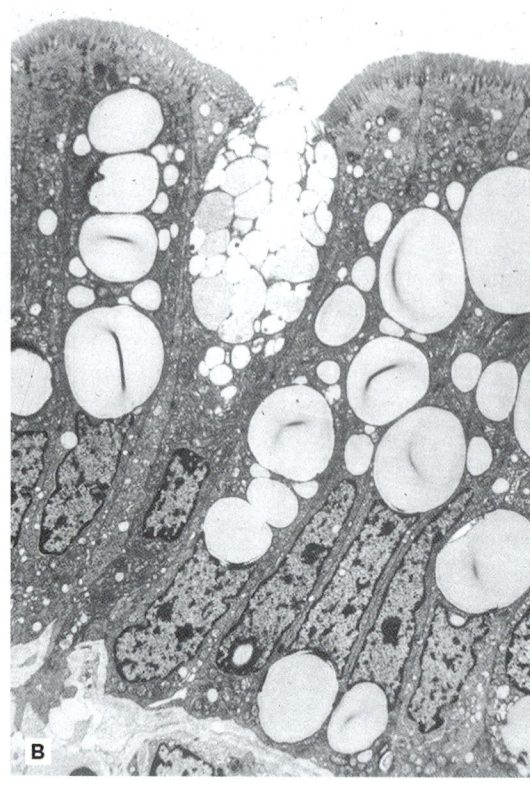

FIGURE 14-32 • Abetalipoproteinemia. **A:** A duodenal biopsy from a 9-month-old boy with failure to thrive and fat malabsorption reveals well-preserved villi with diffuse cytoplasmic vacuolization of the enterocytes 200×. **B:** Electron microscopy reveals numerous non–membrane-bound lipid vacuoles in the cytoplasm. **C:** Schizocytes are noted on the peripheral blood smear.

anti-CD10. The pathognomonic ultrastructural features include absent or small stubby microvilli, and numerous cytoplasmic vesicles near the apex, some of which contain microvilli (Figure 14-33C). Microvillus inclusions have also been reported in the colon, gallbladder, and renal tubular epithelium in these patients (133). A variety of different inclusions has also been noted in patients with this disorder and finding the "typical" inclusions may require a prolonged search (134). "Atypical" inclusions include the presence of numerous small electron-lucent vesicles and accumulation of osmiophilic vermiform structures (135).

Congenital Tufting Enteropathy (CTE, Epithelial Dysplasia)

Patients with tufting enteropathy also present in the neonatal period with a watery diarrhea. Prenatal history is uneventful and the disease appears to be inherited in an autosomal recessive fashion, as suggested by the finding of other affected siblings and frequent parental consanguinity. The incidence is estimated at 1/50,000 to 100,000 live births in Europe and appears to be more frequent in patients of Arabic origin (136). Cases of tufting enteropathy have been described in association with other malformations, including facial dysmorphism, micrognathia and imperforate anus, choanal atresia and hair abnormalities. Superficial punctate keratitis and conjunctival erosions have been observed in about 50% of patients (137). Using single nucleotide polymorphism (SNP) analysis in an affected kindred, Sivagnanam et al. (138) identified the epithelial cell adhesion molecule gene (EpCAM), located on chromosome 2p21, as the mutated gene. EpCAM belongs to a family of cell adhesion receptors, associated with tight junction proteins, and is responsible for cell–cell interaction by recruiting actin filaments to sites of contact. The histologic hallmarks are severe villus atrophy with the formation of "tufts" of rounded, teardrop-shaped enterocytes, which appear to shed into the lumen (Figure 14-34). There may be a mild increase in the lamina propria inflammatory cells, but IELs do not appear to be significantly increased. The brush border is normal by PAS staining, and electron microscopic findings are nonspecific. Dilated crypts have also been described. Epithelial abnormalities typically vary over time and may be subtle or absent in the first biopsy. A helpful feature for diagnosis is the finding that the expression of the antibody to EpCAM in the intestinal tissue of affected individuals is absent by immunohistochemistry (139). Patients are TPN dependent in most cases and may require intestinal transplantation.

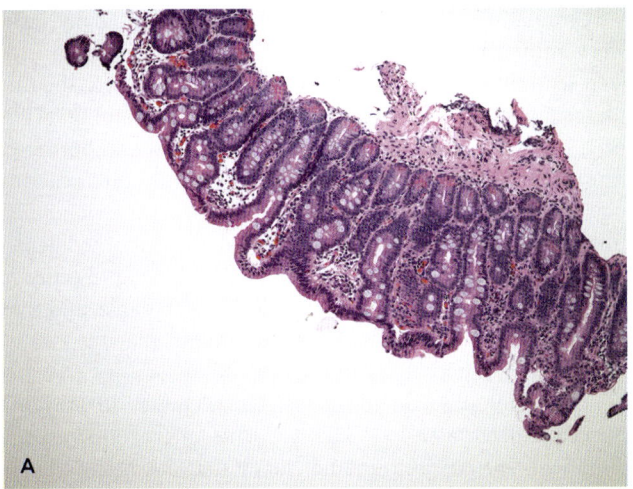
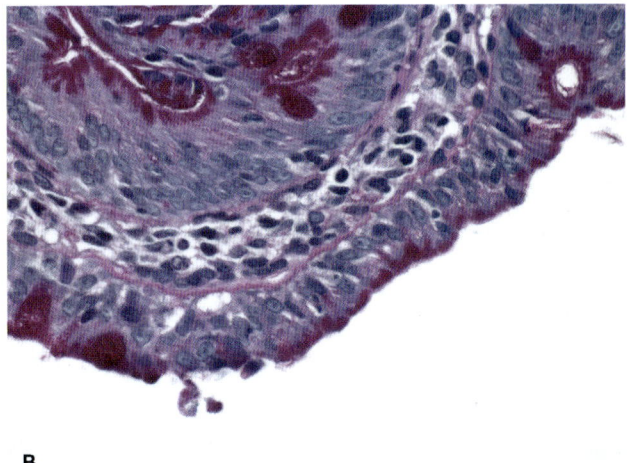
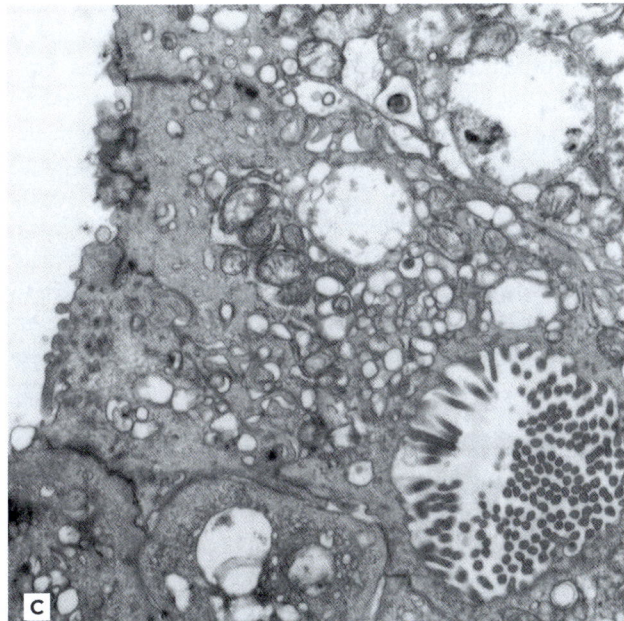

FIGURE 14-33 • Microvillous inclusion disease. **A:** Duodenal biopsy from an 18-day-old male exhibits total villous atrophy, normal-appearing crypts, and no inflammation 100×. **B:** The PAS stain shows lack of a well-defined enterocyte brush border, with periapical cytoplasmic positivity 600×. **C:** Electron microscopy demonstrates absent or stubby microvilli and numerous vesicles in the periapical portion of the enterocyte cytoplasm, some of which contain microvilli.

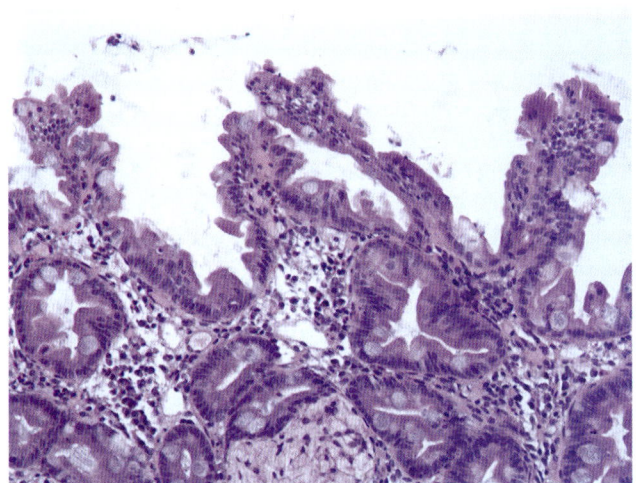

FIGURE 14-34 • Tufting enteropathy. The duodenal biopsy is characterized by coalescence of surface epithelial cells into prominent tufts.

Enteroendocrine Cell Dysgenesis (Enteric Anendocrinosis)

Enteroendocrine cell dysgenesis (ECD) is a recently described autosomal recessive disorder associated with a congenital absence of enteroendocrine cells in the small and large bowel secondary to mutations in the NEUROG3 gene, located on chromosome 10q21.3, required for differentiation of epithelial cells to the endocrine phenotype (140). Affected patients are characterized by a congenital diarrheal syndrome with profound malabsorption of all nutrients from birth. Patients also typically develop insulin-dependent diabetes, some during infancy and others later in childhood (140,141). Pancreatic exocrine function is normal. The intestinal biopsies may be normal or reveal villous atrophy, the severity of the changes perhaps related to different mutations in the NEUROG 3 gene (141). The characteristic absence of enteroendocrine cells in the small bowel and colon is confirmed by immunohistochemistry for chromogranin A. Patients with autoimmune polyglandular syndrome I may have absent or markedly reduced enteroendocrine cells, which may be transient (142,143). Loss of enteroendocrine cells may also be observed in patients with autoimmune enteropathy (AIE), along with loss of goblet and Paneth cells.

Autoimmune Enteropathy

AIE is probably the most frequent disorder leading to infantile intractable diarrhea (144). Most cases occur in infancy or the first year of life. The clinical picture is usually dominated by a secretory diarrhea, dermatitis, and various endocrine disorders. Moreover, these patients also suffer from numerous complications, mainly infectious, related to loss of the functional gut barrier, central lines, underlying immunodeficiency, and immunosuppressive therapy. About 50% of the cases are associated with the immune dysregulation, polyendocrinopathy, enteropathy, X-linked syndrome (IPEX syndrome). Extraintestinal disease in these patients includes insulin-dependent diabetes, thyroiditis, membranous glomerulopathy, and interstitial nephritis. IPEX syndrome has been related to mutations in the *FOXP3* gene (located on Xp11.23), and those bearing this mutation share a very similar phenotype to that of the scurfy mouse, with absence of naturally occurring CD4+ CD25+ regulatory T cells (Tregs). Mutations in the *FOXP3* gene or in its promoter region result in impaired suppression of lymphocyte proliferation by regulatory T cells following an initial inflammatory trigger, resulting in an undampened immune reaction (145). However, about 50% of patients, including older boys and girls, with otherwise typical clinical manifestations of IPEX have no detectable mutations of *FOXP3*, and for whom the term "IPEX-like" has been designated (146). AIE has also been reported in adults, in whom it may be responsible for a proportion of cases previously referred to as "refractory sprue." Akram et al. reported on a series of 15 (7 females) patients, aged 42 to 67 years, in whom celiac disease was excluded by lack of response to gluten-free diet (GFD) or absence of the celiac disease susceptibility HLA genotypes. All patients had protracted diarrhea, weight loss, and malnutrition (147).

The entire GI tract is often involved in AIE, though the histopathologic findings are most severe in the duodenum and small bowel where biopsies are usually characterized by marked villous atrophy, crypt hyperplasia, and a mixed inflammatory infiltrate of the lamina propria (148). Inflammatory destruction of intestinal crypts with extensive apoptosis is a feature noted in many of the cases, similar to those noted in intestinal graft versus host disease (GVHD), and confirms an immune-mediated attack against intestinal epithelium (Figure 14-35A, B). The inflammatory infiltrate in AIE tends to be more abundant than in GVHD. A characteristic feature not routinely observed in other inflammatory intestinal diseases is depletion of goblet and Paneth cells (Figure 14-35C). In contrast to cases of GSE with flat villi, IELs tend to be relatively few in number. A concomitant crypt-destructive colitis and gastritis are present in the majority of cases.

Circulating antienterocyte antibodies, detected by indirect immunofluorescence using the patient's serum on frozen sections of normal bowel, have been noted since the first descriptions of this entity. Positive fluorescent staining results in a linear pattern along the apex and basolateral border of the enterocyte (149) (Figure 14-35D). Antibodies reacting against mucus or goblet cells have also been described, and intestinal biopsies in these cases have shown a marked depletion of goblet cells. However, the role of these antibodies in the pathogenesis and diagnosis of AIE is debatable, and they may represent an epiphenomenon without playing a causative role in mucosal damage.

The differential diagnosis of AIE includes, in addition to celiac disease and GVHD, CD and enterocolitis associated with various immunodeficiency states. A high index of suspicion for AIE should be present when there is a severe inflammatory crypt-destructive process with villous atrophy and increased apoptosis in the base of the crypts, loss of goblet and Paneth cells, or an intestinal inflammatory process in a patient with autoimmune phenomena. Testing for circulating antienterocyte antibodies is useful in the older child and adult but may be of more limited use in the young infant in whom IgG production is limited during the first 3 months of life. Mortality, especially in early cases of this entity, has been high, and the use of immunosuppressants is necessary in most cases. More recently, a good response to tacrolimus and sirolimus has been reported (146). Bone marrow transplantation may be curative.

Celiac Disease (Gluten-Sensitive Enteropathy, GSE)

Celiac disease is a lifelong immune-mediated systemic disorder elicited by gluten, the major protein found in wheat, barley, and rye, in genetically predisposed individuals, resulting in damage to the intestinal mucosa and a variety of clinical manifestations and antibodies. The disease is most prevalent in Western Europe and North America, with reported incidence rates of up to 1:100 but occurs worldwide (150). The increased prevalence reported in more recent epidemiologic studies is likely due to more widespread use of serologic tests in detection and screening, a greater awareness of atypical and silent forms of the disease, and recognition of an increased incidence of GSE in patients with Down syndrome, IgA deficiency, and diabetes. Gluten is digested to the 33-amino acid alcohol-soluble gliadin, which is resistant to further enzymatic degradation. Gliadin appears to induce intestinal epithelial cells to express IL-15, which in turn leads to activation and proliferation of the characteristic intraepithelial CD8+ T lymphocytes. These become cytotoxic and destroy enterocytes with surface MIC-A, an HLA class I–like protein expressed during stress. This results in increased intestinal permeability to gliadin, followed by its deamidation by tissue transglutaminase (tTG), an enzyme normally present in the gut, where it acts to stabilize granulation tissue during

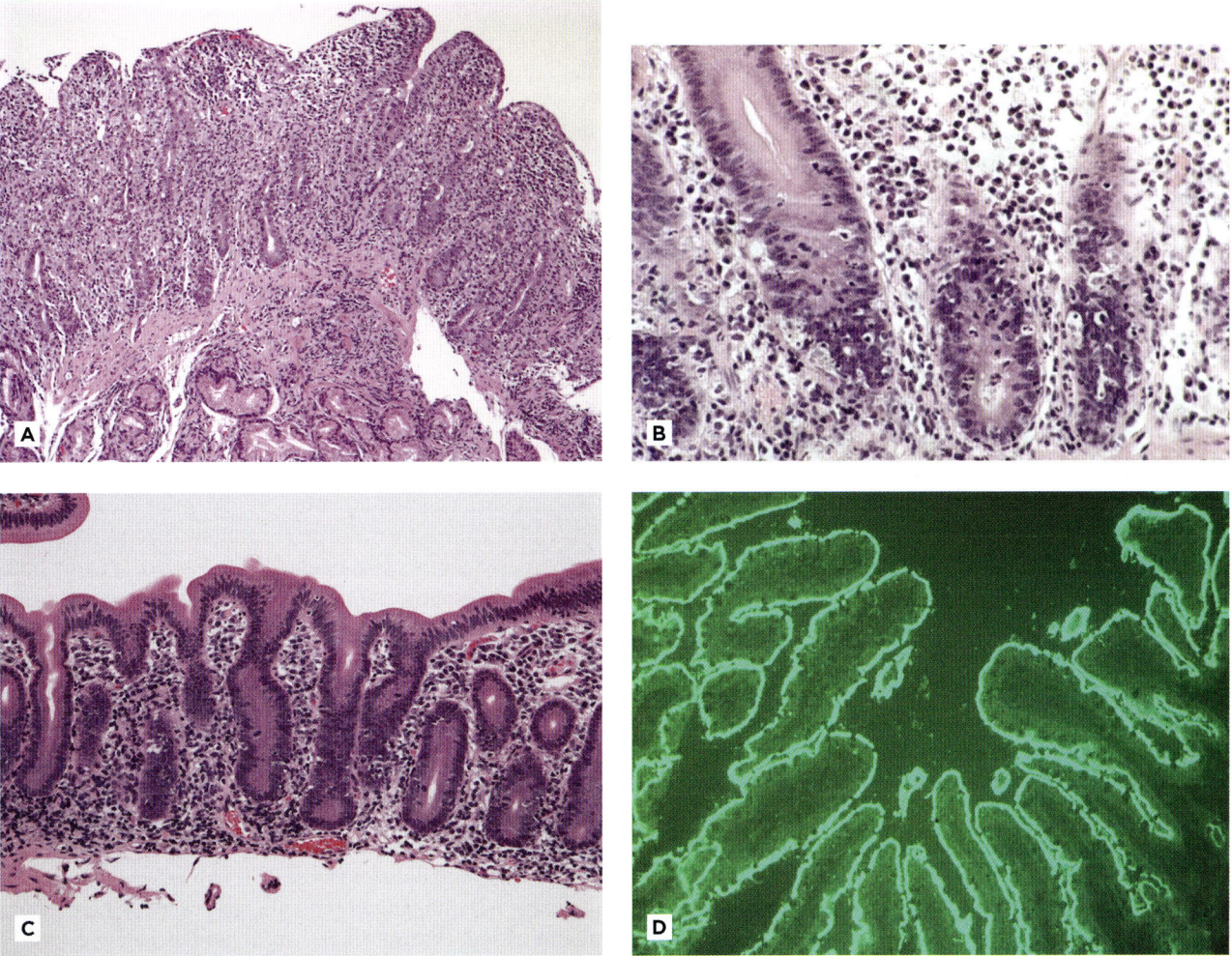

FIGURE 14-35 • Autoimmune enterocolitis. **A:** This duodenal biopsy from a 3-month-old boy with IPEX shows a marked crypt-destructive inflammatory process. **B:** Basal crypt apoptosis is present. **C:** This colonic biopsy from an older child exhibits mild colitis with prominent epithelial cell apoptosis and a complete absence of goblet cells. The serum anti-goblet cell antibody titer was elevated 200×. **D:** Indirect immunofluorescence using the patient's serum from another case reveals linear staining along the apical border of the enterocytes, consistent with the presence of circulating antienterocyte antibodies.

repair processes. Subsequent binding of deamidated gliadin to HLA molecules located on antigen-presenting cells results in activation of CD4+ T lymphocytes with secretion of inflammatory cytokines, production of interferon-γ, and further tissue damage. The principal determinants of genetic susceptibility for CD are major histocompatibility class II genes located on the short arm of chromosome 6. The HLA-DQ2 heterodimer is present in 95% of patients with CD, and most of the remainder have the HLA-DQ8 heterodimer. HLA-DQ2 homozygous individuals have a fivefold greater risk of disease development than HLA-DQ2 heterozygous individuals (151). Expression of these HLA molecules is necessary but not sufficient to cause disease as the HLA-DQ2 haplotype is present in 30% to 40% of the Caucasian population. Outside the HLA region, several genes controlling the immune response have also been related to GSE (151).

The classic presentation occurs in a child 6 to 24 months after gluten ingestion and consists of abdominal distension, diarrhea, and failure to thrive, whereas growth restriction and delayed puberty may be major manifestations in older children. The age at presentation of GSE appears to vary according to the age at introduction of gluten in the diet and to the quantity consumed. A variety of nongastrointestinal symptoms have also been associated with GSE, including dermatitis herpetiformis, short stature, delayed puberty, dental enamel hypoplasia, osteopenia, hepatitis, and iron deficiency anemia unresponsive to iron therapy. The lack of the "classic" symptomatology in older children and adults frequently results in delay of diagnosis.

According to guidelines published in 2005 by the North American Society for Pediatric Gastroenterology, Hepatology and Nutrition (NASPGHAN), the gold standard for diagnosis remains the intestinal biopsy (152). However, a stepwise approach is recommended with serologic testing as the initial step in symptomatic patients. Testing is also recommended for their first-degree relatives and in asymptomatic patients with conditions known to be associated with celiac disease, such as Down syndrome, Turner syndrome, Williams syndrome, autoimmune thyroiditis, and selective IgA deficiency (152). In particular, routine screening of all patients with type 1 diabetes mellitus is recommended, in whom a prevalence rate of GSE up to 8% has been reported (153). Measurements of serum IgA-tTG (tissue transglutaminase) and IgA-EMA (endomysial antibodies) have ranges of sensitivity and specificity of 90% to 100%, provided the subjects are not IgA deficient, and are considered superior to antigliadin antibodies for the diagnosis of GSE (150,154). For subjects with low serum IgA levels, testing with IgG-tTG and IgG-EMA is recommended. It should be noted that antibodies to tTG and EMA are more frequently falsely negative in children less than 2 years of age, in whom additional testing for antigliadin antibodies, or for deamidated gliadin peptides, is recommended (153,155). Detecting celiac disease in individuals who are on a self- or parent-prescribed gluten-free diet (GFD) is challenging as both GSE-specific antibodies and histology may normalize following GFD. In those cases, testing for HLA-DQ2 and HLA-DQ8 may be useful as celiac disease is most unlikely in those who lack these markers (153).

Typical endoscopic findings are scalloping of the duodenal folds. The damage is most severe proximally, but the entire length of the small bowel is sensitive to gluten. Accurate histologic assessment depends on well-oriented multiple biopsies from both the proximal and distal duodenum, as the disease may be patchy, especially in newly diagnosed children. Although it is recommended that biopsies be obtained from the more distal portion of the duodenum, where villi are somewhat longer and which is less subject to nonspecific changes, the bulb may be the more severe site or, in some cases, the only site of involvement (156,157). In a study of 102 pediatric patients by Bonamico, histologic involvement of the duodenum was patchy in 16%, and the bulb was the only site of involvement in 25% of the patients (156). The histologic features of GSE have typically rested on a combination of a flat duodenal mucosa with villus atrophy, crypt hyperplasia, a dense mixed inflammatory infiltrate in the lamina propria, and enterocyte damage with IELs (Figure 14-36A, B). However, a wide range of morphologic alterations, including well-preserved or only mildly atrophic villi, with increased IELs, can be observed (Figure 14-36C, D). There seems to be little association between symptomatology and degree of mucosal damage or with the extent of laboratory abnormalities, though it has been suggested that the length of injured bowel may correlate more closely with symptoms than the severity of villus flattening (158). The Marsh-Oberhuber classification (159) describes the major histologic lesions associated with GSE but is somewhat cumbersome in routine practice and has poor interobserver concordance because of the number of diagnostic categories. More recent classifications, such as that proposed by Corazza and Villanaci (160) and by Ensari (161), limit the number of categories to three:

normal villi with increased IELs, mild to markedly shortened villi with increased IELs and crypt hyperplasia, and a flat mucosa with increased IELs. Increased IELs (>20 to 25 lymphocytes per 100 epithelial cells) are a cardinal feature of intestinal biopsies in patients with GSE and in most cases rarely require enumeration. Counting IELs per 100 enterocytes is impractical in routine practice, but when increased IELs are suspected but not definitive, counting IELs at the tips of 5 well-oriented villi (20 enterocytes at the tip of each) has been proposed as an alternate, equally precise method (162). One study reported that counts of 6 to 12 IELs per 20 epithelial cells at the villus tip correlate with serologic evidence of GSE (162). Loss of the "decrescendo" pattern, in which IELs normally decrease from the base to the tip of the villus, is a useful feature to observe when assessing biopsies for GSE especially when villus morphology is preserved (158). Patients with GSE would have a persistent or increased density of IELs along the sides and especially the tips of the villi. GSE is frequently associated with increased IELs in other parts of the gastrointestinal tract, especially the stomach and colon, indicative of a pan-enteric sensitivity to gluten, which can reverse with a GFD. In one pediatric study, lymphocytic gastritis was found in 13% of patients with GSE and seemed to be associated with greater mucosal damage and more profound laboratory abnormalities (163). The fact that IELs are increased throughout the gut in GSE has led some to propose rectal biopsy following gluten challenge as a way to diagnose GSE, but this has not gained widespread acceptance (161).

The differential diagnosis of GSE in a small-bowel biopsy includes AIE, nongluten food allergy, severe protein-calorie malnutrition (kwashiorkor), immunodeficiency disorders, viral and parasitic infections, and *H. pylori* gastritis. Careful attention to such morphologic features as crypt destruction and increased apoptosis in AIE, and paucity of plasma cells in immunodeficiencies, in addition to clinical and serologic correlation, is essential for proper diagnosis. Refractory sprue is a term used to describe patients with severe villus atrophy, without evidence of lymphoma, which fails to improve on a GFD. In children, major diagnostic considerations would include other non–gluten-related food intolerance and AIE.

Treatment with a lifelong GFD is recommended for all symptomatic children as well as for asymptomatic children belonging to high-risk groups with characteristic intestinal histologic abnormalities (152). The availability of accurate serologic tests for both diagnosis and compliance measurement has greatly reduced the need for second biopsies or for "gluten challenges." However, second biopsies may occasionally be necessary for those who have an unsatisfactory response to treatment (164). Gluten restriction from the diet results in clinical and histologic improvement: enterocytes assume a more columnar appearance, and IELs and lamina propria inflammation decrease. Full restoration of villus architecture may take up to several years in adults and may be sooner in children. After a GFD of 2 years, complete normalization of the intestinal mucosa was observed in two-thirds of pediatric patients but in less than one-third of adults despite normalization of laboratory values (165).

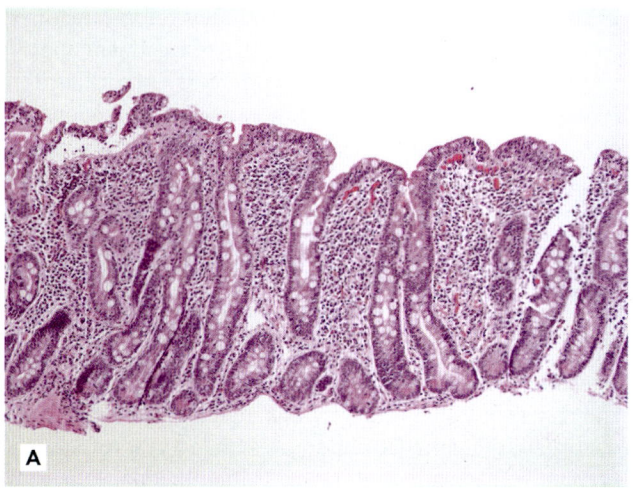
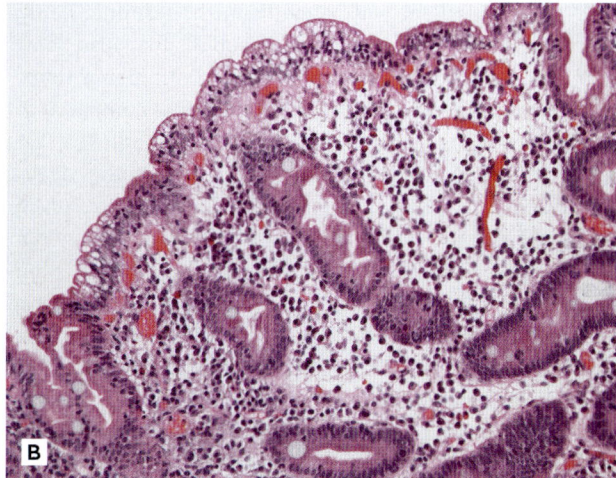
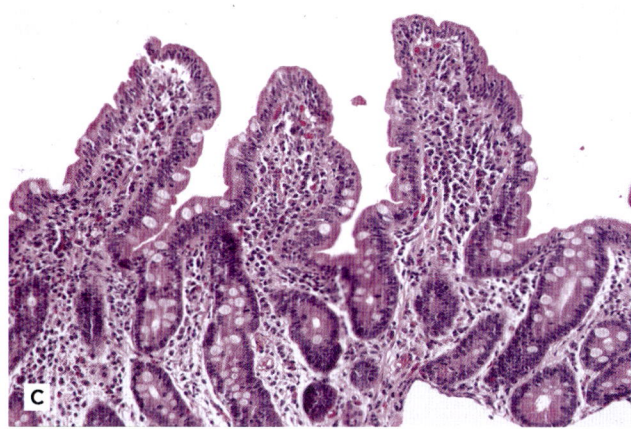
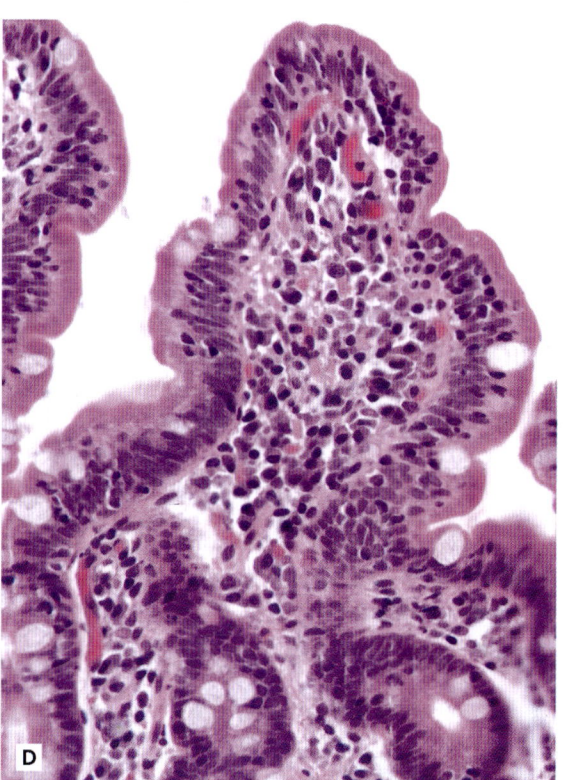

FIGURE 14-36 • Celiac disease. **A:** Villous atrophy with crypt hyperplasia 100×. **B:** Increased intraepithelial lymphocytes in the superficial epithelium and enterocyte injury manifested by vacuolization. **C:** Duodenal biopsy from another patient, a 2-year-old child, with failure to thrive and elevated serum tTG. There is mild villous atrophy 200×. **D:** Increased intraepithelial lymphocytes were noted 400×.

Eosinophilic Gastroenteritis

EG can be broadly defined by the presence of gastrointestinal symptoms with a pathologic eosinophilic infiltrate of one or more segments of the GI tract (typically the stomach and small bowel) without evidence of parasitic infection or other causes of secondary eosinophilic infiltration (166). It appears to be most common in adults during the third and fourth decades but is also observed throughout childhood and adolescence. The foreign antigenic substances are mainly cow's milk in the infant and egg and soy protein in the older child. Cross-reactivity between substances causing GI and respiratory allergic reactions has been demonstrated. Symptoms depend on the location of the infiltrate but most frequently include GI hemorrhage, nausea, vomiting, and diarrhea, though pancreatitis, abdominal mass, intestinal perforation, and duodenal ulcers have also been reported. Some patients may develop a protein-losing enteropathy (PLE). Peripheral eosinophilia is usually, but not always, elevated (166). Confirmation may include supervised food challenges and RAST (radioallergosorbent testing).

Eosinophilic inflammation may involve one or more layers of the GI tract, and in 1970, Klein et al. (167) proposed a pathologic classification linked to the predominant level of eosinophilic infiltration: mucosal, mural, or serosal involvement. Mucosal involvement is by far the most common. As eosinophils are normal residents and part of the innate immune system of the GI tract, determining what constitutes a pathologic elevation in the numbers of eosinophils can be problematic. Eosinophils (and other constituent inflammatory cells) in the bowel appear to follow a bell-shaped gradient with a zenith in the terminal ileum and cecum. Normal numbers of eosinophils may also show geographic variation in the United States, with higher numbers of eosinophils reported in the southern as compared to the northern United States (168), and may also follow a seasonal distribution (169). According to the few studies available in children, mean numbers of eosinophils may reach up to 40 to 50 per HPF in the cecum and ascending colon, decreasing to 10 to 20 eosinophils/HPF in the distal colon and rectum (170,171). Given the absence of clear criteria as to what constitutes pathologic eosinophilia, it is perhaps more prudent for the pathologist to suggest a diagnosis of EG when associated features indicating epithelial damage are also present (172,173). Thus, small-intestinal biopsies in EG usually reveal variable villus atrophy with some blunting, which can be focal (Figure 14-37). Increased numbers of degranulated and intact eosinophils are present in the lamina propria, frequently with infiltration of the epithelium. Often, there is concomitant involvement of other portions of the GI tract, particularly the gastric antrum. Increased numbers of eosinophils without epithelial damage, a situation not infrequently encountered in biopsy material, may nonetheless be evidence of a hypersensitivity-related disease, allowing for the segment of bowel involved and the possibility of normal geographic variation. In that situation, the diagnosis of EG should be used with caution to avoid unwarranted therapy with steroids (172). The differential diagnosis of EG includes parasitic infestation and other infections, drug reactions, CD, some primary immunodeficiencies, connective tissue disorders, inflammatory fibroid polyps, and the hypereosinophilic syndrome. Posttransplant EG has been reported in patients on immunomodulator therapy who developed intestinal symptomatology with peripheral eosinophilia and IgE-positive radioallergosorbent test for milk protein (174). It is postulated that immunosuppressants such as cyclosporine and tacrolimus may play a role in initiating food allergy.

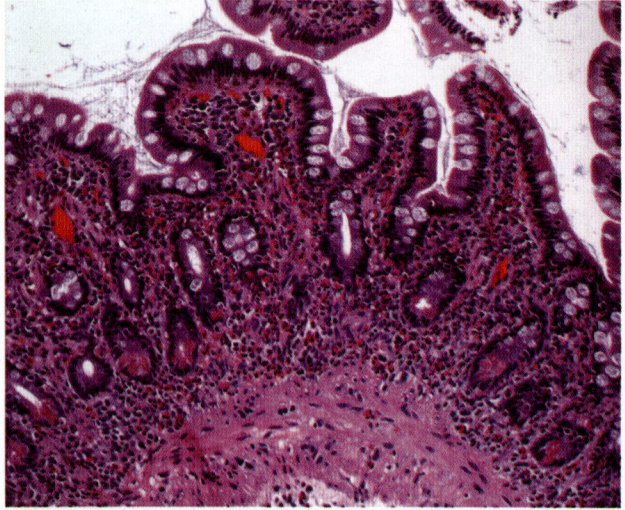

FIGURE 14-37 • Eosinophilic gastroenteritis. This duodenal biopsy demonstrates villous blunting (without crypt hyperplasia) and an intense infiltrate of eosinophils 200×.

There is a paucity of controlled studies on the treatment and outcome of EG, but the mainstay of treatment appears to be dietary therapy and corticosteroids. According to a recent study, about 40% of adult patients had a spontaneous remission, and though a majority responded favorably to steroids, 50% of patients had relapses and a chronic course (166). Children appear to respond to an elemental diet, although food sensitivity persists in most cases (175). Immunosuppression may be required in severe cases.

Intestinal Lymphangiectasia

Intestinal lymphangiectasia may be primary or secondary and results in PLE. Primary lymphangiectasia is a rare disorder usually diagnosed in children less than 3 years of age, who present with diarrhea, PLE, hypoalbuminemia, hypogammaglobulinemia, and lymphopenia, resulting in secondary immunodeficiency. Malabsorption may cause deficiencies in fat-soluble vitamins. Primary disorders appear to result from congenital obstruction to lymph flow or abnormal lymphatic structure and may be essentially limited to intestinal lymphatics, as in primary lymphangiectasia, or may involve multiple organs, as in hereditary lymphedema, also known as Milroy disease, which has been associated with mutations in the gene encoding vascular endothelial growth receptor factor 3 (176). It has been postulated that congenital hypoplasia of lymphatics may also cause PLE in neonates (177).

Secondary lymphangiectasia may be "central," resulting from cardiac disease or from local obstruction to lymphatics due to a variety of causes. In children, secondary immunodeficiency resulting from extensive protein losses in the stools has been reported with intestinal malrotation and cavernous hemangioma of the jejunum. Cardiac causes of lymphangiectasia with PLE usually result from obstruction to systemic venous return or from surgical procedures, which cause increased systemic venous pressure. PLE may occur in up to 5% of patients, who have undergone the Fontan operation for correction of tricuspid atresia and other right-sided cardiac malformations, and carries a poor prognosis (178). This procedure creates a direct communication between the systemic venous return and the pulmonary arterial system, resulting in chronically sustained increased systemic venous pressure.

The endoscopic appearance is usually characteristic, with swollen opaque villi, white nodules, or submucosal elevations. Histologic examination reveals blunted villi with dilated lacteals (Figure 14-38A). The finding of occasional dilated lymphatics in a biopsy of a patient without significant symptoms is not infrequent and of no diagnostic value. Conversely, mucosal biopsies may be nondiagnostic, when the lesions are focal, and will almost always miss lymphangiectasia of the deeper layers of the bowel wall (Figure 14-38B).

Gastroenteritis and Postenteritis Enteropathy

Most cases of acute gastroenteritis in children are caused by viruses. Biopsies are usually not performed during the acute

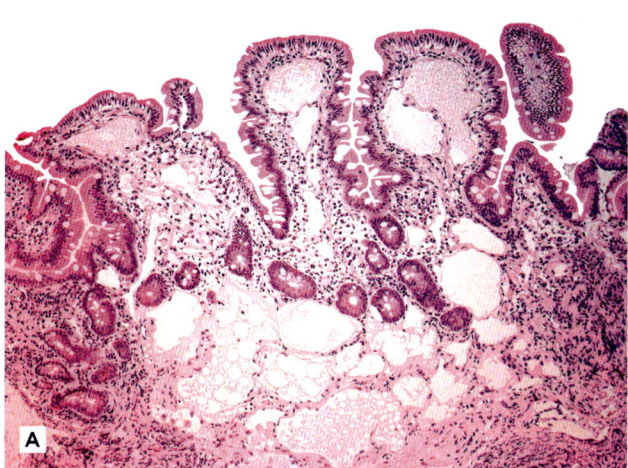 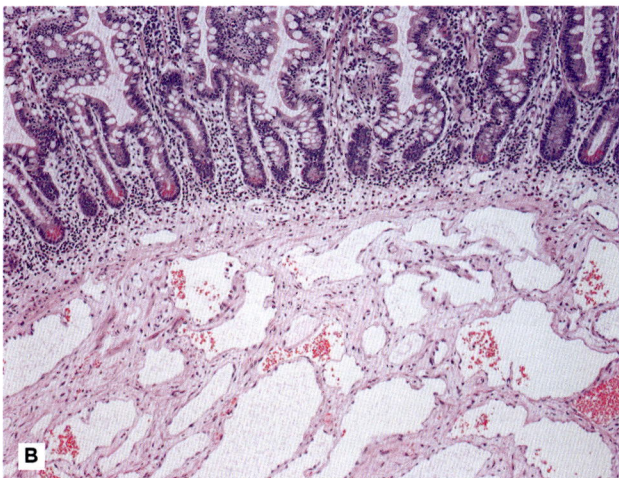

FIGURE 14-38 • Small-bowel lymphangiectasia. **A:** This duodenal biopsy demonstrates dilated lymphatic channels within the lamina propria 200x. **B:** In this resection specimen, the dilated lymphatic vessels are present in the superficial submucosa 100x.

infection. Of more concern is the infant or child who apparently recovers from an episode of acute viral gastroenteritis but then lapses into a malabsorptive state lasting weeks to months. These children may undergo endoscopic examination and their biopsy findings must be distinguished from those of celiac disease. Cow's milk protein intolerance is sometimes unmasked by acute gastroenteritis and should be considered. It has been suggested that persistence of diarrhea may be due to nutritional deficiencies such as zinc, and supplementation with the latter seems to shorten the duration of the diarrhea (179).

Short Bowel Syndrome and Bacterial Overgrowth

Extensive surgical resection of the intestine is the usual cause of short bowel syndrome, defined as malabsorption in the presence of reduced intestinal length, usually 50 cm or less of small intestine in a neonate. The normal small-intestinal length in the term neonate is 239 ± 67 cm (180). Extensive intestinal resection is performed in patients with such conditions as neonatal NEC, malrotation with volvulus, multiple intestinal atresias, and, in older children with Crohn disease. Very rarely, the intestine is congenitally very short. In any case, diarrhea results from a shortened transit time, and malabsorption of nutrients results from an inadequate absorptive surface area. In some patients, a reduction in peristalsis leads to intestinal dilatation. Bacterial overgrowth in the intestinal lumen contributes substantially to malabsorption in many cases of short bowel syndrome. Small-intestinal biopsy specimens often show nonspecific partial villous atrophy, crypt hypertrophy, and inflammation with lymphocytes, plasma cells, and eosinophils. In severe cases of bacterial overgrowth, an acute enteritis with polymorphonuclear leukocytes in the lamina propria or crypts may be present. The colon is often also involved. Bacterial overgrowth can be diagnosed by culture of proximal intestinal fluid; organisms are rarely seen on biopsy specimens. Intravenous alimentation with amino acid and lipid preparations has made long-term survival possible in these patients. Antibiotics often decrease the bacterial overgrowth. Newer bowel-lengthening procedures have been used to correct selected cases, and in the most severe cases, small-bowel transplantation is possible.

Malnutrition

Kwashiorkor and marasmus may both produce villous atrophy and inflammation (Figure 14-39), although this is rare in developed countries. Patients with protein-calorie malnutrition and gastrointestinal symptoms often have a superimposed infection.

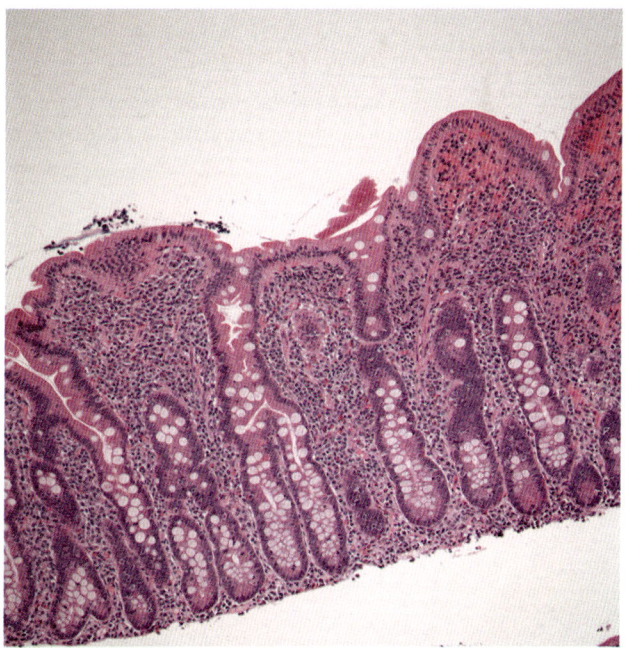

FIGURE 14-39 • Kwashiorkor. Duodenal biopsy from a 12-year-old boy who suffered from long-standing chronic abuse and malnutrition shows villous atrophy and chronic inflammation 100x.

GASTROINTESTINAL MANIFESTATIONS OF IMMUNODEFICIENCY

Gastrointestinal symptoms, infections, and morphologic abnormalities figure prominently in many primary and secondary immunodeficiency syndromes (see Chapter 23). Biopsy specimens from immunodeficient patients may come to the pathologist masquerading as malabsorption, IBD, giardiasis, or lymphoid hyperplasia. The pathologist evaluating an intestinal mucosal biopsy specimen or resected tissue for any of these clinical indications may be the first to suspect AIDS, hypogammaglobulinemia, agammaglobulinemia, or, if plasma cells are absent in the lamina propria, severe combined immunodeficiency or X-linked agammaglobulinemia.

At times, a primary gastrointestinal abnormality may result in a secondary immunodeficiency. Leakage from intestinal lymphatics, as in intestinal lymphangiectasia and CD, may lead to lymphopenia and functional T-cell deficiency. PLE in cow's milk protein intolerance can produce hypogammaglobulinemia and lymphopenia. Structural defects, such as malrotation and cavernous hemangioma of the jejunum, have been associated with defects of both humoral and cellular immunity, postulated to result from intestinal losses of protein and lymphocytes.

Immunosuppression caused by steroids and cytotoxic agents, especially in children with malignancies, increases the risk for fungal or viral infection of the gastrointestinal tract. Necrotizing inflammation of the cecum or typhlitis (neutropenic colitis) is likely to develop in children who are being treated for leukemia.

Primary Immunodeficiencies

Selective IgA deficiency is the most common primary immunodeficiency in the general population, with an incidence of 1 to 2 in 1000. Diarrhea and steatorrhea may occur at any age and are often the initial manifestations of immunodeficiency. The incidence of celiac disease is increased in IgA-deficient patients, and the diagnosis may be more difficult than usual because the serum levels of antigliadin and antiendomysial IgA antibodies are not elevated. Intestinal giardiasis may also cause malabsorption, but malabsorption persists in some IgA-deficient patients even after elimination of gluten from the diet and treatment of *Giardia* infestation. Various chronic IBDs, morphologically identical to CD and UC, have also been reported in IgA-deficient patients. Nodular lymphoid hyperplasia of the small intestine occurs in both selective IgA deficiency and common variable hypogammaglobulinemia but is rare in children.

Common variable immunodeficiency (common variable hypogammaglobulinemia) may also first come to clinical attention with gastrointestinal symptoms in older children. The diagnosis is often delayed because a pattern of recurrent infections involving multiple organs is not recognized. They are susceptible to a host of gastrointestinal complications, which often become the dominant clinical problem. Infections are common, with giardiasis, bacterial infections, and chronic viral infections reported. The diagnosis rests upon the findings of abnormally low serum immunoglobulin (IgA, IgM, and IgG) levels without another explanation. A poor or absent response to immunization is helpful to confirm the diagnosis. Malabsorption states, nonspecific colitis, gastritis, and chronic IBDs resembling CD and UC are also found.

Gastrointestinal plasma cells are absent or markedly decreased in most but not all cases (181). Duodenal biopsies in patients with malabsorption may exhibit villous blunting, crypt hyperplasia, and intraepithelial lymphocytosis, closely resembling the histologic features of celiac disease (Figure 14-40A, B). The proper diagnosis rests on the recognition of the lack of a dense lamina propria infiltrate of lymphocytes and plasma cells, as expected in celiac disease.

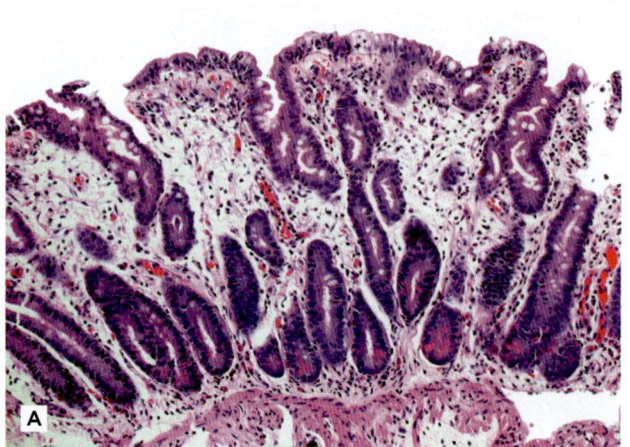 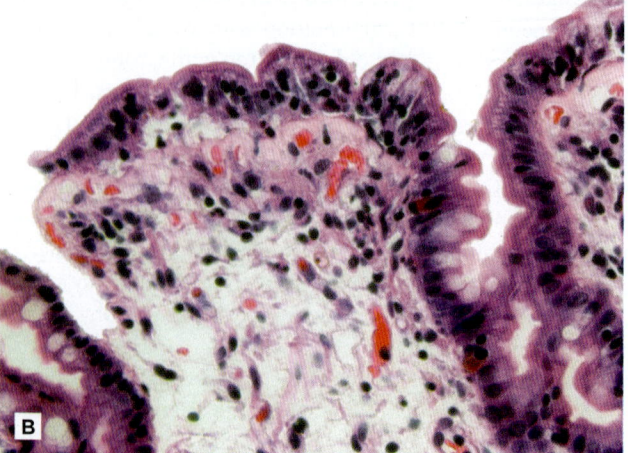

FIGURE 14-40 • Common variable immunodeficiency. **A:** This duodenal biopsy exhibits complete villous blunting and crypt hyperplasia 200×. **B:** There is also a mild intraepithelial lymphocytosis, similar to that seen in celiac disease. However, the complete absence of lamina propria plasma cells suggests the correct diagnosis 400×.

Patients with common variable immunodeficiency are also at particularly increased risk of Giardia infection. In some duodenal biopsies, epithelial apoptosis is prominent, resulting in an appearance similar to severe GVHD or autoimmune enteritis (181). Esophageal biopsies may reveal Candida esophagitis. Severe diffuse nonspecific gastritis may be seen in antral or gastric body biopsies. Colonic biopsies may reveal features consistent with lymphocytic or collagenous colitis or exhibit crypt architectural distortion and active inflammation resembling IBD. Granulomas may also be present. Again, the absence of plasma cells is a clue to the proper diagnosis in most cases.

X-linked agammaglobulinemia presents in the first 6 months of life with severe respiratory infections and meningitis. Diarrhea, malabsorption, giardiasis, and colitis are frequent manifestations and may dominate in any given case. Examination of the lamina propria reveals an absence of plasma cells.

Severe combined immunodeficiency is fatal in the first few months of life unless a bone marrow transplant is successful. Malabsorption, villous atrophy, diarrhea, and severe failure to thrive regularly develop in untreated patients. Gastrointestinal plasma cells are lacking.

Immunodeficient patients are predisposed to gastrointestinal infections by usual and unusual pathogens. *G. lamblia* infection of the small intestine has been found in up to 50% of symptomatic patients with primary immunodeficiency syndromes and is responsible for many of the cases of chronic diarrhea and malabsorption in patients with common variable hypogammaglobulinemia, selective IgA deficiency, and X-linked agammaglobulinemia. Eradication of the parasite usually relieves the symptoms.

Gastrointestinal Involvement in Pediatric HIV infection

Gastrointestinal disorders, especially infections, are the chief cause of morbidity and mortality worldwide in patients infected with HIV. Prior to the use of new HAART therapy, opportunistic infections with such pathogens as *Isospora*, *Mycobacterium avium* complex, microsporidia, *Cryptosporidium*, and CMV were frequent causes of diarrhea. The effective use of HAART therapy in the treatment of HIV has led to a gradual decline in infectious diseases and an increase in HIV-associated malignancy (182).

HIV enteropathy is characterized by relatively mild villous blunting without well-developed crypt hyperplasia. The presence of an opportunistic pathogen such as Cryptosporidium, Microsporidium, Isospora, Giardia, and Mycobacterium must always be ruled out in these patients. Microsporidium is difficult to identify on H&E-stained sections; electron microscopy confirms the presence of the organism in the surface epithelial cells. In mycobacterium avium complex infection, the lamina propria of the intestinal mucosa may be filled with distended macrophages containing the organisms. Stains for acid-fast bacilli are useful in confirming the presence of mycobacterium.

The histology of the colon in HIV enteropathy is less well understood. Increased epithelial cell apoptosis has been reported in association with HIV infection (183); however, it is unclear if this is related to the presence of the virus or other immune mediators or as a result of antiretroviral therapy. Common opportunistic infections include salmonella, *Shigella*, mycobacterium, *Cryptosporidium*, *E. histolytica*, and CMV. Spirochetosis preferentially infects the surface epithelium of the distal colon and rectum. The organisms are dark black with the Warthin-Starry stain, and also identified by IHC. The colonic mucosa is unremarkable in most cases with no increase in chronic inflammation.

A number of atypical proliferations may develop in gastrointestinal lymphoid tissue in HIV-infected patients, including the following: (a) endoscopically visible lymphoid aggregates of duodenal mucosa, (b) a polyclonal lymphoproliferative process resembling posttransplant lymphoproliferative syndrome, and (c) AIDS-related non-Hodgkin lymphoma. More recently EBV-associated SMT, consisting of leiomyomas and leiomyosarcomas, have been described in many HIV-infected children. Leiomyosarcomas have become the second most frequent malignancy in children with HIV infection or other immunodeficiency diseases in the United States, and the prognosis is poor (184).

Graft Versus Host Disease

The intestinal tract is one of the three major target organs in GVHD. The skin and the liver are the other two organs affected when donor lymphoid cells are transfused into an immunosuppressed host. Donor T lymphocytes target epithelial cells in these organs and initiate an immune response that destroys them. GVHD is usually diagnosed following allogeneic bone marrow or stem cell transplant to treat leukemia and other malignant and nonmalignant diseases. It is relatively common in the pediatric setting, reported in 46% of pediatric stem cell transplantation recipients, with hepatic involvement occurring in 39% of children with GVHD (185). It has also been reported following the transfusion of nonirradiated blood into patients with primary or secondary immunodeficiency disorders, although this has become less common with current transfusion practices. GVHD has been traditionally categorized as acute, which begins 1 week to 4 months after transplantation, and chronic, which begins approximately 4 months or more after the transplant. More recent diagnostic criteria distinguishing acute from chronic GVHD and grading of clinical severity have been developed as part of an NIH Consensus Development Project (186).

The gastrointestinal tract is affected in at least half of the patients with acute GVHD. The skin and liver may be involved at the same time, at different times, or not at all. Intestinal GVHD is usually heralded by profuse watery diarrhea, which indicates involvement of the small intestine and colon. Occasionally, the upper gastrointestinal tract will be involved first or exclusively; the symptoms are nausea, vomiting, and anorexia. Acute intestinal GVHD is diagnosed by colonoscopic or upper endoscopic biopsies. The earliest

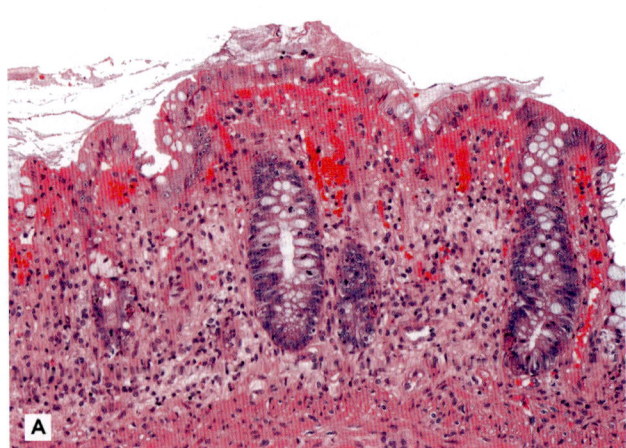
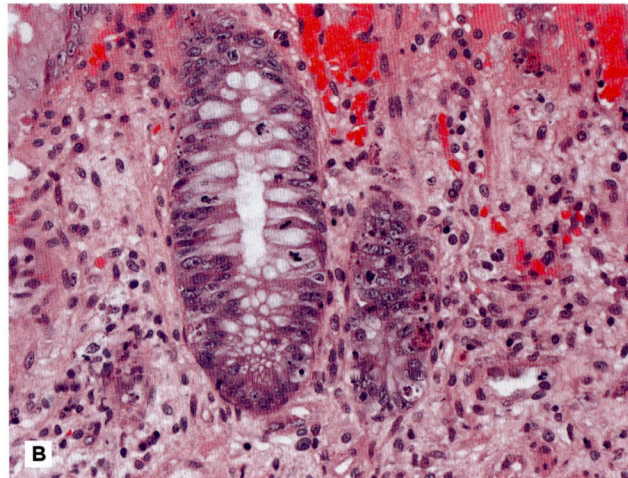

FIGURE 14-41 • Colonic acute graft versus host disease. **A:** Lamina propria cellularity is decreased from normal due to the effect of induction chemotherapy prior to the stem cell transplantation 200×. **B:** Note the characteristic epithelial cell apoptosis 400×.

histologic change is the development of apoptosis of individual epithelial cells in the regenerative (stem cell) compartment, characterized by vacuolization of the cytoplasm and nuclear karyorrhexis (Figure 14-41A, B). The stem cell population in the small bowel and colon resides in the lower portions of the crypts. In the esophageal squamous mucosa, apoptosis is seen in the basal cell layer, similar to that seen in skin involvement. In the stomach, the stem cell population is located in the neck zone of the mucosa. Inflammatory cell infiltrates are typically quite sparse, and lymphocytic infiltration of the epithelium in areas exhibiting apoptosis is usually not apparent. Scattered eosinophils are usually present. Diagnostic histologic features of GVHD are often quite patchy, and many biopsies may be necessary to exclude the diagnosis. Grading schemes for acute GVHD have been proposed, usually based on features best seen in the colonic mucosa, but there is no close relationship between clinical findings and grade. If the process is not arrested by appropriate medical therapy, it progresses to glandular attenuation, destruction, and dropout. Areas of complete glandular loss and extensive mucosal denudation occur in severe GVHD.

Apoptosis can also occur as a consequence of the induction chemoradiation therapy regime used prior to stem cell transplantation. Thus, histologic distinction between therapy-related mucosal damage and GVHD is usually not possible in the first 20 to 30 days after induction therapy is instituted. CMV infection can cause epithelial cell apoptosis, the diagnosis of which relies on identification of viral inclusions. However, because GVHD and CMV infection may occur simultaneously, it may be difficult to separate the effects of each process on the GI tract. In addition, mycophenolate mofetil can cause diarrhea and produce a graft versus host–like appearance in the gastrointestinal mucosa, and this agent is used in some stem cell transplant patients.

Chronic GVHD is a more insidious process that primarily affects skin and liver. The intestinal tract is largely spared except for the esophagus, in which a scleroderma-like fibrosis and dysmotility develop. In the evaluation of all the phases of intestinal GVHD, the differential diagnosis must include infection, particularly with opportunistic organisms.

Henoch-Schönlein Purpura and Other Systemic Vasculitides

HSP is a systemic vasculitis whose cardinal clinical manifestations include a purpuric rash, arthritis, abdominal pain, and nephritis. It occurs worldwide, with seasonal clustering in the winter and early spring. Though it can affect persons of any age, the majority of patients are children, and it is the most common vasculitis in children. The median age at onset is 4 years. Pediatric cases are generally preceded by a viral or bacterial infection; adult cases have also been associated with cancer and drugs. It has also been observed as a complication of anti-TNF (tumor necrosis factor) therapy in CD (187).

The cause of HSP is unknown, but the pathogenic process involves a disordered immune response with the deposition of immune complexes containing IgA and complement factor 3 (C3) in glomerular capillaries and in small blood vessels of the skin, gastrointestinal tract, and other organs. Genetic susceptibility is suggested by increased frequency of the disease in individuals carrying the HLA-B35 haplotype.

Gastrointestinal involvement is frequent and may precede or occur after the rash. Abdominal pain and overt or occult GI bleeding are the most common intestinal symptoms. The duodenum and small bowel are the most frequently involved sites in the gastrointestinal tract, and intussusception is the most significant abdominal complication. Radiologic studies reveal "thumbprinting" of the intestinal wall, as found in other ischemic conditions (188). The underlying gastrointestinal pathology is an acute leukocytoclastic vasculitis of small blood vessels in the submucosa or deep lamina propria (Figure 14-42). However, endoscopic biopsies of the GI lesions are most commonly characterized by nonspecific changes, probably because most mucosal biopsies do not

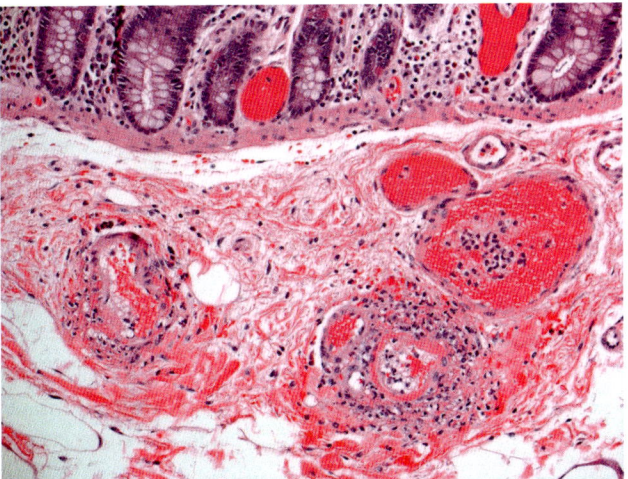

FIGURE 14-42 • Henoch-Schönlein purpura. Leukocytoclastic vasculitis involving small submucosal arterioles of the colon 200×.

include the deeper vessels of the submucosa. In these cases, the value of the biopsy lies in excluding other diseases.

Other forms of vasculitis affecting the intestinal tract include systemic lupus erythematosus, Churg-Strauss syndrome, Wegener granulomatosis, and microscopic polyangiitis. Some cases in the past classified as polyarteritis nodosa affecting the gastrointestinal tract actually represent microscopic polyangiitis using current diagnostic criteria. Some infectious agents, notably enterohemorrhagic strains of *E. coli*, including serotype 0157:H7, and CMV, may target blood vessels and cause small-vessel vasculitis, platelet–fibrin thrombi, and patchy hemorrhage and necrosis.

COLITIS

The numerous causes of colitis in infants and children are listed in Table 14-7.

Inflammatory Bowel Disease

IBD has been recognized with increased frequency in children and adolescents. In fact, approximately 20% to 25% of IBD patients are diagnosed by 20 years of age. On a clinical and histopathologic basis, IBD is commonly classified as either UC or CD. The disease pathogenesis is not fully elucidated by these broadly based phenotypes, which more than likely involve multiple, distinct pathophysiologies. In general, IBD appears to result from an inappropriate immune response to antigens, such as gut microbes or ill-defined food antigens, in a genetically susceptible host. The clinical findings, pattern of involvement in the gastrointestinal tract, radiologic studies, and histopathology must all be integrated before a diagnosis is made. In some cases, the distinction can be elusive, even after surgical resection and careful pathologic examination; in these cases, the designation IBD, indeterminate type, is used (see below.) The symptoms of IBD in children are similar to those in adults, but in addition, growth

TABLE 14-7 CAUSES OF COLITIS IN PEDIATRIC PATIENTS

Idiopathic disorders
    Ulcerative colitis
    Crohn disease
    Lymphocytic/collagenous colitis (rare)
Infections (see Table 14-4)
    Viral (e.g., CMV, adenovirus, and enteric viruses)
    Bacterial (e.g., *Shigella, Salmonella, E. coli, Clostridium difficile*, etc.)
    Fungal (e.g., zygomycosis)
    Parasitic (e.g., Strongyloides)
Autoimmune and immunodeficiency
    Autoimmune enterocolitis
    Common variable immunodeficiency
    Chronic granulomatous disease
    Typhlitis (neutropenic enterocolitis)
Miscellaneous
    Diversion colitis
    Hirschsprung enterocolitis
    Allergic colitis
    Vasculitides

retardation and delayed puberty are commonly encountered, particularly in children with CD. Cessation of growth resulting from steroid therapy is also an important consideration in the treatment of CD and UC in children. The pathology of IBD in children is identical to that in adults in most respects.

Acute Self-Limited Colitis

Early IBD may be difficult to distinguish clinically and pathologically from ASLC, defined as a condition in which diarrhea, often bloody and with a sudden onset, resolves spontaneously after several weeks. It is presumed to be infectious in nature, but since stool cultures are not routinely obtained in every case of diarrhea, a specific causal organism may not be identified in a given patient. On the other hand, microbiologic investigations can reveal a colitis-causing pathogen such as Salmonella, Campylobacter, and Yersinia in up to 15% of patients with IBD. Endoscopic features alone may not reliably distinguish ASLC from IBD. The histologic features of ASLC include neutrophils in the lamina propria, cryptitis, and, in the most severe cases, erosions and microscopic ulcerations, but normal crypt architecture is well maintained. In some cases, the superficial portion of the mucosa is focally necrotic and hemorrhagic (eFigure 14-10). The lamina propria lacks the basal lymphoplasmacytosis seen in chronic IBD. Despite these differences, it has been well documented that initial colonic or rectal biopsies from 10% to 34% of pediatric patients ultimately shown to have UC lacked architectural distortion or other histologic features of chronic colitis. This is seen particularly in younger patients (<10 years) and may be due to shorter duration of symptoms or longer progression to chronicity in children (189). Focal active colitis may be a feature of self-limited colitis but may also be a manifestation of early IBD (190). Close follow-up and repeat biopsies may be necessary in these cases. Increased mucosal eosinophils may be seen in the earliest biopsies of children eventually proven to have IBD, prompting a diagnosis of food allergy. In a recent case series of IBD diagnosed in 16 children less than 2 years of age, 6 children had had an initial diagnosis of allergy (191). On the other hand, histologic features similar to IBD may be seen in patients with primary immunodeficiencies and AIE. These conditions should always merit consideration when clinical manifestations of IBD occur in younger children. Histologic features that may point to a correct diagnosis in these patients include lack or paucity of plasma cells in the inflammatory infiltrate (as in common variable immunodeficiency or severe combined immunodeficiency), extensive crypt apoptotic activity, or absence of goblet and Paneth cells (as in AIE).

Ulcerative Colitis

UC is an idiopathic chronic inflammatory disease that begins in the rectum and extends proximally and contiguously for a variable distance. In a given patient, disease may be limited to the rectum, involve only the left colon, or involve the right colon as well. A fluctuating clinical course with exacerbations and remissions is typical. A fulminant presentation with toxic megacolon is also seen. UC is limited to the colon, although in patients with active pancolitis, mild inflammation may also involve the mucosa of the distal few centimeters of the terminal ileum (the so-called backwash ileitis).

Diarrhea and rectal bleeding are the presenting symptoms in nearly all cases of UC, although abdominal pain, cramping, anorexia, and weight loss are also frequently seen. A small percentage of patients have a fulminant presentation, with acute abdominal signs and toxic megacolon. As many as 20% of children have extraintestinal manifestations, with arthritis of the large joints being the most common; uveitis, growth failure, skin involvement, and liver disease are more unusual. Infections (e.g., with *Shigella*, *Salmonella*, *C. difficile*, *Yersinia*, and *E. histolytica*) must be ruled out, and radiologic investigation, including barium enema and radiography of the upper gastrointestinal tract with small-bowel followthrough, is undertaken to determine the extent and type of disease. Endoscopic features of UC include mucosal hyperemia, friability, and ulceration beginning at the rectum and extending proximally. Biopsy specimens taken at multiple levels during colonoscopy are important in diagnosing the disease, monitoring its progress, and evaluating the response to therapy.

Pathologic findings in the first endoscopic biopsy specimens from a given patient may not be diagnostic by themselves, but they are extremely helpful in arriving at a diagnosis when integrated with clinical and radiologic findings. In most cases of untreated UC, the mucosal biopsy specimen shows diffusely increased numbers of chronic inflammatory cells (plasma cells and lymphocytes) and acute inflammatory cells (polymorphonuclear leukocytes and eosinophils) in the lamina propria. Plasma cells dominate the inflammatory response, often densely packing the lamina propria and extending beneath crypts (basal plasmacytosis). Crypt abscesses and intraepithelial neutrophils may be present at the initial diagnosis and during exacerbations. Superficial ulcerations may be seen, but even in their absence, damage to the surface epithelium is nearly always indicated by the presence of regenerating epithelial cells without goblet cells.

In normal colonic mucosa, the crypts are arranged in straight and evenly spaced rows. Even at the time of the initial presentation of UC, with symptoms of short duration, biopsies of involved segments will usually exhibit distortion of this normal crypt architecture. This is typically manifested by scattered branched and irregularly shaped crypts, as well as crypts that no longer extend all the way down to the muscularis mucosae (Figure 14-43). Assessment of crypt architecture is much easier in well-oriented biopsies. In poorly oriented biopsies, the crypts are usually seen in cross section as doughnut-shaped profiles, which makes it difficult to evaluate branching and foreshortening. However, irregular spacing and variation in crypt diameter may still be observed in tangential sections. A feature often associated with crypt architectural distortion is the presence of Paneth cell metaplasia. Paneth cells are normally present in the mucosa throughout the small intestine but in the colon are limited to crypts of the cecum and ascending colon, except in the infant in whom they can extend to the distal colon. In patients with inactive disease of very long duration, crypt architectural distortion may become very subtle, to the point where the histologic (and endoscopic) appearance may be indistinguishable from normal. In this situation, review of biopsies obtained during previous colonoscopic procedures may be necessary to confirm a diagnosis of IBD.

A number of studies suggest that initial rectal biopsies in children with UC may not demonstrate mucosal architectural

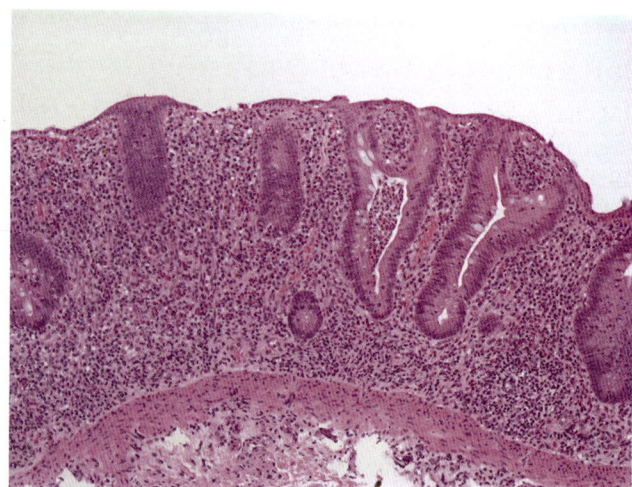

FIGURE 14-43 • Colonic biopsy demonstrating active ulcerative colitis. Note the presence of crypt architectural distortion with a crypt microabscess and a basal infiltrate of lymphocytes and plasma cells between the bases of the crypts and the muscularis mucosae 100×.

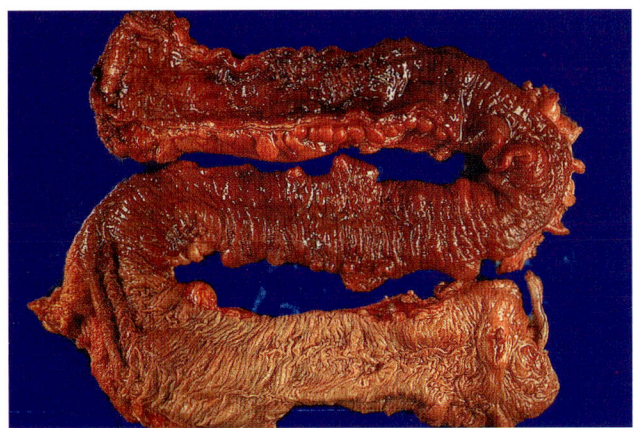

FIGURE 14-44 • Total abdominal colectomy specimen from a patient with ulcerative colitis involving the left colon.

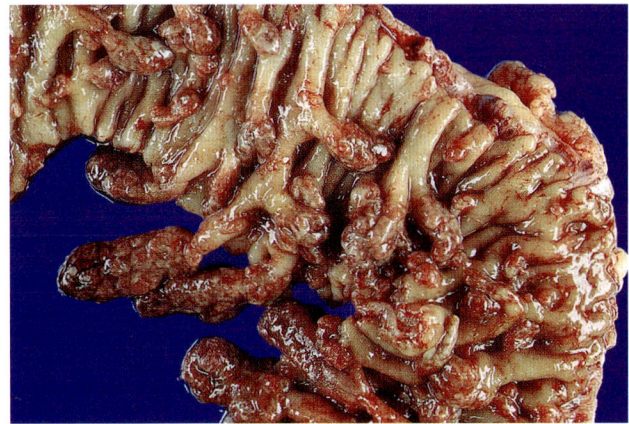

FIGURE 14-45 • Ulcerative colitis with inflammatory polyps.

changes as consistently as in adults or may even be "normal" (rectal sparing) (192). An unequivocal diagnosis of IBD may be more difficult in these cases, as may be distinction between UC and CD. Distinguishing between the two early on, however, may not be critical as the initial medical therapy is similar. No clinical feature appears to separate children who present with rectal sparing from those who do not.

The distinctive features of UC are better visualized in colonic resection specimens. Surgery, usually a total proctocolectomy, cures the disease. Surgery is performed in UC for either acute or chronic indications, including massive bleeding, acute fulminant colitis with megacolon, a chronic course with severe disability or complications of medical therapy, and retardation of growth and sexual maturation. The most commonly performed procedure in children with UC is the ileal pouch anal anastomosis (IPAA). It is imperative to distinguish UC from CD prior to surgical intervention because patients with CD who undergo IPAA often have a poor outcome. UC is most often characterized by uninterrupted mucosal involvement beginning at the rectum and extending proximally in a circumferential and contiguous manner. The mucosa is usually diffusely hyperemic and granular, with areas of superficial or deep ulceration in patients under poor medical control at the time of colectomy (Figure 14-44). Inflammatory polyps may be present and in some cases are numerous (Figure 14-45). The ileal mucosa is generally grossly unremarkable. The rectum and descending colon may show more chronic changes, such as loss of the haustral folds and a smooth or granular mucosal surface. Conspicuously absent are skip (uninvolved) areas, strictures, fistulas, and fibrotic thickening of the colonic wall, all of which are commonly seen in CD.

Histologic examination reveals inflammation that most severely affects the mucosa and submucosa, with lesser severity or sparing of the muscularis layers and serosa. Extensively ulcerated areas show mucosal and submucosal destruction, with replacement by granulation tissue. Inflammatory polyps are composed of islands of surviving mucosa with pronounced glandular distortion, inflammation, and capillary dilatation. After the acute inflammation has subsided and healing has occurred, evidence of UC remains as loss of crypt parallelism, crypt atrophy and shortening, hypertrophy of the muscularis mucosae, and metaplasia of Paneth cells. The appendix is commonly involved in resected specimens even when the cecum is spared, an exception to the diffuse contiguous involvement characteristic of UC. In a recent study, 29 of 367 patients with UC who did not have a pancolitis and had no prior appendectomy were found to have periappendiceal inflammation, the severity of which paralleled that of the distal colon (193). Additionally, discontinuous involvement and rectal healing have been reported during the course of long-standing disease in adults. Microscopic examination of endoscopically normal mucosa in patients with treated UC usually reveals evidence of quiescent disease, as indicated by the presence of (sometimes subtle) crypt architectural distortion. Although UC is classically limited to the colon, some patients with pancolitis may exhibit the so-called backwash ileitis. "Backwash ileitis" generally consists only of scattered neutrophils in the lamina propria and surface epithelium, with relative preservation of the mucosal architecture. However, the spectrum of ileal mucosal damage in backwash ileitis is currently not well defined.

Colonic malignancy is a well-recognized long-term complication of UC, with the risk of cancer increasing over that of the general population by 1% each year after 10 years of disease. However, there is a paucity of prospective data describing long-term IBD with early-onset UC and ultimate cancer risk in pediatric patients. Other less well-characterized risk factors include concomitant sclerosing cholangitis; an excluded, defunctionalized or bypassed segment; and depressed red blood cell folate levels. Children who develop colitis before the age of 10 years should undergo colonoscopy screening during their adolescence, and dysplasia and adenocarcinoma have been documented in adolescents and young adults with long-standing colitis (194). Dysplasia in colitis is generally plaquelike or nodular, frequently referred to as the DALM (dysplasia-associated lesion or mass) lesion. Epithelial dysplasia generally precedes carcinoma; therefore, yearly surveillance colonoscopy is recommended.

Crohn Disease

In contrast to UC, CD may arise anywhere in the gastrointestinal tract, from mouth to anus. In approximately 50% of children with CD, the classic distal ileal and proximal colonic involvement is seen. Approximately 15% of children have only diffuse small-bowel disease, another 15% have only distal ileal involvement, and 10% have isolated colonic disease. The remaining 10% have disease in another site, as in gastroduodenal CD, or a combination of sites.

Symptoms depend on the site of involvement, but in general, the presentation of CD is more insidious than that of UC, so that the diagnosis is often delayed. Vague abdominal pain, diarrhea, growth failure, and anorexia are common. Small-bowel involvement may present as diarrhea and malabsorption. Colonic involvement may present as bloody diarrhea and mimic UC. Diffuse colitis is not an uncommon presentation of CD in the pediatric age group. Endoscopic and radiologic studies of the upper and lower gastrointestinal tract are important in determining the extent of involvement.

Unlike UC, CD is characterized by a segmental or skip pattern, in which involved areas of intestine are often separated by normal intestine. Another important distinguishing feature is that the inflammation in CD is transmural rather than mucosal, so that fissures, fistulas, intramural abscesses, strictures, and fibrous adhesions develop (Figure 14-46). Thickening of the bowel wall as a result of edema and fibrosis occurs at the expense of the lumen and causes intestinal obstruction. Inflammation, edema, and fibrosis of the bowel and regional lymph nodes may cause adjacent structures to mat together and form an ileocecal mass. Perianal fissures, skin tags, and rectal–perineal fistulas and abscesses are common in children with CD.

Endoscopic examination in CD usually confirms the patchy involvement with intervening areas of normal mucosa. Ulcerations are often linear, with intervening preserved mucosal islands, resulting in a cobblestone appearance. Small (<5 mm), round, superficial "aphthoid" ulcerations are common in otherwise normal mucosa at the periphery of more severely involved segments. In Crohn colitis, the right side of the colon is often more severely affected than the left, and the rectum may be completely spared.

Mucosal biopsy specimens in CD show increased numbers of chronic and acute inflammatory cells in the lamina propria, crypt abscesses, and superficial ulcerations, all of which are nondiagnostic in the absence of granulomas. In many cases, the degree of crypt architectural distortion is less severe in CD than is typical of UC, but confident distinction between the two diseases cannot rest on the assessment of this feature. Relative preservation of the mucin content

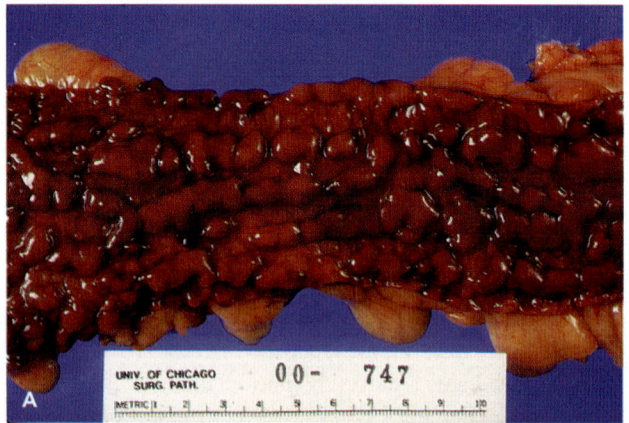
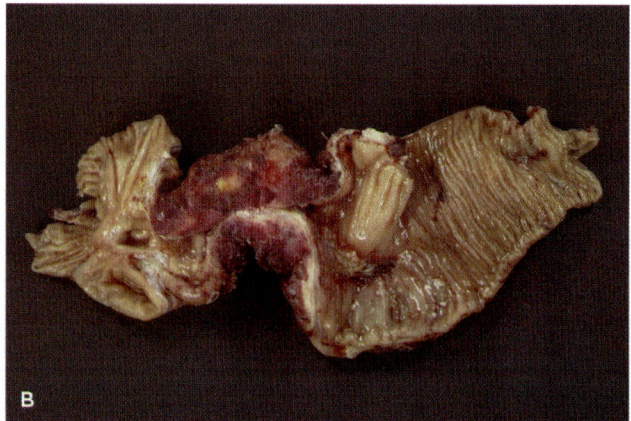
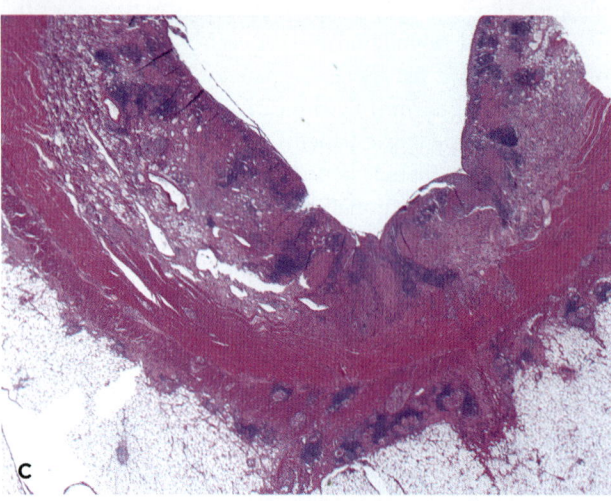

FIGURE 14-46 • **A:** Crohn enteritis with cobblestoned mucosa. **B:** Crohn enteritis with a stricture at the terminal ileum. Note the thickened bowel wall and serpiginous ulcer extending more proximally in the ileum. **C:** Crohn enteritis showing transmural inflammation 10x.

of goblet cells, even in cases of severe inflammation, is also more characteristic of Crohn colitis than UC. The histologic hallmark of CD is the presence of nonnecrotizing epithelioid granulomas (eFigure 14-11). Granulomas are virtually diagnostic of CD when they are well formed, nonnecrotic, basally situated, and remote from areas of active inflammation. Their presence in biopsies may predate radiologic evidence of disease, and prolonged follow-up is necessary when they are observed in the absence of grossly evident disease. The likelihood of finding granulomas is clearly a function of the diligence with which they are sought, increasing with the number of biopsies and sections examined. In a study at The Children's Hospital of Philadelphia, granulomas were identified in 61% of pediatric CD patients undergoing upper and lower endoscopy and were more frequent in untreated patients (195). In nearly half of those patients, granulomas were present in the upper GI tract, in the terminal ileum, or both, but not in the colon. However, colonic granulomas can also be seen in a number of other conditions. Relatively common sources of confusion are the poorly formed granulomas that occur in association with ruptured crypt abscesses in UC, presumably in response to extravasated mucin. Examination of serial sections may be necessary to demonstrate the relationship between the damaged crypt and the granuloma (eFigure 14-12). The granulomas seen in tuberculous infections of the gastrointestinal tract are typically multiple and large and have caseous necrosis (196). Those associated with yersiniosis are also necrotic and frequently present in mesenteric lymph nodes. CGD can present with a colitis similar to CD. Numerous necrotizing granulomas are also observed in this condition; in noninflamed or quiescent cases, collections of pigmented macrophages may be noted in the mucosa. Presentation at a relatively young age and a history of repeated infections are important clues to the diagnosis.

Transmural chronic inflammation is the most helpful histologic feature in a resected intestinal specimen from a patient with CD (Figure 14-46C). Deep knifelike fissures, fistulas lined by granulation tissue, and fibrous strictures are also characteristic. Submucosal fibrosis and the presence of many lymphoid aggregates or follicles also suggest CD rather than UC.

The histologic features of Crohn ileitis are essentially identical to those evident in colonic biopsies. There is usually clear-cut distortion of normal villous architecture at least focally. Mucous (pyloric) gland metaplasia is a reliable marker of long-standing inflammation and is common in ileal biopsies from patients with CD (Figure 14-47). Disease of the upper intestinal tract is well documented in CD and present in 30% of patients, in whom it may cause functional abnormalities such as delayed gastric emptying. More recent studies based on endoscopic biopsies of the upper GI tract in children with IBD have revealed a comparable prevalence of esophagitis, duodenal ulcers, and villus atrophy in both CD and UC (197,198). Recent studies have reported that focally enhanced gastritis, defined as a perifoveolar or periglandular

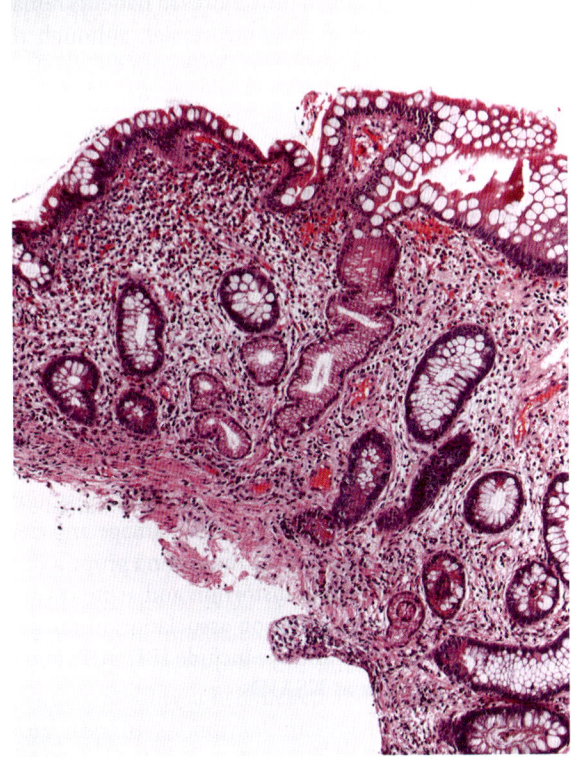

FIGURE 14-47 • Crohn ileitis. Pyloric metaplasia (100×).

mononuclear or neutrophilic infiltrate around gastric crypts, is significantly more common in CD than in UC in patients without *H. pylori* (199,200).

The early medical treatment of CD is similar to that of UC. Surgery is not curative in CD and is generally undertaken only when intestinal obstruction, fistulas, massive hemorrhage, or abscesses supervene. Growth failure while the patient is on medical therapy and failure of medical therapy may also be reasons for a limited surgical resection.

Indeterminate Colitis

The term indeterminate colitis (IC) as originally used by Price (201) was applied to cases presenting in adults as severe or "fulminant" colitis with overlapping features of UC and CD. Gradually, this term has come to describe patients with chronic colitis when definitive features of CD or UC are absent. IC is thus often used as a temporary designation until evolution of the disease provides further clues, such as the development of granulomas, fistulas, or gastroduodenal or perineal involvement in CD. In a small percentage of patients, the distinction between CD and UC is extremely difficult or impossible, even after a chronic course and colonic resection. IC is also encountered in pediatric IBD; in one study, 5% of newly diagnosed cases of pediatric IBD were classified as IC (202). Younger patients, less than 5 years of age, are more likely to be diagnosed with IC (203). In the latter study, after a median follow-up of 7 years, 5 of 19 cases, initially assigned a diagnosis of IC, were reclassified as either CD or UC.

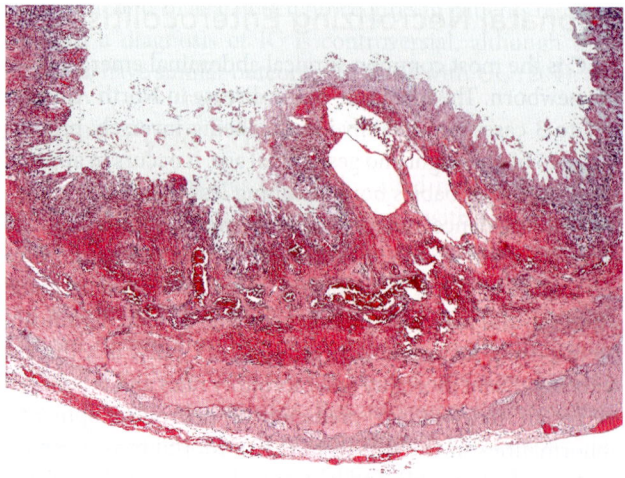

FIGURE 14-49 • Necrotizing enterocolitis. This section from a resected portion of small bowel reveals extensive mucosal necrosis and submucosal hemorrhage. Note the large air spaces in the submucosa consistent with pneumatosis cystoides 40×.

Inflammation, when present, is usually slight. Pneumatosis intestinalis (air in the bowel wall) is found in approximately half of the resected specimens; the air is believed to result from bacterial fermentation and is evidence for the role played by bacterial colonization. Focal reparative changes, such as granulation tissue formation, may also be found. Though some advocate the use of perioperative frozen sections to assess the viability of resection margins, the surgical practice at our institution and many others is to resect only unquestionably necrotic bowel. Major gastrointestinal medium- and long-term complications include strictures in up to one-third of patients (216), short gut syndrome and intestinal malabsorption, and chronic liver disease resulting from TPN. NEC is reported to recur in 4% to 6% of cases, usually within 1 month of the initial episode (216).

Spontaneous Perforation of the Gastrointestinal Tract

Isolated spontaneous perforation of the gastrointestinal tract in premature and term neonates occurs occasionally as a clinical event distinct from neonatal NEC. It is usually an unexpected event in an infant not known to have any prior gastrointestinal compromise. The perforation develops in a single location in almost any part of the stomach, small intestine, or colon, and at laparotomy, the damage to surrounding tissue is inapparent or minimal. Risk factors associated with this disease include early postnatal steroids and use of indomethacin for medical closure of a patent ductus arteriosus (217). In some cases, a localized segmental absence or thinning of the muscularis externa has been observed (218), which could represent either a congenital abnormality or a consequence of excessive distension of muscle fibers or localized ischemia caused by a drug, a transient local decrease in splanchnic circulation, or a combination of these factors. Cases have also been observed as a complication of anorectal malformations (219).

Allergic Colitis (Allergic Proctocolitis)

Allergic proctitis/colitis is a disease of infants, presenting during the first 2 months of life with rectal bleeding shortly after the introduction of cow's milk or soy protein formulae. It also commonly occurs in breast-fed infants, in whom cow's milk protein ingested by the mother is the triggering agent in breast milk (220). Growth is usually not affected, and peripheral eosinophilia is variable. Exclusion of other causes of rectal bleeding, such as infection, NEC, intussusception, and anal fissure, is essential. Biopsies may be performed to rule out Hirschsprung disease in those infants presenting primarily with constipation. Endoscopic features include erythema, mucosal friability, and focal erosions and nodularity, the latter suggestive of nodular lymphoid hyperplasia. Disease is usually limited to the distal colon. Eosinophils may be observed in stool smears, which should also be obtained to rule out parasitic infection. The presence of focal eosinophilic cryptitis with damage to crypt epithelium, eosinophilic crypt abscesses, or infiltration of fibers of the muscularis mucosa are features helpful in confirming the diagnosis when sheets of lamina propria eosinophils are not present (Figure 14-50A, B). The mucosal architecture is well preserved, and significant crypt architectural distortion is distinctly unusual and, if present, should suggest other disorders. Nodular lymphoid hyperplasia is a frequent concomitant finding.

The treatment is dietary change to a "hypoallergenic" formula. The condition is temporary, with most patients able to tolerate milk after 2 years of age.

Solitary Rectal Ulcer Syndrome

Solitary rectal ulcer syndrome (SRUS) is an uncommon disorder, which involves chronic, complete, or incomplete prolapse of the rectum with ulceration. The etiology is unclear; however, SRUS is thought to occur as a result of high intrarectal pressure during voiding, resulting in prolapse of the rectum with subsequent ischemia and ulcer formation (221). Because the symptoms of SRUS overlap with more common pediatric disorders such as constipation and IBD, the diagnosis is often delayed and misdiagnosis is common.

The presenting symptoms of SRUS are highly variable. Perianal pain with defecation is common. Because the symptoms are nonspecific, the diagnosis of SRUS is dependent upon an endoscopic and histologic assessment. Interestingly, the term SRUS is actually a misnomer as less than one-third of patients demonstrate one, single ulcer on endoscopic examination (222); some patients present only with hyperemic rectal mucosa while others present with ulcers of varying size and number. The histologic findings can also be variable. Blackburn and colleagues reported histologic features such as crypt hyperplasia, lamina propria fibrosis, thickening of muscularis mucosa with muscular extension into lamina propria, ulceration, and surface architectural changes with mucin depletion or villous transformation (221).

The treatment of SRUS involves avoidance of constipation with stool softeners and laxatives and also behavioral

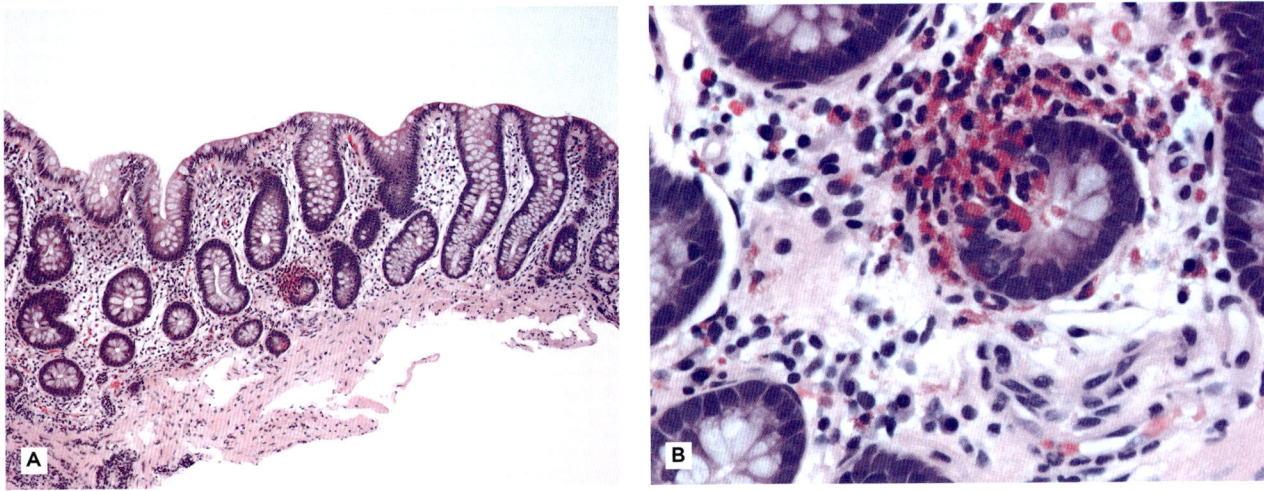

FIGURE 14-50 • Eosinophilic colitis due to food allergy in an infant. **A:** Normal crypt architecture is maintained 100×. **B:** Eosinophilic infiltrates can be quite patchy 400×.

modification. Compliance with behavioral modification has been associated with good outcome (221).

INTESTINAL NEOPLASMS

Primary intestinal tumors are uncommon in children, and most of them are not malignant. Many childhood intestinal masses prove not to be neoplasms but rather inflammatory processes, such as ileocecal CD, or developmental anomalies, such as duplication cyst or pancreatic heterotopia. Except for polyps, epithelial lesions are unusual, in contrast to their frequent occurrence in the adult intestine. Hereditary syndromes should be kept in mind when certain types of gastrointestinal polyps and tumors appear in children as these are associated with an increased risk for gastrointestinal and other malignancies (Table 14-8). Primary intestinal malignancies are rare in children, representing less than 5% of pediatric neoplasms. The most common category of intestinal malignancy in children is non-Hodgkin lymphoma, particularly Burkitt lymphoma. Colorectal carcinoma is the second most common, followed by neuroendocrine tumors.

Juvenile Polyps and Juvenile Polyposis Syndrome

Juvenile (or retention) polyps of the rectosigmoid colon are the most commonly encountered gastrointestinal neoplasms in children. Isolated juvenile polyps occur in about 2% of children ages 1 to 18, with a peak incidence between 2 and 5 years. More than half occur in the rectosigmoid colon, with an approximately equal distribution in the rest of the colon, and about half the patients have more than one polyp at colonoscopy (223). Juvenile polyposis is an autosomal dominant syndrome that occurs at an incidence of approximately 1:100,000 individuals. It is likely when 3 to 5 or more juvenile polyps are found or if any number of juvenile polyps (even one) are found in a patient with a family history of juvenile polyposis (224). In most cases of juvenile polyposis, 50 to 200 polyps may be found; however, the number of polyps can be in the thousands. In addition, the presence of extracolonic juvenile polyps is usually associated with a polyposis syndrome.

There are three major clinical forms of juvenile polyposis: **juvenile polyposis coli**, **juvenile gastrointestinal polyposis**, and **familial juvenile polyposis** of the stomach. Juvenile polyposis coli is the most common of the three and is usually diagnosed in the first decade of life in children with multiple colonic polyps and occasionally small-bowel juvenile polyps, but without polyps elsewhere in the alimentary tract. Juvenile polyposis may be associated with other alimentary tract and extraintestinal anomalies, such as hypertelorism, malrotation, hydrocephalus, undescended testes, and Meckel diverticulum (225). In juvenile gastrointestinal polyposis, polyps are found in the stomach and small bowel, in addition to the colon. In familial juvenile polyposis of the stomach, juvenile polyps are limited to the stomach, where they consist of hyperplastic gastric glands and resemble gastric hyperplastic polyps. All of these forms of juvenile polyposis can be familial. A fourth type, **juvenile polyposis of infancy**, is a rare juvenile polyposis that typically presents before age two and is often associated with PLE and death in the first year of life (225). Approximately 50% to 60% of cases of juvenile polyposis syndrome have been associated with gremline mutations or deletions of two genes of the TGF-beta signaling pathway, the SMAD4 gene located on chromosome 18q21 and the BMPR1a gene on chromosome 10q23. In addition to juvenile polyposis, juvenile polyps are seen in CS, Ruvalcaba syndrome, Cronkhite-Canada syndrome, and Gorlin syndrome.

Colonic juvenile polyps consist of hyperplastic and cystically dilated crypts set in an abundant edematous and markedly inflamed stroma. Isolated juvenile polyps are usually sessile and extensively eroded, resulting in the formation of abundant superficial granulation tissue (Figure 14-51A, B). This produces a highly characteristic strawberry-like

TABLE 14-8 POLYPOSIS SYNDROMES

Syndrome	Gene Defect	Usual Age When Polyps Manifest Clinically	Histology	Polyp Location	Risk of GI Cancer
Juvenile polyposis syndromes	SMAD4 BMPR1A				
Juvenile polyposis coli		Childhood	Juvenile	Colon, occasional small bowel	Increased
Familial juvenile polyposis of the stomach		Childhood	Hyperplastic gastric	Stomach	Low
Juvenile gastrointestinal polyposis		Childhood	Juvenile	Colon, stomach, small bowel	Increased
Juvenile polyposis of infancy		Infancy	Juvenile	Colon, stomach, small bowel	Increased
Peutz-Jeghers syndrome	LKB1 (STK11)	Adolescence	Hamartomatous	Small bowel, colon, stomach	Increased
Cronkhite-Canada syndrome	Unknown, probably not genetic	Adulthood	Juvenile (colon) Hyperplastic (stomach)	Stomach, small bowel, colon, esophagus	Low
PTEN hamartoma syndrome	PTEN	Adulthood	Mixed; juvenile and hamartomatous	Entire GI tract	Low
Cowden syndrome					
Bannayan-Riley-Ruvalcaba syndrome		Adulthood	Mixed; juvenile and hamartomatous	Ileum, colon	Low
Familial adenomatous polyposis (including Gardner and Turcot syndrome)	APC	Adolescence	Adenomatous (colon) Hamartomatous (stomach)	Small bowel, stomach	Extremely high (colon) Increased in small bowel, stomach

From Pawel B. Polyps and tumors of the gastrointestinal tract in children. In: Russo P, Ruchelli E, Piccoli D, eds. *Pathology of Pediatric Gastrointestinal and Liver Disease*. Heidelberg, Germany: Springer; 2014:317–370, with permission.

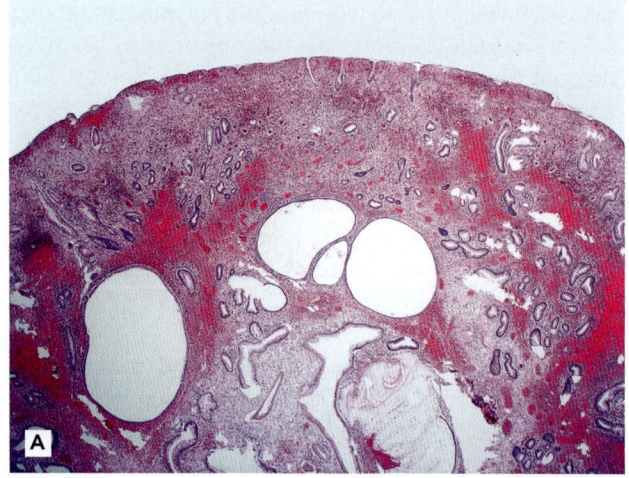
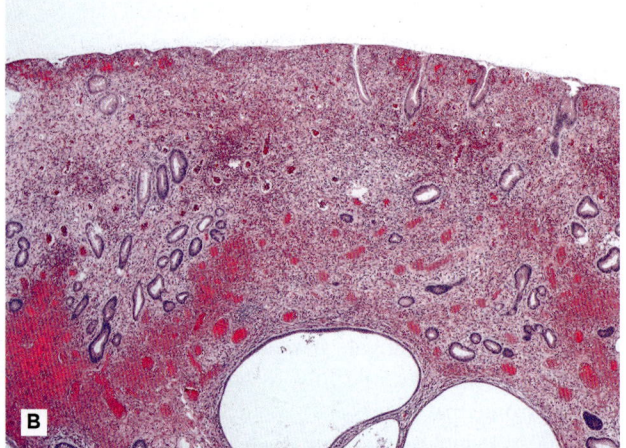

FIGURE 14-51 • A, B: Sporadic juvenile polyps usually exhibit cystically dilated crypts, abundant edematous and inflamed stroma with numerous eosinophils, and surface erosion. **A:** 40×, **B:** 100×.

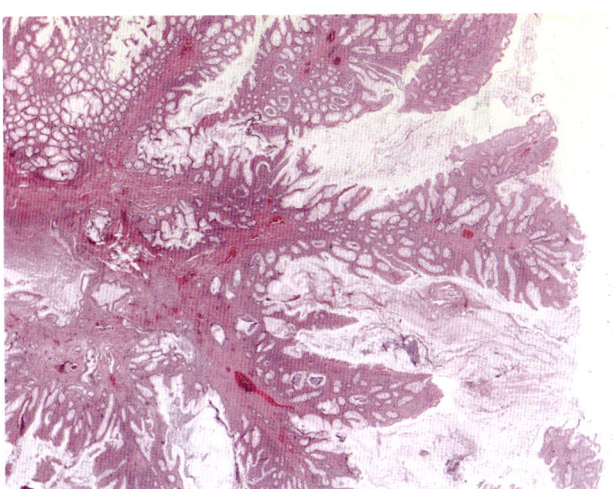

FIGURE 14-52 • Juvenile polyposis syndrome in which the polyps typically exhibit greater epithelial proliferation, less stroma, and an intact surface epithelium 20×.

endoscopic appearance. The polyps in patients with the juvenile polyposis syndrome, in contrast, often lack this extensive surface erosion and may have a more pedunculated configuration. In addition, there is usually a greater amount of the epithelial component and less of the stromal elements in the syndromic polyps (Figure 14-52). In contrast to colonic Peutz-Jeghers polyps, an arborizing core of smooth muscle is usually not present, although a few smooth muscle fibers may be evident if the polyp has been prolapsing. In small polyps, the crypt hyperplasia and stromal edema and inflammation may be minimal, making accurate recognition difficult. Dysplasia does occur rarely in the polyps of patients with colonic juvenile polyposis polyps, but great care must be taken to avoid overcalling reactive changes related to the inflammatory background (Figure 14-53A, B).

Isolated gastric juvenile polyps are rare but are present in up to 25% of patients with generalized juvenile polyposis coli. Gastric juvenile polyps are histologically similar to their colonic counterparts. There is disorganized hyperplasia and cystic dilatation of the gastric foveolar epithelium set in a background of inflamed and edematous stroma (Figure 14-54A, B). Unfortunately, these same features also characterize sporadic gastric hyperplastic polyps, and histologic distinction is generally not possible. Sporadic gastric hyperplastic polyps can be multiple and do not always occur in a background of diffuse gastritis, which makes separation from gastric involvement by juvenile polyposis even more problematic. Furthermore, gastric Peutz-Jeghers polyps often have a very poorly developed core of arborizing smooth muscle fibers and therefore can also closely resemble gastric juvenile polyps. These confounding factors suggest that histologic classification of hamartomatous polyps is best performed by analysis of small-bowel or colonic polyps. If gastric polyps are discovered first, the prudent course for the surgical pathologist is to suggest the possibility of a polyposis syndrome and to recommend examination for small-bowel or colonic polyps. Gastric juvenile polyps may also develop dysplastic changes, but once again, care must be taken not to mistaken reactive epithelial changes due to inflammation for dysplasia.

Involvement of the small bowel by juvenile polyposis is less common than colonic and gastric involvement, and the polyps are less often sampled endoscopically. Small-intestinal juvenile polyps lack the well-developed core of smooth muscle of Peutz-Jeghers polyps and are generally much more inflamed, so accurate distinction is usually not problematic.

Patients with isolated juvenile polyps have no increased risk of carcinoma. There is a significant lifetime risk of malignancy in patients with juvenile polyposis syndrome, including cancers of the pancreas, stomach, small bowel, and colon. One study of the risk of colorectal cancer yielded an absolute risk of 38.7 per 100 affected persons and a relative risk of 34 times compared to the general population (226).

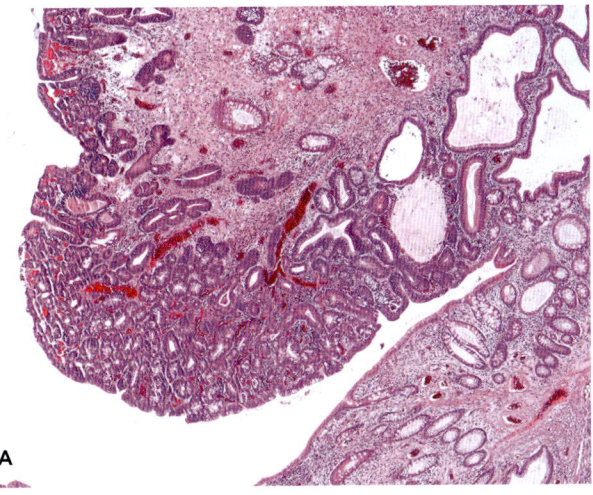
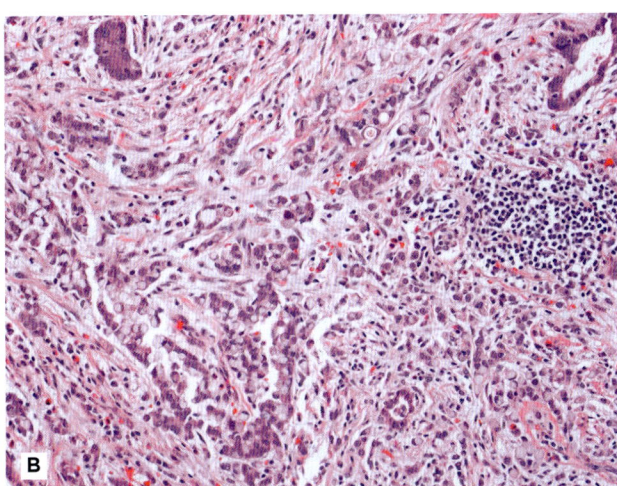

FIGURE 14-53 • Juvenile polyposis syndrome. **A:** Colonic polyp with a focus of high-grade dysplasia 40×. **B:** Focus of invasive signet ring adenocarcinoma in a colonic polyp from an adult patient 200×.

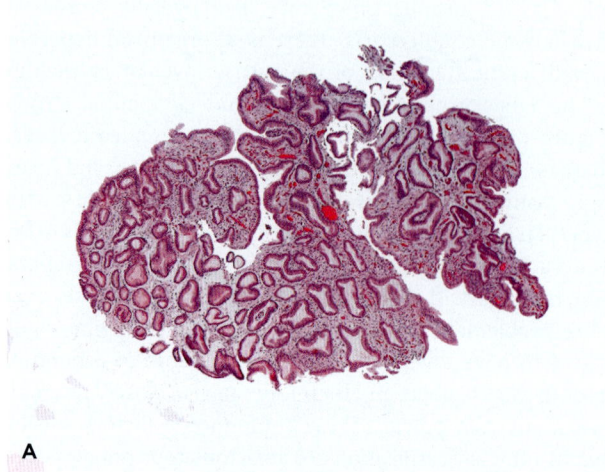 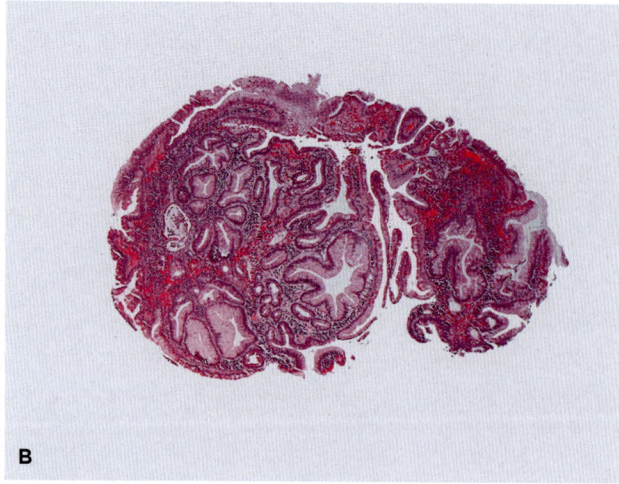

FIGURE 14-54 • Juvenile polyposis syndrome. **A:** The gastric polyps in this syndrome closely resemble sporadic gastric hyperplastic polyps 40x. **B:** This duodenal polyp lacks the central core of smooth muscle typical of small-bowel Peutz-Jeghers polyps 40x.

PTEN Hamartoma Tumor Syndrome

A number of clinical syndromes including hamartomatous gastrointestinal polyps have been linked to mutations in the PTEN (phosphatase and tensin homologue) tumor suppressor gene located on chromosome 10q23.3, including CS, Bannayan-Riley-Ruvalcaba syndrome (BRRS), adult Lhermitte-Duclos disease (LDD), and autism spectrum disorder associated with macrocephaly (227). The best characterized of these disorders is CS, an autosomal dominant disorder with hamartomatous lesions involving multiple organ systems, as well as a substantially increased risk of thyroid, breast, and endometrial cancer. Mucocutaneous lesions, including multiple facial trichilemmomas, acrokeratosis, and papillomas (particularly of the oral cavity), are pathognomonic features of the syndrome. Although it has been reported that PTEN mutations are found in 80% of patients with a clinical diagnosis of CS, the actual number is probably far less. BRRS is clinically characterized by macrocephaly, pigmented penile macules, lipomas, and gastrointestinal hamartomas. Additionally described features include developmental delay, thyroiditis, proximal muscle myopathy, vascular anomalies, and joint hyperextensibility. However, because these lesions can also occur sporadically in the general population, diagnosis requires finding multiple such lesions or additional features of the syndrome. Diagnostic criteria for PTEN hamartoma syndrome have been recently proposed (227).

Because the gastrointestinal hamartomas are usually asymptomatic and documentation of their presence is not necessary to establish a diagnosis of either CS or Bannayan-Ruvalcaba-Riley syndrome, the incidence of polyps in these disorders is not known precisely. In one recent study of patients with CS, gastrointestinal polyps were identified in 93% of patients who underwent endoscopic screening, involving the both upper and lower GI tract in about 20% (228). These polyps are multiple, and the most common type is the juvenile polyp, though other reported types include hamartomatous, adenomatous, ganglioneuromas, and inflammatory polyps. Recent reports have also shown an increased risk for colon cancer. The esophagus in PTEN is characterized by glycogenic acanthosis (see Chapter 24-5 for other PTEN findings).

Peutz-Jeghers Polyposis Syndrome

Peutz-Jeghers syndrome is an autosomal dominant disorder with an estimated incidence of 1:120,000 in the general population. It is characterized by the development of mucocutaneous hyperpigmentation, hamartomatous polyps throughout the gastrointestinal tract, and an increased risk of malignancy at many sites. The median age of onset of symptoms caused by the gastrointestinal polyps is 13 years of age. Presenting symptoms include bowel obstruction, intussusception, and gastrointestinal bleeding or anemia. Recognition of the characteristic hyperpigmented macules can also lead to proper diagnosis. They occur most often on the lips, buccal mucosa, or periorbital skin but can also develop on the skin of the fingers, palms, and soles, genitalia, and perianally. The macules are not present in infancy; they may fade with age, although intraoral lesions tend to persist.

More than 90% of patients have a detectable mutation in the SKT11 gene on chromosome 19p13.3. About 25% of patients present with *de novo* mutations. The protein product is a serine/threonine kinase that is expressed ubiquitously in human tissues. It regulates a number of downstream kinases and has important roles in the cellular response to energy stress and in the establishment of cell polarity.

The hamartomatous polyps occur primarily in the small bowel (92%) but can also develop in the colon (30%) and stomach (25%). Hamartomatous polyps may also occur in the nasal cavity, bladder, and lungs. The burden of gastrointestinal polyps is usually lower than in juvenile polyposis syndrome; often, less than 10 polyps are present. By WHO

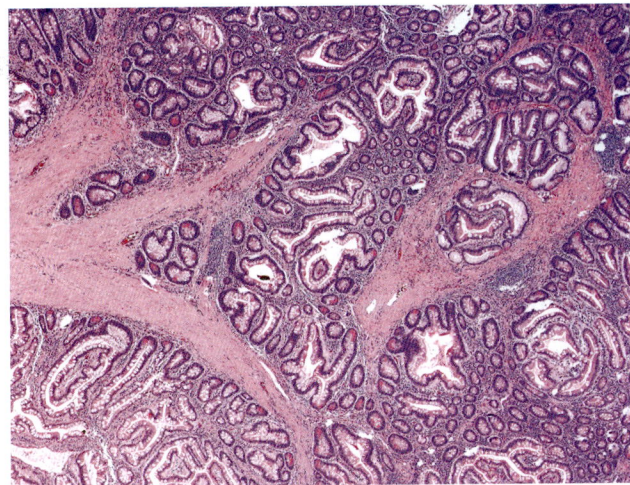

FIGURE 14-55 • Peutz-Jeghers polyp. Jejunal polyp with hyperplastic and disorganized mucosal elements and the characteristic central arborizing core of smooth muscle 40×.

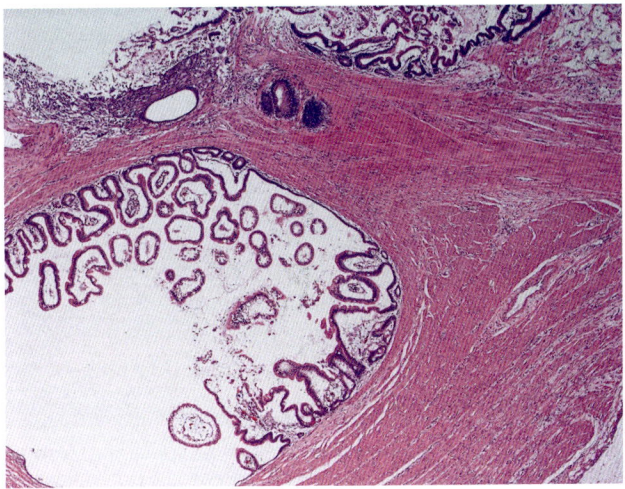

FIGURE 14-56 • Jejunal Peutz-Jeghers polyp. Displacement of epithelial elements into the muscularis can be confused with invasive adenocarcinoma, particularly in frozen sections, but the epithelium is clearly benign 40×.

criteria, in patients with a positive family history, the diagnosis is established by the presence of even one histologically confirmed Peutz-Jeghers polyp or by the presence of the characteristic mucocutaneous pigmentation. In the absence of a family history, the diagnosis can be established by finding three or more histologically confirmed Peutz-Jeghers polyps or by finding even one such polyp in a patient with prominent mucocutaneous pigmentation (225). Peutz-Jeghers polyps are rarely reported outside the setting of this syndrome (229).

The characteristic histologic features are best developed in Peutz-Jeghers polyps of the small intestine. The arborizing central core of haphazardly arranged smooth muscle bundles is the most distinctive feature. The epithelial elements are hyperplastic and disorganized. The inflammatory component is sparse when compared to juvenile polyps, and stromal edema is not prominent (Figure 14-55). Displacement of the hyperplastic epithelial component into the deeper bowel layers is not uncommon, particularly in larger polyps that have caused bowel obstruction or intussusception (Figure 14-56). Herniation of the epithelium into submucosa or muscularis propria can be confused with invasive adenocarcinoma, an error that can be avoided by the recognition of accompanying lamina propria with the displaced glands.

Peutz-Jeghers polyps of the stomach and colon often do not exhibit a prominent central core of arborizing smooth muscle and therefore can be confused with the more common juvenile polyps at these sites. They are less inflamed and edematous than juvenile polyps, but accurate diagnosis is problematic unless small-bowel polyps are also present. While there is a significant increased risk of gastrointestinal malignancy in patients with Peutz-Jeghers syndrome, dysplasia and cancer development within the polyps themselves is rare. Individuals with Peutz-Jeghers syndrome have a significantly increased risk of both benign and malignant neoplasms, with breast cancer having the highest specific disease risk (224). Other associated neoplasms include pancreatic carcinoma, adenoma malignum (minimal deviation adenocarcinoma) of the uterus, testicular Sertoli cell tumor, and ovarian sex cord tumor with annular tubules (SCTAT).

Adenomatous Polyps and Adenocarcinoma

Adenomatous polyps are true neoplasms and are rare in children. When identified in a child, even a single adenomatous polyp should prompt consideration of familial adenomatous polyposis and related syndromes. Familial adenomatous polyposis (adenomatous polyposis coli), the most common of the polyposis syndromes, is an autosomal dominant disorder with an incidence of 1 in 8000 persons. Approximately one-third of the cases are sporadic. FAP is caused by a mutation of the *APC* (adenomatous polyposis coli) gene located at 5q21, with a nearly 100% penetrance of germline mutations. **Gardner syndrome** is a variant of FAP, characterized clinically by the development of osteomas and varied soft tissue tumors, including epidermal cysts, lipomas, fibromas, and desmoids tumors, in addition to intestinal adenomatous polyposis. The APC gene mutation in Gardner syndrome is at a different location than in FAP unassociated with desmoids. **Turcot syndrome** refers to intestinal polyposis coexisting with tumors of the central nervous system, namely, medulloblastomas and glioblastomas.

In patients with familial adenomatous polyposis, hundreds of adenomatous polyps usually carpet the colonic mucosa (Figure 14-57). The disease may become symptomatic in adolescents, usually causing diarrhea and abdominal pain. An adenomatous polyp may be grossly sessile or pedunculated and microscopically exhibit a tubular or villous growth pattern. Microscopically, it exhibits both architectural and cytologic features of dysplasia. Architectural features include crowded crypts or cribriforming. Cytologic features of dysplasia include elongation and stratification of

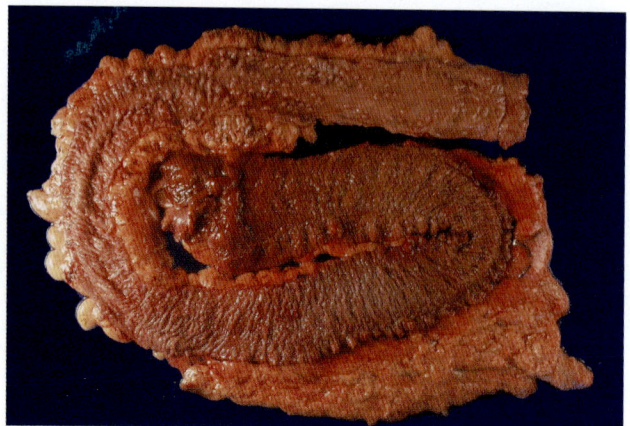

FIGURE 14-57 • Prophylactic colectomy specimen from a 27-year-old female with familial adenomatosis polyposis. No invasive adenocarcinoma was identified.

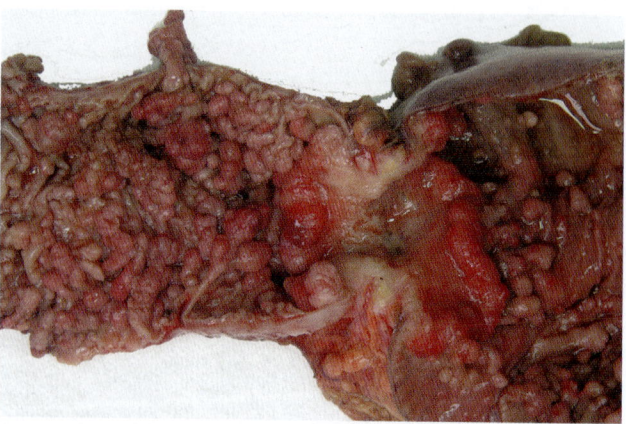

FIGURE 14-58 • Invasive colonic adenocarcinoma arising in an adult patient with familial adenomatosis polyposis. (Courtesy of Richard R. Anderson, M.D., Laboratory & Pathology Diagnostics, LLC.)

nuclei, nuclear contour irregularity, and nuclear hyperchromasia. Adenomas lack the cystic dilatation of crypts and abundant inflammatory stroma of juvenile polyps and the arborizing core of smooth muscle of Peutz-Jeghers polyps. The incidence of colonic adenocarcinoma is very high in patients with familial polyposis, approaching 100% by age 50. Malignancy may occur as early as the second decade. For this reason, colectomy is recommended whenever symptoms develop or in early adulthood. Multiple colonic adenomas also occur in the MUTYH polyposis syndrome, another autosomal recessive disorder with a significantly increased risk of colonic adenocarcinoma. In this condition, however, colonic adenomas are fewer, include serrated adenomas, and almost never develop during childhood (230). The MUTYH gene is involved in repairing DNA as a result of oxidative DNA damage.

After colectomy, continued surveillance is necessary since small-intestinal adenomas will almost always develop, frequently in the area of the ampulla of Vater. Patients also commonly develop gastric fundic gland polyps. Dysplasia has been reported to develop in these polyps, but progression to invasive gastric adenocarcinoma is exceedingly rare.

Patients with familial polyposis coli may exhibit a variety of extraintestinal malignancies, including thyroid and pancreatic carcinomas, hepatoblastoma, and fibromatosis (desmoid tumor). There is also an increased incidence of a variety of benign lesions, including dermatofibroma, lipoma, and bone lesions (e.g., osteoma, exostosis, cortical thickening of long bones, and dental cysts). Congenital hypertrophy of the retinal pigment is the most common extracolonic manifestation of familial adenomatous polyposis and may be detected before the gastrointestinal polyps.

Adenocarcinoma of the colon and rectum remains a rare diagnosis in children, with an incidence of about 1 in 10 million (231). Most, but not all, children and adolescents who develop colon cancer have either FAP or hereditary nonpolyposis colorectal cancer syndrome (HNPCC) (225) (Figure 14-58). Involvement of the right colon where early disease is clinically silent is more frequent in children than in adults. Histologically, the tumor in children tends to show poor differentiation with abundant mucin and often "signet ring" features (225).

In addition to true polyps, other conditions may present as polypoid masses in the gastrointestinal tract. These include inflammatory pseudopolyp in IBD, pancreatic or gastric heterotopia, "cap" polyps and tumors such as leiomyoma, adenocarcinoma, lipoma, neurofibroma, and ganglioneuroma.

Nonepithelial Gastrointestinal Tumors

In children with congenital immunodeficiency or AIDS, SMT may develop in association with EBV infection in either gastrointestinal or extraintestinal sites (184). The tumors are commonly multifocal and are uniformly reactive by *in situ* hybridization with probes to the EBV small noncoding RNAs (EBER). Spindle cell tumors of smooth muscle origin must be distinguished from others with similar histology, including inflammatory myofibroblastic tumor and fibromatosis.

Inflammatory fibroid polyp can occur at any age in the gastric or intestinal wall or adjacent mesentery and can become a large mass. The histologic features are variable but usually includes loose fascicles of bland spindle cells admixed with a mixed inflammatory cell infiltrate with a prominent component of eosinophils (232). The spindle cells often exhibit a perivascular whorling orientation that is characteristic. Because of its large size, a malignancy may be considered clinically, but the low cellularity of the lesion and lack of significant cytologic atypia usually lead to the correct diagnosis. Ganglioneuroma is another intestinal spindle cell tumor that has a frequent polypoid configuration. It is composed of ganglion cells and a Schwannian stroma. The latter may be mistaken for fibrosis in superficial biopsies. The correct diagnosis is supported by a positive reaction with neural immunocytochemical markers.

Mesenteric or omental cysts, although not strictly gastrointestinal tumors, should be considered in the differential diagnosis of abdominal masses in children. Ultrasonography reveals their typical unilocular or multilocular cystic nature.

Most are located in the mesentery immediately adjacent to the small intestine. Mesenteric cyst is lined by a single layer of cells or consists only of fibrous septa. It may be confused with a similar cystic lesion, cystic lymphangioma, which has an endothelial lining (D2-40+) in addition to lymphoid tissue and smooth muscle in its walls. Cystic lymphangioma often spans both the bowel wall and adjacent mesentery, so that a segmental bowel resection is required; in contrast, mesenteric cyst is usually easily separated from the bowel wall.

Lymphoma

The intestine is the most common site of primary extranodal lymphoma, and non-Hodgkin lymphoma is the most common malignant intestinal tumor in children. Boys from 5 to 10 years of age account for most of the affected children, and the usual clinical presentation is abdominal pain and a palpable right lower quadrant mass. Burkitt lymphoma is by far the most common gastrointestinal lymphoma of childhood. It usually arises in the submucosal lymphoid tissue of the ileocecal region and extends transmurally to involve local mesenteric lymph nodes and form a bulky tumor mass. Less advanced cases may present with intussusception or intestinal obstruction. Histologically, the mucosa and submucosa are replaced by sheets of uniform intermediate cells with very regular, round, noncleaved nuclei, usually arranged in a "starry sky" pattern. Appropriate hematopathologic evaluation of Burkitt lymphoma reveals a B-cell lineage; a translocation, t(8;14), is characteristic.

The prognosis is related to the extent of abdominal or systemic tumor spread. If the intestinal and nodal masses are amenable to resection and appropriate chemotherapy is administered, approximately 80% of these children are cured. Other non-Hodgkin lymphoma such as large B-cell lymphoma and anaplastic large-cell lymphoma have been reported in the gastrointestinal tract but are less frequent in otherwise healthy children (225). Some predominantly adult lymphomas that have a propensity for gastrointestinal tract involvement can occasionally present in childhood. *Immunoproliferative small-intestinal disease* (IPSID), or alpha chain disease, is a form of MALT lymphoma, associated with malabsorption, which most often afflicts adolescents and young adults in the developing world, particularly in the Middle East (233). Occasional cases of enteropathy-associated T-cell lymphoma, arising in patients with celiac disease, have been reported in children.

In immunodeficient patients, malignant lymphoma occurs anywhere in the intestinal tract and does not demonstrate a preference for the ileocecal area. Unusual large-cell lymphoproliferative disorders have been reported in the gastrointestinal tract in primary immunodeficiency diseases. A number of lymphoproliferative processes in addition to AIDS-associated non-Hodgkin lymphoma develop in patients with AIDS. A spectrum of posttransplant lymphoproliferative disorders associated with EBV infection, which involves the gastrointestinal tract in many cases, may develop in recipients of solid organ and bone marrow transplants. These include polyclonal and monomorphic B-lineage lymphomas at the most advanced end of the spectrum (234).

Langerhans cell histiocytosis (formerly called histiocytosis X) may affect any portion of the gastrointestinal tract to produce malabsorption, diarrhea, ulceration, or bleeding. Gastrointestinal involvement in children more frequently occurs as a component of widespread systemic infiltration and tends to have a poor prognosis (235). The infiltrate is usually mucosal and consists of the characteristic histiocyte-like cells with grooved nuclei admixed with a mixed inflammatory cell infiltrate including a prominent component of eosinophils (Figure 14-59A, B). Immunohistochemical reactivity for S-100 protein, CD1a, and/or Langerin confirms the diagnosis. Because of the presence of multinucleated giant cells in some cases, this condition may be mistaken for a granulomatous infectious process or CD.

Systemic mastocytosis is one of a group of disorders characterized by abnormal accumulation and proliferation

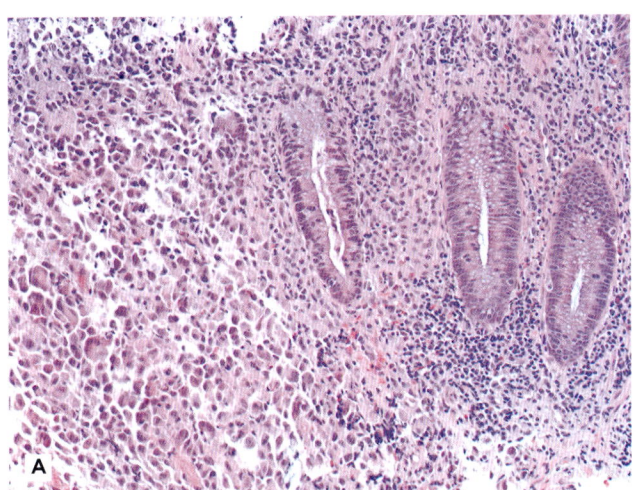
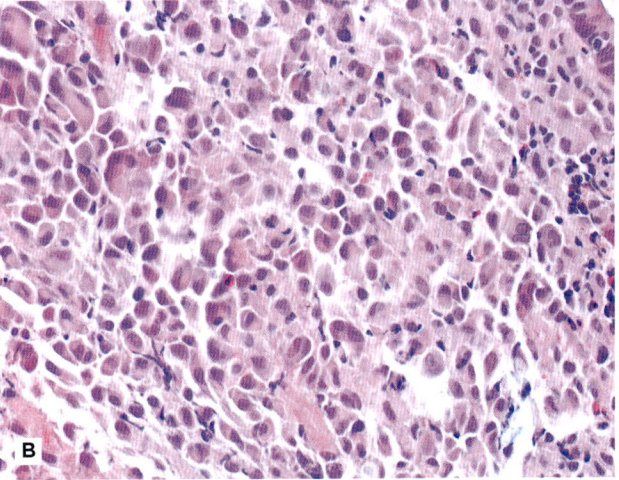

FIGURE 14-59 • Colonic involvement by Langerhans cell histiocytosis. **A:** Histiocytic infiltrate in the lamina propria 200×. **B:** Higher power reveals mixture of histiocytic cells with grooved nuclei, multinucleated giant cells, and a few admixed eosinophils 400×.

of mast cells. Systemic mastocytosis develops due to a specific activating mutation (codon 816) in the *c-kit* gene. Gastrointestinal involvement occurs in about 70% to 80% of patients with systemic mastocytosis (236). Most patients are adults. The stomach and duodenum are the most commonly involved sites. Common symptoms include abdominal pain, diarrhea, and bleeding. Peptic ulcer disease can develop due to hypergastrinemia stimulated by the release of histamine from the mast cells.

Mast cells are cytologically bland and are inconspicuous in H&E sections of normal mucosa. With the use of special stains, scattered mast cells can be seen in the lamina propria. In patients with systemic mastocytosis, endoscopy may be normal or reveal thickened mucosal folds and erosions. In most cases, the infiltrate of mast cells is dense and typically bandlike (eFigure 14-13A, B). Eosinophils are often also increased in number. Mast cells can be highlighted by immunostaining for c-kit and CD25 (eFigure 14-13C).

APPENDIX

Normal Anatomy and Histology

The appendix is present at the tip of the cecum at birth, but as the cecum grows, the appendix moves to a position on the posteromedial wall below the ileocecal valve. However, aberrant takeoff from the cecum is not unusual, and both anterior and retrocecal positions are particularly commonly encountered.

The overall gross anatomy of the appendix is most similar to the colon. There is a serosa, muscularis propria with an outer longitudinal and inner circular layer, submucosa, muscularis mucosae, and mucosa. The mucosa closely resembles its colonic counterpart, although branched crypts are regarded as a normal finding in the appendix. Endocrine cells and Paneth cells are scattered throughout the mucosa. The lymphoid tissue component is also exaggerated in the appendix, more akin to that seen in the terminal ileum. In children, lymphoid follicles may be confluent over large areas of the mucosa. Within the lamina propria, there are numerous ganglion cells, Schwann cells, and nerve fibers, as well as endocrine cells, which may be the origin for carcinoid tumors.

Congenital and Neuromuscular Disorders

Diverticula of the appendix may be congenital or acquired, with acquired lesions being ten times more common (237). Acquired diverticula may easily rupture during bouts of acute appendicitis. Inflammation of the diverticula (akin to sigmoid diverticulitis) may present as a mild form of appendicitis (237). Appendiceal diverticula are particularly common in patients with cystic fibrosis (238). Appendiceal intussusception is usually the result of a pathologic process involving the appendix itself, such as a tumor, endometriosis, cystic fibrosis, or virally induced lymphoid hyperplasia.

Adenovirus infection has specifically been implicated in some cases.

Fibrous obliteration of the appendiceal tip, a common finding in adults, is uncommon in childhood and is of no clinical significance. In some cases, a disorganized hyperplasia of neural elements is evident within the fibrous tissue, including nonmyelinated nerve fibers and Schwann cells, and in some cases endocrine cells. It is unclear whether the presence of these elements is indicative of prior acute appendicitis.

Acute Appendicitis

Acute appendicitis is the most common indication for emergent surgery in the United States, with about 250,000 appendectomies performed each year. The epidemiology, pathogenesis, and clinical features of acute appendicitis have been extensively investigated for many decades, but certain aspects of this very common disorder remain controversial. The peak age of incidence is from 10 to 30 years of age, although cases in infants and the elderly do occur. The lifetime risk of the development of acute appendicitis is about 7% in the United States (239). The rate of appendectomy in which acute appendicitis is not confirmed pathologically is about 15% (240). The rate has not decreased significantly in the past 70 years, despite the use of even more sophisticated and expensive laboratory and imaging techniques.

The classic early symptoms of acute appendicitis include abdominal pain, anorexia, nausea, and vomiting. McBurney described progression from vague periumbilical pain to localized pain in the right lower quadrant more than 100 years ago. Physical examination typically reveals mild tachycardia, low-grade fever, decreased bowel sounds, and tenderness to palpation in the right lower quadrant. Laboratory evaluation usually reveals a mildly elevated white blood cell count with a left shift. The use of abdominal ultrasound and helical computed tomography has been proposed to increase the sensitivity and specificity of the diagnosis of acute appendicitis (239). Appendectomy remains the mainstay of treatment for acute appendicitis. However, when perforation has already occurred at the time of diagnosis, some surgeons advocate delaying surgery until after a course of antibiotics.

The pathogenesis of acute appendicitis is still a matter of debate. Many investigators are convinced that luminal obstruction (usually by a fecalith or lymphoid hyperplasia) leads to distension and ischemia followed by bacterial invasion (239). Alternative hypotheses include primary viral infection or local ischemia producing microscopic ulcers, thus allowing for bacterial invasion. Although ultimately bacterial invasion plays a central role in the pathogenesis of acute appendicitis, microbiologic studies have shown that a variety of enteric organisms could be responsible in an individual case, most frequently *E. coli*.

The gross appearance in acute appendicitis varies depending on the severity of the acute inflammatory process.

In classic cases with transmural involvement, the serosa appears dull, discolored, and shaggy. The wall is edematous and swollen and retracts when incised. Acute inflammatory cell exudate may be evident at the site of a perforation. If the appendix is removed before transmural inflammation has developed, the appendix may grossly appear normal or exhibit only mild serosal hyperemia.

The histologic features of acute appendicitis reflect the gross appearance. In severe acute appendicitis, there may be transmural necrosis with perforation and acute peritonitis.

There is debate, however, regarding the minimal degree of neutrophilic inflammation that is required to render a diagnosis of acute appendicitis. Most authors will accept neutrophilic mucosal infiltrates if associated with at least focal ulceration as diagnostic (241). However, others point to data suggesting that such changes can be present in incidental appendectomies performed in asymptomatic patients. These authors insist that for this reason, a diagnosis of acute appendicitis is not warranted until neutrophilic inflammation extends into the muscularis propria (242). The point has been made that if multiple additional sections are obtained from an appendix that on initial examination exhibits only superficial inflammation, there is a high likelihood of finding involvement of the muscularis propria. There is uniform agreement that luminal neutrophils or focal infiltration of the surface epithelium alone is insufficient for a diagnosis of acute appendicitis (assuming that the entire appendix has been examined). The possibility of an enteric infection (such as *Campylobacter* ileocolitis) should be considered in such patients (239).

Interval Appendectomy

It has become accepted practice in many centers to delay appendectomy in patients in whom perforation and abscess formation have occurred. Instead, the patient is treated conservatively with supportive care and antibiotics, and appendectomy is thus delayed for 4 to 8 weeks, at which time the patient is clinically stable and the complication rate is therefore lower. In fact, some surgeons question the need for appendectomy at all if conservative management is successful (240).

Histologic examination of interval appendectomy specimens most often reveals mural thickening and fibrosis, transmural lymphoid aggregates, and mucosal architectural distortion (Figure 14-60A, B). Not infrequently granulomas are also evident, resulting in a histologic appearance that closely mimics CD. Occasionally, xanthogranulomatous inflammation is evident. In some cases, the appendix is histologically normal or exhibits only mild serosal fibrosis.

Unusual Infections of the Appendix

A variety of viral pathogens can produce inflammation of the appendix and many produce clinical features similar to acute appendicitis. Measles virus infection involving the appendix is very rare but is well described. In most patients, appendectomy is performed during the prodromal stage of the illness, before the diagnosis of measles is established. The histologic hallmark is the presence of Warthin-Finkeldey cells similar to those seen in the tonsillar tissue of infected patients. Lymphoid hyperplasia is also prominent, but there is little evidence of acute inflammation (243). However, if appendectomy is delayed, superimposed bacterial appendicitis of the traditional type may develop. Adenovirus and rotavirus infections have already been mentioned as a cause of appendiceal intussusception. Smudgy-appearing viral inclusions can be identified in epithelial cells with adenovirus, but not rotavirus.

Yersinia, *Campylobacter*, or *Salmonella* infection can cause ileocecitis resulting in symptoms, laboratory test abnormalities, and radiographic findings difficult to distinguish from acute appendicitis. Histologic examination in cases where an appendectomy is performed usually reveals only mild mucosal neutrophilic infiltrates, without involvement of

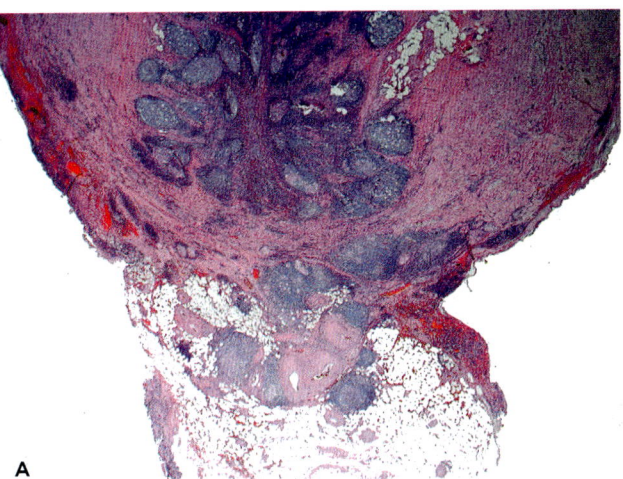
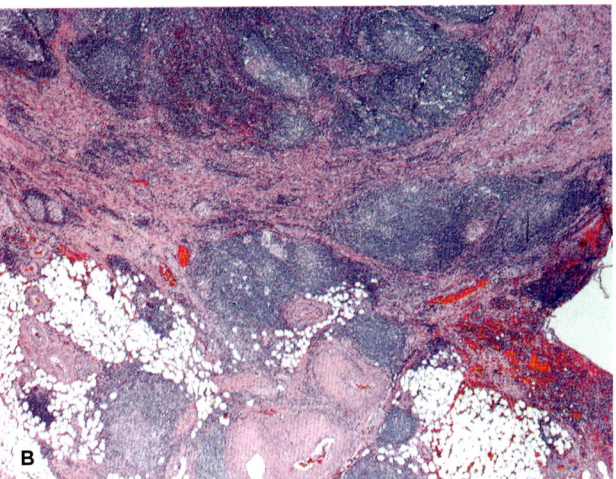

FIGURE 14-60 • Interval appendicitis. **A:** There is fibrosis of the serosa with lymphoid follicles, consistent with resolution of a prior episode of acute appendicitis with perforation 20×. **B:** The acute inflammation has completely resolved 40×.

Goblet cell or adenocarcinoid is a more treacherous neoplasm, but these are most unusual in children.

DISORDERS OF THE ANUS

Congenital Abnormalities

Anorectal anomalies constitute a spectrum of malformations. These range from a thin membrane obstructing an otherwise normal rectum and anus (true imperforate anus) to atresia of the entire distal rectum, in which the proximal rectum ends as a blind pouch in the pelvis. The term imperforate anus is a misnomer because the anomaly usually consists of considerably more than an imperforate anal membrane. The anal canal and rectum are usually both affected. The incidence of these malformations is approximately 1 in 5000 births.

The classification of anorectal malformations has long been confusing and nonstandardized. The malformation is usually classified as high, intermediate, or low, depending on the location of the distal rectum in relation to the levator ani muscle, which can be demonstrated radiologically in relation to bony landmarks (e.g., the pubococcygeal line on a lateral radiograph) (249) (Figure 14-65). Fistulas between the rectal pouch and perineal skin or various locations in the urinary and genital systems are often found. The most common variations are shown in Figure 14-64. Those with a low imperforate anus have an intact anal sphincter and usually a fistula from the rectal pouch to the perineal skin anterior to a covered anal dimple, although in up to 25% of the cases, a fistula is not present. High malformations, formerly known as anorectal agenesis, are associated with absence of the anal sphincter and complex abnormal interval anomalies. A rectourethral fistula is present in most boys with this malformation; girls usually have a fistula between the rectal pouch and the vagina, bladder, or urethra. The term persistent cloaca describes the condition in which a girl has a single perineal opening draining an internal pouch comprised of the terminal portions of rectum, vagina, and urinary tract structures.

Other congenital anomalies are found in as many as 50% of infants with high anorectal malformations. The most frequent associations are genitourinary and skeletal abnormalities (especially of vertebrae and pelvis), congenital heart disease, and esophageal atresia with tracheoesophageal fistula. A diagnosis of VATER syndrome, VATERL syndrome, or caudal regression syndrome should be considered in every infant with an anorectal anomaly (see Chapter 28).

Acquired Diseases

Anogenital Warts

Anogenital warts (condylomata acuminata) are caused by infection with human papillomavirus (HPV). Though HPV types 6 and 11 are responsible for most genital infections, a significant proportion (up to 40%) of AGW in children may be caused by HPV serotypes associated with common skin warts (250). Though sexual abuse should be considered in any child presenting with AGW, these do not always indicate abuse as nonsexual transmission, including perinatal exposure, is well recognized especially in younger children (<4 years of age) (250). In older children and adolescents, AGW are more likely acquired through sexual activity. In boys, they occur in the perianal region, and in girls, they are found in the perianal, vulvar, hymenal, and urethral areas regardless of method of transmission. Histologically, the lesions are

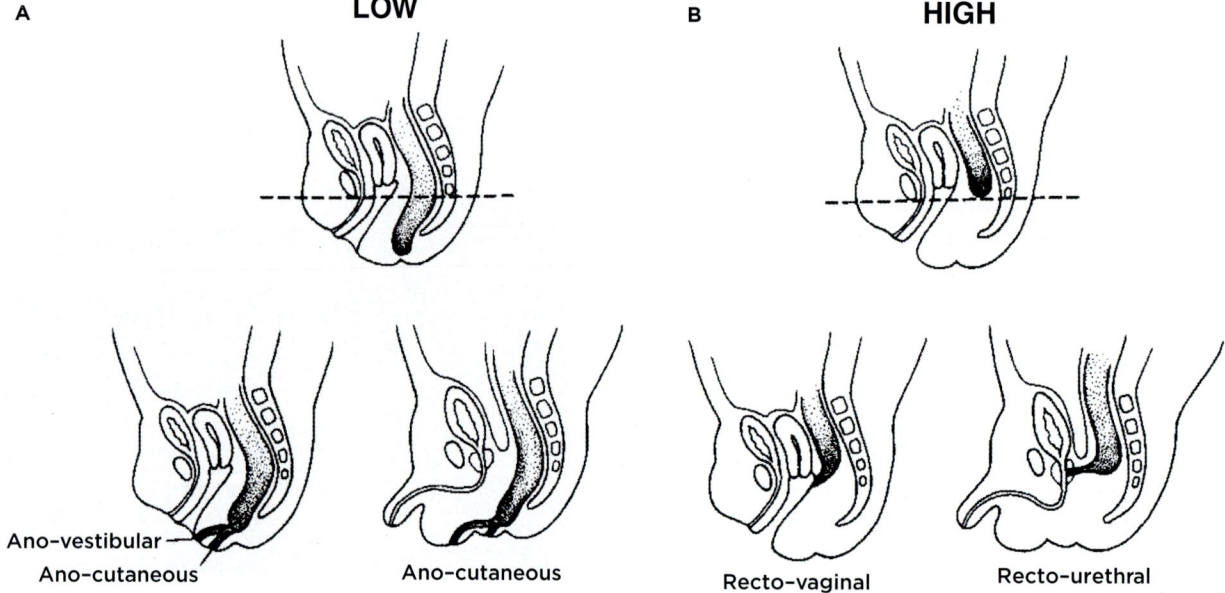

FIGURE 14-65 • Classification of anorectal malformations. Anomalies are classified as low or high depending on their relationship to the pubococcygeal line on x-ray film (*broken line*). Fistula tracts between the rectum and other structures are indicated by stippling. **A:** Low anomalies are usually associated with an external fistula to the vestibule (in girls) or the skin. **B:** In high anomalies, fistulas are internal, usually to the posterior vagina in girls or the proximal urethra in boys.

identical to those seen in adults. Most AGWs in children and adolescents resolve spontaneously and do not need treatment; a variety of medical and surgical options are available for long-lasting cases or for symptomatic patients (251).

Perianal Abscess and Anal Fistula

Perianal abscesses, usually found in infants, result from breaks in the skin or anal mucosa or an infection in the anal glands. Treatment consists of surgical incision and drainage. Anal fistulas between the anal canal and skin may develop secondarily, requiring surgical excision of the fibrous and granulation tissue tract in perianal soft tissues and muscle. Older children with leukemia, CD, and immunodeficiency states are especially susceptible to perianal abscesses and fistulas.

References

1. Akbayir N, et al. Heterotopic gastric mucosa in the cervical esophagus (inlet patch): endoscopic prevalence, histological and clinical characteristics. *J Gastroenterol Hepatol* 2004;19(8):891–896.
2. Dimmick JE, Hardwick DF. Gastrointestinal system and exocrine pancreas. In: Dimmick JE, Kalousek DK, eds. *Developmental Pathology of the Embryo and Fetus*. Philadelphia, PA: J. B. Lippincott Company, 1992:509–544.
3. Superina RA, Ein SH, Humphreys RP. Cystic duplications of the esophagus and neurenteric cysts. *J Pediatr Surg* 1984;19(5):527–530.
4. Michaud L, et al. Characteristics and management of congenital esophageal stenosis: findings from a multicenter study. *Orphanet J Rare Dis* 2013;8:186.
5. Vandenplas Y. Gastroesophageal reflux. In: Wyllie R, Hyams J, eds. *Pediatric Gastrointestinal and Liver Disease*. Philadelphia, PA: Saunders Elsevier; 2006.
6. Dahms BB. Reflux esophagitis: sequelae and differential diagnosis in infants and children including eosinophilic esophagitis. *Pediatr Dev Pathol* 2004;7(1):5–16.
7. Ebach DR, et al. Lymphocytic esophagitis: a possible manifestation of pediatric upper gastrointestinal Crohn's disease. *Inflamm Bowel Dis* 2011;17(1):45–49.
8. Sampliner RE. Updated guidelines for the diagnosis, surveillance, and therapy of Barrett's esophagus. *Am J Gastroenterol* 2002;97(8):1888–1895.
9. Fitzgerald RC, et al. British Society of Gastroenterology guidelines on the diagnosis and management of Barrett's oesophagus. *Gut* 2014;63(1):7–42.
10. Gangopadhyay AN, et al. Adenocarcinoma of the esophagus in an 8-year-old boy. *J Pediatr Surg* 1997;32(8):1259–1260.
11. Liacouras CA, et al. Eosinophilic esophagitis: updated consensus recommendations for children and adults. *J Allergy Clin Immunol* 2011;128(1):3–20e6; quiz 21–2.
12. Furuta GT, et al. Eosinophilic esophagitis in children and adults: a systematic review and consensus recommendations for diagnosis and treatment. *Gastroenterology* 2007;133(4):1342–1363.
13. Kliemann DA, et al. Candida esophagitis: species distribution and risk factors for infection. *Rev Inst Med Trop Sao Paulo* 2008;50(5):261–263.
14. Pandya S, Heiss K. Pyloric stenosis in pediatric surgery: an evidence-based review. *Surg Clin North Am* 2012;92(3):527–539, vii–viii.
15. Serra A, et al. The role of RET genomic variants in infantile hypertrophic pyloric stenosis. *Eur J Pediatr Surg* 2011;21(6):389–394.
16. Krishnamurthy S, et al. Pancreatic acinar cell clusters in pediatric gastric mucosa. *Am J Surg Pathol* 1998;22(1):100–105.
17. Lin CM, et al. Neonatal gastric perforation: report of 15 cases and review of the literature. *Pediatr Neonatol* 2008;49(3):65–70.
18. Koletzko S, et al. Evidence-based guidelines from ESPGHAN and NASPGHAN for *Helicobacter pylori* infection in children. *J Pediatr Gastroenterol Nutr* 2011;53(2):230–243.
19. Jevon GP, et al. Spectrum of gastritis in celiac disease in childhood. *Pediatr Dev Pathol* 1999;2(3):221–226.
20. Aggarwal N, Kuan SF, Fasanella KE. Endoscopic, ultrasonographic, and pathologic correlation of lymphocytic gastritis. *Endoscopy* 2013;45(Suppl 2 UCTN):E145–E146.
21. Nielsen JA, et al. Lymphocytic gastritis is not associated with active *Helicobacter pylori* infection. *Helicobacter* 2014;19(5):349–355.
22. Lamps LW. *Surgical Pathology of the Gastrointestinal System: Bacterial, Fungal, Viral and Parasitic Infections*. New York: Springer, 2009.
23. Dohil R, Hassall E. Gastritis, gastropathy and ulcer disease. In: Wyllie R, Hyams J, eds. *Pediatric Gastrointestinal and Liver Disease*. Philadelphia, PA: Saunders Elsevier,2006:373–408.
24. Dohil R, et al. Gastritis and gastropathy of childhood. *J Pediatr Gastroenterol Nutr* 1999;29(4):378–394.
25. Perme T, et al. Prolonged prostaglandin E1 therapy in a neonate with pulmonary atresia and ventricular septal defect and the development of antral foveolar hyperplasia and hypertrophic pyloric stenosis. *Ups J Med Sci* 2013;118(2):138–142.
26. Ectors NL, et al. Granulomatous gastritis: a morphological and diagnostic approach. *Histopathology* 1993;23(1):55–61.
27. Lenaerts C, et al. High incidence of upper gastrointestinal tract involvement in children with Crohn disease. *Pediatrics* 1989;83(5):777–781.
28. Sharif F, et al. Focally enhanced gastritis in children with Crohn's disease and ulcerative colitis. *Am J Gastroenterol* 2002;97(6):1415–1420.
29. Pascasio JM, Hammond S, Qualman SJ. Recognition of Crohn disease on incidental gastric biopsy in childhood. *Pediatr Dev Pathol* 2003;6(3):209–214.
30. Stolte M, Vieth M, Ebert MP. High-grade dysplasia in sporadic fundic gland polyps: clinically relevant or not? *Eur J Gastroenterol Hepatol* 2003;15(11):1153–1156.
31. Curtis JL, et al. Primary gastric tumors of infancy and childhood: 54-year experience at a single institution. *J Pediatr Surg* 2008;43(8):1487–1493.
32. Pappo AS, Janeway KA. Pediatric gastrointestinal stromal tumors. *Hematol Oncol Clin North Am* 2009;23(1):15–34, vii.
33. Kaemmer DA, et al. The Gist of literature on pediatric GIST: review of clinical presentation. *J Pediatr Hematol Oncol* 2009;31(2):108–112.
34. Stratakis CA, Carney JA. The triad of paragangliomas, gastric stromal tumours and pulmonary chondromas (Carney triad), and the dyad of paragangliomas and gastric stromal sarcomas (Carney-Stratakis syndrome): molecular genetics and clinical implications. *J Intern Med* 2009;266(1):43–52.
35. Pappo AS, et al. Special considerations in pediatric gastrointestinal tumors. *J Surg Oncol* 2011;104(8):928–932.
36. West RB, et al. The novel marker, DOG1, is expressed ubiquitously in gastrointestinal stromal tumors irrespective of KIT or PDGFRA mutation status. *Am J Pathol* 2004;165(1):107–113.
37. Miettinen M, Wang ZF, Lasota J. DOG1 antibody in the differential diagnosis of gastrointestinal stromal tumors: a study of 1840 cases. *Am J Surg Pathol* 2009;33(9):1401–1408.
38. Liegl B, et al. Monoclonal antibody DOG1.1 shows higher sensitivity than KIT in the diagnosis of gastrointestinal stromal tumors, including unusual subtypes. *Am J Surg Pathol* 2009;33(3):437–446.
39. Fletcher CD, et al. Diagnosis of gastrointestinal stromal tumors: a consensus approach. *Hum Pathol* 2002;33(5):459–465.
40. Kelly KB, Ponsky TA. Pediatric abdominal wall defects. *Surg Clin North Am* 2013;93(5):1255–1267.
41. Torfs C, Curry C, Roeper P. Gastroschisis. *J Pediatr* 1990;116(1):1–6.
42. Tovar JA. Chapter 33. Hernias. In: Walker AW, et al., eds. *Pediatric Gastrointestinal Disease*. Hamilton, ON: BC Decker, 2004:573–588.
43. Werler MM, et al. Is there epidemiologic evidence to support vascular disruption as a pathogenesis of gastroschisis? *Am J Med Genet A* 2009;149A(7):1399–1406.
44. Huff DS. Chapter 1: Developmental anatomy and anomalies of the gastrointestinal tract, with involvement in major malformative syndromes. In: Russo P, Ruchelli E, Piccoli D, eds. *Pathology of Pediatric Gastrointestinal and Liver Disease*. New York: Springer, 2004:3–37.
45. Samuels ME, et al. Exome sequencing identifies mutations in the gene TTC7A in French-Canadian cases with hereditary multiple intestinal atresia. *J Med Genet* 2013;50(5):324–329.

46. Bilodeau A, et al. Hereditary multiple intestinal atresia: thirty years later. *J Pediatr Surg* 2004;39(5):726–730.
47. Dalla Vecchia LK, et al. Intestinal atresia and stenosis: a 25-year experience with 277 cases. *Arch Surg* 1998;133(5):490–496; discussion 496–497.
48. Roberts HE, et al. Increased frequency of cystic fibrosis among infants with jejunoileal atresia. *Am J Med Genet* 1998;78(5):446–449.
49. O'Neill J, Grosfeld MRJ. Jejunoileal atresia and stenosis. In: Grosfeld JL, O'Neill JA, Coran AG, Fonkalsrud EW, Caldamone AA, eds. *Pediatric Surgery*. St. Louis, MO: Mosby; 1998:1145–1158.
50. Dehner LP, Scott D, Stocker JT. Meconium periorchitis: a clinicopathologic study of four cases with a review of the literature. *Hum Pathol* 1986;17(8):807–812.
51. Kizer JR, et al. Meconium hydrocele in a female newborn: an unusual cause of a labial mass. *J Urol* 1995;153(1):188–190.
52. Cuenca AG, et al. "Pulling the plug"—management of meconium plug syndrome in neonates. *J Surg Res* 2012;175(2):e43–e46.
53. Farrell PM, et al. Guidelines for diagnosis of cystic fibrosis in newborns through older adults: Cystic Fibrosis Foundation Consensus Report. *J Pediatr* 2008;153(2):S4–S14.
54. Ziegler MM. Meconium ileus. *Curr Probl Surg* 1994;31(9):731–777.
55. Dray X, et al. Distal intestinal obstruction syndrome in adults with cystic fibrosis. *Clin Gastroenterol Hepatol* 2004;2(6):498–503.
56. FitzSimmons SC, et al. High-dose pancreatic-enzyme supplements and fibrosing colonopathy in children with cystic fibrosis. *N Engl J Med* 1997;336(18):1283–1289.
57. Pawel BR, de Chadarevian JP, Franco ME. The pathology of fibrosing colonopathy of cystic fibrosis: a study of 12 cases and review of the literature. *Hum Pathol* 1997;28(4):395–399.
58. Kapur R. Motor disorders. In: Russo P, Ruchelli E, Piccoli D, eds. *Pathology of Pediatric Gastrointestinal and Liver Disease*. Heidelberg, Germany: Springer Verlag; 2014:249–317.
59. Weinberg AG. The anorectal myenteric plexus: its relation to hypoganglionosis of the colon. *Am J Clin Pathol* 1970;54(4):637–642.
60. Monforte-Munoz H, et al. Increased submucosal nerve trunk caliber in aganglionosis: a "positive" and objective finding in suction biopsies and segmental resections in Hirschsprung's disease. *Arch Pathol Lab Med* 1998;122(8):721–725.
61. Barshack I, et al. The loss of calretinin expression indicates aganglionosis in Hirschsprung's disease. *J Clin Pathol* 2004;57(7):712–716.
62. Guinard-Samuel V, et al. Calretinin immunohistochemistry: a simple and efficient tool to diagnose Hirschsprung disease. *Mod Pathol* 2009; 22(10):1379–1384.
63. Kapur RP, et al. Calretinin immunohistochemistry versus acetylcholinesterase histochemistry in the evaluation of suction rectal biopsies for Hirschsprung disease. *Pediatr Dev Pathol* 2009;12(1):6–15.
64. Kapur RP, Calretinin-immunoreactive mucosal innervation in very short-segment Hirschsprung disease: a potentially misleading observation. *Pediatr Dev Pathol* 2014;17(1):28–35.
65. Coe A, et al. Reoperation for Hirschsprung disease: pathology of the resected problematic distal pull-through. *Pediatr Dev Pathol* 2012;15(1):30–38.
66. Coran AG, Teitelbaum DH. Recent advances in the management of Hirschsprung's disease. *Am J Surg* 2000;180(5):382–387. [MEDLINE record in process].
67. Teitelbaum DH, Qualman SJ, Caniano DA. Hirschsprung's disease. Identification of risk factors for enterocolitis. *Ann Surg* 1988;207(3):240–244.
68. Teitelbaum DH, Caniano DA, Qualman SJ. The pathophysiology of Hirschsprung's-associated enterocolitis: importance of histologic correlates. *J Pediatr Surg* 1989;24(12):1271–1277.
69. Hsieh WS, et al. Hirschsprung's disease presenting with diffuse intestinal pneumatosis in a neonate. *Acta Paediatr Taiwan* 2000;41(6):336–338.
70. Teitelbaum DH, Coran AG. Enterocolitis. *Semin Pediatr Surg* 1998;7(3):162–169.
71. Austin KM. The pathogenesis of Hirschsprung's disease-associated enterocolitis. *Semin Pediatr Surg* 2012;21(4):319–327.
72. Knowles CH, et al. The London Classification of gastrointestinal neuromuscular pathology: report on behalf of the Gastro 2009 International Working Group. *Gut* 2010;59(7):882–887.
73. Knowles CH, et al. Quantitation of cellular components of the enteric nervous system in the normal human gastrointestinal tract—report on behalf of the Gastro 2009 International Working Group. *Neurogastroenterol Motil* 2011;23(2):115–124.
74. Dingemann J, Puri P. Isolated hypoganglionosis: systematic review of a rare intestinal innervation defect. *Pediatr Surg Int* 2010;26(11):1111–1115.
75. Schuffler MD, Jonak Z. Chronic idiopathic intestinal pseudo-obstruction caused by a degenerative disorder of the myenteric plexus: the use of Smith's method to define the neuropathology. *Gastroenterology* 1982;82(3):476–486.
76. Navarro J, et al. Visceral neuropathies responsible for chronic intestinal pseudo-obstruction syndrome in pediatric practice: analysis of 26 cases. *J Pediatr Gastroenterol Nutr* 1990;11(2):179–195.
77. Shekitka KM, Sobin LH. Ganglioneuromas of the gastrointestinal tract. Relation to Von Recklinghausen disease and other multiple tumor syndromes. *Am J Surg Pathol* 1994;18(3):250–257.
78. Scharli AF, Meier-Ruge W. Localized and disseminated forms of neuronal intestinal dysplasia mimicking Hirschsprung's disease. *J Pediatr Surg* 1981;16(2):164–170.
79. Meier-Ruge WA, Bruder E, Kapur RP. Intestinal neuronal dysplasia type B: one giant ganglion is not good enough. *Pediatr Dev Pathol* 2006;9(6):444–452.
80. Koletzko S, et al. Rectal biopsy for diagnosis of intestinal neuronal dysplasia in children: a prospective multicentre study on interobserver variation and clinical outcome. *Gut* 1999;44(6):853–861.
81. Gosemann JH, Puri P. Megacystis microcolon intestinal hypoperistalsis syndrome: systematic review of outcome. *Pediatr Surg Int* 2011;27(10):1041–1046.
82. Leon SH, et al. Chronic intestinal pseudoobstruction as a complication of Duchenne's muscular dystrophy. *Gastroenterology* 1986; 90(2):455–459.
83. Kapur RP, et al. Gastrointestinal neuromuscular pathology in Alpers disease. *Am J Surg Pathol* 2011;35(5):714–722.
84. Kapur RP, et al. Diffuse abnormal layering of small intestinal smooth muscle is present in patients with FLNA mutations and x-linked intestinal pseudo-obstruction. *Am J Surg Pathol* 2010;34(10):1528–1543.
85. Ruchti C, Eisele S, Kaufmann M. Fatal intestinal pseudo-obstruction in brown bowel syndrome. *Arch Pathol Lab Med* 1990;114(1):76–80.
86. Young D. Intussusception. In: *Pediatric Surgery*, 5th ed. St. Louis, MO: Mosby, 1998:1185–1198.
87. Peter G, Myers MG. Intussusception, rotavirus, and oral vaccines: summary of a workshop. *Pediatrics* 2002;110(6):e67.
88. Shui IM, et al. Risk of intussusception following administration of a pentavalent rotavirus vaccine in US infants. *JAMA* 2012;307(6):598–604.
89. Caeiro JP, et al. Etiology of outpatient pediatric nondysenteric diarrhea: a multicenter study in the United States. *Pediatr Infect Dis J* 1999;18(2):94–97.
90. Parashar UD, Nelson EA, Kang G. Diagnosis, management, and prevention of rotavirus gastroenteritis in children. *BMJ* 2013;347:f7204.
91. Davidson GP, Barnes GL. Structural and functional abnormalities of the small intestine in infants and young children with rotavirus enteritis. *Acta Paediatr Scand* 1979;68(2):181–186.
92. Agus SG, et al. Acute infectious nonbacterial gastroenteritis: intestinal histopathology. Histologic and enzymatic alterations during illness produced by the Norwalk agent in man. *Ann Intern Med* 1973;79(1):18–25.
93. Troeger H, et al. Structural and functional changes of the duodenum in human norovirus infection. *Gut* 2009;58(8):1070–1077.
94. Yunis EJ, et al. Adenovirus and ileocecal intussusception. *Lab Invest* 1975;33(4):347–351.
95. Dimitroulia E, et al. Frequent detection of cytomegalovirus in the intestine of patients with inflammatory bowel disease. *Inflamm Bowel Dis* 2006;12(9):879–884.

96. Foucar E, et al. Colon ulceration in lethal cytomegalovirus infection. *Am J Clin Pathol* 1981;76(6):788–801.
97. Chhabra P, et al. Etiology of viral gastroenteritis in children <5 years of age in the United States, 2008–2009. *J Infect Dis* 2013;208(5):790–800.
98. Variend S, Phillips AD, Walker-Smith JA. The small intestinal mucosal biopsy in childhood. *Perspect Pediatr Pathol* 1984;8(1):57–78.
99. Pfeiffer ML, DuPont HL, Ochoa TJ. The patient presenting with acute dysentery—a systematic review. *J Infect* 2012;64(4):374–386.
100. Riley MR, Bass D. Infectious diarrhea. In: Piccoli DA, Liacouras C, eds. *Pediatric Gastroenterology*. Philadelphia, PA: Mosby Elsevier; 2008:123–130.
101. Thisyakorn U, Mansuwan P, Taylor DN. Typhoid and paratyphoid fever in 192 hospitalized children in Thailand. *Am J Dis Child* 1987;141(8):862–865.
102. Preziosi MJ, et al. Microbiological analysis of nontyphoidal Salmonella strains causing distinct syndromes of bacteremia or enteritis in HIV/AIDS patients in San Diego, California. *J Clin Microbiol* 2012;50(11):3598–3603.
103. Butler T. Haemolytic uraemic syndrome during shigellosis. *Trans R Soc Trop Med Hyg* 2012;106(7):395–399.
104. Moake JL. Thrombotic microangiopathies. *N Engl J Med* 2002; 347(8):589–600.
105. Dammin G. The acute diarrhea and dysenteries. In: *Pathology of Tropical and Extraordinary Diseases*. Vol. 1. Washington, DC: Armed Forces Institute of Pathology, 1976:135–164.
106. Bell BP, et al. A multistate outbreak of *Escherichia coli* O157:H7-associated bloody diarrhea and hemolytic uremic syndrome from hamburgers. The Washington experience. *JAMA* 1994;272(17):1349–1353.
107. Ostroff SM, Kobayashi JM, Lewis JH, Infections with *Escherichia coli* O157:H7 in Washington State. The first year of statewide disease surveillance. *JAMA* 1989;262(3):355–359.
108. Lamps LW, et al. The role of *Yersinia enterocolitica* and *Yersinia pseudotuberculosis* in granulomatous appendicitis: a histologic and molecular study. *Am J Surg Pathol* 2001;25(4):508–515.
109. Abdel-Haq NM, et al. *Yersinia enterocolitica* infection in children. *Pediatr Infect Dis J* 2000;19(10):954–958.
110. Hansen MG, Pearl G, Levy M. Intussusception due to *Yersinia enterocolitica* enterocolitis in a patient with beta-thalassemia. *Arch Pathol Lab Med* 2001;125(11):1486–1488.
111. Uchiyama T, Kato H. The pathogenesis of Kawasaki disease and superantigens. *Jpn J Infect Dis* 1999;52(4):141–145.
112. Johnson S, et al. Nosocomial *Clostridium difficile* colonisation and disease. *Lancet* 1990;336(8707):97–100.
113. McDonald LC, et al. An epidemic, toxin gene-variant strain of *Clostridium difficile*. *N Engl J Med* 2005;353(23):2433–2441.
114. De Girolami PC, et al. Multicenter evaluation of a new enzyme immunoassay for detection of *Clostridium difficile* enterotoxin A. *J Clin Microbiol* 1992;30(5):1085–1088.
115. Edberg SC, Browne FA, Allen MJ. Issues for microbial regulation: aeromonas as a model. *Crit Rev Microbiol* 2007;33(1):89–100.
116. Current WL, Garcia LS. Cryptosporidiosis. *Clin Microbiol Rev* 1991;4(3):325–358.
117. Mac Kenzie WR, et al. A massive outbreak in Milwaukee of cryptosporidium infection transmitted through the public water supply. *N Engl J Med* 1994;331(3):161–167.
118. Pittman FE, Hennigar GR. Sigmoidoscopic and colonic mucosal biopsy findings in amebic colitis. *Arch Pathol* 1974;97(3):155–158.
119. Logar J, Andlovic A, Poljsak-Prijatelj M. Incidence of *Blastocystis hominis* in patients with diarrhoea. *J Infect* 1994;28(2):151–154.
120. O'Gorman MA, et al. Prevalence and characteristics of *Blastocystis hominis* infection in children. *Clin Pediatr (Phila)* 1993;32(2):91–96.
121. Galantowicz BB, et al. Neonatal *Blastocystis hominis* diarrhea. *Pediatr Infect Dis J* 1993;12(4):345–347.
122. Spencer MJ, Garcia LS, Chapin MR. *Dientamoeba fragilis*. An intestinal pathogen in children? *Am J Dis Child* 1979;133(4):390–393.
123. Cuffari C, Oligny L, Seidman EG. *Dientamoeba fragilis* masquerading as allergic colitis. *J Pediatr Gastroenterol Nutr* 1998;26(1):16–20.
124. Berlin OG, et al. Recovery of Cyclospora organisms from patients with prolonged diarrhea. *Clin Infect Dis* 1994;18(4):606–609.
125. Ortega YR, et al. Cyclospora species—a new protozoan pathogen of humans. *N Engl J Med* 1993;328(18):1308–1312.
126. Veress B, et al. Duodenal intraepithelial lymphocyte-count revisited. *Scand J Gastroenterol* 2004;39(2):138–144.
127. Chillaron J, et al. Heteromeric amino acid transporters: biochemistry, genetics, and physiology. *Am J Physiol Renal Physiol* 2001;281(6):F995–F1018.
128. Heubi JE, et al. Primary bile acid malabsorption: defective *in vitro* ileal active bile acid transport. *Gastroenterology* 1982;83(4):804–811.
129. Peretti N, et al. Guidelines for the diagnosis and management of chylomicron retention disease based on a review of the literature and the experience of two centers. *Orphanet J Rare Dis* 2010;5:24.
130. Jones B, et al. Mutations in a Sar1 GTPase of COPII vesicles are associated with lipid absorption disorders. *Nat Genet* 2003;34(1):29–31.
131. Erickson RP, et al. Navajo microvillous inclusion disease is due to a mutation in MYO5B. *Am J Med Genet A* 2008;146A(24):3117–3119.
132. Muller T, et al. MYO5B mutations cause microvillus inclusion disease and disrupt epithelial cell polarity. *Nat Genet* 2008;40(10):1163–1165.
133. Cutz E, Sherman PM, Davidson GP. Enteropathies associated with protracted diarrhea of infancy: clinicopathological features, cellular and molecular mechanisms. *Pediatr Pathol Lab Med* 1997;17(3):335–368.
134. Iancu TC, et al. The liver in congenital disorders of glycosylation: ultrastructural features. *Ultrastruct Pathol* 2007a;31(3):189–197.
135. Iancu TC, et al. Microvillous inclusion disease: ultrastructural variability. *Ultrastruct Pathol* 2007b;31(3):173–188.
136. Goulet O, et al. Intestinal epithelial dysplasia (tufting enteropathy). *Orphanet J Rare Dis* 2007;2:20.
137. Roche O, et al. Superficial punctate keratitis and conjunctival erosions associated with congenital tufting enteropathy. *Am J Ophthalmol* 2010;150(1):116–121 e1.
138. Sivagnanam M, et al. Identification of EpCAM as the gene for congenital tufting enteropathy. *Gastroenterology* 2008;135(2):429–437.
139. Salomon J, et al. A founder effect at the EPCAM locus in Congenital Tufting Enteropathy in the Arabic Gulf. *Eur J Med Genet* 2011;54(3):319–322.
140. Wang J, et al. Mutant neurogenin-3 in congenital malabsorptive diarrhea. *N Engl J Med* 2006;355(3):270–280.
141. Pinney SE, et al. Neonatal diabetes and congenital malabsorptive diarrhea attributable to a novel mutation in the human neurogenin-3 gene coding sequence. *J Clin Endocrinol Metab* 2011;96(7):1960–1965.
142. Posovszky C, et al. Loss of enteroendocrine cells in autoimmune-polyendocrine-candidiasis-ectodermal-dystrophy (APECED) syndrome with gastrointestinal dysfunction. *J Clin Endocrinol Metab* 2012;97(2):E292–E300.
143. Hogenauer C, et al. Malabsorption due to cholecystokinin deficiency in a patient with autoimmune polyglandular syndrome type I. *N Engl J Med* 2001;344(4):270–274.
144. Montalto M, et al. Autoimmune enteropathy in children and adults. *Scand J Gastroenterol* 2009;44(9):1029–1036.
145. Ochs HD, Gambineri E, Torgerson TR. IPEX, FOXP3 and regulatory T-cells: a model for autoimmunity. *Immunol Res* 2007;38(1–3):112–121.
146. Yong PL, Russo P, Sullivan KE. Use of sirolimus in IPEX and IPEX-like children. *J Clin Immunol* 2008;28(5):581–587.
147. Akram S, et al. Adult autoimmune enteropathy: Mayo Clinic Rochester experience. *Clin Gastroenterol Hepatol* 2007;5(11):1282–1290; quiz 1245.
148. Patey-Mariaud de Serre N, et al. Digestive histopathological presentation of IPEX syndrome. *Mod Pathol* 2009;22(1):95–102.
149. Russo PA, et al. Autoimmune enteropathy. *Pediatr Dev Pathol* 1999;2(1):65–71.
150. Rodrigues AF, Jenkins HR. Investigation and management of coeliac disease. *Arch Dis Child* 2008;93(3):251–254.
151. Husby S, et al. European Society for Pediatric Gastroenterology, Hepatology, and Nutrition guidelines for the diagnosis of coeliac disease. *J Pediatr Gastroenterol Nutr* 2012;54(1):136–160.

152. Hill ID, et al. Guideline for the diagnosis and treatment of celiac disease in children: recommendations of the North American Society for Pediatric Gastroenterology, Hepatology and Nutrition. *J Pediatr Gastroenterol Nutr* 2005;40(1):1–19.
153. Armstrong MJ, Hegade VS, Robins G. Advances in coeliac disease. *Curr Opin Gastroenterol* 2012;28(2):104–112.
154. Giersiepen K, et al. Accuracy of diagnostic antibody tests for coeliac disease in children: summary of an evidence report. *J Pediatr Gastroenterol Nutr* 2012;54(2):229–241.
155. Maglio M, et al. Serum and intestinal celiac disease-associated antibodies in children with celiac disease younger than 2 years of age. *J Pediatr Gastroenterol Nutr* 2010;50(1):43–48.
156. Bonamico M, et al. Patchy villous atrophy of the duodenum in childhood celiac disease. *J Pediatr Gastroenterol Nutr* 2004;38(2):204–207.
157. Levinson-Castiel R, et al. The role of duodenal bulb biopsy in the diagnosis of celiac disease in children. *J Clin Gastroenterol* 2011;45(1):26–29.
158. Goldstein NS. Proximal small-bowel mucosal villous intraepithelial lymphocytes. *Histopathology* 2004;44(3):199–205.
159. Oberhuber G, Granditsch G, Vogelsang H. The histopathology of coeliac disease: time for a standardized report scheme for pathologists. *Eur J Gastroenterol Hepatol* 1999;11(10):1185–1194.
160. Corazza GR, Villanacci V. Coeliac disease. *J Clin Pathol* 2005;58(6):573–574.
161. Ensari A. Gluten-sensitive enteropathy (celiac disease): controversies in diagnosis and classification. *Arch Pathol Lab Med* 2010;134(6):826–836.
162. Jarvinen TT, et al. Villous tip intraepithelial lymphocytes as markers of early-stage coeliac disease. *Scand J Gastroenterol* 2004;39(5):428–433.
163. Bhatti TR, et al. Lymphocytic gastritis in pediatric celiac disease. *Pediatr Dev Pathol* 2011;14(4):280–283.
164. Farrell RJ, Kelly CP. Celiac sprue. *N Engl J Med* 2002;346(3):180–188.
165. Bardella MT, et al. Coeliac disease: a histological follow-up study. *Histopathology* 2007;50(4):465–471.
166. de Chambrun GP, et al. Natural history of eosinophilic gastroenteritis. *Clin Gastroenterol Hepatol* 2011;9(11):950–956 e1.
167. Klein NC, et al. Eosinophilic gastroenteritis. *Medicine (Baltimore)* 1970;49(4):299–319.
168. Pascal RR, et al. Geographic variations in eosinophil concentration in normal colonic mucosa. *Mod Pathol* 1997;10(4):363–365.
169. Polydorides AD, et al. Evaluation of site-specific and seasonal variation in colonic mucosal eosinophils. *Hum Pathol* 2008;39(6):832–836.
170. Lowichik A, Weinberg AG. A quantitative evaluation of mucosal eosinophils in the pediatric gastrointestinal tract. *Mod Pathol* 1996;9:110–114.
171. DeBrosse CW, et al. Quantity and distribution of eosinophils in the gastrointestinal tract of children. *Pediatr Dev Pathol* 2006;9(3):210–218.
172. Collins MH. Histopathology associated with eosinophilic gastrointestinal diseases. *Immunol Allergy Clin North Am* 2009;29(1):109–117, x–xi.
173. Hurrell JM, Genta RM, Melton SD. Histopathologic diagnosis of eosinophilic conditions in the gastrointestinal tract. *Adv Anat Pathol* 2011;18(5):335–348.
174. Saeed SA, et al. Tacrolimus-associated eosinophilic gastroenterocolitis in pediatric liver transplant recipients: role of potential food allergies in pathogenesis. *Pediatr Transplant* 2006;10(6):730–735.
175. Chehade M, et al. Allergic eosinophilic gastroenteritis with protein-losing enteropathy: intestinal pathology, clinical course, and long-term follow-up. *J Pediatr Gastroenterol Nutr* 2006;42(5):516–521.
176. Carver C, et al. Three children with Milroy disease and de novo mutations in VEGFR3. *Clin Genet* 2007;71(2):187–189.
177. Stormon MO, et al. Congenital intestinal lymphatic hypoplasia presenting as non-immune hydrops in utero, and subsequent neonatal protein-losing enteropathy. *J Pediatr Gastroenterol Nutr* 2002;35(5):691–694.
178. Rychik J, et al. End-organ consequences of the Fontan operation: liver fibrosis, protein-losing enteropathy and plastic bronchitis. *Cardiol Young* 2013;23(6):831–840.
179. Bhutta ZA, et al. Therapeutic effects of oral zinc in acute and persistent diarrhea in children in developing countries: pooled analysis of randomized controlled trials. *Am J Clin Nutr* 2000;72(6):1516–1522.
180. Siebert JR. Small-intestine length in infants and children. *Am J Dis Child* 1980;134(6):593–595.
181. Daniels JA, et al. Gastrointestinal tract pathology in patients with common variable immunodeficiency (CVID): a clinicopathologic study and review. *Am J Surg Pathol* 2007;31(12):1800–1812.
182. Huppmann AR, Orenstein JM. Opportunistic disorders of the gastrointestinal tract in the age of highly active antiretroviral therapy. *Hum Pathol* 2010;41(12):1777–1787.
183. Kotler DP, Weaver SC, Terzakis JA. Ultrastructural features of epithelial cell degeneration in rectal crypts of patients with AIDS. *Am J Surg Pathol* 1986;10(8):531–538.
184. Yin X, et al. Treatment for leiomyosarcoma and leiomyoma in children with HIV infection. *Cochrane Database Syst Rev* 2010;5:CD007665.
185. Barker JN, et al. Serious infections after unrelated donor transplantation in 136 children: impact of stem cell source. *Biol Blood Marrow Transplant* 2005;11(5):362–370.
186. Filipovich AH, et al. National Institutes of Health consensus development project on criteria for clinical trials in chronic graft-versus-host disease: I. Diagnosis and staging working group report. *Biol Blood Marrow Transplant* 2005;11(12):945–956.
187. Rahman FZ, et al. Henoch-Schonlein purpura complicating adalimumab therapy for Crohn's disease. *World J Gastrointest Pharmacol Ther* 2010;1(5):119–122.
188. Esaki M, et al. GI involvement in Henoch-Schonlein purpura. *Gastrointest Endosc* 2002;56(6):920–923.
189. Robert ME, et al. Patterns of inflammation in mucosal biopsies of ulcerative colitis: perceived differences in pediatric populations are limited to children younger than 10 years. *Am J Surg Pathol* 2004;28(2):183–189.
190. Xin W, Brown PI, Greenson JK. The clinical significance of focal active colitis in pediatric patients. *Am J Surg Pathol* 2003;27(8):1134–1138.
191. Cannioto Z, et al. IBD and IBD mimicking enterocolitis in children younger than 2 years of age. *Eur J Pediatr* 2009;168(2):149–155.
192. Glickman JN, et al. Pediatric patients with untreated ulcerative colitis may present initially with unusual morphologic findings. *Am J Surg Pathol* 2004;28(2):190–197.
193. Rubin DT, Rothe JA. The peri-appendiceal red patch in ulcerative colitis: review of the University of Chicago experience. *Dig Dis Sci* 2010;55(12):3495–3501.
194. Markowitz J, et al. Endoscopic screening for dysplasia and mucosal aneuploidy in adolescents and young adults with childhood onset colitis. *Am J Gastroenterol* 1997;92(11):2001–2006.
195. De Matos V, et al. Frequency and clinical correlations of granulomas in children with Crohn disease. *J Pediatr Gastroenterol Nutr* 2008;46(4):392–398.
196. Kirsch R, et al. Role of colonoscopic biopsy in distinguishing between Crohn's disease and intestinal tuberculosis. *J Clin Pathol* 2006;59(8):840–844.
197. Abdullah BA, et al. The role of esophagogastroduodenoscopy in the initial evaluation of childhood inflammatory bowel disease: a 7-year study. *J Pediatr Gastroenterol Nutr* 2002;35(5):636–640.
198. Tobin JM, et al. Upper gastrointestinal mucosal disease in pediatric Crohn disease and ulcerative colitis: a blinded, controlled study. *J Pediatr Gastroenterol Nutr* 2001;32(4):443–448.
199. Kundhal PS, et al. Gastral antral biopsy in the differentiation of pediatric colitides. *Am J Gastroenterol* 2003;98(3):557–561.
200. Parente F, et al. Focal gastric inflammatory infiltrates in inflammatory bowel diseases: prevalence, immunohistochemical characteristics, and diagnostic role. *Am J Gastroenterol* 2000;95(3):705–711.
201. Price AB. Overlap in the spectrum of non-specific inflammatory bowel disease—'colitis indeterminate'. *J Clin Pathol* 1978;31(6):567–577.
202. Kugathasan S, et al. Epidemiologic and clinical characteristics of children with newly diagnosed inflammatory bowel disease in Wisconsin: a statewide population-based study. *J Pediatr* 2003;143(4):525–531.
203. Mamula P, et al. Inflammatory bowel disease in children 5 years of age and younger. *Am J Gastroenterol* 2002;97(8):2005–2010.

204. Rogers Boruta MK, Grand RJ, Kappelman MD. Natural history of indeterminate colitis. In: Mamula P, Markowitz J, Baldassano R, eds. *Pediatric Inflammatory Bowel Disease*. New York: Springer, 2013: 79-86.
205. Najarian RM, et al. Clinical significance of colonic intraepithelial lymphocytosis in a pediatric population. *Mod Pathol* 2009;22(1):13-20.
206. Camarero C, et al. Collagenous colitis in children: clinicopathologic, microbiologic, and immunologic features. *J Pediatr Gastroenterol Nutr* 2003;37(4):508-513.
207. Benchimol EI, et al. Collagenous colitis and eosinophilic gastritis in a 4-year old girl: a case report and review of the literature. *Acta Paediatr* 2007;96(9):1365-1367.
208. Fernandez-Banares F, et al. Collagenous and lymphocytic colitis. Evaluation of clinical and histological features, response to treatment, and long-term follow-up. *Am J Gastroenterol* 2003;98(2):340-347.
209. Vujanic GM, Dojcinov SD. Diversion colitis in children: an iatrogenic appendix vermiformis? *Histopathology* 2000;36(1):41-46.
210. Warren BF, et al. Pathology of the defunctioned rectum in ulcerative colitis. *Gut* 1993;34(4):514-516.
211. Bavaro MF. Neutropenic enterocolitis. *Curr Gastroenterol Rep* 2002;4(4):297-301.
212. Newbold KM, Lord MG, Baglin TP. Role of clostridial organisms in neutropenic enterocolitis. *J Clin Pathol* 1987;40(4):471.
213. Caplan MS, Jilling T. New concepts in necrotizing enterocolitis. *Curr Opin Pediatr* 2001;13(2):111-115.
214. Ng S. Necrotizing enterocolitis in the full-term neonate. *J Paediatr Child Health* 2001;37(1):1-4.
215. Neu J, Walker WA. Necrotizing enterocolitis. *N Engl J Med* 2011;364(3):255-264.
216. Albanese CT, Rowe MI. Necrotizing enterocolitis. In: O'Neill JA, et al., eds. *Pediatric Surgery*. St Louis, MO: Mosby, 1998:1297-1330.
217. Gordon PV. Understanding intestinal vulnerability to perforation in the extremely low birth weight infant. *Pediatr Res* 2009;65(2):138-144.
218. Husain AN, et al. Segmental absence of small intestinal musculature. *Pediatr Pathol* 1992;12(3):407-415.
219. Raveenthiran V. Spontaneous perforation of the colon and rectum complicating anorectal malformations in neonates. *J Pediatr Surg* 2012;47(4):720-726.
220. Maloney J, Nowak-Wegrzyn A. Educational clinical case series for pediatric allergy and immunology: allergic proctocolitis, food protein-induced enterocolitis syndrome and allergic eosinophilic gastroenteritis with protein-losing gastroenteropathy as manifestations of non-IgE-mediated cow's milk allergy. *Pediatr Allergy Immunol* 2007;18(4): 360-367.
221. Blackburn C, McDermott M, Bourke B. Clinical presentation of and outcome for solitary rectal ulcer syndrome in children. *J Pediatr Gastroenterol Nutr* 2012;54(2):263-265.
222. Borrelli O, de' Angelis G. Solitary rectal ulcer syndrome: it's time to think about it. *J Pediatr Gastroenterol Nutr* 2012;54(2):167-168.
223. Wang M-L, Rustgi A. Polyps and polyposis syndromes. In: Liacouras C, Piccoli D, eds. *Pediatric Gastroenterology*. Philadelphia, PA: Mosby-Elsevier; 2008:192-199.
224. Gammon A, et al. Hamartomatous polyposis syndromes. *Best Pract Res Clin Gastroenterol* 2009;23(2):219-231.
225. Pawel B. Polyps and tumors of the gastrointestinal tract in children. In: Russo P, Ruchelli E, Piccoli D, eds. *Pathology of Pediatric Gastrointestinal and Liver Disease*. Heidelberg, Germany: Springer; 2014:317-370.
226. Brosens LA, et al. Risk of colorectal cancer in juvenile polyposis. *Gut* 2007;56(7):965-967.
227. Pilarski R, et al. Cowden syndrome and the PTEN hamartoma tumor syndrome: systematic review and revised diagnostic criteria. *J Natl Cancer Inst* 2013;105(21):1607-1616.
228. Heald B, et al. Frequent gastrointestinal polyps and colorectal adenocarcinomas in a prospective series of PTEN mutation carriers. *Gastroenterology* 2010;139(6):1927-1933.
229. Suzuki S, et al. Three cases of Solitary Peutz-Jeghers-type hamartomatous polyp in the duodenum. *World J Gastroenterol* 2008;14(6):944-947.
230. Guarinos C, et al. Prevalence and characteristics of MUTYH-associated polyposis in patients with multiple adenomatous and serrated polyps. *Clin Cancer Res* 2014;20(5):1158-1168.
231. Blumer SL, et al. Sporadic adenocarcinoma of the colon in children: case series and review of the literature. *J Pediatr Hematol Oncol* 2012;34(4):e137-e141.
232. Ozolek JA, et al. Inflammatory fibroid polyps of the gastrointestinal tract: clinical, pathologic, and molecular characteristics. *Appl Immunohistochem Mol Morphol* 2004;12(1):59-66.
233. Al-Saleem T, Al-Mondhiry H. Immunoproliferative small intestinal disease (IPSID): a model for mature B-cell neoplasms. *Blood* 2005;105(6):2274-2280.
234. Parker A, et al. Diagnosis of post-transplant lymphoproliferative disorder in solid organ transplant recipients—BCSH and BTS guidelines. *Br J Haematol* 2010;149(5):675-692.
235. Hait E, et al. Gastrointestinal tract involvement in Langerhans cell histiocytosis: case report and literature review. *Pediatrics* 2006;118(5):e1593-e1599.
236. Sokol H, et al. Gastrointestinal manifestations in mastocytosis: a study of 83 patients. *J Allergy Clin Immunol* 2013;132(4):866-873 e1-3.
237. Lipton S, Estrin J, Glasser I. Diverticular disease of the appendix. *Surg Gynecol Obstet* 1989;168(1):13-16.
238. George DH. Diverticulosis of the vermiform appendix in patients with cystic fibrosis. *Hum Pathol* 1987;18(1):75-79.
239. Shelton T, McKinlay R, Schwartz RW. Acute appendicitis: current diagnosis and treatment. *Curr Surg* 2003;60(5):502-505.
240. Ruffolo C, et al. Acute appendicitis: what is the gold standard of treatment? *World J Gastroenterol* 2013;19(47):8799-8807.
241. Meyers P, Williams R. *Pathology of the Appendix*. London, UK: Chapman & Hall Medical, 1994:180.
242. Carr NJ. The pathology of acute appendicitis. *Ann Diagn Pathol* 2000;4(1):46-58.
243. Stadlmann S, et al. Histopathologic characteristics of the transitional stage of measles-associated appendicitis: case report and review of the literature. *Hum Pathol* 2011;42(2):285-290.
244. Shorter NA, et al. Surgical aspects of an outbreak of *Yersinia enterocolitis*. *Pediatr Surg Int* 1998;13(1):2-5.
245. Kroft SH, Stryker SJ, Rao MS. Appendiceal involvement as a skip lesion in ulcerative colitis. *Mod Pathol* 1994;7(9):912-914.
246. Dudley TH Jr, Dean PJ. Idiopathic granulomatous appendicitis, or Crohn's disease of the appendix revisited. *Hum Pathol* 1993;24(6):595-601.
247. Huang JC, Appelman HD. Another look at chronic appendicitis resembling Crohn's disease. *Mod Pathol* 1996;9(10):975-981.
248. Deschamps L, Couvelard A. Endocrine tumors of the appendix: a pathologic review. *Arch Pathol Lab Med* 2010;134(6):871-875.
249. Santulli TV, Kiesewetter WB, Bill AH Jr. Anorectal anomalies: a suggested international classification. *J Pediatr Surg* 1970;5(3):281-287.
250. Sinclair KA, Woods CR, Sinal SH. Venereal warts in children. *Pediatr Rev* 2011;32(3):115-121; quiz 121.
251. Ornstein A, Hatchette T. Human papillomavirus and anogenital warts in children. *CMAJ* 2012;184(3):321.

CHAPTER 15

The Liver, Gallbladder, and Biliary Tract

Sarangarajan Ranganathan, M.D., and M. John Hicks, M.D., D.D.S., M.S., Ph.D.

DEVELOPMENT

Hepatobiliary morphogenesis occurs during the first 10 weeks of gestation (1). The liver primordium appears in week 3 as a tubular evagination of the future duodenal segment of the foregut endoderm. The hepatic diverticulum differentiates cranially into the proliferating hepatic cords and caudally into the extrahepatic bile ducts and the gallbladder. The hepatic diverticulum branches dichotomously, and thick anastomosing sheets of epithelial cells grow into the mesenchyme of the septum transversum, and the mesenchymal cells form the connective tissue elements of the hepatic stroma and capsule. As the hepatic sheets extend outward in the septum transversum, they are penetrated by the capillary plexus derived from the vitelline veins, which arise from the primitive hepatic sinusoids.

In the 10-mm embryo, bile canaliculi appear as intercellular spaces between sheets of presumptive hepatocytes. The epithelial lining of the extrahepatic bile ducts is continuous with the primitive hepatic sheets that give rise to the epithelium of the intrahepatic bile ducts. The epithelium of the intrahepatic bile ducts is probably generated by interaction of the primitive hepatic epithelium and the mesenchyme surrounding the developing and branching portal vein. The epithelial layer, which is in direct contact with the mesenchyme around the portal vein, transforms into bile duct–like cells, after which a second layer transforms into bile duct epithelial cells. At around 8 weeks' gestation, the ductal plate develops, appearing as a cleft in the shape of a cylinder around the mesenchyme of the progressively developing and branching portal vein. The ductal plate (Figure 15-1) undergoes gradual remodeling to form the interlobular bile ducts in the portal tract, undergoing a balanced process of cell proliferation and apoptosis. Intrahepatic bile ducts are recognized in the 20- to 30-mm embryo. The hepatocytes and bile duct epithelial cells are structurally and functionally distinct. The canals of Hering, which connect the canaliculi to the bile ducts, consist of both typical hepatocytes and bile duct epithelial cells (1,2).

The development of the liver is associated with changes in the primordial vitelline veins, which give rise to the portal, hepatic, and umbilical veins. The definitive pattern of veins within the liver is established in the 10-mm embryo. The proximal end of the right vitelline vein forms the terminal part of the inferior vena cava. The portal vein arises from persistence of segments of both right and left vitelline veins and three anastomotic channels between the two. The right umbilical vein disappears, and all blood from the placenta enters the liver from the left umbilical vein. The coalescence of some of the hepatic sinusoids produces an oblique channel, the ductus venosus, which connects the left umbilical vein to the right vitelline vein, diverting some of the oxygenated blood directly to the heart.

The right side of the liver receives blood predominantly from the portal vein, and the left lobe is supplied mainly by oxygenated blood from the left umbilical vein. This may account for the difference in the appearance of the two lobes. At birth, the left lobe is larger relative to its size in later life. Moreover, the right lobe shows more hematopoiesis, and the hepatocytes contain more glycogen, lipid, and iron pigment than those in the left lobe. Fetal blood flow through the hepatic artery is insignificant compared with that delivered by the umbilical and portal veins.

The caudal part of the hollow diverticulum elongates and presumably becomes the common bile duct, hepatic duct, cystic duct, and the gallbladder between weeks 5 and 7.5. The liver is the site of hematopoiesis between weeks 6 and 7, and erythropoiesis dominates from week 12 until the beginning of the third trimester. During the third trimester, the bone marrow is the dominant site of hematopoiesis, and hepatic erythropoiesis decreases, although it continues in the newborn period and may persist into the first few weeks of life.

HISTOLOGY

The conventional histologic unit of the liver is the hepatic lobule, which consists of a central efferent vein with cords of hepatocytes radiating to several peripheral portal tracts. The portal tract contains the interlobular bile ducts, branches of

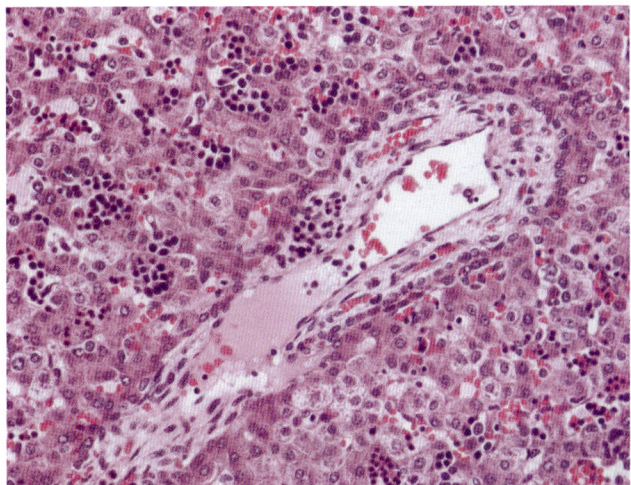

FIGURE 15-1 • Ductal plate in the fetal liver is formed by a collar of epithelial cells at the periphery of the portal tract and abuts against zone 1 hepatocytes. Note the presence of extramedullary hematopoiesis (H&E stain, 200×).

the portal vein, and hepatic artery and lymphatics. The functional unit of the liver is the hepatic acinus (Figure 15-2). The hepatic acinus is a three-dimensional structure with the portal tract as the central point (zone 1) where blood flows from terminal branches of the portal vein and hepatic arteries into the sinusoids and empties into the terminal hepatic venules at the periphery of the acinus (centrilobular/zone 3). Bile is secreted into the canaliculi and flows toward the portal areas into the interlobular bile ducts that are connected to the canaliculi by canals of Hering. The acinus thus includes parts of several adjacent lobules.

The hepatocytes in children older than 5 or 6 years of age are organized into single-cell plates. In younger children, the liver cells are arranged in two-cell-thick plates. In the preterm infant, the lobular structure of the liver is poorly defined and hepatic plates are more than one cell thick. Canaliculi lie between adjacent hepatocytes and, ultrastructurally, tight junctions are present between the hepatocytes surrounding the canaliculus. Microvilli from the hepatocytes project into the canalicular lumen. The hepatocytes in childhood often have nuclear glycogen, and lipofuscin in the cytoplasm is usually scanty. The hepatic sinusoidal lining cells include endothelial and Kupffer cells. The endothelial cells are supported by reticulin fibers, and between the endothelial cells and hepatocytes is the space of Disse. Perisinusoidal cells (cells of Ito) are interstitial fat-storing cells and appear to play a significant role in hepatic fibrogenesis.

CONGENITAL ANOMALIES

Agenesis of the liver is incompatible with life and is usually associated with other severe congenital anomalies in stillborn fetuses. Agenesis of one lobe of the liver, usually the right, is seen infrequently and is rarely associated with clinical symptoms (3,4). In situs inversus totalis, the liver, its peritoneal and vascular connections, and the gallbladder and extrahepatic ducts have a mirror-image configuration to normal situs. In the asplenia–polysplenia syndromes, the liver may be midline and bilaterally symmetrical.

The liver may herniate through defects in the diaphragm (Figure 15-3). Diaphragmatic defects are more common on the left side, and the liver often herniates into the left pleural cavity (4,5). The herniated portion of the liver may be dusky, and a groove often marks the site of compression by the margin of the diaphragm. The right lobe of the liver may bulge into the right pleural cavity in association with eventration of

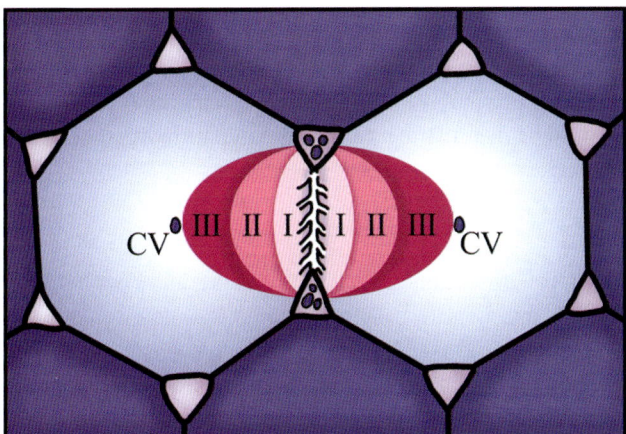

FIGURE 15-2 • Schematic view of hepatic lobule or acinus. The conventional view of the liver consisted of a hepatic lobule with a central vein (CV) surrounded by hepatocyte cords radiating to peripheral portal areas. The functional unit of the liver, the acinus, however, consists of a three-dimensional structure with a central portal tract surrounded by concentric zones of hepatocytes (I, II, and III), with the most peripheral zone (III) lying near the central vein.

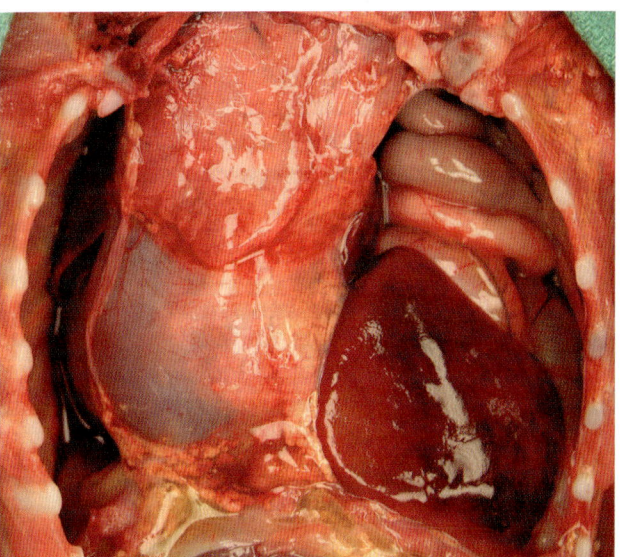

FIGURE 15-3 • Herniation of the liver through diaphragmatic defect. A large defect in the left leaflet of the diaphragm has led to the herniation of the left lobe of the liver and intestines into the left hemithorax, resulting in mediastinal shift to the right and severe pulmonary hypoplasia.

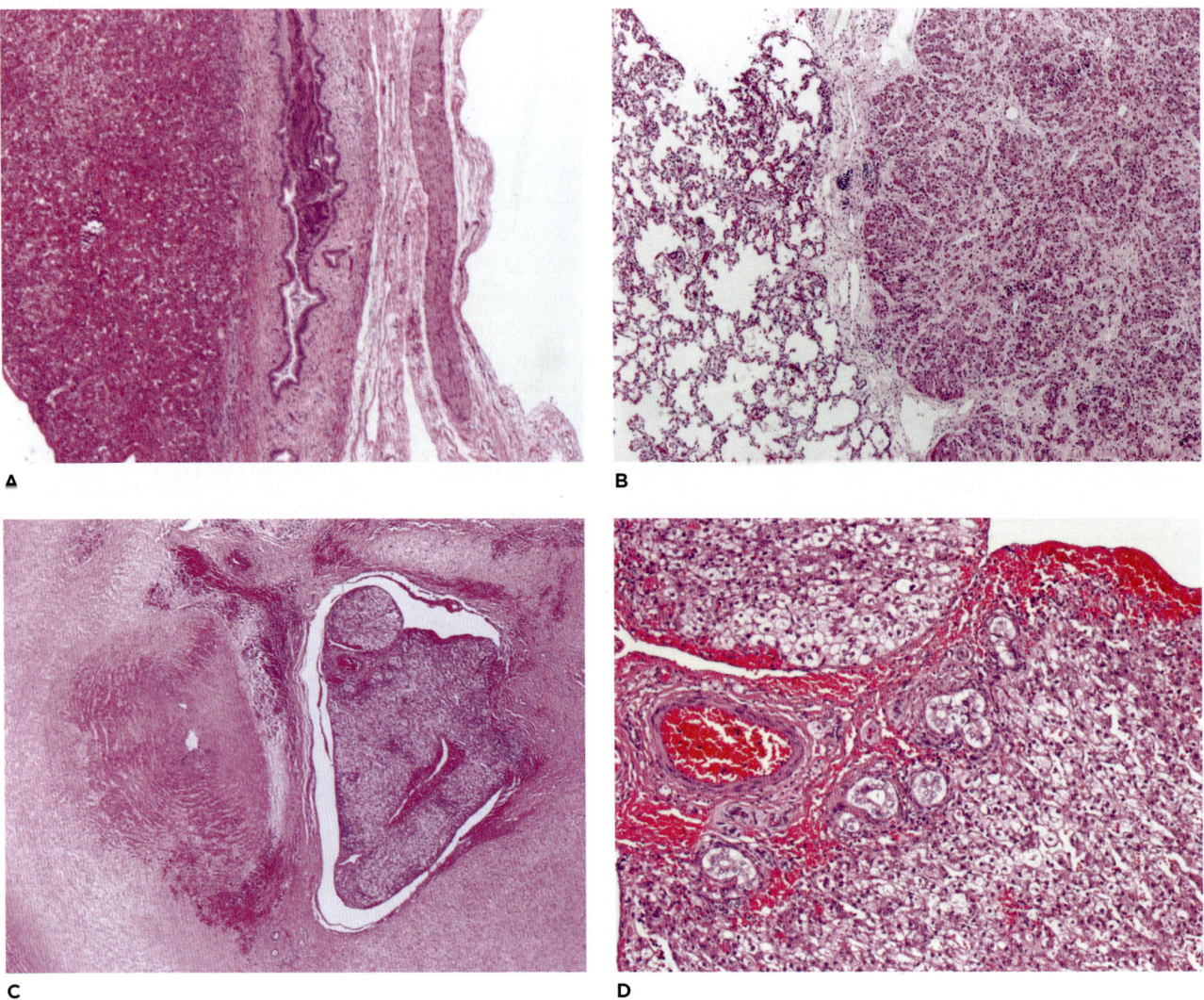

FIGURE 15-4 • **A:** Ectopic liver tissue within the diaphragm **B:** Lung **C:** Umbilical cord (H&E, 40×) **D:** Ectopic liver tissue in the umbilical cord with bile ducts (H&E stain, 200×).

the right hemidiaphragm. In cases of omphalocele, the liver is often herniated into the omphalocele sac. In large omphaloceles, there is often distortion of the liver and its vascular and biliary connections. The liver may have signs of marked congestion and even hemorrhagic necrosis. Intrapericardial herniation of the liver occurs rarely and may result in massive pericardial effusion in neonates. Nearly all cases of the thoracopagus type of conjoined twins show connections between the two livers, ranging from a bridge to a common liver between the two twins.

Hepatic ectopia or heterotopia is extremely unusual, with only rare reports of distinct lobules of hepatic tissue within the gallbladder wall, the substance of the diaphragm, lung, and umbilical cord (6) (Figure 15-4). Often times, this liver tissue is seen in conjunction with congenital diaphragmatic hernias and congenital heart disease. Ectopic pancreatic tissue within the liver or in the porta hepatis may also be seen, occasionally obstructing the common hepatic duct. Adrenal heterotopias are usually the result of adrenal–hepatic adhesion or fusion depending on the presence (adhesion) or absence (fusion) of a capsule between the organs. Liver tissue at these variable sites is at the same risk for viral hepatitis and subsequent hepatocellular carcinoma (HCC) as an orthotopic liver tissue infected with hepatitis viruses.

TISSUE TRIAGING

The most important aspect of providing an accurate diagnosis is appropriate triaging of tissue to allow for optimal evaluation (Figure 15-5). It is imperative that adequate tissue is obtained to perform all necessary tests for an appropriate diagnosis to guide future therapy and to avoid repeat biopsy. Fresh tissue can be obtained for microbiologic and viral cultures, polymerase chain reaction (PCR) testing, and cytogenetic studies. Tissue should be obtained for routine histology (formalin fixation), histochemical stains (frozen in optimal cryomatrix material [OCT] at −20°C and alcohol fixation), electron microscopy (glutaraldehyde), and genetic/molecular evaluation (frozen at −70°C). It is especially important

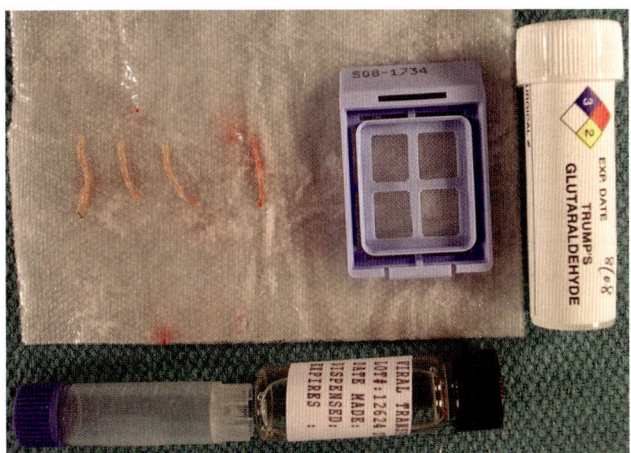

FIGURE 15-5 • Liver biopsy triaging consists of tissue submitted for formalin fixation and paraffin embedding, freezing tissue at −70°C, viral or microbiologic culture submission, and glutaraldehyde fixation for electron microscopy.

with glycogen storage diseases (GSDs) to maintain optimal preservation of glycogen. With formalin fixation, up to 70% of glycogen is lost due to the soluble nature of the predominant form of glycogen in the cytoplasm. Glycogen can be preserved with freezing and/or alcohol fixation, allowing for quantitative evaluation by analytical techniques (frozen tissue) and qualitative assessment by histochemical staining (periodic acid-Schiff [PAS], PAS diastase). Quantitative analysis of enzyme(s) responsible for suspected metabolic and mitochondrial diseases must be done on frozen tissue. Assessment of metals such as copper and iron may require use of metal-free containers to freeze liver tissue for proper quantification. Assessment of gene mutation and sequencing of the gene responsible for the enzyme defect or mitochondrial disease also requires frozen tissue. Preservation of the enzyme, enzyme activity, DNA, and RNA requires cryopreservation at −70°C and maintaining this temperature until the tissue reaches the appropriate reference laboratory. Depending on the testing required for a definitive diagnosis, tissue requirements may dictate an open biopsy of the liver and/or skeletal muscle. Obtaining fibroblast cultures from a skin biopsy may also be necessary for genetic and enzyme studies. The current trend in surgical and interventional radiology practice has been toward needle core biopsies for diagnosis. The pathologist should be aware of necessary tissue requirements (tissue weights and preservation methods) for appropriate testing to be completed. A single tissue core of 20 mm in length from a 16-gauge needle with a 1.5 mm diameter yields about 15 mg of tissue. Several metabolic disease tests require a minimum of 20 mg of tissue. With GSDs, 100 mg or more of tissue will be needed. This may necessitate numerous tissue cores or an open biopsy to obtain adequate tissue for all tests. This emphasizes the importance of active communication between the health care team and the pathologist. Because tissue will be preserved in a steady state with cryopreservation (−70°C), comprehensive workup (histopathology, histochemistry, electron microscopy) by the pathologist to determine which additional testing is most appropriate can be completed prior to performing specialized testing on the frozen tissue.

PHYSIOLOGIC JAUNDICE

Hyperbilirubinemia in the neonatal period is one of the earliest postnatal events that requires clinical assessment to determine its clinical significance (7). In the majority of cases, it is assessed to be physiologic jaundice with an elevated unconjugated bilirubin, which resolves within the first 2 weeks of life. However, in the presence of conjugated hyperbilirubinemia and other concurrent hepatic enzyme abnormalities, a clinically serious underlying disorder must be given consideration. With infants and older children, development of jaundice is a sign of hepatic or biliary tract disease of diverse etiologies; requires thorough clinical, imaging, and laboratory evaluation; and may need liver biopsy to determine the exact nature of the underlying disease.

Physiologic jaundice is characterized by an increase in serum unconjugated bilirubin of 5 to 6 mg/dL by 2 to 4 days of age (8). This is a result of increased bilirubin production following breakdown of fetal red blood cells, combined with transient limitation in the conjugation of bilirubin by the liver. Levels of up to 12 mg/dL may be seen in Chinese, Japanese, Korean, or Native American infants. Other risk factors include maternal diabetes, prematurity, altitude, polycythemia, male sex, trisomy 21, cutaneous bleeding, cephalohematoma, oxytocin induction, and vitamin K use. Additional causes of unconjugated hyperbilirubinemia are listed in Table 15-1. Cholestasis is rarely present in the liver in the absence of other diseases.

HEREDITARY HYPERBILIRUBINEMIAS

Crigler-Najjar syndrome (CNS), an autosomal recessive or dominant disorder, results from a mutation in one of the five exons of the UGT1A1 gene coding for the enzyme bilirubin–UDP–glucuronosyltransferase (8,9). UGT1A1 mutation leads to elevated unconjugated bilirubin levels. In type 1 CNS, enzymatic activity is completely absent and the neonate presents with jaundice and frequently kernicterus with death by 1 year of age. Liver transplantation has been successfully used in management. The liver may show prominent canalicular bile or may appear normal. With type 2 CNS, there is only a partial deficiency of glucuronyl transferase, and this has a milder clinical course with most affected individuals being asymptomatic. Gilbert syndrome is a benign condition with minimal clinical manifestations, owing to greater preservation of enzyme activity. Although the condition is occasionally seen in children, the diagnosis is usually made incidentally in young adults or in later life.

Dubin-Johnson syndrome, an autosomal recessive trait, may present in the neonatal period with conjugated and unconjugated hyperbilirubinemia and severe cholestasis

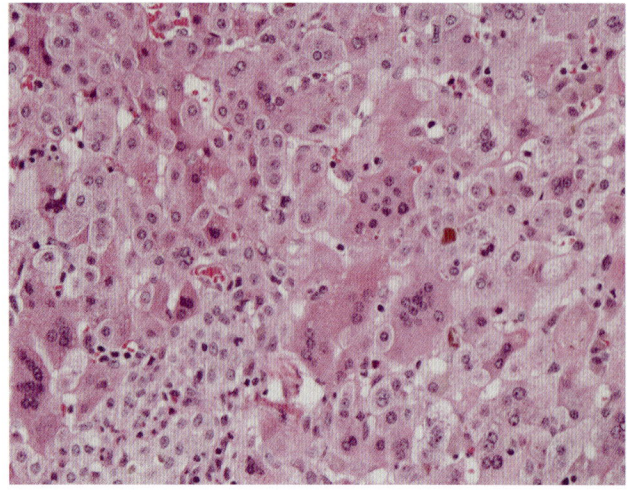
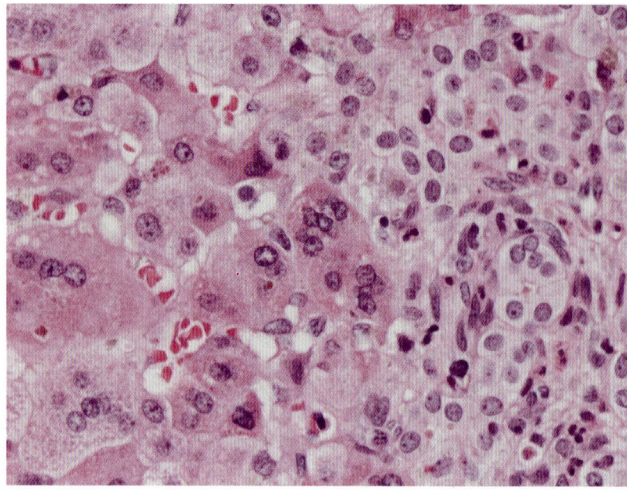
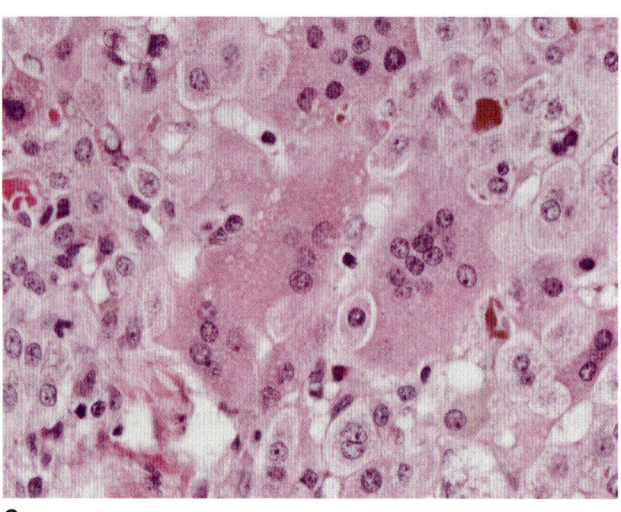

FIGURE 15-6 • **A–C:** Idiopathic neonatal hepatitis. Giant cell transformation with expansion of the portal region by chronic inflammatory cells, prominent bile ducts, and readily identified cholestasis (**A** at 100×, **B** at 200×, **C** at 200×, H&E).

and hydronephrosis) and group 3 is associated with laterality defects with cardiovascular, gastrointestinal, and splenic anomalies. Similar to neonatal hepatitis, EHBA is also considered to be a condition with more than one etiology. In fact, INH and EHBA have been seen as sequential processes in the same infant over a period of several weeks to months (17). While viral theories have been proposed as etiologies for EHBA, recent documentation of a high incidence of autoimmune diseases in first-degree relatives of all BA groups raises the possibility of an autoimmune mechanism (16). Defects in cilia have also been implicated in the pathogenesis of EHBA (18).

TABLE 15-3 COMPARISON OF BILIARY ATRESIA AND NEONATAL HEPATITIS SYNDROME

Features	Biliary Atresia	Neonatal Hepatitis
Giant cell transformation	Usually focal	Diffuse; occasionally focal
Hepatocellular necrosis	Variable	Variable
Lobular disarray	Usually mild	May be marked
Cholestasis	Hepatocytes, canaliculi, and ducts	Hepatocytes and canaliculi; ducts (rare)
Portal fibrosis	In all portal areas	Absent early in the course
Bile ducts	Proliferation typically seen in all portal areas	Normal; rarely focal proliferation
Cellular infiltrate	Variable; mononuclear	Variable; mononuclear
Extramedullary hematopoiesis	Usually present	Usually present
Fat	Typically absent	Typically absent

The liver biopsy remains an integral component in the diagnosis of a neonate or young infant with persistent conjugated hyperbilirubinemia and is a highly reliable means of establishing the diagnosis of EHBA in 85% to 97% of cases (19,20). Most difficulties are encountered in making a definitive diagnosis in the very young (first 4 weeks) or older patients (more than 3 months old). In many instances, the biopsies are open biopsies done at the time of surgical exploration, but needle biopsies if done not too early in the disease may be diagnostic. Ductular proliferation is the most common finding and is considered a diagnostic feature of EHBA, although modest bile duct proliferation may be seen in other causes of neonatal hepatitis (Figures 15-7 to 15-9). The interlobular bile ducts are tortuous and have distorted contours, readily demonstrated with pancytokeratin or cytokeratin AE1/AE3. Resemblance to ductal plate malformation may be noted both in the interlobular bile duct arrangement as well as within the ductular reaction (21). The lining epithelium shows degenerative changes, and periductal reactive fibrosis may occur with plump fibroblasts surrounded by a loose edematous stroma. Lymphocytes and even neutrophils are found within the portal areas, with occasional infiltration of the bile duct epithelium. Portal lymphocytes, which are usually few in number, should not be confused with extramedullary hematopoiesis in younger infants. As the disease progresses in the first few weeks of life, nearly all portal areas are expanded by fibrosis, with type IV collagen deposition. Bridging fibrosis occurs, and early nodular transformation is evident as a prelude to the development of secondary biliary cirrhosis. The progression to cirrhosis varies considerably from one case to another, but there is some direct relationship with age.

Hepatocellular alterations include cholestasis (canalicular, hepatocellular, ductular), feathery (pseudoxanthomatous) degeneration, pseudoacinar transformation, and focal giant cell transformation. These features overlap with those of neonatal hepatitis. Cholestasis in EHBA is usually severe and is most prominent in zone 3, but is also present within the ductules and bile ducts at the zone 1 interface. Hepatocytes may form gland-like structures around bile plugs, imparting a "pseudoacinar" configuration, the so-called cholestatic

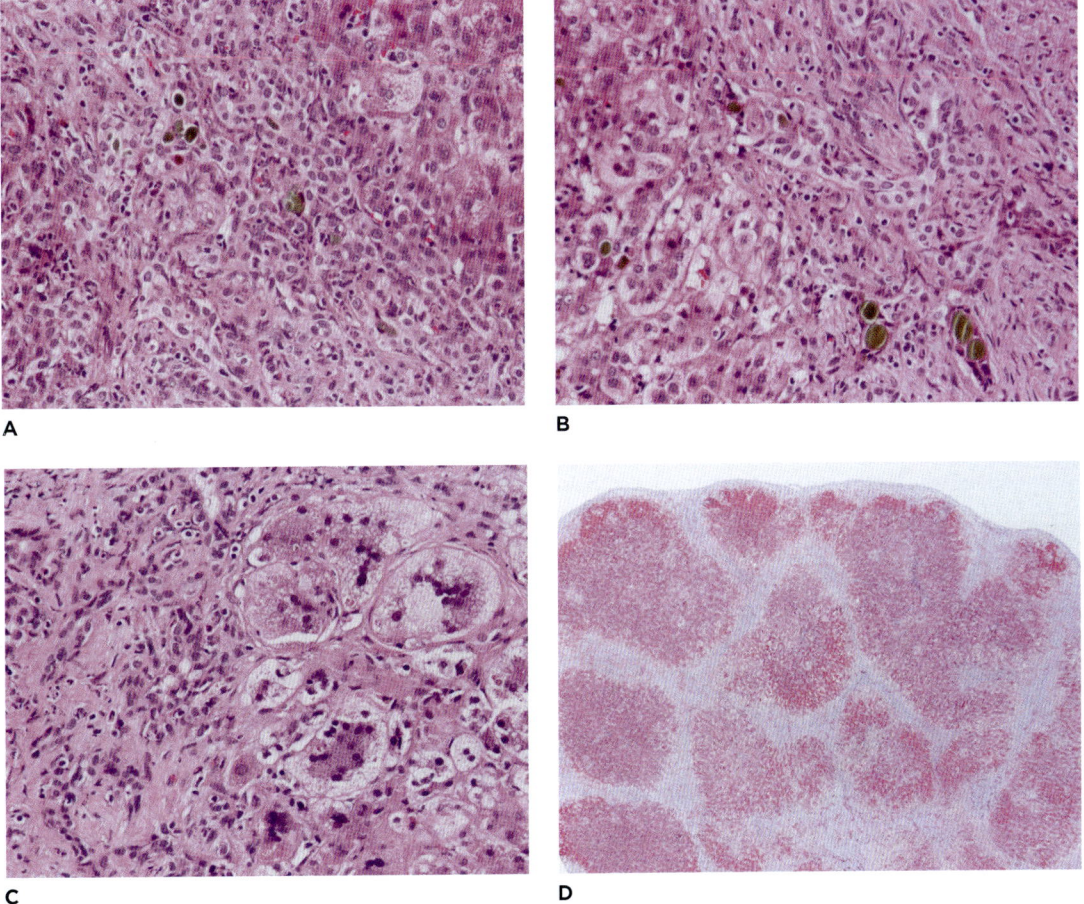

FIGURE 15-7 • **A:** EHBA liver biopsy. Histopathologic features include diffuse bile duct proliferation in expanded portal region with canalicular cholestasis. **B:** Hepatocytes organized into pseudoacinar pattern **C:** Giant cell transformation adjacent to fibrotic portal region **D:** Cirrhosis may occur rapidly without surgical intervention (H&E stains, **A, B, C** at 200×, **D** 40×).

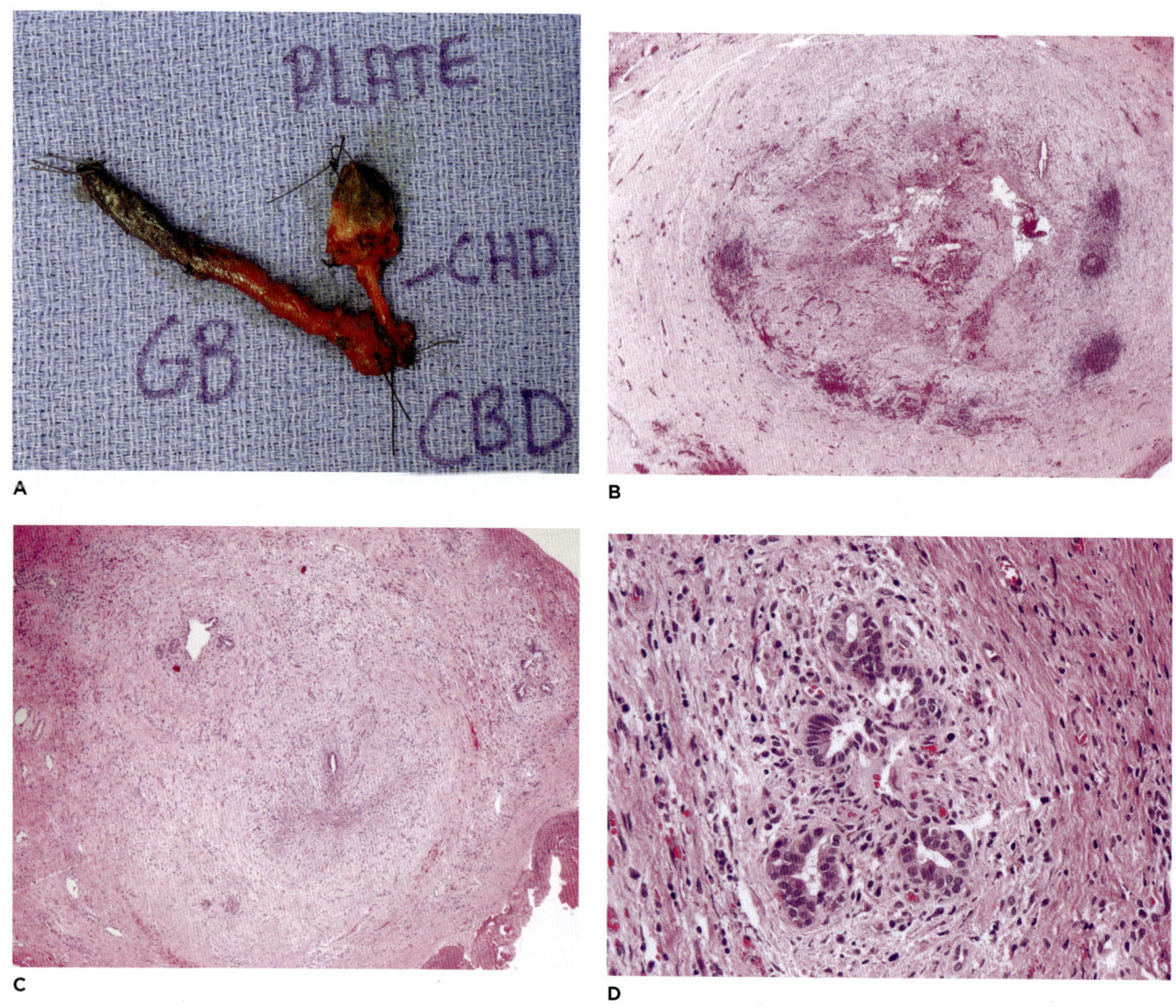

FIGURE 15-8 • Resection of residual common bile duct during Kasai procedure. **A:** Common bile duct remnant with orientation by surgeon. CHD, hepatic duct, GB; gallbladder, CBD; common bile duct; plate, liver plate. **B:** Near-total obliteration of common bile duct lumen with no residual epithelial lining (H&E, 20×). **C:** Microscopic residual common bile duct lumen with epithelial lining (H&E, 20×). **D:** Nests of bile duct epithelium in common bile duct wall (H&E, 200×). The latter side chain structures should not be mistaken as evidence of a patent bile duct.

rosettes. Bile "lakes" consisting of amorphous collections of bile surrounded by inflammatory cells and connective tissue are seen rarely in liver biopsies, unlike in adults with obstruction of the biliary tract. Hepatocytes may display mild enlargement and rarefaction of the cytoplasm (feathery degeneration), but fatty change is rarely seen. Giant cell transformation, if present, is generally restricted to zone 1 at the interface with the expanded portal tracts (Table 15-3). Instances of hepatocyte and giant cell necrosis may be encountered.

The most frequently observed changes within the liver in EHBA are prominent cholestasis, portal fibrosis, and ductal/ductular proliferation. Other causes of obstruction (bile duct stenosis, choledochal cyst, mucous or bile plug) produce similar changes, as will disorders such as alpha-1 antitrypsin deficiency (A1AT) and total parenteral nutrition (TPN)-associated cholestasis. It is important to realize that other disorders can simulate patterns of liver injury similar to those for EHBA.

The extrahepatic ducts may display a wide variety of histopathologic changes, ranging from a mild degree of inflammation to complete obliteration (22,23) (Figure 15-8). The epithelium of large, medium, and small ducts shows nuclear irregularity and pyknosis with cellular degeneration and necrosis. Cellular debris and bile-stained macrophages may be present in the lumen. The duct lining is often infiltrated by neutrophils and is ulcerated, with intraluminal and extraluminal fibrosis distorting the lumen. As the epithelial inflammation and degeneration progresses, fibrosis increases and eventually obliterates the duct. With active ductular

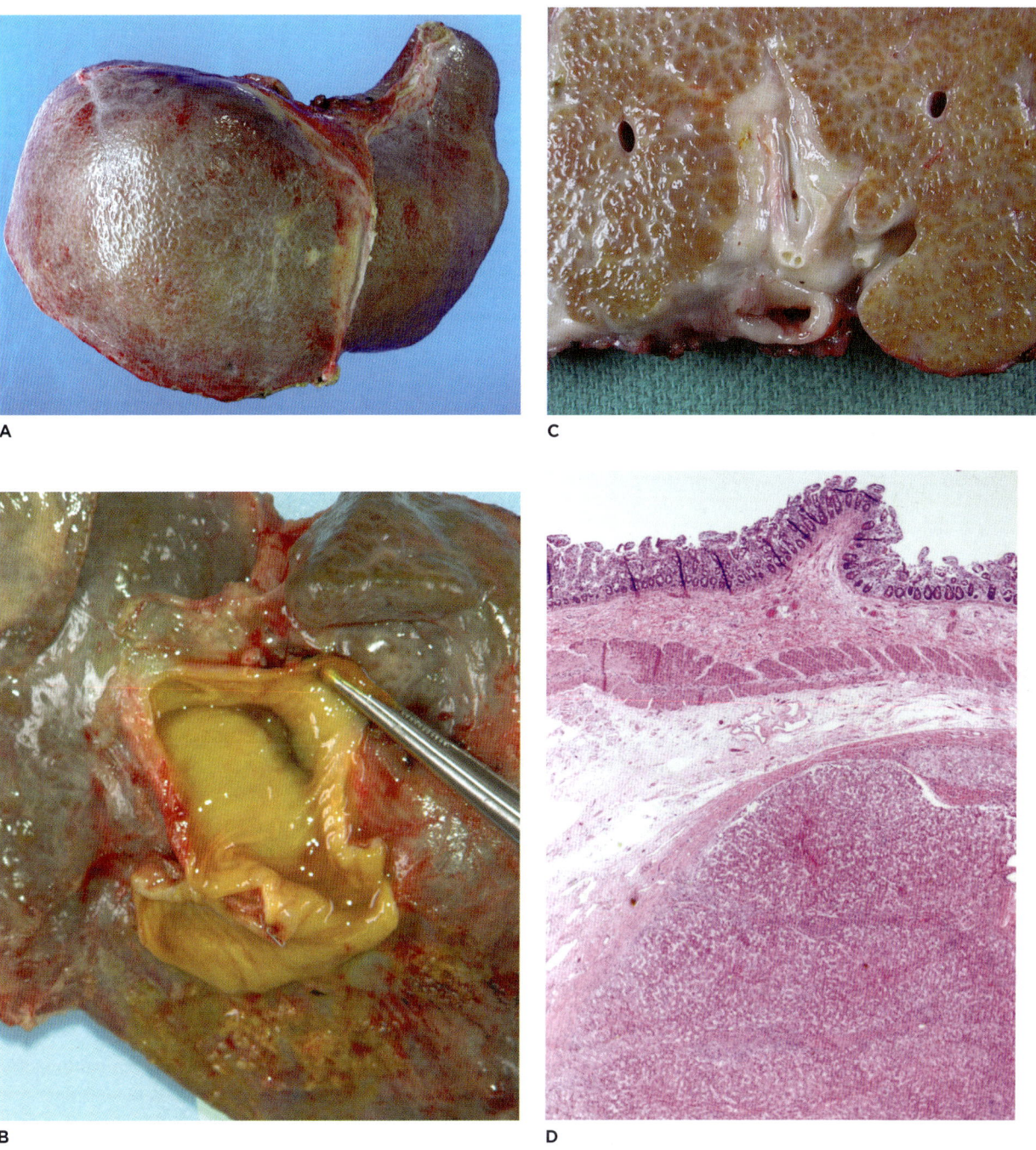

FIGURE 15-9 • Explanted liver with prior Kasai procedure. **A:** Explanted liver with micronodular cirrhosis. **B:** Patent small-bowel anastomosis site at liver hilum. **C:** Liver in cross-section with close apposition of small-bowel anastomosis to liver hilum and micronodular liver parenchyma with diffuse bile staining. **D:** Small-bowel anastomosis separated by muscular wall of small bowel and fibrous tissue from the underlying liver parenchyma (H&E, 10×).

destruction, the stroma around and between ducts becomes infiltrated by neutrophils, lymphocytes, and macrophages, along with a prominent fibroblastic proliferation. As the ductular inflammation diminishes and the ducts are destroyed, the stromal activity is replaced by dense fibrosis, containing a few residual inflammatory cells and remnants of bile ducts. Rarely, islands of hyaline cartilage may be found in the porta hepatis, suggesting a congenital malformation as the cause of the atresia in these selected cases. The gallbladder may be diminutive and exhibit varying degrees of fibrosis, epithelial degeneration and destruction, and luminal compromise.

Biliary remnants have been classified by Gautier and Eliot (22) into three types:

1. Absence of any lumen lined by biliary epithelium, with little or no inflammatory cells in the connective tissue (Figure 15-8).

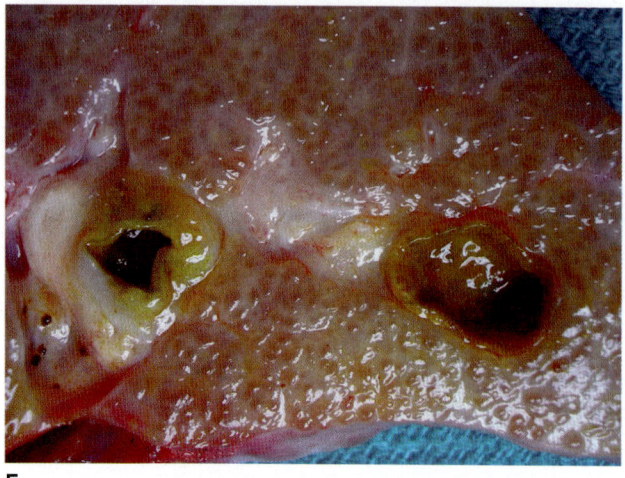
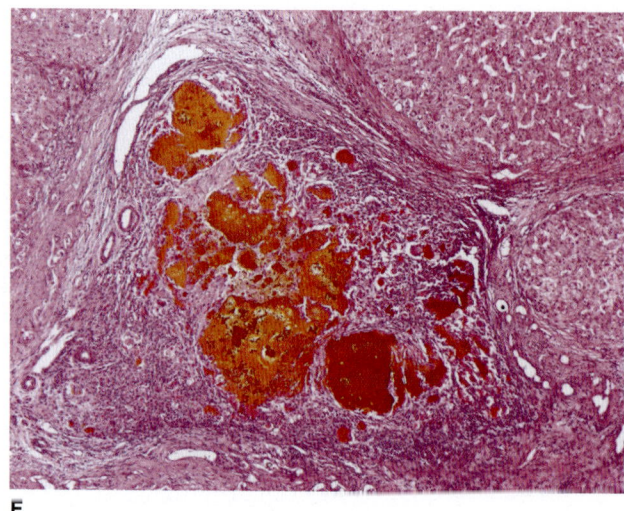

FIGURE 15-9 • (*continued*) **E:** Large bile-filled lakes within the liver parenchyma and micronodular cirrhosis with diffuse bile staining. **F:** Bile plugs distending portal region with adjacent micronodular liver parenchyma (H&E, 40×).

2. Presence of lumina lined by cuboidal epithelium. The remnants may be numerous, have lumens less than 50 μm, and are surrounded by a neutrophilic infiltrate. Cellular debris and bile may be present in the lumen, and epithelial necrosis may be seen in ducts with a diameter exceeding 300 μm.
3. The presence of a central altered bile duct incompletely lined by columnar epithelium, in addition to smaller epithelial structures resembling those in the second type.

The size of the ducts tends to be larger in infants younger than 12 weeks of age, and beyond this age, total obliteration of ducts is the common finding. It has been observed that few or absent ductal remnants at the porta hepatis and absence of portal inflammation were predictors of a poor prognosis (23). Age at Kasai procedure surgery (improved outcome at <60 days of age), the surgical team's experience, and the degree of liver disease are factors associated with prognosis. Liver transplantation is the only option available for children with failed Kasai procedures.

Persistent Intrahepatic Cholestasis

Once the presence of a normal biliary tract has been established through a variety of studies and procedures, the differential diagnosis of persistent conjugated hyperbilirubinemia shifts in the direction of inherited and infectious etiologies. The inherited disorders include those conditions of a primary nature affecting the structure of intrahepatic bile ducts or bile secretion with secondary effects on the intrahepatic ducts. The first category is represented primarily by the Alagille and progressive familial intrahepatic cholestasis (PFIC) syndromes and the second by a diverse group of infectious, metabolic, and inherited disorders.

Alagille Syndrome (Syndromic Paucity of Interlobular Bile Ducts, Arteriohepatic Dysplasia)

Alagille syndrome is an autosomal dominant disorder associated with abnormalities of the liver, heart, eye, skeleton, and a characteristic facial appearance (24,25) (Table 15-4). The genetic defect for this syndrome is the *JAG1* gene locus on chromosome 20p12. JAG1 encodes a ligand for the Notch signaling pathway that is important in early cellular development, particularly in the liver, kidney, and heart (26,27). Alagille syndrome is the most frequent condition associated with paucity of intrahepatic bile ducts and has been referred to as syndromic paucity of interlobular bile ducts. The onset of cholestasis occurs in the first 3 months of life with unconjugated hyperbilirubinemia and an obstructive pattern on laboratory evaluation and hepatobiliary scintigraphy. Cutaneous manifestations occur later in the course and include pruritus (hyperbilirubinemia) and xanthomas (hypercholesterolemia). The typical facies includes a prominent forehead, hypertelorism, flattened malar eminence, and a pointed chin, although the specificity of the abnormal facies has been questioned. Characteristic eye findings include a posterior embryotoxon. The cardiovascular anomaly most often reported is pulmonic stenosis with a heart murmur (95%). Vertebral abnormalities (butterfly vertebrae, 60% to 70%) and foreshortened fingers are skeletal anomalies associated with the syndrome. Renal abnormalities leading to renal failure include interstitial nephritis and membranoproliferative glomerulonephritis with mesangial lipid deposits. Unilateral renal cystic dysplasia, renal hypoplasia, ureteropelvic obstruction, and renal artery stenosis may also be seen. Other features include neurodevelopmental delay, stunted growth, cerebrovascular accidents (15%), pancreatic insufficiency, moyamoya, and middle aortic syndrome. Incomplete forms of the syndrome have been described in which only some of the major features are present. The mortality rate is 17% to 28%, which is largely determined by the presence of cardiovascular disease or progressive liver disease (28).

Liver disease is noted in almost 95% of cases within the first year of life, with progression to cirrhosis. HCC is an infrequent complication. Transplantation has been performed in

TABLE 15-4 FAMILIAL CHOLESTATIC SYNDROMES

Syndrome	Age at Onset	Associated Anomalies	Inheritance	Outcome	Pathologic Features
Alagille	<3 mo	Facies, heart, eye, bone, kidneys	Autosomal dominant	Mild disease, cirrhosis in 12%–14%	Paucity of ducts, cholestasis, giant cells; pigment in Golgi, ER, and lysosomes
Byler	3–12 mo	Diarrhea, malabsorption pancreatitis	Autosomal recessive ATP8B1	Progression to cirrhosis in 2–7 y	Cholestasis, small hepatocytes, fibrosis, Byler bile on EM
BSEP disease	Birth–6 mo	None, development of HCC	Autosomal recessive ABCB11	Progression to cirrhosis 6 mo–10y	Cholestasis, giant cell hepatitis, no coarse bile on EM, absent BSEP stain
MDR3 disease (PFIC3)	1 mo–20 y	None	ABCB4 gene	Progression to cirrhosis 5 mo–20 y	Variable cholestasis, ductular proliferation, mimic atresia
Norwegian	<3 mo	Lymphedema	Autosomal recessive	Mild disease	Cholestasis, portal fibrosis
Benign, recurrent	1–15 y	None	Unknown	No disease	Cholestasis
North American Indian	<3 mo	None	Autosomal recessive	Fatal cirrhosis	Cholestasis, giant cells, actin filament hyperplasia

ER, endoplasmic reticulum; EM, electron microscopy.

approximately 50% of patients in some series, with approximately a 75% survival rate (29).

The characteristic histopathologic feature of Alagille syndrome is absence or paucity of interlobular bile ducts (Figure 15-10). Because normal numbers of bile ducts may be present in early biopsies and even ductal proliferation, it is assumed that the syndrome is characterized by progressive damage and subsequent loss of intrahepatic ducts, as noted in liver biopsies from older children. Loss of ducts through atrophy secondary to decreased bile flow is an alternative explanation for the paucity of bile ducts. An optimal diagnostic liver biopsy should contain 20 portal areas, which may require a wedge biopsy, but a needle biopsy containing at least six portal areas may be adequate. Portal triads may be diminished in size and number and show no or mild fibrosis. Cholestasis is usually present in zone 3, but may be seen in zone 1. Hepatocellular ballooning, pseudoacinar transformation, focal giant cell formation, and lobular disarray are other nonspecific features. A quantitative increase in hepatic copper may occur and is demonstrable by rhodamine or other copper stains in zone 1 hepatocytes, a finding also common in other obstructive or cholestatic hepatopathies. Ultrastructural changes are distinctive with bile pigment retention in the cytoplasm, especially in lysosomes and in vesicles in the outer convex region of the Golgi apparatus. Rarely, bile pigment is present in the bile canaliculi or immediate pericanalicular region, suggesting a block in the bile secretory apparatus (30).

Progressive Familial Intrahepatic Cholestasis

PFIC is a group of severe genetic cholestatic hepatopathies of early life, including the archetypical PFIC1 (Byler disease) first described in Amish children. This autosomal recessive disorder is heralded by infantile cholestasis, which leads to hepatic fibrosis and death (31). Children who have a clinically similar disorder, but are not members of the Amish kindred in which Byler disease was described, are said to have Byler syndrome (now called PFIC2 or BSEP disease). The gene for Byler disease (*FIC1* gene) is at 18q21 locus of the *ATP8P1* gene, which synthesizes an aminophospholipid translocating ATPase on the bile duct epithelium. This same gene mutation is implicated in benign recurrent intrahepatic cholestasis 1 (BRIC1), which is associated with recurrent cholestasis with pruritus, but a mild course. A second form of BRIC is also seen with BSEP gene mutations (BRIC2). PFIC type 1 (*ATP8B1* gene mutation at 18q21) and PFIC type 2 (*ABCB11* gene mutation at 2q24) are characterized by cholestasis and low serum gamma-glutamyltransferase (GGT) activity. With PFIC type 3, serum GGT is elevated and is associated with mutation of the *ABCB4* gene (7q21) (32). This gene encodes the canalicular protein MDR3 responsible for translocation of phospholipids from hepatocytes to canalicular lumens. Intrahepatic cholestasis of pregnancy occurs in heterozygotes with an ABCB4 gene mutation and is associated with elevated aminotransferases, cholestasis with pruritus, and recurrent fetal losses. More recent studies have determined varying mutations within the respective genes causing this

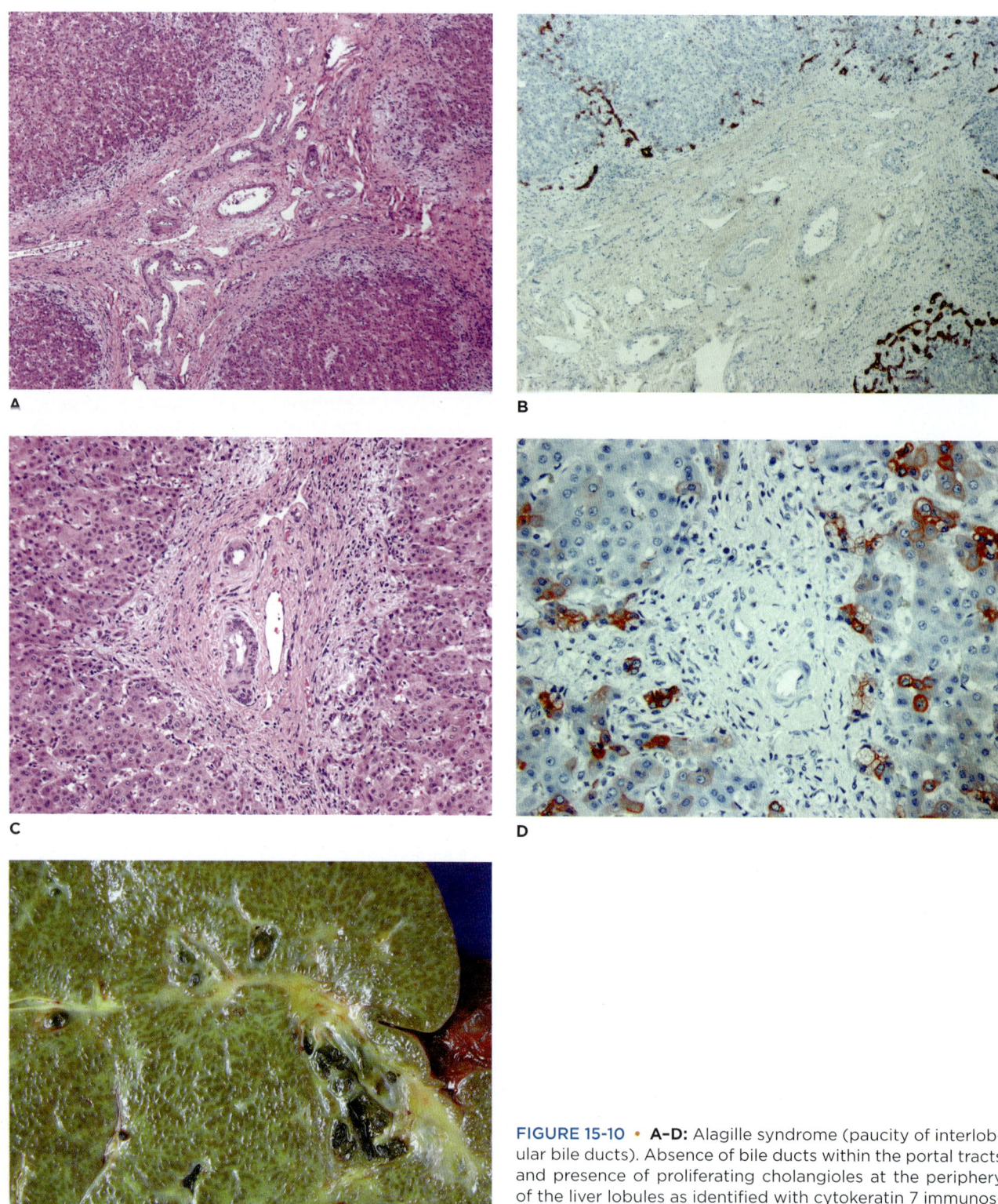

FIGURE 15-10 • **A–D:** Alagille syndrome (paucity of interlobular bile ducts). Absence of bile ducts within the portal tracts and presence of proliferating cholangioles at the periphery of the liver lobules as identified with cytokeratin 7 immunostaining (H&E staining, **A, C:** 20×; cytokeratin 7 immunostaining, **B, D:** 20×). **E:** Micronodular cirrhosis with bile plugs and diffuse bile staining.

familial cholestasis, which may explain the variable presentations and manifestations of the disease (33). There is still a group of familial cholestasis in which the exact genetic defect is still not known, and recent attempts have identified TJP2 and claudin genes as possible candidates (34). PFIC1 disease is associated with extrahepatic disease manifested by diarrhea, pancreatitis, and hearing loss, while BSEP disease (PFIC2) causes progressive liver failure and increased risk of malignancy with no extrahepatic disease (35–37). Gallstones may be seen in some of the BRIC2 patients (36).

Histologically, PFIC1 defect (Byler disease) exhibits small uniform appearing hepatocytes with canalicular and hepatocellular cholestasis and progressive paucity rather than proliferation of bile ducts and no significant fibrosis in these patients (Figure 15-11). Giant cell transformation may be occasionally seen. Immunohistochemical analysis shows normal staining for BSEP and MRP2 with some variation in CD10 staining. The bile has a characteristic coarse granular appearance on electron microscopic examination (38). In contrast, non-Amish children have neonatal hepatitis, amorphous to finely filamentous bile, and a more benign course, but with recurrent cholestasis. PFIC type 2 is characterized by persistent neonatal cholestasis with features of NGCH, feathery degeneration of hepatocytes and progressive biliary cirrhosis that may manifest before 1 year of age.

IHC is useful in the diagnosis due to the absence of staining for BSEP protein in the canaliculi in most cases. HCC and even cholangiocarcinoma have been reported incidentally in these livers at time of transplant (37,39). PFIC type 3 displays periportal inflammation, extensive bile duct proliferation, feathery hepatocyte degeneration, and fibrosis, which progresses to biliary cirrhosis. IHC may be used to facilitate diagnosis and shows alterations or absence of MRP2 protein staining in canaliculi with preservation of BSEP staining. Partial external biliary diversion and transplantation have been helpful in 80% of patients (40). Instances of recurrence of low GGT cholestatic disease in the liver graft posttransplant for BSEP disease have been documented and are thought to be due to *de novo* bile salt exporter protein antibodies (41). Liver biopsies in Amish and Mennonite

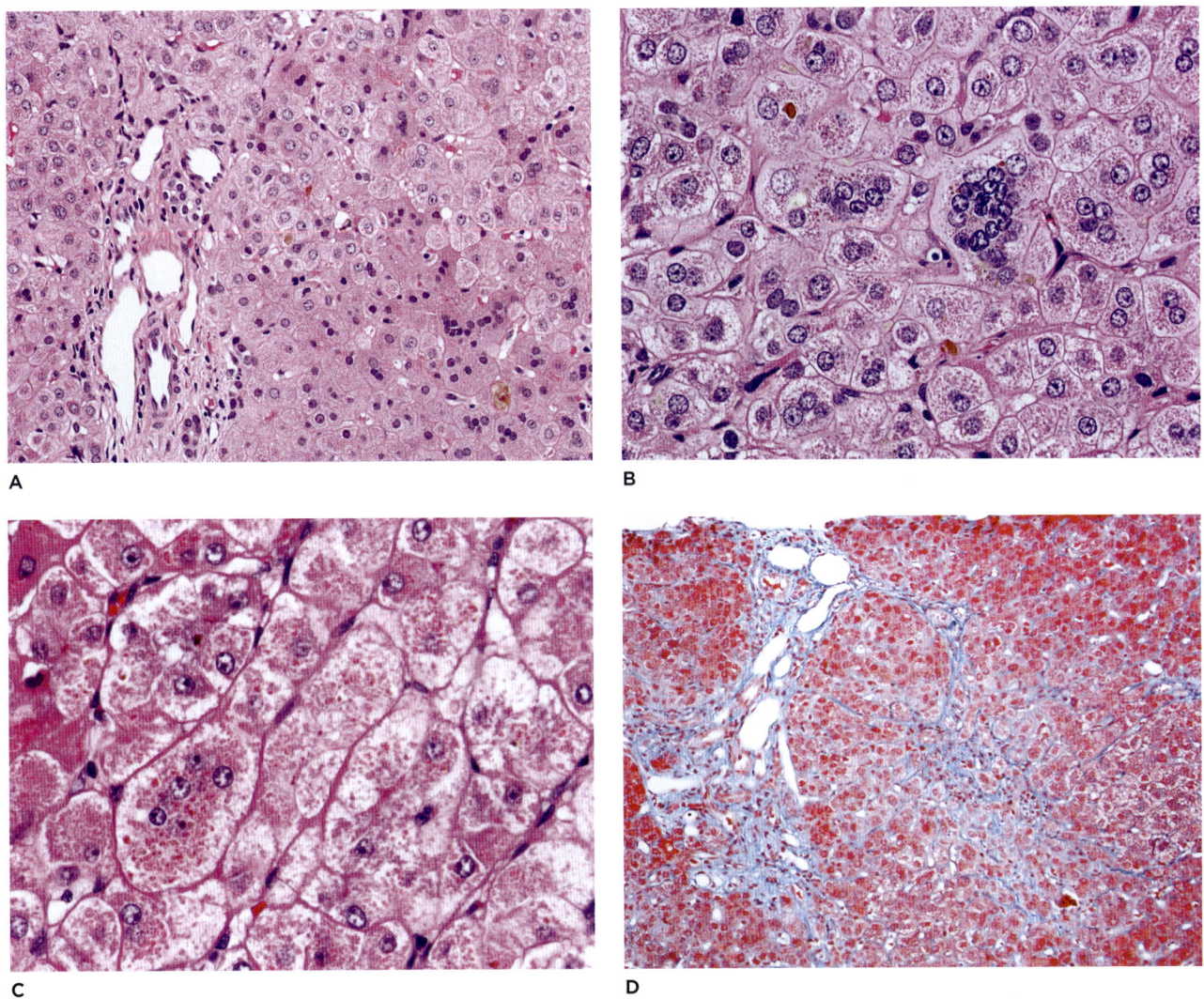

FIGURE 15-11 • **A, B:** Progressive familial intrahepatic cholestasis (PFIC). Hepatic lobular disarray with giant cell transformation and focal canalicular cholestasis (H&E, **A:** 100×, **B:** 400×). **C:** Diffuse cytoplasmic cholestasis of hepatocytes with granular bile (H&E, **C** 400×). **D:** Central lobular fibrosis with fine feathery extension into the peripheral zone toward the portal region (Trichrome, **D:** 100×).

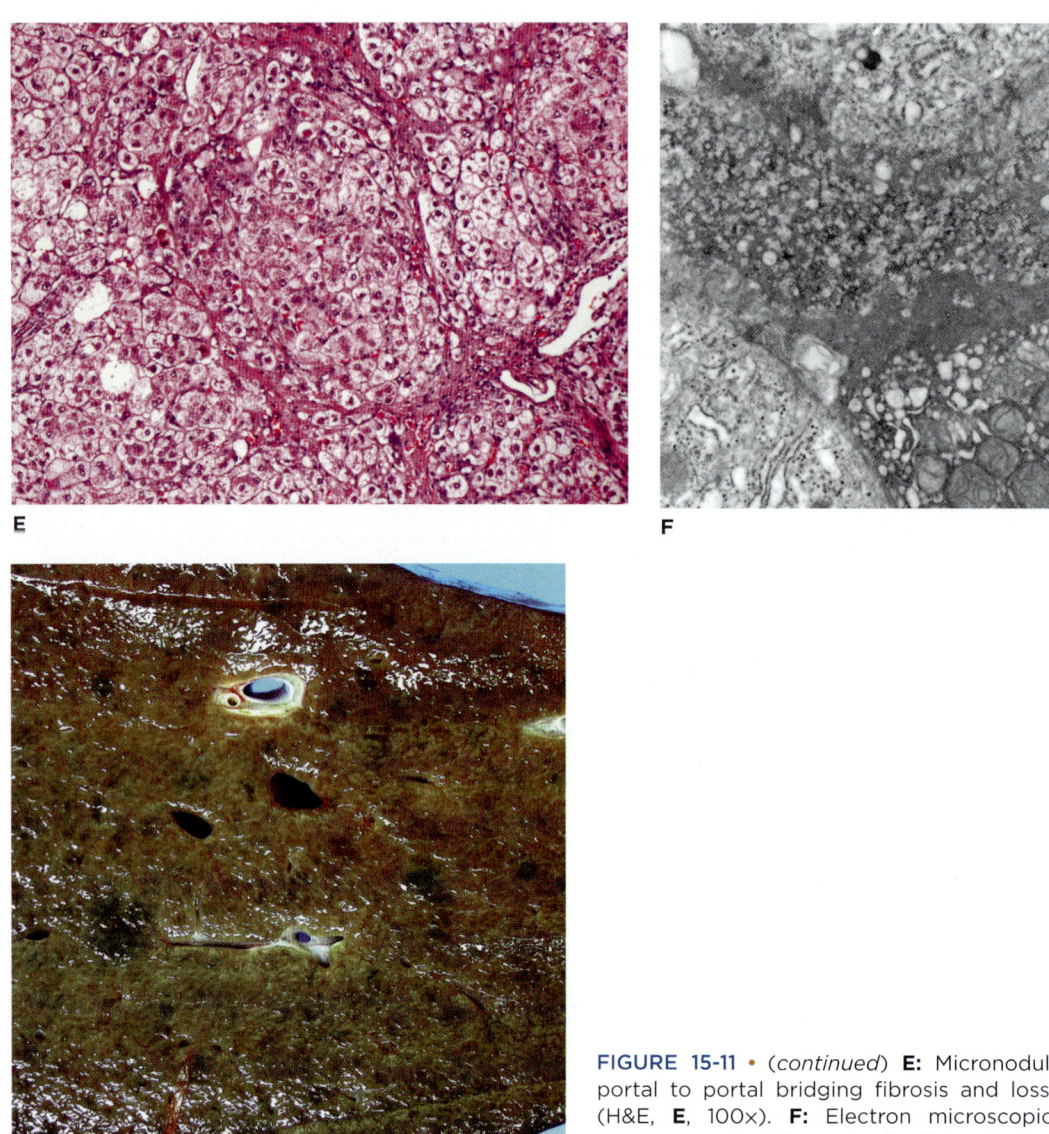

FIGURE 15-11 • (continued) **E:** Micronodular cirrhosis with portal to portal bridging fibrosis and loss of central veins (H&E, **E**, 100×). **F:** Electron microscopic appearance of coarse granular bile markedly distending a canalicular space between hepatocytes (electron microscopy, **F:** 20,000×). **G:** Gross appearance.

children with familial hypercholesterolemia have bland intracanalicular cholestasis and low GGT and improve with ursodeoxycholic acid treatment. The genetic defects in these children are associated with aberrant tight junction proteins (claudin, *TJP2* gene) and a defective bile acid conjugation enzyme (gene *BAAT*) (42). More recent molecular methods have helped elucidate genetic defects in *TJP2* gene in a larger subset of infants with progressive cholestatic liver disease who have low GGT and neither the *ATP8B1* nor *ABCB11* mutations (34).

Other conditions may also present initially with cholestasis and end in cirrhosis. A disease that presents with neonatal cholestasis and may mimic EHBA is North American Indian childhood cirrhosis (43). This disease has progressive fibrosis and usually culminates in cirrhosis early in life. The genetic defect has been localized to a mitochondrial protein CIRHIN (*CIRH1A*, 16q22). A syndrome that is comprised of arthrogryposis, renal tubular dysfunction, and cholestasis (ARC) may present initially as cholestasis with a low GGT and is typically fatal in the first few years of life (44). Another form of progressive cholestatic disease has been associated with microvillus inclusion disease (MVID) mutations in *MYO5B/RAB11A* with low expression of BSEP in these individual by IHC (45). An element of paucity is also reported in this setting of MVID.

Nonsyndromic Paucity of Intrahepatic Ducts

Paucity of intrahepatic bile ducts has been reported in several sporadic cases of neonatal cholestasis with progressive liver disease, but rarely does the condition evolve into cirrhosis (46). A1AT has been associated with paucity of intrahepatic bile ducts in a subgroup of patients. Other conditions include congenital syphilis, Turner syndrome, Down syndrome, cytomegaloviral infection, hepatitis B antigenemia, hypopituitarism, medications, infections, toxins, immune-mediated injury, and graft-versus-host disease (Table 15-5).

TABLE 15-5	CAUSES OF DUCTOPENIA	
Congenital	Immunologic	Others
Syndromic paucity—Alagille	Primary sclerosing cholangitis	Langerhans cell histiocytosis
Extrahepatic biliary atresia	Primary biliary cirrhosis	Hodgkin disease
Alpha-1 antitrypsin deficiency	Acute vanishing bile duct syndrome—posttransplant	Drugs
Peroxisomal disorders	Chronic rejection	Hepatitis C and CMV
Familial cholestasis: MDR3 and Byler	Graft versus host disease	Idiopathic adult ductopenia
CHF and Caroli disease		EBV infection
Cystic fibrosis		Ischemia

Ultrastructural evidence of bile duct destruction in nonsyndromic paucity of bile ducts has been regarded as representing a primary ductal injury.

Hereditary Cholestasis with Lymphedema (Aagenaes Syndrome)

Hereditary intrahepatic cholestasis with lymphedema (Aagenaes syndrome) is an autosomal recessive, inherited syndrome with more than 75% of the cases occurring in Norwegians and is associated with a genetic defect on chromosome 15q (47). Cholestasis with high serum GGT is present before or shortly after birth. With modern treatment, the cholestasis usually improves considerably during the first 2 years of life, but periods of recurrent cholestasis occur later. In some cases, lymphedema is present at birth, but this usually comes to light during childhood. The prognosis for the liver disease is good, but cirrhosis develops in about 15% of Norwegian cases.

Anatomic Anomalies and Disorders of Biliary and Hepatic Ducts

Agenesis of the Common Bile or Hepatic Duct

Agenesis of the common bile duct or hepatic duct is extremely rare. With common duct atresia, the hepatic duct enters directly into the gallbladder, and a long cystic duct drains into the duodenum.

Congenital Bronchobiliary Fistula

Congenital bronchobiliary fistula (CBBF) is a rare anomaly with varied presentations, including aspiration pneumonia and atelectasis, and may be associated with common bile duct abnormalities, including biliary atresia and diaphragmatic hernia (48). CBBF usually arises from the proximal part of the right main bronchus, a short distance below the carina, and joins the biliary system at the level of the left hepatic duct. The intrahepatic portion is usually lined by squamous or columnar epithelium, whereas the proximal section resembles a bronchus with respiratory epithelial lining and cartilage plates in the wall (see Chapter 12).

Ciliated Foregut Cyst

Ciliated hepatic foregut cyst is usually seen in adults, but may rarely present in childhood with abdominal pain or portal hypertension (49). The cyst is thought to arise from the migration of a bronchiolar bud of the foregut through the pleuroperitoneal canal. The cyst is subcapsular, measuring from 1 to 4 cm in diameter, and is composed of a lining of ciliated pseudostratified columnar epithelium overlying the connective tissue, a layer of smooth muscle bundles, and a fibrous capsule.

Congenital Dilatation of the Bile Ducts

Choledochal cyst is a presumed congenital anomaly of the intrahepatic and extrahepatic ducts characterized by segmental ductal dilatation, bile stasis, and hyperbilirubinemia (50–52). An association with malunion of the pancreatic and distal common bile ducts is a common finding. The prevalence of choledochal cysts is 1:15,000 live births and is higher in Asian populations. There is a female predilection. Secondary causes of bile duct dilatation include cholangitis, biliary perforation, biliary tract carcinoma, acute pancreatitis, and biliary cirrhosis. The cysts are classified (Figure 15-12) as follows:

Type Ia—large cystic or saccular dilatation of the choledochus
Type Ib—segmental dilatation with no pancreaticobiliary malunion
Type Ic—diffuse cylindrical or fusiform dilatation
Type II—diverticulum of the common bile duct or gallbladder
Type III—choledochocele of the distal common bile duct that usually extends into the wall of the duodenum
Type IVA—multiple choledochal cysts with intrahepatic and extrahepatic involvement (Caroli disease)
Type IVB—multiple extrahepatic cysts
Type V—single or multiple intrahepatic dilatations (may belong to Caroli disease—see later)

Choledochal cysts present most often with nonspecific symptoms. In 40% of patients, most of whom are children, a classic clinical triad of pain, jaundice, and right upper quadrant mass is seen. Irritability, nausea, vomiting, and a palpable abdominal mass may also be present. Affected infants often have large choledochal cysts, presenting as abdominal masses. Associated atresia or stenosis of the biliary tree is often present and has a greater risk for cirrhosis in infants. Diagnostic imaging studies, including isotope scan, ultrasonography, CT scan, and endoscopic or percutaneous cholangiography, are useful in establishing a preoperative diagnosis. With some, prenatal ultrasound examination may

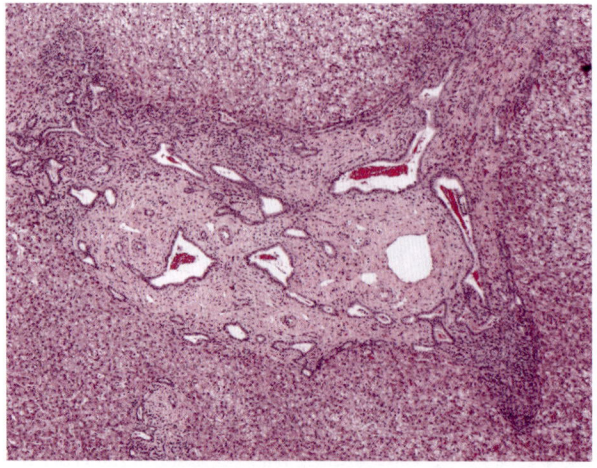
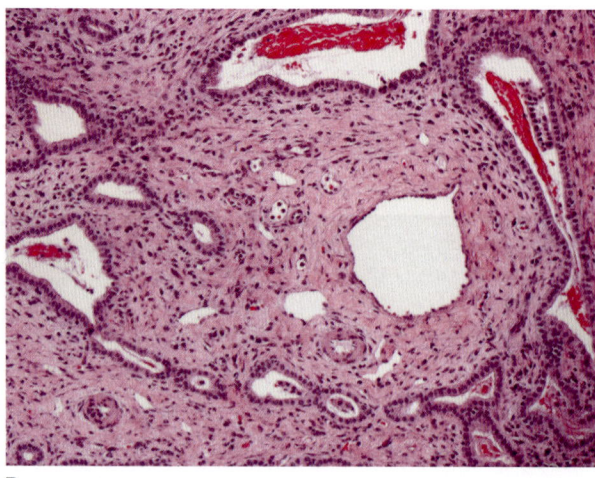
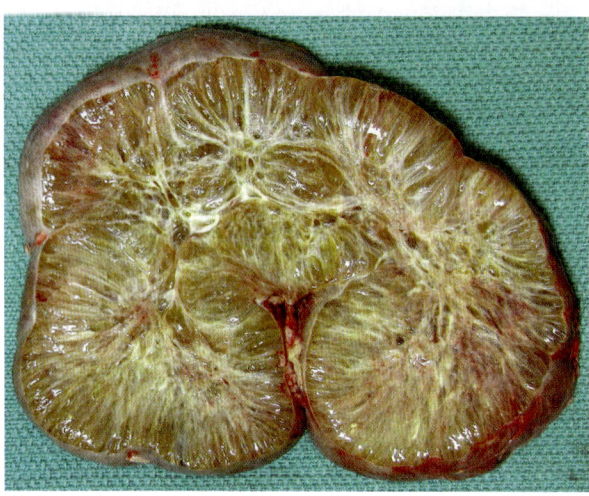

FIGURE 15-14 • CHF associated with autosomal recessive polycystic kidney disease. **A, B:** Ductal plate abnormality with dilated and concentric arrangement of bile ducts in expanded and fibrotic portal regions (H&E, **A:** 20×, **B:** 40×). **C:** Autosomal recessive polycystic kidney disease with markedly enlarged kidney due to numerous thin cysts extending from the cortical to medullary regions.

tendency for progression of the hepatic manifestations over long periods of clinical follow-up.

Several syndromes of inherited renal dysplasia are characteristically associated with hepatic changes that are identical to CHF and carry the designation of biliary dysgenesis (59–61). These include Meckel-Gruber syndrome, chondrodysplasia (short rib-polydactyly), Jeune asphyxiating thoracic dysplasia, trisomy 21, Bardet-Biedl syndrome, Ivemark syndrome (renal–hepatic–pancreatic dysplasia), Zellweger cerebrohepatorenal syndrome, and type II glutaric aciduria. Central nervous system, ocular, and pancreatic abnormalities are additional components of these syndromes. Compared with CHF, the differences in the hepatic lesions in these syndromes are a matter of degree rather than type, with less severe fibrosis and bile duct abnormalities being a general observation. The essential saclike structure of the biliary passages is similar, and ductal dilatation resembling Caroli disease has been seen. Large intrahepatic cysts may be present. A similar hepatic lesion has been described in some cases of vaginal atresia syndrome and tuberous sclerosis (58). Another condition that is associated with CHF is nephronophthisis (mutation in *NPHP1* [nephrocystin], *NPHP2* [inversin], *NPHP3*, or *NPHP4*). Ductal plate abnormalities in the liver and marked tubulointerstitial kidney

TABLE 15-6	CYSTIC LESIONS OF THE LIVER AND ASSOCIATED CONDITIONS
Infantile polycystic disease	
Hereditary renal dysplasia	
Meckel syndrome and congeners	
Chondrodysplasia syndromes	
Majewski and Saldino-Noonan short rib-polydactyly syndromes	
Jeune asphyxiating thoracic dystrophy syndrome	
Ellis-van Creveld chondroectodermal dysplasia	
Elejalde acrocephalopolydactylous dysplasia	
Trisomy 9 syndrome	
Trisomy 13 syndrome	
Zellweger cerebrohepatorenal syndrome	
Ivemark renal–hepatic–pancreatic dysplasia	
Glutaric aciduria, type II	
Hereditary tubulointerstitial nephritis	
Juvenile nephronophthisis	
Bardet-Biedl syndrome	
Adult polycystic disease	
Isolated nonsyndromic disease	

TABLE 15-7	DISTINCTIVE FEATURES IN METABOLIC DISORDERS WITH NEONATAL HEPATITIS-LIKE CHANGES
Disorders	Histologic Features
Galactosemia	Moderate-to-severe fatty change, fibrosis, no other distinctive features
Fructosemia	Moderate-to-severe fatty change, fibrosis, EM shows characteristic "fructose holes"
Tyrosinemia	Moderate-to-severe fatty change and fibrosis; regenerative nodules and hepatocellular dysplasia are suggestive.
A1AT deficiency	Stored A1AT in hepatocytes PAS-positive diastase-resistant globules; IHC and EM are diagnostic aids, especially in the neonate.
Glycogenosis (IV)	Early cirrhosis; stored structurally abnormal glycogen (diastase-resistant PAS-positive material with characteristic fibrillar nonmembrane-bound dense material by EM) in hepatocytes
CF (mucoviscidosis)	"Focal biliary cirrhosis" manifests as proliferated bile ducts with intraluminal inspissated material in expanded and fibrotic portal areas; rarely seen in the newborn
Niemann-Pick disease	Stored sphingolipids in Kupffer cells demonstrable histochemically; EM shows characteristic pleomorphic lamellar inclusions in the lysosomes.
Idiopathic iron storage	Hepatocellular necrosis with collapse; fibrosis; massive amounts of iron in hepatocytes and duct epithelial cells with negligible amounts in Kupffer cells

EM, electron microscopy.

disease are the features of this familial condition. Progressive renal failure occurs during the first two decades of life (62).

METABOLIC DISORDERS

A wide variety of metabolic disorders involve the liver, in addition to other organs, and a number of these disorders may present in the neonatal period as cholestasis and with neonatal hepatitis-like changes (Table 15-7). The overall incidence of metabolic disease is approximately 4 per 10,000 live births (63). The following disorders are considered in some detail because of their association with significant liver disease (see Chapter 5).

Carbohydrate Metabolism Disorders

Galactosemia

Hereditary galactosemia, an autosomal recessive disorder, is most commonly due to deficiency of galactose-1-phosphate uridyl transferase, an enzyme encoded on the *GALT* gene on chromosome 9q13 (64,65). Genetic defects in the enzymes galactokinase and uridyl diphosphate galactose-4-epimerase are less common causes of galactosemia. These three enzymatic defects impair conversion of galactose to glucose. The incidence varies from approximately 1.5 to 4 per 100,000 Whites to 1 per 400,000 in Chinese (63). The disorder exhibits considerable allelic heterogeneity, and more than 150 different mutations have been identified in 24 different populations and ethnic groups in 15 countries. The mutations most frequently cited are Q188R, K285N, S135L, and N314D. Q188R is the most common mutation in European populations or in those predominantly of European descent (65). The clinical features in neonates include hepatomegaly, jaundice, hypoglycemia, generalized aminoaciduria, presence of reducing substances in the urine, diarrhea, and vomiting. The differential diagnosis includes inborn errors of metabolism that manifest as neonatal hepatitis (Table 15-7). Histopathologically, canalicular and intracellular cholestasis, pseudoacinar transformation, bile ductular proliferation, focal giant cell transformation of hepatocytes, and presence of lipid are the notable features (Figure 15-15). These features in the neonatal period are similar to those seen in tyrosinemia and fructosemia. Fibrosis occurs early and progresses to cirrhosis if left untreated within the first 3 to 6 months of life (66). The ultrastructural features are diagnostic, although the individual features are not specific. The diagnosis is made by demonstration of enzyme deficiency in erythrocytes. Neonatal screening tests are available. Liver effects may be reversible with dietary galactose restriction.

Fructosemia

Hereditary fructose intolerance is caused by catalytic deficiency of aldolase B (fructose-1,6-bisphosphate aldolase) in the liver, intestines, and kidneys and is a recessively inherited condition. Aldolase B deficiency inhibits gluconeogenesis and glycogenolysis. Two mutations on chromosome 9q (A149P and A174D) account for more than 70% of cases (67). The disease becomes manifest when fructose is introduced into the diet and presents with vomiting, diarrhea, failure to thrive, jaundice, renal failure, and hepatomegaly. Liver failure may be severe, with hepatic necrosis during the acute phase (66). More commonly, there is variable fibrosis involving the portal and lobular regions as well as microsteatosis and macrosteatosis. Chronic disease may be associated with severe fibrosis, potentially leading to cirrhosis. A neonatal hepatitis-like pattern may be seen with diffuse hepatocellular steatosis, a frequent feature. Electron microscopy of hepatocytes shows endoplasmic reticulum degranulation with membrane profiles. The response to dietary exclusion of fructose is rapid, and when so treated, the disease is compatible with a normal life span (68).

Glycogen Storage Diseases

The GSDs are a group of metabolic disorders with specific enzyme defects resulting in accumulation of abnormal amounts of structurally normal or abnormal glycogen in the

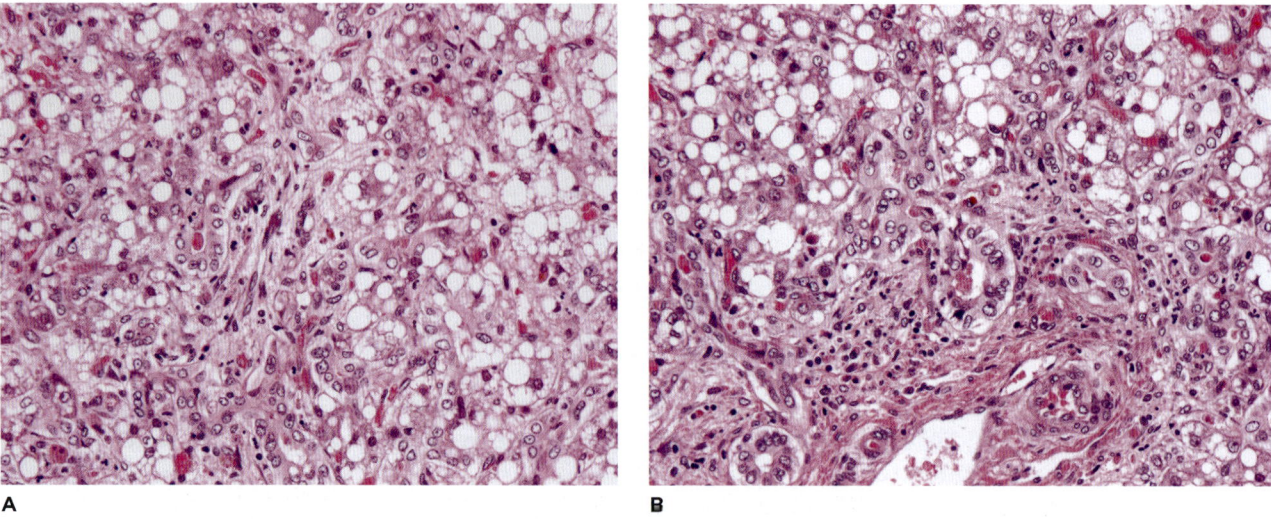

FIGURE 15-15 • Galactosemia. **A, B:** Hepatocytes display medium to large droplet fatty metamorphosis, along with pseudoglandular transformation (H&E, **A:** 100×, **B:** 200×).

liver and other tissues (69,70). The GSDs most frequently associated with hepatic manifestations include types I, II, III, IV, VI, and IX. The mode of inheritance is autosomal recessive in all the types described, with the exception of type IXb, which is inherited as a sex-linked recessive trait. Some forms of the disease present in infancy and others in early childhood, with failure to thrive, developmental delays, acidosis, hypoglycemia, and hepatomegaly. The morphologic changes have been reviewed by McAdams et al. (69), and the ultrastructural features have been illustrated by Phillips et al. (71). Features of those glycogenoses that significantly involve the liver are summarized in Table 15-8.

Type I Glycogenosis (von Gierke Disease)

GSD type I is the most common form of glycogenosis and potentially the most severe (70,72). There is no gender predilection. Children with this disease present in infancy with hypoglycemia and hepatomegaly. There is lactic acidosis, seizures, and failure to thrive. The subsequent course is characterized by the development of hyperlipidemia, xanthomata, hyperuricemia, cyclic neutropenia with recurrent infections, nephropathy, and chronic bowel inflammation with type 1b GSD. Type 1a GSD is due to a deficiency in the enzyme glucose-6-phosphatase (17q21). Type 1b GSD has a deficiency in a transmembrane protein required for glucose-6-phosphate transport (11q23) into microsomes. Type 1c has a deficiency in a phosphatase transporter (11q23-24.2). These deficiencies result in the accumulation of large amounts of normal glycogen in the liver, kidney, and intestine.

Histopathologically, the liver shows marked distension of the hepatocytes with glycogen, resulting in a diffuse mosaic pattern with compression of the sinusoids (Figure 15-16). Intranuclear glycogen is a common feature (70). The glycogen is best demonstrated by PAS stains of unfixed

TABLE 15-8 HEPATIC FINDINGS IN GLYCOGEN STORAGE DISEASE

Disease	Light Microscopic Findings	Electron Microscopic Findings
Type I von Gierke disease	Excess glycogen in enlarged hepatocytes and in nuclei; uniform mosaic pattern; lipid droplets	Accumulation of cytoplasmic glycogen and lipid; nuclear glycogen
Type II Pompe disease	Nonuniform, mild distension, and vacuolation of hepatocytes	Lysosomal monoparticulate glycogen
Type III Cori glycogenosis	Uniform mosaic pattern, resembling type I; portal fibrosis	Similar to type I; lipid and nuclear glycogen less pronounced
Type IV Andersen disease	Inclusions in periportal hepatocytes; cirrhosis	Nonmembrane-bound inclusions of fibrillary material, glycogen, and tubules
Type VI Her disease	Nonuniform enlargement of hepatocytes; periportal fibrosis	Glycogen and finely granular material in cytoplasm
Type VIII	Glycogen deposition	Glycogenosis
Type IX	Glycogen deposition	Glycogen deposition with "starry sky" pattern
Type X	Glycogenosis	Glycogenosis

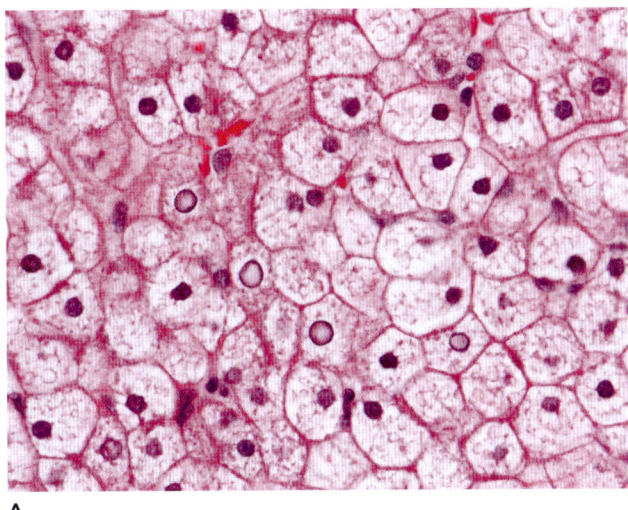
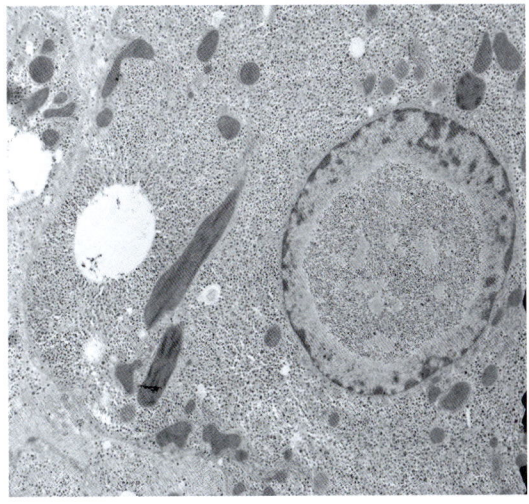

FIGURE 15-16 • Glycogen storage disease, type I. **A:** Hepatocytes distended by glycogen with obliteration of the sinusoids, forming a mosaic pattern, and glycogenated nuclei. (H&E, 400×.) **B:** Hepatocyte with glycogenated nuclei, cytoplasmic monoparticulate glycogen, large lipid droplet, and abnormally shaped mitochondria (electron microscopy, 7500×).

frozen sections or alcohol-fixed tissue. Lipid is also present, while fibrosis is typically absent. Rarely, Mallory bodies may be seen. Ultrastructurally, there are pools of monoparticulate glycogen in the cytoplasm and nuclei of hepatocytes. Lipid vacuoles are found in the cytoplasm. The organelles are displaced, and the size of the mitochondria may be increased. Hepatic adenomas have been reported with some frequency, and cases of HCC and hepatoblastoma have been described in type 1 glycogenosis (73,74). Hepatic transplantation has been used in the treatment of type I, III, and IV GSDs (75).

Type II Glycogenosis (Pompe Disease, Generalized Glycogenosis, or Acid Maltase Deficiency)
GSD type II is classified as a lysosomal storage disorder in contrast to the cytoplasmic storage disorder that occurs in the other GSDs. It is the result of a deficiency in acid maltase caused by mutations in the alpha-1,4-glucosidase (*GAA*, 17q25.2-25.4) gene (76,77). The major manifestations are muscular and cardiac, and the liver shows changes as a component of the generalized involvement. Three clinical types have been described. Infantile or classic Pompe disease manifests in infancy with hypotonia and cardiomyopathy, leading to death in infancy. The second type presents in childhood with predominant involvement of the skeletal musculature, and a third type is described with an onset in the second to fourth decades. Cardiac involvement in these latter variants is minimal. Affected hepatocytes are mildly enlarged and have finely vacuolated cytoplasm (70) (Figure 15-17). Ultrastructural features are characterized by the presence of monoparticulate glycogen within membrane-bound lysosomal vacuoles. Acid phosphatase activity is associated with the lysosomal vacuoles. Currently, enzyme replacement therapy has achieved great success in treatment of these children (76).

Type III Glycogenosis (Cori Disease, Forbes Disease, Limit Dextrinosis, Debranching Enzyme Disease)
GSD type III is the result of a deficiency in the amylo-1, 6-glucosidase (debrancher enzyme, 1p21) activity (70,72). This deficiency leads to abnormal glycogen formation with increased branching points that accumulate in the liver and muscle. Hypoglycemia develops during stress or fasting due to lack of conversion of the abnormal glycogen to glucose. Hepatic morphologic features are very similar to those seen in type I GSD with panlobular cytoplasmic distension by glycogen and a uniform mosaic pattern. Accumulated glycogen is demonstrable by the presence of diastase digestible PAS-positive material in the cytoplasm. Nuclear glycogen is not as prominent as in type I GSD, but is a distinguishing feature from other types of GSD, especially types VI and IX. Hepatomegaly with hepatic fibrosis may be prominent and may progress to cirrhosis by the third or fourth decade of life.

Type IV Glycogenosis (Andersen Disease, Amylopectinosis; Glycogen Branching Enzyme Disease)
GSD type IV manifests at birth or in early infancy with failure to thrive and hepatosplenomegaly (70,72,78). In the absence of transplantation, there is progression to cirrhosis and death in early childhood (79). The brancher enzyme 1,4-1,6-glucon:1-4-glucan, 6-glycosyl transferase (3p12, *GBE1* gene) is absent, resulting in abnormal glycogen with decreased branch points that resembles amylopectin or starch. Deposits of the abnormal glycogen are generalized with significant involvement of the liver, skeletal and cardiac muscles, and intestine. Microscopically, the hepatocytes in the periportal region (zone 1) contain pale eosinophilic hyaline inclusions surrounded by a clear halo, resembling Lafora bodies. These inclusions resist diastase digestion,

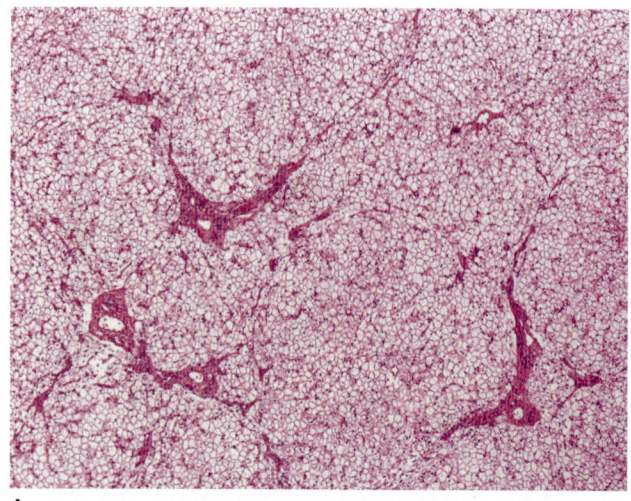
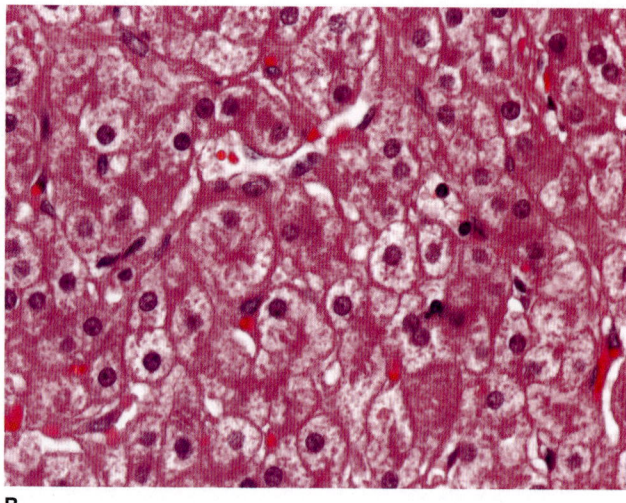
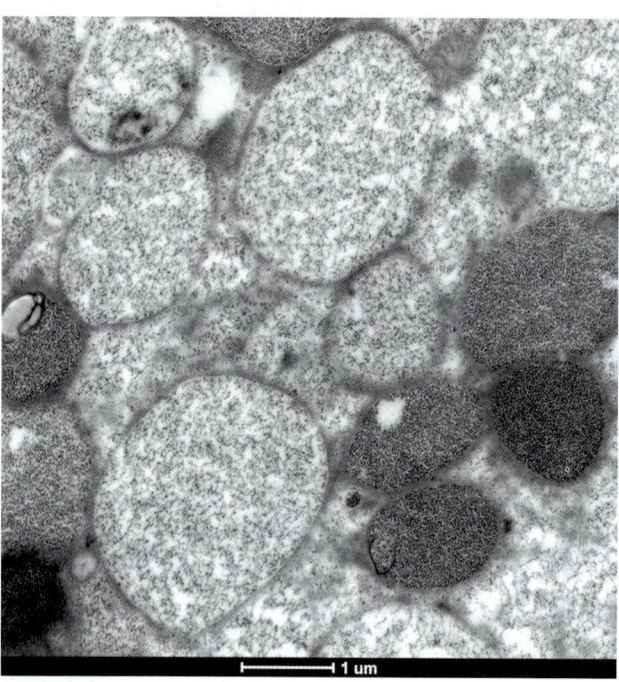

FIGURE 15-17 • Glycogen storage disease, type II. **A:** Hepatocytes demonstrating mosaic pattern with obliteration of sinusoids (H&E, 40×). **B:** Hepatocytes in close proximity to one another, with thickened cell membranes, fine cytoplasmic vacuolization, and indistinct sinusoids (H&E, 400×). **C:** Monoparticulate glycogen within membrane-bound lysosomes (electron microscopy, 20,000×).

but are digestible with pectinase treatment (Figure 15-18). Colloidal iron staining is also seen in the cytoplasmic inclusions. Ultrastructurally, the inclusions consist of central fibrillar glycogen surrounded by polyparticulate glycogen rosettes (69). Rare instances of diffuse reticuloendothelial involvement have also been reported (80). Prenatal diagnosis is possible.

Type VI Glycogenosis (Hers Disease)

GSD type VI, a deficiency in hepatic phosphorylase E activity (14q21-22), presents with hepatomegaly in the absence of the serious complications seen in other glycogenoses (70,72). Histopathologically, there is a mosaic pattern of hepatocellular distension with glycogen in zone 1 hepatocytes. Mild portal fibrosis may be seen. Ultrastructurally, pools of monoparticulate glycogen with interspersed glycogen rosettes displace the cytoplasmic organelles. A finely granular material of low electron density that is devoid of organelles may be scattered in the glycogen aggregates, imparting a starry-sky appearance (70).

Type VIII Glycogenosis

GSD type VIII, a deficiency in phosphorylase kinase (16q12-13), is accompanied by progressive neurologic deterioration leading to death in early childhood secondary to glycogen accumulation within the central nervous system (72,81). Hepatic changes are those of glycogen accumulation with nonspecific features, although a rare case of cirrhosis and adenomatous hyperplasia has been reported.

Type IX, X, and XI Glycogenoses

Other glycogenoses with hepatic manifestations are GSD types IX (phosphorylase b kinase deficiency, Xp22.2-22.1) and X (cyclic 3,5 AMP-dependent kinase deficiency,

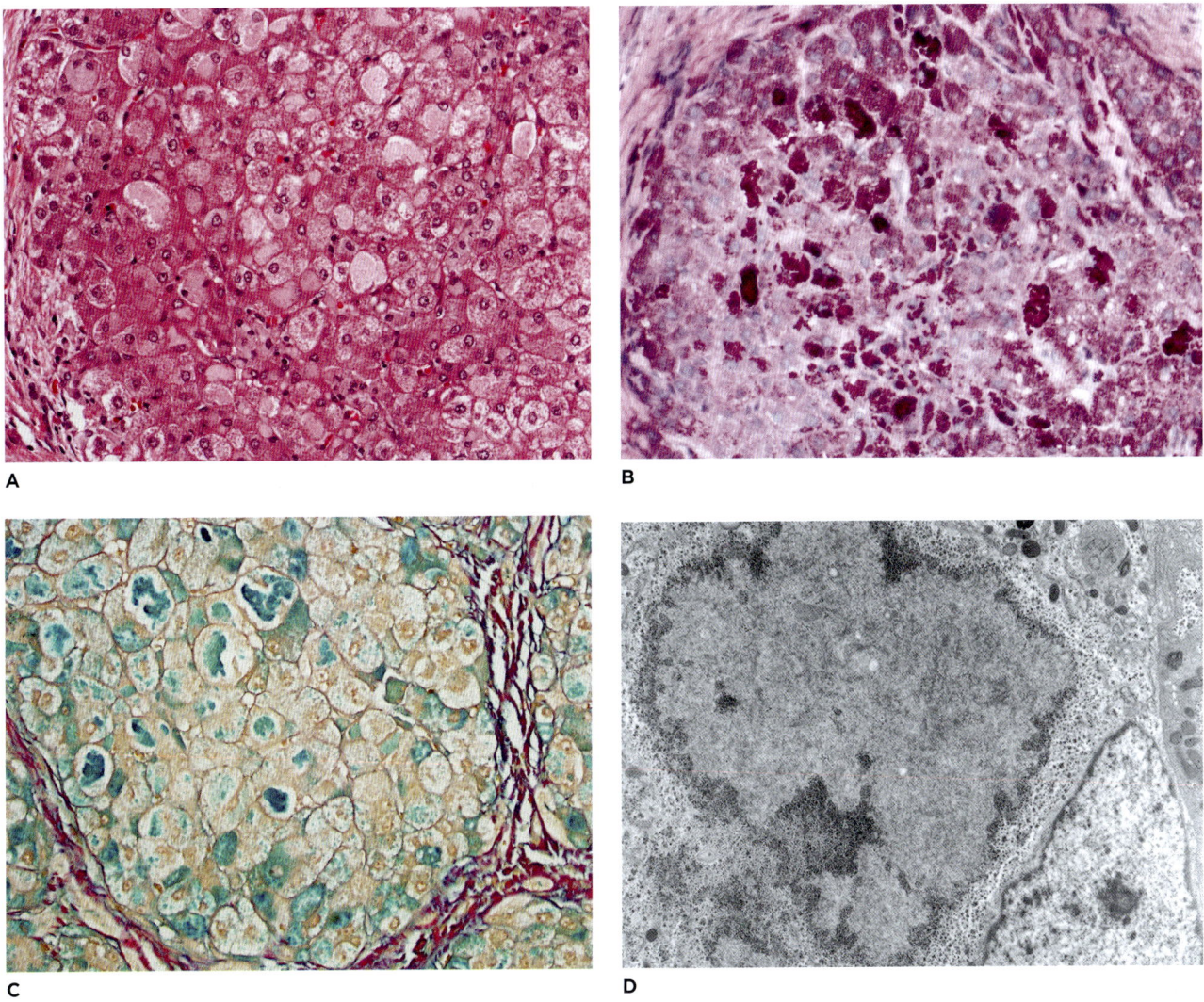

FIGURE 15-18 • **A:** Glycogen storage disease, type IV. Hepatocytes with pale hyaline inclusions surrounded by indistinct halos, resembling Lafora bodies (H&E, 200×). **B, C:** The inclusions stain intensely with PAS (400×) and colloidal iron (400×). **D:** Hepatocyte with hyaline inclusion comprised of fibrillary glycogen (electron microscopy, 6000×).

17q23-24) (72,81). Hepatic glycogenosis with stunted growth (type XI, Fanconi-Bickel syndrome) is associated with renal glycogen deposition. Type XI glycogenosis is caused by mutations in the glucose transporter 2 (*GLUT2*, 3q26.1-26.3) gene (82). Generalized glycogen deposition is accompanied by cirrhosis, but with normal glycogen metabolism.

Other Glycogenoses
Hepatic involvement is not a feature of GSD types V (McArdle disease, muscle glycogen phosphorylase [myophosphorylase], 11q13) and VII (Tarui disease, phosphofructokinase enzyme deficiency, 12q13), in which skeletal muscle is primarily affected (72,81). GSD type 0 (aglycogenosis) is an autosomal recessive disease with a deficiency in glycogen synthase (chromosome 12p12.2) (72,81). Deficiency in glycogen synthase leads to a marked reduction in liver glycogen stores. The symptoms of GSD type 0 are those associated with hypoglycemia and include lethargy, pallor, nausea, vomiting, and, rarely, seizures in the early morning before breakfast. Liver biopsy will demonstrate moderate steatosis and small amounts of glycogen (0.5% versus 1.6% for normal wet liver weight) on quantitative analysis. There have also been reports of liver fibrosis in some GSD type 0 cases.

Amino Acid Metabolism Disorders

Tyrosinemia

Tyrosinemia results from a deficiency of fumarylacetoacetate hydrolase (FAH, 15q23-25) and presents as acute fulminant disease in infancy or as a chronic liver disease later in childhood (83,84). Diagnosis is based upon serologic or urinary determination of succinylacetone level and FAH assays. Liver biopsy in the acute form reveals cholestasis, pseudoacinar transformation of hepatocytes, fatty change, marked intralobular fibrosis, and variable giant cell transformation (Figure 15-19) (66). These features are indicative of a metabolic hepatopathy, but are not specific for tyrosinemia.

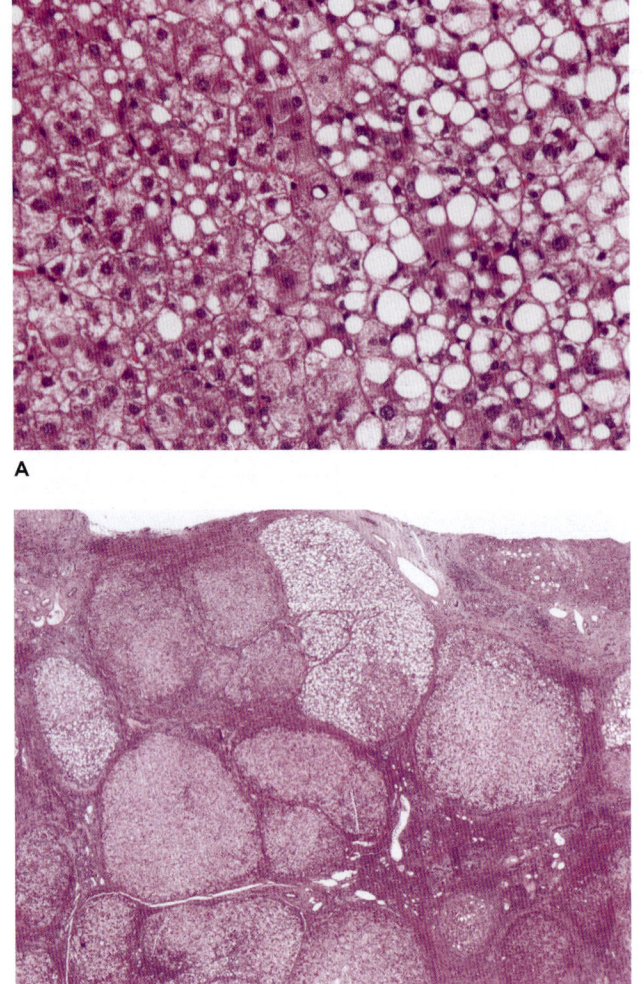

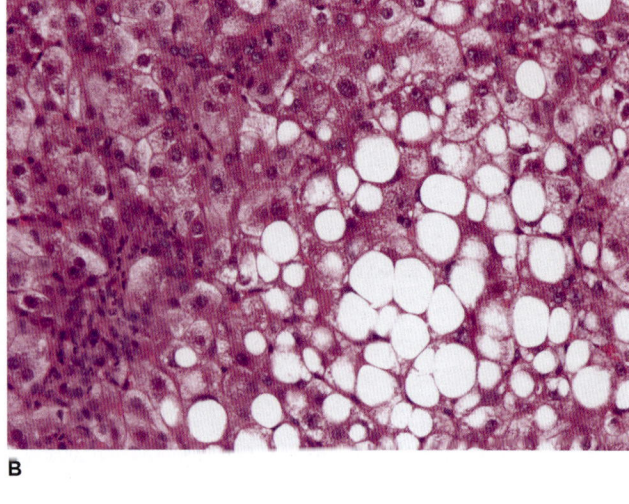

FIGURE 15-19 • Tyrosinemia. **A, B:** Hepatocytes with macrovesicular steatosis and indistinct sinusoid spaces (H&E, **A:** 200×, **B:** 400×). **C:** Micronodular cirrhosis in chronic form of tyrosinemia (H&E, 40×).

Regenerative nodules may already be present in early liver biopsies. The chronic form is characterized by cirrhosis with variable-sized nodules separated by thick bands of fibrous connective tissue with little inflammation or bile duct proliferation. Hepatocytes may demonstrate nuclear hyperchromasia, dysplasia, or adenomatous hyperplasia. The incidence of HCC is quite high with tyrosinemia. Liver transplantation is advisable soon after diagnosis and before 2 years of age, because of the high risk of HCC (85,86). Treatment with NTBC [2(-nitro-4-trifluoromethylbenzoyl)-1-3-cyclohexanedione] prevents the accumulation of the toxic metabolites of FAH and the subsequent liver and neurologic effects, but does not entirely eliminate the risk of HCC (87).

Lysosomal Storage Diseases

Lipidoses

Wolman Disease
Wolman disease and cholesterol ester storage disease (CESD) are rare autosomal recessive lipoprotein-processing disorders caused by mutations in the gene encoding human lysosomal acid lipase (10q24-25; Table 15-9) (88). Wolman disease is fatal in early life, presents with failure to thrive and diarrhea, and is characterized by generalized accumulation of foam cells and adrenal calcifications. Because there is partial enzyme activity, CESD is a milder clinical form of the disorder, generally limited to the gastrointestinal tract and the liver. Liver pathology includes steatosis and numerous foamy macrophages that contain cholesterol and lipid (Figure 15-20) and are similar in both diseases, although cirrhosis may occur in CESD. Cholesterol accumulation is demonstrated with frozen sections using polarized light microscopy. Ultrastructurally, hepatocytes, Kupffer cells, and portal macrophages are engorged with membrane-bound lipid vacuoles with dense membranes. Cholesterol clefts are seen in the cytoplasm (89).

Mucolipidoses

The mucolipidoses are a group of disorders caused by defects of various lysosomal hydrolases and include sialidosis (ML I, neuraminidase gene at 6p21.3), I-cell disease (ML II, *GNPTAB* gene at 12q23.3), pseudo-Hurler disease (ML III, *GNPTAB* gene at 12q23.3), and sialolipidosis (ML IV, mucolipin-1 gene

TABLE 15-9 LYSOSOMAL DISORDERS

Disease	Enzyme Deficiency	Light Microscopic Findings	Electron Microscopic Findings
Gaucher	Glucocerebrosidase	Gaucher cells with striated cytoplasm; fibrosis	Membrane-bound inclusions with twisted tubules in Kupffer cells
Niemann-Pick	Sphingomyelinase	Finely vacuolated cytoplasm of Kupffer cells	Myelin figures in Kupffer cells and hepatocytes
Wolman and cholesterol ester storage	Acid lipase	Steatosis of hepatocytes and Kupffer cells; cholesterol clefts, fibrosis	Lipid droplets and lipolysosomes and cholesterol clefts in hepatocytes and histiocytes
Mucopolysaccharidoses, Hurler, Hunter, Scheie	Iduronidases sulfatases	Swollen clear cytoplasm of hepatocytes and Kupffer cells; fibrosis; cirrhosis	Membrane-bound, sharply delimited, electron-lucent inclusions with some granular material
Mucolipidoses, I-cell disease	Acid hydrolases	Vacuolated hepatocytes, Kupffer cells	Membrane-bound vacuoles with flocculent material
Oligosaccharidoses	Sialidase, mannosidase, fucosidase	Vacuolated hepatocytes and Kupffer cells	Membrane-bound vacuoles with finely granular material
Metachromatic leukodystrophy	Aryl sulfatase A	Metachromatic granules in portal macrophages	Lamellar prismatic inclusions within macrophages, hepatocytes, and Kupffer cells
Farber	Acid ceramidase	Lipogranulomatous infiltrates	Curvilinear lysosomal material
Gangliosidosis GM_1	β-galactosidase	Vacuolated hepatocytes and Kupffer cells	Membrane-bound vacuoles with granular material

at 19p13.3) (90,91). Many of the clinical stigmata of mucopolysaccharidoses may be seen, but mucopolysaccharides are not excreted in the urine. I-cell disease and pseudo-Hurler polydystrophy are autosomal recessive disorders. Coarse facies, skeletal changes, hepatosplenomegaly, and delayed growth and development are some of the clinical features. The primary histopathologic and ultrastructural changes are cytoplasmic vacuolization of hepatocytes, Kupffer cells, and, less frequently, biliary epithelial cells. Inclusions within clear vacuoles can be demonstrated within fibroblasts and peripheral nerves in skin and conjunctival biopsies (71). Glomeruli and renal tubular epithelium contain similar inclusions, and the inclusions are also present in the urine.

Oligosaccharidoses (Glycoproteinoses)

Disorders of glycoprotein degradation resulting from defects in specific lysosomal enzymes lead to the accumulation of oligosaccharides in tissues and urinary excretion of these substances. These are rare autosomal recessive conditions with a phenotypic similarity to the mucopolysaccharidoses (92). These disorders include sialidosis (neuraminidase gene at 6p21.3), mannosidosis (mannosidase 2B1 gene at

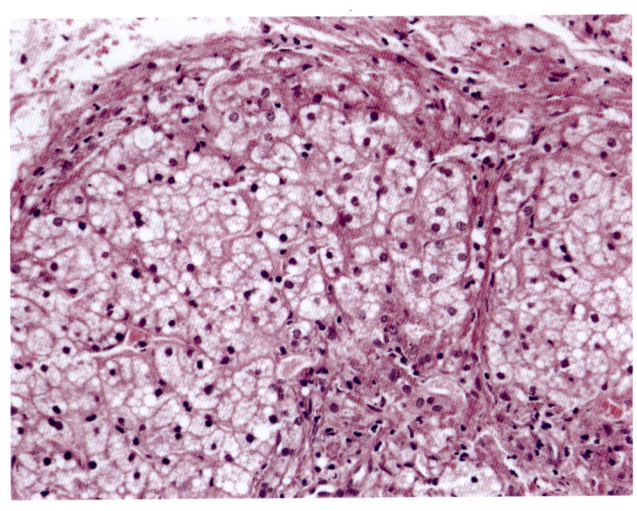
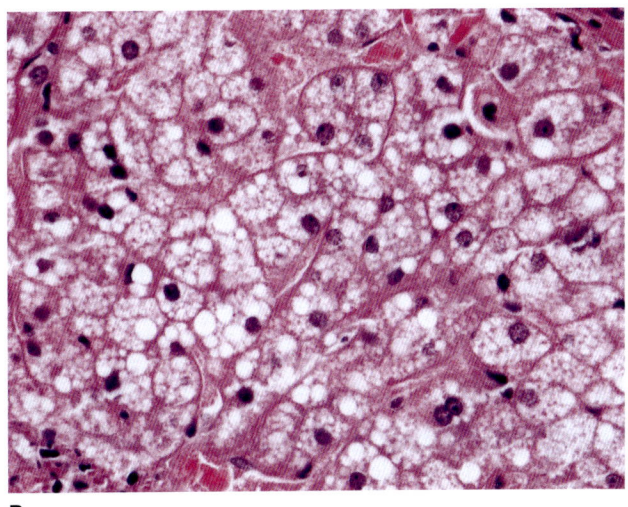

FIGURE 15-20 • **A, B:** Cholesterol ester storage disease. Hepatocytes with diffuse microsteatosis (H&E, **A** 200×, **B** 400×).

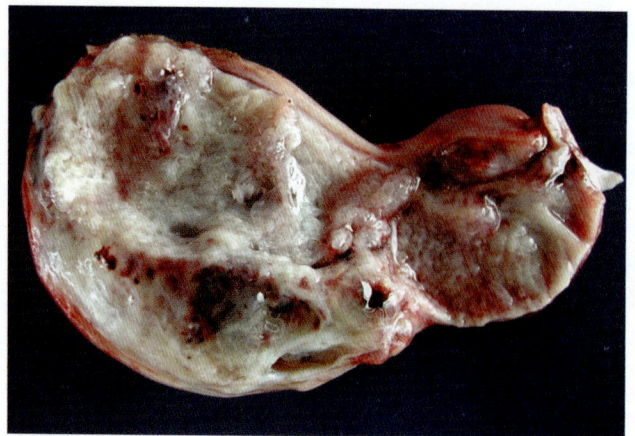
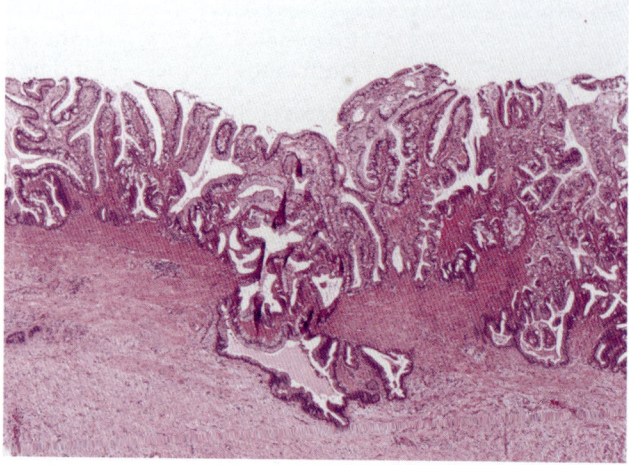
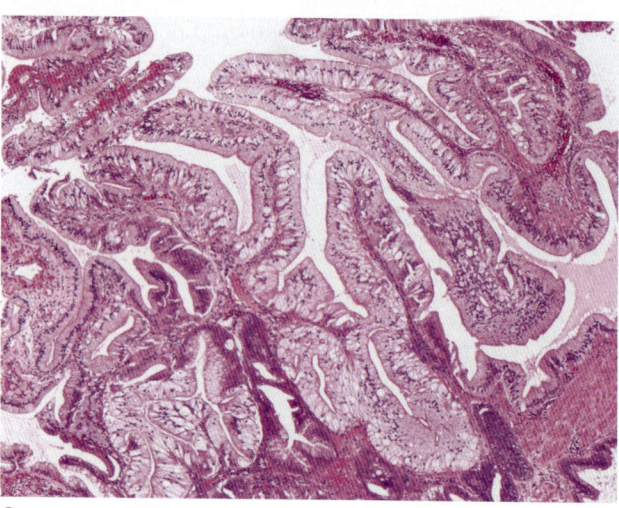
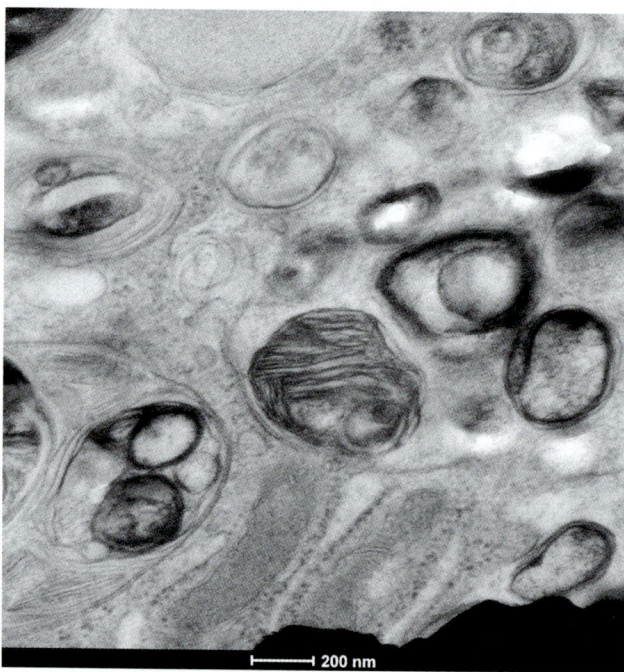

FIGURE 15-21 • Metachromatic leukodystrophy. **A:** Gallbladder with markedly thickened mucosa with fine cobblestone to papillary surface. **B, C:** Papillary fronds lined by columnar epithelial cells with amphophilic cytoplasm (H&E, **B:** 100×, **C:** 200×). **D:** Lysosomal inclusions with closely packed herringbone appearance (electron microscopy, 25,000×).

19cen-q12), fucosidosis (*FUCA1* gene at 1p34), and aspartylglycosaminuria (aspartylglucosaminidase gene at 4q32-33) (93). The liver is involved in all forms and has enlarged vacuolated hepatocytes. Ultrastructurally, the foamy appearance is due to cytoplasmic membrane-bound clear vacuoles (71). The vacuoles are of variable sizes, may be molded by adjacent vacuoles, and fuse to form larger vacuoles. They are composed of finely granular to flocculent material intermingled with membrane material. Kupffer cells, biliary epithelial cells, and endothelial cells show similar vacuoles.

Metachromatic Leukodystrophy

Metachromatic leukodystrophy is an autosomal recessive condition caused by a deficiency in lysosomal aryl sulfatase activity (arylsulfatase A gene at 22q13.31-qter) (93,94). This results in accumulation of galactosyl sulfatide in the tissues and excessive urinary excretion of the metachromatic material.

Demyelination occurs with excess storage of the substrate in the central and peripheral nervous system (93). The storage material is metachromatic and shows brown granules with a characteristic birefringence in cresyl violet–stained, unfixed frozen sections. By light microscopy, foam cells are seen in the nervous system, liver, kidneys, pancreas, adrenal cortex, and gallbladder. The gallbladder may show papillary fronds lined by epithelial cells and with foam cells in the subepithelial stroma (Figure 15-21). Ultrastructurally, the lysosomal inclusions consist of prismatic structures with closely packed periodic leaflets that display a herringbone pattern. In the liver, the inclusions are found in portal macrophages, fibroblasts, and Kupffer cells.

Farber Disease (Farber Lipogranulomatosis)

Farber disease is an autosomal recessive condition in which ceramide, a sphingolipid, accumulates in the tissues due to a deficiency of the lysosomal enzyme acid ceramidase

(*N*-acylsphingosine amidohydrolase gene at 8p22-21.3) (95). Disseminated lipogranulomata are the morphologic findings. The liver is mildly affected, with clear vacuoles in the hepatocytes similar to the membrane-bound vacuoles in mucopolysaccharidoses. The Kupffer cells and portal macrophages have lysosomal comma-shaped, banana-shaped, and curvilinear inclusions in common with other tissues. Death occurs in adolescence or early adulthood (96).

Fabry Disease

Fabry disease is an X-linked recessive disorder caused by mutations in the alpha-galactosidase A gene (*GLA* gene, Xp22) and results in globotriaosylceramide accumulation in the liver and other organs (97). Endothelial cells are the most commonly affected cell type. Ultrastructural findings are characterized by pleomorphic, membrane-bound, osmiophilic lamellar and concentric inclusions (Figure 15-22).

Gangliosidoses

The gangliosidoses are a group of autosomal recessive disorders with impairment of ganglioside metabolism (93,98,99). GM1 and GM2 gangliosidoses have several clinical variants in each group. Five types of GM1 gangliosidosis have been described. The infantile type presents in infancy with coarse facies, skeletal abnormalities, retinal cherry-red spot, hepatosplenomegaly, and progressive deterioration (beta galactosidase-1 at 3p21.33). Lysosomal beta galactosidase is deficient, and the substrate accumulates in the brain and the viscera. Hepatocytes and Kupffer cells are foamy and vacuolated. Ultrastructurally, the cells are distended with large lysosomes that appear as electron lucent vacuoles filled with reticular granular (71). Lamellar, concentric, membrane-bound bodies may also be seen. GM2 gangliosidosis is a group of heterogeneous disorders that includes Tay-Sachs disease (hexosaminidase A gene at 15q23-24) with a hexosaminidase A deficiency and Sandhoff disease with hexosaminidase A and B deficiencies (beta subunit hexosaminidase at 5q13). In Tay-Sachs disease, the central nervous system is primarily affected. The liver appears normal by light microscopy, but concentric membrane-bound inclusions ("zebra bodies") may be seen on electron microscopic examination (Figure 15-23).

Mucopolysaccharidoses

The mucopolysaccharidoses are a group of distinct genetic disorders with accumulation of acid mucopolysaccharides (glycosaminoglycans), dermatan sulfate, heparan sulfate, chondroitin sulfate, and keratin sulfate in the tissues with excretion of these substances in the urine (93,100). Multiple clinical types have been described, each associated with a specific enzyme defect. With the exception of Hunter disease (type II), which is an X-linked recessive condition (Xq28), mucopolysaccharidoses are inherited in an autosomal recessive pattern. The major clinical manifestations are caused by involvement of the brain, skeletal system, liver, cornea, and other organ systems. Because the histopathologic and ultrastructural features are identical, the various syndromes cannot be differentiated on morphologic grounds alone.

The liver is involved in all types with marked cytoplasmic vacuolization of the hepatocytes, Kupffer cells, and Ito cells. Stored acid mucopolysaccharide can be demonstrated with colloidal iron staining, but requires frozen sections or nonaqueous fixatives. Numerous electron lucent membrane-bound vacuoles are seen with electron microscopic examination, corresponding to acid mucopolysaccharides that are extracted with routine tissue processing. Finely granular to flocculent material may be seen in some of the vacuoles arranged in concentric whorls. Hepatic fibrosis may occur.

Sphingolipidoses

Niemann-Pick Disease

Niemann-Pick disease is an autosomal recessive lysosomal disorder associated with a deficiency of sphingomyelinase (type IA and 1B [type A and B], sphingomyelin phosphodiesterase-1 gene at 11p15.4-15.1) or a defect in cholesterol

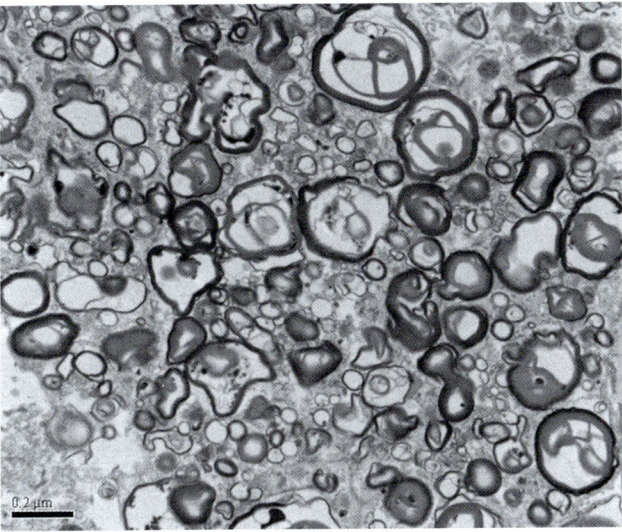

FIGURE 15-22 • Fabry disease. Membrane-bound lysosomal inclusions with lamellar and concentric pattern (electron microscopy, 12,000×).

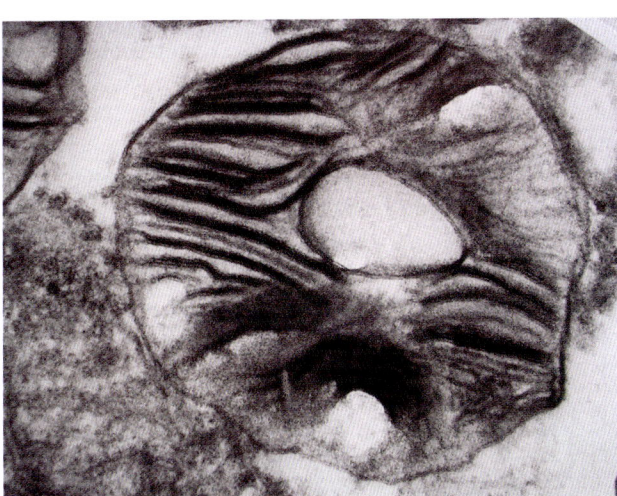

FIGURE 15-23 • Tay-Sachs disease. "Zebra bodies" comprised of concentric membrane-bound lysosomal inclusions (electron microscopy, 20,000×).

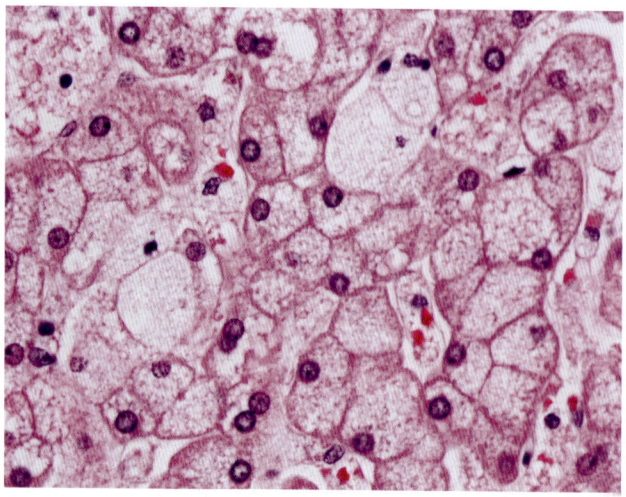 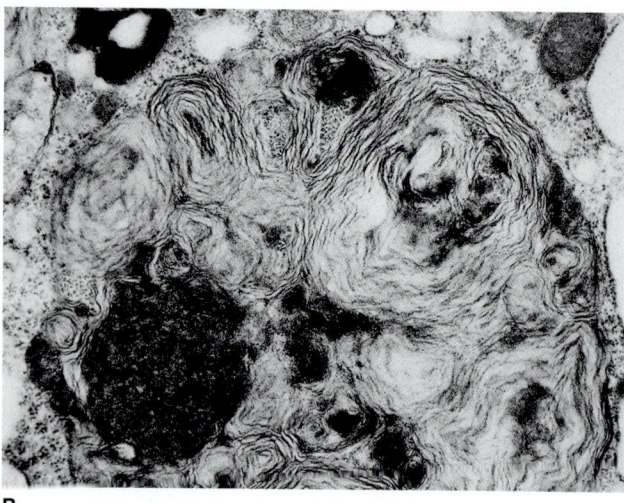

FIGURE 15-24 • Niemann-Pick disease, type C. **A:** Hepatocytes and Kupffer cells with swollen, granular to foamy vacuolated cytoplasm (H&E, 400×). **B:** Large pleomorphic membrane-bound lysosomal inclusions with concentric to parallel lamellae (electron microscopy, 15,000×).

esterification (type II or type C, *NPC* gene at 18q11-12) (70,93). This disease is characterized by sphingomyelin storage in various organs. Sphingomyelin accumulation varies in extent, but it is most pronounced in type A (type 1A), the acute neuropathic form, and in type B (type 1B), the chronic nonneuropathic form. Sea blue histiocytes are seen in the bone marrow. The liver is enlarged and pale on gross examination. The lobular structure of the liver is not disorganized, and fibrosis is generally not a feature. However, cirrhosis may rarely occur.

Type C (type II) disease usually presents with neurologic symptoms between 2 and 4 years of age (70,93,101). However, it may present in the neonatal period with jaundice, hepatosplenomegaly, and failure to thrive and progress to death in months. Foamy macrophages and Kupffer cells may be infrequent initially, but there is progression to the more classic swollen, foamy vacuolated appearance of the cytoplasm (Figure 15-24). Hepatocytes show similar alterations. Ceroid pigment, cholesterol, and phospholipids accumulate in the cells. The stored material is best demonstrated by the Baker hematin reaction for phospholipids. Histochemical staining for acid phosphatase activity reveals a reticular pattern. Ultrastructurally, the appearance is distinctive (71). Large, pleomorphic, membrane-bound inclusions composed of concentric or parallel osmiophilic lamellae are seen in the Kupffer cells and to a lesser extent in the hepatocytes. Bone marrow transplantation has been reported to reverse the amount of storage material in the liver, spleen, lung, and bone marrow, but it does not prevent progression of the neurologic changes.

Gaucher Disease

Gaucher disease is caused by glucocerebrosidase deficiency (acid beta glucosidase gene at 1q21) and leads to glucosylceramide accumulation in various organs (102,103). The disorder is inherited in an autosomal recessive manner, and three clinical types have been described. Type I, the most common, is the adult or chronic nonneuropathic form; type II is the acute neuropathic or infantile form; and type III is the juvenile or subacute neuropathic form. The liver has a similar appearance in all three clinical types. There is massive hepatosplenomegaly with portal hypertension. Gaucher cells are the hallmark. These cells are distended and have a characteristic striated, "wrinkled tissue paper" appearance of the cytoplasm (Figure 15-25). The striations are accentuated with the PAS stain, and acid phosphatase activity can be demonstrated histochemically. Hemosiderin and lipofuscin are frequently present. These macrophages are also seen within the spleen and bone marrow. Clusters of Gaucher cells in the lobule and in portal areas may be associated with fibrosis and cirrhosis in some cases. The ultrastructural features are distinctive with closely apposed, irregular lysosomal inclusions, which correspond to the wrinkled tissue paper light microscopic appearance of Gaucher cells. The inclusions are composed of innumerable tubules with circular profiles on cross-section. "Pseudo-Gaucher" cells have been described in association with benign and malignant hematologic diseases and HIV and mycobacterial infections.

Bile Acid Metabolism Disorders

Bile acid synthesis defects are inherited in an autosomal recessive manner, have low to normal GGT, present in infancy, and are progressive (104). These diseases typically present with neonatal hepatitis and mimic other etiologies for this nonspecific disease process. In older children, there is a more chronic hepatitis-like picture. Clinical signs and symptoms include pruritus with hyperbilirubinemia, difficulty with lipid absorption, and failure to thrive. With some conditions, bile acid substitution will reverse the clinical and histopathologic effects of the bile synthesis deficiencies. The three characteristic clinical findings that distinguish bile acid defects from other causes of neonatal cholestasis are a normal or low serum bile acid levels (as opposed to elevated

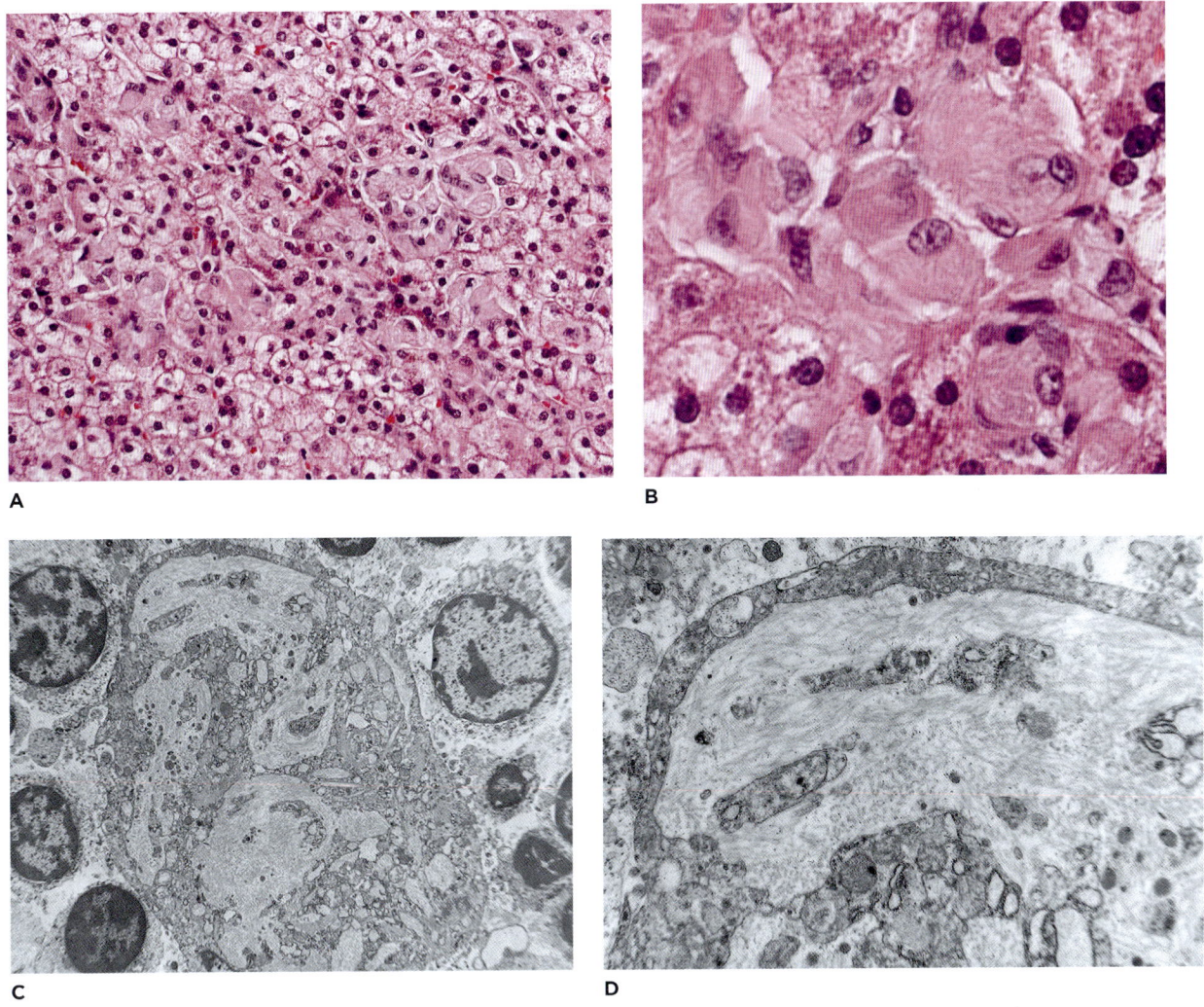

FIGURE 15-25 • Gaucher disease. **A, B:** Markedly enlarged Kupffer cells with cytoplasm with a striated, wrinkled tissue paper appearance (H&E, **A:** 100×, **B:** 800×). **C, D:** Kupffer cells with cytoplasmic tubular inclusions with a circular profile on cross-section (electron microscopy, **C:** 6000×, **D:** 24,000×).

levels in all neonatal cholestasis), normal or only minimally elevated GGT levels, and absence of pruritus. Diagnosis is made by measurement of serum and urinary bile acid levels and detection of specific enzyme defects and/or genetic defects.

Zellweger Syndrome (Cerebrohepatorenal Syndrome)

Zellweger syndrome (cerebrohepatorenal syndrome) is an autosomal recessive disorder characterized clinically by multiple congenital abnormalities, including craniofacial abnormalities, hypotonia, and psychomotor retardation. Renal cortical cysts, cerebral dysgenesis, and hepatic abnormalities are present (105). Several different genes involved in peroxisome biogenesis occur in different forms of Zellweger syndrome, including peroxin-1 (*PEX1* at 7q21-q22), peroxin-2 (*PEX2*, 8q21.1), peroxin-3 (*PEX3* 6q23-q24), peroxin-5 (*PEX5* 12p13.3), peroxin-6 (*PEX6* 6p21.1), peroxin-12 (*PEX12* on chromosome 17), peroxin-14 (*PEX14* 1p36.2),

and peroxin-26 (*PEX26* 22q11.21). Absence of peroxisomes in hepatocytes and renal tubular cells is a distinctive feature (70,104). Death occurs in early infancy. The liver shows hepatocellular disarray, biliary dysgenesis, portal inflammation, and striking iron deposition in Kupffer cells and hepatocytes. Giant cell transformation, steatosis, and hepatic fibrosis or cirrhosis may be seen.

Other Bile Acid Synthesis Defects

Many genetic defects of bile acid synthesis are known (104,106,107). The most common defect among these is 3-beta-hydroxy dehydrogenase deficiency caused by a mutation in the gene encoding 3-beta-hydroxy-delta-5-C27-steroid oxidoreductase (*HSD3B7* gene at 16p12-p11.2). This entity is referred to as congenital bile acid synthesis defect type 1. This leads to neonatal hepatitis and will progress to chronic liver disease without appropriate diagnosis and bile acid substitution. Another form of a congenital defect in bile acid synthesis is due to delta(4)-3-oxosteroid 5-beta-reductase deficiency (congenital bile acid synthesis defect type 2). This is caused by mutation in the *AKR1D1* gene (7q32-33). Congenital bile acid synthesis defect type 4 is caused by mutation in the alpha-methylacyl-CoA racemase (*AMACR*) gene located at 5p13.2-q11.1. Neonatal hepatitis with bile duct proliferation is associated with a bile synthesis defect in oxysterol 7-alpha-hydroxylase (*CYP7B* gene at 6p21.1-p11.2). Cholesterol is converted into one of several oxysterols prior to being 7-alpha-hydroxylated by an oxysterol 7-alpha-hydroxylase. Lack of this enzyme leads to neonatal hepatitis, with the potential for progressive liver disease, that can lead to infantile death. A deficiency in 25-hyroxylase (gene at 10q23) results in a bile acid synthesis defect. This is due to the role of this enzyme in expression of genes involved in cholesterol and lipid metabolism. Liver fibrosis is somewhat variable, with a more prolonged course of fibrosis in affected neonates and children. Early detection of bile acid synthetic defects can prevent progressive liver disease due to the good response to oral bile acid replacement therapy in most defects.

Bile acid conjugation defects such as familial hypercholanemia is characterized by elevated serum bile acid concentrations, itching, and fat malabsorption (*BAAT* gene at 9q22.3) (42). The defect in this condition is associated with the enzyme bile acid CoA amino acid *N*-acyltransferase (BAAT). This enzyme produces *N*-acyl conjugates of cholanoates (C24 bile acids) with glycine or taurine. The resulting bile acid–amino acid conjugates serve as detergents in the gastrointestinal tract. Those affected with bile acid conjugation defects may present as neonatal hepatitis with fibrosis or as mild chronic liver disease. There are several other conditions that may also have bile acid synthesis defects, such as peroxisome diseases (Zellweger syndrome, Refsum disease, hyperpipecolic anemia, adrenolipodystrophies) and cerebrotendinous xanthomatosis (CYP27A1 gene encoding sterol 27-hydroxylase at 2q33-qter).

Alpha-1 Antitrypsin Deficiency

Liver disease associated with A1AT was initially described by Sharp et al. and has been extensively reviewed (81,108,109). This is an autosomal recessive disease caused by mutations in the protease inhibitor gene (Pi) on chromosome 14. Both liver and lung diseases (emphysema) occur due to lack of neutralization of neutrophil elastase secondary to absent or decreased protease inhibitor activity. Liver disease without pulmonary emphysema occurs when a mutant but functional form of protease inhibitor is present that inhibits neutrophil elastase activity. This mutant form of AIAT has a defect that does not allow for proper folding, resulting in failure of the material to be translocated from the endoplasmic reticulum to the Golgi for further processing before release from the hepatocyte. The AIAT continues to accumulate in the rough endoplasmic reticulum, leading to hepatocyte injury and liver disease. Clinical presentations vary from neonatal hepatitis with cholestatic jaundice, to young adults with recurrent hepatitis that may lead to chronic hepatitis and cirrhosis, and to older adults with a silent clinical course and cirrhosis development.

A close association of A1AT deficiency has been noted with neonatal cholestasis, accounting for over 10% of cases of neonatal cholestasis, making it the most common genetic cause of neonatal liver disease (70). Bleeding diathesis, including intracranial hemorrhage, may be the presenting manifestation in the newborn, probably related to an associated vitamin K deficiency.

A1AT is a glycoprotein that is synthesized in the liver and secreted into the serum. Its biosynthesis is controlled by a pair of genes at the protease inhibitor (Pi) locus (81,110). More than 25 alleles have been described and are responsible for A1AT variant molecules. The normal genotype is PiMM. PIZZ is the most clinically significant genotype with respect to liver disease and is due to a point mutation with substitution of Lys for Glu. PiMZ genotype patients have 50% normal A1AT and 50% mutant A1AT. Other mutant gene alleles include PiS with reduced A1AT level and no clinical disease and PiNull with no detectable A1AT. With electrophoresis, PiZ is the slowest of the A1AT variants. In the homozygous (PiZZ) state, there is a marked reduction in the serum A1AT levels. Homozygous PiZZ A1AT has an incidence of 1 in 1600 to 2000 live births, making it nearly as frequent as cystic fibrosis (CF). A few cases of liver disease have been reported in association with PiSZ. Neonatal liver injury has occurred with the PiZ null phenotype. The risk of HCC is increased, especially in homozygous patients, with most cases being reported in adults (111).

Liver morphology varies in the early phase of the disease. Hepatocellular injury is manifested principally as cholestasis, pseudoacinar transformation, and giant cell transformation, similar to other metabolic hepatopathies (Figure 15-26). Extramedullary hematopoiesis is usually seen. Cholestasis is hepatocellular and present in the form of plugs within the canaliculi. Three morphologic patterns with prognostic significance have been described for the early cholestatic phase. In group 1, portal areas show mild portal fibrosis and no bile duct proliferation, which has a neonatal hepatitis-like appearance (Figure 15-26). In group 2, the portal triads are fibrotic and expanded and contain proliferating bile ducts in which bile may be present. This pattern may be mistaken for the obstructive changes seen in EHBA and is associated with persistent hepatic disease leading to cirrhosis with a higher frequency. With group 3, there is a paucity of intrahepatic ducts. The prognosis of this group is uncertain. Extensive hepatocellular necrosis may also occur and lead to fulminant hepatic failure.

The morphologic hallmark of the disease is the presence of A1AT in the hepatocytes, predominantly in zone 1 and occasionally in bile duct epithelium. The stored material appears in the form of eosinophilic hyaline globules that are PAS positive and resist diastase digestion. The globules progressively increase in number and may not be visible by hematoxylin–eosin sections in biopsy specimens obtained in the first

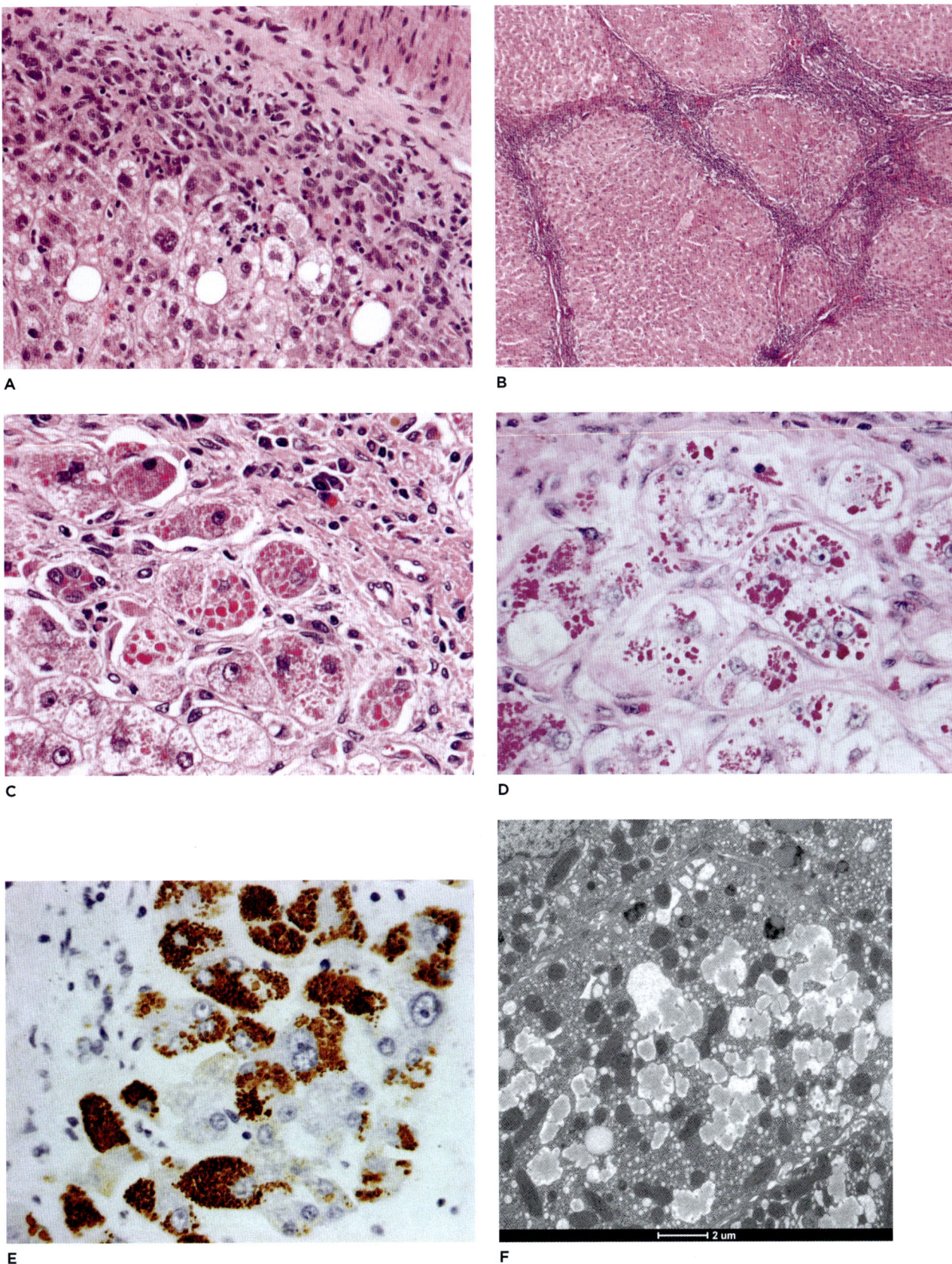

FIGURE 15-26 • **A:** Alpha-1 antitrypsin deficiency. Zone 1 hepatocytes with reactive changes and portal areas with chronic inflammation and mild bile duct proliferation (**A:** H&E, 200×). **B:** Cirrhosis in late stage of disease detection (**B:** H&E, 40×). **C, D:** Zone 1 hepatocytes with PAS-positive (**C:** 400×) cytoplasmic globules that are diastase resistant (**D:** 400×). **E:** Immunostaining for alpha-1 antitrypsin reacts with the cytoplasmic globules (**E:** 400×). **F:** Granular, flocculent material distends cisternae of the rough endoplasmic reticulum (**F:** electron microscopy, 10,000×).

3 months of life (112). The stored material may be demonstrable by IHC, even in the absence of appreciable globules. Ultrastructurally, the stored material appears as flocculent, moderately electron-dense material within dilated cisternae of rough endoplasmic reticulum.

The frequency of progression to cirrhosis after neonatal presentation with prolonged cholestasis is variable. Only about 15% of the PiZZ population develops liver disease in the first 20 years of life. If A1AT deficiency is manifested in the neonatal period, as many as 50% of cases progress to cirrhosis, typically micronodular type (66,70) (Figure 15-26). The presence of PAS-positive diastase-resistant globules is the pathologic hallmark, differentiating micronodular cirrhosis associated with A1AT deficiency from micronodular cirrhosis associated with other disorders. The extrahepatic bile ducts are usually normal. A few cases of hypoplasia of the extrahepatic bile ducts with A1AT deficiency have been described, and this hypoplasia has been ascribed to a low-flow state (20).

Cystic Fibrosis

CF is caused by mutations in the *CFTR* gene (CF transmembrane conductance regulator, 7q31.2) that regulates a cyclic AMP-dependent chloride channel (113). CFTR gene mutation results in decreased sodium and water content of bile with an increase in bile viscosity and reduction in bile low, leading to intrahepatic bile duct obstruction and injury. The incidence of hepatic involvement in CF has increased over the past several decades with increased life expectancy of CF patients. Although pulmonary complications are the predominant clinical manifestations, up to 5% of CF patients may have substantial hepatic dysfunction and an even larger proportion have the typical histologic lesions of CF in the liver without abnormal liver function tests (113,114). The liver may have multiple capsular depressed scars, with a resemblance to hepar lobatum. Histopathologically, there are focal irregular areas of fibrosis with bile duct proliferation and intraluminal inspissated eosinophilic or pale orange secretions (Figure 15-27). This pathognomonic hepatic lesion is the so-called focal biliary cirrhosis. Mononuclear cell infiltration may be seen. Steatosis is confined to zone 3 or shows a panacinar distribution, especially in infants with newly diagnosed CF whose pancreatic enzyme replacement has not yet been initiated.

The disease may present in the neonate with cholestatic changes with giant cell transformation and steatosis as the feature of a metabolic hepatopathy. A liver biopsy in an infant with CF may not show the distinctive bile duct lesion (focal

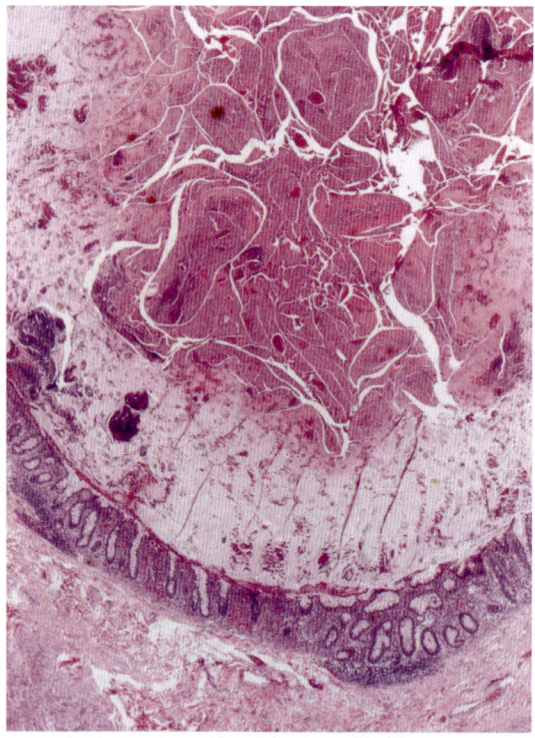
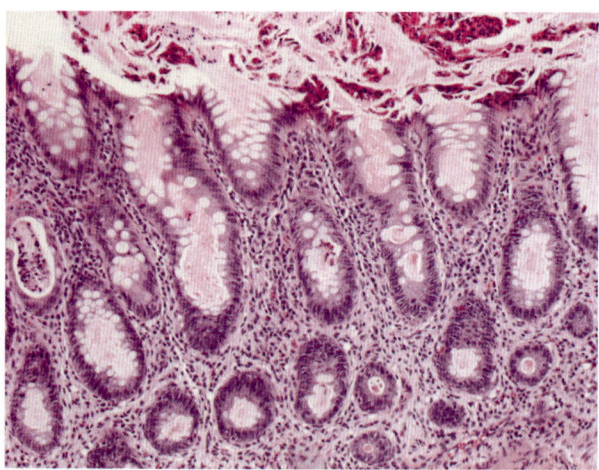
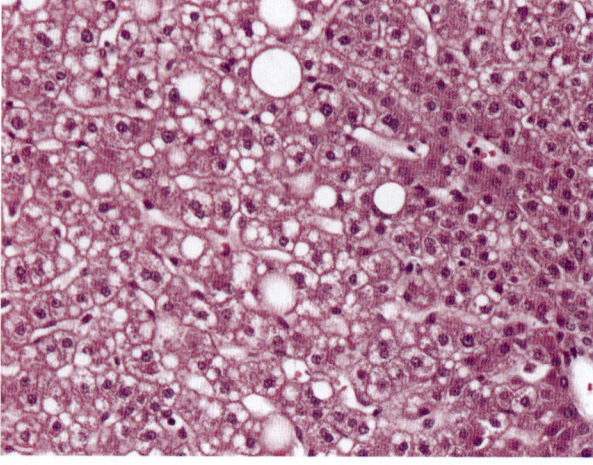

FIGURE 15-27 • Cystic fibrosis. **A:** Appendix with dilated lumen and dense eosinophilic mucin in the lumen (H&E, 20×). **B:** Appendiceal glands with inspissated densely eosinophilic mucin (H&E, 200×). **C:** Hepatocytes with diffuse microsteatosis and focal macrosteatosis (H&E, 200×).

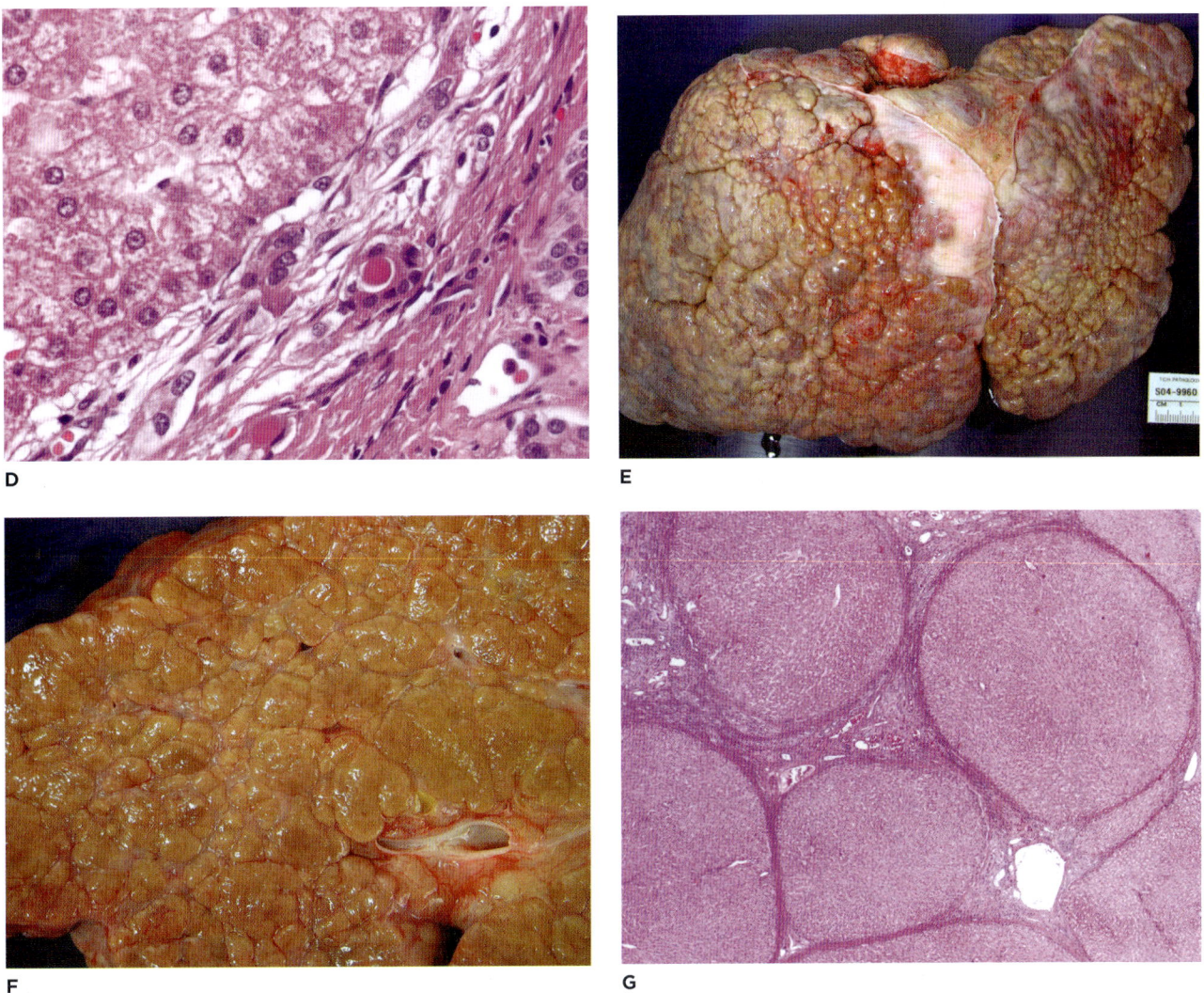

FIGURE 15-27 • (*continued*) **D:** Bile ducts in fibrotic portal region with luminal inspissated densely eosinophilic secretions (H&E, 400×). **E-G:** Explanted liver with macronodular and micronodular cirrhosis (H&E, G 40×).

biliary cirrhosis). The progression from neonatal cholestasis to focal biliary cirrhosis is not clear.

A coarsely nodular cirrhosis is present in 4% to 10% of CF cases, with the prevalence increasing through childhood (113). Interestingly, there is a diminished prevalence of cirrhosis in those surviving to young adulthood, suggesting that liver disease may influence premature respiratory death in teenagers. At the cirrhotic stage, the liver shows multiple, large nodules, with areas between the nodules appearing depressed and presenting a finely nodular appearance. Portal hypertension and its complications may occur, and, rarely, death may ensue acute bleeding from esophageal varices. Combined liver and lung transplantation are necessary in a minority of cases.

The gallbladder is frequently abnormal. The prevalence of gallbladder abnormalities increases with age (115). The gallbladder may be small, with the epithelium frequently having mucinous metaplasia. Diagnostic imaging may show a diminutive or nonfunctioning gallbladder. Cholesterol gallstones are seen in 6% to 12% of patients over 12 years of age, with the risk of developing calculi increasing with age.

Iron Storage Disease

Primary and secondary disorders of iron metabolism are characterized by excessive iron accumulation in the liver (Figure 15-28) as a component of increased total body iron stores (116–118). Secondary iron overload may be the result of multiple transfusions for hemoglobin disorders such as thalassemia and sickle cell disease or may be due to excessive iron intake. Inherited iron storage disease or hemochromatosis is most often an autosomal recessive condition characterized by a defect in the regulation of iron absorption in the intestine and may present in childhood. There are several inherited forms of hemochromatosis caused by different gene mutations. The clinical features of hemochromatosis include cirrhosis of the liver, diabetes, hypermelanotic pigmentation of the skin, and heart failure. Pancreatic deposition of iron leads to diabetes, and congestive cardiomyopathy is the result of iron deposition in the myocardium. Primary HCC, complicating cirrhosis, is responsible for about one-third of deaths in affected homozygotes. Because hemochromatosis is a relatively easily treated disorder if diagnosed

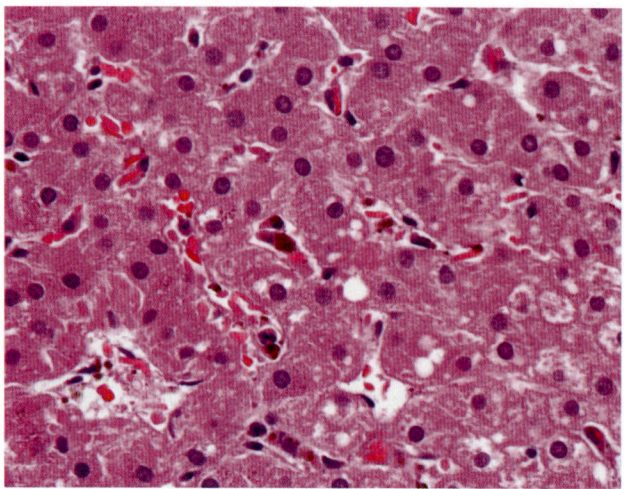 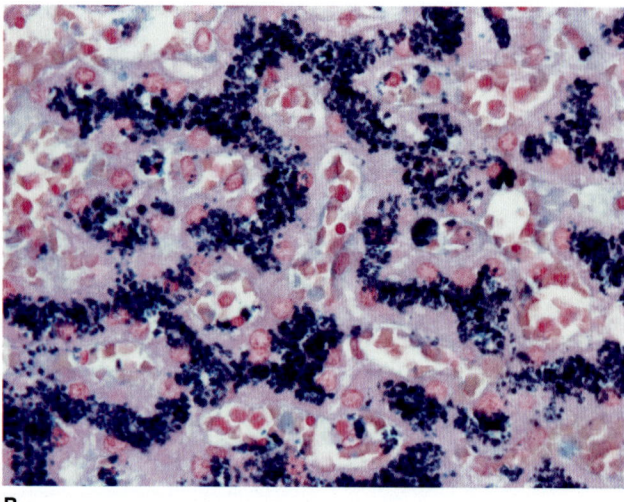

FIGURE 15-28 • Secondary hemosiderosis due to chronic transfusion therapy. **A:** Occasional Kupffer cells with iron pigment in their cytoplasm (H&E, 400×). **B:** Abundant iron storage in Kupffer cells revealed with Prussian blue histochemical stain for iron (400×).

early, this is a form of preventable cancer. At least five iron overload disorders labeled hemochromatosis have been identified on the basis of clinical, biochemical, and genetic characteristics (6,119). Classic hemochromatosis (HFE), an autosomal recessive disorder, is most often caused by a mutation in a gene designated *HFE* on chromosome 6p21.3. It has also been found to be caused by a mutation in the gene encoding hemojuvelin (*HJV*), which maps to 1q21. Juvenile hemochromatosis or hemochromatosis type 2 (HFE2) is also autosomal recessive. One form, designated HFE2A, is caused by a mutation in the *HJV* gene (1q21). A second form, designated HFE2B, is caused by a mutation in the gene encoding hepcidin antimicrobial peptide, which maps to 19q13. Hemochromatosis type 3, also an autosomal recessive disorder, is caused by mutation in the gene encoding transferrin receptor 2 (*TFR2*), which maps to 7q22. Hemochromatosis type 4, an autosomal dominant disorder, is caused by a mutation in the *SLC40A1* gene, which encodes ferroprotein and maps to 2q32. Most affected children and adolescents are asymptomatic with periportal iron accumulations extending toward the central lobule during adolescents. With juvenile hemochromatosis, organ failure with severe iron overload presents before age 30. Both the inherited (hemochromatosis) and secondary (transfusion) forms of iron storage differ from hemosiderosis in that the iron, in addition to being deposited in mononuclear phagocytic cells, is also deposited in the parenchymal cells. Iron deposition in biliary epithelial cells is seen more often in inherited iron storage disease.

Alloimmune Gestational Hepatitis (Neonatal Iron Storage Disease)

Alloimmune gestational hepatitis (AGH), previously known as neonatal iron storage disease (NISD), is a fatal neonatal disorder, characterized by massive iron overload (13,118). The liver is the predominant organ affected, but iron is also deposited in the pancreas, thyroid, adrenals, pituitary, heart, intestinal mucosa, salivary glands, and sweat glands. The condition should be differentiated from other disorders such as tyrosinemia, galactosemia, and Zellweger syndrome, in which excess iron is usually present and is not related to neonatal hemochromatosis. In the last few years, the etiopathogenesis of AGH has been better understood. It is now considered a gestational disease in which maternal IgG antibodies cross the placenta and induce fetal liver injury leading to severe liver disease with a neonatal hepatitis pattern in the neonate. AGH recurrence rate in siblings after the index case is 60% to 80%, implicating maternal alloimmune damage to fetal liver. Pregnant mice injected with human IgG from women with AGH offspring had pups with extensive hepatic injury and liver necrosis. It is now believed that this maternal antibody induces activation of the complement cascade in the neonate with the resultant C5b-9 complex (membrane attack complex, MAC) causing the hepatocyte necrosis and loss (118). Clinical investigations have evaluated treatment of pregnant women with a prior AGH neonate with intravenous immunoglobulin (IV Ig) (120). In these clinical studies, prior gestational histories indicated a high risk for AGH occurrence, with 92% of at-risk pregnancies resulting in intrauterine fetal demise, neonatal death, or liver failure necessitating transplant (121). With IV Ig gestational therapy during pregnancy, there were only three failures, while 52 infants did not experience AGH (118).

In AGH, the hepatic architecture is markedly disorganized with lobular collapse and early fibrosis (Figure 15-29). Scattered nests of hepatocytes with heavy iron deposits, pseudoacinar profiles, and multinucleated hepatocytes are other microscopic features. The diagnosis has now been supported by the diffuse staining of the cytoplasm of hepatocytes with C5b-9 demonstrated by a MAC immunohistochemical stain. This deposition is noted to be prominent in most cases of NGCH and can result in death in the neonatal period. Similar deposition of MAC has not been found in any other causes of neonatal cholestasis or normal livers. Increased iron deposition is noted within the hepatocytes and Kupffer cells as well

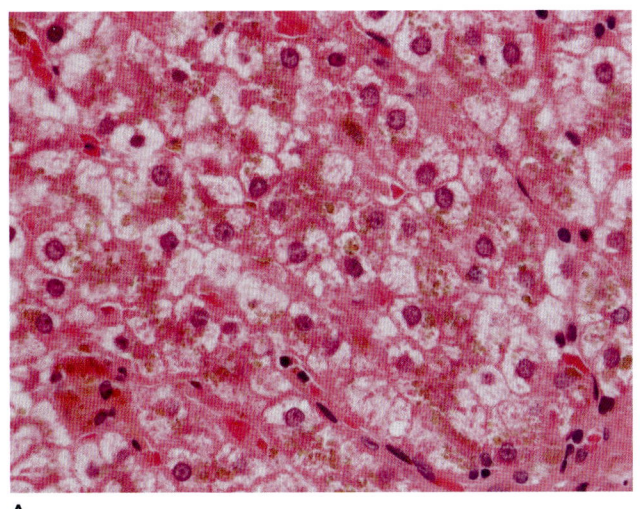
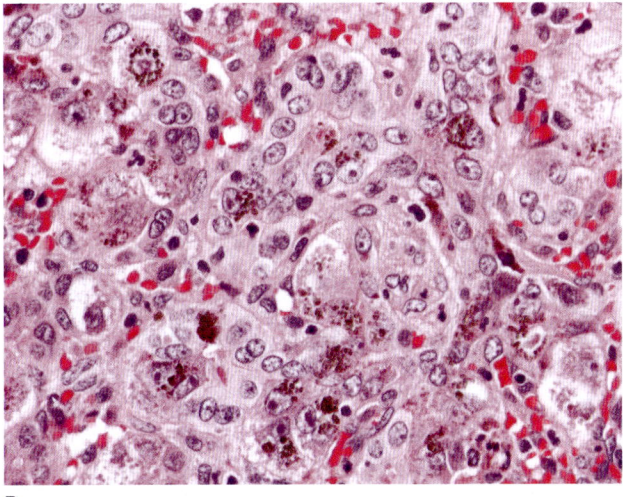
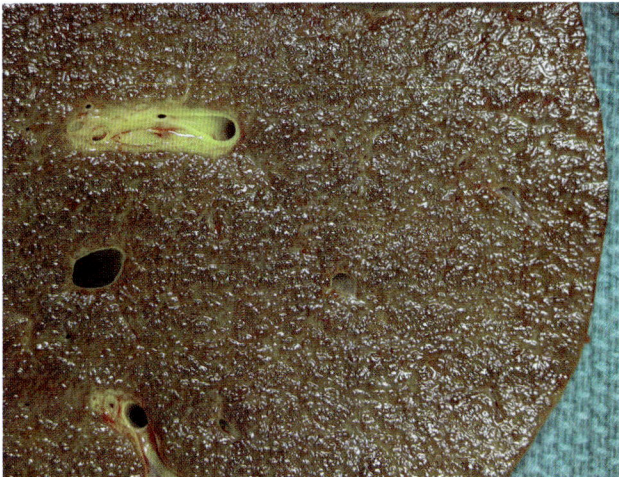

FIGURE 15-29 • Alloimmune gestational hepatitis. **A, B:** Hepatocytes and bile duct epithelium with readily identified iron pigment accumulation in cytoplasm, note giant cell hepatocytes (H&E, 400×). **C:** Explanted liver with micronodular cirrhosis and green and brown pigmentation from bile and iron accumulation, respectively.

as bile duct epithelial cells. With other organ systems, the iron deposits tend to be within the reticuloendothelial system, with sparing of the parenchymal cells. Minor salivary glands in the oral mucosa show iron deposition in AGH and may be biopsied for diagnosis in suspected cases while awaiting genetic testing results for hemochromatosis.

Wilson Disease

Wilson disease is an inborn error of copper metabolism with an autosomal recessive pattern of inheritance. A genetic defect in *ATP7B* on chromosome 13q14-21 has been described. This gene encodes a transmembrane copper-transporting adenosine triphosphatase (ATPase) that is located on the canalicular membrane of hepatocytes and is also homologous with Menkes disease gene (122,123). The genetic defect results in reduced copper excretion in the bile and decreased copper incorporation into ceruloplasmin. There are many different mutations in *ATP7B*, which account for the variable clinical phenotypes.

In normal metabolism, copper is taken up by the stomach and duodenum, weakly bound to albumin, and transferred to hepatocytes (122). Within the hepatocytes, copper is incorporated into the alpha-2-globulin of ceruloplasmin and released into the bloodstream. Senescent ceruloplasmin is reabsorbed by the hepatocytes and undergoes lysosomal degradation and excreted into the bile. In Wilson disease, copper accumulation occurs in the liver, brain, eyes, and other organs. Elevated levels of serum and hepatic copper, increased urinary copper excretion, and diminished levels of serum ceruloplasmin are the common laboratory abnormalities. In some cases, serum ceruloplasmin values may be within normal limits. A normal serum level of copper excludes Wilson disease, but an elevated level is not always diagnostic, because elevations in copper may be seen in other forms of liver disease, especially of cholestatic type, and in chronic hepatitis. Genetic analysis is available for the diagnosis of Wilson disease in patients and their families (123). The mitochondria have been shown to be the main storage house for copper within hepatocytes, and progressive accumulation leads to shutdown of the respiratory cycle and release of reactive oxygen species resulting in cell death and in severe cases acute liver failure (124).

The clinical presentation varies according to the age of the patient and the stage of the disease. The most frequent symptoms are related to hepatic involvement. Liver disease may be chronic, and cirrhosis or chronic hepatitis may be evident at clinical presentation. Acute hepatitis and fulminant hepatic failure may be the presenting features in a minority of cases, especially in the first two decades of life. Hemolytic anemia is frequent. Central nervous system signs, neuropsychiatric symptoms associated with basal ganglia involvement, and Kayser-Fleischer rings develop in the course of the disease. The latter are characterized by green–brown deposits of copper in Descemet membranes of the corneal limbus.

Penicillamine therapy has been reported to alter the natural course of the disease and, when instituted early, can prevent progression of liver disease (122,125). Controversy, however, exists as to the timing of the use of penicillamine in treatment. Treatment using zinc and trientine has also been studied. Transplantation including human hepatocyte transplantation may be necessary in some cases (126,127).

Histopathologic features in the liver vary from mild-to-moderate fatty changes, focal cytoplasmic swelling, glycogenated nuclei, and occasional acidophilic bodies in the early stages (128) (Figure 15-30). Generally, portal tract inflammation, lobular chronic inflammation, and fibrosis are not seen at this stage. Copper is diffusely dispersed in the cytoplasm and usually cannot be demonstrated histochemically. In the symptomatic stage, the liver may have features of chronic hepatitis (interface hepatitis, portal inflammation with plasma cells, fibrosis, and spotty acidophilic necrosis of hepatocytes). Mallory bodies may be seen, especially in the zone 1 hepatocytes. Glycogenated nuclei are a frequent, but nonspecific, feature. A mixed micronodular–macronodular cirrhosis is the consequence of the chronic hepatitis. Rarely, massive liver necrosis is seen.

Copper can be demonstrated histochemically and is most pronounced in the periportal hepatocytes. The rhodamine stain gives a brick red reaction product, while rubeanic acid stains the copper gray–black. The Shikata orcein stain demonstrates associated copper-binding protein. Copper may be irregularly distributed in the hepatocyte nodules and may be absent in the regenerative nodules by histochemical methods. Biochemical quantitation of hepatic copper typically demonstrates marked elevations (>250 µg/g dry weight). This can be performed on fresh tissue collected in metal-free containers or a paraffin block. Ultrastructurally, the mitochondria show characteristic alterations appearing enlarged and pleomorphic. Separation of the inner membranes, widening of the intracristal space with microcystic formations at the tips of the cristae, crystalloid inclusions, disoriented cristae, and increased granules in the matrix of the mitochondria are regarded as diagnostic of the disorder (71,124). Copper deposits are seen in the lysosomes of zone 1 hepatocytes and appear extremely electron dense. Peroxisomal deposition of copper has also been described.

Other copper overload diseases in children include the Indian childhood cirrhosis (ICC), endemic Tyrolean infantile cirrhosis (ETIC), and idiopathic copper toxicosis (ICT) (129). All of these are characterized by elevated liver copper levels, but have normal or elevated ceruloplasmin levels. They are characterized by progressive fibrosis leading to micronodular cirrhosis in the first 2 years of life, especially in ICT. ICC is characterized by variable mixed inflammation, large bands of fibrosis, and hepatocellular damage but not steatosis as in Wilson disease. Mallory hyaline may also be present. Cholestasis may be prominent. A link to dietary copper ingestion has been implicated in these copper-related diseases as opposed to Wilson disease, which usually affects older children.

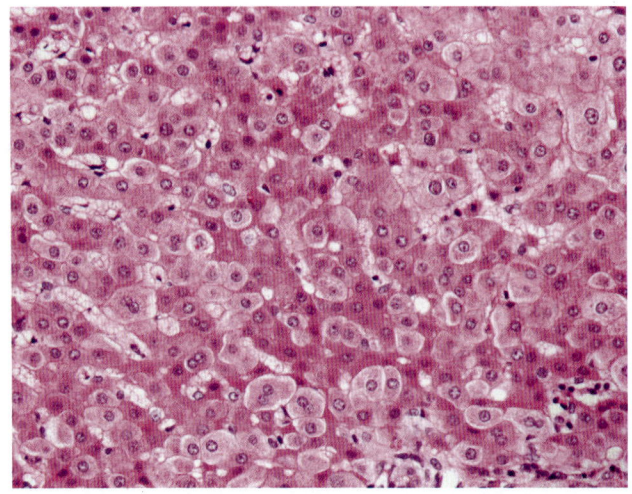
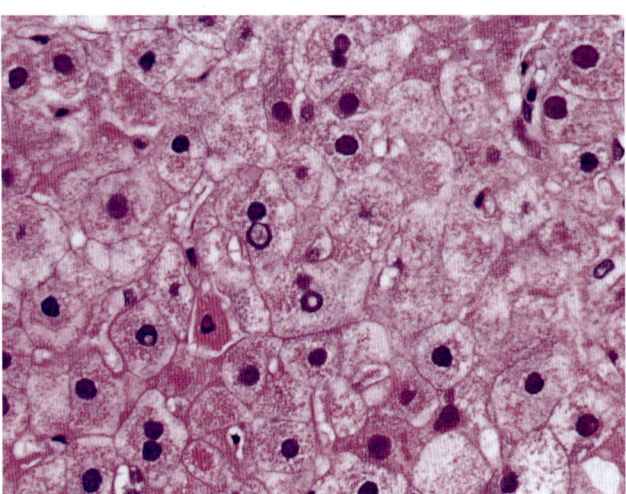

FIGURE 15-30 • Wilson disease. A: Hepatocytes with variable cytoplasmic swelling and decreased cytoplasmic eosinophilia (H&E, 200×). B: Infrequent hepatocytes with glycogenated nuclei, apoptotic (acidophil) bodies, and fine granular cytoplasm with a certain degree of cytoplasmic swelling (H&E, 400×).

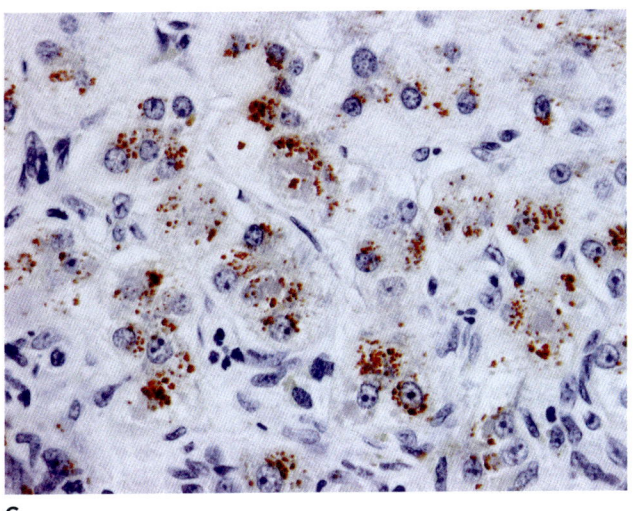

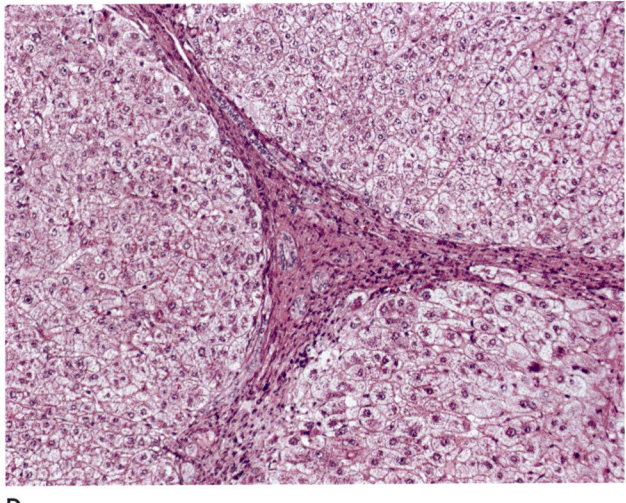

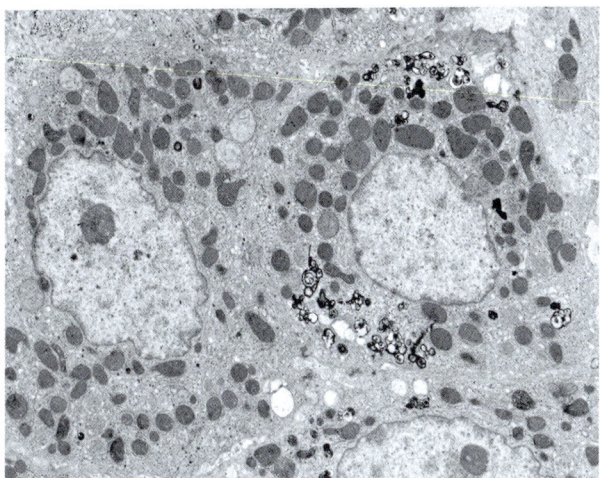

FIGURE 15-30 • (*continued*) **C:** Cytoplasmic copper detection in periportal hepatocytes (Rhodamine stain, 400×). **D:** Wilson disease with cirrhosis of the liver (H&E, 100×). **E:** Variably sized and relatively pleomorphic mitochondria and dense lysosomal deposits in Wilson disease (electron microscopy, 3000×).

Porphyrias

Porphyrias are a group of disorders of porphyrin and heme biosynthesis (93,117). Porphyria may be inherited or acquired and is characterized by increased excretion of porphyrins and storage of abnormal types of porphyrin pigments within tissues. Hepatic abnormalities may be seen in acute intermittent porphyria (hydroxymethylbilane synthase 11q23.3), porphyria cutanea tarda (hemochromatosis gene at 6p21.3, uroporphyrinogen decarboxylase gene at 1p34), and congenital erythropoietic protoporphyria (uroporphyrinogen III synthase gene at 10q25.2-q26.3). The changes in acute intermittent porphyria and porphyria cutanea tarda are similar, although the severity of hepatic injury is greater in porphyria cutanea tarda. Fatty changes and iron overload are evident. Cirrhosis and hepatic failure may occur in porphyria patients, and HCC has been described as a complication in later life. The uroporphyrin crystals are water soluble and needle shaped and have a red fluorescence on examination under ultraviolet light. The needle-shaped inclusions are seen in the hepatic cells by electron microscopy. Additional ultrastructural features include abnormal mitochondria, autophagic vacuoles, and myelin figures. In congenital erythropoietic protoporphyria, the hepatic findings consist of focal accumulation of dark brown pigment in the canaliculi, bile duct epithelium, Kupffer cells, and connective tissue. The pigment is birefringent with bright granules and central Maltese crosses. An intense red fluorescence is seen in frozen sections examined under ultraviolet light. Ultrastructurally, the crystals are electron dense, straight or curved, and arranged singly or in a radiating starburst pattern.

Urea Cycle Disorders

Hyperammonemia is characteristic of this group of disorders and should be differentiated from other conditions with elevated ammonia levels (93,130). In the newborn, hyperammonemia may be found in premature infants or infants with birth asphyxia. *In utero* hepatic necrosis of undetermined cause has been found to be associated with hyperammonemia. Defects of the urea cycle include deficiency of ornithine transcarbamylase (Xp21.1), deficiency of carbamoyl synthetase (2q35), citrullinemia associated with deficiency of

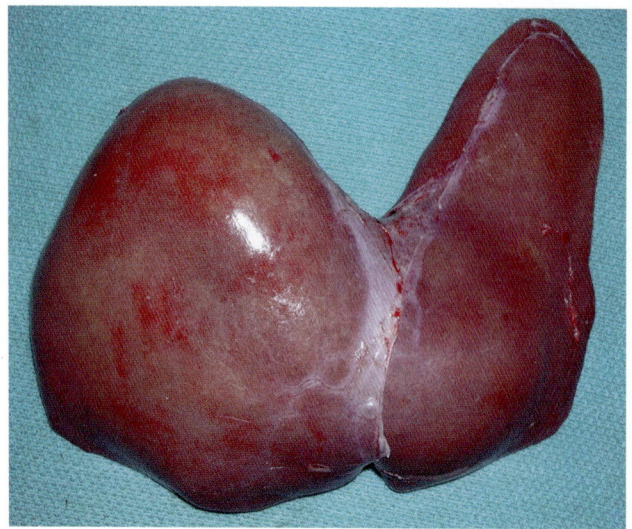
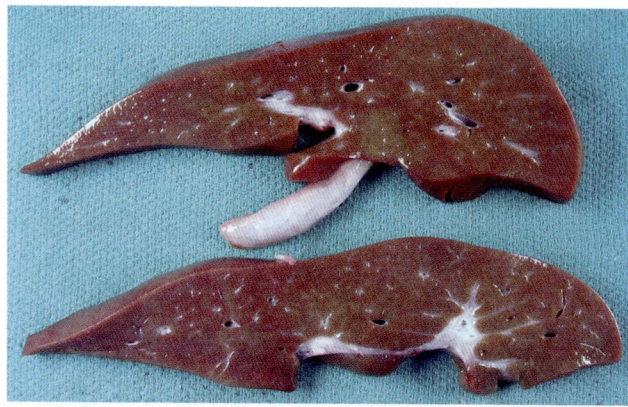
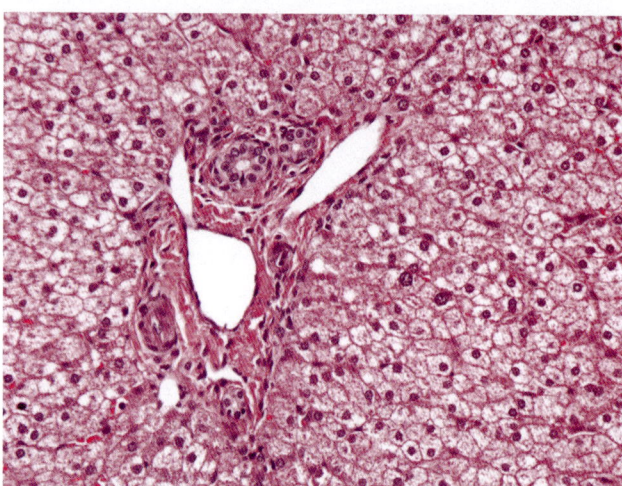

FIGURE 15-31 • Urea cycle disorder—ornithine transcarbamylase deficiency. **A, B:** Explanted liver with no gross abnormalities in ornithine transcarbamylase deficiency. **C:** Portal triad and zone 1 and 2 hepatocytes with no histopathologic abnormalities (H&E, 200×).

argininosuccinic acid synthetase (9q34.1), argininosuccinic aciduria due to deficiency of argininosuccinase lyase (7cen-q11.2), argininemia associated with arginase deficiency (6q23), and deficiency of N-acetyl-glutamate synthetase (17q21.31) (130,131). With the exception of ornithine transcarbamylase deficiency, which is inherited as an X-linked dominant condition, the other conditions have an autosomal recessive pattern of inheritance. Prenatal diagnosis is possible. Liver biopsy in urea cycle defects may be normal or may have only mild nonspecific changes including steatosis, cholestasis, individual cell necrosis, and early fibrosis (132) (Figure 15-31). Liver transplantation may be necessary depending upon the specific urea cycle defect disorder (133). The liver being normal during transplant, these explanted livers can be used as donor organs for other patients with liver disease (domino transplant).

Hepatic Steatosis and Steatohepatitis

Fatty change of the liver is a frequent, nonspecific finding associated with a variety of metabolic and nutritional disorders (134). Diagnosis of the specific metabolic disorder associated with this change requires the demonstration of pathognomonic biochemical and morphologic features of that disease. Disorders of lipid and lipoprotein metabolism include abetalipoproteinemia, hypercholesterolemia, congenital lipodystrophy, and fatty acid oxidation defects. The ultrastructural features of these diseases have been described elsewhere (71). Various chemical agents, drugs (valproate, asparaginase, steroids, amiodarone), and toxins (alcohol) are known to induce hepatosteatosis. Other causes of hepatosteatosis in childhood include protein malnutrition, kwashiorkor, obesity, chronic illnesses, type I diabetes, hepatitis C, TPN, mitochondrial disease, inborn errors of metabolism, and severe infection. In the case of obesity, fatty change may be accompanied by inflammation in the lobules and portal tracts as features of steatohepatitis (135).

This is a reversible form of cellular injury. The lipid may accumulate in the form of small droplets of microvesicular fat or in the form of large (macrovesicular) droplets that occupy most of the cytoplasm and displace the nucleus to the periphery (Figure 15-32). Microvesicular fat leads to a foamy or clear appearance of the hepatocyte cytoplasm, without displacement of the nucleus, and may not be obvious as fat in the usual preparation. Fat stains on frozen sections and electron microscopy conclusively demonstrate the fat.

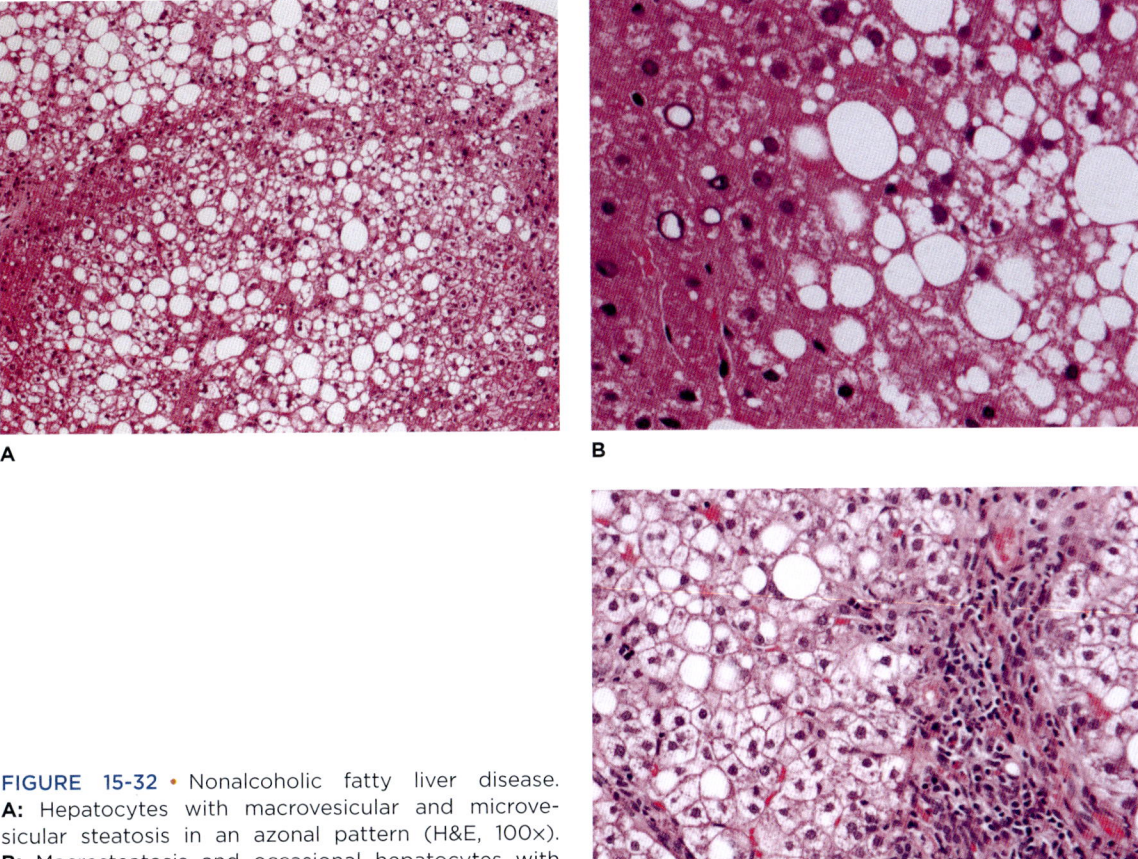

FIGURE 15-32 • Nonalcoholic fatty liver disease. **A:** Hepatocytes with macrovesicular and microvesicular steatosis in an azonal pattern (H&E, 100×). **B:** Macrosteatosis and occasional hepatocytes with glycogenated nuclei (H&E, 400×). **C:** Portal expansion by chronic inflammatory cells with extension into zone 1 (H&E, 200×).

The marked increase in childhood obesity and type II diabetes has significantly increased the prevalence of nonalcoholic fatty liver disease (NAFLD) in the pediatric population (136). In fact, NAFLD has emerged as the leading cause of chronic liver disease in children and adolescents in the United States. Elevated insulin, ALT levels, and hyperlipidemia (increased cholesterol and triglyceride) are commonly present in these children and constitute a metabolic syndrome. Further, cardiovascular risk and morbidity in children and adolescents are associated with fatty liver. Studies have shown that age, gender, and ethnicity are important factors for NAFLD and NASH in children (134,137). There is a higher incidence in male children and also a higher incidence in Asian and Hispanic children than White children and least in African American children.

The characteristic histologic features of NAFLD range from steatosis alone to steatohepatitis (NASH) with or without fibrosis to cirrhosis (Figure 15-32). Liver biopsy remains the gold standard for the diagnosis of NASH. NAFLD grading systems are based upon the proportion of hepatocytes demonstrating macrovesicular steatosis, hepatocyte injury (ballooning degeneration), lobular inflammation, and stage of fibrosis (138). In adults, the histologic features of NAFLD have been well described and include macrovesicular steatosis, perisinusoidal or pericellular fibrosis, foci of lobular inflammation, lipid granulomas, Mallory hyaline, and megamitochondria (138). The combination of macrovesicular steatosis with ballooning change of hepatocytes and/or perisinusoidal fibrosis constitutes a pattern of histology considered diagnostic of NASH in an appropriate clinical context. However, pediatric fatty liver disease often displays a histologic pattern distinct from that found in adults (134,139,140). In a large study of 100 children with biopsy-proven NAFLD, Schwimmer et al. demonstrated two different forms of steatohepatitis. While both types showed steatosis, "type 1" was characterized by ballooning degeneration and perisinusoidal fibrosis (as in adults) affecting 17% of subjects, while "type 2" was more common (affecting 51% of subjects) and was characterized by portal inflammation and portal fibrosis. Boys were significantly more likely to have type 2 NASH than girls. Further, type 1 NASH was more common in White children, whereas type 2 NASH was more common in children of Asian, Native American, and Hispanic ethnicity. In cases of advanced fibrosis, the pattern was generally that of type 2 NASH (139). Recently, attempts have been made to understand the molecular basis of pediatric NAFLD (141). The hedgehog (Hh) pathway has been implicated especially in the prepubertal/adolescent age group and may play an important role in the progression of liver disease with a portal-based pattern leading to liver fibrosis, especially in males. This may explain the prevalence of this disease in the pediatric age group and hence the need to identify and reverse childhood obesity to prevent progressive liver disease.

Reye Syndrome

Reye syndrome (acute encephalopathy with hepatic fatty degeneration) is an acute disease of childhood that presents as an encephalopathy, which may progress rapidly to irreversible coma and death (142). The disease has decreased dramatically since its association with salicylate use was described and warnings issued about the use of salicylates in febrile children. The disease has a biphasic clinical course with an initial febrile illness, usually associated with an upper respiratory viral infection, followed by apparent recovery and the abrupt onset of protracted vomiting, delirium, and stupor. The basic damage appears to be a widespread mitochondrial injury, especially in the liver, brain, and muscle, leading to abnormal metabolism of lipids. Children with symptoms mimicking Reye syndrome may have metabolic disorders, such as organic acid and beta-oxidation defects, and urea cycle disorders. This emphasizes the need to evaluate these children thoroughly, setting aside tissue appropriate for metabolic disorder investigations and molecular genetic studies.

Liver dysfunction is manifested by elevations in transaminases, hypoprothrombinemia, and hyperammonemia (142,143). Hypoglycemia may be present. Serum amino acid and free fatty acid levels may be elevated. Grossly, the liver is enlarged and is yellow to pale due to increased parenchymal lipid. Microscopically, the hepatocytes either appear normal or contain finely vacuolated microvesicular steatosis, which does not displace the nucleus. Oil red O stains on frozen sections reveal the panlobular distribution of lipid, and virtually all hepatocytes contain small droplets of lipid. Characteristically, there is no hepatocellular necrosis or inflammation. Severe decrease or absence of succinate dehydrogenase enzyme activity is demonstrable histochemically.

The ultrastructural features of microvesicular lipid droplets and typical mitochondrial abnormalities are considered virtually diagnostic of the syndrome (71). The changes are reversible, and in children who recover, the liver may show normal morphology, except for the presence of lipid in some hepatocytes and Kupffer cells, and occasional large mitochondria.

Lipid accumulation is also seen in other organs, notably renal tubular epithelium, myocardial and skeletal muscles, lungs, and pancreatic islets. The brain is edematous, and mitochondrial changes similar to those in the liver have been described.

Defects in Fatty Acid Oxidation

Defects in fatty acid oxidation, such as carnitine deficiency (*SLC22A5* gene at 5q31.1) and acyl-CoA-dehydrogenase deficiency (gene locus at 12q22-qter), may be associated with clinical features resembling Reye syndrome. Episodes of a recurrent Reye-like illness or siblings similarly affected should raise the distinct possibility of fatty acid oxidative disorder (see Chapter 5).

Carnitine has a role in the beta-oxidation of fatty acids by aiding in their transport across the inner mitochondrial membranes (144,145). Three clinical types of carnitine deficiency (*SLC22A5* gene at 5q31.1) have been described: myopathic, systemic, and mixed. In the systemic form, carnitine levels are reduced in the serum, liver, and muscle. During the acute episode, often initiated by a relatively minor clinical event such as gastroenteritis, the liver shows microvesicular steatosis with panacinar distribution (Figure 15-33) (93). Ultrastructurally, there is nonmembrane-bound lipid and proliferation of smooth endoplasmic reticulum, increased numbers of lysosomes, and accumulation of lipofuscin. Mitochondria may be abnormal in a nonspecific manner.

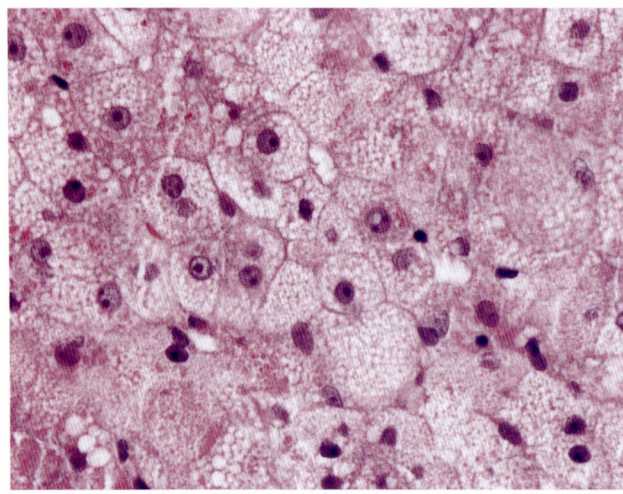
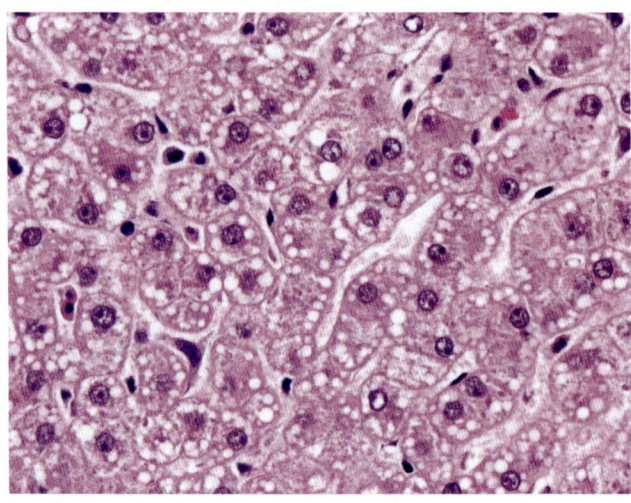

FIGURE 15-33 • Fatty acid oxidation defect—carnitine deficiency. **A–C:** Variable lipid deposition from fine cytoplasmic vacuolization (**A**) to microsteatosis (**B**) to macrosteatosis (**C**) within hepatocytes (H&E, **A:** 400×, **B:** 200×, **C:** 400×). **D:** Nonmembrane-bound lipid droplets within the hepatocyte cytoplasm (electron microscopy, 4000×).

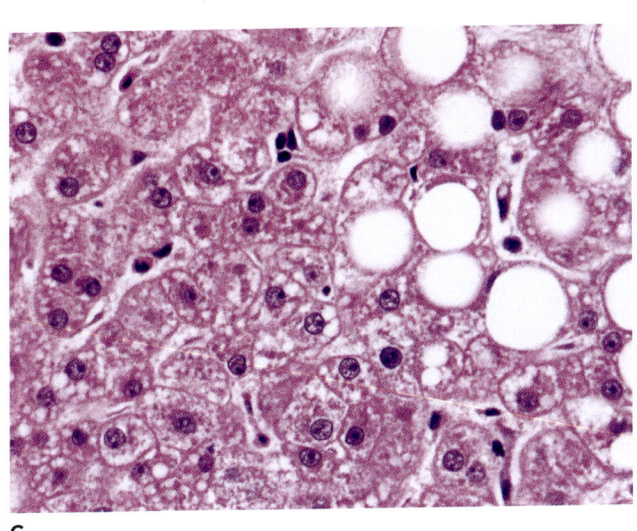
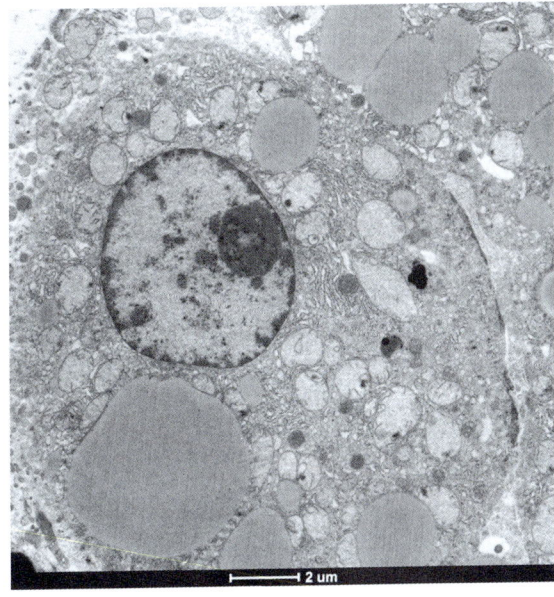

C **D**

FIGURE 15-33 • (continued)

Between clinical episodes, the liver may appear normal. It is important to keep this group of metabolic disorders in mind when a child dies rather abruptly during a seemingly innocuous febrile illness. Tissue and fluids should be obtained at the time of autopsy and be appropriately preserved for possible biochemical and genetic analysis.

Glutaric aciduria type II (type IIA, *ETFA* gene at 15q23-25; type II B, *ETFB* gene at 4q32-qter; type IIC, *ETFDH* gene at 19q13.3) is associated with deficiency of several mitochondrial acyl-CoA-dehydrogenases and is characterized by acidosis, nonketotic hypoglycemia, organic aciduria, hyperammonemia, and accumulation of lipid in the liver, myocardium, and renal tubular epithelium (93,146). One of the unique aspects of this inherited metabolic disorder is the presence of several congenital malformations, including renal cortical and medullary cysts, cerebral pachygyria, pulmonary hypoplasia, and facial dysmorphism. A familial syndrome of hepatosteatosis, jaundice, and kernicterus has been described. Death occurs in the first 3 months of life. Histologically, the liver shows panlobular steatosis with variable cholestasis and portal fibrosis. Lipid is also demonstrable in the renal tubular epithelium and myocardium. The basic mechanism of this disease has not been defined, and there is a possibility that the disease may not be a distinct entity.

Mitochondrial DNA Depletion syndromes

Liver involvement can be the predominant presentation in some of these mitochondrial DNA depletion syndromes (147,148). These are a group of genetic diseases caused by defects in the polymerase genes (*POLG*, *POLG2*, and *PEO1*) or mtDNA maintenance genes such as *TP1*, *TK*, *DGUOK*, and *MPV17*. This group of disease has been known under the rubric of Alpers syndrome, but is now recognized to represent different entities in this group identified by their genetic defect, all causing defects in electron transport chain function. They are frequently associated with cerebral symptoms especially epilepsy. Of these, liver involvement has been most commonly reported with POLG mutations though some of the others can also cause liver involvement. A characteristic feature is the precipitation of liver failure due to valproic acid used for the treatment of epilepsy. Liver pathology in Alpers disease (POLG mutation) is characterized by at least three of the following eight features: microvesicular steatosis, bile ductular proliferation, hepatocyte necrosis or dropout, liver plate collapse, parenchymal disarray, bridging fibrosis or cirrhosis, regenerative changes, and oncocytic change of hepatocytes. Fulminant liver failure may be seen in some cases (149,150).

VIRAL HEPATITIS

Viral hepatitis is the result of primary infection of the liver by specific hepatotropic viruses. These include hepatitis A, B, C, D, E, and possibly G (GB virus C) viruses. Many studies and reviews of clinical findings, the nature of the viruses, morphologic findings, and immunopathology are available that discuss the disease as it affects adult and pediatric age groups (151–153). Some characteristics of these viruses and the associated hepatic diseases are shown in Table 15-10.

Hepatitis A

Infectious hepatitis, or hepatitis A, accounts for one-third of reported pediatric cases. This virus is a single-stranded RNA virus (picornavirus). Transmission is by the fecal–oral route because the virus is resistant to low gastric pH. Epidemics of the disease occur, and there are endemic areas, especially

TABLE 15-10 HEPATITIS VIRUSES AND LIVER DISEASE

Virus	Characteristics	Antigen	Disease	Tissue Markers Nucleus	Tissue Markers Cytoplasm
HAV	27-nm RNA virus found in stool, blood, and liver	Hepatitis A (HAAg)	Acute viral hepatitis	None	+
HBV	42-nm DNA virus with envelope, 27-nm core in nucleus and 22-nm coat found in blood and hepatocyte cytoplasm	Hepatitis B surface (HBsAG)	Acute viral hepatitis	None	None
		Hepatitis B core (HBcAg)	Acute hepatitis with bridging	1+ HBcAg	1+ HBsAg
		Hepatitis E (HBeAg)	Carrier state, no liver disease	None	4+ HBsAg
			CAH	1+ HBcAg	1+ HBsAg
			Chronic hepatitis, immune suppressed	4+ HBcAg	1+ HBsAg
			Carrier state, mild hepatitis	4+ HBcAg	1+ HBsAg
Hepatitis C (non-A, non-B)	Single RNA strand 6 genotypes, 80 subtypes	Hepatitis C	Acute viral hepatitis CAH	None	None
Hepatitis D virus (HDV) delta agent	RNA defective virus; 35–37-nm incomplete virion, requires HBsAg to be infective	Delta	In the presence of coinfection with HBV, implicated in massive hepatic necrosis; and higher frequency of chronic disease	4+ delta	1+ delta
Hepatitis E virus (HEV)	27–30-nm nonenveloped RNA virus	Hepatitis E	Acute self-limiting hepatitis	Immunofluorescence positive in frozen tissue	

in the tropics, with a high rate of infection. Institutionalized children are at risk owing to poor hygienic conditions. In countries with poor sanitary conditions, most children are infected at an early age. Seroepidemiologic studies have routinely shown that up to 100% of preschool children have detectable anti–hepatitis A virus (HAV) antibodies, presumably reflecting previous subclinical infection. The average age of infection is rapidly increasing to 5 years and older, when symptomatic infection is more likely (151). In industrialized countries, there is a low prevalence of HAV infection among children and young adults, possibly related to immunization. Thus, in the United States, the prevalence of anti–HAV antibodies is approximately 10% in children and 37% in adults.

HAV causes acute inflammation of the liver, which resolves without chronic carrier status, chronic hepatitis, or HCC in infected patients. The incubation period is 2 to 4 weeks, rarely up to 6 weeks. Histologically, acute hepatitis manifests as lobular disarray with ballooned hepatocytes, apoptotic (Councilman) bodies, lymphomononuclear inflammation, and zone 3 cholestasis. However, the diagnosis is established on serology and biopsy is not required. Mortality rate is low in previously healthy individuals. The real impact of the disease is in the morbidity it causes, usually a significant problem only in adults and older children. Approximately 11% to 22% of patients with acute HAV require hospitalization (154). Young children (below 2 years of age) are usually asymptomatic with only 20% developing jaundice, whereas most 5-year-old children (80%) develop symptoms. Management includes only general supportive measures. A highly effective vaccine is available and has been approved for use in the United States for children above 12 months (154).

Hepatitis B

The hepatitis B virus (HBV), a partially circular double-stranded DNA virus (hepadnavirus), is usually transmitted perinatally, sexually, and parenterally by means of blood or other body fluids including semen, saliva, and breast milk (151,155). HBV has an incubation period of 6 to 8 weeks. Among children, those at increased risk include hemophiliacs and others who require frequent transfusions, adolescent intravenous drug abusers, institutionalized children, and infants of mothers with chronic HBV infection.

The prevalence of HBV infection varies in different geographic areas. In most high-prevalence areas such as Hong Kong and China, perinatal transmission is the major mode of spread, accounting for 40% to 50% of chronic HBV infection. However, horizontal spread during the first 2 years of life is the major mode of transmission in other endemic areas including Africa and the Middle East. In intermediate-prevalence areas, transmission occurs in all age groups, but early childhood infection accounts for most cases of chronic infection (defined as persistent serum HBsAg for 6 or more months after initial diagnosis). In low-prevalence areas, such as the United States, Western Europe, and Australia, most infections are acquired in early adult life through unprotected sexual intercourse or intravenous drug abuse. Age at infection has a significant impact on the clinical outcome, because chronic infection occurs in approximately 90% of infants infected at birth, in 25% to 50% of children infected between the ages of 1 and 5 years, and in less than 5% of those infected during adult life (151,155).

Acute HBV infection has been estimated to account for 10% to 25% of all cases of childhood acute hepatitis (155). Acute hepatitis B can cause fulminant hepatitis. Acute and chronic hepatitis B morphologically may resemble hepatitis of other etiologies and requires serology for definitive diagnosis. Chronically infected patients may have acute hepatitis B flares; superinfection with hepatitis D virus (HDV) should be considered in this setting. Chronic hepatitis B is an important risk factor for cirrhosis, dysplasia, and HCC.

Anti-HB confers long-term immunity. An effective and safe vaccine has been available since the early 1980s and is now included in the routine pediatric immunization schedule. Following infection, treatment should be instituted as early as possible, before there is irreversible liver damage. Extrahepatic manifestations including arthralgia, arthritis, skin rash, and Gianotti-Crosti syndrome (papular acrodermatitis) are common (in 25% of patients). Many new antiviral and immunomodulatory therapies have become available in recent years; however, these therapies are efficacious in less than 50% of patients. Liver biopsy is also useful in confirming virologic clearance or persistence; a part of the specimen should be routinely preserved for viral DNA quantitation.

Hepatitis C

The hepatitis C virus (HCV) infects over 100 million people worldwide, mostly adults, and is perhaps the most common cause of chronic hepatitis (151,156). Hepatitis C is a single-stranded RNA virus (flavivirus-like). The development of serologic tests has led to donor screening and its decrease in transfusion recipients. A population at risk is injection drug abusers. The most common transmittal route is parenteral, with an incubation period of 6 to 12 weeks. Although transfusions were the most common mode of spread, nucleic acid–based screening of blood and blood products has almost eliminated this route of spread. Intravenous drug abuse is presently the most common route of transmission. Perinatal transmission is known to occur, but the predominant route (transplacental or perinatal) and incidence of transmission are not known (157). Perinatal transmission has been documented only from anti-HCV women who are HCV-RNA positive. Transmission is more efficient if mothers have acute HCV infection during pregnancy, high circulating HCV-RNA levels, and/or HIV coinfection. HCV is not transmitted by breastfeeding. Since maternal HCV antibodies are passively transferred to the neonate, diagnosis requires RNA-based tests.

Eighty percent of patients develop chronic hepatitis, with 20% developing cirrhosis and 20% developing HCC (158). Histopathologically, chronic hepatitis C is characterized by predominant portal lymphomononuclear inflammation with or without lymphoid aggregates and bile duct (Poulsen) lesions, lobular inflammation, and varying degrees of fibrosis. The standard grading and staging systems in use for the histopathologic assessment of most chronic hepatitis were originally developed for evaluating chronic hepatitis C and as such are best standardized in this setting. Transplantation is not curative, and recurrent infection is universal. No vaccine is available, and antiviral therapy is effective in only 25% to 40% of patients until the recent introduction of direct anti-viral agents. Anti-HCV antibody does not confer immunity. Serum transaminases fluctuate markedly and cannot be used as surrogate markers of infection or the degree of hepatic injury.

Hepatitis D

The HDV (or delta agent) is a unique defective passenger RNA virus requiring helper functions provided by the HBV, including provision of the hepatitis B surface antigen coat for virion assembly and penetration into hepatocytes (159). Transmission is via a parenteral route. In about 80% of those affected, chronic hepatitis D progresses to cirrhosis. These individuals are also at risk for HCC. Survival after transplantation is better than for other types of viral hepatitis, and reinfection is rare.

Hepatitis E

The hepatitis E virus (HEV, enterically transmitted non-A, non-B hepatitis) was identified in 1983 and cloned in 1990 (160). HEV is a single-stranded RNA virus (genus Hepevirus, family Hepeviridae) that is waterborne and has an incubation period of 6 weeks. It is responsible for large epidemics of acute hepatitis in parts of Asia, Middle East, Africa, and Mexico. Transmission is fecal–oral, through contaminated water secondary to virion shedding in stools. Young adults are most commonly infected. The illness is usually self-limiting, except in pregnant women who tend to have severe disease and a high mortality rate (up to 25%). Chronic infection is unknown, although there is recent evidence to suggest chronic hep E infection may be the cause of unknown chronic hepatitis in pediatric organ transplants leading to eventual cirrhosis. Diagnosis is based on serologic detection of anti-HEV antibodies and PCR for the virus. Liver biopsy is not usually performed for diagnosis. Biopsy morphology is of acute hepatitis; fatal cases may show submassive to massive necrosis. Chronic hepatitis may be an occasional feature with predominantly low-grade lobular inflammation. No specific treatment or vaccine is available.

Hepatitis G

The hepatitis G virus (HGV or GB virus C) is a flavivirus with global distribution that is transmitted primarily by parental routes, but can also be transmitted sexually and perinatally (161). There is no convincing evidence that HGV is a primary hepatotropic virus, and it has not been known to cause acute or chronic hepatitis. There is controversy as to whether HGV should be included among the well-established hepatitis viruses A through E; however, there is coinfection with HCV in up to 20% of patients with hepatitis E and coinfection in patients with HIV infection.

Pathology of the Viral Hepatitides

Microscopic features of acute viral hepatitis, regardless of specific viral etiology, are characterized by lobular disarray and inflammation (Figure 15-34) (153). Liver injury is manifest by ballooning degeneration, individual cell necrosis with dropout of hepatocytes, and acidophilic (Councilman) bodies. Concomitant regenerative activity is evidenced by mitoses and binucleated or multinucleated cells. The cellular infiltrate is predominantly mononuclear and has a lobular and portal distribution. Portal areas are uniformly infiltrated with lymphocytes. Plasma cells, neutrophils, and eosinophils may be present. The infiltrate may extend into

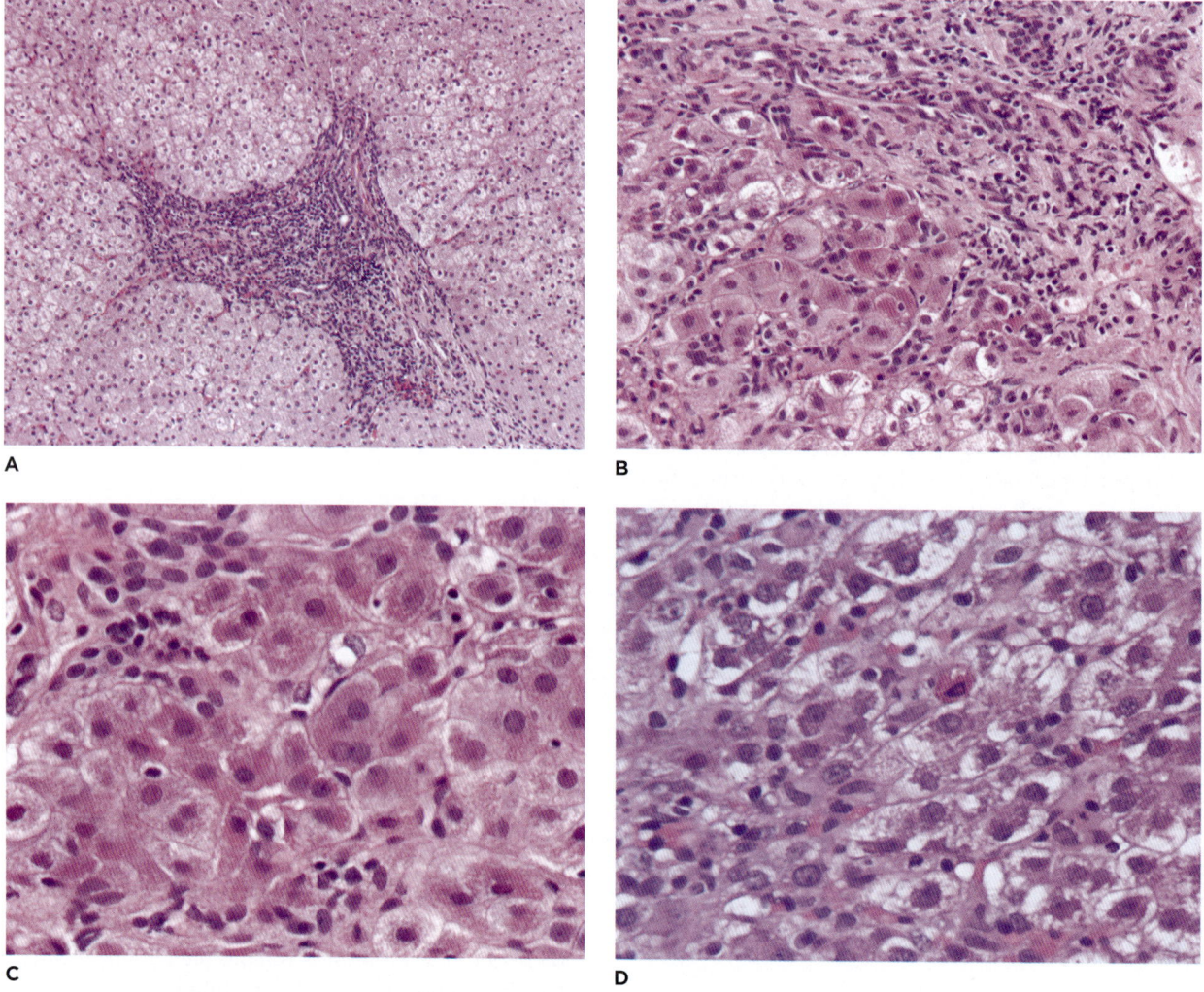

FIGURE 15-34 • Viral hepatitis—hepatitis B. **A:** Expansion of portal region by chronic inflammatory cells with extension into zone 1 by piecemeal necrosis (H&E, 100×). **B, C:** Zone 1 hepatocytes with deeply eosinophilic, glassy cytoplasm, and chronic inflammatory cells extending into zone 1 (H&E, **B:** 200×, **C:** 400×). **D:** Necrotic hepatocytes (apoptotic/acidophil bodies) with pyknotic nuclei and densely eosinophilic cytoplasm (H&E, 400×).

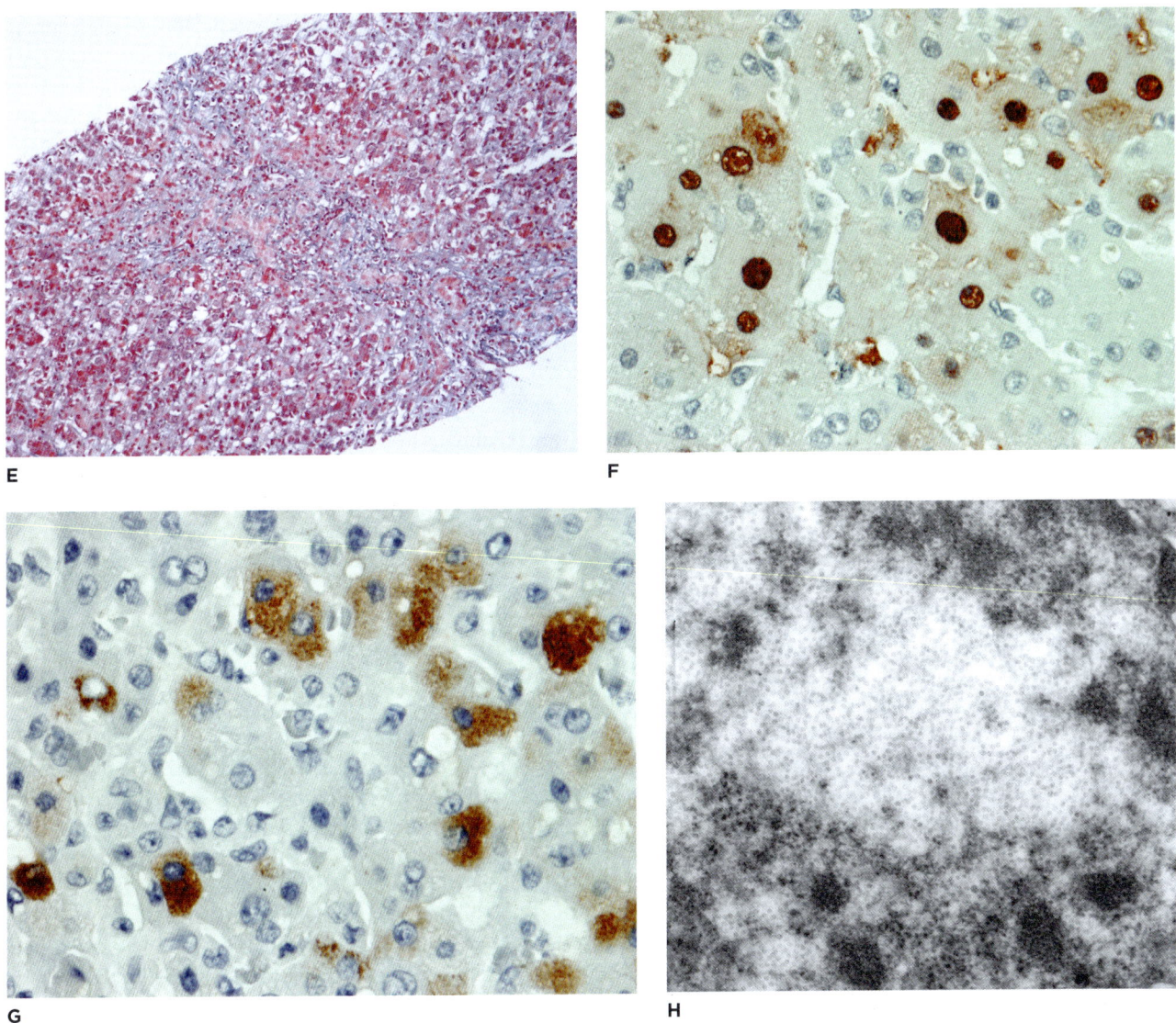

FIGURE 15-34 • (*continued*) **E:** Diffuse fibrosis extending from the portal region into the hepatic lobule (trichrome, 40×). **F, G:** Hepatocytes immunoreact with hepatitis B core antigen in nuclear pattern (**F:** 400×) and with hepatitis B surface antigen in cytoplasmic pattern (**G:** 400×). **H:** Hepatocyte with intranuclear HBV inclusions (electron microscopy, 75,000×).

the periportal lobule, but in contrast to chronic hepatitis with marked activity, periportal necrosis is not usual, and all portal areas are uniformly involved. There is hyperplasia of the sinusoidal lining cells, and Kupffer cells may contain lipofuscin pigment. Cholestasis is variable and usually mild, seen most often in zone 3. In the cholestatic form of hepatitis, prominent cholestasis simulating extrahepatic obstruction may be seen. In subsiding hepatitis, the changes become less prominent and may resemble chronic hepatitis with mild-to-moderate activity. Clusters of macrophages (PAS positive, diastase resistant) may suggest a recent acute hepatitis in these cases. In more severe forms of acute hepatitis, bridging necrosis with loss of hepatocytes may be accompanied by reticulin collapse and the formation of passive septa between central veins and between central veins and portal areas. The presence of bridging necrosis is an adverse prognostic factor that may be associated with a fatal outcome or progression to cirrhosis (162,163). In a few cases, the course may be fulminant with a high mortality rate; at autopsy, submassive necrosis with few surviving hepatocytes is seen in the periportal zones. The major portion of the lobule shows diffuse loss of hepatocytes accompanied by collapse and approximation of the portal areas. Some degree of regenerative activity of the surviving periportal hepatocytes may be evident in the form of pseudoductular or neocholangiolar proliferation. Lymphocytes, plasma cells, neutrophils, and eosinophils are seen in the sinusoids and space of Disse, and an endophlebitis may be seen, particularly if more than 10 days have elapsed since the onset of the process. Inflammation is seen in the portal areas. Kupffer cells contain cell debris and lipofuscin pigment. An etiologic distinction between the acute hepatitis caused by hepatitis A, B, C, D, and E viruses is not possible on morphologic grounds alone, although reports of acute hepatitis caused by hepatitis C describe the presence of lipid in the hepatocytes and a prominent sinusoidal mononuclear cell infiltrate with marked hypertrophy of the sinusoidal lining cells (Figure 15-35) (158). The differences between hepatitis A and B infection are not readily appreciated. Perivenular cholestasis, interface hepatitis with a dense portal infiltrate with frequent plasma cells, and extensive microvesicular steatosis are considered to be more characteristic for HAV-associated acute viral hepatitis. With HBV acute viral infection, hepatocytes with ground-glass cytoplasm are associated with abundant HBsAg production and may be somewhat helpful in differentiating HBV from HAV.

HBV and HCV infection may lead to chronic liver disease. Histopathologic features that predict progression to chronicity include bridging necrosis, prominent portal infiltrate with periportal extension, and distortion of the lamina limitans, lymphoid follicles, and early fibrosis. The concomitant demonstration of the surface and core antigen of HBV by IHC has been associated with progression to chronic liver disease. The histopathology of hepatitis B infection has been recently comprehensively reviewed (163).

Chronic hepatitis is not a single disease, but rather a clinicopathologic syndrome that may have a variety of causes (153,164,165). Traditionally, chronicity has been defined clinically as continuing disease for at least 6 months. This definition still has some practical utility, but asymptomatic disease must also be taken into account; for example, both HCV and autoimmune hepatitis (AIH) may remain asymptomatic for long periods. The terms chronic active hepatitis (CAH), chronic persistent hepatitis (CPH), and chronic lobular hepatitis (CLH) have become obsolete and should not be used.

The chronic hepatitides consist of chronic necroinflammatory diseases in which hepatocytes rather than biliary structures appear to be the main target of attack. Chronic cholestatic diseases, such as primary biliary cirrhosis (PBC) and primary sclerosing cholangitis (PSC), and metabolic disorders, such as Wilson disease and A1AT deficiency, are not always included under the headings of chronic hepatitis (164). However, they may show similar morphologic features, and there is thus practical merit in considering them in the broader spectrum of chronic hepatitis.

Various etiologic types of chronic hepatitis share a number of histopathologic characteristics that may vary over time in an affected individual. Most of these common morphologic features allow the pathologist to assess the grade (severity of inflammatory activity) and stage (degree of fibrosis) of the disease process, but do not always allow a definitive distinction between the various etiologies. In general, lobular inflammation predominates in acute forms of hepatitis, and portal and periportal inflammation predominates in chronic hepatitis. Chronic hepatitis with flares of disease activity commonly shows lobular hepatitis, together with portal and periportal inflammation and fibrosis (153,163,164).

Portal inflammation (Figures 15-34 and 15-35) is common to all forms of chronic hepatitis and is composed mainly of a mixture of lymphocytes, plasma cells, and macrophages. Lymphoid aggregates with or without germinal centers are more often seen in HCV-associated chronic viral hepatitis (Figure 15-35). Periportal inflammation commonly accompanies local hepatocyte damage. This necroinflammatory process is referred to as lymphocytic piecemeal necrosis or interface hepatitis. The composition of these inflammatory infiltrates is identical to those in the portal tracts. As a consequence of the necroinflammatory process, collagen and elastin is deposited. In contrast to portal and periportal inflammation, lobular inflammation usually consists of single small clusters of mononuclear cells rather than confluent sheets. Lobular inflammation is usually accompanied by hepatocellular damage. Hepatocellular damage is generally manifested by scattered necrotic hepatocytes (acidophilic, apoptotic, or Councilman bodies), hepatocellular nuclear disarray (anisonucleosis), mitotic activity, and hepatocellular swelling (ballooning degeneration). Apoptotic hepatocytes are characterized by pyknotic nuclear remnants and dense retracted cytoplasm. Degenerative and regenerative hepatocellular changes are frequently more impressive than the number of inflammatory cells.

Over time, chronic hepatitis leads to progressive fibrosis, which begins in portal areas, extends to periportal zones, and eventually links portal tracts to other portal tracts and

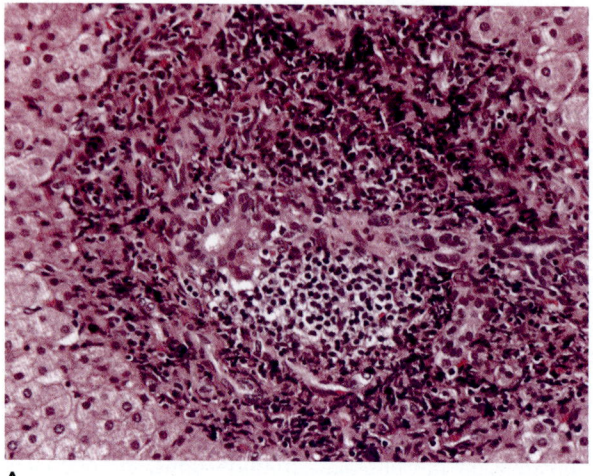
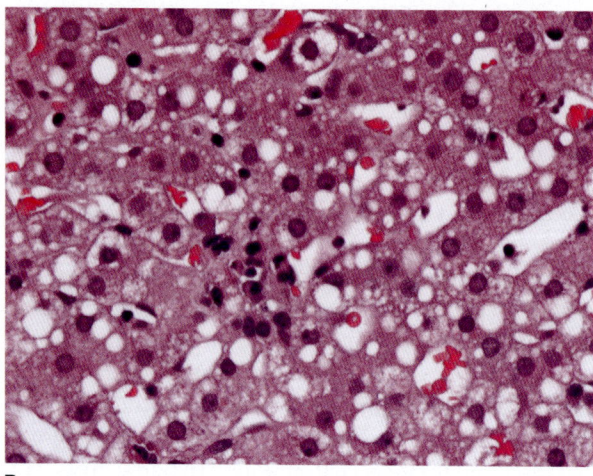

FIGURE 15-35 • Viral hepatitis—hepatitis C. **A:** Portal chronic inflammation with lymphoid aggregate with germinal center (H&E, 200×). **B:** Hepatocytes with microsteatosis and occasional chronic inflammatory cells in sinusoids (H&E, 400×).

TABLE 15-11 GRADING OF DISEASE ACTIVITY IN CHRONIC HEPATITIS[a]

Grading Terminology		Criteria	
Semiquantitative	Descriptive	Lymphocytic Piecemeal Necrosis	Lobular Inflammation and Necrosis
0	Portal inflammation only; no activity	None	None
1	Minimal	Minimal, patchy	Minimal; occasional spotty necrosis
2	Mild	Mild; involving some or all portal tracts	Mild; little hepatocellular damage
3	Moderate	Moderate; involving all portal tracts	Moderate; with noticeable hepatocellular change
4	Severe	Severe; may have bridging fibrosis	Severe; with prominent diffuse hepatocellular damage

[a]When a discrepancy exists between criteria, the more severe lesion should determine the grade.

to terminal hepatic venules. After fibrous septa have formed, regenerative nodules, indicative of cirrhosis, may appear. With the exception of HCV, in which approximately 70% of cases show fatty change, steatosis is uncommon in chronic hepatitis. Steatosis in a liver biopsy may be unrelated to viral hepatitis and may purely reflect of background fatty change. Chronic viral hepatitis is rarely cholestatic.

Pathologic reporting of liver biopsies should include the etiology, grade, and stage of the chronic hepatitis in the final diagnosis (165) (Tables 15-11 and 15-12). Development of cirrhosis may be related to the duration of CAH.

In the asymptomatic patient with chronic hepatitis B, the liver may show no abnormality except for the ground-glass hepatocytes, which represent cells containing HBsAg (Figure 15-34). The ground-glass hepatocyte is larger than the normal hepatocyte and has a smooth, uniform, pale, eosinophilic cytoplasm, often with a clear halo. The nucleus may be displaced to the periphery. These cells show a positive staining reaction with orcein and aldehyde fuchsin. Immunohistochemical staining is more sensitive and specific. The hepatitis B core antigen (HBcAg) is identified predominantly in the nuclei (Figure 15-34) and may correspond with the so-called sanded nuclei seen on hematoxylin–eosin stains. The distribution pattern of the tissue markers varies with the type of hepatic disease and is related to the host's immune response. Immunocytochemical staining for HBsAg and hepatitis B early antigen is also available. Electron microscopic examination may reveal HBsAg in the cytoplasm of hepatocytes, as 22-nm spheres and rods (Figure 15-34).

Nonhepatotropic viruses that may involve the liver as part of a systemic infection include herpes simplex, human herpesvirus 6, varicella, adenovirus, ECHO virus, Epstein-Barr virus (EBV), parvovirus, and cytomegalovirus (CMV) (153). The liver may also be affected in acquired immune deficiency syndrome (AIDS), and a chronic hepatitis-like disorder has been described in children with AIDS. Hepatic involvement can occur in rickettsial diseases. The hepatic lesion in childhood cases of Rocky Mountain spotted fever has been described elsewhere.

FULMINANT HEPATIC FAILURE

Fulminant hepatic failure is characterized clinically by altered mental status and coagulopathy of rapid onset (<8 weeks after jaundice) (166,167). Its etiology is variable around the world and includes viruses (most commonly HBV, EBV, herpes simplex viruses, CMV) (Figure 15-36), drugs (most commonly acetaminophen, other drugs with idiosyncratic reactions), pregnancy induced, metabolic (inborn errors of metabolism), malignancy, and other rare causes. Ten to twenty percent of cases remain cryptogenic. Prognosis depends on age, etiology, and rapidity of onset of disease. A liver biopsy reveals zones of hepatocellular loss, a variable inflammatory reaction, and residual foci of hepatocytes (Figure 15-37). The necrosis may involve the entire lobule (panlobar) or may be zonal (acetaminophen, drugs, shock). Residual hepatocytes have abnormalities ranging from steatosis to ballooning degeneration. Syncytial giant cell formation may be noted in hepatocytes. Inflammation is variable and includes lymphocytes, plasma cells, eosinophils, and many macrophages. Marked biliary proliferation may be noted on biopsies with residual islands

TABLE 15-12 STAGING OF CHRONIC HEPATITIS

Staging Terminology		
Semiquantitative	Descriptive	Criteria
0	No fibrosis	Normal connective tissue
1	Portal fibrosis	Fibrous portal expansion
2	Periportal fibrosis	Periportal or rare portal-portal septa
3	Septal fibrosis	Fibrous septa with architectural distortion; no obvious cirrhosis
4	Cirrhosis	Cirrhosis

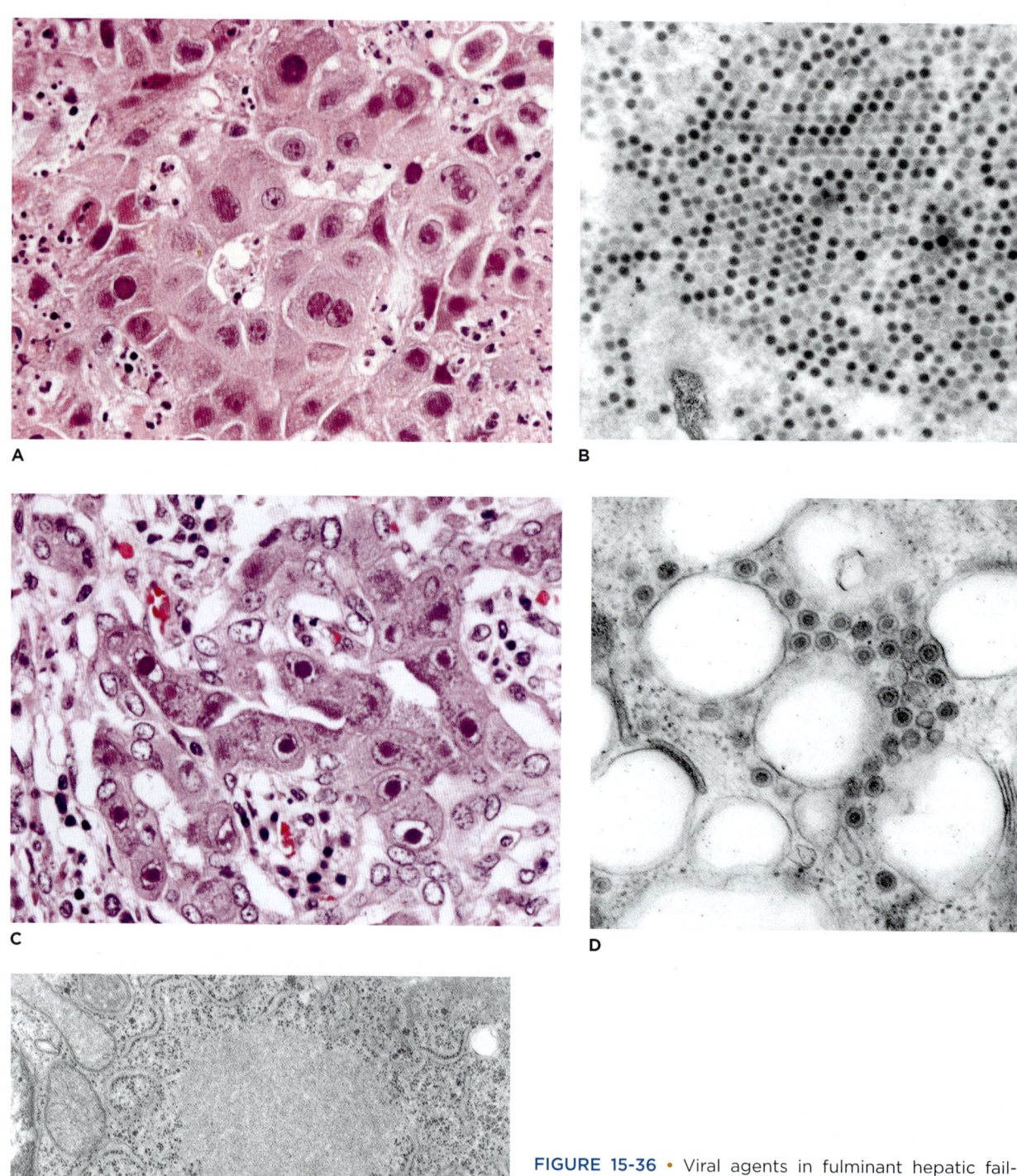

FIGURE 15-36 • Viral agents in fulminant hepatic failure. **A, B:** Adenovirus hepatitis with deeply eosinophilic cherry-red homogenous smudgy inclusions with hepatocytes (H&E, **A:** 400×) and adenovirus particles in nuclei by electron microscopy (**B:** 75,000×). **C, D:** CMV hepatitis with characteristic intranuclear "owl-eye" inclusions with bile duct epithelium (H&E, **C:** 400×) and CMV/herpes viral particles in nuclei by electron microscopy (**D:** 75,000×). **E:** Paramyxoviral particles in the hepatocyte cytoplasm (electron microscopy, 55,000×).

or single hepatocytes with evidence of transdifferentiation as disease progresses. Small regenerative nodules of hepatocytes may be seen at a somewhat later stage in the evolution of the process. In most cases, there are few clues about the etiology in the biopsy findings. The disease is frequently fatal though liver transplantation is often successful. New experimental treatments include use of extracorporeal liver assist devices and hepatocyte transplantation.

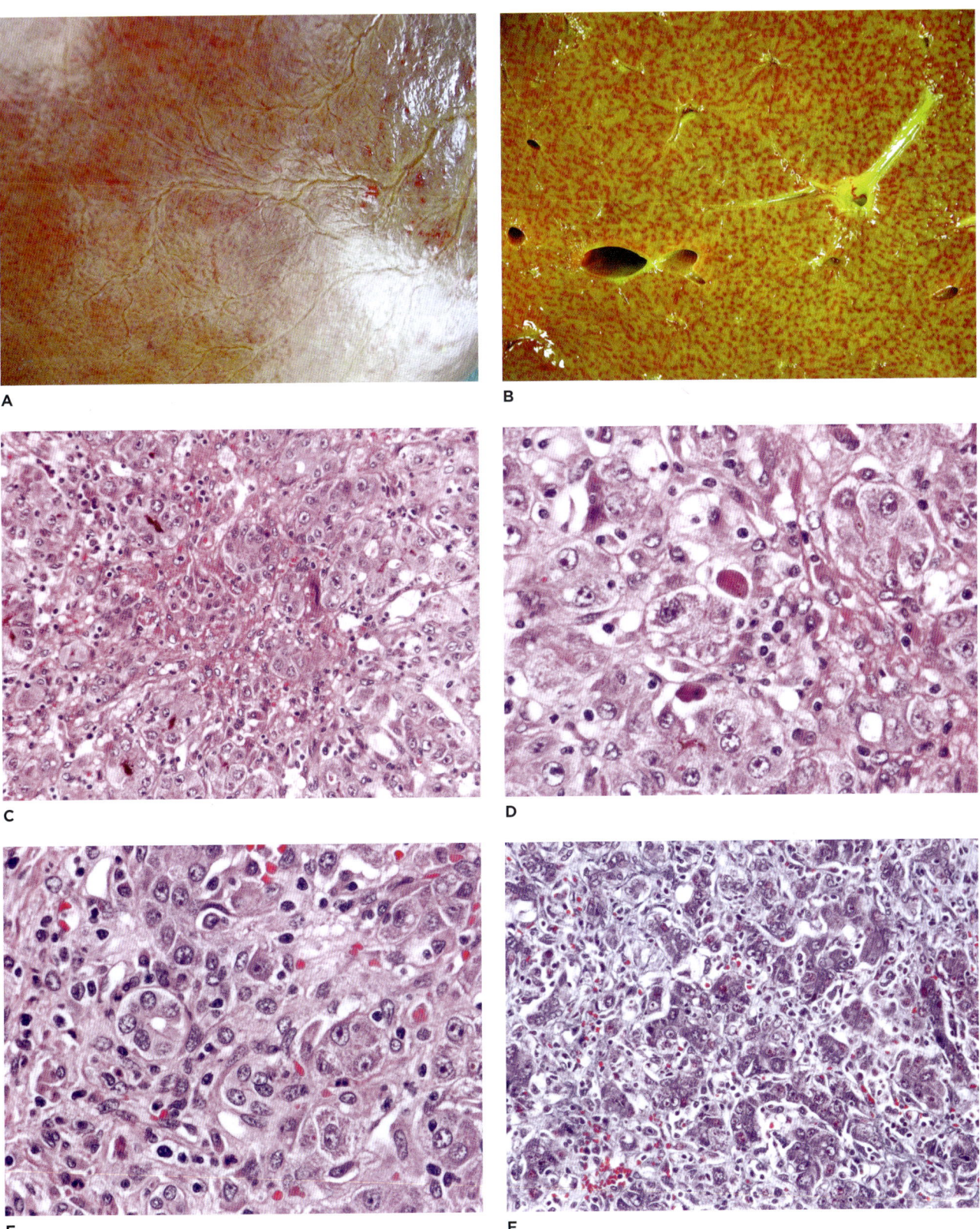

FIGURE 15-37 • Fulminant hepatic failure. **A:** Liver explant with tense, distended liver capsule. **B:** Liver explant cross-section demonstrating diffuse liver necrosis with red-brown fine punctate areas representing viable liver parenchyma. **C:** Central area of hepatocyte necrosis with dense eosinophilia, hemorrhage in the background, and necrotic hepatocytes (H&E, 200×). **D:** Residual bile ducts, hepatocytes organized into pseudoacini, and necrotic hepatocytes (H&E, 400×). **E:** Residual bile ducts with rare hepatocytes and background of chronic inflammatory cells (H&E, 400×). **F:** Trichrome stain highlights residual bile ducts, loss of hepatocytes, and replacement by fibrotic tissue (200×).

PRIMARY SCLEROSING CHOLANGITIS AND AUTOIMMUNE HEPATITIS

PSC is a progressive hepatobiliary disease characterized by a cholestatic syndrome (168,169). Diagnostic imaging abnormalities consist of segmental narrowing and dilatation of intrahepatic and extrahepatic ducts. The disease is seen primarily in young men in the third to fifth decades of life, but it is also seen in the pediatric population including neonates.

The pathogenesis is unknown, but a strong association with ulcerative colitis (UC) has been documented in most cases. Inflammatory bowel disease (UC) has been associated with sclerosing cholangitis in 70% of cases (168). However, PSC is seen in only about 5% of patients with UC. Langerhans cell histiocytosis occurs in 15% of cases of neonatal sclerosing cholangitis, and immunodeficiency is associated with another 10% of children. No apparent underlying disease is present in 24%, including cases of neonatal onset. The clinical presentation of childhood PSC is highly variable and frequently without features of cholestasis. Typically, elevated alkaline phosphatase (ALP), GGTP, and bilirubin are noted. In addition, hypergammaglobulinemia, DRw52a (HLA subtype), perinuclear antineutrophil cytoplasmic antibody (p-ANCA), and IgM elevation may be identified by serologic tests. Clinical similarity to AIH is common (169). Contrast digital imaging of the intrahepatic biliary tree by retrograde endoscopy shows a characteristic beaded appearance. This is due to strictures and secondary dilation of the affected bile ducts.

The histopathologic changes in the liver are not diagnostic in most cases (Figure 15-38). Portal fibrosis, pericholangitis, fibrous obliterative cholangitis, and cirrhosis are the range of microscopic features. Fibrous obliterative cholangitis consisting of concentric whorls of dense collagen, with an onion skin appearance, surrounding the bile ducts is regarded as a characteristic lesion. This is seen only early in the evolution of the disease. Fibroinflammatory stricture of bile ducts may be seen at various sites from the ampulla of Vater to the interlobular bile ducts. Histopathologic staging of PSC is based upon the degree of involvement (stage I—portal;

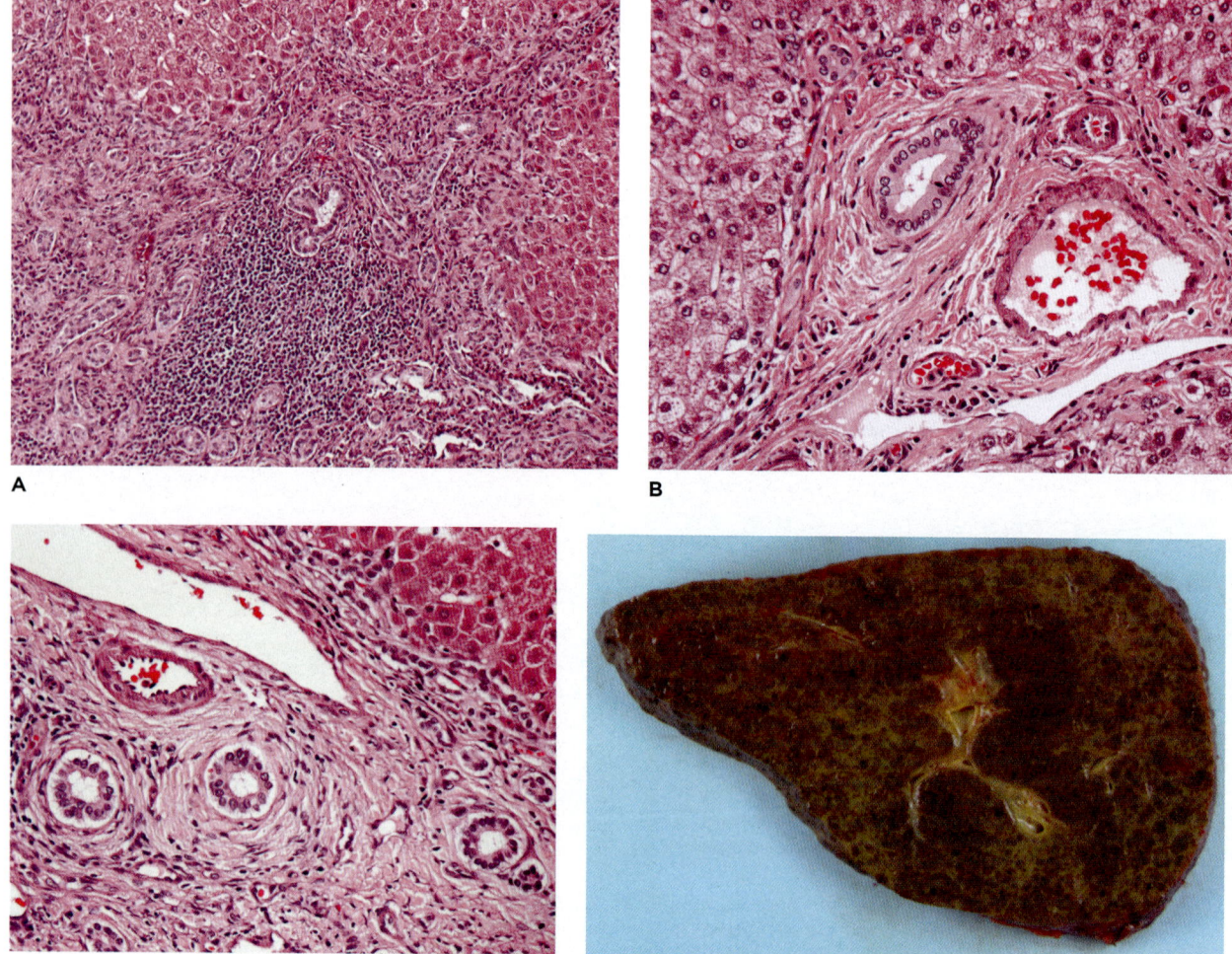

FIGURE 15-38 • Primary sclerosing cholangitis. **A:** Severe portal chronic inflammation with bile duct proliferation, fibrosis, and interface hepatitis (H&E, 100×). **B, C:** Concentric fibrosis around bile ducts (onion skinning) and portal fibrosis (H&E, 200×). **D:** Liver explant for PSC with diffuse bile pigmentation and biliary cirrhotic pattern.

stage II—periportal; stage III—septal; stage IV—cirrhosis). Stage I (portal) has concentric periductal fibrosis with a lymphocytic infiltrate around bile ducts. Stage II (periportal) has fibrosis extending in the periportal tissues with interface hepatitis and reactive bile ducts. Stage III (septal) has obliterated bile ducts and bridging fibrosis. Stage IV (cirrhosis) has biliary-type cirrhosis.

In neonatal sclerosing cholangitis due to LCH, a liver biopsy may not show significant findings since the disease may involve large ducts not sampled in the biopsy and effects of large duct obstruction may be the only findings on biopsy. Immunohistochemical staining for CD1a and langerin (CD207) would help to confirm presence of intraepithelial LCH cells.

Cholangiography is essential for diagnosis to evaluate medium to large intrahepatic ducts, since 40% of children lack extrahepatic duct involvement. The most serious complication is adenocarcinoma of the bile duct and colon in patients with concurrent PSC and UC. The prognosis appears to be more favorable in children than in adults. Liver transplantation is required for children who progress to biliary cirrhosis and hepatic decompensation. Recurrence of PSC may occur in the transplanted liver and may be difficult to differentiate from acute cellular rejection and biliary strictures due to ischemia (170).

AIH may be present in children with signs and symptoms of acute hepatitis (50% to 60%), fulminant liver failure (10%), or a more chronic, insidious onset (30% to 40%) (171,172). This disease is more typically seen in young and middle-aged women. Two types of AIH are recognized: type 1 with antinuclear antibodies (ANA), antismooth muscle antibodies (SMA), antiactin antibodies, soluble liver antigen, and acute asialoglycoprotein receptor and type 2 with anti-LKM1. Younger children present with anti-LKM1 with or without ANA or SMA antibodies. There is no difference in clinical outcome between the types of AIH. Family history of autoimmune disorder is noted in 40% of cases. Affected children may have other autoimmune disorders including lymphocytic (Hashimoto) thyroiditis, rheumatoid arthritis, Sjögren syndrome, and UC. Hyperglobulinemia is a common feature. It is important to ensure that viral serologic markers are negative, for autoimmune disease can occur in conjunction with hepatitis C infection (173). Liver biopsy

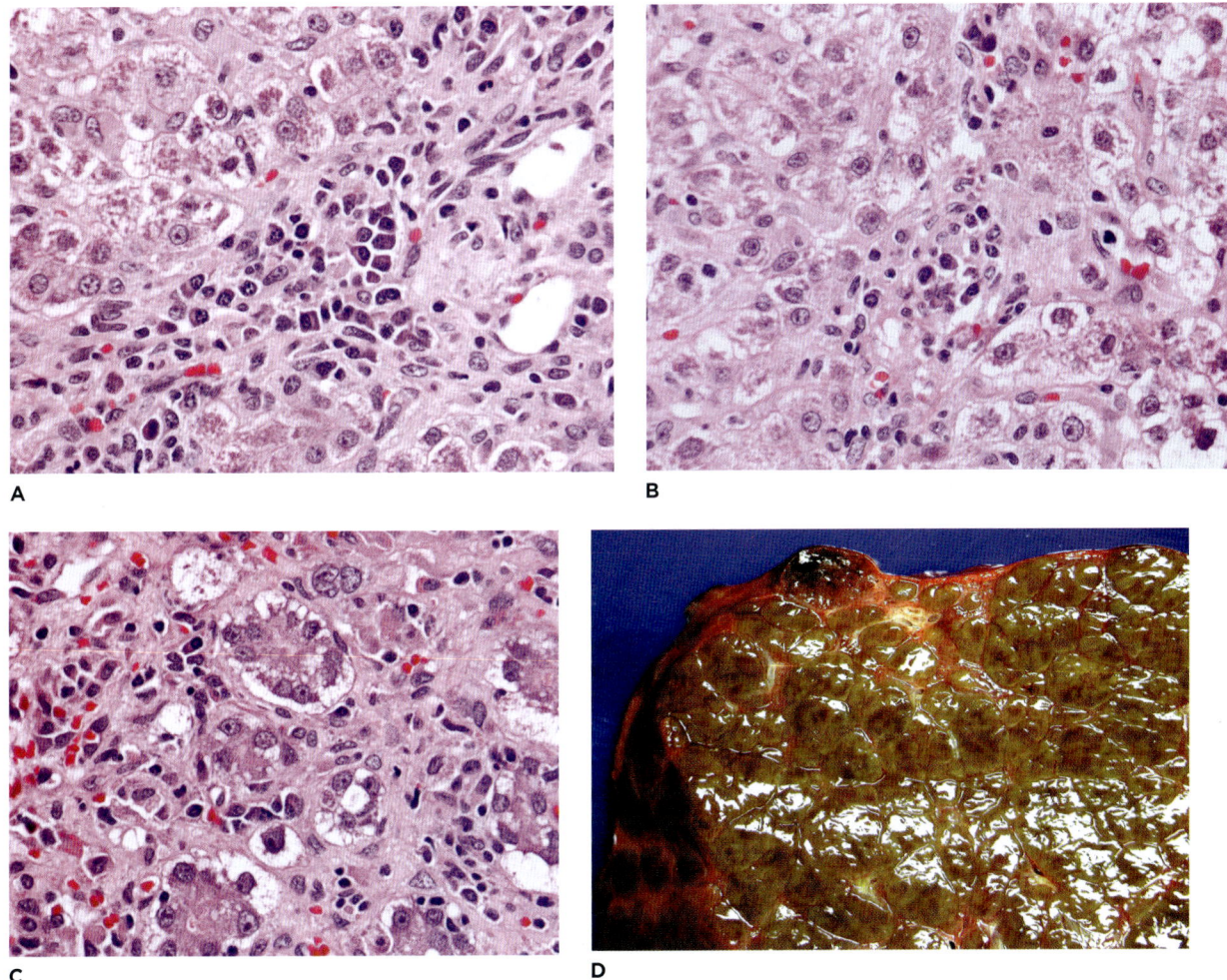

FIGURE 15-39 • Autoimmune hepatitis. **A, B:** Plasma cells within portal regions and within the hepatic lobules (H&E, 400×). **C:** Hepatocytes arranged in pseudoacinar pattern with occasional plasma cells and increased fibrous tissue (H&E, 400×). **D:** Explanted liver for AIH with macronodular pattern of cirrhosis and bile staining.

demonstrates plasma cells within the chronic inflammatory infiltrate in the portal tracts and an aggressive interface hepatitis, which may lead to collapse (Figure 15-39) (165,174). Marked lobular chronic inflammatory infiltrates with plasma cells may be seen. Hepatocellular injury with acinar (rosette) formation and syncytial giant hepatocytes can be features as well. Plasma cells with or without hepatocyte rosette formation are considered to be highly suggestive of AIH. However, one should remember that plasma cells can be seen in other chronic hepatitides as well. Because lymphoid aggregates may be seen in HCV, it is important to eliminate this from consideration. Cirrhosis develops in 90% of cases. In a certain proportion of children, serologic and histologic evidence is supportive of AIH at initial diagnostic evaluation. However, diagnostic imaging and liver biopsy have features that support PSC. When this occurs, the term autoimmune sclerosing cholangitis overlap syndrome is employed (171). These patients appear to respond to immune suppression therapy.

ABSCESSES

Pyogenic abscesses are uncommon in the liver in the pediatric patient and, when they occur, may be single or multiple (175,176). The infection may be hematogenous or ascend via the biliary tract. In the neonate, umbilical vein catheterization complicated by septic omphalitis poses an additional hazard. Ascending cholangitis may be associated with intrahepatic abscesses, especially after a portoenterostomy procedure for EHBA. Hepatic abscess may occur in the setting of a systemic disorder. In patients with congenital or acquired neutropenia or aplastic anemia, hepatic abscesses may show a paucity of neutrophils, and coagulative necrosis without liquefaction may be seen. Hepatic abscesses may be the initial presentation of chronic granulomatous disease (CGD); as many as one-third of hepatic abscesses in children are a complication of CGD. These abscesses show a central area of suppuration, often with a surrounding palisade of macrophages. Pigmented lipid-laden histiocytes in the portal tracts and sinusoidal lining cells are characteristic of this process. Blunt trauma associated with hepatic necrosis may be complicated by abscess formation. Occasional reports have documented hepatic abscess without a predisposing condition. Amebic liver abscess may be seen in areas endemic for amebiasis.

Grossly, the abscesses may be multiple and range from small yellow foci scattered throughout the liver to large cavitary lesions with purulent debris. Microabscesses consist of focal collections of neutrophils with no zonal distribution. Larger abscesses show a central area of liquefaction necrosis in which degenerating neutrophils are seen. At the periphery, there is characteristically a mixed cellular infiltrate consisting of neutrophils and mononuclear cells and a variable fibroblastic proliferation.

Polymicrobial infection is present in about 80% of cases (2.4 isolates per specimen), with anaerobes and microaerophilic streptococci being more common (175). The predominant anaerobes implicated are *Peptostreptococcus*, *Bacteroides* sp., *Fusobacterium* sp., and *Clostridium* sp., whereas common aerobes implicated are *Escherichia coli*, Streptococcus group D, *Klebsiella pneumoniae*, and *Staphylococcus aureus*. Diminutive abscesses consisting of no more than a few neutrophils are seen in CMV hepatitis in immunosuppressed children and adults. The mortality rate for pyogenic liver abscesses has decreased to less than 10% with improved diagnostic imaging, percutaneous draining techniques, and antibiotics.

PARASITIC DISEASES

A variety of parasitic diseases can involve the liver (177). Among the protozoal infections are toxoplasmosis, malaria, leishmaniasis, and amebiasis. Toxoplasma infections have a worldwide distribution. Infection may be transmitted through contact with house pets, such as cats. Congenital infections are an important cause of illness with prominent hepatic manifestations. Giant cell transformation of hepatocytes may be seen. Occasionally, the parasite may be demonstrable.

Acute *Plasmodium falciparum* malaria may be fatal. At autopsy, the liver is enlarged and tense with a dark red or slate gray color. There is marked engorgement of the sinusoids and central veins, and erythrocytes may contain parasites. There is Kupffer cell hyperplasia and phagocytosis of ruptured erythrocytes. Within Kupffer cells, the dark brown malarial pigment is a characteristic cytoplasmic feature. This hemozoin pigment is formed by the trophozoite from the breakdown of hemoglobin and does not give a positive Prussian blue reaction.

In leishmaniasis (kala-azar), hyperplastic Kupffer cells contain the parasites (Leishman-Donovan bodies). Infiltration with lymphocytes, plasma cells, and histiocytes may be seen in portal areas and lobules, and granulomas may form.

Amebic infection of the liver is the most frequent extraintestinal complication of the disease, and it manifests usually as a single abscess, most often involving the right lobe. The abscess cavity contains red–brown, thick ("anchovy sauce-like") material. The abscess wall consists of a layer of necrotic parenchyma, external to which a mixed inflammatory cell infiltrate is seen. A fibrous capsule may be present, and the adjacent liver is compressed. Amoebae may be demonstrable in the necrotic zone or in the compressed parenchyma as PAS-positive round or oval bodies about the size of macrophages.

Liver involvement may also occur in infestation by a variety of helminths. In schistosomiasis, liver injury results through migration of ova in the portal venous system. The ova elicit a granulomatous response, and in severe infection with *Schistosoma japonicum*, diffuse fibrosis and portal hypertension may result. Liver flukes (*Clonorchis sinensis*, *Fasciola hepatica*) inhabit major intrahepatic ducts and cause inflammation and epithelial injury. Biliary hyperplasia, cholangitis, and periductal fibrosis are common findings with liver flukes. Hydatid cyst is caused by infestation with the larval stage of the cestodes *Echinococcus granulosus* and *E. multilocularis*. The right lobe is more frequently involved. The cyst has a thick, white wall and a cavity in which the fluid contains fine granular sediment ("hydatid sand"). The cyst may be unilocular or multilocular. The cyst has a characteristic laminated outer layer and an inner layer containing multiple nuclei. Brood capsules are formed from numerous scolices and arise from the inner germinal layer. Invaginations of the cyst give rise to daughter cysts. Secondary cholangitis may result from intrahepatic bile duct obstruction. Toxocariasis (visceral larva migrans) results from migration of the larvae of *Toxocara canis* or *T. cati* (177). Granulomas containing larval fragments may be seen in the liver. Ascariasis infestation is associated with numerous foul-smelling cavities in the liver upon gross examination. The liver tissue demonstrates necrotic debris with a granulomatous and eosinophil inflammatory response to degenerated parasites.

GRANULOMATOUS HEPATITIS

Granulomas in the liver are associated with the same etiologic agents as granulomas at other sites (178). The frequency of granulomas in the liver varies with geographic location, due to variation in causative agents in different populations. The etiologic associations are shown in Table 15-13. Nevertheless, tuberculosis and sarcoidosis account for the majority of cases.

Histopathologic evaluation includes a search for an etiologic agent with appropriate special stains, especially for acid-fast bacilli and fungi. The auramine O stain for fluorescent microscopy is more sensitive in demonstrating acid-fast bacilli than standard stains. PCR for mycobacteria is also possible from formalin-fixed and paraffin-embedded tissue.

VASCULAR DISORDERS

Cavernous Transformation of the Portal Vein

The most important entity in this group of disorders is portal vein obstruction due to thrombosis and cavernous transformation resulting from recanalization of the thrombus. This is the most frequent cause of noncirrhotic portal hypertension in children (179). Extrahepatic causes of portal hypertension, including portal vein obstruction, are reported in approximately 50% of cases. Umbilical vein catheterization and omphalitis have been incriminated most frequently, with other mechanisms including local infections, portoenterostomy, sepsis, and chemotherapy. Hypercoagulopathy secondary to protein C, protein S, and antithrombin III deficiencies are frequently found in children with portal vein obstruction (180). The liver is histologically normal in most cases of portal vein thrombosis or cavernous transformation of the portal vein. Instances of focal nodular hyperplasia (FNH)-like lesions have been reported.

Budd-Chiari Syndrome

Obstruction of the hepatic veins may occur in the main branches or ostia leading to Budd-Chiari syndrome (181). The lesion occurs most frequently in women in the third and fourth decades of life and is uncommon in childhood. In young women, there is an association with contraceptive medications and pregnancy. Paroxysmal nocturnal hemoglobinuria, sickle cell disease, nephrotic syndrome, TPN, blunt trauma, myeloproliferative disorders, and coagulation abnormalities may also be associated with Budd-Chiari syndrome. Venous occlusion by tumor occurs less frequently in childhood than in adults. Congenital webs and obliteration of the suprahepatic inferior vena cava are see\\n in children. Budd-Chiari syndrome

TABLE 15-13 HEPATIC GRANULOMAS

Bacterial
    Tuberculosis
    Atypical mycobacteria
    Listeriosis
    Tularemia
    Brucellosis
    Rochalimaea henselae (cat scratch disease)
Mycotic
    Candida
    Histoplasmosis
    Cryptococcosis
    Blastomycosis
    Coccidioidomycosis
Rickettsial and spirochetal
    Q fever
    Syphilis
Viral
    Infectious mononucleosis
    Cytomegalovirus
Parasitic and protozoal
    Schistosomiasis
    Visceral larva migrans
    Ascariasis
    Toxoplasmosis
    Leishmaniasis (kala-azar)
Drug related
    Sulfonamides
    Diphenylhydantoin
    Sulfonyl urea compounds
    Allopurinol
Miscellaneous
    CGD of childhood
    Sarcoidosis
    Hodgkin lymphoma
    Crohn disease
    Foreign body
Undetermined etiology

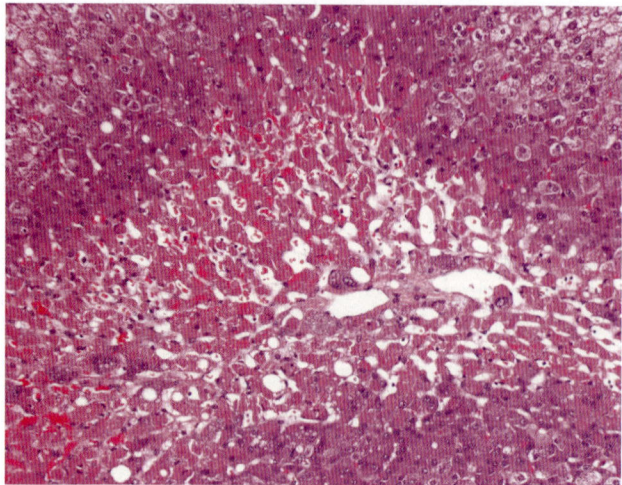

FIGURE 15-40 • Budd-Chiari syndrome. Centrilobular ischemia and hepatocyte degeneration with less affected hepatocytes away from zone 3 (H&E, 200×).

may occur after giant omphalocele repair. Thrombosis of hepatic veins and retrohepatic inferior vena cava may result from direct pressure on the hepatic venous outlet after visceral reduction and final abdominal wall closure. Gaucher disease has also been implicated in rare instances.

Clinical features associated with Budd-Chiari syndrome include ascites and hepatomegaly (181). The liver, in early stages, shows severe centrilobular congestion, hepatocyte degeneration and loss, and erythrocytes in the space previously occupied by the liver cells in zone 3 (Figure 15-40). Central veins are not affected, but sublobular veins may contain thrombi. Pericentral fibrosis with extension into adjacent parenchyma causes distortion of the architecture and may progress to cirrhosis. A few children have been transplanted for this condition (182). Budd-Chiari syndrome can recur in the allograft liver.

Venoocclusive Disease

Venoocclusive disease (VOD) (183) was initially described in Jamaican children and ascribed to pyrrolizidine alkaloids in Senecio tea. Other etiologic associations are cytotoxic agents used for malignant disease therapy and in preparation for bone marrow transplantation, hereditary tyrosinemia, familial immune deficiency disorders, and irradiation. The condition has also been described in newborn infants and following liver transplantation.

Early in the course of the disease, there is massive centrilobular hemorrhage with hepatocyte degeneration or loss. The abnormal central veins have narrowed lumina and widened subendothelial spaces, containing collagen fibers, fragmented cells, cell debris, and hemosiderin-laden macrophages. At this stage, central vein abnormalities are subtle and require special stains to demonstrate collagen deposition. Later in the course of the disease, there is intimal thickening due to reticulin and collagen deposition and presence of foam cells, causing partial or complete obliteration of vessel lumens (Figure 15-41). Central hepatocytes (zone 3) are atrophic, and cholestasis may be seen. Pericentral fibrosis with extension into the adjacent parenchyma distorts the architecture, but true cirrhosis is infrequent. Allograft rejection may resemble VOD, and this needs to be taken into consideration prior to making a diagnosis of VOD.

Peliosis Hepatis

Peliosis hepatis was initially described in adults with chronic debilitating diseases, steroid medications, HIV, mycobacterial infection, and wasting conditions (184). This condition was described in a child with CF who died at the age of 11 years, after which additional reports documented peliosis hepatis in the pediatric age group, including the neonatal period. Two previously healthy young children

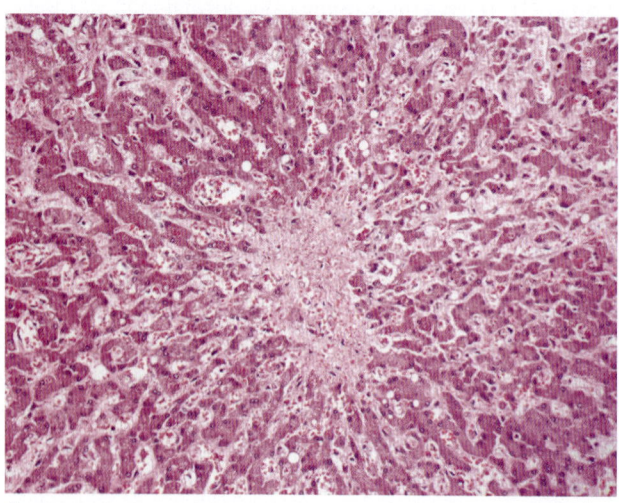

A

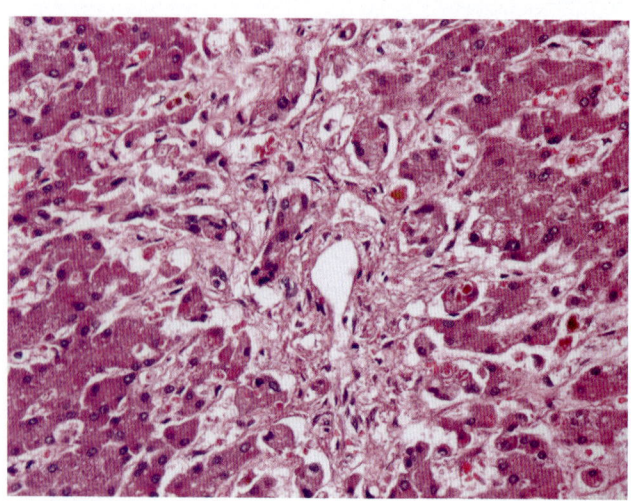

B

FIGURE 15-41 • Venoocclusive disease. **A, B:** Partial to nearly complete obliteration of central veins with pericentral vein fibrosis (H&E, 200× and 400×).

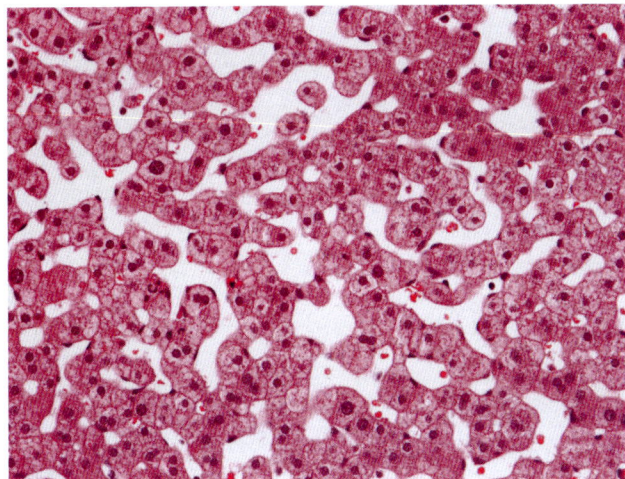

FIGURE 15-42 • Peliosis hepatis. Early lesion of peliosis with widely dilated sinusoids, which tends to be localized due to sinusoidal endothelial injury (H&E, 400×).

in whom peliosis hepatis presented as acute hepatic failure associated with *E. coli* pyelonephritis have also been reported. Both patients had active intraperitoneal hemorrhage from the peliotic liver lesions (185). Focal peliosis hepatis has been found incidentally in five children succumbing to an asphyxiating death. Androgenic anabolic steroids, oral contraceptives, thiopurines, and danazol play a role in development of this lesion. Resolution of the lesion tends to occur after discontinuing such medications. Liver infection by *Bartonella henselae* in HIV-infected patients is known to lead to peliosis hepatis. Also, peliosis hepatis occurs with increased frequency in renal transplant recipients. The liver contains grossly identifiable multiple blood-filled spaces, which, on microscopic examination, consist of pools of erythrocytes in the hepatic lobule with no zonal predilection (Figure 15-42). A definitive endothelial lining is not identified. The early lesion consists of localized areas of sinusoidal dilatation, likely due to disruption and injury to the sinusoidal endothelial cells. Disruption of sinusoidal reticulin fibers may be demonstrated using typical reticulin stains. In HIV-infected patients with Bartonella-associated lesions, there may be myxoid perisinusoidal stroma with granular clumped material. Within the granular material, organisms may be detected with Warthin-Starry staining and PCR. Rupture and hemoperitoneum are potential complications.

Hepatic Hemorrhage

Hepatic hemorrhage may occur as a result of blunt or sharp trauma. Spontaneous subcapsular hemorrhage in the newborn occurs most frequently in premature infants and may be a cause of morbidity. A review of infant autopsies showed a 15% incidence of subcapsular hemorrhage. At-risk infants tend to be premature male infants with chronic problems during gestation and complications during labor and delivery as well as sepsis. Hemoperitoneum due to liver rupture may lead to hypovolemic shock.

TOTAL PARENTERAL NUTRITION–RELATED INJURY

Hepatic abnormalities secondary to TPN were first described in a premature infant. The infant died after 71 days, and the liver at postmortem examination showed cirrhosis, bile duct proliferation, and cholestasis. Subsequent reports have confirmed the association of hepatobiliary dysfunction with TPN (186). The associated cholestasis is seen most frequently in the premature infant, with low birth weight and low gestational age being the greatest risk factors. The incidence and severity of the disease are greater in infants with gastrointestinal disease or intestinal resection.

Cholestasis increases with prolonged TPN infusion. Most infants with TPN-associated cholestasis and subsequent cirrhosis have severe gastrointestinal disease, such as necrotizing enterocolitis, gastroschisis, and volvulus, or have undergone intestinal resection (187). These infants are also subject to infection, cardiopulmonary dysfunction, shock, and hypoxia. Toxicity of the infusate, especially amino acid composition and lipid content, has been considered a factor in liver dysfunction associated with TPN.

The onset of jaundice is insidious, and the infant may manifest no other evidence of hepatic disease. The earliest biochemical abnormality is the elevation of serum bile acid concentration, as early as 5 days after beginning TPN, and routine study of serum bile acids may help in diagnosis. Hyperbilirubinemia is usually seen 3 to 4 weeks after TPN initiation.

Histopathologic changes noted in TPN-associated disease are nonspecific and quite variable (Figure 15-43). Because there is no specific clinical, biochemical, or histopathologic marker, the diagnosis remains one of exclusion although there may be clues on the biopsy (188). Canalicular and hepatocellular cholestasis, most pronounced in zone 3, is the initial finding and a constant feature of TPN. There is lobular disarray with ballooned hepatocytes. Kupffer cell hyperplasia is present, with the Kupffer cells containing lipofuscin pigment, a prominent feature on PASD stains. Iron pigment is demonstrable within hepatocytes. Giant cell transformation, pseudoacinar formation, and scattered foci of hepatocyte necrosis may be present. Extramedullary hematopoiesis may be prominent. Focal inflammation is usually seen and may vary from mild to severe. The cellular infiltrate is predominantly lymphocytic, but neutrophils and eosinophils as well as macrophages with pigment may also be present. A pericholangitis may be seen and may be striking in some cases, along with focal fibrosis of variable degree. A trichrome stain may highlight the portal fibrosis over time and also a characteristic perivenular sinusoidal fibrosis. Ductular reaction seen on cytokeratin 7 stain may be prominent and mimic biliary obstructive pattern. Bile plugs may also be seen. The

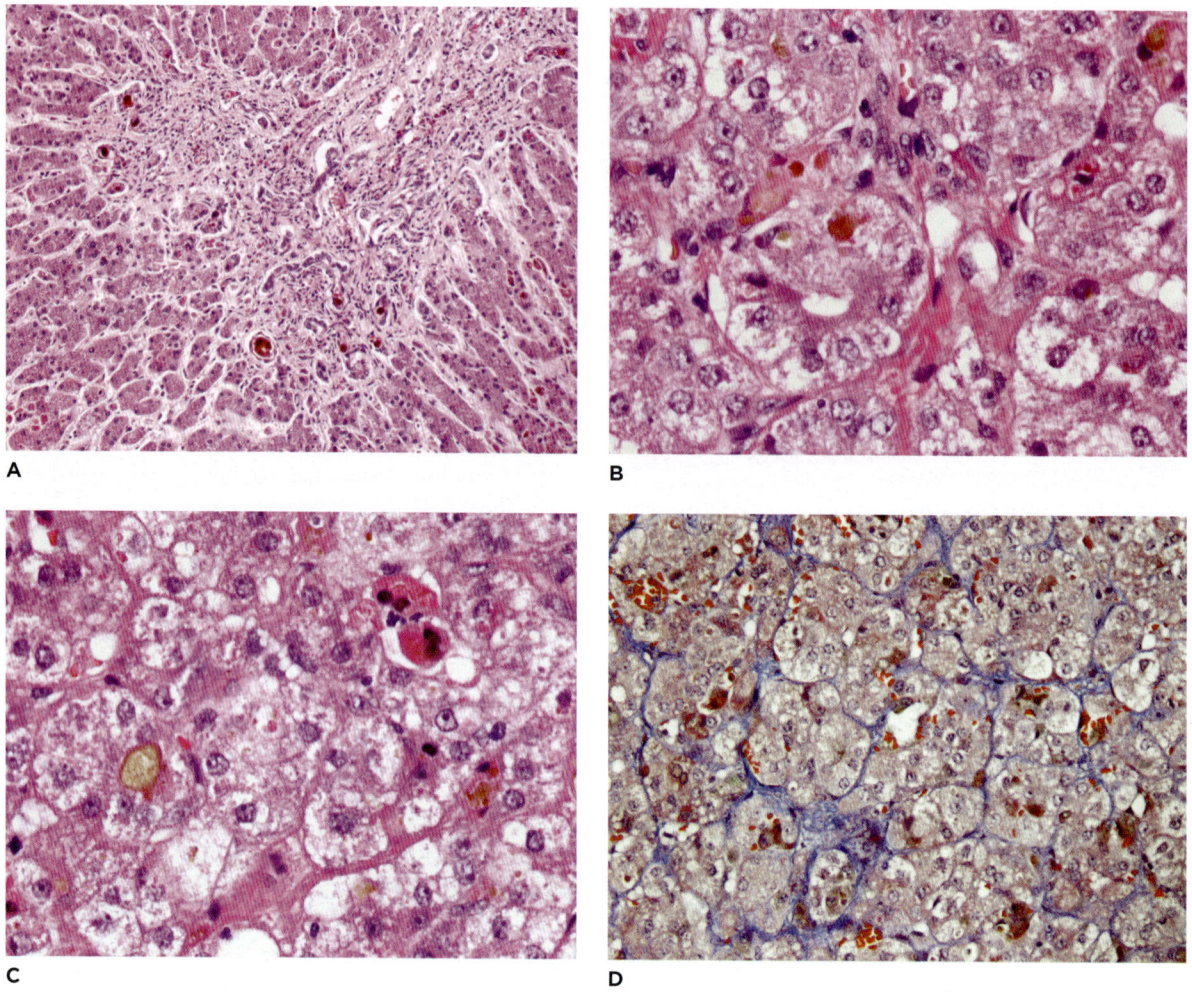

FIGURE 15-43 • Total parenteral nutrition. **A:** Portal tract expansion by fibrous tissue with bile duct proliferation and cholestasis (H&E, 100×). **B, C:** Pseudoacinar arrangement of hepatocytes with obvious cytoplasmic cholestasis, apoptotic hepatocytes (**C**), and increased sinusoidal fibrous tissue (H&E, 400×). **D:** Trichrome staining highlights pseudoacinar pattern and lobular fibrosis (H&E, 200×).

vast majority of patients recover with clearing of the jaundice after cessation of TPN and commencement of enteral feedings. In repeat liver biopsies, cholestasis usually clears. Hepatocyte ballooning, lobular disarray, occasional cholestasis, and perivenular and portal fibrosis may persist. However, cirrhosis with portal hypertension and hepatic failure has been noted in infants receiving TPN. Rare instances of ductopenia have been reported. Liver explants usually show biliary type cirrhosis.

CIRRHOSIS

Cirrhosis has been defined by the Working Group of the World Health Organization as a diffuse process characterized by fibrosis and conversion of normal liver architecture into structurally abnormal nodules (189). Cirrhosis is the end result of hepatic cell necrosis caused by a variety of injurious agents. Necrosis is associated with collapse, fibrosis, and regeneration, resulting in the formation of nodules.

The classification of cirrhosis may be etiologic or morphologic. Cirrhosis has many etiologies. Many metabolic disorders are associated with cirrhosis and have been reviewed elsewhere (79). Alpers disease, a putative mitochondrial disorder, is characterized by progressive neuronal degeneration and cirrhosis in childhood (190). Alcoholic cirrhosis, a common cause of liver injury in adults, may rarely be seen in adolescents. Hepatic changes resembling adult alcohol-associated injury has been described in the fetal alcohol syndrome. Cardiac cirrhosis in the pediatric population occurs most commonly in association with congenital heart disease (191). Hematologic conditions, such as hemophilia, can be associated with progressive liver disease. The role of trace metals in childhood cirrhosis has been detailed elsewhere. Gallbladder duplication has been described in association with childhood obstructive biliary disease and biliary

TABLE 15-14	CIRRHOSIS IN INFANCY AND CHILDHOOD
Causes of Cirrhosis	Related Disorder
Infections	Neonatal viral infection
	Neonatal hepatitis
	Viral hepatitis
	CAH
	Syphilis
Biliary obstruction	EHBA
	Choledochal cyst
	Familial cholestatic syndromes
	Paucity of intrahepatic bile ducts
	Cholangitis
Vascular disease	Hepatic vein occlusion
	VOD
	Constrictive pericarditis
	Chronic congestive cardiac failure
	Rendu-Osler-Weber disease
Hereditary syndromes	Cerebrohepatorenal (Zellweger syndrome)
	CF
	Indian childhood cirrhosis
	CHF
Metabolic abnormalities	Galactosemia
	Fructosemia
	Tyrosinemia
	Glycogenoses, types III and IV
	A1AT deficiency
	Gaucher disease
	Niemann-Pack disease
	Wolman disease
	Cholesterol ester storage disease
	Mucopolysaccharidoses
	Wilson disease
	Hemochromatoses
	Argininosuccinic aciduria
	Cystinosis
	Porphyria
Miscellaneous	TPN
	Malnutrition
	Obesity
	Alcohol
	Sclerosing cholangitis
	Langerhans cell histiocytosis
	Drugs

cirrhosis. Etiologic associations with cirrhosis in childhood are presented in Table 15-14. Establishing the etiology requires demonstration of the specific histopathologic characteristics of a disease, such as A1AT stored in hepatocytes, ground-glass hepatocytes in HBV, or biochemical evaluation in metabolic disorders. As in the adult, cirrhosis in childhood may be cryptogenic, with failure to identify an etiologic agent in the explanted liver.

Morphologic classification is based on nodule size. In micronodular cirrhosis, nodules measure less than 3 mm in diameter and are relatively uniform throughout the liver. Fibrous septa are delicate and extend from portal to central areas or encircle the lobule. Macronodular cirrhosis is characterized by nodules larger than 3 mm, usually with broad bands of fibrous tissue (Figure 15-44). Large nodules contain several lobules in which portal areas and central veins are identifiable. In mixed type cirrhosis, the liver contains an approximately equal proportion of small and large nodules. Transformation of one type to another can occur with continuing necrosis, collapse, and fibrosis. In some conditions, cirrhosis is predominantly macronodular, such as after submassive bridging hepatic necrosis due to hepatitis or toxic agents. A predominantly micronodular cirrhosis is associated with biliary atresia and cholestatic syndromes. However, considerable overlaps exist owing to the transformation that may occur between the various morphologic types of cirrhosis, and the etiology of cirrhosis cannot be ascertained from the morphologic type of cirrhosis in all cases. This morphologic classification has therefore fallen out of favor.

Activity of cirrhosis is evaluated by identifying continuing hepatocellular necrosis and the degree of septal inflammation. Portal hypertension with all its sequelae is a frequent complication, although portal hypertension may also be noncirrhotic in origin. Noncirrhotic portal hypertension may be suspected when the patient presents with portal hypertension without parenchymal dysfunction (as reflected by maintained albumin level and prothrombin time indicating preserved synthetic function) (192). Putative preneoplastic hepatic lesions may be found in cirrhotic livers. Liver cell dysplasia (large cell dysplasia) is characterized by nuclear and cytoplasmic enlargement, nuclear hyperchromasia, prominent nucleoli, and, occasionally, multinucleation (193). Adenomatous hyperplasia (macroregenerative nodule) is a nodular lesion that occurs in cirrhosis and is thought to progress to HCC through an intermediate lesion termed atypical adenomatous hyperplasia (small-cell dysplasia) (194). Atypical adenomatous hyperplasia occurs as an ill-defined nodule within a cirrhotic nodule (the so-called nodule-in-nodule formation), identified by compression of surrounding reticulin fibers and a different orientation of the liver plates. The evidence suggests that this lesion, rather than liver cell dysplasia, is more likely the precursor of HCC in a cirrhotic liver. Although it typically takes many years for HCC to develop, HCC may be associated with cirrhosis even in a neonate.

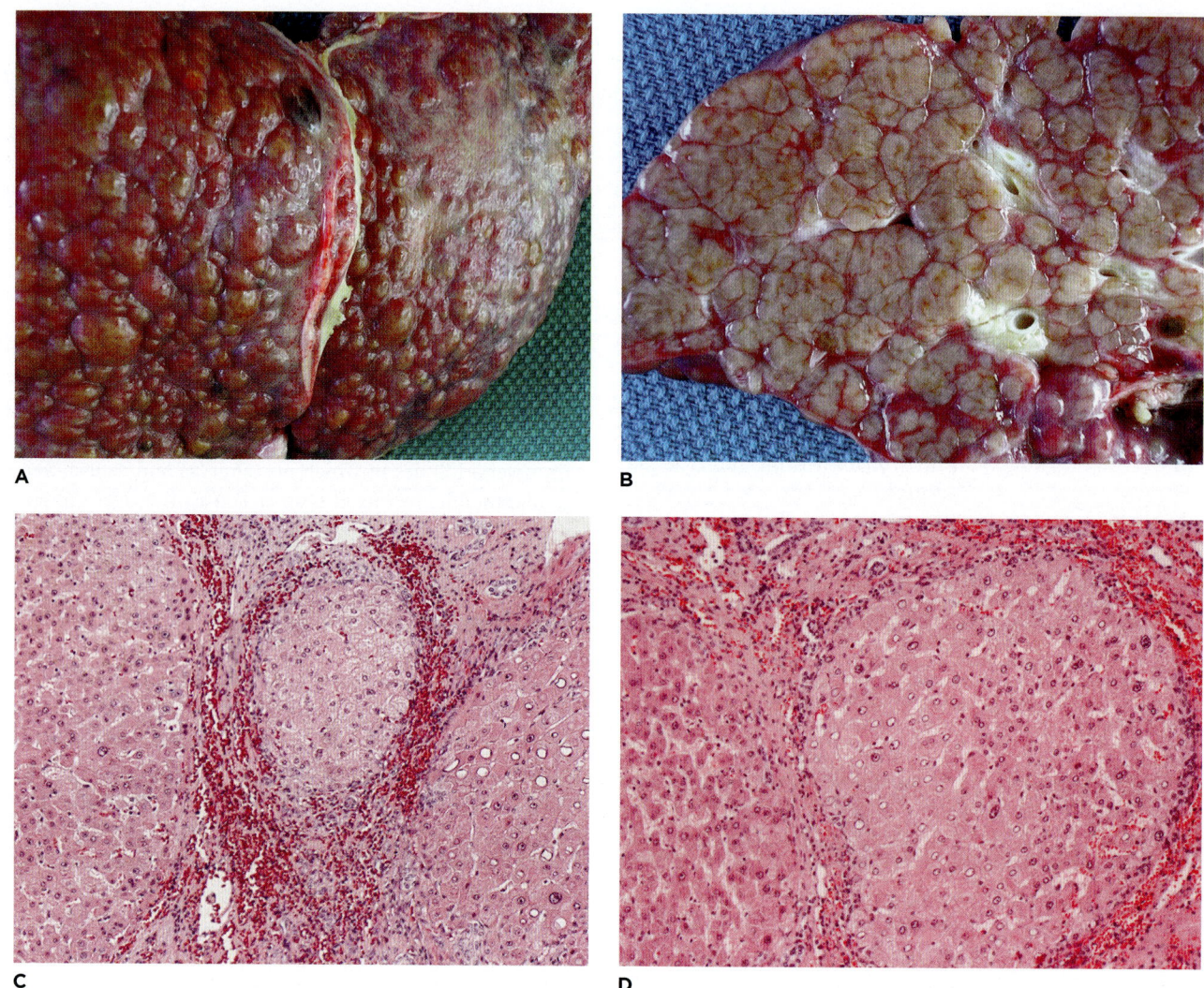

FIGURE 15-44 • Cirrhosis. **A, B:** Liver explant with a cirrhotic surface and cross-section demonstrating numerous macronodules and micronodules. **C, D:** Fibrous tissue separates nodules of hepatocytes lacking central veins from each other. Note the variable size to the nodules (H&E, 100× and 200×).

HEPATIC TUMORS

Primary hepatic neoplasms account for 0.5% to 2.0% of all pediatric neoplasms and comprise a variety of benign and malignant epithelial and mesodermal tumors. Incidences of these tumors change significantly from birth to 20 years of age (Tables 15-15, 15-16, 15-17). Of 716 cases of the 10 most commonly occurring hepatic neoplasms seen at the Armed Forces Institute of Pathology between 1970 and 1999, hepatoblastoma, HCC, and hemangioendothelioma accounted for almost 65% (see Table 15-15).

FOCAL NODULAR HYPERPLASIA

FNH is a benign tumor-like lesion of the liver. Rather than a true neoplasm, it is considered to be the result of a hyperplastic response to hemodynamic disturbance related to vascular abnormalities. Although it most commonly occurs in women

TABLE 15-15 HEPATIC TUMORS IN PEDIATRIC PATIENTS, BIRTH TO 20 YEARS (AFIP 1970–1999)

Type of Tumor	N	%
Hepatoblastoma	198	27.6
Hepatocellular carcinoma	135	18.9
Infantile hemangioma	119	16.5
Focal nodular hyperplasia	72	10.1
Mesenchymal hamartoma	57	8.0
Undifferentiated embryonal sarcoma	52	7.2
Nodular regenerative hyperplasia	32	4.5
Hepatocellular adenoma	27	3.8
Angiosarcoma	17	2.4
Embryonal rhabdomyosarcoma	7	1.0
TOTAL	716	100.0

TABLE 15-16	HEPATIC TUMORS IN PEDIATRIC PATIENTS, BIRTH TO 2 YEARS (AFIP 1970–1999)		
Type of Tumor		N	%
Hepatoblastoma		124	43.5
Infantile hemangioma		103	36.1
Mesenchymal hamartoma		38	13.3
Nodular regenerative hyperplasia		6	2.1
Hepatocellular carcinoma		4	1.4
Angiosarcoma		4	1.4
Focal nodular hyperplasia		3	1.1
Undifferentiated "embryonal" sarcoma		3	1.1
Hepatocellular adenoma		0	0
Embryonal/rhabdomyosarcoma		0	0
TOTAL		285	100.0

TABLE 15-17	HEPATIC TUMORS IN PEDIATRIC PATIENTS, 5–20 YEARS (AFIP 1970–1999)		
Type of Tumor		N	%
Hepatocellular carcinoma		96	36.6
Focal nodular hyperplasia		40	15.3
Undifferentiated embryonal sarcoma		39	14.9
Nodular regenerative hyperplasia		26	9.9
Hepatocellular adenoma		22	8.4
Hepatoblastoma		22	8.4
Angiosarcoma		6	2.3
Mesenchymal hamartoma		5	1.9
Infantile hemangioma		4	1.5
Embryonal rhabdomyosarcoma		2	0.8
TOTAL		262	100.0

of childbearing and middle age, nearly 8% of cases present in the first 15 years of life, with a slightly increased frequency in those 6 to 10 years of age (39%) and a distinct female predominance of more than 3:1 (195) (Figure 15-45A).

Pathogenesis

In 1985, Wanless and collaborators proposed that FNH is a hyperplastic response of the hepatic parenchyma to a preexisting local arterial spider-like malformation, likely with a developmentally abnormal origin (196). FNH is also related to well-known vascular diseases, such as hereditary hemorrhagic telangiectasia or congenital portal vein absence.

[a]Portions of this section were adapted from Stocker, JT. Hepatic tumors in children. In: Suchy FJ, *Liver disease in children*. 2nd ed. Philadelphia: Lippincott Williams and Wilkins, 2000.

Hepatocellular hyperplasia in FNH is thought to be secondary to increased arterial flow and hyperperfusion of localized parenchyma. An association between the use of oral contraceptives in older children and adults and the development of FNH is still under debate. However, some studies suggest that the use of contraceptive pills may increase the size of the nodules or may predispose to bleeding; others have shown no change (197).

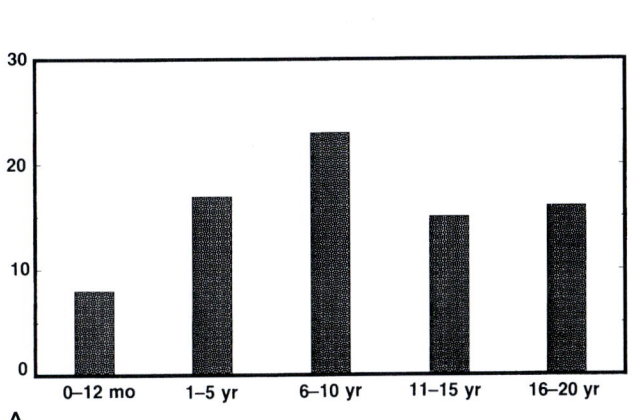
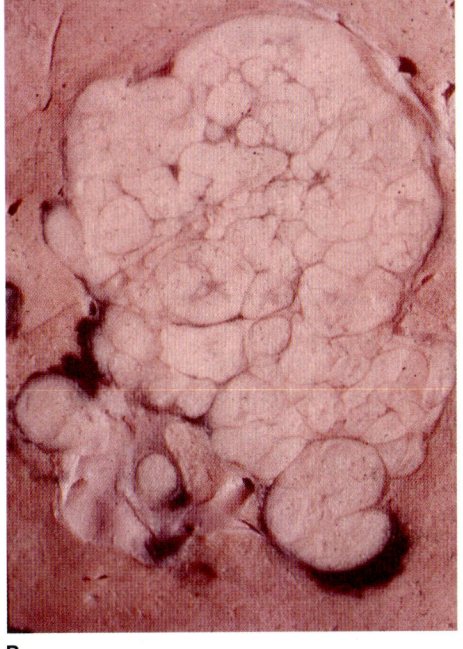

FIGURE 15-45 • Focal nodular hyperplasia. **A:** Age distribution in 79 cases. **B:** A well-circumscribed lesion is subdivided into smaller nodules by bands of connective tissue.

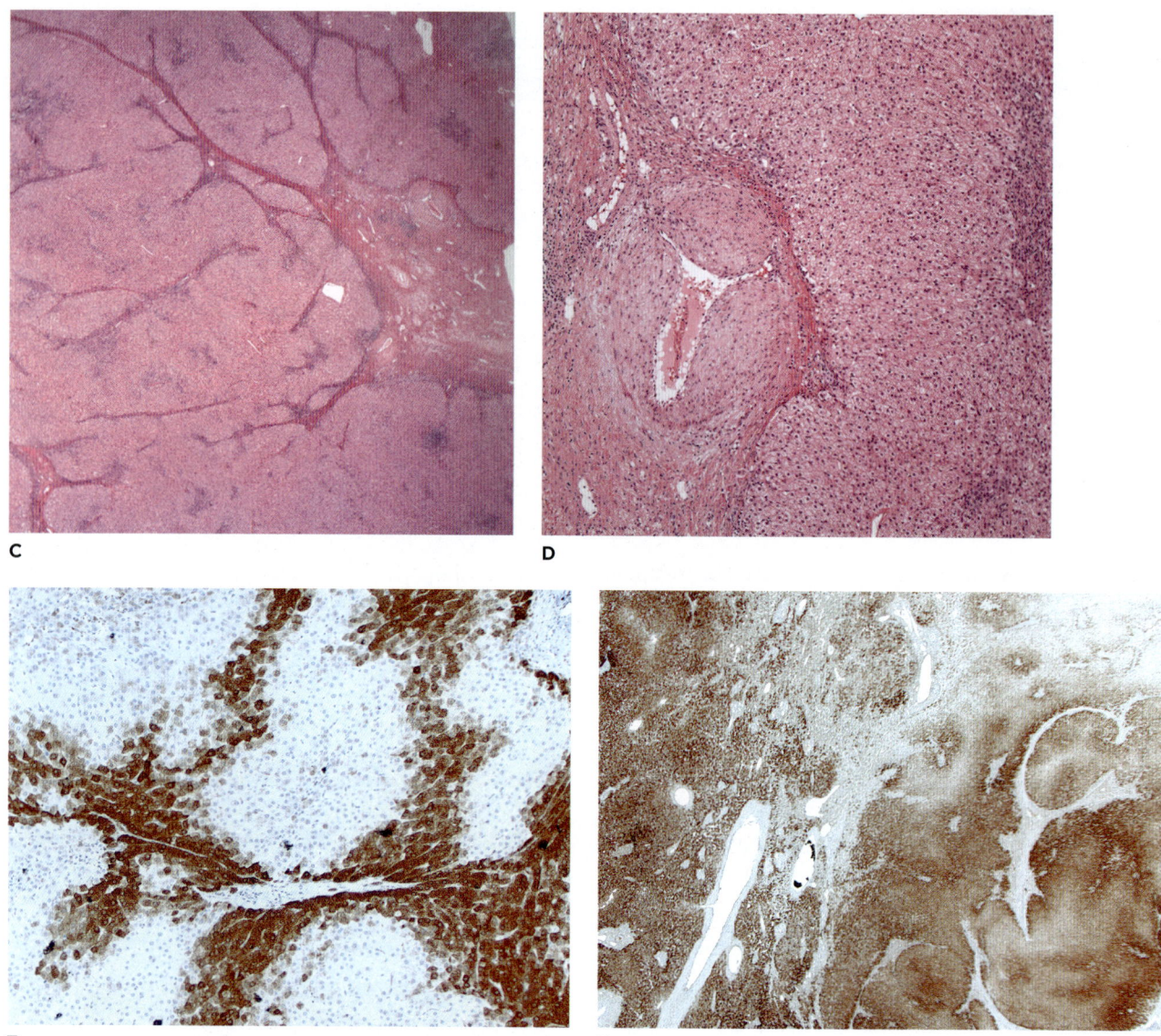

FIGURE 15-45 • (*continued*) **C:** Arborizing septa of fibrous connective tissue surround and subdivide nodules of hepatocytes (reticulin stain, original magnification 15×). **D:** The edges of the fibrous septa contain scattered small ducts along with small to large vessels, some displaying eccentric subintimal thickening (H&E stain, original magnification 60×). **E:** A glutamine synthetase stain highlighting a geographic staining pattern (GS stain 200×). **F:** A liver fatty acid binding protein stain showing normal diffuse staining of lesion (LFABP1 20×).

A variety of associations have been anecdotally noted in children with FNH (Table 15-18). FNH is associated with vascular abnormalities, including hepatic hemangiomas, which supports the concept of a vascular component in the pathogenesis of this lesion. FNH has also been reported in patients with a variety of nonhepatic tumors and tumor-like conditions (198).

Clinical Features

The vast majority of lesions (90%) are asymptomatic, presenting as a mass on routine physical examination or as an incidental finding at surgery or autopsy. Symptomatic cases may present with abdominal pain, weight loss, vomiting, or diarrhea. Laboratory parameters in patients with FNH are rarely abnormal, and alpha-fetoprotein (AFP) is not elevated.

Imaging studies can be extremely helpful in differentiating FNH from other benign or malignant hepatic lesions, especially hypervascular lesions such as hepatocellular adenoma (HCA), HCC, and hypervascular metastases. Color power Doppler allows, in most cases, its distinction from other focal liver lesions. In contrast to adenomas, imaging techniques are sufficient for diagnosis in 70% of cases. Magnetic resonance imaging (MRI) has higher sensitivity and specificity for FNH than does ultrasonography or computed tomography. Typically, FNH is isointense or hypointense on T1-weighted images, is slightly hyperintense or isointense

TABLE 15-18	ASSOCIATED ANOMALIES IN CHILDREN WITH FOCAL NODULAR HYPERPLASIA
Glycogen storage disease	
Gastroschisis, absent gallbladder	
Cardiac hypertrophy, nodular hyperplasia of the thyroid and adrenal cortex	
Ovarian dysgerminoma	
Persistent hypoglycemia	
Multiple telangiectasia on arms and legs	
Hypospadias, bilateral syndactyly of toes, bilateral hydrocele	
Left-sided hemihypertrophy, syndactyly, absent distal phalanges of second and third fingers on left hand, multiple telangiectasia over face and lips, umbilical hernia	
Sickle cell disease	
Biliary atresia with portoenterostomy	
Fibrolamellar HCC	
Adrenocortical tumor	

Modified from Stocker JT, Ishak KG: Focal nodular hyperplasia of the liver: a study of 21 pediatric cases. *Cancer* 1981;48:336–345, with permission.

on T2-weighted images, and has a hyperintense central scar on T2-weighted images. FNH demonstrates intense homogeneous enhancement during the arterial phase of gadolinium-enhanced imaging and enhancement of the central scar during later phases. Arteriography often displays the prominent single or multiple feeder arteries associated with FNH. Centrifugal filling from the feeder artery to the periphery of the lesion may be seen. Ultrasonography may demonstrate a feeding artery with a radial vascular architecture, which, however, may not be present in a lesion smaller than 3 cm in size. Cheon et al. (199), however, noted that children often display a wide spectrum of imaging findings on various radiologic examinations and that the typical centrally placed scar is not always seen. Superparamagnetic iron oxide (SPIO)-enhanced MRI has been shown to be useful in differentiating benign lesions such as FNH and hepatic adenoma from malignant hepatocellular lesions.

Treatment

Symptomatic children are treated with resection of the lesion. However, since morbidity and death have been associated with attempts at resection, it has been suggested that asymptomatic lesions be observed with regular ultrasonography and treated only if they enlarge or become symptomatic. Young girls with FNH should be cautioned on the use of oral contraceptives, because bleeding may occur within the lesion. FNH does not undergo malignant transformation. Although Saul et al. (200) described the association of FNH with fibrolamellar HCC (FL-HCC), they also suggested that the FNH, usually found either in or adjacent to the FL-HCC, is a phenomenon secondary to the highly vascular nature of FL-HCC. There is currently no proof of FL-HCC arising in a pre-existing FNH. However, the radiologist should be cautious about the similar radiographic appearance of FL-HCC and FNH, both of which may contain central scars.

Gross Appearance

FNH occurs most frequently (90%) as a single mass within the right or left lobe (Figure 15-45B). Bilateral involvement by a large lesion may be present in 10% of cases. Multiple lesions within both lobes are seen in 10% of cases and often have a histologic appearance different from that in cases with a single lesion (see later). The single lesions are firm and irregular in outline and range from 1 to 17 cm in greatest diameter with weights as high as 1500 g (195). The lesions often bulge from the surface of the liver and may be pedunculated. On cut section, the lesion is sharply demarcated from the surrounding liver and displays a nodular tan-brown parenchyma subdivided by gray–white septa radiating from a central area of fibrosis. Prominent vessels may be seen near the edge of the lesion arising within the normal liver parenchyma and ramifying within the lesion. Areas of hemorrhage or necrosis may rarely be seen.

Histopathology

The typical histopathologic features of classical FNH include a firm, well-delimited but not encapsulated lesion composed of hepatocellular nodules with normal hepatocytes, a central scar, and radiating fibrous septa. The central scars of the single lesions display broad bands of fibrous connective tissue typically containing large dystrophic arteries (ectatic vessels with eccentric intimal thickening and medial hyperplasia) (Figure 15-45C, D). Frequently, there is a lymphocytic infiltrate. The fibrous septa subdivide, partially or completely enclosing lobules of parenchymal cells arranged in cords, almost imparting an appearance of a focal biliary cirrhosis. Numerous small bile ducts, arterioles, and venules are present within the septa, along with varying numbers of lymphocytes and neutrophils. Bile ductules are usually found at the interface between hepatocytes and fibrous regions. van Eyken et al. (201) demonstrated that hepatocytes within the liver express cytokeratins of bile duct type, suggesting that the ductular proliferation of FNH is derived from ductular metaplasia of hepatocytes. Interlobular bile ducts are usually absent. The cords within the nodules contain hepatocytes in 1- to 2-cell-thick plates that may be slightly larger than those of the normal liver and may contain intracellular fat and variable amounts of glycogen. The cells within the FNH show no evidence of dysplasia. The lesion often compresses the adjacent parenchyma but is separated from it only by a discontinuous fibrous capsule. A large feeder artery is frequently present within this capsule. Wanless et al. (196) demonstrated a connection between this feeder artery and a spiderlike structure of smaller vessels supplying 1-mm nodules within the lesion.

The diagnosis of FNH is usually evident in a liver biopsy specimen. However, some cases of FNH may show atypical clinical and/or histopathologic features, and the diagnosis is difficult in these even in the resected specimen, let alone on a biopsy (198). In atypical FNH, the above key diagnostic features are either lacking or inconspicuous. Differential diagnosis with adenomas may be difficult in these cases, especially when the nodules are small (<10 mm) or associated with significant steatosis. Fabre et al. (202) have proposed a scoring system for the reliable diagnosis of FNH with atypical features. In their study, most radiologically atypical tumors also showed nonclassic histopathology.

Some lesions have histologic features of both adenoma and FNH. These variant lesions have often been classified as the telangiectatic type of FNH (203,204). These tumors are often multiple, and the cut surface displays a spongy telangiectatic appearance with numerous small, blood-filled cavities. Clinical and molecular evidence indicates that telangiectatic FNH should be reclassified as inflammatory hepatocellular adenomas and are discussed in that section. There is however an overlap in histologic features and immunohistochemical profile between these FNH and inflammatory HCA (IHCA) with overlaps in pattern of staining with GS, preserved LFABP1, SAA protein, and CRP (203,205) (Figure 15-45E, F). The typical GS staining pattern in FNH is map-like and is better appreciated on resection specimen rather than biopsies where a pseudo–map-like pattern may be seen. Bile ductular profiles seen by CK7 are common to both lesions. However, no FNH has been reported to show a β-catenin mutation or nuclear staining. A glypican-3 stain is also negative in both lesions.

Molecular Pathology

The molecular pathogenesis of FNH was recently reviewed by Rebouissou et al. (206). Of 33 FNH lesions evaluated by the HUMARA assay in the literature, 9 (27%) showed a uniform pattern of X chromosome inactivation consistent with clonality. Other studies analyzing chromosome gains and losses by comparative genomic hybridization (CGH), allelotyping, or karyotype have identified chromosome alterations indicating a clonal origin in 14% to 50% of cases. Although somatic gene mutations in β-catenin gene (*CTNNB1*), *TP53*, *APC*, or HNF1α have not been identified in FNH, mRNA expression levels of the angiopoietin genes (*ANGPT1* and *ANGPT2*) involved in vessel maturation are altered, with increased ANGPT1 to ANGPT2 ratio (206).

Immunohistochemical assays of extracellular matrix proteins also support the hypothesis that FNH is merely a hyperplastic response of liver parenchyma to local vascular abnormalities and have shown that the lesions of perisinusoidal fibrosis associated with FNH are accompanied by the induction of integrin receptors on hepatocytes and sinusoidal endothelial cells.

NODULAR REGENERATIVE HYPERPLASIA

Nodular regenerative hyperplasia (NRH) of the liver is an uncommon condition characterized by the presence of widely distributed to diffuse parenchymal nodules with little or no fibrosis. The condition is more common in adults than in children and increases with age. In a study of 2500 consecutive autopsies, Wanless (207) found a prevalence of 2.6%, rising to 5.3% above 80 years of age at death. Over 30 cases of NRH have been reported in children, including two cases in fetal livers (208). In the pediatric age group, NRH has been demonstrated in 4.5% of a large series of 716 pediatric liver tumors, but only in 2.1% of liver tumors from birth to 2 years of age. However, since liver tumors are in general rare, NRH remains the fourth most common "liver tumor" from 5 to 20 years of age (Figure 15-46A), after HCC, FNH, and undifferentiated embryonal sarcoma (UES) (209).

Pathogenesis

Originally described as "miliary hepatocellular adenomatosis" in a patient with Felty syndrome, NRH is seen in association with other rheumatologic and autoimmune diseases, hematologic disorders, drug therapy, PBC, congestive heart failure, other hepatic circulatory disorders, metastases, tuberculosis, and CGD (Table 15-19). Three familial cases of NRH have been reported in literature (210). In a series of 16 children with NRH, clinical associations included a history of anticonvulsant drug therapy (four patients), Donohue syndrome, disseminated intravascular coagulation, renal angiomyolipoma, other intra-abdominal tumors, thrombocytopenia, and pancytopenia (208). Other pediatric reports have been associated with congenital heart disease, Krabbe disease, Still disease, chronic inflammation, sacrococcygeal teratoma, autoimmune disorders, celiac disease and inflammatory bowel disease following therapy, and multiple organ malformation in fetuses.

The etiopathogenesis of NRH is not fully understood. NRH may be a hyperproliferative response to an obstructive portal venopathy resulting in an uneven perfusion of the hepatic parenchyma. It is hypothesized that the portal venopathy leads to centrilobular (acinar zone 3) ischemic atrophy with compensatory proliferation of zone 1 hepatocytes. The resultant "regenerative nodules" compress the atrophic hepatocytes, yielding the characteristic pattern highlighted by reticulin stains. This hypothesis is supported by the association of NRH with diseases that are known to cause vascular injury and the frequent histologic finding of portal venous abnormalities in NRH. Vascular abnormalities such as atrial septal defects, ventricular septal defects, abnormal junction of pulmonary veins, congenital absence of portal vein, and other congenital anomalies are reported in children diagnosed with NRH, strengthening the argument that NRH may result from microcirculatory derangements. However, other investigators have not confirmed these findings and suggest

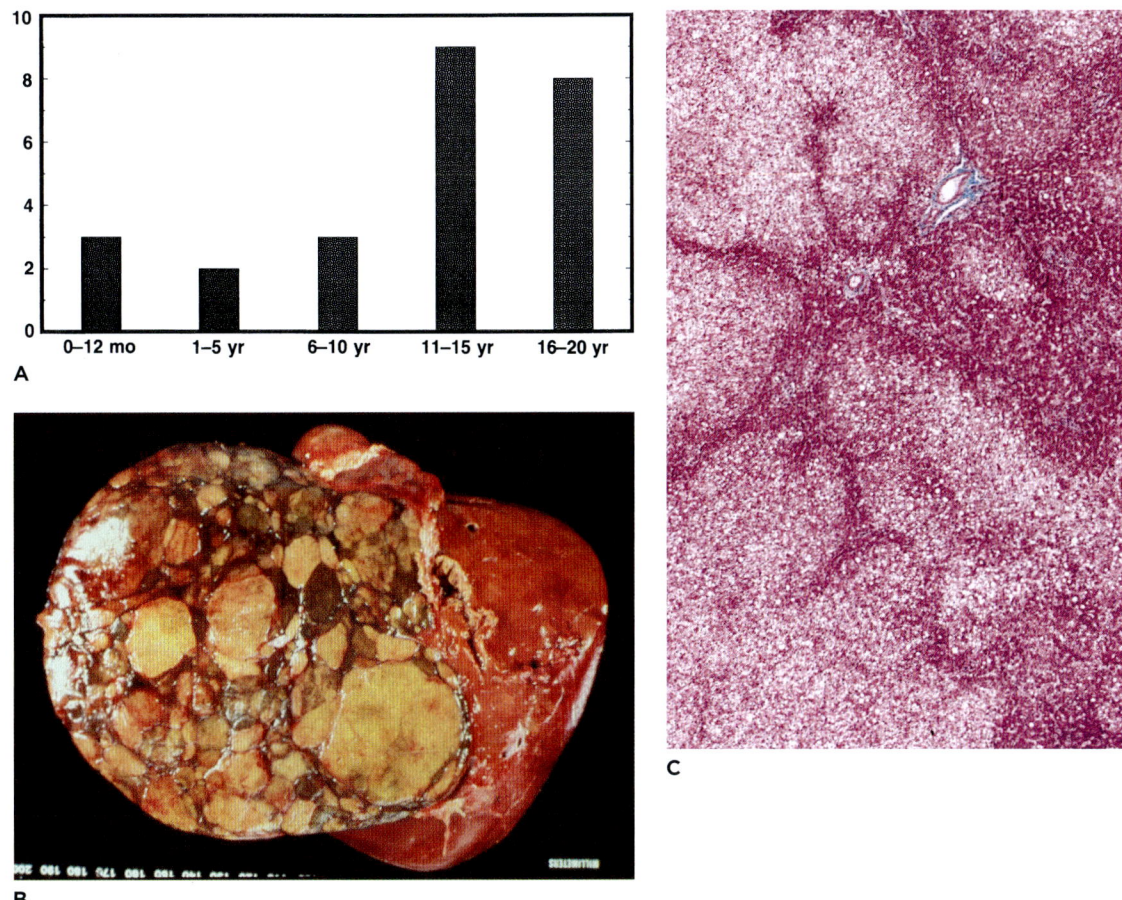

FIGURE 15-46 • Nodular regenerative hyperplasia. **A:** Age distribution in 25 cases. **B:** A large mass of different-sized nodules occupies most of the liver. **C:** The nodules are composed of hyperplasic "regenerative" hepatocytes, which are light staining and compress remnants of atrophic lobules into thin bands. (H&E stain, original magnification 30×).

that NRH is a primary generalized proliferative disorder of the liver. In cases associated with drug therapy, it has been suggested that polymorphisms in genes encoding thiopurine methyltransferase may be linked to development of NRH probably through altered drug metabolism. Some NRH cases have been suggested to result from chronic, cytotoxic CD8+ T lymphocyte targeting of sinusoidal endothelial cells, and NRH has also been postulated to be an organ-specific form of antiphospholipid syndrome. Recent studies have suggested NRH to be an endotheliopathy, and down-regulation of Notch1, Ephrine, and Tek all involved in liver sinusoidal endothelial cell signaling pathways (211).

TABLE 15-19 CONDITIONS ASSOCIATED WITH NODULAR REGENERATIVE HYPERPLASIA IN CHILDREN

Donohue syndrome
Mental retardation
Anticonvulsant therapy
Vater syndrome
Renal angiomyolipoma
Disseminated intravascular coagulopathy
Krabbe disease
Portal hypertension
Wilms tumor
Down syndrome
Still disease

Clinical Features, Diagnosis, and Management

Most patients with NRH may remain asymptomatic for years before coming to clinical attention. The diagnosis of NRH requires a high index of suspicion and awareness of its associations detailed above; NRH should be considered in the differential diagnosis of patients who present with unexplained portal hypertension. NRH may also clinically simulate metastases and should be considered in patients with history of malignancy treated with chemotherapy and/or radiotherapy who develop single or multiple hepatic masses.

In symptomatic patients, portal hypertension and its complications dominate. However, ascites is relatively uncommon since patients typically have normal hepatic synthetic function with normal albumin levels. Although based on the vascular compromise hypothesis, portal hypertension should be presinusoidal in nature (207); portal pressure measurements in a small number of patients have been more consistent with a sinusoidal portal hypertension, possibly due to sinusoidal compression by the regenerating nodules in later stages of the disease (212).

The radiologic findings of NRH reflect clinical observations. Liver size can be normal, reduced, or increased; immense hepatomegaly leading to abdominal deformity is very rare. Nodules range in size from 0.1 to 10 cm in diameter and are often hyperechoic on ultrasound, although they may be even undetectable by this modality. CT scans generally show hypodense nodules with respect to the adjacent liver parenchyma, without significant contrast enhancement (213). On MRI, lesions are described as isointense to normal liver on T2-weighted images and contain foci of high signal intensity on T1-weighted scans. Kobayashi et al. report typical imaging findings to include hyperintensity on T1-weighted MRI, hyperdensity on CT during arterial portography (CTAP), and isointensity to hypointensity on SPIO-enhanced T2-weighted MRI.

Laboratory parameters of liver function are also usually normal in NRH, although approximately 25% of cases reported in the literature note an elevated ALP (212). Liver biopsy is essential for diagnosis. It has been emphasized that the histologic findings of NRH may not be detected by a needle biopsy of the liver and a wedge biopsy may be required. In the case of needle biopsy, the gauge of the needle is an important consideration. Regenerative nodules may be missed if the needle is too narrow, as is often the case with transjugular liver biopsy, thus making the diagnosis of NRH difficult.

The mainstay of treatment is to manage the underlying disease; remove offending drugs, if any; and control portal hypertension. Given the uncommon nature of NRH, there is scant literature on the natural history of this disease and treatment strategies are based on experience with other more common causes of portal hypertension (212). It is not known whether NRH is a reversible process once the presumed cause is removed, such as might occur with stopping a drug. Since the synthetic function of the liver is generally intact in NRH, despite the potential for the development of significant portal hypertension, liver transplantation is not a conventional therapy. The outcome of NRH depends on the presence of portal hypertension, associated systemic disease, and the risk of rupture of a large hyperplastic nodule. Some investigators claim that NRH is a premalignant condition, which may progress to hepatocyte dysplasia and HCC. Nzeako et al. (214) demonstrated that 23 of 342 patients without cirrhosis who had HCC also had NRH and also found that 73.9% of their patients with NRH and HCC had liver cell dysplasia. Liver cell dysplasia is a common finding in NRH and has been noted in 20% to 42% of cases.

The largest pediatric series of NRH (208) comprised 16 patients (10 girls and 6 boys) with a median age of 6 years (range 7 months to 13 years). Nine presented with hepatomegaly or splenomegaly, with and without signs of portal hypertension. Follow-up was available for eight patients; six patients died of causes unrelated to the nodular hyperplasia. Two patients were asymptomatic when last seen 5 and 18 years after the initial diagnosis of nodular hyperplasia.

Pathology

Based on autopsy studies, the liver with NRH shows a diffuse transformation into nodules of 1 to 3 mm in size (Figure 15-46). Unlike cirrhosis, there is no fibrosis separating nodules; each nodule presses directly against its neighbor. Although nodules greater than 15 mm have been described grossly, these are frequently revealed to be composed of smaller nodules when examined microscopically (207).

Histopathology is the only means of definitive diagnosis and is also required to rule out cirrhosis and HCC. By definition, the nodules are less than 3 mm in thickness and perisinusoidal fibrosis is absent to minimal (204,212). At a minimum, to make the diagnosis of NRH, one should see the characteristic nodular zones of widened hepatocyte plates bounded by narrowed and compressed plates. Parenchymal nodularity can be appreciated on scanning magnification with a characteristic pattern of light and dark areas (208). The light areas are comprised of swollen liver cells with empty to clear cytoplasm, whereas the dark areas correspond to compressed liver cell plates between the nodules. The hepatocytes within the nodule may be arranged in plates that are more than one cell thick. The individual hepatocytes may be enlarged and have hypertrophic nuclei. Between individual nodules, the hepatocytes are small and atrophic and are pressed together into thin, parallel plates. This compression is best visualized using a reticulin stain and may be associated with slitlike central veins and sinusoidal dilation (in areas of hepatocellular atrophy). Immunohistochemical granular staining for alpha-1 antitrypsin is reportedly increased in the regenerating (periportal) compartment, and this may help in the histologic evaluation of difficult cases. Whereas the larger portal veins may be widely patent, portal venous structures in smaller radicals may be absent or occluded. Central veins may show venoocclusive changes or may be compressed into narrowed slits. However, no vascular abnormalities were noted in Moran's series (208). Fibrosis typical of chronic liver disease is usually not present, although there may be some degree of periportal fibrosis or perisinusoidal fibrosis, the latter frequently associated with the atrophic areas. There is usually little or no inflammation or cholestasis, and normal bile ducts and arteries can be easily identified. In needle biopsies of the liver, the changes of regeneration and atrophy may be very subtle on routine hematoxylin–eosin stains. Therefore, any "normal" liver biopsy specimens, particularly those from patients with portal hypertension, should be investigated further using reticulin stains (212).

The differential diagnosis of NRH includes hepatic adenoma, FNH, partial nodular transformation, large regenerative nodule, CHF, incomplete cirrhosis, cirrhosis, and HCC. The International Working Party has published guidelines and definitions for these nodular hepatic lesions (204). It is important to remember that more than one type of nodular lesion can coexist in the same liver since clinical portal hypertension may result from NRH, whereas disabling pain or hemorrhage may be due to other pathology such as hepatic adenoma, with different treatment options for each situation. Histologically, patients with portal hypertension not associated with cirrhosis may present with NRH, hepatoportal sclerosis (portal venopathy), central venous obliteration, sinusoidal dilatation, or some combination of these lesions. Histologic findings in these settings may be subtle, and awareness of these will prevent underdiagnosis.

HEPATOCELLULAR ADENOMA

HCA is a rare benign tumor of the liver. In the pediatric age group, it is seen most frequently in teenage girls (Figure 15-47A) but has also been described in younger children with GSD and galactosemia, in infants, and even *in utero* (215). Most patients, however, are older than 10 years of age and, like adults, have a history of oral contraceptive use (216).

Pathogenesis

In addition to oral contraceptive use, HCA has been described in a variety of conditions in children, including GSD types I, III, and IV; galactosemia; Hurler syndrome; severe combined

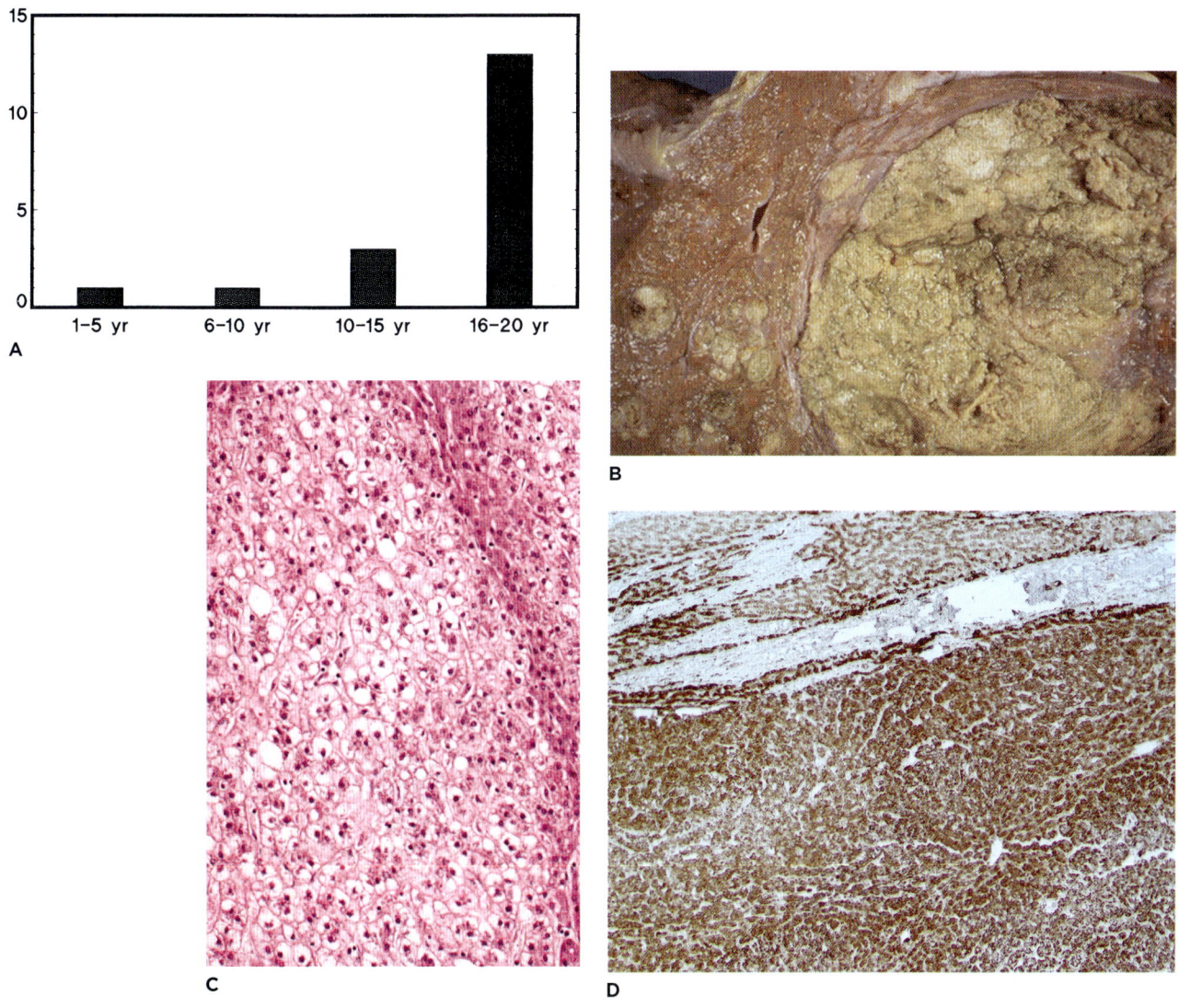

FIGURE 15-47 • Hepatocellular adenoma. **A:** Age distribution in 18 cases. **B:** A poorly circumscribed light yellow–tan mass occupies a large portion of the liver. Note the smaller nodules of similar colored tissue in the adjacent normal liver parenchyma. **C:** The lesion is composed of trabeculae of uniform hepatocytes, some surrounding canaliculi. Note the absence of portal areas and bile ducts. (H&E stain, original magnification 100×). **D:** A glutamine synthetase stain showing diffuse cytoplasmic staining of the lesion (GS stain, original magnification 40×).

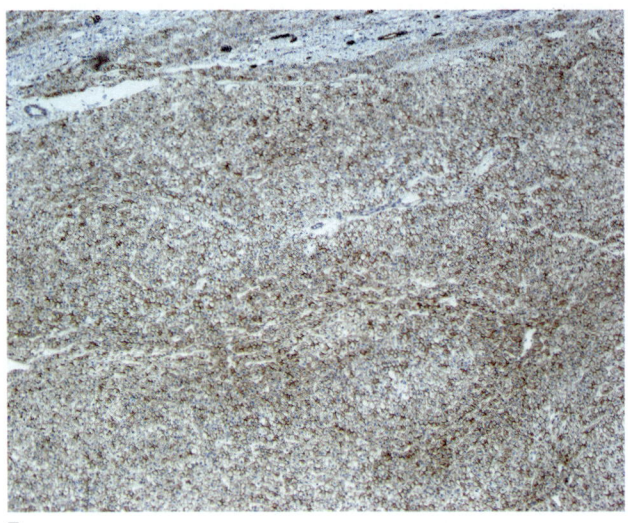
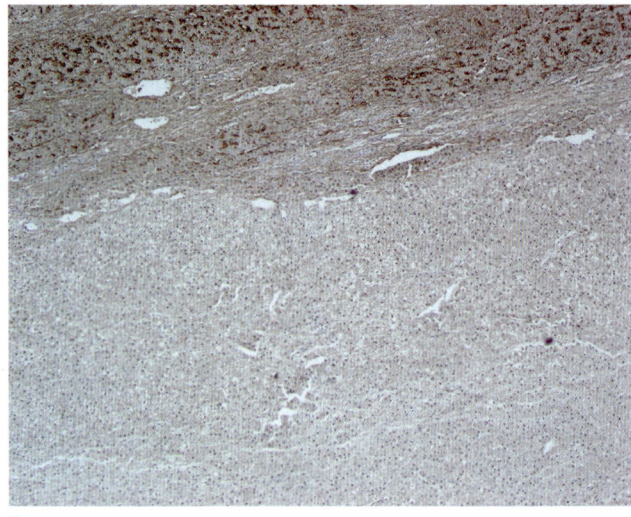

FIGURE 15-47 • (*continued*) **E.** A β-catenin stain showing diffuse membranous staining of an adenoma (β-catenin, original magnification 40x). **F.** A liver fatty acid binding protein stain showing complete loss of staining of adenoma in an HNF-α–mutated lesion (LFABP1, original magnification 40x).

immunodeficiency; diabetes mellitus; and androgen therapy for Fanconi anemia (215,216). Osteoporosis has been noted in some children with HCA. Specific mutations have now been described in various subtypes and are thought to be the defects responsible for adenomas and are discussed below.

Clinical, Laboratory, and Imaging Features

The lesion may be asymptomatic, produce mild episodic abdominal pain, or present as acute abdominal pain due to hemorrhage into the tumor or peritoneal cavity. Laboratory studies are usually not helpful with normal or only mildly elevated serum aminotransferases, ALP, and bilirubin values (215).

Although imaging studies are helpful in demonstrating the large single mass usually seen in this disorder, at present, HCA cannot be conclusively identified by any currently available imaging technique. Arteriography displays hypervascular masses that in some areas are hypovascular, presumably because of intratumor bleeding or necrosis. Ultrasound has detected the lesions *in utero* (215). Imaging findings of HCA and adenomatosis are similar and vary according to the particular characteristics of the lesional tissue: there are fatty patterns, peliotic patterns, and heterogeneous patterns with necrotic and hemorrhagic foci. Currently, imaging techniques are unable to detect early malignant transformation in HCA.

Treatment and Outcomes

HCAs require excision, in view of their propensity to bleed or rupture, association with osteoporosis, and the inability to predict malignant transformation (217). HCAs in girls using contraceptive steroids may regress after discontinuation of their use.

There are, at present, inadequate data regarding the growth and involution of HCAs. Also, the risk of hemorrhage in an HCA is not restricted to larger lesions and is unpredictable. There are no longitudinal studies evaluating transformation of HCA to HCC, although a recent study found malignancy only in adenomas larger than 4 cm and more often in men than in women. β-catenin–mutated HCA has the highest risk for malignant transformation and needs surgical resection (216).

Gross Pathology

HCA is usually a solitary, well-demarcated, globular to ovoid lesion measuring 0.1 to 15 cm in diameter, often with large vessels coursing over its surface (215). The lesion is soft to firm in consistency and has a variegated appearance ranging from light brown to tan, with or without areas of yellow necrosis or reddish–brown hemorrhage. Multiple lesions may be present (Figure 15-47B). By definition, "adenomatosis" requires the presence of at least 10 adenomas in the liver (216). This definition theoretically excludes patients with glycogenosis, or those taking contraceptives, although some authors feel that this may be an unduly restrictive definition.

Histopathology

HCAs can be solitary or multiple. They represent a heterogeneous group of tumors in which histopathologic features may vary according to the etiologic background (216). Microscopically, the tumor is composed of sheets of neoplastic cells in trabeculae that are one to three cells thick, separated by compressed sinusoidal spaces lined by endothelial cells and some Kupffer cells (Figure 15-47C). The tumor cells are the same size as or slightly larger than the normal hepatocytes and may be normal, clear (glycogen rich), or fatty. Some lesions may be almost entirely steatotic, prompting a differential diagnosis including angiomyolipoma. The tumor parenchyma is supplied by thin-walled arteries without other portal tract elements such as significant amounts of connective tissue, bile ducts, or ductular reaction. Bile may be present in intracellular canaliculi. Foci of dilated sinusoids may impart a "pelioid" appearance. Large vessels are often present near the periphery of the lesion, displaying arterial intimal thickening and elastic lamina reduplication. Smooth muscle proliferation may narrow or obliterate the lumen of veins, particularly in cases associated with contraceptive steroid use. Infarcts and hemorrhage are frequent, especially in larger lesions. Hemorrhage may be internal to the lesion, usually admixed with necrotic changes (this type is mostly observed in adenomas larger than 4 cm) or may result in spontaneous rupture with resultant subcapsular hematoma and/or hemoperitoneum. Internal hemorrhage may heal with fibrosis, and this may simulate a central scar of FNH, making it difficult to differentiate the two, particularly in core biopsy material. Hemosiderin-laden macrophages may also be seen. Foci of extramedullary hematopoiesis as seen in cases of hepatoblastoma may be present, sometimes posing difficulty in differentiating the two lesions (150). Foci of dysplastic hepatocytes may be present within the lesion, especially in patients with Fanconi anemia, but malignant transformation is rare (215). Nuclear atypia, mitoses, and acinar ("pseudoglandular") growth pattern are rarely seen; these cases may also be extremely difficult to distinguish from HCC. The term "atypical adenoma" is often used in these settings to indicate that the distinction between HCA and HCC remains problematic and resection and/or close clinical follow-up may be needed (218). Cytogenetic techniques such as FISH and CGH may help distinguish HCA from HCC, since the former usually does not show chromosomal aberrations. Resnick et al. (215) suggest that immunostains for proliferating cell nuclear antigen (PCNA) may be used to help differentiate HCA from hepatoblastoma and HCC; the PCNA labeling index was significantly lower in hepatic adenomas (0.3% to 5.1%) than in HCCs (9.6% to 23.8%) and hepatoblastomas (21.8% to 44.3%) in their study. The range of PCNA labeling is even lower in patients with adenoma who do not have Fanconi anemia (0.3% to 1.7% for adenoma alone versus 3.2% to 5.1% for those with Fanconi anemia). Care must also be taken to distinguish the usual solitary HCA from the multiple nodules of NRH of the liver, which is associated with many other disorders.

As outlined above, the heterogeneous histopathology of HCA raises many differential diagnoses, the greatest overlap being with FNH. Until recently, the presence of bile ductules (characterized immunohistochemically as CK7 positive and usually CK19 negative) in a lesion precluded the diagnosis of HCA. However, molecular studies have shown that HCA may contain bile ductules, especially when associated with sinusoidal dilatation; these lesions traditionally referred to as telangiectatic FNH are being reclassified as adenomas (219). The problem of differentiating HCA and FNH is further compounded by the fact that the two lesions are associated and may occur concurrently. Immunohistochemical stains with antibodies to CD34, cytokeratin 7, or hepatic transporters have been suggested as adjunct techniques to help differentiate between FNH and HCA though there may be overlap especially with the inflammatory HCA.

Molecular Pathology

The past decade and a half has seen numerous advances in understanding the molecular basis of HCA. Based on molecular criteria (hepatocyte nuclear factor 1-α [HNF1-α] mutations and β-catenin mutations) as well as histology and IHC, a molecular/histologic classification correlating the genotype and phenotype of HCAs has been proposed (205,217).

HNF1-α–Mutated HCA (Hepatocyte Nuclear Factor 1-α Mutated) (Figure 15-47 D–F)

This is the first distinct group of HCA identified due to a mutation in a specific gene in 2002. Since then, several molecular studies in large series have confirmed recurrent losses of heterozygosity at chromosome 12q with HNF1-α biallelic somatic mutations in 35% of the HCA cases. These patients are almost always women. There is marked steatosis/clear cells that constitute almost the entire nodule with lack of inflammation or bile ducts within the lesion. They vary in size but are usually less than 5 cm in maximum diameter and may rarely be multiple. IHC reveals a characteristic staining pattern with a lack of expression of liver fatty acid binding protein (LFABP1) on IHC. Glutamine synthetase staining is variable and can be positive in this variant but mainly around vessels, but β-catenin stain is usually negative (membranous only). An HNF1-α germline (constitutional) mutation is observed in less than 5% of HCA cases and is associated with MODY 3 diabetes, familial adenomatosis, and a younger age at presentation (216).

Telangiectatic/Inflammatory HCA

These were previously thought to represent the telangiectatic variant of FNH but have now been recognized to represent HCA despite the presence of bile ductular profiles within the lesion. They have been shown to harbor in-frame somatic mutations in the gp-130 encoding *IL6ST* gene or less frequently in *GNAS* or *STAT3* genes. They show activation of the JAK/STAT pathway. Histologically, they show a prominent mixed inflammatory infiltrate with many atypical vascular profiles and sinusoidal dilatation giving a peliosis-like morphology (hence the name). They constitute 40% to 50% of HCA and are more frequent in women and may be associated with obesity and systemic symptoms. A subgroup has also been associated with the McCune-Albright syndrome (GNAS mutation). IHC shows positive staining for C-reactive protein (CRP) and serum amyloid–associated (SAA) protein with no loss of

LFABP1. GS staining is again variable and may be positive in areas without a diffuse pattern of staining. β-Catenin is usually membranous except in a subset where there may be associated β-catenin mutations characterized by nuclear β-catenin stain and diffuse GS expression (10% of IHCA, bIHCA). This subgroup (double mutation) has an increased risk of progression to HCC, similar to the β-catenin–mutated HCA (216,220).

β-Catenin–Mutated HCA (bHCA)

These constitute about 10% to 15% of adenomas. They are observed in both men and women and are associated with specific risk factors such as male hormone administration or glycogenosis. The activating mutations of β-catenin are mainly located in exon 3 of the CTNNB1 gene and are overlapping with all other subtypes except for the HNF1-α–mutated ones. They are associated with cellular atypia and an acinar pattern with cholestasis and are most likely to progress to HCC (in about two-thirds of bHCAs). Recently, a two-hit hypothesis has been proposed in this transformation with TERT promoter mutations as a possible second hit following an early β-catenin mutation in this adenoma–HCC transition (221). IHC reveals nuclear β-catenin staining, which may be variable in distribution as well as diffuse strong GS staining with normal staining for LFABP1 and no staining for CRP and SAA, except in the combined bIHCA group.

Unclassified

This group consists of 10% of all HCA that do not fit into any of the above groups in that they show no mutations for β-catenin and HNF1-α or inflammatory markers. The exact molecular basis of this group remains to be elucidated.

MESENCHYMAL HAMARTOMA

Hepatic mesenchymal hamartoma (HMH) is an uncommon benign tumor of childhood. Historically, mesenchymal hamartoma has been described in the literature by various names including pseudocystic mesenchymal tumor, giant cell lymphangioma, cystic hamartoma, bile cell fibroadenoma, hamartoma, and cavernous lymphangiomatoid tumor; the unifying term mesenchymal hamartoma was coined by Edmondson in 1956 (209,222). The lesion makes up approximately 8% of all pediatric tumors and, after hemangioma, is the second most common benign hepatic tumor in childhood.

Pathogenesis

The pathogenesis of HMH is still debated. A handful of series have shown an association with placental abnormalities including mesenchymal stem villous hyperplasia of the placenta, thrombosis, or transient honeycombed multicystic placental enlargement (223), raising the possibility of synchronous abnormal mesodermal development rather than a true developmental abnormality (224). Alternatively, placental dysplasia may be secondary to compression of the umbilical vein by the HMH. Given the similarities between the bile duct abnormalities in MHL and those in von Meyenburg complexes, bile duct hamartomas, Caroli disease, and CHF, a primary bile duct plate malformative etiology has also been proposed for MHL. In fact, serial dissection studies have demonstrated a single portal tract as being the source of the lesion. Association with Beckwith-Wiedemann syndrome has also been reported, which together with the placental mesenchymal dysplasia raises the possibility of androgenetic–biparental mosaicism (ABM), which has been reported in HMH (224). A more contemporary view is that HMH is a neoplasm.

Clinical Features, Laboratory Studies, and Imaging

Mesenchymal hamartoma is a lesion of infants; 55% of cases present in the first year of life and nearly 85% by 2 years of age (Figure 15-48A). Rare cases have been reported in children older than 5 years of age, with anecdotal reports in adults. Intrauterine HMHs have been well documented in several reports (222). Cornette et al. (225) reviewed 17 reported cases in the literature, with the earliest case having been incidentally detected on ultrasonography at 15 weeks' gestation. However, only 4 of 17 had been correctly diagnosed antenatally, while in other cases, preoperative diagnoses entertained included ovarian masses, lymphangiomas, pseudocysts, enteric duplication cysts, and choledochal cysts. Mesenchymal hamartomas have also been noted as an incidental finding at autopsy.

Infants usually present with a history of a nontender enlarging abdomen over a period of days to months. Other symptoms that rarely present are vomiting, decreased appetite, and respiratory distress. There is a slight male predominance but no apparent racial predilection. Physical findings are those associated with the abdominal mass, including a protuberant abdomen and dilated superficial veins. Large masses may eventually produce a mass effect such as vena cava compression, feeding difficulties, and respiratory distress secondary to upward pressure on the diaphragm and may be complicated by ascites, jaundice, and even congestive heart failure. Occasionally, the mass will expand rapidly, most likely because of rapid accumulation of fluid within cystic spaces. Stocker and Ishak (222) reported other anomalies or diseases in 5 of 30 patients, including adrenal cytomegaly, neonatal hyperbilirubinemia, endocardial fibroelastosis of the left ventricle, idiopathic thrombocytopenic purpura, and diffuse endocrinopathy.

Laboratory findings are noncontributory; tumor markers including AFP, β-human chorionic gonadotropin (hCG), and vanillylmandelic acid are usually negative, although rare cases may show elevated AFP levels. Ultrasonography, except in the youngest infants, displays an echogenic mass that may be pedunculated and which displays internal septation and

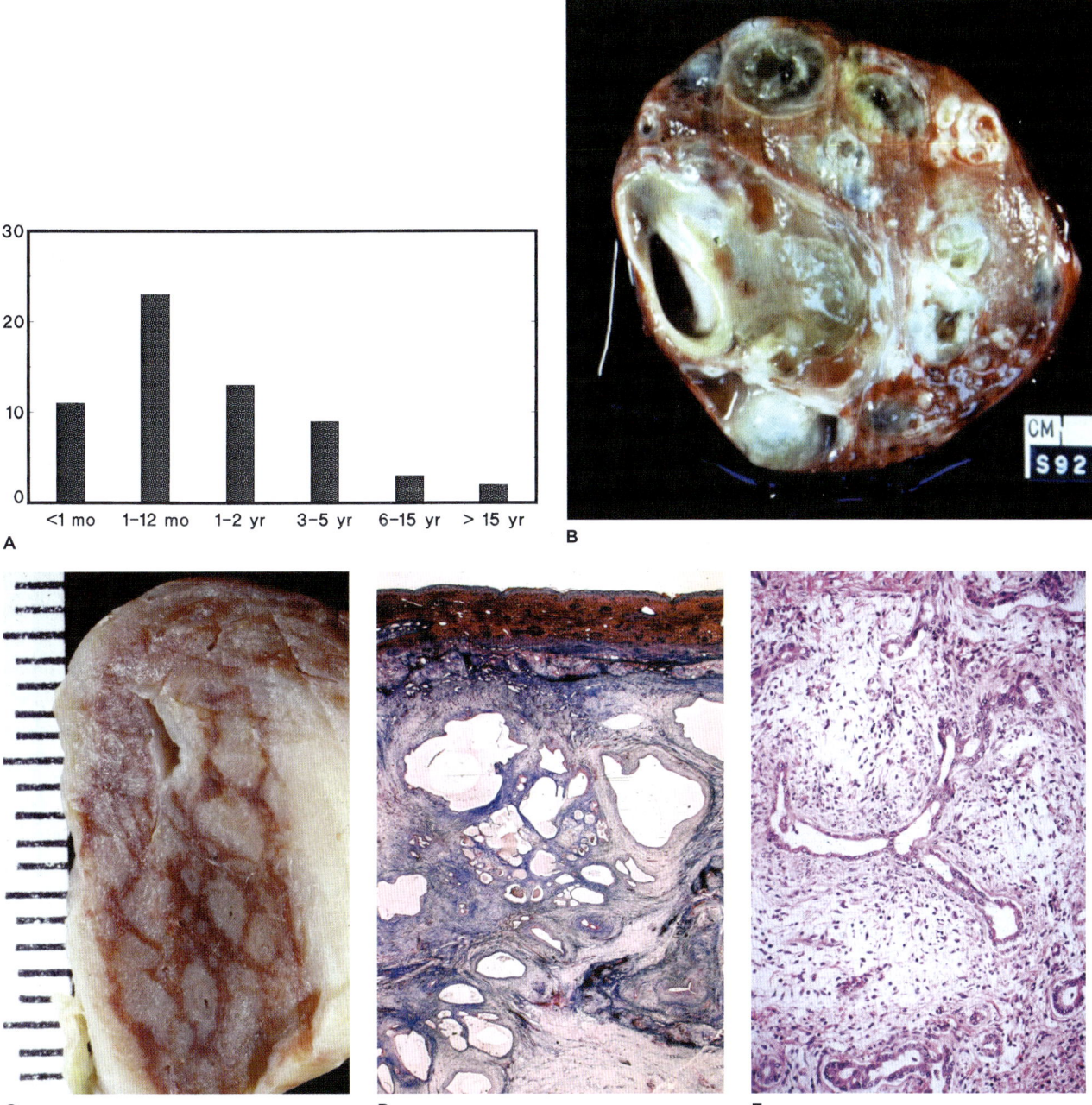

FIGURE 15-48 • Mesenchymal hamartoma. **A:** Age distribution in 71 cases. **B:** Multiple cysts of varying sizes (previously filled with clear yellow fluid) are surrounded by variegated, solid components. **C:** Near the edge of the cystic portion (on the left side of the image), the lesion displays a diffuse infiltration and widening of the portal areas (light tan areas), compressing the intervening hepatocytes lobules into thin brown strips. **D:** The cysts, with no discernible cellular lining, are surrounded by loose to compressed connective tissue, which contains scattered residual bile ducts. Note the compressed liver at top (Masson trichrome stain, original magnification 10×). **E:** Residual bile ducts within the lesion are surrounded by loose mesenchymal tissue containing scattered neutrophils, lymphocytes, and small foci of extramedullary hematopoiesis (H&E stain, original magnification 75×).

cysts. MRI and CT also highlight the multicystic nature of the lesion and can suggest the fluid nature of the cyst contents. The typical CT scan features are that of a well-circumscribed, multilocular, multicystic mass that contains low-density cysts separated by solid septae and stroma. The stroma and septae may be vascular and occasionally show contrast enhancement on CT scan similar to that seen in infantile hemangioma. When the cysts are small, the lesion may appear solid on imaging. Selective arteriography most frequently displays an avascular mass.

Treatment and Outcomes

Surgical resection of the lesion or partial hepatectomy is the treatment of choice. Partial resection with drainage of the cysts and marsupialization has been successful in managing large lesions believed to be impossible to resect completely, but may be associated with recurrence (226). Less invasive techniques, such as laparoscopic fenestration, have also been used successfully. Spontaneous regression of the lesion has been described, prompting some authors to suggest a policy of watchful waiting (227). Others, on the other hand, have used liver transplantation for lesions in those children who are highly symptomatic or are considered to have an unresectable lesion (227).

Prognosis is favorable in patients who undergo complete resection. Of 104 patients who underwent follow-up examination, six had died from intraoperative and postoperative complications; the remaining 98 were alive and well up to 15 years after surgery, except a 4-year-old boy who died of leukemia 2 years after surgery (228). In neonates with large antenatal tumors, vascular compression of great vessels may lead to ischemia complicated by congestive cardiac failure, intraventricular hemorrhage, cystic encephalomalacia, and renal failure. Fluid loss into the cysts and reduced fetal albumin production by the liver can further increase the risk of hydrops. Polyhydramnios is associated with upper intestinal tract obstruction, and elevation of the diaphragm poses the fetus at risk for pulmonary hypoplasia. In their literature review, Cornette et al. (225) observed intrauterine demise or early neonatal mortality in 5 of 17 (29%) antenatally detected cases. In antenatally detected cases, fetal intervention in the form of ultrasound-guided percutaneous cyst aspiration has been reported to dramatically improve outcome. Isaacs reports on 45 patients with mesenchymal hamartoma in the fetal and neonatal period, of which 29 (64%) had surgical resections and 23 (79%) survived (226).

Gross Appearance

The lesions vary in size from a few centimeters, an incidental finding at autopsy, to as large as 30 cm in older patients. The average weight is 1300 to 1900 g, but weights of 5400 g have been reported (222). The right lobe is involved in 75% of cases, the left lobe in 22%, and both lobes in 3%. The tumor may bulge from the surface or even be pedunculated in about 20% of cases, attached to the liver by a thin to broad pedicle.

On cut surface, multiple cysts are present, ranging in size from a few millimeters to 15 cm in over 85% of cases (Figure 15-48B, C). Clear amber to yellow fluid or gelatinous material fills the cyst and is similar to serum, except for lower concentrations of total protein, albumin, immunoglobulin, cholesterol, and glucose. The cysts have gray-tan to yellow linings that may be smooth, long, or ragged. The surrounding tissue is yellow-tan to brown and loose to moderately dense. Only in the youngest patients are the lesions without cysts.

Histopathology

Microscopically, the lesion consists of an admixture of mesenchyme, bile ducts, hepatocyte cords, and variable-sized cysts (Figure 15-48D). The cysts may be no more than a loose, fluid-filled area of mesenchyme or dilated lymphatics or bile ducts. More often, the cysts that are discernible grossly consist of an "unlined" wall of loose to dense mesenchyme. In older patients, however (e.g., those older than 1 to 2 years of age), the cysts may be lined by cuboidal epithelium. The mesenchyme consists of scattered stellate cells in a rich matrix. Collagen in the form of fibrils or small bundles is often associated with vessels and bile ducts within the mesenchyme. Extramedullary hematopoiesis is a consistent finding (more than 85% of cases) (Figure 15-48E), and scattered plasma cells and lymphocytes, although rarely prominent, are seen throughout the lesion. In older patients, more mature collagen bundles may be present. Nodules of mesenchyme may be separated by dense, highly vascular connective tissue. Hepatocytes appear to be a passive component of the lesion, often seen near the periphery of the lesion or as thin compressed strips between collections of mesenchymal tissues within the lesion. Bile ducts, however, appear to be an active or proliferative component, with single ducts or intricately branching ducts primarily near the periphery of the lesion. Bile is rarely present within the ducts. Atypical mitoses and invasion of adjacent liver are absent. Cytologic sampling may result in misdiagnosis due to the heterogeneous nature of the lesion. Although clusters of normal bile duct epithelium and hepatocytes admixed with bland mesenchymal cells in a myxoid background are highly suggestive of HMH on fine-needle aspiration, rare cases with elevated AFP levels have been misdiagnosed as hepatoblastoma due to limited sampling of the hepatocellular component. In a series of 17 cases of HMH, Chang et al. (229) found 7 (41%) to be solid. The solid "variant" was associated with higher serum AFP levels, smaller bile ducts, and more frequent vascular proliferation. Serum AFP level correlated with the proportion of hepatocytes. Two of seven solid cases harbored a larger amount of evenly distributed hepatocytes and proliferation of small ducts with focal hepatocyte–bile duct transition, suggesting that hepatocytes within HMH may be a truly neoplastic rather than an entrapped component.

IHC may be used to rule out other entities. In HMH, bile ducts and hepatocytes are cytokeratin positive, whereas the mesenchyme and pseudocysts are vimentin positive. Myxomatous infantile hemangioendotheliomas (IHEs) can resemble HMH on fine-needle aspiration (FNA) biopsy, but the plump endothelium of the former is positive for factor VIII–related antigen, CD31, and CD34 immunohistochemical stains; however, a localized vascular proliferation within an HMH will stain similarly. Immunostains may not be helpful in differentiating HMH from biphasic hepatoblastomas, and glypican-3 may be positive in the entrapped fetal livers in HMH. However, β-catenin mutations have not been described in HMH, and nuclear staining for β-catenin will help in diagnosis of hepatoblastoma.

Molecular Pathology and Relationship to Undifferentiated Embryonal Sarcoma

Various authors have noted a balanced translocation involving chromosome 11 (band q11, q13, or q15) and chromosome 19 (band 19q13.4) (224). The current understanding is that most HMH represent a neoplastic process with a common t(11;19)(q11;q13.4) breakpoint involving the MALAT1 gene that proximates it with the C19MC microRNA located on chromosome 19q (also known as mesenchymal hamartoma of liver breakpoint 1, MHLB1 locus). Due to this common genetic linkage with UES, it is now believed that recurrences of HMH may actually be due to malignant transformation and/or coexisting UES in these lesions diagnosed as HMH (230). In a case of an undifferentiated (embryonal) sarcoma putatively arising from an HMH, Lauwers et al. (231) demonstrated that the transformed component had the 19q13.4 breakpoint in addition to several other numerical and structural chromosomal abnormalities. Taken together, these findings suggest that a subset of HMH may be truly neoplastic rather than hamartomatous. Shehata et al. (232) have fortified the case reports in the literature suggesting UES arising in an HMH and reported five cases in their series of UES that had transitional areas between HMH and UES, suggesting malignant transformation in HMH as the possible mechanism with acquisition of additional karyotypic defects. Flow cytometric analysis of DNA aneuploidy showed that all three tumor components (HMH, transitional zone, UES) had similar DNA indices, suggesting a common lineage in a study by Begueret et al. (233). While the association of UES and mesenchymal hamartoma is still tenuous, it would be prudent in practice to extensively sample all mesenchymal hamartomas for histologic evaluation, so as not to miss a focus of UES. This may also serve as an indication to resect HMH earlier to prevent possible malignant transformation (227).

VASCULAR TUMORS IN CHILDREN

Vascular tumors in general have undergone a significant change in nomenclature with the new International Society for Study of Vascular Anomalies biology-based classification. The old nomenclature of cavernous hemangioma was changed to a vascular anomaly, and in the liver, the old terminology of IHE has been replaced by congenital and infantile hemangiomas (234). Tumors with the morphology of hemangioendothelioma now represent examples of either epithelioid hemangioendothelioma (EHE) or angiosarcoma of the liver.

Hemangiomas

This group of vascular lesions is the most common types of benign liver tumors accounting for probably up to 17.7% of all liver tumors and 40% of all benign tumors. Most cases are seen in the first year of life.

Congenital Hemangioma

This is a relatively common type of hemangioma that is usually solitary and is present prenatally or noted at birth (226,234). Most lesions are asymptomatic at birth, but can present with features of cardiac failure in the neonatal period. This is due to the presence of high-flow shunts in these lesions. Other clinical manifestations include hepatomegaly and cardiomegaly in an otherwise healthy infant. There may be transient thrombocytopenia (Kasabach-Merrit phenomenon) and anemia. There is no gender predominance, and the lesions frequently undergo spontaneous regression over the first 2 years of life. They may be associated with cutaneous hemangiomas. They are readily visualized on CT and MRI scans as a solitary well-defined spherical tumor, and ultrasonography shows a well-circumscribed vascular lesion with large feeding and draining vessels. In older lesions, calcifications may be noted. They do not demonstrate a growth phase and hence need no active treatment. Histologically, they correspond to the cutaneous congenital hemangiomas and most represent rapidly involuting congenital hemangiomas (RICH). They show lobular or diffuse arrangement of small capillary channels with intervening larger feeding vessels that may be arteries and of venous calibers. They do not show any significant atypia in the endothelial cells and no mitoses are noted. The endothelial cells stain for CD31 and CD34 and are negative for D2-40 and Prox-1 (both lymphatic endothelial markers). They are consistently glucose transporter protein-1 (GLUT-1) negative as opposed to infantile hemangiomas, which eliminates beta blocker therapy as a consideration. Most of these lesions regress over time, but an occasional lesion persists and is thought to represent noninvoluting congenital hemangiomas (NICH) in the Boston series. No effective role for drug therapy has been advocated in this group of lesions (see Chapter 25).

Infantile Hemangioma (IH) (Formerly Called *Infantile Hemangioendothelioma*)

This represents the most common group of lesions in the pediatric age group (234,235). Most cases are seen in the first year of life (Figure 15-49A). None were noted to be present at birth, but do present soon after birth. They are usually multifocal or diffuse large lesions that may occupy a large part of the liver parenchyma. There is a slight female preponderance with more common occurrence in White children. An increased incidence in premature infants has been reported. They are frequently associated with cutaneous hemangiomas that may be multiple. The presence of five cutaneous hemangiomas has been suggested as a marker to evaluate for visceral hemangiomas, especially hepatic lesions. A peculiar presentation of IH is hypothyroidism due to the production of type 3 iodothyronine deiodinase by IH; this converts thyroid hormone into its inactive form leading to progressive hypothyroidism. It has now been recommended to measure TSH levels at diagnosis of hepatic IH. The hypothyroidism can resolve with involution of the IH (235). The diffuse hemangiomas can result in compression of large vessels and abdominal emergencies due to compartment syndrome and acute cardiac failure. These are the ones that require aggressive treatment for stimulation of involution with drugs such as corticosteroids, propranolol (beta blockers), and low-dose vincristine (236). Hepatic transplantation may be necessary in some instances. With multifocal lesions, the more usual outcome is involution following a rapid growth phase. They may be followed by observation alone or treated with chemotherapy depending on the size and symptomatology.

Hemangiomas of the skin have been reported in up to 70% of cases, but in a clinical report of 91 cases, cutaneous hemangiomas were noted in only 11% of cases (237). Isaacs noted cutaneous hemangiomas in 4 (5%) of 76 patients with focal liver tumors, compared to 20 (49%) of 41 patients with multifocal liver lesions (226,235). Associated extrahepatic hemangiomas may also be present in the brain, placenta, lungs, eyes, lymph nodes, pancreas, retroperitoneum, adrenal, or bone as single or multiple lesions (226).

Significant laboratory findings in infantile hemangiomas (IHE) include anemia in about 50% of cases, hyperbilirubinemia in 20% of cases, and elevated aspartate transaminase (over 100 U/dL) in 32% of cases (237). Although in Isaacs' review (226) AFP levels were elevated in 5 fetuses and in 11 neonates (16/117 or 14%) with hemangiomas, the importance of this finding is unclear since even otherwise normal neonates may have elevated AFP levels. Even in the absence of a liver lesion, "adult" levels of AFP (<25 ng/mL) are not reached until 6 months of age, and infants under 1 month of age may normally have levels as high as 2500 ng/mL. When adjusted for the age of the infant, AFP levels are not elevated with infantile hemangioma.

Diagnostic imaging is helpful in the evaluation of infantile hemangiomas (Figure 15-49B). Hepatomegaly with a soft tissue mass is usually visible on plain film of the abdomen, and speckled calcification of the lesion is present in 15% to 37% of cases. Chest radiography may demonstrate cardiomegaly with or without prominent pulmonary vascular markings. Ultrasound examination may show single or multiple hyperechoic, complex, or hypoechoic lesions. If significant arteriovenous shunting is present, a prominent Doppler signal flow is seen. On CT imaging, hepatic hemangiomas manifest as a well-defined, hypoattenuating mass. Contrast enhancement demonstrates peripheral pooling and central enhancement with variable delay. MRI is the most useful single modality because it shows not only the extent of the hemangioma but also the flow characteristics and the surrounding vascular structures (236). Technetium 99m scans display a characteristic early "blush." Imaging studies demonstrate the hepatic origin of the lesion, multifocality, and extrahepatic lesions. Selective arteriography displays diffuse angiomatous lesions with rapid filling of the hepatic vein and can be used to determine the extent of the lesion and possible surgical approaches to the large feeder vessels.

Treatment and Outcomes

Infantile hepatic hemangiomas are benign vascular lesions that show spontaneous involution in most cases. Treatment is determined by the severity of the presenting symptom and whether the lesion is multifocal or diffuse. Patients with congestive heart failure and multifocal lesions are treated with digitalis and diuretics. Although spontaneous regression may occur, steroid therapy is thought by some to hasten the regression of the lesion and improve the platelet count, but is considered by others not to be helpful. Alpha-interferon therapy has also been used as a component of medical management. Radiation therapy has been used in the past, but is infrequently employed now because of the potential long-term side effects. Interventional therapies include hepatic artery ligation or embolization, resectional surgery, or OLT (227). Surgical excision of single lesions, even in the face of congestive heart failure, is frequently successful. Becker and Heitler noted the survival of 46 of 50 infants (92%) who had localized lesions treated with hepatic lobectomy or localized resection (238). For large single lesions or multifocal tumors, success has been achieved through OLT, hepatic artery ligation, or transarterial embolization, often in association with the use of digitalis, diuretics, and steroids (239,240).

Both success and complete failure have been reported variously with many agents including epsilon-aminocaproic acid, tranexamic acid, low-molecular-weight heparin, vincristine, cyclophosphamide, and interferon alpha. A treatment algorithm has been published by the vascular tumors study group at Boston Children's Hospital (234).

Patients with infantile hepatic hemangioma usually have an excellent prognosis, especially with spontaneous regression after the first year of life. Survival in 26 cases reviewed by Becker and Heitler (238) was 65%. Of 71 patients studied at the AFIP who had been followed for at least 6 months, 50 (70%) were alive and well approximately 24 years after diagnosis (mean 7.7 years). Of the 21 deaths, 19 occurred in the first month after diagnosis, and two deaths occurred at 3 and 7 months after diagnosis. Presence of congestive heart failure, jaundice, multiple tumor nodules, and absence of cavernous differentiation were significant predictors of death at 6 months (237). Resection was advocated for the "type 2" infantile hepatic hemangioendothelioma, but these are now considered to represent angiosarcomas in the WHO classification.

Gross Appearance

The tumors are single in about 55% of cases and multiple in 45%. Single tumors measure from smaller than 0.5 cm to as large as 13 cm and are located equally in the right and left lobes, with an occasional single lesion involving both lobes (237). When more than one lesion is present, they may be limited to one lobe but frequently involve large portions of the liver (Figure 15-49B). Lesions near the hepatic surface often show central umbilication. In his review of fetal and neonatal

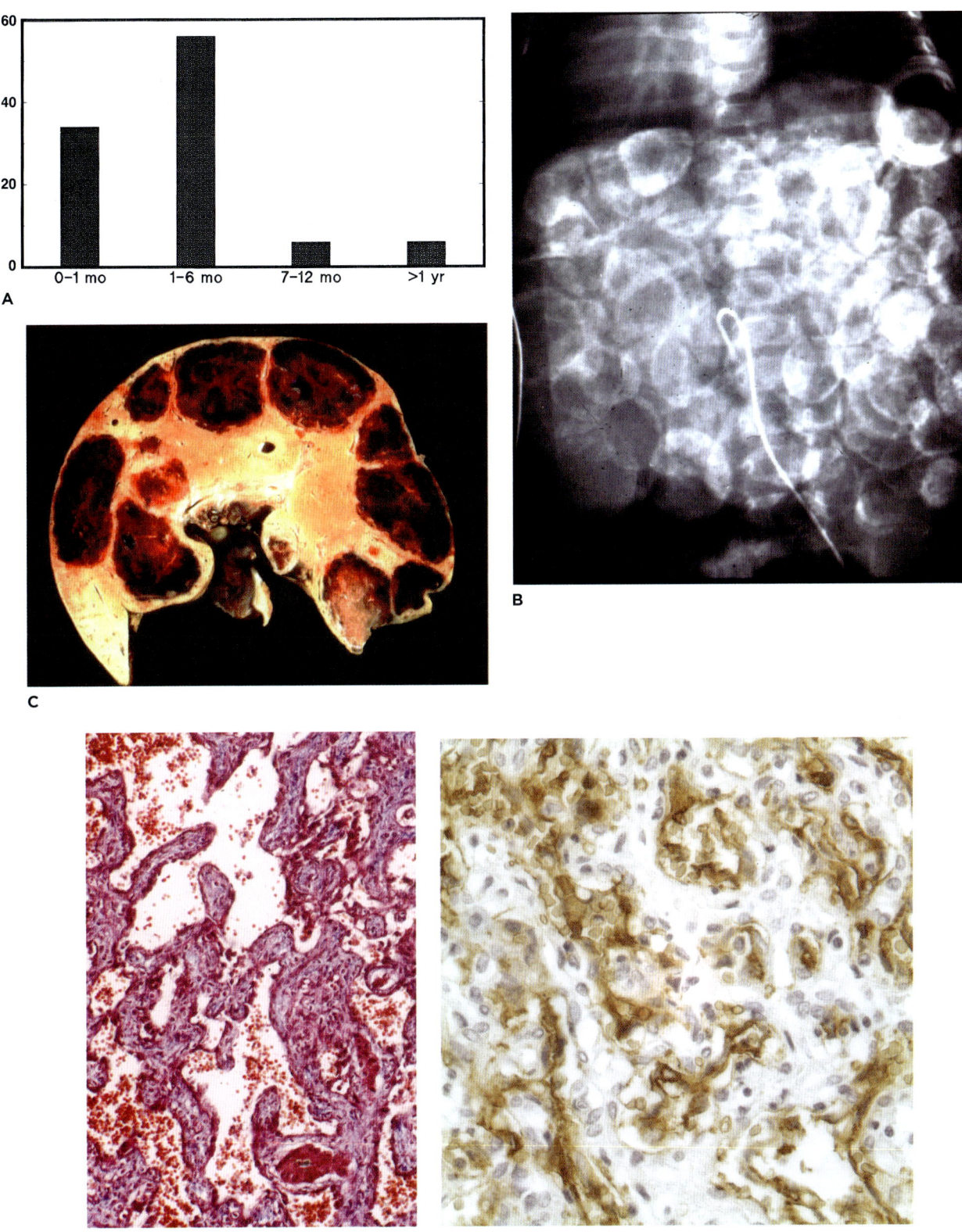

FIGURE 15-49 • Infantile hemangioma. **A:** Age distribution in 102 cases. **B:** Following injection of a radioopaque dye, the liver displays numerous nodules throughout both lobes. **C:** On cut section of the liver, multiple blood-filled nodules are visible. **D:** The lesions of C are composed of trabeculae of loose fibrous connective tissue covered by a single layer of uniform endothelial cells (Masson trichrome stain, original magnification 75×).

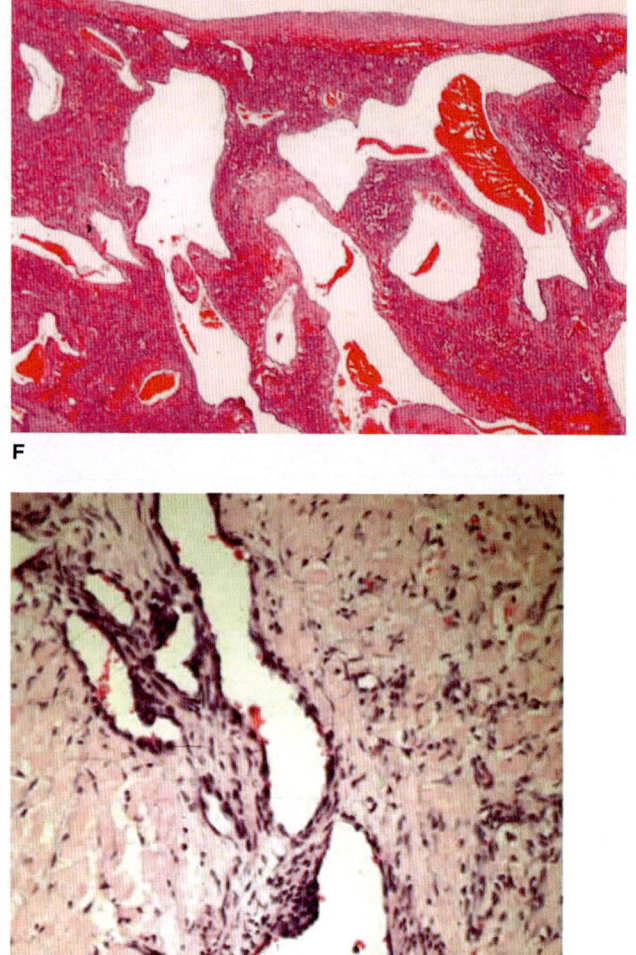

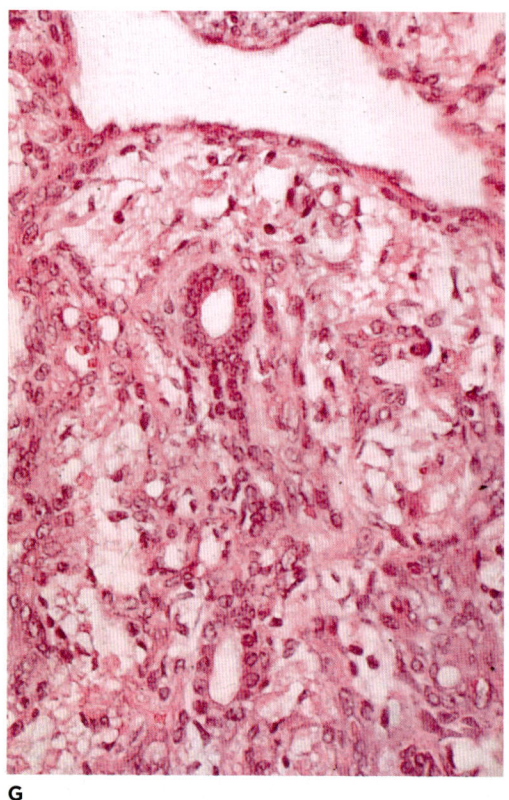

FIGURE 15-49 • (*continued*) **E:** The epithelial cells lining the sinusoid of the lesion stain positively with the GLUT1 stain, a feature of infantile hemangioma (GLUT1 immunoperoxidase stain, original magnification 100×). **F:** Areas of cavernous vascular change are often present at the margin of the hepatic lesion. (H&E stain, original magnification 10×). **G:** Entrapped bile ducts (**center**) can often be found within the fibrous septa. Note the thin covering of endothelial cells at top (H&E stain, original magnification 75×). **H:** Some lesions display dense clusters or "tufts" of endothelial cells felt by many to represent involutional changes within the lesion (H&E stain, original magnification 40×).

cases, Isaacs found 76 solitary and 41 multifocal lesions, the latter also including diffuse lesions. Most focal hemangiomas, 33 (43%) of 76, were found in the right lobe of the liver and 18 (24%) of 76 in the left. Among the 41 multifocal lesions, 11 were limited to the liver, 20 also had cutaneous hemangiomas, and 10 cases showed noncutaneous extrahepatic involvement (226). On cut section, they are well demarcated, reddish brown to light tan, and soft and spongy (Figure 15-49C). In large lesions, central areas of infarction, hemorrhage, fibrosis, and yellowish gritty specks of calcification may be present. In cases preoperatively treated with hepatic artery ligation or embolization, the entire lesion(s) may be infarcted.

Histopathology

Histologically, IHE was traditionally classified as type 1 or type 2 lesion (241). IH (IHE) are composed of vascular channels lined by a single continuous layer of plump endothelial cells in a supporting fibrous stroma (Figure 15-49D–H), reflecting the "type 1" lesion defined by Dehner and Ishak (241). Also, in about 20% of cases, larger pleomorphic and hyperchromatic cells were noted along poorly formed vascular spaces, often displaying tufting or branching, the "type 2" lesion (Figure 15-49H). However, the so-called "type 2" lesions are now grouped together with angiosarcomas (242,243). Well-preserved bile ducts may be present in the supporting stroma, most frequently near the periphery of the lesion. Foci of extramedullary hematopoiesis are noted within the vascular spaces in over 60% of patients. Mitoses are infrequent but rarely may number 5 to 10 per high-power field. Larger vascular channels resembling cavernous hemangioma may be found in 50% to 65% of patients, usually at the periphery of the lesion, and may represent shunt vessels (Figure 15-49F). Areas of hemorrhage, infarction, fibrosis, and calcification may occupy small to large areas of the lesion, occasionally obliterating all but the margin of the lesion. When hemorrhage or fibrovascular reaction dominates the biopsy, it is difficult to differentiate the stroma of an IH from that of a mesenchymal hamartoma. Discussion with the pediatric radiologist may help sort this differential diagnosis (243). One should also remember that hemorrhagic necrosis can be seen in IHE, but is uncommon in mesenchymal hamartoma. The presence of hemorrhagic necrosis in a biopsy should also raise the possibility of a hepatoblastoma. Another vascular lesion with a myxoid stroma is hepatic EHE, albeit rare in children. This is a multifocal tumor, comprised of strands, clusters, and nests of CD31-positive epithelioid cells with intracellular lumina and sinusoidal infiltration (243).

Immunohistochemically, the endothelial cells of IH are positive for CD31, CD34, factor VIII–related antigen, von Willebrand factor, vimentin, and Ulex europaeus I lectin. Cerar et al. (244) noted that the cells beneath the endothelial cells contained cytoplasm that was positive for alpha–smooth muscle actin and antimuscle actin and negative for desmin and were enveloped with basement membrane (BM) that they believed were characteristic of pericytes. Electron microscopy displays vascular channels lined by endothelial cells with irregular fine cytoplasmic processes along the luminal surface. Fibroblasts and collagen fibers are present in the stroma. The "type 2 lesion" with multilayered, hyperchromatic endothelial cells in a tufted or branching pattern is now thought to represent a form of angiosarcoma (see later), but could represent degenerative change.

Mo et al. (245) and others (246) use the presence or absence of GLUT1 immunoreactivity of the endothelial lining in separating the "true infantile hemangioma" (hemangioendothelioma) from a "hepatic vascular malformation with capillary proliferation." Similar phenotype has also been described by the Boston group who term the latter group as RICH. Lymphatic markers such as D2-40 and Prox-1 are negative in both lesions and may highlight a few scattered normal lymphatics at the edges. Presence of large numbers of D2-40 or Prox-1 channels would raise the possibility of a kaposiform hemangioendothelioma or even an EHE involving the liver.

EHE is a rare tumor in childhood, but has been reported in the second decade of life. It is a tumor of intermediate malignant potential and falls between an IH and angiosarcoma. These are characterized by large plump endothelial cells with epithelioid, dendritic, and intermediate characteristics. The cells show vacuolated, signet ring–type cells with cytoplasmic lumina containing erythrocytes. The cells diffusely infiltrate the sinusoids and cause atrophy of the liver cell plates. The mitotic rate is variable and can be low. The tumor cells stain for CD34 and CD31 as well as for keratins. D2-40 may be positive in the tumor cells.

Molecular Pathology

Flow cytometry performed by Selby et al. (237) on 21 cases showed 16 tumors to be diploid, 3 to be aneuploid, and 2 with a wide coefficient of variation. Ito et al. described an interstitial deletion of chromosome 6q in a 6-month-old boy with hepatic infantile hemangioma, microcephaly, hypertelorism, low-set ears, prominent nasal bridge, cubitus valgus, overlapping fingers, cryptorchidism, and micropenis (247). Other anomalies reported in association with infantile hemangioma include trisomy 21, extranumerary digit, hydrocele, and congenital heart disease (237). More recently, a specific translocation t(1;3)(p36;q25) has been found in multifocal hepatic epithelioid HE and other EHE that results in a WWTR1–CAMTA1 fusion protein (248).

TERATOMA

Teratoma involving the liver is a rarely occurring benign neoplasm composed of a mixture of tissue of mesodermal, ectodermal, and endodermal origin. Most pediatric cases occur in the first year of life, presenting as an abdominal mass, which on plain film frequently displays areas of calcification. AFP may be elevated. Associated conditions include anencephaly and trisomy 13. Resection may be curative. Care should be taken not to confuse teratoma with a mixed hepatoblastoma with teratoid features (249). Intrahepatic fetus-in-fetu has been reported.

These lesions are large, with a variegated cut surface reflecting the various tissues of the tumor (Figure 15-50). Microscopically, benign tissues of all three germ cell layers may be found, including well-differentiated squamous epithelium, bone, cartilage, gastrointestinal mucosa and muscularis propria, renal glomeruli and tubules, respiratory epithelium, and neural tissue. The presence of embryonal or fetal hepatoblastoma cells precludes the diagnosis of teratoma and instead favors mixed hepatoblastoma with teratoid features or teratoid hepatoblastoma.

HEPATOBLASTOMA

The prevalence of primary hepatic malignancies in children 0 to 14 years of age is approximately 0.2 per 100,000 children in the United States, with hepatoblastomas accounting for 47% of the malignancies and nearly 27% of all pediatric hepatic tumors (250). By age group, hepatoblastoma accounts for 1% of all pediatric malignancies in children under 15 years age, 1.5% of all malignancies in children younger than 5 years of age, and 3.3% of all malignancies in white and black children under 1 year of age (251). The reported incidence is 11.2 cases per million during the first year of life. Almost 90% of

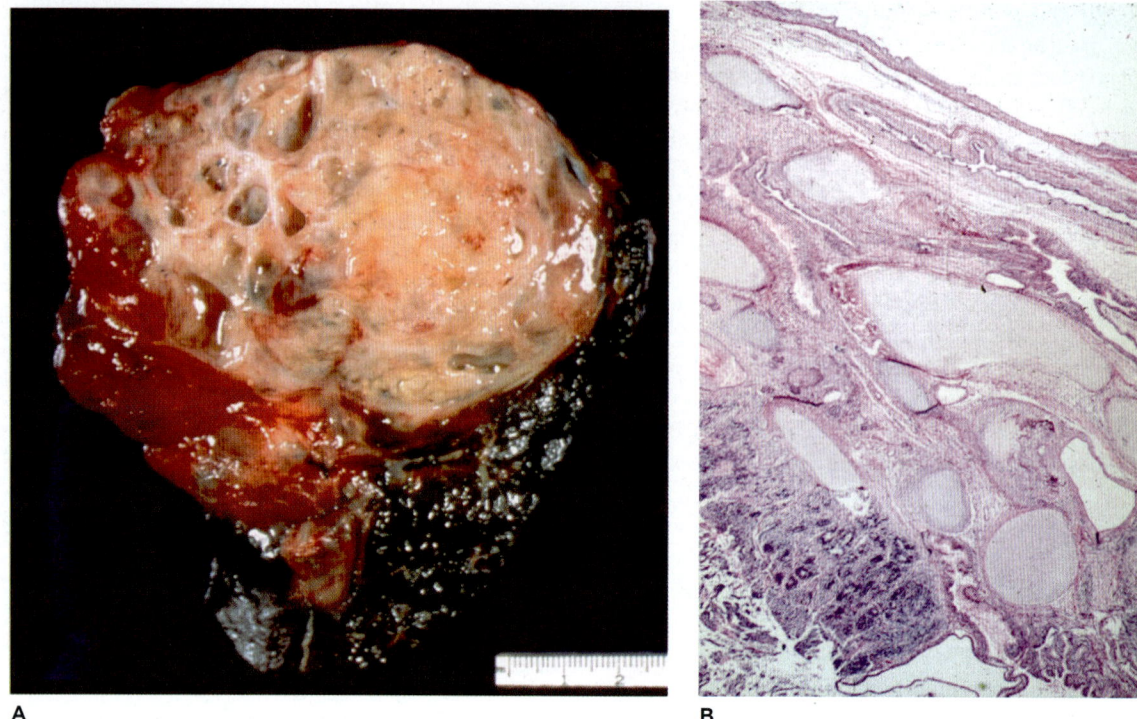

FIGURE 15-50 • Teratoma. **A:** A large irregular mass contains both solid and cystic components of varying color. **B:** Random sampling of the lesion displays tissues of various somatic lines including, in this image, cartilage, epithelial-lined ducts, and "immature" tissue (**lower left**). (H&E stain, original magnification 15×).

hepatoblastomas are seen in the first 5 years of life, with 68% discovered in the first 2 years and 4% present at the time of birth (Figure 15-51). Of 271 primary hepatic malignancies reported in the United States to Surveillance, Epidemiology and End Results (SEER) data between 1973 and 1997 in patients below 20 years of age, 67% and 31% were HB and HCC, respectively. More recent data suggest an overall increase in the incidence of hepatoblastomas in children (252). In the group less than 5 years of age, HB accounted for 91% of malignant liver tumors, whereas among those 15 to 19 years of age, HCC represented 87% of the cases (250). The relative frequency of hepatoblastomas in younger children is most apparent when noting that hepatoblastomas account for over 40% of all hepatic tumors (benign and malignant) in children younger than 2 years of age, but only 7.5% of liver tumors in children 5 to 20 years old. Although there is no racial predilection for hepatoblastoma, there is a distinct male predominance from 1.2:1 to 3.6:1.

Pathogenesis

There appears to be a genetic predisposition to hepatoblastomas, with an increased prevalence in a setting of Beckwith-Wiedemann syndrome (macrosomia, macroglossia, visceromegaly, abdominal wall defects, hemihypertrophy), hemihypertrophy, and familial adenomatous polyposis (FAP). The relative risk for the development of hepatoblastoma in Beckwith-Wiedemann syndrome is 22.80 (253), while that for FAP is 12.20 (254), suggesting a role for genetic aberrations of chromosomes 11 and 5, respectively, in the pathogenesis of hepatoblastoma. Inactivation of the APC tumor-suppressor gene (chromosome 5q21) is found in 67% to 89% of sporadic hepatoblastoma (255,256). This gene is known to regulate β-catenin and modulate the *Wnt* signaling pathway, suggesting a role for this signaling pathway in the development of hepatoblastoma. Additional biologic markers may include trisomies 2, 8, and 20 and translocation of the NOTCH2 gene on chromosome 1. There is also an association of prematurity with low birth weight and hepatoblastoma, with a relative risk of up to 15.64 in patients weighing less than 1000 g, compared with patients weighing 2500 g (251). In Japan, Ikeda et al. (257) have noted an increasing incidence of hepatoblastoma in very low-birth-weight infants from 0.7% of patients with birth weights less than

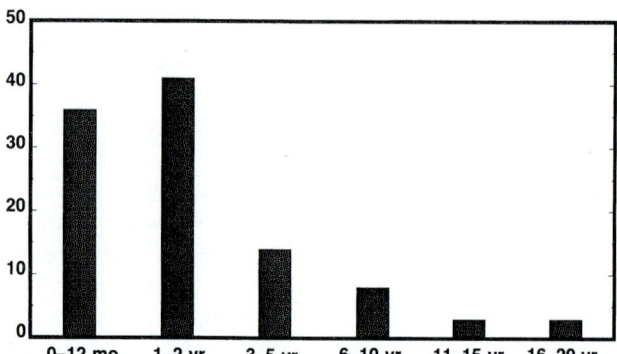

FIGURE 15-51 • Hepatoblastoma. Age distribution in 105 cases.

1500 g with tumors in 1985 to 1989 to 8.6% of patients with similar low birth weights in 1990 to 1993. A similar association has also been well documented in the United States.

Hepatoblastoma has been described in association with trisomy 18, as well as some cases with abdominal wall defects. Hepatoblastoma has been noted in a number of sibling pairs including identical male twins and two siblings with GSD type 1a. There are no known environmental risk factors, although recently an association with parental tobacco smoking has been reported (251).

Clinical Features, Laboratory Studies, and Imaging

Most patients present with an enlarged abdomen noted by a parent or discovered on routine physical examination. Other symptoms such as anorexia, weight loss (less frequently), nausea, vomiting, and abdominal pain may indicate advanced disease. Jaundice is noted in about 5% of cases. Physical examination reveals a firm, often irregular, mass in the right upper abdomen that may cross the midline and extend down to the pelvic rim. A variety of malformations and clinical presentations have been described in patients with hepatoblastoma (Table 15-20). A striking presentation of hepatoblastoma is seen in children (particularly young boys) whose tumors produce hCG, leading to precocious puberty with genital enlargement, the appearance of pubic hair, and a deepening voice. The increased levels of hCG correlate with immunohistochemical staining and are accompanied by increases in serum luteinizing hormone and plasma testosterone (258).

Anemia is common (70%) in patients with hepatoblastoma, as is thrombocytosis (50% of cases). Platelet counts of greater than 500×10^6/L were noted in 35% of 99 cases reported by Shafford and Pritchard (259), with 29% having counts over 800×10^6/L. Along with AFP, thrombocytosis has been used as a measure of disease activity. Approximately 90% of patients demonstrate elevated serum AFP levels, and there is a correlation between AFP levels and extent of disease, with a return to normal levels after complete resection of the tumor and a re-elevation with recurrence (260). AFP levels however may be normal or low (<100 ng/mL) at diagnosis and usually associated with worse outcome possibly due to increased association with small-cell undifferentiated (SCU) histology although similar low levels have been seen with other histologic subtypes. It has been noted that for unresectable or metastatic hepatoblastoma, AFP levels can reliably predict outcome and identify poor responders to treatment. In patients who have undergone initial surgery and chemotherapy, those patients whose AFP fail to decrease by at least two logs have a much poorer prognosis. In contrast, a large early decrease in AFP levels is a strong independent predictor of favorable outcome. It is important to remember, however, that AFP is present at levels of 25,000 to 50,000 ng/mL at birth and does not fall to "adult" levels of less than 25 ng/mL until 5 to 6 months of age. AFP levels in infants with tumors resected in the first 6 months of life may therefore be "appropriately" elevated even though the tumor has been completely resected.

Isaacs reviewed 32 cases of hepatoblastomas reported in fetuses and neonates (226). Nine cases were diagnosed antenatally and 23 at birth, with a female predominance (female to male ratio 1.6). Although the most common presenting

TABLE 15-20 CLINICAL SYNDROMES, CONGENITAL MALFORMATIONS, AND OTHER CONDITIONS ASSOCIATED WITH HEPATOBLASTOMA

Absence of left adrenal gland
Aicardi syndrome
Alcohol embryopathy
Beckwith-Wiedemann syndrome
Beckwith-Wiedemann syndrome with opsoclonus, myoclonus
Bilateral talipes
Budd-Chiari syndrome
Cleft palate, macroglossia, dysplasia of ear lobes
Cystathioninuria
Down syndrome, malrotation of colon, Meckel diverticulum, pectum excavatum, intrathoracic kidney, single coronary artery
Duplicated ureters
Fetal hydrops
Gardner syndrome
Goldenhar syndrome oculoauriculovertebral dysplasia, absence of portal vein
Hemihypertrophy
Heterotopic lung tissue
Heterozygous A1AT deficiency
HIV or HBV infection
Horseshoe kidney
Hypoglycemia
Inguinal hernia
Isosexual precocity
Maternal clomiphene citrate and Pergonal
Meckel diverticulum
Oral contraceptive, mother
Oral contraceptive, patient
Osteoporosis
Persistent ductus arteriosus
Polyposis coli families
Prader-Willi syndrome
Renal dysplasia
Right-sided diaphragmatic hernia
Schinzel-Giedion syndrome
Synchronous Wilms tumor
Trisomy 18
Type 1a GSD
Umbilical hernia
Very low birth weight

From Ishak KG, Goodman Z, Stocker JT. Tumors of the liver and intrahepatic bile ducts. In: Rosai J, Sobin L, eds. *Atlas of tumor pathology*, 3rd series, Washington, DC: Fascicle; Armed Forces Institute of Pathology, 2000.

finding was an elevated AFP, this finding was present only in 50% of the patients, suggesting that AFP levels may not be a reliable indicator of the tumor in the fetus and neonate as compared with older children. Abdominal distension was the second common presenting finding followed in rank by a palpable abdominal mass, hepatic or abdominal mass detected on antenatal sonography, and hepatomegaly. Anemia, fetal hydrops, and respiratory distress were other initial findings. The most common site of origin was the right lobe of the liver (47%) compared with the left lobe (16%), or both lobes (6%). Four patients had more than one hepatic tumor at the time of diagnosis. Most patients were classified as stage 1 (37.5%), none as stage 2, 4 (12.5%) as stage 3, and 6 (18.8%) as stage 4. In 10 patients (31.2%), the stage of disease was not mentioned in the report. Survival rates for stages 1, 3, and 4 were 50%, 50%, and 0%, respectively. Sixty-three percent of the patients were treated by the following modalities: surgical resection alone, surgical resection plus chemotherapy, and surgical resection with hepatic artery embolization and chemotherapy with survival rates being 3 of 9 (33%), 3 of 5 (60%), and 1 of 1 (100%), respectively. Only one of four infants who received chemotherapy alone after a biopsy survived. Fetal survival was slightly less than the neonatal diagnosed cases, 22% and 26%, respectively. All 12 untreated patients died. Of the 20 treated infants, 8 (40%) lived. The overall survival for hepatoblastoma group was poor, with 8 of 32 (25%) surviving. The main cause of death from hepatoblastoma was mass effect by the tumor producing abdominal distension, compression of portal vein and inferior vena cava, fetal hydrops leading to stillbirth, and severe respiratory distress. Metastases to the placenta with occlusion of umbilical vessels and to the lungs were other terminal events. Anemia resulting from bleeding into the tumor and rupture of the tumor during delivery occurred in seven and four patients, respectively. There were a few perioperative deaths related to immaturity and clinical condition of the patients. Female to male ratio was 1.6:1. Of 32 cases, 9 (28%) were diagnosed antenatally and 23 (72%) in the neonatal period. Tumors ranged in size from 3 to 16 cm (mean 8 cm) and weighed from 21 to 429 Gm (mean 160 Gm). The relation of histology and survival was as follows: fetal 3/10 (30%); embryonal 1/6 (17%); fetal and embryonal 1/2 (50%); and fetal, embryonal, and mesenchymal 3/8 (37.5%).

Imaging studies are helpful in diagnosing hepatoblastoma and differentiating it from other liver disorders in young children (261). CT demonstrates a solitary or occasionally multifocal mass(es) with attenuation values between those of water and normal liver parenchyma. Speckled or amorphous calcification may be seen on CT in more than 50% of cases. Ultrasonography displays a mass with increased, nonhomogeneous echogenicity, punctate or amorphous calcifications, and occasional cystic areas. On antenatal ultrasonography, hepatoblastomas are described as well-defined, solid, echogenic lesions, with a "spoked-wheel" appearance. A pseudocapsule gives the lesion(s) a characteristic well-demarcated appearance (226). Differentiation of hepatoblastoma from other childhood hepatic solid, cystic, or vascular lesions, such as mesenchymal hamartoma, infantile hemangioma, and HCC, can be aided by MRI with standard spin-echo T1- and T2-weighted imaging enhanced by the application of advanced sequences, such as gradient-echo, fast spin-echo, and fat suppression techniques (262). The histologic features of hepatoblastomas can be differentiated to a certain extent by MRI as well, with the homogenous character of an "epithelial" lesion contrasting with the heterogeneous character of a "mixed" hepatoblastoma with its fibrotic bands. Decreased signal intensity compared with normal liver is noted on T1-weighted images, whereas increased signal intensity is seen on T2-weighted images. Hypointense bands on MRI identify fibrotic bands, and the presence of vascular invasion may be detected by gradient-echo MRI (261).

Staging

Most patients in the United States are staged postoperatively according to the Children's Cancer Study Group (CCSG) classification (262,263) (see Table 15-21). Other classifications include the TNM or variations of the CCSG staging classification. Based on these classifications, approximately 38% of hepatoblastomas are stage I at the time of initial diagnosis and before any chemotherapy is administered. At this same point, about 9% are stage II, 24% stage III, and 29% stage IV (264). However, this traditional staging system has been criticized for being rather subjective, depending to a large extent on the surgeon rather than the tumor. In 1990, the International Society of Pediatric Oncology Liver Study Group (SIOPEL-1) adopted a new preoperative staging system, Pretreatment Extent of Disease (PRETEXT), based exclusively on images obtained *prior to surgery*, based on the branching pattern of the portal vein, which divides the liver into eight segments. The system divides the liver into four sectors: (a) lateral sector (Couinaud segments 2 and 3), (b) medial sector (segment 4), (c) anterior sector (segments 5 and 8), and (d) posterior sector (segments 6 and 7). Tumors are

TABLE 15-21	STAGING OF HEPATOBLASTOMAS (COG)
Stage I	Complete resection
Stage II	Microscopic residual tumor
	Intrahepatic
	Extrahepatic
Stage III	Gross residual tumor
	Primary completely resected, nodes positive and/or tumor spill
	Primary not completely resected, and/or nodes positive and/or tumor spill
Stage IV	Metastatic disease
	Primary completely resected
	Primary not completely resected

From King D, Ortega J, Campbell J. The surgical management or children with incompletely resected hepatic cancer is facilitated by intensive chemotherapy. *J Pediatr Surg* 1991;26:1074–1081, with permission.

classified as one of four categories (PRETEXT-I to PRETEXT IV) by determining the number of affected liver sector(s) on imaging. Extrahepatic growth of the tumor is indicated by adding a letter (V involvement of hepatic vein, P involvement of portal vein, E for extrahepatic extension, M for the presence of distant metastasis). The PRETEXT system has prognostic value for overall and disease-free survival and is useful in defining treatment (263). Although the PRETEXT system was developed mainly to assess the efficacy of neoadjuvant chemotherapy and to predict surgical resectability, it also had highly prognostic value for both overall survival and event-free survival. Conceptually, both preoperative and postoperative staging systems (POST-TEXT) use the same parameters for staging, namely, size, vascular invasion, extension and complexity of the primary tumor, and the absence or presence of metastases. Metastatic spread of hepatoblastoma is seen most frequently to the lung but may also spread to the bone, brain, eye, and ovaries. Local extension into the hepatic vessels and the inferior vena cava also occurs and is incorporated into the PRETEXT staging system.

Treatment and Outcomes

Although complete resection of hepatoblastoma is the mainstay of treatment and is the only chance of cure, improvements in survival that have occurred over the last three decades have been a function of standardized chemotherapy regimens that reduce tumor size and enable complete tumor excision, even permitting cure in the presence of initially unresectable or metastatic disease. Treatment strategies currently combine surgery, transplantation, and chemotherapy (adjuvant and neoadjuvant), as defined by the PRETEXT stage of the tumor. Surgery remains the mainstay in the treatment of hepatoblastoma, with prognosis directly related to tumor stage. Small, solitary lesions localized to a single lobe can be adequately treated by lobectomy. Larger lesions, including those requiring preoperative chemotherapy to allow resection, may require more extensive surgery or transplantation (252,262,265). Surgical complications, particularly hemorrhage, are noted with primary and second resections. If resection is possible and safely accomplished, an attempt to obtain negative resection margins is essential; positive margins on histopathologic examination warrant a reresection if possible. Although elevated AFP immediately after resection is common, persistently elevated or rising AFP levels indicate the need to evaluate further for disease recurrence or search for distant metastasis. Contraindications to immediate resection include extensive bilateral liver involvement, presence of vascular invasion of major hepatic veins or inferior vena cava, diffuse multifocal disease, and distant metastasis.

At the time of diagnosis, 40% to 60% of hepatoblastomas are considered to be unresectable and 10% to 20% of patients are found to have pulmonary metastases. Preoperative chemotherapy converts nearly 85% of these "unresectable" lesions to ones that can undergo gross total excision, converting the tumors effectively to stage I or II lesion (see Table 15-21), and improve subsequent long-term survival (260,262). Even if unresectable at diagnosis, most hepatoblastomas are unifocal and chemosensitive, with cisplatin and Adriamycin being the most commonly used agents. Chemotherapy has proven effective in both adjuvant and neoadjuvant treatments and can markedly shrink tumors. It makes them less prone to bleed and delineates the tumor from the surrounding normal parenchyma and vascular structures facilitating resection. In rare cases, patients may survive with chemotherapy alone. On the other hand, some tumors may become resistant following prolonged courses of chemotherapy. The highest survival rates have historically been observed in patients with initially resected tumors, although these tumors tend to be the smaller more favorable tumors. The histology of the resected primary tumor also helps in determining adjuvant chemotherapy with a pure fetal low mitotic activity tumor (well-differentiated fetal HB [WDFHB]) currently not requiring chemotherapy (266). Prolonged (>4 cycles) courses of neoadjuvant chemotherapy are discouraged, since this may lead to cumulative chemotherapy toxicity and cause tumor cells to become resistant to chemotherapy.

The 5-year survival rate for hepatoblastomas has improved to over 75% compared with a 5-year survival rate of 35% almost 30 years ago (227). Preoperative chemotherapy has increased resectability of hepatoblastoma from 40% to 60% in the past to 90% currently, with more extensive tumors requiring liver transplantation. In fact, primary liver transplantation with neoadjuvant chemotherapy may result in an 80% 5- to 10-year disease-free survival rate. whereas the 10-year survival falls to 40% in those undergoing liver transplantation as "rescue therapy" (252). The SIOPEL-1 study showed that in patients undergoing transplantation, only macroscopic venous invasion had a significant prognostic effect on survival. A worldwide electronic registry for liver transplant in childhood liver tumors (hepatoblastoma, HCC, hemangioma) has been established; this "pediatric liver unresectable tumor observatory (PLUTO)" registry can be reached at http://transplant.test.cineca.it/. Additional international databases such as the Children's Hepatic Tumor International Collaboration (CHIC) are evaluating outcomes and prognostic factors for HB (262).

Traditionally, tumor stage at the time of initial resection has been the key prognostic factor in determining the survival of children and adults with hepatoblastoma. Data from a recent COG study show 3-year event-free survival of 90% for stages I and II, 50% for stage III, and only 20% for stage IV (227). However, as noted earlier, preoperative and postoperative chemotherapy and aggressive treatment of pulmonary and central nervous system metastases have significantly changed the survival rate in patients with stage IV tumors. Survival is independent of histologic subtype when adjusted for age, sex, and stage. Only SCU hepatoblastoma may have a worse prognosis than others, but the small number of cases makes analysis uncertain (267). More recently, two broad categories of risk stratification have been advocated, namely, standard risk and high risk. Standard risk tumors are PRETEXT I, II, or III. SIOPEL high-risk tumors are defined as tumors involving all four hepatic sectors (PRETEXT IV), or any tumor with metastasis (m), ingrowth of the vena cava (v), ingrowth of the portal vein (p) or contiguous extrahepatic disease (e), and tumors that fail to express AFP (AFP <100 at diagnosis) (260). The Children's Oncology Group (COG) has adopted a 4-tier system with very low-risk, low-risk, intermediate-risk, and high-risk categories in its latest therapeutic trial. The very low-risk category is determined by primary surgical resection of a stage 1 tumor that demonstrates a well-differentiated fetal histology, with no adjuvant chemotherapy given in the current COG trial. There is an attempt to standardize the therapy of HB on a worldwide basis with collaborations among several oncologic groups.

Gross Appearance

Hepatoblastomas are single masses in approximately 80% of cases. They occur in the right lobe in 58% of cases, in the left in 15%, and in both lobes in the remaining 27%, either as a large single lesion extending across the midline or as multiple lesions (209,268). Distant metastasis is present in 20% of patients at the time of diagnosis, with the lung being the most common site of metastasis; other common sites are the brain and bone, and metastasis occurs more commonly with disease relapse.

Tumors may measure 15 cm or more in diameter and weigh in excess of 1000 g. Grossly, they are coarsely lobulated and frequently bulge from the surface of the liver (Figure 15-52A). On cut section, the lesions are tan to light

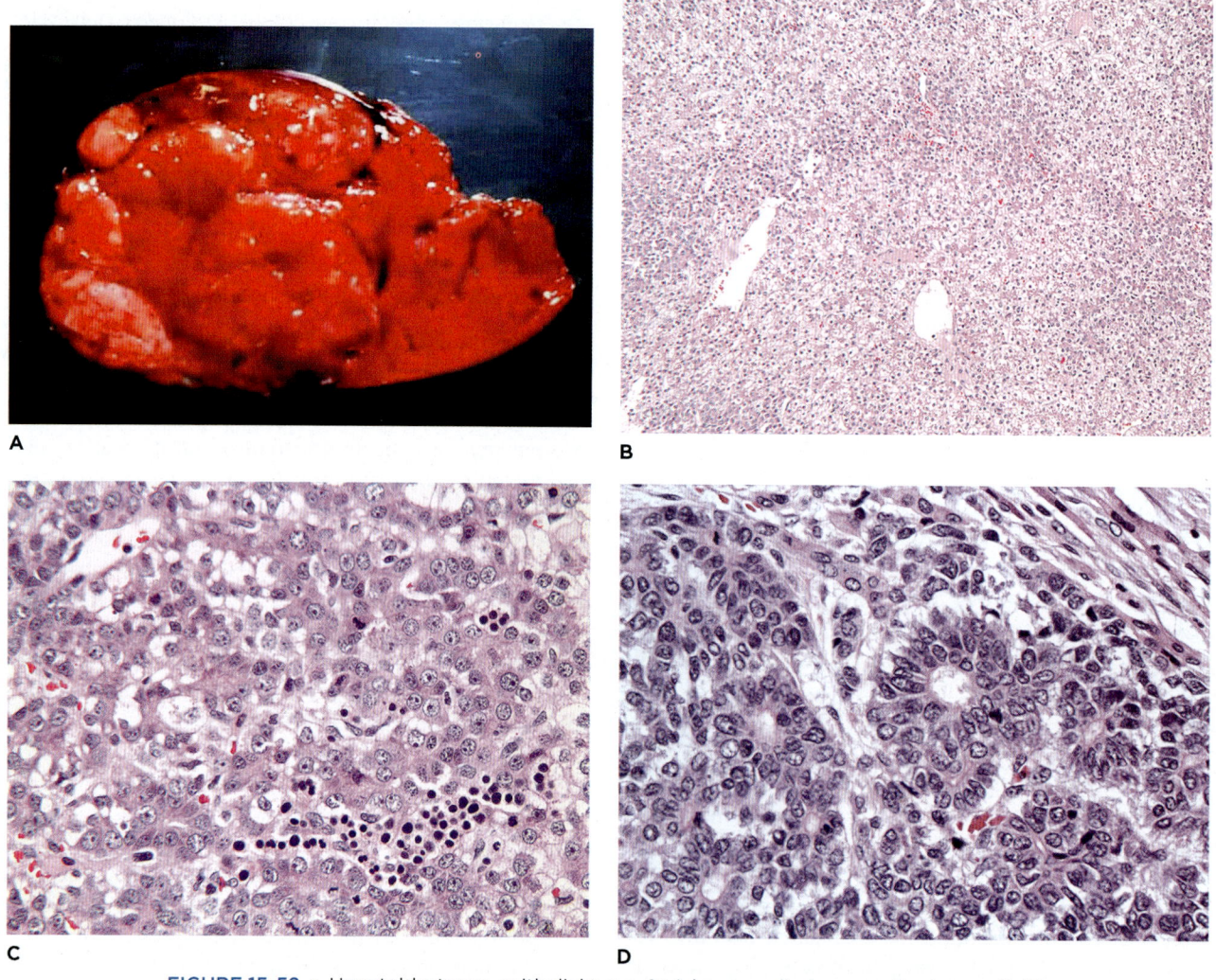

FIGURE 15-52 • Hepatoblastoma, epithelial type. **A:** A large, well-circumscribed mass (**left**) is composed of irregular nodules of tissue resembling normal liver. **B:** A light and dark cell pattern is produced by trabeculae of uniform small hepatocytes with clear (*light*) or granular (*dark*) cytoplasm in this well-differentiated fetal epithelial HB (H&E stain, original magnification 40×). **C:** The fetal mitotically active (crowded fetal) component is composed of polygonal cells with increased N:C ratio, round nucleus with small nucleoli, mitoses, and foci of extramedullary hematopoiesis (H&E stain, original magnification 400×). **D:** An embryonal component of epithelial HB is composed of cells with high N:C ratio, angulated to oval (not round) nuclei with variable nucleoli, mitoses, rosettes and scant cytoplasm (H&E stain, original magnification 400×).

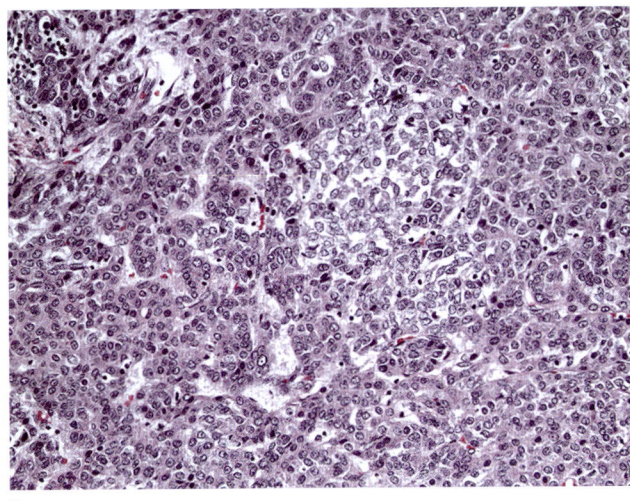
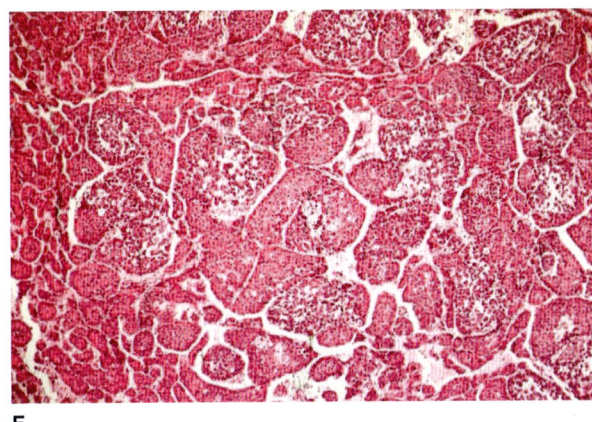

FIGURE 15-52 • (continued) **E:** This image shows an epithelial HB with areas of mitotically active fetal and embryonal cells showing a pale central aggregate of small round to oval cells with no cytoplasm and scant mitosis forming the SCU pattern (H&E stain, original magnification 200×). **F:** A "macrotrabecular" pattern is formed by solid sheets of hepatocytes, some with central areas of necrosis (H&E, original magnification 40×).

brown to green and display frequent areas of hemorrhage and necrosis. Various types of mesenchymal tissues (osteoid, cartilaginous, fibrous) in the mixed type of hepatoblastoma may alter the color and consistency of the gross appearance. Most tumors today are resected after chemotherapy which appreciably alters the classic gross features.

Histopathology

The histology of HB has broadly remained the same over the years with only additional recognition of morphologic variants and patterns that may or may not affect therapy and prognosis (268,269). They were recently updated in the new International Consensus Classification (270) (Table 15-22). The different morphologic subtypes are described below, and salient immunohistochemical features are summarized in Table 15-23. More often than not, most HBs are initially encountered in a biopsy so that the application of this classification is limited as well as in the resected specimen.

Fetal HB

Well-Differentiated Fetal HB (WDFHB)

This variant is frequently present within tumors either as part of an epithelial component or in rare instances may be the sole component in a biopsy or resection specimen. The significance of identifying this subtype is to advocate up-front surgery if possible for total resection of the tumor as the prognosis is favorable in these children with no need for adjuvant therapy. The microscopic features are made up of small uniform-appearing hepatocytes arranged in trabeculae that are 2-cell thick with no nuclear atypia or pleomorphism and small round centrally placed nucleus in abundant pale vacuolated to eosinophilic cytoplasm. This gives the tumor a characteristic "light and dark cell pattern" (Figure 15-52B). The morphologic criterion for this tumor is a low mitotic rate of <2 per 10 high-power fields (hpf). IHC is helpful in identifying these areas as they show a fine stippled pericanalicular pattern of staining with glypican-3 (GPC3), with variable β-catenin staining that is only focal and rarely diffusely nuclear and more often membranous, and strong glutamine synthetase (GS) staining. The tumor cells show low cyclin D1 expression (270).

"Crowded" Fetal or Fetal with Mitoses HB

This variant is the most common subtype of epithelial HB and closely merges with areas of WDFHB and embryonal HB. The tumor cells resemble fetal hepatocytes and have some increase in nuclear to cytoplasmic ratio, but retain the dark, eosinophilic to amphophilic cytoplasm. The nuclei are variable and

TABLE 15-22	HISTOLOGIC CLASSIFICATION OF HEPATOBLASTOMA

I. Epithelial type
  A. Fetal pattern
    Well-differentiated fetal pattern (≤2 mitoses per 10 40× high power fields)
    Fetal with mitoses (>2 mitoses per 10 40× high power fields)
  B. Embryonal
  C. Mixed fetal and embryonal (epithelial) pattern
  D. Pleomorphic epithelial pattern
  E. Macrotrabecular pattern
  F. Small-cell undifferentiated pattern
    INI1 retained
    INI1 lost (mutated), considered a malignant rhabdoid tumor
  G. Other epithelial elements: cholangioblastic, glandular (intestinal), squamous
II. Mixed epithelial and mesenchymal type
  A. Without teratoid features
  B. With teratoid features (neuroepithelium, retinal pigment, melanin)

TABLE 15-23 IMMUNOHISTOCHEMICAL FINDINGS IN HEPATOBLASTOMA

	Fetal Cell Areas	Embryonal Cell Areas	Small-cell Areas	Mesenchymal Areas	"Osteoid" Areas
Keratin	++	++	++	±	+
Alpha-fetoprotein	++	++	−		+
Alpha-1-antitrypsin	++	++	+	+	++
Alpha-1-antichymotrypsin	++	++	+	+	+
Ferritin	++	+	+		+
Carcinoembryonic antigen	++	++	−	−	+
Epithelial membrane antigen		+	−		++
Transferrin	+	++			
Human chorionic gonadotropin	+	+			
Vimentin	−	−	−	++	++
Serotonin	±	±	−	−	−
Somatostatin	±	±	−	−	−
NSE	−	±	−	+	++
Beta-catenin nuclear	+/+++	++/+++	+++	+/++	+/++
Glypican-3	++/+++	+/+++	−	−	−
Glutamine synthetase	+++	++/+++	−	−	−
S-100	±	+	±	+	++
Desmin	−	−		−	−
Chromogranin A	±	±	−	−	+

Symbols: ++, Majority of cases strongly positive; +, moderately or weakly positive in some cases; ±, positive in some reports and negative in others; −, negative in all reports.
Modified from Ishak K, Goodman Z, Stocker J. Tumors of the liver and intrahepatic bile ducts. In: Rosai J, Sobin L, eds. *Atlas of Tumor Pathology*, 3rd series ed. Washington, DC: Armed Forces Institute of Pathology, 2001.

show small, inconspicuous nucleoli. Extramedullary hematopoiesis is prominent, more so than in WDFHB areas. They are characterized by presence of more frequent mitoses with rate of ≥2 mitoses per 10 hpf (Figure 15-52C). IHC shows a strong, coarse cytoplasmic granular staining for GPC3 with more frequent nuclear β-catenin staining and strong GS expression with variable nuclear cyclin D1.

Pleomorphic or Anaplastic Fetal/Epithelial HB

This subtype is to be distinguished from the prior nomenclature wherein anaplastic HB was thought to be synonymous with SCUHB. This component is frequently not present on pretreatment biopsies, but is evident in posttreatment specimen as areas of pleomorphic cells with large nuclei with prominent nucleoli and increased N:C ratio. These cells mimic those seen in HCC, but are present with other areas of more typical HB and show an immunophenotype similar to HB. Atypical mitoses and giant cell formation may be noted in these areas. Occasionally, this may be the predominant histologic pattern in metastatic disease. Presence of such a focus on a biopsy may prompt a diagnosis of HCC unless adequate sampling reveals typical HB areas. GPC3 is usually coarsely positive in these cells, and β-catenin is nuclear.

Embryonal HB

This tumor component mimics embryonal liver morphology and is characterized by smaller cells with oval to angulated nuclei, increased N:C ratio, scant amphophilic cytoplasm, and frequent nucleoli. The tumor cells are arranged in sheets and nests and frequently show pseudorosette formation (Figure 15-52D). These areas are seen merging with areas of "crowded fetal" pattern and may sometimes be difficult to distinguish. Pleomorphism may be noted in these areas and prompt a diagnosis of pleomorphic epithelial HB. While they most often occur with other epithelial or mesenchymal components, occasionally, they may form the dominant component (diagnosed as embryonal HB if >70%). It is interesting to note that the morphology of vascular emboli in HB is most frequently associated with embryonal phenotype.

Small-Cell Undifferentiated HB

This component is most commonly present as a component of an epithelial HB (271). The occurrence of a pure SCUHB is an uncommon phenomenon and warrants INI1 immunostaining (272). If INI1 is not expressed, the tumor is reclassified as malignant rhabdoid tumor. The more common scenario shows sheets of small cells with scant to no cytoplasm aggregating in between nests and sheets of embryonal or "crowded fetal" HB areas that can be easily missed in thick sections, but when present are seen as pale areas (Figure 15-52E). Mitoses are scant in these clusters of cells and atypia is uncommon. The cells are highlighted on IHC, as they are GPC3 negative and show strong nuclear β-catenin in the absence of GS. Cyclin D1 is also expressed strongly with SCU. Most instances of such SCU islands do not show loss of INI1 and may be vimentin and pancytokeratin positive.

Epithelial HB

This terminology is applied when several epithelial patterns are intermixed without any one component dominating the tumor.

Cholangioblastic HB

This component is much less common than the previously described patterns within HB and may be seen toward the periphery of the tumor (273). They need to be distinguished from the profuse bile ductular reaction that may surround a treated HB and are better appreciated in nontreated tumors. They need to be distinguished from the pseudorosettes or tubules in embryonal HB. The cells lining the ductular component are cuboidal with hyperchromatic nuclei. β-Catenin shows nuclear staining of these cells, while GPC3 is negative.

Macrotrabecular HB

This is a pattern of tumor cell arrangement that may have cytologic features of fetal (usually with mitoses) or embryonal HB. The tumor cells are arranged in broad trabeculae that may be more than 5 cell layers in thickness (macrotrabecular) (Figure 15-52F). There can be nuclear pleomorphism, and this tumor pattern needs to be distinguished from HCC (270). Classic HB morphology may be seen in other areas of the tumor, and IHC expression may be similar to crowded fetal or embryonal HB. This pattern can be problematic in HB differentiation from HCC.

Other Epithelial Elements

Rarely, glandular elements and keratin whorls may be seen including squamous epithelium in the absence of teratoid elements. Presence of these components alone would not make the tumor a teratoma or teratoid HB.

Mixed Epithelial and Mesenchymal HB

This is probably the most common histologic variant of HB with intermixing of epithelial and mesenchymal elements that may be seen on biopsy or by imaging and is more prominent in postchemotherapy specimens. The mesenchymal components include bone, cartilage, skeletal muscle, and rarely fat (Figure 15-53A, B). Presence of neural elements including primitive neuroepithelial rosettes or ganglion cells would suggest a teratoid HB. Similarly, while fat may occasionally be seen, presence of melanin pigment would make the tumor a teratoid HB. In some instances, the mesenchymal component may be seen as an immature spindle cell proliferation, suggesting a blastemal pattern. Rare instances of epithelial islands surrounded by primitive oval cells with marked proliferation and nuclear β-catenin immunoreactivity suggests a blastemal component in a mixed HB. The mesenchymal cells, especially the cells rimming osteoid material, are strongly nuclear β-catenin positive and negative for GPC3, suggesting a common progenitor cell for the epithelial and mesenchymal components.

Teratoid HB

This diagnosis is made when primitive neuroepithelium in the form of neuroepithelial rosettes, retinal epithelium, or melanin pigment is present within a mixed HB (249) (Figure 15-54A–C). Glandular and squamous elements may also be seen as part of the lesion as well as heterologous mesenchymal elements (Figure 15-54D, E). The presence of epithelial HB component distinguishes this tumor from a teratoma of the liver. IHC shows the usual staining pattern in the epithelial and mesenchymal component, while β-catenin staining is variable in the neural component. Occasionally, the glandular component may mimic a yolk sac tumor component with subnuclear and supranuclear vacuoles that show GPC3

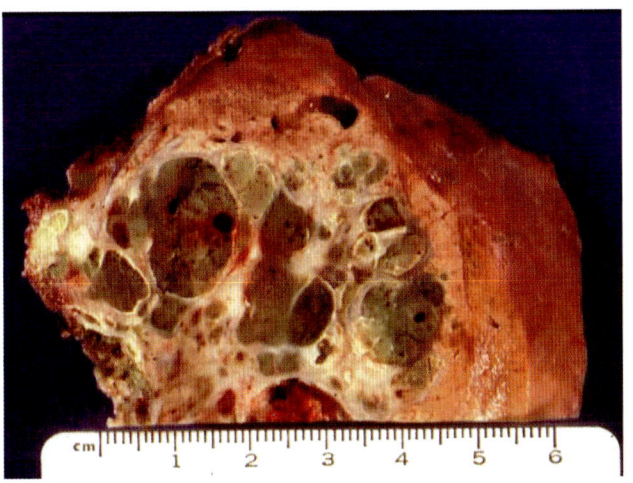
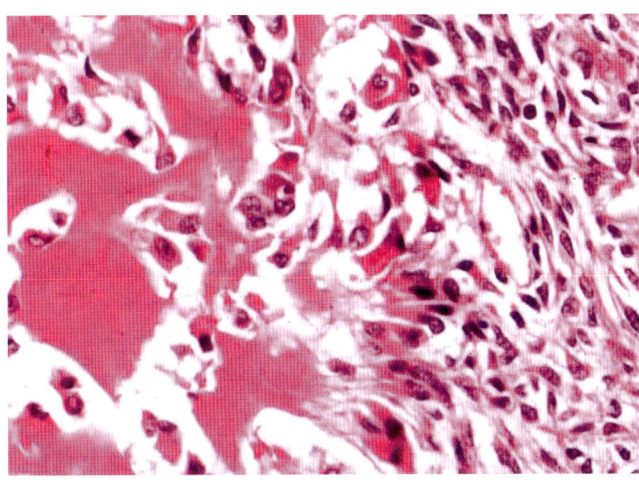

FIGURE 15-53 • Mixed epithelial and mesenchymal hepatoblastoma. **A:** The tumor within the liver displays a highly variegated appearance reflecting the presence of mesenchymal tissue and epithelial cells. **B:** Osteoid-like material (**left**) contains cells similar to the fetal and embryonal epithelial cells (**right**). The cells associated with the "osteoid" are cytokeratin positive (H&E stain, original magnification 125×).

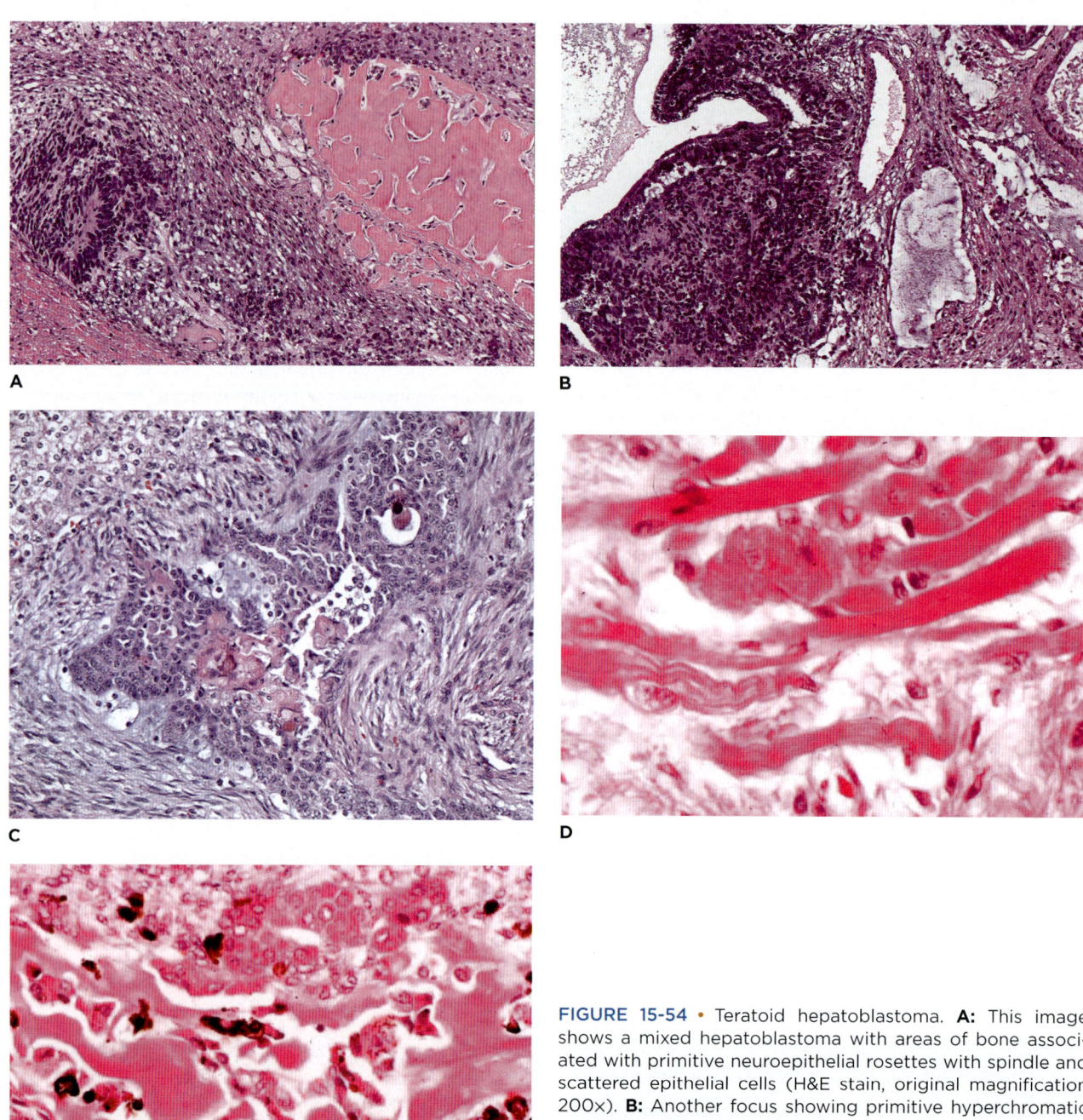

FIGURE 15-54 • Teratoid hepatoblastoma. **A:** This image shows a mixed hepatoblastoma with areas of bone associated with primitive neuroepithelial rosettes with spindle and scattered epithelial cells (H&E stain, original magnification 200×). **B:** Another focus showing primitive hyperchromatic neuroepithelial tissue with many glandular structures containing mucinous material (H&E stain original magnification 200×). **C:** Focus showing stratified squamous epithelium with other epithelial components (H&E stain, original magnification 200×). **D, E:** Striated muscle cells and osteoid-like material containing melanin pigment. (H&E stains, original magnification 300× [**D**], and 200× [**E**]).

staining and nuclear β-catenin staining that confirms this as a component of HB. Rare neuroendocrine areas have also been described in a teratoid HB.

Molecular Pathology

Deregulation of the APC–β-catenin pathway occurs in a substantial proportion of hepatoblastomas, with mutations in the APC and β-catenin genes implicated in FAP-associated and sporadic hepatoblastomas, respectively (255). Mutations of the β-catenin gene are present in over 90% of hepatoblastomas, leading to activating transcription of a number of target genes. β-Catenin is central to the convergence of the Wnt, β-catenin, and cadherin signaling pathways, where it forms a signaling complex with axins, APC tumor suppressor protein, glycogen synthase kinase 3β, and other proteins (274). The Wnt signaling pathway prevents proteasomal degradation of β-catenin and allows β-catenin to translocate to the nucleus and initiate gene transcription. In fact, β-catenin can be immunohistochemically detected in the nucleus, following its translocation. Nuclear staining for β-catenin in hepatoblastomas has been reported to correlate with unfavorable histologic pattern, higher stage disease, and poor survival. Other components of the Wnt signaling pathway including axin gene mutation and loss of APC function have been implicated in hepatoblastoma tumorigenesis. Giardiello et al. identified an APC gene mutation in all eight hepatoblastoma patients of seven FAP kindreds (255). Oda et al. (275) have also noted genetic alterations in the APC (loss of heterozygosity [LOH] or somatic mutations) in 9 of 13 cases of hepatoblastoma in non-FAP patients. Interestingly, a distinct male predominance (nearly 75%) is seen in APC gene-related hepatoblastomas.

A host of other genetic alterations have been described in hepatoblastomas involving cell cycle–related genes, apoptosis pathways, p53 mutations, mismatch repair defects, FOXG1 overexpression, and signal transduction pathways, to name a few (260,276,277). It is possible that many of these molecular aberrations may be late events in the clonal evolution of these tumors that indicate progressive genomic instability rather than primary events (278). López-Terrada et al. have hypothesized that histologic microheterogeneity in hepatoblastoma may correlate with molecular heterogeneity, reflecting different stages of developmental arrest. They found Wnt activation to be most prevalent in embryonal and mixed types, whereas Notch activation needed for cholangiocytic differentiation at a more differentiated state was predominant in pure fetal hepatoblastomas (279). p53 protein expression is seen less frequently in hepatoblastoma than in other childhood tumors. It was suggested that environmental mutagens may be involved in some HB. A recent study has suggested a synergy between β-catenin and Yes-associated protein (YAP) playing a role in tumorigenesis in rats and possibly humans (280).

Many aberrations have also been reported at the chromosomal level in hepatoblastomas. Genome-wide allelotyping of hepatoblastomas has shown frequent allelic losses at many microsatellite loci, implicating chromosome instability as an important factor in the development and progression of hepatoblastoma (281). Trisomy 2, trisomy 20, and 4q structural rearrangement are the most common chromosomal abnormalities in hepatoblastoma (see Table 15-24). A derivative chromosome 4 from an unbalanced translocation between the long arms of chromosomes 1 and 4 has been

TABLE 15-24 CYTOGENETIC FINDINGS IN HEPATOBLASTOMAS

Case No.	Karyotype	Histologic Type
1.	46,XY,-2,der(19)t(4,19),+mar	Epithelial; embryonal
2.	47,XY,+20,dmin	Mixed mesenchymal–epithelial; fetal
3.	47,XY,+20,dmin	Epithelial; primary embryonal, foci of fetal areas
4.	93,XXXX,+I(8q)/93,XXXX,del(1)(p22),+I(8q)	Mixed mesenchymal–epithelial; fetal
5.	50,XY,+2,+8,+20,+dic(1)(p12)	Mixed mesenchymal–epithelial; fetal and embryonal
6.	47,XX,+20,del(1)(q32.2)dup(2)(q21q35),dmin/50, XX,+5,+7,+20,+22,del(1),dup(2),I(8q),dmin	Mixed mesenchymal–epithelial; fetal and embryonal
7.	47,XX,+20,dup(2)(q23q35)/47,XX,+20,dup(2),dup(6)(p11p24)	Mixed mesenchymal–epithelial; fetal
8.	54,Y,der(X)t(X;1)(p22;q21),+2,+6,+8,+8,+12,+15,+17, +20,inv(9)(p11q21)[a]	Mixed mesenchymal–epithelial; fetal and embryonal
9.	46,XYder(4)t(2;4)(q21;q35),t(9;?)(p24;?)/47,XY,+20,der(4),t(9;?)	Mixed mesenchymal–epithelial; fetal
10.	51,XY,+2,+12,+20,+der(5)t(1;5)(q25;q35),+del(6)(q15)	Epithelial; fetal
11.	48,XX,+2,+r/48,XX,+20,+der(2)t(1;2)(q23;p21),inv(5) (q22q35)/49,XX,+20,+der(2),inv(5),+r47,XX,+2	Epithelial; fetal
12.	47,XX,+2	Epithelial; primary fetal, foci of embryonal areas
13.	47,XX,2q+,t(3;5)(p25;q31),dup(4)(q12q26),+20	Mixed mesenchymal-epithelial
14.	46,XY,t(10;22)(q26;q11)	Small-cell undifferentiated
15.	47,XY,+2	Fetal and embryonal, possible macrotrabecular
16.	47,XX,+20	Mixed mesenchymal–epithelial fetal and embryonal
17.	46,XX,del(17)(p12)/46,XX	Mixed with teratoid features

[a]inv(9)(p11q21) was constitutional.
Modified from Stocker J, Conran R, Selby D. Tumor and pseudotumors of the liver. In: Stocker J, Askin F, eds. *Pathology of Solid Tumors in Children*. London, UK: Chapman & Hall, 1998:83–110, with permission.

noted as a recurring abnormality in hepatoblastoma, while it is rarely seen in other types of neoplasms. In 32 cases, Kraus et al. have shown LOH with chromosome 1p in seven cases, LOH with 1q in seven cases, and LOH with both 1p and 1q in three additional cases, suggesting that tumor suppressor genes at the telomeric region of chromosome arm 1p and different regions of chromosome arm 1q may be involved in the pathogenesis of hepatoblastoma (282). DNA analysis by flow cytometry has been reported in more than 70 cases, with a diploid pattern noted in the well-differentiated (fetal) portions of the tumors and an aneuploid pattern present in embryonal portions or in small-cell (anaplastic) tumors. Hata et al. (283) noted an increased incidence of vascular invasion and a poorer prognosis in patients with an aneuploid tumor. By CGH, significant gains of genetic material have been found. The most frequent alterations were gains of Xp (15 cases, 43%) and Xq (21 cases, 60%), while other common alterations were 1p−, 2q+, 2q−, 4q−, and 4q+. There was no difference between different histologic subtypes, suggesting a common clonal origin for the different components.

HEPATOCELLULAR CARCINOMA

HCC is the third most common pediatric liver tumor and represents up to 20% of all pediatric liver neoplasms (284,285). It occurs primarily in older pediatric patients, with over 65% of tumors identified in children >10 years of age (Figure 15-55A) (see Tables 15-15 to 15-17). However, rare cases have been reported in infants. The fibrolamellar variant has not been reported in infants (286). There is a

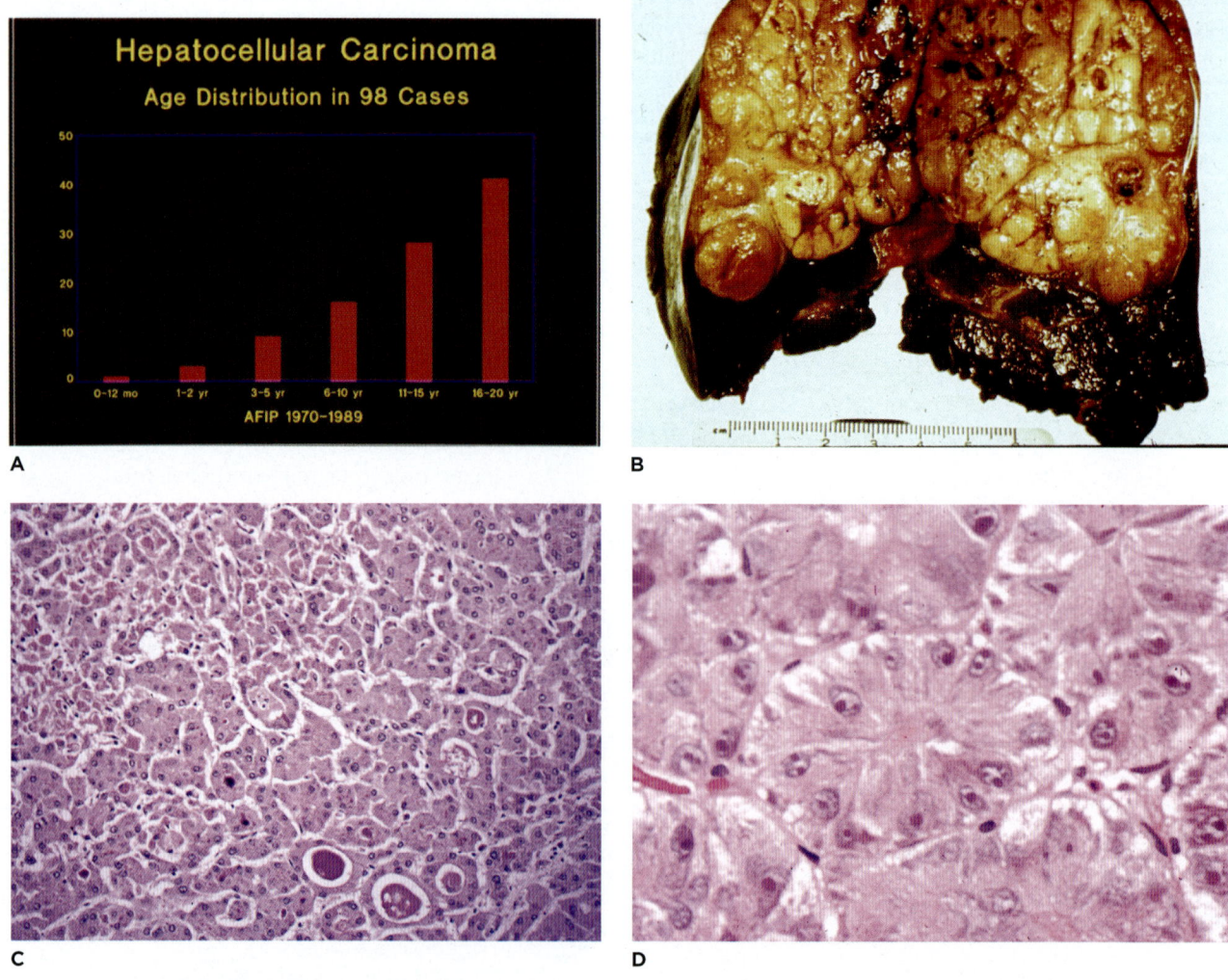

FIGURE 15-55 • Hepatocellular carcinoma. **A:** Age distribution on 98 cases. **B:** A single, large mass displays foci of hemorrhage and necrosis. **C:** The tumor is composed of broad trabeculae of poorly to moderately well-differentiated hepatocytes. Note the pseudogland appearance of some trabeculae with central necrosis of cells (H&E stain, original magnification 40×). **D:** The individual HCC cells may be moderately differentiated and cluster around a canaliculus (**center**), but note the nuclear anisocytosis and multiple nucleoli (H&E stain, original magnification 300×).

slight male predominance, but no specific racial predilection has been detected. There is an increased prevalence in populations with a high number of HBV carriers.

Pathogenesis

Underlying liver conditions, especially viral hepatitis (HBV, HCV) and cirrhosis, are known predisposing conditions. Children are less likely to have HCC-associated chronic liver disease than adults (284). In hyperendemic HBV areas, the vast majority of children with HCC are HBV seropositive (287). In a study of 20 Taiwanese patients aged 8 months to 16 years (only 1 <8 years of age) with HCC, Wu et al. (287) noted HBsAg positivity in all the patients, 70% of their mothers, and 52.9% of their siblings. With these children, HBV was commonly acquired from their mothers, with malignancy developing in 7 to 8 years. However, exposure time may be less in immunocompromised hosts. For example, an exposure time of only 3 years has been described in a 10-year-old boy with HCC who contracted HBV following chemotherapy for acute lymphoblastic leukemia. HBsAg seropositivity is higher in children with the usual histologic type of HCC than in patients with the fibrolamellar variant in whom HBsAg seropositivity is only 5%. Unlike with adults, HBV–DNA integration into the host genome may be a late event in children with chronic HBV infection. Huang et al. found that HBV–DNA integration increased in parallel with the progress of liver disease toward the neoplastic transformation, with 0% in the liver from chronic hepatitis, 22.2% in nontumoral livers from HCC patients, and 66.7% in tumor tissues from HCC patients. Fortunately, the introduction of the hepatitis B vaccine has markedly reduced the prevalence of HCC, especially in males. While becoming more frequently associated with adult HCC, HCV is only occasionally associated with HCC in children (288).

HCC is associated with errors in inborn metabolism, such as A1AT, hereditary tyrosinemia, Gaucher disease, urea cycle defects, CESD, GSD, Alagille syndrome, bile salt export pump deficiency, and congenital biliary atresia (37,74,81,83,85,111,269). Rare instances of HCC and hepatoblastoma have also been described in the setting of TPN injury.

Clinical Features, Laboratory Studies, and Imaging

Most patients (nearly 80%) present with abdominal pain, an abdominal mass, or both. Other symptoms include anorexia, malaise, fever, nausea, vomiting, and jaundice. Symptomatic patients with abdominal discomfort or masses often have advanced-stage disease at presentation. Tumor rupture with hemoperitoneum may be seen rarely. A wide variety of associated conditions are seen in 20% to 25% of cases (228) (Table 15-25), including an association between Gardner syndrome and fibrolamellar HCC. One of the closest associations is with hereditary tyrosinemia, with a 37% incidence of HCC in tyrosinemia patients surviving beyond 2 years of age. Liver transplantation before 2 years of age has been suggested for these patients to avoid HCC development (289).

TABLE 15-25 CONDITIONS ASSOCIATED WITH HEPATOCELLULAR CARCINOMA IN CHILDREN

Acute lymphoblastic leukemia
A1AT deficiency
Ataxia-telangiectasia
Anomalies of the abdominal venous drainage
Arteriohepatic dysplasia
Atypical retinitis pigmentosa
Biliary atresia
CHF
Cystinosis
Familial cholestasis—BSEP disease (PFIC2)
Familial HCC
Familial polyposis
Fanconi anemia
Focal nodular hyperplasia of liver
Galactosemia
Gardner syndrome
Hepatic adenoma
Hepatitis B infection
Hepatitis C infection
Hereditary tyrosinemia
Hyperalimentation
Methotrexate therapy
Neurofibromatosis
Oral contraceptives
Osteogenesis imperfecta
Polycythemia
Soto syndrome
Type I and III glycogenoses
Wilms tumor
Wilson disease

Modified from Stocker JT. Hepatic tumors. In: Balistreri WF, Stocker JT, ed. *Pediatric Hepatology*. New York: Hemisphere Publishing Company, 1990:399–488, with permission.

Laboratory findings in patients with HCC include mild anemia, erythrocytosis, and thrombocytosis. Serum transaminases (ALT, AST), lactate dehydrogenase (LDH), ALP, and lipid levels may be elevated (228). Serum bilirubin levels may be increased in 15% to 20% of cases. Unlike adults with HCC where biochemical liver function tests are often abnormal, ALT, bilirubin, and albumin abnormalities are infrequent in pediatric patients, even with advanced-stage disease. Furthermore, elevated ALP in the presence of a liver mass did not correlate with metastatic disease, in contradistinction to adults. Serum AFP is elevated in 50% to 100% of children with HCC. Of note, AFP may be normal or only mildly elevated in patients with fibrolamellar HCC (286). Elevated AFP levels are especially common in Taiwanese children, attributed to the almost universal association with

HBV. HBV is both carcinogenic and independently reactivates the gene encoding AFP within hepatocytes (287). Alternatively, extremely high AFP levels may be due to advanced HCC tumor stage.

Imaging studies can delineate the mass and are often helpful in determining whether resection is feasible (Figure 15-55B). Soyer et al. (290) employed CT scans to study patients with the fibrolamellar variant and noted a characteristic hypodense single, bilobed, or multilobulated mass with hypervascularity and variable enhancement after injection. Calcification was present in 40% of cases. Fibrolamellar HCC can also be seen as a lobulated heterogeneous mass with a central scar in an otherwise normal liver and could be confused with FNH. Recently, PET/CT scan has been reported to be helpful for preoperative staging, selection of appropriate site for biopsy, identification of occult metastatic disease, follow-up for residual or recurrent disease, and assessment of response to chemotherapy in HCC and other pediatric abdominal neoplasms. Imaging studies may be helpful in differentiating metastatic tumors from primary malignant liver tumors, in that the former are more likely to show hypoechogenicity on abdominal ultrasound examination, while the latter are more likely to show vascular invasion and contrast enhancement on CT scan.

Staging

Multiple staging systems have been proposed for HCC. Lu et al. found the TNM staging system to be superior to the Okuda, Cancer of the Liver Italian Program (CLIP) and the Chinese University Prognostic Index (CUPI) staging systems for prognostication in HCC patients undergoing curative resections (291). In contrast, Seo et al. found the CLIP system to have better predictive power than the TNM and Barcelona Clinic Liver Cancer (BCLC) staging systems (292). In yet another study comparing seven prognostic staging systems (CLIP score, BCLC staging, the Groupe d'Etude et de Traitement du Carcinome Hépatocellulaire [GETCH] classification, CUPI grade, the Japan Integrated Staging [JIS] score, modified JIS [mJIS] score, Tokyo score), Kondo et al. found the JIS score to outperform the other 6 systems in HCC patients undergoing hepatectomy (293). More recently, the PRETEXT system devised for hepatoblastomas (284) has gained popularity with pediatric HCC.

Treatment and Outcome

The typical management strategy for pediatric HCC is the combination of surgery and neoadjuvant chemotherapy. The relative chemoresistance of HCC makes surgery essential (284). Unfortunately, complete tumor resection at the time of diagnosis is possible in only 10% to 30% of cases (227,294). Neoadjuvant chemotherapy may improve tumor resectability. The most frequent chemotherapy regimen used in children is doxorubicin and cisplatin. For unresectable tumors after chemotherapy, locoregional ablative therapies, such as transarterial chemoembolization, have been used.

Tumor size and serum AFP level, alone or in combination, are useful in predicting the presence or absence of vascular invasion before hepatectomy for HCC. Liver transplantation may be helpful when resection is impossible, and transplantation should be considered as early as possible. Extrahepatic disease, nodal involvement, macroscopic vascular invasion, and distant metastases are obvious contraindications to transplantation. The experience with liver transplantation for HCC is still scarce in children. Although Sevmis et al. claim excellent results with both cadaveric and living-donor transplants (295), others have observed relatively poor results, similar to those in adults with HCC. In a recent study, patients with large (3 to 5 cm) tumors, high serum AFP levels (>455 ng/mL), or a high MELD score (≥20) had decreased posttransplantation survival (296).

The prognosis of HCC tends to be poor with an overall survival rate at 3 years of <25% (284,285,294). Despite similar multidisciplinary oncologic management, HCC outcome is notoriously worse than that for hepatoblastoma. Major prognostic factors are metastatic disease and the extent of disease, especially surgical resectability. In an SIOPEL-1 study that included 40 children with HCC, it was reported that 33% were associated with cirrhosis, multifocal tumors were common (56%), as were metastases (31%), and extrahepatic tumor extension, vascular invasion, or both in 39%. Preoperative chemotherapy achieved a partial response in 49% of cases. Complete tumor resection was achieved in 36% of patients, whereas 51% of tumors did not became operable. Overall survival at 5 years was 28%, and event-free survival was 17%. Most deaths resulted from tumor progression. Resectability, metastatic disease, and high PRETEXT score predicted poor outcomes (284). The statistically significant prognostic factors were tumor stage, presence of metastasis, and ability to completely resect tumors.

Childhood hepatoblastoma and HCC differ with respect to age (18 months versus 10.2 years), sex (females versus males), HBsAg status (none versus 64%), tumor stage (low versus high), tendency to rupture (36% versus 9%), chemosensitivity (greater with hepatoblastoma), and tumor respectability (91% versus 45%), with considerably worse survival for HCC than hepatoblastoma. Rare reports of combined hepatoblastoma and HCC, where the HCC component recurred more than 5 years after initial diagnosis, exist, suggesting that prolonged follow-up may be required for these tumors.

In general, fibrolamellar HCC variant of HCC (FL-HCC) is considered to carry a somewhat better prognosis than conventional HCC (286). This is probably true with adults due to lack of association of this histologic form with cirrhosis. In children, FL-HCC may be biologically similar in behavior compared with classic HCC. Controversy does exist whether FL-HCC has a better prognosis than classic HCC. Some series have shown a better survival for FL-HCC than conventional HCC (297,298). This may be due to a larger proportion of localized and resectable FL-HCC cases in these studies. Other clinical reports, including recent studies with children and young adults with FL-HCCs, have not shown favorable outcomes and also reported no difference in surgical resectability compared with classic HCC (284,286). With 46 HCC pediatric cases, Katzenstein et al. reported 10 cases (22%) of FL-HCC. Although the median survival was greater for FL-HCCs than for typical HCCs, the 5-year survival rate was similar for both tumor groups. There was no difference in the number of patients with advanced-stage disease, surgical resectability at diagnosis, or the response to treatment between FL-HCC and typical HCC. Children with resectable HCC at diagnosis had a good prognosis irrespective of histologic subtype. In contrast, outcomes were uniformly poor for children with advanced-stage disease (286). Novel treatment, including targeted c-MET inhibitor therapy, may change the outcome in the future (299).

Gross Appearance

Grossly, HCC may be single or multicentric masses, with both the right and left lobes involved in >70% of cases. The tumors weigh between 800 and 1500 g and vary in size from 2 to 25 cm. The lesions on cut section are tan to red and soft to firm with areas of hemorrhage and necrosis (Figure 15-55B). The surrounding liver may exhibit micronodular or macronodular cirrhosis in up to 60% of cases, which is somewhat less than the 48% to 92% prevalence seen in adults with HCC. The cirrhosis may be related to biliary atresia or hereditary tyrosinemia, among other causes. Fibrolamellar HCC is more often a single mass that is firm and gray. Cirrhosis is less frequent (4%) in patients with fibrolamellar HCC. FNH may be present in or adjacent to tumor in about 4% of patients with the fibrolamellar HCC (200).

Histopathology

Microscopically, the "usual" HCC and the fibrolamellar variant possess distinctly different features. The usual HCC is composed of trabeculae comprised of 2 to 10 or more cell layers in thickness (Figure 15-55C, D). The larger trabeculae may display central necrosis, imparting an acinar or pseudoglandular appearance. Tumor cells are larger than normal hepatocytes, with nuclear hyperchromasia, anisocytosis, multiple nucleoli, and frequent and bizarre mitoses (228). Large, multinucleated osteoclast-like giant cells or "tumor giant" cells (so-called epithelial syncytial giant cells) may also be seen. Bile pigment may be present within the cytoplasm of tumor cells or within the canaliculi between cells. Vascular invasion may be prominent, and metastases to lung and lymph nodes may occur. Children with malignant liver tumors, especially with HCC, may have extensive angiogenesis that induces rapid tumor growth and leads to poor prognosis. Pathologic factors including tumor size greater than 2 cm, multifocality, and vascular invasion have been reported to be independent predictors of decreased survival after resection (294).

The fibrolamellar HCC variant was originally described in 1956 by Edmondson. FL-HCC accounts for 1% of all HCC, but represents 13% to 22% of all HCC in younger patients, as it preferentially occurs in children and young adults (286). It has not been linked with viral infection or other risk factors for classic HCC. FL-HCC patients usually have normal serum AFP levels. FL-HCC is characterized by large, deeply eosinophilic (oncocytic) hepatocytes embedded within lamellar fibrosis (Figure 15-56). Tumor cells vary from polygonal to spindle shaped and often contain discrete, pale eosinophilic bodies. Tumor cell clusters are separated by narrow to broad bands of laminated collagen. Although rare, the most common variant of FL-HCC shows areas of glandular-type differentiation with mucin production (300). Immunohistochemically, the tumor cells immunoreact with fibrinogen, hepar, ferritin, and alpha-1 antitrypsin, but are negative for HBsAg (228). AFP staining has been noted in 21% of fibrolamellar HCCs and in 40% of the classic HCCs. HCCs are positive for HbsAg in 27% of cases.

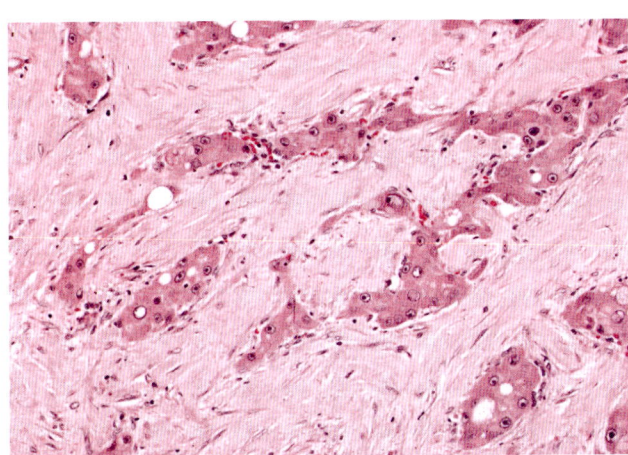
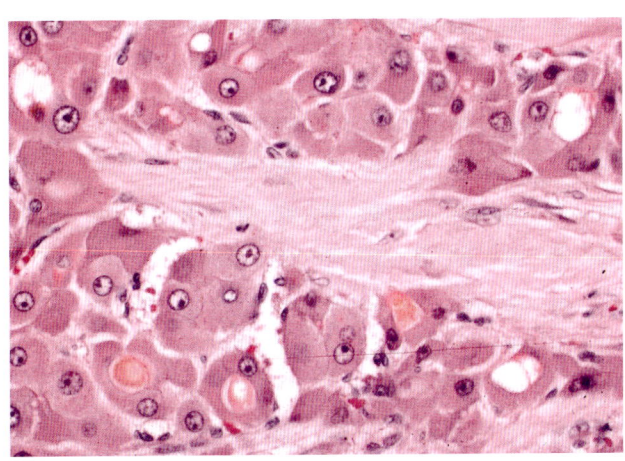

FIGURE 15-56 • Fibrolamellar HCC. **A:** Broad bands of "plump" collagen separate clusters of large hepatocytes with prominent eosinophilic cytoplasm and large nucleoli (H&E stain, original magnification 60×). **B:** The hepatocytes contain abundant smooth to finely granular cytoplasm. Note the bile within the canaliculi between hepatocytes (H&E stain, original magnification 200×).

On occasion, it may be difficult to differentiate the macrotrabecular variant of hepatoblastoma from HCC (278). Computerized image analysis has been claimed to assist in distinguishing hepatoblastoma from HCC. When compared with HCC, hepatoblastoma is rarely multifocal and vascular invasion is uncommon even in advanced-stage tumors. Prokurat et al. have described a novel group of hepatocellular neoplasias in older children and adolescents, with an intermediate histology between HCC and HB and a distinctive β-catenin pattern, that they term "transitional liver cell tumors," now considered as hepatocellular neoplasm, NOS (270).

Recently, glypican-3 has been claimed to be a specific immunomarker for HCC and has been used to distinguish HCC from benign hepatocellular mass lesions, particularly HCA (301). However, the diagnosis of HCC should not rely entirely on glypican-3 immunostaining, because focal immunoreactivity can be detected in a small subset of cirrhotic nodules. Also, glypican-3 expression in HCC can also be focal, and thus, the lack of glypican-3 staining does not exclude the diagnosis of HCC. Furthermore, glypican-3 is also positive in hepatoblastomas. However, in a tissue microarray study of 4387 tissue samples from 139 tumor categories and 36 nonneoplastic and preneoplastic tissue types, glypican-3 expression (using a 10% cut-off score) was detected in 9.2% of nonneoplastic liver samples (11/119), 16% of preneoplastic nodular liver lesions (6/38), 63.6% of HCCs (140/220), and in several nonhepatic tumors including squamous cell carcinoma of the lung (27/50 [54%]), testicular nonseminomatous germ cell tumors (32/62 [52%]), and liposarcoma (15/29 [52%]) (302). A staining panel consisting of glypican-3, glutamine synthetase, and heat shock protein 70 has been suggested to be helpful in distinguishing HCC from benign tumors especially when two or more markers are positive, but others have not been able to duplicate these findings (218,303). HCCs of higher histologic grade have been reported to have loss of E-cadherin, nonnuclear overexpression of β-catenin, and overexpression of osteopontin. Pediatric HCCs have been shown to express nuclear to cytoplasmic β-catenin to variable degrees and range from 20% to 80% but less often than hepatoblastomas, and hence, β-catenin IHC may not be helpful in the diagnosis. EGFR overexpression has been reported in the majority of HCCs, suggesting a role for EGFR antagonists in therapy. However, the increased expression does not correlate with an increase in the EGFR gene copy number (304). Although some have reported that HCCs in children though morphologically similar to those in adults differ due to their expression of CK7, others have not found this to be true (except for fibrolamellar variant) and also noted more frequent expression of EpCAM in pediatric HCCs (305).

Molecular Pathology

In contradistinction to other childhood tumors (neuroblastomas, rhabdomyosarcomas, ganglioneuroblastomas), amplification or overexpression of the oncogenes N-MYC, ERB A, ERB B, N-RAS, or Shb is not seen with HCC or hepatoblastoma. Fibrolamellar HCCs have recently been shown to have the fusion transcript, DNAJB1-PRKACA, in 80% of more tumors (306). The deletion is found on chromosome 19. Abnormalities in chromosomes 7 and 8 have also been detected and their significance is unknown. Usual gene mutations in TP53 and CTNNB1, encountered in HCC, are lacking in FL-HCC (300).

The β-catenin pathway has also been implicated in HCC. MicroRNA profiling may help identify patients with HCC who are likely to develop metastases and recurrences (307). The uniqueness of FL-HCC extends to their molecular findings, as they lack involvement of many of the major pathways and genes that are dysregulated in typical HCC, including AFP, TP53 mutations, and β-catenin mutations. However, much of their molecular biology remains poorly described and awaits future investigation (300). The molecular pathology of pediatric HCCs is probably similar to that in adults.

UNDIFFERENTIATED EMBRYONAL SARCOMA

UES is the fourth or fifth most common pediatric liver tumor (232,308). The term "undifferentiated (embryonal) sarcoma" was given to this lesion by Stocker and Ishak in 1978 and was previously known as embryonal sarcoma, mesenchymoma, primary sarcoma, fibromyxosarcoma, or malignant mesenchymoma.

Pathogenesis

The histogenesis of undifferentiated sarcoma of the liver remains unresolved (309). Suggestions that UES is a sarcomatoid variant of hepatoblastoma have not found acceptance. The observation of UES occurring in association with mesenchymal hamartoma has suggested that the former may arise in a setting of the latter (see discussion section on mesenchymal hamartoma). This concept of malignant transformation occurring in a dysgenetic or hamartomatous lesion is similar to what has been described for other malignancies, such as adenocarcinomas arising in bronchogenic and choledochal cysts, Wilms tumor from perilobar nephrogenic rests, and possibly pleuropulmonary blastoma from presumed congenital lung cysts (controversial).

UES has been associated with Li-Fraumeni syndrome (310). An embryonal or congenital origin has been considered unlikely by some authors, because UES has also been reported in adults. The origin of UES is probably from a mesenchymal lineage. There is no clear differentiation into rhabdomyosarcoma or fibrosarcoma, although myogenic differentiation has been suggested in a few cases based on immunohistochemical findings. The overlap of immunohistochemical staining patterns and ultrastructural features shown by UES and hepatic rhabdomyosarcoma has led Parham et al. to suggest a common histogenesis, perhaps from a multipotential mesenchymal stem cell (309).

Clinical Features, Laboratory Studies, and Imaging

UES occurs primarily in children 6 to 10 years of age (Figure 15-57A), with 88% of cases occurring in those under 15 years of age (269). Others have reported a median age of 9.5 to 12 years, with 63% occurring in children 6 to 10 years of age (209). In most series, there is an almost equal prevalence in both sexes (310). In a large reviewed series of 113 cases in literature, 46 were males and 31 were females. There is no racial predilection.

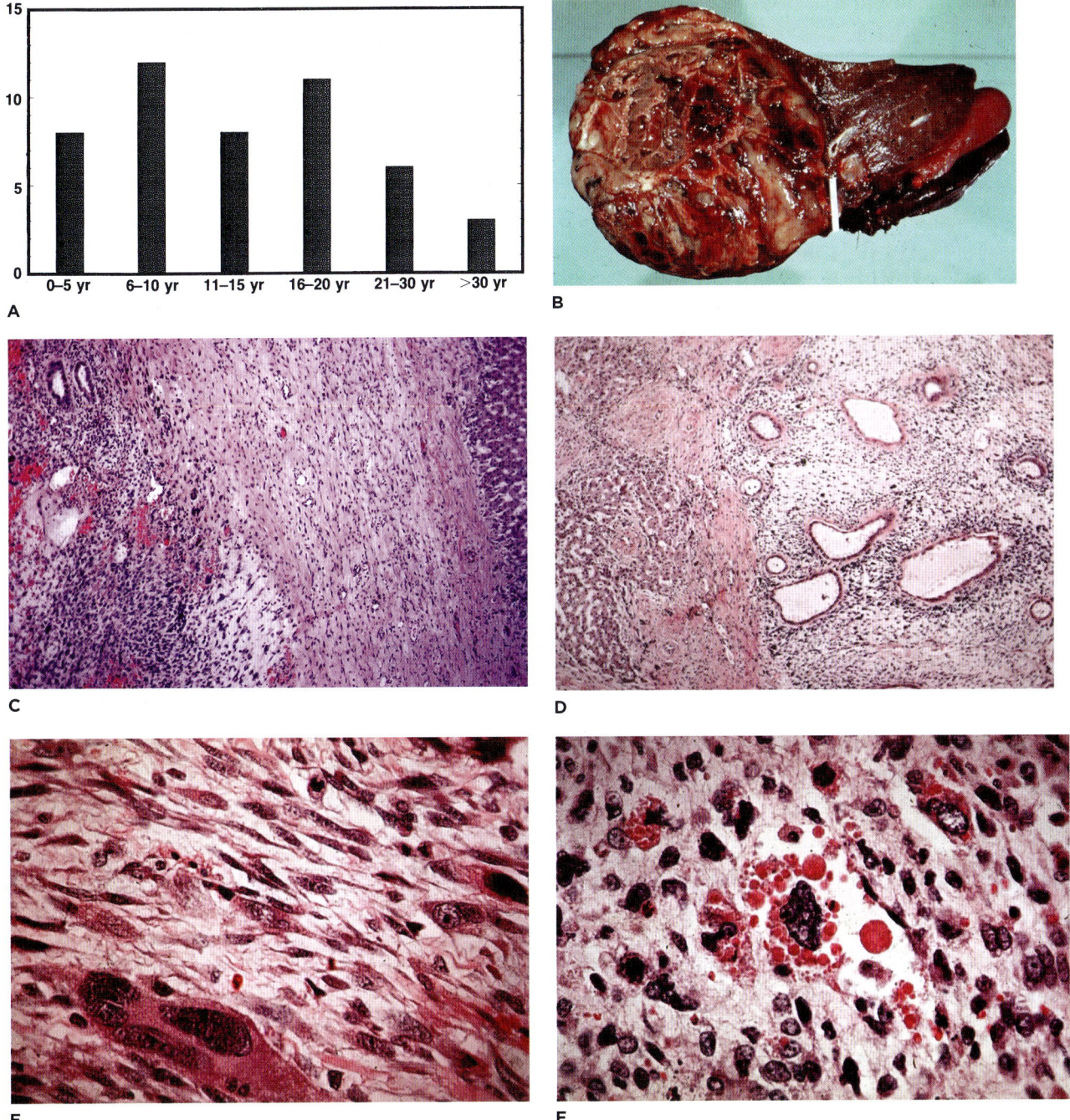

FIGURE 15-57 • Undifferentiated embryonal sarcoma. **A:** Age distribution in 48 cases. **B:** The tumor mass contains multiple cystic areas filled with gelatinous or hemorrhagic material. **C:** Loose and usually incomplete fibrous tissue separates the normal liver (**right**) from the malignant tumor (**left**) (H&E stain, original magnification 30×). **D:** Entrapped and degenerating bile ducts surrounded by anaplastic cells in a loose mesenchymal matrix lie next to the pseudocapsule separating the tumor from the normal liver (**left**) (H&E stain, original magnification 40×). **E:** Bizarre tumor giant cells with large and multiple nuclei are scattered throughout the lesion (H&E stain, original magnification 200×). **F:** Smooth eosinophilic globules are present in the cytoplasm of small and large tumor cells (H&E stain, original magnification 200×).

Abdominal pain or an abdominal mass is seen at presentation in 87% of cases. Unusual presentations include dyspnea, cardiac murmur (due to extension of the tumor through the inferior vena cava into the right atrium and ventricle), jaundice, chest pain, and fever. The abdominal mass and pain are often accompanied by anorexia, vomiting, lethargy, and malaise. Tumor rupture may lead to an acute abdomen (310). Laboratory findings display a variety of abnormalities of elevated SGOT, LDH, and ALP, but serum AFP is uniformly negative and serum bilirubin is rarely elevated (308).

UES appears predominantly as a solid lesion on sonographic studies. The tumor is relatively isoechoic or hyperechoic compared with the surrounding liver parenchyma. Cystic areas comprise an average of 19% of the tumor volume. Sonographic findings are usually in agreement with gross pathologic findings in terms of proportion of solid and cystic components (311). Computed tomographic scans reveal predominantly water attenuation. As determined by unenhanced scans and bolus contrast-enhanced scans, an average of 88% of the tumor volume shows water attenuation. Areas of intermediate or soft attenuation are also noted around the periphery of all lesions. On MRI, the tumor appears predominantly hypointense relative to the liver on T1-weighted images, with areas of high signal intensity present centrally, corresponding to areas of recent hemorrhage. T2-weighted images show predominantly high signal intensity, cystic foci, internal debris, and septations (311). A fibrous pseudocapsule of low signal intensity on T1-weighted and T2-weighted images is sometimes seen. MRI and CT may show a misleading cyst-like appearance with an UES compared with ultrasonography and pathologic findings in which the tumors are predominantly solid (>85% of tissue mass). This discrepancy with gross appearance following tumor resection probably results from the abundant myxoid stroma in these tumors. A cystic appearance on imaging may lead to a misdiagnosis of hydatid disease, especially in areas endemic for this parasitic infestation. On angiography, UES commonly appears as an avascular or hypovascular hepatic mass. Angiograms have shown that the tumor derives its vascular supply from the hepatic arterial system. Angiography has been helpful in delineating hepatic vein invasion and in vascular mapping for surgery (312).

Pachera et al. have reviewed the clinicopathologic features of UES in adults based on 51 cases in the literature. The mean age of affected adults is 31 years (range 15 to 86 years), with a female preponderance (28 F, 19 M). The right lobe is more commonly affected than the left lobe (59% versus 22%), with both lobes involved in 20% of cases. Tumors often exceeded 10 cm in size, with an average weight of 1400 g. Spontaneous rupture was reported in only two cases. Results of liver function tests are usually normal, whereas high AFP levels have been reported in only five adults and elevated CA-12 level in one adult. In adults, the appearance of a cystic lesion on imaging has led to a mistaken diagnosis of a benign lesion with delay in diagnosis in 24% of cases (313).

Treatment and Outcomes

Although UES was uniformly considered to have a very poor prognosis in the past, complete resection and aggressive chemotherapy have changed the outcome favorably in recent years. In their original series, Stocker and Ishak documented an average survival time of only 11 months. Patients who undergo incomplete tumor resection have a tendency toward poorer outcomes (308), and radical complete excision provides the only chance for cure. However, a complete resection was possible in only 65% (33 patients) of the cases reported in the literature (313). Polychemotherapy has been practiced with agents such as doxorubicin, cis-diaminodichloroplatinum, cyclophosphamide, dacarbazine, 5-FU, and vincristine with good reduction in tumor size enabling complete resection (312). The Soft Tissue Sarcoma Italian and German Cooperative Groups treated 17 children with UES using the same multimodal approach as for patients with other sarcomas, including conservative surgery at diagnosis, multiagent chemotherapy, and second-look operation in cases of residual disease, with additional radiotherapy in 2 of 17 patients. Twelve patients (12/17) were alive with follow-up ranging from 2.4 to 20 years. More recently, liver transplantation has improved survival in these patients (312).

The tumor usually spreads by direct extension into adjacent organs and sometimes extends into the right atrium via the inferior vena cava. Rupture of the tumor can occur and massive intraperitoneal spread has sometimes been found (310). Metastases are rare, but have been reported in the lung, bone, pleura, and peritoneum.

Gross Appearance

UES is a large tumor with an average weight of more than 1200 g (range 90 to >4000 g) (310). The tumor ranges from 10 to 35 cm in diameter (308,310). The mass is in the right lobe of the liver in 69% of cases and in the left lobe in 14% and involves both lobes in 17%. Pedunculated or exophytic tumors have been documented. The tumor is well demarcated from the adjacent liver by a compressed incomplete fibrous pseudocapsule. The cut section is variegated and soft. Myxoid gelatinous areas alternate with confluent areas of necrosis and hemorrhage (Figure 15-57B). Foci of hemorrhage or necrosis are present in over 50% of the cases and may constitute up to 80% of the tumor. The tumor is predominantly solid with a mean percentage of the solid component being 83%. An average 17% of cross-sectional areas of the tumor is composed of empty cyst-like cavities. These "cysts" are up to 4 cm in diameter and contain gelatinous brown contents. Calcifications are rare to absent. The uninvolved liver is normal in appearance. Pathologic features are similar in both adults and children (313). With more recent chemotherapy, the response to treatment may be extensive and resections may show mainly necrotic tumor with rare atypical cells at the edges, being the only indication of the aggressive tumor.

Histopathology

Microscopically, the tumor is separated from the normal liver by an incomplete fibrous pseudocapsule of variable thickness (Figure 15-57C). This tumor pseudocapsule and the immediately adjacent tumor may contain remnants of normal-appearing hepatocytes and bile ducts (Figure 15-57D). The bile ducts may extend 0.5 to 1.0 cm into the lesion and show hyperplastic or reactive epithelial changes and may even appear anaplastic. These bile ducts are not present deeper in the tumor, nor within metastases, and are considered to represent entrapped or residual bile ducts rather than neoplastic tumor elements. The major component of the tumor consists of loose to dense foci of stellate or spindle-shaped cells with ill-defined outlines in a myxoid stroma (Figure 15-57D). Multinucleated cells with hyperchromatic nuclei are frequently scattered throughout the lesion (Figure 15-57E) or may only be a minor component. These cells may contain eosinophilic globules that are PAS positive and diastase resistant (Figure 15-57F); these globules may also be seen extracellularly. The histologic appearance may vary due to differing proportions of myxoid stroma, cellularity, hemorrhage, and necrosis. There is marked disparity in individual cell size and anisonucleosis. Mitoses are abundant, with both atypical and bizarre mitotic forms. Proliferation indices range from 30% to 95%. Some densely cellular areas have small round cells with hyperchromatic nuclei without nucleoli. Anaplastic malignant cells occur closer to the duct epithelium elements, as mentioned previously. Numerous reticular fibers surround small groups of cells, and focal collagenization and hyalinization are present. Extramedullary hematopoiesis may be present. In a few tumors, there are foci of direct invasion into the hepatic sinusoids. Patterns mimicking sarcoma as a minor component of the tumor have been recorded, including osteoid-like matrix and "leiomyoblastic" and lipoblastic differentiation. The neoplastic cells may resemble fibroblastic, histiocytoid, fibrohistiocytoid, and myofibroblastic cells, occasionally suggesting a malignant fibrous histiocytoma. Following chemotherapy, resected tumors show central necrosis, fibrosis, and dystrophic calcifications. Histologic dedifferentiation has been described following multiple recurrences. In a comparative study of 14 primary and two recurrent UES, recurrent tumors showed greater cellularity, anaplasia, and pluripotential differentiation compared with primary tumors.

FNA cytology commonly yields a combination of polygonal and spindle cells. Polygonal cells are large with round or lobulated nuclei and occasionally are multinucleated with one or several nucleoli and variable cytoplasm with poorly defined borders. A few intracytoplasmic and extracytoplasmic eosinophilic globules may be observed. Similar cytologic findings have also been described in peritoneal washings. Findings on FNAC have been considered distinctive from other childhood liver tumors, allowing a confident preoperative diagnosis.

IHC shows evidence of widely divergent differentiation into mesenchymal and epithelial phenotypes, suggesting that immunostains have no specific or diagnostic relevance, but may help exclude other tumors. Variable positivity has been described for vimentin, BCL-2, pancytokeratin, CD10, calponin, desmin, smooth muscle actin, muscle-specific actin, p53, alpha-1 antitrypsin, alpha-1 antichymotrypsin, desmin, CD56, and CD68 (232,310,314). The tumors are usually negative for myoglobin, myogenin, muscle-specific actin, h-caldesmon, S100, ALK-1, neuron-specific enolase (NSE), carcinoembryonic antigen (CEA), F-VIII, and AFP, although these could be anecdotally positive. Aberrant cytokeratin expression has been explained on the basis of genetic deregulation rather than differentiation. Glypican-3 staining may be seen in the atypical spindle cells of the lesion (315).

Ultrastructurally, Agaram et al. have described the hallmark features that include dilated RERs and secondary lysosomes with dense precipitates, which correlate with the eosinophilic globules seen on light microscopy (316). Dilated mitochondria and mitochondrial–RER complexes are often seen. Other features include intracytoplasmic fat droplets, scant actin microfilaments, and focal glycogen pools. Primitive fibroblasts, small mesenchymal cells, and membrane-bound bodies that are alpha-1 antitrypsin or alpha-1 antichymotrypsin positive have been described by others.

Molecular Pathology

Leuschner et al. undertook DNA ploidy studies in five cases and found that four tumors were diploid and one was hypodiploid (317). An aneuploid DNA stemline with high proliferative S phases has also been reported in two patients studied with flow cytometry.

Several chromosomal changes have been described in UES. Sowery et al. analyzed six cases of UES by both conventional cytogenetics and CGH. Although CGH demonstrated several chromosomal gains and deletions in each case, there was no specific abnormality seen and no critical event important in tumorigenesis could be identified. Patterns of chromosomal changes included gains of chromosome 1q (four cases), 5p (four cases), 6q (four cases), 8p (three cases), and 12q (three cases) and losses of chromosome 9p (two cases) and 11p (two cases) and chromosome 14 (three cases) (318). Other cytogenetic abnormalities have also been reported in UES, including near-triploid and near-hexaploid clones with several chromosomal rearrangements. A clonal telomeric association (a cytogenetic phenomenon in which chromosome ends fuse to form dicentric, multicentric, and ring chromosomes) has been observed in UES (see hepatic mesenchymal hamartoma).

Mutation of TP53 gene, but not the Wnt or telomerase pathways, has been suggested to be involved in pathogenesis. In fact, Lack et al. (310) described a 9-year-old boy, who was a member of a kindred with a familial cancer syndrome

(Li-Fraumeni syndrome), including a sister with soft tissue sarcoma of the wrist, a father with osteosarcoma of the jaw, a mother with soft tissue sarcoma of the pectoralis muscle, and a half brother with osteosarcoma of the femur.

NESTED STROMAL EPITHELIAL TUMOR OF THE LIVER

Nested stromal epithelial tumor is a recently described extremely rare primary pediatric hepatic neoplasm that has been variably called "ossifying stromal–epithelial tumor," "calcifying nested stromal–epithelial tumor," "desmoplastic nested spindle cell tumor," and "nested stromal–epithelial tumor" (319–321).

Pathogenesis

The tumors are of uncertain histogenesis. However, a possible origin in a hepatic mesenchymal precursor cell with primitive differentiation along the bile duct lineage has been suggested (319).

Clinical Features

Patients have ranged from 2 to 33 years of age; however, most tumors have been described in the first decade of life. Makhlouf et al. noted that four of their nine cases had a history of calcified hepatic nodules since early childhood (321). Ectopic ACTH production can lead to Cushing syndrome that abates following tumor excision. Most patients are asymptomatic and discovered to have tumor incidentally. Meir et al. report a case that was associated with hydronephrosis. The hydronephrosis was discovered on antenatal ultrasound, whereas the hepatic neoplasm was incidentally discovered on routine follow-up abdominal imaging at 2 years of age (322). In the Heerema-McKenney series, one 2-year-old patient subsequently developed nephroblastomatosis and Wilms tumor of the kidney, while another patient had a history of omphalocele, bowel obstruction due to postoperative adhesions, hypoplastic left kidney, and developmental delay (319). A recent case has also been described in the setting of Beckwith-Wiedemann syndrome (323).

Treatment and Outcomes

Partial hepatectomy is probably curative, although local recurrences have been reported in a few patients. Local recurrences are successfully treated with either surgery or radiofrequency ablation (321). Makhlouf et al. have suggested that this tumor is best considered a low-grade malignancy. Long-term prognosis appears to be good, with six of eight patients in one series alive and well, up to 22 years after surgery (321). However, Brodsky et al. have reported a case in a 17-year-old girl with aggressive clinical behavior with multiple hepatic recurrences and extrahepatic lymph node metastasis, suggesting that close follow-up is essential in these patients (324).

Gross Appearance

Based on the reported cases, the tumors are well circumscribed, but not encapsulated and range in size from 4 to 30 cm. The tumors are intrahepatic, but a pedunculated mass has also been described. On cut surface, they appear multinodular, with a homogeneous, tan, granular-appearing cut surface. Variably sized foci of softening, cyst formation, calcifications, or gritty ossification may be observed.

Histopathology

Nested stromal–epithelial tumors have been described as nonhepatocytic, nonbiliary tumors with nests of epithelial and spindle cells, an associated myofibroblastic stroma, as well as variable calcifications and ossifications (319,320). Architecturally, the tumor–liver interface is well defined and the tumors consistently display an organoid arrangement of tumor cell nests comprised of spindled and/or epithelioid cells surrounded by a variably prominent collar of delicate myofibroblasts (Figure 15-58A). The stroma between the nests is usually desmoplastic. The periphery of the tumor shows a bile duct component, most likely due to entrapment. Psammomatous calcifications may be sparse to prominent; when present, they are usually within or adjacent to cellular nests. Focal osteoid formation or ossification is common. The cellular nests have rounded edges and are relatively uniform in size in a given case. Older children may show larger nests, suggesting that the tumor may grow slowly with age. Focal neuroendocrine-appearing architecture has been described in cases with Cushing syndrome. The nests are composed predominantly of plump to fusiform spindled cells with centrally placed or scattered epithelioid cells. Epithelioid cells may predominate in cases with extensive calcification. Both spindle and epithelioid cells have bland oval nuclei with well-defined nuclear membranes, stippled chromatin, and variably conspicuous nucleoli. The cytoplasm is predominantly eosinophilic, with focal cells containing clear cytoplasm. The epithelioid cells have distinct cellular borders. Mitoses are rare to scattered. Delicate osteoid formation may be present between the epithelioid nests. The variably cellular desmoplastic stroma, a prominent feature in all four tumors and composed of cells with morphologic features of myofibroblasts, is seen. Hill et al. specifically mentioned the lack of evidence of a ductal plate abnormality and lack of vascular invasion (320).

Immunohistochemically (Figures 15-58B, C), the tumor cells coexpress vimentin and cytokeratins, at least focally. They also exhibit moderate to strong diffuse nuclear staining for WT-1, using either the C-terminal or N-terminal antibodies (319–321). Beta-catenin stain shows strong nuclear and cytoplasmic staining in the spindle and epithelioid cells (Figure 15-58D). There is variable staining for EMA, CD56, CD57, S100, and other mesenchymal markers.

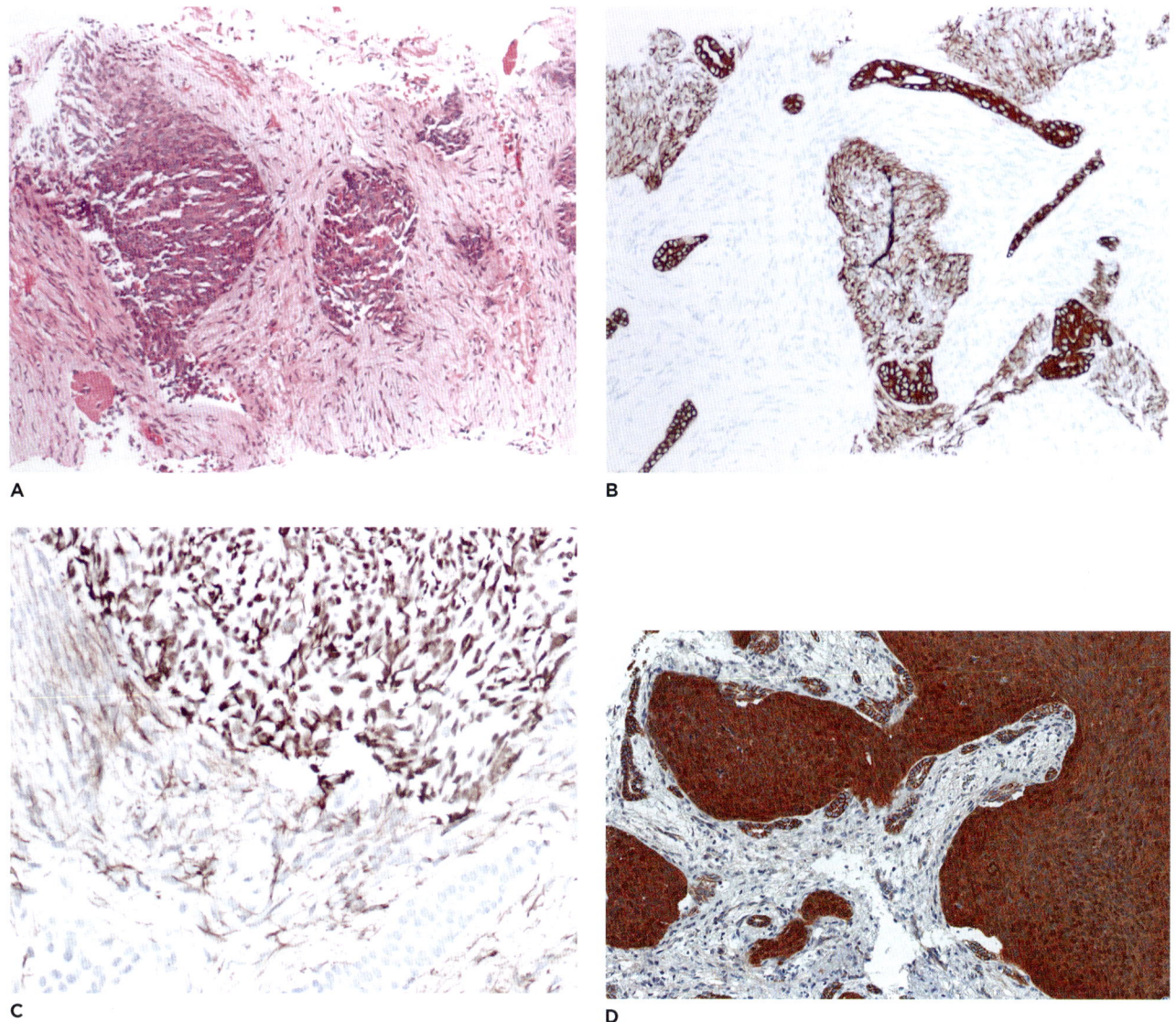

FIGURE 15-58 • Nested stromal epithelial tumor. **A:** The tumor is comprised of variably sized distinct nests of epithelioid cells embedded in variably myofibroblastic to desmoplastic stroma (H&E, 100×). **B, C:** The tumor cells in the nests are positive for cytokeratin (**B:** 100×) and WT-1 (**C:** 200×) immunostains. **D:** The tumor cells show strong nuclear and cytoplasmic staining for β-catenin immunostain (**D:** 200×).

Synaptophysin and chromogranin stains are reportedly negative in all cases. ACTH IHC may be positive in tumors associated with Cushing syndrome (319). The desmoplastic stroma has been reported to prominently display collagen type IV and smooth muscle actin.

Hill et al. performed ultrastructural studies in three cases and observed bland spindled and polygonal cells with focal basal lamina and focally well-developed cell junctions. Few mitochondria and sparse profiles of rough endoplasmic reticulum were seen in the cytoplasm. The polygonal cells contained focal collections of intermediate filaments and had interdigitating cell membranes. No neurosecretory granules were identified (320). On the other hand, Brodsky et al. report an abundance of rough endoplasmic reticulum and mitochondria in a tumor that behaved aggressively with intrahepatic recurrence and lymph node metastasis (324).

Molecular Pathology

Molecular studies for Ewing sarcoma family transcripts and SYT–SSX fusion transcripts have been negative in the cases studied (320,321). Hill et al. found a normal karyotype in the single case that they evaluated. Brodsky et al. report a cytogenetically complex tumor that later recurred and metastasized (324). β-Catenin mutations have been described in the nested tumors including large deletions in exon 3, suggesting a possible link to hepatoblastomas. The epithelial–mesenchymal pathways have been shown to be upregulated in these tumors.

EMBRYONAL RHABDOMYOSARCOMA OF THE BILIARY TRACT

Although it is the most common sarcoma in the pediatric patient, rhabdomyosarcoma of the liver accounts for only 0.8% of all rhabdomyosarcomas and 1.0% of all liver tumors. At the same time, rhabdomyosarcoma is the most common malignant tumor of the biliary tree in childhood. It is difficult to diagnose and delayed diagnosis influences the prognosis. Rhabdomyosarcoma of the liver and biliary tree was first reported in 1875. Almost 85 cases of biliary rhabdomyosarcoma have been reported in the literature, with 75% of patients under 5 years of age (209). The lesion is seen rarely in those older than 15 years (Figure 15-59A) (228).

Jaundice is the presenting symptom in 60% to 80% of cases and may be accompanied by cholemia, pale stools, and hepatomegaly and often confused with infectious hepatitis. Other symptoms include fever, abdominal distension, nausea, and vomiting. The jaundice is reflected in moderate elevations of conjugated and unconjugated bilirubin, with total bilirubin of 1.5 to 9.0 mg/dL. ALP may also be elevated, along with a mild rise in SGOT. Imaging studies, including CT, MRI, ultrasonography (Figure 15-59B), and cholangiography, may clearly demonstrate the site of obstruction within the intrahepatic ductal structures. Due to its rarity, it may be misdiagnosed as a choledochal cyst.

Treatment is aimed at surgical resection, although complete resection is possible in only 20% to 40% of patients because of extension of the tumor into the liver, regional metastasis, and local extension to the duodenum, stomach, and pancreas. Recent preoperative therapy using standard protocols for embryonal rhabdomyosarcoma has proved quite effective. Long-term survival of approximately 20% in previous years has risen for patients treated with preoperative chemotherapy and surgical "second-look" procedures (325).

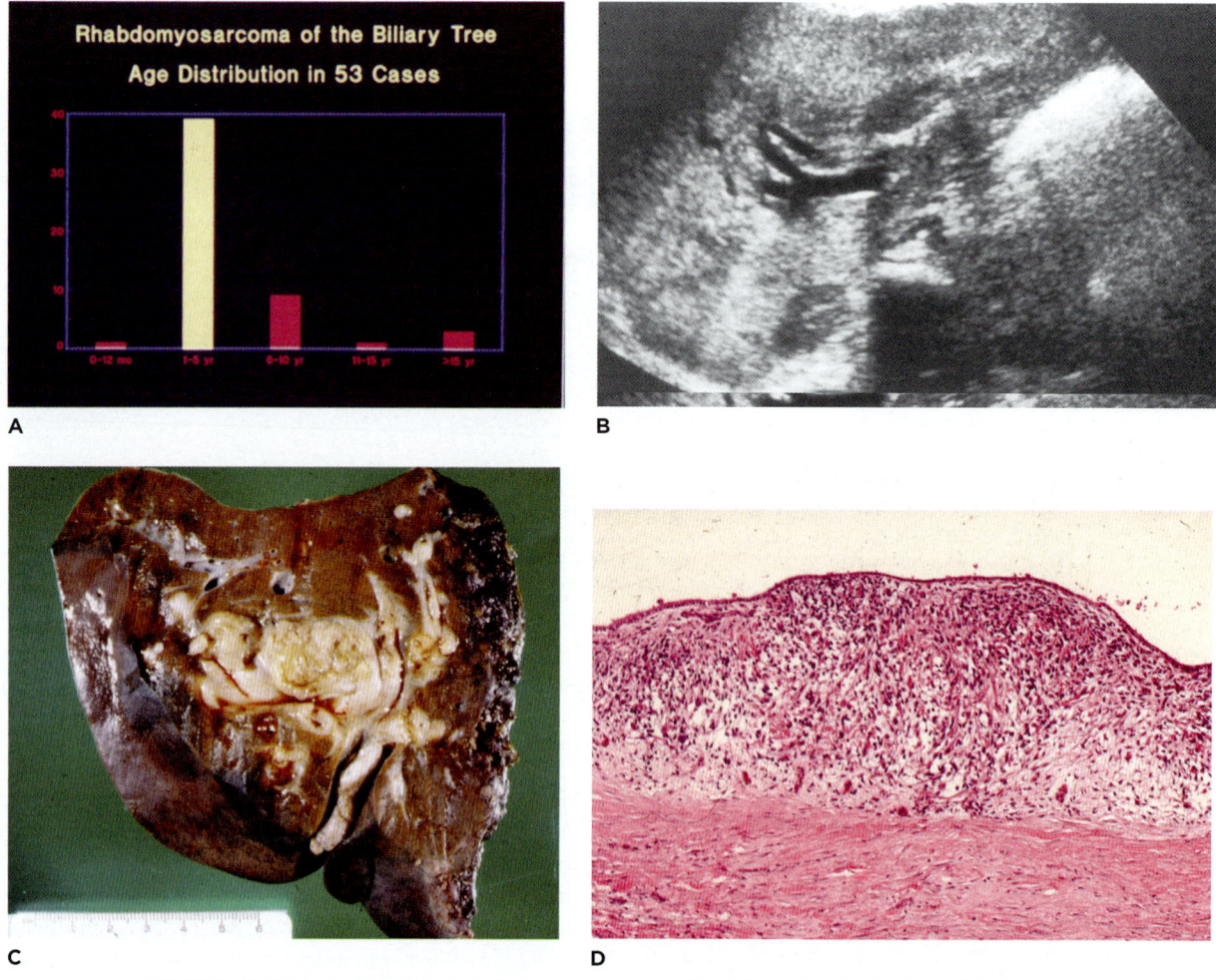

FIGURE 15-59 • Embryonal rhabdomyosarcoma of the biliary tract. **A:** Age distribution. **B:** Ultrasonography displays the dilated ducts proximal to the tumor mass. **C:** The tumor occupies the major ducts within the porta hepatis (**center**) and extends proximally along the intrahepatic ducts. **D:** The tumor cells form a "cambium" layer of rhabdomyoblasts between the bile duct epithelium (**top**) and wall (**bottom**) (H&E stain, original magnification 75×).

Grossly, the tumor often presents as a botryoid, gelatinous mass occluding the lumen of the right and left hepatic ducts or common bile duct (Figure 15-59C). The ducts proximal to the lesion are frequently dilated, and the walls of the duct containing the lesion are thickened. The tumor may extend into the liver as a soft lobulated mass. Occasional cases arise in the intrahepatic bile ducts.

Microscopically, the botryoid masses within the bile ducts are covered by a layer of cuboidal epithelium (bile duct epithelium) that may be inflamed or ulcerated. Beneath the epithelium lies a dense layer of tumor cells, the upper portion of the cambium layer (Figure 15-59D). Cells within this area are small and hyperchromatic, with scant cytoplasm. Deeper to the bile duct epithelium, the cells lie in a loose myxoid stroma and exhibit the typical features of embryonal rhabdomyosarcoma with round, spindle, or straplike shapes; elongate nuclei: scant acidophilic cytoplasm; and frequent mitoses. As with other rhabdomyosarcomas, cross-striations may occasionally be found, but IHC studies are consistently positive for desmin, with myogenin identified in less differentiated cells (228,314). The tumor is usually highly vascular, and areas of recent and remote hemorrhage and acute and chronic inflammation may be found throughout the lesion. The adjacent hepatic parenchyma is often compressed, and bile may be present within canaliculi and hepatocytes.

Nicol et al. have compared the clinicopathologic features of UES and hepatobiliary rhabdomyosarcoma (314). Although similarities do exist between the two lesions, UES has a male to female ratio of 1:1, a median age of occurrence of 10.5 years, and histology showing hyaline globules and diffuse anaplasia. Rhabdomyosarcoma has a male to female ratio of 1.8:1 with a median age of 3.4 years and routinely lacks anaplasia and hyaline globules. Polyclonal desmin and muscle-specific actin are variably immunoreactive in both tumors; however, myogenin and myogenic regulatory protein D1 (MyoD1) is mostly negative in UES, but positive in rhabdomyosarcoma. With a median follow-up of 8 months, 11 of 18 patients with UES were still alive, whereas the estimated 5-year survival for biliary tract rhabdomyosarcoma was 66%. Establishing the correct diagnosis of these distinct clinical and pathologic entities is important, as surgery alone may be curative in UES, whereas initial chemotherapy is often recommended for the treatment of biliary tract rhabdomyosarcoma prior to surgical intervention (see Chapter 24).

ANGIOSARCOMA

Angiosarcoma of the liver accounts for less than 2.5% of liver tumors in children (see Table 15-14). Selby et al. (326) studied 10 patients (six girls, four boys) ranging in age from 18 months to 7 years and three older children (13, 17, and 18 years of age) (Figure 15-60A). There is a reported predominance in females (female to male ratio of 2:1) and a mean age at presentation of nearly 4 years. This is in contrast to infantile hemangioma, which almost always occurs in the first year of life. However, hepatic angiosarcoma has also been reported in neonates. The current nomenclature is that all previously diagnosed type 2 IHEs are considered to be angiosarcomas in the WHO classification (242). The most frequent presenting symptom is a rapidly enlarging abdominal mass, which may be accompanied by jaundice, diarrhea, abdominal pain, or vomiting. Congestive heart failure commonly seen with hepatic hemangiomas is absent with hepatic angiosarcomas. An association with environmental exposure to Thorotrast, vinyl chloride, androgenic and anabolic steroids, oral contraceptives, and diethylstilbestrol, as reported in adults, has not been observed in children. There is also no established syndromic or genetic association. Angiosarcoma arising in a child previously treated for infantile hemangioma has been described, but is unusual and may represent failure to recognize or sample the angiosarcoma component (243).

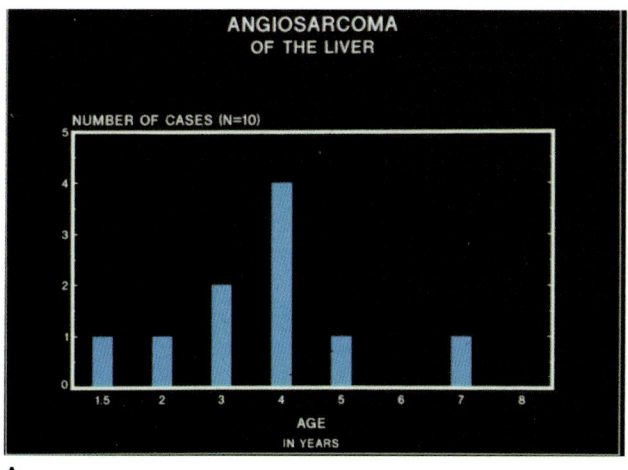
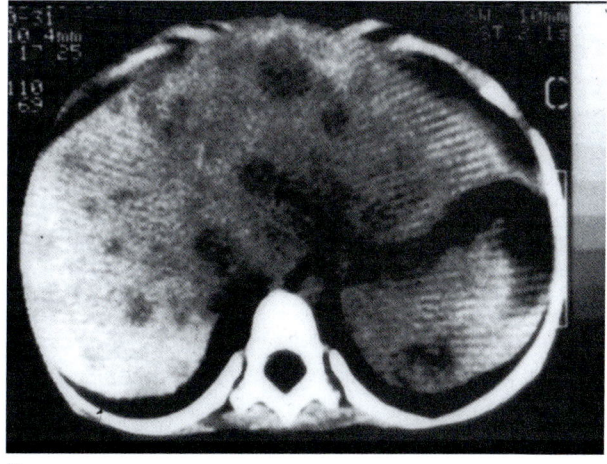

FIGURE 15-60 • Angiosarcoma. **A:** Age distribution in 10 cases. **B:** On CT, multiple hypodense nodules are present in the liver.

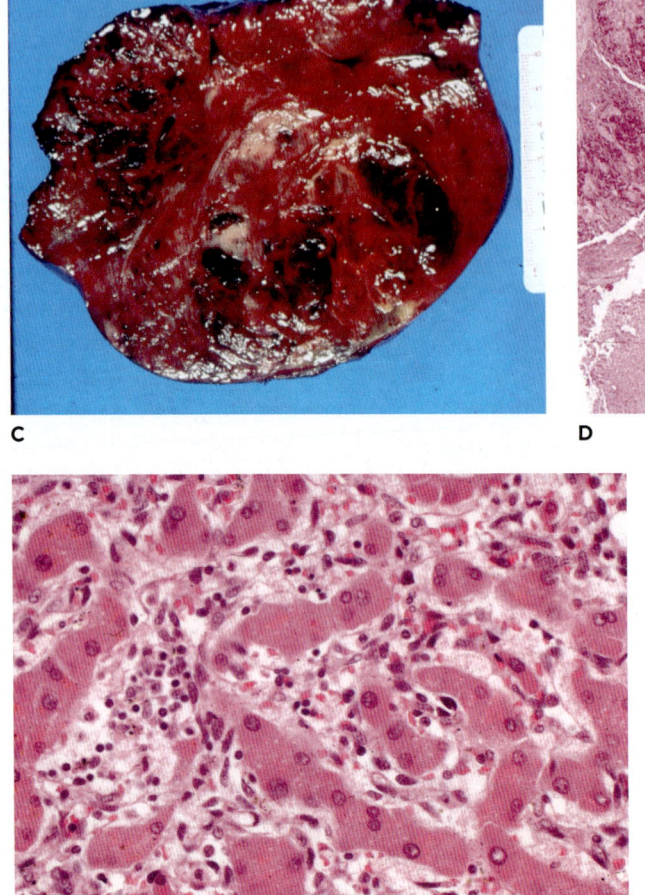

FIGURE 15-60 • (*continued*) **C:** On cut section, the liver displays multiple areas of dense white tissue and areas of hemorrhage. **D:** Foci of spindle cells and hemorrhage are scattered throughout the liver parenchyma (H&E stain, original magnification 40×). **E:** Bizarre endothelial cells fill and greatly distend the sinusoids of the liver, compressing and destroying hepatic trabeculae (H&E stain, original magnification 200×).

Treatment, including resection, radiation, transplantation, and a variety of chemotherapeutic agents, has been unsuccessful, and patients have rarely survived for more than 2 years. More recently, the European Liver Transplant Registry has suggested angiosarcoma as an absolute contraindication for transplantation (327).

Hepatic angiosarcomas are often large multicentric lesions composed of well-demarcated, fleshy, tan nodules usually about 7 cm in diameter displaying areas of hemorrhage and necrosis (Figure 15-60B, C). Microscopically, the tumor is characterized by nodules of spindled cells in a whorled pattern (Figure 15-60D). Larger nodules composed of malignant vascular channels may also be present. Tumor cells are large, with hyperchromatic nuclei and frequent mitoses (Figure 15-60E). Intracytoplasmic and extracellular eosinophilic globules that are PAS positive are present in most cases. Dimashkieh et al. have observed that the histology of pediatric hepatic angiosarcoma is distinct from adult angiosarcoma, with the former displaying hypercellular whorls of sarcomatous cells, or "kaposiform" spindle cells, in addition to the general features of angiosarcoma (328). Immunohistochemical stains are positive with vascular markers, alpha-1 antichymotrypsin, and Ulex europaeus, but negative for keratin and AFP (326). Transcription factor ERG has been reported to be a reliable marker for hepatic angiosarcomas in a recent series (329). Metastases to the lungs, pleura, bone, adrenals, mesentery, and kidney have been described (326).

OTHER NEOPLASMS SEEN IN THE LIVER

Metastatic lesions such as neuroblastoma, Wilms tumor, and lymphoma are the most common neoplasms seen in the liver, but a variety of other primary neoplasms have been described. EBV-associated leiomyosarcoma has been described following liver transplantation in two children—the first, a 9-year-old boy who developed a tumor in his allografted liver 2 years after transplantation and the second, a 12-year-old girl who, after transplantation, developed a leiomyosarcoma in the retroperitoneum involving the superior mesenteric vein (330) (Figure 15-61A–C). Malignant neoplasms that are rarely seen include malignant rhabdoid tumor (Figure 15-61D, E), endodermal sinus (yolk sac) tumor, and lymphoma (228). Examples of

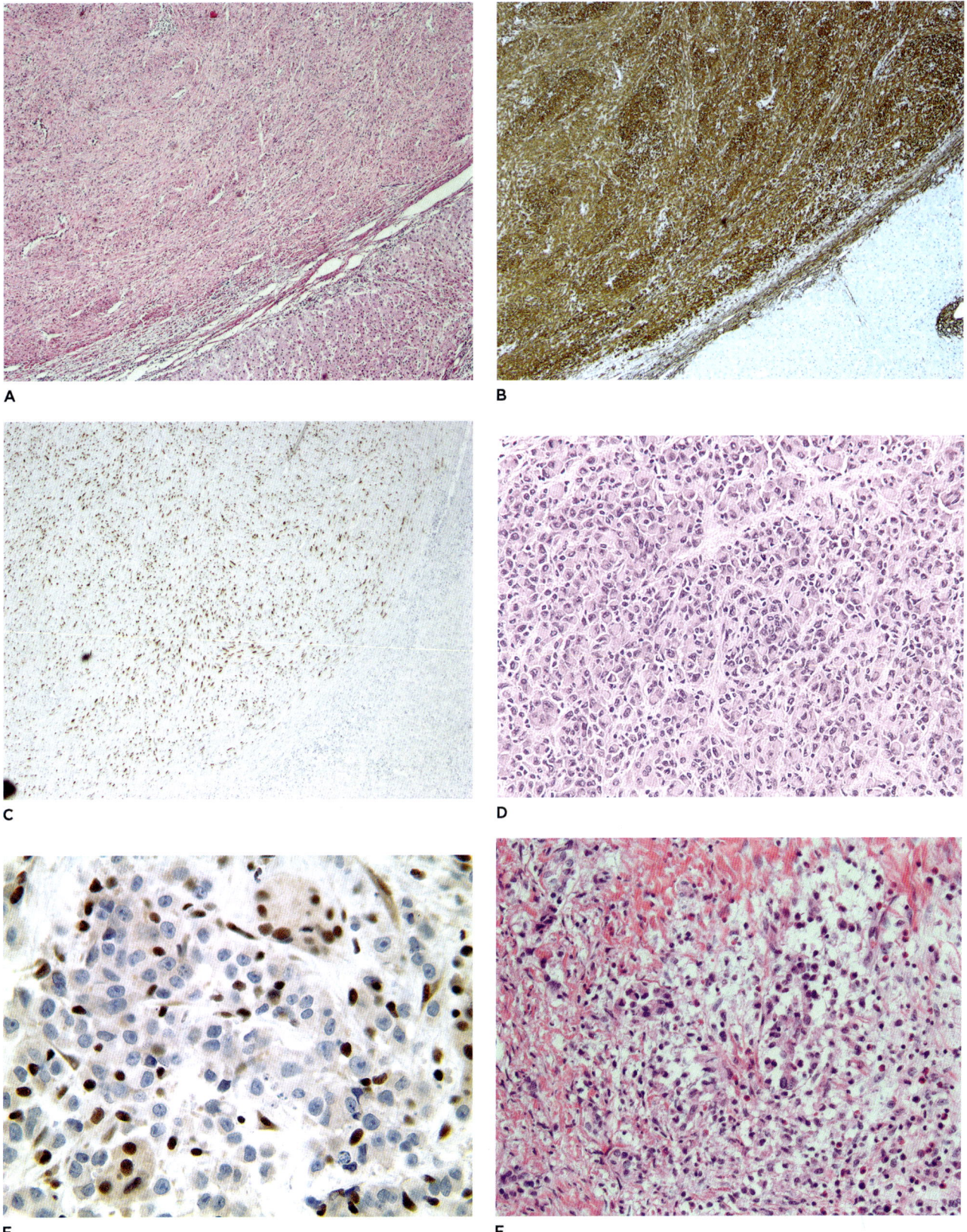

FIGURE 15-61 • Other tumors involving the liver. **A:** Liver showing a large encapsulated lesion composed of interweaving fascicles of smooth muscle cells in this posttransplant allograft (H&E, 40×). **B:** Smooth muscle actin immunostain confirming the diagnosis (SMA 40×). **C:** EBER in situ probe showing diffuse nuclear staining of smooth muscle cells (EBER in situ hybridization, 40×). **D:** An example of malignant rhabdoid tumor of the liver with large polygonal cells with prominent cytoplasmic inclusions (H&E, 100×). **E:** An INI1 immunostain on the same case showing loss of staining of tumor cells with internal positive control of endothelial and inflammatory cells (INI1, 400×). **F:** A mixed inflammatory infiltrate destroying a large bile duct with prominent eosinophils clinically thought to be a liver abscess (H&E, 200×).

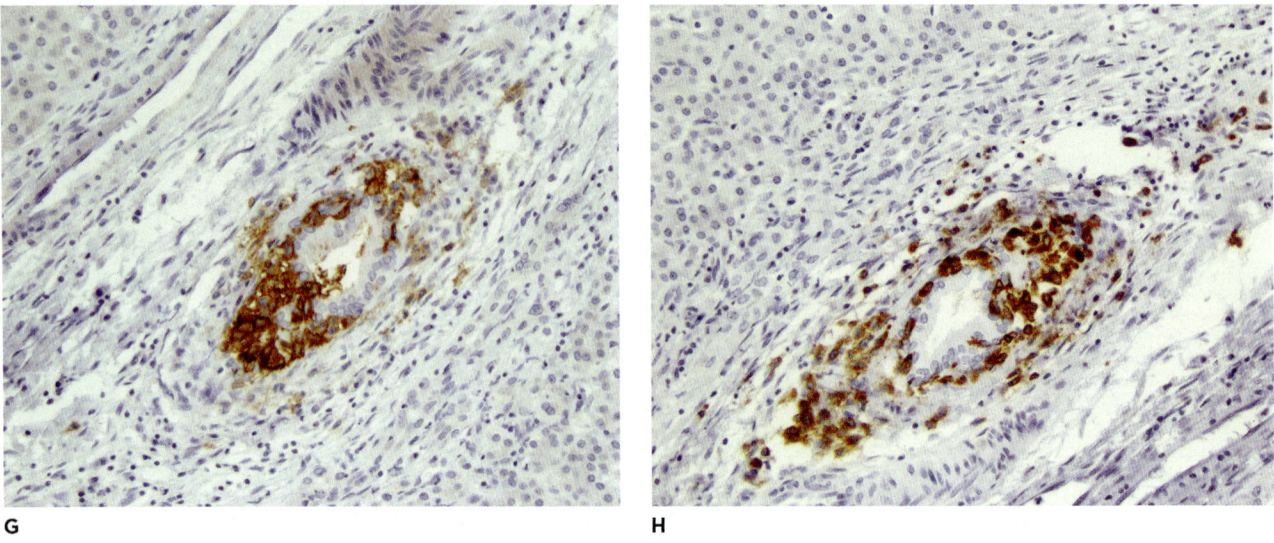

FIGURE 15-61 • (*continued*) **G, H:** A CD1a immunostain showing large positive Langerhans cells in the bile duct epithelium, confirmed with a langerin stain (**G,H:** CD1a and langerin, 200×).

malignant neuroendocrine tumors of the liver and PNET of the biliary tree are also reported. Rare instances of inflammatory myofibroblastic tumor affecting the biliary tree are also reported. While typically part of systemic disease, both Langerhans cell histiocytosis and juvenile xanthogranuloma may give rise to mass lesions in the neonate or young child (Figure 15-61F–H).

GALLBLADDER

Congenital anomalies of the gallbladder include agenesis, duplication, bilobation, multiseptation, diverticula, ectopia, and congenital fistula. Agenesis occurs as an isolated anomaly in the majority of such cases and is an incidental finding at autopsy in childhood (331). The gallbladder may be reduced to a fibrous cord or be diminutive in EHBA. In the neonate, a small or hypoplastic extrahepatic biliary tree may reflect a low-flow state in severe cholestatic liver disease. Alagille syndrome, A1AT, AGH (INH), and familial cholestatic syndromes are some of the conditions in which gallbladder hypoplasia may be seen. In CF, the gallbladder may be small and contain viscid mucus. Rarely, the bile ducts may be obstructed by biliary sludge.

The most common acquired disease of the gallbladder is cholelithiasis (Figure 15-62) (228). This condition may be a complication of hemolytic disease, including congenital spherocytosis, sickle cell disease, and thalassemia. In most cases, the condition is idiopathic. As in adults, there is a female preponderance in childhood cases, and cholecystitis is often associated. Some other conditions predisposing to

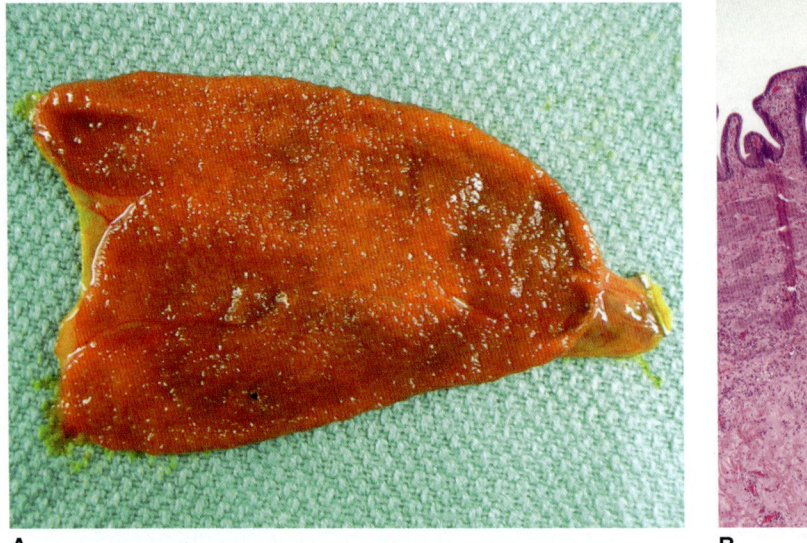
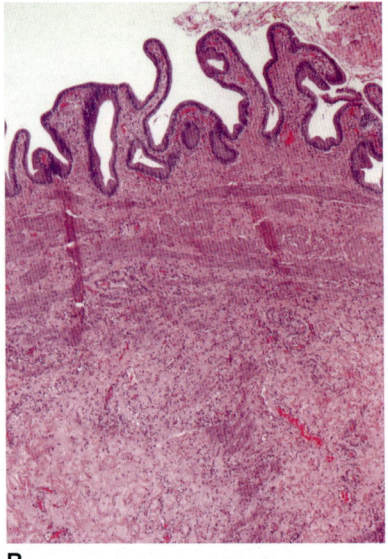

FIGURE 15-62 • Cholecystitis and cholelithiasis. **A:** Gallbladder with red finely granular mucosa. **B:** Chronic cholecystitis with markedly thickened gallbladder wall and scattered chronic inflammatory cells (H&E, 40×).

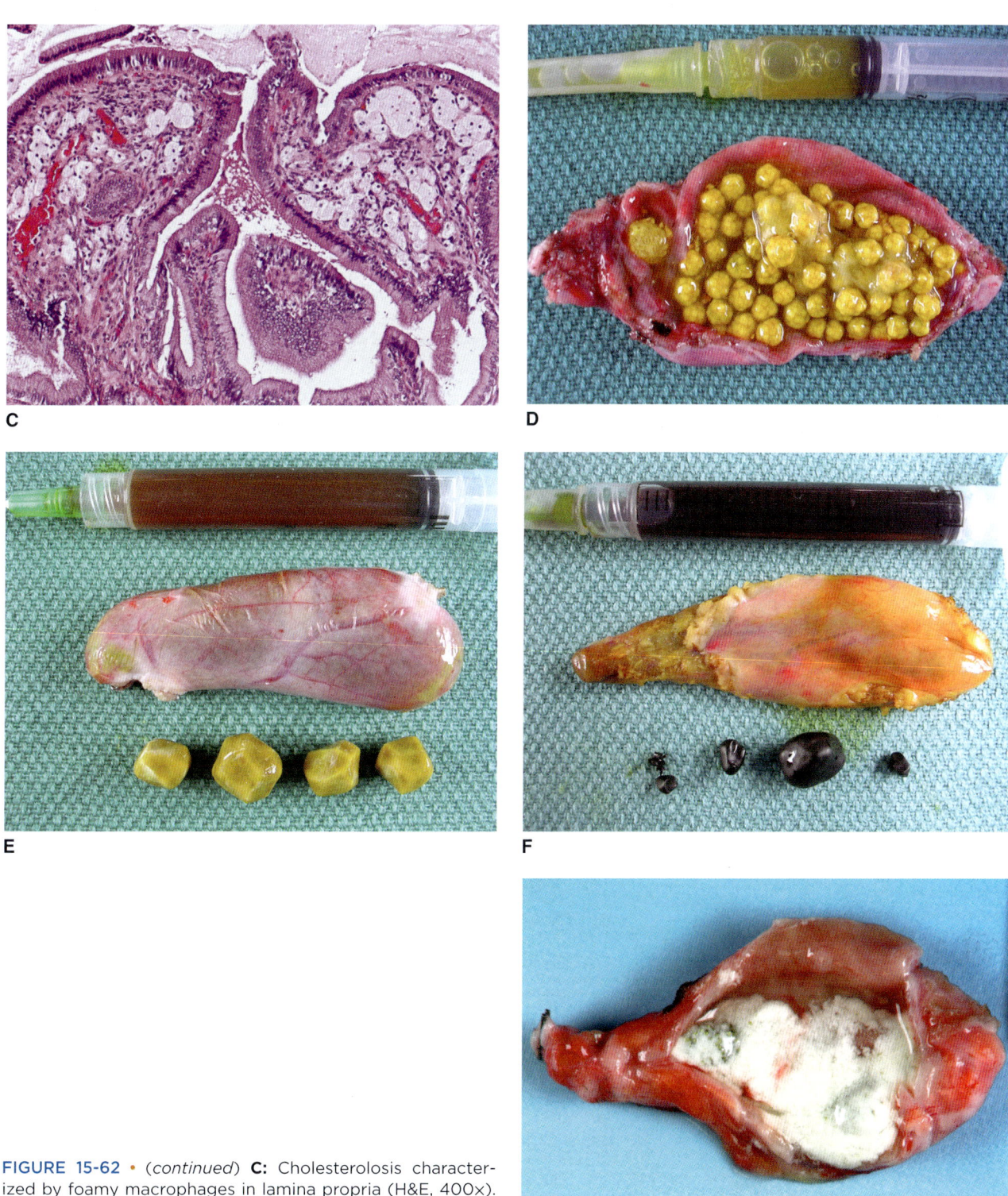

FIGURE 15-62 • *(continued)* **C:** Cholesterolosis characterized by foamy macrophages in lamina propria (H&E, 400×). **D–G:** Cholelithiasis varies from cholesterol choleliths **(D, E)**, ebonized choleliths **(F)**, and calcium choleliths with milklike bile **(G)**.

cholelithiasis include TPN, biliary stasis, ileal disease, sepsis, prolonged fasting, inflammatory bowel disease, short gut syndrome, ileal resection, PSC, prematurity, dehydration, immaturity of the hepatic glucuronyl transferase, ceftriaxone therapy, CF, cirrhosis, Wilson disease, porphyria, biliary dyskinesia, medications, and biliary tract anomalies, such as choledochal cyst. Cholelithiasis with cholesterol stones is seen in obese adolescents, both male and female. Tumors of the gallbladder are extremely rare in children; biliary rhabdomyosarcomas have been discussed above.

ACKNOWLEDGMENT

The contributions to this chapter in the 3rd edition are gratefully acknowledged.

References

1. Roskams T, Desmet V. Embryology of extra- and intrahepatic bile ducts, the ductal plate. *Anat Rec (Hoboken)* 2008;291(6):628–635.
2. Roskams TA, Theise ND, Balabaud C, et al. Nomenclature of the finer branches of the biliary tree: canals, ductules, and ductular reactions in human livers. *Hepatology* 2004;39(6):1739–1745.
3. Prithishkumar IJ, Kanakasabapathy I. Agenesis of the left lobe of liver—a rare anomaly with associated hepatic arterial variations. *Clin Anat* 2010;23(8):899–901.
4. Grisaru-Granovsky S, Rabinowitz R, Ioscovich A, et al. Congenital diaphragmatic hernia: review of the literature in reflection of unresolved dilemmas. *Acta Paediatr* 2009;98(12):1874–1881.
5. Gander JW, Kadenhe-Chiweshe A, Fisher JC, et al. Hepatic pulmonary fusion in an infant with a right-sided congenital diaphragmatic hernia and contralateral mediastinal shift. *J Pediatr Surg* 2010;45(1):265–268.
6. Wax JR, Pinette MG, Cartin A, et al. Ectopic liver: a unique prenatally diagnosed solid umbilical cord mass. *J Ultrasound Med* 2007;26(3):377–379.
7. Reiser DJ. Neonatal jaundice: physiologic variation or pathologic process. *Crit Care Nurs Clin North Am* 2004;16(2):257–269.
8. Gourley GR, ed. *Neonatal Jaundice and Disorders of Bilirubin Metabolism.* 3rd ed. New York: Cambridge University Press, 2007. Suchy FJ, Sokoi RJ, Balisteri WF, ed. Liver disease in children.
9. Erlinger S, Arias IM, Dhumeaux D. Inherited disorders of bilirubin transport and conjugation: new insights into molecular mechanisms and consequences. *Gastroenterology* 2014;146:1625–1538.
10. Ranganathan S. Hereditary hyperbilirubinemia. In: Ferrell L, Kakar, S, ed. *Liver Pathology*. New York: Demos Medical, 2011:153–157.
11. Roberts EA. Neonatal hepatitis syndrome. *Semin Neonatol* 2003;8(5): 357–374.
12. Torbenson M, Hart J, Westerhoff M, et al. Neonatal giant cell hepatitis: histological and etiological findings. *Am J Surg Pathol* 2010;34(10):1498–1503.
13. Whitington PF. Neonatal hemochromatosis: a congenital alloimmune hepatitis. *Semin Liver Dis* 2007;27(3):243–250.
14. Hartley JL, Davenport M, Kelly DA. Biliary atresia. *Lancet* 2009;374(9702):1704–1713.
15. Karrer FM, Bensard DD. Neonatal cholestasis. *Semin Pediatr Surg* 2000;9(4):166–169.
16. Schwarz KB, Haber BH, Rosenthal P, et al. Extrahepatic anomalies in infants with biliary atresia: results of a large prospective North American multicenter study. *Hepatology* 2013;58(5):1724–1731.
17. Balistreri WF, Bezerra JA. Whatever happened to "neonatal hepatitis"? *Clin Liver Dis* 2006;10(1):27–53, v.
18. Karjoo S, Hand NJ, Loarca L, et al. Extrahepatic cholangiocyte cilia are abnormal in biliary atresia. *J Pediatr Gastroenterol Nutr* 2013;57(1):96–101.
19. Russo P, Magee JC, Boitnott J, et al. Design and validation of the biliary atresia research consortium histologic assessment system for cholestasis in infancy. *Clin Gastroenterol Hepatol* 2011;9(4):357–362 e352.
20. Ovchinsky N, Moreira RK, Lefkowitch JH, et al. Liver biopsy in modern clinical practice: a pediatric point-of-view. *Adv Anat Pathol* 2012;19(4):250–262.
21. Desmet VJ. Ductal plates in hepatic ductular reactions. Hypothesis and implications III Implications for liver pathology. *Virchows Arch* 2011;458(3):271–279.
22. Gautier M, Eliot N. Extrahepatic biliary atresia. Morphological study of 98 biliary remnants. *Arch Pathol Lab Med* 1981;105(8):397–402.
23. Mirza Q, Kvist N, Petersen BL. Histologic features of the portal plate in extrahepatic biliary atresia and their impact on prognosis—a Danish study. *J Pediatr Surg* 2009;44(7):1344–1348.
24. Alagille D, Estrada A, Hadchouel M, et al. Syndromic paucity of interlobular bile ducts (Alagille syndrome or arteriohepatic dysplasia): review of 80 cases. *J Pediatr* 1987;110(2):195–200.
25. Kamath BM, Loomes KM, Oakey RJ, et al. Facial features in Alagille syndrome: specific or cholestasis facies? *Am J Med Genet* 2002;112(2):163–170.
26. Kamath BM, Bauer RC, Loomes KM, et al. NOTCH2 mutations in Alagille syndrome. *J Med Genet* 2012;49(2):138–144.
27. Marchetti D, Iascone MR, Pezzoli L. Novel human pathological mutations. Gene symbol: JAG1. Disease: alagille syndrome. *Hum Genet* 2009;126(2):350–351.
28. MacBride Emerick K. Outcome of liver disease in children with Alagille syndrome: a study of 163 patients. *J Pediatr Gastroenterol Nutr* 2002;35(1):103–104.
29. Shneider BL. Liver transplantation for Alagille syndrome: the jagged edge. *Liver Transpl* 2012;18(8):878–880.
30. Byrne JA, Meara NJ, Rayner AC, et al. Lack of hepatocellular CD10 along bile canaliculi is physiologic in early childhood and persistent in Alagille syndrome. *Lab Invest* 2007;87(11):1138–1148.
31. Bull LN, Carlton VE, Stricker NL, et al. Genetic and morphological findings in progressive familial intrahepatic cholestasis (Byler disease [PFIC-1] and Byler syndrome): evidence for heterogeneity. *Hepatology* 1997;26(1):155–164.
32. de Vree JM, Jacquemin E, Sturm E, et al. Mutations in the MDR3 gene cause progressive familial intrahepatic cholestasis. *Proc Natl Acad Sci U S A* 1998;95(1):282–287.
33. Francalanci P, Giovannoni I, Candusso M, et al. Bile salt export pump deficiency: a de novo mutation in a child compound heterozygous for ABCB11. Laboratory investigation to study pathogenic role and transmission of two novel ABCB11 mutations. *Hepatol Res* 2013;43(3):315–319.
34. Sambrotta M, Strautnieks S, Papouli E, et al. Mutations in TJP2 cause progressive cholestatic liver disease. *Nat Genet* 2014;46(4):326–328.
35. Alissa FT, Jaffe R, Shneider BL. Update on progressive familial intrahepatic cholestasis. *J Pediatr Gastroenterol Nutr* 2008;46(3):241–252.
36. Balistreri WF, Bezerra JA, Jansen P, et al. Intrahepatic cholestasis: summary of an American Association for the Study of Liver Diseases single-topic conference. *Hepatology* 2005;42(1):222–235.
37. Knisely AS, Strautnieks SS, Meier Y, et al. Hepatocellular carcinoma in ten children under five years of age with bile salt export pump deficiency. *Hepatology* 2006;44(2):478–486.
38. Morotti RA, Suchy FJ, Magid MS. Progressive familial intrahepatic cholestasis (PFIC) type 1, 2, and 3: a review of the liver pathology findings. *Semin Liver Dis* 2011;31(1):3–10.
39. Scheimann AO, Strautnieks SS, Knisely AS, et al. Mutations in bile salt export pump (ABCB11) in two children with progressive familial intrahepatic cholestasis and cholangiocarcinoma. *J Pediatr* 2007;150(5):556–559.
40. Shneider BL. Liver transplantation for progressive familial intrahepatic cholestasis: the evolving role of genotyping. *Liver Transpl* 2009;15(6):565–566.
41. Siebold L, Dick AA, Thompson R, et al. Recurrent low gamma-glutamyl transpeptidase cholestasis following liver transplantation for bile salt export pump (BSEP) disease (posttransplant recurrent BSEP disease). *Liver Transpl* 2010;16(7):856–863.
42. Carlton VE, Harris BZ, Puffenberger EG, et al. Complex inheritance of familial hypercholanemia with associated mutations in TJP2 and BAAT. *Nat Genet* 2003;34(1):91–96.
43. Chagnon P, Michaud J, Mitchell G, et al. A missense mutation (R565W) in cirhin (FLJ14728) in North American Indian childhood cirrhosis. *Am J Hum Genet* 2002;71(6):1443–1449.
44. Ackermann O, Gonzales E, Keller M, et al. Arthrogryposis, renal dysfunction, and cholestasis syndrome caused by VIPAR mutation. *J Pediatr Gastroenterol Nutr* 2014;58(3):e29–e32.
45. Girard M, Lacaille F, Verkarre V, et al. MYO5B and BSEP contribute to cholestatic liver disorder in microvillous inclusion disease. *Hepatology* 2014;60:301–310.
46. Balistreri WF. Intrahepatic cholestasis. *J Pediatr Gastroenterol Nutr* 2002;35(Suppl 1):S17–S23.

47. Bull LN, Roche E, Song EJ, et al. Mapping of the locus for cholestasis-lymphedema syndrome (Aagenaes syndrome) to a 6.6-cM interval on chromosome 15q. *Am J Hum Genet* 2000;67(4):994–999.
48. DiFiore JW, Alexander F. Congenital bronchobiliary fistula in association with right-sided congenital diaphragmatic hernia. *J Pediatr Surg* 2002;37(8):1208–1209.
49. Vick DJ, Goodman ZD, Deavers MT, et al. Ciliated hepatic foregut cyst: a study of six cases and review of the literature. *Am J Surg Pathol* 1999;23(6):671–677.
50. Singham J, Yoshida EM, Scudamore CH. Choledochal cysts: part 1 of 3: classification and pathogenesis. *Can J Surg* 2009;52(5):434–440.
51. Singham J, Yoshida EM, Scudamore CH. Choledochal cysts: part 2 of 3: Diagnosis. *Can J Surg* 2009;52(6):506–511.
52. Kerkar N, Norton K, Suchy FJ. The hepatic fibrocystic diseases. *Clin Liver Dis* 2006;10(1):55–71, v–vi.
53. Ananthakrishnan AN, Saeian K. Caroli's disease: identification and treatment strategy. *Curr Gastroenterol Rep* 2007;9(2):151–155.
54. Nakanuma Y, Terada T, Ohta G, et al. Caroli's disease in congenital hepatic fibrosis and infantile polycystic disease. *Liver* 1982;2(4):346–354.
55. Gunay-Aygun M. Liver and kidney disease in ciliopathies. *Am J Med Genet C Semin Med Genet* 2009;151C(4):296–306.
56. Desmet VJ. Ludwig symposium on biliary disorders—part I. Pathogenesis of ductal plate abnormalities. *Mayo Clin Proc* 1998;73(1):80–89.
57. Doherty D, Parisi MA, Finn LS, et al. Mutations in 3 genes (MKS3, CC2D2A and RPGRIP1L) cause COACH syndrome (Joubert syndrome with congenital hepatic fibrosis). *J Med Genet* 2010;47(1):8–21.
58. Landing BH, Wells TR, Claireaux AE. Morphometric analysis of liver lesions in cystic diseases of childhood. *Hum Pathol* 1980;11(5 Suppl):549–560.
59. Bernstein J. Hepatic involvement in hereditary renal syndromes. *Birth Defects Orig Artic Ser* 1987;23(1):115–130.
60. Calinescu-Tuleasca AM, Bottani A, Rougemont AL, et al. Caroli disease, bilateral diffuse cystic renal dysplasia, situs inversus, postaxial polydactyly, and preauricular fistulas: a ciliopathy caused by a homozygous NPHP3 mutation. *Eur J Pediatr* 2013;172(7):877–881.
61. Rawat D, Kelly DA, Milford DV, et al. Phenotypic variation and long-term outcome in children with congenital hepatic fibrosis. *J Pediatr Gastroenterol Nutr* 2013;57(2):161–166.
62. Otto EA, Tory K, Attanasio M, et al. Hypomorphic mutations in meckelin (MKS3/TMEM67) cause nephronophthisis with liver fibrosis (NPHP11). *J Med Genet* 2009;46(10):663–670.
63. Applegarth DA, Toone JR, Lowry RB. Incidence of inborn errors of metabolism in British Columbia, 1969-1996. *Pediatrics* 2000;105(1):e10.
64. Fridovich-Keil JL. Galactosemia: the good, the bad, and the unknown. *J Cell Physiol* 2006;209(3):701–705.
65. Tyfield L, Reichardt J, Fridovich-Keil J, et al. Classical galactosemia and mutations at the galactose-1-phosphate uridyl transferase (GALT) gene. *Hum Mutat* 1999;13(6):417–430.
66. Jevon GP, Dimmick JE. Histopathologic approach to metabolic liver disease: part 2. *Pediatr Dev Pathol* 1998;1(4):261–269.
67. Wong D. Hereditary fructose intolerance. *Mol Genet Metab* 2005;85(3):165–167.
68. Pronicka E, Adamowicz M, Kowalik A, et al. Elevated carbohydrate-deficient transferrin (CDT) and its normalization on dietary treatment as a useful biochemical test for hereditary fructose intolerance and galactosemia. *Pediatr Res* 2007;62(1):101–105.
69. McAdams AJ, Hug G, Bove KE. Glycogen storage disease, types I to X: criteria for morphologic diagnosis. *Hum Pathol* 1974;5(4):463–487.
70. Jevon GP, Dimmick JE. Histopathologic approach to metabolic liver disease: Part 1. *Pediatr Dev Pathol* 1998;1(3):179–199.
71. Phillips M, Pucell S, Patterson J. Metabolic liver disease. In: Phillips MJ, Poucell S, Patterson J et al., ed. *The Liver: An Atlas and Text of Ultrastructural Pathology*. New York: Raven Press, 1987:239.
72. Ozen H. Glycogen storage diseases: new perspectives. *World J Gastroenterol* 2007;13(18):2541–2553.
73. Labrune P, Trioche P, Duvaltier I, et al. Hepatocellular adenomas in glycogen storage disease type I and III: a series of 43 patients and review of the literature. *J Pediatr Gastroenterol Nutr* 1997;24(3):276–279.
74. Franco LM, Krishnamurthy V, Bali D, et al. Hepatocellular carcinoma in glycogen storage disease type Ia: a case series. *J Inherit Metab Dis* 2005;28(2):153–162.
75. Boers SJ, Visser G, Smit PG, et al. Liver transplantation in glycogen storage disease type I. *Orphanet J Rare Dis* 2014;9(1):47.
76. Kishnani PS, Beckemeyer AA, Mendelsohn NJ. The new era of Pompe disease: advances in the detection, understanding of the phenotypic spectrum, pathophysiology, and management. *Am J Med Genet C Semin Med Genet* 2012;160C(1):1–7.
77. Remiche G, Ronchi D, Magri F, et al. Extended phenotype description and new molecular findings in late onset glycogen storage disease type II: a northern Italy population study and review of the literature. *J Neurol* 2014;261(1):83–97.
78. Moses SW, Parvari R. The variable presentations of glycogen storage disease type IV: a review of clinical, enzymatic and molecular studies. *Curr Mol Med* 2002;2(2):177–188.
79. Hardwick DF, Dimmick JE. Metabolic cirrhoses of infancy and early childhood. *Perspect Pediatr Pathol* 1976;3:103–144.
80. Magoulas PL, El-Hattab AW, Roy A, et al. Diffuse reticuloendothelial system involvement in type IV glycogen storage disease with a novel GBE1 mutation: a case report and review. *Hum Pathol* 2012;43(6):943–951.
81. Taddei T, Mistry P, Schilsky ML. Inherited metabolic disease of the liver. *Curr Opin Gastroenterol* 2008;24(3):278–286.
82. Santer R, Groth S, Kinner M, et al. The mutation spectrum of the facilitative glucose transporter gene SLC2A2 (GLUT2) in patients with Fanconi-Bickel syndrome. *Hum Genet* 2002;110(1):21–29.
83. Russo PA, Mitchell GA, Tanguay RM. Tyrosinemia: a review. *Pediatr Dev Pathol* 2001;4(3):212–221.
84. Dursun A, Ozgul RK, Sivri S, et al. Mutation spectrum of fumarylacetoacetase gene and clinical aspects of tyrosinemia type I disease. *JIMD Rep* 2011;1:17–21.
85. Romano F, Stroppa P, Bravi M, et al. Favorable outcome of primary liver transplantation in children with cirrhosis and hepatocellular carcinoma. *Pediatr Transplant* 2011;15(6):573–579.
86. Jaffe R. Liver transplant pathology in pediatric metabolic disorders. *Pediatr Dev Pathol* 1998;1(2):102-117.
87. Grompe M. The pathophysiology and treatment of hereditary tyrosinemia type 1. *Semin Liver Dis* 2001;21(4):563–571.
88. Lohse P, Maas S, Elleder M, et al. Compound heterozygosity for a Wolman mutation is frequent among patients with cholesteryl ester storage disease. *J Lipid Res* 2000;41(1):23–31.
89. Boldrini R, Devito R, Biselli R, et al. Wolman disease and cholesteryl ester storage disease diagnosed by histological and ultrastructural examination of intestinal and liver biopsy. *Pathol Res Pract* 2004;200(3):231–240.
90. Gilbert-Barness EF, Barness LA. The mucolipidoses. *Perspect Pediatr Pathol* 1993;17:148–184.
91. Gopaul KP, Crook MA. The inborn errors of sialic acid metabolism and their laboratory investigation. *Clin Lab* 2006;52(3-4):155–169.
92. Xia B, Asif G, Arthur L, et al. Oligosaccharide analysis in urine by maldi-tof mass spectrometry for the diagnosis of lysosomal storage diseases. *Clin Chem* 2013;59(9):1357–1368.
93. Gilbert-Barness E, Barness L. ed *Metabolic Diseases: Foundations of Clinical Management, Genetics and Pathology*. Natick, MA: Eaton Publishing; 2000.
94. Luzi P, Rafi MA, Rao HZ, et al. Sixteen novel mutations in the arylsulfatase A gene causing metachromatic leukodystrophy. *Gene* 2013;530(2):323–328.
95. Alves MQ, Le Trionnaire E, Ribeiro I, et al. Molecular basis of acid ceramidase deficiency in a neonatal form of Farber disease: identification of the first large deletion in ASAH1 gene. *Mol Genet Metab* 2013;109(3):276–281.
96. Antonarakis SE, Valle D, Moser HW, et al. Phenotypic variability in siblings with Farber disease. *J Pediatr* 1984;104(3):406-409.

97. Hoffmann B. Fabry disease: recent advances in pathology, diagnosis, treatment and monitoring. *Orphanet J Rare Dis* 2009;4:21.
98. Brunetti-Pierri N, Scaglia F. GM1 gangliosidosis: review of clinical, molecular, and therapeutic aspects. *Mol Genet Metab* 2008;94(4):391–396.
99. Smith NJ, Winstone AM, Stellitano L, et al. GM2 gangliosidosis in a UK study of children with progressive neurodegeneration: 73 cases reviewed. *Dev Med Child Neurol* 2012;54(2):176–182.
100. Muenzer J. The mucopolysaccharidoses: a heterogeneous group of disorders with variable pediatric presentations. *J Pediatr* 2004;144(5 Suppl):S27–S34.
101. Wraith JE, Baumgartner MR, Bembi B, et al. Recommendations on the diagnosis and management of Niemann-Pick disease type C. *Mol Genet Metab* 2009;98(1–2):152–165.
102. Chen M, Wang J. Gaucher disease: review of the literature. *Arch Pathol Lab Med* 2008;132(5):851–853.
103. Finn LS, Zhang M, Chen SH, et al. Severe type II Gaucher disease with ichthyosis, arthrogryposis and neuronal apoptosis: molecular and pathological analyses. *Am J Med Genet* 2000;91(3):222–226.
104. Sundaram SS, Bove KE, Lovell MA, et al. Mechanisms of disease: Inborn errors of bile acid synthesis. *Nat Clin Pract Gastroenterol Hepatol* 2008;5(8):456–468.
105. Wanders RJ. Peroxisomes in human health and disease: metabolic pathways, metabolite transport, interplay with other organelles and signal transduction. *Subcell Biochem* 2013;69:23–44.
106. Clayton PT. Disorders of bile acid synthesis. *J Inherit Metab Dis* 2011;34(3):593–604.
107. Bove KE, Daugherty CC, Tyson W, et al. Bile acid synthetic defects and liver disease. *Pediatr Dev Pathol* 2000;3(1):1–16.
108. Perlmutter DH. Alpha-1-antitrypsin deficiency: diagnosis and treatment. *Clin Liver Dis* 2004;8(4):839–859, viii-ix.
109. Silverman GA, Pak SC, Perlmutter DH. Disorders of protein misfolding: alpha-1-antitrypsin deficiency as prototype. *J Pediatr* 2013;163(2):320–326.
110. Perlmutter DH. Alpha-1-antitrypsin deficiency: importance of proteasomal and autophagic degradative pathways in disposal of liver disease-associated protein aggregates. *Annu Rev Med* 2011;62:333–345.
111. Rudnick DA, Perlmutter DH. Alpha-1-antitrypsin deficiency: a new paradigm for hepatocellular carcinoma in genetic liver disease. *Hepatology* 2005;42(3):514–521.
112. Perlmutter DH. Liver injury in alpha 1-antitrypsin deficiency. *Clin Liver Dis* 2000;4(2):387–408, vi.
113. Flass T, Narkewicz MR. Cirrhosis and other liver disease in cystic fibrosis. *J Cyst Fibros* 2013;12:116–124.
114. Lewindon PJ, Shepherd RW, Walsh MJ, et al. Importance of hepatic fibrosis in cystic fibrosis and the predictive value of liver biopsy. *Hepatology* 2011;53(1):193–201.
115. Moyer K, Balistreri W. Hepatobiliary disease in patients with cystic fibrosis. *Curr Opin Gastroenterol* 2009;25(3):272–278.
116. Knisely AS, Mieli-Vergani G, Whitington PF. Neonatal hemochromatosis. *Gastroenterol Clin North Am* 2003;32(3):877–889, vi-vii.
117. Batts KP. Iron overload syndromes and the liver. *Mod Pathol* 2007;20(Suppl 1):S31–S39.
118. Whitington PF. Gestational alloimmune liver disease and neonatal hemochromatosis. *Semin Liver Dis* 2012;32(4):325–332.
119. Alexander J, Kowdley KV. Hereditary hemochromatosis: genetics, pathogenesis, and clinical management. *Ann Hepatol* 2005;4(4):240–247.
120. Rand EB, Karpen SJ, Kelly S, et al. Treatment of neonatal hemochromatosis with exchange transfusion and intravenous immunoglobulin. *J Pediatr* 2009;155(4):566–571.
121. Lund DP, Lillehei CW, Kevy S, et al. Liver transplantation in newborn liver failure: treatment for neonatal hemochromatosis. *Transplant Proc* 1993;25(1 Pt 2):1068–1071.
122. Kanwar P, Kowdley KV. Metal storage disorders: Wilson disease and hemochromatosis. *Med Clin North Am* 2014;98(1):87–102.
123. Bennett J, Hahn SH. Clinical molecular diagnosis of Wilson disease. *Semin Liver Dis* 2011;31(3):233–238.
124. Zischka H, Lichtmannegger J. Pathological mitochondrial copper overload in livers of Wilson's disease patients and related animal models. *Ann N Y Acad Sci* 2014;1315(1):6–15.
125. Roberts EA, Schilsky ML. Diagnosis and treatment of Wilson disease: an update. *Hepatology* 2008;47(6):2089–2111.
126. Filippi C, Dhawan A. Current status of human hepatocyte transplantation and its potential for Wilson's disease. *Ann N Y Acad Sci* 2014;1315(1):50–55.
127. Guillaud O, Dumortier J, Sobesky R, et al. Long term results of liver transplantation for Wilson's disease: experience in France. *J Hepatol* 2014;60(3):579–589.
128. Johncilla M, Mitchell KA. Pathology of the liver in copper overload. *Semin Liver Dis* 2011;31(3):239–244.
129. Nayak NC, Chitale AR. Indian childhood cirrhosis (ICC) & ICC-like diseases: the changing scenario of facts versus notions. *Indian J Med Res* 2013;137(6):1029–1042.
130. Burton BK. Urea cycle disorders. *Clin Liver Dis* 2000;4(4):815–830, vi.
131. Vaidyanathan K. Molecular diagnosis of urea cycle disorders: current global scenario. *Indian J Biochem Biophys* 2013;50(5):357–362.
132. Yaplito-Lee J, Chow CW, Boneh A. Histopathological findings in livers of patients with urea cycle disorders. *Mol Genet Metab* 2013;108(3):161–165.
133. Perito ER, Rhee S, Roberts JP, et al. Pediatric liver transplantation for urea cycle disorders and organic acidemias: United Network for Organ Sharing data for 2002-2012. *Liver Transpl* 2014;20(1):89–99.
134. Loomba R, Sirlin CB, Schwimmer JB, et al. Advances in pediatric nonalcoholic fatty liver disease. *Hepatology* 2009;50(4):1282–1293.
135. Roberts EA. Pediatric nonalcoholic fatty liver disease (NAFLD): a "growing" problem? *J Hepatol* 2007;46(6):1133–1142.
136. Chalasani N, Younossi Z, Lavine JE, et al. The diagnosis and management of non-alcoholic fatty liver disease: practice guideline by the American Gastroenterological Association, American Association for the Study of Liver Diseases, and American College of Gastroenterology. *Gastroenterology* 2012;142(7):1592–1609.
137. Patton HM, Yates K, Unalp-Arida A, et al. Association between metabolic syndrome and liver histology among children with nonalcoholic Fatty liver disease. *Am J Gastroenterol* 2010;105(9):2093–2102.
138. Brunt EM. Pathology of nonalcoholic fatty liver disease. *Nat Rev Gastroenterol Hepatol* 2010;7(4):195–203.
139. Schwimmer JB, Behling C, Newbury R, et al. Histopathology of pediatric nonalcoholic fatty liver disease. *Hepatology* 2005;42(3):641–649.
140. Alkhouri N, De Vito R, Alisi A, et al. Development and validation of a new histological score for pediatric non-alcoholic fatty liver disease. *J Hepatol* 2012;57(6):1312–1318.
141. Swiderska-Syn M, Suzuki A, Guy CD, et al. Hedgehog pathway and pediatric nonalcoholic fatty liver disease. *Hepatology* 2013;57(5):1814–1825.
142. Casteels-Van Daele M, Van Geet C, Wouters C, et al. Reye syndrome revisited: a descriptive term covering a group of heterogeneous disorders. *Eur J Pediatr* 2000;159(9):641–648.
143. Glasgow JF, Middleton B. Reye syndrome—insights on causation and prognosis. *Arch Dis Child* 2001;85(5):351–353.
144. Olpin SE. Pathophysiology of fatty acid oxidation disorders and resultant phenotypic variability. *J Inherit Metab Dis* 2013;36(4):645–658.
145. Bonnefont JP, Demaugre F, Prip-Buus C, et al. Carnitine palmitoyltransferase deficiencies. *Mol Genet Metab* 1999;68(4):424–440.
146. Gordon N. Glutaric aciduria types I and II. *Brain Dev* 2006;28(3):136–140.
147. Cohen BH, Naviaux RK. The clinical diagnosis of POLG disease and other mitochondrial DNA depletion disorders. *Methods* 2010;51(4):364–373.
148. Wong LJ, Naviaux RK, Brunetti-Pierri N, et al. Molecular and clinical genetics of mitochondrial diseases due to POLG mutations. *Hum Mutat* 2008;29(9):E150–E172.

149. Muller-Hocker J, Muntau A, Schafer S, et al. Depletion of mitochondrial DNA in the liver of an infant with neonatal giant cell hepatitis. *Hum Pathol* 2002;33(2):247–253.
150. Mandel H, Hartman C, Berkowitz D, et al. The hepatic mitochondrial DNA depletion syndrome: ultrastructural changes in liver biopsies. *Hepatology* 2001;34(4 Pt 1):776–784.
151. Degertekin B, Lok AS. Update on viral hepatitis: 2008. *Curr Opin Gastroenterol* 2009;25(3):180–185.
152. Fishman LN, Jonas MM, Lavine JE. Update on viral hepatitis in children. *Pediatr Clin North Am* 1996;43(1):57–74.
153. White FV, Dehner LP. Viral diseases of the liver in children: diagnostic and differential diagnostic considerations. *Pediatr Dev Pathol* 2004;7(6):552–567.
154. Matheny SC, Kingery JE. Hepatitis A. *Am Fam Physician* 2012;86(11): 1027–1034; quiz 1010–1022.
155. Tovo PA, Lazier L, Versace A. Hepatitis B virus and hepatitis C virus infections in children. *Curr Opin Infect Dis* 2005;18(3):261–266.
156. Mohan N, Gonzalez-Peralta RP, Fujisawa T, et al. Chronic hepatitis C virus infection in children. *J Pediatr Gastroenterol Nutr* 2010;50(2):123–131.
157. Le Campion A, Larouche A, Fauteux-Daniel S, et al. Pathogenesis of hepatitis C during pregnancy and childhood. *Viruses* 2012;4(12): 3531–3550.
158. Goodman ZD, Ishak KG. Histopathology of hepatitis C virus infection. *Semin Liver Dis* 1995;15(1):70–81.
159. Rizzetto M. Hepatitis D: thirty years after. *J Hepatol* 2009;50(5): 1043–1050.
160. Kamar N, Dalton HR, Abravanel F, et al. Hepatitis E virus infection. *Clin Microbiol Rev* 2014;27(1):116–138.
161. Kew MC, Kassianides C. HGV: hepatitis G virus or harmless G virus? *Lancet* 1996;348(Suppl 2):sII10.
162. Ishak KG. Pathologic features of chronic hepatitis. A review and update. *Am J Clin Pathol* 2000;113(1):40–55.
163. Mani H, Kleiner DE. Liver biopsy findings in chronic hepatitis B. *Hepatology* 2009;49(5 Suppl):S61–S71.
164. Desmet VJ, Gerber M, Hoofnagle JH, et al. Classification of chronic hepatitis: diagnosis, grading and staging. *Hepatology* 1994;19(6):1513–1520.
165. Ishak KG. Chronic hepatitis: morphology and nomenclature. *Mod Pathol* 1994;7(6):690–713.
166. Kirsch R, Yap J, Roberts EA, et al. Clinicopathologic spectrum of massive and submassive hepatic necrosis in infants and children. *Hum Pathol* 2009;40(4):516–526.
167. Sundaram V, Shneider BL, Dhawan A, et al. King's College Hospital Criteria for non-acetaminophen induced acute liver failure in an international cohort of children. *J Pediatr* 2013;162(2):319–323 e311.
168. LaRusso NF, Shneider BL, Black D, et al. Primary sclerosing cholangitis: summary of a workshop. *Hepatology* 2006;44(3):746–764.
169. Roberts EA. Primary sclerosing cholangitis in children. *J Gastroenterol Hepatol* 1999;14(6):588–593.
170. Venkat VL, Ranganathan S, Mazariegos GV, et al. Recurrence of Primary Sclerosing Cholangitis (rPSC) in Pediatric Liver Transplant (LTx) Recipients. *Hepatology* 2013;58:810A–810A.
171. Floreani A, Liberal R, Vergani D, et al. Autoimmune hepatitis: contrasts and comparisons in children and adults—a comprehensive review. *J Autoimmun* 2013;46:7–16.
172. Mieli-Vergani G, Vergani D. Paediatric autoimmune liver disease. *Arch Dis Child* 2013;98(12):1012–1017.
173. Molleston JP, Mellman W, Narkewicz MR, et al. Autoantibodies and autoimmune disease during treatment of children with chronic hepatitis C. *J Pediatr Gastroenterol Nutr* 2013;56(3):304–310.
174. Finegold MJ. Common diagnostic problems in pediatric liver pathology. *Clin Liver Dis* 2002;6(2):421–454.
175. Israeli R, Jule JE, Hom J. Pediatric pyogenic liver abscess. *Pediatr Emerg Care* 2009;25(2):107–108.
176. Pereira FE, Musso C, Castelo JS. Pathology of pyogenic liver abscess in children. *Pediatr Dev Pathol* 1999;2(6):537–543.
177. Rana SS, Bhasin DK, Nanda M, et al. Parasitic infestations of the biliary tract. *Curr Gastroenterol Rep* 2007;9(2):156–164.
178. Lamps LW. Hepatic granulomas, with an emphasis on infectious causes. *Adv Anat Pathol* 2008;15(6):309–318.
179. Gioulème O, Theocharidou E. Management of portal hypertension in children with portal vein thrombosis. *J Pediatr Gastroenterol Nutr* 2013;57(4):419–425.
180. Pietrobattista A, Luciani M, Abraldes JG, et al. Extrahepatic portal vein thrombosis in children and adolescents: Influence of genetic thrombophilic disorders. *World J Gastroenterol* 2010;16(48):6123–6127.
181. Zimmerman MA, Cameron AM, Ghobrial RM. Budd-Chiari syndrome. *Clin Liver Dis* 2006;10(2):259–273, viii.
182. Gomes AC, Rubino G, Pinto C, et al. Budd-Chiari syndrome in children and outcome after liver transplant. *Pediatr Transplant* 2012;16(8): E338–E341.
183. Ludwig J, Hashimoto E, McGill DB, et al. Classification of hepatic venous outflow obstruction: ambiguous terminology of the Budd-Chiari syndrome. *Mayo Clin Proc* 1990;65(1):51–55.
184. Tsokos M, Erbersdobler A. Pathology of peliosis. *Forensic Sci Int* 2005;149(1):25–33.
185. Jacquemin E, Pariente D, Fabre M, et al. Peliosis hepatis with initial presentation as acute hepatic failure and intraperitoneal hemorrhage in children. *J Hepatol* 1999;30(6):1146–1150.
186. Klein S, Nealon WH. Hepatobiliary abnormalities associated with total parenteral nutrition. *Semin Liver Dis* 1988;8(3):237–246.
187. Kubota A, Yonekura T, Hoki M, et al. Total parenteral nutrition-associated intrahepatic cholestasis in infants: 25 years' experience. *J Pediatr Surg* 2000;35(7):1049–1051.
188. Naini BV, Lassman CR. Total parenteral nutrition therapy and liver injury: a histopathologic study with clinical correlation. *Hum Pathol* 2012;43(6):826–833.
189. Anthony PP, Ishak KG, Nayak NC, et al. The morphology of cirrhosis. Recommendations on definition, nomenclature, and classification by a working group sponsored by the World Health Organization. *J Clin Pathol* 1978;31(5):395–414.
190. Lee WS, Sokol RJ. Mitochondrial hepatopathies: advances in genetics and pathogenesis. *Hepatology* 2007;45(6):1555–1565.
191. Ghaferi AA, Hutchins GM. Progression of liver pathology in patients undergoing the Fontan procedure: Chronic passive congestion, cardiac cirrhosis, hepatic adenoma, and hepatocellular carcinoma. *J Thorac Cardiovasc Surg* 2005;129(6):1348–1352.
192. Eckhauser FE, Appelman HD, Knol JA, et al. Noncirrhotic portal hypertension: differing patterns of disease in children and adults. *Surgery* 1983;94(4):721–728.
193. Anthony PP. Liver cell dysplasia: a premalignant condition. *J Pathol* 1973;109(1):Pxvii.
194. Nakanuma Y, Terada T, Ueda K, et al. Adenomatous hyperplasia of the liver as a precancerous lesion. *Liver* 1993;13(1):1–9.
195. Stocker JT, Ishak KG. Focal nodular hyperplasia of the liver: a study of 21 pediatric cases. *Cancer* 1981;48(2):336–345.
196. Wanless IR, Mawdsley C, Adams R. On the pathogenesis of focal nodular hyperplasia of the liver. *Hepatology* 1985;5(6):1194–1200.
197. Mathieu D, Kobeiter H, Cherqui D, et al. Oral contraceptive intake in women with focal nodular hyperplasia of the liver. *Lancet* 1998; 352(9141):1679–1680.
198. Bioulac-Sage P, Balabaud C, Wanless IR. Diagnosis of focal nodular hyperplasia: not so easy. *Am J Surg Pathol* 2001;25(10):1322–1325.
199. Cheon JE, Kim WS, Kim IO, et al. Radiological features of focal nodular hyperplasia of the liver in children. *Pediatr Radiol* 1998;28(11):878–883.
200. Saul SH, Titelbaum DS, Gansler TS, et al. The fibrolamellar variant of hepatocellular carcinoma. Its association with focal nodular hyperplasia. *Cancer* 1987;60(12):3049–3055.
201. van Eyken P, Sciot R, Callea F, et al. A cytokeratin-immunohistochemical study of focal nodular hyperplasia of the liver: further evidence that ductular metaplasia of hepatocytes contributes to ductular "proliferation." *Liver* 1989;9(6):372–377.

202. Fabre A, Audet P, Vilgrain V, et al. Histologic scoring of liver biopsy in focal nodular hyperplasia with atypical presentation. *Hepatology* 2002;35(2):414–420.
203. Joseph NM, Ferrell LD, Jain D, et al. Diagnostic utility and limitations of glutamine synthetase and serum amyloid-associated protein immunohistochemistry in the distinction of focal nodular hyperplasia and inflammatory hepatocellular adenoma. *Mod Pathol* 2014;27(1):62–72.
204. International Working Party. Terminology of nodular hepatocellular lesions. *Hepatology* 1995;22(3):983–993.
205. Bioulac-Sage P, Cubel G, Taouji S, et al. Immunohistochemical markers on needle biopsies are helpful for the diagnosis of focal nodular hyperplasia and hepatocellular adenoma subtypes. *Am J Surg Pathol* 2012;36(11):1691–1699.
206. Rebouissou S, Bioulac-Sage P, Zucman-Rossi J. Molecular pathogenesis of focal nodular hyperplasia and hepatocellular adenoma. *J Hepatol* 2008;48(1):163–170.
207. Wanless IR. Micronodular transformation (nodular regenerative hyperplasia) of the liver: a report of 64 cases among 2,500 autopsies and a new classification of benign hepatocellular nodules. *Hepatology* 1990;11(5):787–797.
208. Moran CA, Mullick FG, Ishak KG. Nodular regenerative hyperplasia of the liver in children. *Am J Surg Pathol* 1991;15(5):449–454.
209. Stocker JT. Hepatic tumors in children. *Clin Liver Dis* 2001;5(1):259–281, viii–ix.
210. Albuquerque A, Cardoso H, Lopes J, et al. Familial occurrence of nodular regenerative hyperplasia of the liver. *Am J Gastroenterol* 2013;108(1):150–151.
211. Rothweiler S, Terracciano L, Tornillo L, et al. Downregulation of the endothelial genes Notch1 and ephrinB2 in patients with nodular regenerative hyperplasia. *Liver Int* 2014;34(4):594–603.
212. Reshamwala PA, Kleiner DE, Heller T. Nodular regenerative hyperplasia: not all nodules are created equal. *Hepatology* 2006;44(1):7–14.
213. Ames JT, Federle MP, Chopra K. Distinguishing clinical and imaging features of nodular regenerative hyperplasia and large regenerative nodules of the liver. *Clin Radiol* 2009;64(12):1190–1195.
214. Nzeako UC, Goodman ZD, Ishak KG. Hepatocellular carcinoma and nodular regenerative hyperplasia: possible pathogenetic relationship. *Am J Gastroenterol* 1996;91(5):879–884.
215. Resnick MB, Kozakewich HP, Perez-Atayde AR. Hepatic adenoma in the pediatric age group. Clinicopathological observations and assessment of cell proliferative activity. *Am J Surg Pathol* 1995;19(10):1181–1190.
216. Bioulac-Sage P, Sempoux C, Possenti L, et al. Pathological diagnosis of hepatocellular cellular adenoma according to the Clinical Context. *Int J Hepatol* 2013;2013:253–261.
217. Nault JC, Bioulac-Sage P, Zucman-Rossi J. Hepatocellular benign tumors-from molecular classification to personalized clinical care. *Gastroenterology* 2013;144(5):888–902.
218. Kakar S, Grenert JP, Paradis V, et al. Hepatocellular carcinoma arising in adenoma: similar immunohistochemical and cytogenetic features in adenoma and hepatocellular carcinoma portions of the tumor. *Mod Pathol* 2014;27:1499–1509.
219. Bioulac-Sage P, Rebouissou S, Sa Cunha A, et al. Clinical, morphologic, and molecular features defining so-called telangiectatic focal nodular hyperplasias of the liver. *Gastroenterology* 2005;128(5):1211–1218.
220. Shafizadeh N, Kakar S. Diagnosis of well-differentiated hepatocellular lesions: role of immunohistochemistry and other ancillary techniques. *Adv Anat Pathol* 2011;18(6):438–445.
221. Pilati C, Letouze E, Nault JC, et al. Genomic profiling of hepatocellular adenomas reveals recurrent FRK-activating mutations and the mechanisms of malignant transformation. *Cancer Cell* 2014;25(4):428–441.
222. Stocker JT, Ishak KG. Mesenchymal hamartoma of the liver: report of 30 cases and review of the literature. *Pediatr Pathol* 1983;1(3):245–267.
223. Reed RC, Beischel L, Schoof J, et al. Androgenetic/biparental mosaicism in an infant with hepatic mesenchymal hamartoma and placental mesenchymal dysplasia. *Pediatr Dev Pathol* 2008;11(5):377–383.
224. Kapur RP, Berry JE, Tsuchiya KD, et al. Activation of the chromosome 19q microRNA cluster in sporadic and androgenetic-biparental mosaicism-associated hepatic mesenchymal hamartoma. *Pediatr Dev Pathol* 2014;17:75–84.
225. Cornette J, Festen S, van den Hoonaard TL, et al. Mesenchymal hamartoma of the liver: a benign tumor with deceptive prognosis in the perinatal period. Case report and review of the literature. *Fetal Diagn Ther* 2009;25(2):196–202.
226. Isaacs H Jr. Fetal and neonatal hepatic tumors. *J Pediatr Surg* 2007;42(11):1797–1803.
227. Meyers RL. Tumors of the liver in children. *Surg Oncol* 2007;16(3):195–203.
228. Stocker JT, Conran RM, Selby DM. Tumor and pseudotumors of the liver. In: Askin FB, Stocker JT, eds. *Pathology of Solid Tumors in Children*. London, UK: Chapman & Hall, 1998:83–110.
229. Chang HJ, Jin SY, Park C, et al. Mesenchymal hamartomas of the liver: comparison of clinicopathologic features between cystic and solid forms. *J Korean Med Sci* 2006;21(1):63–68.
230. Mathews J, Duncavage EJ, Pfeifer JD. Characterization of translocations in mesenchymal hamartoma and undifferentiated embryonal sarcoma of the liver. *Exp Mol Pathol* 2013;95(3):319–324.
231. Lauwers GY, Grant LD, Donnelly WH, et al. Hepatic undifferentiated (embryonal) sarcoma arising in a mesenchymal hamartoma. *Am J Surg Pathol* 1997;21(10):1248–1254.
232. Shehata BM, Gupta NA, Katzenstein HM, et al. Undifferentiated embryonal sarcoma of the liver is associated with mesenchymal hamartoma and multiple chromosomal abnormalities: a review of eleven cases. *Pediatr Dev Pathol* 2011;14(2):111–116.
233. Begueret H, Trouette H, Vielh P, et al. Hepatic undifferentiated embryonal sarcoma: malignant evolution of mesenchymal hamartoma? Study of one case with immunohistochemical and flow cytometric emphasis. *J Hepatol* 2001;34(1):178–179.
234. Christison-Lagay ER, Burrows PE, Alomari A, et al. Hepatic hemangiomas: subtype classification and development of a clinical practice algorithm and registry. *J Pediatr Surg* 2007;42(1):62–67; discussion 67–68.
235. Kulungowski AM, Alomari AI, Chawla A, et al. Lessons from a liver hemangioma registry: subtype classification. *J Pediatr Surg* 2012;47(1):165–170.
236. Bosemani T, Puttgen KB, Huisman TA, et al. Multifocal infantile hepatic hemangiomas—imaging strategy and response to treatment after propranolol and steroids including review of the literature. *Eur J Pediatr* 2012;171(7):1023–1028.
237. Selby DM, Stocker JT, Waclawiw MA, et al. Infantile hemangioendothelioma of the liver. *Hepatology* 1994;20(1 Pt 1):39–45.
238. Becker JM, Heitler MS. Hepatic hemangioendotheliomas in infancy. *Surg Gynecol Obstet* 1989;168(2):189–200.
239. Giuliante F, Ardito F, Vellone M, et al. Reappraisal of surgical indications and approach for liver hemangioma: single-center experience on 74 patients. *Am J Surg* 2011;201(6):741–748.
240. Rodriguez JA, Becker NS, O'Mahony CA, et al. Long-term outcomes following liver transplantation for hepatic hemangioendothelioma: the UNOS experience from 1987 to 2005. *J Gastrointest Surg* 2008;12(1):110–116.
241. Dehner LP, Ishak KG. Vascular tumors of the liver in infants and children. A study of 30 cases and review of the literature. *Arch Pathol* 1971;92(2):101–111.
242. Ackermann O, Fabre M, Franchi S, et al. Widening spectrum of liver angiosarcoma in children. *J Pediatr Gastroenterol Nutr* 2011;53(6):615–619.
243. Dehner LP. The challenges of vasoformative tumors of the liver in children. *Pediatr Dev Pathol* 2004;7(5):A5–A7.
244. Cerar A, Dolenc-Strazar ZD, Bartenjev D. Infantile hemangioendothelioma of the liver in a neonate. Immunohistochemical observations. *Am J Surg Pathol* 1996;20(7):871–876.
245. Mo JQ, Dimashkieh HH, Bove KE. GLUT1 endothelial reactivity distinguishes hepatic infantile hemangioma from congenital hepatic vascular malformation with associated capillary proliferation. *Hum Pathol* 2004;35(2):200–209.

246. Hernandez F, Navarro M, Encinas JL, et al. The role of GLUT1 immunostaining in the diagnosis and classification of liver vascular tumors in children. *J Pediatr Surg* 2005;40(5):801–804.
247. Ito H, Yamasaki T, Okamoto O, et al. Infantile hemangioendothelioma of the liver in patient with interstitial deletion of chromosome 6q: report of an autopsy case. *Am J Med Genet* 1989;34(3):325–329.
248. Errani C, Sung YS, Zhang L, et al. Monoclonality of multifocal epithelioid hemangioendothelioma of the liver by analysis of WWTR1-CAMTA1 breakpoints. *Cancer Genet* 2012;205(1-2):12–17.
249. Manivel C, Wick MR, Abenoza P, et al. Teratoid hepatoblastoma. The nosologic dilemma of solid embryonic neoplasms of childhood. *Cancer* 1986;57(11):2168–2174.
250. Darbari A, Sabin KM, Shapiro CN, et al. Epidemiology of primary hepatic malignancies in U.S. children. *Hepatology* 2003;38(3):560–566.
251. Spector LG, Birch J. The epidemiology of hepatoblastoma. *Pediatr Blood Cancer* 2012;59(5):776–779.
252. Cruz RJ, Jr., Ranganathan S, Mazariegos G, et al. Analysis of national and single-center incidence and survival after liver transplantation for hepatoblastoma: new trends and future opportunities. *Surgery* 2013;153(2):150–159.
253. DeBaun MR, Tucker MA. Risk of cancer during the first four years of life in children from The Beckwith-Wiedemann Syndrome Registry. *J Pediatr* 1998;132(3 Pt 1):398–400.
254. Giardiello FM, Offerhaus GJ, Krush AJ, et al. Risk of hepatoblastoma in familial adenomatous polyposis. *J Pediatr* 1991;119(5):766–768.
255. Giardiello FM, Petersen GM, Brensinger JD, et al. Hepatoblastoma and APC gene mutation in familial adenomatous polyposis. *Gut* 1996;39(6):867–869.
256. Jeng YM, Wu MZ, Mao TL, et al. Somatic mutations of beta-catenin play a crucial role in the tumorigenesis of sporadic hepatoblastoma. *Cancer Lett* 2000;152(1):45–51.
257. Ikeda H, Matsuyama S, Tanimura M. Association between hepatoblastoma and very low birth weight: a trend or a chance? *J Pediatr* 1997;130(4):557–560.
258. Heimann A, White PF, Riely CA, et al. Hepatoblastoma presenting as isosexual precocity. The clinical importance of histologic and serologic parameters. *J Clin Gastroenterol* 1987;9(1):105–110.
259. Shafford EA, Pritchard J. Extreme thrombocytosis as a diagnostic clue to hepatoblastoma. *Arch Dis Child* 1993;69(1):171.
260. Czauderna P, Lopez-Terrada D, Hiyama E, et al. Hepatoblastoma state of the art: pathology, genetics, risk stratification, and chemotherapy. *Curr Opin Pediatr* 2014;26(1):19–28.
261. McCarville MB, Roebuck DJ. Diagnosis and staging of hepatoblastoma: imaging aspects. *Pediatr Blood Cancer* 2012;59(5):793–799.
262. Meyers RL, Tiao G, de Ville de Goyet J, Superina R, Aronson DC. Hepatoblastoma state of the art: pre-treatment extent of disease, surgical resection guidelines and the role of liver transplantation. *Curr Opin Pediatr* 2014;26(1):29–36.
263. Meyers RL, Katzenstein HM, Malogolowkin MH. Predictive value of staging systems in hepatoblastoma. *J Clin Oncol* 2007;25(6):737; author reply 737–738.
264. Conran RM, Hitchcock CL, Waclawiw MA, et al. Hepatoblastoma: the prognostic significance of histologic type. *Pediatr Pathol* 1992;12(2):167–183.
265. Meyers RL, Czauderna P, Otte JB. Surgical treatment of hepatoblastoma. *Pediatr Blood Cancer* 2012;59(5):800–808.
266. Malogolowkin MH, Katzenstein HM, Meyers RL, et al. Complete surgical resection is curative for children with hepatoblastoma with pure fetal histology: a report from the Children's Oncology Group. *J Clin Oncol* 2011;29(24):3301–3306.
267. Meyers RL, Rowland JR, Krailo M, et al. Predictive power of pretreatment prognostic factors in children with hepatoblastoma: a report from the Children's Oncology Group. *Pediatr Blood Cancer* 2009;53(6):1016–1022.
268. Finegold MJ. Tumors of the liver. *Semin Liver Dis* 1994;14(3):270–281.
269. Weinberg AG, Finegold MJ. Primary hepatic tumors of childhood. *Hum Pathol* 1983;14(6):512–537.
270. Lopez-Terrada D, Alaggio R, de Davila MT, et al. Towards an international pediatric liver tumor consensus classification: proceedings of the Los Angeles COG liver tumors symposium. *Mod Pathol* 2014;27(3):472–491.
271. Haas JE, Feusner JH, Finegold MJ. Small cell undifferentiated histology in hepatoblastoma may be unfavorable. *Cancer* 2001;92(12):3130–3134.
272. Trobaugh-Lotrario AD, Tomlinson GE, Finegold MJ, et al. Small cell undifferentiated variant of hepatoblastoma: adverse clinical and molecular features similar to rhabdoid tumors. *Pediatr Blood Cancer* 2009;52(3):328–334.
273. Zimmermann A. Hepatoblastoma with cholangioblastic features ('cholangioblastic hepatoblastoma') and other liver tumors with bimodal differentiation in young patients. *Med Pediatr Oncol* 2002;39(5):487–491.
274. Ranganathan S, Tan XP, Monga SPS. beta-Catenin and met deregulation in childhood hepatoblastomas. *Pediatr Develop Pathol* 2005;8(4):435–447.
275. Oda H, Imai Y, Nakatsuru Y, et al. Somatic mutations of the APC gene in sporadic hepatoblastomas. *Cancer Res* 1996;56(14):3320–3323.
276. Luo J-H, Ren B, Keryanov S, et al. Transcriptomic and genomic analysis of human hepatocellular carcinomas and hepatoblastomas. *Hepatology* 2006;44(4):1012–1024.
277. Armengol C, Cairo S, Fabre M, et al. Wnt signaling and hepatocarcinogenesis: the hepatoblastoma model. *Int J Biochem Cell Biol* 2011;43(2):265–270.
278. Zimmermann A. The emerging family of hepatoblastoma tumours: from ontogenesis to oncogenesis. *Eur J Cancer* 2005;41(11):1503–1514.
279. Lopez-Terrada D, Gunaratne PH, Adesina AM, et al. Histologic subtypes of hepatoblastoma are characterized by differential canonical Wnt and Notch pathway activation in DLK+ precursors. *Hum Pathol* 2009;40(6):783–794.
280. Tao J, Calvisi DF, Ranganathan S, et al. Activation of beta-catenin and Yap1 in human hepatoblastoma and induction of hepatocarcinogenesis in mice. *Gastroenterology* 2014;147(3):690–701.
281. Terada Y, Matsumoto S, Bando K, et al. Comprehensive allelotyping of hepatoblastoma. *Hepatogastroenterology* 2009;56(89):199–204.
282. Kraus JA, Albrecht S, Wiestler OD, et al. Loss of heterozygosity on chromosome 1 in human hepatoblastoma. *Int J Cancer* 1996;67(4):467–471.
283. Hata Y, Ishizu H, Ohmori K, et al. Flow cytometric analysis of the nuclear DNA content of hepatoblastoma. *Cancer* 1991;68(12):2566–2570.
284. Czauderna P, Mackinlay G, Perilongo G, et al. Hepatocellular carcinoma in children: results of the first prospective study of the International Society of Pediatric Oncology group. *J Clin Oncol* 2002;20(12):2798–2804.
285. Katzenstein HM, Krailo MD, Malogolowkin MH, et al. Hepatocellular carcinoma in children and adolescents: results from the Pediatric Oncology Group and the Children's Cancer Group intergroup study. *J Clin Oncol* 2002;20(12):2789–2797.
286. Katzenstein HM, Krailo MD, Malogolowkin MH, et al. Fibrolamellar hepatocellular carcinoma in children and adolescents. *Cancer* 2003;97(8):2006–2012.
287. Wu TC, Tong MJ, Hwang B, et al. Primary hepatocellular carcinoma and hepatitis B infection during childhood. *Hepatology* 1987;7(1):46–48.
288. Gonzalez-Peralta RP, Langham MR Jr, Andres JM, et al. Hepatocellular carcinoma in 2 young adolescents with chronic hepatitis C. *J Pediatr Gastroenterol Nutr* 2009;48(5):630–635.
289. Manowski Z, Silver MM, Roberts EA, et al. Liver cell dysplasia and early liver transplantation in hereditary tyrosinemia. *Mod Pathol* 1990;3(6):694–701.
290. Soyer P, Roche A, Levesque M, et al. CT of fibrolamellar hepatocellular carcinoma. *J Comput Assist Tomogr* 1991;15(4):533–538.
291. Lu W, Dong J, Huang Z, et al. Comparison of four current staging systems for Chinese patients with hepatocellular carcinoma undergoing curative resection: Okuda, CLIP, TNM and CUPI. *J Gastroenterol Hepatol* 2008;23(12):1874–1878.
292. Seo YS, Kim YJ, Um SH, et al. Evaluation of the prognostic powers of various tumor status grading scales in patients with hepatocellular carcinoma. *J Gastroenterol Hepatol* 2008;23(8 Pt 1):1267–1275.

293. Kondo K, Chijiiwa K, Nagano M, et al. Comparison of seven prognostic staging systems in patients who undergo hepatectomy for hepatocellular carcinoma. *Hepatogastroenterology* 2007;54(77):1534–1538.
294. Allan BJ, Wang B, Davis JS, et al. A review of 218 pediatric cases of hepatocellular carcinoma. *J Pediatr Surg* 2014;49(1):166–171; discussion 171.
295. Sevmis S, Karakayali H, Ozcay F, et al. Liver transplantation for hepatocellular carcinoma in children. *Pediatr Transplant* 2008;12(1):52–56.
296. Ioannou GN, Perkins JD, Carithers RL, Jr. Liver transplantation for hepatocellular carcinoma: impact of the MELD allocation system and predictors of survival. *Gastroenterology* 2008;134(5):1342–1351.
297. Kakar S, Burgart LJ, Batts KP, et al. Clinicopathologic features and survival in fibrolamellar carcinoma: comparison with conventional hepatocellular carcinoma with and without cirrhosis. *Mod Pathol* 2005;18(11):1417–1423.
298. Lack EE, Neave C, Vawter GF. Hepatocellular carcinoma. Review of 32 cases in childhood and adolescence. *Cancer* 1983;52(8):1510–1515.
299. You H, Ding W, Dang H, et al. c-Met represents a potential therapeutic target for personalized treatment in hepatocellular carcinoma. *Hepatology* 2011;54(3):879–889.
300. Torbenson M. Fibrolamellar carcinoma: 2012 update. *Scientifica (Cairo)* 2012;2012:743–790.
301. Shafizadeh N, Ferrell LD, Kakar S. Utility and limitations of glypican-3 expression for the diagnosis of hepatocellular carcinoma at both ends of the differentiation spectrum. *Mod Pathol* 2008;21(8):1011–1018.
302. Baumhoer D, Tornillo L, Stadlmann S, et al. Glypican 3 expression in human nonneoplastic, preneoplastic, and neoplastic tissues: a tissue microarray analysis of 4,387 tissue samples. *Am J Clin Pathol* 2008;129(6):899–906.
303. Lagana SM, Salomao M, Bao F, et al. Utility of an immunohistochemical panel consisting of glypican-3, heat-shock protein-70, and glutamine synthetase in the distinction of low-grade hepatocellular carcinoma from hepatocellular adenoma. *Appl Immunohistochem Mol Morphol* 2013;21(2):170–176.
304. Buckley AF, Burgart LJ, Sahai V, et al. Epidermal growth factor receptor expression and gene copy number in conventional hepatocellular carcinoma. *Am J Clin Pathol* 2008;129(2):245–251.
305. Zen Y, Vara R, Portmann B, et al. Childhood hepatocellular carcinoma: a clinicopathological study of 12 cases with special reference to EpCAM. *Histopathology* 2014;64(5):671–682.
306. Cornelia H, Alsiner C, Sayoois S, et al. Unique genomic profile of fibrolamellar hepatocellular carcinoma. *Gastroenterology* 2015;148:806–818.
307. Budhu A, Jia HL, Forgues M, et al. Identification of metastasis-related microRNAs in hepatocellular carcinoma. *Hepatology* 2008;47(3):897–907.
308. Stocker JT, Ishak KG. Undifferentiated (embryonal) sarcoma of the liver: report of 31 cases. *Cancer* 1978;42(1):336–348.
309. Parham DM, Kelly DR, Donnelly WH, et al. Immunohistochemical and ultrastructural spectrum of hepatic sarcomas of childhood: evidence for a common histogenesis. *Mod Pathol* 1991;4(5):648–653.
310. Lack EE, Schloo BL, Azumi N, et al. Undifferentiated (embryonal) sarcoma of the liver. Clinical and pathologic study of 16 cases with emphasis on immunohistochemical features. *Am J Surg Pathol* 1991;15(1):1–16.
311. Buetow PC, Buck JL, Pantongrag-Brown L, et al. Undifferentiated (embryonal) sarcoma of the liver: pathologic basis of imaging findings in 28 cases. *Radiology* 1997;203(3):779–783.
312. Walther A, Geller J, Coots A, et al. Multimodal therapy including liver transplantation for hepatic undifferentiated embryonal sarcoma. *Liver Transpl* 2014;20(2):191–199.
313. Pachera S, Nishio H, Takahashi Y, et al. Undifferentiated embryonal sarcoma of the liver: case report and literature survey. *J Hepatobiliary Pancreat Surg* 2008;15(5):536–544.
314. Nicol K, Savell V, Moore J, et al. Distinguishing undifferentiated embryonal sarcoma of the liver from biliary tract rhabdomyosarcoma: a Children's Oncology Group study. *Pediatr Dev Pathol* 2007;10(2):89–97.
315. Levy M, Trivedi A, Zhang J, et al. Expression of glypican-3 in undifferentiated embryonal sarcoma and mesenchymal hamartoma of the liver. *Hum Pathol* 2012;43(5):695–701.
316. Agaram NP, Baren A, Antonescu CR. Pediatric and adult hepatic embryonal sarcoma: a comparative ultrastructural study with morphologic correlations. *Ultrastruct Pathol* 2006;30(6):403–408.
317. Leuschner I, Schmidt D, Harms D. Undifferentiated sarcoma of the liver in childhood: morphology, flow cytometry, and literature review. *Hum Pathol* 1990;21(1):68–76.
318. Sowery RD, Jensen C, Morrison KB, et al. Comparative genomic hybridization detects multiple chromosomal amplifications and deletions in undifferentiated embryonal sarcoma of the liver. *Cancer Genet Cytogenet* 2001;126(2):128–133.
319. Heerema-McKenney A, Leuschner I, Smith N, et al. Nested stromal epithelial tumor of the liver: six cases of a distinctive pediatric neoplasm with frequent calcifications and association with cushing syndrome. *Am J Surg Pathol* 2005;29(1):10–20.
320. Hill DA, Swanson PE, Anderson K, et al. Desmoplastic nested spindle cell tumor of liver: report of four cases of a proposed new entity. *Am J Surg Pathol* 2005;29(1):1–9.
321. Makhlouf HR, Abdul-Al HM, Wang G, et al. Calcifying nested stromal-epithelial tumors of the liver: a clinicopathologic, immunohistochemical, and molecular genetic study of 9 cases with a long-term follow-up. *Am J Surg Pathol* 2009;33(7):976–983.
322. Meir K, Maly A, Doviner V, et al. Nested (ossifying) stromal epithelial tumor of the liver: case report. *Pediatr Dev Pathol* 2009;12(3):233–236.
323. Malowany JI, Merritt NH, Chan NG, et al. Nested stromal epithelial tumor of the liver in Beckwith-Wiedemann syndrome. *Pediatr Dev Pathol* 2013;16(4):312–317.
324. Brodsky SV, Sandoval C, Sharma N, et al. Recurrent nested stromal epithelial tumor of the liver with extrahepatic metastasis: case report and review of literature. *Pediatr Dev Pathol* 2008;11(6):469–473.
325. Ruymann FB, Raney RB Jr, Crist WM, et al. Rhabdomyosarcoma of the biliary tree in childhood. A report from the Intergroup Rhabdomyosarcoma Study. *Cancer* 1985;56(3):575–581.
326. Selby DM, Stocker JT, Ishak KG. Angiosarcoma of the liver in childhood: a clinicopathologic and follow-up study of 10 cases. *Pediatr Pathol* 1992;12(4):485–498.
327. Orlando G, Adam R, Mirza D, et al. Hepatic hemangiosarcoma: an absolute contraindication to liver Transplantation—the European Liver Transplant Registry experience. *Transplantation* 2013;95(6):872–877.
328. Dimashkieh HH, Mo JQ, Wyatt-Ashmead J, et al. Pediatric hepatic angiosarcoma: case report and review of the literature. *Pediatr Dev Pathol* 2004;7(5):527–532.
329. Wang ZB, Yuan J, Chen W, et al. Transcription factor ERG is a specific and sensitive diagnostic marker for hepatic angiosarcoma. *World J Gastroenterol* 2014;20(13):3672–3679.
330. Timmons CF, Dawson DB, Richards CS, et al. Epstein-Barr virus-associated leiomyosarcomas in liver transplantation recipients. Origin from either donor or recipient tissue. *Cancer* 1995;76(8):1481–1489.
331. Keplinger KM, Bloomston M. Anatomy and embryology of the biliary tract. *Surg Clin North Am* 2014;94(2):203–217.

CHAPTER 16

The Pancreas

Mariko Suchi, M.D., Ph.D.

ORGANOGENESIS AND EXOCRINE HISTOGENESIS

During week 4 of gestation, the ventral foregut gives rise to two pancreatic buds at the junction of the hepatic duct. The dorsal primordium develops in the mesentery. The ventral pancreatic bud rotates with the gut and fuses with the larger dorsal anlage and with the duodenum, and the fused primordia take up their normal position against the posterior abdominal wall in the concavity of the duodenum. The ventral bud gives rise to the uncinate process and the inferior portion of the head of the pancreas, and the dorsal primordium gives rise to the body, tail, and superior portion of the head (Figure 16-1). The duct of the dorsal pancreas opens more proximally into the duodenum and the ventral duct more distally, together with the common bile duct. Fusion of the primordia during the middle of week 6 of gestation leads to fusion of the duct systems. The duct of the ventral pancreas becomes the main pancreatic duct of Wirsung. The duct of the dorsal pancreas usually remains patent as the minor duct of Santorini.

During week 7 of gestation, simple, undifferentiated epithelial tubules grow into a loose mesenchyme. The epithelium rapidly forms a ramifying duct system, from which buds of cuboidal cells form the first recognizable acinar units by week 10; endocrine elements are also present by this time. The pancreas, from week 10 to term, continues to ramify and gives rise to exocrine and endocrine elements. Ductal elements, especially the centroacinar cells, can be hard to identify definitively from acinar and endocrine cells at this stage, but they express keratins 7 and 19 in addition to the keratins 8 and 18, which are found on acinar and endocrine cells after week 16 (1).

Complex yet organized gene regulatory networks governing pancreas development are reviewed by Arda et al. (2). Two of the genes are noteworthy as they interact, induce, and are regulated by multiple other gene products and appear to be of vital importance to early pancreatic embryogenesis. They are *PTF1A* (pancreas transcription factor 1 α) and *PDX1* (pancreas and duodenal homeobox 1). Very little is known about the embryologic control of pancreatic duct formations in humans.

Pancreatic exocrine development, like pulmonary alveolar maturation, is largely a postnatal event. The appearance of the pancreas at birth is one of underdeveloped acinar elements in a mesenchymal stroma (Figure 16-2). Acinar tissue increases rapidly after birth. Imrie et al. (3) showed that the ratio of acinar to connective tissue volume increases in a linear manner from 0.5 at week 32 to 2.0 at week 52 after conception. In an assessment of the morphologic maturation of an infant pancreas, the length of postnatal survival is more important than is the gestational age.

CONGENITAL ANOMALIES AND MALFORMATIONS

Agenesis and Hypoplasia

Agenesis of the pancreas refers to a complete absence of the gland, rather than a lack of the endocrine or exocrine portions alone. Recessive mutations in a distal enhancer of one of the organ development regulatory genes mentioned above, *PTF1A*, are the most common cause of isolated pancreatic agenesis. Rare cases of pancreatic agenesis result from *PDX1* mutations. Congenitally absent pancreas may be associated with diaphragmatic hernia. Some infants have also lacked a gallbladder or intrahepatic bile ducts (4).

Functional pancreatic agenesis refers to organ failure without anatomic evidence of gland absence (5). A functionally hypoplastic pancreas may be familial and can also lead to exocrine and endocrine insufficiency. Severe pancreatic hypoplasia has been described in the Wolcott-Rallison syndrome (6).

Partial agenesis has been ascribed to failure of development of the dorsal or ventral primordium and may be familial (7). More commonly, the pancreas is misshapen and described as short, stubby, or globular. These variants are not associated with hypofunction. Short pancreas may be an isolated finding or may be seen with complex congenital heart disease or as part of a wider malformation complex that includes congenital heart disease, multiple spleens, and intestinal malrotation. It has also been observed in complete trisomy 9 (8) and complete trisomy 22 syndromes.

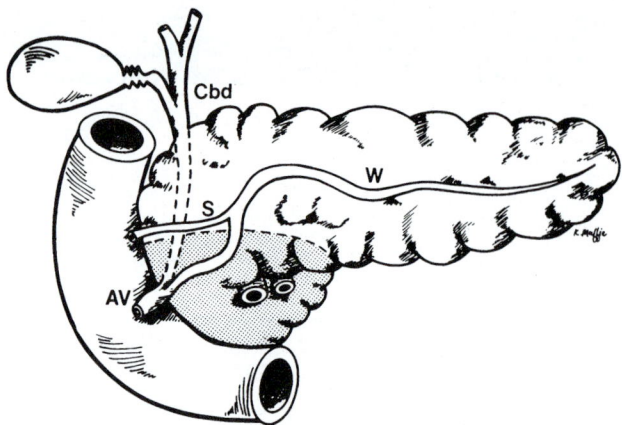

FIGURE 16-1 • Pancreas, ducts, and derivation. The pancreatic duct of Wirsung (*W*) drains most of the pancreas, joining the common bile duct (*Cbd*) proximal to the ampulla of Vater (*AV*). The accessory duct of Santorini (*S*) may drain part of the gland through a separate opening. A portion of the head and the uncinate lobe (stippled area) are derived from the ventral bud of the pancreas.

Figure 16-3 illustrates a short pancreas in association with syndromic extrahepatic biliary atresia.

Pancreatic Enlargement

Infants with Beckwith-Wiedemann syndrome have an enlarged pancreas. Marked fatty replacement of the exocrine portion with preservation of the islets is found in the lipomatous pseudohypertrophy of the Shwachman-Diamond syndrome. Immune and nonimmune hydrops fetalis can lead to pancreatic enlargement through extramedullary hematopoiesis, and infiltration with leukemia can cause massive pancreatic enlargement (Figure 16-4). In congenital syphilis, pancreatomegaly is a consequence of extensive interstitial fibrosis and inflammation (9) (Figure 16-4).

Abnormalities of Position

The pancreas and the duodenum are retroperitoneal and separated from the posterior abdominal wall by an avascular plane. Abnormalities of fixation or position are often associated with left-sided diaphragmatic hernias. Partial situs inversus with normal cardiac situs but inversion of the abdominal viscera, including the pancreas, has been seen with annular pancreas (10).

Annular Pancreas

A ring of pancreatic tissue can encircle the second portion of the duodenum completely or partially (Figure 16-5). Johnston described two forms, extramural and intramural (11). In the extramural form, a flattened band of normal pancreatic tissue can be separated from the duodenum. A duct originating anteriorly runs around the duodenum to join the main pancreatic duct. In the intramural form, ectopic pancreatic tissue is located within the duodenal wall, and small ducts drain directly into the duodenum.

Children and neonates with annular pancreas usually present with duodenal obstruction. Duodenoduodenostomy is the appropriate treatment, with good postsurgical outcome (12). As compared to the adult patients with annular pancreas, children with this anomaly frequently have associated chromosomal anomalies and major congenital malformations (13). The most frequent chromosomal anomaly is trisomy 21. Congenital malformations associated with annular pancreas include tracheoesophageal fistula, Meckel diverticulum, absence of the gallbladder, and imperforate anus. Annular pancreas in a mother and three of her four children and documentation of other familial instances suggest an autosomal dominant inheritance or involvement of an autosomal recessive sex-influenced gene (14).

Annular pancreas may present in the fetus with polyhydramnios or in the neonate with bile-stained vomiting if the constriction is below the ampulla. In older children and adults, it may become symptomatic if duodenal ulceration or pancreatitis develops.

Ectopic Pancreas

Ectopic (heterotopic) pancreas is widely distributed, largely within the gastrointestinal tract. This condition has been discovered in 2% to 15% of all autopsies. Pancreatic tissue is most frequently found in the wall of the stomach, duodenum, or jejunum (15). It is not unusual to find a nodule in the stomach consisting of a centrally ulcerated pit with localized thickening of the gastric wall (Figure 16-6). Ectopic mediastinal pancreas is rare. Pancreatic tissue can be identified within bronchopulmonary foregut malformation (16).

Three types of ectopic pancreatic tissue have been described. The first is similar to normal pancreas showing a full complement of acinar, ductal, and islet constituents with a normal distribution of all cell types as demonstrated by immunohistochemistry. The second is characterized by incomplete lobular arrangement, few acini, many ducts, and an absence of endocrine elements. In the third type of ectopic pancreas, only proliferating ducts are present, without acinar or endocrine elements. This form is usually interpreted as an "adenomyoma" or "myoepithelial hamartoma" of the bowel wall (17).

Pancreatic tissue can be seen in the hilum of the liver or within the liver substance. Although on occasion a metaplastic process has been suggested for microscopic focus of exocrine pancreatic tissue in a posthepatitic cirrhotic liver, it is unlikely to be metaplastic when endocrine cells are seen. The pancreas has also been described in the omentum, mesentery, Meckel diverticulum, vitelline duct, and umbilicus. Ectopic pancreas has been associated with duplication cysts of the gut and has been reported in fallopian tubes, abdominal lymph nodes, and adjacent to the thyroid (18). Intrasplenic islands of pancreas are found in trisomy 13 to 15 syndrome (19). Although heterotopic pancreas is often an incidental finding, it may present clinically as peptic ulceration, massive hemorrhage, biliary obstruction, cholecystitis, pyloric obstruction, intestinal obstruction, intussusception, or cystic degeneration (15). When complicated by pancreatitis, it can present as a

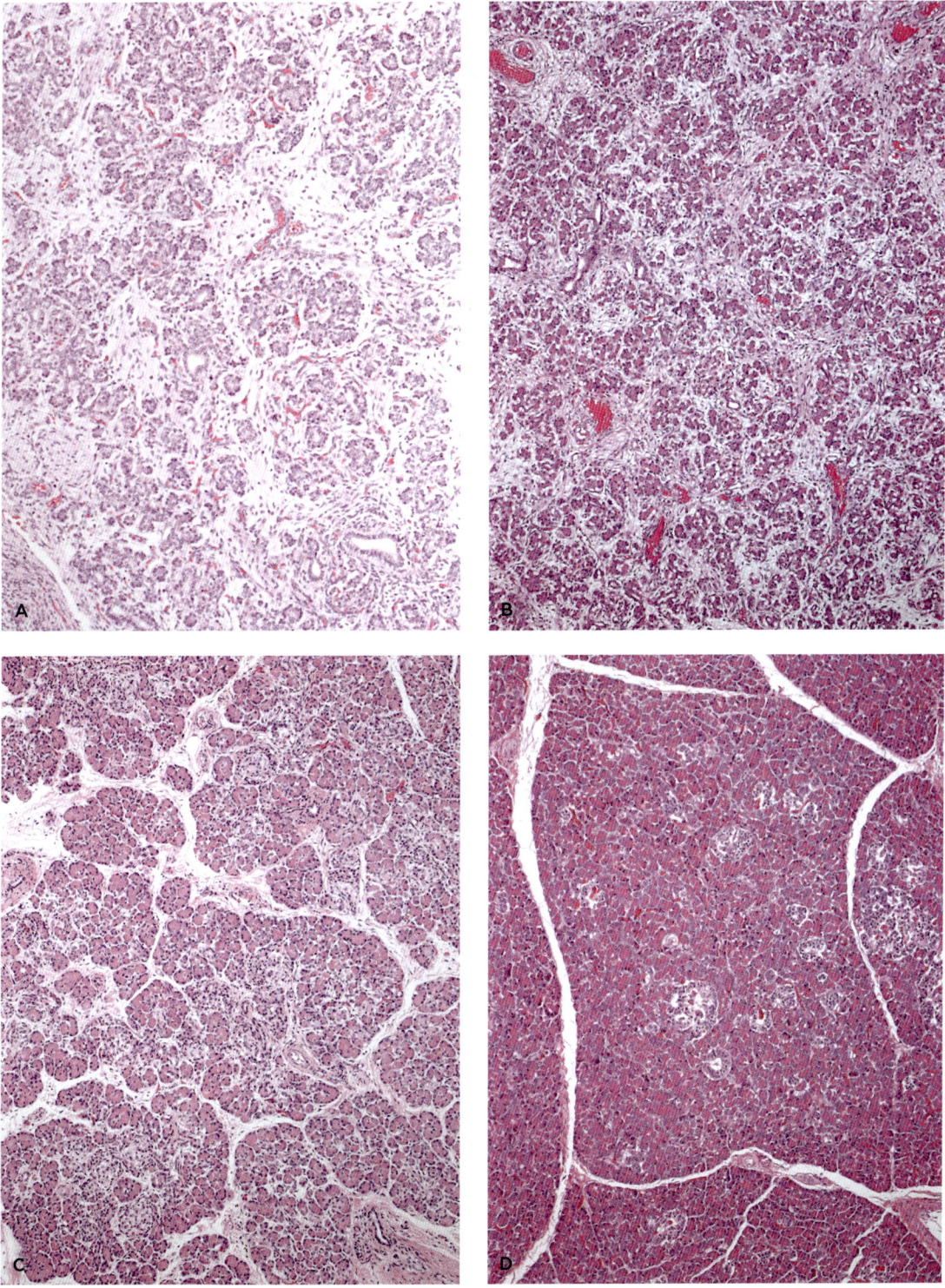

FIGURE 16-2 • Pancreatic development during gestation. **A:** At weeks 12 to 13 of gestation, the pancreas shows ducts and small lobules of acini in a loose mesenchymal stroma. Endocrine cells are demonstrable. (Hematoxylin and eosin stain, original magnification ×155.) **B:** At week 17 of gestation, lobules of acini and islets are more clearly visible. **C:** By week 40 of gestation (in a child who lived 1 day after birth), the endocrine elements lie centrally within the stalk of the lobule, and undeveloped acinar tissue is located peripherally. **D:** At the age of 22 months, the remarkable development of acinar tissue is obvious. (**B–D:** Hematoxylin and eosin stain, original magnification ×100.)

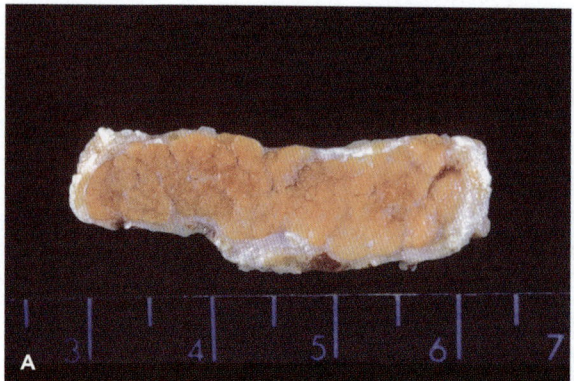
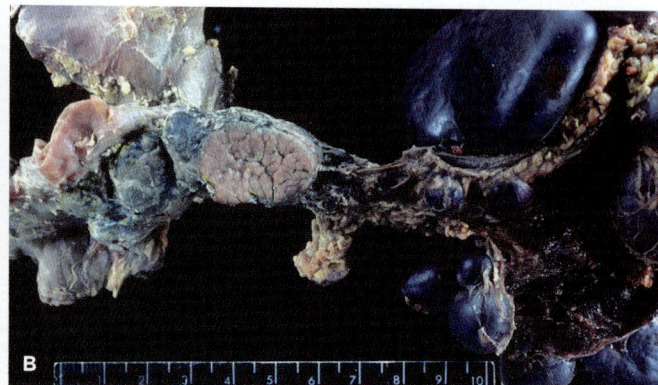

FIGURE 16-3 • Small pancreas. **A:** Hypoplastic pancreas (2.7 g, 3 cm long) from a 5-month-old child with probable tyrosinemia. **B:** Short pancreas (3 cm long) from a 2.5-year-old child with multiple spleens, intestinal malrotation, left bronchopulmonary isomerism, and extrahepatic biliary atresia (heterotaxy).

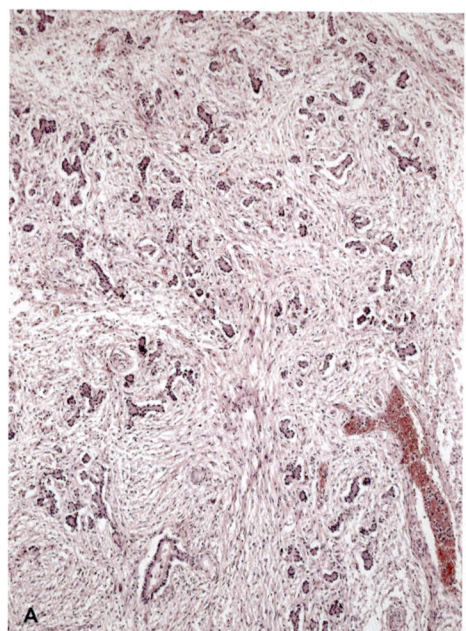
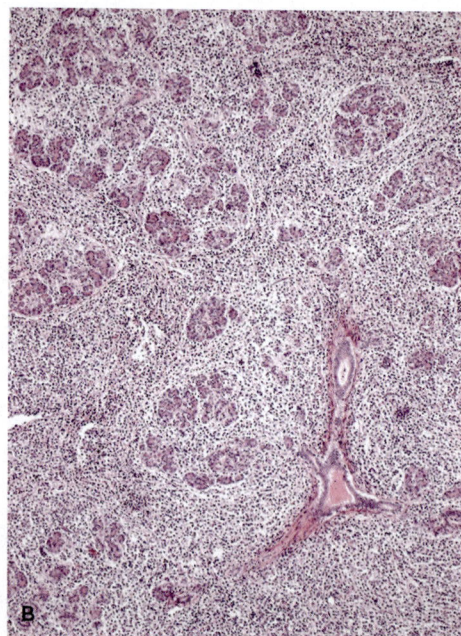

FIGURE 16-4 • Large pancreas. **A:** Congenital syphilis. An extensive, fine fibrosis distorts the pancreas. **B:** Congenital leukemia. Acinar elements are widely separated by the leukemic infiltrate, which is granulocytic in this instance. (**A, B:** Hematoxylin and eosin stain, original magnification ×100.)

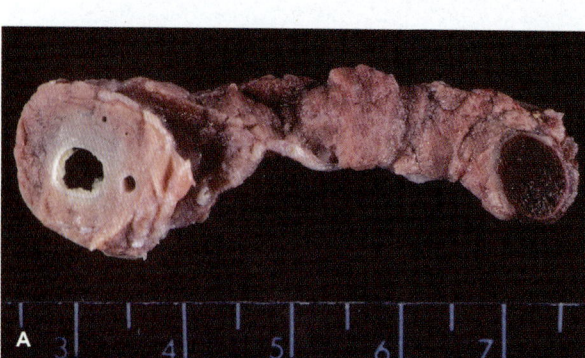
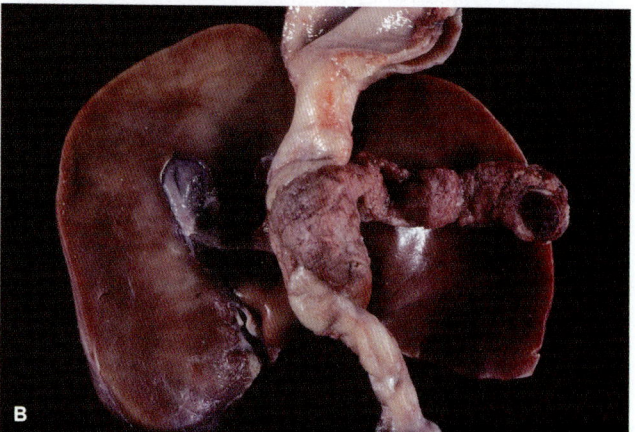

FIGURE 16-5 • Annular pancreas. **A, B:** An annular pancreas completely surrounds the second portion of the duodenum. An accessory spleen is present within the tail of the pancreas (trisomy 6).

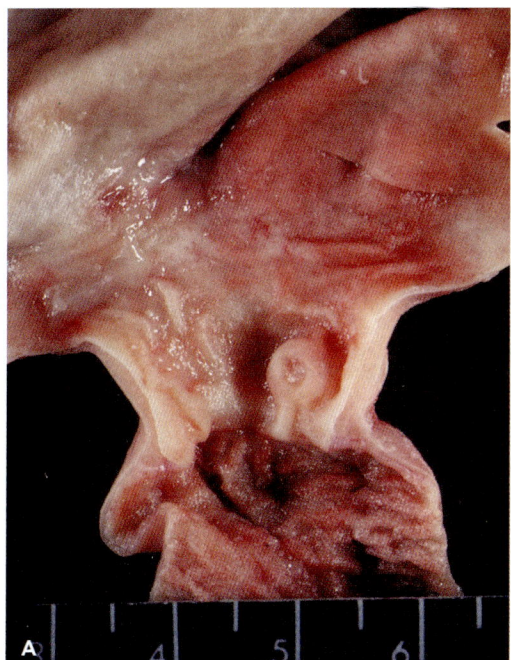
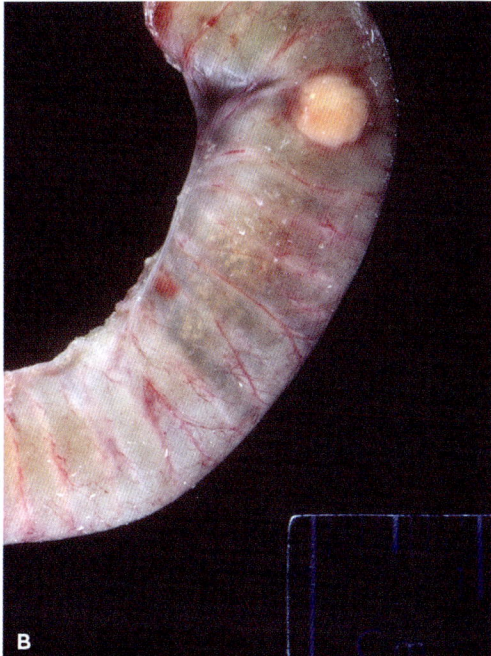
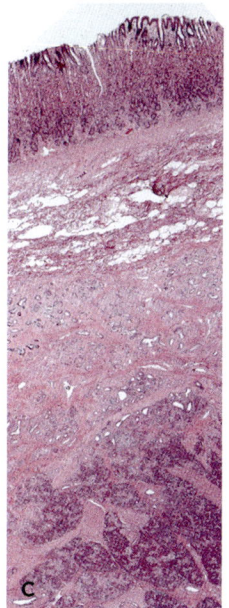
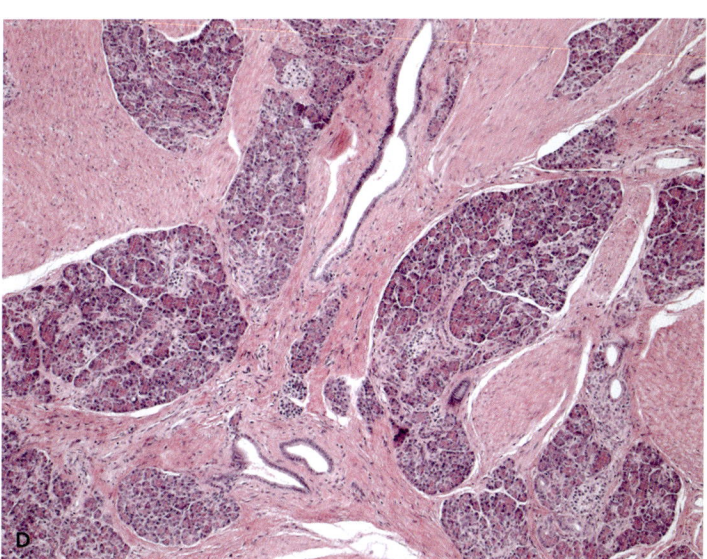

FIGURE 16-6 • Ectopic pancreas. **A:** Umbilicated mucosal nodule of the pyloric area. **B:** A jejunal subserosal nodule. **C:** An ectopic intramural (gastric) pancreas has ducts, exocrine acini, and endocrine component. **D:** Higher magnification of **C**. Islands of pancreatic tissue are separated by smooth muscle bundles. (**C, D:** Hematoxylin and eosin stain, original magnification, ×25 and ×100, respectively.)

mesenteric mass (20). Hyperinsulinism associated with islet cell adenomatous hyperplasia (focal hyperinsulinism) in the ectopic pancreas has been described (21). Solid pseudopapillary neoplasms have been identified in ectopic pancreas (22).

Pancreatic Cysts

Due to increased availability of advanced cross-sectional imaging techniques, congenital and acquired pancreatic cysts are more frequently encountered. They are more likely asymptomatic. True cysts have epithelial lining such as cuboidal epithelium, metaplastic stratified squamous epithelium, and ciliated columnar epithelium (23). "Dermoid cysts" have been also described in children, among which some are mature cystic teratoma upon reviewing the literature. Simple epithelium-lined cysts may be solitary and unassociated with cystic diseases of other organs. On the other hand, the cysts may be associated with a trisomy (19) (Figure 16-7), tuberous sclerosis, von Hippel-Lindau disease,

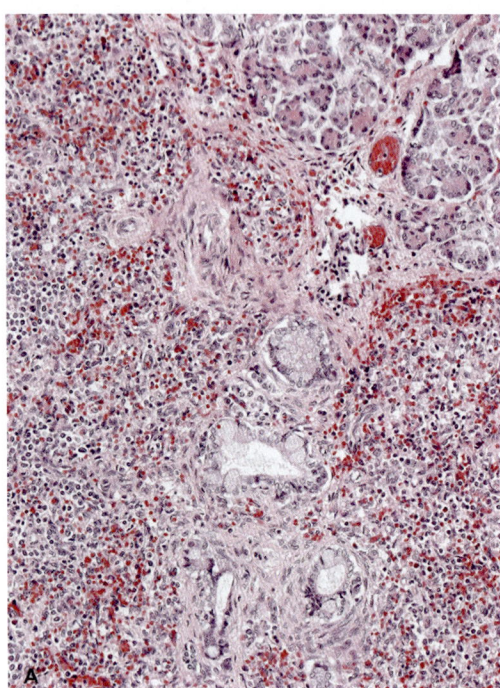 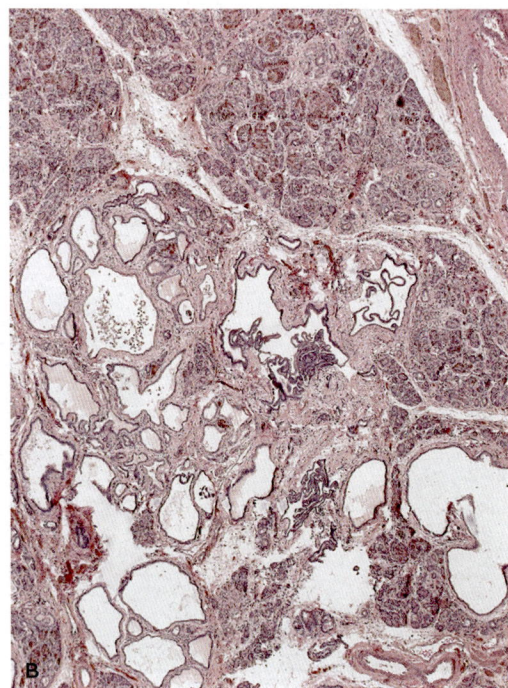

FIGURE 16-7 • Trisomies. **A:** Trisomy 13. Poorly circumscribed areas of splenic stroma extend into the pancreas, entrapping pancreatic ducts with mucoid lining cells. (Hematoxylin and eosin stain, original magnification ×200.) **B:** Trisomy 18. Numerous pancreatic cysts lined by duct-type epithelium are scattered. (Hematoxylin and eosin stain with immunohistochemistry for neuron-specific enolase, original magnification ×50.)

and Beckwith-Wiedemann syndrome (24) (Figure 16-8). The pancreatic lesions in Beckwith-Wiedemann syndrome and von Hippel-Lindau disease are described separately later in the chapter.

In contrast to true cysts, a pancreatic pseudocyst is a collection of pancreatic secretions enclosed in fibrous tissue layer without an epithelial lining. Pseudocysts can arise as a complication of either chronic or acute pancreatitis due to any cause including infections, drugs, genetic predisposition, abdominal trauma, previous surgery, and structural pancreatic duct anomaly. Management options include observation and percutaneous or internal drainage (25). Lymphatic malformation (26) (Figure 16-9) may present as "pancreatic cysts." Pancreatic cysts in cystic fibrosis are pseudocysts and will be discussed separately.

Pancreatic Anomalies in Nonmotile Ciliopathies

Cilia are hairlike structures or organelles that extend from the surface of nearly all mammalian cells. There are two types of cilia, motile and nonmotile. Nonmotile cilia are also known as primary cilia, which play a crucial role as sensory cellular antennae during embryogenesis, guiding developing cells to their ultimate fate. A number of heterogeneous phenotypes and syndromes that manifest with a variety of abnormalities in multiple organ systems including the pancreas have been historically described. The overlapping natures of the syndromes resulted in confusion in diagnostic criteria and classification. Some of these syndromes have been classified as ciliopathies (27) including, but not limited to, autosomal recessive polycystic kidney disease, autosomal dominant polycystic kidney disease, renal–hepatic–pancreatic dysplasias, Meckel-Gruber syndrome, Joubert syndrome–related disorder, and Jeune syndrome. As cilia are present in nearly every cell in the body and mutations of genes encoding ciliary proteins affect multiple organs, including the kidneys, liver, pancreas, retina, central nervous system, and skeletal system, genetic defects will manifest with multiorgan involvement.

The prototype is autosomal dominant kidney disease. This disorder has cysts in the kidney and liver. But cases in this category have been reported to have pancreatic cystic lesions (eFigure 16-1). By ultrasonography, pancreatic cysts are detected in 9% of autosomal dominant polycystic kidney disease patients over 30 years of age.

Renal–hepatic–pancreatic dysplasia 1 (also known as Ivemark II syndrome) is caused by homozygous or compound heterozygous mutation in nephrocystin 3 gene, *NPHP3*, on chromosome 3q22. Pancreatic findings include fibrosis, epithelium-lined cysts, dilated pancreatic ducts, and decrease in parenchymal tissue (28). Endocrine function varies from normal to diabetes mellitus. Another gene, never in mitosis gene A–related kinase 8 gene (*NEK8*), whose homozygous mutation causes another renal–hepatic–pancreatic dysplasia has been discovered recently (renal–hepatic–pancreatic dysplasia 2).

Meckel syndrome, also known as Meckel-Gruber syndrome, shows extensive clinical variability and may include

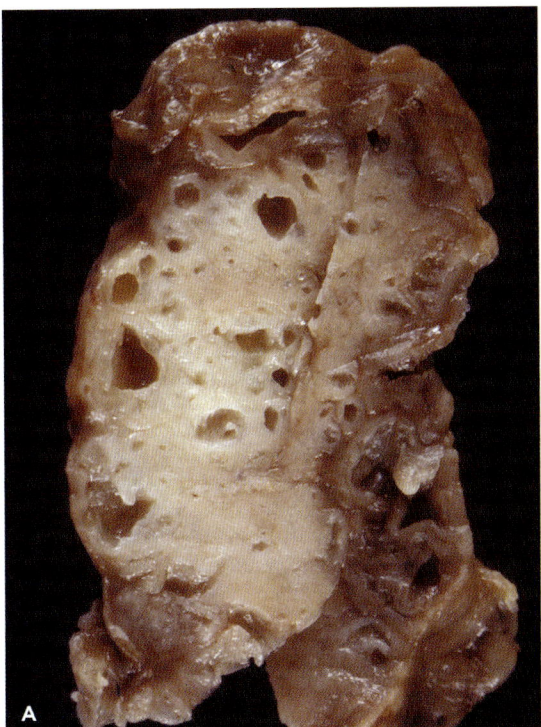
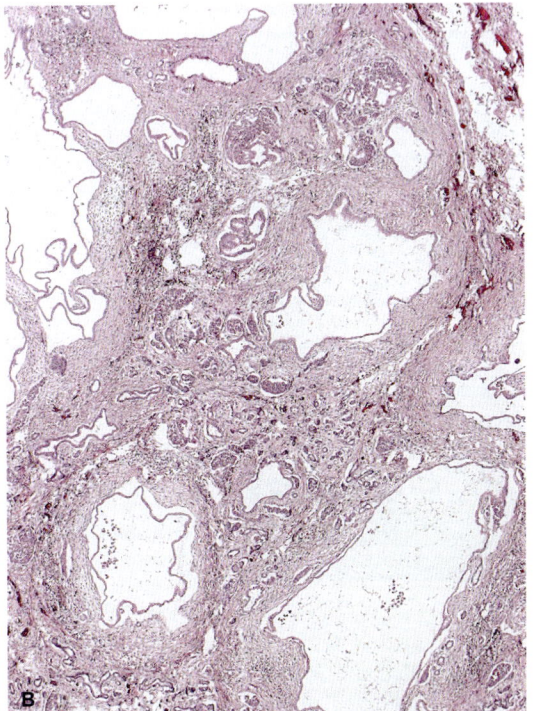
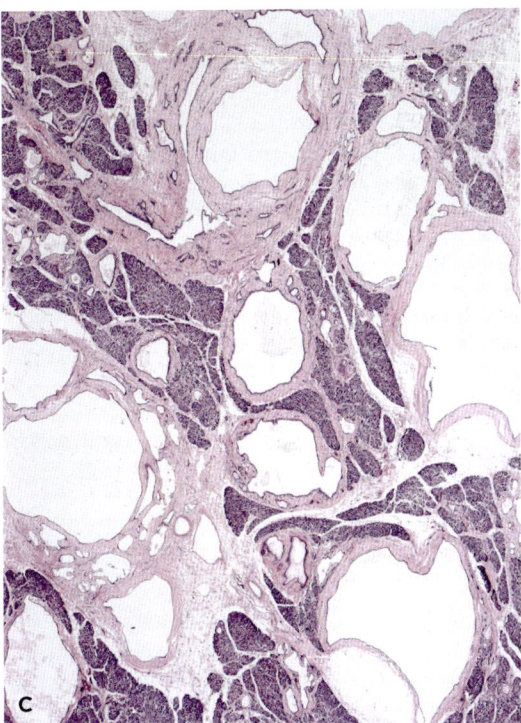

FIGURE 16-8 • Pancreatic cysts. **A:** A large pancreas (120 g) presented as an abdominal mass in a newborn baby with Beckwith-Wiedemann syndrome. Multiple cystic spaces are seen on cut surfaces. (Color version of Copyright 1990 from Beckwith-Wiedemann syndrome with unusual hepatic and pancreatic features: A case expanding the phenotype by Steigman CK, Uri AK, Chatten J, et al. *Pediatr Pathol* 1990;10:593. Reproduced with permission of Taylor & Francis Group, LLC., http://www.taylorandfrancis.com.) **B:** Microphotograph of (**A**). No normal pancreatic tissue is identified. Numerous ectatic ducts, clusters of endocrine cells, and few acini are in loose fibrous connective tissue. (Hematoxylin and eosin stain, original magnification ×50.) **C:** 15-year-old child with oral-facial-digital syndrome type I. Cystically dilated pancreatic ducts with periductal fibrosis. (Hematoxylin and eosin, original magnification ×25.)

pancreatic cystic lesions (eFigure 16-1). This variability is understandable because there are currently 11 types based on the causative gene mutations.

Variations in the Pancreatic Ducts

After the dorsal and ventral pancreatic anlage fuse, the dorsal duct becomes the accessory duct of Santorini, and the ventral duct becomes the main draining duct of the pancreas, the duct of Wirsung. Fusion can occur at a single point proximally or at two points, both proximally and more distally (29). The normal architecture varies widely. The dorsal duct may regress completely, or the dorsal and ventral ducts may not communicate at all (pancreas divisum).

In pancreas divisum, the pancreas is separated into two portions. The pancreatic ducts fail to fuse, and the dorsal duct of Santorini drains most of the gland through the minor

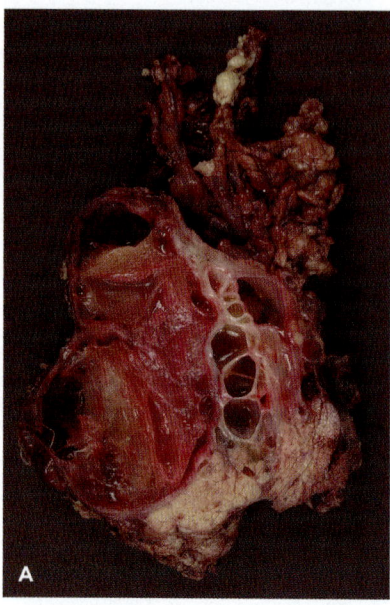
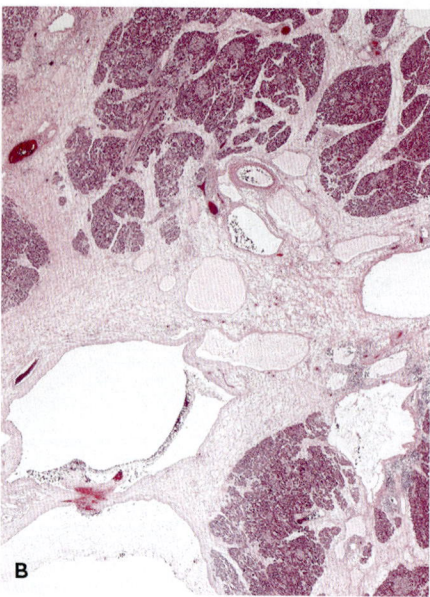

FIGURE 16-9 • Lymphatic malformation. **A:** Lymphatic malformation presented as a cystic pancreatic mass in a 12-year-old child. (Courtesy of Pierre Russo, M.D., Philadelphia, Pennsylvania.) **B:** Lymphatic channels of variable sizes are embedded within the pancreatic lobular septa and parenchyma. A small number of mononuclear cell infiltrates are present in the walls. (Hematoxylin and eosin stain, original magnification ×25.)

papilla. The ventral duct of Wirsung drains only the smaller pancreatic remnant. Because of the recent advances in endoscopic retrograde cholangiopancreatography and magnetic resonance cholangiopancreatography, pancreas divisum is diagnosed with greater frequency. Some investigators believe that pancreas divisum is clinically significant, whereas others are more skeptical.

The anatomy of the pancreaticobiliary junction varies noticeably. The pancreatic duct can join the common bile duct within the duodenal wall, or it can enter the duodenum separately. The common channel can be short or long. If it is longer than 2 cm, the ducts join outside the duodenal wall. Stenosis of the ampulla may present with pancreatitis, but in the newborn, it more commonly manifests as bile duct perforation. Familial cases of pancreaticobiliary anomaly have been reported (30).

Pancreatic Pathology in Trisomies and Triploidy

Lesions of the pancreas characteristic of trisomy 13 were illustrated long before the chromosomal defect was identified. Hashida et al. (19) demonstrated the multiple, poorly demarcated aggregates of splenic tissue in the tail and the body of the pancreas (Figure 16-7). These splenic islands contain pancreatic acini, islets, and knots of ducts lined by tall columnar epithelium rich in goblet cells. Microcystic changes may be focal or quite widespread with inspissations, features that suggest a duct obstruction as the pathogenesis. Ectopic splenic tissue in the gastric fundus and upper pole of the kidney has contained pancreatic elements.

The pancreas in trisomy 18 often exhibits lobular fibrosis (19) and focal fibrotic nodules in which clusters of ducts and atrophic acini are found. An area of serous cystadenomatous changes with back-to-back cysts is seen less frequently (Figure 16-7). These cysts along with inflammatory aggregates suggest an obstructive etiology. Ectopic pancreas in the ileum was reported in a case of trisomy 18 (31).

Annular pancreas occurs in as many as 8% of infants with trisomy 21. Pancreaticobiliary duct anomalies may accompany annular pancreas (32). A short pancreas has been described in trisomy 22. A report of three cases of complete trisomy 9 that survived beyond the first trimester (a rare occurrence) described agenesis or underdevelopment of the body and tail of the pancreas in each of them (8).

Pancreatic anomalies, including agenesis, are described in infants with triploidy. Marked enlargement of the somatostatin-producing D cells has been reported in triploid fetuses (33).

EXOCRINE PANCREAS

Functional Development

Exocrine function of developing pancreas varies significantly among specific enzymes. Immunohistochemical analysis of the fetal pancreas detects pancreatic secretory trypsin inhibitor in developing buds of the pancreas during the 8th gestational week, and proteinases such as trypsin, chymotrypsin, and elastase I are observed in acinar cells during the 14th week of gestation. Morphologically, small zymogen-like granules are present in a few young acinar cells at 12 weeks. During the 12 to 19 fetal week period, there is a gradual increase in the number of mature zymogen granules (34). By week 20 of gestation, basal round granules predominate, and the complex basolateral cell interdigitations are established (eFigure 16-2). These timings coincide with the levels of proteinase activity and immunohistochemical reaction patterns. After 32 weeks of gestation, both preterm and term infants have substantial proteolytic enzyme levels. Chymotrypsin activity is about 50% to 60% of the level found in older children. Trypsin activity, the highest of all enzymes, reaches

90% to 100% of children older than 2 years of age (35). In the adult, pancreozymin is responsible for pancreatic enzyme release, and secretin promotes fluid and electrolyte release. The pancreas of a neonate is unresponsive to exogenous pancreatozymin or secretin before 1 month of age and not fully responsive before 2 years of age.

For lipase and amylase secretion, the pancreas appears to mature through a different time course. Throughout the fetal period studied, mRNA of lipase is shown to be consistently and significantly lower than trypsinogen mRNA level. By immunohistochemistry, while trypsinogen and chymotrypsinogen are observed uniformly in all acinar cells as soon as they appear at 16 weeks of gestation, lipase is detected at 21 weeks in a few acini dispersed in the pancreas and then spreads out progressively to be present in all the acini (36). The duodenal fluid of newborns and infants, nevertheless, contains low levels (5% to 10% of adult values) of lipase, and infants are said to have physiologic steatorrhea (37).

Earlier studies claim that amylase could be detected in the fetal pancreas beginning in the 22nd week of gestation. However, a later study by Fukuyama et al. on fetal pancreas using immunohistochemistry and studies involving postnatal enzyme activity measurements of the duodenal fluid show lack of amylase in the fetal pancreas and early postnatal pancreas of up to 1 month of age (35). The amylase level in the duodenum increases slowly during the first 1 to 2 years of life.

Abnormalities of the Exocrine Pancreas

Isolated Enzyme Deficiencies

Rare pediatric cases of isolated pancreatic exocrine enzyme deficiencies were reported in the 1960s and in the years up to the early 1990s. These patients were without known causes of pancreatic insufficiency such as pancreatitis, tumor, and congenital syndromes. The deficiency is determined by enzymatic activity assays in pancreatic juices. Deficient enzymes include lipase, colipase, and trypsinogen. The pancreatic morphology is not described in these reports except for one case of trypsinogen deficiency whose pancreas showed "immature acini" and lack of zymogen granules. Mutational analysis of the gene encoding pancreatic lipase performed on six members of a consanguineous family identified a missense mutation that shows segregation between the genotype state and the serum pancreatic lipase activity.

Enteropeptidase is a serine protease that activates the pancreatic proenzyme trypsinogen, which, in turn, releases active digestive enzymes from their inactive pancreatic precursors. Therefore, congenital enteropeptidase deficiency may mimic cystic fibrosis manifesting with failure to thrive and diarrhea. But this enzyme is produced from the intestinal brush border in the proximal small intestine, not from the pancreas. Nonsense mutations and a frame shift mutation have been identified in the proenteropeptidase gene.

The maturation of amylase production is normally delayed, and the adult level of amylase activity is reached at the age of 18 months to 2 years. Therefore, alleged cases of isolated amylase deficiency in young children are controversial. Rare adult cases of selective deficiency of pancreatic amylase have been described.

Diseases that Result in Replacement of Exocrine Acini by Adipose Tissue

When the shape of the pancreas is grossly preserved but the exocrine acini are largely replaced by adipose tissue, the condition is termed lipomatous atrophy, lipomatosis, or, when extensive, lipomatous pseudohypertrophy. The pancreas shows relatively preserved endocrine components including islets of Langerhans and scattered small but well-preserved exocrine acinar elements. These acini do not show signs of injury. No fibrosis or fat necrosis is seen. Lipomatosis has been described in a number of pathologic processes (38) including Bannayan syndrome, Shwachman-Diamond syndrome, Johanson-Blizzard syndrome, and rare proteolytic and lipolytic enzyme deficiencies.

Of note, focal replacement of the exocrine pancreas with mature fat is a relatively common histologic change. It usually correlates directly with BMI and presence of diabetes mellitus.

Shwachman-Diamond Syndrome

With an incidence estimated at 1 in 200,000 births, the Shwachman-Diamond syndrome (39) is the most common cause of pancreatic insufficiency after cystic fibrosis. Pancreatic exocrine insufficiency is accompanied by growth restriction, short stature, bone marrow depression with neutropenia, and skeletal changes, predominantly metaphyseal dysostosis (40). Cases with anal atresia, Hirschsprung disease, and possibly asphyxiating thoracic dystrophy have been described (41). The marrow dysfunction, neutropenia in most instances, may be fixed or cyclical and is associated with the development of myelodysplasia and later leukemias, usually acute myelogenous leukemia. The pancreatic insufficiency may be profound and appears shortly after birth; less often, it is mild and improves and normalizes with age in about half of these patients. Replacement of the bulk of the pancreas by fatty tissue gives the appearance of a lipomatous pseudohypertrophy (42). Acinar tissue is absent, without scarring or fibrosis, and the pancreatic ducts and endocrine elements are preserved (Figure 16-10). The characteristic lipomatous pancreas can be demonstrated by magnetic resonance imaging.

Shwachman-Diamond syndrome is an autosomal recessive disorder. The gene involved (*SBDS*) resides at 7q11. Its 1.6-kb transcript encodes a predicted protein of 250 amino acids. A pseudogene copy (*SBDSP*) with 97% nucleotide sequence identity is in a locally duplicated genomic segment. Recurring mutations resulting from gene conversion (substitution of genetic material from another gene) were found in 89% of unrelated individuals of Shwachman-Diamond syndrome. The converted segments include pseudogene-like sequence changes that result in protein truncation. In a study of 23 unrelated patients, molecular genetic and hematologic evaluations demonstrated a poor genotype/phenotype correlation (43).

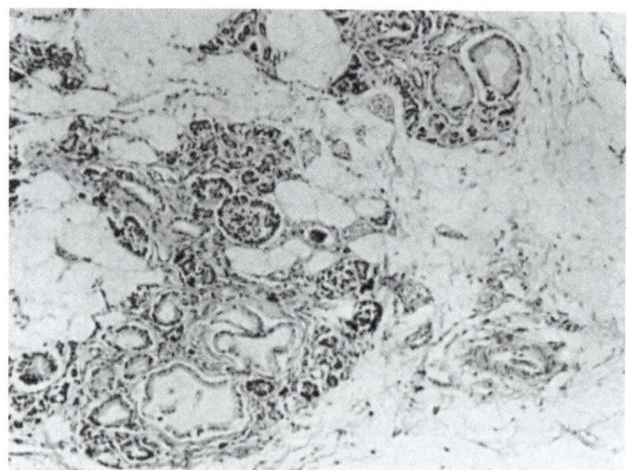

FIGURE 16-10 • Exocrine atrophy in Shwachman-Diamond syndrome. The acinar elements are almost completely replaced by fat (lipomatous pseudohypertrophy), with only small aggregates of endocrine tissue left around ducts. (Hematoxylin and eosin stain, original magnification ×120.)

Johanson-Blizzard Syndrome

First reported in 1971 (44), the Johanson-Blizzard syndrome comprises congenital aplasia of the alae nasi, deafness, hypothyroidism, dwarfism, absence of permanent teeth, and malabsorption resulting from pancreatic insufficiency. Subsequent reports described urogenital abnormalities and imperforate anus associated with this syndrome. Postmortem examination of the pancreas reveals a total absence of acini with complete replacement of the pancreas by adipose tissue and a few remaining islets with connective tissue around the ducts (45). In contrast, an autopsy of a 4-year-old patient showed a pancreas consisting only of the head with immature-appearing acinar cells, centrally placed islets, periductal fibrosis, and ductular squamous metaplasia, but without significant fat replacement (46). A report regarding specimens from 2 fetuses (21 and 34 weeks of gestation) and a newborn baby revealed acinar tissue loss that increased with gestational age, accompanied by inflammatory infiltrates (47). There was no evidence of increased apoptosis in acinar cells by TUNEL assay, suggesting that the pancreatic defect may not be due to perturbed acinar development, but may rather be gradual destruction of previously formed acinar cells. Mutations in the gene *UBR1* have been detected in affected individuals from 12 of 13 families (47). *UBR1* encodes one of E3 ubiquitin ligases of the N-end rule pathway, a conserved proteolytic system. The UBR1 protein substrate, presumably impaired degradation of which causes Johanson-Blizzard syndrome, is not yet known. Using antibody to UBR1 and immunofluorescence microscopy, no UBR1 protein was observed in the pancreas from individuals with Johanson-Blizzard syndrome, while it is readily detectable in the cytosol of acinar cells in the control pancreas. Immunofluorescence pattern for trypsinogen indicated that there was no primary defect of zymogen synthesis. Hypoplasia of the exocrine pancreas in association with facial anomalies, micrognathia, posterior cleft palate, and dental hypoplasia has been referred to as the *Donlan syndrome*, but overlap with the Johanson-Blizzard syndrome seems likely (48).

Pearson Marrow–Pancreas Syndrome

Pearson et al. (49) described a syndrome characterized by pancreatic insufficiency, refractory sideroblastic anemia, and variable neutropenia in which the marrow is normocellular but the cells are vacuolated. A number of mitochondrial DNA deletions have been reported in affected individuals. The pancreatic pathologic features differ from those of the Shwachman-Diamond or Johanson-Blizzard syndrome in that acinar atrophy with fibrosis, not lipomatosis, is present (49,50).

A neonate with Pearson syndrome and diabetes mellitus (50) suggests a connection with Kearns-Sayre syndrome. The features of Kearns-Sayre syndrome, a mitochondrial myopathy, may develop later in life in patients who survive the early manifestations of Pearson syndrome. It has been postulated that a phenotypic shift from a predominantly hematopoietic disorder (Pearson syndrome) to a disease with muscle dysfunction (mitochondrial myopathy) and an eventual evolution to a full picture of Kearns-Sayre syndrome depends on the distribution of deleted mitochondrial DNA (51).

Neonatal Hemochromatosis

Neonatal hemochromatosis is unrelated to adult-type hereditary hemochromatosis. In neonatal hemochromatosis, hemosiderin deposition in the pancreatic acini is massive. The islets are generally spared, at least in the early stages (52) (Figure 16-11). Nevertheless, one case of neonatal diabetes due to neonatal hemochromatosis has been reported. Islets have been described to be increased in size in some cases, but the illustrations are less convincing. Acinar iron deposition in the absence of reticuloendothelial iron deposition is not pathognomonic of hemochromatosis; it was also seen in some control cases (53). Two siblings with a neonatal hemochromatosis phenotype that included pancreatic iron deposition also had hypertelorism and trichomalacia, a trichohepatoenteric syndrome (54).

Cystic Fibrosis

Fanconi et al. in 1936 and then Anderson in 1938, while investigating causes of malabsorption, discovered in some of their patients a condition they termed *cystic fibrosis of the pancreas*. Recognition of the pancreatic lesion preceded the clinical delineation of the disease. Farber (55) proposed mucous plugging of all secretory glands (mucoviscidosis) to be the pathogenetic key in 1944.

Cystic fibrosis is caused by defects in the cystic fibrosis conductance regulator gene (*CFTR*), localized to 7q31.2. Pancreatic insufficiency is not obligatory, and 15% of patients are clinically pancreas "sufficient." The degree of pancreatic disease varies widely at any age, although the disease is progressive and leads to increasingly more severe changes with time. The final stage of cystic fibrosis is characterized by obstruction of the pancreatic ducts by viscous secretion leading to complete acinar atrophy accompanied by fibrosis and lipomatosis (56,57).

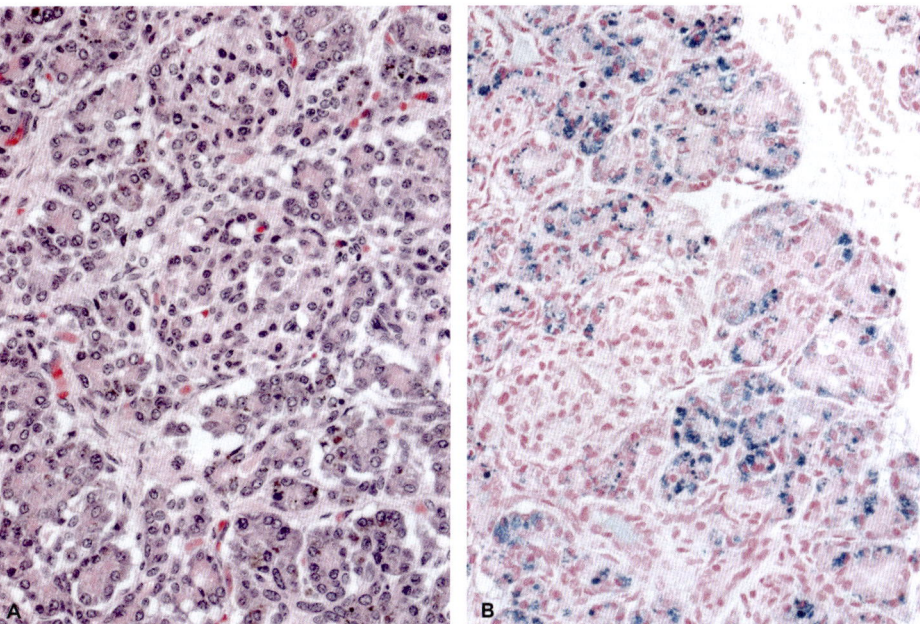

FIGURE 16-11 • Neonatal hemochromatosis. **A:** Exocrine acinar cells contain brown refractile pigment. (Hematoxylin and eosin stain, original magnification ×400.) **B:** The islets are devoid of iron, but acinar lobules have a marked intracytoplasmic iron deposition. (Prussian blue stain, original magnification ×400.)

The tissue alteration can be recognized even before 40 weeks of gestation (3,57,58). The ratio of acinar to connective tissue volume is 0.5 at 32 weeks after conception, increasing to 2.0 at 52 weeks in normal controls (3). In the pancreas, the ratio of acinar to connective tissue, low to begin with, decreases from 0.5 at 35 weeks to 0.3 at 52 weeks after conception. Further degeneration of exocrine tissue supervenes postnatally.

The earliest visible lesions are eosinophilic concretions in acini and ductules, which may lead to acinar or ductular dilation and flattening of the lining epithelium (56). These concretions generally stain with periodic acid–Schiff (PAS) and contain calcium. The changes may be focal in preterm infants and in mildly affected cases. Postnatal acceleration of the pathogenetic train of inspissation, obstruction, dilation, epithelial damage, atrophy, cell destruction, and fibrosis with minimal inflammation leads to progressive acinar loss with replacement by fibrous tissue (Figure 16-12; eFigure 16-3) and adipose tissue.

Cystic fibrosis in the older child can be associated with large single or multilocular cysts (59). The pancreatic pseudocyst, caused by rupture of a duct into the lesser sac or abdominal cavity, consists of a fibroinflammatory wall around an autodigested cavity. In addition to cystic fibrosis, pseudocysts are caused by trauma, surgery, or inflammation (pancreatitis). The fibrous wall of the cyst has no epithelial lining.

Even though acinar tissue may disappear, islet tissue is preserved until very late. The endocrine changes in cystic fibrosis are considered later in this chapter.

Inspissation and Other Changes of Pancreatic Ducts

Baggenstoss (60) described the widespread inspissation of secretions in centroacinar cell-lined ductules in patients with uremia. The finding is not restricted to uremia but is also seen in children dying with acidosis, dehydration, cardiac failure, or sepsis. Inspissation may also be seen in the pancreas of children who have experienced prolonged hyperalimentation, but they usually have many of the other conditions listed.

Striking oncocytic changes of the ducts and centroacinar cells have been observed in an infant with mitochondrial myopathy, lactic acidosis, and "ragged red" muscle fibers (MELAR syndrome). Centroacinar hyperplasia of an impressive degree was observed in a young adult with HIV infection (eFigure 16-4).

Pancreatitis in Childhood

In contrast to pancreatitis in adulthood, which is frequently related to alcohol abuse, the common causes of pancreatitis in children are trauma, multisystemic diseases, medications, infections, and biliary tract diseases. What etiologies are included in the "multisystem" category vary among the studies (61,62). Pancreatitis can also be seen in children with branched-chain organic acidemias, methylmalonic acidemia, isovaleric acidemia, and maple syrup urine disease (63). When all causes are excluded and the etiology remains undetermined, the pancreatitis has been traditionally labeled *idiopathic*. This group accounts for 8% to 34% of cases and leads the "cause" of childhood pancreatitis in some series (61). Except for patients with cystic fibrosis, hereditary pancreatitis, and pancreatitis secondary to congenital structural, syndromic, or metabolic abnormalities, most children have a single, self-limited episode of pancreatitis, and few cases progress to chronicity (62). On the other hand, children with recurrent or so-called idiopathic chronic pancreatitis may possess mutations and sequence variations in modifier genes as discussed below.

Acute pancreatitis of any cause varies from interstitial edema to necrotizing hemorrhagic inflammation depending on the severity and time point of the process. Fat necrosis is the characteristic finding and results from sequential

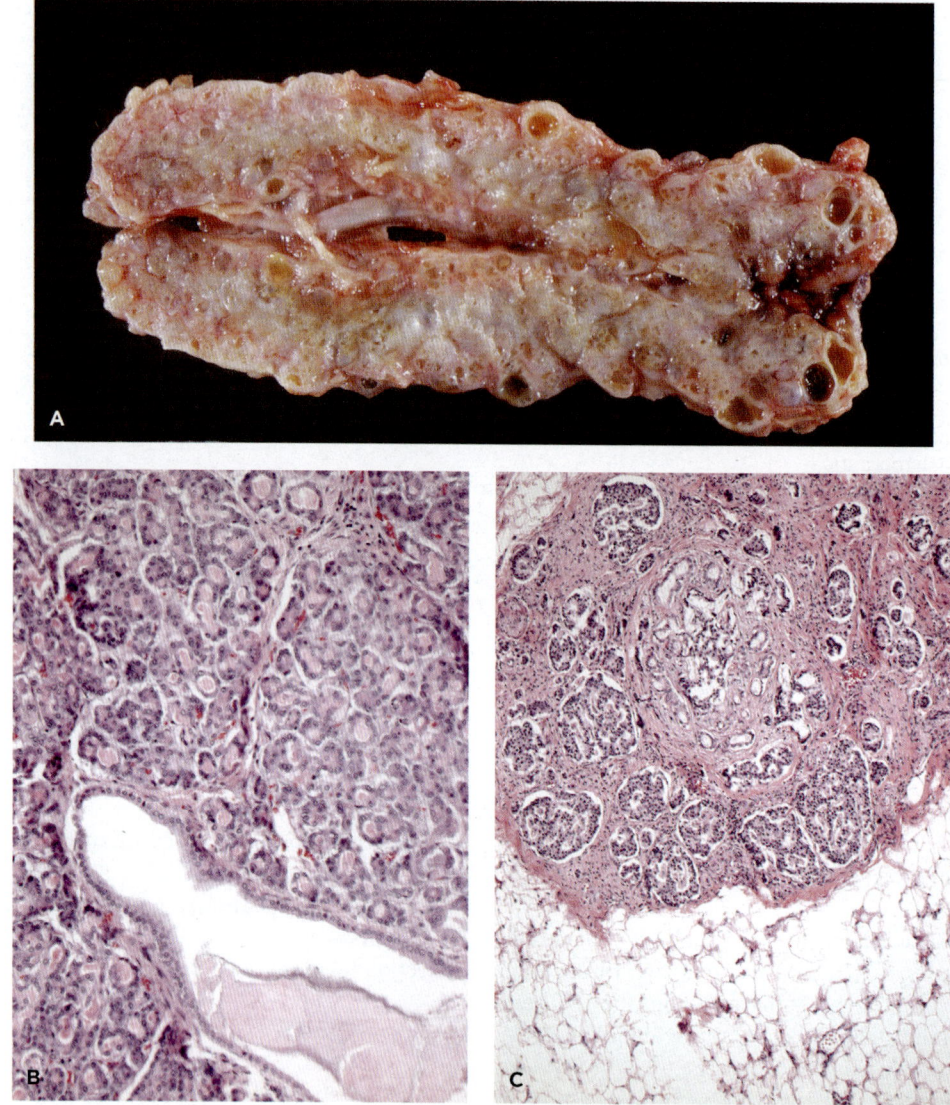

FIGURE 16-12 • Cystic fibrosis. **A:** The pancreas of this 12-year-old child is lipomatous with scattered cysts. **B:** An 8-year-old child with a strong family history of cystic fibrosis was asymptomatic and, at autopsy, had only cystic dilation with inspissation of ducts and acini with minimal fibrosis. (Hematoxylin and eosin stain, original magnification ×200.) **C:** The pancreas of a 10-year-old child shows advanced acinar atrophy, fatty replacement and periductal endocrine overgrowth. (Hematoxylin and eosin stain, original magnification ×100.)

reactions including release of fatty acids from triglyceride esters by lipase and combination of the fatty acids with calcium (saponification). The formed insoluble salts produce grossly visible chalky white to yellow areas. Microscopically, the outlines of degenerated fat cells with basophilic calcium deposits are seen along with acute inflammatory infiltrate (Figure 16-13A).

Recurrent pancreatitis and chronic pancreatitis produce fibroinflammatory changes of the parenchyma (64). The pancreas shows extensive fibrosis, acinar atrophy characterized by reduced number and size of acini, and variable dilatation of ducts with calcification (Figure 16-14). The endocrine islets are generally relatively spared and embedded in fibrotic tissue. They may appear fused and enlarged, but in end-stage disease, they eventually disappear.

Traumatic Pancreatitis

Blunt trauma is recognized as a cause of immediate or delayed pancreatitis in children (Figure 16-13A) and an important cause of pancreatic pseudocyst. A pancreatic pseudocyst may occur as the result of child abuse, but bicycle injuries are the most common cause in children.

Infectious Pancreatitis

The pancreas may be the seat of any disseminated infection, such as herpes simplex, cytomegalovirus infection (Figure 16-13B), or bacterial sepsis, but this may not result in clinically relevant pancreatitis (65,66). In some instances, the late consequences of a previous infectious pancreatitis are serious.

Rubella may cause an interstitial pancreatitis as part of the expanded congenital rubella syndrome, and pancreatic

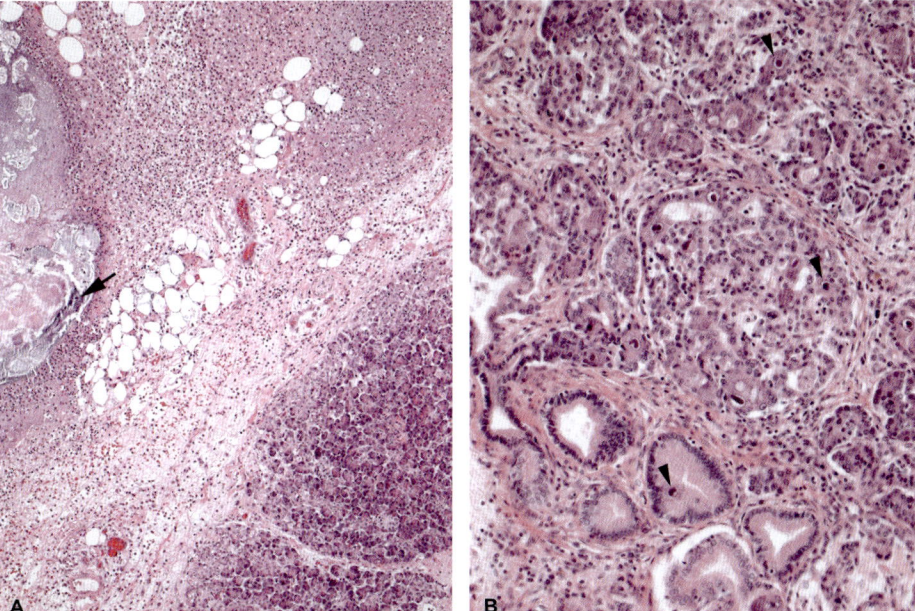

FIGURE 16-13 • Acute pancreatitis. **A:** Traumatic pancreatitis in a 7-year-old child showing fat necrosis with saponification (*arrow*) and acute inflammatory infiltrate. (Hematoxylin and eosin stain, original magnification ×100.) **B:** Cytomegalovirus pancreatitis with inclusions in acinar, ductal, and endocrine cells (*arrow heads*). (Hematoxylin and eosin stain, original magnification ×200; courtesy of James E. Dimmick, M.D., Vancouver, British Columbia.)

insufficiency or even diabetes mellitus can ensue (67). Mumps is a classic cause of pancreatitis in late childhood. Diffuse necrosis and pseudocyst formation has been reported in a surgical specimen (66). Coxsackievirus may selectively involve the exocrine or endocrine components of the pancreas with parenchymal hemorrhage (65,66). Parainfluenza 3 pancreatitis, confirmed by immunohistochemistry, produced multinucleated giant cells in the pancreas of a child with severe combined immunodeficiency. Varicella-zoster infection (chicken pox) resulted in pancreatitis in individuals succumbed to the disease. The postmortem examination revealed focal pancreatic necrosis (66). Chronic coxsackievirus B interstitial pancreatitis in the absence of a meningoencephalomyocarditis in a child with α_1-antitrypsin deficiency has been reported (68). Pancreatitis is a well-recognized consequence of bone marrow transplantation. Adenovirus infection may be the causative agent in some cases. In most cases of pancreatitis in children with acquired immunodeficiency syndrome (AIDS), the disease is mild and reflects systemic disease status. The incidence of opportunistic infections is low, although nonspecific inflammatory changes such as focal lymphoplasmacytic aggregates are common (69). *Escherichia coli* pancreatitis usually accompanies septicemia. Congenital syphilis causes a pancreatitis in which ductular obliteration, acinar loss, and exuberant interstitial fibrosis with concentric perivascular accentuation are noted (70) (Figure 16-4). Gummas are rare.

FIGURE 16-14 • Chronic pancreatitis. **A:** Obstructive pancreatitis with fibrosis, duct ectasia, acinar atrophy, and relative abundance of endocrine islets. Several pancreatic stones were also recovered. (Hematoxylin and eosin stain, original magnification ×50.) **B:** Pancreas of a 79-day-old infant (born at 30 weeks of gestation) with immunodysregulation, polyendocrinopathy, and enteropathy; X-linked inheritance syndrome (IPEX) shows diffuse mononuclear cell infiltrate, fibrosis, and acinar loss. Residual endocrine islets are present.

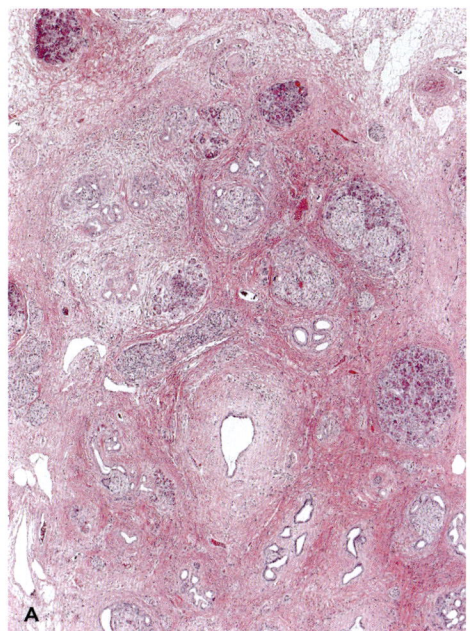
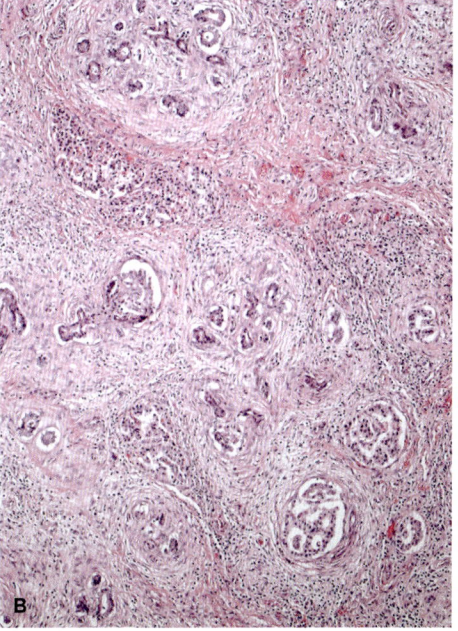

Inflammatory Pancreatitis

Pancreatitis can accompany childhood collagen vascular diseases, such as lupus, but it may be difficult to distinguish between the effects of disease and those of treatment, particularly drugs. Pancreatitis has been described in Henoch-Schönlein purpura, Reye syndrome, hemolytic-uremic syndrome, and Crohn disease.

Immunodysregulation, polyendocrinopathy, enteropathy, X-linked syndrome (IPEX) is a rare X-linked recessive disorder of immune regulation manifesting with neonatal onset diabetes mellitus, severe enteropathy, eczema, anemia, thrombocytopenia, and hypothyroidism. The disorder had been known by alternative names including X-linked polyendocrinopathy, immune dysfunction and diarrhea, and X-linked autoimmunity and allergic dysregulation. A mutant mouse strain, scurfy (*sf*) resembles IPEX, and the disease-causing gene *Foxp3* encoding scurfin was identified. Subsequently, the human IPEX locus was mapped to Xp11.23-q13.3, and mutations have been identified in the human ortholog (*JM2, FOXP3*) (71). Patients with protein-truncating mutations have been reported to demonstrate an absence of FOXP3-nuclear positive lymphocytes in their small and large intestines (72). Postmortem pancreatic histology is almost always abnormal; the findings include mild-to-dense lymphocytic infiltrate, acinar loss with fibrosis (chronic sclerosing pancreatitis), dilated ducts, and cystic changes (Figure 16-14). Islets of endocrine cells are decreased or absent in most cases with severe diabetes mellitus (73).

Biliary/Obstructive Pancreatitis

Some of the causes of biliary/obstructive pancreatitis in children have already been mentioned in the section on congenital malformations, such as annular pancreas, gastric duplications that connect to the pancreatic duct system, and anomalies of the pancreaticobiliary junction. Other causes include choledochal cyst, biliary sludge, and gallstone (74). Children with biliary/obstructive pancreatitis are more likely to present with jaundice and elevated serum levels of amino transferases. Cystic fibrosis is the prototype of a chronic obstructive pancreatitis.

Drug-Induced Pancreatitis

In most studies, medications attribute to less than one quarter of pediatric acute pancreatitis. The 2007 American Gastrointestinal Association Technical Bulletin on Acute Pancreatitis lists and categorizes medications as having "definite," "probable," or "possible" association with acute pancreatitis (75). To be included as drug-associated pancreatitis, the medication needs to be taken before the onset of acute pancreatitis (76). The most common medications in pediatric studies are valproic acid, L-asparaginase, prednisone, 6-mercaptopurine, mesalamine, and trimethoprim/sulfamethoxazole. However, interpretation of the cause-and-effect relation is difficult because many patients who are on the listed medications have systemic illnesses that may predispose to pancreatitis. The comorbidities include seizure disorders, acute lymphocytic leukemia, Crohn disease, ulcerative colitis, transplants/graft versus host disease, AIDS, asthma, renal disorders, and acute myeloid leukemia (76).

Hereditary Pancreatitis

The concept of hereditary pancreatitis was first described by Comfort and Steinberg in 1952 as "chronic relapsing pancreatitis" in a family of three generations. More than 200 kindreds have since been documented, with variable prevalence worldwide. It is an autosomal dominant disorder with an 80% penetrance and variable expressivity. Classically, hereditary pancreatitis diagnosis is defined by the presence of recurrent acute pancreatitis or chronic pancreatitis occurring in two first-degree relatives or three or more second-degree relatives, in two or more generations in the absence of precipitating factors (77). The discovery of mutations within the cationic trypsinogen gene, also referred to as serine protease 1 gene (*PRSS1*), has resulted in the development of genetic testing. Currently, the diagnosis can also be established by the presence of a mutation of the *PRSS1* gene with or without clinical or radiologic manifestations of chronic pancreatitis. Cationic trypsinogen is one of the three isoforms of the digestive proenzyme trypsinogen and represents approximately two-thirds of total trypsinogen in the pancreatic juice. Activation of trypsinogen to trypsin normally occurs in the duodenum by the brush-border localized enterokinase and also by autoactivation by trypsin. The mutations either increase stability or increase autoactivation of trypsin (77).

A major motivation for identifying patients with hereditary pancreatitis is the increased risk for developing pancreatic adenocarcinoma. Despite this increased risk of cancer, however, a national study performed in France demonstrated that hereditary pancreatitis patients do not have an excess mortality risk as compared with the general population, irrespective of gender, tobacco use, or diabetes mellitus (78).

The histopathology of *PRSS1* hereditary pancreases varies among reports. An earlier study of two adult pancreatic specimens described paucicellular thick fibrosis and distorted and dilated ducts, without dysplasia or a mention of fatty replacement (79). Singhi et al. examined 12 total pancreatectomy specimens and suggested a sequential pattern of changes with increasing age (80). In pediatric patients, the pancreas was generally grossly normal, but there was microscopic variation in lobular size and shape, and parenchymal loss in the central portion of the pancreas accompanied by loose perilobular and interlobular fibrosis. The periphery was, however, replaced by mature adipose tissue. With older individuals, the pancreas showed progressive atrophy and extensive replacement by mature adipose tissue with scattered endocrine isles consistent with lipomatous atrophy. Smaller intra- and interlobular ducts were scarred, and the larger interlobular ducts were dilated with intraductal calcification. Pancreatic intraepithelial neoplasia (PanIN), a precursor of infiltrating ductal adenocarcinoma, was identified in only 3 patients. No high-grade PanINs (PanIN-3) was identified. This report is in contrast to a study by Rebours et al. (81), which identified PanIN lesions in 10 of 13 partial pancreatectomy specimens. One 7-year-old boy showed a focus of high-grade dysplasia (PanIN-3).

Genetic Contributing Factors in Chronic Pancreatitis

Identification of genetic alterations in hereditary pancreatitis has provided a significant tool to investigate other pathogenic factors of acute and chronic pancreatitis. Chronic pancreatitis is a persistent inflammation of the pancreas that results in irreversible morphologic changes and impairment of both exocrine and endocrine functions. Genetic studies of familial and so-called idiopathic forms of chronic pancreatitis have characterized four other susceptibility genes. Witt et al. reported a close linkage of sequence alterations in *SPINK1* to chronic pancreatitis. *SPINK1* encodes a natural antagonist of trypsinogens, serine protease inhibitor, Kazal type I, also known as *pancreatic secretory trypsin inhibitor*, which binds reversibly to trypsin and inhibits its activity. Loss-of-function variants in trypsin-degrading enzyme chymotrypsin C gene (*CTRC*) increase the risk of chronic pancreatitis in European and Asian populations. Most recently, variants in the gene encoding carboxypeptidase A1 (*CPA1*) have been shown to be strongly associated with early-onset chronic pancreatitis (82). CPA1 is one of the isoforms of digestive carboxypeptidases that hydrolyzes C-terminal peptide bond. After trypsinogens, proCPA1 is the second largest component of pancreatic juice. Sequence variations of *CFTR*, the gene responsible for cystic fibrosis, are also associated with chronic pancreatitis. *PRSS1*, *SPINK1*, *CTRC*, and *CPA1* are expressed in the acinar cells in the human pancreas, while *CFTR* is expressed in the ductal and centroacinar cells. The expressed protein CFTR is believed to dilute and alkalinize the protein-rich acinar secretions, preventing the formation of protein plugs that predispose to pancreatic injury. There is evidence to support the hypothesis that risk of pancreatitis is related to the balance between degrees of pancreatic acinar preservation and pancreatic ductal obstruction, which are associated with CFTR dysfunction in opposing directions (83). Coinheritance of a *CFTR* mutation that inhibits bicarbonate conductance but maintains chloride conductance and *SPINK1* variants is shown to increase risk of pancreatitis. However, another report argues that the contributions of *CFTR* variants to chronic pancreatitis in transheterozygous status are overestimated (84).

Idiopathic chronic pancreatitis has been a traditional clinical diagnosis describing the lack of an identifiable cause. As more genes and/or more mutations are identified that cause or predispose to chronic pancreatitis, the number of patients with "idiopathic" disease seems to be decreasing. At the same time, the spectrum of diseases associated with the *CTFR* mutant genes keeps expanding.

Exocrine Tumors

Primary exocrine pancreatic tumors are rare in children. Due to the very small number of cases, it has been difficult to predict long-term outcome and develop and optimize therapeutic trials. As a first step, several retrospective and prospective data collections on childhood pancreatic tumors have been undertaken in the last decade in the North America (85,86), Germany (87), Italy, (88), and France (89). The primary exocrine pancreatic tumors listed in these reports are pancreatoblastoma, solid pseudopapillary neoplasm, acinar cell carcinoma, and pancreatic duct carcinoma, and these four are described below. Rare descriptive reports of mucinous cystadenoma and acinar cell cystadenoma appear in the literature (86,90). Tumors and masses that may occur, but are not specific to pancreas, include vascular lesions (26), lymphomas, and other childhood sarcomas (e.g., rhabdomyosarcoma).

Pancreatoblastoma

Pancreatoblastoma (91), also called *pancreaticoblastoma*, is an epithelial neoplasm that exhibits multiple lines of differentiation including acinar differentiation, often with a lesser degree of endocrine and ductal differentiation, and is associated with squamoid corpuscles (92). A distinct mesenchymal component can also be seen. Some view this as the infantile or "blastomatous" form of acinar cell carcinoma. In support of this interpretation, a considerable overlap exists among pancreatoblastoma and acinar cell carcinoma (93). Pancreatoblastomas occur most frequently in young children, but rare congenital cases discovered by prenatal imaging have been reported (94). There is a close association of infantile and congenital pancreatoblastomas with Beckwith-Wiedemann syndrome.

Pancreatoblastomas are usually large, solitary masses (Figure 16-15A), ranging from 1.5 to 20 cm with a mean of 10.6 cm (95) and partially encapsulated. Microscopically, they are highly cellular, and the epithelial tumor cells are arranged in solid sheets and as small acini. The acinar differentiation is demonstrated by immunohistochemical positivity for pancreatic enzymes such as trypsin and chymotrypsin (96) and the presence of zymogen granules by electron microscopy. The tumor usually has a lobular pattern, separated by stromal bands that may be hypercellular. The squamoid corpuscle is the characteristic feature of pancreatoblastoma (Figure 16-15B, C). The structures may be loose aggregates of larger spindle cells, or more frankly squamous, with keratinization. The cells forming squamoid corpuscles are not immunoreactive to antibody against cytokeratin 7, while acinar and solid areas are positively labeled (97) (eFigure 16-5). Alpha-fetoprotein production has been reported (93), a character shared with cases of acinar cell carcinoma in childhood. It is common to detect endocrine and ductal differentiation by immunohistochemistry as a minor component of the tumor (95). Molecular genetic alterations in pancreatoblastomas include a high frequency of allelic loss on chromosome 11p15 and mutations in adenomatous polyposis coli/ β-catenin pathway (eFigure 16-5). Pancreatoblastomas in children are usually detected before developing metastatic diseases and are curable by complete resection (98). For patients with unresectable tumors, multidisciplinary approach including adjuvant chemotherapy is recommended, but no established protocol based on prospective study exists to date (99).

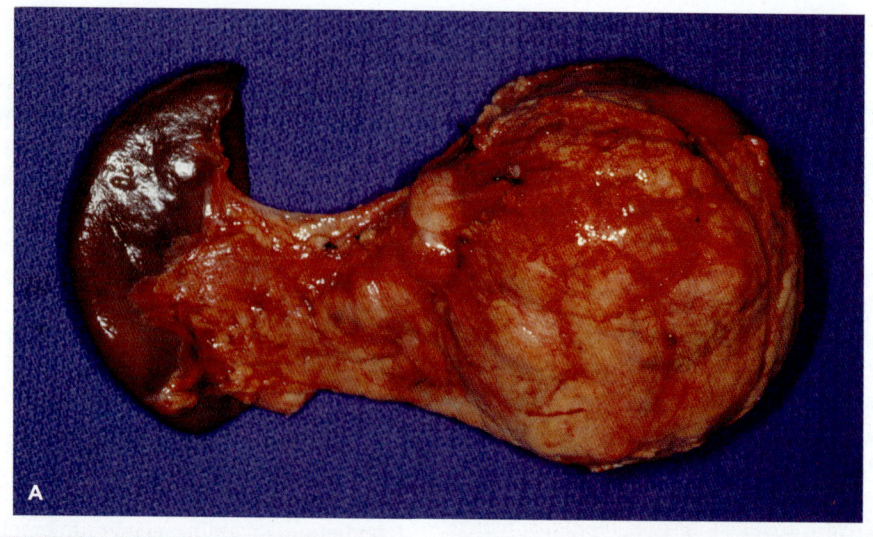
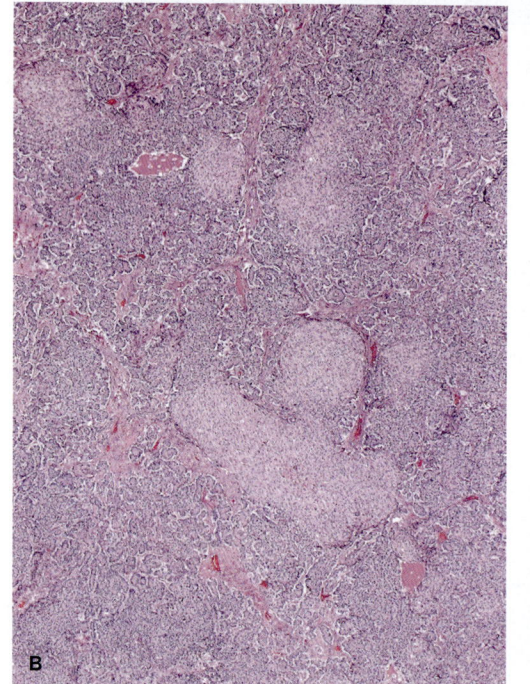
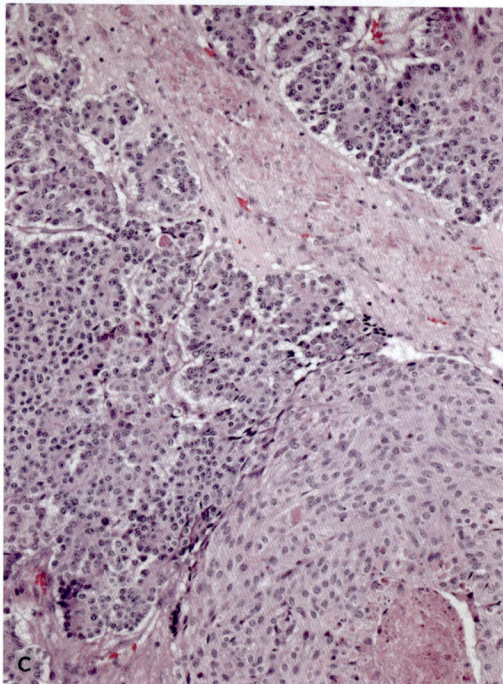

FIGURE 16-15 • Pancreatoblastoma. **A:** A 9.3-cm tumor removed with the tail of pancreas and the spleen from a 4-year-old girl. (Courtesy of James F. Southern, M.D., Milwaukee, Wisconsin.) **B:** Tumor consists of a mixture of areas with acinar arrangement and squamoid corpuscles. **C:** A squamoid corpuscle with central necrosis is on the lower right corner. A stromal band separates the areas of acinar differentiation with pinpoint lumina and cells showing darker cytoplasm and basally located nuclei. (**B, C:** hematoxylin and eosin stain, original magnifications, ×50 and ×200, respectively.)

Acinar Cell Carcinoma

Acinar cell carcinoma is a malignant epithelial neoplasm that shows features of exocrine enzyme production by the neoplastic cells. By definition, endocrine and ductal components are minimal and do not exceed 25% of the neoplastic cells (92). The histology and the clinical behavior in the pediatric population of acinar cell carcinoma are very similar to pancreatoblastoma, and in some cases, the pathologic distinction between the two can be difficult (93,98). Acinar cell carcinomas are usually large, solid, circumscribed tumors that sometimes show necrosis and cystic degeneration (100). They are microscopically highly cellular lesions that characteristically lack the desmoplastic stroma commonly seen with the ductal adenocarcinomas (Figure 16-16, eFigure 16-6). The tumor cells show solid, trabecular, or glandular growth patterns as well as acinar formation. The cytoplasm tends to be abundant and granular. Immunoreactivity for trypsin, lipase, amylase, and chymotrypsin and ultrastructural demonstration of zymogen granules confirm acinar differentiation (101). Electron

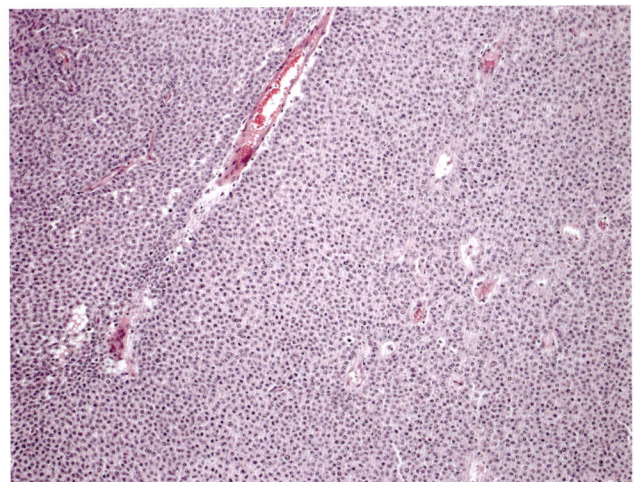

FIGURE 16-16 • Acinar cell carcinoma. The tumor is highly cellular with virtually no stroma. The tumor cells are arranged in solid sheets and nests with small luminal spaces. (Hematoxylin and eosin, original magnification ×100.)

microscopic studies are also helpful in demonstrating epithelial differentiation (102). Vascular invasion and invasion into the tumor capsule are relatively common (102). As both acinar cell carcinoma and pancreatoblastoma share a densely cellular morphology, can exhibit a minor endocrine component, and demonstrate acinar differentiation, it is sometimes impossible to decide whether a tumor is a "squamoid corpuscle-free" pancreatoblastoma or an acinar cell carcinoma (93). It is therefore advised and practical to define pancreatoblastoma as a tumor with the characteristic squamoid corpuscles and distinguish it from acinar cell carcinoma. Genetic alterations in acinar cell carcinomas also point toward the similarity between the two tumors (103). When the tumor is localized to the pancreas, complete surgical resection can result in long-term survival (88). Patients with a higher stage usually receive chemotherapy with variable outcomes (87).

Solid Pseudopapillary Neoplasm

This tumor is also known as *solid pseudopapillary tumor, papillary cystic tumor of the pancreas, solid and papillary epithelial neoplasm, and papillary cystic neoplasm,* but *solid pseudopapillary neoplasm* is currently the preferred term (104). Close to 90% of cases are found in females in the second and third decades of life (105). The number of solid pseudopapillary neoplasms reported in the literature has seen a sevenfold increase since 2000 compared to the years between 1961 and 2000. This increase is accompanied by the increased number of incidentally detected tumors, most likely secondary to improvement in the quality and use of cross-sectional imaging studies.

The tumors are generally large, both solid and cystic (Figure 16-17), and located anywhere in the pancreas. Solid sheets of epithelial cells may have an endocrine appearance, with uniform cells that have sharply defined cell borders. Perivascular pseudopapillae are interspersed with cystic degenerated areas. PAS-positive globules may be present in the cytoplasm (Figure 16-17). The line of differentiation of solid pseudopapillary neoplasm is unknown (96,106). Consistently, positive markers by immunohistochemistry are CD56, vimentin, α_1-antitrypsin, nuclear β-catenin, and CD10 (107) (eFigure 16-7). In addition, a particular dot-like paranuclear cytoplasmic expression of CD99 is characteristic (108). Some tumors show positive labeling for synaptophysin, but chromogranin is negative. The presence of progesterone receptors is frequently reported (109), while there are conflicting results on estrogen receptors. Overall, this neoplasm has a very good prognosis, with over 95% of patients reported as disease free after surgical resection and with less than 2% mortality. However, it should be noted that this tumor is a malignant neoplasm with local and metastatic potential. One single institution study indicates that invasion into muscular vessels and stage are important predictors of disease-specific survival (110).

Pancreatic Ductal Adenocarcinoma

The majority of childhood adenocarcinomas of pancreas are acinar cell carcinomas. However, there are exceptional but documented pancreatic ductal adenocarcinomas in children and young adults. Lüttges et al. (111) reviewed the literature from 1818 to 2001 for patients with pancreatic ductal adenocarcinomas in younger patients (age <40 years). Reevaluation of the tumors in light of the 2000 World Health Organization (WHO) classification system identified 20 fully qualified pancreatic ductal adenocarcinomas. The authors also described three cases from their own files (ages 10, 17, and 20), among whom two showed a mucinous component with MUC2 positivity. The studies by Yu et al. (Boston) (86) and Ellerkamp et al. (Germany) (87) each report two cases of ductal adenocarcinomas, all under 15 years of age. The clinicopathologic findings of ductal adenocarcinomas in younger individuals are reported to be comparable to those in patients older than 40 years except for more frequent associations with genetic factors such as Peutz-Jeghers syndrome.

ENDOCRINE PANCREAS

Histogenesis, Maturation, and Morphology

During weeks 6 and 7 of intrauterine life, the dorsal and ventral pancreatic buds fuse. A simple epithelial tube of endodermal origin grows into the mesenchyme and gives rise to the endocrine and exocrine pancreas. Microdissection studies in the mouse have shown that both the exocrine and endocrine cells of the pancreas develop from foregut endoderm; expression of both acinar enzyme and islet hormone genes is detected. Without mesenchyme, the primordial cells develop into endocrine cells only, but in the presence of mesenchyme, ducts and acini also form (112).

Robb described in 1961 the budding of islet cells from the pancreatic duct into the adjacent mesenchyme, visible after

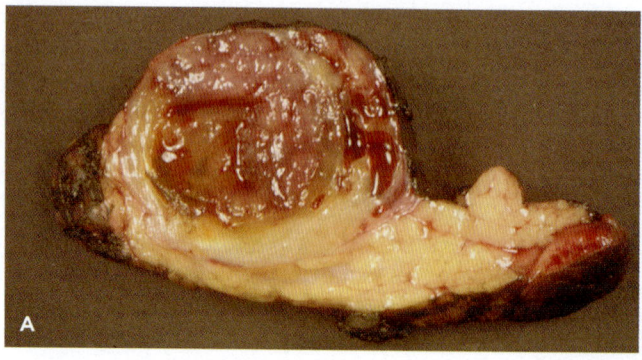
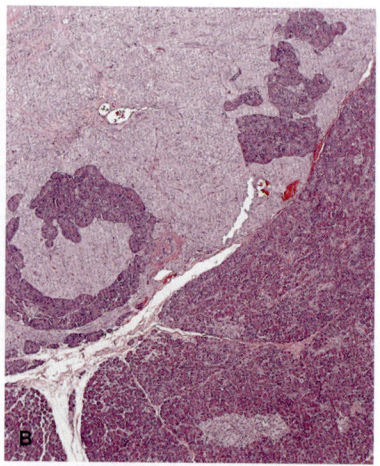
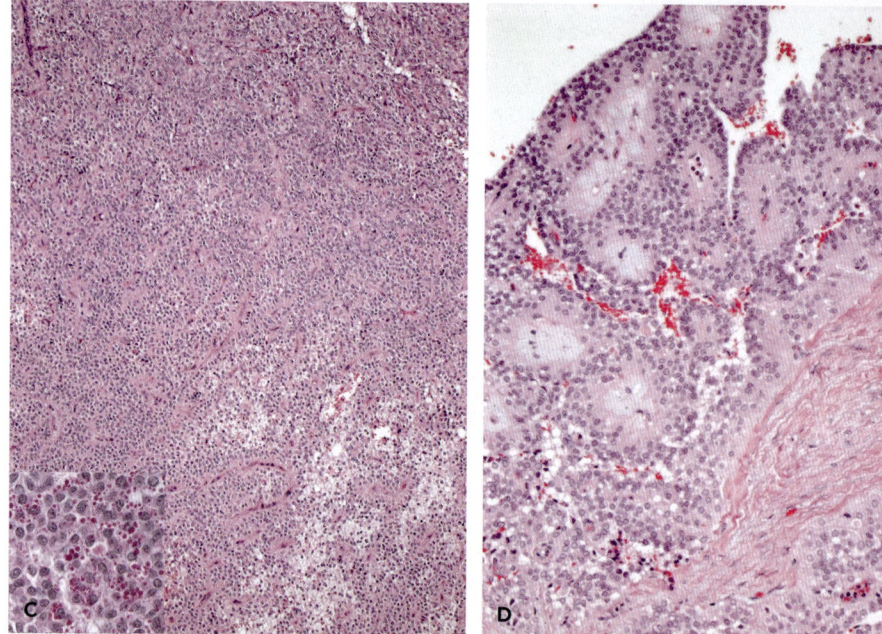

FIGURE 16-17 • Solid pseudopapillary neoplasm. **A:** A 2.5-cm tumor removed from the tail of the pancreas in a 14-year-old girl. (Courtesy of Marta E. Guttenburg, M.D., Philadelphia, Pennsylvania.) **B:** Despite the grossly circumscribed appearance, microscopic infiltrative growth is common, especially into the adjacent nonneoplastic pancreas. (Hematoxylin and eosin stain, original magnification ×50.) **C:** The basic architecture is solid cellular nests with small vessels. Some cells show cytoplasmic vacuolization. (Hematoxylin and eosin stain, original magnification ×100.) **Inset:** Eosinophilic "hyaline globules" are periodic acid–Schiff positive and diastase resistant and typically found in the cytoplasm. (Periodic acid–Schiff with diastase stain, original magnification ×400.) **D:** The tumor cells situated away from the vessels degenerate, resulting in pseudopapillae. (Hematoxylin and eosin stain, original magnification ×200.)

10.5 weeks of gestation. The endocrine cells then lose their connection with the duct and become vascularized by a central capillary. In the study of Stefan and colleagues (113), glicentin-containing cells were the first to appear, becoming detectable at week 8 of gestation in the wall of the developing duct. This pattern virtually disappeared by week 12 or 13 and was replaced by one in which the cells were reactive for adult glucagon and glicentin. By week 9, primitive islets were found to contain insulin (B) cells, somatostatin (D) cells, and glucagon (A) cells; pancreatic peptide (PP) cells were found only in the region of the duct of Wirsung, presumably in the ventral lobe.

Between weeks 16 and 20 of gestation, the bipolar islets of Robb have insulin at one pole and somatostatin or glucagon at the other, except in the ventral lobe, in which PP predominates (113). A central core of insulin cells develops in the mantle islet, surrounded by somatostatin and glucagon cells in the body and the tail and PP cells in the ventral head. The mature islets exhibit a trabecular arrangement, in which inner cells contain insulin and more peripheral cells contain glucagon or somatostatin; this arrangement is thought to be important in paracrine cell-to-cell control. Gap junctions mediate cell-to-cell communication for the biosynthesis, storage, and release of insulin and other hormones.

The distribution of the various cell types is not homogeneous within the pancreas nor are they stable from fetal to adult life. A portion of the head of the pancreas, ostensibly derived from the ventral primordium, is rich in islets containing PP (114). The number of somatostatin-containing D cells is greater in the fetal and neonatal period than later in life, reaching a peak between week 17 of gestation and 5 months of age (113).

The endocrine tissue in the developing pancreas lies centrally within the lobule, close to the ductal system from which it buds. The larger and better formed islets of Langerhans form the stalk of the lobule, and smaller aggregates and single cells bud off within the more peripheral centroacinar tissues, resulting in a greater number of single cells and small clusters of endocrine cells outside the islets (115) (Figure 16-18). At term, the small clusters may be numerous, and the extrainsular endocrine cells may constitute much of the endocrine component. This is often confused with the diffuse form of congenital hyperinsulinism, formerly *diffuse nesidioblastosis*.

A large body of literature has been published on the quantification of the endocrine content of the pancreas at various ages. The endocrine content of the pancreas can be

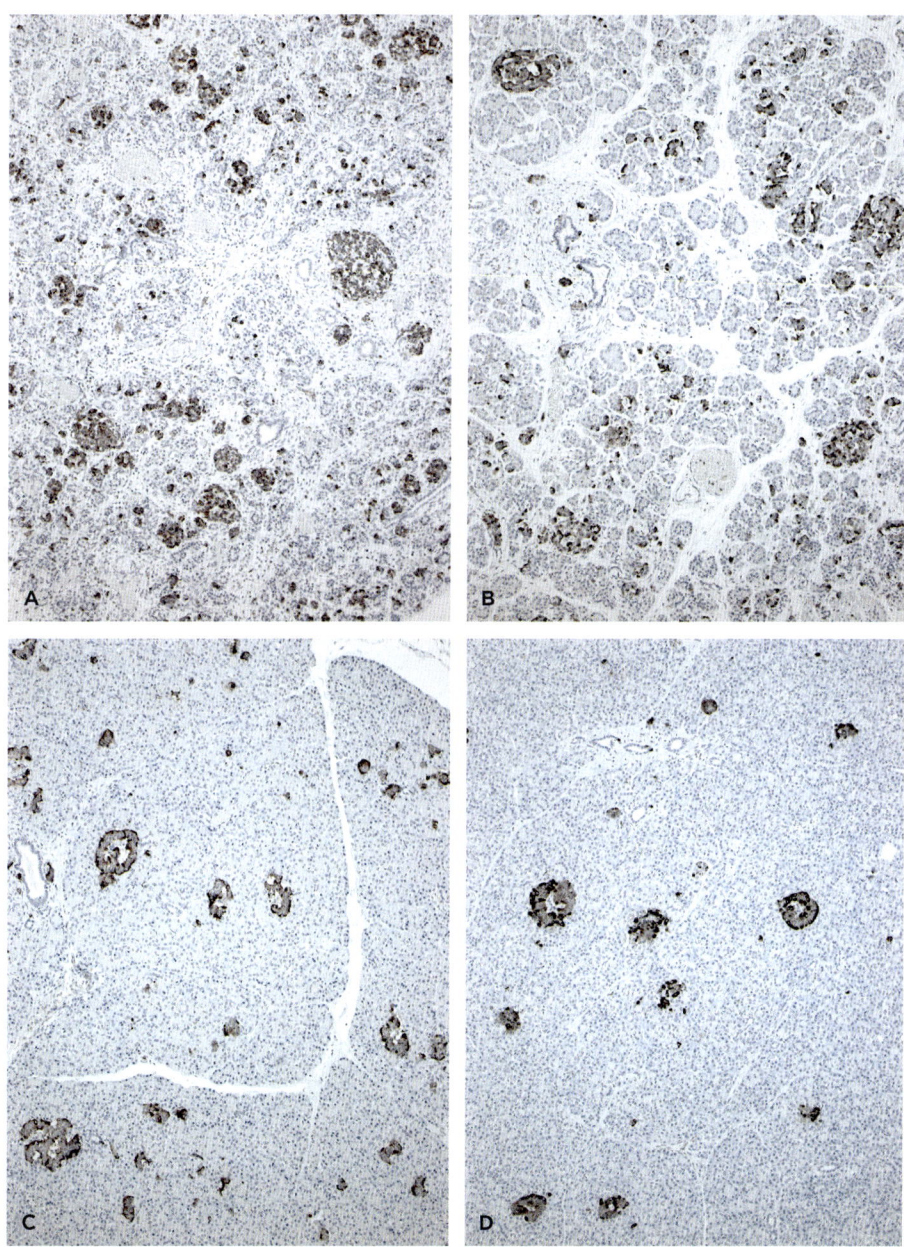

FIGURE 16-18 • Distribution of endocrine cells, which are revealed by immunohistochemistry for chromogranin A. Respective survival dates are as follows: **(A)** Stillbirth at 25 weeks. **(B)** Forty weeks of gestation, 8 days of postnatal survival. **(C)** Twenty-two months. **(D)** Eight years. (**A–D:** original magnifications ×100.)

expressed as a ratio of endocrine to acinar tissue. This is easy to quantify in a mature pancreas, in which confluent acinar tissue is present around islets. It is much more problematic in the pancreas of an infant, which consists mostly of mesenchyme and in which many of the largest islets are "septal" (Figure 16-18).

The amount of endocrine tissue present at birth, in a rough compilation of available estimates, is 10%; this decreases during acinar development to 5% by 6 months of age and then gradually to the adult volumes of 1% to 2% (115,116). Figure 16-19 illustrates histologic features of normal pancreas in children often confused to be abnormal, including abundant endocrine tissue, endocrine cell clusters budding off ducts, and large septal islets.

The amount of endocrine tissue is not fixed. Ductal obstruction, with chronic pancreatitis and fibrosis, may be associated with a resurgence of endocrine development. This situation can mimic an endocrine neoplasm. Because volumetric determinations of endocrine mass are usually expressed relative to the acinar mass and because a decrease in exocrine tissue produces a relative increase in the mass of islet cells, the observer should determine whether an

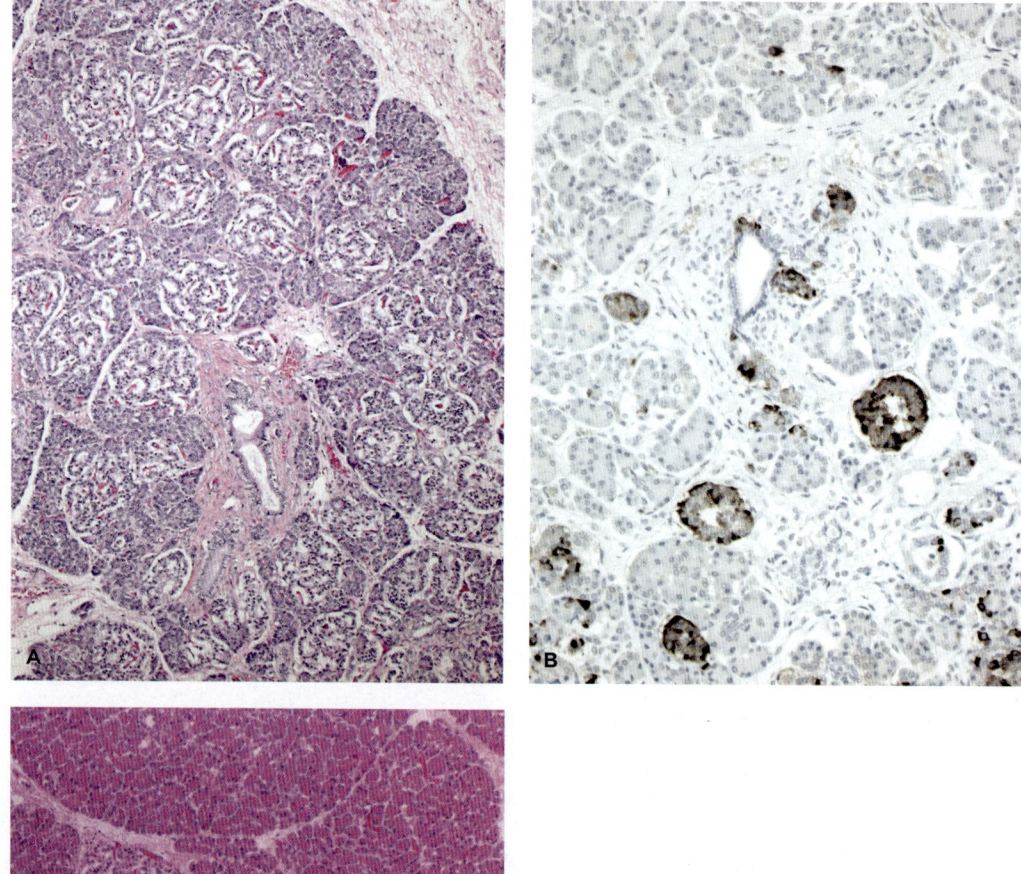

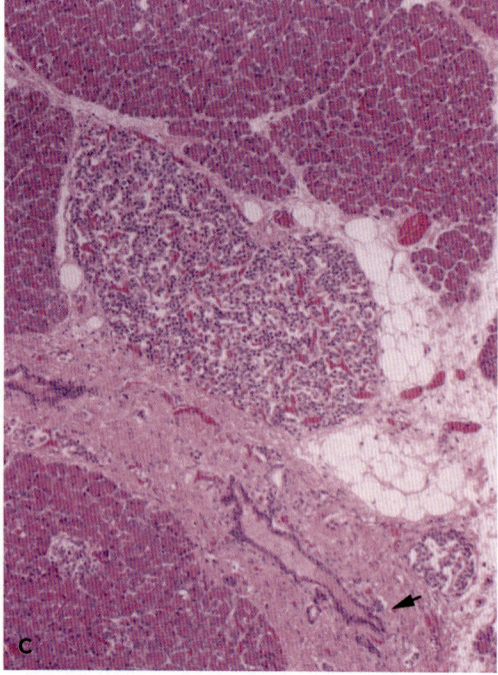

FIGURE 16-19 • Histologic features of pancreas from individuals less than 2 years of age. **A:** Abundant islets/endocrine tissue is seen in the pancreas of a 5-month-old normoglycemic infant, especially in the head. (Hematoxylin and eosin stain, original magnification ×100.) **B:** Endocrine cells budding off a duct (nesidioblastosis) in an 8-day-old infant born at 40 weeks of gestation. (Immunohistochemistry for chromogranin A, original magnification ×200.) **C:** Very large septal islets, such as this one in a 22-month-old child, are not uncommon. A small cluster of endocrine cells is budding off a duct (nesidioblastosis) in the lower right corner (*arrow*). (Hematoxylin and eosin stain, original magnification ×100.)

apparent excess of endocrine cells is absolute or secondary to acinar loss.

Abnormalities of the Endocrine Pancreas

Islet Hypertrophy

Islet size varies with age. Jaffe et al. (115) found that before the age of 2 months, only 3.5% of all islets are larger than 200 μm in diameter. Single septal islets at any age can be much larger, measuring as much as 700 μm in diameter (Figure 16-19). The term *islet hypertrophy* should be used to describe a generalized phenomenon in which the percentage of islets larger than 200 μm is excessive for a particular age. Borchard and Müntefering (117) provide values for islet size at different stages of gestation. True islet hypertrophy is seen in infants of diabetic mothers and, less commonly, in infants with erythroblastosis fetalis (117–119).

Endocrine Aplasia and Hypoplasia

Combined exocrine and endocrine hypoplasia was mentioned previously. A child with metabolic acidosis and diabetes shortly after birth had a pancreas in which exocrine elements appeared normal but no islets were seen on conventional histologic examination; a sibling had a similar clinical story (120). A congenital absence of glucagon cells has been reported (but not illustrated), and an infant with normoinsulinemic hypoglycemia had few glucagon-containing cells (121). A generalized paucity of somatostatin cells has been implicated in some cases of neonatal hypoglycemia (122). Some growth-restricted fetuses have been previously reported to show endocrine paucity, but a more recent study demonstrated no differences between intrauterine growth restriction and control fetuses in insulin-positive areas or islet organization (123).

Infant of the Diabetic Mother

Maternal insulin and glucagon do not cross the placenta, although maternally derived or animal-derived antigen–antibody complexes of insulin do. The changes in the endocrine pancreas of a child born to a diabetic mother are a response to maternal hyperglycemia and anti-insulin antibodies. The various changes in the pancreas of the diabetic offspring are ascribed to variations in the severity of maternal disease, the stringency of the therapeutic control, and the presence or absence of diabetic vascular complications (124). Most infants of diabetic mothers have islet hypertrophy (>10% of islets larger than 200 μm), an increased total islet cell volume, pleomorphism of B-cell nuclei, eosinophilic insulitis (Figure 16-20), and peri-insular or intrainsular fibrosis (118,125). Similar features may be present in the pancreas of infants born to prediabetic mothers.

Hultquist and Olding (118) stated that the pancreas of the infant whose mother is diabetic weighs less than that of a normal infant when corrected for total body weight. This is particularly true of the infants of mothers with the most severe diabetic complications. After week 34 of gestation, infants with a birth weight of 2.25 kg or more have an excess islet cell volume. This correlation was stronger for the offspring of mothers with uncomplicated diabetes because they had the largest babies. No difference was detected between islet cell volume in normal infants and the volume in the offspring of mothers with severely complicated diabetes. Borchard and Müntefering (117) claimed that an increased mean islet diameter is more characteristic of the diabetic infant than an increased number of islets.

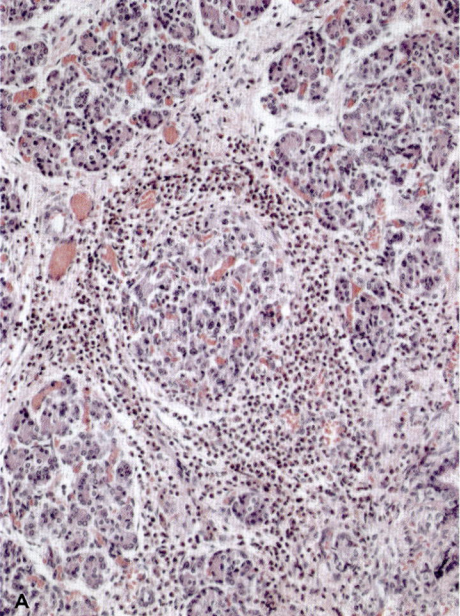 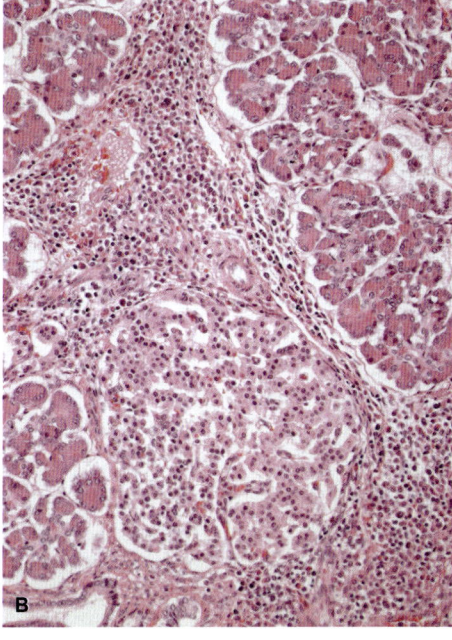

FIGURE 16-20 • Infant of diabetic mother and nonimmune hydrops fetalis. **A:** Eosinophilic insulitis in an infant of a diabetic mother. (Hematoxylin and eosin stain, original magnification ×200.) **B:** In this pancreas from an infant with nonimmune hydrops, an islet is associated with extramedullary hematopoiesis. (Hematoxylin and eosin stain, original magnification ×200.)

The islet cell increase is largely the consequence of expansion of the B-cell mass from 40% of endocrine cells to 63.8% (124). This expansion is observed in the dorsal lobe–derived pancreatic polypeptide–poor portion of the pancreas (e.g., tail) (124) as well as in the pancreatic polypeptide–rich (ventral lobe–derived) region of the pancreas. Milner et al. (116) demonstrated that A-cell and PP-cell increases accompany B-cell hyperplasia in a diabetic pregnancy, with A-cell increase occurring only in the pancreatic polypeptide–poor and PP-cell increase in the pancreatic polypeptide–rich regions. Pleomorphism of B-cell nuclei is seen with increase in endocrine volume and is also marked in the pancreas of infants of mothers with complicated diabetes.

Wellman and Volk (119) reviewed the issue of mesenchymal inflammatory infiltrate. Eosinophilic peri-insulitis, the most characteristic finding, occurs in about 50% of infants of diabetic mothers, whether or not the mother is receiving insulin. The infiltrate is rich in eosinophilic myelocytes, may contain Charcot-Leyden crystals, and is said to disappear within days of birth. Charcot-Leyden crystals can be seen in the macerated pancreas. It has been suggested that the infiltrate is a local reaction to insulin-containing immune complex. Fibrosis within and around islets is seen in association with hypertrophy and eosinophilia, but it is also described as an early *in utero* finding independent of eosinophilic accumulation (118).

Other, less constant findings in the islets of infants of diabetic mothers include an increase in the mitotic rate, degranulation of B cells, islet edema, hydropic swelling of islet cells, ribbon-like transformation of islet cells, necrosis, and thickened extrainsular and intrainsular capillaries. Lymphocytic infiltration is not specific to these children.

A suggestion by Van Assche and Gepts (124) was that an intact hypothalamic–hypophyseal axis is required for the development of pathologic pancreatic changes because they are not seen in the anencephalic offspring of diabetic mothers.

It has been predicted that the prenatally affected islets of infants of diabetic mothers become insufficient through the stress of postnatal life and that infants of diabetic mothers are more likely to develop diabetes mellitus. Several epidemiologic data show that consequences extend to adult life and even to the next generation through the maternal line (126). Family histories secured from consecutive pregnant diabetic women indicated that patients with gestational diabetes are more likely to have a mother with diabetes than gravidas with normal carbohydrate metabolism. The studies on Pima Indians (127) have shown that besides a genetic transmission of diabetes, the diabetic intrauterine milieu can also induce a diabetogenic tendency in the offspring.

Hydrops Fetalis

The accumulation of fluid in the fetus results from various congenital and acquired/maternal conditions. Immune hydrops is caused by blood group incompatibility, mostly of ABO and certain Rh types, between mother and child. The endocrine pancreas of Rh-positive infants born to Rh-negative mother with anti-Rh antibody has been described to partly resemble that of infants of diabetic mother but with some differences. The amount of endocrine tissue is increased in the tail of the pancreas (128), and it is parallel to the increased number of endocrine cells per islet. In contrast to infants of diabetic mothers, the proportion of B cells and the contribution of the different cell types are unchanged. Milner et al. (116) report that the increased volume fraction of B, A, PP-, and D cells is seen only in the pancreatic polypeptide–rich (ventral lobe) part of the pancreas.

Prevention of Rh immunization in at-risk mothers has reduced the incidence of this disorder, and nonimmune hydrops has become more prevalent. The causes of nonimmune hydrops are manifold. Excess endocrine tissue and islet cell hyperplasia (without morphometric confirmation) have been described in nonimmune hydrops fetalis (129). An islet associated with extramedullary hematopoiesis is depicted in Figure 16-20.

Diabetes Mellitus

Diabetes mellitus is a group of metabolic diseases characterized by hyperglycemia resulting from defects in insulin secretion, insulin action, or both. Deficient insulin action is due to diminished tissue responses to insulin at one or more points in the complex pathways of hormone action. The American Diabetes Association is involved in the dissemination of diabetes care standards and guidelines each year, which include diagnostic criteria and an etiologic classification of diabetes mellitus (130). Four main forms are in the classification: type 1 diabetes mellitus, type 2 diabetes mellitus, other specific types, and gestational diabetes mellitus. Patients with any form of diabetes may require insulin treatment at some stage of their disease. Such use of insulin does not, of itself, classify the patient. The third category, other specific types, accounts for less than 10% of all diabetic patients and includes diabetes mellitus caused by monogenetic defects of B-cell function and insulin action, diseases of the exocrine pancreas, endocrinopathies, drugs, infections, uncommon immune-mediated forms, and other genetic syndromes. Some in this category are described elsewhere in this chapter. Provided below are descriptions of type 1 and type 2 diabetes, which are the two principal types of diabetes, followed by neonatal diabetes and maturity-onset diabetes of the young (MODY), which are included in "other specific types" category in the classification.

Type 1 Diabetes Mellitus

Type 1 diabetes mellitus is associated with an absolute insulin deficiency caused by destruction of insulin-producing B cells of the pancreas. This form used to be designated as insulin-dependent diabetes mellitus or juvenile-onset diabetes mellitus and, until recently, was considered the most prevalent type in children. It results from a cellular-mediated autoimmune process. Antibodies detected in 70% to 80% of patients are autoantibodies to islet cells, insulin, glutamic acid decarboxylase, and tyrosine phosphatase IA-2 and IA-2 β.

The rate of B-cell destruction is variable, but when it is rapid as seen in infants and children, severe hyperglycemia and/or ketoacidosis may be the first manifestation. Type 1 diabetes mellitus has a complex pattern of genetic associations, and putative susceptibility genes have been mapped. The most important is the class II MHC (HLA) locus at 6p21. It is influenced by the *DRB* genes, with linkage to the DQA and DQB genes. These *HLA-DR/DQ* alleles can be either predisposing or protective.

Morphologic changes in the pancreas of diabetic individuals are not consistent, and they rarely contribute to diagnosis. The pancreas of classic type 1 diabetes may show a reduction in the number and the size of islets and insulitis (131) (Figure 16-21). Insulitis is characterized by islets infiltrated primarily by T-lymphocytes (132) and is confined to those islets in the recent-onset diabetic that still contain B cells (133). Other early features include cellular vacuolation and nuclear pleomorphism. Later in the course of the disease, insulitis is no longer seen and B cells become sparse (131). Interlobular fibrosis is a feature in some cases. Trophic changes of the exocrine cells can be marked, with diffuse or, in the early stages, patchy, focal acinar atrophy (134) (eFigure 16-8).

Type 2 Diabetes Mellitus
Patients with type 2 diabetes have insulin resistance and usually relative (rather than absolute) insulin deficiency. Relative insulin deficiency implies an inadequate secretory response by the pancreatic B cells to compensate for insulin resistance. The specific etiologies are not known, but autoimmune destruction of B cells does not occur. Patients should not have any of the other causes of diabetes listed under other specific types (130,135). Nevertheless, environmental factors, such as a sedentary life style and dietary habits, play a role in the pathogenesis. Most patients with this form of diabetes are obese, and the link between obesity and diabetes is mediated by insulin resistance. The incidence of type 2 diabetes mellitus, previously considered to be a disease of adult, has recently risen remarkably in children in different geographic areas of the world (136,137). Although type 2 diabetes is often associated with a strong genetic predisposition, more so than type 1 diabetes, its genetics are complex and not clearly defined.

The pancreas generally shows no change other than islet amyloid deposition (138), which becomes more frequent with age in both diabetics and nondiabetics. Islet amyloid is formed from islet amyloid polypeptide, which is secreted with insulin, and is seen in long-standing adult cases of type 2 diabetes (139). Animal studies have shown some evidence of a direct role for amyloid in the pathogenesis of type 2 diabetes (140). Figure 16-22 shows amyloid replacement of islets in a 4.5-year-old boy with diabetes but also with dwarfism and genital hypertrophy. B-cell mass is suggested to be decreased in type 2 diabetes mellitus, but this remains controversial (138,139,141).

Neonatal Diabetes Mellitus
Neonatal diabetes is rare, with a reported incidence of 1 in 400,000 live births, and may be defined as insulin-requiring hyperglycemia that is diagnosed within the first 6 months of life (130,142). It is a heterogeneous group of disorders and has been shown not to be typical autoimmune type 1 diabetes.

The disease may be transient, remitting by 18 months of age but relapsing during adolescence in a significant proportion of patients. Most patients are full-term, but growth-restricted, infants. Three interrelated genetic mechanisms have been ascribed to more than 50% of transient neonatal diabetes mellitus: paternal uniparental isodisomy of chromosome 6, paternal duplication of 6p24, and a methylation defect at a CpG island overlapping exon 1 of *ZAC* (zinc finger protein associated with apoptosis and cell cycle arrest)/*HYMAI* (imprinted in hydatidiform mole). These observations indicate that transient neonatal diabetes results from overexpression of an imprinted gene on 6p24 displaying paternal expression. Pancreatic morphology has not been described specifically for this form.

Permanent neonatal diabetes requires lifelong therapy, and a variety of causes and associations have been identified. Nearly half of all cases of permanent neonatal diabetes are due to activating mutations of the genes encoding two subunits of the adenosine triphosphate (ATP)-sensitive potassium channel of the B cell, *KCNJ11* and *ABCC8* (143). This finding has a significant impact on management because the patients can be treated with oral sulfonylureas. The loss-of-function abnormality in the same channel is responsible for congenital hyperinsulinism discussed later. Heterozygous autosomal dominant mutations in the insulin gene (*INS*) are the second most common cause of permanent neonatal diabetes. *INS* mutations are also found in antibody-negative type 1 diabetes individuals. Another rare cause of isolated neonatal diabetes is recessive mutations in the gene encoding the glycolytis enzyme glucokinase (*GCK*).

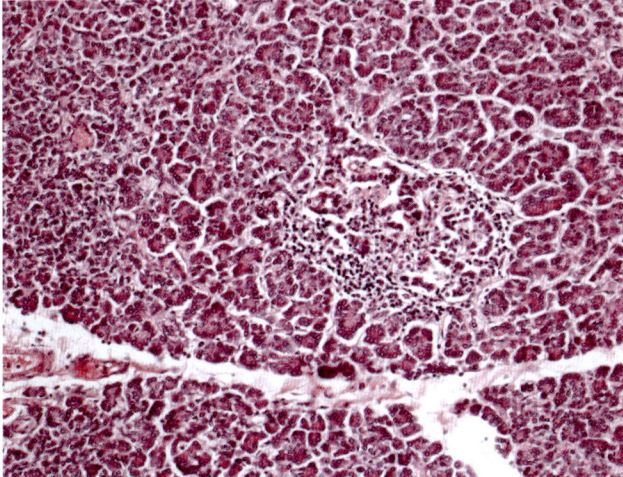

FIGURE 16-21 • Type 1 diabetes mellitus of recent onset. An active insulitis is present within and around an islet. Residual endocrine cells were demonstrable in this islet. (Hematoxylin and eosin stain, original magnification ×200.)

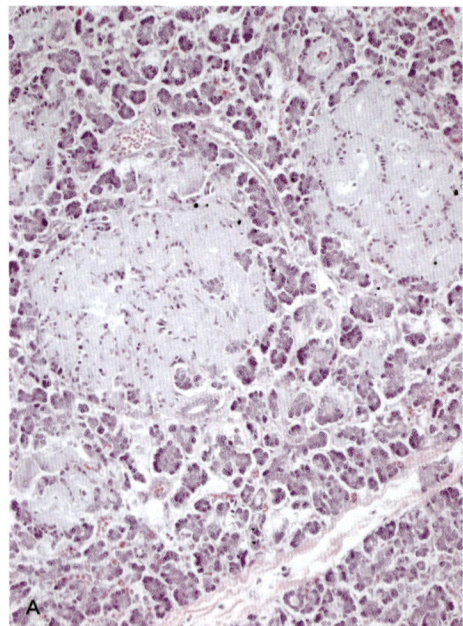 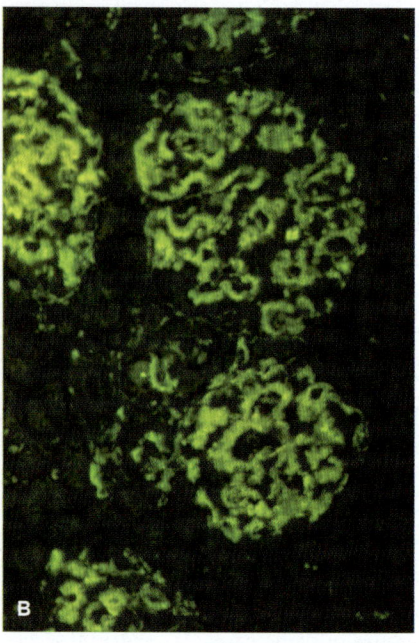

FIGURE 16-22 • Islet amyloid deposition. **A, B:** A 4.5-year-old boy with dwarfism, genital hypertrophy, and diabetes mellitus had amyloid in the islets. (**A:** Hematoxylin and eosin stain, original magnification ×200, **B:** thioflavine T stain, original magnification ×200.)

There are approximately 20 other known monogenic defects that cause neonatal diabetes, usually associated with variable syndromic organ impairments outside glucose metabolism(143). To name a few syndromes/phenotypes with their responsible genes in parentheses (i.e., not a complete list), they are Wolcott-Rallison syndrome (*EIF2AK3*), IPEX syndrome (*FOXP3*), syndrome of neonatal diabetes with cerebellar hypoplasia without pancreatic exocrine dysfunction (*NEUROD1*), syndrome of neonatal diabetes, intestinal atresia, gall bladder hypoplasia and diarrhea (*RFX6*), syndrome of neonatal diabetes with microcephaly and infantile seizures (*IER3IP1*), and Wolfram syndrome (*WFS1*). Pancreatic findings at autopsy from patients with Wolcott-Rallison syndrome and IPEX syndrome are described elsewhere in the chapter.

Maturity-Onset Diabetes of the Young
MODY is characterized by autosomal dominant inheritance and onset of hyperglycemia at an early age (generally before age 25 years). These patients have monogenetic defects resulting in B-cell dysfunction and have impaired insulin secretion with minimal or no defects in insulin action. Childhood type 2 diabetes can be confused with MODY as both have insulin secretion and are not usually insulin dependent or prone to ketoacidosis. Of 112 non–type 1 children reported in a survey performed in the United Kingdom, 25 had type 2 diabetes and 20 had MODY (144). The rest was secondary and unclassifiable due to incomplete data. In contrast to type 2 diabetes, MODY patients were younger (10.8 versus 12.8 years), less likely to be overweight, and none were from ethnic minority groups. Fifty-six percent of type 2 patients were of ethnic minority groups.

To date, at least seven genetic defects that cause MODY have been uncovered (130), five of which correspond to transcription factors expressed in pancreatic B cells: hepatic nuclear factor (HNF)-4α, HNF-1α, PDX1, HNF-1 β, and neurogenic differentiation 1/B-cell E-box transactivation 2 for MODY 1, 3, 4, 5, and 6, respectively. Loss-of-function mutations of glucokinase that catalyzes the first step in glucose metabolism cause MODY 2. Diabetes of the young caused by carboxyl ester lipase was added to the MODY category in 2013. In addition to their effects on B-cell function, deficiency of some of these transcription factors affects function of other organ systems. Patients with HNF-1α mutations have decreased renal reabsorption of glucose and glycosuria. The deficiency of HNF-4α affects triglyceride and apolipoprotein biosynthesis. Families with HNF-1β mutations presenting with renal cysts and diabetes have been described. There is a considerable overlap among the genes encoding transcription factors listed here and the genes responsible for permanent neonatal diabetes.

Hyperinsulinism

Hyperinsulinism is the most common cause of hypoglycemia in infants and children (145). Clinically transient forms of hyperinsulinism are seen in neonates born to diabetic mothers, infants with birth asphyxia, small for gestational age, and Beckwith-Wiedemann infants (146). Persistent hyperinsulinism in children and infants is rarely due to insulinoma (well-differentiated pancreatic endocrine tumor) but most often represents a congenital genetic disorder (Table 16-1).

Insulin levels are not usually dramatically elevated, but there is inadequate suppression of insulin secretion at low plasma concentration of glucose (i.e., hyperinsulinism rather than hyperinsulinemia) (145). The diagnosis is based on evidence of the effects of excess insulin, which includes inappropriate suppression of lipolysis and ketogenesis and an inappropriately positive glycemic response to glucagon at times of hypoglycemia. Uncontrolled hypoglycemia may lead to seizures or permanent brain damage, and immediate medical intervention is required.

Infants with congenital hyperinsulinism were once believed to have abnormal pancreatic development

TABLE 16-1	CONGENITAL HYPERINSULINISM: GENETICS, BIOLOGY, AND PATHOLOGY		
Pathologic Category	Genetics	Biology/Clinical	Histologic Features
	Diazoxide unresponsive		
Diffuse hyperinsulinism	KATP[a], biallelic recessive	KATP channel proteins not trafficking to cell surface	Large islet cell nuclei
	KATP[a], monoallelic dominant	KATP channel proteins trafficking to cell surface but with impaired function	Large islet cell nuclei
	GCK dominant	Low glucose threshold for insulin release	Large islet cell nuclei. The number of large nuclei may be low.
Focal hyperinsulinism	KATP[a], monoallelic recessive, paternal (or de novo), and somatic maternal loss of 11p15.1	KATP channel defect in cells of proliferated endocrine lesion. Surgery may be curative.	Adenomatosis/adenomatous hyperplasia. Lesions are focal, multifocal, or generalized.
	Diazoxide responsive		
NA	*GLUD1*, dominant	Hyperinsulinemia/hyperammonemia syndrome	NA
NA	KATP[a], monoallelic dominant	KATP channel proteins trafficking to cell surface. Channel function impaired but with residual activity responding to diazoxide	NA
NA	Other rare genetic abnormalities (see text)		NA

[a]KATP mutations = mutations of either *ABCC8* encoding sulfonylurea receptor 1 (SUR1) or *KCNJ11* encoding inward rectifier 6.2 (Kir6.2).
NA, not applicable. No or anecdotal pancreatic histology is available as pancreatectomy is not indicated.

associated with persistence of packets of islet cells (B cells) budding off ducts, termed *nesidioblastosis* (147,148). Observations based on immunohistochemical investigations have shown that nesidioblastosis, as defined above, is a common feature of the pancreas in normoglycemic neonates and infants (115,149), and nesidioblastosis by itself is no longer considered the underlying histologic basis of congenital hyperinsulinism (145,150). Congenital hyperinsulinism is a heterogeneous group of diseases that differ with regard to responsiveness to medical treatment with diazoxide, requirement for surgery, histopathology, and molecular etiology. The following sections illustrates histologic findings in pancreases resected from individuals requiring surgery and their molecular etiologies, followed by descriptions of additional hyperinsulinisms that usually do not require pancreatectomy.

Diazoxide-Unresponsive Congenital Hyperinsulinism
Diazoxide is an agonist of the ATP-sensitive potassium (KATP) channels that reside on the plasma membrane of pancreatic B cells. Two adjacent genes located on chromosome 11p15.1, *ABCC8* and *KCNJ11*, encode high-affinity sulfonylurea receptor 1 (SUR1) and its regulated ion pore, potassium inward rectifier 6.2 protein (Kir6.2), respectively. They together form the heterooctamer KATP channel. The loss of KATP channel function leads to persistent membrane depolarization and insulin release, regardless of plasma glucose level. As diazoxide acts to open the channel, it is used to medically manage hyperinsulinism. In a large single institution study ($n = 417$), 72% of cases were diazoxide unresponsive (151). Identification of responsible genetic abnormality is most successful in this group, in which approximately 90% carry KATP mutations and 2% have glucokinase defects. The majority of patients with diazoxide-unresponsive hyperinsulinism undergo pancreatectomy.

Pancreatectomy specimens are histologically categorized into diffuse hyperinsulinism and focal hyperinsulinism, roughly equal in frequency (Table 16-2). There are, in addition, a small number of pancreases that do not fit well with either of these two forms. They include normal histology and pancreases showing large islet cell nuclei only in a confined area (localized islet cell nuclear enlargement). In these cases, no mutations have been detected in the KATP or glucokinase genes in DNA from either peripheral blood or pancreatic tissue (151).

Diffuse Hyperinsulinism
Diffuse hyperinsulinism is characterized by the presence of abnormally large islet cell nuclei that are distributed throughout the pancreas. Frequency and easiness of finding enlarged endocrine cell nuclei vary from case to case. Large nuclei are empirically determined to be nuclei four times that of the nearby acinar cell nuclei (152) or nuclei occupying an area more than three times larger than the surrounding

TABLE 16-2	FINDINGS IN THE PANCREAS RESECTED FROM CHILDREN WITH HYPERINSULINISM (THE CHILDREN'S HOSPITAL OF PHILADELPHIA [1983–2010, n = 321])
Histology of Pancreas	Percentage of Children Affected (%)
Diffuse hyperinsulinism (large islet cell nuclei)	45.5
Focal hyperinsulinism (adenomatosis/adenomatous hyperplasia)	46.5
Insulinoma (well-differentiated pancreatic endocrine tumor)	1.6
Normal	2.8
Equivocal/difficult to classify	3.7

Note: All known and unknown underlying genetic abnormality inclusive.
Reproduced with permission from Suchi M, Bhatti TR, Ruchelli ED. Pancreatic histopathology of hyperinsulinism. In: Stanley CA, De León, eds. *Monogenic Hyperinsulinemic Hypoglycemia Disorders, Front Diabetes*. Vol. 21. Basal: Karger; 2012:57–70.

endocrine nuclei (Figure 16-23). A morphometric analysis revealed that the mean nuclear radius of the 50 largest nuclei of this type is significantly larger than the mean nuclear radius measured in islets that are present outside or away from the adenomatous (focal) lesions in the focal hyperinsulinism (153). The cytologic changes also include "bizarre" crescent-shaped or ovoid nuclei with occasional nuclear pseudoinclusions (intranuclear cytoplasmic invagination). It is important to note that not all islets contain these abnormal nuclei, and the number of islets with characteristic nuclei may be small. Ductuloinsular complex composed of endocrine cells in the epithelium of the ducts and in connection with the endocrine cell clusters may be present (Figure 16-23). The B-cell proliferation rate is not higher when the fraction of Ki-67 positive B cells was compared to a control group (153). Moreover, the mean total endocrine area and the volume density of B cells are not increased in this form (115,149,150). The major source of confusion is lack of familiarity with the histologic features of the normal newborn and infant pancreas, in which endocrine tissue is abundant, and smaller peripheral clusters of endocrine cells may constitute much of the endocrine component (Figures 16-18 and 16-19). These are some of the features that were previously interpreted as excessive "nesidioblastosis."

Mutations of the KATP genes were identified in 89% of children with diffuse hyperinsulinism. Most of these cases are biallelic for recessive KATP mutations, which result in subunit proteins that do not traffic to the cell surface, thus leading to diazoxide unresponsiveness. However, a minority of cases have monoallelic dominant mutations of *ABCC8*, demonstrated to produce channels normally trafficking to the cell surface but with reduced activities.

Dominant activating mutations in glucokinase, encoded by *GCK* located at 7p13-15, are much rarer but are the third most common genetic cause of hyperinsulinism. Within the diazoxide-unresponsive group, they are second most common. Glucokinase, a hexokinase with a low affinity for glucose, controls the rate-limiting step of B-cell glucose metabolism and is responsible for glucose-mediated regulation of insulin secretion. Gain-of-function mutations produce enzymes with a higher affinity for glucose, lower the glucose threshold for insulin release, and are frequently severe enough to interfere with diazoxide treatment. While the pancreases of 4 patients were described as normal in three reports, two more recent reports describe moderately enlarged islet cell nuclei and an increase in the mean islet size compared to the pancreases of age-matched controls and patients with KATP channel hyperinsulinism (154). The single institution study identified two pancreases resected from patients with GCK mutations. They showed islet cell nucleomegaly, but the number of cells with nucleomegaly was lower than in most cases with KATP diffuse hyperinsulinism.

Focal Hyperinsulinism

The pancreatic histology of focal hyperinsulinism is characterized by a lesion formed by the confluence of hyperplastic but apparently normally structured islets occupying greater than 40% of the cross-sectional area of pancreatic lobules (115) (Figure 16-24). The lesion pushes the exocrine elements aside or haphazardly incorporates them. There is recapitulation of islet structure, with peripherally located A and D cells and B cells aggregating more centrally. Other histologic terms frequently used and accepted are *adenomatosis* and *adenomatous hyperplasia*. In contrast to insulinomas (well-differentiated pancreatic endocrine tumor), the lesions are difficult to identify grossly (Figure 16-24) because they do not distort the normal lobular architecture. The boundary between the uninvolved portion of the pancreas and the lesion may be sharp (Figure 16-24) but may also be vague and ill defined (eFigure 16-9). The lesions are generally small, thus their designation as *focal hyperinsulinism*. In one series, 24 of 35 lesions were less than 1 cm in the greatest dimension (155). However, the lesion may be multifocal and/or occupy a large portion of the pancreas to even the entire pancreas (115,156). In these rare cases, the designation *focal lesion* or *focal hyperinsulinism* causes confusion, yet using the word *diffuse* is equally troublesome. A better terminology is being sought and *generalized adenomatosis* may be an option (115). Although there are large nuclei in the confluent islet tissue of the adenomatous focal lesions, the islets in uninvolved portions of pancreas are reported to have a "resting" appearance with B cells showing little cytoplasm and nucleus (152). B-cell nuclear crowding expressed as the number of B-cell nuclei/1000 µm^2 of B-cell cytoplasm is higher in islets

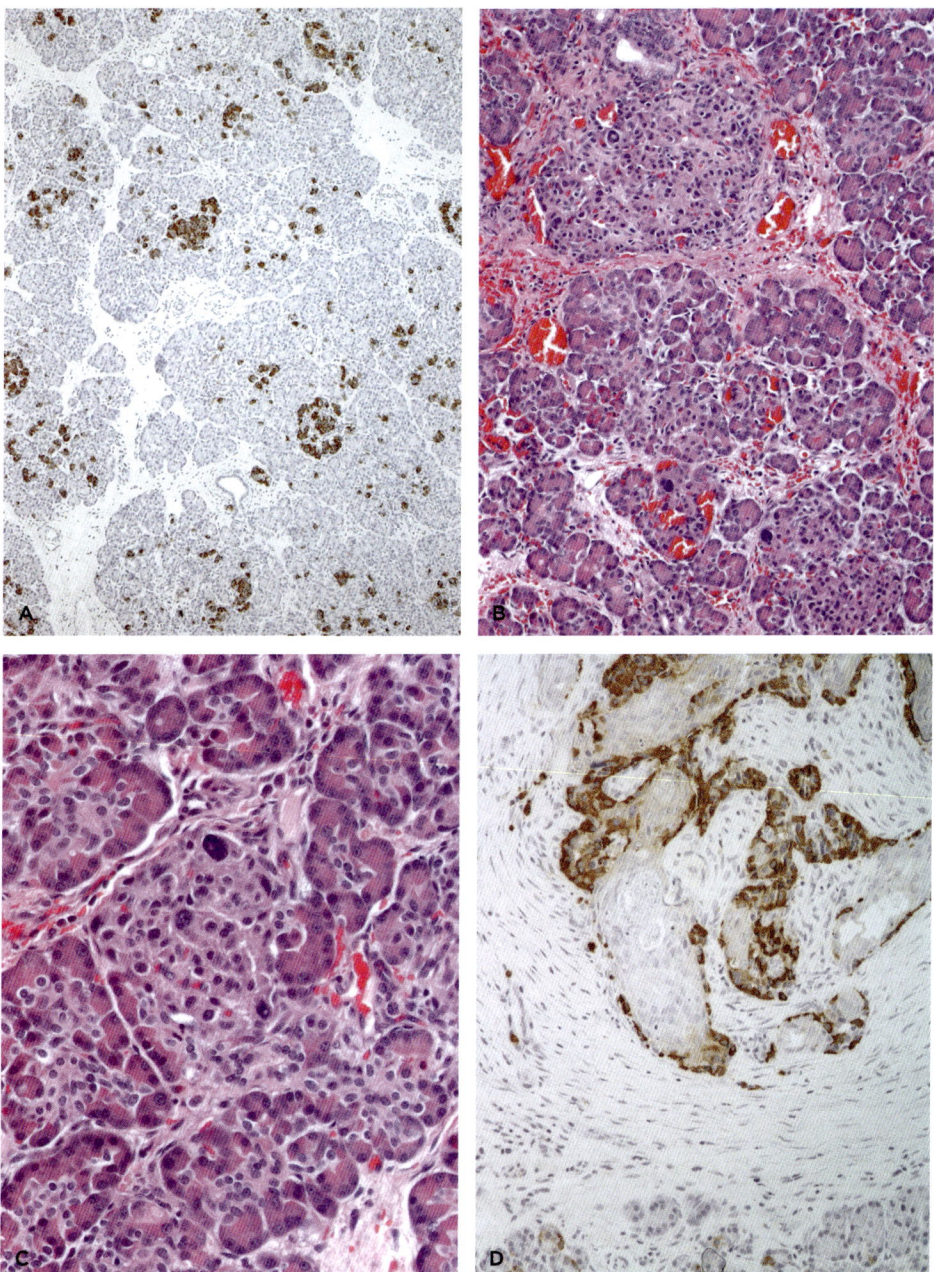

FIGURE 16-23 • Diffuse hyperinsulinism. **A:** Quantity of endocrine component is not significantly different from pancreas of normoglycemic individuals of similar age (2 months). (Immunohistochemistry for insulin. Original magnification ×50.) **B:** On a low-to-medium power field, a few large and hyperchromatic endocrine cell nuclei can be spotted. (Hematoxylin and eosin stain, original magnification ×200.) **C:** Enlarged islet cell nuclei are defined as those occupying an area at least three times larger than the neighboring endocrine nuclei, for diagnostic purposes. (Hematoxylin and eosin stain, original magnification ×400.) **D:** Ductuloinsular aggregates may be present in some cases, but they are seen too seldom to use as a diagnostic criterion. (Immunohistochemistry for chromogranin A, original magnification ×200.)

outside the lesion of focal hyperinsulinism as compared to islets of diffuse hyperinsulinism (157). This difference may be subtle and is not appreciated by other retrospective studies without morphometric measurements.

Focal hyperinsulinism is caused by paternal transmission of a monoallelic recessive KATP channel mutation followed by an embryonic somatic loss of maternal 11p15.1 that contains imprinted genes involved in cell proliferation (158). Rare cases with a putative de novo monoallelic recessive KATP mutation with a maternal 11p15 loss are also reported (151). The unbalanced expression of the imprinted growth factor (*IGF2*) and tumor-suppressor genes (*H19* and

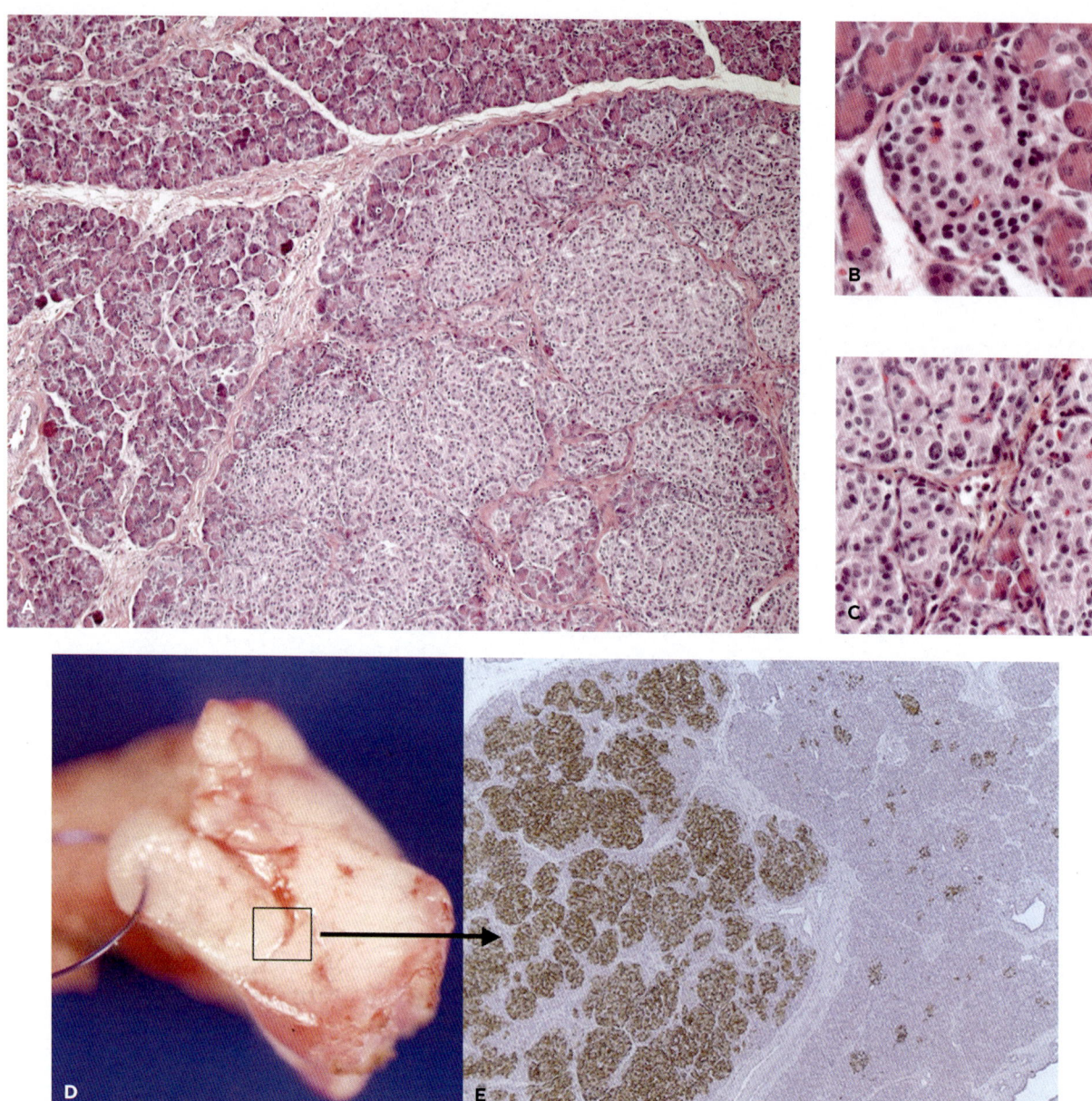

FIGURE 16-24 • Focal hyperinsulinism. **A:** Much of the lobule in the right lower half is occupied by endocrine tissue (adenomatosis). (Hematoxylin and eosin stain, original magnification ×200.) **B:** Islets outside the adenomatous lesion contain nuclei of normal size. **C:** There may be large endocrine cell nuclei within the adenomatosis. (**B, C:** Hematoxylin and eosin stain, original magnification ×400.) **D:** The adenomatous lesion is difficult to distinguish from the neighboring pancreas grossly. **E:** Immunohistochemistry confirms the abundance (>40%) of endocrine elements within the lobules. (Immunohistochemistry for chromogranin A, original magnification ×200.) (**D, E:** Copyright 2004 from A multidisciplinary approach to the focal form of congenital hyperinsulinism by partial pancreatectomy by Adzick NS, Thornton PS, Stanley CA, et al. *J Pediatr Surg* 2004;39:270–275. Reproduced with permission of Elsevier.)

CDKN1C) leads to adenomatous hyperplasia; the expression of the mutated paternal gene causes unregulated insulin secretion from the hyperplastic lesion (158). $p57^{kip2}$ is the product of one of the imprinted genes (*CDKN1C*) that are normally expressed from the maternal allele and is lost in endocrine cells within the adenomatous lesions. The loss of $p57^{kip2}$ expression can be visualized by immunohistochemical labeling (159) (eFigure 16-10).

Accurate and timely diagnosis of focal hyperinsulinism has major clinical implications because the lesion can be surgically excised and cured without near-total pancreatectomy (160). This can be achieved by genetic analysis, imaging studies, and pathology. The sensitivity of mutation analysis for predicting focal hyperinsulinism based on finding a monoallelic recessive KATP mutation is high (97% in one study). However, only 25% of children with KATP mutations carry common founder mutations. Predicting the clinical phenotype of novel missense mutations is complicated by several factors and may not happen in a timely manner. Fluorine-18L-3,4-dihydroxyphenylalanine ([18F]-DOPA) positron emission tomography scan (161) has emerged as a powerful tool to localize focal adenomatous lesions, especially in cases predicted to have focal hyperinsulinism. Multiple lesions within separate foci of ectopic pancreas along the jejunum were detected by this technique (21). However, approximately 15% to 25% of focal lesions are not visualized.

Intraoperative frozen sections can be performed to identify/confirm patients with focal hyperinsulinism and further guide the extent of pancreatic resection (152,156). The presence of islet cell nuclear abnormalities (e.g., enlarged more than three times, "bizarre" shaped) suggests the recessively inherited diffuse form, and a near-total pancreatectomy follows. The absence of nuclear changes *in islets* is indicative of the focal form, and a search for a focal lesion continues until the lesion is identified. Examples of difficult cases are those with an ill-defined border of the focal form, with generalized adenomatosis, and with infrequently encountered and/or localized islet cell nuclear abnormality (156).

Diazoxide-Responsive Congenital Hyperinsulinism
Diazoxide-responsive hyperinsulinism patients do not require pancreatectomy. Therefore, knowledge of pancreatic pathology is very limited. It is also a more diverse group of diseases as compared to the diazoxide-unresponsive hyperinsulinism. Identification of causative gene mutations is less frequently achieved where defects were detected in only half of children. In the single institution study referred above (151), among the mutation-positive patients, 42% were glutamate dehydrogenase mutations, 41 % were KATP channel mutations, and 16% were in rare genes. Each is summarized below.

Hyperinsulinism Caused by Glutamate Dehydrogenase Mutations
Dominant activating mutation in glutamate dehydrogenase, encoded by *GLUD1* on chromosome 10q23.2, is the second most common genetic form of congenital hyperinsulinism following KATP mutations. Glutamate dehydrogenase is a mitochondrial enzyme and catalyzes the reaction converting glutamate to α-ketoglutarate, a substrate for the tricarboxylic acid (TCA) cycle. The genetic abnormality is known as hyperinsulinemia/hyperammonemia syndrome and is distinguished by persistently elevated plasma ammonia concentrations to three to five times normal, as a result of the enzymatic abnormality being expressed in the liver as well as in the pancreas (162). In one report, the pancreas was described as showing unusual islet cells arranged in a ribbon pattern (163). An anecdotal experience consists of one case of an elected a pancreatectomy despite diazoxide control. The pancreas showed diffuse islet cell nucleomegaly similar to that seen in the diffuse hyperinsulinism.

KATP Channel Mutations
This is a category where KATP channels with *ABCC8* or *KCNJ11* mutations manifest with diazoxide-responsive hyperinsulinism. By expression studies, these mutations produce subunit proteins that traffic normally and form KATP channel complexes at the cell surface that have impaired opening in response to MgADP and diazoxide. Depending on the degree of residual channel activity, hyperinsulinism becomes diazoxide responsive. There is no report of cases who underwent pancreatectomy.

Other Rare Genetic Abnormalities
Additional genetic abnormalities associated with diazoxide-responsive hyperinsulinism are mutations in genes encoding short-chain L-3-hydroxylacyl coenzyme A dehydrogenase (*HADH*), uncoupling protein 2 (*UCP2*), HNF-4α (*HNF4A*), and HNF-1α (*HNF1A*) (151). The latter two are mentioned earlier as responsible genes for MODY. No pancreas pathology has been described in these conditions.

Beckwith-Wiedemann syndrome is a congenital overgrowth syndrome that frequently manifest with hypoglycemia in infancy. The pathology of pancreas in this syndrome is described separately later in the chapter.

Insulinoma (Well-Differentiated Pancreatic Endocrine Tumor)
Functioning pancreatic endocrine tumor that secretes insulin (insulinoma) is rare in the pediatric population (Table 16-2). When hyperinsulinism manifests in a noncongenital manner after 6 to 12 months of age, this possibility should be considered. Insulinomas are generally well demarcated and show a diffuse, lobular to trabecular proliferation of endocrine cells (Figure 16-25). The cellular arrangement does not recapitulate islets. The endocrine cells diffusely react with synaptophysin and/or chromogranin and insulin (164) although more than one cell type may be represented.

Sudden Infant Death Syndrome and Hyperinsulinism
In a retrospective review of infants with sudden infant death syndrome (SIDS), examination of the pancreas did not divulge endocrine pathology (165). Klensang et al. (166) reviewed 112 pancreases from patients with SIDS and found no morphologic or morphometric differences between them and 19 controls. It is not unreasonable to assume that some infants or even older children with hyperinsulinism may present as instances of sudden death, but the diagnosis must rely on laboratory documentation of the hyperinsulinism. The morphologic features of normal infant pancreas may appear abnormal or similar to a form of hyperinsulinism if qualitative and quantitative differences from the adult pancreas are not taken into consideration.

Pancreatic Islets in Shock

Bernstein described in 1958 three newborns dying shortly after birth in whom renal tubular and selective pancreatic islet necrosis was found. Asphyxia was implicated. Seemayer

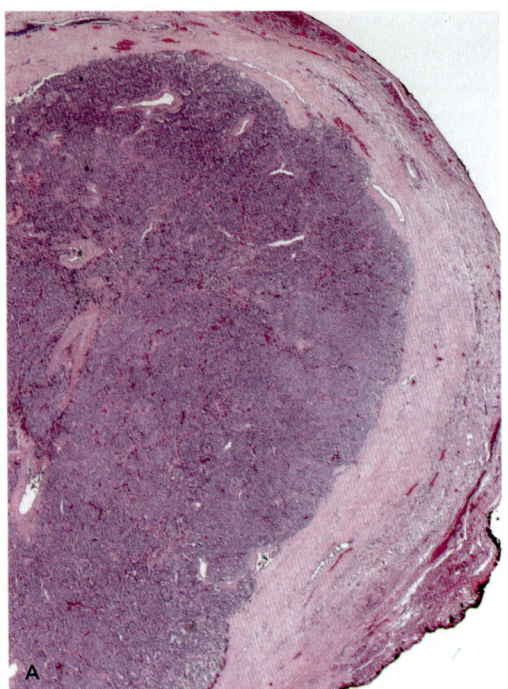 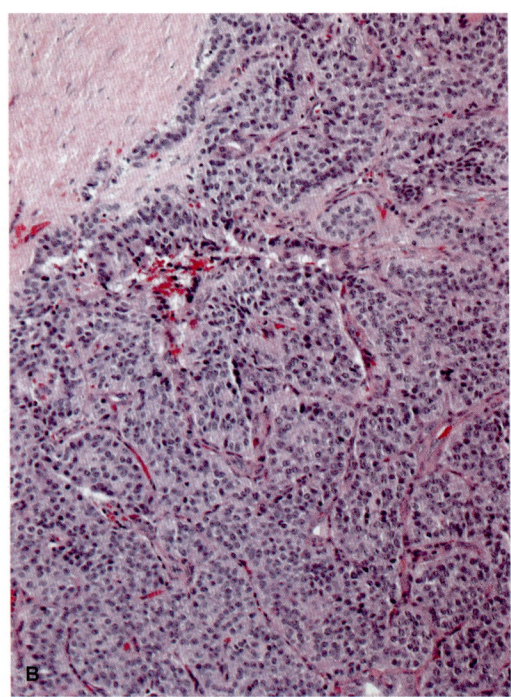

FIGURE 16-25 • Insulinoma from a 10-year-old boy. The tumor is composed of a monotonous population of endocrine cells arranged in trabeculae and cords and has a relatively sharp border. (**A, B:** Hematoxylin and eosin stain, original magnification ×25 and ×200, respectively.)

et al. (167) found the same pattern in only 10% of infants with other severe manifestations of shock.

Viral Infections

Nonselective involvement of the pancreas is seen in disseminated herpesvirus, cytomegalovirus, varicella-zoster virus, and rubella virus infections (65). Selective damage to islet cells has been seen in coxsackievirus B infection (65,168), although caution should be exercised in distinguishing viral effects from the changes of shock, described earlier. The onset of diabetes after coxsackievirus B infection has been documented, although direct evidence for virally induced diabetes is lacking.

Syndromes/Diseases with Endocrine Pancreas Abnormalities

Beckwith-Wiedemann Syndrome

Beckwith-Wiedemann syndrome is a congenital overgrowth syndrome that is clinically and genetically heterogeneous. A number of complex genetic and epigenetic abnormalities resulting in dysregulation of imprinted growth regulatory genes clustered at 11p15 have been demonstrated. Phenotypical features include macrosomia, macroglossia, omphalocele, visceromegaly, and hypoglycemia duo to hyperinsulinism in about one-third to one-half of cases (146). The hypoglycemia is transient in the majority of infants and resolves within the first few days of life. In about 5% of children, the hyperinsulinism persists and extends beyond the neonatal period, requiring either continuous feeding, medical therapy, or partial pancreatectomy.

The available pancreatic histology is, therefore, usually limited to the severe cases in which the patient has died or had partial pancreatectomy. The pathologic changes seen in Beckwith-Wiedemann syndrome are not uniform as the underlying genetic and epigenetic abnormalities are highly variable. There is a significant increase in endocrine tissue relative to the amount of exocrine tissue. The endocrine cells usually have an insular or trabecular arrangement, with or without scattered nucleomegaly. In many cases, the endocrine component is confluent and constitutes a large proportion of the involved lobule (Figure 16-26). In most cases, the abundance of endocrine tissue is distributed throughout the pancreas and is different from focal hyperinsulinism where the increase in endocrine tissue is localized to an affected portion of pancreas. One exceptional Beckwith-Wiedemann syndrome pancreas is described to have the above features in the head and body with tapering to near-normal morphology in the tail (169). By immunohistochemistry, the islet-like aggregates recapitulate islet topography with the insulin-positive B cells residing in the center and the non–B cell being at the periphery of the "macroislets" (170). $p57^{kip2}$ protein expression in the confluent islet cells is preserved in contrast to $p57^{kip2}$ loss seen in focal hyperinsulinism (171). In a Beckwith-Wiedemann patient with a Meckel diverticulum, the heterotopic pancreas within the diverticulum showed numerous enlarged islets or islet-like aggregates, some with a diameter of up to 1600 μm, comprising approximately 15% of the pancreatic tissue (172). In one case with mosaic paternal uniparental disomy for 11p15, $p57^{kip2}$ protein was readily identified within the large islets, which is in contrast to the

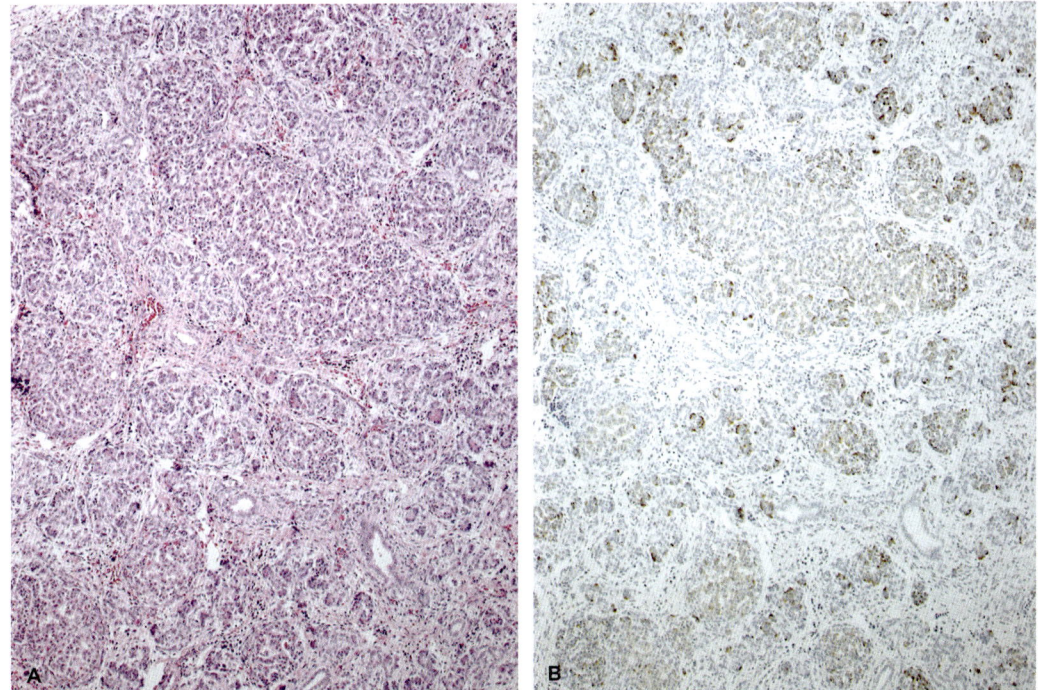

FIGURE 16-26 • Beckwith-Wiedemann syndrome. **A, B:** Much of the pancreatic lobule is formed of complex islet-like aggregates of endocrine cells. Exocrine acini are poorly developed. (**A:** Hematoxylin and eosin stain, **B:** immunohistochemistry for chromogranin A, original magnification ×100.)

loss of p57^{kip2} expression in the B cells within the adenomatous lesions of focal hyperinsulinism (171).

A pancreas examined at 11 months of age at the time of death of a patient with Beckwith-Wiedemann syndrome showed significantly more acinar differentiation and proliferation as compared to the partial pancreatectomy specimen at 1 month of age (173). Another report describes islet cell hyperplasia in five children who died of their disease-associated tumors, even though the earlier hypoglycemia had been transient (174). Steigman et al. (24) reported a 2-day-old autopsy case with an enlarged and solely cystic pancreas containing numerous irregularly shaped ectatic ducts with sparse islands of endocrine tissue and exocrine acini (Figure 16-8). Beckwith-Wiedemann syndrome with hemihypertrophy is associated with a striking tendency toward the development of embryonal tumors in a number of organs, and pancreatoblastoma is one of them (175).

Perlman Syndrome

Beckwith-Wiedemann syndrome and the syndrome of renal hamartomas, nephroblastomatosis, and fetal gigantism overlap to some degree. One-half of the cases are said to have islet cell hyperplasia (176). Hypoglycemia occurs, and hyperinsulinism may be responsible. We have seen a large pancreas associated with Perlman syndrome (Figure 16-27).

von Hippel-Lindau Disease

von Hippel-Lindau disease is a hereditary tumor syndrome that results from a germ-line mutation in the *VHL* tumor suppressor gene on the short arm of chromosome 3 (3p25-26).

The pancreas is involved in 25% to 70% of cases, the majority of which are cystic lesions followed by endocrine tumors.

Asymptomatic pancreatic cysts that occur in the majority of von Hippel-Lindau disease patients rarely need treatment. By WHO classification, these cysts are referred to as von Hippel-Lindau–associated serous cystic neoplasm (177). These lesions are indistinguishable at the histologic level from sporadic serous cystic tumors. A single layer of cuboidal epithelial cells with glycogen-rich clear cytoplasm lines the cysts. The most frequent form is serous microcystic cystadenoma, which is a well-circumscribed spongelike lesion filled by microcysts arranged around a central dense scar. The second form is serous macrocystic or oligocystic cystadenoma without a scar but showing grossly visible cysts.

Endocrine tumors of the pancreas, mostly nonfunctional, are seen in 8% to 17 % of patients (178). Grossly, they are yellow, reflecting a high fat content. Clear cell change is reported in 60 % of the tumors (179). Otherwise, the pathologic features resemble those of other nonfunctional pancreatic endocrine tumors. Although clinically nonfunctional, the cells may react with antibodies against pancreatic and gastrointestinal hormones. Pancreatic endocrine tumors may be accompanied by other visceral tumors such as adrenal pheochromocytomas (180).

Wolcott-Rallison Syndrome

Wolcott-Rallison syndrome is an autosomal recessive disorder that is characterized by permanent neonatal insulin-requiring diabetes mellitus and multiple epiphyseal dysplasia (181). Other features include osteopenia, mental and growth restriction,

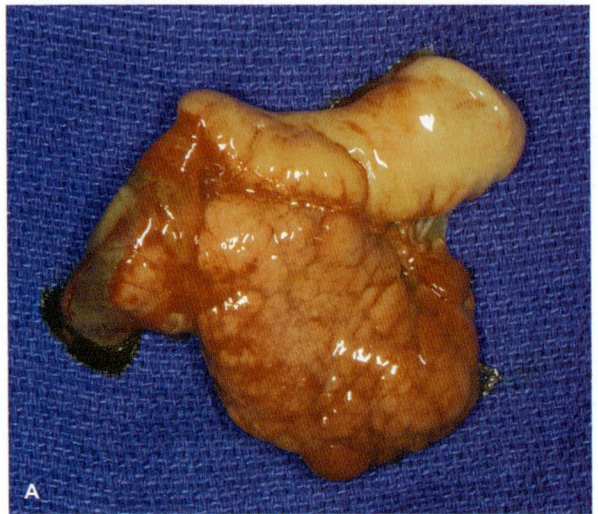

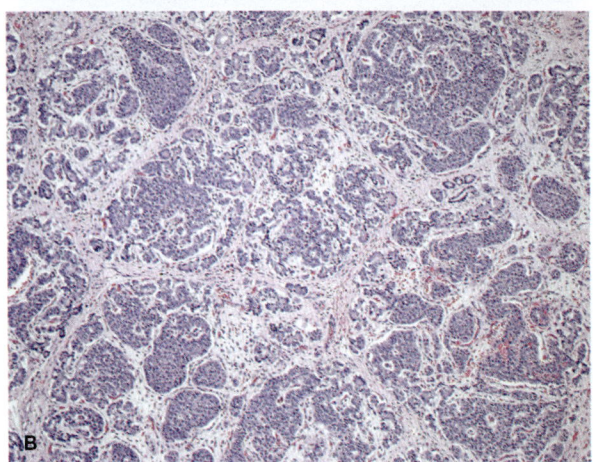

FIGURE 16-27 • Perlman syndrome. **A:** An 11-d-old infant delivered at 30 weeks of gestation presented with hypoglycemia and constellations of malformations consistent with Perlman syndrome. The pancreas was large and weighed 20 g. (Courtesy of Ralph A. Franciosi, M.D., Milwaukee, Wisconsin.) **B:** The pancreatic lobules appear disorganized and are composed of irregularly shaped cords and islands of endocrine cells and poorly developed acini.

hepatic and kidney dysfunction, cardiac abnormalities, exocrine pancreatic dysfunction, and neutropenia (6,182,183). The syndrome results from mutations in the gene encoding the eukaryotic initiation factor 2-α kinase 3 (*EIF2AK3*, also called *PERK*). The transmembrane kinase EIF2AK3 is localized in the endoplasmic reticulum and phosphorylates EIF2A, preventing B-cell death and relieve endoplasmic reticulum stress by reducing the number of unfolded proteins in the endoplasmic reticulum. Autopsy of one case revealed a markedly hypoplastic pancreas with only a narrow cord of tissue (184). Histology showed a reduction of acinar tissue and increased interstitial fibrosis. The islets appeared smaller with more glucagon-staining cells than insulin-staining cells (6).

Leprechaunism (Donohue Syndrome)

Donohue (185) described infants with a characteristic facies, hirsutism, enlarged genitalia, decreased muscle and subcutaneous tissues, and "dysendocrinism." An autosomal recessive defect in the insulin receptor gene (*INSR*) has been documented in some patients. Leprechaunism is listed in the diabetes classification under genetic defects in insulin action (130). On the other hand, intermittent hypoglycemia with hyperinsulinism has been described. Islet hyperplasia is reported in 67% of the cases at autopsy (186). An unusual case described by Szilagyi et al. (187) had the features of lipomatous atrophy with preserved islets.

Cystic Fibrosis

In the pancreas, cystic fibrosis primarily affects the exocrine component causing pancreatic insufficiency. However, diabetes mellitus has been recognized as a complication that commonly develops around 20 years of age. The prevalence increases with age and, with improved survival and prospective screening by glucose tolerance test, approaches 20% in adolescents (188).

Several studies have been published focusing on islet changes in cystic fibrosis (189,190). Although qualitative and quantitative methods differed among the studies and the pathology was always accompanied by exocrine and interstitial alterations, a decrease in the fraction of insulin-positive B cells in islets was generally demonstrated in advanced cystic fibrosis. A "qualitative" islet number (190) and the volume density of endocrine tissue to pancreatic tissue (189) were decreased in cystic fibrosis as compared to the control groups. Endocrine cell composition was not significantly different between pancreases showing predominantly fibrotic pattern and lipoatrophic pattern (189).

In diabetic young adults, islets were described as having a disorganized and lobulated appearance with thin fibrous septa enclosing the capillaries and subdividing the islets. Large amount of amyloid deposition was also demonstrated (191).

In contrast, an early endocrine increase has been also mentioned. Multiple foci of neoformation of islets illustrated by islet cells arising from and around the ductal lumen were reported in all 11 cystic fibrosis patients (age: 3 months to 7 years) as compared to less frequent encounters in the control subjects (192). Neoislet formation from a small duct was present in nondiabetic children, but not in nondiabetic and diabetic young adults in a different series (190).

The morphologic alterations may provide the basis for the glucose intolerance and overt diabetes mellitus eventually developing in some with cystic fibrosis. However, not all patients with advanced cystic fibrosis become diabetic. Other late complications such as liver damage and peripheral insulin resistance might contribute to the changes in glucose metabolism seen in cystic fibrosis patients.

Hereditary Tyrosinemia Type I

Tyrosinemia may be associated with glycosuria and refractory hypoglycemia (193). The pancreas in some infants has been shown to contain many large islets, but this is not a constant feature in this disease (194). The variability likely comes from the difficulty in accurately assessing islet hypertrophy in infants (true increase in the percentage of islets larger than

200 μm for a given age). Mitotic activity within islets and hyalinization of islets have been seen in some cases (195).

Ataxia-Telangiectasia

The familial disease with cerebellar ataxia, oculocutaneous telangiectasia, and immune disorder with IgA deficiency is associated with insulin-resistant diabetes mellitus (196). Islet cell hyperplasia may be impressive; however, the marked nuclear cytomegaly is not confined to islets but is a systemic manifestation of the disease (197).

Pancreatic Endocrine Tumor in Childhood

Pancreatic endocrine tumors are similarly rare as exocrine tumors in children. In the 2004 WHO classification, the term "pancreatic endocrine tumor" replaces earlier terms, for example, pancreatic neuroendocrine tumor, islet cell tumor, and apudoma. One prospective study from Italy registered three (neuro)endocrine neoplasms during the period when four pancreatoblastomas were registered (88). Another single institution retrospective study from North America described five (neuro)endocrine neoplasms, while four solid pseudopapillary neoplasms and three acinar cell carcinoma were identified during the same period (86).

Many of the pancreatic endocrine tumors occur in patients with multiple endocrine neoplasia type 1 (164), von Hippel-Lindau disease (198), and neurofibromatosis 1. In addition, there is an increased risk for certain types of endocrine neoplasms in the tuberous sclerosis complex including pituitary and parathyroid adenomas and gastroenteropancreatic endocrine tumors (199).

Most pancreatic endocrine tumors fall into the well-differentiated category, and it is generally assumed that a lesion designated "pancreatic endocrine tumor" is well differentiated. Only rare examples fit with poorly differentiated endocrine carcinomas having, for example, more than 10 mitoses per 10 high-power fields. When it comes to clinically aggressive endocrine tumors with distant metastasis, the occurrence is even rarer in children (199). On the other hand, endocrine tumors measuring less than 0.5 cm are designated as "endocrine microadenoma" suggesting a completely benign entity. Well-differentiated pancreatic endocrine tumors are subclassified by endocrine functional status. The term functional pancreatic endocrine tumor is applied to those neoplasms associated with clinical endocrine paraneoplastic syndrome. Functional pancreatic endocrine tumors reported in pediatric patients include insulinomas, gastrinoma, and VIPoma (vasoactive intestinal polypeptide). A pancreatic endocrine tumor not associated with a clinical syndrome is designated as a nonfunctional pancreatic endocrine tumor (200).

Pancreatic endocrine tumors generally have a pushing periphery. Nests of neoplastic cells are partially or completely surrounded by a fibrotic pseudocapsule (Figure 16-25). Perineural and vascular invasions occur and are most easily identified in the peritumoral nerves and vessels within the pseudocapsule. The tumor cells are arranged in nesting, trabecular, and gyriform patterns accompanied by a more diffuse growth pattern. The cells have moderately abundant eosinophilic or amphophilic cytoplasm but vary in size. The nuclei have stippled "salt-and-pepper" appearance common to well-differentiated endocrine tumors of other organs. Uncommon histologic features include oncocytic features, clear cell change, and pleomorphic variant.

ACKNOWLEDGMENT

The author would like to acknowledge the contribution of Dr. Ronald Jaffe, Professor, University of Pittsburgh School of Medicine, who authored the chapter in the first and second editions of this book. Portions of the text and many illustrative materials for figures are adapted from the chapters. His generosity and encouragement is deeply appreciated.

References

1. Bouwens L. Cytokeratins and cell differentiation in the pancreas. *J Pathol* 1998;184:234–239.
2. Arda HE, Benitez CM, Kim SK. Gene regulatory networks governing pancreas development. *Dev Cell* 2013;25:5–13.
3. Imrie JR, Fagan DG, Sturgess JM. Quantitative evaluation of the development of the exocrine pancreas in cystic fibrosis and control infants. *Am J Pathol* 1979;95:697–707.
4. Lemons JA, Ridenour R, Orsini EN. Congenital absence of the pancreas and intrauterine growth retardation. *Pediatrics* 1979;64:255–257.
5. Howard CP, Go VL, Infante AJ, et al. Long-term survival in a case of functional pancreatic agenesis. *J Pediatr* 1980;97:786–789.
6. Julier C, Nicolino M. Wolcott-Rallison syndrome. *Orphanet J Rare Dis* 2010;5:29.
7. Yorifuji T, Matsumura M, Okuno T, et al. Hereditary pancreatic hypoplasia, diabetes mellitus, and congenital heart disease: a new syndrome? *J Med Genet* 1994;31:331–333.
8. Ferreres JC, Planas S, Martinez-Saez EA, et al. Pathological findings in the complete trisomy 9 syndrome: three case reports and review of the literature. *Pediatr Dev Pathol* 2008;11:23–29.
9. Judge DM, Tafari N, Naeye RL, et al. Congenital syphilis and perinatal mortality. *Pediatr Pathol* 1986;5:411–420.
10. Adeyemi SD. Combination of annular pancreas and partial situs inversus: a multiple organ malrotation syndrome associated with duodenal obstruction. *J Pediatr Surg* 1988;23:188–191.
11. Johnston DW. Annular pancreas: a new classification and clinical observations. *Can J Surg* 1978;21:241–244.
12. Jimenez JC, Emil S, Podnos Y, et al. Annular pancreas in children: a recent decade's experience. *J Pediatr Surg* 2004;39:1654–1657.
13. Zyromski NJ, Sandoval JA, Pitt HA, et al. Annular pancreas: dramatic differences between children and adults. *J Am Coll Surg* 2008;206:1019–1025; discussion 1025–1027.
14. Lainakis N, Antypas S, Panagidis A, et al. Annular pancreas in two consecutive siblings: an extremely rare case. *Eur J Pediatr Surg* 2005;15:364–368.
15. Ogata H, Oshio T, Ishibashi H, et al. Heterotopic pancreas in children: review of the literature and report of 12 cases. *Pediatr Surg Int* 2008;24:271–275.
16. Ballouhey Q, Abbo O, Rouquette I, et al. Complex communicating bronchopulmonary foregut malformation with pancreatic heterotopy depicted with fetal magnetic resonance imaging: a case report. *J Pediatr Surg* 2012;47:e7–e9.
17. Ryan A, Lafnitzegger JR, Lin DH, et al. Myoepithelial hamartoma of the duodenal wall. *Virchows Arch* 1998;432:191–194.
18. Langlois NE, Krukowski ZH, Miller ID. Pancreatic tissue in a lateral cervical cyst attached to the thyroid gland—a presumed foregut remnant. *Histopathology* 1997;31:378–380.

19. Hashida Y, Jaffe R, Yunis EJ. Pancreatic pathology in trisomy 13: specificity of the morphologic lesion. *Pediatr Pathol* 1983;1:169–178.
20. Ginsburg M, Ahmed O, Rana KA, et al. Ectopic pancreas presenting with pancreatitis and a mesenteric mass. *J Pediatr Surg* 2013;48:e29–e32.
21. Peranteau WH, Bathaii SM, Pawel B, et al. Multiple ectopic lesions of focal islet adenomatosis identified by positron emission tomography scan in an infant with congenital hyperinsulinism. *J Pediatr Surg* 2007;42:188–192.
22. Ishikawa O, Ishiguro S, Ohhigashi H, et al. Solid and papillary neoplasm arising from an ectopic pancreas in the mesocolon. *Am J Gastroenterol* 1990;85:597–601.
23. Chung JH, Lim GY, Song YT. Congenital true pancreatic cyst detected prenatally in neonate: a case report. *J Pediatr Surg* 2007;42:E27–E29.
24. Steigman CK, Uri AK, Chatten J, et al. Beckwith-Wiedemann syndrome with unusual hepatic and pancreatic features: a case expanding the phenotype. *Pediatr Pathol* 1990;10:593–600.
25. Makin E, Harrison PM, Patel S, et al. Pancreatic pseudocysts in children: treatment by endoscopic cyst gastrostomy. *J Pediatr Gastroenterol Nutr* 2012;55:556–558.
26. Vogel AM, Alesbury JM, Fox VL, et al. Complex pancreatic vascular anomalies in children. *J Pediatr Surg* 2006;41:473–478.
27. Chung EM, Conran RM, Schroeder JW, et al. From the radiologic pathology archives: pediatric polycystic kidney disease and other ciliopathies: radiologic-pathologic correlation. *Radiographics* 2014;34:155–178.
28. Larson RS, Rudloff MA, Liapis H, et al. The Ivemark syndrome: prenatal diagnosis of an uncommon cystic renal lesion with heterogeneous associations. *Pediatr Nephrol* 1995;9:594–598.
29. Tadokoro H, Kozu T, Toki F, et al. Embryological fusion between the ducts of the ventral and dorsal primordia of the pancreas occurs in two manners. *Pancreas* 1997;14:407–414.
30. Jaunin-Stalder N, Stahelin-Massik J, Knuchel J, et al. A pair of monozygotic twins with anomalous pancreaticobiliary junction and pancreatitis. *J Pediatr Surg* 2002;37:1485–1487.
31. Su PH, Chen JY, Hsu CH, et al. Trisomy 18 with multiple rare malformations: report of one case. *Acta Paediatr Taiwan* 2007;48:272–275.
32. Urushihara N, Fukumoto K, Fukuzawa H, et al. Recurrent pancreatitis caused by pancreatobiliary anomalies in children with annular pancreas. *J Pediatr Surg* 2010;45:741–746.
33. Rowlands CG, Hwang WS. Cytomegaly of pancreatic D cells in triploidy. *Pediatr Pathol Lab Med* 1998;18:49–55.
34. Laitio M, Lev R, Orlic D. The developing human fetal pancreas: an ultrastructural and histochemical study with special reference to exocrine cells. *J Anat* 1974;117:619–634.
35. Lebenthal E, Lee PC. Development of functional responses in human exocrine pancreas. *Pediatrics* 1980;66:556–560.
36. Carrère J, Figarella-Branger D, Senegas-Balas F, et al. Immunohistochemical study of secretory proteins in the developing human exocrine pancreas. *Differentiation* 1992;51:55–60.
37. Stormon MO, Durie PR. Pathophysiologic basis of exocrine pancreatic dysfunction in childhood. *J Pediatr Gastroenterol Nutr* 2002;35:8–21.
38. Altinel D, Basturk O, Sarmiento JM, et al. Lipomatous pseudohypertrophy of the pancreas: a clinicopathologically distinct entity. *Pancreas* 2010;39:392–397.
39. Shwachman H, Diamond LK, Oski FA, et al. The syndrome of pancreatic insufficiency and bone marrow dysfunction. *J Pediatr* 1964;65:645–663.
40. Ginzberg H, Shin J, Ellis L, et al. Shwachman syndrome: phenotypic manifestations of sibling sets and isolated cases in a large patient cohort are similar. *J Pediatr* 1999;135:81–88.
41. Smith OP, Hann IM, Chessells JM, et al. Haematological abnormalities in Shwachman-Diamond syndrome. *Br J Haematol* 1996;94:279–284.
42. Bodian M, Sheldon W, Lightwood R. Congenital hypoplasia of the exocrine pancreas. *Acta Paediatr* 1964;53:282–293.
43. Kuijpers TW, Alders M, Tool AT, et al. Hematologic abnormalities in Shwachman Diamond syndrome: lack of genotype-phenotype relationship. *Blood* 2005;106:356–361.
44. Johanson A, Blizzard R. A syndrome of congenital aplasia of the alae nasi, deafness, hypothyroidism, dwarfism, absent permanent teeth, and malabsorption. *J Pediatr* 1971;79:982–987.
45. Gould NS, Paton JB, Bennett AR. Johanson-Blizzard syndrome: clinical and pathological findings in 2 sibs. *Am J Med Genet* 1989;33:194–199.
46. Hoffman WH, Lee JR, Kovacs K, et al. Johanson-Blizzard syndrome: autopsy findings with special emphasis on hypopituitarism and review of the literature. *Pediatr Dev Pathol* 2007;10:55–60.
47. Zenker M, Mayerle J, Lerch MM, et al. Deficiency of UBR1, a ubiquitin ligase of the N-end rule pathway, causes pancreatic dysfunction, malformations and mental retardation (Johanson-Blizzard syndrome). *Nat Genet* 2005;37:1345–1350.
48. Guzman C, Carranza A. Two siblings with exocrine pancreatic hypoplasia and orofacial malformations (Donlan syndrome and Johanson-Blizzard syndrome). *J Pediatr Gastroenterol Nutr* 1997;25:350–353.
49. Pearson HA, Lobel JS, Kocoshis SA, et al. A new syndrome of refractory sideroblastic anemia with vacuolization of marrow precursors and exocrine pancreatic dysfunction. *J Pediatr* 1979;95:976–984.
50. Morikawa Y, Matsuura N, Kakudo K, et al. Pearson's marrow/pancreas syndrome: a histological and genetic study. *Virchows Arch A Pathol Anat Histopathol* 1993;423:227–231.
51. Casademont J, Barrientos A, Cardellach F, et al. Multiple deletions of mtDNA in two brothers with sideroblastic anemia and mitochondrial myopathy and in their asymptomatic mother. *Hum Mol Genet* 1994;3:1945–1949.
52. Blisard KS, Bartow SA. Neonatal hemochromatosis. *Hum Pathol* 1986;17:376–383.
53. Silver MM, Valberg LS, Cutz E, et al. Hepatic morphology and iron quantitation in perinatal hemochromatosis. Comparison with a large perinatal control population, including cases with chronic liver disease. *Am J Pathol* 1993;143:1312–1325.
54. Verloes A, Lombet J, Lambert Y, et al. Tricho-hepato-enteric syndrome: further delineation of a distinct syndrome with neonatal hemochromatosis phenotype, intractable diarrhea, and hair anomalies. *Am J Med Genet* 1997;68:391–395.
55. Farber S. Pancreatic function and disease in early life. V. Pathologic changes associated with pancreatic insufficiency in early life. *Arch Pathol* 1944;37:238–250.
56. Oppenheimer EH, Esterly JR. Pathology of cystic fibrosis review of the literature and comparison with 146 autopsied cases. *Perspect Pediatr Pathol* 1975;2:241–278.
57. Sturgess JM. Structural and developmental abnormalities of the exocrine pancreas in cystic fibrosis. *J Pediatr Gastroenterol Nutr* 1984;3(Suppl 1):S55–S66.
58. Szeifert GT, Szabo M, Papp Z. Morphology of cystic fibrosis at 17 weeks of gestation. *Clin Genet* 1985;28:561–565.
59. Toth IR, Lang JN. Giant pancreatic retention cyst in cystic fibrosis: a case report. *Pediatr Pathol* 1986;6:103–110.
60. Baggenstoss AH. The pancreas in uremia. *Am J Pathol* 1947;23:908–909.
61. DeBanto JR, Goday PS, Pedroso MR, et al. Acute pancreatitis in children. *Am J Gastroenterol* 2002;97:1726–1731.
62. Werlin SL, Kugathasan S, Frautschy BC. Pancreatitis in children. *J Pediatr Gastroenterol Nutr* 2003;37:591–595.
63. Kahler SG, Sherwood WG, Woolf D, et al. Pancreatitis in patients with organic acidemias. *J Pediatr* 1994;124:239–243.
64. Klöppel G. Progression from acute to chronic pancreatitis. A pathologist's view. *Surg Clin North Am* 1999;79:801–814.
65. Jenson AB, Rosenberg HS, Notkins AL. Pancreatic islet-cell damage in children with fatal viral infections. *Lancet* 1980;316(8190):354–358.
66. Parenti DM, Steinberg W, Kang P. Infectious causes of acute pancreatitis. *Pancreas* 1996;13:356–371.
67. Bunnell CE, Monif GR. Interstitial pancreatitis in the congenital rubella syndrome. *J Pediatr* 1972;80:465–466.
68. Kennedy JD, Talbot IC, Tanner MS. Severe pancreatitis and fatty liver progressing to cirrhosis associated with Coxsackie B4 infection in a three year old with alpha-1-antitrypsin deficiency. *Acta Paediatr Scand* 1986;75:336–339.
69. Kahn E, Anderson VM, Greco MA, et al. Pancreatic disorders in pediatric acquired immune deficiency syndrome. *Hum Pathol* 1995;26:765–770.
70. Frey C, Redo SF. Inflammatory lesions of the pancreas in infancy and childhood. *Pediatrics* 1963;32:93–102.

71. Wildin RS, Smyk-Pearson S, Filipovich AH. Clinical and molecular features of the immunodysregulation, polyendocrinopathy, enteropathy, X linked (IPEX) syndrome. *J Med Genet* 2002;39:537–545.
72. Heltzer ML, Choi JK, Ochs HD, et al. A potential screening tool for IPEX syndrome. *Pediatr Dev Pathol* 2007;10:98–105.
73. Levy-Lahad E, Wildin RS. Neonatal diabetes mellitus, enteropathy, thrombocytopenia, and endocrinopathy: further evidence for an X-linked lethal syndrome. *J Pediatr* 2001;138:577–580.
74. Choi BH, Lim YJ, Yoon CH, et al. Acute pancreatitis associated with biliary disease in children. *J Gastroenterol Hepatol* 2003;18:915–921.
75. Forsmark CE, Baillie J. AGA Institute technical review on acute pancreatitis. *Gastroenterology* 2007;132:2022–2044.
76. Bai HX, Ma MH, Orabi AI, et al. Novel characterization of drug-associated pancreatitis in children. *J Pediatr Gastroenterol Nutr* 2011;53:423–428.
77. Rebours V, Levy P, Ruszniewski P. An overview of hereditary pancreatitis. *Dig Liver Dis* 2012;44:8–15.
78. Rebours V, Boutron-Ruault MC, Jooste V, et al. Mortality rate and risk factors in patients with hereditary pancreatitis: uni- and multidimensional analyses. *Am J Gastroenterol* 2009;104:2312–2317.
79. Felderbauer P, Stricker I, Schnekenburger J, et al. Histopathological features of patients with chronic pancreatitis due to mutations in the *PRSS1* gene: evaluation of BRAF and KRAS2 mutations. *Digestion* 2008;78:60–65.
80. Singhi AD, Pai RK, Kant JA, et al. The histopathology of PRSS1 hereditary pancreatitis. *Am J Surg Pathol* 2014;38:346–353.
81. Rebours V, Levy P, Mosnier JF, et al. Pathology analysis reveals that dysplastic pancreatic ductal lesions are frequent in patients with hereditary pancreatitis. *Clin Gastroenterol Hepatol* 2010;8:206–212.
82. Witt H, Beer S, Rosendahl J, et al. Variants in CPA1 are strongly associated with early onset chronic pancreatitis. *Nat Genet* 2013;45:1216–1220.
83. Ooi CY, Dorfman R, Cipolli M, et al. Type of CFTR mutation determines risk of pancreatitis in patients with cystic fibrosis. *Gastroenterology* 2011;140:153–161.
84. Rosendahl J, Landt O, Bernadova J, et al. CFTR, SPINK1, CTRC and PRSS1 variants in chronic pancreatitis: is the role of mutated CFTR overestimated? *Gut* 2013;62:582–592.
85. Perez EA, Gutierrez JC, Koniaris LG, et al. Malignant pancreatic tumors: incidence and outcome in 58 pediatric patients. *J Pediatr Surg* 2009;44:197–203.
86. Yu DC, Kozakewich HP, Perez-Atayde AR, et al. Childhood pancreatic tumors: a single institution experience. *J Pediatr Surg* 2009;44:2267–2272.
87. Ellerkamp V, Warmann SW, Vorwerk P, et al. Exocrine pancreatic tumors in childhood in Germany. *Pediatr Blood Cancer* 2012;58:366–371.
88. Dall'igna P, Cecchetto G, Bisogno G, et al. Pancreatic tumors in children and adolescents: the Italian TREP project experience. *Pediatr Blood Cancer* 2010;54:675–680.
89. Muller CO, Guerin F, Goldzmidt D, et al. Pancreatic resections for solid or cystic pancreatic masses in children. *J Pediatr Gastroenterol Nutr* 2012;54:369–373.
90. McEvoy MP, Rich B, Klimstra D, et al. Acinar cell cystadenoma of the pancreas in a 9-year-old boy. *J Pediatr Surg* 2010;45:e7–e9.
91. Horie A, Yano Y, Kotoo Y, et al. Morphogenesis of pancreatoblastoma, infantile carcinoma of the pancreas: report of two cases. *Cancer* 1977;39:247–254.
92. Hruban RH, Pitman MB, Klimstra DS. Pancreatoblastoma. In: *Tumors of the Pancreas, Fascicle 6*. Washington, DC: American Registry of Pathology; 2000:219–229.
93. Cingolani N, Shaco-Levy R, Farruggia A, et al. Alpha-fetoprotein production by pancreatic tumors exhibiting acinar cell differentiation: study of five cases, one arising in a mediastinal teratoma. *Hum Pathol* 2000;31:938–944.
94. Chisholm KM, Hsu CH, Kim MJ, et al. Congenital pancreatoblastoma: report of an atypical case and review of the literature. *J Pediatr Hematol Oncol* 2012;34:310–315.
95. Klimstra DS, Wenig BM, Adair CF, et al. Pancreatoblastoma. A clinicopathologic study and review of the literature. *Am J Surg Pathol* 1995;19:1371–1389.
96. Morohoshi T, Kanda M, Horie A, et al. Immunocytochemical markers of uncommon pancreatic tumors. Acinar cell carcinoma, pancreatoblastoma, and solid cystic (papillary-cystic) tumor. *Cancer* 1987;59:739–747.
97. Nishimata S, Kato K, Tanaka M, et al. Expression pattern of keratin subclasses in pancreatoblastoma with special emphasis on squamoid corpuscles. *Pathol Int* 2005;55:297–302.
98. Shorter NA, Glick RD, Klimstra DS, et al. Malignant pancreatic tumors in childhood and adolescence: the Memorial Sloan-Kettering experience, 1967 to present. *J Pediatr Surg* 2002;37:887–892.
99. Glick RD, Pashankar FD, Pappo A, et al. Management of pancreatoblastoma in children and young adults. *J Pediatr Hematol Oncol* 2012;34(Suppl 2):S47–S50.
100. Klimstra DS, Heffess CS, Oertel JE, et al. Acinar cell carcinoma of the pancreas. A clinicopathologic study of 28 cases. *Am J Surg Pathol* 1992;16:815–837.
101. Hruban RH, Pitman MB, Klimstra DS. Acinar neoplasms. In: *Tumors of the Pancreas, Fascicle 6*. Washington, DC: American Registry of Pathology; 2007:191–218.
102. Tapia B, Ahrens W, Kenney B, et al. Acinar cell carcinoma versus solid pseudopapillary tumor of the pancreas in children: a comparison of two rare and overlapping entities with review of the literature. *Pediatr Dev Pathol* 2008;11:384–390.
103. Abraham SC, Wu TT, Hruban RH, et al. Genetic and immunohistochemical analysis of pancreatic acinar cell carcinoma: frequent allelic loss on chromosome 11p and alterations in the APC/beta-catenin pathway. *Am J Pathol* 2002;160:953–962.
104. Hruban RH, Pitman MB, Klimstra DS. Solid-pseudopapillary neoplasms. In: *Tumor of the Pancreas, Fascicle 6*. Washington, DC: American Registry of Pathology; 2007:231–250.
105. Law JK, Ahmed A, Singh VK, et al. A systematic review of solid-pseudopapillary neoplasms: are these rare lesions? *Pancreas* 2014;43:331–337.
106. Klimstra DS, Wenig BM, Heffess CS. Solid-pseudopapillary tumor of the pancreas: a typically cystic carcinoma of low malignant potential. *Semin Diagn Pathol* 2000;17:66–80.
107. Abraham SC, Klimstra DS, Wilentz RE, et al. Solid-pseudopapillary tumors of the pancreas are genetically distinct from pancreatic ductal adenocarcinomas and almost always harbor beta-catenin mutations. *Am J Pathol* 2002;160:1361–1369.
108. Guo Y, Yuan F, Deng H, et al. Paranuclear dot-like immunostaining for CD99: a unique staining pattern for diagnosing solid-pseudopapillary neoplasm of the pancreas. *Am J Surg Pathol* 2011;35:799–806.
109. Park JY, Kim SG, Park J. Solid pseudopapillary tumor of the pancreas in children: 15-year experience at a single institution with assays using an immunohistochemical panel. *Ann Surg Treat Res* 2014;86:130–135.
110. Estrella JS, Li L, Rashid A, et al. Solid pseudopapillary neoplasm of the pancreas: clinicopathologic and survival analyses of 64 cases from a single institution. *Am J Surg Pathol* 2014;38:147–157.
111. Lüttges J, Stigge C, Pacena M, et al. Rare ductal adenocarcinoma of the pancreas in patients younger than age 40 years. *Cancer* 2004;100:173–182.
112. St-Onge L, Sosa-Pineda B, Chowdhury K, et al. Pax6 is required for differentiation of glucagon-producing alpha-cells in mouse pancreas. *Nature* 1997;387:406–409.
113. Stefan Y, Grasso S, Perrelet A, et al. A quantitative immunofluorescent study of the endocrine cell populations in the developing human pancreas. *Diabetes* 1983;32:293–301.
114. Rahier J, Wallon J, Gepts W, et al. Localization of pancreatic polypeptide cells in a limited lobe of the human neonate pancreas: remnant of the ventral primordium? *Cell Tissue Res* 1979;200:359–366.
115. Jaffe R, Hashida Y, Yunis EJ. Pancreatic pathology in hyperinsulinemic hypoglycemia of infancy. *Lab Invest* 1980;42:356–365.
116. Milner RD, Wirdnam PK, Tsanakas J. Quantitative morphology of B, A, D, and PP cells in infants of diabetic mothers. *Diabetes* 1981;30:271–274.
117. Borchard F, Müntefering H. Beitrag zur quantitativen morphologie der langerhansschen inseln bei früh- und neugeborenen. *Virchows Arch [A]* 1969;346:178–198.
118. Hultquist GT, Olding LB. Endocrine pathology of infants of diabetic mothers. A quantitative morphological analysis including a

118. comparison with infants of iso-immunized and of non-diabetic mothers. *Acta Endocrinol Suppl (Copenhagen)* 1981;241:1–202.
119. Wellman KF, Volk BW. The islets of infants of diabetic mothers. In: Volk BW, Wellman KF, eds. *The Diabetic Pancreas*. New York: Plenum Publishing; 1977:365–380.
120. Dodge JA, Laurence KM. Congenital absence of islets of Langerhans. *Arch Dis Child* 1977;52:411–413.
121. Barresi G, Inferrera C, de Luca F, et al. Persistent neonatal normoinsulinaemic hypoglycaemia. *Histopathology* 1981;5:45–52.
122. Bishop AE, Polak JM, Chesa PG, et al. Decrease of pancreatic somatostatin in neonatal nesidioblastosis. *Diabetes* 1981;30:122–126.
123. Béringue F, Blondeau B, Castellotti MC, et al. Endocrine pancreas development in growth-retarded human fetuses. *Diabetes* 2002;51:385–391.
124. Van Assche FA, Gepts W. The cytological composition of the foetal endocrine pancreas in normal and pathological conditions. *Diabetologia* 1971;7:434–444.
125. D'Agostino A, Bahn RC. A histopathologic study of the pancreas of infants of diabetic mothers. *Diabetes* 1963;12:327–331.
126. Holemans K, Aerts L, Van Assche FA. Lifetime consequences of abnormal fetal pancreatic development. *J Physiol* 2003;547:11–20.
127. Dabelea D, Hanson RL, Lindsay RS, et al. Intrauterine exposure to diabetes conveys risks for type 2 diabetes and obesity: a study of discordant sibships. *Diabetes* 2000;49:2208–2211.
128. Van Assche FA, Aerts L, Holemans K, et al. The endocrine pancreas in nonimmune hydrops fetalis. *Am J Obstet Gynecol* 1994;171:236–238.
129. Mostoufi-Zadeh M, Weiss LM, Driscoll SG. Nonimmune hydrops fetalis: a challenge in perinatal pathology. *Hum Pathol* 1985;16:785–789.
130. American Diabetic Association. Diagnosis and classification of diabetes mellitus. *Diabetes Care* 2014;37(Suppl 1):S81–S90.
131. Gepts W, De Mey J. Islet cell survival determined by morphology. An immunocytochemical study of the islets of Langerhans in juvenile diabetes mellitus. *Diabetes* 1978;27(Suppl 1):251–261.
132. Meier JJ, Bhushan A, Butler AE, et al. Sustained beta cell apoptosis in patients with long-standing type 1 diabetes: indirect evidence for islet regeneration? *Diabetologia* 2005;48:2221–2228.
133. Foulis AK, Liddle CN, Farquharson MA, et al. The histopathology of the pancreas in type 1 (insulin-dependent) diabetes mellitus: a 25-year review of deaths in patients under 20 years of age in the United Kingdom. *Diabetologia* 1986;29:267–274.
134. Rozin L, Perper JA, Jaffe R, et al. Sudden unexpected death in childhood due to unsuspected diabetes mellitus. *Am J Forensic Med Pathol* 1994;15:251–256.
135. Gavin JRI, Alberti KGMM, Davidson MB, et al. Report of the expert committee on the diagnosis and classification of diabetes mellitus. *Diabetes Care* 2003;26(Suppl 1):S5–S20.
136. Kitagawa T, Owada M, Urakami T, et al. Increased incidence of non-insulin dependent diabetes mellitus among Japanese schoolchildren correlates with an increased intake of animal protein and fat. *Clin Pediatr (Phila)* 1998;37:111–115.
137. American Diabetic Association. Type 2 diabetes in children and adolescents. *Diabetes Care* 2000;23:381–389.
138. Sempoux C, Guiot Y, Dubois D, et al. Human type 2 diabetes: morphological evidence for abnormal beta-cell function. *Diabetes* 2001;50(Suppl 1):S172–S177.
139. Clark A, de Koning EJ, Hattersley AT, et al. Pancreatic pathology in non-insulin dependent diabetes (NIDDM). *Diabetes Res Clin Pract* 1995;28(Suppl):S39–S47.
140. Hull RL, Westermark GT, Westermark P, et al. Islet amyloid: a critical entity in the pathogenesis of type 2 diabetes. *J Clin Endocrinol Metab* 2004;89:3629–3643.
141. Butler AE, Janson J, Bonner-Weir S, et al. Beta-cell deficit and increased beta-cell apoptosis in humans with type 2 diabetes. *Diabetes* 2003;52:102–110.
142. Polak M, Shield J. Neonatal and very-early-onset diabetes mellitus. *Semin Neonatol* 2004;9:59–65.
143. Greeley SA, Naylor RN, Philipson LH, et al. Neonatal diabetes: an expanding list of genes allows for improved diagnosis and treatment. *Curr Diab Rep* 2011;11:519–532.
144. Ehtisham S, Hattersley AT, Dunger DB, et al. First UK survey of paediatric type 2 diabetes and MODY. *Arch Dis Child* 2004;89:526–529.
145. Stanley CA. Advances in diagnosis and treatment of hyperinsulinism in infants and children. *J Clin Endocrinol Metab* 2002;87:4857–4859.
146. Elliott M, Bayly R, Cole T, et al. Clinical features and natural history of Beckwith-Wiedemann syndrome: presentation of 74 new cases. *Clin Genet* 1994;46:168–174.
147. Laidlaw GF. Nesidioblastoma, the islet tumor of the pancreas. *Am J Pathol* 1938;14:125–134.
148. Yakovac WC, Baker L, Hummeler K. Beta cell nesidioblastosis in idiopathic hypoglycemia of infancy. *J Pediatr* 1971;79:226–231.
149. Rahier J, Falt K, Muntefering H, et al. The basic structural lesion of persistent neonatal hypoglycaemia with hyperinsulinism: deficiency of pancreatic D cells or hyperactivity of B cells? *Diabetologia* 1984;26:282–289.
150. Rahier J, Guiot Y, Sempoux C. Persistent hyperinsulinaemic hypoglycaemia of infancy: a heterogeneous syndrome unrelated to nesidioblastosis. *Arch Dis Child Fetal Neonatal Ed* 2000;82:F108–F112.
151. Snider KE, Becker S, Boyajian L, et al. Genotype and phenotype correlations in 417 children with congenital hyperinsulinism. *J Clin Endocrinol Metab* 2012;98:E355–E363.
152. Rahier J, Sempoux C, Fournet JC, et al. Partial or near-total pancreatectomy for persistent neonatal hyperinsulinaemic hypoglycaemia: the pathologist's role. *Histopathology* 1998;32:15–19.
153. Sempoux C, Guiot Y, Dubois D, et al. Pancreatic B-cell proliferation in persistent hyperinsulinemic hypoglycemia of infancy: an immunohistochemical study of 18 cases. *Mod Pathol* 1998;11:444–449.
154. Kassem S, Bhandari S, Rodriguez-Bada P, et al. Large islets, beta-cell proliferation, and a glucokinase mutation. *N Engl J Med* 2010;362:1348–1350.
155. Stanley CA, Thornton PS, Ganguly A, et al. Preoperative evaluation of infants with focal or diffuse congenital hyperinsulinism by intraoperative acute insulin response tests and selective pancreatic arterial calcium stimulation. *J Clin Endocrinol Metab* 2004;89:288–296.
156. Suchi M, Thornton PS, Adzick NS, et al. Congenital hyperinsulinism: intraoperative biopsy interpretation can direct the extent of pancreatectomy. *Am J Surg Pathol* 2004;28:1326–1335.
157. Sempoux C, Guiot Y, Jaubert F, et al. Focal and diffuse forms of congenital hyperinsulinism: the keys for differential diagnosis. *Endocr Pathol* 2004;15:241–246.
158. de Lonlay P, Fournet JC, Rahier J, et al. Somatic deletion of the imprinted 11p15 region in sporadic persistent hyperinsulinemic hypoglycemia of infancy is specific of focal adenomatous hyperplasia and endorses partial pancreatectomy. *J Clin Invest* 1997;100:802–807.
159. Suchi M, MacMullen CM, Thornton PS, et al. Molecular and immunohistochemical analyses of the focal form of congenital hyperinsulinism. *Mod Pathol* 2006;19:122–129.
160. Adzick NS, Thornton PS, Stanley CA, et al. A multidisciplinary approach to the focal form of congenital hyperinsulinism leads to successful treatment by partial pancreatectomy. *J Pediatr Surg* 2004;39:270–275.
161. Hardy OT, Hernandez-Pampaloni M, Saffer JR, et al. Diagnosis and localization of focal congenital hyperinsulinism by 18 F-fluorodopa PET scan. *J Pediatr* 2007;150:140–145.
162. Stanley CA. Hyperinsulinism/hyperammonemia syndrome: insights into the regulatory role of glutamate dehydrogenase in ammonia metabolism. *Mol Genet Metab* 2004;81(Suppl 1):S45–S51.
163. Weinzimer SA, Stanley CA, Berry GT, et al. A syndrome of congenital hyperinsulinism and hyperammonemia. *J Pediatr* 1997;130:661–664.
164. Peranteau WH, Palladino AA, Bhatti TR, et al. The surgical management of insulinomas in children. *J Pediatr Surg* 2013;48:2517–2524.
165. Naeye RL. The sudden infant death syndrome: a review of recent advances. *Arch Pathol Lab Med* 1977;101:165–167.
166. Klensang U, Hagemann S, Saeger W, et al. Morphology, immunohistochemistry and morphometry of pancreatic islets in cases of sudden infant death syndrome (SIDS). *Int J Legal Med* 1997;110:199–203.
167. Seemayer TA, Osborne C, de Chadarevian JP. Shock-related injury of pancreatic islets of Langerhans in newborn and young infants. *Hum Pathol* 1985;16:1231–1234.

168. Gladisch R, Hofmann W, Waldherr R. Myokarditis und Insulitis nach Coxsackie Virus-Infekt. *Z Kardiol* 1976;65:837–849.
169. Laje P, Palladino AA, Bhatti TR, et al. Pancreatic surgery in infants with Beckwith-Wiedemann syndrome and hyperinsulinism. *J Pediatr Surg* 2013;48:2511–2516.
170. Stefan Y, Bordi C, Grasso S, et al. Beckwith-Wiedemann syndrome: a quantitative, immunohistochemical study of pancreatic islet cell populations. *Diabetologia* 1985;28:914–919.
171. Hussain K, Cosgrove KE, Shepherd RM, et al. Hyperinsulinemic hypoglycemia in Beckwith-Wiedemann syndrome due to defects in the function of pancreatic beta-cell adenosine triphosphate-sensitive potassium channels. *J Clin Endocrinol Metab* 2005;90:4376–4382.
172. Schier F, Sauerbrey A, Kosmehl H. A Meckel's diverticulum containing pancreatic tissue and nesidioblastosis in a patient with Beckwith-Wiedemann syndrome. *Pediatr Surg Int* 2000;16:124–127.
173. Fukuzawa R, Umezawa A, Morikawa Y, et al. Nesidioblastosis and mixed hamartoma of the liver in Beckwith-Wiedemann syndrome: case study including analysis of H19 methylation and insulin-like growth factor 2 genotyping and imprinting. *Pediatr Dev Pathol* 2001;4:381–390.
174. Sotelo-Avila C, Gooch WM III. Neoplasms associated with the Beckwith-Wiedemann syndrome. *Perspect Pediatr Pathol* 1976;3:255–272.
175. Drut R, Jones MC. Congenital pancreatoblastoma in Beckwith-Wiedemann syndrome: an emerging association. *Pediatr Pathol* 1988;8:331–339.
176. Henneveld HT, van Lingen RA, Hamel BC, et al. Perlman syndrome: four additional cases and review. *Am J Med Genet* 1999;86:439–446.
177. Turcotte S, Turkbey B, Barak S, et al. von Hippel-Lindau disease-associated solid microcystic serous adenomas masquerading as pancreatic neuroendocrine neoplasms. *Surgery* 2012;152:1106–1117.
178. Lonser RR, Glenn GM, Walther M, et al. von Hippel-Lindau disease. *Lancet* 2003;361(9374):2059–2067.
179. Hoang MP, Hruban RH, Albores-Saavedra J. Clear cell endocrine pancreatic tumor mimicking renal cell carcinoma: a distinctive neoplasm of von Hippel-Lindau disease. *Am J Surg Pathol* 2001;25:602–609.
180. Langrehr JM, Bahra M, Kristiansen G, et al. Neuroendocrine tumor of the pancreas and bilateral adrenal pheochromocytomas. A rare manifestation of von Hippel-Lindau disease in childhood. *J Pediatr Surg* 2007;42:1291–1294.
181. Wolcott CD, Rallison ML. Infancy-onset diabetes mellitus and multiple epiphyseal dysplasia. *J Pediatr* 1972;80:292–297.
182. Durocher F, Faure R, Labrie Y, et al. A novel mutation in the EIF2AK3 gene with variable expressivity in two patients with Wolcott-Rallison syndrome. *Clin Genet* 2006;70:34–38.
183. Senée V, Vattem KM, Delépine M, et al. Wolcott-Rallison Syndrome: clinical, genetic, and functional study of EIF2AK3 mutations and suggestion of genetic heterogeneity. *Diabetes* 2004;53:1876–1883.
184. Thornton CM, Carson DJ, Stewart FJ. Autopsy findings in the Wolcott-Rallison syndrome. *Pediatr Pathol Lab Med* 1997;17:487–496.
185. Donohue WL. Dysendocrinism. Clinicopathologic Conference at the Hospital for Sick Children, Toronto, Ontario. *J Pediatr* 1948;32:739–748.
186. Rosenberg AM, Haworth JC, Degroot GW, et al. A case of leprechaunism with severe hyperinsulinemia. *Am J Dis Child* 1980;134:170–175.
187. Szilagyi PG, Corsetti J, Callahan CM, et al. Pancreatic exocrine aplasia, clinical features of leprechaunism, and abnormal gonadotropin regulation. *Pediatr Pathol* 1987;7:51–61.
188. Moran A, Dunitz J, Nathan B, et al. Cystic fibrosis-related diabetes: current trends in prevalence, incidence, and mortality. *Diabetes Care* 2009;32:1626–1631.
189. Löhr M, Goertchen P, Nizze H, et al. Cystic fibrosis associated islet changes may provide a basis for diabetes. An immunocytochemical and morphometrical study. *Virchows Arch A Pathol Anat Histopathol* 1989;414:179–185.
190. Iannucci A, Mukai K, Johnson D, et al. Endocrine pancreas in cystic fibrosis: an immunohistochemical study. *Hum Pathol* 1984;15:278–284.
191. Couce M, O'Brien TD, Moran A, et al. Diabetes mellitus in cystic fibrosis is characterized by islet amyloidosis. *J Clin Endocrinol Metab* 1996;81:1267–1272.
192. Brown RE, Madge GE. Cystic fibrosis and nesidioblastosis. *Arch Pathol* 1971;92:53–57.
193. Baumann U, Preece MA, Green A, et al. Hyperinsulinism in tyrosinaemia type I. *J Inherit Metab Dis* 2005;28:131–135.
194. Russo P, O'Regan S. Visceral pathology of hereditary tyrosinemia type I. *Am J Hum Genet* 1990;47:317–324.
195. Hardwick DF, Dimmick JE. Metabolic cirrhoses of infancy and early childhood. *Perspect Pediatr Pathol* 1976;3:103–144.
196. Claret Teruel G, Giner Muñoz MT, Plaza Martín AM, et al. Variability of immunodeficiency associated with ataxia telangiectasia and clinical evolution in 12 affected patients. *Pediatr Allergy Immunol* 2005;16:615–618.
197. Bar RS, Levis WR, Rechler MM, et al. Extreme insulin resistance in ataxia telangiectasia: defect in affinity of insulin receptors. *N Engl J Med* 1978;298:1164–1171.
198. Tamura K, Nishimori I, Ito T, et al. Diagnosis and management of pancreatic neuroendocrine tumor in von Hippel-Lindau disease. *World J Gastroenterol* 2010;16:4515–4518.
199. Arva NC, Pappas JG, Bhatla T, et al. Well-differentiated pancreatic neuroendocrine carcinoma in tuberous sclerosis—case report and review of the literature. *Am J Surg Pathol* 2012;36:149–153.
200. Breysem L, Kersemans P, Vanbeckevoort D, et al. Nonfunctioning neuroendocrine tumor of the pancreas in an 8-year-old girl. *JBR-BTR* 2007;90:528–531.

CHAPTER 17

The Kidney and Lower Urinary Tract

Laura S. Finn, M.D., and Aliya N. Husain, M.D.

Rapid advances in the field of genetics and molecular biology are leading to a better understanding of normal embryology, congenital malformations, glomerular and tubulointerstitial diseases, and neoplasia of the kidney and lower urinary tract. Approximately one-third of all congenital malformations are found in the urogenital system, many of which are part of complex multisystem anomalies with cumulative effects that are lethal in the neonatal period. Almost 80% of congenital uropathies seen in second trimester fetuses are associated with other anomalies—both chromosomal and nonchromosomal, either syndromic or in casual combination (1). Malformations of the bladder are often accompanied by major anomalies of the male and female genital tract because of the interrelated embryologic development of these organ systems. Glomerular diseases, reflux nephropathy, and infections are important causes of morbidity in childhood. Although cancer of the kidney is relatively uncommon in the pediatric age group, accounting for about 7% of childhood malignancies, 5-year survival from Wilms tumor has increased from 73% in patients diagnosed in 1975 to 1977 to 92% in the period 1996 to 2002, thus establishing a successful model for national multicenter study groups. However, 24% of survivors have severe chronic health conditions 25 years postdiagnosis, thus emphasizing the need to continuously improve treatment protocols (2).

EMBRYOLOGY

Functionally, the urinary and the genital systems can be divided into two entirely separate systems; however, embryologically and anatomically, they are intimately interwoven. Both develop from a common mesodermal ridge (intermediate mesoderm) along the posterior wall of the abdominal cavity, and initially, the excretory ducts of both systems enter a common cavity, the cloaca. In humans, three separate but temporally overlapping renal systems form. The pronephros, which is the most caudal and nonfunctional, regresses completely by the end of the 4th week of gestation, during which time the first excretory tubules of the mesonephros appear that may function for a short period. While the caudal tubules are still differentiating, the cranial tubules and glomeruli show degenerative changes, and by the end of the second month, most have disappeared. In the male, a few of the caudal tubules and the mesonephric duct persist and participate in the formation of the genital system, but they disappear in the female, leaving only a few vestigial structures.

The metanephros, or permanent kidney, appears in the 5th week at the level of the upper sacral segment, with its blood supply coming from the lateral sacral branches of the aorta. By the eighth week, it "ascends" to the lumbar region, mainly secondary to differential growth of the embryo, and derives its blood supply from progressively higher levels of the aorta. In the pelvic ectopic kidney, the renal arteries arise from a lower level of the aorta or from the iliac arteries. The nephrons develop from the caudal end of the metanephric blastema (metanephric mesenchyme), while the renal excretory system (collecting duct, calyces, pelvis, and ureter) develops from the ureteric bud, which is an outgrowth of the mesonephric duct close to its entrance into the cloaca. The proximal tip or the ampulla of the ureteric bud grows dorsally and cranially, pushes the metanephric mesenchyme, and undergoes a series of dichotomous branching; the ampulla of each branch ultimately induces nephron formation. Each division proceeds more rapidly at the poles, so that the kidney acquires its characteristic shape. Ureteric bud branching is complete by 22 weeks of gestation, and the first few generations of branches coalesce to form the renal pelvis and calyces, whereas subsequent generations give rise to collecting ducts (3).

Nephrons form from condensation of the metanephric blastema, which develops a cyst-like cavity, elongates, and folds back to become S-shaped. One end fuses with the ampulla that induced it, while at the other end, a mesh of capillaries develops and invaginates the nephrogenic vesicle to form a glomerulus. The upper and middle limbs of the nephrogenic vesicle elongate and differentiate into the proximal and distal convoluted tubules and the loop of Henle (4).

The process of nephrogenesis can be divided into four periods. From 7 to 14 weeks of gestation, the ureteric bud branches dichotomously for six to eight generations, with each branch inducing the formation of a new nephron.

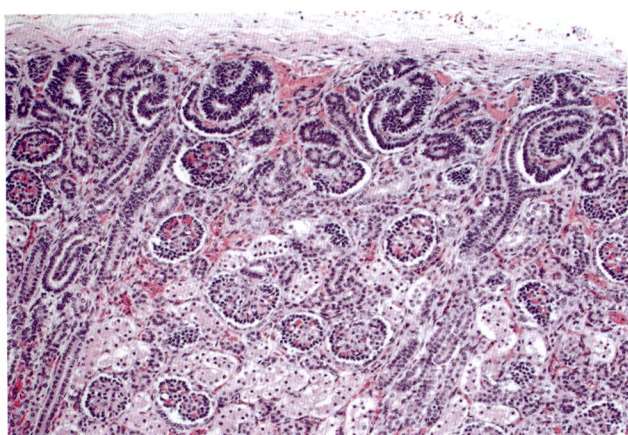

FIGURE 17-1 • Early third trimester kidney with subcapsular nephrogenic zone. (Hematoxylin–eosin stain, original magnification ×100.)

of the ureteric buds, establishing signaling pathways between the two tissues. In turn, the buds induce the mesenchyme via fibroblast growth factor 2 and bone morphogenetic protein 7. Both these growth factors block apoptosis and stimulate proliferation in the metanephric mesenchyme while maintaining production of WT1. Conversion of the mesenchyme to an epithelium for the nephron formation is also mediated by the ureteric buds, in part through modification of the extracellular matrix. Thus, fibronectin, collagen I, and collagen III are replaced with laminin and type IV collagen, characteristic of an epithelial basal lamina. In addition, the cell adhesion molecules, syndecan and E-cadherin, which are essential for condensation of the mesenchyme into an epithelium, are synthesized. Regulatory genes for conversion of the mesenchyme into an epithelium appear to involve *PAX2* and *WNT4* (4).

From 14 to 22 weeks, nephron arcades are formed, with the innermost nephron formed first (juxtamedullary nephron) (eFigure 17-1). From 22 to 36 weeks, no branching of the ureteric bud occurs. The ampulla extends to the subcapsular cortex to induce four to seven nephrons (eFigure 17-2). Thus, the nephrons formed last are subcapsular (the nephrogenic zone seen in sections of fetal kidneys) (Figure 17-1). From 36 weeks of gestation through birth and up to maturity, the nephrons grow, but no new nephrons are formed. In extremely premature infants, nephrogenesis continues after birth until the kidney reaches maturity. However, in this setting, renal maturation appears to be accelerated and associated with an increased number of morphologically abnormal and large glomeruli, suggestive of hyperfiltration and predicting fewer functioning nephrons in postnatal and later life (5).

Studies indicate that nephrons in the developing metanephros may begin functioning as early as the eleventh or 12th week after conception. In fact, it has been suggested that the formation of a tubule fluid is essential to ensure the normal development of the renal pelvis and calyces.

Molecular Regulation of Kidney Development

As with most organs, differentiation of the kidney involves epithelial–mesenchymal interactions, which are under the control of multiple gene regulatory networks that act as inducers or inhibitors. Briefly, epithelium of the ureteric bud from the mesonephros interacts with mesenchyme of the metanephric blastema. The mesenchyme expresses *WT-1*, a transcription factor that makes this tissue competent to respond to induction by the ureteric bud. *WT-1* also regulates production of glial-derived neurotrophic factor (GDNF) and hepatocyte growth factor (HGF or scatter factor) by the mesenchyme, and these proteins stimulate branching and growth of the ureteric buds. The tyrosine kinase receptors RET, for GDNF, and MET, for HGF, are synthesized by the epithelium

CONGENITAL MALFORMATIONS OF THE KIDNEY

If all malformations are considered, ranging from incidental findings with no clinical significance to major lethal anomalies, it is estimated that congenital abnormalities of the kidney and urinary tract are present in 10% of all newborns and interestingly, when unilateral, are more often on the left (6). Worldwide, a substantial percentage of children develop chronic kidney disease early in life, with congenital anomalies of the kidney and urinary tract (CAKUT) such as obstructive uropathy and aplasia/hypoplasia/dysplasia being responsible for almost one-half of all cases (7). Table 17-1 lists the relative frequency of malformations seen in two series of pediatric autopsies—one from a children's hospital and the other from a tertiary care university medical center. Forty-one (38%) of the 107 renal malformations in series No. 2 were associated with major malformations of at least one other organ system.

A wide variety of renal malformations result in the oligohydramnios (Potter) sequence (i.e., characteristic facies, including low-set ears, beaked nose, prominent epicanthic folds, receding chin, limb deformities, growth retardation, and pulmonary hypoplasia) (Figure 17-2). These abnormalities are the result of decreased amniotic fluid rather than renal malformations per se and can result from even a relatively short duration of oligohydramnios, including persistent leakage of amniotic fluid. When these findings are associated with renal agenesis, the term *Potter syndrome* (as initially described by Potter in 1946) is used. Renal findings in children with oligohydramnios sequence are listed in Table 17-2. Most urogenital abnormalities are now diagnosed antenatally on high-resolution ultrasound scans, which have enabled recognition of those that are not compatible with survival and those that can benefit from intervention (8). CAKUT are responsible for approximately 40% to 50% of childhood chronic kidney disease worldwide (9). The classification of congenital and developmental anomalies of

TABLE 17-1 RENAL MALFORMATIONS SEEN IN PEDIATRIC AUTOPSIES

Anomaly	No. of Cases		
	Series 1*	Series 2+	Total (%)
Renal agenesis, bilateral	16	13	29 (12)
Renal agenesis, unilateral	10	6	16 (6.6)
Renal dysplasia, bilateral	45	33	78 (32)
Renal dysplasia, unilateral	4	5	9 (2.1)
Renal dysplasia, unilateral, with contralateral renal agenesis	9	3	12 (5)
Autosomal recessive polycystic kidney disease	5	10	15 (6.2)
Autosomal dominant polycystic kidney disease	1	1	2 (0.8)
Renal fusion	20	12	32 (13.2)
Renal ectopia	4	1	5 (2.1)
Congenital hydronephrosis, bilateral	6	5	11 (4.5)
Congenital hydronephrosis, unilateral	4	8	12 (5)
Ureteral duplication	10	5	15 (6.2)
Renal hypoplasia	1	3	4 (1.7)
Others	0	6	6 (2.5)
Total	135	111	246 (~100)

Series 1* compiled from 1442 consecutive autopsies performed at Minneapolis Children's Medical Center from 1977 to 1987, including stillborn infants and children younger than 1 year of age.
Series 2+ compiled from 1242 pediatric autopsies performed at Loyola University Medical Center from 1978 to 1998, including stillbirths and children up to 18 years (Unpublished data from Aliya N. Husain, M.D.).

the kidney has historically been based on morphologic criteria established decades ago; more recent systems attempt to incorporate new information about nephrogenesis and the pathogenesis of urinary tract malformations (10,11). It is well established that many cases of CAKUT have a genetic basis and many are associated with syndromes; nonsyndromic forms may also be causally linked to several developmental genes. Thus, neither approach is perfect as a given gene can result in a spectrum of anomalies, and the same anomaly can be caused by multiple genes. Nonetheless, it is worthwhile to consider the molecular mechanism of kidney and urinary tract development to better understand the malformation. The diversity of signaling pathways in nephrogenesis likely explains the remarkable locus heterogeneity found in CAKUT. Currently, mutations can be identified in approximately 10% to 20% of children, with *HNF1B* and *PAX2* mutations being the most common (12). Table 17-3 lists the common malformations of the kidney and includes cystic diseases because many of these are inheritable disorders or are secondary to malformations of the kidney parenchyma and lower urinary tract (13).

Renal Ectopia

Permanent malposition of one or both kidneys is seen in 2% of pediatric autopsies (Table 17-1). The incidence is even higher in perinatal autopsies because renal ectopia is commonly associated with multiple other malformations; however, the incidence in screening studies is approximately 1 in 683 infants (14). The ectopic kidney(s) may be located in the pelvis (most common), on the other side (crossed renal ectopia) with or without fusion, or even in the thorax (rare) (15). Prenatal ultrasonographic diagnosis of the pelvic kidney is possible, usually after 24 weeks of gestation, although postnatal ultrasound or CT is more effective at diagnosing

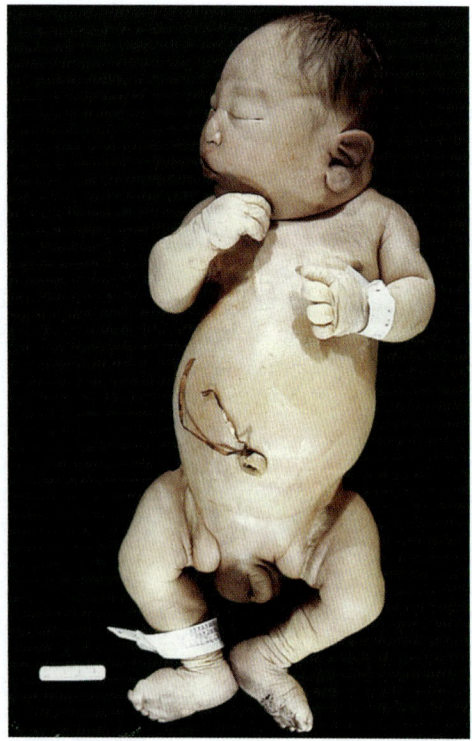

FIGURE 17-2 • Oligohydramnios (Potter sequence) is associated with low-set and deformed ears, beaked nose, receding chin, and lower limb positional deformity.

TABLE 17-2 RENAL FINDINGS IN CHILDREN WITH OLIGOHYDRAMNIOS SEQUENCE

	No. of Cases		
Renal Abnormality	Series 1	Series 2	Total (%)
Bilateral renal agenesis	16	32	48 (30)
Bilateral cystic dysplasia	17	30	47 (29)
Unilateral agenesis with contralateral dysplasia	9	8	17 (10)
Obstructive uropathy	13	—	13 (8)
Autosomal recessive polycystic kidney disease	4	2	6 (4)
Renal ectopia and fusion	1	1	2 (1)
Autosomal dominant polycystic kidney disease	1	1	2 (1)
Others	13	13	26 (16)
Total	74	87	161 (~100)

anomalies of the urinary tract (14). While renal function is normal in the neonatal period in patients with renal ectopia without other associated malformations, vesicoureteral reflux and hydronephrosis have been reported in approximately 20% to 50%, particularly in crossed renal ectopia (16). Pseudocrossed renal ectopia occurs when an enlarging retroperitoneal mass displaces the kidney to the contralateral side of the abdomen.

TABLE 17-3 CLASSIFICATION OF MALFORMATIONS OF THE KIDNEY, INCLUDING CYSTIC DISEASES

I. Renal position and form
   A. Ectopia
   B. Fusion
   C. Supernumerary
II. Renal quantity
   A. Agenesis (bilateral, unilateral)
   B. Hypoplasia, simple, or oligomeganephronic
   C. Renal tubular dysgenesis
   D. Renomegaly
   E. Duplication
III. Hydronephrosis
IV. Renal dysplasia/cystic diseases (gross and/or microscopic)
   A. Renal dysplasia
      1. Sporadic (bilateral, unilateral)
      2. Hereditary
      3. With malformation syndromes
   B. Polycystic kidney disease
      1. Autosomal recessive (infantile type)
      2. Autosomal dominant (adult type)
   C. Medullary cysts
      1. Medullary sponge kidney
      2. Nephronophthisis (Types 1–3)
      3. Medullary cystic disease (Types 1 and 2)
   D. Cortical cysts
      1. Glomerulocystic disease(s)
      2. Simple cysts (acquired)
      3. Microcysts associated with syndromes
   E. Renal cysts with hereditary syndromes

Renal Fusion

Renal fusion, often with ectopia, was seen in 32 (1.2%) of 2684 pediatric autopsies (Table 17-1). The most common fusion anomaly is horseshoe kidney, in which both kidneys are normally lateralized but have fused lower poles (Figure 17-3) and are located in a lower than normal position. The incidence of horseshoe kidney is reported to be 1 in 600 to 700 in the general population (17). One-third of persons with this condition have associated congenital malformations of other organs, including Turner syndrome (18); two-third have a major urologic complication, most of which require surgery, although newer techniques such as laparoscopic robotic-assisted management allow for minimally invasive procedures. Symptomatic hydronephrosis eventually develops in

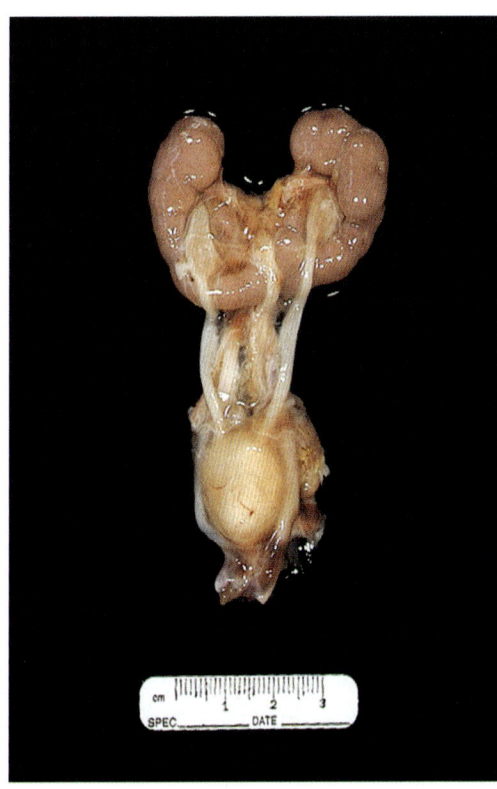

FIGURE 17-3 • Horseshoe kidney with fused lower poles.

more than half of patients with horseshoe kidney, secondary to ureteropelvic junction obstruction, reflux, or malrotation. Individuals with horseshoe kidney are at higher risk for the development of stones (19) and tumors (20). Rare cases of renal–adrenal fusion have been described, which may present as a renal mass in the upper pole (21).

Renal Agenesis/Hypoplasia

Inadequate renal tissue can be considered as a continuum, ranging from renal agenesis to subtle congenital nephron deficits. Renal agenesis (i.e., the complete absence of one or both kidneys) is commonly accompanied by other malformations of the genitourinary tract and various lower body defects and is often the result of one or more genetic mutations that leads to molecular dysregulation of nephrogenesis. Homozygous null mice for *c-Ret*, *Gdnf*, and *Gfrα-1* all exhibit bilateral renal agenesis due to the inhibition of ureteric bud growth and branching morphogenesis; they are less frequently implicated in human renal agenesis (22). Pax2 plays an integral role in the initiation and maintenance of the Ret/Gdnf pathway by not only activating the ligand of the pathway but also enhancing the expression of the pathway receptor Ret (4). Since an exhaustive review is beyond the scope of this chapter, one can focus on Pax2, one of the earliest genes expressed widely during fetal kidney development in the nephric duct, the metanephric mesenchyme, the ureteric bud, and in the S-shaped body. Early failure in the first two developmental stages (e.g., homozygous inactivation of Pax2) precludes formation of metanephric kidneys and causes bilateral renal agenesis, incompatible with life. Interference with the later stages affects the extent of branching morphogenesis (e.g., heterozygous Pax2 mutations). Although the resulting nephron deficits are compatible with life, they may be moderately severe and account for up to 40% of the children in dialysis and transplant units around the world. Finally, the effect of Pax2 on apoptosis in the branching ureteric bud seems to imply a quantitative process that is finely tuned. Modest changes in this program could account for subtle nephron deficits in "normal" humans and increased risk of hypertension or susceptibility to acquired renal disease later in life (23).

Bilateral Renal Agenesis

Uniformly fatal, bilateral renal agenesis, although less common than unilateral renal agenesis (URA), is seen more frequently in pediatric autopsies (1.1% of total autopsies in Table 17-1). The incidence of bilateral renal agenesis varies from 0.1/1000 to 0.3/1000 births (8). It accounts for one-third of births with the oligohydramnios sequence (Table 17-2). The male to female ratio is 2.5:1. It is usually associated with severe oligohydramnios (Potter syndrome), intrauterine growth restriction, extrarenal anomalies, and malpresentation. The ureters and renal arteries are also absent, and the urinary bladder is hypoplastic or absent. The adrenals are disc shaped secondary to lack of molding from the kidneys (eFigure 17-3). Forty percent of affected infants are stillborn, and the remainder die in the immediate postnatal period, generally of pulmonary hypoplasia.

Bilateral renal agenesis is usually sporadic, although familial cases have been described (22). Hereditary renal adysplasia (agenesis/dysplasia syndrome) is defined as URA in association with dysplasia of the contralateral kidney. The term adysplasia is often used more broadly to include dysplasia, absent kidneys, and almost any associated structural or positional defect of the kidney or lower urinary tract. However, hereditary adysplasia should be considered as any combination of unilateral or bilateral agenesis, unilateral or bilateral renal dysplasia, or dysplasia of one kidney and agenesis of the other, in different members of the same family for which autosomal dominant inheritance with varying expression has been suggested (9,24). An increased prevalence of congenital renal anomalies was identified in the relatives of index patients with bilateral renal agenesis/adysplasia (14.7%) compared to controls (2.2%), with a recurrence risk of 6.2 for first-degree relatives (25). But the occasional cases of agenesis or dysplasia affecting siblings with normal parents suggest that there are other types of inheritance. Some patients with adysplasia have *PAX2* mutations. The genetic link between renal agenesis and some types of renal dysplasia points to a common pathogenetic mechanism and may result from varying degrees of failure of induction of the metanephric blastema by the ureteric bud.

Other reported malformations associated with bilateral renal agenesis include congenital pulmonary airway malformation type 2 (cystic adenomatoid malformation), left heart hypoplasia (26), sirenomelia (27), and urorectal septum malformation sequence (28). Limb reduction defects and renal agenesis have been reported in fetuses born to mothers with cocaine addiction and insulin-dependent diabetes (29).

The genetic mechanisms leading to bilateral renal agenesis remain largely unresolved. The absence of kidney development in a large number of mouse knockout models suggests a role for recessive mutations in various genes. Indeed, homozygous mutations in *FGF20* have been shown in fetuses from consanguineous families with bilateral renal agenesis (30). More recently, the same researchers have demonstrated recessive mutations in integrin alpha-8 (*ITGA8*) as being responsible for renal agenesis (31). Integrins are transmembrane receptors expressed in metanephric mesenchyme that mediate biologic processes during organogenesis. Interruption of signaling pathway can thus lead to severe kidney developmental defects.

Unilateral Renal Agenesis

URA is a common developmental defect in humans, occurring at a frequency of approximately 1 in 2000 (32). Although compatible with normal life, URA is still seen twice as often in pediatric autopsies (0.6%) than in the general population (0.3%) owing to its frequent association with other complex malformations (33). The male to female ratio is about 1:1.5.

Long-term follow-up of patients with URA has shown that these patients are at higher risk for the development of proteinuria, hypertension, and renal insufficiency.

Malformations of the genitalia are commonly associated with URA. These include ipsilateral absence of fallopian tube, unicornuate and bicornuate uterus, cysts of the epididymis and seminal vesicle, agenesis of the vas deferens, cystic dysplasia of the testis and rete testis, ectopia of the vas deferens, and urorectal septum malformation sequence (ambiguous genitalia with absence of perineal and anal openings) (28,32,34–36).

Cystic dysplasia of the testis appears to be associated consistently with renal malformations, most frequently ipsilateral renal agenesis; both conditions could be explained by failure of development of the ureteric bud (36).

Genetic factors seem to play a significant role in URA, especially when it is part of a syndrome. Mutations in genes such as *HNF1-β, PAX2, SALL1, WT1, SIX1,* and *EYA1* have been shown to cause some of these rare syndromes; however, a genetic basis for the VATER association, in which URA is a common feature, has not yet been identified (32).

Renal Hypoplasia

Renal hypoplasia, defined as histologically normal kidneys with a weight that is less than two standard deviations below the norm, is extremely rare. In the older literature, any small kidney was labeled *hypoplastic*, irrespective of the cause. Currently, small kidneys that are also dysplastic are considered with the dysplastic group, and those with scarring, inflammation, and hypertensive changes are end-stage kidneys with hypoplasia, or more correctly, atrophy, considered secondary to the underlying disease and thusly categorized. Segmental renal hypoplasia (so-called Ask-Upmark kidney), which may be unilateral or bilateral and is characterized by localized atrophic scarring, was originally regarded as a primary malformation is now known to be secondary to vesicoureteral reflux and considered a form of reflux nephropathy.

In true renal hypoplasia, the absolute number of nephrons is reduced, possibly as a consequence of inadequate branching of the ureteric ducts that may result in a decreased number (<5) of reniculi. Although the volume is reduced, the renal shape and differentiation are normal. Unilateral hypoplasia is a sporadic condition, only rarely associated with lower urinary tract anomalies; patients may present with hypertension and occasionally, when associated with malrotation, may be predisposed to reflux nephropathy. Bilateral hypoplasia results in renal insufficiency and early death in severe cases; less severe cases manifest growth retardation and chronic renal insufficiency likely a consequence of developing secondary focal segmental glomerulosclerosis (FSGS) and tubulointerstitial damage as a consequence of hyperfiltration (37).

Bilateral oligomeganephronic renal hypoplasia is a nonfamilial form of congenitally small kidneys characterized by slowly progressive renal insufficiency. The absolute number of nephrons is reduced. The characteristic feature is glomerulomegaly, unlike the normal glomerular size encountered in simple hypoplasia. Infection, dysplasia, and obstructive uropathy are absent, and patients present with polyuria, polydipsia, and salt wasting; proteinuria may develop. Although several causes, including toxic factors, renal infection, vascular insufficiency, and disseminated intravascular coagulation, have been mentioned, it is not known what factors arrest the development of the metanephric renal blastema, presumably between weeks 14 and 20 of fetal life. Mutations in hepatocyte nuclear factor-1beta (*HNF-1β*) and *PAX2* have been reported in patients with oligomeganephronia (23,38). A nephron deficit has also been reported in premature and low-birth-weight infants and has been linked to the development of hypertension in adults (39).

Renal Tubular Dysgenesis

Familial renal tubular dysgenesis (RTD) is a rare autosomal recessive congenital disorder of the renin–angiotensin system (RAS) that causes the absence or marked reduction in the number of differentiated proximal tubules. Mutations in *AGT*, encoding angiotensinogen; *REN*, encoding renin; *ACE*, encoding angiotensin-converting enzyme; or *AGTR1*, encoding angiotensin 2 receptor type 1 (AT1 receptor) affect the production or efficacy of angiotensin 2 and result in the absence of a functional RAS and abnormal renin expression (40). Oligohydramnios is detected as early as 20 weeks' gestation and persists, resulting in the Potter sequence. Fetuses may die *in utero*, but more often, infants die shortly after birth as a consequence of anuria and respiratory failure secondary to lung hypoplasia. Kidneys are normal or slightly enlarged and lack significant ultrasound abnormalities. Intrauterine growth is normal in the genetic form (41). Associated skull ossification defects, attributed to bone hypoxia, spontaneously improve after birth. In most patients, no proximal tubules can be identified by anti-CD10 or anti-CD15 antibodies and glomeruli are closely packed. The medulla contains few loops of Henle, and collecting ducts are atrophic and collapsed and surrounded by abundant mesenchyme. Interlobular arteries and afferent arterioles show thick and disorganized muscular walls, but larger interlobular arteries are normal.

The lack of proximal tubules is not specific for autosomal recessive RTD and has been seen in animals and humans with reduced renal blood flow of various etiologies, confirming the importance of a functional RAS in the maintenance of fetal blood pressure and renal blood flow (41). Secondary RTD has been described in humans with major cardiac malformations, renal artery stenosis, and extensive ischemic necrosis of the placenta and in conjunction with twin–twin transfusion syndrome, neonatal hemochromatosis, and *in utero* exposure to RAS blockers and nonsteroidal anti-inflammatory drugs (NSAIDs) (41,42). Despite the lack of normal proximal tubules, the major site of water resorption in the kidney, the principal clinical manifestations are caused by fetal and neonatal oliguria.

Renomegaly

The most common form of renal enlargement is compensatory hypertrophy, in which a single functioning kidney may reach twice the normal size and can be detected *in utero*. Bilateral renomegaly secondary to an increased number or size of normally developed nephrons is seen in growth-related disorders such as Beckwith-Wiedemann syndrome, hemihypertrophy, Perlman syndrome, and congenital nephrosis of the Finnish type (43,44).

Renal Duplication (Duplex Kidney)

Duplex kidneys are the most common anomalies of the upper urinary tract in childhood with an estimated incidence of 0.8% (45). The term *renal duplication* denotes the presence of two separate pelves in the same kidney accompanied by complete or partial duplication of the ureter (45) (Figure 17-4). These kidneys usually have greater than normal number of reniculi. The anatomical and functional divisions between upper and lower moieties of duplex kidney are extremely variable. The underlying pathologic condition associated with a lower moiety is usually massive vesicoureteral reflux to the lower collecting system and only rarely, obstruction. The nonfunctioning upper moiety is usually associated with obstructive ectopic ureter (with or without ureterocele) and may show chronic tubulointerstitial injury and hypoplastic or dysplastic changes (46). In mice, a model of congenital kidney and urinary tract anomalies, severe early gestational hypoxia resulted in reduced β-catenin signaling and formation of duplex kidneys. This mirrors the defects caused by suppression of canonical Wnt/β-catenin signaling at that stage of development (47).

Supernumerary Kidney

Supernumerary kidney is one of the rarest of renal malformations with fewer than 100 cases reported so far. In addition to the normal two kidneys, an additional, usually small, kidney is present within the renal fascia caudal to and completely separate from the ipsilateral kidney. Few cases of multiple supernumerary kidneys are described (48,49). Most cases are originally diagnosed as hydronephrosis, or pyelonephritis; thus, the true incidence may be higher than reported. The malformation is thought to result from greater than one ureteric bud divergently arising from different positions in the wolffian duct with induction of metanephric blastema and aberrant divisions resulting in at least two kidneys on one side.

Hydronephrosis

Hydronephrosis may be congenital or acquired, unilateral or bilateral, and mild to severe. Renal dysplasia may or may not be present. Hydronephrosis is readily seen on antenatal ultrasonography but does not necessarily imply obstruction. Although most cases will resolve spontaneously, the probability of a significant pathology is related to the degree of pyelectasis, as seen on the third trimester ultrasound study. Criteria of obstruction are difficult to define with precision, but two that are well accepted are size of the renal pelvis (>15 mm) and relative renal function (50).

Hydronephrosis is the most common cause of an abdominal mass of genitourinary tract origin in neonates (51). It is most frequently caused by obstruction of the ureteropelvic junction, which leads to dilatation of the renal pelvis and calyceal system. Depending on the severity and timing of the obstruction, the appearance of the renal parenchyma varies from relatively normal to markedly atrophic, with fibrosis and a scant chronic inflammatory infiltrate (52). One hypothesis for ureteropelvic obstruction is impaired smooth muscle differentiation, aberrant smooth muscle arrangement, and abnormal pyeloureteral innervation, which results in impaired peristalsis and subsequent hydronephrosis (52,53). *FOXF1* is the only gene so far associated with UPJ obstruction in humans (53).

The specimen most commonly seen in surgical pathology is a portion of the ureteropelvic junction that shows remarkably little pathology on microscopic examination. When end-stage nonfunctioning hydronephrotic kidneys are removed, marked dilatation of the pelvis and calyces with only microscopic foci of residual renal parenchyma can be

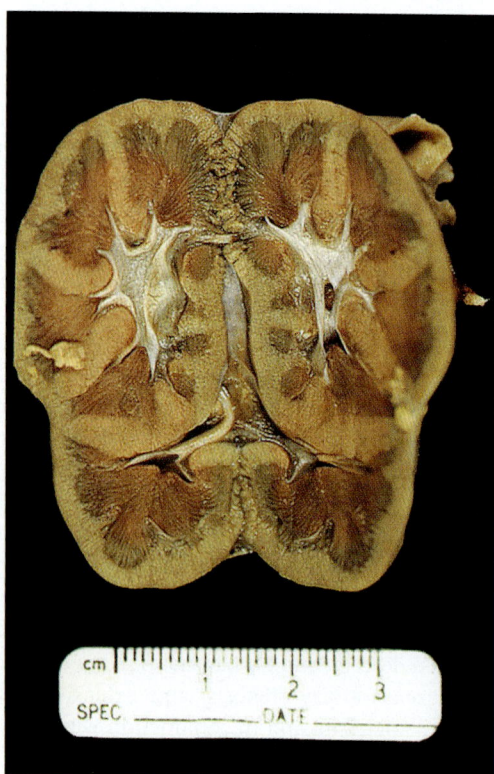

FIGURE 17-4 • Renal duplication (duplex kidney) with two separate pelves in the same kidney and more than the normal number of reniculi.

RENAL DYSPLASIA/CYSTIC DISEASES

Cystic diseases of the kidney are a heterogeneous group of congenital (sporadic and inherited) and acquired disorders characterized by multiple cysts. In view of our better understanding of the genetic basis for some of the cystic renal diseases, the original "Potter classification" with division into types I to IV is no longer widely used (57). There is no universally accepted classification for cystic diseases with categorization dependent upon cyst location, onset (congenital versus acquired), or known etiology (genetic or syndromic association); even renal dysplasia has been variably classified under abnormal renal differentiation or developmental defects or as a unique cystic disease (10).

By convention, the term *multicystic* is reserved for a category of renal dysplasia characterized by multiple unilateral or bilateral cysts, while *polycystic* is conventionally used for hereditary autosomal recessive and autosomal dominant kidney diseases.

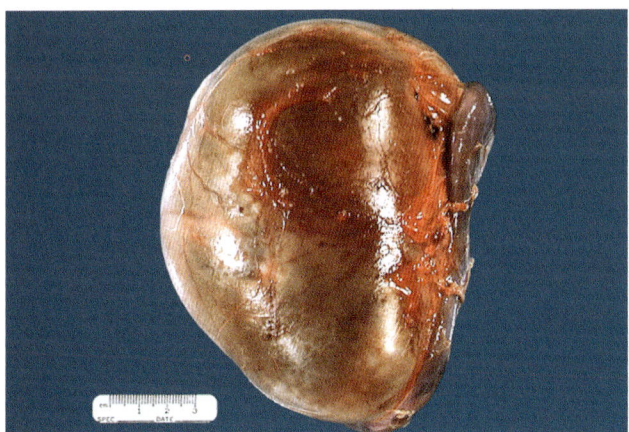

FIGURE 17-5 • Nephrectomy specimen from a 5-year-old who presented with a unilateral renal mass. The kidney appears to be one large cystic structure.

seen (Figures 17-5 and 17-6). Neonatal hydronephrotic kidneys seen at autopsies usually have a histologically normal, although grossly compressed, cortex and medulla.

Hydronephrosis is often associated with renal dysplasia, so that the definition of these two entities often overlaps. Also, because urinary tract obstruction is a common underlying condition, it is best to consider them as the opposite ends of a spectrum. When severe obstruction occurs early in fetal development, it results in renal dysplasia; when it occurs late, one sees hydronephrosis; when it develops in between, both hydronephrosis and dysplasia are apparent to varying degrees. Hydronephrosis associated with reflux disease is discussed later in this chapter in the section on tubulointerstitial diseases (52).

Although the vast majority of cases of hydronephrosis are sporadic, some syndromic associations have been reported (53–55). Hydronephrosis should also be distinguished from the rare disorder of megacalycosis (Puigvert disease), which is characterized by calyceal dilatation, an increased number of calyces, hypoplasia of the pyramids of Malpighi, a normal renal pelvis, and, most importantly, normal renal function (56).

Renal Dysplasia

Multicystic dysplastic kidneys are the most common type of malformed kidneys seen in pediatric autopsies (Table 17-1), with bilateral dysplasia accounting for 32% and unilateral dysplasia (with or without contralateral agenesis) for 7.1% of patients with renal malformations. It may involve one or both kidneys or a portion of one kidney, with or without enlargement of the affected kidney and with or without grossly visible cysts. Thus, the dysplastic kidney may be smaller or larger than normal and grossly misshapen or reniform. Renal dysplasia is one of the most common causes of an abdominal mass in children younger than 1 year; although often diagnosed antenatally, it may present in older children and adulthood (58).

The most common form of dysplasia is sporadic, although genetic causes are being increasingly identified (9,11,33). It is typically associated with obstruction of the ureteropelvic junction and enlarged distorted kidneys that are no longer reniform (Figure 17-7). Cysts of varying sizes can be

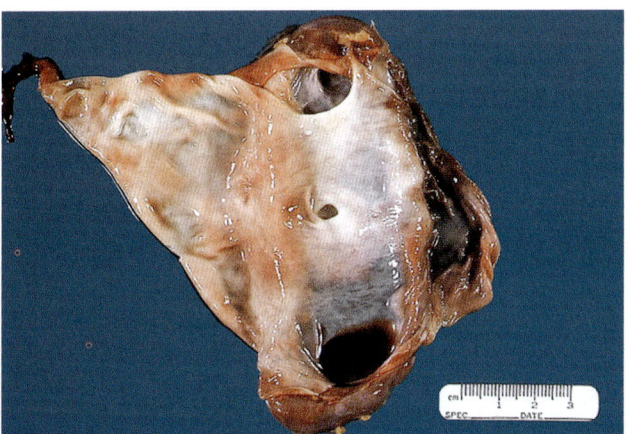

FIGURE 17-6 • Cut section of the kidney in Figure 17-5 shows a markedly dilated pelvis and calyces and very little residual renal parenchyma.

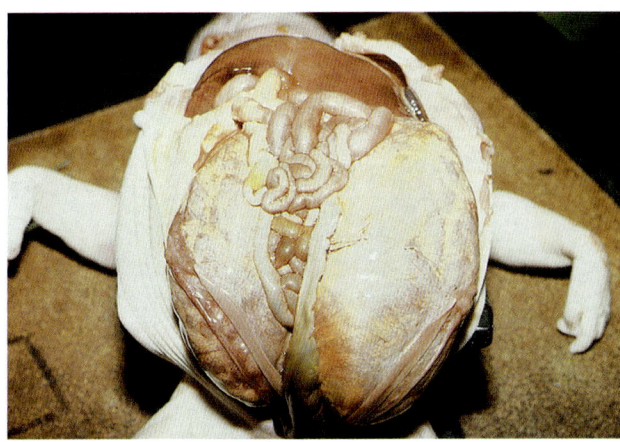

FIGURE 17-7 • Massively enlarged cystic dysplastic kidneys.

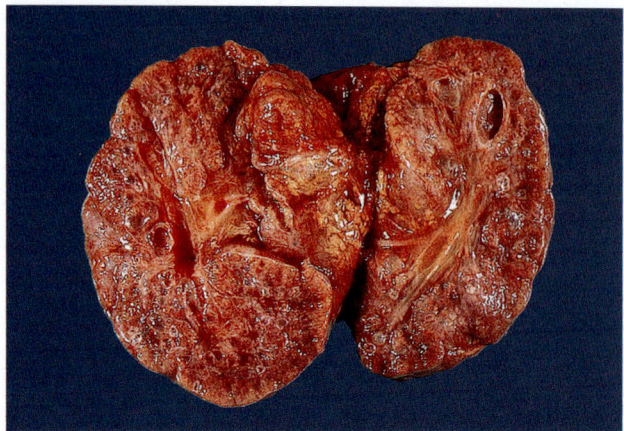

Figure 17-8 • Cut surface of cystic dysplastic kidney with multiple small, variably sized cysts involving both cortex and medulla.

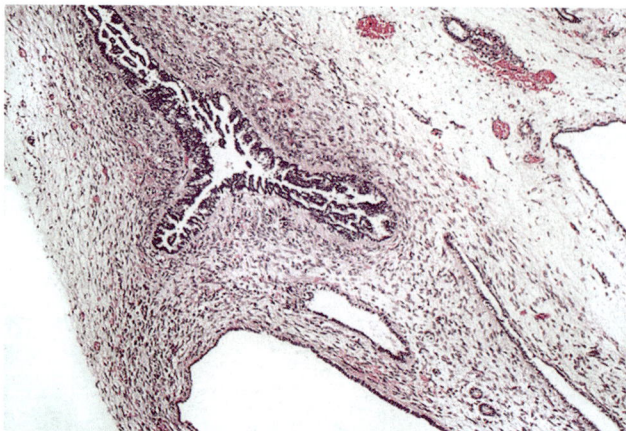

FIGURE 17-10 • Dysplastic tubules with an excessive amount of lining epithelium, which is thrown into papillary folds. (Hematoxylin–eosin stain, original magnification ×40.)

appreciated through the capsule and on sectioning are seen to be irregularly distributed throughout the parenchyma, with no residual identifiable cortex or medulla (Figure 17-8).

The microscopic hallmark is the presence of immature dysplastic-appearing tubules surrounded by collarettes of condensed mesenchyme (Figure 17-9). The tubules are lined by a single layer of primitive undifferentiated cuboidal to columnar epithelium that often appears to be excessive, so that it is folded and may fill the lumen (Figure 17-10). The cells tend to have a relatively high nuclear to cytoplasmic ratio, and the tubular basement membrane may be thick and eosinophilic. A myxoid, moderately cellular condensation of spindle cells encircles the tubules. Ducts and tubules are fewer in number than normal, and the remaining connective tissue is loose and contains many blood vessels, lymphatics, and peripheral nerves. Medullary pyramids often lack vasa recta and loops of Henle. The cortex is usually thin and may contain islands of immature-appearing hyaline cartilage, but their presence is not required for the diagnosis of dysplasia (Figure 17-11). Cysts of varying sizes are formed by the dilated, dysplastic tubules and lined by a markedly flattened, often inapparent, epithelium. Cysts can occur in any part of the nephron. Varying numbers of normal glomeruli and tubules can be identified between the dysplastic areas.

The terms *renal adysplasia (aplastic dysplasia)* and *hypoplastic dysplasia* are used to describe small kidneys with limited nephron development and extensive dysplasia (Figure 17-12) that are totally nonfunctioning or minimally functioning, respectively. The essential histologic features are the same regardless of the size of the kidney or the extent of involvement.

In patients who survive the immediate postnatal period, clinical complications include hypertension, febrile urinary tract infection (UTI), vesicoureteral reflux, progressive scarring, and renal failure. Approximately 50% to 60% of cases undergo involution by 10 years, the rate partly influenced by size on postnatal ultrasound and side (59,60). In 3% to 5% of cases of dysplastic kidney, nodular renal blastema is also present, and although Wilms tumor developing in dysplastic kidney has been reported, a systematic review showed no increased risk of development of WT (61). While the

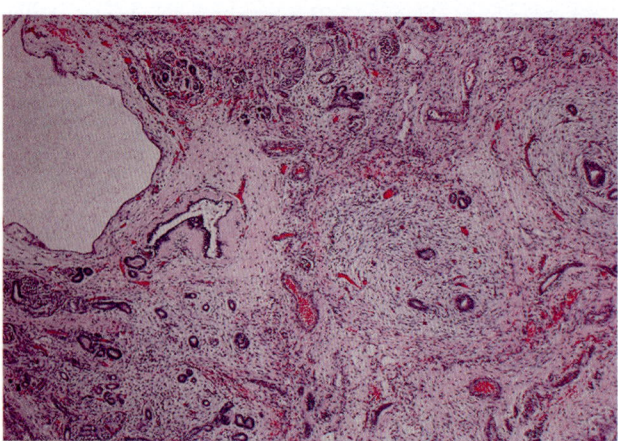

FIGURE 17-9 • Cystic dysplastic kidney with disorganized renal parenchyma in which immature tubules are surrounded by collarettes of condensed mesenchyme. (Hematoxylin–eosin stain, original magnification ×40.)

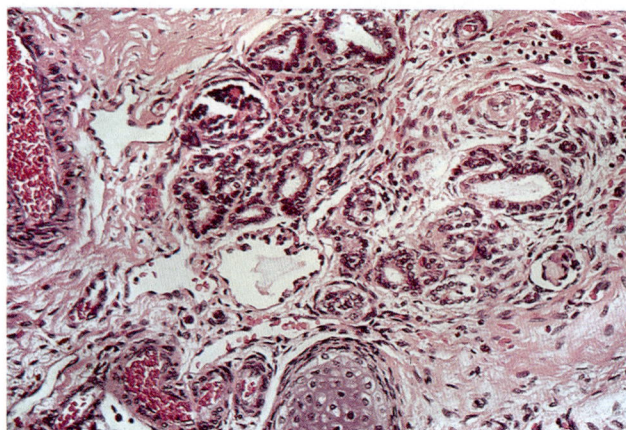

FIGURE 17-11 • Disorganized renal parenchyma and island of immature cartilage in cystic dysplastic kidney disease. (Hematoxylin–eosin stain, original magnification ×100.)

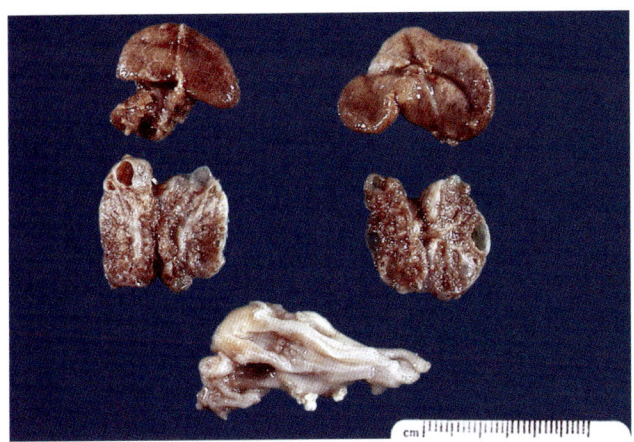

FIGURE 17-12 • Cystic dysplastic kidneys, shown bisected in the middle of the picture, are smaller than the adrenals above.

majority of multicystic dysplastic kidneys (MCDK) can be an isolated finding and is uncommonly bilateral, it is often associated with other (contralateral) anomalies of the kidney and urinary tract. The vast majority of MCDK are associated with congenital urinary tract obstruction, which is often at the ureteropelvic junction but may occur at any level. Several animal models of renal dysplasia after gestational ureteral obstruction have been described (62).

Renal dysplasia is also seen as part of a syndrome in association with extrarenal manifestations. Also, it may be diagnosed sporadically or described with familial aggregation in up to 15% of the cases. When familial, the mode of inheritance is most often autosomal dominant with variable expressivity and reduced penetrance. Epigenetic modifications may explain some of the variability; factors as improbable as maternal diet have been shown to regulate embryonic renal gene expression (63).

Due to the central role of *GDNF–RET* signaling pathway in ureteric budding, it is not surprising that mutations in genes that regulate the pathway, including transcription factors *PAX2*, *EYA1*, and *SALL1*, have been implicated in dysplasia (9,12,24). Mutations in other genes including *DSTYK CHD1L*; *SIX 1, SIX 2*, or *SIX 5*; and *HNF1-β* have also been demonstrated in patients with dysplasia, and a recent large genetic screening study of 749 individuals with various nonsyndromic renal abnormalities identified *SALL1*, *PAX2*, and *HNF1-β* as the most prevalent disease-causing genes (24). An excellent and exhaustive tabulation of these can be found at the end of Chapter 27 in Potter Pathology of the Fetus, Infant, and Child (64). A brief summary is provided in Table 17-4.

Earlier work had shown that apoptosis is prominent in undifferentiated cells around dysplastic tubules, which perhaps explains the tendency of these organs to regress. In contrast, apoptosis was rare in dysplastic epithelia, thought to be ureteric bud malformations. A high rate of proliferation has been demonstrated postnatally in dysplastic tubules, and PAX2, a potentially oncogenic transcription factor, is expressed in these epithelia. In contrast, both cell proliferation and PAX2 are down-regulated during normal maturation of human collecting ducts. Ectopic expression of BCL2, which encodes a protein that prevents apoptosis during renal mesenchymal to epithelial conversion, has been observed in dysplastic kidney epithelia. Thus, dysplastic cyst formation may be understood in terms of aberrant temporal and spatial expression of master genes that are tightly regulated in normal human nephrogenesis.

Polycystic Kidney Disease

According to current concepts, the term *polycystic kidneys* should be used to describe only two forms of inherited disease, autosomal recessive (ARPKD) and autosomal dominant (ADPKD) polycystic kidney disease, and not for any other disease in which multiple renal cysts are present. Despite different patterns of inheritance, clinical presentation, and typical appearance of the kidneys, these two diseases have some similarities. Both diseases are caused by mutations in proteins located in primary cilia, resulting in renal concentrating defect, and both are characterized by increased rates of tubular epithelial proliferation, apoptosis, and secretion as well as elevated levels of tissue cAMP (65). Elucidation of the pathogenic mechanisms of PKDs has been aided by the availability of several animal models. Rodent models have arisen by spontaneous mutation, random mutagenesis, transgenic technologies, or gene-specific targeting. Many of the proteins encoded by these mutated genes are expressed in the primary cilium or the centrosome—indicating the importance of the ciliary–centrosomal axis to normal tubular epithelial cell differentiation—or at sites of cell–cell or cell–matrix adhesion. Cytogenesis is partly the result of loss-of-function mutations in these genes or from loss-of function or gain-of-function mutations in genes that encode downstream signaling molecules and transcription factors in the cystogenic pathway (65,66).

Autosomal Recessive Polycystic Kidney Disease

ARPKD is rare, with an incidence of 1 in 20,000 live births, and shows extreme variability in its severity. It is caused by mutations in the polycystic kidney and hepatic disease (PKHD1) gene, named for the consistent hepatic involvement, located on chromosome 6p21.1-p12 (67). The gene encodes fibrocystin/polyductin that is expressed predominantly in the kidney (mostly collecting ducts and thick ascending loops of Henle), liver (bile duct epithelium), and pancreas. Fibrocystin/polyductin localizes to apical membranes, the primary cilia/basal body, and the mitotic spindle (68).

In ARPKD, nephrogenesis proceeds normally, and the earliest abnormality involves the medullary ducts. Oligohydramnios occurs subsequently (usually before 20 to 21 weeks of gestation). These observations suggest that in severe fetal ARPKD, medullary collecting duct dilatation occurs first and is successively followed by cortical collecting duct dilatation, increased renal echogenicity, and diminution of urine production (67,69–72).

TABLE 17-4 SYNDROMES AND DISEASES ASSOCIATED WITH RENAL DYSPLASIA

Name	Heredity	Chromosomal Defect	Major Features	Congenital Hepatic Fibrosis
Meckel-Gruber syndrome Joubert	AR	MKS1-MKS10, JBTS1-JBTS20	Posterior encephalocele, polydactyly, microcephaly	Yes
Zellweger syndrome	AR	PEX 1–3; 5–6; 10–11; 13;14;16;19; 26	Peroxisomal deficiency, cerebrohepatorenal syndrome	Yes
Ivemark (II) syndrome[a]	AR	NPHP3; NEK8	Renal–hepatic–pancreatic dysplasia	Yes
Jeune syndrome	AR	IFT80 (ATD2), DYNC2H1 (ADT3), ADT1, ADT4, ADT5	Asphyxiating thoracic dystrophy	Yes
Carnitine palmitoyl-transferase deficiency	AR	CPT2	Myopathy	No
Short rib-polydactyly syndrome	AR	NEK1, DYNC2H1	Lethal skeletal dysplasias, multiple anomalies	Yes
Hereditary renal adysplasia	AD, XL	Various; see text	URA with contralateral dysplasia	No
Nail-patella syndrome	AD	LMX1b mutation	Hypoplastic nails, absent patellae, glomerular changes	No
Tuberous sclerosis complex	AD	TSC1:9q34 TSC2:16p13.3	Tumors of the skin, brain, heart, and kidney	No
von Hippel-lindau syndrome carcinoma, pheochromocytoma, pancreatic islet cell tumors	AD mutations	VHL	Retinal and CNS hemangioblastomas, renal cysts–clear cell carcinoma	No
Beckwith-Wiedemann syndrome	Usually sporadic	11p15.5 alterations	Organomegaly, nephroblastomatosis, WT	No
DiGeorge syndrome	Sporadic	DGS1 del(22q11) DGS2 del(10p)	Hypoplasia of thymus and aortic arch defects	No
Prune belly sequence	Sporadic	UK	Deficient abdominal wall musculature, urinary tract dilatation, cryptorchidism	No
Trisomies 13, 18, 21	Risk factor: advanced maternal age	13, 18, 21		No
Fetal alcohol syndrome	*In utero* exposure	UK	CNS dysfunction, growth deficits	No
Diabetic embryopathy	*In utero* exposure	UK	Macrosomia, congenital malformations, stillbirth	No

[a]Not to be confused with asplenia and cardiac malformations, also known as *Ivemark (I) syndrome*.
AR, autosomal recessive; AD, autosomal dominant; XL, X-linked; UK, unknown; CNS, central nervous system.
Hartung EA, Guay-Woodford LM. Autosomal recessive polycystic kidney disease: a hepatorenal fibrocystic disorder with pleiotropic effects. *Pediatrics* 2014;134:e833–e845; Guay-Woodford LM, Bissler JJ, Braun MC, et al. Consensus expert recommendations for the diagnosis and management of autosomal recessive polycystic kidney disease: report of an international conference. *J Pediatr* 2014;165:611–617.

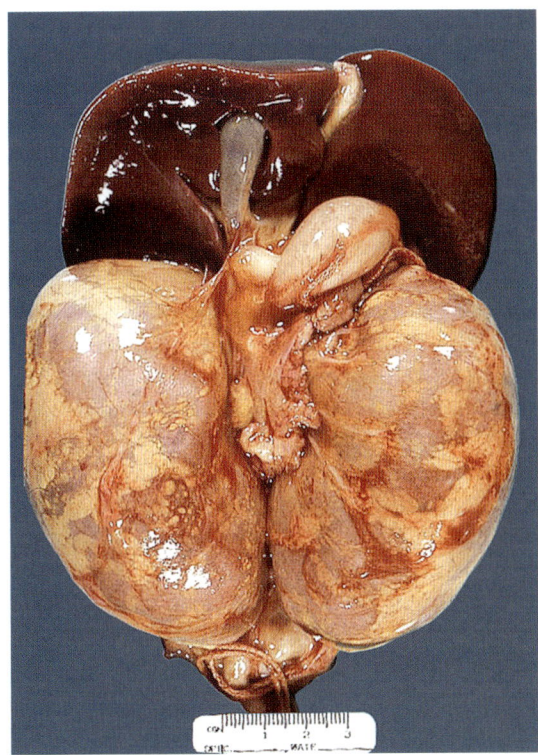

FIGURE 17-13 • Autosomal recessive polycystic kidney disease with massively enlarged symmetric reniform kidneys.

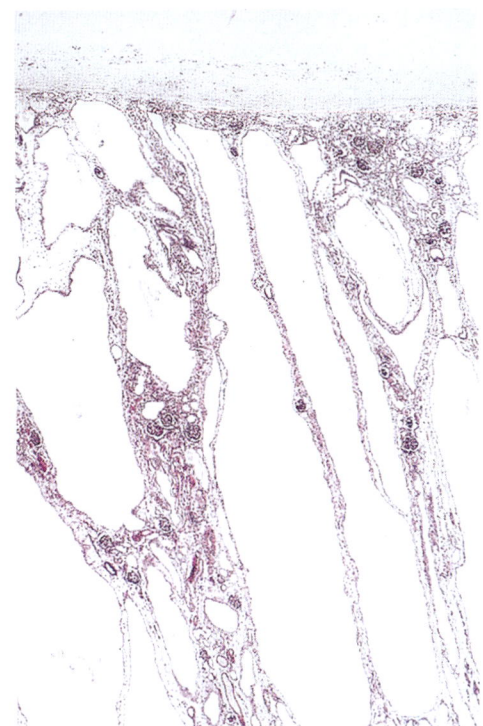

FIGURE 17-15 • Radially arranged cysts of autosomal recessive polycystic kidney disease. Normal glomeruli and tubules are seen between the cysts. (Hematoxylin–eosin stain, original magnification ×40.)

Thirty to fifty percent of patients present with oligohydramnios (Potter sequence): massively enlarged, symmetric, reniform kidneys (Figure 17-13) and pulmonary hypoplasia. Death occurs in the perinatal period. The gross and microscopic hallmark is the presence of tubular cysts with a diameter of 1 to 2 mm arranged radially. The cysts are uniformly distributed and can be appreciated through the capsule of the markedly enlarged kidneys, which retain their shape (Figure 17-14). On cut section, the cortex and the medulla are often unrecognizable. The cysts represent tubular dilatation of presumably normally formed collecting ducts; normal glomeruli

and tubules are seen between the cysts (Figure 17-15). In the medulla, the cysts are more rounded. Significant fibrosis, inflammation, and obstruction are absent (72).

In cases with a later presentation, the degree of renal enlargement is less and the cystic change is less diffuse. However, all forms of ARPKD are associated with congenital hepatic fibrosis (*ductal plate malformation*), although the clinical expression of liver disease varies widely (see Chapter 15). Dilatation of the interlobular bile ducts is associated with a variable degree of portal fibrosis (73). The lobular architecture of the liver is preserved, but all portal areas are expanded and contain tortuous, slightly dilated ducts at the periphery with blood vessels in the middle (Figure 17-16). Stereologic studies have indicated that what appear as ducts on histologic section are in fact cisterns communicating with each other. Similar hepatic changes are seen in Meckel, Zellweger, and Jeune syndromes, medullary cystic disease complex, and tuberous sclerosis (67,71).

Mutational analysis of ARPKD presenting as infants and congenital hepatic fibrosis presenting in later childhood or adulthood with minimal or no renal disease has defined a broader spectrum of ARPKD. Genotype–phenotype correlations for the type of PKHD1 mutation have been shown. Patients with two truncating mutations usually display a severe phenotype with peri- or neonatal demise, whereas patients surviving the neonatal period bear one hypomorphic missense mutation that is expected to allow for the expression of a minimal amount of full-length fibrocystin

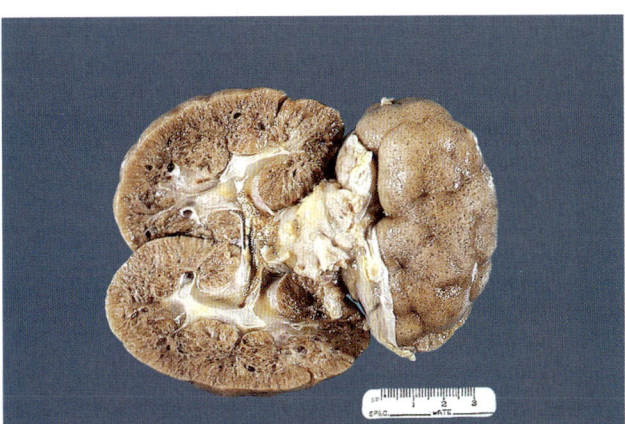

FIGURE 17-14 • Cysts of autosomal recessive polycystic kidney disease can be appreciated on the cortical surface. The cut section shows radially oriented cysts in the cortex and more rounded cysts in the medulla.

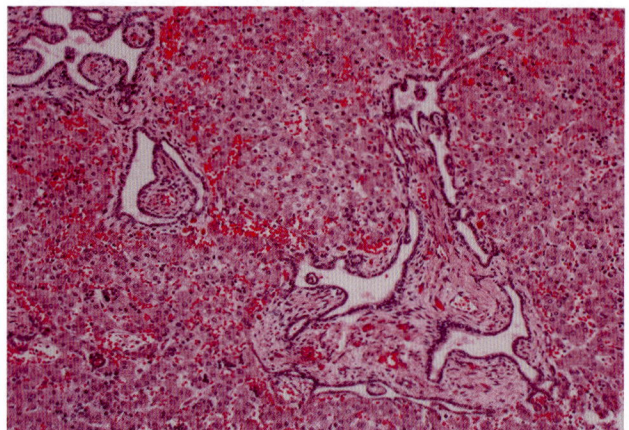

FIGURE 17-16 • Ductal plate malformation of the liver with expanded portal area, peripheral tortuous dilated bile ducts, and blood vessels in the middle. (Hematoxylin–eosin stain, original magnification ×40.)

protein. From these data, researchers have concluded that the milder mutation defines the phenotype. No significant clinical differences have been observed between patients with two missense mutations and those with a truncating mutation in trans to a missense mutation (67).

Up to 30% of patients die in the perinatal period (72). The clinical course of children with ARPKD who survive the neonatal period is variable with ESRD developing in infancy, early childhood, or adolescence. Improved outcomes with kidney and/or liver transplantation are reported (74). A small percentage of long-term survivors are at increased risk of developing benign and malignant liver tumors, particularly cholangiocarcinoma (75). Early detection and appropriate management of renal failure and systemic portal hypertension are important.

Autosomal Dominant Polycystic Kidney Disease

Commonly referred to as *adult PKD* because the vast majority of cases become symptomatic in the fourth and into the fifth decade of life, ADPKD is more common than ARPKD, occurs worldwide, and affects all races with a prevalence estimated to be between 1:400 and 1:1000 (76). ADPKD accounts for about 5% of cases of ESRD.

ADPKD has two disease loci, PKD1 and PKD2, that encode the membrane glycoproteins, polycystin-1 and polycystin-2 (PC1 and PC2, respectively), which have been localized to the primary cilia of the renal epithelial cells (77). The primary cilia are fingerlike projections on the surface of all kidney cells, except acid–base transporting intercalated cells in the collecting duct. Renal cilia bend in response to fluid flow, which activates PC1, that results in activation of PC2, which leads to calcium influx and changes in gene transcription (78). Abnormal cilia structure or function or both may lead to abnormalities in cell proliferation and tubular differentiation, ultimately leading to cyst formation. Recent studies however have highlighted the complexity of cyst formation. Although abnormal or absent cilia are demonstrated in many "ciliopathies," cilia are not required for cyst formation and the presence of intact cilia may actually cause worsening of cystic kidney disease in the presence of abnormal PKD proteins. Noncilia-associated proteins also influence cilia structure and function (77,79,80).

Approximately 85% of affected families have mutations in PKD1 gene, which has been mapped to chromosome 16p13.3, and the remaining 15% have mutations in PKD2, which has been localized to chromosome 4q22. Affected persons in these families appear to have a phenotypic similar to that in PKD1 families, but the onset of cystic disease, hypertension, and renal insufficiency is delayed (66). A third gene, PKD3, has been suspected since approximately 10% of families have disease apparently unlinked to PKD1 or PKD2; recent vigorous re-evaluation of previous "PKD3" families has identified *PKD1* or *PKD2* mutations in four of the five families (81). Mistaken classifications or failure to detect linkage may result from the use of nonflanking markers, the presence of *de novo* mutations, mosaicism, or complex inheritance of hypomorphic alleles (81).

Autosomal dominant polycystic kidney disease diagnosed *in utero* or in the first year of life is associated with more severe renal cystic disease and an increased risk of hypertension and early loss of kidney function. Gross hematuria, truncating *PKD1* mutations, male sex, childhood onset of hyperfiltration, microalbuminuria or frank proteinuria, elevated copeptin levels (surrogate of circulating arginine vasopressin), and elevated total kidney volume have all been associated with rapid ADPKD progression (82).

Although the majority of ADPKD infants survive, they tend to have more significant hypertension and a more rapid decline in renal function than do their affected adult relatives (83). Children can present with acute or chronic abdominal, back or flank pain, hypertension, proteinuria, or hematuria. Urolithiasis is more common in children with ADPKD than the general population. Very extensive structural disease is required for any measurable decrease in eGFR, and the majority of affected children maintain normal eGFR. The kidneys vary in size from normal to enlarged, and rounded cysts range in size from microscopic (in asymptomatic children with disease detected on screening performed because of a positive family history) to about 3 cm in diameter. The kidneys may lose their reniform shape and become distorted by multiple cysts. Some infants and children present with unilateral renal cysts (83). Glomerulocystic disease may be the most common appearance of early-onset ADPKD (84). Residual parenchyma is compressed by the enlarging cysts and eventually becomes atrophic and fibrotic. In contrast to the cysts seen in ARPKD, these cysts occur in any part of the nephron and are present in both the cortex and the medulla (Figure 17-17, eFigure 17-4). Hepatic, pancreatic, and splenic cysts can occur in childhood ADPKD, most commonly teenagers, but usually only as a few small cysts. The prevalence of mitral valve prolapse is about 12% in ADPKD children (83).

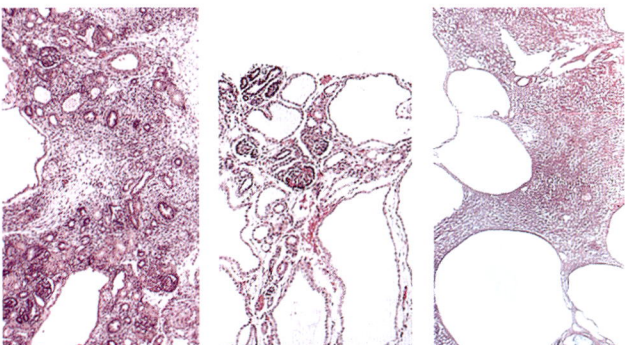

FIGURE 17-17 • Low-power photomicrographs illustrate the differences between cystic dysplastic kidney (**left**), autosomal recessive polycystic kidney disease (**middle**), and autosomal dominant polycystic kidney disease (**right**). (Hematoxylin-eosin stain, original magnification ×40.)

Medullary Cysts

Cysts in the medulla can occur as part of several cystic kidney diseases (e.g., multicystic dysplasia, ARPKD, and ADPKD). The term *medullary cystic disease* generally conjures three clinically and pathologically distinct entities.

Medullary Sponge Kidney

Also referred to as *precalyceal canalicular ectasia*, medullary sponge kidney is generally considered a sporadic disease; however, a few pedigrees have been described with an apparent autosomal dominant inheritance. A recent study demonstrated that 50% of stone-forming patients with MSK have affected relatives with milder forms of the disease (85). Reduced penetrance and variable expressivity imply that the disorder is not an uncommon cause of calcium kidney stones, just uncommonly recognized. It most commonly presents in adults, although some cases have been described in children and even infants. MSK has been associated with other renal and extrarenal malformations supporting the assumption that it is a congenital disorder (86). Medullary sponge kidney is a developmental disorder characterized by ectatic and cystic malformation of the papillary collecting ducts in the renal medulla; the condition is most often bilateral, but it may involve only one kidney or only one or several reniculi. Medullary sponge kidney affects both genders and remains symptomless unless complicated by UTI, renal stones, or hematuria—hence its presentation in later life (86). It is best diagnosed by intravenous pyelography (IVP), which shows dilated medullary tubules and the so-called papillary blush or bouquet of flowers; however, IVP has become an obsolescent test, having been replaced as a screening tool for renal colic by noncontrast CT, which has a low sensitivity for the diagnosis. MSK can be recognized by CT urography with contrast and even ultrasound interpreted by knowledgeable radiologists (87). Heterozygous GDNF mutations have been identified in some patients with MSK in regions of the gene that bind to PAX2, which has a crucial role in nephrogenesis (86,88).

Nephronophthisis

Originally described as two separate diseases, nephronophthisis (NPH) and medullary cystic kidney disease (MCKD) were subsequently considered to be part of the same complex, with similar clinicopathologic features; they are both inherited as progressive tubulointerstitial diseases characterized by medullary cyst formation and secondary glomerular sclerosis. Newer molecular techniques have proven that NPH and MCKD are clearly genetically distinct entities (89).

NPH is an autosomal recessive disease and is one of the most common genetic causes of ESRD in children and adolescents (90). Nearly 20 genes have been implicated and almost all of the gene products, including those of the nephrocystin protein family, are expressed in primary cilia, leading to the classification of NPH as a ciliopathy. NPH occurs as an isolated kidney disease, but approximately 15% of patients have extrarenal manifestations such as retinal degeneration in Senior-Loken syndrome, cerebellar vermis aplasia in Joubert syndrome, cone-shaped epiphyses of the phalanges in Mainzer-Saldino syndrome, or liver fibrosis and situs inversus (91). Several syndromal ciliopathies including Bardet-Biedl syndrome, Meckel-Gruber syndrome (MKS), and Jeune syndrome can present with renal NPH. Gene locus heterogeneity, allelism, and modifier genes influence the phenotype with renal manifestations ranging from isolated "degenerative" (tubulointerstitial damage with progressive medullary cysts) disease to "dysplastic" (perinatal multicystic dysplasia) disease with multiorgan involvement, the latter attributed to ubiquitous expression of NPHP proteins (92).

NPH is characterized by polyuria, polydipsia, salt wasting, secondary enuresis, and anemia and proceeds to end-stage renal disease. Three clinical forms are distinguished as the most common variant, juvenile NPH (type 1) in which ESRD occurs at a mean age of 13 years, but symptoms may present as early as 6 years of age; the rare infantile NPH (type 2) with onset of ESRD prior to 4 years of age; and adolescent NPH (type 3) that has a mean age of ESRD of 19 years. Symptoms in early stages may be subtle, but hypertension, growth retardation, and anemia emerge as renal echogenicity and renal failure progress. With advanced disease, corticomedullary cysts are seen. The cysts, 1 to 15 mm in diameter, are located primarily at the corticomedullary junction and present in only 70% of the patients; the remaining patients have no cysts. All cases have in common nonspecific tubulointerstitial disease with tubular atrophy and basement membrane thinning, thickening, and lamellation plus interstitial fibrosis and inflammation, which is usually more severe than the cystic component. In contrast to types 1 and 3, the kidneys in infantile NPH (type 2) are often enlarged and demonstrate not only tubulointerstitial alterations but widespread cyst development that can mimic polycystic kidney disease (90,91,93).

Medullary Cystic Kidney Disease

In contrast to NPH, MCKD has a dominant inheritance and ESRD usually occurs in adulthood but is extremely variable, ranging from 20 to 70 years. They share the same clinical renal presentation, except for the growth retardation and extrarenal malformations, which are absent in MCKD. Two forms are recognized: MCKD1 and MCKD2, and the genetic defects in both have recently been elucidated. MCKD1 is caused by a mutation in *MUC1*, which encodes mucoprotein 1 that is expressed in skin, breast, lung, and the gastrointestinal tract. In MCKD1, patients develop hyperuricemia (gout) secondary to renal failure, rather than as a primary manifestation of the disease, as seen in MCKD2. The kidney shows marked tubulointerstitial damage but no cysts (94). MCKD2 is caused by mutations in the uromodulin gene, *UMOD*, which encodes uromodulin (Tamm-Horsfall protein), the most abundant protein in human urine. UMOD mutations are responsible for a group of hereditary autosomal dominant tubulointerstitial diseases (often referred to as uromodulin-associated kidney disease), encompassing MCKD2, familial juvenile hyperuricemic nephropathy, and glomerulocystic kidney disease. Patients with MCKD2 develop tubulointerstitial nephritis in adulthood, but the earliest symptoms of hyperuricemia and gout develop in adolescence. Renal imaging demonstrates corticomedullary cysts, and histology shows interstitial fibrosis with tubular atrophy (95–97). New mutations and incomplete penetrance explain the absence of family history in approximately 15% of patients (96).

Cortical Cysts

While cystic dilatation of various parts of the nephron can involve the renal cortex (i.e., cystic change of the collecting ducts in ARPKD), cortical cysts primarily refer to glomerular cysts, characterized as cystic dilatation of Bowman space. The glomerulocystic kidney was recognized in the 1800s (84). The term *disease* is generally reserved for the familial autosomal dominant or sporadic GCK in which a cause is not identified. Bernstein delineated the diagnosis by defining the glomerular cyst as dilatation of Bowman space in the plane of section of two- to threefold that of normal (Figure 17-18) and considered that the presence of glomerular tufts within at least 5% of cysts as evidence to support the diagnosis of glomerulocystic kidney (98). The only evidence of a glomerular tuft may be a cluster of cells adherent to the cyst wall, but the presence of tubular cysts does not preclude the diagnosis. The cysts are usually round, ovoid, or polygonal, range from less than 0.1 cm to greater than 1.0 cm, and can be empty or filled with proteinaceous material or debris.

It is now recognized that GCK is not a single entity but can be categorized as primary or secondary. The former includes (a) autosomal dominant GCKD such as those due to *UMOD*, *REN*, or *TCF2* mutations; (b) GCK associated with familial nonsyndromic cystic disease (ADPKD and ARPKD); (c) GCK associated with heritable syndromes such as tuberous sclerosis (TSC), NPH (*NPHP3* mutations), Jeune syndrome,

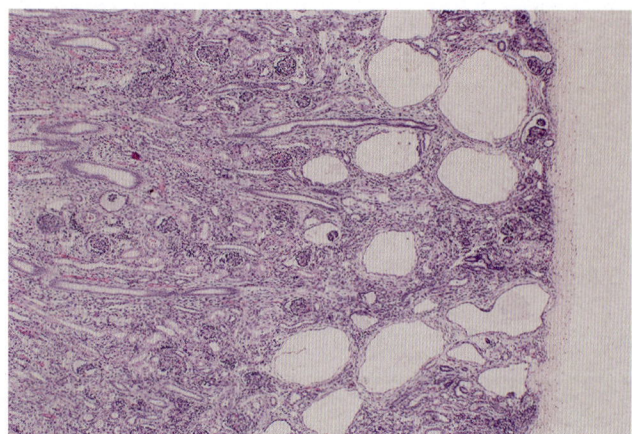

FIGURE 17-18 • GCKD with cystic dilatation of Bowman spaces; the medulla is uninvolved. (Hematoxylin–eosin stain, original magnification ×40.)

orofacialdigital syndrome type 1, glutaric aciduria type 2, Zellweger syndrome, among others; and (d) various genetic abnormalities including trisomies 21, 18, 13, and 9 and monosomy X. In the latter two categories, glomerular cysts are often a minor component, for example, Jeune syndrome and NPH, better known for chronic progressive tubulointerstitial disease, and Zellweger syndrome where glomerular cysts are scattered within the cortex but usually inconsequential and only occasionally serious enough to affect renal function. In all the syndrome and genetic abnormalities, the cysts are inconsistently expressed. Secondary and acquired causes relate to (a) ischemia (postthrombotic microangiopathy—hemolytic–uremic syndrome/thrombotic thrombocytopenic purpura (HUS/TTP), vasculitis, or renal artery stenosis); (b) drugs (lithium, corticosteroids); (c) renal dysplasia; and (d) obstruction (10,84,99).

Most GCKD cases are transmitted according to an autosomal dominant mode of inheritance (84). This disease is often discovered in infants within the context of a familial history of ADPKD. The most common cause in neonates and young children in one series of 20 patients (aged 30 weeks' gestation age to 78 years) was dysplasia (84). Adult presentation has been described along with unilateral disease, both typically associated with secondary etiologies (84). Ultrasonographically, minute cysts, smaller than those occurring in the usual autosomal dominant polycystic kidney disease, are seen in the echogenic renal cortex. No cysts are observed in the renal medulla, in ADGCKD, but may been seen with other etiologies. Kidneys in ADGCKD and ADPKD presenting with a GCK phenotype are bilaterally enlarged and diffusely cystic, in which the main microscopic finding is represented by glomerular cysts, but an asymmetric onset of this disease has also been seen. Kidneys in sporadic GCKD of non-ADPKD phenotype can have either clustered or diffuse cysts and are either slightly larger or normal in size.

Finally, in familial hypoplastic GCKD, the kidneys are smaller than normal and often associated with medullocalyceal abnormalities (100). Familial hypoplastic GCKD is associated with mutations in *TCF2*, which encodes HNF1-β, and is considered the main cause of fetal hyperechoic kidneys (100) and, in some families, is associated with maturity-onset diabetes of the young, type V (MODY5) (101,102). Glomerular cysts in all types of GCKD are less than 1 cm in size and located in the cortex from the subcapsular zone to the inner cortex (eFigure 17-5), and are histologically similar to glomerular cysts seen in other disease conditions.

Simple Cysts

Simple cortical cysts, or retention cysts, which are very common in adults, are rarely seen in children. They are typically asymptomatic and incidentally discovered. They are important because they may present as an abdominal mass, or their appearance ultrasonographic or radiologic images may raise the diagnostic consideration of cystic WT. The diagnosis is established on the basis of typical radiographic findings with surrounding normal renal parenchyma, normal renal function, and the absence of systemic illness or disorders. Simple cysts arise from the cortex, are unilocular, contain yellow clear fluid, and are lined by a single layer of cuboidal epithelium. The cysts may slowly increase in size, at a rate averaging 0.3 mm and 1.0% per year, but can also disappear (103). In addition to excluding malignancy, follow-up should be undertaken to exclude an early presentation of ADPKD, especially when there are bilateral or multiple unilateral cysts (104,105).

Cysts Associated with Syndromes

Cysts of the cortex (sometimes referred to as *pluricystic kidney*), are usually asymptomatic, and have been described as a minor component of multiple malformation syndromes, both inheritable and noninheritable, including tuberous sclerosis; von Hippel-Lindau (VHL) disease; MKS; orofaciodigital syndrome type I; trisomies 9, 13, 18, and 21; short rib-polydactyly syndrome; Jeune asphyxiating thoracic dystrophy syndrome; Zellweger cerebrohepatorenal syndrome; VATER association; lissencephaly; renal-hepatic-pancreatic dysplasia; glutaric aciduria type II; Ellis-van Creveld syndrome; Elejalde syndrome; Peutz-Jeghers syndrome; Robert syndrome; phocomelia syndrome or pseudothalidomide syndrome; and Bardet-Biedl syndrome (13). In the following diseases, the renal cysts are often a dominant feature of the disease and histologically distinct from dysplasia.

Tuberous Sclerosis

Tuberous sclerosis complex is an autosomal dominant systemic malformation syndrome caused by mutations in *TSC1* on chromosome 9q34 (encoding hamartin) and *TSC2* on chromosome 16p13.3 (encoding tuberin). Hamartin and tuberin form a complex that acts as a tumor suppressor by inhibiting mammalian target of rapamycin (mTOR) signaling, which is implicated in proliferation, cell cycle control,

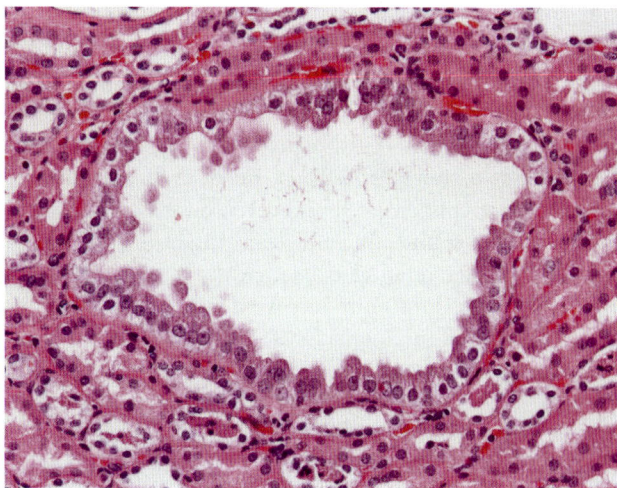

FIGURE 17-19 • Renal cysts of tuberous sclerosis lined by characteristic hyperplastic epithelium with abundant eosinophilic granular cytoplasm. (Hematoxylin–eosin stain, original magnification ×200.) (Courtesy of Dr. John Hicks, Houston, TX).

and regulation of cell size (106). It is characterized by hamartomatous proliferations of the skin, brain, kidney, eye, bone, liver, and lung. In addition to the well-recognized association with renal angiomyolipomas, which occur in 40% to 80% of patients with tuberous sclerosis, characteristic cortical cysts are present in about 50% of patients. Unilateral renal cystic disease has been rarely reported, and glomerulocystic kidney disease is well known (106). The severe, very early-onset polycystic phenotype is associated with mutations that involve the adjacent *TSC2* and PKD1 genes on chromosome 16p13 and accounts for about 2% of patients (107). The extent of involvement varies; small cysts may be diagnosed on imaging, or "polycystic kidneys" may lead to renal failure. The cysts vary in size and are lined by hyperplastic epithelium, which is often multilayered and papillary, with abundant eosinophilic granular cytoplasm (Figure 17-19). The histologic findings are so characteristic as to be virtually diagnostic of tuberous sclerosis when seen in an early biopsy performed before the onset of other stigmata of the disease. Solid nodules of these cells may also form, and nuclear atypia and pleomorphism may be present. Mitotic activity evident in these cells may be related to the increased risk for neoplasia; cystic renal carcinomas with a granular eosinophilic macrocystic morphology have been considered a distinct pattern of TSC (108).

Von Hippel-Lindau Disease

VHL disease is an autosomal dominant multisystem (pre) neoplastic disorder genetically linked to a germline mutation of a tumor-suppressor gene (*VHL* gene) located on chromosome 3p25. The incidence of VHL disease is about one in 36,000 births and the penetrance is high. It is characterized by hemangioblastomas of the retina, brain, and spinal cord, pheochromocytomas, and cysts and tumors of the pancreas, kidneys, and, less frequently, other abdominal organs (69). Multiple renal cysts and tumors develop in approximately two-thirds of patients with VHL disease (109). The most common imaging finding is multiple small unilateral or bilateral renal cysts, although renal function is usually retained (110). Less frequently, the cysts are numerous enough to simulate ADPKD. Renal cysts are lined by flattened clear epithelial cells; however, dysplastic microfoci of hyperplastic epithelium with clear cytoplasm and a "hobnail" appearance, often associated with complex cysts, are associated with a markedly increased risk for the development of renal cell carcinoma (RCC) (111). Multifocal cystic adenocarcinomas develop in 45% to 50% of patients beyond the third decade of life and in about 70% by the fifth decade (69,109). Most RCCs are of the clear cell type although clear cell papillary RCCs have been reported in patients with VHL disease (112).

Meckel-Gruber Syndrome

MKS has an autosomal recessive inheritance and shares significant phenotypic and genotypic overlap with other ciliopathies including the primarily kidney disorder NPH and the neurodevelopmental disorder Joubert syndrome. Patients harboring the same genetic mutation can express a broad range of neurologic and renal involvement; thus, despite the varied clinical presentations, the genotype–phenotype correlations are frequently unclear and there is significant inter- and intrafamilial heterogeneity. These features suggest the operative effects of modifiers and genetic interactions including triallelic inheritance (90). Mutations in at least 16 different genes have been shown to be causative in MKS in humans (113). Many of the genes are linked to ciliary biology, but several are predicted to produce transmembrane proteins or those found in the actin cytoskeleton or influence microtubule organization, vesicle trafficking, and signal transduction. Several of the MKS genes interfere with normal Wnt signaling, which is a key player in the development of cystic kidney disease (114,115). MKS has a reported mean prevalence of 2.6 per 100,000 births, and nowadays, most patients are detected very early in pregnancy (116). It is characterized by cystic kidneys, posterior encephalocele, and polydactyly and frequently associated with other CNS anomalies, fibrocystic changes of the liver, (congenital hepatic fibrosis/ductal plate malformation), and orofacial clefts. The kidneys are always bilaterally involved, although they may occasionally be variably involved. Round cysts arise from any part of the nephron, with microcysts seen in the subcapsular area and larger cysts in the medulla. The cysts are lined by a single layer of low-to-high cuboidal epithelium and are separated by loose, immature mesenchyme that may bulge into the cysts. Metaplastic cartilage is not usually present.
The pathogenesis of renal cysts in Meckel syndrome follows the mechanisms of other ciliopathies and is related to defects in ciliary signaling with perturbation of cell growth, polarity, and cell fate determination (113). Study of midterm fetuses has shown that the kidneys are already enlarged by 11 to 20 weeks of gestation (117). Nephrogenesis may appear normal at the periphery of the kidney, although the nephrogenic zone is often interrupted by dilated ducts and fibrous tissue. Other findings include a thin cortex, poorly demarcated medullary pyramids, and poor caliceal development (118). It also appears that many of the nephrons are formed normally and the tubules and ducts are secondarily converted to cysts.

GLOMERULAR DISEASES

Metanephric blastema condenses around the end of the ureteric bud at about day 32 of development, and elongation, branching, and subsequent fusion of proximal generations of the bud give rise to the pelvicalyceal system and collecting ducts. The first glomerulotubular structures appear during week 8 as a result of the interaction of subcortical blastema with the ampullary ends of the collecting ducts, and glomerulogenesis continues until gestational week 36 when the neogenic (nephrogenic) zone disappears and nine to eleven generations of glomeruli are present. The number of glomeruli in human kidneys varies from 250,000 to 1.8 million. This marked interindividual difference may be genetically programmed or due to perinatal factors such as low birth weight (estimated relation: 250,000 glomeruli per kilogram at birth) and may predispose persons with lesser numbers of glomeruli to renal failure in adulthood (119). Immature (fetal) glomeruli are characterized by their small size and prominent corona of visceral epithelial cells, and normally, this corona disappears during the first year. Mean glomerular diameter increases from 112 μm at birth to 167 μm at 15 years, and enlarged (hypertrophied) glomeruli suggest a compensatory response to reduced nephron mass (120). The thicknesses of the glomerular capillary wall and the lamina densa increase from 169 ± 30 nm and 98 ± 23 nm, respectively, at birth to 285 ± 39 nm and 219 ± 42 nm, respectively, at 11 years (121). More contemporary measurements demonstrate a nearly linear increase in glomerular basement membrane thickness from 1 year to a plateau at 9 years (122). The molecular structure of the glomerular basement membrane also changes with age. Collagen $\alpha1\alpha2\alpha1(IV)$ synthesized by podocytes, endothelial cells, and mesangial cells of immature glomeruli is replaced by collagen $\alpha3\alpha4\alpha5(IV)$ produced exclusively by podocytes (123).

The pathologist most often encounters glomerular diseases in renal biopsy specimens collected with biopsy guns having needles of 18 gauge or less and may be asked to examine the gross specimen for the presence of glomeruli with a magnifying lens or dissecting microscope (Figure 17-20). The presence of renal cortex may be inferred if one sees capsule and fat at one end of the biopsy specimen and architecture consistent with medulla at the other, but the macroscopic recognition of glomeruli requires sufficient blood flow within glomerular capillaries, and this may be reduced by disease.

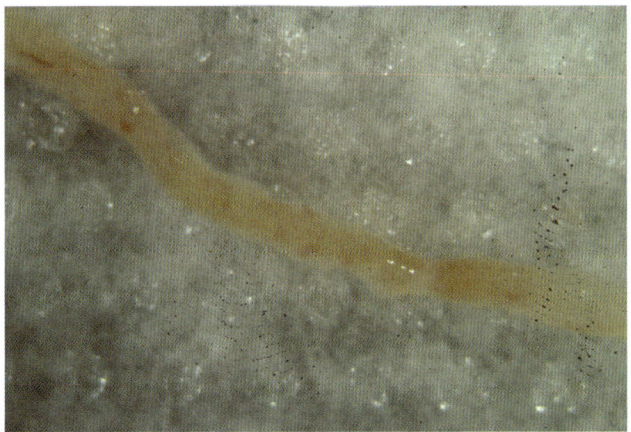

FIGURE 17-20 • Needle biopsy specimen of kidney viewed through a dissecting microscope. Glomeruli appear as red dots in the central region and vasa recta in the outer medulla as linear striations at either end. (Original magnification, 5×.)

Definitive identification of glomeruli may rarely require rapid frozen section, or the pathologist may be asked to perform a rapid frozen section to determine if crescents are present. In either case, the tissue submitted for frozen section can also be utilized for immunofluorescent (IF) studies. Whenever possible, tissue should be sampled for light, IF, and electron microscopy (EM), even if all those studies are not initially requested, and with the smaller-gauge biopsy needles now used by pediatric nephrologists, two or three cores are usually required. The specimen submitted for light microscopy (LM) should contain as much cortex as possible along with the corticomedullary junction, whereas only cortical tissue is ordinarily required in the specimens submitted for IF and EM (124).

Our understanding of pediatric renal pathology has been greatly facilitated by contributions from two multi-institutional collaborative studies, the International Study of Kidney Disease in Children (ISKDC) and the Southwest Pediatric Nephrology Study Group (SPNSG). The terms most commonly used to describe the lesions encountered in renal biopsy specimens are listed in Table 17-5. Children with renal disease usually present with proteinuria or hematuria, alone or in combination, with or without associated systemic disease. Less commonly, patients present with a nephritic syndrome that includes proteinuria, hematuria, red blood cell and white blood cell casts, and decreased plasma levels of complement components, or with acute renal failure, renal concentration defects, or chronic renal failure without known antecedent disease. Isolated proteinuria and hematuria do not usually warrant biopsy study, and most children with nephrotic syndrome responsive to steroid therapy or acute glomerulonephritis attributable to streptococcal disease do not undergo biopsy unless the course is atypical or the response to therapy is suboptimal. Typically, the glomeruli in patients with isolated proteinuria or hematuria are optically normal or show focal and segmental glomerulosclerosis (Figure 17-21A) or mesangial hypercellularity (Figure 17-21B). Diffuse and global mesangial hypercellularity with thickening of capillary walls and obliteration of capillary loops resulting in accentuation of the lobular architecture of the glomerulus (Figure 17-21C) or the presence of crescents and proliferations of parietal epithelial cells and inflammatory cells in Bowman space (Figure 17-21D) are usually associated with a nephritic syndrome or acute renal failure. IF and electron microscopic studies are usually necessary to arrive at a more precise diagnosis. A granular pattern of immunofluorescence—along capillary loops (Figure 17-22A),

TABLE 17-5	TERMS USED IN DESCRIBING GLOMERULAR LESIONS
Focal	Involvement of <50% of all glomeruli
Diffuse	Involvement of ≥50% of all glomeruli
Segmental	Involvement of <50% of a glomerulus
Global	Involvement of ≥50% of a glomerulus
Hyalinosis	Accumulation of eosinophilic, PAS-positive, silver-negative, structureless material that stains red with trichrome stains (glycoproteins and lipids)
Sclerosis	Accumulation of eosinophilic, PAS-positive, silver-positive structureless material that stains blue or green with trichrome stains (collagen IV)
Fibrosis	Accumulation of eosinophilic, PAS-negative, silver-negative fibrillar material that stains blue or green with trichrome stains (collagen I, III)
Mesangial proliferation	More than three mesangial cells per peripheral mesangial area
Mesangiocapillary (membranoproliferative) glomerulonephritis	A combination of mesangial proliferation and capillary wall thickening
Adhesion (synechiae)	Attachment of part or the entire circumference of a glomerular tuft to Bowman capsule. Adhesions may be fibrous or fibrinous
Crescent	A proliferation of glomerular epithelial cells and inflammatory cells that fills part (segmental) or all (circumferential) of Bowman space. Crescents may be cellular, fibrocellular, or fibrous

PAS, periodic acid–Schiff stain.

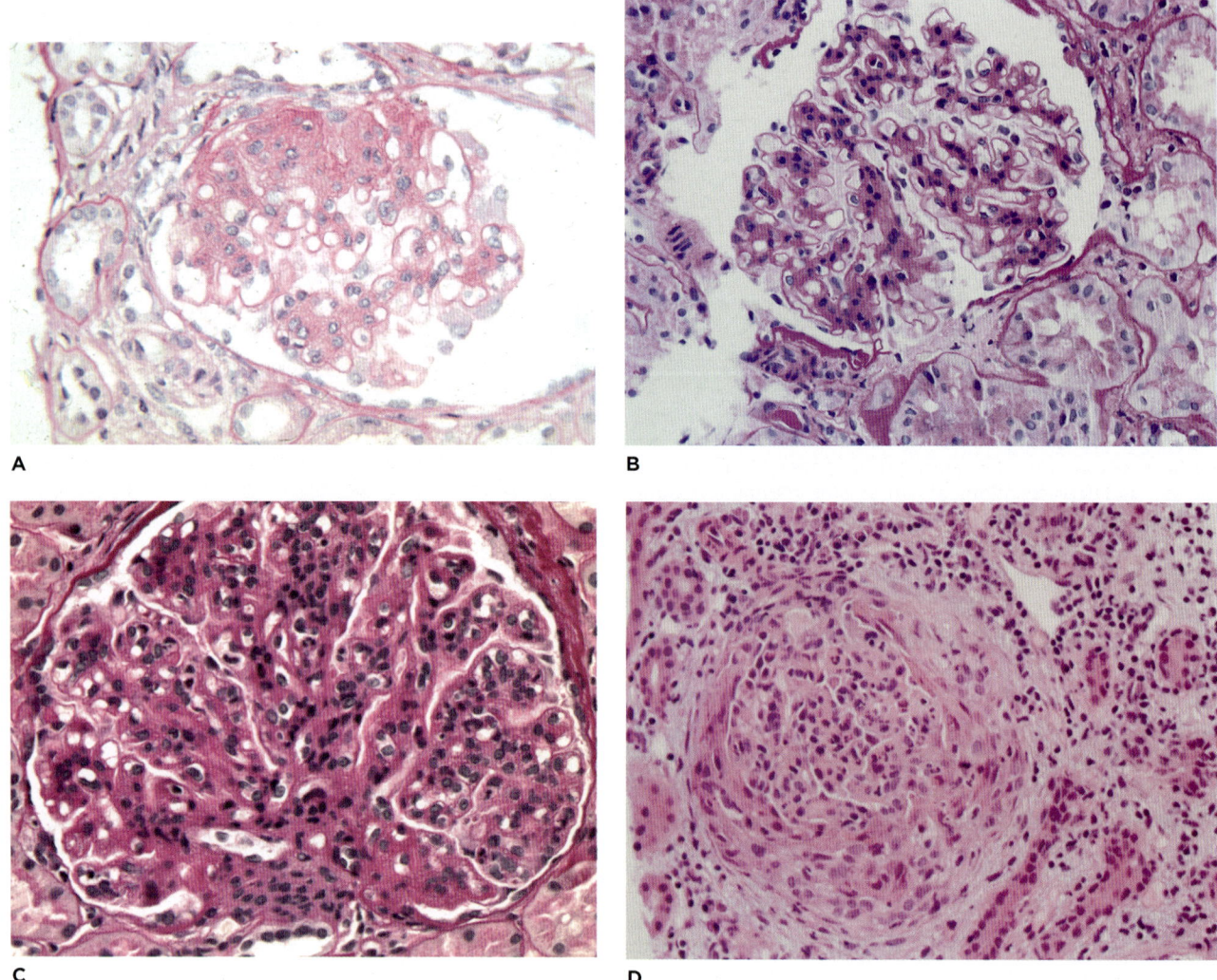

FIGURE 17-21 • Glomerular lesions observed in pediatric renal biopsy specimens. **A:** FSGS with the sclerotic tuft in the 11 o'clock position adherent to Bowman capsule and segmental proliferation of visceral epithelial cells at the 2 o'clock to 4 o'clock position. **B:** Mesangial proliferation is defined as more than three mesangial cell nuclei per peripheral mesangial focus. **C:** Mesangiocapillary or MPGN shows both mesangial proliferation and thickening of capillary loops. **D:** In CGN, a segmental, or in this case, circumferential proliferation of epithelial and inflammatory cells in Bowman space compresses the underlying glomerular tuft. (**D:** hematoxylin–eosin, **A–C** periodic acid–Schiff stain, original magnifications ×400.)

within mesangia (Figure 17-22B), or both (Figure 17-22C)—indicates immune complex (IC) deposition, and the site and the composition of the immunoreactant(s) depend on the disease. Crescents often stain brightly for fibrinogen. Linear staining along the capillary wall may indicate antiglomerular basement membrane disease (usually only IgG). Dense deposit disease, or so-called C3 glomerulopathy, will usually have C3 only or at least C3 predominance (Figure 17-22D). The histologic, IF, and ultrastructural lesions for specific diseases are detailed below, but a careful inventory of the lesions in all renal compartments—glomeruli, tubules, interstitium, and vessels—and correlation of the morphologic findings with the clinical history and the results of renal function tests and serologic studies are necessary for the proper clinicopathologic interpretation of renal biopsy specimens from patients of any age.

Glomerulopathies that Usually Present with Proteinuria or Nephrotic Syndrome

The incidence of idiopathic nephrotic syndrome is two to seven per 100,000 children, 95% of whom respond to steroid therapy, although 60% to 80% of these will experience one or more relapses (125). The distribution of lesions in multiple series of untreated children with nephrotic syndrome was minimal change disease (MCD), 34% to 53%; membranoproliferative glomerulonephritis (MPGN), 2% to 16%; FSGS,

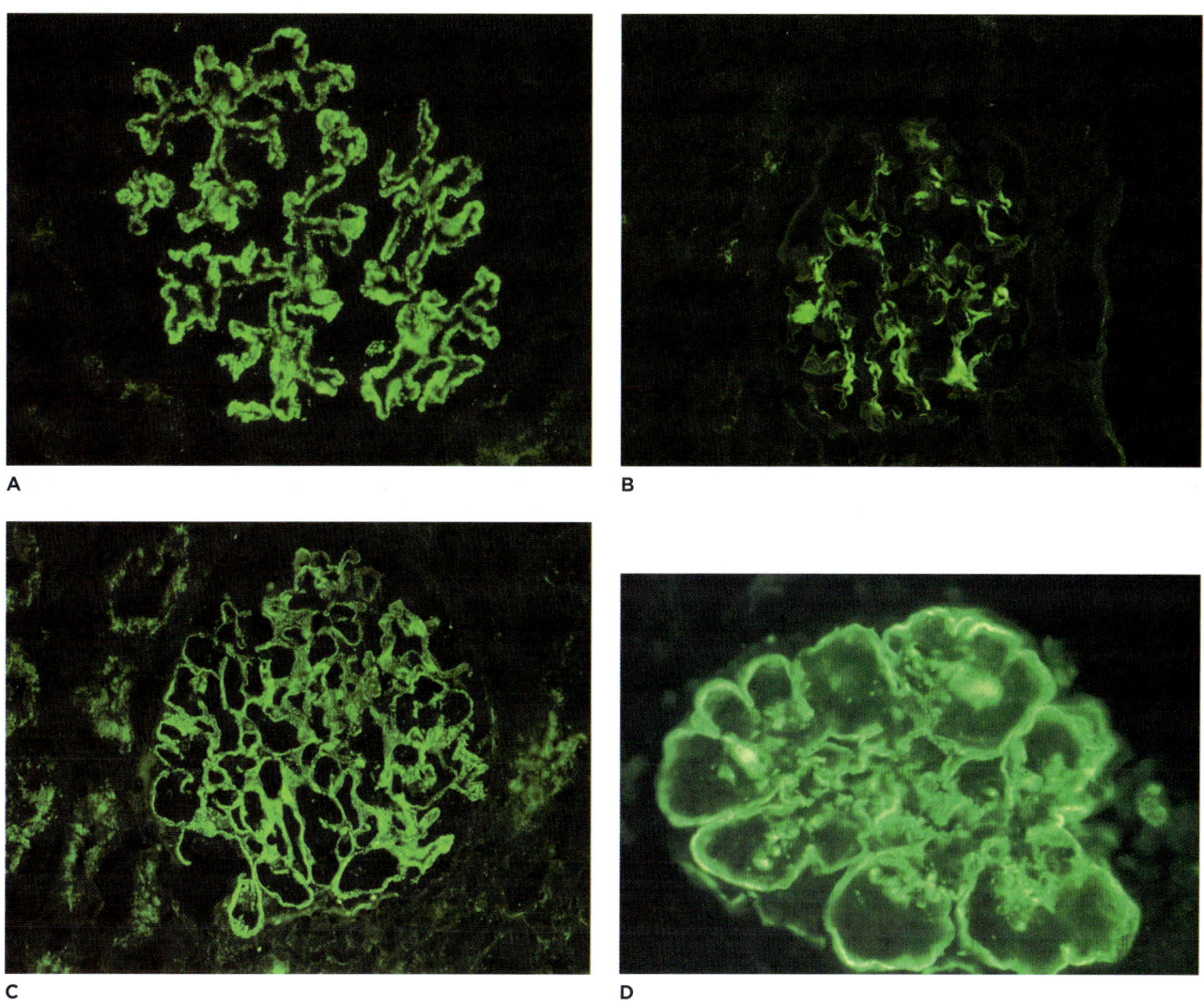

FIGURE 17-22 • Immunofluorescence patterns observed in pediatric renal biopsy specimens. **A:** Granular staining along the capillary loops. **B:** Confluent granular staining in mesangia. **C:** Combination of capillary and mesangial granular staining. **D:** Linear staining for C3 along the capillary wall and bright rings with mesangia in dense deposit disease (type II MPGN). [Fluorescein isothiocyanate-conjugated anti-IgG (**A-C**) or anti-C3 (**D**), original magnifications 400×].

9% to 40%; membranous glomerulonephritis (MGN), 1.5% to 9%; and chronic or unclassified glomerulonephritis, 6% to 17% (126). The incidence of MCD is higher in children under 6 years old at diagnosis (71% versus 24%), more frequent in males (male to female ratios of 60:40), and less often associated with hypertension or hematuria than other causes of nephrotic syndrome. A response to prednisone at 8 weeks was seen in 93% of patients with MCD, 75% with focal global glomerulosclerosis, 30% with FSGS, 56% with diffuse mesangial hypercellularity, 7% with MPGN, and none with MGN. MCD is underrepresented in more recent series, reflecting the current practice of not performing biopsies in children with nephrotic syndrome unless unresponsive or resistant to steroid therapy. However, even allowing for the changes in biopsy practice, the incidence of FSGS in children appears to be increasing in all ethnic groups, becomes more apparent in patients over 6 years of age at presentation, and appears to be more common and more aggressive in African American and possibly Japanese children (127). Familial FSGS has been attributed to mutations that alter slit-diaphragm proteins (nephrin [*NPHS1*], podocin [*NPHS2*], CD2-associated protein [*CD2AP*], short transient receptor potential channel 6 [*TRPC6*]), actin-regulating proteins (alpha-actinin-4 [*ACTN4*], inverted formin-2 [*INF2*], Rho GTPase–activating proteins 24 [*ARHGAP24*], Rho GDP–dissociation inhibitor 1 [*ARHGDIA*]), transcription factors (Wilms tumor protein [*WT1*], LIM homeobox transcription factor 1β [*LMX1B*], WSI/SNF–related matrix-associated actin-dependent regulator of chromatin subfamily A-like protein [*SMARCAL1*]), glomerular basement membrane proteins (laminin subunit β2 [*LAMB2*], integrin β4 [*ITGB4*]), and various mitochondrial and lysosomal proteins. Many of these patients do not present until adulthood, and there is considerable variability in the clinical severity and response to therapy, especially among heterozygotes, implying that other genes or nongenetic triggers may be involved (127,128). Altered expression or distribution of these and other podocyte proteins has been found in studies of nonfamilial FSGS suggesting that reorganization of podocyte proteins in response to injury is a key step in the pathogenesis of proteinuria (129). Gene expression profiling of isolated glomeruli from patients with FSGS, MCD, and normal controls demonstrated numerous significantly differentially regulated genes including some known to be part of the slit-diaphragm complex and previously described in dysregulated podocyte phenotype (130). FSGS, often with lesser (nonnephrotic) levels of proteinuria, is also the lesion seen in cyanotic congenital heart disease, sickle cell anemia, massive obesity, HIV, and other viral infections (parvovirus, SV40, and some cases of hepatitis C). Nephrotic syndrome in the first year of life may be associated with lesions that occur in older children but is more often caused by one of two lesions unique to this age group—congenital nephrotic syndrome (CNS) of the Finnish type (CNF) and diffuse mesangial sclerosis (DMS) that are discussed later. Medical complications of nephrotic syndrome include acute infections and thromboembolic disease related to the nephrotic state and long-term effects on bones, growth, and the cardiovascular system related to the disease and its treatment (125).

Minimal Change Disease, IgM and C1q Nephropathy

Glomerulopathy with minimal change is the most common cause of nephrotic syndrome in children and referred to as minimal change nephrotic syndrome (MCNS) or MCD. The pathogenesis of MCD remains unknown, although it is likely the result of complex interactions among multiple systems including lymphokines that increase glomerular permeability, regulatory T-cell dysfunction, upregulation of CD80 and angiopoietin-like-4 (Ang-4) and Ang-3 by podocytes, or various epigenetic modifications triggered by environmental or immune factors (131,132).

By definition, MCD shows no significant abnormalities by LM. Slight segmental increases in mesangial matrix and cellularity (three or more mesangial cells in most tufts of most glomeruli [Figure 17-21B]) and focal interstitial fibrosis are within the spectrum of "minimal change." The historically termed "diffuse mesangial hypercellularity" is also now considered within the range of MCD (126); some have noted signs of glomerular immaturity in association with hypercellularity (133). The long-term prognosis in these patients is good although there is a trend to initial steroid nonresponsiveness.

The classic light microscopic appearance in MCD includes patent glomerular capillaries that are surrounded by regular walls of expected thickness. Mesangial matrix may show a slight increase, but absent are focal or segmental scarring or collapse, adhesion to Bowman capsule, and endocapillary proliferation. Occasionally, immature glomeruli are seen. IF microscopy is usually negative or reveals only segmentally variable, mesangial staining for IgM with or without C3 or C1q. Ultrastructural findings in patients with the nephrotic syndrome include diffuse retraction of foot processes of visceral epithelial cells, microvillous transformation along the cell membrane, and vacuolization and lipid droplets within visceral epithelial cell cytoplasm. The GBM is usually normal.

Most authors consider any segmental glomerulosclerosis significant, but rare globally sclerotic or hyalinized glomeruli are occasionally seen in otherwise normal infant kidneys. Emery and MacDonald found hyalinized glomeruli in the kidneys of 75 of 200 (38%) infants and children up to 15 years of age (0.5% to 30% of glomeruli in affected kidneys, but in most cases, the range was 1% to 2%) and noted that rare sclerotic glomeruli were present in many of the kidneys that had no such glomeruli in the selected field (134). Global glomerulosclerosis may occur as a part of normal aging and repair in the absence of renal disease. Less than 5% globally sclerosed glomeruli is the expectation up to mid-adulthood. Thus, a rare globally sclerotic glomerulus might be within normal limits but should initiate a search of serial sections through the block for a segmentally sclerotic glomerulus. Examination of serial sections is also recommended if focal tubular atrophy, interstitial fibrosis, enlarged glomeruli, segmental hyalinosis, segmentally positive immunofluorescence, collagen in glomeruli by EM, or an incomplete therapeutic response is found.

The differential diagnosis of MCD is IgM nephropathy, C1q nephropathy, FSGS, and CNS. The latter two are discussed in other sections. Controversy exists as to the definition and significance of IgM nephropathy, as IgM is frequently considered a nonspecific finding due to trapping. The typical light microscopic appearance is normal or mild mesangial hypercellularity with bright mesangial IgM on immunofluorescence; however, various authors have systematically required or excluded the presence of deposits on EM. Several have shown a poorer prognosis or variable responses to steroids, cyclophosphamide, or cyclosporine (135,136).

Jennette et al. described a proliferative glomerulonephritis with mesangial granular C1q as the dominant or codominant immunoreactant and no evidence of systemic lupus erythematosus (SLE) in 15 adolescents and young adults who presented with proteinuria or nephrotic syndrome (137). C1q nephropathy is noted most frequently in children and young adults (age range: 3 to 42 years, mean: 24.2 years) with a female and African American preponderance, and renal biopsies typically show minimal change, mesangial hypercellularity, or FSGS (138). Many authors concluded that C1q nephropathy falls within the spectrum of MCD and FSGS, but recent reports fail to demonstrate significant outcome differences between similar cases with or without C1q (136,139,140).

MCD is most often idiopathic in children and exquisitely sensitive to steroid therapy, such that treatment in most patients is initiated without a biopsy and 90% to 95% of patients respond within 8 weeks, although approximately 60% relapse (126). Less frequent relapse is reported in those who receive extended initial therapy, and supplemental therapies have included calcineurin inhibitors, especially cyclosporine; alkylating agents, particularly cyclophosphamide; and more recent introduction of mycophenolate mofetil (MMF) and rituximab (141). Secondary causes of MCD include NSAIDs, lymphomas, infections, and allergic reaction, and the diagnosis is suspected by clinical history.

Focal Segmental Glomerulosclerosis

Although often considered a spectrum of one disease, with FSGS resulting from progression of MCD, contemporary evidence supports the notion that these two are distinct entities with different pathogeneses (142–145). Most children with primary FSGS present with nephrotic syndrome, and the proportion of pediatric patients with nephrotic syndrome due to FSGS increases with age.

Segmental proliferation of visceral epithelial cells (Figure 17-21A, 2 o'clock to 4 o'clock position) may be the earliest lesion of FSGS. D'Agati et al. (146) have subdivided FSGS into five categories: NOS, cellular, perihilar, tip, and collapsing variants. FSGS-NOS is the most common form seen in children and adults. The collapsing and tip lesion variants are most likely to present with full nephrotic syndrome, which have the lowest and highest rates of remission, respectively, and conversely, the highest and lowest rates of ESRD (147,148). While not all espouse this classification, it can be applied to primary and secondary FSGS and may provide clues to the underlying etiologies.

The classic appearance of FSGS includes segmental tuft sclerosis with adhesion to Bowman capsule in a minority of glomeruli (Figure 17-21A). Juxtamedullary glomeruli are more frequently affected than superficial glomeruli. Mild endocapillary or extracapillary cellular increase may be associated with matrix accumulation in the tuft. IF microscopy is typically negative although nonspecific trapping of IgM or C3 is often noted in sclerotic segments. Podocyte foot process effacement is expected by ultrastructural assessment as well as podocyte swelling, microvillous transformation, and increased organelles; podocytes may be detached from the GBM (148). Proximal tubules often contain resorption droplets, and tubular atrophy is accompanied by interstitial fibrosis. The pathology of primary (idiopathic) and familial FSGS is similar such that clinical and family history may be more significant than the histopathology in determining response to therapy. The treatment approach is similar as with MCD; however, the majority of patients in whom a sustained response is not achieved will eventually progress to ESRD. A recurrence rate after transplant as high as 50% has been reported with initial steroid responsiveness highly predictive of recurrence, while pathogenic genetic mutations are protective of recurrence (149).

Membranous Glomerulonephritis

MGN is seen in 1.5% to 9% of children and 18.5% of adolescents with nephrotic syndrome (126). In children, the age at onset is usually 8 to 16 years, and the sex ratio varies among studies from equal to a male predominance (150). Most patients have microscopic hematuria in addition to proteinuria, but macroscopic hematuria is uncommon. Thirty-five percent of cases of MGN in children are secondary to systemic diseases, whereas the incidence of secondary MGN in adults is 20% (151). The designation of "idiopathic" (primary) may be disappearing as most cases of MGN in adults appear to be mediated by autoantibodies to phospholipase A2 receptor (PLA2R) expressed on podocytes (152). The antibody seems to be relatively specific for primary MGN (153), although other antipodocyte antibodies may be circulating (154). Moreover, primary MGN in the pediatric population must have more etiologies as less than 45% show PLA2R autoantibodies (155). Most cases of secondary MGN are due to SLE with the proportion due to hepatitis B decreasing as vaccination has become routine in many places. Additional secondary causes in children include infection, neoplasia, and other autoimmune disorders.

Following the description in 2002 of a remarkable case of antenatal MGN due to maternal antibodies directed against neutral endopeptidase (NEP), a podocyte and tubular brush border protein, which was present in the fetus but not the mother (156), other cases of MGN in early life attributable to antenatal alloimmunization have been identified (157). This particular disease mechanism bears similarities to the autoimmune form of anti-PLA2R–associated MGN in adults, where autoantibodies bind *in situ* to endogenous podocyte proteins. More recently, the same investigators identified circulating antibodies directed against cationic bovine serum albumin (BSA) and BSA within subepithelial deposits (158). This phenomenon is more analogous to secondary MGN, such as hepatitis B, where planted antigens contribute to an immune complex, which stimulates complement activation and collateral damage to the podocyte.

Histologically, glomeruli in MGN appear large and have uniformly thickened capillary walls but patent capillary lumens (Figure 17-23A). The diagnostic "spikes" seen on silver stains (Figure 17-23B) represent notches along the outer aspect of the normally argyrophilic basement membrane due to immune complexes that do not take up the silver. Spikes cannot be detected when the deposits are small or sparse (Figure 17-23C) or when they have been fully incorporated into the basement membrane (Figure 17-23D). Mesangial hypercellularity, glomerular lobulation, and segmental inflammation, necrosis, or sclerosis are more common in secondary MGN (151). The degree of proteinuria or stage of disease does not correlate with disease course or outcome, although glomerulosclerosis and interstitial fibrosis may portend an unfavorable course (159).

IF microscopy reveals granular staining along capillary walls (Figure 17-22A) and occasionally also within the mesangia (Figure 17-22C). IgG and C3 are very commonly

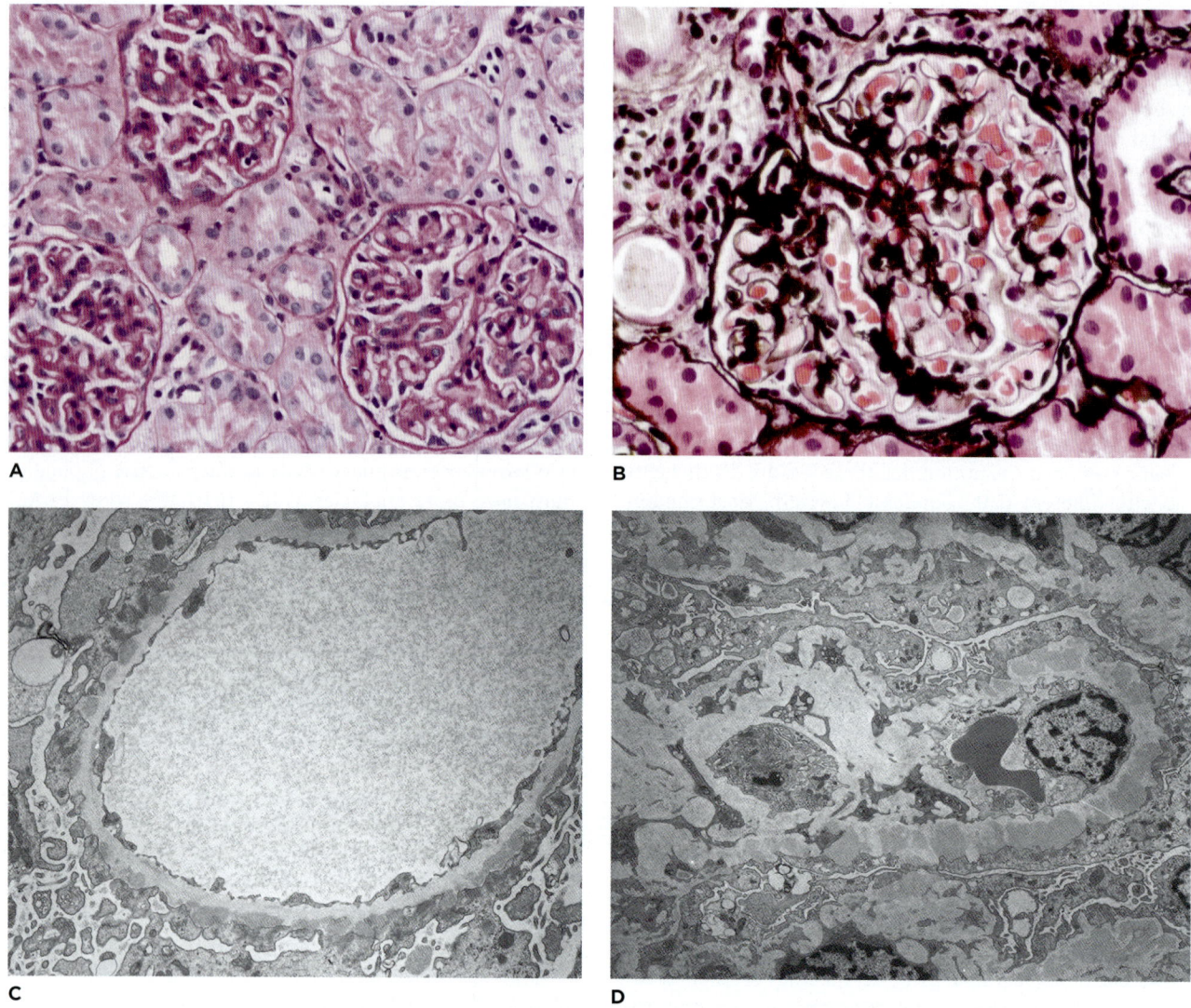

FIGURE 17-23 • **A, B:** MGN with diffuse thickening of the capillary walls that in some stages exhibit short "spikes" extending from the outer surface of the capillary. **C, D:** On Ehrenreich and Churg stage I, small electron-dense deposits are present along the outer aspect of the basement membrane, but in stage III, larger deposits are incorporated into the basement membrane. (**A:** Periodic acid–Schiff stain, original magnification ×400. **B:** Jones methenamine silver stain, original magnification ×600. **C, D:** lead citrate and uranyl acetate.)

present, but a "full house" of immunoreactants suggests lupus or another systemic disease. Mesangial deposits also suggest systemic disease. Four stages have been described in MGN: stage I, small subepithelial deposits (Figure 17-23C); stage II, larger and more numerous deposits bordered by projections of the lamina densa; stage III, incorporation of deposits into the lamina densa (Figure 17-23D); and stage IV, a thickened and irregular basement membrane without recognizable deposits. These observations provide much insight into the morphology of MGN, but they simplify the biologic complexity as the stages do not correlate with proteinuria, outcome, or clinical change and often overlap. Patients may present at any stage and may have deposits characteristic of more than one stage. Foot process retraction is typically extensive in all stages. Treatment is influenced by clinical severity; asymptomatic children with nonnephrotic proteinuria are often managed conservatively with angiotensin-converting enzyme inhibitors or angiotensin receptor blockers, while those with nephrotic syndrome receive various combinations of corticosteroids, alkylating agents, or other immunosuppressants such as calcineurin inhibitors, MMF, and rituximab (150,159).

Diabetic Nephropathy

Diabetic nephropathy develops in 40% to 50% of patients with insulin-dependent diabetes mellitus. Long-standing disease, poor metabolic control, smoking, male sex, non-Caucasian race, and other genetic factors predispose patients to the development of nephropathy (160). There is a higher incidence of renal disease in patients with type 2 diabetes mellitus, and albuminuria appears earlier (161). It is unusual for clinical nephropathy to develop in less than 10 years, but mesangial expansion and tubular and glomerular basement membrane thickening begin to appear within 2 to 5 years and may be apparent before the onset of microalbuminuria. Global glomerulosclerosis and nodular intercapillary glomerulosclerosis (Kimmelstiel-Wilson lesion) have rarely been seen in children with insulin-dependent diabetes mellitus (162). Recent work demonstrates that microalbuminuria, rather than being a specific marker of diabetic kidney disease, may represent reversible endothelial injury; microalbuminuria regression to normoalbuminuria is more common with improved glycemic and blood pressure control (163). Nodular or diffuse glomerulosclerosis and the other glomerular lesions of diabetic nephropathy, hyalinosis fibrin caps and capsular drops, and hyaline arteriolosclerosis may also be seen in kidney biopsy specimens from massively obese adolescents (Figure 17-24). Similar renal pathology has been observed in type 1 and type 2 diabetes, the latter possibly operative in obese adolescents (164). Comorbidities, however, likely contribute to increased heterogeneity in type 2 diabetes, which is disproportionately more common among youths of ethnic minorities (163). Youths with type 2 diabetes experience earlier and more rapid progression of diabetic kidney disease than adults or other youths with type 1 diabetes. IF microscopy shows a characteristic linear staining along the glomerular capillary walls and tubular basement membranes for IgG and albumin, and hyalinotic lesions often stain with IgM and C3. The earliest and most characteristic ultrastructural lesion is thickening of the lamina densa of the glomerular basement membrane, but with time, the width of the membrane varies as thinner areas develop as a result of microaneurysms and the deposition of neomembrane. An imbalance between extracellular matrix synthesis and degradation, mainly regulated by endothelial cells and podocytes, may contribute to GBM abnormalities in diabetes. Other ultrastructural findings include increased mesangial matrix, variable effacement of foot processes, and subendothelial accumulations of electron-dense material that correspond to fibrin caps and should not be confused with the deposits seen in immune complex diseases. These changes have been associated with altered increased and aberrant expression of various matrix proteins including laminin (165).

Nephrotic Syndrome in the First Year of Life

By convention, congenital nephrotic syndrome (CNS) is defined as heavy proteinuria starting *in utero* or within three months after birth. NS appearing later in the first year (4 to 12 months) is referred to as infantile NS and thereafter is called childhood NS. Although these definitions have been used for decades to help guide clinical diagnosis, the rationale is brought into question with recent discoveries demonstrating that a particular gene defect can induce NS at various ages. "Hereditary proteinuria syndromes" may be a more comprehensive term, but, since the clinical features, etiology, and management, on the whole, differ from more common forms of childhood NS, the use of conventional terms may still be practical.

The differential diagnosis of CNS is broad including primary genetic disorders, infectious causes (cytomegalovirus, congenital syphilis, toxoplasmosis, malaria, HIV, etc.), and uncommon miscellaneous disorders (maternal SLE, neonatal alloimmunization against NEP). Most patients have a monogenetic cause of disease with a defect that affects proteins that regulate the glomerular filtration barrier, particularly the slit diaphragm (166), and involve one of five genes, *NPHS1*, *NPHS2*, *LAMB2*, *WT1*, and *PLCE1* (167,168). Genetic testing in nephrotic syndrome is recommended for the following categories of patients: children presenting with CNS, children presenting with infantile nephrotic syndrome associated with other malformations or syndromes, and all patients with a family history of nephrotic syndrome or chronic kidney disease (169). Nonetheless, the cause remains unknown in the majority of cases, even in those with an obvious familial occurrence.

Young patients with nephrotic syndrome should have a thorough investigation of birth and family history, complete physical exam including genitalia and eyes, renal ultrasound, and routine laboratory analysis with TORCH titers. The term *congenital nephrotic syndrome* is often used synonymously with *congenital nephrotic syndrome of the Finnish type* (CNF), a recessively inherited disorder characterized by massive proteinuria at birth, a large placenta, and marked edema. The disease is most frequent in Finland where its incidence is 1 per 8200 newborns, but it is also the most common cause of nephrotic syndrome in the first three months of life in non-Finnish infants (167). In 1998, this autosomal recessive disorder was mapped to the *NPHS1* gene at 19q13.1 that encodes nephrin, a 185-kDa transmembrane protein in the slit diaphragm of podocytes (170).

Affected infants are typically small for gestational age and are born at 35 to 38 weeks of gestation with deformations of the skull, hips, knees, and elbows, which are ascribed to

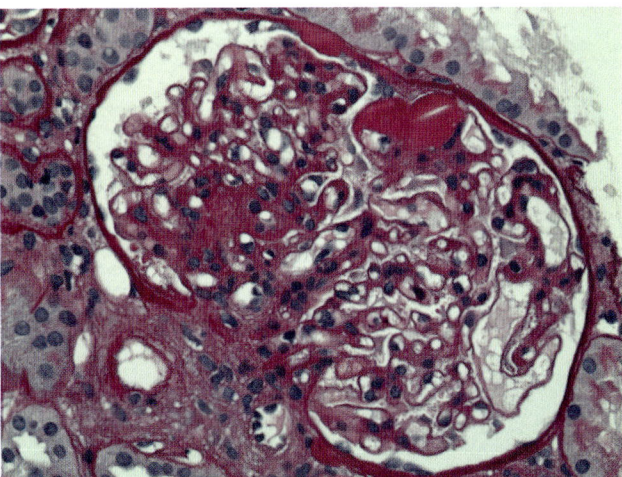

FIGURE 17-24 • Obesity-related glomerulonephritis. Nodular mesangial sclerosis, hyaline caps, capsular drops, and arteriosclerosis, all features of diabetic nephropathy, are also present in this adolescent with obesity-related nephropathy. (Periodic acid–Schiff stain, original magnification ×400.)

the markedly enlarged placenta that weighs more than 25% of the infant's birth weight. Other abnormalities (small nose with low bridge, widely separated cranial sutures, large fontanelles, delayed ossification) may be secondary to hypothyroidism as a consequence of urinary loss of thyroid-binding globulin (171). Proteinuria *in utero* also leads to increased levels of a-fetoprotein in the amniotic fluid and maternal serum. Although proteinuria is present at birth in CNF, renal function is usually normal during the first 6 months, and no extrarenal disorders are present. In contrast, CNS due to other causes typically presents later in the first year of life with less massive proteinuria, extrarenal manifestations are evident in congenital infections and syndromes with urogenital or neurologic components, and the rate of renal deterioration is much faster with DMS or interstitial nephritis (166). The histologic hallmark of CNF is patchy dilatation of the proximal tubules (Figure 17-25A), but this may not be present in biopsy specimens, especially those obtained before 6 months of age, and is neither sensitive nor specific for CNF (126). Glomeruli may show mesangial hypercellularity or crescents, and larger than normal glomeruli appear to be too closely spaced, but no glomerular lesion is diagnostic by light or IF. EM shows extensive foot process effacement with loss of visible slit diaphragms between adjacent processes; nephrin is usually not expressed. An interstitial lymphoid or myeloid infiltrate may be present. Proteinuria recurs in 25% of patients after transplantation, all of whom in one report had the same Fin-major *NPHS1* mutation and may be due to the development of antinephrin antibodies (172).

Mutations in *NPHS2* are the most common cause of nephrotic syndrome in the first year of life and account for a significant portion of those with a congenital presentation (168,173). The pathology in most cases reveals minimal glomerular change or FSGS with few demonstrating mesangial proliferative lesions, although rare cases have shown apparent DMS. As with other nephrotic syndromes, interstitial fibrosis, tubular atrophy, and inflammation increased over time. The autosomal recessive steroid-resistant nephrotic syndrome, which is generally not associated with any extrarenal manifestations, progresses to ESRD but has a very low recurrent rate after transplantation (173).

Just as CNS is often inferred as congenital nephrotic syndrome of the Finnish type, DMS is often considered synonymous with Denys-Drash syndrome. DMS usually presents between 3 and 11 months, somewhat later than CNF, but the characteristic lesion has been reported in fetuses (174). Mesangial sclerosis begins as an increase in fibrillar matrix but not cellularity (Figure 17-25B), and it progresses to transform the entire tuft into a shrunken hyalinized ball surrounded by a rim of visceral epithelium within a prominent Bowman space that may contain crescents. A zonal distribution of small simplified glomeruli and undifferentiated tubules beneath the capsule and relatively normal glomeruli but dilated tubules near the medulla may be present. Immunofluorescence studies may be negative or show mesangial staining for IgM, C3, and C1q in intact glomeruli, and IgM and C3 outline the sclerotic glomeruli. By EM, endothelial and especially mesangial cells appear hypertrophic, and there is a marked increase in mesangial matrix (126,175).

Habib et al. (176) reported DMS as the usual renal lesion in patients with the Denys-Drash syndrome. Initially, only genetic males with pseudohermaphroditism, nephropathy, and WT were included in this syndrome; however, since the recognition of patients who do not express the full syndrome, females with the full syndrome and patients with the characteristic nephropathy who also have either genital abnormalities or WT have been included (177). The genital abnormality in Denys-Drash syndrome is either ambiguous genitalia or normal female genitalia with an XY karyotype, and children in whom WTs develop generally manifest bilateral tumors at a mean age of 18 months (177). Several mutations in the

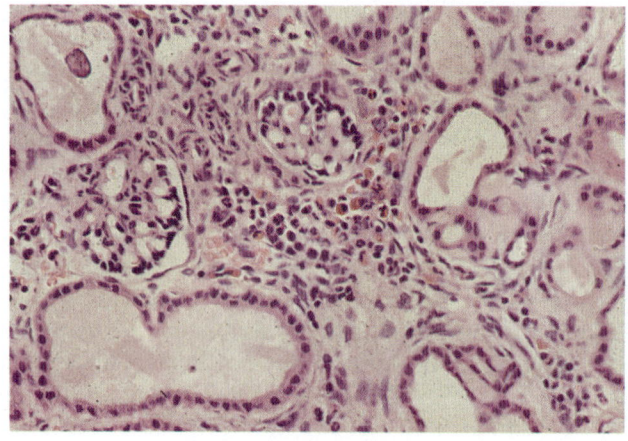 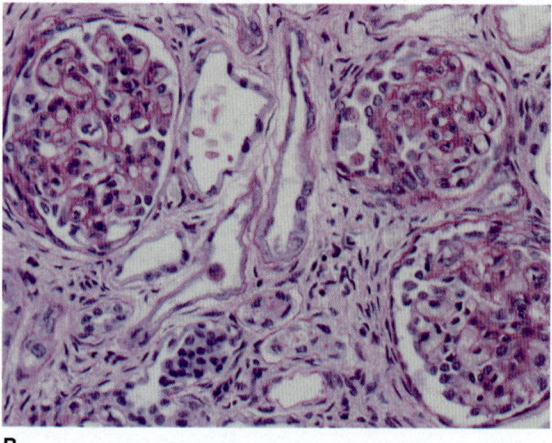

FIGURE 17-25 • Congenital nephropathies. **A:** Tubular ectasia, interstitial inflammation, and variable mesangial hypercellularity are nonspecific features seen in CNF. **B:** Increased mesangial matrix and segmental tuft sclerosis are seen in the early stages of DMS in this newborn infant with Denys-Drash syndrome. (**A:** Hematoxylin–eosin, original magnification 200×, **B:** periodic acid-Schiff stain, original magnification 400×.)

WT suppressor gene, WT1, have been reported in patients with Denys-Drash syndrome. Incomplete forms of the syndrome, consisting of glomerulopathy associated with either genital abnormality or Wilms tumor, have been reported (175). The majority of patients with DDS have mutations in WT1 affecting nucleotides coding for the DNA-binding residues, although KTS mutations in intron 9, characteristic of Frasier syndrome, have been identified in patients with DDS or with isolated DMS. Frasier syndrome described as male pseudohermaphroditism associated with XY gonadal dysgenesis and nephrotic syndrome typically shows FSGS on renal biopsy that progresses to end-stage renal disease during the second or third decade of life (175). Patients with Frasier syndrome are at risk for gonadoblastoma but have a very low risk for WT (177). WT1 mutations characteristic of Frasier or Denys-Drash syndrome have been found in 6% of patients presenting with isolated SRNS; notably, adolescent girls with primary amenorrhea should undergo WT1 screening. Nearly 30% of all patients with a WT1 mutation display isolated sporadic SRNS without any associated comorbidities and extrarenal features, when present can be so subtle that they are only detected retrospectively in light of genetic diagnosis (177).

Nail-Patella Syndrome, Collagen Type III Glomerulopathy, and Pierson Syndrome

Nail–patella syndrome (NPS) may be a cause of proteinuria in infancy, childhood, or adulthood. The cardinal features of this condition are dysplasia of the nails and absent or hypoplastic patellas, but most patients also have iliac horns and dysplasia of the elbows. A nephropathy develops in some kindreds. LM may show patchy tubular atrophy and interstitial fibrosis, but the glomeruli are normal or show only irregular thickening of the capillary wall or mesangial expansion or segmental or global sclerosis. Immunofluorescence studies are usually negative. EM reveals prominent thickening of the glomerular basement membrane, which has a mottled appearance caused by irregular but sharply defined electron-lucent areas containing fibers that have the periodicity of collagen, especially if the grids have been stained with phosphotungstic acid (178). Similar clear zones with collagen are often found in the mesangium. Approximately 40% to 60% of the patients with NPS have renal manifestations, and it is estimated that 15% to 30% progress to renal failure, but the course in an individual patient is unpredictable (178,179). NPS is due to mutations in the LIM–homeodomain protein LMX1B at 9q34 that regulates transcription of collagen IV subtypes α3 and α4, and mutation analysis has shown correlation of mutations in this domain with proteinuria but not to the extrarenal manifestations of the disease (180). Mutations in LMX1B have recently been demonstrated in patients with autosomal dominant FSGS that lacked extrarenal features or ultrastructural features of NPS (181). Collagen type III (collagenofibrotic) glomerulopathy presents with progressive proteinuria in late infancy to adulthood, and most affected children go on to renal failure.

Glomeruli are markedly enlarged and have lobular architecture with expanded mesangia and thick capillary walls due to accumulation of massive amounts of collagen type III, and by EM, the mesangia and the subendothelial space are electron lucent or mottled. Collagen fibers, typically curved rather than straight as in normal interstitial type III collagen, with a periodicity of approximately 60 nm, can be demonstrated with phosphotungstic acid staining, but patients do not have the extrarenal manifestations of NPS (178). Another disorder of the glomerular basement membrane is Pierson syndrome that typically presents with severe nephrosis in early infancy or prenatal onset characterized by a heavy placenta with hydrops fetalis and elevated AFP (mimicking CNF) or even renal failure with intrauterine demise. CNS is often associated with microcoria, but less severe ocular anomalies are described. The autosomal recessive disorder is due to mutations of LAMB2 at chromosome 3p21 that encodes laminin β2 that anchors the podocyte foot process to the basement membrane (182). Pathologically, it may show DMS or glomerular hypercellularity with variable thickening, thinning, rarefaction, and lamination of the glomerular basement membrane on EM (183).

Glomerulopathies that Usually Present with Hematuria with or without Proteinuria

The most important diseases in this category in children include the primary IgA nephropathies—Berger disease and Henoch-Schönlein purpura (HSP) nephritis and the basement membrane nephropathies—Alport syndrome (AS) and thin glomerular basement membrane disease. Hematuria is a well-known complication of hypercalciuria, but no specific pathologic lesion is associated with this condition (184), and the histopathologic abnormalities in loin-pain hematuria syndrome are nonspecific. In all these conditions, the finding of red cell casts or hemosiderin in tubular epithelial cells lends support to a diagnosis of hematuria originating in the kidney rather than in the lower urinary tract. The primary IgA nephropathies are defined by the presence of IgA as the dominant or codominant immunoreactant in the absence of clinical or laboratory features of SLE. Characteristic but not always pathognomonic ultrastructural lesions are observed in many cases of AS, and an ultrastructural lesion defines thin glomerular basement membrane disease.

IgA Nephropathy (Berger Disease)

IgA nephropathy was described by Berger and Hinglais in 1968 (185), but the association of recurrent hematuria and focal glomerulonephritis, often in patients with a recent history of upper respiratory infection, had been recognized many years earlier. Today, IgA nephropathy is the most common glomerulopathy worldwide, accounting for 5% to 10% of cases of glomerular disease in North America, 15% to 30% in Europe, and up to 50% in Japan. Prevalence data garnered from biopsy series should be interpreted with

by immunohistochemical evidence of complete or partial loss of the Alport epitope in glomerular or epidermal basement membranes (Figure 17-26 A, B) or demonstration of a mutation in one of the type IV collagen genes listed above is desired for a diagnosis of AS (199). Hematuria is demonstrable by 5 years of age in affected boys with X-linked AS. The progression to end-stage renal disease in X-linked AS is variable but roughly similar within kindreds and strongly dependent upon the type of mutation. The risk of ESRD by age 30 is 90% for deletions and nonsense mutations of *COL4A5*, 70% for splicing mutations, and 50% for missense mutations (203). Severe mutations are also associated with perimacular dot-and-fleck retinopathy as well as lenticonus and hearing loss (204,205). The effects of *COL4A5* genotype on age of ESRD are not observed in females with X-linked AS due to the significant influence of X inactivation (206,207). Autosomal recessive Alport syndrome (ARAS) accounts for about 15% of individuals and results from two pathogenic mutations in either the *Col4A3* or *COL4A4* gene. Recent data indicate that the nature of the mutation in AR AS affects the clinical phenotype. In general, both males and females with ARAS carry a high risk of ESRD by age 30, but rare cases of mild disease are reported (208). Only about 5% of AS are attributed to autosomal dominant disease, which tends to progress at a relatively slow rate. Recent investigations utilizing next-generation sequencing (NGS), which allows simultaneous assessment of *COL4A3*, *COL4A4*, and *COL4A5*, offer an efficient and cost-effective approach with a sensitivity reported at 99% in one study (209). These authors also noted a higher rate of *COL4A3* and *COL4A4* mutations in their

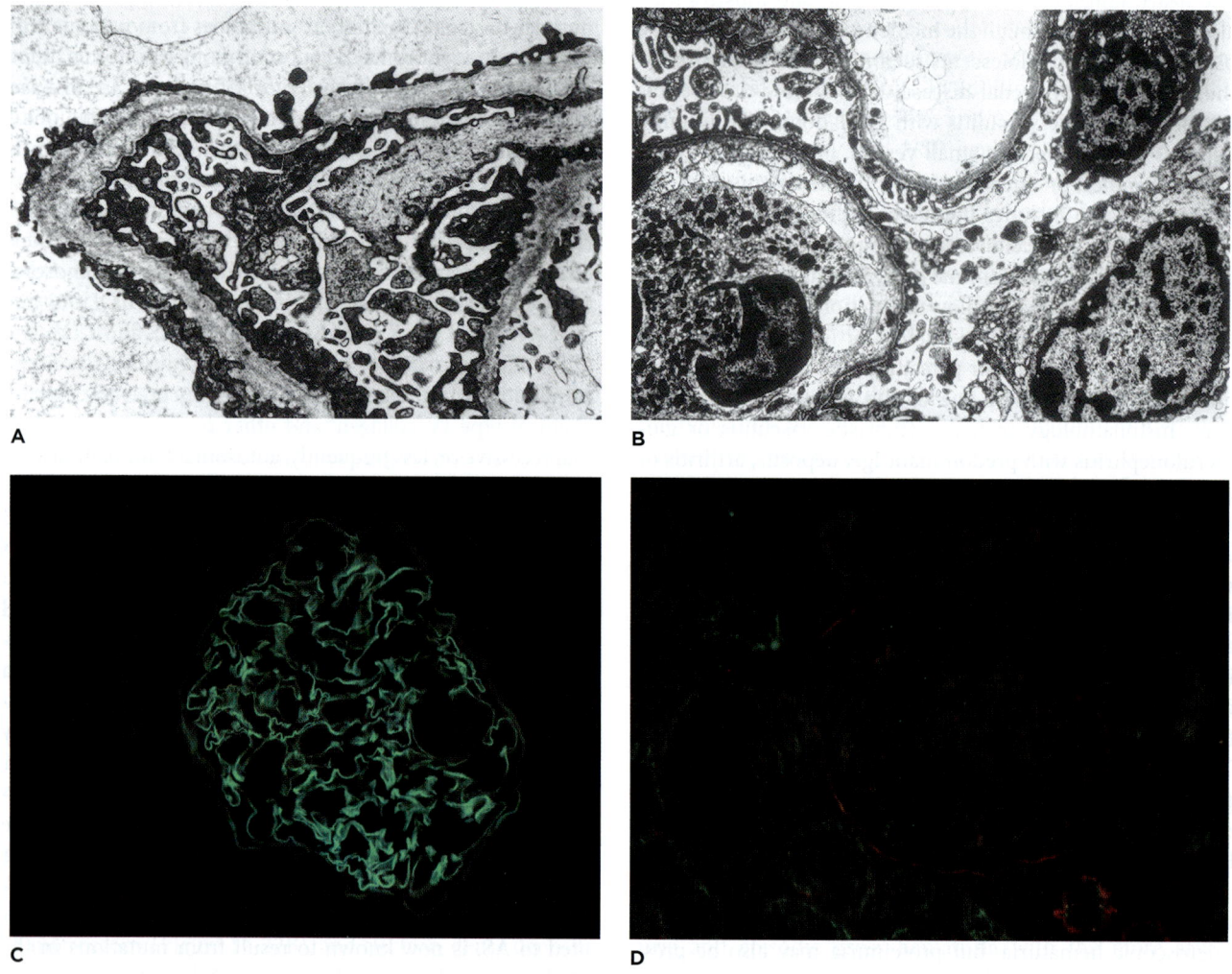

FIGURE 17-26 • Basement membrane nephropathies. **A:** Marked thinning, fraying, intersecting lamination, and granularity of the glomerular capillary basement membrane are characteristics of hereditary nephritis (AS), but are not seen in all cases. **B:** Diffuse thinning of the capillary basement membrane is seen in familial hematuria and may be the only ultrastructural lesion in AS. **C, D:** Staining for collagen IVa5 is seen along the glomerular capillary basement membrane and, to a lesser extent, Bowman capsule in control **(C)** but not patient **(D)** glomeruli. (**A, B:** Lead citrate and uranyl acetate, **C, D:** fluorescein isothiocyanate–conjugated anticollagen IVa5, original magnification 400×.)

WT suppressor gene, WT1, have been reported in patients with Denys-Drash syndrome. Incomplete forms of the syndrome, consisting of glomerulopathy associated with either genital abnormality or Wilms tumor, have been reported (175). The majority of patients with DDS have mutations in WT1 affecting nucleotides coding for the DNA-binding residues, although KTS mutations in intron 9, characteristic of Frasier syndrome, have been identified in patients with DDS or with isolated DMS. Frasier syndrome described as male pseudohermaphroditism associated with XY gonadal dysgenesis and nephrotic syndrome typically shows FSGS on renal biopsy that progresses to end-stage renal disease during the second or third decade of life (175). Patients with Frasier syndrome are at risk for gonadoblastoma but have a very low risk for WT (177). WT1 mutations characteristic of Frasier or Denys-Drash syndrome have been found in 6% of patients presenting with isolated SRNS; notably, adolescent girls with primary amenorrhea should undergo WT1 screening. Nearly 30% of all patients with a WT1 mutation display isolated sporadic SRNS without any associated comorbidities and extrarenal features, when present can be so subtle that they are only detected retrospectively in light of genetic diagnosis (177).

Nail-Patella Syndrome, Collagen Type III Glomerulopathy, and Pierson Syndrome

Nail–patella syndrome (NPS) may be a cause of proteinuria in infancy, childhood, or adulthood. The cardinal features of this condition are dysplasia of the nails and absent or hypoplastic patellas, but most patients also have iliac horns and dysplasia of the elbows. A nephropathy develops in some kindreds. LM may show patchy tubular atrophy and interstitial fibrosis, but the glomeruli are normal or show only irregular thickening of the capillary wall or mesangial expansion or segmental or global sclerosis. Immunofluorescence studies are usually negative. EM reveals prominent thickening of the glomerular basement membrane, which has a mottled appearance caused by irregular but sharply defined electron-lucent areas containing fibers that have the periodicity of collagen, especially if the grids have been stained with phosphotungstic acid (178). Similar clear zones with collagen are often found in the mesangium. Approximately 40% to 60% of the patients with NPS have renal manifestations, and it is estimated that 15% to 30% progress to renal failure, but the course in an individual patient is unpredictable (178,179). NPS is due to mutations in the LIM–homeodomain protein LMX1B at 9q34 that regulates transcription of collagen IV subtypes α3 and α4, and mutation analysis has shown correlation of mutations in this domain with proteinuria but not to the extrarenal manifestations of the disease (180). Mutations in LMX1B have recently been demonstrated in patients with autosomal dominant FSGS that lacked extrarenal features or ultrastructural features of NPS (181). Collagen type III (collagenofibrotic) glomerulopathy presents with progressive proteinuria in late infancy to adulthood, and most affected children go on to renal failure.

Glomeruli are markedly enlarged and have lobular architecture with expanded mesangia and thick capillary walls due to accumulation of massive amounts of collagen type III, and by EM, the mesangia and the subendothelial space are electron lucent or mottled. Collagen fibers, typically curved rather than straight as in normal interstitial type III collagen, with a periodicity of approximately 60 nm, can be demonstrated with phosphotungstic acid staining, but patients do not have the extrarenal manifestations of NPS (178). Another disorder of the glomerular basement membrane is Pierson syndrome that typically presents with severe nephrosis in early infancy or prenatal onset characterized by a heavy placenta with hydrops fetalis and elevated AFP (mimicking CNF) or even renal failure with intrauterine demise. CNS is often associated with microcoria, but less severe ocular anomalies are described. The autosomal recessive disorder is due to mutations of LAMB2 at chromosome 3p21 that encodes laminin β2 that anchors the podocyte foot process to the basement membrane (182). Pathologically, it may show DMS or glomerular hypercellularity with variable thickening, thinning, rarefaction, and lamination of the glomerular basement membrane on EM (183).

Glomerulopathies that Usually Present with Hematuria with or without Proteinuria

The most important diseases in this category in children include the primary IgA nephropathies—Berger disease and Henoch-Schönlein purpura (HSP) nephritis and the basement membrane nephropathies—Alport syndrome (AS) and thin glomerular basement membrane disease. Hematuria is a well-known complication of hypercalciuria, but no specific pathologic lesion is associated with this condition (184), and the histopathologic abnormalities in loin-pain hematuria syndrome are nonspecific. In all these conditions, the finding of red cell casts or hemosiderin in tubular epithelial cells lends support to a diagnosis of hematuria originating in the kidney rather than in the lower urinary tract. The primary IgA nephropathies are defined by the presence of IgA as the dominant or codominant immunoreactant in the absence of clinical or laboratory features of SLE. Characteristic but not always pathognomonic ultrastructural lesions are observed in many cases of AS, and an ultrastructural lesion defines thin glomerular basement membrane disease.

IgA Nephropathy (Berger Disease)

IgA nephropathy was described by Berger and Hinglais in 1968 (185), but the association of recurrent hematuria and focal glomerulonephritis, often in patients with a recent history of upper respiratory infection, had been recognized many years earlier. Today, IgA nephropathy is the most common glomerulopathy worldwide, accounting for 5% to 10% of cases of glomerular disease in North America, 15% to 30% in Europe, and up to 50% in Japan. Prevalence data garnered from biopsy series should be interpreted with caution as there are wide regional differences in ascertainment (186). For example, children of school age in Japan undergo an annual screening urinalysis, and three quarter of cases of IgA nephropathy in Japan are detected when only microscopic hematuria is present. In Europe and North America, 75% of children with IgA nephropathy present with gross hematuria. The annual incidence of IgA nephropathy among children in the United States is about 0.5 cases per 100,000; however, the incidence is 10 times as high in Japan (186). Besides biopsy practices, race seems to influence the geographic differences in the frequency of IgA nephropathy. A considerably lower incidence is reported among African American and Black Africans compared to Caucasians. A high incidence has been reported in Native Americans (187). The male to female ratio is about 2:1 in North American cohorts but approaches 1:1 in Asia (186). Many cases of IgA nephropathy occur within a few days after an upper respiratory or a gastrointestinal infection; in contrast, several weeks usually separate the antecedent infection from the onset of postinfectious glomerulonephritis. Serum levels of IgA are significantly elevated in up to 50% of adults but in only 8% to 16% of children with IgA nephropathy, but serum levels of IgA or of IgA–fibronectin cannot be used in lieu of renal biopsy for the diagnosis of these conditions (186). Recent studies have implicated aberrant glycosylation of the hinge region of the IgA1 molecule in the pathogenesis of IgA nephropathy. The abnormal molecule has a galactose deficiency in some carbohydrate side chains (*O*-glycans) and mostly affects polymeric IgA1 produced in mucosal tissues. Nearly all circulating galactose-deficient IgA1 is within immune complexes bound to a glycan-specific antibody, thus not cleared by the reticuloendothelial system, and able to reach the glomerulus, bind to mesangial cells, and activate complement. The formation of immune complexes is critical for the nephritogenicity of the abnormal IgA1 via the alternative and lectin pathways. Despite frequent serum elevation of galactose-deficient IgA1, it has low sensitivity and specificity in diagnosis; however, the level of glycan-specific IgG antibodies correlates with urinary protein excretion and risk of progression to end-stage renal disease, thus may prove a useful biomarker of disease activity and response. Additional consideration has been proposed for genetic profiling, miRNAs, and CD89–IgA complex levels, although specificity remains suspect (186,188,189).

Classically, IgA nephropathy is characterized by focal segmental to global mesangial hypercellularity by LM (Figure 17-21B), confluent granular mesangial deposits that stain more brightly for IgA than for other immunoglobulins by IF microscopy (Figure 17-22B), and electron-dense deposits within and especially along the periphery of mesangia and adjacent to mesangial cells. However, the histologic picture is quite variable. Biopsies from pediatric patients usually show greater mesangial and endocapillary hypercellularity and crescent formation than adults, who typically have more glomerulosclerosis, matrix expansion, and interstitial damage, perhaps reflecting earlier detection in children. Nonetheless, the histology in IgA nephropathy is highly variable with 8% to 55% of biopsies showing minimal abnormalities (190). This proportion may reflect biopsy practice where investigations of patients with isolated microscopic hematuria have a higher incidence of normal findings. Endocapillary hypercellularity, usually focal, is evident in about one-third of cases. A similar percentage contains extracapillary proliferative lesions, although the proportion of glomeruli with crescents is typically low (190). Segmental glomerulosclerosis, characterized by occlusion of capillary lumina by extracellular matrix in part of a glomerulus, is a frequent finding in IgA nephropathy. High levels of proteinuria are associated with protein resorption droplets in tubular epithelium and can lead to tubular injury that results in fibrosis and mononuclear cell infiltration. Interstitial fibrosis with tubular atrophy is one of the most reliable markers of adverse outcomes (187,190).

The diagnosis of IgA nephropathy requires the demonstration of IgA dominant or codominant glomerular staining involving the mesangium with or without involvement of peripheral capillary walls. In addition, IgG was present in 43%, C3 in 93%, IgM in 54%, and C1q in 10%. In addition to IgA nephropathy and HSP nephritis (which cannot be distinguished from IgA nephropathy on a renal biopsy), the differential diagnosis of dominant or codominant mesangial IgA deposits includes lupus nephritis (LN), C1q nephropathy, HIV-associated glomerulonephritis, poststaphylococcal glomerulonephritis, and combinations of mesangial IgA deposits with MCD, MGN, and ANCA-associated glomerulonephritis (187). Mesangial electron-dense immune complex deposits are detected in nearly all instances, and the typical location is in the paramesangium (immediately beneath the basement membrane as it crosses the mesangium). They are typically unstructured and uniform; occasional deposits are noted deep within the mesangial matrix. Approximately one-third of cases also have capillary wall deposits, usually small and subendothelial, but intramembranous and rarely subepithelial deposits are noted (190). In an ultrastructural study of 34 patients with IgA nephropathy, Vogler et al.(191) noted focal and segmental attenuation, splitting, duplication, paramesangial microaneurysms, and subepithelial protrusions of the glomerular basement membrane—features that were more marked in specimens with relatively severe lesions by LM and capillary wall deposits by IF microscopy. Such structural abnormalities are relatively common in IgA nephropathy and may be to the degree that they resemble AS.

Historical analyses have found a correlation of proteinuria and episodic gross hematuria with the more severe histologic and ultrastructural lesions and correlated the development of end-stage disease with more significant cellularity and crescents. A recent study of 250 adults and children with IgA nephropathy followed for a median of 5 years found that mesangial and intracapillary hypercellularity, segmental glomerulosclerosis, and tubular atrophy and interstitial fibrosis independently predicted renal outcome, but crescents did not, possibly because patients with more severe disease were excluded (192). Validation studies of the Oxford Classification focusing on pediatric populations have shown variable results partly influenced by inclusion criteria, particularly the fraction of patients with mild disease and minimal hypercellularity. Nonetheless, with univariant and multivariant analysis, tubular atrophy and interstitial fibrosis consistently predicted poor outcome, mesangial and endocapillary cellularity and segmental sclerosis usually had prognostic significance, but crescents, not a significant predictor in some analysis, may have predictive value in patients with severe disease (i.e., low glomerular filtration rate [GFR]) (193,194).

Henoch-Schönlein Purpura Nephritis

HSP is a clinical syndrome involving the skin, joints, gastrointestinal tract, and, in 20% to 50% of cases, the kidneys. The heart, lungs, central nervous system, and muscles may also be affected. Although the incidence peaks at 4 to 5 years, older children and adolescents seem to be at higher risk for the development of renal disease. HSP is now classified as a form of systemic vasculitis with IgA1-dominant immune deposits (IgAV) affecting small vessels, predominantly capillaries, venules, or arterioles (195); the justification for the change in name includes the likely pathogenic significance of IgA deposits while conversely recognizing that syndromic features of purpura, abdominal pain, arthralgias, and nephritis are not so unique as to allow distinction from other small-vessel vasculitides. Updated criteria for IgAV (HSP) include the presence of purpura or petechiae with a lower limb predominance plus at least one of the following: abdominal pain, histopathology of leukocytoclastic vasculitis or glomerulonephritis with predominant IgA deposits, arthritis or arthralgia, and renal involvement as evidenced by hematuria and/or proteinuria (196). Glomerulonephritis indistinguishable from IgA nephropathy may occur. The incidence of renal involvement varies among studies, based on definition, ranges from 20% to 56% (average 34%), and is lower than in adults (187). Also shared are the male predominance, lower incidence in African Americans than Caucasians, and onset during or shortly following an upper respiratory infection; the majority of cases arise within the fall or winter months. There are no specific laboratory tests for HSP, but titers for galactose-deficient IgA are elevated if renal disease is present, and serologic studies are useful in excluding the other leading causes of rash and renal disease in children—lupus and microscopic polyarteritis nodosa (polyangiitis). Renal involvement in HSP is heralded by asymptomatic gross or microscopic hematuria, but proteinuria may also be present, and in some series from referral centers, a nephrotic syndrome is present in 30% of patients with renal disease. Persistent renal involvement (hypertension, reduced renal function, nephrotic or nephritic syndrome) occurs in approximately 2% of children overall, but the incidence varies with the severity of kidney disease at presentation, occurring in 5% of children with isolated hematuria and/or proteinuria but 20% who had acute nephritis and/or nephrotic syndrome during the acute phase (197).

The renal lesions in HSP are similar to those in IgA nephropathy by light, IF, and EM, but the glomerular disease tends to be more severe and to more often include crescents than in IgA nephropathy. As in IgA nephropathy, the outcome is worse in patients with severe segmental lesions and crescents (187). The skin lesion in HSP is a leukocytoclastic vasculitis, and deposits of IgA are seen in the walls of blood vessels in biopsies of fresh purpuric lesions, but they are not seen in skin specimens from patients with IgA nephropathy and may disappear in later stages of HSP (198).

Alport Syndrome

AS includes various combinations of abnormalities of the kidney, inner ear, eye, skin, and smooth muscle that are caused by mutations in genes coding for type IV collagen (199). Proceeding from the observation that the antiglomerular basement membrane antibodies from patients with Goodpasture syndrome did not stain glomeruli from patients with AS, it was learned that type IV collagen in all basement membranes is made up of a triple helix of two alpha-1 chains and one alpha-2 chain, but that with maturation in certain basement membranes, this structure is replaced by a triple helix composed of various combinations of four other chains, alpha-3 through alpha-6 and that the genes for these chains are arranged in head-to-head pairs on chromosome 13 (*COL4A1* and *COL4A2*), chromosome 2 (*COL4A3* and *COL4A4*), and the X chromosome (*COL4A5* and *COL4A6*) (200). Eighty to 85% of cases of AS are X linked secondary to mutations in the gene at Xq22 that encodes the alpha-5 chain of type IV collagen, and other patients have autosomal recessive or, less frequently, autosomal dominant disease secondary to mutations in the alpha-3 and alpha-4 genes on chromosome 2 (199). The distribution of the alpha-3 through alpha-6 isomers in the body accounts for the organs involved in AS.

The typical symptoms of AS involve the kidney, eye, and ear; therefore, a diagnosis is suggested after a careful examination. Most authorities recommend that several criteria be met before a diagnosis of AS is assigned to an individual or a family (201). Pertinent clinical and family history includes persistent unexplained hematuria, nephritis, or gradual progression to end-stage renal disease in a first-degree relative; bilateral sensorineural hearing loss in the 2000- to 8000-Hz range; and anterior lenticonus or other characteristic ocular lesions. The finding of macrothrombocytopenia or granulocyte inclusions, previously attributed to AS, is now known to result from mutations in the *MYH9* gene, which encodes nonmuscle myosin heavy chain IIA, and results in the May-Hegglin anomaly and Sebastian, Fechtner, and Epstein syndromes, the latter two of which share renal, ocular, and auditory symptoms that overlap with AS; GBM splitting is also evident (202). Diagnostic support by demonstration of widespread ultrastructural alterations in the glomerular basement membrane and confirmation by immunohistochemical evidence of complete or partial loss of the Alport epitope in glomerular or epidermal basement membranes (Figure 17-26 A, B) or demonstration of a mutation in one of the type IV collagen genes listed above is desired for a diagnosis of AS (199). Hematuria is demonstrable by 5 years of age in affected boys with X-linked AS. The progression to end-stage renal disease in X-linked AS is variable but roughly similar within kindreds and strongly dependent upon the type of mutation. The risk of ESRD by age 30 is 90% for deletions and nonsense mutations of *COL4A5*, 70% for splicing mutations, and 50% for missense mutations (203). Severe mutations are also associated with perimacular dot-and-fleck retinopathy as well as lenticonus and hearing loss (204,205). The effects of *COL4A5* genotype on age of ESRD are not observed in females with X-linked AS due to the significant influence of X inactivation (206,207). Autosomal recessive Alport syndrome (ARAS) accounts for about 15% of individuals and results from two pathogenic mutations in either the *Col4A3* or *COL4A4* gene. Recent data indicate that the nature of the mutation in AR AS affects the clinical phenotype. In general, both males and females with ARAS carry a high risk of ESRD by age 30, but rare cases of mild disease are reported (208). Only about 5% of AS are attributed to autosomal dominant disease, which tends to progress at a relatively slow rate. Recent investigations utilizing next-generation sequencing (NGS), which allows simultaneous assessment of *COL4A3*, *COL4A4*, and *COL4A5*, offer an efficient and cost-effective approach with a sensitivity reported at 99% in one study (209). These authors also noted a higher rate of *COL4A3* and *COL4A4* mutations in their

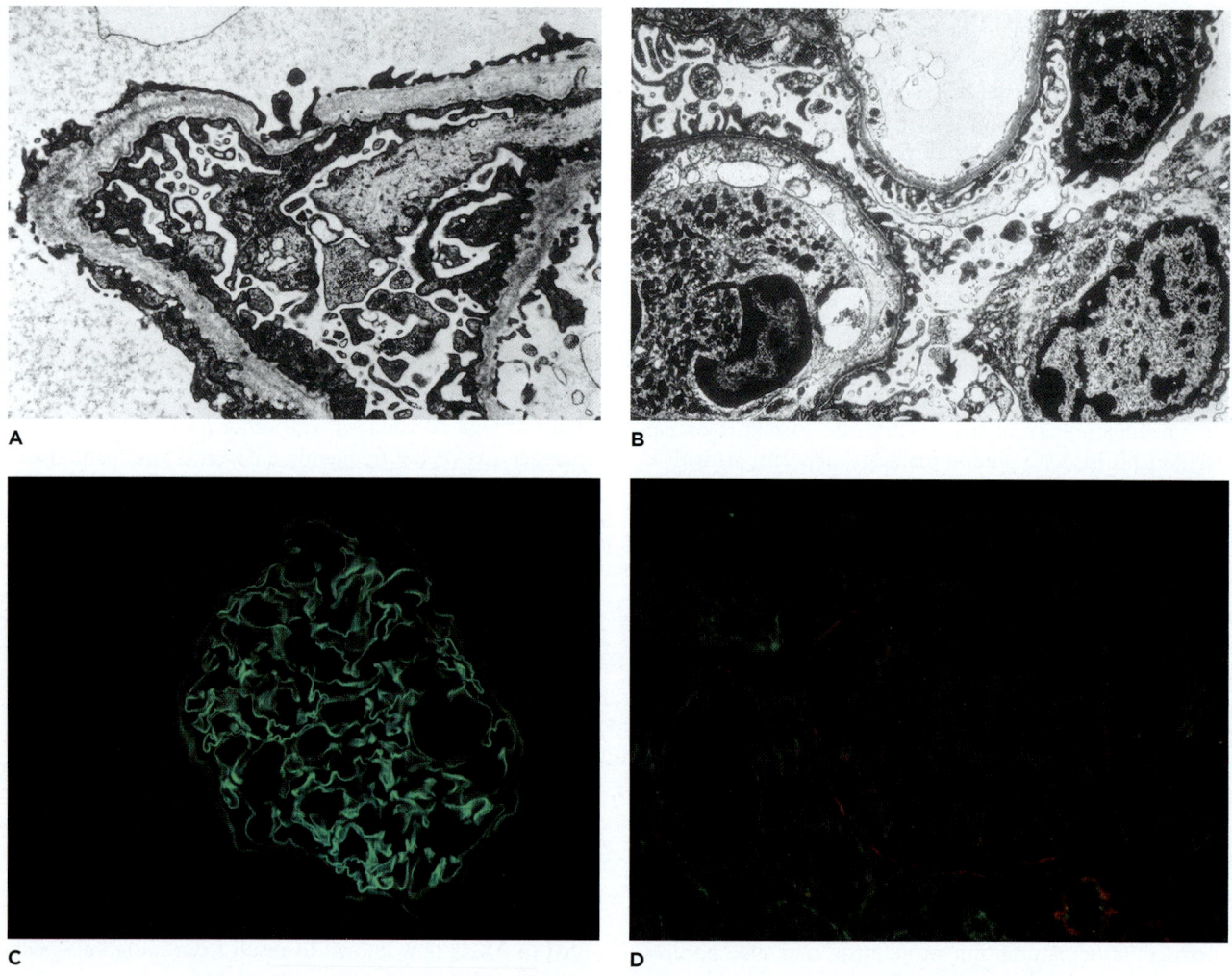

FIGURE 17-26 • Basement membrane nephropathies. **A:** Marked thinning, fraying, intersecting lamination, and granularity of the glomerular capillary basement membrane are characteristics of hereditary nephritis (AS), but are not seen in all cases. **B:** Diffuse thinning of the capillary basement membrane is seen in familial hematuria and may be the only ultrastructural lesion in AS. **C, D:** Staining for collagen IVa5 is seen along the glomerular capillary basement membrane and, to a lesser extent, Bowman capsule in control **(C)** but not patient **(D)** glomeruli. (**A, B:** Lead citrate and uranyl acetate, **C, D:** fluorescein isothiocyanate-conjugated anticollagen IVa5, original magnification 400×.)

cohort of over 100 patients, 10% of whom were considered to have benign familial hematuria, implying that autosomal dominant forms of AS are more frequent than previously reported and thus validating the need to interrogate beyond *COL4A5* sequencing, which is a common approach in many laboratories based on presumed frequency and ambiguous transmission.

Histologic findings in children under 10 may be minimal, and at any age, they are nonspecific. The number of fetal glomeruli may be increased, and there may be variable degrees of segmental or global mesangial hypercellularity, thickening of capillary walls, tuft sclerosis, patchy tubular atrophy, red cell casts or hemosiderin in tubular epithelial cells, and aggregates of foam cells in the interstitium (210). Results of the standard immunofluorescence studies are negative, an important finding in ruling out IgA nephropathy or an immune complex glomerulonephritis; nonspecific staining with IgM, IgG, C3, and C1q may accumulate with progressive tuft sclerosis. Monoclonal analysis of type IV collagen chain expression in kidney and skin basement membranes is often informative; analogous results can be achieved using fluorescein-tagged antiglomerular basement membrane antibodies obtained from patients with Goodpasture syndrome. In about 70% to 80% of males with X-linked AS, examination of the kidney reveals lack of alpha-3, alpha-4, and alpha-5 in the GBM and distal tubular basement membranes in conjunction with expanded expression of alpha-1 throughout the glomerulus (Figure 17-26C, D). There is also loss of alpha-5 (and alpha-6) in Bowman capsule and collecting duct membranes as well as epidermal basement membranes assessed in skin punch biopsies (199). Renal and cutaneous expression in female carriers is often segmental due to random inactivation of the X chromosome, but can appear normal or completely absent due to patchy distribution (206). Renal expression of the alpha-3 or alpha-4 chains is altered in patients with ARAS.

The characteristic ultrastructural abnormalities of AS include irregular thinning, thickening, splitting, and a wavy intersecting lamellation known as the *basket weave* pattern (Figure 17-26A), often with 50-nm-diameter electron-dense granules between lamellae. However, renal specimens obtained early in life may show no abnormalities, and the most common observation in children is thinning of the basement membrane to less than 150 nm (Figure 17-26B) (210). The immunofluorescence studies and variable ultrastructural findings support the hypothesis that the Alport GBM is defective not only because of an absence of collagen-4-alpha-3, alpha-4, and alpha-5 and prolonged presence of collagen 4 alpha-1 and alpha-2, which is more susceptible to proteolysis, but because of the dysregulation of laminins, which may represent a compensatory response. The resulting abnormal GBM likely conveys inappropriate signals to the adherent endothelial cells and podocytes, which leads to progressive disease (123).

Thin Glomerular Basement Membrane Disease

The only significant abnormality in the renal biopsy specimens of 20% to 25% of children or adults evaluated for isolated hematuria is thinning of the glomerular basement membrane on ultrastructural study (Figure 17-26B). The incidence is difficult to ascertain because its demonstration depends upon the definition of abnormal thinning and the indication for renal biopsy. The term *thin glomerular basement membrane disease* describes a pathologic finding that may be familial or sporadic and may be associated with a benign or progressive course. The term *benign familial hematuria* is applied when thin GBM is the only abnormality, the family has a history of isolated hematuria that follows an autosomal dominant pattern, and the affected person has persistent or recurrent microscopic hematuria (rarely macroscopic); no significant proteinuria, hypertension, or progressive renal disease; and no extrarenal manifestations of AS. Some favor abandoning this term as familial hematuria is not always benign and benign hematuria is not always familial (211). Heterozygous mutations in the *COL4A3* and *COL4A4* genes have been found in 40% to 50% of kindreds with benign familial hematuria (212). Furthermore, thinning of the glomerular basement membrane may be the only abnormality in a renal specimen from patients with typical X linked, autosomal recessive, or autosomal dominant and is especially common in children and females with X-linked AS, even after a careful search for proteinuria, extrarenal lesions, and abnormal collagen distribution in the biopsy, underscoring the need for close clinical follow-up and consideration of type IV collagen mutation analysis (209). Diffuse thinning of the glomerular basement membrane has also been described in IgA nephropathy and other glomerulopathies including MCD and FSGS (213). The latter is significant as thin GBM due to Col4A3 or Col4A4 mutations associated with FSGS is more likely to have renal outcome that resembles FSGS than thin glomerular basement membrane disease (214).

Almost by definition, renal specimens with thin glomerular basement membrane disease are normal by light and IF microscopy. Focal immature or globally sclerotic glomeruli, areas of tubular atrophy, and variable staining for immunoglobulin or complement components along the glomerular capillary loop have been reported (183). The cardinal finding in this group of diseases is diffuse thinning of the glomerular basement membrane by EM (Figure 17-26B). The widths of the lamina densa and capillary wall increase throughout childhood, but reported measurements of these structures have shown considerable interlaboratory variation, emphasizing the need for each facility to establish its own reference range (122). The mean thicknesses of the glomerular basement membranes in published reports of thin basement membrane disease have ranged from 150 to 300 nm, but most pediatric series have used a cutoff of 250 nm (122). Recent assessment has found no correlation between the degree of GBM thinning and the presentation or clinical outcome (215).

Loin Pain Hematuria Syndrome

Gross hematuria is accompanied by loin pain in many adults with IgA nephropathy, but such pain is encountered less often in children with IgA nephropathy (216). *Loin pain hematuria syndrome*, a controversial diagnosis, refers to gross or microscopic hematuria accompanied by unilateral or bilateral loin pain, often severe enough that opiates are required. Whether it is a discrete entity or a collection of unrelated disorders with common symptoms remains to be determined. Most patients are women between 20 and 40 years of age, but adolescent boys and girls and an occasional younger child are included in reported series. Subtle biochemical or renovascular lesions have been described in some reports, and several reports have included patients with psychiatric disorders or an altered perception of pain (217). By LM, a renal biopsy specimen may show a slight segmental proliferation of mesangial cells; mild interstitial fibrosis, especially near the corticomedullary junction; and minimal thickening of the walls of the intracortical arteries and arterioles; increased RBC casts, pointing to a glomerular origin of RBCs, have been noted in kidney biopsies from patients with loin pain hematuria. Immunofluorescence often reveals linear or flecklike staining for C3 in the walls of the arterioles, but not in the glomeruli. However, such staining in the arterioles is not uncommon in specimens from patients with hematuria of many causes. EM shows no electron-dense deposits or diagnostic abnormality of the glomerular capillary basement membrane, although variations in GBM thickness have been noted (218). Since none of these findings have any diagnostic specificity, the pathologist's role in the evaluation of these patients is to confirm, if possible, the renal origin of hematuria and exclude other conditions that might present with hematuria. Various approaches to treatment including analgesics, capsaicin, ACE inhibitors, acupuncture, or surgery such as kidney autotransplantation, renal denervation, or nephrectomy have had mixed and usually temporary results. Although hematuria and pain often persist, the kidney function remains good.

Glomerulopathies that Usually Present with a Nephritic Syndrome of Hypertension, Impaired Renal Function, Hypocomplementemia, and Cellular Casts, Protein, and Blood in the Urine

The most important causes of the "nephritic syndrome" in children include postinfectious glomerulonephritis, MPGN, and LN. These three conditions constitute the differential diagnosis of mesangiocapillary or endocapillary proliferative glomerulonephritis because they can produce a similar histologic lesion characterized by marked glomerular hypercellularity with accentuation of the lobular architecture and thickened capillary walls (Figure 17-21C). However, variations related to the stage or age of the lesion do exist. A similar clinical picture can be seen in crescentic glomerulonephritides (Figure 17-21D). Although crescents can occasionally be seen in almost any glomerulopathy, the major differential diagnosis of crescentic glomerulonephritis (CGN) in children and adolescents includes immune complex diseases, such as postinfectious glomerulonephritis, LN, and MPGN, particular dense deposit disease, and pauci-immune (ANCA-associated glomerulonephritis), which are discussed in this section; the small-vessel vasculitides, which are discussed in the section on renovascular diseases; and IgA nephropathy and HSP nephritis, discussed previously.

Postinfectious Glomerulonephritis

The incidence of acute glomerulonephritis following throat or skin infections with group A streptococci in the United States and Europe has been declining for nearly 50 years, but poststreptococcal glomerulonephritis (PIGN) is still a relatively common disease worldwide, especially in tropical countries (219). Renal biopsies are usually obtained only if gross hematuria persists beyond 1 month; hypocomplementemia persists beyond 6 weeks; hypertension persists beyond 2 months; progressive deterioration of renal function or evidence of extrarenal disease is present; nephritis occurred within 48 hours of pharyngitis; age is less than 2 years, or there is a family history of renal disease (220). Infections with organisms other than group A streptococci can produce morphologic features similar to that seen in poststreptococcal acute glomerulonephritis (hence the more generic term *postinfectious glomerulonephritis*), but many of these organisms can also elicit other forms of glomerular disease (221).

Histologically, PIGN evolves over several weeks from an endocapillary proliferative (mesangiocapillary) (Figure 17-21C) and exudative (increased neutrophils within tufts) glomerulonephritis to a mesangial proliferative glomerulonephritis (Figure 17-21B) with patent capillary loops and normally thin capillary walls. The immunofluorescence pattern also evolves from a coarse capillary granular (Figure 17-22A) staining for IgG and C3, with lesser amounts of other immunoreactants, to a mesangial granular (Figure 17-22B) staining for C3, typically without staining for other immunoreactants; however, isolated C3 has also been shown early in the disease course (219). Specimens obtained within 2 weeks of the onset of symptoms often show a capillary granular pattern, termed *starry sky*, and a mesangial pattern is seen when a biopsy occurs later. A third immunofluorescence pattern—confluent lumpy staining along the capillary loops and lesser staining within and around mesangia—termed *garland* is observed in both early and later biopsy specimens. The pattern does not correlate with the degree of proteinuria (219). Ultrastructurally, patients with the capillary wall (starry sky) pattern by immunofluorescence showed domed electron-dense deposits on the epithelial side of the basement membrane over which the foot processes of visceral epithelial cells characteristically arch (Figure 17-27). These subepithelial "humps" can be sparse to numerous and were flattened and focally confluent in specimens that showed the garland pattern by immunofluorescence. Basement membrane deposits may persist for years in some patients, but few if any humps are typically seen

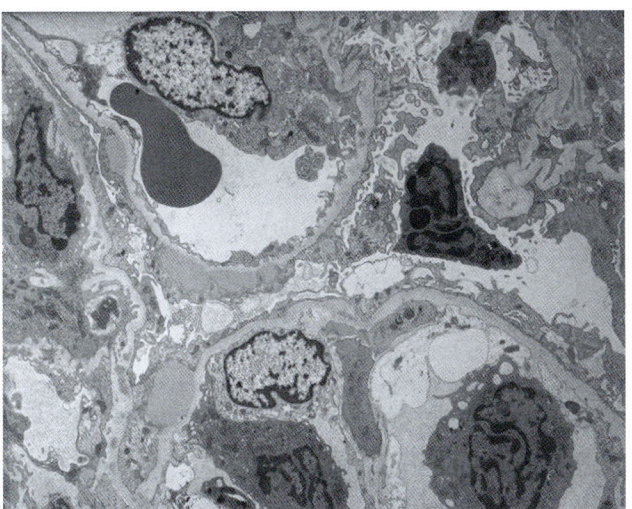

FIGURE 17-27 • Postinfectious glomerulonephritis. The foot processes of an epithelial cell arch over large subepithelial "humps." (Lead citrate and uranyl acetate.)

in later biopsy specimens from children. Thus, the absence of humps in a later specimen does not exclude the diagnosis of postinfectious glomerulonephritis, and because structures consistent with humps have been described in other conditions, the finding of a rare hump, typically above the junction of the capillary loop and mesangium, suggests (222), but does not necessarily establish, this diagnosis.

The majority of children with well-documented acute PIGN have a good prognosis and recover completely (219). A recent series showed that ESRD was more prevalent in crescentic postinfectious glomerulonephritis and did not occur in any of the children without crescents; an estimated 2% of patients with PIGN have a clinical course severe enough to even warrant a biopsy (223).

Not unexpectedly, nonstreptococcal postinfectious glomerulonephritides manifest a more varied morphology. Staphylococcal infections often show a predominance of mesangial deposits with IgA as the dominant immunoreactant. The glomerulonephritis associated with subacute bacterial endocarditis may be diffuse and proliferative, but the classic lesion is a focal and segmental fibrinoid necrosis or thrombosis that evolves to similarly distributed sclerotic lesions in glomeruli by LM, but diffuse global, predominantly mesangial and subendothelial deposits by immunofluorescence and EM. Acute bacterial endocarditis can produce a variety of renal lesions ranging from a proliferative glomerulonephritis, often with crescents, to interstitial inflammation to infarction, and glomeruli show mesangial and intramembranous deposits as well as subepithelial humps that seem to persist longer than those in PIGN. The glomerulonephritis associated with infected ventriculoatrial shunts is similar to that seen in acute PIGN, including the presence of increased numbers of neutrophils, but typically shows mesangial and subendothelial rather than subepithelial deposits. It is worth noting that patients with "atypical postinfectious glomerulonephritis" defined as no recognizable antecedent infection, persistent hematuria and proteinuria, and characteristic light and electron microscopic pathology including "humps" and C3-dominant IF with or without Ig may have an underlying defect in the alternative pathway of complement (224).

Membranoproliferative Glomerulonephritis

MPGN is a morphologic pattern of injury characterized by an expanded mesangium with hypercellularity, mesangial interposition, and duplication of GBMs that occurs in reaction to deposition of immunoglobulins and/or complement and can appear in association with a heterogeneous group of disorders such as with infected shunts or valves; hepatitis C and other viral, bacterial, or protozoal infections; sickle cell disease; autoimmune disease; and α1-antitrypsin deficiency and other liver diseases; it is considered "idiopathic" or "primary" in the absence of an underlying cause. Historically, MPGN has been classified into three different types, based on light and electron microscopic findings.

Type I MPGN was initially described in children, but it also occurs in adults, and the median age at onset is 21 years. Type II MPGN, or preferably dense deposit disease, is more common in children than adults, with a median age at onset of 11.5 years. The designation type III MPGN has been applied to several lesions over the years including discrete subendothelial, intramembranous, and subepithelial deposits with features that overlapped with MPGN I and membranous glomerulopathy but is now generally reserved for the disorder with subepithelial, subendothelial, and complex ill-defined intramembranous deposits associated with disruption of the glomerular basement membrane. This lesion is probably lumped with type I disease in most reports.

MPGN in pediatrics most commonly affects older children and adolescents. The incidence of MPGN is influenced by age and region, but the overall rate appears to be declining in childhood (225). Up to 70% of children with idiopathic MPGN present with nephrotic syndrome or mild proteinuria, and macrohematuria is noted in about 20% (226), but a persistent nephrotic syndrome is a poor prognostic sign. Extrarenal abnormalities, especially partial lipodystrophy and densities in the retinal epithelium, are seen in patients with dense deposit disease (226). Decreased levels of the third component of complement (C3) are seen in all forms of MPGN, but C4 is usually normal in DDD.

Histologically, type I MPGN is the most common and shows uniformly enlarged and hypercellular glomeruli with expanded and hypercellular mesangia (Figure 17-21C), compressed capillary lumens, and thickened capillary walls with segmental double contours ("tram tracks") on silver stains. Increased numbers of neutrophils are seen in glomeruli in 25% of cases and crescents in 10%. Hyaline "thrombi," large eosinophilic globules in glomerular capillaries, raise the question of cryoglobulinemia and hepatitis C. The interstitium shows edema, lymphocytic infiltrates, and patchy fibrosis. The three types of idiopathic MPGN are defined by their ultrastructure. In type I, the lamina densa of the glomerular capillary wall is normal, but numerous electron-dense deposits and cytoplasmic processes (interposition) are seen in the subendothelial space (Figure 17-28A). The two lines of the histologic "tram track" are the original lamina densa and the new membrane deposited between the interposed material and the endothelial cell. Mesangial deposits are noted, and subepithelial deposits are seen in 30% to 50% of cases (227). Type II disease shows more variable cellularity but more uniformly thickened capillary walls. It has a distinctive EM appearance, characterized by extensive ribbonlike extremely electron-dense material in the glomerular basement membrane (Figure 17-28B), mesangia, and, in some cases, the basement membranes of tubules and Bowman capsule; similar deposits have been observed in extrarenal locations. Type III MPGN generally has a less pronounced and more variable cellularity. Ultrastructural analysis of MPGN III shows a thickened basement membrane with subendothelial and subepithelial deposits that are less electron dense than those in MPGN I, and silver impregnation reveals a frayed and laminated basement membrane (227).

Immunofluorescence microscopy shows coarse granular staining along the capillary loops and the periphery of expanded mesangia, the "peripheral pattern" for immunoglobulins (usually IgG or IgM) and C3, occasionally associated with C1q and C4. Type II MPGN shows a linear or a ribbonlike staining of capillary walls and hollow rings in mesangia for C3 (Figure 17-22D) and, uncommonly and less intensely, for other immunoreactants. Type III MPGN shows finely granular to confluent capillary wall and central mesangial staining for immunoglobulins and C3 (227). However, as early as the 1970s, it was apparent that C3-positive but immunoglobulin-negative examples of MPGN I and MPGN III exist. As understanding of etiology has increased over the past decades, there has been a major shift toward categorization based on immunofluorescence rather than morphology (228,229). Those with substantial deposits of Ig are considered immune complex mediated, deserving of investigation of etiology (as above), while the term C3 glomerulopathy (C3G) was proposed for cases with deposition of C3 only, including DDD and MPGN I and III with predominant C3, that also lacked early components of the classical pathway of complement (C1q and C4).

C3G results from aberrant control of the alternate complement pathway, and abnormalities have included genetic deficiencies in regulators of the alternative complement cascade (i.e., complement factors H, HR1-5 and I, and CD46) or acquired autoantibodies to factors H and B and C3 convertase (C3 nephritic factor [C3NeF]) (228–230). Proposals for diagnosis, including C3 dominant (C3 at least two orders of magnitude more intense than any Ig), appear reproducible and may help to guide therapy and predict outcome (230–233).

Early reports of treatment and outcome predate use of angiotensin-converting enzyme (ACE) inhibitors and angiotensin II receptor blockers but predicted worse outcomes in patients with crescents, sclerotic glomeruli, extensive double contours, and tubulointerstitial disease as well as those with nephrotic syndrome, macroscopic hematuria, and decreased renal function at the time of presentation. There is a suggestion of benefit from long-term alternate-day glucocorticoid therapy for idiopathic MPGN in children (234). A pragmatic approach includes treatment of underlying infection or autoimmune disease where appropriate, replacement of factor deficiency with plasma infusion, and the potential use of anticomplement drugs (235,236).

In summary, a practical approach to MPGN is to consider it as an immune complex (IC)-mediated disorder (typically MPGN types I and III) resulting from deposition of ICs in glomeruli that develop from persistent antigenemia secondary to chronic infections, autoimmune diseases, or paraproteinemias, with activation of the classic complement pathway, or as a complement-mediated disorder (classically MPGN II—DDD, and some MPGN I and III—C3G) owing

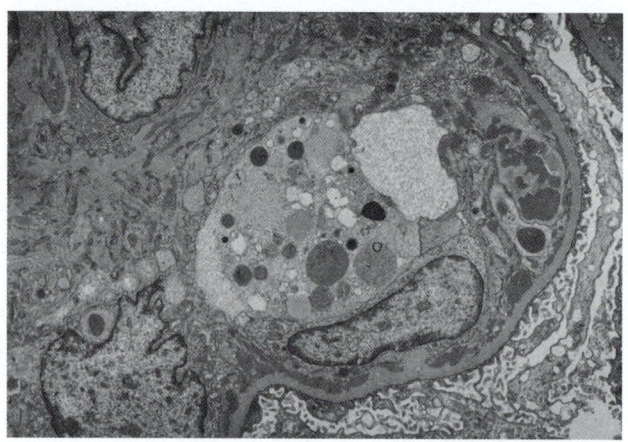
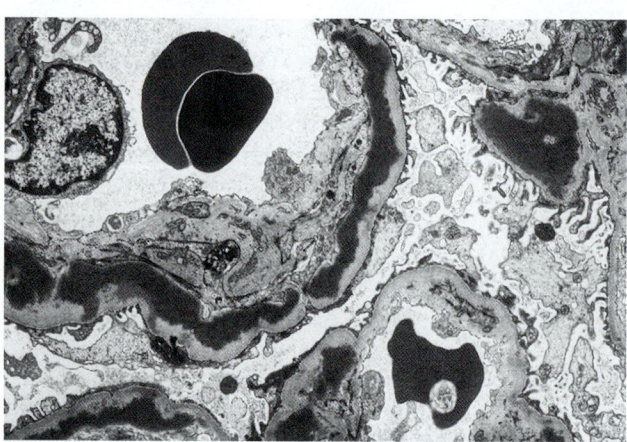

FIGURE 17-28 • **A:** Type I MPGN with subendothelial electron-dense deposits and interposed mesangial cell cytoplasm. **B:** Type II MPGN (dense deposit disease) is defined by irregular ribbons of electron-dense material along the glomerular capillary basement membrane (**A, B**, lead citrate and uranyl acetate stain, original magnifications ×3000.)

to dysregulation of alternative pathway because of mutations or autoantibodies.

Lupus Nephritis

Pediatric onset of SLE accounts for 10% to 20% of all patients with SLE (237). The most common presenting complaints in children with SLE are arthritis, arthralgia, rash, and fever, but renal, cardiac, and central nervous system involvement becomes evident as the disease progresses, and urinary or renal function abnormalities develop in 60% to 80% of children with SLE, usually within 2 years from the onset of disease (237–239). Renal involvement in childhood SLE is more common and more severe than in adult SLE (238). Most patients are girls, but the female predominance may be less pronounced than in adults, especially in patients diagnosed before puberty (237). The frequency of SLE is increased in Hispanic, Asian, and African American children, and the course of LN is more severe in Hispanics and African Americans, possibly because of socioeconomic as well as biologic factors (240). Renal involvement in SLE is heralded by hematuria, proteinuria, and hypertension, and these findings may prompt a renal biopsy before the diagnosis of SLE has been made. In children with an established diagnosis, renal biopsy may be performed to characterize the extent of renal disease or response to therapy.

LN is generally categorized by some variation on the World Health Organization (WHO) classification originally formulated in 1974 coupled with an indication of the activity and the chronicity of the disease. The 2003 International Society of Nephrology/Renal Pathology Society (ISN/RPS) classification maintains the emphasis on the appearance of glomeruli but incorporates information from IF and EM and includes subdesignations for activity and chronicity (241). In class I, minimal mesangial LN, glomeruli are normal by LM but have mesangial immune deposits by IF. In class II in the ISN/RPS scheme, mesangial proliferative LN, glomeruli show mesangial hypercellularity or matrix expansion and allow for very rare small subendothelial or subepithelial deposits by IF or EM. Class III, focal LN, and class IV, diffuse LN, show focal (<50% of glomeruli) or diffuse glomerulonephritis, respectively, typically with subendothelial immune deposits by IF and EM, and the lesions may be active (A) or chronic (C) (or both—A/C) and, in class IV, segmental (IV-S) or global (IV-G) to indicate whether the majority (≥50%) of affected glomeruli show segmental or global involvement. Class V, membranous LN, is diagnosed, alone or in combination with class III or IV, when there are subepithelial immune deposits or their sequelae over greater than 50% of the capillary wall. Class VI indicates global sclerosis of 90% or more of glomeruli without evidence of activity. Lesions indicative of active disease include endocapillary hypercellularity, leukocyte infiltration, subendothelial hyaline material, fibrinoid necrosis, karyorrhexis, cellular crescents, and interstitial inflammation. Lesions indicative of chronic disease include glomerulosclerosis, fibrous crescents, tubular atrophy, and interstitial fibrosis. Since its publication, studies

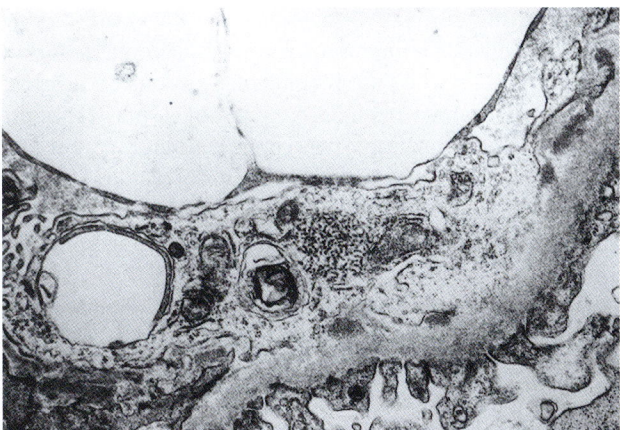

FIGURE 17-29 • LN may show tubuloreticular aggregates within endothelial cells. (Lead citrate and uranyl acetate stain, original magnification ×5000.)

in comparison with the WHO classifications show superior standardization and reproducibility (242).

The incidence of the various categories in published reports depends on the population studied, the indications for biopsy, and the specific criteria used for classification. Applying the INS/RPS criteria to a group of 39 children, Marks et al. (243) found class I in 2%, class II in 13%, class III in 15%, class IV in 51%, and class V in 20% with 12% of cases overlapping between classes III or IV and class V. Electron-dense deposits with curvilinear patterning, so-called fingerprint deposits, and tubuloreticular aggregates in the cytoplasm of glomerular endothelial cells (Figure 17-29) are characteristics of LN and easiest to find in class IV disease. Immunofluorescence microscopy reveals IgG in nearly all cases of LN, regardless of the class, and IgM and IgA in most (coexpression of these three immunoreactants is referred to as a "full house"). C3 is detected in most and C1q or C4 in many cases. Unlike IgA staining in IgA nephropathy, that in LN is generally less intense than IgG staining. In patients without an established diagnosis, a "full house" of immunoreactants, numerous mesangial deposits in an otherwise typical MGN, immune deposits along tubular basement membranes or in tubular nuclei, "fingerprint deposits," or tubuloreticular aggregates raise the possibility of SLE.

Crescentic Glomerulonephritis

Glomerular crescents have long been recognized to correlate frequently with poor outcome, in part due to their association with the standard clinical designation of "rapidly progressive glomerulonephritis" where patients present with proteinuria, hematuria, and renal insufficiency. The heterogeneity of diseases that cause crescents became evident as IF and EM became routine. Therefore, a pathologic diagnosis of CGN requires further disease categorization as outcome may be dependent on rapid institution of immunosuppressive agents.

CGN is divided by immunofluorescence into immune complex CGN, anti-GBM CGN with linear GBM staining, and pauci-immune CGN where there is little or no staining for complement or immunoglobulins. The contribution of each to patients with CGN is influenced by age and region. In contrast to adults, the most common cause of CGN in the pediatric population is immune complex disease, accounting for 45% to 85%, followed by small-vessel vasculitides associated with antineutrophil cytoplasmic antibodies (ANCAs) (i.e., pauci-immune CGN) (5% to 40%) and, uncommonly, anti-GBM disease (6% to 15%) (244,245).

During the influenza pandemic of 1919, Goodpasture described the development of hemoptysis and renal failure in an 18-year-old young man (246), and the role of antiglomerular basement membrane antibody in the pathogenesis of this form of glomerulonephritis was elucidated in the 1960s. Anti-GBM disease is the generic term for any clinical presentation of the disease caused by anti-GBM antibodies, including isolated glomerulonephritis, pulmonary hemorrhage, or Goodpasture syndrome, the use of which is restricted to the pulmonary–renal syndrome (195). In patients of all ages, >95% of biopsy specimens from patients with antiglomerular basement membrane disease contain some crescents, and an average of >75% of glomeruli are involved. Comparable figures for other glomerulopathies are 90% of specimens and 50% of glomeruli for antineutrophil cytoplasmic antibody-associated vasculitides, 57% of specimens and 31% of glomeruli for classes III and IV LN, 61% of specimens and 27% of glomeruli for HSP nephritis, 33% of specimens and 21% of glomeruli for IgA nephropathy, 33% of specimens and 19% of glomeruli in PIGN, 24% of specimens and 25% of glomeruli in type I MPGN, 44% of specimens and 48% of glomeruli in type II MPGN (DDD), and 3% of specimens and 15% of glomeruli in MGN (195). The presence of crescents portends a worse prognosis regardless of underlying disease.

Glomerular tufts beneath crescents may be compressed, necrotic, or sclerotic, but the better-preserved tufts in antiglomerular basement membrane disease and the pauci-immune glomerulonephritis secondary to small-vessel vasculitis are generally normal, whereas in immune complex glomerulonephritis, they may show mesangial hypercellularity and thickening of the capillary wall. Extensive disruptions of the capillary wall and Bowman capsule may be seen in the vicinity of the crescents, and the interstitium can show a mixed cellular infiltrate of varying intensity and distribution or patchy tubular atrophy and interstitial fibrosis in cases of longer duration. Crescents stain brightly with labeled antibody to fibrin in all forms of CGN, but the staining pattern observed in the underlying glomerulus depends on the primary disease. In antiglomerular basement disease, there is linear staining along the glomerular capillary walls for IgG and usually C3, but only rarely for IgA or IgM. In immune complex–mediated diseases, there is granular staining characteristic of the underlying disease, and in vasculitis-related CGN, there is absent or very weak staining. By EM, all forms of CGN can show endothelial cell swelling, expansion of the subendothelial space, disruptions of the glomerular basement membrane and Bowman capsule, and effacement of the foot processes of visceral epithelial cells, and in immune complex–mediated disease, there are dense deposits.

Crescents are initially cellular (Figure 17-21D) and resolve or organize into fibrocellular or fibrous forms. The constituent cells are predominantly macrophages or epithelial cells, and the proportion of each appears to be a function of the age of the lesion and the cause of the glomerulonephritis. Epithelial cells predominate in older lesions and in those caused by immune complex diseases. The origin of epithelial cells in crescents has been controversial, but contributions from parietal epithelial cells, podocytes, and progenitor cells within the Bowman capsule have been demonstrated (247).

TUBULOINTERSTITIAL DISEASES

The renal tubule, consisting of the proximal convoluted tubule, loop of Henle, and distal convoluted tubule, is derived from the metanephric blastema through a process of elongation between the developing glomerulus and the collecting duct. The renal interstitium is composed of extracellular matrix and two or three types of interstitial cells whose function is poorly understood. Ordinarily, the interstitium is inapparent in the cortex, comprising less than 10% of the volume, but it occupies progressively more volume as one proceeds through the medulla to the papillary tip. In addition to the diseases that primarily affect the tubules and interstitium, tubular injury and atrophy and interstitial inflammation and fibrosis are components of many glomerular and vascular diseases, and an increasing interstitial volume, which reflects tubular loss and interstitial fibrosis, is the best morphologic correlate of deteriorating renal function and progressive renal failure (248,249).

Acute Tubular Necrosis

Isolated acute tubular necrosis (ATN) is seen infrequently in biopsy specimens because a biopsy is not performed if the diagnosis can be established clinically, where patients present with rising creatinine and dropping GFR and urine output (250). However, it is not unusual to see ATN in conjunction with other lesions, especially in allograft biopsies performed because of a sudden decline in renal function. The two classic categories of ATN are ischemic and toxic. The former, also known as *acute vasomotor nephropathy*, follows renal hypoperfusion of any cause, and in children, it most often occurs in conditions associated with massive fluid shifts, such as shock, sepsis, and trauma. Hospitalized children are at increased risk where acute kidney injury is found in one in three children with acute illness and often in association with major surgery. Extremely young infants are also vulnerable (251). Toxic ATN is defined as dose-dependent toxic renal injury, and in children, it is most often caused by an antibiotic, such as an aminoglycoside or amphotericin B, or an antineoplastic agent, such as cisplatin or ifosfamide (252). However, clinically, many patients have risk factors for both types, and though the two types of ATN differ in

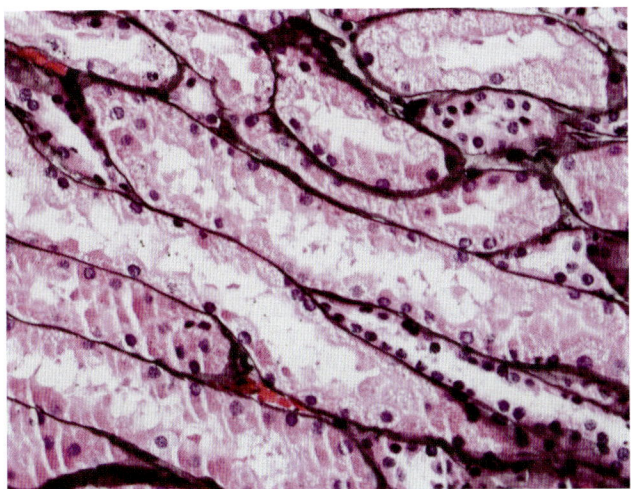

FIGURE 17-30 • ATI is characterized by variable ectasia of lumina and necrosis and desquamation of epithelial cells. (Jones methenamine silver, original magnification 40×.)

the extent and the location of injury along the tubule, it can be difficult to make this distinction on a biopsy specimen. Injury from toxins is typically associated with more severe tubular epithelial damage, including actual necrosis. In renal biopsy specimens, one initially sees swelling and vacuolation of the tubular epithelial cells and loss of the brush border in the proximal tubules (best appreciated in sections stained with periodic acid–Schiff); this is more accurately termed acute tubular injury (ATI) as it is sublethal with little to no frank necrosis. Cell death is indicated by nuclear dropout, hypereosinophilia, and apoptosis, and the cells exfoliate into the lumen along with proteinaceous material (Figure 17-30). Two key histopathologic clues to ATN are mitotic figures in tubular epithelial cells, rarely seen if there is no tubular injury, and ectasia of the tubular lumens. One may also see casts and refractile crystals in distal tubules, mild interstitial edema, mononuclear cell infiltration, and accumulation of nucleated cells in the vasa recta.

Interstitial Nephritis

Inflammation of the renal interstitium is known as *interstitial nephritis* or *tubulointerstitial nephritis* because extension of inflammatory cells into the epithelium of the tubules (tubulitis) and associated tubular injury are frequently present. Such inflammation is most often caused by infection or a drug, but it is also the renal lesion in obstructive and reflux uropathies and in several immunologically mediated, metabolic, and familial diseases as well a cellular rejection of a renal allograft (253). Clinically, acute tubulointerstitial nephritis has a relatively acute onset, and chronic tubulointerstitial nephritis has an insidious presentation and chronic occasionally silent progression. Unfortunately, there is clinical and temporal overlap, and the use of either term is arbitrary. Pathologically, acute interstitial nephritis is characterized by interstitial edema and an infiltrate of activated lymphocytes, predominantly T cells, variably admixed with neutrophils and eosinophils. This condition is uncommon in childhood and historically dominated by an infectious etiology, but more current series show an increased prevalence of medication induces hypersensitivity, especially in developed countries, where it is responsible for over two-thirds of the cases, and often related to the use of NSAIDs (254,255). Approximately 5% to 10% of cases are considered "idiopathic" including tubulointerstitial nephritis with uveitis (TINU syndrome), and another 5% to 10% are associated with systemic diseases (i.e., SLE, sarcoidosis). Presenting symptoms include fatigue, fever, gastrointestinal disturbances, and weight loss, laboratory studies document acute renal failure with low urinary specific gravity or glucosuria suggesting tubular dysfunction, and in many of the cases, the diagnosis is initially made on the renal biopsy. Pyelonephritis is a subset of interstitial nephritis, caused by hematogenous or ascending bacterial infection of the kidney, in which the collecting system is involved in addition to the interstitium. Chronic interstitial nephritis is characterized pathologically by interstitial fibrosis, tubular atrophy, and an infiltrate of small lymphocytes. Plasma cells, macrophages, and granulomas may be seen in acute or chronic interstitial nephritis (255). Renal biopsy is necessary to establish the diagnosis of interstitial nephritis, but because the histologic response is not specific, clinical and laboratory findings must be correlated to determine a cause.

Interstitial Nephritis Caused by Infectious Agents

It seems that almost any organism can cause acute interstitial nephritis. Many including *Brucella*, *Legionella*, *Yersinia*, Epstein-Barr virus, HIV, *Leishmania donovani*, and *Toxoplasma gondii* are examples of reactive interstitial nephritis in which organisms do not directly infect the kidney, but generate a cytokine-mediated reaction that leads to injury (256). In contrast, *Escherichia coli*, *Staphylococcus aureus*, invasive streptococci, *Leptospira*, fungi, mycobacteria, rickettsiae, cytomegalovirus, herpes simplex virus, Asian and European Hantaviruses, BK polyomavirus, and adenovirus do infect the kidney. *Escherichia coli* may cause acute pyelonephritis (see below) or, in rare circumstances, malakoplakia of the kidney. Bacteria and fungi can be demonstrated with histologic stains; cytomegalovirus, herpes simplex virus, BK polyomavirus, and adenovirus produce characteristic inclusions and can be identified with specific immunohistochemical stains or molecular probes. Rickettsiae require specific staining, and hantavirus infection is typically diagnosed serologically, although immunohistochemistry and reverse transcriptase PCR are recently employed.

Acute pyelonephritis is a clinical diagnosis made in an infant with fever and evidence of a UTI or in an older child with significant bacteriuria, systemic symptoms, or renal tenderness. Hematogenous infection may occur in the first 2 months of life, but thereafter, acute pyelonephritis results from ascending infection. The usual pathogen is *E. coli*, but *Klebsiella*, *Proteus*, *Pseudomonas*, *Enterobacter*, and *Enterococcus* species, group B or group A streptococci, and coagulase-negative staphylococci can also cause UTIs in infants and children (257). The pathologic features of acute pyelonephritis include patchy interstitial infiltrates of neutrophils that may form abscesses and eventually involve tubules with the formation of white blood cell casts in the urine. However, because prompt clinical diagnosis and treatment typically lead to resolution, these lesions are only rarely encountered in pathology specimens.

Chronic pyelonephritis is characterized by inflammation and fibrosis that involves the pelvicalyceal system in addition to the interstitium, features shared with the analgesic and sickle cell nephropathies but not other forms of interstitial nephritis. The risk of scar development from febrile UTIs is difficult to assess and has likely been exaggerated. It is becoming evident that UTIs are overcredited for renal scarring where retrospective investigations, which are fraught with referral bias, suggest a rate of approximately 60% with development of chronic renal disease in approximately 20%; recent and prospective studies support a rate of permanent scarring in about 15% or less and a low rate of long-term consequences (258). The relationship between vesicoureteral reflux and renal scarring has also been called into question. Scans performed with technetium 99mTc dimercaptosuccinic acid (DMSA), which are sensitive and specific for histologically confirmed pyelonephritis, are positive in 50% to 85% of children with a clinical diagnosis of acute pyelonephritis, but half of these lesions resolve on imaging studies in 4 to 6 months, and the remainder appears to develop into segmental parenchymal scars. However, renal scarring occurred as often in patients without vesicoureteral reflux as in patients with vesicoureteral reflux. In addition, the renal scarring conformed to the distribution of composite papillae, which have a more patulous pore than simple papillae, supporting the notion that scarring is caused by intrarenal reflux. Moreover, many children have parenchymal scarring at the time of their first imaging study, which suggests that they had an earlier unrecognized infection or that damage might have occurred *in utero*. With improved antenatal ultrasound, studies have found congenital renal anomalies and reflux in increasing numbers in children, which is likely the most common cause of chronic kidney disease rather than acquired pyelonephritis (258–260). Sclerotic glomeruli are seen in scarred areas, and FSGS can develop in the remaining glomeruli as a result of hyperperfusion injury. Of note, congenital or acquired intrarenal reflux, rather than segmental hypoplasia, is the etiology for the segmental scarring in "Ask-Upmark" kidney.

Complications of acute pyelonephritis that are unusual in children include pyonephrosis and perinephric abscess. In pyonephrosis, an acute inflammatory exudate fills the renal calyces and pelvis because of a high-grade obstruction, and perinephric abscesses develop when the inflammation penetrates the renal capsule. Complications of chronic UTI that are also uncommon in children are xanthogranulomatous pyelonephritis and malakoplakia. Xanthogranulomatous pyelonephritis, which occurs in the setting of urinary obstruction or stone disease, presents clinically in affected children with abdominal pain, fever, weight loss, and anorexia, often with a palpable flank mass, and is characterized by orange–yellow foci or distinct masses that are composed of foamy macrophages, neutrophils, lymphocytes, plasma cells, and multinucleated giant cells with frequent calcification (261). Malakoplakia, in which yellow–brown nodules composed of foamy macrophages contain round laminated Michaelis-Gutmann bodies, has been described in the urinary bladder, kidney, and other tissues in children (262,263).

Drug-Induced Interstitial Nephritis

While infection used to be the most common cause of tubulointerstitial nephritis, but presently, immunoallergenic mechanisms due to drugs is the primary cause (253,255,264). Many commonly used therapeutic agents can cause an acute interstitial nephritis. This allergic reaction is generally unpredictable and may be associated with other systemic symptoms, such as fever, rash, and eosinophilia, although this "classic triad" is seen in less 10% to 20% of patients (253). The clinical presentation, however, is quite variable, ranging from nearly asymptomatic to rapidly progressive renal failure. Antibiotics, especially β-lactams and NSAIDs, are most often implicated, but other antibacterial and antiviral agents, anticonvulsants, and diuretics have produced interstitial nephritis (264). 5-Aminosalicylates for the treatment of inflammatory bowel disease and proton pump inhibitors are increasingly implicated (254). Other drugs, including some of the above-listed agents, can produce glomerular, tubular, or renovascular lesions. Direct toxic effects of anticancer drugs are well known, but their significant role in acute and chronic tubulointerstitial nephritis is underrecognized (265). Only a minority of patients with drug-induced interstitial nephritis has eosinophilia of blood or urine, and eosinophils, if present, usually constitute 10% or fewer of the infiltrating cells in biopsy specimens. They are most often seen in reactions to β-lactam antibiotics, especially methicillin, and least often in reactions to NSAIDs and cimetidine. The majority of infiltrating cells are T lymphocytes admixed with few monocytes. Neutrophils and basophils are rare (264). Epithelioid granulomas were initially observed in reactions associated with sulfonamides but have subsequently been reported in association with numerous drugs (266) and have been described in children (267). Interstitial inflammation is usually accompanied by tubulitis, which is associated with degenerative changes. Effective therapy includes elimination of the suspected agent. Corticosteroids are widely used in the treatment of drug-induced interstitial nephritis, but their efficacy has not been tested in randomized, controlled trials (254).

Immune-Mediated/Idiopathic Tubulointerstitial Nephritis

TINU is characterized by interstitial nephritis in association with acute onset of bilateral anterior uveitis. The median age of onset is 15 years, and female predominance was initially reported but not confirmed in recent data

(268). Urinary beta-2-microglobulin levels are usually increased. Ocular symptoms precede urinary symptoms in about 20% of cases but may develop late (up to 14 months) and are often initially asymptomatic; therefore, ophthalmologic investigation should be considered in all children with idiopathic interstitial nephritis (269). Renal outcome is usually good. The pathogenesis of TINU is unclear but is thought to result from an autoimmune phenomenon. The pathogenic role of autoantibodies against modified C-reactive protein (mCRP) has been postulated (270). HLA-associated alleles are noted in some populations (271). Lymphocytic interstitial infiltrates and tubulitis are the usual pathology. A small group of patients with idiopathic TIN have antibodies directed against tubular basement membranes. Circulating antibodies can react to proximal tubules and are detected as linear IgG along tubular basement membranes by IF (255). Anti-TBM interstitial nephritis is occasionally manifested with membranous nephropathy. Tubulointerstitial nephritis is sometimes associated with other diseases that have immune-mediated mechanisms such as SLE, sarcoidosis, and Sjögren syndrome or secondary to other systemic diseases including malignancies (253,255).

RENOVASCULAR DISEASES

Thrombotic Microangiopathy Syndrome

Thrombotic microangiography (TMA) syndromes are a diverse group of disorders that are acquired or inherited, have rapid or gradual onset, and affect both children and adults. The most common etiology in children is Shiga toxin–mediated TMA (Shiga toxin–related HUS) with the highest incidence in adults attributed to acquired TTP. They share clinical features of microangiopathic hemolytic anemia, thrombocytopenia, and organ injury as well as pathologic features of vascular damage (272).

Recent scientific progress has led to the understanding of the pathogenesis, which is attributed to a deficiency of the von Willebrand factor (VWF) cleaving protease, ADAMTS 13 (**A D**isintegrin **A**nd **M**etalloproteinase with **T**hrombo**S**pondin-1-like motifs, member **13**) (273). Hereditary TTP is caused by homozygous or compound heterozygous *ADAMTS13* mutations, and acquired TTP results from autoantibodies that inhibit its activity, which has a much higher incidence in adults than children. TTP is unique among TMA syndromes in that it rarely causes kidney injury (274). Hereditary TTP is treated with plasma infusions to replace ADAMTS 13, and plasma exchange has greatly improved the outcome for acquired TTP along with glucocorticoids and other immunosuppressive agents, which may be required in complicated cases (274).

The term *HUS* was introduced to describe the disease reported in children with hemolytic anemia, thrombocytopenia, and acute renal failure. An infectious etiology was long suspected and now well established. Multiple *Escherichia coli* strains produce Shiga toxin (ST), but *E. coli* O157:H7 is the most common pathogen associated with ST-HUS in America and Europe (272). *Shigella dysenteriae type 1* remains an endemic cause in other countries. ST-HUS is most common among children (mean age, 2 years) in whom mortality is 3%. Despite appearance, ST-HUS is most typically sporadic rather than associated with large outbreaks. An uncommon but unique form of HUS may occur after infection with *Streptococcus pneumoniae* (SPA-HUS) where children present with septicemia, meningitis, and pneumonia and suffer more severe renal and hematologic disease and mortality than HUS associated with Shiga toxin (275). Microangiopathic hemolytic anemia, thrombocytopenia, and acute renal failure constitute the diagnostic criteria for HUS, and approximately 90% of pediatric cases are preceded by a diarrheal prodrome (275,276). It is the most common cause of acute renal failure in childhood. Enteropathogenic *E. coli* have been linked to 75% of cases of postdiarrheal HUS. These organisms asymptomatically inhabit the intestines of cattle, and consumption of undercooked beef, unpasteurized milk, or contaminated drinking water is the primary cause of infection. Damage to colonic tissue is enhanced by an influx of neutrophils attracted by the release of cytokines from colonic epithelial cells where the toxin binds. The toxin, absorbed into the bloodstream, binds to the receptor Gb3 (globotriaosylceramide) on susceptible cells and is then internalized and causes the cell's death. Toxin binds to endothelial cells, and in the cortex of the kidney, where the Gb3 is found in high concentrations, it binds to glomerular endothelial as well as mesangial cells, podocytes, and tubular epithelial cells. Cell death results from endocytosis, retrograde transport, cytosolic translocation of Shiga toxin, and subsequent ribosomal inactivation. The toxin is also prothrombotic and facilitates thrombosis by inducing endothelial secretion of VWF, thus inducing TMA (272). Involvement of the brain, liver, pancreas, heart, lung, skeletal muscle, skin, parotid gland, and retina has been reported in HUS, but central nervous system dysfunction occurs in one-third of cases, and central nervous system hemorrhage is the most common cause of death (277). Interindividual variations in the presence or density of receptors, especially in the brain, may account for the seemingly unpredictable extrarenal complications of HUS.

Three major categories of pathologic lesions have been described in the kidney in HUS—cortical necrosis, glomerular TMA, and arterial TMA. Tubular and interstitial injury are most likely secondary, possibly through endothelial injury in peritubular capillaries, and striking degrees of apoptosis have been described in tubular epithelial cells (278). Cortical necrosis is discussed in a subsequent section of this chapter, but the histologic lesion noted in the noninfarcted portions of the renal cortex in patients with cortical necrosis associated with HUS is usually glomerular TMA. In glomerular TMA, obliteration of the capillary loops by a combination of fibrin and platelet thrombi result

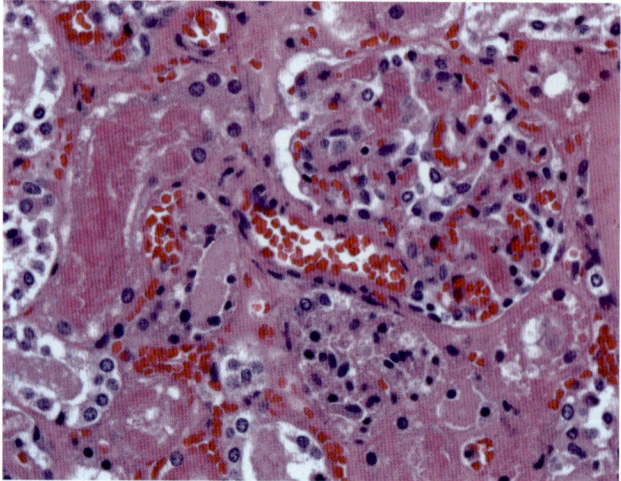

FIGURE 17-31 • Hemolytic uremic syndrome. Fibrin thrombi and fragmented red blood cells occlude glomerular capillaries, and fibrin is seen in an arteriole. (Hematoxylin–eosin, original magnification 400×.)

in the fragmentation of red blood cells (Figure 17-31) and swelling, necrosis, and detachment of endothelial cells and expansion of the subendothelial space by electron-lucent "fluff." Neomembrane beneath the endothelial cell and the normal lamina densa on the other side of the fluffy material may impart a double contour to the capillary wall in histologic sections stained with silver methenamine. IF microscopy shows granular deposits of fibrin-reactive antigen, apparently within the capillary loops. Mesangia often show a decreased amount of matrix (mesangiolysis) but are usually normocellular. Early arterial TMA is characterized by narrowing of the lumens of interlobular (intracortical) arteries and arterioles by endothelial cell swelling and fibrinoid mural necrosis, and later, lesions show intimal fibrosis or laminar proliferation ("onion skinning"). Red blood cells and fibrin thrombi may accumulate in the lumina and walls of affected vessels at any stage. Glomerular and arterial TMA can be present in the same biopsy specimen, but usually one or the other predominates, and the most common glomerular lesions seen with arterial TMA are collapse or retraction of the glomerular tuft, mostly involving superficial glomeruli, and "paralysis" (exaggerated congestion) of capillary loops, presumably reflecting obstructive lesions in afferent and efferent arterioles, respectively. The prevalence of one or another pathologic lesion may be a function of the age of the patient and the evolution of the disease. Lack of diarrheal prodrome and lack of Shiga toxin–producing infectious organism are associated with a poor renal prognosis. Oliguria and hypertension occur whether glomerular or arterial TMA predominates but are more severe with arterial TMA. Anuria is usually only observed if glomerular TMA is present. The prognosis is worst in patients with predominantly arterial involvement, which affects children and adults more commonly than infants. Severe glomerular endothelial injury and subsequent renal ischemia might result in permanent renal capillary damage that could lead to hypoxia-induced fibrosis (279).

Atypical HUS, historically used in reference to TMA that developed in the absence of Shiga toxin, has been described as a complication of other glomerulopathies, several drugs, pregnancy, bone marrow transplantation, neoplasms, collagen vascular disorders, and HIV infection and rare metabolic diseases (272). Many of these patients have loss-of-function mutations in the complement regulatory genes that encode complement factor H (CFH) and factor I (CIF) or membrane cofactor protein/CD46 or a gain-of-function mutation in complement effector genes such as *CFB* or *C3*. Additionally, a functional deficiency in CFH may develop from antibodies to complement, which are responsible for about 10% of complement-mediated TMA (280). A review of recurrence risk after renal transplantation showed that approximately 0.8% of 118 children with diarrhea-associated HUS had recurrence with graft loss while 21% of the 63 children without a diarrheal prodrome had recurrence with graft loss, demonstrating the significance of genetic predisposition (281).

Renal Involvement in Systemic Vasculitides

Renal involvement in vasculitis in children is seen most often in HSP, microscopic polyarteritis (polyangiitis), Wegener granulomatosis (granulomatosis with polyangiitis), Churg-Strauss syndrome (eosinophilic granulomatosis with polyangiitis), and medium-vessel vasculitis including polyarteritis nodosa; kidney disease can also occur in Kawasaki disease and Takayasu arteritis (282). Jennette noted that no classification of the systemic vasculitides has been universally accepted but outlined a functional approach to the diagnosis of those that involve the kidney (195). Giant cell arteritis and Takayasu arteritis cause granulomatous inflammation in larger arteries and may involve the aorta and main renal artery, with subsequent luminal narrowing and development of hypertension. Macroscopic polyarteritis nodosa and Kawasaki disease cause segmental necrosis in medium-sized vessels, including the interlobar and the arcuate arteries in the kidney, which can result in renal hemorrhage, ischemia, or infarction. Small-vessel vasculitis is characterized by a focal and segmental glomerulonephritis, often with segmental necrosis of the glomerular tuft and segmental cellular crescents. Such glomerular lesions are further categorized by IF microscopy. If immunoglobulin and complement components are deposited in the glomeruli, the likely diagnosis is lupus or another immune complex–mediated vasculitis, HSP nephritis, or cryoglobulinemic vasculitis. If immunoglobulin or complement components are not present, the so-called pauci-immune glomerulonephritides include microscopic polyangiitis (microscopic polyarteritis nodosa), Wegener granulomatosis, and Churg-Strauss syndrome and usually have detectable antineutrophilic cytoplasmic autoantibodies (ANCAs) (283).

Macroscopic polyarteritis nodosa can occur in children, and Kawasaki disease is a childhood illness with a peak incidence in the first year of life. Kawasaki disease preferentially involves the coronary arteries, but medium-sized renal arteries are the next most frequently affected site, and it can also cause renal artery stenosis (282). The early histologic lesion in renal arteries in both these diseases involves the media, but in polyarteritis nodosa, it is characterized by fibrinoid necrosis, whereas in Kawasaki disease, medial edema with myocyte degeneration, subintimal edema, and leukocytic infiltration are seen. Microscopic polyangiitis, Wegener granulomatosis, and Churg-Strauss syndrome share many clinical features, and most affected patients have ANCA. Recent studies suggest a contribution of both genetic and environmental factors to the development of ANCA and associated vasculitis (284). Evidence for genetic contributions is strengthened by familial associations, and links to environmental triggers, such as air pollutants, infections, and drugs, are considered to arise through molecular mimicry where antibodies develop against epitopes on bacteria cross-react with complementary human peptides (i.e., anti-hLAMP2 antibody has 100% homology to Fim H in gram-negative bacteria) (284). A single case report of pulmonary hemorrhage and renal disease in a newborn infant has been attributed to transplacental passage of ANCA antibodies, whereas a second case demonstrated high levels of ANCA (MPO antibodies) in the newborn without development of the disease, suggesting that clinical vasculitis requires more than the presence of antibodies (285,286).

Ear, nose, and throat involvement is more common in Wegener granulomatosis and Churg-Strauss syndrome than microscopic polyangiitis and is characterized by allergic rhinitis or asthma and peripheral blood eosinophilia. Histopathologically, all three conditions produce segmental fibrinoid necrosis that can involve glomerular and alveolar capillaries, arterioles in many organs, and venules in the skin and sinuses (283). As noted above, the most common lesion in renal biopsy specimens is segmental necrosis of the glomerular tuft with crescent formation, and fluorescent antibody and ultrastructural studies show no immune complexes, a key negative that excludes the immune complex vasculitides that may have similar histologic features. A minority of specimens shows fibrinoid necrosis of interlobular arteries, and the predominant tubulointerstitial lesion is periglomerular inflammation. Interstitial eosinophils suggest, but are not diagnostic of, Churg-Strauss syndrome (283).

Renal Vein Thrombosis

Renal vein thrombosis occurs in the fetus or the neonate under conditions of dehydration, sepsis, maternal diabetes, birth asphyxia, or polycythemia and less frequently in the infant or the older child with nephrotic syndrome (287) or leukemic hyperleukocytosis (288). It has been suggested that neonates are especially prone to thrombosis due to naturally low levels of anticoagulants, such as protein C, protein S, and antithrombin, as well as low fibrinolytic components, such as plasminogen. Low renal perfusion pressure may also be contributory; inherited thrombophilia may increase the risk (289). Renal vein thrombosis may present as a flank mass or with hematuria, hypertension, or renal failure, and it can be readily diagnosed by renal ultrasonography. Entrapment of the left renal vein between the aorta and the superior mesenteric artery (nutcracker phenomenon) may be a cause of renal congestion and postural proteinuria (290). Grossly, the involved kidney is enlarged, hemorrhagic, and friable. Histology reveals intense congestion of veins and capillaries in the interstitium, interstitial edema or hemorrhage, variable degrees of necrosis of the tubular epithelial cells, and margination of leukocytes in glomerular capillaries.

Renal Artery Stenosis

Renal artery stenosis in children is most often caused by fibromuscular dysplasia (291). It has also been reported in neurofibromatosis, Takayasu arteritis, William syndrome, Kawasaki disease, and Alagille syndrome (292–295). In addition, renal artery thrombosis has been reported in a dehydrated infant (296,297). Fibromuscular dysplasia, or renal artery dysplasia, typically affects girls and women in the second or the third decade but can be seen in younger children. It is classified according to the layer of the vessel wall that is affected, but nearly 90% of cases show medial fibroplasia with aneurysms in which a longitudinal section of the artery shows thickened fibrotic ridges alternating with almost full-thickness defects resulting from a loss of smooth muscle and elastic laminae or perimedial fibroplasia in which much of the outer portion of the media is fibrotic (291). Renal artery stenosis in neurofibromatosis may be caused by compression by an encircling neurofibroma, adventitial or intimal compression in larger vessels by a proliferation of Schwann cells, or mesodermal dysplasia by nodular proliferations of smooth muscle cells in the intima or media of the smaller vessels (298).

Renal Cortical Necrosis and Papillary Necrosis

Renal cortical necrosis occurs in response to a sudden and sustained loss of renal perfusion caused by arterial thrombosis, as in the HUS, or shock, as in acute blood loss, overwhelming sepsis, or severe perinatal asphyxia. It is characterized by coagulative necrosis. Thrombi in glomeruli suggest that a TMA, such as disseminated intravascular coagulation or HUS, may be present, but correlation with clinical information is usually necessary to determine a cause.

Papillary necrosis in adults is usually a complication of analgesic abuse (299) or diabetes, but it has been reported, often in conjunction with renal cortical necrosis, in neonates following asphyxia or shock, infants following gastroenteritis, and children with sickle cell disease, disseminated candidiasis, Wegener granulomatosis, and meningococcal sepsis (300). The affected papillary tips are grossly yellow and show coagulative necrosis with a neutrophilic infiltrate at the junction with viable tissue, and necrotic papillae may slough into the collecting system and cause acute obstruction.

Radiation Nephritis

Radiation therapy can cause acute or chronic renal injury. Fibrinoid necrosis in the arteries and arterioles progresses to subintimal fibrosis, which may be the only clue that the associated glomerulosclerosis, tubular atrophy, and interstitial fibrosis were caused by radiation (301).

Bartter Syndrome

Bartter syndrome (BS) is a hereditary hypokalemic renal salt-wasting disorder with secondary hyperaldosteronism in which the patients have hypokalemic alkalosis with hypercalciuria and hyperreninemia but normal or low blood pressure, secondary to mutations in renal electrolyte transporters and channels. In neonates (BS types I and II), it can present with polyhydramnios, growth retardation, severe electrolyte derangements, and hypercalciuria leading to nephrocalcinosis. Classic BS (type III) presents in infancy with polyuria, growth retardation, and failure to thrive. BS type IV is similar to the antenatal presentation, but hypercalciuria is only transient to patients who develop chronic kidney disease. Patients also have complete sensory deafness. The hypocalciuric, hypomagnesemic variant (Gitelman syndrome) presents in early adulthood usually with musculoskeletal symptoms (302). The characteristic renal lesion is hyperplasia of the juxtaglomerular apparatus in the hilum of the glomerulus, which is markedly enlarged and shows more than the allowable eight cells. The autosomal recessive disorder is due to numerous different mutations in genes that affect the function of ion channels and transporters including *CLCNKB, CLCNKA, NKCC2,* and *ROMK* with Gitelman syndrome attributed to mutations in the *NCCT* gene.

RENAL NEOPLASMS

During the past 45 years, cooperative groups have been remarkably successful at targeting pediatric renal tumors that comprise only 7% of all childhood cancers. They have enabled the development of accurate diagnostic criteria, stage and histology-based therapeutic stratifications, and appropriate surgical techniques. In addition, they have demonstrated that irradiation in conjunction with several active chemotherapeutic agents is effective. The overall result has been a dramatic improvement in the prognosis for most patients with WT (the most common pediatric renal tumor), from approximately 8% at the beginning of the century to approximately 50% in 1960 to greater than 90% in 2000. Most children in European countries are registered as patients in the International Society of Pediatric Oncology cooperative group protocols, which rely on the use of preoperative neoadjuvant chemotherapy and the provision of postoperative chemotherapy based on pathologic response.

TABLE 17-6 PRIMARY RENAL TUMORS OF CHILDHOOD

Tumors	Relative Percentage
WT, favorable histology[a]	80
Anaplastic WT	5
Mesoblastic nephroma	5
Clear cell sarcoma	4
Rhabdoid tumor	2
Miscellaneous	4
Neuroblastoma	
Peripheral neuroectodermal tumor	
Synovial sarcoma	
Renal cell carcinoma	
Angiomyolipoma	
Lymphoma[b]	<1

[a]Includes cystic, partially differentiated nephroblastoma, and cystic nephroma, which together comprise fewer than 5% of cases of favorable WT cases.
[b]Includes only cases presenting as renal tumors. In many patients with leukemia/lymphoma, renal lesions develop later.

In contrast, the pediatric cooperative groups centered in North America have favored primary nephrectomy, with postoperative chemotherapy based on pathologic analysis of untreated tumors. Although these two approaches are difficult to compare, both have met with similar success in treating children with WT. During the 45 years of its existence, the former National Wilms Tumor Study Group (NWTSG) and its successor the Children's Oncology Group (COG) Renal Tumors Committee, enrolling 85% of all new cases diagnosed in North America, have contributed greatly to the increase in long-term survivorship. The results of the NWTSG/COG clinical trials are widely published, and many complete detailed reviews are available. The pathologist seeking guidelines for managing pediatric renal tumor specimens is referred to any of the recommendations by Perlman (303,304).

The classification of pediatric renal tumors and their relative percentages are given in Table 17-6. As more is being discovered about the underlying genetic defects in these tumors, classifications based on gene expression provide diagnostic confidence and accuracy greater than that of pathologic analysis alone; however, these have to be used in the appropriate histopathologic context (305). This chapter only summarizes the salient features of these rare neoplasms, the study of which has answered many questions also relevant to other neoplasms.

Nephroblastoma (Wilms Tumor)

Nephroblastoma is one of the most common malignant, solid, extracranial tumors of childhood, with an incidence of 1/10,000 White children (the incidence is higher among Blacks and lower in Orientals). The estimated yearly occurrence of WT is 400 to 500 cases in the United States with only 15 cases a year in the Chicago area, for instance (303,304). It is slightly more common in girls, in whom it tends to present at an older age (mean age, 36 months in boys versus 42 months in girls). It is uncommon in neonates and infants and is only occasionally reported in adults. Most cases of "adult WT" are primitive neuroectodermal tumors, synovial sarcomas, or metanephric adenomas. Approximately 10% of nephroblastomas develop in association with one of several well-characterized dysmorphic syndromes (e.g., WT; aniridia; genitourinary malformation; mental retardation; the WAGR syndrome; Denys-Drash syndrome, a syndrome characterized by mesangial sclerosis, pseudohermaphroditism; Beckwith-Wiedemann syndrome, characterized by hemihypertrophy, macroglossia, omphalocele, and visceromegaly). Five percent of cases are bilateral, with the bilateral tumors more likely to be associated with one of these syndromes as well as with nephrogenic rests. A positive family history is found in 1% to 2% of patients with WT (304).

WT is believed to originate from the metanephric blastema and is histopathologically characterized by a triphasic pattern of blastemal, epithelial, and stromal elements that can show a wide variety of patterns and differentiation. Loss of heterozygosity (LOH) and clonality studies have shown that the different histologic components are of tumor origin (306).

Molecular and Cellular Biology

Advances in the genetics of renal tumors are driving diagnosis, staging, therapy stratification, and future research (2). The genetics of WT are very complex with multiple genetic events (some mutually exclusive) leading to tumor formation, the more common of which are discussed below.

WT1: WT1 is an important regulatory molecule involved in cell growth and development. It is expressed in a tissue-specific manner. In the developing embryo, WT1 expression is found primarily in the urogenital system. In adult tissues, WT1 expression is found in the urogenital system, central nervous system, mesothelium, and in tissues involved in hematopoiesis, including the bone marrow and the lymph nodes. The WT1 gene is located in the p13 region of chromosome 11. *WT1* encodes a zinc finger DNA-binding transcription factor that is essential for normal genitourinary development. Mutations in WT1 were first identified in patients with the WAGR syndrome, which carries a 30% risk of developing WT (304). Abnormalities involving WT1 are consistently found in the tumors of WAGR patients as well as in patients with Denys-Drash syndrome, which carries a 90% risk of nephroblastoma. Different WT1 abnormalities are associated with these different syndromes. Additionally, mutations or deletions are found in 20% of sporadic WT. The uncontrolled growth of cancer cells can be due to the loss of function of tumor suppressors and/or the activation of oncogenes. Although these are opposite functions that would be intuitively mutually exclusive for a single protein, evidence is emerging that one protein can exhibit both properties under different cellular conditions. An example of this is the oncogene Myc1. The WT1 protein has a similar dual behavior depending upon the cell type in which it is expressed. There is evidence that WT1 can behave either as a tumor suppressor or an oncogene in the development of the malignancies (307). In addition to protein–protein interactions, other mechanisms that can affect the function of WT1 include alternate splicing, usage of alternate promoters, and posttranslational modification of WT1 (307,308). Adding to the complexity of WT1 is the fact that it has multiple layers of regulatory activity that are both DNA and RNA mediated (309). Identical WT1 mutations and LOH patterns have been reported in both nephroblastomas and their associated nephrogenic rests. This suggests that WT1 inactivation may result in the formation of a nephrogenic rest and that at least some nephroblastomas are the result of subsequent genetic events occurring in a nephrogenic rest (304).

CTNNB1: β-Catenin is a cellular adhesion molecule that promotes overexpression of the c-myc and cyclin D1. Inframe deletions and missense mutations in the β-catenin gene (CTNNB1 on chromosome 3p22) leading to the stabilization of protein have been detected in 15% to 35% of patients with WT (2). There is a strong correlation between reduced expression of the WT1 gene and the β-catenin mutation (310). However, the majority of WT express wild-type WT1, sometimes to high levels. Furthermore, in WT that express wild-type WT1, it is not known whether the persistent expression of WT1 contributes to the development of the disease or is just a reflection of tumor ontogeny (311).

WTX: A gene located at Xq11.1, and named WTX, was shown to be inactivated in WTs (312). WTX inactivation appears to follow a "one-hit hypothesis" since males only have one copy and females only need to lose the copy on the active X chromosome. One-hit inactivation of a tumor-suppressor gene on the X chromosome is a departure from the traditional biallelic Knudson model and has been postulated but never documented until this study. A more recent study assessed 125 tumors and showed that WTX alterations were approximately equally frequent in WTs with mutations in WT1 and/or CTNNB1 and in tumors with no mutation in either WT1 or CTNNB1 and that WTX mutations occurred with about the same frequency as WT1 mutations. Thus, about one-third of tumors carry mutations at WT1, CTNNB1, and/or WTX (313). It encodes a protein reported to negatively regulate the Wnt pathway (314). WTX appears to participate in the WNT signaling pathway and to promote the ubiquitination and degradation of β-catenin (315,316). Whole or partial gene deletion or nonsense mutations are found in about

20% of WT. The truncation mutations result in loss of most or all of the β-catenin binding region. Truncated WTX results in an increase in nuclear β-catenin, suggesting that these mutations stabilize β-catenin.

TP53: Approximately 5% of WT have missense mutations in this well-known tumor-suppressor gene, leading to inactivation of protein. The high correlation of p53 mutations and anaplastic WT (75% of anaplastic WT have p53 mutations) suggests that p53 alterations are required for progression to the anaplastic phenotype (317). They have also been shown to correlate with recurrence/metastasis in tumors that are not anaplastic (318).

11p15: LOH or loss of imprinting on 11p15 occurs in up to 70% of tumors. This region is known to harbor genes for the somatic overgrowth syndrome, Beckwith-Wiedemann syndrome, one feature of which is a predisposition to embryonal tumors, including a 5% risk of developing WT (319). BWS families with WT carry germline mutations that alter the imprinting (methylation) of the insulin-like growth factor 2 (*IGF2*)-H19 gene cluster and result in biallelic expression of *IGF2*, which is normally expressed solely from the paternally derived allele (314). IGF2 upregulation is also observed in WT with 11p15 LOH or LOI, strongly suggesting that epigenetic upregulation of *IGF2* can be an important, but not sufficient, alteration for tumorigenesis. LOH, as determined by 11p15 methylation analysis, was significantly associated with relapse in very low risk WT as were *WT1* abnormalities (2).

LOH 1p and 16q: Tumor-specific LOH for both chromosomes 1p and 16q identifies a subset of favorable histology WT patients who have a significantly increased risk of relapse and death. This is an independent prognostic factor, which guides intensity of therapy together with other risk factors (320).

Other loci, including 1q, 2q, 7p, 9q, 14q, and 22, have also been implicated in the etiology of Wilms tumor through the studies of LOH, loss of imprinting, and constitutional chromosomal defects (313). Several studies have shown that there is 1q gain in 25% of favorable histology WT and a strong association between 1q gain and relapse (2).

Continuing advances in understanding the biology of WT are leading to better therapies with fewer long-term consequences (2,321). Also, newer prognostic markers are being identified, which will also modify therapy; one recent example is accumulation of phosphorylated Yes-associated protein 1 (p-YAP1) as a biomarker of unfavorable histology (322).

Gross Features

Nephroblastoma commonly presents as a solitary, more or less rounded, mass arising from any part of the kidney. The tumor origin is multicentric in 7% of cases (Figure 17-32), and 5% of cases are bilateral (304). The tumor kidney specimen weight ranges from 60 to 6350 g, with a median of 550 g. The bulging cut surface is pale gray, soft, friable, and lobulated, and areas of hemorrhage, necrosis, and cyst formation are often apparent (Figure 17-33). The tumor is sharply demarcated from the adjacent renal tissue by a pseudocapsule (eFigure 17-6). The tumor may protrude into the calyces and sometimes the ureter, forming polypoid excrescences resembling botryoid rhabdomyosarcoma. It often invades the renal vein, from which it may extend up through the vena cava to the right atrium.

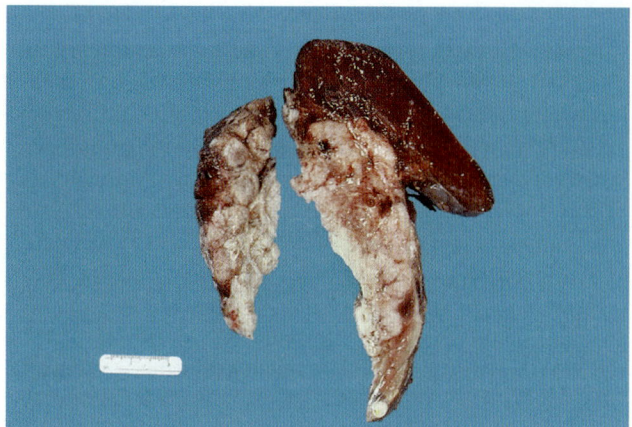

FIGURE 17-32 • Multicentric WT, cut surface. The larger, dominant mass invaded the spleen, and a second small round tumor is seen in the lower pole.

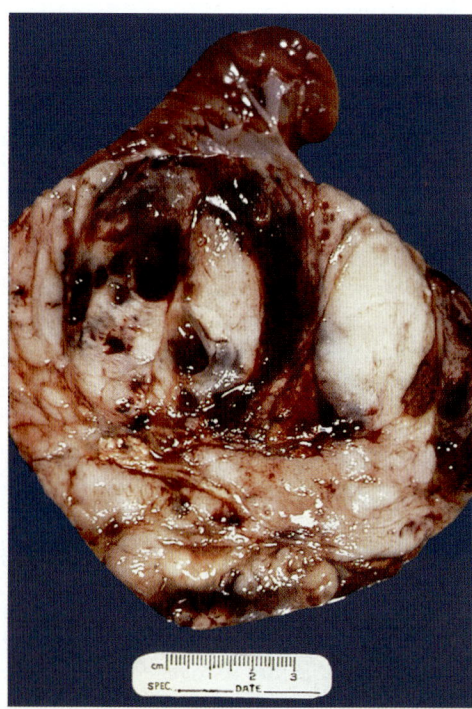

FIGURE 17-33 • Cut surface of WT is bulging, soft, and friable and has a nodular variegated appearance with areas of hemorrhage and necrosis. Normal kidney can be identified at the one pole.

Adequate sampling is critical. One tissue block for each centimeter in the maximal dimension is recommended. Evaluation of the renal pelvis and sinus, vein, capsule, and all lymph nodes is needed for staging. Beckwith and Perlman's suggestions for handling pediatric renal tumors include the following: receiving the specimen intact, avoiding frozen sections, not stripping the capsule, inking the surface, bivalving to demonstrate the relationship of tumor to kidney and renal sinus, taking initial sections for diagnosis and special studies (cytogenetic, molecular, and ultrastructural), fixing overnight in refrigerator, taking most of the sections from the periphery, including any areas that appear different (eFigure 17-7), documenting the exact source of each section, and generously sampling uninvolved kidney. In addition, submit sections that include the triangular interface between the intrarenal tumor pseudocapsule, the extrarenal tumor pseudocapsule, and the renal capsule. Careful consideration must be given to the renal sinus, which extends into the kidney following its medial contour and carries blood vessels and nerves within its fat and connective tissue (303).

Microscopic Features

The type of histologic pattern seen in WTs was of prognostic significance before the era of modern chemotherapy. Within the same specimen, the pattern tends to be uniform; however, it varies greatly from tumor to tumor. Classical triphasic WT is composed of blastemal, epithelial, and stromal components (Figure 17-34, eFigure 17-8), but biphasic and monophasic tumors are not uncommon. When one component comprises more than two-third of the tumor, the tumor is designated accordingly. The mixed type, in which no component predominates, is most common (41%), followed by blastema predominant (39%) and epithelium predominant (18%). Stroma-predominant WT is rare (1.4%). With adequate sampling, microscopic foci of all three components can be recognized in most cases.

Metanephric blastema is the most primitive cell type in WT and is characterized by densely packed primitive

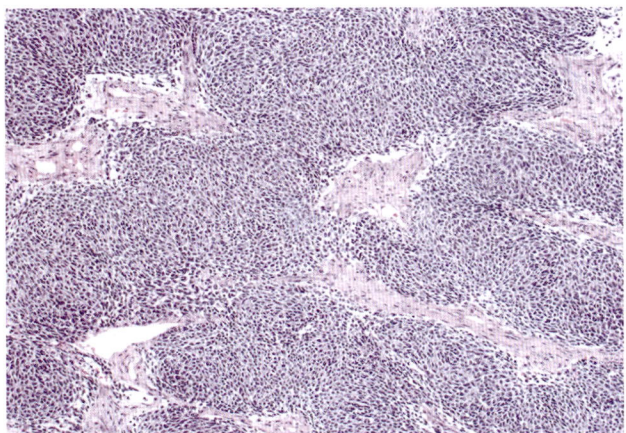

FIGURE 17-35 • Classic WT showing a predominantly blastemic appearance. (Hematoxylin–eosin stain, original magnification ×100.)

cells lacking identifiable features of differentiation by LM (Figure 17-35). Tumors with a diffuse blastemal pattern and noncohesive, infiltrative margins are highly aggressive but usually respond to current therapy. The organoid blastemal patterns (serpentine, nodular, and basaloid) are characterized by regularly defined aggregates of blastemal cells set in a myxoid mesenchymal background, without aggressive infiltration and with a clearly demarcated edge, as is usual in all WT patterns.

The epithelial component of WT is most often of nephrogenic type, in which various stages of tubular and glomeruloid differentiation are seen (Figures 17-36 and 17-37). Heterologous epithelial patterns include mucinous, squamous, and neuroepithelial and neuroendocrine cells. Similarly, stromal patterns may be nephrogenic (myxoid, fibrous, smooth muscle, and adipose cells) or heterologous (skeletal muscle, which is most common, cartilage, and bone) (Figure 17-38).

Anaplastic nuclear change is the only marker of "unfavorable histology" in WT. Other pediatric renal tumors with an unfavorable histology or in the high-risk category of the

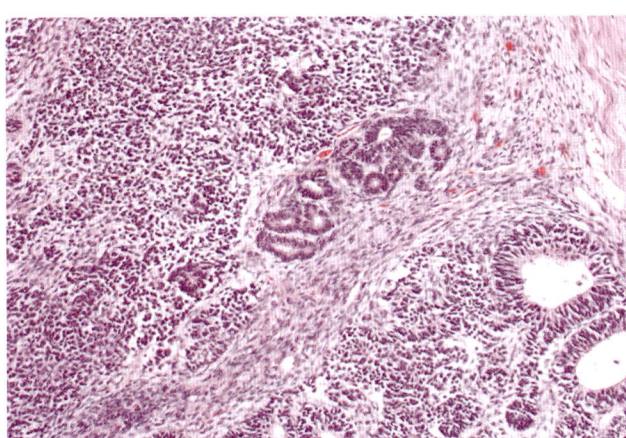

FIGURE 17-34 • Classic WT showing a triphasic pattern of blastema, tubules, and a glomerulus. (Hematoxylin–eosin stain, original magnification ×200.)

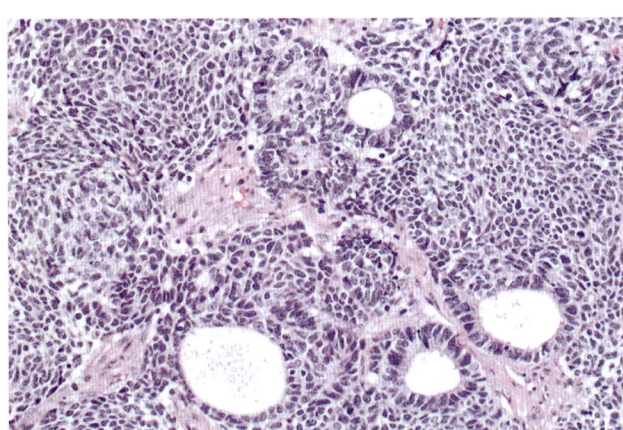

FIGURE 17-36 • Classic WT showing neoplastic tubules in a blastemal background. (Hematoxylin–eosin stain, original magnification ×200.)

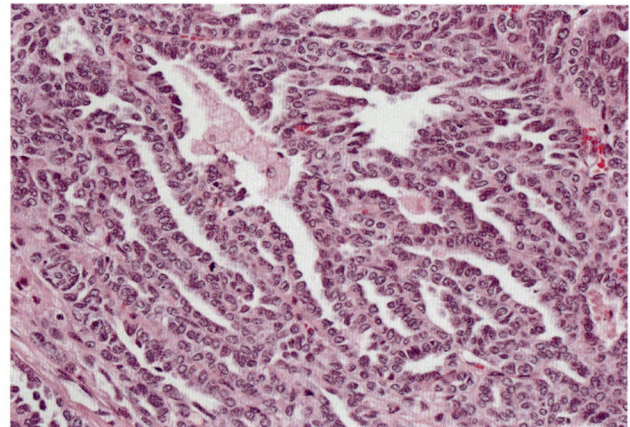

FIGURE 17-37 • WT showing a predominantly tubular or epithelial pattern. (Hematoxylin–eosin stain, original magnification ×200.)

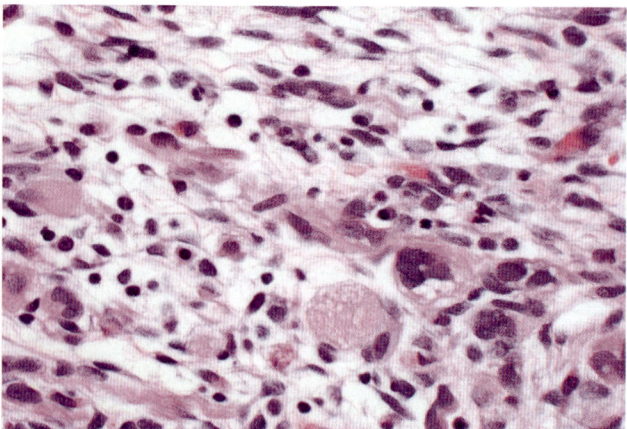

FIGURE 17-38 • WT with area of skeletal muscle differentiation in the stromal component. (Hematoxylin–eosin stain, original magnification ×400.)

International Society of Pediatric Oncology, such as clear cell sarcoma and rhabdoid tumor, are separate neoplastic entities and not variants of WT. Anaplastic nuclear changes refer to extreme cytologic atypia, not minor variations in nuclear shape or size. Anaplasia is defined as a threefold increase in nuclear diameter, hyperchromasia of the enlarged nuclei, and multipolar mitotic figures (Figure 17-39A, B). These changes are severe enough to be detected when scanned with a 10× objective.

Anaplastic nuclear changes are a marker of resistance to therapy and do not imply aggressiveness. All patients are staged irrespective of presence or absence of anaplasia. Patients with anaplastic stage I WT generally do well with conventional therapy (Table 17-7). Anaplasia is currently designated as focal when it is limited to one or a few discretely demarcated foci within the primary tumor and limited to the kidney. An adverse prognosis for anaplastic nuclear changes is associated only with stages II through IV tumors with diffuse anaplasia.

Therapy neither obscures nor produces anaplasia. WT can be accurately staged in nephrectomy specimens obtained following chemotherapy. Staging based on the extent of viable tumor cells is directly related to outcome. Posttherapy specimens may have extensive residual mature skeletal muscle (eFigure 17-9).

Regional lymph node metastasis is the most common site of noncontiguous spread of a WT. Benign inclusions in regional lymph nodes should not be misinterpreted as metastatic WT. Peritoneum, liver, and lung are the other common metastatic sites. Peritoneal metastases with desmoplasia can simulate a desmoplastic small round-cell tumor. Bone marrow and skeletal metastases are rare; fewer than 2% of classic WTs metastasize to bone.

Bilateral Wilms tumors occur in 5% of patients and are designated as *stage V disease*, but the prognosis depends on the substage, that is, the stage of the largest tumor and presence or absence of anaplasia. The largest clinical experience is that of the NWTS (323). Several clinical and pathologic features characterize this group of tumors; genitourinary tract anomalies (16%), younger age at diagnosis, presence of nephroblastomatosis (67%), multicentricity (61%), and

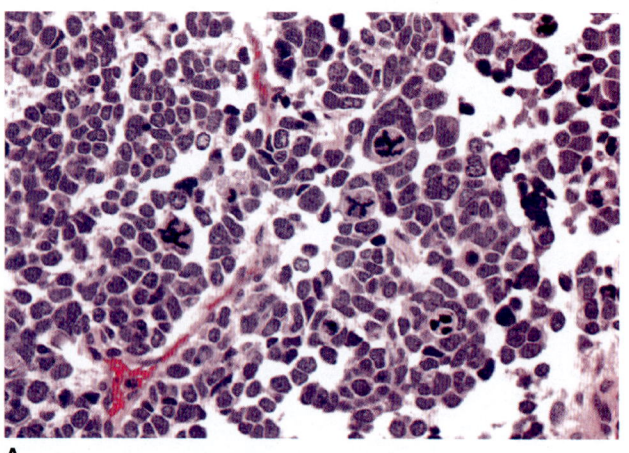
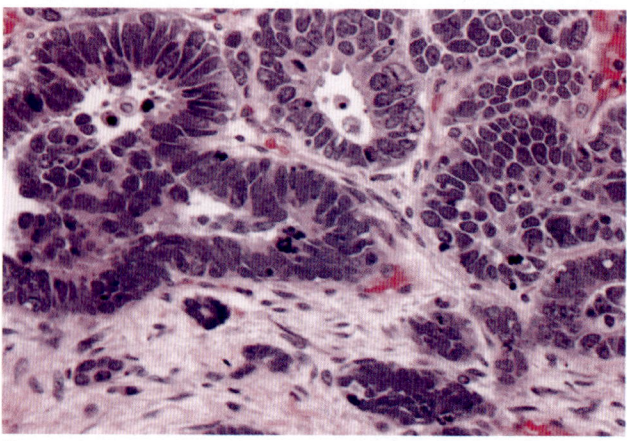

A B

FIGURE 17-39 • WT showing anaplasia in the form of atypical multipolar mitotic figures; **A:** Within the blastomatous component and **B:** within the epithelial component. (Hematoxylin–eosin stain, original magnification ×400.) (Courtesy of Dr. John Hicks.)

TABLE 17-7 NATIONAL WILMS TUMOR STUDY STAGING DEFINITIONS

Stage	Definition
I	Tumor confined to kidney parenchyma and completely resected. Renal capsule intact, not penetrated by tumor. No involvement of vessels of renal sinus. No biopsy before nephrectomy (fine-needle aspiration biopsy is acceptable)
II	Tumor extends beyond kidney parenchyma but is completely resected. Tumor penetration of renal capsule into vessels of the renal sinus, including the renal vein, extensive renal sinus soft tissue invasion or localized spillage confined to the flank. Specimen margins uninvolved by tumor
III	Residual nonhematogenous tumor confined to the abdomen. Tumor in abdominal nodes, tumor spillage involving the peritoneum, peritoneal implants, tumor involvement of resection margin
IV	Hematogenous metastases or nodal deposits outside the abdomen
V	Bilateral renal tumors. In such cases, whenever possible, the lesions on each side should be staged individually, with a substage designation according to the highest individual tumor stage (e.g., stage V, substage 1).

From Perlman EJ. Pediatric Renal Tumors: Practical Update for the Pathologist. *Ped Dev Pathol*. 2005;8:320–338, with permission.

favorable histology (90%) are findings that tend to differentiate the stage V cases from all others. The overall 3-year survival was 76% in the NWTS.

Immunohistochemistry, EM, and molecular cytogenetics are useful in those cases in which the diagnostic material is limited, predominantly in differentiating Wilms tumor from other childhood small blue cell tumors (e.g., PNET, rhabdomyosarcoma, and neuroblastoma).

Cystic Variants of Nephroblastic Tumors

Cystic nephroma, previously considered to be the benign end of the spectrum of nephroblastoma, has recently been shown to have *DICER1* mutations as the major genetic event in its development (324). Rare cases of renal sarcoma have been reported to develop from cystic nephroma. This has led to its comparison with pleuropulmonary blastoma (see Chapter 12). Both cystic nephroma and pleuropulmonary blastoma have similar *DICER1* loss-of-function and "hotspot" missense mutation rates, which involve specific amino acids in the RNase IIIb domain. Thus, an alternative pathway has been proposed with the genetic pathogenesis of cystic nephroma and *DICER1*–renal sarcoma paralleling that of type I to type II/III malignant progression of pleuropulmonary blastoma (324).

Cystic partially differentiated nephroblastoma is a benign neoplasm, which is still considered to be a part of the spectrum of nephroblastoma (304,325). Both cystic nephroma and cystic partially differentiated nephroblastoma are well-circumscribed tumors composed entirely of cystic spaces separated by delicate septa (Figure 17-40A). The solid

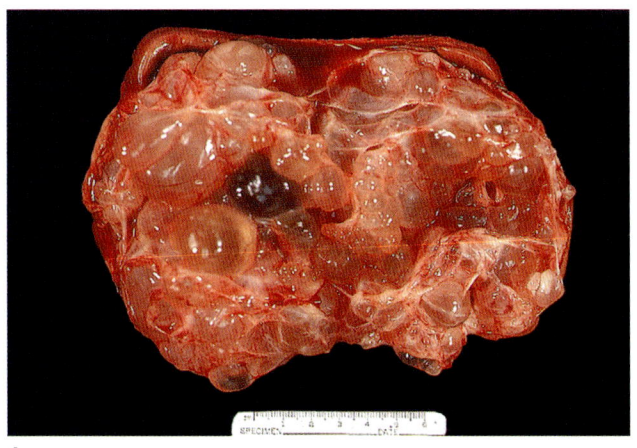
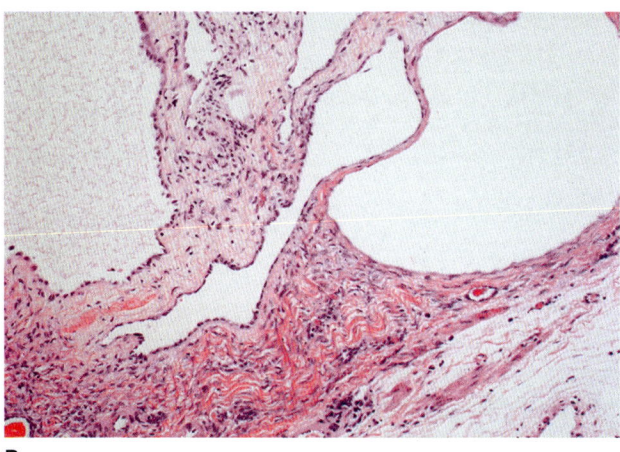

FIGURE 17-40 • Cystic nephroma (unilateral multilocular cyst) of the kidney. **A:** Gross picture of the cut surface shows multiple thin-walled cysts. Only a small amount of residual kidney present at the top. **B:** Typical cysts are lined by cuboidal or flat cells and a nondescript spindle cell stroma. (Hematoxylin–eosin stain, original magnification ×200.)

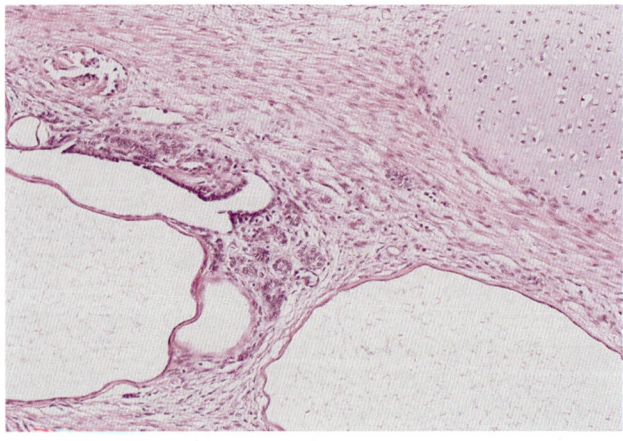 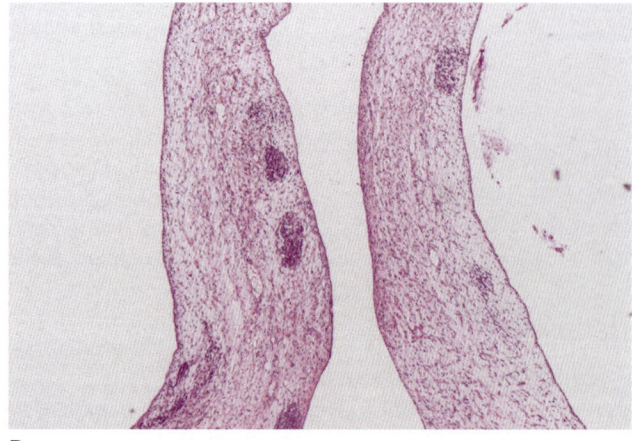

FIGURE 17-41 • Cystic partially differentiated WT. Cysts have features very similar to those of cystic nephroma, but the surrounding stroma has immature tubules and cartilage in **(A)** and islands of blastoma in **(B)**. (Hematoxylin–eosin stain, original magnification ×200.) (**B**: Courtesy of John Hicks. M.D. Houston, TX).

component conforms to the contours of the cystic spaces. In cystic nephroma (formerly known as *unilateral multilocular cyst*), it is composed of mature cell types (Figure 17-40B), whereas in cystic partially differentiated nephroblastoma, the cystic septa contain embryonal cell types without anaplasia (Figure 17-41A, B). If larger, solid, expansile regions are present, the tumor should be considered a conventional cystic WT.

Nephrogenic Rests and Nephroblastomatosis

Nephrogenic rests are abnormally persistent foci of embryonal cells with the potential of developing into WT. They are encountered in 25% to 40% of WT and in 1% of routine postmortem examinations in infants (304,326). When these are multifocal or diffuse, the term *nephroblastomatosis* is used (Figure 17-42). They are classified into perilobar (Figure 17-43) and intralobar types (eFigure 17-10), which exhibit different biologic behaviors and have been shown to be genetically different, which may explain the ethnic differences in the epidemiology of WT (327,328). They consist of variable amounts of blastemal, epithelial, and stromal components but do not show the same potential to evolve into WT. The rests may be dormant, sclerosing, or hyperplastic (eFigure 17-11). The majority regresses and becomes fibrotic, and some give rise to WT, with the remnants of nephrogenic rest visible at the periphery of the neoplasm.

Perilobar rests occur in hemihypertrophy (Figure 17-44) and Beckwith-Wiedemann syndrome and also in

FIGURE 17-42 • Perilobar nephroblastomatosis in an infant with massive enlargement of the kidneys. The compact, uniform blastema with a nodular configuration and the discrete interface with the adjacent parenchyma are characteristic features. (Hematoxylin–eosin stain, original magnification ×40.)

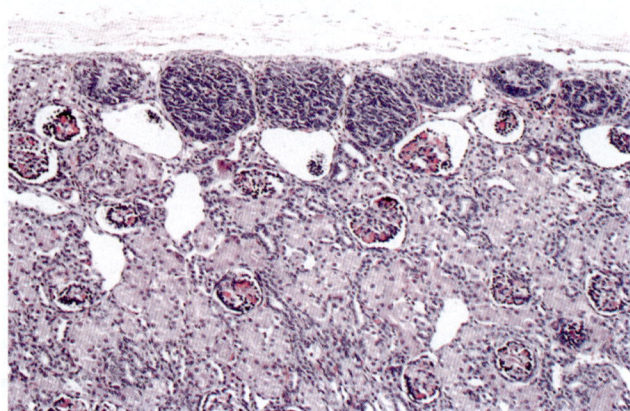

FIGURE 17-43 • Typical appearance of perilobar nephrogenic rests. (Hematoxylin–eosin stain, original magnification ×100.)

OTHER CHILDHOOD NEOPLASMS

Congenital Mesoblastic Nephroma

Congenital mesoblastic nephroma (CMN) is a stromal neoplasm of infancy, composed of myofibroblasts, and is most commonly diagnosed in the first 3 months of life. Initially thought to be a variant of WT but, based on the cytogenetic data available currently, it is now known to be distinct from WT. The classic variant of CMN shows no consistent genetic abnormality and probably represents infantile fibromatosis of the kidney. In contrast, the cellular variant is identical to infantile fibrosarcoma with the same t(12;15)(p13;q25) chromosomal translocation resulting in ETV6–NTRK3 gene fusion. CMN is the most common renal tumor of infancy, with no sex predilection and only an occasional association with Beckwith-Wiedemann syndrome. Most cases are detected because of an abdominal mass (eFigure 17-12), although polyhydramnios, premature delivery, and nonimmunologic hydrops have been reported. Hypertension secondary to renin production by entrapped renal elements, which may be immature and dysplastic, is not uncommon (304).

Grossly, the tumor is solitary, unilateral, characteristically whorled or trabeculated, and gray–white to yellow, with a rather indistinct tumor–kidney interface and a softly bulging cut surface (Figure 17-46). Cysts, hemorrhage, and necrosis are common and have no prognostic significance. The tumor tends to arise centrally within the kidney and extensively involves the renal sinus; thus, the medial margin needs to be carefully sampled.

Microscopically, classic, cellular, and mixed patterns are recognized with frequencies of 24%, 66%, and 10%, respectively, and a mean age at presentation of 7 days, 4 months, and 2 months, respectively. The classic pattern is characterized by intersecting bundles of spindle cells with minimal atypia and infrequent mitoses (Figure 17-47). At the periphery, the tumor infiltrates extensively into the renal parenchyma, so that wide margins of excision are necessary

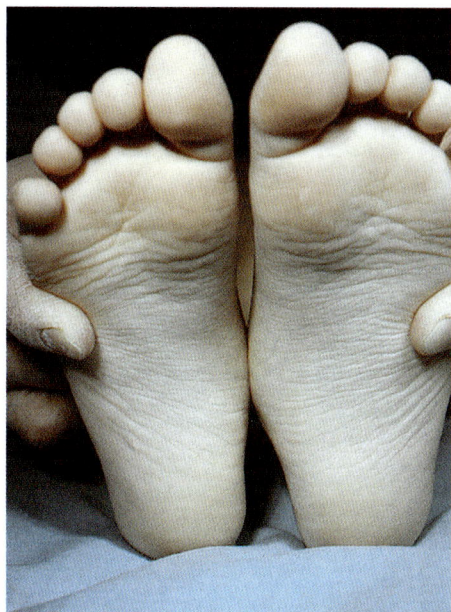

FIGURE 17-44 • Seven-year-old boy with hemihypertrophy that was diagnosed only after he was found to have a large WT (Figure 17-36). (Courtesy of David Hatch, M.D., Loyola University Medical Center, Maywood, IL.)

association with some sporadic tumors. Perilobar rests are occasionally seen in cystic renal dysplasia and are rarely associated with mesoblastic nephroma. Intralobar rests are seen with the WAGR and Denys-Drash syndromes (Figure 17-45). Hyperplastic rests and Wilms tumors comprise a morphologic continuum that cannot be distinguished cytologically. Hyperplastic perilobar rests tend to preserve the original shape of the rest and have a distinct interface with the adjacent renal parenchyma, whereas the intralobar rest intermingles with the adjacent kidney.

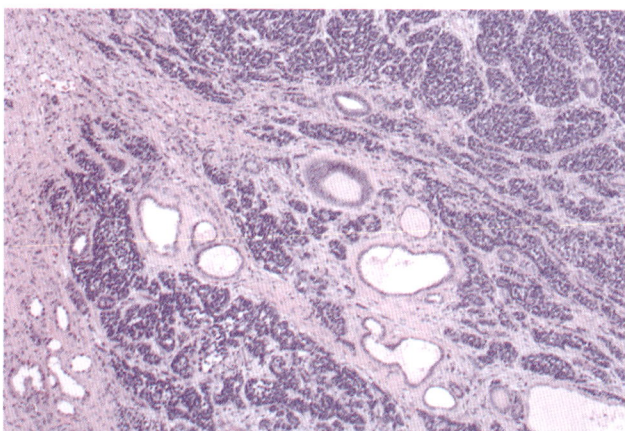

FIGURE 17-45 • Intralobar nephroblastomatosis with blastema and immature tubules blending into the surrounding kidney. (Hematoxylin–eosin stain, original magnification ×100.)

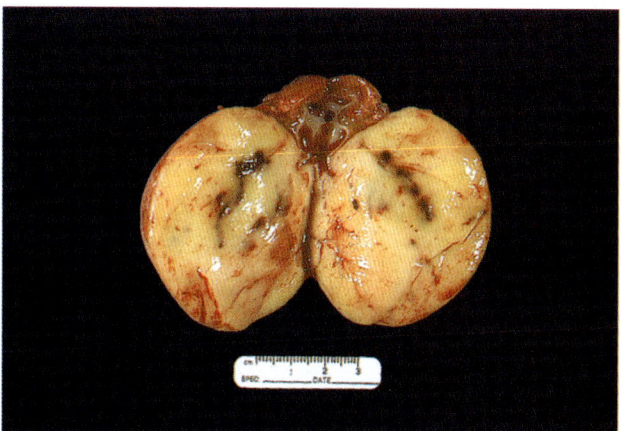

FIGURE 17-46 • Cut surface of CMN shows yellow–white bulging cut surface with focal hemorrhage.

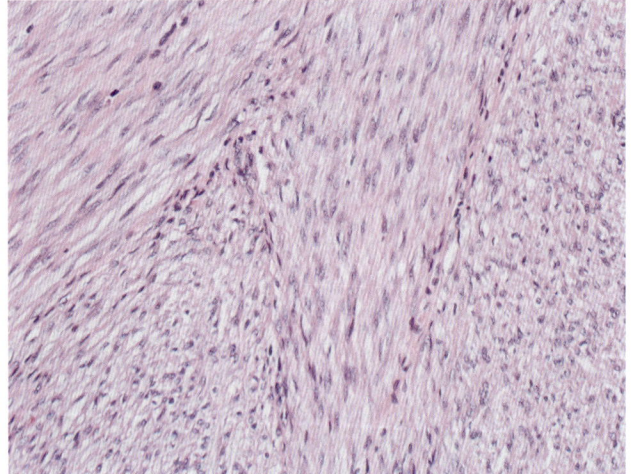

FIGURE 17-47 • Classic pattern of CMN with intersecting bundles of uniform, bland spindle cells with minimal atypia. (Hematoxylin–eosin stain, original magnification ×200.)

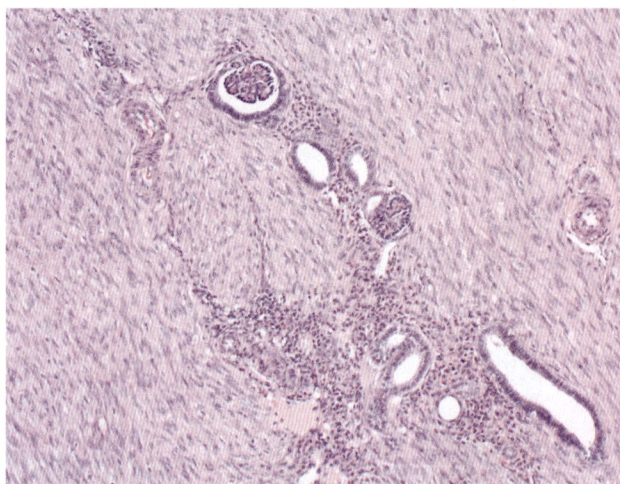

FIGURE 17-48 • CMN infiltrates and overgrows renal elements. (Hematoxylin–eosin stain, original magnification ×200.)

(Figure 17-48). Dysplastic entrapped tubules and islands of cartilage are often seen. The cellular mesoblastic nephroma has a distinct pushing border and is characterized by dense cells, mitoses, and a "sarcomatous" appearance (Figure 17-49A, B). Areas of cellular mesoblastic nephroma may be seen in an otherwise classic tumor, with eventual overgrowth of the former evidenced by the finding of compressed remnants of the classic pattern at the periphery of a cellular mesoblastic nephroma. However, all mixed tumors studied so far have shown no ETV6–NTRK3 gene fusion (329). By immunohistochemistry, both types of tumors react with antibodies directed toward myofibroblasts. Recurrences and metastases occur in about 5% to 10% of patients, risk factors for which are cellular histology, stage III or higher, and involvement of intrarenal or sinus vessels (304,330).

Clear Cell Sarcoma of the Kidney

Although a rare tumor (approximately 20 cases occur in the United States every year), the diagnosis of clear cell sarcoma of the kidney (CCSK) is clinically important because it is a tumor with "unfavorable histology" that responds to chemotherapeutic regimens containing doxorubicin, actinomycin, and vincristine. In addition, it has been called the *great masquerader* because it can mimic or be mimicked by every other pediatric renal neoplasm. The age distribution is similar to that of Wilms tumor, with a peak incidence during the second year of life; however, the age ranges from 2 months to 54 years (331). There is no association with any anomaly or syndrome. A genetic alteration specific for CCSK has not been discovered yet. Recently, t(10;17), *YWHAE-FAM22*

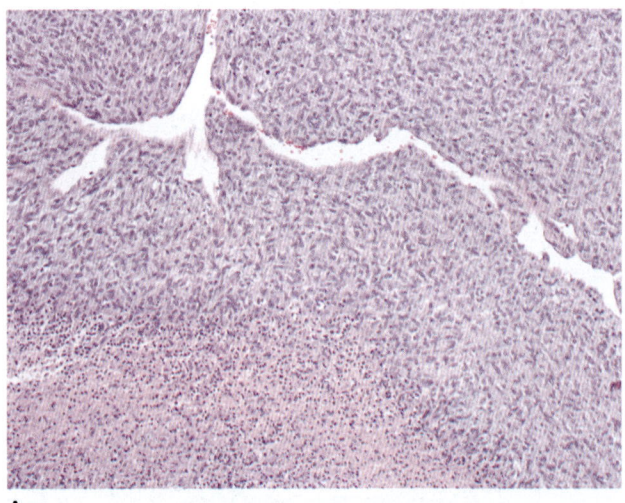

A

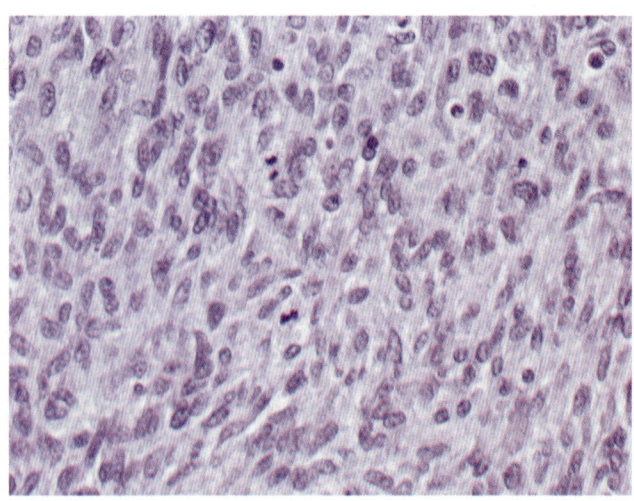

B

FIGURE 17-49 • Cellular mesoblastic nephroma. **A:** Low power shows high cellularity with hemangiopericytoma-like vessel and area of necrosis. **B:** High power shows mitoses and some pyknotic cells. (Hematoxylin–eosin stain, original magnification: **A**, ×200; **B**, ×400.)

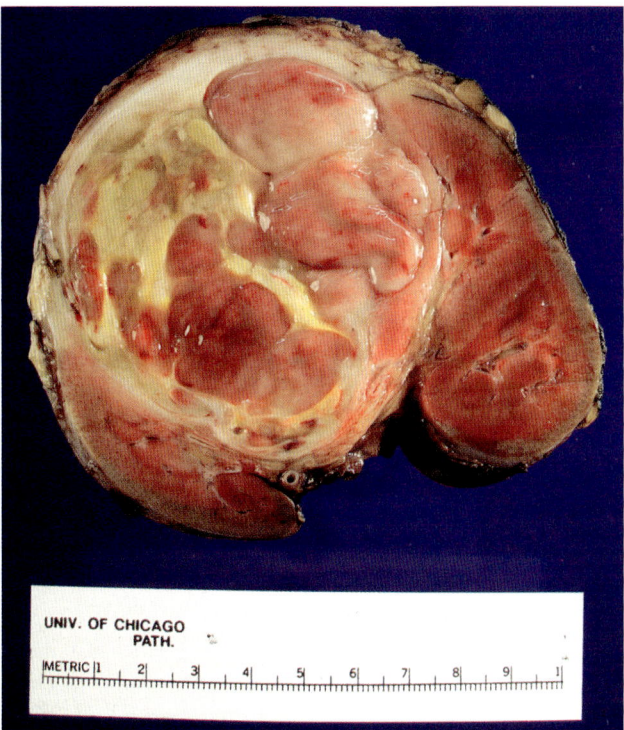

FIGURE 17-50 • CCSK showing distinct tumor–kidney junction, gelatinous nodular cut surface, and yellow areas of necrosis. (Courtesy of Christopher Weber, M.D., Ph.D., University of Chicago, Chicago, IL).

Microscopically, various patterns can be seen; however, most tumors are quite monomorphous with a characteristic tumor–kidney interface. At low magnification, this appears scalloped and irregular but usually sharp. Under high magnification, the interface is less sharp because the tumor infiltrates between and around renal structures (eFigure 17-13), which may show metaplastic changes. In the classic pattern, an evenly distributed network of vascular septa with parallel capillary-sized vessels subdivides the tumor into cords and nests that are 6 to 10 cells wide (Figure 17-51A). The tumor cells are polygonal, with indistinct cell–cell borders, finely granular nuclear chromatin (hence the pale nuclei), and small or absent nucleoli (Figure 17-51B). Mitoses are variable but less than in other renal malignancies. The cytoplasm usually consists of delicate tendrils surrounding intercellular space (hence the "clear cell" appearance), although it is important to recognize that not all CCSKs are clear. Histologic variations include epithelioid (eFigure 17-14), spindle cell (eFigure 17-15), sclerosing, myxoid, cystic, pericytomatous, palisading, and monstrocellular patterns. However, most CCSKs exhibit the classic pattern, and even in those with a variant pattern, some areas with the classic pattern can be found.

CCSKs are strongly positive for vimentin (eFigure 17-16), and vascular markers highlight the typical distribution of small vessels. Positivity for CD99 (MIC2) (eFigure 17-17) and CD56 (eFigure 17-18) may also be seen. The differential diagnosis includes WT, rhabdoid tumor, and cellular variant of mesoblastic nephroma.

Almost 40% of cases metastasize to the bone, hence the original term *bone-metastasizing renal tumor of childhood*. It can also metastasize to other unusual sites, including skeletal muscle, orbit, brain, meninges, and spinal cord. Late recurrences may occur as many as 5 to 8 years after diagnosis. In contrast to WTs, even stage I CCSKs have relatively high recurrence rates, presumably because of occult micrometastases at

fusion transcript, p53/c-kit overexpression, deletion of 14q/19p, and loss of imprinting of IGF2 have been described in CCSK (332).

CCSK is always unilateral, unicentric, and generally irregularly shaped with a distinct tumor–kidney junction. It has a variable color and a glistening gelatinous surface (Figure 17-50). Cysts are often present. It seems to arise deep within the renal parenchyma.

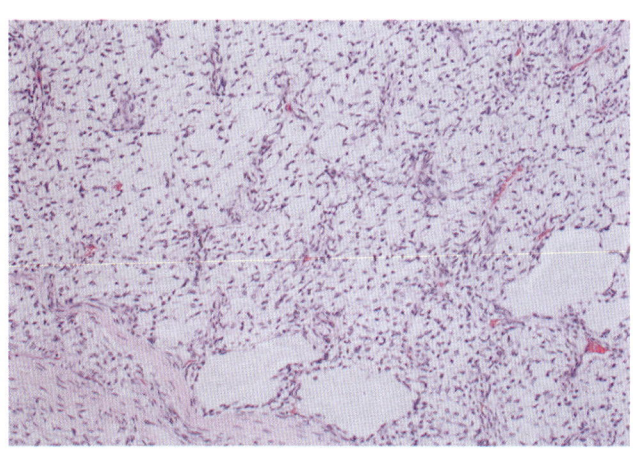
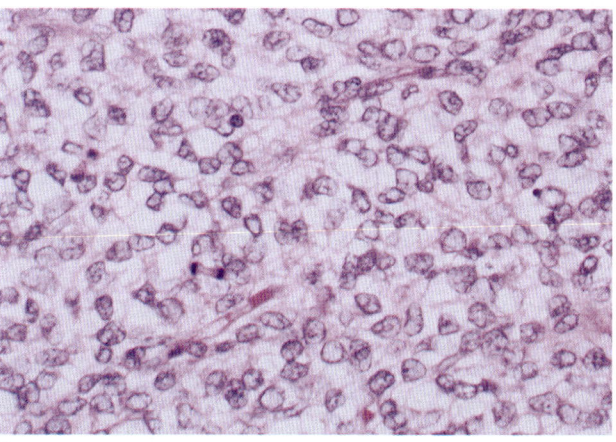

A **B**

FIGURE 17-51 • **A:** CCSK showing a characteristic vascular or plexogenic pattern in which ill-defined groups of uniform tumor cells are separated by a capillary network of vessels. (Hematoxylin–eosin stain, original magnification ×100.) **B:** The nuclei often have an optically clear appearance, as in papillary carcinoma of the thyroid. (Hematoxylin–eosin stain, original magnification ×300.)

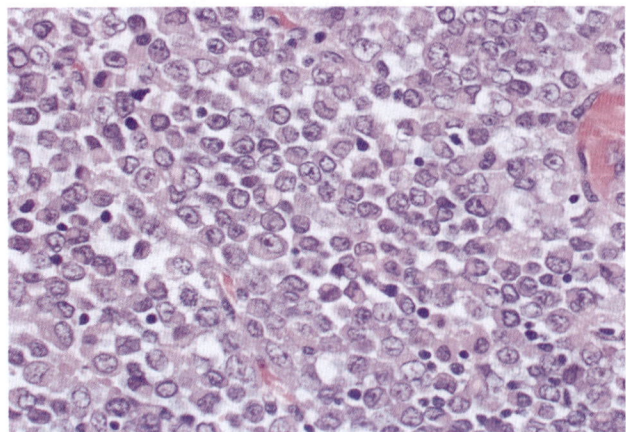

FIGURE 17-52 • Rhabdoid tumor of the kidney showing sheets of large, atypical mononuclear cells with a prominent nucleolus in each nucleus. There are characteristic intracytoplasmic hyaline inclusions indenting some of the nuclei. (Hematoxylin–eosin stain, original magnification ×300.)

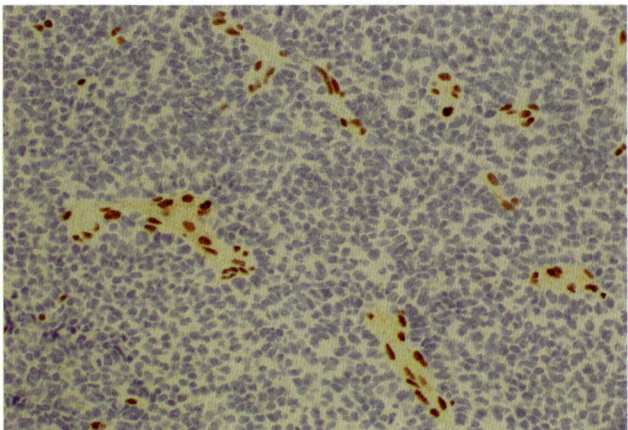

FIGURE 17-53 • Rhabdoid tumor of the kidney showing lack of immunoreactivity for BAF47. Note normally positive endothelial cells and scattered lymphocytes. (Peroxidase–antiperoxidase stain, original magnification ×200.)

the time of diagnosis. Prognosis varies with stage at presentation: 97% 6-year survival for stage I to 50% for stage IV (331).

Rhabdoid Tumor of the Kidney

This is a rare (2.5% of NWTS cases) and highly malignant (50%, 67%, and 80% mortality for stages I, II/III, and IV, respectively) tumor of the infantile kidney that it is not related to WT or to any syndrome except the familial rhabdoid tumor predisposition syndrome. The only known associations are with hypercalcemia in a few cases and, in 15% of cases, primitive neuroectodermal tumor of the brain. It is seen in infants and children, with a 1.5:1 male to female ratio. Metastases are generally widespread at the time of diagnosis.

Grossly, rhabdoid tumor is usually round, pale, soft, and unencapsulated. Satellite tumors may be present. Microscopically, the pattern is monomorphous; sheets of large, loosely cohesive tumor cells are characterized by intracytoplasmic hyaline inclusion and vesicular nuclei containing prominent central nucleoli (Figure 17-52). These features may be focal and should be looked for carefully in any undifferentiated tumor of the kidney. The finding of rhabdoid features in other tumors, such as Wilms tumor and mesoblastic nephroma, does not imply the same poor prognosis.

Immunohistochemically, the tumor cells consistently show loss of INI1 staining (Figure 17-53) and are positive for vimentin with frequent coexpression of cytokeratin (eFigures 17-19 and 17-20), epithelial membrane antigen, desmin, and neurofilament. The staining pattern is characteristically patchy and strong, with small clusters of positive cells in a background of nonreactive tumor cells, seen in over 90% of cases. Other markers, including CD99 and CD56 (eFigure 17-21), have been reported but are not found consistently. They may represent nonspecific antibody entrapment by the filamentous arrays seen ultrastructurally to correspond to the cytoplasmic inclusion.

Primary extrarenal rhabdoid tumors can be seen in both children and adults, particularly in the central nervous system (see Chapter 10) and in the soft tissues (see Chapter 25). The unifying feature at all sites is the presence of a mutation or deletion of the *SMARCB1 (also referred to as INI1, BAF47, and SNF5)* gene located at chromosome 22q11. These tumors have altered expression of members of the p16^{INK4A}/cyclinD1/E2F pathway, which regulates cell cycle (2). All rhabdoid tumors contain mutations or deletions that inactivate the *hSNF5/INI1* gene, whose role is to alter the conformation of the DNA–histone complex so that transcription factors have access to target genes. Immunohistochemical staining using antibody to hSNF5/INI1, BAF47 is very sensitive and highly specific for the detection of hSNF5/INI1 loss of function, which correlates well with the biallelic inactivation of this tumor-suppressor gene (333) (Figure 17-53).

Renal Cell Carcinoma

Malignant epithelial tumors are rare in children (2% of all new renal tumors) and biologically different than those in adults. Clear cell RCC is exceedingly rare in the absence of a predisposing genetic condition such as VHL syndrome.

The most common RCC in children are the translocation-associated renal tumors, which are defined by their genetic features (majority have translocations involving the TFE3 gene located at Xp11.2 and a number of variant partner genes). These tumors have a nested or a tubulopapillary pattern composed of cells with voluminous clear-to-acidophilic cytoplasm and distinct cell borders separated by thin fibrovascular septa (Figure 17-54). The tumor cells are frequently positive for PAX8 and PAX2 and, in contrast to other RCCs, are negative or only focally positive for EMA, cytokeratin CAM5.2, and vimentin, but show nuclear reactivity for TFE3 or TFEB proteins (eFigure 17-22) (334).

Renal medullary carcinoma is a rare highly malignant tumor associated with sickle cell trait that occurs in adolescents and young adults. It typically demonstrates loss of the INI-1 protein, a finding almost never seen in the more common RCC subtypes (335). Presenting symptoms are

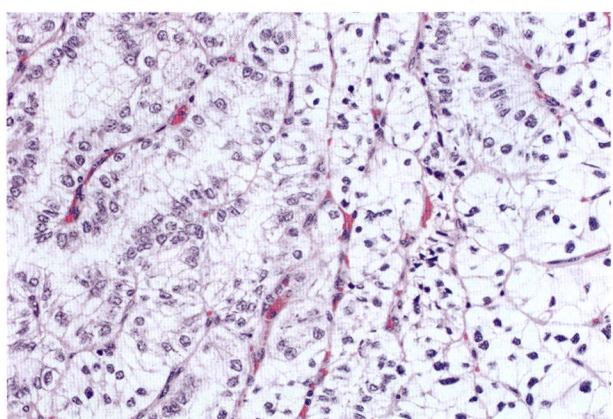

FIGURE 17-54 • RCC with translocation at Xp11.2. There are distinct cell borders and abundant clear cytoplasm. (Hematoxylin–eosin stain, original magnification ×200.)

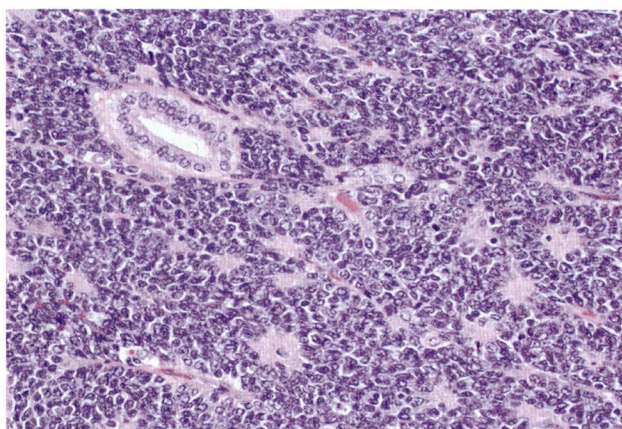

FIGURE 17-56 • Primitive neuroendocrine tumor of kidney showing pseudorosettes and an entrapped tubule. (Hematoxylin–eosin stain, original magnification ×200.)

flank pain, hematuria, and a palpable abdominal mass. It is usually a lobulated neoplasm arising in the renal medulla. Histologically, it often shows cribriform and reticular growth patterns, reminiscent of yolk sac tumor (eFigure 17-23). The cells have dark cytoplasm, clear nuclei, and prominent nucleoli (Figure 17-55). Focally, rhabdoid features (eFigure 17-24) and intracytoplasmic lumens may be present. The stroma is often prominently desmoplastic, and marked acute and chronic inflammation is characteristic (eFigure 17-25). It is widely metastatic at diagnosis, is unresponsive to chemotherapy and radiotherapy, and has a mean survival of only 4 months.

Other Rare Renal Tumors

Ossifying renal tumor of the kidney is a rare neoplasm, characteristically seen in infant boys, that presents with hematuria. A calcified mass in the renal pelvis grossly resembles calculi and is microscopically composed of proliferating spindle cells admixed with partially calcified osteoid matrix. The prognosis is excellent, with no known recurrences or metastases.

Metanephric tumors are rare benign tumors that have a pathologic spectrum from adenoma (most common of the group, occurring mainly in females with a mean age of 41 years) to adenofibroma (containing both epithelial and stromal components, occurring at a mean age of 82 months with 2:1 male to female ratio) to stromal tumor (mean age of 2 years) (304). All are unencapsulated and show distinctive morphology (eFigures 17-26 and 17-27).

Primitive neuroectodermal tumor occasionally occurs in the kidney in older children and adults. It is a small blue cell tumor, the diagnosis of which rests on the findings of pseudorosettes (Figure 17-56), CD99 and FLI-1 positivity, and t(11;22).

Angiomyolipomas and oncocytomas may occur in children, almost always in association with tuberous sclerosis. Primary neuroblastoma and lymphoma of the kidney also occur rarely.

DISEASES OF THE URETERS, BLADDER, AND URETHRA

Congenital Malformations of the Ureter

Malformations of the ureter are common and often occur in combination (e.g., duplication and ectopia or ectopia and ureterocele with or without obstruction).

Ureteral Agenesis

Unilateral or bilateral ureteral agenesis is almost always seen with renal agenesis. Whenever a ureter is present, some renal tissue can usually be identified.

Ureteral Duplication

The vast majority of cases of ureteral duplication are sporadic, although a few cases have been reported with syndromic associations. All types of ureteral duplication are much more common in girls (male to female ratio of 6:1) (336). Duplication of the upper part of the ureter and renal pelvis occurs in association with premature branching of the ureteric bud; complete duplication occurs when two ureteric buds form.

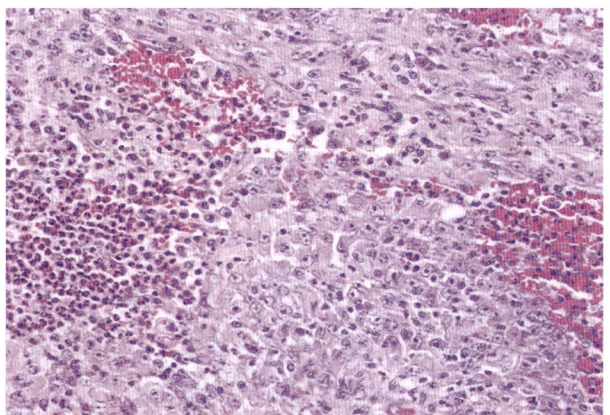

FIGURE 17-55 • Renal medullary carcinoma. Tumor cells have dark cytoplasm, clear nuclei, and very prominent nucleoli. Note acute inflammation and sickled red blood cells. (Hematoxylin–eosin stain, original magnification ×200.)

Partial unilateral duplication is the most common form and is associated with duplication of the renal pelvis and a duplex kidney. Often, the upper pole is smaller and dysplastic, with the associated ureter tortuous and dilated. In cases with complete duplication, the upper pole ureter inserts ectopically.

Ureteral Ectopia

Ureteral ectopia is more common in girls, often associated with ureteral duplication, and frequently presents with symptoms of UTI. In boys, the ectopic orifice is located more often in the urinary tract than in the seminal tract. That part of the kidney drained by the ectopic ureter is often dysplastic. The severity of the dysplasia is apparently determined by the position of the ectopic ureteric orifice; the more lateral the ectopia, the more severe the degree of dysplasia and hypoplasia of the kidney. Nonfunctioning renal segments are treated by laparoscopic nephroureterectomy of the upper pole (337), and functioning renal segments are conservatively treated, usually with ureterovesical reimplantation (338).

Ureterocele

Ureterocele is a congenital cystic dilatation of the intravesical portion of the distal ureter. It is commonly detected by prenatal ultrasound (339). In childhood, it usually presents with symptoms of vesicoureteral reflux and chronic infection. The ureteral orifice may be normally positioned or ectopic at the neck of the bladder or ureter, in which case it is most often associated with the upper pole of a duplex kidney (336).

Ureteral Obstruction

Intrinsic ureteral obstruction, bilateral in 20% of cases, is most often seen at the ureteropelvic junction, causing hydronephrosis (Figure 17-57), or associated with multicystic dysplasia, in which case the ureter(s) may be atretic. The obstruction of the ureteropelvic junction may be caused by stenosis, valves, or functional constriction (340). Extrinsic obstruction is seen in retrocaval ureters and less often in retroiliac ureters. In obstruction of the vesicoureteral junction, there is an additional smooth muscle collar surrounding the terminal ureter. It appears that the younger the age of the patient at the time of unilateral ureteral obstruction, the more severe the growth impairment of the ipsilateral kidney and the greater the compensatory growth of the opposite kidney.

Vesicoureteric Reflux

Vesicoureteric reflux is a congenital defect of the urinary tract that causes urine to flow retrogradely from the bladder to the kidneys due to short intravesical ureter(s), poorly developed trigone, and ectopic abnormally large ureteral orifice(s). It is associated with recurrent UTIs, hypertension, and renal failure (third most common cause in children). Prevention of recurrent UTIs is believed to significantly reduce the risk of reflux nephropathy. However, despite medical and surgical therapy, the incidence of renal failure in these patients has not decreased. Thus, it is proposed that the renal damage

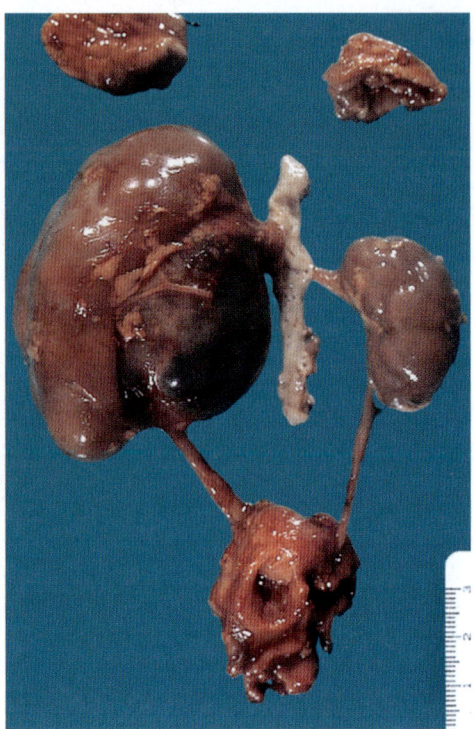

FIGURE 17-57 • Left hydronephrosis secondary to unilateral ureteropelvic junction obstruction.

associated with reflux is congenital and arises from a defect that affects both renal and urinary tract development (341).

Acquired Lesions of the Ureter

Inflammation and neoplasia primarily involving the ureter are rarely, if ever, seen by the pediatric pathologist. Chronic inflammation and fibrosis may be seen in association with pyelonephritis and vesicoureteral reflux. The ureter may be secondarily involved by rhabdomyosarcoma arising in the urinary bladder and other retroperitoneal tumors. Transitional cell carcinoma of the ureter is seen only in adults.

Congenital Lesions of the Bladder and Urethra

Most patients with bilateral agenesis of the kidneys also have agenesis of the bladder, although a small, contracted bladder may be identified in some. Agenesis is also seen as part of severe malformations (e.g., sirenomelia, caudal regression syndrome, and limb-body wall defects). Hypoplasia of the bladder is commonly seen with bilateral multicystic dysplastic kidneys. Duplication of the bladder is uncommon and rarely occurs as an isolated anomaly; rather, it is generally part of a complex malformation, as in the VACTERL (vertebrae, anal, tracheoesophageal, renal, and limb) association (Chapter 4).

Bladder Exstrophy

Bladder exstrophy is an uncommon anomaly with an even sex ratio (342). Epispadias, exstrophy of the bladder, and cloacal exstrophy are a spectrum of related malformations

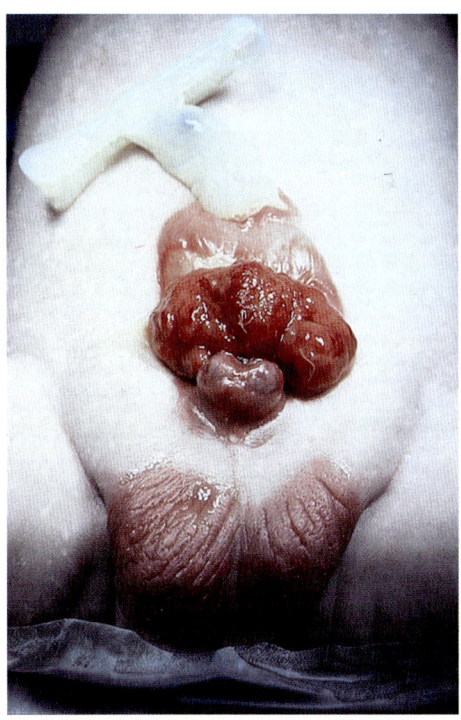

FIGURE 17-58 • Newborn boy with bladder exstrophy. (Courtesy of David Hatch, M.D., Loyola University Medical Center, Maywood, Illinois.)

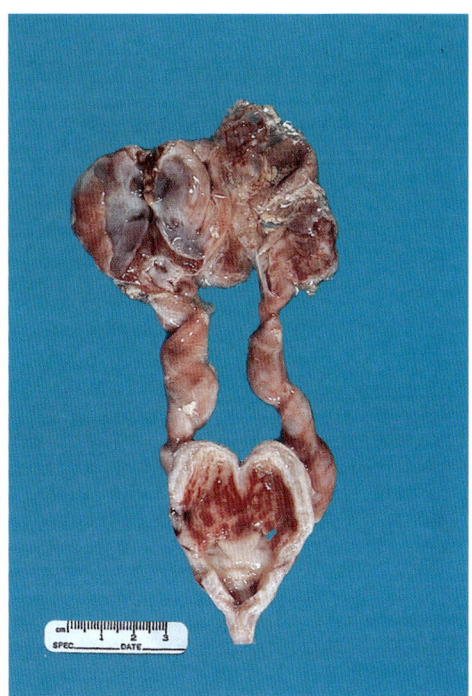

FIGURE 17-59 • Severe obstruction secondary to posterior urethral valve was diagnosed *in utero* and a vesicoamniotic shunt placed. A thick-walled, dilated bladder, bilateral hydroureters, and hydronephrosis were found at autopsy in this newborn boy, who died of pulmonary hypoplasia.

that result from a failure of the primitive streak mesoderm to invade the anterior part of the cloacal membrane (343). The size of the exstrophic bladder varies from patient to patient, ranging from a small hole in the anterior abdominal wall through which the bladder trigone protrudes on straining at micturition to a large defect through which the entire posterior wall of the bladder is exposed (Figure 17-58). The pubic symphysis remains open. Epispadias, in which the opening of the urethra is on the upper surface of the penis, is present in males and bifid clitoris in females. In cloacal exstrophy, the bladder is separated into two halves by the central exstrophic bowel; other urogenital anomalies are also present.

Even after surgical repair, bladder function is often not normal. Complications include vesicoureteral reflux, cystitis cystica, squamous metaplasia, and an increased risk for the development of squamous cell carcinoma or adenocarcinoma.

Obstructive Lesions

Obstruction of the urinary tract results in a series of changes referred to as *obstructive uropathy*, which is a leading cause of renal failure in childhood and adolescence. It accounts for 16.3% of pediatric renal transplantations (344). The obstruction can occur at multiple levels of the urinary tract, including the urethra, bladder outlet, and ureters. Renal lesions in obstructive uropathy vary from bilateral hydronephrosis to severe and diffuse hypodysplasia in which variably sized cysts mimic polycystic disease. A less severe renal change, characterized by the conservation of normal renal structure and the presence of subcapsular cysts (Potter type IV), is seen less frequently.

The causes of bladder outlet obstruction include posterior urethral valves in males, urethral stenosis or atresia, and functional neck obstruction. Posterior urethral valves are the most common cause of lower urinary tract obstruction in male infants with an incidence of 1 in 5,000 to 8,000 live births (344). Severe obstruction can be detected *in utero* and treated by vesicoamniotic shunt placement, the efficacy of which decreases in the latter part of gestation (Figure 17-59).

Prune Belly Syndrome

Also called *abdominal muscle deficiency syndrome* or *Eagle-Barrett syndrome*, prune belly syndrome is rare, with an incidence of 3.8/100,000 live male births (345), and often fatal. It predominantly affects boys and consists of absence or hypoplasia of the abdominal wall musculature, cryptorchism, and urinary tract anomalies. Findings include hypoplasia of the prostate, urethral obstruction in many but not all cases, markedly distended bladder, megaureters, bilateral hydronephrosis with atrophy, and often renal dysplasia and cyst formation. The condition is named for the characteristically lax and wrinkled appearance of the abdominal wall (Figure 17-60). The earliest manifestations are fetal ascites and Potter syndrome.

The pathogenesis of prune belly syndrome is not known; it may simply arise from the effects of early urethral obstruction or else from a basic defect of the mesoderm from which the triad of abnormalities develop. It is associated with a genomic HNF1-β (hepatocyte nuclear factor) mutation in 3% of cases. It is thought that posterior urethral valves cause obstruction

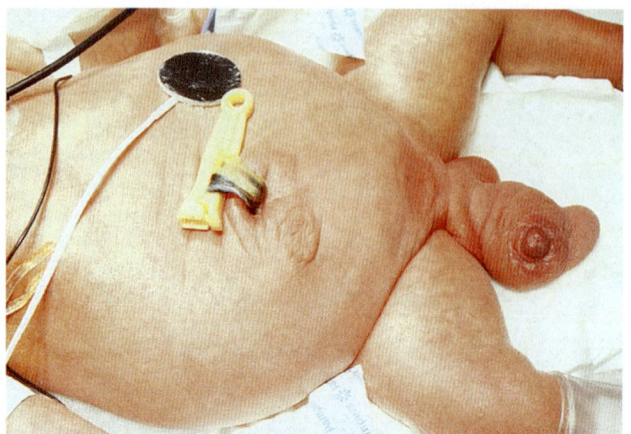

FIGURE 17-60 • Newborn boy with prune belly syndrome; note the lax anterior abdominal wall and redundant scrotal skin. (Courtesy of David Hatch, M.D., Loyola University Medical Center, Maywood, IL.)

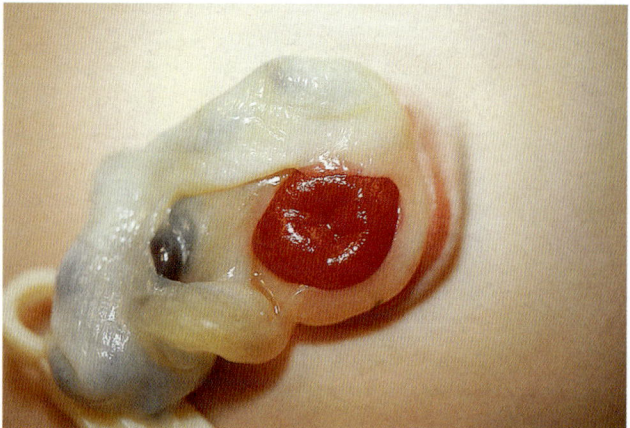

FIGURE 17-61 • Patent urachus with sinus opening into the umbilicus. (Courtesy of Preston Black, M.D., Loyola University Medical Center, Maywood, IL.)

of the lower urinary tract leading to oligohydramnios and massive dilatation of the bladder. This then leads to bilateral hydronephrosis and renal dysplasia, and pressure over the abdomen causes atrophy of the anterior abdominal muscles. The survival of these patients depends on the degree of pulmonary hypoplasia, which is fatal in severe cases. They also have undescended testis and intestinal malrotation secondary to the distended urinary bladder that does not allow for normal bowel positioning or testicular descent. If the obstruction is not treated *in utero*, these children develop oligohydramnios sequence with low-set ears, flat nose, folds under the eyes, and club feet. Treatment options include *in utero* vesicoamniotic shunts and drainage and reconstruction after birth (345).

Megacystis–Microcolon–Intestinal Hypoperistalsis Syndrome

Megacystis–microcolon–intestinal hypoperistalsis syndrome (MMIHS) is a rare congenital disorder characterized by a massively enlarged urinary bladder without mechanical outlet obstruction, microcolon, and a hypoperistaltic bowel with normal ganglion cells in a majority of cases (346). Absence of interstitial cells of Cajal, vacuolar degeneration of smooth muscle, neuronal dysplastic changes associated with increased laminin and fibronectin, and excessive smooth muscle cell glycogen storage with severely reduced contractile fibers displaced to the extreme periphery of cells have been reported (346). Heterozygous de novo and inherited mutations in the smooth muscle actin (*ACTG2*) gene have recently been demonstrated and are likely to be the cause of this syndrome (347).

Urachal Remnants

The patent urachus, which connects the developing urinary bladder with the allantoic duct, normally becomes a solid cord by month 4 of gestation. Patency may persist either completely, so that a fistula forms between the umbilicus and the bladder, or partially, in which case a sinus forms that usually opens into the umbilicus (Figure 17-61). A cyst develops if the urachus remains partially patent anywhere along its length. Persistence of the distal urachus where it joins the bladder produces a variably sized diverticulum. These remnants can be lined by transitional, intestinal, or squamous epithelium. There is a membrane to an ostomy site. Symptoms and complications include persistent umbilical discharge, infections, and development of carcinoma in adulthood.

ACQUIRED LESIONS OF THE BLADDER AND URETHRA

Cystitis

Cystitis in children can be broadly classified into two main categories: specific, in which the cause is known (e.g., bacteria, fungi, viruses, drugs, or radiation), and nonspecific, in which the cause is unknown (e.g., proliferative, interstitial, and eosinophilic cystitis and malakoplakia).

The etiology of UTIs is affected by underlying host factors such as age, diabetes, spinal cord injury, or catheterization. Consequently, complicated UTI has a more diverse etiology than uncomplicated UTI, and organisms that rarely cause disease in healthy patients can cause significant disease in hosts with anatomic, metabolic, or immunologic underlying disease. Most uncomplicated UTIs in children are caused by enterobacteria, mainly *E. coli*, 90% of which possess P fimbriae that allow the bacteria to adhere to the uroepithelial cell lining. *S. aureus* is more commonly seen among children with indwelling catheters. Coagulase-negative staphylococci and *Candida* app. are commonly associated with infections after instrumentation of the urinary tract. In nosocomial UTI, half of whom have had prior instrumentation; the organisms are *E. coli* (28%), *Candida* spp. (18%), *Enterococcus* (13%), gram-negative fermenters (13%), *Enterobacter* (10%), and *Pseudomonas* (10%). Although there have been minimal changes in the predominant uropathogens over the past decades, there have been significant changes in resistance patterns to antimicrobials that need to be considered when determining the most appropriate empiric therapy (348).

Granulomatous Cystitis

Granulomatous cystitis may be idiopathic or associated with a specific infection (e.g., tuberculosis, schistosomiasis, fungal infections in the immunocompromised). It may also be seen as part of chronic granulomatous disease of childhood, which is a rare congenital abnormality of the phagocyte reduced nicotinamide adenine dinucleotide phosphate (NADPH) oxidase system.

Cystitis Cystica and Glandularis

Cystitis cystica and cystitis glandularis are two forms of chronic proliferative cystitis, cystitis cystica being more common, that are often seen together in patients with chronic inflammation of the bladder. Proliferative cystitis eventually develops in patients with bladder exstrophy and may be a preneoplastic change, which would explain the increased risk for adenocarcinoma in these patients (349).

Cystoscopically, small rounded projections of the bladder mucosa are seen. Microscopically, cystic structures are apparent in the submucosa, composed of transitional and glandular epithelium (eFigure 17-28). When the lining resembles intestinal epithelium and the cysts become dilated with mucin, the condition is called *cystitis glandularis*. Chronic inflammatory infiltrate is usually minimal. A case with a 15-cm botryoid-like polyp has been described (350).

Interstitial Cystitis

Interstitial cystitis (IC) is a chronic noninfectious, probably inflammatory disorder of the bladder that primarily affects female adults. Occasionally, it can be seen in adolescent girls (351). Classic IC is characterized by frequency, nocturia, and suprapubic pain with ulceration (Hunner ulcer); in the nonclassic form, ulceration does not occur. The etiology and the pathogenesis are still undetermined, and the pathologic diagnosis is essentially one of the exclusion. IC appears to be a syndrome with neural, immune, and endocrine components in which activated mast cells play a central role. The bladder transitional cell epithelium is normally covered by a mucin layer composed of glycosaminoglycans. This layer is thought to be almost impermeable, thereby preventing urine solutes from diffusing into the subepithelial components of the bladder. IC might affect this layer by increasing solute permeability, possibly leading to irritation, inflammation, and sensory nerve sensitization of the bladder. Potassium could be the main offending substance and its diffusion across the permeable transitional epithelium the primary irritant, hence the development of the potassium sensitivity test for the diagnosis of IC (352).

Eosinophilic Cystitis

Eosinophilic cystitis is a rare disorder. In children, it may be associated with parasites, food allergens, or drugs. Associated risk factors include bronchial asthma, atopic diseases, and environmental allergens (353). It has also been reported in association with chronic granulomatous disease (354). The bladder mucosa may be markedly polypoid, so that embryonal rhabdomyosarcoma must be included in the differential diagnosis (355). Histologically, extensive eosinophilic inflammation of the bladder wall is present.

Malakoplakia

Malakoplakia is a chronic inflammatory disease that was originally described in the urinary bladder but can involve many other organs and soft tissues. It is rarely seen in children (262,356). Histologically, it is characterized by chronic inflammation, histiocytes, and poorly formed granulomas. A diagnostic feature is the Michaelis-Gutmann body, which is a laminated calcospherite present in the cytoplasm or extracellularly (Figure 17-62). It stains with periodic acid–Schiff, iron, and von Kossa stains and may represent bacterial degradation products (357).

Hemorrhagic Cystitis

Acute hemorrhagic cystitis may be infectious or sterile. BK virus has been shown to be the main cause of viral hemorrhagic cystitis in bone marrow transplant patients (358). BK virus cystitis has also been reported in nonimmunocompromised hosts. In patients receiving hematopoietic stem cell transplantation, older age at transplant, allogeneic transplant, cyclophosphamide-containing conditioning, moderate-to-severe acute graft-versus-host disease (GVHD), and hepatic GVHD were associated with higher risks of HC (359). Adenovirus type 11 is responsible for acute, self-limiting

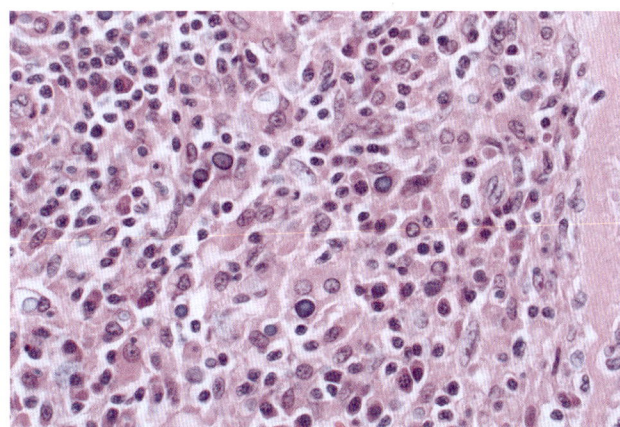

FIGURE 17-62 • Malakoplakia of the bladder in a child with a surgically repaired exstrophy. The inflammatory infiltrate is composed of lymphocytes, plasma cells, and macrophages, some with purple stained Michaelis-Gutmann bodies. (Hematoxylin–eosin stain, original magnification ×200.)

cystitis with the sudden onset of gross hematuria, dysuria, and urinary frequency. *E. coli* and occasionally *Candida albicans* may also cause hemorrhagic cystitis.

Cyclophosphamide therapy is complicated by ulceration of the bladder mucosa and massive hemorrhage into the submucosa in 7% of patients receiving the drug. During high-dose therapy, up to 35% of patients have severe hemorrhagic cystitis. Ifosfamide produces hemorrhagic cystitis even more commonly, which is its main dose-limiting toxicity. The cytokines, tumor necrosis factor-α, and interleukin-1, nitric oxide, nitric oxide synthetase, and platelet-activating factor have been shown to be involved in the pathogenesis of hemorrhagic cystitis. The blood loss may be so severe that blood transfusions and even surgical intervention are warranted. Marked cytologic atypia can be seen in the regenerating epithelium. The incidence of urothelial neoplasms is increased in patients receiving long-term cyclophosphamide therapy. Mesna is a drug that protects urothelium and prevents hemorrhagic cystitis and may even decrease the risk for urothelial carcinoma.

Tumors of the Bladder and Urethra

All tumors of the bladder and urethra are rare in children; benign tumors are even more infrequent. Benign tumors in children described in case reports include polyps, papilloma, hemangioma (350,360), neurofibroma, leiomyoma (361), paraganglioma (362), granular cell tumor, nephrogenic adenoma (eFigure 17-29) (363), and inverted papilloma (364).

Rare cases of transitional cell carcinoma and leiomyosarcoma and secondary involvement by leukemia, lymphoma, and WT have been reported.

Inflammatory Myofibroblastic Tumor (Pseudosarcomatous Tumor)

Inflammatory myofibroblastic tumor (IMT) is occasionally seen in the bladder. Myxoid, leiomyomatous, and sclerosing matrix patterns are seen, with the myxoid type being most common (eFigures 17-30 and 17-31). The proliferating cells stain with vimentin, muscle-specific actin, smooth muscle actin, desmin, and occasionally keratin and, rarely, Epstein-Barr virus (365). Although this tumor was long considered a benign proliferative response to inflammation, the frequent anaplastic lymphoma kinase gene alterations indicate that it is a neoplastic process (366). Some of the pathologic aspects occurring in a few of these tumors that support this view include local recurrence, development of multifocal noncontiguous tumors, infiltrative local growth, vascular invasion, and, rarely, malignant transformation (367). However, a recent review of 35 pediatric cases showed no recurrence or metastasis (368). IMT should be regarded as a soft tissue mesenchymal tumor with an indeterminate or low potential for malignancy (see Chapter 25).

Rhabdomyosarcoma

Although the term *rhabdomyosarcoma* indicates a mesenchymal tumor differentiating toward striated muscle, rhabdomyosarcoma typically arises in sites lacking striated muscle. Approximately 250 new cases of rhabdomyosarcoma are diagnosed in the United States each year, 15% to 30% of which are found in the genitourinary tract. Thus, although rhabdomyosarcoma is the most common tumor of the lower genitourinary tract in the first two decades of life, only a handful of cases occurring in the bladder are seen in the United States each year. The majority of cases are sporadic; however, rhabdomyosarcoma has an association with the familial cancer syndromes, including Li-Fraumeni, Beckwith-Wiedemann, neurofibromatosis type 1, and Gorlin syndrome (369). The mean age at diagnosis is 5 years, with a male to female ratio of 3:2. Symptoms include hematuria, signs of bladder outlet obstruction (abdominal pain and distension, dysuria), and, occasionally, abdominal mass (370).

The vast majority of cases of rhabdomyosarcoma of the bladder are of the botryoid subtype of embryonal rhabdomyosarcoma. The gross configuration in most cases is grapelike. The tumor cells form a distinct layer with a thickness of several cells, at least focally, near the epithelium. The superficial stroma next to the epithelium is loose. The condensed tumor cells or cambium layer of Nicholson varies in thickness and extent (Figure 17-63). Some grossly grapelike lesions do not show the cambium layer under the epithelium. By this definition, these would not be called *botryoid rhabdomyosarcoma*, but rather *embryonal rhabdomyosarcoma*. Cytogenetic and molecular features are discussed in the soft tissue chapter (Chapter 25).

In the vast majority of cases, the stroma of the botryoid lesion consists of a very loosely cellular tissue with a myxoid appearance. In the remainder, the stroma is more cellular. The appearance of the tumor cells also varies. In about 50% of the cases, the tumor cells are small and primitive, show very little myogenesis, and often demonstrate stellate cytoplasmic processes. In the remainder, the tumor cells are somewhat larger and more definitive myogenesis is present, consistent with rhabdomyoblasts. The cytoplasm of the rhabdomyoblasts varies from slight to abundant with cross-striations.

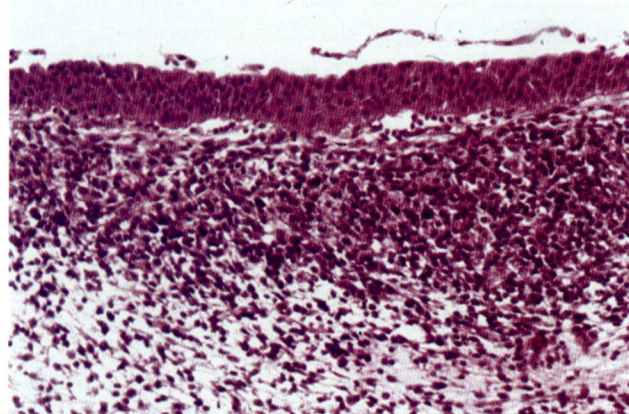

FIGURE 17-63 • Embryonal rhabdomyosarcoma as a polypoid urethral mass from an 8-week-old girl. The concentration of small, primitive tumor cells beneath the mucosal surface is typical of sarcoma botryoides. (Hematoxylin–eosin stain, original magnification ×200.)

The importance of recognizing the botryoid subtype lies in the fact that these patients have a very good prognosis (95% survival at 5 years); in contrast, patients with embryonal rhabdomyosarcoma have a 5-year survival of 67%, and those with alveolar and undifferentiated sarcoma have 5-year survival rates of 54% and 47%, respectively.

The goal of multimodality therapy is to improve outcome while preserving organ and function; therapy is intensified according to a risk-based study design. Bladder rhabdomyosarcoma is responsive to chemotherapy and radiotherapy. A complete loss of tumor cells was observed in 12 of 26 patients after induction therapy. Cystectomy specimens showed diminished tumor cells with varying degrees of cellular maturation. There is lack of agreement concerning the significance of mature-appearing cells in posttreatment biopsies.

References

1. Sanna-Cherchi S, Sampogna RV, Papeta N, et al. Mutations in DSTYK and dominant urinary tract malformations. *N Engl J Med* 2013;369:621–629.
2. Dome JS, Fernandez CV, Mullen EA, et al. Children's Oncology Group's 2013 blueprint for research: renal tumors. *Pediatr Blood Cancer* 2013;60:994–1000.
3. Faa G, Gerosa C, Fanni D, et al. Morphogenesis and molecular mechanisms involved in human kidney development. *J Cell Physiol* 2012;227:1257–1268.
4. Little MH, McMahon AP. Mammalian kidney development: principles, progress, and projections. *Cold Spring Harb Perspect Biol* 2012;4:1–18.
5. Sutherland MR, Gubhaju L, Moore L, et al. Accelerated maturation and abnormal morphology in the preterm neonatal kidney. *J Am Soc Nephrol* 2011;22:1365–1374.
6. Schreuder MF. Unilateral anomalies of kidney development: why is left not right? *Kidney Int* 2011;80:740–745.
7. Harambat J, van Stralen KJ, Kim JJ, et al. Epidemiology of chronic kidney disease in children. *Pediatr Nephrol* 2012;27:363–373.
8. Dias T, Sairam S, Kumarasiri S. Ultrasound diagnosis of fetal renal abnormalities. *Best Pract Res Clin Obstet Gynaecol* 2014;28:403–415.
9. Vivante A, Kohl S, Hwang DY, et al. Single-gene causes of congenital anomalies of the kidney and urinary tract (CAKUT) in humans. *Pediatr Nephrol* 2014;29:695–704.
10. Bonsib SM. The classification of renal cystic diseases and other congenital malformations of the kidney and urinary tract. *Arch Pathol Lab Med* 2010;134:554–568.
11. Song R, Yosypiv IV. Genetics of congenital anomalies of the kidney and urinary tract. *Pediatr Nephrol* 2011;26:353–364.
12. Copelovitch L, Furth SL. Genetics and urinary tract malformations. *Am J Kidney Dis* 2014;63:183–185.
13. Bisceglia M, Galliani CA, Senger C, et al. Renal cystic diseases: a review. *Adv Anat Pathol* 2006;13:26–56.
14. Caiulo VA, Caiulo S, Gargasole C, et al. Ultrasound mass screening for congenital anomalies of the kidney and urinary tract. *Pediatr Nephrol* 2012;27:949–953.
15. Adam A, De Villiers M, Van Biljon G. Quest for the missing kidney in the "treasure chest": report of a thoracic kidney in a child with recurrent diaphragmatic hernia. *Urology* 2013;82:922–924.
16. Arena F, Arena S, Paolata A, et al. Is a complete urological evaluation necessary in all newborns with asymptomatic renal ectopia? *Int J Urol* 2007;14:491–495.
17. Natsis K, Piagkou M, Skotsimara A, et al. Horseshoe kidney: a review of anatomy and pathology. *Surg Radiol Anat* 2014;36:517–526.
18. Carvalho AB, Guerra Junior G, Baptista MT, et al. Cardiovascular and renal anomalies in Turner syndrome. *Rev Assoc Med Bras* 2010;56:655–659.
19. Saussine C, Lechevallier E, Traxer O. Urolithiasis and congenital renoureteral malformations. *Prog Urol* 2008;18:997–999.
20. Dhillon J, Mohanty SK, Kim T, et al. Spectrum of renal pathology in adult patients with congenital renal anomalies—a series from a tertiary cancer center. *Ann Diagn Pathol* 2014;18:14–17.
21. Ye H, Yoon GS, Epstein JI. Intrarenal ectopic adrenal tissue and renal-adrenal fusion: a report of nine cases. *Mod Pathol* 2009;22:175–181.
22. Jeanpierre C, Mace G, Parisot M, et al. RET and GDNF mutations are rare in fetuses with renal agenesis or other severe kidney development defects. *J Med Genet* 2011;48:497–504.
23. Harshman LA, Brophy PD. PAX2 in human kidney malformations and disease. *Pediatr Nephrol* 2012;27:1265–1275.
24. Hwang DY, Dworschak GC, Kohl S, et al. Mutations in 12 known dominant disease-causing genes clarify many congenital anomalies of the kidney and urinary tract. *Kidney Int* 2014;85:1429–1433.
25. Schwaderer AL, Bates CM, McHugh KM, et al. Renal anomalies in family members of infants with bilateral renal agenesis/adysplasia. *Pediatr Nephrol* 2007;22:52–56.
26. Loo CK, Algar EM, Payton DJ, et al. Possible role of WT1 in a human fetus with evolving bronchial atresia, pulmonary malformation and renal agenesis. *Pediatr Dev Pathol* 2012;15:39–44.
27. Chikkannaiah P, Mahadevan A, Gosavi M, et al. Sirenomelia with associated systemic anomalies: an autopsy pathologic illustration of a series of four cases. *Pathol Res Pract* 2014;210:444–449.
28. Jain D, Sharma MC, Kulkarni KK, et al. Urorectal septum malformation sequence: a report of seven cases. *Congenit Anom (Kyoto)* 2008;48:174–179.
29. Kashiwagi M, Chaoui R, Stallmach T, et al. Fetal bilateral renal agenesis, phocomelia, and single umbilical artery associated with cocaine abuse in early pregnancy. *Birth Defects Res A Clin Mol Teratol* 2003;67:951–952.
30. Barak H, Huh SH, Chen S, et al. FGF9 and FGF20 maintain the stemness of nephron progenitors in mice and man. *Dev Cell* 2012;22:1191–1207.
31. Humbert C, Silbermann F, Morar B, et al. Integrin alpha 8 recessive mutations are responsible for bilateral renal agenesis in humans. *Am J Hum Genet* 2014;94:288–294.
32. Westland R, Schreuder MF, Ket JC, et al. Unilateral renal agenesis: a systematic review on associated anomalies and renal injury. *Nephrol Dial Transplant* 2013;28:1844–1855.
33. Renkema KY, Winyard PJ, Skovorodkin IN, et al. Novel perspectives for investigating congenital anomalies of the kidney and urinary tract (CAKUT). *Nephrol Dial Transplant* 2011;26:3843–3851.
34. Wang S, Lang JH, Zhu L, et al. Duplicated uterus and hemivaginal or hemicervical atresia with ipsilateral renal agenesis: an institutional clinical series of 52 cases. *Eur J Obstet Gynecol Reprod Biol* 2013;170:507–511.
35. Schwarzer JU, Schwarz M. Significance of CFTR gene mutations in patients with congenital aplasia of vas deferens with special regard to renal aplasia. *Andrologia* 2012;44:305–307.
36. Camassei FD, Francalanci P, Ferro F, et al. Cystic dysplasia of the rete testis: report of two cases and review of the literature. *Pediatr Dev Pathol* 2002;5:206–210.
37. Carmody JB, Charlton JR. Short-term gestation, long-term risk: prematurity and chronic kidney disease. *Pediatrics* 2013;131:1168–1179.
38. Thomas R, Sanna-Cherchi S, Warady BA, et al. HNF1B and PAX2 mutations are a common cause of renal hypodysplasia in the CKiD cohort. *Pediatr Nephrol* 2011;26:897–903.
39. Abitbol CL, Rodriguez MM. The long-term renal and cardiovascular consequences of prematurity. *Nat Rev Nephrol* 2012;8:265–274.
40. Gribouval O, Moriniere V, Pawtowski A, et al. Spectrum of mutations in the renin-angiotensin system genes in autosomal recessive renal tubular dysgenesis. *Hum Mutat* 2012;33:316–326.
41. Gubler MC. Renal tubular dysgenesis. *Pediatr Nephrol* 2014;29:51–59.
42. Bonilla SF, Melin-Aldana H, Whitington PF. Relationship of proximal renal tubular dysgenesis and fetal liver injury in neonatal hemochromatosis. *Pediatr Res* 2010;67:188–193.
43. Neri G, Martini-Neri ME, Katz BE, et al. The Perlman syndrome: familial renal dysplasia with Wilms tumor, fetal gigantism and multiple congenital anomalies. 1984. *Am J Med Genet A* 2013;161A:2691–2696.

44. Mussa A, Peruzzi L, Chiesa N, et al. Nephrological findings and genotype-phenotype correlation in Beckwith-Wiedemann syndrome. *Pediatr Nephrol* 2012;27:397–406.
45. Ma R, Wu RD, Liu W, et al. A new classification of duplex kidney based on kidney morphology and management. *Chin Med J (Engl)* 2013;126:615–619.
46. Meneghesso D, Castagnetti M, Della Vella M, et al. Clinico-pathological correlation in duplex system ectopic ureters and ureteroceles: can preoperative work-up predict renal histology? *Pediatr Surg Int* 2012;28: 309–314.
47. Wilkinson LJ, Neal CS, Singh RR, et al. Renal developmental defects resulting from in utero hypoxia are associated with suppression of ureteric beta-catenin signaling. *Kidney Int* 2015;87:975–983.
48. Afrouzian M, Sonstein J, Dadfarnia T, et al. Four miniature kidneys: supernumerary kidney and multiple organ system anomalies. *Hum Pathol* 2014; 45:1100–1104.
49. Sureka B, Mittal MK, Mittal A, et al. Supernumerary kidneys—a rare anatomic variant. *Surg Radiol Anat* 2014;36:199–202.
50. Swords KA, Peters CA. Neonatal and early infancy management of prenatally detected hydronephrosis. *Arch Dis Child Fetal Neonatal Ed* 2015 (epub ahead of print).
51. Vemulakonda V, Yiee J, Wilcox DT. Prenatal hydronephrosis: postnatal evaluation and management. *Curr Urol Rep* 2014;15:430.
52. Klein J, Gonzalez J, Miravete M, et al. Congenital ureteropelvic junction obstruction: human disease and animal models. *Int J Exp Pathol* 2011;92:168–192.
53. Rasouly HM, Lu W. Lower urinary tract development and disease. *Wiley Interdiscip Rev Syst Biol Med* 2013;5:307–342.
54. Kupferman JC, Druschel CM, Kupchik GS. Increased prevalence of renal and urinary tract anomalies in children with Down syndrome. *Pediatrics* 2009;124:E615–E621.
55. Johnston JJ, Sapp JC, Turner JT, et al. Molecular analysis expands the spectrum of phenotypes associated with GLI3 mutations. *Hum Mutat* 2010;31:1142–1154.
56. Pieretti-Vanmarcke R, Pieretti A, Pieretti RV. Megacalycosis: a rare condition. *Pediatr Nephrol* 2009;24:1077–1079.
57. Osathanondh V, Potter EL. Pathogenesis of polycystic kidneys. Type 1 due to hyperplasia of interstitial portions of collecting tubules. *Arch Pathol* 1964;77:466–473.
58. Takeuchi M, Kamishima Y, Hara M, et al. Segmental multicystic dysplastic kidney in an adult: usefulness of enhanced CT in excretory phase. *Abdom Imaging* 2013;38:603–607.
59. Eickmeyer AB, Casanova NF, He C, et al. The natural history of the multicystic dysplastic kidney—is limited follow-up warranted? *J Pediatr Urol* 2014;10:655–661.
60. Tiryaki S, Alkac AY, Serdaroglu E, et al. Involution of multicystic dysplastic kidney: is it predictable? *J Pediatr Urol* 2013;9:344–347.
61. Psooy K. Multicystic dysplastic kidney in the neonate: the role of the urologist. *Can Urol Assoc J* 2010;4:95–97.
62. Pringle KC, Kitagawa H, Seki Y, et al. Development of an animal model to study congenital urinary obstruction. *Pediatr Surg Int* 2013;29: 1083–1089.
63. Welham SJ, Riley PR, Wade A, et al. Maternal diet programs embryonic kidney gene expression. *Physiol Genomics* 2005;22:48–56.
64. Gilbert-Barness E. Renal system. In: Gilbert-Barness E ed. *Potter's Pathology of the Fetus, Infant and Child*. Philadelphia, PA: Mosby Elsevier, 2007:1356–1373.
65. Torres VE, Harris PC. Strategies targeting cAMP signaling in the treatment of polycystic kidney disease. *J Am Soc Nephrol* 2014;25:18–32.
66. Harris PC, Torres VE. Genetic mechanisms and signaling pathways in autosomal dominant polycystic kidney disease. *J Clin Invest* 2014;124: 2315–2324.
67. Hartung EA, Guay-Woodford LM. Autosomal recessive polycystic kidney disease: a hepatorenal fibrocystic disorder with pleiotropic effects. *Pediatrics* 2014;134:e833–e845.
68. Zhang J, Wu M, Wang S, et al. Polycystic kidney disease protein fibrocystin localizes to the mitotic spindle and regulates spindle bipolarity. *Hum Mol Genet* 2010;19:3306–3319.
69. Kurschat CE, Muller RU, Franke M, et al. An approach to cystic kidney diseases: the clinician's view. *Nat Rev Nephrol* 2014;10:687–699.
70. Bergmann C. ARPKD and early manifestations of ADPKD: the original polycystic kidney disease and phenocopies. *Pediatr Nephrol* 2015; 30:15–30.
71. Guay-Woodford LM, Bissler JJ, Braun MC, et al. Consensus expert recommendations for the diagnosis and management of autosomal recessive polycystic kidney disease: report of an international conference. *J Pediatr* 2014;165:611–617.
72. Buscher R, Buscher AK, Weber S, et al. Clinical manifestations of autosomal recessive polycystic kidney disease (ARPKD): kidney-related and non-kidney-related phenotypes. *Pediatr Nephrol* 2014;29: 1915–1925.
73. Rock N, McLin V. Liver involvement in children with ciliopathies. *Clin Res Hepatol Gastroenterol* 2014;38:407–414.
74. Jalanko H, Pakarinen M. Combined liver and kidney transplantation in children. *Pediatr Nephrol* 2014;29:805–814; quiz 12.
75. Telega G, Cronin D, Avner ED. New approaches to the autosomal recessive polycystic kidney disease patient with dual kidney-liver complications. *Pediatr Transplant* 2013;17:328–335.
76. Cornec-Le Gall E, Audrezet MP, Meur YL, et al. Genetics and pathogenesis of autosomal dominant polycystic kidney disease: 20 years on. *Hum Mutat* 2014;35:1393–1406.
77. Watnick TJ, Germino GG. Polycystic kidney disease: polycystin-1 and polycystin-2–it's complicated. *Nat Rev Nephrol* 2013;9:249–250.
78. Paul BM, Vanden Heuvel GB. Kidney: polycystic kidney disease. *Wiley Interdiscip Rev Dev Biol* 2014;3:465–487.
79. Ma M, Tian X, Igarashi P, et al. Loss of cilia suppresses cyst growth in genetic models of autosomal dominant polycystic kidney disease. *Nat Genet* 2013;45:1004–1012.
80. Dell KM. The role of cilia in the pathogenesis of cystic kidney disease. *Curr Opin Pediatr* 2015;27:212–218.
81. Paul BM, Consugar MB, Ryan Lee M, et al. Evidence of a third ADPKD locus is not supported by re-analysis of designated PKD3 families. *Kidney Int* 2014;85:383–392.
82. Schrier RW, Brosnahan G, Cadnapaphornchai MA, et al. Predictors of autosomal dominant polycystic kidney disease progression. *J Am Soc Nephrol* 2014;25:2399–2418.
83. Cadnapaphornchai MA. Autosomal dominant polycystic kidney disease in children. *Curr Opin Pediatr* 2015;27(2):193–200.
84. Lennerz JK, Spence DC. Iskandar SS, et al. Glomerulocystic kidney: one hundred-year perspective. *Arch Pathol Lab Med* 2010;134:583–605.
85. Fabris A, Lupo A, Ferraro PM, et al. Familial clustering of medullary sponge kidney is autosomal dominant with reduced penetrance and variable expressivity. *Kidney Int* 2013;83:272–277.
86. Fabris A, Anglani F, Lupo A, et al. Medullary sponge kidney: state of the art. *Nephrol Dial Transplant* 2013;28:1111–1119.
87. Goldfarb DS. Evidence for inheritance of medullary sponge kidney. *Kidney Int* 2013;83:193–196.
88. Torregrossa R, Anglani F, Fabris A, et al. Identification of GDNF gene sequence variations in patients with medullary sponge kidney disease. *Clin J Am Soc Nephrol* 2010;5:1205–1210.
89. Renkema KY, Stokman MF, Giles RH, et al. Next-generation sequencing for research and diagnostics in kidney disease. *Nat Rev Nephrol* 2014;10:433–444.
90. Wolf MT. Nephronophthisis and related syndromes. *Curr Opin Pediatr* 2015;27:201–211.
91. Benzing T, Schermer B. Clinical spectrum and pathogenesis of nephronophthisis. *Curr Opin Nephrol Hypertens* 2012;21:272–278.
92. Chaki M, Hoefele J, Allen SJ, et al. Genotype-phenotype correlation in 440 patients with NPHP-related ciliopathies. *Kidney Int* 2011;80:1239–1245.
93. Halbritter J, Porath JD, Diaz KA, et al. Identification of 99 novel mutations in a worldwide cohort of 1,056 patients with a nephronophthisis-related ciliopathy. *Hum Genet* 2013;132:865–884.
94. Bleyer AJ, Kmoch S, Antignac C, et al. Variable clinical presentation of an MUC1 mutation causing medullary cystic kidney disease type 1. *Clin J Am Soc Nephrol* 2014;9:527–535.

95. Ekici AB, Hackenbeck T, Moriniere V, et al. Renal fibrosis is the common feature of autosomal dominant tubulointerstitial kidney diseases caused by mutations in mucin 1 or uromodulin. *Kidney Int* 2014;86:589–599.
96. Scolari F, Izzi C, Ghiggeri GM. Uromodulin: from monogenic to multifactorial diseases. *Nephrol Dial Transplant* 2014 (epub ahead of print).
97. Iorember FM, Vehaskari VM. Uromodulin: old friend with new roles in health and disease. *Pediatr Nephrol* 2014;29:1151–1158.
98. Bernstein J. Glomerulocystic kidney disease—nosological considerations. *Pediatr Nephrol* 1993;7:464–470.
99. Bissler JJ, Siroky BJ, Yin H. Glomerulocystic kidney disease. *Pediatr Nephrol* 2010;25:2049–2056; quiz 56–59.
100. Decramer S, Parant O, Beaufils S, et al. Anomalies of the TCF2 gene are the main cause of fetal bilateral hyperechogenic kidneys. *J Am Soc Nephrol* 2007;18:923–933.
101. Faguer S, Chassaing N, Bandin F, et al. The HNF1B score is a simple tool to select patients for HNF1B gene analysis. *Kidney Int* 2014; 86:1007–1015.
102. Clissold RL, Hamilton AJ, Hattersley AT, et al. HNF1B-associated renal and extra-renal disease-an expanding clinical spectrum. *Nat Rev Nephrol* 2015;11:102–112.
103. Bayram MT, Alaygut D, Soylu A, et al. Clinical and radiological course of simple renal cysts in children. *Urology* 2014;83:433–437.
104. Reed B, Nobakht E, Dadgar S, et al. Renal ultrasonographic evaluation in children at risk of autosomal dominant polycystic kidney disease. *Am J Kidney Dis* 2010;56:50–56.
105. Pei Y, Obaji J, Dupuis A, et al. Unified criteria for ultrasonographic diagnosis of ADPKD. *J Am Soc Nephrol* 2009;20:205–212.
106. Siroky BJ, Yin H, Bissler JJ. Clinical and molecular insights into tuberous sclerosis complex renal disease. *Pediatr Nephrol* 2011;26:839–852.
107. Kozlowski P, Roberts P, Dabora S, et al. Identification of 54 large deletions/duplications in TSC1 and TSC2 using MLPA, and genotype-phenotype correlations. *Hum Genet* 2007;121:389–400.
108. Guo J, Tretiakova MS, Troxell ML, et al. Tuberous sclerosis-associated renal cell carcinoma: a clinicopathologic study of 57 separate carcinomas in 18 patients. *Am J Surg Pathol* 2014;38:1457–1467.
109. Bausch B, Jilg C, Glasker S, et al. Renal cancer in von Hippel-Lindau disease and related syndromes. *Nat Rev Nephrol* 2013;9:529–538.
110. Northrup BE, Jokerst CE, Grubb RL, et al. Hereditary renal tumor syndromes: imaging findings and management strategies. *Am J Roentgenol* 2012;199:1294–1304.
111. Montani M, Heinimann K, von Teichman A, et al. VHL-gene deletion in single renal tubular epithelial cells and renal tubular cysts: further evidence for a cyst-dependent progression pathway of clear cell renal carcinoma in von Hippel-Lindau disease. *Am J Surg Pathol* 2010;34:806–815.
112. Williamson SR, Zhang S, Eble JN, et al. Clear cell papillary renal cell carcinoma-like tumors in patients with von Hippel-Lindau disease are unrelated to sporadic clear cell papillary renal cell carcinoma. *Am J Surg Pathol* 2013;37:1131–1139.
113. Barker AR, Thomas R, Dawe HR. Meckel-Gruber syndrome and the role of primary cilia in kidney, skeleton, and central nervous system development. *Organogenesis* 2014;10:96–107.
114. O'Brien LL, McMahon AP. Induction and patterning of the metanephric nephron. *Semin Cell Dev Biol* 2014;36:31–38.
115. Abdelhamed ZA, Wheway G, Szymanska K, et al. Variable expressivity of ciliopathy neurological phenotypes that encompass Meckel-Gruber syndrome and Joubert syndrome is caused by complex de-regulated ciliogenesis, Shh and Wnt signalling defects. *Hum Mol Genet* 2013;22:1358–1372.
116. Barisic I, Boban L, Loane M, et al. Meckel-Gruber syndrome: a population-based study on prevalence, prenatal diagnosis, clinical features, and survival in Europe. *Eur J Hum Genet* 2015;23:746–752.
117. Eckmann-Scholz C, Jonat W, Zerres K, et al. Earliest ultrasound findings and description of splicing mutations in Meckel-Gruber syndrome. *Arch Gynecol Obstet* 2012;286:917–921.
118. Guay-Woodford LM, Galliani CA, Musulman-Mroczek E, et al. Diffuse renal cystic disease in children: morphologic and genetic correlations. *Pediatr Nephrol* 1998;12:173–182.
119. Dotsch J, Plank C, Amann K. Fetal programming of renal function. *Pediatr Nephrol* 2012;27:513–520.
120. Fong D, Denton KM, Moritz KM, et al. Compensatory responses to nephron deficiency: adaptive or maladaptive? *Nephrology (Carlton)* 2014;19:119–128.
121. Vogler C, McAdams AJ, Homan SM. Glomerular basement membrane and lamina densa in infants and children: an ultrastructural evaluation. *Pediatr Pathol* 1987;7:527–534.
122. Haas M. Alport syndrome and thin glomerular basement membrane nephropathy: a practical approach to diagnosis. *Arch Pathol Lab Med* 2009;133:224–232.
123. Abrahamson DR. Role of the podocyte (and glomerular endothelium) in building the GBM. *Semin Nephrol* 2012;32:342–349.
124. Chang A, Gibson IW, Cohen AH, et al. A position paper on standardizing the nonneoplastic kidney biopsy report. *Hum Pathol* 2012;43: 1192–1196.
125. Eddy AA, Symons JM. Nephrotic syndrome in childhood. *Lancet* 2003;362:629–639.
126. Olson JL. The nephrotic syndrome and minimal change disease. In: Jennette JC, Olson JL, Silve FG, et al. eds. *Heptinstall's Pathology of the Kidney*. Philadelphia, PA: Wolters Kluwer; 2015:173–205.
127. Laurin LP, Lu M, Mottl AK, et al. Podocyte-associated gene mutation screening in a heterogeneous cohort of patients with sporadic focal segmental glomerulosclerosis. *Nephrol Dial Transplant* 2014; 29:2062–2069.
128. Pollak MR. Familial FSGS. *Adv Chronic Kidney Dis* 2014;21:422–425.
129. Agrawal V, Prasad N, Jain M, et al. Reduced podocin expression in minimal change disease and focal segmental glomerulosclerosis is related to the level of proteinuria. *Clin Exp Nephrol* 2013;17:811–818.
130. Hodgin JB, Borczuk AC, Nasr SH, et al. A molecular profile of focal segmental glomerulosclerosis from formalin-fixed, paraffin-embedded tissue. *Am J Pathol* 2010;177:1674–1686.
131. Clement LC, Mace C, Avila-Casado C, et al. Circulating angiopoietin-like 4 links proteinuria with hypertriglyceridemia in nephrotic syndrome. *Nat Med* 2014;20:37–46.
132. Ishimoto T, Shimada M, Gabriela G, et al. Toll-like receptor 3 ligand, polyIC, induces proteinuria and glomerular CD80, and increases urinary CD80 in mice. *Nephrol Dial Transplant* 2013;28:1439–1446.
133. Ostalska-Nowicka D, Zachwieja J, Nowicki M, et al. Is mesangial hypercellularity with glomerular immaturity a variant of glomerulosclerosis? *Pediatr Nephrol* 2007;22:674–683.
134. Emery JL, Macdonald MS, Involuting and scarred glomeruli in the kidneys of infants. *Am J Pathol* 1960;36:713–723.
135. Geier P, Roushdi A, Skalova S, et al. Is cyclophosphamide effective in patients with IgM-positive minimal change disease? *Pediatr Nephrol* 2012;27:2227–2231.
136. Kanemoto K, Ito H, Anzai M, et al. Clinical significance of IgM and C1q deposition in the mesangium in pediatric idiopathic nephrotic syndrome. *J Nephrol* 2013;26:306–314.
137. Jennette JC, Hipp CG, C1q nephropathy: a distinct pathologic entity usually causing nephrotic syndrome. *Am J Kidney Dis* 1985;6:103–110.
138. Markowitz GS, Schwimmer JA, Stokes MB, et al. C1q nephropathy: a variant of focal segmental glomerulosclerosis. *Kidney Int* 2003;64: 1232–1240.
139. Gunasekara VN, Sebire NJ, Tullus K. C1q nephropathy in children: clinical characteristics and outcome. *Pediatr Nephrol* 2014;29:407–413.
140. Vintar Spreitzer M, Vizjak A, Ferluga D, et al. Do C1q or IgM nephropathies predict disease severity in children with minimal change nephrotic syndrome? *Pediatr Nephrol* 2014;29:67–74.
141. Samuel S, Morgan CJ, Bitzan M, et al. Substantial practice variation exists in the management of childhood nephrotic syndrome. *Pediatr Nephrol* 2013;28:2289–2298.
142. D'Agati VD. Pathobiology of focal segmental glomerulosclerosis: new developments. *Curr Opin Nephrol Hypertens* 2012;21:243–250.
143. Gellermann J, Schaefer F, Querfeld U. Serum suPAR levels are modulated by immunosuppressive therapy of minimal change nephrotic syndrome. *Pediatr Nephrol* 2014;29:2411–2414.

144. Huang J, Liu G, Zhang YM, et al. Plasma soluble urokinase receptor levels are increased but do not distinguish primary from secondary focal segmental glomerulosclerosis. *Kidney Int* 2013;84:366–372.
145. Jefferson JA, Shankland SJ. The pathogenesis of focal segmental glomerulosclerosis. *Adv Chronic Kidney Dis* 2014;21:408–416.
146. D'Agati V. Pathologic classification of focal segmental glomerulosclerosis. *Semin Nephrol* 2003;23:117–134.
147. D'Agati VD, Alster JM, Jennette JC, et al. Association of histologic variants in FSGS clinical trial with presenting features and outcomes. *Clin J Am Soc Nephrol* 2013;8:399–406.
148. Stokes MB, D'Agati VD. Morphologic variants of focal segmental glomerulosclerosis and their significance. *Adv Chronic Kidney Dis* 2014;21:400–407.
149. Ding WY, Koziell A, McCarthy HJ, et al. Initial steroid sensitivity in children with steroid-resistant nephrotic syndrome predicts posttransplant recurrence. *J Am Soc Nephrol* 2014;25:1342–1348.
150. Ayalon R, Beck LH, Jr. Membranous nephropathy: not just a disease for adults. *Pediatr Nephrol* 2015;30:31–39.
151. Markowitz GS, D'Agati VD. *Membranous Glomerulonephritis*. 7th ed. Philadelphia, PA: Wolters Kluwer; 2015.
152. Beck LH, Jr, Bonegio RG, Lambeau G, et al. M-type phospholipase A2 receptor as target antigen in idiopathic membranous nephropathy. *N Engl J Med* 2009;361:11–21.
153. Larsen CP, Messias NC, Silva FG, et al. Determination of primary versus secondary membranous glomerulopathy utilizing phospholipase A2 receptor staining in renal biopsies. *Mod Pathol* 2013;26:709–715.
154. Murtas C, Bruschi M, Candiano G, et al. Coexistence of different circulating anti-podocyte antibodies in membranous nephropathy. *Clin J Am Soc Nephrol* 2012;7:1394–1400.
155. Cossey LN, Walker PD, Larsen CP. Phospholipase A2 receptor staining in pediatric idiopathic membranous glomerulopathy. *Pediatr Nephrol* 2013;28:2307–2311.
156. Debiec H, Guigonis V, Mougenot B, et al. Antenatal membranous glomerulonephritis due to anti-neutral endopeptidase antibodies. *N Engl J Med* 2002;346:2053–2060.
157. Debiec H, Nauta J, Coulet F, et al. Role of truncating mutations in MME gene in fetomaternal alloimmunisation and antenatal glomerulopathies. *Lancet* 2004;364:1252–1259.
158. Debiec H, Lefeu F, Kemper MJ, et al. Early-childhood membranous nephropathy due to cationic bovine serum albumin. *N Engl J Med* 2011;364:2101–2110.
159. Menon S, Valentini RP. Membranous nephropathy in children: clinical presentation and therapeutic approach. *Pediatr Nephrol* 2010;25:1419–1428.
160. Collins AJ, Foley RN, Chavers B, et al. US Renal Data System 2013 annual data report. *Am J Kidney Dis* 2013;63:A7.
161. Dart AB, Sellers EA, Martens PJ, et al. High burden of kidney disease in youth-onset type 2 diabetes. *Diabetes Care* 2012;35:1265–1271.
162. Caramori ML, Parks A, Mauer M. Renal lesions predict progression of diabetic nephropathy in type 1 diabetes. *J Am Soc Nephrol* 2013;24:1175–1181.
163. Afkarian M. Diabetic kidney disease in children and adolescents. *Pediatr Nephrol* 2015;30:65–74.
164. Mazzucco G, Bertani T, Fortunato M, et al. Different patterns of renal damage in type 2 diabetes mellitus: a multicentric study on 393 biopsies. *Am J Kidney Dis* 2002;39:713–720.
165. Setty S, Michael AA, Fish AJ, et al. Differential expression of laminin isoforms in diabetic nephropathy and other renal diseases. *Mod Pathol* 2012;25:859–868.
166. Rheault MN. Nephrotic and nephritic syndrome in the newborn. *Clin Perinatol* 2014;41:605–618.
167. Machuca E, Benoit G, Nevo F, et al. Genotype-phenotype correlations in non-Finnish congenital nephrotic syndrome. *J Am Soc Nephrol* 2010;21:1209–1217.
168. Hinkes BG, Mucha B, Vlangos CN, et al. Nephrotic syndrome in the first year of life: two thirds of cases are caused by mutations in 4 genes (NPHS1, NPHS2, WT1, and LAMB2). *Pediatrics* 2007;119:e907–e919.
169. Gbadegesin RA, Winn MP, Smoyer WE. Genetic testing in nephrotic syndrome—challenges and opportunities. *Nat Rev Nephrol* 2013;9:179–184.
170. Kestila M, Lenkkeri U, Mannikko M, et al. Positionally cloned gene for a novel glomerular protein–nephrin—is mutated in congenital nephrotic syndrome. *Mol Cell* 1998;1:575–582.
171. Dagan A, Cleper R, Krause I, et al. Hypothyroidism in children with steroid-resistant nephrotic syndrome. *Nephrol Dial Transplant* 2012;27:2171–2175.
172. Holmberg C, Jalanko H. Congenital nephrotic syndrome and recurrence of proteinuria after renal transplantation. *Pediatr Nephrol* 2014;29:2309–2317.
173. Bouchireb K, Boyer O, Gribouval O, et al. NPHS2 mutations in steroid-resistant nephrotic syndrome: a mutation update and the associated phenotypic spectrum. *Hum Mutat* 2014;35:178–186.
174. Mark K, Reis A, Zenker M. Prenatal findings in four consecutive pregnancies with fetal Pierson syndrome, a newly defined congenital nephrosis syndrome. *Prenat Diagn* 2006;26:262–266.
175. Niaudet P, Gubler MC. WT1 and glomerular diseases. *Pediatr Nephrol* 2006;21:1653–1660.
176. Habib R, Loirat C, Gubler MC, et al. The nephropathy associated with male pseudohermaphroditism and Wilms' tumor (Drash syndrome): a distinctive glomerular lesion—report of 10 cases. *Clin Nephrol* 1985;24:269–278.
177. Lipska BS, Ranchin B, Iatropoulos P, et al. Genotype-phenotype associations in WT1 glomerulopathy. *Kidney Int* 2014;85:1169–1178.
178. Cohen AH. Collagen type III glomerulopathies. *Adv Chronic Kidney Dis* 2012;19:101–106.
179. Marini M, Bocciardi R, Gimelli S, et al. A spectrum of LMX1B mutations in Nail-Patella syndrome: new point mutations, deletion, and evidence of mosaicism in unaffected parents. *Genet Med* 2010;12:431–439.
180. Witzgall R. How are podocytes affected in nail-patella syndrome? *Pediatr Nephrol* 2008;23:1017–1020.
181. Boyer O, Woerner S, Yang F, et al. LMX1B mutations cause hereditary FSGS without extrarenal involvement. *J Am Soc Nephrol* 2013;24:1216–1222.
182. Matejas V, Hinkes B, Alkandari F, et al. Mutations in the human laminin beta2 (LAMB2) gene and the associated phenotypic spectrum. *Hum Mutat* 2010;31:992–1002.
183. Kashtan CE, Segal Y. Genetic disorders of glomerular basement membranes. *Nephron Clin Pract* 2011;118:c9–c18.
184. Lee JH, Choi HW, Lee YJ, et al. Causes and outcomes of asymptomatic gross haematuria in children. *Nephrology (Carlton)* 2014;19:101–106.
185. Berger J, Hinglais N. [Intercapillary deposits of IgA-IgG]. *J Urol Nephrol (Paris)* 1968;74:694–695.
186. Wyatt RJ, Julian BA. IgA nephropathy. *N Engl J Med* 2014;368:2402–2414.
187. Haas M. IgA nephropathy and IgA vasculitis (Henoch-Schonlein Purpura) nephritis. In: Jennette JC, Olson JL, Silve FG, et al. eds. *Heptinstall's Pathology of the Kidney*. Philadelphia, PA: Wolters Kluwer; 2015:463–523.
188. Canetta PA, Kiryluk K, Appel GB. Glomerular diseases: emerging tests and therapies for IgA nephropathy. *Clin J Am Soc Nephrol* 2014;9:617–625.
189. Szeto CC, Li PK. MicroRNAs in IgA nephropathy. *Nat Rev Nephrol* 2014;10:249–256.
190. Roberts IS. Pathology of IgA nephropathy. *Nat Rev Nephrol* 2014;10:445–454.
191. Vogler C, Eliason SC, Wood EG. Glomerular membranopathy in children with IgA nephropathy and Henoch Schonlein purpura. *Pediatr Dev Pathol* 1999;2:227–235.
192. Cattran DC, Coppo R, Cook HT, et al. The Oxford classification of IgA nephropathy: rationale, clinicopathological correlations, and classification. *Kidney Int* 2009;76:534–545.
193. Edstrom Halling S, Soderberg MP, Berg UB. Predictors of outcome in paediatric IgA nephropathy with regard to clinical and histopathological variables (Oxford classification). *Nephrol Dial Transplant* 2012;27:715–722.

194. Shima Y, Nakanishi K, Hama T, et al. Validity of the Oxford classification of IgA nephropathy in children. *Pediatr Nephrol* 2012;27:783–792.
195. Jennette JC, Falk RJ, Bacon PA, et al. 2012 revised International Chapel Hill Consensus Conference nomenclature of vasculitides. *Arthritis Rheum* 2013;65:1–11.
196. Ozen S, Pistorio A, Iusan SM, et al. EULAR/PRINTO/PRES criteria for Henoch-Schonlein purpura, childhood polyarteritis nodosa, childhood Wegener granulomatosis and childhood Takayasu arteritis: Ankara 2008. Part II: Final classification criteria. *Ann Rheum Dis* 2010;69:798–806.
197. Brogan P, Eleftheriou D, Dillon M. Small vessel vasculitis. *Pediatr Nephrol* 2010;25:1025–1035.
198. Micheletti RG, Werth VP. Small vessel vasculitis of the Skin. *Rheum Dis Clin North Am* 2015;41:21–32.
199. Kruegel J, Rubel D, Gross O. Alport syndrome—insights from basic and clinical research. *Nat Rev Nephrol* 2013;9:170–178.
200. Hudson BG, Tryggvason K, Sundaramoorthy M, et al. Alport's syndrome, Goodpasture's syndrome, and type IV collagen. *N Engl J Med* 2003;348:2543–2556.
201. Hanson H, Storey H, Pagan J, et al. The value of clinical criteria in identifying patients with X-linked Alport syndrome. *Clin J Am Soc Nephrol* 2011;6:198–203.
202. Han KH, Lee H, Kang HG, et al. Renal manifestations of patients with MYH9-related disorders. *Pediatr Nephrol* 2011;26:549–555.
203. Bekheirnia MR, Reed B, Gregory MC, et al. Genotype-phenotype correlation in X-linked Alport syndrome. *J Am Soc Nephrol* 2010;21:876–883.
204. Tan R, Colville D, Wang YY, et al. Alport retinopathy results from "severe" COL4A5 mutations and predicts early renal failure. *Clin J Am Soc Nephrol* 2010;5:34–38.
205. Wang Y, Sivakumar V, Mohammad M, et al. Clinical and genetic features in autosomal recessive and X-linked Alport syndrome. *Pediatr Nephrol* 2014;29:391–396.
206. Rheault MN. Women and Alport syndrome. *Pediatr Nephrol* 2012;27:41–46.
207. Rheault MN, Kren SM, Hartich LA, et al. X-inactivation modifies disease severity in female carriers of murine X-linked Alport syndrome. *Nephrol Dial Transplant* 2010;25:764–769.
208. Storey H, Savige J, Sivakumar V, et al. COL4A3/COL4A4 mutations and features in individuals with autosomal recessive Alport syndrome. *J Am Soc Nephrol* 2013;24:1945–1954.
209. Moriniere V, Dahan K, Hilbert P, et al. Improving mutation screening in familial hematuric nephropathies through next generation sequencing. *J Am Soc Nephrol* 2014;25:2740–2751.
210. Heidet L, Gubler MC. The renal lesions of Alport syndrome. *J Am Soc Nephrol* 2009;20:1210–1215.
211. Vivante A, Calderon-Margalit R, Skorecki K. Hematuria and risk for end-stage kidney disease. *Curr Opin Nephrol Hypertens* 2013;22:325–330.
212. Rana K, Wang YY, Powell H, et al. Persistent familial hematuria in children and the locus for thin basement membrane nephropathy. *Pediatr Nephrol* 2005;20:1729–1737.
213. Haas M. Thin glomerular basement membrane nephropathy: incidence in 3471 consecutive renal biopsies examined by electron microscopy. *Arch Pathol Lab Med* 2006;130:699–706.
214. Malone AF, Phelan PJ, Hall G, et al. Rare hereditary COL4A3/COL4A4 variants may be mistaken for familial focal segmental glomerulosclerosis. *Kidney Int* 2014;86:1253–1259.
215. Szeto CC, Mac-Moune Lai F, Kwan BC, et al. The width of the basement membrane does not influence clinical presentation or outcome of thin glomerular basement membrane disease with persistent hematuria. *Kidney Int* 2010;78:1041–1046.
216. Dube GK, Hamilton SE, Ratner LE, et al. Loin pain hematuria syndrome. *Kidney Int* 2006;70:2152–2155.
217. Coffman KL. Loin pain hematuria syndrome: a psychiatric and surgical conundrum. *Curr Opin Organ Transplant* 2009;14:186–190.
218. Taba Taba Vakili S, Alam T, Sollinger H. Loin pain hematuria syndrome. *Am J Kidney Dis* 2014;64:460–472.
219. Eison TM, Ault BH, Jones DP, et al. Post-streptococcal acute glomerulonephritis in children: clinical features and pathogenesis. *Pediatr Nephrol* 2011;26:165–180.
220. Stratta P, Musetti C, Barreca A, et al. New trends of an old disease: the acute post infectious glomerulonephritis at the beginning of the new millenium. *J Nephrol* 2014;27:229–239.
221. Nasr SH, Radhakrishnan J, D'Agati VD. Bacterial infection-related glomerulonephritis in adults. *Kidney Int* 2013;83:792–803.
222. Haas M. Incidental healed postinfectious glomerulonephritis: a study of 1012 renal biopsy specimens examined by electron microscopy. *Hum Pathol* 2003;34:3–10.
223. Wong W, Morris MC, Zwi J. Outcome of severe acute post-streptococcal glomerulonephritis in New Zealand children. *Pediatr Nephrol* 2009;24:1021–1026.
224. Sethi S, Fervenza FC, Zhang Y, et al. Atypical postinfectious glomerulonephritis is associated with abnormalities in the alternative pathway of complement. *Kidney Int* 2012;83:293–299.
225. Kawamura T, Usui J, Kaseda K, et al. Primary membranoproliferative glomerulonephritis on the decline: decreased rate from the 1970s to the 2000s in Japan. *Clin Exp Nephrol* 2013;17:248–254.
226. Licht C, Schlotzer-Schrehardt U, Kirschfink M, et al. MPGN II—genetically determined by defective complement regulation? *Pediatr Nephrol* 2007;22:2–9.
227. Cook HT, Pickering MC. Histopathology of MPGN and C3 glomerulopathies. *Nat Rev Nephrol* 2015;11:14–22.
228. Sethi S, Fervenza FC. Membranoproliferative glomerulonephritis: pathogenetic heterogeneity and proposal for a new classification. *Semin Nephrol* 2011;31:341–348.
229. Fakhouri F, Fremeaux-Bacchi V, Noel LH, et al. C3 glomerulopathy: a new classification. *Nat Rev Nephrol* 2010;6:494–499.
230. Nicolas C, Vuiblet V, Baudouin V, et al. C3 nephritic factor associated with C3 glomerulopathy in children. *Pediatr Nephrol* 2014;29:85–94.
231. Medjeral-Thomas NR, O'Shaughnessy MM, O'Regan JA, et al. C3 glomerulopathy: clinicopathologic features and predictors of outcome. *Clin J Am Soc Nephrol* 2014;9:46–53.
232. Hou J, Markowitz GS, Bomback AS, et al. Toward a working definition of C3 glomerulopathy by immunofluorescence. *Kidney Int* 2013;85:450–456.
233. Pickering MC, D'Agati VD, Nester CM, et al. C3 glomerulopathy: consensus report. *Kidney Int* 2013;84:1079–1089.
234. Sethi S, Fervenza FC. Membranoproliferative glomerulonephritis—a new look at an old entity. *N Engl J Med* 2012;366:1119–1131.
235. Bomback AS. Eculizumab in the treatment of membranoproliferative glomerulonephritis. *Nephron Clin Pract* 2014;128:270–276.
236. Vivarelli M, Emma F. Treatment of C3 glomerulopathy with complement blockers. *Semin Thromb Hemost* 2014;40:472–477.
237. Malattia C, Martini A. Paediatric-onset systemic lupus erythematosus. *Best Pract Res Clin Rheumatol* 2013;27:351–362.
238. Vachvanichsanong P, McNeil E. Pediatric lupus nephritis: more options, more chances? *Lupus* 2013;22:545–553.
239. Barsalou J, Levy DM, Silverman ED. An update on childhood-onset systemic lupus erythematosus. *Curr Opin Rheumatol* 2013;25:616–622.
240. Sestak AL, Nath SK, Kelly JA, et al. Patients with familial and sporadic onset SLE have similar clinical profiles but vary profoundly by race. *Lupus* 2008;17:1004–1009.
241. Weening JJ, D'Agati VD, Schwartz MM, et al. The classification of glomerulonephritis in systemic lupus erythematosus revisited. *Kidney Int* 2004;65:521–530.
242. Haas M, Rastaldi MP, Fervenza FC. Histologic classification of glomerular diseases: clinicopathologic correlations, limitations exposed by validation studies, and suggestions for modification. *Kidney Int* 2013;85:779–793.
243. Marks SD, Sebire NJ, Pilkington C, et al. Clinicopathological correlations of paediatric lupus nephritis. *Pediatr Nephrol* 2007;22:77–83.
244. Jennette JC. Rapidly progressive crescentic glomerulonephritis. *Kidney Int* 2003;63:1164–1177.

245. Dewan D, Gulati S, Sharma RK, et al. Clinical spectrum and outcome of crescentic glomerulonephritis in children in developing countries. *Pediatr Nephrol* 2008;23:389–394.
246. Goodpasture EW. The significance of certain pulmonary lesions in relation to the etiology of influenza. *Am J Med Sci* 1919;158:863–870.
247. Singh SK, Jeansson M, Quaggin SE. New insights into the pathogenesis of cellular crescents. *Curr Opin Nephrol Hypertens* 2011;20:258–262.
248. Farris AB, Alpers CE. What is the best way to measure renal fibrosis? A pathologist's perspective. *Kidney Int Suppl* 2014;4:9–15.
249. Zoja C, Abbate M, Remuzzi G. Progression of renal injury toward interstitial inflammation and glomerular sclerosis is dependent on abnormal protein filtration. *Nephrol Dial Transplant* 2015;30:706–712.
250. Ricci Z, Cruz DN, Ronco C. Classification and staging of acute kidney injury: beyond the RIFLE and AKIN criteria. *Nat Rev Nephrol* 2011;7:201–208.
251. Rewa O, Bagshaw SM. Acute kidney injury-epidemiology, outcomes and economics. *Nat Rev Nephrol* 2014;10:193–207.
252. Patzer L. Nephrotoxicity as a cause of acute kidney injury in children. *Pediatr Nephrol* 2008;23:2159–2173.
253. Ulinski T, Sellier-Leclerc AL, Tudorache E, et al. Acute tubulointerstitial nephritis. *Pediatr Nephrol* 2012;27:1051–1057.
254. Praga M, Sevillano A, Aunon P, et al. Changes in the aetiology, clinical presentation and management of acute interstitial nephritis, an increasingly common cause of acute kidney injury. *Nephrol Dial Transplant* 2014 (epub ahead of print).
255. Praga M, Gonzalez E. Acute interstitial nephritis. *Kidney Int* 2010;77:956–961.
256. Tanaka T, Nangaku M. Pathogenesis of tubular interstitial nephritis. *Contrib Nephrol* 2011;169:297–310.
257. Ragnarsdottir B, Svanborg C. Susceptibility to acute pyelonephritis or asymptomatic bacteriuria: host-pathogen interaction in urinary tract infections. *Pediatr Nephrol* 2012;27:2017–2029.
258. Montini G, Tullus K, Hewitt I. Febrile urinary tract infections in children. *N Engl J Med* 2011;365:239–250.
259. Paintsil E. Update on recent guidelines for the management of urinary tract infections in children: the shifting paradigm. *Curr Opin Pediatr* 2013;25:88–94.
260. Koyle MA, Shifrin D. Issues in febrile urinary tract infection management. *Pediatr Clin North Am* 2012;59:909–922.
261. Li L, Parwani AV. Xanthogranulomatous pyelonephritis. *Arch Pathol Lab Med* 2011;135:671–674.
262. Shah A, Chandran H. Malakoplakia of bladder in childhood. *Pediatr Surg Int* 2005;21:113–115.
263. Yigiter M, Ilgici D, Celik M, et al. Renal parenchymal malacoplakia: a different stage of xanthogranulomatous pyelonephritis? *J Pediatr Surg* 2007;42:E35–E38.
264. Perazella MA, Markowitz GS. Drug-induced acute interstitial nephritis. *Nat Rev Nephrol* 2010;6:461–470.
265. Airy M, Raghavan R, Truong LD, et al. Tubulointerstitial nephritis and cancer chemotherapy: update on a neglected clinical entity. *Nephrol Dial Transplant* 2013;28:2502–2509.
266. Colvin RB, Traum AZ, Taheri D, et al. Granulomatous interstitial nephritis as a manifestation of Crohn disease. *Arch Pathol Lab Med* 2014;138:125–127.
267. Tong JE, Howell DN, Foreman JW. Drug-induced granulomatous interstitial nephritis in a pediatric patient. *Pediatr Nephrol* 2007;22:306–309.
268. Mandeville JT, Levinson RD, Holland GN. The tubulointerstitial nephritis and uveitis syndrome. *Surv Ophthalmol* 2001;46:195–208.
269. Saarela V, Nuutinen M, Ala-Houhala M, et al. Tubulointerstitial nephritis and uveitis syndrome in children: a prospective multicenter study. *Ophthalmology* 2013;120:1476–1481.
270. Tan Y, Yu F, Qu Z, et al. Modified C-reactive protein might be a target autoantigen of TINU syndrome. *Clin J Am Soc Nephrol* 2011;6:93–100.
271. Perasaari J, Saarela V, Nikkila J, et al. HLA associations with tubulointerstitial nephritis with or without uveitis in Finnish pediatric population: a nation-wide study. *Tissue Antigens* 2013;81:435–441.
272. George JN, Nester CM. Syndromes of thrombotic microangiopathy. *N Engl J Med* 2014;371:654–666.
273. Chapman K, Seldon M, Richards R. Thrombotic microangiopathies, thrombotic thrombocytopenic purpura, and ADAMTS-13. *Semin Thromb Hemost* 2012;38:47–54.
274. Loirat C, Coppo P, Veyradier A. Thrombotic thrombocytopenic purpura in children. *Curr Opin Pediatr* 2013;25:216–224.
275. Scheiring J, Rosales A, Zimmerhackl LB. Clinical practice. Today's understanding of the haemolytic uraemic syndrome. *Eur J Pediatr* 2010;169:7–13.
276. Scheiring J, Andreoli SP, Zimmerhackl LB. Treatment and outcome of Shiga-toxin-associated hemolytic uremic syndrome (HUS). *Pediatr Nephrol* 2008;23:1749–1760.
277. Spinale JM, Ruebner RL, Copelovitch L, et al. Long-term outcomes of Shiga toxin hemolytic uremic syndrome. *Pediatr Nephrol* 2013;28:2097–2105.
278. Porubsky S, Federico G, Muthing J, et al. Direct acute tubular damage contributes to Shigatoxin-mediated kidney failure. *J Pathol* 2014;234:120–133.
279. Deshmukh AB, Patel JK, Prajapati AR, et al. Perspective in chronic kidney disease: targeting hypoxia-inducible factor (HIF) as potential therapeutic approach. *Ren Fail* 2012;34:521–532.
280. Meri S. Complement activation in diseases presenting with thrombotic microangiopathy. *Eur J Intern Med* 2013;24:496–502.
281. Loirat C, Fremeaux-Bacchi V. Hemolytic uremic syndrome recurrence after renal transplantation. *Pediatr Transplant* 2008;12:619–629.
282. Dillon MJ, Eleftheriou D, Brogan PA. Medium-size-vessel vasculitis. *Pediatr Nephrol* 2010;25:1641–1652.
283. Vanoni F, Bettinelli A, Keller F, et al. Vasculitides associated with IgG antineutrophil cytoplasmic autoantibodies in childhood. *Pediatr Nephrol* 2010;25:205–212.
284. Furuta S, Jayne DR. Antineutrophil cytoplasm antibody-associated vasculitis: recent developments. *Kidney Int* 2013;84:244–249.
285. Bansal PJ, Tobin MC. Neonatal microscopic polyangiitis secondary to transfer of maternal myeloperoxidase-antineutrophil cytoplasmic antibody resulting in neonatal pulmonary hemorrhage and renal involvement. *Ann Allergy Asthma Immunol* 2004;93:398–401.
286. Silva F, Specks U, Sethi S, et al. Successful pregnancy and delivery of a healthy newborn despite transplacental transfer of antimyeloperoxidase antibodies from a mother with microscopic polyangiitis. *Am J Kidney Dis* 2009;54:542–545.
287. Kerlin BA, Ayoob R, Smoyer WE. Epidemiology and pathophysiology of nephrotic syndrome-associated thromboembolic disease. *Clin J Am Soc Nephrol* 2012;7:513–520.
288. Crespo-Solis E. Thrombosis and acute leukemia. *Hematology* 2012;17(Suppl 1):S169–S173.
289. Brandao LR, Simpson EA, Lau KK. Neonatal renal vein thrombosis. *Semin Fetal Neonatal Med* 2011;16:323–328.
290. He Y, Wu Z, Chen S, et al. Nutcracker syndrome—how well do we know it? *Urology* 2014;83:12–17.
291. Persu A, Touze E, Mousseaux E, et al. Diagnosis and management of fibromuscular dysplasia: an expert consensus. *Eur J Clin Invest* 2012;42:338–347.
292. Park HS, Do YS, Park KB, et al. Long term results of endovascular treatment in renal arterial stenosis from Takayasu arteritis: angioplasty versus stent placement. *Eur J Radiol* 2013;82:1913–1918.
293. Duan L, Feng K, Tong A, et al. Renal artery stenosis due to neurofibromatosis type 1: case report and literature review. *Eur J Med Res* 2014;19:17.
294. Bouchireb K, Boyer O, Bonnet D, et al. Clinical features and management of arterial hypertension in children with Williams-Beuren syndrome. *Nephrol Dial Transplant* 2010;25:434–438.
295. Salem JE, Bruguiere E, Iserin L, et al. Hypertension and aortorenal disease in Alagille syndrome. *J Hypertens* 2012;30:1300–1306.
296. Demirel N, Aydin M, Zenciroglu A, et al. Neonatal thrombo-embolism: risk factors, clinical features and outcome. *Ann Trop Paediatr* 2009;29:271–279.

297. Unal S, Arhan E, Kara N, et al. Breast-feeding-associated hypernatremia: retrospective analysis of 169 term newborns. *Pediatr Int* 2008;50:29–34.

298. Srinivasan A, Krishnamurthy G, Fontalvo-Herazo L, et al. Spectrum of renal findings in pediatric fibromuscular dysplasia and neurofibromatosis type 1. *Pediatr Radiol* 2011;41:308–316.

299. Broadis E, Barbour L, O'Toole S, et al. Bilateral ureteric obstruction secondary to renal papillary necrosis. *Pediatr Surg Int* 2010;26: 867–869.

300. Gordon M, Cervellione RM, Postlethwaite R, et al. Acute renal papillary necrosis with complete bilateral ureteral obstruction in a child. *Urology* 2007;69:575 e11–575 e12.

301. Bolling T, Ernst I, Pape H, et al. Dose-volume analysis of radiation nephropathy in children: preliminary report of the risk consortium. *Int J Radiat Oncol Biol Phys* 2011;80:840–844.

302. Shaer AJ. Inherited primary renal tubular hypokalemic alkalosis: a review of Gitelman and Bartter syndromes. *Am J Med Sci* 2001; 322:316–332.

303. Perlman EJ. Pediatric renal tumors: practical updates for the pathologist. *Pediatr Dev Pathol* 2005;8(3):320–338.

304. Perlman EJ. Tumors of the kidney, bladder, and related urinary structures. In: Murphy WM, Grignon DJ, Perlman EJ, eds. *AFIP Atlas of Tumor Pathology*. Washington, DC: American Registry of Pathology; 2004:10–90.

305. Huang CC, Cutcliffe C, Coffin C, et al. Classification of malignant pediatric renal tumors by gene expression. *Pediatr Blood Cancer* 2006;46(7):728–738.

306. Guertl B, Leuschner I, Harms D, et al. Genetic clonality is a feature unifying nephroblastomas regardless of the variety of morphological subtypes. *Virchows Arch* 2006;449(2):171–174.

307. Yang L, Han Y, Suarez Saiz F, et al. A tumor suppressor and oncogene: the WT1 story. *Leukemia* 2007;21(5):868–876.

308. Morrison AA, Viney RL, Ladomery MR. The post-transcriptional roles of WT1, a multifunctional zinc-finger protein. *Biochim Biophys Acta* 2008;1785(1):55–62.

309. Ehrlich PF. Wilms tumor: progress and considerations for the surgeon. *Surg Oncol* 2007;16(3):157–171.

310. Varan A. Wilms' tumor in children: an overview. *Nephron Clin Pract* 2008;108(2):c83–c90.

311. Rivera MN, Haber DA. Wilms' tumour: connecting tumorigenesis and organ development in the kidney. *Nat Rev Cancer* 2005;5(9):699–712.

312. Rivera MN, Kim WJ, Wells J, et al. An X chromosome gene, WTX, is commonly inactivated in Wilms tumor. *Science* 2007;315(5812):642–645.

313. Ruteshouser EC, Robinson SM, Huff V. Wilms tumor genetics: mutations in WT1, WTX, and CTNNB1 account for only about one-third of tumors. *Genes Chromosomes Cancer* 2008;47(6):461–470.

314. Huff V. Wilms' tumours: about tumour suppressor genes, an oncogene and a chameleon gene. *Nat Rev Cancer* 2011;11(2):111–121. doi: 10.1038/nrc3002.

315. Major MB, Camp ND, Berndt JD, et al. Wilms tumor suppressor WTX negatively regulates WNT/beta-catenin signaling. *Science* 2007;316(5827):1043–1046.

316. Nusse R. Cancer. Converging on beta-catenin in Wilms tumor. *Science* 2007;316(5827):988–989.

317. Peres EM, Savasan S, Cushing B, et al. Chromosome analyses of 16 cases of Wilms tumor: different pattern in unfavorable histology. *Cancer Genet Cytogenet* 2004;148(1):66–70.

318. Hill DA, Shear TD, Liu T, et al. Clinical and biologic significance of nuclear unrest in Wilms tumor. *Cancer* 2003;97(9):2318–2326.

319. Sparago A, Russo S, Cerrato F, et al. Mechanisms causing imprinting defects in familial Beckwith-Wiedemann syndrome with Wilms' tumour. *Hum Mol Genet* 2007;16(3):254–264.

320. Grundy PE, Breslow NE, Li S, et al. Loss of heterozygosity for chromosomes 1p and 16q is an adverse prognostic factor in favorable-histology Wilms tumor: a report from the National Wilms Tumor Study Group. *J Clin Oncol* 2005;23(29):7312–7321.

321. Hamilton TE, Shamberger RC. Wilms tumor: recent advances in clinical care and biology. *Semin Pediatr Surg* 2012;21(1):15–20. doi: 10.1053/j.sempedsurg.2011.10.002.

322. Murphy AJ, Pierce J, de Caestecker C, et al. Aberrant activation, nuclear localization, and phosphorylation of Yes-associated protein-1 in the embryonic kidney and Wilms tumor. *Pediatr Blood Cancer* 2014;61(2):198–205. doi: 10.1002/pbc.24788.

323. Shamberger RC, Haase GM, Argani P, et al. Bilateral Wilms' tumors with progressive or nonresponsive disease. *J Pediatr Surg* 2006;41(4):652–657; discussion 652–657.

324. Doros LA, Rossi CT, Yang J, et al. DICER1 mutations in childhood cystic nephroma and its relationship to DICER1-renal sarcoma. *Mod Pathol* 2014;27(9):1267–1280. doi: 10.1038/modpathol.2013.242.

325. Luithle T, Szavay P, Furtwangler R, et al. Treatment of cystic nephroma and cystic partially differentiated nephroblastoma—a report from the SIOP/GPOH study group. *J Urol* 2007;177(1):294–296.

326. Beckwith JB. Management of incidentally encountered nephrogenic rests. *J Pediatr Hematol Oncol* 2007;29(6):353–354.

327. Breslow NE, Beckwith JB, Perlman EJ, et al. Age distributions, birth weights, nephrogenic rests, and heterogeneity in the pathogenesis of Wilms tumor. *Pediatr Blood Cancer* 2006;47(3):260–267.

328. Fukuzawa R, Reeve AE. Molecular pathology and epidemiology of nephrogenic rests and Wilms tumors. *J Pediatr Hematol Oncol* 2007;29(9):589–594.

329. Gadd S, Beezhold P, Jennings L, et al. Mediators of receptor tyrosine kinase activation in infantile fibrosarcoma: a Children's Oncology Group study. *J Pathol* 2012;228(1):119–130. doi: 10.1002/path.4010.

330. Furtwaengler R, Reinhard H, Leuschner I, et al. Mesoblastic nephroma—a report from the Gesellschaft fur Padiatrische Onkologie und Hamatologie (GPOH). *Cancer* 2006;106(10):2275–2283.

331. Argani P, Perlman EJ, Breslow NE, et al. Clear cell sarcoma of the kidney: a review of 351 cases from the National Wilms Tumor Study Group Pathology Center. *Am J Surg Pathol* 2000;24(1):4–18.

332. Furtwängler R, Gooskens SL, van Tinteren H, et al. Clear cell sarcomas of the kidney registered on International Society of Pediatric Oncology (SIOP) 93-01 and SIOP 2001 protocols: a report of the SIOP Renal Tumour Study Group. *Eur J Cancer* 2013;49(16):3497–3506. doi: 10.1016/j.ejca.2013.06.036.

333. Agaimy A. The expanding family of SMARCB1(INI1)-deficient neoplasia: implications of phenotypic, biological, and molecular heterogeneity. *Adv Anat Pathol* 2014;21(6):394–410. doi: 10.1097/PAP.0000000000000038.

334. Tan PH, Cheng L, Rioux-Leclercq N, et al; ISUP Renal Tumor Panel. Renal tumors: diagnostic and prognostic biomarkers. *Am J Surg Pathol* 2013;37(10):1518–1531. doi: 10.1097/PAS.0b013e318299f12e.

335. Smith NE, Deyrup AT, Mariño-Enriquez A, et al. VCL-ALK renal cell carcinoma in children with sickle-cell trait: the eighth sickle-cell nephropathy? *Am J Surg Pathol* 2014;38(6):858–863. doi: 10.1097/PAS.0000000000000179.

336. Siomou E, Papadopoulou F, Kollios KD, et al. Duplex collecting system diagnosed during the first 6 years of life after a first urinary tract infection: a study of 63 children. *J Urol* 2006;175(2):678–681; discussion 681–672.

337. Piaggio L, Franc-Guimond J, Figueroa TE, et al. Comparison of laparoscopic and open partial nephrectomy for duplication anomalies in children. *J Urol* 2006;175(6):2269–2273.

338. Nakai H, Asanuma H, Shishido S, et al. Changing concepts in urological management of the congenital anomalies of kidney and urinary tract, CAKUT. *Pediatr Int* 2003;45(5):634–641.

339. Direnna T, Leonard MP. Watchful waiting for prenatally detected ureteroceles. *J Urol* 2006;175(4):1493–1495; discussion 1495.

340. Pontincasa P, Bartoli F, Di Ciaula A, et al. Defective in vitro contractility of ureteropelvic junction in children with functional and obstructive urine flow impairment. *J Pediatr Surg* 2006;41(9):1594–1597.

341. Murawski IJ, Gupta IR. Vesicoureteric reflux and renal malformations: a developmental problem. *Clin Genet* 2006;69(2):105–117.

342. Nelson CP, Dunn RL, Wei JT, et al. Surgical repair of bladder exstrophy in the modern era: contemporary practice patterns and the role of hospital case volume. *J Urol* 2005;174(3):1099–1102.
343. Sadler TW(editor). Urogenital system. In: *Langman's Medical Embryology*, 10th ed. Philadelphia, PA: Lippincott Williams & Wilkins; 2006:229–239.
344. Becker A, Baum M. Obstructive uropathy. *Early Hum Dev* 2006;82(1):15–22.
345. Rodriguez MM. Congenital anomalies of the kidney and the urinary tract (CAKUT). *Fetal Pediatr Pathol* 2014;33(5–6):293–320. doi: 10.3109/15513815.2014.959678.
346. Puri P, Shinkai M. Megacystis microcolon intestinal hypoperistalsis syndrome. *Semin Pediatr Surg* 2005;14(1):58–63.
347. Wangler MF, Gonzaga-Jauregui C, Gambin T, et al; Baylor-Hopkins Center for Mendelian Genomics. Heterozygous de novo and inherited mutations in the smooth muscle actin (ACTG2) gene underlie megacystis-microcolon-intestinal hypoperistalsis syndrome. *PLoS Genet* 2014;10(3):e1004258. doi: 10.1371/journal.pgen.1004258.
348. Ronald A. The etiology of urinary tract infection: traditional and emerging pathogens. *Am J Med* 2002;113(Suppl 1A):14S–19S.
349. Novak TE, Lakshmanan Y, Frimberger D, et al. Polyps in the exstrophic bladder. A cause for concern? *J Urol* 2005;174(4 pt 2):1522–1526; discussion 1526.
350. Al-Ahmadie H, Gomez AM, Trane N, et al. Giant botryoid fibroepithelial polyp of bladder with myofibroblastic stroma and cystitis cystica et glandularis. *Pediatr Dev Pathol* 2003;6(2):179–181.
351. Newsome G. Interstitial cystitis. *J Am Acad Nurse Pract* 2003;15(2):64–71.
352. Phatak S, Foster HE Jr. The management of interstitial cystitis: an update. *Nat Clin Pract Urol* 2006;3(1):45–53.
353. van den Ouden D. Diagnosis and management of eosinophilic cystitis: a pooled analysis of 135 cases. *Eur Urol* 2000;37(4):386–394.
354. Barese CN, Podesta M, Litvak E, et al. Recurrent eosinophilic cystitis in a child with chronic granulomatous disease. *J Pediatr Hematol Oncol* 2004;26(3):209–212.
355. Redman JF, Parham DM. Extensive inflammatory eosinophilic bladder tumors in children: experience with three cases. *South Med J* 2002;95(9):1050–1052.
356. Minor L, Lindgren BW. Malacoplakia of the bladder in a 16-year-old girl. *J Urol* 2003;170(2 Pt 1):568–569.
357. Weiss M, Liapis H, Tomaszewski JE, et al. Pyelonephritis and other infections, reflux nephropathy, hydronephrosis, and nephrolithiasis (chapter 22). In: Jennette JC, Olson JL, Schwartz MM, et al., eds. *Heptinstall's Pathology of the Kidney*. Philadelphia, PA: Lippincott Williams & Wilkins; 2007:991–1081.
358. Gorczynska E, Turkiewicz D, Rybka K, et al. Incidence, clinical outcome, and management of virus-induced hemorrhagic cystitis in children and adolescents after allogeneic hematopoietic cell transplantation. *Biol Blood Marrow Transplant* 2005;11(10):797–804.
359. Cheuk DK, Lee TL, Chiang AK, et al. Risk factors and treatment of hemorrhagic cystitis in children who underwent hematopoietic stem cell transplantation. *Transpl Int* 2007;20(1):73–81.
360. Isaac J, Lowichik A, Cartwright P, et al. Inverted papilloma of the urinary bladder in children: case report and review of prognostic significance and biological potential behavior. *J Pediatr Surg* 2000; 35(10):1514–1516.
361. Moyano Calvo JL, Maqueda Marin Mde L, Davalos Casanova G, et al. Bladder leiomyoma in a 17-year-old male patient. *Arch Esp Urol* 2005;58(9):954–956.
362. Naqiyah I, Rohaizak M, Meah FA, et al. Phaeochromocytoma of the urinary bladder. *Singapore Med J* 2005;46(7):344–346.
363. Vemulakonda VM, Kopp RP, Sorensen MD, et al. Recurrent nephrogenic adenoma in a 10-year-old boy with prune belly syndrome: a case presentation. *Pediatr Surg Int* 2008;24(5):605–607.
364. Xambre L, Prisco R, Carreira F, et al. Inverted papillomas—cases at our service and review of the literature. *Actas Urol Esp* 2003;27(8):605–610.
365. Mergan F, Jaubert F, Sauvat F, et al. Inflammatory myofibroblastic tumor in children: clinical review with anaplastic lymphoma kinase, Epstein-Barr virus, and human herpesvirus 8 detection analysis. *J Pediatr Surg* 2005;40(10):1581–1586.
366. Montgomery EA, Shuster DD, Burkart AL, et al. Inflammatory myofibroblastic tumors of the urinary tract: a clinicopathologic study of 46 cases, including a malignant example inflammatory fibrosarcoma and a subset associated with high-grade urothelial carcinoma. *Am J Surg Pathol* 2006;30(12):1502–1512.
367. Harik LR, Merino C, Coindre JM, et al. Pseudosarcomatous myofibroblastic proliferations of the bladder: a clinicopathologic study of 42 cases. *Am J Surg Pathol* 2006;30(7):787–794.
368. Houben CH. Pseudosarcomatous myofibroblastic proliferations of the bladder: a clinicopathologic study of 42 cases. *Am J Surg Pathol* 2007;31(4):642; author reply 642.
369. Parham DM, Ellison DA. Rhabdomyosarcomas in adults and children: an update. *Arch Pathol Lab Med* 2006;130(10):1454–1465.
370. Lott S, Lopez-Beltran A, Montironi R, et al. Soft tissue tumors of the urinary bladder Part II: malignant neoplasms. *Hum Pathol* 2007; 38(7):963–977.

CHAPTER 18

The Female Reproductive System

Michael K. Fritsch, M.D., Ph.D., and Mariana M. Cajaiba, M.D.

Abnormalities confined to the genital tract are quite unusual in prepubertal girls, and such disorders seldom come to the attention of pediatricians or pediatric pathologists. Major developmental abnormalities affecting the reproductive system are often eclipsed by concomitant urinary tract abnormalities, which are more immediately clinically significant. Abnormal gonadal development is an important group of diseases that may also result in abnormal development of secondary sexual characteristics. The most frequent acquired diseases of the female genital tract are infections and neoplasms. Infections confined to the female reproductive tract are seldom life threatening in childhood, yet they may result in reproductive sequelae during adulthood. Neoplasms are dominated by those arising from germ cells.

ANATOMY AND EMBRYOLOGY

The female reproductive tract consists of the gonads, a ductal system (fallopian tubes, uterus, cervix, vagina), and the external genitalia (clitoris, labia majora, labia minora, vestibule, mons pubis). The process of sexual differentiation can be divided into various phases. Chromosomal (genetic) sex is determined by the XY or XX genotype, with the potential for abnormal deletion or addition of sex chromosomal material such as in Turner (45,X) and Klinefelter syndromes (47,XXY). Gonadal sex refers to gonadal differentiation into testis or ovary and is predominantly dependent on the expression of the sex-determining region on Y gene (SRY). SRY begins a cascade of molecular signals, resulting in male gonadal differentiation; the inhibition of these male-specific signals and the presence of several female-specific molecular signals result in female gonad differentiation. Phenotypic sex refers to the differentiation of the ductal system and of the external genitalia, a process that is regulated by production of the antimüllerian hormone (AMH) by the Sertoli cells of the testis and steroid hormone production by the testis (testosterone/dihydrotestosterone) and the ovary (estrogen/progesterone). Lastly, the assigned or adopted sex is usually determined by the chromosomal, gonadal, and phenotypic sex at birth but may be altered postnatally in a variety of *disorders of sex development* (DSD, see below). These processes occur predominantly *in utero*, with the final phenotypic changes being initiated by the onset of puberty. Previously, it was thought that sex determination involved the initiation of molecular and cellular events leading to male gonad development and that if this pathway failed, there was a default to a female gonadal phenotype. We now know that there are specific male and female molecular pathways that are needed to initiate, complete, and maintain the respective sex phenotypes as well as pathways that prevent the other sex from developing. Specific alterations in these pathways during development can result in partial male and female gonads (e.g., ovotestis) and/or ambiguous genitalia.

Primordial Germ Cells

The primordial germ cells (PGCs) first appear in the wall of the yolk sac at about 3 to 4 weeks after fertilization and migrate through the hindgut and mesonephric ridge to the genital ridge beginning about week 4 to 5, a process mediated by a number of molecular factors (1–4). Germ cells that do not reach the genital ridge are thought to undergo apoptosis, but they have also been proposed as the cell of origin of extragonadal germ cell tumors. PGCs are bipotential, and complete differentiation into oogonia or prospermatogonia depends upon the local environment. The initial events in testicular and ovarian differentiation are independent of the presence or genotype of PGCs in the gonad. However, completion of appropriate ovarian development depends upon the presence of meiotic germ cells. In the absence of meiotic germ cells, the ovarian structure degenerates leaving streak ovaries (5,6). Germ cell sexual dimorphism begins at about 11 to 12 weeks of gestation. Male PGCs (prospermatogonia) enter mitotic arrest, whereas ovarian PGCs (oogonia) enter the first meiotic prophase and then arrest. We now know that retinoic acid produced locally by the ovary induces PGC entry into meiosis beginning in the medulla and slowly radiating out to the cortex. Male germ cells produce the retinoic acid–degrading enzyme CYP26B1 via paracrine FGF9 signaling from male support cells to prevent entry into meiosis.

Early Gonadal Development

The gonadal ridge develops at the ventromedial aspect of the mesonephros by a proliferation of mesodermal cells and thickening of the overlying coelomic epithelium at 4 to 5 weeks' gestation. Between 4.5 and 6 weeks, the indifferent gonad is indistinguishable as male or female (Figure 18-1). A number of critical genes have been identified in regulating normal genital ridge development including SF1, WT1, LHX9, CITED2, IGF signaling, and potentially EMX2 and PBX1. In humans and mice, the Wilms tumor gene isoform WT1-KTS as well as the steroidogenic factor 1 (previously referred to as SF1 and now officially designated NR5A1) genes are important in maintaining the indifferent gonad. Mutations in SF1 can lead to adrenal–gonadal failure, mostly affecting male gonad development, as maintenance of SF1 expression is also critical in testis development. The WT-KTS isoform is required for cell survival and proliferation within the bipotential gonad in both males and females (5). WT1+KTS isoform is critical later for male development, and the ratio of +KTS/−KTS seems critical for appropriate gonadal differentiation. Mutations in WT1 are associated with three syndromes characterized by gonadal dysgenesis (Wilms tumor/aniridia/gonadal dysgenesis/retardation—WAGR [OMIM 194072], Denys-Drash [OMIM 194080], and Frasier [OMIM 136680]) (see www.omim.org or www.ncbi.nlm.nih.gov/omim). The phenotype of affected individuals includes genital and kidney defects as well as an increased risk for the development of Wilms tumors. Insulin signaling occurs via IGF1 and IGF2 and is critical for cell proliferation during early gonadal development. In the absence of proper insulin signaling, the gonads can be very small or absent. At about 7 weeks' gestation, in XY embryos, a Y-linked genetic switch, SRY, is expressed by pre-Sertoli cells (1–5). The expression of SRY is necessary and sufficient to trigger male testis development; however, both the timing and the level of SRY expression are critical for normal testis development. In an XY embryo, the lack of SRY results in ovarian development. The SRY protein contains a highly conserved DNA-binding domain that allows specific genes to be turned on or off. The primary target is SOX9, which is thought to be the key Sertoli cell differentiation factor. Both SRY and SF1 bind upstream of SOX9 to initiate transcription. Once SOX9 transcription is initiated, there is a feedforward loop whereby SOX9 itself replaces SRY and binds upstream to maintain its own transcription. SOX9 also induces FGF9, which stimulates more SOX9 production. SOX9 is essential for production of the first male-specific cell type, the Sertoli cell. Mutation in SOX9 leads to the human dwarfism syndrome camptomelic dysplasia (OMIM 114290), which is often associated with XY sex reversal (7). Duplication of SOX9 causes XX female-to-male sex reversal. SF1 expression in the developing testis regulates expression of several male-specific genes, including AMH (see Chapter 28). It has been recently discovered that SOX9 activation results in increased prostaglandin D2 (PGD2) production, which is essential for maintenance of the testis phenotype by facilitating Sox9 transportation into the nucleus. In animal models, there are well-documented examples of both male and female maintenance factors (e.g., PGD2), which if disrupted even postnatally can result in gonadal transdifferentiation to the alternative gonad. Leydig cells are derived from mesenchymal precursors via desert hedgehog (DHH) signaling (1–4).

Ovarian Differentiation

Ovarian development is thought to be characterized by active ovarian determination pathways as well as by inhibition of testis-specific pathways. In addition, it is now clear that once established, maintenance of the ovarian phenotype occurs via FOXL2 and estrogen receptor alpha and beta signaling. The early formation of the ovary can be thought of as involving three major processes: (a) entrance of oogonia into prophase of meiosis I to form primary oocytes, (b) granulosa cells surrounding these primary oocytes to form primordial follicles, and (c) differentiation of the steroid-producing theca cells. By 6 weeks of development, primordial sex cords form. The ovary can be identified at 7 to 8 weeks' gestation by the absence of true testicular cords and possessing PGC nests. After their arrival in the gonad, germ cells in the female continue to undergo active mitotic cell division, a process that diminishingly continues into the third trimester at least in the cortex. It is estimated that approximately 3 to 4 million germ cells are present in each ovary by 20 weeks' gestation, and then the number decreases to about 0.5 to 1 million at term. The mechanism leading to the loss of oocytes remains poorly understood. At approximately 12 weeks' gestation, the first germ cells begin to enter into meiosis via retinoic acid signaling, a process first seen close to the medullary region (Figure 18-2). On entering meiosis, the primary oocyte will arrest at the diplotene stage of the first meiotic prophase and become enclosed by follicular cells to form primordial follicles. Follicular or granulosa cells are in direct contact with the germ cells and are thought to

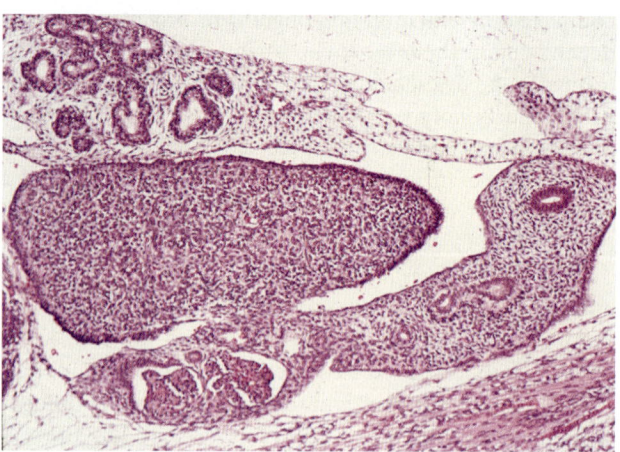

FIGURE 18-1 • The undifferentiated gonad lies adjacent to the mesonephros and the wolffian and müllerian ducts. The mesonephros has a profound effect on normal gonadal differentiation.

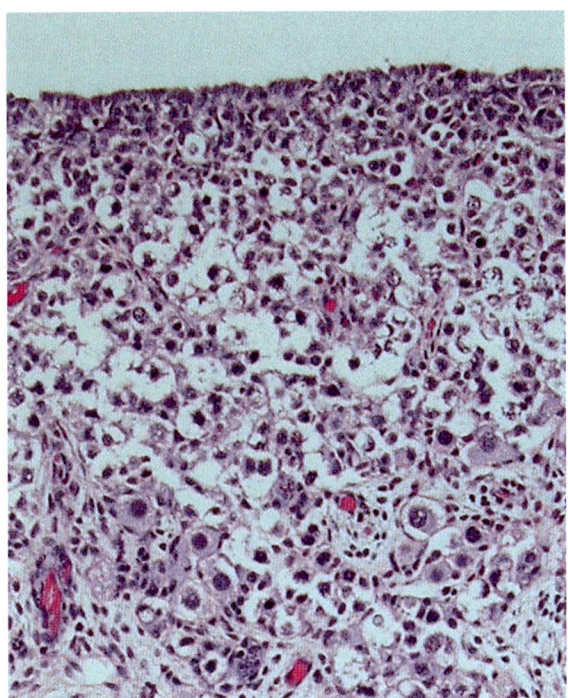

FIGURE 18-2 • Developing ovary at approximately 22 weeks' gestation showing formation of primordial follicles containing oocytes arrested in meiosis I in the deep ovarian cortex and premeiotic oogonia in the superficial cortex. Germ cell proliferation continues within the premeiotic oogonia until term.

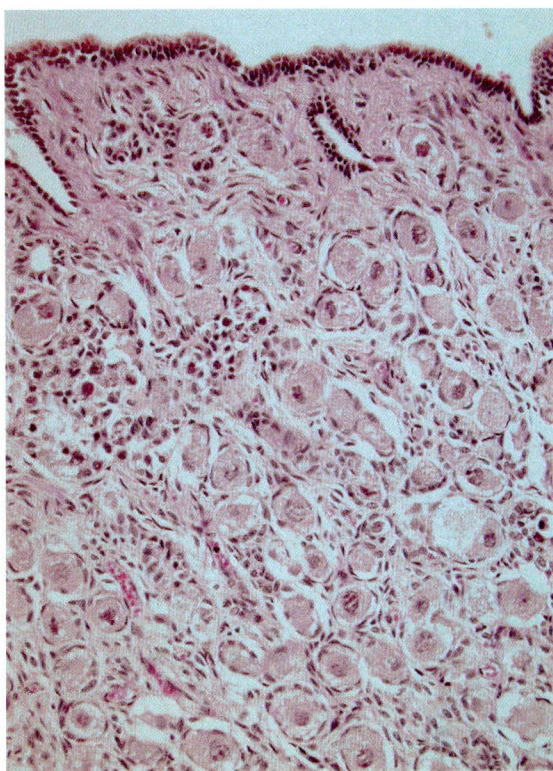

FIGURE 18-3 • Developing ovary at term showing numerous primordial follicles, and early development of the subepithelial stromal layer that will become more prominent with age. The number of germ cells will decrease progressively with age.

play a role in regulating continued meiotic arrest in the germ cells. Oogenesis is a gradual process that is generally complete by the third trimester, and there is no further increase in the number of primary oocytes thereafter (Figure 18-3). However, in the mouse germ or stem cell, replication may continue into adulthood. In addition to the germ cells, the ovary is populated by stromal cells that continue to remodel during the early first trimester, resulting in the formation of the ovarian cortex and the medulla. During the second trimester, a subepithelial collagenous connective tissue layer develops within the ovarian cortex beneath the basement membrane. The interstitial (thecal) cells, of unknown origin, can be detected during the first half of the second trimester, although estrogen production may begin as early as 8 to 10 weeks' gestation. The importance of the production of estrogen by the developing fetus remains somewhat controversial with some evidence that significant ovarian estrogen production does not occur until following birth (6). The histology of the developing ovary has been previously described in detail (8).

While many of the molecular details of testis development have been clearly established, the details regulating molecular ovarian development are now coming to light. The NR0B1 gene, previously designated DAX-1, is a dosage-sensitive gene locus on the X chromosome that encodes an orphan nuclear receptor protein. This gene was initially thought to be a specific ovary-determining gene but has since been shown to be more essential for normal testicular development and not required for normal ovarian development. NR0B1 is expressed in the normally developing ovary but turned off in the developing testis (5,6). Mutations of NR0B1 in XY males lead to hypogonadotropic hypogonadism with primary testicular defects and are associated with adrenal insufficiency (X-linked adrenal hypoplasia congenita). Loss of function of NR0B1 in XX females does not alter normal ovarian development. Overexpression of NR0B1, however, leads to ovarian development in males even if SRY is expressed. NR0B1 therefore appears to be more important in normal testis development. Unlike the SRY gene and testis development, there does not appear to be a single ovarian determining gene. The canonical WNT signaling pathway is specifically activated in XX gonads and diminished in XY gonads. WNT4 is expressed in both early gonads but is then up-regulated in ovarian somatic cells, and down-regulated in the testis. WNT4 expression seems critical for some portions of ovarian development, but not all. Constitutive activation of beta-catenin in XY gonads results in sex reversal with a XY female gonad. Without WNT4 expression in XX individuals, male-specific changes occur that include the presence of steroid-producing cells within the ovary, persistence of the wolffian ducts, loss of the müllerian ducts, and the development of a male-specific coelomic blood vessel to the ovary. In the absence of WNT4, germ cells can still enter meiosis, but there is massive apoptosis of the germ cells prior to birth. Another recently identified gene that is involved in activating the WNT/beta-catenin pathway is a pro-ovarian gene, RSPO1 (R-spondin-1). Homozygous mutation in RSPO1 results in female-to-male sex reversal in XX individuals. It would seem that activation of the canonical WNT signaling pathways is required to fully suppress the testis-determining pathway. WNT4 signaling appears to be necessary for (a) normal development of the müllerian duct, (b) suppression of the Sertoli cell lineage in the developing ovary, and (c) oocyte maintenance (1–4,6). Another gene proposed to be involved in ovary-specific development is FOXL2. FOXL2 seems to be critical for maintenance of the ovarian phenotype by repressing SOX9 expression and therefore preventing testicular differentiation. Mutations in the forkhead transcription factor 2 (FOXL2) gene in humans are associated with eyelid defects and premature ovarian failure (blepharophimosis, ptosis, and epicanthus inversus syndrome—BPES [OMIM 110100]). FOXL2 is expressed by pregranulosa cells (9). While estrogen secretion *in utero* does not appear to be important for sex determination, estrogen signaling does appear to be critical in the maintenance of the maturing ovary later during puberty. Blocking estrogen signaling in puberty results in transdifferentiation of the ovary and expression of Sertoli cell markers. Estrogen signaling appears to be critical in maintaining the mature ovarian structure by suppressing testicular development during early adult development. Estrogen signaling seems to antagonize activation of the transcriptional enhancer site for SOX9, thereby helping prevent SOX9 expression. It would seem that the gonadal phenotype is maintained early and throughout life by repression of the molecular pathways of the opposite sex. This helps to explain the wide variety of gonadal and genital anomalies including ovotestis.

The ovary differs from the testis in that the presence of germ cells is essential for normal ovarian development. In the developing testis, the male germ cells do not play a significant role in the structural development of the organ. Female germ cells appear to follow an intrinsic clock to enter the first meiosis and arrest prior to completion. Once female germ cells have entered meiosis, they have committed to the oocyte fate. During fetal development, the oocyte becomes surrounded by a single layer of granulosa cells to form the primordial follicle. Early primordial follicle formation and maintenance involve several complex molecular pathways acting sequentially and together (reviewed in (4,10,11)). Maturation of these follicles can proceed under hormonal signaling, especially during the third trimester of pregnancy.

At birth, the ovary is tan, flat, and elongated and measures about 1.3 × 0.5 × 0.3 cm. and weighs less than 0.3 g. Before birth, some primordial follicles can develop further. The ovum enlarges, and the surrounding follicular cells become more cuboidal to columnar and thereby form a primary follicle. This may be followed by stratification of the granulosa cells and increased granulosa cell proliferation, resulting in a preantral follicle (Figure 18-4). The graafian follicle demonstrates a cavity within the granulosa cell layer. The granulosa cells in these follicles have scant cytoplasm and often surround cavities filled with deeply eosinophilic material,

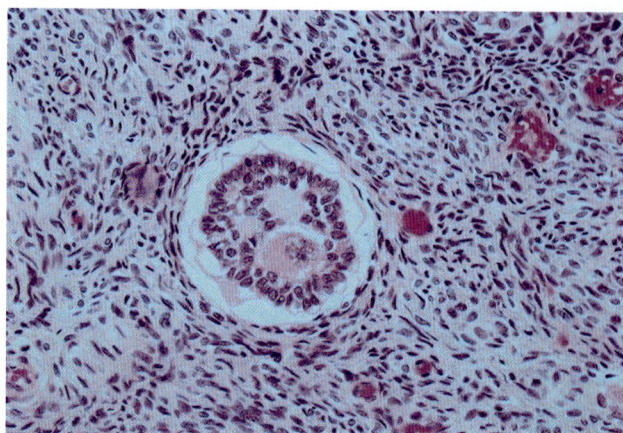

FIGURE 18-4 • Primary follicle, preantral stage, showing a thick layer of granulosa cells surrounding the oocyte. Several Call-Exner bodies containing acellular hyaline material are present.

known as *Call-Exner bodies* that may result in microscopic structures resembling gonadoblastoma or annular tubule-like profiles. These likely represent abnormal folliculogenesis. Thecal cells, which differentiate from the stromal cells at the periphery of developing follicles, may be seen. Throughout childhood, the ovaries enlarge to reach the size and the shape of an adult ovary (4 × 2 × 1 cm, 5 to 8 g). During the prepubertal period, the number of oocytes and primordial follicles continues to decrease, and the amount of ovarian stroma increases. Like the testicular Leydig cells, ovarian hilus cells disappear during childhood and reappear during puberty.

The Ductal System

The development of the urinary and reproductive systems is highly interdependent, which explains the high incidence of coexisting genital and urinary tract anomalies in several syndromes. Early in development (approximately week 4), paired mesonephric (wolffian) ducts arise from the intermediate mesoderm and nephrogenic cord (Figure 18-5). In the female embryo, the mesonephric duct is needed for induction of paramesonephric (müllerian) duct development from invaginations of the coelomic epithelium. The mesonephric and the paramesonephric ducts are enclosed in a peritoneal fold that gives rise to the broad ligament of the uterus. In the male embryo, AMH produced by fetal Sertoli cells leads to regression of the ipsilateral paramesonephric duct between weeks 8 and 10. AMH is proposed to have multiple functions in women (12). After the sensitivity of the paramesonephric ducts to AMH has disappeared, the ovarian granulosa cells begin to produce AMH with increasing levels that peak at about 10 years of age. AMH is thought to maintain meiotic arrest in the oocyte of the developing follicle in prepubertal females (10,11).

In the female embryo, the paramesonephric ducts fuse caudally before reaching the urogenital sinus, a process that is completed by week 10 (Figure 18-5). The unfused paramesonephric ducts become fallopian tubes and the fused portions the uterus and the upper vagina. The distal tip of the müllerian duct abuts the posterior wall of the urogenital sinus

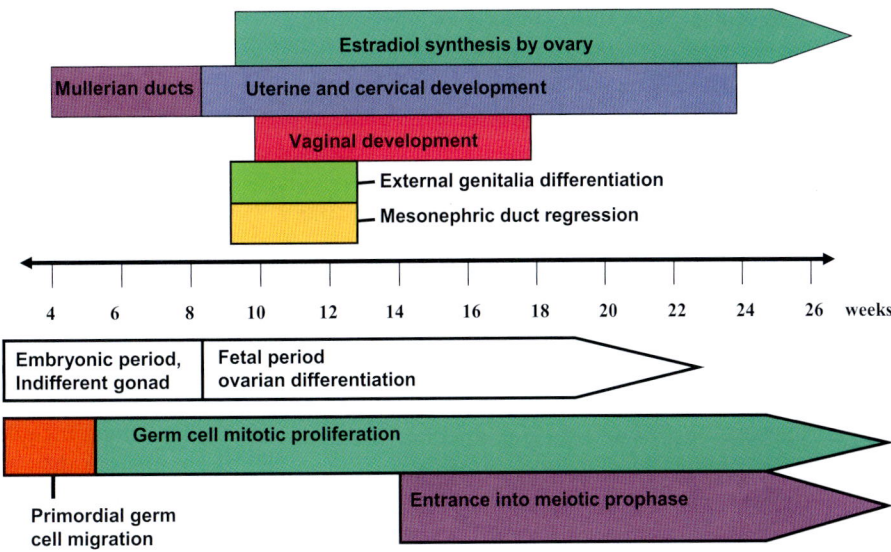

FIGURE 18-5 • Diagram indicating the gestational period of development of the ovary, ducts, and external genitalia.

Time Line of Female Reproductive Tract Development

within a patch of mesoderm. This point is the future site of the hymenal membrane. The patch of mesodermal urogenital sinus epithelium begins to proliferate, forming a column of squamous cells called the *vaginal plate* that eventually gives rise to the vaginal epithelium. The vaginal plate and the müllerian duct become patent by canalization early in the second trimester (by week 18). Mesonephric ducts in the female embryo begin to regress if not stimulated by testosterone by about week 10; however, mesonephric remnants in the broad ligament and lateral wall of the uterus and vagina can persist as Gartner ducts. By 13 weeks' gestation, the body (corpus) of the uterus and the cervix begin to be distinguished. In the fetus and the newborn, the cervix is twice as long as the corpus, whereas in the adult, the corpus is about two times longer than the cervix. At birth, the cervix and uterus together measure about 4 cm in length. The effects of maternal hormones (estrogens and progestins) result in a proliferative-to–weakly secretory endometrium at birth and cervical squamous cell maturation. These changes rapidly disappear after birth. During childhood, the endometrium is usually thin, with inactive glands in a spindled inactive stroma. The uterus reaches a plateau of growth in the 2nd year of life, until the premenarchal uterine growth increase. The final adult (nulliparous) uterus measures 7 to 8 cm in longest dimension and weighs between 40 and 80 g. The final maturation of the female reproductive tract is at the beginning of uterine bleeding (menarche), which occurs between 11 and 15 years of age. The early menstrual cycles are often anovulatory and can result in disordered proliferative endometrium. By mid-adolescence, regular menstrual cycles should be occurring, along with the monthly histologic changes that are well described for the adult female reproductive tract.

A number of genes have been reported as important in regulating normal internal female genital development. WNT signaling is essential for normal müllerian duct development. Spatial and temporal expression patterns of members of the HOXA gene locus are essential for normal development of the fallopian tubes (HOXA9), uterus (HOXA10), cervix (HOXA11), and upper vagina (HOXA13). In mice, many transcription factors have been implicated in normal müllerian duct formation including Lim1, Pax2, Emx2, several Wnt members (Wnt4, Wnt5a, Wnt7a, Wnt7b, Wnt11), and members of the retinoic acid receptor family (Rar-alpha, beta, and gamma) (13). Estrogen receptors alpha and beta are highly expressed in the female internal genital tract and are important for attaining the final functional phenotype especially for the uterus. Knocking out both ERa and ERb results in a hypoplastic uterus (reviewed in (13–16)).

Female External Genitalia

The external female genitalia begin to form during the 4th week of embryonic development. The genital tubercle forms ventral to the cloacal plate as two stromal elevations of the ectoderm. Lateral to the cloacal plate on each side, two parallel folds develop, which will give rise to the labia majora and the minora. As the labioscrotal folds extend cranially around the genital tubercle, they fuse and become the mons pubis (17,18). Sonic hedgehog signaling is an important regulator of genital tubercle formation, as well as other downstream genes including WNT5a and FGF8. The role of estrogen in the development of the entire female reproductive tract is unknown. Androgen production in the male is a critical regulator of penis and scrotum formation. If a female fetus is exposed to elevated androgens before 10 to 12 weeks of gestation, the external genitalia may become ambiguous or resemble a phenotypic male and the vagina will often open into the membranous portion of the urethra. If androgens become elevated after week 20, the only effect will be an enlarged clitoris. Similarly, androgen insensitivity due to mutations in the androgen receptor in XY males results in female external genitalia (16,17).

The entire vulva, with the exception of the vestibule, is lined by keratinized, stratified squamous epithelium. The vestibule and the vagina are lined by nonkeratinizing squamous epithelium, which becomes glycogenated in women of reproductive years, and should not be confused with koilocytotic change. The vaginal vestibule contains the orifices of the paraurethral (Skene) glands, the major (Bartholin) and minor vestibular glands, and the urethral meatus. The paired paraurethral glands are located on either side of the urethral meatus, are composed of pseudostratified mucus-secreting columnar epithelium, and are drained by ducts lined by transitional epithelium. The vestibular glands contain acini composed of simple columnar, mucus-secreting epithelium. The major vestibular (Bartholin) glands are drained by ducts lined proximally by mucus-secreting epithelium epithelium and more distally by transitional epithelium with terminal lining by squamous epithelium on their exit just external to the hymenal ring. The minor vestibular glands are located close to the surface and ring the vestibule.

STRUCTURAL ABNORMALITIES OF THE FEMALE REPRODUCTIVE ORGANS

The phenotypic abnormalities that can occur in the development of the female reproductive tract are numerous. These may represent isolated poorly understood variations in normal development, or they may be associated with major malformation syndromes; either may be related to chromosomal abnormalities or defects in known and unknown genes. Additionally, teratogens have been associated with abnormalities of the reproductive tract. DSDs are discussed separately.

The Ductal System

Müllerian duct anomalies are frequently associated with DSD. In patients with normal ovaries, müllerian duct malformations occur in about 0.5% of women and are frequently accompanied by anomalies of the urinary tract. These müllerian duct anomalies include lateral and vertical fusion defects, hypoplasia, or absence of fallopian tubes, the uterus, or the upper vagina. Uterine abnormalities can be structurally and morphologically divided into three categories. These include (a) complete failure of formation of the müllerian duct unilaterally (resulting in unicornuate uterus) or bilaterally (absent uterus), (b) arrested müllerian duct development (hypoplastic uterus), or (c) abnormal lateral fusion of the müllerian ducts to varying extents, resulting in paired uteri and cervices, accompanied by a vaginal septum (uterus didelphys), paired uteri and one cervix (bicornuate uterus), or a uterine septum (septate uterus) (19). The American Fertility Society classification scheme is shown in Figure 18-6 (20,21). A newer classification scheme to describe müllerian anomalies has been recently proposed; however, its clinical utility remains under study (22). Patients with müllerian anomalies may be asymptomatic or may present with infertility, repeated abortions, breech delivery, preterm delivery, dyspareunia, or dysmenorrhea. Because the wolffian ducts are essential for inducing the müllerian ducts, defects in wolffian duct development may likewise lead to uterine abnormalities. Isolated abnormalities of the fallopian tubes (duplication or absence) are rare. Abnormalities of the cervix are

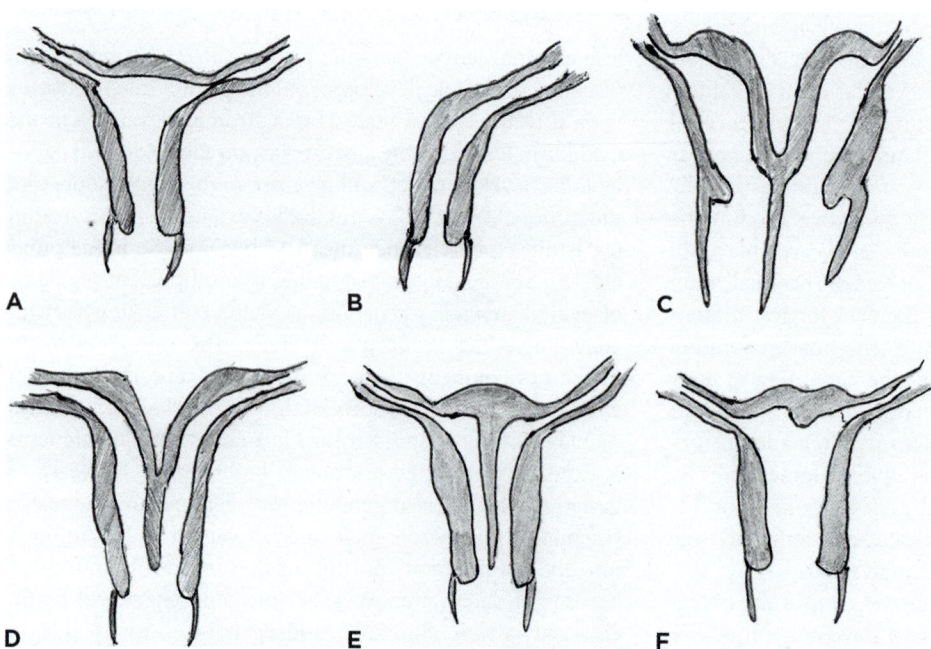

FIGURE 18-6 • American Fertility Society classification of müllerian duct abnormalities. Class I (not shown) müllerian aplasia consists of hypoplastic or absent uterus and other müllerian structures. **(A)** Normal uterus; **(B)** class II, unicornuate uterus; **(C)** class III, uterus didelphys (complete failure of midline fusion of müllerian ducts with duplication of uterus and cervix +/− vagina); **(D)** class IV, bicornuate uterus (defect in fusion at level of uterus only); **(E)** class V, septate uterus (incomplete (partial) resorption of uterine septum); **(F)** class VI, arcuate uterus (mildest form with small residual septum in superior portion of uterus). Artwork by RB Fritsch.

also very rare and include atresia or hypoplasia, which is due to failure of canalization of the müllerian ducts. The molecular events regulating lateral fusion remain largely unknown.

Absence of the vagina occurs in 1 in 4000 to 5000 women and is often associated with müllerian anomalies. In müllerian agenesis, also known as Mayer-Rokitansky-Kuster-Hauser (MRKH) sequence, there is an absent vagina and often an absent or poorly formed uterus and fallopian tubes (19,23). These patients are genotypic (46,XX) and phenotypic (normal external genitalia) females with normal endocrine status, and they often present with amenorrhea. Some cases are associated with upper urinary tract abnormalities and/or spine and skeletal abnormalities. MURCS (Müllerian, renal, cervical, somite) association appears to be an extreme presentation of these clustered anomalies (OMIM 601076). It has been suggested that this sequence may be due to abnormal development of the wolffian duct, with resulting abnormal müllerian duct development. MRKH sequence is thought to have a heterogeneous molecular basis with candidate genes proposed to include those involved in normal uterine development such as WT1, PAX2, HOX genes, WNT2, WNT4, and PBX1. The MRKH sequence usually occurs in a sporadic manner, and therefore, temporally altered aberrant gene expression may be related to exogenous factors rather than to mutations. Other anomalies of the vagina result from developmental defects involving the cloaca or urogenital sinus. As previously discussed, the lower third of the vagina and the hymen are thought to be derived from the ectoderm. If the urogenital sinus develops normally, the vagina can be present as a blind pouch even in the absence of normal müllerian duct development. A variety of miscommunications between the urethra, rectum, and vagina have been described (24). Vaginal obstruction can result from absence of communication between the introitus and the vaginal canal, related to defects in vertical fusion. Etiologies include imperforate hymen, atresia of the lower vagina, or a transverse vaginal septum (failure of vertical canalization of the vaginal plate at the site of fusion between the urogenital sinus and the müllerian ducts). Imperforate hymen, formed where the urogenital sinus and canalized fused sinuvaginal bulbs meet, is the most common cause, and if there is complete obstruction, this leads to a marked dilatation of the vagina and the uterus (hydrometrocolpos—retention of secreted mucous). If the person is asymptomatic until the onset of menses, the obstruction can result in hematocolpos.

The External Genitalia

Abnormalities in the development of the perineum, labia, and clitoris are not uncommon. The normal variations and structural abnormalities of the vulva have been extensively reviewed (25). Complete absence of the external genitalia is rare and occurs as part of malformation syndromes such as sirenomelia, limb–body wall defects, Robinow syndrome, multiple pterygia syndrome, Fryns syndrome, or CHARGE association. Vulvar duplication is rare and is associated with multiple congenital anomalies. Abnormalities of the clitoris and labia may cause problems in assigning the correct sex at birth. Clitoral hypertrophy may resemble male hypospadias. Exposure of the female fetus to excess androgens, such as in congenital adrenal hyperplasia, a maternal or fetal virilizing tumor, or maternal medication, can result in clitoral hypertrophy and may result in partial fusion of the posterior portion of the labia. Complete absence of the clitoris is rare.

DISORDERS OF SEX DEVELOPMENT

DSDs, previously referred to as intersex disorders, are defined as any congenital condition presenting with aberrant development of gonads and/or genitalia resulting in discordant chromosomal (genetic) and anatomic sex, associated or not with chromosomal anomalies. An early diagnosis is warranted not only for potential early gender assignment but also for identification of patients at risk for the development of gonadal neoplasms. DSDs encompass several conditions with significant clinicopathologic overlap, and the diagnosis of a specific entity requires a multidisciplinary approach with correlation of several clinical and laboratory features, including phenotypic features (external and internal genitalia), endocrine profile, karyotype, molecular studies, and histopathology. In addition, both the lack of uniformity in the existing literature and the confusing nomenclature represent a challenge to the diagnosis of these conditions. A revised nomenclature and classification system (Table 18-1) had been proposed in an attempt to provide a more descriptive approach to DSD (26); however, this classification system is still limited in terms of overcoming all the subtleties and overlapping features associated with these conditions.

Despite these limitations, the etiologies of DSD can be broadly characterized into chromosomal, molecular, or endocrine. Chromosomal abnormalities result from numerical aberrations in sex chromosomes and include aneuploidies (Chapter 3), such as 45,X (Turner syndrome), 47,XXY (Klinefelter syndrome), or mosaic aneuploidies, such as 45,X/46,XY (mixed gonadal dysgenesis) and 46,XX/47,XY. The molecular aberrations resulting in DSD include numerous defects in genes involved in testicular development such as SRY, WT1, SOX9, DHH, AMH, or the AMH receptor, among others (2,3,27–29). Endocrine causes are divided into undervirilization syndromes (including androgen insensitivity syndrome and defects in androgen biosynthesis) and hypervirilization syndromes (examples include congenital adrenal hyperplasia and excess exogenous androgens) (30).

Most patients with DSD present with a wide spectrum of clinical manifestations, and significant clinical overlap is

TABLE 18-1 CLASSIFICATION OF DSD

I. Normal sex chromosomes
  A. Female pseudohermaphroditism (excess androgens in females)—**(46,XX DSD)**
    1. Adrenogenital syndrome (21-hydroxylase deficiency, 11-β-hydroxylase deficiency)
    2. Maternal ingestion of androgenic hormones
    3. Maternal virilization
  B. Male pseudohermaphroditism (deficient androgens in males)—**(46,XY DSD)**
    1. Testicular regression syndrome
    2. Gonadotropin-Leydig cell defects
    3. Steroid enzyme deficiencies (testosterone/dihydrotestosterone)
    4. Androgen insensitivity syndromes
    5. Persistent müllerian duct syndrome

II. Abnormal sex chromosomes
  A. Sexual ambiguity frequently present
    1. Mixed gonadal dysgenesis—**(45,X/46,XY MGD)**
    2. True hermaphroditism—**(ovotesticular DSD)**
  B. Sexual ambiguity infrequently present
    1. Pure gonadal dysgenesis—**(46,XY complete gonadal dysgenesis)**
    2. Klinefelter syndrome—**(47,XXY)**
    3. Turner syndrome—**(45,X)**
    4. XX male syndrome—**(46,XX testicular DSD)**

Shown in **bold** is the new nomenclature.
From Lee PA, Houk CP, Ahmed SF, et al. Consensus statement on management of intersex disorders. International Consensus Conference on Intersex. *Pediatrics* 2006;118:e488–e500.

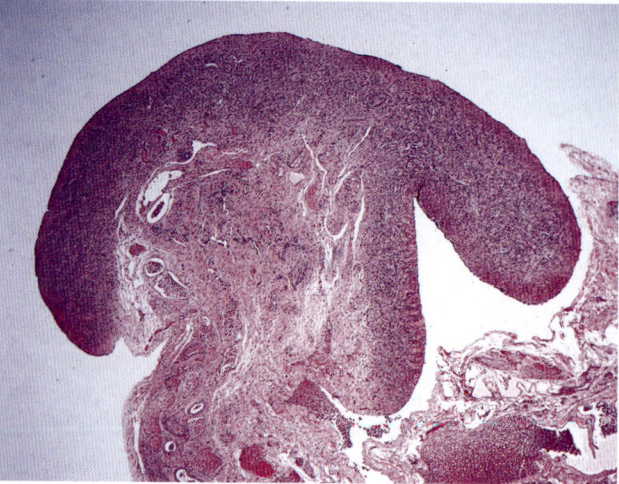

FIGURE 18-7 • Streak gonad composed of wavy ovarian stroma with no identifiable follicular structures.

seen among distinct entities. The clinical presentation in DSD reflects the extent of gonadal maldevelopment. The external genitalia phenotype typically is a direct result of the degree of virilization achieved by androgen exposure during fetal development. Ambiguous genitalia, usually resulting from partial virilization, is the most common presentation of DSD and encompasses a broad range of phenotypic abnormalities including hypospadias, clitoral hypertrophy, micropenis, bifid scrotum, and fused labia majora. Internal genitalia development is mostly determined by exposure to antimüllerian hormone (AMH) and androgens. AMH is responsible for regression of the müllerian (paramesonephric) structures that will give rise to the uterus and fallopian tubes. Androgens are implicated in the development of the wolffian (mesonephric) structures that will give rise to the epididymis, vas deferens, and seminal vesicles. Other clinical presentations of DSD include precocious puberty, delayed puberty, primary amenorrhea, and complete sex reversal. As an example, bilateral streak gonads in a 46,XY patient often result in a female phenotype due to absence or minimal production of androgens and AMH by the undifferentiated gonadal tissue. A female phenotype in a 46,XY individual is also usually seen in cases of complete androgen insensitivity syndrome.

Gonadal Pathology in DSD

Morphologically, the gonads in DSD can be divided into well or maldeveloped (dysgenetic gonads). Well-developed gonads can be anatomically normal but functionally abnormal, resulting in a DSD phenotype due to inadequate hormone production and are usually associated with endocrine etiologies of DSD such as congenital adrenal hyperplasia (adrenogenital syndrome). In contrast, dysgenetic (or maldeveloped) gonads are often associated with chromosomal, molecular, or unknown etiologies of DSD. Morphologically, dysgenetic gonads usually fall into one of the following patterns: streak gonads, dysgenetic testes, and ovotestes. Streak gonads consist of variable degrees of ovarian stroma and dense fibrous tissue and an absent tunica albuginea (31); primordial follicles/germ cells are usually scant or absent, and primitive cord-like structures are often present (Figure 18-7). In Turner syndrome patients (45,X), streak gonads are thought to represent regressive changes within ovarian tissue, whereas in patients with a 46,XY cell line, the streak gonads are thought to represent abortive testicular development. Dysgenetic testes occur in patients with a 46,XY cell line (examples include mixed gonadal dysgenesis and a few cases of gonadal dysgenesis due to germline mutations in genes involved in testicular development) and are thought to represent a milder phenotype of abortive testicular development, containing variable amounts of well-developed seminiferous cords (31). However, these seminiferous cords contain subtle abnormalities such as irregular contours and aberrant distribution of germ cells; in addition, dysgenetic testes show a poorly developed tunica albuginea with irregular thickness and deficient collagenization, occasionally penetrated by seminiferous cords, and foci of ovarian stroma (Figure 18-8). Ovotestis is the rarest type of dysgenetic gonad, characterized by recognizable testicular (containing well-formed seminiferous cords with spermatogonia) and ovarian (containing numerous follicles at various degrees of

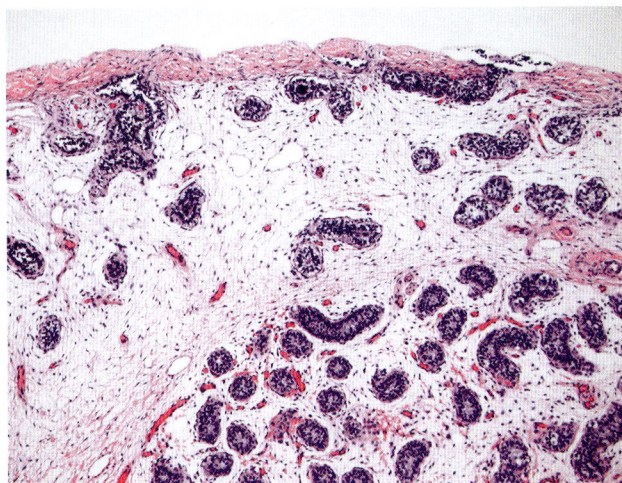

FIGURE 18-8 • Dysgenetic testis demonstrating abnormal branching of seminiferous tubules, some of which invade the tunic albuginea. The tunica can be of variable (often thin) thickness.

maturation) parenchyma occurring within the same gonad (Figure 18-9) (32,33). This gonadal phenotype characterizes ovotesticular DSD (true hermaphroditism), for which different etiologies have been implied, including numerical anomalies in sex chromosomes (such as 46,XX/46,XY mosaicism) and molecular defects in genes involved in gonadal development (34).

Tumors Associated with Gonadal Dysgenesis

Patients with dysgenetic gonads containing Y chromosome material in their genome, specifically the GBY region encoding the *TSPY* gene, are at increased risk for the

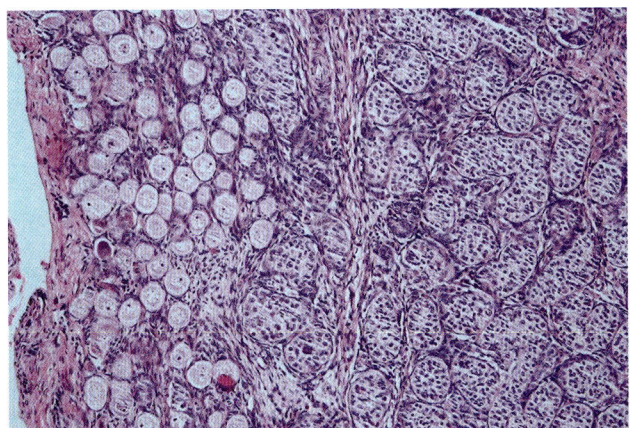

FIGURE 18-9 • Ovotestis removed from a 6-year-old child with ambiguous genitalia and an undescended left testicle. Peripheral lymphocyte karyotype 46,XY. The gonad demonstrates two distinct regions: the area on the left composed of ovarian stroma and numerous primordial follicles, and the area on the right lower corner showing normally developed seminiferous tubules with reduced numbers of germ cells.

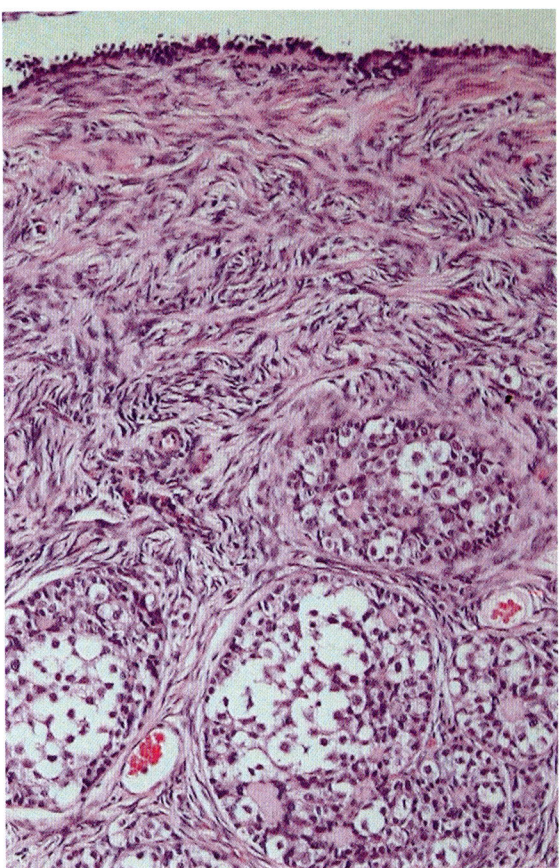

FIGURE 18-10 • Small, streak gonad from a 46,XY phenotypic female that is composed of wavy ovarian-type stroma and no primordial follicles. Deep within the cortex, well-defined nests composed of a mixture of germ cells and granulosa-like cells, consistent with gonadoblastoma.

development of neoplasms (35). The presence of SRY or other sex-determining genes is irrelevant in this context. More than 50% of neoplasms arising in these gonads are gonadoblastomas (Figure 18-10). The frequency of occurrence of gonadoblastoma in these patients correlates with the frequency of an intact Y chromosome containing the GBY region. Gonadoblastoma is seen in approximately 30% of patients with mixed gonadal dysgenesis, less than 3% of individuals with true hermaphroditism, and over 50% of patients with 46,XY pure (complete) gonadal dysgenesis (36). The pathology of gonadoblastoma is described later. The significance of the development of gonadoblastoma is that it is associated with a very high frequency of concurrent or future development of a malignant germ cell tumor, most commonly dysgerminoma. Other less common gonadal tumors in patients with DSD include other types of germ cell tumors, juvenile granulosa cell tumor (JGCT), Sertoli-Leydig cell tumor, and epithelial tumors. DSD patients with a 46,XX karyotype and patients with Turner syndrome without 45,X/46,XY mosaicism only rarely develop gonadal tumors; however, hilus cell hyperplasia and hilus cell tumors have been reported.

NONNEOPLASTIC LESIONS OF THE LOWER GENITAL TRACT

Infections

Infections of the lower genitourinary tract account for the majority of genital lesions in premenarchal girls. These infections are most commonly due to a variety of bacterial organisms that do not penetrate the mucosa and are not related to specific pathologic findings. Infections common in sexually active females, such as Gardnerella vaginalis and molluscum contagiosum, are quite rare in young children and should raise the suspicion of sexual abuse (Chapter 7). Specific infections of the vulvovagina include human papillomavirus (HPV), herpes simplex virus, syphilis, and molluscum contagiosum.

Human Papillomaviruses

Condyloma acuminata are sexually transmitted lesions caused by papillomaviridae, most commonly the HPV types 6 or 11, although HPV 2 may also be seen. It is now recommended that condyloma acuminata be referred to as low-grade squamous intraepithelial lesions (LGSILs) (37). The modes of transmission of HPV include perinatal, autoinoculation, heteroinoculation, and sexual abuse. These lesions may involve the vulva, vagina, cervix, urethra, and/or perianal skin. Vulvar and vaginal lesions are commonly papillary and are almost always multiple; cervical lesions are often flat, white lesions surrounded by hyperemic mucosa. Uncommonly, the involved epithelium may extend into the endocervical glands and, therefore, have an endophytic appearance. Most lesions are asymptomatic unless secondarily infected. Histologically, parakeratosis, acanthosis, hyperkeratosis, and dyskeratosis are evident (Figure 18-11). The typical koilocytic cells with perinuclear cytoplasmic halos surrounding irregularly contoured ("raisinoid") nuclei may be seen in the more superficial or intermediate layers. The development of high-grade intraepithelial neoplasia—HGSIL—(associated with high-risk HPV genotypes 16 and 18) is an uncommon finding in females under 21 years of age. Most cases in this age group correspond to LGSILs, whereas high-grade lesions and progression to carcinoma are rare occurrences (38). LGSIL may at times be difficult to distinguish from HGSIL or vulvar intraepithelial neoplasia. The presence of a flat, macular growth pattern, abnormal mitoses, atypical nuclei, marked variation in nuclear size and shape, and hyperchromasia are all characteristics of vulvar intraepithelial neoplasia. In addition, immunohistochemistry can be helpful as Ki67 will show increased staining up into the epidermis in LGSIL and all the way to the surface epidermis in HGSIL. Also, p16 is extremely helpful as LGSILs show only weak staining, whereas HGSIL demonstrate strong staining in the epidermis. Identification of the specific HPV genotype may be indicated in some circumstances, but is not considered routine in children.

Herpes Simplex

Patients with genital infection with herpes simplex virus types I or II can present with dysuria and vulvar pain, often accompanied by generalized malaise and fever. The clinical picture is dominated by the appearance of vesicles and shallow ulcers that are often secondarily infected. Only two-thirds of culture-positive women show diagnostic genital lesions. Histologically, the ulcers typically demonstrate extension deep into the epidermis, with the characteristic intranuclear inclusions present at the periphery of the lesion. Late in the evolution of the ulcer, the infected cells undergo karyorrhexis and lysis, and therefore, infected cells may not be identifiable in biopsy material. Cytologic evaluation of scrapings from a fresh ulcer or freshly opened vesicle will usually show the characteristic viral cytopathic effects. Recurrent episodes of herpetic vulvitis are common; however, these episodes decrease in frequency over time whether or not acyclovir is given. Anogenital herpes in children raises the concern of sexual abuse, but is not definitive evidence. Varicella infection of the lower genital tract is rare in children and more commonly detected in postmenopausal women.

Syphilis

The primary lesion of syphilis is the chancre, a painless, shallow ulcer with raised edges that usually presents within 10 to 90 days of initial contact. These lesions often occur on inconspicuous surfaces, such as the cervix, and in about 50% of patients, the primary lesion is never seen (39). Histologically, the chancre is characterized by ulceration of the epidermis with acute and chronic inflammation within the dermis. There is a marked perivascular inflammatory response with a large number of plasma cells. The lack of specificity of these findings raises the importance of considering syphilis in the differential diagnosis of inflammatory lesions. Lymphadenopathy may develop 3 to 4 days after the

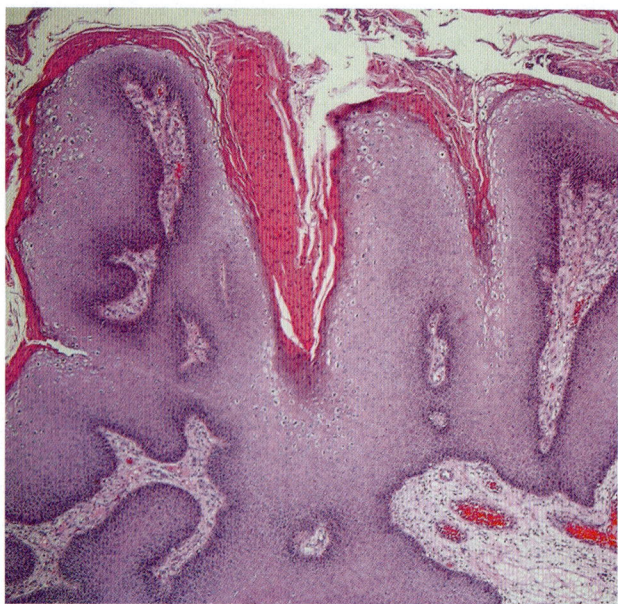

FIGURE 18-11 • Condyloma acuminatum showing parakeratosis, acanthosis, and numerous koilocytic cells with nuclear irregularity and prominent perinuclear vacuolization. No dysplasia is present.

chancre appears. If the primary stage is left untreated, the secondary stage of the disease will become evident within 6 weeks to 6 months when the patient will show elevated plaques measuring up to 3 cm, especially on the vulva. These plaques are known as *condylomata lata* and demonstrate marked acanthosis, epithelial hyperplasia, and hyperkeratosis. The inflammatory response within the dermis is similar to that seen in the chancre. Both the chancre and the condyloma lata are rich in spirochetes, which may be detected by the Dieterle or Warthin-Starry silver stains. However, these stains may be negative even with active infection. Serologic studies should be performed if syphilis is considered clinically or pathologically; even these studies may be negative for weeks after the presentation of the primary chancre. Other methods used for detecting spirochetes include dark field examination of serum expressed from the base of the ulcer or by a fluorescent-conjugated antibody technique. These methods are more sensitive and specific than the silver stain on paraffin-embedded tissue (39).

Molluscum Contagiosum

Molluscum contagiosum is usually an asymptomatic infection caused by a moderately contagious virus often passed through sexual contact. The lesions are generally multiple, small, smooth 3- to 6-mm papules with a central umbilication. Diagnosis rarely requires biopsy. Cytologic identification of the typical intracytoplasmic inclusion bodies (molluscum bodies) within scrapings or in biopsy material is adequate to confirm the diagnosis (Figure 18-12).

Chlamydia trachomatis

The most common sexually transmitted disease in adolescent girls is *Chlamydia trachomatis*. Approximately 32% of asymptomatically reported cases of *Chlamydia* infection occurred in people aged 15 to 19 years (40). The organism most commonly infects the columnar and immature squamous cells of the endocervix; however, salpingitis and endometritis may be seen, which often leads to infertility. Nucleic acid amplification test (NAAT) performed on either urine, urethral, vaginal, or cervical samples has the highest sensitivity and specificity in establishing the presence of disease and is the preferred diagnostic test (40). Infected patients show lymphocytic inflammation and reactive epithelial changes by cytology. Some observers have reported cytoplasmic inclusion bodies in infected cells; however, others interpret these bodies as nonspecific cytoplasmic vacuoles. Therefore, the finding of lymphocytes, reactive epithelial cells, often dyskeratotic cells, and vacuolization of metaplastic cells should be considered suggestive but not diagnostic for chlamydial infection. Chlamydial infection of the vulva or vagina may result in lymphogranuloma venereum, a skin lesion characterized first by painless skin erosion, followed by lymphadenitis involving superficial groin lymph nodes, which may ulcerate and rupture. Over time, the chronic inflammatory process and chronic lymphatic obstruction may result in stricture, fibrosis, and nonpitting edema of the vagina and rectum.

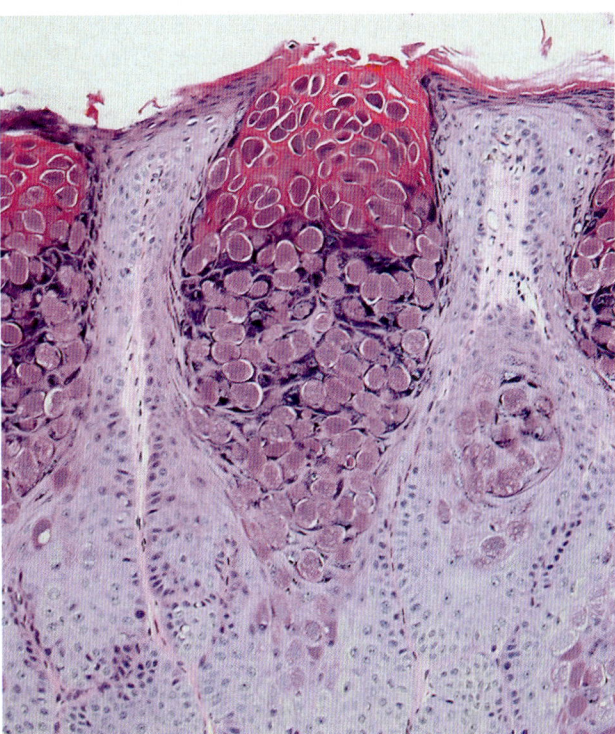

FIGURE 18-12 • Molluscum contagiosum with numerous epidermal cells containing large intracytoplasmic inclusion bodies, the so-called molluscum bodies, which are typically found in the lower cells of the stratum malpighii. The molluscum body compresses the nucleus, which appears as a thin crescent at the periphery of the cell.

Miscellaneous Infectious Diseases

Cytomegalovirus, Epstein-Barr virus, Candida, and other fungal and bacterial infections may cause acute or chronic inflammatory lesions of the lower genital tract, most commonly without ulceration. Chancroid is a rare infection characterized by a genital ulcer caused by *Haemophilus ducreyi*, which is identified by culture. Histologically, chancroid shows granulomatous inflammation with Gram-negative organisms. Tuberculosis of the vulva is rare and is usually associated with the disease at other sites. Sexual transmission is uncommon in the absence of immunosuppression. Enterobius vermicularis (pinworm) may cause a severe vulvovaginal pruritus in infected children. Granuloma inguinale is caused by *Klebsiella granulomatis* (previously known as *Calymmatobacterium granulomatous*), a Gram-negative encapsulated rod with primary lesions presenting anywhere in the lower genitourinary tract as painless papules or necrotizing ulcers. The diagnosis depends on the identification of large, vacuolated histiocytes containing the characteristic cytoplasmic encapsulated bacilli called *Donovan bodies*, demonstrated by Warthin-Starry or Giemsa stains.

Noninfectious Inflammatory Diseases

Behçet Disease

Behçet disease is characterized by the triad of recurrent oral ulcers, vulvar ulcers, and various ophthalmologic inflammations (OMIM 109650). Acne, cutaneous nodules, thrombophlebitis, encephalopathy, and colitis may also be present. The vulvar ulcers, seen in postmenarchal females, may be deep and characteristically relapse. Healing of the ulcers may result in severe scarring. Histologic examination reveals chronic inflammation and necrotizing vasculitis, which is considered a cardinal finding. Vascular endothelial cell swelling may result in arteriolar occlusions and venous thrombosis. Behçet disease is presumed to be autoimmune in etiology (41).

Crohn Disease

Vulvar involvement by Crohn disease is rare and characterized by papules, nodules, or ulcerations that are often multiple, deep, and secondarily infected. The diagnosis may be difficult, particularly if this is the presenting site of the disease. Genital lesions are the most common presentation of metastatic/cutaneous Crohn disease in children. Histology demonstrates noncaseating granulomatous inflammation with extensive granulation tissue within the dermis (Chapter 14).

Lichen Sclerosus

Lichen sclerosus is a dermatosis of unknown etiology characterized pathologically by thinning of the epithelial layer, blunting or loss of the rete ridges, and a homogeneously collagenized or edematous subepithelial layer in the dermis with a band of chronic inflammatory cells beneath (Chapter 26). There is an absence of melanosomes and disappearance of the melanocytes, resulting in a hypopigmented patch that may be pruritic. The microscopic findings may vary considerably, depending on the age of the lesions, excoriation, and treatment. Lichen sclerosus is not limited to the elderly population and may be seen in the reproductive years, and between 5% and 15% of all cases occur in prepubertal girls (42). In children, symptoms include dysuria, painful defecation, and rectal bleeding. This may lead to anal fissures and genital and perianal ulcers, which may be confused with sexual abuse, trauma, and infections. Although lichen sclerosus is sometimes associated with vulvar squamous carcinoma, it is not considered to be a premalignant condition.

Bullous Diseases

The vulva may be involved with virtually any dermatologic disease; however, some of the bullous diseases (see Chapter 26) may have their first manifestations in the vulva and in childhood. Darier-White disease (keratosis follicularis) is an autosomal dominant skin disorder that frequently involves the vulva (OMIM 124200). Hailey-Hailey disease (familial benign pemphigus or benign chronic pemphigus) is an autosomal dominant disease that may also be sporadic (OMIM 169600). Onset often occurs during adolescence, and several cases confined exclusively to the vulva have been reported. Benign chronic bullous disease of childhood (linear IgA bullous dermatosis) commonly involves the genital region of children. It presents as clusters of annular pruritic lesions that evolve into tense bullae, which may then ulcerate. Patients may have fever and anorexia, and a preceding infection is identified in 50% the cases. Vulvar involvement may be seen in Stevens-Johnson syndrome, the severe form of erythema multiforme. This disease may be associated with herpes virus or mycoplasma infection, drug therapy, malignancy, or radiotherapy and is characterized by involvement of the mouth, eyes, and skin with associated fever and other systemic symptoms.

CYSTIC LESIONS OF THE FEMALE REPRODUCTIVE TRACT

Benign Cystic Lesions of the Lower Genital Tract

Müllerian Cysts

Of uncertain genesis, müllerian cysts can be located anywhere within the vagina with a predilection for the anterolateral wall and are lined by any of the epithelia of the müllerian duct, including mucinous, endocervical, endometrial, and ciliated tubal types. Squamous metaplasia may also be observed. The majority of vaginal cysts represent müllerian remnant cysts or epidermal inclusion cysts.

Bartholin Cysts

Bartholin glands produce a clear mucoid secretion that continually lubricates the vestibular surface. The ducts of Bartholin glands are prone to obstruction, resulting in cystic dilatation of the duct and secondary infection. The epithelium lining the cyst may be squamous, transitional, or low cuboidal mucinous and is immunoreactive for carcinoembryonic antigen.

Vulvar Mucous Cysts

Vulvar mucous cysts are lined by tall-to-cuboidal Alcian blue–positive mucus-secreting epithelium. Squamous metaplasia may be present. Mucous cysts likely arise from the urogenital sinus epithelium, and they lack both myoepithelial cells and muscle fibers.

Gartner Duct Cysts

Commonly seen remnants of the mesonephric (wolffian) duct mostly within the anterolateral wall of the vagina are known as *Gartner duct cysts*. They are thin-walled cysts lined by low cuboidal epithelium that may or may not be ciliated, without mucinous differentiation. A basement membrane and smooth muscle may be present in the submucosal region. However, both müllerian and wolffian duct remnants can be surrounded by variable amounts of smooth muscle. Associated ipsilateral urinary tract malformations have been reported in a few cases. CD10 immunohistochemistry can be helpful as mesonephric-derived remnants show strong apical staining of the epithelium and paramesonephric-derived remnant epithelium is negative (43).

Cysts of the Canal of Nuck (Peritoneal Lined Cysts)

These cysts are found in the superior aspect of the labia majora or inguinal canal and are believed to arise from inclusions of the peritoneum at the inferior insertion of the round ligament into the labia majora, analogous to the hydrocele of the spermatic cord. They may get quite large and must be distinguished from an inguinal hernia.

Skene Duct Cysts

Skene duct cysts result from congenital or acquired obstruction of paraurethral or Skene glands in the distal urethra. They can be asymptomatic or present as a mass at the vaginal introitus and are lined by squamous epithelium, reflecting their proposed urogenital sinus origin.

Nonneoplastic Ovarian Cysts

The most common ovarian lesions detected radiographically are cysts derived from follicles at different stages of maturation in prepubertal girls (44). Congenital ovarian cysts may be diagnosed in utero by ultrasound and are associated with resolution; however, their evolution is variable and may require intervention (45). Complications such as torsion and rupture usually occur in cysts larger than 5 cm in diameter. Cysts that develop in utero are most often lined by luteinized cells, whereas those in older children prior to menarche are more often lined by granulosa cells. Premature infants born before the 30th week of gestation may have multiple follicular cysts. These cysts are secondary to elevated follicle-stimulating hormone (FSH) and luteinizing hormone (LH) secretion, and they may be associated with relative insensitivity of the hypothalamus and anterior pituitary to negative feedback by estradiol.

Follicular cysts are commonly found in the ovaries of prepubertal females as an incidental finding. Follicular cysts are usually greater than 2.5 cm in diameter and can occur in both pre- and postpubertal females. Rarely, multiple follicular cysts may be the cause of pseudoprecocious puberty, although more often they are the result of central causes of pseudoprecocity. As many as 75% of girls with juvenile hypothyroidism have multicystic ovaries, and rarely, the ovarian enlargement may be the presenting sign leading to a diagnosis of hypothyroidism. Clinically, affected patients may show varying degrees of sexual precocity and galactorrhea due to increased secretion of pituitary gonadotropins and prolactin. Treatment with thyroxin results in regression of the ovarian cysts as well as the other symptoms.

Multiple follicular cysts should be distinguished from polycystic ovary syndrome (PCOS), which affects 3% to 8% of the female population. PCOS is responsible for 25% of cases of primary amenorrhea and is the most common cause of delayed puberty and heavy anovulatory bleeding in adolescent females (46). It is characterized by inappropriate gonadotropin secretion (especially LH), hyperandrogenemia, increased peripheral conversion of androgens to estrogens, chronic anovulation, and sclerocystic ovaries. The diagnostic criteria for PCOS in adults were established in 2004 by the Rotterdam criteria, although this has been heavily debated. These criteria include the presence of 2 of the following 3: (a) oligo- or anovulatory cycles, (b) hyperandrogenism (confirmed biochemically or clinically), and (c) polycystic ovaries by ultrasound. Definitive diagnostic criteria in adolescents are more difficult to apply due to common anovulatory cycles (47). Other common features of PCOS include obesity and insulin resistance. See (46,47) for recent reviews. Affected patients often have a history of premenarcheal obesity, secondary amenorrhea or oligomenorrhea, infertility, and hirsutism. These features may occur alone or in any combination and the clinical spectrum is broad. The unopposed estrogenic stimulation may cause menometrorrhagia and endometrial hyperplasia. Currently, the underlying etiology of PCOS is widely debated; however, the resulting clinical manifestations are known to be heavily impacted by environmental factors. While several genes have been linked with PCOS, the evidence supporting this linkage is weak (16). Grossly, the ovaries of PCOS are enlarged two- to fivefold and have smooth or nodular white surfaces, with multiple cysts located beneath the thickened cortex. Histologically, multiple follicle cysts, atretic follicles, a prominent theca interna with luteinization, and medullary stromal overgrowth are the principal histologic features. The superficial cortex is fibrotic and hypocellular. Maturing follicles up to midantral stage and atretic follicles showing prominent luteinization of the theca interna may be twice as numerous as in normal ovaries. Primordial follicles are often decreased in number. It is important to remember that these findings are not specific and may accompany adrenal lesions such as Cushing syndrome, congenital adrenal hyperplasia, virilizing adrenal tumors, primary hypothalamic disorders, ovarian lesions that produce excessive quantities of estrogens or androgens, and hypothyroidism. Long-term sequelae of PCOS include infertility, endometrial carcinoma, an increased risk for cardiovascular disease due to type II diabetes mellitus, dyslipidemia, and systolic hypertension.

Other types of cysts that involve the ovary include corpus luteal cysts, paramesonephric- or mesonephric-derived developmental cysts (including paratubal cysts) and endometrial cysts related to endometriosis (see below).

OTHER NONNEOPLASTIC OVARIAN LESIONS

Endometriosis

Endometriosis or endometrioma of the ovary may cause an adnexal mass in reproductive age females (16). Pigmented foci on an otherwise normal ovary or a large solitary hemorrhagic cyst are the gross findings. Histologic findings include columnar-to-plump cuboidal epithelium with condensed subepithelial stroma, hemosiderin-laden macrophages, fibrosis, and inflammation (Figure 18-13). Rare cases may also contain smooth muscle. Patients with uterine anomalies may develop severe endometriosis. Acute torsion of the adnexal structures is an uncommon event but is a surgical emergency. The severity of the symptoms varies widely and includes fever, nausea or vomiting, and

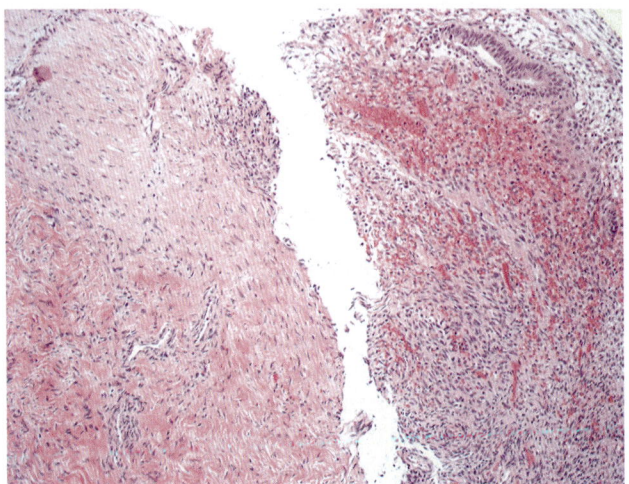

FIGURE 18-13 • Removal of an ovarian cyst with a significant solid component revealed endometriosis attached to the ovary. There is edematous endometrial stroma and small collections of glands. Definitive hemosiderin was not seen in the tissue examined.

abdominal pain. The correct diagnosis is rarely made preoperatively. The preoperative radiograph commonly shows a pelvic mass with a cystic or solid texture, often with thin internal septae, and may simulate an ovarian mass. Because the sigmoid colon cushions and secures the left adnexa, the right adnexa are more often affected than the left. The fallopian tube and ovary have usually undergone hemorrhagic necrosis by the time of the surgery, often with secondary calcification. As a result, the cause of the torsion is not clear in most cases.

Massive Ovarian Edema

Massive ovarian edema is an unusual clinical entity most often occurring in adolescence. It is characterized by marked enlargement of one or both ovaries due to marked accumulation of edema fluid in the ovarian stroma. Massive ovarian edema may result from partial or intermittent torsion of the mesovarium, interfering with venous and lymphatic drainage, but not with arterial blood flow obstruction (48).

NEOPLASMS OF THE LOWER FEMALE GENITAL TRACT

Benign Tumors of the Lower Female Genital Tract

Hidradenoma Papilliferum

Papillary hidradenoma is a benign tumor of apocrine sweat gland origin that presents as an asymptomatic small mass in the labia majora or the lateral labia minora. This tumor has not been described before puberty and almost all cases have occurred in white women (49). Histologically, papillary hidradenoma is composed of tubules and acini lined by cuboidal epithelial cells with an outer layer of myoepithelial cells. These cells may simulate a well-differentiated adenocarcinoma, and entrapped epithelial cells may create a pseudoinfiltrative appearance. Mitotic figures are rare, and only mild nuclear pleomorphism is present.

Prepubertal Vulval Fibroma

This entity has been reported in prepubertal girls, affecting the labia majora in most cases (50). It presents as a painless, ill-defined mass and is characterized by a nonencapsulated proliferation of cytologically bland spindle cells embedded in a variably collagenized and edematous stroma. Entrapped adipose tissue, vessels, nerves, and adnexal structures are often seen. Local recurrence has been demonstrated in a subset of patients.

Müllerian or Mesonephric Papilloma

Several tumors that are composed of complex, arborizing papillae with a fibrovascular core supporting bland-appearing epithelial cells have been reported within the vagina of young girls (51). In some areas, the tumor either may appear as a solid mass or may contain glandular lumina and eosinophilic hyaline globules. Their embryologic origin remains uncertain.

Fibroepithelial Polyp (Mesodermal Stromal Polyp)

Fibroepithelial polyps are uncommon hamartomatous polypoid masses of the vagina that are of interest to pathologists because of their inclination to show bizarre stromal cells that may be confused with embryonal rhabdomyosarcoma (52). The age at presentation ranges from 16 to 75 years, and while the majority of the lesions arise in the vagina, they may be found in the cervix and the vulva. The lesions are usually asymptomatic and discovered incidentally. They resemble an acrochordon and microscopically show a stratified squamous epithelium covering an edematous stroma with variable numbers of fibroblasts. The lesions often demonstrate marked hypercellularity, pleomorphism, mitotic counts of more than ten mitoses per ten high-power fields, and atypical mitoses. The immunolocalization of steroid receptors in these bizarre cells and the frequent relationship to pregnancy raise the possibility that these may be hormonally induced.

Miscellaneous Lesions

As with virtually all other soft tissue neoplasms, capillary and cavernous hemangiomas and lymphangiomas may occur in the lower female genitourinary tract and are similar to those in other anatomic sites. These lesions should be distinguished from entities such as Kaposi sarcoma (which may have a hemangioma-like appearance) and bacillary angiomatosis. Angiokeratomas are variants of hemangiomas that occur almost exclusively in the scrotum and the vulva. Histologically, the dilated vascular channels are separated by strands of squamous epithelial cells growing down from the overlying epithelium. This may be accompanied by various degrees of acanthosis and papillomatosis. Neurofibromas, leiomyomas, lipomas, granular cell tumors, hemangiopericytomas, inflammatory pseudotumors, nodular fasciitis, fibrous hamartoma of infancy, Langerhans cell histiocytosis, mastocytosis, cutaneous adnexal tumors, and alveolar soft part sarcoma have likewise been described (53).

Malignant Tumors of the Lower Female Genital Tract

Malignancies of the lower female genital tract are rare, with an incidence of about 0.5 cases per million female children per year. The majority of these malignancies (more than 80%) are sarcomas, most commonly rhabdomyosarcoma; approximately 10% are carcinomas and 5% extragonadal germ cell tumors.

Rhabdomyosarcoma

Embryonal rhabdomyosarcoma is the most common malignancy of the lower genital tract in girls. Although these lesions may arise in the vulva and the uterus, by far the most common genital site is the vagina. Most patients present before the age of 5 years, with a peak incidence between 1 and 2 years (54). Patients often present with vaginal bleeding or discharge, a palpable abdominal mass, or gross protrusion of a polypoid mass at the introitus. The site of origin is often the anterior vaginal wall, with extension into the bladder and the rectum. The initial size of the tumor has little prognostic significance (see Chapters 17 and 25).

The most common histologic appearance of female genital rhabdomyosarcomas is that of the botryoid embryonal subtype, with round-to-spindled cells of varying size in a loose, myxoid stroma (Figure 18-14). Eosinophilic cytoplasm may or may not be apparent, and cytoplasmic cross-striations may occasionally be seen. The tumor cells often crowd around blood vessels, and a cambium layer may be present with condensation of tumor cells beneath the vaginal epithelium. The myxoid stroma may in some cases be rather hypocellular, resulting in a tumor mass that may resemble a benign polyp. Rhabdomyosarcomas of the cervix provide a greater diagnostic challenge histologically owing to the presence of islands of mature metaplastic cartilage in more than 40% of the cases. This histologic manifestation appears to be unique to cervical rhabdomyosarcomas a DICER1-related neoplasm (54A). An uncommon histologic pattern in the genital tract is the diffuse form of embryonal rhabdomyosarcoma. The differential diagnosis of rhabdomyosarcoma in the female genital tract includes fibroepithelial polyps, müllerian papillomas, and rhabdomyomas. Immunohistochemical analysis in the diagnosis of embryonal rhabdomyosarcoma is discussed elsewhere (Chapter 25).

The clinical presentation and prognosis vary with the site of involvement. The majority of patients with vaginal rhabdomyosarcomas present before the age of 5, and the lesions are localized. These tumors are treated by chemotherapy, which provides a high overall survival rate. There is now a broad consensus that primary chemotherapy after an initial biopsy is the recommended therapeutic plan, followed by local excision (55). Rhabdomyosarcomas of the uterus and cervix are rare and have been considered to be distinct from those of the vagina, with a mean age of presentation of greater than 14 years and a seemingly better prognosis. However, more conservative management using preoperative chemotherapy and radiotherapy has resulted in increased survival in vaginal tumors.

Yolk Sac Tumor (Endodermal Sinus Tumor)

The lower female genital tract is one of the more common sites for extragonadal, nonsacral yolk sac tumor (YST). This is presumably due to abnormal migration of PGCs early in gestation; however, this does not explain the predilection for the vagina. These tumors present in children younger than 3 years of age, with the peak incidence between 8 and 11 months of age. Presenting symptoms usually include bloody vaginal discharge and a polypoid tumor filling the vagina. Microscopically, these tumors show the same histologic patterns as those seen in the sacral region, infantile testis, and ovary (Figure 18-15). Although reports before 1970 indicate an aggressive tumor with poor outcome, current chemotherapeutic regimens containing cyclophosphamide,

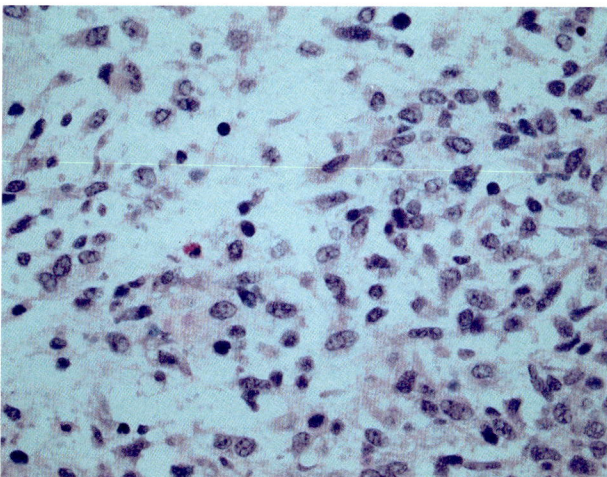

FIGURE 18-14 • Embryonal rhabdomyosarcoma of the genitourinary tract may be deceptively hypocellular, with inapparent cytoplasm.

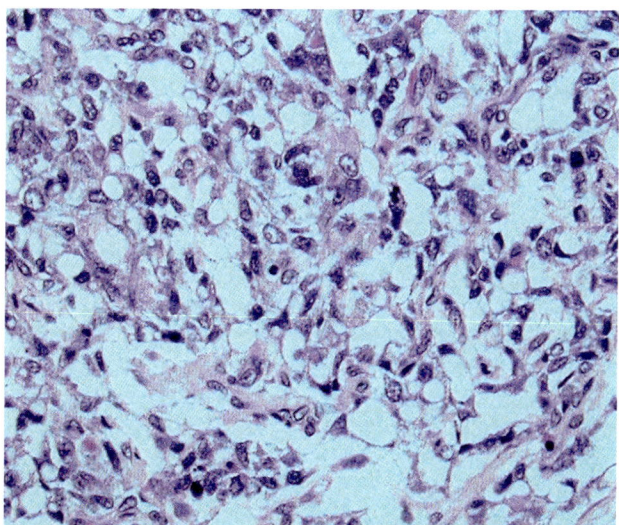

FIGURE 18-15 • YST of the vagina may demonstrate the entire histologic spectrum, similar to that seen in the ovary and testis. Many lack the characteristic Schiller-Duval bodies and other architectural features, such as the tumor illustrated. The histologic clues are the reticular pattern, the course chromatin, and the occasional cytoplasmic pink globules.

vincristine, and actinomycin have resulted in a 95% disease-free survival. Several reports of children treated only with chemotherapy with complete response suggest that surgery may not always be required (56).

OVARIAN NEOPLASMS

Ovarian neoplasms account for approximately 1% of all childhood cancers. Although the most common ovarian cancers in adults are epithelial, the distribution of histologic tumor types differs in children, with the majority being derived from PGCs (Table 18-2). Ovarian tumors are most frequently found from 10 to 14 years of age, suggesting that hormonal factors may play a role in many. The most common symptoms at presentation include abdominal pain that often simulates acute appendicitis, resulting in emergency laparotomy. Advances in the management of these tumors have led to increased cure rates as well as preservation of future fertility. Examples include new disease-specific chemotherapeutic regimens as well as the advent of surgical staging (Table 18-3).

Ovarian Germ Cell Tumors

The ovary is the site of approximately 30% of all germ cell tumors. Ovarian germ cell tumors are composed of both benign and malignant types. Ovarian germ cell tumors in children show a higher frequency of malignancy than those in adults. The vast majority are diagnosed in postpubertal adolescents. Germ cell tumors at extragonadal sites in females are more common in younger children, and malignant germ cell tumors in the ovaries of very young children are exceedingly rare. Ovarian germ cell tumors show a biologic and clinical heterogeneity not seen in their testicular or extragonadal counterparts, with at least four distinct subgroups. These include mature teratomas, immature teratomas, malignant germ cell tumors, and germ cell tumors arising in dysgenetic gonads. The molecular characteristics of each malignant ovarian germ cell tumor have recently been reviewed in detail (57,58).

Mature Teratoma

Teratomas are defined as benign neoplasms containing a haphazard growth of one or more types of tissue derived from the three embryonic layers (ectoderm, mesoderm, and

TABLE 18-2 RELATIVE FREQUENCY OF OVARIAN NEOPLASMS IN CHILDREN AND ADOLESCENTS

Histogenetic Category	No. (%)
Germ cell	205 (58)
Coelomic epithelium	67 (19)
Sex cord-stromal	62 (18)
Supportive stroma and miscellaneous	19 (5)
Total	353 (100)

TABLE 18-3 FEDERATION OF INTERNATIONAL GYNECOLOGISTS AND OBSTETRICIANS (FIGO) STAGING OF OVARIAN CARCINOMA (2014)

I. Tumor limited to ovaries
  A. Tumor limited to one ovary, capsule intact, no tumor on surface, negative washings
  B. Tumor limited to both ovaries; similar to IA
  C. Tumor limited to one or both ovaries
    IC1 Surgical spill
    IC2 Capsule rupture before surgery or tumor on ovarian surface
    IC3 Malignant cells in the ascites or peritoneal washings
II. Tumor involves one or both ovaries with pelvic extension (below the pelvic brim) or primary peritoneal cancer.
  A. Extension and/or implant on uterus and/or fallopian tubes
  B. Extension to other pelvic intraperitoneal tissues
III. Tumor involves one or both ovaries with cytologically or histologically confirmed spread to the peritoneum outside the pelvis and/or metastasis to the retroperitoneal lymph nodes.
  A1. Positive retroperitoneal lymph nodes only
    A1i. Metastasis ≤10mm
    A1ii. Metastasis >10mm
  A2. Microscopic, extrapelvic (above the brim) peritoneal involvement +/- positive retroperitoneal lymph nodes
  B. Macroscopic, extrapelvic, peritoneal metastasis ≤2 cm +/− positive retroperitoneal lymph nodes. Includes extension to capsule of liver/spleen
  C. Macroscopic, extrapelvic, peritoneal metastasis > 2 cm +/− positive retroperitoneal lymph nodes. Includes extension to capsule of liver/spleen
IV. Distant metastasis excluding peritoneal metastasis
  A. Pleural effusion with positive cytology
  B. Hepatic and/or splenic parenchymal metastasis, metastasis to extra-abdominal organs (including inguinal lymph nodes and lymph nodes outside of the abdominal cavity)

Zeppernick F, Meinhold-Heerlein I. The new FIGO staging system for ovarian, fallopian tube, and primary peritoneal cancer. *Arch Gynecol Obstet* 2014;290:839–842.

endoderm). Tumors predominantly arising from a single or two germ layers can also occur. Mature ovarian teratomas represent 40% to 60% of all childhood ovarian neoplasms, and patients with these tumors most commonly present at 13 to 15 years of age (59). There is a 10% incidence of bilaterality. Mature teratomas can be subdivided into those that are predominantly cystic and those that are predominately solid. Cystic teratomas characteristically contain copious hair and sebaceous material characteristic of those in adults; however,

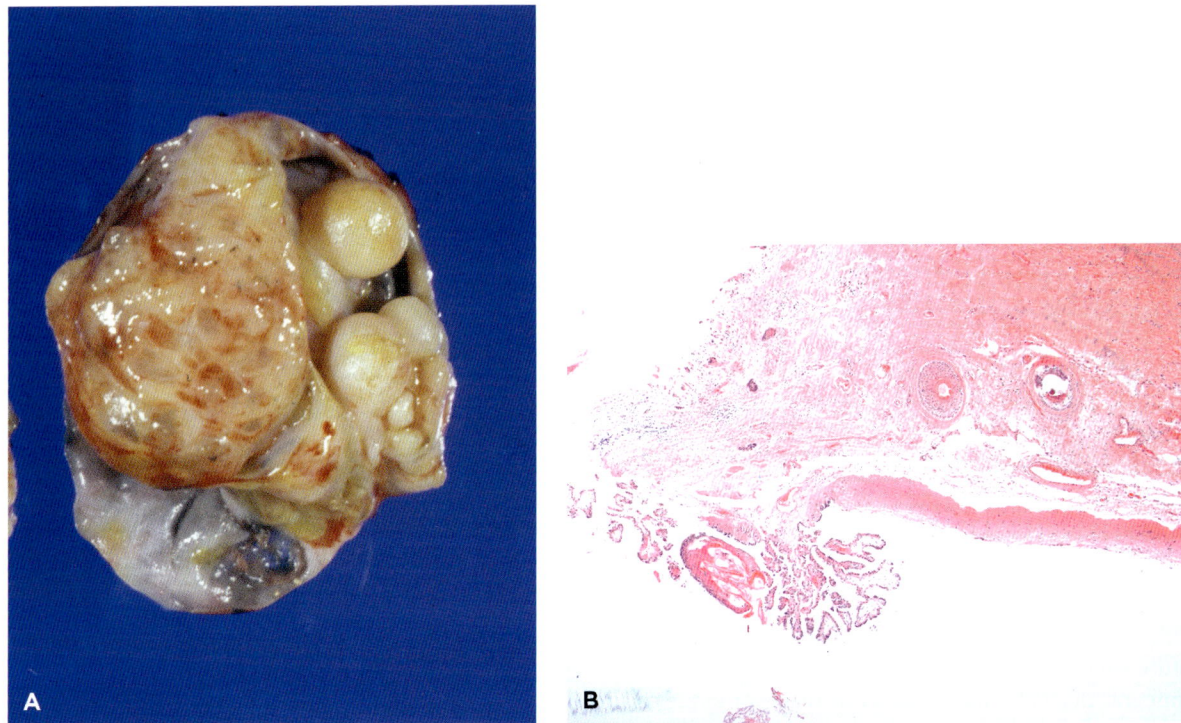

FIGURE 18-16 • Gross specimen of mature teratoma demonstrating multiple large and small cysts separated by heterogeneous solid nodules **(A)**. Microscopy reveals multiple well-differentiated tissue types, mostly ectodermal (skin, neural, and choroid plexus) in this photomicrograph (endoderm and mesoderm components were present on other slides) **(B)**.

this type is less common in children (Figure 18-16A, B). Immature elements are rarely found in predominantly cystic teratomas, and the malignant potential of cystic teratomas in children is minimal unless the child has a constitutional genetic abnormality resulting in increased risk of development of neoplasms (such as Li-Fraumeni syndrome). The solid mature teratoma, which is more common in children, may show a closer biologic relationship to immature teratomas than to cystic mature teratomas, and it should be carefully sectioned to exclude immature elements. Neuroglial tissue is the predominant component in these lesions.

The development of a somatic malignancy within a teratoma is a rare event in childhood. This malignant transformation is thought to occur within differentiated teratomatous elements rather than from totipotent embryonal cells. Within childhood ovarian teratomas, 7/246 tumors developed somatic malignancies (60). The types of nongerm cell malignancies most commonly encountered were epithelial, glial, and embryonal. Such nongerm cell malignancies are associated with a worse prognosis owing to poor response to therapy. In the past, these events were referred to as *teratocarcinoma* or *malignant teratoma*, terms that are confusing and best avoided.

Ovarian mature teratomas have been the most thoroughly studied biologically owing to their abundant numbers. More than 325 cases have been cytogenetically analyzed, demonstrating 95% to be karyotypically normal and the remainder to show nonrecurring numeric abnormalities (61). Studies of molecular loci show that the majority of mature ovarian teratomas have entered, but have not completed, meiosis (61). These studies suggest that mature ovarian teratomas arise from germ cells arrested in meiosis I.

Immature Teratoma

Immature teratomas (ITs) are the third most common germ cell tumor seen in the adolescent female ovary. These are considered to be of intermediate malignancy, a concept that is controversial. Although immature teratomas have rarely been reported to metastasize, those that do so almost invariably contain endodermal sinus tumor (EST) components in the original tumor. Small amounts of EST do not alter prognosis for IT if the amount of EST is less than 3 foci of less than 3 mm each. This raises the possibility that the metastasizing component is the EST, which subsequently undergoes differentiation. ITs are predominately unilateral solid tumors that may be quite large and are most often confined to the ovary. ITs can be graded histologically according to the quantity of immature elements, most commonly the quantity of immature neuroectoderm (Figure 18-17). Many variants of this grading system have been proposed; however, the differences between these systems are not substantive. Grade 1 lesions are those with immature neuroectoderm limited to rare low magnification fields, with not more than one field in any one slide. Grade 2 lesions contain immature neuroectoderm not exceeding three low-power fields (10× objective, with a 4× to 10× ocular for a total magnification of 40× to 100× per slide). Grade 3 tumors show extensive immature neural epithelium in more than three low-power fields

and cytology of YSTs vary widely, often causing difficulty in diagnosis (58,66,67). Several histologic subtypes of YST have been described; most tumors contain several subtypes, and none of these subtypes have prognostic implication (Figures 18-22, 18-23 to 18-24). The two most common are the endodermal sinus and microcystic (reticular) patterns. The endodermal sinus pattern consists of columnar tumor cells with ample clear to pink cytoplasm and hyperchromatic nuclei, often with a single small nucleolus, aligned in intertwined anastomosing glands and papillae. The microcystic pattern is composed of flat to cuboidal tumor cells with similar cytology lining loose collections of microcystic spaces. PAS-positive eosinophilic globules are frequently present in YSTs, especially in these two common histologic subtypes. The prototypic Schiller-Duval bodies of YST (Figure 18-24) are present in 50% to 75% of tumors. Syncytiotrophoblast-like cells are only rarely present. YSTs are commonly associated with highly elevated serum AFP levels, which may be monitored clinically for recurrence and/or metastasis. Aggressive monitoring of serum AFP levels constitutes one of the important improvements in the management of patients with germ cell tumor, particularly those with YST. The AFP should fall into the normal range 5 to 7 weeks following surgery if resection of the tumor is complete. By immunohistochemistry, tumor cells are positive for AFP, glypican-3 (cytoplasmic or membranous), and SALL4 (nuclear). YSTs can show variable positivity for CD117 or AE1/AE3. Negative stains include OCT4, CD30, EMA, and CK7. Rarely bilateral, YSTs are rapidly growing, yet most present as stage Ia tumors. YSTs are highly responsive to surgery and especially to combination chemotherapy, with patients with stage I disease having an overall survival of greater than 80%.

Other Histologic Types of Germ Cell Tumors

Pure *embryonal carcinomas* (EC) are rare ovarian neoplasms (4%) that should be differentiated from the more common YST. These are more commonly seen as a minor component

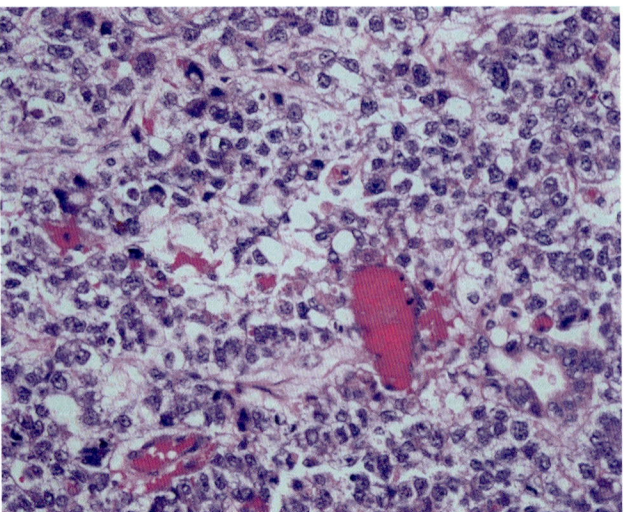

FIGURE 18-23 • Solid regions may be seen within YSTs; however, they are usually a minority component. The cells may contain large intracellular vacuoles. Hyaline bodies are occasionally seen.

of a mixed germ cell tumor. Like YSTs, embryonal carcinomas may show papillary, glandular, and solid areas. The cells are large, epithelioid, and often anaplastic with large nucleoli, abundant mitotic activity, hemorrhage, apoptosis, and necrosis (Figure 18-25). Syncytiotrophoblastic giant cells are usually present and produce hCG. Serum hCG levels are elevated in most patients with EC and its decrease can be monitored to measure response to therapy or to document possible relapse. ECs show immunoreactivity for cytokeratin AE1/AE3, but not for EMA, a feature that may help to distinguish EC from other epithelial neoplasms. A minority of embryonal carcinomas show focal, weak immunoreactivity for PLAP, as well as for AFP. It has been noted that embryonal carcinomas, but not other germ cell tumor histologic types, show immunopositivity for membranous CD30, a marker more conventionally utilized for Hodgkin lymphoma. Embryonal carcinomas are reliably positive for

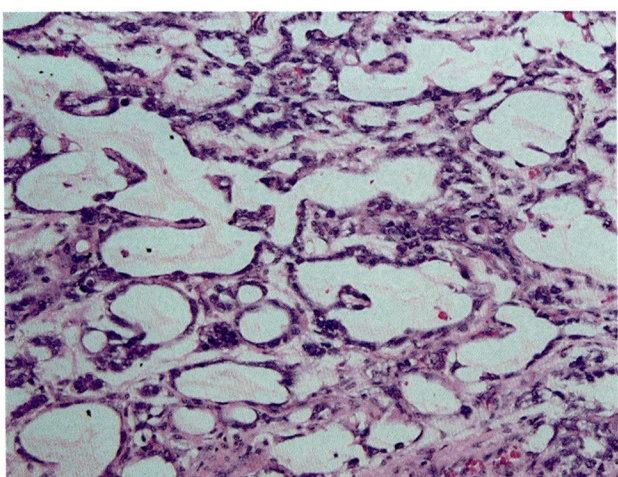

FIGURE 18-22 • YSTs often show a mixture of histologic types. The reticular pattern shows a network of communicating spaces.

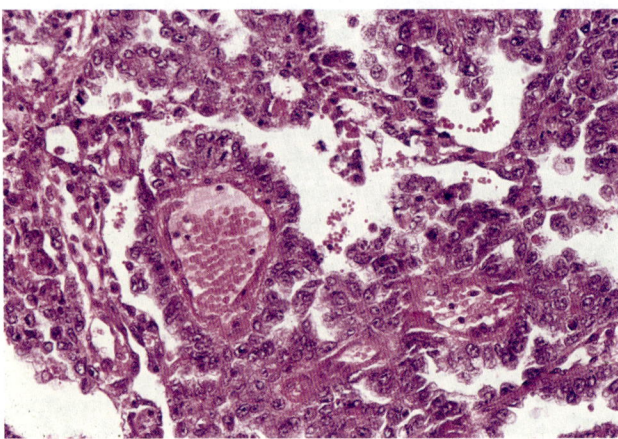

FIGURE 18-24 • Schiller-Duval bodies are present in many YSTs. These bodies are composed of a central vascular core lined by tumor cells, a space, and then an outer rim of tumor cells.

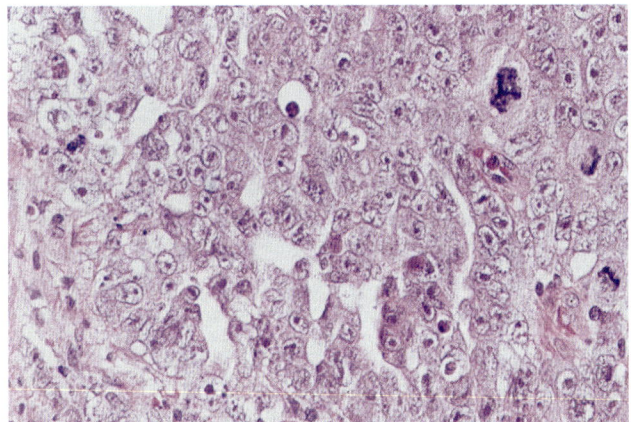

FIGURE 18-25 • Embryonal carcinoma is composed of large, overlapping nuclei with very large, prominent nucleoli and prominent individual cell necrosis. The cytoplasm is characteristically amphophilic.

OCT4, SALL4, and SOX2 and negative for CD117 and D2-40 (67). Treatment with surgery and chemotherapy yields long-term survival in greater than 90% of patients.

Ovarian choriocarcinoma is rarely seen as the sole histologic type but may constitute a minor component within a mixed germ cell tumor. Choriocarcinomas are composed of both medium-sized cytotrophoblastic tumor cells with abundant cytoplasm and vesicular nuclei with large nucleoli and multinucleated syncytiotrophoblastic cells with frequent evidence of hemorrhage (Figure 18-26). Immunohistochemical stains for hCG identify syncytiotrophoblastic cells, with unreliable staining of cytotrophoblasts. Both cell types are positive for cytokeratins. Trophoblast cells also stain positive for alpha-inhibin, glypican-3, and CD10. Treatment involves surgery and chemotherapy. Choriocarcinoma as part of mixed germ cell tumor responds poorly to the chemotherapy regimen used for gestational choriocarcinoma, thereby making distinction between these two forms of choriocarcinoma important in a young woman of childbearing age. DNA testing for paternal markers may be necessary.

The prognosis of nongerminomatous malignant germ cell tumors prior to the chemotherapy era was dismal. With the advent of bleomycin, etoposide, and cisplatin protocols, survival rates of 70% to 90% have been reported.

Genetic studies of malignant ovarian germ cell tumors involving normal gonads show no difference from their testicular counterparts. Most malignant ovarian germ cell tumors are aneuploid or near-tetraploid. Most contain the i(12p) by classic cytogenetics or amplification of 12p by comparative genomic hybridization (64,68). As previously mentioned, ESTs frequently develop in the context of immature teratomas. The biologic changes associated with this histologic transformation have not been established; however, ploidy analyses have suggested a genetic change is associated with the histologic transformation (57). The absence of the i(12p) in immature teratomas and the presence of the i(12p) in ESTs associated with immature teratomas suggest that one genetic change may be the acquisition of the i(12p) (57,64).

Gonadoblastoma

Gonadoblastoma is a rare "benign tumor" that arises in the dysgenetic gonads of phenotypic females having Y chromosomal material (90%). Gonadoblastomas are usually quite small and recognizable only on microscopic examination. The average age of diagnosis is 18 years and they can be bilateral in up to 40% of patients. Histologically, gonadoblastomas are characterized by nests containing both germ cells and sex cord–stromal cells of granulosa type, recently proven by strong nuclear FOXL2 staining and no staining for the Sertoli marker SOX9 (69) (Figures 18-27 and 18-28). These nests may be separated by stroma that often contains Leydig cells. Gonadoblastomas often show extensive hyalinization. A common feature is the presence of laminated calcific concretions. Numerous calcifications identified within a dysgerminoma should suggest the possibility that the patient

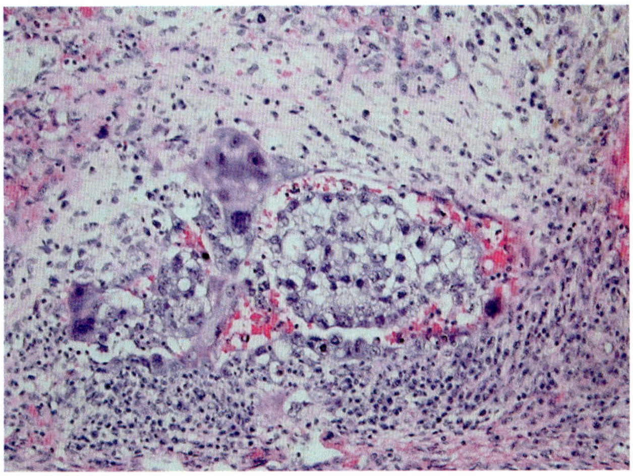

FIGURE 18-26 • Choriocarcinoma is composed of both multinucleate syncytiotrophoblastic cells and cytotrophoblastic cells. This histologic subtype can often be found associated with areas of hemorrhage.

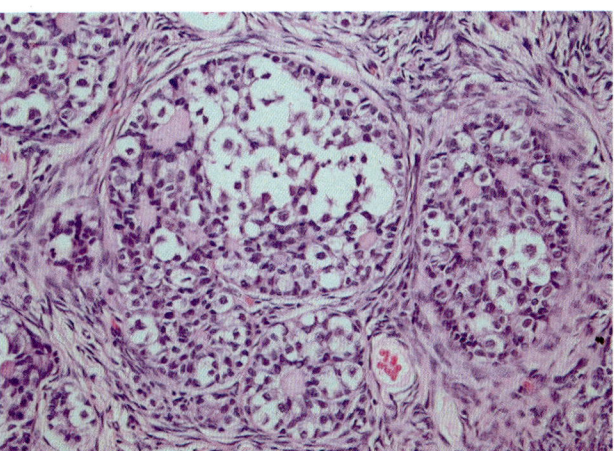

FIGURE 18-27 • Gonadoblastomas are seen as small nodules within streak gonads that contain eosinophilic hyaline bodies composed of basement membrane material. Calcifications are frequent.

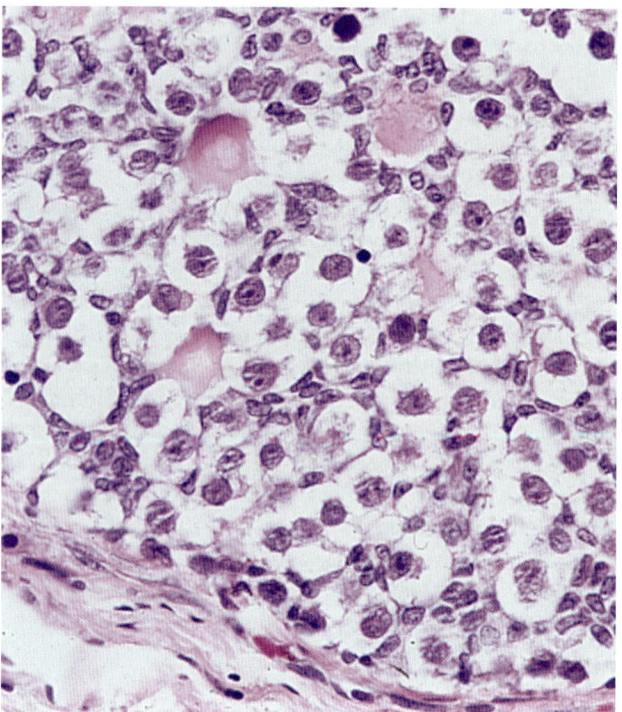

FIGURE 18-28 • Nodules of gonadoblastoma contain both germ cells and stromal cells, in varying proportions.

may have gonadal dysgenesis and may be at a high risk for developing a contralateral dysgerminoma. While dysgerminoma is the most common histologic subtype of malignancy following gonadoblastoma, YST and EC are also reported (35,58,70,71). Testis-specific protein Y encoded (TSPY) has been reported as a candidate gene involved in the development of gonadoblastoma (72). The germ cells express many of the same markers as dysgerminomas including OCT4, SALL4, NANOG, CD117, PLAP, and D2-40 as well as the TSPY protein. The stromal cells show positivity for inhibin, vimentin, SF1, FOXL2, and WT1.

Serologic Markers

Serum and CSF concentrations of AFP and hCG are useful as markers of some germ cell tumors. AFP is expressed at high levels by over 85% of YSTs and at lower levels in other histologic types. The predominant utility is for monitoring for recurrence or metastasis in AFP-secreting tumors. The half-life of AFP is 5 to 7 days. Other neoplastic and nonneoplastic disorders may result in elevation of AFP, for example, hepatitis, cirrhosis, and other malignancies. The beta subunit of hCG is secreted by the syncytiotrophoblastic cells of the placenta and thus is characteristically markedly elevated in choriocarcinomas. However, virtually all histologic subtypes of malignant germ cell tumors may show rare or scattered syncytiotrophoblastic cells that may result in mildly elevated hCG but do not indicate a worse prognosis. Elevations above 100 ng/mL are unusual and suggest the true presence of choriocarcinoma. The half-life of hCG is approximately 20 to 30 hours.

Hematologic Malignancies Associated with Germ Cell Tumors

The association between germ cell tumors and hematologic malignancy is well established but uncommon. The vast majority of germ cell tumors that subsequently develop hematologic malignancies are malignant mediastinal germ cell tumors in men (73). The associated hematologic abnormalities have included erythroleukemia, histiocytic sarcoma, acute nonlymphocytic leukemia, myelodysplasia, and systemic mast cell disease. Three ovarian germ cell tumors have been reported in association with hematologic abnormalities; two of these were in 46,XY phenotypic females. The median interval between the diagnosis of the germ cell tumor and that of the hematologic malignancy is 6 months, much shorter than the 25- to 60-month interval commonly seen in chemotherapy-related hematologic malignancies. Primary resections of germ cell tumors that show proliferating hematopoietic cells should raise the suspicion of an associated hematologic abnormality; however, more often this process is not detected at the initial resection.

Ovarian Sex Cord–Stromal Tumors

In addition to germ cells, the ovary is populated by granulosa cells, theca cells, interstitial (hilus) cells, and stromal fibroblasts. Each of these components may give rise to a neoplasm, and such lesions are grouped together as sex cord–stromal tumors. They account for 10% of all ovarian neoplasms in children and adolescents. Most are composed of ovarian cell types, but some contain only elements of testicular type (such as Sertoli cell tumors). Precocious puberty and virilization are the major clinical manifestations. Before 9 years of age, most sex cord–stromal tumors are feminizing, and after 9 years of age, there is a predominance of virilizing neoplasms. On occasion, it may be difficult or impossible to accurately identify a lesion as a stromal tumor or to determine to which of the stromal tumor categories a tumor belongs. Younger age and early-stage disease are important predictors for improved survival in patients with ovarian sex cord–stromal tumors (74). Immunohistochemistry has been used to verify the diagnosis of sex cord–stromal tumors. Inhibin, calretinin, and CD99 are useful markers that positively mark the majority of sex cord–stromal tumors, while most are negative for epithelial membrane antigen (75).

Juvenile granulosa cell tumor (JGCT) constitutes the most common type of functioning ovarian neoplasm. Although these are commonly composed almost entirely of granulosa cells, they may also contain theca cells or fibroblasts singly or in any combination. Fewer than 10% of all granulosa cell tumors are diagnosed in the first two decades of life. The majority (80% to 85%) of granulosa cell tumors in children are histologically and genetically distinct from the adult-type granulosa cell tumors (AGCTs) described later. JGCTs typically present with precocious pseudopuberty or virilization in a child younger than 10 years old, although infants and elderly patients have been reported (76). A few cases have been associated with Ollier disease, Potter

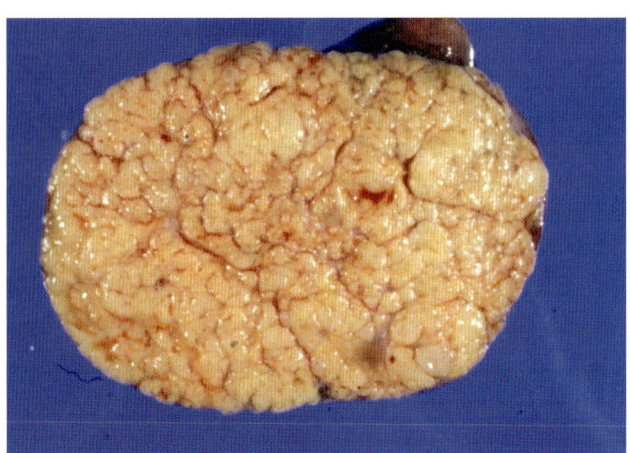

FIGURE 18-29 • JGCT in a 7-year-old girl who presented with precocious puberty and a pelvic mass.

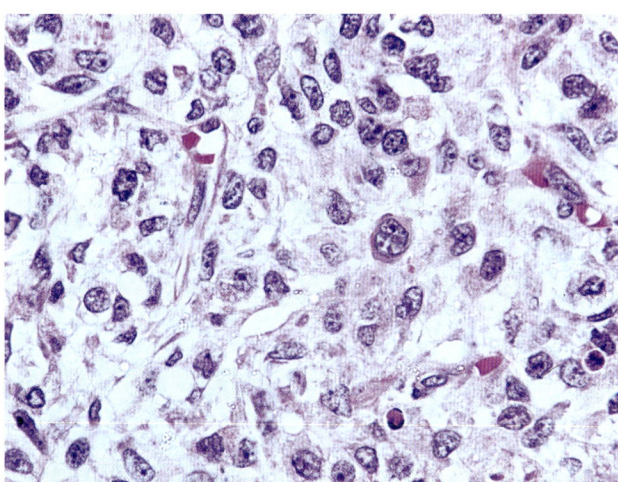

FIGURE 18-31 • JGCT of the ovary with ovoid-to-elliptical cells with pale eosinophilic cytoplasm and polygonal cells with clear cytoplasm are found in the nodules. Nuclear atypia and mitoses are often present.

syndrome, Maffucci syndrome, and other forms of dysmorphisms and more recently in patients with germ-line mutations in *DICER1*. Grossly, JGCTs are solid with fibrous bands separating yellow nodules and are usually confined to the ovary (Figure 18-29). Microscopically, JGCTs have a rather complex growth pattern with nodules of incompletely luteinized cells. Follicles may be present that are irregular and resemble large graafian follicles (Figure 18-30). The luminal contents contain mucicarmine-positive secretions. The stromal cells resemble fibroblasts or have polygonal outlines and pale cytoplasm containing abundant lipid (Figure 18-31). Luteinization is commonly greater, and the nuclei are more hyperchromatic and immature than those in the AGCTs. Call-Exner bodies are not a feature of these tumors, and the nuclear grooves typical of AGCTs are infrequent. Mitotic activity and nuclear atypia are often present and are more pronounced than that seen in AGCTs, resulting in their frequent misdiagnosis as malignant germ cell tumors (Figure 18-31). JGCTs lack the FOXL2 mutation seen in over 90% of AGCTs. Immunohistochemical studies reveal that the tumor cells are positive for inhibin, calretinin, FOXL2, SF1, CD56, CD99, and often WT1 and vimentin. Variable staining for low molecular weight keratins is reported. JGCTs are negative for EMA. Histologic distinction of JGCT from small cell carcinoma of the ovary can be difficult, but small cell carcinoma is usually EMA positive and inhibin and CD99 negative. Although JGCTs commonly present as stage 1, it is not uncommon for these tumors to rupture (76). Low-stage tumors have an excellent prognosis; however, the outcome for patients with nonconfined tumors may be poor. Although the AGCT has a local recurrence of 20%, 92% of patients with JGCTs are free of disease following surgical removal. However, those that recur tend to do so within 3 years and have a rapid course. The benefits from adjuvant chemotherapy or radiotherapy are limited (75,76).

Adult-type granulosa cell tumors (AGCTs) may also occur in the first two decades of life. These tumors are characterized by rounded follicles of varying sizes, minimal luteinization, and rare mitoses. The most differentiated forms show Call-Exner bodies, which consist of granulosa cells in a radial arrangement around a small cystic cavity containing a central rounded mass of eosinophilic material. AGCTs may demonstrate a wide range of histologic appearances, which are commonly mixed within a single specimen, often making their diagnosis a challenge. Different patterns include microfollicular, macrofollicular, trabecular, insular solid-tubular, diffuse (sarcomatous), and luteinized. Some show branching columns of cells, whereas others are more diffuse; all show characteristic nuclear grooves (Figure 18-32). Over 90% of AGCTs have a mutation in FOXL2 (9,77,78). Immunohistochemical expression pattern is similar to JGCTs. These tumors are commonly estrogenic and may cause endometrial hyperplasia and carcinoma in 5% to 25% of women of reproductive age. Serum markers include inhibin, AMH, and estradiol. Most tumors are confined to the ovary at presentation, and surgery is the treatment of choice. Higher-stage tumors or those that recur have a dismal prognosis due to poor response to chemotherapy.

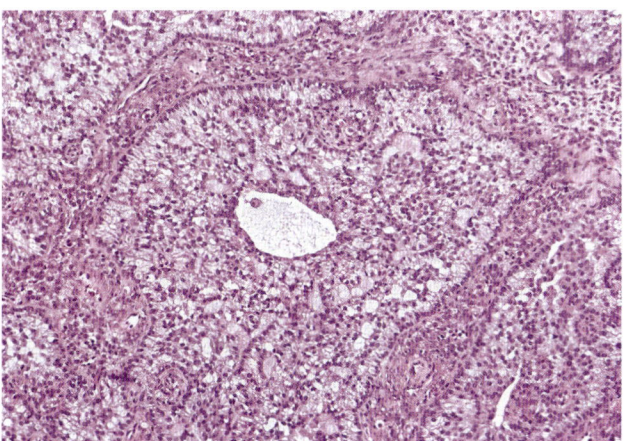

FIGURE 18-30 • JGCT of the ovary showing a smaller cyst lined by clear cells and resembling a large, irregular graafian follicle.

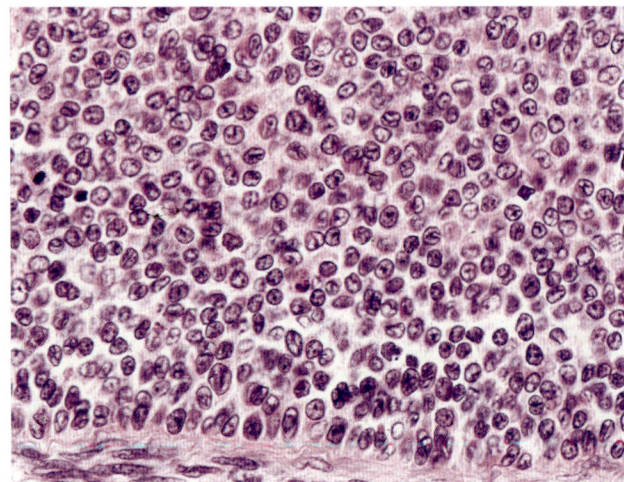

FIGURE 18-32 • AGCTs at times show a predominately solid pattern, which may cause diagnostic difficulty. However, the prominent nuclear groves are seen in all tumors.

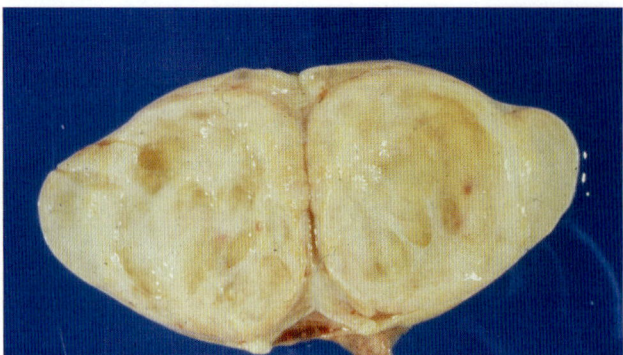

FIGURE 18-34 • Sclerosing stromal tumors show pseudolobulation at low power due to areas with differing cellularity, collagen, and edema.

Sex cord tumors with annular tubules (SCTATs) are distinctive ovarian neoplasms of unknown origin with morphologic features intermediate between granulosa cell tumor and Sertoli cell tumor. SCTATs demonstrate multifocal cortical stromal tumors that contain epithelial nests with single or multiple PAS-positive hyaline bodies, representing annular tubules (Figure 18-33). These bodies may resemble the hyaline bodies seen in gonadoblastomas; however, the cells of the annular tubules have more abundant, pale, and vacuolated cytoplasm and lack germ cells. The tumor cells are positive for inhibin, calretinin, vimentin, WT1, SF1, CD56, and cytokeratins but negative for EMA. Hyperestrinism is common. Approximately one-third of patients with SCTATs have Peutz-Jeghers syndrome. Occasional metastases of nonsyndromic SCTATs have been reported. The treatment of choice is surgery (79).

Sclerosing stromal tumors are rare benign neoplasms that most commonly present in younger women (14 to 19 years of age) with irregular menses and abdominal pain (80). Occasionally, these tumors present with Meigs syndrome.

Grossly, the tumors are unilateral, firm, and gray to white; areas of edema, necrosis, and cystic degeneration are common (Figure 18-34). Microscopic features include spindled cells arranged in lobules separated by edematous stroma. Polygonal cells are scattered among the spindle cells and may have signet ringlike features; however, these cells contain oil red O–positive lipid and not mucin (Figure 18-35). These tumors yield positive immunohistochemical staining for vimentin, calretinin, inhibin, melan-A, SF1, and FOXL2. Associated myoid cells are positive for SMA and desmin. Steroid hormone receptors may also be detected. None of these tumors has behaved in a malignant fashion.

Sertoli cell tumors of the ovary are exceedingly rare in children. These tumors are composed of Sertoli cells with the predominant pattern being tubular, with a minority of tumors demonstrating retiform or diffuse patterns. Immunohistochemical staining for vimentin, cytokeratin, inhibin, calretinin, CD99, WT1, and SF1 is usually present. The tumor cells are negative for EMA. Interestingly, only about 50% of tumors will show positive nuclear staining for the Sertoli-specific marker SOX9. The tumors are most often virilizing but may produce estrogen. Only about 10% will behave in a malignant manner. Surgery is the treatment of choice (81).

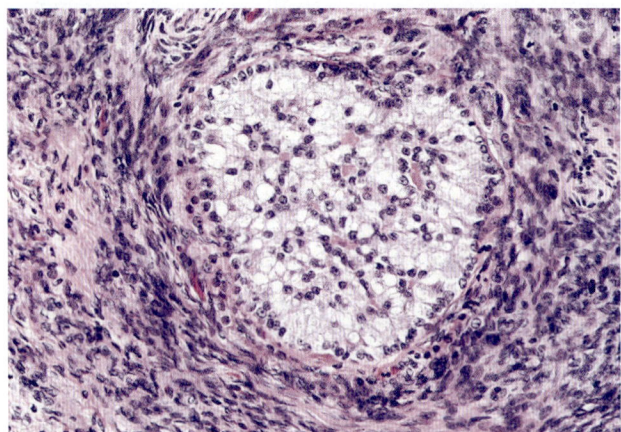

FIGURE 18-33 • Sex cord tumor with annular tubules is composed of rounded epithelial units containing cells with abundant eosinophilic cytoplasm that surrounds multiple hyaline bodies.

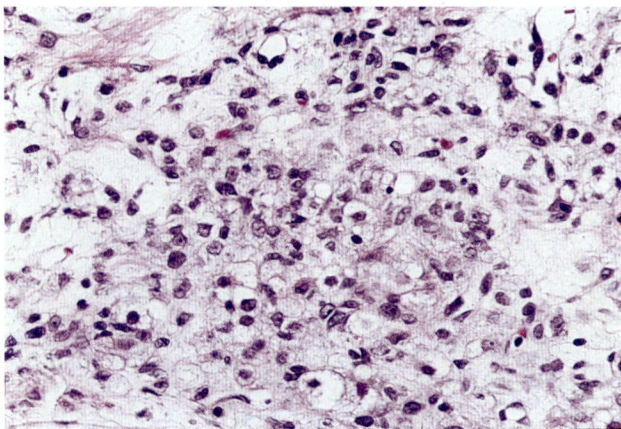

FIGURE 18-35 • Sclerosing stromal tumors are composed of an admixture of spindle cells forming collagen and lipid-laden theca-like cells with shrunken nuclei.

Sertoli-Leydig cell tumors contain various proportions of Sertoli, Leydig, and indifferent stromal cells, often similar to that seen in various phases of testicular development. These represent only 0.5% of ovarian neoplasms and are the most commonly virilizing of all ovarian tumors (79,82). They are the second most common sex cord–stromal tumor in children after JGCTs. Half have symptoms of androgen excess or virilization, but a few have estrogenic manifestations. Survival is excellent, with tumor-related deaths in only 5%, likely due to the fact that they are stage I at presentation in over 97% of patients (82). Sertoli-Leydig cell tumors have been classified on the basis of degree of differentiation and the presence or absence of heterologous elements. The well-differentiated or pure Sertoli cell tumors are the least common. These are composed of well-developed tubules or solid cords of cells with or without Leydig cells. Intermediate tumors comprise poorly formed tubules in a cellular stroma with a nodular or a diffuse configuration (Figure 18-36). Poorly differentiated or sarcomatoid tumors are composed of undifferentiated mesenchyme, poorly formed cords of Sertoli cells, and a paucity of Leydig cells. Sertoli-Leydig cell tumors with heterologous elements comprise 25% of all Sertoli-Leydig cell tumors and may contain cysts or glands with intestinal-type mucosa, carcinoid tumor, rhabdomyoblasts, cartilage, or neuroblastoma. These seem to be more common in Sertoli-Leydig cell tumors of younger patients and may be difficult to distinguish from immature teratomas. The retiform pattern has received increased attention due to the younger age at presentation (median age of 15 years), and they often lack androgenic manifestations, increasing the risk of misdiagnosis. Occasional retiform Sertoli-Leydig cell tumors may be associated with elevated serum levels of AFP. The Sertoli cells are usually positive for cytokeratins, CD99, WT1, CD56, SF1, and steroid receptors but negative for EMA. The Leydig and stromal cells stain for vimentin. Both the Leydig cells and Sertoli cells are positive for inhibin and calretinin. Most tumors are confined to the ovary at diagnosis. Poor prognostic factors include tumor rupture or spread outside the ovary, poorly differentiated histology with increased stromal mitoses, and heterologous elements. Surgical removal is the current treatment and chemotherapy may be beneficial in those patients with recurrence. Overall 5-year survival exceeds 90% even in intermediate and poorly differentiated tumors (75,83–85). These tumors occur with increased incidence in patients with germ-line DICER1 mutations.

Rare Tumors

A few examples of mixed germ cell–sex cord–stromal tumors have been described but are quite rare. Thecomas and fibromas are very rare in children and predominantly affect older women. Other abdominal soft tissue tumors have presented in the ovary, including desmoplastic small round cell tumor, peripheral neuroectodermal tumors, and alveolar soft part sarcoma, to name a few. Adenomatoid tumors are also very rare in the ovary.

Epithelial Neoplasms

While previously thought to arise from the surface epithelium of the ovary, ovarian epithelial neoplasms are now proposed to arise from Müllerian structures (86,87). Low- and high-grade serous neoplasms are proposed to arise from fallopian tube epithelium, endometrioid, and clear cell carcinoma from endometriosis resulting from retrograde menstruation, and mucinous and transitional cell neoplasms may arise from the endocervical epithelium. These tumors comprise about 15% of ovarian neoplasms of patients younger than 20 years of age, and in this population, they occur after menarche and are virtually exclusively mucinous or serous, with mucinous tumors comprising the majority (77%). The majority are unilateral and benign; approximately 15% are malignant. The pathologic categorization of these epithelial lesions is based on an evaluation of epithelial proliferative changes. These subgroups are benign, atypically proliferating ("borderline" tumors), and malignant. The intermediate group is defined as showing greater proliferation (including epithelial budding and nuclear stratification, mitotic activity, and nuclear atypia) but showing no destructive invasion of the stromal component. The criteria for inclusion into the intermediate group, and the nomenclature used, remain controversial (88,89).

Serous neoplasms are usually composed of multiple cysts with watery and clear contents. Characteristic is the presence of nodular papillary excrescences scattered over the lining of the cysts. These may be few and barely visible or numerous. Microscopically, the cysts are lined by papillary processes covered by a single layer of columnar-to-cuboidal cells (Figure 18-37). Intermediate neoplasms show more extensive and complex papillary patterns with stratification of the epithelial lining. The neoplastic cells show loss of polarity, nuclear pleomorphism, and increased mitotic activity. Most

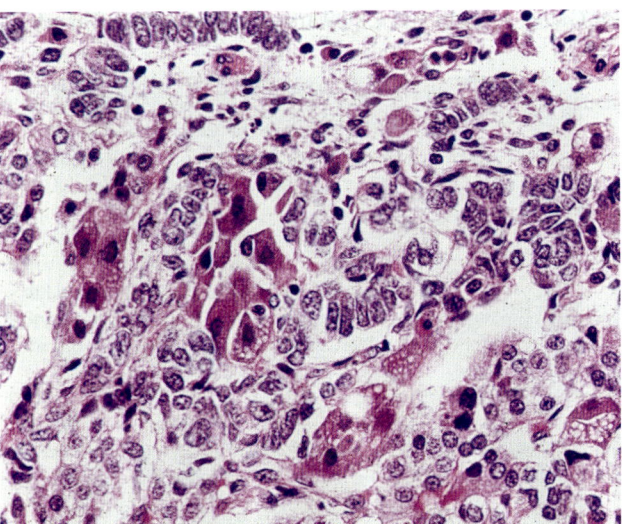

FIGURE 18-36 • Sertoli-Leydig cell tumor composed of irregular poorly formed tubules and cords lined by cells containing moderate amounts of cytoplasm; occasional clusters of Leydig cells demonstrating atypia and eosinophilic cytoplasm are seen.

45. Zachariou Z, Roth H, Boos R, et al. Three years' experience with large ovarian cysts diagnosed in utero. *J Pediatr Surg* 1989;24:478–482.
46. Bremer AA. Polycystic ovary syndrome in the pediatric population. *Metab Syndr Relat Disord* 2010;8:375–394.
47. Dewailly D, Lujan ME, Carmina E, et al. Definition and significance of polycystic ovarian morphology: a task force report from the Androgen Excess and Polycystic Ovary Syndrome Society. *Hum Reprod Update* 2014;20:334–352.
48. Yilmaz Y, Turkyilmaz Z, Sonmez K, et al. Massive ovarian oedema in adolescents. *Acta Chir Belg* 2005;105:106–109.
49. Virgili A, Marzola A, Corazza M. Vulvar hidradenoma papilliferum: a review of 10.5 years' experience. *J Reprod Med* 2000;45:616–618.
50. Iwasa Y, Fletcher CDM. Distinctive prepubertal vulvar fibroma. A hitherto unrecognized mesenchymal tumor of prepubertal girls: analysis of 11 cases. *Am J Surg Pathol* 2004;28:1601–1608.
51. Mierau GW, Lovell MA, Wyatt-Ashmead J, et al. Benign Mullerian papilloma of childhood. *Ultrastruct Pathol* 2005;29:209–216.
52. Nucci MR, Young RH, Fletcher CD. Cellular pseudosarcomatous fibroepithelial stromal polyps of the lower female genital tract: an underrecognized lesion often misdiagnosed as sarcoma. *Am J Surg Pathol* 2000;24:231–240.
53. Baker GM, Selim MA, Hoang MP. Vulvar adnexal lesions. A 32-year, single institution review from Massachusetts General Hospital. *Arch Pathol Lab Med* 2013;137:1237–1246.
54. Leuschner I, Harms D, Mattke A, et al. Rhabdomyosarcoma of the urinary bladder and vagina: a clinicopathologic study with emphasis on recurrent disease—a report from the Kiel Pediatric Tumor Registry and the German CWS Study. *Am J Surg Pathol* 2001;25:856–864.
54a. Dehner LP, Jarzembowski JA, Hill DA. Embryonal rhabdomyosarcoma of the uterine cervix: a report of 14 cases and a discussion of its unusual clinicopathological associations. *Mod Pathol* 2012;25:602-614.
55. Walterhouse DO, Meza JL, Breneman JC, et al. Local control and outcome in children with localized vaginal rhabdomyosarcoma: a report from the Soft Tissue Sarcoma Committee of the Children's Oncology Group. *Pediatr Blood Cancer* 2011;57:76–83.
56. Lacy J, Capra M, Allen L. Endodermal sinus tumor of the infant vagina treated exclusively with chemotherapy. *J Pediatr Hematol Oncol* 2006;28:768–771.
57. Kraggerud SM, Hoei-Hansen CE, Alagaratnam S, et al. Molecular characteristics of malignant ovarian germ cell tumors and comparison with testicular counterparts: implications for pathogenesis. *Endocr Rev* 2013;34:339–376.
58. Mosbech CH, Rechnitzer C, Brok JS, et al. Recent advances in understanding the etiology and pathogenesis of pediatric germ cell tumors. *J Pediatr Hematol Oncol* 2014;36:263–270.
59. De Backer A, Madern GC, Oosterhuis JW, et al. Ovarian germ cell tumors in children: a clinical study of 66 patients. *Pediatr Blood Cancer* 2006;46:459–464.
60. Biskup W, Calaminus G, Schneider DT, et al. Teratoma with malignant transformation: experiences of the cooperative GPOH protocols MAKEI 83/86/89/96. *Klin Padiatr* 2006;218:303–308.
61. Surti U, Hoffner L, Chakravarti A, et al. Genetics and biology of human ovarian teratomas. I. Cytogenetic analysis and mechanism of origin. *Am J Hum Genet* 1990;47:635–643.
62. O'Connor DM, Norris HJ. The influence of grade on the outcome of stage I ovarian immature (malignant) teratomas and the reproducibility of grading. *Int J Gynecol Pathol* 1994;13:283–289.
63. Lu KH, Gershenson DM. Update on the management of ovarian germ cell tumors. *J Reprod Med* 2005;50:417–425.
64. Riopel MA, Spellerberg A, Griffin CA, et al. Genetic analysis of ovarian germ cell tumors by comparative genomic hybridization. *Cancer Res* 1998;58:3105–3110.
65. Ferguson AW, Katabuchi H, Ronnett BM, et al. Glial implants in gliomatosis peritonei arise from normal tissue, not from the associated teratoma. *Am J Pathol* 2001;159:51–55.
66. Ulbright TM. Germ cell tumors of the gonads: a selective review emphasizing problems in differential diagnosis, newly appreciated, and controversial issues. *Mod Pathol* 2005;18:S61–S79.
67. Nogales FF, Dulcey I, Preda O. Germ cell tumors of the ovary. An update. *Arch Pathol Lab Med* 2014;138:351–362.
68. Hoffner L, Deka R, Chakravarti A. Cytogenetics and origins of pediatric germ cell tumors. *Cancer Genet Cytogenet* 1994;74:54–58.
69. Buell-Gutbrod R, Ivanovic M, Montag A, et al. FOXL2 and SOX9 distinguish the lineage of the sex cord-stromal cells in gonadoblastomas. *Pediatr Dev Pathol* 2011;14:391–395.
70. Pena-Alonso R, Nieto K, Alvarez R, et al. Distribution of Y-chromosome-bearing cells in gonadoblastoma and dysgenetic testis in 45,X/46,XY infants. *Mod Pathol* 2005;18:439–445.
71. Bergeron MB, Lemieux N, Brochu P. Undifferentiated gonadal tissue, Y chromosome instability, and tumors in XY gonadal dysgenesis. *Pediatr Dev Pathol* 2011;14:445–459.
72. Hertel JD, Huettner PC, Dehner LP, et al. The chromosome Y-linked testis-specific protein locus TSPY1 is characteristically present in gonadoblastoma. *Hum Pathol* 2010;41:1544–1549.
73. Nichols CR, Roth BJ, Heerema N, et al. Hematologic neoplasia associated with primary mediastinal germ-cell tumors. *N Engl J Med* 1990;322:1425–1429.
74. Zhang M, Cheung MK, Shin JY, et al. Prognostic factors responsible for survival in sex cord stromal tumors of the ovary: an analysis of 376 women. *Gynecol Oncol* 2007;104:396–400.
75. Schneider DT, Janig U, Calaminus G, et al. Ovarian sex cord-stromal tumors—a clinicopathological study of 72 cases from the Kiel Pediatric Tumor Registry. *Virchow's Arch* 2003;443:549–560.
76. Young RH, Dickersin GR, Scully RE. Juvenile granulosa cell tumor of the ovary: a clinicopathological analysis of 125 cases. *Am J Surg Pathol* 1984;8:575–596.
77. Shah SP, Kobel M, Senz J, et al. Mutation of FOXL2 in granulosa-cell tumors of the ovary. *N Engl J Med* 2009;360:2719–2729.
78. D'Angelo E, Mozos A, Nakayama D, et al. Prognostic significance of FOXL2 mutation and mRNA expression in adult and juvenile granulosa cell tumors of the ovary. *Mod Pathol* 2011;24:1360–1367.
79. Roth LM. Recent advances in the pathology and classification of ovarian sex cord-stromal tumors. *Int J Gynecol Pathol* 2006;25:199–215.
80. Saitoh A, Tsutsumi Y, Osamura RY, et al. Sclerosing stromal tumor of the ovary: immunohistochemical and electron-microscopic demonstration of smooth-muscle differentiation. *Arch Pathol Lab Med* 1989;113:372–376.
81. Oliva E, Alvarez T, Young RH. Sertoli cell tumors of the ovary: a clinicopathologic and immunohistochemical study of 54 cases. *Am J Surg Pathol* 2005;29:143–156.
82. Young RH, Scully RE. Ovarian Sertoli-Leydig cell tumors: a clinicopathological analysis of 207 cases. *Am J Surg Pathol* 1985;9:543–569.
83. Gui T, Cao D, Shen K, et al. A clinicopathological analysis of 40 cases of ovarian Sertoli-Leydig cell tumors. *Gynecol Oncol* 2012;127:384–389.
84. Cecchetto G, Ferrari A, Bernini G, et al. Sex cord stromal tumors of the ovary in children: a clinicopathological report from the Italian TREP project. *Pediatr Blood Cancer* 2011;56:1062–1067.
85. Schneider DT, Calaminus G, Harms D, et al. Ovarian sex cord-stromal tumors in children and adolescents. *J Reprod Med* 2005;50:439–446.
86. Kurman RJ, Shih IM. Molecular pathogenesis and extraovarian origin of epithelial ovarian cancer—shifting the paradigm. *Hum Pathol* 2011;42:918–931.
87. Nik NN, Vang R, Shih IM, et al. Origin and pathogenesis of pelvic (ovarian, tubal and primary peritoneal) serous carcinoma. *Ann Rev Pathol Mech Dis* 2014;9:27–45.
88. Grapsa D, Kairi-Vassilatou E, Kleanthis C, et al. Epithelial ovarian tumors in adolescents: a retrospective pathologic study and critical review of the literature. *J Pediatr Adolesc Gynecol* 2011;24:386–388.
89. Hazard FK, Longacre TA. Ovarian surface epithelial neoplasms in the pediatric population. *Am J Surg Pathol* 2013;37:548–553.
90. Hart WR. Mucinous tumors of the ovary: a review. *Int J Gynecol Pathol* 2004;24:4–25.
91. Riopel MA, Ronnett BM, Kurman RJ. Evaluation of diagnostic criteria and behavior of ovarian intestinal-type mucinous tumors: atypical proliferative (borderline) tumors and intraepithelial, microinvasive, invasive, and metastatic carcinomas. *Am J Surg Pathol* 1999;23:617–635.

92. Tagawa T, Morgan R, Yen Y, et al. Ovarian cancer: opportunity for targeted therapy. *J Oncol* 2012;2012:682480.
93. Harrison ML, Hoskins P, du BA, et al. Small cell of the ovary, hypercalcemic type: analysis of combined experience and recommendation for management. A GCIG study. *Gynecol Oncol* 2006;100:233–238.
94. Young RH, Oliva E, Scully RE. Small cell carcinoma of the ovary, hypercalcemic type: a clinicopathological analysis of 150 cases. *Am J Surg Pathol* 1994;18:1102–1116.
95. Clement PB. Selected miscellaneous ovarian lesions: small cell carcinomas, mesothelial lesions, mesenchymal and mixed neoplasms, and non-neoplastic lesions. *Mod Pathol* 2005;18:S113–S129.
96. Distelmaier F, Calaminus G, Harms D, et al. Ovarian small cell carcinoma of the hypercalcemic type in children and adolescents: a prognostically unfavorable but curable disease. *Cancer* 2006;107: 2298–2306.
97. Penson RT, Dizon DS, Birrer MJ. Clear cell cancer of the ovary. *Curr Opin Oncol* 2013;25:553–557.
98. del Carmen MG, Birrer M, Schorge JO. Clear cell carcinoma of the ovary: a review of the literature. *Gynecol Oncol* 2012;126:481–490.
99. DeLair D, Oliva E, Kobel M, et al. Morphologic spectrum of immunohistochemically characterized clear cell carcinoma of the ovary: a study of 155 cases. *Am J Surg Pathol* 2011;35:36–44.

CHAPTER 19

The Male Reproductive System, Including Intersex Disorders

Hikmat A. Al-Ahmadie, M.D., and Rohit Mehra, M.D.

THE TESTIS

Testicular Development and Disorders

Normal sexual development and differentiation are the result of a complex interplay of genetic, molecular, and endocrine factors necessary for the development of the genitourinary system including the kidneys as well as the adrenals. Embryologically, the urogenital ridges appear at around the 4th week of gestation and are initially devoid of germ cells. By the 5th week, primordial germ cells have migrated to the genital ridge and are arranged into the seminiferous cords. Up to the 6th week, both male and female gonads appear relatively similar. By the 7th week of gestation, the testes are formed with recognizable short, straight cellular tubules and are functioning with the synthesis of anti-müllerian hormone (AMH), müllerian inhibiting substance, or müllerian inhibiting factor (MIF) by the Sertoli cells, which develop from the somatic sex cord cells and subsequently the synthesis of testosterone by the Leydig cells, which develop from the intercordal gonadal mesenchyme in the 8th week (1,2). The intercordal mesenchyme is composed of cells that migrate from the mesonephric stroma and eventually differentiate into testicular stromal cells, and blood vessels in addition to Leydig cells. The produced hormones are essential as AMH plays a major role in the process of regression of the müllerian ducts, whereas testosterone is crucial for the differentiation of the wolffian ducts, which develop into the epididymis, vas deferens, and seminal vesicles. The rete testis develops from the mesonephric remnants in proximity to the seminiferous cords. Development of a dense fibrous tunica albuginea in the 8th week of gestation is definitive for testis formation. Testosterone synthesis peaks at 12 to 16 weeks of gestation, allowing for male secondary sexual development (3). The remaining structures of the male genital system are derived from the urogenital sinus through the differentiation of the endoderm-derived epithelium into prostate, urethra, bulbourethral, and periurethral glands. In contrast, the wolffian duct derivatives are of mesodermal origin. The differentiation of the wolffian ducts occurs under the influence of testosterone secreted by the ipsilateral testis. The differentiation of the urogenital sinus into male external genitalia occurs under the influence of dihydrotestosterone (DHT), which is derived from testosterone by enzymatic conversion by 5α-reductase. Two additional hormones, FSH (follicle-stimulating hormone) and LH (luteinizing hormone), play important roles in the development of the male genital system mainly in the last months of gestation, regulating androgen production and Sertoli cell activity (4,5). The actions and the timing of these hormones are closely and precisely coordinated during development (6). After birth, the testis continues to develop until puberty with changes affecting all testicular components until puberty.

Chromosomal sex (genotype) is established at fertilization, and from the bipotential gonads, the male genotype (46,XY) leads to the development of the testis through a series of sex chromosome–linked and autosomal genes–mediated functions. As described earlier, the testis in turn secretes essential hormones for the development of the external male genitalia (phenotype) (7). In a normal 46,XX female, ovarian and müllerian duct development occurs because of absence of the Y chromosome, which is instrumental in the suppression of the female genitalia and reproductive organs.

Of the genes involved in the formation of the bipotential gonads, *WT1* (Wilms tumor gene), *NR5A1* (nuclear receptor subfamily 5, which encodes the steroidogenic factor 1, *SF-1*), and *LIM1* are perhaps the most important (7,8). These events are triggered by *SRY* (sex-determining region of the Y) located on the distal tip of the short arm of the Y chromosome (8,9). The *SRY* gene encodes a protein that acts on the HMG (high mobility group) DNA-binding domain in somatic cells in the urogenital ridge to differentiate into Sertoli cells, the first differentiated cell type of the testis (7). Although *SRY* is the essential determinant of testicular development, various autosomal genes, downstream from *SYR*, are involved in this process including *WT1*, *SF-1*, *DAX-1* (dosage-sensitive sex reversal, adrenal hypoplasia critical region, on chromosome X, gene 1), and *SOX9* (SRY-box 9) (10).

Congenital and Developmental Anomalies

Congenital or developmental anomalies affecting the testis may be an isolated finding or may be associated with a sexual maldevelopment syndrome that may or may not be associated with an underlying cytogenetic defect. Clinically, these conditions most commonly present as an "undescended" testis or ambiguous external genitalia.

Monorchidism, or the presence of a single testicle, may be due to a testicular regression syndrome (TRS) (discussed later), vascular injury, cryptorchidism, or another congenital anomaly. Polyorchidism (or duplication of the testis), defined as the presence of more than two testes, is a rare condition with about 100 cases reported in the literature. This condition usually manifests as triorchidism, but bilateral duplication has been also reported (11). Clinically, two masses within the hemiscrotum, inguinal swelling and an undescended testis (UDT), or pain are the usual presentations. Associated conditions include those related to anomalies in the processus vaginalis (hernia, hydrocele), testicular maldescent, intermittent torsion, epididymitis and varicocele, as well as malignant neoplasms (12). The exact mechanisms behind this condition are unknown, but the supernumerary or duplicate testis is suggested to result from an abnormal division of the urogenital ridge before the 8th week of gestation (13). According to Leung's anatomical classification, the most common variant (type II) is that of a supernumerary testis draining into the epididymis of the primary or usual testis, and hence, they share a common vas. Other variants include a supernumerary testis without any epididymis or vas and with no attachment to the usual testis (type I), supernumerary testis that has its own epididymis and both epididymides of the ipsilateral testes drain into one vas (type III), and a completely independent supernumerary testis with its own epididymis and vas (type IV) (13). The supernumerary testis is often smaller than a normal testis, and its torsion is more frequent. The histologic appearance of the supernumerary testis ranges from normal testicular tissue with intact spermatogenesis to disorganized seminiferous tubules with diminished spermatogenesis. Rare associated chromosomal anomalies have also been reported (12).

Cystic dysplasia of the testis (CDT) is a rare congenital malformation, presenting as testicular enlargement due to cystic dilation of the rete testis (14). It is thought to result from an embryologic defect around the 5th week of gestation preventing the connection of the rete testis (afferent seminiferous tubule derived) with the efferent tubules (mesonephric or wolffian derived), which further drain into the epididymis. The failure of this anastomotic connection leads to cystic dilatation of rete testis in the mediastinum testis with progressive dilation of cysts compressing and replacing the adjacent testicular parenchyma. A second alternative theory of overproduction of fluid by rete testis epithelium has also been proposed (14). Ipsilateral renal agenesis and multicystic dysplasia of the kidney are the most common associated findings with CDT. Histopathologic features of CDT include multiple, anastomosing, irregular cystic spaces of varying sizes and shapes predominantly located in the region of the mediastinum testis but also displacing the testicular parenchyma, which becomes subsequently compressed under the tunica albuginea. The cystic lining is flat epithelium resembling that of the rete testis (15). Spontaneous regression of this lesion after conservative management has very rarely been reported in the literature (14).

Prepubertal macroorchidism is an idiopathic condition in most cases but has also been associated with McCune-Albright syndrome, juvenile hypothyroidism, continuous splenogonadal fusion, and fragile X syndrome. Histopathologic findings may include some enlargement of the seminiferous tubules and thickening of the tubular basement membrane. The tubules contain Sertoli cells, and scattered Leydig cells are usually present in the interstitium. Focal mild interstitial fibrosis, occasional tubules containing only Sertoli cells, and focal paucity of Leydig cells are some of the pathologic findings. Some have attributed the testicular enlargement in the absence of other findings to interstitial edema and obstruction.

Vascular anomalies of the testis are rare and include angiomatous malformations and congenital lymphangiectasis. Angiomatous malformation is a rare cause of testicular enlargement and consists of numerous thin-walled vascular channels. Congenital lymphangiectasis has been reported in association with bilateral cryptorchidism and with Noonan syndrome, manifested by numerous ectatic and irregular lymphatic channels with frequent anastomoses among and around the seminiferous tubules. The seminiferous tubules may have smaller diameter, immature Sertoli cells, reduced spermatogenesis, and peritubular fibrosis (16). Similar findings, however, have also been reported in the testes of infants without other abnormalities at autopsy.

Cryptorchidism or UDT, where either one or both testes fail to migrate to the base of the scrotum, is one of the most common genitourinary disorders in male children. The exact incidence of this condition has been reported as 1% to 5% of full term and 9% to 30% of premature males at birth (17–19). Based on many recently published series, there has been an increase in the incidence of cryptorchidism over recent decades in North America and Europe (20). The cryptorchid testis can be found in any position along its usual line of descent including intra-abdominally; however, approximately 80% will be located in the inguinal region, just outside the inguinal canal, and 20% to 27% of cryptorchid testes are not palpable. Rarely, ectopic locations outside the normal line of descent have been reported that included the perineum, base of the penis, abdominal wall, pubic region, and upper thigh. The majority of undescended testes will achieve full spontaneous descent by 1 year of age, predominantly within the first 3 months, and only 0.8% of infants would have incomplete descent 12 months after birth. Spontaneous testicular descent after the first year is very unlikely (19). A number of studies have reported an increased rate of UDT with low birth weight, maternal preeclampsia, mild gestational diabetes, and breech presentation (21). Bilateral testicular maldescent was reported in as high as 39% of babies with cryptorchidism, which was also more likely to occur in babies with low birth weights.

In addition to the presence of a patent processus vaginalis in most cryptorchid testes other abnormalities can occur in these patients especially those pertaining to the genitourinary tract, which include dysgenetic testis, duplication of the ureter, hypospadias, renal dysplasia, and inguinal hernia (22). Of the most common associations with cryptorchidism are malformations in the paratesticular structures such as the epididymis and its attachment to the vas deferens and gubernaculum. Epididymal abnormalities have been reported in less than 5% of normal male fetuses compared to 35% in children with cryptorchidism. The most common of these anomalies is detachment between the epididymis and the testis followed by separation of the epididymis from the vas deferens and the long looping epididymis.

Outside the genitourinary tract, abnormalities may include gastroschisis, omphalocele, imperforate anus, cardiac anomalies, lower limb anomalies, and caudal spinal malformations. It has been reported that the etiologies of cryptorchidism and hypospadias are partly shared, and the presence of both conditions simultaneously is associated with increased risk for ambiguous external genitalia and intersex disorders (22).

Multiple causes for testicular maldescent have been suggested including an abnormal differentiation of the male sexual organs, midline abnormalities, anatomical anomalies of the gubernaculum testis, hormonal dysfunction affecting the hypothalamic–pituitary–testicular axis (hypogonadotropic hypogonadism), mechanical impairment (insufficient intraabdominal pressure, short spermatic cord, underdeveloped processus vaginalis), and heredity.

The prepubertal UDT is usually smaller than the contralateral one, and the difference becomes even more significant with progressive lesions. Generally, there is correlation between the age at the time of orchiopexy or orchiectomy and the severity of the histologic alterations seen in the testis. The isolated cryptorchid testis in the prepubertal child has only subtle quantitative abnormalities such as decreased percentage of tubules containing germ cells (low tubular fertility index), decreased mean tubular diameter, apparent tubular loss, and early interstitial fibrosis (23) (Figure 19-1). The postpubertal and adult cryptorchid testis usually exhibits abnormalities in all testicular structures characterized by tubular sclerosis, maturational arrest in spermatogenesis, and interstitial fibrosis. Tubules with immature Sertoli cells only (Sertoli cell nodules) may also be found (Figure 19-2), and areas of Leydig cell hyperplasia are frequent. Granular transformation and degeneration of Sertoli cells have been reported in the cryptorchid testis as well as in other testicular disorders (24). Similar histopathologic features may also be found in retractile testis (which is essentially a suprascrotal testis but can be easily manipulated into the

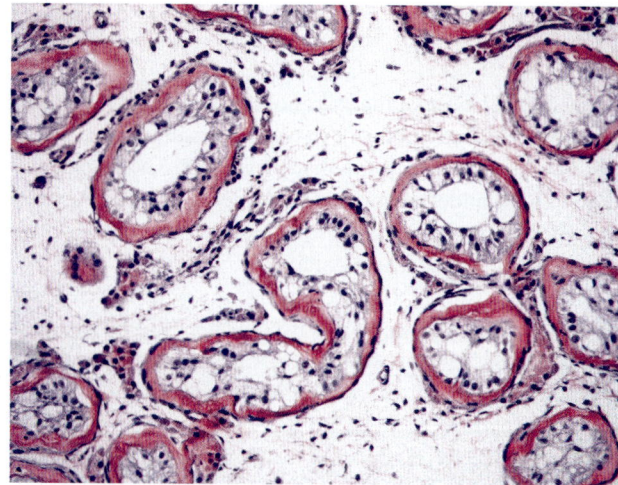

FIGURE 19-1 • Cryptorchid testis. Atrophic seminiferous tubules characterized by irregular contour, thickened basement membrane, and lack of spermatogenesis with Sertoli-only pattern. Loose fibrous interstitial stroma is evident.

scrotum), indicating that these conditions may share some causal relationships and that they may require similar management approach (25). Some changes in the rete testis have been reported particularly in postpubertal cryptorchid testis including adenomatous features or dysgenesis with hypoplastic changes.

The relationship between cryptorchidism and male infertility has been extensively studied, and links between the two conditions have been made in a number of series. Cryptorchidism has been reported as the cause of infertility in up to 9% of cases. Biopsies from cryptorchid testes may reveal lack of germ cells as early as 18 months of age, the incidence of which increases with advanced age and with bilaterality (26). Similar trends were observed even in patients who underwent orchiopexy, implying that the actual development of germ cells in cryptorchidism might also be impaired (26). Some authors, however, cast some doubt on the level of certainty of this causative relationship between cryptorchidism and infertility and advocate that while it is certain that untreated men with bilateral abdominal testes will be infertile, the levels of fertility are unpredictable in other less severe scenarios (unilateral cryptorchidism, inguinal testes, postorchiopexy).

Another important association with cryptorchidism is the increased risk of developing testicular germ cell tumors (GCT), especially seminoma, compared with normally descended testes (18). The relative risk of GCT in a cryptorchidism patient is approximately 2.75 to 8. The relative risk of GCT is between 2 and 3 in patients who undergo orchiopexy by ages 10 to 12 years. However, patients who undergo orchiopexy after age 12 years or no orchiopexy might be two to six times as likely to have GCT as those who undergo orchiopexy at a prepubertal stage. Multiple studies in literature demonstrate conflicting opinions, but overall, it seems that a contralateral, normally descended testis in a patient with cryptorchidism carries no increased risk of GCT. It has

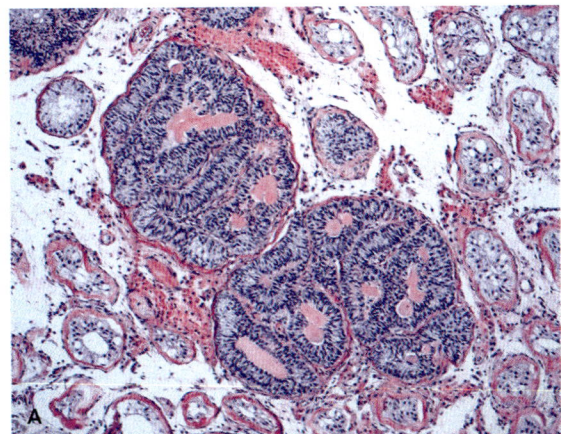 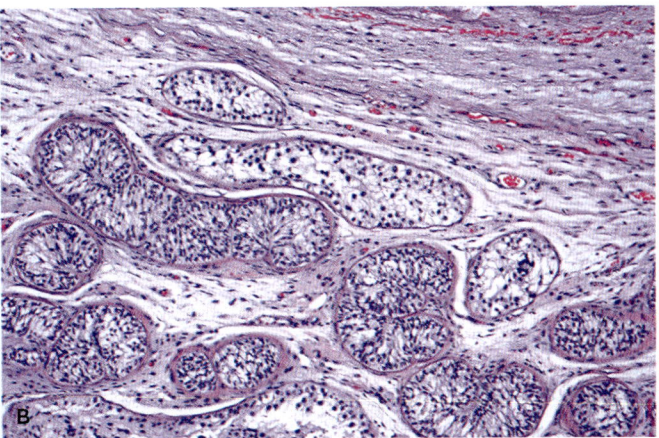

FIGURE 19-2 • **A:** Sertoli cell nodule in a cryptorchid testis. A well-circumscribed, nodular proliferation of immature Sertoli cells filling the seminiferous tubules with central hyaline foci. The surrounding testicular tissue is atrophic. Note the presence of Leydig cells in the interstitial area. **B:** We have encountered similar proliferation adjacent to a malignant germ cell tumor in an adolescent.

been demonstrated that the risk of developing a malignancy increases with an abdominal testis location compared with an inguinal testis and also with those treated with orchiopexy postpubertally (26). In the latter case, the tubules are arrested in maturation. Interestingly, persistently cryptorchid testes at inguinal and abdominal locations might be at higher risk for development of seminoma, while corrected cryptorchid or scrotal testes might be at higher risk of developing GCT of the nonseminomatous type (18).

Disorders of Sex Development (Intersex Disorders)

The term *intersex disorders* has been largely used to refer primarily to a clinical scenario of an infant born with external genitalia sufficiently ambiguous that sex assignment is not possible. However, the mechanisms underlying such a clinical scenario are variable, and some disorders in sex development do not necessarily present with genital ambiguity. It has been recently recommended to use the term disorders of sex development (DSD) to replace such terms as *intersex*, *hermaphrodite*, and *pseudohermaphrodite* (27). DSD represents a congenital condition characterized by discordance between phenotypic sex and chromosomal sex and in which development of chromosomal, gonadal, or anatomic sex is atypical. Recent advances in molecular biology have enabled us to further our understanding of the processes involving normal sexual differentiation and the inborn errors that result in sexual ambiguity, which has led to improvement in diagnosing and managing patients with DSD (27,28). It is estimated that two-thirds of sexually ambiguous neonates are female pseudohermaphrodites with congenital adrenal hyperplasia. The remaining DSD are associated with some abnormality in male gonadal development or persistence of the müllerian tract with or without an abnormal constitutional karyotype.

Currently, the classification of DSD can be organized by broader categories in which the intersexual disorders are divided into "abnormalities of genital differentiation," due largely to the abnormal production or sensitivity of a single hormone, or "abnormalities in sex determination," due to abnormal gonadal differentiation, usually testicular, with or without chromosomal aberration (see Table 19-1) (27) (see Chapter 18).

Disorders of Genital Differentiation

These disorders are generally associated with a normal chromosomal composition and normal gonads. This includes female and male pseudohermaphroditism.

Female pseudohermaphroditism occurs as a result of relative androgen excess *in utero* in an individual with two ovaries and a 46,XX genotype. The elevated levels of androgen present during embryogenesis usually result in genital ambiguity and may result in a male phenotype. The most common cause is the **adrenogenital syndrome** (AGS, congenital adrenal hyperplasia). The manifestations of AGS in genotypically female patients are related to defects in the biosynthetic pathways of mineralocorticoid, glucocorticoid, and sex steroids. In males with AGS, usually there is no evidence of genital ambiguity, but they may have an enlarged phallus. They may also develop clinically detectable bilateral testicular nodules during childhood or young adulthood that may be confused with true Leydig cell tumors (LCTs) and are designated as testicular *tumors* of the AGS (29) (see Chapters 18 and 21).

A rare condition, **placental aromatase deficiency**, causes maternal virilization during pregnancy and pseudohermaphroditism of the female fetus. Due to mutations in the aromatase gene *CYP19* and the resulting lack of aromatase activity, fetal androstenedione cannot be converted to estrogen by the placenta and instead is converted to testosterone peripherally, resulting in virilization of both fetus and mother.

TABLE 19-1 DISORDERS OF SEXUAL DEVELOPMENT

Disorders of genital differentiation	Female pseudo-hermaphroditism (female intersex)	Adrenogenital syndrome 　—21 α-hydroxylase deficiency 　—11 β-hydroxylase deficiency Placental aromatase defect Maternal ingestion of progestins or androgens Maternal virilizing lesions
	Male pseudoher-maphroditism (male intersex)	Testicular regression syndrome Leydig cell deficiency (defective hCG–LH receptor) Defects in testosterone synthesis: a. Testosterone and adrenocorticoid insufficiency 　—Defect in cholesterol synthesis (Smith-Lemli-Opitz syndrome) 　—Congenital lipoid adrenal hyperplasia (defect StAR gene) 　—Congenital adrenal hyperplasia (3 β-hydroxylase dehydrogenase deficiency, 17 α-hydroxylase deficiency) b. Testosterone insufficiency only 　—17, 20-desmolase deficiency 　—17 β-hydroxysteroid (17-ketosteroid reductase) dehydrogenase deficiency Defect in müllerian inhibiting system End-organ defects: a. Androgen receptor disorders (androgen insensitivity syndromes) 　—Complete testicular feminization (androgen receptor insufficiency) 　—Partial androgen receptor insufficiency b. Disorder of peripheral testosterone metabolism 　—5-α-reductase type 2 deficiency
Disorders of sex determination		Klinefelter syndrome (47 XXY) Turner syndrome and Turner-like (45 XO and X mosaicism) XX male and XY female syndrome (sex reversal) Pure gonadal dysgenesis (bilateral) Defect in the Wilms tumor suppressor (WT1) gene 　—Denys-Drash syndrome 　—Frasier syndrome Mixed gonadal dysgenesis (Turner-like, dysgenetic male pseudohermaphroditism, gonadoblastoma) True hermaphroditism

Adapted with modification from Robboy SJ, Jaubert F. Neoplasms and pathology of sexual developmental disorders (intersex). *Pathology* 2007;39(1):147–163.

Other conditions that might be associated with female pseudohermaphroditism are related to maternal factors such as **maternal ingestion of synthetic progestins or androgens** or the presence of **maternal virilizing lesions** during pregnancy including a luteoma of pregnancy (27).

Male pseudohermaphroditism represents a heterogeneous group of intersex conditions that occur in individuals with normal 46,XY karyotype and either identifiable testes or evidence that testes were present during fetal development but the external genitalia are usually female or ambiguous (30). The responsible defect may be (a) at the gonad level, leading to disorders of testosterone biosynthesis and metabolism or testosterone receptor abnormalities, or deficiency in MIS gene or (b) at the end organ level, where the developing tissues are unresponsive to androgen stimulation leading to an abnormal phenotype. Other less well-defined causes may also be responsible.

Gonadal defects responsible for male pseudohermaphroditism include TRS, agenesis or deficiency of the Leydig cells, defects in specific enzymes in the pathway of testosterone or DHT biosynthesis or receptors to these hormones, or a defect in elaboration or action of MIS.

Testicular regression syndrome (TRS, congenital anorchia, vanishing testis) is a condition in which a testis is thought to have once existed but has atrophied and disappeared during early development (31,32). The testis is clinically impalpable, and no normal testicular tissue can be identified following exploration. Generally, congenital absence of the testis, or testicular agenesis, is an uncommon anomaly as it was detected in less than 1% of testes both in fetuses and cryptorchid patients. This condition results from the irreversible destruction of one or both testes during fetal life in an XY individual, resulting in variable hormonal deficiencies and developmental anomalies based on the stage at which testicular damage occurred (33). Unilateral testicular destruction does not result in TRS. By histopathologic examination, the testis may be completely absent or represented by only a microscopic remnant. In addition to having no gonadal tissue, pathologic findings include a collection of vascularized fibroconnective tissue (85%), hemorrhage or hemosiderin deposition (70%), calcification (60%), or giant cells near the residual vas deferens or epididymis, the expected site of the gonad (31–33). The vas deferens ends blindly, and a small circumscribed nodule of tissue may be located in the retroperitoneum, in the iliac fossa, or in the scrotum. By definition, no evidence of preserved remnants of seminiferous tubules should be present.

The clinical presentation of individuals with TRS is variable and is reflective of the specific stage of fetal development during which the testes were damaged. Generally, at one end of the spectrum, when gonadal regression occurs early in embryonic life before the testes release androgenic or antimüllerian hormones, the testes are absent and the phenotype is female. At the other end, regression occurring later and through fetal life would allow for a male phenotype with infantile to nearly normal male genitalia and differentiated wolffian-derived structures. Affected individuals commonly have ambiguous genitalia. A number of etiologies have been proposed for TRS including inherited genetic defect, intrauterine infection, and infarction-torsion (27).

It is presumed that testicular regression develops late in the fetal period after the müllerian structures regressed under the influence of the müllerian inhibitory substance and the male gonads and genitalia developed under the influence of the androgens. Despite the familial occurrences of TRS suggesting a genetic etiology, no specific genes have been identified to be associated with it and in particular those related to the opening reading frame sequence of SRY. Unlike cryptorchidism, there is no increased risk of gonadal neoplasia, because there is little, if any, residual gonadal tissue.

Leydig cell deficiency (agenesis or hypoplasia) is a rare condition of male pseudohermaphroditism thought to be due to a defect in the human chorionic gonadotropin–LH receptor, primary agenesis or hypoplasia of the Leydig cells, or an abnormal LH receptor molecule. Affected individuals are genotypically males (46,XY) with female phenotype and unremarkable or ambiguous external genitalia. Bilateral, slightly small to normal-sized cryptorchid testes are present with fully or partially developed epididymides and vasa deferentia, indicating that testosterone production by Leydig cells was intact early in embryonic development. The testes exhibit interstitial fibrosis, but no mature Leydig cells are present and no testosterone production is noted. LH levels are elevated in affected individuals. Tubules with Sertoli cells are found, and müllerian structures are typically absent, indicating appropriate testicular production of MIS by Sertoli cells during fetal life (27).

Familial occurrence of this condition has been reported, and a number of mutations in the transmembrane domain of LH receptor gene, resulting in Leydig cell deficiency, have been identified (34).

Defects in testosterone synthesis may be due to inborn errors of the enzymes involved in testosterone biosynthesis in the testis or the adrenal gland that may result in subnormal levels of testosterone and DHT during embryogenesis (relative estrogen excess) resulting in female or ambiguous external genitalia. These defects may involve cholesterol synthesis (mutations in 7-dehydrocholesterol reductase gene) as in Smith-Lemli-Opitz syndrome or mutations in the steroidogenic enzymes responsible for the conversion of cholesterol to testosterone and DHT, which include (a) steroidogenic acute regulatory protein (*StAR*) gene responsible for congenital lipoid adrenal hyperplasia, (b) 17α-hydroxylase and 3β-hydroxylase dehydrogenase responsible for congenital adrenal hyperplasia, and (c) 17-ketosteroid reductase.

The degree to which the external genitalia develop depends upon the type and the severity of the defect. The microscopic features of testes in patients with these conditions vary and may show large clusters of Leydig cells surrounding seminiferous tubules. Germ cells (spermatogonia) are often normal in children but disappear by puberty resulting in Sertoli-only syndrome. Some germ cells, however, can persist and rarely develop into intratubular germ cell neoplasia. Müllerian-derived structures are absent, but wolffian duct structures may be present (27).

Defect in müllerian inhibiting system or the **persistent müllerian duct syndrome (PMDS)**, also referred to as *hernia uteri inguinale*, is a rare form of male pseudohermaphroditism characterized by the presence of müllerian duct structures in 46,XY phenotypic males. The age at diagnosis ranges from a neonate to the fourth decade. Most patients have unilateral or bilateral cryptorchid testes, normal or almost normal male external genitalia, and an inguinal hernia containing a prolapsed infantile uterus and fallopian tubes (35). The testes may be histologically normal, and the wolffian duct structures are developed with the vas deferens embedded in the wall of the upper vaginal structure in most cases. Inguinal hernias occur in almost 40% of cases. Malignant testicular tumors such as intratubular germ cell neoplasia and seminoma have been rarely reported in cases of adult PMDS patients with uncorrected cryptorchid testis. More recently, rare examples of clear-cell adenocarcinoma of the müllerian duct and uterine adenosarcoma in a boy with PMDS have been reported. PMDS has been reported with a familial occurrence and rarely in identical male twins.

PMDS is currently considered a heterogeneous group of disorders caused by at least two different defects in the müllerian inhibiting system. The most common is a defect in the *MIS* (müllerian inhibiting substance) gene, also known as *AMH* (antimüllerian hormone) gene preventing it from producing any biologically functional MIS. The second defect involves an abnormal AMH type II receptor resulting in end-organ insensitivity to MIS despite the presence of biologically active MIS. In other patients, an abnormality in the timing of MIS secretion may exist.

End-Organ Defects

As mentioned earlier, responsiveness to androgen is required for the normal development of the external genitalia and wolffian duct–derived structures. The presence of the enzyme 5α-reductase in the anlage of the prostate and external genitalia is also required for the conversion of testosterone to DHT. An absent or unstable androgen receptor in 46,XY individuals leads to impaired development of both wolffian duct–derived structures and external genitalia. If only 5α-reductase is absent or defective, abnormalities confined to the external genitalia and prostate will be observed.

Androgen receptor disorders (androgen insensitivity syndromes) result in variable phenotypes ranging from a female phenotype with intra-abdominal testes to ambiguous genitalia to a male phenotype with minimal clinical abnormalities.

Complete testicular feminization due to **complete androgen insensitivity** (e.g., testicular feminization, Goldberg-Maxwell-Morris syndrome, hairless women, androgen receptor insufficiency) is the most common form of male pseudohermaphroditism occurring in 1 of 20,000 newborns. It is caused by failure of androgen receptor binding despite its production and secretion by the fetal testis. The underlying mechanisms have been identified as mutations in the androgen receptor gene including point mutations resulting in amino acid substitutions or premature stop codons, frameshift mutations by nucleotide insertions or deletions, complete or partial gene deletion, or intronic mutations affecting the splicing of the androgen receptor RNA.

Due to the presence of phenotypically female external genitalia (Figure 19-3), the condition is rarely diagnosed before puberty unless an inguinal hernia or labial mass is encountered or unless the disorder is known to be familial. Primary amenorrhea is the most common complaint leading to evaluation and subsequent diagnosis. The wolffian tract involutes resulting in cystic epididymides that are usually not connected to the testes. The vasa differentia, seminal vesicles, and prostate are absent. As a rule, both the cervix and the uterine corpus are absent. A fragment of fallopian tube may be found in up to one-third of cases (27).

The testes are cryptorchid and may be intra-abdominal or inguinal, or in the labia majora, and 50% are found in inguinal hernias. Overall, the testes in androgen insensitivity

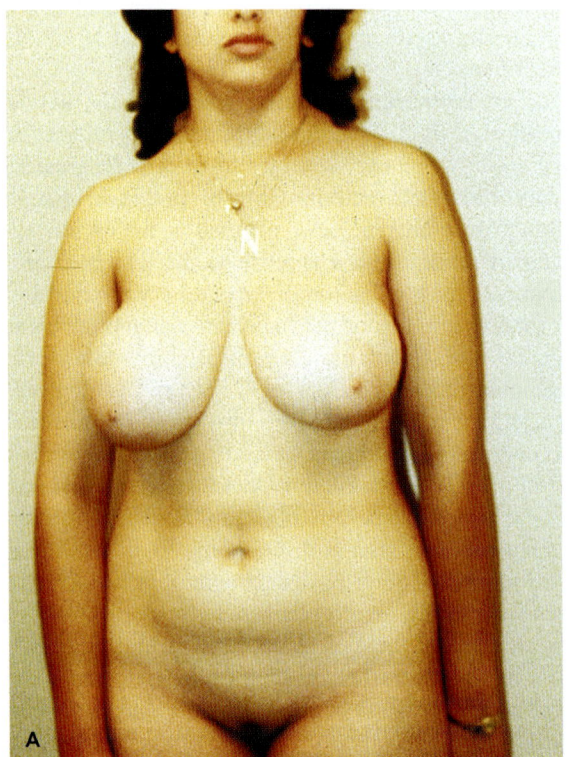

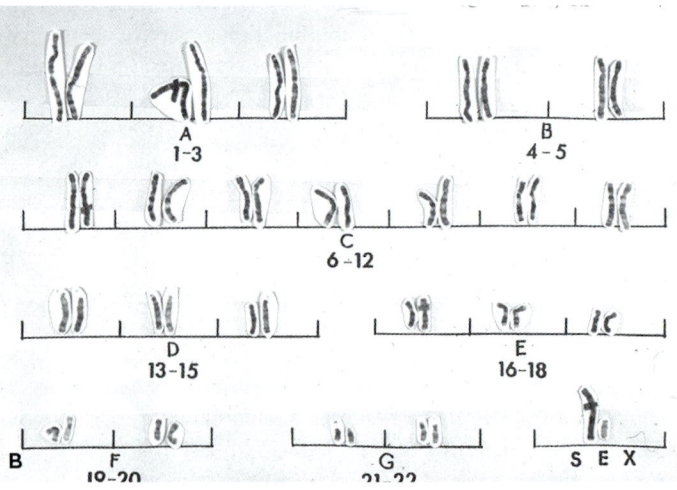

FIGURE 19-3 • Testicular feminization. **A:** In this example of complete testicular feminization, a fully developed female phenotype is evident. **B:** The karyotype is that of a male (Contributed by Dr. Jerome Taxy, Chicago, IL).

syndrome are histologically similar to the cryptorchid testis except that the tubules are less mature with possible spermatogonia but no spermatogenesis. Leydig cells are absent or replaced by collagenized interstitial tissue in portions of the gonad, whereas sheets of Leydig cells may be found near the hilus and nerves. Ovarian-like stroma replaces the testicular interstitium. Hamartomas and Sertoli cell adenomas were reported in the majority of cases in the postpubertal testis. These hamartomatous nodules are multiple, bilateral, tan, yellow, or white in appearance with bulging cut surface and may be composed of immature Sertoli cells, germ cells, Leydig cells, ovarian-type stroma, nonspecific fibrous stroma, and smooth muscle. The typical size varies from 1 to 10 mm, but may occasionally be up to 40 mm. Sertoli cell adenomas consist of nodules of predominantly or exclusively packed seminiferous tubules with immature Sertoli cells that are 3 cm in average size but range up to 25 cm. A rare example of a testicular tumor resembling the sex cord with annular tubules has been reported. GCT, particularly seminoma and less commonly intratubular germ cell neoplasia, can sometimes be encountered in patients with this syndrome, and, rarely, sex cord–stromal tumors have been reported (27). The development of malignant gonadal tumors in patients with testicular feminization usually occurs later in adulthood.

Partial androgen insensitivity syndrome due to partial androgen receptor insufficiency accounts for 10% of all cases of androgen insensitivity and encompasses several different phenotypes, ranging from individuals with a predominantly female appearance to persons with ambiguous genitalia or individuals with a predominantly male phenotype. Affected patients typically present at birth with genital ambiguity, but severe hypospadias, micropenis, bifid scrotum, and bilateral cryptorchidism are also common. Alternatively, the external genital phenotype may be predominantly female with partial labial fusion and clitoromegaly. The underlying mechanism involves a qualitative defect in the androgen receptor. Additionally, a number of syndromes and conditions are characterized by partial androgen insensitivity including Reifenstein, Lubs, Gilbert-Dreyfus, Rosewater, and the infertile male syndromes and Kennedy disease.

A disorder of peripheral testosterone metabolism is caused by mutation in the enzyme 5α-reductase type 2, which is responsible for converting testosterone to DHT to exert its effect on differentiating the urogenital sinus into external male genitalia and prostate. Affected males usually have female to ambiguous external genitalia at birth. The penis is small (clitoris-like) and lacks a urethral orifice. A blind vaginal pouch and inguinal or labial testes may be observed. Wolffian-derived structures are normal but no müllerian-derived structures are present. Due to activation of type 1 isoenzyme, some virilization occurs at puberty demonstrated by penile enlargement, scrotal rugation and hyperpigmentation, and testicular enlargement and descent. Microscopic findings of testicular tissue may include spermatogenesis, tubular atrophy, no spermatogenesis, or Leydig cell hyperplasia. The prostate remains rudimentary, and the seminal vesicles remain underdeveloped (27).

Disorders of Sexual Determination

These disorders are generally associated with sex chromosome abnormalities resulting in abnormal gonad formation. Affected individuals characteristically have additions, deletions, or mosaicism of the sex chromosomes, and the appearance of the gonads is variable, ranging from a streak gonad to a nearly normal female or male both grossly and microscopically.

Mixed gonadal dysgenesis (MGD) is one of the most frequent causes of male sexual ambiguity in individuals usually with a 45,X/46,XY or 46,XY karyotype. In one series, MGD was the diagnosis in approximately 8% of children with intersex conditions. It represents a heterogeneous group of abnormalities characterized by persistent müllerian duct structures, a dysgenetic testis, and a contralateral streak gonad (30). The phenotypical heterogeneity of MGD is attributed to the presence of a variety of different genetic abnormalities causing the syndrome mostly related to deletions of both the short and the long arms of chromosome Y.

The loss of testicular functions leads to incomplete inhibition of müllerian development, incomplete differentiation of wolffian duct structures, and incomplete male development of the external genitalia. Testicular maldescent may also occur, and some patients have phenotypical features of a Turner-like syndrome. An infantile or rudimentary uterus and at least one fallopian tube are found on the side with the uncommitted streak gonad. An intra-abdominal or inguinal cryptorchid testis or fibrous streak dysgenetic testis without an accompanying fallopian tube is present on the contralateral side. Organs of wolffian duct derivation may be present with variable frequency. An epididymis is identified in two-thirds of cases and is usually present on the side where there is a testis. The vas deferens is encountered less frequently, and the seminal vesicle is identified only rarely.

The gonad may be a testis or a streak gonad (Figure 19-4). Streak gonads may show partial differentiation into testicular phenotype, or may exhibit features toward ovarian differentiation with the characteristic ovarian-type stroma and rare primordial follicles. However, no true ovary is present, which requires the presence of differentiation with follicles in at least the antral stage (27). A unilateral macroscopic testis is found in 60% of cases, whereas bilateral testes may be seen in about 15% of cases usually with an asynchronous degree of maturity.

The testicular architecture is consistently abnormal in these individuals as the region of the tunica albuginea or cortex contains widely spaced seminiferous tubules with ovarian-like stroma or immature primary sex cords indeterminate between female and male structures. The medullary region may contain normal seminiferous tubules and interstitium, but in some cases, it is difficult to distinguish between female and male structures. Occasional narrow closed seminiferous tubules are lined by Sertoli cells, and in other examples, the germ cells may be seen directly lining the basement membrane of the seminiferous tubule without the Sertoli cell layer that usually normally surrounds them. Leydig cells may be present in small clusters of varying size.

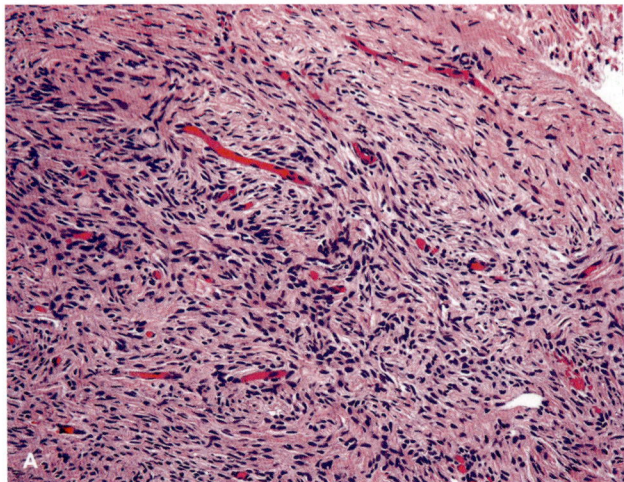
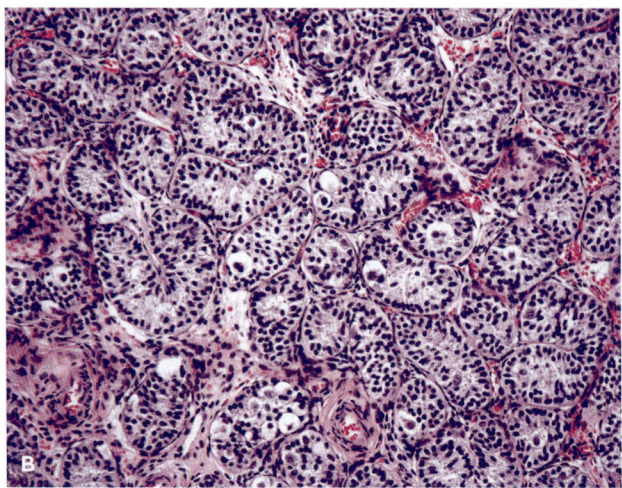
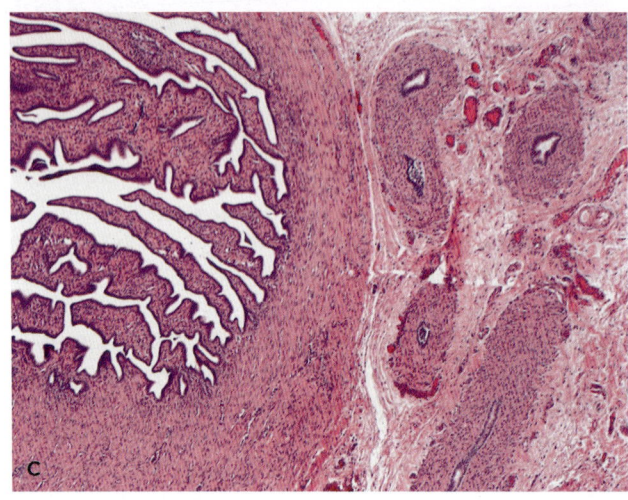

FIGURE 19-4 • Mixed gonadal dysgenesis in a 3-year-old patient with a female phenotype. **A:** On one side, an intra-abdominal streak gonad was present consisting of vascularized fibrous stroma. **B:** The contralateral side contained an immature cryptorchid testis with predominant Sertoli cells and only occasional spermatogonia. **C:** Bilaterally, structures of both wolffian (vas deferens) and müllerian (fallopian tube) origins were present.

Occasionally, broad zones of the cortex may exhibit a degree of differentiation toward streak-like ovary, even displaying rare primordial follicles. By puberty, the germ cells present in a streak gonad may degenerate and disappear, resulting in a gonad composed exclusively of fibrous tissue and a few rete tubules. The hilar region of the streak gonad or streak testis is populated by hilus cells and rete or mesonephric tubules. Hyperplasia of the hilus cells in response to pituitary gonadotropins may result in clinical virilization. Tumors develop in about 10% of those with MGD and the dysgenetic gonads of which 25% to 30% are malignant, the most common of which is gonadoblastoma accounting for 75% to 80% of all germ cell neoplasms in this disorder. However, other GCTs have been also reported including germinoma, yolk sac tumor (YST), teratoma, embryonal carcinoma (EC), and choriocarcinoma. These tumors may be unilateral or bilateral. Occasionally, Sertoli cell tumor (SCT) and SCT-like proliferations of sex cord elements have been also reported. Early gonadal resection is recommended in order to avoid the development of an invasive GCT and to avoid the consequences of onset of virilization in a patient who has been raised as a female.

Pure gonadal dysgenesis (PGD) refers to phenotypically female individuals with streak gonads and internal genitalia that include müllerian structures (uterus and fallopian tubes). It occurs with both 46,XX and 46,XY karyotypes and has both familial and sporadic patterns of inheritance. The stroma of the gonads has an ovarian-like appearance, and primary amenorrhea is the usual clinical presentation. PGD patients with 46,XX karyotype only rarely develop gonadal tumors, examples of which include GCT and mucinous epithelial tumors. Some have hilus cell hyperplasia and hilus cell tumors with the usual associated virilizing effects.

PGD patients with 46,XY karyotype are at higher risk for gonadoblastoma and other GCTs that may develop in 10% to 25% of cases and can be unilateral or bilateral (36,37).

True hermaphroditism (TH) is a disorder of gonadal differentiation defined by the concurrence of both ovarian and testicular tissue, with coexistent ovarian follicles (not just connective tissue stroma) and seminiferous tubules (not just Leydig cells). The gonads may be ovary and testis separately or combined in an ovotestis (27,38). Affected individuals may have either a female or a male phenotype with variable degrees of sexual ambiguity. The clinical manifestations are variable and depend on the gonadal tissue present and the age at the time of diagnosis. TH is a rare condition both in North American and Europe but is more commonly encountered in Africa, especially in South Africa.

The architecture and the distribution of gonadal tissues in TH take several forms with asymmetry of the gonads in the majority of cases. An ovotestis represents the most frequently encountered type of gonad in this condition (38–40). Patterns of gonadal development include an ovary on one side and a testis on the other (30% of cases) or an ovary on one side and a contralateral ovotestis (30%). Bilateral ovotestes are found in 20% or more of true hermaphrodites, and a testis–ovotestis combination is found in 10% of cases. In the majority of cases (approximately 80%), the ovarian and the testicular tissues are arranged in an end-to-end fashion with a distinct line demarcating the two tissues. The ovary, which is the second most common gonad in TH, preferentially develops on the left side, whereas the testis, which is the least common gonad encountered in TH, develops preferentially on the right (27). The location of the gonad is influenced by the type and the quantity of gonadal tissue present. Increasing amounts of ovarian tissue heightens the probability that the gonad will be in an ovarian position, and as a result, it is very unlikely for female gonadal tissue (either ovary or ovotestis) to be situated in the inguinal canal or in the labioscrotal fold. The position of the testis is less constant as most reside in the scrotum but can be encountered in the inguinal region or in the normal ovarian position. The nature of the genital structure adjacent to a gonad in TH follows that of the ipsilateral gonad, which is characterized by having a fallopian tube adjacent to an ovary and an epididymis or vas deferens adjacent to a testis. Either a müllerian (more commonly) or wolffian structure, but not both, is adjacent to an ovotestis.

In young patients, the microscopic appearance of the gonadal tissue is often normal with the ovarian tissue containing numerous follicles, whereas the testicular parenchyma has normal-appearing seminiferous tubules with spermatogonia. In older patients, ovarian tissue with structures indicative of ovulation (follicles, corpora lutea, and corpora albicantia) may be seen, but the testicular tissue (in testis or ovotestis) is usually abnormal with incomplete development, lack of spermatogenesis, loss of germ cells, and tubular sclerosis. Scrotal testes in these patients show less severe changes, sometimes showing faulty spermatogenesis (27).

The prevalence of gonadal neoplasms, mainly gonadoblastoma and other types of malignant germ cell neoplasms, is estimated at 2% to 3% of cases (41). A rare case of juvenile granulosa cell tumor (JGCT) in this setting has been reported.

The causes of TH are probably as varied as the karyotypic expressions, and genetic aberrations appear to play a key role in its development. Patients with a "Y" chromosome have a two- to threefold increased frequency of having a testis as opposed to an ovotestis, and nearly 75% of true hermaphrodites with an ovary and an ovotestis have a 46,XX karyotype. A 46,XX/46,XY karyotype represents true genetic chimerism, whereas the 46,XX karyotype is very likely to represent a crossing over of the X and Y chromosome during first meiotic division in the primary spermatocyte, or the presence of hidden mosaicism for *SRY* (42). There are examples where the patients were 46,XX and lacked the *SRY* gene in usual cells examined (leukocytes), but cells from the gonad itself demonstrated *SRY*. Autosomal dominant mutations that mimic *SRY* have been suggested as one possibility where *SRY* was absent. The 46,XY karyotype probably contains a hidden 46,XX cell line or that *SRY*, if present, may act at a time too late to stimulate the development of a testis, hence permitting ovarian tissue to develop.

Klinefelter syndrome (KS) is one of the most common causes of prepubertal delay and primary hypogonadism in males, occurring in about 1 of every 500 to 1 of every 1000 live newborn males and accounting for about 3% of infertile males (27,43,44). In the majority of cases, the karyotype is 47,XXY, which usually results from nondisjunction occurring during meiosis of either paternal or maternal gametes. The clinical picture varies depending on the age when the diagnosis is first suspected. Men with KS present with sequels of androgen deficiency like infertility, low testosterone, erectile dysfunction, and low bone mineral density. They typically are tall men with narrow shoulders, broad hips, sparse body hair, gynecomastia, small testicles, and azoospermia. Infants with KS may have normal external male genitalia at birth, which may cause a delay in its discovery. However, in some individuals, other findings may be indicative of this syndrome such as hypospadia, micropenis, and small, soft testes or cryptorchidism. In adults with KS, the testes are small and rarely exceed 2 cm in greatest dimension. Histologically, the seminiferous tubules may show some degenerative changes during fetal life, which increases with age to the point that by late childhood, the primary spermatogonia are greatly decreased in number. This degenerative process may dramatically accelerate shortly before the expected time of puberty. In adults, the testes are largely atrophic with hyalinized seminiferous tubules and prominence of Leydig cells. Some tubules may be preserved, but lined only by Sertoli cells. Functionally, the Leydig cells are abnormal, as evidenced by low levels of serum testosterone with elevated levels of serum LH and FSH.

A variety of neoplasms have been associated with KS including both gonadal and extragonadal GCTs. Most extragonadal tumors occur in the mediastinum as teratoma and EC, but rare examples of primary intrapelvic seminoma have been reported. In the testis, seminoma, teratoma, and EC have been encountered. LCTs are rare. Men with KS are at a higher risk of developing breast carcinoma than men without KS (45). Additionally, various hematologic malignancies have been reported in individuals with KS, including acute leukemia, chronic myeloid leukemia, and malignant lymphoma.

Turner syndrome is a disorder of sexual differentiation that is discussed in detail elsewhere in the book, whereas **Turner-like** mosaicism (45,X/46,XY) is part of the MGD discussed earlier (see Chapter 18).

XX MALE AND XY FEMALE SYNDROME (SEX REVERSAL)

The XX male syndrome is one of the rarest of all sex chromosome anomalies, occurring in about 1 of 24,000 newborn males, and is characterized by a nearly normal but infertile phenotypical male with a 46,XX karyotype. Genotypically, XX males share many characteristics of men with KS as both groups have a generally masculine appearance, normal or near-normal external genitalia, and azoospermia with associated small testes, prominent Leydig cells, and tubules lined only by Sertoli cells. XX males, however, are generally shorter in height, and the frequency of hypospadias and gynecomastia is higher. Prenatal diagnosis of this syndrome is currently possible due to the increasing application of prenatal ultrasonography and genetic analyses. In some cases, the mechanism underlying this disorder has been identified as translocation of the *SRY* gene from the Y chromosome to the X chromosome during meiosis.

Rare cases of male-to-female sex reversal have been identified in which phenotypically female individuals with 46,XY karyotype are identified, with some of these cases involving duplication and translocations of the short arm of the "Y" chromosome.

Defects in the Wilms Tumor (WT1) Suppressor Gene

Syndromic male pseudohermaphroditism with gonadal dysgenesis and other genitourinary tract anomalies is intertwined with several genes that are active in male sexual differentiation, and one of these is *WT1* on chromosome 11p13. The product of *WT1* is a zinc finger transcriptional factor for many growth factor genes and is expressed in the developing kidney, especially in the condensing mesenchyme, and elsewhere in the genital ridge, in particular the Sertoli cells of the fetal gonad and mesothelium (46). Constitutional mutations in *WT1* are found in the following syndromes: Denys-Drash syndrome (90% or more of cases), Frasier syndrome, and WAGR syndrome (47).

Patients with **Denys-Drash syndrome** have the clinical triad of early renal failure secondary to diffuse mesangial sclerosis, Wilms tumor in most cases (20% bilateral), and male pseudohermaphroditism in children with a 46,XY karyotype (i.e., dysgenetic testes, cryptorchidism, and severe hypospadias with micropenis). Multiple gonadal abnormalities are reported in association with this syndrome and include normal ovaries with signs of early ovarian failures, normal müllerian and wolffian ducts, and normal to dysgenetic testes. Gonadoblastoma(s) is known to develop in the dysgenetic gonads of a child with a 46,XY karyotype. Constitutional heterozygosity in *WT1* represents missense point mutations within exons 8 and 9 in this gene.

Frasier syndrome is rare and results from a mutated *WT1* gene, specifically mutation of intron 9 resulting from abnormal splicing that leads to an unbalanced ratio of the WT1 isoforms needed for normal development of the glomeruli and gonads. It is phenotypically similar to Denys-Drash syndrome with male pseudohermaphroditism (normal female external genitalia, streak gonads, and XY karyotype) and progressive nephropathy. The nephropathy is usually focal segmental glomerulosclerosis, which differs from the diffuse mesangial sclerosis seen in Denys-Dash syndrome. As a rule, Wilms tumors do not develop in the Frasier syndrome patients because the loss of KTS-positive isoform of the WT1 protein retains its tumor suppressor function, but gonadoblastoma develops in the dysgenetic testis in the child with a 46,XY karyotype. Mutations in the donor splice site in intron 9 of *WT1* distinguish Frasier syndrome from Denys-Drash syndrome.

WAGR syndrome, which includes Wilms tumor, aniridia, genitourinary anomalies, and mental retardation, is the phenotypic expression of the constitutional chromosomal deletion within the short arm of one copy of chromosome 11p13 that includes both *WT1* and *PAX6*.

Acquired Abnormalities and Other Lesions

Torsion of the testis or its appendage occurs with a yearly incidence of approximately one in 4000 males younger than 25 years and accounts for 60% to 90% of cases of acute scrotal pain and swelling in men up to 18 years of age (48). Torsion of the testicular appendages may be more common than actual torsion of the testis, especially in prepubertal males. Torsion of the testis itself is seen more often in adolescence, when acute epididymoorchitis also becomes an important consideration in the differential diagnosis (48). Torsion of the testis in infancy is rare but is well documented, including its detection in the prenatal period. Testicular torsion should be suspected clinically in every young patient with testicular pain and must be diagnosed quickly and accurately in order not to risk testicular viability. Imaging studies, including color Doppler ultrasonography and scintigraphy, can be very helpful especially in clinically equivocal cases (48). Torsion usually occurs in the absence of any precipitating event. However, in 4% to 8% of cases, it may be associated with trauma or other possible predisposing factors including an increase in testicular volume (often associated with puberty), testicular tumor, testicles with horizontal lie, a history of cryptorchidism, and a spermatic cord with a long intrascrotal portion.

The pathology of testicular torsion is that of testicular ischemia, the degree of which depends on the duration of torsion and the degree of rotation of the spermatic cord. Ischemia can occur as soon as 4 hours after torsion and is almost certain after 24 hours. It has been reported that testicular salvage can be achieved in approximately 90% of cases if treated within 6 hours from the onset of symptoms, but this rate falls to 50% after 12 hours and to less than 10% after

24 hours. Greater degrees of rotation, as expected, lead to a more rapid onset of ischemia (48). Intermittent testicular torsion with spontaneous resolution within 2 hours or less is a known clinical event. Chronic intermittent torsion may lead to the development of testicular hemorrhage, necrosis, and vasculopathy, which can clinically potentially mimic a testicular neoplasm (49).

Grossly, the testis is enlarged with a tense, bluish tunica albuginea and a dark, hemorrhagic appearance on cross-sections (Figure 19-5). The epididymis has a similar appearance, and a spiral twist may or may not be seen in the spermatic cord. Little if any testicular parenchyma is appreciated through the hemorrhage. There is a sequence of microscopic changes in the testis that precede the final acute stage of near-total hemorrhagic infarction, starting with interstitial edema and hemorrhage and premature sloughing of germinal cells into the tubular lumina followed by diffuse interstitial hemorrhage and necrosis of germinal cells except for some viable seminiferous tubules beneath the tunica albuginea. Total necrosis of the testis is present in almost all cases of continuous torsion after 24 hours. Torsion of the testicular appendage, on the other hand, results in a hemorrhagic cystic structure measuring up to 5 mm in diameter.

Two types of testicular torsion are recognized, with different ages at clinical presentation and anatomic location of the torsion. Extravaginal torsion (neonatal torsion, torsion of the spermatic cord) involves the testis, epididymis, and peritoneal coverings and results from spiraling on a vertical axis in the area of the external inguinal ring. This type accounts for approximately 6% of all torsion cases in childhood and occurs predominantly in neonates since the testis and the gubernaculum are free to rotate. Most cases are unilateral, but some may occur bilaterally and may present as neonatal testicular enlargement if it occurred *in utero*. Intravaginal torsion (adolescent torsion) occurs when the testis, usually accompanied by the epididymis, is abnormally suspended and twists within the tunica vaginalis. This is caused by an abnormality of the processus vaginalis in which the tunica vaginalis covers not only the testis and the epididymis but also the spermatic cord. This creates a bell-clapper deformity, present in approximately 10% of all men, which allows the testis to rotate freely within the tunica vaginalis (48). The peak age of incidence of this type of torsion is between 12 and 18 years of age, and it accounts for up to 90% of torsions in later childhood and adolescence (48). Testicular torsion in neonates and infants demonstrates similar features like testicular parenchymal necrosis, calcifications, hemosiderin-laden macrophages, and fibrosis; complete testicular regression might be evident in neonatal cases (50).

Epididymoorchitis can produce symptoms very similar to those of torsion and generally manifests in adolescence. Acute scrotal pain on the basis of acute epididymoorchitis is found in 15% to 35% of cases in various pediatric series with this clinical presentation. Epididymoorchitis is uncommon in prepubertal boys, but has been reported in association with urinary tract infections with reflux or with an accompanying anorectal or related anomaly. A gram-negative organism, such as *Salmonella* or *Escherichia coli*, may be identified as the causative pathogen. Tuberculous epididymoorchitis has been reported in children in the less developed regions of the world. Viral orchitis, especially mumps orchitis, has diminished as a result of vaccination practices. Testicular pain related to a vasculitis-associated orchitis has been reported in up to 22% of boys with Henoch-Schönlein purpura.

Testicular microliths and calcified nodules are more frequently identified due to the increased use of ultrasound as they produce hyperechogenic signals in up to 5% of healthy individuals. Histologically, there are concentric calcifications and their presence has been linked to cryptorchidism, testicular regression, silent torsion, and testicular GCT.

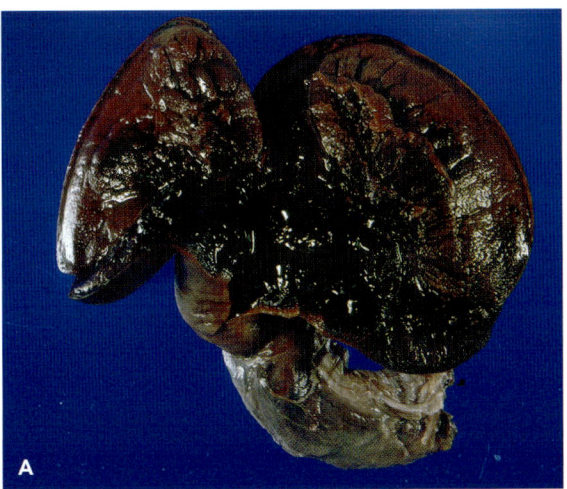
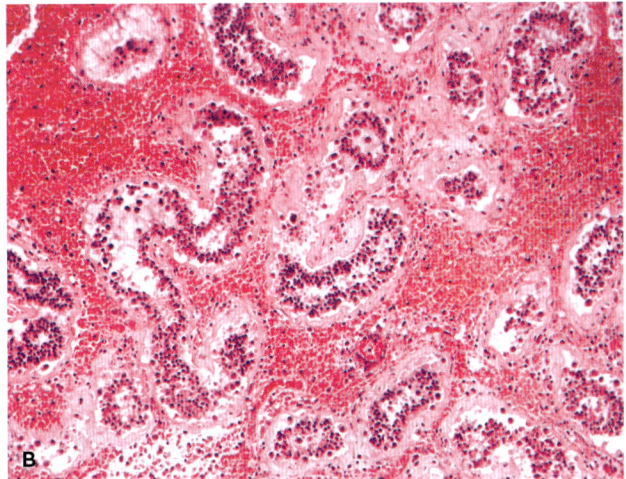

FIGURE 19-5 • Testicular torsion. **A:** The testis is congested with hemorrhagic cut section (Courtesy: Dr. Jerome Taxy, Chicago, IL). **B:** Microscopically, ischemic changes and features of hemorrhagic infarction are evident with sloughing of the seminiferous tubules and interstitial edema and hemorrhage.

Toxic injury to the testis in childhood can result in loss of germ cells, atrophy, and possible subfertility. Systemic chemotherapy and radiation of the testes or central nervous system are significant causes of testicular damage in survivors of childhood malignancy and in children who receive cyclophosphamide for renal diseases (51). The prepubertal state of the testis does not protect the gonad from the late effects of treatment. Decreased or absent spermatogenesis with Sertoli-only tubules, interstitial fibrosis, and testicular atrophy are the principal histologic findings. The effects of these medications are related to their cumulative doses. Decreased testicular size correlates with decreased sperm production and inhibin B levels and increased levels of LH and FSH (51). It has been suggested that despite these histologic effects, there is some recovery of spermatogenesis following aggressive chemotherapy when pharmacologic protection has been instituted. Additionally, testicular tissue cryopreservation in prepubertal boys before chemotherapy and radiotherapy is now possible. Children with renal failure may experience a significant loss of spermatogonia per seminiferous tubule, which tends to increase with age but is not seen in all children with renal failure.

Neoplasms of the Testis

Prepubertal testicular tumors are rare with an incidence of only between 0.5 and 2 per 100,000 children, accounting for approximately 1% to 2% of all pediatric solid neoplasms (52). They represent a heterogeneous group of tumors of germ cell as well as non–germ cell origins (Table 19-2). Some of these tumors are associated with sexual maldevelopment syndromes with dysgenetic gonads, or cryptorchidism. As a result of the rarity of such tumors, the Section of Urology of the American Academy of Pediatrics established the Prepubertal Testicular Tumor Registry (PTTR) in order to compile clinical and pathologic data from multiple institutions. Data from this registry have been published in a number of excellent studies and review papers (65). It was reported that approximately 30% of these tumors occur in the first year of life and about 7% occur in the neonatal period (65). In earlier studies, the age of distribution was reported to be bimodal, with a peak in the first 5 years of life and then a gradually increasing frequency in late adolescence.

The majority of pediatric testicular tumors are of germ cell origin followed in frequency by gonadal stromal tumors (53). Rhabdomyosarcoma (RMS), on the other hand, represents the most common tumor of the spermatic cord and paratesticular soft tissues. In the newborn, however, the most frequent testicular tumor is JGCT (66,67). A painless nontender scrotal mass is the presentation of the majority of prepubertal testicular neoplasms although, less commonly, the presentation may be that of testicular pain or trauma. Incidental testicular tumors during workup for gynecomastia or precocious puberty have been reported in up to 10% of patients in one institution. Adequate workup of a testicular mass is important to determine the nature of the process, to select the appropriate management approach, and to avoid misinterpretation as a nonneoplastic condition. It has been reported that 5% to 23% of pediatric testicular tumors were misdiagnosed as torsion or hydrocele. Other conditions to be included in the differential diagnosis of a scrotal mass include hernia, hydrocele, hematoma/trauma, torsion, epididymitis, mumps orchitis, Henoch-Schönlein purpura, and paratesticular tumors.

The protocol for the examination of specimens from patients with malignant germ cell and sex cord–stromal tumors of the testis, exclusive of paratesticular malignancies, is useful in selected pediatric cases (68).

TABLE 19-2 TESTICULAR TUMORS IN CHILDREN

Germ cell tumors	Yolk sac tumor	856
	Teratoma	439
	Epidermoid cyst	48
	Mixed germ cell tumor[a]	51
	Embryonal carcinoma	20
	Seminoma	7
	Dermoid cyst	5
	Choriocarcinoma	1
Gonadal-stromal tumors	Leydig cell tumor	27
	Sertoli cell tumor	29
	Juvenile granulosa cell tumor (JGCT)	12
	Stromal tumors, unspecified	37
Gonadoblastoma		5
Paratesticular tumors	Rhabdomyosarcoma	115
	Other sarcomas	5
	Other tumors, unspecified	26
Miscellaneous tumors		34
Total		1717

Compiled data from 12 series (53–64).
[a]Some of these tumors were designated *teratocarcinoma* in their original reports.

Germ Cell Tumors

GCTs are the most common primary tumors of the testis in the first two decades of life, 50% to 60% of which occur in the first 2 years. Significant differences exist between prepubertal testicular GCTs and their adult (postpubertal) counterparts. While adult tumors usually comprise a mixed histology of seminomatous and nonseminomatous components, are most often malignant and are almost always associated with intratubular germ cell neoplasia (ITGCNU), prepubertal tumors typically contain only one histologic type (either teratoma or yolk sac tumor [YST]), may be either benign or malignant, do not usually occur in undescended testes, and lack the association with ITGCNU (69,70). These differences are also reflected in their respective genetic abnormalities. Prepubertal GCTs are diploid (teratoma) or aneuploid (YST). Postpubertal GCTs are hypertriploid (seminoma) or hypotriploid (nonseminoma) and consistently have one or more copies of the short arm of chromosome 12 [i(12p)] or other forms of 12p amplification (69). Staging of pediatric GCTs is distinct from that of the adult counterparts (Table 19-3) (71,72).

The most current World Health Organization (WHO) classification of testicular GCTs divides them into tumors of one histologic type, which includes seminoma, EC, YST, trophoblastic tumors, and teratoma, and tumors with more than one histologic type, which can contain any combination of any proportions of the pure forms (71). Consensus has now been reached concerning the prognostic factors that determine the outlook for patients with metastatic disease (72,73).

Despite the weak correlation of most etiologic factors with testicular GCTs, it is generally believed that these tumors are associated with abnormal conditions in fetal life. A number of contributing factors are recognized including cryptorchidism, prior testicular GCT, family history of testicular GCT, and certain somatosexual ambiguity syndromes. Most of these factors, however, are important only in postpubertal boys and adults.

GCTs of the testis generally encompass three clinicopathologic entities: the teratomas–YSTs of the infantile testis, the seminomas and nonseminomas of adolescents and adults, and the spermatocytic seminomas. This chapter will focus on the former most entity with highlights on the other two as they relate to the pediatric population.

Yolk Sac Tumor

Formerly known as *endodermal sinus tumor*, YST is characterized by numerous growth patterns that recapitulate the yolk sac, allantois, and extraembryonic mesenchyme. The nosology has evolved from the concept of infantile adenocarcinoma, orchioblastoma, EC, and infantile EC to the current concept of a neoplasm with morphologic features recapitulating the extraembryonic yolk sac or endodermal sinus.

YST is the most common testicular GCT in childhood, accounting for as much as 75% of prepubertal testicular GCTs (52). Despite its occurrence in all races, it is much more common in Caucasians than in African Americans, Native Americans, and Indians and may be more common in Asians when compared to Caucasians. The median age at presentation is 16 to 19 months (52). YST occurs more commonly in the right testis, and the most common presenting symptom is a painless scrotal mass. Other possible symptoms include a history of trauma, acute onset of pain, and hydrocele. At least one case has been previously reported in an intra-abdominal testis. Serum α-fetoprotein (AFP) levels are elevated in more than 90% of tumors in a number of studies including those that are based on data from the PTTR (52). It is very important to remember that normal AFP ranges in young infants are higher than those in older patients. Usually, YST is not hormonally active rendering precocious puberty an unlikely presentation. Most tumors are not associated with cryptorchidism or a dysgenetic gonad. ITGCNU is not observed in the adjacent testis in children with pure YST in contrast to its ubiquitous presence in testicular GCT in adolescents and young adults (74). By ultrasonography, YST is typically solid, hypoechoic, and devoid of cystic structures, which, when present within the mass, argues against the diagnosis of YST. Approximately 10% to 20% of children with YST will present with metastases (52,75), which can occur hematogenously or via lymphatic drainage, unlike adult YST that metastasizes predominantly through lymphatics. Hematogenous spread alone can occur in up to 40% of cases (75). YST metastases to the lung occur in 20% of cases compared with 4% to 6% to the retroperitoneal lymph nodes (75). The lungs represent the most common site of metastasis followed by retroperitoneal lymph nodes, liver, and bones (76). When metastases develop, they usually appear within 14 months of initial presentation (52,75).

Grossly, pure YST is often solid and soft with a pale gray to pale yellow cut surface, which can sometimes be gelatinous or mucoid (52,77). Hemorrhage and necrosis may be observed in large tumors; however, their presence (and/or that of cysts) should raise the possibility of a mixed GCT, especially in adolescents.

Microscopically, the histopathologic appearance of YST is similar in both the prepubertal and the postpubertal age groups. Several patterns are recognized that are usually admixed in variable proportions (Figure 19-6). It is not unusual for one pattern to predominate; however, it is rare that an entire tumor comprises a pure single histologic pattern (52,77). The most common histologic pattern is the *microcystic or reticular pattern*, which consists of meshwork of vacuolated cells producing a honeycomb appearance, often with hyaline globules. Tumor cells are usually small and may contain pale eosinophilic secretions. The *endodermal sinus*

TABLE 19-3	STAGING OF PEDIATRIC GCT BY THE PEDIATRIC ONCOLOGY GROUP
Stage I	Tumor limited to the testis
	No clinical, radiographic, or histologic evidence of disease beyond the testis
	Appropriate decline in serum AFP (AFP half-life = 5 d)
Stage II	Microscopic disease located in scrotum or high in spermatic cord (≤0.5 cm from proximal end)
	Retroperitoneal lymph node involvement (≤2 cm)
	Serum AFP persistently elevated
Stage III	Retroperitoneal lymph node involvement (>2 cm)
	No visceral or extra-abdominal involvement
Stage IV	Distant metastases

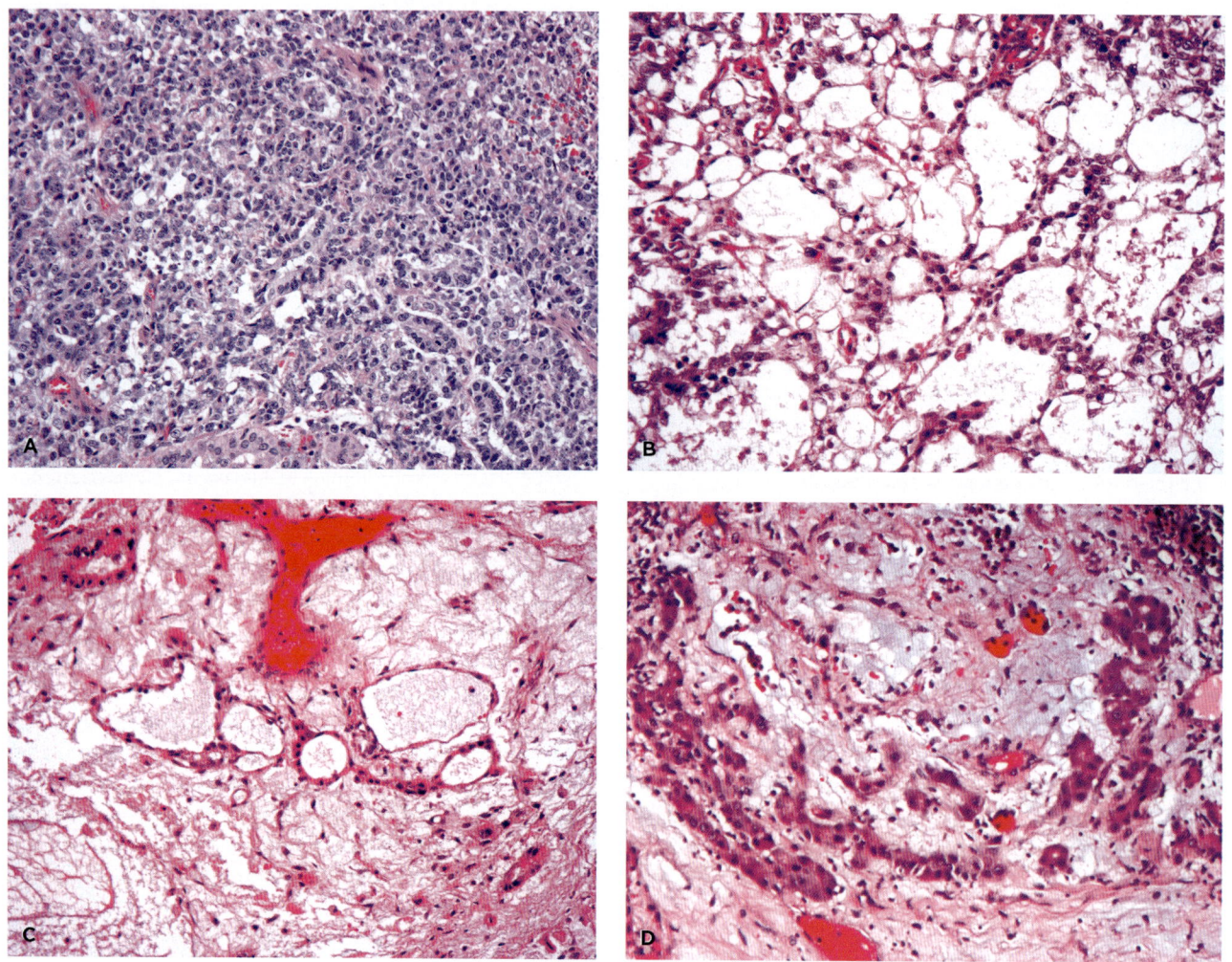

FIGURE 19-6 • Yolk sac tumor. **A-D:** Predominantly solid and focal glandular pattern (**A**), microcystic pattern (**B**), tubular/macrocystic pattern (**C**), and hepatoid pattern (**D**). Note the myxoid and hypocellular background (**C**, **D**).

pattern consists of papillary structures known as *Schiller-Duval bodies*, which are considered the hallmark of YST, even though they are not required for the diagnosis and are actually identified only in a minority of cases. These structures consist of a stalk of connective tissue with thin-walled blood vessels lined on the surface by a layer of cuboidal cells with clear cytoplasm and prominent nucleoli. Other recognized microscopic patterns include *solid, macrocystic, glandular–alveolar, papillary, myxomatous, polyvesicular vitelline, hepatoid,* and *enteric* patterns (Figure 19-6). Mitotic activity can be brisk in any of these patterns. Hyaline globules may be identified especially in the hepatoid and enteric patterns. By immunohistochemistry, AFP expression is helpful but can be variable and sometimes weak. Its absence, however, does not exclude the diagnosis of YST. Low molecular weight cytokeratins are usually strongly expressed, and a SALL4-positive/OCT4-negative profile can also be helpful in diagnostically challenging cases (78). A number of proteins, usually present in the fetal liver, may also be expressed in YST such as α-1-antitrypsin, albumin, and ferritin. Genetic analysis of infantile YST did not identify a specific gene or genes involved in the pathogenesis of this tumor. However, a number of recurrent genetic anomalies are known to occur including losses of the short arm of chromosome 1 (particularly the 1p36 region), the long arm of chromosomes 6 (6q21–26) and 16 and gains in the long arms of chromosomes 1 and 20 (20q13), the short arm of chromosome 3 (3p21-pter), and the complete chromosome 22 (79).

The treatment of choice for prepubertal YST is surgical excision (i.e., radical orchiectomy). Metastatic workup is required for adequate staging of tumor, and serum AFP is important in establishing the preoperative diagnosis and also as a follow-up postoperatively for possible tumor recurrence.

Teratoma

Teratoma is a tumor composed of several types of tissue representing different germinal layers (endoderm, mesoderm, and ectoderm), forming somatic-type tissue in various stages of maturation and differentiation (80) for which the term *mature* or *immature* (fetal-like) apply. However, based on findings of genetic studies, it is now recommended to consider teratoma as a single entity regardless of the degree of maturation and differentiation of the tissue comprising it (71). Tumors consisting of ectoderm, mesoderm, or endoderm derivatives only are classified as monodermal teratomas. In its pure form, teratoma comprises approximately 3% of testicular GCT in adults and up to 38% of the prepubertal GCT (80) with a reported incidence that ranges from 0.5 to 2.0 cases per 100,000 boys. Teratoma is the second most common testicular tumor in children and adolescents following YST with a relative frequency ranging from 13% to 60% (54). About 65% of prepubertal teratomas occur in the first 2 years of life with a mean age of 20 months and represent 50% of GCT seen in the first decade of life.

Most patients present with a firm, irregular, nodular, and nontender scrotal mass that usually does not transilluminate. Approximately 2% to 3% of prepubertal teratomas may be associated with or misdiagnosed as hydroceles, especially if the tumor has a cystic component. Teratomas usually present as a unilateral scrotal mass, but rare examples of bilaterality in infancy and childhood have been reported (81).

Teratomas in undescended, intra-abdominal testes may present with abdominal pain due to torsion, as calcification or ossification on imaging studies, or as an abdominal mass. Prenatal sonographic diagnosis might be possible in cases of a fetal abdominal mass, especially when the testis cannot be detected in the scrotum by the 8th month. Teratomas are hormonally inactive; hence, precocious puberty is not a common presentation and serum AFP levels are helpful in distinguishing them from YST (75).

By imaging studies, teratomas are generally well-circumscribed and heterogeneous masses and a cystic component is commonly demonstrated (82). On gross examination, teratomas are usually nodular and firm with a variably cystic and solid cut surface (Figure 19-7A). The cysts may be filled with keratinous material or clear serous or mucoid fluid. The solid areas may contain translucent, gray–white nodules representing cartilage. Rarely, hair or melanin-containing tissue may also be evident. Areas of immature tissue are mostly solid and may have an encephaloid, hemorrhagic, or necrotic appearance.

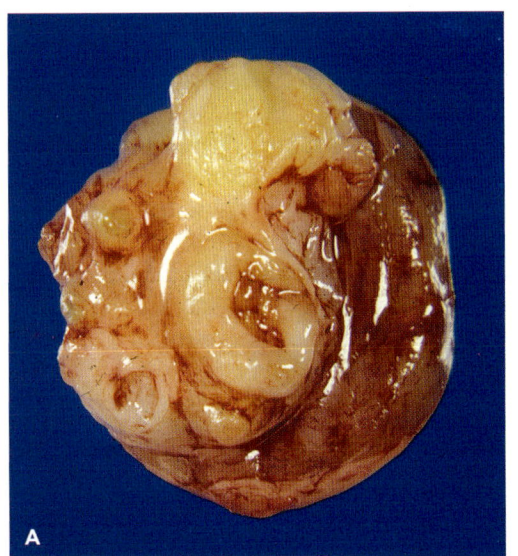
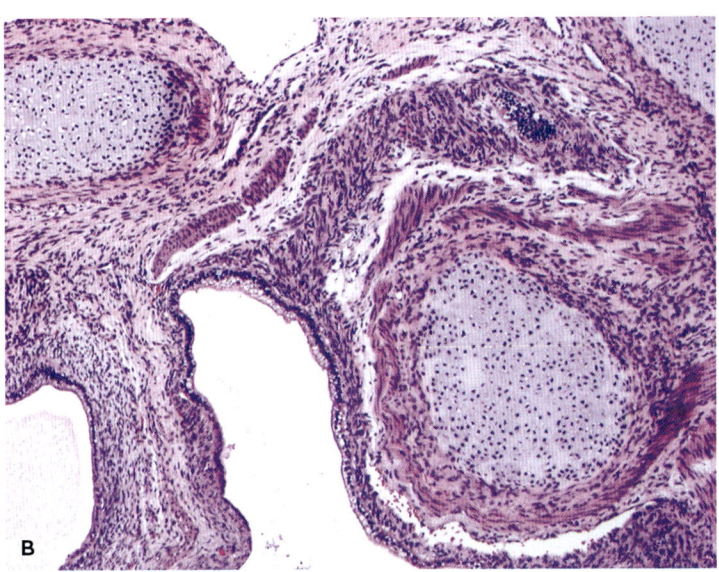
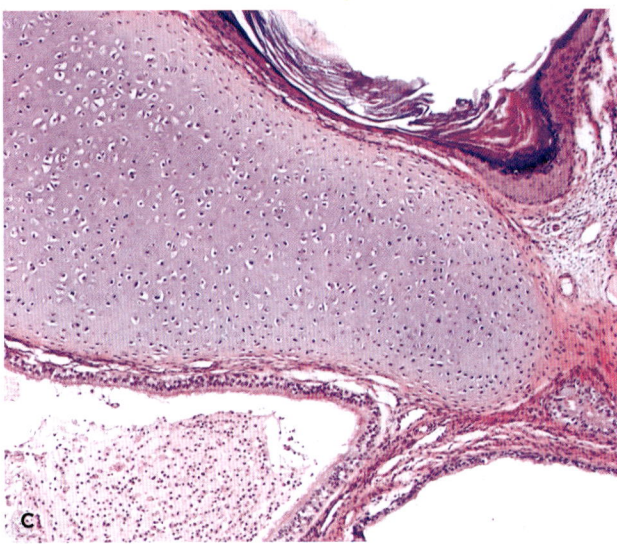

FIGURE 19-7 • Teratoma in a prepubertal testis. **A:** Grossly, the tumor has a heterogeneous multinodular appearance with cystic and solid areas. (Courtesy: Dr. Jerome Taxy, Chicago, IL). **B, C:** Microscopically, a mixture of mature structures derived from ectoderm, mesoderm, and endoderm is noted, characterized by keratinizing squamous epithelium, ciliated respiratory-type epithelium, and mature cartilage.

Microscopically, mature elements resemble normal postnatal tissue and typically include structures derived from the three germ layers (Figure 19-7B). Structures of ectodermal origin are usually manifested by nests of squamous epithelium with or without cyst formation and keratinization. Neural tissue may be encountered as foci of neuroglia. Structures of endodermal origin are represented by glandular epithelium of enteric or respiratory type. Other glandular tissue such as pancreas, mucus-producing epithelium, prostate, and thyroid may be found. Mesodermal elements are represented by cartilage, bone, adipose tissue, fibrous tissue, and, most commonly, muscle. Attempts at organ formation are frequently identified with smooth muscle encircling glands of respiratory or enteric morphology. Immature, fetal-type tissue may also consist of ectodermal, endodermal, and/or mesodermal elements. It usually occurs as islands of immature neuroepithelium resembling that of the developing embryonic neural tube. Immature tissue may also have an organoid arrangement with blastomatous and primitive tubular structures resembling that of the developing kidney or lung. Embryonic skeletal muscle, cartilage, and nonspecific cellular stroma may also be encountered (77,80). The so-called fetus in fetu is an expression of extreme maturation and organization of a teratoma or a form of pathologic monozygotic twinning. A number of somatic-type malignancies have developed in testicular teratomas, some of which developed following irradiation for a testicular teratoma with metastases. These included Wilms tumor, leiomyosarcoma, angiosarcoma, and RMS (83,84).

Infantile teratomas are diploid. Genetic studies (karyotyping and comparative genomic hybridization) have failed to demonstrate chromosomal changes in these tumors. In contrast, teratomas in adult testes are hypotriploid and have genetic changes similar to those seen in other components of adult GCT (73,79,85).

The prognosis is excellent in children since teratomas are universally benign tumors, unlike their adult counterpart (80). Pure teratoma of the prepubertal testis has not been reported to metastasize and does not develop, at least in the overwhelming majority of cases, from the lesion recognized as intratubular germ cell neoplasia, unclassified (69). Although orchiectomy has been considered the treatment of choice for prepubertal testicular teratomas, recent studies with long-term follow-up have demonstrated the safety and efficacy of testis-sparing surgery (86).

Epidermoid Cyst

Epidermoid cyst is a benign tumor of ectodermal origin, characterized by its keratin-producing epithelium and lack of other germinal layer components, thus differentiating it from a teratoma. It accounts for less than 1% of all testicular tumors and 3% to 14% of pediatric testicular tumors with 25% occurring in the first two decades of life (53,87). The nosology and the pathogenesis are uncertain. A germ-cell origin is most likely; however, intratubular germ cell neoplasia is not an accompanying feature. This lesion usually presents as a firm, well-defined intratesticular nodule, with or without symptoms. On ultrasonography, it appears as a central hypoechoic mass with an echogenic rim. Grossly, the cyst is confined to the testicular parenchyma and is filled with flaky yellow–white keratinous material (Figure 19-8A). Orderly, stratified squamous epithelium, a dense fibrous tissue wall, focal calcifications, and acellular keratinous debris are the classic histologic findings (Figure 19-8B). The cyst and the surrounding tissue should be examined carefully for presence of teratomatous or dermal adnexal elements, a testicular scar (which could potentially represent a regressed GCT component) or ITGCNU, the presence of which should lead to reclassification of the lesion as a mature teratoma (87).

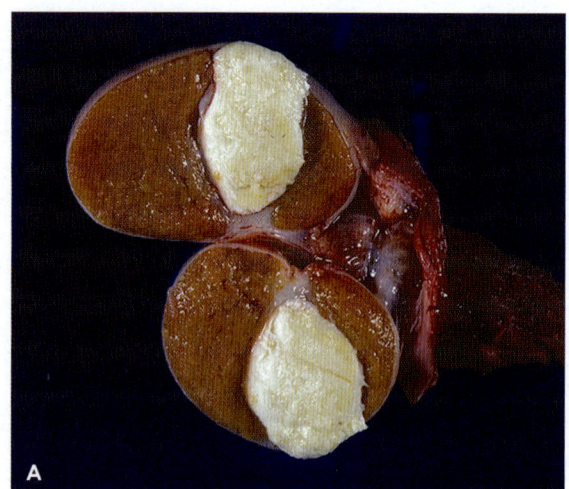
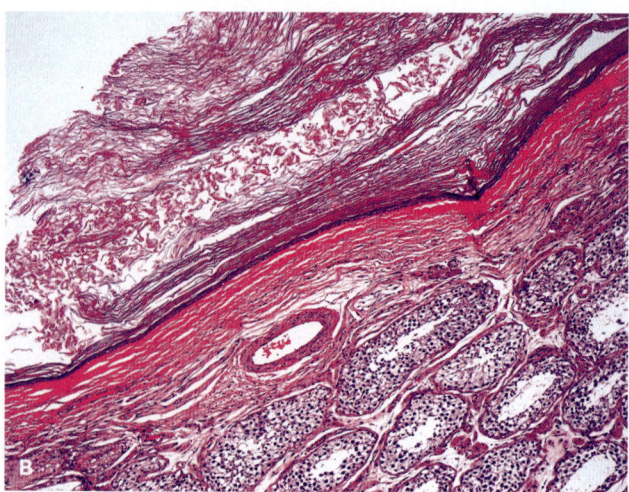

FIGURE 19-8 • Epidermoid cyst. **A:** The cyst is well circumscribed and completely intratesticular. It contains flaky yellow-white keratinous material (Courtesy: Dr. Jerome Taxy, Chicago, IL). **B:** Microscopically, abundant lamellated keratinous material is filling the cyst with a fibrous wall separating it from the adjacent testicular parenchyma. No intratubular germ cell neoplasia is noted in the adjacent seminiferous tubules.

A conservative surgical approach with simple enucleation has been advocated for this benign lesion.

Intratubular Germ Cell Neoplasia, Unclassified Type

Intratubular germ cell neoplasia, unclassified type (IGCNU or ITGCN) is a microscopic precursor lesion composed of malignant germ cells within the seminiferous tubules with abundant clear cytoplasm, large irregular nuclei, and prominent nucleoli. This term refers to the lesion initially described by Skakkebaek as "carcinoma *in situ*" as well as to other "differentiated" forms of intratubular germ cell neoplasia. IGCNU is present in up to 4% of cryptorchid testes, in up to 5% of contralateral gonads in patients with unilateral GCT, and in up to 1% of biopsies from oligospermic infertile men (69). Additionally, it can be found in virtually all cases adjacent to invasive GCT in adult testes when residual testicular parenchyma is present. In contrast, its association with GCT arising in prepubertal testes is still a source of controversy and its true incidence is difficult to assess (70,74). It is generally believed, however, that IGCNU is not associated with teratomas and pure YST in early childhood, in keeping with a different pathogenesis for this subset of testicular GCT (88). Rarely, IGCNU has been described in association with maldescended testes, intersex states, and rare infantile YST and teratoma. In one series, IGCNU was reported in four patients with gonadal dysgenesis (89). In 12 patients with androgen insensitivity (testicular feminization), three were found to have unexpected IGCNU when no tumor was clinically apparent (90). In another study of 102 cases of various intersex states, the authors reported IGCNU in 0 of 23 patients with androgen insensitivity syndrome (testicular feminization), 3 of 38 with gonadal dysgenesis, 1 of 12 with TH, 1 of 22 with male pseudohermaphroditism, and 1 of 7 with multiple congenital anomalies and ambiguous genitalia (91).

IGCNU is not reliably detected in the prepubertal at-risk patients. Conversely, the identification of atypical germ cells in prepubertal biopsies does not correlate with tumor risk. Although abnormal germ cell morphology has been described in prepubertal patients with cryptorchidism (23), the findings are different from IGCNU, and their significance is not established, unlike the known significance of IGCNU. One large study found no intratubular germ cells adjacent to GCT in prepubertal children were positive for PLAP or c-kit; five of seven were positive for PCNA, and p53 was present in the two examined cases. These results indicate that germ cells adjacent to infantile GCT are proliferative but not neoplastic and offer additional evidence that intratubular germ cells and GCT in prepubertal boys are different from those of adolescents and adults (88). Similar studies have reported morphologic and immunohistochemical features of normal prepubertal germ cells that resemble those of IGCNU that can persist up to 1 year of life. Therefore, little or no benefit is derived from the routine biopsy of cryptorchid testes at the time of orchidopexy in prepubertal boys, and, if biopsy is to be performed, it should be delayed until after puberty. The assessment of risk by testicular biopsy in most prepubertal patients is not currently possible. An important exception to this general rule applies to prepubertal patients with intersex syndromes in whom the reliable identification of IGCNU or gonadoblastoma can be accomplished in early childhood (89).

Microscopically, the seminiferous tubules are partially or completely lined by large cells with round nuclei, coarse chromatin, mitoses, and abundant clear cytoplasm (Figure 19-9A). A PAS stain demonstrates abundant glycogen. Immunohistochemical markers that are positive include PLAP, CD117, OCT4, and SALL4 (78) (Figure 19-9B, C). In contrast to invasive GCT in adult testis, the presence of i(12p) in IGCNU has not been universally confirmed with most investigators suggesting it is not present (69).

Embryonal Carcinoma

EC is a rare tumor in the first decade of life and has a peak incidence in the 15- to 34-year-old age group. Although very common in mixed GCT, occurring in greater than 80% of cases, pure EC is rare with a rate of approximately 2.5%. An adolescent or young adult may present with an enlarging painful scrotal mass or metastases in the regional lymph nodes, abdomen, or mediastinum. The testis often contains a gray, focally necrotic, and hemorrhagic mass. The tumor is often poorly demarcated and the cut surface bulges markedly. Microscopically, sheets of large, pleomorphic undifferentiated cells with enlarged irregular and vesicular nuclei, distinct nuclear membranes, prominent nucleoli, and frequent mitoses are seen (Figure 19-10). Tumor necrosis is evident. Primitive gland formation and papillary structures with or without fibrovascular cores may be encountered. The characteristic immunohistochemical profile is cytokeratin positive, CD30 positive, SALL4 positive, OCT4 positive, PLAP positive (focal), and epithelial membrane antigen (EMA) negative (78,92). EC shares similar genetic abnormalities with other adult GCT. Tumor stage is the single most important prognostic indicator, and pure or predominant EC in a testicular tumor is associated with increased risk of advanced disease.

Seminoma

Seminoma is a malignant GCT composed of relatively uniform cells, typically with clear cytoplasm, well-defined cell borders, and large regular nuclei with one or more prominent nucleoli; the cells resemble primitive germ cells. There is almost always an associated lymphoid infiltrate and frequently a granulomatous inflammatory response (68). While seminoma is the most common primary testicular tumor in adults, it is rare in prepubertal boys but is found more frequently in late adolescence. In pediatric cases, the average age of presentation is 9.7 years. It remains crucial to distinguish seminoma from other (nonseminomatous) forms of GCT because of different therapeutic approaches.

Grossly, a seminoma characteristically forms a gray, cream to pale pink, soft, homogeneous, lobulated, and well-defined

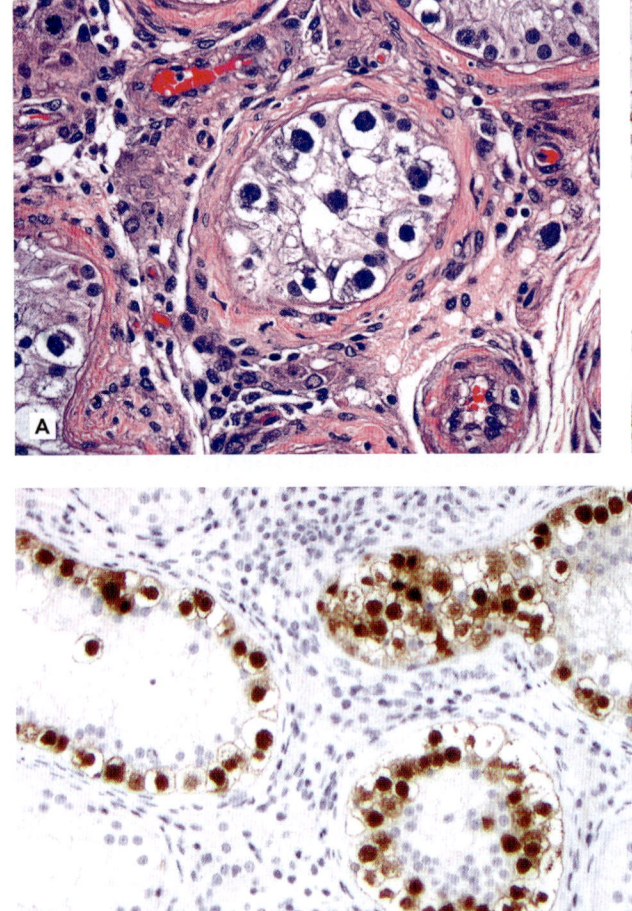
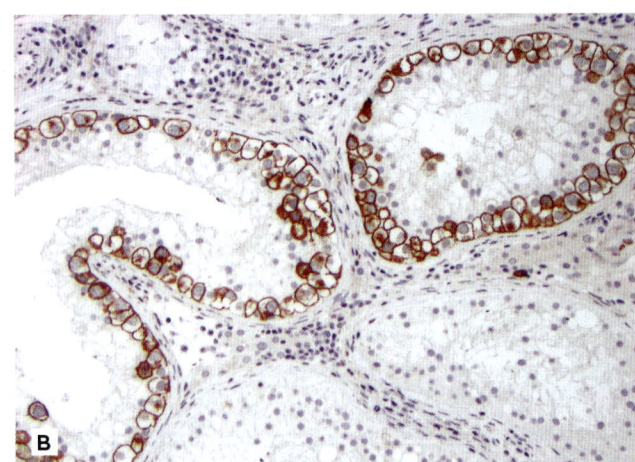

FIGURE 19-9 • Intratubular germ cell neoplasia, unclassified type. **A:** The lesion consists of large cells with round-to-irregular nuclei, coarse chromatin, and occasional nucleoli. A mitotic figure is present. The cytoplasm is abundant and clear. **B, C:** The presence of lesional cells can be further facilitated by membranous expression of CD117 and nuclear labeling by OCT4.

mass that may have irregular yellow foci of necrosis. The tumor may occasionally present as multiple macroscopically distinct nodules. Microscopically, the uniform cells of seminoma are arranged in sheets, clusters, or columns and associated with lymphocytic infiltrates of variable density. Pseudoglandular, tubular, and cribriform morphologic patterns have been reported, but the basic cellular morphology of seminoma remains the same. The immunohistochemical profile of seminoma classically includes expression of vimentin, PLAP, CD117, OCT4, and SALL4 (78,92).

Choriocarcinoma, as a pure form, almost never occurs in childhood, but maybe found as a component of mixed GCT, especially in adolescents. The pathologic features and treatment are similar to those as in adults. Metastatic choriocarcinoma rarely occurs in infants from a primary tumor in the mother.

Mixed Germ Cell Tumor

Mixed germ cell tumor (MGCT) includes tumors containing two or more GCT components (68,71). The individual components are microscopically identical to those seen in pure GCT. While accounting for up to 54% of tumors in the adult testis, MGCT is rarely seen in prepubertal children and becomes increasingly common in the second and third decades of life. In one study, it accounted for 3% of prepubertal testicular tumors (55). A common pattern is EC with one or more components of teratoma, seminoma, and YST, but virtually, any combination of GCT components can be seen. For diagnostic reporting, similar to tumors of the adult testis,

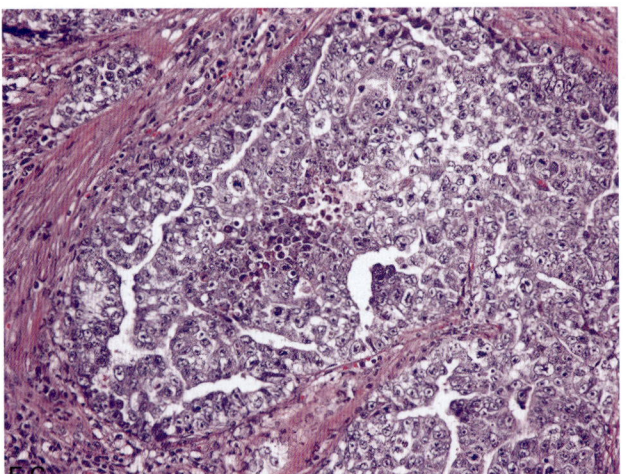

FIGURE 19-10 • Embryonal carcinoma. Tumor cells are large and pleomorphic with enlarged irregular and vesicular nuclei, distinct nuclear membranes, prominent nucleoli, and frequent mitoses. Numerous apoptotic cells are present. Necrosis is a common finding.

these tumors should be termed "mixed germ cell tumor, composed of…" followed by a tabulation of their percentages. The adjacent testis usually exhibits intratubular germ cell neoplasia. The combination of EC and teratoma has been previously termed *teratocarcinoma*, but it is currently recommended to include these under the MGCT category and list the components separately.

Sex Cord–Stromal Tumors

Sex cord–stromal tumors are composed of cells that recapitulate the specialized supportive structures of the male or the female gonad and include LCTs, SCT, granulosa cell tumors, and tumors of the theca/fibroma group (71). They account for 4% to 6% of tumors of the adult testis and up to 12% of prepubertal testicular tumors (93). Sex cord–stromal tumors are generally benign (94) with only rare cases of SCT reportedly behaving in a malignant fashion (95). Additionally, a number of sex cord-stromal tumors have been reported without demonstrable evidence of differentiation toward any of the specific entities mentioned here and are referred to as *undifferentiated sex cord–stromal tumors*. Some of these tumors have occurred in pediatric age patients, and some also developed metastasis.

Leydig Cell Tumor

LCT, also known as *interstitial cell tumor*, is rare in children, accounting for up to 8% of pediatric testicular tumors and 14% of sex cord–stromal tumors (71). Generally, approximately 20% of LCTs occur in the first decade of life. In this patient population, the tumor is most common between 3 and 9 years with a mean age at presentation of 7 years. Although it typically presents with a painless testicular mass, patients usually display signs of precocious puberty and elevated levels of serum testosterone and androstenedione and dehydroepiandrosterone. Gynecomastia may be seen in 10% to 15% of patients. LCT may be seen in patients with KS, and 5% to 10% of patients with LCT may have a history of cryptorchid testis. By ultrasonography, these tumors are typically small, solid, well defined, and hypoechoic. Grossly, the tumor is well circumscribed and may be encapsulated. The cut surface is homogeneous yellow–brown, with possible areas of hyalinization and calcification. Microscopically, the tumor is composed of large polygonal or round cells with abundant granular, eosinophilic cytoplasm, forming sheets, trabeculae, and cords that displace seminiferous tubules (Figure 19-11). Nuclei may vary in size and shape, but atypia and mitoses are not reliable for predicting aggressive behavior of LCT. Two other cell types seen occasionally are small round cells with scanty cytoplasm and an eccentric, hyperchromatic nucleus and clear cells resembling the adrenal zona fasciculata. Occasional spindling of tumor cells may be present. Lipofuscin pigment may be seen in up to 15% of cases. Crystals of Reinke are present only in 30% to 40% of cases. Abundant smooth endoplasmic reticulum and lipid are identified ultrastructurally. By immunohistochemistry, LCT is generally positive for vimentin, inhibin, calretinin, and melan-A (A103) and exhibits variable expression of cytokeratins, EMA, desmin, S-100 protein, chromogranin, and synaptophysin. Immunostains for carcinoembryonic antigen and PLAP are consistently negative. LCT in prepubertal patients is benign and can be adequately treated by either radical orchiectomy or testis-sparing surgery.

In contrast to LCT, Leydig cell hyperplasia occurs in neonates, is bilateral, and shows a transition between nodular and diffuse Leydig cell proliferation (96). Normal seminiferous tubules intermingle with Leydig cells throughout, and spermatogenesis is evident in tubules adjacent to nodules. An important differential diagnosis to consider is the testicular "tumor" of the AGS. These lesions are usually discovered in early adult life in patients with congenital adrenal hyperplasia, but in up to one-third of cases may be detected in

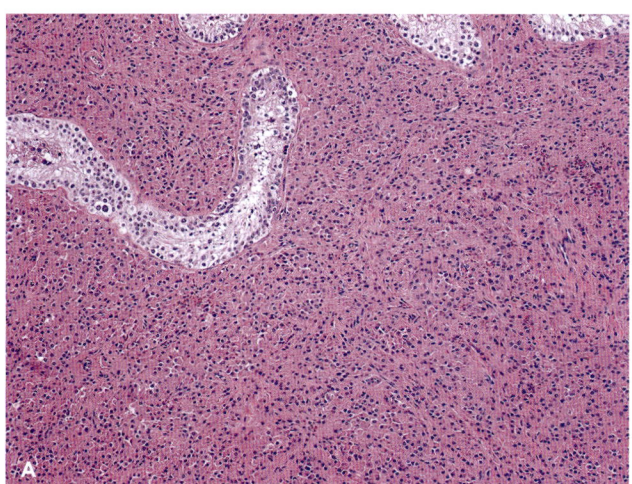
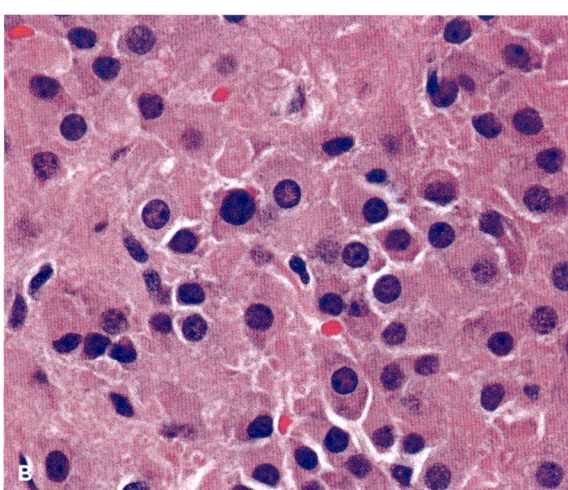

FIGURE 19-11 • Leydig cell tumor. **A:** Sheets of polygonal or round cells with abundant granular, eosinophilic cytoplasm are evident, displacing seminiferous tubules. **B:** The cytoplasm is typically finely granular and eosinophilic with mild variation in nuclear size and shape.

children where they occur as small nodules. Similar lesions are typically seen in Nelson syndrome (97). This condition consists of bilateral, dark brown nodules with pleomorphic pigmented cells and hyalinized fibrotic stroma. Although small lesions may involve the testicular hilum only, larger nodules almost always involve the testicular parenchyma (29). Awareness of this entity is important since these lesions usually decrease in size following corticosteroid therapy and may be managed conservatively. Surgical removal, either by tumor enucleation or orchiectomy, however, may become necessary in refractory cases.

Sertoli Cell Tumor

SCT is a sex cord–stromal tumor of the testis composed of cells recapitulating features of Sertoli cells at variable degrees of development. This is a rare neoplasm accounting for less than 1% of all testicular tumors and typically occurring in adults and only exceptionally reported in males younger than 20 (98). Some variant forms, however, are more common in infants and children, especially those with syndromic and/or genetic associations such as androgen insensitivity syndrome (99), Carney syndrome, and Peutz-Jeghers syndrome (98,100).

Painless and slow testicular enlargement is a common presentation (98). Elevated estradiol levels, sexual precocity, and gynecomastia may occur in patients with SCT associated with the Peutz-Jeghers syndrome. Although this tumor is usually unilateral, those associated with syndromic conditions may be multiple and bilateral. By ultrasonography, SCT is generally hypoechoic but can demonstrate variable echogenicity with possible cystic areas. In general, no imaging characteristics would allow distinction from a GCT. An exception is the large cell calcifying variant (see below), which is characterized by large areas of calcifications that can be readily suspected by ultrasound, especially when this tumor presents as multiple and bilateral masses.

The gross appearance of the enlarged testis with SCT is variable, ranging from a firm, circumscribed, lobulated, gritty, tan or yellow nodule to a multicystic mass. Foci of hemorrhage may be seen but necrosis is uncommon. Microscopically, SCT may vary in appearance ranging from tubular arrangement to retiform or solid growth pattern to cords of tumor cells (Figure 19-12). The intervening stroma is fibrotic, moderately to sparsely cellular or hyalinized. Tumor cells have round, oval, or elongated nuclei. The chromatin pattern is vesicular; nucleoli are not prominent and nuclear grooves or inclusions may be seen. The cytoplasm can be pale to eosinophilic, clear, or vacuolated due to the presence of lipids. Mild nuclear pleomorphism and atypia may be seen in the minority of cases. By immunohistochemistry, SCT is consistently reactive with antibodies against vimentin and cytokeratins with variable expression reported with antibodies against inhibin and S-100 (98). SCT is typically negative for placental alkaline phosphatase, α-fetoprotein, and EMA. Frequent mutations of β-catenin were detected in a recent series of SCT with strong nuclear and diffuse cytoplasmic β-catenin immunohistochemical expression in tumors harboring mutations (101). None of the studied cases in that series however was from a pediatric patient, and it remains unknown whether such aberrations would be detected in SCT in the pediatric age group. Electron microscopy reveals the characteristic features of Sertoli cells: tubular structures with well-defined basement membrane, complex cytoplasmic interdigitations, numerous intercellular junctions, prominent Golgi apparatus, large lipid droplets, abundant smooth endoplasmic reticulum, and Charcot-Böttcher crystals in some examples.

In children, SCTs typically follow a benign course. However, metastatic potential does exist especially in older children. Radical orchiectomy is the preferred treatment. In older boys when the tumor is suspected of behaving in a malignant fashion, patients should undergo evaluation for metastatic disease. The latter condition should be treated aggressively with a combination of chemotherapy, radiation therapy, and retroperitoneal lymph node dissection (86).

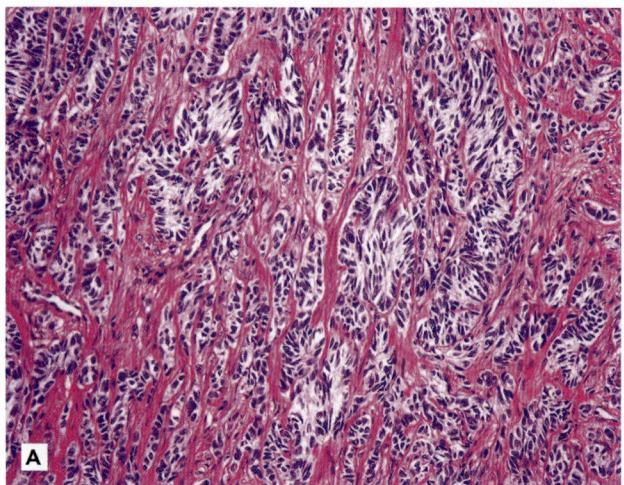
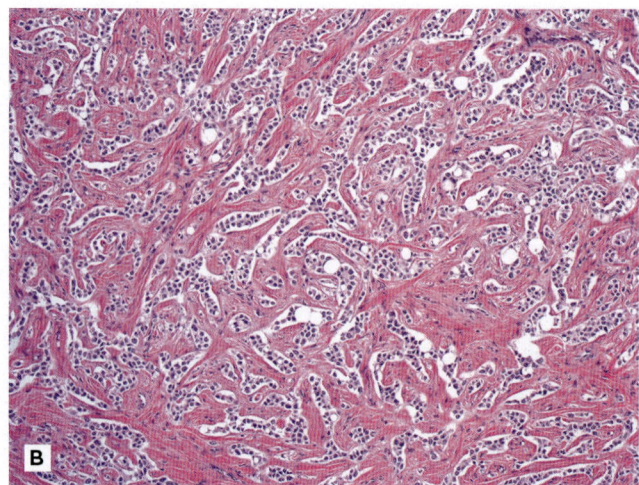

FIGURE 19-12 • Sertoli cell tumor. **A, B:** This tumor exhibits variable morphology characterized by solid nests in a dense fibrotic background, compressed tubular arrangement (trabecular) with a resemblance to a carcinoid.

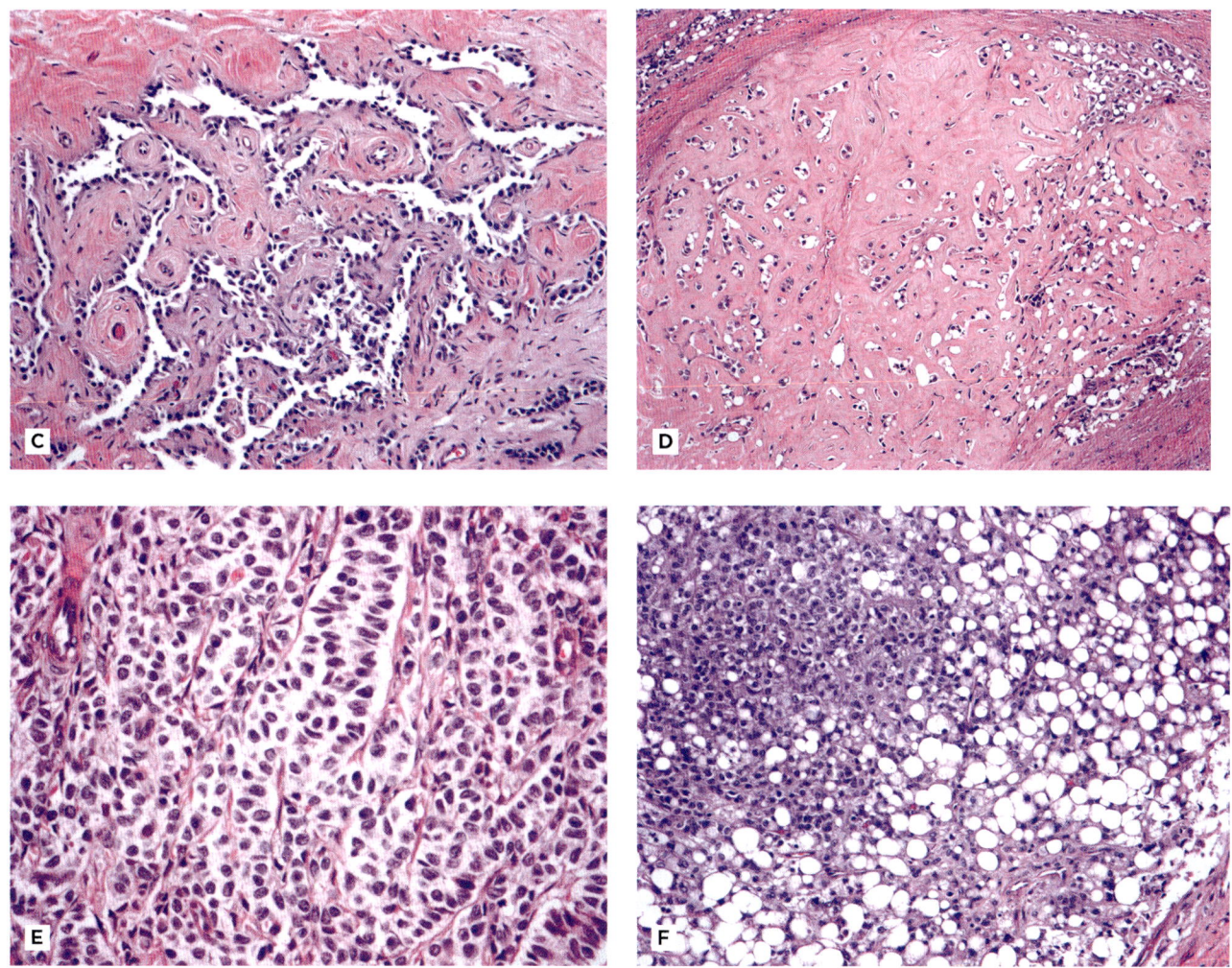

FIGURE 19-12 • *(Continued)* **C:** Complex and anastomosing tubular structures "retiform," or cordlike structures in a sclerotic to hyalinized stroma. **D, E:** Tumor cells with round, oval, or elongate nuclei, vesicular chromatin pattern, occasional grooves, and inconspicuous nucleoli. **F:** The cytoplasm is pale to eosinophilic but can also exhibit prominent clearing or vacuolization.

Large cell calcifying SCT (LCCSCT), as mentioned above, is a unique variant of SCT that can be sporadic (60%), but can also be part of Peutz-Jeghers and Carney syndromes (40%). This variant tends to occur in young individuals with an average age of 16 years and can be bilateral in 40% of cases. Associated features include multiple endocrine disorders manifested by precocious puberty, gynecomastia, acromegaly, bilateral primary adrenocortical hyperplasia, and pituitary adenomas. Cardiac myxomas and mucocutaneous pigmentations are other reported features in Carney syndrome. Microscopically, LCCSCT consists of nests, trabeculae, small clusters, and cords of large polygonal cells with abundant eosinophilic finely granular cytoplasm embedded in a myxohyaline stroma, which typically contains large areas of calcifications (Figure 19-13). The nuclei are round to oval with vesicular chromatin pattern and inconspicuous nucleoli. Intratubular spread of tumor cells is usually present.

Interestingly, multifocal intratubular proliferations of Sertoli cells distinct from those observed in LCCSCT have been recently reported in patients with Peutz-Jeghers syndrome in two separate studies. Eleven of the 14 patients from both studies did not have an associated SCT (102,103).

Juvenile Granulosa Cell Tumor

JGCT is a rare tumor consisting of structures resembling Graafian follicles. Despite its rarity, this tumor is the most frequent congenital testicular neoplasm and most common tumor in the first 6 months of life (66,67). The reported incidence ranges from 3% to 6.6% of all prepubertal testicular tumors (93), with 50% of tumors occurring in the neonatal period and 90% within the first year of life (67,104), making it exceptional to observe this tumor after the first year of life. Most of these tumors present as painless testicular mass and typically are not hormonally active. JGCT can be associated with abnormal karyotypic mosaicism and structural abnormalities in chromosome Y, especially in patients with ambiguous external genitalia (105). Other associated abnormalities include MGD and hypospadias. JGCT can occasionally occur

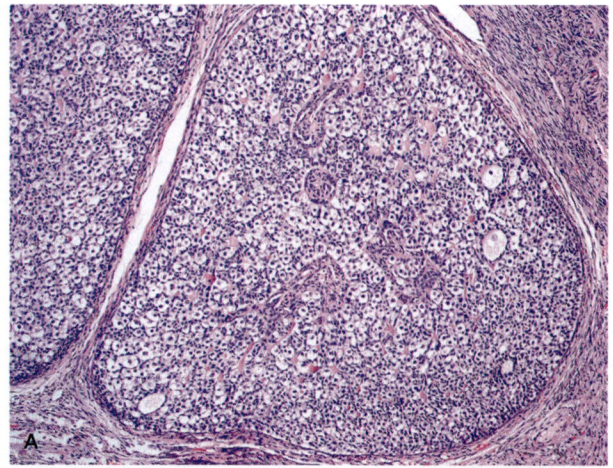
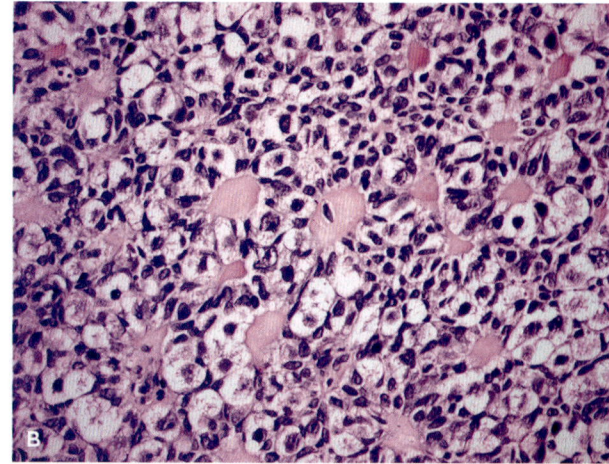
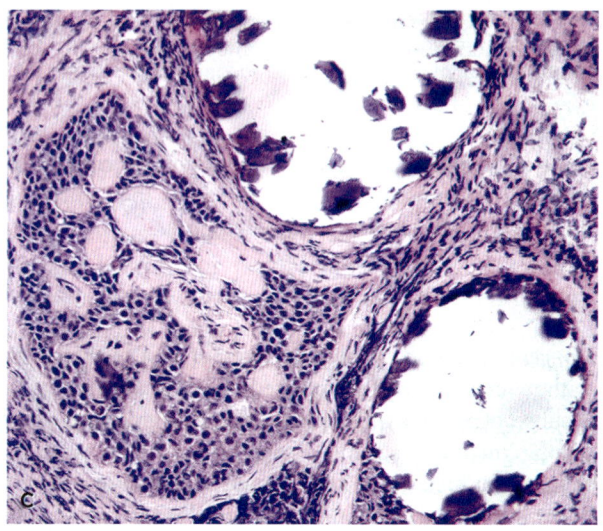

FIGURE 19-15 • Gonadoblastoma. **A:** Nodules of tumor consisting of a mixture of nests of large and pale seminoma-like cells admixed with sex cord cells with small, dark, angular nuclei. **B:** Hyalinized nodules of basement membrane material are surrounded by tumor cells. **C:** A focus with prominent calcifications.

supporting the view that testicular infiltration is indicative of widespread disease (112). Although testicular involvement by ALL may be clinically evident in about 8% of cases, microscopic involvement may be as high as 21%. The testis may also be the site of relapse after bone marrow remission is established and may signal a systemic relapse. In clinically evident cases, the testis has a bulging, pale tan surface with diffuse and nodular pattern of infiltration. Microscopically, there is diffuse interstitial infiltrate of small cells with scanty cytoplasm, surrounding and infiltrating the seminiferous tubules. The diagnosis can be established by needle or open-wedge testicular biopsy.

Juvenile xanthogranuloma rarely occurs in the testis of infants.

EPIDIDYMIS, SPERMATIC CORD, AND PARATESTICULAR TISSUES

Congenital and Developmental Anomalies

A number of congenital anomalies of the mesonephric duct system can occur. These anatomic defects are usually identified either at the time of orchidopexy for an UDT or during an investigation for infertility. The spectrum of morphologic manifestations ranges from total absence of the epididymis, vas deferens, seminal vesicles, and ejaculatory ducts to selective atresia, cysts, diverticula, and ectopias (113). Complete absence of the vas deferens is the most common congenital obstructive abnormality of the male mesonephric duct system and is found in 3.5% to 8% of males evaluated for infertility (113); cystic fibrosis should be considered in the differential diagnosis. Absence of the seminal vesicles and ejaculatory ducts often accompanies absence of the vas deferens. Epididymal abnormalities are present in 36% to 43% of patients with maldescent of the testis. These include agenesis; atresia of the head, body, or tail; and a loop or an elongated epididymis. This association is especially common in the presence of an UDT and a complete hernia sac (114). Seminal vesicle cysts may simulate prostatitis clinically and are associated with ipsilateral upper urinary tract abnormalities. Spermatic cord cysts may be of mesothelial or mesonephric origin. Those of mesothelial origin are typically unilocular and lined by flat poorly cohesive epithelium with chronic inflammation and hyalinization in the wall, while mesonephric cysts are multilocular and lined by cohesive attenuated or columnar epithelium and may contain spermatozoa if in continuity with the sperm excretory ducts. In approximately 10% of cases, the origin of spermatic cord cysts maybe indeterminate due to the lack of recognizable epithelium.

Small glandular or tubular inclusions, which probably represent embryonal remnants of müllerian ducts, are found in 0.53% to 6% of hernia sacs from males in the first two decades (115). The ciliated low columnar epithelial cells have eosinophilic cytoplasm and basal nuclei and are surrounded by a mantle of fibrous tissue without smooth muscle. Due to their morphologic overlap, it is important to distinguish these embryonal remnants in hernia sacs from the true vas deferens or epididymis because of the implications for fertility and potential medicolegal ramifications (116,117). These embryonal tubular structures have a smaller diameter than the vas deferens, often lack smooth muscle, and do not increase in diameter with advancing age. Tortuous blood vessels and tangentially oriented, mesothelial-lined spaces are other pseudoglandular structures observed in hernia sacs.

Abnormalities of the epididymis and spermatic cord structures can also occur as a result of prenatal conditions. Exposure to diethylstilbestrol *in utero* is associated with epididymal cysts and varicoceles in addition to hypotrophic testes and capsular induration. Congenital rubella, in addition to causing cryptorchidism, may be associated with absence or obstruction of the vas deferens or epididymis. Cystic fibrosis is a condition that, in addition to other manifestations/complications in other organs, contributes to infertility in adult males. The disease may additionally be associated with aplasia or hypoplasia of the vas deferens or epididymis. Moreover, congenital bilateral absence of the vas deferens has been linked to defects in the cystic fibrosis transmembrane conductance regulator (*CFTR*) gene (118).

A number of heterotopic tissues may be encountered in the paratesticular region such as in splenogonadal fusion, ectopic immature renal tissue, ectopic adrenal rests, and rarely ectopic prostatic tissue. These lesions should be considered in the differential diagnosis of a scrotal mass (119). Splenogonadal fusion consists of a spectrum of malformations of unknown etiology involving abnormal fusion between the spleen and the gonad or mesonephric derivatives such as the epididymis and vas deferens. There are two main morphologic types of this malformation: the continuous and the discontinuous type, depending on the presence or the absence of a structural connection between the regular spleen and the ectopic splenic tissue that is fused to the gonad. Splenogonadal fusion occurs much more frequently in males than females and is almost always left sided. Patients, typically younger than 20 years, usually present with left scrotal swelling, left inguinal hernia, or cryptorchidism. About one-third of reported cases have additional congenital defects, predominantly in the continuous type. The most common of these anomalies is cryptorchidism and other associated anomalies bilateral absent legs, imperforate anus, spina bifida, diaphragmatic hernia, and hypospadias. Microscopically, normal splenic tissue and testicular tissue are identified, but atrophy or immaturity may be seen. The cordlike structure present in the continuous type is composed of an admixture of splenic and fibrous tissues.

Nodules of ectopic immature renal tissue, ectopic adrenocortical tissue (adrenal rests), and rarely ectopic prostatic tissue may be found incidentally along the spermatic cord and adjacent to the epididymis (Figure 19-16).

Acquired Abnormalities and Other Lesions

A variety of acquired disorders of the epididymis and spermatic cord may present as an "acute scrotum" and may simulate testicular torsion or neoplasia. *Acute nonspecific epididymitis* in prepubertal and early adolescent boys presents with slow onset of scrotal pain, erythema, and edema. Although coexistent anatomic anomalies with this condition

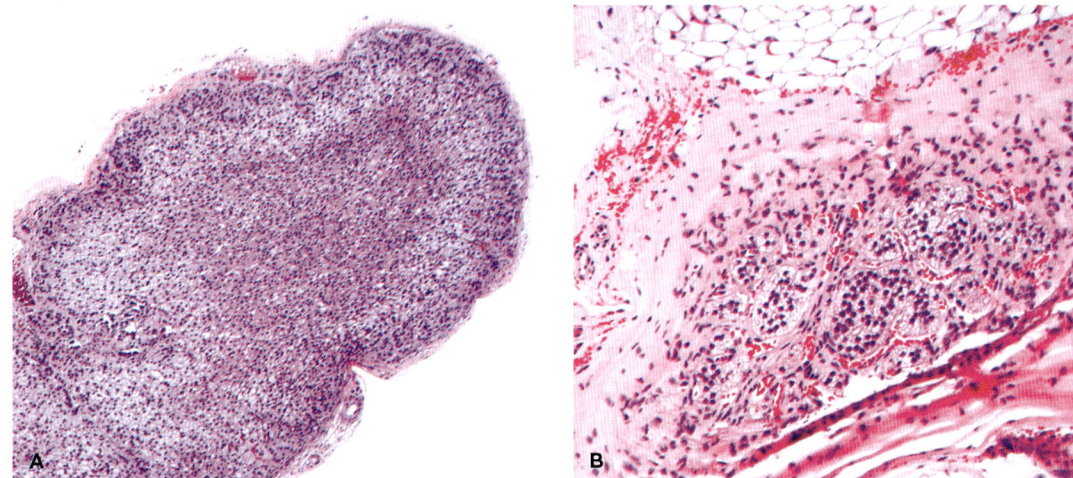

FIGURE 19-16 • Ectopic adrenal tissue. **A:** One example of adrenocortical tissue presented as a palpable paratesticular nodule. The lesion is well circumscribed and encapsulated and exhibits zonation similar to the normal adrenal cortex. **B:** Another example of ectopic adrenal tissue incidentally discovered in an inguinal hernia sac.

are rare in the pediatric age group, further workup may be warranted if this condition recurs. Infants have a higher rate of associated acute epididymitis and genitourinary malformations than older children. *Tuberculous epididymitis*, probably due to hematogenous spread of infection, mimics malignancy because of the combination of painless testicular swelling and an abnormal chest radiograph. This condition should be included in the differential diagnosis of testicular swelling in endemic regions. *Epididymal sarcoidosis* causes granulomatous epididymitis and scrotal swelling mimicking a neoplasm. Spermatic vein thrombosis may simulate intermittent testicular torsion, with acute pain and swelling of the scrotum, spermatic cord, and epididymis.

Henoch-Schönlein purpura may cause acute scrotum and scrotal swelling in up to 38% of patients and usually resolves spontaneously and does not require surgery. If the scrotum is explored, edema, petechiae, and purpura of the scrotum, epididymis, and testis are the morphologic manifestations. Scrotal abscess formation has been reported following appendectomy performed by both laparoscopic and open approaches.

Varicocele results from dilatation of veins of the pampiniform plexus of the spermatic cord and is found in 16% of boys between 10 and 15 years, and uncommon in boys younger than 10 years. In order to prevent progressive and irreversible damage to the testis, surgical correction of varicocele should be performed soon after diagnosis regardless of the degree of severity and the presence or absence of symptoms. The pathogenesis is venous stasis and reflux with vascular insufficiency and consequent progressive tubular damage. Hydrocele is a lower abdominal and scrotal cystic mass resulting from accumulation of fluid in the processus vaginalis or tunica vaginalis.

Meconium periorchitis presents as a large solitary paratesticular mass or several small nodules along the spermatic cord and is frequently associated with a hydrocele. It may be the rare initial manifestation of cystic fibrosis or result from volvulus, intestinal atresia, or ischemia. A rare case of scrotoschisis associated with meconium periorchitis has been also reported (120). For this condition to occur, it requires an *in utero* perforation of the gastrointestinal tract, allowing meconium to leak into the peritoneal cavity and then into the tunica vaginalis via the processus vaginalis. The perforation may resolve antenatally with the scrotal lesion as the only clue and manifestation of the process. Scrotal and abdominal calcifications on plain films and hyperechogenic areas on scrotal ultrasound are the imaging abnormalities. The gross appearance is a yellowish green, gritty mass with focal dystrophic calcifications. Microscopically, the lesion consists of loose myxoid to irregular fibrous connective tissue. Aggregates of macrophages with multinucleated giant cells containing brown bile pigment or cholesterol clefts and scattered calcifications may be seen. The mass may spontaneously resolve without surgery. A case of barium peritonitis secondarily causing an acute scrotal lesion in an infant has also been reported.

Tumors of the Paratesticular Structures

Mesothelial proliferations have been reported in the paratesticular region in the pediatric age group ranging from mesothelial hyperplasia to malignant mesothelioma.

Nodular mesothelial hyperplasia is a benign reactive process that may mimic a malignant process. It is typically encountered in hernia sacs as an incidental finding, the majority of which occur in the pediatric age group. It could also be associated with hydrocele or hematocele. The persistent irritation may easily result in histology that mimics malignant mesothelioma such as papillae and small tubules, solid nests, and cords extending into the underlying reactive connective tissue simulating invasion. However, the overall morphology is devoid of overtly malignant features.

Malignant mesothelioma of the paratesticular region is rare and even rarer in young patients with only 10% occurring in patients younger than 25 years. Grossly, the tumor typically presents as thickening of the tunica vaginalis with multiple friable nodular lesions. The histopathologic features are variable with the majority of tumors showing pure epithelial phenotype. The biphasic tumors contain a variable proportion of sarcomatoid morphology, basically resembling their pleural and intra-abdominal peritoneal counterparts. The entire spectrum of differentiation may be seen ranging from well-differentiated tumors characterized by tubulopapillary architecture and variably invasive tubules to poorly differentiated tumors with solid sheets, cords, and nests of highly infiltrative epithelioid cells with necrosis.

Rarely, tumors of the ovarian epithelial types have been reported in the paratesticular region of adolescent patients. Their histopathologic features and classification are similar to their ovarian counterparts.

Desmoplastic small round cell tumor (DSRCT) consists of proliferation of small round cells with an epithelial growth pattern and a desmoplastic stroma. Although typically affecting the pelvic and abdominal cavities of adolescent males, involvement of the paratesticular region is not uncommon. It may present in the paratesticular soft tissue, serosal surfaces, and the epididymis near the junction with the rete testis. Grossly, the tumor is firm and has a white-to-tan appearance. Microscopically, it consists of nests and anastomosing cords of uniformly small blue cells with scant cytoplasm embedded in a densely fibrotic stroma. Focal tubular formation may be seen. Mitoses are readily seen and tumor necrosis is commonly present. By immunohistochemistry, the tumor typically exhibits dual reactivity with keratin and desmin. Additionally, neuron-specific enolase (NSE), EMA, and vimentin are expressed. DSRCT is typically nonreactive for muscle common actin, myogenin, and chromogranin and is variably reactive for MIC2 (CD99) and p53 (121). DSRCT is characterized by a specific chromosomal abnormality, t(11;22)(p13;q12), resulting in the fusion of the Ewing sarcoma gene *EWS* on 22q12 and the Wilms tumor gene *WT1* on 11p13. The detection of this gene fusion EWS-WT1 is both a sensitive and a specific marker of DSRCT (121), and its EWS-WT1 chimeric protein product is expressed in over 90% of tumors. Most patients with DSRCT develop metastasis to regional lymph nodes or to distant sites.

Mesenchymal paratesticular tumors in infants and children are rare and include a variety of neoplasms such as hemangioma, juvenile xanthogranuloma, and RMS.

Paratesticular RMS is one of the relatively common tumors that involve the scrotal contents that are not of germ cell origin and is the most common paratesticular sarcoma in children (122). The mean age of occurrence in one large study was 6.6 years. Most paratesticular RMS are of embryonal subtype including the spindle cell variant, although alveolar subtype has been also reported. Their histopathologic features are identical to their soft tissue counterpart. Metastases have been reported from these tumors to retroperitoneal lymph nodes and distant sites (see chapter 25).

Of the vascular tumors, cavernous hemangioma predominates and usually follows a benign course. A case involving the testis of a stillborn has been reported (123). Bilateral testicular **hemangiomas** in neonates have been associated with cystic hygromas and may regress spontaneously. **Juvenile xanthogranuloma** presents as a hard, irregularly enlarged testis with a circumscribed yellow nodule on cut surface.

Other tumors of the connective tissue surrounding the testicle include benign (leiomyoma, fibroma, lipoma, calcifying fibrous tumor/pseudotumor) as well as malignant entities (leiomyosarcoma, fibrosarcoma, liposarcoma, rhabdoid tumor, and malignant peripheral nerve sheath tumor). These tumors are extremely rare, being mostly the subject of case reports, and their morphologic features are similar to those of their soft tissue counterparts (124).

Melanotic neuroectodermal tumor (*retinal anlage tumor*) is a rare melanin-containing tumor typically affecting the facial and skull bones. This tumor, however, has been reported in the epididymis and is seen mainly in infants (125). Grossly, these are circumscribed firm epididymal tumors with a white-to-gray cut surface that may show darker areas of pigmentation. Microscopically, the tumor consists of two components: the melanin-containing epithelioid cells arranged in cords, nests, or glandular structures and the small neuroblast-like cells in a variably cellular stroma. These two components are usually intermixed. This tumor generally follows a benign clinical course but may recur locally. No distant metastases have been reported, but regional lymph nodes (inguinal, retroperitoneal) have been rarely involved.

Adenomatoid tumor, the second most common tumor of the epididymis and cord in adults, can rarely be found in children as a scrotal nodule. The mass is gray, dense, and homogeneous, with a mucoid cut surface. Microscopically, tubules and cords of flattened or cuboidal eosinophilic mesothelial cells in a fibrous stroma are characteristic of this tumor.

Papillary cystadenoma of the epididymis is a rare benign epithelial tumor of the epididymal ducts and, rarely, the spermatic cord. This tumor can be associated with von Hippel-Lindau disease especially when it is bilateral, which can happen in about 30% to 40% of cases. The tumor is solid and cystic with occasional papillary formation and is composed of cuboidal-to-columnar cells with clear or vacuolated cytoplasm.

THE PENIS

Most congenital abnormalities of the penis are related to defects in urethral closure, such as hypospadia and epispadia and meatal stenosis. Hypospadia, with an incidence of 1:300 male newborns, is an anomaly involving the ventral aspect of the penis in the form of an abnormal ventral opening of the urethral meatus, an abnormal ventral curvature of the penis (chordee), and/or an abnormal distribution of the foreskin. The extent of the malformation is variable as the ectopic urethral opening (meatus) can be located anywhere from the tip of the glans penis, along the penile shaft and scrotum, to the perineum. The form and the extent of the malformed urethral opening can be variable but is rarely stenotic. Epispadia refers to the congenital absence of the dorsal aspect of the urethra, resulting in a urethral opening on the dorsum of the penis. The most frequent location of the opening is penopubic but can be penile or glanular. The incidence of male epispadia is 1 in 117,000 live male births. Associated urinary incontinence is frequently observed with penopubic epispadias and occasionally with penile type, but is not associated with glanular epispadias. Congenital anomalies that have been associated with epispadias include diastasis of the pubic symphysis, bladder exstrophy, renal agenesis, and ectopic pelvic kidney.

Other rare malformations of the penis include penile agenesis, or aphallia, diphallia, accessory scrotum, and transposition of the penis and scrotum (penoscrotal transposition). Some of these conditions may have familial predisposition and may be associated with other anomalies mostly in organs of the genitourinary tract.

Cutaneous viral infections and balanitis xerotica obliterans (BXO) are the principal acquired penile lesions in children and adolescents. The presentation of human papillomavirus (HPV) infection is variable ranging from asymptomatic infection to condyloma acuminata to bowenoid papulosis. Although DNA from certain known pathogenic HPV strains was detected in foreskins from newborns undergoing routine circumcision, there was no correlation with their respective mothers who had abnormal cervicovaginal cytologic smears (126). In young children with clinically evident condyloma acuminata, a sexual etiology was determined in more than half of them, and occasionally, these patients were found to have a mother with extensive condylomata observed at the time of childbirth. It has been also noted that condylomata acuminata in young people are associated with the same HPV types found in anogenital lesions in adults. Bowenoid papulosis, histologically identical to preinvasive squamous carcinoma, is usually a condition of young adults but may affect young children and is associated with HPV-16.

BXO is a chronic dermatitis of unknown etiology most often involving the glans and prepuce but sometimes extending into the urethra. BXO is relatively common in children and occurs in approximately 9% of all circumcised foreskins and in 19% to 40% of circumcisions performed for phimosis. It may be seen in boys as young as 2 years of age and appears clinically as a thick, white plaque on the prepuce, with occasional involvement of the glans and meatus. The gross pathologic findings are subtle ranging from loss of skin wrinkling to change in skin color and texture (thick and white or thin and pink) compared with the adjacent skin. The microscopic features are identical to those of lichen sclerosus et atrophicus, which is characterized by a thick subepidermal zone of acellular eosinophilic hyaline material underlying the keratotic and atrophic epidermis. Slight basal liquefaction is characteristic, with occasional formation of bullae or ulcers. A dense bandlike or patchy lymphoid infiltrate is present toward the deep border of the hyalinized zone, and clusters of plasma cells are sometimes seen.

Fournier disease is a form of necrotizing fasciitis affecting the penis and has been reported in children only rarely. Staphylococcal and streptococcal infections are responsible for the condition.

Overall, neoplasms of the penis are exceptionally rare in the first two decades of life. Squamous cell carcinoma is rare in children in the United States but has been reported in several adolescents who were not circumcised during childhood. Rare examples of endodermal sinus tumor of the penis have been reported, with histopathologic features identical to their testicular counterpart. Benign and malignant mesenchymal tumors such as cavernous hemangioma, neurofibroma, dermatofibroma, glomus tumor, malignant lymphoma, malignant peripheral nerve sheath tumor, embryonal RMS, and clear-cell sarcoma have been also rarely reported in the penis. The histopathologic features of these tumors are identical to their soft tissue counterparts. Malignant peripheral nerve sheath tumor in this site has been usually reported in the clinical setting of von Recklinghausen neurofibromatosis.

THE PROSTATE

Congenital and Developmental Anomalies

Congenital abnormalities of the prostate are rare. Hypoplasia and dilation of the prostate are consistent findings in the prune-belly syndrome. The epithelium of the prostatic glands and ducts, prostatic utricle, and prostatic urethra can undergo squamous metaplasia, in response to maternal estrogenic stimulation, during prenatal life. This histologic feature gradually disappears in the early postnatal months. Focal hyperplasia of glandular epithelium, cystic dilatation of tubules, and intraluminal secretions are other histologic changes that are observed in the fetal and neonatal prostate. Congenital abnormalities of the prostate are rare. Cysts of the prostatic utricle (müllerian duct cyst) are an unusual cause of lower urinary tract obstruction and inflammation in boys.

Fibroepithelial polyps of the urethra have been reported typically in males younger than 10 years but can also occur in older men. These benign growths can cause a variety of symptoms in young boys including obstructive uropathy, infection, and/or hematuria. They typically occur in the posterior urethra near the verumontanum and consist of a fibrovascular core with loose stroma covered by urothelial lining. Surface ulceration, reactive atypia, and squamous metaplasia may develop in these polyps, which are considered developmental anomalies and are treated by simple transurethral resection.

Acquired Abnormalities and Other Lesions

Overall, lesions and tumors of the prostate are rare in infants and children. A few reports of periprostatic abscesses or hematomas appeared in the literature in which a midline pelvic mass was present accompanied by scrotal abscess and fever and caused lower urinary tract obstruction in infants (127,128). *Staphylococcus aureus* and *E. coli* were implicated as causative organisms in these cases.

RMS is by far the most common neoplasm of the prostate in children and adolescents. Approximately 5% of all pediatric RMS primarily involve the prostate. RMS can occur anytime from infancy to early adulthood but has a peak incidence during the first 4 years of life (54) and a mean age of presentation of 5.3 years. Overall, genitourinary involvement by RMS was found to more commonly affect infants younger than 1 year compared to older children. Like soft tissue RMS, another peak of incidence may be observed during adolescence at 15 to 19 years. The presenting symptoms include bladder outlet obstruction, hematuria, incontinence, infection, and a pelvic or an abdominal mass. Large tumors can be difficult to assign a prostatic or a bladder origin, especially since both structures are frequently involved (129). An association between RMS in genitourinary sites and neurofibromatosis type 1(NF1) has been rarely reported in one study.

In the pretreatment clinical staging for pediatric RMS, prostatic or bladder involvement, unlike the favorable overall genitourinary location, is regarded as unfavorable site of involvement and assigned a higher clinical stage. Regional lymph nodal metastasis (usually iliac and para-aortic) can occur in up to 20% of prostate and bladder RMS, necessitating adequate nodal sampling for proper staging of the tumor.

Microscopically, the majority of prostatic RMS is of the embryonal type and is considered as favorable histology (Figure 19-17). It remains important, however, to identify the rare cases of alveolar RMS in this location due to its unfavorable histologic subtype and the additional need for more aggressive chemotherapy. For further review, please refer to the soft tissue section for detailed histopathologic, immunohistochemical, and molecular and genetic evaluation of

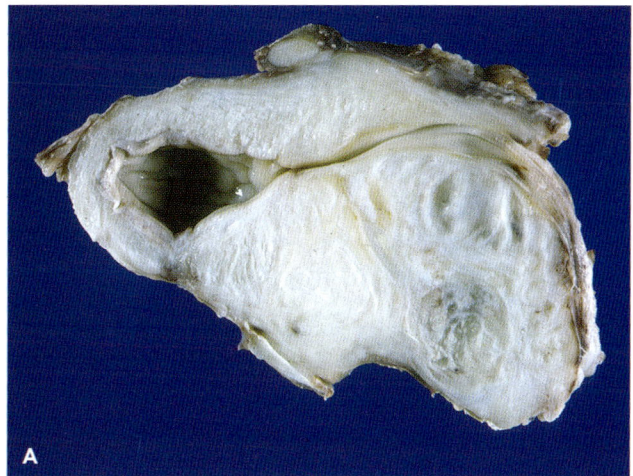
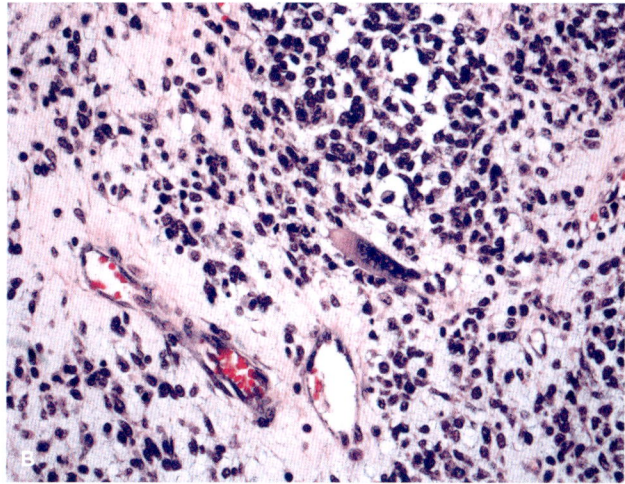
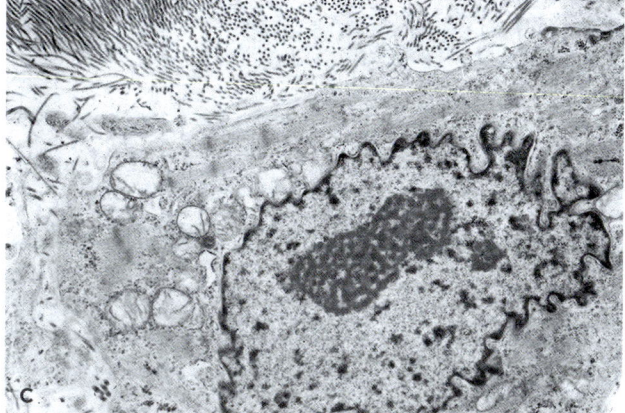

FIGURE 19-17 • Embryonal RMS. **A:** The tumor involves the prostatic and the bladder region. **B:** The tumor has variable cellularity with small hyperchromatic cells and scant cytoplasm in a loose stroma. **C:** An occasional giant cell with abundant eosinophilic cytoplasm is depicted. By ultrastructural examination, the cytoplasm contains thin and thick filaments with densities representing the z-bands (Courtesy of Dr. Jerome Taxy, Chicago, IL).

RMS. Multimodality treatment combining surgery, chemotherapy, and radiation therapy is currently applied to pediatric RMS and has greatly improved the prognosis (130) (see Chapter 25).

Rare examples of other tumors occurring in the prostate or prostatic region have been the subject of case reports only. These include a malignant rhabdoid tumor, an undifferentiated carcinoma with disseminated metastasis, non-Hodgkin lymphomas, a pheochromocytoma, a teratoma with angiosarcoma component, and a case of fibromatosis. Conventional prostatic adenocarcinoma was not detected before the fourth decade in a study of 152 young male patients (131).

References

1. Blyth B, Duckett JW, Jr. Gonadal differentiation: a review of the physiological process and influencing factors based on recent experimental evidence. *J Urol* 1991;145:689–694.
2. Byskov AG. Differentiation of mammalian embryonic gonad. *Physiol Rev* 1986;66:71–117.
3. Rey R, Picard JY. Embryology and endocrinology of genital development. *Baillieres Clin Endocrinol Metab* 1998;12:17–33.
4. Dufau ML, Khanum A, Winters CA, et al. Multistep regulation of Leydig cell function. *J Steroid Biochem* 1987;27(1–3):343–350.
5. Eskola V, Nikula H, Huhtaniemi I. Age-related variation of follicle-stimulating hormone-stimulated cAMP production, protein kinase C activity and their interactions in the rat testis. *Mol Cell Endocrinol* 1993;93(2):143–148.
6. Cunha GR, Alarid ET, Turner T, et al. Normal and abnormal development of the male urogenital tract. Role of androgens, mesenchymal-epithelial interactions, and growth factors. *J Androl* 1992;13:465–475.
7. Hiort O, Holterhus PM. The molecular basis of male sexual differentiation. *Eur J Endocrinol* 2000;142:101–110.
8. Lim HN, Hawkins JR. Genetic control of gonadal differentiation. *Baillieres Clin Endocrinol Metab* 1998;12:1–16.
9. Fechner PY. The role of SRY in mammalian sex determination. *Acta Paediatr Jpn* 1996;38:380–389.
10. Parker KL, Schimmer BP, Schedl A. Genes essential for early events in gonadal development. *Cell Mol Life Sci* 1999;55:831–838.
11. Khedis M, Nohra J, Dierickx L, et al. Polyorchidism: presentation of 2 cases, review of the literature and a new management strategy. *Urol Int* 2008;80:98–101.
12. de Buys Roessingh AS, El Ghoneimi A, Enezian G, et al. Triorchidism and testicular torsion in a child. *J Pediatr Surg* 2003;38:E13–E14.
13. Tonape T, Singh G, Koushik P, et al. Triorchidism: a rare genitourinary abnormality. *J Surg Tech Case Rep* 2012;4:126–128.
14. Jeyaratnam R, Bakalinova D. Cystic dysplasia of the rete testis: a case of spontaneous regression and review of published reports. *Urology* 2010;75:687–690.
15. Glantz L, Hansen K, Caldamone A, et al. Cystic dysplasia of the testis. *Hum Pathol* 1993;24:1142–1145.
16. Nistal M, Paniagua R, Bravo MP. Testicular lymphangiectasis in Noonan's syndrome. *J Urol* 1984;131:759–761.
17. Thong M, Lim C, Fatimah H. Undescended testes: incidence in 1,002 consecutive male infants and outcome at 1 year of age. *Pediatr Surg Int* 1998;13:37–41.

18. Wood HM, Elder JS. Cryptorchidism and testicular cancer: separating fact from fiction. *J Urol* 2009;181:452–461.
19. Cryptorchidism: a prospective study of 7500 consecutive male births, 1984-8. John Radcliffe Hospital Cryptorchidism Study Group. *Arch Dis Child* 1992;67:892–899.
20. Thonneau PF, Gandia P, Mieusset R: Cryptorchidism: incidence, risk factors, and potential role of environment; an update. *J Androl* 2003;24:155–162.
21. Jones ME, Swerdlow AJ, Griffith M, et al. Prenatal risk factors for cryptorchidism: a record linkage study. *Paediatr Perinat Epidemiol* 1998;12:383–396.
22. Weidner IS, Moller H, Jensen TK, et al. Risk factors for cryptorchidism and hypospadias. *J Urol* 1999;161:1606–1609.
23. Nistal M, Paniagua R, Diez-Pardo JA. Histologic classification of undescended testes. *Hum Pathol* 1980;11:666–674.
24. Rune GM, Mayr J, Neugebauer H, et al. Pattern of Sertoli cell degeneration in cryptorchid prepubertal testes. *Int J Androl* 1992;15:19–31.
25. Han SW, Lee T, Kim JH, et al. Pathological difference between retractile and cryptorchid testes. *J Urol* 1999;162:878–880.
26. Cortes D, Thorup JM, Visfeldt J. Cryptorchidism: aspects of fertility and neoplasms. A study including data of 1,335 consecutive boys who underwent testicular biopsy simultaneously with surgery for cryptorchidism. *Horm Res* 2001;55:21–27.
27. Robboy SJ, Jaubert F. Neoplasms and pathology of sexual developmental disorders (intersex). *Pathology* 2007;39:147–163.
28. Lee PA, Houk CP, Ahmed SF, et al. Consensus statement on management of intersex disorders. International Consensus Conference on Intersex. *Pediatrics* 2006;118:e488–e500.
29. Rutgers JL, Young RH, Scully RE. The testicular "tumor" of the adrenogenital syndrome. A report of six cases and review of the literature on testicular masses in patients with adrenocortical disorders. *Am J Surg Pathol* 1988;12:503–513.
30. Borer JG, Nitti VW, Glassberg KI. Mixed gonadal dysgenesis and dysgenetic male pseudohermaphroditism. *J Urol* 1995;153:1267–1273.
31. Hegarty PK, Mushtaq I, Sebire NJ. Natural history of testicular regression syndrome and consequences for clinical management. *J Pediatr Urol* 2007;3:206–208.
32. Law H, Mushtaq I, Wingrove K, et al. Histopathological features of testicular regression syndrome: relation to patient age and implications for management. *Fetal Pediatr Pathol* 2006;25:119–129.
33. Merry C, Sweeney B, Puri P. The vanishing testis: anatomical and histological findings. *Eur Urol* 1997;31:65–67.
34. Kremer H, Kraaij R, Toledo SP, et al. Male pseudohermaphroditism due to a homozygous missense mutation of the luteinizing hormone receptor gene. *Nat Genet* 1995;9:160–164.
35. Buchholz NP, Biyabani R, Herzig MJ, et al. Persistent Mullerian duct syndrome. *Eur Urol* 1998;34:230–232.
36. Seraj IM, Chase DR, Chase RL, et al. Malignant teratoma arising in a dysgenetic gonad. *Gynecol Oncol* 1993;50:254–258.
37. Uehara S, Funato T, Yaegashi N, et al. SRY mutation and tumor formation on the gonads of XP pure gonadal dysgenesis patients. *Cancer Genet Cytogenet* 1999;113:78–84.
38. Yordam N, Alikasifoglu A, Kandemir N, et al. True hermaphroditism: clinical features, genetic variants and gonadal histology. *J Pediatr Endocrinol Metab* 2001;14:421–427.
39. Aaronson IA. True hermaphroditism. A review of 41 cases with observations on testicular histology and function. *Br J Urol* 1985;57:775–779.
40. Krob G, Braun A, Kuhnle U. True hermaphroditism: geographical distribution, clinical findings, chromosomes and gonadal histology. *Eur J Pediatr* 1994;153:2–10.
41. Levin HS. Tumors of the testis in intersex syndromes. *Urol Clin North Am* 2000;27:543–551, x.
42. Hadjiathanasiou CG, Brauner R, Lortat-Jacob S, et al. True hermaphroditism: genetic variants and clinical management. *J Pediatr* 1994;125:738–744.
43. Lanfranco F, Kamischke A, Zitzmann M, et al. Klinefelter's syndrome. *Lancet* 2004;364:273–283.
44. Paduch DA, Fine RG, Bolyakov A, et al. New concepts in Klinefelter syndrome. *Curr Opin Urol* 2008;18:621–627.
45. Swerdlow AJ, Schoemaker MJ, Higgins CD, et al. Cancer incidence and mortality in men with Klinefelter syndrome: a cohort study. *J Natl Cancer Inst* 2005;97:1204–1210.
46. Pritchard-Jones K, Fleming S, Davidson D, et al. The candidate Wilms' tumour gene is involved in genitourinary development. *Nature* 1990;346:194–197.
47. Clericuzio CL: Clinical phenotypes and Wilms tumor. *Med Pediatr Oncol* 1993;21:182–187.
48. Ringdahl E, Teague L. Testicular torsion. *Am Fam Physician* 2006;74:1739–1743.
49. Kao CS, Zhang C, Ulbright TM. Testicular hemorrhage, necrosis, and vasculopathy: likely manifestations of intermittent torsion that clinically mimic a neoplasm. *Am J Surg Pathol* 2014;38:34–44.
50. Mneimneh WS, Nazeer T, Jennings TA. Torsion of the gonad in the pediatric population: spectrum of histologic findings with focus on aspects specific to neonates and infants. *Pediatr Dev Pathol* 2013;16:74–79.
51. Siimes MA, Rautonen J. Small testicles with impaired production of sperm in adult male survivors of childhood malignancies. *Cancer* 1990;65:1303–1306.
52. Kaplan GW, Cromie WC, Kelalis PP, et al. Prepubertal yolk sac testicular tumors—report of the testicular tumor registry. *J Urol* 1988;140:1109–1112.
53. Metcalfe PD, Farivar-Mohseni H, Farhat W, et al: Pediatric testicular tumors: contemporary incidence and efficacy of testicular preserving surgery. *J Urol* 2003;170:2412–2415; discussion 5–6.
54. Cangir A. Malignant genital tract tumors in children. *Curr Probl Cancer* 1986;10:301–341.
55. Lee SD. Epidemiological and clinical behavior of prepubertal testicular tumors in Korea. *J Urol* 2004;172:674–678.
56. Abell MR, Holtz F. Testicular neoplasms in infants and children. I tumors of germ cell origin. *Cancer* 1963;16:965–981.
57. Ciftci AO, Bingol-Kologlu M, Senocak ME, et al. Testicular tumors in children. *J Pediatr Surg* 2001;36(12):1796–1801.
58. Fernandes ET, Etcubanas E, Rao BN, et al. Two decades of experience with testicular tumors in children at St Jude Children's Research Hospital. *J Pediatr Surg* 1989;24(7):677–681; discussion 682.
59. Green DM. Testicular tumors in infants and children. *Semin Surg Oncol* 1986;2(3):156–162.
60. Kay R. Prepubertal testicular tumor registry. *Urol Clin North Am* 1993;20(1):1–5.
61. Leonard MP, Schlegel PN, Crovatto A, et al. Burkitt's lymphoma of the testis: an unusual scrotal mass in childhood. *J Urol* 1990;143(1):104–106.
62. Pohl HG, Shukla AR, Metcalf PD, et al. Prepubertal testis tumors: actual prevalence rate of histological types. *J Urol* 2004;172(6 Pt 1):2370–2372.
63. Ross JH, Rybicki L, Kay R. Clinical behavior and a contemporary management algorithm for prepubertal testis tumors: a summary of the Prepubertal Testis Tumor Registry. *J Urol* 2002;168(4 Pt 2):1675–1678; discussion 1678–1679.
64. Sugita Y, Clarnette TD, Cooke-Yarborough C, et al. Testicular and paratesticular tumours in children: 30 years' experience. *Aust N Z J Surg* 1999;69(7):505–508.
65. Levy DA, Kay R, Elder JS. Neonatal testis tumors: a review of the Prepubertal Testis Tumor Registry. *J Urol* 1994;151:715–717.
66. Harms D, Kock LR. Testicular juvenile granulosa cell and Sertoli cell tumours: a clinicopathological study of 29 cases from the Kiel Paediatric Tumour Registry. *Virchows Arch* 1997;430:301–309.
67. Lawrence WD, Young RH, Scully RE: Juvenile granulosa cell tumor of the infantile testis. A report of 14 cases. *Am J Surg Pathol* 1985;9:87–94.
68. Ulbright TM. Protocol for the examination of specimens from patients with malignant germ cell and sex cord-stromal tumors of the testis, exclusive of paratesticular malignancies: a basis for checklists. Cancer Committee, College of American Pathologists. *Arch Pathol Lab Med* 1999;123:14–19.
69. Reuter VE. Origins and molecular biology of testicular germ cell tumors. *Mod Pathol* 2005;18(Suppl 2):S51–S60.

70. Looijenga LH, Oosterhuis JW. Pathogenesis of testicular germ cell tumours. *Rev Reprod* 1999;4:90–100.
71. JL E. *Tumors of the Testis and Paratesticular Tissue*, Chapter 4. Lyon, France: IARC Press; 2004.
72. International Germ Cell Consensus Classification: a prognostic factor-based staging system for metastatic germ cell cancers. International Germ Cell Cancer Collaborative Group. *J Clin Oncol* 1997;15:594–603.
73. Perlman EJ, Hu J, Ho D, et al. Genetic analysis of childhood endodermal sinus tumors by comparative genomic hybridization. *J Pediatr Hematol Oncol* 2000;22:100–105.
74. Manivel JC, Simonton S, Wold LE, et al. Absence of intratubular germ cell neoplasia in testicular yolk sac tumors in children. A histochemical and immunohistochemical study. *Arch Pathol Lab Med* 1988;112:641–645.
75. Grady RW, Ross JH, Kay R. Patterns of metastatic spread in prepubertal yolk sac tumor of the testis. *J Urol* 1995;153:1259–1261.
76. Skoog SJ. Benign and malignant pediatric scrotal masses. *Pediatr Clin North Am* 1997;44:1229–1250.
77. Harms D, Janig U. Germ cell tumours of childhood. Report of 170 cases including 59 pure and partial yolk-sac tumours. *Virchows Arch A Pathol Anat Histopathol* 1986;409:223–239.
78. Cao D, Li J, Guo CC, et al. SALL4 is a novel diagnostic marker for testicular germ cell tumors. *Am J Surg Pathol* 2009;33:1065–1077.
79. Veltman I, Veltman J, Janssen I, et al. Identification of recurrent chromosomal aberrations in germ cell tumors of neonates and infants using genomewide array-based comparative genomic hybridization. *Genes Chromosomes Cancer* 2005;43:367–376.
80. Carver BS, Al-Ahmadie H, Sheinfeld J. Adult and pediatric testicular teratoma. *Urol Clin North Am* 2007;34:245–251; abstract x.
81. Taskinen S, Fagerholm R, Aronniemi J, et al. Testicular tumors in children and adolescents. *J Pediatr Urol* 2008;4:134–137.
82. Garrett JE, Cartwright PC, Snow BW, et al. Cystic testicular lesions in the pediatric population. *J Urol* 2000;163:928–936.
83. Ulbright TM, Clark SA, Einhorn LH. Angiosarcoma associated with germ cell tumors. *Hum Pathol* 1985;16:268–272.
84. Ulbright TM, Loehrer PJ, Roth LM, et al. The development of non-germ cell malignancies within germ cell tumors. A clinicopathologic study of 11 cases. *Cancer* 1984;54:1824–1833.
85. Mostert M, Rosenberg C, Stoop H, et al. Comparative genomic and in situ hybridization of germ cell tumors of the infantile testis. *Lab Invest* 2000;80:1055–1064.
86. Ross JH, Kay R. Prepubertal testis tumors. *Rev Urol* 2004;6:11–18.
87. Umar SA, MacLennan GT. Epidermoid cyst of the testis. *J Urol* 2008;180:335.
88. Hawkins E, Heifetz SA, Giller R, et al. The prepubertal testis (prenatal and postnatal): its relationship to intratubular germ cell neoplasia: a combined Pediatric Oncology Group and Children's Cancer Study Group. *Hum Pathol* 1997;28:404–410.
89. Muller J, Skakkebaek NE, Ritzen M, et al. Carcinoma in situ of the testis in children with 45,X/46,XY gonadal dysgenesis. *J Pediatr* 1985;106:431–436.
90. Muller J. Morphometry and histology of gonads from twelve children and adolescents with the androgen insensitivity (testicular feminization) syndrome. *J Clin Endocrinol Metab* 1984;59:785–789.
91. Ramani P, Yeung CK, Habeebu SS. Testicular intratubular germ cell neoplasia in children and adolescents with intersex. *Am J Surg Pathol* 1993;17:1124–1133.
92. Emerson RE, Ulbright TM. The use of immunohistochemistry in the differential diagnosis of tumors of the testis and paratestis. *Semin Diagn Pathol* 2005;22:33–50.
93. Kaplan GW, Cromie WJ, Kelalis PP, et al. Gonadal stromal tumors: a report of the Prepubertal Testicular Tumor Registry. *J Urol* 1986;136:300–302.
94. Hofmann M, Schlegel PG, Hippert F, et al. Testicular sex cord stromal tumors: analysis of patients from the MAKEI study. *Pediatr Blood Cancer* 2013;60:1651–1655.
95. Silberstein JL, Bazzi WM, Vertosick E, et al. Clinical outcomes for local and metastatic testicular sex cord-stromal tumors. *J Urol* 2014;192:415–419.
96. Nistal M, Gonzalez-Peramato P, Paniagua R. Congenital Leydig cell hyperplasia. *Histopathology* 1988;12:307–317.
97. Johnson RE, Scheithauer B: Massive hyperplasia of testicular adrenal rests in a patient with Nelson's syndrome. *Am J Clin Pathol* 1982;77:501–507.
98. Young RH, Koelliker DD, Scully RE. Sertoli cell tumors of the testis, not otherwise specified: a clinicopathologic analysis of 60 cases. *Am J Surg Pathol* 1998;22:709–721.
99. Rutgers JL. Advances in the pathology of intersex conditions. *Hum Pathol* 1991;22:884–891.
100. Wilson DM, Pitts WC, Hintz RL, et al. Testicular tumors with Peutz-Jeghers syndrome. *Cancer* 1986;57:2238–2240.
101. Perrone F, Bertolotti A, Montemurro G, et al. Frequent mutation and nuclear localization of beta-catenin in sertoli cell tumors of the testis. *Am J Surg Pathol* 2014;38:66–71.
102. Ulbright TM, Amin MB, Young RH. Intratubular large cell hyalinizing sertoli cell neoplasia of the testis: a report of 8 cases of a distinctive lesion of the Peutz-Jeghers syndrome. *Am J Surg Pathol* 2007;31:827–835.
103. Venara M, Rey R, Bergada I, et al. Sertoli cell proliferations of the infantile testis: an intratubular form of Sertoli cell tumor? *Am J Surg Pathol* 2001;25:1237–1244.
104. Crump WD. Juvenile granulosa cell (sex cord-stromal) tumor of fetal testis. *J Urol* 1983;129:1057–1058.
105. Cortez JC, Kaplan GW. Gonadal stromal tumors, gonadoblastomas, epidermoid cysts, and secondary tumors of the testis in children. *Urol Clin North Am* 1993;20:15–26.
106. Nistal M, Redondo E, Paniagua R. Juvenile granulosa cell tumor of the testis. *Arch Pathol Lab Med* 1988;112:1129–1132.
107. Al-Agha OM, Huwait HF, Chow C, et al. FOXL2 is a sensitive and specific marker for sex cord-stromal tumors of the ovary. *Am J Surg Pathol* 2011;35:484–494.
108. Shah SP, Kobel M, Senz J, et al. Mutation of FOXL2 in granulosa-cell tumors of the ovary. *N Engl J Med* 2009;360:2719–2729.
109. Lima JF, Jin L, de Araujo AR, et al. FOXL2 mutations in granulosa cell tumors occurring in males. *Arch Pathol Lab Med* 2012;136:825–828.
110. Krasna IH, Lee ML, Smilow P, et al. Risk of malignancy in bilateral streak gonads: the role of the Y chromosome. *J Pediatr Surg* 1992;27:1376–1380.
111. Scully RE. Gonadoblastoma. A review of 74 cases. *Cancer* 1970;25:1340–1356.
112. Reid H, Marsden HB: Gonadal infiltration in children with leukaemia and lymphoma. *J Clin Pathol* 1980;33:722–729.
113. Cromie WJ. Congenital anomalies of the testis, vas epididymis, and inguinal canal. *Urol Clin North Am* 1978;5:237–252.
114. Elder JS. Epididymal anomalies associated with hydrocele/hernia and cryptorchidism: implications regarding testicular descent. *J Urol* 1992;148:624–626.
115. Cerilli LA, Sotelo-Avila C, Mills SE. Glandular inclusions in inguinal hernia sacs: morphologic and immunohistochemical distinction from epididymis and vas deferens. *Am J Surg Pathol* 2003;27:469–476.
116. Gill B, Favale D, Kogan SJ, et al. Significance of accessory ductal structures in hernia sacs. *J Urol* 1992;148:697–698.
117. Tolete-Velcek F, Leddomado E, Hansbrough F, et al. Alleged resection of the vas deferens: medicolegal implications. *J Pediatr Surg* 1988;23:21–23.
118. Casals T, Bassas L, Ruiz-Romero J, et al. Extensive analysis of 40 infertile patients with congenital absence of the vas deferens: in 50% of cases only one CFTR allele could be detected. *Hum Genet* 1995;95:205–211.
119. Kocher NJ, Tomaszewski JJ, Parsons RB, et al. Splenogonadal fusion: a rare etiology of solid testicular mass. *Urology* 2014;83:e1–e2.
120. Chun K, St-Vil D. Scrotoschisis associated with contralateral meconium periorchitis. *J Pediatr Surg* 1997;32:864–866.

121. Gerald WL, Ladanyi M, de Alava E, et al. Clinical, pathologic, and molecular spectrum of tumors associated with t(11;22)(p13;q12): desmoplastic small round-cell tumor and its variants. *J Clin Oncol* 1998;16:3028–3036.
122. Loughlin KR, Retik AB, Weinstein HJ, et al. Genitourinary rhabdomyosarcoma in children. *Cancer* 1989;63:1600–1606.
123. Suriawinata A, Talerman A, Vapnek JM, et al. Hemangioma of the testis: report of unusual occurrences of cavernous hemangioma in a fetus and capillary hemangioma in an older man. *Ann Diagn Pathol* 2001;5:80–83.
124. Agarwal PK, Palmer JS. Testicular and paratesticular neoplasms in prepubertal males. *J Urol* 2006;176:875–881.
125. Henley JD, Ferry J, Ulbright TM. Miscellaneous rare paratesticular tumors. *Semin Diagn Pathol* 2000;17:319–339.
126. Roman A, Fife K. Human papillomavirus DNA associated with foreskins of normal newborns. *J Infect Dis* 1986;153:855–861.
127. Heyman A, Lombardo LJ, Jr. Metastatic prostatic abscess with report of a case in a newborn infant. *J Urol* 1962;87:174–177.
128. Williams DI, Martins AG. Periprostatic haematoma and prostatic abscess in the neonatal period. *Arch Dis Child* 1960;35:177–181.
129. El-Sherbiny MT, El-Mekresh MH, El-Baz MA, et al. Paediatric lower urinary tract rhabdomyosarcoma: a single-centre experience of 30 patients. *BJU Int* 2000;86:260–267.
130. McLean TW, Castellino SM. Pediatric genitourinary tumors. *Curr Opin Oncol* 2008;20:315–320.
131. Sakr WA, Haas GP, Cassin BF, et al. The frequency of carcinoma and intraepithelial neoplasia of the prostate in young male patients. *J Urol* 1993;150:379–385.

CHAPTER 20

Breast

Louis P. Dehner, M.D.

The breast shares a similar sequence of developmental–morphologic events with the skin, salivary gland, tooth, kidney, and lung. There is an initial proliferation of surface epithelium that subsequently projects into the underlying mesenchyme. Molecular interaction between the epithelium and mesenchyme results in the branching of the epithelium that in the female breast gives rise to a network of ducts and terminal duct lobular units, which only develop with puberty. The first vestige of the breast is seen in the 4th week of gestation when small mounds of surface ectoderm form as placodes; these paired structures are found along a line from the anterior thorax into the inguinal region. The eventual number of mammary glands as functional structures varies among the mammalian species and correlates with number of offspring in the litter (1). During the 5th week of gestation, the placode in a cap of pseudostratified epithelium proliferates into the stroma where the epithelium and mesenchyme interact through an intricate series of subcellular programs (2). The mammary buds remain as solid structures until approximately the 10th week when branching is initiated and secondary buds are formed; this process of lengthening and branching continues throughout gestation (3). There is also narrowing of the neck of the bud with the transformation of the solid epithelial structures into structures with a central lumen during the 20th week of gestation; the latter structures are the lactiferous ducts, which are recognized by 32 weeks when they open to the surface of the skin. By 28 weeks, the two primary cell types of the ducts and acini have differentiated into a basal myoepithelial cell and luminal cell.

The mesenchyme is the other central component not just from the perspective of forming supporting structures like blood vessels, but it has an early inductive effect upon the overlying ectoderm during the phase of placode and bud formation via paracrine and endocrine receptors (4). The sprouting of the bud by parathyroid hormone–related peptide signaling and its receptor is a function of mesenchyme. The adipose tissue of the breast is a necessary component for the mediation of future growth also through signaling cascades (5). A complex molecular network is in place in both the stroma and epithelium to interpret and coordinate cytokines and growth factors including hormones and hormone receptors (6).

Several signaling pathways are involved in the earliest stages of placode and bud formation (2). These same pathways are activated in the regulation of development in virtually all organ systems; these pathways include hedgehog, Wnt/β-catenin, TGF-β, and FGG pathways (7–9).

A term male or female newborn often has subareolar nodules measuring 2 to 3 cm in greatest dimension (Figure 20-1). Galactorrhea may be noted as well. As placental–maternal hormones and prolactin from the infant decline in the first month, the epithelial proliferation ceases and the stroma regresses with the resolution of the nodules. Until the onset of puberty, the breast tissue remains in a resting or quiescent state in the absence of a functioning neoplasm of the adrenal cortex, ovary (juvenile granulosa cell tumor), testis (Leydig cell tumor), or pituitary (prolactinoma).

With puberty, the female breast with its rudimentary ductal network develops an extensive network of ducts through the mechanism of branching morphogenesis (10). There is penetration of the stroma where the process is continuously monitored and constrained through the various signaling pathways. Unlike the earlier stages of breast development, estrogen and insulin-like growth factor 1 (IGF1) are critical in the growth of breasts at puberty and with the formation of the terminal duct lobular unit (5,7,11). The inhibition of IGF1 by its binding protein results in apoptosis of ductal epithelial cells, whereas IGF1 facilitates the growth in the number of terminal end buds (7,12). Other molecular agents important in breast organogenesis and growth include growth hormone, TGF-α, TGF-β, tenascin-c, and collagen type IV (13).

Morphologic events at thelarche with progressive growth of the breast through its five Tanner stages involve the network of ducts as they branch and form acinar–lobular units from the terminal ducts (11,14). Fibrous stroma and adipose tissue constitute 25% or more of the total breast volume. There is progressive proliferation and condensation of fibrous stroma around the ducts, a process initially recognized in the embryo–fetal stage of breast development (11,15).

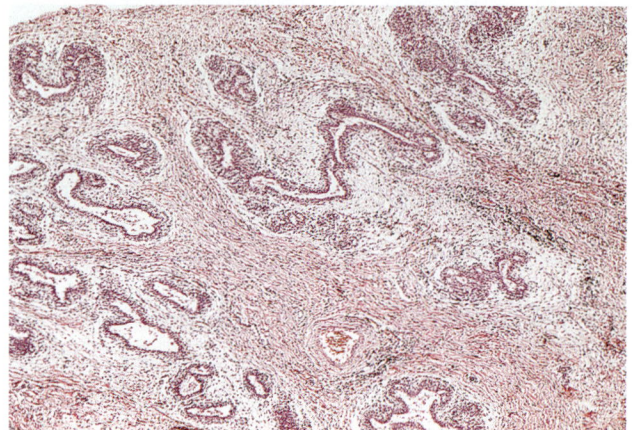

FIGURE 20-1 • Neonatal breast tissue forms a subareolar nodule composed of small ducts with epithelial proliferative features. A resemblance to gynecomastia is not surprising given that changes are driven by maternal–placental hormones in the one and endogenous hormones in the other.

CONGENITAL ANOMALIES

Abnormalities in breast development may or may not be accompanied by defects in the chest wall. There are several categories of breast anomalies based upon complete absence or reduction in the breast volume (amastia or hypoplasia to varying degrees) that may be unilateral or bilateral, defects in the nipple and/or areolar complex (polythelia or athelia), accessory breast tissue in the axillary tail or vulva, and abnormal shape and anomalies in the chest wall. If one reviews the development of the normal breast, it is possible to associate the particular abnormality with a perturbation in one of the sequence of events in normal mammary gland embryology. Several reviews were found helpful for those with a particular interest in this topic (15–19).

Congenital Absence of the Breast

Absence of the breast is defined as total absence of breast parenchyma or amastia, which includes both the nipple–areolar complex and underlying mammary tissue (amastia), and absence of the nipple (athelia) and mammary gland tissue (amazia) (16). Although most cases are sporadic and may be unilateral or bilateral, there are several syndromic associations, of which the Poland syndrome may be the most familiar (16,20,21). These children have aplasia/hypoplasia of the pectoralis major and minor muscles, and the nipple and breast tissue are absent (22). Yet another syndrome is characterized by congenital choanal atresia and bilateral amastia (23). Scalp–ear–nipple syndrome (Finlay-Marks syndrome), an ectodermal dysplasia–like disorder, has a missense mutation in the *KCTD1* gene (24). Athelia and/or amastia is present in these children, which would be anticipated in a gene that is involved in ectodermal development. Meier-Gorlin syndrome with mutations in ORC1, ORC4, ORC6, CDT1, and CDC6 genes is accompanied by amazia in 100% of cases (25,26). The topic of bilateral congenital amazia has been thoroughly reviewed elsewhere (27).

Athelia with a congenital absence of the nipple–areolar complex is invariably syndromic and usually a manifestation of one of the ectodermal dysplasias; there is also absence of glandular mammary tissue (25,28). Limb–mammary syndrome in addition to congenital amastia, but unlike the p63 syndrome, does not have mullerian tract abnormalities (29). A lack of breast development has been reported in the genetic disorder, 17-alpha-hydroxylase/17, 20-lyase deficiency (30). The absence of breast development should initiate studies, if not already started, on one of several possible genetic disorders. In the case of an ectodermal dysplasia, there is not only absence of mammary breast tissue but also cutaneous adnexal structures that are absent or severely miniaturized (31–33).

Breast Displacement

Breast displacement on the anterior chest wall resulting in asymmetry is yet another anomaly. It is probably not true that the distance between the nipples is increased in Turner or monosomy 45X0 syndrome. By contrast, congenital symmastia is a disorder in which the breasts are displaced medially by the presence of fibrous bands (34).

Polythelia and Supernumerary Breast Tissue

Polythelia, also known as supernumerary nipples, is relatively common with a frequency of 0.2% to 5.6% and may be unilateral or bilateral (10% of cases) and is found along the embryonic milk line to the level of the vulva (35). Newborn males are found with polythelia somewhat more commonly than are females. Urinary tract abnormalities have been reported in association with polythelia, but there is still some question as to the strength of this relationship in some quarters (36). Yet another association of polythelia is with various genodermatoses (37). These are also reported kindreds with polythelia (38). Microscopically, the supernumerary nipple has a somewhat papillomatous epidermis and has a resemblance to an epidermal nevus, in addition to hyperpigmentation of the basal layer, lactiferous ductlike structures with or without epithelial hyperplasia, pilosebaceous units with or without keratin accumulation, and cyst formation resembling a keratinous cyst of infundibular type.

Supernumerary or accessory breast tissue is found in 1% to 2% of the population where the two most common sites are the axilla and vulva, and bilateral accessory breast tissue is found in approximately 40% to 45% of these cases (39). Accessory breast tissue may remain occult until pregnancy with the development of an axillary or vulvar mass. The ductal lobular tissue is indistinguishable from orthotopic breast tissue. Fibroadenomas (FA) may arise in accessory breast in the adolescent female or a hidradenoma papilliferum in the vulva of a comparably aged female.

ACQUIRED BREAST PATHOLOGY

This section is concerned with a variety of pathologic processes, both common and uncommon and usually presenting as a discrete mass or as diffuse swelling in the breast. Most of these lesions make their clinical appearance in pubertal females as a FA or gynecomastia in the adolescent male. Together, these two entities account for 50% or more of all breast pathology in patients 20 years old or less (40). Beyond these two entities, a number of other lesions present in the breast of children and adolescents, but usually as single examples. An important point to keep in mind is that only 2% to 3% of all breast lesions in children are malignant (41).

Benign Fibroepithelial Neoplasms

Fibroepithelial neoplasms are biphasic tumors of the breast that arise from terminal duct lobular units and the intra- and extralobular stroma. The various individual entities among the fibroepithelial neoplasms are recognized morphologically as the FA with and without distinctive histologic features mainly in the appearance of the stroma (cellular, myxoid, and atypical stromal cells), benign phyllodes tumor (PT), low-grade malignant or borderline PT, and high-grade malignant PT (42). Sarcomatous overgrowth of a malignant PT with residual foci of the latter is considered as a tumor type in this spectrum of neoplasms. Yang et al. (43) have discussed and illustrated the overlap of these various fibroepithelial tumors. Carcinomas of lobular or ductal type are known to occur rarely in or around FAs, but these cases are restricted almost exclusively to adults (44).

Fibroadenomas

FA is the most common neoplasm of the breast in the first two decades of life, and the overwhelming majority of cases are diagnosed in the interval from early puberty into late adolescence and beyond. There is a predilection for these tumors to occur in young African and African American females in whom the tumor commonly presents as a rapidly enlarging mass, which may be multifocal and even bilateral (45). Both FA and PT are seemingly more common in several tumor predisposition syndromes including Li-Fraumeni, Maffucci, and Beckwith-Wiedemann syndromes and Carney complex (40,46).

In most cases, there are relatively few difficulties in the histopathologic recognition of an FA in a young patient, but there is a thicket of largely semantic issues in the distinction, if any, among the juvenile, cellular, and giant FA from the FA, ordinary, and benign PT since the clinical and pathologic criteria are seemingly not burdened by a consensus or established criteria (47,48). Such qualifications as "increased stromal cellularity," "massive," and "juvenile" are both vague and subjective in their application to FAs in young individuals between the ages of 12 and 20 years (49).

Most FAs are well circumscribed from the surrounding breast parenchyma with a seeming cleft between the tumor

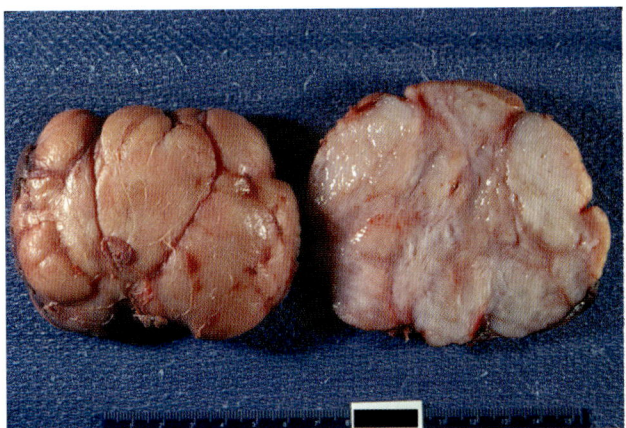

FIGURE 20-2 • Fibroadenoma of the juvenile type is a multinodular, circumscribed mass measuring 6 cm. The individual nodules are separated by depressed clefts, raising the possibility of a phyllodes tumor.

and adjacent soft tissues. A true capsule is not present in most cases. The external surfaces often have a bosselated appearance that corresponds to the bulging multinodular or lobulated cut surface (Figure 20-2). A glistening, mucoid yellowish-tan to whitish surface characterizes most tumors although extensive hemorrhage may indicate the presence of infarction (50). The majority of tumors measure 2 to 5 cm in greatest dimension although some have applied the designation of "giant" to those tumors measuring 5 cm or greater (up to 20 cm). Some of the larger FAs can ulcerate the overlying skin and present as a fungating mass (49). Two basic histologic patterns are recognized in FAs: an intracanalicular pattern with a prominent stroma compressing strands of epithelium in various configurations including the phyllodes or leaflike pattern of a benign PT (Figure 20-3) and the periductal or pericanalicular pattern whose stroma separates individual terminal ductal lobular units (Figure 20-4). One or the other of these patterns is exclusive in any one

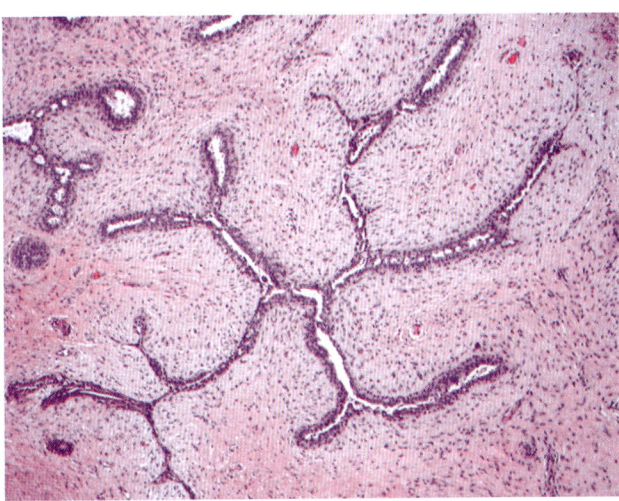

FIGURE 20-3 • Fibroadenoma with the intracanalicular pattern of stroma compressing the epithelial profiles.

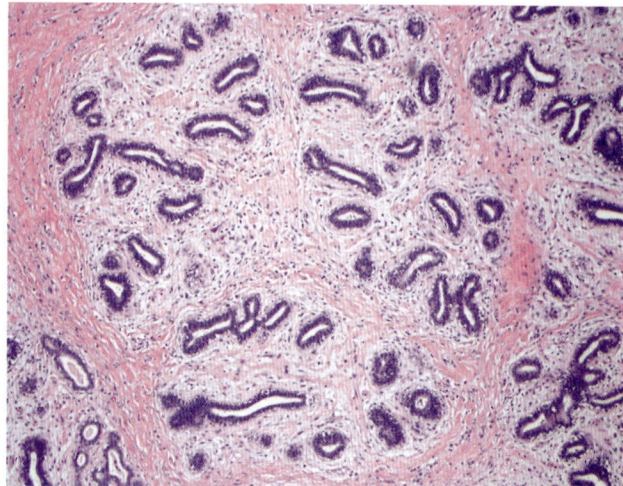

FIGURE 20-4 • Fibroadenoma with the pericanalicular pattern with tubular-like glands separated and surrounded by a fibrous and fibromyxoid stroma. Exclusive proliferation of these tubular-like glands results in the tubular adenoma pattern.

FA, or alternatively, there are FAs with a mixed pattern of phyllodes-like profiles and intracanalicular and/or pericanalicular patterns. The cellularity of the stroma is the usual source of concern in FAs in young individuals. In most cases, the stroma has a bland fibrous appearance with or without edema or a predominant myxoid stroma (Figure 20-5). The stroma adjacent to the epithelium is typically more cellular and less fibrotic than is the more remote, fibrous stroma. The occasional mitotic figure can be found in the stroma adjacent to the epithelium. When the stroma is more uniformly cellular, attention is directed to the presence or absence of mitotic figures since the latter separates the so-called cellular or juvenile FA from the borderline or low-grade PT (Figure 20-6A, B). Mitotic activity generally should not exceed 2 mitoses

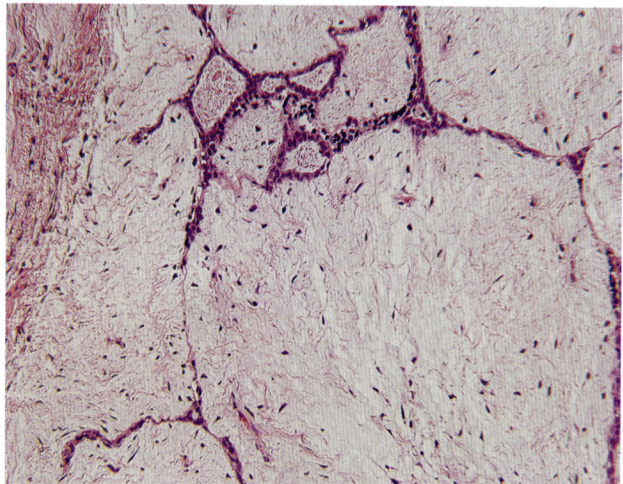

FIGURE 20-5 • Fibroadenomas of the left breast in a 17-year-old female, measuring 3.7 cm and having a gelatinous cut surface. The stroma has a diffuse myxoid appearance and represents a myxoid intracanalicular FA. The possibility of Carney syndrome of multiple myxomas was raised at the time.

per 10 high-power (400×) fields (HPF) nor the leaflike phyllodes epithelial pattern, but in a needle core biopsy, the latter epithelial configuration may be difficult to appreciate (51). Mitotic figures become a concern when they are found in the stroma without difficulty, which usually translates into 10 mitoses in 10 HPF. An infiltrating stromal border at the periphery should be viewed with concern. Pleomorphic stromal giant cells are found infrequently, similar in some respects, to those stromal cells in nasal polyps or lamina propria of the bladder (52).

While there is considerable focus on the stroma of FAs, the epithelium may be quite hyperplastic with a degree of complexity and papillary profiles, which are especially notable in those tumors from adolescent or young adult women. Fibrocystic changes with cysts, apocrine metaplasia, and sclerosing adenosis are seen in some FAs in young individuals though they are more commonly observed in FAs from older women (Figure 20-7A, B). As a final note, there are examples of intraductal papillary lesions with FA-like features in young females (Figure 20-8) (53,54). Some have questioned the relationship in younger individuals between the intraductal papilloma and FA.

Immunohistochemistry has a very limited role in the diagnosis of FA. Those cases with an unsettling degree of cellularity and mitotic activity may benefit with Ki-67 and p53 staining (55). The stroma cells in FAs are rich in CD34+ fibroblasts, factor XIIIa+ dendrocytes, and smooth muscle actin + myofibroblasts (56). It has been noted that CD10+ stromal cells are uncommon in cellular FAs (57).

A recurrence rate of 10% to 15% is reported after resection of an FA in young patients; however, the "recurrence" may represent a new lesion. There are rare examples, principally in adults, of malignant progression of a recurrent FA to a malignant PT (58).

Benign PT is basically defined as a fibroepithelial neoplasm whose architecture is defined by the leaflike epithelial-lined structures and a stroma with a variable degree of cellularity (Figure 20-9). The periductal stroma is usually more cellular than in the stroma of the FA. An isolated mitotic figure in the mesenchymal cells adjacent to the epithelial component is permissible, which is also the case in an FA.

Adenomas

Adenomas constitute at least two general categories of breast lesions: one a monotypic fibroepithelial neoplasm arising from the terminal duct lobular unit in the absence of an intralobular stroma. The tubular and lactational adenomas are examples of the latter category (59,60). Tubular or pure adenoma is uncommon compared to FA, but is seen in the same young age group and is undistinguishable clinically from the FA (Figure 20-10). The distinctive histologic features are those of a multinodular tumor, which is composed of small uniform tubuloglandular structures with a variably prominent stroma in the background (Figure 20-11). In fact, some fibroepithelial neoplasms have a mixed pattern of tubular adenoma and FA. Lactational or secretory changes are the

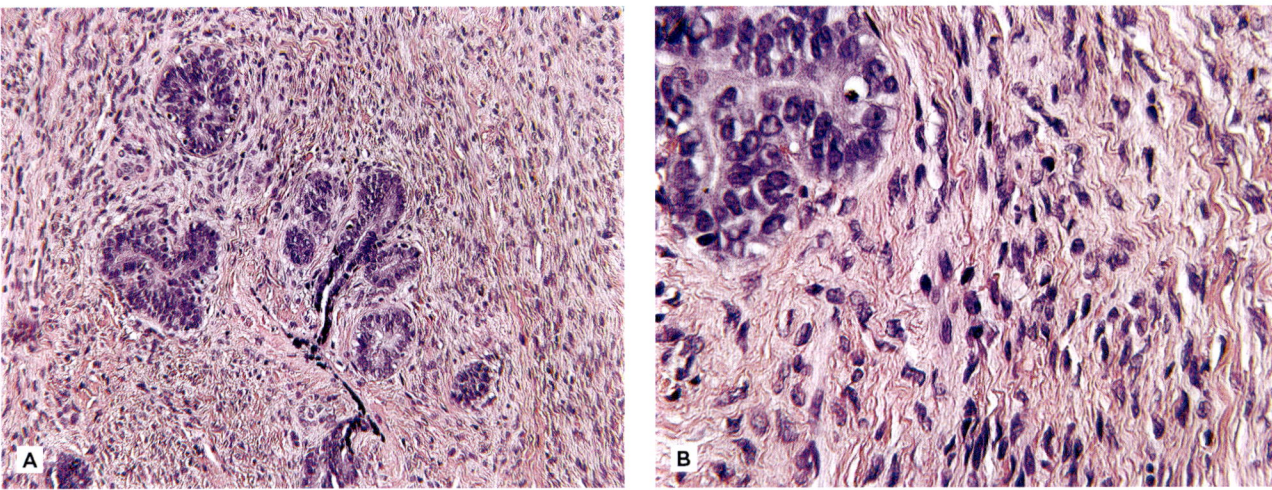

FIGURE 20-6 • **A:** Fibroadenoma of the cellular or juvenile type in a 12-year-old female. The stroma is notably hypercellular and displays a pericanalicular pattern. **B:** Despite the hypercellular appearance, mitotic activity is inapparent.

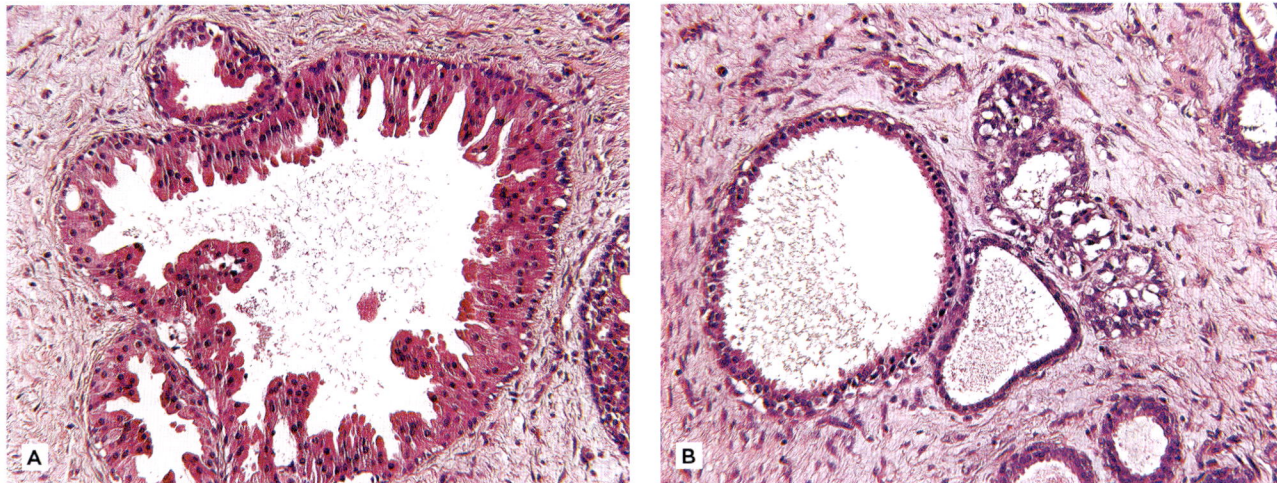

FIGURE 20-7 • **A:** Fibroadenoma of the right breast in a 16-year-old female shows the presence of papillary apocrine metaplasia. **B:** Elsewhere in the FA, cysts and foci of usual ductal hyperplasia are seen.

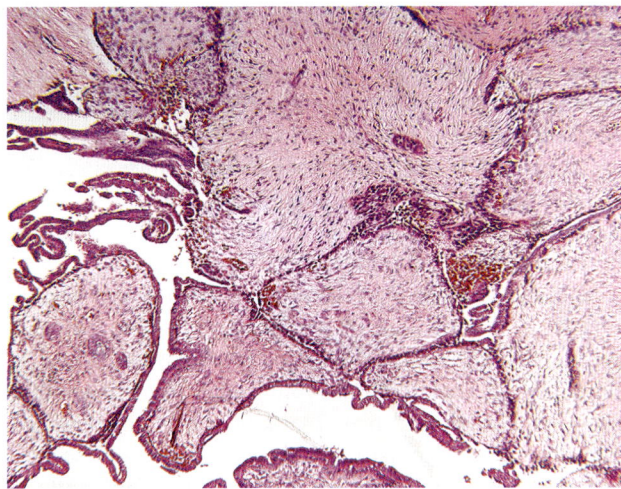

FIGURE 20-8 • Fibroadenoma-like features are seen in this intraductal papillary lesion in the right breast of an 11-year-old female.

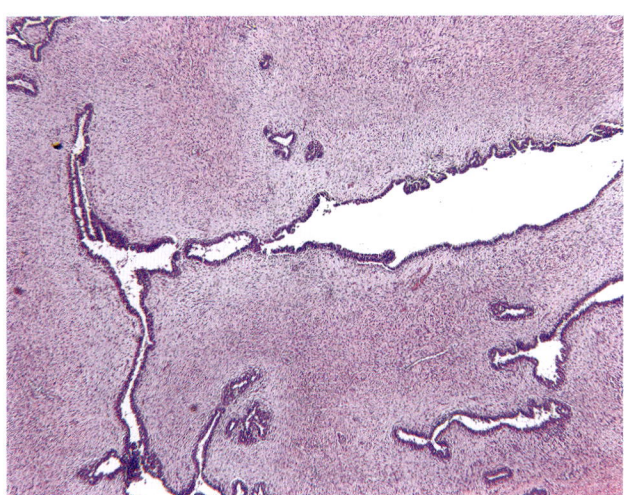

FIGURE 20-9 • Benign phyllodes tumor in the left breast of a 16-year-old female. The leaflike epithelial profiles are surrounded by a pale hypocellular and fibrous stroma.

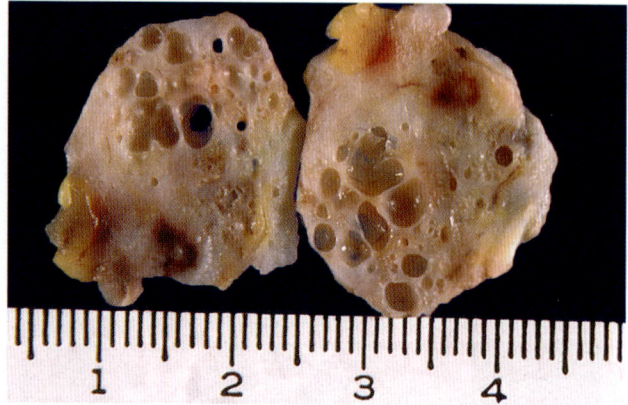

FIGURE 20-15 • Juvenile papillomatosis or so-called Swiss cheese disease presents as a mass, and the cut surface exposes numerous cysts within a sclerotic stroma.

overlapping microscopic features were present leading to some diagnostic semantic improvisation. Another pathologic process is subareolar sclerosing duct hyperplasia whose features overlap with the nipple duct adenoma or florid nipple duct papillomatosis.

The various papillary lesions of the breast can be accompanied by fibrocystic changes, which encompass several histologic patterns including sclerosing adenosis, variably sized cysts, apocrine metaplasia, small and intermediate usual duct hyperplasia, interlobular fibrosis, and pseudoangiomatous stromal hyperplasia (PASH). Some of these lesions can be found in FAs, but infrequently in breast biopsies from adolescent females.

Gynecomastia and Juvenile Macromastia

This section is concerned with two overgrowth processes of otherwise normal breast tissues mainly in the fibrous stromal component; both are seen at puberty or in the postpubertal

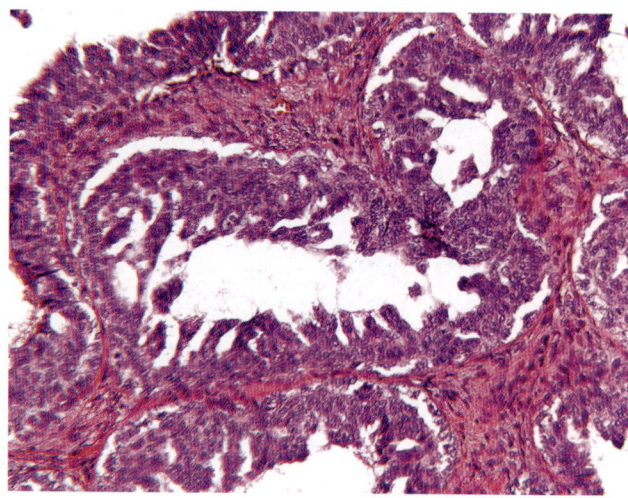

FIGURE 20-17 • Papillary duct hyperplasia presented in the left breast of a 16-year-old female. Rather than cysts intermixed with papillary proliferations as in juvenile papillomatosis, the ducts are relatively uniform with papillomatous excrescences.

adolescent years. In both cases, surgical intervention with reduction in breast tissue is generally indicated for cosmesis and postural and back problems in the case of macromastia.

Gynecomastia occurs in 50% or more of adolescent males (73). Young obese prepubertal males develop breast enlargement on the basis of pure adipose tissue deposition (pseudogynecomastia) rather than growth of glandular–stromal breast tissue (Figure 20-18). Another form of pseudogynecomastia is the presence of diffuse or plexiform neurofibroma (NF) in a child with NF1. The so-called physiologic gynecomastia is contrasted clinically from "pathologic" gynecomastia with an underlying disorder or neoplasm including aromatase excess syndrome (74) (Table 20-1). Prepubertal gynecomastia should be regarded as "pathologic" in nature.

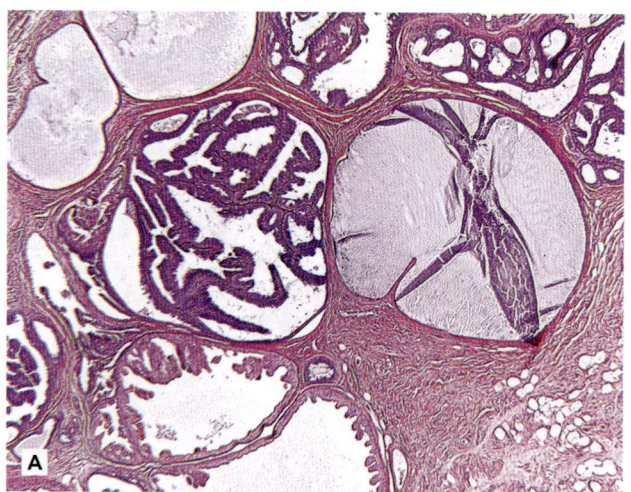
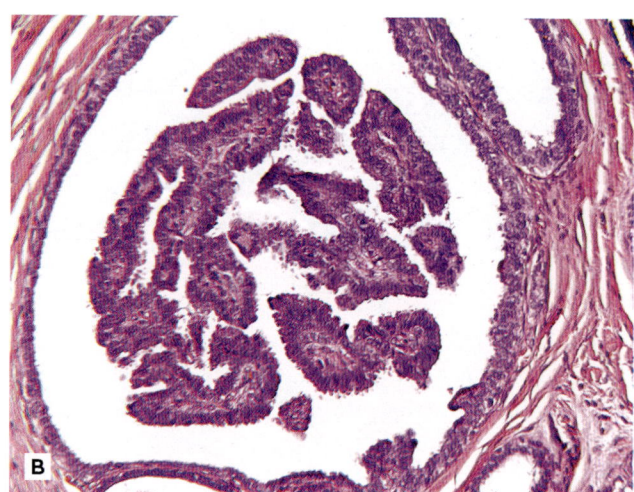

FIGURE 20-16 • **A:** Juvenile papillomatosis in the right breast of a 17-year-old female presented as a mass. Numerous cysts are found in the midst of ducts with papillary and hyperplastic features. **B:** This papillary proliferation is one of many different papillomatous patterns.

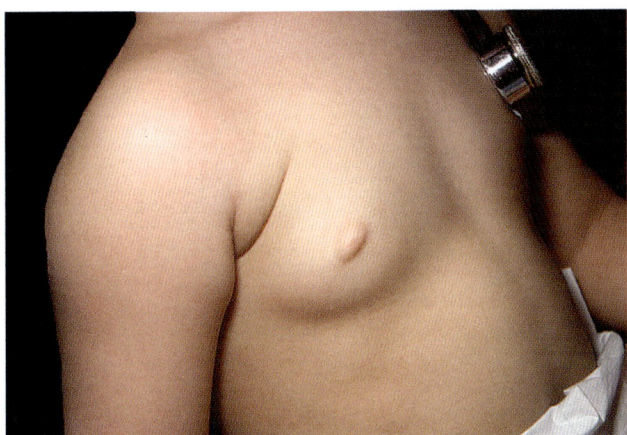

FIGURE 20-18 • Gynecomastia in a prepubertal boy is cause for concern about a possible functioning neoplasm of the pituitary, adrenal, or testis.

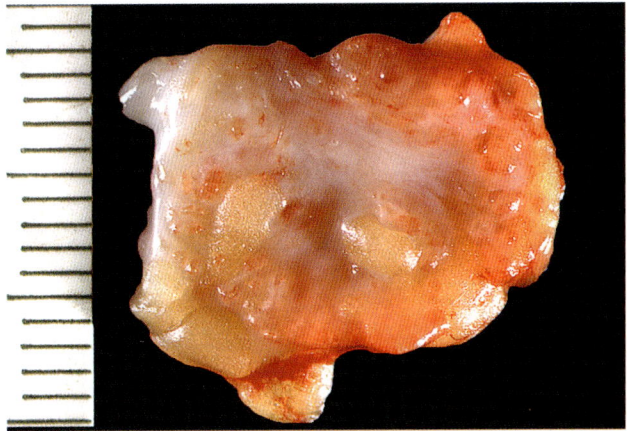

FIGURE 20-19 • Gynecomastia specimen is an ill-defined dense fibrofatty, rubbery tissue.

Rubbery fibrous or fibrofatty tissue is the rather nondescript appearance of the gross specimen (Figure 20-19). Dense fibrous tissue with edema in some cases and the presence of circular and elongated ducts without lobules in most cases are the microscopic features (Figure 20-20). The degree of epithelial proliferation ranges from minimal to impressively exuberant or florid. In the latter category, there are reported examples of ductal carcinoma in situ arising in gynecomastia in adolescent males (75–77). Since the epithelial proliferation can be striking, there is the diagnostic conundrum of florid hyperplasia, atypical ductal hyperplasia, and ductal carcinoma in situ with low-grade cytologic features.

Juvenile macromastia (juvenile or virginal hypertrophy or gigantomastia) is an uncommon disorder in breast growth with rapid enlargement of one or both breasts at menarche. Unilateral or bilateral reduction mammoplasty is the management of choice (78,79). Several attempts have been made to define the disorder, but one criterion is the need to resect over 1500 gm of breast tissue per breast (80). There is a microscopic similarity to gynecomastia except for the presence of terminal duct lobular units separated by edematous or dense fibrous tissue (Figure 20-21). In some cases, residual lactational changes are present in those cases whose onset or acceleration in the size of the breasts occurred during pregnancy. Another complication is breakdown or ulceration of the taut skin when there is compromise of blood supply and pyoderma in some cases.

Primary Malignant Neoplasms

Low- and High-Grade Malignant Phyllodes Tumor

Low-grade and high-grade malignant PT importantly must be differentiated from those fibroepithelial neoplasms with the branching, leaflike pattern of the benign PT and cellular

TABLE 20-1 SPECIFIC CONDITIONS ASSOCIATED WITH GYNECOMASTIA IN CHILDREN AND ADOLESCENTS

Adrenocortical adenoma and carcinoma
Choriocarcinoma and other gonadotropin-producing germ cell neoplasms
Congenital adrenal hyperplasia
Familial gynecomastia with aromatase excess
Fibrolamellar hepatocellular carcinoma with aromatase excess
Growth hormone therapy
Hepatoblastoma
Hypergonadotropic hypogonadism
Large-cell calcifying Sertoli cell tumor with and without Peutz-Jeghers syndrome
Prolactinoma
Pseudohermaphroditism (5-α-reductase deficiency)
Spinal cord disorders
von Recklinghausen neurofibromatosis
X-linked mental retardation
Drugs

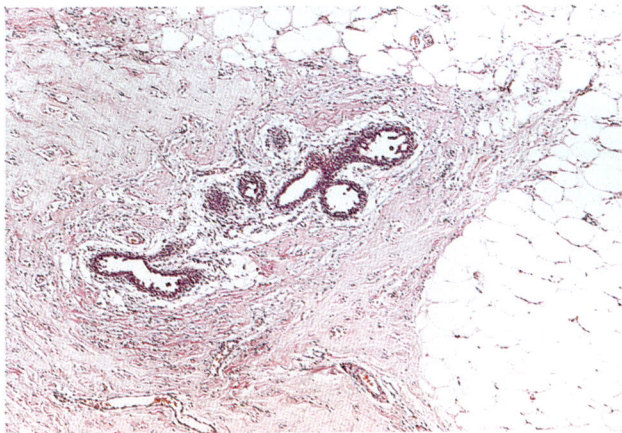

FIGURE 20-20 • Gynecomastia is characterized by the presence of small elongated and tubular ducts without lobules and a zone of edematous stroma or "halo" surrounded by fibrous and fibrofatty stroma.

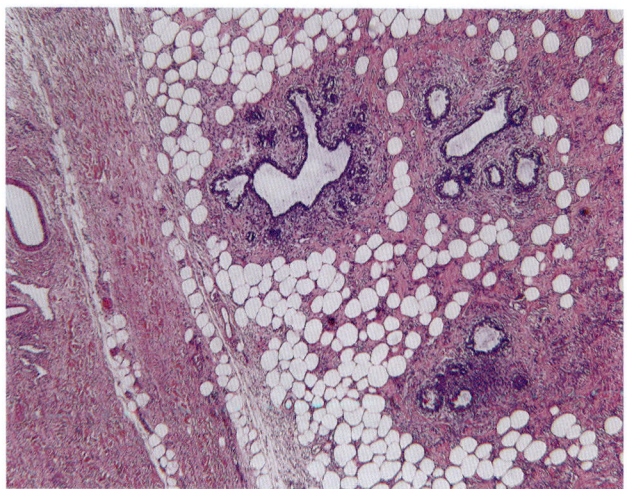

FIGURE 20-21 • Juvenile macromastia has a somewhat variable histologic appearance with a resemblance to gynecomastia. Herein, a fibrofatty stroma contains several ductlike structures with smaller ducts at the periphery.

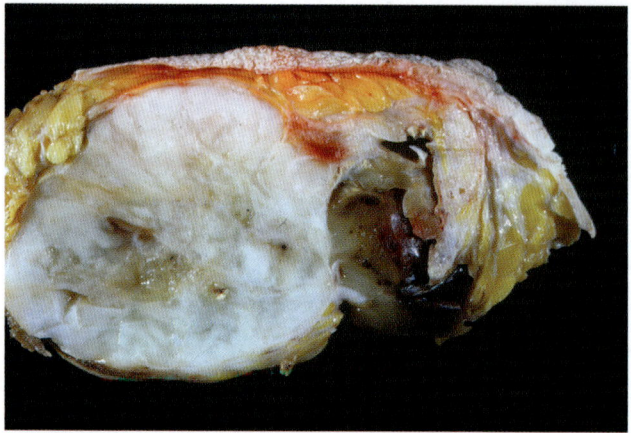

FIGURE 20-22 • Phyllodes tumor seen in this mastectomy specimen is sharply demarcated from the surrounding tissues. The multinodularity of the mass is accentuated by the clefted and branching epithelial-lined structures.

FA. It has been estimated that 30% to 40% of primary malignancies of the breast in the first two decades of life are malignant PTs (42,69). It is notable that almost 20% or more of PTs in some larger series are examples of benign PT (81,82). Less than 10% of all PTs of "benign," low-grade, and high-grade malignant subtypes are diagnosed in the second decade of life. Among 34 sarcomas arising in the breast in individuals between 12 and 19 years old at diagnosis, 29 (85%) were "phyllodes tumors"; there were no details about the pathologic features in this group of cases collected from the data of the Surveillance, Epidemiology and End Results (SEER) (83).

PTs, like FAs, are not seen until puberty, and most are diagnosed well beyond adolescence. Overall, the mean and median ages at diagnosis including all age groups are 35 to 45 years, and the incidence increases through the third decade of life (84).

Grossly, the tumor is well circumscribed in most cases and generally measures in excess of 15 cm in diameter (Figure 20-22). The cut surface is lobulated with discernible clefts or has a more homogeneous surface that may indicate the presence of stromal overgrowth; stromal or overt sarcomatous overgrowth may be accompanied by infiltration of the tumor into the adjacent breast tissue. Hemorrhage and necrosis are uncommon in the low-grade malignant PT. Stromal hypercellularity, nuclear enlargement and atypia, increased mitotic activity in excess of 2 to 5 mitoses per 10 HPF, and stromal overgrowth with loss of clefted or leaflike epithelial-lined structures in at least one low-power microscopic field are the histologic features of a low-grade malignant PT (Figure 20-23A, B). There is a lack of consensus on the upper numeral limit of mitotic figures per 10 HPFs in the differentiation between the low-grade and high-grade malignant PT (Figure 20-23C) (42). Invasion into the adjacent breast parenchyma may be microscopic or obvious from the gross examination. Invasion at the borders, stroma with high-grade nuclear features, and mitotic activity generally in excess of 10 mitoses per 10 HPF are the features of the high-grade malignant PT. The sarcomatous component can have various patterns including fibrosarcoma, rhabdomyosarcoma (RMS), and liposarcoma. Those tumors with high-grade sarcomatous and locally aggressive features have the potential for metastatic behavior in 1% to 2% of cases in general, but even rarer in young individuals (85).

The differential diagnosis is cellular FA with or without a phyllodes pattern. When mitotic figures are found in a cellular FA, they are usually identified adjacent to an epithelial-lined space and do not exceed 2 mitoses per 10 HPF. There is no question about the existence of those borderline fibroepithelial tumors where the only consensus is the need to re-excision if the surgical margins are in doubt. The periductal stromal tumor is a rare neoplasm, which presents as a nodule with a hypercellular cuff of spindle cells with atypia around ducts in the absence of the phyllodes architecture and stroma (86). A case has been reported in a 14-year-old male (87). The spindle cells are variably positive for CD10, CD34, and CD117.

Mammary Carcinoma

Mammary carcinoma in the first two decades of life is very uncommon yet well documented; carcinoma of the breast accounts for approximately 50% of primary malignancies among adolescents and young adults (88,89). The SEER data recorded 75 breast malignancies in females 19 years old or less; 41 (55%) cases were carcinomas of several pathologic subtypes (83). Approximately 15% of carcinomas in the latter study were diagnosed between the ages of 11 and 14 years and the remainder at or before 19 years of age. Infiltrating ductal carcinoma was reportedly the most common subtype, which is coincidental with the adult experience.

The subject of mammary carcinoma in younger age individuals is not an entirely remote one given that 5% to 10% of cases are hereditary; Li-Fraumeni (TP53) and hereditary breast and ovarian carcinoma (BRAC1/BRAC2) syndromes

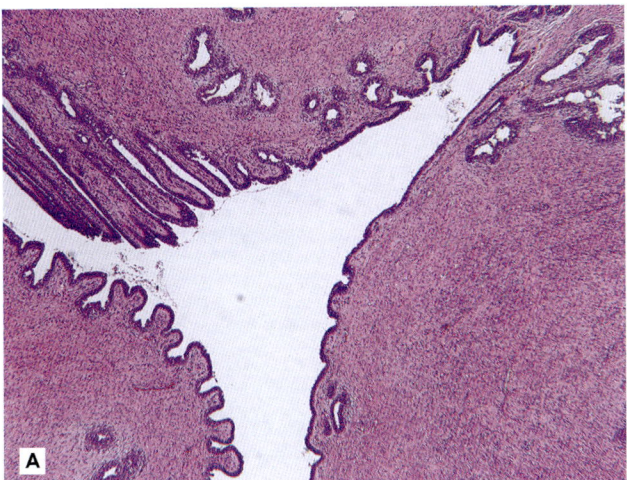
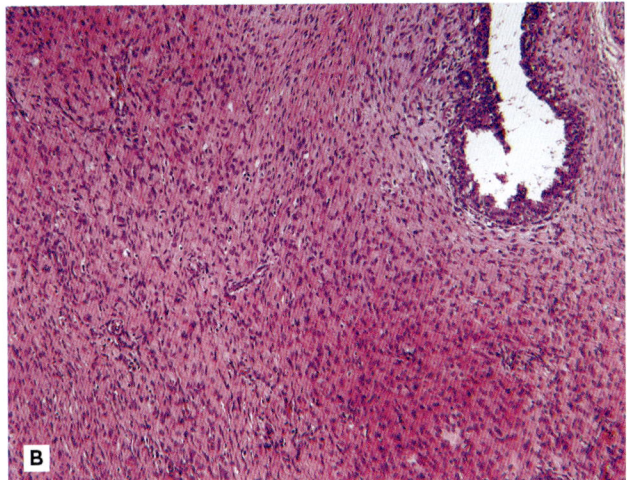
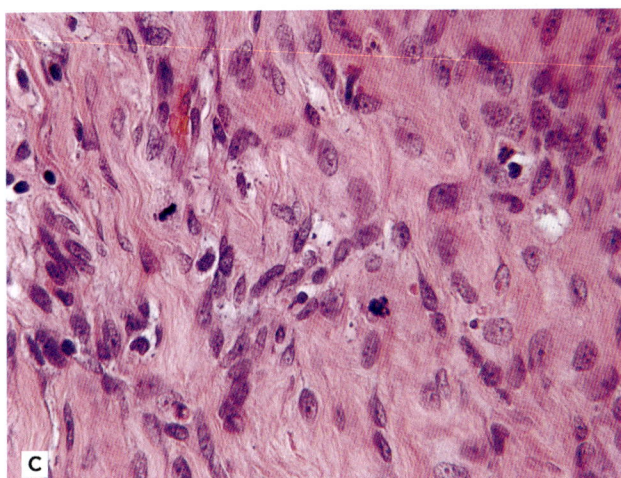

FIGURE 20-23 • **A:** Low-grade malignant phyllodes tumor in the left breast of a 14-year-old female measured 2.5 cm in greatest dimension. This low magnification shows the clefted epithelial-lined structure of the phyllodes type. **B:** This field demonstrates the stromal expansion or overgrowth. **C:** At least two mitotic figures are seen in high-power microscopic field, but overall, the mitotic activity was low.

are associated with a high risk for the development of breast cancer (90–92). However, other germline mutations in PTEN, STK1, NBS1, and BRIP/FANKJ are accompanied by an intermediate risk for breast cancer. There is no apparent increased risk of childhood malignancies in BRAC1/BRAC2 syndrome, but there is a need to begin the process of appropriate genetic counseling in affected pedigrees as children progress through their adolescent years (93–95). By contrast, the initial suspicion about the possibility of Li-Fraumeni syndrome may be heralded by the occurrence of RMS, adrenocortical neoplasm, or choroid plexus tumor in childhood (96,97).

Secretory (Juvenile) Carcinoma

Secretory (juvenile) carcinoma (SC) of the breast is unique in that approximately 30% to 35% of cases are diagnosed between the ages of 3 and 19 years (98). The remaining patients are adults at diagnosis so that "juvenile carcinoma" is a misnomer in a sense. Though the majority of tumors are found in females, SC occurs in young males (99). Juvenile papillomatosis has been reported in a minority of children with SC (100). This neoplasm has the same t (12; 15) translocation (ETV6-NTRK3 fusion gene) as congenital infantile fibrosarcoma, cellular mesoblastic nephroma, and the mammary analog SC of the salivary gland (101,102).

Pathologically, this tumor is typically well circumscribed with a firm to soft consistency and has a grayish white cut surface. The size infrequently exceeds 3 cm in greatest dimension. These tumors have several patterns from solid to microcysts, to cribriform, and to papillary; most have a ductal architecture and tumor cells with abundant eosinophilic to vacuolated cytoplasm (98,102) (Figure 20-24A–D). The nuclei have low- to intermediate-grade features. The presence of eosinophilic luminal secretions accounts for the appellation of the neoplasm, but is not present in all cases. The tumor has a triple-negative phenotype for estrogen and progesterone receptors and Her-2/neu and has the immunophenotype of basal cells (cytokeratin 5/cytokeratin 6, cytokeratin 14, cytokeratin 17, EGFR, and vimentin) (103,104).

Despite the "unfavorable" triple-negative status of SC, the prognosis is quite favorable in most cases in childhood, but the tumor is seemingly more aggressive in adults (105,106). Sentinel lymph node biopsy is usually performed and is negative for tumor in most cases.

One note of caution is the development of premature thelarche presenting as a subareolar nodule, which can be mistaken for a neoplasm like SC (107). A small incisional biopsy should settle any diagnostic concerns.

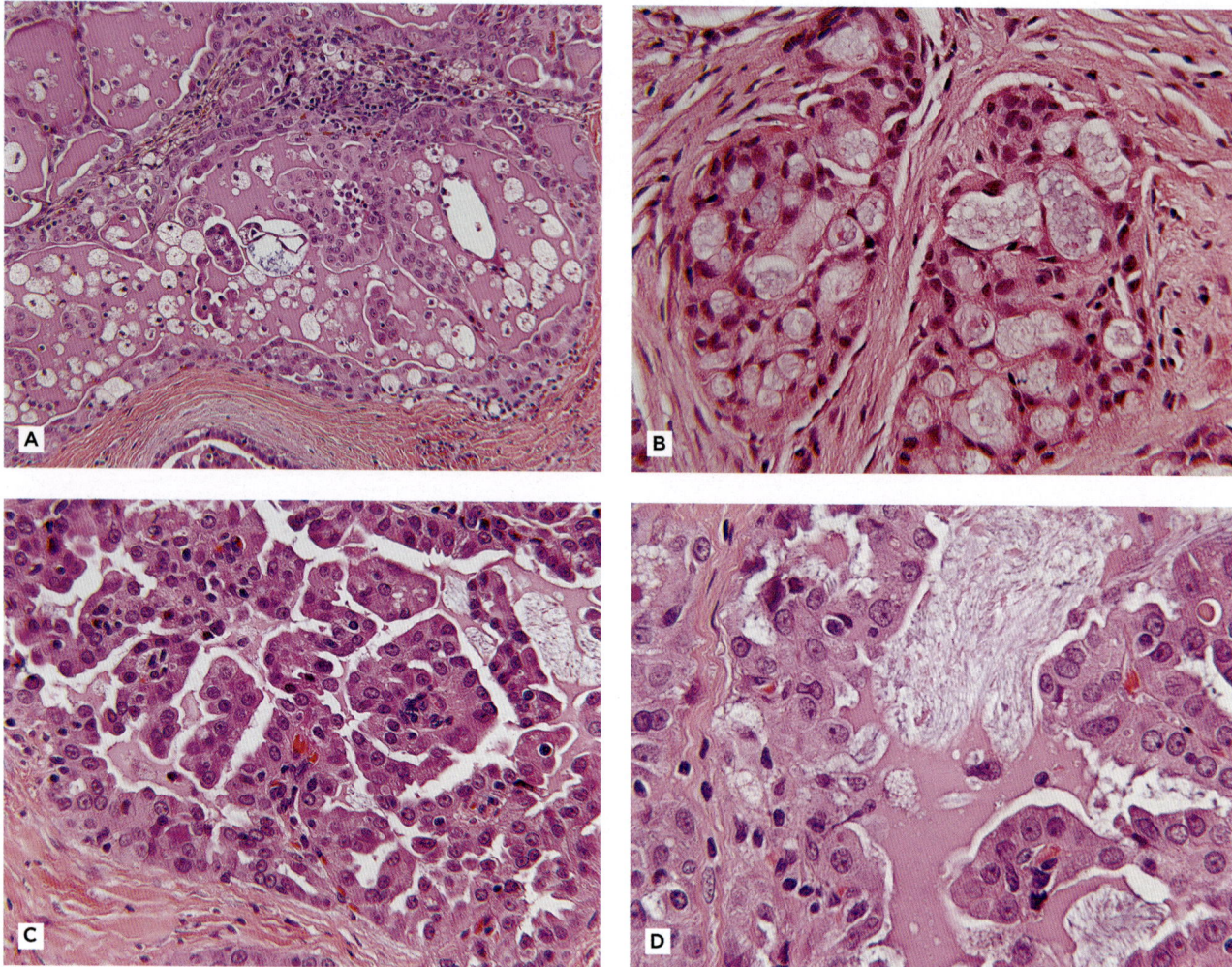

FIGURE 20-24 • **A:** Secretory carcinoma in the right breast of this 4-year-old female had the t(12;15) translocation. One of the many circumscribed nests of tumor is showing a microcystic cribriform pattern. **B:** These nests have a cribriform pattern and luminal secretions. **C:** A papillary focus in secretory carcinoma. **D:** Luminal secretions and tumor cells with abundant eosinophilic cytoplasm. The tumor cells have low- to intermediate-grade nuclei.

Soft Tissue and Secondary Tumors

Soft tissue and secondary tumors constitute a diverse and uncommon to rare category of neoplasms in the breast of children. Many of the mesenchymal or soft tissue tumors presenting in the breast are more commonly encountered in nonmammary sites except for the myofibroblastoma.

Neurofibroma

NF may arise in the skin overlying the breast as a solitary lesion, which is not associated with neurofibromatosis 1. However, the presence of a diffuse and infiltrating NF within the breast tissue in a child is a manifestation of NF1 (108). Approximately 3% to 4% of patients with NF1 have breast involvement (109). In a prepubertal female with NF1, premature thelarche or in a similarly aged male, the possibility of gynecomastia may be the clinical impression (96,97,110). NF with a plexiform and/or diffuse features is diagnostic of NF1. Juvenile papillomatosis and PASH are other reported lesions of the breast in NF1 (111,112).

Granular Cell Tumor

Granular cell tumor (GCT) is presumably a Schwann cell–derived neoplasm in most cases with an anatomic distribution of ubiquitous proportions from the pituitary to the skin of the lower extremity. The breast, in addition to the oral cavity (tongue, lip) and vulva, is one of the more common sites (5% to 15% of all cases) of GCT (113). Most cases are diagnosed in the 4th to 5th decades of life, with a minority of cases presenting in the breast of adolescents (113,114). A firm mass in the breast measuring 2 to 4 cm is a cause for concern about a possible carcinoma (Figure 20-25). Nests and strands of polygonal to somewhat spindle cells with abundant granular eosinophilic cytoplasm have an infiltrating poorly circumscribed growth (Figure 20-26). The central nuclei are generally not atypical, but mitotic activity should be viewed with some concern. The stroma accounts for the firmness of these tumors. The granular cytoplasm is due to lysosomes, which account for the immunopositivity for CD68; these tumors are also positive for vimentin and S-100 proteins (Figure 20-26B).

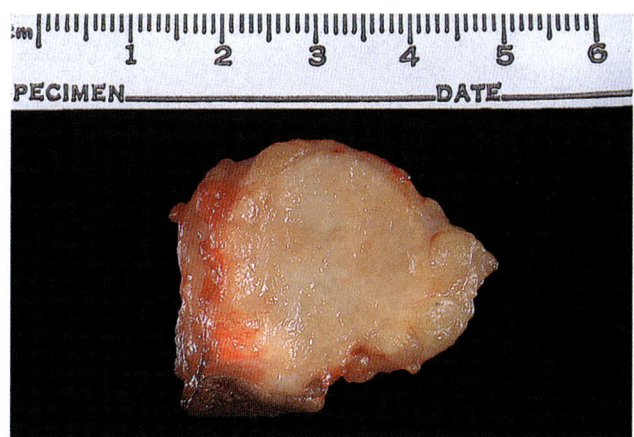

FIGURE 20-25 • Granular cell tumor in the breast presenting as a firm mass with a pale yellow cut surface and infiltrating borders.

Lipomatous Tumors

Lipomatous tumors of the breast are exceedingly rare, as evidenced by the first case of lipoblastoma in the left breast of a 13-month-old boy (115). If multiple lipomatous tumors are present in addition to the breast, a PTEN overgrowth syndrome should be considered.

Vascular Tumors

Vascular lesions, one of the most common benign mesenchymal tumors in childhood, are known to occur infrequently in the skin of the breast (116,117). Infantile hemangioma presents in the dermis and/or subcutis and displays the multilobulated architecture, and the cellularity is related to early proliferative phase in contrast to the latter involutional phase with the presence of patent capillaries. The endothelial cells are consistently immunoreactive for GLUT1 (118). Another more common vascular lesion, lymphangioma or lymphatic malformation, has been reported in the breast of a 6-year-old boy (119). Another lymphatic lesion, kaposiform hemangioendothelioma, is known to occur on the chest and may involve the soft tissues in the region of the breast (120,121). Angiosarcoma of the breast was diagnosed with one case among 34 (3%) sarcomas of the breast detected between the ages of 12 and 19 years (83). Van Geel et al. (122) reported bilateral angiosarcomas of the breast in a 14-year-old female. Two (4%) of 49 patients with angiosarcoma of the breast were 15 and 17 years old at diagnosis in one series (123). There is a distinction made between the parenchymal angiosarcoma and the cutaneous angiosarcoma in women who have radiation therapy to the breast (124).

Fibrous and Myofibroblastic Tumors

Fibrous and myofibroblastic tumors of several specific pathologic types are recognized in the breast across a broad age group. The three familiar fibrous lesions of the breast are fibromatosis, nodular fasciitis, and myofibroblastoma, but these three tumors do not exhaust the list, which also includes the hamartoma and PASH (125–127).

Fibromatosis of the breast tends to occur in women beyond the fourth decade of life with the uncommon sporadic case seen in late adolescence and into the third decade (128). A firm mass measuring 10 cm or less and having deceptively circumscribed borders is the gross appearance. Interlacing bundles and fascicles of spindle cells within an edematous and/or densely collagenized stroma are the principal histologic features (Figure 20-27A). Nuclear atypia and mitotic activity are generally inconspicuous (Figure 20-27B). In addition to smooth muscle actin immunopositivity, 70% to 80% of cases display nuclear positivity for β-catenin, reflecting the mutation in CTNNB1 (Figure 20-27C) (129,130). Staining for β-catenin is useful in the differential diagnosis of desmoid fibromatosis from other spindle cell tumors (131). Fibromatosis also arises from the chest wall beneath the breast (132). Fibrous hamartoma of infancy is seen more commonly in the axilla, but in this cases presented in a 1-year-old female (Figure 20-28A, B).

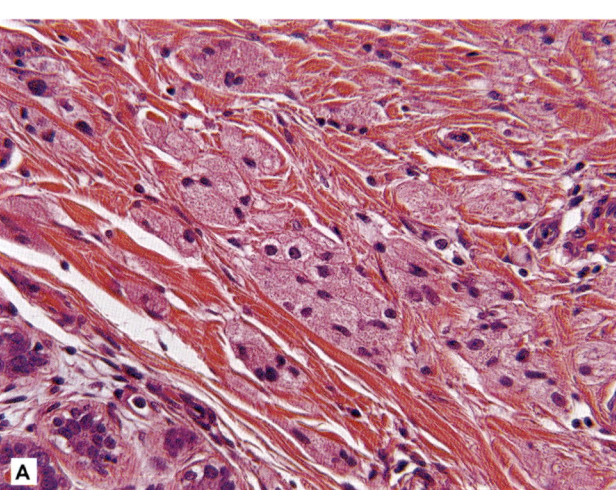
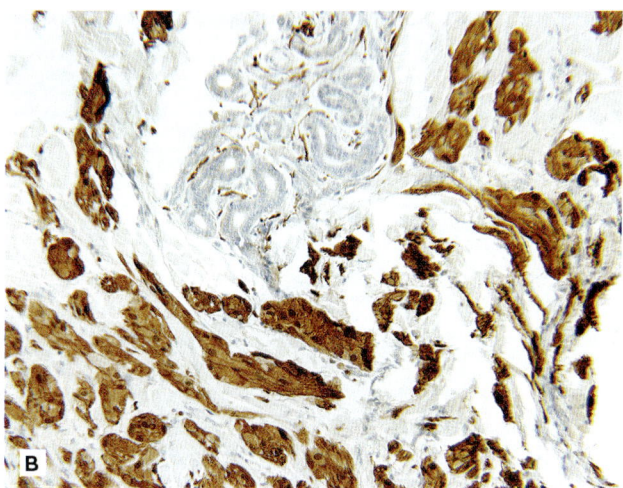

FIGURE 20-26 • **A:** Granular cell tumor presented in the right breast of a 15-year-old female. The granular cells infiltrate through the stroma adjacent to a lobule. **B:** Diffuse S-100 positivity is seen in the tumor cells that surround a lobule.

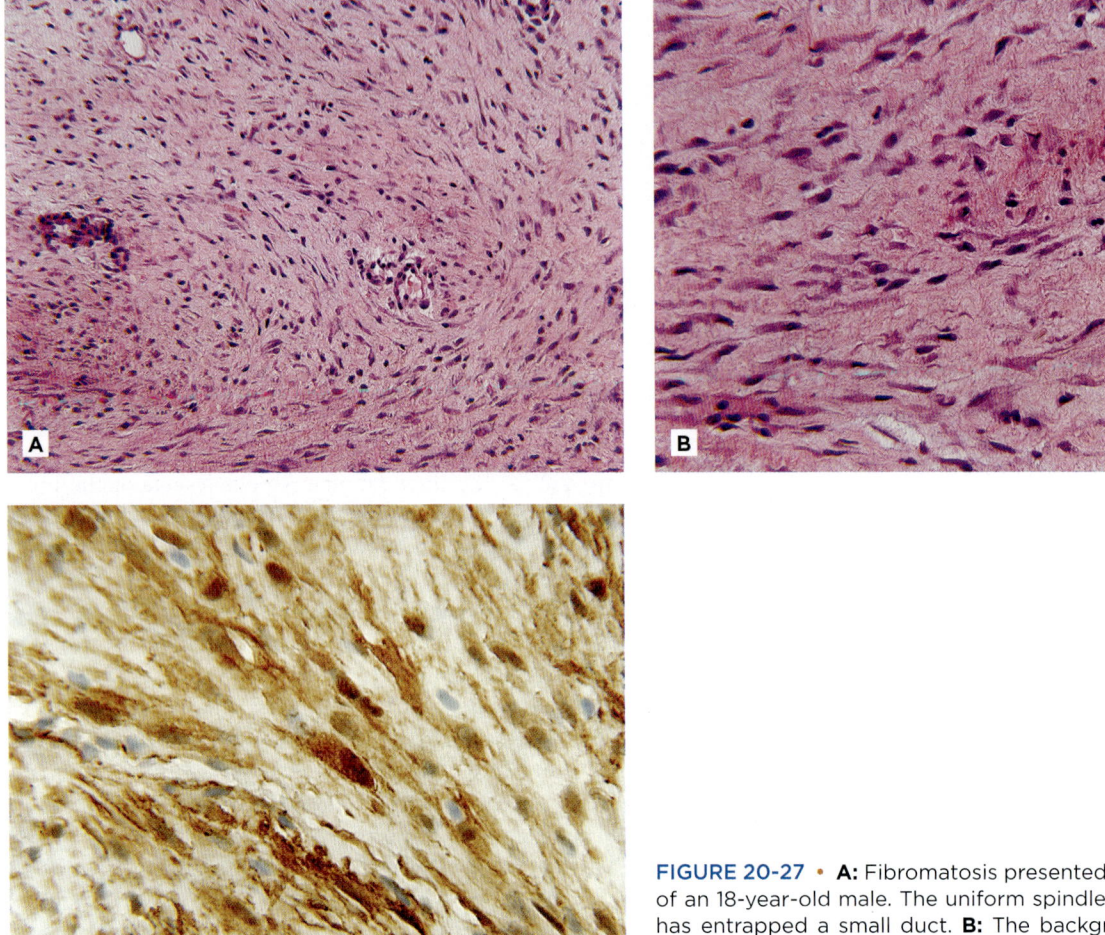

FIGURE 20-27 • **A:** Fibromatosis presented in the left breast of an 18-year-old male. The uniform spindle cell proliferation has entrapped a small duct. **B:** The background has a pale eosinophilic appearance and hemorrhage. **C:** The nuclei of the tumor cells are immunoreactive for β-catenin.

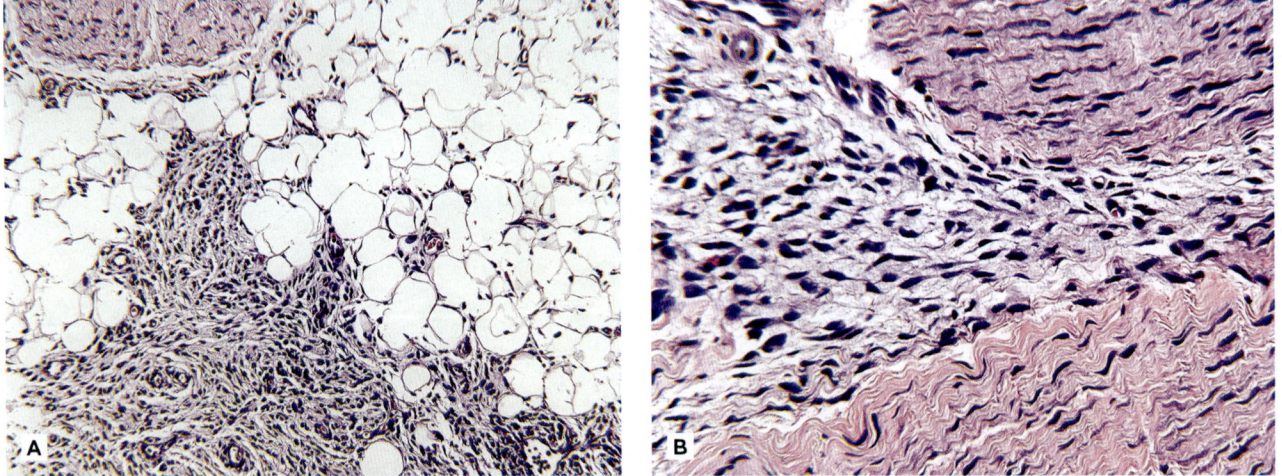

FIGURE 20-28 • **A:** Fibrous hamartoma of infancy presented in the right breast of a 1-year-old female. The background of adipose tissue is occupied by immature-appearing spindle cells. **B:** A focus of immature spindle cells in adjacent to more mature fibroblasts with a collagenized background.

Nodular fasciitis presents rarely in the breast, and the two of the younger examples occurred in 15 and 21 years old (133–135). These lesions typically arise in the underlying stroma beneath the dermis as a circumscribed spindle cell proliferation, which may be quite mitotically active, but foci of red cell extravasation and mucoid microcysts are useful features to assist in avoiding a diagnosis of a low-grade sarcoma. The mucoid microcysts of nodular fasciitis are differentiated from nodular mucinosis (136).

PASH is another myofibroblastic proliferation like nodular fasciitis and myofibroma, which may present as a mass or as an incidental histologic finding in association with a FA or gynecomastia; its presence has been documented mainly in adolescent females (137,138). Bundles of dense collagen are separated by slitlike spaces lined by spindle cells without atypia (Figure 20-29) (139). These lesions can be nodular as they were in a 12-year-old female (140). The stromal cells are immunoreactive for smooth muscle actin and CD34 (141).

Myofibroblastoma is a spindle cell tumor with an intermixture of mature adipose tissue, which is typically diagnosed in the breast of adult males (142). At least one case has been reported in a 10-month-old male (98). There is some resemblance to the spindle cell lipoma, in addition to several other morphologic variants (143). The myofibroblasts are immunopositive for smooth muscle actin, desmin, and CD34 like the spindle cells in PASH and dermatofibrosarcoma protuberans (DESP)–giant cell fibroblastoma (144).

Hamartoma presents as a discrete nodule and, like the FA, is reported in adolescent females (145). A spindle cell stroma surrounds somewhat disorganized lobules and can be overlooked without difficulty without an appreciation that the clinical presentation is that of a mass (Figure 20-30) (146).

Inflammatory myofibroblastic *tumor* is a neoplasm of the lung, mesentery, and intestinal tract of children. There are very few reports in the breast, and one of the youngest was in a 23-year-old female (147).

DFSP–giant cell fibroblastoma is a well-documented neoplasm of the breast and is seen in young children (148,149).

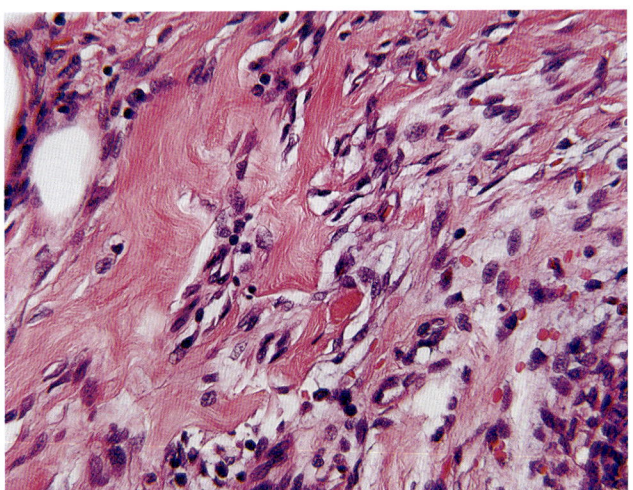

FIGURE 20-29 • PASH is present in a reduction mammoplasty for juvenile macromastia.

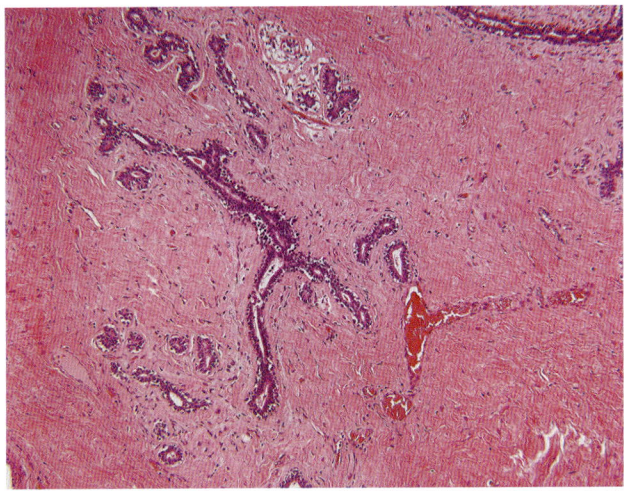

FIGURE 20-30 • Hamartoma of the breast in a 16-year-old female is a sometimes subtle lesion composed of well-circumscribed, somewhat enlarged lobules surrounded by stroma presenting as a mass.

The histologic features can be variable from those tumors with a predominant infiltrative pattern of uniform spindle cells in a myxoid background or a more collagenized stroma resembling a fibromatosis (Figure 20-31A, B) (148–150). GCF foci have a more fibrogenic appearance with scattered "smudged" giant cells (Figure 20-31C, D) (150).

Sarcomas

Primary sarcoma of the breast is rare in adults and even more so in children. Some cases may represent malignant PT with near total sarcomatous overgrowth. Angiosarcoma is one of the more common sarcomas arising in the breast, but among 15 cases of angiosarcoma in individuals 19 years old or less, two (13%) presented in the breast (151). Ewing sarcoma-primitive neuroectodermal tumor, and extraosseous osteosarcoma have been reported in the breast of young individuals (152,153).

Metastatic and Hematolymphoid Neoplasms

Even in adults, metastatic or secondary malignant tumors to the breast are very rare occurrences. Less than 1% of all of malignancies in the breast originated in extramammary sites in an adult series (154). Hematolymphoid neoplasms of various subtypes can account for 30% to 35% of secondary neoplasms in addition to melanoma and a broad array of carcinomas including neuroendocrine carcinoma in individual cases (155). With the exception of hematolymphoid malignancies, an entirely different group of neoplasms are seen in the breasts of children and adolescents.

RMS, especially the alveolar subtype, is seemingly the most common nonhematopoietic malignancy in childhood to metastasize to the breast and is seen in approximately 4% to 6% of cases (156). The breast is generally one of multiple sites of metastatic RMS. Primary alveolar RMS of the breast has been reported in a 13-year-old female (157). A biopsy shows the presence of a diffuse infiltrating high-grade and

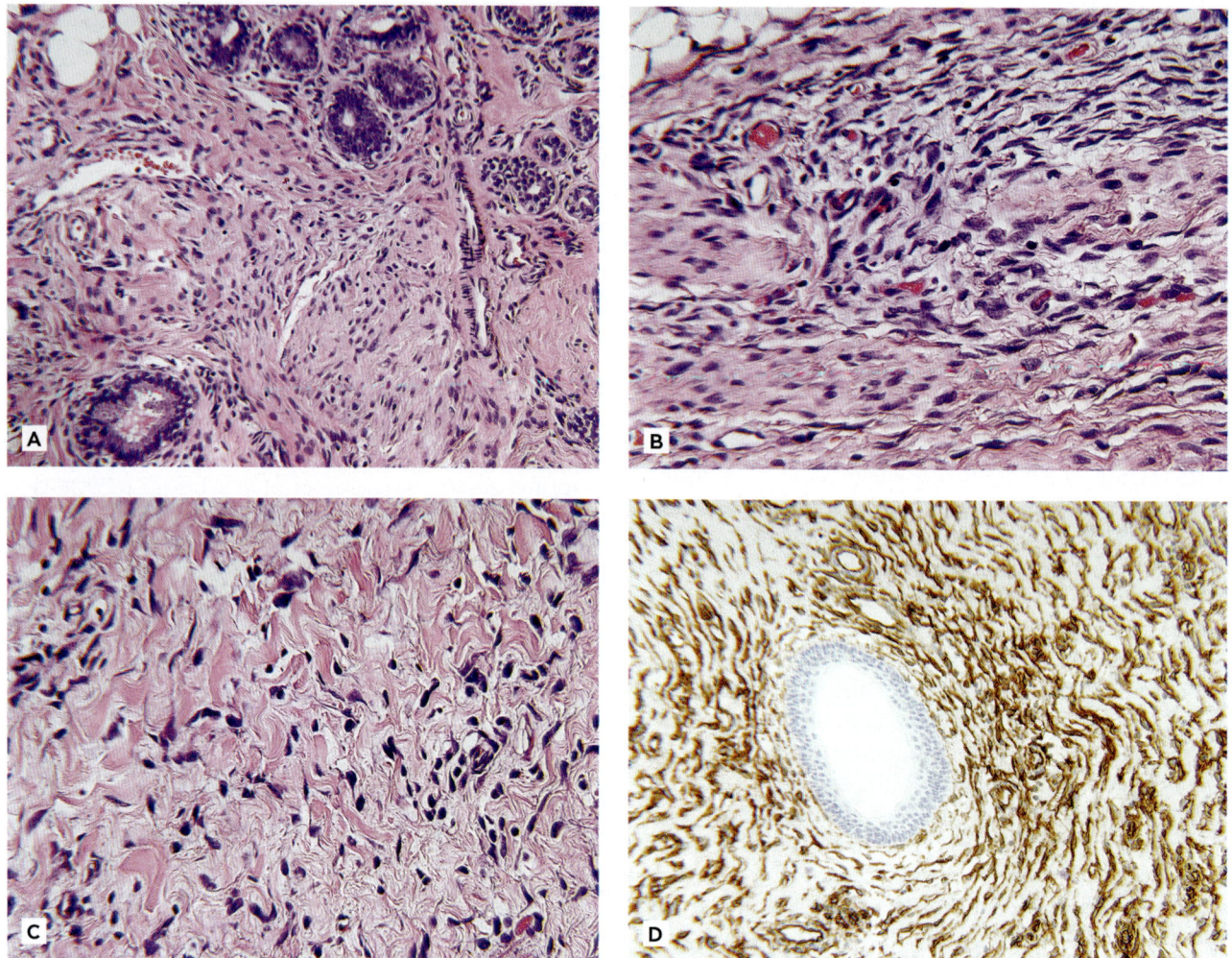

FIGURE 20-31 • **A:** Dermatofibrosarcoma protuberans presented in the right breast of a 1-year-old male. The spindle cell proliferation infiltrates and replaces the normal stroma. **B:** Uniform spindle cells are intermixed with more fibroblastic cells. **C:** A fibrogenic focus with a pseudoangiectoid appearance and "smudged" giant cells. **D:** CD34 immunopositivity in the spindle cells surrounding a small duct.

uniform round cell sarcoma with intensely hyperchromatic nuclei, frequent mitoses, and individually necrotic cells. The background of the tumor is devoid of a myxoid appearance, which is commonly present in the background of an embryonal RMS. Without a clinical history, the differential diagnosis is a broad one including several other round cell malignancies of childhood. Diffuse cytoplasmic staining for desmin and an equally diffuse nuclear positivity for myogenin establish the diagnosis of alveolar RMS.

Hematolymphoid malignancies rarely present in the breast of children and adolescents, and like alveolar RMS, most cases are examples of a relapse with disseminated sites of involvement (158,159). Most leukemias and lymphomas with involvement of the breast(s) in children and adults are B cell in lineage and in children specifically are pre-B acute lymphoblastic leukemia or Burkitt lymphoma, whereas in adults, diffuse large B-cell lymphoma and extranodal marginal lymphoma are seen more commonly (160). Anaplastic large cell lymphoma of T-cell lineage with breast involvement is the one exception to the predilection of B-cell lymphoid neoplasms (161,162). Acute myelocytic leukemia is more likely to present as a primary breast mass or as a site of relapse than the acute lymphocytic leukemia (163–165). It is important to include granulocytic sarcoma in the differential diagnosis of a malignant round cell neoplasm in a child without a prior history of a malignancy. In such cases, CD45, CD43, CD20, lysozyme, CD68, CD117, and myeloperoxidase should be performed with consistent positivity for CD45, CD43, lysozyme, CD68, and CD117 (165).

Metastatic and secondary neoplasms of the breast of children exclusive of RMS and hematolymphoid neoplasms include a number of case studies of individual cases: serous papillary carcinoma of ovary (166), Ewing sarcoma (167), neuroendocrine tumor of pancreas (168), osteosarcoma (169), and renal cell carcinoma (170).

Most children, who present with widely disseminated disease, and the breast as one of multiple sites of involvement, have either alveolar RMS or a hematopoietic neoplastic

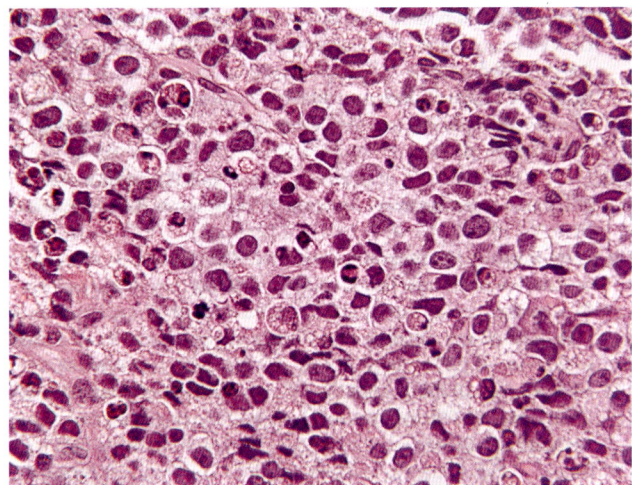

FIGURE 20-32 • Malignant round cell neoplasm in a 12-year-old female presented as multiple nodules in both breasts. This tumor was immunoreactive for cytokeratin and vimentin. Though designated as small cell carcinoma of ovary, these neoplasms are composed of large cells when compared to neuroblasts.

process. One exception in our experience was a 12-year-old female with the latter clinical presentation whose breast biopsy showed a malignant round cell neoplasm, which was a small cell carcinoma of the ovary (Figure 20-32). A similar case to ours was reported in a 14-year-old female (171)

References

1. Oftedal OT, Dhouailly D. Evo-devo of the mammary gland. *J Mammary Gland Biol Neoplasia* 2013;18:105–120.
2. Biggs LC, Mikkola ML. Early inductive events in ectodermal appendage morphogenesis. *Semin Cell Dev Biol* 2014;25–26:11–21.
3. Gabriel A, Maxwell G, Long JN, et al. The embryologic breast. http://www.emedicine.medscape.com/article/1275146-overview
4. Sakakura T, Suzuki Y, Shiurba R. Mammary stroma in development and carcinogenesis. *J Mammary Gland Biol Neoplasia* 2013;18:189–197.
5. Hassiotou F, Geddes D. Anatomy of the human mammary gland: current status of knowledge. *Clin Anat* 2013;26:29–48.
6. Macias H, Hinck L. Mammary gland development. *Wiley Interdiscip Rev Dev Biol* 2012;1:533–557.
7. Kleinberg DL, Barcellos-Hoff MH. The pivotal role of insulin-like growth factor 1 in normal mammary development. *Endocrinol Metab Clin North Am* 2011;40:461–471.
8. Iber D, Menshykau D. The control of branching morphogenesis. *Open Biol* 2013;3:130088.
9. Boras-Granic K, Hamel PA. Wnt-signalling in the embryonic mammary gland. *J Mammary Gland Biol Neoplasia* 2013;18:15–163.
10. Sternlicht MD. Key stages in mammary gland development: the cues that regulate ductal branching morphogenesis. *Breast Cancer Res* 2006;8:201.
11. Javed A, Lteif A. Development of the human breast. *Semin Plast Surg* 2013;27:5–12.
12. Yee D, Wood TL. The IGF system in mammary development and breast cancer. *J Mammary Gland Biol Neoplasia* 2008;13:351–352.
13. Anbazhagan R, Osin PP, Bartkova J, et al. The development of epithelial phenotypes in the human fetal and infant breast. *J Pathol* 1998;184:197–206.
14. Colvin CW, Abdullatif H. Anatomy of female puberty: the clinical relevance of developmental changes in the reproductive system. *Clin Anat* 2013;26:115–129.
15. Ellis H, Colborn GL, Skandalakis JE. Surgical embryology and anatomy of the breast and its related anatomic structures. *Surg Clin North Am* 1993;73:611–632.
16. Van Aalst JA, Phillips JD, Sadove AM. Pediatric chest wall and breast deformities. *Plast Reconstr Surg* 2009;124:39e–49e.
17. Merlob P. Congenital malformations and developmental changes of the breast: a neonatological view. *J Pediatr Endocrinol Metab* 2003;16:471–485.
18. Latham K, Fernandez S, Iteld L, et al. Pediatric breast deformity. *J Craniofac Surg* 2006;17:454–467.
19. Kulkarni D, Dixon JM. Congenital abnormalities of the breast. *Womens Health (Lond Elgl)* 2012;8:75–88.
20. Nso-Roca AP, Aquirre-Balsalobre FJ, Juste Ruiz M. Isolated unilateral amazia: an exceptional breast anomaly. *J Pediatr Adolesc Gynecol* 2012;25:e147–e148.
21. Caquette-Laberge L, Borsuk D. Congenital anomalies of the breast. *Semin Plast Surg* 2013;27:36–41.
22. Baban A, Torre M, Costanzo S, et al. Familial Poland anomaly revisited. *Am J Med Genet A* 2012;158A:140–149.
23. Papadimitriou A, Karapanou O, Papadopoulou A, et al. Congenital bilateral amazia associated with bilateral choanal atresia. *Am J Med Genet A* 2009;149A:1529–1531.
24. Marneros AG, Beck AE, Turner EH, et al. Mutations in KCTD1 cause scalp-ear-nipple syndrome. *Am J Hum Genet* 2013;92:621–626.
25. De Munnik SA, Otten BJ, Schoots J, et al. Meier-Gorlin syndrome: growth and secondary sexual development of a microcephalic primordial dwarfism disorder. *Am J Med Genet A* 2012;158A:2733–2742.
26. De Munnik SA, Bicknell LS, AFtimos S, et al. Meier-Gorlin syndrome genotype-phenotype studies: 35 individuals with pre-replication complex gene mutations and 10 without molecular diagnosis. *Eur J Hum Genet* 2012;20:598–606.
27. Dreifuss SE, Macisaac ZM, Grunwaldt LJ. Bilateral congenital amazia: a case report and systematic review of the literature. *J Plast Reconstr Aesthet Surg* 2014;67:27–33.
28. Ishida LH, Alves HR, Munhoz AM, et al. Athelia: case report and review of the literature. *Br J Plast Surg* 2005;58:833–837.
29. Guazzarotti L, Caprio C, Rinne TK, et al. Limb-mammary syndrome (LMS) associated with internal female genitalia dysgenesis: a new genotype/phenotype correlation? *Am J Med Genet A* 2008;146A:2001–2004.
30. Athanasoulia AP, Auer M, Riepe FG, et al. Rare missense P450c17 (CYP17A1) mutation in exon 1 as a cause of 46, XY disorder of sexual development: implications of breast tissue 'unresponsiveness' despite adequate estradiol substitution. *Sex Dev* 2013;7:212–215.
31. Lindfors PH, Voutilainen M, Mikkola ML. Ectodysplasin/NF-kB signaling in embryonic mammary gland development. *J Mammary Gland Biol Neoplasia* 2013;18:165–169.
32. Visinoni AF, Lisboa-Costa T, Pagnan NA, et al. Ectodermal dysplasias: clinical and molecular review. *Am J Med Genet A* 2009;149A:1980–2002.
33. Garcia-Martin P, Hernandez-Martin A, Torrelo A. Ectodermal dysplasias: a clinical and molecular review. *Actas Dermosifiliogr* 2013;104:451–470.
34. Sillesen NH, Holmich LR, Siersen HE, et al. Congenital symmastia revisited. *J Plast Reconstr Aesthet Surg* 2012;65:1607–1613.
35. Galli-Tsinopoulou A, Stergidou D. Polythelia: simple atavistic remnant or a suspicious clinical sign for investigation? *Pediatr Endocrinol Rev* 2014;11:290–297.
36. Ferrara P, Giorgio V, Vitelli O, et al. Polythelia: still a marker of urinary tract anomalies in children. *Scand J Urol Nephrol* 2009;43:47–50.
37. Cohen PR, Kurzrock R. Miscellaneous genodermatoses: Beckwith-Wiedemann syndrome, Birt-Hogg-Dube syndrome, familial atypical multiple mole melanoma syndrome, hereditary tylosis, incontinentia pigmenti, and super numerary nipples. *Dermatol Clin* 1995;13:211–229.
38. Galli-Tsinopoulou A, Krohn C, Schmidt H. Familial polythelia over three generations with polymastia in the youngest girl. *Eur J Pediatr* 2001;160:375–377.
39. Aydogan F, Baghaki S, Celik V, et al. Surgical treatment of axillary accessory breasts. *Am Surg* 2010;76:270–272.

137. Shehata BM, Fishman I, Collings MH, et al. Pseudoangiomatous stromal hyperplasia of the breast in pediatric patients: an underrecognized entity. *Pediatr Dev Pathol* 2009;12:450–454.
138. Baker M, Chen H, Latchaw L, et al. Pseudoangiomatous stromal hyperplasia of the breast in a 10-year-old girl. *J Pediatr Surg* 2011;46:e27–e31.
139. Stoinicu S, Moldovan C, Podoleanu C, et al. Mesenchymal tumor and tumor-like lesions of the breast: a contemporary approach review. *Ann Pathol* 2014;pii:210–217.
140. Singh KA, Lewis MM, Runge RL, et al. Pseudoangiomatous stromal hyperplasia. A case for bilateral mastectomy in a 12-year-old girl. *Breast J* 2007;13:603–606.
141. Virk RK, Khan A. Pseudoangiomatous stromal hyperplasia: an overview. *Arch Pathol Lab Med* 2010;134:1070–1074.
142. Magro G, Bisceglia M, Michal M, et al. Spindle cell lipoma-like tumor, solitary fibrous tumor and myofibroblastoma of the breast: a clinicopathological analysis of 13 cases in favor of a unifying histogenetic concept. *Virchows Arch* 2002;440:249–260.
143. Soyer T, Ayva S, Senyucel MF, et al. Myofibroblastoma of breast in a male infant. *Fetal Pediatr Pathol* 2012;31:164–168.
144. Magro G. Mammary myofibroblastoma: a tumor with a wide morphologic spectrum. *Arch Pathol Lab Med* 2008;132:1813–1820.
145. Chang HL, Lerwill MF, Goldstein AM. Breast hamartomas in adolescent females. *Breast J* 2009;15:515–520.
146. Daya D, Trus T, D'Souza TJ, et al. Hamartoma of the breast, an underrecognized breast lesion. A clinicopathologic and radiographic study of 25 cases. *Am J Clin Pathol* 1995;103:685–689.
147. Bosse K, Ott C, Biegner T, et al. 23-year-old-female with an inflammatory myofibroblastic tumour of the breast: a case report and a review of the literature. *Geburtshilfe Frauenheilkd* 2014;74:167–170.
148. Perry DA, Schultz LR, Dehner LP. Giant cell fibroblastoma with dermatofibrosarcoma protuberans-like transformation. *J Cutan Pathol* 1993;20:451–454.
149. Soto L, Jie T, Saltzman DA. Giant cell fibroblastoma of the breast in a child—a case report and review of the literature. *J Pediatr Surg* 2004;39:229–230.
150. Jha P, Moosavi C, Fanburg-Smith JC. Giant cell fibroblastoma: an update and addition of 86 new cases from the Armed Forces Institute of Pathology, in honor of Dr. Franz M Enzinger. *Ann Diagn Pathol* 2007;11:81–88.
151. Deyrup AT, Miettinen M, North PE, et al. Angiosarcomas arising in the viscera and soft tissue of children and young adults: a clinicopathologic study of 15 cases. *Am J Surg Pathol* 2009;33:264–269.
152. Majid N, Amrani M, Ghissassi I, et al. Bilateral Ewing sarcoma/primitive neuroectodermal tumor of the breast: a very rare entity and review of the literature. *Case Rep Oncol Med* 2013;2013:964568.
153. Zils K, Ebner F, Ott M, et al. Extraskeletal osteosarcoma of the breast in an adolescent girl. *J Pediatr Hematol Oncol* 2012;34:e261–e263.
154. Georgiannos SN, Chin J, Goode AW, et al. Secondary neoplasms of the breast: a survey of the 20th Century. *Cancer* 2001;92:2259–2266.
155. Vaughan A, Dietz JR, Moley JF, et al. Metastatic disease to the breast: the Washington University experience. *World J Surg Oncol* 2007;5:74.
156. D'Angelo P, Carli M, Ferrari A, et al. Breast metastases in children and adolescents with rhabdomyosarcoma: experience of the Italian Soft Tissue Sarcoma Committee. *Pediatr Blood Cancer* 2010;55:1306–1369.
157. Nogi H, Kobayashi T, Kawase K, et al. Primary rhabdomyosarcoma of the breast in a 13-year-old girl: report of a case. *Surg Today* 2007;37:38–42.
158. Aksu G, Inan N, Corapcioglu F, et al. Breast involvement in nodular lymphocyte predominant type Hodgkin lymphoma in childhood. *Pediatr Hematol Oncol* 2008;25:159–161.
159. Talwalkar SS, Miranda RN, Valbuena JR, et al. Lymphomas involving the breast: a study of 106 cases comparing localized and disseminated neoplasms. *Am J Surg Pathol* 2008;32:1299–1309.
160. Mandal S, Jain S, Khurana N. Breast lump as an initial manifestation in acute lymphoblastic leukemia: an unusual presentation. A case report. *Hematology* 2007;12:45–47.
161. Daneshbod Y, Oryan A, Khojasteh HN, et al. Primary ALK-positive anaplastic large cell lymphoma of the breast: a case report and review of the literature. *J Pediatr Hematol Oncol* 2010;32:e75–e78.
162. Gualco G, Bacchi CE. B-cell and T-cell lymphomas of the breast: clinical–pathological features of 53 cases. *Int J Surg Pathol* 2008;16:407–413.
163. Cunningham I. A clinical review of breast involvement in acute leukemia. *Leuk Lymphoma* 2006;47:2517–2526.
164. Monteleone PM, Steele DA, King AK, et al. Bilateral breast relapse in acute myelogenous leukemia. *J Pediatr Hematol Oncol* 2001;23:126–129.
165. Chen J, Yanuck RR III, Abbondanzo SL, et al. c-Kit (CD117) reactivity in extramedullary myeloid tumor/granulocytic sarcoma. *Arch Pathol Lab Med* 2001;125:1448–1452.
166. Kolwijck E, Boss EA, van Altena AM, et al. Stave IV epithelial ovarian carcinoma in an 18 year old patient presenting with a Sister Mary Joseph's nodule and metastasis in both breasts: a case report and review of the literature. *Gynecol Oncol* 2007;107:583–585.
167. Orguc S, Basara I, Pocan T, et al. Ewing's sarcoma metastasis into the breast. *Diagn Interv Radiol* 2012;18:167–170.
168. Judson K, Argani P. Intraductal spread by metastatic islet cell tumor (well-differentiated pancreatic endocrine neoplasm) involving the breast of a child, mimicking a primary mammary carcinoma. *Am J Surg Pathol* 2006;30:912–918.
169. Roebuck DJ, Sato JK, Fahmy J. Breast metastasis in osteosarcoma. *Australas Radiol* 1999;43:108–110.
170. Pursner M, Petchprapa C, Haller JO, et al. Renal carcinoma: bilateral breast metastases in a child. *Pediatr Radiol* 1997;27:242–243.
171. Cheng Z, Yin H, Du J, et al. Bilateral breast metastasis from small cell carcinoma of the ovary. *J Clin Oncol* 2008;26:5129–5130.

CHAPTER 21

The Pineal, Pituitary, Parathyroid, Thyroid, and Adrenal Glands

M. John Hicks, M.D., D.D.S., M.S., Ph.D., Nicole Cipriani, M.D., Peter Pytel, M.D., and Hiroyuki Shimada, M.D., Ph.D., F.R.C.P.A.

PINEAL GLAND

Anatomy and Physiology

The pineal gland is a small, cone-shaped midline structure that is attached to the superior–posterior border of the third ventricle. This 50- to 150-mg tan-brown structure sits just rostral to the quadrigeminal plate. It develops at approximately 7 weeks' gestation from an evagination of the ependymal lining covering the caudal portion of the roof of the third ventricle (1). Based on magnetic resonance (MR) imaging studies, the pineal gland increases in size from birth through 2 years of age, at which time it remains constant in size through adolescence. No size difference has been noted between male and female children. In children older than 2 years of age, the average pineal gland measures 6.5 × 4.8 × 4 mm. At approximately 5 years of age, calcifications, in the form of corpora arenacea, develop. These calcifications increase with age, giving the pineal gland a hyperdense appearance on computed tomography (CT) imaging starting around at puberty. Pineal calcifications are observed in 8% of children by age 10, 20% at puberty, and 40% by age 20.

Histologically, the pineal gland is composed of nests of cells in lobular profiles, with a resemblance to the "zellballens" of paraganglia, surrounded by connective tissue septa containing blood vessels and nerve fibers (2–4). The pinealocytes, or chief cells, have basophilic cytoplasm with large irregular nuclei and prominent nucleoli and are arranged in cords or follicles within the lobules. Randomly distributed throughout the pineal gland in perivascular areas and between pinealocytes are astrocytes as the second main cell population of the pineal gland. In the late third-trimester fetus and neonate, two populations of pineal parenchymal cells are identified with the small cell population disappearing with advancing age. The pinealocytes are immunoreactive for synaptophysin (SYN), chromogranin (CHR), and neurofilament protein (NFP), and the interstitial astrocytes are immunoreactive for S100 and glial fibrillary acidic protein (GFAP) (1).

In lower vertebrates, the pineal gland is located more superficially and directly photosensitive. In higher vertebrates, the pineal receives afferent connections from the retina (5). The major hormone produced by the pineal gland is the indoleamine, melatonin, which plays a role in circadian rhythm regulation and gonadal steroidogenesis. Other physiologic functions attributed to the pineal gland include a role in modulating the hypothalamic–pituitary–gonadal axis, hormonal rhythms, sleep cycle, and body temperature. Destruction of the pineal gland by a benign cyst or tumor has led to precocious puberty. Interference with the inhibitory effect of melatonin on gonadal steroidogenesis represents one mechanism. Melatonin levels have been reported elevated in some children with primary pineal tumors (6). Melatonin levels may be useful in determining the adequacy of pineal tumor resection when the level was increased before surgery. Other aspects of the anatomy and function of the pineal gland are discussed in more detail by Reiter (1).

Developmental Disorders

Pineal agenesis has been reported as a component of other midline central nervous system developmental syndromes with absence of the corpus callosum, such as in Aicardi syndrome (7). The contrasting abnormality, *pineal gland hyperplasia*, has been reported in children with genital enlargement (7).

Pineal cysts (glial cyst) are a relatively common radiologic finding on MR and an incidental finding in 25% to 40% of autopsies. There is a female predilection (eFigure 21-1) (2,4,6). On CT and MRI imaging, the content of pineal cysts exhibits similar properties as CSF. A pineal cyst larger than 1 cm in diameter may cause headache, vertigo, and visual disturbances (1). Symptomatic cysts have been treated by surgical excision (8,9). Possible mechanisms for pineal cyst development include persistence of the ependymal-lined pineal diverticulum, secondary cavitation within the pineal gland, or development secondary to prior hemorrhage in the gland (1). An ependymal lining accompanied by reactive-appearing astrocytes can be seen (eFigure 21-2). Typically cases show a wall that exhibits features of piloid gliosis. Approximately 5% of children with hereditary retinoblastomas have pineal cyst (10). Cyst formation is also seen in pineal neoplasms (6,11).

Acquired Disorders

Neoplasms of the pineal gland region account for 2% or less of all primary CNS tumors in children and are discussed in more detail by Burger and Scheithauer (2) and in Chapter 10. They may present with features including hydrocephalus from aqueductal obstruction, Parinaud syndrome, ataxia, or diplopia. Classically, there are three histogenetic categories: tumors of pineal parenchyma, gliomas, and germ-cell tumors (12). Overall gliomas account for about 17% of pineal neoplasms and include pilocytic astrocytomas, diffuse astrocytomas, and anaplastic astrocytomas (13). In children, they are proportionally less common than in adults. Germ-cell tumors account for about 27% of cases (eFigure 21-3) overall. They are typically said to be more common in East Asian populations, but one recent study did not confirm this finding (14,15). They include the same morphologic spectrum found in gonadal germ-cell tumors (eFigures 21-4 to 21-6) (16,17). A recent study found frequent mutations leading to KIT/RAS pathway activation (15). The mentioned calcifications that form with normal aging are typically not seen in children under age 10 to 12 years on CT imaging studies. In younger children, calcification can be a feature worrisome for a germ-cell tumor because pineal germ-cell neoplasms often appear on CT as solid masses with dense calcifications (eFigure 21-7A to C). On MR, the solid portion is isodense to brain on T1-weighted images and hyperintense to brain on T2-weighted images, while calcifications are hypointense on both pulse sequences.

Pineal parenchymal tumors (PPTs) also account for some 27% of pineal tumors (12). These include pineocytoma, pineoblastoma, and PPT of intermediate differentiation (2,18–20). Pineoblastomas, like germ-cell tumors, preferentially occur in the first decade of life in contrast to pineocytomas, which are seen in the second decade and into adulthood. In the pediatric population, almost 60% of PPTs are pineoblastomas (mean age, 2 to 3 years) and another 10% are pineocytomas (mean age 10 to 12 years) (16,21). The M:F gender ratio for pineoblastomas varies among series from 5:1 to 1:2 for children 16 years of age or younger (16,19). Pineal tumors may compress the tectum and aqueduct of Sylvius causing findings of hydrocephalus (eFigure 21-7). On imaging studies, pineocytomas are hypo- to isointense to brain on T1-weighted images and hyperintense to brain on T2-weighted images (eFigure 21-8). Pineoblastomas are variable in their MR appearance. They may be large and lobulated and have areas of necrosis (Figure 21-1A) causing a heterogeneous appearance. PPTs generally enhance markedly after intravenous gadolinium contrast administration. These tumors are assigned to the following grades: pineocytoma (WHO grade I), pineoblastoma (WHO grade IV), PPT of intermediate differentiation (WHO grade II or III) (18–21). Prognosis of PPTs is dependent on stage, tumor volume, histologic type, and NFP immunostaining (19,21). Pineocytoma has a favorable survival (85% to 90%, 5 years), whereas the 5-year survival in pineoblastoma is less than 25% (18,19,21). Among pineoblastomas, tumors with mutated *Rb1* gene are more aggressive with decreased survival when compared to sporadic pineoblastomas without *RB1* mutation.

Pineoblastoma is a high-grade primitive embryonal tumor akin to other central primitive neuroectodermal tumors (cPNET). Grossly, they are tan–gray, soft, infiltrative tumors that may exhibit hemorrhage, necrosis, and extension into the leptomeninges (2) (Figure 21-1B). Sheets of primitive round to slightly ovoid cells with irregular, hyperchromatic nuclei and scant cytoplasm are observed on histologic examination. Mitotic figures and apoptotic bodies are readily identified (Figure 21-1C, D, eFigures 21-9 and 21-10). Focal necrosis and Homer Wright rosettes are present in some cases, but pineocytomatous rosettes found in pineocytomas are lacking. Infrequently, photoreceptor differentiation is indicated by the presence of Flexner-Wintersteiner–like rosettes. Tumor cells are immunoreactive for SYN (Figure 21-1E, eFigure 21-11), to CHR and NFP to a lesser degree, and to retinal S antigen in about 50% of cases (2,22). Trilateral retinoblastoma syndrome is defined by the development of a pineoblastoma as a midline intracranial malignancy in the setting of hereditary retinoblastoma (2,10).

Pineocytoma, unlike pineoblastoma, has a lobular appearance like other examples of endocrine or neuroendocrine neoplasms, is well circumscribed, and displaces surrounding structures. The tumor cells are uniform with small central nuclei and conspicuous eosinophilic cytoplasm with an absence of pleomorphism, necrosis, and mitotic figures. Homer Wright and Flexner-Wintersteiner rosettes and large GFAP-positive fibrillary areas, referred to as pineocytomatous rosettes, are observed in these tumors (eFigures 21-12A, B and 21-13). Like pineoblastoma, tumor cells are immunoreactive for SYN, CHR, NFP, and neuron-specific enolase (NSE), in addition to retinal S antigen in approximately 30% of cases (eFigure 21-14) (22). Neurosecretory granules are identified ultrastructurally in contrast to their usual absence in pineoblastomas. PPT of intermediate differentiation shows histologic features of both pineoblastoma and pineocytoma. Some atypia and mitotic activity may be seen, but their prominence does not reach that seen in pineoblastomas.

Other rare tumors described in this location include papillary tumor of the pineal region (PPTR) (23), atypical teratoid/rhabdoid tumor (AT/RT) (24), pleomorphic xanthoastrocytoma (PXA) (25), Langerhans cell histiocytosis (LCH), lipoma, and meningioma. Pineal involvement with acute lymphocytic leukemia has been reported. Infections, vascular malformations, epidermoid cyst, hemorrhage, and apoplexy are nonneoplastic lesions of the pineal gland in children.

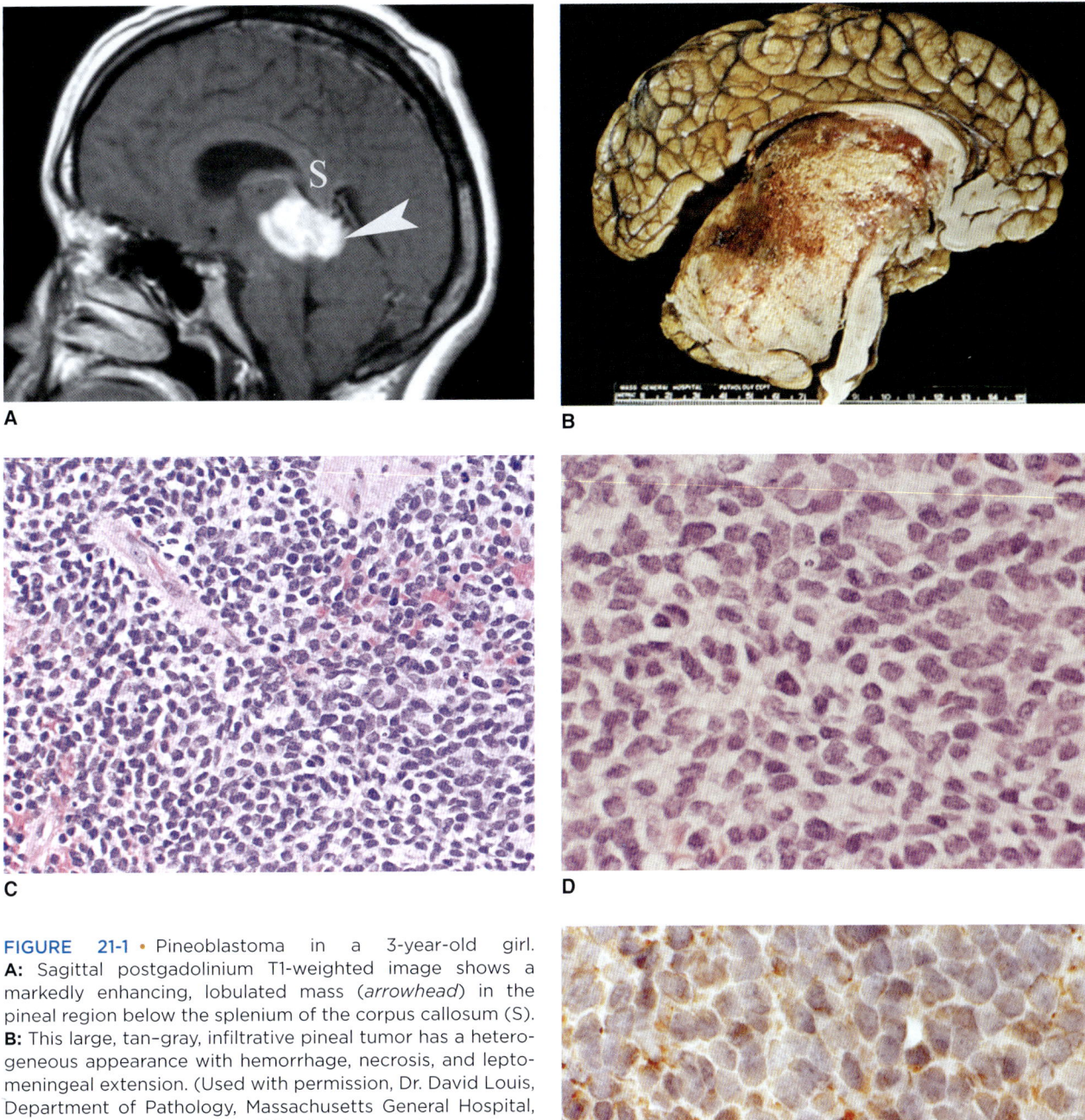

FIGURE 21-1 • Pineoblastoma in a 3-year-old girl. **A:** Sagittal postgadolinium T1-weighted image shows a markedly enhancing, lobulated mass (*arrowhead*) in the pineal region below the splenium of the corpus callosum (S). **B:** This large, tan–gray, infiltrative pineal tumor has a heterogeneous appearance with hemorrhage, necrosis, and leptomeningeal extension. (Used with permission, Dr. David Louis, Department of Pathology, Massachusetts General Hospital, Boston, Massachusetts.) **C:** This pineal tumor is composed of sheets of primitive round to slightly ovoid cells (H&E stain, original magnification 200×). (Courtesy of Dr. Joe Parisi, Mayo Clinic, Rochester, Minnesota.) **D:** The tumor cells have irregular, hyperchromatic nuclei and scant cytoplasm. Mitotic figures were also present (H&E stain, original magnification 400×). (Courtesy of Dr. Joe Parisi, Mayo Clinic, Rochester, Minnesota.) **E:** The tumor cells demonstrate immunoreactivity with SYN (immunostain for SYN, original magnification 400×). (Courtesy of Dr. Joe Parisi, Mayo Clinic, Rochester, Minnesota.)

PITUITARY GLAND

Anatomy and Physiology

The pituitary regulates key physiologic processes including growth, metabolism, reproduction, and homeostasis. The pituitary gland extends by a narrow stalk from the hypothalamus into the sella turcica within the sphenoid bone (26–28). The pituitary gland is a small ovoid structure that is divided into a red–brown anterior lobe (adenohypophysis), a gray–white posterior lobe (neurohypophysis), and an indistinct intermediate lobe. The pituitary gland weighs approximately 100 mg at birth and increases in weight during adolescence to its adult weight of 500 to 600 mg. The adenohypophysis accounts for 80% of the gland (26,27). The neonatal pituitary gland is especially prominent, owing to its stimulation by maternal hormones, but it undergoes some involution in the postnatal period, followed by increased growth through the age of 3 years. A notable increase in the size of the gland occurs with menarche and pregnancy. Generally, the pituitary gland in women after puberty weighs more than the gland in men. Suprasellar extension of the pituitary gland during puberty has been reported as a normal variant.

The pituitary gland receives its vascular supply from two hypophyseal arteries that branch from the internal carotid arteries and give rise to two anastomosing networks of capillaries that surround the stalk and adenohypophysis. The hypophyseal portal circulation, which arises from the second capillary plexus, supplies the adenohypophysis (26,27). A thin diaphragm, arising from the dura, covers the opening to the sella turcica, but in the center of the diaphragm, the pituitary stalk passes through an aperture. The pituitary gland is not covered by meninges. The periosteal dura lines the sella turcica.

The adenohypophysis is composed of three cell types on histologic examination: the chromophobes, acidophils, and basophils, accounting for 50%, 40%, and 10% of adenohypophyseal cells, respectively (eFigure 21-15). Five main hormonally active cell types are identifiable in the adult gland, which express six different hormones. The cell types and their respective hormones are the somatotrophs (growth hormone), lactotrophs (prolactin), corticotrophs (ACTH), gonadotrophs (FSH/LH), and thyrotrophs (TSH), accounting for 40% to 50%, 10% to 30%, 10% to 20%, 5% to 10%, and 5% of the adenohypophyseal cells, respectively (27,28). Stimulating and inhibitory hypothalamic factors released into the hypophyseal–portal circulation regulate the release of these hormones from the adenohypophysis (eFigure 21-16).

The folliculostellate cells are agranular; immunostain for S100, GFAP, and vimentin (VIM); and extend between the other adenohypophyseal cells. These cells are thought to have a paracrine regulatory function on the hormone-producing cells (27). Calcified concretions are an incidental finding in the anterior pituitary of ostensibly normal fetuses and neonates.

The posterior pituitary (neurohypophysis) contains the axonal processes of neurosecretory neurons that originate in the supraoptic and paraventricular nuclei of the hypothalamus to secrete vasopressin and oxytocin, respectively. Vasopressin and oxytocin are stored in secretory granules (Herring bodies) in the nerve endings (27). The intermediate lobe contains melanotrophs. These produce proopiomelanocortin (POMC), a precursor for endorphins as well as melanocyte-stimulating factor (MSH).

The development of the pituitary is complex and depends on a series of signals that are expressed in distinct spatial and temporal patterns. Defects in these signals can lead to developmental defects as outlined below. The anterior and intermediate lobes develop from oral ectoderm, while the posterior lobe arises from neuroectoderm through an evagination of tissue from the base of the developing diencephalon. During the 4th week of gestation, an outpouching of ectoderm from the roof of the stomatodeum (primitive oral cavity) grows dorsally toward the diencephalon as Rathke pouch. Along this route of migration, progenitor cells of the future adenohypophysis may lag behind as potential sources of ectopic anterior pituitary. Constriction and disappearance of Rathke pouch during the 5th to 6th gestational week separate the adenohypophysis from the stomatodeum. Concurrently, the elongating Rathke pouch passes between the developing presphenoid and basisphenoid bones of the skull and joins with the infundibulum, a diverticulum arising from the diencephalon, as the future neurohypophysis. The first vestiges of the hypothalamic–hypophyseal portal circulation are seen at 7 weeks' gestation, with the process being complete at 18 to 20 weeks' gestation.

Somatotrophs and corticotrophs are identified immunohistochemically in the adenohypophysis between the 5th and 12th gestational week. By 12 to 13 weeks' gestation, thyrotrophs and gonadotrophs are seen. At 13 to 16 weeks' gestation, lactotrophs first appear. During the sixth gestational month, innervation of the neurohypophysis with axonal processes from the supraoptic and paraventricular nuclei takes place.

The differentiation of the oral ectoderm into the terminal anterior pituitary cell types with expression of hormones and receptors is under the control of a large complement of genes and transcription factors (eFigure 21-17). Several excellent reviews discuss the role of these factors in pituitary organogenesis in more detail (29–32). The physiology of the different cell types, their specific hormones, and mechanisms of action of these hormones are beyond the scope of this chapter, but is detailed by others (26,27,30,32,33).

Imaging

Due to its small size and location within the bony sella, the pituitary is best evaluated with dedicated MR imaging. The adenohypophysis is isointense to gray matter and has a flat superior margin until puberty, when the margin becomes slightly convex, especially in females. The neurohypophysis is hyperintense compared to brain on T1-weighted images, producing the posterior pituitary "bright spot." The pituitary stalk (infundibulum) is normally midline and no larger than the basilar artery on axial images. Developmental lesions may be detected on imaging. Posterior pituitary ectopia is seen as an abnormal location of the posterior pituitary as a bright spot along the infundibulum or near the infundibular recess of the third ventricle (eFigure 21-18). Rathke cleft cysts are well circumscribed, round or lobulated, and isodense to CSF on CT. The signal intensity of the cyst content is variable on MR, depending on the protein content of the fluid. The cyst contents are generally isointense to slightly hyperintense to CSF on T1-weighted images and isointense to slightly hypointense to CSF on T2-weighted images (eFigure 21-19).

Inflammatory or infiltrative disorders are optimally demonstrated on MR images. Lymphocytic and granulomatous hypophysitis and LCH appear similar on imaging studies. With these conditions, the hypothalamus and infundibulum appear enlarged, with usually uniform enhancement following intravenous administration of gadolinium (eFigures 21-20 to 21-23). Primary pituitary tumors are best evaluated by MRI studies with and without contrast. Microadenomas do not distort the gland, but are hypointense to the normal gland on T1-weighted images and enhance less than the normal gland on early dynamic postgadolinium imaging (eFigure 21-24). Macroadenomas distort the gland and the infundibulum and enhance uniformly and intensely.

Developmental Disorders

Anomalies in pituitary gland development are outlined in Table 21-1 (34). Agenesis, complete absence, of the pituitary gland is rare as an isolated finding. Isolated agenesis of the pituitary has been noted in infants of diabetic mothers, as a presumed form of diabetic embryopathy. Pituitary dysfunction in neural tube defects is well documented. Agenesis can be associated with other midline and craniofacial abnormalities (27). In most cases of human holoprosencephaly, a hypoplastic gland can still be found in contrast to findings in animal studies (35). In the presence of pituitary agenesis, the thyroid gland, the adrenal glands, and gonads are expectedly diminutive. The posterior pituitary or neurohypophysis may be present.

Hypopituitarism, defined as diminution or absence of one or more anterior pituitary hormones, is estimated to occur in 1:4,000 to 10,000 live births. In general, isolated hormone deficiencies and combined pituitary hormone deficiencies (CPHDs) can be distinguished. Hypopituitarism can be the result of developmental defects or a rare secondary effect of traumatic brain injury, treatment for childhood cancer, or meningitis (5,36–38). Hypopituitarism can also be the result of neoplastic and inflammatory processes discussed in detail below. The complex development of the pituitary with contribution of two separate embryonic tissues is guided by a number of cellular signals (Table 21-2). Disruption in signals that regulate the early steps of this development results in syndromic defects with variably associated CNS, eye, and peripheral manifestations. This is in contrast to defects in signals guiding later steps of development, differentiation, and function that may cause selective hormone deficiencies.

Early signals include *Lhx3*, *Lhx4*, and the sonic hedgehog (SHH) signaling pathway (Table 21-2). Mutations in *Lhx3* and *Lhx4* result in aplasia or hypoplasia of the anterior pituitary and the intermediate lobe as well as other manifestations. These may include a short rigid spine and hearing loss (*Lhx3*) or cerebellar abnormalities and Chiari malformation (*Lhx4*). Holoprosencephaly can be the result of many different mutations (Chapter 10—Nervous System). Disruption of SHH signaling is a common cause. Mutations in *GLI2*, a factor in the SHH pathway, have been shown to cause congenital hypopituitarism in isolation or in association with other craniofacial anomalies and polydactyly (39,40). The importance of *SHH* mutations as the cause of hypopituitarism in humans is less clear than it appears to be in animal studies (40).

Mutations in *HSEX1*, *SOX2*, and *SOX3* are linked to septo-optic dysplasia with pituitary hypoplasia, midline forebrain defects, and optic nerve hypoplasia. *OTX2* mutations can cause anophthalmia and pituitary defects (41). The transcription factors PROP1 and POU1F1 are expressed during pituitary development. Mutations in either of these result in CPHD. Some mutations disrupt isolated pituitary hormones. Isolated GH (growth hormone) deficiency has been linked to mutations in the *GH1* gene encoding growth hormone or the gene encoding the GHrH receptor, but also *SOX3* and *HESX1*. Congenital deficiency of ACTH has been linked to *TBX19* mutations. Kallmann syndrome results from *FEZH* mutations causing failure of GnRH neurons to develop (42).

Other syndromes with hypopituitarism include MELAS syndrome, Rieger syndrome, trisomy 18, trisomy 13, Pallister-Hall syndrome, neurofibromatosis, Fanconi anemia, and ataxia–telangiectasia.

Anencephaly is characterized by the presence of anterior pituitary tissue within the mass of cerebrovascular tissue (eFigure 21-25A, B). The presence of somatotrophs, lactotrophs, and gonadotrophs is demonstrated by immunohistochemistry. Corticotrophs and thyrotrophs present in the pituitary in the second trimester disappear owing to lack of hypothalamic stimulation during the third trimester. A distinct neurohypophysis is absent. The adrenal glands are hypoplastic at birth (eFigure 21-25C, D).

Ectopia of anterior pituitary type tissue is common and invariably an incidental finding typically in the roof of the nasopharynx or as a pharyngeal pituitary. Persistence of

TABLE 21-1 CONGENITAL AND DEVELOPMENTAL ANOMALIES OF THE PITUITARY GLAND

Agenesis
Hypoplasia
Ectopic pituitary
Duplication
Rathke cleft cysts
Pars intermedia cyst
Dermoid cyst
Empty sella syndrome
Hamartoma
Teratoma
Isolated growth hormone deficiency
Combined pituitary hormone deficiency (CPHD)
Cranial vault abnormalities involving sella turcica
    Transsphenoidal encephalocele
    Persistent craniopharyngeal canal

Modified from Parks JS, Felner EI. Hypopituitarism. In: Kliegman RM, Behrman RE, Jenson HB, Stanton BF, eds. *Nelson textbook of pediatrics*, 18th ed. Philadelphia, PA: Elsevier, 2007; Chapter 558.

TABLE 21-2	MANIFESTATIONS ASSOCIATED WITH MUTATIONS IN SELECTED GENES INVOLVED IN PITUITARY DEVELOPMENT	
Gene	Function	Manifestations
LHX3, LHX4	Development and maintenance of adenohypophysis	CPHD, IPHD, pituitary hypoplasia, ectopia of neurohypophysis, Arnold-Chiari I malformation, cerebellar abnormalities, short rigid spine, hearing loss
HESX1	Early development of pituitary gland	CPHD, IPHD, pituitary hypoplasia, ectopia of neurohypophysis, septo-optic dysplasia
SOX2		
SOX3		
POU1F1(PIT 1)	Differentiation of the somatotrophs, lactotrophs, and thyrotrophs	Growth hormone, prolactin and TSH deficiency
PROP 1	Differentiation of the somatotrophs, lactotrophs, thyrotrophs, and gonadotrophs	30%–50% of cases of familial CPHD
Tpit	Differentiation of corticotrophs	ACTH deficiency
Gli 2, Gli3		Holoprosencephaly and panhypopituitarism, Hall-Pallister syndrome
PTX2		Rieger syndrome

CPHD, combined pituitary hormone deficiency; IPHD, isolated pituitary hormone deficiency; ACTH, adrenocorticotropic hormone; TSH, thyroid-stimulating hormone.
Based on data from Lap-Yin Pang A, Martin MM, Martin ALA, et al. Molecular basis of diseases of the endocrine system. In: Coleman WB, Tsongalis GJ, eds. *Molecular Pathology: The Molecular Basis of Human Disease*. Amsterdam, The Netherlands: Elsevier, 2009:435–463.

Rathke pouch in the roof of the oronasopharynx, the source of the pharyngeal pituitary gland, has been reported in a number of conditions, including the anencephalic fetus, spina bifida, trisomy 18, and Meckel syndrome. Ectopia of the posterior pituitary has been associated with mutations in genes responsible for pituitary organogenesis (eFigure 21-18) (43). Ectopic pituitary adenomas (PAs) are documented in the suprasellar region, clivus, nasopharynx, and paranasal sinuses mainly in adults, but also in children.

Rathke cleft cysts may become symptomatic because of compression of intrasellar or suprasellar structures. Rare cases present with growth retardation in children (the so-called pituitary dwarfism) (eFigure 21-19) or central precocious puberty. Morphologically, these exhibit similar morphologic features as those found with colloid cysts: the cyst is filled with thickened mucoid secretions or dark fluid (eFigure 21-26) and lined by ciliated columnar or low cuboidal epithelium. Microscopic incidental cystic rests with similar morphologic features are a common incidental finding in the pars intermedia in 2% to 26% of autopsies. Other cystic lesions in the region of the pituitary include craniopharyngioma (CRP) and intrasellar arachnoid cyst. A distinguishing feature of the CRP is mixed cystic and solid areas with the palisading and squamoid-type epithelium (Figure 21-2A, B). Because CRP and Rathke cleft cyst have a shared histogenesis, ciliated columnar epithelium may be seen on occasion in a CRP. Abscess formation and hypophysitis are rare complications in Rathke cleft cysts.

Pituitary duplication is a rare disorder that is ascribed to a duplication of the prechordal plate and anterior aspect of the notochord. Two distinct pituitaries, each with its own stalk, are the typical presentation. This anomaly has been seen with partial twinning, median cleft facial syndrome, precocious puberty, and fetal exposure to meclizine (teratogenic effect). A midline hypothalamic mass of disorganized neurons is accompanied by other midline developmental anomalies, including a duplicated sella, cleft palate, hypertelorism, agenesis of corpus callosum, and vertebral anomalies. Nasopharyngeal teratomas have been reported in association with pituitary duplication in infancy.

Empty sella syndrome (ESS) is usually an incidental finding in young children in contrast to adults. The primary form of ESS results from a defect in the diaphragm covering the opening to the sella turcica, with arachnoid tissue extending through the diaphragmatic defect. Increased CSF pressure leads to enlargement of the sella turcica and compression of the pituitary gland along the floor of the sella turcica, giving the appearance of an empty sella turcica (eFigures 21-27 and 21-28). Pituitary infarction, pituitary atrophy from a tumor, other mass lesion, and prior hypophysectomy account for secondary ESS.

Acquired Disorders

Inflammatory and infiltrative disorders are known to involve the pituitary gland including infections, noninfectious inflammatory conditions, and infiltrative processes. Examples of these diseases are congenital syphilis, mycobacteriosis, lymphocytic–granulomatous hypophysitis, LCH, sarcoidosis (44), Wegener granulomatosis (45), iron overload, storage disorder, Rosai-Dorfman disease (RDD), and Hurler syndrome.

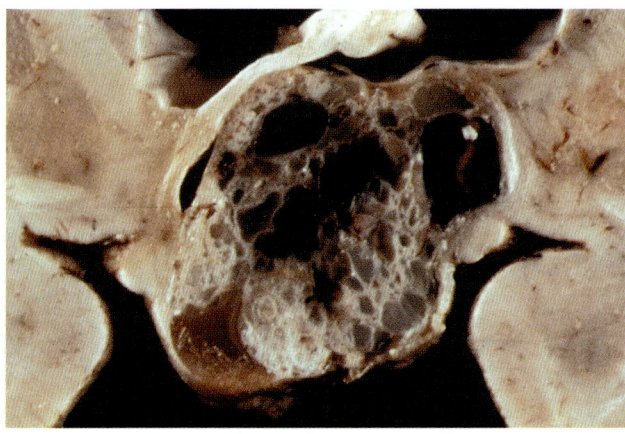 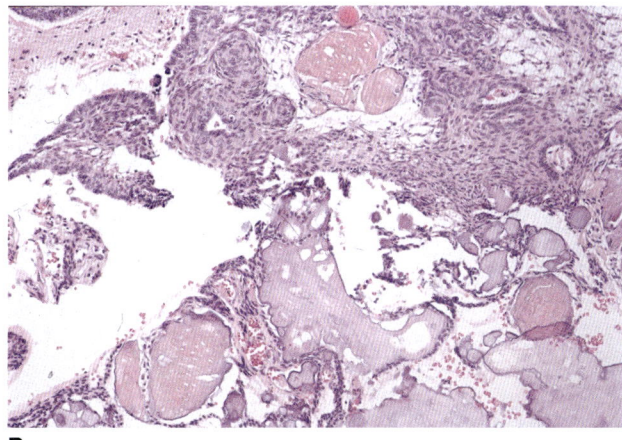

FIGURE 21-2 • Craniopharyngioma. **A:** This gross brain image shows a suprasellar cystic lesion filled with a dark brown fluid containing cholesterol debris. **B:** This adamantinomatous variant consists of ribbons of epithelial cells with pseudopalisaded nuclei at the periphery of the lobules surrounding cystic spaces. The inner cells in the more solid areas have a loose, stellate appearance. The so-called wet keratin is seen as intermixed stacks of necrobiotic squames. This image is from a 7-year-old girl, who presented with headaches and decreased visual acuity and was found to have a suprasellar mass (H&E stain).

Lymphocytic hypophysitis was first described as a disease of pregnant woman presenting with hypopituitarism. This condition is now recognized as occurring in other settings, including children as young as 9 years of age, but is generally uncommon in children. It is regarded as an autoimmune condition, because of its association with Hashimoto or chronic lymphocytic thyroiditis (CLT). The adenohypophysis (lymphocytic adenohypophysitis) and neurohypophysis (lymphocytic infundibuloneurohypophysitis) may be involved. In general, the designation of lymphocytic hypophysitis is used to describe both conditions. The pituitary is enlarged with a firm consistency and contains an inflammatory infiltrate of small lymphocytes intermixed with plasma cells (eFigure 21-29A to C). Eosinophils and some macrophages are also seen. Fibrosis is common, but may not be apparent in a small biopsy. Hypopituitarism, diabetes insipidus, and mass lesion symptoms are the usual clinical manifestations in both children and adults. Because the pituitary and sella are enlarged, a PA is often the clinical impression.

Granulomatous hypophysitis with epithelioid or caseous granulomas has the differential diagnosis of infection (tuberculosis), sarcoidosis, rupture of Rathke cleft cyst, LCH, and idiopathic granulomatous hypophysitis. Granulomas are not a feature of lymphocytic hypophysitis, although a nosologic and etiologic relationship may exist between these idiopathic inflammatory disorders.

Xanthogranulomatous inflammation (cholesterol granuloma) of the sellar region is an inflammatory reaction characterized by cholesterol clefts, lymphoplasmacytic infiltrates, hemosiderin deposits, fibrosis, foreign body giant cells, histiocytes, and eosinophilic necrotic debris. Although xanthogranulomatous inflammation may be associated with an adamantinomatous craniopharyngioma (CRP), this pattern has also been observed in idiopathic cases primarily in adolescents and young adults lacking a CRP component.

Vascular lesions with hypopituitarism are uncommon in children, but hemorrhagic infarction of a pituitary macroadenoma, referred to as pituitary apoplexy or pituitary tumor apoplexy, is one such example (Figure 21-3A, B) (46). Pediatric cases of pituitary apoplexy may be milder than in adults, having a more indolent course and associated with a more favorable outcome (47). Sheehan syndrome is the result of severe maternal intrapartum hypotension leading to pituitary infarction in the postpartum period. Presumed ischemia of the pituitary in sickle cell crisis is associated with decreased growth hormone secretion and impaired growth in affected children. Some cases of septo-optic dysplasia, classified as a developmental anomaly, are thought to represent a vascular disruption of the anterior cerebral artery. Vascular lesions due to stalk transection may occur secondary to trauma.

Nonneoplastic cysts identified in children on radiologic studies are not clinically evident unless the sella turcica is expanded, which leads to hypopituitarism and diabetes insipidus. Cystic dilatation of Rathke pouch remnants is common; however, these cysts are usually less than 5 mm in diameter (eFigures 21-19 and 21-26). Rathke cleft cysts arise from the squamous epithelium of the Rathke cleft and infrequently become enlarged with symptoms resembling a CRP. Arachnoid and dermoid cysts are also regarded by some as congenital defects. An intrasellar arachnoid cyst must also be distinguished from a CRP.

Pituitary hyperplasia is a nonneoplastic proliferation of one of the functional adenohypophyseal cell types. It is a polyclonal proliferation leading to pituitary enlargement and may produce a suprasellar mass. In children, somatotroph hyperplasia is reported in the McCune-Albright syndrome (MAS) and gigantism. Pituitary hyperplasia has also been reported in primary hypothyroidism. During pregnancy, the pituitary gland doubles in size due to the proliferation

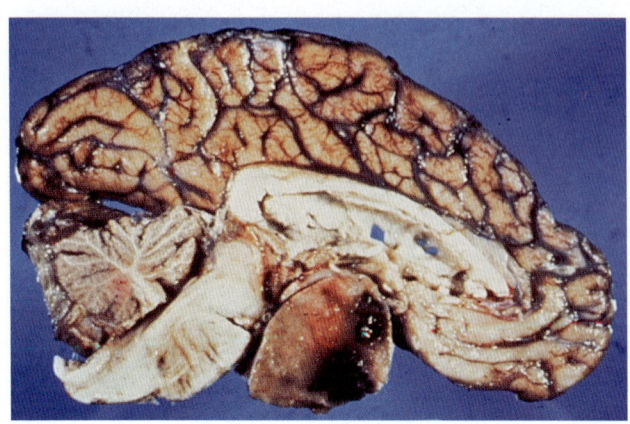 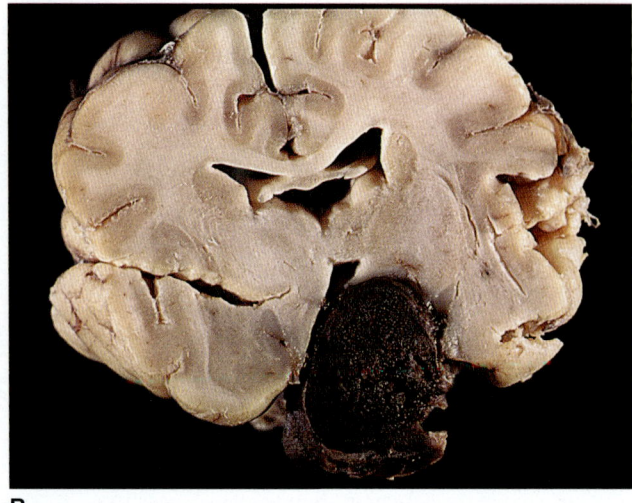

FIGURE 21-3 • Pituitary apoplexy. **A:** Sagittal section of brain showing hemorrhage within a pituitary macroadenoma. **B:** Coronal section showing hemorrhagic infarction of a 2-cm diameter well-circumscribed pituitary macroadenoma.

of the lactotrophs (responsible for prolactin secretion) and decreases in size postpartum (27).

Pituitary adenoma (PA) is a monoclonal neoplasm of the adenohypophysis. Up to 10% of all PAs present in the first two decades of life. Over 90% of these are diagnosed in the second decade, and less than 10% before 10 years of age. Between 15 and 19 years of age, PAs are the most common CNS tumor, being twice as common in girls as boys (26,46,48,49). Reports of adenomas occurring in children less than 4 years of age are uncommon. The youngest example of an ACTH-secreting PA occurred in a 7-month-old infant with Cushing disease. Most PAs are sporadic, but a number of cases are linked to familial mutations (Table 21-3). About 20% of PAs in the pediatric populations are the result of *AIP* mutations (50–52). Most of the AIP-associated PAs express growth hormone with or without prolactin. Other cases are linked to germline mutations in *MEN1, VHL, SDHB, SDHC, SDHD,* and *PRKAR1A* (Carney complex) (50,53,54,55). Cases with *SDH* subunit mutations typically exhibit prominent cytoplasmic vacuolation (55).

In terms of function, the majority of PAs in children are prolactinomas (53%). The remaining tumors are ACTH-secreting tumors (31%), growth hormone–secreting tumors (9%), and endocrine-inactive (null cell tumors) (3%) (48,56,57). ACTH-secreting adenomas are more common before puberty, in contrast to prolactinomas and growth hormone–secreting tumors, which are more common after puberty.

The clinical manifestations of PAs in children are variable. Headaches and visual field defects are the most common clinical manifestations of mass effect. Prolactinomas may result in amenorrhea and galactorrhea in girls and gynecomastia and hypogonadism in boys. Children with ACTH-secreting adenomas present with Cushing disease. Children with somatotropin or growth hormone–secreting adenomas present with gigantism.

Most prolactinomas, growth hormone–secreting tumors, and endocrine-inactive PAs are macroadenomas (>10-mm tumors in diameter) (Figure 21-4A, B). In contrast, ACTH-secreting adenomas are more often microadenomas (<10-mm tumor in diameter) (eFigures 21-30 and 21-31) (58). Macroadenomas are more common than microadenomas in children, consistent with the fact that prolactinomas are more common than ACTH-secreting tumors. PAs are classified on the basis of five-tiered features: endocrine activity, imaging studies and operative findings, histology, immunohistochemistry, and ultrastructure (59). PAs are soft and gray–red and measure less than or equal to 2 cm. On the basis of imaging criteria, four grades of tumors are recognized: grade I (<1 cm in diameter), grade II (intrasellar lesion >1 cm in diameter or with suprasellar expansion without invasion), grade III (small or large locally invasive tumor with bony invasion of the sella turcica), and grade IV (large invasive tumor involving the bone, hypothalamus, or cavernous sinus) (26). Larger aggressive tumors are more likely to be cystic, hemorrhagic, and necrotic (Figure 21-3A, B). One or more concurrent histologic patterns (diffuse, trabecular, papillary) may be evident. The degree of cellularity is variable from highly cellular to more scantily cellular tumors with hyalinized or amyloid-like stroma. The tinctorial quality of the cytoplasm has given rise to the characterization of PAs as basophilic, acidophilic, or chromophobic with some limitations. The tumor cells are generally rounded with some occasional spindling with the rounded central or eccentric nuclei. The tumor cells may have plasmacytoid qualities in the presence of an eccentric nucleus and prominent basophilic, acidophilic, or amphophilic cytoplasm. Prolactinomas are typically composed of chromophobes or slightly acidophilic cells with a solid or papillary pattern and hyalinized stroma with or without microcalcifications (Figure 21-4C, D, eFigure 21-32). PAs tend to lack a capsule (eFigure 21-30). Electron microscopy

TABLE 21-3 ENDOCRINE ORGANS INVOLVED IN SELECTED FAMILIAL TUMOR SYNDROMES

Syndrome	Inheritance	Gene	Pituitary	Parathyroid	Thyroid	Adrenal	Other Endocrine Organ Manifestations
Beckwith-Wiedemann	paternal uniparental disomy	CDKN1C/NSD1				ACN	Pancreatoblastoma, adrenal cytomegaly, neuroblastoma
Carney complex (LAMB and NAME syndromes)	AD	PRKAR1A	Adenoma		PTC	ACN	
Cowden	AD	PTEN			FTC/PTC		
Familial adenomatous polyposis coli	AR/AD	APC			PTC, cribriform-morula variant		
Gardner's syndrome							
Familial medullary thyroid carcinoma	AD	RET Exons 10 and 11 Codons 618, 620, 209, 611			MTC		
Familial paraganglioma-pheochromocytoma		SDHD (PLG1), SDHAF2 (PLG2), SDHC (PLG3), SDHB (PLG4)			Non-MTC in SDHB, SDHD	PHEO	Paraganglioma
Hyperparathyroidism–jaw tumor	AD	HRPT2		Adenoma/carcinoma			
Li-Fraumeni	AD	TP53, CHEK2				can	
McCune-Albright		GNAS	Adenoma		Hyperplasia	Hyperplasia/adenoma	
MEN 1 (Wermer syndrome)	AD	MEN1 (Menin, 11q13)	Adenoma	Adenoma/hyperplasia		ACN	Islet cell neoplasia
MEN 2A (Sipple syndrome)	AD	RET, Exons 10 and 11, Codons 609, 611, 618, 620, 634		Adenoma/hyperplasia	MTC	PHEO	Paraganglioma, enteric ganglia

(Continued)

TABLE 21-3 ENDOCRINE ORGANS INVOLVED IN SELECTED FAMILIAL TUMOR SYNDROMES (continued)

Syndrome	Inheritance	Gene	Pituitary	Parathyroid	Thyroid	Adrenal	Other Endocrine Organ Manifestations
MEN 2B (Wagenmann-Froboese syndrome	AD	RET Exon 16, Codon 918			MTC	PHEO	Mucosal neuromas, enteric ganglioneuromatosis
Neurofibromatosis type 1	AD	NF1				PHEO	Paraganglioma
Von Hippel-Lindau	AD	VHL1, VHL2A, VHL2B, VHL2C				PHEO	Islet cell neoplasia Paraganglioma
Peutz-Jeghers	AD	STK11/LKB1			Non-MTC		
Werner	AR	WRN			Non-MTC		
Papillary renal neoplasia		PTCPRN t(2;3;8)			PTC		
Familial papillary thyroid carcinoma with clear cell renal carcinoma					PTC		
Familial papillary carcinoma with or without oxyphilia		TCO			PTC		
Familial papillary thyroid carcinoma		NMTC1			PTC		
Familial multinodular goiter with papillary thyroid carcinoma		MNG1, MNG3			PTC		
Familial papillary thyroid carcinoma		PTC1			PTC		
Familial follicular thyroid carcinoma		NMCT1			PTC		

ACN, adrenocortical neoplasm; AD, autosomal dominant; FTC, follicular thyroid carcinoma; MTC, medullary thyroid carcinoma; non-MTC, nonmedullary thyroid carcinoma; PHEO, pheochromocytoma; PTC, papillary thyroid carcinoma.

Modified from Table 5.01. Eng C. Inherited tumor syndromes. Introduction. In: DeLellis RA, Lloyd RV, Heiz PU, eds. *World Health Organization Classification of Tumors: Pathology and Genetics. Tumors of Endocrine Organs.* Lyon, France: IARC, 2004:210.

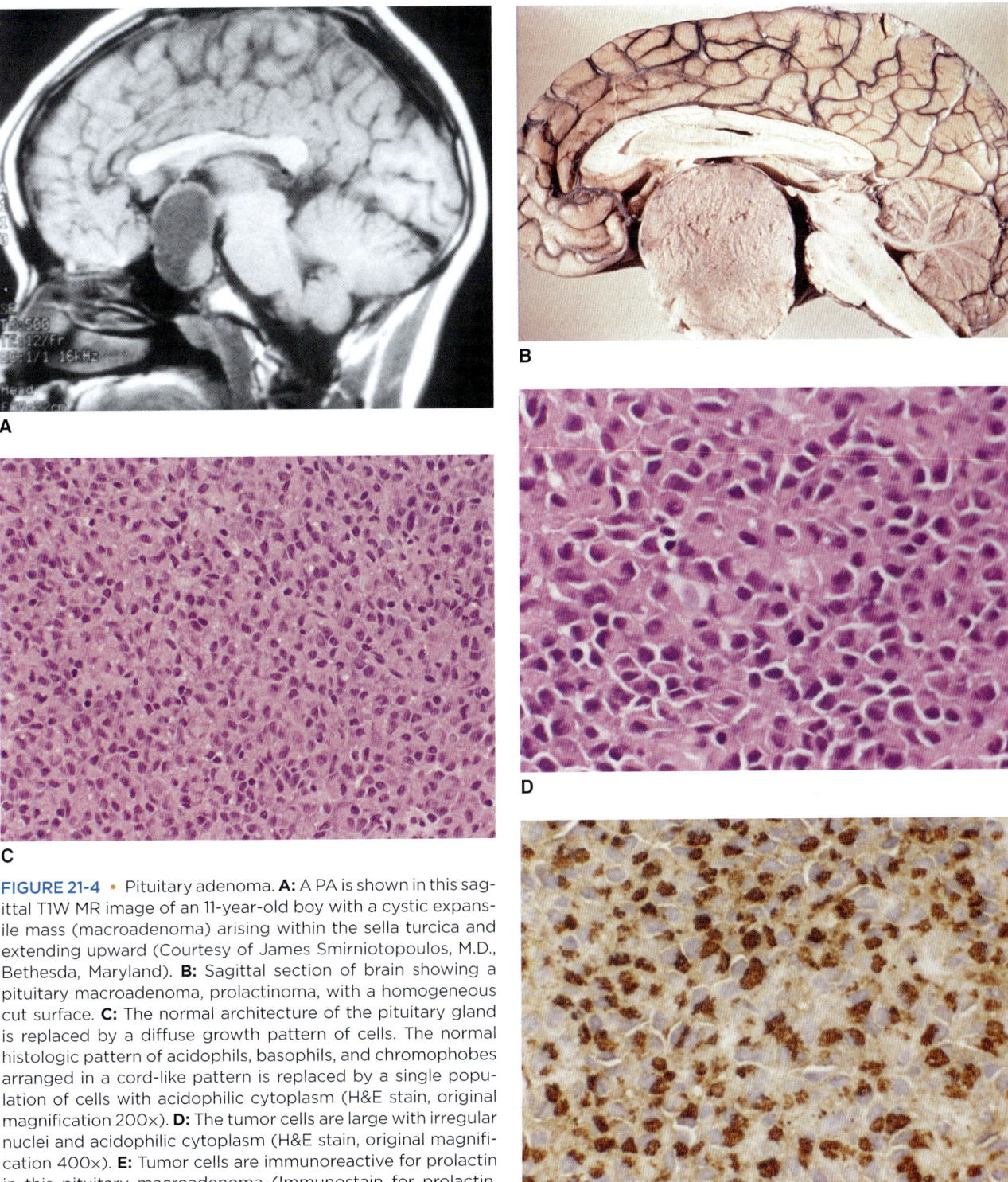

FIGURE 21-4 • Pituitary adenoma. **A:** A PA is shown in this sagittal T1W MR image of an 11-year-old boy with a cystic expansile mass (macroadenoma) arising within the sella turcica and extending upward (Courtesy of James Smirniotopoulos, M.D., Bethesda, Maryland). **B:** Sagittal section of brain showing a pituitary macroadenoma, prolactinoma, with a homogeneous cut surface. **C:** The normal architecture of the pituitary gland is replaced by a diffuse growth pattern of cells. The normal histologic pattern of acidophils, basophils, and chromophobes arranged in a cord-like pattern is replaced by a single population of cells with acidophilic cytoplasm (H&E stain, original magnification 200×). **D:** The tumor cells are large with irregular nuclei and acidophilic cytoplasm (H&E stain, original magnification 400×). **E:** Tumor cells are immunoreactive for prolactin in this pituitary macroadenoma (Immunostain for prolactin, original magnification 400×). (Images **C–E**, courtesy of Dr. Joe Parisi, Mayo Clinic, Rochester, Minnesota.)

and immunohistochemistry are adjuncts to characterize these tumors (Figure 21-4E, eFigure 21-33). In addition to specific hormonal immunostaining, PAs are positive for SYN, CHR, and NSE (30).

In terms of clinical behavior, macroadenomas are more likely to be invasive in contrast to the smaller expansile microadenomas. It is debatable whether PAs in children are more aggressive than their adult counterparts. Invasive adenomas are characterized by extension into dura, bone, and cavernous sinus. These features are generally not well documented in the pathologic examination. There is a certain degree of correlation between proliferative activity, as determined by MIB-1 (Ki67) nuclear immunostaining, and observed invasiveness of the tumor.

Pituitary blastoma is a rare pediatric lesion linked to germline mutations in *DICER1*, composed of various cell types, including primitive Rathke-type epithelium, and folliculostellate and secretory adenohypophyseal cells (60,61). *Pituicytoma* is a rare neoplasm arising from specialized glial cells, pituicytes, in the neurohypophysis, presenting as a low-grade spindle cell lesion with glial differentiation (62).

Craniopharyngiomas (CRPs) are thought to be derived from remnants of the Rathke pouch and account for 3% to 4% of primary CNS tumors in children (63). Generally, the tumor is found in the suprasellar region (Figure 21-2A, eFigures 21-34 to 21-36). Rare cases may be parasellar or ectopic in the pineal gland region. The differential diagnosis includes PA, infection, inflammatory processes, vascular malformations, and Rathke cleft cyst. Imaging is helpful in distinguishing among CRPs, PAs, and Rathke cleft cysts.

CRPs in children are most commonly diagnosed between 5 and 14 years of age with no gender predilection (63). Tumors occurring during infancy are uncommon. Compressive symptoms, including pituitary dysfunction with retarded growth, are the principal clinical manifestations (64). Diabetes insipidus due to posterior pituitary involvement is infrequent. A calcified cystic suprasellar mass is characteristic on CT and MR scans (eFigure 21-36). Surgical resection may be followed by a recurrence (2). The gross specimen consists of cyst fragments with a yellow to dark brown appearance. Fluid contents have a dark oily appearance (crankcase) with cholesterol crystals and fragments of keratinous debris. In children, the histologic features are typically adamantinomatous or ameloblastic. A papillary squamous pattern is seen more often in adults (26,29). Beta-catenin mutations are seen in the adamantinomatous pattern (26,29), while the papillary squamous pattern is linked to BRAF mutations (65). In adamantinomatous CRPs, epithelial lobules are arranged in a cloverleaf-like pattern. Palisading of the cells adjacent to the randomly distributed fluid-filled cyst-like spaces is a characteristic feature. Aggregates of necrotic, keratinized cells, or "wet" keratin accompanied by dystrophic calcification, are other features (Figure 21-2B, eFigure 21-37). Fibrosis, chronic inflammation, and cholesterol clefts are observed in the solid areas. A xanthogranulomatous reaction is prominent in some cases, especially with a ruptured cyst. Although CRPs are regarded as clinically benign, adherence to the hypothalamus and extension into the surrounding brain parenchyma occur in some cases. Cytokeratin expression has been used to distinguish CRP from Rathke cleft cyst. An uncommon CRP variant is one with adamantinomatous features together with elements of a PA, a so-called collision tumor. In many of these "collision tumors," the adenoma is nonfunctional; however, immunohistochemistry displays gonadotropin, prolactin, ACTH, and TSH staining.

Other tumefactive lesions of the pituitary and sellar region include the ganglion cell tumor (so-called gangliocytoma), LCH, granular cell tumor, RDD, and salivary gland hamartoma. Gangliocytomas are regarded as neoplasm by most observers, but hamartoma by others. These may be found in association with PAs, pituitary hyperplasia, or as a distinct mass. These lesions have been classified as either mixed adenoma–gangliocytoma or pure gangliocytoma.

In addition to PA and CRP, the midline region of the sella and suprasellar area is another common anatomic site besides the pineal region for intracranial germ-cell tumors. 60% to 70% of all primary intracranial germ-cell tumors arise in the pineal region and 30% to 40% in the sellar or suprasellar area. Cases associated with prominent inflammatory infiltrates may be mistaken for an inflammatory disease process if the neoplastic cells are not appreciated. Visual field defects, diabetes insipidus, and panhypopituitarism are the principal clinical manifestations of suprasellar germ-cell tumors.

Langerhans cell histiocytosis (LCH) is well documented in the CNS with involvement of brain parenchyma and/or the hypothalamic–pituitary axis, causing central diabetes insipidus (66). The pituitary stalk is thickened on imaging studies (eFigures 21-21 to 21-23). Almost 15% of those with multisystem LCH have hypothalamic–pituitary involvement. There is limited documentation of the pathology in such cases because the diagnosis is usually established on the basis of a biopsy from a more accessible site. A mixture of Langerhans cell histiocytes, characterized by large, convoluted, and indented nuclei, that are CD207 (langerin, more specific) and CD1a (less specific) positive, mixed with lymphocytes, plasma cells, and eosinophils, is diagnostic for LCH (Figure 21-5A, B, eFigure 21-38A to C).

RDD has craniospinal manifestations in a minority of cases, including the sellar–suprasellar region. In 50% of cases, RDD is limited to this site.

Salivary gland rest or heterotopia is an incidental microscopic finding on the surface of the posterior pituitary. Other neoplasms of presumed salivary gland type, granular cell tumor of the pituitary and pituitary stalk, leukemia, lymphoma, and metastatic involvement of the pituitary are restricted to adults in most cases. Both primary and metastatic germ-cell neoplasms also occur in the pituitary.

PARATHYROID GLANDS

Anatomy/Physiology

The parathyroid glands, usually four in number, are pink–red, oval 4 to 6 mm in diameter glands located in proximity (usually posterior) to the thyroid gland or even embedded within the thyroid (intrathyroidal). The inferior and superior parathyroid glands arise as endodermal outpouchings from the dorsal bulbar portion of the third and fourth pharyngeal pouches, respectively, during the fifth gestational week in the 8- to 9-mm-stage embryo as bilateral cellular clusters. Concurrently, the thymus arises from the ventral aspect of the third pharyngeal pouches. Both the thymus and inferior parathyroid glands initially migrate together caudally with the heart. During the descent, the thymus and inferior

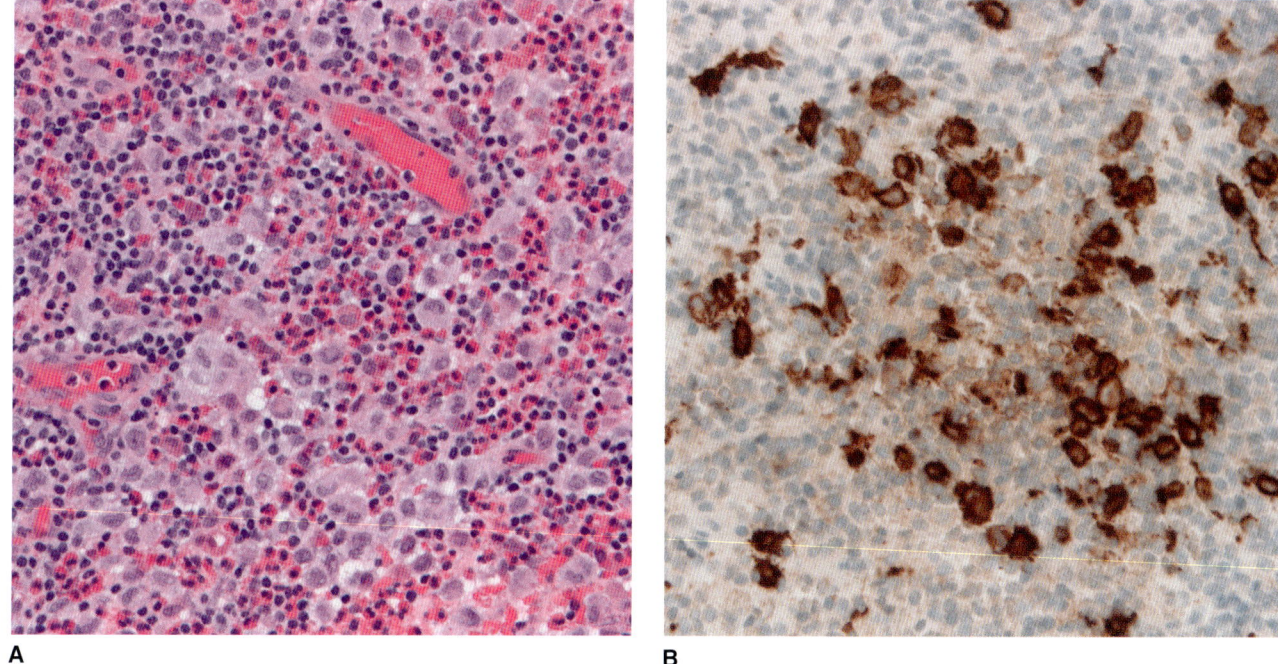

FIGURE 21-5 • Langerhans cell histiocytosis. **A:** Biopsy from the pituitary stalk in an adolescent with diabetes insipidus. The infiltrate is composed of foamy histiocytes that were immunoreactive with CD1a, in a background of lymphocytes, eosinophils, and plasma cells (H&E stain, original magnification, 400×). (Courtesy of Dr. Joe Parisi, Mayo Clinic, Rochester, Minnesota.) **B:** CD1a positivity in histiocytic cells in a patient with LCH (immunostain for CD1a, original magnification 400×). (Courtesy of Dr. Joe Parisi, Mayo Clinic, Rochester, Minnesota.)

parathyroid glands separate and the inferior parathyroid glands localize to the inferior aspect of the thyroid gland. Formation of the parathyroid glands is associated with the genes EOLVO and GCM2 on chromosome 6 (6p24.2). Other genes associated with parathyroid development and migration include HOX3a (12q13), PAX1 (7q36), EYA1 (8q13.3, branchiootorenal syndrome 1), SIX1 (14q23, branchiootorenal syndrome), and TBX1 (22q11.2, DiGeorge syndrome). Dysregulation or mutation in these genes results in absence, hypoplasia, or ectopic parathyroid glands.

In children, the combined weight for all four parathyroid glands increases with age from a mean weight of 5 to 10 mg each in the neonatal period to a combined weight of 120 mg for adult males and 140 mg for adult females by age 30 years. In children less than 10 years of age, the mean weight of all four glands is less than 60 mg. Between the ages of 11 and 20 years, the mean weight of all four glands has been recorded as less than 100 mg. A more recent study of parathyroid gland weight in children 9 to 19 years of age indicated individual gland weights can range between 10 and 80 mg.

The parathyroid glands in children tend to be solid and cellular with minimal fat. A connective tissue capsule encloses the gland. Chief cells are the predominant cell type. Blood vessels are intermixed among the parenchymal cells, and small delicate capillaries are present between the cells. The polyhedral chief cells have a small central nucleus and pale to clear cytoplasm. Oxyphil (oncocytic) cells are not observed generally until puberty, if at all. Adipocytes within the gland initially appear around puberty with fatty change gradually accounting for 25% to 30% of the total gland weight after age 18 years (67).

Calcium homeostasis is regulated by the interaction of parathyroid hormone (PTH), calcitonin, and vitamin D (eFigure 21-39) (68,69). In response to hypocalcemia, PTH is released from the chief cells, which is accompanied by an increase in PTH mRNA within hours of the onset of hypocalcemia. Hyperplasia of chief cells occurs within weeks. In contrast, hypercalcemia inhibits the release of PTH by activation of the chief cell calcium receptor (Table 21-4). Serum phosphate levels, independent of vitamin D_3, also affect PTH release (68,69). The anatomy and physiology of the parathyroid glands is discussed in more detail elsewhere (70).

Imaging

The parathyroid glands are small and difficult to appreciate on imaging studies when not enlarged. Patients with hyperparathyroidism (HPT) are best evaluated with ultrasonography (US) and/or radionuclide scintigraphy. In children, high-resolution US should be the first-line imaging modality. Enlarged parathyroid glands in the neck are typically identified posterior to the thyroid gland. As parathyroid glands are best identified based on proximity to the thyroid gland, ectopic glands pose a diagnostic challenge. Radionuclide scintigraphy is more accurate than US (87% versus 80%), particularly for ectopic glands. The combination of nuclear

TABLE 21-4	PRIMARY HYPERPARATHYROIDISM ETIOLOGY IN CHILDHOOD

Parathyroid adenoma
   Sporadic (nonsyndromic)
   HPT–jaw tumor syndrome
Parathyroid hyperplasia
   Sporadic (nonsyndromic)
   Neonatal HPT
Familial isolated HPT
   MEN1
   MEN2a
Parathyroid carcinoma

Differential Diagnosis of Hypercalcemia in Children

Elevated parathyroid hormone
   Hyperparathyroidism, primary, secondary, or tertiary
      Parathyroid hyperplasia
      Parathyroid adenoma
      Parathyroid carcinoma
   Ectopic parathyroid hormone production
Hypervitaminosis D
Sarcoidosis
Subcutaneous fat necrosis of newborn
Familial hypocalciuric hypercalcemia
Idiopathic hypercalcemia (Williams syndrome)
Thyrotoxicosis
Hypervitaminosis A
Hypophosphatasia
Prolonged immobilization
Thiazide diuretics

MEN, multiple endocrine neoplasia.
Based on data from DeLellis RA, Mazzaglia P, Mangray S. Primary hyperparathyroidism: a current perspective. *Arch Pathol Lab Med* 2008;132:1251–1262.

scintigraphic studies and US provides the highest accuracy for preoperative localization of hyperfunctioning glands.

Nuclear medicine studies utilize ^{99m}Tc sestamibi, which localizes to hyperfunctioning parathyroid glands, as well as the thyroid gland and salivary glands. Sestamibi scans can be performed in several ways. In dual-isotope single-phase imaging, the patient is administered and labeled with sestamibi and ^{123}I and ^{99m}Tc pertechnetate, which are taken up by the thyroid gland. The images are subtracted to show the activity only in the hyperfunctioning parathyroid glands (eFigure 21-40). Alternatively, a single-isotope dual-phase technique may be employed. Sestamibi washes out of the thyroid and salivary glands faster than the parathyroid glands, so delayed images show relatively greater uptake in the hyperfunctioning parathyroid gland. Single-photon emission computed tomography (SPECT) imaging in addition to planar imaging helps to localize the abnormality in the anterior–posterior plane. Fusion of SPECT imaging to x-ray–based CT adds additional anatomic information that aids in precise localization of the parathyroid gland, which may be particularly useful in tumor recurrence after surgery.

Parathyroid adenomas may also be demonstrated on CT and MR, but the accuracy of these studies for preoperative localization is no greater than for US. Parathyroid adenomas may be present at the typical gland location or located anywhere from the mandible to cervical thymus to mediastinal thymus or within the substance of the thyroid gland (intrathyroidal). On CT, adenomas are usually well defined and enhance intensely following intravenous contrast administration (eFigure 21-41). On MR, adenomas are generally of intermediate signal on T1-weighted images and of high signal intensity on T2-weighted images and enhance intensely following intravenous administration of gadolinium chelate (Figure 21-6A). Prior to the advent of laboratory screening, patients with undiagnosed, prolonged HPT developed characteristic findings on bone radiographs as well as nephrocalcinosis and nephrolithiasis. These findings are now rarely encountered (eFigures 21-42 and 21-43).

Developmental Disorders

Supernumerary parathyroid glands are found in up to 16% of the population, with an additional single gland being the most common presentation. Supernumerary glands, with as many as 12 glands, may be of normal size or rudimentary. Parathyroid adenomas and carcinoma have been reported in ectopic parathyroid glands in children (eFigure 21-41) (71).

Ectopic parathyroid tissue or a normally formed gland is relatively common within the thyroid or thymus. Ectopic parathyroid tissue has also been observed as scattered small nests in the soft tissues of the neck and mediastinum owing to aberrant migration or premature separation of parathyroid primordia during fetal development. Not surprisingly, nests of parathyroid tissue may be accompanied by equally diminutive nests of thymic tissue. Aberrant parathyroid and thymus are known to present as a recurrent lateral neck mass in children. Heterotopic parathyroid tissue has also been observed at remote sites, including the vagina.

Agenesis–hypoplasia of the parathyroids, due to a defect in pharyngeal pouch development or defective neural crest migration, is uncommon as an isolated finding with associated congenital hypoparathyroidism. Agenesis–aplasia is more frequently associated with other syndromes, including 22q11.2 deletion syndrome (DiGeorge anomaly, DiGeorge syndrome), Smith-Lemli-Opitz syndrome type II, X-linked recessive hypoparathyroidism, Kenny syndrome, Kearns-Sayre syndrome, and trisomy 18. The parathyroid glands may be absent in up to 50% of patients with 22q11.2 deletion syndrome. Anomalies of the aortic arch, thymus, thyroid, and C-cells in addition to abnormal facial development are also observed. Parathyroid hemorrhage is reported in osteogenesis imperfecta and refractory hypocalcemia (see Chapter 3).

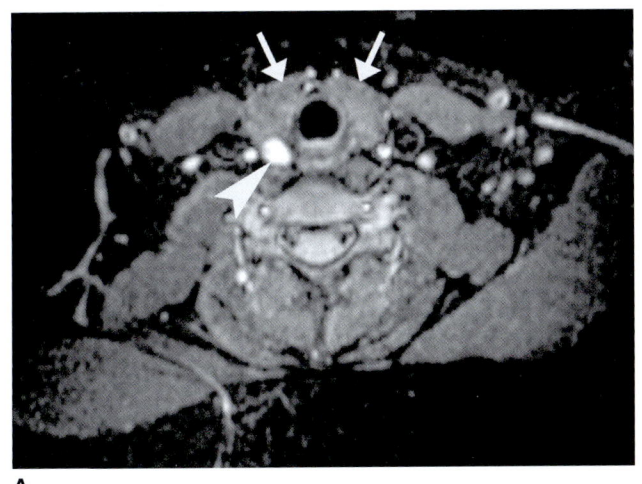
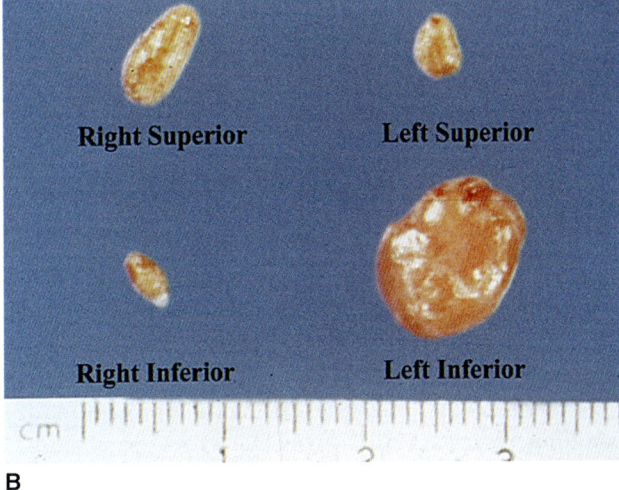
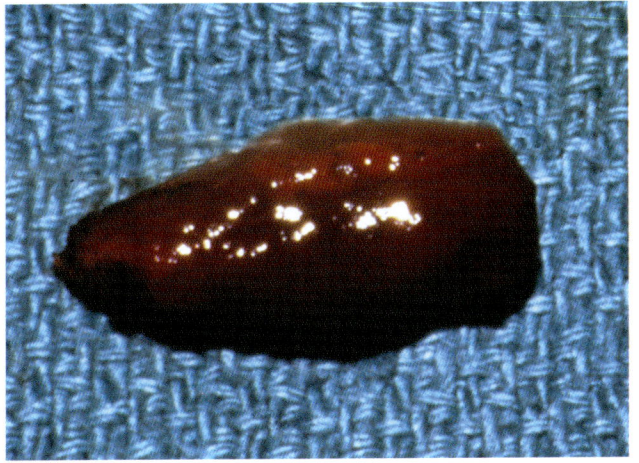
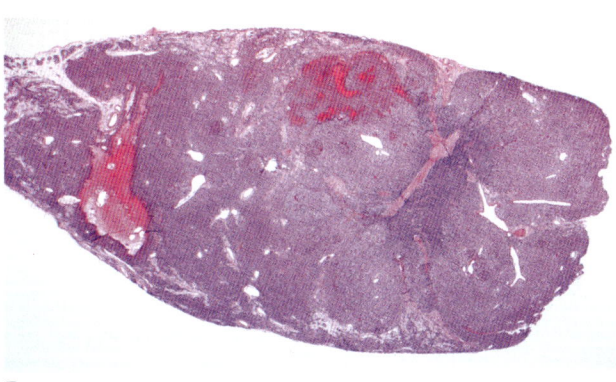

FIGURE 21-6 • Parathyroid adenoma. **A:** Axial T2-weighted MR image shows the hyperintense parathyroid adenoma (*arrowhead*) posterior to the thyroid gland (*arrows*) in a 14-year-old girl. **B:** Parathyroid adenoma in a child with primary HPT is seen as a solitary enlargement of the left inferior gland. (Courtesy of Robert Dufour, M.D., Washington, DC.) **C:** Parathyroid adenoma in a 16-year-old girl who presented with flank pain due to nephrolithiasis, elevated serum calcium, decreased phosphate, and increased parathormone levels. The parathyroid gland was enlarged and red–brown on gross examination. **D:** The enlarged parathyroid gland shows a hypercellular parenchyma composed of chief cells without intraglandular fat on low power. Necrosis was absent (H&E stain). **E:** The parathyroid gland is composed of a monotonous population of chief cells with no intraglandular fat. Mitotic figures were absent (H&E stain).

Cyst(s) of the parathyroid are rare in children and usually asymptomatic. These cysts may represent cystic degeneration of an adenoma or result from a presumed aberration in development. Other cysts in the neck may contain both parathyroid and thymic tissues, as developmental cysts derived from the third pharyngeal pouch. Parathyroid cysts are classified as functional or nonfunctional, based upon whether elevated PTH levels or symptoms of HPT are identified. These lesions account for as many as 10% of HPT cases and account for about 1% of all thyroid and parathyroid masses. These cysts are often mistaken for thyroid cysts, because there is no radiologic or ultrasound method that differentiates parathyroid cysts from thyroid cysts. These cysts may be located anywhere from the mandible to the mediastinum. The cysts typically contain clear colorless fluid when aspirated, compared with the cloudy, gelatinous to bloody aspirate fluid from thyroid cysts. The aspirate material tends to be acellular or paucicellular with rare histiocytes or parathyroid cells. Resection of the cysts shows a smooth, glistening semitransparent to fibrous wall, which maybe loosely attached to adjacent thyroid tissue and surrounding soft tissue. Microscopic examination shows a fibrous to fibromembranous cyst wall with parathyroid tissue embedded within the cyst wall. Only rarely have parathyroid cysts been associated with MEN syndromes.

Acquired Disorders

Hypercalcemia in childhood may be a manifestation of (a) increased PTH secretion by an adenoma or hyperplasia (primary HPT); (b) PTH-related peptide-induced hypercalcemia of malignancy; (c) mutations involving the calcium-sensing receptor gene (*CASR*) (familial hypocalciuric hypercalcemia [FHH], neonatal HPT) or PTH receptor; (d) conditions associated with vitamin D excess (sarcoidosis, tuberculosis, granulomatous disorders); (e) medications; (f) immobilization; or (g) other endocrine disorders (69,72,73). Anorexia, fatigue, constipation, weight loss, weakness, and mental status changes are some of the clinical manifestations. Metastatic calcifications in various organs may result in organ damage if the hypercalcemia is not recognized (73).

Primary HPT is uncommon in children with a prevalence of two to five cases per 100,000 (Table 21-4) (74). Most children are greater than 10 years of age at diagnosis, with a male predilection in contrast to a female predilection in adults (Figure 21-6B) (74,75). A solitary adenoma is the etiology in 80% to 90% of cases. The serum calcium level is usually elevated greater than 12 mg/dL. Hereditary syndromes contribute to about 25% of cases with parathyroid hyperplasia.

In neonatal HPT and MEN syndromes, four gland hyperplasia is a common finding (eFigure 21-44). Other heredofamilial settings with HPT are HPT with or without fibroossseous tumor of the jaws, MEN1, and MEN2a (Chapter 28).

MEN1, an autosomal dominant disorder, is characterized by parathyroid gland hyperplasia, pituitary adenoma, pancreatic endocrine tumors, extrapancreatic neuroendocrine tumors, adrenocortical neoplasms (ACNs), angiofibromas, and lipomas (Table 21-2) (76). The *MEN1* gene, a tumor-suppressor gene, has been mapped to chromosome 11q13 and encodes the protein menin, which is involved in transcriptional regulation, genome stability, and cell division (43). In addition to parathyroid gland hyperplasia, medullary thyroid carcinoma (MTC) and pheochromocytoma (PHEO) are the other associated tumors in MEN2a, an autosomal dominant disorder, with *RET* gene (10q11.2) mutation, which encodes a tyrosine kinase receptor. HPT–jaw tumor (HPT–JT) syndrome, an autosomal dominant disorder, is associated with inactivating mutations in the tumor-suppressor gene *HRPT2* (1q25–32), which encodes parafibromin. Solitary or multiple enlarged parathyroid glands are accompanied by fibroosseous lesions of the mandible or maxilla (43). Parathyroid carcinoma is reportedly more common in this syndrome. Renal cysts, hamartomas, renal cell carcinoma, and Wilms tumor (WT) are other associated lesions and tumors. Isolated familial HPT, distinct from HPT–JT syndrome, is a rare disorder without other associated endocrinopathies, but with germline mutations involving *CASR*, *MEN1*, and *HRPT2* genes. All four glands show chief cell hyperplasia.

Osteopenia, subperiosteal phalangeal bone resorption, bone cyst formation, and genu valgum are skeletal anomalies in long-standing unrecognized HPT (eFigures 21-43 and 21-45). Hypercalciuria and nephrolithiasis are frequent manifestations of primary HPT in childhood (75). Pulmonary calcinosis has also been observed. Measurement of intact serum PTH distinguishes primary HPT from other causes of hypercalcemia in most cases; however, cases of HPT with apparent normal PTH levels have been reported. Preoperative US and radionuclide scan may be helpful in the localization of enlarged glands, but are more limited in small adenomas or multigland hyperplasia. Intraoperative PTH testing has an important role in the differentiation of a solitary adenoma from multiglandular hyperplasia in primary HPT (74).

Neonatal primary HPT is an uncommon disorder associated with FHH. Hypotonia, failure to thrive, and respiratory distress are clinical manifestations. Severe hypercalcemia and elevated PTH levels are present. Osteopenia, subperiosteal bone resorption, and multiple pathologic fractures of long bones are some of the overlapping skeletal findings with osteogenesis imperfecta. FHH, an autosomal dominant condition, has an estimated prevalence of 1:15,000 to 30,000 individuals. It is usually asymptomatic with hypercalcemia, normal PTH levels, and decreased urine calcium excretion (75). Mutations in the *CASR* gene, which encodes for the calcium-sensing receptor in the parathyroid gland and renal tubular epithelium, are found in FHH and neonatal primary HPT.

Secondary HPT is a multiglandular hyperplasia of the parathyroid to hypocalcemia (70). Chronic renal failure is the major cause, with malabsorption, vitamin D deficiency, and X-linked hypophosphatemic rickets being less common causes. Secondary HPT is also a feature of mucolipidosis type II and maternal hypoparathyroidism. Multiglandular hyperplasia is additionally seen in tertiary HPT, an uncommon entity in children, which is characterized by hypercalcemia with renal function restoration following renal transplantation in children with secondary HPT.

Parathyroid adenomas account for 80% of parathyroid tumors in primary HPT in children, being somewhat lower than the adult experience once familial HPT and other inherited endocrinopathies are included. Several different genetic alterations involving PTH, *RET*, *MEN1*, *PRAD1*, *p53*, *HRPT2*, and G protein genes are responsible for different pathogenetic mechanisms (67,68,76). Clonal analysis of sporadic parathyroid adenomas reveals a monoclonal cell population in contrast to the polyclonal population seen in diffuse hyperplasia, except for certain cases of hyperplasia in secondary HPT due to chronic renal failure (68). It is usually not possible to morphologically distinguish a single gland adenoma from multigland hyperplasia without examination of additional glands. This differentiation can be accomplished with an intraoperative PTH level, which normalizes within a few minutes in the case of a single gland adenoma, whereas it initially falls and returns to an elevated level in the presence of hyperplasia (74). An enlarged gland may be occult within the thymus, thyroid, or paraesophageal. Ultrasound and nuclear medicine scans are important in localizing abnormal glands prior to surgery.

Parathyroid adenomas and hyperplasia have similar gross features, including red–brown appearance, weight greater than 60 mg, and 1 to 2 cm in greatest dimension (Figure 21-6B, C). Any parathyroid gland greater than 40 mg in a child should be considered abnormal (67). In a single pediatric study, the mean weight of adenomas was 597 mg, with a range between 170 and 1,550 mg (75). A nodular or diffuse pattern of chief cells with minimal interstitial fat interspersed is the usual microscopic finding (Figure 21-6D, E, eFigure 21-46). Cellular pleomorphism, necrosis, and increased mitotic activity are usually not present, but some mitotic activity should not be viewed with any undue concern. A well-formed capsule is usually not present, but the adenomatous portion of the gland is distinguishable from remnants of compressed and suppressed parathyroid gland at the periphery if present. The chief cells often contain glycogen, which is demonstrable by a periodic acid–Schiff stain with diastase digestion. They are also positive for PTH and CHR by immunohistochemistry. Normal glands demonstrate greater immunoreactivity to PTH compared with hyperplastic glands and adenomas (77). These benign tumors are monoclonal, with loss of 1p a common finding. The genetic mutations associated with inherited syndromes are found with parathyroid adenomas, which are found in Table 21-2. More than 1 adenoma may occur in 7% to 15% of affected patients and are more frequent in children with HPT–JT syndrome (75,76).

Parathyroid carcinoma is a rare cause of primary HPT in adults and even more so in children. These malignant tumors typically present with moderate to very high serum calcium levels with associated clinical symptoms, such as a palpable cervical mass and hoarseness. Screening for germline *HRPT2* mutations should be undertaken in any child with either a personal or family history of parathyroid carcinoma. Other important molecular features include tumor-suppressor gene mutations, in particular Rb and MEN1 genes, and frequent somatic loss of heterozygosity of *HRPT2* gene (parafibromin protein loss on immunostaining) in sporadic cases. Unlike smaller adenomas, carcinomas infiltrate into the soft tissues of the neck and have vascular and capsular invasion. Other features of malignancy are relatively nonspecific and include broad bands of fibrosis, increased mitoses, high proliferative index, nuclear pleomorphism, and atypia. The features, which ultimately confirm the diagnosis of parathyroid carcinoma, are invasion of adjacent tissues, peritumoral lymphovascular and/or perineural invasion, and metastatic disease. An atypical adenoma may be diagnosed in the presence of extensive fibrous bands dissecting through irregular nests of cells in the absence of tissue destructive, or vascular or capsular invasion.

Hypocalcemia in children is multifactorial. It is due to (a) decreased PTH production (hypoparathyroidism); (b) PTH receptor defects; (c) pseudohypoparathyroidism as in Albright hereditary osteodystrophy; (d) mitochondrial DNA mutations as in the Kearns-Sayre syndrome; (e) dietary imbalances with vitamin D, calcium, and magnesium; or (f) increased inorganic phosphate consumption (70,72). Hypocalcemia is also observed with pancreatitis, sepsis, increased serum phosphate levels, renal failure, and antineoplastic therapy. Impaired renal and bone response to PTH accounts for the hypocalcemia seen in premature infants.

Hypoparathyroidism is due to a developmental anomaly of the parathyroid glands as in 22q11.2 microdeletion syndrome and 10p13 deletion as well as autoimmune disorders, infiltrative disorders, prior thyroidectomy, or parathyroidectomy (70). Clinically, children may be either asymptomatic or symptomatic with paresthesias, tetany, muscle cramps, or seizures. Polyglandular autoimmune syndrome type I is an autosomal recessive multisystem autoimmune disorder due to a mutation in the autoimmune regulatory gene (*AIRE*) on chromosome 21q22.3. It presents during infancy, childhood, or adolescence with hypoparathyroidism in 80% to 85% of patients, hypoadrenalism (Addison disease), and chronic mucocutaneous candidiasis (78). Parathyroid autotransplantation is effective in preventing hypoparathyroidism associated with total thyroidectomy.

THYROID GLAND

The thyroid gland is the first endocrine organ to develop as a proliferation of endodermal cells in the floor of the oropharynx (base of tongue) at approximately 3 weeks' gestation. Two small lateral and a larger median anlagen are formed at the foramen cecum. Through a process of elongated cephalad embryonic growth rather than active descent, the thyroid diverticulum comes to reside between the first pharyngeal pouches. The median thyroid anlage elongates ahead of the thyroid gland to allow for descent into the neck and forms the thyroglossal duct. Through the thyroglossal duct, the thyroid gland descends anterior to the eventual location of the hyoid bone and into the midline of the lower neck. The thyroglossal duct becomes obliterated by the 5th week of gestation, but leaves behind the foramen cecum at the base of the tongue as a proximal remnant. Persistence of the thyroglossal duct occurs if it fails to become obliterated before the mesodermal anlage of the hyoid bone is formed. This may result in a thyroglossal duct cyst (TDC) in the affected child. The TDC is one of the most common anomalies of the neck. The endodermal cells differentiate into follicular cells in the eighth gestational week. Diminutive follicles without colloid are identifiable by 8 to 9 weeks' gestation. Well-defined follicles containing colloid are observed by the end of the first trimester.

The pharyngeal pouch-derived ultimobranchial body incorporates into the thyroid, carrying neural crest-derived C-cells, which disseminate into the thyroid follicles. Interstitial solid cell nests are ultimobranchial body remnants. In addition to the TDC, the pyramidal lobe is a second potential remnant of the thyroglossal duct. This lobe is a narrow ribbon of thyroid tissue that is attached to the superior isthmus and is present in 40% to 65% of individuals. More detailed discussion of the embryology of the thyroid gland is found elsewhere (79,80). In addition to *POU1F1*, several distinct genes, TTF1, TTF2, *PAX8*, *TSH*, and *TSHR*, are involved in thyroid gland development and migration (79–83).

The thyroid gland is a bilobed structure connected by an isthmus at the level of the trachea, located in the midanterior neck, and adherent to the larynx and trachea (84,85). The weight of the thyroid varies with gender and age through fetal, infantile, and childhood periods. There are also geographic differences in thyroid weight within the United States and elsewhere. The thyroid gland at birth weighs 1 to 2 g. By 2 years of age, it approaches 3 g, and at 4 years of age 4 to 5 g, and by 15 years of age 15 to 20 g, which is near the adult weight of the gland.

Thyroid follicles are the basic morphologic and functional unit of the thyroid gland and comprise the majority of the thyroid parenchyma. Follicular cells are responsible for the synthesis of thyroid hormone. Both the growth and synthetic functions of the thyroid gland are under the control of thyroid-stimulating hormone (TSH) synthesized by the thyrotrophs of the anterior pituitary gland, which in turn is under the control of thyrotropin-releasing hormone (TRH) from the hypothalamus. TSH mediates its action via cyclic AMP following attachment to receptor sites on the follicular cell membrane. Through a classic feedback mechanism, peripheral levels of thyroxine (T4) have a positive or negative effect on hypothalamic TRH (84) (eFigure 21-47). Excess TSH as a response to low T4 is the mechanism by which hyperplasia of the thyroid gland is mediated in congenital hypothyroidism.

Stimulation or activation of the follicular cells by TSH results in the production of thyroid hormone from thyroglobulin. Several enzymes localized to the follicular cell are required for thyroid hormone synthesis, and loss of one of these enzymes on the basis of an autosomal recessive defect leads to dyshormonogenic goiter (Figure 21-7). There are numerous genes involved in thyroid development and function, which may be mutated in dyshormonogenic goiter-thyroglobulin (8q24), thyroperoxidase (2p25), sodium-iodide symporter (19p13), GNAS 1 (20q13), pendrin (7q31), DUOX2 (15q15), DUOXA2 (15q15), and DHAL1 (6q24). The physiology and biochemistry of the thyroid gland in the context of the various inherited disorders and clinical manifestations of congenital hypothyroidism or hereditary hyperthyroidism have been reviewed by others (79,81,84).

The C-cell (parafollicular cell) is the other hormonally active cell of the thyroid, representing less than 0.5% of the

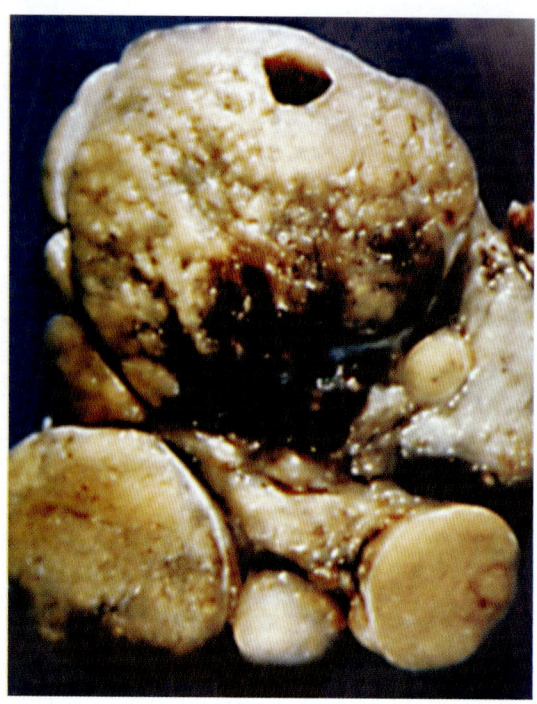

FIGURE 21-7 • Dyshormonogenic goiter. This image is a section through the thyroid gland of an individual who presented with a dyshormonogenic goiter. The thyroid parenchyma has a nodular pattern with retrogressive and hyperplastic changes including hemorrhage and fibrosis. (From Lloyd RV, Douglas BR, Young WF. *Endocrine diseases. Atlas of Nontumor Pathology*. Washington, DC: American Registry of Pathology, 2001. Originally published in *Atlas of tumor pathology, tumors of the thyroid gland*, Fascicle 5, Third Series. Washington, DC: Armed Forces Institute of Pathology).

total epithelial population. These neuroendocrine cells may be identified immunohistochemically by their reactivity for CHR, SYN, and calcitonin (84). Like the follicular cell, the C-cell is enclosed within the basement membrane of the follicle, but is located at the periphery without contact with the colloid. Unlike the endodermally derived follicular cell, the C-cell progenitor migrates from the vagal or cephalic region of the neural crest to the fourth and fifth pharyngeal pouches, one of whose derivatives is the ultimobranchial body (84). The greatest number of C-cells is found in the upper two-thirds of the lateral lobes of the thyroid, along the central axis (84). The neonatal gland contains a tenfold increase in C-cells compared to the adult thyroid. The number of C-cells diminishes with age. A paucity of C-cells in the thyroid is reported in DiGeorge anomaly (syndrome) on the presumed basis of a developmental field defect in the formation of pharyngeal pouch derivatives. Hyperplasia of C-cells in children is divided into physiologic hyperplasia in neonates, after a hemithyroidectomy, in the presence of autoimmune (Hashimoto) thyroiditis, and in association with MEN2a or MEN2b and neoplastic hyperplasia (84). Hyperplasia is defined as the presence of 50 or more C-cells in one 10× objective field. MTC in MEN2a, MEN2b, and familial (non-MEN) MTC (FMTC) is the consequence of germline *RET* gene mutations (Table 21-2). These syndromes are characterized by multifocal C-cell hyperplasia and often multifocal MTCs (84,86,87).

Solid epithelial cell nests, a remnant of the ultimobranchial body, are the third cell type identified in the thyroid gland. They are localized to the upper and middle third of the thyroid gland with a parafollicular or intrafollicular location. These squamoid to transitional appearing cells may be solid or demonstrate microcystic change and are immunoreactive to low molecular weight keratin and carcinoembryonic antigen. Cells with follicular or C-cell differentiation are present within these nests and may account for the rare mixed follicular–medullary carcinoma.

More detailed comprehensive reviews of the functional and morphologic aspects of the thyroid gland have been detailed elsewhere (83,84,88–90).

Imaging

Imaging studies are an integral component of the diagnostic evaluation of a child with an enlarged thyroid or other mass-producing process in the neck. US is a basic modality and provides for a confident diagnosis of TDC, which appears as a midline or paramedian cyst, possibly with debris when complicated by infection or hemorrhage (91) (Figure 21-8A, B). TDCs are usually near the hyoid bone. Branchial cleft cysts have a similar imaging appearance but are positioned in the lateral neck away from the midline (eFigure 21-48).

Ultrasound is useful in depicting thyroid nodules in patients with thyroid dysfunction or goiter. Complex cases may require MR. CT is less desirable for the evaluation of thyroid lesions because the use of iodinated contrast may preclude later radioactive thyroid ablation therapy if necessary for several weeks. Thyroid carcinomas appear well defined and heterogeneous on US, CT, or MR. Papillary thyroid carcinoma (PTC) is more likely to contain cystic-appearing, necrotic areas compared to follicular thyroid carcinoma (FTC) (Figure 21-9A). Most MTCs are solid and may contain coarse calcifications (Figure 21-9B).

Radionuclide scintigraphy with ^{99m}Tc pertechnetate or ^{123}I is very useful in the evaluation of thyroid dysfunction and nodules or in the localization of ectopic thyroid tissue (eFigure 21-49A to C). Nodules with decreased radiotracer uptake ("cold" nodules) are more likely to be malignant than nodules that are similar to surrounding normal thyroid or take up more radiotracer than normal thyroid ("hot," hyperfunctioning nodules). When ectopic thyroid tissue is identified, it is important to evaluate the neck base and base of the tongue for orthotopic thyroid gland (Figure 21-10A, B, eFigure 21-49A to C).

Developmental Disorders

Dysmorphism of the thyroid gland is a structural phenomenon with several morphologic variations including absence or incomplete formation of a normal gland, failure of the normal anatomic localization of the gland, or persistence of embryologic remnants with a branching lobular pattern of immature follicles rather than dense formation of individual follicles (Table 21-5). Recessively inherited defects in enzymes responsible for thyroid hormone synthesis are other developmental disorders that are not characterized by primary structural anomalies of the thyroid gland (eFigure 21-50); however, elevated TSH levels lead to multinodular hyperplasia in the form of dyshormonogenic goiter (Figure 21-7). Clinically, these various developmental disorders present with congenital hypothyroidism, a mass at the base of the tongue or in the neck, or congenital hypothyroidism with development of a goiter. Many of these developmental anomalies also affect first-degree relatives, indicating a familial component.

Dysgenesis of the thyroid is a generic designation for various developmental anatomic anomalies that include complete failure in gland formation (agenesis), decreased amount

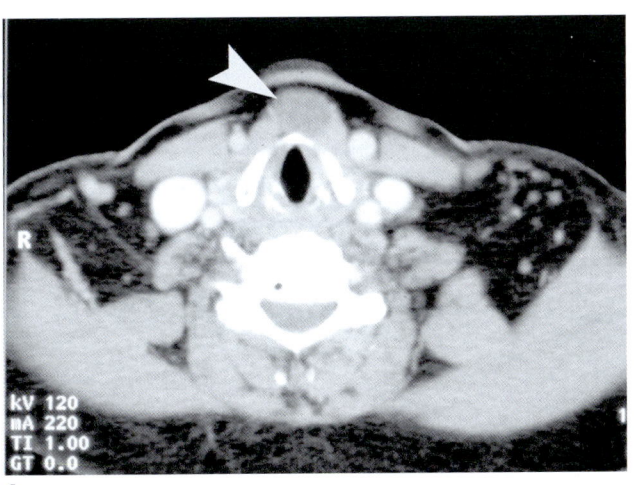
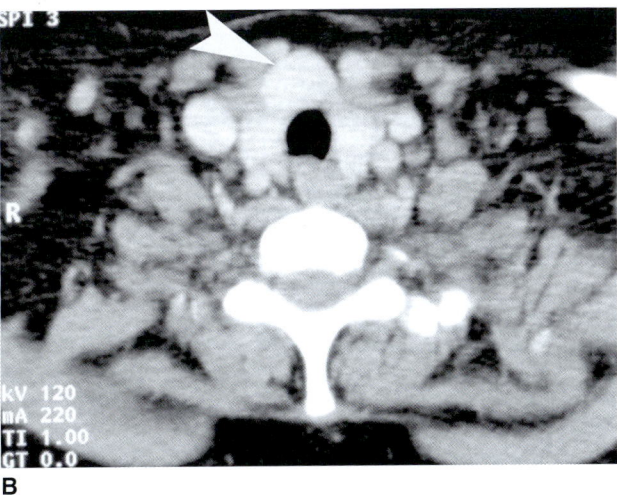

FIGURE 21-8 • Thyroglossal duct cyst in an adult complicated by PTC. **A:** Axial contrast-enhanced CT image shows a midline cyst (*arrowhead*). **B:** Axial CT image caudal to (a) shows markedly enhancing, midline mass (*arrowhead*).

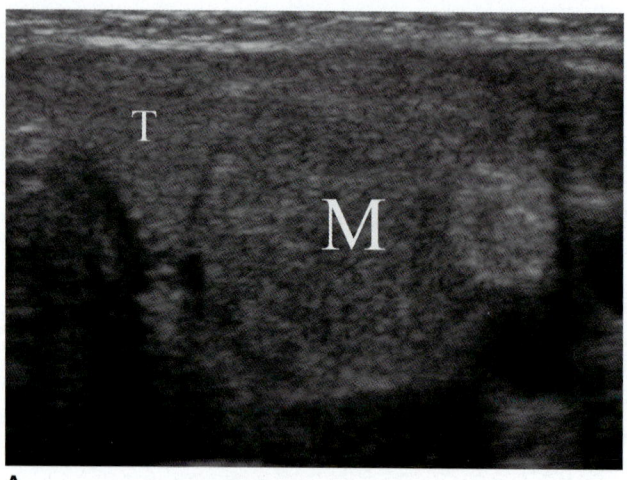
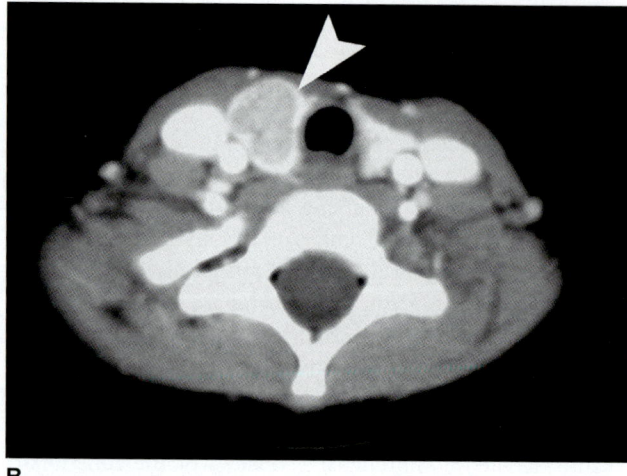

FIGURE 21-9 • Papillary thyroid carcinoma in 15-year-old girl. **A:** Transverse sonographic image showing a heterogeneous mass (M) within the homogeneous thyroid gland (T). **B:** MTC in an 8-year-old girl with family history of MEN2a. Axial contrast-enhanced CT shows a mass within the left thyroid lobe, which enhances less than the surrounding thyroid gland (*arrowhead*).

of thyroid tissue (hypoplasia), absence of a lobe (hemiagenesis), or ectopic location. Dysgenesis is an important etiology of congenital hypothyroidism, with prevalence in the United States of 1:3000 to 5000 live births. Most causes of congenital hypothyroidism are due to dysgenesis or inherited defects in thyroid hormone synthesis (Table 21-5). Congenital hypothyroidism has been also been observed in Williams and Down syndromes.

Congenital hypothyroidism in 80% to 85% of cases is associated with one of several types of dysgenesis. The prevalence of hypothyroidism in the neonatal period is 1:4000 live births with thyroid dysgenesis, 1:30,000 live births with dyshormonogenesis, 1:40,000 live births with transient hypothyroidism, and 1:100,000 live births with central hypothyroidism or hypothalamic–pituitary defect (81,89). In a study of 230 children with congenital hypothyroidism, scintigraphy revealed the following findings: ectopia in 61%, goiter in 18%, agenesis in 16%, normal in 4%, and hemiagenesis in less than 1%. In a series of 800,000 neonates with increased TSH and normally positioned thyroid glands, an enlarged gland or goiter was observed in 55% of cases, a normal gland in 29% of cases, and hypoplasia in 16% of cases. If the thyroid

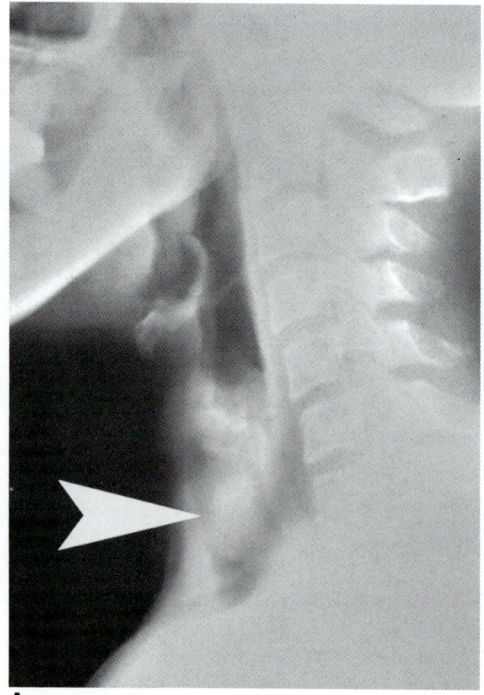
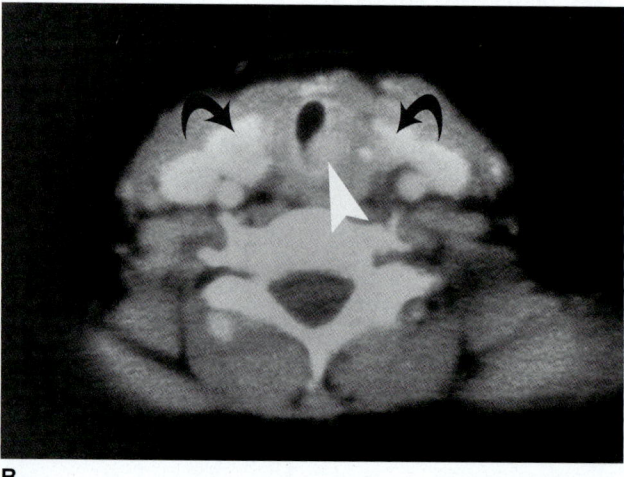

FIGURE 21-10 • Ectopic thyroid gland in the trachea of an adult. **A:** Lateral tomogram shows an ovoid mass within the tracheal air column (*arrowhead*). **B:** Axial CT image shows markedly enhancing eccentric mass in the trachea (*arrowhead*) and normal thyroid lobes in the orthotopic location (*curved arrows*).

TABLE 21-5	ETIOLOGIC CLASSIFICATION OF CONGENITAL HYPOTHYROIDISM

I. Primary hypothyroidism
   A. Dysgenesis (85%) (1:4,000)
      Idiopathic or genetic (*TTF-1, TTF-2, FOXE1, PAX-8,* and *TSHR* defects)
         Agenesis
         Hemiagenesis
         Hypoplasia
         Ectopia
            Lingual thyroid (90% of thyroid ectopia) (1:10,000)
   B. Dyshormonogenesis (10–15%) (1:30,000)
      Iodide transport (sodium-iodide symporter defect (*NIS* gene)
      Iodide organification and coupling defect
         Thyroid peroxidase defect (*TPO* gene) (Pendred defect)
         Thyroid oxidase 2 defect (*DUOX1/THOX1 DUOX/THOX2* genes)
      Defect in thyroglobulin synthesis or transport (*Tg* gene)
      Iodotyrosine deiodinase defect (*DEHAL1* gene)
   C. Others (5%)
II. Secondary/tertiary hypothyroidism (hypothalamic-pituitary-thyroid axis dysfunction) (1:100,000)
      Genetic defects involving *LHX3, LHX4, PROP 1, POU1F1, HESX1, TRHR, TSHB*
III. Peripheral thyroid hormone resistance
      Genetic defects involving *MCT8, THRB*
IV. Transient hypothyroidism (1:40,000)
      Maternal antithyroid antibodies, goitrogenic drugs, iodine deficiency

Based on data from Peter, F, Muzsnai A. Congenital disorders of the thyroid: hypo/hyper. *Endocrinol Metab Clin North Am.* 2009;38:491-507; LaFranchi S. Section 2: Disorders of the thyroid gland. In: Kliegman RM, Behrman RE, Jenson HB, Stanton BF, eds., *Nelson Textbook of Pediatrics,* 18th ed. Philadelphia, PA: Elsevier, 2007; Bettendorf M. Thyroid disorders in children from birth to adolescence. *Eur J Nucl Med Mol Imaging.* 2002;29(Suppl 2):S439-S446.

gland is anatomically orthotopic in the presence of congenital hypothyroidism, a defect exists in thyroid hormone biosynthesis with the development of a dyshormonogenic nodular goiter or an inability of the gland to respond to TSH. Dysgenesis is more common in females than in males (3:1) and is sporadic in most cases (85%) (79). Affected infants with agenesis or hypoplasia have permanently elevated levels of TSH and low levels of circulating thyroid hormone. A number of mutations have been identified in the genes responsible for thyroid development, including *PAX8, TTF-1* (thyroid transcription factor-1), *TTF-2* (thyroid transcription factor-2), *TSHR* (TSH receptor), thyroglobulin (8q24), thyroperoxidase (2p25), sodium-iodide symporter (19p13), GNAS 1 (20q13), pendrin (7q31), DUOX2 (15q15), and DUOXA2 (15q15) and DHAL1 (6q24) and are pathogenetically involved in thyroid dysgenesis (79–83,92). These genetic defects and their association with other diseases are reviewed elsewhere (79).

Hemiagenesis is another form of dysgenesis with failure in the formation of the left lobe in most cases. This anomaly occurs in less than 0.5% of the population and is more common in females. Thyroid function is within normal limits (93).

Ectopia of the thyroid gland is more thoroughly documented on a morphologic basis than the other types of dysgenesis, as judged by the descriptions in the literature (eFigure 21-51). Ectopia has a female predominance. Lingual thyroid (base of tongue) occurs in approximately 1:10,000 individuals and is detected in most cases during a diagnostic evaluation for congenital hypothyroidism or as an incidentally discovered mass (Figure 21-11A, eFigure 21-49). Lingual thyroid accounts for approximately 90% of all thyroid ectopias. Most lingual thyroids are accompanied by an orthotopic thyroid; however, a minority of lingual thyroids constitutes the only site of thyroid tissue. Some cases classified as agenesis have a lingual remnant. Ectopic thyroid tissue including dual ectopia (location at different sites), with exclusion of occurrence in a teratoma, has been documented in the submandibular region, trachea, heart, mediastinum, and various intra-abdominal sites. The presence of thyroid follicles in lymph nodes as so-called lateral aberrant thyroid is controversial and is favored to represent metastatic thyroid carcinoma in most, if not all, cases (84). Thyroid neoplasia arising in ectopic thyroid, usually in a TDC, is recognized in children.

Ectopic thyroid may be represented by individual microfollicles or small foci of multiple microfollicles or solid nests of follicular cells without apparent colloid formation. The follicles are interspersed between bundles of skeletal muscle in the tongue or within the tissues of the other ectopic sites (Figure 21-11B, eFigure 21-52). In some instances, the epithelial structures are not readily identifiable as thyroid tissue and may require immunohistochemical staining for thyroglobulin, thyroid transcription factor 1, or PAX-8. In addition to the immature or nonfunctioning appearance of ectopic follicles, the ectopia is also hypoplastic because the total tissue volume of thyroid is less than normal for the age and gender.

Another form of thyroid dysgenesis is an enlarged lobe composed of immature lobules of fetal-appearing follicles separated by an immature mesenchyme. Nodules of immature cartilage or other heterologous tissues present within the lobule may suggest a teratoma.

Thyroglossal duct cyst (TDC) is the consequence in the failure of the thyroglossal duct to undergo complete obliteration and regression during fetal life (56). Approximately 15% of all neck masses in children are TDCs, presenting as a midline anterior neck mass overlying the hyoid bone (56,94). Rather than a midline location, 10% to 25% of TDCs are found

autoimmune diathesis. Approximately 4% of children with type I diabetes mellitus have CLT. Trisomy 21 syndrome, Klinefelter syndrome, and Turner syndrome are three chromosomal disorders associated with CLT. Approximately 25% of young individuals with Turner syndrome have antithyroid antibodies and 10% have enlarged thyroids.

The pathologic diagnosis of CLT is more often established by FNAB than by histologic examination. Surgical resection is reserved for specific clinical circumstances, such as a possible thyroid neoplasm. The thyroid is symmetrically enlarged and weighs more than 25 to 30 g. A pale, vaguely nodular, tan–gray appearance with a resemblance to lymph nodal tissue is noted on cross-section after fixation (Figure 21-13A). On occasion, one or the other lateral lobe or the pyramidal lobe is larger with the loss of symmetry. Any areas of discrete firmness, sclerosis, or nodularity may indicate the presence of PTC or scarring as in the fibrosing stage of CLT. Microscopically, lymphoid follicles with reactive germinal centers are interspersed throughout the gland with destructive replacement of parenchyma (Figure 21-13B, eFigure 21-58B, C). An intermixture of mature plasma cells is also apparent in a predominant population of B and T lymphocytes. The follicles are typically small and uniform, although some larger follicles with papillary infoldings may be seen. Some of the intact thyroid follicles may contain intrafollicular histiocytes and giant cells, as evidence of so-called palpation thyroiditis or the presence of giant cells and lymphoid aggregates where follicles once resided. The diminutive follicles are lined by cuboidal or flattened epithelial cells or by epithelial cells with optically clear nuclei and grooves as seen in PTC. The diagnosis of PTC is made in the presence of a discrete lesion(s). Classic Hurthle or oncocytic follicular cells as a diffuse finding are uncommon in CLT in children and, in this respect, do not fulfill the classic morphologic definition of Hashimoto thyroiditis (eFigure 21-59). However, CLT and Hashimoto thyroiditis are pathogenetically identical forms of autoimmune thyroiditis in all other respects. Mizukami et al. found no morphologic difference in the types of chronic thyroiditis between adults and children less than 10 years old.

The fibrosing or end stage of CLT with marked loss and atrophy of follicles, fibrosis with a finely nodular pattern, and a diminution of the lymphocytic infiltrate are infrequently encountered in children. As noted earlier, the morphologic diagnosis of CLT is usually based on FNAB. The typical cytologic finding is a mixture of individual and small nonpapillary groups of benign-appearing follicular epithelial cells in a background of many dispersed small lymphocytes, some plasma cells, and histiocytes. Hurthle cells are infrequent, and even less common are papillae, whose presence should raise the possibility of PTC. Approximately 30% of cases of CLT in children had distinct nodules and 3% had a PTC.

Other types of thyroiditis, infectious and noninfectious, occur infrequently in children. Abscess of the thyroid has been reported in children, and opportunistic infections are seen in the immunocompromised setting. Recurrent acute suppurative thyroiditis with or without abscess formation should suggest the presence of a branchial pouch anomaly, such as a pyriform sinus cyst or TDC remnant (56). Most cultures demonstrate a mixed flora, containing a *Streptococcus* species. Common features of acute suppurative thyroiditis include a painful/tender neck mass associated with fever. Involvement of the left lobe is more common. A left hemithyroidectomy may need to be performed for recurrent infections. An infectious etiology should be excluded in granulomatous thyroiditis in a child, because subacute giant cell or de Quervain thyroiditis is extremely rare in childhood.

Hyperplasia of the thyroid gland is either diffuse or multinodular. Diffuse hyperplasia is often associated with hyperthyroidism or thyrotoxicosis. The so-called simple goiter is defined clinically as diffuse or nodular enlargement of the

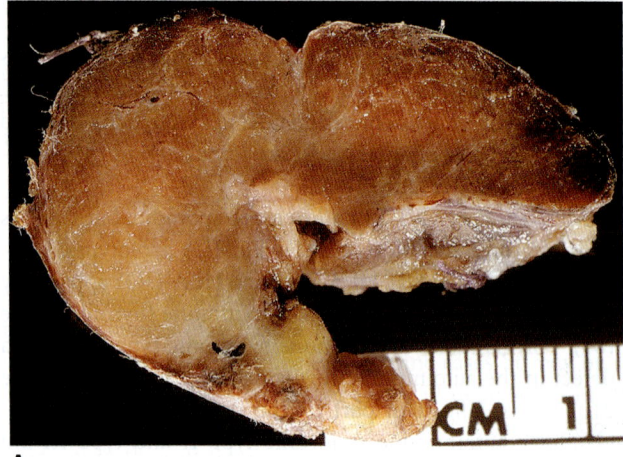
A

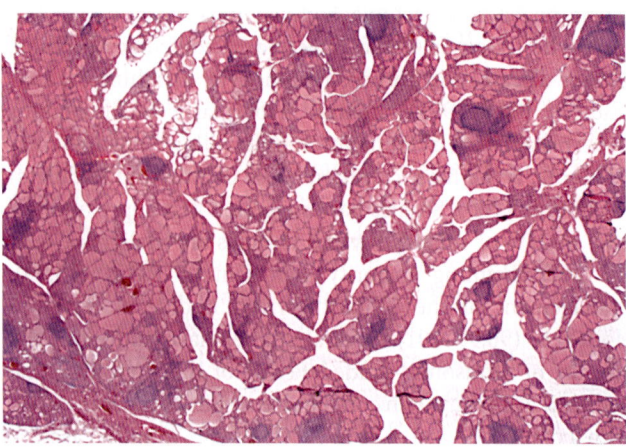
B

FIGURE 21-13 • Chronic lymphocytic thyroiditis. **A:** This specimen shows the characteristic diffuse thyroid gland enlargement seen in CLT on gross examination. A vaguely nodular pattern corresponding to the presence of lymphoid follicles is seen in this cut section. **B:** CLT in this low-power magnification image shows prominent lymphoid aggregates interspersed between the thyroid follicles. Plasma cells and lymphocytes were present in the interstitium (H&E stain).

thyroid gland without obvious evidence of hyperthyroidism. Children with a simple goiter are predominantly young adolescent females and do not experience any further gland enlargement. A small percentage, however, may develop CLT.

The simple or colloid goiter is a more or less symmetrically enlarged thyroid gland with a diffuse or multinodular appearance (eFigure 21-60). The follicles vary in size with one or more colloid-filled macrofollicles lined by a flattened layer of epithelial cells (eFigure 21-61). Formation of colloid cysts occurs in some cases. Conversely, nodular hyperplasia or adenomatous nodules manifest as multiple variably sized follicular nodules with or without dense fibrous bands, cystic degeneration, hemorrhage, and nonspecific chronic inflammation. Papillary hyperplasia is a source of concern in areas of degeneration, but the follicular cells usually do not have well-developed nuclear features of PTC. A peripheral (so-called parasitic or exophytic) nodule may be found in the perithyroidal soft tissues and even embedded in skeletal muscle, especially at the isthmus.

Multinodular hyperplasia is the pathologic finding associated with dyshormonogenic goiter (Figure 21-7). One example is Pendred syndrome, manifesting as goiter and hearing loss in adolescence due to a defect in the *PDS* gene (*SLC26A4* gene) on chromosome 7 that encodes for the protein pendrin, which is involved in iodide transport across the cell membranes, and whose absence results in decreased organification of iodide with disruption in thyroid hormone synthesis. The follicular nodules of a dyshormonogenic goiter tend to be hypercellular due to the formation of microfollicles, trabeculae, and papillae (eFigure 21-62). Cytologic atypia may be present, usually in the form of "random" endocrine atypia, rather than PTC-like atypia. Endocrine-type atypia includes isolated nuclear enlargement, hyperchromasia, and mitotic activity without diffuse enlargement, clearing, or grooves. Well-differentiated thyroid carcinoma has been reported in dyshormonogenic goiters, but it is difficult to determine whether the risk of malignancy is increased in these glands.

Diffuse hyperplasia with clinical hyperthyroidism (Graves disease) is an autoimmune disorder of the thyroid, with some overlapping immunologic and pathologic findings with CLT. Hyperthyroidism also occurs infrequently on the basis of "toxic" nodular hyperplasia, functioning follicular adenoma, autosomal dominant nonimmune hyperthyroidism, and congenital hyperthyroidism. The latter two disorders have been reported with activating germline mutations in the TSH receptor gene. Sporadic congenital hyperthyroidism occurs in the presence of maternal autoimmune thyroid disease with the transplacental passage of maternal thyroid-stimulating immunoglobulins. Only 1% of neonates whose mothers have active Graves disease during pregnancy have evidence of hyperthyroidism at birth. Most cases of hyperthyroidism in children are on the basis of Graves disease (81). Other etiologies of hyperthyroidism in children have been tabulated by LaFranchi (82,89).

A screening study of school-aged population children between 11 and 18 years of age revealed that almost 4% had clinical or laboratory evidence of "thyroid abnormalities" and approximately 5% of those with abnormalities had hyperthyroidism. This figure compares with other studies in which 10% to 15% of all pediatric thyroid disease is diagnosed as hyperthyroidism. Juvenile hyperthyroidism typically presents in girls (6:1, female to male ratio) who are usually 11 years of age and older (11 to 18 years) and have diffuse enlargement of the thyroid (95% of cases) or less often have a dominant "toxic" or autonomous nodule (81). Hyperthyroidism occurs in families and is associated with MAS activating mutations in the stimulatory G protein domain. Germline mutations in the TSH receptor account for cases of toxic multinodular goiter and toxic thyroid adenoma.

Graves disease (diffuse toxic goiter) is characterized by hyperthyroidism, ophthalmopathy (exophthalmos), and dermopathy (pretibial myxedema) in the pediatric population. Its peak prevalence is in adolescence (11 to 15 years of age) and is three to five times more common in girls (81). The clinical symptoms include weight loss, heat intolerance, sweating, palpitations, emotional lability, nervousness, and intellectual decline. Congenital diffuse toxic goiter occurs in a small percentage of infants (1%) born to mothers with active Graves disease. The thyroid on physical examination is goiterous, smooth, firm, and nontender. The pathogenesis of Graves disease involves T- and B-cell dysregulation leading to the production of several anti-TSH receptor, thyroid-stimulating, thyroid growth–stimulating, and TSH-binding inhibitor antibodies (eFigure 21-57). Thyroid-stimulating immunoglobulin mimics TSH and binds to the follicular cell TSH receptor leading to hypersecretion of thyroid hormones. The thyroid growth-stimulating immunoglobulin also binds to the TSH receptor and stimulates follicular cell hyperplasia with the development of increased serum levels of thyroxine or triiodothyronine and decreased TSH. The presence of anti-TSH receptor antibodies confirms the diagnosis of Graves disease versus other causes of hyperthyroidism. Total or subtotal thyroidectomy is performed in cases of medical failure or intolerance. The clinical management of Graves disease in children is the subject of continued study and controversy.

Pathologically, the thyroid gland is symmetrically enlarged without apparent nodules in most cases (Figure 21-14A, eFigure 21-63A). A red–brown color without an appreciation of translucent colloid is noted on cut surface. The weight of the gland is generally more than 25 to 30 g, but this varies somewhat with the age of the patient. In the unsuppressed gland, the follicular cells have a tall columnar appearance. Crowding of these cells leads to intrafollicular papillary infoldings on histologic examination (Figure 21-14B, eFigure 21-63B). Marked follicular cell pleomorphism can be seen in pretreated glands. The colloid has a pale watery appearance and is absent in some follicles. Those follicles with colloid often show peripheral scalloping of the colloid. These latter findings are usually attenuated with preoperative suppression to diminish the function and vascularity of the gland (eFigure 21-64). Epithelial hyperplasia through the action of TSH, leading to more prominent intrafollicular papillary

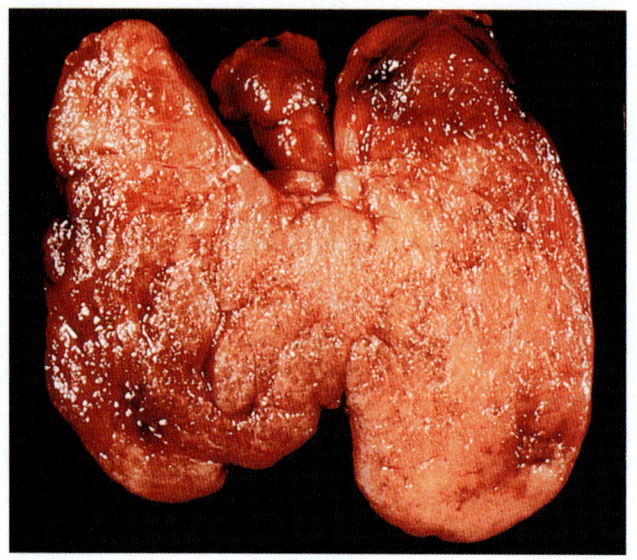
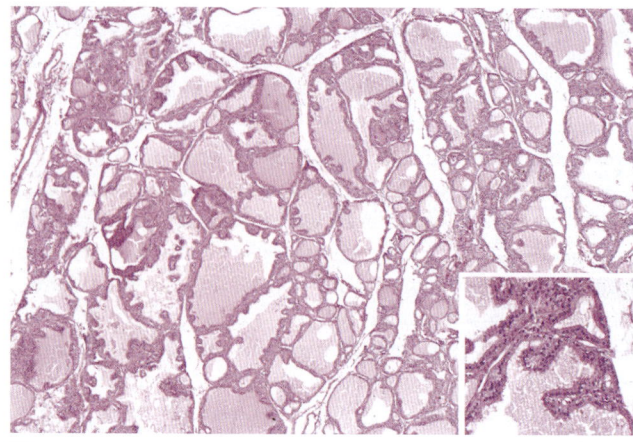

FIGURE 21-14 • Graves disease. **A:** This image shows diffuse symmetrical enlargement of the thyroid gland from a patient with Graves disease. The parenchyma has a deep red color due to increased vascularity within the gland. (Reprinted with permission from Lloyd RV, Douglas BR, Young WF. *Endocrine Diseases. Atlas of Nontumor Pathology*. Washington, DC: American Registry of Pathology, 2001.) **B:** This section of thyroid gland from a patient with untreated Graves disease shows follicles with hyperplastic epithelium and papillary infoldings. Pale watery colloid and an interstitial lymphocytic infiltrate (not pictured) were observed. The papillary infoldings (inset) lack the optically clear nuclei seen in PTC (H&E stain).

infoldings, is seen in the gland treated by thiouracil. Iodine administration before surgery results in the accumulation of colloid and the formation of macrofollicles, often with associated accentuation of thyroid lobules by thin fibrous bands. Rather than cuboidal to columnar epithelium, flattened epithelial cells cover the slender papillae.

Lymphocytic infiltrates in the interstitium and lymphoid nodules with reactive germinal centers are prominent in some glands. Without the clinical history of Graves disease, a diagnosis of CLT may be the preferred interpretation based on histologic examination. The intrafollicular papillae may cause concern about PTC; however, the follicular cells lack the well-developed nuclear atypia of PTC. At least in the pediatric age population, PTC is rarely found in the midst of diffuse toxic hyperplasia.

Neoplasms

The World Health Organization classification of thyroid tumors contains a number of histologic types, but the overwhelming majority of differentiated carcinomas of the thyroid in children are PTC. Institutional referral patterns may affect the proportion of MTC in children with *RET* mutations in affected kindreds with MEN2a or MEN2b. Almost 30% of children with differentiated carcinomas at St. Louis Children's Hospital are MTCs because of MEN2 referrals to the institution. FTC and MTC comprise less than 10% of thyroid carcinomas in the experience of most other institutions. Undifferentiated (anaplastic) carcinomas are rare in children in contrast to adults.

Differentiated carcinomas of the thyroid gland account for only 1% to 3% of all malignant neoplasms in the pediatric age group in North America. It has an annual incidence of 2.4:100,000 children, less than 19 years of age (102). The most common histologic type is PTC, representing approximately 85% to 90% of all thyroid malignancies in children. The follicular variant of PTC accounts for approximately 25% of PTCs (59). Other than thyroid carcinomas, follicular adenomas, hemangiomas, lymphangiomas, teratomas, mucoepidermoid carcinoma, lymphoma, and plexiform neurofibromas are other types of tumors involving the thyroid in children. FTC and follicular adenoma have been observed in patients with congenital goitrous hypothyroidism. Follicular adenoma is a relatively frequent cause of a solitary thyroid nodule in children (97). RDD, LCH, and hematolymphoid malignancies are examples of infiltrative processes involving the thyroid in children.

Most carcinomas of the thyroid in children are diagnosed between 13 and 16 years of age, but individual cases have been reported throughout childhood, even in the newborn. The female to male ratio is approximately 1:1 in carcinomas diagnosed prior to adolescence, but with a 3–6:1 female predominance during adolescence. The risk for developing thyroid cancer in nodules is much higher in childhood than in adulthood. Malignancy is identified in only 5% to 10% of thyroid nodules in adults, whereas cancer is present in thyroid nodules in children in 30% to 50%. Children are also more likely to present with disseminated disease at diagnosis than adults. Almost 80% of children with PTC have cervical lymph node involvement, 20% will have extrathyroidal extension, and 5% will have pulmonary metastases. Although children present at more advanced stage of disease than adults, children rarely die of disease with a mortality of only 1% to 2% being most commonly reported. With children with distant metastases, it was found over a 10-year period that overall survival was 100% with persistent, stable disease in 30% to 45%. Risk factors for thyroid cancer development include radiation therapy and treatment of a prior malignancy. The latency period for cancer development is 4 to 6 years. Thyroid cancer represents almost 10% of second malignancies, with Hodgkin lymphoma being the most common primary malignancy in affected children.

Many recent studies have examined the molecular events underlying the development of thyroid cancer (Table 21-6) (86). A number of somatic mutations involving the *RET* gene have been identified in sporadic PTC (59,86); *RET/PTC1* and the *RET/PTC3* gene arrangements are found in a variable proportion of PTCs in children. In children not exposed to radiation, the *RET/PTC1* rearrangement is more frequent than the *RET/PTC3* rearrangement, which is more common in radiation-induced thyroid cancer (59,100). The "classic" papillary pattern is associated with *RET/PTC1* rearrangement, whereas the *RET/PTC3* is found more often in the follicular variant of PTC. In terms of behavior, PTCs with the *RET/PTC3* gene rearrangement appear to have a somewhat more aggressive course than PTCs with the *RET/PTC1* rearrangement. Mutations involving *BRAF* are uncommon in PTCs in children less than 15 years of age at diagnosis (86). FTC and follicular adenoma are associated with *RAS* and *PAX8–PPARγ* (peroxisome proliferator–activated receptor gamma) mutations, but these mutations do not distinguish adenoma from carcinoma (86,100).

MTCs, in contrast, demonstrate distinct mutations in the *RET* gene (Table 21-6). Mutations in the RET protooncogene in the pericentromeric region of chromosome 10q11.2 have been identified in three autosomal dominant syndromes, MEN2a, MEN2b, and FMTC (59,86,87). The *RET* gene codes for a transmembrane receptor tyrosine kinase that is involved in the development of the kidney and nervous system. The gene spans 21 exons. Each of these syndromes involves mutations with different codons (eFigure 21-65). MEN2a and FMTC more frequently involve missense mutations in exons 10 and 11 involving codons 609, 611, 618, 620, and 634. MEN2b has a characteristic mutation in exon 16 (codon 918) in 95% of cases and in codon 883 in exon 15 (59).

PTC presents with a painless or tender mass in the thyroid gland. Palpable cervical adenopathy at diagnosis is common since regional lymph node metastasis is present in 30% to 80% of children at diagnosis (96,100,103). Most cases of PTC are sporadic, but a family history should be sought because there are several familial-associated tumor predisposition syndromes (Table 21-2). There is an increased incidence of PTC in children who have received radiation therapy for a

TABLE 21-6 MOLECULAR PATHOLOGY AND CYTOGENETICS OF THYROID ADENOMAS AND CARCINOMAS

<u>Follicular adenomas</u>
RAS (RAS–RAF–MEK–MAPK pathway)
H-RAS
K-RAS
N-RAS
Clonal cytogenetic aberrations (45%)
 Trisomy 7 and other trisomies
 t(2;19)(p21;q13)
 Deletions of 3p, 10, 13, 19
<u>Atypical follicular adenoma (tumor of uncertain malignant potential)</u>
N-RAS codon 61 mutation
PAX8/PPAR-gamma rearrangements
<u>Microfollicular adenoma</u>
RET/PTC rearrangements
<u>Papillary thyroid carcinomas: translocations</u>

RET/PTC1-H4	inv(10)(q11.2;q21)
RET/PTC2-PRKAR1A	t(10;17)(q11.2;q23)
RET/PTC3-NCOA4	inv(10)(q11.2;q10)
RET/PTC4-NCOA4	inv(10)(q11.2;q10)
RET/PTC5-GOLGA5	t(10;14;)(q11.2;q32)
RET/PTC6-HTIF1	t(7;10)(q32-34;q11.2)
RET/PTC7-TIF1G	t(1;10)(p13;q11.2)
RET/PTC8-KTN1	t(10;14)(q11.2;q22.1)
RET/PTC9-RFG9	t(10'18)(q11.2;q21-22)
ELKS/RET	t(10;12)(q11.2;q13.3)
PCM1/RET	t(8;10)(p21-22;q11.2)
RFP/RET	t(6;10)(p21;q11.2)
HOOK3/RET	t(8;10)(p11.21;q11.2)
TRK/T1	TPR (1q25)
TRK/T2	TPR (1q25)
TRK/TPM3	TPM3 (1q22-23)
TRK/T3	TFG (3q11-12)

<u>Follicular carcinoma</u>

PAX8/PPAR-gamma	t(2;3)
FTCF/PPAR-gamma	t(3;7)
X/PPAR-gamma	t(1;3)

Chromosomal Imbalances
2, 3p, 6, 7q, 8, 9, 10q, 11, 13q, 17p, 22
<u>Prevalence of genetic mutations in thyroid cancer</u>
Papillary carcinoma

BRAF	45%
RET/PTC	20%
RAS	10%
TRK	<5%

Follicular Carcinoma

RAS (N-RAS, H-RAS)	45%
PAX8-PPARgamma	25%–50%
PIK3CA	<10%
PTEN	<10%

(Continued)

TABLE 21-6	MOLECULAR PATHOLOGY AND CYTOGENETICS OF THYROID ADENOMAS AND CARCINOMAS (continued)	
Poorly differentiated carcinomas		
RAS	35%	
Beta-Catenin (CTNNB1)	20%	
TP53	20%	
BRAF	20%	
AKT1	15%	
Anaplastic carcinoma		
TP53	70%	
Beta-Catenin (CTNNB1)	60%	
RAS	50%	
BRAF	20%	
PIK3CA	20%	
PTEN	>10%	
Medullary carcinoma		
Familial forms:	RET	>95%
Sporadic forms:	RET	50%

prior neoplasm in the head and neck. In one study, the average interval between the delivery of radiation and the diagnosis of carcinoma was 8.5 years, with approximately 75% of patients exposed between 3.5 and 14 years before the development of the carcinoma. An increased prevalence of thyroid cancer with the signature *RET/PTC* gene rearrangement was detected in children as early as 4 years after exposure to radiation fallout from the Chernobyl nuclear reactor explosion in 1986. Ten to thirty percent of children with PTC and no history of radiation exposure demonstrate *RET/PTC* gene rearrangement in contrast to 50% to 70% in children with a history of radiation exposure (86). Nonneoplastic abnormalities such as multinodularity, fibrosis, and lymphocytic infiltrates have also been reported in the thyroid gland after prior neck irradiation.

PTC, as well as follicular adenoma and carcinoma, is found in association with MAS and MEN1 (parathyroid hyperplasia, islet cell hyperplasia, and pituitary adenoma) but not with MEN2a or MEN2b, in which MTC is the rule (Table 21-2). Other familial settings of non-MTC are Carney complex, familial adenomatous polyposis (FAP), and Cowden syndrome (Table 21-2) (59).

The gross features of PTC are variable from one or more solid, gray–tan nodules; dense, poorly circumscribed areas of fibrosis; cyst(s) with a mural nodule; or solid, red glistening nodule(s) with a fibrous capsule (Figure 21-15A, B). Calcifications or ossification may be present. The classic type and follicular variant of PTC usually present as relatively well-circumscribed tumors, whereas the diffuse sclerosing variant may manifest as dense tumor and fibrosis, replacing the majority of the thyroid parenchyma and often extending into the surrounding soft tissues including skeletal muscle. This variant, though uncommon, is seen more often in children than in adults. Among PTCs in children, the classic type, follicular variant, and sclerosing variant were present in 11%, 35%, and 8% of cases, respectively, and among adolescents, 26%, 28%, and 2% of cases, respectively.

Classic PTC is composed of branching fronds or papillae with fibrovascular cores lined by neoplastic follicular epithelial cells (Figure 21-15C, eFigure 21-66). Classically, nuclei are enlarged, elongated, crowded, and overlapping, often with prominent nuclear grooves or folds, peripheral margination of chromatin with central clearing (optically clear or "Orphan Annie" nuclei), and cytoplasmic invaginations or intranuclear cytoplasmic pseudoinclusions (Figure 21-15D, eFigure 21-67). Small concentric whorls of calcification (psammoma bodies) are present more commonly in the classic type and sclerosing variant of PTC than in other variants, especially follicular variant (Figure 21-15E). Multifocal gross lesions, but more commonly multiple microscopic foci of PTC, are identified in the ipsilateral and the contralateral lobe in 20% to 25% of cases. The latter finding is the rationale for subtotal to total thyroidectomy.

Squamous metaplasia is a feature of PTC in the pediatric age group, especially in the diffuse sclerosing and cribriform–morular variants (59). The diffuse sclerosing variant is also characterized by a desmoplastic or sclerotic stroma, lymphovascular invasion, diffuse psammoma bodies, and lymphocytic thyroiditis. Although diffuse involvement of the thyroid gland is common, it is not required for diagnosis, and a dominant nodule may be present (104). Despite high rates of extrathyroidal extension and regional lymph node metastases, prognosis remains good (>90% 5-year survival) following treatment with total thyroidectomy, bilateral lymph node dissection, and, in some cases, radioactive iodine. Cribriform–morular variant, as its name suggests, is characterized by a cribriform follicular architecture as well as squamous morules. Beta-catenin mutation appears to play a role in tumorigenesis, both in FAP and sporadic cases (105). Nuclear reactivity for beta-catenin may assist in the diagnosis and prompt screening for FAP.

The follicular variant of PTC is comprised exclusively of follicles with nuclear features of PTC. It can be encapsulated, well circumscribed but unencapsulated, or invasive (vascular, capsular, or intrathyroidal invasion). The encapsulated and well-circumscribed types tend to behave in an indolent manner in the absence of any invasive growth. The invasive type is more likely to have hematogenous rather than lymphatic metastases, similar to follicular carcinoma. These tumors tend to harbor RAS mutations, also similar to FTC (106,107).

Lymphocytic infiltration of nonneoplastic thyroid is a common feature in PTC regardless of age, and its presence has been associated with an improved prognosis (100). Regional lymph node metastasis varies from 30% to 80% of cases. Pulmonary metastasis is found in 6% to 8% of pediatric cases at diagnosis (96,100), although some series report a higher incidence (96).

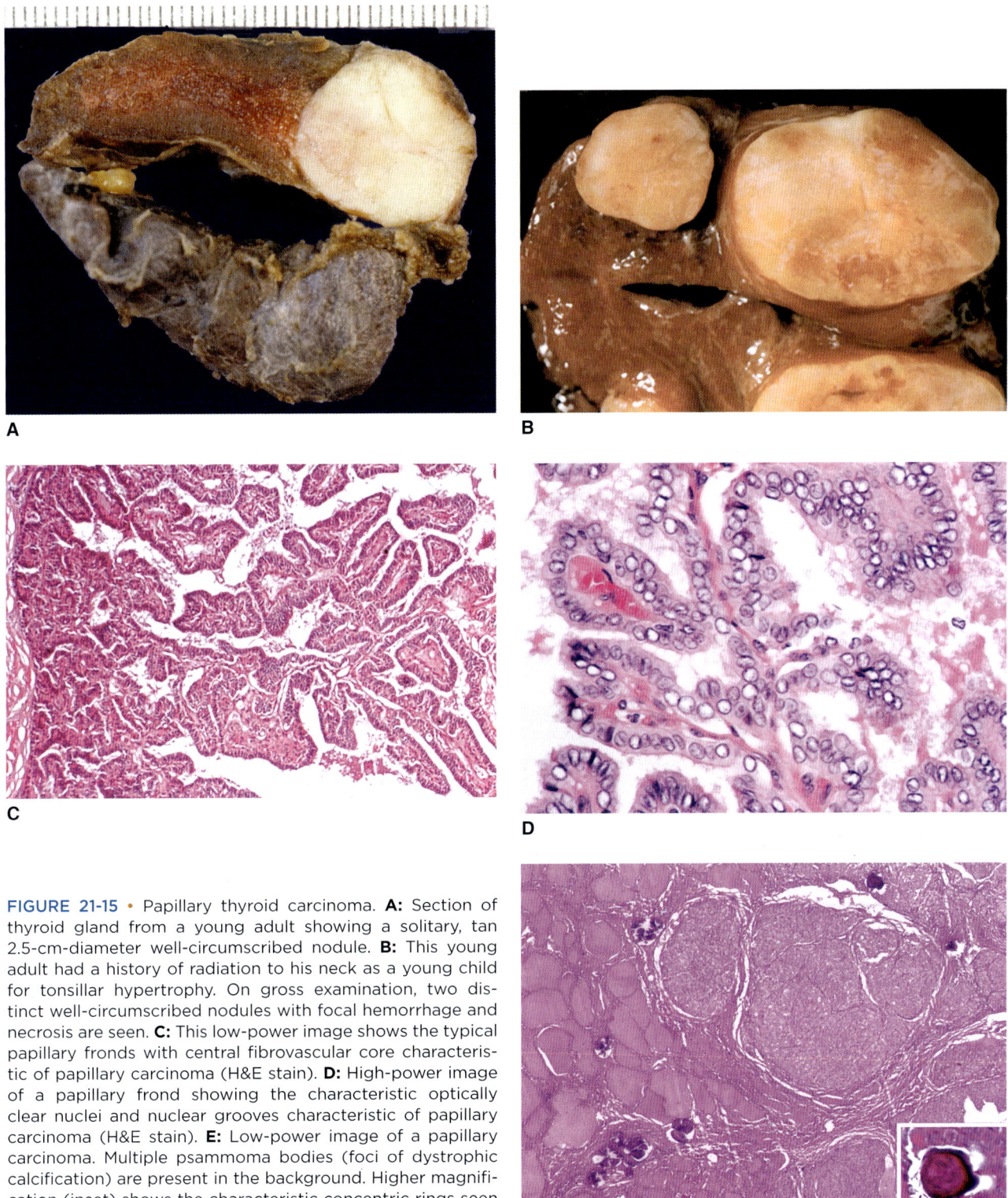

FIGURE 21-15 • Papillary thyroid carcinoma. **A:** Section of thyroid gland from a young adult showing a solitary, tan 2.5-cm-diameter well-circumscribed nodule. **B:** This young adult had a history of radiation to his neck as a young child for tonsillar hypertrophy. On gross examination, two distinct well-circumscribed nodules with focal hemorrhage and necrosis are seen. **C:** This low-power image shows the typical papillary fronds with central fibrovascular core characteristic of papillary carcinoma (H&E stain). **D:** High-power image of a papillary frond showing the characteristic optically clear nuclei and nuclear grooves characteristic of papillary carcinoma (H&E stain). **E:** Low-power image of a papillary carcinoma. Multiple psammoma bodies (foci of dystrophic calcification) are present in the background. Higher magnification (inset) shows the characteristic concentric rings seen in a psammoma body. Their presence strongly suggests a diagnosis of papillary carcinoma (H&E stain).

The diagnosis of pediatric thyroid cancer is made for the most part on specific histopathologic criteria. Immunohistochemistry is not usually necessary in most cases of non-MTC although the occasional solid PTC or FTC may require differentiation from MTC. The tumor cells in PTC are immunoreactive for cytokeratins, thyroglobulin, TTF-1 (thyroid transcription factor-1), and PAX-8 (59). Additional immunostaining for high molecular weight cytokeratins (including CK-19), thyroglobulin, galectin-3, HBME1, and RET may be helpful in difficult cases. Staining for RET/PTC rearrangements has been utilized, but availability of sensitive antibodies is a limiting factor (59).

The prognosis in children with PTC is excellent despite the presence of local extrathyroidal spread (40% to 50% of cases) and lymph node metastasis. The presence of invasion in the soft tissues of the neck from the primary or extranodal site contributes substantially to the local morbidity of the disease.

The extent of disease and age at diagnosis are important prognostic features. Management is surgical resection in most cases with additional modalities in some cases (96). Prognostically unfavorable histologic variants of PTC are uncommon in children, such as tall cell and poorly differentiated variants. Postoperative staging is based on a combination of factors. The MACIS (metastasis–age–completeness of resection–invasion–size) system has been found useful in children (96). In children less than 10 years of age, PTC is more locally aggressive and more likely to have pulmonary metastasis. Overall, the long-term survival rate for PTC is excellent in children with a 98% 10-year survival, regardless of the pathologic stage.

Follicular neoplasms of the thyroid present several problems in pathologic diagnosis without regard for age. One of the less consequential ones is the differentiation of a follicular adenoma from a dominant nodule of multinodular or adenomatous hyperplasia. In some cases, it is a distinction without a difference in terms of prognosis. Follicular lesions diagnosed pathologically as an adenoma have a delicate continuous or interrupted fibrous capsule (eFigure 21-68). Follicular adenoma is a sporadically occurring tumor in most cases in children, but is reported in young individuals with Cowden syndrome (PTEN mutation) and pleuropulmonary blastoma familial tumor predisposition syndrome (DICER1 mutation).

FTC is less common in children (3% to 20%) than in adults (5% to 10%). In the past, follicular carcinoma (25% to 40%) accounted for a higher proportion of thyroid cancers in endemic regions with iodine deficiency. FTC is diagnosed pathologically, not on the basis of nuclear features, which are often quite bland, but on the presence of a well-defined, thickened fibrous capsule with preferably more than one focus of transcapsular invasion as a "mushroom" of neoplastic follicles protruding through the capsule. Intracapsular "trickling" of tumor cells does not count as true capsular invasion, but may be confused with minimally invasive FTC. Vascular invasion in the capsule is another diagnostic feature, but there should be endothelialization of tumor cells with adherence of tumor cells to the endothelium or associated thrombosis. Free floating tumor cells within the vascular space or subendothelial bulging into a vascular space should not count as true vascular invasion (Figure 21-16A–C to C, eFigure 21-69). It is common to

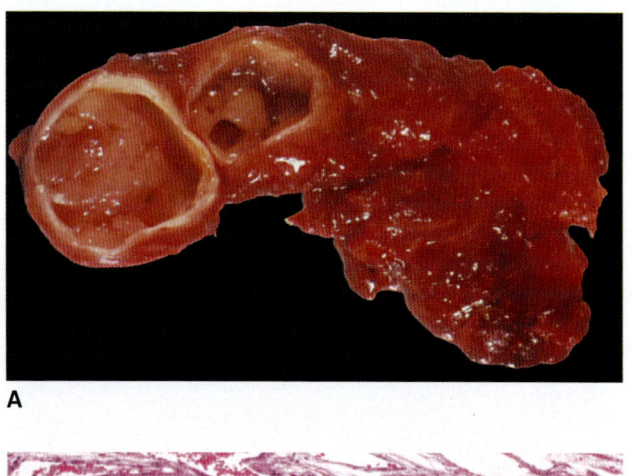

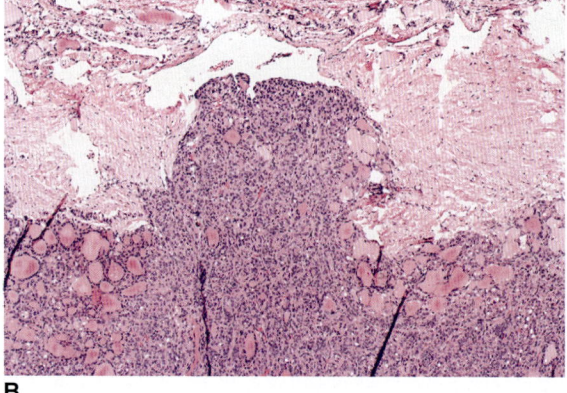

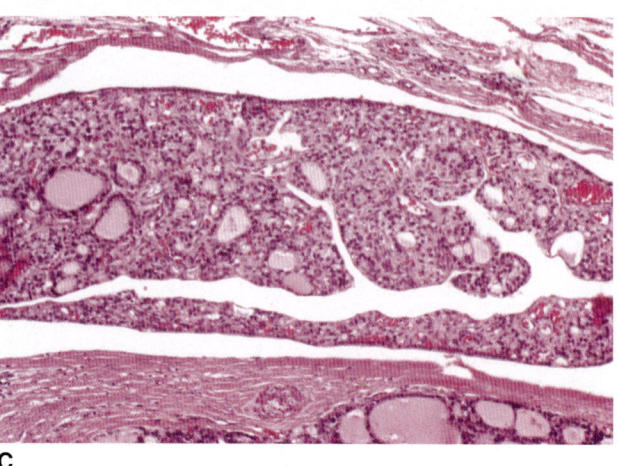

FIGURE 21-16 • Follicular thyroid carcinoma. **A:** This section of thyroid gland shows a well-circumscribed nodule with a thick irregular capsule within the thyroid parenchyma. The neoplasm was composed of small well-defined follicles on histologic examination. No well-formed papillae or psammoma bodies were present. The nuclei did not have the optically clear appearance or nuclear grooves characteristic of the follicular variant of papillary carcinoma. **B,C:** Invasion of the adjacent capsule and blood vessels was present (H&E stain).

identify groups of follicles pressing on vascular spaces in a follicular adenoma or dominant adenomatous nodule, which should not be interpreted as vascular invasion. An accurate diagnosis of an encapsulated, well-differentiated FTC often requires sampling of the entire fibrous capsule with well-oriented sections and the use of deeper levels to evaluate suspicious foci and confirm true capsular or vascular invasion. FTCs have been divided into minimally invasive and widely invasive tumors. Minimally invasive follicular cancers have a gross appearance that is similar to follicular adenomas, except for possessing irregular, thickened capsules. These tumors demonstrate focal capsular and/or vascular invasion. This term has also been used for tumor with only focal vascular invasion (<4 vessels). Another term that may be used for this tumor is grossly encapsulated angioinvasive follicular carcinoma, when only vascular invasion outside the capsule is present. FTC is immunoreactive for low molecular weight cytokeratins, thyroglobulin, TTF-1, and PAX-8 (108).

Poorly differentiated carcinomas are distinct yet uncommon neoplasms in children. They are defined by (a) solid, trabecular, or insular growth, (b) absence of papillary nuclei, and (c) presence of at least one of the following: "convoluted" (or dark and wrinkled) nuclei, mitotic activity greater than or equal to 3 per 10 HPF, or necrosis (109). These tumors usually present as well-defined neoplasms with invasion often appreciated during gross examination.

In general, intraoperative frozen section examination to diagnose carcinoma is not recommended and often adds no additional information to that gained by preoperative fine-needle aspiration (110). The characteristic nuclei of PTC are often destroyed by freezing artifact. If frozen section is requested for a thyroid nodule, smears or touch preparations are integral to identify nuclear features of the lesion. Nuclear enlargement, grooves, clearing, and pseudoinclusions seen on cytology may provide support to a suspicious frozen section. Furthermore, the distinction between follicular adenoma and FTC requires evaluation of multiple blocks of tumor with capsule and often multiple levels through individual blocks, which is unsuitable for frozen section analysis.

MTC in children occurs almost exclusively in the familial setting (Tables 21-2 and 21-6) with or without the other features of MEN2a (diffuse parathyroid hyperplasia and PHEO) or MEN2b (PHEO, intestinal ganglioneuromatosis, and mucosal neuromas). Medullary carcinomas are derived from the C-cells or parafollicular cells, which secrete calcitonin. The C-cells originate from the lateral thyroid anlage of the 4th branchial pouch, whereas the follicular cells of the thyroid are derived from the median anlage. C-cell hyperplasia occurs as a precursor lesion in hereditary syndromes that have predisposition to medullary carcinoma and other endocrine and nonendocrine tumors.

Only 1% to 3% of differentiated thyroid carcinomas in children are MTCs, except in some specialized medical centers (73,86). Sporadic MTCs, which are palpable, unifocal neoplasms without C-cell hyperplasia, account for 80% to 90% of all MTCs in the general population; however, they are uncommon in children. The aggressive nature of MTC is evident in adults who have regional lymph node metastasis in at least 50% of cases and distant metastasis (lung, liver) in 15% of cases at diagnosis (59). It is noteworthy that approximately 20% of adults with apparent sporadic MTCs have germline *RET* mutations with its obvious familial implications (96). In addition, loss of heterozygosity of 11p (40%), 3p (30%), 3q (40%), 11p (11%), 13q (10%), 17p (8%), and 22q (30%) has been shown by cytogenetics and comparative genomic hybridization with sporadic tumors.

Syndromic-associated MTCs in children are typically small, often microscopic, multifocal tumors in association with diffuse C-cell hyperplasia in the upper two-thirds of the lateral lobes (e493). The small size of the tumor or tumors in syndromic MTC is in part a reflection of genetic screening of children in affected kindreds using molecular diagnostic techniques. Virtually, all resected thyroids in the setting of MEN2a, MEN2b, and FMTC have microscopic multifocal C-cell hyperplasia, if not microscopic or grossly visible tumors.

On gross examination, MTCs present as well-circumscribed or infiltrative masses that are gray–white to tan. The individual tumors range from 1 mm or less to 4 to 5 cm in diameter (Figure 21-17A, B). Histologic architecture varies from nested or trabecular to solid. Whether the tumor cells are epithelioid or spindled, nuclei are usually round to oval with finely dispersed chromatin and a prominent nucleolus. There are also small-cell and pigmented variants of MTC. Mitotic activity and anaplasia are inapparent in most cases. Intersecting bands of fibrosis and/or amyloid stroma are generally found in tumors larger than 2 cm in diameter (Figure 21-17C, eFigure 21-70).

One of the challenges in syndromic cases is the differentiation between C-cell hyperplasia and microscopic MTC. The degree and extent of C-cell hyperplasia can vary markedly from one prophylactic thyroidectomy to another. Foci of C-cell hyperplasia (defined as 50 C-cells per low-power field) can be relatively inconspicuous without the assistance of immunohistochemistry. In other cases, the C-cell hyperplasia is not only apparent but also extensive to the degree that there is concern about microscopic MTC. Hyperplasia is recognized by a collection of C-cells partially filling the colloid space of the follicle and/or bulging into the perifollicular, interstitial space without breaching of the basement membrane of the follicle, which is not always readily apparent. A microscopic MTC has a similar bulging growth pattern from the follicle as C-cell hyperplasia. More importantly, there is interstitial infiltration and the displacement of contiguous follicles or coalescence of aggregates of enlarged atypical cells. The tumor cells are larger than those of the surrounding smaller hyperplastic C-cells, and the nucleoli are prominent in comparison to the inapparent or micronucleoli of the hyperplastic C-cells.

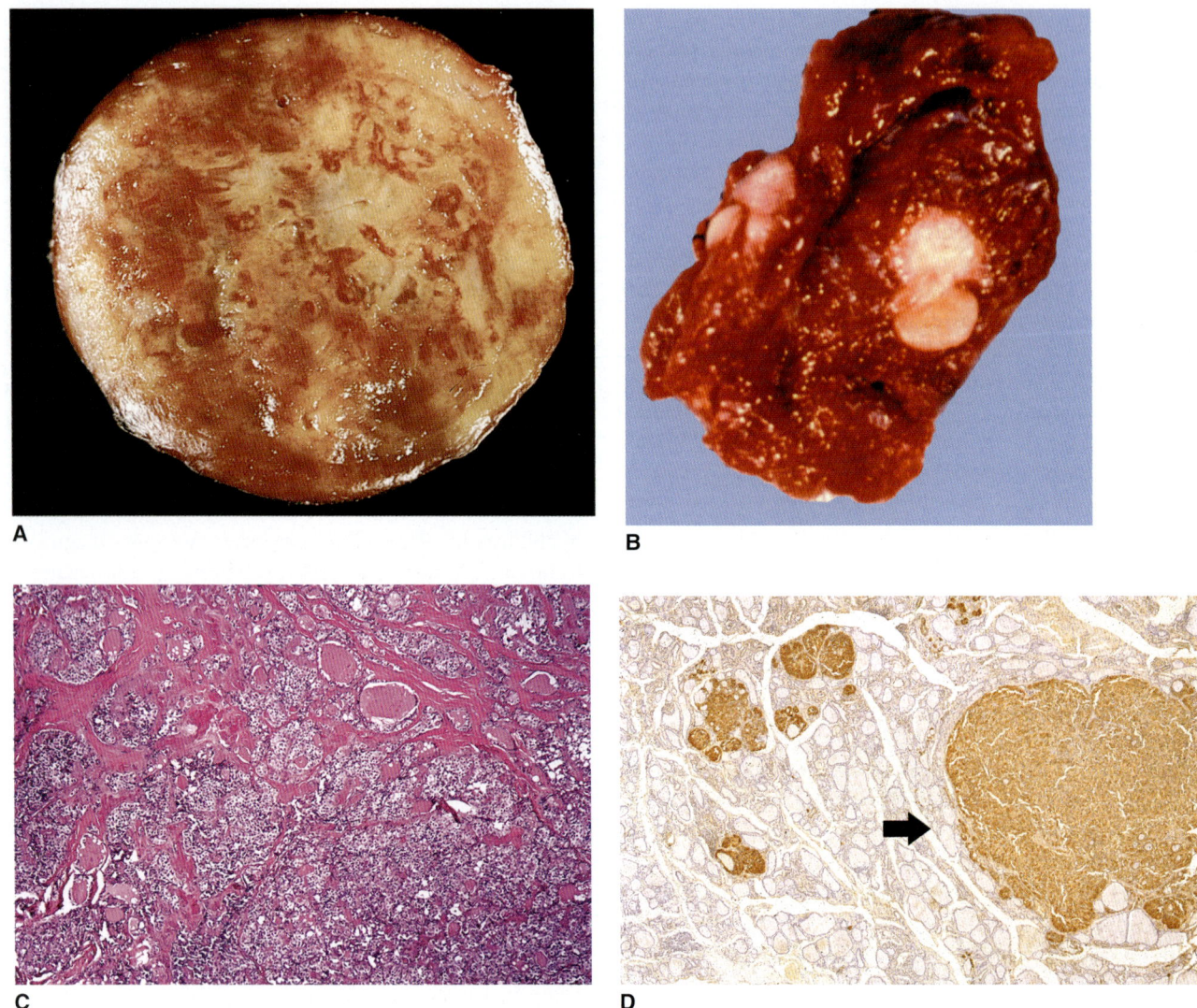

FIGURE 21-17 • Medullary thyroid carcinoma. **A:** This image from a sporadic (nonsyndromic) medullary carcinoma shows a large tan–yellow, nonencapsulated mass that had a firm gritty consistency on sectioning. **B:** Syndromic medullary carcinoma tends to be small and multifocal. This 0.4 cm in diameter tumor nodule (**right**) in a patient with MEN2 is demarcated from the red–brown thyroid parenchyma. A smaller nodule of medullary carcinoma (**left**) is also seen. **C:** This tumor on low power demonstrates the characteristic lobular pattern. Nests of tumor cells with round nuclei were surrounded by bands of connective tissue. The round to polygonal tumor cells has an abundant eosinophilic or clear cytoplasm. The nuclei are predominantly round to oval with coarse chromatin. The cells were immunoreactive for calcitonin (H&E stain). **D:** This section of thyroid gland from a child with MEN2 shows a small focus of medullary carcinoma (arrow) and several foci of C-cell hyperplasia that were immunoreactive for calcitonin (immunostain for calcitonin).

Immunohistochemical staining for calcitonin is helpful in the identification of inconspicuous foci of C-cell hyperplasia or in the confirmation of the thyroid carcinoma as MTC (Figure 21-17D, eFigure 21-71). C-cells and MTC are also immunoreactive for SYN, CHR, and CEA (84). TTF-1 and PAX-8 can be weakly positive in a subset of MTCs, in contrast to the strong positivity in tumors of follicular cell origin (111). In keeping with the distribution of C-cells in the thyroid, hyperplasia and MTC have a predilection for the upper two-thirds of the lateral lobes. It is helpful to submit multiple sections consecutively from the superior to the inferior pole of the resected gland.

Early prophylactic thyroidectomy with lymph node dissection and serum calcitonin levels in children with germline *RET* mutations is the recommended management (87). Based on the specific *RET* codon involved, specific risk groups have been established with recommended surgical intervention dependent on the risk group (87,96). In young children, most cases of MTC are associated with MEN2b. For this reason, thyroidectomy is recommended as soon as possible in MEN2b *RET*-positive infants, whereas in MEN2a, surgery is recommended between 3 and 5 years of age (87). For children with constitutional (germline*)* *RET* oncogene mutations, thyroidectomy is recommended at specific ages as follows: at 6 months of age for mutations in codon 883, 918, and 922; by age 5 years for mutations in codons 611, 618, 620, and 634; and between 5 and 10 years of age for mutations in codons 609,630, 768, 790,791, 804, and 891. Prognosis is dependent on stage and postoperative calcitonin levels. Syndromic MTC with total thyroidectomy and negative postoperative serum calcitonin levels at 6 and 12 months postsurgery have a recurrence rate of 5% and a 10-year survival rate of 98% (96). Poor prognostic risk factors are older age, male gender, and degree of local invasion. Individuals with sporadic microcarcinomas (<1 cm) have improved survival compared with individuals with tumors greater than 1cm in diameter. With MTC, the serum markers calcitonin and CEA may be followed to evaluate for residual or recurrent disease. Molecular targeted therapy may prove to be of benefit for those with residual or recurrent disease in the future.

Cervical–thyroidal teratoma (CTT) accounts for up to 3% of thyroid resections in children especially in the infancy period. Approximately 2% to 5% of germ-cell neoplasms in children present in the head and neck region, and the anterior portion of the neck including the thyroid gland is one of several specific sites in this anatomic region. There is an equal male to female ratio (112,113). These tumors are typically congenital and are not subtle clinically given their size. Byard et al. reported that 6 of 14 (43%) of cases were detected in stillborn infants or neonates who died within 2 days of birth. Compression of the upper airway is the major complication requiring early surgical intervention. A minority of cases are known to present beyond infancy. The mass fills the soft tissues of the anterior and lateral portions of the neck. Attachment to the thyroid is not always demonstrable due to the size and extensive replacement of normal tissues. Grossly, these tumors are soft and often cystic, measuring several centimeters in greatest dimension and microscopically are composed of a range of immature and mature somatic elements. Immature neuroepithelium with primitive neural tubules and sheets of neuroblasts are often the dominant microscopic pattern and should not be mistaken for neuroblastoma (NB), which can present in the cervical region but more lateral and with an exclusive neuroblastic appearance, usually poorly differentiated NB. One confounding aspect is the presence of immature or mature teratoma in regional lymph nodes in some cases, which may be referred to as "nodal gliomatosis" or nodal "deposits" rather than metastases. The excellent clinical outcome of CTT is usually not affected by the presence of nodal deposits. As in sacrococcygeal teratomas, microscopic foci of endodermal sinus may be detected. If these foci of endodermal sinus tumor represent only a minor component and are not in regional lymph nodes, an excellent prognosis may be affected in only a marginal fashion, but the decision about further management is complex.

ADRENAL GLANDS

The cortex of the adrenal gland is derived from the adrenogonadal primordium that develops from the urogenital ridge (43,57). WT1 and WNT4 genes play an early role in development, along with steroidogenic factor 1 (transcription factor) and a nuclear hormone receptor gene (DAX1, Xp21). Growth and maturation of the gland is also dependent on ACTH stimulation. The fetal cortex zone develops and is followed by the more peripheral definitive adult cortex zone. During the first 3 months of life, the fetal zone undergoes apoptosis and is replaced entirely by the adult zone. The adult zone forms the zona glomerulosa (mineralocorticoids, aldosterone), zona fasciculata (glucocorticoids, cortisol), and zona reticularis (androgens). Zonation is complete by the second decade of life. The medulla is derived from neural crest cells that migrate into the developing medial portion of the adrenocortical primordium during the 8th week. The neural crest cells are sympathetic postganglionic cells of the autonomic nervous system. The medulla is comprised of pheochromocytes. These are polygonal cells with eosinophilic granular cytoplasm and possess neurosecretory granules containing epinephrine and norepinephrine. The endocrine nature of the adrenal medulla is demonstrated by the rich capillary network that is closely associated with the clusters of pheochromocytes. These cells are concentrated in the head of the adrenal gland and not uniformly distributed throughout the medulla.

The adrenal glands are composed of an outer cortex and an inner medulla. Functionally, they are two separate endocrine organs, with the cortex responsible for steroid hormone synthesis and the medulla for catecholamine production. In children and adolescents, the pyramidal-shaped right and crescent-shaped left adrenal glands have an average combined weight of 4 to 6 g, similar to adults with combined adrenal weights ranging between 2 and 8 g (114,115). There is no difference in the weight of the adrenals between male and female children. A coarse connective tissue capsule with attached periadrenal fat surrounds the gland. The fat in the vicinity of the adrenals has immature features of finely vacuolated adipocytes in infants resembling those of a lipoblastoma. On sectioning, the adrenal cortex consists of a yellow subcapsular layer that corresponds to the zona glomerulosa and zona fasciculata. A thin brown layer, the zona reticularis, separates the zona fasciculata from the gray–white central medulla. The adrenals receive their blood supply from the inferior phrenic artery, aorta, and renal artery.

In the fetus, a prominent provisional (fetal) cortex is present. Adrenal weight ranges upward with the gestational age. There is rapid growth of the provisional cortex during the third trimester. The average combined weight of the adrenals is about 2 g at 30 weeks' gestation compared to 6 g at birth in a term infant. Following birth, the provisional cortex involutes and rapidly disappears, leaving the permanent cortex and central medulla (114) (see Appendices: *Weights of Organs of 1- to 12-Month-old Girls* and *Weights of Organs of 1- to 12Month-old Boys*). The involuted remnant of the fetal cortex can be observed throughout the first 6 months of life. In the newborn, the adrenal gland on sectioning has a dark red–brown appearance beneath a thin yellow cortical rim due to degeneration of the provisional cortex. The adrenal medulla, which makes up less than 1% of the fetal adrenal compared with 10% of the adult adrenal, is generally not recognized on gross examination.

The definitive adrenal cortex is divided into three distinct zones. The zona glomerulosa, which accounts for approximately 10% of the adult adrenal gland, consists of islands of haphazardly distributed cells beneath the connective tissue capsule. Individual cells contain small amounts of eosinophilic cytoplasm and have rounded nuclei. The zona fasciculata located beneath the zona glomerulosa accounts for 70% to 80% of the adult adrenal cortex and consists of large polyhedral, lipid-laden cells arranged in columns 1- to 2-cells thick separated by thin sinusoidal capillaries in the nonstressed adrenal gland. The nuclei are round, pale staining, and occasionally binucleated. The zona reticularis, which accounts for less than 10% of the cortex, consists of anastomosing cords of small eosinophilic cells with deeply staining closely apposed nuclei. The adrenal medulla, which occupies the center of the gland, consists of large, pale staining, polyhedral cells, known as chromaffin cells (pheochromocytes), which are arranged in cords and small islands. These cells are innervated by preganglionic sympathetic nerve fibers and are modified postganglionic neurons.

In the fetus, the provisional (fetal) zone accounts for 70% to 80% of the total weight of the gland (eFigure 21-72). The fetal zone is composed of cords of large eosinophilic cells surrounded by sinusoidal capillaries and located beneath the permanent cortex. A distinct adrenal medulla is not identifiable in the fetal gland. Chromaffin cells are haphazardly scattered throughout the fetal cortex. In fact, neuroblastic cells from the neural crest migrate through the cortex as individual and small nests of primitive-appearing cells. These cells should not be interpreted as evidence of congenital NB.

The adrenal cortex is responsible for the synthesis of three classes of steroids, glucocorticoids, mineralocorticoids, and androgens. A series of cytochrome P450 enzymes are involved in adrenal steroid synthesis (eFigure 21-73). The rate-limiting step is the transfer of cholesterol from the cytosol across the mitochondrial membrane. Several proteins, including the steroidogenic acute regulatory protein (StAR) induced by ACTH, are involved in this rate-limiting step. In response to ACTH stimulation, cholesterol is metabolized through a series of enzymatic steps in the zona fasciculata and reticularis into cortisol, the major glucocorticoid (eFigure 21-74). Once secreted, cortisol provides negative feedback on the pituitary gland to inhibit further ACTH secretion. Aldosterone is synthesized in the zona glomerulosa and is a mineralocorticoid. Dihydroepiandrosteindione sulfate is the primary androgen and is synthesized in the zona reticularis. During early fetal development, androgens of adrenal origin are responsible for differentiation of the male external genitalia.

The catecholamines, epinephrine, and norepinephrine are formed from tyrosine and secreted in response to sympathetic neural stimulation by the chromaffin cells. Extensive reviews of adrenal steroidogenesis and catecholamine production are beyond the scope of this chapter, but reviewed elsewhere (90,114,116).

Adrenal glands may have many different types of lesions originating from either the cortical component or the medullary component. In children, the most common diagnosis is neuroblastoma (45%) followed by adrenal cortical neoplasms (27%), benign adrenal cysts (12%), WT by direct extension or intra-adrenal location (4%), and PHEO (3%). Other uncommon primary adrenal tumors include soft tissue tumors (3%), teratoma (1%), pigmented micronodular hyperplasia (1%), and hemangioma (1%) (43,57).

Imaging

The visualization of the adrenal glands in infants is accomplished optimally by US. In older children, US is useful as a screening method for an adrenal mass. If an adrenal mass is discovered, further imaging with MR or CT is indicated.

The normal adrenal glands of an infant on US are Y- or V-shaped on longitudinal images. The medulla is seen as an echogenic (bright) central line surrounded by the thin hypoechoic (dark) cortex. A long straight adrenal gland may be seen in cases of renal agenesis or ectopia. In the presence of congenital adrenal hyperplasia (CAH), the adrenal glands are enlarged with an abnormal undulating surface and/or replacement of the central echogenic line by a stippled pattern throughout the gland (117). An adrenal mass in the neonate tends to be a hemorrhagic mass, congenital cystic or solid NB, or cystic mass. In the case of adrenal hemorrhage, US provides the most useful modality in the follow-up period without the need for CT or MR (118). The echogenicity of the hemorrhage varies with the age of the hemorrhage and is usually heterogeneous. No flow is demonstrated to the mass on Doppler evaluation. On follow-up examination, the mass becomes smaller and more hypoechoic (dark) over time. The adrenal gland may become calcified, appearing as a dense focus with posterior acoustic shadowing (118). NB should be suspected if the mass fails to decrease in size on short-interval follow-up. It should be noted that NBs in neonates are more likely to be cystic than in older children. Cystic NBs may become smaller over time, but do not entirely resolve as does cystic hemorrhage. Calcifications may be identified in

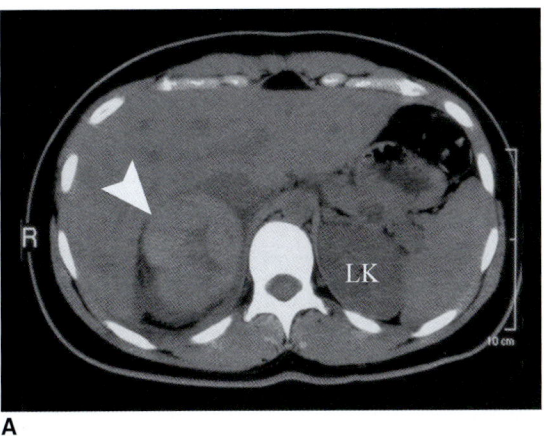
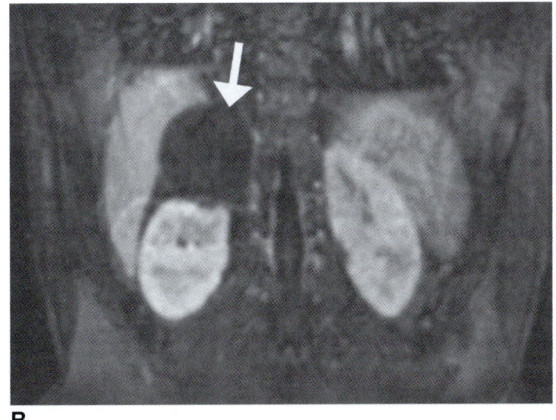
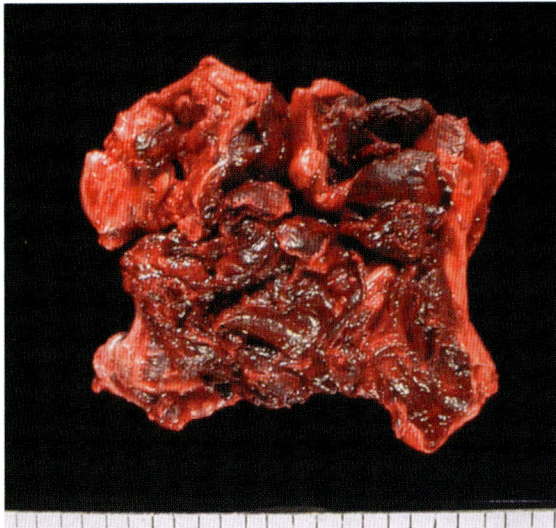

FIGURE 21-18 • **A:** Hemorrhagic adrenal cyst in an 18-year-old girl. Axial unenhanced CT image shows a mass in the right suprarenal region (*arrowhead*), which is denser than the left kidney (LK) indicating acute hemorrhage. **B:** Coronal postgadolinium T1-weighted image showing no enhancement of the cyst (*arrow*) above the enhancing right kidney. **C:** Image of the sectioned resected specimen showing hemorrhage.

both lesions. The neonate may present with the characteristic pattern of metastases of stage 4S disease with diffuse involvement of the liver, skin nodules, and bone marrow infiltration. Adrenal cysts have a varied appearance on imaging depending on the presence or absence of hemorrhage or infection. Simple cysts are anechoic (black) on US and show fluid attenuation on CT or MR. Hemorrhage or infection causes a heterogeneous appearance to the internal structure of the cyst, and the wall of the cyst may be calcified (Figure 21-18A–C).

If an adrenal mass is initially discovered by US, further imaging with CT or MR is necessary to further characterize the mass. The imaging appearance of adrenocortical tumors on US, CT, and MR depends on their size (119). Small tumors tend to appear homogeneous, whereas with larger tumors, central necrosis, calcification, or scar causes a heterogeneous appearance (Figure 21-19, eFigure 21-75). Local spread or metastatic disease may indicate an aggressive tumor. Evaluation for extension into the vena cava is necessary.

NB typically appears as a greater than 2-cm mass in most cases (Figure 21-20). Calcifications are relatively frequent, which is particularly evident on CT, but may also be seen on US as echogenic foci possibly with posterior acoustic shadowing. Cystic areas from old hemorrhage or cystic or

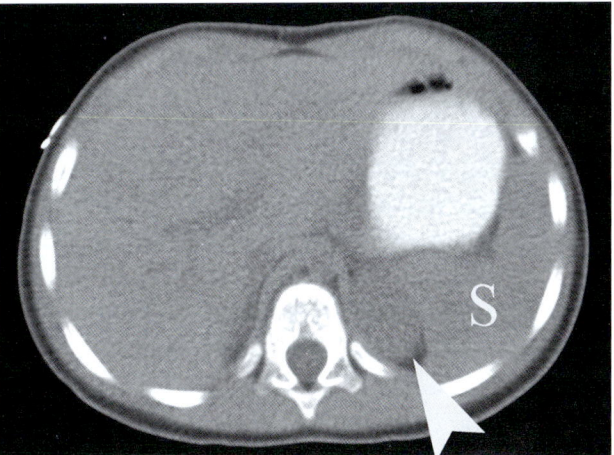

FIGURE 21-19 • Adrenal cortical tumor in 18-month-old girl with virilization. CT image without intravenous contrast material shows a mass in the region of the left adrenal fossa (*arrowhead*) adjacent to the spleen (S).

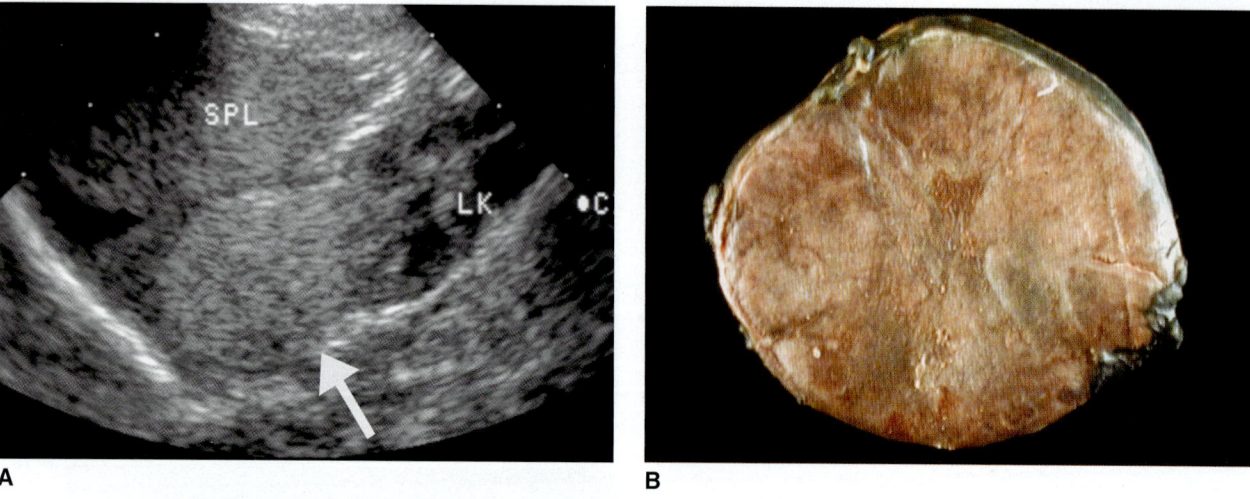

FIGURE 21-20 • Neuroblastoma in 2-month-old boy. **A:** Longitudinal ultrasound image demonstrating a homogeneous mass (arrow) between the upper pole of the left kidney (LK) and the spleen (SPL). **B:** The sectioned gross specimen shows a homogeneous yellowish–tan tumor and calcifications.

necrotic changes are anechoic (black) on US and have fluid attenuation on CT and MR. With contrast material, the tumor generally enhances heterogeneously. CT and MR are useful in evaluating the extent of disease. The primary tumor frequently crosses the midline and surrounds the aorta and other vessels (Figure 21-21). Adjacent organ involvement may be seen and enlarged lymph nodes and liver metastases may be identified (Figure 21-22). MR is particularly useful in demonstrating neural foramen and spinal canal invasion (eFigure 21-76). PHEO appears as a soft tissue mass on CT with homogeneous, heterogeneous, or rim-like enhancement postcontrast (119). On MR, PHEOs are hypointense (dark) on T1-weighted images and hyperintense on T2-weighted images. Postgadolinium images typically show intense enhancement with slow washout (Figure 21-23) (120). As lesions are frequently multiple, the radionuclide scan using ^{131}I-MIBG may be helpful in the preoperative localization of lesions.

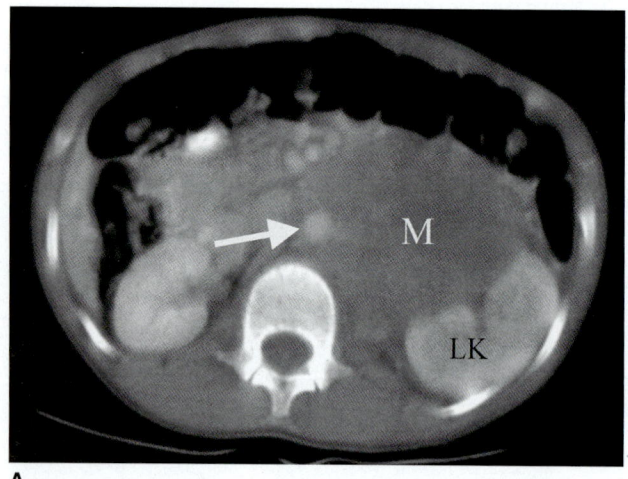

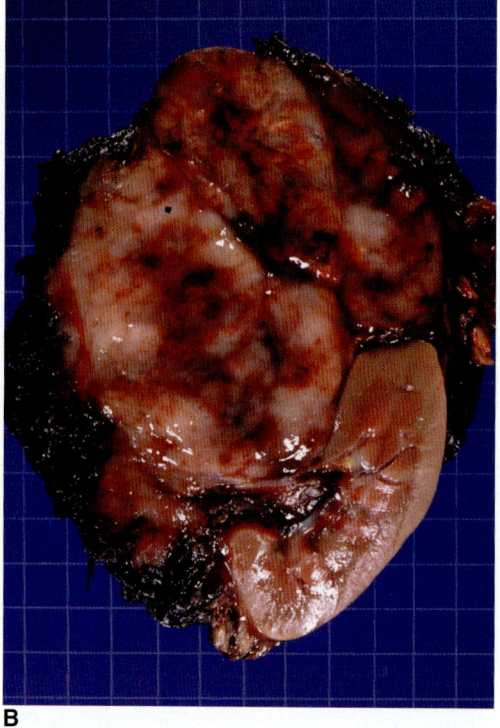

FIGURE 21-21 • Neuroblastoma in 9-month-old boy. **A:** Contrast-enhanced CT image of the abdomen demonstrates a mass (M) pushing the left kidney (LK) laterally and surrounding the aorta (arrow). **B:** The sectioned gross specimen shows a multinodular, whitish–tan tumor with hemorrhage.

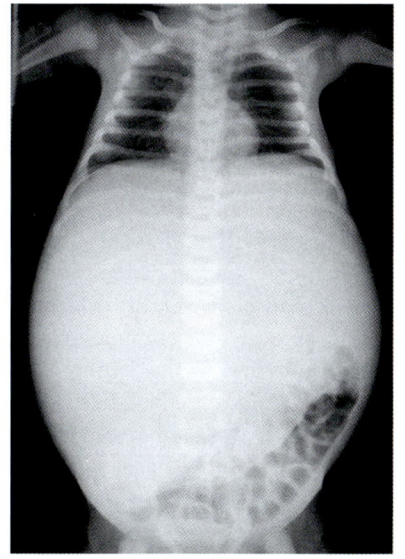
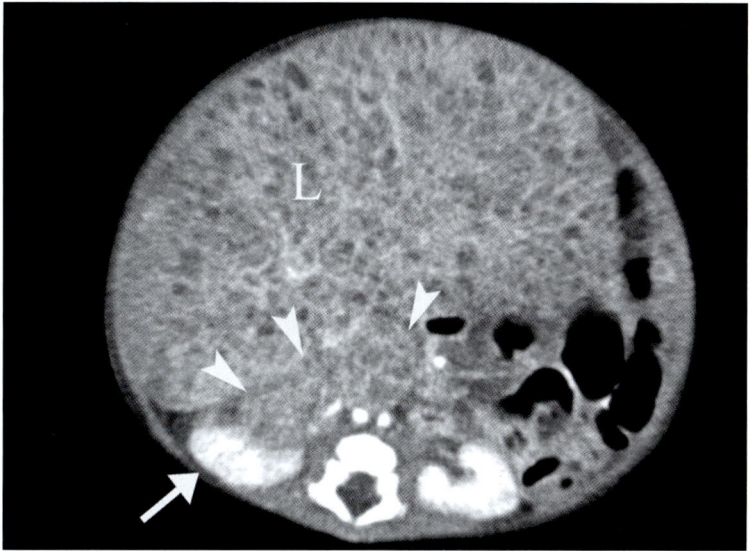
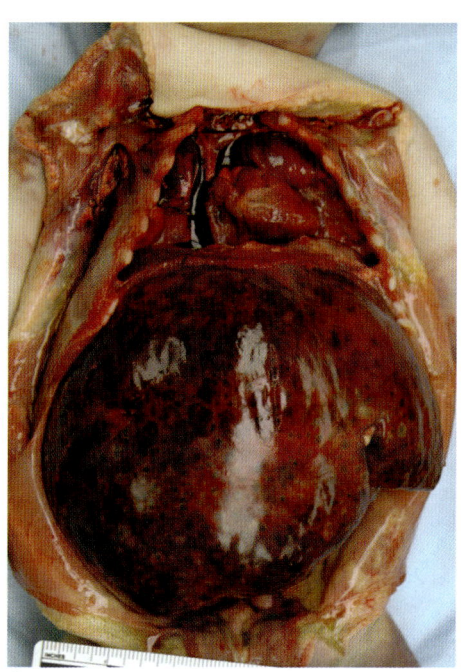

FIGURE 21-22 • Congenital stage 4 neuroblastoma with Pepper syndrome. **A:** KUB shows marked enlargement of the liver pushing up on the hemidiaphragms and pushing the air-filled bowel to the left lower quadrant. **B:** Contrast-enhanced CT scan of the abdomen shows a markedly enlarged liver diffusely infiltrated with small hypoattenuating masses (L). Anterior to the right kidney (*arrow*) is an adrenal mass (*arrowheads*). **C:** Massive hepatomegaly reflects the diffuse infiltration by neuroblastoma.

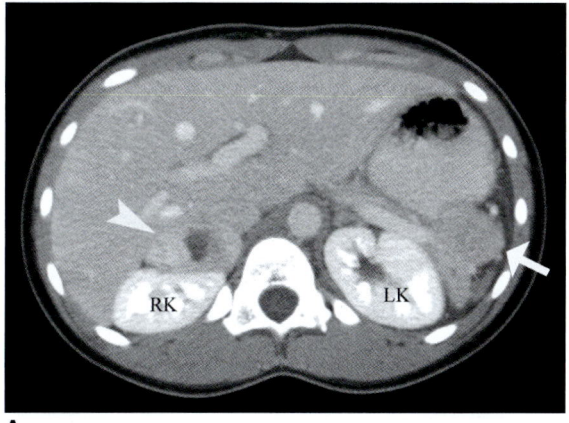
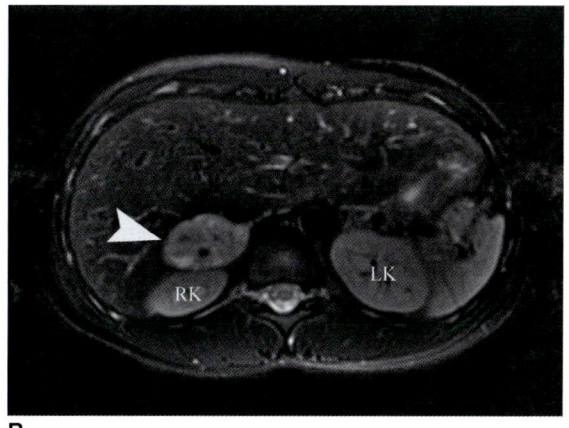

FIGURE 21-23 • Pheochromocytoma in a 12-year-old girl with hypertension. **A:** Axial contrast-enhanced CT image shows a heterogeneous mass (*arrowhead*) anterior to the right kidney (RK). Also noted is a mass of the pancreatic tail, which was a neuroendocrine tumor (*arrow*). **B:** Axial T2-weighted MR image demonstrates a heterogeneous, predominantly hyperintense mass in the right suprarenal fossa (*arrowhead*).

TABLE 21-7	CONGENITAL DISORDERS OF THE ADRENAL GLAND

Agenesis
Adrenal cytomegaly
Adrenal fusion
Congenital adrenal hypoplasia
    Anencephalic form
    Cytomegalic form (*NROB1* gene defect, DAX1 mutation)
    Miniature form
Congenital adrenal hyperplasia
    21-hydroxylase deficiency (*CYP21A2* gene defect)
    11 β-hydroxylase deficiency (*CYP11B1* gene defect)
    17 α-hydroxylase deficiency (*CYP17A1* gene defect)
    3β-hydroxysteroid dehydrogenase deficiency (*HSD3β2* gene defect)
    Cholesterol desmolase deficiency (StAR protein defect) (congenital lipoid adrenal hyperplasia)
Ectopia
Metabolic disorders
    Adrenoleukodystrophy
    Wolman disease

Developmental Disorders

Agenesis, congenital adrenal hypoplasia (CAHP), CAH, and adrenal gland heterotopia are the major structural and biochemical disorders of a congenital or developmental nature (Table 21-7). Except in the setting of anencephaly or other syndromes in which there is adenohypophyseal dysfunction or absence, bilateral adrenal agenesis is rare. *Unilateral adrenal agenesis* may be seen in combination with other malformational syndromes and in the setting of unilateral renal agenesis. *Adrenal fusion*, characterized by midline fusion of adrenal glands imparting a horseshoe or butterfly shape, is rare and associated with other congenital anomalies (Figure 21-24A). Renal–adrenal fusion (accreta) and hepatic–adrenal and renal–adrenal union, characterized by intermingling of parenchymal cells of both organs, are uncommon in childhood (Figure 21-24B, eFigure 21-77) (121). Adrenal shape alteration occurs in renal agenesis with the adrenal gland acquiring a flat disk shape in contrast to its normal triangular appearance (eFigure 21-78).

Ectopic adrenal tissue is usually observed in the abdominal cavity along the celiac axis or along the gonadal descent pathway (122). Intrarenal ectopia can simulate renal cell carcinoma or an invasive adrenal neoplasm (123). Adrenal ectopia is found in up to 10% of orchiopexies and in approximately 4% of inguinal herniorrhaphies (see Chapter 19). Ectopic adrenal occurs in the lung, liver, brain, ovary, and

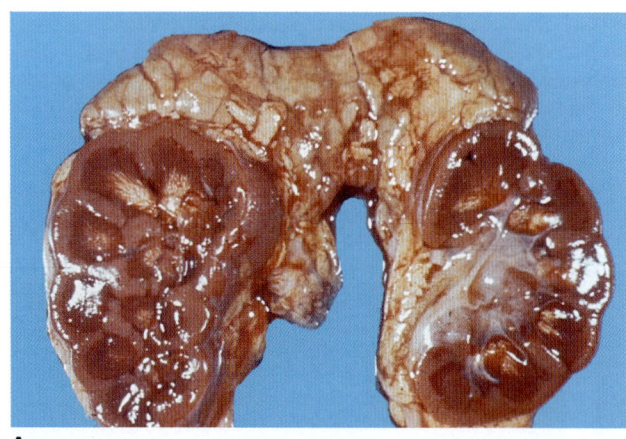

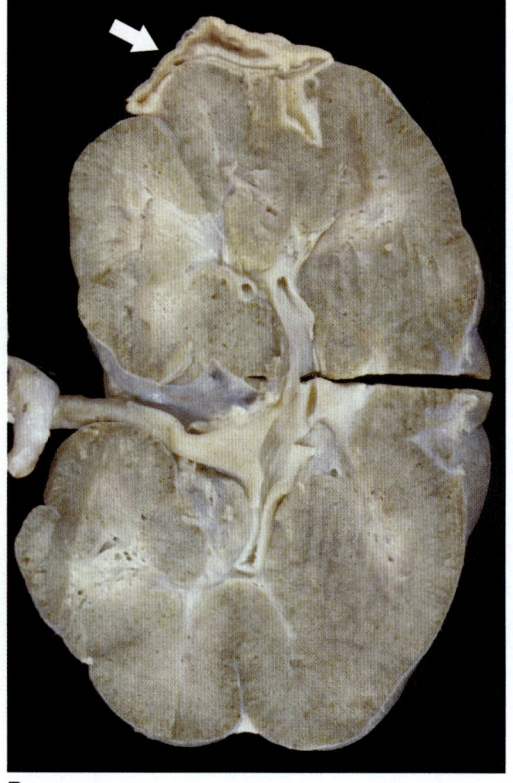

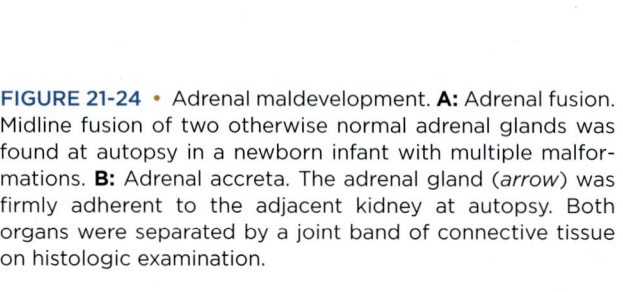

FIGURE 21-24 • Adrenal maldevelopment. **A:** Adrenal fusion. Midline fusion of two otherwise normal adrenal glands was found at autopsy in a newborn infant with multiple malformations. **B:** Adrenal accreta. The adrenal gland (*arrow*) was firmly adherent to the adjacent kidney at autopsy. Both organs were separated by a joint band of connective tissue on histologic examination.

placenta as a rare isolated event (eFigure 21-79). Most ectopic adrenal tissue, especially at distant sites, includes only adrenocortical tissue with distinct cortical zonation in some instances. Small islands or nodules of adrenocortical tissue can be found with some frequency in the fat surrounding the orthotopic adrenal gland. True adrenal gland heterotopia, in which the adrenal gland is absent from its normal location and an adrenal gland with both cortex and medulla is identified, is usually present in the vicinity of the celiac axis, but has also been found at distant sites including the brain.

Wolman disease together with the related cholesterol ester storage disease is a heritable disorder characterized by an inborn error of acid lipase A deficiency (10q23.2–q23.3). Vomiting, steatorrhea, failure to thrive, hepatosplenomegaly, and adrenomegaly with bilateral adrenal calcifications visible radiographically occur in the neonatal period (Figure 21-25A) (124–126). Cholesterol and triglycerides

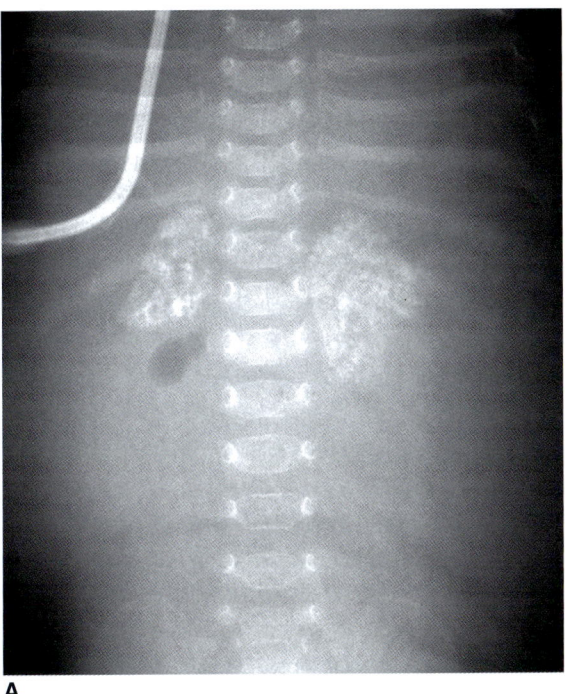
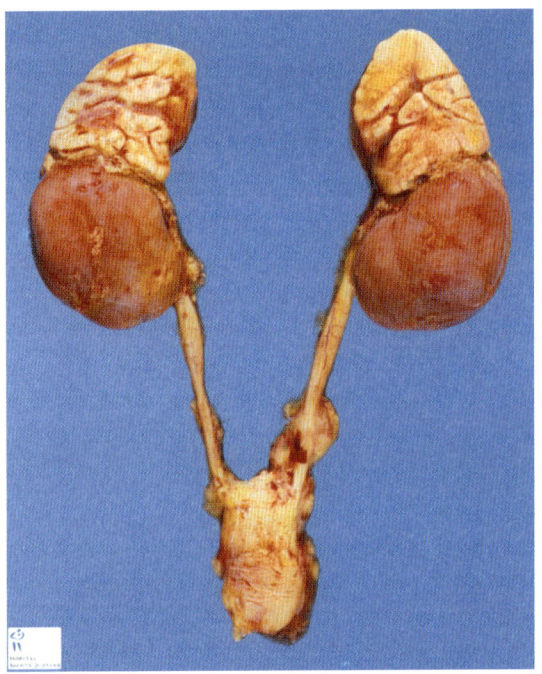
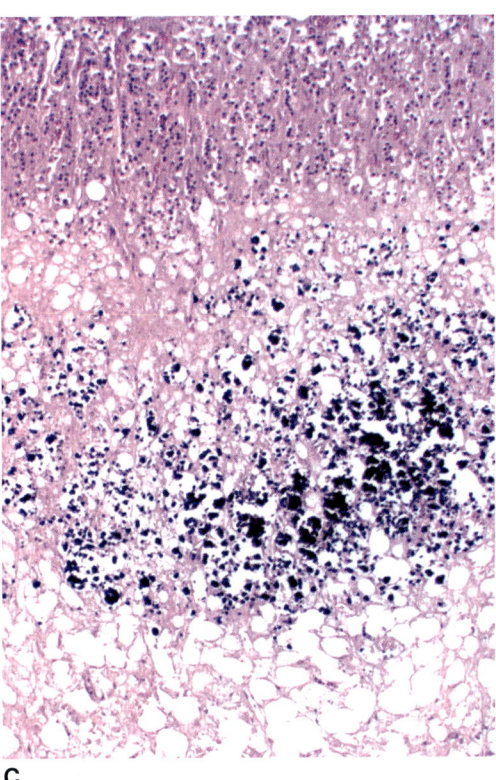

FIGURE 21-25 • Wolman disease. **A:** Plain radiograph of the abdomen reveals triangular-shaped collections of mottled calcifications in the expected location of the adrenal glands. **B:** Both adrenals are enlarged and deep yellow in color due to accumulation of cholesterol esters within the adrenal cortex in this autosomal recessive inherited disease. Image from www.humpath.com. (Reprinted with permission, Dr. Jean-Christophe Fournet, CHU Sainte-Justine, Montreal, Canada.) **C:** Wolman disease was diagnosed in this 3-month-old boy with bilateral adrenal calcifications. The cortical cells of the zona reticularis and inner zona fasciculata are swollen with vacuolated cytoplasm due to cholesterol ester accumulation. Dystrophic calcification is present in the foci of necrosis. (Reprinted with permission from Lack EE. Tumors of the adrenal glands and extraadrenal paraganglia. In: *AFIP Atlas of Tumor Pathology*, 4th Series. Washington, DC: American Registry of Pathology.)

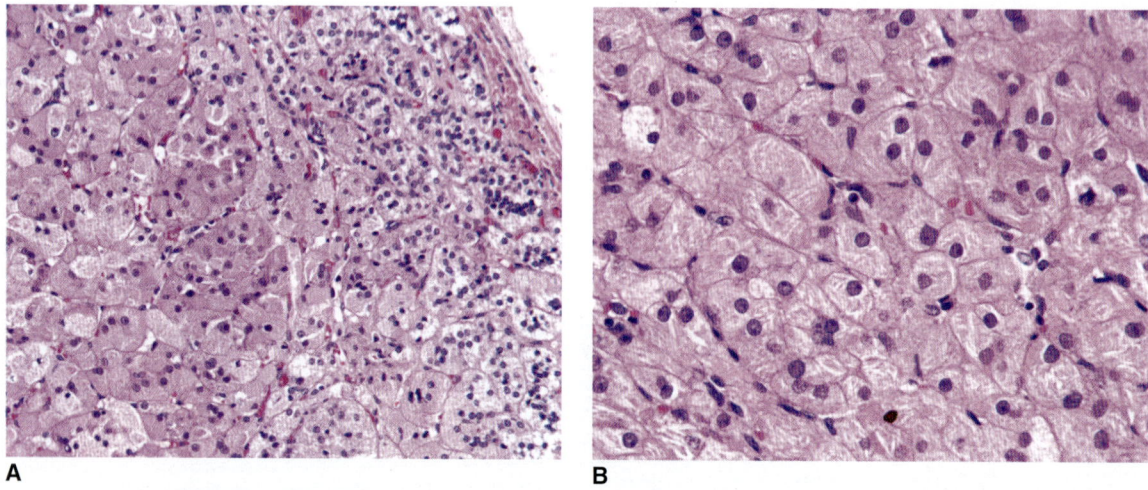

FIGURE 21-26 • X-linked adrenoleukodystrophy in a young male child. **A:** There was prominent atrophy of the adrenal cortex at autopsy. The inner cortical cells are enlarged with abundant pale cytoplasm (H&E stain, original magnification 100×). **B:** Cortical nodules of ballooned cells with a waxy cytoplasm and faint striations are observed in this peroxisomal disorder with defective fatty acid β-oxidation leading to accumulation of very-long-chain saturated fatty acids within cells (H&E stain, original magnification 200×).

accumulate in the lysosomes of the liver, spleen, adrenal glands, gastrointestinal tract, hematopoietic organs, and brain. The adrenal glands are symmetrically enlarged, yellow, and firm. There is a prominent yellow cortical rim and gray–white center (Figure 21-25B). The zona glomerulosa and outer zona fasciculata are histologically unremarkable, but the fetal zone, zona reticularis and inner zona fasciculata, are replaced by haphazardly arranged foamy cells, which are accompanied by focal areas of necrosis and calcification (Figure 21-25C). Cholesterol clefts may be identified as well (eFigure 21-80) (see Chapter 5).

Adrenoleukodystrophy (ALD), a peroxisomal disorder with defective fatty acid β-oxidation leading to accumulation of very-long-chain saturated fatty acids, is associated with inflammatory demyelination of axons and loss of oligodendrocytes and atrophy of the adrenal glands (127,128). A neonatal autosomal recessive form with hypotonia and seizures and a childhood X-linked recessive form are recognized. The adrenals are atrophic and normal cortical zonation is absent (Figure 21-26A, B, eFigure 21-81). The adrenal medulla appears unremarkable (129). Cortical nodules of ballooned cells with waxy cytoplasm are observed, and between the nodules are macrophages with phagocytized lipid and mild fibrosis. Membrane-bound lipid vacuoles with cholesterol clefts are seen on ultrastructural examination (eFigure 21-82) (129) (see Chapter 5).

X-linked form of ALD (ABCD1 gene mutations at Xp28 encoding transporter protein [ALDP] in peroxisome membrane) is estimated to occur in 1:17,000 male infants in both hemizygotes and heterozygotes. The affected adrenal glands usually weigh less than or equal to 2 g (128,129). Quantitative (absence) and qualitative defects in ALDP lead to the accumulation of very-long-chain saturated fatty acids (129). There are greater than 400 mutations leading to variable clinical presentation. Likewise, the morphologic appearance of the adrenal gland is variable. All cortical zones are decreased in thickness. However, both the zona fasciculata and reticularis are markedly reduced in thickness so that the zona glomerulosa occupies about half of the adrenal cortex thickness. The medulla is otherwise normal.

Adrenal cytomegaly is either an incidental focal or diffuse finding within the fetal cortex and occurs in approximately 6% of normal adrenal glands (130). It is more frequently seen in stillborn, premature, and newborn infants; however, it may be observed in older children. The cytomegalic cells are 2 to 3 times normal size and have hyperchromatic pleomorphic nuclei, often with prominent nucleoli, cytoplasmic pseudoinclusions, and abundant vacuolated eosinophilic cytoplasm (Figure 21-27A, B). Mitoses are absent. These cells are seen in association with malformation syndromes including trisomies 13 and 18 and in various perinatal–maternal conditions, including hemolytic disease of the newborn, nonimmune hydrops, eclampsia, intrauterine infection, sepsis, multifetal gestations, congenital lupus erythematosus, and polyhydramnios (131,132). It has also been associated with Rh incompatibility and *in utero* fetal distress and as an incidental finding in approximately 1% of pediatric autopsies (133). Adrenal cytomegaly may be present in Beckwith-Wiedemann syndrome (BWS), which is characterized by exomphalos, macroglossia, and hemihypertrophy. The estimated frequency is 1:13,000 live births. Dysregulation of several genes encoded on chromosome 11p15.5 is thought to be the pathogenetic mechanism (115). Most cases are sporadic (85%); however, an autosomal dominant inheritance with variable expressivity is reported in familial cases. WT, hepatoblastoma, ACNs, NB, pancreaticoblastoma, and PHEO are some of the childhood neoplasms associated with BWS (115). The adrenal glands in BWS are enlarged and may have a combined weight of greater than or equal to 16 g. Grossly, the glands have cerebriform contours due to cortical

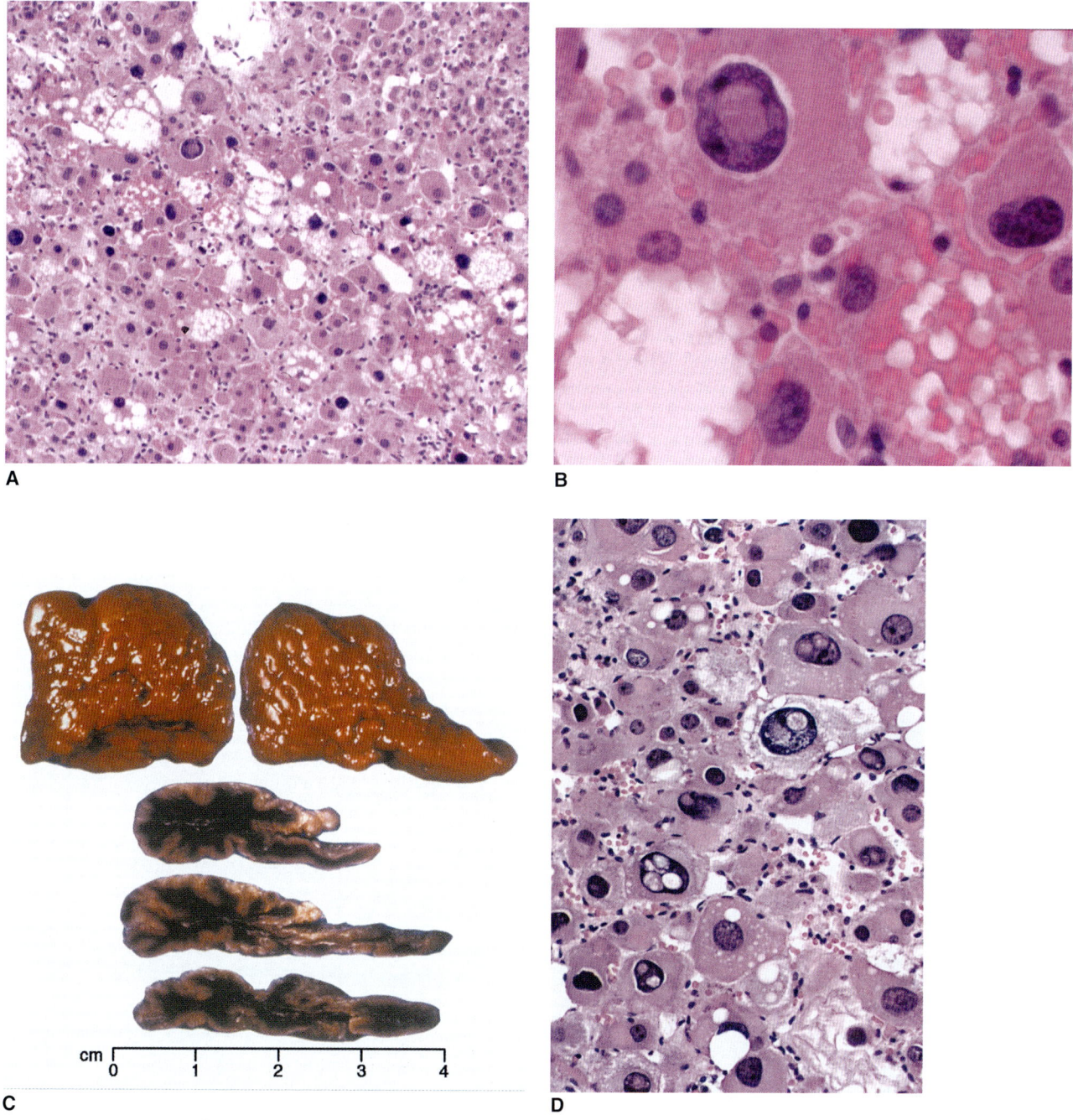

FIGURE 21-27 • Adrenal cytomegaly. **A:** Cytomegaly of the fetal adrenal cortex characterized by large cells with hyperchromatic nuclei is seen in this term infant with in utero fetal demise due to a cord accident (H&E stain). **B:** Nuclear pseudoinclusion (cytoplasmic invagination into the nucleus) is seen in this image of adrenal cytomegaly from a term infant with in utero fetal demise (H&E stain). **C:** The adrenal glands from a 3-week-old infant with BWS are hyperplastic with increased cortical nodularity and redundant folds. **D:** There is marked cytomegaly with nuclear enlargement, hyperchromasia, and nuclear "pseudoinclusions" in this section of fetal cortex from an infant with BWS on histologic examination (H&E stain). (Reprinted with permission from Lack EE. Tumors of the adrenal glands and extraadrenal paraganglia. In: *AFIP Atlas of Tumor Pathology*, 4th Series. Washington, DC: American Registry of Pathology.)

hyperplasia (Figure 21-27C, eFigure 21-83). Large cells with bizarre nuclei (adrenal cytomegaly) are a prominent feature. Diffuse sheets of such cells cause marked expansion of the fetal zone (Figure 21-27D, eFigure 21-84). Hemorrhagic cysts may occur and present as an abdominal mass in the neonate (134,135).

Congenital adrenal hypoplasia (CAHP) is an uncommon condition with an estimated prevalence of 1:12,500 births.

Three distinct histologic patterns (cytomegalic, anencephalic, miniature) have been described (136). A combined adrenal weight of less than 2 g in a term infant defines hypoplasia. Use of a combined adrenal weight:body weight ratio of less than 1:1000 improves diagnostic accuracy. Utilizing these criteria, CAHP is present in 2% of fetopsies and perinatal autopsies. Prenatally, maternal plasma levels of dehydroepiandrosterone sulfate and estriol are useful in detecting CAHP in families at risk. Decreased maternal estriol levels are an important diagnostic clue. X-linked, autosomal recessive, and variable or sporadic inheritances are reported (137). CAHP may present with signs of adrenocortical insufficiency and be associated with sudden infant death syndrome.

The cytomegalic type is the most common pattern and has X-linked inheritance. It is due to deletion or inactivating mutation of *NROB1* (Xp21.3-p21.2) that encodes for DAX-1, which is critical for adrenal gland development. Over 100 *NROB1* gene mutations have been reported accounting for the phenotypic variability (43,138). *NROB1* (DAX-1) mutations have been reported in about 60% of 46,XY phenotypic males with adrenal hypoplasia and in 100% of males with hypogonadotropic hypogonadism and a family history of adrenal failure (139). The cytomegalic pattern has also been reported in association with other inheritance patterns (e654). As part of a contiguous gene syndrome, some affected males also have glycerol kinase deficiency and Duchenne muscular dystrophy without any CNS anomalies (e246). Grossly, the adrenals are small and lack a definitive cortex (Figure 21-28A). The fetal cortex has a disorganized architectural pattern consisting of clusters of large adrenocortical cells with variable nuclear hyperchromasia. The eosinophilic cytoplasm is vacuolated and intranuclear cytoplasmic inclusions may be seen (Figure 21-28B).

The anencephalic type with autosomal recessive inheritance in many cases resembles the adrenal glands of anencephalic infants (eFigure 21-25C, D) (140). The pituitary and CNS either are normal or may have developmental anomalies. Adrenal insufficiency is noted at birth, and hypogonadism may develop at puberty with survival beyond infancy. The small adrenal glands have a definitive, but attenuated, cortex, and the fetal zone is markedly diminished.

The miniature type with a sporadic pattern or autosomal recessive inheritance is seen in infants without any karyotypic abnormalities or developmental anomalies. This type has also been reported in association with triploidy and trisomies 13 and 18 (141). Clinical manifestations are dependent upon the degree of hypoplasia. The miniature pattern is associated with the onset of pregnancy-induced hypertension (142). Grossly, the adrenals are small with a definitive cortex, but with a diminutive or absent fetal cortex.

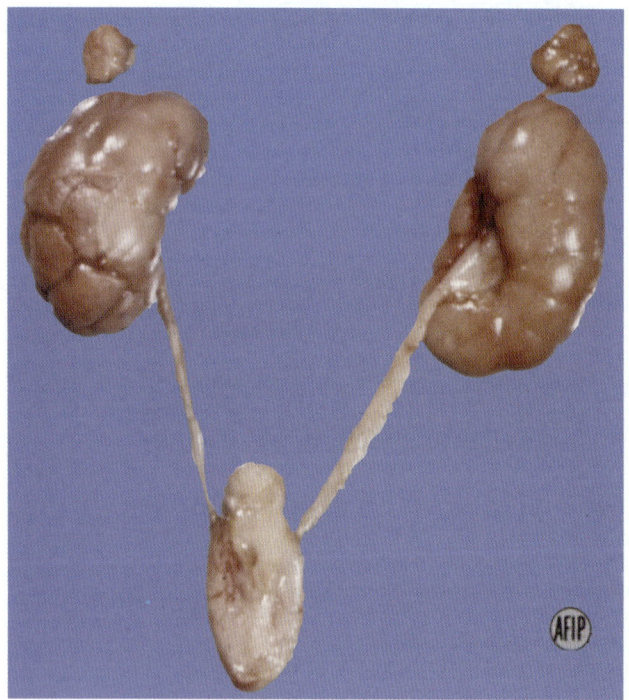
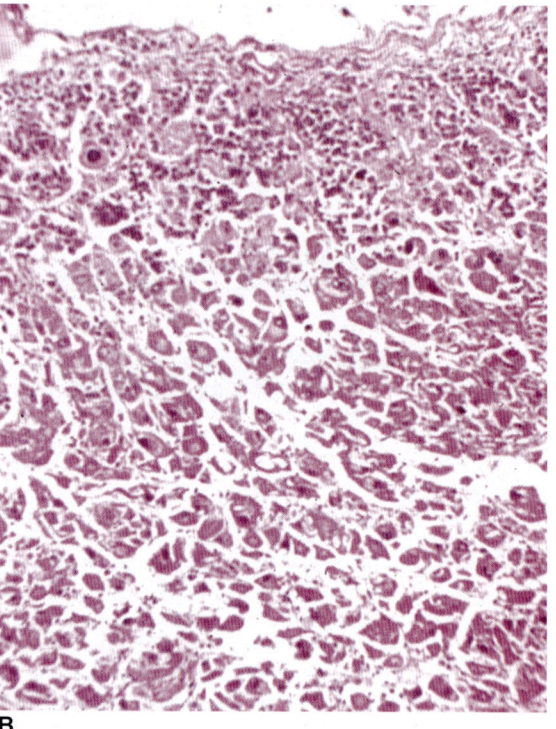

FIGURE 21-28 • Congenital adrenal hypoplasia. **A:** Section of bladder, kidneys, and adrenals from a 470-g preterm male infant. The combined adrenal weight was 0.147 g (versus expected of 2.5 g). The brain and pituitary were normal on gross examination. A normal component of acidophilic cells was present in the pituitary. **B:** The adrenal glands consisted of large cells with abundant eosinophilic cytoplasm. The nuclei were large and bizarre with eosinophilic inclusions similar to adrenal cytomegaly. (From James A, Luther Y. *Pediatric Pathology: Congenital Malformations* [Slide collection, 1966]. Washington, DC: The Armed Forces Institute of Pathology.)

There is normal zonation and an absence of any cellular abnormalities (eFigure 21-85). Unresponsiveness to ACTH due to mutations involving the ACTH receptor gene may mimic CAHP (43,57).

Congenital adrenal hyperplasia (CAH, adrenogenital syndrome) is a group of autosomal recessive disorders of adrenal steroid biosynthesis with similar morphologic features (43,57,143–145). The prevalence is 1:500 to 1:16,000 live births. CAH is the most frequent cause of ambiguous genitalia in the neonate and/or of primary adrenal insufficiency in children (43,57,143–145). Approximately 95% of CAH cases are due to 21-hydroxylase deficiency and 5% due to 11 β-hydroxylase deficiency (43,57,143–145). Decreased cortisol production interrupts normal feedback inhibition on the pituitary gland, leading to persistent ACTH secretion and continued synthesis of cortisol precursors up to the level of the enzymatic defect in the cortisol synthesis pathway. Symptoms and laboratory findings are dependent on which enzyme is absent. The diagnosis of CAH can be made prenatally by chorionic villus sampling during the first trimester (143–145). Many states have neonatal screening programs for 17-hydroxyprogesterone to detect 21-hydroxylase deficiency. Dexamethasone administration, which crosses the placenta before 8 weeks' gestation, has been helpful in preventing virilization of the external genitalia *in utero* (143–145). The clinical, laboratory, and genetic features are beyond the scope of this chapter, but are reviewed elsewhere (57,143–145).

The 21-hydroxylase deficiency (21-OHD) is the most common form of CAH (43,57,143–145). Clinical manifestations vary with the enzymatic deficiency severity (e1120). The affected gene (*CYP21A2*) is located in the major histocompatibility complex III region (6p21.3) (43,143–145). Intergenic recombinations occur between *CYP21A2* and the pseudogene *CYP21A1P*. These recombinant events account for most mutations (80%), with the remainder being deletions in *CYP21* (143–145). Three distinct clinical patterns of 21-OHD are recognized—classic salt wasting, simple virilizing (70% and 30% of classic subtypes, respectively), and nonclassic milder subtypes (43,57,143–145). These three types represent a continuum from mild to severe rather than three distinct phenotypes. Greater than 50 *CYP21A2* mutations have been described and these determine the particular phenotypic expression (145). The prevalence for classic salt-wasting form is 1:10,000 to 1:16,000 live births. The milder form may be as frequent as 1:500 to 1:1000 individuals, which makes this one of the most common autosomal recessive disorders (57,143–145). In the classic form, failure to convert progesterone to the mineralocorticoids, deoxycorticosterone and aldosterone, leads to decreased sodium reabsorption by the kidney, resulting in hyponatremia, hyperkalemia, acidosis, shock, and death. Decreased glucocorticoid production due to the failure to convert 17-hydroxyprogesterone to 11-deoxycortisol leads to lack of negative feedback on the pituitary gland and subsequent unimpeded ACTH secretion. Increased adrenal androgen production causes virilization of the external genitalia, with fusion of the labioscrotal fold in the most severe form in with female infant with male-appearing external genitalia at birth. Fetal stem villi hydrops has been reported in CAH (146). Signs of androgen excess characterize the nonclassic form at puberty with premature adrenarche, menstrual irregularities, acne, hirsutism, and sclerocystic ovaries (143,144). Mineralocorticoid activity is adequate. An attenuated pattern with biochemical abnormalities only is also recognized.

The 11-β-hydroxylase deficiency is the second most frequent pattern and accounts for 5% to 8% of cases. The prevalence is approximately 1:100,000 to 1:200,000 live births. Greater than 50 different inactivating mutations involving the 11 β-hydroxylase gene (*CYP11B1*, 8q21) have been identified (43,57,143–145). Failure to convert 11-deoxycortisol to cortisol and 11-deoxycorticosterone to corticosterone results in increased mineralocorticoid activity, leading to hypernatremia, hypokalemia, and hypertension. Lack of negative feedback inhibition by cortisol leads to increased androgen production. Female pseudohermaphroditism and virilization of male and female infants postnatally are the other major manifestations (see Chapter 18).

The 17-α-hydroxylase deficiency (*CYP17A1*) accounts for approximately 1% of cases. Deficiency leads to failure to hydroxylate pregnenolone and progesterone, resulting in decreased synthesis of androgens and cortisol. Increased synthesis of corticosterone may cause hypertension. Affected females may present at puberty with primary amenorrhea and males with incomplete masculinization (43,57,143–145).

The 3-β-hydroxysteroid dehydrogenase deficiency and StAR (cholesterol desmolase deficiency) are rare causes of CAH. The 3-β-hydroxysteroid dehydrogenase (*HSD3β2*) deficiency leads to salt wasting and female pseudohermaphroditism and precocious masculinization in male infants. The so-called congenital lipoid adrenal hyperplasia is the only one in this group of disorders that is not caused by a defective steroidogenic enzyme. It is caused by a StAR protein defect, which is required for the transport of cholesterol to the inner mitochondrial membrane for conversion to pregnenolone. Greater than 34 mutations occur in the gene encoding for the StAR protein. Korean and Japanese populations are notably affected with these mutations. These infants have adrenal insufficiency and a female phenotype (57,143–145). Bilateral hyperplasia of the adrenal glands, with weights two to four times normal size, is the typical finding; however, normalized glands may be present (115) (Figure 21-29A, B). The external surfaces have a cerebriform appearance. Depletion of the lipid-rich cells of the zona fasciculata leading to compact eosinophilic cells, identical to those observed normally in the zona reticularis, gives the glands a dark, tan–brown color on sectioning (Figure 21-29C, D, eFigure 21-86). The exception occurs in the adrenals of those individuals who have been partially treated with steroids. The zone fasciculata under ACTH stimulation shows the greatest degree of hyperplasia among the three zones of the cortex.

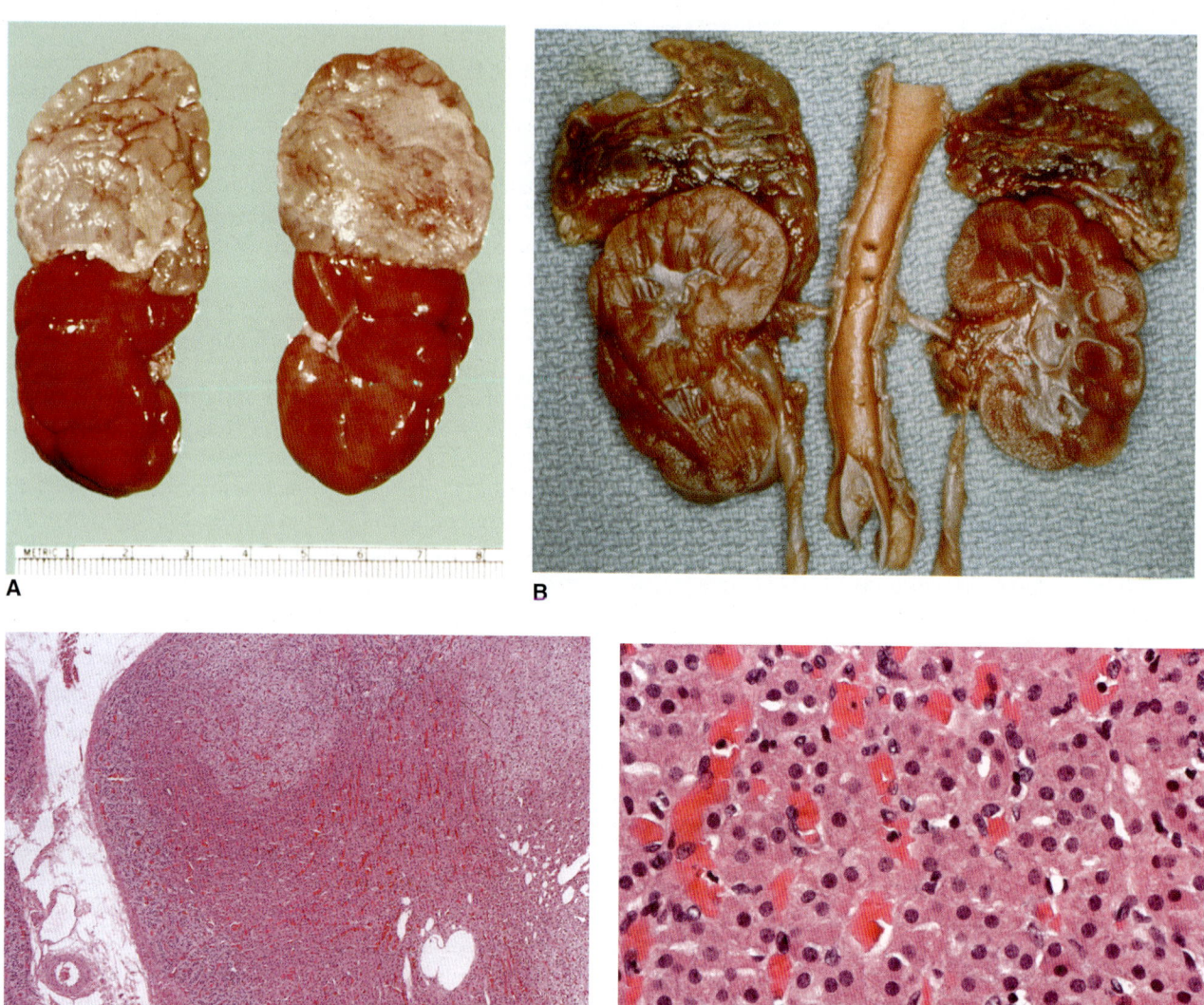

FIGURE 21-29 • Congenital adrenal hyperplasia in a 7-week-old boy who had signs of intestinal obstruction. **A:** The kidneys and adrenal glands are shown, and the enlarged adrenals (combined weight 16.8 g) have a convoluted cerebriform appearance due to the hyperplastic cortex. (From James A, Luther Y. *Pediatric Pathology: Congenital Malformations Slide Collection, 1966*. Washington, DC: The Armed Forces Institute of Pathology.) **B:** This image of kidneys, adrenals, and aorta is from another child with congenital adrenal hyperplasia showing enlarged cerebriform adrenals. **C:** The adrenal cortex is enlarged due to marked expansion of the zona fasciculata in CAH. The cortex is predominantly characterized by a pattern of compact cells with focal collections of clear cells with lipid-rich cytoplasm interspersed (H&E stain). **D:** High-power image showing lipid depletion of zona fasciculata cells with compact eosinophilic cytoplasm in CAH (H&E stain). (Figures C and D reprinted with permission from Lloyd RV, Douglas BR, Young WF. *Endocrine Diseases. Atlas of Nontumor Pathology*. Washington, DC: American Registry of Pathology, 2001.)

In contrast to the other forms of CAH, cholesterol accumulated in the cytoplasm of the cortical cells imparts a bright yellow, nodular appearance to the cortex in congenital lipoid adrenal hyperplasia (115). Lipid-rich cells, cholesterol clefts, foreign body giant cells, and calcifications are the principal histologic features. There is some resemblance in the latter respect to the adrenals in Wolman disease. The presence of bilateral adrenal incidentaloma (unsuspected, nonhyperfunctional adrenal nodule) and adrenal adenomas and the development of adrenocortical carcinoma have been reported in association with CAH (147,148).

Bilateral nodular hyperplasia of testicular adrenal rests (testicular adrenal rest tumors [TARTs]) is reported with some frequency in CAH in greater than 90% of affected adult males (147,149). Male infertility secondary to primary gonadal failure is associated with TART. The testis has a firm multilobular, tan–brown appearance on cross-section, and the lesional tissue is commonly localized in the rete testis (eFigure 21-87). Confluent sheets of polygonal cells with eosinophilic cytoplasm resembling adrenocortical tissue are present on microscopic examination (eFigure 21-88). These cells have the biochemical attributes of adrenocortical cells. Morphologic differentiation of TART from the Leydig cell tumor is difficult, but TART tends to be bilateral in contrast to Leydig cell tumor. Reinke crystals are absent in TART, but present in up to 35% of Leydig cell tumors. These nodules can be locally resected in an attempt to preserve testicular parenchyma (150) (see Chapter 19). Bilateral ovarian steroid cell tumors and malignant Leydig cell tumors have also been reported in the setting of CAH (see Chapters 18 and 19).

Primary pigmented nodular adrenal disease (PPNAD) is associated with Cushing syndrome, and 25% to 35% of cases have the manifestations of Carney complex with myxomas, spotty skin pigmentation, and endocrine hyperactivity (115,148). In addition to PPNAD in 45% of cases, growth hormone–secreting PAs are present in about 10% of cases (151). Two affected genetic loci in this autosomal recessive disorder have been mapped to chromosomes 2p16 and 17q22,24 (*PRKAR1A*) (115,148). The adrenal glands may be decreased, normal, or slightly increased in size. Multiple pigmented nodules less than 4 mm in diameter occupy an otherwise atrophic appearing cortex with loss of normal zonation (eFigure 21-89). Nodules may also be present in the periadrenal fat. The enlarged cortical cells have eosinophilic cytoplasm with abundant lipofuscin pigment (eFigure 21-90). These cells are immunoreactive for SYN, but fail to stain for CHR (152). In this respect, the cortical nodules of PPNAD react in a similar manner to ACNs.

Adrenocortical hyperplasia is also seen in BWS, MAS, and MEN1. Cushing syndrome in the setting of MAS is associated with autonomously functioning multinodular hyperplasia of the adrenals (153). Cushing syndrome is present in 30% to 40% of cases of MEN1 (154).

Adrenocortical insufficiency can be congenital or acquired (57). ALD, CAHP, and CAH are the primary adrenal disorders with accompanying adrenal insufficiency. Other inherited syndromes with adrenal insufficiency include Smith-Lemli-Opitz syndrome, Kearns-Sayre syndrome, and ACTH insensitivity syndrome. Infections, autoimmune disorders, adrenal hemorrhage, and drugs represent acquired etiologies. In children, autoimmune involvement can be isolated or part of an autoimmune syndrome. Autoimmune polyglandular syndrome type 1 is a multisystem autoimmune disease associated with adrenal insufficiency and hypoparathyroidism. Pituitary and other CNS diseases, as discussed previously, are secondary causes. CAH is the most common etiology of adrenal insufficiency accounting for about 70% of cases, with autoimmune adrenalitis being the second most common etiology (155). These findings are similar to the study by Osuwannaratana et al. who observed that greater than 85% of cases were examples of CAH, with panhypopituitarism as the most common cause of secondary adrenal insufficiency.

Acquired Disorders

Adrenal cysts are relatively uncommon in children (115). There are four histopathogenetic types: epithelial, endothelial, pseudocystic, and parasitic. Adrenal neoplasms can undergo cystic necrosis and simulate a large benign cyst or cystic NB in the infant. Cystic cortical degeneration with microcysts may be seen in stillborn infants exposed to substantial stress *in utero*. Adrenal cysts are also present in a number of syndromes including BWS, autosomal recessive polycystic kidney disease, prune belly syndrome, and Gorlin-Goltz syndrome. Idiopathic adrenal cysts are reported from the neonatal period into adolescence (156).

Bacterial, fungal, parasitic, and viral infections can involve the adrenal glands. Adrenal infections with or without necrosis are found in congenital intrauterine infections (*Herpes simplex* with necrosis, cytomegalovirus with adrenalitis or necrosis, *varicella-zoster*) and congenital or acquired immunodeficiency disorders (eFigures 21-91 and 21-92). Histoplasmosis and tuberculosis are also recognized causes of Addison disease. Paracoccidioidomycosis has been observed in children in South America (see Chapter 6).

Adrenal hemorrhage occurs in a wide spectrum of lesions in children and adults. The hemorrhage may range from massive involvement of the gland to focal segmental necrosis. Unilateral or bilateral involvement is dependent in some cases on the etiology. Fetal adrenal hemorrhage occurs with some frequency and has been observed as early as the second trimester (157). Although many lesions in the perinatal period are ascribed to birth trauma and *in utero* asphyxia, the etiology for most adrenal hemorrhages is uncertain. Trauma, sepsis, shock, underlying coagulopathy, arterial thrombosis secondary to umbilical artery catheterization, extracorporeal membrane oxygenation (ECMO), neonatal stress, and renal vein thrombosis have been associated with neonatal adrenal hemorrhage (eFigure 21-93). Massive adrenal hemorrhage is one of several sources of an abdominal mass in an infant. Imaging studies are helpful in the diagnosis. Resolution of a hemorrhage with progressive calcifications is well documented (eFigure 21-94). One should keep in mind the possibility of NB. Spontaneous resolution after birth is a feature of adrenal hemorrhage in contrast to an adrenal tumor. Transient adrenocortical insufficiency has been observed. Rarely, adrenal abscess formation complicates adrenal hemorrhage (158).

Trauma, adrenal tumors, stress, and infection are important considerations in the differential diagnosis of adrenal hemorrhage in older children and adolescents. Trauma-associated adrenal hemorrhage is unilateral with a preference for the right adrenal gland (eFigure 21-95) (159). Child abuse must be considered in the differential diagnosis of traumatic adrenal hemorrhage. Unilateral involvement of the right adrenal gland with adrenal medullary hemorrhage on histologic examination has been reported in child abuse cases (160). Bilateral adrenal hemorrhagic necrosis in the setting of sepsis with rapid onset of circulatory collapse, petechial rash (noninflammatory microangiopathy), and coagulopathy

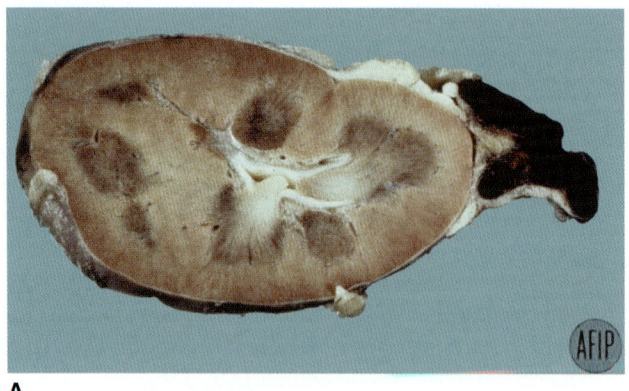 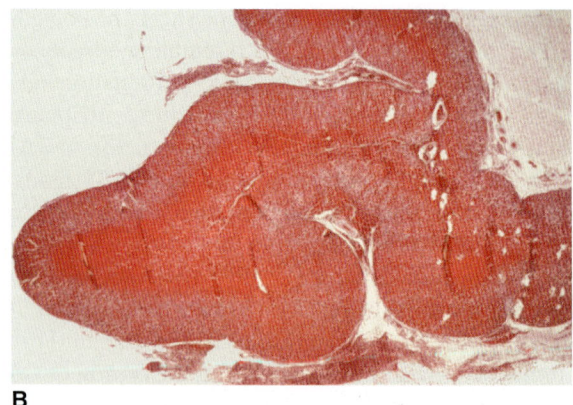

FIGURE 21-30 • **A and B:** Waterhouse-Friderichsen syndrome in a young child who died of meningococcal sepsis is manifested by adrenal hemorrhage on gross examination and diffuse hemorrhage throughout the cortex and medulla on histologic examination (H&E stain).

is known as the Waterhouse-Friderichsen syndrome (WFS) and most commonly associated with meningococcemia. Other common infectious agents in children associated with WFS include group A β-*hemolytic streptococci* and *Haemophilus influenza*. Congenital asplenia or splenic atrophy in the setting of sickle cell anemia is a risk association for bacterial septicemia and development of WFS in children (161,162). Acute adrenal insufficiency is common. Adrenal hemorrhage in WFS begins in the adrenal reticular plexus and extends toward the capsule (Figure 21-30A). There is a loss of the adrenal cortical parenchyma with hemorrhage and partial or complete cortical necrosis (Figure 21-30B). Subcapsular hematomas may form, extend into the periadrenal fat, and surround tissues in severe cases. Histologic examination reveals compression of the sinusoidal capillaries with occasional rupture. Small fibrin thrombi may be seen in the sinusoidal capillaries as features of microangiopathy (163).

Calcifications of the adrenal glands are found in several defined settings, but most notably in Wolman disease and resolving adrenal hemorrhage (eFigure 21-94) (115). There are also individual reports of adrenal calcifications in association with congenital nephrotic syndrome, as a sequela to congenital infections, congenital heart disease, and BWS (eFigure 21-91B) (115).

Adrenocortical neoplasms (ACNs) include adrenocortical adenoma (AA) and carcinoma (ACC) and are rare in the pediatric age group (164,165). The clinicopathologic features of ACN in children, their behavior, and epidemiology contrast nominally with the same neoplasms in adults. However, one of the consistent observations is that these neoplasms in children, though having several morphologic features associated with ACC in adults, do not have the same unfavorable prognostic implications, especially in children less than 6 years of age (164,166). Because atypical histologic features are commonly found in ACNs in children, they are disproportionately interpreted as ACCs. The prevalence of cases classified as ACCs in children in the United States is 0.2 cases:1,000,000 individuals less than 19 years of age (167). ACC accounts for less than 0.5% of all pediatric malignancies, but is the third most common carcinoma in children, with PTC and salivary gland carcinomas being more common (164,166).

There is a bimodal age distribution of ACNs, and they are more common in females in the pediatric population. In a report of 256 cases from the International Pediatric Adrenocortical Tumor Registry (IPATR), the male to female ratio was 1:1.6 (168). Two age distributions were noted by the IPATR, an infantile group with a peak in the first year of life and an adolescent group with a peak between 9 and 16 years. Female predilection with a mean age at diagnosis of 4.6 years and about 50% of cases diagnosed in the first 4 years of life has been documented (166). In a review of 39 cases, ACN presented in children between 7 days and 12 years of age with a mean age of 3 years and median of 2 years (166). Seventy-six percent of children were less than 4 years of age. The male to female ratio was 1:2.5. Others have reported similar findings. There are congenital examples of ACNs (164). One of the highest occurrences of purported ACCs in children (4.7:1,000,000) has been identified in southern Brazil, where a distinct germline *p53* mutation has been identified in this population, but whose other features are not those of classic Li-Fraumeni syndrome. ACNs have also been seen in the setting of CAH. Bilateral ACNs, often seen in syndromic-associated cases, and ectopic ACNs are uncommon (166).

ACNs may be seen in certain genetic predisposition syndromes. There are several syndromic associations with ACNs including BWS (hemihypertrophy, splanchnomegaly, macroglossia, and intra-abdominal neoplasms), Li-Fraumeni syndrome, and Carney complex (164,166). Adrenal hyperplasia and ACN have been reported in MEN1 syndrome, MAS, and neurofibromatosis type 1 (169). Mutations in the tumor-suppressor gene p53, seen in Li-Fraumeni syndrome and in a cohort of children in a specific region of Brazil, predispose children to the development of ACNs. The tumors in Brazilian children have specific p53 mutations (p53-R337H; p53-R175L). Children with BWS (11p15.5 imprinted gene cluster) are at high risk for the development of ACNs. IGF2 is found to be overexpressed in 80% of tumors associated with this syndrome. *BRAF*(6%), *N-RAS* (3%), *K-RAS* (3%), and *EGFR* (11%) mutations have been found in a limited number or cases, but may provide potential treatment targets in tumor with these specific gene mutations. Rare mutations in *RET* and *ATR1* have been reported. Expression profiles have been carried out on tumors from Brazilian children and compared with adult tumors. Decreased expression of histocompatibility class II genes was more common in pediatric tumors. The pediatric tumors had increased *FGFR4* and *IGF2* gene expression and decreased *KCNQ1, CDKN1C, p57/KIP2,* and *HSD3B2* gene expression, when compared with normal adrenal cortical cells. IGF2, KCNQ1, p57/KIP2, and CDKN1c are localized to the imprinting region on chromosome 11p15. This implies an imprinting defect with adrenocortical tumors similar to that observed in BWS. The lower expression of KCNQ1 and HSD3B2 supports the idea that the tumors originate from the fetal cortex during embryogenesis or the zona fasciculata or reticularis during the first few years of life. Of interest was the overall similarity between the gene expression profile of adult and pediatric tumors. This may imply that there is an adrenal stem cell that gives rise to development of tumors in adults similar to that in children, with respect to gene expression.

ACNs in children account for 50% to 70% of cases of Cushing syndrome, in contrast to only 20% of cases in adults (170). Less often does an ACN present with feminizing and masculinizing manifestations in children. Conn syndrome, due to an aldosterone-producing ACN, is rare in childhood. Most tumors in Conn syndrome are benign and characterized by lipid-rich clear cells.

The most important initial step in the pathologic examination of an ACN in childhood is weighing the tumor, because all other gross and histopathologic features are of less importance, if the tumor is confined to the gland, and does not have evidence of metastatic spread to regional lymph nodes or to more distant sites, such as the liver and lungs. In some cases, it may be difficult to judge whether a circumscribed mass in the adrenal is part of multinodular hyperplasia of the cortex or even a PHEO (eFigure 21-96).

ACNs, not only in children but also in adults, vary in size, weight, coloration, consistency (solid and/or cystic), presence or absence of hemorrhage, and presence or absence of necrosis (Figures 21-31 to 21-33, eFigure 21-97). A complete or incomplete fibrous capsule may be apparent at the periphery of the tumor, or the tumor may appear to compress the adjacent parenchyma without a capsule. As noted earlier, the size

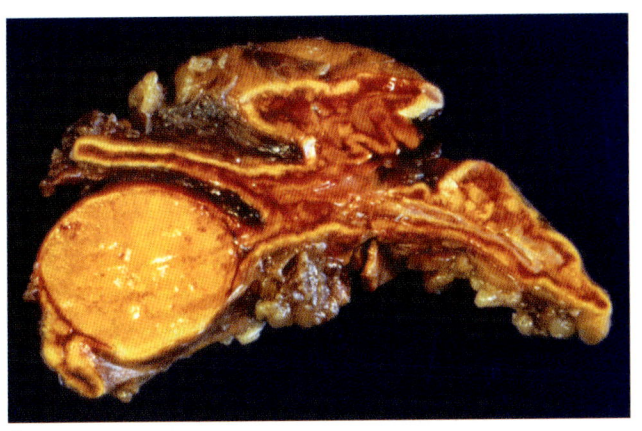

A

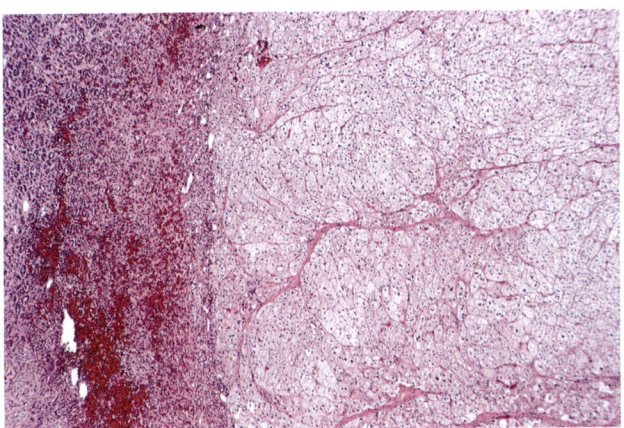

B

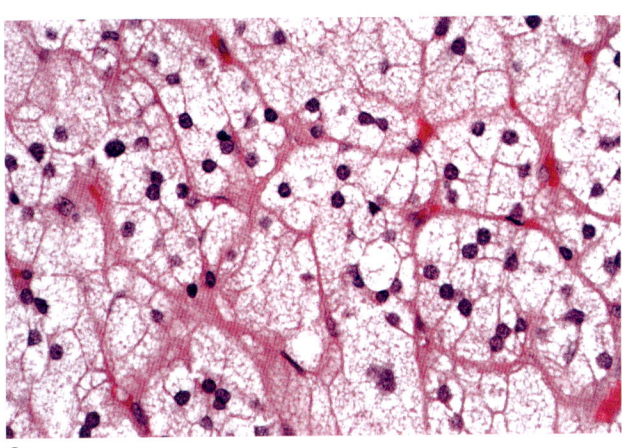

C

FIGURE 21-31 • Adrenal adenoma. **A:** This adrenalectomy specimen that weighed 35 g was from a 17-year-old male who presented with hypertension. A 2-cm-diameter yellow cortical nodule surrounded by a thin rim of stretched uninvolved adrenocortical tissue is present. The remainder of the adrenal gland shows the typical zonation and was unremarkable. **B:** Low-power magnification demonstrating an adrenal adenoma with lipid-laden cells (balloon cells) arranged in small clusters that are surrounded by a thin delicate vascular network. A rim of uninvolved (nonneoplastic) adrenocortical tissue compressed by the mass with focal hemorrhage is on the left (H&E stain). **C:** High-power magnification shows the typical clear lipid-laden cells arranged in small clusters. Cellular and nuclear pleomorphism is not present. Mitotic figures are absent (H&E stain). This tumor would be classified as an ACN, low risk in Dehner and Hill's proposed classification (see Table 21-7 reproduced from Dehner LP, Hill A. Adrenal cortical neoplasms in children: Why so many carcinomas and yet so many survivors? *Pediatr Dev Pathol* 2009;12:284–291).

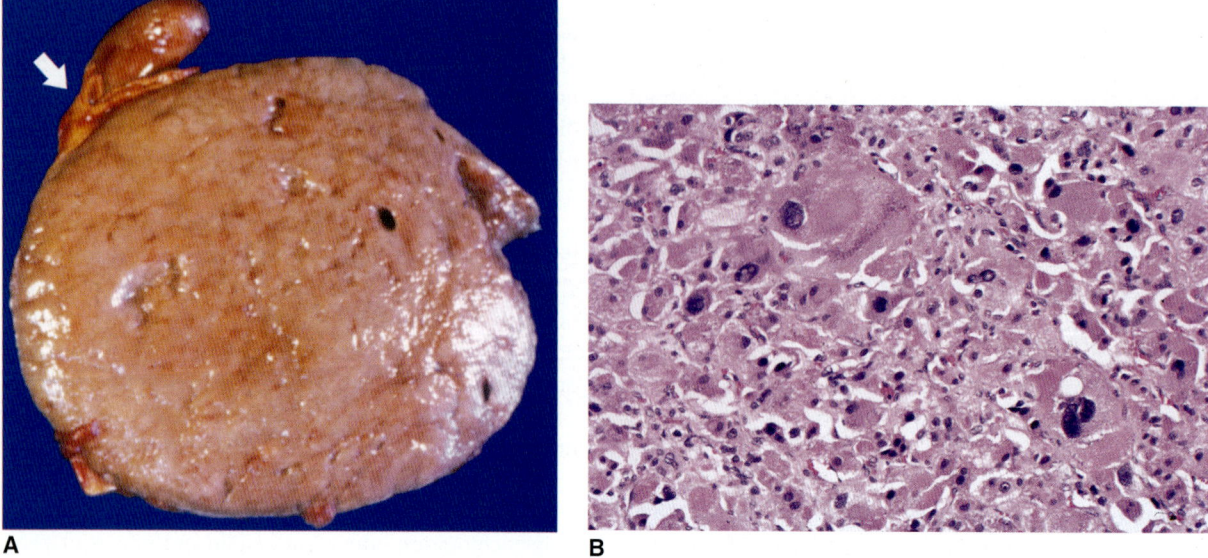

FIGURE 21-32 • Adrenocortical neoplasm. **A:** This 250 g adrenal gland from an adolescent who presented with hypertension and signs of virilization had a homogenous tan appearance on gross examination. A small portion of normal adrenal gland (*arrow*) is present. **B:** On histologic examination, there is prominent cellular pleomorphism with enlarged atypical nuclei. Occasional mitotic figures are present. There is no capsular or vascular invasion. There were no signs of metastatic disease at the time of surgery. This lesion is diagnosed as an atypical adenoma. This tumor would be classified as an ACN, intermediate risk in Dehner and Hill's proposed classification. (See Table 21-7 reproduced from Dehner LP, Hill A. Adrenal cortical neoplasms in children: Why so many carcinomas and yet so many survivors? *Pediatr Dev Pathol* 2009;12:284–291.)

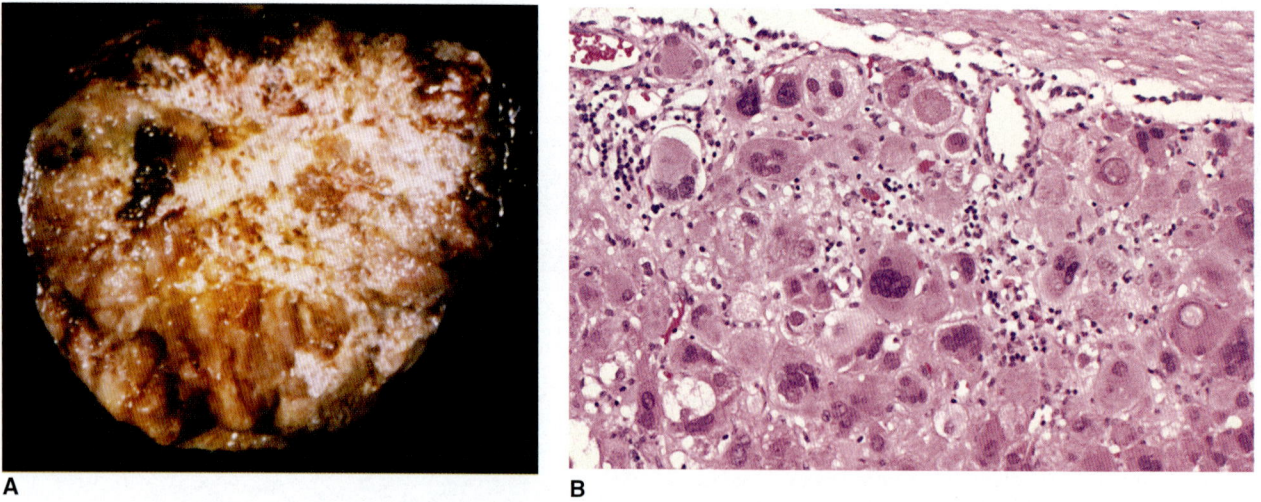

FIGURE 21-33 • Adrenocortical neoplasm. **A:** A 2-year-old-male child with precocious puberty and accelerated bone age was found to have a 9.6- × 8- × 6.2-cm mass arising from the right adrenal gland. There was no sign of metastatic disease at the time of surgery. The 215-g adrenal gland had extensive necrosis and calcification on gross examination. **B:** On histologic examination, the tumor was composed of large, pleomorphic, eosinophilic cells. Nuclear enlargement with hyperchromasia, intranuclear inclusions, and increased mitotic rate were present. Capsular invasion (not shown) was also observed. This tumor was classified as an adrenocortical carcinoma. This tumor would be classified as an ACN, intermediate risk in Dehner and Hill's proposed classification. (See Table 21-7 reproduced from Dehner LP, Hill A. Adrenal cortical neoplasms in children: Why so many carcinomas and yet so many survivors? *Pediatr Dev Pathol* 2009;12:284–291.)

and weight, especially the latter, are closely correlated with the clinical outcome of ACN in children. The cut surface in the absence of hemorrhage and necrosis often has a pale to bright yellow to yellow–brown appearance, which may or may not be uniform throughout because of cystic changes (Figure 21-31A, eFigure 21-97). Uncommonly, the tumor may have a brown–black appearance due to lipofuscin accumulation in the cytoplasm of tumor cells, similar to PPNAD. A hemorrhagic mass may be difficult to differentiate from NB.

A number of studies have examined the microscopic features of ACN for their predictive prognostic value, but most of the studies have consisted principally of tumors in adults where cytologic atypia, mitotic activity, zonal necrosis, and transecting fibrous bands have predictive value in terms of outcome when several of these features are present. Some of these histologic features are found with some frequency in ACNs in children, yet lack definitive significant correlation with prognosis. The classic histologic pattern for ACN is a neoplasm composed of clear or pale polygonal cells with abundant lipid-rich cytoplasm, or cells with homogeneous eosinophilic cytoplasm, arranged in short cords or trabecular profiles (Figure 21-31B, C, eFigure 21-98). The nuclei are uniform and centrally positioned in the cell. The adjacent cortex is often compressed and atrophic (eFigure 21-99). Other histologic patterns include diffuse sheets of polygonal cells, alveolar pattern with loosely cohesive cells, glandular profiles, a yolk sac tumorlike pattern, and delicate ribbons of cells in a hyaline myxoid stroma, either as an exclusive pattern or as an component of the ACN (165,166). Polymorphism is the theme for the various patterns in ACNs in children.

The individual cellular features of ACN in children demonstrate considerable pleomorphism (Figures 21-32 and 21-33, eFigure 21-100). In some ACNs, monomorphism is present with uniform tumor cells. More often with ACNs in children less than or equal to 4 years of age, there is pleomorphism with tumor giant cells, bizarre nuclear forms, and marked hyperchromatism. The pleomorphic tumor cell population may be either a minor or major component of the tumor (Figure 21-33).

Immunocytochemical stains that may be helpful with the diagnosis of adrenal cortical neoplasms include α subunit of inhibin, vimentin, CK5/CK6, CEA, and melan-A. Of these immunostains, inhibin is most helpful. Negative reactivity to neuroendocrine markers, such as SYN, CHR A, and S100 protein, is helpful as well. Overexpression of p53 by immunocytochemistry is more common in clinically aggressive tumors (malignant behavior). There are no immunophenotypic differences between an adenoma and carcinoma (171). However, adenomas may demonstrate immunoreactivity for cytokeratin, whereas ACCs are usually nonreactive (172). Ploidy analysis has limited value in distinguishing adenomas from carcinomas. With 29 pediatric ACNs, 73% of tumors with aneuploidy remained disease-free (173,174).

The distinction between a cortical neoplasm and PHEO is not clear in all cases, especially in tumors with large bizarre cells, granular basophilic cytoplasm, and a nested zellballen growth pattern. Serologic tests for PHEO markers may not be available to correlate with histopathologic findings at the time of diagnosis. In such cases, immunohistochemistry is helpful with the diagnosis. SYN and NSE are commonly immunoreactive in both PHEOs and adrenocortical tumors. CHR is nonreactive in adrenocortical tumors, but is consistently expressed in PHEOs and paragangliomas (often inappropriately referred to as extra-adrenal PHEO) (172). Cytokeratin is typically not found in either PHEOs or paragangliomas with rare exceptions, but these tumors are often immunoreactive for VIM (172). S100 protein and HMB-45 staining is useful in the labeling of sustentacular cells in PHEOs. Inhibin is positive in ACNs and is useful.

ACNs may have marked mitotic activity, including bizarre mitotic figures, and still be small tumors (<100 g) confined to the gland. ACNs in children may demonstrate individual cell, focal, or diffuse necrosis. The tumors may have intratumoral lymphovascular invasion and microscopic evidence of capsular invasion. Because of the tendency of pediatric ACNs to have features that in adults would be diagnosed as ACC, many children with these tumors have been classified as ACC based upon adult criteria for malignancy. In contrast to adults with ACC, pediatric tumors that would qualify as ACC using previously established criteria for adult tumors have favorable outcomes. The event-free survival after 5 years for children less than 5 years of age diagnosed with ACCs using adult criteria is 70% to 80% (166).

Concerted efforts have been expended to determine diagnostic and prognostic factors in pediatric ACNs (Table 21-8) (166). Vascular invasion, tumor necrosis, tumor weight, and high stage of disease are more prevalent in pediatric tumors with malignant histology and benign clinical behavior and malignant histology and malignant clinical behavior categories compared with benign histology and benign clinical behavior category. Based upon extensive evaluation of histologic and clinical behavior characteristics, AFIP criteria for malignancy and a scoring system have been established for pediatric ACNs (Table 21-8). Tumor weight greater than 400 g, tumor size greater than 10.5cm, soft tissue extension or invasion of adjacent organs, venal caval invasion, venous invasion, capsular invasion, tumor necrosis, greater than 15 mitoses per 20 high-power fields, and atypical mitotic figures are assessed for determining benign, indeterminate, and malignant nature of the tumors. Each item that is present is given a score of 1. The total score determines if the tumor is classified as benign (score = 0 to 2), indeterminate (score = 3), or malignant (score = 4 to 9). Obviously, metastatic disease to lymph nodes or distant sites provides a diagnosis of malignancy. Guidelines for risk group assessment in children have also been proposed (Table 21-8) based upon tumor confinement to the adrenal gland or not, tumor weight, microscopic or gross invasion or extension into adjacent organs, resection status, and metastatic disease status. Based upon these criteria, children may be placed into low-, intermediate-, and high-risk categories.

Staging systems for children have been established by the International Adrenal Pediatric Tumor Registry (IAPTR) and the Armed Forces Institute of Pathology (AFIP) (Table 21-8). Compared with adults, children tend to be at lower

TABLE 21-8 CRITERIA FOR ASSIGNING RISK GROUPS AND STAGING FOR PEDIATRIC ADRENOCORTICAL NEOPLASMS

AFIP criteria for malignancy of adrenal cortical neoplasms in pediatrics
(1 point for each feature present in tumor)
    Tumor weight of >400 g
    Tumor size of >10.5 cm
    Extension into periadrenal soft tissues and /or adjacent organs
    Vena cava invasion
    Venous invasion
    Capsular invasion
    Tumor necrosis present
    Mitoses of >15 per 20 high-power fields
    Atypical mitotic figures

Good long-term clinical outcome (benign):	Score of 0–2
Indeterminate for malignancy	Score of 3
Poor clinical outcome (malignant)	Score of 4–9

IAPTR proposed risk groups for adrenal cortical neoplasms in children

Low risk	Tumor confined to adrenal gland
	<200 g tumor weight
	No microscopic invasion of surrounding soft tissue
	Completely resected
	No metastatic spread
Intermediate Risk	Tumor confined to adrenal gland
	200–400 g tumor weight
	Microscopic invasion of surrounding soft tissue
	Completely resected
	No metastasis
High Risk	>400 g tumor weight or
	Gross invasion of adjacent organs (liver, spleen, kidney)
	Or metastatic disease

Staging of pediatric adrenal cortical neoplasms (IAP: International Adrenal Pediatric Tumor Registry; AFIP: Armed Forces Institute of Pathology)

Stage I:	AFIP:	Tumor ≤5 cm with No Invasion (T1)
	AFIP:	Tumor >5 cm (T2)
	IAPTR:	Tumor completely resected with negative margins,
		Weight ≤200 g and no metastasis
Stage II:	AFIP:	Tumor of any size with local invasion without adjacent
		Organ involvement (T3)
	AFIP:	Tumor of any size with adjacent organ invasion (T4)
	IAPTR:	Tumor completely resected with negative margins,
		Weight >200 g
		No metastasis
Stage III:	AFIP:	Any tumor with regional lymph node metastasis
	IAPTR:	Residual gross or microscopic tumor or inoperable tumor
Stage IV:	AFIP:	Any tumor with distant metastasis.
	IAPTR:	Hematogenous metastasis at presentation

Adrenal cortical neoplasms staging

	IAPTR children	AFIP children	Adults
Stage I	44%	82%	3%
Stage II	32%	18%	29%
Stage III	10%	0%	19%
Stage IV	15%	0%	49%

stages (stage I and II IAPTR and AFIP) when tumors are detected. This may provide a more favorable outcome for children with adrenocortical tumors compared with adults. Event-free survival for children with IAPTR stage I and II diseases has been evaluated for various factors. Factors associated with better survival include younger age, virilization symptoms, normal blood pressure, stage I disease, no tumor spillage during surgery, no intravenous tumor thrombus, and tumor weight less than or equal to 200 g. With all children with ACNs, overall survival and event-free survival at 5 years were over 50%. Children less than or equal to 3 years of age had an 80% survival rate compared with only 20% for the 12- to 20-year age group. Stage I had a 90% survival rate compared with only 40% for stage II and about 20% for stages III and IV.

Three risk groups based on tumor localization and weight have been proposed as an alternative method for predicting clinical behavior with pediatric ACNs (166) (Table 21-8). ACNs greater than 200 g and confined to the gland are considered at low risk for malignant behavior and classified as adenomas (Figure 21-31, eFigures 21-98 and 21-99). ACNs greater than 400 g are considered at high risk of malignant behavior. These pediatric ACNs often share histopathologic features associated with adult ACCs and are classified as pediatric ACCs. ACNs with weights between 200 and 400 g and confined to the adrenal gland are considered at intermediate (indeterminate) risk for malignant behavior and classified as atypical AAs (Figures 21-32 and 21-33, eFigure 21-100). Most atypical ACNs have favorable outcomes (166). However, certain "atypical" adenomas demonstrate soft tissue invasion and/or major vessel invasion, declaring malignant behavior.

When adrenocortical carcinomas occur in children, these tumors usually are greater than 400 g. These tumors have irregular contours, extensive hemorrhage, necrosis, and invasion beyond the tumor capsule into soft tissues and other organs. Histopathologic features associated with ACCs in adults are present with these pediatric ACCs (165,166). These obviously malignant neoplasms are found in children greater than 10 years of age whose 5-year event-free survival ranges from 20% to 35%. These tumors metastasize to the liver (>90%), lungs (80%), retroperitoneal soft tissues, and regional lymph nodes with less common spread to the bone and brain (165). Most children with "bona fide" ACCs usually die from their disease within 2 years following diagnosis. As another measure that putative ACCs in young children behave in a different fashion compared to adults are the observations that BWS-associated ACCs are not aggressive neoplasms and that a congenital ACC is reported to have undergone spontaneous regression (175). Recent treatment protocols for children and adults with recurrent or advanced-stage malignant adrenal cortical tumors have incorporated mitotane as a therapeutic agent. In limited trials, this agent has shown promise. Preliminary data indicate that stable disease or a certain degree of tumor response to mitotane therapy may be observed in patients with recurrent and/or advanced stage disease.

Peripheral Neuroblastoma (NB) Group Tumors

Classic or peripheral neuroblastic tumors are represented by NB, ganglioneuroblastoma (GNB), and ganglioneuroma (GN) as a group of histogenetically related neoplasms of neural crest origin (eFigure 21-101). These tumors are histogenetically distinct from the cPNET and Ewing sarcoma–peripheral primitive neuroectodermal tumor (EWS–PPNET), despite the presence of overlapping morphologic and immunophenotypic features (see Chapters 10 and 25).

Epidemiology

NB is the most common extracranial solid neoplasm of childhood and is surpassed in prevalence only by acute leukemias and primary brain tumors, principally astrocytoma and medulloblastoma; SEER Program from 1975 to 2000 reported that NB accounted for 7.2% of all cancers among children less than 15 years of age in the United States, and the total prevalence was 10.2 to 10.3:1,000,000 for males and 10.1 for females (176). The prevalence rates by age are the following: 19.6:1,000,000 for ages 1 to 4 years, 2.9 for ages 5 to 9 years, and 0.7 for 10 to 14 years. The prevalence rates by race and ethnicity are the following: 10.8:1,000,000 for whites, 8.4 for blacks, and 7.5 for children in other racial/ethnic groups. In the United States, approximately 650 children are newly diagnosed each year (177). Based on the SEER data, the 5-year relative survival rate is 65%, a figure that has remained more or less static for the past several decades.

In the past, NB was referred to as "enigmatic" because of its unpredictable behavior, because these tumors manifest a wide range of clinical courses from an excellent prognosis due to complete resectability, tumor involution, spontaneous regression, and/or maturation to a fatal outcome due to tumor progression despite intensive treatment. Now, NB is believed to be biologically heterogeneous and is composed of at least two subgroups, clinically favorable and unfavorable. These two subgroups have distinct molecular genetic attributes closely correlated with their clinical behaviors. Several epidemiologic studies in the past have not identified any causal factors for NB; however, it may be necessary to analyze neuroblastic tumors in each biologic subgroup separately to elucidate any possible extrinsic factors.

Familial or hereditary NB, first recognized in 1945, is a rare entity (178) and has offered an opportunity to identify any hereditary NB predisposition genes: Maris et al. have reported a hereditary NB predisposition gene (*HNB1*) on the distal short arm of chromosome 16p (16p12-13) (179). Perri et al. have identified another gene on the distal short arm of chromosome 4p (4p16) (180). Recently, activating mutations in the anaplastic lymphoma kinase (*ALK*) oncogene (2p23) have been found in hereditary NB cases, as well as a smaller subset of sporadic tumors (181–185). The same gene has an important oncogenic role in anaplastic large cell lymphoma and inflammatory myofibroblastic tumor.

Beckwith and Perrin used the term of NB *in situ* to describe an exclusively microscopic finding in neonatal and infant autopsies, histologically identical to NB, as an incidental finding in or around the adrenal medulla. The prevalence of these lesions has been calculated as 40 to 100 times that of clinically overt NBs. Most NBs *in situ* are asymptomatic. Because similar neuroblastic nodules are seen during the fetal development of the adrenal medulla, some have questioned the neoplastic potential if any of NB *in situ*. It has not yet been demonstrated whether these lesions are clonal proliferations of genetically abnormal cells. Therefore, the premalignant or neoplastic nature of these lesions remains unproven.

The anatomic sites of predilection for NB are related to the distribution of neural crest cells. They include the paravertebral region from the neck to the pelvis (3% to 5% of cases), the adrenal medulla (35% of cases), the extra-adrenal retroperitoneum (30% to 35% of cases), and the posterior mediastinum (20% of cases) (186). Less common primary sites include the cephalic, paratesticular or paraovarian tissues, and the inguinal region. A concern about these various sites of tumor is whether they represent a primary tumor or metastasis (113,181,187,188). Rarely, NB presents as multifocal tumors (189). A primitive-appearing neuronal tumor may occur as the only or predominant element of a sacrococcygeal or ovarian teratoma, in which case, the neuroblastic cells usually have the characteristics of the central nervous system rather than the peripheral nervous system or neural crest.

Occasionally, some difficulty is encountered in distinguishing an adrenal or perirenal NB from WT. Most WTs are well-demarcated intrarenal masses. Biologically favorable perirenal NB usually grows outside of the kidney, while biologically unfavorable perirenal NB often shows direct invasion into the renal parenchyma, especially when *MYCN* oncogene is amplified. The blastema-predominant WT may frequently require immunohistochemical differentiation from NB. Blastemal cells of WT are positive for VIM and WT-1 and are negative for CHR and SYN. In the case of EWS-PNET, the tumor may be positive for neuroendocrine markers as well as MIC2 (CD99) and FLI-1, but is negative for WT-1 and TH (tyrosine hydroxylase [TH]) (190).

Clinical Features

Signs and symptoms at presentation are related to the location of the primary tumor and the extent of disease. The most common presentation of NB is an abdominal mass in which radiologic imaging studies demonstrate a suprarenal or retroperitoneal mass with or without calcification. Orbital metastasis also causes periorbital ecchymosis and edema with the so-called raccoon or panda eyes. Invasion or circumscription of the kidney by NB in the adrenal gland, retroperitoneum, or the perihilar region can mimic a WT. NB may cause renal artery stenosis due to compression leading to systemic hypertension.

Patients with localized disease are often asymptomatic. A localized NB may be discovered incidentally in a routine well-baby examination or by the caregiver. Metastatic spread is seen in patients with "progressive" stage 4 disease and "regressive" stage 4S (S = "special") disease (Table 21-9). Major metastatic sites in stage 4 disease include bone marrow and bone. To find a metastatic nodule in the brain parenchyma

TABLE 21-9 INTERNATIONAL NEUROBLASTOMA STAGING SYSTEM

Stage	Description
Stage 1	Localized tumor with complete gross excision, with or without microscopic residual disease; representative ipsilateral lymph nodes negative for tumor microscopically (nodes attached to and removed with the primary tumor may be positive)
Stage 2A	Localized tumor with incomplete gross excision; representative ipsilateral nonadherent lymph nodes negative for tumor microscopically
Stage 2B	Localized tumor with or without complete gross excision, with ipsilateral nonadherent lymph nodes positive for tumor. Enlarged contralateral lymph nodes must be negative microscopically.
Stage 3	Unresectable unilateral tumor infiltrating across the midline,[a] with or without regional lymph node involvement; or localized unilateral tumor with contralateral regional lymph node involvement; or midline tumor with bilateral extension by infiltration (unresectable) or by lymph node involvement
Stage 4	Any primary tumor with dissemination to distant lymph nodes, bone, bone marrow, liver, skin, and/or other organs (except as defined for stage 4S)
Stage 4S	Localized primary tumor (as defined for stage 1, 2A, or 2B), with dissemination limited to skin, liver, and/or bone marrow[b] (limited to infants <1 year of age)

Multifocal primary tumors (e.g., bilateral adrenal primary tumors) should be staged according to the greatest extent of disease, as defined previously, followed by a subscript "M" (e.g., 3_M).

[a]The midline is defined as the vertebral column. Tumors originating on one side and "crossing the midline" must infiltrate to or beyond the opposite side of the vertebral column.

[b]Marrow involvement in stage 4S should be minimal, that is, <10% of total nucleated cells identified as malignant on bone marrow biopsy or on marrow aspirate. More extensive marrow involvement would be considered to be stage 4. The MIBG scan (if done) should be negative in the marrow.

(International Neuroblastoma Staging System. Reproduced with permission from Brodeur GM, Hogarty MD, Mosse YP, Maris, JM. Neuroblastoma. In: Pizzo PA, Poplack DG, editors. *Principles and Practice of Pediatric Oncology*, 6th ed. Philadelphia, PA: Lippincott-Williams & Wilkins Publishers, 2011; 886–922.)

is rare. When present, CNS metastasis often shows a form of diffuse meningeal spread. Lung metastasis at initial diagnosis is also extremely rare (191). In stage 4S disease, liver, skin, and bone marrow (without bone destruction) are the sites of metastasis. Congenital NB can be diagnosed perinatally by ultra sound and placental examination. Most congenital NBs are stage 1 or 4S with an excellent clinical outcome (192,193). It is interesting to note that neuroblastic cells may be found in the fetal capillaries of the chorionic villi in the presence of a congenital NB, suggesting that neuroblastic cell dissemination takes place through the placenta (eFigure 21-102) (194). Another presentation is nonimmune fetal hydrops. Placental metastasis is often present in these cases (184). Spinal cord compression is caused by a paravertebral tumor growing into the spinal canal through the neural foramina ("dumbbell lesion") or osteolytic metastasis with vertebral collapse (195). Neurologic abnormalities include motor deficit, radicular or back pain, sphincter abnormalities, and sensory deficit.

Other uncommon clinical manifestations of NB are listed in Table 21-10. A small proportion of cases may have a paraneoplastic syndrome including the opsoclonus–myoclonus–ataxia (OMA) syndrome (Kinsbourne syndrome) with "dancing eyes" (rapid and irregular movement of the eyes) and/or myoclonus and ataxia of the limbs, trunk, and eyelids (196–198). An immune-mediated pathogenesis is suggested by the presence of a prominent lymphocytic infiltrate and lymphoid follicle formation in the primary site. It is believed that this paraneoplastic syndrome is an immune-mediated disease with the neuroblasts possessing antigens recognized by the host's immune system, resulting in normal neural tissue at other sites being targets for cytotoxic T cells or production of antibodies against neuroblasts and normal neurons by B cells. Anti-Hu and antineuronal antibodies have been reported in neuroblastoma patients with OMA. The prognosis in terms of tumor behavior itself is generally excellent, but cognitive and motor developmental delay and language deficit often persist even after complete resection of the NB. Immune suppressive therapy and intravenous immunoglobulin administration may provide some degree of resolution of the acute symptoms. Horner syndrome (ptosis, miosis, enophthalmos) and heterochromia (difference in color) of the iris may occur in the presence of an NB involving the cervical sympathetic ganglia. Intractable diarrhea with hypokalemia and dehydration are the manifestations of vasoactive intestinal peptide (VIP) producing neuroblastic tumor with differentiating neuroblasts or a GN. Differentiating neuroblasts may also produce somatostatin and other neuropeptides. Cushing syndrome and systemic hypertension are other clinical manifestations (199). Extremely rare cases of virilizing adrenal GN with Leydig cell hyperplasia have been reported. The so-called neuroblastic "leukemia" in the peripheral blood with extensive bone marrow involvement is an uncommon hematologic event. Another hematopathologic finding is myelofibrosis in the absence of demonstrable metastatic NB in the bone marrow.

There are several distinct associations of NB with other disorders including neurofibromatosis, BWS, Hirschsprung disease, musculoskeletal and cardiovascular malformations, and Turner syndrome (Table 21-11). Molecular studies of cases of familial NB have failed to provide any linkage with the genes responsible for neurofibromatoses 1 and 2 (179). The relationship of congenital NB to the syndrome of central failure of ventilation (incorrectly referred to as Ondine curse—the curse involves loss of all autonomic and perceptive function) often accompanied by Hirschsprung disease has been explained on the basis of a widespread abnormality of neural crest cell development and migration (200,201) due to *PHOX2B* mutation. Increased risk for thyroid cancer is reported in individuals who received radiation therapy for NB, similar to that seen in other pediatric cancers requiring radiation. An unusual type of renal cell carcinoma with oncocytoid features is reported as a second primary neoplasm in survivors of NB (202,203). *Biochemical Markers:* NB is characterized biochemically by catecholamine synthesis with metabolites that are detected in the serum and urine. This property is utilized in the initial diagnosis and clinical follow-up as a measure of therapeutic response. The precursor amino acids for catecholamine synthesis are phenylalanine and tyrosine. A series of enzymes, such as TH, DOPA decarboxylase, dopamine β-hydroxylase, and phenylethanolamine N-methyltransferase, are involved in

TABLE 21-10 UNCOMMON AND UNUSUAL CLINICAL MANIFESTATIONS OF NEUROBLASTOMA

Opsoclonus–myoclonus ataxia syndrome
Horner syndrome and heterochromia of the iris
Intractable watery diarrhea with hypokalemia and dehydration (VIP secretion)
Cushing syndrome
Systemic hypertension
Virilizing, masculinization (ganglioneuroma)
Neuroblastoma "leukemia"
Myelofibrosis
Fetal hydrops with placental involvement

VIP, vasoactive intestinal peptide.

TABLE 21-11 ASSOCIATION OF NEUROBLASTOMA WITH OTHER DISORDERS

von Recklinghausen neurofibromatosis
Beckwith-Wiedemann syndrome
Hirschsprung disease
Musculoskeletal and cardiovascular malformations
Turner syndrome
Central failure of ventilation ("Ondine curse")
Increased incidence of thyroid carcinoma in irradiated neuroblastoma patients (in comparison with patients irradiated for other childhood neoplasms)
Renal cell carcinoma (oncocytoid variant)

the pathway of catecholamine catabolism and production of norepinephrine and epinephrine. NB cells usually lack the last enzyme, phenylethanolamine N-methyltransferase, which is present in adrenal chromaffin cells and PHEOs. Degradation of L-DOPA and dopamine by catechol-O-methyltransferase and norepinephrine by monoamine oxidase is primarily responsible for production of the metabolites, homovanillic acid (HVA) and vanillylmandelic acid (VMA). The metabolites VMA and HVA are the most widely measured serum and urinary products for the diagnosis of NB and GNB. GN is not a biochemically active neoplasm in most cases. When the VMA/HVA ratio is less than 1, these tumors seem to have a less favorable clinical outcome than those with a ratio of greater than or equal to 1. Elevated tissue levels of the neuropeptides, VIP, and somatostatin have been correlated with cellular differentiation and low-stage disease. An elevated serum level of neuron-specific enolase is reported not only in NB but also in other tumors such as EWS–PPNET, small-cell neuroendocrine carcinoma, PHEO, acute lymphoblastic leukemia, and non-Hodgkin lymphoma (204). Although detecting NSE in serum is less specific for the diagnosis of NB, high levels at diagnosis have been correlated with a poor clinical outcome in several studies. This marker has some value for monitoring of recurrent tumor (205). Elevated serum ferritin levels are also observed in NB, Hodgkin lymphoma, leukemia, histiocytic disorders, and breast cancer (204). Higher serum ferritin levels at diagnosis are associated with metastatic NB and poor prognosis. Ferritin is not suitable for monitoring disease activity, because it becomes elevated from frequent blood transfusions during the course of clinical treatment. High serum lactate dehydrogenase (LDH) has some prognostic value; although LDH is not tumor specific, elevated levels reflect tumor load and rapid cell turnover (206,207). Other tumor markers reported to correlate with disease stage and/or prognosis include serum CHR A (112) and neuropeptide Y levels. Recently, detection of circulating *MYCN* DNA in serum has shown some promise in unmasking *MYCN*-amplified NBs (208).

Morphologic Features

Bone marrow (BM) biopsy is one of the essential procedures in the staging of a newly diagnosed NB, but it is also important in the monitoring of disease activity (209). It is generally recognized that both BM needle and aspiration biopsies have their complimentary value (210). An adequate aspirate may be difficult to obtain when the marrow is densely replaced by tumor or with fibrosis after therapy. Paratrabecular nests of metastatic NB are the characteristic findings in the involved biopsy, but micrometastatic disease may require immunohistochemistry, flow cytometry, and even RT-PCR in an attempt to establish the presence of tumor cells in a posttreatment specimen (211–213). TH, PGP9.5, CD56 (NCAM), NB84, and MAP2 immunostaining are useful with limitations on the basis of specificities and sensitivities for detecting the rare neuroblastoma cell. Recently PHOX2B is reported as a specific and stable immunohistochemical marker for detecting neuroblastoma cells (301). Metastatic NB in BM from a newly diagnosed case typically demonstrates collections of poorly differentiated neuroblasts with only a hint of neuropil in the background. On the other hand, differentiating neuroblasts, individually distributed or forming small clusters, with abundant neuropil are often seen in the BM after chemotherapy. Schwannian stroma is rarely encountered in BM biopsies.

The International Neuroblastoma Pathology Committee (INPC) made recommendations in 1999 for terminology and morphologic criteria of neuroblastic tumors by adopting and modifying the original Shimada classification (214–216). The recommendations were based on the hypothesis that these tumors provided one of the better models for analyzing the biologic relationship between molecular/genomic alterations and morphology. As outlined below, peripheral neuroblastic tumors are classified into four categories:

TABLE 21-12 CATEGORY AND SUBTYPES RECOMMENDED BY THE INTERNATIONAL NEUROBLASTOMA PATHOLOGY COMMITTEE

Category	Subtype
Neuroblastoma (Schwannian stroma poor)[a]	Undifferentiated Poorly differentiated Differentiating
Ganglioneuroblastoma, intermixed (Schwannian stroma rich) Ganglioneuroma (Schwannian stroma dominant)	Maturing Mature
Ganglioneuroblastoma, nodular[b] (Schwannian stroma dominant/stroma rich and stroma poor)	

[a]MKI (mitosis–karyorrhexis index; low, intermediate, or high) is assigned along with subtype of each neuroblastic tumor.
[b]Subtype (undifferentiated, poorly differentiated, or differentiating) and MKI are assigned to the neuroblastomatous nodule of each ganglioneuroblastoma, nodular tumor.
(From Peuchmaur M, d'Amore ESG, Joshi VV, et al. Revision of the international neuroblastoma pathology classification: confirmation of favorable and unfavorable prognostic subsets in ganglioneuroblastoma, nodular. *Cancer.* 2003;98:2274-2281; Shimada H, Ambros IM, Dehner LP, et al. Terminology and morphologic criteria of neuroblastic tumors: recommendation by the International Neuroblastoma Pathology Committee. *Cancer.* 1999;86:349-363.)

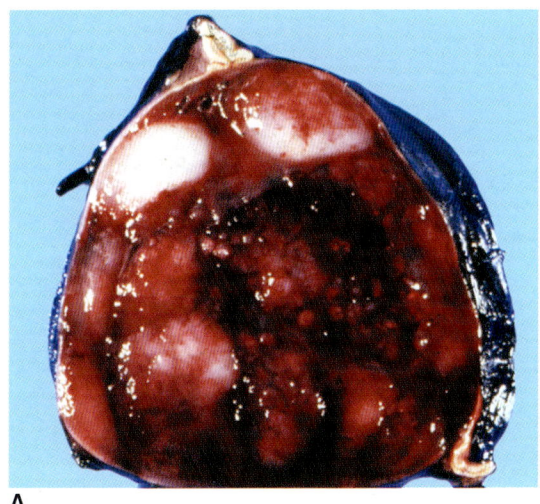
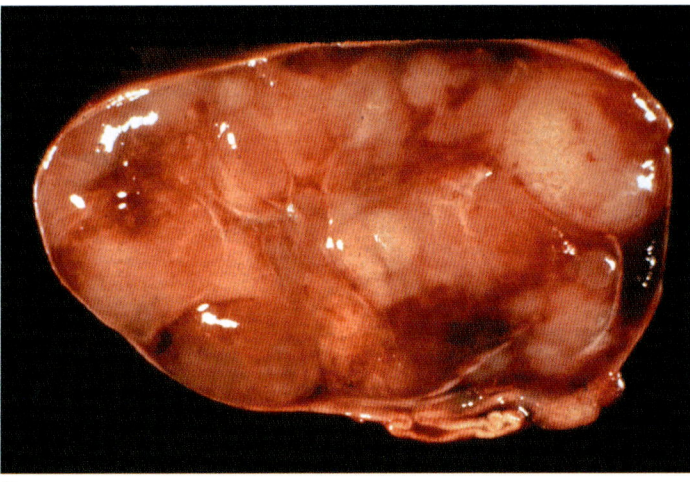

FIGURE 21-34 • Neuroblastoma. **A:** Adrenal neuroblastoma (Schwannian stroma poor), poorly differentiated subtype, measuring 5 cm × 4.5 cm in the greatest dimension, shows a friable and hemorrhagic appearance. **B:** Adrenal neuroblastoma (Schwannian stroma poor), differentiating subtype, measuring 6 cm × 4 cm in the greatest dimension, shows a soft and less hemorrhagic appearance.

(Table 21-12) NB, GNB—intermixed, GNB—nodular, and ganglioneuroma (GN).

NBs are further subclassified into undifferentiated, poorly differentiated, and differentiating subtypes. Grossly (Figure 21-34A, B, eFigure 21-103), NB usually presents as a solid circumscribed and often lobulated mass, measuring less than or equal to 10 cm greatest dimension, with considerable variation in appearance, depending on the anatomic location, histologic subtype, and secondary changes. A deep purple–red hemorrhagic appearance with or without scattered foci of glistening gray–white tissue is a common gross presentation for NB of the undifferentiated or poorly differentiated subtype. Punctate or coarse calcifications or yellow areas of coagulative necrosis are other relatively common macroscopic features in these two subtypes. Cystic degeneration with or without hemorrhage is another feature. Cystic NB, commonly arising in the adrenal gland, may require extensive sampling to identify microscopic foci of tumor. On the other hand, NB of the differentiating subtype is usually tan–yellow and less hemorrhagic with only limited areas of necrosis, if any.

NBs are further defined as Schwannian stroma poor and composed of neuroblasts forming lobules, which are completely or incompletely separated by delicate fibrovascular septa. Putative Schwannian blasts may be detected as slender S100-positive cells in the septal area (217). The typical neuroblast is round or slightly ovoid with a round to oval nucleus with finely granular (salt and pepper) chromatin and scanty cytoplasm. With the formation of neurites, an eosinophilic fibrillary network (neuropil) becomes apparent, but is not regarded as "stroma." Homer Wright rosettes are arranged around a central tangle of neurofibrillary processes without a central lumen or canal. Differentiating neuroblasts, a transitional form of neuroblastic differentiation toward ganglion cells, are characterized by synchronous changes in both the nucleus (enlarged, eccentrically located with vesicular chromatin pattern, and a single prominent nucleolus) and cytoplasm (eosinophilic/amphophilic with a diameter usually two or more times larger than the nucleus). Differentiating neuroblasts tend to produce more neuritic processes or neuropil.

The undifferentiated subtype of NB is composed of undifferentiated neuroblasts (small round-cell appearance) without clearly identifiable neuropil or rosettes (Figure 21-35). In fact, it is difficult for the pathologists to differentiate these tumor cells from the nonneuroblastic round-cell neoplasms of childhood without the assistance of immunohistochemistry, ultrastructural, molecular, and cytogenetic studies. Preliminary data suggest that undifferentiated neuroblasts lack the potential for differentiation. S100 protein staining demonstrates no or very few putative Schwannian blasts in the septal areas of the tumor when septation is present. Some tumors in this subtype show a diffuse growth pattern without a lobular architecture.

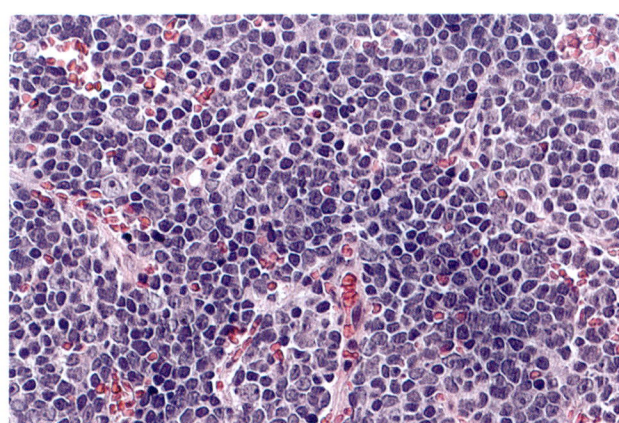

FIGURE 21-35 • Neuroblastoma (Schwannian stroma poor), undifferentiated subtype is composed of primitive cells without clearly recognizable neurite formation. Tumor cells in this case often have one or few prominent nucleoli. Note that tumor cells are irregularly demarcated by thin fibrovascular septal tissue.

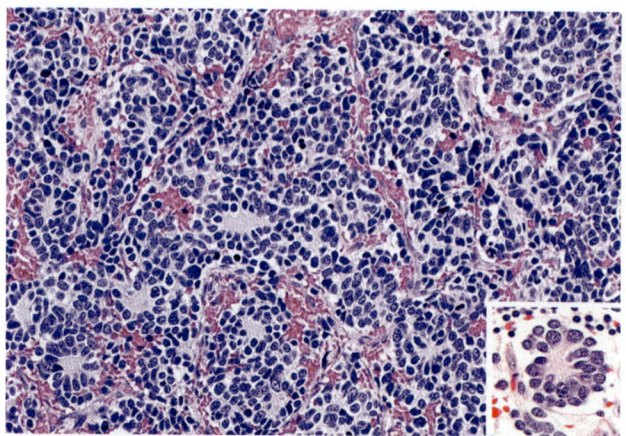

FIGURE 21-36 • Neuroblastoma (Schwannian stroma poor), poorly differentiated subtype is the most common form of tumor in the neuroblastoma group. Neuroblastoma cells produce neurites and can show rosette formations. Inset: typical Homer Wright rosette.

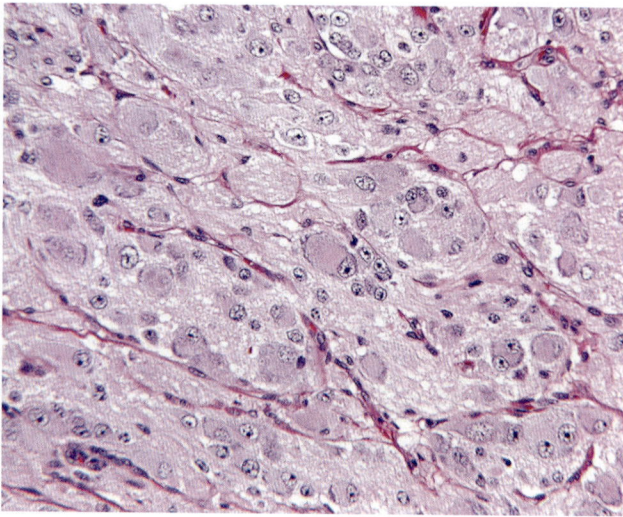

FIGURE 21-37 • Neuroblastoma (Schwannian stroma poor), differentiating subtype (containing more than 5% of the tumor cells showing an appearance of differentiating neuroblast by definition) is often characterized by abundant neuropil formation. Tumor cells are irregularly separated by thin fibrovascular septa, but significant Schwannian stromal development is not observed.

The poorly differentiated subtype is the most common pattern of NB in this group and is diagnosed in most cases without difficulty because neuropil and/or Homer Wright rosettes are commonly present (Figure 21-36) (eFigure 21-104). Most tumor cells are typical neuroblasts, and less than 5% of the population is pursuing ganglionic differentiation. Lobular formations of neuroblasts with thin fibrovascular septa are evident in many of these tumors. S100 protein–positive slender Schwann cells or putative Schwannian blasts can be detected, especially in the biologically favorable tumors of this subtype. It has been postulated that Schwann cells/Schwannian blasts are recruited into the tumor by the biologically favorable neuroblasts, rather than as end-stage differentiation from the neural crest cells.

NB differentiating subtype contains greater than or equal to 5% tumor cells with the features of differentiating neuroblasts (Figure 21-37). These tumors also have a prominent neuropil. It is thought that biologically favorable NBs of the poorly differentiated subtype can either regress or mature in the direction of the differentiating subtype. To date, among the biologically favorable NBs, there is no clear distinction in molecular characteristics between tumors with a potential for regression and those with presumed potential for maturation. In fact, during the process of tumor maturation from a poorly differentiated subtype to a differentiating subtype, the vast majority of neuroblasts undergo programmed cell death or apoptosis before or after attaining a certain degree of neuroblastic differentiation.

Some NBs have unique morphologic features including diffuse proliferation of anaplastic-appearing tumor cells, which are characterized by the presence of enlarged, bizarre cells and atypical mitotic figures (218). There is also a large cell type of NB characterized by open or vesicular nuclear morphology with few prominent nucleoli (219,220) that are sometimes referred to as bull's-eye nuclei. These rare tumors are known for their aggressive clinical course and often fatal outcome (221).

Ganglioneuroblastoma intermixed is defined as a Schwannian stroma-rich tumor whose Schwannian component occupies greater than 50% of the tumor area (Figure 21-38). The histologic features imply that there is incomplete transition to a fully mature GN, as evidenced by the presence of scattered "residual" microscopic foci or collections in neuroblasts in varying stages of differentiation within a background of neuropil. These neuroblasts, many with differentiating features toward immature ganglion cells, are in a process of either apoptosis or continuous maturation to mature ganglion cells. Individually distributed mature and

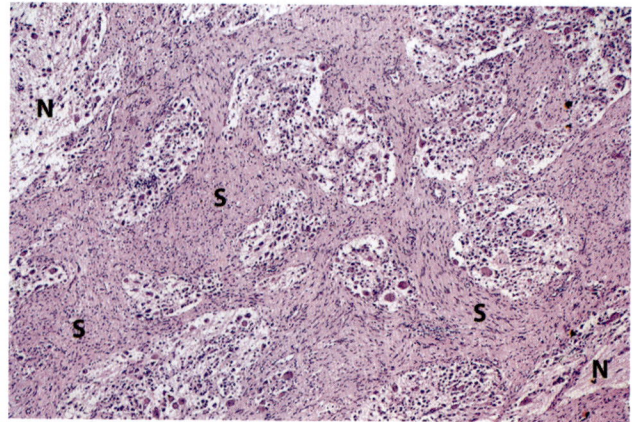

FIGURE 21-38 • Ganglioneuroblastoma, intermixed (Schwannian stroma rich) is characterized by an extensive Schwannian stromal development (S) occupying more than 50% of tumor tissue. Pockets of naked neuropil (N) area containing tumor cells in various stages of neuronal differentiation are found. Tumor cells in those pockets are composed of a mixture of differentiating neuroblasts and maturing ganglion cells with or without poorly differentiated neuroblasts.

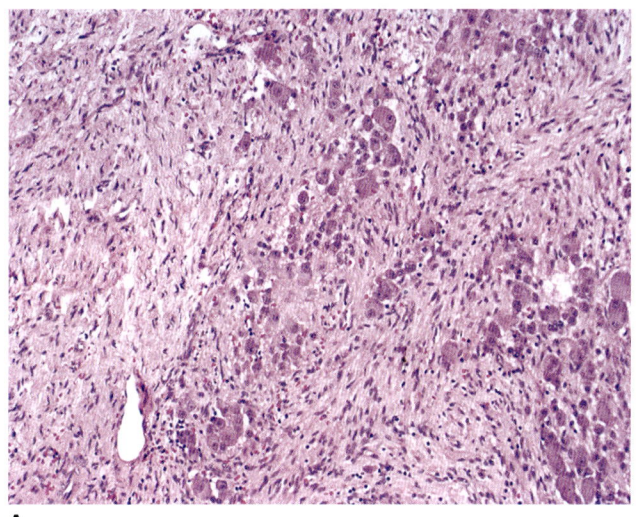
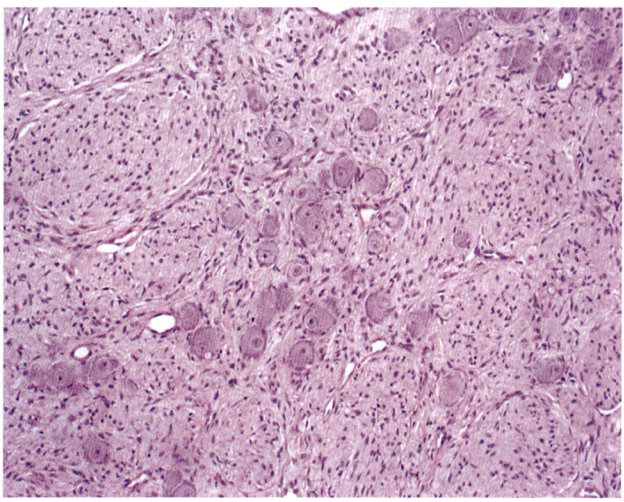

FIGURE 21-39 • **A:** Ganglioneuroma (Schwannian stroma dominant), maturing in a tumor predominantly composed of Schwannian stromal tissue. Differentiating neuroblasts and maturing/mature ganglion cells are distributed without clearly recognizable pockets of neuropil. **B:** Ganglioneuroma (Schwannian stroma dominant), mature, is a completely mature form in the neuroblastoma group. Fully mature ganglion cells are covered with satellite cells. Stroma component is well organized and shows multiple fascicular formations composed of Schwann cells of unmyelinated type surrounded by perineurial cells.

maturing ganglion cells are also found in the Schwannian stroma with the pattern of GN.

Ganglioneuroma is a Schwannian stroma-dominant neoplasm without any aggregates of neuroblasts in a neuropil background. The exclusive cellular elements are Schwann cells with accompanying individually distributed or small groups of maturing/mature ganglion cells. Two subtypes, GN maturing (Figure 21-39A) and GN mature (Figure 21-39B), are included in this category. The GN maturing, previously designated as "GNB, well differentiated" in the original Shimada classification (216), contains scattered individual immature ganglion cells in addition to mature ganglion cells. The mature GN (GN mature) is the fully mature peripheral neuroblastic tumor and is composed of Schwannian stroma and mature ganglion cells, which are surrounded by satellite cells. Fully developed Schwannian stroma is seen in GNs and focally in the GNB intermixed. Mature unmyelinated types of Schwann cells characteristically forming multiple fascicles covered with perineurial cells are present. These areas of a mature GN without ganglion cells resemble a schwannoma. A well-formed capsule is more characteristic of schwannoma, whereas GN tends to blend into the adjacent soft tissues with some circumscription at the peripheral margins.

Both the GNB intermixed and GN have similar gross features with a firm consistency and a cut surface with a tan-yellow, homogenous appearance with or without fibrous bands (Figure 21-40).

Ganglioneuroblastoma nodular is a composite tumor characterized by the presence of one or more grossly visible, often hemorrhagic/necrotic neuroblastic nodule(s) coexisting with GNB intermixed or GN (Figure 21-41A, B). There is typically an abrupt demarcation (pushing border or pseudocapsular formation) between the neuroblastic nodule(s) and the ganglioneuromatous component (GNB intermixed or GN). Some neuroblastic nodules may not be clearly demarcated, but rather there is neuroblastic infiltration into the Schwannian stromal component of GNB intermixed or GN component. It is possible that some neuroblastic nodules are intratumoral metastasis into the ganglioneuromatous areas. Infrequently, a neuroblastic nodule grows so large that the ganglioneuromatous component (GNB intermixed or GN) can only

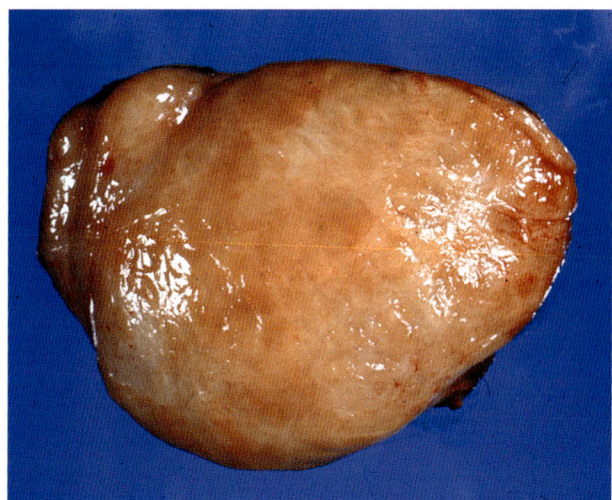

FIGURE 21-40 • Ganglioneuroblastoma, intermixed (Schwannian stroma rich), in the mediastinum measuring 9 cm × 7 cm in the greatest dimension, is rubbery in consistency and has no grossly visible nodule of neuroblastomatous growth. Tumors in both ganglioneuroblastoma, intermixed (Schwannian stroma rich) and ganglioneuroma (Schwannian stroma dominant) category present a gross appearance similar to a schwannoma.

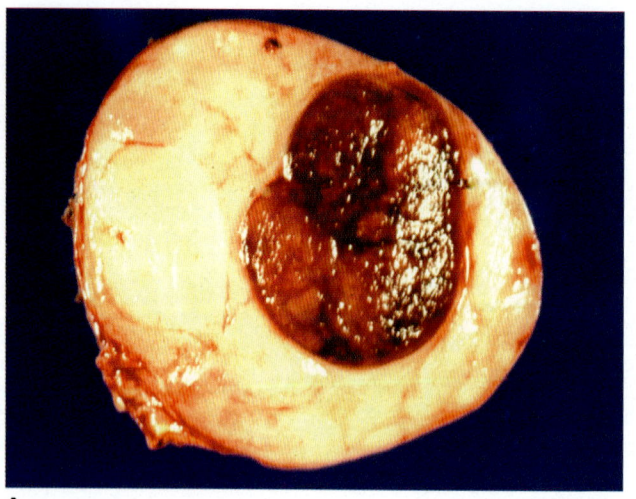 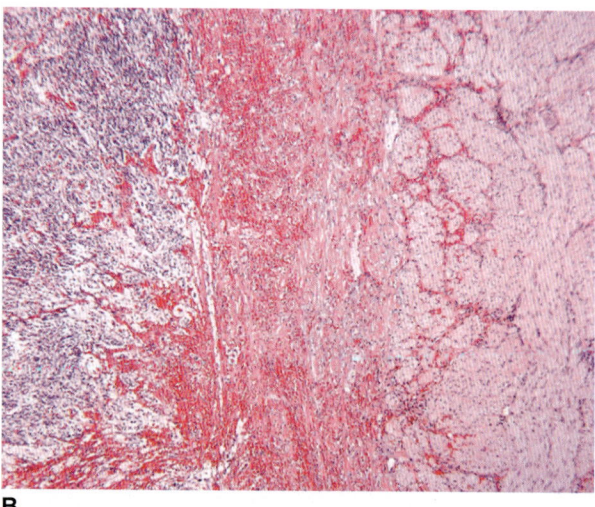

FIGURE 21-41 • Ganglioneuroblastoma, nodular (composite, Schwannian stroma dominant/stroma rich and stroma poor) arising the retroperitoneum. **A:** The tumor measuring 8 cm × 7 cm in the greatest dimension, is tan–yellow and rubbery in consistency, and contains a grossly visible hemorrhagic nodule. There are two (or multiple) distinct tumor types/clones coexisting in the same tumor tissue of this category. **B:** As shown in this example, one tumor type (**left side**) has an appearance of neuroblastoma (Schwannian stroma poor) forming a grossly visible and often hemorrhagic nodule, and the other (**right side**) has a feature of ganglioneuroma (Schwannian stroma dominant).

be recognized microscopically, often at the periphery of the tumor, as a narrow ribbon of GN. Neuroblastic nodules are usually evident in the gross examination of the primary tumor; however, they may be overlooked. For that reason, those primary tumors with the features of GNB intermixed or GN, but with metastatic NB to lymph node, bone, or other sites, are also included in the category of GNB nodular (222).

As a component of the pathologic evaluation of an NB, the INPC has recommended a determination of the mitotic and karyorrhectic activities by the mitosis–karyorrhexis index (MKI). MKI has been defined by three semiquantitative levels: low (<2% or <100 mitotic and karyorrhectic cells per 5,000 neuroblasts), intermediate (2% to 4% or 100 to 200 mitotic and karyorrhectic cells per 5,000 neuroblasts), and high (>4% or >200 mitotic and karyorrhectic cells per 5,000 neuroblasts). The MKI is determined by counting the number of tumor cells in mitosis and in the process of karyorrhexis and should reflect an average for all tumor sections available. Cells in karyorrhexis, one of the apoptotic processes and individual cell death due to severe genomic instability, are characterized by condensed and fragmented nuclear chromatin without nuclear membrane, usually accompanied by condensed eosinophilic cytoplasm. Hyperchromatic nuclei without chromatin fragmentation are not included in the MKI count. It has been reported that increased mitotic and karyorrhectic activity is correlated with *MYCN* amplification and excess production of *MYCN* protein (223,224).

Ultrastructure, Immunohistochemistry, and Molecular Diagnostics

Ultrastructural features characteristic of neuroblastic cells include the presence of membrane-bound neurosecretory granules in the cytoplasm and neuritic processes with typically arranged microtubules, which are parallel to each other. Rudimentary attachment structures are found between adjacent neuroblasts. These features, however, are also detectable in EWS–PNETs. Nissl bodies composed of rough endoplasmic reticulum and free ribosomes are found in the periphery of the cytoplasm of differentiating neuroblasts and ganglion cells. Neuromelanin can be detected in some of the differentiating neuroblasts. Mature Schwannian cells found in the GNB intermixed and GN are the unmyelinated form and contain multiple neurites in the individual cell bodies.

Immunohistochemically, neuroblastic cells are positive for PHOX2B, NSE, NB84, PGP9.5, SYN, CHR, Leu 7 (CD57), a variety of NFPs, NCAMs, and other neural antigens (225). TH is a useful marker for identifying neural crest cells and is positive in NB, PHEO, and paraganglioma (so called extra-adrenal pheochromocytomas) (226). In most cases, application of immunohistochemistry is more adjunctive to the histologic examination, because the accumulative data of clinical and laboratory findings generally support a straightforward diagnosis of NB on routine staining. In practice, PHOX2B, PGP9.5, TH, CD56, MIC2 (CD99), desmin, MyoD1, myogenin, and lymphoid markers are applied as the immunohistochemical panel for distinguishing an undifferentiated NB from other malignant round-cell neoplasms of childhood. Undifferentiated NBs are diffusely positive for PHOX2B and PGP9.5, often sporadically positive for TH, and negative for the other markers. While EWS–PNET is positive for PGP9.5 and MIC2 (CD99), it is negative for PHOX2B and TH. Rhabdomyosarcoma is positive for desmin, MyoD1, and myogenin. Hematolymphoid malignancies can be screened with CD43 and CD45 to be followed by additional specific lineage markers as appropriate. When only VIM is immunoreactive, one should think in terms of an undifferentiated

NB or a hematolymphoid malignancy. Putative Schwannian blasts are positive for S100 (monoclonal antibody for β-chain recommended) and located in the thin fibrovascular septa demarcating groups and clusters of NB cells especially the biologically favorable NB tumors (217). Ganglioneuroblastoma and GN are characterized by S100-positive Schwannian stromal development. Satellite cells surrounding the fully mature ganglion cells are also positive for S100.

Frequently used molecular markers include *EWS–ETS* translocation (*EWS–FLI1*, *EWS–ERG*, etc.) and *PAX–FOXO1* translocation with undifferentiated NBs to exclude other small round-cell tumors. NBs are negative for those translocations. Demonstrating *EWS–ETS* translocation or EWS rearrangement by FISH and detecting its chimeric protein are diagnostic of EWS–PPNET (227,228). The presence of *PAX–FOXO1* translocation, detectable in around 80% alveolar rhabdomyosarcomas (229), is reported to indicate an aggressive clinical behavior of the disease (230).

International NB Pathology Classification

A morphologic classification designed to be prognostically significant and biologically relevant was established by the INPC in 1999 (214,215) and revised in 2003 (Table 21-12) (222). This classification distinguishes two pathologic–prognostic groups: favorable histology (FH) and unfavorable histology (UH) group (Table 21-13) (231–240). This

TABLE 21-13 PROGNOSTIC DISTINCTION ACCORDING TO THE INTERNATIONAL NEUROBLASTOMA PATHOLOGY CLASSIFICATION

Age	Favorable Histology Group	Unfavorable Histology Group
Any	Ganglioneuroma (Schwannian stroma dominant) Maturing Mature Ganglioneuroblastoma, intermixed (Schwannian stroma rich)	
		Neuroblastoma (Schwannian stroma poor) Undifferentiated and any MKI
Less than 1.5 years	Neuroblastoma (Schwannian stroma poor) Poorly differentiated and low or intermediate MKI Differentiating and low or intermediate MKI	Neuroblastoma (Schwannian stroma poor) Poorly differentiated and high MKI Differentiating and high MKI
1.5 years up to less than 5 years	Neuroblastoma (Schwannian stroma poor) Differentiating and low MKI	Neuroblastoma (Schwannian stroma poor) Poorly differentiated and any MKI Differentiating and intermediate or high MKI
Equal to or greater than 5 years		Neuroblastoma (Schwannian stroma poor) Any subtype and any MKI
	Ganglioneuroblastoma, nodular (composite, Schwannian stroma rich/stroma dominant and stroma poor), favorable subset[a]	Ganglioneuroblastoma, nodular (composite, Schwannian stroma rich/stroma dominant and stroma poor), unfavorable subset[a]

[a]All tumors in the category of ganglioneuroblastoma, nodular were once classified into an unfavorable histology group according to the original Shimada classification (216) and the original International Neuroblastoma Pathology Classification (INPC) (214). However, the revised INPC distinguishes two prognostic subsets, favorable, and unfavorable, by applying the same age-linked histopathology evaluation to the nodular (neuroblastoma) components of the tumors in this category (222).
MKI, Mitosis-karyorrhexis index.
(From Peuchmaur M, d'Amore ESG, Joshi VV, et al. Revision of the International Neuroblastoma Pathology Classification: confirmation of favorable and unfavorable prognostic subsets in ganglioneuroblastoma, nodular. *Cancer.* 2003;98:2274–2281; Shimada H, Ambros IM, Dehner LP, et al. Terminology and morphologic criteria of neuroblastic tumors: Recommendation by the International Neuroblastoma Pathology Committee. *Cancer.* 1999;86:349–363.)

classification is age linked and utilizes three morphologic indicators: status of Schwannian stromal development (stroma poor, stroma rich, stroma dominant), grade of neuroblastic differentiation (undifferentiated, poorly differentiated, differentiating), and MKI (low, intermediate, high). The histologic features should be evaluated on a resected specimen or biopsy before the initiation of chemotherapy and/or radiation therapy. Metastatic sites, except for bone marrow, are eligible for the evaluation of all these histologic features. BM biopsy is not informative for MKI determination. FH NBs fall within the conceptual framework of an age-appropriate maturational sequence starting with NB (Schwannian stroma poor), poorly differentiated subtype (up to 1.5 years of age at diagnosis) to NB-differentiating subtype (up to 5 years of age at diagnosis) to GNB intermixed (Schwannian stroma-rich) to GN (Schwannian stroma dominant). All GNs, the final end of tumor maturation, are thought to have had a neuroblastic component in their early developmental stage. In this regard, most GNs are diagnosed in later childhood, adolescence, and even into adulthood. FH neuroblastic tumors should have a low MKI when diagnosed less than 5 years of age, or an intermediate MKI when diagnosed less than 1.5 years of age. In contrast, the histologic features of UH neoplasms are immature or inappropriate for the age at diagnosis and include NB, undifferentiated subtype (at any age), poorly differentiated NB ($\geq$1.5 years of age), and all NB subtypes ($\geq$5 years of age). Among tumors in the NB category, those with high MKI at any age, or an intermediate MKI at greater than or equal to 1.5 years of age, are also assigned to the UH group. Ganglioneuroblastoma intermixed and GN, usually diagnosed in older children, are examples of FH tumors with an excellent prognosis (241). Tumors in the GNB nodular (composite, Schwannian stroma-rich/stroma-dominant and stroma-poor) category are further subclassified into two subsets, favorable and unfavorable, by application of the same criteria of age-linked evaluation of histologic features (grade of neuroblastic differentiation, MKI) to the nodular (NB and Schwannian stroma-poor) component (222,242).

Ganglioneuroblastoma intermixed or GN is usually resected surgically. These tumors may encase the great vessels and/or organs, making complete surgical excision with tumor-free margins often difficult and unnecessary in most cases. Because of the non-infiltrative nature of such tumors, local recurrences are uncommon. When only a biopsy is available and shows features of GNB intermixed or GN, the pathologic diagnosis should be qualified by the comment "the diagnosis is made based on review of limited material and may not be representative of the tumor as a whole." In this circumstance, careful reassessment of the primary tumor site as well as a metastatic workup is recommended. This is because of the possibility of GNB nodular in which a nonsampled neuroblastic nodule may exist. A nonsampled neuroblastic nodule, if present, is often hemorrhagic and necrotic or may show invasive growth into the surrounding tissues, which may be apparent on imaging studies. Metastatic foci may be demonstrable as well. Catecholamine determination is also advisable.

Histologic changes after chemotherapy and/or radiation therapy especially in the UH tumors do not provide any reliable information in predicting clinical outcome. These changes include extensive necrosis, hemorrhage, hemosiderin deposition, fibrosis, and calcification along with varying degrees of tumor maturation, often presenting different histologic features from area to area. With FH tumors, chemotherapy often facilitates uniform tumor maturation without extensive necrosis, hemorrhage, and marked hemosiderin deposition. According to the Children's Oncology Group (COG) Neuroblastoma Study, the INPC evaluation of either FH or UH, once determined based on the review of prechemotherapy specimen, will not be altered during the clinical course of individual cases.

Molecular/Genetic Alterations

The remarkable aspect of NB is the biologic heterogeneity, which is reflected in its tumorigenesis and diverse clinical behaviors. Structural genetic alterations often detected in NB include genomic amplification of *MYCN* oncogene on chromosome 2p24, allelic deletion of the short arm of chromosome 1p36 (del 1p) (243,244), allelic deletion of the long arm of chromosome 11q23 (del 11q) (243,245,246), and unbalanced gain of genetic material of the long arm of chromosome 17q21 (17q-gain). In addition, allelic losses of genetic material on 3p, 4p, 9p, 14q, 16p, and 19q as well as segmental gains of 1q, 5q, and 18q have been detected in varying numbers of NBs (247). Most of these alterations are associated with unfavorable clinical behavior. Among these changes, 17q gain is the most frequent alteration in about two-thirds of NBs and may be related to tumorigenesis. However, the prognostic impact of 17q gain in children with NB has not been identified (248). PHOX2B transcription factor (homeobox gene important in development of normal autonomic nervous system) is mutated in a small proportion of NBs (249–251).

MYCN amplification, one of the strongest indicators for aggressive tumor progression, is observed in 15% to 20% of all NBs, resulting in overproduction of MYCN protein. MYCN–MAX heterodimer formation in the tumor nuclei prevents cellular differentiation, promotes cellular proliferation, and affects genomic instability. A reproducible correlation is present between the molecular event of *MYCN* amplification and the morphologic features of NB. Those tumors with amplified *MYCN* typically have undifferentiated or poorly differentiated features with a high MKI, reflecting increased cellular proliferation and apoptosis due to genomic instability (Figure 21-42) (223,224). Prominent nucleoli in neuroblastic cells of undifferentiated or poorly differentiated tumor cells appear to be an additional hallmark of *MYCN* amplification (220,252,253).

MYCN status of tumors is determined by fluorescent *in situ* hybridization (FISH) analysis in many institutions. The International Neuroblastoma Risk Group (INRG) Biology Committee has defined *MYCN* amplification by FISH

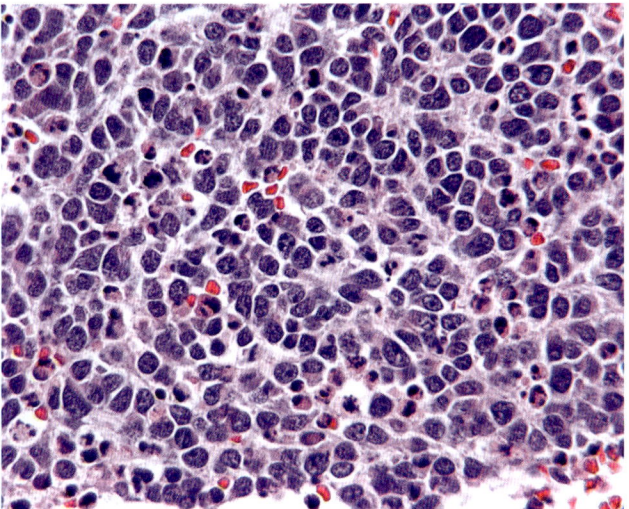

FIGURE 21-42 • Neuroblastoma. Typical histologic features of the MYCN amplified neuroblastoma include no Schwannian stroma development, no or limited neuroblastic differentiation, and markedly increased mitotic and karyorrhectic activities (high MKI—mitosis–karyorrhexis index).

analysis as greater than fourfold increase in *MYCN* signal number compared with the reference probe located on chromosome 2q. Furthermore, *MYCN* gain has been defined as a signal increase, but not up to the amplified status, whose clinical significance is yet to be determined (254). It is also noted that *MYCN*-amplified status usually remains unchanged after chemotherapy. Recent studies report that MYCN protein expression rather than *MYCN* oncogene amplification provides a measure of aggressive clinical behavior (255,256). MYC (C-myc) protein overexpression is a relatively new prognostic indicator of poor prognosis (257,302).

Activating ALK oncogene mutations appear to be responsible for many hereditary NBs and may be relevant for certain sporadic NBs. Interestingly, 20% to 25% of primary NBs have increased *ALK* (2p23) copy numbers, and elevated ALK gene expression levels occur in aggressive neuroblastic tumors (182–185,258). Genetic variation at chromosome 6p22 has been identified for NB susceptibility. Additionally, patients whose tumors are homozygous for the risk alleles at 6p22 are likely to have metastatic disease, *MYCN* amplification, and decrease relapse (259). Also reported is ATRX gene mutation detected in older children and young adults with stage 4 NB (260).

Gene expression–based analyses show that elevated levels of TrkA, CD44, and CAMTA1 correlate with favorable clinical outcome (261,262), while elevated levels of expression of survivin, repp86, and PRAME are reported to correlate with adverse outcome (263–265). However, anyone of those candidates alone cannot sufficiently explain the diverse clinical behaviors of NBs and is not considered as an independent prognostic factor in clinical trials.

DNA ploidy patterns, diploid ("near diploid") or hyperdiploid ("near triploid"), are reported to distinguish prognostic categories (266,267). A near-triploid DNA content due to whole chromosomal gain (lack of structural chromosomal aberration) has been reported as a favorable prognostic indicator. In contrast, a near-diploid DNA content predicts a poor clinical outcome, especially for infants.

Both familial and sporadic neuroblastomas may have mutations in several members of the neuroblastoma breakpoint family gene (*NBPF*) and neuroblastoma susceptibility gene (*NBLST*), neuroblastoma amplified sequence gene (*NBAS*), neuroblastoma candidate region suppression of tumorigenicity gene (*NBL1*), and *BRACA1*-associated ring domain 1 (*BARD1*). A regulator of autonomic nervous system development (*PHOX2B*) has been identified as playing a major role in neuroblastoma in both hereditary and sporadic neuroblastomas. Single nucleotide polymorphism variations may be associated with neuroblastoma development (FLJ22536, *BARD1*). Other well-known genetic abnormalities with neuroblastoma include loss of tumor-suppressor genes at 1p and 3p and deletion of a regulator of the cell cycle on chromosome 9 (*CDKN2A*). Silencing of gene function by methylation is another common mechanism for neuroblastoma development in children. Methylation of genes associated with regulation of apoptosis (caspase 8, *TMS1*) and the cell cycle (*CDKN2A*, *CCND2*, *SFN*) have been shown to participate in genesis of neuroblastomas. In addition, dysregulation of retinoic acid receptor genes and cell adhesion molecules (cadherin 1) participate in the neoplastic process. Small nonencoding RNAs (miRNA) play an important role as negative regulators. Certain miRNAs participate in sporadic and familial neuroblastomas by affecting *MYCN* amplification. In the past few years, attention has been directed toward genome-wide analysis of pediatric and adult tumors. It has been shown that certain chromosomal aberrations (translocations, amplifications, deletions, regional chromosomal losses and gains) are associated with aggressive neuroblastomas. In contrast, whole chromosomal gains (hyperdiploidy, chromosomal duplications) are associated with "benign" or less aggressive neuroblastomas. Based upon genome wide association studies, it has been possible to stratify neuroblastomas and relate these to established low-, intermediate-, and high-risk categories as well as those that fall into the very favorable category of stage 4S. In the not-too-distant future, genome-wide association studies may be utilized to determine treatment, prognosis, event-free survival, and overall survival of individual patients. A limited gene expression signature (59 genes) may distinguish between low- and high-risk patients with respect to overall survival, progression-free survival, risk of dying of disease, and disease relapse. A 144 gene expression signature has distinguished patients that have favorable versus unfavorable clinical courses, *MYCN*-amplified versus nonamplified tumors, favorable versus unfavorable survival over a 5-year period, and clinical low- versus intermediate- versus high-risk categories. This 144 gene expression signatures act as an independent prognostic marker for event-free and overall survival. The availability of "designer" gene microarray technology allows the neuroblastoma gene expression signature to be a prognostic test that can be readily applied within the

dren is different than those for adults. With adults, the adrenal medulla is the primary site in about 80% of cases. With children, about one-third of tumors arise from the adrenal medulla, whereas the majority arise from paraganglia, with the most common site being para-aortic. Tumors are larger in malignant tumors (8.6 cm) when compared with benign tumors (4.5 cm). There are nearly an even proportion of benign and malignant tumors in children. Local invasion occurs in 23%. Metastatic disease occurs in 27% with involvement of lymph nodes, lung, liver, and mediastinum. Although the tumors are considered to be resectable in about 90% of cases, surgical resection provides negative margins in only about two-thirds of cases. Chemotherapy and radiation therapy are employed in 15% to 18% of affected patients. Tumor recurrence is seen in 26%, with a mean time to recurrence of 2 years. Benign paragangliomatous tumors have a 15-year survival rate of 100%, while malignant tumors have only a 31% 15-year survival rate. With children, certain risk factors are more commonly associated with malignant paragangliomatous tumors. These include genetic mutation or familial history of paragangliomatous tumors, tumor size of greater than or equal to 6 cm, and extra-adrenal location.

Sporadic PHEO is typically a solitary, well-circumscribed mass with either a true capsule or a pseudocapsule related to the tumor expansion and compression of adjacent connective tissue. Most tumors range in size from 3 to 5 cm, and the average weight is about 100 g (Figure 21-43A). Periadrenal brown fat is often seen. Because medullary tissue is concentrated in the head and body of the adrenal, the smaller PHEO arises in the latter locations (Figure 21-44A). On cut section, the tumor is firm and gray or dark red or is extensively hemorrhagic with cystic degeneration and friability. The chromaffin reaction is a manifestation of the catecholamines in the tissue and produced by exposure of the unfixed specimen to a dichromate solution, which leads to a deep brown coloration (Figure 21-43B).

Three principal histologic patterns are found in PHEO: a trabecular pattern with anastomosing cords of cells, an alveolar or nesting pattern with "zellballen" formation, and a diffuse or solid growth pattern (Figure 21-44B, eFigure 21-105). Spindle cells, angiomatoid foci, prominent interstitial and perivascular sclerosis, pseudopapillary formations, and small spaces filled with eosinophilic proteinaceous debris are focal or generalized features in any one tumor (286). Nuclear pseudoinclusions and eosinophilic hyaline intracytoplasmic globules are common. The cytoplasm of the tumor cells ranges from eosinophilic and granular to intense basophilia.

These tumors are typically immunoreactive for VIM, CHR, VIP, and, infrequently, HMB-45 (172). CHR A and TH are the most reliable markers for distinguishing this tumor from adrenal cortical neoplasms and neuroendocrine tumors, respectively. Lack of EMA staining helps to differentiate this tumor from renal cell carcinoma. SYN staining is quite variable. S100 protein staining highlights sustentacular cells at the periphery of cell clusters (alveolar

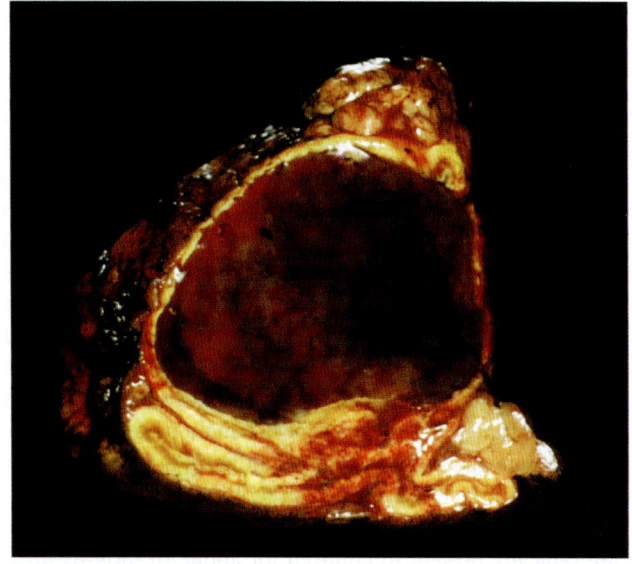

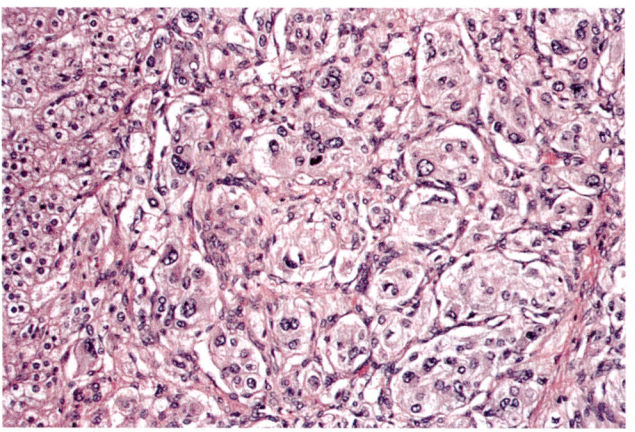

A B

FIGURE 21-44 • Pheochromocytoma. **A:** This adrenal gland demonstrates a central brown 3-cm-diameter tumor replacing the adrenal medulla. The adrenal cortex (*yellow*) is seen at the periphery of this tumor. This tumor was resected from a patient with a chief complaint of paroxysmal attacks of headache, blurred vision, tachycardia, and diaphoresis. **B:** The tumor cells are arranged in a characteristic alveolar "zellballen" or nesting pattern. They are surrounded by thin fibrovascular septa. The polyhedral tumor cells vary in shape and size. Most cells have an eosinophilic granular cytoplasm. The ovoid nuclei have a dispersed stippled chromatin pattern with inconspicuous nucleolus. Mitotic figures were infrequent in this tumor (H&E stain).

or zellballen pattern). More recently, immunocytochemical staining for SDHB, SDHC, and SDHD has become available. Lack of immunocytochemical staining of the tumor cells for one of these components is helpful in directing appropriate genetic testing for somatic and constitutional mutations in the succinate dehydrogenase genes. Electron microscopy reveals cells with interdigitating borders and poorly formed cells junctions. Membrane-bound dense core neurosecretory granules are prominent. These granules appear to contain norepinephrine with a prominent eccentric electron-lucent space surrounding the dense core, are associated with paragangliomatous tumors, and differentiate this tumor from renal cell carcinoma, adrenal cortical neoplasms, and neuroblastoma.

The prevalence of malignancy in childhood PHEOs is difficult to ascertain due to the inclusion of paragangliomas in many studies; however, it is estimated that 2% to 12% of these tumors behave in a malignant fashion (287). With inclusion of paragangliomas, the prevalence is even higher, because paragangliomas especially in sites other than in the head and neck region are more prone to malignant behavior. When paragangliomas are included in the assessment of prognosis, the prevalence of malignancy approaches 50% in some series, inclusive of pediatric series (288,289). Except for the presence of metastasis, no single histologic feature of the tumor itself, including local invasion, is definitively predictive of malignant behavior (eFigure 21-106) (290,291). Risk factors for malignancy include the diagnosis of paraganglioma and tumor size greater than 6 cm. However, tumor size is not always predictive of malignancy (292). Although not diagnostic of malignancy, the features more commonly seen with malignant tumors include (a) capsular invasion; (b) vascular invasion; (c) extension into periadrenal soft tissue; (d) expanded, large, and confluent cell nests; (e) diffuse growth; (f) necrosis, usually confluent; (g) increased cellularity; (h) tumor cell spindling; (i) marked cellular and nuclear pleomorphism; (j) cellular monotony; (k) nuclear hyperchromasia; (l) macronuclei; (m) increased mitotic figures; (n) atypical mitoses; (o) absence of hyaline globules; (p) extraadrenal location; and (q) coarse nodularity. An increased MIB-1 index (nuclear immunopositivity) correlated with malignant behavior in some, but not all studies (290,291). The 5-year and 10-year survival rates for malignant tumors are 78% and 31%, respectively (288).

Adrenal medullary hyperplasia occurs in the setting of MEN2 syndromes as the presumed precursor of PHEOs. It has also been reported as an isolated finding in the nonfamilial setting of hypertension and biochemical studies suggesting PHEO; however, no discrete adrenal medullary tumor is found at surgery, implying an occult PHEO/paraganglioma (115,293). Criteria for the diagnosis of adrenal medullary hyperplasia include increase in adrenal weight accompanied by diffuse or nodular extension of the medulla into the alae (294,295). Morphometric criteria include a decrease in the overall ratio of cortex to medulla (normal is 10:1) and an increase in the calculated medullary weight and volume (eFigures 21-107 and 21-108).

Composite adrenal medullary neoplasms are rare entities that are composed in part by PHEO, neuroblastic tumor, or peripheral nerve sheath neoplasm. Most of these tumors have been reported in adults, but have been infrequently observed in children. Other tumor and tumorlike lesions of the adrenal gland include a variety of cysts of a presumed vascular nature. Extramedullary hematopoiesis in the setting of β-thalassemia may present as an adrenal incidentaloma in childhood (e949). Myelolipoma is a more common "incidentalomas" of the adrenal gland in adults and extremely unusual in children and slightly more frequent than the lipoma and leiomyoma. Hemangioma or hemangioendothelioma of the adrenal has been observed in infancy. Extrarenal WT of the adrenal gland has been reported in a 4-year-old boy (296). A primitive epithelial and mesenchymal neoplasm of the adrenal gland in an infant with virilizing signs has been reported and interpreted as an adrenal blastoma (164). PNET family tumor has also been reported in the adrenal gland of children (297,298). Though not an adrenal lesion per se, subdiaphragmatic extralobar sequestration may simulate an adrenal tumor when it presents as a suprarenal mass (see Chapter 12) (299).

References

1. Reiter RJ. The pineal gland. In: Lechago J, Gould VE, eds. *Bloodworth's Endocrine Pathology*, 3rd ed. Baltimore, MD: Lippincott Williams & Wilkins, 1997:153–170.
2. Burger PC, Scheithauer BW. *AFIP Atlas of Tumor Pathology, Series 4, Tumors of the Central Nervous System*. Washington, DC: American Registry of Pathology, 2007:295–308.
3. Jouvet A, Fevre-Montange M, Besancon R, et al. Structural and ultrastructural characteristics of human pineal gland, and pineal parenchymal tumors. *Acta Neuropathol* 1994;88:334–348.
4. Tapp E, Huxley M. The histological appearance of the human pineal gland from puberty to old age. *J Pathol* 1972;108:137–144.
5. Sapède D, Cau E. The pineal gland from development to function. *Curr Top Dev Biol* 2013;106:171–215. doi: 10.1016/B978-0-12-416021-7.00005-5
6. Mandera M, Marcol W, Bierzynska-Macyszyn G, et al. Pineal cysts in childhood. *Childs Nerv Syst* 2003;19:750–755.
7. Schimke RN. The endocrine glands. In: Stevenson RE, Hall JG, Goodman RM, eds. *Human Malformations and Related Anomalies*. New York: Oxford University Press, 1993:1017–1029.
8. Michielsen G, Benoit Y, Baert E, et al. Symptomatic pineal cysts: clinical manifestations and management. *Acta Neurochir (Wien)* 2002;144:233–242.
9. Wisoff JH, Epstein F. Surgical management of symptomatic pineal cysts. *J Neurosurg* 1992;77:896–900.
10. Popovic MB, Diezi M, Kuchler H, et al. Trilateral retinoblastoma with suprasellar tumor and associated pineal cyst. *J Pediatr Hematol Oncol* 2007;29:53–56.
11. Engel U, Gottschalk S, Niehaus L, et al. Cystic lesions of the pineal region—MRI and pathology. *Neuroradiology* 2000;42:399–402.
12. Mottolese C, Szathmari A, Beuriat PA. Incidence of pineal tumours. A review of the literature. *Neurochirurgie* 2015;61(2–3):65–69. pii: S0028-3770(14)00078-2. doi: 10.1016/j.neuchi.2014.01.005
13. Magrini S, Feletti A, Marton E, et al. Gliomas of the pineal region. *J Neurooncol* 2013;115(1):103–111. doi: 10.1007/s11060-013-1200-9
14. McCarthy BJ, Shibui S, Kayama T, et al. Primary CNS germ cell tumors in Japan and the United States: an analysis of 4 tumor registries. *Neuro Oncol* 2012;14(9):1194–1200. doi: 10.1093/neuonc/nos155

112. Hsiao RJ, Seeger RC, Yu AL, et al. Chromogranin A in children with neuroblastoma. Serum concentration parallels disease stage and predicts survival. *J Clin Invest* 85:1555–1559.
113. van den Berg H, Caron HN. Paratesticular neuroblastoma: a case against metastatic disease? *J Pediatr Hematol Oncol* 2007;29:187–189.
114. Lack EE. Tumors of the adrenal gland and extra-adrenal paraganglia. In: *AFIP Atlas of Tumor Pathology*, Ser. 4. Washington, DC: American Registry of Pathology, 2007:1–37.
115. Lloyd RV, Douglas BR, Young WF. *Endocrine Diseases: Atlas of Nontumor Pathology*, Fascicle 1. Washington, DC: American Registry of Pathology, 2001:171–258.
116. Auchus RJ, Miller WL. The principles, pathways, and enzymes of human steroidogenesis. In: DeGroot LJ, Jameson JL, eds. *Endocrinology*, 5th ed. Philadelphia, PA: Elsevier, 2006.
117. Al-Alwan I, Navarro O, Daneman D, et al. Clinical utility of adrenal ultrasonography in the diagnosis of congenital adrenal hyperplasia. *J Pediatr* 1999;135:71–75.
118. Mittelstaedt CA, Volberg FM, Merten DF, et al. The sonographic diagnosis of neonatal adrenal hemorrhage. *Radiology* 1979;131:453–457.
119. Paterson A. Adrenal pathology in childhood: a spectrum of disease. *Eur Radiol* 2002;12:2491–2508.
120. Shady KL, Brown JJ. MR imaging of the adrenal glands. *Magn Reson Imaging Clin N Am* 1995;3:73–85.
121. Honma K. Adreno-hepatic fusion. An autopsy study. *Zentralbl Pathol* 1991;137:117–122.
122. Graham L. Celiac accessory adrenal glands. *Cancer* 1953;6:149–152.
123. Ye H, Yoon GS, Epstein JI. Intrarenal ectopic adrenal tissue and renal-adrenal fusion: a report of nine cases. *Mod Pathol* 2009;22:175–181.
124. Gilbert-Barness E, Barness LA. *Metabolic Diseases. Foundations of Clinical Management, Genetics and Pathology*. Natick, MA: Eaton Publishing, 2000.
125. Assmann G, Seedorf U. Acid lipase deficiency. Wolman disease and cholesteryl ester storage disease. In: Scriver CR, Beaudet AL, Sly WS, et al., eds. *The Metabolic and Molecular Basis of Inherited Diseases*. New York: McGraw-Hill inc., 1995:2563–2587.
126. Mayatepek E, Seedorf U, Wiebusch H, et al. Fatal genetic defect causing Wolman disease. *J Inherit Metab Dis* 1999;22:93–94.
127. Berger J, Gartner J. X-linked adrenoleukodystrophy: clinical, biochemical and pathogenetic aspects. *Biochim Biophys Acta* 2006;1763:1721–1732.
128. Bezman L, Moser AB, Raymond GV, et al. Adrenoleukodystrophy: incidence, new mutation rate, and results of extended family screening. *Ann Neurol* 2001;49:512–517.
129. Berger J, Gartner J. X-linked adrenoleukodystrophy: clinical, biochemical and pathogenetic aspects. *Biochim Biophys Acta* 2006;1763:1721–1732.
130. Atkinson GO, Jr., Zaatari GS, Lorenzo RL, et al. Cystic neuroblastoma in infants: radiographic and pathologic features. *AJR Am J Roentgenol* 1986;146:113–117.
131. Aterman K, Kerenyi N, Lee M. Adrenal cytomegaly. *Virchows Arch A Pathol Pathol Anat* 1972;355:105–122.
132. Nakamura Y, Komatsu Y, Yano H, et al. Nonimmunologic hydrops fetalis: a clinicopathological study of 50 autopsy cases. *Pediatr Pathol* 1987;7:19–30.
133. Favara BE, Steele A, Grant JH, et al. Adrenal cytomegaly: quantitative assessment by image analysis. *Pediatr Pathol* 1991;11:521–536.
134. Anoop P, Anjay MA. Bilateral benign haemorrhagic adrenal cysts in Beckwith-Wiedemann syndrome: case report. *East Afr Med J* 2004;81:59–60.
135. McCauley RG, Beckwith JB, Elias ER, et al. Benign hemorrhagic adrenocortical macrocysts in Beckwith-Wiedemann syndrome. *AJR Am J Roentgenol* 1991;157:549–552.
136. Burke BA, Wick MR, King R, et al. Congenital adrenal hypoplasia and selective absence of pituitary luteinizing hormone: a new autosomal recessive syndrome. *Am J Med Genet* 1988;31:75–97.
137. Binder G, Wollmann H, Schwarze CP, et al. X-linked congenital adrenal hypoplasia: new mutations and long-term follow-up in three patients. *Clin Endocrinol (Oxf)* 2000;53:249–255.
138. Phelan JK, McCabe ER. Mutations in NR0B1 (DAX1) and NR5A1 (SF1) responsible for adrenal hypoplasia congenita. *Hum Mutat* 2001;18:472–487.
139. Lin L, Gu WX, Ozisik G, et al. Analysis of DAX1 (NR0B1) and steroidogenic factor-1 (NR5A1) in children and adults with primary adrenal failure: ten years' experience. *J Clin Endocrinol Metab* 2006;91:3048–3054.
140. Gray ES, Abramovich DR. Morphologic features of the anencephalic adrenal gland in early pregnancy. *Am J Obstet Gynecol* 1980;137:491–495.
141. Kalousek DK. Case 6. Adrenal hypoplasia in triploidy. *Pediatr Pathol* 1984;2:359–362.
142. Brown W, Singer DB. Pregnancy-induced hypertension and congenital adrenal hypoplasia. *Obstet Gynecol* 1988;72:190–194.
143. Collett-Solberg PF. Congenital adrenal hyperplasia: from genetics and biochemistry to clinical practice, part 1. *Clin Pediatr (Phila)* 2001;40:1–16.
144. Collett-Solberg PF. Congenital adrenal hyperplasia: from genetics and biochemistry to clinical practice, part 2. *Clin Pediatr (Phila)* 2001;40:125–132.
145. Kroner N, Art W. Genetics of congenital adrenal hyperplasia. *Best Pract Res Clin Endocrinol Metab* 2009;23:181–192.
146. Furuhashi M, Oda H, Nakashima T. Hydrops of placental stem villi complicated with fetal congenital adrenal hyperplasia. *Arch Gynecol Obstet* 2000;264:101–104.
147. Lack EE. Tumors of the adrenal gland and extra-adrenal paraganglia. In: *AFIP Atlas of Tumor Pathology*, Ser. 4. Washington, DC: American Registry of Pathology, 2007:39–55.
148. Lack EE. Tumors of the adrenal gland and extra-adrenal paraganglia. In: *AFIP Atlas of Tumor Pathology*, Series 4. Washington, DC: American Registry of Pathology, 2007:57–97.
149. Claahsen-van der Grinten HL, Otten BJ, Stikkelbroeck MM, et al. Testicular adrenal rest tumours in congenital adrenal hyperplasia. *Best Pract Res Clin Endocrinol Metab* 2009;23:209–220.
150. Srikanth MS, West BR, Ishitani M, et al. Benign testicular tumors in children with congenital adrenal hyperplasia. *J Pediatr Surg* 1992;27:639–641.
151. Pack SD, Kirschner LS, Pak E, et al. Genetic and histologic studies of somatomammotropic pituitary tumors in patients with the "complex of spotty skin pigmentation, myxomas, endocrine overactivity and schwannomas" (Carney complex). *J Clin Endocrinol Metab* 2000;85:3860–3865.
152. Stratakis CA, Carney JA, Kirschner LS, et al. Synaptophysin immunoreactivity in primary pigmented nodular adrenocortical disease: neuroendocrine properties of tumors associated with Carney complex. *J Clin Endocrinol Metab* 1999;84:1122–1128.
153. Kirk JM, Brain CE, Carson DJ, et al. Cushing's syndrome caused by nodular adrenal hyperplasia in children with McCune-Albright syndrome. *J Pediatr* 1999;134:789–792.
154. Ezzat S, Asa SL. The multiple endocrine neoplasia syndromes. In: Kovacs K, Asa SL, eds. *Functional Endocrine Pathology*. Malden, MA: Blackwell Science, Inc., 1998:952–966.
155. Pidasheva S, D'Souza-Li L, Canaff L, et al. CASRdb: calcium-sensing receptor locus-specific database for mutations causing familial (benign) hypocalciuric hypercalcemia, neonatal severe hyperparathyroidism, and autosomal dominant hypocalcemia. *Hum Mutat* 2004;24:107–111.
156. Broadley P, Daneman A, Wesson D, et al. Large adrenal cysts in teenage girls: diagnosis and management. *Pediatr Radiol* 1997;27:550–552.
157. Felc Z. Ultrasound in screening for neonatal adrenal hemorrhage. *Am J Perinatol* 1995;12:363–366.
158. Atkinson GO Jr, Kodroff MB, Gay BB Jr, et al. Adrenal abscess in the neonate. *Radiology* 1985;155:101–104.
159. Sivit CJ, Ingram JD, Taylor GA, et al. Posttraumatic adrenal hemorrhage in children: CT findings in 34 patients. *AJR Am J Roentgenol* 1992;158:1299–1302.
160. Nimkin K, Teeger S, Wallach MT, et al. Adrenal hemorrhage in abused children: imaging and postmortem findings. *AJR Am J Roentgenol* 1994;162:661–663.

161. Kanthan R, Moyana T, Nyssen J. Asplenia as a cause of sudden unexpected death in childhood. *Am J Forensic Med Pathol* 1999;20:57–59.
162. Lobel JS, Bove KE. Clinicopathologic characteristics of septicemia in sickle cell disease. *Am J Dis Child* 1982;136:543–547.
163. Bohm N. Adrenal, cutaneous and myocardial lesions in fulminating endotoxinemia (Waterhouse-Friderichsen syndrome). *Pathol Res Pract* 1982;174:92–105.
164. Lack EE. Tumors of the adrenal gland and extra-adrenal paraganglia. In: *AFIP Atlas of Tumor Pathology*, Series 4. Washington, DC: American Registry of Pathology, 2007:161–179.
165. Wieneke JA, Thompson LD, Heffess CS. Adrenal cortical neoplasms in the pediatric population: a clinicopathologic and immunophenotypic analysis of 83 patients. *Am J Surg Pathol* 2003;27:867–881.
166. Dehner LP, Hill A. Adrenal cortical neoplasms in children: Why so many carcinomas and yet so many survivors? *Pediatr Dev Pathol* 2009;12:284–291.
167. Horner MJ, Ries LAG, Krapcho M, et al., eds. *Table 29.1: Age-Adjusted and Age-Specific SEER Cancer Incidence Rates, 2002–2006*. Bethesda, MD: National Cancer Institute. http://seer.cancer.gov/csr/1975_2006/, based on November 2008 SEER data submission, posted to the SEER web site, 2009.
168. Michalkiewicz E, Sandrini R, Figueiredo B, et al. Clinical and outcome characteristics of children with adrenocortical tumors: a report from the International Pediatric Adrenocortical Tumor Registry. *J Clin Oncol* 2004;22:838–845.
169. Calender A, Morrison CD, Komminoth P, et al. Multiple endocrine neoplasia, type 1. In: DeLellis RA, Lloyd RV, Heiz PU, et al., eds. *World Health Organization Classification of Tumors Pathology and Genetics Tumors of Endocrine Organs*. Lyon, France: IARC, 2004:218–227.
170. Bornstein SR, Stratakis CA, Chrousos GP. Adrenocortical tumors: recent advances in basic concepts and clinical management. *Ann Intern Med* 1999;130:759–771.
171. Favara BE, Franciosi RA, Miles V. Idiopathic adrenal hypoplasia in children. *Am J Clin Pathol* 1972;57:287–296.
172. Dabbs D. *Diagnostic Immunohistochemistry*, 2nd ed. Philadelphia, PA: Elsevier, 2006:278–283.
173. Venara M, Sanchez Marull R, Bergada I, et al. Functional adrenal cortical tumors in childhood: a study of ploidy, p53-protein and nucleolar organizer regions (AgNORs) as prognostic markers. *J Pediatr Endocrinol Metab* 1998;11:597–605.
174. Moore L, Bramwell NH, Byard RW. DNA analysis and clinical outcome in pediatric adrenal cortical tumors. *Pathology* 1993;25:144–147.
175. Saracco S, Abramowsky C, Taylor S, et al. Spontaneously regressing adrenocortical carcinoma in a newborn. A case report with DNA ploidy analysis. *Cancer* 1988;62:507–511.
176. SEER. *Surveillance, Epidemiology, and End Results Program, SEER*Stat Data-base: Incidence – SEER 9 Regs, Nov 2002 Sub (1973–2000)*. National Cancer Institute, DCCPS, Surveillance Research Program, Cancer Statistics Branch, released April 2003, based on the November 2002 submission, www.seer.cancer.gov.
177. Goodman MT, Gurney JG, Smith MA, et al. Sympathetic nervous system tumors, chap IV. In: Ries LAG, Smith MA, Gurney JG, et al., eds. *Cancer Incidence and Survival Among Children and Adolescents: United States SEER Program 1975–1995, National Cancer Institute, SEER Program*. Bethesda, MD: 1999.
178. Dodge HJ, Brenner MC. Neuroblastoma of the adrenal medulla in siblings. *Rocky Mt Med* 1945;42:35–38.
179. Maris JM, Weiss MJ, Mosse Y, et al. Evidence for hereditary neuroblastoma predisposition locus at chromosome 16p12–13. *Cancer Res* 2002;62:6651–6658.
180. Perri P, Longo L, Cusano R, et al. Weak linkage at 4p16 to predisposition for human neuroblastoma. *Oncogene* 2002;21:8356–8360.
181. Akramipour R, Zargooshi J, Rahimi Z. Infant with congenital presence of hernia/hydrocele and primary paratesticular neuroblastoma: a diagnostic and therapeutic challenge. *J Pediatr Hematol Oncol* 2009;31:349.
182. Chen Y, Takita J, Choi YL, et al. Oncogenic mutations of ALK kinase in neuroblastoma. *Nature* 2008;455;971–974.
183. Mosse YP, Laudenslager M, Longo L, et al. Identification of ALK as a major familial neuroblastoma predisposition gene. *Nature* 2008;455:930–935.
184. Oberthuer A, Kaderali L, Kahlert Y, et al. Subclassification and individual survival time prediction from gene expression data of neuroblastoma patients by using CASPAR. *Clin Cancer Res* 2008;14:6590–6601.
185. Osajima-Hakomori Y, Miyake I, Ohira M, et al. Biological role of anaplastic lymphoma kinase in neuroblastoma. *Am J Pathol* 2005;167:213–222.
186. Brodeur GM, Maris JM. Neuroblastoma. In: Pizzo PA, Poplack DG, eds. *Principles and practice of pediatric oncology*, 4th ed. Philadelphia, PA: Lippincott-Williams & Wilkins, 2002;895–937.
187. Calonge WM, Heitor F, Castro LP, et al. Neonatal paratesticular neuroblastoma misdiagnosed as in utero torsion of testis. *J Pediatr Hematol Oncol* 2004;26:693–695.
188. Hua X, Mao-Sheng X, Hong-Quan G, et al. Primary paratesticular neuroblastoma: a case report and review of literature. *J Pediatr Surg* 2008;43:E5–E7.
189. Hiyama E, Yokoyama T, Hiyama K, et al. Multifocal neuroblastoma: biologic behavior and surgical aspects. *Cancer* 2000;88:1955–1963.
190. Parham DM, Roloson GJ, Feely M, et al. Primary malignant neuroepithelial tumors of the kidney: a clinicopathological analysis of 146 adult and pediatric cases from the National Wilms' Tumor Study Group Pathology Center. *Am J Surg Pathol* 2001;25:133–146.
191. DuBois S, London W, Zhang Y, et al. Lung metastases in neuroblastoma at initial diagnosis: a report from the International Neuroblastoma Risk Group (INRG) Project. *Pediatr Blood Cancer* 2008;51:589–592.
192. Isaacs H. Fetal and neonatal neuroblastoma: retrospective review of 271 cases. *Fetal Pediatr Pathol* 2007;26:177–184.
193. Schiavetti A, Foco M, Ingrosso A, et al. Congenital stage 1 neuroblastoma evolved into stage 4s. *J Pediatr Hematol Oncol* 2009;31:59–60.
194. Ohyama M, Kobayashi S, Aida N, et al. Congenital neuroblastoma diagnosed by placental examination. *Med Pediatr Oncol* 1999;33:430–431.
195. DeBernardi B, Pianca C, Pistamiglio P, et al. Neuroblastoma with symptomatic spinal cord compression at diagnosis: treatment and results with 76 cases. *J Clin Oncol* 2001;19:183–190.
196. Cooper R, Khakoo Y, Matthay KK, et al. Opsoclonus-myoclonus-ataxia syndrome in neuroblastoma: histopathologic features—a report from the Children's Cancer Group. *Med Pediatr Oncol* 2001;36:623–629.
197. Gambini C, Conte M, Bernini G, et al. Neuroblastic tumors associated with opsoclonus-myoclonus syndrome: histological, immunohistochemical and molecular features of 15 Italian cases. *Virchows Arch* 2003;442:555–562.
198. Rudnick E, Khakoo Y, Antunes N, et al. Opsoclonus-myoclonus-ataxia syndrome in neuroblastoma: clinical outcome and antineuronal antibodies—a report from the Children's Cancer Group Study. *Med Pediatr Oncol* 2001;36:612–622.
199. Espinasse-Holder M, Defachelles AS, Weill J, et al. Paraneoplastic Cushing syndrome due to adrenal neuroblastoma. *Med Pediatr Oncol* 2000;34:231–233.
200. Schor NF. Neuroblastoma as a neurobiological disease. *J Neurooncol* 1999;41:159–166.
201. Trochet D, O'Brien LM, Gozal D, et al. PHOX2B genotype allows for prediction of tumor risk in congenital central hypoventilation syndrome. *Am J Hum Genet* 2005;76:421–426.
202. Bassal M, Mertens AC, Taylor L, et al. Risk of selected subsequent carcinomas in survivors of childhood cancer: a report from the Childhood Cancer Survivor Study. *J Clin Oncol* 2006;24:476–483.
203. Fleitz JM, Wootton-Gorges SL, Wyatt-Ashmead J, et al. Renal cell carcinoma in long-term survivors of advanced neuroblastoma in early childhood. *Pediatr Radiol* 2003;33:540–545.
204. Hann HW, Bombardieri E. Serum markers and prognosis in neuroblastoma: Ferritin, LDH, NSE. In Brodeur G, Sawada T, TSuchida Y, et al., eds. *Neuroblastoma*. Amsterdam, The Netherlands: Elsevier, 2000;371–381.
205. Simon T. Tumour markers are poor predictors for relapse or progression in neuroblastoma. *Eur J Cancer* 2003;39:1899–1903.

206. Lau L. Neuroblastoma: a single institution's experience with 128 children and an evaluation of clinical and biological prognostic factors. *Pediatr Hematol Oncol* 2002;19:79–89.
207. Shuster JJ, McWilliams NB, Castleberry R, et al. A Pediatric Oncology Group recursive partitioning study. Serum lactate dehydrogenase in childhood neuroblastoma. *Am J Clin Oncol* 1992;15:295–303.
208. Combaret V, Bergeron C, Noguera R, et al. Circulating MYCN DNA predicts MYCN-amplification in neuroblastoma. *J Clin Oncol* 2005;23:8919–8920.
209. Shono K, Tajiri T, Fujii Y, et al. Clinical implications of minimal disease in the bone marrow and peripheral blood in neuroblastoma. *J Pediatr Surg* 2000;35:1415–1420.
210. Aronica PA, Pirrotta VT, Yunis EJ, et al. Detection of neuroblastoma in the bone marrow: biopsy versus aspiration. *J Pediatr Hematol Oncol* 1998;20:330–334.
211. Beiske K, Burchill SA, Cheung IY, et al. Consensus criteria for sensitive detection of minimal neuroblastoma cells in bone marrow, blood and stem cell preparations by immunocytology and QRT-PCR: recommendations by the International Neuroblastoma Risk Group Task Force. *Br J Cancer* 2009;100:1627–1637.
212. Komada Y, Zhang XL, Zhou YW, et al. Flow cytometric analysis of peripheral blood and bone marrow for tumor cells in patients with neuroblastoma. *Cancer* 1998;82:591–599.
213. Seeger RC, Reynolds CP, Gallego R, et al. Quantitative tumor cell content of bone marrow and blood as a predictor of outcome in Stage IV neuroblastoma: a Children's Cancer Group study. *J Clin Oncol* 2000;18:4067–4076.
214. Shimada H, Ambros IA, Dehner LP, et al. Establishment of the International Neuroblastoma Pathology Classification (Shimada System). *Cancer* 1999;86:364–372.
215. Shimada H, Ambros IM, Dehner LP, et al. Terminology and morphologic criteria of neuroblastic tumors: recommendation by the International Neuroblastoma Pathology Committee. *Cancer* 1999;86:349–363.
216. Shimada H, Chatten J, Newton WA Jr, et al. Histopathologic prognostic factors in neuroblastic tumors: definition of subtypes of ganglioneuroblastoma and an age-linked classification of neuroblastoma. *J Natl Cancer Inst* 1984;73:405–416.
217. Shimada H, Aoyama C, Chiba T, et al. Prognostic subgroups for undifferentiated neuroblastoma: immunohistochemical study with anti-S-100 protein antibody. *Hum Pathol* 1985;16:471–476.
218. Navarro S, Noguera R, Pellin A, et al. Pleomorphic anaplastic neuroblastoma. *Med Pediatr Oncol* 2000;35:498–502.
219. Tornoczky T, Kalman E, Kajtar PG, et al. Large cell neuroblastoma: a distinct phenotype with aggressive clinical behavior. New entity? *Cancer* 2004;100:390–397.
220. Tornoczky T, Semjen D, Shimada H, et al. Pathology of peripheral neuroblastic tumors: significance of prominent nuclei in undifferentiated/poorly differentiated neuroblastoma. *Pathol Oncol Res* 2007;13:269–275.
221. Ikegaki N, Shimada H, Fox AM, et al. Transient treatment with epigenetic modifiers yields stable neuroblastoma stem cells resembling aggressive large-cell neuroblastomas. *Proc Natl Acad Sci U S A* 2013;110:6097–6102.
222. Peuchmaur M, d'Amore ESG, Joshi VV, et al. Revision of the International Neuroblastoma Pathology Classification: confirmation of favorable and unfavorable prognostic subsets in ganglioneuroblastoma, nodular. *Cancer* 2003;98:2274–2281.
223. Goto S, Umehara S, Gerbing RB, et al. Histopathology and MYCN Status in peripheral neuroblastic tumors: a report from the Children's Cancer Group. *Cancer* 2001;92:2699–2708.
224. Shimada H, Stram D, Chatten J, et al. Identification of subsets of neuroblastomas combined histopathologic and N-myc analysis. *J Natl Cancer Inst* 1995;87:1470–1476.
225. Wirnsberger GH, Becker H, Ziervogel K, et al. Diagnostic immunohistochemistry for neuroblastic tumors. *Am J Surg Pathol* 1992;16:49–57.
226. Iwase K, Nagasaka A, Nagatsu I, et al. Tyrosine hydroxylase indicates cell differentiation of catecholamine biosynthesis in neuroendocrine tumors. *J Endocrinol Invest* 1994;17:235–239.
227. Arvand A, Danny CT. Biology of EWS/ETS fusions in Ewing's family tumors. *Oncogene* 2001;20:5747–5754.
228. Janknecht R. EWS-ETS oncoproteins: the linchpins of Ewing's tumors. *Gene* 2005;363:1–14.
229. Parham DM, Qualman SJ, Teot L, et al. Soft Tissue Sarcoma Committee of the Children's Oncology Group: correlation between histology and PAX/FKHR fusion status in alveolar rhabdomyosarcoma: a report from the Children's Oncology Group. *Am J Surg Pathol* 2007;31:895–901.
230. Davicioni E, Anderson MJ, Finckenstein FG, et al. Molecular classification of rhabdomyosarcoma—genotypic and phenotypic determinants of diagnosis: a report from the Children's Oncology Group. *Am J Pathol* 2009;174:550–564.
231. Altungoz O, Aygun N, Tumer S, et al. Correlation of modified Shimada classification with MYCN and 1p36 status detected by fluorescence in situ hybridization in neuroblastoma. *Cancer Genet Cytogenet* 2007;172:113–119.
232. Ambros IM, Hata J, Joshi VV, et al. Morphologic features of neuroblastoma (Schwannian stroma-poor tumors) in clinically favorable and unfavorable groups. *Cancer* 2002;94:1574–1583.
233. Burgues O, Navarro S, Noguera R, et al. Prognostic value of the International Neuroblastoma Pathology Classification in Neuroblastoma (Schwannian stroma-poor) and comparison with other prognostic factors: a study of 182 cases from the Spanish Neuroblastoma Registry. *Virchows Arch* 2006;449:410–420.
234. George RE, Variend S, Cullinane C, et al.; United Kingdom Children Cancer Study Group. Relationship between histopathological features, MYCN amplification, and prognosis: a UKCCSG study. *Med Pediatr Oncol* 2001;36:169–176.
235. Ikeda H, Iehara T, Tsuchida Y, et al. Experience with international neuroblastoma staging system and pathology classification. *Br J Cancer* 2002;86;1110–1116.
236. Lastowska M, Cullinane C, Variend S, et al., United Kingdom Children Cancer Study Group and United Kingdom Cancer Cytogenetics Group. Comprehensive genetic and histopathologic study reveals three types of neuroblastoma tumors. *J Clin Oncol* 2001;19:3080–3090.
237. Munchar MJ, Sharifah NA, Jamal R, et al. CD44s expression correlates with the International Neuroblastoma Pathology Classification (Shimada system) for neuroblastic tumours. *Pathology* 2003;35:125–129.
238. Navarro S, Amann G, Beiske K, et al. European Study Group 94.01 Trial and Protocol. Prognostic value of International Neuroblastoma Pathology Classification in localized resectable peripheral neuroblastic tumors: a histopathologic study of localized neuroblastoma European Study Group 94.01 Trial and Protocol. *J Clin Oncol* 2006;24:695–696.
239. Sano H, Bonadio J, Gerbing RB, et al. International Neuroblastoma Pathology Classification adds independent prognostic information beyond the prognostic contribution of age. *Eur J Cancer* 2006;42:1113–1119.
240. Shimada H, Umehara S, Monobe Y, et al. International Neuroblastoma Pathology Classification for prognostic evaluation of patients with peripheral neuroblastic tumors: a report from the Children's Cancer group. *Cancer* 2001;92:2451–2461.
241. Okamatsu C, London WB, Naranjo A, et al. Clinicopathological characteristics of ganglioneuroma and ganglioneuroblastoma: a report from the CCG and COG. *Pediatr Blood Cancer* 2009;53:563–569.
242. Umehara S, Nakagawa A, Matthay KK, et al. Histopathology defines prognostic subsets of ganglioneuroblastoma, nodular: a report from the Children's Cancer Group. *Cancer* 2000;89:1150–1161.
243. Attiyeh EF, London WB, Mosse YP, et al. Chromosome 1p and 11q deletions and outcome in neuroblastoma. *N Engl J Med* 2005;353:2243–2253.
244. Spitz R, Hero B, Westermann F, et al. Fluorescence in situ hybridization analysis of chromosome band 1p36 in neuroblastoma detect two classes of alterations. *Genes Chromosomes Cancer* 2002;34:299–305.
245. Spitz R, Hero B, Ernestus K, et al. Deletions in chromosome arms 3p and 11q are new prognostic markers in localized and 4s neuroblastoma. *Clin Cancer Res* 2003;9:52–58.
246. Spitz R, Hero B, Simon T, et al. Loss in chromosome 11q identifies tumors with increased risk for metastatic relapses in localized and 4s neuroblastoma. *Clin Cancer Res* 2006;12:3368–3373.

247. Schwab M, Westermann F, Hero B, et al. Neuroblastoma: biology and molecular and chromosomal pathology. *Lancet Oncol* 2003;4: 472–480.
248. Spitz R, Hero B, Ernestus K, et al. Gain of distal chromosome arm 17q is not associated with poor prognosis in neuroblastoma. *Clin Cancer Res* 2003;9:4835–4840.
249. Mosse YP, Laudenslager M, Khazi D, et al. Germline PHOX2B mutations in hereditary neuroblastoma. *Am J Hum Genet* 2004;75: 727–730.
250. Trochet D, Bourdeaut F, Janoueix-Lerosey I, et al. Germline mutations of the paired-like homeobox 2B (PHOX2B) gene in neuroblastoma. *Am J Hum Genet* 2004;74:761–764.
251. van Limpt V, Schramm A, van Lakemen A, et al. The Phox2B homeobox gene is mutated in sporadic neuroblastomas *Oncogene* 2004; 23:9280–9288.
252. Kobayashi C, Monforte-Munoz HL, Gerbing RB, et al. Enlarged and prominent nucleoli may be indicative of MYCN amplification: a study of neuroblastoma (Schwannian stroma-poor), undifferentiated /poorly differentiated subtype with high mitosis-karyorrhexis index. *Cancer* 2005;103:174–180.
253. Thorner PS, Ho M, Chilton-MacNeill S, et al. Use of chromogenic in situ hybridization to identify MYCN gene copy number in neuroblastoma using routine tissue sections. *Am J Surg Pathol* 2006;30: 635–642.
254. Ambros PF, Ambros IM, Brodeur GM, et al. International consensus for neuroblastoma molecular diagnostics: report from the International Neuroblastoma Risk Group (INRG) Biology Committee. *Br J Cancer* 2009;100:1471–1482.
255. Suganuma R, Wang LL, Sano H, et al. Peripheral neuroblastic tumors with genotype-phenotype discordance: a report from the Children's Oncology Group and the international neuroblastoma pathology committee. *Pediatr Blood Cancer* 2013;60:363–370.
256. Valentijin LJ, Koster J, Haneveld F, et al. Functional MYCN signature predicts outcome of neuroblastoma irrespective of MYCN amplification. *Proc Natl Acad Sci U S A* 2012;109:19190–19195.
257. Wang LL, Suganuma R, Ikegaki N, et al. Neuroblastoma—undifferentiated subtype, prognostic significance of prominent nucleolar formation and MYC/MYCN protein expression: a report from the Children's Oncology Group. *Cancer* 2013;119:3718–3726.
258. Wang Q, Diskin S, Rappaport E, et al. Integrative genomics identifies distinct molecular classes of neuroblastoma and shows that multiple genes are targeted by regional alterations in DNA copy number. *Cancer Res* 2006;66:6050–6062.
259. Maris JM, Mosse YP, Bradfield JP, et al. Chromosome 6p22 locus associated with clinically aggressive neuroblastoma. *N Engl J Med* 2008;358:2585–2593.
260. Cheung N-KV, Zhang J, Lu C, et al. Association of age at diagnosis and genetic mutations in patients with neuroblastoma. *JAMA* 2012;307:1062–1071.
261. Henrich KO, Fischer M, Mertens D, et al. Reduced expression of CAMTA1 correlates with adverse outcome in neuroblastoma patients. *Clin Cancer Res* 2006;12:131–138.
262. Shimada H, Nakagawa A, Peters J, et al. TrkA expression in peripheral neuroblastic tumors: prognostic significance and biological relevance. *Cancer* 2004;101:1873–1881.
263. Krams M, Heidebrecht HJ, Hero B, et al. Repp86 expression and outcome in patients with neuroblastoma. *J Clin Oncol* 2003;21:1810–1818.
264. Miller MA, Ohashi K, Zhu X, et al. Survivin mRNA levels are associated with biology of disease and patient survival in neuroblastoma: a report from the Children's Oncology Group. *J Pediatr Hematol Oncol* 2006;28:412–417.
265. Oberthuer A, Hero B, Spitz R, et al. The tumor-associated antigen PRAME is universally expressed in high-stage neuroblastoma and associated with poor outcome. *Clin Cancer Res* 2004;10(13) 4307–4313.
266. Ladenstein R, Ambros IM, Potschger U, et al. Prognostic significance of di-tetraploidy in neuroblastoma. *Med Pediatr Oncol* 2001;36: 83–92.
267. Spitz R, Betts DR, Simon T, et al. Favorable outcome of triploid neuroblastomas: a contribution to the special oncogenesis of neuroblastoma cells. *Cancer Genet Cytogenet* 2006;167:51–56.
268. Monclair T, Brodeur GM, Ambros PF, et al. The International Neuroblastoma Risk Group (INRG) Staging System: an INRG Task Force Report. *J Clin Oncol* 2009;27:298–303.
269. Cohn SL, Pearson ADJ, London WB, et al. The International Neuroblastoma Risk Group (INRG) Classification System: an INRG Task Force Report. *J Clin Oncol* 2009;27:289–297.
270. Schilling F, Oberrauch W, Schanz F, et al. Evaluation of a rapid and reliable method for mass screening for neuroblastoma in infants. *Prog Clin Biol Res* 1991;366:579–583.
271. Sawada T, Takeda T. Screening for neuroblastoma in infancy in Japan. In: Brodeur GM, Sawada T, Tsuchida Y, et al., eds. *Neuroblastoma*. Amsterdam, The Netherlands: Elsevier, 2000:245–264.
272. Woods WG, Gao R, Shuster J, et al. Screening of infants and mortality due to neuroblastoma. *N Engl J Med* 2002;346:1041–1046.
273. Schilling F, Spix C, Berthold F, et al. Neuroblastoma screening at one year of age. *N Engl J Med* 2002;346:1047–1053.
274. Tsubono Y, Hisamichi S. A halt to neuroblastoma screening in Japan. *N Engl J Med* 2004;350:2010.
275. Hiyama E, Iehara T, Sugimoto T, et al. Effectiveness of screening for neuroblastoma at 6 months of age: a retrospective population-based cohort study. *Lancet* 2008;371:1173–1180.
276. Hiyama E. Neuroblastoma screening in Japan: population-based cohort study and future aspects of screening. *Ann Acad Med Singapore* 2008;37(12 suppl):88–94.
277. McNicol AM, Young WF Jr, Kawashima A, et al. Benign phaeochromocytoma. In: DeLellis RA, Lloyd RV, Heiz PU, et al., eds. *World Health Organization Classification of Tumors Pathology and Genetics Tumors of Endocrine Organs*. Lyon, France: IARC, 2004:151–155.
278. Loh KC, Shlossberg AH, Abbott EC, et al. Phaeochromocytoma: a ten-year survey. *QJM* 1997;90:51–60.
279. Neumann HP, Bausch B, McWhinney SR, et al. Germ-line mutations in nonsyndromic pheochromocytoma. *N Engl J Med* 2002;346:1459–1466.
280. Havekes B, Romijn JA, Eisenhofer G, et al. Update on pediatric pheochromocytoma. *Pediatr Nephrol* 2009;24:943–950.
281. Beltsevich DG, Kuznetsov NS, Kazaryan AM, et al. Pheochromocytoma surgery: epidemiologic peculiarities in children. *World J Surg* 2004;28: 592–596.
282. Ein SH, Shandling B, Wesson D, et al. Recurrent pheochromocytomas in children. *J Pediatr Surg* 1990;25:1063–1065.
283. Bhansali A, Rajput R, Behra A, et al. Childhood sporadic pheochromocytoma: clinical profile and outcome in 19 patients. *J Pediatr Endocrinol Metab* 2006;19:749–756.
284. Dagartzikas MI, Sprague K, Carter G, et al. Cerebrovascular event, dilated cardiomyopathy, and pheochromocytoma. *Pediatr Emerg Care* 2002;18:33–35.
285. Kizer JR, Koniaris LS, Edelman JD, et al. Pheochromocytoma crisis, cardiomyopathy, and hemodynamic collapse. *Chest* 2000;118: v1221–1223.
286. Lamovec J, Frkovic-Grazio S, Bracko M. Nonsporadic cases and unusual morphological features in pheochromocytoma and paraganglioma. *Arch Pathol Lab Med* 1998;122:63–68.
287. Lack EE. Tumors of the adrenal gland and extra-adrenal paraganglia. In: *AFIP Atlas of Tumor Pathology*, Series 4. Washington, DC: American Registry of Pathology, 2007:241–282.
288. Pham TH, Moir C, Thompson GB, et al. Pheochromocytoma and paraganglioma in children: a review of medical and surgical management at a tertiary care center. *Pediatrics* 2006;118:1109–1117.
289. Coutant R, Pein F, Adamsbaum C, et al. Prognosis of children with malignant pheochromocytoma. Report of 2 cases and review of the literature. *Horm Res* 1999;52:145–149.
290. Tischler AS, Kimura N, McNicol AM. Pathology of pheochromocytoma and extra-adrenal paraganglioma. *Ann N Y Acad Sci* 2006; 1073:557–570.
291. Tischler AS. Pheochromocytoma and extra-adrenal paraganglioma updates. *Arch Pathol Lab Med* 2008;132:1272–1284.

292. Shen WT, Sturgeon C, Clark OH, et al. Should pheochromocytoma size influence surgical approach? A comparison of 90 malignant and 60 benign pheochromocytomas. *Surgery* 2004;136:1129–1137.
293. Qupty G, Ishay A, Peretz H, et al. Pheochromocytoma due to unilateral adrenal medullary hyperplasia. *Clin Endocrinol (Oxf)* 1997;47:613–617.
294. Lack EE. Adrenal medullary hyperplasia and multiple endocrine neoplasia (MEN) syndrome type 2. In: *AFIP Atlas of Tumor Pathology Series 4 Tumors of the Adrenal Glands and Extraadrenal Paraganglia*. Washington, DC: American Registry of Pathology, 2007:231–240.
295. Padberg BC, Garbe E, Achilles E, et al. Adrenomedullary hyperplasia and phaeochromocytoma. DNA cytophotometric findings in 47 cases. *Virchows Arch* 1990;416:443–446.
296. Santonja C, Diaz MA, Dehner LP. A unique dysembryonic neoplasm of the adrenal gland composed of nephrogenic rests in a child. *Am J Surg Pathol* 1996;20:118–124.
297. Kato K, Kato Y, Ijiri R, et al. Ewing's sarcoma family of tumor arising in the adrenal gland—possible diagnostic pitfall in pediatric pathology: histologic, immunohistochemical, ultrastructural, and molecular study. *Hum Pathol* 2001;32:1012–1016.
298. Maddock IR, Moran A, Maher ER, et al. A genetic register for von Hippel-Lindau disease. *J Med Genet* 1996;33:120–127.
299. Karadag-Oncel E, Cakir M, Kara A, et al. Evaluation of hypothalamic-pituitary function in children following acute bacterial meningitis. *Pituitary* 2015;18(1):1-7. doi: 10.1007/s11102-013-0547-4
300. Amar L, Bertherat J, Baudin E, et al. Genetic testing in pheochromocytoma or functional paraganglioma. *J Clin Oncol* 2005;23:8812–8818.
301. Hata JL, Correa H, Krishnan C, et al. Diagnostic utility of PHOX2B in primary and treated neuroblastoma and in neuroblastoma metastatic to the bone marrow. *Arch Pathol Lab Med* 2014;139:543–546.
302. Wang LL, Teshiba R, Ikegaki N, et al. Augmented expression of MYC and/or MYCN protein defines highly aggressive MYC-driven neuroblastoma: a Children's Oncology Group study. *Br J Cancer* 2015;113:57–63.

CHAPTER 22

Oral, Maxillofacial, Head and Neck Pathology in Pediatrics

M. John Hicks, M.D., D.D.S., M.S., Ph.D.

INTRODUCTION

The oral and maxillofacial and head and neck region is composed of vastly different tissue types and experience many of the conditions afflicting specific tissues. However, this region also has unique lesions that are not seen at other body sites or with other organ systems. This chapter will review those entities that are unique to the oral and maxillofacial and head and neck region. These include infectious, reactive, congenital, autoimmune, and benign and malignant neoplastic processes that occur in the pediatric age group.

NASOPHARYNGEAL ANGIOFIBROMA (JUVENILE NASOPHARYNGEAL ANGIOFIBROMA)

Nasopharyngeal angiofibroma (NPA) is a rare tumor representing less than 1% of all head and neck tumors. It occurs exclusively in males in the second decade of life and is uncommon after 25 years of age (1–8). If NPA is diagnosed in a phenotypic female, chromosomal studies are indicated to determine if gonadal dysgenesis is present. The most common symptoms are nasal congestion and epistaxis. Nasal discharge, sinusitis, headache, midface and nasal bridge swelling, proptosis, visual distortion, anosmia, and cranial nerve deficits, including hearing loss, may also occur. Symptoms may be long-standing (1 year or more), but without pain. The most common site of involvement is the posterolateral nasal roof near the sphenopalatine foramen. The tumor may extend anteriorly into the nasal cavity, posteriorly into the oropharynx and nasopharynx, through the sphenopalatine foramen into the pterygomaxillary and infratemporal fossa, and into the middle cranial fossa.

The overwhelming predilection for male gender with NPA is related to the presence of androgen receptors and lack of estrogen receptors, with dependency on testosterone for tumor growth and inhibition by estrogen (1–8). This tumor is also associated with familial adenomatous polyposis syndrome with a 25-fold increased risk. Beta-catenin–activating mutations in the stromal cells are noted within tumors associated with FAP; however, in certain sporadic cases, these mutations may also be present. This emphasizes the need for constitutional testing for beta-catenin mutation if this mutation is detected in the tumor. NPA stromal cells may also express neural growth factor and CD117 (see Chapter 25).

Diagnostic imaging typically shows a soft tissue tumor (Figure 22-1) that is markedly hypervascular with prominent arteries. The feeding vessels for this tumor are most often from the maxillary artery. The vascularity is best appreciated on angiography. Because of the prominent vascularity, embolization of the tumor is often performed prior to biopsy or surgical intervention to avoid excessive blood loss and also to avoid consumptive coagulopathy. The tumor typically shows impingement on and bowing of the posterior wall of the maxillary sinus and posterior displacement of the pterygoid plates (Holman-Miller sign).

NPAs may have several different clinical appearances, such as sessile, lobulated, polypoid, or pedunculated (1–8). Typically, the specimen submitted for gross examination is markedly fragmented and the clinical appearance cannot be appreciated. Microscopic examination shows a tumor with no apparent capsule that is comprised of stroma that is typically of low cellularity with collagen in the background with variably sized thin vessels (Figure 22-1). The vessels have lumens that vary from gaping to stellate to staghorn to poorly visible due to compression by the stromal component. The vessels are lined by typical endothelial cells and have an inconspicuous to incomplete smooth muscle layer. Tumors of long duration tend to have increased collagen content and fewer vessels.

Treatment of NPAs is usually surgical, since spontaneous regression is rare (1–8). Use of testosterone receptor inhibitors, estrogen therapy, and irradiation have been utilized as nonsurgical therapies, especially in nonresectable tumors. Recurrence rates vary from 5% to 25% being higher for those involving the skull base and with extension into the cranium.

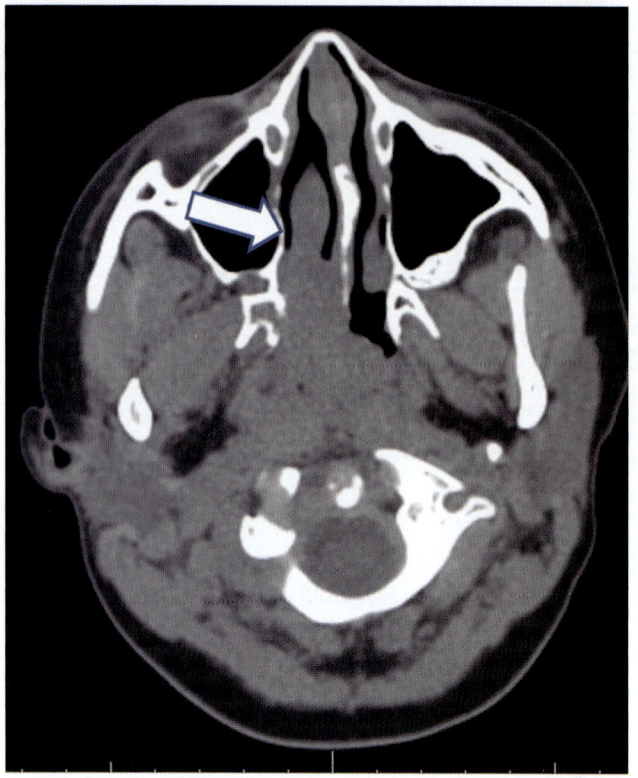
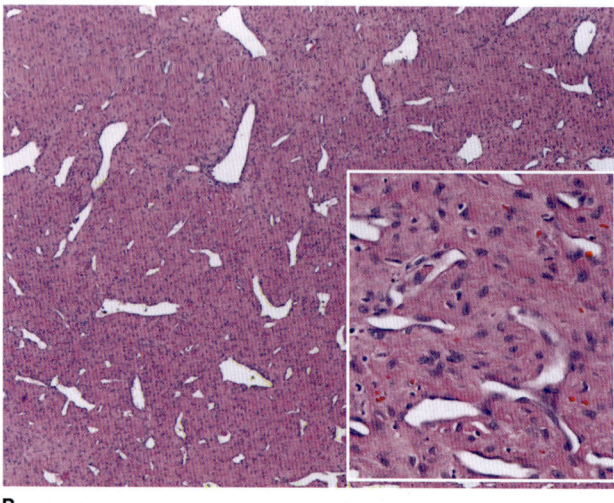

FIGURE 22-1 • Nasopharyngeal angiofibroma. **A:** Soft tissue mass (*arrow*) obstructing nasal cavity and extending into nasopharynx on CT scan. **B:** Low-cellularity tumor with abundant stroma, prominent gaping vessels lacking muscular walls, and bland slightly spindled stromal cells.

There is some degree of mortality associated with NPAs (2% to 10%). Irradiation of these tumors has been rarely associated with sarcomatous transformation and usually with massive radiation dosages.

NASOPHARYNGEAL CARCINOMA, TYPE II NONKERATINIZING, UNDIFFERENTIATED (WHO GRADE TYPE II UNDIFFERENTIATED)

The WHO classification system divides nasopharyngeal carcinoma (NPC) into keratinizing type I, nonkeratinizing type II differentiated, and nonkeratinizing type II undifferentiated (9–18). This tumor arises from the nasopharyngeal mucosa and there is evidence of squamous differentiation. The most common population affected by this tumor is Asian (southern China and Taiwan) and with decreased risk with immigration to low prevalence areas. However, Chinese descent still carries an increased risk compared with non-Chinese descent. Other ethnic groups commonly afflicted with this tumor include Southeast Asians, central and northern Africans, and Arctic natives. In China, NPC accounts for almost 20% of all cancers. Nonkeratinizing type II undifferentiated NPC represents greater than 60% of cases, while type 1 keratinizing NPC (25%) and type II nonkeratinizing differentiated NPC (<15%) are less frequent. HLA types A2, B17, Bw46, and BW58 may be predisposing factors in NPC tumorigenesis. Pediatric NPCs account for less than 20% of all type II undifferentiated subtypes, with only 2% of NPCs occurring in children in China and up to 20% of NPCs occurring in children in central and northern Africa. In contrast, NPC in the United States accounts for less than 0.5% of all cancers. With the pediatric population, only type II nonkeratinizing undifferentiated tumors occur and have a strong association with Epstein-Barr virus. There is a trend to rename this tumor as Epstein-Barr virus–associated carcinoma.

The tumor is more common in males and typically involves the lateral wall of the nasal cavity (Rosenmüller fossa) and the superior–posterior wall (9–18). Often, the tumor presents as a neck mass involving the posterior cervical or superior jugular lymph node chain. The nasopharynx mass may be discovered after needle core biopsy (Figure 22-2) or excisional biopsy of a neck lymph node, because presentation is usually at an advanced clinical stage, with some having cranial nerve involvement (up to 25%). The nasopharyngeal mass may cause nasal obstruction, epistaxis, otitis media, hearing loss, and nasal discharge.

Type II undifferentiated NPCs are characterized by large islands of tumor cells surrounded by a lymphocytic infiltrate in the background (9–18). The nonkeratinizing

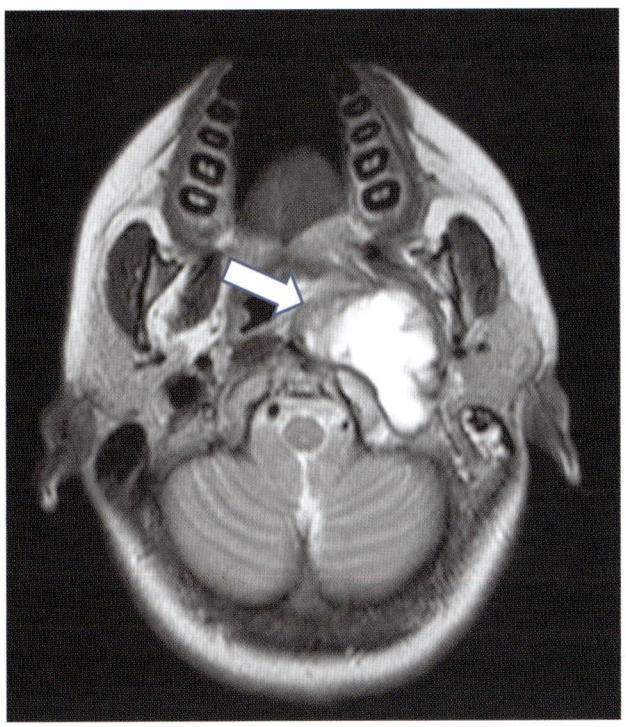
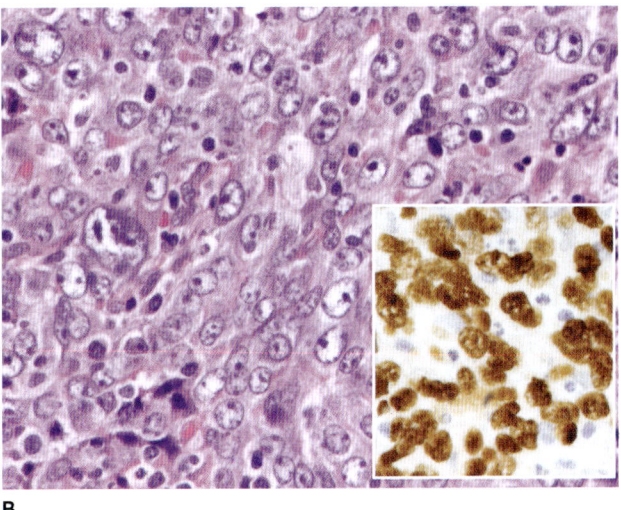

FIGURE 22-2 • Nasopharyngeal carcinoma, type II nonkeratinizing, undifferentiated. **A:** Soft tissue mass (*arrow*) involving and expanding into posterolateral aspect of nasopharynx on CT scan. **B:** Malignant tumor cells with vesicular nuclei, prominent nucleoli, and moderate cytoplasm. *Inset*: Tumor cells with diffuse nuclear reactivity for EBV (*in situ* hybridization for EBER-1).

undifferentiated tumor cells have minimal cytoplasm with indistinct borders, imparting a syncytial appearance (Figure 22-2). The tumor cells have large oval vesicular nuclei with prominent nucleoli. The tumor cells immunoreact with EBER-1, while the adjacent lymphocytes are negative. The tumor is also negative for p16. The tumor is also positive for pancytokeratin and high molecular weight keratins. EBV of a clonal nature can be identified, indicative of a strong oncogenic association between EBV and nonkeratinizing NPC, especially the undifferentiated subtype. Serology is positive for EBV viral capsid antigen (VCA) and EBV early antigen in 90% of cases. In addition, circulating EBV DNA in both plasma and serum is noted in over 95% of those affected by nonkeratinizing NPC. Oncologic management involves radiation therapy and adjuvant chemotherapy. Clinical stage at diagnosis is the primary factor in survival. Stage I disease has a 98% 5-year survival rate, while stage IV disease has only a 73% 5-year survival rate.

NASAL CHONDROMESENCHYMAL HAMARTOMA

Nasal chondromesenchymal hamartoma (NCMH) is a rare neoplasm involving the sinonasal region and is comprised of chondroid and stromal components (19–21). This lesion is most commonly identified in the neonatal period and usually by 3 months of age. It is more commonly seen in males. The presenting symptom is respiratory difficulty associated with facial swelling and a sinonasal mass, with involvement of the septum and middle turbinate being most common (Figure 22-3). The tumor may erode the cribriform plate and extend into the cranial cavity, and this may mimic a meningoencephalocele. The mean size is 3.6 cm with some tumors of up to 8 cm.

The tumor is characterized by nodules and irregular islands of hyaline and fibrocartilage that are surrounded by bland stromal spindle cells (19–21). The stroma may have a myxoid to loose to dense to fibrous character. There is an abrupt transition from the stromal spindle cells to the cartilaginous nodules. These cartilaginous nodules may vary from chondromyxomatous (vaguely resembling chondromyxoid fibroma) to well-differentiated cartilage. There may be several patterns present, such as myxoid spindle cell stroma, fibroosseus proliferation with cellular stroma and immature woven bone mimicking fibrous dysplasia, trabecular and ossicle-like bone formation, and cyst-like blood-filled spaces mimicking aneurysmal bone cyst. Immunohistochemical studies show S100 positivity with the cartilaginous component and smooth muscle actin (SMA) and vimentin reactivity with the stromal spindle cell component.

More recently, there has been an association with DICER-1 mutations and DICER-1 tumor predisposition syndromes, such as familial pleuropulmonary blastoma predisposition

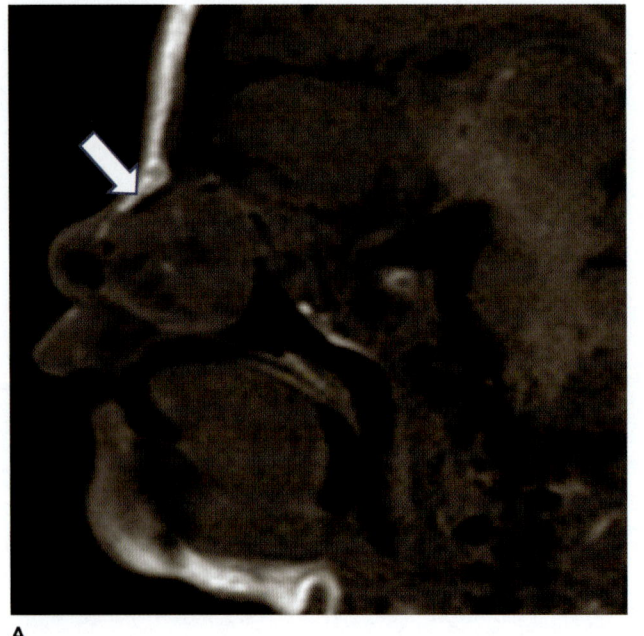
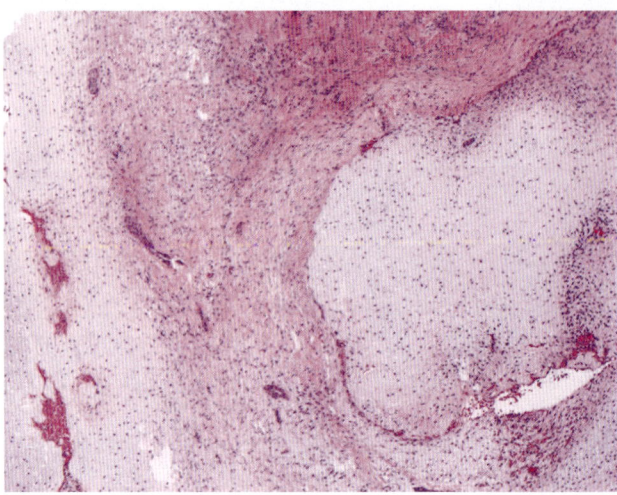
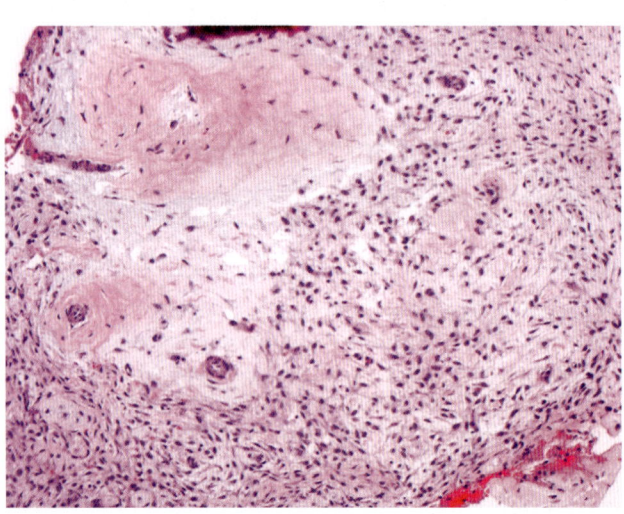

FIGURE 22-3 • Nasal chondromesenchymal hamartoma. **A:** Well-defined soft tissue mass (*arrow*) occupying the nasal cavity on CT scan. **B, C:** Moderately cellular myxofibrous stroma with abrupt transition into cartilaginous nodules.

syndrome (19–21). The majority of NCMH are nonsyndromic in nature; however, constitutional DICER-1 mutation analysis should be performed in the affected individual.

Treatment is surgical with complete surgical resection indicated (19–21). Due to the extent of the tumor, both intranasal and neurosurgical approaches may be necessary. With complete surgical resection, either primary or staged resection, no recurrences have been noted.

NASAL-ASSOCIATED LESIONS

Sinonasal Inflammatory Polyps

With sinonasal inflammatory polyps in general, these polyps most often arise from the lateral nasal wall or from the ethmoid sinus (22–39). These polyps can be single, unilateral, bilateral, or multiple. The typical symptoms are rhinorrhea, nasal cavity obstruction, and headache. Allergies, cystic fibrosis, infections, diabetes, and aspirin sensitivity are often associated with sinonasal polyps. Most occur in individuals older than 20 years of age and infrequently in young children (<5 years of age). However, nasal polyps may be the first sign of **cystic fibrosis** in young children and typically present in the first or second decade of life in about 20% of affected individuals (Figure 22-4). Polyps in cystic fibrosis contain fewer eosinophils and lack basement membrane thickening. The inspissated mucin in cystic fibrosis is acidic in nature and may be highlighted with PAS–Alcian blue with the mucin staining blue to purple compared with typical mucin that stains pink to magenta.

Sinonasal polyps have a myxoid to gelatinous stroma with a mixed acute and chronic inflammatory infiltrate comprised predominantly of lymphocytes and eosinophils. There is a markedly thickened basement membrane beneath the respiratory epithelium, which may demonstrate squamous metaplasia. Charcot-Leyden crystals may be seen with

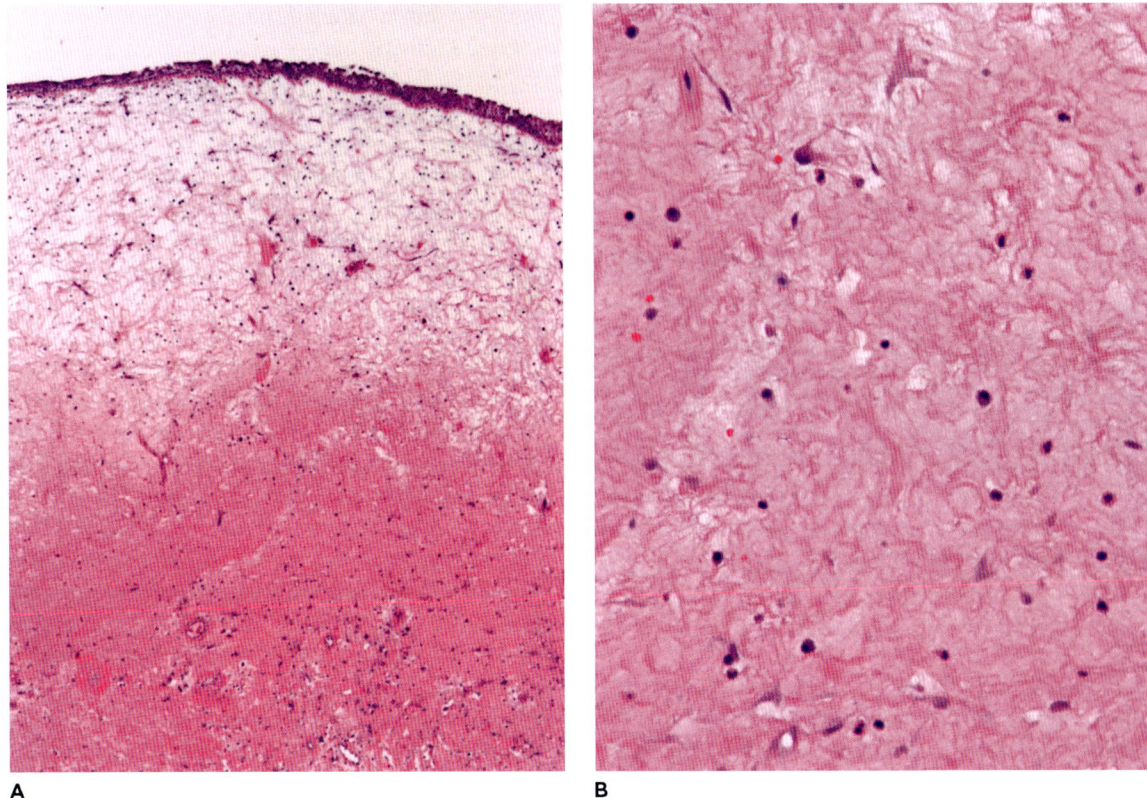

FIGURE 22-4 • Sinonasal polyp in cystic fibrosis. **A and B:** Intact respiratory mucosa overlying submucosa with abundant deeply eosinophilic mucinous stroma.

abundant eosinophils. Treatment is surgical excision with identification of the underlying cause in order to avoid recurrence.

Antrochoanal polyps (AP) arise from the maxillary antrum and are considered sinonasal polyps, which are inflammatory, noninfectious polyps (22–39). APs represent about 5% of sinonasal polyps. Males are more often affected than females and most occur at a young age. Most are unilateral, single polyps (90%) and result in nasal cavity obstruction; and if the AP extends posteriorly, the nasopharynx may be obstructed. These polyps are often seen in conjunction with maxillary sinusitis as well as allergic conditions (up to 40%). Antrochoanal polyps typically show prominent vascular spaces in a fibromyxoid to fibrous background without an inflammatory infiltrate (Figure 22-5). The treatment of APs is surgical with excision of the stalk in order to avoid recurrence.

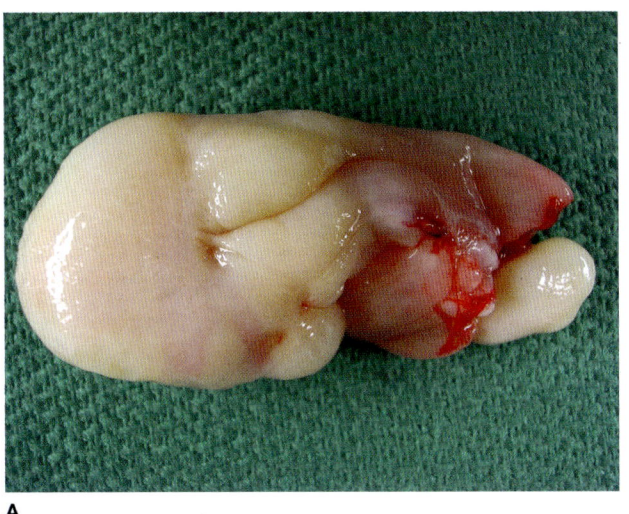
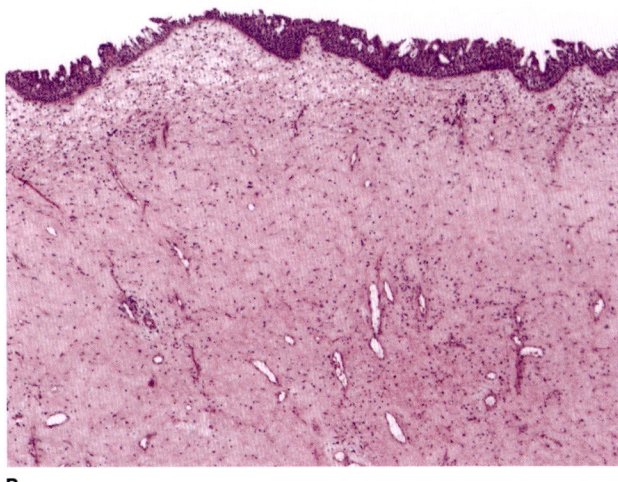

FIGURE 22-5 • Antrochoanal polyp. **A:** Polyp with intact mucosa and irregular surface contour. **B:** Intact respiratory mucosa with underlying submucosa comprised of fibromyxoid tissue with prominent vessels.

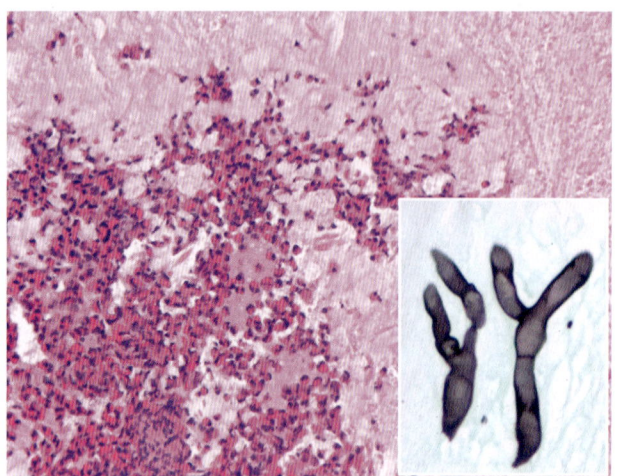

FIGURE 22-6 • Allergic sinusitis. Abundant eosinophilic mucin with aggregates of numerous eosinophils. *Inset*: Hyphae with 45-degree branching and septations (MSN-silver histochemical stain).

Sinonasal Mycotic Sinusitis

Sinonasal mycotic sinusitis may be subtyped as acute fulminant, angioinvasive sinusitis, chronic noninvasive indolent sinusitis, mycetoma, or allergic sinusitis. The most common fungal sinusitis is allergic in nature (22–39). **Allergic sinusitis** occurs in immunocompetent individuals and is a noninvasive fungal sinusitis. The affected individual typically has elevated IgE, peripheral eosinophilia, and a history of a long-standing allergic condition (atopy). This condition is caused by dichotomous fungal hyphae with most organisms in the Dematiaceae family (Bipolaris, Curvularia, Exserohilum, Alternaria, Cladosporium). Microscopic examination shows abundant pale eosinophilic to basophilic mucin with a laminated appearance with numerous eosinophils and other chronic inflammatory cells (Figure 22-6). Fungal organism with 45 degree branching and rare yeast forms may be seen on silver or PAS staining. Mycotic cultures are necessary to determine the precise organisms responsible for the sinusitis. With noninvasive sinusitis, curettage of involved sinus mucosa with systemic antimycotic agents is necessary.

Acute fulminant angioinvasive mycotic sinusitis is associated with immunocompromised or immunosuppressed hosts, often affecting individuals with hematologic malignancies (22–39). These mycotic infections are characterized by mucosal ulceration, tissue necrosis, acute inflammatory infiltrates, and angioinvasion by organisms (Figure 22-7). *Zygomycetes* (Mucor), *Aspergillus, Candida, Cryptococcus, Curvularia,* and

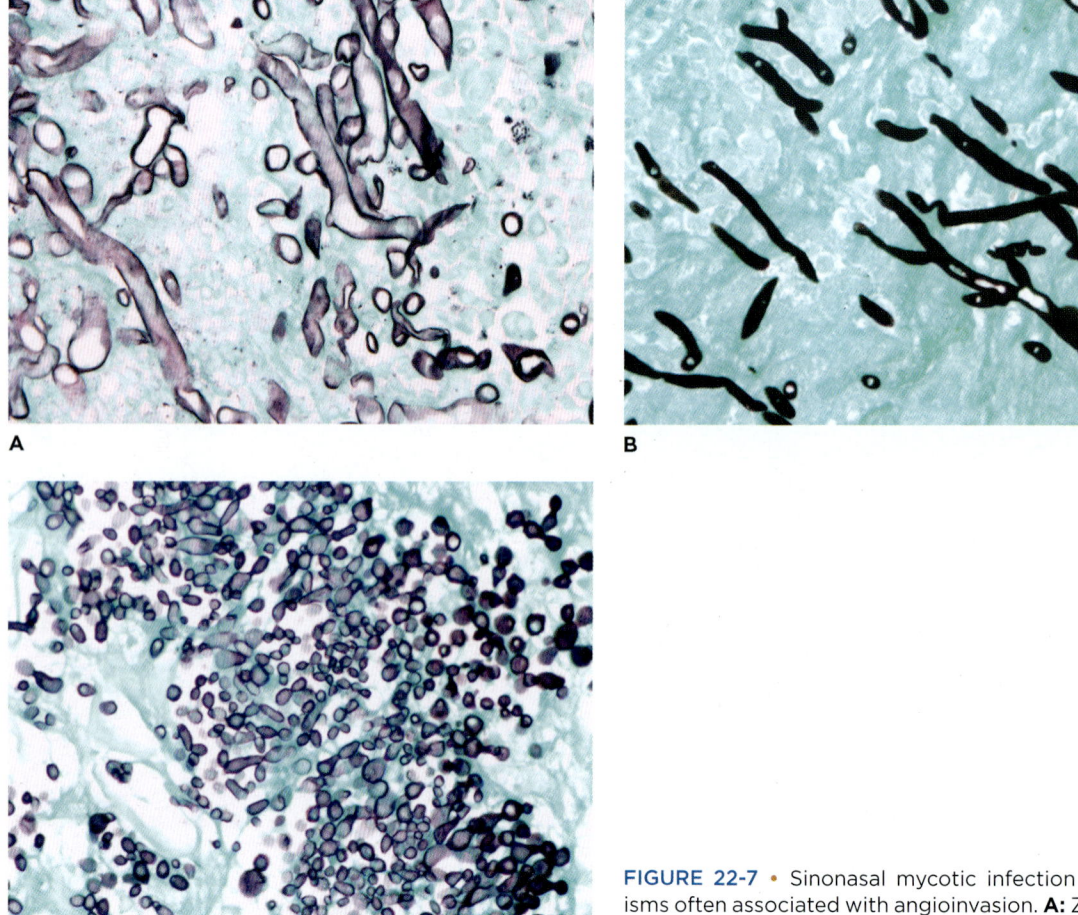

FIGURE 22-7 • Sinonasal mycotic infection with organisms often associated with angioinvasion. **A:** Zygomycetes species. **B:** Aspergillus. **C:** Candida (MSN-silver histochemical stain).

Alternaria may be the invasive mycotic agents. Treatment involves aggressive sinonasal debridement and intravenous antimycotic agents. Survival for invasive mycotic infections is variable from 75% for individuals with no underlying disease to 20% for individuals with leukemia or renal disease. With diabetic patients, the survival rate is almost 80% when appropriate antimycotic agents are utilized.

NASAL GLIAL HETEROTOPIA (NASAL GLIOMA)

Glial heterotopia is a nonneoplastic, congenital displacement of neuroglial tissue at an extracranial site (40–44). It is often considered to be an encephalocele variant without communication with the central nervous system and not a neoplasm. This entity presents at birth or within the first few weeks of life and is most common in nasal subcutaneous tissues (60%), within the nasal cavity (30%) and less often in the sinuses, palate, middle ear, tonsils, or pharynx. Diagnostic imaging is mandatory to exclude communication with the central nervous system and exclude encephalocele with cranial bony defect. These lesions may present as red to blue area on the nasal bridge. The nasal cavity lesions present with symptoms of obstruction, epistaxis, respiratory distress, deviation of the septum, rhinorrhea from CSF fluid, or even meningitis. The tissue is comprised of an admixture of neuroglial elements, including astrocytes, gemistocytic astrocytes, glial fibers, and fibrovascular tissue (Figure 22-8). Neuronal elements tend to be rare to absent, but some cases have shown abundant neuronal elements. Fibrosis may be more pronounced with long-standing lesions. Immunohistochemical staining is positive for S100 protein and glial fibrillary acidic protein. Treatment is simple surgical resection. If the lesion is determined to be an encephalocele, craniotomy with repair of the bony defect is also necessary. Recurrence is rare if the lesion is completely excised.

SQUAMOUS PAPILLOMATOSIS, LARYNGOTRACHEAL TYPE (RESPIRATORY PAPILLOMATOSIS)

Laryngeal squamous papillomatosis is associated with multiple lesions involving most commonly the larynx (95%) and less commonly the tracheobronchial tree (5%) (45–50).

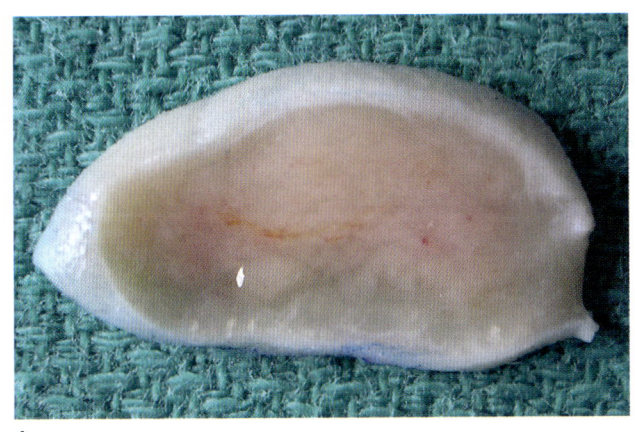
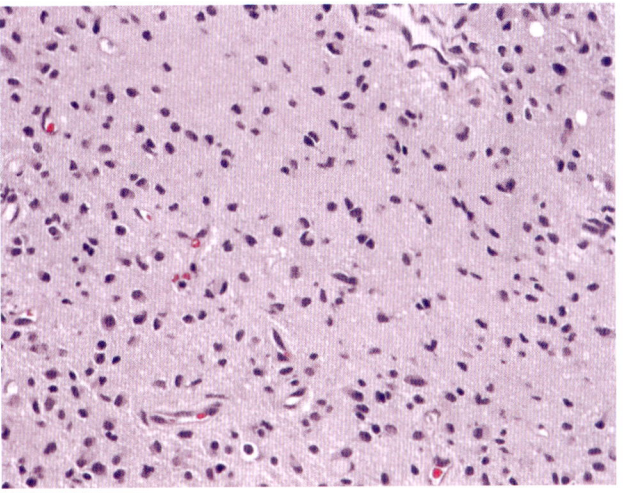
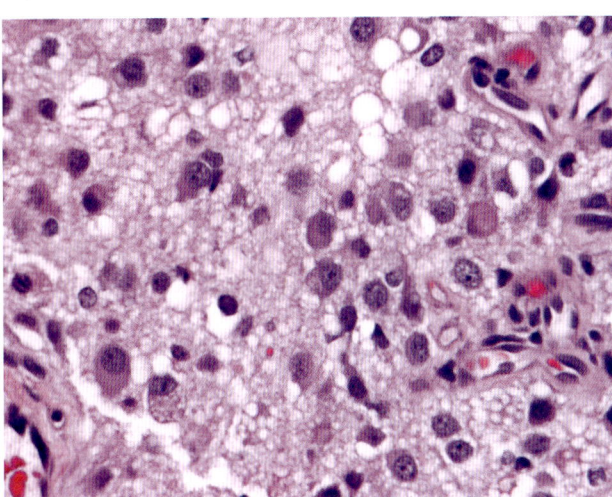

FIGURE 22-8 • Nasal glial heterotopia. **A:** Sectioning of lesion with intact overlying skin and underlying myxoid tissue. **B:** Neuroglial tissue with prominent neuropil. **C:** Neurons within a vacuolated neuroglial background.

The association with human papillomavirus (HPV) types 6 and 11 is well known. HPV type 11 is more often associated with more extensive involvement. These lesions occur in two separate forms: juvenile form before 5 years of age and adult form between 20 and 40 years of age. The juvenile form is associated with HPV transmission from the genital lesions of the mother during vaginal delivery. Of note, HPV infection is not completely obviated by cesarean section delivery. There is no gender bias with the juvenile form; however, the adult form affects males more often. The presenting signs and symptoms include inspiratory stridor, hoarseness, and less often obstructive symptoms. With the juvenile form, the lesions tend to recur and grow rapidly even after surgery. The lesions may undergo spontaneous regression during puberty.

The lesions occur as papillomatous exophytic, pedunculated, or sessile 1- to 5-mm masses along the respiratory mucosa (45–50). There is a tendency to bleed upon manipulation and trauma. Microscopic examination shows papillary lesions lined by stratified squamous epithelium with basal cell hyperplasia and with an underlying fibrovascular core (Figure 22-9). Koilocytic changes secondary to HPV infection are noted in the more superficial layers of the epithelium. The surface of the epithelium may demonstrate minimal parakeratinization. Only rarely is dysplasia of the squamous epithelial cells noted (50).

Extralaryngeal spread does occur in about one-third of children, and this is most common to the oral cavity and tracheobronchial tree (45–50). Endobronchial and lung involvement is noted in about 5% of individuals. Rarely invasive squamous cell carcinoma involving the lung develops in the pediatric age group (Figure 22-9). A poor prognostic factor is development of squamous papillomatosis in the

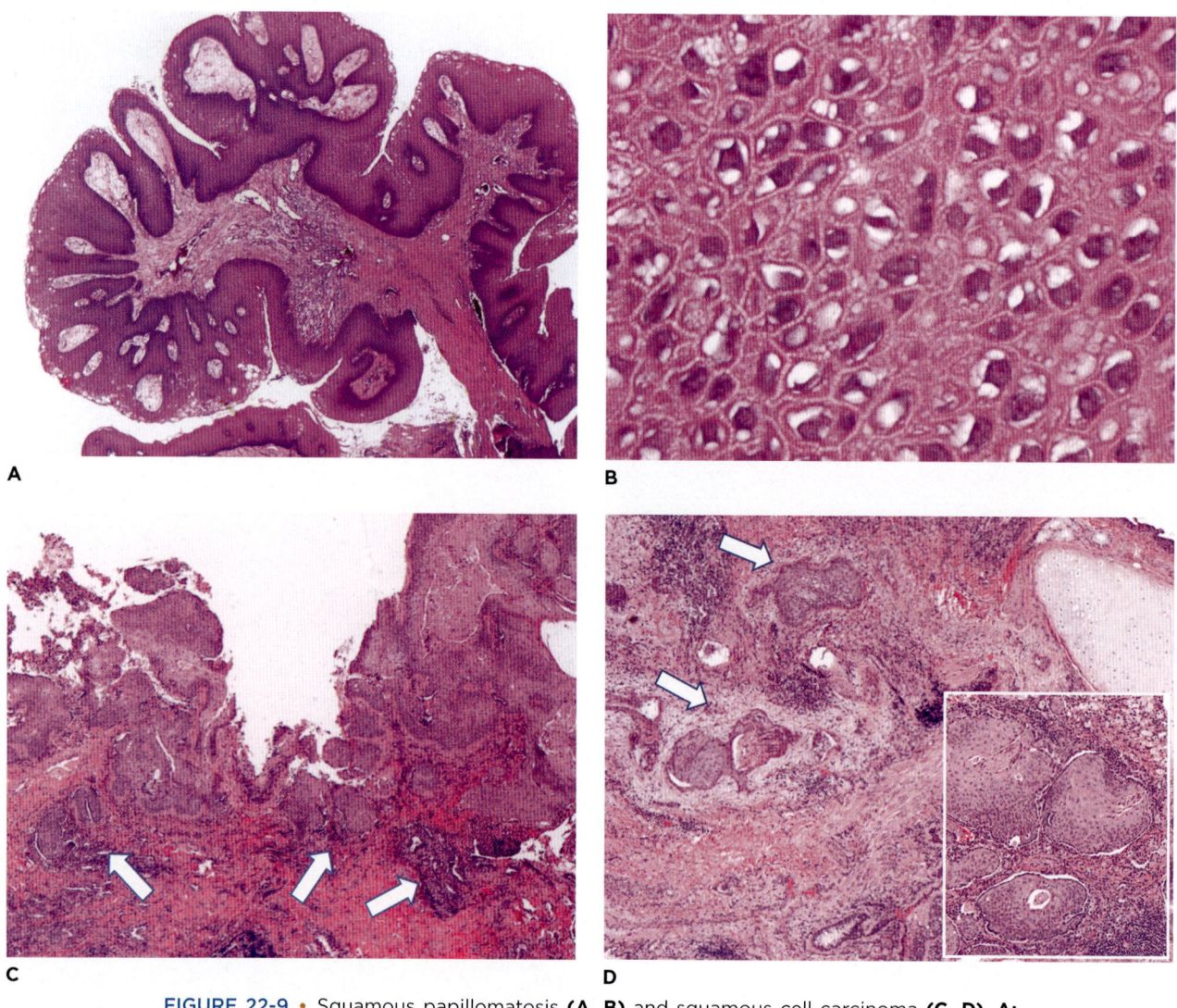

FIGURE 22-9 • Squamous papillomatosis (A, B) and squamous cell carcinoma (C, D). A: Squamous papilloma with marked squamous cell proliferation with fibrovascular core. B: Koilocytic change with squamous epithelial cells, indicative of HPV infection. C: Squamous papillomatous lesion with superficial squamous cell carcinoma invasion (arrows) into underlying tissue. D: Invasive squamous cell carcinoma infiltrating peribronchial (arrows) and lung tissue.

neonatal period, often necessitating tracheotomy, and may result in demise of the child. There are no other prognostic clinical or pathologic factors that predict the clinical course. Of note, radiation therapy is associated with an increased risk for malignant transformation (see Chapter 12).

CONGENITAL EPULIS OF THE NEWBORN (GINGIVAL GRANULAR CELL TUMOR OF INFANCY, NEUMANN TUMOR)

Congenital epulis of the newborn is a rare mucosal tumor that is predominantly located on the anterior alveolar ridge of newborns with the maxilla more commonly involved (75%) (51–53). The vast majority occur in female neonates (90%) with multiple lesions occurring in 10% of affected neonates. This tumor is typically pedunculated and varies in maximum dimension (0.5 to 9 cm, most 0.5 to 2 cm). The lesion is painless and does not increase in size after being discovered. Some small lesions tend to regress spontaneously over time. Microscopic examination shows intact squamous mucosa with the underlying submucosa filled with markedly enlarged polygonal-shaped tumor cells (Figure 22-10). These tumor cells have abundant granular eosinophilic cytoplasm with bland nuclei. The tumor cells are closely apposed with minimal fibrous stroma and occasional fine vascular channels. The granular cells are negative for S100 protein, CD57, cytokeratin, actin, desmin, estrogen and progesterone receptors, and neuron-specific enolase. Other neural markers are also negative. The granular cells react with vimentin and CD68. Ultrastructural examination shows lysosome, lipid, and variably sized dense granules. The overlying squamous mucosa is intact but lacks pseudoepitheliomatous hyperplasia, which is seen in adult granular cell tumors. Odontogenic epithelial rests interspersed among the granular cells may be seen in up to 50% of these lesions. The tumor cells are believed to be derived from primitive mesenchyme from the neural crest; however, there is no convincing evidence for this belief. Treatment is surgical excision in order to provide a definitive diagnosis and eliminate other entities from concern. Recurrence is extremely rare after even incomplete excision. This is no doubt due to the tendency for some lesions to undergo spontaneous regression (see Chapter 25).

GIANT CELL LESION OF JAW (CENTRAL AND PERIPHERAL GIANT CELL GRANULOMA)

Giant cell lesion of the jaw is histopathologically and immunohistochemically indistinguishable from its long bone counterpart (54–58). This tumor may occur within the maxilla, mandible, or oral soft tissues without bony involvement.

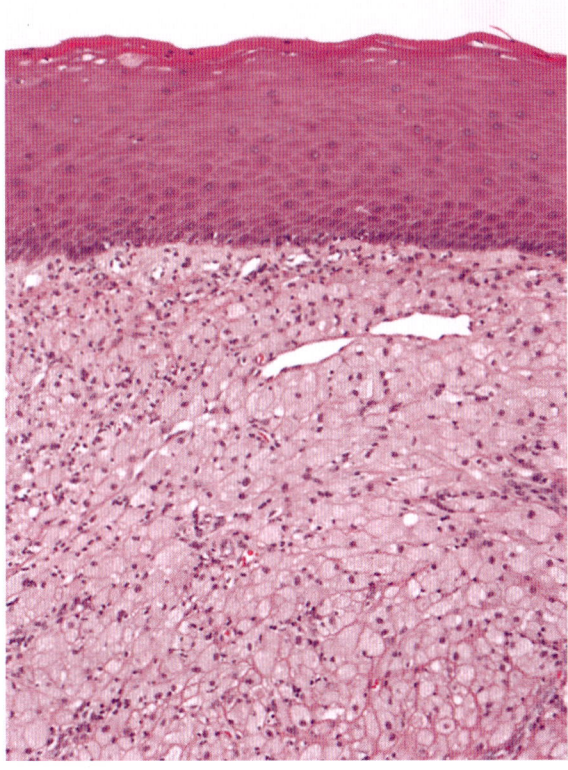
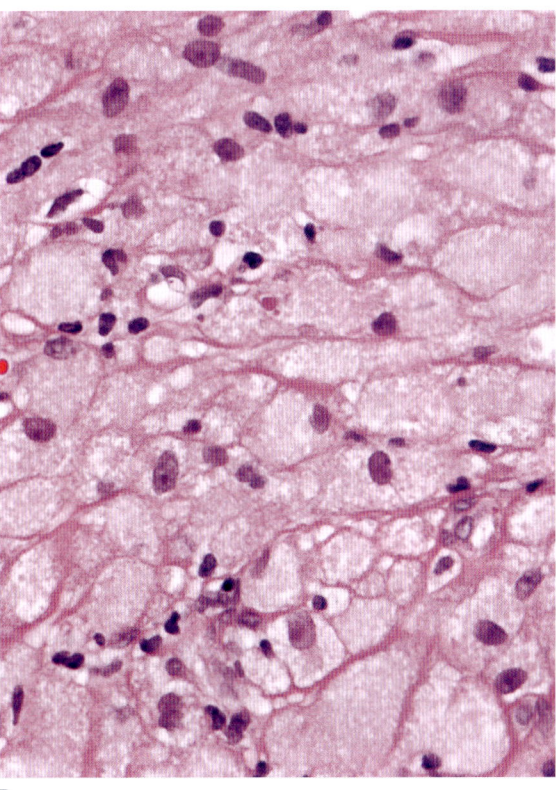

FIGURE 22-10 • Congenital epulis of newborn. **A and B:** Gingiva with intact stratified squamous mucosa overlies a proliferation of markedly enlarged polygonal cells with lightly eosinophilic granular cytoplasm.

Although not proven by cytogenetic or molecular techniques, this tumor is most likely a neoplastic one, similar to giant cell tumor of bone. Clonality with t(1;17;18) and other random numerical chromosomal changes have been reported in isolated cases. The age range for this tumor is wide, but about two-thirds occur before age 30 years with a peak in the second decade of life during mid to late adolescence. There is a female predilection. The anterior mandible is most commonly involved and often crosses the midline of the mandibular symphysis. Most tumors are asymptomatic and are discovered during routine dental radiologic examination or because of painless bony expansion. The minority of tumors are rapidly growing aggressive lesions with bone perforation, tooth root resorption and displacement, and paresthesia. Based upon these clinical features, the tumors have been divided into nonaggressive and aggressive lesions.

Biopsy of the lesion is performed prior to surgical intervention (54–58). The tumor is comprised of giant cells of variable sizes and shapes with varying numbers of nuclei per cells (up to 20 per cell), resembling osteoclast-like giant cells (Figure 22-11). In the background are mononuclear stromal cells, which vary from round to oval or spindle shaped. The stromal cell nuclei are similar in appearance to the giant cell nuclei. The mononuclear stromal cells may be seen merging and fusing with the giant cells. Immunohistochemical staining with CD68 highlights the cytoplasm of both the stromal cells and giant cells, suggesting a common histiocytic derivation. There is also a fine vascular pattern within the stroma. Cytogenetic and molecular genetic studies have not been analyzed thoroughly with this tumor. However, the *SH3BP2* gene mutation, which leads to RANKL-induced activation of calcineurin and NFAT proteins responsible for the giant cell lesion phenotype in cherubism, has not been identified in giant cell lesions of the jaw (59). This indicates that giant cell lesions of the jaw are a distinct entity from the lesions associated with cherubism and have a different pathogenesis. Ramon, Noonan, Schimmelpenning, and neurofibromatosis type 1 syndromes are inherited conditions that have been associated with giant cell lesions of the jaw (54–58) (see Chapter 28).

These jaw tumors are typically treated with aggressive curettage and less often with formal resections (54–58). Soft tissue lesions not involving bone are conservatively excised. Treatment for aggressive tumors may involve intralesional administration of corticosteroids, interferon-α-2A, or subcutaneous or nasal spray calcitonin. Recurrence rates vary from 10% to 35%. Curettage of recurrent tumors is usually performed with good outcomes. Aggressive and/or recurrent tumors tend to possess large giant cells that are evenly distributed throughout the lesion. Prior to surgical treatment, the patients should be evaluated for cherubism, hyperparathyroidism, and the solid variant of aneurysmal bone cyst, which may have similar giant cell lesions involving the jaws.

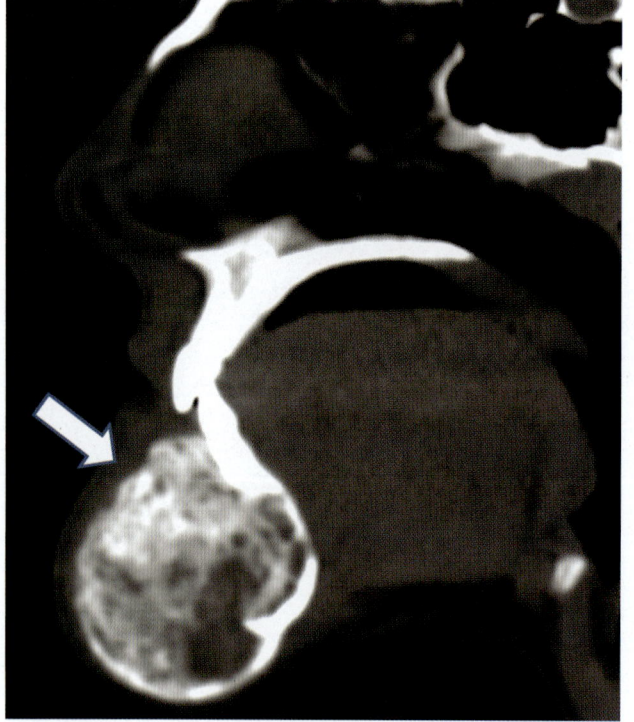
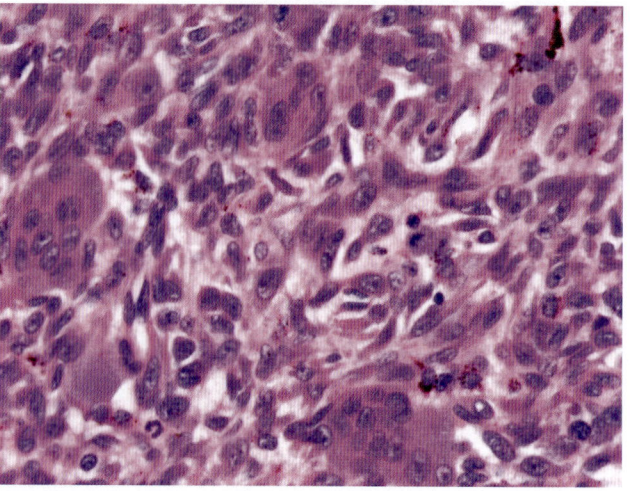

FIGURE 22-11 • Giant cell lesion of jaw. **A:** Anterior mandible markedly expansile lesion (*arrow*) on CT scan. **B:** Numerous osteoclast-like giant cells with variable numbers of nuclei and cellular stroma with mononuclear cells. Note the nuclear features of the giant cells and mononuclear cells are similar.

CRANIOFACIAL OSTEOMA

Craniofacial osteomas (CFO) are typically found incidentally and are asymptomatic (60–66). With larger CFOs, the tumors may present as facial swelling or asymmetry. Sinus obstruction may also occur with mucocele formation and sinus discharge. When involving the orbital bones, there may be exophthalmos and inflammation of the tear duct (dacryocystitis). CFOs typically develop on the surface of the craniofacial bones and tend to more commonly involve the frontal and paranasal sinuses and the orbit. Although the tumor may arise on the surface of the frontal or paranasal sinus, the tumor may involve and obliterate the sinus (Figure 22-12). These tumors vary considerably in maximum dimension but are typically 0.5 to 2 cm in diameter. The osteoma is comprised of dense bone that merges with cortical

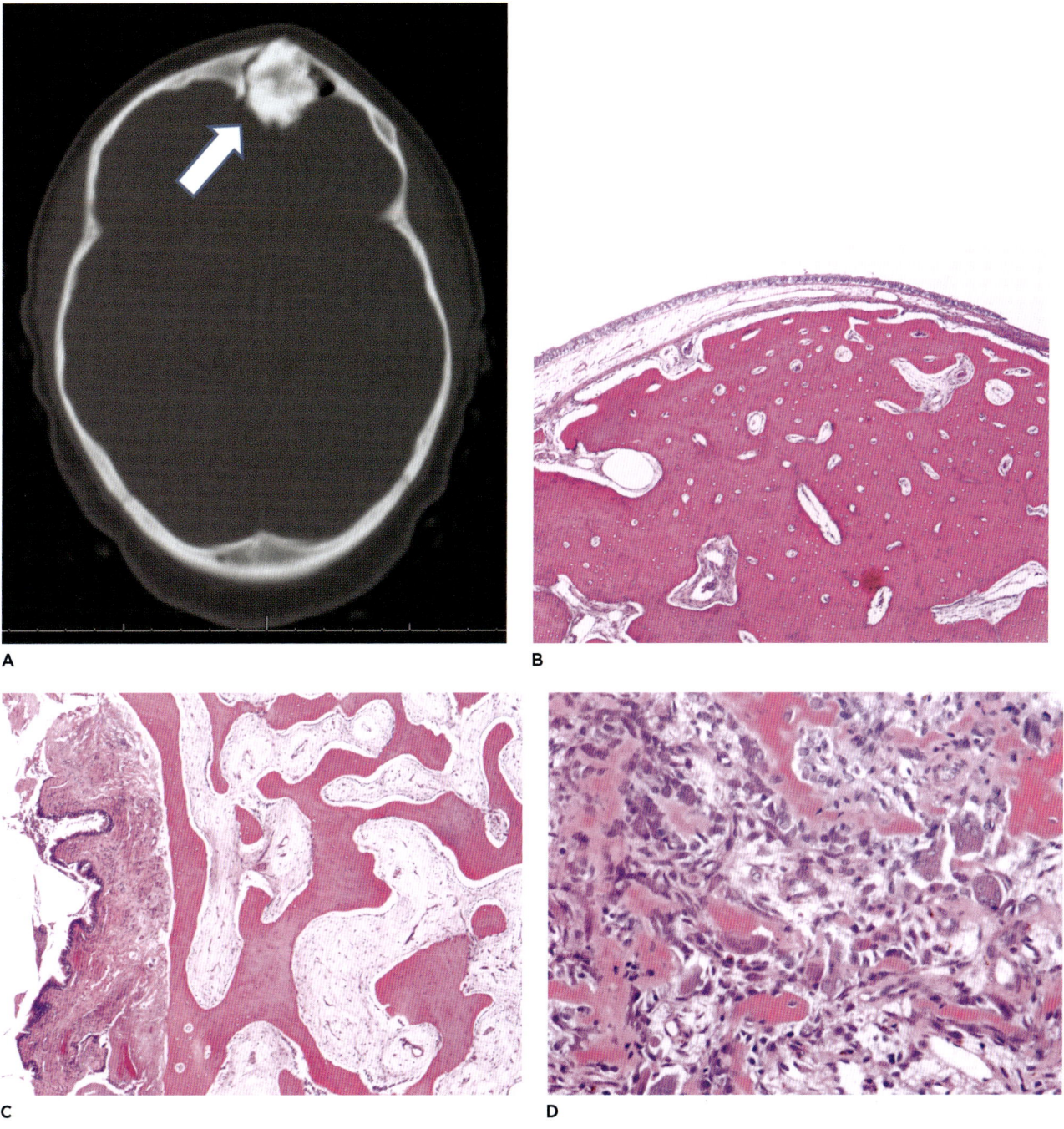

FIGURE 22-12 • Craniofacial osteoma. **A:** Expansile bone-forming lesion involving frontal bone (*arrow*) on CT scan. **B:** Respiratory mucosa from frontal sinus overlies dense cortical bone. **C:** Thin cortex and trabecular bone with fibrotic marrow from frontal sinus lesion. **D:** Cellular area resembling nidus for osteoid osteoma or osteoblastoma may occur with this entity.

bone. With the craniofacial region, surgical removal consists of curettage with fragmentation of the lesion, making it difficult to determine the cortical surface from the underlying lesional tissue. Microscopic examination of the fragmented specimen demonstrates an admixture of lamellar and woven bone (Figure 22-12). The cancellous component shows intersecting broad trabeculae of bone. It is not unusual to note a more cellular component resembling osteoblastoma or a nidus usually associated with osteoid osteoma. Osteomas tend to be slow growing. Osteomas in a young individual necessitate elimination of Gardner syndrome from consideration. This can be done based upon clinical findings and/or constitutional genetic testing for APC gene mutations. Treatment of CFOs is surgical with curettage being the most common procedure with close follow-up for evaluating recurrence. There is no evidence that malignant transformation occurs (see Chapter 28).

JUVENILE OSSIFYING FIBROMA (JUVENILE ACTIVE/AGGRESSIVE OSSIFYING FIBROMA)

Juvenile ossifying fibroma (JOF) is divided into two distinct entities: trabecular JOF (TJOF) and psammomatoid JOF (PJOF) (66–73). The majority of TJOF affects children and adolescents (mean age ranges from 8.5 to 12 years), with only 20% of affected individuals over 15 years of age. Both genders are equally affected. The maxilla and mandible (gnathic bones) are most commonly involved, with other extragnathic craniofacial bones representing a minority of lesions. Although pain is rarely associated with TJOF, the lesions tend to be progressive and may rapidly expand. With maxillary involvement, there may be epistaxis and nasal obstruction. Diagnostic imaging identifies a relatively well-demarcated expansile lesion (Figure 22-13) that may show cortical thinning and even cortex perforation. The lesion may be radiolucent or radiodense depending upon the degree of calcification. Trabecular JOF is comprised of a markedly cellular stroma with immature osteoid trabeculae without obvious osteoblasts or osteoclast rimming (Figure 22-13). The stroma contains spindled to polygonal cells with a paucity of collagen. Typical mitotic figures may be seen and these tend to be sparse. The immature osteoid trabeculae vary from long and slender to broad. Irregular, disorderly calcifications may be seen at the center of the trabeculae. Lamellar bone is not appreciated. Cystic changes may be seen in infrequent cases. Conservative excision or curettage is the treatment. Recurrence is not unusual due to the inability to perform a complete resection without considerable morbidity in most cases. Malignant transformation does not occur.

In contrast to TJOF, PJOF involves primarily extragnathic cranial bones, such as those in periorbital, frontal, and ethmoid regions, and less frequently the calvarium, maxilla, and mandible (66–73). Affected individuals tend to be young, but the age range spans from 3 months to 72 years. There is no gender predilection. These tumors present as expansile lesions. With orbital tumors, there may be proptosis, blindness, nasal obstruction, ptosis, and papilledema. Diagnostic imaging tends to show an ovoid, well-demarcated osteolytic lesion with a cystic character.

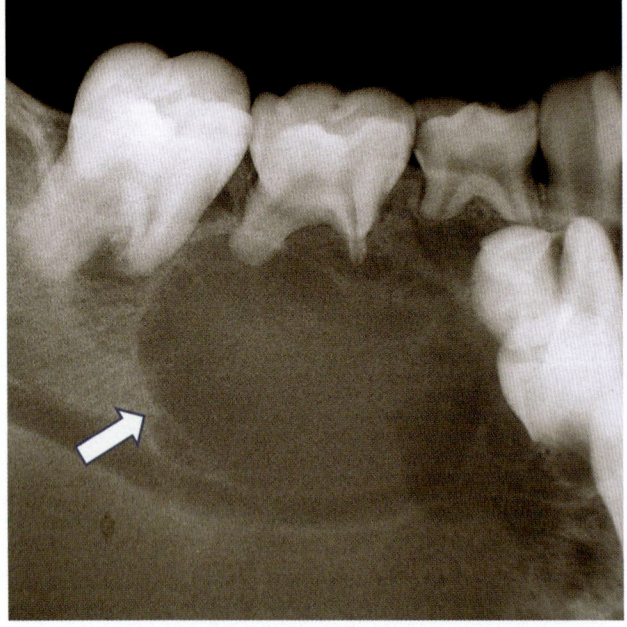
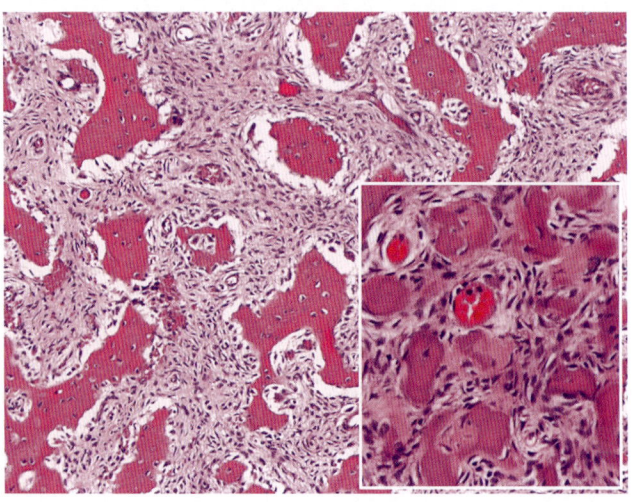

FIGURE 22-13 • Juvenile ossifying fibroma. **A:** Relatively well-defined radiolucent lesion (*arrow*) in mandible with tooth root resorption of primary teeth and displacement of developing permanent teeth on panoramic radiograph. **B:** Cellular trabecular pattern. *Inset*: Psammomatoid pattern.

The tumor varies in size from 2 to 8 cm. Gross examination of the lesional tissue demonstrates yellow–white and gritty tissue. Microscopic examination identifies numerous round, ossicle-like, psammomatoid bodies embedded in a cellular stroma (Figure 22-13). The psammomatoid bodies resemble dental cementum. At the periphery of the lesion, the psammomatoid bodies tend to fuse to form irregular thin trabeculae. The stroma is composed of bland spindle cells and matrix that lacks a collagenous background. Of note, cystic degeneration and aneurysmal bone cyst-like areas have been described with some lesions. Treatment is surgical excision or curettage. Recurrence rates are variable and depend upon whether complete eradication of the lesional tissue is accomplished. There is no evidence of malignant transformation. Of note, cytogenetic studies have been performed in a minority of PJOF cases. However, a translocation involving Xq26 and 2q33 has been identified (see Chapter 28).

PERIPHERAL OSSIFYING FIBROMA (CEMENTO-OSSIFYING FIBROMA) OF THE ORAL CAVITY

This benign reactive proliferation is derived from pluripotential cells of the periodontal ligament and periosteum that attach the cementum root surface to the alveolar bone (74–79). These pluripotential mesenchymal cells have the ability to undergo differentiation to osteoblasts, cementoblasts, and fibroblasts. This differentiation is a reactive process to inflammation and not considered to be a true neoplastic process, such as the ossifying fibroma involving the bony structures of the head and neck region. Peripheral ossifying fibroma (POF) occurs in the submucosa subjacent to gingival tissue. This reactive lesion is typically a 1- to 2-cm lobulated painless mass that is covered by gingiva, which may undergo erosion secondary to trauma and may be associated with long-standing calculus and plaque accumulation, poor oral hygiene, orthodontic appliances, and ill-fitting dentures. The lesion may resemble a traumatic or irritation fibroma; however, POF contains spicules of bone or cementum. Adolescents and young adults are most commonly affected. Females are more commonly affected than males. Fine scattered calcifications and opacities may be seen on routine radiographic examination. Microscopic examination may be somewhat variable with some POFs showing a submucosal cellular proliferation of ovoid to spindled mesenchymal cells or paucicellular fibrotic tissue with occasional typical fibroblasts (Figure 22-14). The hallmark of this lesion that differentiates it from a traumatic or irritation fibroma is the presence of dystrophic calcifications and/or spicules and trabecula of bone and/or cementum. The bone may have either a woven or lamellar pattern. The overlying gingiva may show reactive features, such as areas of erosion and submucosal inflammation. The lesion tends to be relatively well demarcated. Treatment

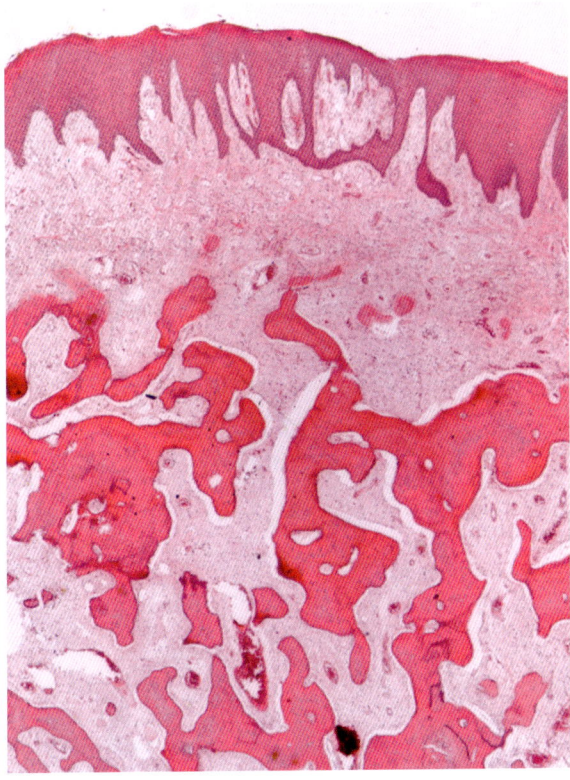
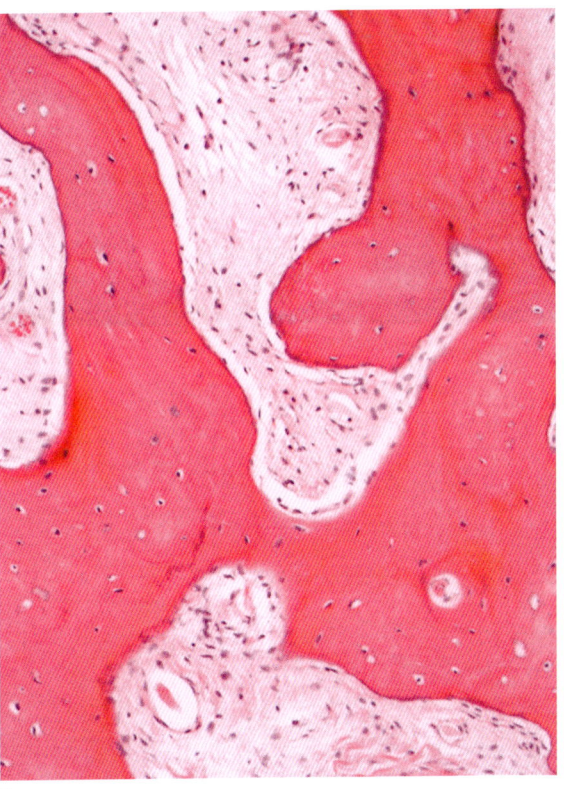

FIGURE 22-14 • Peripheral ossifying fibroma. **A and B:** Gingiva with intact stratified squamous epithelium **(A)** and underlying submucosa with bony trabeculae **(A, B)** with a background of low-cellularity fibrous tissue.

involves surgical excision, deep surgical site curettage, as well as root planning of the associated teeth.

DESMOPLASTIC FIBROMA

Desmoplastic fibroma (juvenile aggressive fibromatosis) is a benign intraosseous fibroblastic proliferation that is locally infiltrative and aggressive (80–84). This lesion occurs primarily in children and young adults, with 85% of cases occurring before age 30 years and a mean age of 14 years. Typically, the tumor involves the body–ramus of the mandible, less often the maxilla, and often erodes the bone and extends into the soft tissues (Figure 22-15). The size of the tumor varies from 3 to 9 cm and often has a lobulated soft tissue surface, and the cut surface has a firm tan–white fibrous character (Figure 22-15). The tumor is comprised of spindle cells with varying cellularity and may have a somewhat fascicular pattern with interspersed areas of collagen (Figure 22-15). Cytologic atypia, mitoses, and bone formation are absent within this tumor. The cellularity tends to be greatest at the periphery of the tumor. In contrast to desmoid tumor associated with Gardner syndrome and familial adenomatous polyposis syndrome, nuclear beta-catenin expression on immunohistochemistry is rare. The etiology of desmoplastic fibroma is unknown; however, it has been suggested that this lesion may be an exuberant reactive process. Treatment consists of complete excision with negative surgical margins. Recurrence is about 5% with complete excision and about 30% with curettage only (see Chapter 28).

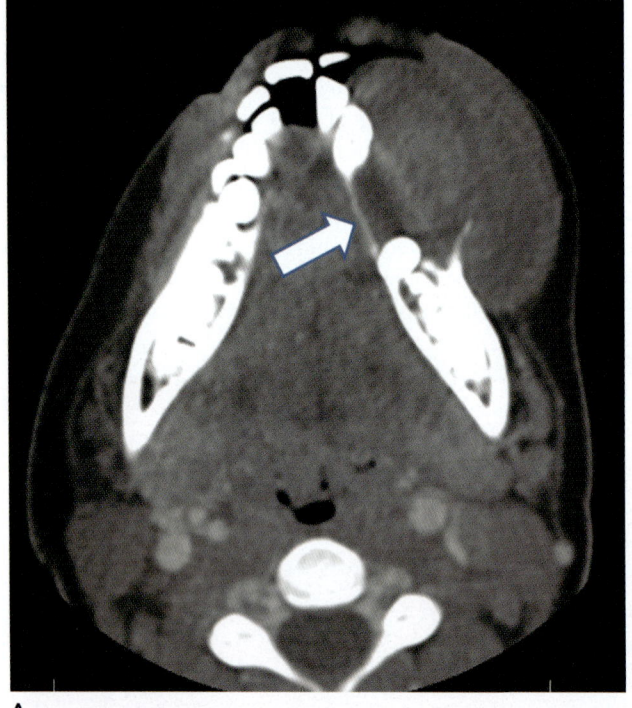
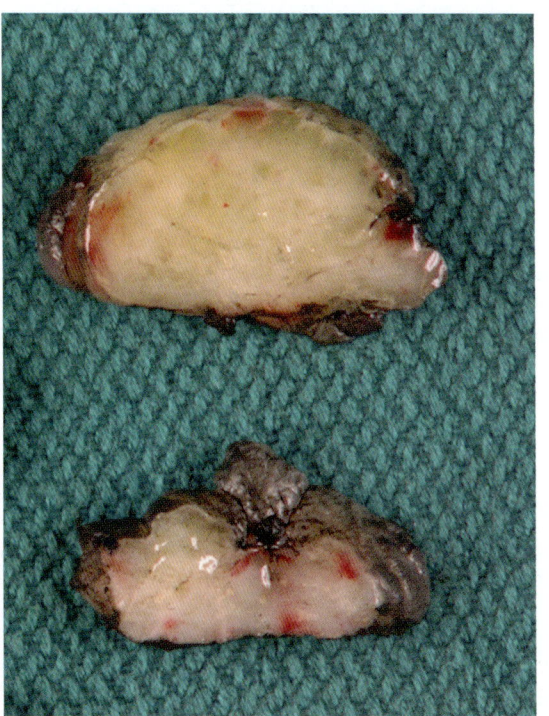
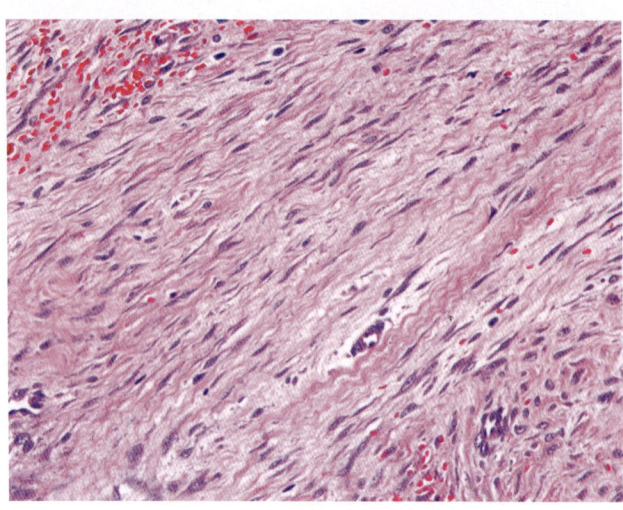

FIGURE 22-15 • Desmoplastic fibroma. **A:** Destructive mandibular soft tissue lesion (*arrow*) with expansion into the adjacent soft tissues on CT scan. **B:** Gross appearance of soft tissue mass with firm cut surface. **C:** Low to moderately cellular spindle cell tumor with interspersed collagen deposition and no cytologic atypia.

MELANOTIC NEUROECTODERMAL TUMOR OF INFANCY (PIGMENTED EPULIS OF INFANCY; MELANOTIC PROGONOMA OF ORAL CAVITY; RETINAL ANLAGE TUMOR)

Melanotic neuroectodermal tumor of infancy (MNTI) is a congenital/infantile neoplasm that most likely arises from neural crest tissue (85–95). In addition to involving the maxillofacial area, this tumor has also been reported in the mediastinum, central nervous system, anterior fontanelle, epididymis/spermatic cord, and soft tissue of the arm. The vast majority of MNTIs present during the first year of life (95%) with female predilection (67%). The anterior maxillary alveolus is the most common craniofacial site (80% of tumors) with the mandible (10%) and skull (10%) being less common. MNTI occurs as a pedunculated to sessile blue–black mass and usually is 2 to 4 cm in maximum dimension. The tumor has rapid growth with displacement of teeth. Diagnostic imaging shows a poorly circumscribed, infiltrative, and destructive radiolucent lesion (Figure 22-16). Laboratory evaluation may show high vanillylmandelic acid levels (VMA) similar to those in other neural crest

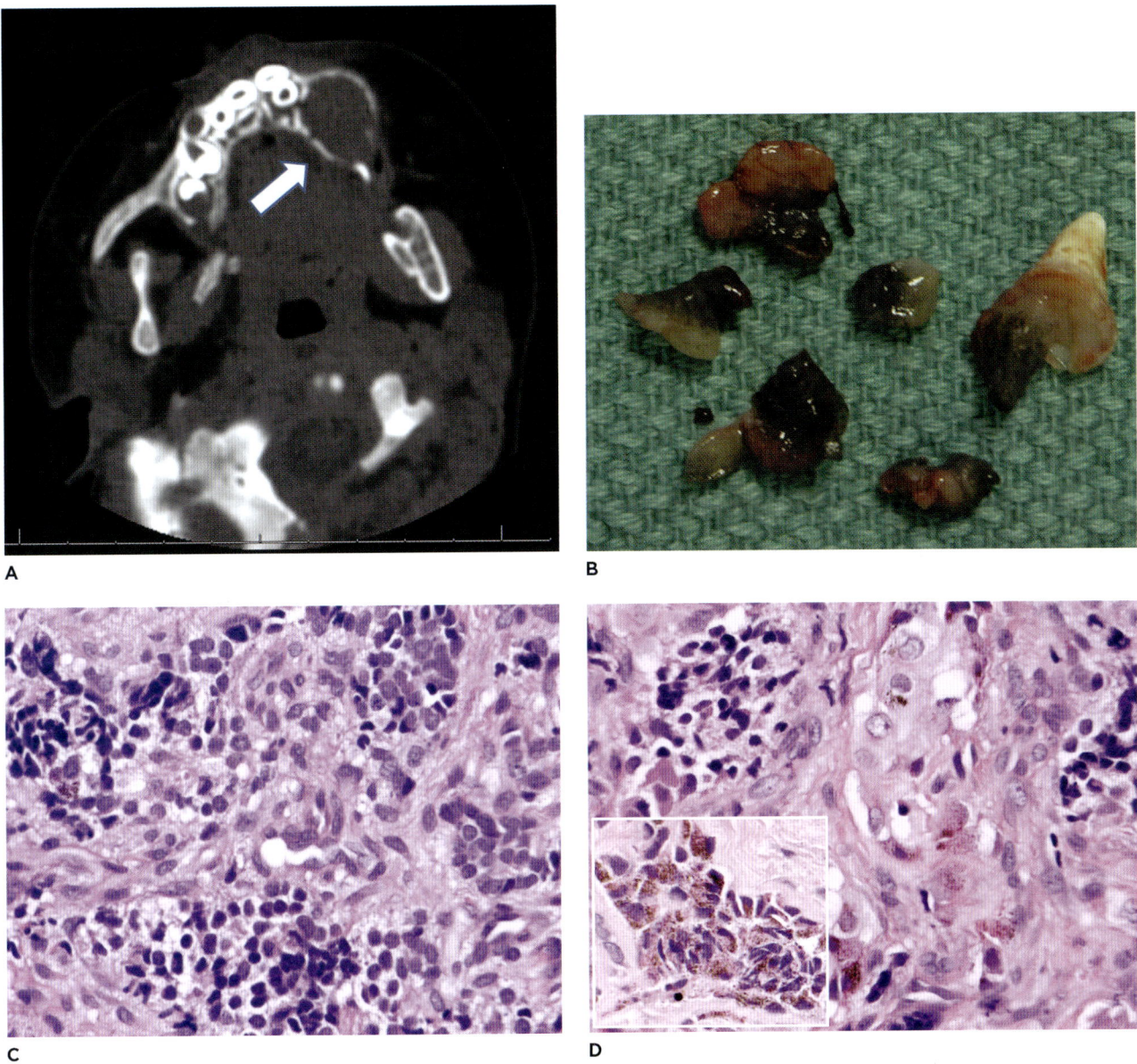

FIGURE 22-16 • Melanotic neuroectodermal tumor of infancy. **A:** Expansile soft tissue mass (*arrow*) arising in the maxilla with residual thin cortex on CT scan. **B:** Gross appearance of mass with deeply pigmented somewhat gelatinous soft tissue. **C:** Admixture of larger epithelioid cells and smaller neuroblasts with dense nuclei. **D:** Epithelioid tumor cells with abundant slight eosinophilic cytoplasm with fine melanin pigment and smaller neuroblasts at periphery of epithelioid cell nest. *Inset*: Tumor cells with prominent melanin pigment.

tumors. Gross examination shows a firm, mottled lesion with white–gray to blue–black coloration (Figure 22-16). Upon microscopic examination, the tumor demonstrates a biphasic pattern with epithelioid cells with melanin pigment arranged in an alveolar to tubular pattern and with small round neuroblast-like cells with fine granular chromatin and scant cytoplasm arranged in nests (Figure 22-16). When the epithelioid cells are in close proximity to the neuroblast-like cells, prominent neuropil may be appreciated imparting a glial fibrillary character. There is intervening vascularized fibrotic stroma. Mitotic figures are rare to absent. Hemorrhage and necrosis are not apparent. Immunohistochemical studies show the epithelioid cells to react with cytokeratin, vimentin, HMB-45, NSE, and CD57, while the neuroblast-like cells react with synaptophysin, GFAP, NSE, and CD57. Ultrastructural examination shows the neuroblast-like cells to have dense core neurosecretory granules and elongated cell process, while the epithelioid cells possess premelanosomes. The tumor infiltrates the adjacent bone and may displace developing tooth buds and reactive bone. Although malignant variants represent 5% of cases, there are no histopathologic distinguishing features for malignancy other than dysplastic change, numerous mitotic figures, or atypical mitotic figures. Wide local excision is necessary due to the infiltrative nature of MNTI. With wide local excision, recurrence is about 15%, and 50% for those not treated with wide resection. Metastatic disease occurs in less than 10% of cases. VMA levels should return to normal after resection and serve as serologic marker for recurrence.

OLFACTORY NEUROBLASTOMA (ESTHESIONEUROBLASTOMA)

Olfactory neuroblastoma (ONB) arises from a basal reserve cell (olfactory stem cell) that differentiates into neuronal, epithelial, and sustentacular cells (96–106). There is no gender predilection, and this tumor has a wide age distribution (2 to 90 years) with a bimodal peak at 15 years and 50 years. The presenting signs and symptoms are epistaxis, nasal obstruction, headache, rhinorrhea, and anosmia. The tumor arises in the superior nasal cavity as a polypoid mass. Occasionally, secretion of ectopic adrenocorticotropic and antidiuretic hormones may occur. Radiologic imaging typically shows a bilobed (dumbbell) mass with the lower portion in the superior nasal cavity and the upper portion extending through the cribriform plate of the ethmoid sinus into the cranium (Figure 22-17). The Kadish staging system is based upon extent of tumor (A, limited to nasal cavity with survival of 90%; B, limited to sinonasal area with survival of 70%; C, extending beyond sinonasal cavity with survival of <50%). Pathology grading system has been developed (Hyams grade I to IV; I, lobular, syncytial, neurofibrillary matrix, vesicular chromatin, no mitosis or necrosis; II, less neurofibrillary matrix, scattered mitoses; III, more pleomorphic cells, Flexner-Wintersteiner rosettes, possible necrosis; IV, anaplasia, high mitotic rate, necrosis) with 5-year survival of 80% for low-grade tumors and 25% for high-grade tumors.

The histopathologic features vary according to the differentiation of the tumor (96–106). The tumor may have a lobular pattern, syncytial pattern with haphazard neuropil,

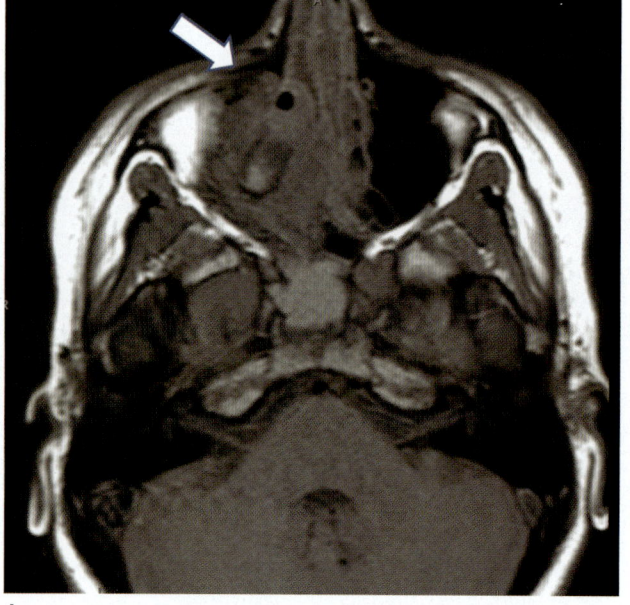
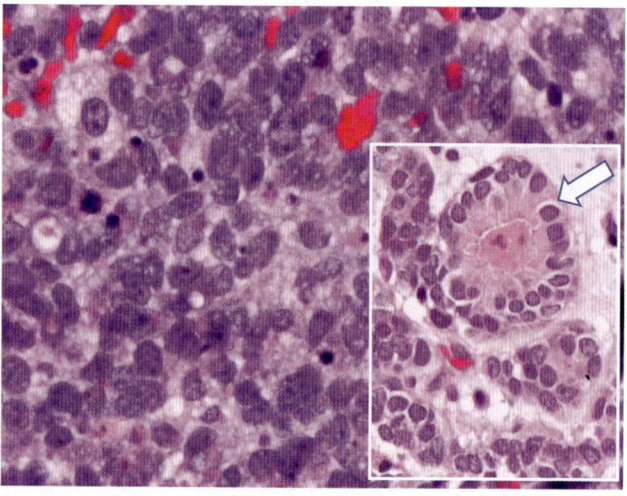

FIGURE 22-17 • Olfactory neuroblastoma. **A:** Soft tissue mass (*arrow*) obstructing nasal cavity on CT scan. **B:** Lobular pattern with neuroblast-like cells with fine chromatin pattern and indistinct neuropil in background. *Inset:* True rosette formation (*arrow*) of tumor cells with more primitive neuroepithelial cells in background.

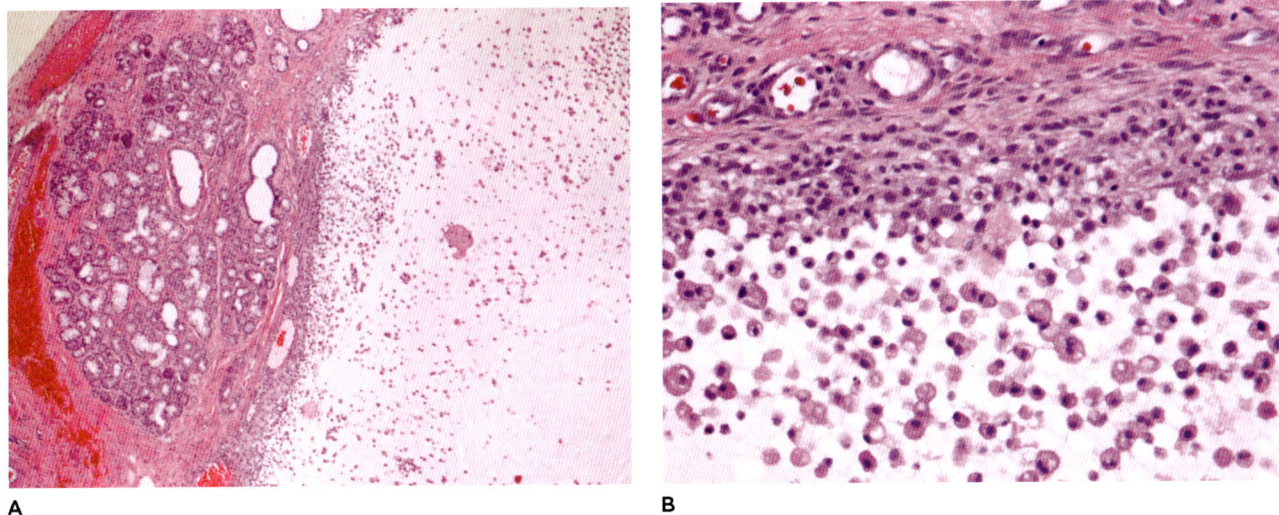

FIGURE 22-18 • Mucocele. **A:** Cystlike cavity engorged with mucus separated by fibroinflammatory wall from adjacent minor salivary gland lobule. **B:** Numerous muciphages reacting to extravasated mucin.

small round cell pattern, pseudorosette (Homer-Wright) pattern, or true rosette (Flexner-Wintersteiner) pattern (Figure 22-17). The tumor cells immunoreact with a variety on neuroendocrine antibodies (CD56, NSE, synaptophysin, chromogranin, NFP, GFAP). The sustentacular cells at the periphery of cell nests immunoreact with S100 protein. The tumor cells may be focally positive for cytokeratin CAM5.2, especially in area with epithelial differentiation. The tumor cells are negative for LCA, CD99, desmin, and myogenin. Rearrangement of hASH1 (human achaete-scute homolog) may be tumor defining in ONB. Poor outcome and metastatic disease are associated with chromosome 11 deletion and 1p gain. ONBs lack the EWS-FLI1 translocation, which is tumor defining for Ewing sarcoma.

Optimal treatment is with the combination of surgical excision with accomplishment of negative margins and radiotherapy (overall 5-year survival of 80%) (96–106). Local recurrence (30%) is quite common due to difficulty with obtaining negative surgical margins. Local metastatic disease in about one-quarter of patients and distant metastases (10%) predicts a poor outcome. Poor prognosis is also associated with age less than 20 years and greater than 50 years are also associated with poor outcome, female gender, high tumor grade, and extensive intracranial tumor.

MUCOCELE (MUCUS RETENTION PHENOMENON)

Mucocele occurs when there is rupture of minor salivary glands with extravasation of mucus into the surrounding tissues creating pseudocysts (107–111). This is the most common salivary gland lesion and is most common in the first three decades of life, arising at any intraoral location that possesses minor salivary glands. The most common site is the lower lip. These painless masses have a blue-white appearance. Microscopic examination shows a cyst-like space containing mucinous material with associated muciphages (Figure 22-18). The wall of the cyst-like space is comprised of granulation tissue with variable numbers of muciphages and inflammatory cells. Adjacent residual salivary gland tissue may demonstrate dilated ducts, inflammatory infiltrates, and even fibrosis if long-standing. Treatment is surgical excision with removal of adjacent lobules of minor salivary glands in order to avoid recurrence.

Of note, ranula is also formed by extravasation of mucosa into the floor of the mouth superficial to the mylohyoid muscle secondary to trauma to sublingual or submandibular glands (107–111). Simple ranula is confined to the floor of the mouth, whereas the deep (plunging) ranula extends beneath the mylohyoid muscle into the cervical tissues and even extending into the mediastinum. The histopathologic findings are similar to those of a mucocele with a pseudocyst, mucous extravasation, muciphages, and granulation tissue. Treatment is surgical excision with removal of the offending major salivary gland. Excision of the ranula alone results in recurrence in 25% to 35%.

SJÖGREN SYNDROME SIALADENITIS (MIKULICZ DISEASE, SICCA SYNDROME)

Sjögren syndrome (SS) is an autoimmune-mediated disease associated with lymphocytic infiltration of exocrine glands, most commonly involving salivary and lacrimal glands (111–115). Affected individuals are typically female in the fifth to seventh decades; however, a juvenile form exists and is more common in males. Typical presentation is xerostomia and xerophthalmia with painless parotid and/or

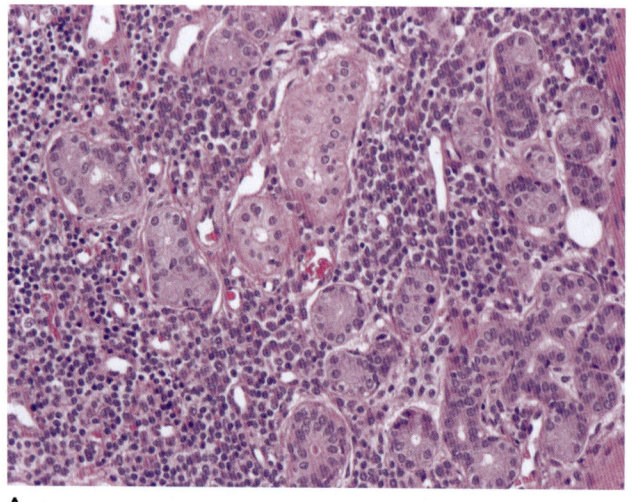
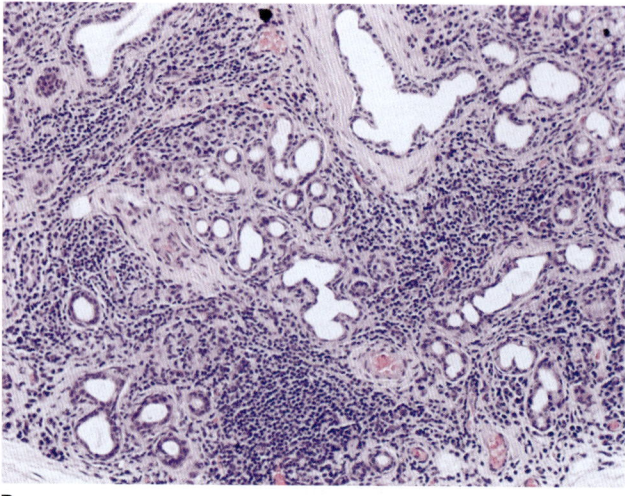

FIGURE 22-19 • Sjögren syndrome sialadenitis. **A and B:** Minor salivary gland lobules with diffuse chronic inflammatory infiltrate.

lacrimal gland enlargement. The disease may be primary SS (HLA-B8, HLA-Dw3) affecting mainly parotid and lacrimal glands or may be secondary SS (HLA-DRw4) associated with other autoimmune conditions, such as systemic lupus erythematosus and rheumatoid arthritis. Serologic testing is typically positive for anti-SSA, anti-SSB, rheumatoid factor, and antinuclear antibody.

Minor salivary gland biopsy (from the lip) may be the initial step in diagnosis of primary or secondary SS (111–115), which shows infiltration by lymphocytes and plasma cells (Figure 22-19). A scoring system has been developed and requires a minimum of 4 mm^2 of minor salivary gland tissue (5 to 10 minor salivary glands). A focus of greater than 50 lymphocytes is required for diagnosis. The lymphocytes cannot be periductal aggregates. The certainty of SS diagnosis increases with increasing number of foci. There is a high CD4:CD8 lymphocyte ratio in SS in contrast to a high CD8:CD4 lymphocyte ratio with HIV-associated diffuse lymphocytic infiltration of salivary glands. In patients with lymphocytic infiltration of salivary glands and without SS, other considerations are EBV, coxsackievirus, HTLV-1, measles, lymphoepithelial cysts and carcinoma, chronic sialadenitis, and B-cell lymphoma.

PLEOMORPHIC ADENOMA (MIXED TUMOR)

Pleomorphic adenoma (PA) is a benign tumor affecting major and minor salivary glands and is comprised of epithelial cells, myoepithelial cells, and mesenchymal stroma cells with myxoid, chondroid, and mucoid components (Figure 22-20) (116–121). PA has a wide age range but peaks in the fourth to sixth decades. However, this is the most common benign salivary gland tumor in the pediatric population. In children, males

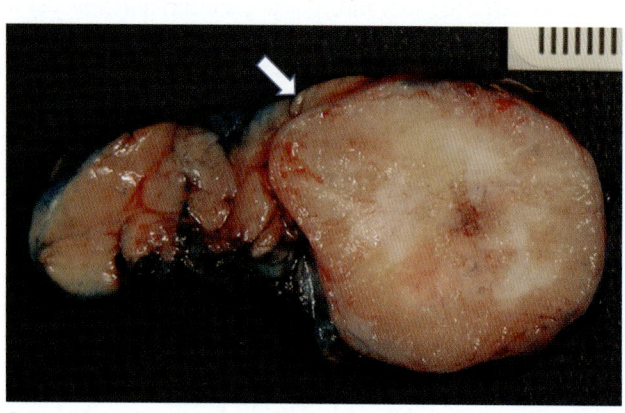
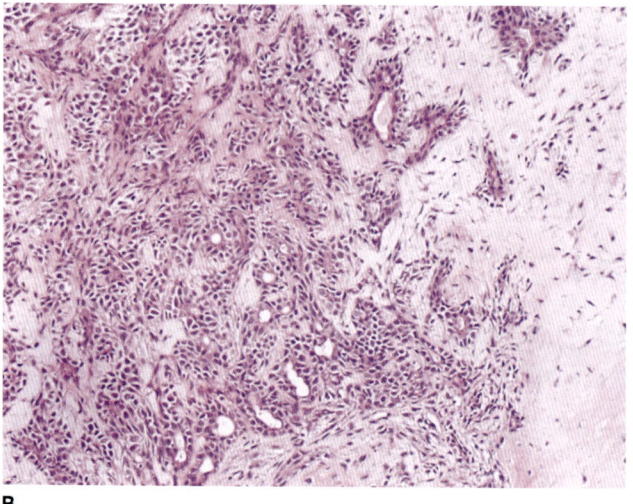

FIGURE 22-20 • Pleomorphic adenoma. **A:** Gross appearance of tumor (*arrow*) involving the parotid gland. **B-D:** Chondroid matrix background with varying tubular and trabecular patterns comprised of epithelial and myoepithelial cells.

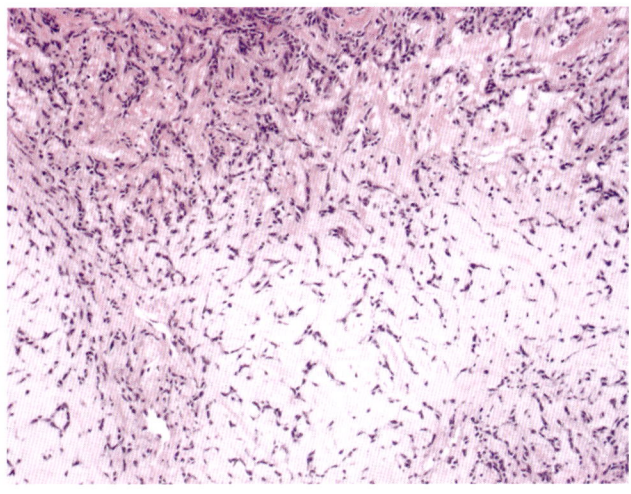
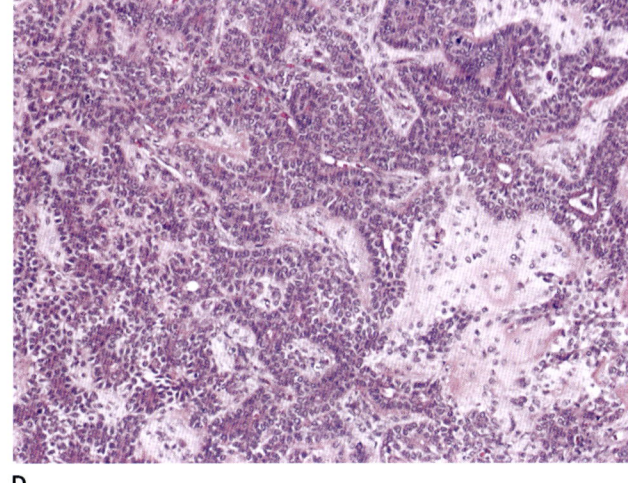

FIGURE 22-20 • (Continued)

are more commonly affected than females, with the opposite being true for adults. The superficial lobe of the parotid is the most common location for this tumor, with palatal minor salivary gland being the second most common site. It may also affect the tracheobronchial tree, nasal cavity, orbit, larynx, ear, and gastrointestinal tract. This painless, mobile mass is slow growing, firm, and without mucosal ulceration. PAs tend to have an irregular surface and variable fibrous capsule within major salivary glands and lack of a capsule within minor salivary glands. Sectioning reveals a tan to white, relatively homogenous surface. Hemorrhage and hemosiderin deposition may be present if the lesion has undergone fine-needle biopsy. The tumor is comprised of many architectural patterns (solid, tubular, trabecular, cystic), epithelial cell diversity (spindled, clear, squamous, basaloid, plasmacytoid, sebaceous), numerous mesenchymal components (myxoid, chondroid, hyalinized, ossified, adipocytic), and cuboidal and columnar epithelial-lined ducts. The tumor cells stain with cytokeratins, p63, GFAP, calponin, S100, CD10, and SMA. Translocations involving either PLAG1 at 8q12 or HMGA2 at 12q13-15 occur in about 50% of tumors. Other sporadic clonal rearrangements occur in about 20%. However, no chromosomal changes are noted in 30% of tumors. Treatment is complete surgical resection with negative margins. Recurrence occurs in about 2.5% of cases. Malignant transformation occurs in less than 10% of tumors and is associated with long-standing tumors, multiple recurrences, older age, deep lobe involvement, parotid gland tumor, and male gender.

MUCOEPIDERMOID CARCINOMA

Mucoepidermoid carcinoma (MEC) is the most common malignant salivary gland tumor in children (117–127). This tumor may occur as a primary neoplasm or secondary to radiation therapy for other childhood malignancies. It is comprised of malignant mucous, intermediate epithelial cells, and squamous epidermoid cells. The tumor may be pure cystic, partially cyst and partially solid, or pure solid with an epidermoid carcinoma appearance (Figure 22-21). The parotid is the most common site. Minor salivary glands and the mandible and maxilla may be primary sites as well. Typically, MEC is a slow-growing painless mass. With rapid growth, there may be facial pain, facial nerve paralysis, and numbness, especially with parotid tumors. Minor salivary gland tumors may be initially considered to be inflammatory reactive lesions. Intraosseous MECs appear as radiolucent masses and may be associated with facial asymmetry, trismus, and referred pain from the involved intraosseous nerves. The tumor has variable circumscription, demonstrates variable cystic areas, and may be quite small to massive in size (Figure 22-21). Microscopic examination shows a variable appearance with some tumor being predominantly cystic with mucous cells and a few intermediate cells; other tumors are partially cystic and partially solid areas with a mixture of mucous cells and intermediate cells with less frequent epidermoid cells, whereas other tumors have a solid pattern with infrequent to rare mucous cells with no cysts and predominantly epidermoid and intermediate cells (Figure 22-21). Grading of mucoepidermoid tumors (123–126) is based upon a scoring system: intracystic component less than 20% (2 points), neural invasion (2 points), necrosis (3 points), ≥4 mitotic figures per 10 high-power fields (3 points), and anaplasia (4 points). The 3-tiered grading system is as follows: low grade 0 to 4 points, intermediate grade 5 to 6 points, and high grade ≥7 points. Others have simply graded MECs as low (cystic with mucus and intermediate cells), intermediate (cystic and solid with intermediate and mucus cells), and high (solid with epidermoid and intermediate cells) grade. Histochemical stains, such as mucicarmine and Alcian blue, may be of utility in identifying cells containing mucin when the tumor is predominately comprised of intermediate and/or epidermoid tumor cells. Immunohistochemical profile is nonspecific, with immunoreactivity with p63 and a variety of cytokeratins. The tumors may be strongly positive for HER2, which may provide a

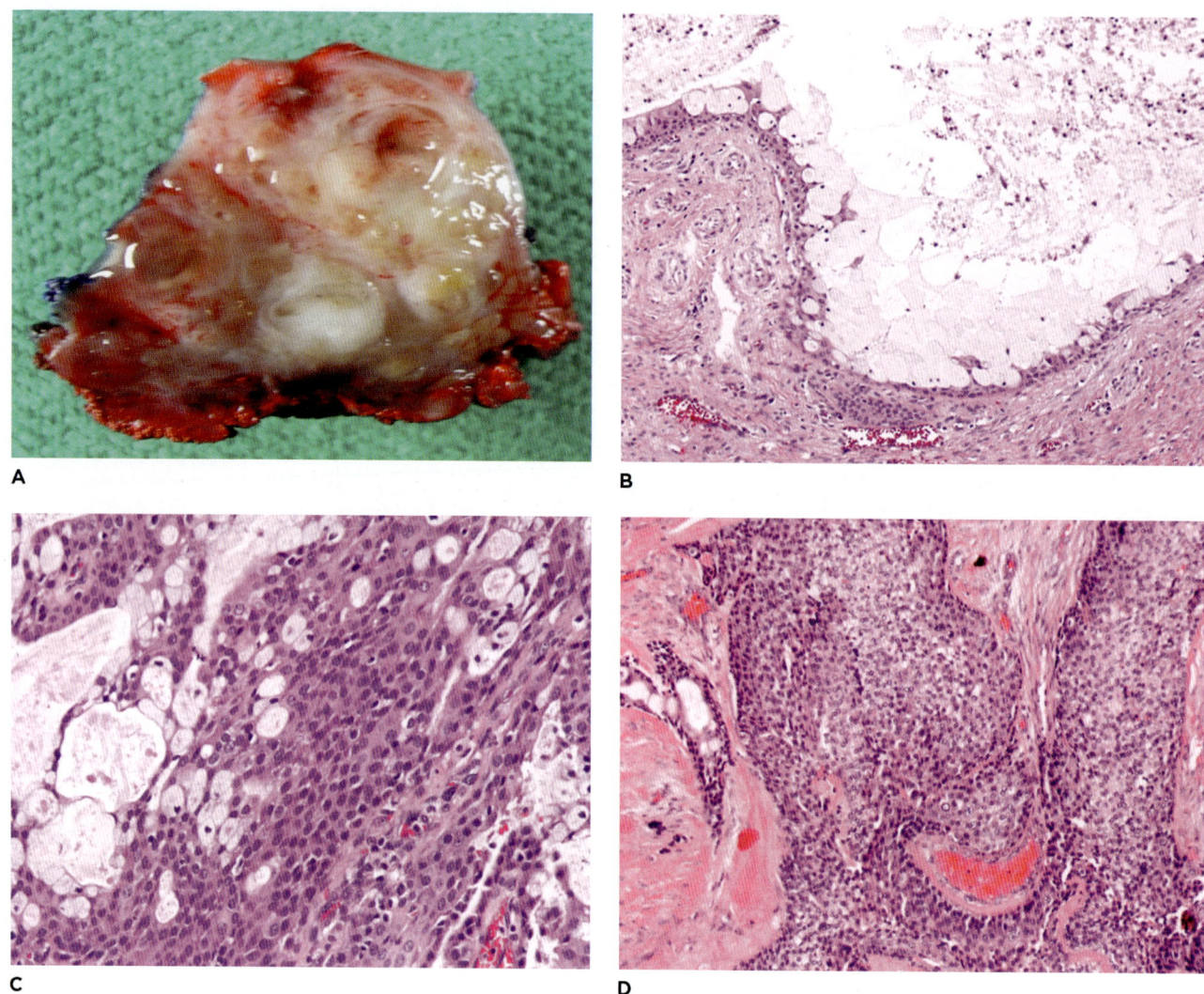

FIGURE 22-21 • Mucoepidermoid carcinoma. **A:** Gross appearance of tumor with predominant solid pattern with focal cystic areas. **B:** MEC pattern with predominance of cysts lined by mucin-producing cells and intermediate cells. **C:** MEC pattern with predominance of intermediate cells and less frequent mucous cells. **D:** MEC pattern with solid sheets of epidermoid cells in a sclerotic background.

target for therapy. Cytogenetic and molecular analyses have identified several translocations and alterations (127). The most common translocation (40%) is t(11;19)(q21;p13) [CRTC1-MAML2], which disrupts the Notch signaling pathway. Both CRTC1 and MAML2 are involved in cyclic AMP regulation. CRTC1 is also known as MECT1, TORC1, or WAMP1. Of interest is the fact that MECs with a CRTC1-MAML2 fusion or a novel CRTC3-MAML2 (t[11;15][q21;q26]) fusion comprise a favorable tumor subset that is distinct from fusion-negative cases. A less common (20% to 30%) translocation is t(1;11)(p22;q13), which involves cyclin D1 (11q13), leading to increased cyclin D1 expression and cell cycle dysregulation. There are several other translocations reported that most frequently involve chromosomes 1, 5, 7, and 11. There are also other reciprocal translocations that have been identified, including t(11;19), t(1;16), t(6;8), t(3;15), and t(7;15). The differential diagnosis includes other malignant salivary gland malignancies, conventional squamous cell carcinoma, and sialometaplasia. Treatment is primarily surgical resection with sampling of cervical lymph nodes. Radiotherapy and chemotherapy are reserved for unresectable and high-grade tumors.

ACINIC CELL CARCINOMA

Acinic cell carcinoma (ACC) is the second most common malignant salivary gland tumor in childhood and usually occurs in the second decade (117–121,128–133). This tumor is comprised of malignant epithelial cells with serous acinar differentiation with zymogen granules and ductal differentiation. The tumor is thought to arise from the intercalated ducts. The parotid gland (80%) is most often involved followed by minor salivary glands (up to 15%) at various sites in the oral cavity. This tumor can be bilateral. The tumor is typically slowly growing with vague pain in about 50% of those affected and facial nerve involvement in up to 10%. Gross examination usually reveals a well-circumscribed, solitary, firm to rubbery tumor that may have hemorrhagic to cystic areas (Figure 22-22). The average size is 1 to 3 cm but ranges up to 13 cm. There are many histologic patterns, with the most common being comprised of polygonal serous cells with basophilic granular cytoplasm and dense deeply basophilic zymogen granules, which are PAS positive and diastase resistant (Figure 22-22). This is referred to as a solid lobular pattern. There are also less frequent microcystic, papillary cystic, and follicular patterns. Immunohistochemistry is of very limited diagnostic utility. Ultrastructural examination reveals zymogen granules within acinar tumor cells, ductal cells lacking zymogen granules, and basement membrane material lining the basal aspect of the tumor cells. Cytogenetics and molecular genetics have not identified specific alterations or translocations. There is loss of heterozygosity, most frequently with 4p15-16, 6p25-qter, and 17p11. The differential includes other malignant salivary gland tumors with similar histopathologic patterns. With complete excision, overall 5-year (80% to 90%) and 10-year (66%) survival is favorable. The tumor recurs in about one-third of cases within 5 years. Clinical stage is more predictive of outcome than histologic grade or growth pattern. There are certain poor prognostic factors, including local and regional metastatic disease, residual tumor after surgery, recurrences, increased mitotic rate or proliferation fraction (>10% mib-1 staining), submandibular gland tumor, deep lobe of parotid tumor, or perineural involvement. Complete surgical excision is the recommended treatment. Radiation therapy is employed for incompletely excised tumors and advanced stage and metastatic disease that cannot be resected.

SIALOBLASTOMA

Sialoblastoma is considered to be a low-grade epithelial and myoepithelial malignancy (117,120,121,134–145). This exceedingly rare tumor resembles the anlage of salivary glands during embryonic development (12 weeks gestation) and has also been termed embryoma, and congenital basal cell adenoma in the past. This congenital tumor may be discovered *in utero*, at birth or during the neonatal period, and rarely in children over 2 years of age. There is an equal gender ratio. The parotid gland is most commonly involved. Presentation is usually with an obvious mass in the region of the parotid or submandibular gland, which may undergo rapid growth. Gross examination shows a somewhat circumscribed, lobular mass, which may have focal hemorrhage and necrosis. These tumors vary from 2 to 8 cm in size. The tumor cells have a blastemal character, similar to many of the small round cell tumors of childhood. The tumor has both epithelial and myoepithelial components, arising from reserve basal cells. The tumor tends to be multilobular with basaloid blastemal cells with minimal cytoplasm predominating, with myoepithelial cells at the periphery of the lobules (Figure 22-23). There may

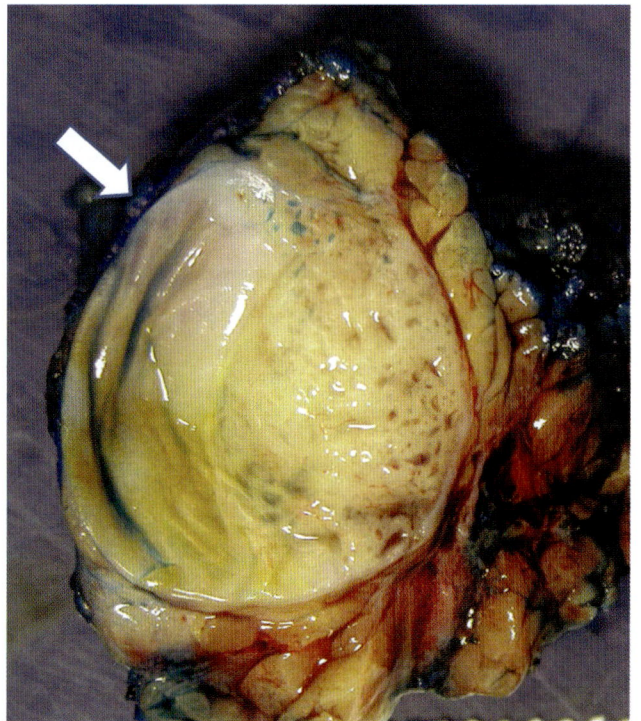

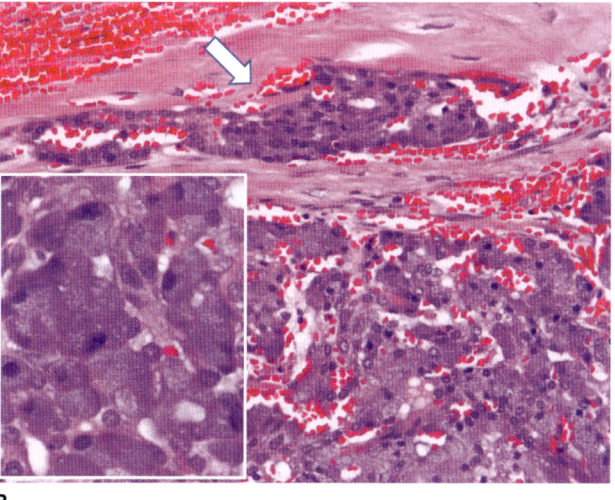

FIGURE 22-22 • Acinic cell carcinoma. **A:** Gross appearance of well-circumscribed tumor (*arrow*) involving parotid gland. **B:** Polygonal tumor cells with abundant basophilic granular cytoplasm (**inset**) and bland nuclei. Note vascular invasion (*arrow*) by tumor.

be peripheral palisading along the lobules. There also may be ductule formation with a cuboidal epithelial lining. There is myxoid stroma surrounding individual lobules, which shows collagenization away from the basaloid lobule. Unfavorable features are perineural or vascular invasion, infiltrative or broad pushing borders, and anaplasia with the basaloid cells. A tumor with remarkably similar histopathologic features is the pancreatoblastoma. The immunohistochemical profile is nonspecific and highlights the ductal epithelial, basaloid, and myoepithelial cells (cytokeratin, p63, S100, SMA, calponin). Of interest is HER2 expression in some of the tumor cells, perhaps representing a therapeutic target for this tumor. High proliferative index (mib-1) and p53 overexpression are associated with more aggressive tumors. Cytogenetic and molecular features have not been evaluated for this exceedingly rare tumor. There are infrequent case reports with sialoblastoma associated with hepatoblastoma and nevus sebaceous. Hepatoblastoma are known to have dysregulation of the Wnt signaling pathway with translocation of beta-catenin from the cytoplasm to the nucleus. This is also seen in pancreatoblastoma, a similar tumor as sialoblastoma. It would be assumed that beta-catenin and the WNT signaling pathway may be dysregulated in sialoblastoma. While pancreatoblastoma and hepatoblastoma are tumors associated with Beckwith-Wiedemann syndrome, this association has not been reported with sialoblastoma. Treatment is usually complete surgical excision. Chemotherapy and radiation therapy are reserved for unresectable tumors in these very young patients who may have significant short-term and long-term effects of such therapy. Recurrences are noted in about one-third and metastatic locoregional disease in about 10%.

DENTIGEROUS CYST (FOLLICULAR CYST)

Following tooth development, the enamel organ epithelium undergoes atrophy to form a thin layer of flattened reduced enamel epithelium overlying the crown of the tooth that is still undergoing root development prior to eruption into the oral cavity. A dentigerous (follicular) cyst may form if fluid accumulates between the crown of the tooth and the reduced enamel epithelium (146–151). This is the most common odontogenic cyst (25%). Other developmental odontogenic cysts include eruption cyst, odontogenic keratocyst, orthokeratinized odontogenic cyst, gingival cysts of newborn and

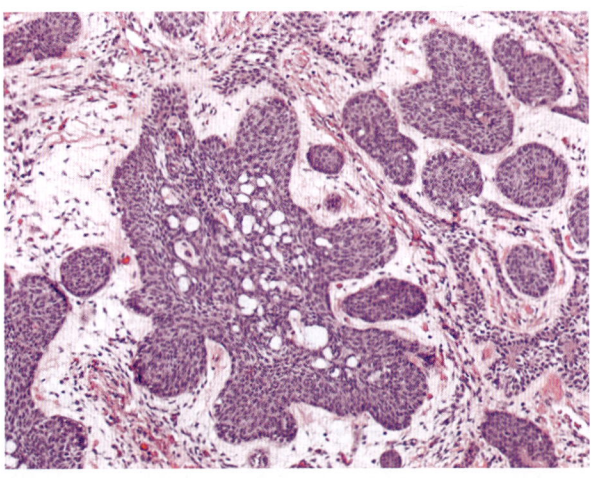
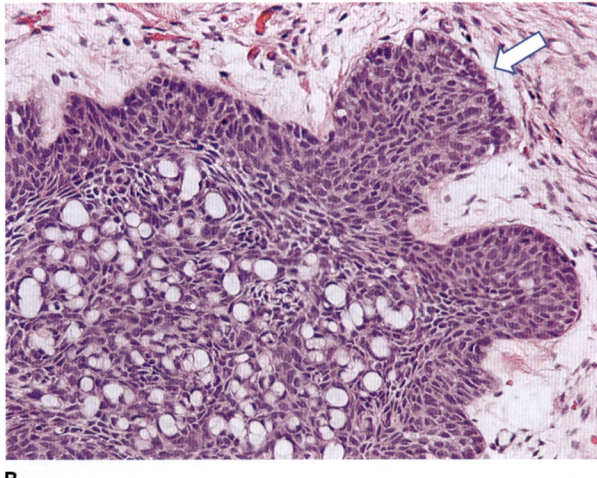
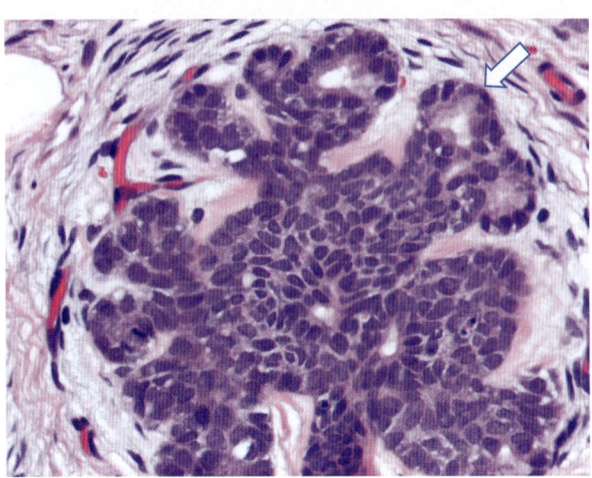

FIGURE 22-23 • Sialoblastoma. **A:** Numerous variably sized nest tumor cells in fibromyxoid stroma background. **B:** Predominance of basaloid cells with central area demonstrating tubule formations and peripheral palisading (*arrow*). **C:** Ductule formation with cuboidal to low columnar epithelial cells.

adult, lateral periodontal cysts, and glandular odontogenic cyst. In addition, inflammatory cysts such as periapical cyst and residual cyst also occur in the jaws.

Dentigerous cysts occur with unerupted teeth, with impacted mandibular and maxillary third molars, maxillary canines, and mandibular second premolars being most commonly affected (146–151). Although this entity may be identified at any age, the most common age of discovery is the second and third decades. Most cysts are asymptomatic and painless. With large dentigerous cysts, there may be bony expansion, and pain may be present if the cyst becomes secondarily infected. The cyst is well-demarcated and unilocular and surrounds the crown of the tooth, and only the crown of the tooth is noted within the cyst on radiologic examination (Figure 22-24). The cyst less commonly extends along the root surface. Displacement of the affected tooth and resorption of the roots of adjacent teeth may occur. Microscopic examination of a noninflamed dentigerous cyst shows a relatively thin, flattened, nonkeratinized epithelium without rete pegs and a cyst wall composed of loose fibromyxoid to

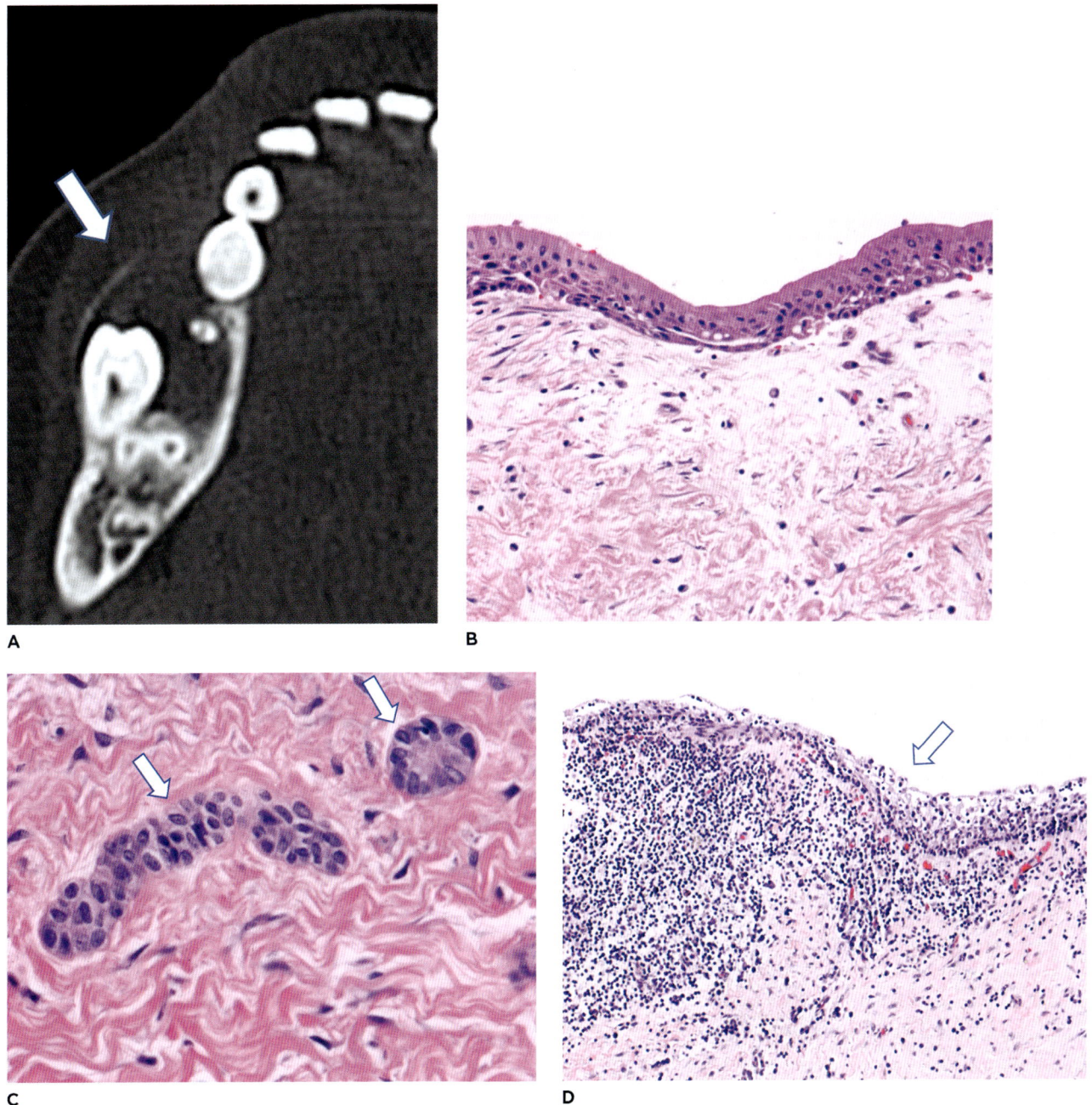

FIGURE 22-24 • Dentigerous cyst. **A:** Cystic expansion (*arrow*) with impacted permanent molar tooth in mandible on CT scan. **B:** Cyst lined by nonkeratinized stratified squamous epithelium and underlying fibromyxoid cyst wall. **C:** Odontogenic epithelial rests (*arrows*) in cyst wall. **D:** Inflamed dentigerous cyst with reactive attenuated epithelial lining and chronic inflammation in cyst wall.

fibrous stroma (Figure 22-24). Scattered odontogenic epithelial rests may also be present in the cyst wall. With inflammation, the epithelium may become reactive and also possess rete pegs. Oftentimes, the inflamed dentigerous cyst will either have lost its epithelial lining or have a thin atrophic epithelial layer with chronic inflammatory cells present in the cyst wall. Rarely, mucinous cells and ciliated cells may be seen. Treatment is enucleation of the cyst. With large cysts, marsupialization may be used in order to decrease the size of the cyst prior to definitive removal. It is important to perform a biopsy on the cyst prior to marsupialization in order to confirm the clinical and radiologic diagnosis.

ODONTOGENIC KERATOCYST (KERATOCYSTIC ODONTOGENIC TUMOR)

Odontogenic keratocyst (OKC; WHO terminology keratocystic odontogenic tumor) is derived from the dental lamina epithelium or from the basal cell layer of oral epithelium (146,147,152–163). OKC may occur at any site within the jaws and has also been reported as a soft tissue cyst involving the gingiva. Most of these cysts occur in the mandible (70%) with a predilection for the posterior mandible and ramus. An unerupted tooth is often seen in association with the OKC and this may mimic a dentigerous cyst. The majority of OKCs occur from 10 to 40 years of age, with a peak during the second and third decades. Similar to dentigerous cysts, small OKCs may be an incidental finding, whereas large OKCs lead to bony expansion and less commonly pain and cyst fluid drainage. Radiologic examination shows small OKCs to be well-demarcated, unilocular radiolucencies with a sclerotic border (Figure 22-25). In contrast, large OKCs may be multilocular. Gross examination of OKCs shows a thin cyst wall and a lumen with keratinaceous debris. Oftentimes, the keratinaceous debris has been removed during the surgical procedure. Keratin debris is not specific for OKC. Microscopic examination shows stratified squamous epithelium with a corrugated, wavy surface with parakeratinization (Figure 22-25). Rete pegs are usually absent and the basal

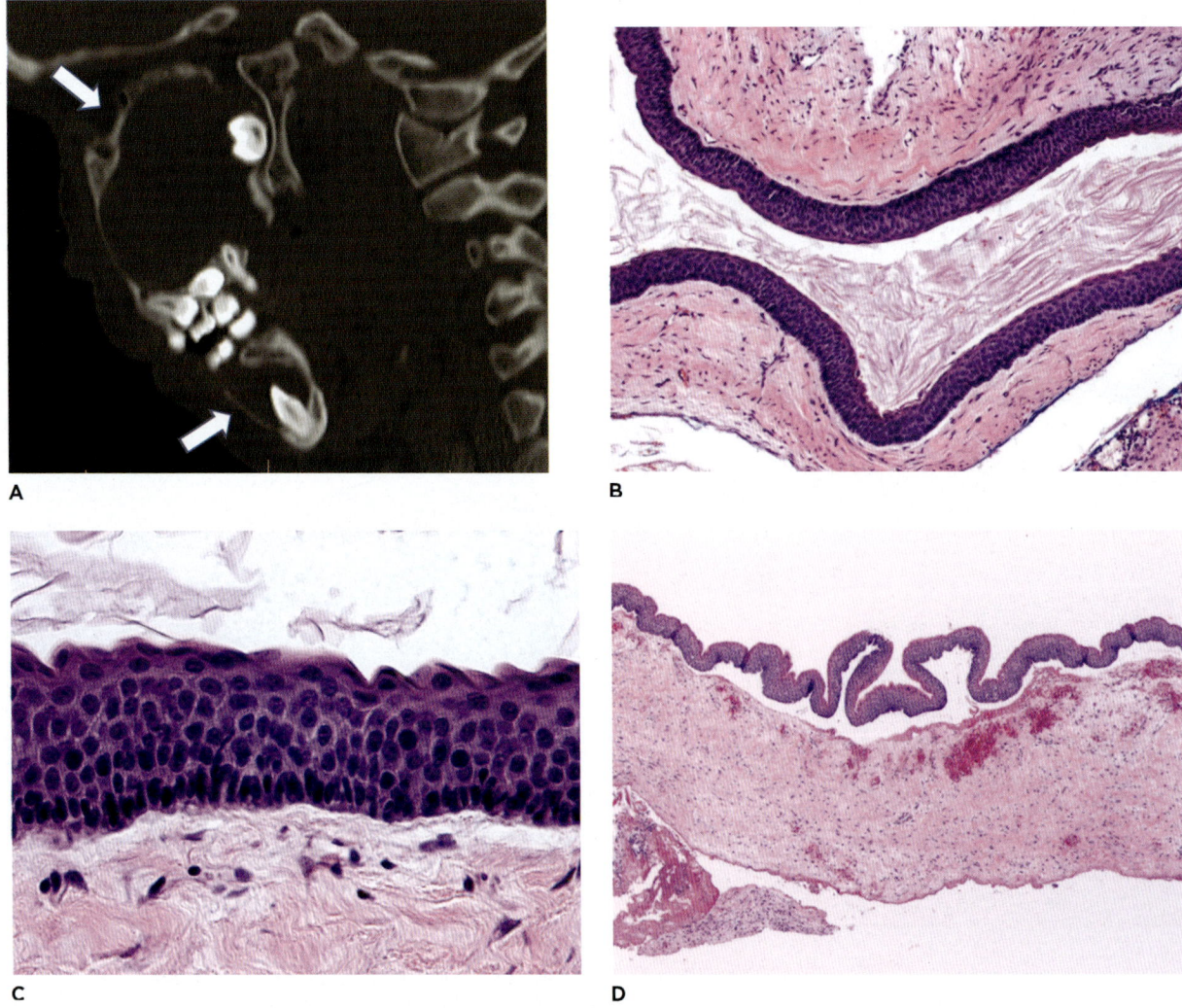

FIGURE 22-25 • Odontogenic keratocyst (keratogenic odontogenic tumor). **A:** Cystic lesions (*arrows*) with impacted, displaced teeth involving maxilla and mandible in Gorlin syndrome. **B:** Cyst containing readily identified keratin debris. **C:** Characteristic corrugated, wavy epithelial surface, parakeratinization, basal cell palisading, and keratin debris in lumen. **D:** Characteristic lifting and separation of epithelium from cyst wall, usually focal to multifocal.

cell epithelial layer has a palisading appearance comprised of cuboidal to low columnar cells. The epithelium lining the cyst is often detached or has fine separation from the underlying cyst wall. The cyst wall may show invagination of the epithelium and separate isolated cysts (daughter cysts, satellite cysts).

Of great importance is the association of odontogenic keratocysts with Gorlin syndrome (nevoid basal cell carcinoma syndrome) (151,152,154,155,162,163). Gorlin syndrome is autosomal dominant and is associated with multiple keratocysts in 75% of affected individuals. Other features include basal cell carcinoma at young age in atypical sites, bifid ribs, kyphoscoliosis, mandibular prognathism, falx cerebri calcifications, ovarian fibroma, soft tissue and adnexal tumors, medulloblastoma, and hypertelorism. This syndrome is associated with constitutional and lesional PTCH (9q22.3-q31) gene mutation in the sonic hedgehog pathway, which results in bcl-2 and TP53 overexpression. OKC is often the first indication of Gorlin syndrome. OKCs in Gorlin syndrome tend to have more prominent epithelial proliferation, foci of calcification, and satellite cysts in the cyst wall. Of note, sporadic nonsyndromic OKCs may also have PTCH mutations and loss of heterozygosity for other tumor suppressor genes. Hence, this is the reasoning behind the WHO introducing the term keratocystic odontogenic tumor.

Treatment of choice is complete removal of the cyst with ostectomy using a bone bur (152–163). However, most OKCs are not suspected and are most likely initially treated with curettage or enucleation similar to dentigerous cysts. The need for ostectomy is based upon the recurrence rate of up to 30%. If the cyst has perforated bone, removal of the affected soft tissue and potentially the overlying mucosa is warranted. With aggressive, large cysts, resection of the involved area with reconstruction and bone grafting may be necessary. Rarely, malignant transformation has been reported.

PERIAPICAL CYST AND GRANULOMA

This lesion consists of granulation tissue that develops at the tip of the root or along the root surface with nonvital teeth in response to inflammation due to caries, trauma, large restorations, prior root canal therapy, or periodontal disease (164–170). Epithelial odontogenic rests associated with root development within the periodontal ligament (rests of Malassez) may form the epithelium lining the periapical cyst. The epithelial lining may also be derived from crevicular epithelium where the gingiva attaches to the root surface, from epithelium lining a sinus tract due to the inflammatory process, or from an adjacent maxillary sinus. When there is no epithelial lining, the granulation tissue response is termed a periapical granuloma. This lesion is the most common odontogenic lesion and represents about 50% of oral cavity cysts. Periapical cyst or granulomas occur more commonly in young adults and especially with the anterior maxillary incisors. Symptoms include pain, swelling, and drainage in the area of a nonvital tooth. With maxillary anterior teeth, there may be an ascending infection that if untreated could extend maxillofacial soft tissues and potentially into the cavernous sinus. Radiologic examination shows bone destruction (radiolucency) at the apex or less often at the lateral aspect of the root with loss of the typical lamina dura surrounding a vital tooth. Microscopic examination of a periapical cyst (Figure 22-26) shows areas with an irregular stratified squamous epithelium lining and a cyst wall comprised of fibrous connective tissue

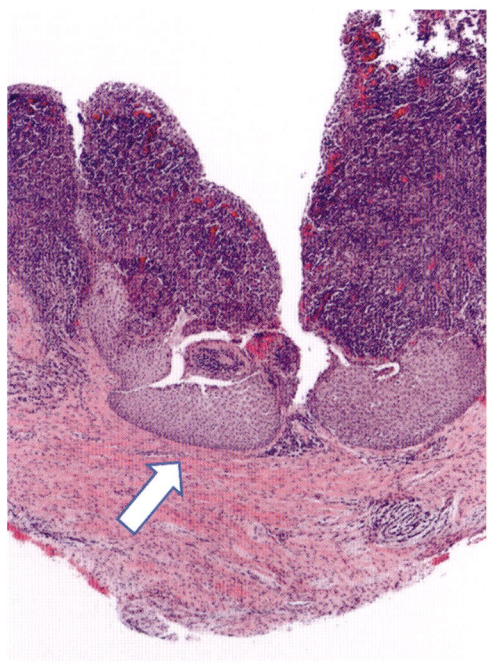 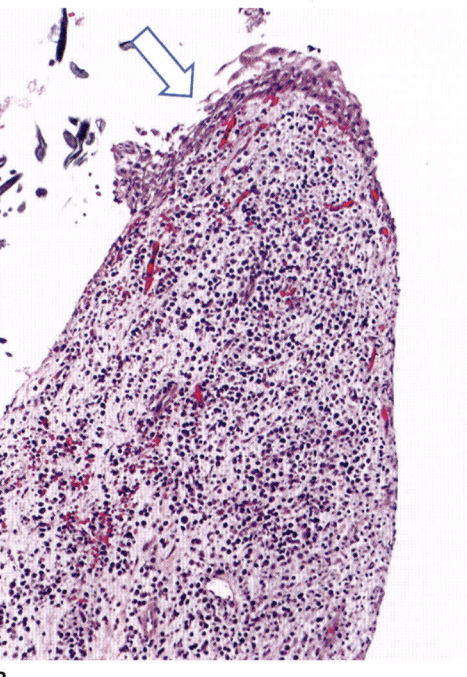

FIGURE 22-26 • Periapical cyst. **A:** Cyst with portions of retained stratified squamous epithelial lining (arrow), intraluminal inflammation, and fibrotic cyst wall. **B:** Markedly inflamed cyst wall with focal retention of reactive epithelium (arrow).

with a mixed inflammatory infiltrate. Some periapical lesions will resemble granulation tissue and perhaps having only focal areas with a thin reactive epithelial lining.

Tooth extraction and removal of the lesion are necessary with nonrestorable teeth (164–170). Root canal therapy with antibiotic therapy is required for restorable teeth. On occasion, the periapical lesion does not resolve and a residual periapical cyst may be present and may require surgical excision. Most lesions resolve with restoration of normal bone formation; however, some lesions may show dystrophic calcifications.

TUMORS DERIVED FROM ODONTOGENIC EPITHELIUM AND ECTOMESENCHYME

Odontoma

This is the most common odontogenic "tumor" and is more prevalent than all other odontogenic tumors combined (161,171–175). Rather than being a true tumor, this entity is considered to be a developmental hamartoma of odontogenic epithelium and ectomesenchyme that typically forms the tooth buds. Odontomas are divided into compound (comprised of multiple tooth-like structures, denticles; Figure 22-27A) and complex (irregular aggregates of enamel, dentin, and cementum that do not form structures resembling denticles). Most often, odontomas occur within the jaws and rarely only within gingival soft tissues. Odontomas are identified during the first and second decades often when there is failure of a tooth to erupt into the oral cavity or painless jaw swelling or with routine radiologic examination. The anterior maxilla is more commonly affected. Radiologic examination shows a unilocular radiolucency with poorly formed teeth with a compound odontoma and radiopaque amorphous material with a complex odontoma. Microscopic examination of the soft tissue and associated mineralized tissue shows enamel protein matrix with typical prism (fish scale; Figure 22-27B) or

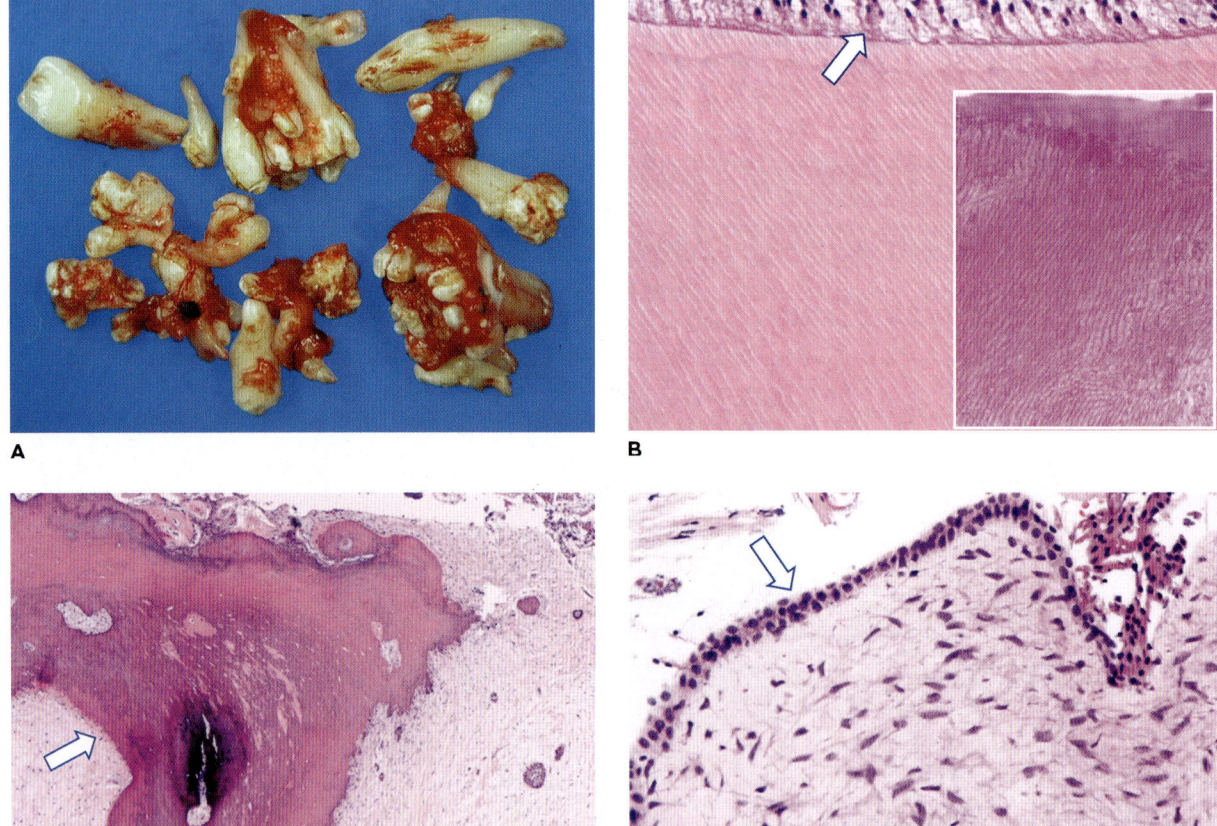

FIGURE 22-27 • Odontoma. **A:** Compound odontoma with toothlike structures and odontogenic soft tissue intermixed with teeth requiring removal during surgery. **B:** Dentin matrix, noncalcified with associated odontoblasts (*arrow*). *Inset:* Enamel matrix protein, noncalcified. **C:** Irregular mass of cementum and dentin (*arrow*), focally calcified. **D:** Dental papilla with odontoblasts and papillary cells at periphery (*arrow*).

netlike appearance, dentinal matrix with tubular arrays and sometimes with associated odontoblasts (Figure 22-27B), and irregular cementum and cementicles (Figure 22-27C). Dental papilla (Figure 22-27D) that forms the dental pulp may also be seen and confused with an odontogenic myxoma. Treatment consists of conservative excision by enucleation of the lesion.

Ameloblastic Fibroma

In contrast to odontoma, ameloblastic fibroma (AF) is a true neoplasm of odontogenic epithelium and ectomesenchyme and is important to recognize in order to avoid confusion with ameloblastoma (161,176–179). Typically, this tumor occurs in the first and second decades with a slight male predilection, and most are located in the posterior mandible. These tumors are typically painless and discovered either due to localized swelling or on routine dental radiographic examination. Large AFs may cause a certain degree of discomfort and may cause impaction of adjacent teeth. The typical lesion is a well-demarcated radiolucency with or without a sclerotic border on radiologic examination. Microscopic examination shows delicate strands and islands of odontogenic epithelium in a myxoid background resembling cellular dental papilla (Figure 22-28A). The cells at the periphery of the odontogenic epithelium tend to be columnar and resemble ameloblasts. The more central cells may appear similar to stellate reticulum. The stroma may have areas with a more hyalinized appearance (Figure 22-28B). Treatment varies from aggressive curettage to wide local resection depending upon the extent of the tumor. Recurrence is approximately 20%; however, recurrence may be up to 90% with conservative management compared with 10% with more aggressive treatment. Malignant transformation to ameloblastic fibrosarcoma does occur in a certain percentage of ameloblastic fibromas (up to 10%) and is most often associated with recurrent ameloblastic fibromas. This necessitates close clinical follow-up to assess for recurrence of this tumor.

Ameloblastic Fibro-Odontoma (Odontoameloblastoma, Ameloblastic Odontoma)

Ameloblastic fibro-odontoma possesses histopathologic features of ameloblastic fibroma and an admixture of hard tissue components, such as enamel, dentinal, and cementum matrix, usually found in complex odontomas (161,179–187). This tumor is most common in the first and second decades and occurs more commonly in the mandible. The affected individual is asymptomatic unless the tumor is of large size. Radiologic examination shows a well-demarcated lesion, which shows variably radiopacities and is often associated with an impacted tooth (Figure 22-29). Gross examination shows an admixture of soft tissue and irregular portions of hard tissue with no evidence of poorly formed tooth-like structures (Figure 22-29). Microscopic examination demonstrates areas resembling ameloblastic fibroma in close association with portions of hard tissue matrix (dentin, cementum, enamel; Figure 22-29). The proportion of the two components is quite variable from tumor to tumor. In contrast to ameloblastic fibroma, treatment for ameloblastic fibro-odontoma is conservative with only rare recurrences.

Adenomatoid Odontogenic Tumor

Adenomatoid odontogenic tumor (AOT) is most commonly discovered by the second decade with 75% to 90% of cases in individuals less than age 20 years (188–191). This tumor occurs more commonly in females (70%) and usually involves the anterior maxilla or mandible. Failure of tooth

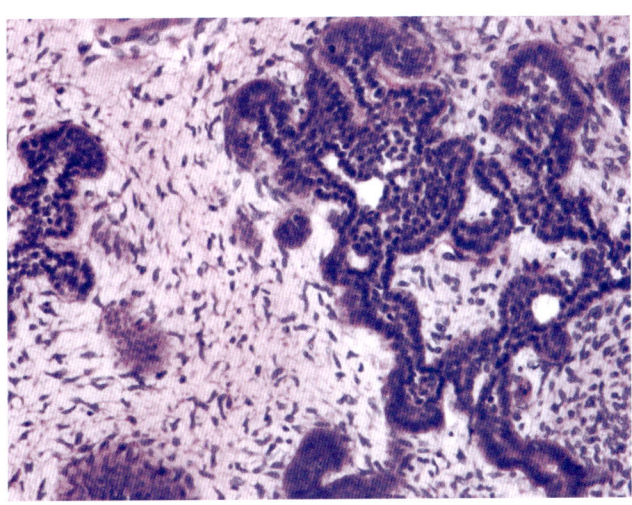
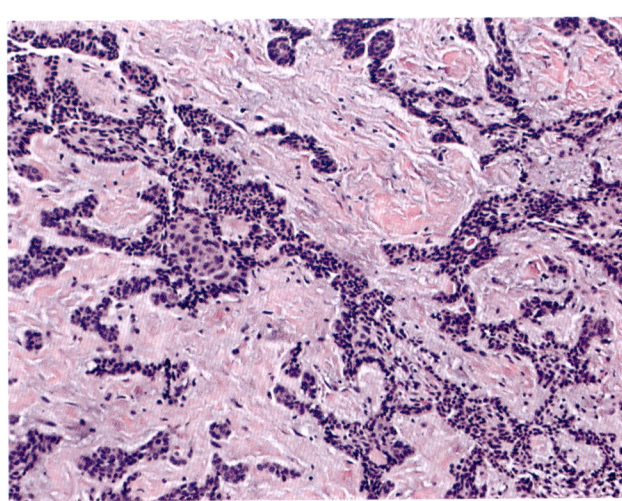

FIGURE 22-28 • Ameloblastic fibroma. **A:** Cords and strands of odontogenic epithelium in an abundant cellular myxoid background. **B:** Ameloblastic fibroma with hyalinized stroma.

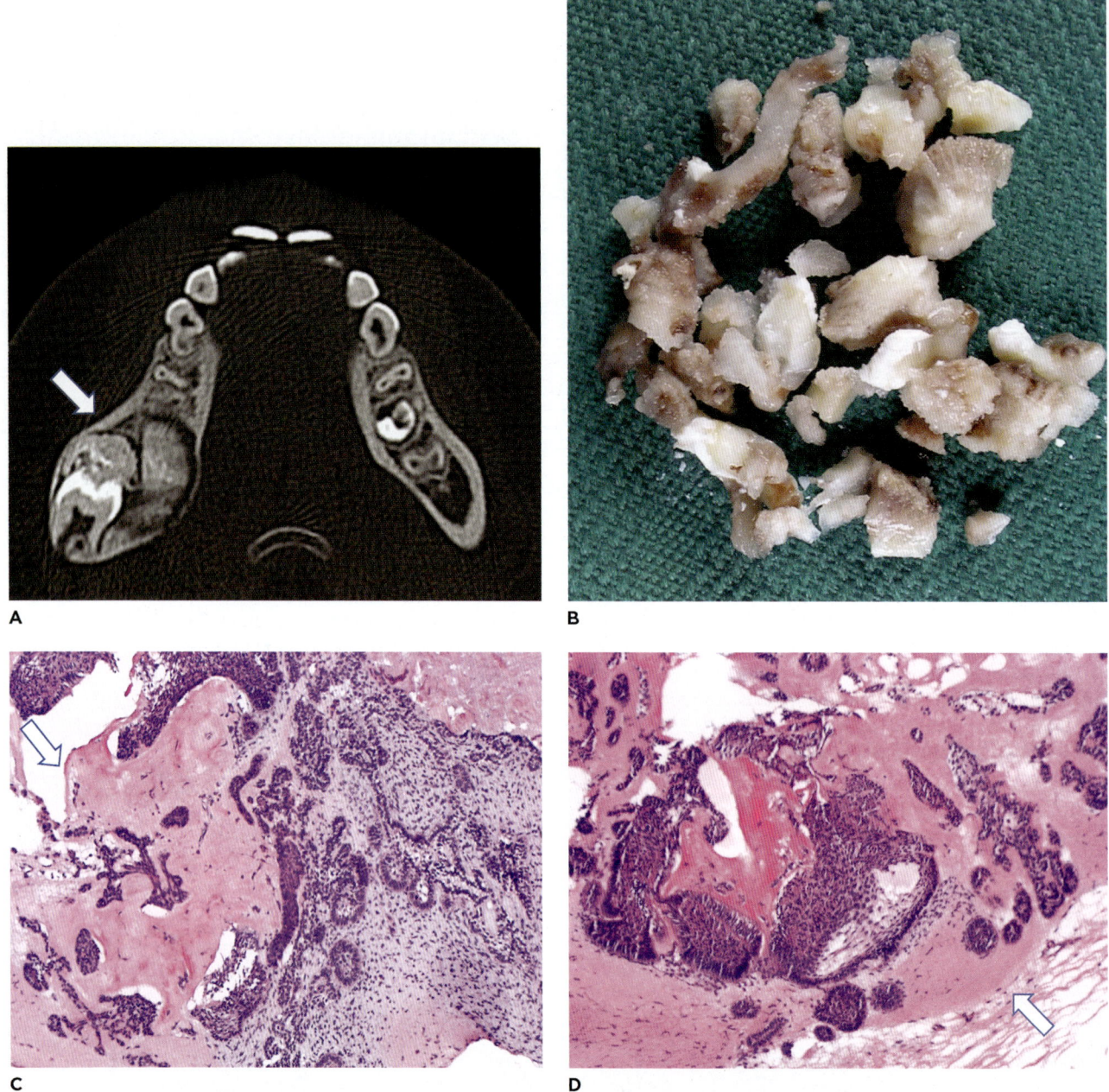

FIGURE 22-29 • Ameloblastic fibro-odontoma. **A:** Expansile mandibular mass (*arrow*) with impacted permanent tooth and mass containing material of similar density as tooth structure on CT scan. **B:** Morcellated contents of mass with partially calcified tissue and firm soft tissue. **C and D:** Firm soft tissue comprised of noncalcified cementum-like tissue (*arrow*) with associated ameloblastic fibroma component.

eruption due to impaction by this tumor is often the presenting sign in this asymptomatic odontogenic tumor. Radiologic examination shows a well-circumscribed, radiolucent lesion, which sometimes may have fine calcifications (Figure 22-30). If there is an impacted tooth, the cystic lesion surrounds the crown and a portion of the root impacted tooth. This finding is in contrast to dentigerous cysts where the lesion only surrounds the crown of the tooth. Microscopic examination demonstrates a partially encapsulated tumor comprised of stromal spindle-shaped cells arranged in swirling to nodular patterns sometimes with focal basophilic dystrophic calcifications often with lamination (Figure 22-30). In addition, there are duct-like structures lined by cuboidal to columnar epithelial cells. Amyloid-like material in the stroma and cytoplasmic melanin pigment may be present. Treatment is enucleation with only very rare recurrences reported.

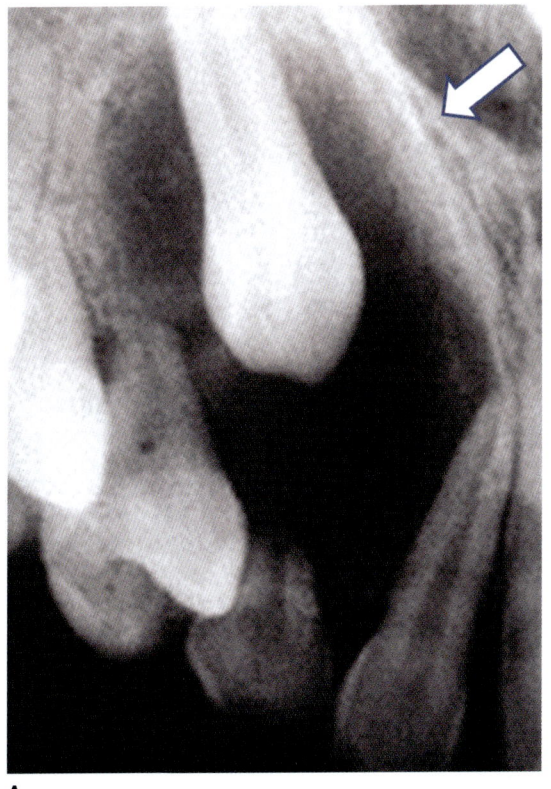
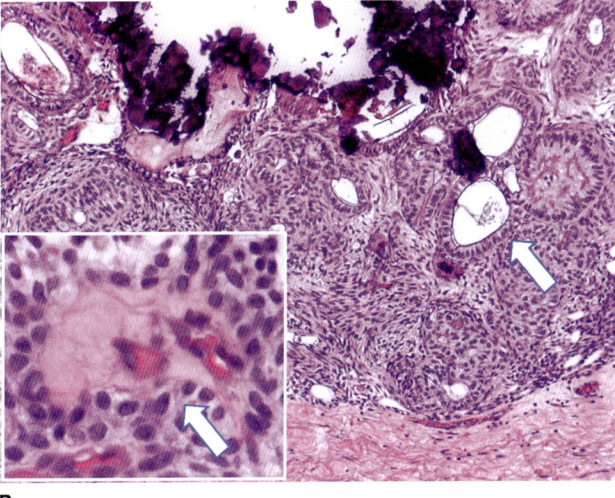

FIGURE 22-30 • Adenomatoid odontogenic tumor. **A:** Expansile cyst (*arrow*) with impaction of maxillary canine tooth. Note the cyst extends along the root surface of the impacted canine tooth. **B:** Tumor with well-defined interface, swirling stromal spindle cells, focal duct-like structures, and dystrophic calcification. *Inset*: Amyloid-like material focally in stroma (*arrow*).

ODONTOGENIC MYXOMA: TUMOR OF ODONTOGENIC ECTOMESENCHYME

Odontogenic myxoma (OM) occurs as a centrally placed lesion in the jaws without a soft tissue origin (192–199). This tumor occurs in wide age range from childhood into later adulthood and affects the mandible more frequently with no gender predilection. This radiolucent lesion may be unilocular with small tumors and multilocular with large tumors on radiologic examination (Figure 22-31). Gross examination shows a homogeneously gelatinous tumor. Microscopic examination demonstrates spindle to stellate to sometimes ovoid bland fibroblastic-like tumor cells in a myxoid background (Figure 22-31). More aggressive lesions may have increased cellularity (Figure 22-31). Odontogenic epithelial rests may be seen in some OMs. The adjacent bone tends to be infiltrated by the tumor and makes it difficult to define the surgical margin on radiologic features alone. When there is substantial collagen present, the term fibromyxoma or myxofibroma may be used depending upon whether the fibrous or myxoid components predominate. Because of the myxoid nature, this tumor may be mistaken for dental papilla from removal of a developing tooth during the surgery (199). Dental papilla can be differentiated from OM by searching for the presence of odontoblasts at the periphery of the dental papilla (Figure 22-27D). Treatment is aggressive curettage for small OMs and en bloc or segmental resection for large OMs because of the infiltrative growth pattern (192–199). With conservative surgery, about one-third of OMs recur. There are reports of transformation to myxosarcoma.

AMELOBLASTOMA: TUMOR OF ODONTOGENIC EPITHELIUM WITHOUT ODONTOGENIC MESENCHYME

Ameloblastoma is the most common of odontogenic neoplasms, since odontoma is considered to be a developmental hamartoma rather than a true neoplasm (200–222). The origin of this tumor is most likely from dental lamina rests within the gingiva, alveolar bone, and follicles of unerupted teeth. Other possible sources include enamel organ cell rests, odontogenic cyst epithelial lining, and oral mucosa basal cells. Ameloblastoma has tumor cells that are similar to ameloblasts and stellate reticulum and recapitulate these

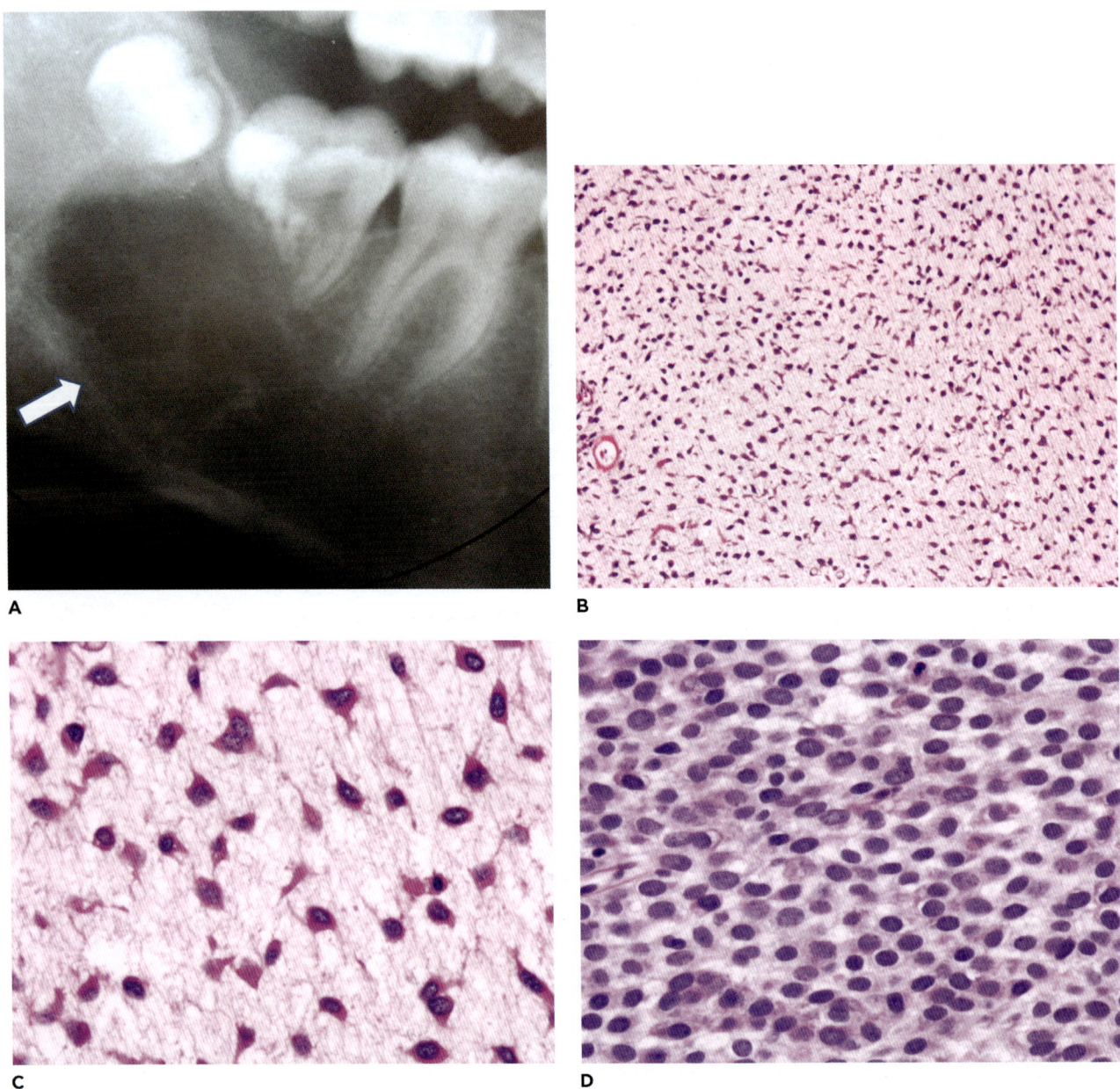

FIGURE 22-31 • Odontogenic myxoma. **A:** Radiolucent lesion (*arrow*) without sclerotic border causing root resorption of mandibular second molar. **B and C:** Abundant myxoid stroma with scattered spindle to stellate stromal cells. **D:** Cellular stroma associated with more aggressive tumor.

components of the enamel organ. However, ameloblastomas do not have the stratum intermedium that is an essential component of the enamel organ. The lack of this component is attributed to the inability of ameloblastoma to produce enamel matrix.

Ameloblastoma is divided into three types: unicystic ameloblastoma (Figure 22-32), conventional ameloblastoma (Figure 22-33), and extraosseous ameloblastoma (Figure 22-34) (200–222). Unicystic ameloblastoma accounts for only about 5% of all ameloblastomas, with the vast majority of ameloblastomas being the conventional type. Extraosseous ameloblastoma is rare (2%) with most involving the gingiva.

Unicystic Ameloblastoma

Unicystic ameloblastoma occurs in younger patients with a mean age of 22 years and is seen much more commonly in the pediatric age group compared with conventional ameloblastoma (200–214). About 50% of unicystic ameloblastomas occur during the second decade of life with no gender predilection. These tumors are noted on radiologic examination to be predominantly unilocular and infrequently multilocular (Figure 22-32) and mimic a dentigerous cyst. However, it may or may not be associated with an unerupted tooth. Microscopic examination shows a cystic lesion lined by epithelium with a plexiform to columnar basal cell layer,

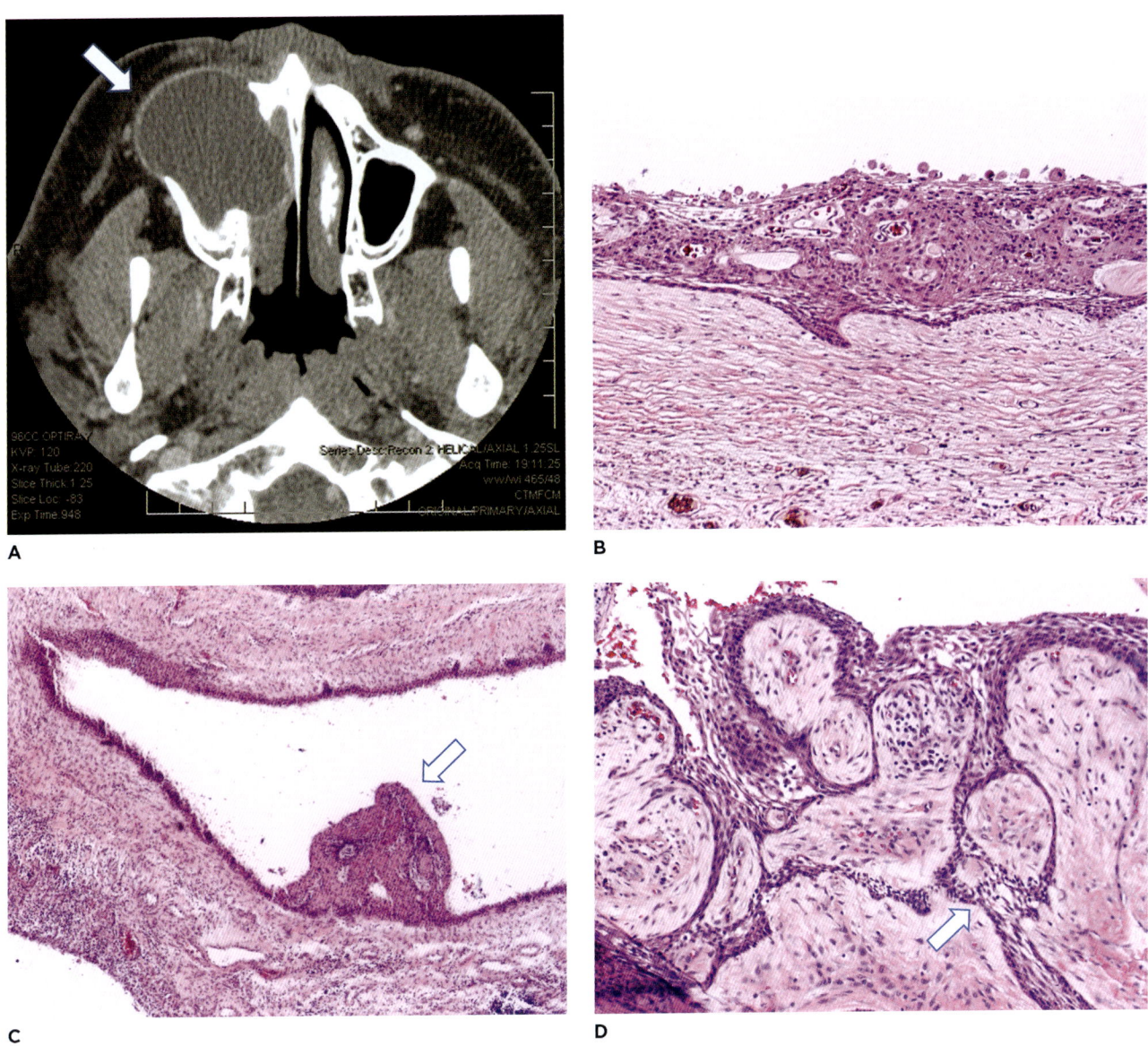

FIGURE 22-32 • Unicystic ameloblastoma. **A:** Cystic lesion (*arrow*) markedly expanded maxilla and obstructing nasal cavity. **B:** Cyst lined by proliferation of odontogenic epithelium with ameloblastic plexiform pattern—note basal cell layer palisading. **C:** Intraluminal nodular extension (*arrow*) in unicystic ameloblastoma. **D:** Mural invasion (*arrow*) of cyst wall in unicystic ameloblastoma.

often with reverse polarization of the nuclei. The underlying cyst wall has a hyalinized to fibrotic appearance. The luminal subtype lacks intraluminal extension or mural invasion of the cyst wall (Figure 22-32). The intraluminal subtype of unicystic ameloblastoma shows one or more nodules of tumor extending into the lumen (Figure 22-32). The nodular extension may also have a plexiform appearance without typical ameloblasts. There is also an intramural subtype, which demonstrates superficial mural invasion of the cyst wall (Figure 22-32). Extensive sampling of the lesion is important to determine if mural invasion is present and the degree of invasion. If there is diffuse invasion of the cyst wall, the diagnosis of conventional ameloblastoma should be considered. It is important to emphasize that the diagnosis of unicystic versus conventional ameloblastoma requires examination of the entire cystic structure. Biopsy only of a cystic lesion may lead to a misleading diagnosis and inappropriate surgical management.

Treatment of luminal or intraluminal subtypes of unicystic ameloblastoma requires removal of the cyst by enucleation and does not require more extensive surgery (200–214). With the intramural subtype, there is invasion of the cyst wall and this requires removal of the cyst and an adequate portion of the adjacent bone. Some oral and maxillofacial surgeons prefer to enucleate the intramural subtype with ostectomy with a bone bur rather than removing a rim of adjacent bone. With all unicystic ameloblastomas, close follow-up is required to assess for local recurrence. A recurrence rate of about 15%

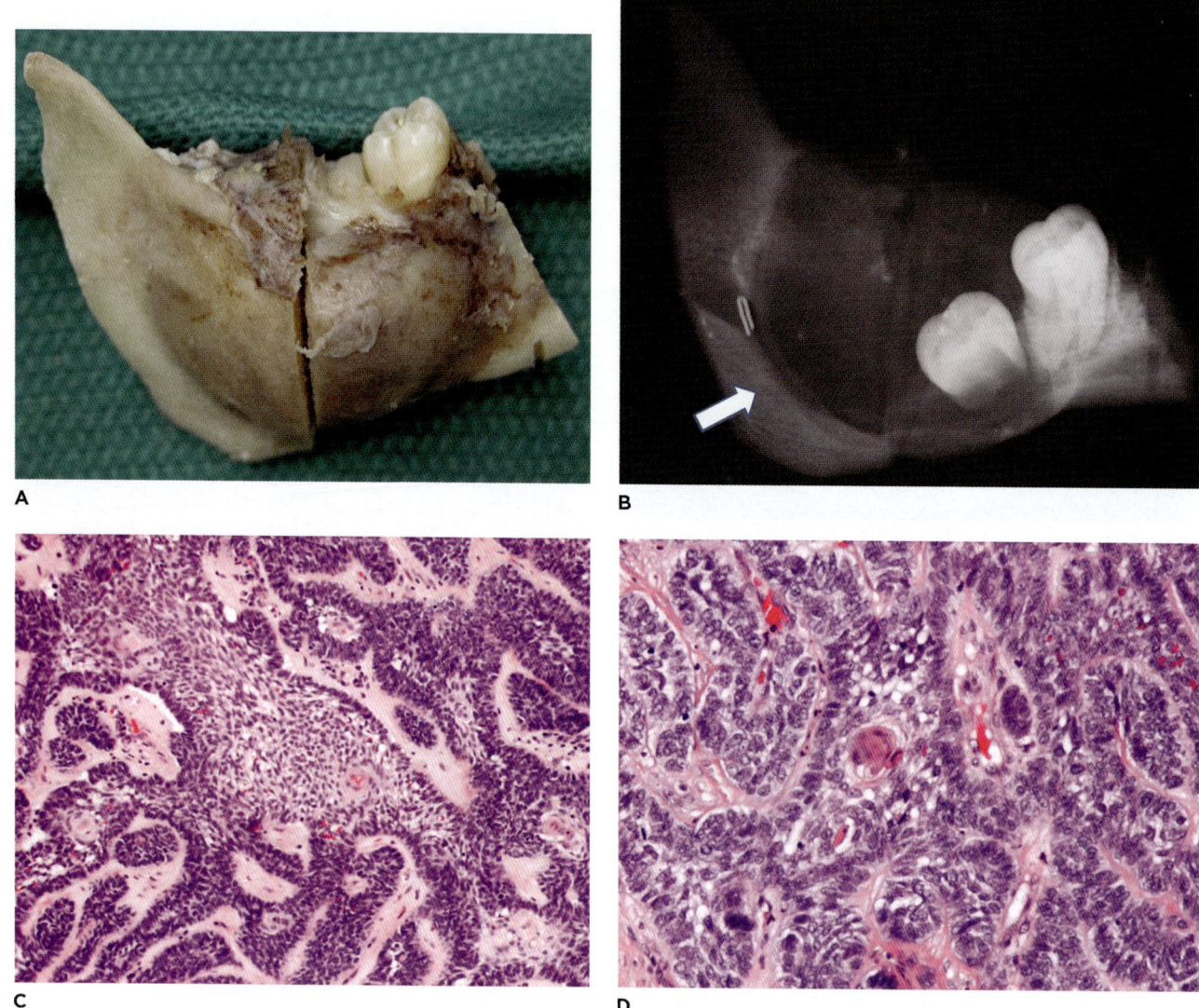

FIGURE 22-33 • Conventional ameloblastoma. **A:** Segmental mandibular resection—note marked tumoral expansion of mandible. **B:** Radiologic examination of resection specimen demonstrates lesion to be radiolucent, poorly demarcated, and associated with impacted teeth. **C:** Plexiform pattern with tumor cell nests with peripheral palisading and central areas mimicking stellate reticulum of tooth buds. **D:** Basal cell pattern of ameloblastoma.

has been reported and most likely is secondary to incomplete removal of the lesions.

Conventional Ameloblastoma

Conventional ameloblastoma typically involves the posterior mandible (85%; Figure 22-33) and has a mean age around 35 years with no gender bias (200–214). The pediatric age group is rarely affected by this type of ameloblastoma (<2%). These tumors tend to be asymptomatic and are most often unilocular. Up to 40% of conventional ameloblastomas are associated with an impacted tooth. Tooth root resorption of adjacent erupted teeth, tooth displacement, and cortical expansion with possible perforation are not uncommon. Microscopic examination shows an infiltrative pattern but may also undergo cystic degeneration (Figure 22-33).

In some tumors, derivation from a cystic structure may be appreciated. Several patterns may be present, including plexiform, follicular, basal cell, acanthomatous, granular cell, and desmoplastic. In general, the periphery of the cell nests and islands is formed by columnar cells with usually reverse nuclear polarization and basement membrane surrounds the peripherally placed epithelial cells. The central portion of the islands may have a stellate reticulum-like character and may contain acanthomatous or granular cells. The intervening stroma may vary from loose myxoid to fibrotic tissue of a low cellularity. The desmoplastic subtype is characterized to be relatively few widely spaced islands of compressed odontogenic epithelium with abundant sclerotic stroma, which is paucicellular.

Because conventional ameloblastoma diffusely infiltrates the adjacent bone and radiologic examination cannot define

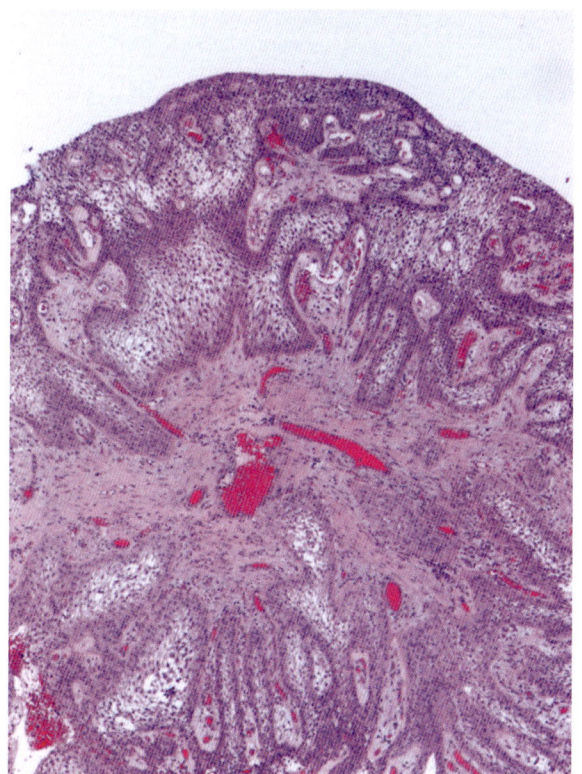

FIGURE 22-34 • Extraosseous ameloblastoma. Tumor arising from the basal cell layer of gingiva with invasion of underlying submucosa.

the precise tumor borders, conservative surgery is not performed (200–214). Marginal or en bloc surgical excision with at least 1-cm surgical margins beyond the radiologic extent of the tumor is typically utilized. Recurrence with conservative surgery is almost 40%, whereas it is about 15% with less conservative surgery. The extent of tumor involving the maxillary region is more difficult to define and requires radical surgery in order to avoid local recurrence that may involve vital structures. Unfortunately, chemotherapy and radiation therapy have no appreciable effect on these tumors, making surgery necessary. Rare cases of malignant transformation do occur and these are associated with metastatic disease and a poor prognosis.

Extraosseous Ameloblastoma

These rare tumors arise more commonly within the gingiva as soft tissue masses with intact overlying epithelium and are not derived from the jaws (215–222). Many of these tumors occur within the anterior mandibular soft tissue along the lingual aspect. The mean age is around 50 years. Radiologic examination is helpful in determining that there is no intraosseous derivation of the tumor. Microscopic examination shows similar histopathologic patterns (Figure 22-34) as those for conventional ameloblastoma. Many of the tumors are contiguous with the overlying epithelium. Although dental lamina rests in the gingiva are often considered to be the source, it is also thought that the basal cell layer of gingiva may give rise to these peripheral ameloblastomas. Treatment is conservative excision because these tumors tend to not be aggressive. This is attested to by a local recurrence rate of less than 10%. Long-term follow-up is indicated to assess for recurrence. Rare cases of malignant transformation have also been reported.

Possible Therapeutic Targets for Ameloblastoma

During recent years, molecular genetics have identified several potential therapeutic targets for ameloblastoma (223–228). Ameloblastomas have been found to have V600E BRAF mutations in a high proportion of tumors, and BRAF inhibitors may play a role in treatment of large nonresectable tumors. BRAF inhibitors are currently employed in treatment of melanoma, thyroid carcinoma, and Langerhans cell histiocytosis, as well as other tumors. Epithelial growth factor receptor (EGFR) has been shown in immortalized ameloblast cell cultures to influence expression of EGF and also metalloprotease, both of these are factors in proliferation, and targeted therapy is available. Interleukins 6 and 8 production is important in ameloblastic growth and inhibitors of interleukins may be employed for possible treatment. The AKT pathway has also been implicated in tissue invasion by ameloblasts, and AKT pathway inhibitors are currently used in certain tumors clinically. The MAP (mitogen-activated protein) kinase pathway is also up-regulated by fibroblastic growth factors 7 and 10 produced by ameloblastoma. MAP kinase pathway inhibitors are available for therapy. With the discovery of targetable factors via molecular genetics, it would appear that in the near future, ameloblastoma may be treated to a certain extent by precision/personalized medicine approaches in addition to surgical management.

References

1. Tsai EC, Santoreneos S, Rutka JT. Tumors of the skull base in children: review of tumor types and management strategies. *Neurosurg Focus* 2002;12(5):e1 [review].
2. Fletcher CD. Distinctive soft tissue tumors of the head and neck. *Mod Pathol* 2002;15(3):324–330 [review].
3. Yi Z, Fang Z, Lin G, et al. Nasopharyngeal angiofibroma: a concise classification system and appropriate treatment options. *Am J Otolaryngol* 2013;34(2):133–141. doi: 10.1016/j.amjoto.2012.10.004
4. Blount A, Riley KO, Woodworth BA. Juvenile nasopharyngeal angiofibroma. *Otolaryngol Clin North Am* 2011;44(4):989–1004, ix. doi: 10.1016/j.otc.2011.06.003
5. Nonogaki S, Campos HG, Butugan O, et al. Markers of vascular differentiation, proliferation and tissue remodeling in juvenile nasopharyngeal angiofibromas. *Exp Ther Med* 2010;1(6):921–926.
6. Stokes SM, Castle JT. Nasopharyngeal angiofibroma of the nasal cavity. *Head Neck Pathol* 2010;4(3):210–213. doi: 10.1007/s12105-010-0181-7
7. Mohammadi M, Saedi B, Basam A. Effect of embolisation on endoscopic resection angiofibroma. *J Laryngol Otol* 2010;124(6):631–635. doi: 10.1017/S0022215109992726
8. Riggs S, Orlandi RR. Juvenile nasopharyngeal angiofibroma recurrence associated with exogenous testosterone therapy. *Head Neck* 2010;32(6):812–815. doi: 10.1002/hed.21152
9. Thompson LD. Update on nasopharyngeal carcinoma. *Head Neck Pathol* 2007;1:81–86.

10. Brennan B. Nasopharyngeal carcinoma. *Orphanet J Rare Dis* 2006;1:23.
11. Wei WI, Sham JS. Nasopharyngeal carcinoma. *Lancet* 2005;365:2041–2054.
12. Wenig BM. Nasopharyngeal carcinoma. *Ann Diagn Pathol* 1999;3:374–385.
13. Afqir S, Ismaili N, Alaoui K, et al. Nasopharyngeal carcinoma in adolescents: a retrospective review of 42 patients. *Eur Arch Otorhinolaryngol* 2009;266:1767–1773.
14. Tao Q, Chan AT. Nasopharyngeal carcinoma: molecular pathogenesis and therapeutic developments. *Expert Rev Mol Med* 2007;9:1–24.
15. Tsao SW, Tsang CM, To KF, et al. The role of Epstein-Barr virus in epithelial malignancies. *J Pathol* 2015;235(2):323–333. doi: 10.1002/path.4448 [review].
16. Xiao L, Xiao T, Wang ZM, et al. Biomarker discovery of nasopharyngeal carcinoma by proteomics. *Expert Rev Proteomics* 2014;11(2):215–225. doi: 10.1586/14789450.2014.897613 [review].
17. Colaco RJ, Betts G, Donne A, et al. Nasopharyngeal carcinoma: a retrospective review of demographics, treatment and patient outcome in a single centre. *Clin Oncol (R Coll Radiol)* 2013;25(3):171–177. doi: 10.1016/j.clon.2012.10.006 [review].
18. Chan AT. Nasopharyngeal carcinoma. *Ann Oncol* 2010;21(Suppl 7):vii308–vii312. doi: 10.1093/annonc/mdq277 [review].
19. Schultz KA, Yang J, Doros L, et al. DICER1-pleuropulmonary blastoma familial tumor predisposition syndrome: a unique constellation of neoplastic conditions. *Pathol Case Rev* 2014;19(2):90–100.
20. Wang T, Li W, Wu X, et al. Nasal chondromesenchymal hamartoma in young children: CT and MRI findings and review of the literature. *World J Surg Oncol* 2014;12:257. doi: 10.1186/1477-7819-12-257
21. Priest JR, Williams GM, Mize WA, et al. Nasal chondromesenchymal hamartoma in children with pleuropulmonary blastoma—a report from the International Pleuropulmonary Blastoma Registry. *Int J Pediatr Otorhinolaryngol* 2010;74(11):1240–1244. doi: 10.1016/j.ijporl.2010.07.022
22. Wooles N, Bell P, Adair R. A review of the management of 84 cases of nasal polyposis in a Tertiary Otorhinolaryngology Centre. *Clin Otolaryngol* 2015. doi: 10.1111/coa.12415 [Epub ahead of print].
23. Kang SH, Dalcin Pde T, Piltcher OB, et al. Chronic rhinosinusitis and nasal polyposis in cystic fibrosis: update on diagnosis and treatment. *J Bras Pneumol* 2015;41(1):65–76. doi: 10.1590/S1806-37132015000100009 [review].
24. Hulse KE, Stevens WW, Tan BK, et al. Pathogenesis of nasal polyposis. *Clin Exp Allergy* 2015;45(2):328–346. doi: 10.1111/cea.12472
25. Mygind N. Allergic rhinitis. *Chem Immunol Allergy* 2014;100:62–68. doi: 10.1159/000358505
26. Chaaban MR, Walsh EM, Woodworth BA. Epidemiology and differential diagnosis of nasal polyps. *Am J Rhinol Allergy* 2013;27(6):473–478. doi: 10.2500/ajra.2013.27.3981 [review].
27. Jiang N, Kern RC, Altman KW. Histopathological evaluation of chronic rhinosinusitis: a critical review. *Am J Rhinol Allergy* 2013;27(5):396–402. doi: 10.2500/ajra.2013.27.3916 [review].
28. Settipane RA, Schwindt C. Chapter 15: Allergic rhinitis. *Am J Rhinol Allergy* 2013;27(Suppl 1):S52–S55. doi: 10.2500/ajra.2013.27.3928 [review].
29. Laury AM, Wise SK. Chapter 7: Allergic fungal rhinosinusitis. *Am J Rhinol Allergy* 2013;27(Suppl 1):S26–S27. doi: 10.2500/ajra.2013.27.3891 [review].
30. Settipane RA, Peters AT, Chiu AG. Chapter 6: Nasal polyps. *Am J Rhinol Allergy* 2013;27(Suppl 1):S20–S25. doi: 10.2500/ajra.2013.27.3926 [review].
31. Segal N, Gluk O, Puterman M. Nasal polyps in the pediatric population. *B-ENT* 2012;8(4):265–267 [review].
32. Georgy MS, Peters AT. Chapter 7: Nasal polyps. *Allergy Asthma Proc* 2012;33(Suppl 1):S22–S23. doi: 10.2500/aap.2012.33.3537 [review].
33. Cingi C, Demirbas D, Ural A. Nasal polyposis: an overview of differential diagnosis and treatment. *Recent Pat Inflamm Allergy Drug Discov* 2011;5(3):241–252 [review].
34. Jeong WJ, Lee CH, Cho SH, et al. Eosinophilic allergic polyp: a clinically oriented concept of nasal polyp. *Otolaryngol Head Neck Surg* 2011;144(2):241–246. doi: 10.1177/0194599810421738
35. Casale M, Pappacena M, Potena M, et al. Nasal polyposis: from pathogenesis to treatment, an update. *Inflamm Allergy Drug Targets* 2011;10(3):158–163 [review].
36. Pakdaman MN, Corry DB, Luong A. Fungi linking the pathophysiology of chronic rhinosinusitis with nasal polyps and allergic asthma. *Immunol Invest* 2011;40(7–8):767–785. doi: 10.3109/08820139.2011.596876 [review].
37. Sarafraz M, Niazi A, Araghi S. The prevalence of clinical presentations and pathological characteristics of antrochoanal polyp. *Niger J Med* 2015;24(1):12–16.
38. Caimmi D, Matti E, Pelizzo G, et al. Nasal polyposis in children. *J Biol Regul Homeost Agents* 2012;26(1 Suppl):S77–S83.
39. Nikakhlagh S, Rahim F, Saki N, et al. Antrochoanal polyps: report of 94 cases and review the literature. *Niger J Med* 2012;21(2):156–159 [review].
40. Ramadass T, Narayanan N, Rao P, et al. Glial heterotopia in ENT-two case reports and review of literature. *Indian J Otolaryngol Head Neck Surg* 2011;63(4):407–410.
41. Pereyra-Rodríguez JJ, Bernabeu-Wittel J, Fajardo M, et al. Nasal glial heterotopia (nasal glioma). *J Pediatr* 2010;156(4):688–688.e1. doi: 10.1016/j.jpeds.2009.09.015
42. Riffaud L, Ndikumana R, Azzis O, et al. Glial heterotopia of the face. *J Pediatr Surg* 2008;43(12):e1–e3. doi: 10.1016/j.jpedsurg.2008.08.009
43. Sun LS, Sun ZP, Ma XC, et al. Glial choristoma in the oral and maxillofacial region: a clinicopathologic study of 6 cases. *Arch Pathol Lab Med* 2008;132(6):984–988. doi: 10.1043/1543-2165(2008)132[984:GCITOA]2.0.CO;2
44. Husein OF, Collins M, Kang DR. Neuroglial heterotopia causing neonatal airway obstruction: presentation, management, and literature review. *Eur J Pediatr* 2008;167(12):1351–1355. doi: 10.1007/s00431-008-0810-2
45. Silva L, Gonçalves CP, Fernandes AM, et al. Laryngeal papillomatosis in children: the impact of late recognition over evolution. *J Med Virol* 2015. doi: 10.1002/jmv.24181 [Epub ahead of print].
46. Sittel C. Pathologies of the larynx and trachea in childhood. *GMS Curr Top Otorhinolaryngol Head Neck Surg* 2014;13:Doc09. doi: 10.3205/cto000112. eCollection 2014 [review].
47. Szydłowski J, Jonczyk-Potoczna K, Pucher B, et al. Prevalence of human papillomavirus (HPV) in upper respiratory tract mucosa in a group of pre-school children. *Ann Agric Environ Med* 2014;21(4):822–824. doi: 10.5604/12321966.1129940
48. Knepper BR, Eklund MJ, Braithwaite KA. Malignant degeneration of pulmonary juvenile-onset recurrent respiratory papillomatosis. *Pediatr Radiol* 2014. [Epub ahead of print].
49. Marsico M, Mehta V, Chastek B, et al. Estimating the incidence and prevalence of juvenile-onset recurrent respiratory papillomatosis in publicly and privately insured claims databases in the United States. *Sex Transm Dis* 2014;41(5):300–305. doi: 10.1097/OLQ.0000000000000115
50. Sajan JA, Kerschner JE, Merati AL, et al. Prevalence of dysplasia in juvenile-onset recurrent respiratory papillomatosis. *Arch Otolaryngol Head Neck Surg* 2010;136(1):7–11. doi: 10.1001/archoto.2009.179
51. Liang Y, Yang YS, Zhang Y. Multiple congenital granular cell epulis in a female newborn: a case report. *J Med Case Rep* 2014;8:413. doi: 10.1186/1752-1947-8-413
52. Conrad R, Perez MC. Congenital granular cell epulis. *Arch Pathol Lab Med* 2014;138(1):128–131. doi: 10.5858/arpa.2012-0306-RS [review].
53. Childers EL, Fanburg-Smith JC. Congenital epulis of the newborn: 10 new cases of a rare oral tumor. *Ann Diagn Pathol* 2011;15(3):157–161. doi: 10.1016/j.anndiagpath.2010.10.003
54. Triantafillidou K, Venetis G, Karakinaris G, et al. Central giant cell granuloma of the jaws: a clinical study of 17 cases and a review of the literature. *Ann Otol Rhinol Laryngol* 2011;120:167–174.
55. Ferretti C, Muthray E. Management of central giant cell granuloma of mandible using intralesional corticosteroids: case report and review of literature. *J Oral Maxillofac Surg* 2011;69:2824–2829.
56. Suárez-Roa Mde L, Reveiz L, Ruíz-Godoy Rivera LM, et al. Interventions for central giant cell granuloma (CGCG) of the jaws. *Cochrane Database Syst Rev* 2009;(4):CD007404. doi: 10.1002/14651858.CD007404.pub2

57. de Lange J, van den Akker HP, van den Berg H. Central giant cell granuloma of the jaw: a review of the literature with emphasis on therapy options. *Oral Surg Oral Med Oral Pathol Oral Radiol Endod* 2007;104:603–615.
58. Mighell AJ, Robinson PA, Hume WJ. Peripheral giant cell granuloma: a clinical study of 77 cases from 62 patients, and literature review. *Oral Dis* 1995;1:12–19.
59. Lietman SA, Yin LG, Levine MA. SH3BP2 mutations potentiate osteoclastogenesis via PLC-gamma. *J Orthop Res* 2010;28:1425–1430.
60. Gundewar S, Kothari DS, Mokal NJ, et al. Osteomas of the craniofacial region: a case series and review of literature. *Indian J Plast Surg* 2013;46(3):479–485. doi: 10.4103/0970-0358.121982
61. Halawi AM, Maley JE, Robinson RA, et al. Craniofacial osteoma: clinical presentation and patterns of growth. *Am J Rhinol Allergy* 2013;27(2):128–133. doi: 10.2500/ajra.2013.27.3840
62. Herford AS, Stoffella E, Tandon R. Osteomas involving the facial skeleton: a report of 2 cases and review of the literature. *Oral Surg Oral Med Oral Pathol Oral Radiol* 2013;115(2):e1–e6. doi: 10.1016/j.oooo.2011.09.033
63. Nah KS. Osteomas of the craniofacial region. *Imaging Sci Dent* 2011;41(3):107–113. doi: 10.5624/isd.2011.41.3.107
64. McHugh JB, Mukherji SK, Lucas DR. Sino-orbital osteoma: a clinicopathologic study of 45 surgically treated cases with emphasis on tumors with osteoblastoma like features. *Arch Pathol Lab Med* 2009;133(10):1587–1593. doi: 10.1043/1543-2165-133.10.1587
65. Larrea-Oyarbide N, Valmaseda-Castellón E, Berini-Aytés L, et al. Osteomas of the craniofacial region. Review of 106 cases. *J Oral Pathol Med* 2008;37(1):38–42.
66. Perry KS, Tkaczuk AT, Caccamese JF Jr, et al. Tumors of the pediatric maxillofacial skeleton: a 20-year clinical study. *JAMA Otolaryngol Head Neck Surg* 2015;141(1):40–44. doi: 10.1001/jamaoto.2014.2895
67. Ojo MA, Omoregie OF, Altini M, et al. A clinico-pathologic review of 56 cases of ossifying fibroma of the jaws with emphasis on the histomorphologic variations. *Niger J Clin Pract* 2014;17(5):619–623. doi: 10.4103/1119-3077.141429
68. Ranganath K, Kamath SM, Munoyath SK, et al. Juvenile psammomatoid ossifying fibroma of maxillary sinus: case report with review of literature. *J Maxillofac Oral Surg* 2014;13(2):109–114. doi: 10.1007/s12663-013-0479-6 [review].
69. Phattarataratip E, Pholjaroen C, Tiranon P. A clinicopathologic analysis of 207 cases of benign fibro-osseous lesions of the jaws. *Int J Surg Pathol* 2013;22(4):326–333.
70. Slootweg PJ. Juvenile trabecular ossifying fibroma: an update. *Virchows Arch* 2012;461(6):699–703. doi: 10.1007/s00428-012-1329-5
71. Urs AB, Kumar P, Arora S, et al. Clinicopathologic and radiologic correlation of ossifying fibroma and juvenile ossifying fibroma—an institutional study of 22 cases. *Ann Diagn Pathol* 2013;17(2):198–203. doi: 10.1016/j.anndiagpath.2012.06.003
72. Malathi N, Radhika T, Thamizhchelvan H, et al. Psammomatoid juvenile ossifying fibroma of the jaws. *J Oral Maxillofac Pathol* 2011;15(3):326–329. doi: 10.4103/0973-029X.86710
73. Sarode SC, Sarode GS, Waknis P, et al. Juvenile psammomatoid ossifying fibroma: a review. *Oral Oncol* 2011;47(12):1110–1116. doi: 10.1016/j.oraloncology.2011.06.513 [review].
74. Mergoni G, Meleti M, Magnolo S, et al. Peripheral ossifying fibroma: a clinicopathologic study of 27 cases and review of the literature with emphasis on histomorphologic features. *J Indian Soc Periodontol* 2015;19(1):83–87. doi: 10.4103/0972-124X.145813
75. Hotwani K. A pediatric viewpoint on peripheral ossifying fibroma: a case report. *Gen Dent* 2015;63(2):e6–e8.
76. de Matos FR, Benevenuto TG, Nonaka CF, et al. Retrospective analysis of the histopathologic features of 288 cases of reactional lesions in gingiva and alveolar mucosa. *Appl Immunohistochem Mol Morphol* 2014;22(7):505–510. doi: 10.1097/PAI.0b013e31829ea1c5
77. Verma E, Chakki AB, Nagaral SC, et al. Peripheral cemento-ossifying fibroma: case series literature review. *Case Rep Dent* 2013;2013:930870. doi: 10.1155/2013/930870. Erratum in: *Case Rep Dent* 2013;2013:827247.
78. Hunasgi S, Raghunath V. A clinicopathological study of ossifying fibromas and comparison between central and peripheral ossifying fibromas. *J Contemp Dent Pract* 2012;13(4):509–514.
79. Mishra MB, Bhishen KA, Mishra S. Peripheral ossifying fibroma. *J Oral Maxillofac Pathol* 2011;15(1):65–68. doi: 10.4103/0973-029X.80023
80. Arya AN, Saravanan B, Subalakshmi K, et al. Aggressive fibromatosis of the mandible in a two-month old infant. *J Maxillofac Oral Surg* 2015;14(Suppl 1):235–239. doi: 10.1007/s12663-012-0460-9
81. Flucke U, Tops BB, van Diest PJ, et al. Desmoid-type fibromatosis of the head and neck region in the paediatric population: a clinicopathological and genetic study of seven cases. *Histopathology* 2014;64(6):769–776. doi: 10.1111/his.12323
82. Nedopil A, Raab P, Rudert M. Desmoplastic fibroma: a case report with three years of clinical and radiographic observation and review of the literature. *Open Orthop J* 2013;8:40–46. doi: 10.2174/1874325001307010040
83. Averna R, De Filippo M, Ferrari S, et al. Desmoplastic fibroma of the mandible. *Acta Biomed* 2011;82(1):69–73.
84. Said-Al-Naief N, Fernandes R, Louis P, et al. Desmoplastic fibroma of the jaw: a case report and review of literature. *Oral Surg Oral Med Oral Pathol Oral Radiol Endod* 2006;101(1):82–94 [review].
85. Gupta R, Gupta R, Kumar S, et al. Melanotic neuroectodermal tumor of infancy: review of literature, report of a case and follow up at 7 years. *J Plast Reconstr Aesthet Surg* 2015;68(3):e53–e54. doi: 10.1016/j.bjps.2014.12.014 [review].
86. Chaudhary S, Manuja N, Ravishankar CT, et al. Oral melanotic neuroectodermal tumor of infancy. *J Indian Soc Pedod Prev Dent* 2014;32(1):71–73. doi: 10.4103/0970-4388.127064
87. Reddy ER, Kumar MS, Aduri R, et al. Melanotic neuroectodermal tumor of infancy: a rare case report. *Contemp Clin Dent* 2013;4(4):559–562. doi: 10.4103/0976-237X.123091
88. Majumdar K, Batra VV, Tyagi I, et al. Embryonal tumor with abundant neuropil and true rosettes with melanotic (retinal) differentiation. *Fetal Pediatr Pathol* 2013;32(6):429–436. doi: 10.3109/15513815.2013.799250
89. Bangi BB, Tejasvi ML. Melanotic neuroectodermal tumor of infancy: a rare case report with differential diagnosis and review of the literature. *Contemp Clin Dent* 2012;3(1):108–112. doi: 10.4103/0976-237X.94559
90. Mendis BR, Lombardi T, Tilakaratne WM. Melanotic neuroectodermal tumor of infancy: a histopathological and immunohistochemical study. *J Investig Clin Dent* 2012;3(1):68–71. doi: 10.1111/j.2041-1626.2011.0086.x
91. Rustagi A, Roychoudhury A, Karak AK. Melanotic neuroectodermal tumor of infancy of the maxilla: a case report with review of literature. *J Oral Maxillofac Surg* 2011;69(4):1120–1124. doi: 10.1016/j.joms.2010.01.017 [review].
92. Chaudhary A, Wakhlu A, Mittal N, et al. Melanotic neuroectodermal tumor of infancy: 2 decades of clinical experience with 18 patients. *J Oral Maxillofac Surg* 2009;67(1):47–51. doi: 10.1016/j.joms.2007.04.027
93. Slootweg PJ. Lesions of the jaws. *Histopathology* 2009;54(4):401–418. doi: 10.1111/j.1365-2559.2008.03097.x [review].
94. Fowler DJ, Chisholm J, Roebuck D, et al. Melanotic neuroectodermal tumor of infancy: clinical, radiological, and pathological features. *Fetal Pediatr Pathol* 2006;25(2):59–72.
95. Kruse-Lösler B, Gaertner C, Bürger H, et al. Melanotic neuroectodermal tumor of infancy: systematic review of the literature and presentation of a case. *Oral Surg Oral Med Oral Pathol Oral Radiol Endod* 2006;102(2):204–216 [review].
96. Tajudeen BA, Arshi A, Suh JD, et al. Esthesioneuroblastoma: an update on the UCLA experience, 2002–2013. *J Neurol Surg B Skull Base* 2015;76(1):43–49. doi: 10.1055/s-0034-1390011
97. Tajudeen BA, Arshi A, Suh JD, et al. Importance of tumor grade in esthesioneuroblastoma survival: a population-based analysis. *JAMA Otolaryngol Head Neck Surg* 2014;140(12):1124–1129. doi: 10.1001/jamaoto.2014.2541
98. König MS, Osnes T, Meling TR. Treatment of esthesioneuroblastomas. *Neurochirurgie* 2014;60(4):151–157. doi: 10.1016/j.neuchi.2014.03.007
99. Bell D, Saade R, Roberts D, et al. Prognostic utility of Hyams histological grading and Kadish-Morita staging systems for esthesioneuroblastoma

100. El Kababri M, Habrand JL, Valteau-Couanet D, et al. Esthesioneuroblastoma in children and adolescent: experience on 11 cases with literature review. *J Pediatr Hematol Oncol* 2014;36(2):91–95. doi: 10.1097/MPH.0000000000000095
101. Rimmer J, Lund VJ, Beale T, et al. Olfactory neuroblastoma: a 35-year experience and suggested follow-up protocol. *Laryngoscope* 2014;124(7):1542–1549. doi: 10.1002/lary.24562
102. Kaur G, Kane AJ, Sughrue ME, et al. The prognostic implications of Hyam's subtype for patients with Kadish stage C esthesioneuroblastoma. *J Clin Neurosci* 2013;20(2):281–286. doi: 10.1016/j.jocn.2012.05.029
103. Ow TJ, Bell D, Kupferman ME, et al. Esthesioneuroblastoma. *Neurosurg Clin N Am* 2013;24(1):51–65. doi: 10.1016/j.nec.2012.08.005 [review].
104. Bak M, Wein RO. Esthesioneuroblastoma: a contemporary review of diagnosis and management. *Hematol Oncol Clin North Am* 2012;26(6):1185–1207. doi: 10.1016/j.hoc.2012.08.005 [review].
105. Kondo N, Takahashi H, Nii Y, et al. Olfactory neuroblastoma: 15 years of experience. *Anticancer Res* 2012;32(5):1697–1703.
106. Fukushima S, Sugita Y, Niino D, et al. Clinicopathological analysis of olfactory neuroblastoma. *Brain Tumor Pathol* 2012;29(4):207–215. doi: 10.1007/s10014-012-0083-3
107. Carlson ER. Diagnosis and management of salivary lesions of the neck. *Atlas Oral Maxillofac Surg Clin North Am* 2015;23(1):49–61. doi: 10.1016/j.cxom.2014.10.005 [review].
108. More CB, Bhavsar K, Varma S, et al. Oral mucocele: a clinical and histo-pathological study. *J Oral Maxillofac Pathol* 2014;18(Suppl 1):S72–S77. doi: 10.4103/0973-029X.141370
109. Khandelwal S, Patil S. Oral mucoceles—review of the literature. *Minerva Stomatol* 2012;61(3):91–99 [review].
110. Martins-Filho PR, Santos Tde S, da Silva HF, et al. A clinicopathologic review of 138 cases of mucoceles in a pediatric population. *Quintessence Int* 2011;42(8):679–685.
111. Mandel L. Salivary gland disorders. *Med Clin North Am* 2014;98(6):1407–1449. doi: 10.1016/j.mcna.2014.08.008 [review].
112. Luciano N, Valentini V, Calabrò A, et al. One year in review 2015: Sjögren's syndrome. *Clin Exp Rheumatol* 2015;33(2):259–271 [review].
113. Llamas-Gutierrez FJ, Reyes E, Martínez B, et al. Histopathological environment besides the focus score in Sjögren's syndrome. *Int J Rheum Dis* 2014;17(8):898–903. doi: 10.1111/1756-185X.12502
114. Lida Santiago M, Seisdedos MR, García Salinas RN, et al. Frequency of complications and usefulness of the minor salivary gland biopsy. *Reumatol Clin* 2012;8(5):255–258.
115. Haldorsen K, Moen K, Jacobsen H, et al. Exocrine function in primary Sjögren syndrome: natural course and prognostic factors. *Ann Rheum Dis* 2008;67(7):949–954 [review].
116. Ito FA, Jorge J, Vargas PA, et al. Histopathological findings of pleomorphic adenomas of the salivary glands. *Med Oral Patol Oral Cir Bucal* 2009;14:E57–E61.
117. da Cruz Perez DE, Pires FR, Alves FA, et al. Salivary gland tumors in children and adolescents: a clinicopathologic and immunohistochemical study of fifty-three cases. *Int J Pediatr Otorhinolaryngol* 2004;68:895–902.
118. Eveson JW, Cawson RA. Salivary gland tumours. A review of 2410 cases with particular reference to histological types, site, age and sex distribution. *J Pathol* 1985;146:51–58.
119. Eveson JW, Cawson RA. Tumours of the minor (oropharyngeal) salivary glands: a demographic study of 336 cases. *J Oral Pathol* 1985;14:500–509.
120. Sultan I, Rodriguez-Galindo C, Al-Sharabati S, et al. Salivary gland carcinomas in children and adolescents: a population-based study, with comparison to adult cases. *Head Neck* 2011;33:1476–1481.
121. Guzzo M, Ferrari A, Marcon I, et al. Salivary gland neoplasms in children: the experience of the Instituto Nazionale Tumori of Milan. *Pediatr Blood Cancer* 2006;47:806–810.
122. Guzzo M, Andreola S, Sirizzotti G, et al. Mucoepidermoid carcinoma of the salivary glands: clinicopathologic review of 108 patients treated at the National Cancer Institute of Milan. *Ann Surg Oncol* 2002;9:688–695.
123. Bai S, Clubwala R, Adler E, et al. Salivary mucoepidermoid carcinoma: a multi-institutional review of 76 patients. *Head Neck Pathol* 2013;7:105–112.
124. Brandwein MS, Ivanov K, Wallace DI, et al. Mucoepidermoid carcinoma: a clinicopathologic study of 80 patients with special reference to histological grading. *Am J Surg Pathol* 2001;25:835–845.
125. Goode RK, Auclair PL, Ellis GL. Mucoepidermoid carcinoma of the major salivary glands: clinical and histopathologic analysis of 234 cases with evaluation of grading criteria. *Cancer* 1998;82:1217–1224.
126. Auclair PL, Goode RK, Ellis GL. Mucoepidermoid carcinoma of intra-oral salivary glands. Evaluation and application of grading criteria in 143 cases. *Cancer* 1992;69:2021–2030.
127. Okumura Y, Miyabe S, Nakayama T, et al. Impact of CRTC1/3-MAML2 fusions on histological classification and prognosis of mucoepidermoid carcinoma. *Histopathology* 2011;59:90–97.
128. Al-Zaher N, Obeid A, Al-Salam S, et al. Acinic cell carcinoma of the salivary glands: a literature review. *Hematol Oncol Stem Cell Ther* 2009;2:259–264.
129. Munteanu MC, Mărgăritescu C, Cionca L, et al. Acinic cell carcinoma of the salivary glands: a retrospective clinicopathologic study of 12 cases. *Rom J Morphol Embryol* 2012;53:313–320.
130. Schwarz S, Zenk J, Müller M, et al. The many faces of acinic cell carcinomas of the salivary glands: a study of 40 cases relating histological and immunohistological subtypes to clinical parameters and prognosis. *Histopathology* 2012;61:395–408.
131. Cha W, Kim MS, Ahn JC, et al. Clinical analysis of acinic cell carcinoma in parotid gland. *Clin Exp Otorhinolaryngol* 2011;4:188–192.
132. Thompson LD. Salivary gland acinic cell carcinoma. *Ear Nose Throat J* 2010;89:530–532.
133. Seethala RR. Histologic grading and prognostic biomarkers in salivary gland carcinomas. *Adv Anat Pathol* 2011;18:29–45.
134. Brown MM, Walsh EJ, Shetty A, et al. Sialoblastoma: an unexpected diagnosis. *J Am Acad Dermatol* 2012;67:e276–e277.
135. Kattoor J, Baisakh MR, Mathew A, et al. Sialoblastoma: a rare salivary gland neoplasm. *Indian J Cancer* 2010;47:219–220.
136. Ellis GL. What's new in the AFIP fascicle on salivary gland tumors: a few highlights from the 4th Series Atlas. *Head Neck Pathol* 2009;3:225–230.
137. Saffari Y, Blei F, Warren SM, et al. Congenital minor salivary gland sialoblastoma: a case report and review of the literature. *Fetal Pediatr Pathol* 2011;30(1):32–39.
138. Vidyadhar M, Amanda C, Thuan Q, et al. Sialoblastoma. *J Pediatr Surg* 2008;43:e11–e13.
139. Williams SB, Ellis GL, Warnock GR. Sialoblastoma: a clinicopathologic and immunohistochemical study of 7 cases. *Ann Diagn Pathol* 2006;10:320–326.
140. Verret DJ, Galindo RL, DeFatta RJ, et al. Sialoblastoma: a rare submandibular gland neoplasm. *Ear Nose Throat J* 2006;85:440–442.
141. Tatlidede S, Karsidag S, Ugurlu K, et al. Sialoblastoma: a congenital epithelial tumor of the salivary gland. *J Pediatr Surg* 2006;41:1322–1325.
142. Brandwein M, Al-Naeif NS, Manwani D, et al. Sialoblastoma: clinicopathological/immunohistochemical study. *Am J Surg Pathol* 1999;23:342–348.
143. Batsakis JG, Frankenthaler R. Embryoma (sialoblastoma) of salivary glands. *Ann Otol Rhinol Laryngol* 1992;101:958–960.
144. Hsueh C, Gonzalez-Crussi F. Sialoblastoma: a case report and review of the literature on congenital epithelial tumors of salivary gland origin. *Pediatr Pathol* 1992;12:205–214. Erratum in: *Pediatr Pathol* 1992;12:631.
145. Taylor GP. Congenital epithelial tumor of the parotid-sialoblastoma. *Pediatr Pathol* 1988;8:447–452.
146. Johnson NR, Gannon OM, Savage NW, et al. Frequency of odontogenic cysts and tumors: a systematic review. *J Investig Clin Dent* 2014;5(1):9–14. doi: 10.1111/jicd.12044 [review].
147. Al Sheddi MA. Odontogenic cysts. A clinicopathological study. *Saudi Med J* 2012;33(3):304–308 [review].

148. Wali GG, Sridhar V, Shyla HN. A study on dentigerous cystic changes with radiographically normal impacted mandibular third molars. *J Maxillofac Oral Surg* 2012;11(4):458–465. doi: 10.1007/s12663-011-0252-7
149. Tegginamani AS, Prasad R. Histopathologic evaluation of follicular tissues associated with impacted lower third molars. *J Oral Maxillofac Pathol* 2013;17(1):41–44. doi: 10.4103/0973-029X.110713
150. Noffke CE, Chabikuli NJ, Nzima N. Impaired tooth eruption: a review. *SADJ* 2005;60(10):422, 424–425 [review].
151. Baykul T, Saglam AA, Aydin U, et al. Incidence of cystic changes in radiographically normal impacted lower third molar follicles. *Oral Surg Oral Med Oral Pathol Oral Radiol Endod* 2005;99(5):542–545.
152. Tarakji B, Baroudi K, Hanouneh S, et al. Possible recurrence of keratocyst in nevoid basal cell carcinoma syndrome: a review of literature. *Eur J Dent* 2013;7(Suppl 1):S126–S134. doi: 10.4103/1305-7456.119090 [review].
153. Cabay RJ. An overview of molecular and genetic alterations in selected benign odontogenic disorders. *Arch Pathol Lab Med* 2014;138(6):754–758. doi: 10.5858/arpa.2013-0057-SA [review].
154. Nayak MT, Singh A, Singhvi A, et al. Odontogenic keratocyst: what is in the name? *J Nat Sci Biol Med* 2013;4(2):282–285. doi: 10.4103/0976-9668.116968 [review].
155. Finkelstein MW, Hellstein JW, Lake KS, et al. Keratocystic odontogenic tumor: a retrospective analysis of genetic, immunohistochemical and therapeutic features. Proposal of a multicenter clinical survey tool. *Oral Surg Oral Med Oral Pathol Oral Radiol* 2013;116(1):75–83. doi: 10.1016/j.oooo.2013.03.018 [review].
156. Pogrel MA. The keratocystic odontogenic tumor. *Oral Maxillofac Surg Clin North Am* 2013;25(1):21–30, v. doi: 10.1016/j.coms.2012.11.003 [review].
157. Johnson NR, Batstone MD, Savage NW. Management and recurrence of keratocystic odontogenic tumor: a systematic review. *Oral Surg Oral Med Oral Pathol Oral Radiol* 2013;116(4):e271–e276. doi: 10.1016/j.oooo.2011.12.028 [review].
158. Jurisic M, Andric M, dos Santos JN, et al. Clinical, diagnostic and therapeutic features of keratocystic odontogenic tumors: a review. *J BUON* 2012;17(2):237–244 [review].
159. Kaczmarzyk T, Mojsa I, Stypulkowska J. A systematic review of the recurrence rate for keratocystic odontogenic tumour in relation to treatment modalities. *Int J Oral Maxillofac Surg* 2012;41(6):756–767. doi: 10.1016/j.ijom.2012.02.008 [review].
160. Bhargava D, Deshpande A, Pogrel MA. Keratocystic odontogenic tumour (KCOT)—a cyst to a tumour. *Oral Maxillofac Surg* 2012;16(2):163–170. doi: 10.1007/s10006-011-0302-9 [review].
161. Morgan PR. Odontogenic tumors: a review. *Periodontol 2000* 2011;57(1):160–176. doi: 10.1111/j.1600-0757.2011.00393.x [review].
162. Gomes CC, Diniz MG, Gomez RS. Review of the molecular pathogenesis of the odontogenic keratocyst. *Oral Oncol* 2009;45(12):1011–1014. doi: 10.1016/j.oraloncology.2009.08.003 [review].
163. Lo Muzio L. Nevoid basal cell carcinoma syndrome (Gorlin syndrome). *Orphanet J Rare Dis* 2008;3:32. doi: 10.1186/1750-1172-3-32 [review].
164. García CC, Sempere FV, Diago MP, et al. The post-endodontic periapical lesion: histologic and etiopathogenic aspects. *Med Oral Patol Oral Cir Bucal* 2007;12(8):E585–E590 [review].
165. Lin LM, Ricucci D, Lin J, et al. Nonsurgical root canal therapy of large cyst-like inflammatory periapical lesions and inflammatory apical cysts. *J Endod* 2009;35(5):607–615. doi: 10.1016/j.joen.2009.02.012 [review].
166. Lin LM, Huang GT, Rosenberg PA. Proliferation of epithelial cell rests, formation of apical cysts, and regression of apical cysts after periapical wound healing. *J Endod* 2007;33(8):908–916 [review].
167. Nair PN. On the causes of persistent apical periodontitis: a review. *Int Endod J* 2006;39(4):249–281 [review].
168. Chogle SM, Goodis HE, Kinaia BM. Pulpal and periradicular response to caries: current management and regenerative options. *Dent Clin North Am* 2012;56(3):521–536. doi: 10.1016/j.cden.2012.05.003 [review].
169. JOE Editorial Board. Periradicular lesions not of endodontic origin: an online study guide. *J Endod* 2008;34(5 Suppl):e205–e208. doi: 10.1016/j.joen.2007.12.010 [review].
170. Graunaite I, Lodiene G, Maciulskiene V. Pathogenesis of apical periodontitis: a literature review. *J Oral Maxillofac Res* 2012;2(4):e1. doi: 10.5037/jomr.2011.2401 [review].
171. Owosho AA, Potluri A, Bilodeau EA. Odontomas: a review of diagnosis, classification, and challenges. *Pa Dent J (Harrisb)* 2013;80(5):35–37 [review].
172. Kulkarni VK, Deshmukh J, Banda NR, et al. Odontomas—silent tormentors of teeth eruption, shedding and occlusion. *BMJ Case Rep* 2012;2012. doi: 10.1136/bcr-2012-007666 [review]. Retraction in: *BMJ Case Rep* 2013;2013. doi: 10.1136/bcr-2012-007666rp
173. Troeltzsch M, Liedtke J, Troeltzsch M, et al. Odontoma-associated tooth impaction: accurate diagnosis with simple methods? Case report and literature review. *J Oral Maxillofac Surg* 2012;70(10):e516–e520. doi: 10.1016/j.joms.2012.05.030 [review].
174. Soluk Tekkesin M, Pehlivan S, Olgac V, et al. Clinical and histopathological investigation of odontomas: review of the literature and presentation of 160 cases. *J Oral Maxillofac Surg* 2012;70(6):1358–1361. doi: 10.1016/j.joms.2011.05.024 [review].
175. Acton CH, Savage NW. Odontomes and their behaviour: a review. *Aust Dent J* 1987;32(6):430–435 [review].
176. Buchner A, Vered M. Ameloblastic fibroma: a stage in the development of a hamartomatous odontoma or a true neoplasm? Critical analysis of 162 previously reported cases plus 10 new cases. *Oral Surg Oral Med Oral Pathol Oral Radiol* 2013;116(5):598–606. doi: 10.1016/j.oooo.2013.06.039 [review].
177. Abughazaleh K, Andrus KM, Katsnelson A, et al. Peripheral ameloblastic fibroma of the maxilla: report of a case and review of the literature. *Oral Surg Oral Med Oral Pathol Oral Radiol Endod* 2008;105(5):e46–e48. doi: 10.1016/j.tripleo.2008.01.012 [review].
178. Chen Y, Wang JM, Li TJ. Ameloblastic fibroma: a review of published studies with special reference to its nature and biological behavior. *Oral Oncol* 2007;43(10):960–969 [review].
179. Takeda Y. Ameloblastic fibroma and related lesions: current pathologic concept. *Oral Oncol* 1999;35(6):535–540 [review].
180. Boxberger NR, Brannon RB, Fowler CB. Ameloblastic fibro-odontoma: a clinicopathologic study of 12 cases. *J Clin Pediatr Dent* 2011;35(4):397–403 [review].
181. Pontes HA, Pontes FS, Lameira AG, et al. Report of four cases of ameloblastic fibro-odontoma in mandible and discussion of the literature about the treatment. *J Craniomaxillofac Surg* 2012;40(2):e59–e63. doi: 10.1016/j.jcms.2011.03.020 [review].
182. De Riu G, Meloni SM, Contini M, et al. Ameloblastic fibro-odontoma. Case report and review of the literature. *J Craniomaxillofac Surg* 2010;38(2):141–144. doi: 10.1016/j.jcms.2009.04.009 [review].
183. Atwan S, Geist JR. Ameloblastic fibro-odontoma: case report and review of the literature. *J Mich Dent Assoc* 2008;90(11):46–49 [review].
184. Martín-Granizo-López R, López-García-Asenjo J, de-Pedro-Marina M, et al. Odontoameloblastoma: a case report and a review of the literature. *Med Oral* 2004;9(4):340–344 [review: English, Spanish].
185. Fregnani ER, Fillipi RZ, Oliveira CR, et al. Odontomas and ameloblastomas: variable prevalences around the world? *Oral Oncol* 2002;38(8):807–808 [review].
186. Mosqueda-Taylor A, Carlos-Bregni R, Ramírez-Amador V, et al. Odontoameloblastoma. Clinico-pathologic study of three cases and critical review of the literature. *Oral Oncol* 2002;38(8):800–805 [review].
187. Kaugars GE, Zussmann HW. Ameloblastic odontoma (odonto-ameloblastoma). *Oral Surg Oral Med Oral Pathol* 1991;71(3):371–373 [review].
188. Becker T, Buchner A, Kaffe I. Critical evaluation of the radiological and clinical features of adenomatoid odontogenic tumour. *Dentomaxillofac Radiol* 2012;41(7):533–540. doi: 10.1259/dmfr/19253953 [review].
189. Ide F, Mishima K, Kikuchi K, et al. Development and growth of adenomatoid odontogenic tumor related to formation and eruption of teeth. *Head Neck Pathol* 2011;5(2):123–132. doi: 10.1007/s12105-011-0253-3 [review].

190. Philipsen HP, Reichart PA, Zhang KH, et al. Adenomatoid odontogenic tumor: biologic profile based on 499 cases. *J Oral Pathol Med* 1991;20(4):149–158 [review].
191. Philipsen HP, Samman N, Ormiston IW, et al. Variants of the adenomatoid odontogenic tumor with a note on tumor origin. *J Oral Pathol Med* 1992;21(8):348–352 [review].
192. Kawase-Koga Y, Saijo H, Hoshi K, et al. Surgical management of odontogenic myxoma: a case report and review of the literature. *BMC Res Notes* 2014;7:214. doi: 10.1186/1756-0500-7-214 [review].
193. Kansy K, Juergens P, Krol Z, et al. Odontogenic myxoma: diagnostic and therapeutic challenges in paediatric and adult patients—a case series and review of the literature. *J Craniomaxillofac Surg* 2012;40(3):271–276. doi: 10.1016/j.jcms.2011.04.009 [review].
194. Gomes CC, Diniz MG, Duarte AP, et al. Molecular review of odontogenic myxoma. *Oral Oncol* 2011;47(5):325–328. doi: 10.1016/j.oraloncology.2011.03.006 [review].
195. Noffke CE, Raubenheimer EJ, Chabikuli NJ, et al. Odontogenic myxoma: review of the literature and report of 30 cases from South Africa. *Oral Surg Oral Med Oral Pathol Oral Radiol Endod* 2007;104(1):101–109 [review].
196. Rotenberg BW, Daniel SJ, Nish IA, et al. Myxomatous lesions of the maxilla in children: a case series and review of management. *Int J Pediatr Otorhinolaryngol* 2004;68(10):1251–1256 [review].
197. Barker BF. Odontogenic myxoma. *Semin Diagn Pathol* 1999;16(4):297–301 [review].
198. Kaffe I, Naor H, Buchner A. Clinical and radiological features of odontogenic myxoma of the jaws. *Dentomaxillofac Radiol* 1997;26(5):299–303 [review].
199. Suarez PA, Batsakis JG, El-Naggar AK. Don't confuse dental soft tissues with odontogenic tumors. *Ann Otol Rhinol Laryngol* 1996;105(6):490–494 [review].
200. Hasegawa T, Imai Y, Takeda D, et al. Retrospective study of ameloblastoma: the possibility of conservative treatment. *Kobe J Med Sci* 2013;59(4):E112–E121.
201. Suma MS, Sundaresh KJ, Shruthy R, et al. Ameloblastoma: an aggressive lesion of the mandible. *BMJ Case Rep* 2013;2013:200483. doi: 10.1136/bcr-2013-200483
202. Seintou A, Martinelli-Kläy CP, Lombardi T. Unicystic ameloblastoma in children: systematic review of clinicopathological features and treatment outcomes. *Int J Oral Maxillofac Surg* 2014;43(4):405–412. doi: 10.1016/j.ijom.2014.01.003 [review].
203. Bansal S, Desai RS, Shirsat P, et al. The occurrence and pattern of ameloblastoma in children and adolescents: an Indian institutional study of 41 years and review of the literature. *Int J Oral Maxillofac Surg* 2015;44(6):725–731. doi: 10.1016/j.ijom.2015.01.002
204. Dhanuthai K, Chantarangsu S, Rojanawatsirivej S, et al. Ameloblastoma: a multicentric study. *Oral Surg Oral Med Oral Pathol Oral Radiol* 2012;113(6):782–788. doi: 10.1016/j.oooo.2012.01.011
205. Castro-Silva II, Israel MS, Lima GS, et al. Difficulties in the diagnosis of plexiform ameloblastoma. *Oral Maxillofac Surg* 2012;16(1):115–118. doi: 10.1007/s10006-011-0265-x
206. Singh T, Wiesenfeld D, Clement J, et al. Ameloblastoma: demographic data and treatment outcomes from Melbourne, Australia. *Aust Dent J* 2015;60(1):24–29. doi: 10.1111/adj.12244
207. Hertog D, Bloemena E, Aartman IH, et al. Histopathology of ameloblastoma of the jaws; some critical observations based on a 40 years single institution experience. *Med Oral Patol Oral Cir Bucal* 2012;17(1):e76–e82.
208. Chaudhary Z, Krishnan S, Sharma P, et al. A review of literature on ameloblastoma in children and adolescents and a rare case report of ameloblastoma in a 3-year-old child. *Craniomaxillofac Trauma Reconstr* 2012;5(3):161–168. doi: 10.1055/s-0032-1313358
209. Zhang J, Gu Z, Jiang L, et al. Ameloblastoma in children and adolescents. *Br J Oral Maxillofac Surg* 2010;48(7):549–554. doi:10.1016/j.bjoms.2009.08.020 [review].
210. Gomes CC, Duarte AP, Diniz MG, et al. Review article: current concepts of ameloblastoma pathogenesis. *J Oral Pathol Med* 2010;39(8):585–591. doi: 10.1111/j.1600-0714.2010.00908.x
211. Krishnapillai R, Angadi PV. A clinical, radiographic, and histologic review of 73 cases of ameloblastoma in an Indian population. *Quintessence Int* 2010;41(5):e90–e100.
212. Andrade NN, Shetye SP, Mhatre TS. Trends in pediatric ameloblastoma and its management: a 15 year Indian experience. *J Maxillofac Oral Surg* 2013;12(1):60–67. doi: 10.1007/s12663-012-0387-1
213. Tamme T, Tiigimäe J, Leibur E. Mandibular ameloblastoma: a 28-years retrospective study of the surgical treatment results. *Minerva Stomatol* 2010;59(11–12):637–643.
214. Slater LJ. Diagnostic criteria for unicystic ameloblastoma: ameloblastic versus ameloblastomatous epithelium. *Oral Surg Oral Med Oral Pathol Oral Radiol Endod* 2011;111(5):536; author reply 536–538. doi: 10.1016/j.tripleo.2010.12.025
215. Bhat V, Bhandary SK, Bhat SP. Extraosseous ameloblastoma of maxillary gingiva—a case report. *Indian J Surg Oncol* 2014;5(3):211–213. doi: 10.1007/s13193-014-0328-1
216. Nonaka CF, de Oliveira PT, de Medeiros AM, et al. Peripheral ameloblastoma in the maxillary gingiva: a case report. *N Y State Dent J* 2013;79(1):37–40 [review].
217. Kato H, Ota Y, Sasaki M, et al. Peripheral ameloblastoma of the lower molar gingiva: a case report and immunohistochemical study. *Tokai J Exp Clin Med* 2012;37(2):30–34.
218. Beena VT, Choudhary K, Heera R, et al. Peripheral ameloblastoma: a case report and review of literature. *Case Rep Dent* 2012;2012:571509. doi: 10.1155/2012/571509
219. Isomura ET, Okura M, Ishimoto S, et al. Case report of extragingival peripheral ameloblastoma in buccal mucosa. *Oral Surg Oral Med Oral Pathol Oral Radiol Endod* 2009;108(4):577–579. doi: 10.1016/j.tripleo.2009.06.023. Erratum in: *Oral Surg Oral Med Oral Pathol Oral Radiol Endod* 2010;109(2):324. Yamada, Tomoaki [corrected to Yamada, Chiaki].
220. Vanoven BJ, Parker NP, Petruzzelli GJ. Peripheral ameloblastoma of the maxilla: a case report and literature review. *Am J Otolaryngol* 2008;29(5):357–360. doi: 10.1016/j.amjoto.2007.10.002 [review].
221. Pekiner FN, Ozbayrak S, Sener BC, et al. Peripheral ameloblastoma: a case report. *Dentomaxillofac Radiol* 2007;36(3):183–186.
222. Buchner A, Merrell PW, Carpenter WM. Relative frequency of peripheral odontogenic tumors: a study of 45 new cases and comparison with studies from the literature. *J Oral Pathol Med* 2006;35(7):385–391.
223. Kurppa KJ, Catón J, Morgan PR, et al. High frequency of BRAF V600E mutations in ameloblastoma. *J Pathol* 2014;232(5):492–498. doi: 10.1002/path.4317
224. da Rosa MR, Falcão AS, Fuzii HT, et al, EGFR signaling downstream of EGF regulates migration, invasion, and MMP secretion of immortalized cells derived from human ameloblastoma. *Tumour Biol* 2014;35(11):11107–11120. doi: 10.1007/s13277-014-2401-3
225. Fuchigami T, Kibe T, Koyama H, et al. Regulation of IL-6 and IL-8 production by reciprocal cell-to-cell interactions between tumor cells and stromal fibroblasts through IL-1α in ameloblastoma. *Biochem Biophys Res Commun* 2014;451(4):491–496. doi: 10.1016/j.bbrc.2014.07.137
226. Cecim RL, Carmo HA, Kataoka MS, et al. Expression of molecules related to AKT pathway as putative regulators of ameloblastoma local invasiveness. *J Oral Pathol Med* 2014;43(2):143–147. doi: 10.1111/jop.12103
227. Siar CH, Ng KH. Differential expression of transcription factors Snail, Slug, SIP1, and Twist in ameloblastoma. *J Oral Pathol Med* 2014;43(1):45–52. doi: 10.1111/jop.12065
228. Nakao Y, Mitsuyasu T, Kawano S, et al. Fibroblast growth factors 7 and 10 are involved in ameloblastoma proliferation via the mitogen-activated protein kinase pathway. *Int J Oncol* 2013;43(5):1377–1384. doi: 10.3892/ijo.2013.2081

CHAPTER 23

The Lymph Nodes, Spleen, and Thymus

Kamran M. Mirza, M.D., Ph.D., Choladda V. Curry, M.D., and Andrea N. Marcogliese, M.D.

LYMPH NODES

The lymph node is a remarkable structure that serves as (a) a meeting place for antigen, antigen-presenting cells, and naive B and T cells to initiate the adaptive immune response and (b) the site of clonal expansion and differentiation of effector B and T lymphocytes (1). These processes so essential to normal immune function also require a number of genetic events (DNA replication, class switching, somatic mutation, receptor editing, etc.) that, when deranged, lead to mutations and translocations that underlie most lymphomas (both Hodgkin and non-Hodgkin) (2).

Lymph Nodes (Normal Structure and Function)

The normal lymph node is a round or an ovoid encapsulated structure. It is usually small (2 to 3 mm) to modest (approximately 1 cm) in size, but it may attain dramatic dimensions if the lymph draining into it is particularly rich in immunogenic material. Macroscopically, normal or reactive lymph nodes are tan or creamy white in color, and the cut surface may be homogeneous or vaguely nodular (Figure 23-1). In reactive lymph nodes, the hilum may be visible on gross examination. Microscopically, three anatomic compartments can be recognized: cortex, paracortex, and medulla (3) (Figure 23-2). Residing in the cortex are the primary and/or secondary follicles, which are spherical collections of small and large B lymphocytes. The primary follicles are composed primarily of aggregates of small lymphocytes (naive B cells). The secondary follicles, formed through the process of antigen stimulation, are composed of germinal centers surrounded by mantle zones. The former is composed of a dark zone, consisting primarily of large B cells (centroblasts) and tingible body macrophages, where proliferation (clonal expansion) and somatic mutation occur, and an adjacent light zone, consisting primarily of small B cells (centrocytes), where selection of high-affinity B cells and differentiation to plasma cells (PC) and memory B cells occur (Figure 23-3). Although rich in B cells, the follicles also contain T helper cells and follicular dendritic cells. Surrounding the germinal center is a rim of uniformly sized small lymphocytes, known as the mantle, which is polarized toward the subcapsular sinus and blends imperceptibly into the cortex. Like the germinal center, the mantle is composed largely of B cells. The paracortex is a T-cell–rich zone, which contains a heterogeneous population of cells, including macrophages, interdigitating reticulum cells, scattered B cells, and abundant T cells in various stages of activation. High endothelial venules in this area serve as the site of entry for naive T cells and B cells. The medulla (not always evident in tissue sections as a discrete zone) is located in the central portion of the lymph node, composed of the medullary cords and medullary sinuses. The sinuses, endothelium-bounded spaces containing PCs, effector T cells, macrophages, and antigen-presenting cells, converge on the hilum from multiple points along the subcapsular sinus.

Clinical Significance of Lymphadenopathy in Children

Palpable lymphadenopathy is more common in children and adolescents than in adults. The most common cause of adenopathy in children is a benign lymphoid proliferation, and in many patients, some evidence of a self-limiting infectious or inflammatory process can be found to explain the enlarged nodes. The presence of certain clinical factors suggests that biopsy may disclose a condition requiring specific treatment, including fevers unresponsive to antibiotics, generalized adenopathy or massive localized adenopathy, mediastinal disease, weight loss, peripheral blood cytopenias, and elevated serum levels of lactate dehydrogenase. Slap et al. (4) defined three simple variables that identify lymph nodes that should be biopsied: (a) size greater than 2 cm in diameter, (b) abnormalities on chest x-ray, and (c) absence of symptoms of recent otolaryngologic disease in patients with cervical adenopathy. Soldes et al. (5) reported that the risk of malignancy in childhood peripheral lymphadenopathy increased with age and increasing size and number of locations of adenopathy. Other factors included supraclavicular location, an abnormal chest x-ray, and fixed nodes. A lymph node biopsy is warranted to exclude malignancy if there is

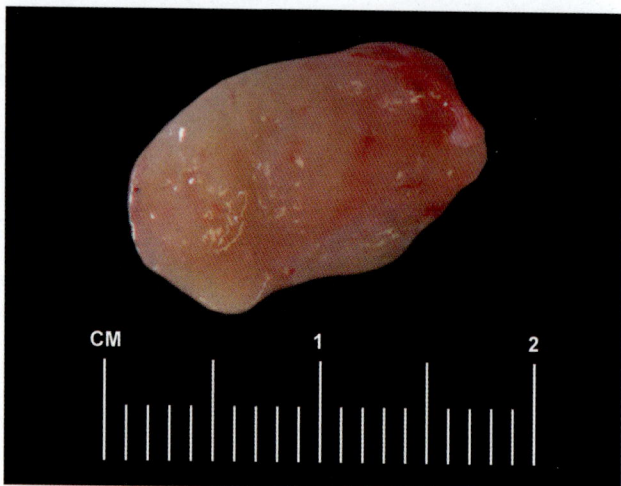

FIGURE 23-1 • Gross examination of a reactive lymph node in a child shows tan vaguely nodular cut surface.

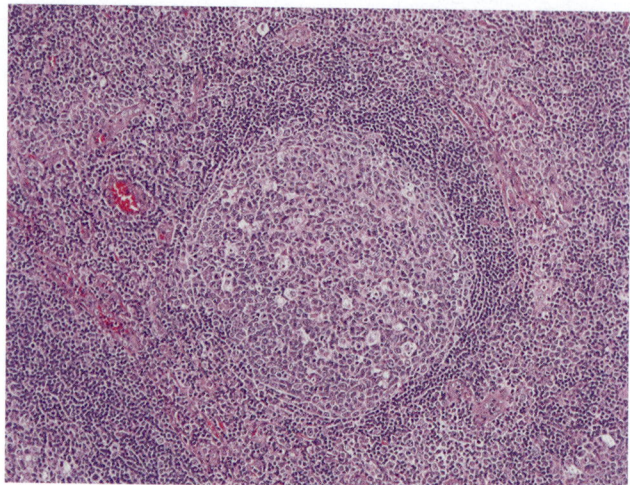

FIGURE 23-3 • The secondary follicles show a reactive germinal center, surrounded by a well-demarcated mantle zone. Polarization of the benign germinal center reflects the segregation of centrocytes to the light zone and mitotically active centroblasts to the dark zone. (Hematoxylin and eosin stain 10× magnification.)

no response to antibiotic therapy or a failure to regress after 6 weeks without identification of an infectious etiology (6).

Approach to Diagnosis in Patients with Lymphadenopathy

The availability of a broad array of new diagnostic techniques in hematopathology offers the opportunity for making faster diagnoses with more precision on smaller samples using less invasive procedures such as fine needle aspiration (FNA) cytology and core needle biopsy. The success of such efforts (if they are to be cost effective) depends in part on the quality of communication between hematologists and hematopathologists so that the most appropriate studies are ordered in a timely fashion.

In our practice, we examine touch preps or smears on biopsies or aspirates of lymph nodes immediately after staining (Table 23-1). Since the most common pediatric non-Hodgkin hematopoietic lymphoid neoplasms are recognizable as malignant on touch preps/smears (anaplastic large-cell lymphoma [ALCL], diffuse large B-cell lymphoma [DLBCL], Burkitt lymphoma, lymphoblastic lymphoma), these entities can be quickly triaged to flow cytometry and cytogenetic analysis. Similarly, most reactive proliferations, metastatic tumors, and Hodgkin lymphoma (HL) would not benefit from flow cytometry but may require cultures, cytogenetics, or other studies. This approach often allows the definitive diagnosis of many malignancies within hours and prevents substantial waste in resources.

Immunophenotypic Studies of Lymph Node Biopsy Specimens

Flow cytometry is an essential part of the diagnosis and classification of non-Hodgkin lymphoma (NHL) involving lymph nodes. The rapid availability of results (1 to 3 hours) allows triage to appropriate ancillary genetic studies while viable material is still available (7). In HL and in cases of NHL in which flow cytometry is not performed, the wide variety of antibody reagents that recognize most clinically relevant CD markers, which mark well in fixed tissue, allow immunohistochemical characterization of most hematopoietic lymphoid neoplasms (Table 23-2).

Cytogenetic Studies of Lymph Node Biopsy Specimens

For routine cytogenetic analysis, which is helpful in securing an accurate diagnosis in some cases, viable, fresh tissue must be taken by sterile technique at the time of biopsy and placed into culture so that metaphase spreads can be

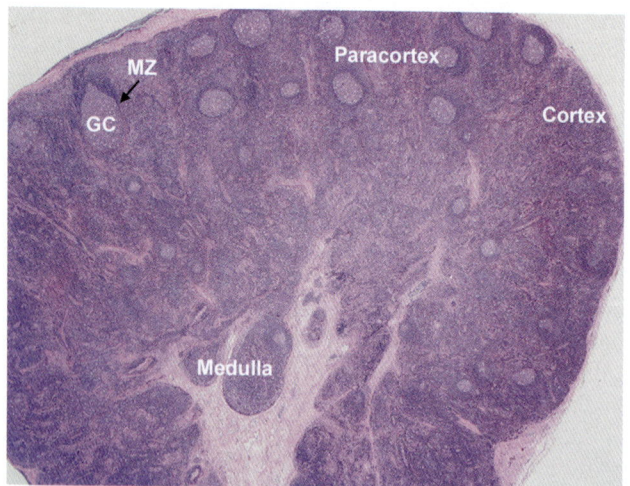

FIGURE 23-2 • The lymph node consists of three recognizable compartments: cortex (B-cell–rich zone), paracortex (T-cell–rich zone), and medulla. The secondary follicles located in the cortical areas show germinal center (GC) and well-demarcated mantle zone (MZ). (Hematoxylin and eosin stain 1.25× magnification.)

TABLE 23-1 APPROACH TO DIAGNOSIS AT THE TIME OF BIOPSY

Clinical input with likely diagnosis based on history and imaging studies
↓
Examination of biopsy touch preps or smears from FNA
↓

Numerous dyshesive atypical lymphoid cells (blasts, large cells, etc.)	Mixed population of small lymphocytes and only occasional or no large atypical lymphoid cells	Cohesive clumps of tumor cells suggestive of small blue cell tumor
↓	↓	↓
Flow cytometry, defer to histology	Consider cultures and decisions about immunohistochemistry for further diagnosis	Cytogenetics; Immunohistochemistry
↓		
Confirmation of neoplastic lymphoid phenotype		
↓		
Triage to cytogenetics and appropriate FISH studies based on phenotype		

TABLE 23-2 MARKERS USEFUL IN DIAGNOSIS OF HEMATOLYMPHOID NEOPLASMS

Cluster Designation/Antigen	Utility
General markers (not lineage specific)	
CD45 (LCA)	Leukocyte common antigen (+ in almost all NHL, negative/dim in most acute leukemias, negative in CHL and many ALCL)
TdT	Terminal deoxynucleotidyl transferase (+ >95% LBL, 20% AML, negative in all mature NHL)
CD34	Human progenitor cell antibody (50% of blasts in ALL/AML), endothelial cells
CD30	Activation marker, positive in CHL, ALCL, PMBCL
ALK	Positive in ALK+ ALCL and ALK+ DLBCL, negative in all other hematopoietic tumors
BCL2	Antiapoptotic protein, negative in normal germinal centers, positive in T-cells and mantle zone B cells; negative in BL and most pediatric FL, positive in subset of DLBCL
Ki-67 (MIB-1)	Proliferation marker, >95% positivity in BL
B-cell lineage markers	
CD10	CALLA; positive in germinal center B-cells (+ >95% B-ALL, 100% BL, 25%–80% of DLBCL)
CD19	Pan B-cell marker (present in all B-cell NHL including B-LBL)
CD20	Mature B-cell marker (present in DLBCL and BL, negative/dim in most B-LBL); + in NLPHL, variable positivity in CHL
CD22	Pan B-cell marker (present in all B-cell NHL including B-LBL)
PAX-5	B-cell transcription factor (present in all B-cell NHL including B-LBL), weak positivity in HRS cells
CD79a	Pan B-cell marker (present in all B-cell NHL including B-LBL)
CD23	Activated B cells; follicular dendritic cells, low-affinity FcR for IgE, + in most PMBCL
BCL6	Germinal center B-cells, + in BL and most DLBCL
T-/NK-cell lineage markers	
CD1a	Thymic T cells, Langerhans cells, T-LBL
CD2	T cells and NK cells; E-rosette receptor, + in some AML
CD3	T cells; TcR complex component NK cells (cytoplasm only)
CD4	Helper/suppressor T cells; MHC class II receptor, monocyte/macrophages, 60% of AML
CD5	Preferential T-cell marker, B-cell subset
CD7	T cells and NK cells; FcR for IgM, 25% of AML
CD8	Cytotoxic T cells and some NK cells; MHC class I receptor
CD16	NK cells, granulocytes; IgG FcR III
CD43	Pan T-cell marker, macrophages, monocytes blasts in AML, T-LBL and B-LBL

(Continued)

TABLE 23-2 MARKERS USEFUL IN DIAGNOSIS OF HEMATOLYMPHOID NEOPLASMS (continued)

Cluster Designation/Antigen	Utility
CD45RO	T cells, some macrophages
CD56	NK cells and cytotoxic T cells; N-CAM isoform, neuroendocrine tumors
CD57	Cytotoxic T cells and NK cells
Myeloid/monocytic/histiocytic markers	
CD1a	Immature T cells, Langerhans cells
CD15	Granulocytes, also positive in HRS cell in classic Hodgkin lymphoma
CD21	Follicular dendritic cells some B cells; C3d/EBV receptor
CD23	Follicular dendritic cells, mature B cells, macrophages low-affinity FcR for IgE
CD68 (KP-1)	Macrophages, monocytes, myeloid cells, blasts in AML
CD163	Macrophages, monocytes
S100	Langerhans cells, melanoma, other cell types; + in SHML
CD207	Langerin; positive on Langerhans cells
Myeloperoxidase	Positive in myeloid cells; useful to establish myeloid lineage in acute leukemias

ALCL, anaplastic large-cell lymphoma; AML, acute myeloid leukemia; BL, Burkitt lymphoma; B-LBL, B-cell lymphoblastic lymphoma; CALLA, common acute lymphoblastic leukemia antigen; CHL, classical Hodgkin lymphoma; EBV, Epstein-Barr virus; FcR, Fc receptor; MHC, major histocompatibility complex; NHL, non-Hodgkin lymphoma; NK, natural killer; PMBCL, primary mediastinal large B cell lymphoma; TcR, T-cell receptor; T-LBL, T lymphoblastic lymphoma.

generated. In the appropriate clinical setting, some karyotypic abnormalities may be pathognomonic for certain types of malignancies (Table 23-3) and can therefore be used for diagnostic/classification purposes (8,9). In other settings, especially precursor B-cell lymphoblastic lymphoma/leukemia, the results of cytogenetic studies can also be used for prognostic purposes (10). The most common karyotypic changes related to lymphoproliferative disorders in children

TABLE 23-3 KARYOTYPIC AND GENETIC CHANGES ASSOCIATED WITH NON-HODGKIN LYMPHOMA

Disease	Abnormality	Implicated Genes
B-cell LBL/B-cell ALL (see Chapter 24 on Bone Marrow for further discussion)	t(1;19)(q23;p13)	PBX-E2A
	t(4;11)(p21;q23)	AF4-MLL
	Hyperdiploidy (>50 chr)	
	Hyperdiploidy (47/50 chr)	
	Hypodiploidy	
	t(12;21)	ETV6-RUNX1
	t(5;14)	IL-3-IgH
	t(9;22)	BCR-ABL1
	iAMP21	
Diffuse large B-cell lymphoma	t(3q27;var)	BCL6
Burkitt lymphoma	t(2;8) (p11;q24)	IgL-lambda-myc
	t(8;14) (q24; q32)	c-myc-IgH
	t(8;22) (q24;q11)	c-myc-IgL-kappa
T-cell LBL/T-cell ALL	t(1;14-15)(p12;q11)	TAL1;TcR gamma
	t(1;14)(p32;p14-15)	TAL1;TcR delta
	t(1;7)(p32;q34)	TAL1;TcR beta
	t(10;11)(p13;q14)	CALM-AF10
	t(7;10)(q34;q24), t(10;14)(q24;q11)	HOX11
ALK+ anaplastic large-cell lymphoma	t(2;5)(p23;q35)	NPM-ALK, most cases of ALK+ ALCL
	t(2;var)	Variety of other partners described; all result in ALK positivity by IHC

ALL, acute lymphoblastic leukemia; IgH, immunoglobulin heavy chain; IgL, immunoglobulin light chain; LBL, lymphoblastic lymphoma; TcR, T-cell receptor, IHC, immunohistochemistry.

include translocations of immunoglobulin and T-cell receptor loci, which are frequently paired with loci involved in normal development and hematopoiesis (11,12). A major advance in diagnostic cytogenetics is the widespread availability of fluorescent in situ hybridization (FISH) studies for these translocations. Two major advantages of FISH techniques over routine cytogenetics are (a) rapid turnaround (<24 hours) and (b) ability to utilize fixed tissues including touch preparations, cytospin preparations, or sections of paraffin-embedded tissues (13,14).

Reactive Lymphadenopathy

The two major patterns of reactive lymphadenopathy are usually dominated either by follicular hyperplasia or by interfollicular expansion (immunoblastic, granulomatous, or histiocytic). Occasional reactive processes produce diffuse alteration of architecture and may mimic a lymphoma (Table 23-4). In practice, a single lymph node is constantly exposed to a diversity of immunogens and therefore exhibits more than one pattern of response; however, when the degree of adenopathy is sufficient to warrant a biopsy, a single pattern usually dominates. Additional factors that assist in the differential diagnosis include the age-specific nature of some disorders; certain reactive processes affecting lymph nodes are rare in children (e.g., luetic lymphadenitis, Kikuchi disease), whereas others affect them primarily (e.g., acute infectious mononucleosis, autoimmune lymphoproliferative disorder [ALPS]).

FOLLICULAR HYPERPLASIAS

Nonspecific Reactive Follicular Hyperplasia

Nonspecific reactive follicular hyperplasia is the most common pattern of reactive lymphadenopathy. The lymph node shows increased follicular density with variable sizes and shapes of follicles. The germinal centers show polarization and contain small, intermediate, and large mitotically active lymphocytes, tingible body macrophages, and apoptotic cells. Well-demarcated mantle zones surround germinal centers. The hyperplastic follicles tend to remain in the cortical regions, but in particularly robust cases, the paracortex and the medulla may be compressed by the process. Immunophenotypic studies show that the secondary follicles contain a predominance of $CD20^+$, $CD10^+$, $BCL6^+$ B cells that are negative for BCL2. Differential diagnostic considerations in children are few but include Castleman disease, HIV-related adenopathy, progressive transformation of germinal centers (PTGC), and rarely pediatric type follicular lymphoma (15).

HIV-Related Adenopathy

Most series treating the subject of HIV-related persistent generalized lymphadenopathy are based on a patient population of homosexual young adult men at risk for HIV (16,17). Reports of this condition in children at risk for HIV because of maternal–fetal transmission or hemophilia present similar data (18). A spectrum of histologic findings may be seen in this context, with two clearly recognizable extremes. Florid follicular hyperplasia, the earliest change of HIV-related persistent generalized lymphadenopathy, has many features in common with nonspecific follicular hyperplasia, although the germinal centers are larger and often serpiginous and tend to fuse with focal follicular lysis (Figure 23-4). Regressively transformed germinal centers typify late persistent generalized lymphadenopathy and are characterized by small size, lymphoid depletion, and numerous dendritic cells, vessels, and amorphous eosinophilic deposits (19). The mantle is absent or very poorly formed, and the paracortex is proportionally rich in histiocytes, PCs, and high endothelial venules because

TABLE 23-4 REACTIVE LYMPHADENOPATHY IN CHILDREN

Follicular Pattern
Nonspecific Reactive Follicular Hyperplasia
HIV
Progressive transformation of follicular centers
Toxoplasmosis
Castleman disease/angiofollicular hyperplasia
Interfollicular Pattern
Paracortical immunoblastic reactions
EBV
Hypersensitivity reactions (phenytoin)
Juvenile rheumatoid arthritis 1
Systemic lupus erythematosus 1,3
Kikuchi histiocytic necrotizing lymphadenitis 1,3
Autoimmune lymphoproliferative syndrome (ALPS) 1
Kawasaki disease
Granulomatous
Mycobacterial infection (MTB and atypical mycobacterial) 1,2
Cat-scratch disease 1,2,4
Fungal infection
Histiocytic
Sinus histiocytosis
Lysosomal storage disorders
Hemophagocytic syndromes (hemophagocytic lymphohistiocytosis)
Rosai-Dorfman
Dermatopathia
Langerhans cell histocytosis
Diffuse alteration of architecture
Sarcoidosis
Posttransplant lymphoproliferative disorder
Notations for other features
  1. Follicular hyperplasia
  2. Necrosis with neutrophils
  3. Necrosis with apoptosis
  4. Capsulitis

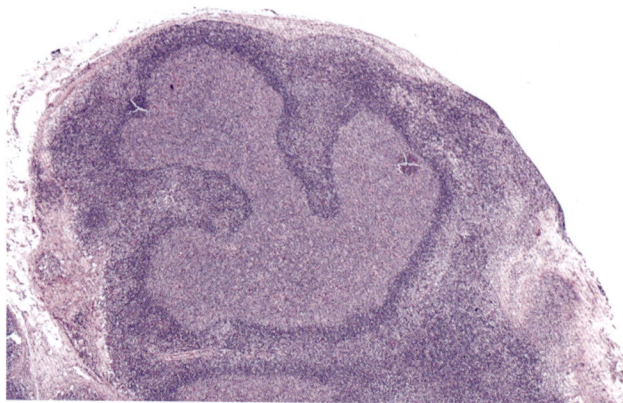

FIGURE 23-4 • Serpentine follicular center in a patient with HIV infection and persistent generalized lymph adenopathy. (Hematoxylin and eosin stain 4× magnification.)

of the paucity of lymphocytes. The morphologic features associated with persistent generalized lymphadenopathy (i.e., large and irregularly shaped follicles, follicular lysis, follicular involution) are distinctive but not specific for HIV infection, as they have been seen in 5% to 10% of otherwise entirely unremarkable lymph nodes obtained as part of carcinoma staging before the beginning of the AIDS era (20).

Progressive Transformation of Germinal Centers

For unknown reasons, when clinically significant lymphadenopathy develops in some patients, the biopsy specimen shows PTGC. Most patients are asymptomatic male adolescents or young adults with isolated inguinal or cervical adenopathy (21,22). The bulk of the lymph node, which can be up to 5 cm in size, exhibits florid reactive follicular hyperplasia with focal involvement by very large (three to five times the size of surrounding reactive follicles) nodules that are dramatically expanded by an influx of small lymphocytes (Figure 23-5) with mantle cell-like morphology and phenotype (IgM+, IgD+) (23,24). Relative to normal follicles, the transformed follicles exhibit a disrupted and dispersed dendritic cell network on CD21 or CD23 staining (21). Clusters of epithelioid histiocytes are more commonly identified in children than adults (22,25). The main malignant counterpart differential diagnosis is nodular lymphocyte–predominant Hodgkin lymphoma (NLPHL), which typically demonstrates neoplastic nodules replacing the entire lymph nodes, and the presence of neoplastic lymphocyte–predominant (LP) cells (also known as "popcorn" or "L&H" cells). Two studies of PTGC that focus on the pediatric population found that HL, particularly NLPHL, occasionally may precede, follow, or be concurrent with PTGC (22,25). Approximately one-third of patients will have recurrent PTGC (25), and approximately one-fourth have associated immune disorders including immune thrombocytopenia (ITP), lupus, Castleman disease, and ALPS (22).

Toxoplasmosis

Acute toxoplasmosis, an infectious disease, is often accompanied by lymphadenopathy. This is usually limited to the cervical lymph nodes, although occasionally patients with typical histology and serologic confirmation have isolated inguinal or axillary lymph node enlargement. Florid follicular hyperplasia dominates the histology at low power and is invariably accompanied by clusters of epithelioid histiocytes and patches of monocytoid B cells. The epithelioid histiocytic aggregates, randomly distributed throughout, abut and even infiltrate the germinal centers. The triad of florid follicular hyperplasia, monocytoid B-cell hyperplasia, and perifollicular and intrafollicular clusters of epithelioid histiocytic aggregates (variably encroaching on follicular centers) has a high degree of sensitivity and specificity for diagnosis of toxoplasmosis (Figure 23-6) (26,27).

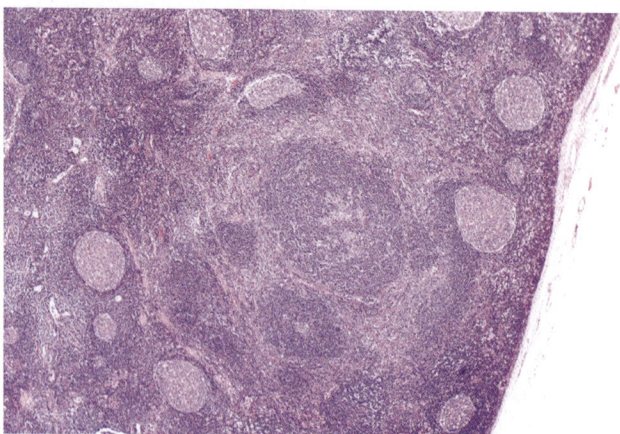

FIGURE 23-5 • Progressively transformed germinal center (with disrupted follicle infiltrated by small mantle zone lymphocytes) in a background of follicular hyperplasia. (Hematoxylin and eosin stain 4× magnification.)

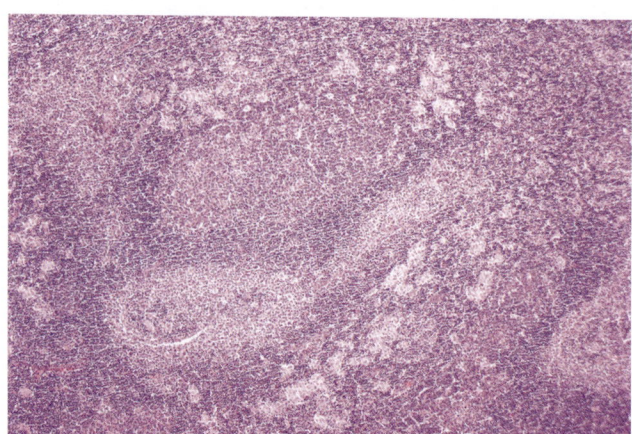

FIGURE 23-6 • Low power of toxoplasmosis demonstrating the triad of hyperplastic follicles, monocytoid B-cell proliferation, and histiocytic aggregates encroaching of follicles. (Hematoxylin and eosin stain 4× magnification.)

Castleman Disease

Castleman disease is a heterogenous group of diseases with variable clinical presentations and prognosis. The disease mainly affects adults and rarely occurs in children. Castleman disease has been previously classified based on histology into hyaline vascular (HV) type and PC type and based on clinical presentation into localized (unicentric) and multicentric (28). Human herpes virus-8 (HHV-8) has also been found to play a role in the pathogenesis of Castleman disease, and there has been a proposal to update the classification of Castleman disease to incorporate HHV-8 status (29). The entity has been recently reviewed by Talat et al. (30) In hyaline vascular Castleman disease (HV-CD), which is usually unicentric, there are increased small and involuted lymphoid follicles surrounded by broad mantle zones throughout the node ("bag of marbles") (Figure 23-7). The expanded mantle zones are composed of tightly packed small lymphocytes often in a laminated (orbiting) or "onion-skin" pattern; this feature together with radially penetrating hyalinized sclerotic blood vessels passing into the germinal centers creating "lollipop" appearance (Figure 23-8) is characteristic of the disease (28,29). The germinal centers appear atrophic and are depleted of lymphocytes and contain both extracellular matrix and abundant follicular dendritic cells. The interfollicular areas are highly vascular with hyalinization. Large clusters or sheets of PCs are not present. The plasma cell variant of Castleman disease (PC-CD), usually multicentric, is extremely rare in children (31–34). The majority of follicles in PC-CD appear reactive, but some may show a few with hyaline vascular–like follicles. Marked interfollicular plasmacytosis is present (28,29). Castleman disease in children has different characteristics than in adults. Pediatric Castleman disease is usually unicentric and has a more favorable course. HV-CD is also more common than PC-CD. Mesenteric location of unicentric CD is relatively more common in children than in adults, who

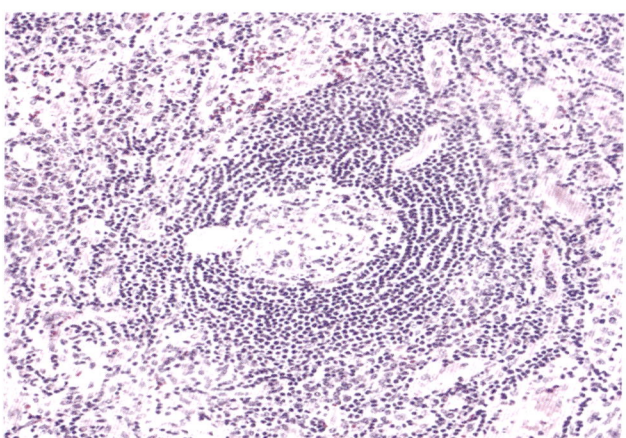

FIGURE 23-8 • The mantle zone has a laminated or "onion-skin" appearance in the hyaline vascular type of Castleman disease. Note the radially penetrating vessel. (Hematoxylin and eosin stain 10× magnification.)

usually have intrathoracic (mediastinal) localization. Head and neck location is also uncommon in children. Similar to adults, anemia and hypergammaglobulinemia are more often present in PC variant rather than the HV variant (32,33). HHV-8-associated CD typically occurs in immunosuppressed and/or HIV-positive adults and has rarely been reported in an immunosuppressed child related to a possible inborn error of immunity to HHV-8 (35).

INTERFOLLICULAR/PARACORTICAL REACTIONS: IMMUNOBLASTIC

Epstein-Barr Virus Infection (Infectious Mononucleosis)

Acute illness secondary to Epstein-Barr virus (EBV) infection (acute infectious mononucleosis) is common in young children and is usually self-limited. In those few cases that culminate in biopsy, the clinical features are often atypical—advanced age, the presence of "B" symptoms, a negative monospot test [uncommon except in very young children (<4 years) or early in infection], localized adenopathy or persistent adenopathy, hepatosplenomegaly, or splenic rupture. Patients with X-linked lymphoproliferative disorder (Duncan syndrome) present with rapidly progressive and usually fatal disease because of an inability to mount a successful immune response against EBV-infected cells.

At low power, the architecture is obscured but generally preserved with moth-eaten follicles and prominent paracortical expansion (Figure 23-9) by immunoblasts, PCs, and plasmacytoid lymphocytes (Figure 23-10). Similar large cells pack the sinusoids. Occasionally, large cells with bilobed or multilobed nuclei and prominent nucleoli are present, reminiscent of Hodgkin/Reed-Sternberg (HRS) cells. Histiocytes may be scattered singly or in small clusters, and increased numbers of capillaries and high endothelial venules also contribute to the polymorphic appearance of the paracortex.

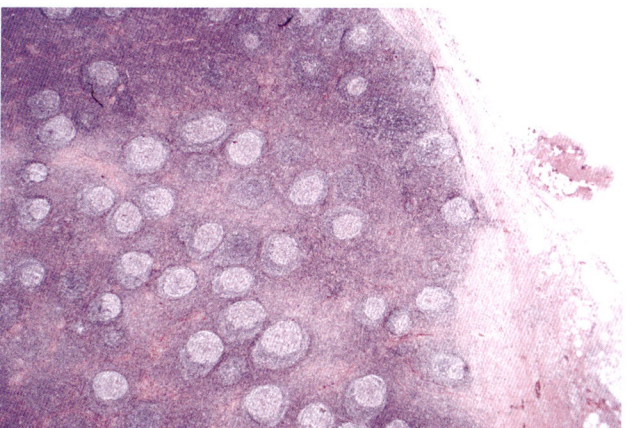

FIGURE 23-7 • Low power of hyaline vascular Castleman disease with "bag of marbles": small uniform follicles evenly dispersed throughout the cortex and the medulla. (Hematoxylin and eosin stain 4× magnification.)

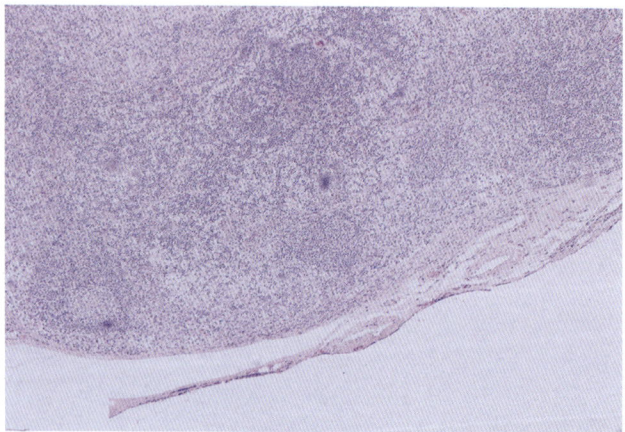

FIGURE 23-9 • The immunoblastic proliferation in acute infectious mononucleosis localizes to the paracortex and may compress or distort residual germinal centers. (Hematoxylin and eosin stain 4× magnification.)

Normal landmarks—germinal centers and subcapsular and paratrabecular sinuses—are generally present but may be compressed or distorted by the immunoblastic proliferation. In very early cases of EBV infection, monocytoid B-cell proliferation may be prominent (36). Staining with CD20 and CD3 highlights the presence of a mixture of interfollicular B and T immunoblasts, respectively, and a polytypic pattern of light-chain expression is always seen. The Reed-Sternberg–like cells are characteristically CD20+ and CD15− and show variable reactivity for the activation antigen CD30 as well as markers of EBV infection such as latent membrane protein (LMP1) or EBV-encoded RNA transcripts (EBER) (37). Difficult cases may exhibit sheet-like arrays of immunoblasts, a brisk mitotic rate, or extensive necrosis and may closely mimic large-cell lymphoma. In such cases, examination of the peripheral blood smear for atypical lymphocytes, viral serology, and immunohistochemistry to better define architectural preservation and establish the presence of EBV is helpful.

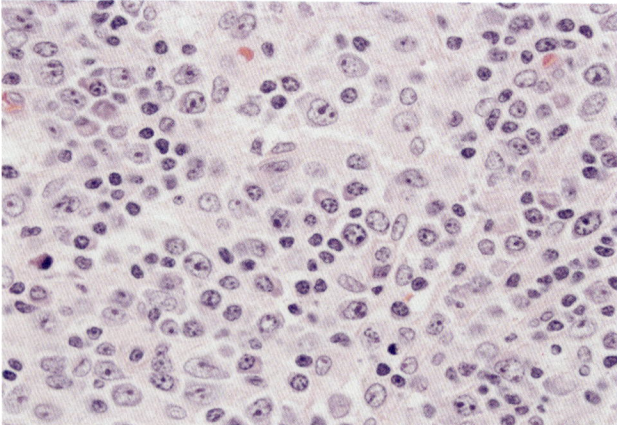

FIGURE 23-10 • Small, intermediate, and large cells fill the paracortex in acute infectious mononucleosis, often with a predominance of immunoblasts. (Hematoxylin and eosin stain 40× magnification.)

Non-EBV Viral Adenopathy

Lymphadenopathy may occur as a result of herpes simplex or cytomegalovirus infection and is seen most often in children with some form of immune deficiency. Paracortical hyperplasia with discrete foci of necrosis is the typical histologic finding in these cases. In comparison with acute EBV-related lymphadenopathy, the proportion of immunoblasts is less, and interfollicular areas are expanded by a mixture of mature lymphocytes, PCs, histiocytes, plasmacytoid monocytes, and fewer numbers of immunoblasts. Viral inclusions appearing as smudged (38) or hyperchromatic alterations of the nucleus (herpes simplex virus) or very large eosinophilic structures within the nucleus (cytomegalovirus) can be identified and may be most numerous adjacent to zones of necrosis. Immunohistochemistry is helpful in excluding neoplasia and can also document the presence of infected cells. Of note, the viral inclusions in the enlarged cells of cytomegalovirus lymphadenitis are CD15+, a potential pitfall in the exclusion of HL. Attention to clinical parameters will assist in discriminating viral lymphadenitis from other causes of necrotizing lymphadenitis, which include Kikuchi-Fujimoto disease and lupus erythematosus.

Hypersensitivity Reactions, Emphasizing Phenytoin (Dilantin) Reactions

Hypersensitivity-related lymphadenopathy is quite rare and has been associated most commonly with phenytoin (Dilantin) therapy and vaccines (small pox, measles, tetanus) but can be seen associated with a variety of drug classes. In phenytoin hypersensitivity, the architecture of the lymph node is distorted by a paracortical proliferation of immunoblasts, lymphocytes, PCs, and eosinophils. Germinal centers persist, and in some cases, a florid follicular hyperplasia may accompany the immunoblastic reaction. Rarely, a granulomatous lymphadenopathy secondary to phenytoin therapy has been reported (39). Purely diffuse architectural effacement is rare. The immunoblasts represent a mixture of CD20+ B cells and CD3+ T cells. Progression to lymphoma is well described. A similar pattern of paracortical expansion may be seen in T-cell lymphomas such as angioimmunoblastic T-cell lymphoma (40), which can be a major problem in differential diagnosis. A detailed history as well as immunophenotypic studies is usually helpful.

Juvenile-Onset Rheumatoid Arthritis Emphasizing Still Disease

Several different histologies have been described in juvenile rheumatoid arthritis (JRA), including the classic findings associated with adult RA of follicular hyperplasia, interfollicular PCs, and intrasinusoidal neutrophils. In Still disease, a pattern of paracortical immunoblastic proliferation mimicking lymphoma is occasionally described as well as interfollicular necrosis similar to that seen in Kikuchi-Fujimoto disease (41,42).

Systemic Lupus Erythematosus

Systemic lupus erythematosus (SLE) is an autoimmune disease that affects both adolescents and young adults. Lymphadenopathy is frequently observed in children with SLE and may occasionally be the presenting feature. When lymphadenopathy is part of the clinical picture, it is typically peripheral and multifocal or generalized (43). Classically, follicular hyperplasia with patchy paracortical necrosis dominates the low-power appearance of the lymph node. The germinal centers are well formed with a discrete mantle zone, and they are separated by an expanded paracortex in which pockets of necrosis are randomly distributed. The necrotic foci are composed of amorphous eosinophilic material and apoptotic debris. Neutrophils and PCs are scarce. In addition, "hematoxylin bodies" (round or oblong blue structures, 5 to 15 μm long, which stain with periodic acid–Schiff and the Feulgen method) and vascular encrustations (Azzopardi effect) may be present (44). Less commonly, necrosis dominates the morphology, and follicles may be few and more widely spaced; in these circumstances, the lymph node findings may resemble those of Kikuchi-Fujimoto disease. Other patterns described in SLE include follicular hyperplasia without necrosis resembling Castleman disease. SLE presenting with granulomatous changes has also been reported (45).

Histiocytic Necrotizing Lymphadenitis/ Kikuchi-Fujimoto Disease

Kikuchi-Fujimoto disease (histiocytic necrotizing lymphadenitis) is a self-limited regional lymphadenopathy with prolonged fever that is uncommon in children. The median age is in the third decade in most large series, although the age range is wide. Rare fatal cases in children have been reported, often associated hemophagocytic syndrome. Recurrent Kikuchi-Fujimoto disease has been reported in the pediatric population (46). Histologically, these nodes exhibit follicular hyperplasia, but the histologic hallmark of this disease is zonal karyorrhexis with scant neutrophil response. At low power, the paracortex is distorted by pale-staining patchy zones of necrotic debris with a cellular rim composed of apoptotic cells, histiocytes, small lymphocytes, plasmacytoid dendritic cells, and immunoblasts. The areas of necrosis may coalesce, but a serpiginous contour rarely develops. Beyond the necrotic zone is a mottled paracortex, rich in small lymphocytes, immunoblasts, apoptotic debris, plasmacytoid dendritic cells, and high endothelial venules (Figure 23-11). In children, the differential diagnostic considerations for the early proliferative lesions of histiocytic necrotizing lymphadenitis include NHL and mixed cellularity Hodgkin lymphoma (MCHL). Fully developed lesions may mimic Kawasaki disease or herpetic lymphadenitis, and lupus-related lymphadenitis may be difficult or even impossible to exclude. A third pattern is characterized by dominance of foamy histiocytes. Immunophenotypic characterization of the large cells at the periphery of karyorrhectic areas shows that they represent CD8+ T cells and

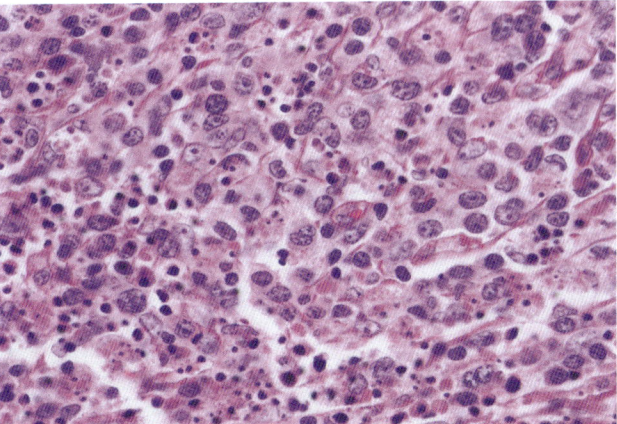

FIGURE 23-11 • The border of necrosis shows apoptotic debris admixed with histiocytes, small lymphocytes, plasmacytoid dendritic cells, and immunoblasts in Kikuchi disease. (Hematoxylin and eosin stain 40× magnification.)

plasmacytoid dendritic cells (47). One report suggests that the sparsity of CD8+ T cells in SLE may be helpful in differential diagnosis (48).

Autoimmune Lymphoproliferative Syndrome

Lymphadenopathy secondary to loss of Fas or Fas ligand-mediated apoptosis is a rare cause of nonneoplastic lymphadenopathy, known as *autoimmune lymphoproliferative disorder* (*ALPS*). Patients with ALPS present within the first 2 years of life with bulky generalized adenopathy and hepatosplenomegaly and chronic multilineage cytopenias due to autoimmune peripheral destruction or splenic sequestration and have an increased risk of B-cell lymphoma (49–51). Enlarged lymph nodes show generally intact architecture with follicles ranging from floridly hyperplastic to small involuting follicles with compressed mantle zones like those seen in HV-CD. The proliferation that occurs in the interfollicular areas consists of immunoblasts and transformed large cells with scant-to-moderate cytoplasm (52). Small lymphocytes, PCs, and histiocytes may be present. Some studies have found an overlap of histologic features with sinus histiocytosis with massive lymphadenopathy (SHML) (Rosai-Dorfman disease) (53) and sarcoidosis (54)

On flow cytometry, CD2+, CD3+, CD4−, CD8− T cells with an α-β T-cell receptor are increased ("double-negative T cells" or DNT), and increased DNT in the peripheral blood (>1% of T cells) is one of the diagnostic criteria. B cells are phenotypically normal. On tissue sections, the immunoblasts in the interfollicular zones are virtually all CD3+, double-negative T cells, with only a few showing reactivity for CD4, CD8, or CD20 (55). Peripheral T-cell lymphoma may mimic ALPS, but the former typically contains more small-to-intermediate cells and rarely has a CD4−, CD8− phenotype. Gene sequencing is necessary to confirm the diagnosis of ALPS, which may be caused by mutations in Fas, Fas ligand, or the caspase 10 gene (50,56).

Kawasaki Disease

Kawasaki disease is endemic in Japan but rare in Western countries. A slight male predominance has been noted, and the peak incidence is in children 3 to 4 years old. Histologic descriptions are quite variable, and lymph node biopsy seldom leads to a firm diagnosis of Kawasaki disease without correlation with clinical parameters. The main findings are patchy paracortical necrosis with phlebitis and fibrin microthrombi. Germinal centers are inconstantly present, as is an immunoblast-rich paracortical expansion. If perinodal tissues are present for review, an acute necrotizing arteritis similar to infantile polyarteritis nodosa may be identified even in early phases; in established cases, a measure of luminal dilation is also present in larger-caliber vessels, with medial destruction (see Chapter 13).

INTERFOLLICULAR GRANULOMATOUS PROCESSES

Cat-Scratch Disease

Cat-scratch disease frequently affects children and adolescents, although in large, population-based studies, nearly half of all patients have been over the age of 20 (57). The adenopathic phase of the disease is dominated by follicular hyperplasia, capsulitis, paracortical monocytoid B-cell hyperplasia, and small, neutrophil-rich microabscesses. As the lesions develop, the microabscesses coalesce, forming serpiginous and stellate zones of eosinophilic necrosis (Figure 23-12). In the late stage, the microabscesses take on a granulomatous appearance, with a well-formed rim of palisading histiocytes and scattered multinucleated giant cells (Figure 23-13). Warthin-Starry staining may highlight pleomorphic and bow-shaped rods and cocci, both in the center of the abscesses and around blood vessels in the early phases of disease. However, Warthin-Starry staining is technically difficult and often problematic to interpret. Additionally, patients may be seronegative. Therefore, PCR techniques that detect the organism in the tissue with a high degree of specificity are preferred for confirmation of diagnosis (58). Histologically, similar lesions may also be seen in Yersinia infection, lymphogranuloma venereum, tularemia, and infection with *Mycobacterium avium–intracellulare* (MAI) in young children (59–61).

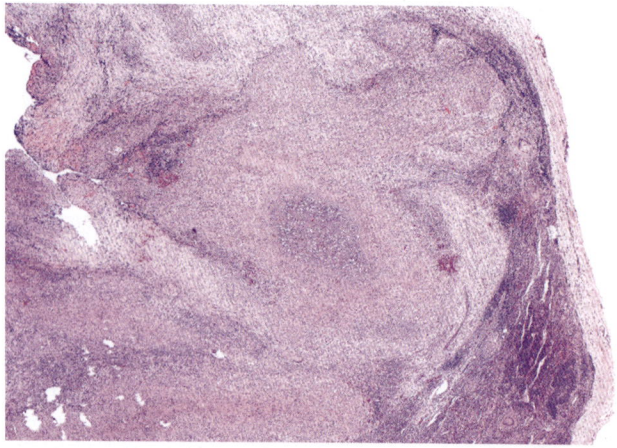

FIGURE 23-12 • The microabscesses in cat-scratch disease have a serpiginous or stellate contour. (Hematoxylin and eosin stain 4× magnification.)

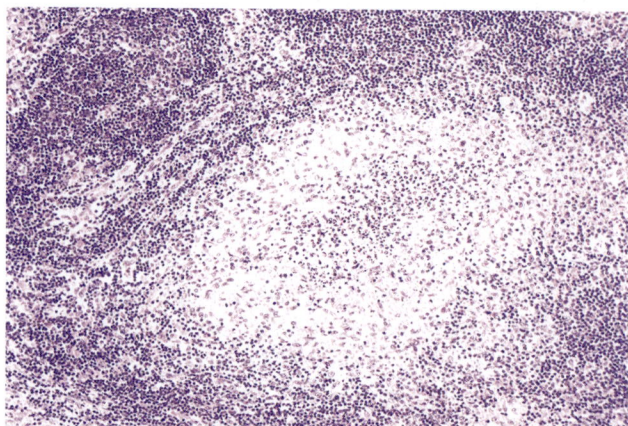

FIGURE 23-13 • In well-developed cases, the abscesses of cat-scratch disease have a broad rim of palisading histiocytes surrounding abundant neutrophils forming a so-called pyogranuloma. (Hematoxylin and eosin stain 10× magnification.)

Mycobacterial Infections

The most common cause of granulomatous lymphadenitis in small children (1- to 5-year old) is infection by nontuberculous "atypical" mycobacteria (NTM), most commonly MAI or *Mycobacterium scrofulaceum* (62,63). Diagnosis may be made by FNA or excisional lymph node biopsy. Cytologically, smears show epithelioid histiocytes and granulomata with reactive lymphocytes and PCs in the background as well as amorphous necrosis or necrosis associated with abundant neutrophils. Histologically, the nodal architecture is partially distorted or entirely effaced by follicular hyperplasia with well-formed granulomata composed of epithelioid histiocytes and multinucleated giant cells, which rim central areas of caseous necrosis (eFigures 23-1 and 23-2) or necrosis containing abundant neutrophils similar to lesions in cat-scratch disease (eFigures 23-3 and 23-4) (64). Although there is significant overlap between *Mycobacterium tuberculosis* (MTB) and NTM lymphadenopathy, some studies suggest that well-defined granulomata with caseous necrosis and numerous giant cells are more characteristic of MTB, while microabscesses are more predictive of NTM. Small lymphocytes are evenly distributed throughout lesional areas, and immunoblasts are rare or absent. Immunocompromised patients may not be able to mount responses to the infection and lack the classical granulomata, instead showing looser aggregates of histiocytes with a foamy appearance and more abundant organisms on special stains (eFigures 23-5 and 22-6) (63). Rare cases in immunocompetent patients may show mycobacterial organisms on acid-fast stain, although greater sensitivity may be obtained using fluorescence microscopy using auramine orange (65) or immunohistochemistry against the MPT64 mycobacterial antigen (more specific for the *Mycobacterium tuberculosis complex*) (66,67). The remainder of cases may be diagnosed via one of several polymerase chain reaction–based techniques (68–72) or microbiologic culture. Most of these techniques, except for culture, have the advantage of being applicable to fresh as well as paraffin-embedded tissue and may be performed using cytology specimens, core needle biopsies, or whole lymph node biopsies. Other causes of caseating and noncaseating granulomatous lymphadenitis include nonmycobacterial infections and neoplastic disease, including peripheral T-cell lymphoma, NLPHL, and classical Hodgkin lymphoma (CHL).

Chronic Granulomatous Disease

Chronic granulomatous disease (CGD) of childhood is a congenital disorder caused by defective components of the NADPH (reduced nicotinamide adenine dinucleotide phosphate) oxidase pathway (73). This extremely rare form of granulomatous lymphadenitis presents with lymph nodes and other tissues that are extensively infiltrated by granulomata and neutrophil-rich abscess-like foci. Catalase-positive organisms, specifically *Staphylococcus aureus,* gram-negative bacilli, and *Aspergillus*, are the most common agents to be recovered in culture (73). A test for nitroblue tetrazolium reduction or other assessment of the respiratory burst by peripheral blood leukocytes using either chemiluminescence or flow cytometry should be performed in suspected cases. Molecular diagnostic testing may be performed to confirm the gene involved (74) (see Chapter 6).

In 11% to 25% of cases, a careful review of clinical, radiologic, histologic, and laboratory data fails to identify a cause of the granuloma formation (75), and a diagnosis of idiopathic granulomatous lymphadenitis is rendered. In such circumstances, with all secondary causes excluded, sarcoidosis can be considered a possibility (76) (Chapter 12).

Although occasionally seen in adolescents, sarcoidosis is rare in children and more commonly occurs in young adults. Lymph node architecture is often totally effaced with few or no residual follicles. Necrosis is rare but when present is more commonly fibrinoid than caseating. Recent studies have demonstrated an increased CD4+ FoxP3+ regulatory T-cell (Treg) population both in the peripheral blood and lymph nodes of patients with sarcoidosis (77,78). Noncaseating granulomatous lymphadenitis may also be seen in benign lymph nodes draining organs involved by tumor, and histiocytic proliferations mimicking granulomas may be present in lymph nodes involved by lymphoma (79).

INTERFOLLICULAR PROCESSES WITH HISTIOCYTIC PROLIFERATION (NONGRANULOMATOUS)

Sinus histiocytosis is a nonspecific reactive pattern that may be seen in lymph nodes draining either inflammatory or malignant processes of the skin, bowel, or lungs. In particularly striking cases, only compressed primary follicles are seen, and germinal centers are either diminutive or absent. The subcapsular and paratrabecular sinuses are expanded by a cellular infiltrate composed of large polygonal cells with bland nuclei and abundant pale eosinophilic cytoplasm, some with phagocytosed debris (80). These histiocytes can be distinguished from Langerhans cells and Rosai-Dorfman cells by their CD68+, lysozyme-positive, S100−, CD1a−, CD207− phenotype.

Sinus Histiocytosis with Massive Lymphadenopathy (Rosai-Dorfman Disease)

SHML, also known as *Rosai-Dorfman disease*, affects young patients (81). Germinal centers are atrophic, compressed, or lacking in most cases, and the paracortex is diminished secondary to the compressive effects of the expanded sinusoids (Figure 23-14). A polymorphous array of lymphocytes, PCs, histiocytes, xanthoma cells, and "SHML" cells distend the sinusoids, with the proportions varying from case to case. The SHML cells, which are the hallmark of this disorder, have oval nuclei with condensed chromatin and abundant eosinophilic to xanthomatous cytoplasm (Figure 23-15 and eFigure 23-7). Engulfed lymphocytes ("emperipolesis") are pathognomonic, although this feature may be focal in some cases. Several groups have demonstrated the utility of FNA in the diagnosis of SHML. Smears generally demonstrate the presence of small lymphocytes, PCs, neutrophils (few), and SHML cells (82–85). The phenotype of the SHML cell is S100+ and CD68+, but the cells lack markers for Langerhans cells (CD1a and CD207) or dendritic cells (DRC, CD23, CNA42) (86). SHML has been seen in association with neoplasms, including mixed cellularity and lymphocyte-predominant HL as well as NHLs, and in patients with immune dysregulation such as post–bone marrow transplant or in the setting of

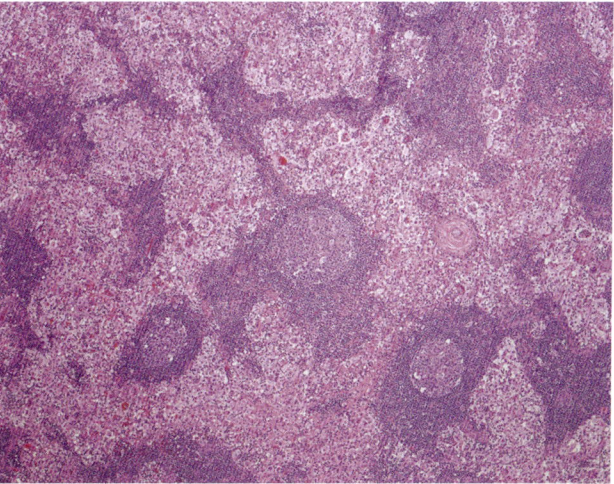

FIGURE 23-14 • As a result of massive sinusoidal expansion by histiocytes, germinal centers are compressed in Rosai-Dorfman disease (SHML). (Hematoxylin and eosin stain 4× magnification.)

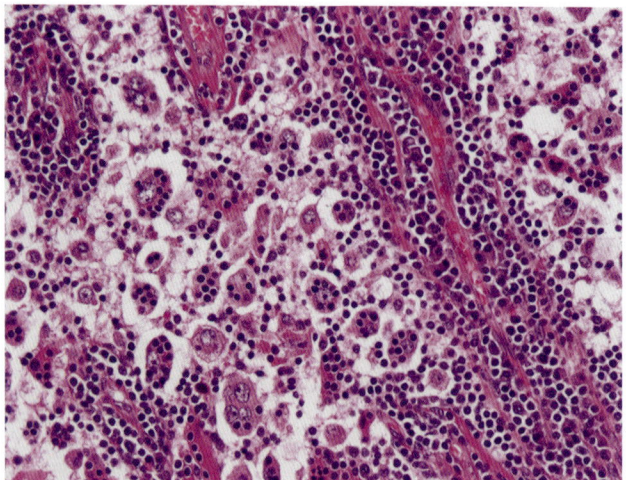

FIGURE 23-15 • The lesional cell in Rosai-Dorfman disease (SHML) has a small, cytologically bland nucleus and abundant eosinophilic cytoplasm containing one or more lymphocytes (emperipolesis). Although obvious in this case, emperipolesis may be difficult to detect on routine sections. (Hematoxylin and eosin stain 20× magnification.)

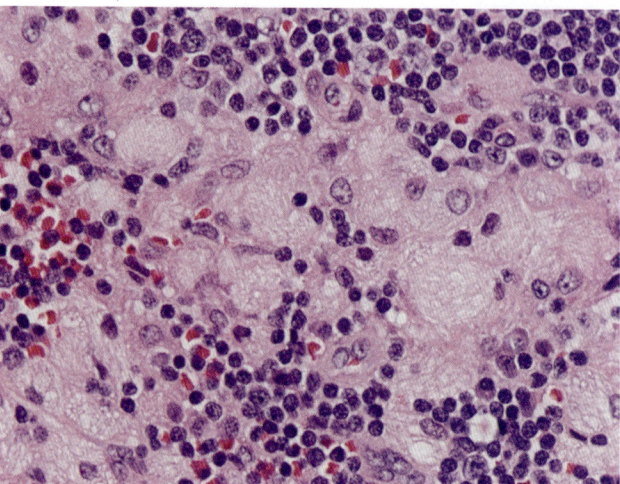

FIGURE 23-16 • Histiocytic proliferations caused by congenital storage disorders have a sinusoidal, often paracortical distribution in lymph nodes. The histiocytes seen in storage disorders often have coarsely vacuolated, ("bubbly") or fibrillar ("crumpled tissue paper") cytoplasm, as seen in this case of Gaucher disease. (Hematoxylin and eosin stain 40× magnification.)

ALPS, which should be taken into account in the evaluation of unusual cases (53,87–89). A subset of SHML shows features of IgG4-related disease, and an overlap between certain aspects of the two diseases has been suggested (90).

Foreign Body Sinusoidal Histiocytic Reactions

Histiocytic lymphadenopathy secondary to foreign (nonnodal) material occurs in the setting of primary metabolic disease, in lymph nodes draining tumors or ulcerated areas, adjacent to joint prostheses, or after lymphangiography (although current radiographic techniques have largely replaced lymphangiography). The adenopathy in these patients is rarely worrisome. In cases of accumulated contrast media, the sinusoids are dilated by foamy macrophages, histiocytes, and multinucleated giant cells containing large lipid vacuoles (eFigure 23-8). A similar pattern may be seen in cases of lymphadenopathy due to silicone from leaking or ruptured implants (eFigures 23-9 to 23-11). In the case of joint replacement, sinuses contain pale-staining vacuolated macrophages with refractile or birefringent material that may be Oil Red O positive, depending on whether metallic particles or polyethylene particles are present. Associated granulomata, giant cells, and fibrosis may be seen in some cases (91). Similar findings may be noted in patients with Gaucher disease or other metabolic storage diseases (Figure 23-16). In such cases, histiocytes resemble those seen in the bone marrow in storage diseases with either fibrillar "crumpled tissue paper" or bubbly foamy macrophages (see Chapter 24). Little of the material is found outside the sinusoids, and the remainder of the lymph node, although compressed or atrophic, is normal. Morbidity and mortality may be associated with the primary process causing the accumulation of foreign material, but not with the adenopathy itself.

Dermatopathic Lymphadenopathy

Children with dermatopathic lymphadenopathy commonly have eczema or another chronic exanthematous disorder, and they present with enlarged axillary or inguinal lymph nodes. Because of the age distribution of the predisposing dermatologic conditions (mycosis fungoides, psoriasis, eczema) (92), dermatopathic lymphadenopathy is more frequently seen in adults. At low power, involved lymph nodes show a mixed pattern of follicular hyperplasia and often marked paracortical expansion caused by an influx of histiocytes, Langerhans cells (93), and variable numbers of eosinophils (usually few) (Figure 23-17 and eFigure 23-12). The paracortical expansion

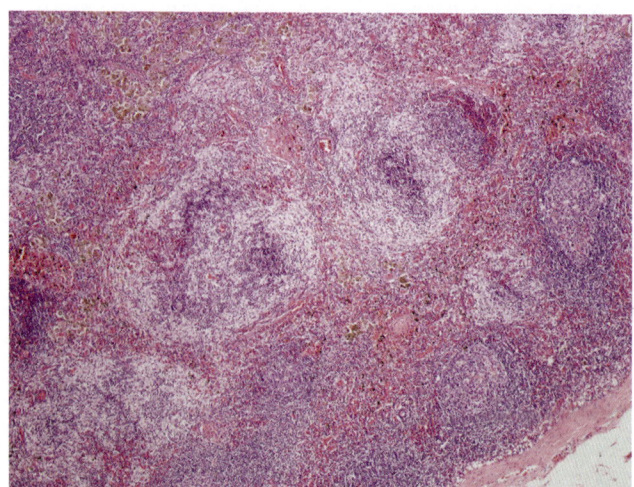

FIGURE 23-17 • The paracortical regions in dermatopathic lymphadenitis are expanded and show a pale pink swirled appearance due to the collections of abundant histiocytes and Langerhans cells admixed with small lymphocytes. Some histiocytes contain brown melanin pigment. (Hematoxylin and eosin stain 4× magnification.)

may have a pink mottled appearance because of infiltrating histiocytes and Langerhans cells (S100+, CD1a+, CD207+), some of which may contain coarsely granular brown–black melanin pigment (melanophages) that is positive on Fontana-Masson staining. Occasional hemosiderin pigment is also seen. FNA of lymph nodes with dermatopathia shows large clusters of histiocytes, histiocytes with melanin pigment, few tingible body macrophages, and histiocytes with elongated or grooved nuclei (94).

Hemophagocytic Lymphohistiocytosis

Hemophagocytic lymphohistiocytosis (HLH) may be idiopathic, familial, infection-related (95,96), rheumatologic, malignancy related (97,212), related to antineoplastic therapy (98), or rarely preceded by Kikuchi disease (99,100). HLH results from uncontrolled activation of CD8+ T cells, macrophages, and histiocytes associated with decreased NK cell function and increased levels of circulating proinflammatory cytokines (97,101). HLH is diagnosed according to HLH-2004 guidelines established by the Histiocyte Society when specific clinical, laboratory, and histopathologic criteria are met (102). Clinically significant lymphadenopathy is uncommon in primary HLH, and when present, lymph node biopsy is generally performed to exclude lymphoma.

Histologically, follicles are usually small and germinal centers few in number. The paracortex is depleted and has a mottled appearance because of the presence of increased numbers of pale-staining histiocytes. The sinusoids are distended by histiocytes, many of which are phagocytic. The nuclear features are bland, and the cells have abundant eosinophilic cytoplasm containing variable numbers of red blood cells and red blood cell fragments (eFigure 23-13). Leukophagocytosis is uncommon relative to erythrophagocytosis in this condition, and in further contrast to SHML cells, the histiocytes in HLH exhibit a CD68+, S100−, CD1a−, CD207− phenotype. Erythrophagocytosis and hemophagocytosis can be seen as a secondary phenomenon outside the context of primary HLH, and all these conditions must be considered as part of the differential diagnostic assessment. For instance, it has been reported in patients with a robust autoimmune hemolytic anemia, active SLE (103), X-linked lymphoproliferative disease, ehrlichiosis (104), typhoid fever (105), the accelerated phase of Chediak-Higashi disease (101), SHML, acute myelogenous leukemia (AML), acute lymphoblastic leukemia (106,212), juvenile myelomonocytic leukemia (99,107), and peripheral T-cell lymphoma (108,109). In some cases, there may be a spectrum of histiocytic disorders with macrophage activation syndrome (MAS) or secondary hemophagocytic syndrome seen in patients with Langerhans cell histiocytosis (LCH) (110). Patients with T lymphoblastic leukemia have rarely shown subsequent involvement by LCH or HLH (111,112).

Langerhans Cell Histiocytosis

LCH most commonly presents in children and may involve a single site, single organ system, or multiple organ systems. Children with systemic multiorgan disease may present with palpable adenopathy. Common sites of involvement include the bone, skin, lung, liver, spleen, bone marrow, and pituitary (113,114). In most cases, the disease is accurately diagnosed after biopsy of a painful bone lesion or skin biopsy (114). When biopsied, lymph nodes may show a spectrum of involvement from subtle focal sinus or paracortical involvement to total effacement of the nodal architecture involving the sinuses and/or the paracortex (115) (eFigure 23-14). The sinuses, when involved, are expanded by an array of Langerhans cells, non-Langerhans histiocytes, multinucleated giant cells, dendritic cells, lymphocytes, eosinophils, and actively phagocytic macrophages (eFigures 23-15 and 23-16). Older lesions may have a proportional increase in non–Langerhans-type histiocytes and xanthoma cells, and eosinophils may be scarce. It is important to distinguish LCH from dermatopathic lymphadenitis, which will also have Langerhans cells present but does not involve the sinuses and is less confluent.

By immunohistochemical analysis, Langerhans cells are reactive for CD1a and S100 but less so for CD68. They are negative for factor 13a. CD207, or Langerin, has been shown to be more specific for Langerhans cells than CD1a (116,117). Ultrastructural demonstration of Birbeck granules is pathognomonic, although often unnecessary if characteristic morphologic and immunohistochemical features (CD1a+ CD207+) are present. By molecular genetic analysis, it has been shown that approximately 50% of cases harbor a *BRAF* V600E mutation, with a recent study showing a high prevalence of *MAP2K1* mutations in the *BRAF* V600E-negative cases (118).

MALIGNANT LYMPHADENOPATHY

The most common nodal malignancies in children are of lymphoid lineage, although mesenchymal, histiocyte/macrophage, and metastatic tumors may also present initially as lymph node–based disease. Immunophenotypic analysis is always required for an accurate diagnosis, and cytogenetic studies in NHLs are frequently helpful. Like its benign counterparts, malignant adenopathy can be categorized morphologically by the architectural changes seen in affected lymph nodes (Table 23-5). The most widely accepted current classification from the World Health Organization (WHO) adopts a diagnostic and biologically meaningful approach based on the lineage of the malignant cell. Within each lineage of the WHO classification, distinct diseases are defined based on a combination of clinical, morphologic, immunophenotypic, and molecular genetic features (Table 23-6) (119).

The vast majority of pediatric cases of NHL fall into one of the four categories: DLBCL, Burkitt lymphoma, lymphoblastic lymphoma (T-cell or B-cell), and ALK+ ALCL. Indolent lymphomas composed of small lymphocytes (e.g., marginal zone lymphoma and follicular lymphoma) are extremely rare in children, and they should be diagnosed with caution.

TABLE 23-5	MALIGNANT CAUSES OF LYMPH NODE ENLARGEMENT CLASSIFIED ACCORDING TO HISTOLOGIC PATTERNS

Nodular proliferations
Classical Hodgkin lymphoma, nodular sclerosis type
Classical Hodgkin lymphoma, lymphocyte-rich type
Nodular lymphocyte–predominant Hodgkin lymphoma
Follicular lymphoma
Diffuse and paracortical proliferations
Myeloid sarcoma (chloroma, granulocytic sarcoma)
Lymphoblastic lymphoma
Burkitt lymphoma
Diffuse large B-cell lymphoma
Primary mediastinal (thymic) large B-cell lymphoma
Peripheral T-cell lymphoma
Marginal zone lymphoma
Classical Hodgkin lymphoma, mixed cellularity type
Classical Hodgkin lymphoma, lymphocyte-depleted type
Post transplant lymphoproliferative disorders (polymorphic, monomorphic)
Partial nodal involvement by lymphoma (any type)
Solid tumor metastasis
Posttransplant lymphoproliferative disorders (early lesions)
Necrotizing proliferations
Nodal infarction secondary to lymphoma or leukemia
Granulomatous or histiocyte-rich proliferations
Classical Hodgkin lymphoma, mixed cellularity type (some cases)
Sinusoidal proliferations
Hepatosplenic T-cell lymphoma
Anaplastic large-cell lymphoma (ALK+, ALK–)
Solid tumor metastasis

TABLE 23-6	ABBREVIATED WHO LYMPHOMA CLASSIFICATION AS APPLIED TO PEDIATRICS

Precursor B- and T-cell neoplasms
B lymphoblastic leukemia/lymphoma
T lymphoblastic leukemia/lymphoma
Mature B-cell neoplasms
Burkitt lymphoma
Diffuse large B-cell lymphoma
Mediastinal (thymic) large B-cell lymphoma
Pediatric follicular lymphoma (rare)
Pediatric marginal zone lymphoma (rare)
Mature T-cell and NK-cell neoplasms
Anaplastic large-cell lymphoma, ALK+
Hepatosplenic T-cell lymphoma[a]
Enteropathy-associated peripheral T-cell lymphoma[a]
Subcutaneous panniculitis like T-cell lymphoma[a]
Extranodal NK-/T-cell lymphoma, nasal type[a]
Angioimmunoblastic T-cell lymphoma[a]
Peripheral T-cell lymphoma, unspecified
EBV+ lymphoproliferative diseases of childhood[a]
Primary cutaneous CD30+ T-cell lymphoproliferative disorders[a]
    Primary cutaneous anaplastic large-cell lymphoma (C-ALCL)
    Lymphomatoid papulosis
Hodgkin lymphoma
Classical Hodgkin lymphoma
    Nodular sclerosing Hodgkin lymphoma
    Mixed cellularity Hodgkin lymphoma
    Lymphocyte-depleted Hodgkin lymphoma
    Lymphocyte-rich classical Hodgkin lymphoma
Nodular lymphocyte–predominant Hodgkin lymphoma

[a]Not discussed in this chapter.

B Lymphoblastic Lymphoma

B-cell lymphoblastic lymphoma, which represents approximately 15% of all cases of lymphoblastic lymphoma, is most common in older children and young adults. Patients typically present with rapidly enlarging lymph nodes or soft tissue masses. In contrast to T-cell lymphoblastic lymphoma, B lymphoblastic lymphoma rarely involves the mediastinum. Distinction between B lymphoblastic *lymphoma* and B acute lymphoblastic *leukemia* depends on the degree of peripheral blood and bone marrow involvement. By convention, cases with fewer than 25% bone marrow blasts should be diagnosed as B lymphoblastic *lymphoma*. One feature typical of lymphoblastic lymphoma (both B-cell and T-cell) is infiltration through perinodal fat and linear infiltrates in capsular collagen (Figure 23-18). The nodal architecture is effaced by a diffuse proliferation of small- and intermediate-sized cells (12 to 14 mm) with fine or speckled chromatin, small or indistinct nucleoli, and scant cytoplasm (Figure 23-19). The mitotic rate is frequently elevated, and tingible body macrophages and necrosis may be present. A CD45 (dim-to-negative), terminal deoxynucleotidyl transferase–positive (TdT+), CD19+, CD20−, sIg− phenotype sets these tumors apart from lymphomas composed of mature B cells, including Burkitt lymphoma and DLBCL (Figure 23-19, Table 23-7). Almost all cases are positive for CD10 (common acute lymphocytic leukemia antigen or CALLA) (120). Important in the differential diagnosis in children are other small blue cell tumors, including granulocytic sarcoma/chloroma, Ewing sarcoma/primitive neuroectodermal tumor (121), and alveolar rhabdomyosarcoma, which can be distinguished by phenotype, although care should be taken not to overvalue results from any single stain. For example, like Ewing sarcoma, lymphoblastic lymphomas are often CD45− and CD99+.

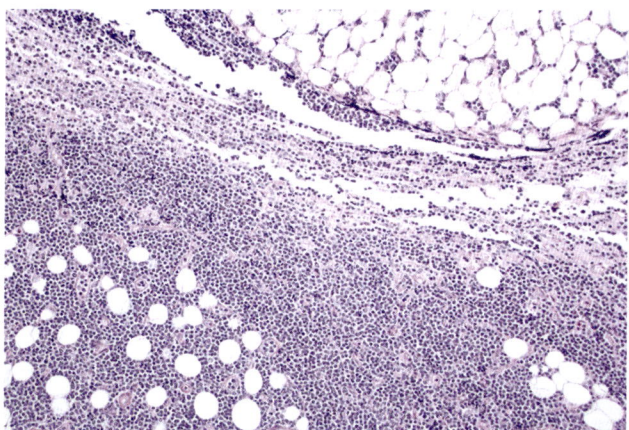

FIGURE 23-18 • B lymphoblastic lymphoma demonstrating diffuse architectural effacement of the node and infiltration into adjacent perinodal fat with linear infiltrates along the capsular collagen. (Hematoxylin and eosin stain 10× magnification.)

Diffuse Large B-Cell Lymphoma

Patients with DLBCL may present with steadily enlarging peripheral lymphadenopathy or extranodal disease (soft tissue, bone, gastrointestinal tract, and oropharynx). Although rare, primary mediastinal (thymic) diffuse large B-cell lymphoma (PMBCL) can also be seen in children (see Thymus section). DLBCL is disproportionately common relative to other types of lymphoma in patients with congenital, iatrogenic, or acquired immunodeficiency states. DLBCL has a diffuse growth pattern and may have intermixed fibrosis (particularly in the mediastinum). Lymphoma cell cytoplasm is abundant and may be amphophilic or densely eosinophilic. The cytology of the tumor cells ranges from that of reactive immunoblasts (round nucleus, thick nuclear membrane, single large eosinophilic nucleolus, abundant cytoplasm) to polylobate and even frankly anaplastic multilobate cells. Immunophenotypically (Table 23-7), tumor cells mark with pan B-cell markers (CD19, CD20, CD79a, CD22) and are surface Ig+ (except in PMBCL—see section under

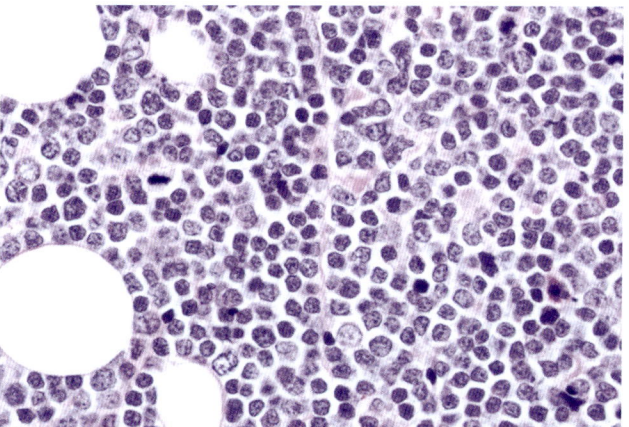

FIGURE 23-19 • The chromatin is fine and nucleoli are indistinct in lymphoblastic lymphoma. (Hematoxylin and eosin stain 40× magnification.)

Thymus for further discussion). CD10 is often positive, and positivity for BCL6 or BCL2 is variable.

Burkitt Lymphoma

Burkitt lymphoma takes three epidemiologic forms (122). *Endemic* Burkitt lymphoma most commonly affects children and exhibits a male predominance. Strongly associated with EBV infection, it is common in equatorial Africa and New Guinea. *Sporadic* Burkitt lymphoma is less commonly related to EBV infection and affects both children and adults, with a bimodal age distribution. *Immunodeficiency-related* Burkitt lymphoma is seen in the setting of congenital immunodeficiency, HIV infection, and posttransplant states. Burkitt lymphoma is one of the most rapidly replicating of all human tumors, and patients frequently present with the sudden development of large tumor masses (123). In endemic Burkitt lymphoma, the tumor shows an unexplained predilection for areas of growth, including the sockets around deciduous teeth of young (2- to 4-year-old) children, and hormonally responsive locations, such as the breasts of pubertal and pregnant women, ovaries, testes, and thyroid. In sporadic and immunodeficiency-associated Burkitt lymphoma, visceral involvement, particularly of the small bowel, is common, with initial symptoms related to obstruction or perforation.

Histologically, Burkitt lymphoma diffusely effaces nodal architecture. A monomorphic proliferation of intermediate-sized cells is seen (nuclear size similar to that of histiocytes or endothelial cells); the round or oval nuclei have a thick nuclear membrane and two to four nucleoli, and the cytoplasm is moderately amphophilic. Many Burkitt lymphomas have a somewhat cohesive appearance, and the cell borders maintain a slightly molded and "squared off" contour, particularly at the periphery. The mitotic rate is very high (MIB-1/KI-67 is positive in >95% of cells), and necrosis is often present. Evenly distributed tingible body macrophages containing cellular debris give a mottled ("starry sky") appearance to Burkitt lymphoma at low power. The immunophenotype is that of a mature surface Ig+ B-cell, and both CD19 and CD20 are expressed. CD10 and BCL6 are positive. BCL2 and TdT expression are absent (Table 23-7). Differential diagnostic considerations include lymphoblastic lymphoma and rapidly replicating large-cell lymphomas. Cytogenetic analyses play a key role in confirming the diagnosis. FISH studies are very helpful in demonstrating translocations that deregulate expression of the proto-oncogene c-myc (chromosome 8) paired with either the heavy-chain locus (chromosome 14) or the light-chain loci (chromosomes 2 and 22) (Table 23-3).

Other Rare B-Cell Lymphoma in Children

Two small B-cell lymphomas are worthy of note but only rarely seen in children—follicular lymphoma and nodal marginal zone lymphoma. Follicular lymphoma in children affects males more than females and, unlike their

TABLE 23-7 IMMUNOPHENOTYPE OF COMMON PEDIATRIC LYMPHOMAS

Lymphoma	Usually positive	Negative
Classical HL	HRS cells: CD30, CD15, PAX-5 (weak), +/−CD20, +/−, CD79a−/+, EBV+/−	HRS cells: CD45, CD3, ALK
NLPHL	LP cells: CD45, CD20 (strong), PAX-5 (strong), CD79a+, EMA+/−, BCL6+; background nodules: usually CD20, CD21, CD4+ and CD57+ T-cell rosettes around LP cells	LP cells: CD15, CD30, EBV
DLBCL	Pan B-cell markers (CD19, CD20, PAX-5, CD79a, surface Ig), CD10 +/−, BCL6+/−, BCL2+/−, Ki-67 variable	TdT, CD34
BL	Pan B-cell markers (CD19, CD20, CD79a, PAX-5, surface Ig), CD10+, BCL6+, Ki-67 >95%, EBV−/+	BCL2, TdT, CD34
B-LBL	CD19, CD22, CD79a, PAX-5, CD20 (variable −/+), CD34+/−, TdT	Surface Ig (usually), CD45 (negative to weak)
T-LBL	Cytoplasmic CD3, CD2, CD7, CD5, CD4 (variable), CD8 (variable), TdT, CD34−/+, CD1a+/−, CD10+/−	Surface CD3 (often, may be variably+)
ALCL	CD30, ALK, CD43, CD4, TIA-1+, perforin+, T-cell markers variable (CD3, CD2, CD5, CD7), CD45 (variable)	CD8 (may be positive in some cases), EBV, CD15

adult counterparts, often presents with limited-stage disease. Even though most are grade 2 or 3, many are curable. Morphologically, they range from the typical low-power pattern of crowded monomorphic small-to-medium size follicles to large expansive follicles and even the "floral variant." Phenotypically like adults, most cases are CD10+ and BCL6+ but, unlike adults, are often BCL2−, and most do not have the underlying BCL2/IgH t(14;18) translocation. The small minority with BCL2 translocations appear to have a worse prognosis (124). Given the indolent nature of BCL2 rearrangement negative pediatric follicular lymphoma and that cases with similar features and biology can occur outside the pediatric population, the term pediatric-type follicular lymphoma has been suggested (125).

Pediatric nodal marginal zone lymphoma, like its adult counterpart, can be particularly difficult to diagnose in that these lymphomas often only partially efface architecture with an interfollicular distribution. The neoplastic cells are frequently a mix of classic monocytoid B cells with small somewhat folded nuclei and abundant cytoplasm, small lymphocytes with little cytoplasm, large lymphocytes, and variable numbers of PCs and plasmacytoid lymphocytes. Follicular colonization may be present as well as follicles resembling those of PTGC. Most cases have a CD5− CD10− phenotype with monotypic surface Ig. Many have monotypic cytoplasmic immunoglobulin in PCs on paraffin immunoperoxidase stains. Like pediatric follicular lymphoma, these patients are predominantly males with limited stage disease (usually cervical nodes) and have an apparently good prognosis (126).

T Lymphoblastic Lymphoma

Although a rare type of lymphoma in the adult population, T lymphoblastic lymphoma represents approximately 30% of all pediatric NHLs. Like B-cell lymphoblastic lymphoma, T-cell lymphoblastic lymphoma is distinguished from T-cell lymphoblastic leukemia by the demonstration of limited bone marrow disease (<25% involvement). T-cell lymphoblastic lymphoma is commonly seen in adolescents and young adults. Because it is frequently located in the mediastinum, a rapidly growing T-cell lymphoblastic lymphoma may compress the heart and great vessels and cause pleural or pericardial effusions. The morphology of T-cell lymphoblastic lymphoma is identical in every respect to B-cell lymphoblastic lymphoma, and the immunophenotype is that of an immature T-cell with CD45 (dim), TdT+, cytoplasmic CD3+, usually surface CD3−, CD2+, CD7+ with variable expression of CD1a, CD4, CD5, and CD8 (Table 23-7). HLA-DR is negative. CD10 is expressed in 25% of cases. Other entities in the differential diagnosis, including B lymphoblastic lymphoma, Ewing sarcoma/primitive neuroectodermal tumor, and alveolar rhabdomyosarcoma, can be excluded with immunophenotypic studies. Tumor karyotype is less helpful in the prognosis of T-cell lymphoblastic lymphoma than B-cell lymphoblastic lymphoma (127). Many (although not all) translocations involve either the alpha/delta T-cell receptor locus at 14q11.2, the beta locus at 7q35, or the gamma locus at 7p14-15.

ALK-Positive ALCL

ALK-positive ALCL, a special type of peripheral T-cell lymphoma, affects patients of all ages, from children to the elderly, but is one of the more common lymphoma types seen in children. Cervical lymphadenopathy is particularly common in some series, and the skin, bone, and soft tissue may be secondarily involved. Involved lymph nodes may exhibit either a diffuse or a sinusoidal pattern (Figure 23-20) of tumor cell infiltration, and the latter may be mistaken for metastases of a solid tumor. The tumor cells of ALCL are often very large (>20 mm) and have bizarre, lobulated, or wreath-like nuclei (hallmark cells) with small-to-large nucleoli and abundant eosinophilic cytoplasm (Figure 23-21). Pleomorphic, sarcomatoid, lymphocyte/histiocyte-rich, neutrophil-rich (128,129), and even monomorphic/small-cell variants (130) have been described. The common denominator in the vast

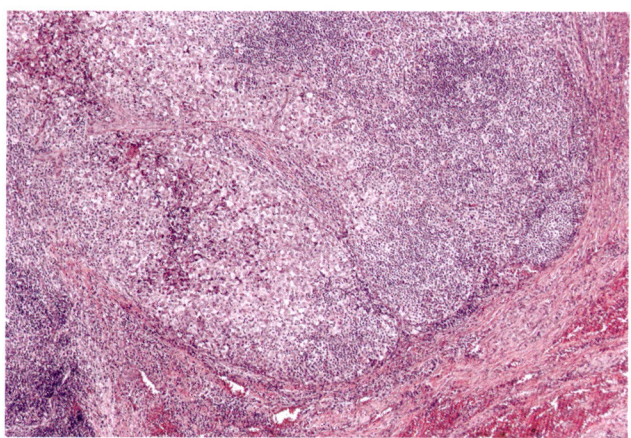

FIGURE 23-20 • Anaplastic large-cell lymphoma may resemble metastatic carcinoma when it remains localized to the sinusoids. (Hematoxylin and eosin stain 4× magnification.)

majority of pediatric cases is the chromosomal rearrangement of ALK and resultant ALK positivity, with the most common translocation being the t(2;5) NPM-ALK. This results in nuclear and cytoplasmic ALK positivity on immunohistochemical stain. A variety of other translocations have been described, many of which will results in alternate patterns of ALK positivity. Membranous staining (usually associated with Golgi positivity) for CD30 is uniformly diffusely strong and required for the diagnosis. ALCL exhibits variable expression of pan T-cell markers CD3, CD7, and CD5. Epithelial membrane antigen (EMA) and CD45 are usually but not always positive (9). CD4, CD2, CD43, and CD45RO are often positive. Most cases are positive for cytotoxic molecules like TIA-1, granzyme B, and perforin (Table 23-7). Only a minority are CD8$^+$. Stains for EBV (LMP1 and EBER) are consistently negative (131,132).

Peripheral T-Cell Lymphoma

Peripheral T-cell lymphomas, including angioimmunoblastic T-cell lymphoma, represent only a small fraction of lymphomas in children. Heterogeneity is their histologic hallmark. At low power, lymph node architecture either is diffusely effaced or shows interfollicular expansion. Thick-walled vessels are more prominent in peripheral T-cell lymphomas than in B-cell NHLs, and the even mixture of atypical small, intermediate, and large lymphoid elements is another clue to the lineage of this type of lymphoma. Irregularity of the nuclear contour may be particularly prominent, and these tumors in many cases may have cells with clear cytoplasm. Scattered eosinophils, histiocytes, and PCs may also be seen in the background. Detailed phenotypic studies have shown that peripheral T-cell lymphomas are uniformly TdT−, CD45+ with most having a CD3+, CD45RO+, CD4+, CD8− helper T-cell phenotype. Other T-cell antigens (e.g., CD2, CD5, CD7, BCL-2) are variably expressed, and the loss of one or more of these T-cell antigenic markers is characteristic of peripheral T-cell lymphoma. Virally mediated or drug hypersensitivity immunoblastic reactions may mimic peripheral T-cell lymphoma, as can HL, large B-cell lymphomas rich in T cells ("T-cell/histiocyte-rich diffuse large B-cell lymphoma"), and Fas mutation-related lymphoproliferations (ALPS).

Hodgkin Lymphoma

HL is a primary nodal tumor of B-cell lineage (133,134). Microdissected tissue and single-cell polymerase chain reaction methods have shown that the HRS cells in most cases of HL have clonal rearrangements of the immunoglobulin heavy-chain locus and exhibit intraclonal point mutations, indicative of ongoing somatic hypermutation. These findings have allowed assignment to a B-cell lineage and germinal center status to the cell of origin of HRS cells (133).

HL manifests a bimodal age distribution, with peaks in young adults and older adults, and is more common overall in males than in females. The key pathologic characteristic of HL is that the bulk of the tumor is composed of reactive leukocytes and histiocytes, with very few neoplastic cells (usually <5% of the tumor mass) (135). The diagnosis of HL requires (a) the presence of neoplastic HRS cells of appropriate immunophenotype and (b) an appropriate cytologically bland inflammatory background. The WHO divides these lymphomas into NLPHL and CHL, which includes nodular sclerosing, mixed cellularity, lymphocyte-rich, and lymphocyte-depleted subtypes (Figure 23-22).

In CHL, typical HRS cells are very large (20 to 40 μm), with a range of appearances. The classic type has a bilobed or a multilobed nucleus, with a thick nuclear membrane and one or several very large eosinophilic macronucleoli, and abundant eosinophilic cytoplasm (136). In the mononuclear type (Hodgkin cell), the nucleus has a single lobe and often a single central large nucleolus, which may be so large that it mimics a cytomegalovirus inclusion. The lacunar type of HRS cell characteristic of nodular sclerosing HL (NSHL) has a single-lobed or a multilobed nucleus, usually with small nucleoli and a water-clear cytoplasm that is retracted from the surrounding cells (Figure 23-23). Phenotypically, the HRS cells of the different subtypes of CHL all share a

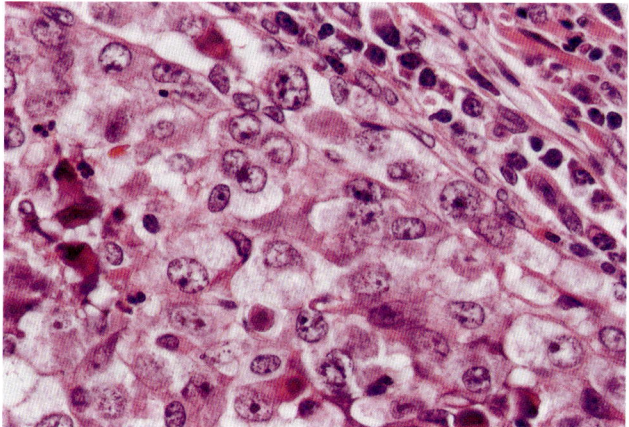

FIGURE 23-21 • Anaplastic large-cell lymphoma with large bizarre tumor cells with multilobated nuclei with small-to-large nucleoli and abundant cytoplasm. (Hematoxylin and eosin stain 40× magnification.)

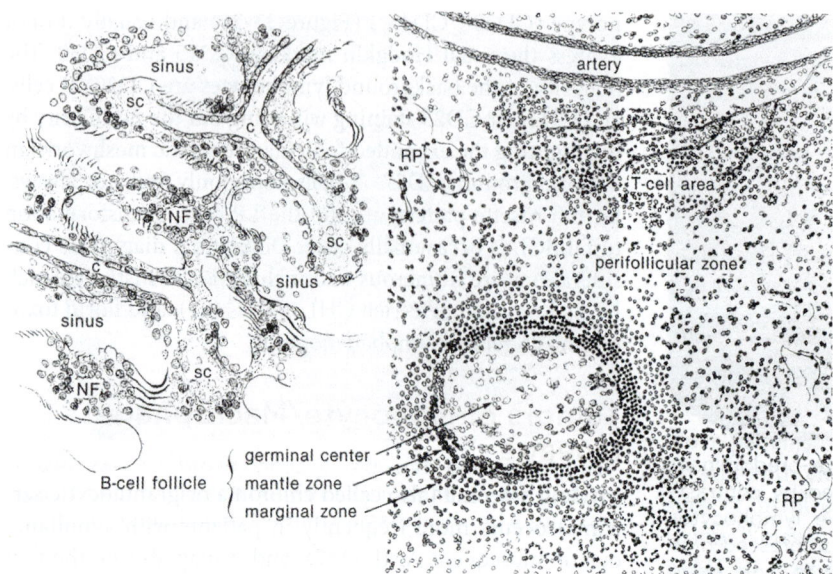

FIGURE 23-26 • Schematic representation of the splenic red pulp (**left**) and white pulp (**right**) showing the main compartments and structures of the human spleen. (From Van Krieken JH, Orazi A. Spleen. In: Mills SE, ed. *Histology for Pathologists*, 3rd ed. Philadelphia, PA: Lippincott Williams & Wilkins; 2007:783–798.

are removed. The spleen is also a major site of removal of red cells with decreased flexibility, increased fragility, or other defects. The filtering function of the spleen is a dual-edged sword. Although the spleen protects against life-threatening infections caused by encapsulated bacteria, the destruction of antibody-coated platelets or red blood cells makes it necessary to remove the spleen in certain diseases when other means fail to maintain peripheral counts.

The spleen is subdivided into the areas of red and white pulp (Figure 23-26). This division is useful for surgical pathologists because most diseases primarily affect one compartment or the other. The red pulp comprises most of the splenic volume and is the major site of removal of senescent and antibody-coated red cells and platelets and of red cell inclusions, such as Howell-Jolly bodies (nuclear fragments) and Pappenheimer bodies (siderotic granules). Blood enters the spleen via splenic arteries. The splenic arteries branch into progressively smaller arteries and arterioles that ultimately empty into a network of thin-walled, endothelium-lined capillaries. These terminate in sheathed capillaries that are lined not by endothelium but by specialized phagocytic mononuclear cells (littoral cells) that express CD8. Blood cells traverse the sheathed capillaries and basement membrane to enter the splenic sinuses and ultimately drain into the splenic veins. While crossing the sheathed capillaries, red blood cells with decreased flexibility become trapped in the splenic cords (cords of Billroth) and are destroyed by the phagocytic lining cells.

The white pulp of the spleen, which grossly appears as numerous gray-white spots within the red pulp, is composed of masses of T and B lymphocytes. The T lymphocytes surround the arterioles, so-called periarteriolar lymphoid sheaths or PALS, and become less plentiful around the more distant arteriolar branches. Within the PALS are the B-cell areas, which may contain germinal centers, particularly in the spleens of children and persons with autoimmune disorders. Germinal centers in the spleen, as in other sites, are surrounded by a mantle zone. This in turn is surrounded by a marginal zone of cells with relatively abundant pale cytoplasm that is usually appreciable only in the spleen or mesenteric lymph nodes. In a retrospective review of splenic histopathology from 205 children dying unexpectedly, there was a significant increase in reactive germinal centers in the spleen of children dying unexpectedly in comparison to other children of the same age. Germinal centers in the spleen develop in response to immunologic stimulation. The existence of a high number of germinal centers in the spleen is evidence that an immune reaction has occurred. The histology of the normal spleen is described in greater detail by van Krieken and te Velde (146).

Examination of the Spleen

Many pathologic processes affect the spleen of children, including congenital anomalies, benign cysts, trauma, infection, malignancies, and other hematologic disorders (147). Splenectomies in children are performed for many reasons. The most common reasons for splenectomy include hereditary spherocytosis, chronic hemolytic anemias, chronic ITP, hypersplenism, and trauma. Splenectomies to stage HL, once the most common indication, have become rare as advances in imaging modalities have provided accurate staging information. Common causes of splenomegaly are listed in Table 23-8.

Regardless of the indication for splenectomy, all surgically removed spleens should be measured and weighed (148). It is noted, however, that gross examination of the spleen can be challenging as laparoscopic splenectomy has become commonplace, resulting in specimens that have been largely fragmented prior to arrival at the surgical pathology bench, making accurate measurements of size or weight difficult. After the capsule has been examined for color, irregularities, and tears, as best can be ascertained depending on the surgical procedure performed, the spleen is sliced transversely

TABLE 23-8	CAUSES OF SPLENOMEGALY IN CHILDHOOD
Nonspecific infections	
Acute splenitis	Hodgkin lymphoma
Autoimmune disorders	Malaria
Autoimmune hemolytic anemia	Myeloproliferative neoplasms (CML, JMML, chronic myelofibrosis)
Acute leukemias (AML, ALL)	Niemann-Pick disease
Brucellosis	Non-Hodgkin lymphoma
Cardiac failure	Portal or splenic vein thrombosis
Congestion	Rheumatoid arthritis
Cytomegalovirus infection	Schistosomiasis
Echinococcosis	Sickle cell anemia
Gaucher disease	Storage diseases
Hematologic malignancies	Systemic lupus erythematosus
Hemolytic anemias	Thalassemias
Hepatic cirrhosis	Toxoplasmosis
Hereditary elliptocytosis	Trypanosomiasis
Hereditary spherocytosis	Tuberculosis
Histoplasmosis	Typhoid fever
Other causes	
Vascular tumors (hemangioma, lymphangioma, angiosarcoma)	
Myofibroblastic tumor (inflammatory pseudotumor)	
Metastatic tumors	
Hamartomas	
Cysts	

AML, acute myeloid leukemia; ALL, acute lymphoblastic leukemia; CML, chronic myelogenous leukemia; JMML, juvenile myelomonocytic leukemia.

into thin sections. The sections of abnormal-appearing areas should be taken (typically six to eight sections) in addition to a section of normal-appearing spleen. Periodic acid–Schiff staining of the section of normal spleen may be helpful, as this highlights the splenic cords and makes it easier to recognize other hematopoietic elements. If hilar lymph nodes are present, these should be dissected off and processed as a regular fresh lymph node biopsy.

CONGENITAL ANOMALIES

Asplenia

Asplenia, congenital absence of the spleen, occurs in about 1/40,000 live births. It is more common in boys and is often associated with cardiac anomalies, such as dextrocardia, transposition of the great vessels, and bilateral superior venae cavae, and development defects in other organs, including the liver, lungs, and intestines. Primarily because of these associated defects, the prognosis of patients with congenital asplenia is poor. In one series, nearly 80% of the patients died in infancy of cardiac failure or complications of surgery (149). Asplenia of any cause is associated with characteristic peripheral blood findings, including Howell-Jolly bodies, Pappenheimer bodies, and dysmorphic and nucleated red blood cells.

Polysplenia

In contrast to asplenia, polysplenia is more common in girls (149). The multiple small splenic masses are located in the right upper quadrant and are often associated with dextrocardia, a right-sided aortic arch, and pulmonary and hepatic defects. The histology of the splenic tissue is normal. Although less likely to die of cardiopulmonary defects in infancy, patients with polysplenia nonetheless have a high mortality rate. In one series, only 25% of patients were alive at 5 years (150).

Accessory Spleen

Accessory spleen is the most common congenital anomaly, encountered in about 16% of pediatric splenectomies. Accessory spleens are usually solitary and are most commonly located in the splenic hilum, although they may be found in the omentum, gastrosplenic and splenocolic ligaments, or retroperitoneum. The primary importance of accessory spleens is that they must be removed along with the spleen in therapeutic splenectomies for diseases such as immune thrombocytopenic purpura to prevent recurrence.

Fusion

Most cases of splenic fusion occur in white males, and most often, the spleen is fused with the left testis. Very rare cases of splenorenal or splenohepatic fusion have also been reported.

Hamartoma

Hamartomas of the spleen are uncommon benign tumors located primarily within the red pulp (151). They are usually discovered incidentally after a splenectomy or at autopsy. Most are reported in the adult population, but recent reviews suggest that 20% of reported hamartomas occur in children (151). The lesions are associated with congenital abnormalities such as tuberous sclerosis. Often, patients present with hematologic conditions including refractory microcytic anemia, sickle cell anemia, hereditary spherocytosis, and dyserythropoietic hemolytic anemia.

A recent report of four pediatric patients with splenic hamartomas described children ranging in age from 4 to 11 years, who presented with splenomegaly and hematologic abnormalities. In each case, the spleen was enlarged (315 to 724 g). On cut surface, single or multiple discrete bulging nodules ranging from 1.3 to 7 cm were identified. In other studies, the nodules have been reported as large as 15 cm in diameter. Microscopically, the lesions are composed of vascular channels that resemble splenic sinusoids and lack Malpighian corpuscles. They are usually associated with histiocytic proliferations, extramedullary hematopoiesis (EMH), lymphoplasmacytosis, fibrosis, and siderotic–calcific deposits.

Cysts

Congenital splenic cysts are rare. Hydatid or echinococcal cysts are the most common splenic cysts worldwide but are very rare in the United States. True or primary cysts are lined by epithelium, whereas false cysts or pseudocysts lack a cellular lining and are thought to arise after trauma. Splenic cysts can become quite large (>20 cm) and are typically filled with serous fluid. Although most congenital cysts are asymptomatic, cases of rupture associated with granulomatous peritonitis have been reported.

ACQUIRED ABNORMALITIES

Congestion

Chronic passive congestion of the spleen is commonly the result of portal hypertension or right-sided cardiac failure. The spleen is grossly enlarged, and microscopically, the findings are nondescript. The splenic sinuses are distended with red cells, and the capsule and splenic cords may be thickened and fibrotic. Splenic congestion is also common in hereditary hemolytic anemias and hemoglobinopathies, which are discussed in the following sections.

Immune Thrombocytopenia

ITP is an autoimmune-mediated condition, resulting from autoimmune destruction of platelets and suppression of megakaryocyte platelet production (152). A standardization of terminology, definitions, and outcome criteria in ITP of both adults and children was published in 2009 by an International Working Group of recognized expert clinicians (153,154). The diagnosis of ITP requires a platelet count less than 100×10^9/L and is subdivided into primary or secondary ITP (associated with other autoimmune or medical conditions). ITP may be further classified based on disease duration into newly diagnosed (<3 months), persistent (3 to 12 months), and chronic (>12 months) (152,153). The spleen is the major site of both antiplatelet antibody production and platelet removal from the bloodstream. Splenectomy, therefore, is an established method to achieve a sustained improvement of platelet count in children with chronic ITP, particularly, in those with persistent severe bleeding symptoms who have not responded to conventional-dose corticosteroids, IVIG, anti-D, or other immunosuppressive therapies (155). Splenectomy offered nearly 85% of patients an immediate platelet response and close to 70% a durable remission at 5 years. While it is also relatively safe and an effective treatment for severe and nonresponsive ITP, the increasing number of available treatment options and potential complications of splenectomy has caused both physicians and patients to consider other alternatives (152,155). International guidelines for the management of ITP have been recently reviewed (156).

Surgically removed spleens from patients with ITP are usually of normal size or mildly enlarged. Grossly, they are unremarkable with no significant congestion, unlike spleens from patients with autoimmune hemolytic anemia or hereditary spherocytosis. The white pulp is unremarkable or in some cases may show more prominent micronodularity than normal due to follicular lymphoid hyperplasia. Microscopically, the white pulp is usually prominent; numerous well-developed germinal centers surrounded by attenuated mantle zones and hyperplastic marginal zones are present. The red pulp shows increased neutrophilic granulocytes and precursors and increased numbers of foamy histiocytes containing platelets and phospholipid debris. Erythroid precursors and megakaryocytes are less frequently seen (157). After corticosteroid treatment, the spleen may demonstrate reduction and shrinkage of the B-cell regions of splenic white pulp resulting in germinal centers that are decreased in size and number or are absent. Typically, there is no change in the T-cell zone of PALS. Red pulp congestion with foamy macrophages is often reduced (Figure 23-27A, B) (157).

Hereditary Hemolytic Anemias

Common inherited causes of hemolytic anemia include hereditary spherocytosis and elliptocytosis and hemoglobinopathies such as the thalassemias and sickle cell anemia. Many of the clinical problems of more severe hereditary hemolytic disorders can be controlled by splenectomy. However, the use of splenectomy in a young child exposes the patient to a lifelong risk of overwhelming infections and other complications.

Most patients with **hereditary spherocytosis and elliptocytosis** have splenomegaly. The erythrocytes in these conditions are inflexible and become trapped as they attempt to pass through the splenic cords. Spleens removed for these diseases typically weigh from 250 to 500 g and are firm and dark red as a result of congestion. Microscopically, the venous sinuses are distended with red cells and are surrounded by hemosiderin-laden macrophages and endothelial cells. Often, the splenic white pulp is hyperplastic, with increased numbers of germinal centers. Patients usually respond well to splenectomy. Refractory cases are most commonly the result of an unrecognized accessory spleen.

Splenomegaly is also present in the majority of young children with **sickle cell anemia**. In patients more than 10 years old, however, the spleen is usually decreased in size as a result of infarction and scarring. Acute rapid enlargement of the spleen, due to sudden massive pooling of red blood cells in the spleen, may result in a sequestration crisis. Ultimately, the organ undergoes "autosplenectomy," and only a fibrotic remnant is left. Since sequestration crisis recurs in half of the

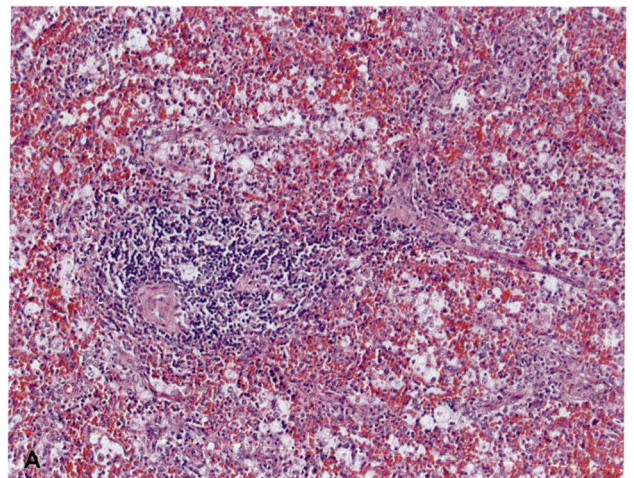
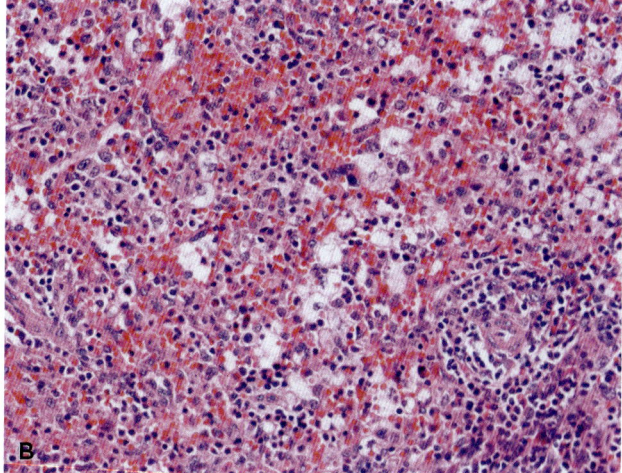

FIGURE 23-27 • Splenectomy from a child who was previously treated with IVIG, anti-D, and corticosteroid treatment for immune thrombocytopenic purpura. **A:** Secondary lymphoid follicles are absent, but the PALS is preserved. (hematoxylin and eosin stain 10× magnification) **B:** Red pulp shows increased foamy macrophages and neutrophilic granulocytes and precursors. (hematoxylin and eosin stain 20× magnification)

cases, splenectomy is usually performed after the acute episode subsides. Therefore, most of the spleens received as pathology specimens are from patients who experience acute sequestration crisis (158). Grossly, splenic infarcts are commonly seen. Gamna-Gandy bodies, old fibrotic infarcts containing multicolored deposits of minerals, iron (hemosiderin), and calcium, as well as foreign body giant cells, may be present. Microscopically, in acute sequestration, the red pulp is congested due to the stasis of sickled red blood cells within the splenic cords and focal hemorrhagic necrosis. In many patients, the erythrocytes tend to be sequestrated in the marginal zone of the white pulp, resulting in atrophy of the lymphoid follicles. This observation may help explain the increased susceptibility to infection in individuals with sickle cell disease (158).

Patients with **thalassemia** syndromes who develop severe anemia may undergo splenectomy. The microscopic findings of the spleen show prominent sequestration of red blood cells in the red pulp. EMH, primarily erythropoiesis, is common. Hemosiderosis may be pronounced in transfusion-dependent patients, and fibrosis may be present in advanced disease (158,159).

Infection

Acute splenitis can arise as a result of many blood-borne infections. The spleen typically becomes congested, with infiltration of the red and white pulp by neutrophils and PCs. Sometimes, necrotic foci develop. Abscess formation is uncommon. Granulomatous inflammation may be seen in disseminated fungal or mycobacterial infections. As previously mentioned echinococcal infections, although rare in the United States, are the most common cause of splenic cysts worldwide.

Bartonella henselae infection usually results in self-limited lymphadenitis, cat-scratch disease, primarily a disease of children (160,161). Bartonella species are small, intracellular gram-negative rods. Bacillary infection can also result in an unusual vascular lesion called *bacillary angiomatosis*. Bacillary angiomatosis usually occurs in the skin, the bone, and the brain, but a related proliferative lesion called *vascular peliosis* occurs in the liver and the spleen. Bacillary angiomatosis–peliosis was first identified in HIV-infected patients with AIDS. In most children and adolescents with intact immune systems, cat-scratch disease is confined to the lymph nodes. But numerous examples of the systemic manifestation have been reported in immunosuppressed patients (160,161).

Splenomegaly is seen in about half of patients with *infectious mononucleosis* and is occasionally complicated by fatal splenic rupture. Microscopically, the red pulp cords and sinuses are infiltrated by a polymorphic population of T and B immunoblasts that may include large multinucleated forms resembling HRS cells. The clinical setting is most helpful in avoiding a misdiagnosis of HL. Immunohistochemically, the immunoblasts in acute EBV infection may be CD30$^+$ but are usually CD15$^-$ and positive for leukocyte common antigen.

Inborn Errors of Metabolism

Splenomegaly is a common feature of a variety of inborn errors of metabolism, including diseases ranging from sphingolipidosis to glucocerebrosidosis. The accumulation of storage histiocytes engorged with storage products within the spleen causes progressive enlargement (162). The etiology and classification of the inborn errors of metabolism, including storage diseases, which affect the spleen, are discussed in detail in Chapter 5. **Gaucher disease**, which encompasses a spectrum of autosomal recessive disorders that result from glucocerebrosidase deficiency, is the most common metabolic cause of splenomegaly in childhood and the most prevalent lysosomal storage disorder (163). Of the three clinical types, type I (chronic nonneuropathic) is the most common, particularly in individuals of

European Jewish descent. Although traditionally referred to as the "adult type," 66% of individuals with type I Gaucher disease present in childhood as hypersplenism develops. In this form of Gaucher disease, macrophages containing glucosylceramide-laden lysosomes accumulate primarily in the bone marrow and spleen without involving the central nervous system. Hepatosplenomegaly is also seen in type II disease (acute neuropathic), but involvement of the central nervous system leads to death in early childhood. The spleen is also involved in type III disease (subacute neuropathic), where neurologic manifestations begin in early adult life. Microscopic evaluation of the spleen shows that the sinuses are diffusely expanded by clusters and sheets of large macrophages. The storage macrophages or Gaucher cells are two to six times the size of a normal macrophage but maintain the cytologically bland, round, oval, vesicular nuclei. There is abundant cytoplasm with a wrinkled or a striated appearance, so-called "wrinkled or crumpled tissue paper" appearance. The cytoplasm stains with both periodic acid–Schiff and iron. Of note, pseudo-Gaucher cells can be seen in a number of disorders associated with hematopoietic cell turn over or destruction such as chronic myelogenous leukemia. In these cases, the macrophage cytoplasm contains insoluble lipid pigment that stains intensely blue ("sea-blue histiocytes") (see Chapter 5).

Niemann-Pick disease is an autosomal recessive deficiency of sphingomyelinase that leads to the accumulation of sphingomyelin within cells and tissues. Splenomegaly is the most common presenting manifestation, and most extensively involved in type IA and IS. The spleen becomes significantly enlarged. Splenic volume directly correlates with liver volume and the patient's triglyceride level and inversely correlates with the patient's HDL level, their height, hemoglobin concentration, and white cell count. Microscopically, the red pulp shows infiltration by foam cells or Niemann-Pick cells, which have finely vacuolated cytoplasm. The Niemann-Pick cells are yellow–green in hematoxylin and eosin-stained sections and blue–green in Wright-Giemsa-stained smears, thus the term "sea-blue histiocytes." The cells are usually positive for period acid–Schiff (PAS) and lipid stains, such as Sudan black B (performed on air-dried smears or frozen tissue), but negative for iron stains (see Chapter 5).

Extramedullary Hematopoiesis

The spleen is a common site of EMH, which describes proliferations of bone marrow elements outside the marrow (158). EMH should be used to describe benign proliferations of bone marrow elements, but should not be used when referring to neoplastic extramedullary myeloid proliferations such as myeloid sarcomas or other myeloproliferative neoplasms (158).

EMH in infants is not uncommon, and the typical locations are liver, spleen, and lymph node. As the infant gets older, EMH would be expected to regress. Prematurity or a perinatal period associated with physiologic stress may cause persistence of EMH. Possible causes include bleeding,

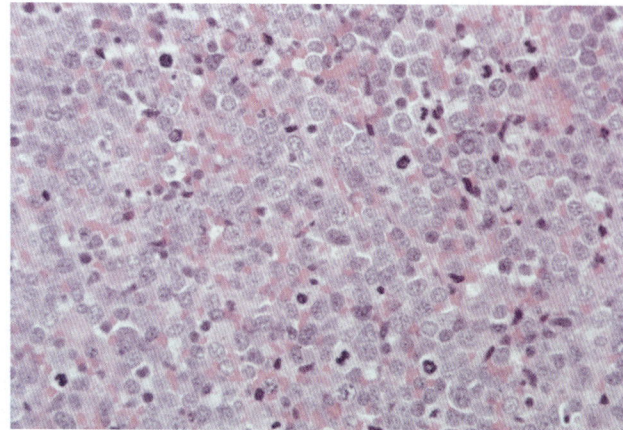

FIGURE 23-28 • Immature myeloid and megaloblastic erythroid progenitors effacing red pulp in spleen from a 2-year-old boy with juvenile myelomonocytic leukemia. Rapid splenic enlargement prompted splenectomy. (Hematoxylin and eosin stain, original magnification 20× magnification.)

infection, hypoxia, and a wide variety of congenital defects of the heart, lungs, kidneys, and other organs. Some well-known benign hematologic disorders that cause EMH include thalassemia, hereditary spherocytosis, sickle cell anemia, congenital dyserythropoietic anemia, and ITP (164). The pathologic findings of EMH in some of these conditions are described above. Moreover, some degree of EMH may be seen in the storage diseases described above.

Spleens with extensive EMH usually primarily involve the red pulp and grossly show a "beefy"-red appearance like other splenic red pulp disorders (158). In focal EMH, a mass lesion may be seen. Microscopic findings of EMH in the spleen show variable findings, partly depending on the underlying cause of EMH. Trilineage hematopoietic elements in varying proportions mimicking those seen in the normal bone marrow are generally seen. In hemolytic anemias and other anemias, erythroid elements predominate, whereas in cytokine-induced proliferations, as in G-CSF, granulocytic components predominate. Significant dysplasia in granulocytic elements (high nuclear to cytoplasmic ratio, scant cytoplasm) or dysplastic megakaryocytes (unilobated, small-size, bizarre chromatin or nuclei) should raise the possibility of an underlying neoplastic extramedullary myeloid proliferation (158,165) (Figure 23-28).

Vascular Tumors

Vascular neoplasms are the most common nonhematopoietic proliferations to involve the spleen. Vascular neoplasms are usually easily distinguished from histiocytic proliferations, inflammatory myofibroblastic tumors, and hematomas. Vascular tumors that involve the spleen include hemangiomas, lymphangiomas, littoral cell angiomas, hemangioendotheliomas, angiosarcomas, and myoid angioendotheliomas (see Table 23-9).

Lymphangiomas and **hemangiomas** are closely related benign vascular tumors that may involve the spleen, either as

TABLE 23-9	IMMUNOPHENOTYPE OF SPLENIC VASCULAR TUMORS
Tumor	Immunophenotype
Hemangioma	CD31+, CD34+, Factor VIII+, CD8−
Lymphangioma	CD31+, D2-40 (podoplanin) +, LYVE+, CD34−, factor VIII+
Littoral cell angioma	CD31+, factor VIII+, CD34−, CD68+/−, lysozyme+/−, CD21+/−, CD8− (occasionally +)
Myoid angioendothelioma	stromal cells: SMA+, desmin− vascular spaces: CD31+, CD34+, CD8−
Angiosarcoma	CD31+, factor VIII+/−, CD34+/−, CD8−/+, CD68−/+

a solitary mass or as part of a disseminated disease. Splenic hemangiomas are usually solitary and less than 2 cm in diameter. Although most are asymptomatic, larger hemangiomas are prone to rupture or may result in a consumptive coagulopathy or thrombocytopenia. Microscopically, splenic hemangiomas are composed of masses of dilated, endothelium-lined spaces filled with erythrocytes. By convention, tumors consisting of vessels filled with hypocellular proteinaceous fluid are considered lymphangiomas. In some cases, it is not possible to distinguish a hemangioma from a lymphangioma definitively on morphologic grounds alone, and for such cases, immunohistochemistry can be very helpful. Although both will express endothelial-related antigen CD31, hemangiomas are typically CD34+ and D2-40 (podoplanin) negative, while the opposite is true for lymphangiomas (see Table 23-9). **Peliosis** of the spleen is usually associated with peliosis of the liver. In contrast to the dilated spaces of hemangiomas, the dilated blood-filled spaces in peliosis lack an endothelial lining and are diffusely dispersed throughout the spleen.

Littoral cell angiomas are benign vascular tumors composed of specialized tall endothelial cells that express both endothelial and histiocytic markers (CD31+, factor VIII+, CD68+, CD34−, CD8−). The sinusoidal spaces of littoral cell angiomas are lined by tufts and papillary arrays of littoral cells that project into the lumen. The youngest reported patient was a 3-year-old boy. Other vascular tumors that involve the spleen include epithelioid hemangioendothelioma and epithelioid and spindle cell hemangioendothelioma.

Myoid angioendothelioma is a distinct vascular entity with features that differ from the other vascular neoplasms (166). This is a benign tumor as originally described as a composite tumor with areas of vascular stasis intermixed with stromal cells with myoid features (SMA+, desmin−). In the original description of three patients by Kraus and Dehner, two of the patients were children, 3 and 7 years of age (167). The one remaining patient was a 43-year-old patient. A recent publication describes a 51-year-old man with similar morphology. The reported lesions vary in size but were otherwise histologically quite similar and all were well circumscribed. There were scattered rounded or tubular spaces lined by cytologically bland cells throughout that documented the vascular nature of these lesions (CD34+, CD8−). The predominant cell was a large, polygonal-shaped epithelioid cell with abundant eosinophilic cytoplasm and indistinct cell borders. Nuclear configuration ranged from rounded to elongated or twisted and hyperchromatic, and eosinophilic nucleoli were present and occasionally prominent. In many cases, the fibroblastic-rich stroma was interspersed with chronic inflammatory cells.

Angiosarcomas of the spleen are extraordinarily rare in children and do not show the association with exposure to vinyl chloride, arsenic, or Thorotrast established for angiosarcomas involving the liver. Distinction from benign vascular tumors rests primarily on the presence of cytologic atypia and mitoses among the endothelial cells, in addition to an infiltrative pattern of growth. CD31 positivity is also helpful to confirm the diagnosis. The prognosis is poor (168).

Other Nonhematopoietic Tumors

A variety of mesenchymal tumors or proliferations, including Kaposi sarcoma (169), mycobacterial spindle cell tumors, and smooth muscle tumors, tend to develop in patients infected with HIV.

Inflammatory myofibroblastic tumor, also known as *inflammatory pseudotumor*, is most common in the lungs or mesentery but also occasionally involves the spleen. Inflammatory pseudotumors are well-circumscribed gray masses composed microscopically of spindle cells that on immunophenotyping are of myofibroblastic origin (positive for smooth muscle and muscle-specific actin, positive for cytokeratin). Although inflammatory pseudotumors are usually clinically benign, in rare cases, they may undergo malignant transformation (170). Metastatic tumors to the spleen in children are uncommon. Direct invasion of the spleen is occasionally seen in neuroblastoma, hepatoblastoma, or Wilms tumor.

Follicular Hyperplasia

Splenic follicular hyperplasia is common in children and especially prominent in autoimmune diseases, including rheumatoid arthritis, SLE, autoimmune hemolytic anemia or immune thrombocytopenic purpura, and HIV infection.

Localized Lymphoid Hyperplasia

In localized lymphoid hyperplasia, proliferations of lymphocytes form solitary nodules that are suspicious for lymphoma. Two forms were originally described by Burke and Osborne (171). In the first, the nodules are composed of aggregates of reactive germinal centers. In the other form, the aggregates are composed of small lymphocytes, immunoblasts, and PCs. The principal features distinguishing lymphoid hyperplasia from NHL are the polymorphic nature of the infiltrate and the absence of cytologic or immunophenotypic atypia.

abnormalities in the development and maturation of the immune system. Significant advances in understanding the defects underlying many subtypes of primary immunodeficiency have identified specific blocks in the normal schema of lymphoid maturation. Each block in lymphoid maturation results in a distinct immunodeficiency state, with increasing numbers of unique entities described every year (currently >180). The current classification by the International Union of Immunological Societies (IUIS) and most recent advances in the field have recently been reviewed by Al-Herz et al. (185). Perez-Atayde and Rosen (186) have described the pathology of primary immunodeficiencies and provided the diagnostic pathologist with a readily usable system for evaluating the spleen, lymph nodes, and thymus of a child with a suspected or confirmed immunodeficiency state (186). The outline encompasses immunologic defects resulting from combined immunodeficiencies (i.e., deficiencies of both B cells and T cells) either with or without associated or syndromic features; predominant antibody (B-cell) deficiencies; diseases of immune dysregulation; congenital defects of phagocyte number, function, or both; defects in innate immunity; autoinflammatory disorders; and complement deficiencies (185). Disorders resulting in a primary T-cell deficiency are caused either by a defect in primary thymic maturation or by secondary thymic abnormalities associated with altered T-cell development. Some examples of primary immunodeficiencies that affect thymocyte maturation include DiGeorge syndrome, reticular dysgenesis, combined immunodeficiency disease, and ataxia–telangiectasia (Table 23-11).

DiGeorge anomaly was first identified as thymic agenesis associated with abnormalities of T-cell maturation (175). DiGeorge syndrome results from a failure of the normal development of the third and fourth branchial arches, which results in abnormalities in multiple organs during the fourth to 6th weeks of embryogenesis. The clinical features vary, and there is considerable overlap with velocardiofacial syndrome. The major defects observed include aplasia or hypoplasia of the thymus and parathyroid glands, type I truncus arteriosus, and dysmorphic facies with micrognathia. Other associated conditions include esophageal atresia, thyroid aplasia/hypoplasia, absence of calcitonin-containing cells of the thyroid, and endocardial cushion defects. Likewise, the degree of T-cell immunodeficiency is variable, ranging from near normal T-cell numbers and function to near complete absence. Although a small percentage (5%) of cases are familial and rare cases result from *in utero* exposure to teratogens, the vast majority result from an unknown defect occurring *in utero* during the first trimester of pregnancy (187).

In cases of "complete" DiGeorge syndrome, both the thymus and the parathyroid glands are completely absent. Most patients manifest a "partial" or "incomplete" DiGeorge syndrome, in which the thymus is hypoplastic and otherwise histologically normal. The degree of thymocyte hypoplasia is variable, but in most instances, thymic lobation is normal, corticomedullary differentiation is detected, and Hassall corpuscles are present. Although not all the genetic defects are defined, most patients have a deletion at chromosome 22q11 with a smaller subset having an abnormality at 10p (187). Recent progress has been made in treating the athymia by thymus transplantation (188). Markert et al. (188,189) report that transplantation of cultured postnatal thymus successfully restored many of the immune abnormalities in patients with complete DiGeorge syndrome.

Severe combined immunodeficiency diseases (SCID) are represented by several distinctive disorders with similar clinical manifestations, severe naive T-cell deficiency, and distinct genetic bases. These include the lymphoid stem cell type (Swiss type) with autosomal recessive or X-linked modes of inheritance. Infants with SCID usually present by 3 months of age with thrush, monilial rashes, intractable diarrhea, and *Pneumocystis jiroveci* pneumonia. In some neonates, the symptoms are similar to those of graft-versus-host disease. Hecht giant cell pneumonia, resulting from measles infection or live measles or smallpox vaccination, is lethal to the immunocompromised host. Death results from overwhelming infection and uniformly occurs without early intervention and treatment, often with hematopoietic stem cell transplant or, in some cases, gene therapy. The T-cell receptor excision circle (TREC) assay has been introduced into newborn screening in many states, allowing early diagnosis and intervention in cases of SCID (190). Laboratory evaluation of infants with SCID reveals a marked lymphopenia (<1000 lymphocytes per cubic millimeter). At least ten different genetic defects have been identified in cases of SCID.

TABLE 23-11 IMMUNODEFICIENCY DISEASES ASSOCIATED WITH THYMIC ABNORMALITIES

	T-Cell Areas (Lymphocytes in Paracortex or Periarteriolar Lymphoid Sheath)	Germinal Centers	Plasma Cells
DiGeorge syndrome	A	NL	NL
Severe combined immunodeficiency	↓	↓	↓
Autosomal recessive	A	A	A
X-linked	↓-A	↓-A	↓-A
Thymic hypoplasia	↓	↓	↓
Ataxia–telangiectasia	↓-A	NL-↓	NL-↓

↓, decreased; A, absent, NL, normal

In the X-linked form, the number of B cells is normal, but the B cells fail to mature properly. T cells are rare and of maternal origin. One genetic defect responsible for X-linked SCID is a mutation of the gene coding for the γ-chain of interleukin (IL) receptor, mapped to Xq13, representing approximately 50% of cases of SCID. The γ-chain is a component of several IL receptors, including IL-4, IL-7, IL-11, and IL-16. Normal lymphocyte progenitors fail to differentiate because of a lack of appropriate growth factor stimulation. Other types of SCID are recessive in inheritance. The most common enzyme defects that result in immunodeficiency are of enzymes in the purine degradation pathway. The accumulation of toxic metabolites in adenosine deaminase deficiency and purine nucleoside phosphorylase deficiency results in lymphocyte defects (173). The symptomatology is essentially identical to that in children with AIDS.

The difference in the lymphoid tissue among the various types of SCID is minimal. The lymphocytes are generally depleted in all lymphoid tissues, including the thymus, spleen, lymph nodes, tonsils, adenoids, and mucosa-associated lymphoid tissue. The thymus is small and dysplastic. A variable number of T cells at the corticomedullary junction and scattered Hassall corpuscles are found early in most cases. Because of progressive lymphoid depletion, the thymic epithelium becomes prominent and may appear disorganized or acquire an organoid and pseudoglandular architecture (186). The morphology of the thymus in other well-characterized immunodeficiencies, including ataxia–telangiectasia, Wiskott-Aldrich syndrome, and chronic mucocutaneous candidiasis, is variable. The thymus histology can be normal or show slight lymphocytic depletion or complete atrophy.

The Thymus in AIDS

Changes in the thymus in patients with AIDS have been controversial. In a report of 11 infants with AIDS, Joshi (191) described histologic changes similar to those in patients subjected to severe stress. The thymus was located in the correct anatomic site and the lobation and blood vessels were normal, but the size, weight, and number of lymphocytes were reduced. In some cases, more severe abnormalities were noted, including complete involution or inflammatory changes. Animal studies suggest that transmission of the virus early in fetal development results in more severe immune destruction. A recent study demonstrated that HIV infection results in a high rate of spontaneous abortions and that the thymus in spontaneously aborted fetuses demonstrates severe abnormalities of lymphocytic differentiation and corticomedullary demarcation and an absence of Hassall corpuscles (191). The more severe thymic abnormalities develop earlier in gestation.

Thymic Tumors

The majority of tumors that occur in the mediastinum of children are lymphomas (41%) or tumors of neurogenic origin. True thymic lesions including cysts, thymolipomas, thymic hyperplasia, and thymic tumors represent approximately 2.5% of all mediastinal masses in children (192). *Hyperplasia of the thymus* is the most common anterior mediastinal mass found in infants. Histologically, two types of thymic hyperplasia are recognized. True thymic hyperplasia is characterized by increases in both the size and the depth of the gland with retention of the normal microscopic appearance. In the second type, lymphoid hyperplasia, reactive lymphoid follicles appear within the thymus. The reactive germinal centers are identical to those seen in normal lymph nodes. Follicular hyperplasia of the thymus can occur *de novo* or in association with autoimmune diseases and chronic inflammatory states, most commonly myasthenia gravis. Approximately 70% to 80% of patients with myasthenia gravis have follicular hyperplasia of the thymus, and in other cases, the thymus may be atrophic or have thymoma (193). Although myasthenia is usually a disease of older persons, Somnier (194) identified a bimodal male and female age distribution. The incidence of early-onset myasthenia gravis peaked at 21 to 30 years, but persons as young as 5 to 10 years of age were affected. The peak for early-onset disease was approximately 10 years later in males than in females. Other autoimmune diseases, including Graves disease, Addison disease, SLE, scleroderma, and rheumatoid arthritis, are associated with thymic hyperplasia.

True thymic hypertrophy, enlargement of the thymus, has been reported in neonates and children up to 14 years of age. In most cases, an enlarged thymus is an incidental finding. In other cases, the mediastinal enlargement causes respiratory or gastrointestinal symptoms (194). In some cases, the hypertrophy represents regeneration following stress. The thymus in cases of hypertrophy is normal, with a normal cortical–medullary junction and Hassall corpuscles. The diagnosis is based on the weight of the thymus at resection. Because the thymic weight varies widely, the thymus must weigh more than approximately 100 g to be considered hypertrophic.

Neoplastic Proliferation of the Thymus

Thymic tumors account for only 1.5% of all mediastinal masses in children and include thymomas, thymic carcinomas, and thymic carcinoids (192). Lymphomas are neoplastic proliferations of the lymphoid cells within the thymus and will be discussed separately. Thymomas are neoplastic proliferations of the thymic epithelium. Although thymomas are the most common primary neoplasms of the anterior mediastinum, they are the least frequent mediastinal tumors in children. Fewer than 2% of all thymomas are diagnosed in the first two decades of life. Small series of childhood cases occurring between 9 months and 15 years of life have been reported in the literature (192,195–199). Myasthenia gravis and other autoimmune disorders occur in 30% of adults with thymoma but are less frequent in children.

Morphologically, although thymomas are composed of neoplastic epithelial cells and lymphocytes, there is great morphologic heterogeneity. The role of histology in prognosis has been hotly debated. The WHO in 1999 defined the histologic criteria for distinct subtypes of thymic epithelial tumors (192,195–198), which was later updated in 2004. Thymic neoplasms are now subdivided into six entities: types A, AB, B1, B2, and B3 thymomas and thymic carcinomas (formerly thymoma type C), although Suster and Moran have proposed that the classification system could be simplified into thymoma (types A, AB, B1, B2), atypical thymoma (type B3), and thymic carcinoma (200,201). The classification is still largely based on the extent of lymphocytic infiltration. It is important to recognize the possibility of a thymoma because the lymphocytes express the antigens of immature thymocytes. These normal thymocytes can be confused with the lymphoblasts of lymphoblastic lymphoma, especially on a small biopsy. A variety of distinct cellular features may be seen within the typical thymoma, including thymic cysts that may form papillary structures, germinal centers, squamous differentiation, and keratin pearls (202). As would be expected, the typical epithelial component of a thymoma expresses epithelium-associated antigens, including cytokeratin and EMA. The lymphocytes in a typical thymoma express the markers of normal cortical thymocytes, medullary thymocytes, or mixtures. Immature thymocytes express CD1a, CD2, CD5, CD7, variable CD3, coexpress CD4 and CD8, and express TdT. The maturation patterns of marker expression, best observed by flow cytometry, can be very helpful and reassuring to rule out lymphoma, as is the use of epithelial markers, which would be negative in lymphoblastic lymphoma.

Thymic carcinomas represent 5% to 15% of all thymic neoplasms. In contrast to thymoma, thymic carcinoma shows cytologically malignant epithelial cells with nuclear prominence, increased mitotic activity, and areas of necrosis. Thymic carcinomas can present with squamous cell, basaloid, adenosquamous, small-cell, clear cell, sarcomatoid, and anaplastic large-cell features. Significant numbers of immature intraepithelial thymocytes are lacking. Thymic carcinoma is usually indistinguishable from a carcinoma observed elsewhere (203). These malignant lesions are more likely to invade and metastasize.

Thymic carcinoma is very rare in children. In a current literature review by Yaris et al., only 14 cases of thymic carcinoma in patients younger than 18-year old were reported. In this series of children, the median age was 13 years and there was a male predominance. Although myasthenia gravis is frequently associated with thymoma, myasthenia gravis and other paraneoplastic disorders are rarely associated with thymic carcinomas (204,205). Dehner et al. reported that the mortality for children with thymoma is much higher than that for adults (206). In this series, only 3 of 11 children survived for 6 months after diagnosis.

A number of the diseases associated with thymomas are similar to those associated with thymic hyperplasia, and they resolve following removal of the mass. Both thymic hyperplasia and thymomas are associated with numerous autoimmune diseases: myasthenia gravis, hypogammaglobulinemia, polymyositis, SLE, Hashimoto thyroiditis, and a variety of cytopenias, including pure red cell aplasia. A recent study reports the case of a 7-year-old child with a thymoma. The child presented with facial muscle weakness without ophthalmoplegia or ptosis. The patient had a thymoma. Following thymic resection, the patient became asymptomatic (207). Of the patients reported by Dehner et al., three presented with signs of superior vena cava syndrome (206). Thymomas or thymic carcinomas outside the thorax are seen in children when metastasis to the lungs, bone, liver, and lymph nodes has occurred.

Lymphomas

Hodgkin and NHLs account for approximately one-third of all childhood cancers, and lymphomas are the third most common group of cancers in children. Of all the tumors that occur in the mediastinum, lymphomas (Hodgkin and non-Hodgkin) represent the second most common malignancy. Although any lymphoma may present in the mediastinum, only three are encountered with any significant frequency: NSHL, T lymphoblastic lymphoma (Figure 23-30), and

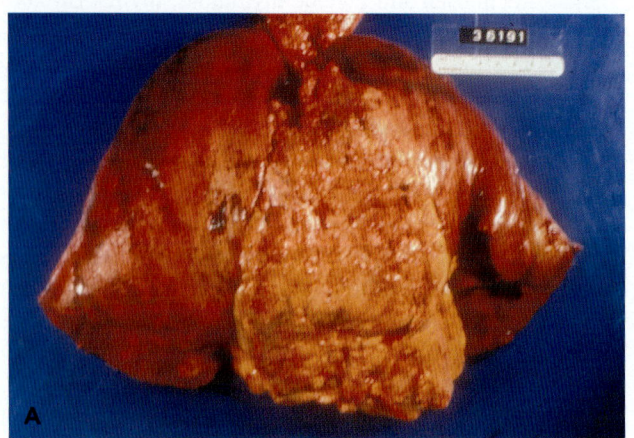 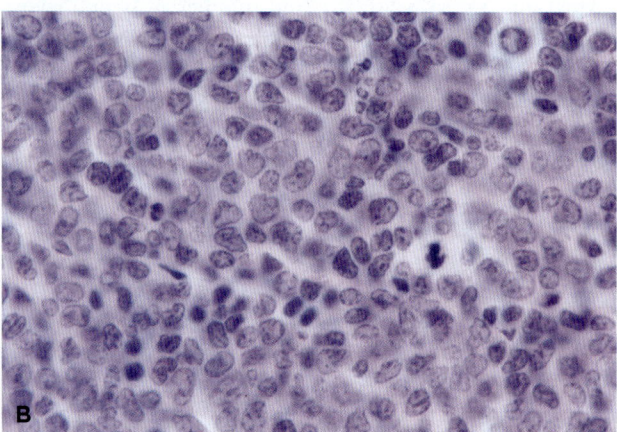

FIGURE 23-30 • **A:** T lymphoblastic lymphoma results in massive enlargement of the thymus. **B:** T lymphoblastic lymphoma effaces the normal thymic architecture with sheets of uniform malignant lymphoid small- to medium-sized lymphocytes with very scant cytoplasm, irregular, convoluted, and inconspicuous nuclei. (Hematoxylin and eosin stain, original magnification 40× magnification.)

PMBCL. The WHO classification of lymphoma, with particular attention to the specific entities that more commonly occur in children, has been discussed in detail earlier in the Lymph Node section and therefore discussion of HL and T lymphoblastic lymphoma will not be repeated here.

PMBCL is a tumor that derives from a thymic B-cell of germinal center or postgerminal center origin. Although the morphology and immunophenotype overlap with other types of DLBCLs, there are unique clinical, immunophenotypic, and molecular genetic features that merit its characterization as a unique clinicopathologic entity. PMBCL usually presents in adolescents or young adults with a large anterior mediastinal mass. Symptoms due to the mass lesion, such as superior vena cava syndrome, are common. There is a female predominance. The lymphoma usually remains localized to the mediastinum but may invade adjacent structures or the chest wall. Nodal or bone marrow involvement is uncommon. PMBCL may spread more extensively at relapse but tends to involve other extranodal sites rather than lymph nodes. Histologic sections show sheets of medium to large lymphoid cells with clear cytoplasm. Some may be multinucleated or mimic Hodgkin/Reed-Sternberg cells. Fine compartmentalizing reticular fibrosis is common, which can be accentuated using a reticulin stain. These lymphomas express CD45 and pan B-cell markers (CD19, CD20, CD79a, PAX-5, Oct2, BOB.1) but not surface immunoglobulin. CD30 is commonly expressed but is usually weaker or more focal than in NSHL. CD15 is negative. Expression of BCL2 and BCL6 is common, but genetic rearrangements are rare. CD10 expression is uncommon. Unlike other types of DLBCL, PMBCL more commonly expresses CD200, CD23, MAL, TRAF, and REL (208,209). Molecular genetic studies using gene expression profiling, whole genome, or whole transcriptome sequencing have shown a closer genetic relationship between PMBCL and NSHL than between PMBCL and other DLBCL (210,211). Some patients may have both PBCML and NSHL presenting at the same time or may present with one and relapse or recur with the other. Gray-zone lymphomas with features intermediate between PMBCL and NSHL are well recognized and suggest that these lymphomas may arise from a common thymic B-cell precursor.

References

1. Janeway CA, Travers P, Walport M, et al. The generation of lymphocyte antigen receptors. In: *Immunobiology*. London, UK: Taylor & Francis; 2004:136–164.
2. Kuppers R, Klein U, Hansmann ML, et al. Cellular origin of human B-cell lymphomas. *N Engl J Med* 1999;341(20):1520–1529.
3. Campo E, Jaffe JS, Harris NL. Normal lymphoid organs and tissues. In: Jaffe ES, ed. *Hematopathology*. Philadelphia, PA: Saunders, an imprint of Elsevier Inc; 2011:97–119.
4. Slap GB, Brooks JS, Schwartz JS. When to perform biopsies of enlarged peripheral lymph nodes in young patients. *JAMA* 1984;252(10):1321–1326.
5. Soldes OS, Younger JG, Hirschl RB. Predictors of malignancy in childhood peripheral lymphadenopathy. *J Pediatr Surg* 1999;34:1447–1452.
6. Twist CJ, Link MP. Assessment of lymphadenopathy in children. *Pediatr Clin N Am* 2002;49:1009–1025.
7. Dunphy CH. Applications of flow cytometry and immunohistochemistry to diagnostic hematopathology. *Arch Pathol Lab Med* 2004;128(9):1004–1022.
8. Coventry S, Punnett HH, Tomczak EZ, et al. Consistency of isochromosome 7q and trisomy 8 in hepatosplenic gammadelta T-cell lymphoma: detection by fluorescence In situ hybridization of a splenic touch-preparation from a pediatric patient. *Pediatr Dev Pathol* 1999;2(5):478–483.
9. Kinney MC, Kadin ME. The pathologic and clinical spectrum of anaplastic large cell lymphoma and correlation with ALK gene dysregulation. *Am J Clin Pathol* 1999;111(1 Suppl 1):S56–S67.
10. Green E, McConville CM, Powell JE, et al. Clonal diversity of Ig and T-cell-receptor gene rearrangements identifies a subset of childhood B-precursor acute lymphoblastic leukemia with increased risk of relapse. *Blood* 1998;92(3):952–958.
11. Antillon F, Behm FG, Raimondi SC, et al. Pediatric primary diffuse large cell lymphoma of bone with t(3;22)(q27;q11). *J Pediatr Hematol Oncol* 1998;20(6):552–555.
12. Kramer MH, Hermans J, Wijburg E, et al. Clinical relevance of BCL2, BCL6, and MYC rearrangements in diffuse large B-cell lymphoma. *Blood* 1998;92(9):3152–3162.
13. Buno I, Nava P, Alvarez-Doval A, et al. Lymphoma associated chromosomal abnormalities can easily be detected by FISH on tissue imprints: an underused diagnostic alternative. *J Clin Pathol* 2005;58(6):629–633.
14. Cook JR. Paraffin section interphase fluorescence in situ hybridization in the diagnosis and classification of non-Hodgkin lymphomas. *Diagn Mol Pathol* 2004;13(4):197–206.
15. Agrawal R, Wang J. Pediatric follicular lymphoma: a rare clinicopathologic entity. *Arch Pathol Lab Med* 2009;133:142–146.
16. Baroni CD, Uccini S. The lymphadenopathy of HIV infection. *Am J Clin Pathol* 1993;99(4):397–401.
17. Ioachim HL, Cronin W, Roy M, et al. Persistent lymphadenopathies in people at high risk for HIV infection. Clinicopathologic correlations and long-term follow-up in 79 cases. *Am J Clin Pathol* 1990;93(2):208–218.
18. Chadburn A, Metroka C, Mouradian J. Progressive lymph node histology and its prognostic value in patients with acquired immunodeficiency syndrome and AIDS-related complex. *Hum Pathol* 1989;20(6):579–587.
19. Ioachim HL, Lerner CW, Tapper ML. The lymphoid lesions associated with the acquired immunodeficiency syndrome. *Am J Surg Pathol* 1983;7(6):543–553.
20. O'Murchadha MT, Wolf BC, Neiman RS. The histologic features of hyperplastic lymphadenopathy in AIDS-related complex are nonspecific. *Am J Surg Pathol* 1987;11(2):94–99.
21. Nguyen PL, Ferry JA, Harris NL. Progressive transformation of germinal centers and nodular lymphocyte predominance Hodgkin lymphoma: a comparative immunohistochemical study. *Am J Surg Pathol* 1999;23(1):27–33.
22. Shaikh F, Ngan BY, Alexander S, et al. Progressive transformation of germinal centers in children and adolescents: an intriguing cause of lymphadenopathy. *Pediatr Blood Cancer* 2013;60(1):26–30.
23. Ferry JA, Zukerberg LR, Harris NL. Florid progressive transformation of germinal centers. A syndrome affecting young men, without early progression to nodular lymphocyte predominance Hodgkin's disease. *Am J Surg Pathol* 1992;16(3):252–258.
24. Osborne BM, Butler JJ. Clinical implications of progressive transformation of germinal centers. *Am J Surg Pathol* 1984;8(10):725–733.
25. Osborne BM, Butler JJ, Gresik MV. Progressive transformation of germinal centers: comparison of 23 pediatric patients to the adult population. *Mod Pathol* 1992;5:135–140.
26. Eapen M, Mathew CF, Aravindan KP. Evidence based criteria for the histopathological diagnosis of toxoplasmic lymphadenopathy. *J Clin Pathol* 2005;58(11):1143–1146.
27. Lin MH, Kuo TT. Specificity of the histopathological triad for the diagnosis of toxoplasmic lymphadenitis: polymerase chain reaction study. *Pathol Int* 2001;51(8):619–623.
28. Ramsay AD. Reactive lymph nodes in pediatric practice. *Am J Clin Pathol* 2004;122(Suppl 1):S87–S97.

29. Cronin DM, Warnke RA. Castleman disease: an update on classification and the spectrum of associated lesions. *Adv Anat Pathol* 2009;16:236–246.
30. Talat N, Schulte KM. Castleman's disease: systemic analysis of 416 patients from the literature. *Oncologist* 2011;16:1316–1324.
31. Baserga M, Rosin M, Schoen M, et al. Multifocal Castleman disease in pediatrics: case report. *J Pediatr Hematol Oncol* 2005;26:666–669.
32. Karapinar TH, Tufekci O, Gozmen S, et al. Multicentric plasma cell type of Castleman disease in a child: difficulty in diagnosis and treatment. *J Pediatr Hematol Oncol* 2013;35(7):e306–e308.
33. Parez N, Pader-Meunier B, Roy CC, et al. Pediatric Castleman disease: report of seven cases and review of the literature. *Eur J Pediatr* 1999;158:631–637.
34. Smir BN, Greiner TC, Weisenburger DD. Multicentric angiofollicular lymph node hyperplasia in children: a clinicopathologic study of eight patients. *Mod Pathol* 1996;9:1135–1142.
35. Leroy S, Moshous D, Cassar O, et al. Multicentric Castleman disease in an HHV-8-infected child born to consanguineous parents. *Pediatrics* 2012;129:e199–e203.
36. Anagnostopoulos I, Hummel M, Falini B, et al. Epstein-Barr virus infection of monocytoid B-cell proliferates: an early feature of primary viral infection? *Am J Surg Pathol* 2005;29(5):595–601.
37. Niedobitek G, Hamilton-Dutoit S, Herbst H, et al. Identification of Epstein-Barr virus-infected cells in tonsils of acute infectious mononucleosis by in situ hybridization. *Hum Pathol* 1989;20(8):796–799.
38. Villa D, Skinnider B. Herpes simplex virus lymphadenitis. *Blood* 2014:123(1):12.
39. Ovallath S, Remya RK, Kumar C, et al. Granulomatous lymphadenopathy secondary to phenytoin therapy. *Seizure* 2013;22(3):240–241.
40. Ree HJ, Kadin ME, Kikuchi M, et al. Angioimmunoblastic lymphoma (AILD-type T-cell lymphoma) with hyperplastic germinal centers. *Am J Surg Pathol* 1998;22(6):643–655.
41. Kim YM, Lee YJ, Nam SO, et al. Hemophagocytic syndrome associated with Kikuchi's disease. *J Korean Med Sci* 2003;18(4):592–594.
42. Kojima M, Nakamura S, Morishita Y, et al. Reactive follicular hyperplasia in the lymph node lesions from systemic lupus erythematosus patients: a clinicopathological and immunohistological study of 21 cases. *Pathol Int* 2000;50(4):304–312.
43. Smith LW, Petri M. Diffuse lymphadenopathy as the presenting manifestation of systemic lupus erythematosus. *J Clin Rheumatol* 2013;19(7):397–399.
44. Fox R, Rosahn P. The lymph nodes in disseminated lupus erythematosus. *Am J Pathol* 1943;19:70–100.
45. Shrestha D, Dhakal AK, Shiva RK, et al. Systemic lupus erythematosus and granulomatous lymphadenopathy. *BMC Pediatr* 2013;13:179. doi: 10.1186/1471-2431-13-179.
46. Yoo IH, Na H, Bae EY, et al. Recurrent lymphadenopathy in children with Kikuchi-Fujimoto disease. *Eur J Pediatr* 2014;173:1193–1199.
47. Lin C-W, Liu T-Y, Lin C-J, et al. Oligoclonal T cells in histiocytic necrotizing lymphadenopathy are associated with TLR$_9^+$ plasmacytoid dendritic cells. *Lab Invest* 2004;85:267–275.
48. Hu S, Kuo T-t, Hong H-S. Lupus lymphadenitis simulating Kikuchi's lymphadenitis in patients with systemic lupus erythematosus: a clinicopathological analysis of six cases and review of the literature. *Pathol Int* 2003;54(4):221.
49. Canale VC, Smith CH. Chronic lymphadenopathy simulating malignant lymphoma. *J Pediatr* 1967;70(6):891–899.
50. Drappa J, Vaishnaw AK, Sullivan KE, et al. Fas gene mutations in the Canale-Smith syndrome, an inherited lymphoproliferative disorder associated with autoimmunity. *N Engl J Med* 1996;335(22):1643–1649.
51. Price S, Shaw PA, Seitz A, et al. Natural history of autoimmune lymphoproliferative syndrome associated with FAS gene mutations. *Blood* 2014;123(13):1989–1999.
52. Lim MS, Straus SE, Dale JK, et al. Pathological findings in human autoimmune lymphoproliferative syndrome. *Am J Pathol* 1998;153(5):1541–1550.
53. Maric I, Pittaluga S, Dale JK, et al. Histologic features of sinus histiocytosis with massive lymphadenopathy in patients with autoimmune lymphoproliferative syndrome. *Am J Surg Pathol* 2005;29(7):903–911.
54. Müllauer L, Emhofer J, Wohlfart S, et al. Autoimmune lymphoproliferative syndrome (ALPS) caused by Fas (CD95) mutation mimicking sarcoidosis. *Am J Surg Pathol* 2008;32(2):329–334.
55. Kraus MD, Shenoy S, Chatila T, et al. Light microscopic, immunophenotypic, and molecular genetic study of autoimmune lymphoproliferative syndrome caused by fas mutation. *Pediatr Dev Pathol* 2000;3(1):101–109.
56. Wang J, Zheng L, Lobito A, et al. Inherited human Caspase 10 mutations underlie defective lymphocyte and dendritic cell apoptosis in autoimmune lymphoproliferative syndrome type II. *Cell* 1999;98(1):47–58.
57. Zangwill KM. Cat scratch disease and other Bartonella infections. *Adv Exp Med Biol* 2013;764:159–166.
58. Shin OR, Kim YR, Ban TH, et al. A case report of seronegative cat scratch disease, emphasizing the histopathologic point of view. *Diagn Pathol* 2014;9:62. doi: 10.1186/1746-1596-9-62.
59. Kojima M, Morita Y, Shimizu K, et al. Immunohistological findings of suppurative granulomas of Yersinia enterocolitica appendicitis: a report of two cases. *Pathol Res Pract* 2007;203(2):115–119. Epub 2006 Dec 26.
60. Lamps LW, Havens JM, Sjostedt A, et al. Histologic and molecular diagnosis of tularemia: a potential bioterrorism agent endemic to North America. *Mod Pathol* 2004;17(5):489–495.
61. Pahwa R, Hedau S, Jain S, et al. Assessment of possible tuberculous lymphadenopathy by PCR compared to non-molecular methods. *J Med Microbiol* 2005;54:873–878.
62. Albright JT, Pransky SM. Nontuberculous mycobacterial infections of the head and neck. *Pediatr Clin North Am* 2003;50(2):503–514.
63. Jarzembowski JA, Young MB. Nontuberculous mycobacterial infections. *Arch Pathol Lab Med* 2008;132(8):1333–1341.
64. Tang YW, Procop GW, Zheng X, et al. Histologic parameters predictive of mycobacterial infection. *Am J Clin Pathol* 1998;109(3):331–334.
65. Cheng AG, Chang A, Farwell DG, et al. Auramine orange stain with fluorescence microscopy is a rapid and sensitive technique for the detection of cervical lymphadenitis due to mycobacterial infection using fine needle aspiration cytology: a case series. *Otolaryngol Head Neck Surg* 2005;133(3):381–385.
66. Mustafa T, Wiker HG, Mfinanga SG, et al. Immunohistochemistry using a *Mycobacterium tuberculosis* complex specific antibody for improved diagnosis of tuberculous lymphadenitis. *Mod Pathol* 2006;19(12):1606–1614.
67. Purohit MR, Mustafa T, Wiker HG, et al. Immunohistochemical diagnosis of abdominal and lymph node tuberculosis by detecting *Mycobacterium tuberculosis* complex specific antigen MPT64. *Diagn Pathol* 2007;2:36.
68. Baek CH, Kim SI, Ko YH, et al. Polymerase chain reaction detection of *Mycobacterium tuberculosis* from fine-needle aspirate for the diagnosis of cervical tuberculous lymphadenitis. *Laryngoscope* 2000;110(1):30–34.
69. Bruijnesteijn Van Coppenraet ES, Lindeboom JA, Prins JM, et al. Real-time PCR assay using fine-needle aspirates and tissue biopsy specimens for rapid diagnosis of mycobacterial lymphadenitis in children. *J Clin Microbiol* 2004;42(6):2644–2650.
70. Patzina RA, de Andrade HF Jr, de Brito T, et al. Molecular and standard approaches to the diagnosis of mycobacterial granulomatous lymphadenitis in paraffin-embedded tissue. *Lab Invest* 2002;82(8):1095–1097.
71. Purohit MR, Mustafa T, Sviland L. Detection of *Mycobacterium tuberculosis* by polymerase chain reaction with DNA eluted from aspirate smears of tuberculous lymphadenitis. *Diagn Mol Pathol* 2008;17(3):174–178.
72. Vago L, Barberis M, Gori A, et al. Nested polymerase chain reaction for *Mycobacterium tuberculosis* IS6110 sequence on formalin-fixed paraffin-embedded tissues with granulomatous diseases for rapid diagnosis of tuberculosis. *Am J Clin Pathol* 1998;109(4):411–415.
73. Seger RA. Modern management of chronic granulomatous disease. *Br J Haematol* 2008;140(3):255–266.
74. Stasia MJ, Li XJ. Genetics and immunopathology of chronic granulomatous disease. *Semin Immunopathol* 2008;30(3):209–235.
75. Moore SW, Schneider JW, Schaaf HS. Diagnostic aspects of cervical lymphadenopathy in children in the developing world: a study of 1,877 surgical specimens. *Pediatr Surg Int* 2003;19(4):240–244.
76. Shetty AK, Gedalia A. Childhood sarcoidosis: a rare but fascinating disorder. *Pediatr Rheumatol Online J* 2008;6:16.

77. Miyara M, Amoura Z, Parizot C, et al. The immune paradox of sarcoidosis and regulatory T cells. *J Exp Med* 2006;203(2):359–370.
78. Taflin C, Miyara M, Nochy D, et al. FoxP3+ regulatory T cells suppress early stages of granuloma formation but have little impact on sarcoidosis lesions. *Am J Pathol* 2009;174(2):497–508.
79. Corapcioglu F, Basar EZ, Demirel A, et al. Granulomatous reaction in mediastinal B-cell non-Hodgkin lymphoma and intracardiac thrombosis. *Pediatr Hematol Oncol* 2008;25(3):217–226.
80. De Petris G, Lev R, Siew S. Peritumoral and nodal muciphages. *Am J Surg Pathol* 1998;22(5):545–549.
81. Rosai J, Dorfman RF. Sinus histiocytosis with massive lymphadenopathy. A newly recognized benign clinicopathological entity. *Arch Pathol* 1969;87(1):63–70.
82. Das DK, Gulati A, Bhatt NC, et al. Sinus histiocytosis with massive lymphadenopathy (Rosai-Dorfman disease): report of two cases with fine-needle aspiration cytology. *Diagn Cytopathol* 2001;24(1):42–45.
83. Deshpande AH, Nayak S, Munshi MM. Cytology of sinus histiocytosis with massive lymphadenopathy (Rosai-Dorfman disease). *Diagn Cytopathol* 2000;22(3):181–185.
84. Kumar B, Karki S, Paudyal P. Diagnosis of sinus histiocytosis with massive lymphadenopathy (Rosai-Dorfman disease) by fine needle aspiration cytology. *Diagn Cytopathol* 2008;36(10):691–695.
85. Ruggiero A, Attina G, Maurizi P, et al. Rosai-Dorfman disease: two case reports and diagnostic role of fine-needle aspiration cytology. *J Pediatr Hematol Oncol* 2006;28(2):103–106.
86. Bernacer-Borja M, Blanco-Rodriguez M, Sanchez-Granados JM, et al. Sinus histiocytosis with massive lymphadenopathy (Rosai-Dorfman disease): clinico-pathological study of three cases. *Eur J Pediatr* 2006;165(8):536–539.
87. Ambati S, Chamyan G, Restrepo R, et al. Rosai-Dorfman disease following bone marrow transplantation for pre-B cell acute lymphoblastic leukemia. *Pediatr Blood Cancer* 2008;51(3):433–435.
88. Lu D, Estalilla OC, Manning JT Jr, et al. Sinus histiocytosis with massive lymphadenopathy and malignant lymphoma involving the same lymph node: a report of four cases and review of the literature. *Mod Pathol* 2000;13(4):414–419.
89. Sachdev R, Shyama J. Co-existent Langerhans cell histiocytosis and Rosai-Dorfman disease: a diagnostic rarity. *Cytopathology* 2008;19(1):55–58.
90. Zhang X, Hyjek E, Vardiman J. A subset of Rosai-Dorfman disease exhibits features of IgG4-related disease. *Am J Clin Pathol* 2013;139(5):622–632.
91. Urban RM, Jacobs JJ, Tomlinson MJ, et al. Dissemination of wear particles to the liver, spleen, and abdominal lymph nodes of patients with hip or knee replacement. *J Bone Joint Surg Am* 2000;82(4):457–476.
92. Winter LK, Spiegel JH, King T. Dermatopathic lymphadenitis of the head and neck. *J Cutan Pathol* 2007;34(2):195–197.
93. Geissmann F, Dieu-Nosjean MC, Dezutter C, et al. Accumulation of immature Langerhans cells in human lymph nodes draining chronically inflamed skin. *J Exp Med* 2002;196(4):417–430.
94. Iyer VK, Kapila K, Verma K. Fine needle aspiration cytology of dermatopathic lymphadenitis. *Acta Cytol* 1998;42(6):1347–1351.
95. Imashuku S, Ueda I, Teramura T, et al. Occurrence of haemophagocytic lymphohistiocytosis at less than 1 year of age: analysis of 96 patients. *Eur J Pediatr* 2005;164(5):315–319.
96. Lin MT, Chang HM, Huang CJ, et al. Massive expansion of EBV+ monoclonal T cells with CD5 down regulation in EBV-associated haemophagocytic lymphohistiocytosis. *J Clin Pathol* 2007;60(1):101–103.
97. Filipovich AH. Hemophagocytic lymphohistiocytosis and related disorders. *Curr Opin Allergy Clin Immunol* 2006;6(6):410–415.
98. Lackner H, Urban C, Sovinz P, et al. Hemophagocytic lymphohistiocytosis as severe adverse event of antineoplastic treatment in children. *Haematologica* 2008;93(2):291–294.
99. Gerritsen A, Lam K, Marion Schneider E, et al. An exclusive case of juvenile myelomonocytic leukemia in association with Kikuchi's disease and hemophagocytic lymphohistiocytosis and a review of the literature. *Leuk Res* 2006;30(10):1299–1303.
100. Lim GY, Cho B, Chung NG. Hemophagocytic lymphohistiocytosis preceded by Kikuchi disease in children. *Pediatr Radiol* 2008;38(7):756–761.
101. Janka GE. Familial and acquired hemophagocytic lymphohistiocytosis. *Eur J Pediatr* 2007;166(2):95–109.
102. Henter JI, Horne A, Arico M, et al. HLH-2004: diagnostic and therapeutic guidelines for hemophagocytic lymphohistiocytosis. *Pediatr Blood Cancer* 2007;48(2):124–131.
103. Qian J, Yang CD. Hemophagocytic syndrome as one of main manifestations in untreated systemic lupus erythematosus: two case reports and literature review. *Clin Rheumatol* 2007;26(5):807–810.
104. Dierberg KL, Dumler JS. Lymph node hemophagocytosis in rickettsial diseases: a pathogenetic role for CD8 T lymphocytes in human monocytic ehrlichiosis (HME)? *BMC Infect Dis* 2006;6:121.
105. Silva-Herzog E, Detweiler CS. Intracellular microbes and haemophagocytosis. *Cell Microbiol* 2008;10(11):2151–2158.
106. Menasce LP, Banerjee SS, Beckett E, et al. Extra-medullary myeloid tumour (granulocytic sarcoma) is often misdiagnosed: a study of 26 cases. *Histopathology* 1999;34(5):391–398.
107. Shin HT, Harris MB, Orlow SJ. Juvenile myelomonocytic leukemia presenting with features of hemophagocytic lymphohistiocytosis in association with neurofibromatosis and juvenile xanthogranulomas. *J Pediatr Hematol Oncol* 2004;26(9):591–595.
108. Sevilla DW, Choi JK, Gong JZ. Mediastinal adenopathy, lung infiltrates, and hemophagocytosis: unusual manifestation of pediatric anaplastic large cell lymphoma: report of two cases. *Am J Clin Pathol* 2007;127(3):458–464.
109. Shimada A, Kato M, Tamura K, et al. Hemophagocytic lymphohistiocytosis associated with uncontrolled inflammatory cytokinemia and chemokinemia was caused by systemic anaplastic large cell lymphoma: a case report and review of the literature. *J Pediatr Hematol Oncol* 2008;30(10):785–787.
110. Favara BE, Jaffe R, Egeler RM. Macrophage activation and hemophagocytic syndrome in Langerhans cell histiocytosis: report of 30 cases. *Pediatr Dev Pathol* 2002;5(2):130–140.
111. Rodig SJ, Payne EG, Degar BA, et al. Aggressive Langerhans cell histiocytosis following T-ALL: clonally related neoplasms with persistent expression of constitutively active NOTCH1. *Am J Hematol* 2008;83(2):116–121.
112. Trebo MM, Attarbaschi A, Mann G, et al. Histiocytosis following T-acute lymphoblastic leukemia: a BFM study. *Leuk Lymphoma* 2005;46(12):1735–1741.
113. Narula G, Bhagwat R, Arora B, et al. Clinico-biologic profile of Langerhans cell histiocytosis: a single institutional study. *Indian J Cancer* 2007;44(3):93–98.
114. Satter EK, High WA. Langerhans cell histiocytosis: a review of the current recommendations of the Histiocyte Society. *Pediatr Dermatol* 2008;25(3):291–295.
115. Edelweiss M, Medeiros LJ, Suster S, et al. Lymph node involvement by Langerhans cell histiocytosis: a clinicopathologic and immunohistochemical study of 20 cases. *Hum Pathol* 2007;38(10):1463–1469.
116. Chikwava K, Jaffe R. Langerin (CD207) staining in normal pediatric tissues, reactive lymph nodes, and childhood histiocytic disorders. *Pediatr Dev Pathol* 2004;7(6):607–614.
117. Lau SK, Chu PG, Weiss LM. Immunohistochemical expression of Langerin in Langerhans cell histiocytosis and non-Langerhans cell histiocytic disorders. *Am J Surg Pathol* 2008;32(4):615–619.
118. Brown NA, Furtado LV, Betz BL, et al. High prevalence of somatic MAP2K1 mutations in BRAF V600E negative Langerhans cell histiocytosis. *Blood* 2014;124(10):1655–1658.
119. Harris NL, Jaffe ES, Stein H, et al. Tumours of haematopoietic and lymphoid tissues: introduction. In: Jaffe ES, Harris NL, Stein H, et al., ed. *World Health Organization Classification of Tumours Pathology and Genetics.* Lyon, France: IRAC Press; 2001:12–13.
120. Reaman GH, Sposto R, Sensel MG, et al. Treatment outcome and prognostic factors for infants with acute lymphoblastic leukemia treated on two consecutive trials of the Children's Cancer Group. *J Clin Oncol* 1999;17(2):445–455.
121. Ozdemirli M, Fanburg-Smith JC, Hartmann DP, et al. Precursor B-Lymphoblastic lymphoma presenting as a solitary bone tumor and mimicking Ewing's sarcoma: a report of four cases and review of the literature. *Am J Surg Pathol* 1998;22(7):795–804.

CHAPTER 24

The Bone Marrow

Xiangdong Xu, M.D., Ph.D., and Anjum Hassan, M.D.

Acute lymphoblastic leukemia (ALL) is the most common malignancy in children and classically presents with pancytopenia, bleeding, and signs of anemia or infection. Characterized by an almost complete loss of normal hematopoietic elements, this disease tragically illustrates the fragility of the otherwise harmonically orchestrated "fluid–organ," the bone marrow. Ultimately forming approximately 3% to 6% of the total body weight and reconstructing the peripheral blood throughout life, this organ undergoes a fascinating embryologic development. From midfetal development on and extending throughout life, the bone marrow is the site of origin of peripheral blood hematopoietic elements, specialized dendritic cells of monocyte–macrophage lineage, mast cells lymphocytes, natural killer (NK) cells, platelets, and osteoclasts (1). At this point, we know that the potency of some of the stem cells extends beyond this spectrum and through bone marrow mesenchymal stem cells; the bone marrow also contributes to endothelial cells, adipocytes, fibroblasts, osteoblasts, myofibroblasts, and reticular cells.

DEVELOPMENT

Mesenchymal-derived primitive erythroblasts in the yolk sac are the earliest signs of hematopoiesis in the embryo at a crown rump length of 95 mm (2). While the presence of lymphoid elements in the yolk sac is controversial, it has been shown that the aorta (aorta-gonad-mesonephros [AGM]) (3) and the placenta contribute in this earliest phase to the lymphomyeloid stem cell pool (4,5). The proposed candidates for hematopoietic stem cells (HSCs) in the AGM express CD34, CD45, CD117 (c-kit), and the transcription factor *GATA-2* (6). The cells arising in the yolk sac show myeloid restriction (7). At weeks 10 to 24, the liver is the primary hematopoietic organ with production of red cells, granulocytes, and megakaryocytes in the primitive sinusoids. At this time, the spleen also contributes with approximately 20% to hematopoiesis. Slowly, the production within the bone marrow takes over, and at 4 to 5 months, it becomes the primary site of hematopoiesis. Typically by term, liver and spleen show minimal myelopoiesis. This switch is often referred to as *embryo-to-fetal-to-adult-type hematopoieses* (8). The development of the bone marrow continues in a topographically organized fashion. Hematopoiesis changes from the axial and radial skeleton (newborns) to the flat bones of the central skeleton by 12 to 16 years. Microscopically, the bone marrow is an inhomogeneous organ, which is often illustrated by higher cellularity within deeper areas of the medullary cavity than in subcortical zones. Due to the relatively short lifespan of peripheral blood elements, the production rates within the bone marrow are astronomic (9). The turnaround time of neutrophils (approximately 2 hours) requires the production of approximately 700,000 cells per second to maintain the normal value of 5000/μL; exponentially higher values are needed in neutrophilia or sepsis, illustrating the dynamics of this system.

Significant age-related normal variations are seen in overall bone marrow cellularity with approximately 80% cellularity until 9 years, approximately 50% until 70 years, and less than 30% beyond. Relative proportions of various cell types also change. Hematopoiesis is a developmental continuum of HSCs and progenitor cells, which are very rare in normal bone marrow accounting for less than 0.001% of nucleated cells (Table 24-1). It is an exquisitely regulated, dynamic, and highly complicated system that involves complex interaction with diverse bone marrow microenvironment, coordinated expression of many genes, progressive loss of proliferative capacity, differentiation commitment, and maturation with specific biochemical, functional, and morphologic features (10,11).

BONE MARROW STRUCTURE

Encased and protected by cortical bone, traversed and supported by trabecular bone, the bone marrow consists of a highly organized thin-walled capillary network, venous sinuses, and surrounding extracellular matrix. The capillary–venous

TABLE 24-1	GENERAL FEATURES OF THE BONE MARROW AND HEMATOPOIESIS

- Microenvironment with regulatory factors for stem/progenitor cells and structural support via stromal framework and surrounding liquid matrix
- Stem/progenitor cells localize to specific niches based on complementary adhesion molecule expression between hematopoietic cells, microenvironment, and stromal cells
- Stem/progenitor cell proliferation and maturation under exquisite regulatory control; regulated "cross talk" between stromal cells and hematopoietic cells maintains steady state.
- Stimulatory and suppressive factors within microenvironmental matrix; regulatory factors consist of CSFs, ILs, and inhibitory cytokines.
- Stem cells[a] are capable of self-renewal and multilineage differentiation.
- Committed progenitor cells[a] are destined to a specific lineage.

[a]Not morphologically distinct.

sinuses, which result from bifurcations of the nutrient or medullary arteries, are the basic structural unit of the bone marrow (12). Within this histologic compartment, HSC and progenitor cells are exposed to the extracellular matrix that comprises the bone marrow microenvironment (Figure 24-1). The outer adventitial reticular cells (ARCs) add connective tissue elements and form the outer sinusoidal wall and synthesize collagen, laminin, fibronectin, and proteoglycans. All regulatory factors, adhesion molecules, and other proteins necessary for the regulation of hematopoiesis are contained within this matrix (1,13). Furthermore, the ARCs are phagocytic and can become lipocytes. As outlined before, the fat/hematopoietic ratio ("marrow cellularity") is variable and a rough estimate can be calculated as cellularity = 100% − age (see below). Mitotically active cells are normally found around the supporting bone, typically paratrabecular and perivascular from where cells mature progressively into the medullary cavity. All newly formed mature hematopoietic cells are released into the bone marrow capillary–venous sinuses. Most cells pass through the sinus wall, but megakaryocytes reside adjacent to sinuses and extend pseudopodia directly into the vascular space (14,15). The capillary–venous sinuses coalesce into the venules and ultimately become veins that carry newly formed hematopoietic cells to the systemic circulation (12).

STEM CELLS AND PROGENITOR CELLS

HSC can be defined by their ability to regenerate long-term multilineage hematopoiesis in myeloablated recipients. Although not morphologically recognizable, stem cells can be detected by either functional features (the simultaneous capability of sustained self-renewal and multilineage differentiation potential) or immunophenotype ($CD34^+$, $Thyr-1^+$, $c-kit^+$, $CD38^-$, cytokine receptor, and adhesion molecule expression) (1,16) (Figure 24-2). HSCs are estimated to constitute 1 in 10^4 nucleated marrow cells. In contrast, progenitor cells are progressed stem cells with lineage commitment. The process of lineage commitment is incompletely understood; however, the resulting committed stem/progenitor cells are also morphologically unrecognizable but immunophenotypically defined by CD34, c-kit, and CD38 expression (16,17). Further, maturation is characterized by the acquisition of morphologic and immunophenotypic properties of the corresponding hematopoietic lineages. Both proliferation and lineage maturation are regulated by the synergistic

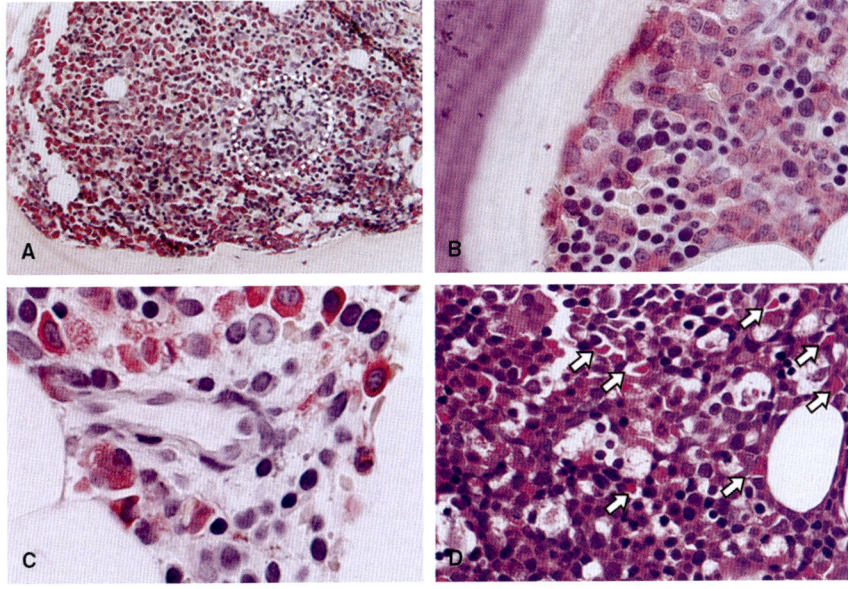

FIGURE 24-1 • Bone marrow microarchitecture. A: Bone marrow biopsy from a 1-day-old boy showing hematopoietic tissue that occupies approximately 90% of the marrow space. Only few regions of bone marrow fat are seen. The myeloid lineage is highlighted in red (Leder stain), and the *perivascular region* (*circle*) shows lack of myeloid cells. B: The *paratrabecular region* shows myeloid and erythroid precursors. C: Perivascular distribution of precursors in a bone marrow biopsy from an 18-year-old girl; note the delicate reticulum and extracellular matrix derived from *ARCs*. D: Highly cellular (>90%) bone marrow biopsy in a preterm girl shows numerous capillaries (*arrows*) interspersed between the hematopoietic cells and extracellular matrix.

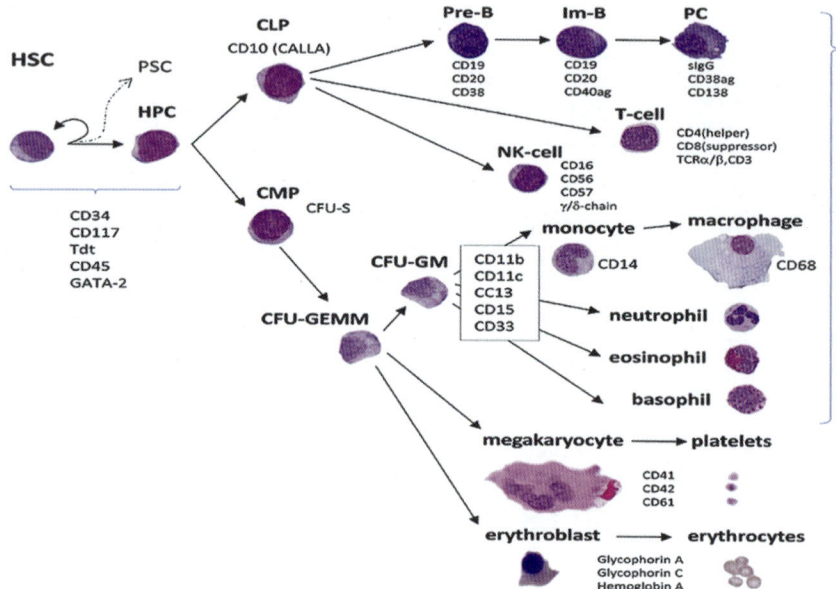

FIGURE 24-2 • Selected aspects of hematopoiesis. See text for details. CLP, committed lymphoid progenitor; CMP, committed myeloid progenitor (e.g., CFU-S: colony-forming unit—spleen); GEMM, granulo–erythro–megakaryo–monocytic; GM, granulo-monocytic (= myelomonocytic); HPC, hematopoietic progenitor committed; HSC, hematopoietic stem cell; Im-B, immature B-lymphocyte; PC, plasma cell; PSC, peripheral stem cell.

stimulatory activities of colony-stimulating factors (CSFs) and interleukins (ILs), whereas antagonistic effects are driven by inhibitory factors that include tumor necrosis factor (18,19). It is known that mature hematopoietic elements play a role in the regulation of lineage production and in maintaining steady-state hematopoiesis. In addition to the complicated molecular pathways, endocrine, paracrine, mesenchymal, and autonomic nervous system regulations have been implicated for homeostasis (18,19).

HEMATOPOIETIC LINEAGES

A detailed discussion of all hematopoietic lineages is beyond the scope of this chapter; however, some selected lineages are described below.

Granulopoiesis

The process of granulocytic maturation is characterized by a progressive nuclear segmentation, simultaneous decrease in the nuclear-to-cytoplasmic (N/C) ratio, as well as acquisition and increase of primary and later secondary cytoplasmic granules. The earliest morphologically recognizable cell in the granulocytic lineage is the myeloblast (20 μm; N/C ratio >85%); the subsequent arbitrary stages of this continuous maturation process include promyelocytes (the largest granulocytic cell), myelocytes, metamyelocytes, band neutrophils, and segmented neutrophils (Figure 24-3). The last maturation stage with a proliferative potential is a myelocyte. The key regulatory factors involved in granulopoiesis are granulocyte–macrophage colony–stimulating factor (GM-CSF), granulocyte colony-stimulating factor (G-CSF), and interleukin-3 (IL-3) (20). G-CSF is an 813 amino acid membrane protein that functions by binding to its specific cell surface receptor (G-CSFr) and activates cytoplasmic tyrosine kinases (21). Granulopoiesis is also under the control of retinoic acid receptors (RAR), which bind to all-trans retinoic acid (ATRA) and 9-cis-retinoic acid (21). The combination of four otherwise non–myeloid-restricted transcription factors is unique to the granulocyte lineage: C/EBPa (restricted to CD34+/CD33+ myeloid cells), PU.1 (Ets family member), CBF (AML1), and c-Myb (22–25). Other transcription factors (e.g., WT-1, Rb, and Hox) have also been implicated in granulopoiesis (25). Granulopoiesis occurs predominantly in paratrabecular and perivascular regions within the bone marrow (13). Thus, in normal bone marrow biopsy sections, immature granulocytic precursors selectively localize to the paratrabecular and, less conspicuously, the perivascular regions. This distribution may be altered after cytokine treatment, after chemotherapy, as well as after bone marrow transplantation (see below). Normal localization can be highlighted by immunoperoxidase staining for myeloperoxidase (MPO). Metamyelocytes, bands,

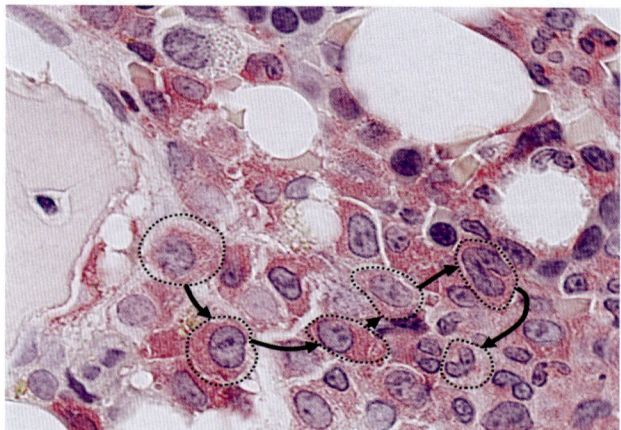

FIGURE 24-3 • Granulopoiesis. Immature granulocytic precursors (Leder positive) localize to the paratrabecular regions. Subsequent arbitrary stages are indicated (circles) and maturation progresses to, for example, band neutrophils.

and neutrophils comprise the largest maturation storage compartment of the bone marrow, which can be released into the peripheral blood in response to multiple host-mediated challenges.

Erythropoiesis

The earliest morphologically recognizable cell in the erythroid lineage is the erythroblast (normoblast). The subsequent maturation has been arbitrarily divided into the basophilic normoblast, polychromatophilic normoblast, orthochromic normoblast, reticulocyte, and mature erythrocyte stages (Figure 24-4). The maturational process is characterized by progressive nuclear condensation with ultimate extrusion of the pyknotic nucleus at the end of the orthochromic normoblastic stage, which results in the young erythrocyte (reticulocyte). Simultaneously, the cytoplasm gradually changes from a deeply basophilic, organelle-rich substance to one that consists almost entirely of hemoglobin. In addition to the general growth factors (GM-CSF, IL-3, and IL-11), the primary growth factor responsible for red blood cell (RBC) production is erythropoietin (EPO), a 30.4-kDa glycoprotein that induces proliferation and maturation of committed erythroid progenitor cells by binding to its specific cell receptor (R-EPO), which inhibits apoptosis and thereby regulates the rate of red cell production (26,27). EPO does not cross the placenta, and therefore, the fetus primarily controls erythropoiesis (27). Although erythroid and megakaryocytic lineages share several transcription factors such as *GATA-1* and *NF-E2* (28,29), specific growth factors act selectively and allow committed cells to differentiate and proliferate. Erythropoiesis occurs in small colonies (erythroblast islands), and even though related to vascular structures, they appear randomly dispersed throughout the hematopoietic cavity. They are neither paratrabecular nor perivascular in distribution (30). Erythroid architecture can be highlighted by immunohistochemistry utilizing E-cadherin, hemoglobin A, or glycophorin (Figure 24-4).

Megakaryopoiesis

Megakaryocytes are the largest nucleated cell (50 to 150 µm) in the bone marrow. Unlike the maturation of the other lineages, megakaryocyte maturation from the blast to the mature cell stage is not associated with mitotic divisions. Megakaryocyte differentiation occurs via endomitosis, resulting in increasing nuclear lobulations without cell division (31), controlled via thrombopoietin (TPO) (32,33). The earliest megakaryocyte precursor identified in cell culture studies is the promegakaryoblast. Subsequent maturational stages have been arbitrarily designated as megakaryoblast, basophilic megakaryocyte, granular megakaryocyte, and platelet-producing megakaryocyte. The maturational sequence is characterized by a progressive increase in the overall size, an increase in nuclear lobulations ($n = 8$, 16 or 32), without nucleoli, and the development of demarcation membranes and multiple types of (purple–red or pink) cytoplasmic granules. Megakaryocyte production is regulated by a variety of factors, including multilineage growth factors such as GM-CSF, stem cell factor, IL-3, IL-6, and lineage-selective factors such as IL-11 and TPO (32–34). TPO binds to c-Mpl and acts in synergy with other cytokines (see above, EPO, IFN-α, IFN-β) (35). Even though megakaryocytes appear randomly distributed in biopsy sections, they are localized selectively to the parasinusoidal regions within the bone marrow microanatomy. Megakaryocytes project pseudopodia into the vascular space, and proplatelets are directly released into the blood stream by this mechanism.

Monopoiesis and Dendritic Cell Development

Monocytes, the largest leukocyte (12 to 20 µm), are derived from the same precursor cells that give rise to neutrophils. Macrophage colony-stimulating factor (M-CSF) is instrumental in influencing the progenitor cells to differentiate into monocyte–macrophages (36). Gradual nuclear folding

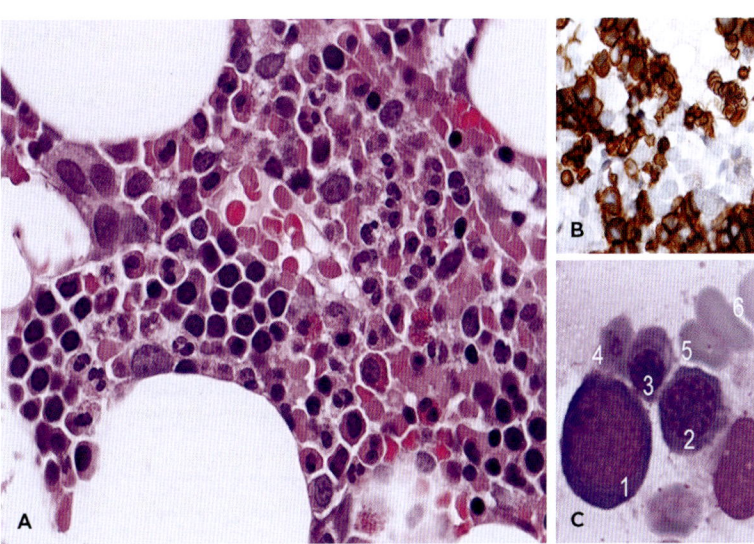

FIGURE 24-4 • **A:** Erythropoiesis occurs in small colonies (erythroblast islands) related to vascular structures. **B:** Glycophorin A; marker of erythroid differentiation. **C:** Subsequent stages of erythroid differentiation.

and the acquisition of cytoplasmic granules characterize the stages of maturation, designated as monoblast, promonocyte, and mature monocyte. Although characteristically, monocytes have fewer and smaller granules than neutrophils, neither monoblasts nor promonocytes are generally recognizable in normal bone marrow. Monocytes circulate in the blood and subsequently migrate to solid tissues and become macrophages or various types of immune accessory cells. Due to this accessory role and evidence that these cells play an integrated, multifaceted role in humoral and cellular immunity beyond simple phagocytosis, the former designation *mononuclear phagocyte system* (37) has been replaced. Foucar and Foucar (38) proposed the alternative name *mononuclear phagocyte and immunoregulatory effector* (M-PIRE) system as a more accurate descriptor. The M-PIRE system includes monocytes, macrophages, multiple dendritic cells (e.g., Langerhans and dendritic reticulum cells), and their bone marrow precursors. Some evidence suggests a common cell of origin (39). Because the constituent cells show unique immunophenotypic and functional properties, the M-PIRE designation remains controversial. Regardless of the name, both macrophages (histiocytes) and dendritic cells are inconspicuous normal constituents of virtually all organ systems, and mature cells of monocyte–macrophage lineage also remain as a major constituent of the bone marrow microenvironment.

Lymphopoiesis

T and B lymphocytes are derived from the same HSCs that give rise to all hematopoietic elements. Regulatory molecules known to influence B-cell proliferation, differentiation, and function include IL-1, IL-2, IL-4, IL-10, adhesion molecules, and IFN-γ. In comparison, regulatory factors of T-cell development and function include IL-1 through IL-9 (40). The bone marrow microenvironment serves as the "bursal equivalent" in humans and is the primary site of postnatal B-cell development, whereas T-cell precursors migrate from the marrow to the thymus for maturation and differentiation. Antigenetically mature T and B cells can proliferate in response to a variety of cytokines.

The stages of maturation of both B and T lymphocytes are generally defined by the surface antigen profile rather than by morphologic features (Figure 24-2). The earliest immunologically recognizable B cells express nuclear terminal deoxynucleotidyl transferase (TdT), surface CD34, CD79a, and HLA-DR; CD10 expression is variable but common (41,42). Further maturation is characterized by the acquisition of cytoplasmic mu heavy chain and, later, surface immunoglobulin. B-cell precursors are generally infrequent in normal bone marrow, although these immature cells are much more prominent in specimens from infants and young children. When they are abundant, the term *hematogones* has been applied to immature lymphocytes (see below).

T-cell maturation is characterized by the presence of cytoplasmic and, later, surface CD3 together with the expression of many other antigens associated with T cells (43). Terminal maturation is defined by the development of either a helper (CD4+) or a cytotoxic (CD8+) suppressor T cell.

Although the terms *lymphoblast* and *prolymphocyte* have been applied to developing lymphoid cells and are utilized in leukemia classification, the distinction is not easy in normal bone marrow specimens. Lymphocytes migrate from blood to specific tissue sites throughout the body, selectively homing to B- or T-cell regions of lymph node, spleen, and thymus, and to widespread extranodal regions. T lymphocytes are characteristically long-lived and periodically recirculate.

Development of Natural Killer Cells

NK cells are morphologically indistinguishable from CD8+ cytotoxic T cells, both of which are large granular lymphocytes. NK cells were initially defined by a functional activity, that is, major histocompatibility complex (MHC)-nonrestricted cytotoxicity (44). These cells were subsequently found to perform many other functions (43–45). Evidence suggests a common T/NK progenitor cell, and the thymus may be an additional site of NK-cell maturation.

On immunophenotype analysis, NK cells are defined by the expression of adhesion molecules such as CD56, CD57, and CD16. However, the expression of these adhesion molecules is not restricted to NK cells. The fact that true NK cells lack surface CD3 and CD8 expression facilitates their distinction from cytotoxic suppressor T cells.

Cells with NK activities (both cytotoxic suppressor T cells and true NK cells) are concentrated within the large granular lymphocyte population of peripheral blood. The mature cells have round nuclei, condensed chromatin, inconspicuous nucleoli, and moderate amount of pale blue cytoplasm that contains a small number of coarse, azurophilic granules. The granules contain cytolytic perforin and associated granule proteases (e.g., granzyme) essential for their cytolytic activity.

NORMAL HEMATOPOIETIC PARAMETERS

The peripheral blood and bone marrow profiles are characterized by prominent age-related physiologic variations (Table 24-2 and Table 24-3). As previously outlined, bone marrow cellularity decreases with age (46) and is classically best evaluated on biopsy sections or imprints. Particle sections are the next best choice, and aspirate smears may be difficult to evaluate; however, section imprints and aspiration smears are all reported as equally reliable (47). While earlier references specified 100% cellularity at birth, more recent studies show that bone marrow cellularity is somewhat lower than previously estimated (48); therefore, the percentage should be taken as a representative figure. The distribution of erythroid and lymphoid elements also varies by age, whereas the proportion of bone marrow devoted to granulopoiesis is

TABLE 24-2	NORMAL VALUES FOR BONE MARROW AND DIFFERENTIAL CELL COUNTS					
Parameter (Unit)	Cord Blood	Week 1	Week 4	1 Year	Child	Adult
Hemoglobin (g/dL)	16.5	17	14	12	13.5	M: 16 F: 14
Hematocrit (%)	53	54	43	37	40	M: 47 F: 41
RBC (×10^6/μL)	5.3	5	4	4.6	4.6	M: 5.2 F: 4.6
MCV (fL)	115	100	98	80	84	90
MCHC (g/dL)	32	33	33	34	34	34
Reticulocytes (% of RBC)	3-7	0-1	0	0-1	0-1	0-1
Nucleated RBC (per 100 WBC)	500	0	0	0	0	0
WBC (×10^9/L)	20	12	10	10	7	6
Absolute neutrophil count (×10^9/L)	13	5	4	4	3	3
Absolute lymphocyte count (×10^9/L)	5	5	6	6-8	4	3
Platelet count (×10^9/L)	290	250	250	250	250	250

Cell Type	Normal Range (%)	Cell Type	Normal Range (%)
Myeloblasts	0-3	Basophils and precursors	0-1
Promyelocytes	2-8	Monocytes	0-1
Myelocytes	10-13	Erythroblasts	0-2
Metamyelocytes	10-15	Other erythroid elements	10-25
Band/neutrophils	25-40	Lymphocytes	10-35
Eosinophils and precursors	1-3	Plasma cells	0-1

TABLE 24-3	HEMATOLOGIC PROFILE DURING THE FIRST MONTH OF LIFE AND IN YOUNG INFANTS

I. Term infants to 1 month
- Hgb and Hct drop from 16.5 g/dL and 53% at birth to 14 g/dL and 43% at 1 mo of age, respectively.
- MCV declines from 115 fL at birth to about 98 fL at 1 mo.
- Reticulocyte count drops from 5% to 7% at birth to ~0% at 1 mo.
- Nucleated RBCs are present at birth but disappear in the first week of life.
- Marked leukocytosis with neutrophilia is normal at birth and lymphocytes predominate by 1 mo.

II. Preterm infants
- Lower Hgb and Hct levels at birth than term neonates
- Higher MCV, more nucleated RBCs, and higher reticulocyte counts compared with term neonates
- More rapid and pronounced physiologic nadir
- Lower leukocyte counts than term neonates

III. Young infants
- Neonatal assessment complex because of dramatic physiologic variations in conjunction with potential maternal, familial, obstetric, and other fetal and neonatal factors
- Maternal factors: infections, medications, obstetrical complications, and underlying illnesses
- For example, maternal and paternal incompatibility for RBC antigens can result in hemolysis (hemolytic disease of the newborn).
- Numerous constitutional hereditary disorders of hematopoietic cell production and survival including:
  - Diamond-Blackfan anemia (red cell aplasia)
  - Thalassemias (hemoglobinopathy)
  - Congenital neutropenia (granulocyte aplasia)
  - Thrombocytopenia with absent radii (megakaryocyte aplasia)
- Constitutional disorders can manifest at birth or in early infancy.
- Fetomaternal hemorrhage or internal hemorrhage can produce neonatal anemia.
- Other causes include various congenital malformations and congenital neoplasms.

Hct, hematocrit; Hgb, hemoglobin; MCV, mean corpuscular volume.

TABLE 24-4 INDICATIONS FOR BONE MARROW EXAMINATION IN CHILDREN

- Peripheral blood abnormality (undetermined after regular workup)
- Evaluation of possible constitutional hematopoietic disorder
- Evaluation for leukemia, myelodysplasia, myeloproliferative/myelodysplastic disorders, and myeloproliferative neoplasms
- Evaluation for fever of unknown origin, storage diseases, and unexplained splenomegaly
- Staging and management of patients with certain types of neoplasms (e.g., Hodgkin and non-Hodgkin lymphoma, various other solid tumors)
- Evaluation of patient with atypical but nondiagnostic lymphoreticular process in other sites
- Evaluation of patient who does not follow predicted course of initial diagnosis (e.g., patient with presumed idiopathic thrombocytopenic purpura who does not respond to therapy)
- Ongoing monitoring of response to therapy in patients with a variety of hematologic and lymphoreticular disorders
- Bone marrow assessment prior to autologous bone marrow transplantation

generally stable. A dramatic decline in erythroid elements parallels the drop in EPO levels that occurs after birth in full-term neonates (49). Erythropoiesis returns to normal steady-state levels following resolution of this so-called physiologic anemia of infancy. Likewise, dramatic age-related variations occur in the proportion of bone marrow lymphoid cells, with up to 40% lymphocytes in bone marrow specimens of very young children and infants (50). The proportion of lymphocytes decreases in bone marrow specimens, and B-cell production in general declines with age (51).

Age-related variations in peripheral blood values are well delineated (Table 24-4), and the most dramatic changes are found in erythrocyte, neutrophil, and lymphocyte parameters (52).

HEMATOLOGIC PROFILE OF THE NEONATE

The 1st month of life is characterized by remarkable physiologic changes in erythrocyte and white blood cell (WBC) parameters (Table 24-5), and these parameters vary between full-term and preterm neonates (52). In the full-term neonates, the hematocrit, mean corpuscular volume (MCV), RBC, and WBC counts are higher than those in later life. The neonatal period is also the only time when circulating erythroid precursors are physiologic. The nucleated RBCs are cleared rapidly from the blood and do not normally persist

TABLE 24-5 SPECIALIZED TECHNIQUES IN BONE MARROW EXAMINATIONS

Technique	Specimen Required	Indications
Culture	Aspirate, sterile	Workup for infection
Cytochemical stains	Air-dried aspirate smears	Lineage identification of immature cells
Immunohistochemical stains	FFPE tissues	Numerous antibodies available to assess for lymphoid, myeloid, erythroid, and megakaryocytic antigens as well as to determine lineage of metastatic processes
		Selected antibodies to assess immaturity (e.g., CD34, TdT) also available
Immunophenotyping (by flow cytometry)	Aspirate, sterile	Useful in determining immunophenotypic profile of wide variety of neoplastic disorders (e.g., leukemias and lymphomas) as well as benign infiltrates (e.g., hematogones)
Cytogenetics	Aspirate, sterile	Yield prognostic and diagnostic information in acute leukemias, myeloid neoplasms, and lymphoma
		Essential in the evaluation of acute leukemias
Fluorescence in situ hybridization	Air-dried smears, cell culture smears, or FFPE tissues	Assess for specific cytogenetic abnormality if probe available
		Useful in minimal residual disease assessment
Molecular analysis	FFPE tissues (PCR)	Useful in determining B- and T-cell clonality as well as gene rearrangements and other genetic aberrations
	Aspirate, sterile (other methods)	Useful in detecting gene amplifications in metastatic neuroblastoma

FFPE: formalin-fixed, paraffin-embedded

beyond the first 3 to 4 days of life (53). In healthy neonates, the relative hypoxia *in utero* is reversed at birth, so that a marked, transient, abrupt decline in erythropoiesis (so-called physiologic anemia of infancy) occurs. These physiologic changes are exaggerated in preterm infants (49).

The neonate assessment for a hematologic disorder is uniquely challenging because of the complex interplay between possible maternal, familial, and obstetric factors in conjunction with the normal and dramatic physiologic variations (53), all of which must be considered in the workup of any hematologic aberration.

EXAMINATION OF THE BONE MARROW IN CHILDREN

Indications for bone marrow examination in children are listed in Table 24-4. The decision to examine the bone marrow is made on an individual basis by correlating laboratory and hematologic findings with the clinical history. While the posterior iliac crest is the preferred site for the evaluation in older children, aspirates and even biopsy specimens can be obtained from the tibia in young infants (54). Before performing a bone marrow examination, careful consideration must be given to the types of specimens necessary for optimal evaluation of the most likely differential diagnosis (Table 24-5). Except for cultures, as a general rule, all specialized studies should be delayed until the bone marrow aspirate smears have been reviewed as adequate. Flow cytometry is one of the routine techniques for immunophenotyping and aids in determining the lineage and maturation of neoplastic infiltrates. Cytogenetic evaluation provides essential diagnostic and prognostic information not only in acute leukemias but also in other myeloid disorders and nonhematopoietic malignancies. Other ancillary techniques are also useful to assess for minimal residual disease in patients with leukemias/lymphomas and to evaluate metastatic processes (Table 24-5).

Inherited Bone Marrow Failure Syndromes and Constitutional Disorders

Bone marrow biopsies for constitutional/inherited hematologic disorders may be encountered in clinical practice. The different entities represent a heterogeneous group of diseases and involve individual lineage with defects of, for example, erythroid, megakaryocytic, and/or histiocytic elements (Table 24-6). Many of these disorders (e.g., thrombocytopenia with absent radii; see below) are evident at birth or shortly thereafter, whereas the multilineage abnormalities that characterize the constitutional aplastic anemias usually develop gradually, sometimes not until adulthood (62,63). Another interesting pattern is that these hematologic disorders are frequently associated with a variety of abnormalities in other organ systems (Table 24-6), while the bone marrow picture is largely one of single lineage aplasia or multilineage failure without distinctive morphologic aberrations (62). Exceptions include marked dyserythropoiesis in congenital dyserythropoietic anemia and erythroid hyperplasia in various constitutional erythrocyte survival disorders (64,65).

The related group of storage diseases typically occurs as a consequence of lysosomal enzyme defects, affecting mainly histiocytes. Various tissues throughout the body could be involved, and the affected cells exhibit distinctive morphologic abnormalities caused by the accumulation of substrate proteins. Although not a primary hematologic disorder, the accumulation of abnormal histiocytes in the bone marrow produces secondary hematologic effects (62) (see Chapter 5).

TABLE 24-6 CONSTITUTIONAL HEMATOLOGIC DISORDERS

Fanconi anemia
DNA repair defect (autosomal/X-linked recessive) with increased incidence of AML
Aplastic anemia in >90%, prominent neonatal cytopenia, pancytopenia by midchildhood
Gradual development of single and multilineage aplasia
Associated congenital anomalies of bone, skin, kidney; mental retardation

15 genes (A-P) identified—most common:	*FANCA* (16q24.3; exon 43) 60%–70%
	FANCC (9q22.3; exon 14) ~14%
	FANCG (9p13; exon 14) ~10%

Dyskeratosis congenita
DNA repair defect, unable to maintain telomere complex (uncharacterized genetic subtype in 50%)
Gradual development of pancytopenia and aplastic anemia (~80%)
Initial hypercellularity common
Associated with congenital anomalies of skin, nails, mucosa; frequent mental retardation

Four genes identified:	X-linked recessive (~30%)	*DKC1*/dyskerin (Xq28; exon 15)
	Autosomal dominant (10%)	*TERC* (3q26; exon1)
		TERT (5p15; exon16)
	Autosomal recessive (~1%)	*NOP10* (15q14; exon 2)
		TERT (5p15; exon 16)

TABLE 24-6 CONSTITUTIONAL HEMATOLOGIC DISORDERS (continued)

Diamond-Blackfan anemia[a]

90% cases are sporadic. Inherited forms are <10%, due to autosomal inheritance and haplodeficiency.
Likely intrinsic progenitor cell defect
Constitutional red cell aplasia (rare erythroblasts present)
Some patients develop marrow failure.
Associated with congenital anomalies, especially skeletal (30%–40%)

Nine genes identified: (*RPS19, RPL5, RPL11, RPL35A, RPS24, RPS17, RPS7, RPS10,* and *RPS26*) 50%–60% cases carry at least one of these mutants.	Autosomal dominant	*RPS19* (19q13.2), 25%, 129 distinct mutations
		RPL5 (1p22.1), 6.6%, 39 mutations
		RPS10 (6p21.31), 6.4%, 3 mutations

Congenital dyserythropoietic/idiopathic aplastic anemia[a]

Erythroid hyperplasia/aplasia
Associated with distinctive bone marrow abnormalities including multinucleation, nuclear bridging, and megaloblastic changes/bone marrow failure
Chromosomal instability and increased incidence of malignancy (repair defect)
Heterozygous mutations in *TERC* and *TERT* are risk factors for some cases.

Shwachman-Diamond syndrome[b]

Constitutional neutropenia with frequent development of aplasia (~20%)
Associated with congenital anomalies including exocrine pancreas insufficiency

One gene identified:	Autosomal recessive (~90%)	*SBDS* (7q11; exon 5)

Thrombocytopenia with absent radii[c] **(TAR)**

Constitutional thrombocytopenic disorder with reduced megakaryocytes and bone anomalies

Compound inheritance (biallelic) of a low-frequency noncoding SNP and a rare null mutation in *RBM8A* (55)	*RBM8A* (1q21)

Congenital amegakaryocytic thrombocytopenia[c]

Isolated thrombocytopenia with decreased/no megakaryocytes
50% patients develop aplastic anemia at the age of 5.
Can evolve into MDS

Genetically heterogeneous; one autosomal recessive subtype characterized	*C-MPL* (1p34.2)

Lysosomal enzyme defects/storage disorders (multiple types):

Over 40 genetic disorders (~1 in 7000 live births) with mostly secondary hematologic manifestations
Accumulation of substrate protein within histiocytes/macrophages
Increased bone marrow histiocytes with distinctive morphology

Classification into six groups:	*Lipid storage disorders* (Gaucher, Niemann-Pick)
	Gangliosidosis (Tay-Sachs disease)
	Leukodystrophies (ADL, MLD, Krabbe, Refsum, Pelizaeus-Merzbacher)
	Mucopolysaccharidosis (Hunter syndrome, Hurler disease)
	Glycoprotein storage disorders (mucolipidosis, pseudoHurler)
	Mucolipidoses (ML type I-IV; sialidosis)

[a]Considered a *constitutional erythrocyte disorder;* this group also includes hemoglobinopathies, membrane defects, and enzyme defects; for example, thalassemias, sickle cell disorders, hereditary spherocytosis, and pyruvate kinase deficiency (not discussed here).

[b]Considered a *constitutional granulocyte disorder*; this group also includes Kostmann agranulocytosis syndrome, cyclic neutropenia, and Chediak-Higashi syndrome (see Table 24-5).

[c]Considered a constitutional megakaryocytic disorder.

ALD, adrenal leukodystrophy; MLD, metachromatic leukodystrophy.

Aplastic Anemia in Children

Aplastic anemia in children can be separated into constitutional/inherited versus acquired (66). This heterogeneous group of disorders, characterized by bone marrow failure with/without somatic abnormalities, typically presents with bone marrow failure in childhood. Eventually, severe trilineage hypoplasia develops; however, despite the name (aplastic), initial presentation is often trilineage hyperplasia, megaloblastic changes, or single lineage aplasia. It is noteworthy that some cases may not present until adulthood, highlighting the importance not only for pediatric pathologists. Since cloning of the first aplastic anemia–related gene in 1992 [*Fanconi anemia (FA)*-gene], considerable advances in the syndromic entities have been made (62). It is clear that approximately 20% of bone marrow failure syndromes in children are inherited and approximately 10% represent secondary causes. The latter includes radiation, chemicals and drugs (typically busulfan, chloramphenicol, nonsteroids), viruses (e.g., hepatitis), and immunologic causes (e.g., systemic lupus erythematosus). The classic diepoxybutane/mitomycin C–induced chromosome fragility testing in cytogenetics has been complemented by targeted molecular approaches (67). The former test assayed the underlying constitutional DNA repair defect in FA, which represents the most common genetic aplastic anemia (Table 24-6). Our current understanding of the molecular mechanisms underlying this group of diseases is convergence in the DNA repair–FBRCA pathway (62). The diseases affect telomere complex maintenance in dyskeratosis congenita–related genes (e.g., *DKC1/dyskerin*, *TERC*, *TERT*, *NOP10*), ribosome biogenesis in Shwachman-Diamond syndrome (SBDS) and Diamond-Blackfan anemia genes (nine genes including *RPS19* and *RPL5*) (68,69), or TPO receptor (*C-MPL*) in congenital amegakaryocytic thrombocytopenia (62,67). Despite the availability of mutational information and mode of inheritance (Table 24-6), the majority (approximately 70%) of "classical" bone marrow failures are "idiopathic" or uncharacterized, and therefore, the main/primary pathogenesis remains unknown (62,70). The peak incidence for secondary and idiopathic aplastic anemia in children is 3 to 5 years of age, and the morphologic features in the bone marrow are generally severely reduced or absent hematopoiesis.

Benign Erythroid Disorders in Children

Nonneoplastic erythroid disorders (also known as *pure red cell aplasia*) consist primarily of congenital and acquired anemias (Table 24-6) (71). The congenital form is induced by intrauterine damage to early erythroid precursors (65). Although the uncommon familial or tumor-associated polycythemia/erythrocytosis can be seen in the neonatal period, the most common neonatal polycythemia is physiologic, resulting from intrauterine hypoxia. The prevalence of specific types of anemia varies by patient age and ethnicity. In neonates, anemias secondary to blood loss predominate, followed by immune and nonimmune hemolytic processes. Anemias secondary to either maturation or proliferation defects are uncommon in infants and include constitutional red cell aplasia and congenital dyserythropoietic anemias (65).

Depending on the ethnic composition in a given practice area, constitutional erythrocyte survival disorders, including hemoglobinopathies and erythrocyte membrane disorders (72), could be relatively common causes of anemia in infants. However, bone marrow examination is generally not required for diagnosis.

A relatively common diagnostic challenge in bone marrow biopsies in children is the classification of red cell aplasia. The three primary causes of red cell aplasia in young children are Diamond-Blackfan anemia, transient erythroblastopenia of childhood, and red cell aplasia secondary to parvovirus infection (73). The latter (also-called acquired pure red cell aplasia) is typically transient and self-limited. If a variety of clinical, laboratory, hematologic, and bone marrow morphologic findings are integrated, the types of red cell aplasia in young children can generally be distinguished. In all types of constitutional and acquired red cell aplasia, the bone marrow is characterized by a profound decrease in maturing erythroid elements, although usually a variable number of erythroblasts are apparent. In addition, distinctive intranuclear inclusions within the residual enlarged erythroblasts are the hallmark of parvovirus infection, but these may not be readily apparent in all cases, and immunohistochemistry can be helpful (Figure 24-5). Consequently, acute parvovirus infection should always be excluded by serologic or molecular studies in cases of red cell aplasia, even when the

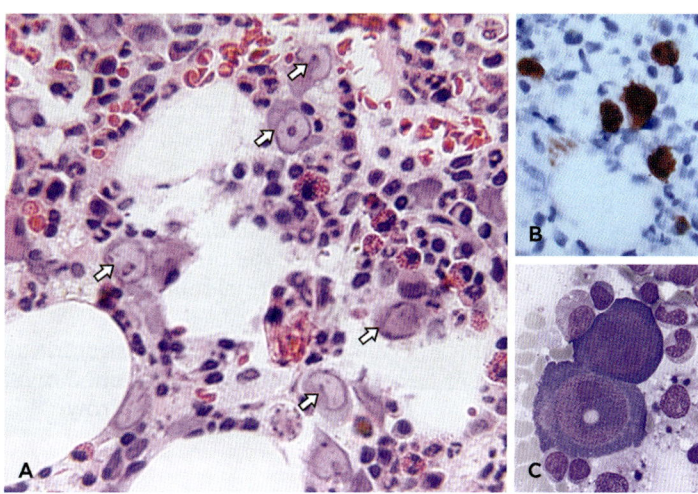

FIGURE 24-5 • Parvovirus. **A,B:** Intranuclear viral inclusions in a patient with parvo B19–induced red cell aplasia (*arrows*) and corresponding parvovirus immunohistochemistry. **C:** Morphology of intranuclear inclusion on smear (Wright-Giemsa stain).

TABLE 24-8	SELECTED CONSTITUTIONAL HEMATOLOGIC DISORDERS INVOLVING B CELLS AND T CELLS	
Antibody deficiency disorders		
Combined variable immunodeficiency (86,87)	Heterogeneous group of disorders with intrinsic B lymphocyte defect; T lymphocyte defects described in some; lymphadenopathy with hyperplastic germinal centers, no plasma cells	Recurrent sinopulmonary infections, malabsorption; complications like chronic lung disease, chronic gastroenteritis, or liver failure
X-linked (Bruton) agammaglobulinemia (87,88)	Mutations in B lymphocyte–specific tyrosine kinase gene; hypoplastic lymphoid organs with atretic germinal centers; decreased B lymphocytes, absent plasma cells	Sinopulmonary, GI, skin, and joint infections caused by pyogenic bacteria and enteroviruses
Selective IgA deficiency (89)	Most common and mildest; varying modes of inheritance; nonspecific findings of villous blunting and follicular hyperplasia in GI biopsies	Heterogeneous clinical presentation; mostly no significant illness; recurrent sinopulmonary infections; food allergy; celiac disease
Hyper IgM syndromes (90)	Mostly X linked; inapparent germinal centers; B lymphocytes are present with abundant plasma cells.	Similar clinical findings to other antibody deficiency disorders
Predominantly T-cell deficiency disorders		
Severe combined immunodeficiency (91)	X linked; defects in all stages of T-cell development; B lymphocytes affected in some types; involuted thymus; decreased lymphocytes	Several subtypes with varied presentations; severe and recurrent systemic infections
Ataxia telangiectasia (92)	A single genetic defect localized to chromosome 11q22–23; loss of cerebellar Purkinje cells and granular layer; pneumonia; chronic hepatitis; hypoplastic lymph nodes	Sinopulmonary infections, telangiectasia; progressive ataxia, and hypersensitivity to ionizing radiation
Wiskott-Aldrich syndrome (93)	Deletions on Xp11.22–23; varying degrees of lymphoid depletion in lymphoid organs; poorly formed or absent germinal centers	Thrombocytopenia with petechiae or bleeding; recurrent infections, eczema; immunodeficiency

include maternal illnesses, maternal drug therapy, maternal alloimmunization against fetal platelets, fetal or neonatal infections, and chromosomal abnormalities. If a bone marrow biopsy is deemed necessary, megakaryocytes are usually slightly increased in number and morphologically normal. Decreased number of bone marrow megakaryocytes is usually seen in constitutional disorders such as thrombocytopenia with absent radii or X-linked amegakaryocytic thrombocytopenia (Table 24-6). Down syndrome (DS) is associated with multiple platelet and megakaryocytic abnormalities including giant platelets, circulating megakaryocytes, and thrombocytopenia in some cases (96,97).

NEOPLASTIC DISORDERS IN BONE MARROW

Myeloproliferative Disorders in Down Syndrome

Transient abnormal myelopoiesis (TAM) and myeloid leukemia associated with Down syndrome (MLADS) are the two most common myeloid disorders encountered in DS. Somatic mutations of the GATA-1 gene have been detected in TAM and MLADS and are considered pathognomonic findings (98,99).

Transient Abnormal Myelopoiesis

TAM is the most frequently encountered myeloproliferative disorder in neonates. TAM generally occurs in the neonatal period but has been documented *in utero* (100). It affects up to 10% of the newborns with DS or trisomy 21 mosaicism (100,101). Although it resembles congenital acute leukemia (102) and can show up to 50% blasts and a clonal chromosome X inactivation in all lineages, it resolves spontaneously before 3 months (102). The WBC count is characteristically markedly elevated, exceeding $50 \times 10^9/L$ and shows normal-appearing neutrophils with an otherwise variable hemogram. The hallmark of TAM is the striking number of circulating heterogeneous blasts. Morphologic, cytochemical, and immunophenotypic studies show a predominance of erythroblasts and megakaryoblasts (103,104) (Figure 24-8).

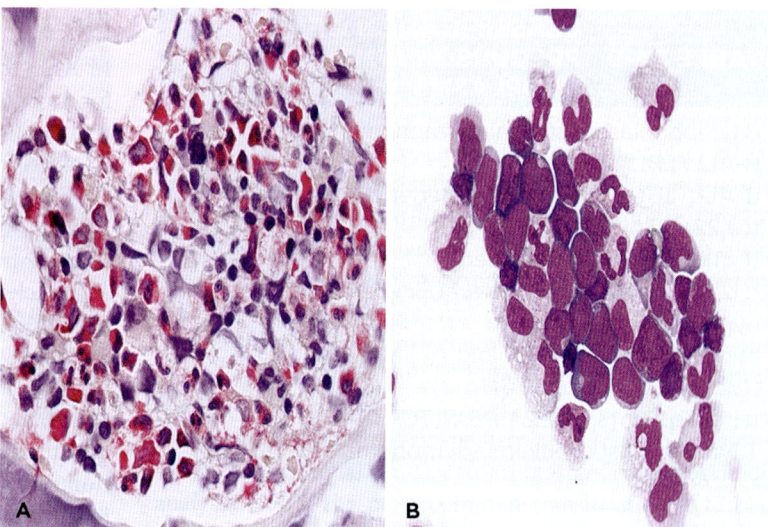

FIGURE 24-8 • **A, B:** Bone marrow in a newborn with TAM associated with DS, showing myeloid left shift **(A)** and prominence of immature cells including blasts **(B)**.

Despite spontaneous resolution, approximately 20% of TAM patients develop MLADS, which is usually acute megakaryoblastic leukemia (AMKL) (103–105).

Acute Leukemia

The incidence of overt acute leukemia is markedly increased in children with DS irrespective of an antecedent TAM (103,106,107). The affected children are generally older and present with evidence of severe bone marrow failure and hepatosplenomegaly. The types of acute leukemia seen in DS children are age dependent. In children less than 3 years of age, AMKL generally develops with an admixed erythrocytic component, whereas ALL predominates in older children (106,108). In an overt acute leukemia, the bone marrow is replaced by blasts, which are generally cytochemically, morphologically, and phenotypically homogeneous. Additional clonal chromosomal abnormalities along with trisomy 21 are more common in acute leukemias than in TAM (106).

Congenital Acute Leukemias

Congenital leukemias are by definition acute leukemias presenting at birth until 1 month of age. Likely to have originated *in utero*, these are extremely rare and described with rates of one in 5 million births (109). Congenital leukemias are predominantly myeloid; however, lymphoid types have been described in biologic subsets associated with translocations involving 11q23 (MLL gene) (110–114). The myeloid leukemias typically demonstrate a prominent monoblastic component, marked leukocytosis, and extramedullary disease; hepatosplenomegaly and skin lesions are especially prominent (113,114). Distinctive features of 11q23-associated congenital ALL include central nervous system disease and a CD10$^-$ and CD15$^+$ B-cell precursor phenotype with frequent myeloid antigen coexpression (110,111). The second biologic subset of congenital acute leukemias are associated with t(1;22)(p13;q13). This subtype is AMKL that occurs in infants less than 1 year of age (115), and the clinical picture resembles a solid tumor. Both bone marrow and extramedullary infiltrates are extremely fibrotic, and tumor cells often appear as isolated nests (116,117). On the hemogram, t(1;22)-associated leukemia presents typically with severe pancytopenia, while in contrast, the 11q23-associated leukemia is characterized by marked leukocytosis. Although the prognosis is poor in all subtypes of congenital leukemia, those cases that present within the first month have the worst prognosis. Lineage switch in congenital acute leukemias is characterized by MLL gene rearrangements with t(4;11), t(9;11) and other translocation partners (118,119).

Acute Lymphoblastic Leukemia

ALL is a clonal B- or T-cell neoplasm characterized by a loss of normal hematopoietic elements and the predominance of immature B or T cells demonstrating minimal, if any, maturation. ALL represents the most prevalent of pediatric leukemias with an incidence of approximately 3/100,000 children annually. ALL predominates in children between 2 and 9 years of age, and 75% of all ALL patients are younger than 15 years (120,121). Boys are affected more often, and a substantially increased incidence of ALL has been documented in patients with genetic disorders such as DS and 11q23 abnormalities (108).

Patients typically present with fever, bleeding, splenomegaly, or hepatosplenomegaly. In infants, remarkable organomegaly, high white cell count, and central nervous system involvement predominate. In older children, the

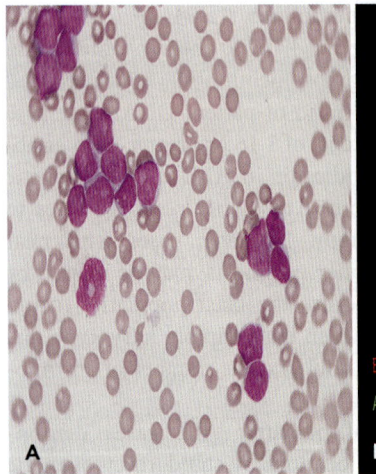
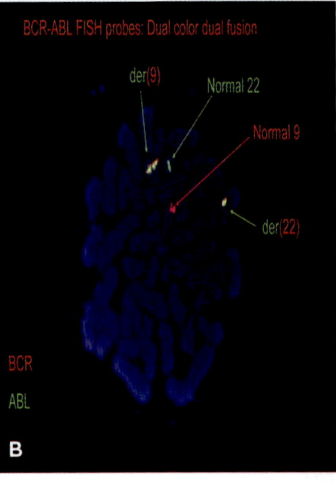

FIGURE 24-12 • **A,B:** Precursor B-acute lymphoblastic leukemia with translocation t(9;22) as demonstrated by dual color fusion FISH probes.

alternative therapies including bone marrow transplant (136,137). With few exceptions, the prognosis in ALL can be determined by integrating age, WBC count, sex, genotype, response to therapy, and other parameters (Table 24-10). The clinical, immunophenotypic, and prognostic significance of a variety of these chromosomal translocations is summarized in Table 24-11.

Acute Myeloid Leukemia

Acute myeloid leukemia (AML) is a clonal hematopoietic disorder characterized by a predominance of immature cells capable of minimal, if any, maturation. AML can be derived from progenitors of any lineage, and hence, multilineage differentiation can be noted. AML occurs in patients of all ages but is more prevalent in adults. Nevertheless, most congenital leukemias are myeloid in origin. The incidence of AML is low throughout childhood and early adulthood, but the proportion steadily increases during these years. Factors linked to an increased incidence of AML include constitutional genetic disorders, acquired bone marrow diseases, smoking, occupational/environmental exposures, and therapeutic agents (108,138,139). Numerous studies have documented an increased incidence of AML in patients receiving chemotherapy, especially alkylating agents or topoisomerase II inactivators (109,138,140).

The most widely accepted classification system for AML is used to be the FAB system. Subsequently, WHO classification published in 2001 and 2008 has integrated traditional approaches (morphology, cytochemistry, and immunophenotyping) with emerging knowledge of molecular and cytogenetic abnormalities (Table 24-12). The goal of WHO classification is to provide the first "evidence-based" classification system, which serves the needs of daily practice and also provides a flexible framework for integration of new data in the future (123). Among the major proposed changes, some are summarized below:

1. 20% of more blasts are required for diagnosing AML.
2. AML with recurrent genetic abnormalities with new additions as of 2008 (Table 24-12):
3. "AML with myelodysplasia-related changes" replacing the old term "AML with multilineage dysplasia"
4. Therapy-related myeloid neoplasms that are no longer subclassified based on chemotherapeutic agents

Morphologic and Immunophenotypic Basis of AML Classification

The morphologic diagnosis of AML depends on the identification of a variety of types of blasts and other immature cells that define the subtype of AML. Accordingly, cytochemical stains are still valuable in delineating specific types of immature myeloid cells and greatly enhance accuracy in the diagnosis of AML (Table 24-13). Flow cytometry is useful in determining the lineage and stage of maturation in many cases of AML; immunophenotyping is also critical in the successful identification of both undifferentiated myeloid leukemias and AMKL (115). In addition, paraffin immunoperoxidase techniques

TABLE 24-10 CLINICAL AND LABORATORY POOR PROGNOSTIC FEATURES IN PEDIATRIC ALL

Clinical features
Age at diagnosis: <1 yr or >10 yr old
Gender: Male
CNS involvement at the time of presentation
Response to therapy
Suboptimal response to induction chemotherapy: (>25% blasts on day 15)
Minimal residual disease postinduction: >5% blasts by morphology or >0.1% blasts by flow cytometry or PCR
Laboratory and genetic features
High WBC count (>50 × 10^9/L)
Blast immunophenotype (T cell, or CD10−)
Genetic abnormalities: hypodiploidy, *BCR-ABL1*+, *MLL-AFF1*+ (see also Table 24-9)

TABLE 24-11 INCIDENCE AND CLINICAL FEATURES ASSOCIATED WITH GENOTYPIC ABNORMALITIES IN PEDIATRIC ALL

Numerical Abnormalities	Incidence	Comments/Prognosis
Hypodiploid	2%–8%	Older than 10, poor risk by NCI criteria, poor prognosis
Hyperdiploid	25%–40%	Most frequently seen genetic abnormality; low risk by NCI criteria, favorable response to antimetabolite therapy; further improved outcome is associated with "triple trisomies" (trisomies 4, 10, and 17).
Structural abnormalities		
t(12;21)(p13;q22); *TEL-AML1* (*ETV6-RUNX1*)	20%–40%	The most common translocation; good prognosis
t(9;22)(q34;q11); *BCR-ABL1*	3%–5%	May be cryptic; may be associated with additional abnormalities; poor response to therapy
t(1;19)(q23;p13); *E2A-PBX1*(*TCF3-PBX1*)	≤5% by routine cytogenetics; 20%–25% if molecular techniques are employed	Mostly in neonates and infants; high-risk disease at presentation; usually pre-B with cytoplasmic μ chain; intensive chemotherapy had improved survival.
t(v;11q23); *MLL* rearranged	2%–11%	High-risk presentation; inferior treatment outcome; predominates in therapy-related and congenital leukemias
t(11;14)(p15;q11), t(1;14)(p32;q11), and t(1;7)(p32;q35)	30% of T-ALL by molecular techniques	*TAL1* dysregulation on chromosome 1p32 or TCR gene dysregulation; usually older patients; prominent extramedullary disease
t(5;14)(q31;q32); *IL3-IGH*	Rare	Older patients; aggressive disease course; neural and cardiovascular complication due to striking eosinophilia secondary to *IL-3*-related stimulation

Modified from Lennerz JKM, Hassan A. The bone marrow. In: Stocker JT, Dehner LP, eds. *Pediatric Pathology*, 3rd ed. Philadelphia, PA: Lippincott Williams & Wilkins; 2010;1010–1039.

can be used to assess for immaturity (CD34, TdT), myeloid/monocytic maturation (MPO, CD43, lysozyme, CD68, CD15, CD4, CD14, CD64), erythroid maturation (hemoglobin A, glycophorin, CD71), and megakaryocyte maturation (CD61, CD41, CD42, factor VIII) (Figure 24-13A,B).

TABLE 24-12 SUMMARY OF WHO CLASSIFICATION OF ACUTE MYELOID LEUKEMIA[a]

AML with recurrent genetic abnormalities
AML with myelodysplasia-related changes
Therapy-related myeloid neoplasms
AML, not otherwise specified
Myeloid sarcoma
Myeloid proliferations related to Down syndrome
Transient abnormal myelopoiesis
Myeloid leukemia associated with Down syndrome
Blastic plasmacytoid dendritic cell neoplasms

[a]Adapted from WHO Classification of Hematopoietic and Lymphoid Tissues, 2008; Also see Table 24-13 for AML subtypes.

Biologic Basis of AML Classification

Because of the implications for diagnosis, treatment, and prognosis, cytogenetic analysis and molecular studies are now a standard of care for patients with AML and are recommended for initial workup. In addition to meeting the requirement of diagnosing genetically defined entities, cytogenetic and molecular abnormalities also help provide a baseline for monitoring disease progression. Clonal cytogenetic abnormalities in childhood AML are identified less frequently than in ALL, approximating 50% to 80% of cases (133). In the 2008 WHO classification of AML, the traditional lineage-based classification is retained (as "AML—not otherwise specified" category) and distinct biologic subtypes based on genotype are integrated (Table 24-14). Cases of AML characterized by reciprocal translocations occur more commonly in children than in adults (132,133).

AML with t(8;21)(q22;q22); *RUNX1–RUNX1T1*

The fusion gene *RUNX1–RUNX1T1* (or *AML1-ETO*) produced by t(8;21)(q22;q22) accounts for 10% to 15% of childhood AML cases and is diagnostic of AML regardless of blast count. AML with t(8;21) usually shows myeloid maturation (132,133), and patients may present with

TABLE 24-13 MORPHOLOGIC FEATURES OF BLASTS AND OTHER IMMATURE CELLS

Type of Cell	Key Morphologic Features	Cytochemistry	Immunophenotypic Features
Myeloblast	Large nucleus with finely dispersed chromatin and variably prominent nucleoli. Relatively high nuclear-to-cytoplasmic ratio		
	Variable number of cytoplasmic granules, may be concentrated in limited portion of cytoplasm	SBB+, MPO+	HLA-DR, CD33, CD13, anti-MPO, CD34
Promyelocyte	Nuclear chromatin slightly condensed; nucleoli variably prominent; nucleus often eccentric and Golgi zone may be apparent.	SBB+, MPO+	CD33, CD13, anti-MPO, CD117
	Numerous cytoplasmic granules that may be more dispersed throughout cytoplasm		
	In APL, intense cytoplasmic granularity usually present, and nuclear configuration variable, but nuclear folding and lobulation characteristic of microgranular variant of APL		
Monoblast	Moderate-to-low nuclear-to-cytoplasmic ratio, nuclear chromatin finely dispersed with variably prominent nucleoli; nuclei round to folded	NSE+	HLA-DR, CD33, CD13, vCD14, CD4
	Abundant, slightly basophilic cytoplasm containing fine granulation and occasional vacuoles		
Promonocyte	Slightly condensed nuclear chromatin; variably prominent nucleoli	NSE+	HLA-DR, CD33, CD13, CD14, CD4
	Abundant finely granular blue/gray cytoplasm that may be vacuolated		
	Very monocytic appearance with nuclear immaturity		
Erythroblast	Relatively high nuclear-to-cytoplasmic ratio	PAS+	Glycophorin A, Hgb A, CD71
	Nucleus round with slightly condensed chromatin; nucleoli variably prominent		
	Moderate amounts of deeply basophilic cytoplasm that may be vacuolated		
Megakaryoblast	Highly variable morphologic features	PAS+	CD41, CD61, v factor VIII
	Often not recognizable without special studies		
	May be lymphoid appearing with high nuclear-to-cytoplasmic ratio		
	Nuclear chromatin fine to variably condensed		
	Cytoplasm may be scant to moderate, is usually agranular, or contains a few granules; blebbing or budding of cytoplasm may be evident.		

SBB, Sudan black B; MPO, myeloperoxidase; APL, acute promyelocytic leukemia; NSE, neuron-specific esterase; PAS, periodic acid-Schiff; Hgb, hemoglobin.

extramedullary myeloid tumors. The bone marrow is characteristically effaced by myeloblasts and maturing myeloid elements, which may exhibit an odd, salmon-colored cytoplasm with a peripheral basophilic rim. Dysplastic findings may lead to a mistaken diagnosis of myelodysplasia, especially if the blast count is less than 20%. Auer rods with tapered ends are typically readily apparent (141). Coexpression of CD19 and CD56 has been noted in cases of AML with t(8;21) (142,143). AML with t(8;21) has a favorable prognosis in adults; however, the presence of KIT-activating mutation and CD56 expression confers poor prognosis.

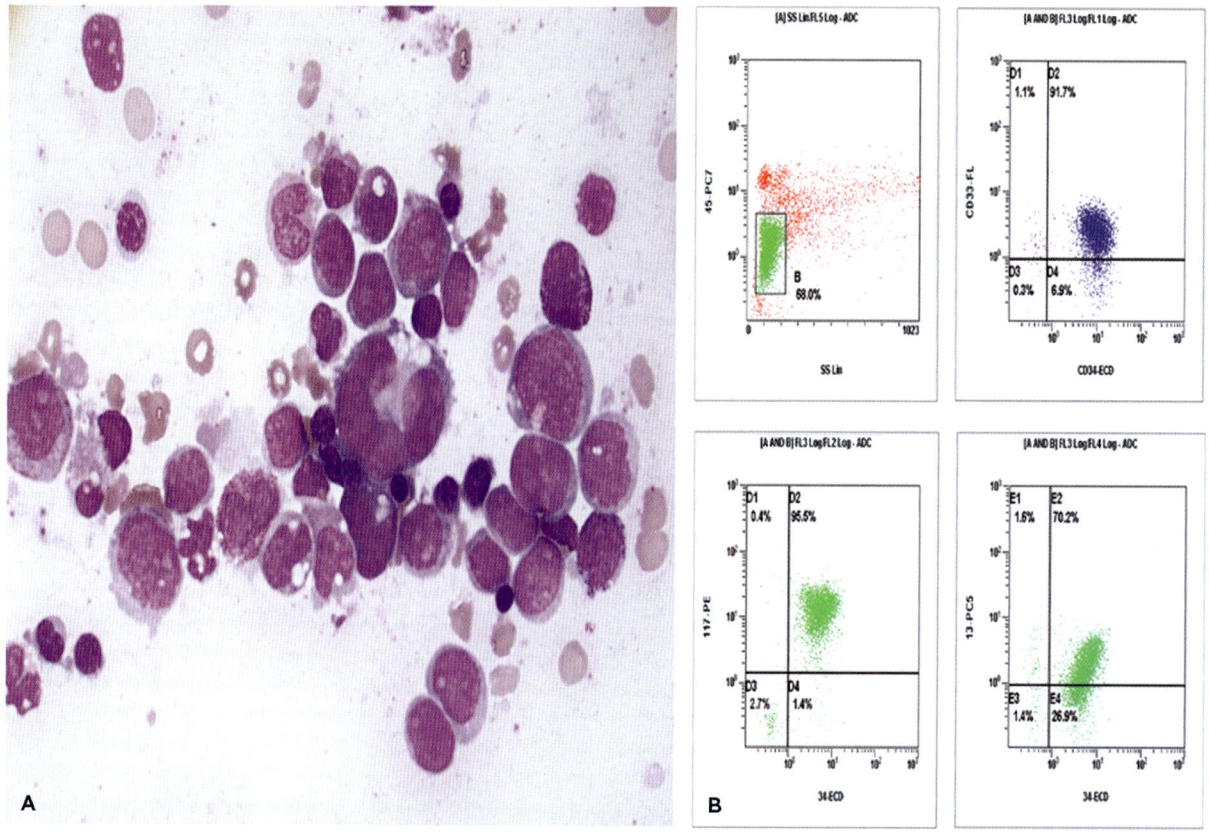

FIGURE 24-13 • **A:** Acute myeloid leukemia with maturation. **B:** Flow cytometry histograms show a dim CD45 population, coexpressing CD34, CD33, CD13, and CD117.

Acute Promyelocytic Leukemia with t(15;17)(q22;q12); *PML–RARa*

Acute promyelocytic leukemia (APL) is a distinct clinicopathologic entity with t(15;17)(q22;q12) resulting in a *PML–RARa* fusion gene (132,133) (Figure 24-14). t(15;17)(q22;q12) is considered as AML regardless of blast count. Older children and young adults are most commonly affected and present with pancytopenia, profound thrombocytopenia, and marked coagulopathy. In the common, hypergranular subtype, promyelocytes are inconspicuous in blood, whereas the bone marrow is effaced by intensely granulated promyelocytes (Figure 24-15). Auer rods are numerous and often stacked in bundles (Figure 24-15, inset). A microgranular variant accounts for about one-fourth of cases and is characterized by leukocytosis and hypogranular promyelocytes exhibiting marked nuclear folding. Intense staining with Sudan black B and MPO characterizes both the hypergranular and the microgranular subtypes. Immunophenotypic studies usually show a CD34- and HLA-DR–negative phenotype that indicates maturity, but is not diagnostic of APL. The clinical outcome is good with ATRA induction. Several other chemotherapeutic agents could be used during induction, based on risk stratification (144,145).

AML with inv(16)(p13.1q22) or t(16;16)(p13.1;q22); *CBFB-MYH11*

AML with inv(16) or t(16;16) is the third AML entity without a required minimal blast count. It often shows myelomonocytic differentiation and eosinophilia (Figure 24-16). AML with inv(16) is more common than AML with t(16;16), and, together, these account for approximately 10% of pediatric AMLs. This subtype may be associated with extramedullary myeloid cell tumors (myeloid sarcoma). The bone marrow eosinophils often exhibit mixed eosinophil–basophil granules (146) (Figure 24-17). However, not all cases with this cytogenetic abnormality exhibit eosinophilia or myelomonocytic morphology. Prognosis is good with a high likelihood of cure by chemotherapy and prolonged disease-free course (147,148). The presence of *KIT* mutation is associated with poor prognosis.

AML with t(9;11)(p22;q23); *MLLT3-MLL* or Other Balanced Translocations Involving 11q23

This AML subtype results from a balanced translocation targeting the mixed lineage leukemia gene (*MLL*) and any one of over 50 partner genes located at other chromosomal loci. The most common partner gene is AF9 located at chromosome 9p22. In children, four translocations, t(9;11)(p22;q23), t(11;19)(q23;p13.1), t(11;19)(q23;p13.3), and t(10;11)

TABLE 24-14 SUMMARY OF THE 2008 WHO CLASSIFICATION OF ACUTE MYELOID LEUKEMIAS

Disease	Clinical	Morphology	Immunophenotype	Prognosis
A. AML with Recurrent Genetic Abnormalities				
AML with t(8;21)(q22;q22); *RUNX1-RUNX1T1*	Often presents with extramedullary disease	Blasts with long slender Auer rods, abnormal granulation	CD13+, CD33+, MPO+, CD19+, CD34+, CD56+	Favorable
AML with inv(16) (p13.1q22) or t(16;16) (p13.1q22);*CBFB-MYH11*	Occasionally presents with extramedullary disease	Abnormal eosinophils with large basophilic granules, decreased lobation	CD13+, CD33+, MPO+; frequently CD4+, CD14+, CD11b+, CD11c+, CD64+, CD36+, lysozyme+	Favorable
Acute promyelocytic leukemia with t(15;17) (q22;q12); *PML-RARA*	Coagulopathy, normal/low WBC (hypergranular variant) or high WBC (hypogranular variant)	Abnormal promyelocytes with multiple Auer rods predominate	CD13+ (heterogeneous), CD33+ (bright), HLA-DR–, CD34–	Favorable
AML with t(9;11) (p22;q23); *MLLT3-MLL*	Frequently occurs in children	Monocytic blasts predominate	Variable CD13 and CD33+, CD4+, CD14+, CD11b+, CD11c+, CD64+, CD36+, lysozyme+	Intermediate
AML with t(6;9) (p23;q34); *DEK-NUP214*	In both children and adults; cytopenias,	Marrow and PB basophilia; multilineage dysplasia	CD34, CD117, MPO, CD13, CD33, CD38, HLA-DR, and CD15	Poor
AML with inv(3) (q21q26.2) or t(3;3) (q21;q26.2); *RPN1-EVI1*	Usually anemia, normal platelet counts	Multilineage dysplasia	CD13, CD33, HLA-DR, CD34 and CD38	Poor
AML(megakaryoblastic) with t(1;22)(p13;q13); *RBM15-MKL1*	<1% of all AML; commonly in infants without Down syndrome, with a female predominance; hepatosplenomegaly	Similar to those of AMKL (M7)	Platelet glycoproteins (CD41, CD61, CD13, CD33, CD36; CD34 (–), CD45(–),HLA-DR(–)	Respond well to intensive AML chemotherapy with long disease-free survival
AML with mutated *NPM1* (provisional)	2%–8% of childhood AML; with a female predominance	Frequently has myelomonocytic or monocytic features	Myeloid markers (CD13, CD33, MPO) and monocytic markers (CD11b, CD14, CD68)	Favorable in absence of a *FLT3*-ITD mutation Poorer with coexistent *FLT3*-ITD mutation
AML with mutated *CEBPA* (provisional)	6%–15% of *de novo* AML and in 15%–18% of AML with normal karyotypes	No distinctive morphologic features	CD34, HLA-DR, myeloid markers	Favorable

B. AML with myelodysplasia-related changes
- Morphologic features of myelodysplasia
- A prior history of an MDS or MDS/MPN
- MDS-related cytogenetic abnormalities; exclusion of AML with recurrent genetic abnormalities

C. Therapy-related myeloid neoplasms
- Including t-AML, t-MDS, t-MDS/MPN; as late complications of cytotoxic chemotherapy and/or radiation therapy; exclusion of transformed MPN

D. AML, not otherwise specified (NOS)

AML with minimal differentiation	Usually presents in adulthood, cytopenias	<3% of blasts MPO+, <3% of blasts NBE+	Often CD13+, CD33+, CD117+, CD34+, CD38+, HLA-DR+	Unfavorable
AML without maturation	Usually presents in adulthood, cytopenias, occasionally with markedly increased WBC	Blasts comprise ≥90% of nonerythroid cells; ≥3% of blasts MPO+, ≥3% of blasts NBE+	Often CD13+, CD33+, CD34+, CD117+, MPO+	Unfavorable
AML with maturation	Variable age range and symptomatology	≥3% of blasts MPO+, ≤3% of blasts NBE+	Usually CD13+, CD33+, CD15+; variable CD117+, CD34+, HLA-DR+	Variable
Acute myelomonocytic leukemia	Anemia, fever, fatigue; WBC usually elevated	>20% blasts; ≥ monocytes and precursors; ≥neutrophils and precursors; ≥3% of blasts MPO+, ≥3% of blasts usually NBE+*	Usually CD13+, CD33+; Often CD4+, CD14+, CD11b+, CD11c+, CD64+, CD36+, lysozyme+	Variable
Acute monoblastic leukemia	Most common in children, often presents with extramedullary disease, bleeding disorders	≥80% monocytic cells, of which ≥80% are monoblasts, <20% neutrophils and precursors, <3% of blasts MPO+, ≥3% of blasts NBE+	Variable CD13+, CD33+, CD117+; often CD14+, CD4+, CD11b+, CD11c+, CD64+, CD68+, CD36+, lysozyme+	Unfavorable
Acute monocytic leukemia	Most common in adults, often presents with extramedullary disease, bleeding disorders	≥80% monocytic cells, of which the majority are promonocytes, <20% neutrophils and precursors, <3% of blasts MPO+, ≥3% of blasts NBE+	Variable CD13+, CD33+, CD117+; Often CD14+, CD4+, CD11b+, CD11c+, CD64+, CD68+, CD36+, lysozyme+	Unfavorable
Erythroleukemia (erythroid/myeloid)	Adults; anemia	≥50% of entire nucleated population is erythroid and ≥20% myeloblasts in nonerythroid population; >3% of blasts may be MPO+.	Erythroblasts are glycophorin A+ and hemoglobin A+; myeloblasts are CD13+, CD33+, CD117+, and MPO+.	Unfavorable
Pure erythroid leukemia	Extremely rare	>80% of cells are immature erythroid cells; no significant myeloblast component; <3% of blasts MPO+, ≥3% of blasts NBE+	Blasts are sometimes glycophorin A+ and hemoglobin A+.	Unfavorable
Acute megakaryoblastic leukemia	Cytopenias	Dysplastic megakaryocytes, blasts often have cytoplasmic pseudopods. Abnormal platelets and megakaryocyte fragments in peripheral blood; usually <3% of blasts MPO+ and <3% of blasts NBE+	Usually CD41+, CD61+; occasionally CD13+, CD33+; CD34−, CD45−, HLA-DR−	Poor
Acute basophilic leukemia	Very rare	Blasts are toluidine blue+; usually <3% of blasts MPO+, <3% of blasts NBE+.	Usually CD13+, CD33+, CD34+, HLA-DR+, CD9+	Difficult to predict due to low number of reported cases, probably poor
Acute panmyelosis with myelofibrosis	Very rare, adults, pancytopenia with no/minimal splenomegaly	Panhyperplasia, dysplastic megakaryocytes; increased reticulin fibrosis	CD13+, CD33+, CD117+, MPO+; some cases express erythroid or megakaryocytic antigens	Poor

MPO, myeloperoxidase; NBE, naphthyl butyrate esterase; WBC, white blood count.

Modified from Humphrey P, Dehner L, Pfeifer J. Bone marrow pathology. *The Washington Manual of Surgical Pathology*, 1st ed. Philadelphia, PA: Lippincott Williams & Wilkins; 2008:573–588.

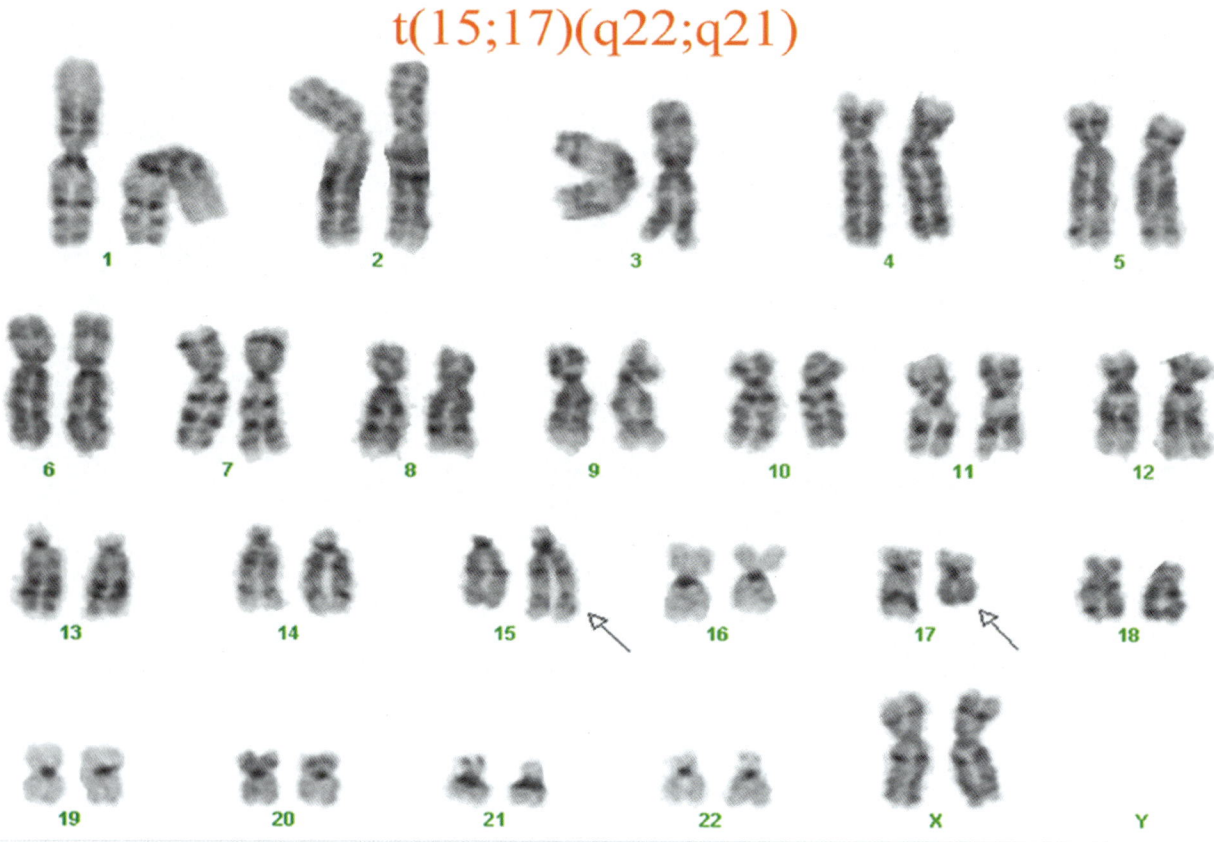

FIGURE 24-14 • The translocation (15;17) is exclusively observed in APL; *arrows* indicate breakpoints.

(p12;q23), account for majority of *MLL*-AMLs. As a group, these AMLs comprise 15% to 20% of all pediatric AMLs and, as such, are the most common cytogenetic AML subtypes (149,150). The frequency of *MLL* translocation is very high in both ALL and AML arising during infancy, and they are detected in over 50% of the cases. Most *MLL*-AMLs show some degree of monocytic differentiation and are classified as either acute myelomonocytic leukemia or acute monocytic leukemia using FAB criteria. Cases containing t(9;11) are frequently classified as acute monocytic leukemias. Clinical evidence of extramedullary infiltration is frequently seen as hepatosplenomegaly, gingival hypertrophy, and leukemia cutis.

Therapy-Related AML/MDS (t-AML/t-MDS)

These neoplasms arise as late complications of cytotoxic and radiation therapy for prior neoplastic or nonneoplastic

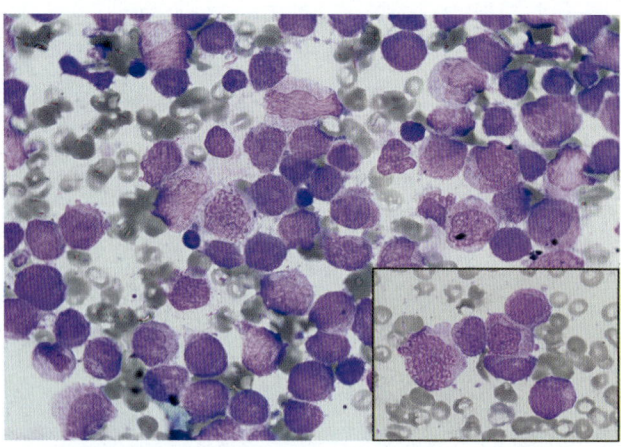

FIGURE 24-15 • Several intensely granular promyelocytes are evident in the aspirate smear showing APL; Auer rods can be seen **(inset)**.

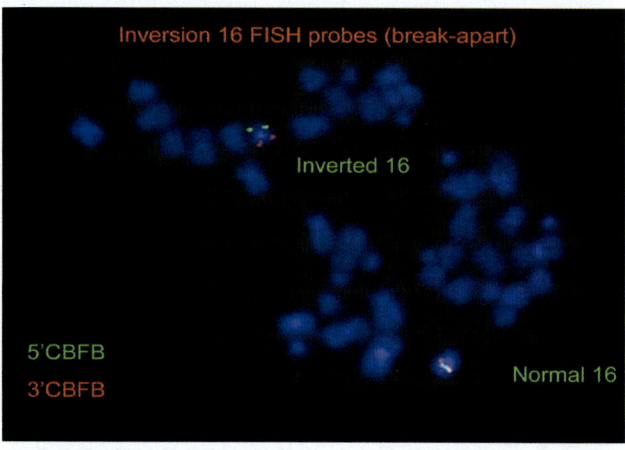

FIGURE 24-16 • Florescent *in situ* hybridization (FISH) analysis of the AMML cells demonstrates inversion of chromosome 16 utilizing break-apart FISH probes (*two green, two red signals*).

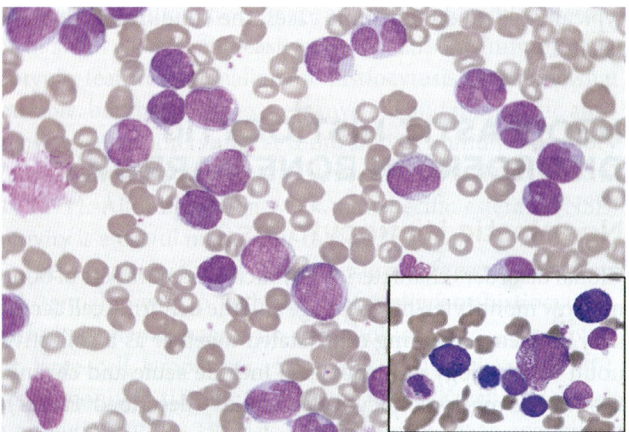

FIGURE 24-17 • AMML demonstrates myeloid blasts and immature monocytic cells; scattered cells with eo–baso granules were evident **(inset)**.

AML WITH MYELODYSPLASIA-RELATED CHANGES (AML-MRC)

According to the WHO criteria, AML-MRC has 20% or more blasts and one of the following associations: (a) previous history of MDS or MDS/MPN, (b) presence of MDS-related cytogenetic abnormalities, or (c) morphologic features of MDS. For example, monosomy 7 detected in approximately 5% to 7% of pediatric *de novo* AML cases (155) meets the criteria of AML–MRC based on the current WHO recommendations.

Myelodysplastic and Myeloproliferative Neoplasms in Children

In young children, a myelodysplastic/myeloproliferative neoplasm is characterized by leukocytosis with both neutrophilia and monocytosis, a left shift to blasts, multilineage dyspoiesis, anemia, and thrombocytopenia (Figure 24-19; Table 24-15). Typically, hepatosplenomegaly and skin lesions also develop (156–158). In some children, a constitutional monosomy 7 has been identified, and the term *infantile monosomy 7 syndrome* has been utilized to describe such cases. In other infants, a very similar blood, bone marrow, and clinical picture develops in conjunction with increased levels of hemoglobin F and various RAS or NF1 gene mutations (156,159). The latter disease, originally termed *juvenile chronic myelogenous leukemia* and later called *juvenile myelomonocytic leukemia*, is differentiated from CML by lacking the Philadelphia chromosome breakpoint cluster region–abl gene rearrangement (160–162). Despite the disparate terminology, so-called infantile monosomy 7 syndrome and juvenile myelomonocytic leukemias are currently thought to comprise a spectrum of infantile myelodysplastic/myeloproliferative processes that are frequently associated with monosomy 7/del(7q) (157,158). The WHO Working Group placed these disorders into a hybrid "myelodysplastic/myeloproliferative neoplasm" category to distinguish them from

conditions. The risk with alkylating agent therapy and radiation usually increases with age. Those treated with topoisomerase II inhibitors show no age-related increase in incidence (151). Childhood therapy-related myeloid neoplasms tend to occur most frequently within 6 years of primary diagnosis of Hodgkin lymphoma, osteogenic sarcoma, ALL, non-Hodgkin lymphoma, and Ewing sarcoma. They can also occur following autologous or allogeneic bone marrow transplant (152–154). Over 90% of cases show an abnormal karyotype. The most common cytogenetic abnormality associated with alkylating agents is unbalanced chromosomal alterations such as complete or partial loss of chromosome 5 and/or 7. These are often associated with one or more additional chromosomal abnormalities. For topoisomerase II inhibitors, balanced translocations that involve rearrangements of 11q23, 21q22, and other abnormalities are commonly seen (Figure 24-18). The prognosis is dismal and generally related to the associated karyotypic abnormalities, comorbidities of underlying disease, and performance status.

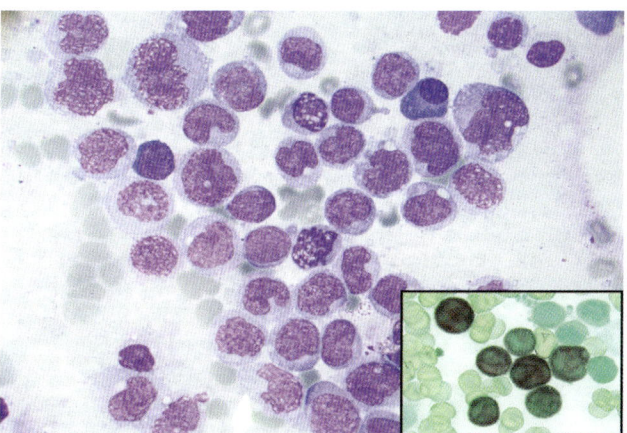

FIGURE 24-18 • 11q23-associated acute monocytic leukemia evolving in posttherapy setting; the monocytic nature is confirmed by NSE staining **(inset)**.

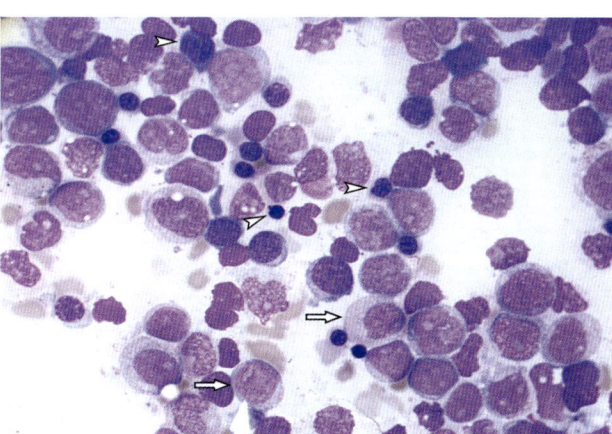

FIGURE 24-19 • Acute myeloid leukemia evolved from myelodysplastic syndrome. Note dyserythropoiesis (*arrowheads*) and abnormally granular myelocytes with nuclear cytoplasmic asynchrony (*arrows*).

apparent on aspirate smears or biopsy sections, a variety of immunologic techniques can be used to distinguish these metastatic lesions conclusively from a primary hematologic neoplasm. Immunoperoxidase staining for various solid tumor-associated antigens can be employed, and bone marrow biopsies are considered more effective in the diagnosis of metastatic disease as the aspirates are often "aspicular" due to fibrosis (188).

Bone Marrow/Hematopoietic Stem Cell Transplantation

Bone marrow/hematopoietic stem cell transplantation (BMT/HSCT) is currently a therapeutic option for a variety of neoplastic and nonneoplastic disorders (189,190). It is particularly considered as an option in refractory acute leukemias, lymphomas, and untreatable solid tumors (191,192). Two kinds of bone marrow transplants are usually available: autologous and allogeneic (HLA-matched donor). The concept behind allogeneic BMT is reconstitution of normal bone marrow elements after giving very high doses of chemotherapy, which in other circumstances would be lethal owing to the effects on the bone marrow. In diseases involving clonal stem cell abnormalities, particularly poor-risk acute leukemias, relapsed or unresponsive lymphomas, and some solid tumors, an allogeneic transplant offers the best chance for cure. Allogeneic BMT usually follows intense chemotherapy with or without total body irradiation to eradicate the bone marrow and immune cells as well as the neoplastic cells followed by an infusion of HSCs from an HLA-matched donor. In patients with solid tumors, stem cells may be harvested from the patients' own bone marrow or peripheral blood and infused as an autologous transplant (192). This does not require marrow ablation and can be performed if the bone marrow is free of neoplastic process. Autologous BMT does not carry the risk of serious complications associated with allogeneic transplants such as graft versus host disease, posttransplant lymphoproliferative disorders, secondary hematologic malignancies, solid tumors, and graft rejection (193). The aim of the autologous BMT is to ablate the abnormal cells in the marrow and to reconstitute hematopoiesis with the patient's own normal stem cells.

Bone Marrow Findings in Post-BMT Samples

In the immediate posttransplant period (1 to 7 days), the bone marrow findings are similar to those of chemotherapy-ablated bone marrow, such as transient fibrosis, serous atrophy, nonspecific edema, hemosiderin-laden macrophages with a predominance of stromal cells, and small, nonspecific granulomas (194). Bone marrow engraftment starts as early as day 7 and is characterized by small nonparatrabecular colonies of erythroid precursors (which usually appear first), followed by granulocytic precursors, and megakaryocytes (195,196). During weeks 3 and 4, the hematopoietic colonies are stably expanding and the marrow cellularity is expected to be half of the normal at the end of week 4. Simultaneously, there is stromal recovery with resolving fibrosis. Complete engraftment with normal level hematopoiesis is expected in 2 to 3 months (Table 24-16). The process of marrow engraftment is slower in recipients of allogeneic transplant when compared to autologous transplant recipients. The blood counts also reflect the above\mentioned sequence of engraftment. There is profound pancytopenia early on, followed by increasing red cell counts, then by increasing white cell counts, which usually normalize by day 21. Increasing platelet counts usually normalize by days 25 to 30 after transplant. Hematogone levels are often increased in BMT recipients, and extensive transfusion therapy may increase storage iron levels, resulting in ringed sideroblasts.

Failure to engraft (failure of transplanted cells to engraft by day 28) is a dismal complication of BMT. Several factors contribute to graft failure, such as inadequate numbers of the transplanted stem cells, immunologic destruction of stem cells, infection, and drug toxicity to name a few (197). Signs heralding graft failure include failure of marrow cellularity to normalize (50% of normal cellularity expected by day 21) and persistent peripheral cytopenias. On the other hand, significant increase in peripheral blood counts may be a sign of recurrence of primary disease (198). Bone marrow morphology, combined with ancillary studies such as flow cytometry and cytogenetic and molecular studies, is needed to monitor graft status and residual/recurrent disease. In particular, the popular engraftment analysis is PCR-based short tandem repeat (STR) DNA test, which is sensitive and informative (199). In addition, sex-mismatched BMT can

TABLE 24-16 BONE MARROW MORPHOLOGY POST–BONE MARROW TRANSPLANTATION

Time after BMT	Morphologic Findings
Week 1	Markedly hypocellular, cell death, stromal edema, serous atrophy, transient fibrosis, hemosiderin-laden macrophages
Week 2	Early small colonies of erythroid and granulocytic precursors; megakaryocytes appear later
Week 3–4	Hematopoietic colonies keep expanding; marrow cellularity is expected to be 50% of normal; evidence of stromal recovery and fibrosis resolution
Months 2–3	Complete recovery of trilineage hematopoiesis to normal level

BMT, bone marrow transplantation.
Adapted from Foucar, et al. *Bone Marrow Pathology*, 3rd ed.; 2010.

also be analyzed using FISH for sex chromosome complement (199). Most patients after BMT are on protocols that dictate marrow sampling at specific intervals usually after 100 days and after 1 year. Additional marrow examination may be performed as deemed clinically necessary to assess possibility of infection and/or relapse.

References

1. Evans T. Developmental biology of hematopoiesis. *Hematol Oncol Clin North Am* 1997;11(6):1115–1147.
2. Chen LT, Weiss L. The development of vertebral bone marrow of human fetuses. *Blood* 1975;46(3):389–408.
3. Tavian M, Peault B. Embryonic development of the human hematopoietic system. *Int J Dev Biol* 2005;49(2–3):243–250.
4. Mikkola HK, Gekas C, Orkin SH, et al. Placenta as a site for hematopoietic stem cell development. *Exp Hematol* 2005;33(9):1048–1054.
5. Zambidis ET, Sinka L, Tavian M, et al. Emergence of human angiohematopoietic cells in normal development and from cultured embryonic stem cells. *Ann N Y Acad Sci* 2007;1106:223–232.
6. Marshall CJ, Thrasher AJ. The embryonic origins of human haematopoiesis. *Br J Haematol* 2001;112(4):838–850.
7. Tavian M, Cortes F, Charbord P, et al. Emergence of the haematopoietic system in the human embryo and foetus. *Haematologica* 1999;84(Suppl EHA-4):1–3.
8. Dame C, Juul SE. The switch from fetal to adult erythropoiesis. *Clin Perinatol* 2000;27(3):507–526.
9. Lyman SD, Jacobsen SE. c-kit ligand and Flt3 ligand: stem/progenitor cell factors with overlapping yet distinct activities. *Blood* 1998;91(4):1101–1134.
10. Charbord P, Moore K. Gene expression in stem cell-supporting stromal cell lines. *Ann N Y Acad Sci* 2005;1044:159–167.
11. Weisel KC, Moore MA. Genetic and functional characterization of isolated stromal cell lines from the aorta-gonado-mesonephros region. *Ann N Y Acad Sci* 2005;1044:51–59.
12. Wickramasinghe SN. Bone marrow. In: *Histology for Pathologists*. New York: Raven Press, 1992:1–31.
13. Naeim F. Topobiology in hematopoiesis. *Hematol Pathol* 1995;9(2):107–119.
14. Peterson P, Ellis J. The development, morphology, and function of normal bone marrow: a review. In: *Polycythemia Vera and the Myeloproliferative Disorders*. Philadelphia, PA: WB Saunders, 1995:1–13.
15. Sieff C, Nathan D, Clark S. The anatomy and physiology of hematopoiesis. In: *Hematology of Infancy and Childhood*. Philadelphia, PA: WB Saunders, 1998:161–236.
16. McKinstry WJ, Li CL, Rasko JE, et al. Cytokine receptor expression on hematopoietic stem and progenitor cells. *Blood* 1997;89(1):65–71.
17. Metcalf D. Lineage commitment and maturation in hematopoietic cells: the case for extrinsic regulation. *Blood* 1998;92(2):345–347; discussion 352.
18. Katayama Y, Battista M, Kao WM, et al. Signals from the sympathetic nervous system regulate hematopoietic stem cell egress from bone marrow. *Cell* 2006;124(2):407–421.
19. Maestroni GJ. Sympathetic nervous system influence on the innate immune response. *Ann N Y Acad Sci* 2006;1069:195–207.
20. Sawai N, Koike K, Mwamtemi HH, et al. Thrombopoietin augments stem cell factor-dependent growth of human mast cells from bone marrow multipotential hematopoietic progenitors. *Blood* 1999;93(11):3703–3712.
21. Chambon P. A decade of molecular biology of retinoic acid receptors. *FASEB J* 1996;10(9):940–954.
22. Ess KC, Witte DP, Bascomb CP, et al. Diverse developing mouse lineages exhibit high-level c-Myb expression in immature cells and loss of expression upon differentiation. *Oncogene* 1999;18(4):1103–1111.
23. Klemsz MJ, McKercher SR, Celada A, et al. The macrophage and B cell-specific transcription factor PU.1 is related to the ets oncogene. *Cell* 1990;61(1):113–124.
24. Levanon D, Negreanu V, Bernstein Y, et al. AML1, AML2, and AML3, the human members of the runt domain gene-family: cDNA structure, expression, and chromosomal localization. *Genomics* 1994;23(2):425–432.
25. Ward AC, Loeb DM, Soede-Bobok AA, et al. Regulation of granulopoiesis by transcription factors and cytokine signals. *Leukemia* 2000;14(6):973–990.
26. Freyssinier JM, Lecoq-Lafon C, Amsellem S, et al. Purification, amplification and characterization of a population of human erythroid progenitors. *Br J Haematol* 1999;106(4):912–922.
27. Orkin SH, Weiss MJ. Apoptosis. Cutting red-cell production. *Nature* 1999;401(6752):433, 435–436.
28. Andrews NC, Erdjument-Bromage H, Davidson MB, et al. Erythroid transcription factor NF-E2 is a haematopoietic-specific basic-leucine zipper protein. *Nature* 1993;362(6422):722–728.
29. Martin DI, Zon LI, Mutter G, et al. Expression of an erythroid transcription factor in megakaryocytic and mast cell lineages. *Nature* 1990;344(6265):444–447.
30. Brown DC, Gatter KC. The bone marrow trephine biopsy: a review of normal histology. *Histopathology* 1993;22(5):411–422.
31. Vitrat N, Cohen-Solal K, Pique C, et al. Endomitosis of human megakaryocytes are due to abortive mitosis. *Blood* 1998;91(10):3711–3723.
32. Kaushansky K. The molecular mechanisms that control thrombopoiesis. *J Clin Invest* 2005;115(12):3339–3347.
33. Patel SR, Hartwig JH, Italiano JE Jr. The biogenesis of platelets from megakaryocyte proplatelets. *J Clin Invest* 2005;115(12):3348–3354.
34. Wang Z, Skokowa J, Pramono A, et al. Thrombopoietin regulates differentiation of rhesus monkey embryonic stem cells to hematopoietic cells. *Ann N Y Acad Sci* 2005;1044:29–40.
35. Miyazaki R, Ogata H, Kobayashi Y. Requirement of thrombopoietin-induced activation of ERK for megakaryocyte differentiation and of p38 for erythroid differentiation. *Ann Hematol* 2001;80(5):284–291.
36. Hashimoto S, Suzuki T, Dong HY, et al. Serial analysis of gene expression in human monocytes and macrophages. *Blood* 1999;94(3):837–844.
37. Lasser A. The mononuclear phagocytic system: a review. *Hum Pathol* 1983;14(2):108–126.
38. Foucar K, Foucar E. The mononuclear phagocyte and immunoregulatory effector (M-PIRE) system: evolving concepts. *Semin Diagn Pathol* 1990;7(1):4–18.
39. Goordyal P, Isaacson PG. Immunocytochemical characterization of monocyte colonies of human bone marrow: a clue to the origin of Langerhans cells and interdigitating reticulum cells. *J Pathol* 1985;146(3):189–195.
40. Sanchez M, Alfani E, Visconti G, et al. Thymus-independent T-cell differentiation in vitro. *Br J Haematol* 1998;103(4):1198–1205.
41. Foucar K. Hematopoiesis. In: *Bone Marrow Pathology*. Chicago, IL: ASCP Press, 2010:3–28.
42. Lucio P, Parreira A, van den Beemd MW, et al. Flow cytometric analysis of normal B cell differentiation: a frame of reference for the detection of minimal residual disease in precursor-B-ALL. *Leukemia* 1999;13(3):419–427.
43. Moore TA, Zlotnik A. T-cell lineage commitment and cytokine responses of thymic progenitors. *Blood* 1995;86(5):1850–1860.
44. Caligiuri MA. Human natural killer cells. *Blood* 2008; 112:461–469.
45. Bendelac A, Savage PB, Teyton L. The biology of NKT cells. *Annu Rev Immunol* 2007;25:297–336.
46. Marley SB, Lewis JL, Davidson RJ, et al. Evidence for a continuous decline in haemopoietic cell function from birth: application to evaluating bone marrow failure in children. *Br J Haematol* 1999;106(1):162–166.
47. Moid F, DePalma L. Comparison of relative value of bone marrow aspirates and bone marrow trephine biopsies in the diagnosis of solid tumor metastasis and Hodgkin lymphoma: institutional experience and literature review. *Arch Pathol Lab Med* 2005;129(4):497–501.

48. Friebert SE, Shepardson LB, Shurin SB, et al. Pediatric bone marrow cellularity: are we expecting too much? *J Pediatr Hematol Oncol* 1998;20(5):439–443.
49. Palis J, Segel GB. Developmental biology of erythropoiesis. *Blood Rev* 1998;12(2):106–114.
50. Brunning R. Normal bone marrow. In: *Tumors of the Bone Marrow. Atlas of Tumor Pathology*. Washington, DC: Armed Forces Institute of Pathology, 1994:2–18.
51. Allman D, Miller JP. B cell development and receptor diversity during aging. *Curr Opin Immunol* 2005;17(5):463–467.
52. Brugnara C. Reference values in infancy and childhood. In: *Hematology of infancy and childhood*. Philadelphia, PA: WB Saunders, 1998.
53. Reichard K. Bone marrow examination in children. In: *Bone Marrow Pathology*. Chicago, IL: ASCP Press, 2010:703–726.
54. Sola MC, Rimsza LM, Christensen RD. A bone marrow biopsy technique suitable for use in neonates. *Br J Haematol* 1999;107(2):458–460.
55. Albers CA, Newbury-Ecob R, Ouwehand WH, et al. New insights into the genetic basis of TAR (thrombocytopenia-absent radii) syndrome. *Curr Opin Genet Dev* 2013;23(3):316–323.
56. Stasia MJ, Li XJ. Genetics and immunopathology of chronic granulomatous disease. *Semin Immunopathol* 2008;30:209–235.
57. Hanna S, Etzioni A. Leukocyte adhesion deficiencies. *Ann N Y Acad Sci* 2012;1250:50–55.
58. Kaplan J, De Domenico I, Ward DM. Chediak-Higashi syndrome. *Curr Opin Hematol* 2008;15(1):22–29.
59. Dale DC, Bolyard AA, Aprikyan A. Cyclic neutropenia. *Semin Hematol* 2002;39(2):89–94.
60. Boxer L, Dale DC. Neutropenia: causes and consequences. *Semin Hematol* 2002;39:75–81.
61. Cham B, Bonilla MA, Winkelstein J. Neutropenia associated with primary immunodeficiency syndromes. *Semin Hematol* 2002;39:107–112.
62. Dokal I, Vulliamy T. Inherited aplastic anaemias/bone marrow failure syndromes. *Blood Rev* 2008;22(3):141–153.
63. Memon S, Shaikh S, Nizamani MA. Etiological spectrum of pancytopenia based on bone marrow examination in children. *J Coll Physicians Surg Pak* 2008;18(3):163–167.
64. Heimpel H, Wilts H, Hirschmann WD, et al. Aplastic crisis as a complication of congenital dyserythropoietic anemia type II. *Acta Haematol* 2007;117(2):115–118.
65. Steiner LA, Gallagher PG. Erythrocyte disorders in the perinatal period. *Semin Perinatol* 2007;31(4):254–261.
66. Shimamura A. Inherited bone marrow failure syndromes: molecular features. *Hematology Am Soc Hematol Educ Program* 2006:63–71.
67. Tamary H, Alter BP. Current diagnosis of inherited bone marrow failure syndromes. *Pediatr Hematol Oncol* 2007;24(2):87–99.
68. Ganapathi KA, Shimamura A. Ribosomal dysfunction and inherited marrow failure. *Br J Haematol* 2008;141(3):376–387.
69. Boria I, Garelli E, Gazda HT, et al. The ribosomal basis of Diamond-Blackfan Anemia: mutation and database update. *Hum Mutat* 2010; 31(12):1269–1279.
70. Keohane EM. Acquired aplastic anemia. *Clin Lab Sci* 2004;17(3):165–171.
71. Perkins SL. Pediatric red cell disorders and pure red cell aplasia. *Am J Clin Pathol* 2004;122 (Suppl):S70–S86.
72. Delaunay J. Red cell membrane and erythropoiesis genetic defects. *Hematol J* 2003;4(4):225–232.
73. Giri N, Kang E, Tisdale JF, et al. Clinical and laboratory evidence for a trilineage haematopoietic defect in patients with refractory Diamond-Blackfan anaemia. *Br J Haematol* 2000;108(1):167–175.
74. Jelic TM, Raj AB, Jin B, et al. Expression of CD5 on hematogones in a 7-year-old girl with Shwachman-Diamond syndrome. *Pediatr Dev Pathol* 2001;4(5):505–511.
75. Klupp N, Simonitsch I, Mannhalter C, et al. Emergence of an unusual bone marrow precursor B-cell population in fatal Shwachman-Diamond syndrome. *Arch Pathol Lab Med* 2000;124(9):1379–1381.
76. Federman N, Sakamoto KM. The genetic basis of bone marrow failure syndromes in children. *Mol Genet Metab* 2005;86(1–2):100–109.
77. Young NS, Scheinberg P, Calado RT. Aplastic anemia. *Curr Opin Hematol* 2008;15(3):162–168.
78. Sawada K, Fujishima N, Hirokawa M. Acquired pure red cell aplasia: updated review of treatment. *Br J Haematol* 2008;142(4):505–514.
79. Erslev AJ, Soltan A. Pure red-cell aplasia: a review. *Blood Rev* 1996;10(1):20–28.
80. Longacre TA, Foucar K, Crago S, et al. Hematogones: a multiparameter analysis of bone marrow precursor cells. *Blood* 1989;73(2):543–552.
81. Vogel PB, Frank AB. Sternal marrow of children in normal and in pathologic states. *Am J Dis Child* 1939;57:245–268.
82. Mandel M, Rechavi G, Neumann Y, et al. Bone marrow cell populations mimicking common acute lymphoblastic leukemia in infants with stage IV-S neuroblastoma. *Acta Haematol* 1991;86(2):86–89.
83. Rimsza LM, Larson RS, Winter SS, et al. Benign hematogone-rich lymphoid proliferations can be distinguished from B-lineage acute lymphoblastic leukemia by integration of morphology, immunophenotype, adhesion molecule expression, and architectural features. *Am J Clin Pathol* 2000;114(1):66–75.
84. Rimsza LM, Viswanatha DS, Winter SS, et al. The presence of CD34+ cell clusters predicts impending relapse in children with acute lymphoblastic leukemia receiving maintenance chemotherapy. *Am J Clin Pathol* 1998;110(3):313–320.
85. Wedgewood RA, Primary immunodeficiency disease. *Clin Exp Immunol* 1995; 99 (suppl 1):1–24.
86. Cunningham-Rundles C, Bodian C. Common variable immunodeficiency: clinical and immunological features of 248 patients. *Clin Immunol* 1999;92:34–48.
87. Hermaszewski RA, Webster AD. Primary hypogammaglobulinaemia: a survey of clinical manifestations and complications. *Q J Med* 1993;86:31–42.
88. Zhu Q, Zhang M, Winkelstein J, et al. Unique mutations of Bruton's tyrosine kinase in fourteen unrelated X-linked agammaglobulinemia families. *Hum Mol Genet* 1994;3:1899–1900.
89. Yel L. Selective IgA deficiency. *J Clin Immunol* 2010;30(1):10–16.
90. Etzioni A, Ochs HD. The hyper IgM syndrome—an evolving story. *Pediatr Res* 2004;56(4):519–525.
91. van der Burg M, Gennery AR. The expanding clinical and immunological spectrum of severe combined immunodeficiency. *Eur J Pediatr* 2011;170(5):561–571.
92. Chun HH, Gatti RA. Ataxia-telangiectasia, an evolving phenotype. *DNA Repair (Amst)* 2004;3:1187–1196.
93. Zhu Q, Zhang M, Blaese RM, et al. The Wiskott-Aldrich syndrome and X-linked congenital thrombocytopenia are caused by mutations of the same gene. *Blood* 1995;86:3797–3804.
94. Dreyfus M, Kaplan C, Verdy E, et al. Frequency of immune thrombocytopenia in newborns: a prospective study. Immune Thrombocytopenia Working Group. *Blood* 1997;89(12):4402–4406.
95. Newland A, Evans T. ABC of clinical haematology. Haematological disorders at the extremes of life. *Br Med J* 1997;314:1262–1265.
96. Beardsley D. Platelet abnormalities in infancy and childhood. In: *Hematology of Infancy and Childhood*. Philadelphia, PA: WB Saunders, 1993:216.
97. Bussel J, Corrigan JJ. Platelet and vascular disorders. In: *Blood Disease of Infancy and Childhood*. St. Louis, MO: Mosby; 1995:866.
98. Hitzler JK, Cheung J, Li Y, et al. GATA1 mutations in transient leukemia and acute megakaryoblastic leukemia of Down syndrome. *Blood* 2003;101(11):4301–4304.
99. Greene ME, Mundschau G, Wechsler J, et al. Mutations in GATA1 in both transient myeloproliferative disorder and acute megakaryoblastic leukemia of Down syndrome. *Blood Cells Mol Dis* 2003;31(3):351–356
100. Foucar K, Friedman K, Llewellyn A, et al. Prenatal diagnosis of transient myeloproliferative disorder via percutaneous umbilical blood sampling. Report of two cases in fetuses affected by Down's syndrome. *Am J Clin Pathol* 1992;97(4):584–590.
101. Zipursky A, Brown EJ, Christensen H, et al. Transient myeloproliferative disorder (transient leukemia) and hematologic manifestations of Down syndrome. *Clin Lab Med* 1999;19(1):157–167, vii.

102. Kurahashi H, Hara J, Yumura-Yagi K, et al. Monoclonal nature of transient abnormal myelopoiesis in Down's syndrome. *Blood* 1991;77(6):1161–1163.
103. Avet-Loiseau H, Mechinaud F, Harousseau JL. Clonal hematologic disorders in Down syndrome. A review. *J Pediatr Hematol Oncol* 1995;17(1):19–24.
104. Litz CE, Davies S, Brunning RD, et al. Acute leukemia and the transient myeloproliferative disorder associated with Down syndrome: morphologic, immunophenotypic and cytogenetic manifestations. *Leukemia* 1995;9(9):1432–1439.
105. Massey GV, Zipursky A, Chang MN, et al. A prospective study of the natural history of transient leukemia (TL) in neonates with Down syndrome (DS): Children's Oncology Group (COG) study POG-9481. *Blood* 2006;107(12):4606–4613.
106. Creutzig U, Ritter J, Vormoor J, et al. Myelodysplasia and acute myelogenous leukemia in Down's syndrome. A report of 40 children of the AML-BFM Study Group. *Leukemia* 1996;10(11):1677–1686.
107. Tchernia G. Erythroblastic and/or megakaryoblastic leukemia in Down's syndrome. *J Pediatr Hematol Oncol* 1996;18:59.
108. Horwitz M. The genetics of familial leukemia. *Leukemia* 1997;11(8):1347–1359.
109. Pui CH, Kane JR, Crist WM. Biology and treatment of infant leukemias. *Leukemia* 1995;9(5):762–769.
110. Cimino G, Rapanotti MC, Rivolta A, et al. Prognostic relevance of ALL-1 gene rearrangement in infant acute leukemias. *Leukemia* 1995;9(3):391–395.
111. Greaves MF. Infant leukaemia biology, aetiology and treatment. *Leukemia* 1996;10(2):372–377.
112. McCoy Jr, Overton WR. Immunophenotyping of congenital leukemia. *Cytometry* 1995;22(2):85–88.
113. Pui CH, Ribeiro RC, Campana D, et al. Prognostic factors in the acute lymphoid and myeloid leukemias of infants. *Leukemia* 1996;10(6):952–956.
114. Satake N, Maseki N, Nishiyama M, et al. Chromosome abnormalities and MLL rearrangements in acute myeloid leukemia of infants. *Leukemia* 1999;13(7):1013–1017.
115. Washio S, Ido M, Azuma E, et al. Acute megakaryoblastic leukemia with translocation t(1;22)(p13;q13) in a 10-week-old infant. *Am J Hematol* 1992;39(1):56–60.
116. Carroll A, Civin C, Schneider N, et al. The t(1;22)(p13;q13) is nonrandom and restricted to infants with acute megakaryoblastic leukemia: a Pediatric Oncology Group Study. *Blood* 1991;78(3):748–752.
117. Lion T, Haas OA, Harbott J, et al. The translocation t(1;22)(p13;q13) is a nonrandom marker specifically associated with acute megakaryocytic leukemia in young children. *Blood* 1992;79(12):3325–3330.
118. Krawczuk-Rybak M, Zak J, Jaworowska B. A lineage switch from AML to ALL with persistent translocation t(4;11) in congenital leukemia. *Med Pediatr Oncol* 2003;41(1):95–96.
119. Shimizu H, Culbert SJ, Cork A, et al. A lineage switch in acute monocytic leukemia. A case report. *Am J Pediatr Hematol Oncol* 1989;11(2):162–166.
120. Alexander FE, Chan LC, Lam TH, et al. Clustering of childhood leukaemia in Hong Kong: association with the childhood peak and common acute lymphoblastic leukaemia and with population mixing. *Br J Cancer* 1997;75(3):457–463.
121. Krajinovic M, Labuda D, Richer C, et al. Susceptibility to childhood acute lymphoblastic leukemia: influence of CYP1A1, CYP2D6, GSTM1, and GSTT1 genetic polymorphisms. *Blood* 1999;93(5):1496–1501.
122. Harris NL, Jaffe ES, Diebold J, et al. World Health Organization classification of neoplastic diseases of the hematopoietic and lymphoid tissues: report of the Clinical Advisory Committee meeting-Airlie House, Virginia, November 1997. *J Clin Oncol* 1999;17(12):3835–3849.
123. Swerdlow SH, Campo E, Harris NL, et al. *WHO Classification of Tumours of Haematopoietic and Lymphoid Tissue*. Lyon, France: IARC Press; 2008.
124. Borowitz MJ, Chan JKC. B lymphoblastic leukaemia/lymphoma, not otherwise specified. In: Swerdlow SH, Campo E, Harris NL, et al., eds. *WHO Classification of Tumours of Haematopoietic and Lymphoid Tissue*. Lyon, France: IARC Press; 2008:168–170.
125. Leoncini L, Raphaël M, Stein H, et al. Burkitt lymphoma. In: Swerdlow SH, Campo E, Harris NL, et al., eds. *WHO Classification of Tumours of Haematopoietic and Lymphoid Tissue*. Lyon, France: IARC Press; 2008:262–264.
126. Cerezo L, Shuster JJ, Pullen DJ, et al. Laboratory correlates and prognostic significance of granular acute lymphoblastic leukemia in children. A Pediatric Oncology Group study. *Am J Clin Pathol* 1991;95(4):526–531.
127. Geijtenbeek TB, van Kooyk Y, van Vliet SJ, et al. High frequency of adhesion defects in B-lineage acute lymphoblastic leukemia. *Blood* 1999;94(2):754–764.
128. Griesinger F, Piro-Noack M, Kaib N, et al. Leukaemia-associated immunophenotypes (LAIP) are observed in 90% of adult and childhood acute lymphoblastic leukaemia: detection in remission marrow predicts outcome. *Br J Haematol* 1999;105(1):241–255.
129. Borowitz MJ, Guenther KL, Shults KE, et al. Immunophenotyping of acute leukemia by flow cytometric analysis. Use of CD45 and right-angle light scatter to gate on leukemic blasts in three-color analysis. *Am J Clin Pathol* 1993;100(5):534–540.
130. Davis BH, Foucar K, Szczarkowski W, et al. U.S.-Canadian Consensus recommendations on the immunophenotypic analysis of hematologic neoplasia by flow cytometry: medical indications. *Cytometry* 1997;30(5):249–263.
131. Faderl S, Kantarjian HM, Talpaz M, et al. Clinical significance of cytogenetic abnormalities in adult acute lymphoblastic leukemia. *Blood* 1998;91(11):3995–4019.
132. Martinez-Climent JA. Molecular cytogenetics of childhood hematological malignancies. *Leukemia* 1997;11(12):1999–2021.
133. Rubnitz JE, Look AT. Molecular genetics of childhood leukemias. *J Pediatr Hematol Oncol* 1998;20(1):1–11.
134. Harrison CJ, Haas O, Harbott J, et al. Detection of prognostically relevant genetic abnormalities in childhood B-cell precursor acute lymphoblastic leukaemia: recommendations from the Biology and Diagnosis Committee of the International Berlin-Frankfurt-Munster study group. *Br J Haematol* 2010;151(2):132–142.
135. Meeker TC, Hardy D, Willman C, et al. Activation of the interleukin-3 gene by chromosome translocation in acute lymphocytic leukemia with eosinophilia. *Blood* 1990;76(2):285–289.
136. Ribeiro RC, Abromowitch M, Raimondi SC, et al. Clinical and biologic hallmarks of the Philadelphia chromosome in childhood acute lymphoblastic leukemia. *Blood* 1987;70(4):948–953.
137. Schlieben S, Borkhardt A, Reinisch I, et al. Incidence and clinical outcome of children with BCR/ABL-positive acute lymphoblastic leukemia (ALL). A prospective RT-PCR study based on 673 patients enrolled in the German pediatric multicenter therapy trials ALL-BFM-90 and CoALL-05-92. *Leukemia* 1996;10(6):957–963.
138. Bhatia S, Neglia JP. Epidemiology of childhood acute myelogenous leukemia. *J Pediatr Hematol Oncol* 1995;17(2):94–100.
139. Fircanis S, Merriam P, Khan N, et al. The relation between cigarette smoking and risk of acute myeloid leukemia: an updated meta-analysis of epidemiological studies. *Am J Hematol* 2014;89(8):E125–E132.
140. Pedersen-Bjergaard J, Pedersen M, Roulston D, et al. Different genetic pathways in leukemogenesis for patients presenting with therapy-related myelodysplasia and therapy-related acute myeloid leukemia. *Blood* 1995;86(9):3542–3552.
141. Nucifora G, Dickstein JI, Torbenson V, et al. Correlation between cell morphology and expression of the AML1/ETO chimeric transcript in patients with acute myeloid leukemia without the t(8;21). *Leukemia* 1994;8(9):1533–1538.
142. Hurwitz CA, Raimondi SC, Head D, et al. Distinctive immunophenotypic features of t(8;21)(q22;q22) acute myeloblastic leukemia in children. *Blood* 1992;80(12):3182–3188.
143. Porwit-MacDonald A, Janossy G, Ivory K, et al. Leukemia-associated changes identified by quantitative flow cytometry. IV. CD34 overexpression in acute myelogenous leukemia M2 with t(8;21). *Blood* 1996;87(3):1162–1169.

144. Adès L, Sanz MA, Chevret S, et al. Treatment of newly diagnosed acute promyelocytic leukemia (APL): a comparison of French-Belgian-Swiss and PETHEMA results. *Blood* 2008;111(3):1078–1084.
145. Sanz MA, Montesinos P, Rayón C, et al. Risk-adapted treatment of acute promyelocytic leukemia based on all-trans retinoic acid and anthracycline with addition of cytarabine in consolidation therapy for high-risk patients: further improvements in treatment outcome. *Blood* 2010;115(25):5137–5146.
146. Arthur DC, Bloomfield CD. Partial deletion of the long arm of chromosome 16 and bone marrow eosinophilia in acute nonlymphocytic leukemia: a new association. *Blood* 1983;61(5):994–998.
147. Le Beau MM, Larson RA, Bitter MA, et al. Association of an inversion of chromosome 16 with abnormal marrow eosinophils in acute myelomonocytic leukemia. A unique cytogenetic-clinicopathological association. *N Engl J Med* 1983;309(11):630–636.
148. Marlton P, Keating M, Kantarjian H, et al. Cytogenetic and clinical correlates in AML patients with abnormalities of chromosome 16. *Leukemia* 1995;9(6):965–971.
149. Forestier E, Heim S, Blennow E, et al. Cytogenetic abnormalities in childhood acute myeloid leukaemia: a Nordic series comprising all children enrolled in the NOPHO-93-AML trial between 1993 and 2001. *Br J Haematol.* 2003;121(4):566–577.
150. Raimondi SC, Chang MN, Ravindranath Y, et al. Chromosomal abnormalities in 478 children with acute myeloid leukemia: clinical characteristics and treatment outcome in a cooperative pediatric oncology group study-POG 8821. *Blood* 1999;94(11):3707–3716.
151. Leone G, Mele L, Pulsoni A, et al. The incidence of secondary leukemias. *Haematologica* 1999;84(10):937–945.
152. Aguilera DG, Vaklavas C, Tsimberidou AM, et al. Pediatric therapy-related myelodysplastic syndrome/acute myeloid leukemia: the MD Anderson Cancer Center experience. *J Pediatr Hematol Oncol* 2009;31(11):803–811.
153. Meadows AT, Baum E, Fossati-Bellani F, et al. Second malignant neoplasms in children: an update from the Late Effects Study Group. *J Clin Oncol* 1985;3(4):532–538.
154. Neglia JP, Friedman DL, Yasui Y, et al. Second malignant neoplasms in five-year survivors of childhood cancer: childhood cancer survivor study. *J Natl Cancer Inst* 2001;93(8):618–629.
155. Luna-Fineman S, Shannon KM, Lange BJ. Childhood monosomy 7: epidemiology, biology, and mechanistic implications. *Blood* 1995;85(8): 1985–1999.
156. Emanuel PD. Myelodysplasia and myeloproliferative disorders in childhood: an update. *Br J Haematol* 1999;105(4):852–863.
157. Luna-Fineman S, Shannon KM, Atwater SK, et al. Myelodysplastic and myeloproliferative disorders of childhood: a study of 167 patients. *Blood* 1999;93(2):459–466.
158. Martinez-Climent JA, Garcia-Conde J. Chromosomal rearrangements in childhood acute myeloid leukemia and myelodysplastic syndromes. *J Pediatr Hematol Oncol* 1999;21(2):91–102.
159. Baumann I, Bennett JM, Niemeyer CM, et al. Juvenile myelomonocytic leukaemia. In: Swerdlow SH, Campo E, Harris NL, et al., eds. *WHO Classification of Tumours of Haematopoietic and Lymphoid Tissue.* Lyon, France: IARC Press, 2008:82–84.
160. Foucar K. Chronic leukemias in childhood. In: *Pediatric Hematopathology.* New York: Churchill Livingstone, 2001.
161. Foucar K. Myelodysplastic syndrome. In: *Bone Marrow Pathology.* Chicago, IL: ASCP Press, 2010:331–362.
162. Foucar K. Neonatal hematopathology: special considerations. In: *Pediatric Hematopathology.* New York: Churchill Livingstone, 2001.
163. Savage DG, Szydlo RM, Goldman JM. Clinical features at diagnosis in 430 patients with chronic myeloid leukaemia seen at a referral centre over a 16-year period. *Br J Haematol* 1997;96(1):111–116.
164. Dror Y, Zipursky A, Blanchette VS. Essential thrombocythemia in children. *J Pediatr Hematol Oncol* 1999;21(5):356–363.
165. Kapoor G, Correa H, Yu LC. Essential thrombocythemia in an infant. *J Pediatr Hematol Oncol* 1996;18(4):381–383.
166. Sekhar M, Prentice HG, Popat U, et al. Idiopathic myelofibrosis in children. *Br J Haematol* 1996;93(2):394–397.
167. Cline MJ. Histiocytes and histiocytosis. *Blood* 1994;84(9):2840–2853.
168. Arico M, Egeler RM. Clinical aspects of Langerhans cell histiocytosis. *Hematol Oncol Clin North Am* 1998;12(2):247–258.
169. Schmitz L, Favara BE. Nosology and pathology of Langerhans cell histiocytosis. *Hematol Oncol Clin North Am* 1998;12(2):221–246.
170. Gogusev J, Nezelof C. Malignant histiocytosis. Histologic, cytochemical, chromosomal, and molecular data with a nosologic discussion. *Hematol Oncol Clin North Am* 1998;12(2):445–463.
171. Takeshita M, Kikuchi M, Ohshima K, et al. Bone marrow findings in malignant histiocytosis and/or malignant lymphoma with concurrent hemophagocytic syndrome. *Leuk Lymphoma* 1993;12(1–2):79–89.
172. Egeler RM, Schmitz L, Sonneveld P, et al. Malignant histiocytosis: a reassessment of cases formerly classified as histiocytic neoplasms and review of the literature. *Med Pediatr Oncol* 1995;25(1):1–7.
173. Murase T, Nakamura S, Tashiro K, et al. Malignant histiocytosis-like B-cell lymphoma, a distinct pathologic variant of intravascular lymphomatosis: a report of five cases and review of the literature. *Br J Haematol* 1997;99(3):656–664.
174. Bitter MA, Franklin WA, Larson RA, et al. Morphology in Ki-1(CD30)-positive non-Hodgkin's lymphoma is correlated with clinical features and the presence of a unique chromosomal abnormality, t(2;5) (p23;q35). *Am J Surg Pathol* 1990;14(4):305–316.
175. Bucsky P, Egeler RM. Malignant histiocytic disorders in children. Clinical and therapeutic approaches with a nosologic discussion. *Hematol Oncol Clin North Am* 1998;2(2):465–471.
176. Lauritzen AF, Ralfkiaer E. Histiocytic sarcomas. *Leuk Lymphoma* 1995;18(1–2):73–80.
177. Bucsky P, Favara B, Feller AC, et al. Malignant histiocytosis and large cell anaplastic (Ki-1) lymphoma in childhood: guidelines for differential diagnosis—report of the Histiocyte Society. *Med Pediatr Oncol* 1994;22(3):200–203.
178. Malone M. The histiocytoses of childhood. *Histopathology* 1991;19(2): 105–119.
179. Calverly DC, Wismer J, Rosenthal D, et al. Xanthoma disseminatum in an infant with skeletal and marrow involvement. *J Pediatr Hematol Oncol* 1995;17(1):61–65.
180. Favara BE, Feller AC, Pauli M, et al. Contemporary classification of histiocytic disorders. The WHO Committee On Histiocytic/Reticulum Cell Proliferations. Reclassification Working Group of the Histiocyte Society. *Med Pediatr Oncol* 1997;29(3):157–166.
181. Delta BG, Pinkel D. Bone marrow aspiration in children with malignant tumors. *J Pediatr* 1964;64:542–546.
182. Reid MM, Hamilton PJ. Histology of neuroblastoma involving bone marrow: the problem of detecting residual tumour after initiation of chemotherapy. *Br J Haematol* 1988;69(4):487–490.
183. Reid MM, Roald B. Adequacy of bone marrow trephine biopsy specimens in children. *J Clin Pathol* 1996;49(3):226–229.
184. Almanaseer IY, Trujillo YP, Taxy JB, et al. Systemic rhabdomyosarcoma with diffuse bone marrow involvement. Case report of an unusual presentation. *Am J Clin Pathol* 1984;82(3):349–353.
185. DuBois SG, Kalika Y, Lukens JN, et al. Metastatic sites in stage IV and IVS neuroblastoma correlate with age, tumor biology, and survival. *J Pediatr Hematol Oncol* 1999;21(3):181–189.
186. Head DR, Kennedy PS, Goyette RE. Metastatic neuroblastoma in bone marrow aspirate smears. *Am J Clin Pathol* 1979;72(6):1008–1011.
187. Pollak E, Miller H, Vye M. Medulloblastoma presenting as leukemia. *Am J Clin Pathol* 1981;76:98–103.
188. Westerman MP. Bone marrow needle biopsy: an evaluation and critique. *Semin Hematol* 1981;18(4):293–300.
189. Mehta PA, Davies SM. Allogeneic transplantation for childhood ALL. *Bone Marrow Transplant* 2008;41(2):133–139.
190. Shenoy S, Smith FO. Hematopoietic stem cell transplantation for childhood malignancies of myeloid origin. *Bone Marrow Transplant* 2008;41(2):141–148.
191. Bhatia M, Walters MC. Hematopoietic cell transplantation for thalassemia and sickle cell disease: past, present and future. *Bone Marrow Transplant* 2008;41(2):109–1017.

192. Barrett D, Fish JD, Grupp SA. Autologous and allogeneic cellular therapies for high-risk pediatric solid tumors. *Pediatr Clin North Am* 2010;57(1):47–66.
193. Thomas ED. A history of haemopoietic cell transplantation. *Br J Haematol* 1999;105(2):330–339.
194. Sale GE, Buckner CD. Pathology of bone marrow in transplant recipients. *Hematol Oncol Clin North Am* 1988;2(4):735–756.
195. Dick F, Gingrich RD. Biopsy analysis in bone marrow transplantation. In: *Transplant Pathology*. Chicago, IL: ASCP Press, 1994: 281–292.
196. Van den Berg H, Kluin PM, Vossen JM. Early reconstitution of haematopoiesis after allogeneic bone marrow transplantation: a prospective histopathological study of bone marrow biopsy specimens. *J Clin Pathol* 1990;43(5):365–369.
197. Donohue J, Homge M, Kernan NA. Characterization of cells emerging at the time of graft failure after bone marrow transplantation from an unrelated marrow donor. *Blood* 1993;82(3):1023–1029.
198. Byrne JL, Haynes AP, Russell NH. Use of haemopoietic growth factors: commentary on the ASCO/ECOG guidelines. American Society of Clinical Oncology/Eastern Co-operative Oncology Group. *Blood Rev* 1997;11(1):16–27.
199. Antin JH, Childs R, Filipovich AH, et al. Establishment of complete and mixed donor chimerism after allogeneic lymphohematopoietic transplantation: recommendations from a workshop at the 2001 Tandem Meetings. *Biol Blood Marrow Transplant* 2001;7(9):473–485.
200. Humphrey P, Dehner L, Pfeifer J. Bone marrow pathology. In: *The Washington Manual of Surgical Pathology*, 1st ed. Philadelphia, PA: Lippincott Williams & Wilkins, 2008:573–588.

CHAPTER 25

Soft Tissue

Louis P. Dehner, M.D., D. Ashley Hill, M.D., and Jason A. Jarzembowski, M.D., Ph.D.

The pediatric surgical pathologist who is presented with a "soft tissue tumor" from a child may be confronted with a wide spectrum of pathology ranging from an enlarged lymph node, fibroinflammatory process in the superficial soft tissues, vascular malformation (VM) or a true neoplasm. Some soft tissue tumors (STTs) arise in the skin (infantile myofibroma) with involvement of the subcutis (infantile subcutaneous fibromatosis or lipofibromatosis), or at the level of the fascia and the deep soft tissues. Some of the soft-tissue sarcomas (STSs) in children may be organ based as in the case of embryonal rhabdomyosarcoma (ERMS) of the bladder or prostate gland, or congenital infantile fibrosarcoma (CIFS) of the small intestine, whereas others such as Ewing sarcoma-primitive neuroectodermal tumor (EWS-PNET), alveolar rhabdomyosarcoma (ARMS), and synovial sarcoma (SS), have the more familiar pattern of presenting in the deep soft tissues of the extremities. However, EWS-PNET is known to present in the kidney and SS can arise in the lung. Immunohistochemistry (IHC) and molecular diagnostic studies have facilitated the diagnostic evaluation of STSs in children of malignant and benign types (1). The fusion proteins from the various translocations among the STSs provide potential molecular targets for therapy (2).

One of the more common clinical diagnoses accompanying a pediatric surgical specimen from the superficial soft tissues is "ruleout soft-tissue tumor." If this is the case, the neoplasm is benign in the majority of cases and more often than not is either a vascular anomaly of one type or another or a nonneoplastic process such as deep granuloma annulare. Of course, there is the dilemma in the case of some vascular tumors whether they are true neoplasms or malformations, which could have some bearing upon the surgical management. Vascular, neurogenic, fibrous myofibroblastic and myogenic tumors account for the majority (70% to 85%) of all STTs in children (3). Most of these tumors are benign (60% to 70% of cases) and have a predilection for the trunk, extremities, and head and neck regions in descending order of frequency; most of the benign STTs come to clinical attention at or before 10 years of age. Some of the more aggressive STSs, such as EWS-PNET, ARMS and SS, are usually diagnosed in the second decade of life; however, like all generalizations, there are exceptions and each one of these neoplasms has been diagnosed in children less than 5 years of life (4). Arguably one of the most malignant and treatment-resistant STSs of childhood is the malignant rhabdoid tumor (MRT) with its many organ-based primary sites (kidney, liver, and central nervous system), in addition to various nonvisceral soft-tissue locations such as the head and neck and mediastinum. Congenital STTs are mainly restricted to vascular anomalies, benign fibrous tumors of various types and teratomas arising in the sacrococcygeal soft tissues, retroperitoneum, and head and neck. Other less common STTs presenting at birth or in the first month of life are CIFS, myofibroma–myofibromatosis, granular cell tumor (GCT), primarily the congenital epulis of the oral cavity, ERMS, dermatofibrosarcoma protuberans (DFSP) and rarely ARMS. However, again, one should be prepared for the unanticipated when the clinical impression is a STT in a child.

The classification of STTs in children is accommodated for the most part by the World Health Organization (WHO) classification (5). Traditionally, STTs are classified on the basis of tissue differentiation and phenotype as determined by IHC. Molecular genetics has come to occupy an increasingly important role in the diagnosis of both benign and malignant STTs in children and adults for that matter (1,6) (Table 25-1). One of the first STS-specific, nonrandom chromosomal abnormalities, t(11;22)(q24;q12) translocation, was identified in EWS-PNET, the second most common STS of childhood (7). Emerging from this initial observation over the succeeding years has been the appreciation that there is a "family" of STSs with a predilection for children, adolescents, and young adults whose specific tumor types have nonrandom chromosomal translocations with the *EWS* gene on chromosome 22q as one of the fusion partners. This concept of families of tumors sharing a common

TABLE 25-1 SOFT TISSUE NEOPLASMS IN CHILDREN AND THEIR RECURRING CYTOGENETIC ABNORMALITIES

Tumor Type	Cytogenetic Abnormality	LOCI
EWS-PNET[a]	t(11;22)(q24;q12)	EWSR1-FLI1 (85%)
	t(21;22)(q22;q12)	EWSR1-ERG (10%)
	t(7;22)(p22;q12)	EWSR1-ETV1
	t(17;22)(q21;q12)	EWSR1-ETV4
	t(2;22)(q35;q12)	EWSR1-FEV
	t(16;21)(p11;q22)	FUS-ERG
	t(2;16)(q35;p11)	FUS-FEV
	t(20;22)(q13;q12)	EWSR1-NFATC2
	t(6;22)(p21;q12)	EWSR1-POU5F1
	t(4;22)(q31;q12)	EWSR1-SMARCA5
	t(1;22)(q36.1;q12)	EWSR1-PATZ1
	t(2;22)(q31;q12)	EWSR1-SP3
DSRCT[a]	t(11;22)(q13;q12)	EWSR1-WT1
CCS of soft tissue (melanoma of soft parts)[a]	t(12;22)(q13;q12)	EWSR1-ATF1
CCS-like GI tumor[a]	t(2;22)(q33;q12)	EWSR1-CREB1
EMC[a]	t(9;22)(q22;q12)	EWSR1-CHN/TEC
	t(9;17)(q22;q11)	TAF15-NR4A3
	t(9;15)(q22;q21)	TCF12-NR4A3
	t(3;9)(q12;q22)	TFG-NR4A3
AFH[a]	t(12;22)(q13;q12)	EWSR1-ATF1
	t(2;22)(q33;q12)	EWSR1-CREB1
	t(12;16)(q13;p11)	FUS-ATF1
Primary pulmonary myxoid sarcoma	t(2;22)(q33;q12)	EWSR1-CREB1
Myxoid LPS[a]	t(12;16)(q13;p11)	FUS-DDIT3 (90%)
	t(12;22)(q13;q12)	EWSR1-DDIT3
Angiosarcoma	t(12;22)(q13;q12)	EWSR1-ATF1
Myoepithelial tumor[a]	t(12;22)(q13;q12)	EWSR1-ATF1
	t(6;22)(p21;q12)	EWSR1-POU5F1
	t(1;22)(q23;q12)	EWSR1-PBX1
	t(19;22)(q13;q12)	EWSR1-ZNF444
ERMS	LOH at 11p15, gains 2+, 7+, 8+, 11+, 12+, 20+, 21+, 13q 21+, 20+; Losses 1p35-36−, 3−, 7−, 6−, 9q22−, 14q 21-32−, 17−	
ARMS	t(2;13)(q35;q14)	PAX 3-FOXO1 (FKHR)
	t(1;13)(p36;q14)	PAX7-FOXO1 (FKHR)
CIFS	t(12;15)(p13;q25)	ETV6-NTRK3
SS	t(X;18)(p11;q11)	SYT-SSX1(biphasic)
		SYT-SSX2(monophasic)
		SYT-SSX4
ASPS	der(17)t(X;17)(p11.2;q25)	ASPL-TFE3
MRT, ES	Deletion and mutation in 22q11	SMARCB1/INI1 (hSNF5/INI1)
Lipoblastoma	8q11-13	PLAG1
IMT	Translocations involving 2p23	ALK-CLTC
	t(2;17)(p23;q23)	
	t(1;2)(q21;p23)	ALK-TPM3
	t(2;19)(p23;p13)	ALK-TPM4
	t(2;11)(p23;p15)	ALK-CARS
	t(2;2)(p23;q12)	ALK-RANBP2
	t(2;2)p23;q35)	ALK-ATIC

TABLE 25-1 SOFT TISSUE NEOPLASMS IN CHILDREN AND THEIR RECURRING CYTOGENETIC ABNORMALITIES (continued)

Tumor Type	Cytogenetic Abnormality	LOCI
	t(2;4)(p23;q21)	ALK-SEC31L
	t(6;17)(q22;p13.3)	YWHE-ROS1
	t(3;6)(q12.2;q22)	TFG-ROS1
LGFS—SEF[a]	t(7;16)(q32–34;p11)	FUS-CREB3L2
	t(11;16)(p11;p11)	FUS-CREB3L1
	t(16;22) (p11;q12)	EWSR1-CREB3L1
NF	t(17;22)(p13;q13)	USP6-MYH9
EWS-like	t(4;19)(q35;q13.1)	CIC-DUX4
	t(x;19)(q13;q13.3)	CIC-FOXO4
NF	t(17;22)(p13;q13)	USP6-MYH9
EHE	t(1;3)(p36.23;q25.1)	CAMTA1-WWTR1
DFSP	t(17;22)(q22;q13)	COL1A1-PDGF
Mesenchymal chondrosarcoma	t(1;5)(q42;q32)	HEY1-NC0A2
Solitary fibrous tumor		NAB2-STAT6

[a]Extended EWS family of tumor.

fusion partner has evolved in the case of EWS, ALK, FUS and INI1 (8). These chromosomal perturbations can be detected by multiple techniques including (in approximate order of increasing sensitivity) conventional karyotyping, fluorescent in situ hybridization (FISH) on nuclear preparations from fresh or cultured tumor cells or formalin-fixed, paraffin-embedded tissue sections, DNA sequencing, or polymerase chain reaction (PCR).

The approach to the pathologic diagnosis of a STT from a child has the same starting point as one in an adult—a careful gross examination followed by the selection of representative tissue blocks based on the macroscopic features of the tumor (if one has digital photographic capability, a gross illustration can often substitute for a long narrative description; a picture is indeed worth a thousand words). The decision about the number of tissue blocks to submit is guided by the size of the specimen and the heterogeneity of gross features ranging from viable areas to those with a necrotic or hemorrhagic appearance. Many blocks may be required to identify any residual tumor in those cases with prior adjuvant therapy. If the specimen is submitted as a gross resection, the peripheral margins and any attached organs or bony structures should be identified and the margins tattooed with India ink or other dyes that will survive processing in order to evaluate the adequacy of the surgical margins. Margins of surgical resection are generally reported as "free of tumor" or not. Determining the distance between the tumor and the tumor-free margin by gross and microscopic examination is difficult in many cases. Some margins are limited by the constraints of the anatomy as it relates to neurovascular bundles or bony structures. The margins can be even more challenging in an infant or small child.

If the specimen is a small biopsy and submitted for intraoperative frozen section consultation, very little tissue may remain for permanent sections, let alone ancillary studies; thus, another tissue sample should be requested, if at all possible, as a contingency. Once the biopsy has been examined, it should be marked with an appropriate dye and placed in a small tea bag before tissue processing. If facilities are available and the tissue sample is judged to be more than adequate for histologic examination and molecular studies, tissue banking should be considered as well. Often times, the safest course of action is to snap-freeze a sugar cube–sized (approximately 1 cm^3) piece of viable-appearing tissue and wait for the histologic examination to guide the selection of additional studies, most of which can be performed on a frozen specimen.

The world of STTs in children can be divided into three morphologic spheres: vascular tumors of varying morphology, spindle cell tumors, and small and not-so-small round cell tumors (Table 25-2). Various spindle cell tumors are listed in this tabulation and many of these are familiar to the pediatric pathologist. Some of the diagnoses are made with relative ease through one's own experience with the appreciation of specific histologic details, which separate that particular round cell or spindle cell proliferation from all of the other similar appearing tumors. As one peruses Table 25-2, it becomes apparent that some of these STTs occur almost exclusively in the first two decades of life whereas others are seen more often in adolescence or young adulthood. Again, while the patient's age should facilitate the crafting of a differential diagnosis, it should never be the sole cause for excluding a particular diagnosis.

Ancillary IHC studies have had a profound, impact upon the practice of surgical pathology over the past 25 years, but especially so in the diagnosis of soft tissue and hematopoietic neoplasms; the same can be said about the role of molecular genetics for these two phenotypic

TABLE 25-2	MORPHOLOGIC THEMES IN SSTS IN CHILDREN SOME DIFFERENTIAL DIAGNOSTIC CONSIDERATIONS
Morphology	Tumor Types
Round and not so "rounded" small cells	RMS (both ERMS and ARMS)
	EWS-PNET
	EWS-like sarcoma
	Mononuclear histiocytic tumors (LCH, JXG, Rosai-Dorfman disease, DC tumor, giant cell tumor of tendon sheath, LCH and JXG
	Non-histiocytic hemato-lymphoid neoplasms (lymphoma, granulocytic sarcoma)
	MRT
	ASPS
	PEComa
	Epithelioid vascular tumor
	Epithelioid sarcoma
	Myoepithelial tumor
Spindle cells	Fibrous-myofibroblastic tissue reaction
	NF
	Fibrous tumors—fibromatosis
	CIFS
	SS
	IMT
	DFSP
	Schwannoma
	KHE
	LGFS
	MPNST
	Spindle cell RMS
Blood vessels and lymphatics	Hemangiomas of diverse subtypes and hemangioendothelioma
	Vascular malformations
	Lymphatic malformations
	Cystic hygroma

categories. In the case of malignancies in children, several of the more common neoplasms, soft tissue or otherwise, are morphologically similar from the perspective of their more or less uniform composition of small or large malignant round cells (Table 25-2). There are other accompanying features, which should be incorporated into the construction of the differential diagnosis without the need to utilize every commercially available antibody in one's IHC laboratory (it does become necessary in some cases). However, it is acknowledged that there are those occasional cases in which successive waves of newly ordered IHC becomes necessary in order to arrive at a final diagnosis or the realization for the need of consultation. In the meantime, the titer of anxiety is on the rise for all concerned in the care of the patient. A difficult case is difficult for no other reason than that it is a difficult case as an existential reality or one simply does not appreciate the diagnosis. The most difficult diagnosis in the world to make is the one that we do not consider or it has yet to be described. Attention to the clinical aspects including clinical laboratory studies can be helpful in crafting the differential diagnosis and guiding the selection of stains. Table 25-3 summarizes the immunophenotype of malignant round cell tumors seen in children and should be familiar to most pathologists with some level of experience with the malignant round cell tumors of childhood. Each of these tumor types, less the ever diminishing category of "undifferentiated round cell sarcoma," has one or more molecular aberrations, often with diagnostic and prognostic implications. One emerging category of malignant round cell neoplasms is the EWS-like sarcomas with their unique translocations, but with the morphology and immunophenotype of EWS-PNET.

There are other "round cell" neoplasms presenting in childhood, though chiefly in adults, which are not included in Table 25-2. Some of the round cell neoplasms have the added characterization of "epithelioid" whose cytomorphologic features are polygonal contours, a central nucleus, prominent nucleolus and abundant eosinophilic to clear cytoplasm. Alveolar soft part sarcoma (ASPS), perivascular epithelioid cell tumor, epithelioid vascular neoplasms, MRT and epithelioid sarcoma (ES) are among the more familiar tumor types in this category.

GRADING OF SOFT TISSUE SARCOMAS

STSs in adults are commonly graded pathologically on the basis of mitotic activity [mitoses per 10 or 50 high power fields (×400)], nuclear pleomorphism, and necrosis. Pleomorphic undifferentiated sarcoma (PUS) (formerly many of these sarcomas were interpreted as "malignant fibrous histiocytomas"), liposarcoma (LPS) and leiomyosarcoma are the three most common STSs in adults, which lend themselves to this traditional grading scheme (9). Pathologic grading of nonrhabdomyosarcomatous soft tissue tumors (NRMSTS) in the Children's Oncology Group (COG) system (modified National Cancer Institute system) relies on a combination of morphologic type and histologic features: CIFS and myxoid LPS are grade 1, mesenchymal chondrosarcoma (MCS) and alveolar soft part sarcoma are grade 3, and other tumors are assigned either grade 2 or grade 3 depending on the mitotic activity and extent

TABLE 25-3 MALIGNANT ROUND CELL TUMORS AND THEIR IMMUNOPHENOTYPE

Tumor	VIM	CK	DES	MYOD1-MYOG	CD99	CD43	WT1	CHR	CD31	BAF47-INI1 retained (+) or lost (−)
RMS	+	−	+	+	−	−	−	−	−	+
NB	±	−	−	−	−	−	−	+	−	+
EWS/PNET	+	±	−	−	+	−	−	−	−	+
WT-BL	+	−	±	−	−	−	+	−	−	+
DSRCT	+	±	+	−	±	−	+	±	−	+
SS-PD	+	+	−	−	±	−	−	−	−	+
MRT	+	+	−	−	±	−	−	−	−	−
UDS-EWS-like	+	±	−	−	±	−	−	−	−	+
HPN	+	−	−	−	±	+	−	−	−	+
ES	+	+	−	−	±	−	−	−	−	−
EHE	+	±	−	−	−	−	−	−	+	+

RMS, rhabdomyosarcoma; NB, neuroblastoma; EWS/PNET, Ewing sarcoma—primitive neuroectodermal tumor; WT-BL, Wilms tumor—blastemal predominant; DSRCT, desmoplastic small round cell tumors; SS—PD, synovial sarcoma—poorly differentiated; MRT, malignant rhabdoid tumor; UDS, undifferentiated sarcoma; ES, epithelioid sarcoma; EHE, epithelioid hemangioma-hemangioendothelioma; HPN, hematopoietic neoplasm to include lymphoid and non-lymphoid tumors; ES, epithelioid sarcoma; VIM, vimentin; CK, cytokeratin; DES, desmin; MyoD1-Myog, MyoDI—myogenin; WT1, Wilms tumor1; CHR, chromogranin.

of necrosis (>5 mitoses per 10 high-powered fields (40× objective and/or >15% surface area necrosis indicate grade 3). Needless to say, differences in pathologic grading may arise between observers in a particular STS. A comparison between the COG and Fédération Nationale des Centre de Lutte Contre le Cancer (FNCLCC) systems of grading of STSs demonstrated that these systems were equally predictive for 5-year event free survivals except for the intermediate prognosis groups (9). Pathologic staging of STSs in children differs in several respects from sarcomas in adults and especially so in the case of RMSs in children where the primary site has a significant impact upon the stage and thus the prognosis as in the case of one unfavorable site, the perianal–perineal location.

Some important developments in regard to STTs in children in the recent past include the reclassification of nodular fasciitis (NF) as a transient fibrous neoplasm on the basis of its molecular genetics, the stratification of RMSs on the basis of the presence or absence of PAX3 or PAX7 fusion partners with FOXO1 (FKHR) and the recognition of EWS-like round cell sarcomas with unique translocations other than an EWS fusion transcript (10–12).

VASCULAR TUMORS

Vascular anomalies, including both neoplasms and malformations, are the most common STTs in children, account for 20% to 30% of all cases and are among the most frequently recognized tumors at or shortly after birth and as many as one-third of cases are diagnosed in the first year of life (3,13–15). Cutaneous and even deep organ vascular anomalies are seen with multifocal sites of involvement in infants.

Traditionally, vasoformative lesions (or tumors) have been divided morphologically on the basis of their resemblance to blood vessels or lymphatics. A pathologic distinction is also made between a vascular neoplasm and malformation, which has been incorporated into the general classification of "vascular anomalies" (16). The International Society for the study of Vascular Anomalies (ISSVA) classification is more widely utilized by clinicians whereas the WHO classification of vascular tumors is more familiar to most general pathologists but the pediatric pathologist is generally expected to be conversant with the ISSVA classification and its application to vascular lesions in children (5) (Table 25-4). If one turns to the standard dermatopathology reference, the number of individual vascular lesions expands to another level (17).

Hemangioma with any number of qualifying prefixes is the most common pathologic diagnosis of STTs seen in the first two decades of life (3,13). The most common site is the skin where 25% or more of all vascular anomalies are encountered. There is a preference for the head and neck region in the case of skin and soft tissue involvement. Other sites include the deep soft tissues, bone, orbit, parotid gland, skeletal muscle, and upper air passages including the nasal cavity and larynx. The overwhelming majority (70% to 90%) of hemangiomas in children are initially recognized at or before 6 months of age (18). It is difficult in reviewing studies from the past to determine the proportion of infantile hemangiomas relative to VMs, also considered "hemangiomas" in many cases before the current conceptualization of the pathogenesis of vascular anomalies. However, one study

TABLE 25-4	CLASSIFICATION OF VASCULAR ANOMALIES	
	ISSVA	WHO, 2013
Tumors		
	Hemangioma	Hemangiomas (benign)
	Infantile – (GLUT-1+)	Synovial
	Congenital (GLUT-1–)	Venous
	Tufted angioma (D2-40+)	Arteriovenous
	Epithelioid	Intramuscular
	Spindle cell (D2-40+)	
	Capillary	
	Lobular capillary (pyogenic granuloma)	
	HE	
	Kaposiform (D2-40+)	Epithelioid
	Papillary intralymphatic (Dabska tumor)	Angiomatosis
	Retiform	Lymphangioma
	Spindle cell	Intermediate, locally aggressive
	Epithelioid	Kaposiform HEA
	Angiosarcoma	Retiform HEA
		Intermediate (rarely metastasizing)
		Papillary intralymphatic angioendothelioma
		Composite HEA
		KS
		Malignant
		Epithelioid HEA
		Angiosarcoma
Malformations		
	Simple (slow flow)	Arteriovenous malformations/hemangiomas
	Capillary (portwine, angiokeratoma)	
	Lymphatic (lymphangioma)	
	Venous (cavernous hemangiomas)	
	Simple (fast flow)	
	Arterial (arteriovenous hemangiomas)	
	Combined	
	AVM	
	Capillary—venous	
	Capillary—lymphatic venous	
	Lymphatic—venous	
	Capillary AVM	

noted that among 932 children with vascular anomalies, two-thirds were hemangiomas and the remainder were VMs (19).

INFANTILE AND CONGENITAL HEMANGIOMAS

Infantile hemangioma (IH) is the most common vascular anomaly in children, excluding lobular capillary hemangioma–pyogenic granuloma (LCH-PG) from the current discussion (19). A prospective study of 578 pregnant women and their 594 infants revealed that 29 (4.5%) infants had IHs (20). In the latter study, only two infants (0.3%) had congenital hemangiomas (CH) which are differentiated from IH on the basis of clinical behavior, pathologic features and the expression of glucose transporter-1 (GLUT-1) (21). The latter marker is expressed in virtually all IHs whereas all other vascular anomalies and malformations, including CHs, are GLUT-1 immunonegative (22,23). The study of IHs has provided opportunities to better understand the morphogenetic mechanisms of angiogenesis and vasculogenesis and their signaling pathways (24–26). A placenta-derived vascular stem cell has been postulated as the progenitor of IH (27,28). Immunohistochemical studies have shown that IHs express stem cell, neural crest and pericyte phenotypes (29).

There is a female prediction and a preference for the head and back region (40% to 60% of all cases) for IHs (30,31).

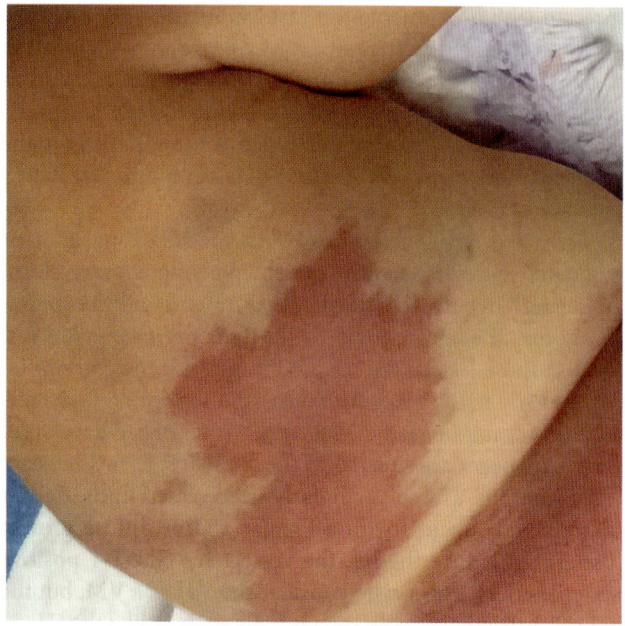
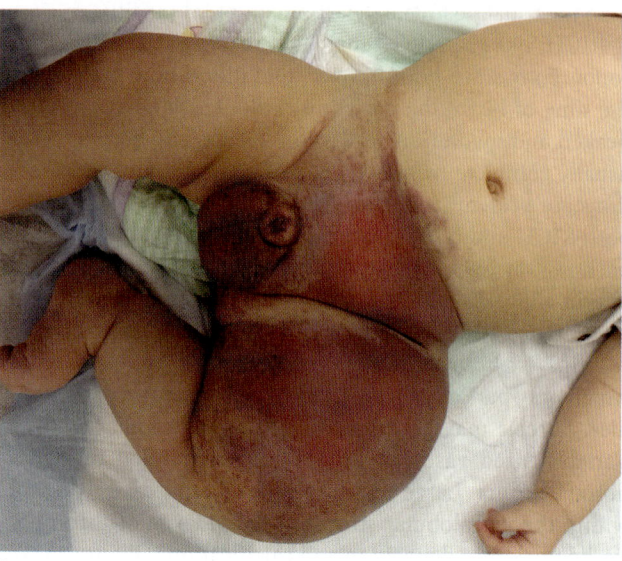

FIGURE 25-4 • Kaposiform hemangioendothelioma. **A:** This infant presented initially with erythematous slightly raised plaques. **B:** Only a few weeks later, the two lesions had coalesced into the bluish mass occupying the entire thigh (Contributed by Adam Vogel, M.D., St. Louis, MO).

erythrocytes and hyaline globules like Kaposi sarcoma (KS) (Figure 25-5). However, the tumor cells have a more bland appearance, mitotic activity is sparse and hemosiderin is less conspicuous in the KHE. Like KS, the tumor cells are positive for CD31 and D2-40, but unlike KS, there is absence of human herpesvirus 8 (HHV8) by IHC (Table 25-5).

Kaposiform lymphangiomatosis (KLA) is a vascular anomaly which may also present with consumptive coagu-lopathy, and/or hemoptysis, pleural and pericardial effusions due to intrathoracic involvement of the mediastinum and lungs (50). The median age at diagnosis is 6.5 years which is considerably older than in the case of KHE. The spleen and bones may be involved unlike KHE (Figure 25-6A, B). Microscopically, spindle cells and lymphatic endothelial cells like those seen in KHE are present, but there are accompanying ectatic lymphatic spaces of a lymphatic malformation or

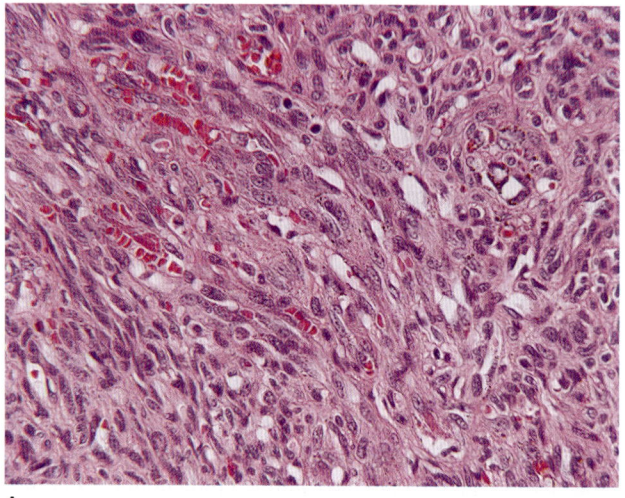
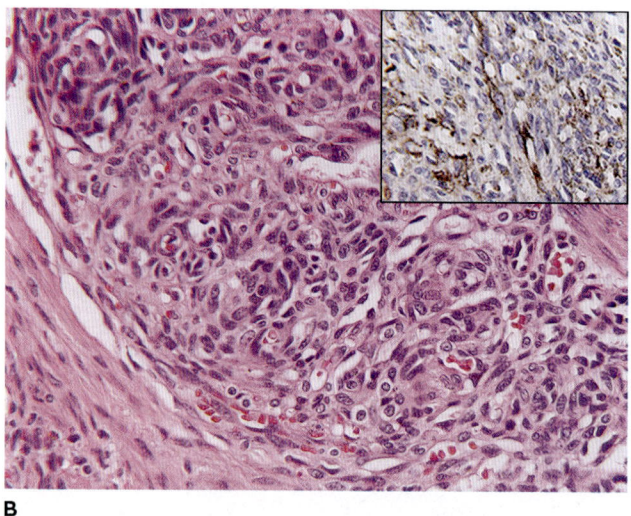

FIGURE 25-5 • KHE presented as multiple masses in the intestinal tract and retroperitoneum in a 7-year-old female. **A:** Many of the nodules are composed of compact spindle cells with interposed erythrocytes resembling KS. **B:** Other nodules had a more lobulated and tufted appearance. **Inset:** Factor VIII–related antigen immunostaining labeled the spindle cells.

TABLE 25-5	KAPOSIFORM VASCULAR LESION AND KAPOSI SARCOMA		
	KHE	KLA	KS
Age	Infants	Early-late childhood and few adults	Adults except lymphadenopathic form in children
Distribution	Solitary, but locally extensive, soft tissue, retroperitoneum	Multifocal	Solitary skin or multifocal (HIV-associated)
IHC	CD31+, D2-40+	CD31+, D2-40+	CD31+, D2-40+, HHV8+

KHE, kaposiform hemangioendothelioma; KLA, kaposiform lymphangiomatosis; KS, Kaposi sarcoma; IHC, immunohistochemistry; HHV8, Human herpes virus 8.

"lymphangioma" (Table 25-5). A small biopsy may not show the spindle cell component. Morphologically, there are subtle distinctions from KHE, but lymphatic spaces are apparent in KLA (Figure 25-7). The overall survival is only 35% or so (50).

Epithelioid hemangioma (EH) and *hemangioendothelioma* (EHE) are similar appearing vascular neoplasms composed of plump endothelial cells with abundant eosinophilic cytoplasm and intracytoplasmic vacuoles representing luminal formation (Figure 25-8). Though there remains some confusion in the pathologic distinction between EH and EHE, the latter is regarded as malignant together with angiosarcoma. Even in aggregate, EH and EHE are very uncommon in children. *Angiolymphoid hyperplasia with eosinophilia* is one cutaneous presentation of EH; most cases present in the head and neck region (51–53). Erythematous papules are composed of lymphoid aggregates in the dermis with accompanying eosinophils which may obscure the small vessels lined by plump endothelial cells; these vessels have a vague lobular architecture (54). Bone, soft tissue and blood vessels are other sites of EH in children. EHE lacks the lobular architecture of EH and is composed of nests, cords and strands of epithelioid cells with vacuoles resembling signet ring cells (55) (Figure 25-9). A myxoid or myxohyaline stroma is often prominent in the background. There is an angiocentric orientation of this tumor in the soft tissues whereas those arising in the bone, liver and lung are multifocal in 50% or more of cases (56). The liver is seemingly the most common site of EHE in children, usually in the adolescent years. There is a *CAMTA1-WWTR1* fusion transcript with the t(1;3)(p36.23;q25.1) translocation; the latter is found in all EHEs regardless of primary site and is not found in other vascular neoplasms (57).

The differential diagnosis of EH and EHE includes other epithelioid vascular and nonvascular neoplasms. One of these is the *cutaneous epithelioid angiomatous nodule* (CEAH) which resides in the dermis as a well circumscribed nodule with some overlapping features with EH except for the less intense inflammation in CEAH (58–60). This vascular lesion is seen in older children and adolescents. *Epithelioid sarcoma–like hemangioendothelioma (pseudomyogenic EHE)* is a keratin-positive and INI1-retained vascular neoplasm occurring in the skin, soft tissues, or bones of children and young adults (61–63). There is a predilection for the extremities (lower greater than upper) and multifocal lesions are present in some cases. In addition to spindle cells, the predominant

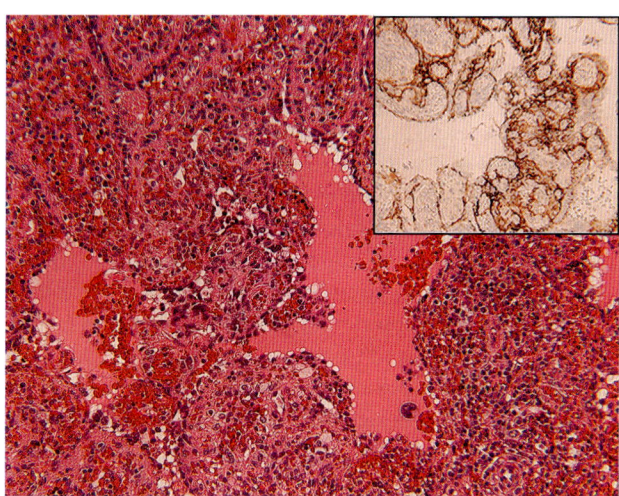

FIGURE 25-6 • Kaposiform lymphangiomatosis involving the spleen and other sites in a 3-year-old female. Branching and anastomosing vascular spaces, some with a pale coagulum representing lymph. **Inset:** D2-40 immunostain highlights the endothelial-lined spaces.

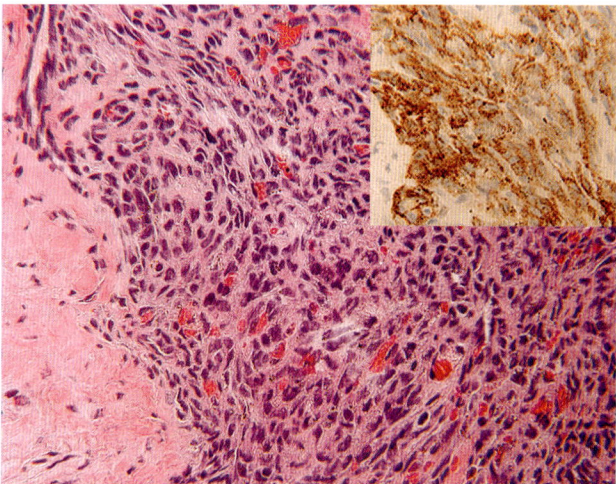

FIGURE 25-7 • Kaposiform lymphangiomatosis. This bone biopsy shows a lobule of spindle cells with a resemblance to SCH and KHE. **Inset:** D2-40 immunostain reacts with lymphatic endothelial cells.

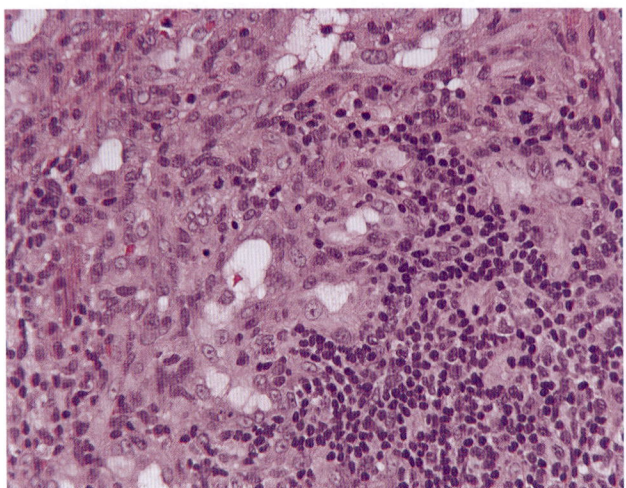

FIGURE 25-8 • Epithelioid hemangioma presented as a cutaneous mass on the arm of a 3-year-old male. Compact small vessels lined by epithelioid or histiocytoid endothelial cells, some with vacuolated cytoplasm and an accompanying lymphocytic infiltrate characterize this lesion.

cell type has rhabdoid or epithelioid features. Vascular spaces are readily apparent and eosinophils and neutrophils may be seen in the background. Local recurrence or the development of new lesions is seen in 50% to 60% of cases. This neoplasm has a *t(7;19)(q22;q13)* translocation representing a *SERPINE1-FOSB* fusion transcript (64).

Angiosarcoma (AS) is a rare malignancy at any age let alone childhood. EHE is the low-grade variant of AS whereas epithelioid and classic ASs are both high-grade malignant neoplasms. The skin is the most common site of AS in adults, but in children, even infants, this tumor presents in the liver, spleen, and superficial and deep soft tissues (65,66) (Figure 25-10A–D). Epithelioid AS may not suggest that diagnosis initially in either a child or an adult in the absence

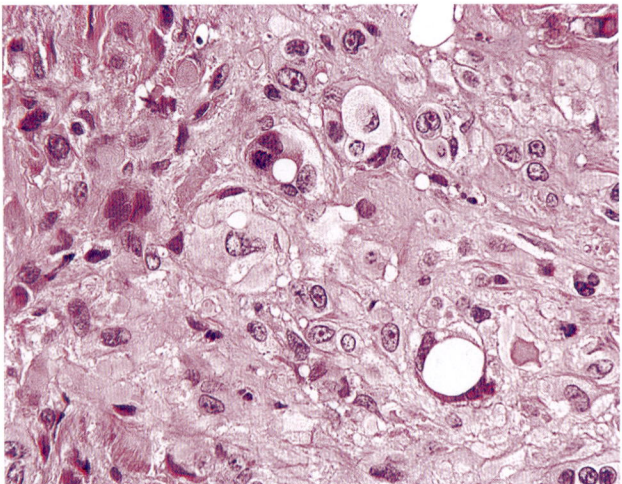

FIGURE 25-9 • Epithelioid hemangioma. This tumor contained both epithelioid cells with a moderate degree of cytologic atypia and cells with a prominent intracytoplasmic vacuole.

of recognizable neoplastic vascular structures, but the presence of hemorrhagic background and eosinophils is a clue to the diagnosis. Classic AS is composed of high grade round or spindle cells and is often accompanied by a hemophagocytic background. Papillary profiles may be present creating the so-called type II pattern of infantile EHE of the liver which we and others now believe is AS. In the latter case, retiform profiles with prominent endothelial cells assume a pattern resembling the retiform EHE.

Retiform hemangioendothelioma (RHE) is a rare vascular neoplasm of the dermis and subcutis which presents in children as a reddish plaque or mass with infiltrative borders (67,68). Though its histologic features have been likened to the rete testis with aggregates of small vascular structures, its growth through the dermis and into the subcutis resembles AS except for the absence of marked unclear atypia and mitotic figures. The vascular channels tend not to have an infiltrative pattern, but a more arborizing one. These cases can be challenging regardless of the age of the patient. A lymphangioma-like component and small glomeruloid profiles within the vascular channels are other features to suggest the diagnosis of RHE.

Papillary intralymphatic angioendothelioma (PILA, Dabska tumor) was first recognized in children, but is also seen in adults (69). There are some overlapping features between the PILA and RHE. Variably sized vascular spaces are immunoreactive for the lymphatic marker, D2-40, and a subset contain the characteristic intraluminal papillary endothelial-lined structures. Unlike RHEs, PILAs generally do not locally recur.

Composite hemangioendothelioma (CHE) is another low grade vascular neoplasm which like several of the other tumors in this section is rare, and rarer still in children (70,71). There is a predilection for the distal extremities where the CHE has patterns of EH, RHE, SCH, cavernous hemangioma, EHE and AS-like foci (72). A sheet-like growth of epithelioid and spindle cells may appear to occupy a lymph node (71). This tumor has been observed in the setting of Maffucci syndrome (72). The polymorphous EHE is regarded as a distinct entity from CHE (73).

Spindle cell hemangioma (SCH, spindle cell EHE), once thought to be a low grade vascular neoplasm, is now considered a benign tumor; this tumor occurs in older children and young adults in the more superficial soft tissues of the distal extremities as a circumscribed mass (74). More than 50% of SCHs are intravascular where the pattern is a mixture of spindle cells and vascular structures with cavernous and epithelioid features (Figure 25-11A–D). Approximately 5% of cases are diagnosed in the clinical setting of Maffucci syndrome. In addition to immunoreactivity for CD31 and CD34, this tumor is also D2-40 positive (Figure 25-11D). Somatic hotspot heterozygous mutations on *IDH1* (2q34) and *IDH2* (15q26.1) have been detected in the enchondromas of Maffucci syndrome and Ollier disease as well as in the SCH (75,76).

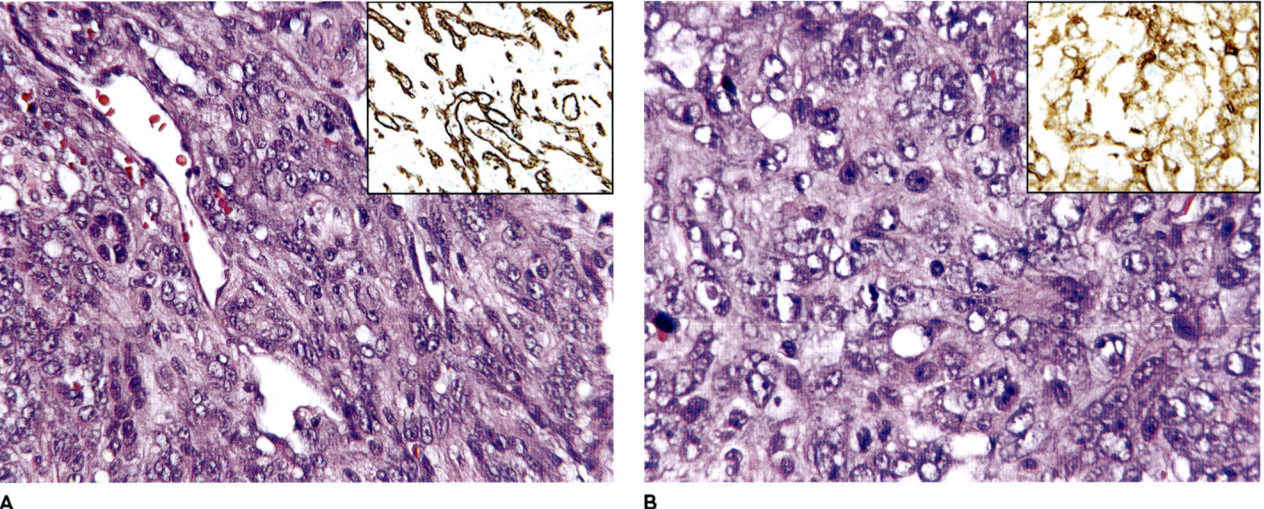

FIGURE 25-10 • Angiosarcoma of the liver in a 3-year-old boy with a 15–cm hepatic mass and pulmonary nodules. **A:** Foci of this neoplasm have retained the pattern of an infantile hemangioma. **Inset:** GLUT-1 immunopositivity is present. **B:** Other areas show a more solid pattern of atypical polygonal cells. **Inset:** GLUT-1 immunopositivity is partially lost.

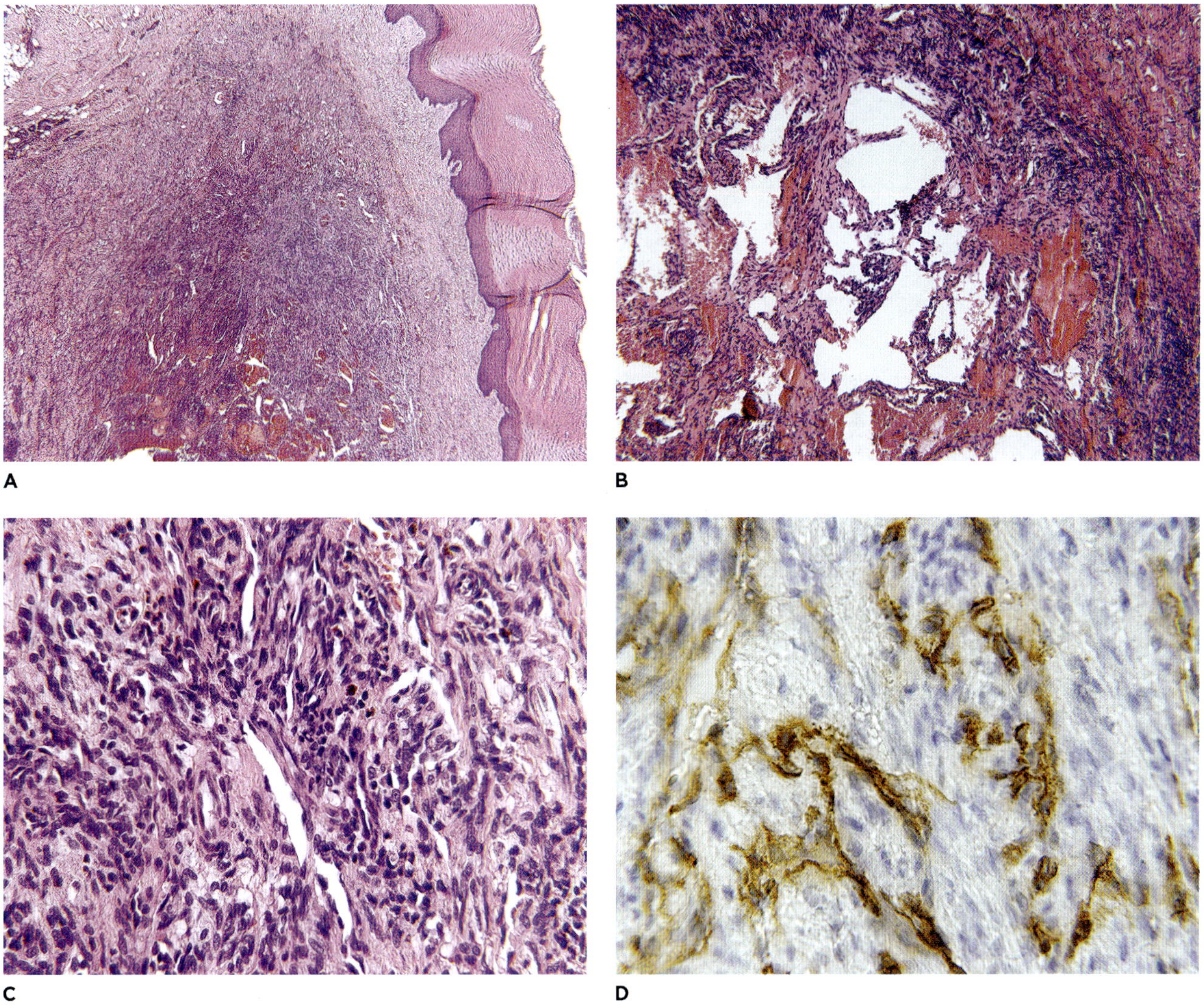

FIGURE 25-11 • SCH presenting on the palmar surface of the hand of a 9-year-old male. **A:** Low magnification of this circumscribed mass filling the dermis. **B:** The circumscribed mass has a variable pattern of uniform spindle cells and irregular ectatic vascular spaces. **C:** The spindle cells are uniform and do not display any worrisome atypia. **D:** The tumor is immunoreactive for CD31, CD34, and D2-40 (shown).

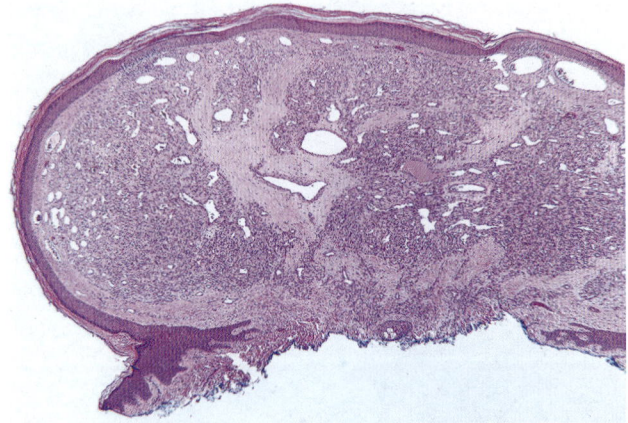
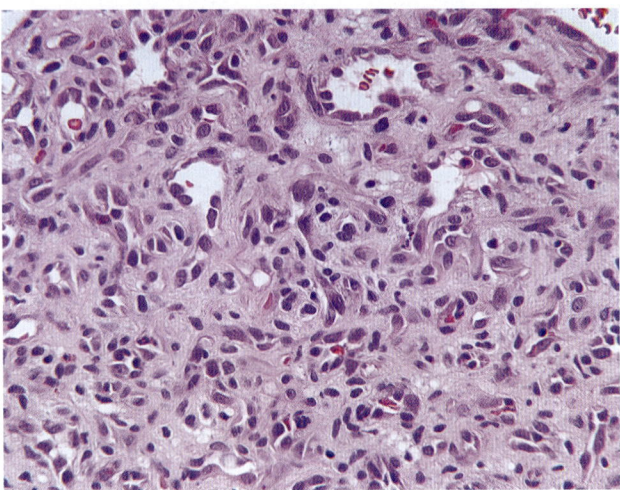
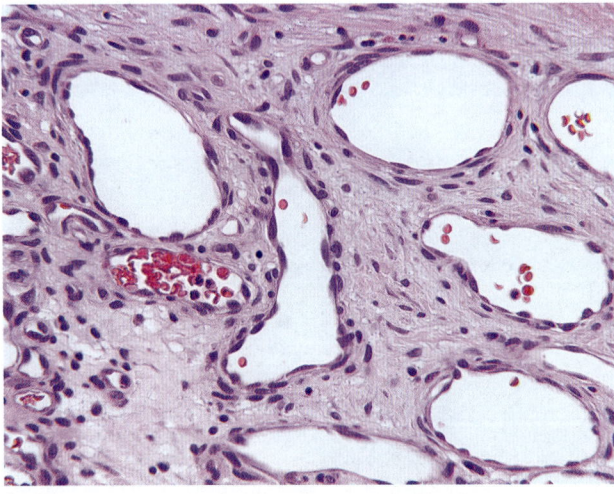

FIGURE 25-12 • Lobular capillary hemangioma presented on the shoulder of this young female. **A:** A polypoid mass is composed of lobules of capillary-sized vascular spaces. **B:** In the more cellular or proliferating areas, vascular spaces are difficult to appreciate, and mitotic figures are found with ease. **C:** The involuting areas are characterized by well-formed, patent capillaries. Some CH do not involute.

Kaposi sarcoma in children is most commonly seen as the endemic/African subtype which typically presents with regional and generalized lymphadenopathy in the absence of cutaneous lesions (77). A substantial proportion of children with KS are HIV positive, but examples are reported in children who are transplant recipients (78). As in virtually all other cases of KS, HHV-8 is positive (77) (Table 25-5).

Lobular capillary hemangioma–pyogenic granuloma is one of the most common vascular tumors in childhood whose pathogenesis as either a neoplasm or a reactive process remains somewhat ambiguous; recent studies tend to favor a reaction to tissue injury (79). This tumor occurs throughout childhood and adolescence as a rapidly evolving polypoid or pedunculated lesion, often in the head and neck region (including the oral and nasal cavity) or the finger, but has a ubiquitous distribution and may also present as multiple lesions. LCH-PG often ulcerates, bleeds and forms a crust of red cells, neutrophils and fibrin to the extent that the undergoing histologic features may be substantially obscured. Capillary-sized vascular spaces are arranged as lobules beneath the intact or ulcerated epidermis. Collarettes of epidermis wrap beneath the peripheral vascular lobules in most, but not all cases (Figure 25-12A–C). A central vessel is often present at the base of each lobule. A similar appearing lobular vascular lesion can be seen in the subcutis or within the lumen of a small blood vessel. LCH-PG seemingly evolves from a proliferative to involutional phase in a manner similar to IH. A cautionary note is that rarely KS and more often *bacillary angiomatosis* (BA) cases both have LCH-PG–like features. However, BA does not have the exquisite multilobulation of LCH-PG and the intervening stroma contains neutrophils and amorphous granular material representing either *Bartonella henselae* or *B. quintana* and macrophages. Both immunocompromised and immunocompetent children can develop BA (80,81).

VASCULAR MALFORMATIONS

The other major category of vascular anomalies in children is VMs which accounted for 33% of cases in a retrospective study of children with vascular lesions (19). "Low flow" VMs are composed of veins, capillaries or lymphatics in contrast to "high flow" VMs of arterial derivation. The remaining VMs are complex anomalies of veins, capillaries, arteries and lymphatics (82–84). Additionally, VMs occur in the settings of several syndromes (Table 25-6). The low flow VMs comprise almost 40% of all VMs whereas the isolated capillary VMs represent another 30% (19). High flow arterial–arteriolar–venous VMs constitute less than 5% of all cases. It is notable that the various syndrome-associated VMs have a distinctive morphologic composition of vessels; examples include the arteriovenous VMs in hereditary hemorrhagic telangiectasia (Rendu-Osler-Weber

TABLE 25-6 REGIONAL AND DIFFUSE SYNDROMES ASSOCIATED WITH VASCULAR MALFORMATIONS

Syndrome	Malformation
Regional syndromes with slow-flow VMs	
Sturge-Weber	Facial and intracranial capillary malformation, venous malformation, or AVM
Kippel-Tenaunay	Limb, trunk capillary, or venous-lymphatic malformation and overgrowth
Regional syndromes with fast-flow VMs	
Parkes-Weber	Capillary AVM with overgrowth; lymphatic malformation
Diffuse syndromes with slow-flow VMs	
Blue rubber bleb nevus (Bean)	Multiple venous malformations of the skin, musculoskeletal system, and GI tract
Proteus	Capillary or venous malformations, hamartomas, asymmetric limb or digit overgrowth in various body parts, lipoma, pigmented nevi
Gorham-Stout	Spontaneous osteolysis and lymphatic malformations; intercranial
Maffucci	Enchondromatosis, multiple venous-lymphatic malformations
Epidermal nevus (Solomon)	AVM; epidermal nevi; and varied abnormalities of eyes, skin, nervous, skeletal, cardiac, and genitourinary systems
Bannayan-Riley-Ruvalcaba	Skin, intracranial malformations, macrocephaly, ectoderm dysplasia, fatty masses, GI hamartomas, PTEN mutation
Diffuse syndromes with fast-flow VMs	
Hereditary hemorrhagic telangiectasia	Skin, mucous membrane, and GI telangiectasias; AVM of lungs, liver, brain, and spinal cord
Wyburn-Mason	AVM or AVF of brain or retina with same-segment facial malformations
Cobb	AVM or AVF of spinal cord with same-segment skin VM

AVM, arteriovenous malformation; PTEN, phosphatase and tensin homology suppressor gene; AVF, =arteriovenous fistula.
From Kollipara R, Dinneen L, Rentas KE, et al. Current classification and terminology of pediatric vascular anomalies. *AJR Am J Roentgenol* 2013;201(5): 1124–1135.

syndrome), capillary malformations the macrocephaly–capillary malformation disorder and the mixed VM–connective tissue elements of the PTEN hamartoma tumor syndrome (85–88).

No one single description is sufficient to characterize VMs from the perspective of their morphologic features (Figure 25-13). The pure lymphatic VM, also known as a cystic hygroma or lymphangioma, is composed of thin-walled vascular structures which are empty or contain a pale coagulum (lymph) or red cells as a result of venous efflux of blood (84,85). Lymphoid nodules residing beneath lymphatic endothelium or prolapsed into the vessel lumen are seen in some but not all cases (Figure 25-14). Smooth muscle beneath endothelium may indicate the presence of veins and thus a lymphovenous malformation (Figure 25-15). Immunostaining for D2-40 is helpful in the identification of lymphatic component when it is not apparent from the microscopic examination. Prior surgery often results in a marked fibrous tissue reaction which substantially alters the appearance of the malformation; a similar change may be seen in large VMs in a site like the mediastinum.

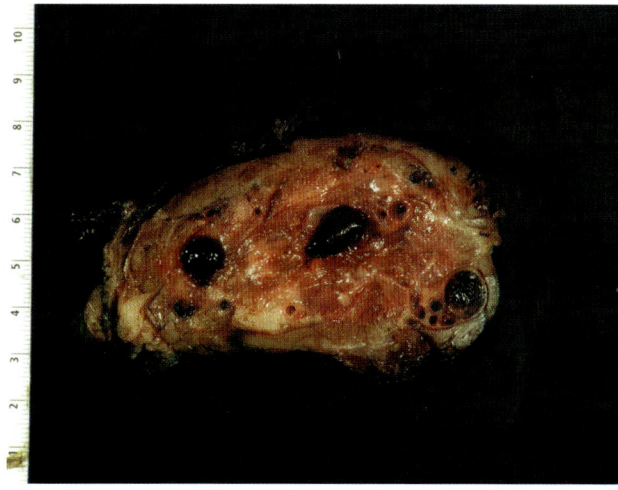

FIGURE 25-13 • VM from the posterior thigh of a 15-year-old male. This deceptively well-circumscribed mass has a range of gross findings from the presence of thrombosed vessels in various stages of formation and organization. Several foci of dystrophic calcification, mainly in vessels, are noted.

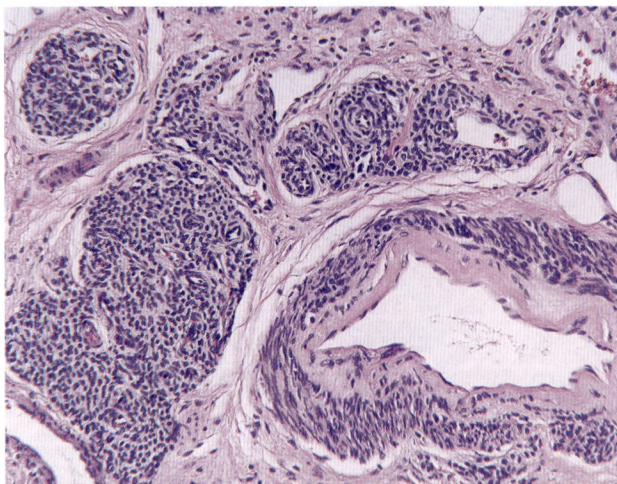

FIGURE 25-18 • Glomangioma (glomuvenular malformation) in a 20-year-old female presented as paraspinal and retroperitoneal masses. The vascular spaces are accompanied by a circumferential population of small, basophilic-appearing cells beneath the endothelium.

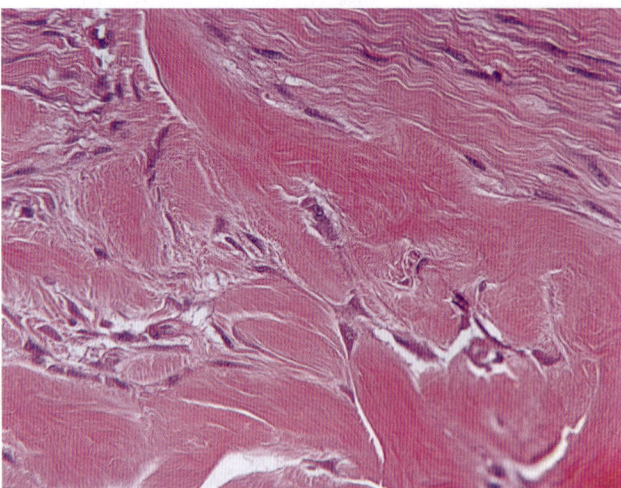

FIGURE 25-19 • Keloid presented as a mass in the posterior auricular region of a 5-year-old female. Dense acellular bundles of collagen are separated by fibroblasts.

that is usually immunopositive for alpha-smooth muscle actin and vimentin, but usually negative for desmin (90). Cuffs of small uniform, basophilic cells are present beneath an intact, inconspicuous endothelium (Figure 25-18).

FIBROUS, MYOFIBROBLASTIC, AND PERICYTIC TUMORS

This section is focused on the category of non–neoplastic and neoplastic entities which have in common a spindle cell with the morphologic and phenotypic features of a fibroblast, and/or a transitional type mesenchymal cell, the myofibroblast, with the composite attributes of a fibroblast and smooth muscle cell which has a smooth muscle phenotype and vascular perithelial localization (91,92). In the setting of one of the unique fibrous tumors of childhood, infantile myofibromatosis–myofibroma, the proliferating subintimal myofibroblasts have the capacity to differentiate into cells with the morphology and immunophenotype of pericytes with contractile attributes of smooth muscle.

SCAR AND KELOID

Scars are reactive fibrous and myofibroblastic proliferations that occur in all tissue types and organs (brain excepted with its reactive gliosis) and are a programmed process of repair. It is not always clear as to the cause when a scar is submitted as a "tumor" in a child. Morphologically, the myofibroblasts and fibroblasts can acquire a significant degree of atypia, especially in a radiation field or site of inflammation which can be a source of concern about its benign or malignant nature.

Keloids and hypertrophic scars are similar in many respects with the formation of nodules of reactive fibroblasts in the dermis, whose presence has obliterated or replaced the normal microanatomy; both are regarded as manifestations of abnormal wound healing (93). Both processes may have a predilection in some families and are more common in individuals of African descent (94). The ear lobe is a particular site of predilection for keloids in young women after ear piercing. Keloids are additionally characterized by groups of thickened, intensely eosinophilic bundles of collagen (Figure 25-19). Similar bundles of collagen may be seen in a desmoid tumor, mesenteric fibromatosis, and NF. Both COX-1 and COX-2 are important mediators in the pathogenesis of abnormal wound healing (95–97).

FIBROBLASTIC AND MYOFIBROBLASTIC TUMORS

Nodular fasciitis (NF) is now regarded as a self-limiting neoplasm rather than a reactive process and is classified among fibrous/myofibroblastic tumors (5). It is unclear at the present whether the other "pseudosarcomas" are neoplastic in the same sense as NF. NF remains a problematic lesion in its differentiation from a true sarcoma (98). It is generally underappreciated that NF occurs in children with some frequency including very young children (99). One of the more dramatic examples of a fasciitis in infancy is cranial fasciitis presenting as a large mass with compression of the underlying brain in some cases (100). In our experience, approximately 40% of all cases of NF present in the first two decades, particularly in the first decade of life, as a mass with a predilection for the head and neck region in over 50% of our cases where involvement of the parotid gland is seen (101) (Table 25-7). The subcutis of the extremity (upper more common than lower) and chest wall are the more common presenting sites of NF in older children and young adults. There are also examples of intravascular and intra-articular NF (102). In the head and neck region of children, ERMS may arise in the differential diagnosis. The myxoid background and mitotic figures are the

TABLE 25-7 NODULAR FASCIITIS PRESENTING IN FIRST TWO DECADES OF LIFE[a]

Anatomic Region	No (%)	Sex (M:F)	Age Range	Mean Age	Median Age
Head and neck, Total	92 (53)	60:32	2 m–20 y	6 y	5 y
Scalp	25 (27)				
Neck	19 (21)				
Face	17 (18)				
Nasal cavity[b]	15 (16)				
Periorbital	7 (8)				
Ear	5 (5)				
Parotid	4 (4)				
Extremity, Total	45 (26)	22:23	2 m–20 y	12 y	13 y
Arm	21 (47)				
Leg	20 (44)				
Hand	3 (6)				
Foot	1 (2)				
Trunk, Total	36 (21)	23:13	3 m–20 y	10 y	10 y
Chest wall	18 (50)				
Back	13 (36)				
Abdominal wall	4 (11)				
Trunk	1 (3)				
Perineum, Total	2 (1)	1:1	1 y and 3 y		
Vulva	1				
Scrotum	1				
Total:	175	106:69			

[a]Cases of NF from the Lauren V. Ackerman Laboratory of Surgical Pathology, St. Louis Children's Hospital, Washington University Medical Center, St. Louis, MO. between the years of 1989 and 2014.
[b]Includes cases from nasal cavity, paranasal sinus, oral cavity and lip.
m, month; y, year; m, male; f, female.

findings of concern in a NF. The subcutis is the tissue level of origin for most NFs, followed by the fascia, lower dermis and skeletal muscle. Grossly, a circumscribed, nonencapsulated nodule, measuring 3 cm or less in most cases, has a glistening mucoid appearance. The periphery has nodular contours with an abrupt transition to the adjacent soft tissues. Several histologic patterns coexist in the nodule with dense, spindle cell areas forming short fascicles adjacent to less cellular foci with separation of the spindle cells by mucoid–myxoid extracellular material (so-called tissue culture pattern) and transitional areas with both patterns (Figure 25-20). Mitotic figures are readily identified with some nuclear atypia (absent atypical mitotic figures and anaplasia). Microcysts with mucin and a variable number of histiocytes, foci of interstitial hemorrhage (so-called "extravasated red cells"), and scattered inflammatory cells in the background are the constellation of histologic features (Figure 25-21). Scattered multinucleated cells and a storiform-like pattern may suggest a fibrohistiocytic proliferation. The compact spindle cell proliferation with mitotic figures serves to raise concern for "fibrosarcoma" or leiomyosarcoma. Immature, often stellate fibroblasts in the tissue culture-like foci are the features most like an ERMS. Metaplastic bone is seen infrequently. The myofibroblasts of NF express vimentin and SMA but desmin, h-caldesmon, myoD1, and myogenin are all nonreactive by IHC. In general, NF is regarded as a nonrecurring process and with the potential for spontaneous regression. The difficulty in the differentiation of cranial fasciitis from a fibromatosis is presented in a study reporting β-catenin expression in the nuclei of a putative recurring cranial fasciitis (100). The USP6 is the fusion partner of MYH9 gene to form the t(17; 22) (p13; q13) translocation in over 90% of cases (103). Aneurysmal bone cyst (ABC) also has a USP6 translocation, but with different fusion partners than NF. The stroma of an ABC has many similarities to NF. Proliferative fasciitis and myositis are regarded as related entities in a morphologic sense to the NF (104,105). There is no evidence to date that the latter two lesions have a similar translocation as NF. The epithelioid cells in proliferative fasciitis can be mistaken for rhabdoid cells (105).

Myositis ossificans (MO), as the solitary (circumscripta), sporadically occurring soft-tissue mass or the multifocal fibrodysplasia ossificans progressiva (FOP), has its own potential for diagnostic miscues. Most cases of MO may or may not be accompanied by a history of trauma to possibly explain the male predominance (106). It is seen uncommonly in the first decade of life and more often in later childhood or adolescence in which case there may be a history of incidental or organized (sports) blunt trauma. The classic presentation is a circumscribed intramuscular mass, or alternatively the formation of a parosteal, calcified mass, or a mass attached to the surface of the bone by a pedicle. The sites of predilection are the thigh, buttock, and abdominal wall (107). In

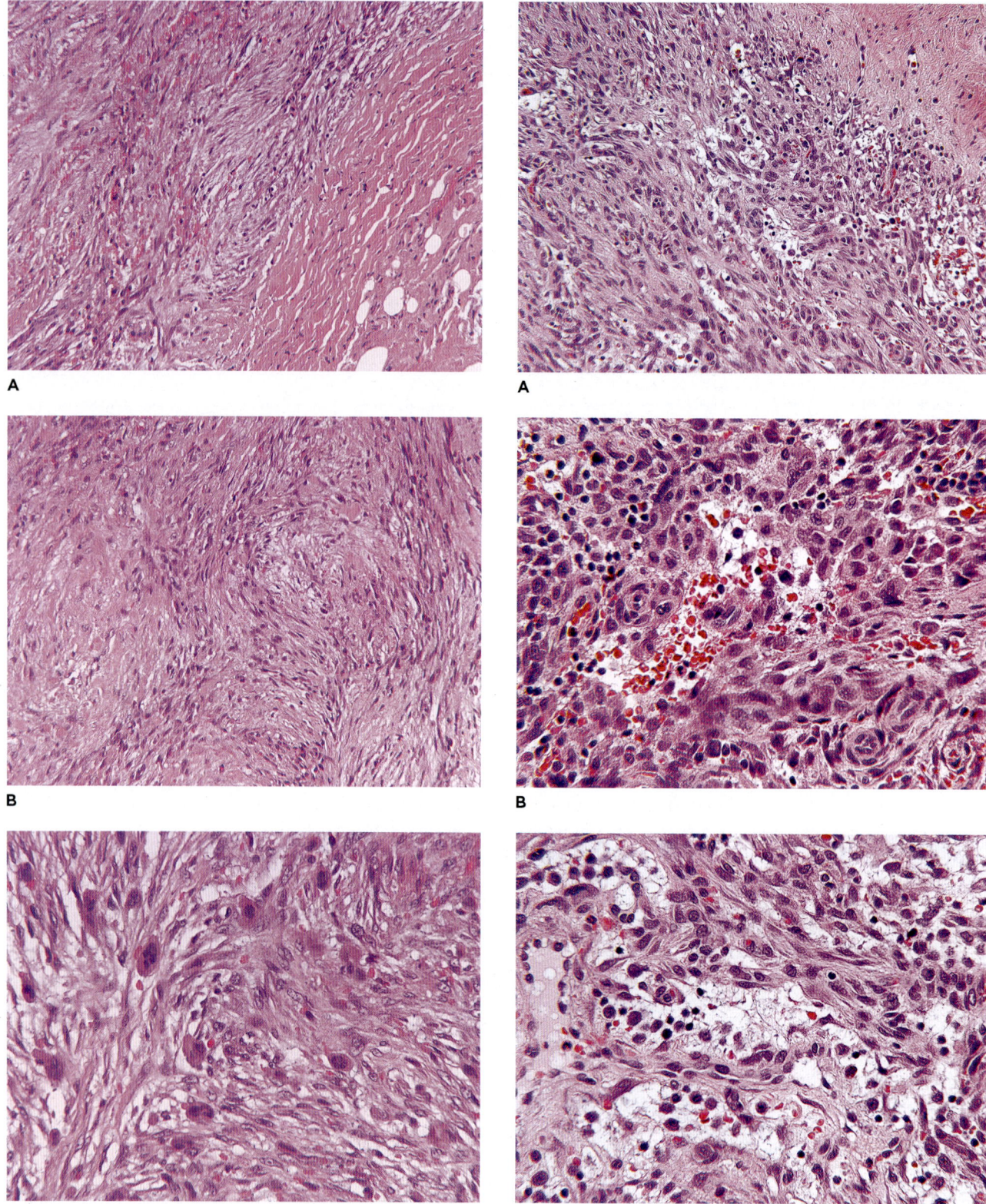

FIGURE 25-20 • Nodular faciitis in a 10-year-old female presented as a 2-cm mass in the posterior triangle of the neck. **A:** The abrupt interface exists between the spindle cells and the adjacent nonlesional collagen. Note the presence of interstitial hemorrhage. **B:** Intersecting fascicles and nodules of loosely arranged spindle cells and interstitial mucin are some of the characteristic features. The nuclei failed to immunostain for β-catenin. **C:** The presence of multinucleated cells may cause confusion with a fibrohistiocytic lesion.

FIGURE 25-21 • Nodular fasciitis presenting in the periorbital region of a 4-year-old female. **A:** Note the circumscribed periphery of the mass from the adjacent soft tissues and without infiltration as in the case of fibromatosis. **B:** Red cell extravasation is present in the interstitium. **C:** Several microcysts with histiocytes and mucin in the background are useful clues to the diagnosis.

terms of size, MO can measure in excess of 10 to 15 cm. The inner portion of the three-zone mass is composed of plump spindle and polygonal myofibroblasts, blood vessels and histiocytes, which are surrounded by a zone of immature osteoid and an outer shell of mature bone (Figure 25-22). The diagnostic trap is set if a biopsy is obtained from the central, proliferating zone. Despite the initial concern for the presence of marked cellularity and some degree of atypia in a biopsy or excision, the paucity of mitotic figures, especially atypical mitoses, and the lack of anaplasia should prompt the likelihood of at least a nonmalignant process.

Heterotopic ossification with fibro-osseous features has been reported in the auditory canal of young individuals. Cutaneous osteoma occurs sporadically or may be a manifestation of Albright hereditary osteodystrophy (AHO) or pseudohypoparathyroidism type Ia with or without the AHO phenotype. There are inactivating mutations of the GNAS gene (20q13).

FOP is an autosomal dominant disorder which is characterized by the progressive transformation of soft tissues and skeletal muscle to heterotopic bone (108). The mutation has been mapped to chromosome 2q23-24, the site of activin A type I receptor/activin-like kinase 2 (ACVR1/ALK2), a bone morphogenetic protein type I receptor. In addition to the characteristic great toe malformations, there is the development of soft-tissue swelling or masses on the back, which are described as "spreading" through the subcutaneous tissues and deeper. A biopsy reveals a spindle cell and myxoid transformation of the subcutis with a resemblance to infantile subcutaneous fibromatosis or lipofibromatosis and even more so to NF. A biopsy site may enlarge due to metaplastic ossification, which appears to accelerate in foci of trauma.

Other forms of so-called *pseudosarcomatous proliferations* of the soft tissues and periosteum are florid reactive periostitis, fibrous pseudotumor of the digit, a form of localized MO, and bizarre parosteal osteochondromatous proliferation (Nora lesion) (107). These various lesions are problematic if the specimen is a biopsy without adequate clinical information and characterization of the imaging features. The theme is again an atypical histology which is not accompanied by overtly malignant features, as discussed in the previous sections on NF and MO, in particular as it relates to the absence of atypical mitoses and anaplasia.

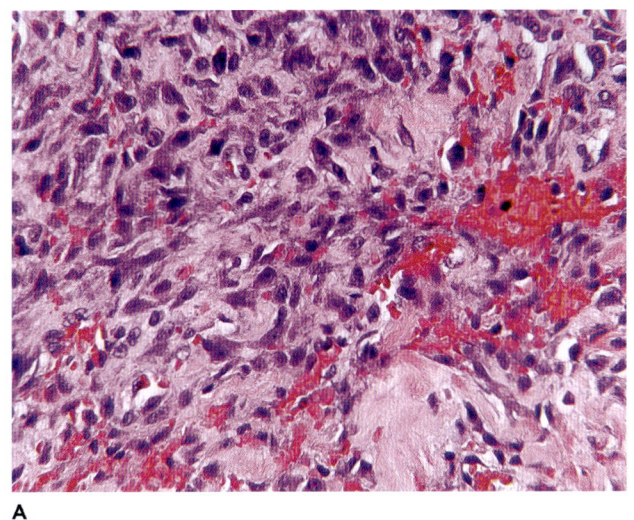

A

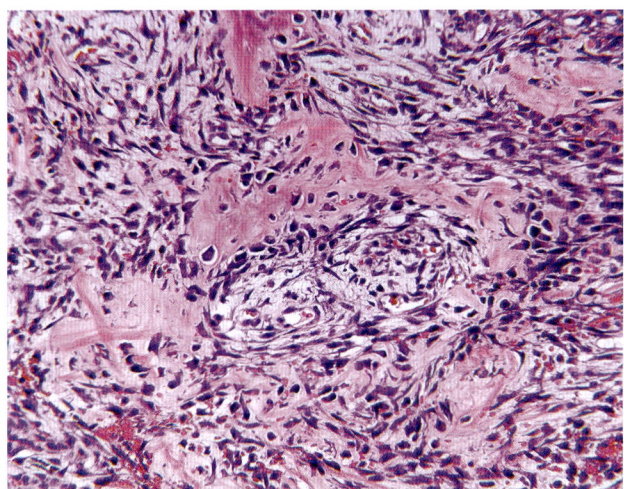

B

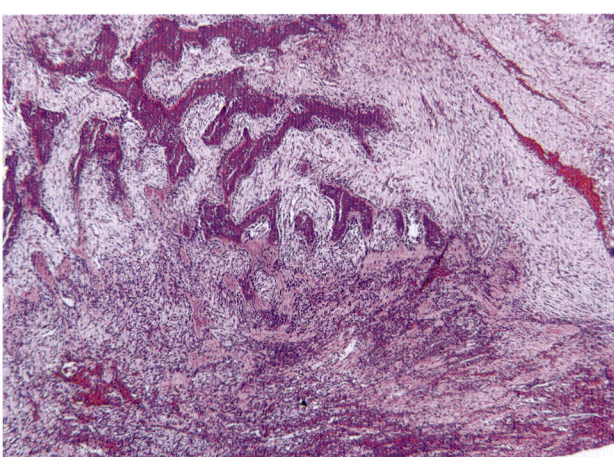

C

FIGURE 25-22 • MO presenting as a soft tissue mass in the posterior neck of a 10-year-old male. **A:** The center of this mass is composed of compact spindle cells with some nuclear atypia but in the absence of atypical mitotic figures. **B:** The transition zone is between the central spindle cells and osteoid formation. **C:** The peripheral zone is represented by the active new bone formation.

Fibroblastic–myofibroblastic tumors of childhood with some exceptions are recognized in the first 5 years of life and many at or before 2 years of age (109). These fibrous tumors of childhood or juvenile fibromatoses include the following: fibromatosis colli, myofibroma–myofibromatosis, fibrous hamartoma of infancy (FHI), inclusion body fibromatosis (infantile digital fibroma), infantile fibromatosis (lipofibromatosis and other subtypes), Gardner-nuchal fibroma, juvenile aponeurotic fibroma and nasopharyngeal angiofibroma (109). Palmar and plantar fibromatoses (superficial fibromatosis) and desmoid-type fibromatosis (deep fibromatosis) are seen in all age groups. Desmoid-type fibromatosis or desmoid tumor, Gardner fibroma, and nasopharyngeal angiofibroma are known manifestations of familial adenomatous polyposis (FAP) syndrome including Gardner syndrome (110).

Infantile myofibroma (myofibromatosis), the most common of various fibrous tumors of childhood, accounts for 20% to 25% of all cases (109). A solitary cutaneous or subcutaneous nodule (90% of cases) measures less than 3 cm in most cases, presents in the first 5 years of life and may be noted at birth and has a predilection for the head and neck region (40% to 60% of cases) followed by the trunk and extremities (111). However, the bone and various organs including the brain, dura, liver, intestinal tract, lung, and testicle are some of the other less common solitary sites, but all of these locations may be involved in congenital generalized myofibromatosis (CGM). The cardiac fibroma occurring in infancy may be a related lesion. Virtually no site is immune to the development of a myofibroma. Multifocal lesions, usually restricted to the skin–subcutis and/or bone, are seen in 5% to 8% of cases, and in 1% to 2% of cases, there are more widespread skin, soft tissue, and visceral lesions, typically recognized in an infant less than 6 months old, comprising the entity of CGM. The clinical outcome is poor in these infants with CGM because of pulmonary venous occlusion by the formation of intravascular myofibromas. On the other hand, solitary lesions are known to undergo spontaneous regression. Another aspect of infantile myofibroma is its familial presentation with autosomal dominant or recessive inheritance with germline mutations in PDGFRB, (5q33.1) or NOTCH 3 (19p13.2–p13.1).

A firm nodular non–encapsulated mass measuring 1 to 3 cm in greatest dimension may also be accompanied by calcifications, cysts, and central hemorrhage with a microscopic pattern of a hemangiopericytoma (HPC) with coagulative type necrosis. The cellularity is most apparent toward the periphery where the compact spindle cells are arranged in short fascicles or within hyaline–myxoid, almost chondroid-appearing stroma, which separates or largely replaces the spindle cells (Figure 25-23). If the nodule is located in the dermis, there are often multiple discrete nodules with normal intervening cutaneous structures and dermal collagen and if in the subcutis, there is overgrowth and entrapment of fat. A more infiltrative pattern may be seen in the dermis, but the small, SMA-positive nodules are best seen in the superficial dermis. The myofibroma does not have the infiltrative growth of a desmoid-type fibromatosis but rather an expansile type growth. At the periphery of some nodules, a compressed vessel is a hallmark feature of the myofibroma and can be identified in many cases (Figure 25-24). The associated HPC-like pattern can be dominant in some tumors with only peripheral, nodular myofibromatous foci (Figure 25-25). Central degeneration without overt necrosis is yet another feature. Cells within the myofibromatous pattern are immunopositive for SMA whereas those in the HPC-like foci are positive for CD34. In addition to the HPC-like areas, dense spindle cell foci can simulate congenital

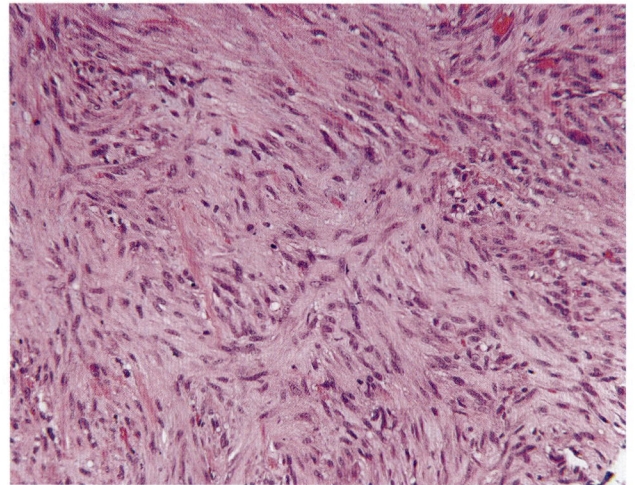
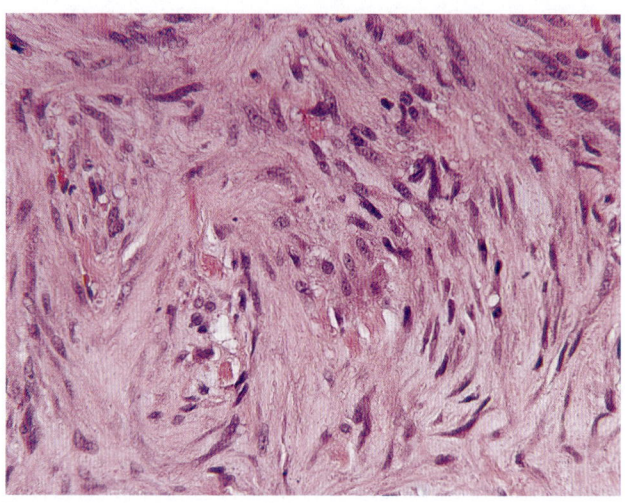

FIGURE 25-23 • Infantile myofibroma (myofibromatosis) presented as deep mass in the posterior neck of a 3-month-old female. **A:** The sharply demarcated mass measuring 3.0 cm is composed of uniform spindle cells in a pale eosinophilic stroma. **B:** Sweeping arrays of spindle cells are present in a fibrohyaline stroma with a small vascular space that has been compressed by spindle cells.

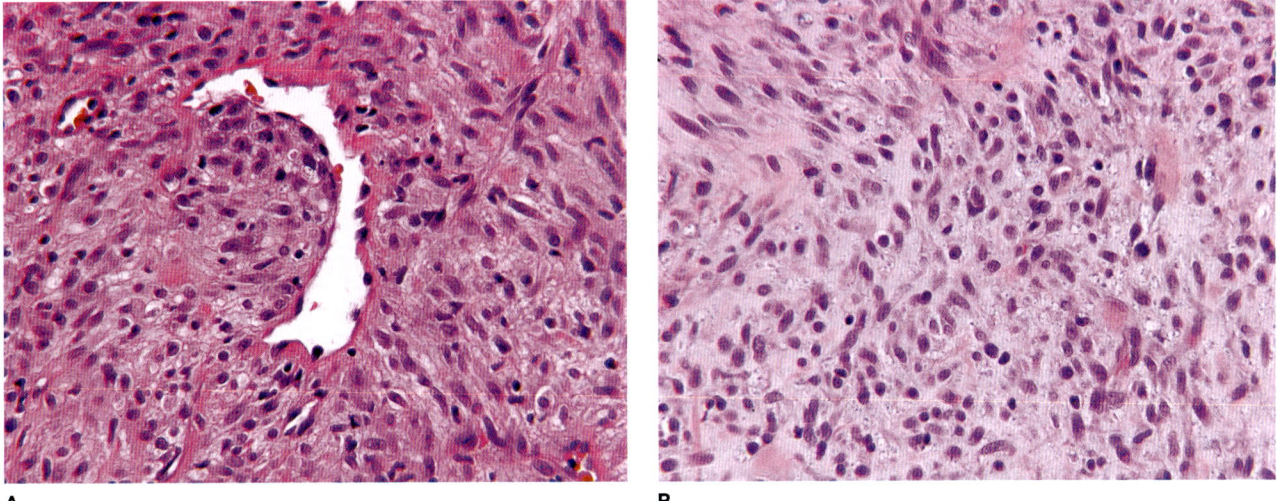

FIGURE 25-24 • Infantile myofibroma (myofibromatosis) presented as a soft tissue mass in the neck of a 3-month-old boy. **A:** The smaller nodules of spindle cells are associated with a compressed vessel at the periphery that is useful in the recognition of a myofibroma. **B:** Other fields are composed of fascicles and nodules with a fibromyxoid appearance.

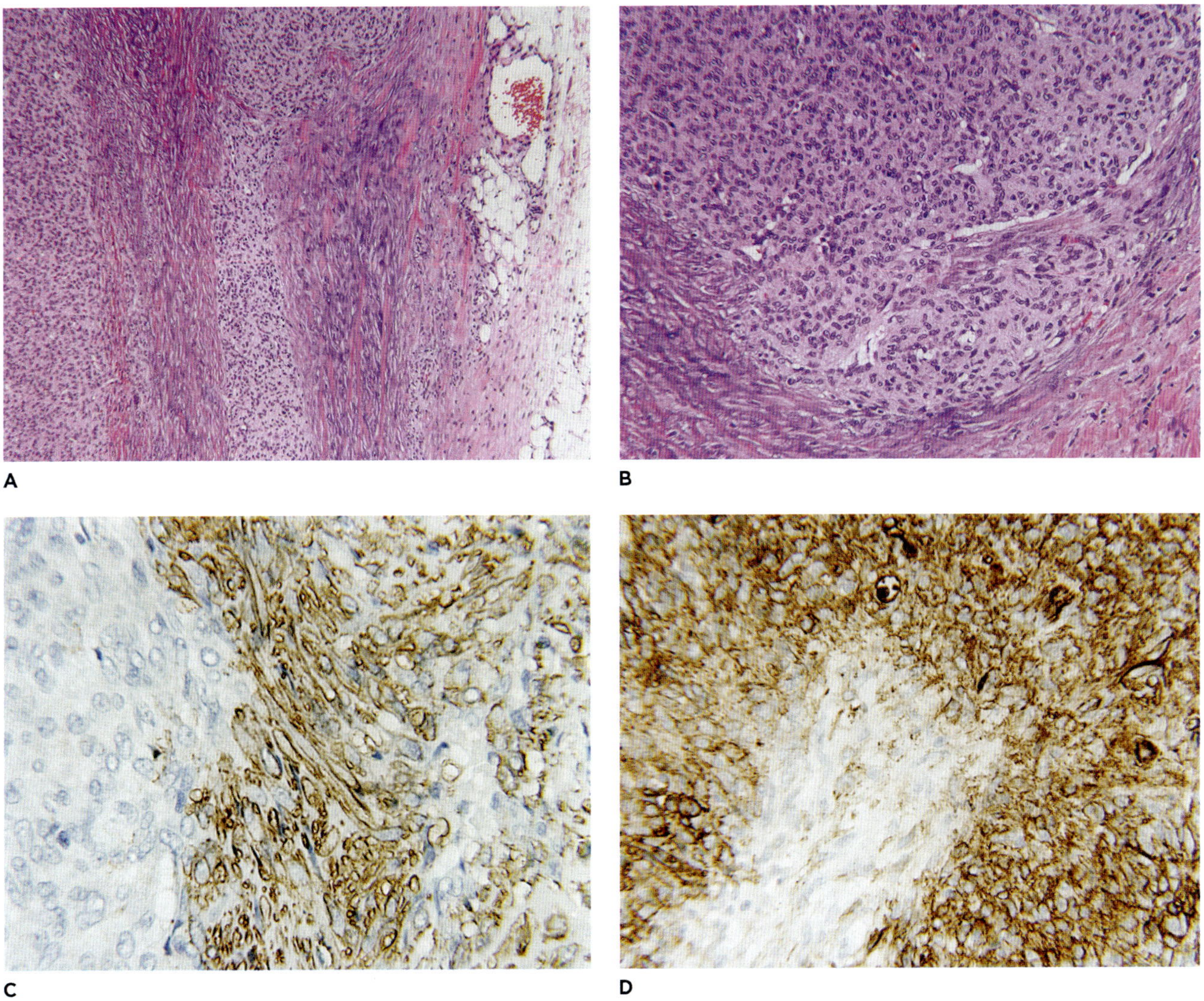

FIGURE 25-25 • Infantile myofibroma (myofibromatosis) presented as a mass in the groin of a 4-month-old male. **A:** This tumor has a mixed pattern of myofibroma and HPC which in this field has the former features. **B:** The HPC areas are usually present centrally with more ovoid cells surrounding small, clefted vascular spaces. **C:** Immunohistochemical staining for SMA highlights the myofibromatous pattern without reactivity in the contiguous HPC-like foci. **D:** A contrasting pattern of immunoreactivity for CD34 is seen in the CD34-positive HPC-like foci and absence of staining in myofibromatous focus.

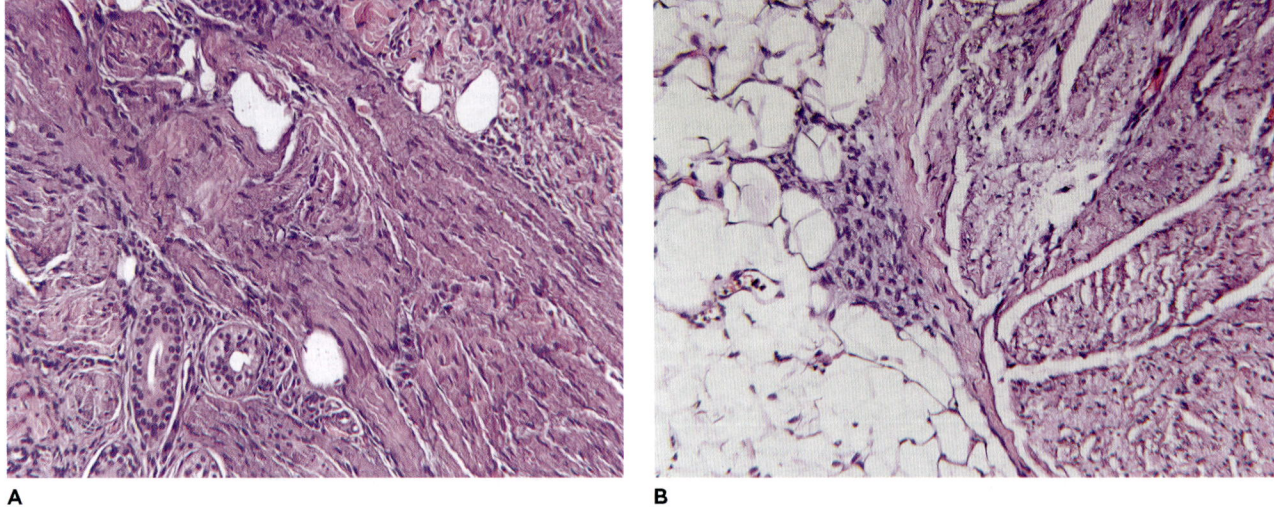

FIGURE 25-30 • FHI presented in the axillary region of a 4-month-old boy. **A:** The pattern of subcutaneous infiltration by bland-appearing spindle cells resembles ISF. **B:** The presence of small bundles of immature spindle cells at the periphery or within the midst of the more mature fibroblasts is the diagnostic feature.

nantly in the first 2 to 3 years of life—even in slightly older children—but most commonly in the first few months where the trunk (60% to 65%), axilla, inguinal, and perineal region (vulva and scrotum), and extremities are the sites of predilection in descending order (109,124–126). The subcutaneous, poorly circumscribed fibrofatty tumor generally measures less than 5 cm. It shares many of the same gross and microscopic features with the ISF except for the small nodules of immature, spindled mesenchymal cells in a pale basophilic background (Figure 25-30). These may be found as isolated structures in the fat or along the periphery or within bundles of more mature-appearing spindle cells. Focal extension may be found into the dermis where secondary changes in the eccrine sweat glands have been observed (127). Pseudoangiomatous foci have been described with accompanying bcl-2 reactivity (126). Both smooth muscle actin and CD34 are expressed in the more fibrous areas of a FHI (125). If the lobules of fat have an immature appearance, lipoblastoma (LPB) may arise in the differential diagnosis. The local recurrence rate is only 10% to 15%, which is low in light of the fact that FHI is incompletely resected in most cases.

Inclusion body fibromatosis (infantile digital fibroma) presents on the lateral and/or dorsal aspect of a finger and/or toe, though usually sparing the thumb and great toe, as a firm nodule(s) in an infant or child 5 years of age or less at diagnosis (128). Multiple digits are involved in 25% to 30% of cases. This tumor measures 1 to 2 cm in most cases and has a uniform white, fibrous appearance similar to a desmoid-type fibromatosis. The dermis is commonly effaced by a uniform spindle cell proliferation, forming short fascicles, and with a prominent collagenous background entrapping isolated hair follicles or sweat glands (129) (Figure 25-31). Confluent,

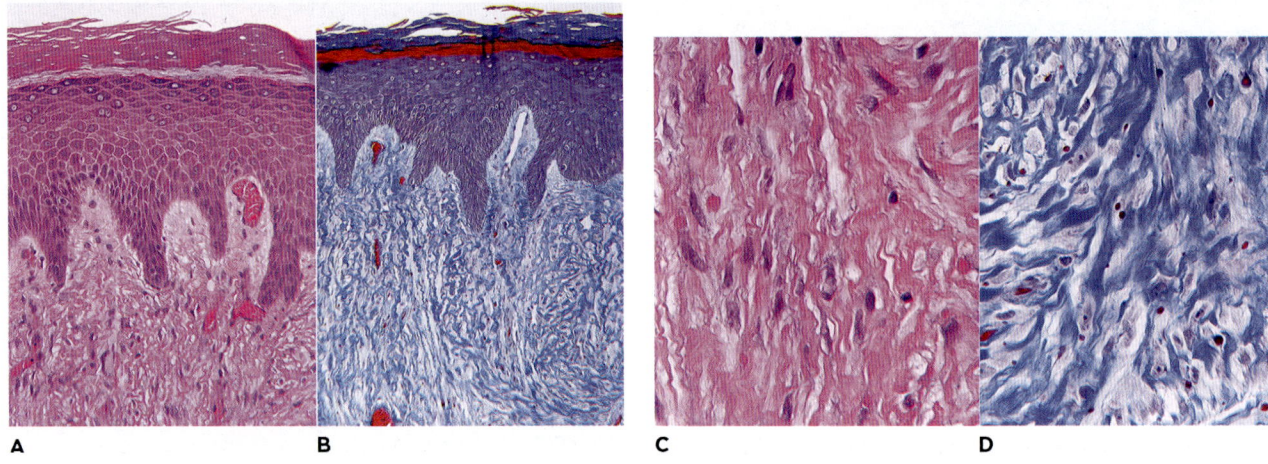

FIGURE 25-31 • Inclusion body fibromatosis (infantile digital fibroma) presented on the fifth toe of a 7-month-old female. **A:** The dense, relatively hypocellular spindle cell proliferation has effaced the dermis. **B:** Trichrome stain demonstrates uniform pattern of collagen deposition. **C:** Paranuclear eosinophilic bodies are best seen at higher magnification. **D:** These filamentous bodies of actin are better demonstrated in the trichrome stain.

contiguous extension into the subcutis is associated with overgrowth of fat with features resembling macrodactyly. There is a microscopic resemblance to the desmoid-type fibromatosis, except for the presence of eosinophilic, paranuclear inclusions in variable numbers; these inclusions are usually more readily identified in a trichrome stain. The eosinophilic inclusions are pathognomonic of this entity when present in a digital lesion, but the inclusions have also been observed in rare extradigital fibroblastic lesions and in fibroepithelial tumors of the breast (130). The infiltrative growth around and through neurovascular structures in the digit limits complete resection in most cases, which accounts for a local recurrence rate in excess of 50% (131). There are uncommon examples of spontaneous regression (132).

Dermatomyofibroma is described in children between the ages of 2 and 16 years as a plaque or nodule, typically in the neck or upper trunk (133). A spindle cell proliferation is found in the lower dermis and subcutis with a pattern which tends to parallel the overlying epidermis (134). Smooth muscle actin is commonly positive, but CD34 positivity is seen which promotes diagnostic confusion with DFSP and the fibroblastic connective tissue nevus (135).

A small subset of fibroblastic–myofibroblastic tumors, typically presenting in the first 2 years of life, demonstrates a collage of more than one histologic pattern of the various fibrous tumors of childhood (composite fibrous tumor). The most common example is the infantile myofibromatosis—HPC with concurrent patterns of both which is regarded as a spectrum phenomenon in the infantile myofibroma. Other combinations are the infantile subcutaneous fibromatosis with CIFS-like foci and infantile myofibroma (112). These tumors demonstrate the morphologic plasticity of the fibroblast–myofibroblast and its capacity to simultaneously express itself as several microscopic patterns and in a sense reflects the relationship of these seemingly disparate fibrous tumors of childhood (Figure 25-32). We have seen examples of composite fibrous tumor behave in the fashion of multifocal or generalized infantile myofibromatosis.

Desmoid-type fibromatosis (desmoid tumor, musculo-aponeurotic fibromatosis) is the most common fibrous neoplasm presenting in the first two decades of life (60% to 70% of all fibrous tumors) and occurring throughout childhood and adolescence with a bimodal age distribution in the first 2 years and later in older children (3,109,136). The

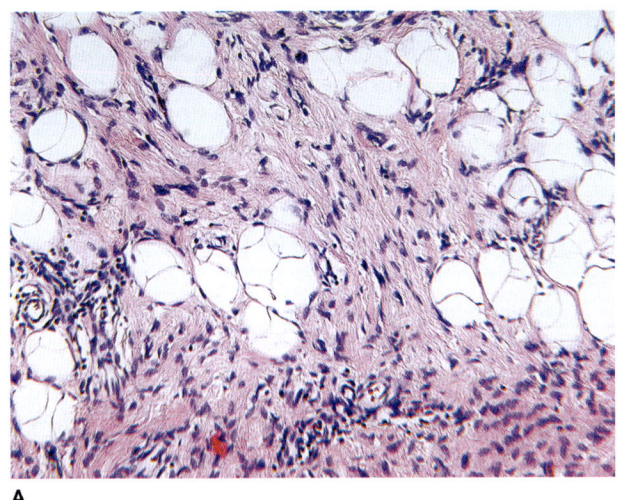
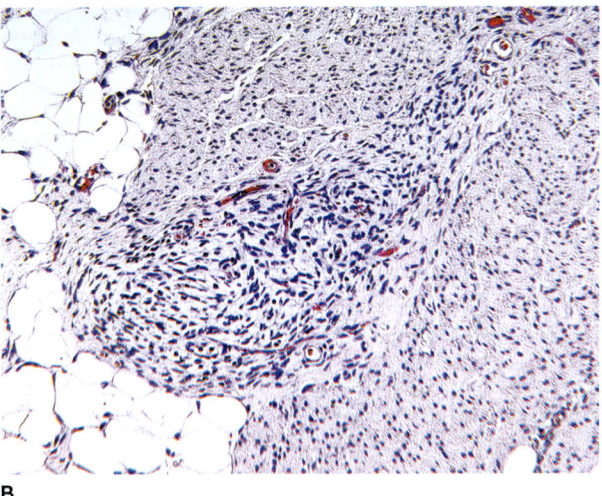
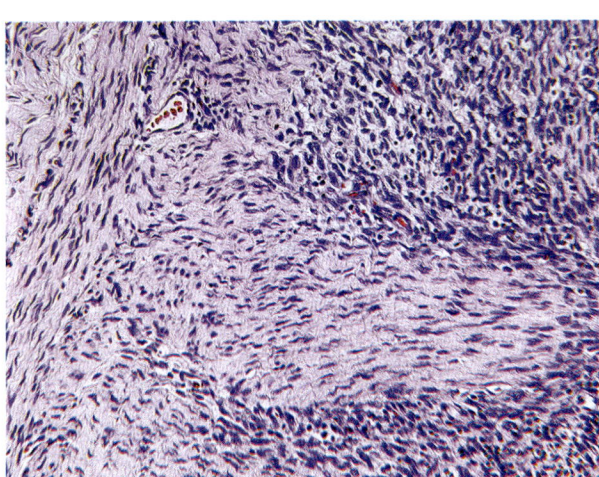

FIGURE 25-32 • Composite fibrous tumor in a 1-year-old male who presented with a mass in the arm, and then developed masses in the paraspinal and retroperitoneal regions. **A:** The tumor has areas of ISF. **B:** This is a focus resembling FHI. **C:** A third pattern with the features of myofibroma and CIFS.

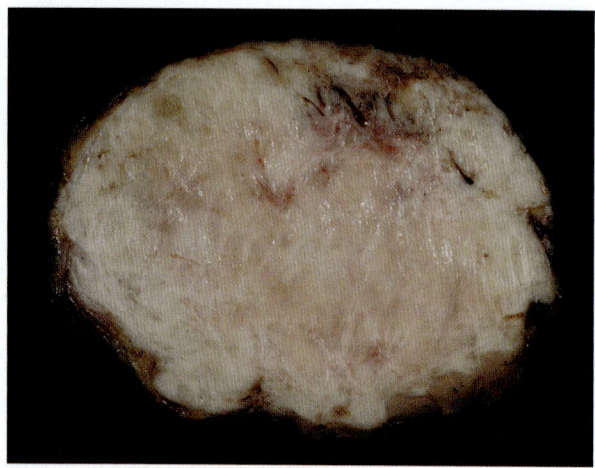

FIGURE 25-33 • Desmoid fibromatosis (desmoid tumor) presented as a deep soft tissue mass in the posterior thigh of a 15-year-old female. The cut surface of this 12-cm circumscribed mass has a tan-white trabecular appearance. Note the pushing growth into the skeletal muscle at the periphery.

extremities (including brachial plexus) (40%) and trunk (35% to 40%) are the sites of predilection in older children, but these tumors are also seen in the head and neck (15% to 20%) and abdominal (mesentery and pelvis) sites (10%). Desmoid tumors arising in the shoulder–axilla or gluteal–thigh region have a local recurrence rate of 30% or greater (136,137). Most tumors occur sporadically (90% to 97% of cases), but there is an association with Gardner syndrome—FAP in less than 5% of cases; there is an increased risk for Gardner syndrome in those with FAP who have mutations between exons 1310 and 2011 (138).

A small incisional or needle biopsy can be challenging since other non–neoplastic and neoplastic fibrous proliferations are considerations in the differential diagnosis given the limitations of a small specimen. Could this rather bland fibrous proliferation represent a scar or low grade fibromyxoid sarcoma (LGFS)? An operative resection yields a gray-white mass with a uniform mucoid to trabeculated appearance whose dimensions range from a few centimeters to >10 cm (Figure 25-33). When skeletal muscle is present at the periphery of the resection, irregular infiltration by the usually bland spindle cell proliferation into the muscle is a common feature. The periphery of the mass should be tattooed with India ink (or other appropriate dye) to document the invariably positive surgical margins. Fascicles of variably dense spindle cells or a loosely organized pattern of spindle cells are accompanied by a pale, myxoid to edematous or more collagenized background. The spindle cells may have the features of mature fibroblasts or display variation in the size and configuration of the stromal cells to reflect their less mature, more myofibroblastic features, which is manifested by cytoplasmic immunopositivity for SMA and nuclear positivity for β-catenin (Figure 25-34). Mitotic figures can be identified among the myofibroblasts but atypical mitotic figures should be viewed with wariness. A myxoid background, proliferating myofibroblasts, some interstitial hemorrhage and edema portray a more NF-like appearance. The infiltrative margins rather than peripheral nodularity characterize the desmoid tumor in contrast to NF and LGFS. The same infiltrative pattern of spindle cells into infant skeletal muscle can risk the diagnosis of spindle cell rhabdomyosarcoma. Scattered lymphoid nodules at the interface with the surrounding normal soft tissues also usefully distinguish a desmoid tumor from other fibrous proliferations. There is little to differentiate a recurrent desmoid tumor from the newly diagnosed tumor except for the findings of earlier surgery including dense scarring, foreign body giant cells, and a more circumscribed margin than in the primary tumor. Immunostaining for β-catenin is helpful in those cases when

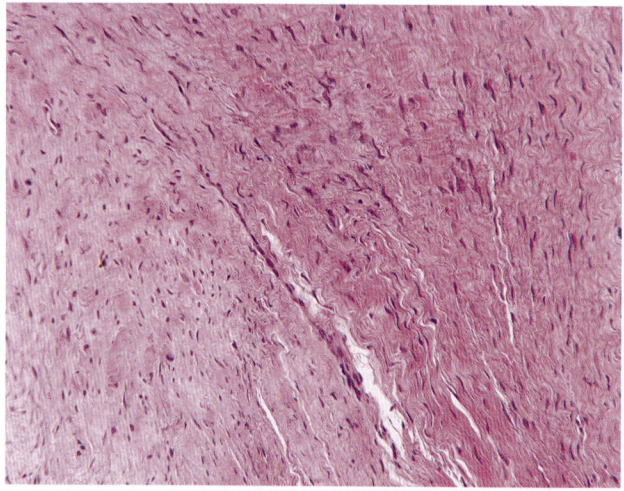
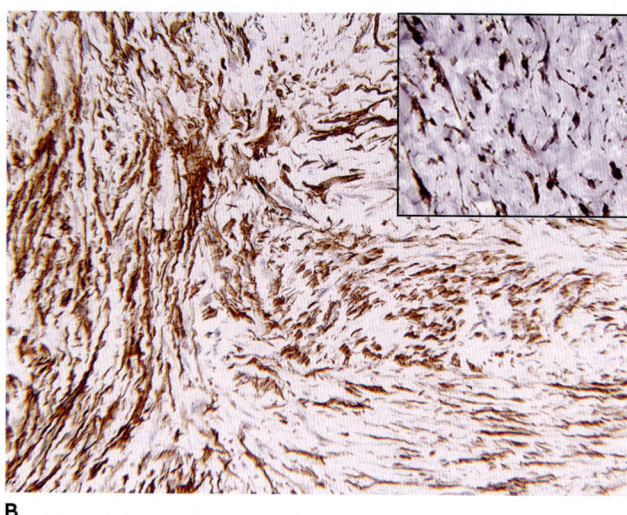

FIGURE 25-34 • Desmoid fibromatosis (desmoid tumor) presented in the posterior thigh of a 15-year-old female. **A:** A bland proliferation of fibroblasts is seen in a nonhomogeneous collagenous background. **B:** The fibroblasts maintain their myofibroblastic phenotype with immunostaining for SMA. **Inset:** Most desmoids express nuclear β-catenin by IHC.

there is uncertainty whether the particular fibrous tumor is a desmoid or not; there is diffuse nuclear positivity in the desmoid tumor (139,140). There is also the disputed role of β-catenin as a prognostic marker for recurrence (141,142).

The local recurrence of the desmoid tumor is 35% to 70%, which has given rise to reconsideration as to the approach in follow-up care. Some have advocated a "wait and see" approach since positive surgical margins, though predictive of recurrence, are not always associated with recurrent disease (136,137,143–145). Some have even called into question the desirability of primary surgery in those cases with the likelihood of serious functional or cosmetic morbidity in a child (146).

The relationship of the desmoid tumor to FAP has provided the opportunity to understand some of the molecular pathology of this neoplasm. Sporadic desmoid tumors have somatic mutations in the β-catenin gene (CTNNB1 on 3p21), which regulates the Wnt signaling pathway whereas the FAP-associated desmoids have an APC (5q22) germline mutation (138). Nuclear expression of β-catenin is a useful marker to differentiate the sporadic and familial desmoid tumors from other fibrous tumors, but some of the other fibrous tumors may also have nuclear positivity for β-catenin so that it is not absolutely specific for desmoid tumors. Nonetheless, greater than 80% of desmoid tumors express nuclear β-catenin.

Gardner-nuchal fibroma is a distinctive paucicellular, densely collagenized mass presenting in the first decade of life with a predilection for the posterior truncal–paraspinal region (147,148). Other sites of involvement include the head and neck and extremities. Approximately 70% of affected individuals have a family history of FAP or represent a new mutation. The tumor is poorly circumscribed with a plaque-like growth in the subcutis or deeper soft tissues, and there is overgrowth of the subcutis with entrapment of adipose tissue. It can be difficult to distinguish between the peripheral margins of a fibroma and the normal fibrous connective tissues. A desmoid tumor may accompany a fibroma or evolve from a recurrent fibroma. There is nuclear positivity for β-catenin but in a less consistent fashion than in the desmoid tumor (3,148). Cyclin-D1 is expressed in the nuclei in virtually all cases. These tumors are immunopositive for vimentin and CD34. Nuchal and Gardner fibromas have virtually identical pathologic features.

Palmar–plantar fibromatosis is seen in children but more commonly in adults. These are poorly circumscribed fibrous tumors with a pattern of spindle cell foci separated by bland hypocellular collagenized stroma (149).

Juvenile hyaline fibromatosis (JHF) is an autosomal recessive disorder, which is allelicallyrelated to *infantile systemic hyalinosis (ISH)* with a loss of function mutation in the capillary morphogenesis gene-2 (CMG2 on 4q21) (150,151). Large, painful nodules in the head and neck region (including marked gingival hypertrophy) and around joints evolve from small cutaneous papules, which are first noted in infancy and accelerate in growth throughout childhood.

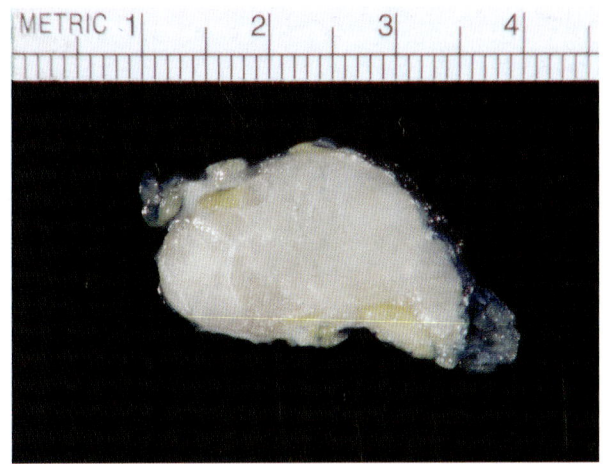

FIGURE 25-35 • JHF presented as a firm mass around the knee of a 17-year-old female who had several other similar masses excised previous to this one. This well-circumscribed mass had a glistening, slightly nodular appearance on cut surface. The consistency of the mass was described as firm with a chondroid-like quality.

Osteolytic bone lesions develop, as well as joint contractures. Firm, white nodules in the soft tissues and dense fibrous effacement of the dermis, resembling to some extent morphea–scleroderma, are some of the pathologic features (Figure 25-35). The nodules are circumscribed and consist of homogeneously dense hyaline collagen with both paucicellular and hypercellular foci, consisting of ovoid stromal cells residing in apparent lacunae with a chondrocyte-like appearance (Figure 25-36). Unlike JHF, ISH has visceral involvement in addition to papulonodular lesions of the skin and soft tissues. The heart, intestinal tract, spleen, and skeletal muscle are infiltrated by the fibrohyaline tissue with a

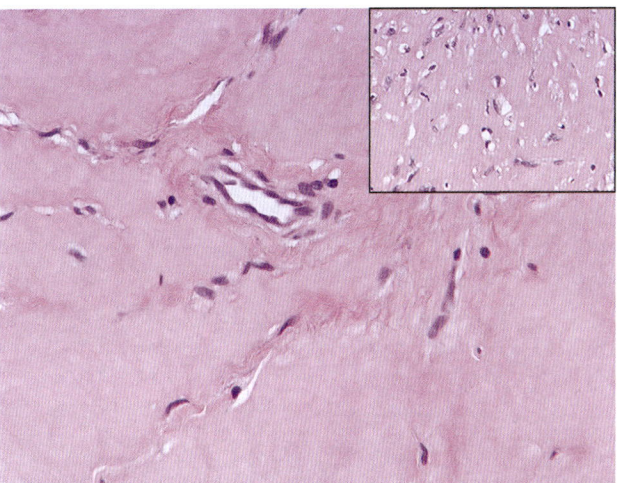

FIGURE 25-36 • JHF presented as multiple masses in this 17-year-old female. The dense, hypocellular nodules of collagen are characteristic of this tumor. **Inset:** Rounded stromal cells within lacunar spaces resembling chondrocytes is another histologic feature. No other fibrous lesion in childhood approaches this degree of dense, uniform hyalinization with the possible exception of a Gardner fibroma which lacks nodularity.

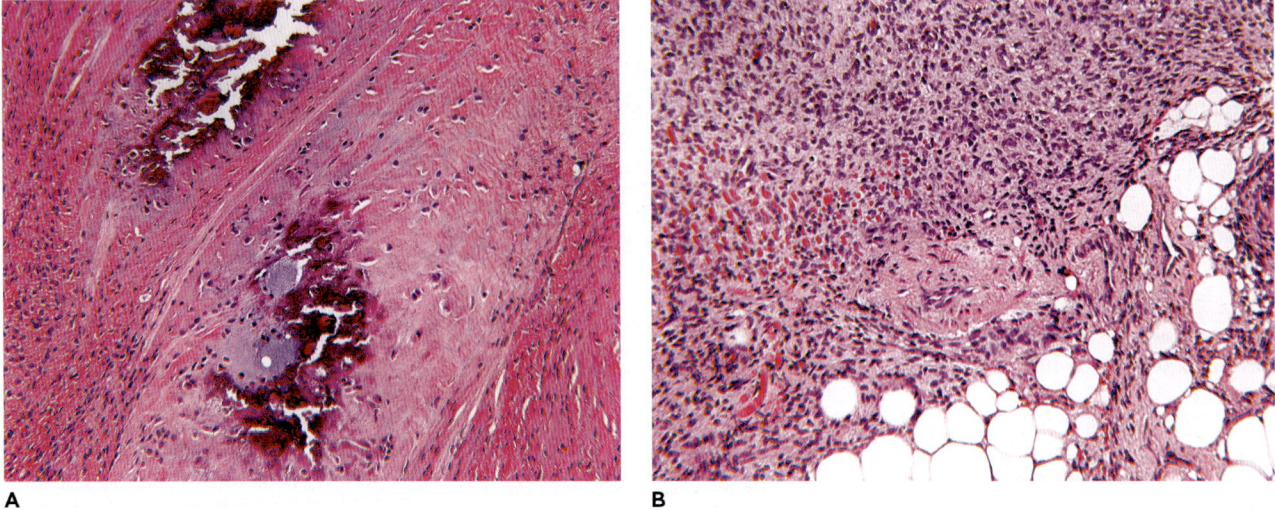

FIGURE 25-37 • Calcifying aponeurotic fibroma in a 5-year-old male along the biceps tendon. **A:** Foci of dystrophic calcification within a nodular hyaline focus. **B:** Elsewhere the tumor had an infiltrative spindle cell pattern.

resemblance to amyloid. Protein-losing enteropathy can be a complication of small intestinal hyalinosis. Only infantile myofibromatosis among the other fibrous proliferations has visceral involvement by a more cellular, vasocentric nodular proliferation than the diffuse interstitial hyalinosis of ISH.

Calcifying aponeurotic fibromatosis (juvenile aponeurotic fibroma) is one of the least common of the fibrous tumors of childhood (1% to 2% of all cases) and has a predilection for the distal extremities (109). Usually, older children and adolescents present with a mass in the ankle or wrist in the deep subcutis, fascia, or tendon. A poorly circumscribed mass measuring less than 5 cm has a firm, gritty, gray-white appearance of cut surface. An infiltrative process of spindle cells (fibroblasts) is accompanied by less cellular, hyalinized areas in which foci of granular calcifications are found (Figure 25-37). Without the calcifications, there is a resemblance to infantile subcutaneous fibromatosis. Recurrences are reported in 50% or more of cases. Because of the distal, periarticular localization, monophasic SS may be briefly considered in the differential diagnosis.

Juvenile nasopharyngeal angiofibroma (JNA) is a fibrovascular tumor which is more fibrous than vascular in terms of histogenesis. Most cases present in pubertal-aged males with epistaxis (152). These tumors are seen in the setting of FAP, and like desmoid-type fibromatosis, the nuclei of JNA express β-catenin and androgen receptor (153) (Figure. 25-38). Another susceptibility gene in the development of JNA is GSTM1 (1p13.3) in a Brazilian study (154).

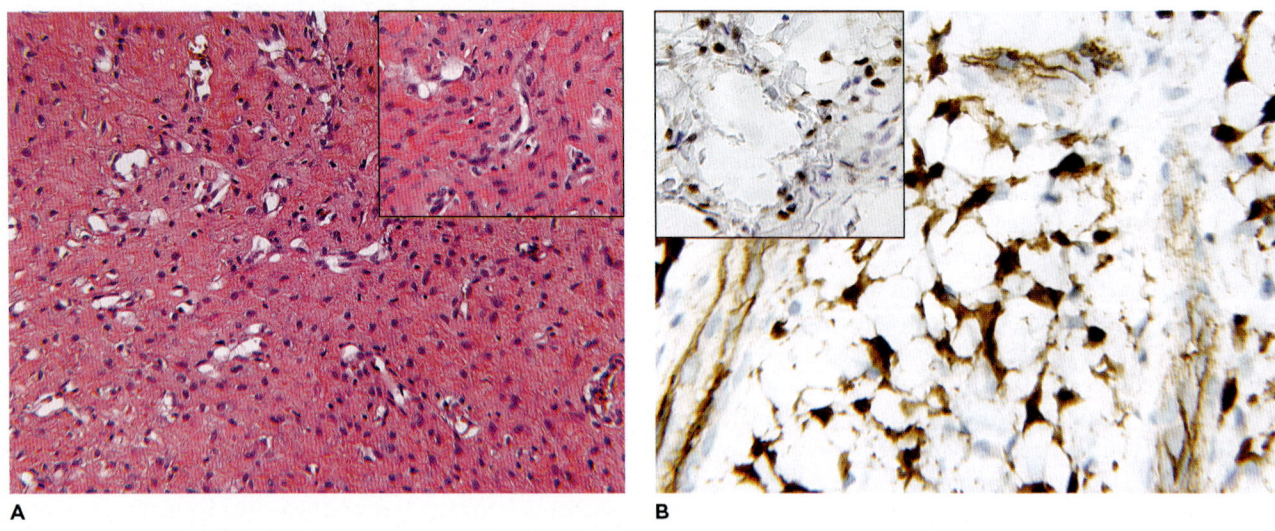

FIGURE 25-38 • JNA in an 11-year-old male with a large skull-based mass. **A:** This field shows the presence of regularly distributed vascular spaces in a dense fibrous stroma with uniform cellularity. **Inset:** The stromal cells have indistinct cellular borders. **B:** β-Catenin immunostain shows intense nuclear positivity. **Inset:** There is nuclear positivity for androgen receptor as well.

A firm lobulated or pedunculated mass measuring 5 to 10 cm is the gross appearance. A uniform population of spindled to stellate fibroblasts lacks a fasciculated pattern, but appears more diffuse and is interrupted by evenly distributed thin-walled vascular spaces. Mast cells are commonly distributed within the background. These tumors have pushing rather than the infiltrating borders of desmoid-type fibromatosis, but despite this difference, JNAs are known to recur locally (155).

Fibromatosis colli is infrequently seen as a surgical specimen though it is one of the more common fibrous tumors of childhood. There is a predilection for the right neck and spontaneous regression occurs in more than 90% of cases (109,156). A firm, white lobulated fibrous mass measuring 1 to 3 cm typically arises in the lower one-third of the sternocleidomastoid muscle where it has infiltrative borders like the desmoid-type fibromatosis. However, fibromatosis colli is usually more cellular than desmoid-type fibromatosis and has a less collagenized stroma. There is some similarity to NF, which infrequently arises in skeletal muscle.

Calcifying fibrous pseudotumor (CFP) is a fibroinflammatory tumefaction which is recognized in children and adults alike and has a broad anatomic distribution with a predilection for the extremities in children (157,158). Virtually no anatomic site is immune from CFP (153). A well circumscribed, firm fibrous mass can measure in excess of 20 cm or as small as 2 to 3 cm. Dense collagen with scattered lymphoplasmacytic infiltrates and small calcific deposits, some with psammoma-like features, are the characteristic microscopic features. The spindle cells are immunoreactive for CD34, and nonreactive for smooth muscle actin and ALK, unlike the inflammatory myofibroblastic tumor (IMT) (159). A CFP of the neck in a 5-week-old girl was immunopositive for factor XIIIa, raising the question whether these tumors are dendritic cell (DC) in origin and possibly related to juvenile xanthogranuloma (JXG) (160).

Inflammatory myofibroblastic tumor (IMT) is a distinctive clinicopathologic entity, which has emerged from the somewhat poorly defined group of idiopathic fibroinflammatory processes collectively known as inflammatory pseudotumors (161). In the WHO classification, the IMT is regarded as an "intermediate, rarely metastasizing" neoplasm, together with DFSP, SFT, low grade myofibroblastic sarcoma, myxoinflammatory fibroblastic sarcoma (MIFS) and CIF (5). IMT is typically seen in the first three decades with cases occurring as early as the first year of life and into early adulthood with a mean age at diagnosis between 10 and 15 years without the inclusion of older adults (3,109). The lung, gastrointestinal (GI) tract, mesentery, liver, and bladder are the principal primary sites, which in aggregate account for 70% to 75% of all cases in children (Table 25-8). This tumor is also ubiquitous in terms of its other less common sites of presentation including the dura, orbit, kidney, uterus, and

TABLE 25-8	SITES OF INFLAMMATORY MYOFIBROBLASTIC TUMOR IN THE FIRST TWO DECADES OF LIFE			
Sites	No.	Mean Age and Range	Sex (M/F)	Total (%)
Abdomen				61 (50)
Small Intestine Omentum-mesentery	36	9 y (3 mo–17 y)	13/23	
Liver	11	4 y (2 mo–9 y)	6/5	
Stomach	5	9 y (6–14 y)	2/3	
Retroperitoneum	5	7 y (4 mo–14 y)	3/2	
Pancreas	2	12 y, 7 y	1/1	
Spleen	2	16 y, 9 y	2/0	
Genitourinary Tract				16 (13)
Bladder	13	11 y (4–17 y)	6/7	
Scrotum	2	7 y, 15 y	2/0	
Prostate	1	17 y	1/0	
Thorax				32 (26)
Lung	17	10 y (2–20 y)	13/4	
Larynx-Trachea	6	7 y (12 days–12 y)	3/3	
Heart	9	2½ y (1 mo–12 y)	6/3	
Superficial and Deep Soft Tissues				12 (10)
Extremities-trunk	5	6 y (1 mo–13 y)	3/2	
Head and neck	3	2 y (1 y–3 y)	2/1	
Perirectal-pelvic	4	8 y (3 y–13 y)	1/3	
Brain				2 (2)
	2	1 y, 15 y	0/2	123 (~100)

From the files of the Lauren V. Ackerman Laboratory of Surgical Pathology, St. Louis Children's Hospital, Washington University Medical Center, St. Louis, MO.

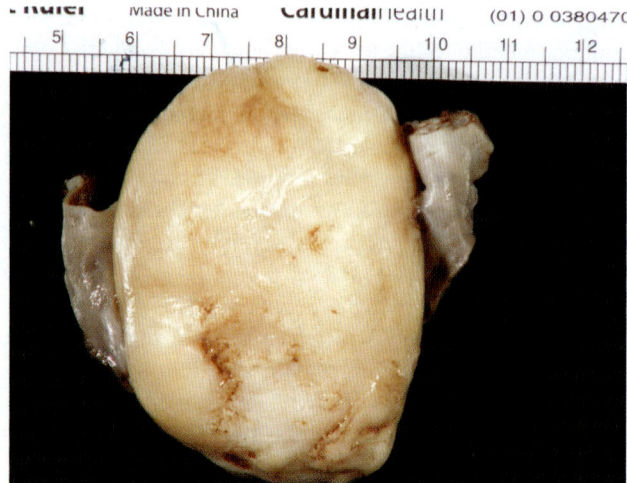

FIGURE 25-39 • IMT in a 19-year-old male arising in the region of the inferior vena cava. The mass measures almost 7 cm in greatest dimension (51 g) and has a homogenous pale tan-white cut surface.

upper respiratory tract. Peripheral soft tissues and bones are infrequently affected. In a small proportion of cases, multiple lesions may be detected at presentation or develop over the evolving clinical course. It is not always clear whether multiple IMTs are metastases or independently developing multifocal tumors (162). Constitutional or B-symptoms with fever, failure to thrive, and weight loss together with microcytic hypochromic anemia and polyclonal gammopathy are present in 5% to 15% of cases; these children may be a diagnostic dilemma for weeks to months. There is IL-6 production in association with IMTs, which often falls to normal levels after surgical resection.

The tumors range in size from less than 1 to 15 cm in greatest dimension, with the larger IMTs arising in the abdomen. In the lung, IMT measures 4 to 6 cm, but in the mesentery or retroperitoneum, IMT is generally in excess of 10 cm. A well-circumscribed, non–encapsulated tumor has a glistening tan-white to gray-tan homogeneous and nodular appearance, with minimal hemorrhage and absence of necrosis in most cases (Figure 25-39). Calcifications are seen more often in the pulmonary IMTs (where it is one of the more common primary neoplasms of the lung in childhood) (163,164). Microscopically, three basic patterns are recognized; they are not necessarily in equal proportions nor is each represented in every tumor. The first of these is characterized by a dense spindle cell proliferation with the formation of fascicles and a variably prominent population of lymphocytes and mature plasma cells in the background. Adjacent foci may be composed of loosely arranged spindled to plump stromal cells in a myxoid and edematous background resembling NF to yet a third pattern of paucicellular dense fibrosis with some inflammatory cells in the background (Figure 25-40A–D). Dystrophic calcifications, osseous metaplasia, and collections of histiocytes are other features. Mitotic figures are found in the spindle cell foci; however, atypical mitotic figures and anaplasia should suggest a high-grade pleomorphic sarcoma. Necrosis is present in those IMTs which have undergone sarcomatous transformation and may be accompanied by overt nuclear pleomorphism and hyperchromatism. Those IMTs arising in the abdomen which are multifocal and are composed of polygonal or epithelioid cells tend to behave in an aggressive manner, more so than those tumors with the typical histologic features (161). Most IMTs are immunoreactive for vimentin and SMA (Figure 25-40C), as well as cytokeratin in a minority of cases in children. Approximately 50% to 60% of IMTs are ALK-1 positive with a membranous and/or cytoplasmic pattern reflecting a specific ALK-1 translocation (Figure 25-40D) (161,162) (Table 25-1). Coffin and associates (165) found that ALK-1–positive IMTs pursue a less aggressive course than those which are ALK-1 negative

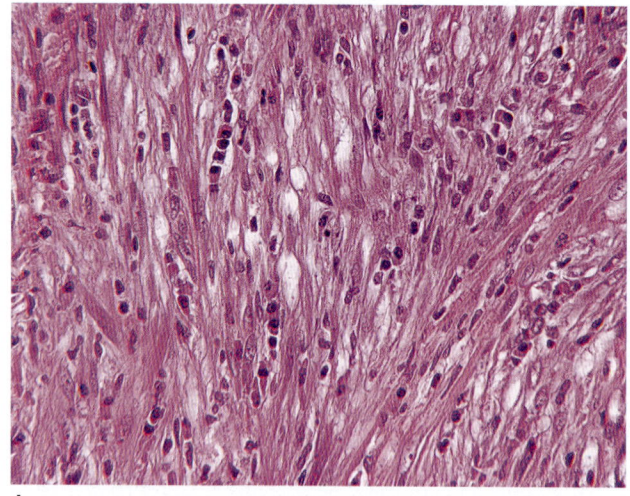
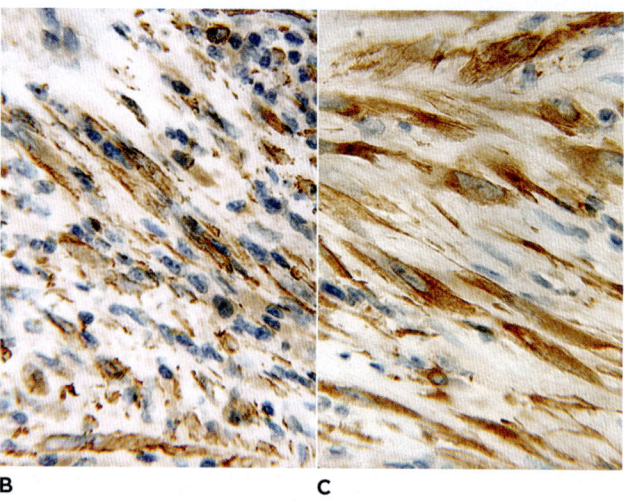

FIGURE 25-40 • IMT in a 19-year-old male (see Figure 25-39). **A:** A uniform spindle cell proliferation is seen with few inflammatory cells (mainly plasma cells) in the background. **B:** The spindle cells are immunopositive for smooth muscle actin and also note the inflammatory cells in the background. **C:** Intense ALK-1 cytoplasmic positivity is shown.

and may represent another tumor type. Those IMTs with a prominent epithelioid or round cell population are seemingly more aggressive (166). Attention has also been directed to the relationship, if any, between IMT with its often prominent population of polyclonal plasma cells and the IgG4-related sclerosing disorders (167). Surgical resection is the treatment of choice with a recurrence-free survival of 80% or greater. It is now recognized that there is an ALK-positive family of neoplasms beyond anaplastic large cell lymphoma and IMT (168). In a minority of IMTs, ROS-1 translocation has been reported (169).

The differential diagnosis includes low-grade myofibroblastic sarcoma, NF, inflammatory leiomyosarcoma, myxofibrosarcoma and CFP, desmoid-type fibromatosis, and gastrointestinal stromal tumor (GIST). The latter two neoplasms, when arising in the mesentery or intestine, display β-catenin (nuclear) and CD117 immunopositivity, respectively.

Myxoinflammatory fibroblastic sarcoma (MIFS) is an uncommon neoplasm with a predilection for the distal extremities mainly in adults, but is documented in older children and adolescents in nonacral sites (170,171). A sharply demarcated, lobulated or nodular tumor has a fibrous or fibromyxoid appearance. There is considerable microscopic variation in the stroma and spindled and epithelioid cells (Figure 25-41). These tumors are immunoreactive for D2-40, CD34, and CD68. It is thought that MIFS is one in a spectrum of related tumors including the hemosiderotic fibrolipomatous tumor and pleomorphic hyalinizing angiectatic tumor; these tumors appear to share a translocation involving rearrangements of TGFBR3 and/or MGEA5.

Low-grade myofibroblastic sarcoma is a rare sarcoma with many overlapping morphologic and immunohistochemical features in common with myofibroma and IMT (172). There is a preference for the head and neck region in children (113). A superficial biopsy can be misleading especially given the resemblance to myofibroma or fibromatosis.

Fibrosarcoma (FS) with the exception of some specific histologic types is largely a diagnosis of exclusion and in children as such is uncommon (172). Monophasic SS, spindle cell RMS and malignant peripheralnerve sheath tumor are the three STS in children with FS-like spindle cell morphology.

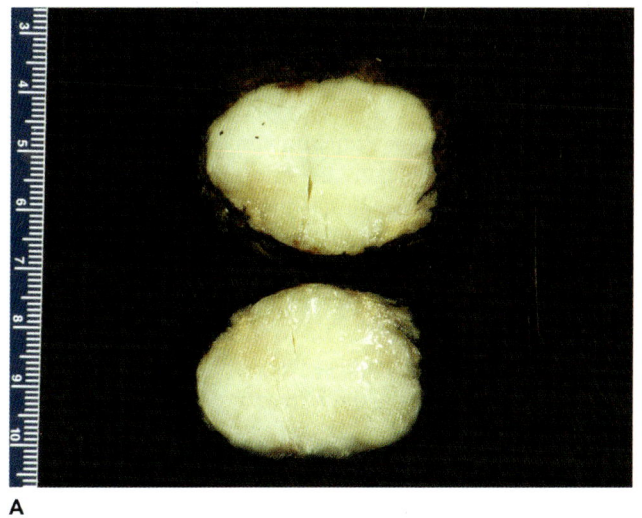
A

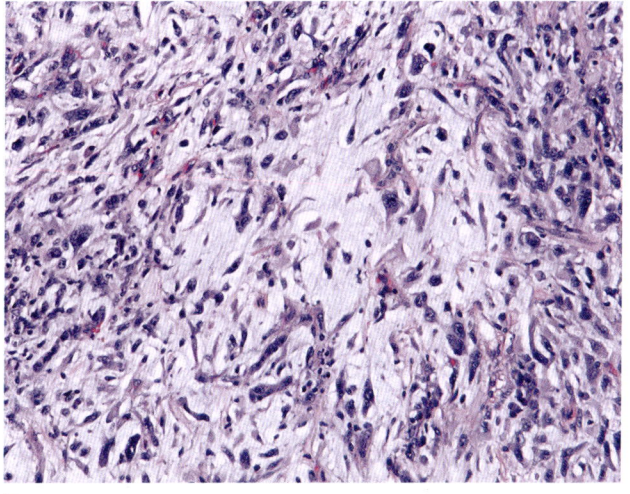
B

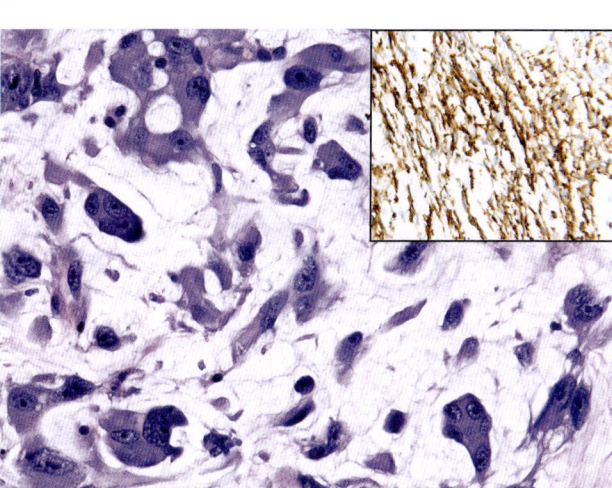
C

FIGURE 25-41 • MIFS presenting in the left axilla of a 10-year-old male. **A:** The mass is well circumscribed, measuring 6 × 5 × 4.5 cm, and has a glistening, firm tan surface. **B:** Spindle- and polygonal-shaped tumor cells are accompanied by lymphocytes, plasma cells, and a myxoid background. **C:** Ganglion-like cells and polygonal cells with vacuoles are seen. **Inset:** CD34 (shown), S100 protein, smooth muscle actin, and CD68 were expressed by the tumor cells.

TABLE 25-9	CONGENITAL-INFANTILE FIBROSARCOMA[a]
20 Cases	
11 Males: 9 Females	
Age range at diagnosis: 5 day-25 months (mean, 7.3 months; median, 5 months)	
Sites:	
Lower extremity	5
Trunk	5
Small intestine	3
Gluteal region	2
Intraabdominal	2
Upper extremity	1
Intrathoracic	1
Neck	1
Lung metastasis	2

[a]From the files (1989–2014) of the Lauren V. Ackerman Laboratory of Surgical Pathology, St. Louis Children's Hospital, Washington University Medical Center, St. Louis, MO.

Congenital infantile fibrosarcoma (CIFS) is discussed in this section though it resides in the intermediate category of rarely metastasizing fibrous neoplasms. In general, there is a preference for the extremities (lower greater than upper) where the tumor presents either proximally or distally as a rapidly enlarging mass (173,174). Our own experience revealed 20 cases, virtually all presenting before 2 years of age, and 5 cases were diagnosed in the first month of life; the extremities including the gluteal region and trunk accounted for 60% of our cases (Table 25-9). We have also seen a few examples arising in the small or large intestine (Figure 25-42). These tumors can be quite hemorrhagic and may be mistaken for a vascular tumor clinically. Resected tumors are generally examined after preoperative chemotherapy which substantially alters the gross features including the size of the mass.

A circumscribed, but non–encapsulated mass measuring 6 to 15 cm in greatest dimension has either a uniform, glistening tan-white cut surface or a cystic, hemorrhagic, and friable character in those cases without adjuvant therapy before surgery. Fascicles of uniform spindle cells with or without the so-called herringbone pattern are the classical features, but we have been impressed by the histologic diversity of these tumors with a poorly organized pattern of immature and even primitive mesenchymal cells. Whether in skeletal muscle or small intestine, the highly infiltrative character of the tumor can be appreciated (Figure 25-43A–D). The hemorrhagic appearance reflects the absence of a supporting stroma and the presence of pooled erythrocytes has a resemblance to peliosis. The individual tumor cells have elongated uniform nuclei, and mitotic figures are found without difficulty (Figure 25-43B). If there are an appreciable degree of pleomorphism and atypical mitotic figures, the tumor may represent something other than CIFs such as a spindle cell RMS. If the tumor is especially primitive with a myxoid background, ERMS, primitive myxoid mesenchymal tumor of infancy (PMMTI), MRT, and undifferentiated round cell sarcoma with Ewing-like features are other considerations in the differential diagnosis in a child less than 2 years old. CIFS has the ETV6-NTRK3 fusion transcript, t(12;15)(p13;q25), in some 70% of cases (173–175). If the translocation is not identified, but the tumor otherwise satisfies the morphologic features then a diagnosis of CIFS should be made (175). These tumors have an immunophenotype restricted to vimentin positivity (Figure 25-43D). Foci resembling CIFS may be found in other fibrous tumors of childhood including infantile myofibroma, but the characteristic translocation is not present in these cases (176,177). The other neoplasms with the t(12;15) translocation are cellular mesoblastic nephroma or infantile FS of the kidney, juvenile or secretory carcinoma of the breast and salivary gland. After chemotherapy, the resected specimen may have minimal residual tumor

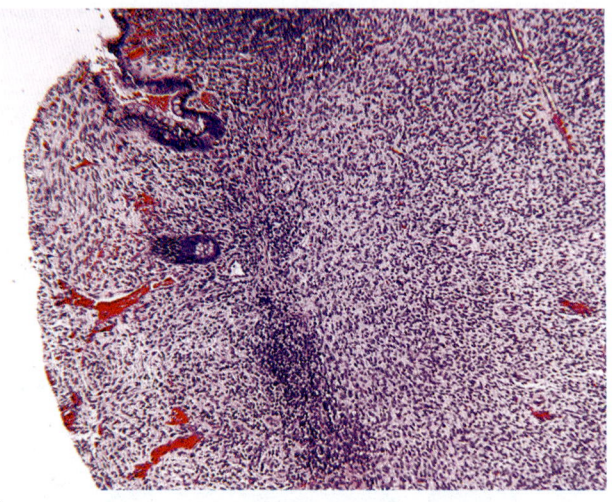
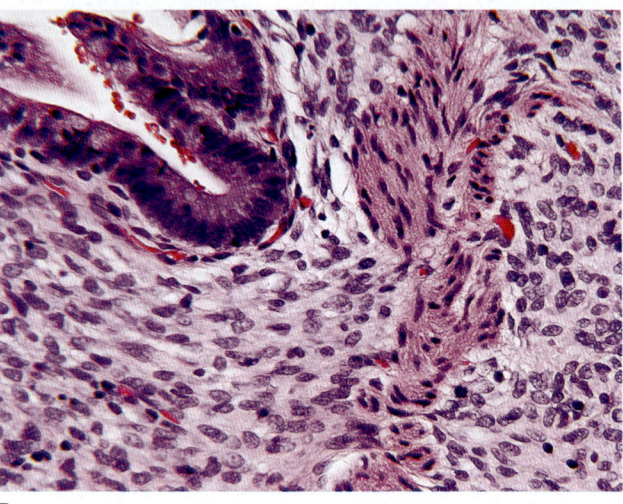

FIGURE 25-42 • CIFS of the jejunum in a 10-day-old male who presented with intestinal obstruction. **A:** A uniform spindle cell proliferation involves the entire thickness of the bowel wall. **B:** The spindle cells infiltrate into the lamina propria.

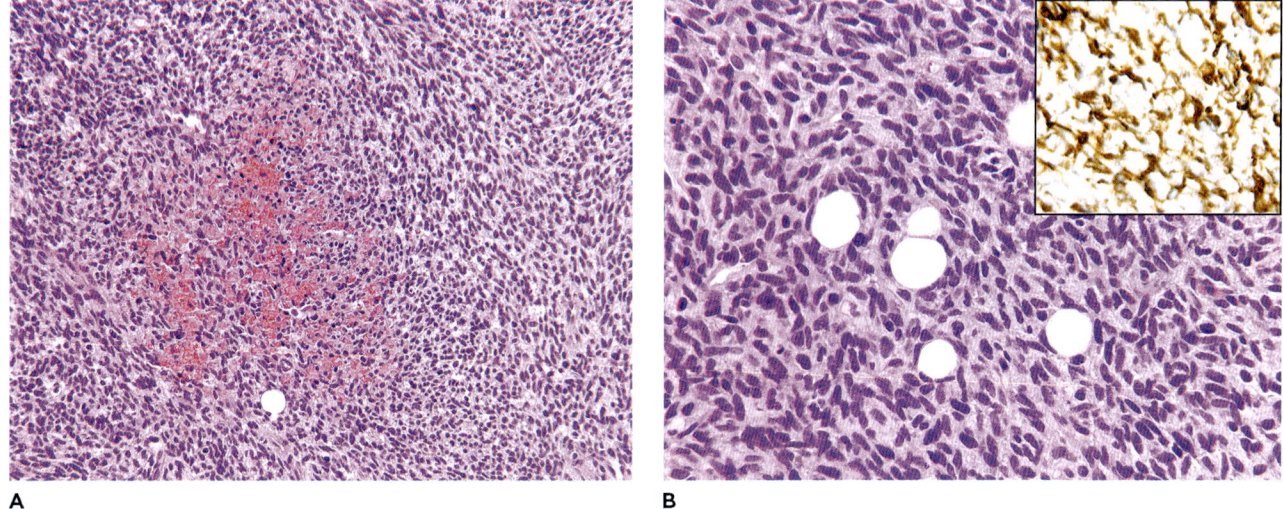

FIGURE 25-43 • CIFS presenting in the soft tissues of the posterior trunk in a 4 month-old female. **A:** The spindle cell pattern forming short fascicles presents the differential diagnosis of spindle cell rhabdomyosarcoma. Focal areas of hemorrhage resulted in the clinical impression of a hemangioma. **B:** The infiltrative character of the tumor is seen in this focus of residual adipose tissue in the background. **Inset:** All muscle markers were nonreactive with only immunopositivity for vimentin.

with only fibrosis, histiocytes, and hemosiderin deposition. Metastasis occurs in less than 5% of cases. In the lung, the infantile peribronchial myofibroblastic tumor has a histologic resemblance to CIFS but lacks the signature translocation of the latter tumor (178). *Primitive myxoid mesenchymal tumor of infancy* is represented by less than 15 cases in the literature of a soft tissue neoplasm on the trunk or extremities mainly in infants to the age of 15 months (179). These soft, often gelatinous tumors are composed of uniform spindle cells in a myxoid matrix except at the periphery where the tumor is more cellular and has a collagenized stroma (180). There is some resemblance to CIF, but with an absence of the t(12;15) translocation. PMMTI should be regarded as a low grade malignant neoplasm with the potential to progress to a high grade sarcoma (181).

Low-grade fibromyxoid sarcoma (LGFS, Evans tumor) is a generally slow-growing soft-tissue neoplasm with a preference for the lower extremity and trunk but has a wide anatomic distribution (182,183). Approximately 20% of cases are discovered before the age of 20 years and have been seen as early as 4 years of age (184). A well-circumscribed, fibrous-appearing tumor with a sharply demarcated pseudocapsule has a distinctive microscopic appearance of bland spindle cells with an alternating pale myxoid background to a more collagenous stroma (Figure 25-44A–D). Foci of epithelioid cells are found in those tumors with a hyalinized

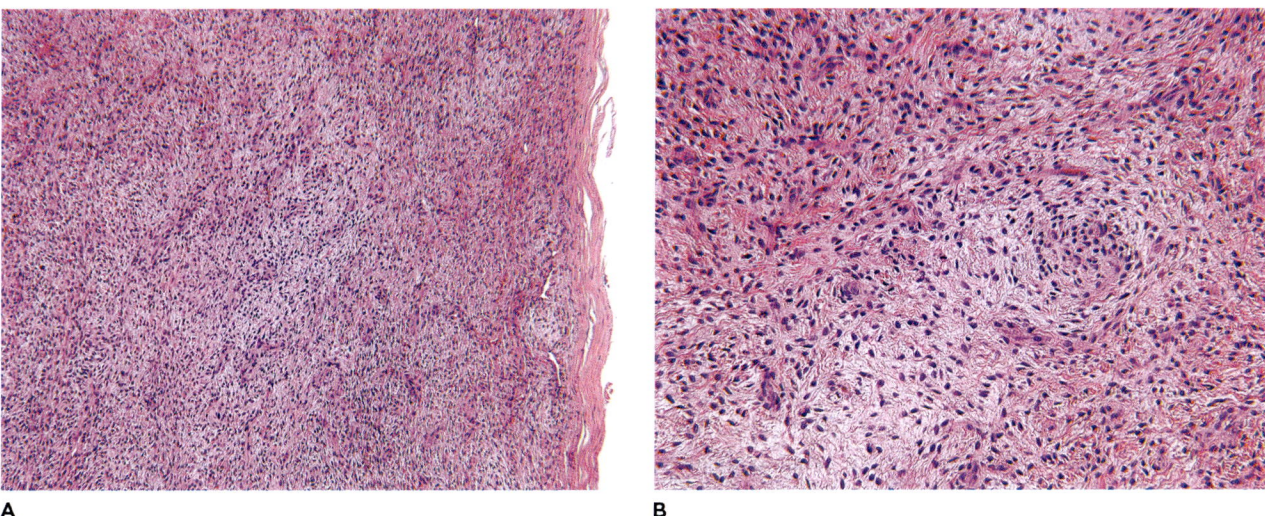

FIGURE 25-44 • LGFS of the lower extremity in a 10-year-old male. **A:** The tumor measuring 3.5 cm in greatest dimension was well circumscribed with a delicate capsule as seen in this low-magnification field. **B:** An alternating myxoid and more cellular focus.

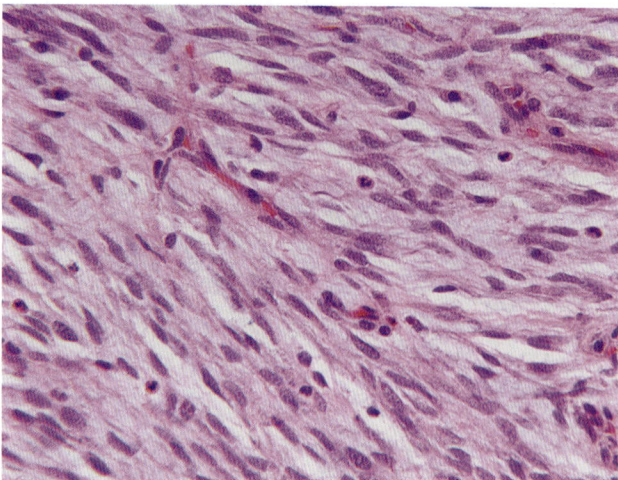

FIGURE 25-48 • DFSP presented as a soft tissue mass in the breast of a 2-year-old female. Uniform spindle cells with pale staining nuclei are arranged in broad fascicles.

(203). One such tumor is the *CD34-positive dermal fibroma*; also known as the medallion-like dermal dendrocyte hamartoma; it is a lesion of the dermis in children with a horizontal layer of fusiform spindle cells in the superficial papillary dermis (204). Another CD34-positive spindle cell lesion is the *fibroblastic connective tissue nevus* found in the deep reticular dermis and contiguous subcutis; this plaque-like lesion, occurring in children, is found on the trunk and head and neck region (135). *Superficial CD34-positive fibroblastic tumor*, a more recent entry, is found in the deep dermis and subcutis as a somewhat pleomorphic, fasciculated spindle cell proliferation with minimal mitotic activity (205). *Dermatomyofibroma and FHI* are also composed of CD34-positive spindle cells. CD34-positive SFT has been reported in the superficial soft tissue and skin in children (206).

FIBROHISTIOCYTIC TUMORS

WHO classification of fibrohistiocytic tumors conveys a certain element of histogenetic skepticism and legitimacy in still referring to them as the "so-called fibrohistiocytic tumors (5)." The pathway to this state of affairs was the result of the decline and fall of the malignant fibrous histiocytoma (MFH) as it reemerged as the "pleomorphic undifferentiated sarcoma (PUS)," which was premised on the argument that MFH is a pattern representing the final common morphologic pathway for several specific types of STSs mainly in adults (207–209). PUS is uncommonly encountered in children and some have presented as a second malignant neoplasm in a survivor of a first childhood malignancy (210,211). A study of STSs exclusive of RMS, revealed that 11% of cases were diagnosed as "MFHs" in addition to the more common SS (24% of cases) and malignant peripheral nerve sheath tumor (MPNST) (15% of cases) (212). A mixed histologic pattern of large pleomorphic and anaplastic tumor cells arranged into fascicles of spindle and/or irregularly shaped (some polygonal) cells with a fibrous and/or myxoid background are just some of microscopic features (211) (Figure 25-49A, B).

Though fibrohistiocytic tumors have been diminished in a sense, life must go on with the acknowledgment of their existence (213). The category of fibrohistiocytic tumors has been truncated in the latest WHO classification to include the benign entities of tenosynovial giant cell tumor and deep benign fibrous histiocytoma, and the "intermediate,

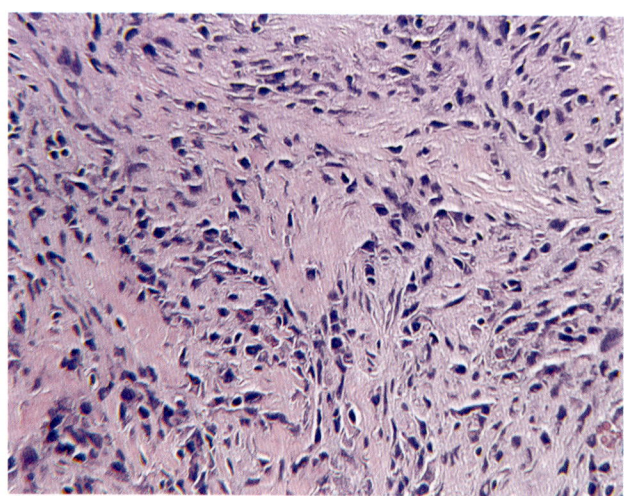

A

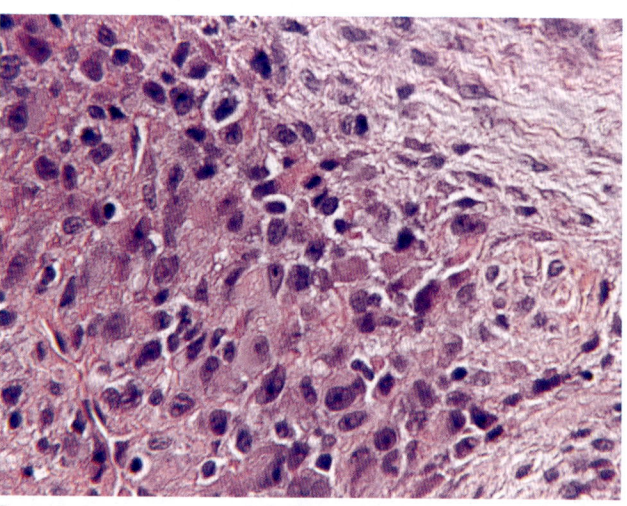

B

FIGURE 25-49 • PUS arising in the pelvic soft tissues of an 11-year-old female. **A:** Pleomorphic and hyperchromatic spindled and epithelioid cells in a collagenous stroma. Rhabdomyosarcoma, proximal ES, and leiomyosarcoma were ruled out with nonreactive muscle markers (myogenin negative) and retained INI1. **B:** This focus of tumor cells has a more epithelioid appearance; the tumor cells were positive for vimentin (diffuse) and cytokeratin (focal). There was no bone involvement.

rarely metastasizing" entities of plexiform fibrohistiocytic tumor (PFHT) and giant cell tumor of soft tissues (5). In the interim, AFH has migrated into the category of "tumors of uncertain differentiation" but for the sake of semantic consistency, it remains in the present discussion (5).

Dermatofibroma (DF, benign or common fibrous histiocytoma) is encountered with some frequency among skin biopsies in older children or adolescents and may be the most common fibrohistiocytic tumor overall in all age groups (214). In general, this solitary lesion is first encountered in the second decade with a predilection for the lower extremity (40% to 45% of cases) followed by the arm (25% to 30% of cases), but few body surfaces are spared. One rare presentation is the multiple clustered and eruptive DFs (215). One of the challenges in the pathologic diagnosis is the multiplicity of histologic patterns (Figure 25-50) (216). A dermocentric, poorly circumscribed (especially at the lateral borders), plump to fusiform spindle cell proliferation is the usual appearance of the common DF. Within the background, dense hyalinized stroma may be present to the extent that the lesion appears largely sclerotic. In those DFs with extension into the deep reticular dermis, the border may push into the subcutis, but without the overgrowth and infiltration of the subcutis as seen in DFSP, deep dermal NF, congenital melanocytic nevus with neurotization and some other examples of fibrous tumors in children. There are several morphologic variants with hemosiderin deposition, aneurysmal or angiomatoid blood-filled spaces, lipidized histiocytes, epithelioid histiocytes and giant cells, including those with Touton giant. Some tumors with xanthomatous or lipidized histiocytes and Touton giant cells are a conundrum in terms of the distinction from JXG since both express factor XIIIa, CD68, CD34 and CD163. This may reflect the common histogenetic origin of DF and JXG from dermal dendrocytes.

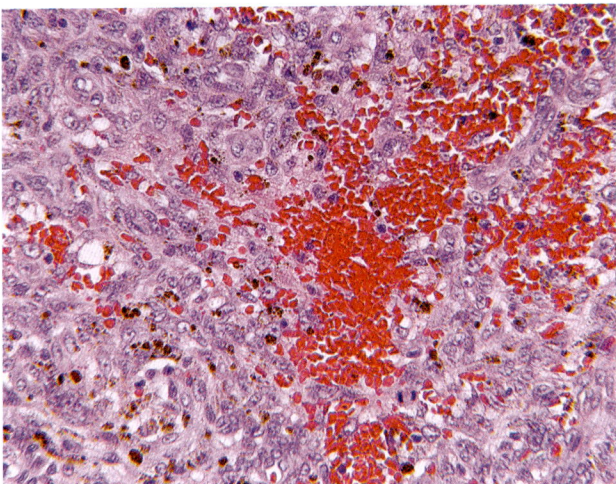

FIGURE 25-50 • Hemosiderotic DF in the lower extremity of a 16-year-old male. The tumor is composed of plump spindle cells with interstitial hemorrhage and hemosiderin.

Benign cutaneous fibrous histiocytoma (BCFH, cellular DF) is a neoplasm of the dermis, often with extension into the subcutis (Figure 25-51). BCFH is more cellular than the common DF and has the architecture of short fascicles and storiform profiles (217,218). The presence of some unsettling cytomorphology including atypical multinucleated cells is one of the principal features of an *atypical fibrous histiocytoma* of skin (219). Older children and young adults present with a nodular mass on an extremity or the face. Mitotic figures in the absence of appreciable atypia, and central necrosis are present in some cases. Marked pleomorphism and anaplasia are typically not present. These are often immunopositive for smooth muscle actin (approximately 95% of cases), desmin (30%) and CD34 (5%). Unlike DFSP, CD34 displays only patchy positivity in BCFH (220). Whether a BCFH or atypical fibrous histiocytoma, these lesions should be completely resected since 15% to 20% of these tumors may locally recur, and even rarely metastasize (221). Pleomorphic dermal sarcoma (PDS) is rarely encountered in children (222). It is somewhat difficult to judge from reports in the literature, but "atypical fibroxanthoma of skin," possibly representing PDS, has been seen infrequently in children and usually in the setting of hereditable defective DNA repair (223,224).

Tenosynovial giant cell tumor is the encompassing designation for three presumably related lesions involving the tendon sheath (giant cell tumor of tendon sheath or nodular tenosynovitis), intra-articular synovium (pigmented villonodular synovitis) and extra-articular soft tissues (diffuse type giant cell tumor or diffuse type pigmented villonodular synovitis) (225,226). *Giant cell tumor of tendon sheath* is seen in older children and adolescents (10 to 19 years), representing approximately 5% to 10% of all such tumors and presenting on the volar surface of the finger, but also around the knee and foot. A circumscribed nodule measuring 2 cm or less is composed predominantly of brownish yellow mononuclear histiocytes with or without xanthomatized cytoplasm, variable number of giant cells, spindled stromal fibroblasts and stromal hyalinization (Figure 25-52). Collections of mononuclear cells may have dyscohesive features. Hemosiderin may or may not be prominent. Local recurrence is seen in 20% to 25% of cases.

Pigmented villonodular synovitis (intra-articular) is reported in children, typically over the age of 10 years, presenting in the knee joint (75% to 80% of cases) with a chronic joint effusion (227,228). Papillary-appearing hemorrhagic tissues are characterized by synovial cell hyperplasia with a hypercellular stroma and hemosiderin-laden mononuclear cells (Figure 25-53). The local recurrence rate is in excess of 50% (229). Chronic hemarthropathy of hemophilia and synovial hemangiomatosis are other considerations in the differential diagnosis.

Diffuse-type giant cell tumor typically presents in the juxta-articular soft tissues of the knee, ankle and hip/gluteal region. The growth pattern is diffuse through the soft tissues and

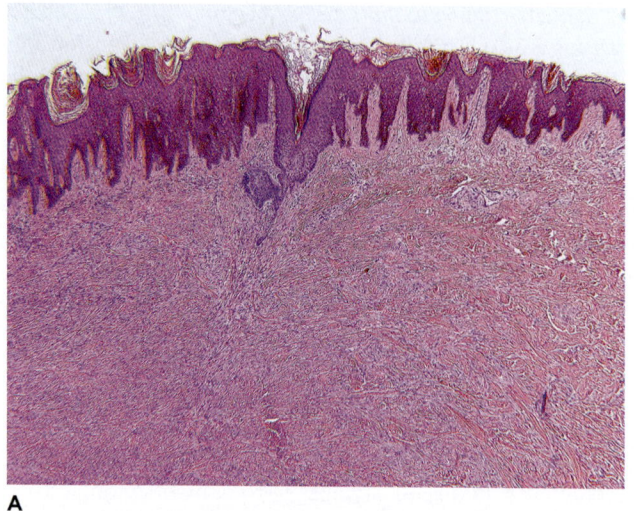
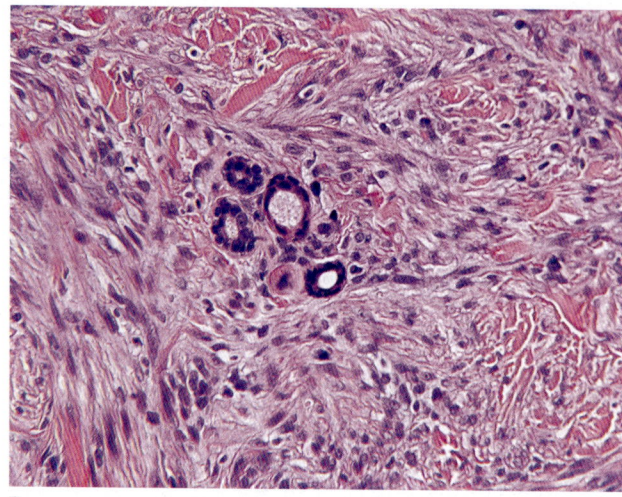
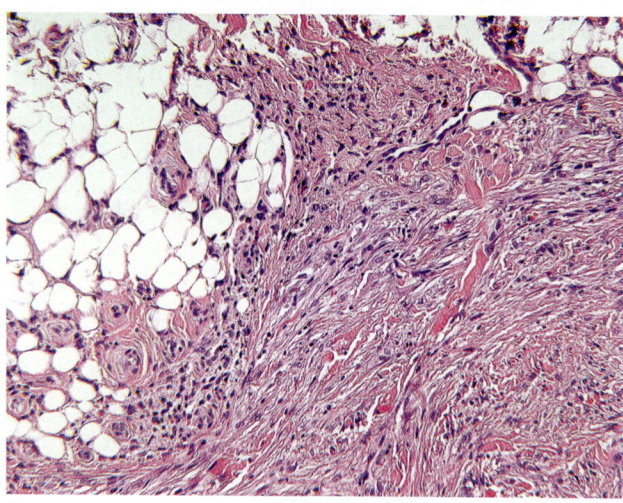

FIGURE 25-51 • Benign cutaneous fibrous histiocytoma in the shoulder of a 10-year-old female. **A:** The low-magnification field demonstrates total replacement of the dermis. **B:** Nuclear enlargement with atypia and occasional mitotic figures are present. **C:** Infiltration into the subcutis is present. CD34 positivity was confined to the cells at the periphery of the tumor. Re-excision was recommended because of positive margins.

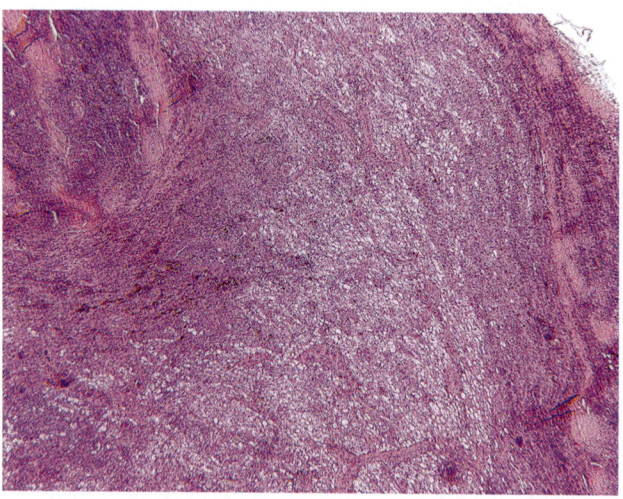
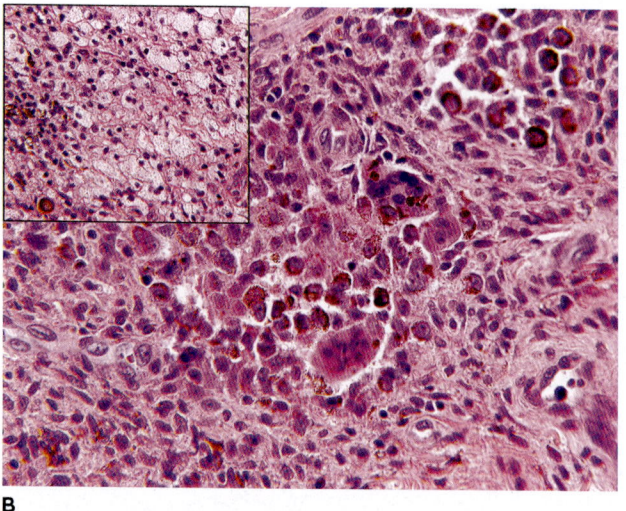

FIGURE 25-52 • Giant cell tumor of tendon sheath presenting on the left ankle of a 13-year-old female. **A:** This low-magnification field shows the nodularity of the lesion, also known as nodular tenosynovitis. **B:** Giant cells are generally less prominent than the mononuclear cells, but their numbers can vary from one tumor to another. **Inset**: Foamy macrophages also tend to vary from tumor to tumor.

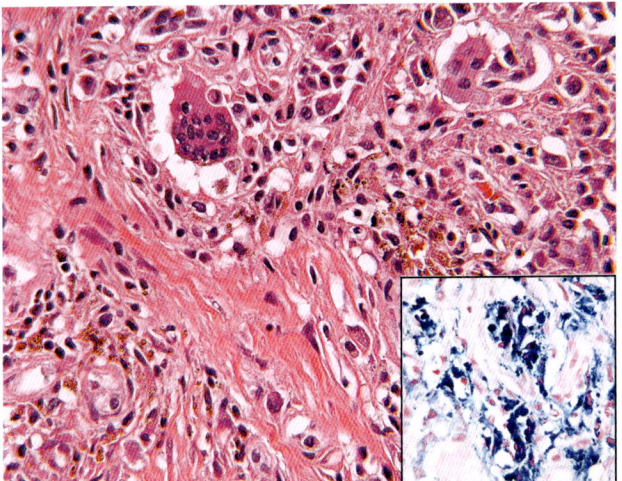

FIGURE 25-53 • Pigmented villonodular synovitis presenting in the left knee of an 18-year-old female. A multinucleated giant cell is surrounded by mononuclear cells with hemosiderin. **Inset:** Hemosiderin deposition is shown in this Prussian blue stain.

skeletal muscle as sheets of rounded mononuclear cells with abundant eosinophilic cytoplasm with or without osteoclast-like giant cells (230,231). In the absence of the latter, a histiocytic or other type of mononuclear cellular neoplasm with innocuous cytologic features also arises in the differential diagnosis. These tumors may express desmin in addition to "histiocytic" markers including CD163 as well as clusterin (232). Both t(1;2)(p13;q35) and t(1;1)(q21;p11) chromosomal translocations have been detected in tenosynovial giant cell tumors (233).

PFHT and giant cell tumor of soft tissues are the two remaining "intermediate, rarely metastasizing," fibrohistiocytic tumors in the WHO classification (5).

Angiomatoid fibrous histiocytoma (AFH) is one of several soft tissue neoplasms which is characterized by rearrangements of the *EWSR1* gene (234,235). Two of the three translocations in AFH are *EWSR1-CREB1* [t(2;22)(q33;q12)] and *EWSR-ATF1* [t(12;22)(q13;q12)] (236). The third translocation is t(12;16)(q13;p11) with the fusion transcript, *FUS-ATF*. CREB1 and ATF1 are partnered with EWSR1 in clear cell sarcoma (CCS) of soft parts or gastrointestinal tract (CREB1), LGFMS (CREB1), myoepithelial tumor (ATF1), primary pulmonary myxoid sarcoma (CREB1) and hyalinizing clear cell carcinoma of salivary gland (ATF1) (236). Although the majority of AFHs present as a mass in the extremities or trunk in children older than 10 years and in those individuals less than 40 years, it has been reported in the trachea, hard palate, pulmonary artery, bone, vulva and retroperitoneum. Constitutional or B symptoms and membranous nephropathy have been reported in a small number of cases (237). A sharply demarcated mass measuring 8 cm or less has a gross resemblance to a lymph node with or without cystic areas of hemorrhage, without germinal centers and with a fibrous pseudocapsule (Figure 25-54A to D). The lymph node-like areas encircle one or more nodules composed of ovoid, histiocytoid and less often spindle-shaped cells with pale staining cytoplasm with minimal atypia and only occasional mitotic figures (238). In a minority of tumors the pleomorphism and mitotic activity, including atypical mitotic figures, can be extreme. Other uncommon variations in the morphology include myxoid and/or sclerotic features (239). These tumors may also have a striking round cell appearance with a resemblance to EWS-PNET. AFH has an immunophenotype that includes positivity for CD99 (almost 100%), CD68 (75% to 80%), epithelial membrane antigen (70% to 75%) and desmin (45% to 50%) (Figure 25-54D). The differential diagnosis includes myoepithelial tumor, EWS-PNET, perineurioma and IMT (when plasma cells and lymphocytes are prominent), osteosarcoma (when sclerosis and calcification are present), and even granulomatous lymphadenitis. AFH has a local recurrence rate of 10% to 15% and metastasis in 5% or less of cases (240).

Plexiform fibrohistiocytic tumor (PFHT) is a distinctive neoplasm of the dermis and/or subcutis whose morphologic variability contributes to some of the difficulties in pathologic diagnosis (241). A firm nodule on the forearm, lower extremity, or trunk in a child over 10 years of age and into early adulthood is the clinical presentation. At least one case has been reported in the bone (242). The multinodular growth pattern at low magnification is characteristic but does overlap with cellular neurothekeoma. The nodules are composed of fibroblast-like cells and/or mononuclear cells with osteoclast-like giant cells whose numbers can vary from inapparent to several in the midst of the mononuclear cells (Figure 25-55A to D). In some cases, the nodules with mononuclear and giant cells can convey the impression of a granulomatous process. In those PFHTs with a predominant fibroblastic pattern, an inflammatory component is often present. Infiltration of the subcutaneous fat has some similarities to infantile subcutaneous fibromatosis and DFSP. Most tumors have a locally non-aggressive appearance in contrast to a fibromatosis. There is minimal mitotic activity in most cases. A background of hyalinized collagen can accentuate the nested character of the tumor and can have some resemblance to the CCS of soft tissue (CCS). The mononuclear cells of PFHT are immunoreactive for CD68 whereas the tumor cells in the CCS express S100 protein and HMB-45 (Figure 25-55D) (243). The fibroblastic cells of PFHT are strongly and diffusely positive for smooth muscle actin. Other considerations in the differential diagnosis when the dermis is involved by multiple nodules of histiocytic cells are melanocytic proliferation (Spitz or cellular blue nevus) and a cellular neurothekeoma especially in those PFHTs with myxoid features. One histogenetic perspective is that PFHT and cellular neurothekeoma may be related neoplasms. Like several other fibrohistiocytic neoplasms, PFHT has a local recurrence rate of 15% to 40%, and a metastatic rate of 2% or more especially to regional

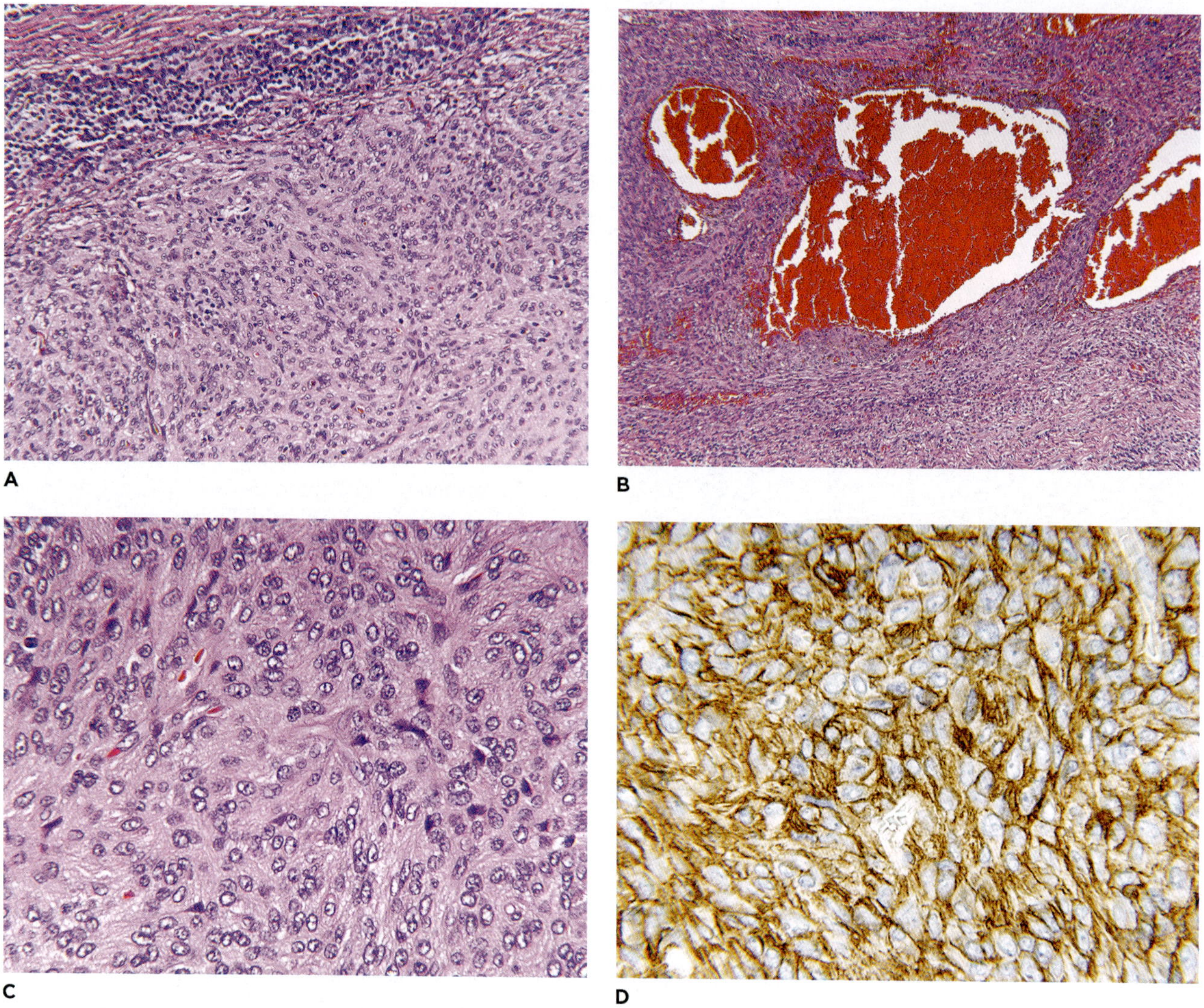

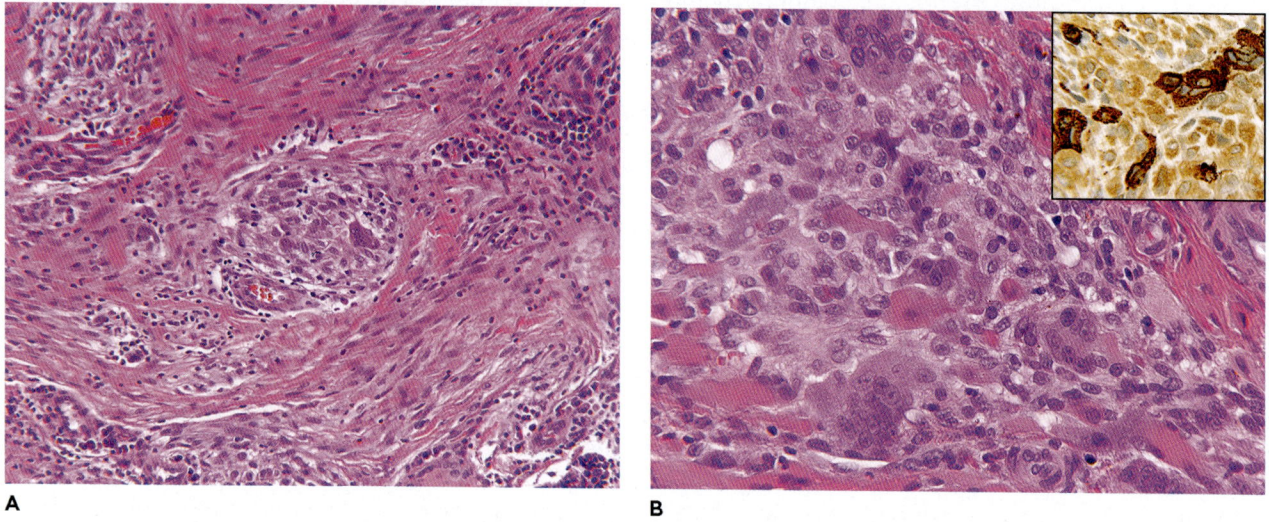

FIGURE 25-54 • AFH in a 14-year-old male presented in the upper arm. **A:** A lymphocytic infiltrate is present at the periphery of the mass in addition to lymphoid follicles can be mistaken for a lymph node–based neoplasm. **B:** The angiomatoid characterization of this tumor is based upon the presence of red cell–filled spaces. These spaces are seen in most but not all cases that can lead to diagnostic difficulties. **C:** The tumor cells have ovoid to polygonal-shaped nuclei and eosinophilic cytoplasm. The cell borders are poorly defined. Scattered mitotic figures are present and in some cases, atypical mitotic figures may be seen. **D:** Immunohistochemical staining for CD99 shows diffuse membrane positivity. This tumor had an EWS breakapart by FISH.

FIGURE 25-55 • PFHT arising in the posterior thigh of a 4-month-old female. **A:** This tumor was comprised in part of multiple nodules surrounded by spindle cells that impart a fibrous tumor-like appearance. **B:** Several multinucleated giant cells present within a nodule of mononuclear cells. **Inset:** CD68 immunostain highlights the multinucleated cells.

lymph nodes and lungs (244). To date, no signature cytogenetic abnormality has been detected (245).

Dendritic cell (DC) neoplasms are composed of mononuclear cells which are presumably derived from a common DC precursor cell; these cells are found in nonlymphoid organs and sites and migrate into lymphoid sites in order to stimulate T lymphocytes (246,247). The four categories of DC include the follicular DC, interdigitating DC, Langerhans cell and histiocytic fibroblastic cell (246). The latter cell may serve as the neoplastic progenitor for the DF and JXG. The Langerhans cell and Langerhans cell histiocytosis (LCH) are familiar topics in pediatric pathology. DCs have also been alternatively divided into conventional and nonconventional DCs (246).

Juvenile xanthogranuloma (JXG) is best known as a cutaneous lesion in a young child, but approximately 5% of cases of JXG in children present as a mass in the subcutis or within the skeletal muscle (248,249). These children are often less than 1-year-old at diagnosis and the mass may even be present at birth. The head, neck and trunk are the sites of predilection for a nodule measuring 3 cm or less. A well-circumscribed, nonencapsulated proliferation may be composed predominantly of mononuclear cells, a combination of mononuclear and spindle cells or infrequently only of bland appearing spindle cells (Figure 25-56A to D). The presence of xanthomatized mononuclear cells should alert to the possibility of JXG since classic Touton giant cells are often not present or inconspicuous in numbers, in the extracutaneous lesions. Eosinophils can be prominent and their presence may lead to the alternative interpretation of LCH, but the cells of JXG do not express CD1a; however, like most DC proliferations, there is often S100 protein reactivity. JXGs are immunopositive for CD68 and factor XIIIa (Figure 25-56D). Pseudorheumatoid nodule or deep granuloma annulare, a nonneoplastic lesion of the soft tissues of the head and lower

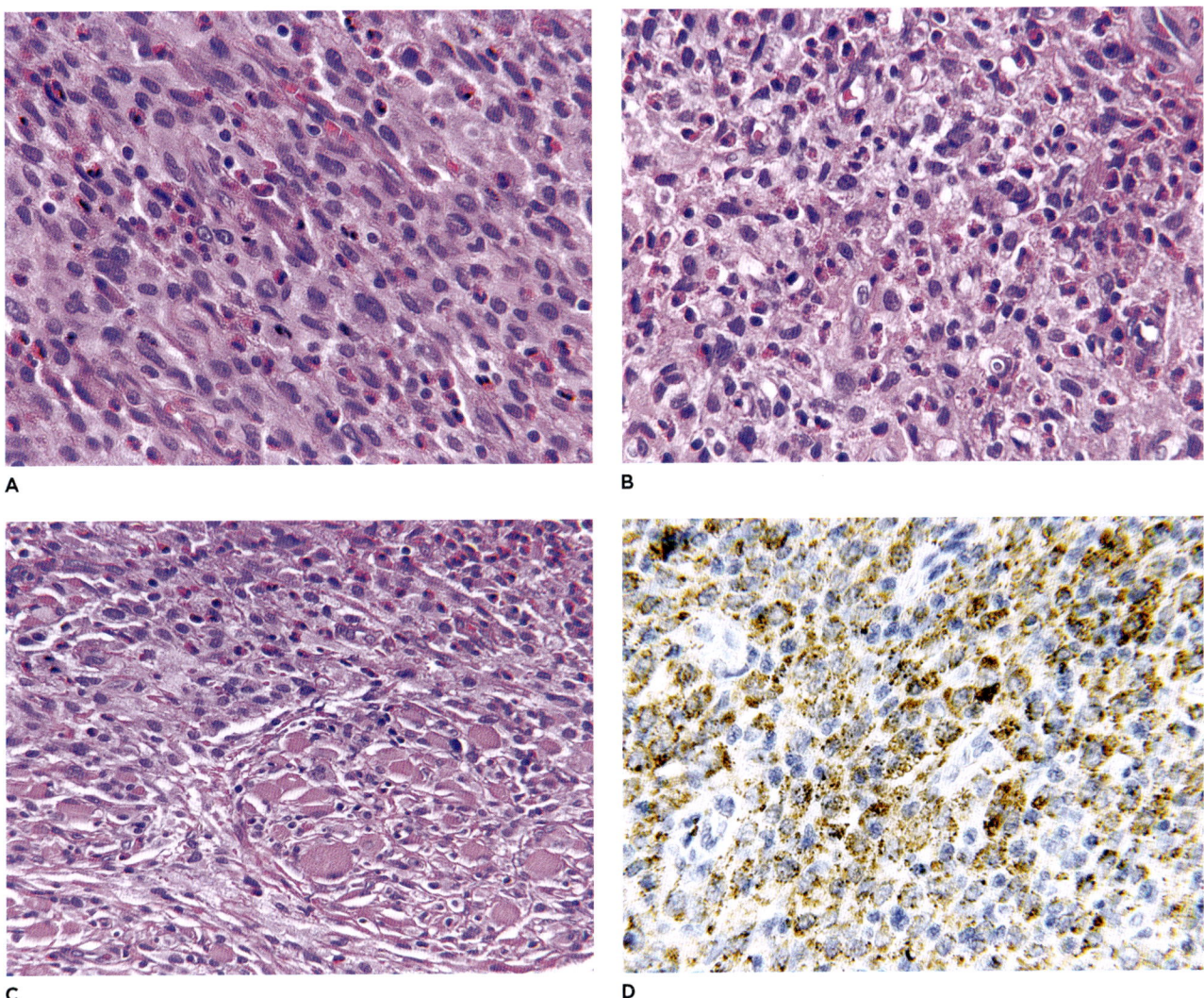

FIGURE 25-56 • JXG presented as a soft tissue mass in the posterior thigh of a 10-week-old male. **A:** Mononuclear, pale staining histiocyte-like cells and Touton giant cells are the classic microscopic features. **B:** Other foci are composed of xanthoma-like cells. **C:** A spindle cell component is infiltrating into the skeletal muscle. **D:** Factor XIIIa and CD68 (shown) are expressed by the tumor cells that are immunonegative for CD1a.

extremities in young children, can be mistaken for a histiocytic or vascular proliferation.

Follicular DCs are found in the germinal centers where they are characterized by CD21, CD35, CD138, D2-40 and clusterin positivity, less often S100 protein positivity, and CD1a nonreactivity. These mononuclear and spindle cell tumors with concentric whorls of cells can be mistaken for a fibrohistiocytic neoplasm of unspecified type or IMT. Though a rare neoplasm, follicular DC tumor is recognized in children (250,251).

Interdigitating DC tumor is seemingly less common than the follicular DC tumor and has also been documented in children (252). These tumors may be composed of highly pleomorphic large polygonal cells whose features have some resemblance to the cells of the MRT. Multinucleated giant cells have been observed as well. The tumor cells are reactive for vimentin, CD68, and S100 protein but are nonreactive for CD30 or ALK-1 (positive in anaplastic large cell lymphoma), CD1a, or CD21.

Blastic plasmacytoid DC neoplasm (BPDCN) is rare, is seen in children, but is more common in adults with spreading cutaneous nodules or unexplained purpura (253,254). At one time, BPDCN was known as blastic NK-cell lymphoma or CD4+/CD56+ hematodermic neoplasm (255). The dermal infiltrate is immunoreactive for CD4, CD56, CD123, CD303, and less frequently S100 protein.

LIPOMATOUS TUMORS

Lipomatous tumors constitute less than 10% of all soft tissue neoplasms in the first two decades of life (256). In fact, some of the lipomatous tumors are hamartomatous overgrowths occurring as a manifestation of several well-characterized syndromes in which the soft tissue mass is not just another "lipoma" (Table 25-10). Each of these syndromes is associated with multiple lipomatous tumors.

TABLE 25-10 SYNDROMIC-ASSOCIATED LIPOMA-LIPOMATOSIS

Congenital infiltrating lipomatosis (Slavin-Cols)
Encephalocraniocutaneous lipomatosis (Haberland)
Congenital lipomatous overgrowth, VMs and epidermal nevi (Sapp)
PTEN (10q23.3) hamartoma tumor syndromes
　Cowden syndrome
　Bannayan-Kiley-Ruvaleaba syndrome
　Proteus and proteus-like syndrome
Bannayan-Zonana syndrome
Multiple familial lipomatosis
Macrodystrophia lipomatosa
Hemihypertrophy-multiple lipomatosis syndrome
Familial angiolipomatosis
Plantar lipomatosis (Pierpont syndrome)
Michelin tire baby syndrome

LIPOMATOUS HAMARTOMAS

Lipomatosis in *encephalocraniocutaneous lipomatosis* (ECCL) is a diffuse overgrowth of subcutaneous fat of the scalp and intracranial and intraspinal lipomas (257,258). It has been questioned whether ECCL is a variant of the Proteus syndrome and is related to oculocerebral syndrome. There is also the possible relationship of congenital infiltrating lipomatosis to multiple familial lipomatosis. Recently, many of the sporadic and hereditary lipomatosis syndromes including congenital lipomatosis overgrowth with vascular, epidermal, and skeletal anomalies (CLOVES), Klippel-Trenaunay syndrome, hemimegalencephaly, and facial infiltrating lipomatosis have been shown to be associated with mutations in the phosphatidylinositide-3-kinase (PI3K) signaling pathway (259).

PTEN-hamartoma syndromes (PTHS) comprise at least two entities, Bannayan-Riley-Ruvalcaba and Cowden syndromes, which are characterized by a germline mutation in the tumor suppressor gene PTEN on 10q23.3 (260,261). Another disorder, Lhermitte-Duclos disease (LDD) may be associated with Cowden's syndrome (262). Dysplastic gangliocytoma of the cerebellum is the hallmark lesion of LDD (263).

Proteus (PS) and proteus-like syndromes are characterized by disproportionate overgrowth of one or more mesenchymal derived tissues (fat, blood vessels, bone) (264–266). Both syndromes are regarded as PTEN-related, but PS is caused by a somatic activation mutation in AKT1 (265). Both PTEN and AKT1 are active in the P13KCA/AKT pathway so that phenotypic overlap is not unexpected. Lipomatous tumors with or without a vascular component are one manifestation of the PTEN hamartoma of soft tissue (87,267) (see Figure 25-17). Hypertrophied nerves and a myxofibrous stroma are other features of the group of PTEN-related disorders. In PS, lipomatous tumors with either the circumscribed features of the mature lipoma or diffuse overgrowth of fatty tissues are present in 90% of cases. Fibrous septa are often prominent in the latter setting. The hamartomas are composed of other differentiated mesenchymal tissue elements.

Other overgrowth syndromes with a distinct phenotype from PS, are perturbations in the same RTK/P13K/CA/AKT/mTOR pathway with segmental overgrowth (259). Unlike PS, these segmental, asymmetric overgrowths are congenital and in some cases, there is minimal progression after birth, but in others there is continued growth. In addition to the multiple lipomatosis, lymph VMs, epidermal nevi and skeletal and spinal anomalies are present to the complete the phenotype of CLOVES syndrome (268). The latter syndrome is one of many others which are characterized by the presence of epidermal nevi (269,270). Michelin tire baby syndrome is characterized symmetric circumferential rings of folded skin; the features of nevus lipomatosis or smooth muscle hamartoma (271,272).

Megalencephaly or hemimegalencephaly and cutaneous capillary malformations, another PIK3CA-related segmental overgrowth, may also be accompanied by fibroadipose masses, syndactyly and/or polydactyly (273).

Macrodystrophia lipomatosa (MDL) and *lipofibromatous hamartoma* (LFH) or type 1 macrodactyly (LFH) are linked by the fact that there is localized overgrowth of adipose tissue. In the case of LFH, there is preference for the median nerve in which bundles of nerve are embedded in adipose tissue and in 25% to 30% of cases, there is accompanying macrodactyly (274). An overgrowth of predominantly fibrofatty tissue is the distinguishing feature of MDL and for that reason; some have regarded it as a localized expression of PS. Even after debulking of the adipose tissue, local recurrence is reported in 30% to 60% of cases (275,276). Neither MDL nor LFH is apparently hereditary.

Other types of lipomatosis in children have been reviewed elsewhere (256). One distinctive disorder is congenital infiltrating lipomatosis of the face.

Congenital spinal lipoma ("cord lipoma," CSL) is seen with some frequency in those institutions with an active neural tube defect—spinal dysgraphia (NTD-SD) program (277,278). One-third to one-half of all lipomas in children in our own experience are diagnosed in NTD-SD. Muthukumar (279,280) has divided CSLs into two anatomic groups: those without and with a dural defect. Those without a dural defect are found in the filum terminale or within the spinal cord. A mass in the subcutis is detected in the midline of the lower back. A circumscribed, multinodular mass of pale tan to yellow tissue is composed predominantly of lobules of mature adipose tissue with neural elements and a variety of other tissues indigenous to this site including bone and cartilage; those lipomas with disorganized neural tissues are accompanied with a dural defect and are examples of lipomyelomeningoceles or lipomyeloceles. Microscopic foci of immature nephrogenic tissue and enteric- and/or respiratory-lined cysts offer the possibility of a teratoma as an alternative interpretation, but the context of a spinal defect and the predominance of adipose tissue should be kept in mind before a diagnosis of a sacral teratoma is made. The differential diagnosis also includes the Currarino syndrome (point mutations in the *HLXB9* homeobox gene at 7q36) with sacral anomalies, tethered spinal cord or lipoma, anorectal malformations and presacral teratoma (281). The spinal lipoma should be distinguished from a mature teratoma with a substantial component of mature adipose tissue.

NEOPLASMS

Lipomas are neoplasms and perhaps more hyperplasias or hamartomas in some cases which in either instance are circumscribed masses of lobules of mature adipocytes. In adults, lipomas comprise 50% or more of all STTs whereas in children lipomas constitute 10% or less of all STTs compared to vascular tumors at 30% in this age group (Figure 25-57) (3). Given the infrequency of lipomas in children, one should question whether the tumor is a lipoma-like LPB or a manifestation of one or another syndrome such as an overgrowth syndrome or nasopalpebral lipoma–coloboma syndrome or Pai syndrome (282). Sporadic lipomas in children have a preference for the superficial soft tissues of the head and neck and trunk. However, vulvar and perineal lipomas have been reported in children (283). Deep and intramuscular lipomas are uncommon in children. Angiolipoma presents in the subcutis of the extremities (forearm predilection) or trunk, usually in adolescents and young adults. There are any number of sites other than the subcutis where these tumors have been reported. Multiple angiolipomas, often tender, may have an autosomal dominant or recessive pattern of inheritance. Angiolipoma, like the common lipoma, is composed of one or more lobules of mature adipose tissue

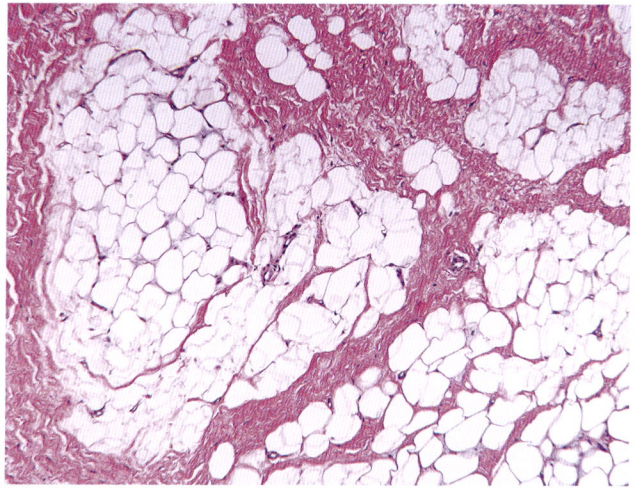
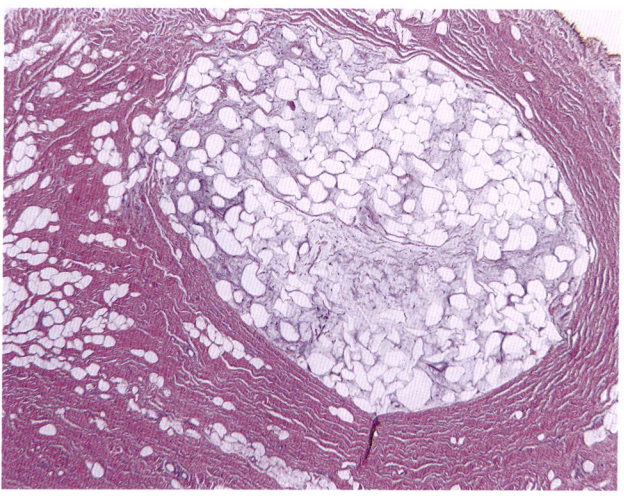

FIGURE 25-57 • Lipoma with myxofibrous features presented as a soft tissue mass on the foot of an 8-year-old male. **A:** Lobules of mature lipocytes are separated by prominent fibrous septa. **B:** Some of the lobules of fat have a myxomatous appearance. In the presence of immature lipocytes, it may support the interpretation of a lipoma-like LPB.

but with small peripheral capillaries, which are congested or contain fibrin thrombi. A cellular variant of angiolipoma has been described (284). Although rarely performed as an ancillary study, cytogenetic analysis of the true lipoma demonstrates supernumerary rings and giant rod chromosomes reflecting amplification of 12q14-15, the site of the *MDM2* oncogene (285).

Hibernoma is a rare adipocytic neoplasm in adults and even rarer in children (286,287). However, hibernomatous fat especially in the retroperitoneum is commonly observed in infants. Approximately 5% of hibernomas are diagnosed in individuals 18 years old or less (288). The thigh is the most common site overall. Eosinophilic to pale staining adipocytes with multivacuolated to granular cytoplasm are the characteristic cellular components of these tumors which can also have a myxoid, spindle cell or lipoma-like features in a minority of cases.

Lipoblastoma (LPB) is the distinctive lipomatous neoplasm of childhood, presenting between infancy to 10 years of age (one-third of cases at or before 1 year old) with a predilection for the extremities (60% to 65% of cases) (Table 25-11). However, LPB has a wide anatomic distribution from the soft tissues of neck, mediastinum, mesentery, retroperitoneum and scrotum. Individual cases have been detected *in utero* by fetal ultrasonography. There are two growth patterns, localized and diffuse (so-called lipoblastomatosis), but most LPBs are well-circumscribed masses in the subcutis rather than diffusely infiltrating through the deep soft tissues (289,290). A well-circumscribed, lobulated yellow-tan to grayish mucoid mass measures from 1 to 10 cm in greatest dimension (Figure 25-58). The distinctive multilobulated appearance of the gross specimen is reflected in the microscopic examination as well formed fibrous septa separating the rounded lobules. Within any one LPB, the lobules of adipocytes may display a range in maturity from those indistinguishable from a mature lipoma to those with a myxoid

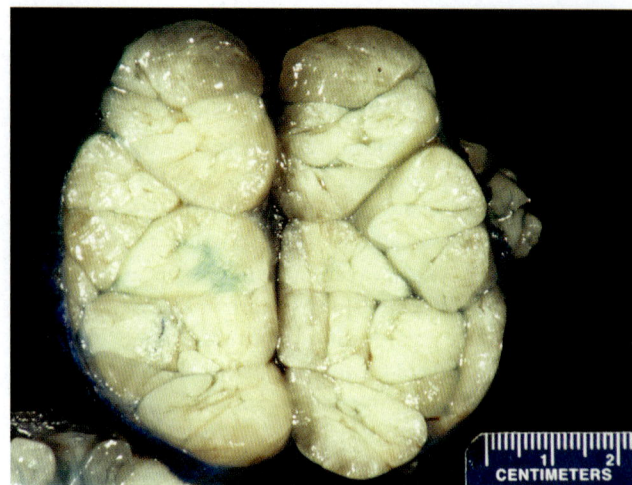

FIGURE 25-58 • LPB presenting in the posterior neck of a 2-year-old male. The mass measured 6.5 cm in greatest dimension and had a well-defined multilobular appearance.

stroma, immature multivacuolated lipoblasts and a network of delicate capillaries (Figure 25-59A,B). Some LPBs with lipoma-like features have lobules with centrally mature adipocytes and a peripheral residual population of lipoblasts with a myxoid stroma (Figure 25-59A). Pools of acellular, basophilic mucoid material are seen in both LPB and myxoid LPS, but the lobules in the latter neoplasm are less distinct in formation. In those cases with doubts about the distinction between a LPB and myxoid LPS, the demonstration of desmin-positive spindle cells at the periphery of the lobules is a useful differentiating feature of LPB and very uncommon in myxoid LPS (Figure 25-60A to C) (291). A desmin-positive spindle cell overgrowth of LPB is an uncommon feature. LPB is characterized by PLAG1 (8q12) rearrangements with at least five different fusion partners (292,293). There is also a polysomy 8 (70% to 80% of cases). Low level PLAG1 rearrangements have been identified in hepatoblastoma as well.

TABLE 25-11 SITES AND AGE AT PRESENTATION OF LIPOBLASTOMAS FROM THE FILES OF LAUREN V ACKERMAN LABORATORY OF SURGICAL PATHOLOGY (1989–2009)

Site	No. (%)	Age (Range and Mean)	Sex (Male:Female)
Lower extremity[a]	16 (32)	1–10 y (3.5 y)	8 M/8 F
Trunk	10 (20)	3 mo–9 y (2.7 y)	6 M/4 F
Neck[b]	6 (12)	1–5 y (3 y)	2 M/4 F
Axilla—upper extremity	6 (12)	6 mo–4 y (2 y)	2 M/4 F
Retroperitoneum—omentum	3 (6)	1–2 y (1.6 y)	1 M/2 F
Scrotum	3 (6)	2 y–6 y (5 y)	1 M/2 F
Mediastinum	2 (4)	8 mo, 6 y	1 M/1 F
Orbit	2 (4)	1 y, 1 y	2 M
Scalp	1 (2)	1 y	1 M
Vulva	1 (2)	1 y	1 F
	50 (100)	Mean (2.8 y)	26 M/24 F

[a]Gluteal region, thigh, foot.
[b]Parotid (1 case).
From the files of the Lauren V. Ackerman Laboratory of Surgical Pathology, St. Louis Children's Hospital, Washington University Medical Center, St. Louis, MO.

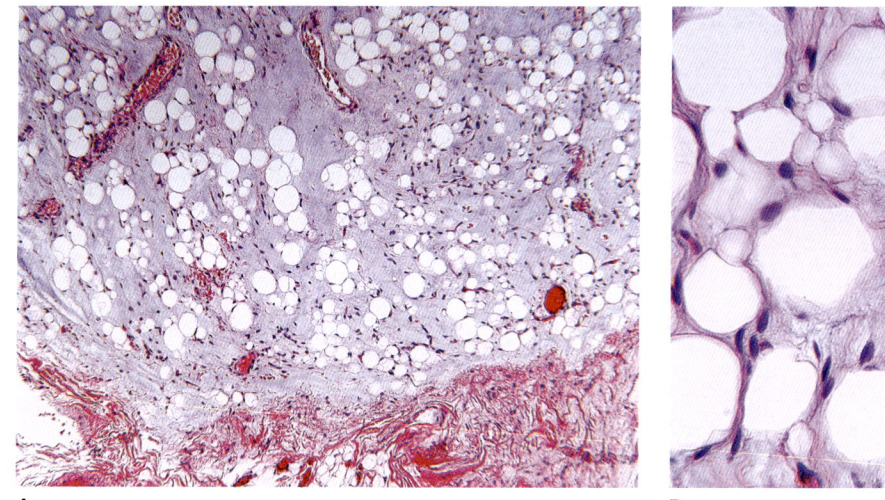
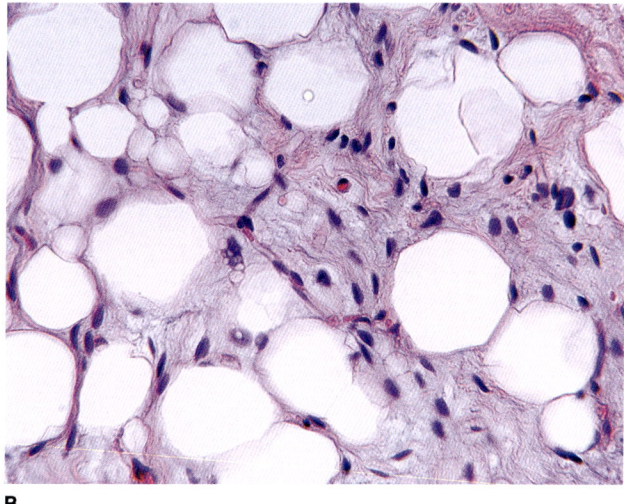

FIGURE 25-59 • LPB in a 2-year-old male. **A:** This low-magnification field shows a lobule with a pale myxoid background. The pattern of arborizing capillaries has a resemblance to myxoid LPS. **B:** A pale myxoid background with a delicate arborizing network of capillaries separate both immature and more mature lipocytes.

An HMGA-2 rearrangement rather than PLAG1 has been reported in a LPB (294). LPB has a local recurrence rate of 15% to 20% (290).

Liposarcoma (LPS) is seen in childhood, but only accounts for approximately 3% of all STSs in children (3). By contrast, LPS constitutes 20% of STSs in adults and less than 5% of all LPSs are diagnosed in the first two decades of life (295). LPS in children typically presents in the second decade (average age of 15 to 17 years), has a female predilection (2F:1M), and has a preference for the lower extremity (60% to 70% of cases) (296,297). Myxoid LPS accounts for 80% to 90% of cases in children and most of these tumors are conventional myxoid-round cell types (Figure 25-61). Our own experience also reflected the female predilection, lower extremity predilection and myxoid type (Table 25-12). The presence of a round cell component is correlated with a worse prognosis, but most myxoid LPSs in young individuals are devoid of this primitive pattern. Variations in the morphology of LPS in children and adolescents include spindle cell foci and pleomorphic features (296–298). Lipoma-like or well-differentiated and pleomorphic LPSs that together account for 65% to 70% of LPSs in adults represent 15% or less of cases in children. There are rare examples of dedifferentiated LPS in children (299). Cytogenetics is available to corroborate a diagnosis of myxoid LPS and to resolve any concerns about a possible

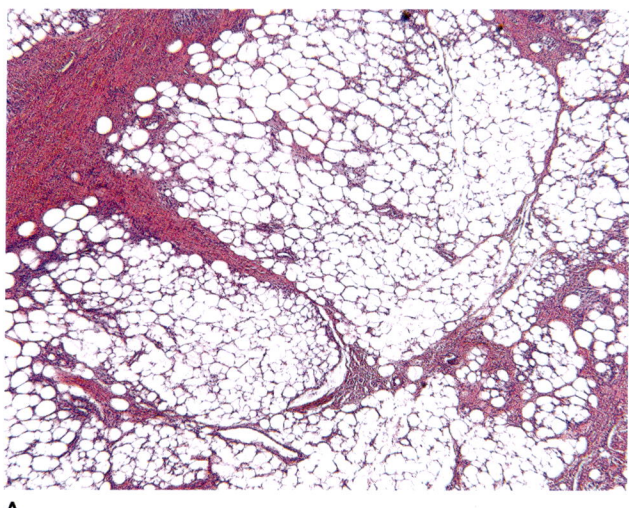
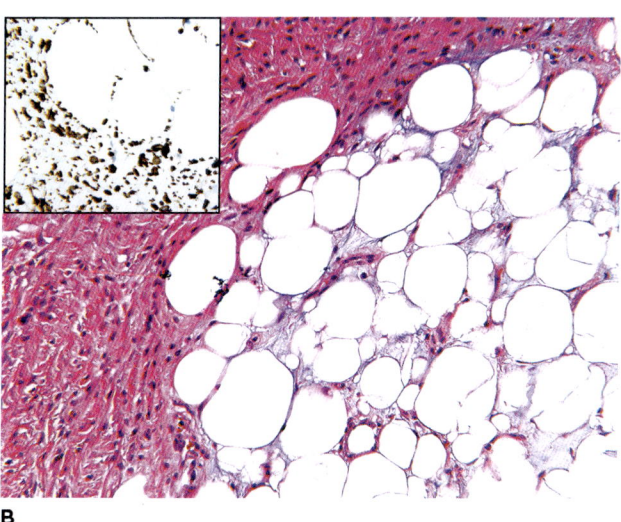

FIGURE 25-60 • LPB presenting in the soft tissues of the knee in a 1-year-old male. **A:** This low-magnification field shows several lobules of mature lipocytes demonstrating the maturation from the center of the lobule to the periphery with the lipoblasts. **B:** Residual lipoblasts are present at the periphery of lobule adjacent to more spindle cell fibrous area. **Inset**: The mature and immature stromal cells showing immunopositivity for desmin.

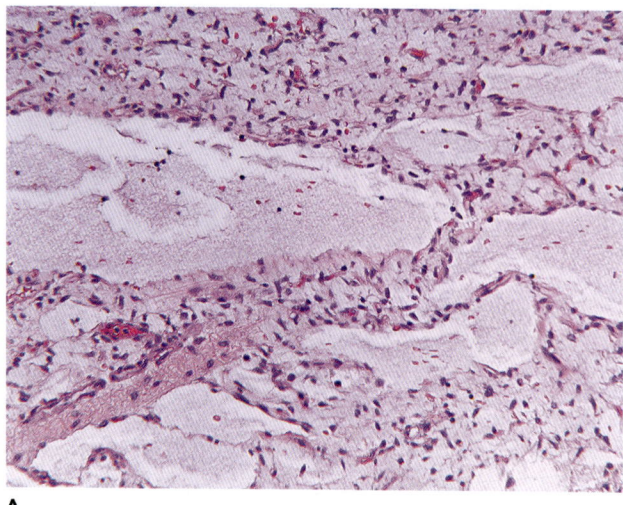 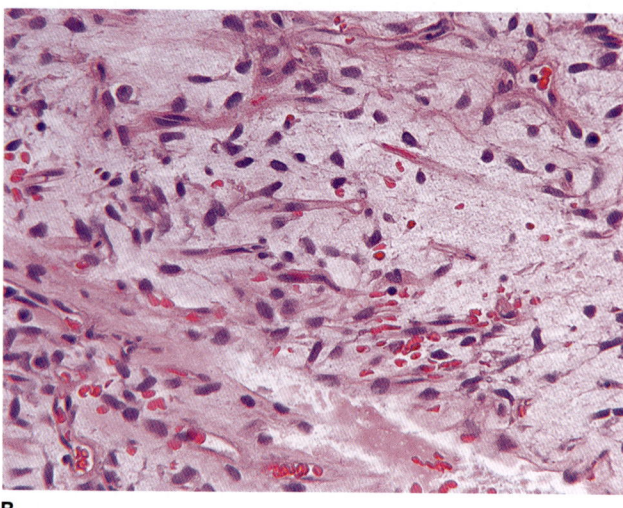

FIGURE 25-61 • Myxoid LPS presented on the anterior abdominal wall of a 13-year-old male. **A:** Mucinous-filled cysts are separated by moderately cellular foci with a myxoid and vascularized background. **B:** The individual tumor cells have enlarged nuclei that are moderately hyperchromatic. The delicate network of capillaries is present in the background.

LPB with the demonstration of the t(12;16)(q13;p11) (*FUS-CHOP* or DDIT3 fusion transcript in 95% of cases) or t(12; 22)(q13; p12) *EWSR1-CHOP* rearrangement (300). The prognosis of LPS in children and young adults is excellent with an overall survival of 90% (290,297). As a final note, LPS in a young individual may be the initial manifestation of Li-Fraumeni syndrome (301).

Lipomatous lesion of the heart constitutes a clinical and genetic group of disorders (302–304). One of the latter is arrhythmogenic right ventricular cardiomyopathy/dysplasia which is responsible for 10% of sudden cardiac deaths in individuals 18 years or less. There are 12 genes to date implicated in the defective formation of cardiac desmosomes (302,305). The pathologic findings are those of fibrofatty replacement of the right ventricle with eventual full thickness involvement of the apical, inferior and infundibular wall. The process seemingly begins in the epicardium or midmyocardium.

PERIPHERAL NERVE SHEATH TUMORS

This category of tumor accounts for 5% to 15% of all STTs in childhood with NF and schwannoma as the two most common types (306). There are several morphologic subtypes in the latter two categories reflecting variability in the histologic features from the growth pattern (localized, diffuse, and plexiform in the case of NF) to cellular and regressive atypia (in the case of the schwannoma). Both NF and schwannoma have pigmented variants; the psammomatous melanotic schwannoma arises in spinal nerve roots, bone, skin, and upper intestinal tract and may be a manifestation of the Carney complex. Also included among the peripheral nerve sheath tumors (PNSTs) are the perineurioma, GCT, and neurothekeoma or nerve sheath myxoma (5). MPNST presents as a sporadically occurring neoplasm or in the setting of NF1 in children and adults alike (307,308).

TABLE 25-12	SITES AND AGE OF PRESENTATION OF LIPOSARCOMAS IN CHILDREN FROM THE FILES OF LAUREN V. ACKERMAN LABORATORY OF SURGICAL PATHOLOGY (1990–2014)				
Site	No (%)	Age	Sex	Pathologic Type	No (%)
Lower extremity	6 (45)	11–22 yrs, mean and median, 14 yrs	7 M/15 F	Myxoid LPS	19 (80)
Head and neck	4 (18)			Pleomorphic LPS	3 (14)
Inguinal region	2 (9)				
Trunk	2 (9)				
Axilla	1 (5)				
Pelvis	1 (5)				
Mediastinum	1 (5)				
Upper extremity	1 (5)				
Total	22 (100)				22

In children, MPNST is the second or third most common nonrhabdomyosarcomatous STS, accounting for 15% of all sarcomas compared to SS that represents 25% of cases in the pediatric age group (3). There is also a category of tumefactions of a reparative-reactive type, which includes the traumatic neuroma, postamputation nerve hypertrophy, and presumed hamartomatous lesions such as the neuromuscular hamartoma and the neural fibrolipomatous hamartoma arising most commonly in the median nerve (309).

Neurofibroma (NF), the most common PNST in children, accounts for almost 70% of all such phenotypic STTs (306). Localized NF is restricted to the dermis whereas the diffuse NF with involvement of the dermis and subcutis as well as the deeper plexiform NF are invariably a manifestation of NF1 with multiple cutaneous, subcutaneous, and deep soft-tissue masses. NF1 is characterized by mutations in the neurofibromin gene, which is involved in RAS pathway signaling, on chromosome 17 (310,311) (Table 25-13). In fact, there are other neurodevelopmental syndromes with germline mutations in the RAS/MAPK signaling pathway (so-called RASopathies) including Noonan, neurofibromatosis-Noonan, Leopard, Costello, cardiofaciocutaneous syndromes, capillary–arteriovenous malformation and Legius syndromes (312–314). Plexiform NF in NF1 is detected in 40% to 50% of children by 5 years of age with a anatomic preference for the trunk and extremities, although the infiltrative plexiform NF may involve deep anatomic structures in the head and neck region and urinary tract (315,316). In addition to the plexiform NF in NF1, there is the diffuse NF involving the dermis and subcutis. NFs are less common in NF2, where the characteristic tumor type is the schwannoma, which can have plexiform features and should be differentiated from the plexiform NF. NF2 is characterized by truncated mutations in the Merlin gene on chromosome 22 (317–319) (Table 25-13).

Diffuse NF is composed of uniform, bland appearing spindle cells in a pale staining eosinophilic background. There is often overgrowth of the dermis with contiguous growth into the subcutis. Plexiform NF is composed of rounded to more serpentine nodules of spindle cells in a pale staining myxoid background. These nodules are found in the skin and/or subcutis with or without an accompanying pattern of diffuse NF (Figure 25-62). The nodules can be found in and around salivary glands in the head and neck region and appear grossly as thickened and tortuous peripheral nerves. The smaller plexiform NF is less readily traceable to a peripheral nerve. The presence of enlarged, pleomorphic nuclei and even a few mitotic figures should be viewed with concern about sarcomatous transformation of a plexiform NF; but the diagnosis of MPNST should be made in our estimation in the presence of compact spindle cell pattern and accompanying mitotic activity. Nuclear pleomorphism as an individual cell change in a background of otherwise typical NF can be acknowledged with the interpretation of "atypical NF" (320). If the biopsy has been obtained because of the recent onset of pain and/or increasing enlargement of a previously stable NF, a rebiopsy may be indicated since overtly sarcomatous changes may not be apparent in a uniform fashion within any given NF until there is substantial replacement of the benign component (321). Immunostaining for p53 and CD34 have limitations, but Ki-67 (Mib-1) may provide a context for the nuclear atypism (322,323). These biopsies are often problematic and may not yield a diagnostic consensus as to the typical versus sarcomatous nature of the findings.

TABLE 25-13	GENETICS AND MANIFESTATIONS OF NEUROFIBROSIS TYPE 1 AND 2 AND SCHWANNOMATOSIS		
	NF Type 1	NF Type 2	Schwannomatosis
Incidence	1:3000	1:30–40,000	1:1.7 million (Finnish)
Gene	NF1: 17q11.2	NF2: 22q12.2	22q 11 harboring SMARCB1/INI1
	Neurofibromin, negative regulator of RAS-MAPK	Merlin, inhibits cell proliferation in response to cellular adhesion	
Phenotype	Café au lait macules (infancy)	Schwannomas	Two or more schwannomas without VIII nerve schwannomas
	Diffuse and plexiform NFs	Bilateral VIII nerve schwannomas	
	Optic nerve glioma (pilocytic astrocytoma)	Ependymoma	
	MPNST (lifetime risk 8%–13%)		
	Pseudarthrosis		
	Vascular dysplasias		

Compiled from Yohay, K. *Neurologist* 2006;12:86–93; McClatchey AI. Neurofibromatosis. *Annu Rev Pathol* 2007;2:191–216; MacCollin M, Chiocca EA, Evans DG, et al. Diagnostic criteria for schwannomatosis. *Neurology* 2005;64(11):1838–1845; Hadfield KD, Newman WG, Bowers NL, et al. Molecular characterisation of SMARCB1 and NF2 in familial and sporadic schwannomatosis. *J Med Genet* 2008;45(6):332–339; Brems H, Beert E, de Ravel T, et al. Mechanisms in the pathogenesis of malignant tumours in neurofibromatosis type 1. *Lancet Oncol* 2009;10(5):508–515.

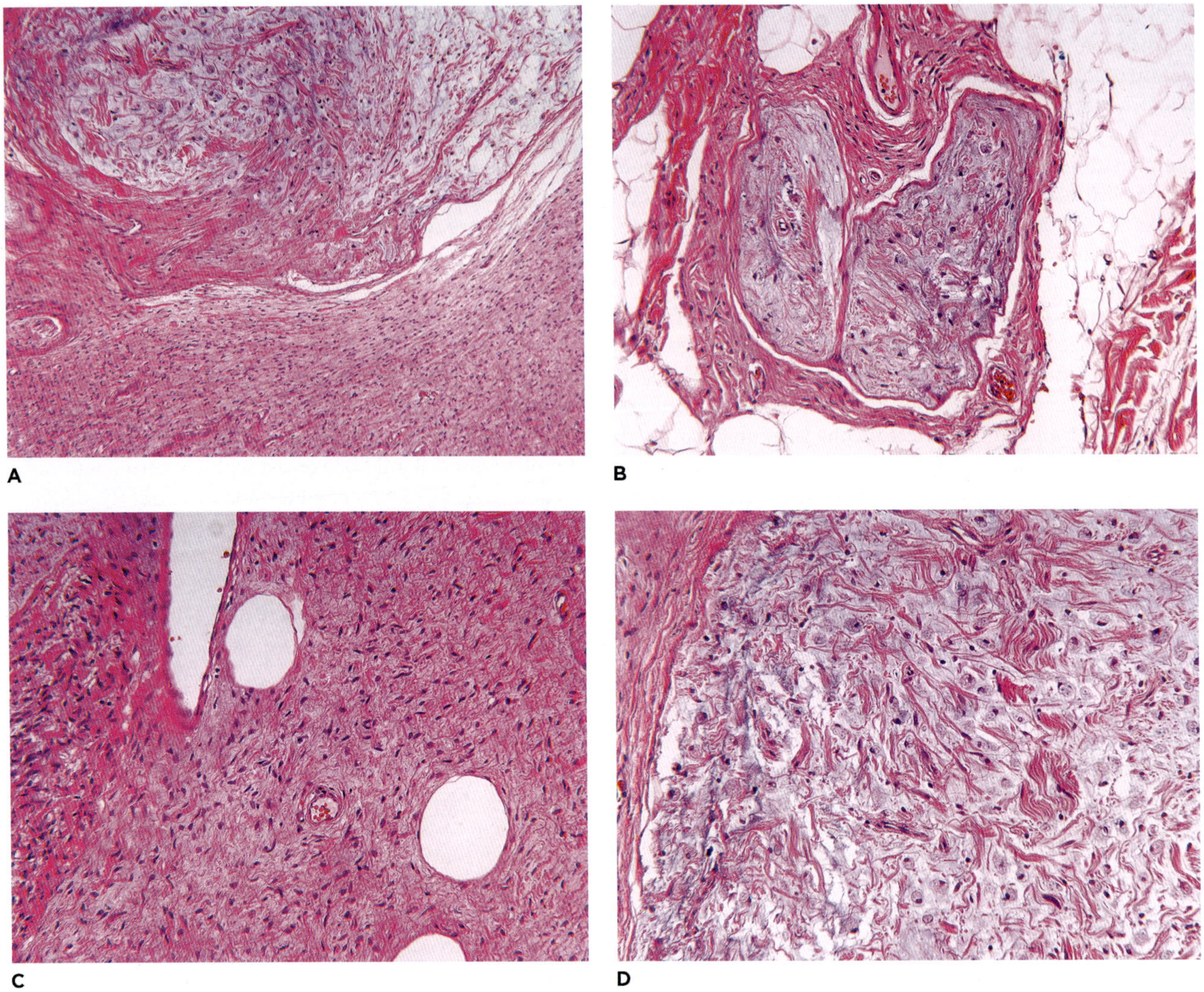

FIGURE 25-62 • Plexiform NF arose in soft tissues of the lower back in a 14-year-old female with a history of NF1. **A:** This field discloses both the plexiform and diffuse pattern of growth, both characteristic of NF1. **B:** Plexiform transformation occurs in peripheral nerves at all levels of the nerve. **C:** Diffuse pattern is often found in association with plexiform tumors. **D:** The plexiform nodules are usually hypocellular with or without coarse eosinophilic bundles. Increased cellularity and mitotic figures should be viewed with concern about malignant progression.

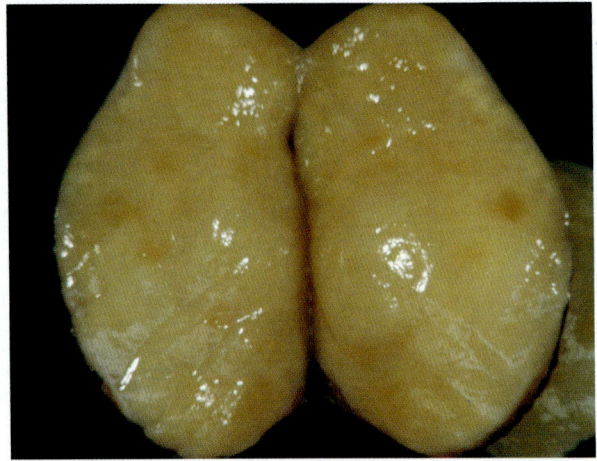

FIGURE 25-63 • Schwannoma presented as a paraspinal mass in a 17-year-old male. This encapsulated tumor measured 10 cm in greatest dimension and had a uniform, glistening yellowish-tan cut surface.

Schwannoma is a neoplasm with morphologic and immunophenotypic features of Schwann cells forming the nerve sheath (5,306,324,325). There is a predilection for the head and neck region and upper extremity in the case of the sporadic schwannoma in a child (306,326,327). It is unusual for a schwannoma to present before the age of 10 years. In children with NF2, nodular or plaque lesions in the skin or subcutis are well circumscribed, encapsulated spindle cell neoplasms with or without plexiform features; these tumors show strong diffuse S100 protein and collagen IV positivity unlike the less uniform pattern of positivity for these two markers in a NF. Grossly, the schwannoma varies in size from 1 to 10 cm in greatest dimension, is encapsulated, and has a glistening, mucoid, and pale tannish to yellowish tan appearance (Figure 25-63). Schwannomas arising in deep soft tissues in and around the head and neck region often do not have an apparent capsule, but has a circumscribed, noninfiltrating interface with adjacent tissues. Hemorrhage, cystic

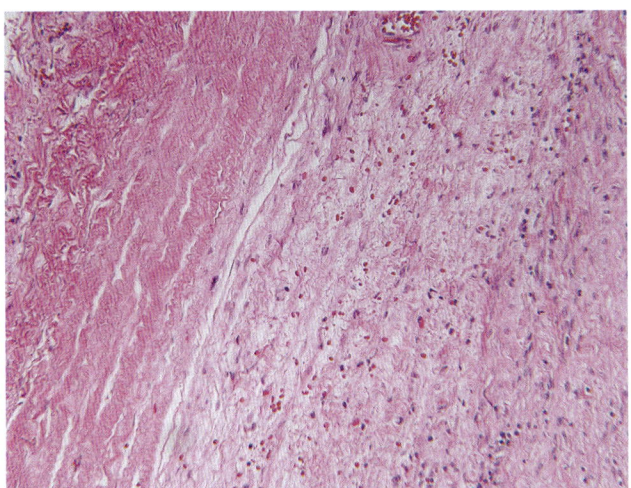

FIGURE 25-64 • The encapsulated Schwannoma (see Figure 25-63) had a predominant Antoni B pattern of loosely arrayed spindle cells in an edematous to myxoid background.

degeneration, and fibrosis are uncommon secondary features in schwannomas in children in contrast to these changes in schwannomas in adults. The challenge in the pathologic diagnosis is the variability in the histologic patterns, but the two basic ones are the spindle cell pattern with or without Verocay body formation (Antoni A) and the alternating less cellular myxoid foci (Antoni B) (Figure 25-64). Foci resembling a NF may be seen in some cases, but keep in mind the presence of a capsule in the schwannoma. Lymphocytes, foamy histiocytes and thickened vessels may be more or less apparent in a schwannoma from a child where secondary changes are uncommon. Mast cells are present in variable numbers, as they can be in an NF. Nuclear enlargement and hyperchromatism are present in some cases and should not be viewed with concern about potential malignancy since true malignant schwannomas are diminishingly rare.

The sporadic schwannoma can have a hypercellular spindle cell pattern, and mitotic figures can be seen (generally less than 20%) in the cellular variant (328). In the setting of NF2, caution is advisable with a diagnosis of MPNST when the schwannoma is both cellular and mitotically active to some degree. Rather than a diffuse pattern, a multinodular pattern also occurs in children and these tumors can be mistaken for a NF (329). Bilateral schwannomas of cranial nerve VIII are a virtually pathognomonic feature of NF2 and may be one of the first manifestations in a young child with NF2 (330,331). (Table 25-13). Finally without the presence of ganglion cells, a ganglioneuroma with its predominant neuromatous–stromal component has a convincing resemblance to a schwannoma or NF (Figure 25-65).

Schwannomatosis, the third "neurofibromatosis" is characterized clinically by the presence of two or more schwannomas typically peripheral, unlike NF2 with its vestibular-based tumors (332–334) (Table 25-13). Some 15% of affected individuals develop schwannomas in the first two decades of life. The germline SMARCB1 mutation in the INI1 gene is the predisposing oncogenic site (334). Familial multiple meningiomas with a preference for the falx cerebri is another SMARCB1 associated disorder (335).

Malignant peripheral nerve sheath tumor (MPNST) presents as a sporadic neoplasm or as a complication of NF1 with a lifetime risk of approximately 10% (308). Most MPNSTs in the first two decades of life occur after 6 years of age. The other STS seen in the setting of NF1 is ERMS in 1% to 6% of cases, which presents earlier in life than does the MPNST. It is rare for a MPNST in NF1 to develop before 5 years of age, but exceptions exist (336–339). Most MPNSTs generally measure in excess of 5 cm and have a gelatinous grayish tan to white surface with or without necrosis and hemorrhage. When the MPNST arises as a plexiform NF, as it often does in NF1, there is often widespread sarcomatous involvement

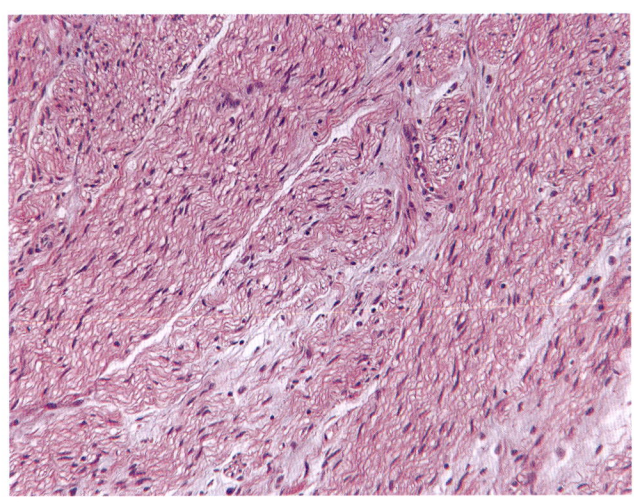

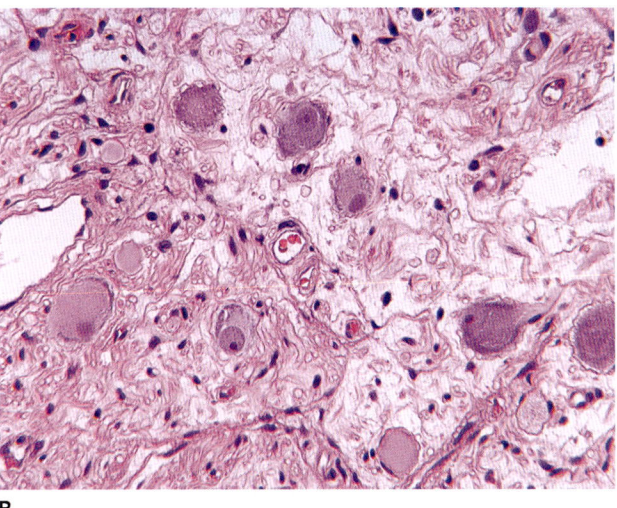

FIGURE 25-65 • Ganglioneuroma presented in the lumbosacral region of a 12-year-old female. **A:** The tumor is well circumscribed with a capsule or pseudocapsule and is composed of bundles of fusiform spindle cells with a resemblance to a schwannoma. **B:** Other microscopic fields contain individual or small groups of mature ganglion cells.

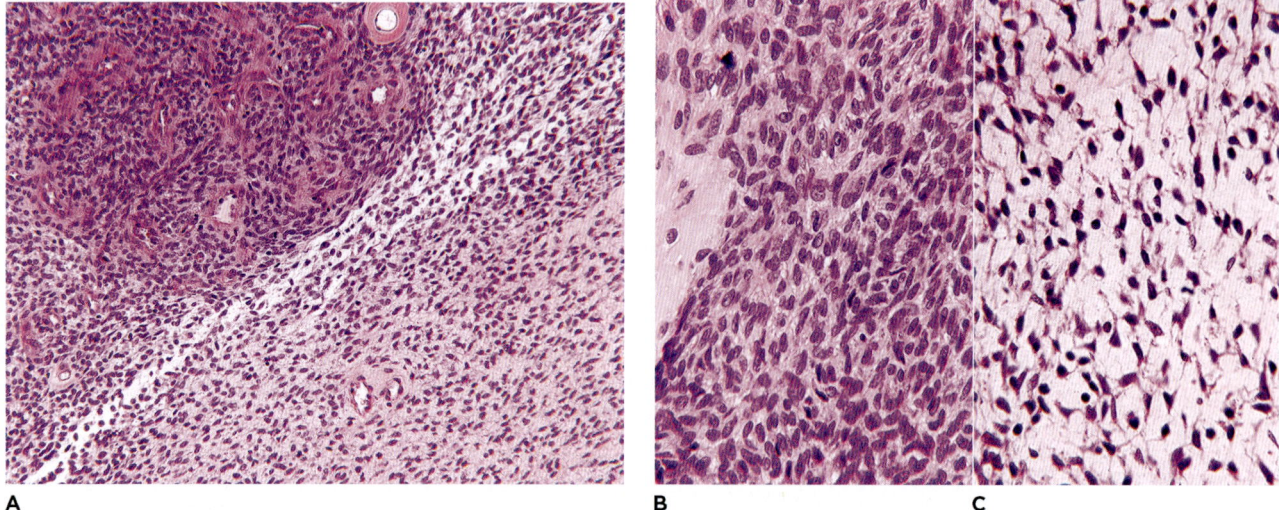

FIGURE 25-66 • MPNST arising in the thigh of an 18-year-old female with NF1. **A:** This focus shows adjacent hypo- and hypercellular areas. **B:** Cellular focus of compact spindle cells. **C:** A myxoid focus composed of spindle cells in pale loosely textured background.

of the nerve with the formation of one or more masses. The mass(es) is usually not sharply demarcated from the plexiform component. The basic histologic pattern of a MPNST is a spindle cell sarcoma with fascicular profiles of interweaving cells. At low magnification, the fascicles may have an alternating "light cell–dark cell" quality due to more cellular and less cellular foci with lucency between the cells, often with a pale mucoid to myxoid appearance (Figure 25-66A to C). Fusiform to more ovoid nuclei display varying degrees of hyperchromatism and mitotic activity. Anaplasia is generally uncommon but can be extensive in some cases. Residual foci of plexiform NF are often present in NF1-associated MPNSTs; overgrowth or infiltration by the sarcoma is appreciated in these transitional zones with residual NF. It is for this reason that a biopsy may yield equivocal findings for MPNST other than scattered atypical spindle cells intermixed within a background of plexiform NF. Though the biopsy may not be satisfactory for an unequivocal diagnosis of MPNST, atypical histologic features in a plexiform NF should prompt a rebiopsy especially in the presence of an enlarging, previously stable deep soft-tissue mass. In addition to the features of a spindle cell sarcoma, other less common findings include individual and small collections of rhabdomyoblasts (Triton tumor), gland-like structures, a multinodular pattern with overgrowth of a plexiform NF, an epithelioid pattern with tumor cells resembling those of a MRT, nodules of cartilage or a small cell, rosette-like pattern with a resemblance to EWS-PNET, or neuroblastoma (Figure 25-67). Formations

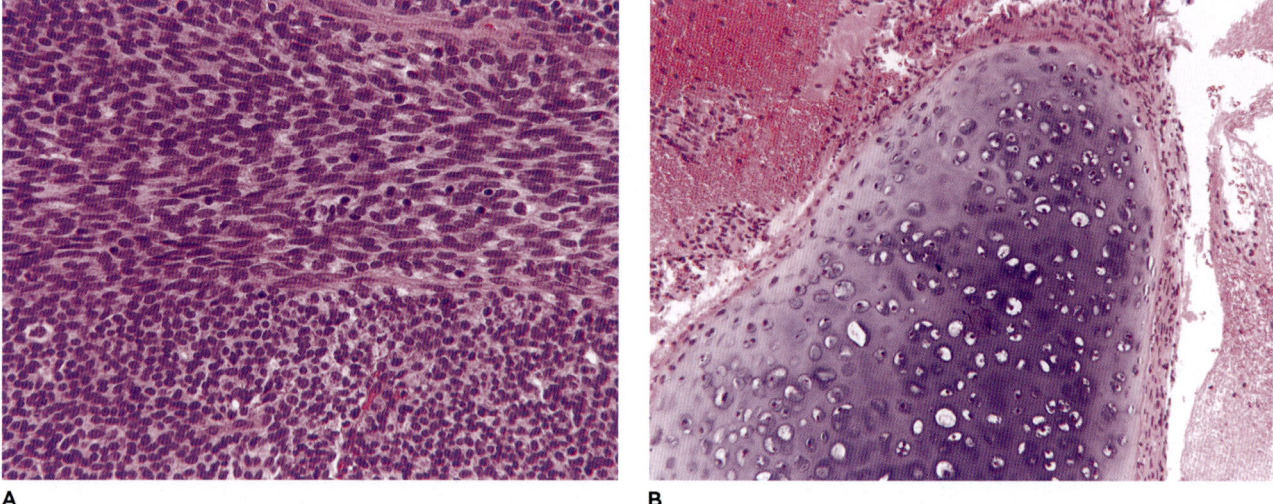

FIGURE 25-67 • MPNST presented in a 5-year-old male with NF1 with an intracranial presentation of a large mass arising in the region of the frontal lobe. **A:** A high-grade spindle cell sarcoma consists of uniform cells with enlarged, elongated hyperchromatic nuclei. **B:** Nodules of hypercellular cartilage are present focally.

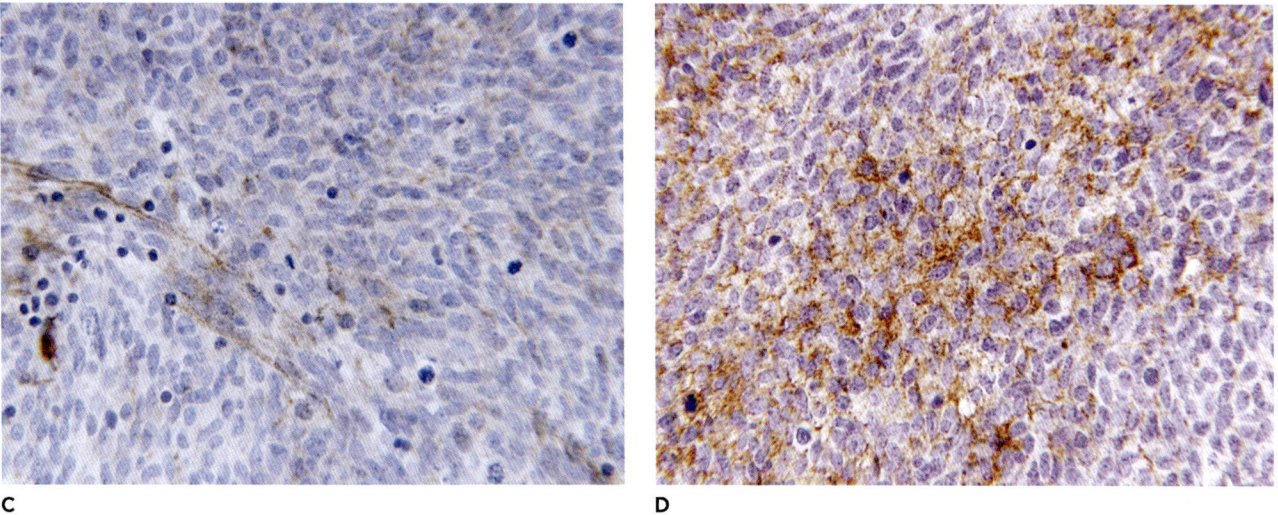

FIGURE 25-67 • (*continued*) **C:** The tumor cells are uniformly reactive for vimentin, but only focally for S100 protein. **D:** The CD57 immunostaining is diffuse throughout all microscopic fields.

resembling tactile bodies (Meissner corpuscles) are found in both NFs and MPNSTs (but not in the schwannoma). Sporadically occurring MPNSTs are more difficult to diagnose with certainty when major nerve involvement is either not present or inapparent. IHC is not always helpful but may be useful in the differentiation of MPNST from monophasic SS or LGFMS. In addition to vimentin, MPNST is variably immunoreactive for S100, CD56, and collagen type IV (Figure 25-68). Another issue in the prognostic assessment of MPNST is the histologic grade; the prevailing opinion is that all MPNSTs should be viewed as high-grade sarcomas regardless of their individual pathologic features even in the presence of "low-grade" histology but this is a subject without a consensus (340). More relevant is the adequacy of the surgical resection, which can be problematic when a major nerve is the primary site. The cytogenetics of MPNST is best characterized as complex and without a signature balanced translocation (341). BRAFV600E mutation has recently been reported in sporadic and NF1 associated MPNSTs (342).

Other types of PNSTs of the soft tissues include the perineurioma, nerve sheath myxoma, and neurothekeoma (340). *Perineurioma* is an uncommon neoplasm, which is seen in children and adults alike (263). Extraneural and intraneural variants are recognized (343). A well-circumscribed subcutaneous mass measuring less than 7 cm is composed of spindle cells or more epithelioid appearing cells in a fibrous appearing background. Tight whorls of spindle cells and storiform profiles have some resemblance to DFSP. These tumors may be immunoreactive for CD34 (like DFSP and SFT) but are also positive for EMA and vimentin (both markers are positive in meningiomas) as well as collagen type IV. Unlike the schwannoma, the perineurioma does not express S100 protein. Intraneural perineurioma is even less common than extraneural or soft-tissue variant. Over 50% of cases are diagnosed by 20 years of age as a soft-tissue mass arising in a major nerve or the brachial plexus (344). There is some resemblance to a plexiform NF in terms of gross involvement. The spindle cell areas like those in the extraneural perineuriomaare EMA-positive and S100 protein–negative.

Nerve sheath myxoma is largely a myxoid neoplasm of the dermis and subcutis (345). It is composed of spindled and epithelioid cells arranged in cords and nests. These Schwann-like cells are immunoreactive for S100 protein, glial fibrillary acidic protein, and CD57 with some EMA-positive, presumed perineural cells. *Neurothekeoma* is a neoplasm of young individuals with 60% of cases presenting before the age of 20 years, and also a tumor whose features overlap with the nerve sheath myxoma (346). These tumors have been histologically subtyped as cellular, myxoid, and mixed (347).

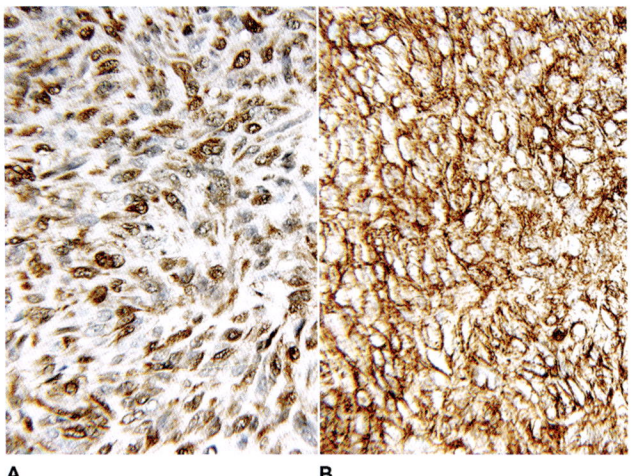

FIGURE 25-68 • MPNST in an 18-year-old female (see Figure 25-66). **A:** S100 protein immunostaining. **B:** Collagen type IV immunostaining. The immunoreactivity for these two markers varies from one MPNST to another.

Multiple, small nodules of spindled to epithelioid cells with or without a prominent myxoid matrix are accompanied by osteoclast-like giant cells. The immunophenotype of these tumors includes expression of NK1-C3 (CD63), neuron-specific enolase, CD10, and CD68 whereas they are nonreactive for S100 protein. Quite frankly, some of these cases are difficult to distinguish from the plexiform fibrohistiocytic tumor (348). An emerging category of PNSTs is represented by those tumors with hybrid or overlap features as in the case of a perineurioma–schwannoma, neurofibroma–schwannoma in the setting of schwannomatosis or congenital melanocytic nevus with perineurioma–schwannoma as the ultimate expression of the neural crest pathology (349–351). Additional examples of the latter are melanocytic differentiation in diffuse NFs and schwannoma is a congenital melanocytic nevus (352–354).

Granular cell tumor (GCT) is one of the ubiquitous neoplasms in terms of its anatomic distribution whose phenotype characterizes it as either neural (S100 protein positive) or nonneural (S100 negative) in type. Two examples of the latter are the so-called congenital epulis or GCT presenting on the anterior alveolar border of the maxilla or mandible of a neonate and the so-called primitive polypoid GCT of the dermis (Figure 25-69A to D) (355–358). There is a report of an S100 protein positive congenital GCT of the tongue (359). The skin, oral cavity, and upper respiratory tract are among the more frequent primary sites in children (Table 25-14). Multifocal GCTs can occur in the presence

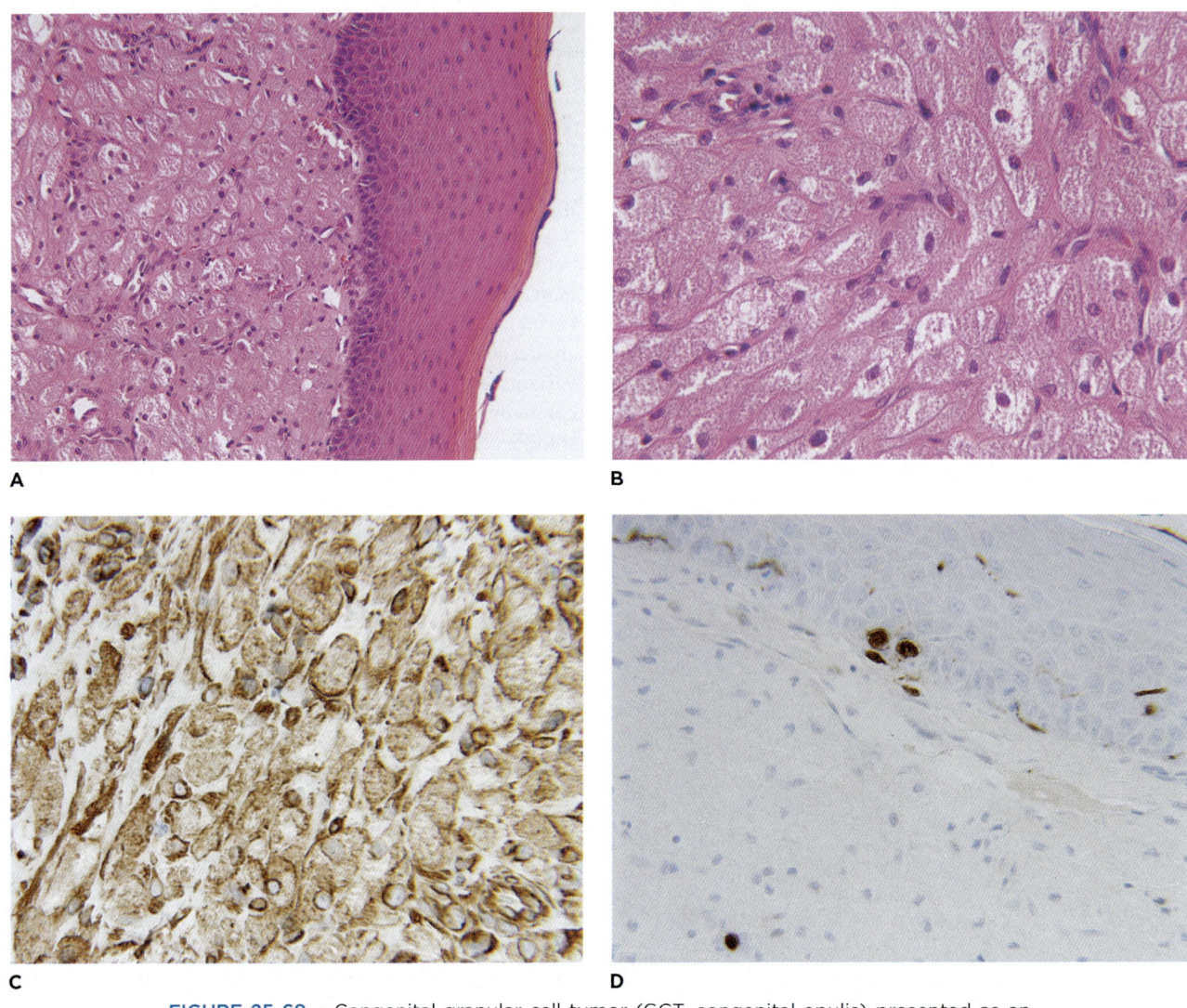

FIGURE 25-69 • Congenital granular cell tumor (GCT, congenital epulis) presented as an intraoral mass attached to maxillary gingival ridge in a neonatal female. **A:** The tumor cells are compactly arranged against the overlying squamous mucosa. **B:** The individual tumor cells are characterized by the pale eosinophilic granular cytoplasm. **C:** The tumor cells are immunoreactive for CD68 with a granular pattern of positivity. **D:** This tumor is regarded as a "nonneural" type of GCT since the S100 protein is nonreactive in the tumor cells. Note the positivity of the Langerhans and DCs in the mucosa.

TABLE 25-14 GRANULAR CELL TUMORS IN CHILDREN AND ADOLESCENTS

Site	No. (%)	Age Range (Mean)	M:F
Solitary skin	21 (34)	2–16 y (10 y)	7/14
Soft tissue[a]	9 (15)	11–17 y (12.5 y)	4/5
Oral cavity (congenital)[b]	9 (15)	1 day–1 mo (10 days)	0/9
Breast	5 (8)	14–18 y (17 y)	0/5
Orbit	4 (7)	15–17 y (16 y)	1/3
Lip	4 (7)	9–14 y (12 y)	2/2
Multiple skin	4 (7)	5–16 y (13 y)	2/2
Larynx	3 (5)	4–18 y (11 y)	1/2
Tongue	1 (2)	10 y	0/1
Esophagus	1 (2)	16 y	1/0
	61 (~100)		18:43

[a]One case in the thigh of 13M with regional lymph node metastasis.
[b]Anterior maxilla (five cases), anterior mandible (two cases), hard palate (one case), frenulum of tongue (one case).
From the files of the Lauren V. Ackerman Laboratory of Surgical Pathology, St. Louis Children's Hospital, Washington University Medical Center, St. Louis, MO.

of a positive family history or in the setting of Noonan syndrome. A firm, poorly demarcated yellowish tan to white mass measuring less than 2 cm is the usual gross appearance in most cases. Nests of granular cells of varying sizes and shapes are composed of polygonal to more ovoid cells with prominent eosinophilic cytoplasm and a central nucleus (Figure 25-70). The cytoplasm contains eosinophilic or granular bodies representing lysosomes; these bodies account for the CD68 granular positivity (Figure 25-69C). Nuclear pleomorphism is present in some cases without immediate implications about behavior, but mitotic figures should be viewed with concern. Perineural involvement with plexiform features is seen in a small minority of cases. With the noted exceptions, most GCTs are diffusely immunoreactive for S100 protein as well as inhibin A (360). Malignancy in GCT is rare, especially in children. Mitotic activity, nuclear pleomorphism, spindle cell morphology, and deep invasion of soft tissues should alert to the possibility of malignancy. We have seen malignant GCT in the vulva of a 4-year-old female and in the thigh of a 17-year-old female.

Glioneuronal heterotopia (nasal glioma), usually presents in the head and neck region as a polypoid intranasal or midline subcutaneous mass at the root of the nose or intranasally (361). However, glial heterotopias may present in the tongue, beneath the mucous membranes of the oral cavity, lip and middle ear (362,363). Islands of mature neurogliastroma are typically embedded in fibrous stroma. Glial heterotopias have been described on the trunk as an example of a soft-tissue glioma.

Rudimentary meningocele (meningothelial hamartoma, soft tissue meningioma) is a mass lesion, typically in the occipital region, which is discovered in infants and young children.

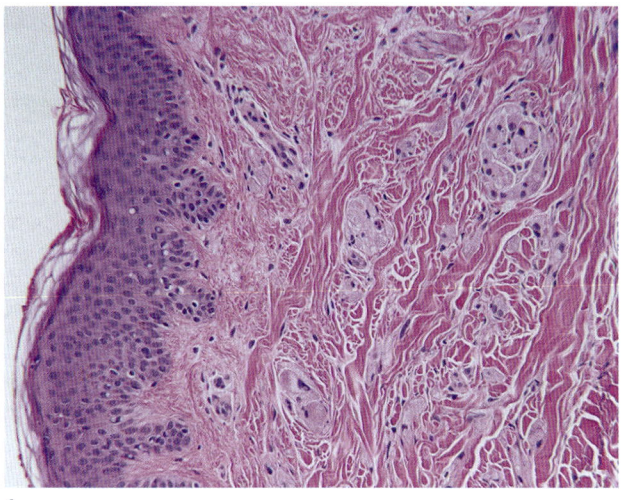
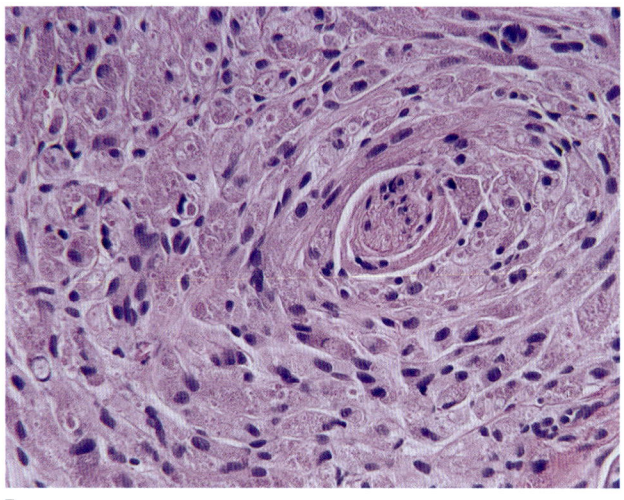

FIGURE 25-70 • GCT presented on the arm of a 7-year-old female. **A:** Small collections of granular cells are seen in the superficial dermis. **B:** This tumor also had a plexiform growth pattern with its intraneural and perineural involvement (see *J Cutan Pathol* 2009;36:1174–1176).

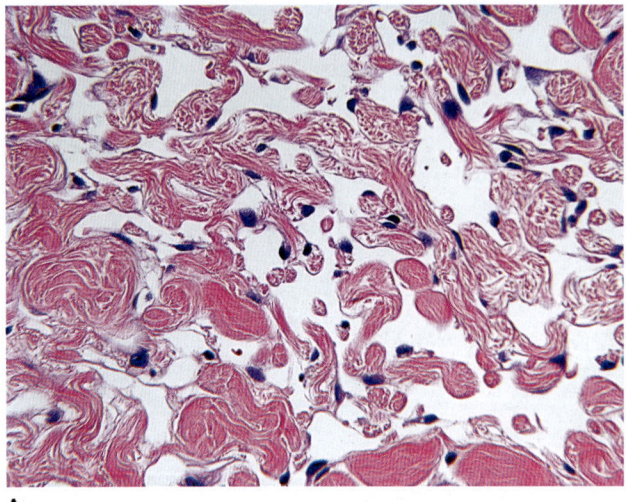
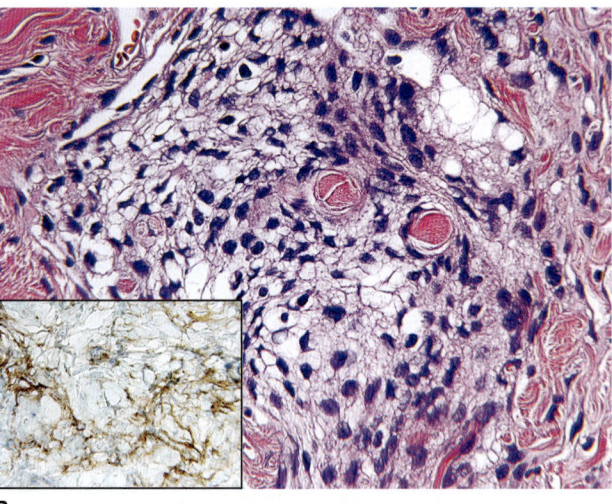

FIGURE 25-71 • Rudimentary meningocele or meningothelial hamartoma presenting as a soft mass of the scalp in a 2-year-old male. **A:** The mass in part has a sieve-like or angiomatoid pattern. **B:** Accompanying the angiomatoid pattern are small circumscribed meningioma-like nodules. **Inset**: Both the angiomatoid foci (shown) and nodules are immunopositive for epithelial membrane antigen (shown) and vimentin.

The soft midline lesion occupies the lower dermis and subcutis and is composed of small meningothelial nodules in association with a pattern resembling vascular spaces dissecting through the collagen (Figure 25-71).

PERIVASCULAR EPITHELIOID CELL NEOPLASM (PEComa)

This category of neoplasms represents in a sense a histogenetic concept since the perivascular epithelioid cell has no known recognized normal or phenotypic counterpart to account for these tumors (364,365). What has emerged from the concept is a group of neoplasms designated as perivascular epithelioid cell neoplasm (PEComa), to include angiomyolipoma (AML) or epithelioid AML of the kidney or liver, so-called sugar tumor, lymphangiomyomatosis of the lung, myomelanocytic tumor of the falciform ligament and PEComas arising in a variety of organs such as the uterus. Although these tumors lack morphologic homogeneity, they share a unique immunophenotype of smooth muscle (SMA, calponin) and melanocytes (HMB-45, Melan-A, and microphthalmic transcription factor). The S100 protein is non-reactive in most but not all cases as well as TFE3, especially in PEComas from younger individuals (364,366,367).

PEComa arises in soft tissues, bone and various visceral structures and organs including the falciform ligament, uterus, vagina, intestinal tract, and liver, where the epithelioid AML can be mistaken for a hepatic adenoma (Figure 25-72) (368,369). Collectively, these neoplasms present far more often in adults, but Alaggio et al. (370) identified some 40 malignant PEComas presenting in the first two decades, mainly in the second decade. The ligamentum teres/broad ligament and wall of the intestine accounted for almost 50% of cases in children. AML of the kidney is also one of the more common sites of a PEComa in children (368). The tumor cells of the PEComa can have a predominantly clear cell appearance or as large epithelioid cells with abundant eosinophilic cytoplasm (Figure 25-73). The histologic features of malignancy include atypism, mitotic activity, and necrosis like other sarcomas. These tumors are infrequently pigmented so that malignant melanoma is more than a serious consideration. The differential diagnosis includes alveolar soft part sarcoma and CCS of soft tissues. MUM-1 expression in malignant melanoma and CCS differentiates these tumors from PEComa (371). There is also the conundrum of the histogenetic relationship of the PEComa to the Xp11.2 translocation renal cell and extrarenal carcinoma

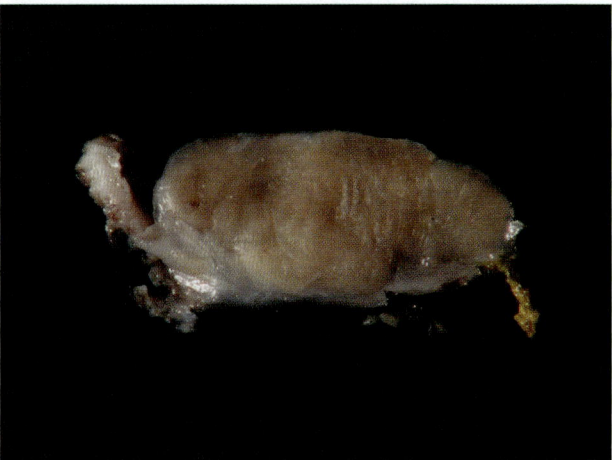

FIGURE 25-72 • PEComa presented as a mass in the abdominal mid-line and was associated with the umbilical vein-ligamentum teres in a 4-year-old female. The tumor on cut surface has a well-circumscribed appearance with a slightly nodular tannish-brown appearance. It measured 3.5 cm in greatest dimension.

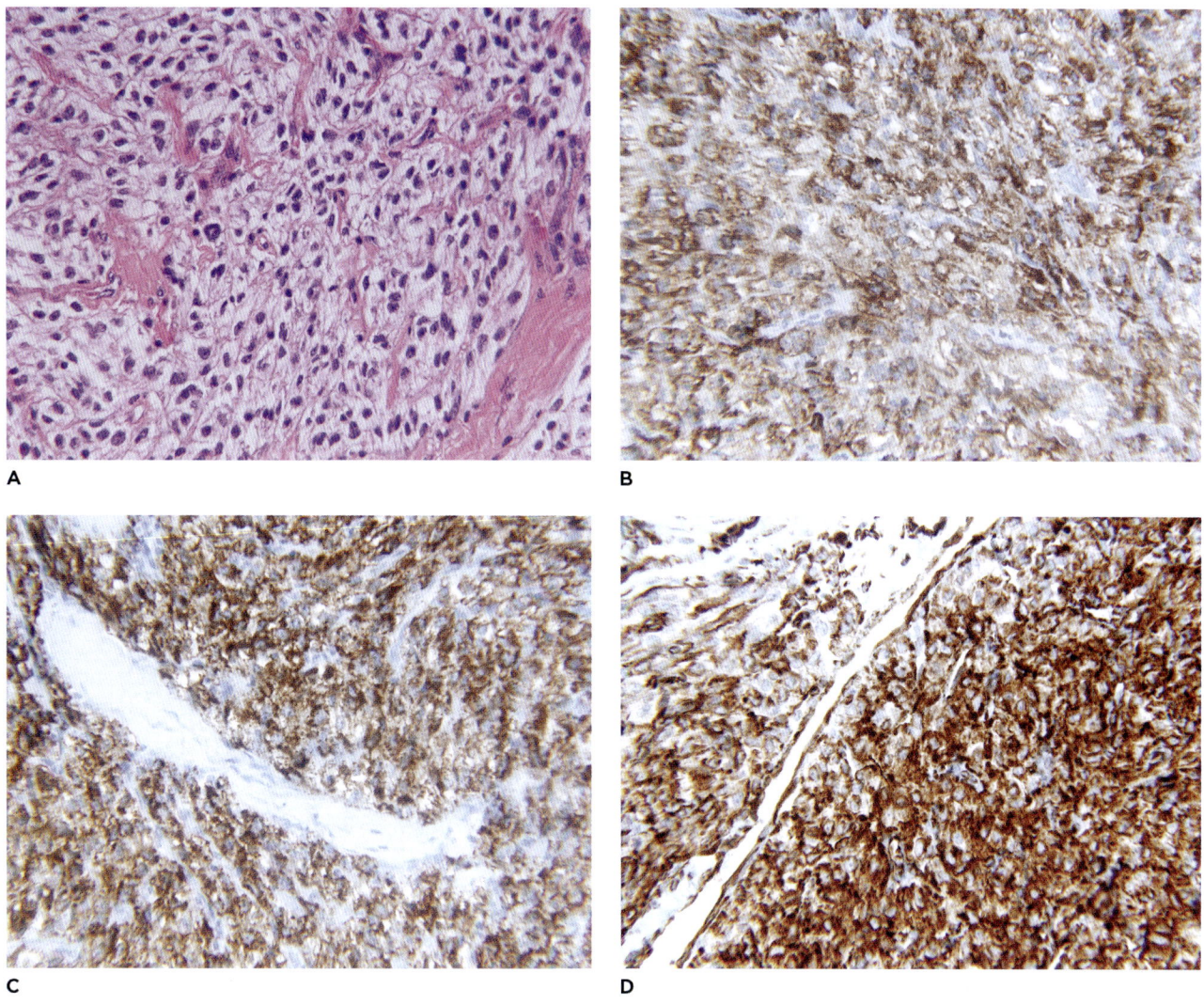

FIGURE 25-73 • PEComa has characteristic microscopic and immunophenotypic features. **A:** A uniformly nested neoplasm is composed of rounded to ovoid tumor cells with uniform clear cytoplasm. **B:** The immunohistochemical profile included positivity for vimentin. **C:** The tumor cells are immunoreactive for SMA. **D:** A similar diffuse pattern of positivity is seen for HMB-45.

with its TFE3 gene fusion and alveolar soft part sarcoma (der TFE3 fusion) (372,373). Approximately 80% of PEComas have a translocation in the TSC2 gene, and the remaining examples have a TFE3 translocation. The PBK/mTOR pathway is affected in these translocations.

GASTROINTESTINAL STROMAL TUMOR

GIST is a well-established clinicopathologic entity with its signature activating pathway mutations of KIT (type III tyrosine receptor kinase) or PDGFRA (platelet-derived growth factor receptor α) on 4q12 with resulting immunohistochemical positivity for CD117 (c-kit) and CD34 (374,375). It is estimated that 10% to 15% of GISTs in adults and 80% to 85% of cases in children do not have either of these signature mutations (wild type) (376). The so-called wild-type GISTs are further classified into those with SDH-deficiency (Carney-Stratakis syndrome), those without SDHx mutations (Carney triad), and the SDH deficient tumors with NF1 or BRAF mutations (376,377). Only 1% to 2% of GISTs present in the first two decades of life and the majority of these in children beyond 10 years of age (378). There are rare examples in neonates (379,380); one infant also had jejunal atresia (380). The general experience with sporadic GISTs in all age groups is that the stomach (50% to 60% of cases) and small intestine (20% to 30%) are the two most common primary sites. In individuals 21 years of age or less, there is a female predilection and the presence of multiple gastric tumors and lymph node metastasis (381). The stomach is the preferred site of presentation in children (>80% of cases). A small subset of GISTs in children (usually over the age of 10 years at diagnosis) is a manifestation of the Carney triad (pulmonary chondroma, paraganglioma, and GISTs), Carney-Stratakis syndrome, or NF1 (375,382–385). Histopathologically, GISTs in children more often have a plexiform, multinodular and epithelioid pattern (386). This same pattern has been in "pediatric" type GISTs in adults (387). The latter pattern appears to correlate with loss of SDHB (388). In the absence of CD117 immunostaining in mild type GISTs, there is positivity for CD34 and DOG1 (389). Spread into the peritoneal cavity and regional lymph node metastases are reportedly more common in children, but paradoxically the clinical course is more indolent despite the more malignant behavior of these tumors. The risk assessment based upon the size of the tumor and mitotic rate loses some of its predictive value in GISTs in children (390). Separate risk stratification criteria have not been developed for pediatric GISTs so by default, the adult criteria are generally utilized. As a final note, GISTs have been reported in extraintestinal sites such as the liver, adrenal, pancreas, prostate, and bladder but mainly in adults. There are some overlapping histologic features among PNSTs, PEComas, fibromatosis, and GISTs.

SKELETAL AND SMOOTH MUSCLE NEOPLASMS

Not surprisingly, the subject of myogenic tumors in children is dominated by one neoplasm, rhabdomyosarcoma (RMS), which accounts for 40% to 60% of all STSs in the first two decades of life (3,5). Benign myogenic tumors represented by the adult, fetal, and cardiac rhabdomyomas and leiomyoma are uncommon in children by any measure.

Rhabdomyoma in children presents either in the heart or as a mass in the subcutis of the head and neck region or chest wall in children in the first 2 years of life (391). Over 50% of cardiac tumors in children are rhabdomyomas and 90% of these cases are associated with the tuberous sclerosis complex (392,393). *Cardiac rhabdomyoma* is diagnosed *in utero* in 0.1% to 0.2% of prenatal ultrasounds. Fetal hydrops, findings to suggest hypoplastic left heart syndrome, arrhythmias and outflow obstruction are among some of the clinical presentations (394,395). Most single or multiple well-circumscribed, pale tan masses are present in either or both ventricles. Histologically, the enlarged myocytes have clear to vacuolated to eosinophilic cytoplasm with scattered cells having strands of cytoplasm from the nuclear to cell membrane, producing the so-called spider cell (Figure 25-74).

Fetal rhabdomyoma (FRM) is a rare, sporadic tumor in most cases (also known to occur in the basal cell carcinoma syndrome) and has two histologic patterns: myxoid and cellular (396–398). Unlike RMS with its presentation in deep soft tissue sites, or visceral organs, most FRMs present in the deep dermis and/or subcutis. A vague multinodular pattern is composed of an orderly, almost layered, arrangement of small immature cells with interposed immature myotubes (Figure 25-75). The nuclei of both cell types are uniform and are neither enlarged nor hyperchromatic. The cellular foci have a more spindle cell pattern and myotubes may be less apparent (Figure 25-76). The presence of any mitotic figures or atypical appearing rhabdomyoblasts should serve as a warning that tumor is probably a well-differentiated ERMS.

Adult rhabdomyoma is a rare tumor overall, but even more so in children (283). Over 90% of all cases present in the head and neck region and are known to form multifocal masses occurring almost exclusively in males (399). These tumors have some resemblance to the cardiac rhabdomyoma.

Focal myositis (FM) presents as a mass or masses in the deep soft tissues of the extremities (400,401). This inflammatory process forms a well-circumscribed mass in the skeletal muscle with a combination of inflammatory and myopathic

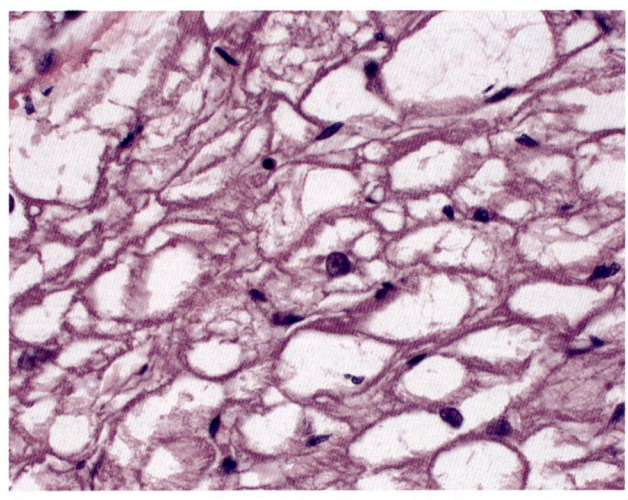
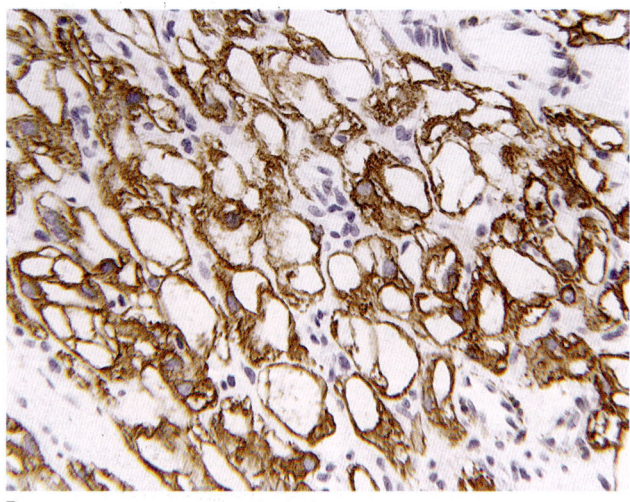

FIGURE 25-74 • Cardiac rhabdomyoma in a 3-week-old female presented as an obstructing mass in the left ventricle. **A:** Large tumor cells with abundant clear cytoplasm are accompanied by interspersed cells with strands of cytoplasm producing the features of the so-called spider cells. **B:** The tumor cells are strongly immunopositive for desmin.

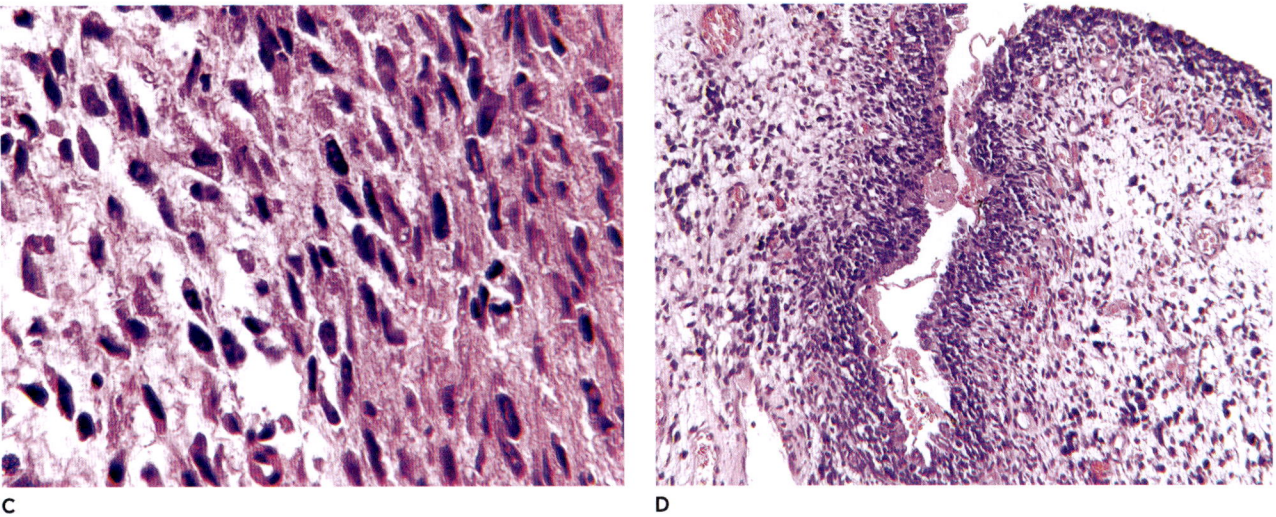

FIGURE 25-81 • (continued) **C:** This focus is composed predominantly of differentiated rhabdomyoblasts. **D:** Classic cambium layer pattern of sarcoma botyroides.

diversity of individual tumor cells is an important clue to the diagnosis of ERMS. The nuclei are densely hyperchromatic, and mitotic figures are variably prominent. Scattered among the smaller tumor cells, larger individual cells with eosinophilic cytoplasm may be present; these latter cells are usually the clues to the diagnosis of ERMS. The small primitive tumor cells are diffusely positive for vimentin, but desmin may demonstrate a similar diffuse pattern of staining to the vimentin or is restricted to scattered tumor cells as dot positivity. Nuclear staining for myogenin (our preferred stain) or myo-D1 is also quite variable and may also be restricted to a small fraction of tumor cells (Figure 25-82) (430,431). The dense round cell pattern of ERMS may be difficult to differentiate from ARMS histologically, but the results of IHC and molecular studies resolve the issue between ERMS and ARMS in most cases (432–435). Other microscopic patterns of ERMS include condensation of small primitive cells beneath an epithelial-lined surface (cambium layer) in the sarcoma botyroides or solid sheets of tumor cells interspersed by nested collections of primitive tumor cells resembling the blastemal pattern of Wilms tumor. The latter pattern is composed predominantly of polygonal-shaped tumor cells with scattered rhabdomyoblasts with clear to eosinophilic cytoplasm. A spindled population can be seen in association with the blastemal-like pattern, but the pure spindle cell/sclerosing RMSs are regarded by some as separate category of RMS, despite the focal presence of embryonal and alveolar like-foci (Figure 25-83) (436). In the uterine cervix, ERMS is often seen in association with heterologous cartilage (40% to 50% of cases) and may be associated with the DICER1-familial PPB tumor syndrome (437) (Figure 25-84). Unlike ERMS of the vagina occurring in infants as a polypoid mass (sarcoma botryoides) from the anterior vaginal wall, cervical RMS is seen in older children, adolescents and young adults. When the primary site is the paratesticular region, ERMS often is associated with spindle cell features.

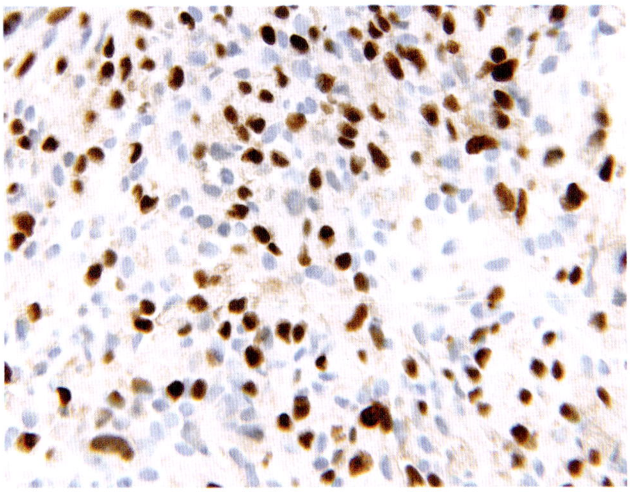

Anaplasia may be seen on occasion and if the suspected ERMS is a tumor in or near the chest or lung, it is likely that the neoplasm is a PPB especially in the presence of a collage of high-grade sarcomatous patterns including nodules of malignant-appearing cartilage.

The molecular genetics of ERMS is different from those of alveolar RMS in that there is no signature or non–random translocations. There is loss of heterozygosity on 11p15.5 in the region of IGF-2. Gains and losses of chromosomes or chromosomal regions have also been identified, often trisomy 8 (Table 25-1). There are individual examples of ERMS with a unique balanced translocation.

Alveolar RMS is the less common of the two subtypes and in our series accounted for 19% of cases with the soft tissues

FIGURE 25-82 • Embryonal rhabdomyosarcoma. Myogenin nuclear immunostaining is generally restricted to a minority of tumor cells in contrast to ARMS with myogenin positivity in the vast majority of tumor cells.

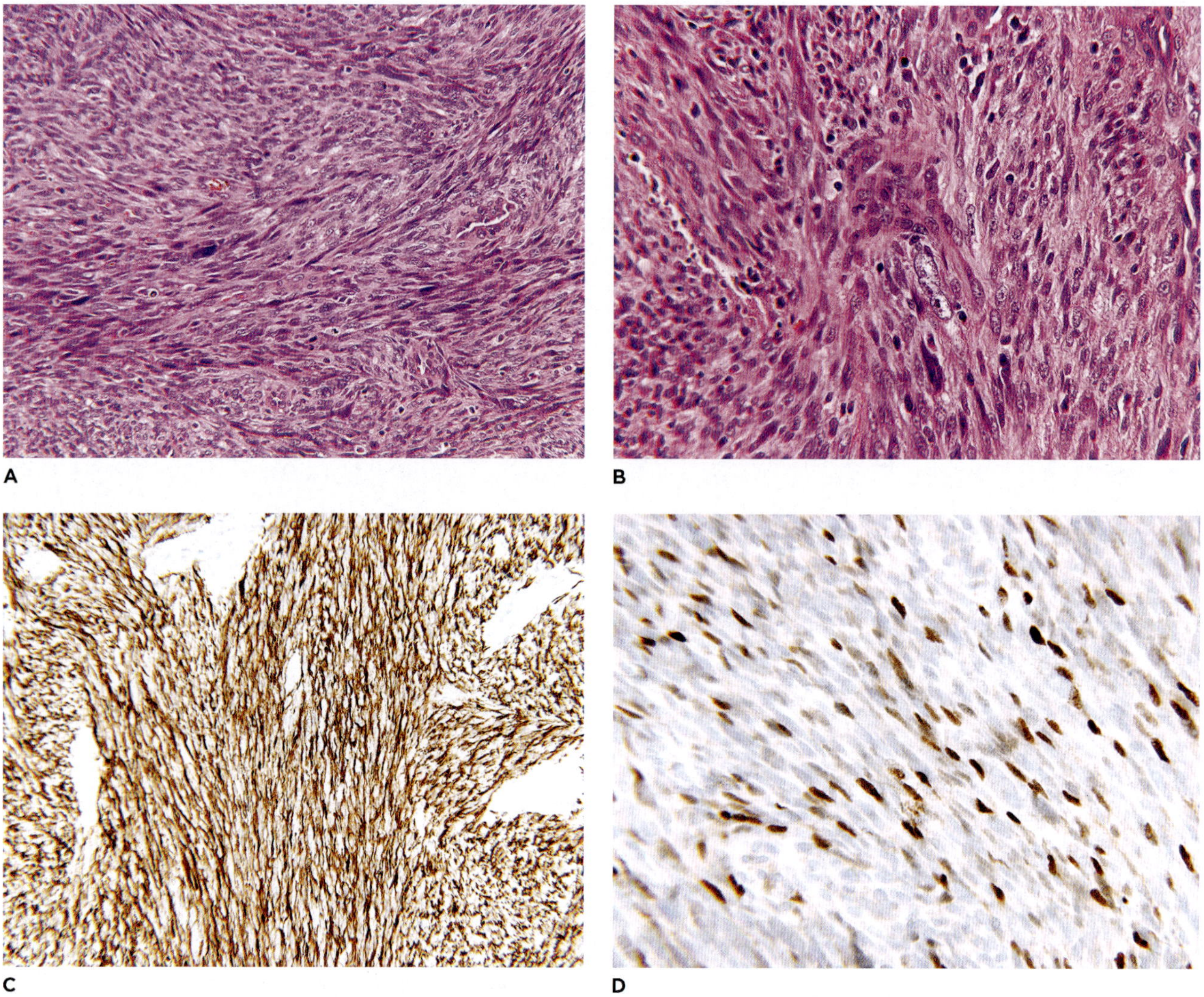

FIGURE 25-83 • Spindle cell rhabdomyosarcoma presenting in the arm of a 1-year-old male. **A:** Fascicles of spindle cells with features resembling CIFS, monophasic SS or MPNST. **B:** The tumor cells are uniform and primitive or differentiated rhabdomyoblasts are not seen. **C:** The tumor is diffusely immunopositive for desmin. **D:** Myogenin immunoreactive in many but not all tumor cell nuclei.

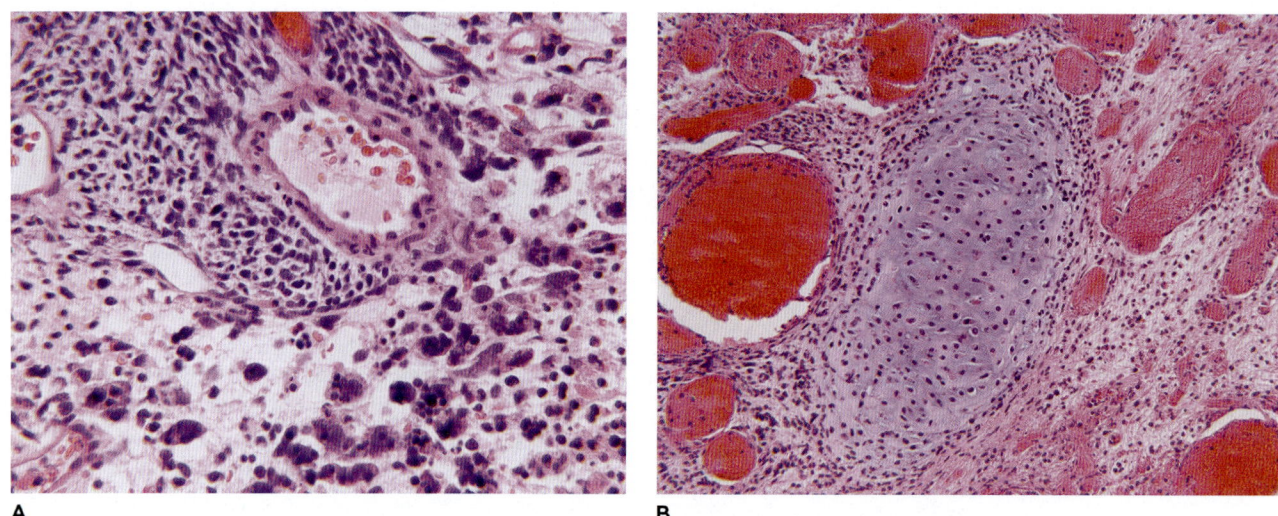

FIGURE 25-84 • ERMS presented as a polypoid mass arising from the uterine cervix of a 15-year-old female. **A:** Primitive-appearing rhabdomyoblasts are present with population of enlarged, more pleomorphic malignant cells. **B:** Unique among ERMS is the presence of nodules of cartilage when this tumor presents in the cervix. There is the question of the relationship of this tumor to the adenosarcoma of the uterus. This tumor may be found in association with the PPB complex with DICER1 mutation.

of the extremities (lower greater than upper) as the preferred primary site in 40% or more of our cases (Table 25-14). In the perianal region, ARMS accounted for 50% of cases where the prognosis is particularly unfavorable even in those cases of ERMS (438).

More so than ERMS, ARMS accommodates to the characterization of a malignant round cell neoplasm in that the cells are largely polygonal with high-grade, intensely hyperchromatic nuclei and variably prominent cytoplasm (Figure 25-85A to C). Mitotic figures and nuclear debris are more prominent than in ERMS and are reminiscent of the high MKI poorly differentiated or undifferentiated neuroblastoma. The tumor cells may form solid sheets of non-overlapping cells and/or foci of tumor cells that tend to fall away from each other, producing the nascent or overt alveolar pattern (Figure 25-85B). When the biopsy is a more generous one with stroma in the background, the tumor cells are more likely to have a nested-septal pattern in which the alveolar pattern of central disaggregated individual tumor cells is surrounded by individual tumor cells still attached to the septal stroma. A similar alveolar pattern is seen in some cases of EWS-PNET. The presence of large multinucleated tumor cells with prominent eosinophilic cytoplasm ("wreath" cells) among the mononuclear tumor cells in these solid or more obvious septal-alveolar foci is a relatively specific feature of ARMS. One may encounter foci of an ARMS-like pattern in ERMS which has been characterized as the "dense pattern"; these cases probably account for the examples of fusion-negative ARMS (Figure 25-86).

Most ARMSs are consistently immunopositive for vimentin and desmin as well as myoD1 and myogenin (Figure 25-87). The latter three markers are diffusely positive in most

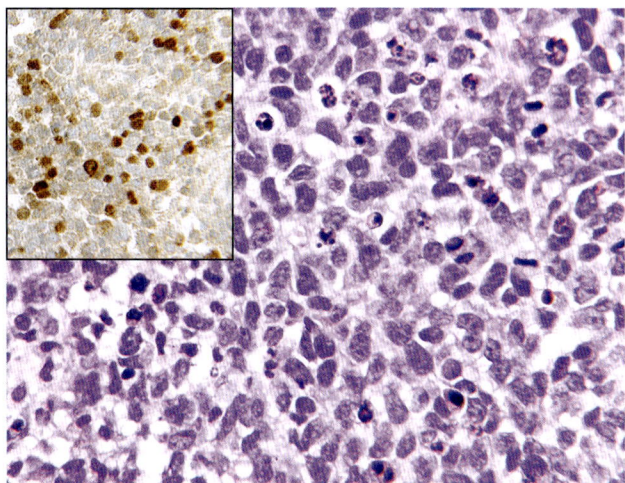

FIGURE 25-86 • ERMS presenting in the parotid gland of a 9-year-old female. The so-called dense pattern can be mistaken for ARMS. **Inset:** Myogenin immunostain shows that 25% or so of tumor cells show nuclear positivity.

cases of ARMS in contrast to ERMS in which myogenin and myoD1 have a more patchy pattern of positivity. Diffuse nuclear staining for myogenin in ARMS has been described as a useful discriminating reaction from the more limited nuclear positivity in ERMS; the diffuse nuclear staining for myogenin has been characterized as a surrogate marker for the fusion-positive RMS (433).

There are two well-documented translocations in ARMS involving PAX3-FOXO1 (formerly FKHR) and PAX7-FOXO1 gene fusions, t(2;13) (q35;q14) and t(1;13) (p36;q14) in 60% and 20% of fusion-positive cases, respectively (424,425). The t(1;13) ARMS is seen more often in younger

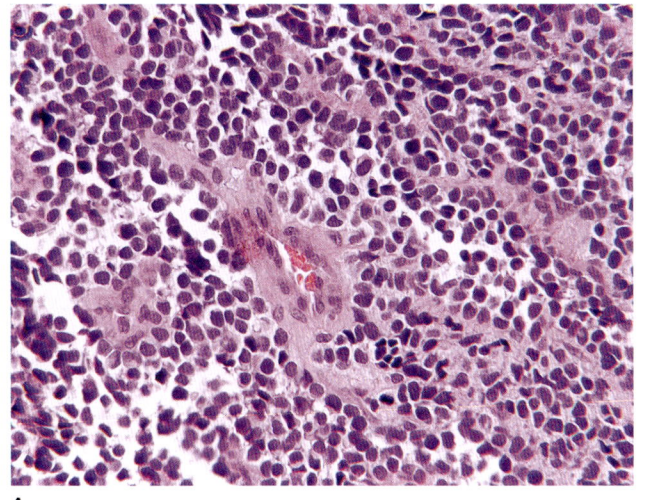
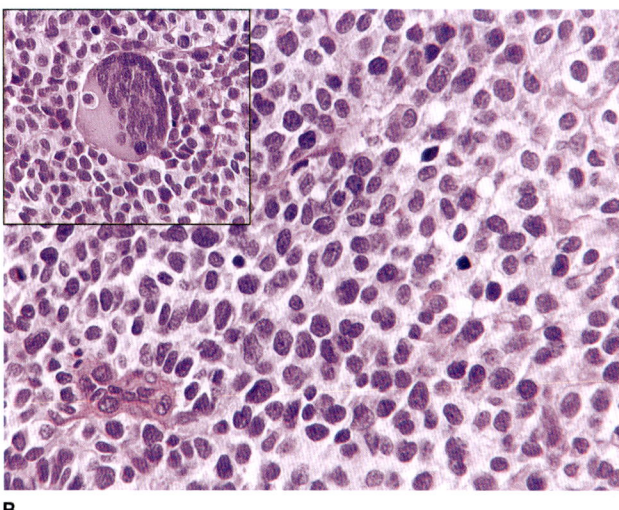

A   B

FIGURE 25-85 • ARMS present in the foot of a 3-month-old female. The tumor demonstrates the three histologic features of this neoplasm. **A:** Most areas had the septal growth of uniform malignant round cells attached to fibrovascular stroma and the remaining individual tumor cells seemingly suspended in space. **B:** Other foci display the individual tumor cells in loose sheets with the so-called nascent alveolar pattern. **Inset:** Large, multinucleated tumor cells are seen in a background of monotonous round cells. FISH studies identified a FKHR breakapart.

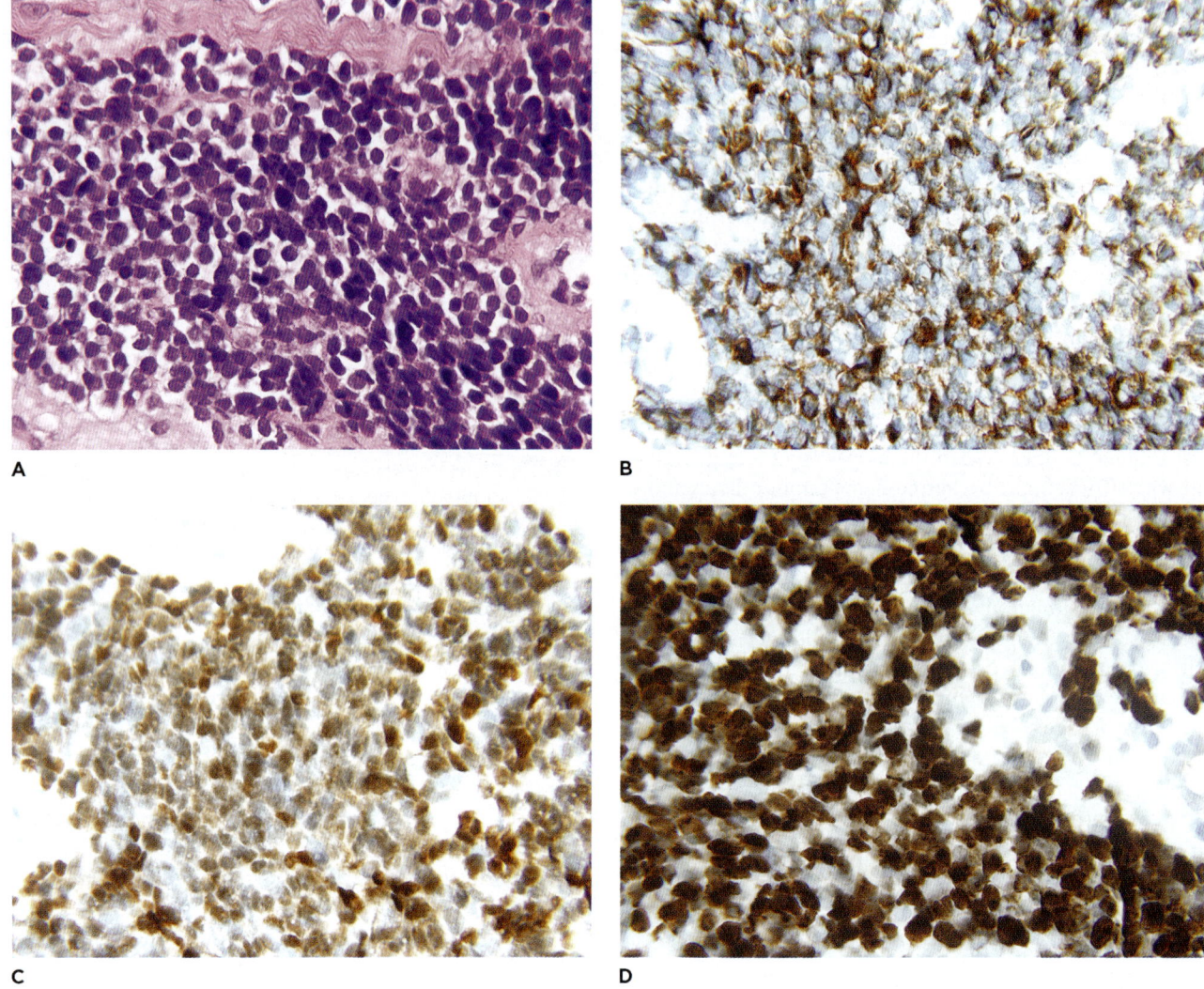

FIGURE 25-87 • ARMS presenting in the orbit of a 9-year-old female. **A:** So-called nascent pattern is seen as tumor cells fall away from each other. **B:** The tumor cells are diffusely positive for desmin. **C:** Virtually 100% of tumor cells are positive for myogenin. **D:** Ki-67 is intensely positive in 100% of tumor cells.

children. PAX3-FOXO1-positive ARMS is associated with a poorer outcome than the PAX7-FOXO1-positive and fusion-negative ARMS. Amplification of 12q13-q14 has an adverse effect upon prognosis.

The morphologic characterization of RMS into an ERMS and ARMS subtypes (and sometimes "mixed") has traditionally been an inexact exercise, as evidenced by high discrepancy rates between the diagnoses rendered by the "poor, but well intentioned" local pathologist versus the expert pathologist performing central review for collaborative studies. Recent data from both SIOP and COG, though, have shown that the presence of *PAX3/PAX7-FOXO1* translocations, not the presence of alveolar morphology, is the key biologic and prognostic finding. Fusion gene-positive ARMS has a worse prognosis than both fusion-negative ARMS and ERMS; the tumors in the latter two groups behave in a similarly favorable manner (423,432). Thus, genetic testing for the PAX-FOXO1 translocation by FISH in most cases should be part of the pathology workup of RMS. Overexpression of ALK mRNA is yet another unfavorable biologic marker in ARMS (439).

What is clear about ARMS is that it is prognostically unfavorable. Because ARMS can present with a lymph node metastasis or as disseminated disease in bones and bone marrow, the pathologic diagnosis can be challenging if ARMS is not considered in the differential diagnosis. A nonlymphoid hematopoietic neoplasm, MRT, EWS-PNET, and neuroblastoma are other childhood malignancies which are candidate neoplasms with some qualified clinical and pathologic overlap with ARMS.

Other patterns of RMS include the spindle, epithelioid, anaplastic and pleomorphic types. The latter type of RMS is rare enough in adults and much less in children (440). These tumors have features of a high grade sarcoma with myogenin and/or myoD1 positivity. Spindle/sclerosing RMS is regarded as an entity separate from ERMS and ARMS

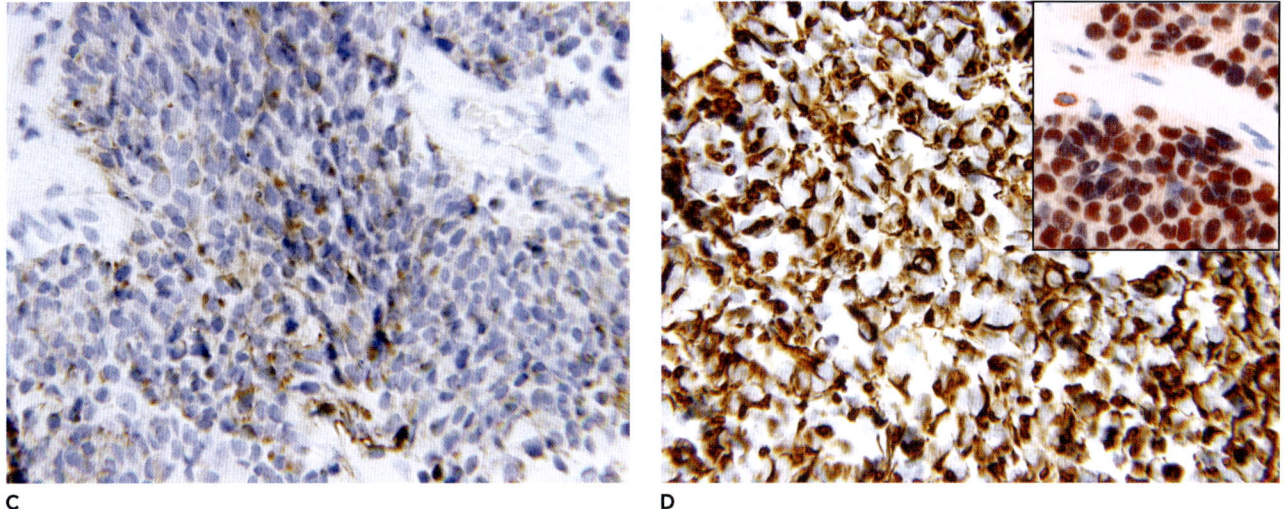

FIGURE 25-92 • (continued) **C:** Scattered tumor cells show dot-like and perinuclear pattern of cytokeratin positivity. **D:** Desmin expression may be strong and diffuse as in this case or may be more limited. These tumors also show strong nuclear positivity for WT1 (**Inset**). The EWS breakapart was identified by FISH.

children 5 years old or less. A mass in the region of a tendon or aponeurosis, measuring 5 cm or less, is firm and well-circumscribed with a grayish-tan surface. Like the cutaneous melanoma, the spindled or more epithelioid cells are arranged in cohesive groups with a delicate fibrous stromal network in the background or with a more prominent hyalinized stroma and can be highly infiltrative (478,479). Other patterns have a resemblance to the disaggregated cells of an ARMS or EWS-PNET when the tumor cells are more polygonal in appearance. Multinucleated giant cells are seen with some frequency. Clear to eosinophilic cytoplasm can add to the EWS-like appearance. The rounded to ovoid nuclei are modestly hyperchromatic and vesicular with amphophilic nucleoli (Figure 25-93). Pseudoinclusions are more or less prominent in any one case. Mitotic figures are not especially numerous. Other immunophenotypic attributes include the expression of CD99, CD57, bcl-2, CD56, EMA, synaptophysin and neuron-specific enolase (475,479). Tumors in excess of 5 cm and those with necrosis are features correlated with an unfavorable prognosis. Regional lymph node metastasis is a common mode of spread. Overall survival is approximately 50% (479). The differential diagnosis includes SS (common sites of presentation), PEComa (similarities in immunophenotype, but without EWSR1-BA), paraganglioma (similar immunophenotype, but absence of HMB-45 or Melan-A expression) and cutaneous melanoma, especially the clear cell type (similar immunophenotype, but absence of EWSR1-BA) (480).

Two "apparent" neoplasms arising in the GI tract, and both having EWSR1 rearrangements and both demonstrating the presence of osteoclast-like giant cells are recognized; one is designated CCS-like GI tumor and the other malignant GI neuroectodermal tumor (481,482). In addition to osteoclast-like giant cells, these tumors are similar with a cellular composition of nests and fascicles of spindled and epithelioid cells, resembling malignant melanoma and PEComa. Neither of these tumors (or this tumor) are immunoreactive for the melanocyte markers, in contrast to the "true" CCS with osteoclast-like of GI tract whose immunophenotype is similar to CCS of soft tissues (483). MUM-1 immunopositivity in malignant melanoma is useful in the differentiation from PEComa and CCS (371).

NUT midline carcinomas are undifferentiated tumors of uncertain origin that primarily occur in the upper aerodigestive tract in children, but can also affect any midline soft tissue site (484). This is a rare entity, affected fewer than 50 children a year, usually teenagers (median age 17 years), and the prognosis is dismal, with a mean survival of less than 9 months. Microscopically, the tumor consists of sheets of primitive- or undifferentiated-appearing cells which focally form islands of epithelial cells with or without squamous differentiation; the latter foci can mimic Hassall corpuscles in the thymus. The cells are immunohistochemically positive for various cytokeratins, p63, CEA, and CD34. These tumors have a canonical t(15;19) translocation which fuses the BRD3 or BRD4 protein with the NUT protein, and while not yet widely available, NUT immunopositivity is diagnostic (485).

Extraskeletal myxoid chondrosarcoma (EMC) is seemingly the least common representative of the extended EWS family tumors and is infrequent in children and adolescents. The fusion transcript, EWSR1-NR4A3 [(t9;22)(q22;q12)] is present in approximately 75% cases (486). However, another translocation has been identified with FUS rather than EWSR1 (487). A large combined institutional experience revealed no cases in the first decade and only 2 (2%) of 87 cases in individuals between 11 and 20 years old, though the individual case has been seen in younger children (488). Four translocations have been identified to date and one of these is an EWSR1 fusion partner (Table 25-1). The proximal

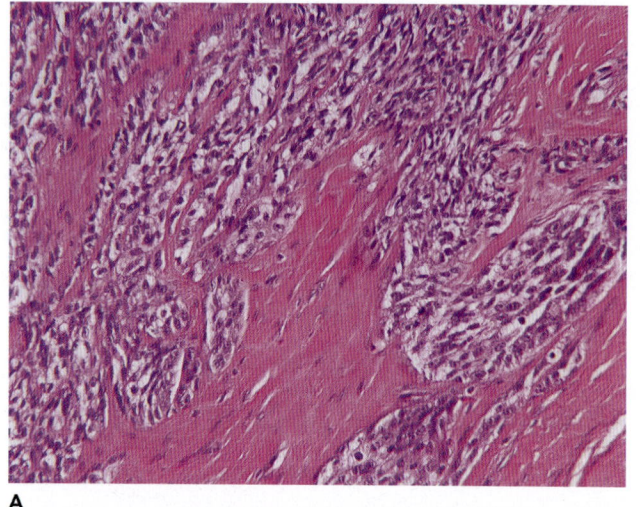
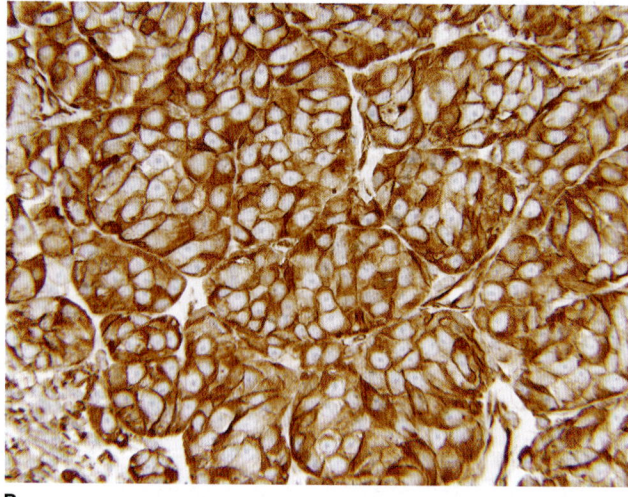
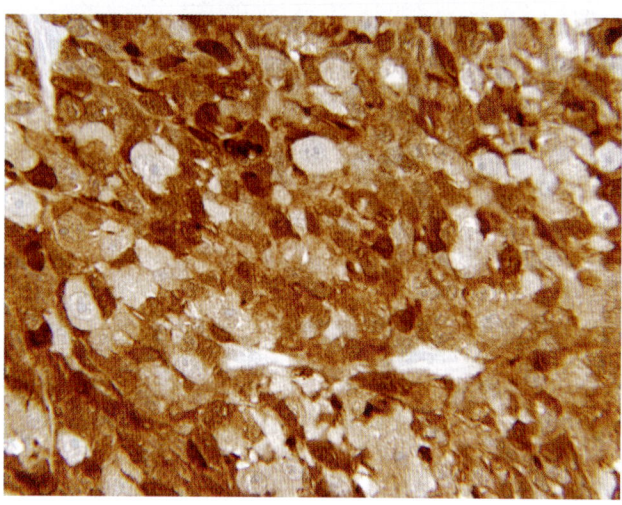

FIGURE 25-93 • CCS of tendon sheath (melanoma of soft part) presented as a mass over the clavicle in a 10-year-old male. **A:** A nodular tan-white mass measuring 2.5 cm consisted of ill-defined nests of rounded to spindled-shaped tumor cells in a background of fibrous stroma. **B:** Immunohistochemical staining showed strong positivity for HMB-45. **C:** The tumor cells are also positive for S100 protein. An EWS breakapart was demonstrated by FISH.

lower extremity is the most common site of presentation in all age groups. These tumors arise in the subcutis or deeper soft tissues as a well-circumscribed, multinodular mass with a complete or incomplete fibrous capsule, usually less than 10 cm in diameter and a gelatinous whitish-tan to tannish appearance. Cartilage is generally not identified grossly or microscopically leading to question whether EMC should be regarded as chondrosarcoma since it is also inconsistently immunoreactive for S100 protein. Fibrous septa separate the tumor into lobules, which are composed of delicate lacelike strands, more solid-appearing nests, spindle cells, and high-grade round cells. The background has a variable myxoid or mucoid appearance. In some cases, it is the multilobulated architecture at low magnification, which provides the subtle clue to the diagnosis while other STSs are under consideration in the differentiated diagnosis like poorly differentiated or monophasic SS, MRT (rhabdoid cells in EMC), neurothekeoma, myoepithelial tumor of soft tissues, chordoma, parachordoma (if it exists as a distinct entity), and EWS-PNET (489). Immunohistochemically, EMC is reactive for vimentin (75% to 80% of cases), neuron-specific enolase (50% to 95%), EMA (10% to 15%), S100 protein (15% to 20%), synaptophysin (40% to 50%), and glial fibrillary acidic protein (2% to 5%) (325). These tumors are generally nonreactive for CD99, c-MET, and CAM 5.2 (the two latter markers are also positive in chordomas) and have retained expression of BAF47 (INI1). A tumor similar to EMC is reported in the lung that has an EWSR1 breakapart, but the transfusion transcript is EWSR1-CREB1 (490).

Mesenchymal chondrosarcoma (MCS), like myxoid chondrosarcoma and EWS-PNET, has a primary soft tissue and skeletal presentation (491,492). Its relationship to the other extended EWS family of tumors is not entirely clear, but the HEY1-NCOA2 would appear to be the diagnostic gene fusion in MCS (493). Most MCSs present in children beyond the age of 10 years and into the third decade. Very rarely, MCS is seen in the neonate (494,495). Approximately 60% to 70% of MCSs arise in the soft tissues or nonosseous sites including the dura, orbit, pelvis, sinonasal tract, peripheral soft tissues, and kidney. The tumor is characterized microscopically by nodules or islands of atypical hyaline cartilage and an accompanying population of primitive round cells resembling EWS or a more spindle cell stroma with clefted vascular spaces resembling HPC. We have seen cases of MCS in which the two patterns appeared to segregate from each other. These tumors are immunopositive for vimentin, CD99, and reportedly desmin and myogenin (496). The 5-year survival is 40% to 50%. MCSs arising in the soft tissues and with the HPC-like pattern seem to fare worse than tumors arising in the bone and with EWS-like features.

Myoepithelial tumor (myoepithelioma MET) is a rare and thus challenging neoplasm, which presents predominantly in the soft tissues of the extremities, but in a number of other sites including the skin, bone and viscera (497). Both benign and malignant types are recognized; the latter is seen in children (498). Approximately 20% of METs are diagnosed before the age of 20 years. There is a considerable spectrum in the morphology from those tumors with a lobulated growth with a mixture of epithelioid and spindle cells, cord-like structures with and without duct-like structures or a diffuse round cell proliferation with a myxoid background (497,499). Those tumors with tubuloductal profiles may be PLAG1 positive (500). Nuclear positivity for p63 is also helpful in the diagnosis (501). Other sensitive markers include EMA, calponin, GFAP, and CD10 (502); EWSR1 rearrangement is present in 45% to 50% of cases; the fusion partners include POUSF1, PBX1, PBX3, ZNF444 and ATF-1, (503). There is also a subset of METs with homozygous deletions in SMARCB1/ZIN11 (504). An interesting point has recently been made about the identifications of an EWSR1 rearrangement in a variety of tumors and its diagnostic utility, but obviously the morphologic and immunophenotypic context remains a critical factor.

Synovial sarcoma (SS) is one of the most common non-RMSs in the first two decades of life together with the MPNST (505). Approximately 15% to 30% of SSs are diagnosed at or before 20 years of age but less than 15% of all SSs in children occur before the age of 10 years (506,507). In our own experience with SSs, there were 57 cases, in individuals between 4 and 20 years of age at diagnosis (mean age, 14 years) with 12 (20%) of the cases seen in children 10 years old or less. Some 60% of cases presented in the extremities, which is in accord with other large series, which have reported up to 70% of tumors in the extremities (Table 25-19). Various sites in the head and neck region accounted for 10% of our cases. With molecular genetic testing for the t(X;18) translocation, SS has been documented in any number of non-soft tissue sites from the lung-pleura, kidney dura, brain and heart, intestinal tract as just some examples. Several cases of pleuropulmonary SS were originally submitted for review as possible examples of type I or cystic PPBs, but four of the patients were adolescents between 13 and 15 years of age whereas the median age for type I PPB is 9 months. A firm, well-circumscribed fibrous appearing mass may be accompanied by focal hemorrhagic cysts and dystrophic calcifications or metaplastic bone (Figure 25-94). In those tumors with minimal fibrous stroma, the consistency of the tumor is soft and the cut surface has a glistening, mucoid appearance resembling an ERMS or CIFS. Attention to the dimensions of the tumor is important since there is a correlation between size (> or <5 cm) and outcome; those tumors in excess of 5 cm have a significantly poorer prognosis (non-RMSs in children, regardless of pathologic type, have a poor outcome if the tumor measures greater than 5 cm in greatest dimension) (508,509).

There are two basic histologic patterns of SS: monophasic spindle cell proliferation and biphasic spindle-glandular type (Figure 25-95). A third, poorly differentiated SS, constitutes 5% or less of cases, has some similarities to EWS-

TABLE 25-19	SYNOVIAL SARCOMA IN CHILDREN AND ADOLESCENTS	
Anatomic Site	No.	(%)
Lower extremity	22	(39)
Proximal	14	
Distal	8	
Upper extremity	11	(19)
Proximal	6	
Distal	5	
Chest wall	7	(12)
Lung-Pleura	5	(9)
Abdominal wall	3	(5)
Retroperitoneum	2	(3)
Neck	2	(3)
Paranasal sinus—pharynx	2	(3)
Scalp	1	(2)
Orbit	1	(2)
Posterior mediastinum	1	(2)
	57	(100)

37 males, 20 females (mean age, 14 years).
From the files of the Lauren V. Ackerman Laboratory of Surgical Pathology, St. Louis Children's Hospital, Washington University Medical Center, St. Louis, MO.

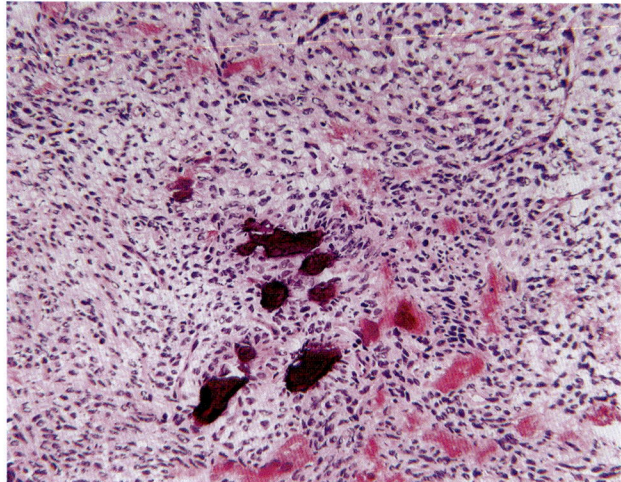

FIGURE 25-94 • This SS presented in the ankle of an 8-year-old male. Some tumors are associated with dystrophic calcifications.

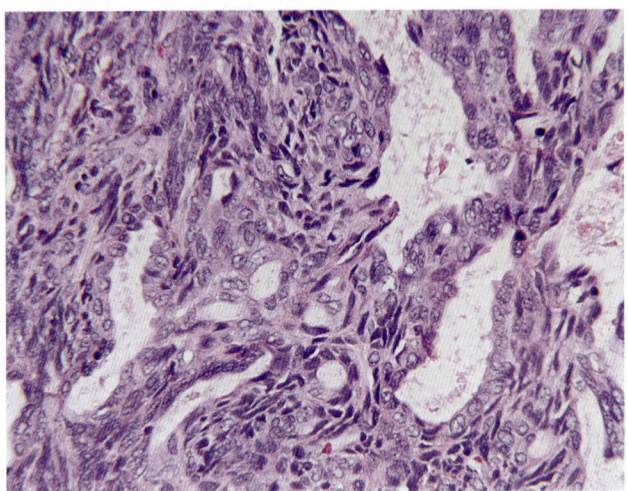

FIGURE 25-95 • SS presented in the left foot of this 18-year-old male. This neoplasm had a classic biphasic pattern of gland formation in a spindle cell background.

PNET including a similar immunophenotype of vimentin, cytokeratin, and CD99 positivity and an SYT-SSX fusion instead of one involving EWSR1. Approximately 60% of SS in children have monophasic features (509). Epithelial differentiation may represent de-repression of E-cadherin transcription by either one of the translocations (510). The fourth purely glandular pattern resembling well-differentiated adenocarcinoma is very rare. Necrosis and rhabdoid cells are other features of poorly differentiated SS. Uniform spindle cells with either ovoid or fusiform contours are arranged in dense sheets or short fascicles (Figure 25-96). The nuclei have a pale, finely granular chromatin, and the cytoplasm is inconspicuous. Mitotic figures are not prominent. Like the MPNST, which the monophasic spindle cell SS resembles, there may be alternating "light cell-dark cell" areas reflecting variable cellular density. A HPC-like pattern is another useful clue to the diagnosis. In addition, myxoid foci convey an impression of MPNST or DFSP. Mast cells are nonspecific, but their presence should raise the question concern about SS, MPNST or SFT in the appropriate clinical setting. The glandular profiles are either subtle, residing as small tubular structures interspersed in a predominant spindle cell background or are overly obvious large glands or cysts. Immunohistochemically, SS is diffusely positive for vimentin in the spindle cell component whereas the epithelial component expresses cytokeratin AE1/AE3, CK7, and EMA; the cytokeratins may be limited to individual tumor cells or entirely nonreactive (Figure 25-97). The EMA is more likely to stain small groups of tumor cells with a membranous pattern. Both CD99 and bcl-2 are consistently expressed in SS. An antibody to TLE1 has shown diagnostic value in cases of SS. SS is also known to occasionally be immunopositive for S100 protein. Though most SSs have the t(X;18) translocation, whether it is the fusion transcript SYT-SSX1 (present more often in biphasic SS) or SYT-SSX2 (more often monophasic SS) does not seem to have prognostic significance though circumstantial evidence suggests that the latter fusion transcript is correlated with a less favorable outcome. All SSs are at least grade 2 sarcomas but increased mitotic activity and necrosis are grade 3 features. However, COG regards all SSs as grade 3 based upon the tumor type. A spindle cell sarcoma with marked nuclear pleomorphism, anaplasia, and extensive necrosis is unlikely to represent a SS. The overall survival of children and adolescents is approximately 80%, whereas it is lower in adults (60%) (507).

Malignant rhabdoid tumor (MRT) and its counterpart in the brain and spinal cord, atypical teratoid/rhabdoid tumor (AT/RT), are the archetypes of the INI1-deficient

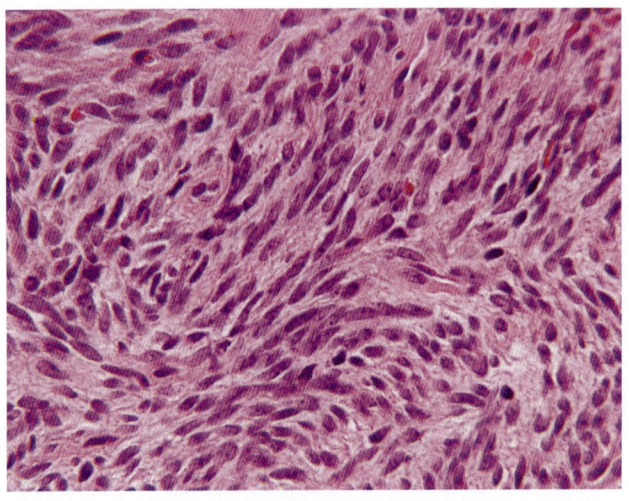
A

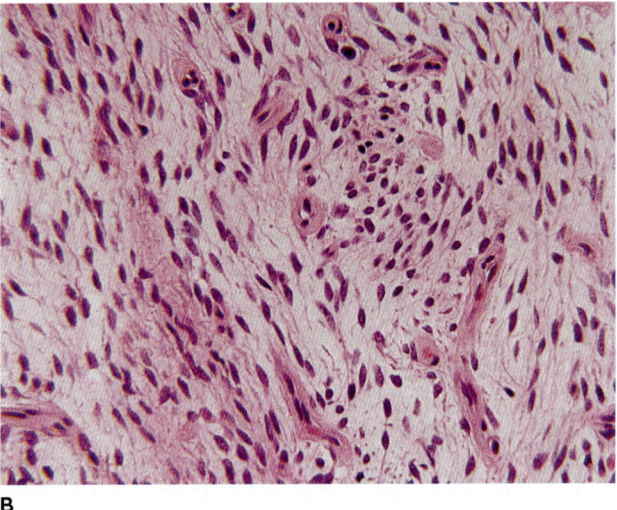
B

FIGURE 25-96 • SS presented in the wrist of an 11-year-old male. **A:** A monotonous population of uniform spindle cells characterizes this monophasic neoplasm. **B:** Some areas had a more myxoid appearance with the separation of tumor cells.

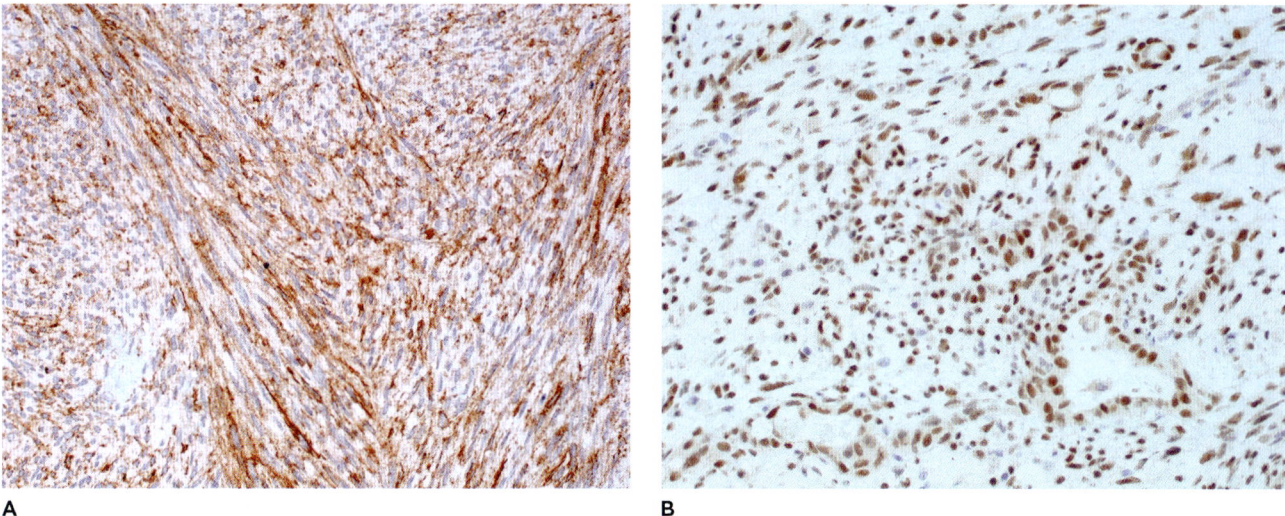

FIGURE 25-97 • Most SSs have a characteristic immunophenotype. **A:** There is diffuse positivity for epithelial membrane antigen (EMA) in this case. **B:** Another useful marker is TLE1 that is a nuclear stain. With this immunophenotype, one can then move on to FISH studies to evaluate for the t(X;18) breakapart.

TABLE 25-20	EXTRARENAL AND RENAL MALIGNANT RHABDOID TUMORS IN CHILDREN (1989–2009)	
	No.	(%)
Soft tissue (1 week–16 years, mean 3.9 years)	47	(48)
Neck (16)		
Paraspinal region (11)		
Axilla (5)		
Abdominal wall (3)		
Arm (3)		
Back (2)		
Other (7)		
Central nervous system (1 year–18 years, mean 5 years)	15	(15)
Kidney (3 days–5 years, mean 1.3 years)	12	(12)
Liver (3 months–8 years, mean 1.6 years)	11	(11)
Abdomen (2 months–2 years, mean 1 year)	4	(4)
Mediastinum (7 months–3 years, mean 1.2 years)	4	(4)
Dessiminated (3 days–3 weeks, mean 1.5 weeks)	3	(3)
Bladder (5 years, 10 years)	2	(2)
	98	(100)

53 males and 45 females.
From the files of the Lauren V. Ackerman Laboratoryears of Surgical Pathology, St. Louis Children's Hospital, Washington University Medical Center, St. Louis, MO.

neoplasms which are characterized by biallelic inactivation of the hSNF5/INI1/SMARCB1 gene on 22q11.2 through deletion or mutation (EWSR1 gene is located on 22q12) (511,512). Though the MRT was initially described in the kidney, our experience has been that almost 50% of cases presented in a variety of extrarenal sites in the soft tissues with a preference for the neck and paraspinal region (Table 25-20). Three neonates had disseminated disease including the soft tissues of the head and neck and multiple organs. Like congenital neuroblastoma, the placenta may contain micrometastases in the fetal capillaries of the chorionic villi. The AT/RTs presented as a supratentorial (nine cases), posterior fossa (four cases), and spinal cord (two cases) mass. The MRT, regardless of its primary site, is a neoplasm of early childhood and 53 (54%) of our cases presented in children 1-year-old or less with the youngest, a 3-day-old female with a renal MRT and another neonate with disseminated MRT with disfiguring facial masses and widespread metastases including the placenta. Approximately 80% of our cases were diagnosed at or before 5 years of age.

The gross features of a MRT are optimally demonstrated in a resected mass from the kidney or liver; these tumors are soft and have a bosselated, glistening tan-white surface. In the soft tissues, fibrous stroma can accompany these tumors so that there is a nesting pattern or a fibromyxoid alteration with remote resemblance to chondroid matrix. The number and prominence of rhabdoid cells with intensely eosinophilic filamentous inclusions in the cytoplasm can vary considerably from one MRT to another and from one microscopic field to another in the same tumor. Small biopsies can be especially problematic without appropriate immunohistochemical stains and/or molecular studies

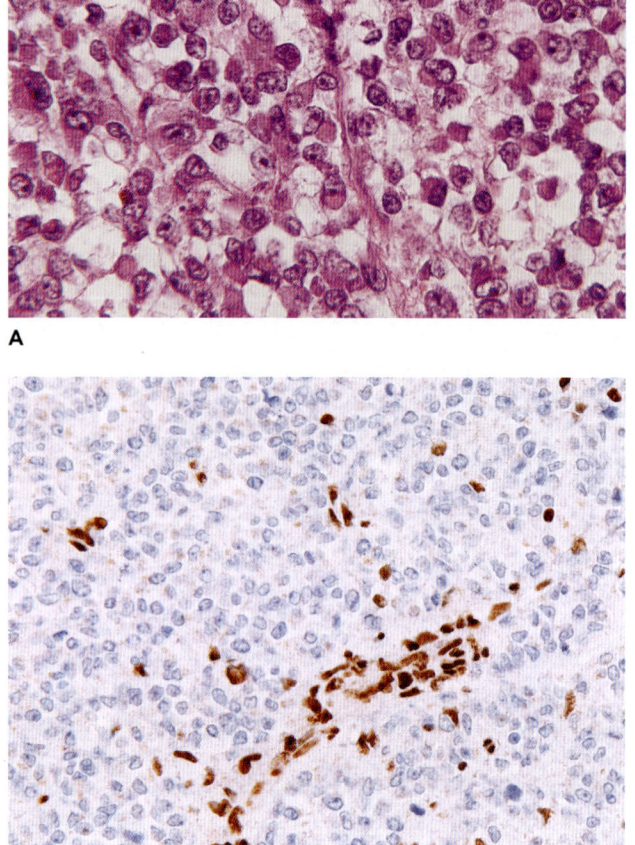
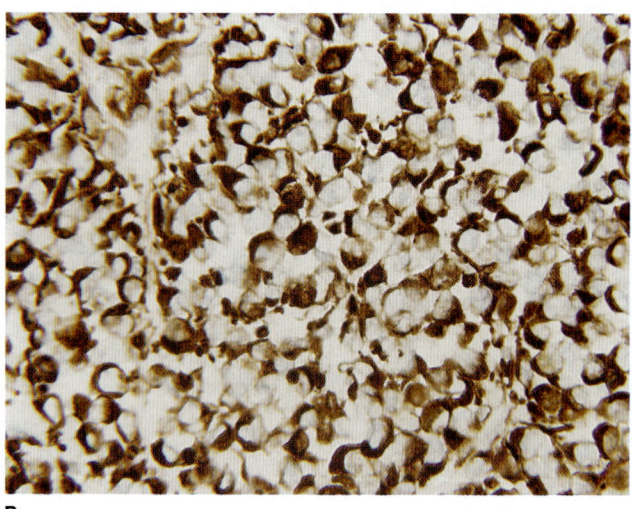

FIGURE 25-98 • MRT presenting as a rapidly enlarging mass in the neck of a 5-month-old female. **A:** This focus shows the presence of a relatively monotonous population of malignant-appearing round cells, several with rhabdoid inclusions. **B:** Vimentin immunostain highlights the rhabdoid inclusions. **C:** INI1 (BAF47) showing immunopositivity in the nuclei of the small stromal cells and lymphocytes in the background (retained INI1), in contrast to the absence of nuclear staining in the tumor cells.

(Figure 25-98A to C). Another important morphologic attribute is the large, eccentric vesicular nucleus with its prominent nucleolus resembling ganglion cells. Rhabdoid cells may be inconspicuous in a background of more epithelioid appearing cells without inclusions to populations of smaller, lymphoid-like cells, which are seen with some frequency in ATRTs, leading to a diagnosis of a central PNET or medulloblastoma in the past. It is advisable to consider MRT in the differential diagnosis of a malignant round cell neoplasm in a young child before settling on an interpretation of "undifferentiated round cell sarcoma." IHC for vimentin and cytokeratin demonstrates intense cytoplasmic positivity in the configuration of a spherical inclusion that totally occupies the cytoplasm (Figure 25-98C). In general, vimentin staining produces the more diffuse pattern of positivity, but the cytokeratin staining of the rhabdoid inclusions often stands out in a background of non-reactive tumor cells (513). Membrane-cytoplasmic positivity for CD99 is often focal and less intense than the diffuse, intense pattern of EWS-PNET. SMA positivity is consistently present in the ATRT in contrast to nonneural MRTs. The nuclei fail to stain for BAF47 to reflect the inactivated INI1 gene, but the interpretation can be complicated by the presence of numerous inflammatory cells or fibroblasts with their functioning INI1 gene with intense nuclear staining as the internal control, but these cells may also obscure small groups of non-reactive tumor cells in the background (Figure 25-98C). Originally reported as INI1-negative small cell hepatoblastoma, these tumors are considered by some as primary MRTs of the liver (514). Other malignant round cell neoplasms of infancy and young children with INI1 loss but without the dire clinical outcome of MRT have been reported (515).

Epithelioid sarcoma (ES) is a rare STS regardless of age at diagnosis. It accounts for 1% to 2% of all STSs overall, but because it has a predilection for adolescents and young adults, it may represent as many as 5% to 8% of non-RMSs STSs in the first two decades of life (516,517). Approximately 10% to 15% of ESs present in individuals 20 years old or less at diagnosis, and typically in the second decade of life (517,518). There is a male predilection. There are two clinical expressions of ES: the classic or the distal type presenting as a slow-growing nodule or nodules in the hand or forearm in almost 50% of cases and the proximal or axial presenting type. The classic or distal ES is a more superficial neoplasm in the dermis or subcutis in contrast to the proximal ES arising in the deep soft tissues of the proximal extremities or perineum. Classic ES has a multinodular or diffuse pattern of uniform epithelioid cells with abundant eosinophilic or clear, but vacuolated cytoplasm with or without a spindle cell component to resemble an epithelioid vascular neoplasm. The nodules are composed of a mantle of epithelioid cells with central necrosis or hyalinization; the latter alteration may be subtle or not present in some cases. In the presence of nodules with central necrosis, necrobiotic granulomas of the granuloma annulare type may arise in the differential diagnosis, both clinically and pathologically. IHC can settle the diagnostic dilemma in that the histiocytes of granuloma annulare are CD68-positive whereas the cells of ES coexpress vimentin, pancytokeratin, EMA and CD34 in 50% of cases (517–519). There is loss of nuclear staining for BAF-47/INI1 as a reflection of the inactivation of INI1 which is hallmark of the INI1-deficient neoplasms (513). Over 90% of distal and proximal ESs have a loss of function of INI1, and in 80% of cases, there is a homozygous deletions of the gene (504,520–522). Despite the considerable overlap between ES and MRT, these two neoplasms have different microRNA expression profiles (523).

Alveolar soft part sarcoma (ASPS) is a neoplasm, which occurs in a similar age group as ES and also represents only 1% of all STSs in the first two decades of life. Like EWS-PNET and MRT, ASPS is a molecular genetic archetype which in this case is the presence of TFE3 as a fusion partner in other neoplasms including the translocation renal cell carcinoma (xp11.2), epithelioid EHE, GCTs and PEComa (57,366,524,525). ASPS may present in early childhood as other STSs such as ERMS, ARMS, and CIFS. The head and neck region is the preferred site for the presentation of ASPS in younger children whereas the deep soft tissue of the proximal lower extremity (60% to 70%) is the single most common primary site (526–528). There are a number of diverse sites in which ASPS has been documented including the heart, lung, bone, orbit, kidney, retroperitoneum and uterus as a sampling of some of the non–soft tissue primary sites (529). The average age at diagnosis in first two decades is 13 to 15 years and there is a female predilection in most series in contrast to the other STSs in childhood (530). Although the histogenesis of ASPS remains uncertain, it has a non–random unbalanced translocation, der(17)t(x;17)(p11.2;q25), representing the fusion gene, ASPL-TFE3; these same fusion partners are present in the Xp11.2 renal cell carcinoma (nonmelanotic and melanotic types) of childhood (531–535).

Grossly, a circumscribed mass with a grayish to yellowish to hemorrhagic cut surface is the rather nonspecific appearance. The alveolar characterization refers to distinct collections of uniform polygonal cells with eosinophilic to granular cytoplasm surrounding a central nucleus with a variably sized nucleolus, which is surrounded by delicate vascular envelopes like the paraganglioma (Figure 25-99). Larger groups of tumor cells may be separated by dense, hyaline stroma or the overall pattern may be one of sheets of tumor cells without the alveolar architecture. The latter appearance has been seen with some frequency in ASPSs in children in our experience and can be the source of a diagnostic conundrum. Other variations include the presence of more gigantiform rounded or elongated tumor cells in a background of smaller but more typical appearing cells identifiable by routine histology or PAS staining after diastase digestion. Vascular invasion is commonly observed and has a unique pattern of CD31 envelopment of tumor nests. Necrosis, hemorrhage, and an inflammatory infiltrate are other secondary findings. In the presence of a classic alveolar pattern, the diagnosis is reasonably straightforward together with corroborating IHC, which includes reactivity for vimentin, muscle specific actin, and desmin. On the other hand, the only immunoreactivity is for vimentin, which outlines the delicate vascular envelope around groups of tumor cells and tumor cells may or may not be positive. The most specific diagnostic marker is TFE3 nuclear positivity. The differential diagnosis of ASPS includes ARMS, but in most cases, the distinction is made without difficulty given the absence of true organized alveolar pattern, the presence of marked nuclear hyperchromatism, and mitotic activity in the ARMS; these features contrast with those of ASPS. Desmin is diffusely positive in ARMS and only focally so, if at all, in ASPS. If the cells of ASPS have vacuolated cytoplasm and a less than obvious alveolar pattern, diffuse GCT of tendon sheath is worthy of consideration. The PEComa is another neoplasm in the differential diagnosis, but the immunophenotypic profile of PEComa should resolve the problem since TFE3 staining occurs in both neoplasms. The short-term survival is relatively favorable, but ASPS is known for its delayed metastatic behavior to the brain and/or lung with an interval of 5 to 10 years after the original diagnosis. This tumor is an example of a grade 3 sarcoma in the COG grading scheme based on its pathologic type rather than individual pathologic features, which are commonly low grade.

Malignant ectomesenchymoma is a neoplasm of childhood with the composite morphologic and immunophenotypic features of ERMS and a neuroectodermal component (5): neuroblasts with or without rosettes, Schwann cells or ganglion cells in various combinations. These tumors typically occur in infants or young children with a predilection for the perineum and head and neck region that parallels the distribution of ERMS (536,537). Neuroblasts with or without Homer Wright rosettes intermingled in a background of ERMS are the distinctive histologic features (Figure 25-100). As a reflection of the morphology, these tumors are immunoreactive for desmin, myogenin, chromogranin, synaptophysin and CD56. Cytogeneticstudies have demonstrated

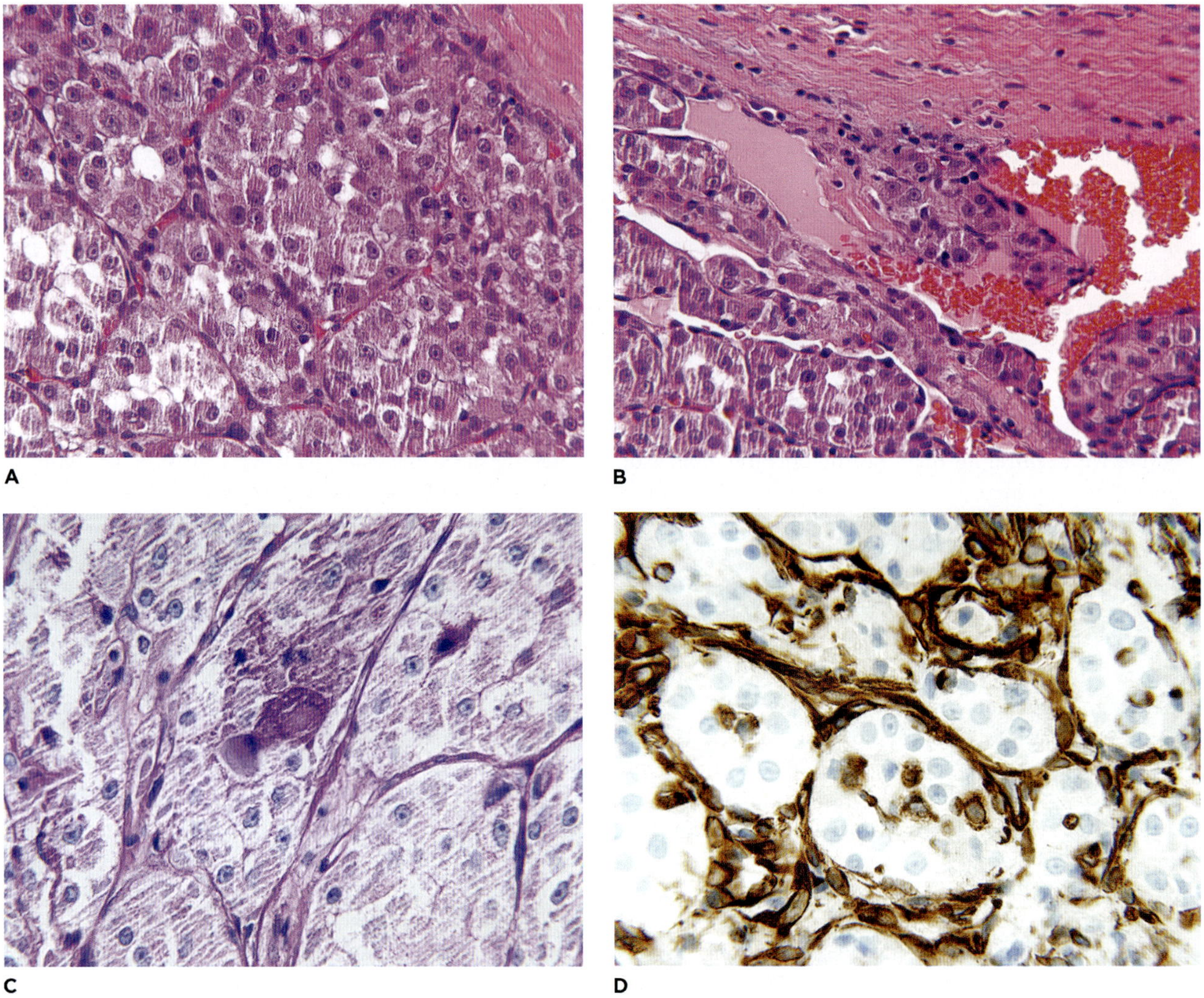

FIGURE 25-99 • ASPS presented as a soft tissue mass in the lower leg of a 9-year-old male. **A:** The circumscribed 7 cm tumor is composed of uniform polygonal cells with prominent nucleoli surrounded by delicate stromal envelopes. **B:** Microvascular invasion is found at the periphery of the tumor. **C:** Pale granular cytoplasmic staining was present in the PAS stain. **D:** Only isolated tumor cells are immunoreactive for vimentin. Note the prominent staining of the stromal envelopes.

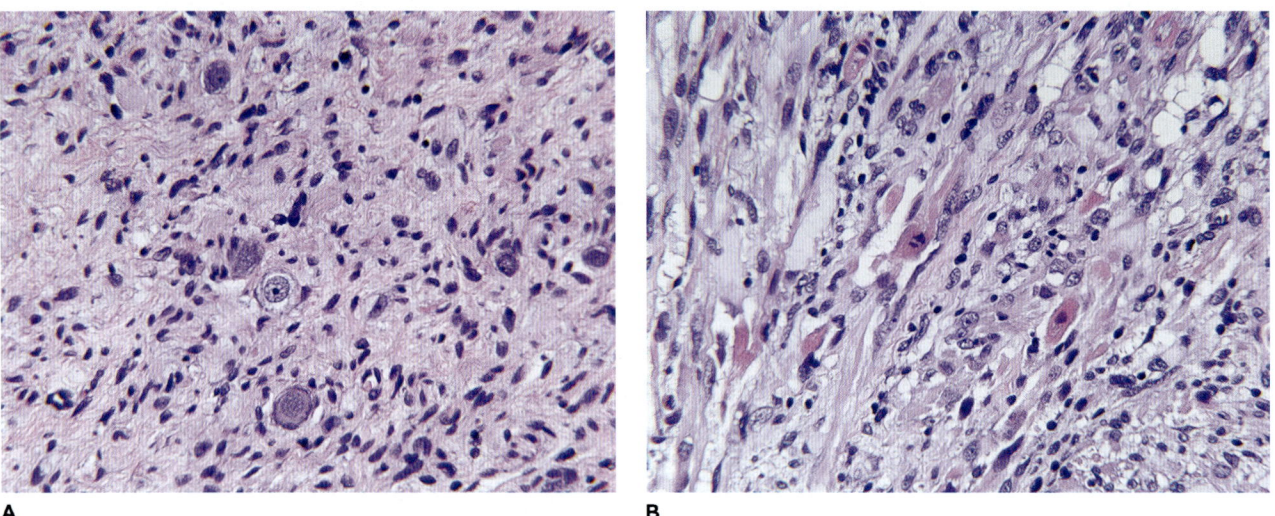

FIGURE 25-100 • Malignant ectomesenchymoma presented as an extratesticular scrotal mass in a 2-year-old boy. **A:** Focal areas of the tumor are composed in part of immature ganglion cells in a background with a neuromatous appearance. **B:** Other foci show an ERMS with differentiated rhabdomyoblasts accompanied by less mature-appearing malignant cells.

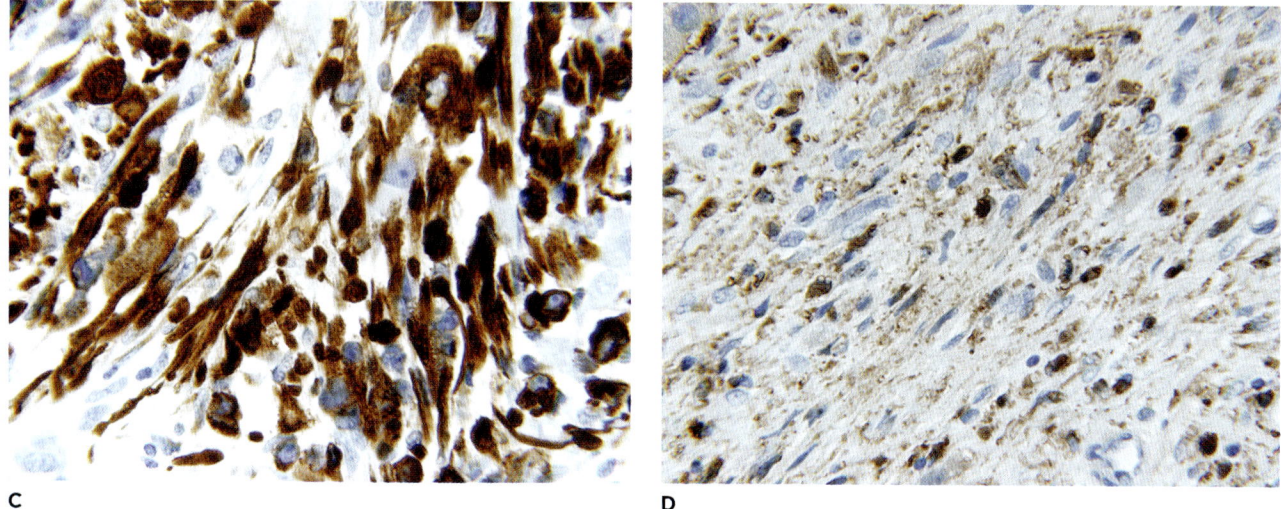

FIGURE 25-100 • (*continued*) **C:** Desmin immunostaining is shown in the rhabdomyosarcomatous areas. **D:** The neuromatous stroma is strongly positive for S100 protein.

some of the same chromosomal numerical abnormalities as ERMS (538).

Sacrococcygeal teratoma (SCT) and those arising in the presacral space or retroperitoneum may be the largest STT proportionately since these neoplasms are usually diagnosed in infancy, if not, as a prenatally discovered mass (539). These tumors are typically in excess of 6 cm and have a soft consistency. The cut surface is often solid and cystic or purely solid with a greyish-white and hemorrhagic appearance in some cases. We have found the surgical margin difficult to access since these tumors often have an indistinct interface with uninvolved soft tissues of which there may be minimal. As a general observation, those tumors whose somatic tissue components are appropriately mature as defined by the appearance of these same tissues in the patient are less likely to have any malignant elements. By contrast, those teratomas with foci of embryo-fetal neural tubules are the ones to be examined carefully for the various patterns of yolk sac tumor (540). The latter foci are recognized by lacy or reticulated, tubular or solid patterns of vacuolated malignant cells which may be surrounded or seemingly suspended in a myxoid to mucoid background (Figure 25-101). These microscopic foci are often multifocal and localized to the most embryo-fetal-like areas of the tumor. Microscopic nodules and gross nodules of tumor are uncommon especially in those teratomas diagnosed and treated before the age of 6 months. Like ovarian and testicular teratomas in prepubertal children, SCT lacks 12p gains, including the i12p (541).

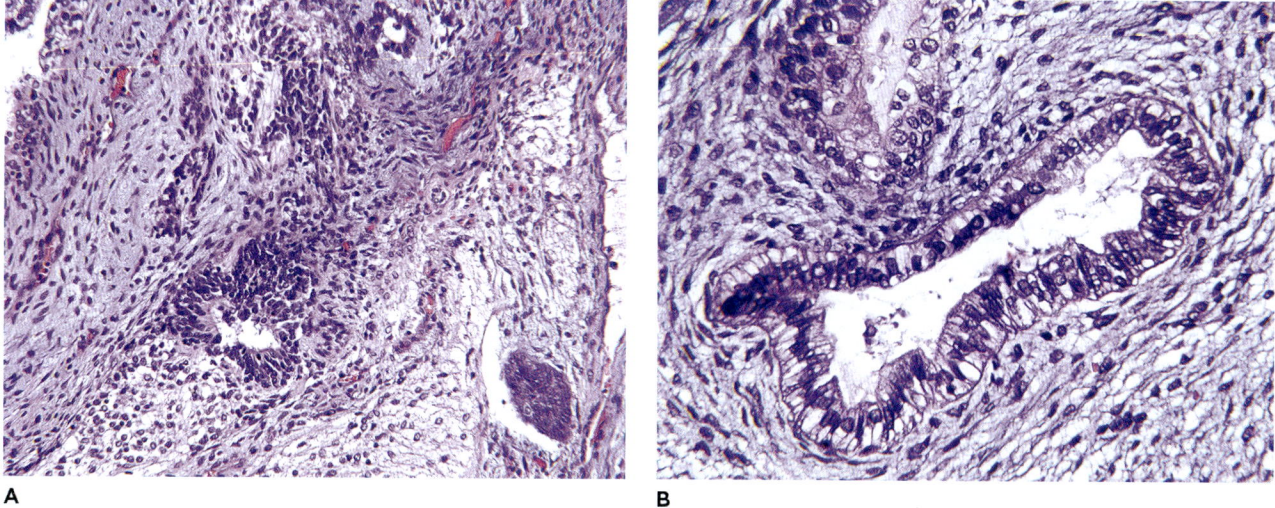

FIGURE 25-101 • Sacrococcygeal teratoma in a 9-day-old female. **A:** Pale myxoid focus with immature neural tube in association with smaller enteric-like profiles. **B:** A focus of yolk sac tumor with enteric-like tubule.

References

1. Bridge JA. The role of cytogenetics and molecular diagnostics in the diagnosis of soft-tissue tumors. *Mod Pathol* 2014;27:S80–S97.
2. Anderson JL, Denny CT, Tap WD, et al. Pediatric sarcomas: translating molecular pathogenesis of disease to novel therapeutic possibilities. *Pediatr Res* 2012;71:112–121.
3. Coffin CM, Alaggio R, Dehner LP. Some general considerations about the clinicopathogic aspects of soft tissue tumors in children and adolescents. *Pediatr Dev Pathol* 2012;15:11–25.
4. Meyer WH, Spunt SL. Soft tissue sarcomas of childhood. *Cancer Treat Rev* 2004;30:269–280.
5. Fletcher CDM, Bridge JA, Hogendorn PCW, et al. *WHO Classification of Tumours*. Lyon, France: Soft Tissue and Bone IARC, 2013.
6. Nishio H. Updates on the cytogenetics and molecular cytogenetics of benign and intermediate soft tissue tumors. *Oncol Lett* 2013;5:12–18.
7. Harms D. Soft tissue malignancies in childhood and adolescence. Pathology and clinical relevance based on data from the Kiel Pediatric Tumor Registry. *Handchir Mikrochir Plast Chir* 2004;36:268–274.
8. Fletcher CD. The evolving classification of soft tissue tumours—an update based on the new 2013 WHO classification. *Histopathology* 2014;63:2–11.
9. Khoury JD, Coffin CM, Sprunt SL, et al. Grading of nonrhabdomyosarcoma soft tissue sarcoma in children and adolescents: a comparison of parameters used for the Federation Nationale des Centers de Lutte Contre le Cancer and Pediatric Oncology Group Systems. *Cancer* 2010;116:2266–2274.
10. Erickson-Johnson MR, Chou MM, Evers BR, et al. Nodular fasciitis: a novel model of transient neoplasia induced by MYH9-USP6 gene fusion. *Lab Invest* 2011;91:1427–1433.
11. Parham DM, Barr FG. Classification of rhabdomyosarcoma and its molecular basis. *Adv Anat Pathol* 2013;20:387–397.
12. Antonescu C. Round cell sarcomas beyond Ewing: emerging entities. *Histopathology* 2014;64:26–37.
13. Bruder E, Alaggio R, Kozakewich HP, et al. Vascular and perivascular lesions of skin and soft tissues in children and adolescents. *Pediatr Dev Pathol* 2012;15:26–61.
14. Thacker MM. Benign soft tissue tumors in children. *Orthop Clin North Am* 2013;44:433–444.
15. Coffin CM, Dehner LP. Soft tissue tumors in first year of life: a report of 190 cases. *Pediatr Pathol* 1990;10:509–526.
16. Mulliken J. Classification of vascular anomalies. In: Mulliken JB, Burrows PE, Fishman SJ. *Mulliken & Young's Vascular Anomalies, Hemangiomas and Malformations*. 2nd ed. Oxford: Oxford University Press, 2013; 2:22–39.
17. Weeden D. *Weeden's Skin Pathology*. 3rd ed. Churchill Livingstone, 2010;888–925.
18. Chiller KG, Passaro D, Frieden IJ. Hemangiomas of infancy: clinical characteristics, morphologic subtypes, and their relationship to race, ethnicity, and sex. *Arch Dermatol* 2002;138: 1567–1576.
19. Fraulin FO, Flannigan RK, Sharma VK, et al. The epidemiological profile of the Vascular Birthmark Clinic at the Alberta Children's Hospital. *Can J Plast Surg* 2012;20:67–70.
20. Munden A, Butschek R, Tom WL, et al. Prospective study of infantile haemangiomas: incidence, clinical characteristics and association with placental anomalies. *Br J Dermatol* 2014;170:907–913.
21. North PE, Waner M, Buckmiller L, et al. Vascular tumors of infancy and childhood: beyond capillary hemangioma. *Cardiovasc Pathol* 2006;15:303–317.
22. Ahrens WA, Ridenour RV 3rd, Caron BL, et al. GLUT-1 expression in mesenchymal tumors: an immunohistochemical study of 247 soft tissue and bone neoplasms. *Hum Pathol* 2008;39:1519–1526.
23. Kollipara R, Dinneen L, Rentas KE, et al. Current classification and terminology of pediatric vascular anomalies. *AJR Am J Roentgenol* 2013;201:1124–1135.
24. Mulliken JB, Bischoff J. Pathogenesis of infantile hemangiomas. In: Mulliken JB, Burrows PE, Fishman SJ, eds. *Mulliken & Young's Vascular Anomalies. Hamangioma and Malformations*, 2nd ed. Oxford: Oxford University Press, 2013:43–67.
25. Ji Y, Chen S, Li K, et al. Signaling pathways in the development of infantile hemangioma. *J Hematol Oncol* 2014;7:13.
26. Boye E, Olsen BR. Signaling mechanisms in infantile hemangioma. *Curr Opin Hematol* 2009;16:202–208.
27. Barnes CM, Christison-Lagay EA, Folkman J. The placenta theory and the origin of infantile hemangioma. *Lymphat Res Biol* 2007;5: 245–255.
28. Lo K, Mihm M, Fay A. Current theories on the pathogenesis of infantile hemangioma. *Semin Ophthalmol* 2009;24:172–177.
29. Spock CL, Tom LK, Canadas K, et al. Infantile hemangiomas exhibit neural crest and pericyte markers. *Ann Plast Surg* 2015;74(2):230–236.
30. Mulliken JB, Diagnosis and natural history of hemangiomas. In: Mulliken JB, Burrows JE, Fishman SJ, eds. *Mulliken and Young's Vascular Anomalies*, 2nd ed. Oxford: Oxford University Press, 2013:68–110.
31. Hemangioma Investigator Group; Haggstrom AN, Drolet BA, et al. Prospective study of infantile hemangiomas: demographic, prenatal, and perinatal characteristics. *J Pediatr* 2007;150;291–294.
32. Horii KA, Drolet BA, Frieden IJ, et al. Prospective study of the frequency of hepatic hemangiomas in infants. *Pediatr Dermatol* 2011;28: 245–253.
33. Mo JQ, Dimashkieh HH, Boye KE. GLUT1 endothelial reactivity distinguishes hepatic infantile hemangioma from congenital hepatic vascular malformation with associated capillary proliferation. *Hum Pathol* 2004;35:200–209.
34. Haggstrom AN, Garzon MC, Baselga E, et al. Risk for PHACE syndrome in infants with large facial hemangiomas. *Pediatrics* 2010;126: e418–e426.
35. Bayer ML, Frommelt PC, Blei F, et al. Congenital cardiac, aortic arch, and vascular bed anomalies in PHACE syndrome (from the International PHACE Syndrome Registry). *Am J Cardiol* 2013;112:1948–1952.
36. Puttgen KB, Lin DD. Neurocutaneous vascular syndromes. *Childs Nerv Syst* 2010;26:1407–1415.
37. Hoeger PH, Colmenero I. Vascular tumours in infants. Part I: benign vascular tumours other than infantile haemangioma. *Br J Dermatol* 2014;171:466–473.
38. Mulliken JB, Enjolras O. Congenital hemangiomas and infantile hemangioma: missing links. *J Am Acad Dermatol* 2004;50:875–882.
39. Krol A, MacArthur CJ. Congenital hemangiomas: rapidly involuting and noninvoluting congenital hemangiomas. *Arch Facial Plast Surg* 2005;7:307–311.
40. Nasseri E, Piram M, McCuaig CC, et al. Partially involuting congenital hemangiomas: a report of 8 cases and review of the literature. *J Am Acad Dermatol* 2014;70:75–79.
41. Berenguer B, Mulliken JB, Enjolras O, et al. Rapidly involuting congenital hemangioma: clinical and histopathologic features. *Pediatr Dev Pathol* 2003;6:495–510.
42. Lee PW, Frieden IJ, Streicher JL, et al. Characteristics of noninvoluting congenital hemangioma: a retrospective review. *J Am Acad Dermatol* 2014;70:899–903.
43. Le Huu AR, Jokinen CH, Rubin BP, et al. Expression of prox1, lymphatic endothelial nuclear transcription factor, in kaposiform hemangioendothelioma and tufted angioma. *Am J Surg Pathol* 2010;34:1563–1573.
44. Picard A, Boscolo E, Khan ZA, et al. IGF-2 and FLT-1/VEGF-R1 mRNA levels reveal distinctions and similarities between congenital and common infantile hemangioma. *Pediatr Res* 2008;63:263–267.
45. Arai E, Kuramochi A, Tsuchida T, et al. Usefulness of D2-40 immunohistochemistry for differentiation between kaposiform hemangioendothelioma and tufted angioma. *J Cutan Pathol* 2006;33:492–497.
46. Drolet BA, Trenor CC III, Brandao LR, et al. Consensus-derived practice standards plan for complicated kaposiform hemangioendothelioma. *J Pediatr* 2013;163:285–291.
47. Croteau SE, Liang MK, Kozakewich HP, et al. Kaposiform hemangioendothelioma: atypical features and risks of Kasabach-Merritt phenomenon in 107 referrals. *J Pediatr* 2013;162:142–147.
48. Osio A, Fraitag S, Hadj-Rabia S, et al. Clinical spectrum of tufted angiomas in childhood: a report of 13 cases and a review of the literature. *Arch Dermatol* 2010;146:758–763.
49. Herron MD, Coffin CM, Vanderhooft SL. Tufted angiomas: variability of the clinical morphology. *Pediatr Dermatol* 2002;19:394–401.

50. Croteau SE, Kozakewich HP, Perez-Atayde AR, et al. Kaposiform lymphangiomatosis: a distinct aggressive lymphatic anomaly. *J Pediatr* 2014;164:383–388.
51. Shevchenko L, Aaberg T Jr, Grossniklaus HE. Conjunctival angiolymphoid hyperplasia with eosinophilia in a child. *J Pediatr Ophthalmol Strabismus* 2012;49:e66–e69.
52. Park J, Hwang SR, Song KH, et al. Angiolymphoid hyperplasia with eosinophilia affecting the scrotum of a child. *Eur J Dermatol* 2013;23:423–424.
53. Zarrin-Khameh N, Spoden JE, Tran RM. Angiolymphoid hyperplasia with eosinophilia associated with pregnancy: a case report and review of the literature. *Arch Pathol Lab Med* 2005;129:1168–1171.
54. Abrahim MJ, Gregory ND, Chennupati SK. Epithelioid hemangioma of the internal carotid artery: a case report supporting the reactive pathogenesis hypothesis of this vascular tumor. *Int J Pediatr Otorhinolaryngol* 2014;78:1186–1189.
55. Mehrabi A, Kashfi A, Fonouni H, et al. Primary malignant hepatic epithelioid hemangioendothemioma: a comprehensive review of the literature with emphasis on the surgical therapy. *Cancer* 2006;107:2108–2121.
56. Guiteau JJ, Cotton RT, Karpen SJ, et al. Pediatric liver transplantation for primary malignant liver tumors with a focus on hepatic epithelioid hemangioendothelioma: the UNOS experience. *Pediatr Transplant* 2010;14:326–331.
57. Antonescu CR, Le Loarer F, Mosquera JM, et al. Novel YAP1-TFE3 fusion defines a distinct subset of epithelioid hemangioendothelioma. *Genes Chromosomes Cancer* 2013;52:775–784.
58. Sangueza OP, Walsh SN, Sheehan DJ, et al. Cutaneous epithelioid angiomatous nodule: a case series and proposed classification. *Am J Dermatopathol* 2008;30:16–20.
59. Brenn T, Fletcher CD. Cutaneous epithelioid angiomatous nodule: a distinct lesion in the morphologic spectrum of epithelioid vascular tumors. *Am J Dermatopathol* 2004;26:14–21.
60. Goh SG, Calonje E. Cutaneous vascular tumours: an update. *Histopathology* 2008;52:661–673.
61. Billings, SD, Folpe AL, Weiss SW. Epithelioid sarcoma-like hemangioendothelioma. *Am J Surg Pathol* 2003;27:48–57.
62. Billings SD, Folpe AL, Weiss SW. Epithelioid sarcoma-like hemangioendothelioma (pseudomyogenic hemangioendothelioma). *Am J Surg Pathol* 2011;35:1088.
63. Hornick JL, Fletcher CD. Pseudomyogenic hemangioendothelioma: a distinctive, often multicentric tumor with indolent behavior. *Am J Surg Pathol* 2011;35:190–201.
64. Walther C, Tayebwa J, Lilljebjorn H, et al. A novel SERPINE1-FOSB fusion gene results in transcriptional up-regulation of FOSB in pesudomyogenic haemangioendothelioma. *J Pathol* 2014;232:534–540.
65. Bien E, Kazanowska B, Dantonello T, et al. Factors predicting survival in childhood malignant and intermediate vascular tumors: retrospective analysis of the Polish and German cooperative paediatric soft tissue sarcoma study groups and review of the literature. *Ann Surg Oncol* 2010;17:1878–1889.
66. Ackermann O, Fabre M, Franchi S, et al. Widening spectrum of liver angiosarcoma in children. *J Pediatr Gastroenterol Nutr* 2011;53:615–619.
67. Albertini AF, Brousse N, Bodemer C, et al. Retiform hemangioendothelioma developed on the site of an earlier cystic lymphangioma in a six-year-old girl. *Am J Dermatopathol* 2011;33:e84–e87.
68. Sanz-Trelles A, Rodrigo-Fernandez I, Ayala-Carbonero A, et al. Retiform hemangioendothelioma. A new case in a child with diffuse endovascular papillary endothelial proliferation. *J Cutan Pathol* 1997;24:440–444.
69. Fanburg-Smith JC, Michal M, Partanen TA, et al. Papillary intralymphatic angioendothelioma (PILA): a report of twelve cases of a distinctive vascular tumor with phenotypic features of lymphatic vessels. *Am J Surg Pathol* 1999;23:1004–1010.
70. Reis-Filho JS, Paiva ME, Lopes JM. Congenital composite hemangioendothelioma: case report and reappraisal of the hemangioendothelioma spectrum. *J Cutan Pathol* 2001;29:226–231.
71. McNab PM, Quigley BC, Glass LF, et al. Composite hemangioendothelioma and its classification as a low-grade malignancy. *Am J Dermatopathol* 2013;35:517–522.
72. Fukunaga M, Suzuki K, Saegusa N, et al. Composite hemangioendothelioma: report of 5 cases including one with associated Maffucci syndrome. *Am J Surg Pathol* 2007;31:1567–1572.
73. Tadros M, Rizk SS, Opher E, et al. Polymorphous hemangioendothelioma of the neck. *Ann Diagn Pathol* 2003;7:165–168.
74. Perkins P, Weiss SW. Spindle cell hemangioendothelioma. An analysis of 78 cases with reassessment of its pathogenesis and biologic behavior. *Am J Surg Pathol* 1996;20:1196–1204.
75. Pansuriya TC, van Eijk R, d'Adamo P, et al. Somatic mosaic IDH1 and IDH2 mutations are associated with enchondroma and spindle cell hemangioma in Ollier disease and Maffucci syndrome. *Nat Genet* 2011;43:1256–1261.
76. Kurek KC, Pansuriya TC, van Ruler MA, et al. R132C IDH1 mutations are found in spindle cell hemangiomas and not in other vascular tumors or malformations. *Am J Pathol* 2013;182:1494–1500.
77. Radu O, Pantanowitz L. Kaposi sarcoma. *Arch Pathol Lab Med* 2013;137:289–294.
78. Arkin LM, Cox CM, Kovarik CL. Kaposi's sarcoma in the pediatric population: the critical need for a tissue diagnosis. *Pediatr Infect Dis J* 2009;28:426–428.
79. Godfraind C, Calicchio ML, Kozakewich H. Pyogenic granuloma, an impaired wound healing process, linked to vascular growth driven by FLT4 and the nitric oxide pathway. *Mod Pathol* 2013;26:247–255.
80. Zarraga M, Rosen L, Herschthal D. Bacillary angiomatosis in an immunocompetent child: a case report and review of the literature. *Am J Dermatopathol* 2011;33:513–515.
81. Rostad CA, McElroy AK, Hilinski JA, et al. Bartonella henselae-mediated disease in solid organ transplant recipients: two pediatric cases and a literature review. *Transpl Infect Dis* 2012;14:E71–E81.
82. Mulligan PR, Prajapati HJ, Martin LG, et al. Vascular anomalies: classification, imaging characteristics and implications for interventional radiology treatment approaches. *Br J Radiol* 2014;87:20130392.
83. Garzon MC, Huang JT, Enjolras O, et al. Vascular malformations: part I. *J Am Acad Dermatol* 2007;56:353–370.
84. Garzon MC, Huang JT, Enjolras O, et al. Vascular malformations: part II. *J Am Acad Dermatol* 2007;56:541–564.
85. Giordano P, Lenato GM, Suppressa P, et al. Hereditary hemorrhagic telangiectasia: arteriovenous malformations in children. *J Pediatr* 2013;163:179–186.
86. Martinez-Glez V, Romanelli V, Mori MA, et al. Macrocephaly-capillary malformations: analysis of 13 patients and review of the diagnostic criteria. *Am J Med Genet A* 2010;152A:3101–3106.
87. Kurek KC, Howard E, Tennant LB, et al. PTEN hamartoma of soft tissue: a distinctive lesion in PTEN syndromes. *Am J Surg Pathol* 2012;36:671–687.
88. Richert B, Lecerf P, Caucanas M, et al. Nail tumors. *Clin Dermatol* 2013;31:602–617.
89. Boon LM, Vikkula M. Molecular genetics of vascular malformations. In: Mulliken JB, Burrows PE, Fishman SJ. *Mulliken & Young's Vascular Anomalies, Hemangiomas and Malformations*, 2nd ed. Oxford: Oxford University Press, 2013;9:327–375.
90. Kaye VM, Dehner LP. Cutaneous glomus tumor. A comparative immunohistochemical study with pseudoangiomatous intradermal melanocytic nevi. *Am J Dermatopathol* 1991;13:2–6.
91. Hinz B, Phan SH, Thannickal VJ, et al. Recent developments in myofibroblast biology: paradigms for connective tissue remodeling. *Am J Pathol* 2012;180:1340–1355.
92. Hu B, Phan SH. Myofibroblasts. *Curr Opin Rheumatol* 2013;25:71–77.
93. Slemp AE, Kirschner RE. Keloids and scars: a review of keloids and scars, their pathogenesis, risk factors, and management. *Curr Opin Pediatr* 2006;18:396–402.
94. Seifert O, Mrowietz U. Keloid scarring: bench and bedside. *Arch Dermatol Res* 2009;301:259–272.
95. Profyris C, Tziotzios C, Do Vale I. Cutaneous scarring: pathophysiology, molecular mechanisms, and scar reduction therapeutics part I. The molecular basis of scar formation. *J Am Acad Dermatol* 2012;66:1–10.
96. Tziotzios C, Profyris C, Sterling J. Cutaneous scarring: pathophysiology, molecular mechanisms, and scar reduction therapeutics part II.

Strategies to reduce scar formation after dermatologic procedures. *J Am Acad Dermatol* 2012;66:13–24.
97. Abdou AG, Maraee AH, Saif HF. Immunohistochemical evaluation of COX-1 and COX-2 expression in keloid and hypertrophic scar. *Am J Dermatopathol* 2014;36:311–317.
98. Rosenberg AE. Pseudosarcomas of soft tissue. *Arch Pathol Lab Med* 2008;132:579–586.
99. Pandian TK, Zeidan MM, Ibrahim KA, et al. Nodular fasciitis in the pediatric population: a single center experience. *J Pediatr Surg* 2013;48:1486–1489.
100. Rakheja D, Cunningham JC, Mitui M, et al. A subset of cranial fasciitis is associated with dysregulation of the Wnt/beta-catenin pathway. *Mod Pathol* 2008;21:1330–1336.
101. Gibson TC, Bishop JA, Thompson LD. Parotid gland nodular fasciitis: a clinicopathologic series of 12 cases with a review of 18 cases from the literature. *Head Neck Pathol* 2014;Dec 4 [epub ahead of print].
102. Gans I, Morrison MJ 3rd, Chikwava KR, et al. Intra-articular nodular fasciitis of the knee in a pediatric patient. *Orthopedics* 2014;37:e313–e316.
103. Oliveira AM, Chou MM. USP6-induced neoplasms: the biologic spectrum of aneurysmal bone cyst and nodular fasciitis. *Hum Pathol* 2014;45:1–11.
104. Meis JM, Enzinger FM. Proliferative fasciitis and myositis of childhood. *Am J Surg Pathol* 1992;16:364–372.
105. Rosa G, Billings SD. A report of three cases of pediatric proliferative fasciitis. *J Cutan Pathol* 2014;41(9):720–723.
106. Micheli A, Trapani S, Brizzi I, et al. Myositis ossificans circumscripta: a paediatric case and review of the literature. *Eur J Pediatr* 2009;168:523–529.
107. de Silva MV, Reid R. Myositis ossificans and fibroosseous pseudotumor of digits: a clinicopathological review of 64 cases with emphasis on diagnostic pitfalls. *Int J Surg Pathol* 2003;11: 187–195.
108. Pignolo RJ, Shore EM, Kaplan FS. Fibrodysplasia ossificans progressive: diagnosis, management, and therapeutic horizons. *Pediatr Endocrinol Rev* 2013;10:437–448.
109. Coffin CM, Alaggio R. Fibroblastic and myofibroblastic tumors in children and adolescents. *Pediatr Dev Pathol* 2012;15(1 Suppl):127–180.
110. Coffin CM, Davis JL, Borinstein SC. Syndrome-associated soft tissue tumours. *Histopathology* 2014;64:68–87.
111. Stanford D, Rogers M. Dermatological presentations of infantile myofibromatosis: a review of 27 cases. *Australas J Dermatol* 2000;41:156–161.
112. Alaggio R, Barisani D, Ninfo V, et al. Morphologic overlap between infantile myofibromatosis and infantile fibrosarcoma: a pitfall in diagnosis. *Pediatr Dev Pathol* 2008;11:355–362.
113. Cai C, Dehner LP, El-Mofty SK. In myofibroblastic sarcomas of the head and neck, mitotic activity and necrosis define grade: a case study and literature review. *Virchows Arch* 2013;463(6):827–836.
114. Eyden B, Banerjee SS, Shenjere P, et al. The myofibroblast and its tumours. *J Clin Pathol* 2009;62:236–249.
115. Mentzel T, Dei Tos AP, Sapi Z, et al. Myopericytoma of skin and soft tissues: clinicopathologic and immunohistochemical study of 54 cases. *Am J Surg Pathol* 2006;30:104–113.
116. Wu WW, Chu JT, Romansky SG, et al. Pediatric renal solitary fibrous tumor: report of a rare case and review of the literature. *Int J Surg Pathol* 2015;23(1):34–47.
117. Wang H, Shen D, Hou Y. Malignant solitary tumor in a child: a case report and review of the literature. *J Pediatr Surg* 2011;46:e5–e9.
118. Gengler C, Guillou L. Solitary fibrous tumour and haemangiopericytoma: evolution of a concept. *Histopathology* 2006;48:63–74.
119. Fisher C. Low-grade sarcomas with CD34-positive fibroblasts and low-grade myofibroblastic sarcomas. *Ultrastruct Pathol* 2004;28:291–305.
120. Doyle LA, Vivero M, Fletcher CD, et al. Nuclear expression of STAT6 distinguishes solitary fibrous tumor from histologic mimics. *Mod Pathol* 2014;27:390–395.
121. Goldblum JR, Folpe AL, Weiss SW. *Enzinger and Weiss's Soft Tissue Tumors*, 6th ed. Philadelphia, PA: Mosby Elsevier, 2014;256–287.
122. Fetsch JF, Miettinen M, Laskin WB, et al. A clinicopathologic study of 45 pediatric soft tissue tumors with an admixture of adipose tissue and fibroblastic elements, and a proposal for classification as lipofibromatosis. *Am J Surg Pathol* 2000;24:1491–1500.
123. Coffin CM, Dehner LP. Fibroblastic-myofibroblastic tumors in children and adolescents: a clinicopathologic study of 108 examples in 103 patients. *Pediatr Pathol* 1991;11:569–588.
124. Carretto E, Dall'Igna P, Alaggio R, et al. Fibrous hamartoma of infancy: an Italian multi-institutional experience. *J Am Acad Dermatol* 2006;54:800–803.
125. Saab ST, McClain CM, Coffin CM. Fibrous hamartoma of infancy: a clinicopathologic analysis of 60 cases. *Am J Surg Pathol* 2014;38:394–401.
126. Monajemzadeh M, Vasei M, Kalantari M, et al. Vulvar fibrous hamartoma of infancy: a rare case report and review of literature. *J Low Genit Tract Dis* 2013;17:92–94.
127. Grynspan D, Meir K, Senger C, et al. Cutaneous changes in fibrous hamartoma of infancy. *J Cutan Pathol* 2007;34:39–43.
128. Laskin WB, Miettinen M, Fetsch JF. Infantile digital fibroma/fibromatosis. A clinicopathologic and immunohistochemical study of 69 tumors from 57 patients with long-term follow-up. *Am J Surg Pathol* 2009;33:1–13.
129. Grenier N, Liang C, Capaldi L, et al. A range of histologic findings in infantile digital fibromatosis. *Pediatr Dermatol* 2008;25:72–75.
130. Dey D, Nicol A, Singer S. Benign phyllodes tumor of the breast with intracytoplasmic inclusion bodies identical to infantile digital fibromatosis. *Breast J* 2008;14:198–199.
131. Girgenti V, Restano L, Arcangeli F, et al. Infantile digital fibromatosis: a rare tumour of infancy. Report of five cases. *Australas J Dermatol* 2012;53:285–287.
132. Niamba P, Leaute-Labreze C, Boralevi F, et al. Further documentation of spontaneous regression of infantile digital fibromatosis. *Pediatr Dermatol* 2007;24:280–284.
133. Tardop KC, Azprom D, Jermamdez-Nunez A, et al. Dermatomyofibromas presenting in pediatric patients: clinicopathologic characteristics and differential diagnosis. *J Cutan Pathol* 2011;38:967–972.
134. Mentzel T, Kutzner H. Dermatomyofibroma: clinicopathologic and immunohistochemical analysis of 56 cases and reappraisal of a rare and distinct cutaneous neoplasm. *Am J Dermatopathol* 2009;31: 44–49.
135. deFeraudy S, Fletcher CD. Fibroblastic connective tissue nevus: a rare cutaneous lesion analyzed in a series of 25 cases. *Am J Surg Pathol* 2012;36:1509–1515.
136. Buitendijk S, van de Ven CP, Dumans TG, et al. Pediatric aggressive fibromatosis: a retrospective analysis of 13 patients and review of the literature. *Cancer* 2005;104:1090–1099.
137. Soto-Miranda MA, Sandoval JA, Rao B, et al. Surgical treatment of pediatric desmoid tumors. A 12-year, single-center experience. *Ann Surg Oncol* 2013;20:3387–3390.
138. Half E, Bercovich D, Rozen P. Familial adenomatous polyposis. *Orphanet J Rare Dis* 2009;12:22.
139. Bhattacharya B, Dilworth HP, Iacobuzio-Donahue C, et al. Nuclear beta-catenin expression distinguishes deep fibromatosis from other benign and malignant fibroblastic and myofibroblastic lesions. *Am J Surg Pathol* 2005;29:653–659.
140. Carlson JW, Fletcher CDM. Immunohistochemistry for beta-catenin in the differential diagnosis of spindle cell lesions: analysis of a series and review of the literature. *Histopathology* 2007;51:509–514.
141. Mullen JT, DeLaney TF, Rosenberg AE, et al. β-Catenin mutation status and outcomes in sporadic desmoid tumors. *Oncologist* 2013; 18:1043–1049.
142. Colombo C, Miceli R, Lazar AJ, et al. CTNNB1 45F mutation is a molecular prognosticator of increased postoperative primary desmoid tumor recurrence: an independent, multicenter validation study. *Cancer* 2013;119:3696–3702.
143. Devata S, Chugh R. Desmoid tumors: a comprehensive review of the evolving biology, unpredictable behavior and myriad of management options. *Hematol Oncol Clin North Am* 2013;27:989–1005.
144. Woltsche N, Gilg MM, Frassler L, et al. Is wide resection obsolete for desmoid tumors in children and adolescents? Evaluation of histological margins, immunohistochemical markers and review of literature. *Pediatr Hematol Oncol* 2015;32:60–69.

145. Briand S, Barbier O, Biau D, et al. Wait-and-see policy as a first-line management for extra-abdominal desmoid tumors. *J Bone Joint Surg Am* 2014;96:631–638.
146. Oudot C, Defachelles AS, Minard-Colin V, et al. [Desmoid tumors in children: current strategy]. *Bull Cancer* 2013;5:518–528.
147. Michal M, Fetsch JF, Hes O, et al. Nuchal-type fibroma: a clinicopathologic study of 52 cases. *Cancer* 1999;85:156–163.
148. Coffin CM, Hornick JL, Zhou H, et al. Gardner fibroma: a clinicopathologic and immunohistochemical analysis of 45 patients with 57 fibromas. *Am J Surg Pathol* 2007;31:410–416.
149. Fetsch JF, Laskin WB, Miettinen M. Palmar-plantar fibromatosis in children and preadolescents. A clinicopathologic study of 56 cases with newly recognized demographics and extended follow-up information. *Am J Surg Pathol* 2005;29:1095–1105.
150. Lindvall LE, Kormeili T, Chen E, et al. Infantile systemic hyalinosis: case report and review of the literature. *J Am Acad Dermatol* 2008;58:303–307.
151. Deuquet J, Lausch E, Superti-Furga A, et al. The dark sides of capillary morphogenesis gene 2. *EMBO J* 2012;31:3–13.
152. Blount A, Riley KO, Woodworth BA. Juvenile nasopharyngeal angiofibroma. *Otolaryngol Clin North Am* 2011;44:989–1004.
153. Ponti G, Losi L, Pellacani G, et al. Wnt pathway, angiogenetic and hormonal markers in sporadic and familial adenomatous polyposis-associated juvenile nasopharyngeal angiofibromas (JNA). *Appl Immunohistochem Mol Morphol* 2008;16:173–178.
154. Maniglia MP, Ribeiro ME, Costa NM, et al. Molecular pathogenesis of juvenile nasopharyngeal angiofibroma in Brazilian patients. *Pediatr Hematol Oncol* 2013;30:616–622.
155. Boghani Z, Husain Q, Kanumuri VV, et al. Juvenile nasopharyngeal angiofibroma: a systematic review and comparison of endoscopic, endoscopic-assisted and open resection in 1047 cases. *Laryngoscope* 2013;123:859–869.
156. Skelton E, Howlett D. Fibromatosis colli: the sternocleidomastoid pseudotumour of infancy. *J Paediatr Child Health* 2014;50:833–835.
157. Cao KX, Rosenberg AE, Hakim J, et al. Axillary calcifying fibrous tumor (CFT) in an 8 year old girl. *J Pediatr Surg* 2012;47:2341–2344.
158. Nascimento AF, Ruiz R, Hornick JL, et al. Calcifying fibrous 'pseudotumor': clinicopathologic study of 15 cases and analysis of its relationship to inflammatory myofibroblastic tumor. *Int J Surg Pathol* 2002;10:189–196.
159. Sigel JE, Smith TA, Reith JD, et al. Immunohistochemical analysis of anaplastic lymphoma kinase expression in deep soft tissue calcifying fibrous pseudotumor: evidence of a late sclerosing stage of inflammatory myofibroblastic tumor? *Ann Diagn Pathol* 2001;5:10–14.
160. Hill KA, Gonzalez-Crussi F, Omeroglu A, et al. Calcifying fibrous pseudotumor involving the neck of a five-week-old infant. Presence of factor XIIIa in the lesional cells. *Pathol Res Pract* 2000;196:527–531.
161. Gleason BC, Hornick JL. Inflammatory myofibroblastic tumours: where are we now? *J Clin Pathol* 2008;61:428–437.
162. Morotti RA, Legman MD, Kerkar N, et al. Pediatric inflammatory myofibroblastic tumor with late metastasis to the lung: case report and review of the literature. *Pediatr Dev Pathol* 2005;8:224–229.
163. Dishop MK, Kuruvilla S. Primary and metastatic lung tumors in the pediatric population: a review and 25-year experience at a large children's hospital. *Arch Pathol Lab Med* 2008;132:1079–1103.
164. Yu DC, Grabowski MJ, Kazakewich HP, et al. Primary lung tumors in children and adolescents: a 90-year experience. *J Pediatri Surg* 2010;45:1090–1095.
165. Coffin CM, Hornick JL, Fletcher CDM. Inflammatory myofibroblastic tumor: comparison of clinicopathologic, histologic and immunohistochemical features including ALK expression in atypical and aggressive cases. *Am J Surg Pathol* 2007;31:509–520.
166. Marino-Enriquez A, Wang WL, Roy A, et al. Epithelioid inflammatory myofibroblastic sarcoma: an aggressive intra-abdominal variant of inflammatory myofibroblastic tumor with nuclear membrane or perinuclear ALK. *Am J Surg Pathol* 2011;35:135–144.
167. Yamamoto H, Yamaguchi H, Aishima S, et al. Inflammatory myofibroblastic tumor versus IgG4-related sclerosing disease and inflammatory pseudotumor: a comparative clinicopathologic study. *Am J Surg Pathol* 2009;33:1330–1340.
168. Minoo P, Wang HY. ALK-immunoreactive neoplasms. *Int J Clin Exp Pathol* 2012;5:397–410.
169. Hornick JL, Sholl LM, Dal Cin P, et al. Expression of ROS1 gene rearrangement in inflammatory myofibroblastic tumors. *Mod Pathol* 2015;28:732–739.
170. Weiss VL, Antonescu CR, Alaggio R, et al. Myxoinflammatory fibroblastic sarcoma in children and adolescents: clinicopathologic aspects of a rare neoplasm. *Pediatr Dev Pathol* 2013;16:425–431.
171. Laskin WB, Fetsch JF, Miettinen M. Myxoinflammatory fibroblastic sarcoma: a clinicopathologic analysis of 104 cases, with emphasis on predictors of outcome. *Am J Surg Pathol* 2014;38:1–2.
172. Folpe AL. Fibrosarcoma: a review and update. *Histopathology* 2014;64:12–25.
173. Rizkalla H, Wildgrove H, Quinn F, et al. Congenital fibrosarcoma of the ileum: case report with molecular confirmation and literature review. *Fetal Pediatr Pathol* 2011;30:329–337.
174. Steelman C, Katzenstein H, Parham D, et al. Unusual presentation of congenital infantile fibrosarcoma in seven infants with molecular-genetic analysis. *Fetal Pediatr Pathol* 2011;30:329–337.
175. Gadd S, Beezhold P, Jennings L, et al. Mediators of receptor tyrosine kinase activation in infantile fibrosarcoma: a Children's Oncology Group study. *J Pathol* 2012;228:119–130.
176. Alaggio R, Barisani D, Ninfo V, et al. Morphologic overlap between infantile myofibromatosis and infantile fibrosarcoma: a pitfall in diagnosis. *Pediatr Dev Pathol* 2008;44:355–362.
177. Linos K, Carter JM, Gardner JM, et al. Myofibromas with atypical features: expanding the morphologic spectrum of a benign entity. *Am J Surg Pathol* 2014;38:1649–1654.
178. Calvo-Garcia MA, Lim, FY, Stanek J, et al. Congenital peribronchial myofibroblastic tumor: prenatal imaging clues to differentiate from other fetal chest lesions. *Pediatr Radiol* 2014;44:479–483.
179. Cipriani NA, Ryan DP, Nielsen GP. Primitive myxoid mesenchymal tumor of infancy with rosettes: a new finding and literature review. *Int J Surg Pathol* 2014;22:647–651.
180. Alaggio R, Ninfo V, Rosolen A, et al. Primitive myxoid mesenchymal tumor of infancy: a clinicopathologic report of 6 cases. *Am J Surg Pathol* 2006; 30:388–394.
181. Guilbert M, Rougemont A, Samson Y, et al. Transformation of a primitive myxoid mesenchymal tumor of infancy to an undifferentiated sarcoma: a first reported case. *J Pediatr Hematol Oncol* 2015;37:e118–e120.
182. Folpe AL, Lane KL, Paull G, et al. Low-grade fibromyxoid sarcoma and hyalinizing spindle cell tumor with giant rosettes. A clinicopathologic study of 73 cases supporting their identity and assessing the impact of high-grade areas. *Am J Surg Pathol* 2000;24:1353–1360.
183. Oda Y, Takahira T, Kawaguchi K, et al. Low-grade fibromyxoid sarcoma versus low-grade myxofibrosarcoma in the extremities and trunk. A comparison of clinicopathological and immunohistochemical features. *Histopathology* 2004;45:29–38.
184. Vernon SE, Bejarano PA. Low-grade fibromyxoid sarcoma: a brief review. *Arch Pathol Lab Med* 2006;130:1358–1360.
185. Doyle LA, Moller E, Dal Cin P, et al. MUC4 is a highly sensitive and specific marker for low-grade fibromyxoid sarcoma. *Am J Surg Pathol* 2011;35:733–741.
186. Lau PP, Lui PC, Lau GT, et al. EWSR1-CREB3L1 gene fusion: a novel alternative molecular aberration of low-grade fibromyxoid sarcoma. *Am J Surg Pathol* 2013;37:734–738.
187. Ossendorf C, Studer GM, Bode B, et al. Sclerosing epithelioid fibrosarcoma: case presentation and a systematic review. *Clin Orthop Relat Res* 2008;466:1485–1491.
188. Wojcik JB, Bellizzi AM, Dal Cin P, et al. Primary sclerosing epithelioid fibrosarcoma of bone: analysis of a series. *Am J Surg Pathol* 2014;38:1538–1544.
189. Doyle LA, Wang WL, Dal Cin P, et al. MUC4 is a sensitive and extremely useful marker for sclerosing epithelioid fibrosarcoma: association with FUS gene rearrangement. *Am J Surg Pathol* 2012;36:1444–1451.

190. Arbajian E, Puls F, Magnusson L, et al. Recurrent FrEWSR1-CREB3L1 gene fusions in sclerosing epithelioid fibrosarcoma. *Am J Surg Pathol* 2014;38:801–808.
191. Guillou L, Benhattar J, Gengler C, et al. Translocation-positive low-grade fibromyxoid sarcoma: clinicopathologic and molecular analysis of a series expanding the morphologic spectrum and suggestion potential relationship to sclerosing epithelioid fibrosarcoma: a study from the French Sarcoma Group. *Am J Surg Pathol* 2007;31:1387–1402.
192. Kuzel P, Metelitsa AI, Dover DC, et al. Epidemiology of dermatofibrosarcoma protuberans in Alberta, Canada, from 1988 to 2007. *Dermatol Surg* 2012;38:1461–1468.
193. Tsai YJ, Lin PY, Chew KY, et al. Dermatofibrosarcoma protuberans in children and adolescents: clinical presentation, histology, treatment, and review of the literature. *J Plast Reconstr Aesthet Surg* 2014;67:1222–1229.
194. Jha P, Moosavi C, Fanburg-Smith JC. Giant cell fibroblastoma: an update and addition of 86 new cases from the Armed Forces Institute of Pathology, in honor of Dr. Franz M. Enzinger. *Ann Diagn Pathol* 2007;11:81–88.
195. Llombart B, Serra-Guillen C, Monteagudo C, et al. Dermatofibrosarcoma protuberans: a comprehensive review and update on diagnosis and management. *Semin Diagn Pathol* 2013;30:13–28.
196. Gerlini G, Mariotti G, Urso C, et al. Dermatofibrosarcoma protuberans in childhood: two case reports and review of the literature. *Pediatr Hematol Oncol* 2008;25:559–566.
197. Lee DW, Yang JH, Won CH, et al. A case of congenital pigmented dermatofibrosarcoma protuberans (Bednar tumor) in a patient with Fanconi anemia. *Pediatr Dermatol* 2011;28:583–585.
198. Kesserwan C, Sokolic R, Cowen EW, et al. Multicentric dermatofibrosarcoma protuberans in patients with adenosine deaminase-deficient severe combined immune deficiency. *J Allergy Clin Immunol* 2012;129:762–769.
199. Kumar R, Rodriguez V, Khan SP, et al. Postradiation dermatofibrosarcoma protuberans in a patient with Wilms tumor. *J Pediatr Hematol Oncol* 2011;33:635–636.
200. King L, Lopez-Terrada D, Jakacky J, et al. Primary intrathoracic dermatofibrosarcoma protuberans. *Am J Surg Pathol* 2012;36:1897–1902.
201. Liang CA, Jambusaria-Pahlajani A, Karia PS, et al. A systematic review of outcome data for dermatofibrosarcoma protuberans with and without fibrosarcomatous change. *J Am Acad Dermatol* 2014;71:781–786.
202. Reis-Filho JS, Milanezi F, Ferro J, et al. Pediatric pigmented dermatofibrosarcoma protuberans (Bednar tumor): case report and review of the literature with emphasis on the differential diagnosis. *Pathol Res Pract* 2002;198:621–626.
203. Tardio JC. CD34-reactive tumors of the skin. An updated review of an ever-growing list of lesions. *J Cutan Pathol* 2009;36:89–102.
204. Kutzner H, Mentzel T, Palmedo G, et al. Plaque-like CD34-positive dermal fibroma ("medallion-like dermal dendrocyte hamartoma"): clinicopathologic, immunohistochemical, and molecular analysis of 5 cases emphasizing its distinction from superficial, plaque-like dermatofibrosarcoma protuberans. *Am J Surg Pathol* 2010;34:190–221.
205. Carter JM, Weiss SW, Linos K, et al. Superficial CD34-positive fibroblastic tumor: report of 18 cases of a distinctive low-grade mesenchymal neoplasm of intermediate (borderline) malignancy. *Mod Pathol* 2014;27:294–302.
206. Rakheja D, Wiulson KS, Meehan JJ, et al. Extrapleural benign solitary fibrous tumor in the shoulder of a 9-year-old girl: case report and review of the literature. *Pediatr Dev Pathol* 2004;7:653–660.
207. Dei Tos AP. Classification of pleomorphic sarcomas: where are we now? *Histopathology* 2006; 48:51–62.
208. Al-Agha OM, Igbokwe AA. Malignant fibrous histiocytoma: between the past and the present. *Arch Pathol Lab Med* 2008;132:1030–1035.
209. Delisca GO, Mesko NW, Alamanda VK, et al. MFH and high-grade undifferentiated pleomorphic sarcoma-what's in a name? *J Surg Oncol* 2015;111:173–177.
210. Incesoy Özdemir S, Balkaya E, et al. A rare type of secondary cancer in a child with acute lymphoblastic leukemia: malignant fibrous histiocytoma. *J Pediatr Hematol Oncol* 2014;36:e121–e124.
211. Alaggio R, Collini P, Randall RL, et al. Undifferentiated high-grade pleomorphic sarcomas in children: a clinicopathologic study of 10 cases and review of literature. *Pediatr Dev Pathol* 2010;13:209–217.
212. Hayes-Jordan AA, Spunt SL, Poquette CA, et al. Nonrhabdomyosarcoma soft tissue sarcomas in children: is age at diagnosis an important variable? *J Pediatr Surg* 2000;35:948–953.
213. Black J, Coffin CM, Dehner LP. Fibrohistiocytic tumors and related neoplasms in children and adolescents. *Pediatr Dev Pathol* 2012;15:181–210.
214. Han TY, Chang HS, Lee JH, et al. A clinical and histopathological study of 22 cases of dermatofibroma (benign fibrous histiocytoma). *Ann Dermatol* 2011;23:185–192.
215. Pinto-Almeida T, Caetano M, Alves R, et al. Congenital multiple clustered dermatofibroma and multiple eruptive dermatofibromas—unusual presentations of a common entity. *An Bras Dermatol* 2013;88:63–66.
216. Alves JV, Matos DM, Barreiros HF, et al. Variants of dermatofibroma—a histopathological study. *An Bras Dermatol* 2014;89:472–477.
217. Gleason BC, Fletcher CD. Deep "benign" fibrous histiocytoma: clinicopathologic analysis of 69 cases of a rare tumor indicating occasional metastatic potential. *Am J Surg Pathol* 2008;32:354–362.
218. Luzar B, Calonje E. Cutaneous fibrohistiocytic tumours—an update. *Histopathology* 2010; 56:148–165.
219. Kaddu S. McMenamin ME, Fletcher CD. Atypical fibrous histiocytoma of the skin: clinicopathologic analysis of 59 cases with evidence of infrequent metastasis. *Am J Surg Pathol* 2002;26:35–46.
220. Volpicelli ER, Fletcher CD. Desmin and CD34 positivity in cellular fibrous histiocytoma: an immunohistochemical analysis of 100 cases. *J Cutan Pathol* 2012;39:747–752.
221. Doyle LA, Fletcher CD. Metastasizing "benign" cutaneous fibrous histiocytoma: a clinicopathologic analysis of 16 cases. *Am J Surg Pathol* 2013;37:484–495.
222. Miller K, Goodlad JR, Brenn T. Pleomorphic dermal sarcoma: adverse histologic features predict aggressive behavior and allow distinction from atypical fibroxanthoma. *Am J Surg Pathol* 2012;36:1317–1326.
223. Boukari F, Butori C, Cardot-Leccia N, et al. [Atypical histiocytoma in a child]. *Ann Dermatol Venereol* 2014;141:279–284.
224. Shao L, Newell B, Quintanilla N. Atypical fibroxanthoma and squamous cell carcinoma of the conjunctiva in xeroderma pigmentosum. *Pediatr Dev Pathol* 2007;10:149–152.
225. Van der Heijden L, Gibbons CL, Hassan AB, et al. A multidisciplinary approach to giant cell tumors of tendon sheath and synovium—a critical appraisal of literature and treatment proposal. *J Surg Oncol* 2013;107:433–445.
226. Lucas DR, Tenosynovial giant cell tumor: case report and review. *Arch Pathol Lab Med* 2012;136:901–906.
227. Verspoor FG, van der Geest IC, Vegt E, et al. Pigmented villonodular synovitis: current concepts about diagnosis and management. *Future Oncol* 2013;9:1515–1531.
228. Garner HW, Bestic JM. Benign synovial tumors and proliferative processes. *Semin Musculoskelet Radiol* 2013;17:177–188.
229. O'Connell JX. Pathology of the synovium. *Am J Clin Pathol* 2000;114:773–784.
230. Yun SJ, Hwang SY, Jin W, et al. Intramuscular diffuse-type tenosynovial giant cell tumor of the deltoid muscle in a child. *Skeletal Radiol* 2014;43:1179–1183.
231. Somerhausen NS, Fletcher CD. Diffuse-type giant cell tumor: clinicopathologic and immunohistochemical analysis of 50 cases with extraarticular disease. *Am J Surg Pathol* 2000;24:479–492.
232. Boland JM, Folpe AL, Hornick JL, et al. Clusterin is expressed in normal synoviocytes and in tenosynovial giant cell tumors of localized and diffuse types: diagnostic and histogenetic implications. *Am J Surg Pathol* 2009;33:1225–1229.
233. Panagopoulos I, Brandal P, Gorunova L, et al. Novel CSF1-S100A 10 fusion gene and CSF1 transcript identified by RNA sequencing in tenosynovial giant cell tumors. *Int J Oncol* 2014;44:1425–1432.
234. Romeo S, Dei Tos AP. Soft tissue tumors associated with EWSR1 translocation. *Virchows Arch* 2010;456:219–234.

235. Fischer C. The diversity of soft tissue tumours with EWSR1 gene rearrangements: a review. *Histopathology* 2014;64:134–150.
236. Thway K, Fisher C. Tumors with EWSR1-CREB1 and EWSR1-ATF1 fusions: the current status. *Am J Surg Pathol* 2012;36:e1–e11.
237. Kohorst MA, Tran CL, Folpe AL, et al. Membranous nephropathy associated with angiomatoid fibrous histiocytoma in a pediatric patient. *Pediatr Nephrol* 2014;29:2221–2224.
238. Bohman SL, Goldblum JR, Rubin BP, et al. Angiomatoid fibrous histiocytoma: an expansion of the clinical and histological spectrum. *Pathology* 2014;46:199–204.
239. Schaefer IM, Fletcher CD. Myxoid variant of so-called angiomatoid "malignant fibrous histiocytoma": clinicopathologic characterization in a series of 21 cases. *Am J Surg Pathol* 2014;38:816–823.
240. Thway K, Stefanaki K, Papadakis V, et al. Metastatic angiomatoid fibrous histiocytoma of the scalp, with EWSR1-CREB1 gene fusions in primary tumor and nodal metastasis. *Hum Pathol* 2013;44:289–293.
241. Moosavi C, Jha P, Fanburg-Smith JC. An update of plexiform fibrohistiocytoma tumor and addition of 66 new cases from the Armed Forces Institute of Pathology, in honor of Franz M. Enzinger, MD. *Ann Diagn Pathol* 2007;11:313–319.
242. Yalcinkaya U, Uz Unlu M, Bilgen MS, et al. Plexiform fibrohistiocytic tumor of bone. *Pathol Int* 2013;63:554–558.
243. Taher A, Pushpanathan C. Plexiform fibrohistiocytoma tumor: a brief review. *Arch Pathol Lab Med* 2007;131:1135–1138.
244. Lynnhtun K, Achan A, Shingde M, et al. Plexiform fibrohistiocytic tumour: morphological changes and challenges in assessment of recurrent and metastatic lesions. *Histopathology* 2012;60:1156–1158.
245. Leclerc-Mercier S, Pedeutour F, Fabas T, et al. Plexiform fibrohistiocytic tumor with molecular and cytogenetic analysis. *Pediatr Dermatol* 2011;28:26–29.
246. Kushwah R, Hu J. Complexity of dendritic cell subsets and their function in the host immune system. *Immunology* 2011;133:409–419.
247. Schraml BU, Reis e Sousa C. Defining dendritic cells. *Curr Opin Immunol* 2015;32:13–20.
248. Dehner LP. Juvenile xanthogranulomas in the first two decades of life: a clinicopathologic study of 174 cases with cutaneous and extracutaneous manifestations. *Am J Surg Pathol* 2003;27:579–593.
249. Janssen D, Harms D. Juvenile xanthogranuloma in childhood and adolescence: a clinicopathologic study of 129 patients from the Kiel Pediatric Tumor Registry. *Am J Surg Pathol* 2005;29:21–28.
250. Bradshaw EJ, Wood KM, Hodgkinson P, et al. Follicular dendritic cell tumour in a 9-year-old child. *Pediatr Blood Cancer* 2005;45:725–727.
251. Silver AL, Faquin WC, Caruso PA, et al. Follicular dendritic cell sarcoma presenting in the submandibular region in an 11-year-old. *Laryngoscope* 2010;120(Suppl 4):S183.
252. Pillay K, Solomon R, Daubenton JD, et al. Interdigitating dendritic cell sarcoma: a report of four paediatric cases and review of the literature. *Histopathology* 2004;44:283–291.
253. Julia F, Dalle S, Duru G, et al. Blastic plasmacytoid dendritic cell neoplasms: clinicoimmunohistochemical correlations in a series of 91 patients. *Am J Surg Pathol* 2014;38:673–680.
254. Jegalian AG, Buxbaum NP, Facchetti F, et al. Blastic plasmacytoid dendritic cell neoplasm in children: diagnostic features and clinical implications. *Haematologica* 2010;95:1873–1879.
255. Shi Y, Wang E. Blastic plasmacytoid dendritic cell neoplasm: a clinicopathologic review. *Arch Pathol Lab Med* 2014;138:564–569.
256. Coffin C, Alaggio R. Adipose and myxoid tumors of childhood and adolescence. *Pediatr Dev Pathol* 2012;15(1 Suppl):239–254.
257. Moog U. Encephalocraniocutaneous lipomatosis. *J Med Genet* 2009;46:721–729.
258. Delfino L, Fariello G, Quattrocchi C, et al. Encephalocraniocutaneous lipomatosis [ECCL]: neuroradiological findings in three patients and a new association with fibrous dysplasia. *Am J Med Genet* 2010;155A:1690–1696.
259. Keppler-Noreuil K, Sapp J, Lindhurst M, et al. Clinical delineation and natural history of the PIK3CA-related overgrowth spectrum. *Am J Med Genet* 2014;164A:1713–1733.
260. Pilarski R, Burt R, Kohlman W, et al. Cowden syndrome and the PTEN hamartoma tumor syndrome: systematic review and revised diagnostic criteria. *J Natl Cancer Inst* 2013;105:1607–1616.
261. Piccione M, Fragapane T, Antona V, et al. PTEN hamartoma tumor syndromes in childhood: description of two cases and a proposal for follow-up protocol. *Am J Med Genet* 2013; 161A:2902–2908.
262. Prabhu S, Aldape K, Bruner J, et al. Cowden disease with Lhermitte-Duclos disease: case report. *Can J Neurol Sci* 2004;31:542–549.
263. Abel TW, Baker SJ, Fraser MM, et al. Lhermitte-DUclos disease: a report of 31 cases with immunohistochemical analysis of the PTEN/AKT/mTOR pathway. *J Neuropathol Exp Neurol* 2005;64:341–349.
264. Pagon R, Adam M, Ardinger H, et al. *PTEN Hamartoma Tumor Syndrome (PHTS). GeneReviews* [Internet]. Seattle, WA: University of Washington, Seattle; 1993–2014. 2001 Nov 29 [updated 2014 Jan 23].
265. Cohen MM Jr. Proteus syndrome review: molecular, clinical and pathologic features. *Clin Genet* 2014;85:111–119.
266. Jelsig A, Qvist N, Brusgaard K, et al. Hamartomatous polyposis syndromes: a review. *Orphanet J Rare Dis* 2014;9:101.
267. Thomason J, Abramowsky C, Rickets R, et al. Proteus syndrome: three case reports with a review of the literature. *Fetal Pediatr Pathol* 2012;31:145–153.
268. Bloom J, Upton J III. CLOVES syndrome. *J Hand Surg Am* 2013;38:2508–2512.
269. Happle R. The group of epidermal nevus syndromes Part I. Well defined phenotypes. *J Am Acad Dermatol* 2010;63:1–22.
270. Happle R. The group of epidermal nevus syndromes part II. Less well defined phenotypes. *J Am Acad Dermatol* 2010;63:25–30.
271. Rothman I. Michelin tire baby syndrome: a review of the literature and a proposal for diagnostic criteria with adoption of the name circumferential skin folds syndrome. *Pediatr Dermatol* 2014;31:659–663.
272. Janicke E, Nazareth Mrothman I. Generalized smooth muscle hamartoma with multiple congenital anomalies without the "Michelin tire baby" phenotype. *Pediatr Dermatol* 2014;31:731–733.
273. Mirzaa G, Rivière JB, Dobyns W. Megalencephaly syndromes and activating mutations in the PI3K-AKT pathway: MPPH and MCAP. *Am J Med Genet C Semin Med Genet* 2013;163C:122–130.
274. Tahiri Y, Xu L, Kanevsky J, et al. Lipofibromatous hamartoma of the median nerve: a comprehensive review and systematic approach to evaluation, diagnosis and treatment. *J Hand Surg Am* 2013;38:2055–2067.
275. Rohilla S, Jain N, Sharma R, et al. Macrodystrophia lipomatosa involving multiple nerves. *J Orthop Traumatol* 2012;13:41–45.
276. van der Meer S, Nicolai J, Meek M. Macrodystrophia lipomatosa: macrodactyly related to affected nerves and a review of the literature. *Handchir Mikrochir Plast Chir* 2007;39:414–417.
277. Oi S, Nomura S, Nagasaka M, et al. Embryopathogenetic surgico-anatomical classification of dysraphism and surgical outcome of spinal lipoma: a nationwide multicenter cooperative study in Japan. *J Neurosurg Pediatr* 2009;3:412–419.
278. Xenos C, Sgouros S, Walsh R, et al. Spinal lipomas in children. *Pediatr Neurosurg* 2000;32:295–307.
279. Muthukumar N. Congenital spinal lipomatous malformations: part I—classification. *Acta Neurochir (Wien)* 2009;151:179–188.
280. Muthukumar N. Congenital spinal lipomatous malformations: part II—clinical presentation, operative findings and outcome. *Acta Neurochir (Wien)* 2009;151:189–197.
281. Kole MJ, Fridley JS, Jea A, et al. Currarino syndrome and spinal dysraphism. *J Neurosurg Pediatr* 2014;13:685–689.
282. Abdelmaaboud M, Nimeri N. Pai syndrome: first reported in Qatar and review of literature of previously published cases. *BMJ Case Rep* 2012; pii: bcr0220125940.
283. Mifsud W, Sambandan N, Humphries P, et al. Perineal lipoma with accessory labioscrotal fold and penislike phallus in a female infant with unilateral renal agenesis. *Urology* 2014;84:209–212.
284. Sheng W, Lu L, Wang J. Cellular angiolipoma: a clinicopathological and immunohistochemical study of 12 cases. *Am J Dermatopathol* 2013;35:220–225.

285. Hameed M. Pathology and genetics of adipocytic tumors. *Cytogenet Genome Res* 2007;118:138–147.
286. Beals C, Rogers A, Wakely P, et al. Hibernomas: a single-institution experience and review of literature. *Med Oncol* 2014;31:769.
287. Guidry CA, McGahren ED, Rodgers BM, et al. Pediatric cervicomediastinal hibernoma: a case report. *J Pediatr Surg* 2013;48:258–261.
288. Furlong MA, Fanburg-Smith J, Miettinen M. The morphologic spectrum of hibernoma: a clinicopathologic study of 170 cases. *Am J Surg Pathol* 2001;25:809–814.
289. Hicks J, Dilley A, Patel D, et al. Lipoblastoma and lipoblastomatosis in infancy and childhood: histopathologic, ultrastructural, and cytogenetic features. *Ultrastruct Pathol* 2001;25:321–333.
290. Coffin C, Lowichik A, Putnam A. Lipoblastoma (LPB): a clinicopathologic and immunohistochemical analysis of 59 cases. *Am J Surg Pathol* 2009;33:1705–1712.
291. Kubota F, Matsuyama A, Shibuya R, et al. Desmin-positivity in spindle cells: under-recognized immunophenotype of lipoblastoma. *Pathol Int* 2013;63:353–357.
292. Yoshida H, Miyachi M, Ouchi K, et al. Identification of COL3A1 and RAB2A as novel translocation partner genes of PLAG1 in lipoblastoma. *Genes Chromosomes Cancer* 2014;53:606–611.
293. Choi J, Bouron Dal Soglio D, Fortier A, et al. Diagnostic utility of molecular and cytogenetic analysis in lipoblastoma: a study of two cases and review of the literature. *Histopathology* 2014;64:731–740.
294. Pedeutour F, Deville A, Steyaert H, et al. Rearrangement of HMGA2 in a case of infantile lipoblastoma without Plag1 alteration. *Pediatr Blood Cancer* 2012;58:798–800.
295. Conyers R, Young S, Thomas DM. Liposarcoma: molecular genetics and therapeutics. *Sarcoma* 2011;2011:483154.
296. Alaggio R, Coffin CM, Weiss SW, et al. Liposarcomas in young patients: a study of 82 cases occurring in patients younger than 22 years of age. *Am J Surg Pathol* 2009;33:645–658.
297. Huh W, Yuen C, Munsell M, et al. Liposarcoma in children and young adults: a multi-institutional experience. *Pediatr Blood Cancer* 2011;57:1142–1146.
298. Rudzinski E, Mawn L, Kuttesch J, et al. Orbital pleomorphic liposarcoma in an eight-year-old boy. *Pediatr Dev Pathol* 2011;14:339–344.
299. Okamoto S, Machinami R, Tanizawa T, et al. Dedifferentiated liposarcoma with rhabdomyoblastic differentiation in an 8-year-old girl. *Pathol Res Pract* 2010;206:191–196.
300. Dei Tos A. Liposarcomas: diagnostic pitfalls and new insights. *Histopathology* 2014;64:38–52.
301. Debelenko LV, Perez-Atayde AR, Debois SG, et al. p53+/mdm2-atypical lipomatous tumor/well-differentiated liposarcoma in young children: an early expression of Li-Fraumeni syndrome. *Pediatr Dev Pathol* 2010;13:218–224.
302. Saffitz JE. The pathobiology of arrhythmogenic cardiomyopathy. *Annu Rev Pathol* 2011;6:299–321.
303. Asimaki A, Kléber A, MacRae C, et al. Arrhythmogenic cardiomyopathy—new insights into disease mechanisms and drug discovery. *Prog Pediatr Cardiol* 2014;37:3–7.
304. Vassalini M, Verzeletti A, Restori M, et al. An autopsy study of sudden cardiac death in persons aged 1-40 years in Brescia (Italy). *J Cardiovasc Med (Hagerstown)* 2015; Jan 7 [Epub ahead of print].
305. Lazzarini E, Jongbloed JD, Pilichou K, et al. The ARVD/C genetic variants database: 2014 update. *Hum Mutat* 2015;30:403–410.
306. Cates JMM, Coffin CM. Neurogenic tumors of soft tissues. *Pediatr Dev Pathol* 2012;15(1 Suppl):62–107.
307. Furniss D, Swan MC, Morritt DG, et al. A 10-year review of benign and malignant peripheral nerve sheath tumors in a single center: clinical and radiographic features can help to differentiate benign from malignant lesions. *Plast Reconstr Surg* 2008;121:529–533.
308. Ferrari A, Bisogno G, Macaluso A, et al. Soft-tissue sarcomas in children and adolescents with neurofibromatosis type 1. *Cancer* 2007;109;1406–1412.
309. Philp L, Naert KA, Ghazarian D. Fibrolipomatous hamartoma of the nerve arising in the neck: a case report with review of the literature and differential diagnosis. *Am J Dermatopathol* 2014; Jul 15 [Epub ahead of print].
310. Abramowicz A, Gos M. Neurofibromin in neurofibromatosis type 1—mutations in NF1 gene as a cause of disease. *Dev Period Med* 2014;18:297–306.
311. Hirbe AC, Gutmann DH. Neurofibromatosis type 1: a multidisciplinary approach to care. *Lancet Neurol* 2014;13:834–843.
312. Bezniakow N, Gos M, Obersztyn E. The RASopathies as an example of RAS/MAPK pathway disturbances—clinical presentation and molecular pathogenesis of selected syndromes. *Dev Period Med* 2014;18:285–296.
313. Niemeyer CM. RAS disease in children. *Haematologica* 2014;99:1653–1662.
314. Rauen KA. The RASopathies. *Annu Rev Genomics Hum Genet* 2013;14:355–369.
315. Tucker T, Friedman JM, Friedrich RE, et al. Longitudinal study of neurofibromatosis 1 associated plexiform neurofibromas. *J Med Genet* 2009;46:81–85.
316. Tucker T, Wolkenstein P, Revuz J, et al. Association between benign and malignant peripheral nerve sheath tumors in NF1. *Neurology* 2005;65:205–211.
317. Korf BR. Neurofibromatosis. *Handb Clin Neurol* 2013;111:333–340.
318. Lloyd SK, Evans DG. Neurofibromatosis type 2 (NF2): diagnosis and management. *Handb Clin Neurol* 2013;115:957–967.
319. Cooper J, Giancotti FG. Molecular insights into NF2/Merlin tumor suppressor function. *FEBS Lett* 2014;588:2743–2752.
320. Valeyrie-Allanore L, Ortonne N, Lantieri L, et al. Histopathologically dysplastic neurofibromas in neurofibromatosis 1: diagnostic criteria, prevalence and clinical significance. *Br J Dermatol* 2008;158:1008–1012.
321. Valeyrie-Allanore L, Ismaïli N, Bastuji-Garin S, et al. Symptoms associated with malignancy of peripheral nerve sheath tumors: a retrospective study of 69 patients with neurofibromatosis 1. *Br J Dermatol* 2005;153:79–82.
322. Liapis H, Marley EF, Lin Y, et al. p53 and Ki-67 proliferating cell nuclear antigen in benign and malignant peripheral nerve sheath tumors in children. *Pediatr Dev Pathol* 1999;2:377–384.
323. Naber U, Friedrich RE, Glatzel M, et al. Podoplanin and CD34 in peripheral nerve sheath tumours: focus on neurofibromatosis 1-associated atypical neurofibroma. *J Neurooncol* 2011;103:239–245.
324. Kurtkaya-Yapicier O, Scheithauer B, Woodruff JM. The pathobiologic spectrum of schwannomas. *Histol Histopathol* 2003;18:925–934.
325. Hilton DA, Hanemann CO. Schwannomas and their pathogenesis. *Brain Pathol* 2014;24:205–220.
326. Kim DH, Murovic JA, Tiel RL, et al. A series of 397 peripheral neural sheath tumors: 30-year experience at Louisiana State University Health Sciences Center. *J Neurosurg* 2005;102:246–255.
327. Knight DM, Birch R, Pringle J. Benign solitary schwannomas. A review of 234 cases. *J Bone Joint Surg Br* 2007;89:382–387.
328. Pekmezci M, Reuss DE, Hirbe AL, et al. Morphologic and immunohistochemical features of malignant peripheral sheath tumor and cellular schwannomas. *Mod Pathol* 2015;28:187–200.
329. Woodruff JM, Scheithauer BW, Kurtkaya-Yapicier O, et al. Congenital and childhood plexiform (multinodular) cellular schwannoma: a troublesome mimic of malignant peripheral nerve sheath tumor. *Am J Surg Pathol* 2003;27:1321–1329.
330. Ruggieri M, Iannetti P, Polizzi A, et al. Earliest clinical manifestations and natural history of neurofibromatosis type 2 (NF2) in childhood: a study of 24 patients. *Neuropediatrics* 2005;36:21–34.
331. Ruggieri M, Gabriele AL, Polizzi A, et al. Natural history of neurofibromatosis type 2 with onset before the age of 1 year. *Neurogenetics* 2013;14:89–98.
332. McClatchey AI. Neurofibromatosis. *Annu Rev Pathol* 2007;2:191–216.
333. MacCollin M, Chiocca EA, Evans DG, et al. Diagnostic criteria for schwannomatosis. *Neurology* 2005;64:1838–1845.
334. Merker VL, Esparza S, Smith MJ, et al. Clinical features of schwannomatosis: a retrospective analysis of 87 patients. *Oncologist* 2012;17:1317–1322.

SECTION II ORGAN SYSTEM PATHOLOGY 1215

TABLE 26-1 ALGORITHMIC APPROACH TO CUTANEOUS PATHOLOGY

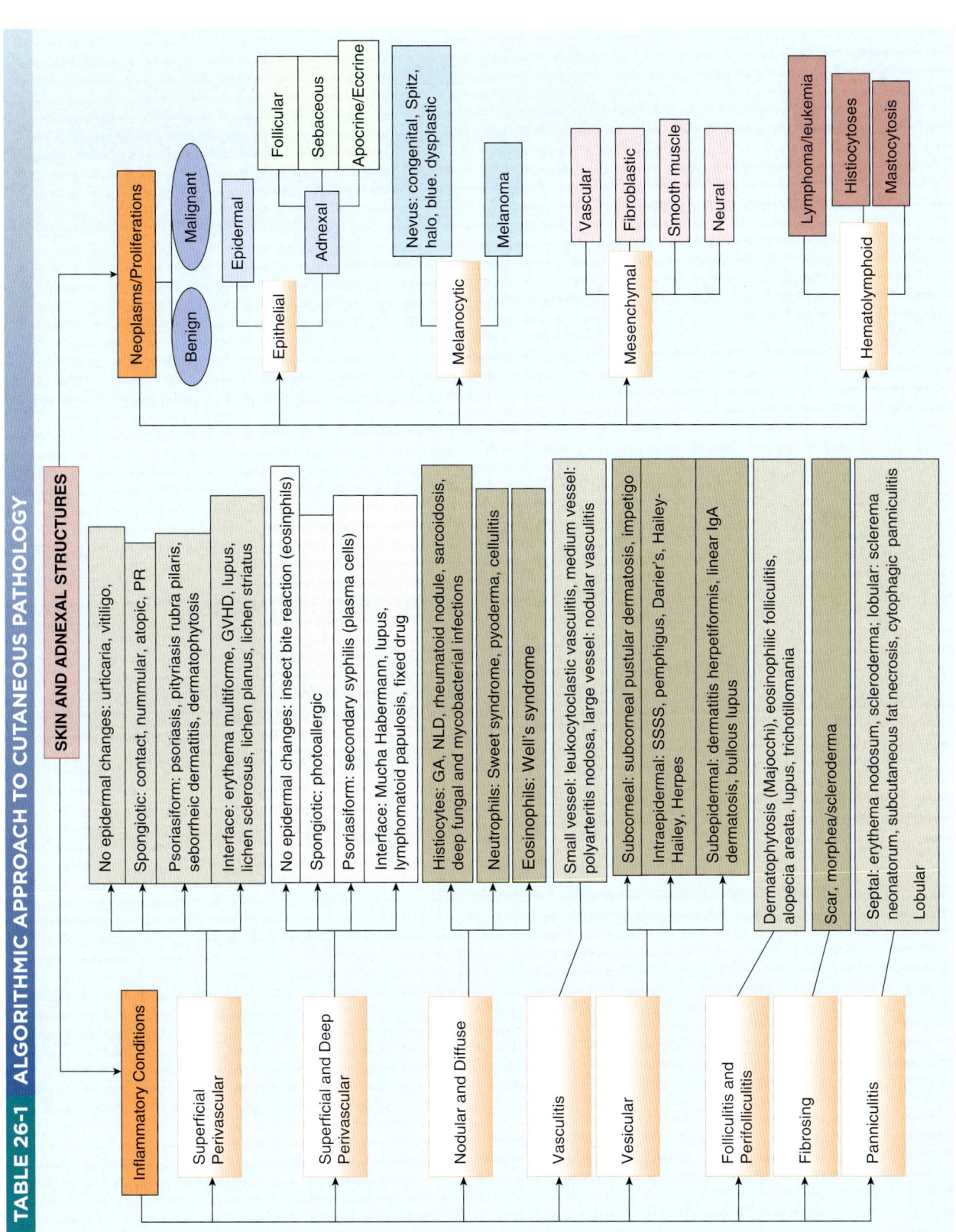

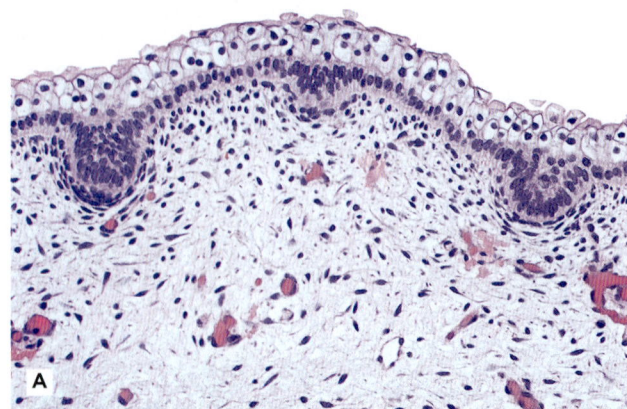 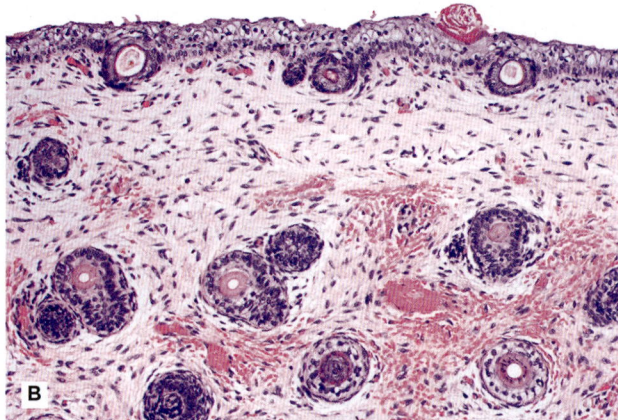

FIGURE 26-1 • **A:** Skin of an early, second trimester fetus showing stratification of epidermis, beginning of the follicular germs, and immature dermis. **B:** Skin from a 28-week fetus with stratum corneum and adnexal structures in a collagenized dermis. (Hematoxylin and eosin stain, original magnifications ×200.)

BIOPSY TECHNIQUES

Skin samples can be obtained using various biopsy techniques, including punch, shave, excision, and curettage. Selection of the appropriate biopsy method depends on the clinical impression and the kind of information anticipated by the clinician.

Punch biopsy is generally the best choice for evaluation of inflammatory dermatoses. This technique allows the histologic examination of the full thickness of the skin including the subcutaneous fat. A 4-mm punch biopsy provides an adequate sample. In small children and cosmetically important areas, a 3-mm punch may be substituted. The area selected for biopsy should be a well-developed lesion and representative of the pathologic process.

Shave biopsy is the technique used in the evaluation of lesions that appear to be confined to the epidermis and superficial dermis and is best for the clinical diagnosis of keratoses and other benign neoplastic lesions. This technique is also used for suspected benign melanocytic lesions as well as for diagnostic confirmation of basal cell or squamous cell carcinoma prior to undertaking definitive surgical procedure.

Excisional biopsy is the technique of choice for suspected malignancies or atypical pigmented lesions. It generally allows for the evaluation of surgical margins, and as such, the lateral and deep margins should be inked before sectioning. Excisional biopsy or an incisional biopsy can also be used when panniculitis is clinically suspected.

Curettage is the technique some clinicians employ in examining clinically benign lesions. From a pathologist's point of view, this is not a preferred method because the fragments of tissue so obtained are often small and superficial, precluding accurate analysis. Furthermore, if a clinically benign lesion turns out to be malignant on histologic examination, vital prognostic information such as invasion and thickness cannot be obtained since curetted fragments are difficult to orient.

Scrape preparation is useful in evaluation of viral vesicles, when cells are scraped off a vesicular or pustular lesion and analyzed after a quick stain.

Fine-needle aspiration biopsy is a popular method of biopsy in the evaluation of subcutaneous bumps and lumps. However, it requires an experienced cytopathologist for proper handling and interpretation of the material obtained.

SPECIMEN HANDLING

Routine Processing

Biopsy specimens should be placed immediately in a fixative. The fixative of choice for the majority of the specimens is 10% buffered formalin. Punch and shave biopsies larger than 3 mm in diameter should be bisected for optimal fixation as well as for appropriate plane of sectioning through the lesion, which is usually located in the center of the specimen. Excisional biopsies should be inked and sectioned at 2- to 3-mm intervals. Histologic sections cut at 3 to 5 μm are routinely stained with hematoxylin and eosin.

Special Processing

Specimens for direct immunofluorescence (IF) testing of bullous diseases are ideally obtained by biopsy of perilesional skin. A well-established lesion is best for suspected cases of lupus, whereas an early lesion is ideal for suspected case of vasculitis. Michel fixative is a good transport medium because the specimen can be safely tested for IF for up to 7 days. Alternatively, the specimen can be placed in normal saline and transported immediately to the laboratory. Frozen sections are incubated with fluorescein-labeled antibodies typically against IgG, IgA, IgM, C3, C1q, and fibrinogen and evaluated with IF microscope.

Electron microscopy may be of use in the diagnosis of undifferentiated neoplasms and can be invaluable in establishing the diagnosis of various types of epidermolysis bullosa and also in metabolic disorders like Fabry disease.

Specimens for electron microscopy should be fixed immediately in 2% glutaraldehyde or paraformaldehyde.

Skin and subcutaneous tissue may be used for cytogenetic analysis. Sterile specimens should be placed in a transport medium such as RPMI.

ALGORITHMIC APPROACH TO SPECIFIC DIAGNOSES

A systematic approach in analysis of biopsy sections allows for a smooth and accurate diagnosis. The pattern analysis method, which was introduced by Wallace H. Clark Jr., popularized by A. Bernard Ackerman and followed widely by most dermatopathologists today, involves the evaluation of sections at a scanning magnification. Examination at scanning magnification can be highly informative and usually helps in classifying a disease process as either proliferation/neoplastic or inflammatory. Table 26-1 is rather simplistic but offers the flavor for an algorithmic approach and includes representative dermatoses that occur in the pediatric patient. The following is a brief description of diseases grouped according to etiology and pathogenesis.

CONGENITAL DISEASES (GENODERMATOSES)

Genodermatoses are a large and diverse group of disorders presenting with cutaneous involvement and an underlying genetic defect. Only those genodermatoses that can be diagnosed in the fetus, neonate, or child will be discussed. It must be emphasized that some of these will be rarely seen by the pathologist, while others are not uncommon and are frequently included in the differential diagnosis.

Aplasia Cutis Congenita

Aplasia cutis congenita, or localized absence of skin, presents as a single or multiple skin defects typically involving the scalp. It presents at birth with a deep ulcer-like lesion, in which the subcutaneous fat is exposed. If the lesion occurs *in utero*, it manifests as a healed scar at birth. A sporadic lesion of aplasia cutis has no significant clinical consequences. More often, aplasia cutis may be a part of a variety of inheritable or noninheritable syndromes including trisomy 13, amniotic bands, and cardiac anomalies (1,2).

A histologic section of aplasia cutis shows a full-thickness skin defect with healing at the edges. A fully healed lesion shows scar with absence of adnexal structures. Formerly considered as synonymous, congenital absence of skin, characterized by absence of epidermis only, is now regarded as part of the epidermolysis bullosa group of disorders.

Ichthyosis

Ichthyoses are a heterogeneous group of disorders of epidermal cornification that are characterized by dryness and scaling of the skin. Ichthyoses are generally inherited, although acquired forms are described, especially in association with hematopoietic malignancies. The hereditary forms are divided into (a) the primary forms, which include ichthyosis vulgaris, recessive X-linked ichthyosis, epidermolytic hyperkeratosis (bullous congenital ichthyosiform erythroderma), classical lamellar ichthyosis, and nonbullous congenital ichthyosiform erythroderma; (b) ichthyosiform disorders such as Harlequin ichthyosis, erythrokeratoderma variabilis, and CHILD (congenital hemidysplasia with ichthyosiform erythrodermal and limb defects) syndrome; and (c) other related disorders of differentiation such as Darier disease, Hailey-Hailey disease, and porokeratosis (3).

Ichthyosis vulgaris is a common disorder, inherited in an autosomal dominant pattern that presents with fine white to larger scales involving large areas of the body but most prominent on the extensor surfaces of the extremities with relative sparing of the flexural areas. Histologically, there is moderate hyperkeratosis with a decreased or an absent granular layer and follicular plugging (Figure 26-2).

X-linked ichthyosis inherited as a recessive disorder presents early in infancy with large brown scales involving the entire body with accentuation on the neck and behind ears and relative sparing of the flexural areas. Histologically, there is hyperkeratosis with normal or thickened granular layer.

Bullous congenital ichthyosiform erythroderma or epidermolytic hyperkeratosis has an autosomal dominant pattern of inheritance and presents with generalized erythema and blistering at birth. Microscopic features include hyperkeratosis, a characteristic vacuolization of the cells in spinous and granular layers and prominent keratohyaline granules (Figure 26-3).

Lamellar ichthyosis is inherited as an autosomal recessive disorder and characterized by large platelike scales involving face, trunk, and extremities with a predilection for flexor areas. Microscopic changes are nonspecific and include hyperkeratosis with or without foci of parakeratosis and mild

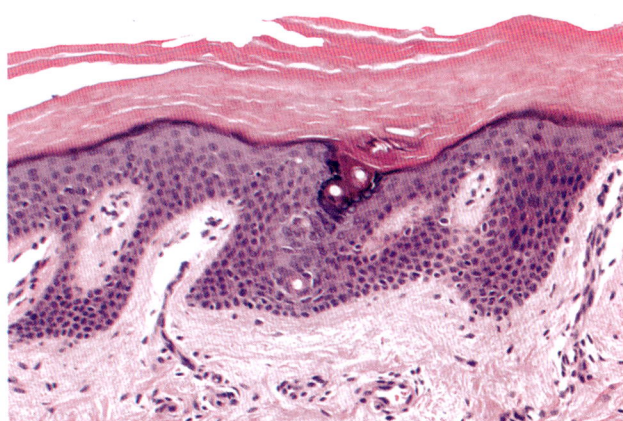

FIGURE 26-2 • Ichthyosis vulgaris showing hyperkeratosis and a prominent stratum corneum with a diminished granular cell layer. (Hematoxylin and eosin stain, original magnification ×200.)

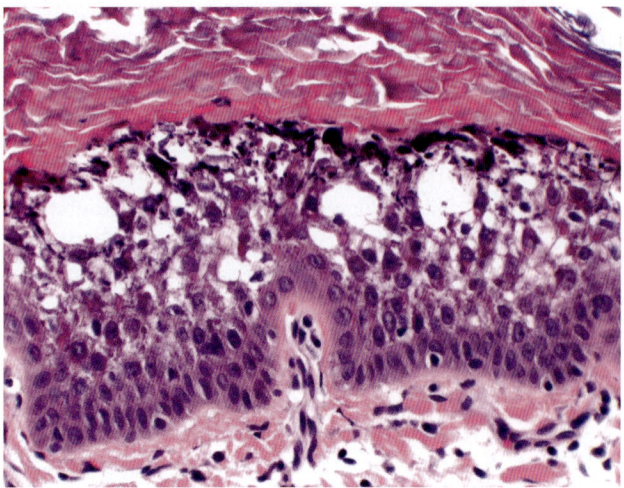

FIGURE 26-3 • Congenital bullous ichthyosiform erythroderma showing marked hyperkeratosis and epidermolytic hyperkeratosis with vacuolar degeneration of the stratum spinosum and granulosum, which is responsible for the formation of bullae. (Hematoxylin and eosin stain, original magnification ×200.)

epidermal hyperplasia (Figure 26-4). Lamellar ichthyosis can present as a collodion baby, in which the infant is encased in a keratinous membrane and superficially resembles a harlequin fetus. However, the membrane is usually shed in 10 to 14 days, following which the clinical features of lamellar ichthyosis become apparent.

Nonbullous congenital ichthyosiform erythroderma is inherited as autosomal recessive disorder, is milder than lamellar ichthyosis, and has a more prominent erythrodermic component.

Fetal harlequin ichthyosis is an autosomal recessive disorder that can be fatal. Fetal skin biopsy can be diagnostic and shows massive hyperkeratosis. *In utero*, the massive hyperkeratosis interferes with normal development. At birth, the child is encased in a thick, fissured, scaly cast, associated with ectropion.

Darier Disease

Darier disease, also known as *keratosis follicularis*, is a relatively uncommon disease that is inherited in an autosomal dominant pattern. Darier disease gene has been localized to chromosome 12 (4). It typically presents in children aged 5 to 15 years as keratotic papules distributed in the seborrheic areas such as face, neck, and upper trunk (5). Oral mucosa and nails can also be involved (6,7). The histopathologic findings are characterized by suprabasal acantholysis covered by dyskeratotic cells (corps ronds) and parakeratosis (corps grains), in addition to papillomatous epidermal hyperplasia and hyperkeratosis (Figure 26-5). Occasionally, these lesions are centered on the hair follicles.

Most cases of Darier disease have a benign but protracted course with exacerbations during summer.

Hailey-Hailey Disease

Hailey-Hailey disease is an autosomal dominant genodermatosis that initially manifests typically only after puberty (late teens or early 20s). It is characterized by recurrent vesicles and erosions on the neck, axillae, and groin. Mucosal involvement is uncommon. Histologic features include suprabasal acantholysis resulting in a dilapidated brick wall-like appearance (Figure 26-6). Most cases of Hailey-Hailey disease have a fairly stable course. The cutaneous lesions are exacerbated by heat, humidity, and bacterial and candidal infections.

Porokeratosis

Porokeratosis is inherited as an autosomal dominant disorder that manifests in childhood and infancy as asymptomatic keratotic papules that enlarge progressively to form plaques with peripheral keratotic ridges. Four variants of porokeratosis can be seen in the pediatric population and include the classic plaque type of Mibelli, linear porokeratosis, porokeratosis palmaris, plantaris et disseminata, and punctate

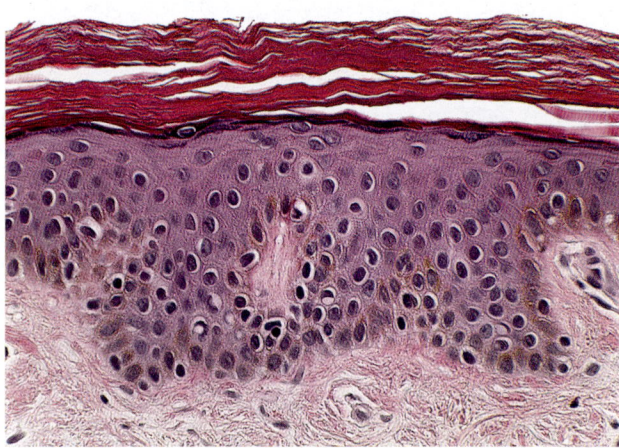

FIGURE 26-4 • Lamellar ichthyosis showing hyperkeratosis and mild psoriasiform changes. (Hematoxylin and eosin stain, original magnification ×200.)

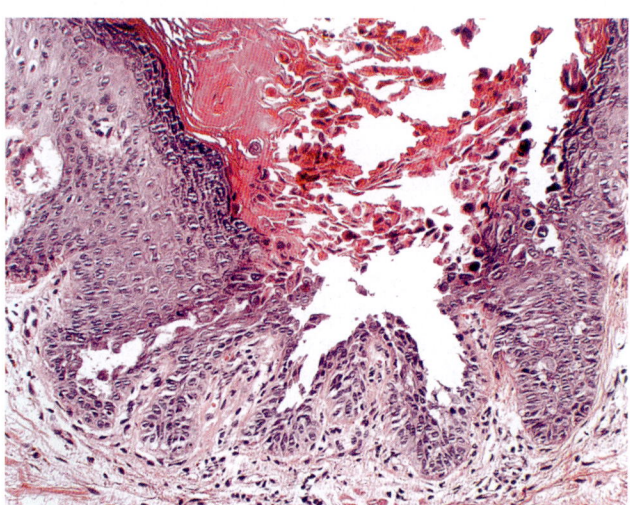

FIGURE 26-5 • Darier disease with focal intraepidermal acantholysis, dyskeratosis, and hyperkeratosis. (Hematoxylin and eosin stain, original magnification ×200.)

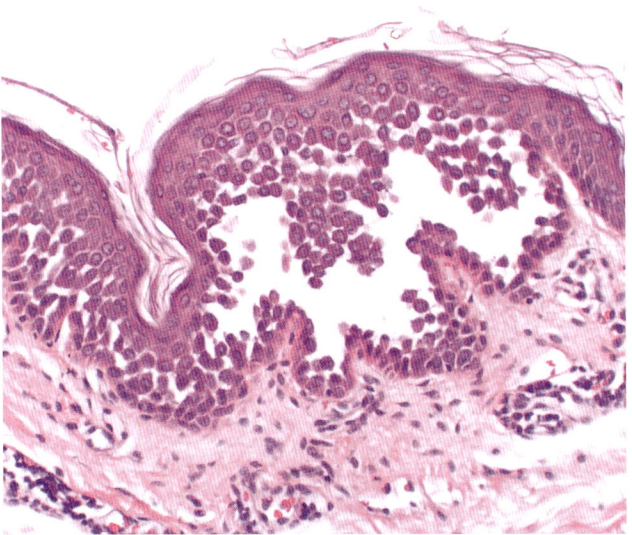

FIGURE 26-6 • Hailey-Hailey disease showing intraepidermal acantholysis with a dilapidated brick wall-like appearance. There is no significant dyskeratosis, which helps in the differential diagnosis from Darier disease.

porokeratosis that is limited to palms and soles. A fifth type, disseminated superficial actinic porokeratosis, is a disease of adulthood (8–11). Histopathologic features common to all types of porokeratoses include a cornoid lamella, which is a column of parakeratosis that corresponds to the peripheral keratotic ridges seen clinically (Figure 26-7). The cornoid lamella overlies an area of epidermal invagination where there is a diminished granular zone and vacuolated and dyskeratotic keratinocytes that correspond to an abnormal clone of keratinocytes. In porokeratosis of Mibelli, the epidermal invagination is more pronounced and deep compared with other types of porokeratosis.

In addition to the inherited form, porokeratosis has been described in various immunosuppressive states including Crohn disease, renal transplantation, and HIV infection. Squamous cell carcinoma has been reported to develop in lesions of porokeratosis.

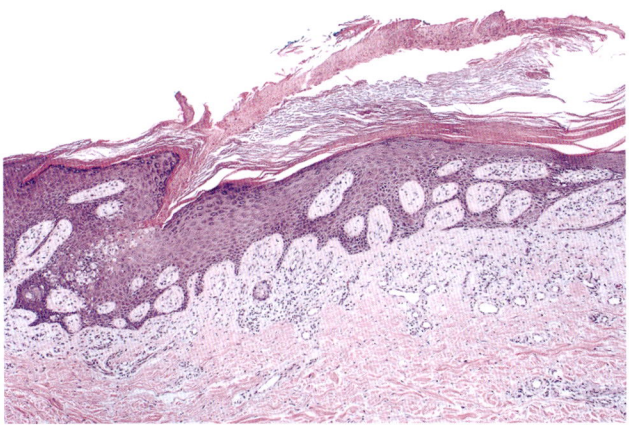

FIGURE 26-7 • Porokeratosis showing a column of parakeratosis that is inclined toward the center (cornoid lamella). Dyskeratotic keratinocytes may be seen at the base of the column. (Hematoxylin and eosin stain, original magnification ×100.)

Restrictive Dermopathy

Restrictive dermopathy is an uncommon autosomal recessive disorder that presents with prematurity; rigid and tense skin with erosions, denudations, and multiple joint contractions; fixed facial expression; and perineal anomalies (Figure 26-8). Histologic features include a thickened epidermis with flattening of rete ridges and hyperkeratosis. The dermis is thin with absent elastic fibers, collagen bundles oriented parallel to the surface, and poorly developed adnexal structures (Figure 26-9). The disease is fatal, with most infants dying within weeks after birth. Abnormalities in collagen and abnormal synthesis of keratin have been proposed as the underlying defects.

Ectodermal Dysplasia

Ectodermal dysplasias form a large and heterogeneous group of genetic disorders that are characterized by developmental abnormalities in two or more major structures of ectodermal origin including hair, nails, teeth, sweat glands, and sebaceous glands. Ectodermal dysplasia syndromes are associated with abnormalities of nonectodermally derived structures with more than 100 syndromes encompassing all forms of Mendelian inheritance described clinically. The different disorders are differentiated based on the type of ectodermal defect (hair, teeth, nails, etc.), associated nonectodermal abnormalities, mode of inheritance, and underlying genetic defect. The two classic forms of ectodermal dysplasia include hidrotic and anhidrotic/hypohidrotic. The hidrotic form, with typically an autosomal dominant pattern of inheritance, is primarily a disorder of keratinization. It is characterized by hypotrichosis, dystrophic nails, and palmoplantar hyperkeratosis. The anhidrotic/hypohidrotic form is most commonly inherited as an X-linked recessive disorder localized to the Xq12-q13.1 region of X chromosome with full expression occurring only in men, who show the tetrad of anhidrosis or hypohidrosis, hypotrichosis, dental hypoplasia, characteristic facies, and frequently dystrophy of nails. In addition to aplasia and hypoplasia of sweat glands, the submucosal glands of the trachea and bronchus may be affected, leading to frequent respiratory infections. Histologically, both forms show hypoplasia of hair follicles and sebaceous glands. In addition, the anhidrotic form shows aplasia or hypoplasia of eccrine glands and occasionally of apocrine glands.

Focal Dermal Hypoplasia

Focal dermal hypoplasia was originally described by Libermann (12) as part of ectodermal and mesodermal dysplasia in association with osseous defects. The cutaneous aspects were first detailed by Goltz et al. (13). Because a majority of the patients are female, it has been assumed to have X-linked dominant mode of inheritance. Focal dermal hypoplasia is a multisystem condition in which developmental defects of skin are associated with ocular, dental, and skeletal system abnormalities. The clinical course is dictated by the extent of systemic involvement. The skin findings, which

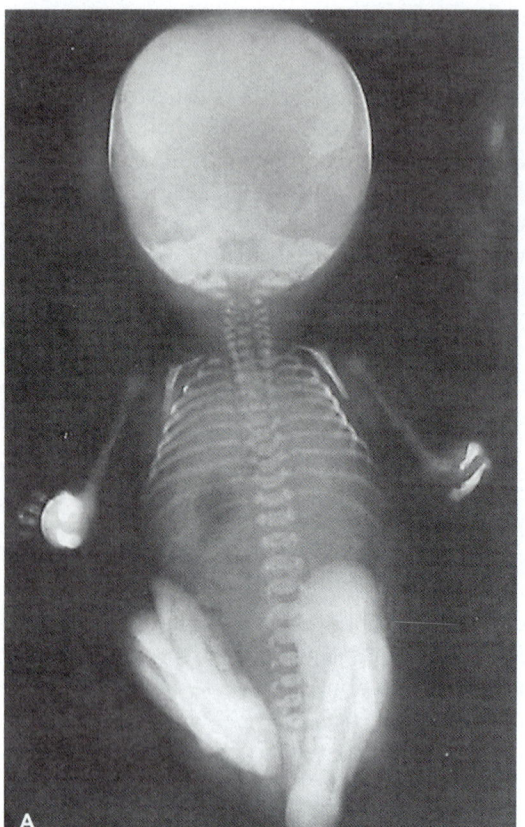
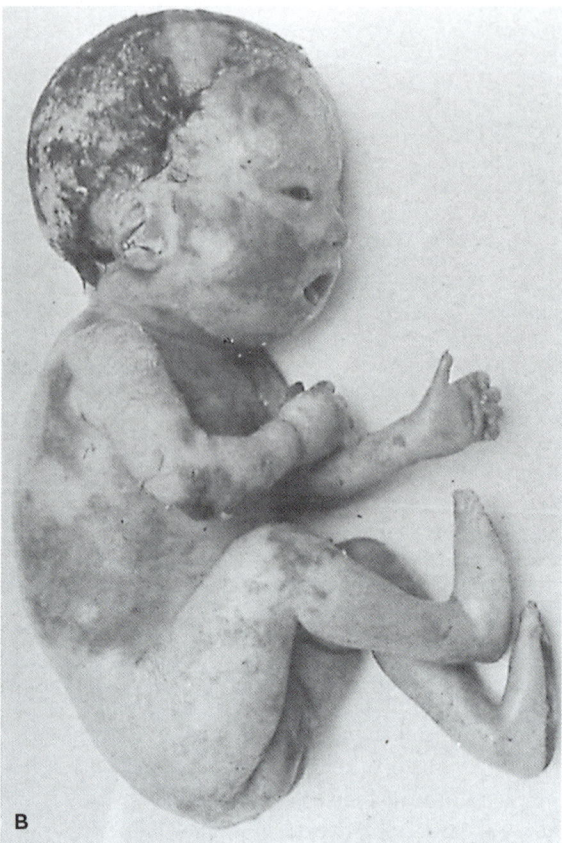
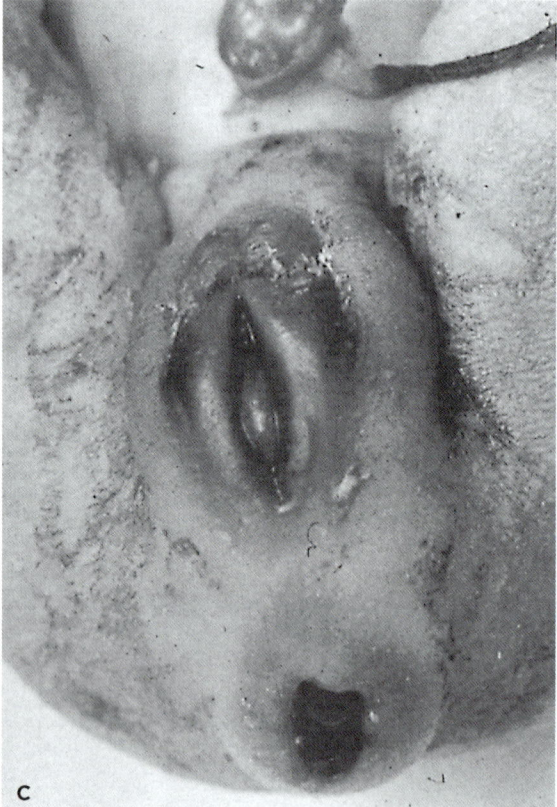

FIGURE 26-8 • **A:** Restrictive dermopathy showing severe contractures in the absence of overt bony abnormalities. **B, C:** The tight, shiny skin and characteristic fixation of the mouth and perineum.

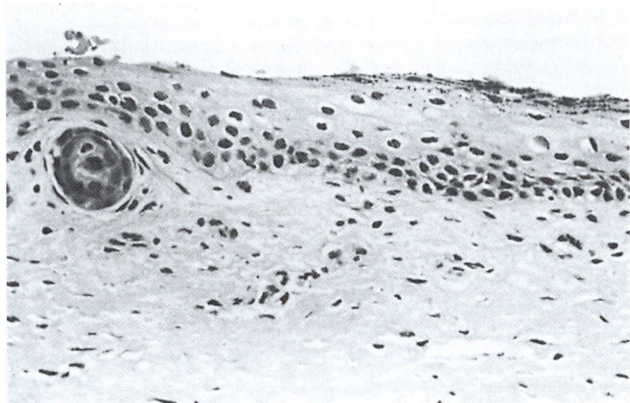

FIGURE 26-9 • Restrictive dermopathy without a stratum corneum, but the granular layer is prominent, indicating that the stratum corneum may have been lost in the postmortem interval. The rete ridges are flattened and most of the adnexal structures are atrophic. (Hematoxylin and eosin stain, original magnification ×250.)

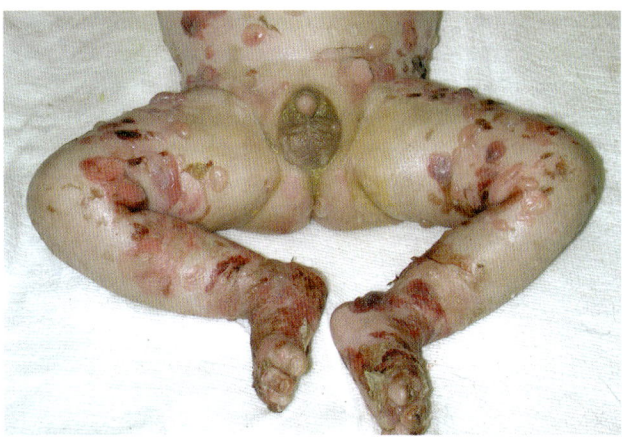

FIGURE 26-10 • Junctional epidermolysis bullosa in a 6-week-old infant showing extensive blistering and sloughing of the skin. (Courtesy of Sarah Stein, M.D., Department of Medicine, University of Chicago Medical Center.)

are present from birth, consist of widely distributed asymmetric linear streaks of atrophy or hypoplasia of the skin, often with associated telangiectasia that follows Blaschko lines. Some lesions may present as soft yellow nodular outpouchings caused by herniation of fat through an atrophic dermis in linear array. Various mutations in X-linked PORCN, a putative regulator of Wnt signaling, have been identified in focal dermal hypoplasia (14,15).

Histologic features of focal dermal hypoplasia include a marked decrease in the thickness of the dermis, with collagen distributed as thin fibrils rather than bundles, which may be interrupted by presence of adipocytes. The latter corresponds to the clinically apparent soft yellow nodules. The frequent presence of adipocytes high up in the dermis raises the possibility of nevus lipomatosus in the differential diagnosis. Nevus lipomatosus, however, lacks the collagen abnormalities and the frequent X-linked chromosomal abnormalities of focal dermal hypoplasia.

Epidermolysis Bullosa

Epidermolysis bullosa is a heterogeneous group of inherited disorders with variable modes of transmission, characterized by bullous lesions that develop spontaneously or secondary to minor trauma and include approximately 20 subtypes (16). Based on the presence or absence of scarring, mode of inheritance, cleavage plane of the blister, and the presence or absence of structural elements of skin, epidermolysis bullosa is traditionally divided into three major forms: simplex, junctional, and dystrophic (17,18).

Epidermolysis bullosa simplex, including Cockayne and Dowling-Meara forms, is typically transmitted in an autosomal dominant pattern, and is generally associated with good prognosis because the blisters heal without scar formation. Histologic sections show intraepidermal separation, generally within the basal cell layer. A periodic acid–Schiff (PAS) stain is helpful in localizing the level of cleavage above the basement membrane zone. Gene defects of keratins 5 and 14 are implicated and may be identified with IF mapping.

Junctional epidermolysis bullosa is inherited as an autosomal recessive disorder and includes the fatal Herlitz type, in which blistering begins at birth and death occurs within the first 2 years (Figure 26-10), and the non-Herlitz type, which manifests similar to the Herlitz type but with a generally better overall prognosis. The cleavage plane occurs in the lamina lucida of the basement membrane at the dermoepidermal junction. Similar changes may involve the gastrointestinal, respiratory, and urinary tracts. Gene defects involving laminin 5 chain and collagen are identified.

Dystrophic epidermolysis bullosa includes the dominant form, which has a good prognosis, and the recessive form, which has a poor prognosis due to extensive erosions and ulcerations that heal with scarring. The level of cleavage is in the papillary dermis below the basement membrane (Figure 26-11). The principal gene defect involves collagen VII.

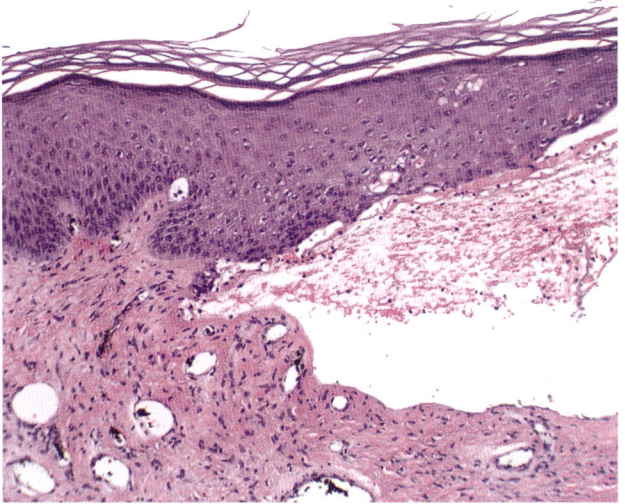

FIGURE 26-11 • Epidermolysis bullosa dystrophica has a subepidermal blister with mild dermal inflammation. (Hematoxylin and eosin stain, original magnification ×200.)

Immunomapping studies are useful in localizing the cleavage plane and determining the presence, increase, or absence of the structural protein for which the gene is mutated in epidermolysis bullosa. These studies are essential for accurate classification of the type of epidermolysis bullosa, which in conjunction with clinical presentation forms the basis of prognostic information and genetic counseling. Furthermore, fetal skin biopsies during the third trimester can be diagnostic in the most severe forms of epidermolysis bullosa.

Incontinentia Pigmenti

Incontinentia pigmenti (Bloch-Sulzberger syndrome) is an X-linked dominant dermatosis that affects mostly women (19,20). Affected hemizygous male fetuses are generally thought to die *in utero* although recent literature suggests that some male individuals may show cutaneous and extracutaneous features of incontinentia pigmenti in a limited distribution that allow survival (21). The characteristic cutaneous manifestations evolve from crops of vesicles and bullae on the extremities arranged in linear or whorled pattern at birth or shortly thereafter that heal with hyperkeratotic verrucous lesions. As the verrucous lesions subside, characteristic streaks and whorls of hyperpigmentation develop, being most pronounced on the trunk. Faint hypochromic or atrophic lesions in a linear pattern may be seen on the lower extremities in some women and rarely in children (22).

Histologically, the vesicular stage is characterized by eosinophilic spongiosis and intraepidermal vesicle formation and eosinophil-rich dermal inflammatory cell infiltrate (Figure 26-12). The verrucous stage is characterized by hyperkeratosis and papillomatous epidermal hyperplasia with focal dyskeratosis. The hyperpigmented stage corresponds to numerous melanophages in the dermis as in any other postinflammatory pigmentary change.

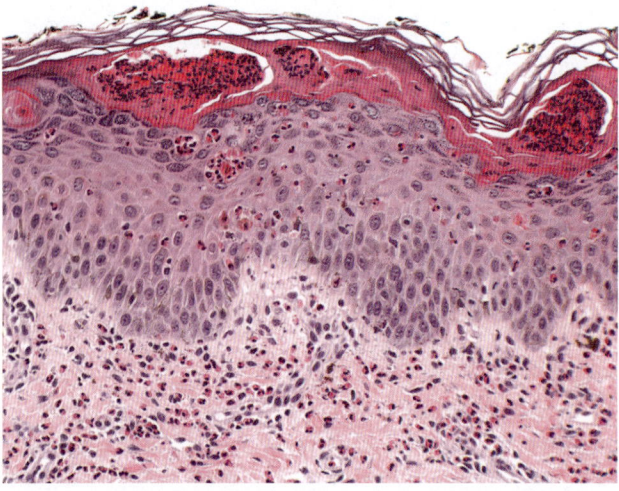

FIGURE 26-12 • Incontinentia pigmenti showing the initial skin changes with an intense eosinophilic infiltration within mildly spongiotic epidermis and the dermis. (Hematoxylin and eosin stain, original magnification ×200.)

In approximately 80% of patients, systemic involvement, particularly of the central nervous system and the eye, and teeth abnormalities may be present. Although the skin manifestations are self-limiting, the clinical course is guided by the extent of systemic involvement.

Acrodermatitis Enteropathica

Acrodermatitis enteropathica is an autosomal recessive disorder characterized by defective intestinal absorption of zinc presenting with the triad of dermatitis, diarrhea, and alopecia in infancy at the time of weaning (23). Acquired acrodermatitis enteropathica–like syndromes can occur in exclusively breastfed preterm infants, infants who are fed on breast milk low in zinc, infants with organic acid urea, and any other acquired zinc deficiency states including human immunodeficiency virus infection. Cutaneous manifestations are characterized by vesiculobullous lesions with acral and periorificial distribution. The histopathologic findings include intraepidermal bulla with epidermal necrosis or spongiosis and superficial perivascular mixed inflammatory cell infiltrate. A well-established lesion shows parakeratosis, marked pallor and ballooning of keratinocytes, and a markedly diminished granular zone. The histologic changes can be identical to those seen in glucagonoma syndrome and pellagra, conditions associated with nutritional deficiencies of factors essential for normal maturation and metabolism of epidermal keratinocytes.

NONINFECTIOUS ACQUIRED VESICULOBULLOUS DISEASES

Linear IgA Bullous Dermatosis

Linear IgA bullous dermatosis, also known as *chronic bullous dermatosis of childhood*, presents with large tense bullae in prepubertal children often younger than 5 years of age. The lesions are widespread in distribution and vesicles and bullae, sometimes arranged like a string of pearls, occur at the periphery of a healing lesion. Areas of predilection include the lower part of the trunk, including the groin and genitalia and perioral areas. Rare cases have been described in neonates. Microscopic features are essentially indistinguishable from dermatitis herpetiformis and consist of neutrophilic microabscesses at the tips of dermal papillae in early lesions and subepidermal bulla filled with neutrophils or eosinophils in well-established lesions (Figure 26-13). Direct IF testing shows a distinct linear pattern of staining at the basement membrane zone with IgA, in sharp contrast to the granular IgA deposits seen in dermatitis herpetiformis. Direct IF testing is crucial in differentiating lupus erythematosus and chronic bullous dermatosis of childhood from other childhood bullous diseases like bullous pemphigoid and lichen planus. Chronic bullous disease of childhood generally has a benign course with spontaneous remission before puberty. Rare cases heal with scarring when the

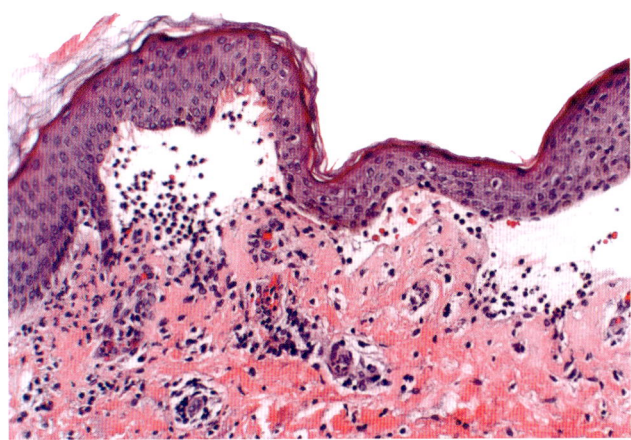

FIGURE 26-13 • Linear IgA dermatosis with a subepidermal blister with neutrophils.

disease process seems to overlap with childhood cicatricial pemphigoid, which some consider to be another morphologic expression of linear IgA dermatosis of childhood and adults. Linear IgA dermatosis of both children and adults are also similar, both IgA1-mediated diseases (24) with some cases of chronic bullous dermatosis of childhood relapsing into adulthood. Distinction of linear IgA bullous disease from dermatitis herpetiformis is important because the former is not typically associated with gluten-sensitive enteropathy.

Dermatitis Herpetiformis

Dermatitis herpetiformis presents as an intensely pruritic papulovesicular eruption that is typically distributed on the scalp, the extensor aspects of extremities, and the back. The lesions may be grouped in herpetiform fashion and symmetrical in distribution. They are characterized by small papules and tense vesicles that rupture easily (25).

Although dermatitis herpetiformis generally manifests as a skin disease, approximately 75% to 90% of the children with this disorder have an associated gluten-sensitive enteropathy and a high frequency of HLA antigens, including HLA B8, DR3, and DqW2 (26,27). Histologic sections of a papular lesion show the characteristic neutrophilic microabscesses at the tips of the dermal papillae (Figure 26-14). Sections of a clinically apparent vesicle show a subepidermal bulla filled with neutrophils and a varying mixture of eosinophils and fibrin. Microabscesses are present at the edge of the blister. Direct IF testing is positive for granular deposits of IgA at the tips of dermal papillae in almost all patients (28). A gluten-free diet is effective in controlling the intestinal and cutaneous manifestations in most children.

Herpes Gestationis

Pemphigoid gestationis (herpes gestationis) is a rare acquired autoimmune bullous disease that affects pregnant women most commonly during the second trimester (29) and, in a small percentage of cases, can be transmitted to the neonates born to these women. The affected neonate may present with macules or papulovesicular or bullous lesions at birth or shortly thereafter. In neonates, the condition is transient, with complete resolution of the lesions occurring within a month, and it is attributed to the transplacental transfer of maternal antibodies (30). Studies have failed to show significant association between pemphigoid gestationis and increased incidence and risk of fetal morbidity or mortality. Histopathologic and IF findings may be identical to those seen in bullous pemphigoid and consist of subepidermal bulla with eosinophils and linear deposits of C3 and IgG at the basement membrane zone. Additionally, sera from patients with pemphigoid gestationis like those with bullous pemphigoid are positive for antibodies against a 180-kD epidermal antigen (31).

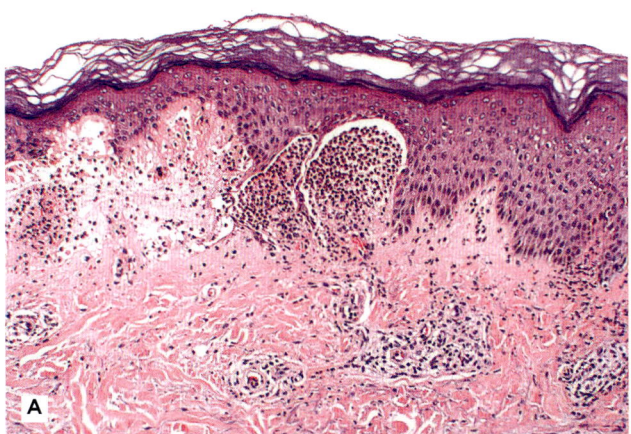
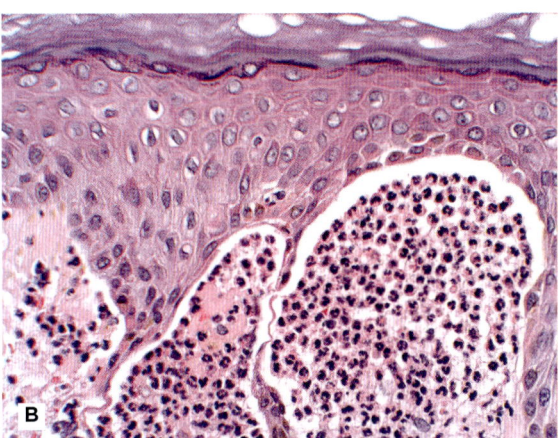

FIGURE 26-14 • Dermatitis herpetiformis. **A, B:** Subepidermal separation with neutrophilic microabscesses at the tips of dermal papillae. Differentiation from linear IgA dermatosis is possible only on IF studies. (Hematoxylin and eosin stains, original magnification ×200 **(A)**, ×400 **(B)**.)

Epidermolysis Bullosa Acquisita

Epidermolysis bullosa acquisita is an acquired form of epidermolysis bullosa that is seen more commonly in adults but can sometimes be seen in children (32,33). Clinically, it may resemble the autosomal dominant dystrophic type of epidermolysis bullosa manifesting with tense blisters on the extensor aspects that heal with scarring and milia formation. However, epidermolysis bullosa acquisita is an autoimmune disease characterized by IgG antibodies to type VII collagen of the basement membrane (34,35).

Light microscopic and IF findings are indistinguishable from bullous pemphigoid, which can also be seen in children (36). Both conditions are characterized by subepidermal bulla with linear deposits of IgG and C3 at the basement membrane zone. Indirect IF studies localize the IgG deposits to the roof of salt-split skin, in which the cleavage runs through the lamina lucida of the basement membrane in pemphigoid and the floor (beneath the lamina lucida) in epidermolysis bullosa acquisita.

Erythema Multiforme, Stevens-Johnson Syndrome, and Toxic Epidermal Necrolysis

Erythema multiforme, Stevens-Johnson (S-J) syndrome, and toxic epidermal necrolysis (TEN) (Lyell syndrome) form the clinical and histopathologic spectrum of a potentially life-threatening group of disorders characterized by epidermal necrosis with formation of bullae, which can involve a large part of the skin surface and mucosa. The high mortality rate in patients with TEN is directly related to the resultant fluid loss and sepsis. S-J syndrome is more common in childhood than erythema multiforme or TEN.

Erythema multiforme is distinguished clinically by the characteristic iris or targetoid lesions that can occur on any part of the body but most commonly on the palms and soles. Erythematous and purpuric macules that progress to flaccid bullae and detach from the underlying dermis are characteristic of S-J syndrome and TEN. The detachment is extensive in TEN while mucosal involvement is more prominent in S-J syndrome.

The majority of cases of erythema multiforme in children are etiologically related to herpes simplex virus (HSV) infection; other viral infections including Epstein-Barr virus and orf and mycoplasma infections have also been implicated (37). Drugs such as sulfonamides and penicillins play an important role, especially in the more severe S-J syndrome and TEN (38,39). No cause can be identified in a significant number of cases.

Histopathologic features include interface dermatitis with vacuolar alteration of the basal cell layer and mild perivascular infiltrate of lymphocytes, which are also present along the dermoepidermal junction. The histologic hallmark of this group of diseases is the necrotic keratinocyte, which may be few in milder forms and numerous

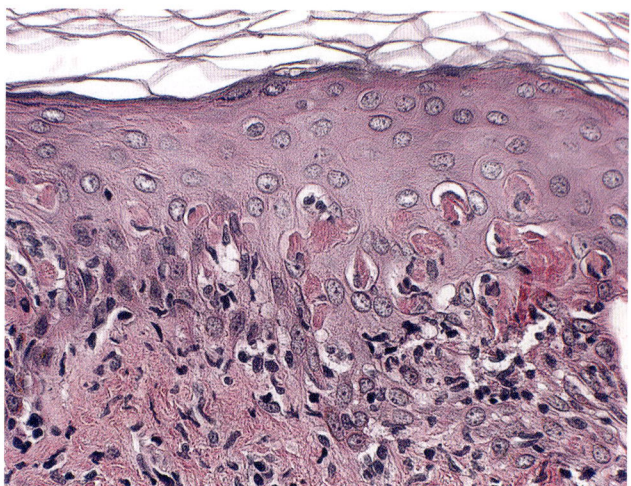

FIGURE 26-15 • Erythema multiforme with basket-weave orthokeratosis, vacuolar alteration of the basal cell layer, necrotic keratinocytes, and mild superficial perivascular inflammation. (Hematoxylin and eosin stain, original magnification ×400.)

with confluent areas of necrosis in more established lesions (Figure 26-15). In TEN, full-thickness epidermal necrosis leads to subepidermal separation and loss of epidermal surface with the eroded clinical appearance of skin originally described by Lyell (Figure 26-16). An unaltered stratum corneum in skin biopsies attests to the acute nature of the assault on the skin. Immune complex–mediated reactions of types III and IV and helper T-cell–mediated immunoreactions are believed to play a role in the pathogenesis of erythema multiforme/TEN (40). Erythema multiforme/S-J syndrome/TEN are potentially life-threatening disorders that require hospitalization, withdrawal of recent drugs, and supportive care. Potential infectious causes should be sought and treated. The benefits of specific treatment

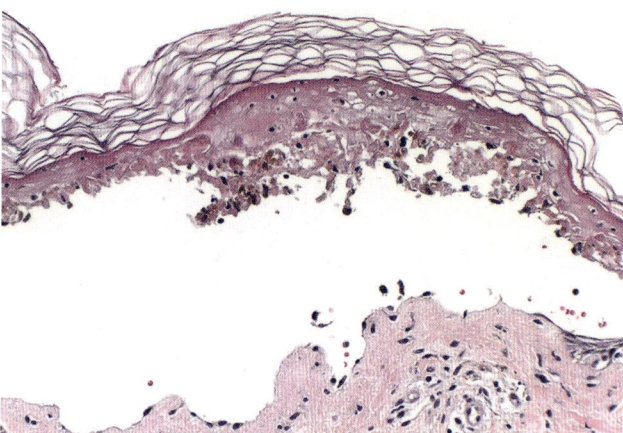

FIGURE 26-16 • TEN with full-thickness epidermal necrosis with separation at the dermoepidermal junction and sparse inflammatory cell infiltrate. An unaltered cornified layer attests to the acuteness of the event. (Hematoxylin and eosin stain, original magnification ×400.)

including corticosteroids and intravenous administration of immunoglobulin are still under debate and further investigation (41–44).

MISCELLANEOUS NONINFECTIOUS VESICULOPUSTULAR DISEASES

A variety of benign vesiculopustular diseases are commonly seen in neonates and infants. It is important to differentiate these conditions from the more serious vesiculopustular diseases that can affect children (45).

Erythema Toxicum Neonatorum

Erythema toxicum neonatorum (toxic erythema of newborn) is an asymptomatic, transient, self-limiting, common eruption that occurs in the first 24 to 48 hours of life of full-term newborns. The lesions are characterized by macules, papules, and tiny pustules that can affect any part of the body but favor the trunk and proximal extremities. Classical clinical presentation rarely requires a skin biopsy that would reveal eosinophils in the pilosebaceous units and differentiate erythema toxicum neonatorum from other neonatal pustular dermatoses including incontinentia pigmenti (46,47).

TRANSIENT NEONATAL PUSTULAR MELANOSIS

Transient neonatal pustular melanosis is a benign, self-limiting condition that predominantly affects black infants. The skin eruption begins as superficial sterile pustules that rupture easily and typically heal with hyperpigmented macules with collarettes of fine scale. Similarities between transient neonatal pustular melanosis and erythema toxicum neonatorum are emphasized by some authors who proposed "sterile transient neonatal pustulosis" as a unifying term (48). However, the pustules in transient neonatal pustular melanosis show abundance of neutrophils.

Acropustulosis of Infancy

Acropustulosis of infancy presents as recurrent crops of pruritic vesicles and pustules on distal extremities with predilection for palms and soles, primarily in black infants during the first year of life. Most cases show spontaneous resolution by the age of 2 years (49). Smears from the pustule and histologic sections of the subcorneal pustules show abundant neutrophils.

ECZEMATOUS DERMATITIS

"Eczema" is the term often used to describe erythematous, scaling vesicular lesions with serum crust. Eczematous dermatitis is characterized histologically by epidermal spongiosis and, therefore, is often referred to interchangeably as spongiotic dermatitis. A specific diagnosis is based on clinical history, morphologic appearance, and distribution of lesions. This group of disorders includes nummular dermatitis, contact dermatitis, dyshidrotic dermatitis, and atopic dermatitis.

Nummular Dermatitis

Nummular dermatitis is characterized by coin-shaped, pruritic, erythematous, scaly crusted plaques on the extensor aspect of the extremities. It is believed to be a manifestation of xerosis and is more commonly seen in older patients.

Atopic Dermatitis

Atopic dermatitis is an inherited chronic pruritic skin disease and is the most common skin disease seen in children, with an estimated incidence of as high as 20% (50). About one-third of the cases are diagnosed before the age of 1 year and before 5 years of age in vast majority of patients (51). Sites of predilection are the face in young infants, extensor surfaces of extremities in children younger than 1 year of age, and the popliteal and antecubital fossae, face, and neck in older children and adolescents. The major abnormality in this disease appears to be the overproduction of allergen-specific IgE, and some authors suggest that demonstration of such antibodies be a requisite for the diagnosis of atopic dermatitis (52). Cytokines, T cells, and antigen-presenting cells in addition to abnormalities of skin barrier appear to play a role in the pathogenesis (53).

Contact Dermatitis

Contact dermatitis includes primary irritant dermatitis and allergic contact dermatitis. Primary irritant dermatitis is frequently seen in children on the cheeks caused by saliva, extremities in response to harsh soaps or detergents, and the diaper area from toiletries (54). Allergic contact dermatitis presents with pruritic, edematous papules, plaques, and occasionally vesicles 12 to 24 hours after exposure to an allergen such as poison ivy, fragrances, nickel, and rubber compounds (55). Allergic contact dermatitis occurs more frequently in children with atopic tendencies (56).

Dyshidrotic Dermatitis

Dyshidrotic dermatitis (pompholyx) typically presents with numerous, pinpoint, recurrent, pruritic vesicles along the sides of the fingers and toes and on palms and soles that usually last a few weeks and frequently relapse.

Histopathology of Spongiotic Dermatitis

Irrespective of the specific type of disease, spongiotic dermatitis shows a similar spectrum of changes. In the acute phase, there is epidermal spongiosis, sometimes marked, with vesiculation (Figure 26-17). In the subacute phase, the spongiosis is milder, but associated parakeratosis with plasma cells, neutrophils, eosinophils, and epidermal hyperplasia may be present. In the chronic phase, the spongiosis is mild to absent, but changes of chronicity are reflected in a

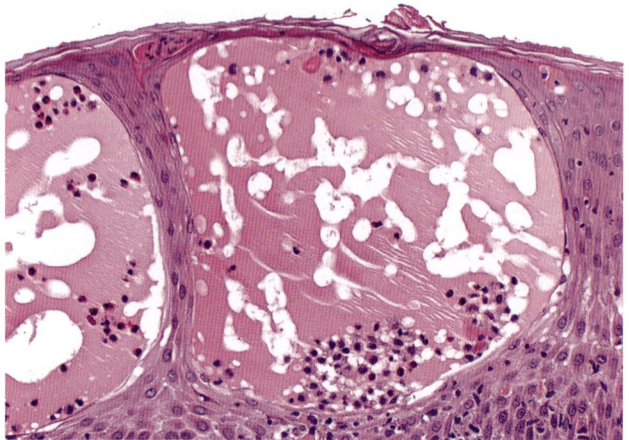

FIGURE 26-17 • Eczematous dermatitis showing marked epidermal spongiosis with formation of intraepidermal vesicles and moderate perivascular mixed inflammation. (Hematoxylin and eosin stain, original magnification ×400.)

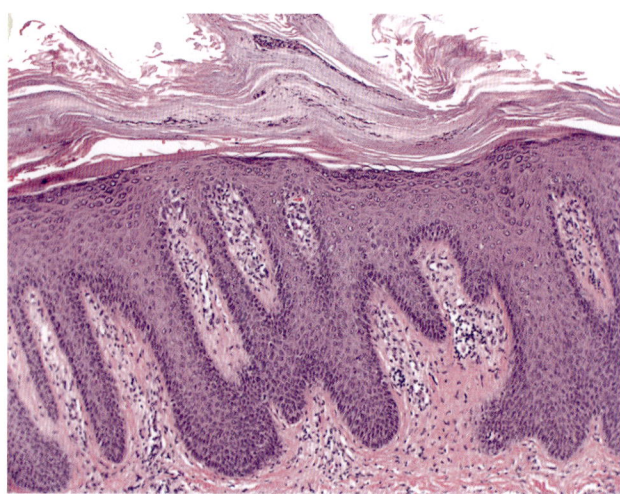

FIGURE 26-18 • Psoriasis is characterized by confluent parakeratosis and regular epidermal hyperplasia. (Hematoxylin and eosin stain, original magnification ×200.)

hyperkeratotic cornified layer, marked epidermal hyperplasia, and fibrotic papillary dermis. Superficial perivascular lymphohistiocytic infiltrate is present to varying degrees in all the phases of spongiotic dermatitis.

NONINFECTIOUS PAPULOSQUAMOUS DERMATOSES

This includes a group of diverse disorders characterized by papular and scaling lesions and associated epidermal proliferation. Approximately 10% of the patients seen in a pediatric dermatology clinic present with papulosquamous skin disorders (57). The following is a brief discussion of the more common dermatoses traditionally regarded as the papulosquamous dermatoses.

Psoriasis Vulgaris

Psoriasis vulgaris accounts for 4% of all dermatoses encountered in children younger than the age of 16 years, (58) and in about 30% of the patients, psoriasis manifests in the first or the second decade of life (59). Of the various forms of psoriasis, namely, plaque type, guttate, pustular and erythrodermic psoriasis, plaque type is the most common one seen in children followed by guttate psoriasis (60). Pustular psoriasis and psoriatic arthropathy are less common in children (61). The clinical presentation is characterized by asymptomatic scaly erythematous plaques in the plaque type and by slightly pruritic small red drop-like scaly lesions in guttate psoriasis. Silvery scales that, on scraping, leave pinpoint areas of bleeding (Auspitz sign) are typical of psoriasis. Lesions are distributed in a bilaterally symmetrical pattern with predilection for scalp and extensor aspects of extremities. Involvement of face is more common in children than in adults and needs to be distinguished from atopic dermatitis. Similarly, psoriasis may involve the diaper area in up to 13% of patients where it must be differentiated from infantile seborrheic dermatitis and other causes of diaper dermatitis (62). Classic histologic features of psoriasis include confluent parakeratosis with neutrophils (Munro microabscesses), regular elongation of epidermal rete with thin suprapapillary plates, dilated vessels in dermal papillae, and mild superficial perivascular inflammation (Figure 26-18). Dermatophytes can produce psoriasiform dermatitis.

Psoriasis, a multifactorial disorder with a genetic basis, typically runs a chronic course with remissions and flare-ups.

Seborrheic Dermatitis

A chronic dermatosis of unknown cause, seborrheic dermatitis is quite common in infants aged 2 to 10 weeks and in adolescents. In infants, seborrheic dermatitis begins as an erythematous scaly rash typically involving the scalp, face, and diaper area. In adolescents, it appears as a dry fine exfoliation of the scalp (dandruff) and expands to the face with the clinical features sometimes overlapping with those of psoriasis.

Histopathologic features overlap with psoriasis and spongiotic dermatitis and consist of epidermal hyperplasia and spongiosis with exocytosis and patchy parakeratosis, which is often present at the openings of the follicular infundibula. A mild superficial perivascular lymphohistiocytic inflammation is present in the dermis.

Infantile seborrheic dermatitis may clinically mimic Langerhans cell histiocytosis (LCH), which is a potentially serious disorder.

Lichen Planus

More commonly a disease of adulthood, lichen planus, generally a self-limiting pruritic eruption, is generally considered uncommon in children (63). However, children of South Asian subcontinent appear to be more susceptible to developing lichen planus (64). The clinical appearance of the eruption is distinctive and consists of flat-topped violaceous papules involving flexor aspects of the extremities and lower back. Lichen planus can also involve hair, nails, and mucous membranes in a significant number of cases. The histologic features are distinctive and consist of hyperkeratosis,

The characteristic lesion is a well-demarcated, slightly indurated, dusky red area with an advancing border, typically on the face and recently more commonly seen on legs, especially in association with chronic lymphatic obstruction (94). Histologic sections show marked dermal edema with diffuse infiltrate of predominantly neutrophils. Dilated lymphatics and capillaries are present. Gram stain is positive for gram-positive cocci. Septicemia, abscess formation, and, rarely, necrotizing fasciitis may complicate some cases of erysipelas.

Viral Infections

Human Papillomavirus

HPV, a member of the Papoviridae family, is a group of DNA viruses. With advances in molecular biology techniques, more than 100 types of HPV have been identified, some with specific tissue tropism. Transmission of HPV is by direct contact. Clinical patterns of HPV infection include verruca vulgaris or common wart, verruca plantaris or palmaris, verruca plana, and condyloma acuminatum. Certain HPV types manifest with characteristic type of lesions such as HPV types 2, 4, and 7 in verruca vulgaris; HPV type 3 in verruca plana; HPV types 1, 2, and 4 in palmoplantar warts; and HPV types 6 and 11 in condyloma acuminatum in children (95). However, more than one type can share the same tissue tropism.

The characteristic histologic changes of HPV infection, irrespective of the clinical pattern, are epithelial hyperplasia, which can be papillomatous, hyperkeratotic, and parakeratotic, especially at the tips of the papillary projections. The cytopathic effect of HPV is manifested as an irregular and hyperchromatic nucleus surrounded by a halo of clear cytoplasm or koilocyte (Figure 26-27).

In children, verruca vulgaris is the most common pattern of HPV infection seen. In most immunocompetent hosts, spontaneous regression is the expected course. In immunocompromised patients, including patients with epidermodysplasia verruciformis (both autosomally inherited and acquired forms), widespread infection with HPV and progression to squamous cell carcinoma can occur. Oncogenetic types of HPV, such as HPV type 16, can be identified by DNA hybridization in these lesions. Sexual abuse can be a source of condyloma acuminatum in children and requires careful evaluation of the clinical findings and history (96,97). However, most cases of anogenital warts in children are likely to be the result of nonsexual transmission, that is, prenatal mode, maternal history of warts, or autoinoculation may be obtained in a many number (98).

Molluscum Contagiosum

Molluscum contagiosum is a common pediatric cutaneous infection caused by a DNA poxvirus that spreads through person-to-person contact or autoinoculation. It most commonly presents in children younger than 5 years of age with discrete, dome-shaped umbilicated waxy papules varying in size from 1 to 5 mm, involving the face, neck, axilla, abdomen, and thighs.

The histologic findings are classic and consist of epidermal hyperplasia with surface invaginations. Within the epidermal cells, there are large intracytoplasmic inclusion bodies—called *molluscum bodies*—that compress the nuclei to a thin crescent at the periphery of the cell (Figure 26-28). The molluscum bodies increase in size as the infected cells move toward the surface. Basophilic molluscum bodies are found along with the cornified layer within the invaginations. Occasionally, molluscum contagiosum can rupture into the dermis and induce an inflammatory response.

In most immunocompetent hosts, spontaneous regression of the lesions is seen without treatment. In the context of immunosuppressed states, especially HIV infection, hundreds of lesions of molluscum contagiosum may be seen

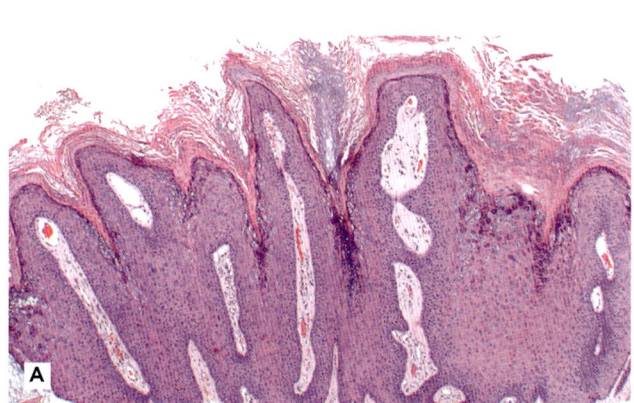
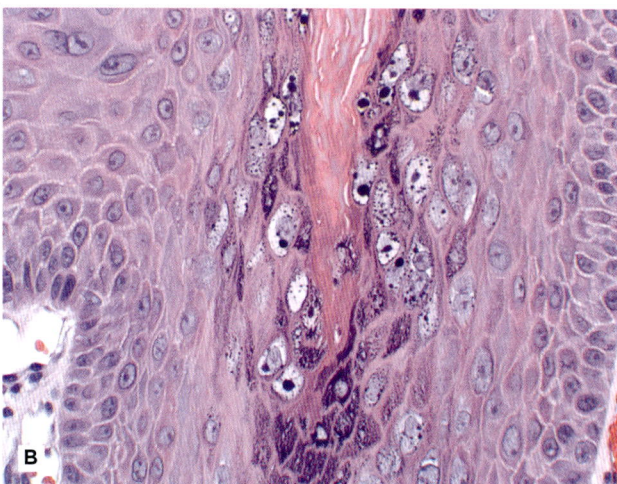

FIGURE 26-27 • Verruca vulgaris. **A:** Hyper- and parakeratosis and papillomatous epidermal hyperplasia. **B:** Hypergranulosis and koilocytosis typical of papillomavirus infection. As warts involute, koilocytes and papillomatosis become less apparent. (Hematoxylin and eosin stain, original magnification ×100 **(A)**, ×400 **(B)**.)

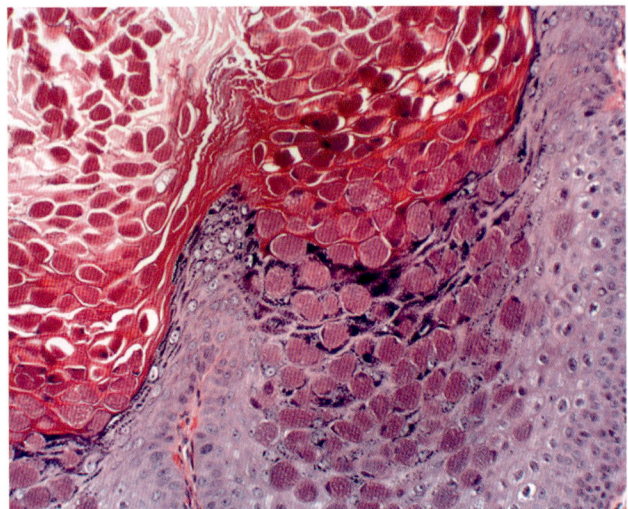

FIGURE 26-28 • Molluscum contagiosum with characteristic eosinophilic round intranuclear and intracytoplasmic inclusions is seen within the hyperplastic epithelium of the follicular infundibula. (Hematoxylin and eosin stain, original magnification ×400.)

with no tendency toward resolution. Hundreds of lesion in a child is cause for concern about immunodeficiency.

Herpes Virus Infection

Herpes viruses are a family of large DNA viruses that include HSV, varicella-zoster virus, cytomegalovirus, Epstein-Barr virus, and human herpes viruses 6, 7, and 8.

Herpes Simplex

Two forms of HSV infections are recognized—orofacial type caused by HSV type 1 and genital type caused by herpes simplex type 2—and both can present as primary or recurrent infections. Primary infection with HSV-1 is largely a childhood disease that can manifest as gingivostomatitis and rarely as Kaposi varicelliform eruption and keratoconjunctivitis. HSV-2 is primarily acquired through sexual contact and can rarely be seen in infants owing to *in utero* infection or direct contact in the birth canal. Most primary HSV infections are asymptomatic. Recurrent HSV infection occurs in people with previous infections and is characterized by repeated episodes of lesions at the same site.

Varicella and Herpes Zoster

Herpes zoster virus commonly manifests in children as chicken pox due to primary infection with *varicella-zoster* infection. Chicken pox is a highly contagious generalized vesiculopustular eruption that spreads centrifugally, with lesions in different stages of development. *Herpes zoster* is caused by reactivation of latent *varicella-zoster* virus that resides in a dorsal root ganglion and presents as grouped vesicles in a dermatomal distribution. *Herpes zoster* can develop any time after a primary infection and is often triggered by immunocompromised state. Because varicella vaccine is a live attenuated virus, *herpes zoster* can develop in a vaccine recipient. In young children, *herpes zoster* has a predilection for areas supplied by the cervical and sacral dermatomes (99).

The histologic findings are identical in herpes simplex and varicella-zoster infections. Intraepidermal vesicles with acantholysis are the characteristic feature. Balloon degeneration and multinucleated keratinocytes with eosinophilic intranuclear inclusions are seen (Figure 26-29). Epidermal necrosis with neutrophilic scale crust characterizes older lesions. Vascular damage with microthrombi and hemorrhage are more pronounced in varicella-zoster infection than in herpes simplex infection.

Human Immunodeficiency Virus

In the acute stage, HIV can present with a transient viral exanthem not unlike other viral exanthems. More commonly, the cutaneous manifestations in HIV are related to immunocompromise and opportunistic infections. Mucocutaneous candidiasis, severe seborrheic dermatitis, eosinophilic pustular folliculitis, and lichenoid dermatitis of AIDS are some

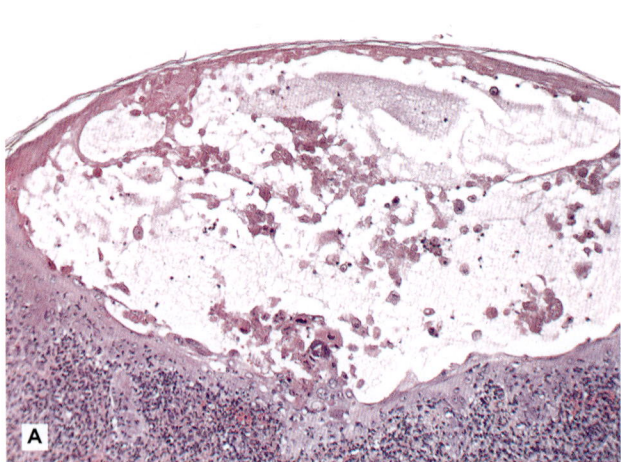
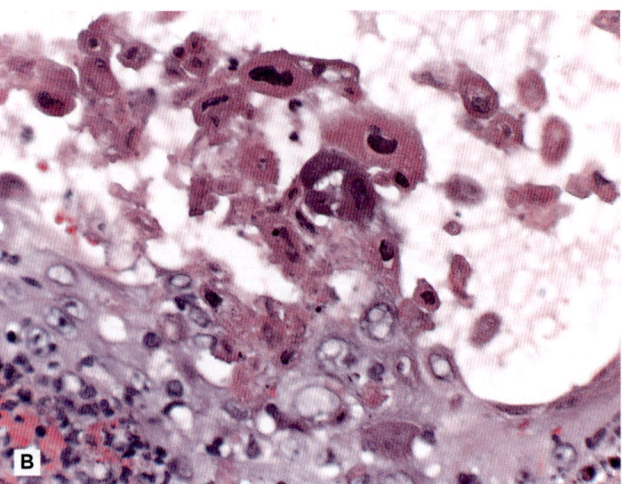

FIGURE 26-29 • Herpes. **A:** An intraepidermal vesicle surrounded by multinucleated keratinocytes. **B:** Characteristic intranuclear inclusions are present at the margins of the vesicle. (Hematoxylin and eosin stain, original magnification ×200 **(A)**, ×400 **(B)**.)

of the manifestations (100). In addition, a range of persistent infections including fungal infections, prolonged varicella, severe cases of herpes zoster, herpes gingivostomatitis, verrucae or condyloma acuminatum, and molluscum contagiosum can be seen in HIV-infected patients (101).

Fungal Infections

Fungal infections of the skin can be classified as superficial and deep forms.

Superficial fungal infections of the skin include dermatophytosis (Tinea) typically caused by three genera, namely, *Trichophyton*, *Microsporum*, and *Epidermophyton*. In addition, *Pityrosporum* and *Candida* can also cause superficial fungal infections of the skin (102).

Tinea capitis is a fungal infection of the scalp and hair that is common in prepubertal children and is most often caused by *Tinea tonsurans* in the United States (103). Tinea capitis presents as one or more scaly patches of alopecia. With some species, such as *T. verrucosum* or *Microsporum canis*, large boggy swellings called *kerion* can develop in the infected areas. Tinea corporis is also common in children and characteristically presents with annular scaly lesions with an active inflammatory border (ringworm). The lesions can be seen anywhere on the body.

Tinea versicolor caused by *Pityrosporum ovale* involves upper trunk with areas of brownish discoloration that later appear hypopigmented.

Primary cutaneous infection with Candida is often seen in the diaper area of infants and characteristically presents as an eczematous dermatitis. Oral candidiasis (thrush) is not uncommon in infants, especially those born to HIV-positive mothers. The diagnosis of superficial fungal infections is best accomplished by demonstration of the organism by culture. KOH preparation offers a rapid method of diagnosis if the organism can be demonstrated. A biopsy of the lesion and demonstration of the organism is another reliable method of establishing diagnosis (104).

Histologically, dermatophytoses generally show mild nonspecific superficial perivascular inflammation and occasionally subcorneal pustules. Fungal hyphae, best seen with PAS stain, are present in the cornified layer in tinea corporis, and within the cornified layer as well as the follicle and hair shaft in tinea capitis (Figure 26-30). In kerion celsi, a marked, mixed inflammatory response with formation of dermal abscesses is seen. A granulomatous response to disrupted hair shafts may also be present.

Histologic sections from a biopsy of pityriasis versicolor show minimal inflammatory reaction. However, the short nonbranching hyphae and spores of Malassezia are easily identified within the cornified layer, even on hematoxylin and eosin–stained sections.

Deep mycosis can be primarily a cutaneous fungal infection with a propensity to involve deeper tissues or be part of systemic infections such as those involving the respiratory system or reticuloendothelial system. Primary subcutaneous mycoses often caused by saprophytic organisms include sporotrichosis, chromoblastomycosis, histoplasmosis, coccidioidomycosis, blastomycosis, and cryptococcosis. Most of these infections manifest with suppurative and granulomatous inflammation of the dermis and subcutis, with frequent pseudoepitheliomatous epidermal hyperplasia. PAS and silver stains often reveal the characteristic morphology of the fungal organism (Figure 26-31). Deep mycosis may be part of a systemic infection, especially in immunocompromised children. Necrotizing skin lesions with vasculitis and granulomas can be seen with disseminated aspergillosis, mucormycosis, and fusarial infection. A deep necrotizing process in the subcutis should suggest a deep angioinvasive infection.

Infestations

Scabies is a highly contagious pruritic papulovesicular and pustular eruption caused by *Sarcoptes scabiei* (105). Children are often affected with rapid spread through person-to-person contact. The adult female mite lays eggs within

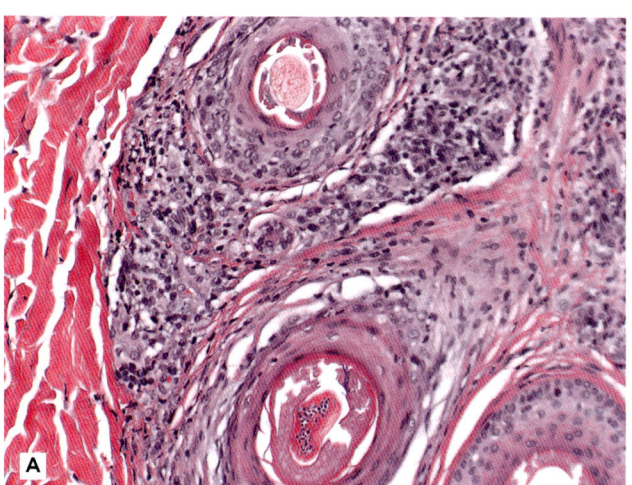 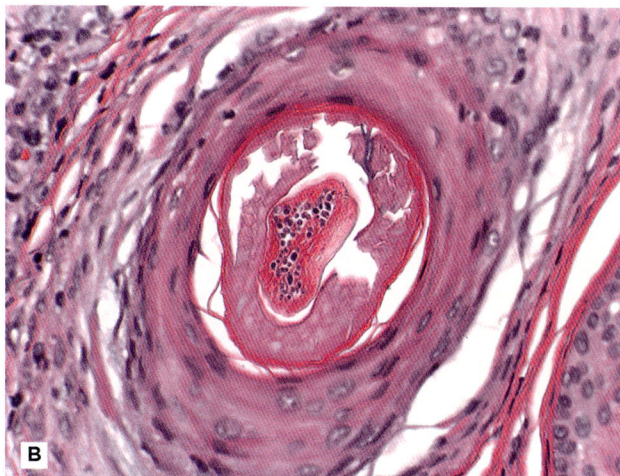

FIGURE 26-30 • **A, B:** Tinea capitis showing involvement of a hair follicle and shaft by numerous spores. (Hematoxylin and eosin stain, original magnification ×200.)

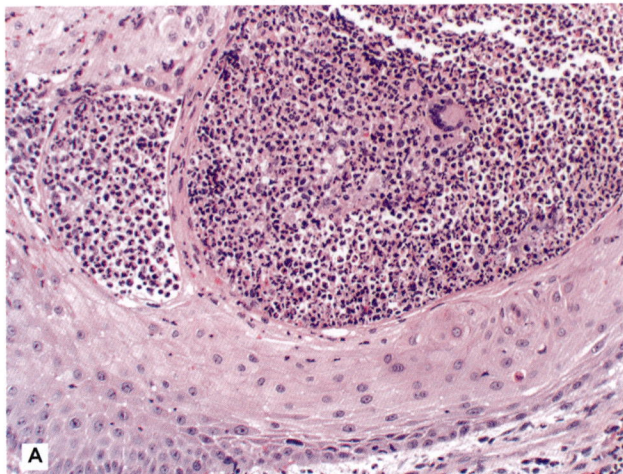 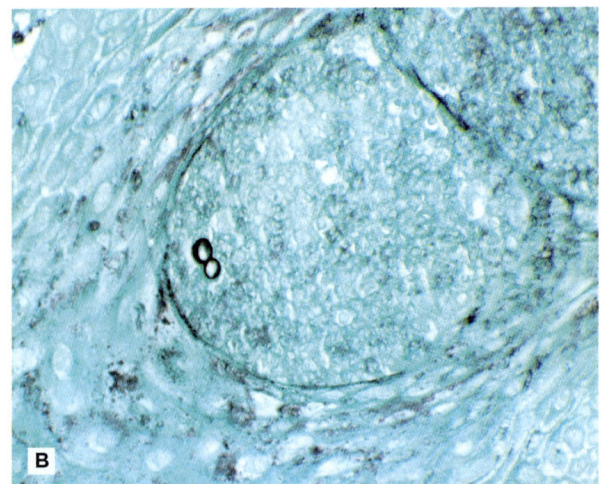

FIGURE 26-31 • Blastomycosis. **A:** Pseudoepitheliomatous hyperplasia with suppurative and granulomatous inflammation. Broad-based budding yeast forms of blastomycosis can be seen within the cytoplasm of multinucleated giant cells or within the microabscesses or both. (Hematoxylin and eosin stain, original magnification ×400.) **B:** GMS stain highlights the characteristic broad-based budding yeast form.

burrows in the superficial epidermis, most commonly involving the soles, wrists, interdigital spaces, thenar eminences, and genitalia. Erythematous papules and pustules with intense pruritus and multiple excoriations characterize the clinical presentation. A positive diagnosis can be made by scraping a burrow and examining the scrapings under a drop of mineral oil. A more aggressive approach is to biopsy a suspected lesion. Histologic sections show a superficial and deep perivascular mixed inflammatory cell infiltrate with frequent eosinophils suggestive of a hypersensitivity reaction. A definite diagnosis can be made only when the mite or eggs of *S. scabiei* are identified within the parakeratotic cornified layer.

NONINFECTIOUS INFLAMMATORY DERMATOSES

Acute Febrile Neutrophilic Dermatosis

Acute febrile neutrophilic dermatosis (Sweet syndrome) is generally a disease of adults characterized by fever; leukocytosis; violaceous plaque-like lesions on the face, trunk, and extremities; and a diffuse dermal neutrophilic infiltrate without vasculitis. Although the condition is rare, several reports of Sweet syndrome in children have been documented (106–108), and as in adults, many of these cases are associated with underlying malignancies or inflammatory diseases, which most often dictate the overall clinical prognosis.

Eosinophilic Cellulitis

Eosinophilic cellulitis, or Well syndrome, originally described in adults, is a rare, recurrent inflammatory dermatosis of uncertain pathogenesis. Cases of eosinophilic cellulitis have been reported in children (109) in association with various precipitating events such as viral infections and insect bites. A possible genetic factor is also suggested. Histologic features include a dense diffuse dermal infiltrate of eosinophils. Foci of collagen degeneration deposited with eosinophilic granules, referred to as *flame figures*, may be present.

Neutrophilic Eccrine Hidradenitis and Idiopathic Palmoplantar Hidradenitis

Neutrophilic eccrine hidradenitis is a generally self-limiting inflammatory dermatosis often seen in association with chemotherapy for various malignancies. Neutrophilic eccrine hidradenitis has been reported in children in association with chemotherapy for non-Hodgkin lymphoma and acute myelogenous leukemia (110). The condition is characterized by the appearance of numerous erythematous papules and plaques on the trunk and extremities within several weeks of beginning chemotherapy. Histologic sections show a dense neutrophilic infiltrate within and around the coils of eccrine glands and ducts.

Idiopathic palmoplantar hidradenitis was first described by Stahr et al. (111) primarily in otherwise healthy children and young people. It is characterized by the abrupt onset of tender erythematous papules, plaques, and nodules on the soles and, less often, palms of young patients. The ages of the patients range from 1.5 to 15 years, with increased prevalence in autumn and spring (112,113). Skin biopsy shows a dense neutrophilic infiltrate with abscess formation in and around the eccrine coil. However, special stains and microbiologic cultures are generally negative for organisms. The presence of neutrophilic abscesses and absence of squamous syringometaplasia in idiopathic palmoplantar hidradenitis aids in differentiation from neutrophilic eccrine hidradenitis. There is complete resolution of the lesions within 2 to 3 weeks with supportive therapy alone. Approximately 50% of the patients may experience a relapse that resolves spontaneously (114).

Pyoderma Gangrenosum

Pyoderma gangrenosum is an uncommon idiopathic ulceronecrotic skin disease, in the family of neutrophilic dermatoses, which can present in children 4% to 5% of the time (115). A systemic illness, most often inflammatory bowel disease or hematologic disorder, is present in 50% to 74% of the patients (116). As in adults, the lower extremities are often involved. In addition, head and neck and anogenital areas appear to be more commonly involved in infants and children. A typical lesion of pyoderma gangrenosum consists of ulceration with a necrotic center, mucopurulent exudate, a violaceous undermined border, and an erythematous periphery. Histologic findings are nonspecific and vary depending on the area biopsied from a typical ulcer with necrosis and neutrophilic abscesses in the center of the lesion to endothelial swelling, fibrinoid necrosis, thrombosis, and extravasated red cells and a lymphocytic infiltrate at the erythematous periphery. Biopsy of the undermined edge shows mixed inflammatory cell infiltrate and early neutrophilic abscesses. A lymphocytic or a leukocytoclastic vasculitis was observed at the border of the lesion by some authors (117).

NONINFECTIOUS GRANULOMATOUS DERMATOSES

Granulomatous reaction may be seen in response to a variety of agents including infections, foreign body, and degenerative changes of collagen. In some cases, as in sarcoidosis, the inciting agent is not apparent. An infectious process should be appropriately excluded in all cases. Some granulomatous reactions such as those seen in response to ruptured cyst contents, degenerating collagen (necrobiotic granulomas), and sarcoidosis are so characteristic that a specific diagnosis can usually be rendered.

Granuloma Annulare

Granuloma annulare is a benign disorder of unknown etiology associated with degenerated collagen and is often seen in children. It is characterized by a single or multiple asymptomatic ringed papules most commonly on the dorsa of hands and feet and often mistaken for tinea.

Histologic findings are diagnostic of granuloma annulare. They consist of zones of degeneration of collagen within the upper half of the dermis, sometimes with mucinous deposits. These zones are surrounded by a palisade of histiocytes (Figure 26-32). Perivascular lymphocytic infiltrates may also be present. A subcutaneous form of granuloma annulare, also known as *pseudorheumatoid nodule*, is more commonly seen in children than in adults. This form presents commonly on the pretibial area or lower legs and head and neck as asymptomatic deep dermal or subcutaneous nodules. Histologic sections show large foci of myxoid degeneration of collagen surrounded by palisades of histiocytes within the deep dermis and subcutaneous tissue (118). Although mucinous degeneration rather than fibrinoid degeneration

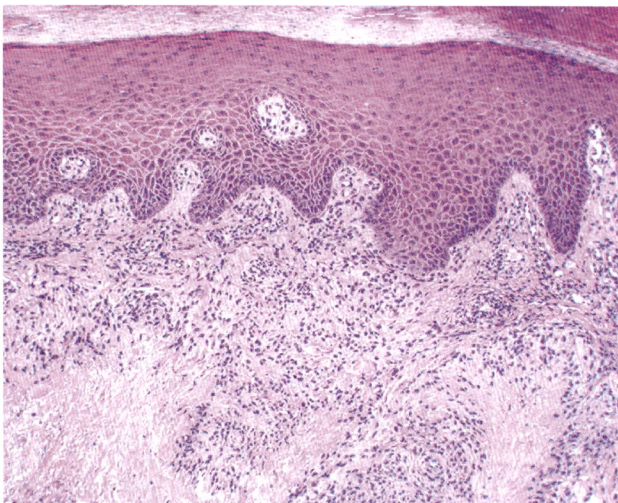

FIGURE 26-32 • Granuloma annulare as an upper dermal granuloma showing central myxoid degeneration of the collagen surrounded by a palisade of histiocytes. (Hematoxylin and eosin stain, original magnification ×200.)

of the collagen and the absence of arthritis help differentiate subcutaneous granuloma annulare from rheumatoid nodule, this distinction is not always possible. However, the majority of patients with granuloma annulare show no serologic evidence of IgM rheumatoid factor. Deep granuloma annulare in a child may present as a soft tissue tumor.

Although an association of granuloma annulare with systemic diseases such as diabetes, lymphoma and other malignancies, and sarcoidosis has been suggested in adult patients, most of the children are otherwise healthy and progression to systemic disease of any kind is not common (119). Rare cases of underlying immune defects, such as IgA–IgG2 deficiency, have been reported in children (120). The clinical course of granuloma annulare is spontaneous regression with occasional recurrences.

Necrobiosis Lipoidica

Necrobiosis lipoidica is a degenerative disease of the dermal collagen often seen in association with diabetes. It is a disease of young adults and is rarely reported in children (121,122). Clinically, it is characterized by oval plaques, most commonly on the shins. The center of the plaque may later become atrophic with a distinctive yellow waxy hue. Histologic sections show a palisading granulomatous inflammation surrounding zones of degenerated collagen. The process may involve the entire dermis and extend up to the subcutaneous fat. Plasma cells are a frequent component of the inflammatory cell infiltrate. Late lesions show marked sclerosis and deposits of fat in the epidermis.

Rheumatoid Nodule

Juvenile rheumatoid arthritis is a chronic debilitating disease of childhood. Classic rheumatoid nodules are, however, uncommon in this form of rheumatoid arthritis.

Rheumatoid nodules occur as subcutaneous nodules over the extensor surfaces. Histologically, the lesions are characterized by palisading granulomas surrounding large zones of fibrinoid degeneration of collagen. These lesions occur in patients with rheumatoid arthritis and elevated rheumatoid factors. Similar lesions occurring in the absence of rheumatoid arthritis and more commonly seen in children and referred to as *pseudorheumatoid nodule* most likely represent subcutaneous granuloma annulare (123).

Sarcoidosis

Sarcoidosis is a multisystem disorder characterized by noncaseating granulomas (Chapters 12 and 22). Although rare, sarcoidosis can be seen in children younger than the age of 15 years (124). Skin involvement is seen in approximately a 25% of the patients with sarcoidosis and up to 50% of patients have eye involvement. A subgroup of childhood sarcoidosis manifests in preschool children younger than 6 years of age with skin, joint, and eye involvement without any pulmonary lesions, which may be confused with juvenile rheumatoid arthritis (125). The cutaneous lesions of sarcoidosis are red to yellow or violaceous papules and plaques that, on histologic examination, show typical noncaseating epithelioid granulomas with little or no necrosis, similar to lesions seen in other organs. Sarcoidosis must be differentiated from infectious conditions particularly mycobacterial and deep fungal infections (126).

PANNICULITIS

Inflammation of the fat may predominantly involve either the lobules of the fat, that is, lobular panniculitis, or the fibrous septa, that is, septal panniculitis. It is important to recognize that, on histologic examination, considerable overlap may exist. Panniculitis may be a manifestation of underlying systemic disease, most notably connective tissue diseases such as lupus, dermatomyositis, polyarteritis nodosa, and juvenile rheumatoid arthritis. The histologic changes are typical and diagnostic in some entities, like erythema nodosum, whereas in others, they are nonspecific and require extensive clinical, microbiologic, and often serologic support.

Erythema Nodosum

Patients with erythema nodosum present with sudden onset of symmetric, tender, erythematous subcutaneous nodules on the extensor aspects of lower legs. A prodrome of sore throat and respiratory symptoms may be seen in some children. Histologic sections that contain subcutaneous fat show a predominantly septal pattern of inflammation with acute and chronic inflammation and thickening of the septa with some involvement of the periphery of lobules. In older lesions, granulomatous inflammation with multinucleated giant cells may be present (Figure 26-33). Necrosis within the granulomatous foci should prompt a search for microorganisms. Overt fat necrosis and vasculitis are uncommon findings.

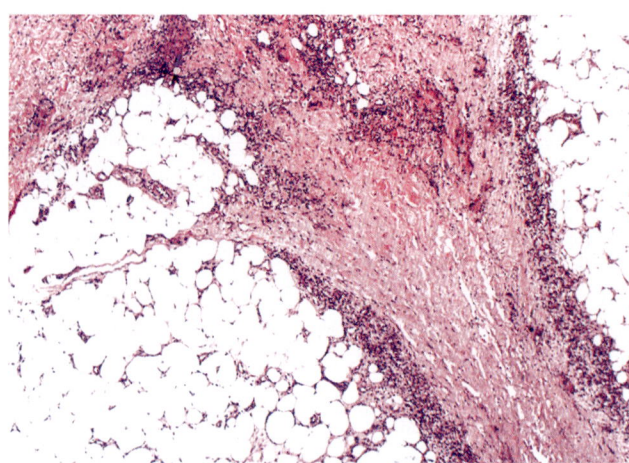

FIGURE 26-33 • Erythema nodosum with a septal pattern of panniculitis and marked fibrous thickening of the septa and granulomatous inflammation. (Hematoxylin and eosin stain, original magnification ×200.)

Erythema nodosum–like reaction patterns can be seen in a variety of infections including tuberculosis, streptococcal infection, histoplasmosis, coccidioidomycosis, and occasionally mumps. Another well-recognized association is with inflammatory bowel disease.

In children, erythema nodosum is a self-limiting disease, with resolution of the lesions occurring within a few weeks. Elimination of the precipitating factor and treatment of infection, if identified, are generally sufficient (127).

Subcutaneous Fat Necrosis of the Newborn

Subcutaneous fat necrosis of the newborn is a relatively uncommon, painless, self-limiting disease that affects full-term and postterm infants (128). It manifests at 1 to 6 weeks of age as asymptomatic, firm nodules on cheeks, shoulder, back, buttocks, and thighs.

Histologic sections show a predominantly lobular involvement with foci of fat necrosis and infiltration by macrophages and multinucleated giant cells. Within the cytoplasm of the macrophages and giant cells, lipid is present as needle-shaped crystals arranged in a radial array (Figure 26-34). Deposits of calcium may be seen. The etiology of subcutaneous fat necrosis is largely unknown. Maternal factors and obstetric trauma are implicated in some cases. Spontaneous resolution of the lesions occurs within the first few months of life. Hypercalcemia is a rare complication, which, if present, should be actively treated (129).

Sclerema Neonatorum

Sclerema neonatorum is a rare, rapidly spreading, diffuse hardening of the subcutaneous tissue of back, shoulders, and buttocks usually affecting premature, ill newborns. Histologic features include diffuse involvement of fat lobules by fat cells containing radially arranged crystals of lipid. Inflammation is minimal or absent, a feature that histologically distinguishes

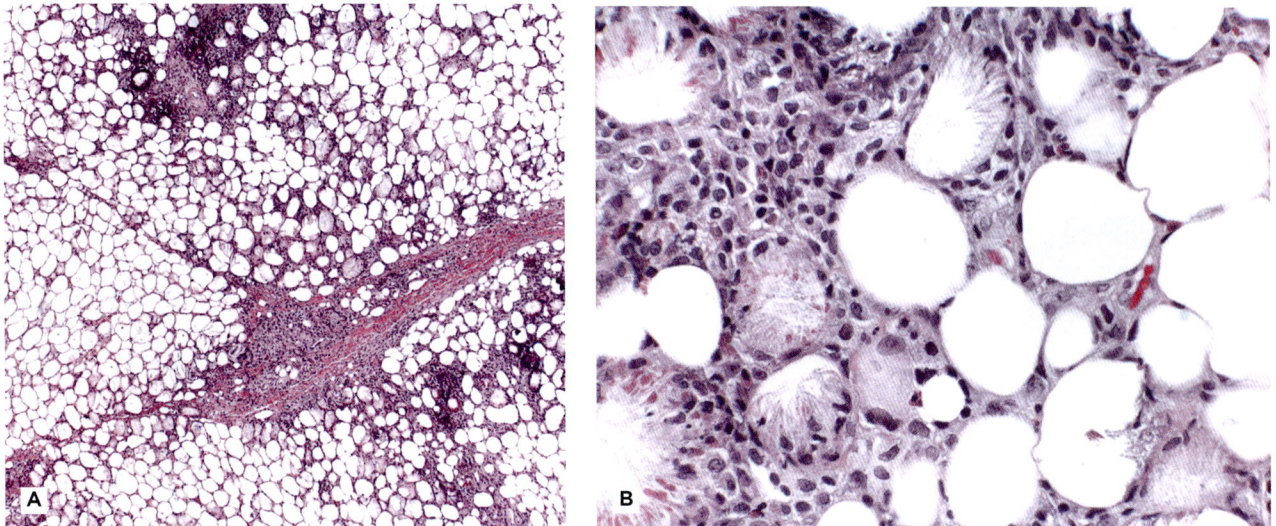

FIGURE 26-34 • Subcutaneous fat necrosis. **A:** Lobular pattern of panniculitis with lymphohistiocytic infiltrate. **B:** Multinucleated histiocytes contain characteristic needle-shaped crystals of lipid. Histologic differential diagnosis includes sclerema neonatorum. (Hematoxylin and eosin stain, original magnification ×200 **(A)**, ×400 **(B)**.)

sclerema neonatorum from subcutaneous fat necrosis of newborn (130). The prognosis is generally poor, with a fatal outcome in most cases. In a case–control study of neonates with sepsis and sclerema, exchange transfusion has been shown to improve survival (131).

VASCULITIS

Cutaneous vasculitis may be a primary disorder, but more commonly, it is a manifestation of an underlying systemic disease such as collagen vascular disease. A simple classification of vasculitis considers the type of blood vessel involved, namely, capillary, venule, or artery, and the type of inflammatory cell infiltrate involved, namely, lymphocytes and neutrophils. Although there is some debate regarding the actual classification schemes, it is generally agreed that the minimum criteria for the diagnosis of vasculitis include demonstration of actual damage to the vessel wall in the form of fibrinoid necrosis, a perivascular inflammatory cell infiltrate and red cell extravasation.

Leukocytoclastic Vasculitis

Henoch-Schönlein Purpura

Henoch-Schönlein purpura, a form of leukocytoclastic vasculitis, is the most common type of vasculitis seen in children (132,133), typically following streptococcal infection of upper respiratory tract, with a peak incidence between 4 and 8 years of age. In addition to palpable purpura on buttocks and lower extremities, affected children often have arthralgias and arthritis, abdominal pain, and hematuria. A skin biopsy is of great value in the diagnostic workup of these patients. Histologic features typical of leukocytoclastic vasculitis are usually present and include superficial perivascular infiltrates of neutrophils, neutrophilic nuclear dust (leukocytoclasia), and extravasated red blood cells (Figure 26-35). The vessels show endothelial swelling and deposits of fibrin within the walls. IF studies are of help in differentiating other causes of leukocytoclastic vasculitis from Henoch-Schönlein purpura. Deposits of IgA in association with C3 and fibrinogen are present within the vessel walls (134).

Henoch-Schönlein purpura is a self-limiting immune complex disorder, with complete resolution occurring within 6 to 16 weeks (135).

Leukocytoclastic vasculitis may be seen secondary to infections due to either direct invasion of vessels or immune-mediated mechanisms. Meningococcal infection is a frequent cause of infectious leukocytoclastic vasculitis in children (136), in whom meningococci can be found within the endothelial cells and neutrophils. Leukocytoclastic vasculitis can also be seen in association with autoimmune diseases and secondary to use of certain drugs. An unusual variant of leukocytoclastic vasculitis, acute hemorrhagic edema of childhood (Finkelstein disease), generally affects children younger than 3 years of age (137) and has many similarities to Henoch-Schönlein purpura (138). However, the lesions are larger and not associated with systemic symptoms. IgA may not be detected by IF studies. Leukocytoclastic vasculitis in children has a relatively benign course, especially in those cases associated with infection and drugs.

Lymphocytic Vasculitis

A histologic diagnosis of lymphocytic vasculitis with authentic vascular damage and infiltration of the vessel walls with lymphocytes is only rarely documented. A lymphocytic vasculitis may be seen in insect bite reactions, PLEVA, lymphomatoid papulosis, and collagen vascular diseases. Lichen aureus and Schamberg-Majocchi purpura represent benign pigmented purpuras characterized by chronic petechiae on

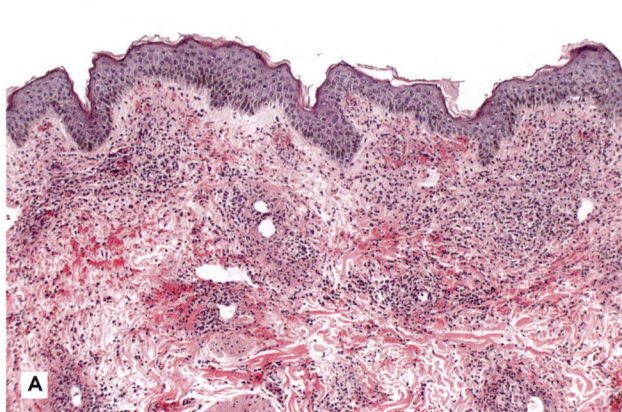
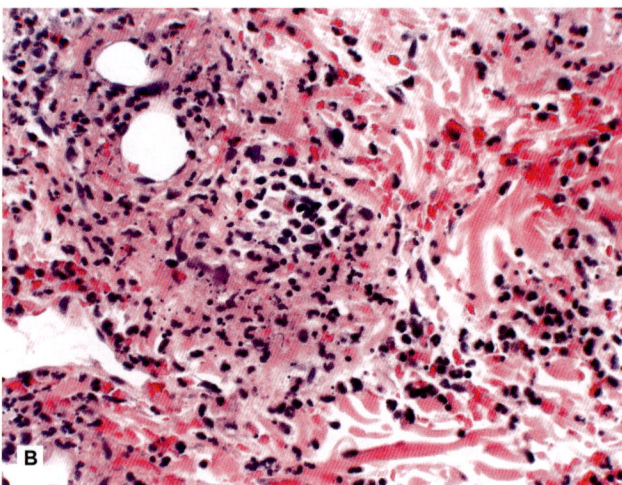

FIGURE 26-35 • Henoch-Schönlein purpura. **A:** Superficial perivascular and interstitial infiltrate of neutrophils and extravasated red cells. **B:** Neutrophils, extravasated red blood cells, and neutrophilic dust are present. Fibrinoid necrosis of the vessel wall is seen only in later lesions. (Hematoxylin and eosin stain, original magnification ×200 **(A)**, ×400 **(B)**.)

legs and elsewhere. Histologically, there is a superficial perivascular lymphocytic infiltrate and extravasated red cells. In older lesions, hemosiderin-laden macrophages may be seen that give the characteristic pigmented appearance. The lesions are asymptomatic and may last for months to years.

Other rare causes of childhood vasculitis include polyarteritis nodosa, Wegener granulomatosis, and Churg-Strauss syndrome, which can rarely present with cutaneous symptoms (139,140). Some cases are a manifestation of a drug reaction.

FOLLICULITIS AND PERIFOLLICULITIS

Acne

Acne is a common cause of visits to the physician's office, especially among adolescents. Acne vulgaris is most common on the face and anterior and posterior trunk, where there are abundant sebaceous glands that produce more sebum in response to androgens. The primary lesion is intrafollicular hyperkeratosis, together with collection of desquamating cells and sebum with subsequent obstruction of the follicular infundibula leading to the formation of a comedone. Open comedones (blackheads) appear as large pores with central black–brown cores. Closed comedones (whiteheads) are often associated with inflammation and rupture to produce a pustule or nodule when the inflammation is deep. Nodulocystic acne and acne conglobata are severe expressions of acne vulgaris, whereas neonatal acne is a transient eruption in newborns secondary to maternal and infant androgen response (141). Persistent acne in an infant should raise suspicion of a possible androgen-producing neoplasm (142).

Eosinophilic Pustular Folliculitis

Eosinophilic pustular folliculitis, or Ofuji disease, originally described in healthy Japanese adults, can present in infancy with white–yellow pustules on the scalp and upper forehead (143). However, it is more likely that this is simply a histologic pattern that can be seen in association with a variety of diseases including scabies and insect bite reactions rather than a specific entity (144).

Histologic findings include eosinophilic spongiosis, subcorneal pustule with eosinophils, and a dense perifollicular inflammation with frequent eosinophils. Microbiologic cultures are generally negative for organisms. The eruption resolves without scarring. Eosinophilic pustular folliculitis may occur in association with HIV infection and other immunocompromised states.

SYSTEMIC DISEASES WITH CUTANEOUS MANIFESTATIONS

Collagen Vascular Diseases

Lupus erythematosus is the most common collagen vascular disease to present in childhood, followed by juvenile rheumatoid arthritis and dermatomyositis (145). Polyarteritis nodosa, scleroderma, and other collagen vascular diseases are less common.

Lupus Erythematosus

Although all forms of lupus can affect children, systemic lupus erythematosus is the most common form. Childhood systemic lupus erythematosus peaks in early adolescence, with about 60% of cases occurring between the ages of 11 and 15 years. Cutaneous manifestations are the second most frequent finding (77%) next to renal involvement (84%) in pediatric patients with systemic lupus erythematosus. Discoid lupus erythematosus without clinical and serologic evidence of systemic disease can occur rarely in children (146). However, discoid lupus erythematosus may be a part of systemic lupus erythematosus syndrome. Cutaneous changes of lupus erythematosus include malar rash, oral ulcerations, photosensitivity, alopecia, and discoid lupus erythematosus (147).

Neonatal lupus erythematosus is seen in newborn infants born to anti-Ro (SS-A) antibody–positive mothers (148), with the development of skin lesions and/or heart block at birth to 2 months of age (149). The skin lesions consist of erythematous, nonscaling, sharply demarcated lesions with a predilection for involvement around the eyes and sometimes annular polycyclic type of lesions commonly seen in subacute cutaneous lupus erythematosus.

Sections from early lesions of systemic lupus erythematosus corresponding to the erythematous malar rash show only nonspecific changes. The histologic changes seen in well-established systemic lupus erythematosus, subacute cutaneous lupus erythematosus, neonatal lupus erythematosus, and discoid lupus erythematosus are essentially similar, varying only in degree. The characteristic changes are those of interface dermatitis with marked vacuolar alteration of the basal cell layer, where there is also a lymphocytic infiltrate that obscures the dermoepidermal junction. Additional findings include hyperkeratosis with epidermal atrophy and follicular plugging, most prominent in discoid lesions, and perivascular and periadnexal lymphocytic infiltrate. A thickened basement membrane, best seen with PAS stain, and separation at the dermoepidermal junction are seen in older lesions (Figure 26-36). Interstitial dermal mucin is also seen. Direct IF reveals continuous granular deposits of C3, IgG, and, occasionally, IgM along the dermoepidermal junction in involved and uninvolved skin in systemic lupus erythematosus and only in involved skin in discoid lupus erythematosus (lupus band test).

Neonatal lupus erythematosus is a transient disorder, and prognosis is generally good in the absence of heart block (150). Some of these infants may develop systemic lupus erythematosus as young adults. The prognosis in childhood systemic lupus erythematosus, like that in adults, has improved with aggressive therapy. Renal complications generally dictate the survival (see Chapter 17).

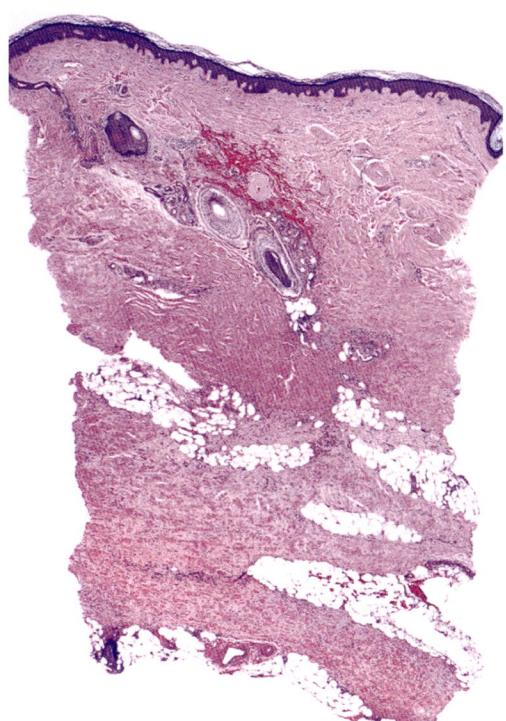

FIGURE 26-37 • Scleroderma demonstrates the characteristically rectangular biopsy with dense dermal sclerosis and thickening of the septa in the subcutaneous fat. (Hematoxylin and eosin stain, original magnification ×200.)

Scleroderma

Scleroderma or progressive systemic sclerosus in children shows a significantly less frequent involvement of all organs, a higher prevalence of arthritis and myositis, and a better outcome than in adults (151). The localized form of scleroderma or morphea is a disease of children and young adults. It can present as plaque, linear, guttate, or generalized forms. Histologic findings vary according to the duration of the lesion. In active lesions, there is a superficial and deep perivascular and interstitial lymphocytic infiltrate that extends into the subcutaneous tissue associated with thickened collagen bundles. In older lesions, the inflammatory component is mild or absent, and hyalinized collagen bundles replace the entire dermis and extend into the septa of the subcutaneous fat (Figure 26-37). The prognosis of morphea is generally good, with the lesions healing with atrophy and eventual cessation of new lesions occurring. Sclerodermoid skin changes may occur in chronic graft versus host disease.

GRAFT VERSUS HOST DISEASE

Graft versus host disease is a response seen in immunocompromised hosts to immunocompetent donor cells. In children, this is most often seen as a complication of hematopoietic stem cell transplantation in the treatment of acute leukemia or following a nonirradiated blood transfusion in an immunocompromised infant (152). The cutaneous findings of acute graft versus host disease include a pruritic

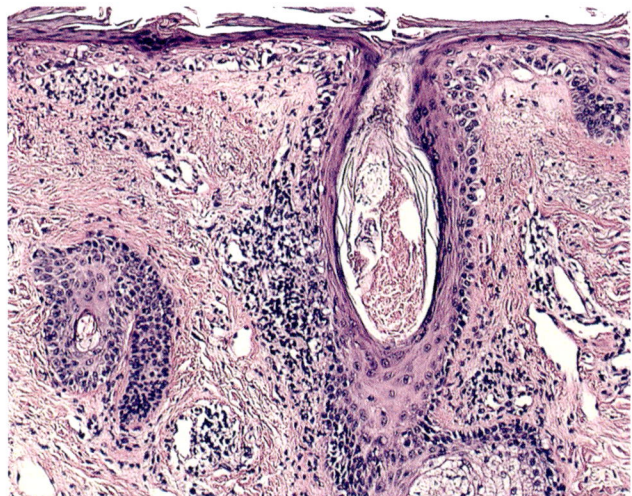

FIGURE 26-36 • Lupus erythematosus: mild hyperkeratosis, atrophy of the epidermis with vacuolar alteration of the basal cell layer, smudging of the basement membrane, and interface dermatitis extending around the hair follicle. (Hematoxylin and eosin stain, original magnification ×400.)

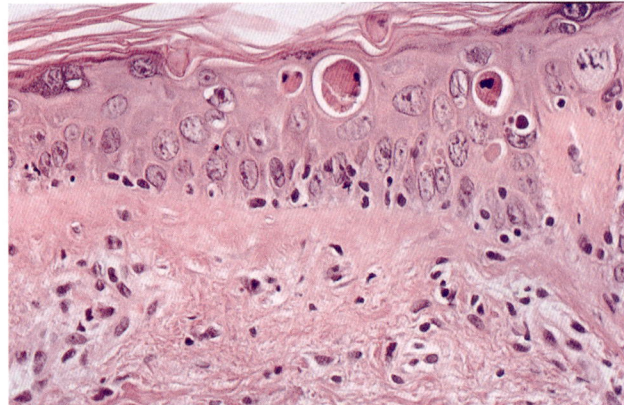

FIGURE 26-38 • Acute graft versus host disease characterized by vacuolar alteration of the basal cell layer with scattered "apoptotic" keratinocytes surrounded by few lymphocytes. The changes are those of interface dermatitis. (Hematoxylin and eosin stain, original magnification ×400.)

maculopapular eruption, which can become exfoliative. The histologic findings in acute graft versus host disease closely resemble those of erythema multiforme and TEN and consist of vacuolar alteration of the basal cell layer with necrotic keratinocytes, some of which are surrounded by lymphocytes, the so-called satellite necrosis (Figure 26-38). In severe cases, there is marked epidermal necrosis with formation of subepidermal bulla. A subacute lesion of graft versus host disease resembles lichen planus, with a dense band-like lymphocytic infiltrate that obscures the dermoepidermal junction. In the chronic form, the histologic changes closely resemble those of scleroderma, with hyalinization of collagen bundles. Vacuolar alteration at the basal cell layer and satellite necrosis, if present, may help in the diagnosis of graft versus host disease in all stages.

The prognosis for graft versus host disease is generally good when the disease is limited to skin. Early treatment may be of help in preventing joint contractures and disability associated with chronic graft versus host disease. In recent reports, a significantly higher mortality was observed in children with sclerodermatous graft versus host disease (153). The clinical differential diagnosis of graft versus host disease includes host lymphocyte recovery and drug reaction in the first 30 days posttransplantation.

METABOLIC DISORDERS

Calcinosis Cutis

Cutaneous calcifications may be of the localized dystrophic type or systemic metastatic type. One type of localized calcinosis is subepidermal calcific nodules seen on the heels of infants following repeated heel sticks (Figure 26-39) (154). Idiopathic subepidermal calcific nodules can be seen at birth. Calcinosis may be a manifestation of systemic disease such as dermatomyositis and, rarely, scleroderma and renal failure (155). Tumoral calcinosis seen around joint areas is mainly a disease of children, which presents as a soft tissue tumor.

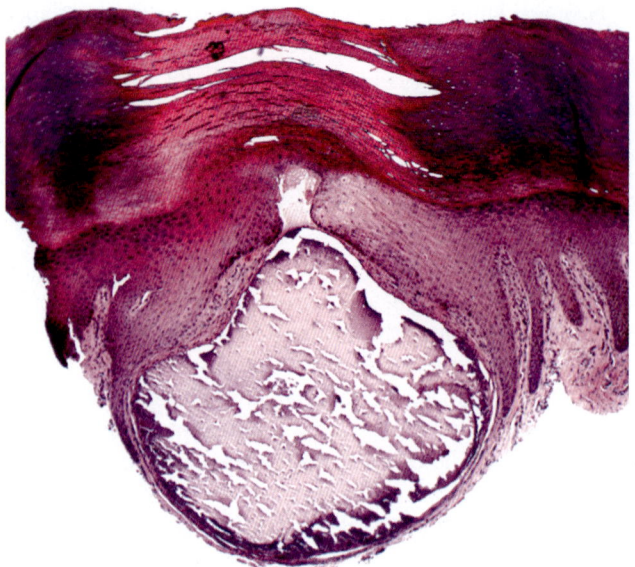

FIGURE 26-39 • Subepidermal calcified nodule at the site of a heel stick. (Hematoxylin and eosin stain, original magnification ×40.)

Other metabolic diseases like amyloidosis, porphyrias, and mucinoses can involve the skin but are not common in pediatric age groups.

Mucopolysaccharidoses

Mucopolysaccharidoses are lysosomal enzyme deficiency disorders that manifest with abnormal accumulations of mucopolysaccharides in many organs including the skin. In all types of mucopolysaccharidoses, the skin may appear thickened and inelastic. Biopsy sections stained with Giemsa stain show metachromatic granules within fibroblasts. By electron microscopy, membrane-bound finely granular deposits can be seen in the cytoplasm of fibroblasts (Figure 26-40) (see Chapter 5).

CYSTS, NEOPLASMS, AND HAMARTOMAS

Epidermal Nevi

Epidermal nevi are proliferations of epidermal keratinocytes that present as rough-surfaced lesions at birth or shortly thereafter. Clinically, they may be localized to palms and soles, widespread or segmental in distribution. Clinical patterns of expression include linear, zosteriform, and whorled. Histologic sections usually show a single pattern throughout the lesion. Various histologic patterns that are seen in epidermal nevi include epidermolytic hyperkeratosis, focal acantholytic dyskeratosis, verrucous hyperkeratosis, psoriasiform (inflammatory linear verrucous epidermal nevus), and seborrheic keratosis-like (Figure 26-41) (156). Abnormally formed pilosebaceous units, often in excess numbers, are characteristic of nevus sebaceous of Jadassohn.

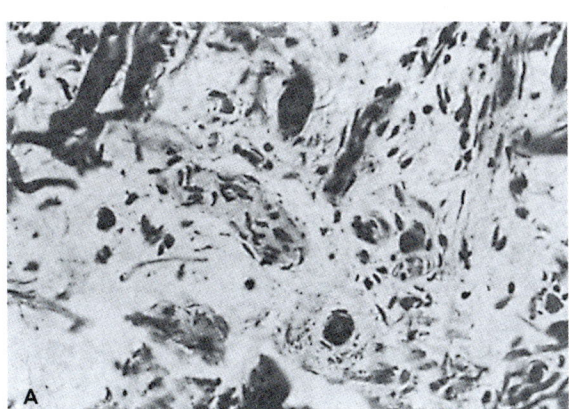
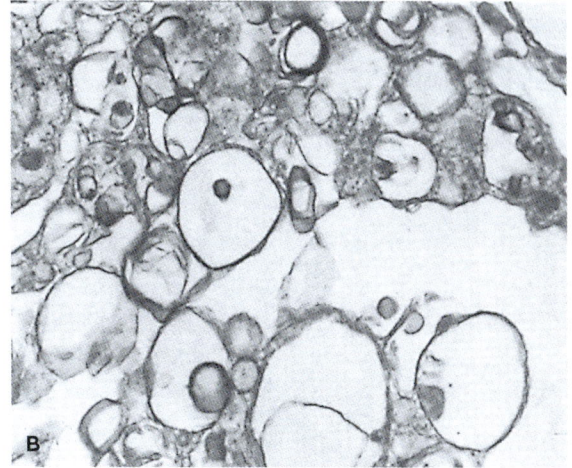

FIGURE 26-40 • **A:** Hurler syndrome showing a skin biopsy specimen with questionable increase in dermal metachromasia. (Toluidine blue stain, original magnification ×400.) **B:** Electron microscopy of fibroblasts, endothelial cells, and macrophages disclosed numerous membrane-bound vacuoles, some with granular and lamellar electron-dense contents. (Uranyl acetate and lead citrate stain, original magnification ×40,000.)

Epidermal nevi are generally stable benign lesions, and transformation to benign or malignant neoplasms is rare but well described in adults. Some epidermal nevi are associated with extracutaneous manifestations, notably of the central nervous, skeletal, and renal systems, and are called *epidermal nevus syndromes* that are likely due to specific genetic defects (157,158).

Nonneoplastic epithelial cysts are among the most common tumorous lesions seen in children.

Epidermal Inclusion Cyst

Epidermal inclusion cyst or keratinous cyst presents as a single firm dermal nodule that shows a keratinizing stratified squamous epithelial-lined cyst filled with laminated keratin or pilar keratin in the case of a trichilemmal cyst. Multiple epidermal inclusion cysts are seen in Gardner syndrome (159). Milia that can be seen occasionally on the face of a neonate are small epidermal inclusion cysts, which are not associated with a formed hair follicle.

Dermoid Cyst

Dermoid cysts are developmental in origin and arise along lines of embryonic suture closures. Common sites of involvement are the periorbital region, midline of nose, scalp, and anterior neck (160). Dermoid cysts are lined by keratinizing squamous epithelium. In contrast to epidermal inclusion cysts, the lining also contains folliculosebaceous and apocrine units, and sebum and hair are seen in addition to laminated keratin in the cyst contents. There is a resemblance to a steatocystoma. Simple excision is the treatment of choice. Midline dermoid cysts may be accompanied by a sinus tract and should be evaluated radiologically before surgery.

Eruptive Vellus Hair Cyst

Eruptive vellus hair cysts occur as multiple soft asymptomatic follicular papules of sudden onset in children and young adults. The sites of predilection are anterior chest, extremities, face, neck, and posterior trunk. Histologic sections show a squamous epithelial-lined cyst filled with laminated keratin and numerous hairs cut transversely and obliquely. An autosomal dominant developmental abnormality of vellus hair follicles is believed to be the underlying etiology.

Steatocystoma Multiplex

Steatocystoma multiplex is an autosomal dominant disorder seen as multiple small cystic lesions most commonly in the axillae, sternal region, and on the arms. The cysts are lined by stratified squamous epithelium, with only two to three cell layers, and covered with a thick homogeneous eosinophilic cuticle (Figure 26-42). Flattened sebaceous lobules can be seen in the vicinity. It is generally believed that eruptive vellus hair cysts and steatocystoma multiplex are variable expressions of the same disorder with overlapping clinical and histologic features (161,162).

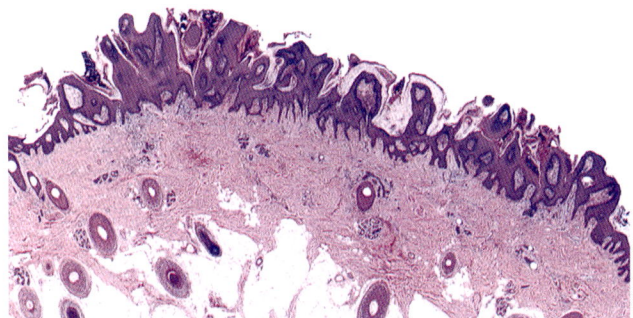

FIGURE 26-41 • Epidermal nevus: hyperkeratosis and papillomatous epidermal hyperplasia. Note that the adnexal structures are normal. (Hematoxylin and eosin stain, original magnification ×200.)

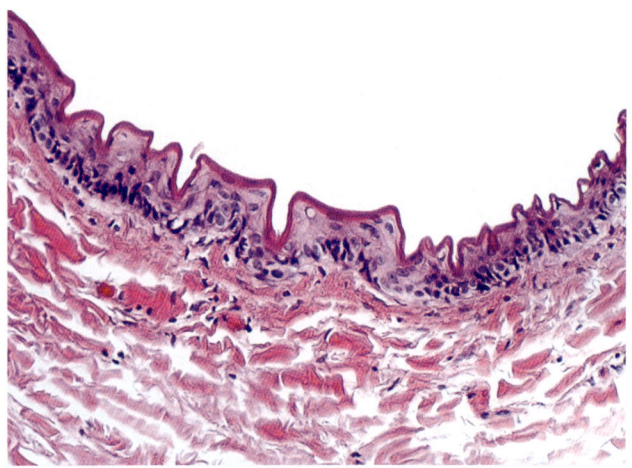

FIGURE 26-42 • Steatocystoma: cyst lined by stratified squamous epithelium with only two to three cell layers and a thick homogeneous eosinophilic cuticle. (Hematoxylin and eosin stain, original magnification ×200.)

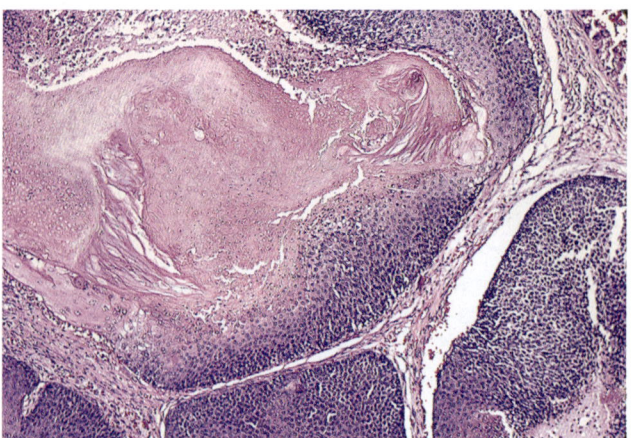

FIGURE 26-43 • Pilomatrixoma is a well-circumscribed cyst-like lesion with proliferation of basaloid cells that cornify in a peculiar pattern resulting in formation of shadow or ghost cells. (Hematoxylin and eosin stain, original magnification ×40.)

ADNEXAL TUMORS

Adnexal tumors occur in children less commonly than in adults. Of the adnexal tumors, tumors with follicular differentiation account for the majority. Pilomatrixoma, also known as *calcifying epithelioma of Malherbe*, is perhaps the most common adnexal neoplasm seen in the pediatric age group (163). *Pilomatrixomas* present with increased frequency in the first and the sixth decades, with the head and neck area being the most common site. Clinically, they present as a hard dermal or a subcutaneous nodule (164). Familial occurrences and multiple lesions are documented (165,166).

Histologic changes follow a distinct chronologic sequence. Early lesions begin as cystic structures lined by matrical and supramatrical cells similar to those in the bulb of normal hair follicles. As the cells mature, the nuclei disappear and leave ghosts of completely cornified cells, or the "shadow cells." Fully developed lesions show irregularly shaped and sized lobules of matrical and supramatrical cells. Each lobule shows maturation toward the center in the form of masses of "shadow cells" (Figure 26-43). With time, the lesion shows signs of regression in the form of less apparent or even absent peripheral epithelial elements and consists mostly of the shadow cells, which may be surrounded by granulation tissue and granulomatous inflammation. Late lesions show no epithelial component and consist only of masses of cornified cells with extensive calcification and occasionally ossification (167).

At all times, the benign nature of the neoplasm is apparent from the sharp circumscription seen at the periphery. In early lesions, mitotic figures may be frequent in keeping with the proliferative phase of the neoplasm and do not imply malignancy.

Trichoepithelioma often presents as solitary, flesh-colored papules occurring on the face. Less commonly, it presents as multiple lesions, transmitted as an autosomal dominant disorder.

Histologically, the silhouette is that of a benign neoplasm composed of germinative cells embedded in a cellular fibrocytic stroma. The germinative cells can be arranged as nodules or cribriform and retiform patterns and are usually encircled by mesenchymal cells like those of the embryonic perifollicular sheath. Infundibulocystic structures filled with cornified cells may be prominent in trichoblastoma, a less differentiated follicular neoplasm composed of germinative cells, which is another expression of trichoepithelioma.

Eccrine Neoplasms

Syringoma is a relatively common adnexal neoplasm that differentiates toward the acrosyringium of the eccrine duct. It is seen in children with greater frequency in association with trisomy 21 syndrome (168). It can present as a sudden-onset eruption of small papules, usually on the face and sometimes on the vulva (169,170). Histologically, the lesions are characterized by multiple, small epithelial structures that may be solid or tubular. The tubular structures may contain granular material within the lumina. Some of the epithelial nests may have elongated or tadpole-like shapes. An important histologic feature is the confinement of the neoplasm to the upper half of the dermis, a feature helpful in distinguishing syringoma from microcystic adnexal carcinoma, especially in adults.

Other eccrine neoplasms such as eccrine poroma and eccrine acrospiroma occur infrequently in children.

Sebaceous and apocrine neoplasms: True sebaceous and apocrine neoplasms are uncommon in children. Nevus sebaceus of Jadassohn is a hamartoma that contains most elements of normal skin and subcutaneous fat and is best designated as an organoid nevus. Nevus sebaceus commonly occurs as a yellowish round-to-oval hairless plaque on the scalp, forehead, and lateral portions of the face. The clinical and histologic appearances vary considerably and follow a chronologic sequence. The yellowish pebbly appearance of

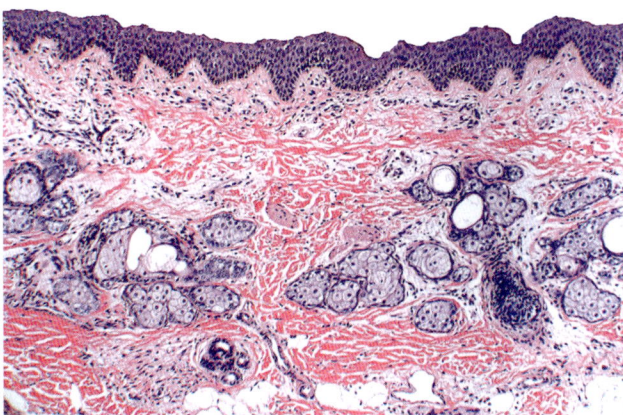

FIGURE 26-44 • Nevus sebaceus of Jadassohn is a broad lesion characterized by epidermal hyperplasia, numerous sebaceous lobules, poorly formed hair follicles, and apocrine glands. (Hematoxylin and eosin stain, original magnification ×100.)

Melanocytic Nevi

Melanocytic nevi are of two main types, namely, congenital and acquired, and both types can be junctional, compound, or intradermal. Although melanocytic nevi may be present at birth in 1.5% to 2.0% of the population, the majority of the nevi are acquired during the first two decades of life.

Congenital Melanocytic Nevi

Congenital melanocytic nevi are first noticed at birth or shortly thereafter as variably sized pigmented lesions. Depending on the size, congenital melanocytic nevi have been classified as giant (>20 cm), large (1.5 to 20 cm), and small (<1.5 cm). The bathing trunk–type giant congenital nevi are rare and are characterized by an uneven verrucous surface, variations in shades of brown and blue, and moderate growth of hair throughout the lesions (Figure 26-45). Scattered similar but smaller satellite lesions are often present. Giant congenital nevi, when present on the head and neck region, may be associated with leptomeningeal melanocytosis and neurologic disorders (neurocutaneous melanosis). There is an increased risk of primary leptomeningeal melanoma in these cases. Large congenital nevi show mild-to-moderate variation in color and epidermal hyperplasia. Small congenital nevi are seen as solitary light tan to brown uniformly pigmented macules. Congenital nevi change with age with development of darker areas, nodules, and coarse hair.

Similar to acquired nevi, congenital nevi may be junctional, compound, or intradermal. It is believed that all nevi begin with increased numbers of melanocytes at the dermoepidermal junction with subsequent dropping down into the dermis. Eventually, the junctional component disappears and only the dermal component is left behind. Congenital

these lesions at birth corresponds to prominent sebaceous lobules, a result of the effects of maternal hormones.

After infancy, the appearance and development of the sebaceous lobules in the lesions follow the growth of sebaceous units elsewhere. They are small and the epidermis is flat until puberty, when sebaceous lobules become greatly increased in number and arranged as clusters. The epidermis also becomes papillomatous. After puberty, the number of sebaceous lobules decreases but their size increases. The epidermis remains hyperplastic and verrucous (171). Rudimentary hair follicles and apocrine glands are common findings (Figure 26-44). In the postpubertal stage, nevus sebaceus can be the site of a variety of adnexal neoplasms, the most common being trichoblastoma, followed by syringocystadenoma papilliferum and sebaceous tumors (172,173).

CARCINOMA

Carcinomas of the skin are extremely uncommon in childhood and usually are seen in association with hereditary syndromes. Based cell nevus syndrome, also known as *Gorlin* and *Gorlin-Goltz syndromes*, is an autosomal dominant disorder characterized by multiple jaw cysts, skeletal anomalies, intracranial calcifications, and multiple basal cell carcinomas that commonly appear after puberty (174). Medulloblastoma can occur in early childhood. Survivors face the problem of repeated cutaneous and internal malignancies. Many other patients affected with nevoid basal cell carcinoma can suffer from disfigurement secondary to multiple surgeries.

MELANOCYTIC NEOPLASMS

In normal skin, melanocytes are located within the basal cell layer, where they are separated by four to ten keratinocytes. A proliferation of these melanocytes may give rise to a variety of melanocytic lesions.

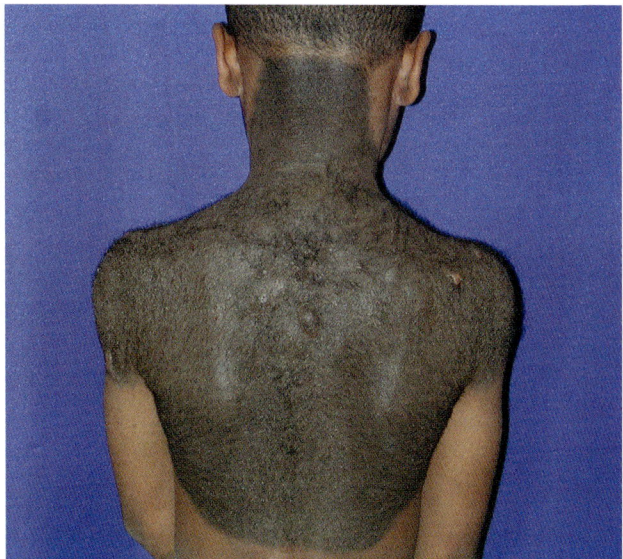

FIGURE 26-45 • Congenital melanocytic nevus typified by a diffuse involvement of the upper trunk, arms, and neck. (Courtesy of Sarah Stein, M.D., Department of Medicine, University of Chicago Medical Center.)

nevi are histologically distinguished from acquired nevi by the presence of melanocytic nests and individual melanocytes around the adnexal and vascular structures as well as infiltration between the collagen bundles as individual cells. Deep infiltration into the reticular dermis, often with extension into the septa of subcutaneous fat, is a feature seen in giant congenital nevi (Figure 26-46). In smaller congenital nevi, the nests of melanocytes are located more superficially and have led some authors to classify congenital nevi on histologic grounds into superficial and deep types. Nests of larger melanocytes may be seen closer to the dermoepidermal junction with maturation to smaller monomorphous melanocytes toward the base.

Congenital Nevus and Malignant Melanoma

One of the complications of giant congenital nevus, especially when associated with leptomeningeal melanosis, is the development of malignant melanoma and other primitive malignancies such as rhabdomyosarcoma within the nevus. The estimated incidence of malignant transformation is between 4% and 12% in various reports (175), although a more recent study suggests a much lower overall risk of 0.7% (176). In one study, the relative risk of development of malignant melanoma in giant congenital nevi was 1000 times greater than that in the general population, which supports a multistage excision approach in the treatment of giant congenital nevi. The incidence of melanoma in other congenital nevi correlates with the size of the lesion. When melanoma develops in a congenital nevus, it generally begins at the dermoepidermal junction. In some instances, especially in association with giant congenital nevus, it may begin deep in the dermis comprising of a nodule of undifferentiated cells, which must be distinguished from "proliferative nodules." Heterologous differentiation and cytologic anaplasia do not necessarily imply poor prognosis.

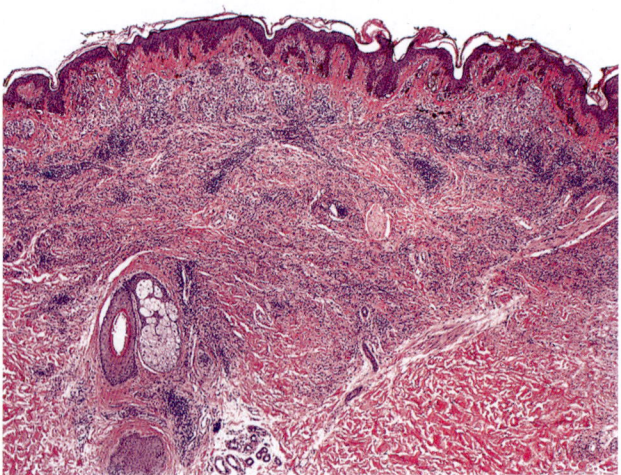

FIGURE 26-46 • Compound congenital melanocytic nevus with nests of melanocytes at the dermoepidermal junction and deep in the dermis, where they infiltrate between the collagen bundles and surround the blood vessels and adnexal structures as individual cells. (Hematoxylin and eosin stain, original magnification ×100.)

Melanoma can appear at any time but occurs most often before puberty in giant congenital nevi and after puberty when associated with smaller congenital nevi.

Acquired Melanocytic Nevi

Most melanocytic nevi are acquired and appear within the first two decades of life and only rarely in midlife. Nevi generally begin as junctional nevi, characterized clinically by small tan to tan–brown macules and histologically by increased basal melanocytes that nest eventually at the dermoepidermal junction (177). This is followed by dermal migration of some melanocytes characteristic of a compound nevus that results in a papule formation. With progression, the junctional component eventually disappears, leaving only the dermal component of an intradermal nevus.

The number and distribution of acquired melanocytic nevi are influenced by genetics, sex, and hormonal and environmental factors. Clinically, acquired melanocytic nevi are characterized by small size, uniform color, and well-defined borders and histologically by a symmetric, well-circumscribed proliferation of monomorphous melanocytes that show well-formed nests and maturation with progressive descent into the dermis. The following variations of acquired melanocytic nevi deserve special attention because some may have clinical or histologic features that make distinction from malignant melanoma difficult.

Spitz Nevus

Spitz nevus, also known as *spindle* and *epithelioid cell nevus* (178), was originally described by Sophie Spitz in 1948 (179) as a juvenile form of malignant melanoma with good prognosis. Although it is now apparent that Spitz nevus is a distinct type of nevus, distinguishing Spitz nevus from melanoma continues to be a challenge (180). Spitz nevus occurs more commonly in children before the age of 14 years as an acquired nevus and only rarely as a congenital nevus. Most Spitz nevi are solitary, small (<1 cm), and pink and clinically mimic hemangioma or pyogenic granuloma. In rare instances, multiple lesions can occur (154). Histologically, Spitz nevus is symmetric and well circumscribed and shows maturation, features characteristic of a nevus. However, cytologically, the melanocytes are large, spindle shaped, and/or epithelioid, with considerable cytologic and nuclear pleomorphism. Pagetoid spread of melanocytes into the epidermis and frequent mitotic figures further make distinction from melanoma difficult and sometimes impossible. Eosinophilic hyaline globules (Kamino bodies), often present in significant numbers, are more commonly seen in Spitz nevi. Pseudoepitheliomatous epidermal hyperplasia, hyperkeratosis and parakeratosis, patchy perivascular lymphohistiocytic inflammation, and papillary dermal vascular ectasia are other features commonly seen in Spitz nevus (Figure 26-47). Like other melanocytic nevi, Spitz nevus can be junctional, compound, or intradermal.

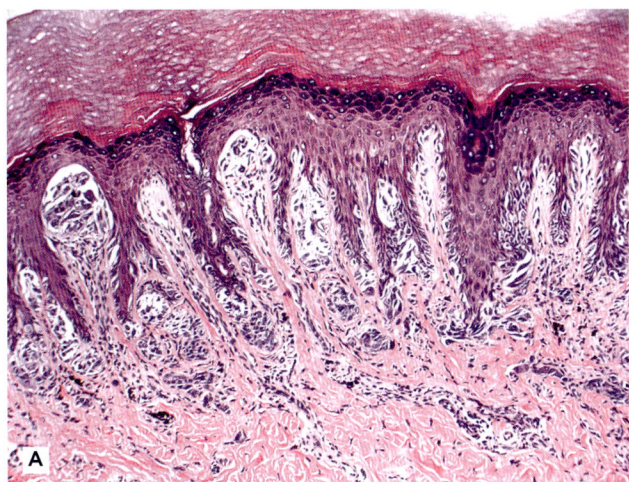
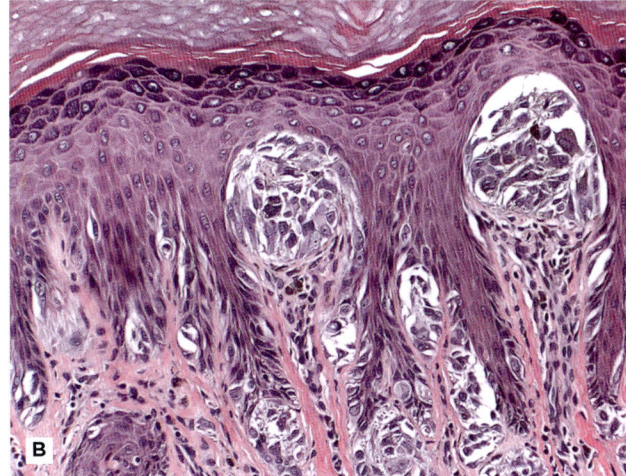

FIGURE 26-47 • **A:** Spindle–epithelioid (Spitz) nevus characterized by junctional and dermal nests of spindle- and epithelioid-shaped cells amelanocytes. The overlying epidermis is hyperkeratotic and somewhat hyperplastic. **B:** Clefts surround the vertically oriented nests of epithelioid melanocytes. (Hematoxylin and eosin stain, original magnification ×40.)

Halo Nevus

Halo nevus has a clinically distinct appearance characterized by the appearance of a zone of depigmentation surrounding a previously present nevus. A majority of halo nevi are seen on the back of children and young adults. Complete regression of the pigmented lesion may occur, leaving a depigmented macule. Histologically, halo nevi are characterized by the presence of dense lymphocytic inflammation with destruction of melanocytes. Destruction of the normal melanocytes at the periphery of the nevus results in the initial halo formation. Eventually, all melanocytes within the nevus may disappear and the inflammation subsides. In the earlier stage of inflammation, the melanocytes of the nevus may be enlarged and cytologically atypical and rare mitotic figures may be present. However, the overall architecture is that of a nevus, and pagetoid spread of melanocytes is generally absent. Halo nevi are common in patients with vitiligo suggesting a common underlying immune-mediated mechanism. Occasionally, halo phenomenon may be observed around Spitz nevi and congenital nevi.

Blue Nevus

Blue nevi are rarely seen in children younger than 10 years of age. Clinically, blue nevi present as blue–gray papules. Histologically, dendritic melanocytes with melanin pigment are present as nests and fascicles extending into the deep reticular dermis. Cellular blue nevus is a variant of blue nevus, which often presents as a blue nodule on the scalp and lumbosacral region, and is histologically characterized by cellular islands of large oval cells with pale cytoplasm, in addition to the dendritic melanocytes (Figure 26-48). A variant of this nevus, the epithelioid blue nevus composed

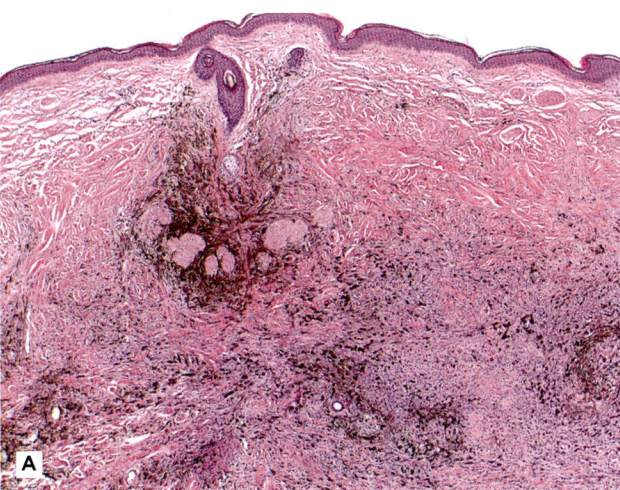
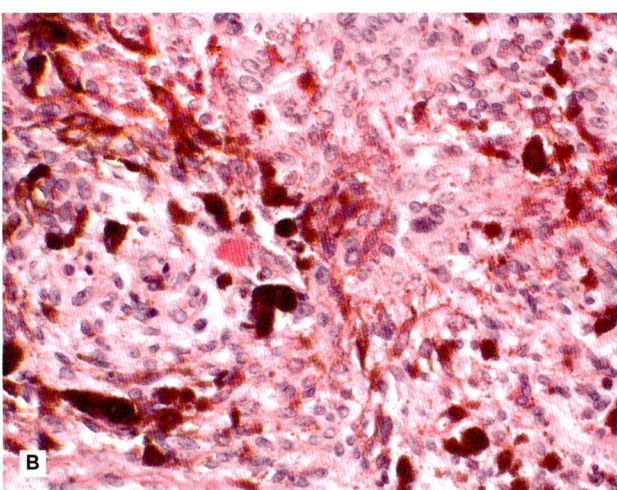

FIGURE 26-48 • Cellular blue nevus from the lumbosacral region of a 14-year-old girl. **A:** Interlacing spindle cells and nodular foci of cells with clear cytoplasm are shown. **B:** Pigmented spindle-shaped cells with dendritic processes are scattered throughout the lesion. (Hematoxylin and eosin stain, original magnification ×100.)

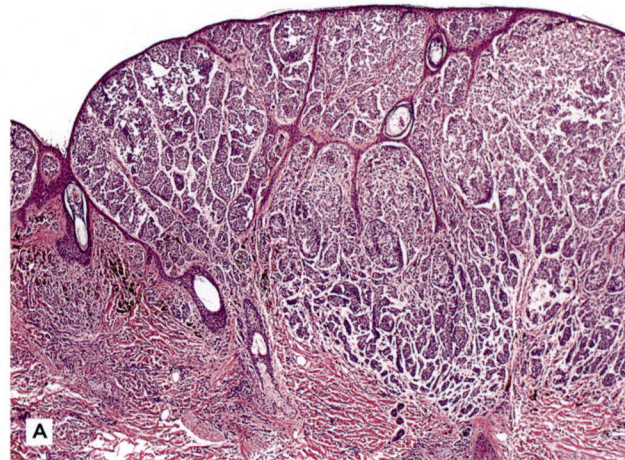
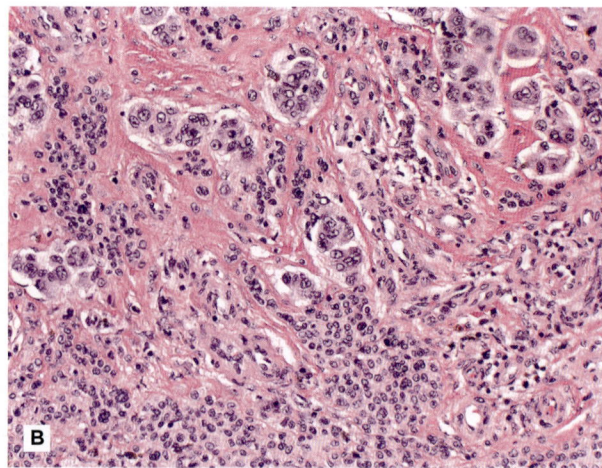

FIGURE 26-49 • Malignant melanoma in association with congenital nevus. **A:** A nodular proliferation of large atypical melanocytes arranged in a sheetlike pattern. **B:** Atypical melanocytes of melanoma adjacent to smaller monomorphous nevus cells. Beware that this pattern may represent a nonmalignant proliferation nodule.

of deeply pigmented spindle-shaped cells and lightly pigmented oval to polygonal melanocytes, were described in patients with Carney complex (181). Combined nevi, with features of both blue nevus and Spitz nevus, may fall within the spectrum of epithelioid blue nevus and more recently described *pigmented epithelioid melanocytoma* (182,183). However, a combined nevus can have various patterns.

Clark Dysplastic Nevus

Originally described by Reimer et al. (184) dysplastic nevus has been the subject of considerable controversy for a long time. It is now generally agreed that a subgroup of population with a family history of melanoma and multiple clinically atypical-appearing nevi has a genetic predisposition to developing malignant melanoma. The histologic features of dysplastic nevi include a broad junctional or compound nevus, with nests of melanocytes bridging the adjacent rete ridges, concentric and lamellar fibroplasia, and melanocytic atypia to include large size, enlarged nuclei, and abundant dusty melanin-laden cytoplasm. It must be emphasized that histologic diagnosis of dysplastic nevus is relevant only in the context of appropriate clinical findings. Nevi when biopsied in very young children, particularly shortly after birth and those on genital skin, conjunctiva, palms, and soles, and recurrent nevi are notorious simulators of malignant melanoma and should be interpreted with caution in these circumstances (185).

Malignant Melanoma

Less than two percent of malignant melanomas are diagnosed in children and, in the absence of congenital nevus, are rare in the first decade of life (186). Congenital melanoma is a rare event (187,188) and can occur as a de novo process or as transplacental metastases. Malignant melanoma in children has similar clinical and histologic features as that in adults and is characterized clinically by large size, asymmetry, and irregular color and borders. Histologic features include asymmetry, poor circumscription, pagetoid melanocytes in a pagetoid pattern, lack of maturation, and cytologic atypia with mitotic figures (Figure 26-49). Prognostic factors are likewise similar to those in adults and include maximum thickness (depth of invasion) and presence of ulceration.

In addition, a distinct type of melanoma (childhood/Spitzoid type) with capability for metastasis and features overlapping with Spitz nevus has been reported in prepubescent children (189). These lesions are characterized clinically by rapid growth and histologically by a vertical growth of large epithelioid melanocytes that fail to mature with progressive descent into the dermis. Presence of mitotic figures including atypical forms, particularly in the deep dermal component, may be helpful in making the correct diagnosis. Despite the usually deep invasion, this type has been reported to carry a better prognosis than a conventional melanoma.

MESENCHYMAL NEOPLASMS

Neurothekeoma

Neurothekeoma are benign tumors of nerve sheath origin. In a recently published large series, 24% of the patients were 10 years old or less. The tumor presents as a solitary, superficial slow-growing mass measuring 0.3 to 2 cm, most commonly involving the head and neck area and upper extremities (190). Histologically, the tumor is characterized by multinodular dermal mass composed of whorls of spindle-shaped and epithelioid cells with varying amounts of myxoid matrix in the background. The tumor cells are positive for vimentin, NKI/C3, and CD10 and negative for S-100 protein. Although the exact lineage of these tumors is uncertain, nerve sheath differentiation, as initially suggested, is not supported by the recent literature (191) (see Chapter 25).

Other neurogenic tumors in children include solitary neurofibroma and plexiform neurofibroma of von Recklinghausen

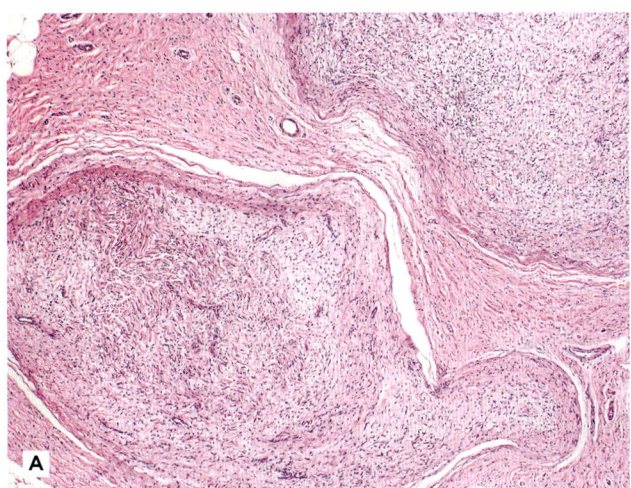
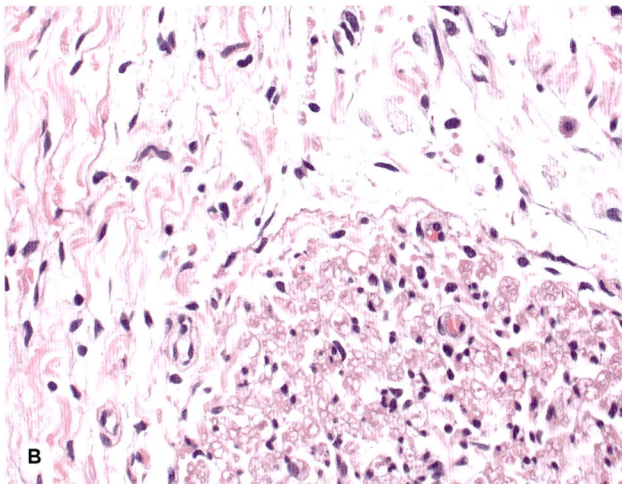

FIGURE 26-50 • **A:** Plexiform neurofibroma from the forearm of an adolescent male showing multiple myxoid nodules in the dermis. (Hematoxylin and eosin stain, original magnification ×100.) **B:** Some cytologic atypia is present and should be further evaluated for possible sarcomatous transformation. (Hematoxylin and eosin stain, original magnification ×200.)

disease (Figure 26-50). Rare complex neural tumors with heterologous elements have been described in neonates and infants. In children with neuroblastoma, metastasis to skin may occur (see Chapter 21).

Vascular Tumors

True neoplasms with vascular differentiation as well as malformations of the vessels are common in children.

Hemangioma

Hemangioma is one of the most common benign tumors of childhood and can be superficial, deep, or mixed. It may present as a single or multiple lesions, which vary in size from 10 mm to several centimeters. The head and neck area is the most common site, with one-third being present at birth. Spontaneous regression occurs in most cases. Rarely, the large size of the lesion may cause distortion and dysfunction of neighboring structures (see Chapter 25).

Histologic changes vary from dilated thin-walled vessels in the superficial dermis in superficial hemangioma (portwine stain) to lobular clusters of spindle cells with barely recognizable vascular spaces in cellular hemangioma of infancy. In the latter, the endothelial cells are also large and mitotically active, which may lead to a mistaken diagnosis of malignancy.

Pyogenic Granuloma

Pyogenic granuloma, also known as *lobular capillary hemangioma*, is common in children and presents as a rapidly growing elevated bright red papule on the hand, finger, lip, or gum. Histologically, the lesion is a polypoid mass of vascular proliferation with myxoid and edematous stroma. Surface ulceration, acute and chronic inflammatory cell infiltrate, and a collarette of epidermis surrounding the lesion are other features. After an initial phase of rapid growth, the lesion persists as a stable mass unless surgically removed.

Tufted Hemangioma

Tufted hemangioma presents as angiomatous papules and plaques in children aged 1 to 5 years, most commonly on the upper trunk, neck, and extremities. In some patients, lesions may be present at birth (192). Histologically, the lesion is characterized by well-defined foci of closely set capillaries, discrete ovoid angiomatous lobules, or tufts within the dermis and occasionally the subcutis. Most of the lesions progress slowly over years, whereas some show spontaneous regression (193) (see Chapter 25).

Myofibroblastic/Fibroblastic Tumors

Smooth muscle hamartoma and rhabdomyoma can be seen in children. Rhabdomyosarcomas infrequently metastasize to skin.

Congenital/Infantile Myofibromatosis

Congenital/infantile myofibromatosis generally presents as a solitary cutaneous or subcutaneous mass at birth or within the first year of life. A generalized or systemic variant with a poor prognosis is also recognized, and in some cases, a familial pattern of inheritance is reported (194). Histologically, both the solitary and the systemic variants show a nodular proliferation with biphasic pattern consisting of a central vascular area reminiscent of hemangiopericytoma surrounded by peripheral fascicles of spindle-shaped myofibroblasts and fibroblasts.

Cutaneous myofibroma has identical histologic features but presents as a well-circumscribed solitary mass in older children and adults (Figure 26-51) (see Chapter 25).

Infantile Digital Fibromatosis

Infantile digital fibromatosis is a distinctive benign tumor that occurs in the fingers and the toes of infants. It presents as a single or multiple dome-shaped lesions on the lateral or the dorsal aspect of the distal or middle phalangeal joint, most often in the fingers, sparing the thumb and the

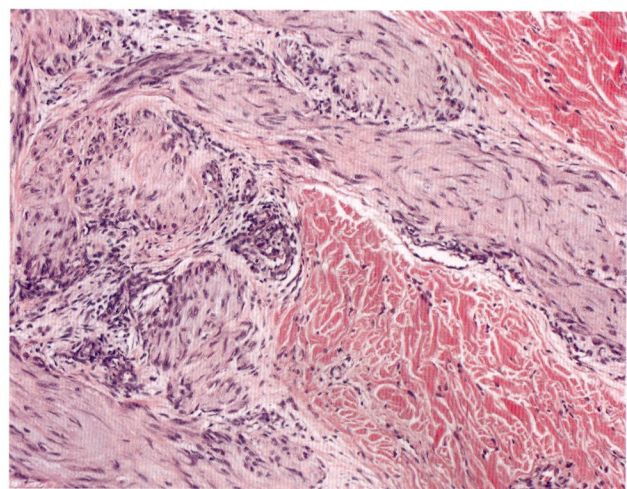

FIGURE 26-51 • Cutaneous myofibroma: myofibroblastic nodules of loosely arrayed spindle cells within the dermis often noted in an infant. (Hematoxylin and eosin stain, original magnification ×100.)

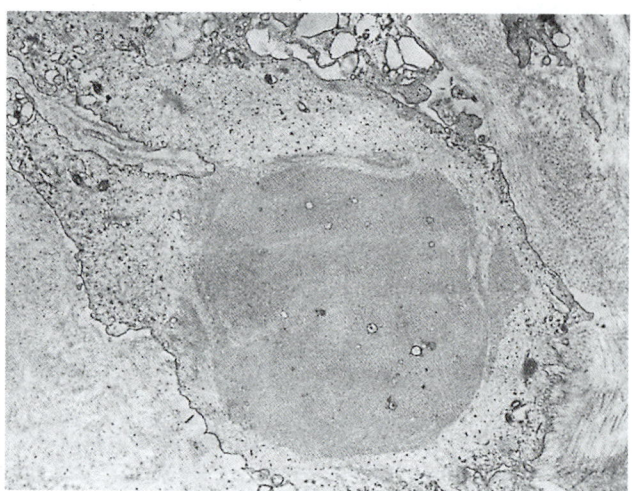

FIGURE 26-53 • Infantile digital fibromatosis showing an inclusion composed of a tangled network of filaments. (Uranyl acetate and lead citrate stain, original magnification ×14,400.)

greater toes. The tumor consists of a uniform proliferation of fibroblasts surrounded by a dense collagenous stroma. Characteristic inclusion bodies, first described by Reye in 1965 (195), are present in the fibroblast cytoplasm, separated from the nucleus by a narrow clear zone (Figure 26-52). The inclusions vary in number and range from 3 to 15 mm in diameter. They are round and eosinophilic and resemble erythrocytes. They stain a deep red with Masson trichrome and are PAS negative. Ultrastructurally, the tumor cells are identified as fibroblasts and myofibroblasts. The inclusion bodies consist of fibrillary and granular material, which is often actin positive (Figure 26-53). Local recurrence is common; however, the vast majority of infantile digital fibromas regress over time (196) (see Chapter 25).

Giant Cell Fibroblastoma

Giant cell fibroblastoma, first described by Shmookler and Enzinger in abstract form in 1992, is now considered to be the juvenile form of dermatofibrosarcoma protuberans, as supported by the frequent presence of giant cell fibroblastoma–like areas in examples of conventional dermatofibrosarcoma protuberans (197). Furthermore, immunohistochemical studies have shown both areas to be reactive with CD34 (197–199) and CD99 (200). It presents at a median age of 3 years as a painless nodule or mass in the dermis or subcutis of the back of the thigh, inguinal region, or chest wall. Two-thirds of the patients are boys. The lesion is poorly circumscribed and measures from 1 to 8 cm. Histologically, giant cell fibroblastoma is composed of spindle cells with moderate nuclear pleomorphism, infiltrating the deep dermis and subcutis. Cellularity varies with the formation of characteristic pseudovascular spaces lined by a discontinuous row of multinucleated cells that are the basic proliferating tumor cells (Figure 26-54). Both giant cell fibroblastoma and dermatofibrosarcoma protuberans share the same cytogenetic abnormality, which include reciprocal

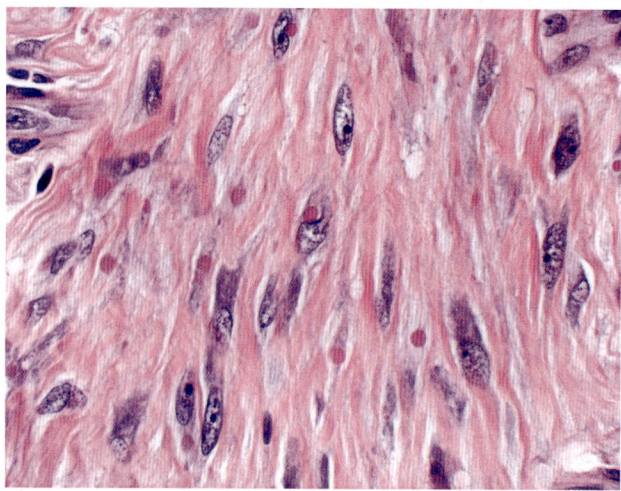

FIGURE 26-52 • Infantile digital fibromatosis characterized by paranuclear inclusions. (Hematoxylin and eosin stain, original magnification ×400.)

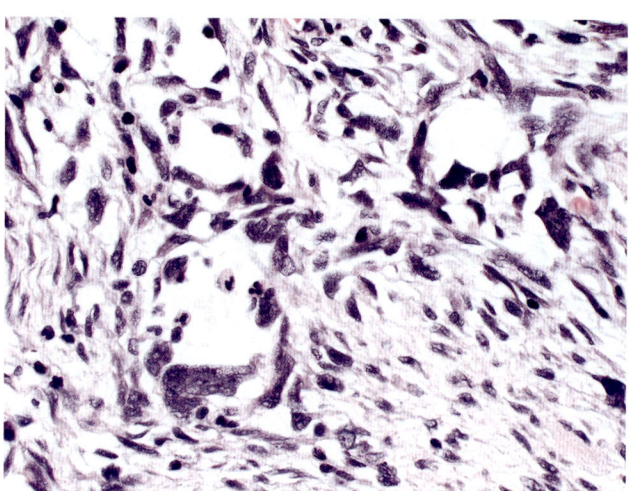

FIGURE 26-54 • Giant cell fibroblastoma is a spindle-cell lesion with pseudovascular spaces, multinucleated giant cells, and occasional mitoses. (Hematoxylin and eosin stain, original magnification ×400.)

translocation t(17;22) (q22;q13) resulting in formation of supernumerary ring chromosomes containing sequences from chromosomes 17 and 22. The tumor recurs locally in half the cases but is not known to metastasize (200).

HEMATOPOIETIC

Mast Cell Diseases

Mastocytosis in children is generally a benign self-healing condition characterized by abnormal proliferation of mast cells, most often presenting as cutaneous lesions (201). Cutaneous mastocytosis can manifest as solitary mastocytoma usually present at birth, urticaria pigmentosa presenting as maculopapular eruption in children between the ages of 3 to 9 months, or as diffuse mastocytosis that presents with diffuse thickening of the skin in infants and is associated with a poor prognosis owing to systemic involvement. Of these lesions, urticaria pigmentosa is the most common manifestation and includes the telangiectatic form.

All variants of cutaneous mastocytosis are generally marked by wheal formation in response to rubbing, which is known as *Darier sign*. Occasional blister formation is also seen. A skin biopsy is diagnostic in all cases and demonstrates an infiltrate of monomorphous mononuclear cells (Figure 26-55) with oval bland nuclei and abundant amphophilic to pale cytoplasm. Eosinophils are present in varying numbers. The infiltrate may be of varying density depending on the clinical appearance, with most cells being present in a nodule of solitary mastocytoma and least in telangiectasia macularis eruptiva perstans. Special stains such as Giemsa, toluidine blue, and Leder stain or immunohistochemical stains for mast cell tryptase and CD117 can be helpful in confirming the diagnosis.

The prognosis is generally good for cutaneous mastocytosis, with solitary mastocytomas regressing spontaneously in a few years and urticaria pigmentosa resolving before puberty in the majority of patients. Diffuse mastocytosis has a guarded prognosis and may be complicated by tachycardia and shock.

Histiocytoses

Histiocytoses are a complex group of disorders best divided into Langerhans cell and non-LCH.

Langerhans Cell Histiocytosis

LCH is characterized by a proliferation of Langerhans histiocytes that are immunoreactive with S100 protein, langerin, and CD1a and contain Birbeck granules by electron microscopy. Three clinical classes are traditionally recognized: an acute disseminated form with visceral involvement known as *Letterer-Siwe disease* presenting in the first year of life, a chronic multisystem disease with osseous involvement but less visceral involvement known as *Hand-Schüller-Christian syndrome* presenting in early childhood, and the chronic focal disease presenting with one or more bone lesions known as *eosinophilic granuloma* seen in late childhood and adults. Cutaneous involvement is encountered in all forms but is most common in the acute disseminated form, and a skin biopsy is often diagnostic. Cutaneous lesions may consist of petechiae, papules, and often diffuse eruption, particularly of the scalp and the anogenital areas, resembling seborrheic dermatitis. Occasionally, the lesions may be vesicular, ulcerated, or urticarial. Langerhans histiocytes are present in the papillary dermis, obscuring the dermoepidermal junction (Figure 26-56) and often extending into the overlying epidermis. The cells are characterized by abundant pale cytoplasm and characteristic reniform nucleus. Multinucleated histiocytes and eosinophils are present in varying numbers. Several dermatoses are associated with hyperplasia of Langerhans cells, which should not be diagnosed as LCH.

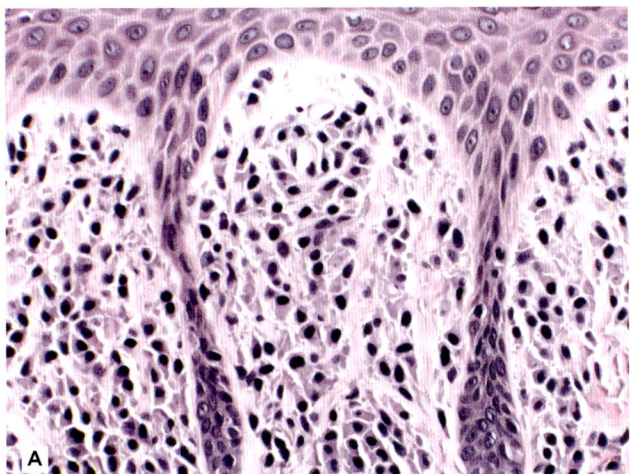
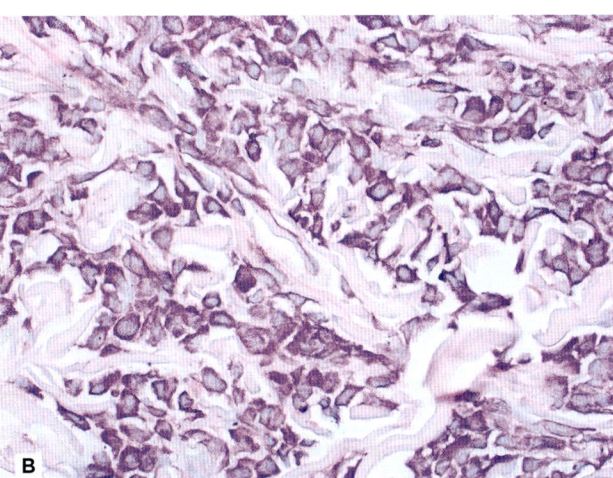

FIGURE 26-55 • Urticaria pigmentosa. **A:** Dense dermal infiltrate of monomorphic cells, which are mast cells. (Hematoxylin and eosin stain, original magnification ×400.) **B:** Giemsa stain shows the mast cells with purple, metachromatic granules. Most cells are also c-kit (CD117) positive.

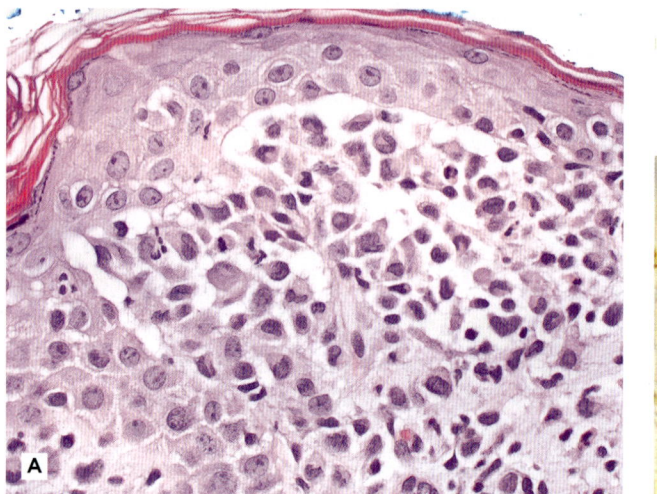 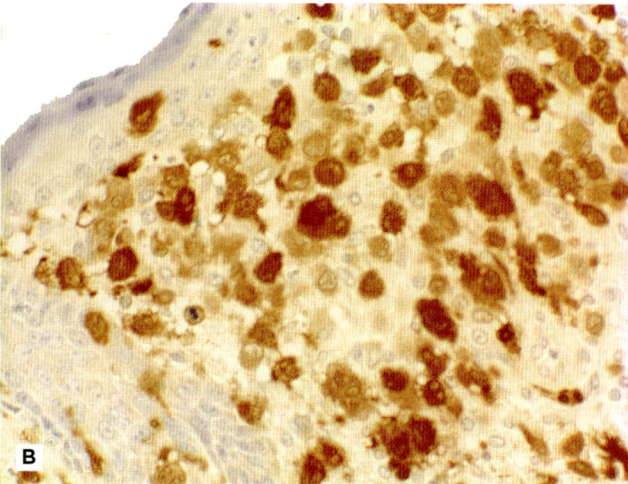

FIGURE 26-56 • Langerhans cell histiocytosis. **A:** Dense diffuse dermal infiltrate of atypical histiocytic cells with grooved nuclei and multinucleation, admixed with eosinophils. (Hematoxylin and eosin stain, original magnification ×400.) **B:** The histiocytic cells are positive for S100 protein and CD1a (not illustrated) by immunohistochemistry.

Congenital self-healing reticulohistiocytosis is considered to be on the benign end of the spectrum of LCH, presenting at birth or shortly after and resolving spontaneously (203). Microscopically, the histiocytes in this condition are distinguished by the presence of abundant eosinophilic cytoplasm with a ground-glass appearance.

Non-Langerhans Cell Histiocytoses

These histiocytoses are characterized by a proliferation of histiocytic cells that express a variety of macrophage markers but not langerin, CD1a, or S100 protein.

Juvenile xanthogranuloma is the most common form of non-LCH seen in children. The clinical appearance is that of a solitary or multiple red–yellow papules or nodules appearing during the first year of life. Histologically, the lesions show a dense dermal infiltrate of histiocytes with varying degrees of lipidization, a variety of multinucleated cells including Touton giant cells, and an admixture of lymphocytes and eosinophils (Figure 26-57). Older lesions show proliferation of fibroblasts with fibrosis replacing the infiltrate. Deep forms with involvement of the subcutaneous tissue or muscle can occur.

Although juvenile xanthogranuloma is generally a benign disorder, several systemic complications, including ocular involvement, oral lesions, central nervous system, and bone involvement, are seen in rare cases.

Benign cephalic histiocytosis is a clinically distinct self-healing disorder of children characterized by small papular eruptions on the face. Histologic features overlap with juvenile xanthogranuloma and eruptive histiocytoma of adults (202,203).

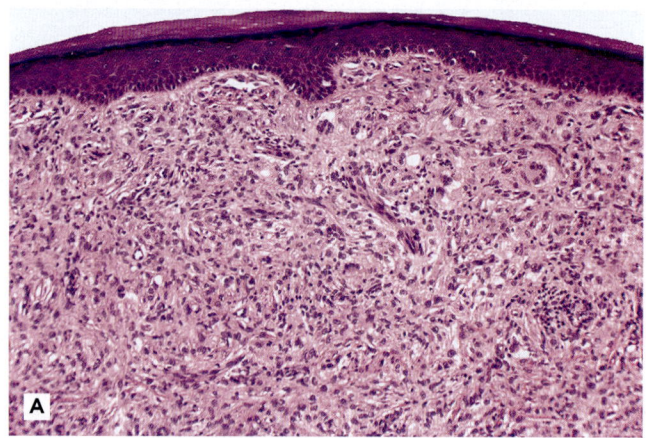 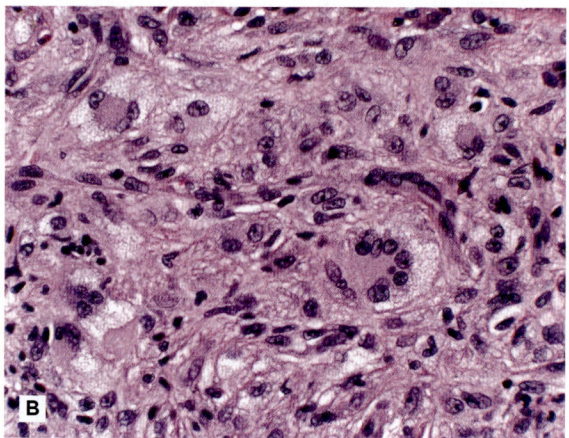

FIGURE 26-57 • Juvenile xanthogranuloma. **A:** A well-circumscribed dome-shaped papule. **B:** Diffuse infiltrate of histiocytic cells, many of which are multinucleated with nuclei arranged in a wreath-like pattern. Note also the lipidized features of the cytoplasm. (Hematoxylin and eosin stain, original magnification ×25 **(A)**, ×400 **(B)**.)

Sinus Histiocytosis with Massive Lymphadenopathy (Rosai-Dorfman Disease)

Skin involvement may be seen in approximately 10% of Rosai-Dorfman disease cases and presents as papules or nodules that on biopsy show histiocytes with abundant cytoplasm and occasional multinucleation with emperipolesis of lymphocytes.

Leukemia and Lymphoma

Cutaneous involvement by leukemia and lymphoma is uncommon in childhood. Congenital monocytic leukemia has been reported in some patients (204). Anaplastic large T-cell lymphoma may present with cutaneous involvement with or without lymph node involvement. Involvement of mediastinum, viscera, and skin is associated with increased risk of progression/relapse (205). The histologic features include a dense diffuse infiltrate of anaplastic mononuclear cells that are typically CD30 positive. The skin lesion may be ALK negative. Lymphomatoid papulosis may show a population of cells identical to those seen in anaplastic large T-cell lymphoma but is generally regarded as a self-limiting benign disorder. Rare cases have shown progression to anaplastic large T-cell lymphoma and, therefore, require close follow-up.

A subset of lymphomatoid papulosis, which is likely to progress to malignant lymphoma and clinically resembles hydroa vacciniforme and histologically shows typical features of lymphomatoid papulosis, has also been described in children (206). A related entity is angiocentric cutaneous T-cell lymphoma of childhood that presents with a vesiculopapular eruption mimicking hydroa vacciniforme. Most of these children are from Asia and Latin America (207–208). Patients present with vesicles, necrotic areas, and scars on the face and dorsa of the hands, forearms, and legs. Unlike hydroa vacciniforme, the lesions are not related to sun exposure and are larger and deeper. Histologically, atypical lymphoid infiltrates are present in the dermis and subcutaneous tissue with a tendency for angiocentricity and vascular destruction. Epstein-Barr virus has been detected in several cases, suggesting a possible etiologic role. These lymphomas are graded as any other angiocentric T-cell lymphoma. The prognosis correlates with grade and extent of disease. Higher grade and systemic involvement are associated with a high mortality rate.

References

1. Caksen H, Kurtoglu S. Our experience with aplasia cutis congenita. *J Dermatol* 2002;29(6):376–379.
2. Rodrigues RG. Aplasia cutis congenita, congenital heart lesions, and frontonasal cysts in four successive generations. *Clin Genet* 2007;71(6):558–560.
3. Paller AS, Mancini AJ, eds. Hereditary disorders of cornification. In: *Hurwitz Clinical Pediatric Dermatology*. Philadelphia, PA: Elsevier, 2006:107.
4. Wakem P, Ikeda S, Haake A, et al. Localization of the Darier disease gene to a 2-cM portion of 12q23-24.1. *J Invest Dermatol* 1996;106(2):365–367.
5. Burge SM, Wilkinson JD. Darier-White disease: a review of the clinical features in 163 patients. *J Am Acad Dermatol* 1992;27(1):40–50.
6. Gorlin RJ, Chaudhry AP. The oral manifestation of keratosis follicularis. *Oral Surg Oral Med Oral Pathol* 1959;12:1468–1470.
7. Zaias N, Ackerman AB. The nail in Darier-White disease. *Arch Dermatol* 1973;107(2):193–199.
8. Chernosky ME. Porokeratosis. *Arch Dermatol* 1986;122(8):869–870.
9. Himmelstein R, Lynfield YL. Punctate porokeratosis. *Arch Dermatol* 1984;120(2):263–264.
10. Otsuka F, Shima A, Ishibashi Y. Porokeratosis as a premalignant condition of the skin. Cytologic demonstration of abnormal DNA ploidy in cells of the epidermis. *Cancer* 1989;63(5):891–896.
11. Sasaki S, Urano Y, Nakagawa K, et al. Linear porokeratosis with multiple squamous cell carcinomas: study of p53 expression in porokeratosis and squamous cell carcinoma. *Br J Dermatol* 1996;134(6):1151–1153.
12. Libermann S. Atrophoderma linearis maculosa et papillomatosis congenita. *Acta Derm Venereol* 1935;16:476.
13. Goltz RW, Peterson WC, Gorlin RJ, et al. Focal dermal hypoplasia. *Arch Dermatol* 1962;86:708–717.
14. Grzeschik KH, Bornholdt D, Oeffner F, et al. Deficiency of PORCN, a regulator of Wnt signaling, is associated with focal dermal hypoplasia. *Nat Genet* 2007;39(7):833–835.
15. Wang X, Reid Sutton V, Omar Peraza-Llanes J, et al. Mutations in X-linked PORCN, a putative regulator of Wnt signaling, cause focal dermal hypoplasia. *Nat Genet* 2007;39(7):836–838.
16. Fine JD, Eady RA, Bauer EA, et al. The classification of inherited epidermolysis bullosa (EB): Report of the Third International Consensus Meeting on Diagnosis and Classification of EB. *J Am Acad Dermatol* 2008;58(6):931–950.
17. Bergman R. Immunohistopathologic diagnosis of epidermolysis bullosa. *Am J Dermatopathol* 1999;21(2):185–192.
18. Uitto J, Richard G. Progress in epidermolysis bullosa: genetic classification and clinical implications. *Am J Med Genet C Semin Med Genet* 2004;131C(1):61–74.
19. Poziomczyk CS, Recuero JK, Bringhenti L et al. Incontinentia pigmenti. *An Bras Dermatol* 2014;89(1):26–36.
20. Phan TA, Wargon O, Turner AM. Incontinentia pigmenti case series: clinical spectrum of incontinentia pigmenti in 53 female patients and their relatives. *Clin Exp Dermatol* 2005;30(5):474–480.
21. Pacheco TR, Levy M, Collyer JC, et al. Incontinentia pigmenti in male patients. *J Am Acad Dermatol* 2006;55(2):251–255.
22. Berlin AL, Paller AS, Chan LS. Incontinentia pigmenti: a review and update on the molecular basis of pathophysiology. *J Am Acad Dermatol* 2002;47(2):169–187.
23. Maverakis E, Fung MA, Lynch PJ, et al. Acrodermatitis enteropathica and an overview of zinc metabolism. *J Am Acad Dermatol* 2007;56(1):116–124.
24. Wojnarowska F, Bhogal BS, Black MM. Chronic bullous disease of childhood and linear IgA disease of adults are IgA1-mediated diseases. *Br J Dermatol* 1994;131(2):201–204.
25. Safai B, Rappaport I, Matsuoka L, et al. Childhood dermatitis herpetiformis. Review of the new aspects and report of a case. *J Am Acad Dermatol* 1981;4(4):435–441.
26. Karpati S, Kosnai I, Verkasalo M, et al. HLA antigens, jejunal morphology and associated diseases in children with dermatitis herpetiformis. *Acta Paediatr Scand* 1986;75(2):297–301.
27. Katz SI, Hall RP III, Lawley TJ, et al. Dermatitis herpetiformis: the skin and the gut. *Ann Intern Med* 1980;93(6):857–874.
28. Alonso-Llamazares J, Gibson LE, Rogers RS III. Clinical, pathologic, and immunopathologic features of dermatitis herpetiformis: review of the Mayo Clinic experience. *Int J Dermatol* 2007;46(9):910–919.
29. Castro LA, Lundell RB, Krause PK, et al. Clinical experience in pemphigoid gestationis: report of 10 cases. *J Am Acad Dermatol* 2006;55(5):823–828.
30. Aoyama Y, Asai K, Hioki K, et al. Herpes gestationis in a mother and newborn: immunoclinical perspectives based on a weekly follow-up of the enzyme-linked immunosorbent assay index of a

30. bullous pemphigoid antigen noncollagenous domain. *Arch Dermatol* 2007;143(9):1168–1172.
31. Di Zenzo G, Calabresi V, Grosso F, et al. The intracellular and extracellular domains of BP180 antigen comprise novel epitopes targeted by pemphigoid gestationis autoantibodies. *J Invest Dermatol* 2007;127(4):864–873.
32. Callot-Mellot C, Bodemer C, Caux F, et al. Epidermolysis bullosa acquisita in childhood. *Arch Dermatol* 1997;133(9):1122–1126.
33. Trigo-Guzman FX, Conti A, Aoki V, et al. Epidermolysis bullosa acquisita in childhood. *J Dermatol* 2003;30(3):226–229.
34. Mayuzumi M, Akiyama M, Nishie W, et al. Childhood epidermolysis bullosa acquisita with autoantibodies against the noncollagenous 1 and 2 domains of type VII collagen: case report and review of the literature. *Br J Dermatol* 2006;155(5):1048–1052.
35. Woodley DT, Briggaman RA, Gammon WR. Acquired epidermolysis bullosa. A bullous disease associated with autoimmunity to type VII (anchoring fibril) collagen. *Dermatol Clin* 1990;8(4):717–726.
36. Edwards S, Wakelin SH, Wojnarowska F, et al. Bullous pemphigoid and epidermolysis bullosa acquisita: presentation, prognosis, and immunopathology in 11 children. *Pediatr Dermatol* 1998;15(3):184–190.
37. Lam NS, Yang YH, Wang LC, et al. Clinical characteristics of childhood erythema multiforme, Stevens-Johnson syndrome and toxic epidermal necrolysis in Taiwanese children. *J Microbiol Immunol Infect* 2004;37(6):366–370.
38. Forman R, Koren G, Shear NH. Erythema multiforme, Stevens-Johnson syndrome and toxic epidermal necrolysis in children: a review of 10 years' experience. *Drug Saf* 2002;25(13):965–972.
39. Khalili B, Bahna SL. Pathogenesis and recent therapeutic trends in Stevens-Johnson syndrome and toxic epidermal necrolysis. *Ann Allergy Asthma Immunol* 2006;97(3):272–280.
40. Villada G, Roujeau JC, Clerici T, et al. Immunopathology of toxic epidermal necrolysis. Keratinocytes, HLA-DR expression, Langerhans cells, and mononuclear cells: an immunopathologic study of five cases. *Arch Dermatol* 1992;128(1):50–53.
41. Fromowitz JS, Ramos-Caro FA, Flowers FP. Practical guidelines for the management of toxic epidermal necrolysis and Stevens-Johnson syndrome. *Int J Dermatol* 2007;46(10):1092–1094.
42. Hughey LC. Approach to the hospitalized patient with targetoid lesions. *Dermatol Ther* 2011;24:196.
43. Schneck J, Fagot JP, Sekula P, et al. Effects of treatments on the mortality of Stevens-Johnson syndrome and toxic epidermal necrolysis: a retrospective study on patients included in the prospective EuroSCAR Study. *J Am Acad Dermatol* 2008;58(1):33–40.
44. Stella M, Clemente A, Bollero D, et al. Toxic epidermal necrolysis (TEN) and Stevens-Johnson syndrome (SJS): experience with high-dose intravenous immunoglobulins and topical conservative approach. A retrospective analysis. *Burns* 2007;33(4):452–459.
45. Wagner A. Distinguishing vesicular and pustular disorders in the neonate. *Curr Opin Pediatr* 1997;9(4):396–405.
46. Posso-De Los Rios CJ, Pope E. New insights into pustular dermatoses in pediatric patients. *J Am Acad Dermatol* 2014;70(4):767–773.
47. Nanda S, Reddy BS, Ramji S, et al. Analytical study of pustular eruptions in neonates. *Pediatr Dermatol* 2002;19(3):210–215.
48. Ferrandiz C, Coroleu W, Ribera M, et al. Sterile transient neonatal pustulosis is a precocious form of erythema toxicum neonatorum. *Dermatology* 1992;185(1):18–22.
49. Dorton DW, Kaufmann M. Palmoplantar pustules in an infant. Acropustulosis of infancy. *Arch Dermatol* 1996;132(11):1365–1366, 1368–1369.
50. Peroni DG, Piacentini GL, Bodini A, et al. Prevalence and risk factors for atopic dermatitis in preschool children. *Br J Dermatol* 2008;158(3):539–543.
51. Hanifin JM, Reed ML. A population-based survey of eczema prevalence in the United States. *Dermatitis* 2007;18(2):82–91.
52. Somani VK. A study of allergen-specific IgE antibodies in Indian patients of atopic dermatitis. *Indian J Dermatol Venereol Leprol* 2008;74(2):100–104.
53. Totri CR, Diaz L, Eichenfield LF. 2014 update on atopic dermatitis in children. *Curr Opin Pediatr* 2014;26:466–471.
54. Shin HT. Diagnosis and management of diaper dermatitis. *Pediatr Clin North Am* 2014;61(2):367–382.
55. Beattie PE, Green C, Lowe G, et al. Which children should we patch test? *Clin Exp Dermatol* 2007;32(1):6–11.
56. Hogeling M, Pratt M. Allergic contact dermatitis in children: the Ottawa hospital patch-testing clinic experience, 1996 to 2006. *Dermatitis* 2008;19(2):86–89.
57. Schachner L, Ling NS, Press S. A statistical analysis of a pediatric dermatology clinic. *Pediatr Dermatol* 1983;1(2):157–164.
58. Seyhan M, Coskun BK, Saglam H, et al. Psoriasis in childhood and adolescence: evaluation of demographic and clinical features. *Pediatr Int* 2006;48(6):525–530.
59. Benoit S, Hamm H. Childhood psoriasis. *Clin Dermatol* 2007;25(6):555–562.
60. Fan X, Xiao FL, Yang S, et al. Childhood psoriasis: a study of 277 patients from China. *J Eur Acad Dermatol Venereol* 2007;21(6):762–765.
61. Rogers M. Childhood psoriasis. *Curr Opin Pediatr* 2002;14(4):404–409.
62. Bowcock AM, Barker JN. Genetics of psoriasis: the potential impact on new therapies. *J Am Acad Dermatol* 2003;49(2 Suppl):S51–S56.
63. Luis-Montoya P, Dominguez-Soto L, Vega-Memije E. Lichen planus in 24 children with review of the literature. *Pediatr Dermatol* 2005;22(4):295–298.
64. Balasubramaniam P, Ogboli M, Moss C. Lichen planus in children: review of 26 cases. *Clin Exp Dermatol* 2008;33(4):457–459.
65. Chuang TY, Ilstrup DM, Perry HO, et al. Pityriasis rosea in Rochester, Minnesota, 1969 to 1978. *J Am Acad Dermatol* 1982;7(1):80–89.
66. Broccolo F, Drago F, Careddu AM, et al. Additional evidence that pityriasis rosea is associated with reactivation of human herpesvirus-6 and -7. *J Invest Dermatol* 2005;124(6):1234–1240.
67. Allison DS, El-Azhary RA, Calobrisi SD, et al. Pityriasis rubra pilaris in children. *J Am Acad Dermatol* 2002;47(3):386–389.
68. Ersoy-Evans S, Greco MF, Mancini AJ, et al. Pityriasis lichenoides in childhood: a retrospective review of 124 patients. *J Am Acad Dermatol* 2007;56(2):205–210.
69. Khachemoune A, Blyumin ML. Pityriasis lichenoides: pathophysiology, classification, and treatment. *Am J Clin Dermatol* 2007;8(1):29–36.
70. Kempf W, Kazakov DV, Palmedo G, et al. Pityriasis lichenoides et varioliformis acuta with numerous CD30(+) cells: a variant mimicking lymphomatoid papulosis and other cutaneous lymphomas. A clinicopathologic, immunohistochemical, and molecular biological study of 13 cases. *Am J Surg Pathol* 2012;36(7):1021–1029.
71. Magro C, Crowson AN, Kovatich A, et al. Pityriasis lichenoides: a clonal T-cell lymphoproliferative disorder. *Hum Pathol* 2002;33(8):788–795.
72. Weinberg JM, Kristal L, Chooback L, et al. The clonal nature of pityriasis lichenoides. *Arch Dermatol* 2002;138(8):1063–1067.
73. Gelmetti C, Rigoni C, Alessi E, et al. Pityriasis lichenoides in children: a long-term follow-up of eighty-nine cases. *J Am Acad Dermatol* 1990;23(3 Pt 1):473–478.
74. Brandt O, Abeck D, Gianotti R, et al. Gianotti-Crosti syndrome. *J Am Acad Dermatol* 2006;54(1):136–145.
75. Powell J, Wojnarowska F. Childhood vulvar lichen sclerosus: an increasingly common problem. *J Am Acad Dermatol* 2001;44(5):803–806.
76. Drut RM, Gomez MA, Drut R, et al. Human papillomavirus is present in some cases of childhood penile lichen sclerosus: an in situ hybridization and SP-PCR study. *Pediatr Dermatol* 1998;15(2):85–90.
77. Poindexter G, Morrell DS. Anogenital pruritus: lichen sclerosus in children. *Pediatr Ann* 2007;36(12):785–791.
78. Adachi J, Endo K, Fukuzumi T, et al. Increasing incidence of streptococcal impetigo in atopic dermatitis. *J Dermatol Sci* 1998;17(1):45–53.
79. Hedrick J. Acute bacterial skin infections in pediatric medicine: current issues in presentation and treatment. *Paediatr Drugs* 2003;5(Suppl 1):35–46.
80. Bernard P. Management of common bacterial infections of the skin. *Curr Opin Infect Dis* 2008;21(2):122–128.

81. Handler MZ, Schwartz RA. Staphylococcal scalded skin syndrome: diagnosis and management in children and adults. *J Eur Acad Dermatol Venereol* 2014;28:1418–1423.
82. Amagai M. Desmoglein as a target in autoimmunity and infection. *J Am Acad Dermatol* 2003;48(2):244–252.
83. Yamasaki O, Yamaguchi T, Sugai M, et al. Clinical manifestations of staphylococcal scalded-skin syndrome depend on serotypes of exfoliative toxins. *J Clin Microbiol* 2005;43(4):1890–1893.
84. Iwatsuki K, Yamasaki O, Morizane S, et al. Staphylococcal cutaneous infections: invasion, evasion and aggression. *J Dermatol Sci* 2006;42(3):203–214.
85. Chi CY, Wang SM, Lin HC, et al. A clinical and microbiological comparison of *Staphylococcus aureus* toxic shock and scalded skin syndromes in children. *Clin Infect Dis* 2006;42(2):181–185.
86. Hurwitz RM, Ackerman AB. Cutaneous pathology of the toxic shock syndrome. *Am J Dermatopathol* 1985;7(6):563–578.
87. Martin JM, Green M. Group A streptococcus. *Semin Pediatr Infect Dis* 2006;17(3):140–148.
88. Chan YH, Chong CY, Puthucheary J, et al. Ecthyma gangrenosum: a manifestation of *Pseudomonas* sepsis in three paediatric patients. *Singapore Med J* 2006;47(12):1080–1083.
89. Zomorrodi A, Wald ER. Ecthyma gangrenosum and multiple nodules: cutaneous manifestations of Pseudomonas aeruginosa sepsis in a previously healthy infant. *Pediatr Dermatol* 2011;28(2): 204–205.
90. Dorff GJ, Geimer NF, Rosenthal DR, et al. Pseudomonas septicemia. Illustrated evolution of its skin lesion. *Arch Intern Med* 1971;128(4):591–595.
91. Khalil BA, Baillie CT, Kenny SE, et al. Surgical strategies in the management of ecthyma gangrenosum in paediatric oncology patients. *Pediatr Surg Int* 2008;24(7):793–797.
92. Eriksson B, Jorup-Ronstrom C, Karkkonen K, et al. Erysipelas: clinical and bacteriologic spectrum and serological aspects. *Clin Infect Dis* 1996;23(5):1091–1098.
93. Celestin R, Brown J, Kihiczak G, et al. Erysipelas: a common potentially dangerous infection. *Acta Dermatovenerol Alp Panonica Adriat* 2007;16(3):123–127.
94. Grosshans EM. The red face: erysipelas. *Clin Dermatol* 1993;11(2):307–313.
95. Sinclair KA, Woods CR, Sinal SH. Venereal warts in children. *Pediatr Rev* 2011;32:115.
96. Marcoux D, Nadeau K, McCuaig C, et al. Pediatric anogenital warts: a 7-year review of children referred to a tertiary-care hospital in Montreal, Canada. *Pediatr Dermatol* 2006;23(3):199–207.
97. Syrjänen S. Current concepts on human papillomavirus infections in children. *APMIS* 2010;118:494.
98. Jones V, Smith SJ, Omar HA. Nonsexual transmission of anogenital warts in children: a retrospective analysis. *Sci World J* 2007;7:1896–1899.
99. Leung AK, Robson WL, Leong AG. Herpes zoster in childhood. *J Pediatr Health Care* 2006;20(5):300–303.
100. Rennert WP. Noninfectious cutaneous manifestations of HIV infection in children. *AIDS Read* 2006;16(2):103–105.
101. Gottschalk GM. Pediatric HIV/AIDS and the skin: an update. *Dermatol Clin* 2006;24(4):531–536, vii.
102. Hawkins DM, Smidt AC. Superficial fungal infections in children. *Pediatr Clin North Am* 2014;61(2):443–455.
103. Elewski BE. Tinea capitis: a current perspective. *J Am Acad Dermatol* 2000;42(1 Pt 1):1–20; quiz 21–24.
104. Abraham AG, Kulp-Shorten CL, Callen JP. Remember to consider dermatophyte infection when dealing with recalcitrant dermatoses. *South Med J* 1998;91(4):349–353.
105. Hengge UR, Currie BJ, Jager G, et al. Scabies: a ubiquitous neglected skin disease. *Lancet Infect Dis* 2006;6(12):769–779.
106. Uihlein LC, Brandling-Bennett HA, Lio PA, et al. Sweet syndrome in children. *Pediatr Dermatol* 2012;29(1):38–44.
107. Herron MD, Coffin CM, Vanderhooft SL. Sweet syndrome in two children. *Pediatr Dermatol* 2005;22(6):525–529.
108. Howard R, Tsuchiya A. Adult skin disease in the pediatric patient. *Dermatol Clin* 1998;16(3):593–608.
109. Powell JG, Ramsdell A, Rothman IL. Eosinophilic cellulitis (Wells syndrome) in a pediatric patient: a case report and review of the literature. *Cutis* 2012;89(4):191–194.
110. Katsanis E, Luke KH, Hsu E, et al. Neutrophilic eccrine hidradenitis in acute myelomonocytic leukemia. *Am J Pediatr Hematol Oncol* 1987;9(3):204–208.
111. Stahr BJ, Cooper PH, Caputo RV. Idiopathic plantar hidradenitis: a neutrophilic eccrine hidradenitis occurring primarily in children. *J Cutan Pathol* 1994;21(4):289–296.
112. Rubinson R, Larralde M, Santos-Munoz A, et al. Palmoplantar eccrine hidradenitis: seven new cases. *Pediatr Dermatol* 2004;21(4):466–468.
113. Shih IH, Huang YH, Yang CH, et al. Childhood neutrophilic eccrine hidradenitis: a clinicopathologic and immunohistochemical study of 10 patients. *J Am Acad Dermatol* 2005;52(6):963–966.
114. Simon M Jr, Cremer H, von den Driesch P. Idiopathic recurrent palmoplantar hidradenitis in children. Report of 22 cases. *Arch Dermatol* 1998;134(1):76–79.
115. Bhat RM, Shetty SS, Kamath GH. Pyoderma gangrenosum in childhood. *Int J Dermatol* 2004;43(3):205–207.
116. Meissner PE, Jappe U, Niemeyer CM, et al. Pyoderma gangraenosum, a rare, but potentially fatal complication in paediatric oncology patients. *Klin Padiatr* 2007;219(5):296–299.
117. von den Driesch P. Pyoderma gangrenosum: a report of 44 cases with follow-up. *Br J Dermatol* 1997;137(6):1000–1005.
118. Stefanaki K, Tsivitanidou-Kakourou T, Stefanaki C, et al. Histological and immunohistochemical study of granuloma annulare and subcutaneous granuloma annulare in children. *J Cutan Pathol* 2007;34(5):392–396.
119. Felner EI, Steinberg JB, Weinberg AG. Subcutaneous granuloma annulare: a review of 47 cases. *Pediatrics* 1997;100(6):965–967.
120. Kutukculer N, Tutuncuoglu S, Yilmaz D, et al. Subcutaneous granuloma annulare and IgA-IgG2 deficiency. *Turk J Pediatr* 1998;40(2):279–281.
121. Pestoni C, Ferreiros MM, de la Torre C, et al. Two girls with necrobiosis lipoidica and type I diabetes mellitus with transfollicular elimination in one girl. *Pediatr Dermatol* 2003;20(3):211–214.
122. Verrotti A, Chiarelli F, Amerio P, et al. Necrobiosis lipoidica diabeticorum in children and adolescents: a clue for underlying renal and retinal disease. *Pediatr Dermatol* 1995;12(3):220–223.
123. Evans MJ, Blessing K, Gray ES. Pseudorheumatoid nodule (deep granuloma annulare) of childhood: clinicopathologic features of twenty patients. *Pediatr Dermatol* 1994;11(1):6–9.
124. Milman N, Hoffmann AL. Childhood sarcoidosis: long-term follow-up. *Eur Respir J* 2008;31(3):592–598.
125. Shetty AK, Gedalia A. Pediatric sarcoidosis. *J Am Acad Dermatol* 2003;48(1):150–151.
126. Mangas C, Fernandez-Figueras MT, Fite E, et al. Clinical spectrum and histological analysis of 32 cases of specific cutaneous sarcoidosis. *J Cutan Pathol* 2006;33(12):772–777.
127. Moraes AJ, Soares PM, Zapata AL, et al. Panniculitis in childhood and adolescence. *Pediatr Int* 2006;48(1):48–53.
128. Fretzin DF, Arias AM. Sclerema neonatorum and subcutaneous fat necrosis of the newborn. *Pediatr Dermatol* 1987;4(2):112–122.
129. Mahe E, Girszyn N, Hadj-Rabia S, et al. Subcutaneous fat necrosis of the newborn: a systematic evaluation of risk factors, clinical manifestations, complications and outcome of 16 children. *Br J Dermatol* 2007;156(4):709–715.
130. Zeb A, Darmstadt GL. Sclerema neonatorum: a review of nomenclature, clinical presentation, histological features, differential diagnoses and management. *J Perinatol* 2008;28(7):453–460.
131. Sadana S, Mathur NB, Thakur A. Exchange transfusion in septic neonates with sclerema: effect on immunoglobulin and complement levels. *Indian Pediatr* 1997;34(1):20–25.
132. Golitz LE. The vasculitides and their significance in the pediatric age group. *Dermatol Clin* 1986;4(1):117–125.
133. Yang YH, Yu HH, Chiang BL. The diagnosis and classification of Henoch-Schönlein purpura: an updated review. *Autoimmun Rev* 2014;13(4-5):355–358.
134. Yang YH, Chuang YH, Wang LC, et al. The immunobiology of Henoch-Schönlein purpura. *Autoimmun Rev* 2008;7(3):179–184.

135. Trnka P. Henoch-Schönlein purpura in children. *J Paediatr Child Health* 2013;49(12):995–1003.
136. Edwards MS, Baker CJ. Complications and sequelae of meningococcal infections in children. *J Pediatr* 1981;99(4):540–545.
137. Gonggryp LA, Todd G. Acute hemorrhagic edema of childhood (AHE). *Pediatr Dermatol* 1998;15(2):91–96.
138. Crowe MA, Jonas PP. Acute hemorrhagic edema of infancy. *Cutis* 1998;62(2):65–66.
139. Dillon MJ. Childhood vasculitis. *Lupus* 1998;7(4):259–265.
140. Sheth AP, Olson JC, Esterly NB. Cutaneous polyarteritis nodosa of childhood. *J Am Acad Dermatol* 1994;31(4):561–566.
141. Bekaert C, Song M, Delvigne A. Acne neonatorum and familial hyperandrogenism. *Dermatology* 1998;196(4):453–454.
142. Jansen T, Burgdorf WH, Plewig G. Pathogenesis and treatment of acne in childhood. *Pediatr Dermatol* 1997;14(1):17–21.
143. Hernández-Martín Á, Nuño-González A, Colmenero I, et al. Eosinophilic pustular folliculitis of infancy: a series of 15 cases and review of the literature. *J Am Acad Dermatol* 2013;68(1):150–155.
144. Ziemer M, Boer A. Eosinophilic pustular folliculitis in infancy: not a distinctive inflammatory disease of the skin. *Am J Dermatopathol* 2005;27(5):443–455.
145. See Y, Koh ET, Boey ML. One hundred and seventy cases of childhood-onset rheumatological disease in Singapore. *Ann Acad Med Singapore* 1998;27(4):496–502.
146. Sampaio MC, de Oliveira ZN, Machado MC, et al. Discoid lupus erythematosus in children—a retrospective study of 34 patients. *Pediatr Dermatol* 2008;25(2):163–167.
147. Hiraki LT, Benseler SM, Tyrrell PN, et al. Clinical and laboratory characteristics and long-term outcome of pediatric systemic lupus erythematosus: a longitudinal study. *J Pediatr* 2008;152(4):550–556.
148. Wisuthsarewong W, Soongswang J, Chantorn R. Neonatal lupus erythematosus: clinical character, investigation, and outcome. *Pediatr Dermatol* 2011;28(2):115–121.
149. Monari P, Gualdi G, Fantini F, et al. Cutaneous neonatal lupus erythematosus in four siblings. *Br J Dermatol* 2008;158(3):626–628.
150. Robles DT, Jaramillo L, Hornung RL. Neonatal lupus. *Dermatol Online J* 2006;12(7):25.
151. Zulian F. Systemic sclerosis and localized scleroderma in childhood. *Rheum Dis Clin North Am* 2008;34(1):239–255; ix.
152. Jacobsohn DA. Acute graft-versus-host disease in children. *Bone Marrow Transplant* 2008;41(2):215–221.
153. Tolland JP, Devereux C, Jones FC, et al. Sclerodermatous chronic graft-versus-host disease—a report of four pediatric cases. *Pediatr Dermatol* 2008;25(2):240–244.
154. Rho NK, Youn SJ, Park HS, et al. Calcified nodule on the heel of a child following a single heel stick in the neonatal period. *Clin Exp Dermatol* 2003;28(5):502–503.
155. Tan O, Atik B, Kizilkaya A, et al. Extensive skin calcifications in an infant with chronic renal failure: metastatic calcinosis cutis. *Pediatr Dermatol* 2006;23(3):235–238.
156. Su WP. Histopathologic varieties of epidermal nevus. A study of 160 cases. *Am J Dermatopathol* 1982;4(2):161–170.
157. Rogers M, McCrossin I, Commens C. Epidermal nevi and the epidermal nevus syndrome. A review of 131 cases. *J Am Acad Dermatol* 1989;20(3):476–488.
158. Sugarman JL. Epidermal nevus syndromes. *Semin Cutan Med Surg* 2007;26(4):221–230.
159. Gardner EJ, Richards RC. Multiple cutaneous and subcutaneous lesions occurring simultaneously with hereditary polyposis and osteomatosis. *Am J Hum Genet* 1953;5(2):139–147.
160. Pryor SG, Lewis JE, Weaver AL, et al. Pediatric dermoid cysts of the head and neck. *Otolaryngol Head Neck Surg* 2005;132(6):938–942.
161. Cho S, Chang SE, Choi JH, et al. Clinical and histologic features of 64 cases of steatocystoma multiplex. *J Dermatol* 2002;29(3):152–156.
162. Patrizi A, Neri I, Guerrini V, et al. Persistent milia, steatocystoma multiplex and eruptive vellus hair cysts: variable expression of multiple pilosebaceous cysts within an affected family. *Dermatology* 1998;196(4):392–396.
163. Cigliano B, Baltogiannis N, De Marco M, et al. Pilomatricoma in childhood: a retrospective study from three European paediatric centres. *Eur J Pediatr* 2005;164(11):673–677.
164. Julian CG, Bowers PW. A clinical review of 209 pilomatricomas. *J Am Acad Dermatol* 1998;39(2 Pt 1):191–195.
165. Avci G, Akan M, Akoz T. Simultaneous multiple pilomatrixomas. *Pediatr Dermatol* 2006;23(2):157–162.
166. Pujol RM, Casanova JM, Egido R, et al. Multiple familial pilomatricomas: a cutaneous marker for Gardner syndrome? *Pediatr Dermatol* 1995;12(4):331–335.
167. Ackerman AB, Reddy VB, Soyer HP. Pilomatricoma and matricoma (Chapter 20). In: *Neoplasms with follicular differentiation*. New York: Ardor Scribendi, 2001:349–388.
168. Schepis C, Siragusa M, Palazzo R, et al. Palpebral syringomas and Down's syndrome. *Dermatology* 1994;189(3):248–250.
169. Garman M, Metry D. Vulvar syringomas in a 9-year-old child with review of the literature. *Pediatr Dermatol* 2006;23(4):369–372.
170. Soler-Carrillo J, Estrach T, Mascaro JM. Eruptive syringoma: 27 new cases and review of the literature. *J Eur Acad Dermatol Venereol* 2001;15(3):242–246.
171. Steffen C, Ackerman AB. Neoplasms with sebaceous differentiation. In: Steffen C, Ackerman AB, eds. *Nevus sebaceus*. Philadelphia, PA: Lea & Febiger, 1994:89.
172. Cribier B, Scrivener Y, Grosshans E. Tumors arising in nevus sebaceus: a study of 596 cases. *J Am Acad Dermatol* 2000;42(2 Pt 1): 263–268.
173. Kazakov DV, Calonje E, Zelger B, et al. Sebaceous carcinoma arising in nevus sebaceus of Jadassohn: a clinicopathological study of five cases. *Am J Dermatopathol* 2007;29(3):242–248.
174. Friedrich RE. Diagnosis and treatment of patients with nevoid basal cell carcinoma syndrome [Gorlin-Goltz syndrome (GGS)]. *Anticancer Res* 2007;27(4A):1783–1787.
175. Marghoob AA, Schoenbach SP, Kopf AW, et al. Large congenital melanocytic nevi and the risk for the development of malignant melanoma. A prospective study. *Arch Dermatol* 1996;132(2):170–175.
176. Krengel S, Hauschild A, Schafer T. Melanoma risk in congenital melanocytic naevi: a systematic review. *Br J Dermatol* 2006;155(1):1–8.
177. Elder DE, Clark WH Jr. Developmental biology of malignant melanoma. *Pigment Cell Res* 1987;8:1.
178. Paniago-Pereira C, Maize JC, Ackerman AB. Nevus of large spindle and/or epithelioid cells (Spitz's nevus). *Arch Dermatol* 1978;114 (12):1811–1823.
179. Spitz S. Melanomas of childhood. 1948. *CA Cancer J Clin* 1991;41 (1):40–51.
180. Mooi WJ, Krausz T. Spitz nevus versus spitzoid melanoma: diagnostic difficulties, conceptual controversies. *Adv Anat Pathol* 2006;13 (4):147–156.
181. Carney JA, Ferreiro JA. The epithelioid blue nevus. A multicentric familial tumor with important associations, including cardiac myxoma and psammomatous melanotic schwannoma. *Am J Surg Pathol* 1996;20(3):259–272.
182. Groben PA, Harvell JD, White WL. Epithelioid blue nevus: neoplasm Sui generis or variation on a theme? *Am J Dermatopathol* 2000;22(6):473–488.
183. Zembowicz A, Carney JA, Mihm MC. Pigmented epithelioid melanocytoma: a low-grade melanocytic tumor with metastatic potential indistinguishable from animal-type melanoma and epithelioid blue nevus. *Am J Surg Pathol* 2004;28(1):31–40.
184. Reimer RR, Clark WH Jr, Greene MH, et al. Precursor lesions in familial melanoma. A new genetic preneoplastic syndrome. *JAMA* 1978;239(8):744–746.
185. Ackerman AB. Melanocytic proliferations that simulate malignant melanoma histopathologically. *Monogr Pathol* 1988;30:153–173.
186. Hawryluk EB, Liang MG. Pediatric melanoma, moles, and sun safety. *Pediatr Clin North Am.* 2014;61(2):279–291.
187. Prose NS, Laude TA, Heilman ER, et al. Congenital malignant melanoma. *Pediatrics* 1987;79(6):967–970.
188. Schneiderman H, Wu AY, Campbell WA, et al. Congenital melanoma with multiple prenatal metastases. *Cancer* 1987;60(6):1371–1377.

189. Mones JM, Ackerman AB. Melanomas in prepubescent children: review comprehensively, critique historically, criteria diagnostically, and course biologically. *Am J Dermatopathol* 2003;25(3): 223–238.
190. Fetsch JF, Laskin WB, Hallman JR, et al. Neurothekeoma: an analysis of 178 tumors with detailed immunohistochemical data and long-term patient follow-up information. *Am J Surg Pathol* 2007;31(7):1103–1114.
191. Hornick JL, Fletcher CD. Cellular neurothekeoma: detailed characterization in a series of 133 cases. *Am J Surg Pathol* 2007;31(3):329–340.
192. Herron MD, Coffin CM, Vanderhooft SL. Tufted angiomas: variability of the clinical morphology. *Pediatr Dermatol* 2002;19(5):394–401.
193. Browning J, Frieden I, Baselga E, et al. Congenital, self-regressing tufted angioma. *Arch Dermatol* 2006;142(6):749–751.
194. Arcangeli F, Calista D. Congenital myofibromatosis in two siblings. *Eur J Dermatol* 2006;16(2):181–183.
195. Reye RD. Recurring digital fibrous tumors of childhood. *Arch Pathol* 1965;80:228–231.
196. Grenier N, Liang C, Capaldi L, et al. A range of histologic findings in infantile digital fibromatosis. *Pediatr Dermatol* 2008;25(1):72–75.
197. Shmookler BM, Enzinger FM, Weiss SW. Giant cell fibroblastoma. A juvenile form of dermatofibrosarcoma protuberans. *Cancer* 1989;64(10):2154–2161.
198. Harvell JD, Kilpatrick SE, White WL. Histogenetic relations between giant cell fibroblastoma and dermatofibrosarcoma protuberans. CD34 staining showing the spectrum and a simulator. *Am J Dermatopathol* 1998;20(4):339–345.
199. Diwan AH, Skelton HG III, Horenstein MG, et al. Dermatofibrosarcoma protuberans and giant cell fibroblastoma exhibit CD99 positivity. *J Cutan Pathol* 2008;35(7):647–650.
200. Jha P, Moosavi C, Fanburg-Smith JC. Giant cell fibroblastoma: an update and addition of 86 new cases from the Armed Forces Institute of Pathology, in honor of Dr. Franz M Enzinger. *Ann Diagn Pathol* 2007;11(2):81–88.
201. Frieri M, Quershi M. Pediatric mastocytosis: a review of the literature. *Pediatr Allergy Immunol Pulmonol* 2013;26(4):175–180.
202. Kapur P, Erickson C, Rakheja D, et al. Congenital self-healing reticulohistiocytosis (Hashimoto-Pritzker disease): ten-year experience at Dallas Children's Medical Center. *J Am Acad Dermatol* 2007;56(2):290–294.
203. Gianotti R, Alessi E, Caputo R. Benign cephalic histiocytosis: a distinct entity or a part of a wide spectrum of histiocytic proliferative disorders of children? A histopathological study. *Am J Dermatopathol* 1993;15(4):315–319.
204. Francis JS, Sybert VP, Benjamin DR. Congenital monocytic leukemia: report of a case with cutaneous involvement, and review of the literature. *Pediatr Dermatol* 1989;6(4):306–311.
205. Le Deley MC, Reiter A, Williams D, et al. Prognostic factors in childhood anaplastic large cell lymphoma: results of a large European intergroup study. *Blood* 2008;111(3):1560–1566.
206. Tabata N, Aiba S, Ichinohazama R, et al. Hydroa vacciniforme-like lymphomatoid papulosis in a Japanese child: a new subset. *J Am Acad Dermatol* 1995;32(2 Pt 2):378–381.
207. Sangueza M, Plaza JA. Hydroa vacciniforme-like cutaneous T-cell lymphoma: clinicopathologic and immunohistochemical study of 12 cases. *J Am Acad Dermatol* 2013;69(1):112–119.
208. Quintanilla-Martinez L, Ridaura C, Nagl F, et al. Hydroa vacciniforme-like lymphoma: a chronic EBV+ lymphoproliferative disorder with risk to develop a systemic lymphoma. *Blood* 2013;122(18):3101–3110.

CHAPTER 27

Neuromuscular Diseases

Kevin E. Bove, M.D., and Lili Miles, M.D.

NORMAL MUSCLE DEVELOPMENT

Detailed reviews of skeletal muscle development provide a basis for understanding early events in myogenesis (1,2). In the first few weeks of embryonic life (Figure 27-1), primitive mesenchyme, under the influence of *MyoD*, *Myf*, and *PAX* genes, differentiates to muscle progenitor cells. Myofibrils form under the influence of myogenin. Myoblasts with disorganized sarcomeres fuse to form multinucleate myotubes in which oriented sarcomeres surround a central core that is rich in organelles but devoid of contractile filaments (Figure 27-2A). At this stage, muscle nuclei are centrally located, and there are no definable histochemical or structural subtypes. Prominent peripheral nuclei are those of satellite cells, located within the sarcolemmal basement membrane, or residual unfused myoblasts. Desmin and myogenin are strongly expressed in fetal myotubes: this immunohistochemical reactivity is markedly reduced by late gestation (3). Further growth and development of muscle are influenced by workload, growth factors such as myostatin, and steroid hormones.

The transition from myotubes, which average 8 to 10 μm in diameter, to larger muscle fibers with peripheral nuclei is completed between 22 and 26 weeks of gestation when most are typeable as IIc fetal fibers containing fetal myosin. During the third trimester (Figure 27-2B), type IIc fibers are replaced by type I fibers, type IIa fibers, and type IIb fibers (4). Type IIc fibers, defined as those with an intermediate level of myosin ATPase reactivity at low pH, evolve to mature subtypes and finally disappear during early infancy. Abnormal persistence of type IIc fibers occurs in both myopathic and neuropathic disorders of infancy and may indicate a maturation disturbance. Myofibers containing fetal myosin may transiently reappear during regeneration after muscle fiber injury at all ages.

A few widely scattered, relatively large type I fibers (the Wohlfart B fibers) with an uncertain role in development make a brief appearance during late gestation and then rapidly regress. Most type I fibers are smaller than type IIc fibers until birth or slightly later in normal infants (5). Underlying the progressive disappearance of fetal fibers and appearance of mature fiber subtypes are poorly understood determinants of structural, enzymatic, and contractile proteins and of organelle populations including links between muscle and central nervous system maturation.

Brooke and Engel published a useful review of muscle fiber subtype profiles for normal and abnormal muscle in children (6). They identified disproportionately small type I muscle fibers as a major finding in childhood neuromuscular disease, defining this state as a difference in diameter of type I and type II fibers of greater than 12%. Their nomogram relating normal muscle fiber diameter to age is valuable but falls short of the ideal because data for several muscles and for fiber subtypes were pooled and because of the paucity of data from young infants. A nomogram derived from frozen postmortem specimens of thigh muscles (Figure 27-3) is useful for assessment of fiber size in infants (5). Muscle fiber diameter in formalin-fixed paraffin sections is about 70% to 80% of that in sections of fresh frozen muscle.

MUSCLE APLASIA AND HYPOPLASIA

Determination of whether muscles are small because of primary failure to develop or because of regression is always problematic for the pathologist. The best documented examples of primary muscle aplasia or hypoplasia are secondary to spinal cord abnormalities. In the Poland anomaly, familial absent pectoralis muscle is associated with local soft tissue and skeletal defects and syndactyly (7). Möbius syndrome may coexist with the Poland anomaly, suggesting that a primary lesion may exist in the central nervous system and interfere with development of specific muscles in some cases (8). Chromosome abnormalities influence muscle development in trisomy syndromes, but it is uncertain whether this is a defect in muscle specification from primitive mesenchyme or the result of abnormal organization at

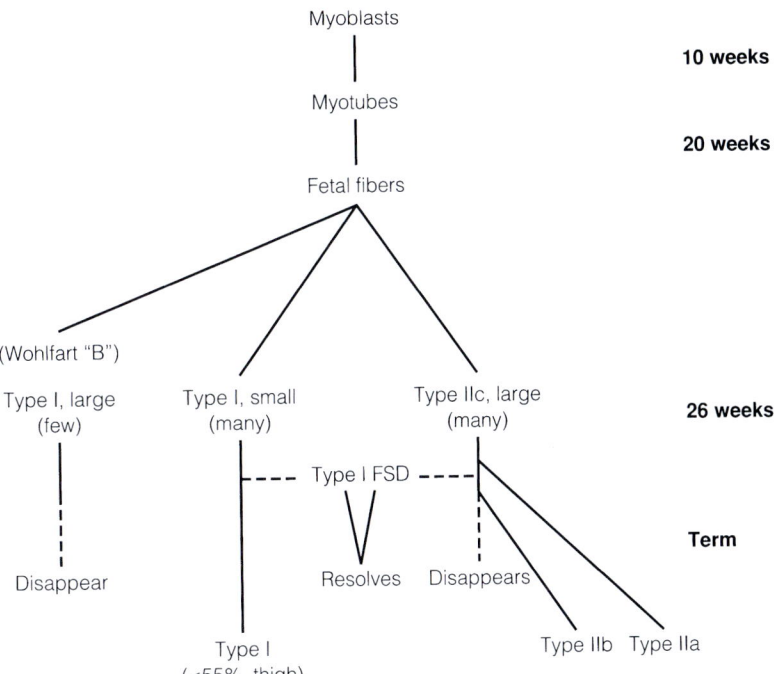

FIGURE 27-1 • Steps involved in prenatal and perinatal muscle fiber maturation. Fsd, fiber size disproportion.

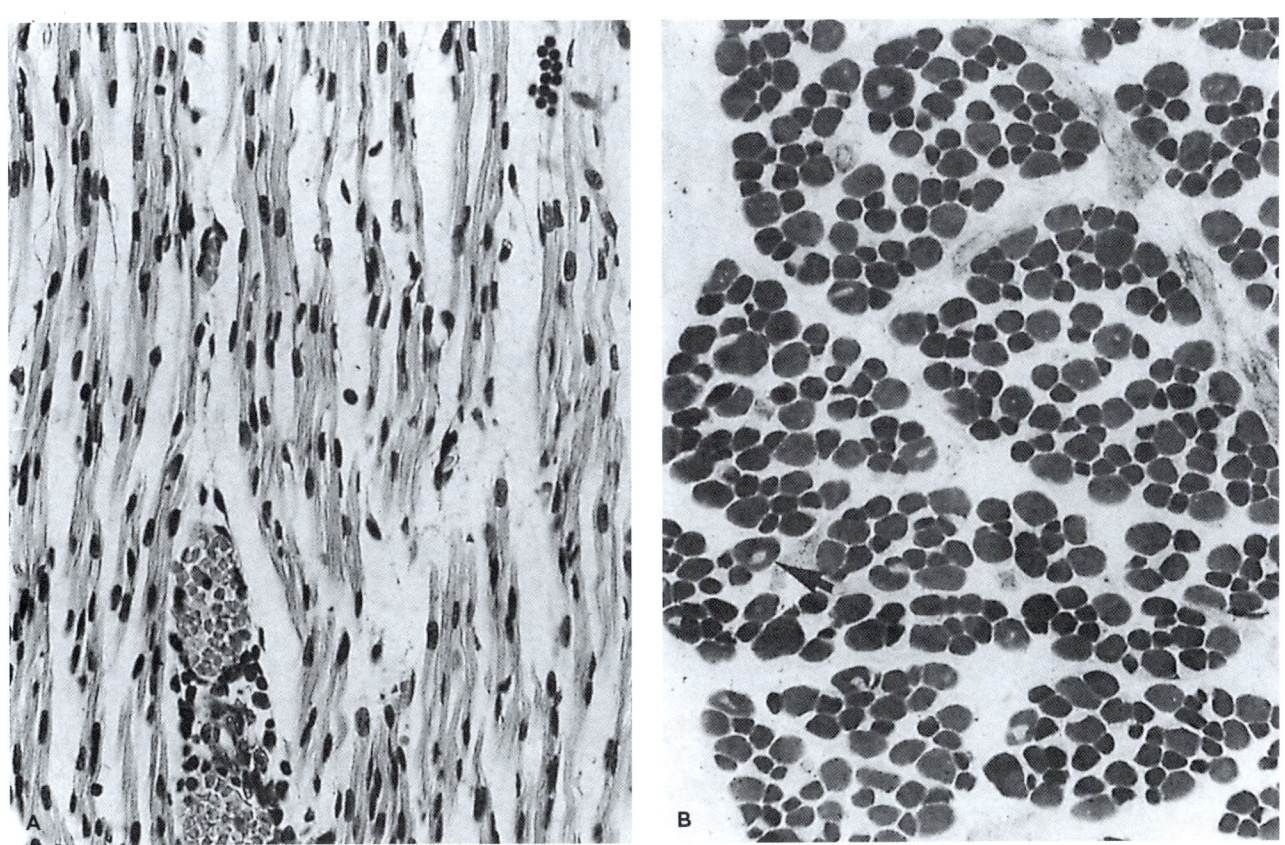

FIGURE 27-2 • **A:** Myotubular configuration of muscle fibers in a 19-week-old fetus. (Hematoxylin and eosin stain; original magnification ×400.) **B:** Normal deltoid muscle in a 29-week-old fetus contains small, dark, type I fibers and larger, intermediate-stained, type IIc fibers, many retaining central nuclei (*arrow*). (Myosin ATPase stain with preincubation at pH 4.3; original magnification ×250.)

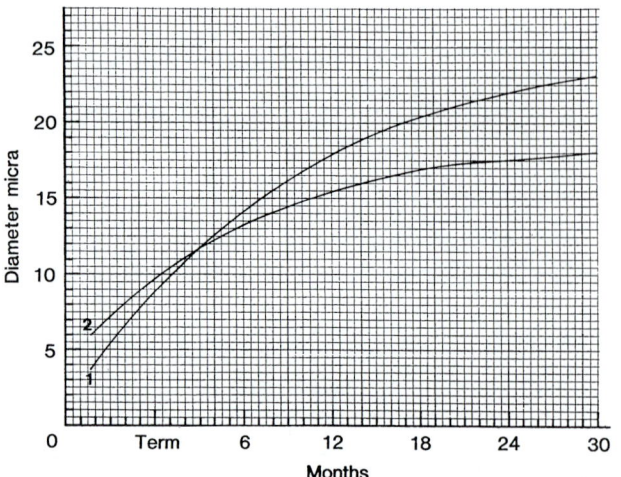

FIGURE 27-3 • Diameter of normal type I (1) and type II (2) fibers at various ages in young children.

the level of the spinal cord (9–11). The alleged normality of the spinal cord in most patients with urinary tract dilatation and deficient abdominal wall musculature (so-called prune belly syndrome) requires reexamination but focuses attention on alternate hypotheses for deficient numbers of fibers (Figure 27-4A), such as a mesodermal field defect, favored by the character of associated anomalies, and linkage to trisomy 18 (12). Compression secondary to abdominal distension may contribute to muscle atrophy by direct pressure, by limiting blood supply, or by interfering with innervation (Figure 27-4B, C).

Congenital diaphragmatic hernia is either an open defect or one covered only by a thin membrane lacking muscle fibers. Typically, located on the left, the phrenic nerve and the cervical spinal cord are normal. This form of hernia is thought to result from a primary defect in mesenchymal precursors involved in closure of the pleuroperitoneal canal. Eventration of the diaphragm is a unilateral or bilateral thin diaphragm that is a consequence of neuromuscular disease, such as birth trauma to the spinal cord or brachial plexus, anterior horn cell disease, phrenic nerve agenesis, myotonic dystrophy, or congenital myopathy (13). Diaphragm muscle usually displays the lesion of the primary disorder (see Chapter 12) (14–16).

ARTHROGRYPOSIS

Congenital joint contractures involving more than one area of the body (Figure 27-5A) usually result from intrauterine disorders that restrict fetal movement, also known as fetal akinesia deformation sequence (17–19). The etiology is heterogeneous and includes oligohydramnios, chromosome abnormalities of various types (20), teratogens, neurogenic and myogenic disorders, and rare restrictive skin and skeletal diseases (see Chapters 25, 26, and 28) (21,22). Most cases are sporadic and of unknown etiology. A tentative pathogenic classification (Table 27-1) of arthrogryposis congenita includes subtypes due to external compression, primary muscle disease, primary or secondary disorders of the central nervous system, such as dysgenesis or disruption of the motor centers of the brain or spinal cord, or deficiencies in

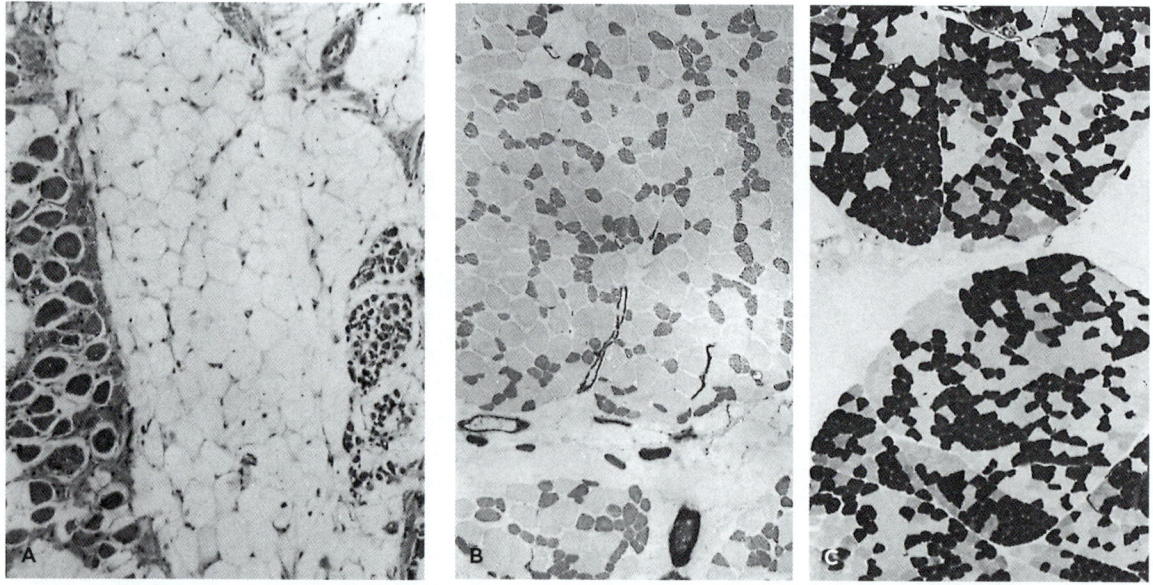

FIGURE 27-4 • **A:** Severely hypoplastic abdominal wall muscle in an infant with prune belly syndrome typically contains few fibers and abundant fat. (Hematoxylin and eosin stain; original magnification ×70.) **B:** Thin rectus abdominis muscle in a 19-year-old patient with prune belly syndrome exhibits type I FSD. (Myosin ATPase stain with preincubation at pH 4.3; original magnification ×80.) **C:** Thin rectus abdominis muscle in a 13-year-old child with prune belly syndrome. Homogeneous-type groups suggest reinnervation. (Myosin ATPase stain with preincubation at pH 4.6; original magnification ×400.)

Table 27-3 outlines the primary neuromuscular diseases presenting in infancy and childhood. Six generic categories are delineated:

1. Disorders of innervation
2. Congenital myopathy (CM)
3. Metabolic myopathy
4. Skeletal and cardiomyopathy
5. Muscular dystrophy
6. Inflammatory myopathy

TABLE 27-3 NEUROMUSCULAR DISEASES
Disorders of innervation
• Spinal cord dysplasia
• Motor neuron disease
• Peripheral neuropathy
• Combined central and peripheral neuropathy
• Nutritional disorders
• Disorders of neuromuscular transmission
Congenital myopathy
• Central nuclear and myotubular myopathy
• Nemaline myopathy
• Central core disease
• Minicore–multicore disease
• Congenital myopathy with small type I fibers
• Congenital myopathy with fingerprint bodies
• Congenital myopathy, other
Metabolic myopathy
• Lysosomal storage diseases
• Glycogen storage diseases
• Triglyceride storage diseases
• Mitochondriopathies
• Metabolic myopathy, other
• Episodic myoglobinuria
• Malignant hyperthermia syndrome
• Drug-induced myopathy
Muscular dystrophy
• Dystrophinopathies, X-linked
• Duchenne muscular dystrophy
• Becker muscular dystrophy
Muscular dystrophies, autosomal recessive
• Adhalin deficiency (dystrophin-associated complex)
• Other limb-girdle types
Muscular dystrophies, dominant
• Facioscapulohumeral type
Congenital muscular dystrophy
• Merosin normal
• Merosin absent
• Fukuyama type
• Walker-Warburg type
Inflammatory myopathy
• Infectious myositis
• Local myositis
• Idiopathic inflammatory myopathy, childhood dermatomyositis
Skeletal myopathy and cardiomyopathy

TABLE 27-4 MAJOR CHILDHOOD DENERVATING DISORDERS
Spinal cord hypoplasia or dysplasia
Spinomuscular atrophy
• Type I (infantile, Werdnig-Hoffmann)
• Type II (late infantile)
• Type III (juvenile, Kugelberg-Welander)
• Infantile spinomuscular atrophy, X-linked
Bulbar muscular atrophy (Fazio-Londe)
Scapuloperoneal spinal muscular atrophy
Hereditary sensory motor neuropathies, all types
Acquired myelopathy or neuropathy
• Traumatic
• Ischemic
• Infectious (enterovirus)
• Postinfectious (Guillian-Barré)
• Toxic/drug-induced
• Nutritional

DISORDERS OF INNERVATION

Denervation is expressed in all of the muscle fibers of an affected motor unit, producing clusters of hypotonic atrophic muscle fibers. Denervated fibers often exhibit angulated contours due to molding by normotonic neighbors. The appearance of denervated muscle has no specificity for the underlying neurologic disorder (Table 27-4) and may depend on the chronologic relation of the biopsy to the onset of the disease (Figure 27-10A, B). Findings are further modified by expression in utero or during early infancy, a time when impairment of muscle maturation may be added to the effect of denervation (Figure 27-10C, D). Reinnervation occurs unpredictably as the distal nerve twigs of an intact motor unit expand to make new junctions with adjacent denervated fibers, resulting in abnormally large groups of fibers of one subtype (Figure 27-9B). Recognition of clusters of reinnervated fibers in muscle that normally contains mostly one type of fiber may require a quantitative approach. Other helpful features of chronic denervation are target and targetoid fibers, and central nuclei (49).

Spinal Cord Diseases

Deficiency of spinal neurons results from developmental deficiency (dysplasia or hypoplasia) or may result from degeneration or loss caused by genetic motor neuron diseases, trauma, ischemia, and viral infections (e.g., enterovirus) with affinity for spinal motor neurons. Microscopic dysplasia or malformation of the spinal cord is typically sporadic and may be generalized or limited to the distal cord, causing segmental deficiency of lower motor units, muscle hypoplasia, and contractures (27).

Spinal cord trauma occurs during difficult deliveries or as a result of accidents, and it does not selectively damage the anterior horn regions. Diaphragmatic paralysis in newborns

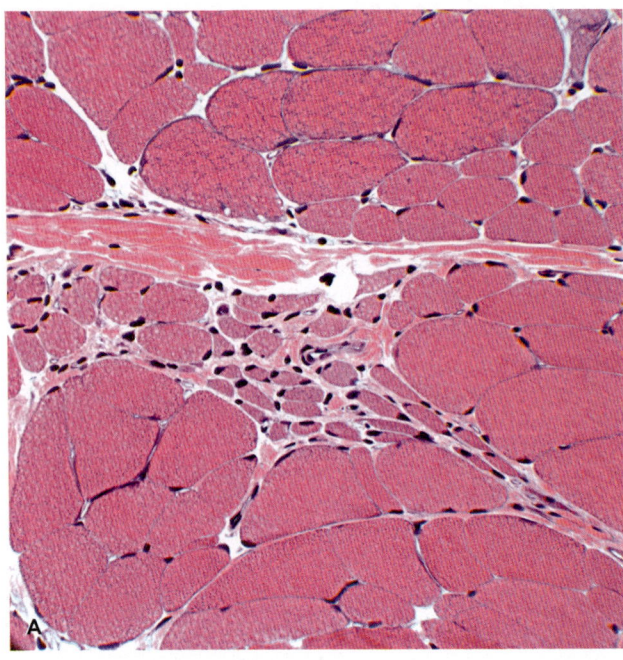
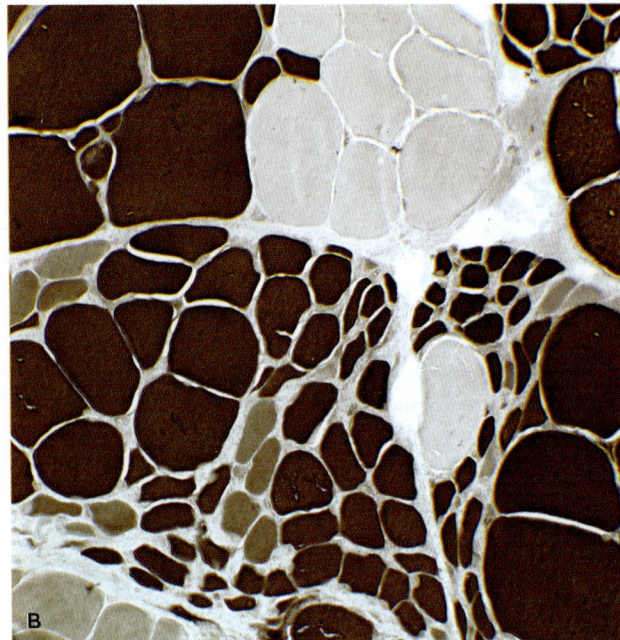
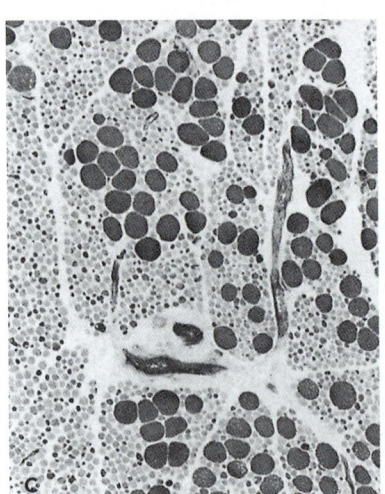
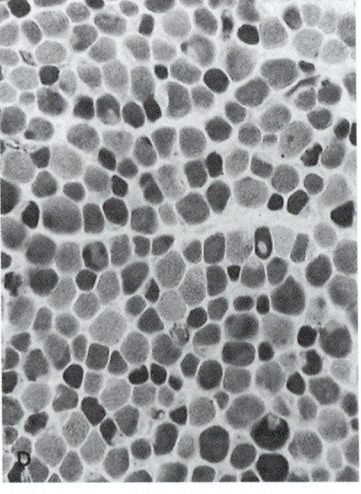

FIGURE 27-10 • **A:** Active denervation involves fibers of each subtype that causes atrophy, often with angulated profiles. (Hematoxylin and eosin stain; original magnification ×400.) **B:** Reinnervation produces clusters of fibers of similar type in chronic peripheral neuropathy. (Myosin ATPase stain with preincubation at pH 4.6; original magnification ×400.) **C:** Infantile spinomuscular atrophy (ISMA). Subtotal or panfascicular fiber atrophy with clusters of hypertrophied type I fibers. (Myosin ATPase stain with preincubation at pH 4.6; original magnification ×64.) **D:** Atrophic fibers in ISMA exhibit features of delayed maturation. (Myosin ATPase stain with preincubation at pH 4.3; original magnification ×640.)

is more often the result of unilateral brachial plexus injury than of spinal cord injury. Cervical spine instability or a narrow cervical canal, as in skeletal dysplasia or other developmental disorders involving the spine, predisposes to hyperextension injury of the spinal cord. Acute selective upper spinal motor neuron necrosis occasionally accompanies widespread perinatal ischemic injury to brain stem nuclei (50). Spinal cord injury from compromise of the spinal arterial circulation is a recognized complication of surgical procedures near the aorta.

MOTOR NEURON DISEASE

Hereditary motor neuron diseases of children are characterized by progressive degeneration of the motor neurons of the spinal cord. Typically, sensory and upper motor neurons are not involved. Classification is based on factors such as age at presentation, rate of progression, milestones achieved, and distribution of neuronal lesions (51). The following clinical classification enjoys wide usage:

Type 1: never able to sit, onset before 6 months (Werdnig-Hoffman disease)
Type 2: able to sit but not to walk, onset 6 to 18 months (Dubowitz disease)
Type 3: able to walk, onset in childhood beyond 18 months (Kugelberg-Welander disease)
Type 4: adult onset

Infantile SMA is characterized by rapid progression and may be recognized at birth, or the onset may be delayed. Weakness is generalized but mainly proximal; respiratory muscles are spared; diaphragmatic involvement is rarely observed at onset. Onset in utero (proposed Type 0) with fetal akinesia syndrome or arthrogryposis is very rare.

Infantile SMA has an incidence of 1/10000 and long has been considered an autosomal recessive trait. Linkage studies have now mapped the gene to a 5q deletion in greater than 95% of cases of type 1 SMA, including many families with a pattern of later onset (52,53). Important deletions have been identified in the survival motor neuron gene (SMN). Deletions in SMN are found in more than 90% of children with types 1 and 2 SMA and about 80% with type 3 SMA but are absent in patients with type 4 SMA. SMN1-negative variants of infantile SMA include a diaphragmatic form with early respiratory failure and distal muscle atrophy (SMARD1) due to mutation of a gene on 11p13 (54) and an X-linked arthrogrypotic form that also lacks the 5q/SMN deletion (55).

Genetic testing is a diagnostic tool in SMA, eclipsing the role of muscle biopsy, except when clinical findings are unusual or loss of function SMN1 mutations are negative. A cautionary note: the SMN gene deletion may be deleted in normal siblings. SMN deletion negative cases, though a small minority, when studied with next-generation sequencing technologies, have shown remarkable clinical and genetic diversity (53).

Muscle biopsy discloses groups or entire fascicles composed of small rounded fibers displaying poor delineation of fiber subtypes, small immature type I fibers, variable persistence of type IIc fibers, and small clusters of hypertrophied type I fibers (see Figure 27-10C, D). Features of infantile SMA in muscle may be confused with the incomplete muscle maturation that prevails in late gestation. SMA presenting in older children exhibits features similar to denervation in adults, including clusters of angulated atrophic fibers and groups of hypertrophied reinnervated type I and type II fibers. In older children, proximal muscle involvement in SMA may simulate muscular dystrophy. In addition to denervation atrophy, focal myopathic changes may be observed, as is true in other chronic denervating diseases. Single-fiber electromyography may help resolve the issue of pathogenesis in patients with mixed neuromyopathic biopsy findings by identifying enlarged motor units, a consequence of reinnervation.

PERIPHERAL NEUROPATHY

The diagnosis of the peripheral neuropathies in children is facilitated by electrophysiologic studies that distinguish myelinopathies from axonopathies, by evaluation of individual teased axons, by light and electron microscopy of sural nerve specimens, and by genetic testing for more than 70 genes that have been linked to Charcot-Marie-Tooth disease with weak phenotype–genotype correlation (56,57).

Hereditary sensory motor neuropathies (HSMN) are far more common in children than acquired chronic neuropathies. Classic phenotypes include the usually autosomal dominant hypertrophic peroneal neuropathies of Charcot-Marie-Tooth (types I and II hereditary sensory motor neuropathy), the autosomal recessive hypertrophic hypomyelinating infantile neuropathy of Dejerine-Sottas (type III hereditary sensory motor neuropathy), and Refsum disease (type IV hereditary sensory motor neuropathy).

Schwann cell proliferation that results in "onion bulb" formation (Figure 27-11A, B) is most prominent in type III,

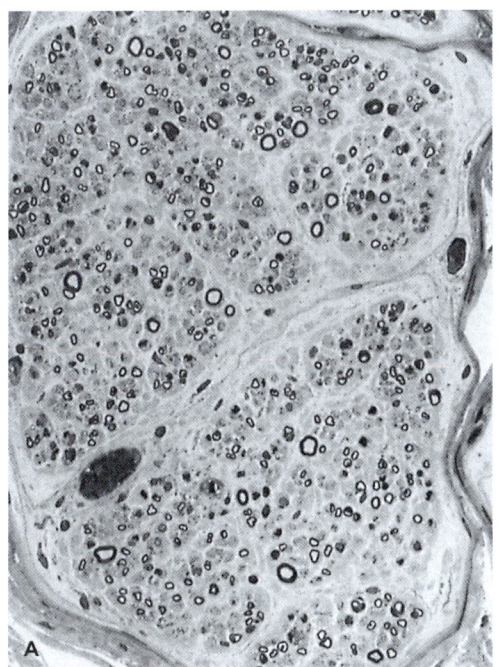 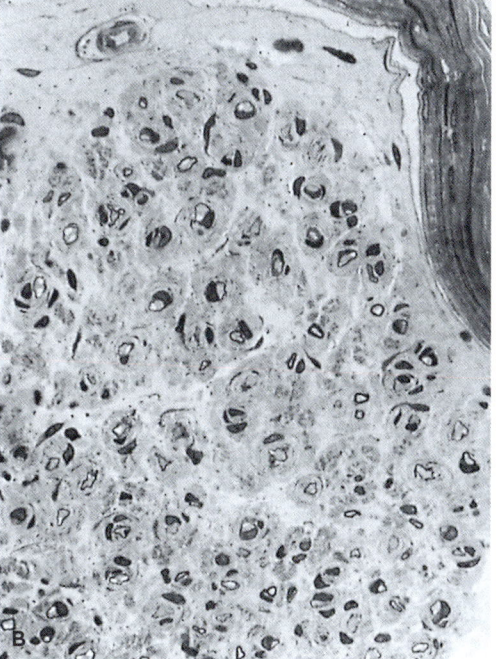

FIGURE 27-11 • **A:** Sural nerve in idiopathic childhood neuropathy, possibly type I hereditary sensory motor neuropathy (HSMN), with scattered "onion bulbs" and variable myelin thickness. (Methylene blue and azure II stain; original magnification ×400.) **B:** Sural nerve in type III HSMN with prominent "onion bulbs" and uniform severe defect in myelin thickness. (Methylene blue and azure II stain; original magnification ×640.)

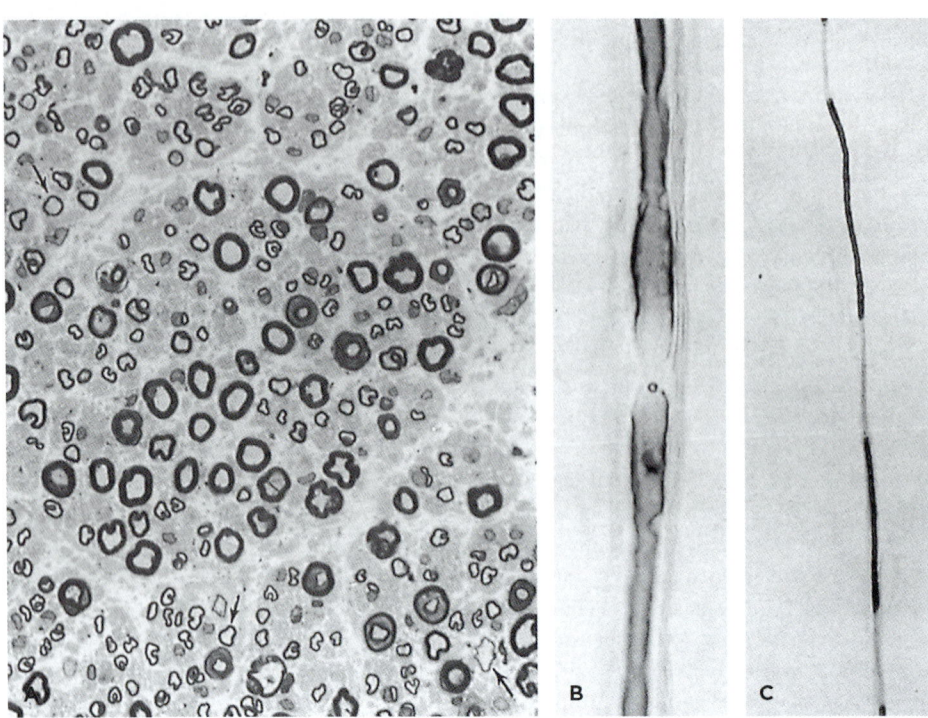

FIGURE 27-12 • **A:** Sural nerve in prolonged Guillain-Barré syndrome. Thin myelin sheaths are inconspicuous. There is no inflammation. (Methylene blue and azure II stain; original magnification ×640.) **B:** Teased isolated myelinated fiber. Demyelination begins at nodes of Ranvier. **C:** Teased isolated myelinated fibers with segmental demyelination, typical of postinfectious polyneuropathy.

but it is not a specific feature for genetic disorders. Delayed nerve conduction velocity related to myelination disorder is a feature of all except type II. Denervation of muscle may occur with axonopathy. Genetic analyses have disclosed extreme heterogeneity with defects in different steps in myelin formation producing overlapping phenotypes. Neuropathy in infants with extreme hypomyelination and Schwann cell proliferation associates with multiple gene defects. Congenital absence of peripheral myelin is described in a lethal form of arthrogryposis congenita (58) and has also been observed in some infants with congenital muscular dystrophy (59).

Acquired demyelinating diseases of peripheral nerves include acute postinfectious polyneuritis (Guillain-Barré syndrome) and chronic idiopathic inflammatory polyneuropathy (60,61). Both cause hypotonia, weakness, hyporeflexia, and slow nerve conduction, more commonly in older children or adults and rarely in infancy. In both conditions, segmental demyelination and remyelination are accompanied by Schwann cell proliferation and mononuclear infiltrates of variable severity (Figure 27-12). Inflammation is often scanty, making distinction from genetic forms of peripheral neuropathy difficult. Perivascular infiltrates of macrophages may be helpful (62). In chronic cases, muscle wasting probably is due more to disuse than to denervation, which typically is lacking. Peripheral neuropathy caused by drugs, heavy metal intoxication (e.g., lead), or bacterial toxins (e.g., diphtheria) may be due to axonal degeneration alone or combination with demyelination.

COMBINED CENTRAL AND PERIPHERAL NEUROPATHY

Complex multisystem metabolic diseases and genetically determined diseases of central neurons or central white matter usually do not involve peripheral nerves, but exceptions are noteworthy. Rare patients with mitochondrial myopathy and peripheral neuropathy have complex crystalline inclusions in Schwann cell cytoplasm (Figure 27-13) (63). Lower motor

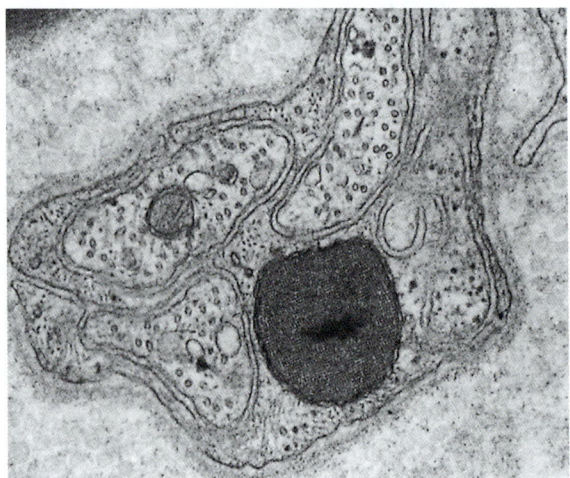

FIGURE 27-13 • A Schwann cell, enclosing several unmyelinated nerves, contains crystalline inclusion with double mitochondroid outer membrane. Patient had abnormal mitochondria in heart, skeletal muscle, and peripheral nerves. (Uranyl acetate and lead citrate stain; original magnification ×20,000.)

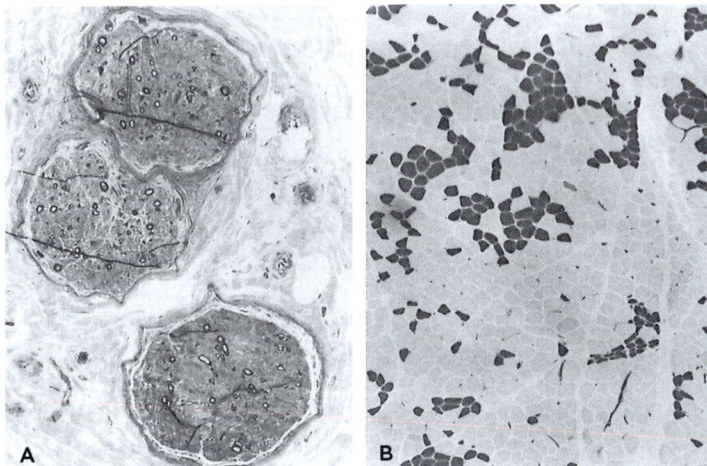

FIGURE 27-14 • **A:** Marked reduction of fascicular area and number of myelinated axons in the sural nerve from an older child with Friedreich ataxia. (Original magnification ×200.) **B:** Denervation atrophy with type groups indicating reinnervation in Friedreich ataxia. (Myosin ATPase stain with preincubation at pH 4.3; original magnification ×64.)

neuron involvement in olivospinocerebellar atrophy, Friedreich ataxia, and ataxia–telangiectasia leads to axonal loss and muscle denervation and reinnervation (Figure 27-14), which usually is overshadowed clinically by the peripheral and central sensory deficits. Neuroaxonal dystrophy involves central and peripheral axons in which focal expansile lesions accumulate complex tubulomembranous inclusions. Among the leukodystrophies, the metachromatic subtypes are most likely to involve peripheral nerves and may cause muscle denervation; peripheral neuropathy also occurs in Krabbe disease (see Chapters 5 and 10).

NUTRITIONAL DISORDERS

Neuropathies due to malnutrition are rare in industrialized societies. However, deficient absorption of fat-soluble vitamins may produce neuropathy in infants with chronic cholestasis, in cystic fibrosis, or in abetalipoproteinemia. Areflexia or progressive ataxia due to central dysfunction due to vitamin E deficiency complicates unrelenting cholestasis in early infancy (64). In these children, muscle fiber-type groups develop, residual bodies accumulate in muscle fibers (Figure 27-15) and in

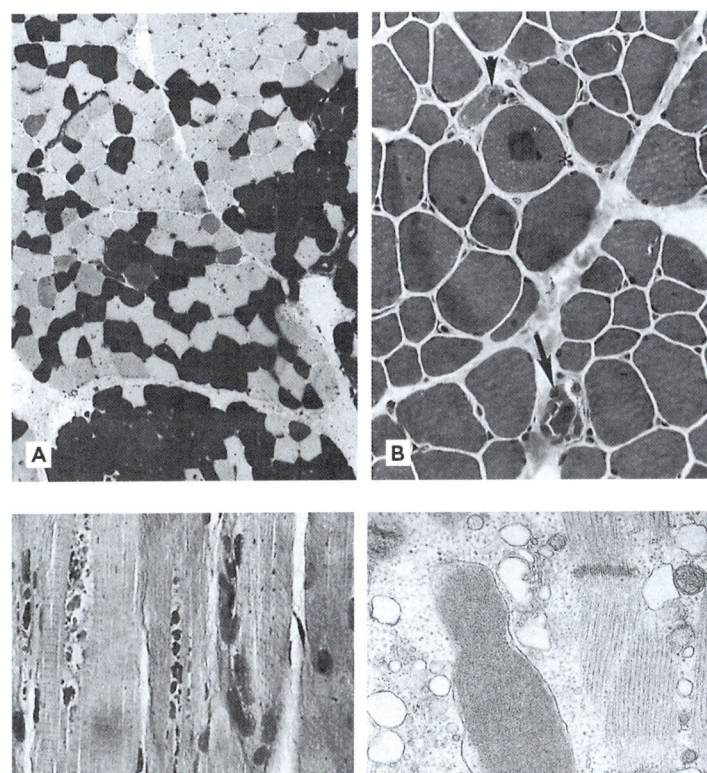

FIGURE 27-15 • **A:** Reinnervation (type groups) in a child with chronic cholestasis from infancy causing central and peripheral neuropathy due to low levels of vitamin E. (Myosin ATPase stain with preincubation at pH 4.6; original magnification ×160.) **B:** Mixed neuromyopathic change in a child with prolonged vitamin E deficiency. Fiber necrosis (*arrow*), degeneration (*arrowhead*), and target fibers (*asterisk*) are shown. (Trichrome stain; original magnification ×500.) **C:** Massive deposition of residual bodies in a child with chronic cholestasis and low vitamin E levels. (Methylene blue and azure II stain; original magnification ×1,000.) **D:** Dense monomorphous residual body, typical of infantile vitamin E deficiency myopathy. (Uranyl acetate and lead citrate stain; original magnification ×10,500.)

Schwann cells, and serum creatine kinase may be elevated. This mixed neuromyopathy can be arrested with parenteral vitamin E therapy (65).

DISORDERS OF NEUROMUSCULAR TRANSMISSION

The neuromuscular junction is the target of many toxic, infectious, or autoimmune insults and the locus of several rare genetically transmitted defects. The specific site of impairment may be presynaptic or postsynaptic. The differential diagnosis of these conditions requires evaluation of response to acetylcholine esterase inhibition, detailed electromyography, measurement of circulating antibodies to acetylcholine receptors, and in selected cases, morphologic studies of motor end plates, which are best sampled in external intercostal muscle specimens. Muscle may be normal or show selective type II fiber atrophy or overt signs of denervation.

Neonatal myasthenia gravis is a transient condition expressed within the first few days after birth and continuing for several weeks thereafter in babies born to mothers with myasthenia gravis. Affected infants are otherwise normal, although the rare coexistence of congenital contractures suggests the possibility of in utero injury. The mediator of the disease is thought to be transplacental maternal IgG antibody to acetylcholine receptors on the postsynaptic muscle membrane. High maternal levels of pathologic antibody increase the risk. Myasthenia gravis, similar to that in adults, also occurs in older children. Antibody to acetylcholine receptor is usually demonstrable, and acetylcholine esterase inhibitors relieve symptoms. Congenital myasthenia syndromes are rare heterogeneous genetic disorders of neuromuscular transmission that cause hypotonia, weakness, ptosis, respiratory problems, and motor delay (66). Diagnosis is challenging and often delayed. Muscle biopsy is usually not helpful.

Acquired disorders of neuromuscular transmission in children are caused by neurotoxins associated with diphtheria or the infantile form of botulism, drugs such as magnesium sulfate or aminoglycoside antibiotics, and neoplasms or autoimmune disorders that cause motor conduction changes typical of the Eaton-Lambert syndrome. Infantile botulism is of particular interest because it results from endogenous production of a neurotoxin by gastrointestinal flora rather than ingestion of preformed toxin. Early signs may be constipation and various degrees of failure to thrive. In protracted cases, dysphagia, loss of head control, and progressive flaccid paralysis develop. A few infants with sudden unexplained death have had clostridial endotoxin detected in the gut. The basis for transient susceptibility of infants to endogenous toxin production is unknown. Morphologic studies of terminal motor nerves in affected infants have not been reported.

Serious neuromuscular sequelae to intensive care may be due to excessive use of curare-like drugs, to concomitant exposure to aminoglycoside antibiotics or to corticosteroid drugs, or to severe underlying illness, such as sepsis. In all age groups, a few patients supported by prolonged exposure to curare-like drugs during mechanical ventilation develop persistent weakness or after withdrawal (67). The consequences may be profound, especially in infants (68,69). Autopsy evaluation of psoas muscle fiber diameter in infants who had been paralyzed for extended periods indicated smaller average muscle fiber diameter than expected, suggesting the possibility of muscle fiber growth retardation (68). Muscle biopsy may help exclude antecedent neuromuscular disease and identify the basis for prolonged weakness. Clinically overlapping disorders include critical illness polyneuropathy and critical illness myopathy.

CONGENITAL MYOPATHY

The congenital myopathies (CMs) are static or slowly progressive disorders of muscle of genetic origin that exhibit substantial clinical overlap. Definitions based on distinctive morphology may be supplemented by knowledge of mutations in proteins such as alpha-actin, alpha-actinin, nebulin, beta-tropomyosin, or myotubularin (70,71). Clinical severity correlates imperfectly with morphologic features and specific gene defects. Weakness, first detected at any age, is associated with normal serum levels of creatine kinase, absence of electrophysiologic or morphologic evidence for denervation, and no other definable primary muscle diseases, such as a dystrophy or myositis. Subtypes with most distinctive morphologic features are myotubular–centronuclear myopathy, nemaline myopathy, central core disease, minicore–multicore disease, type I FSD myopathy, and myofibrillar myopathy.

Severity of CM is highly variable from patient to patient and within affected families. Infants with CM may have prenatal hypokinesia, deceptively low Apgar scores, and may be weaned from mechanical ventilatory support with great difficulty. Muscles with cranial nerve innervation are sometimes involved, resulting in ptosis, ophthalmoplegia, facial weakness, and dysphagia. Muscle contractures may be congenital or may develop during infancy, but they are usually not severe. In less-affected infants, modest motor progress may occur, but ambulation and acquisition of motor skills are delayed. Older children with CM usually are thin, have reduced muscle bulk and strength, and tend to avoid strenuous activity, but are able to perform ordinary tasks. Recurrent pneumonia or progressive scoliosis is frequent. Regardless of age at presentation, cerebral function is usually intact. Family studies have often identified minimally impaired or asymptomatic relatives with similar morphologic abnormalities in a muscle biopsy.

Although myotonic dystrophy is not in the strict sense a CM, central nervous system injury is unusually prevalent in affected infants (Figure 27-16) and may overshadow the natural history of the primary myopathy, the principal early manifestations of which are delayed muscle maturation

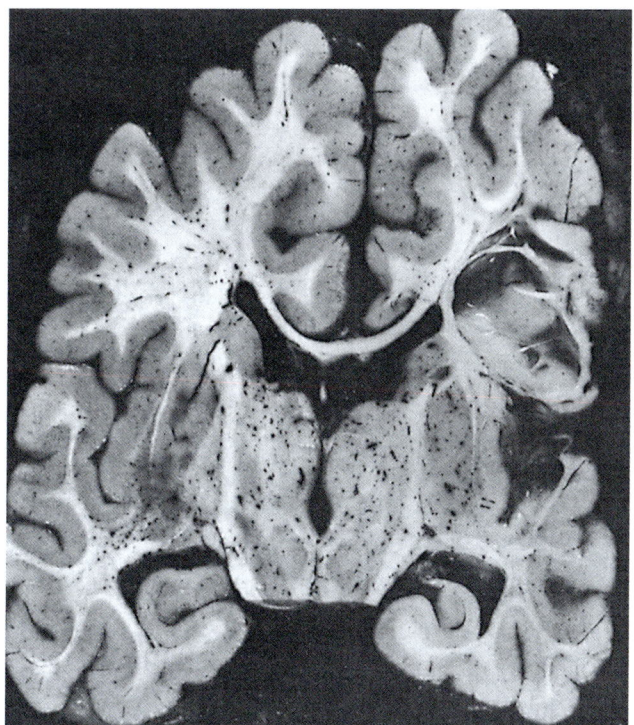

FIGURE 27-16 • Acquired porencephaly in a 2-year-old child who had symptomatic myotonic dystrophy with documented muscle maturation delay as an infant.

and weakness (see Figure 27-8). Maternal weakness or fetal hypotonia may prolong labor. Myotonia in the mother is a helpful diagnostic sign.

Identification and classification of the patient with CM is often challenging. Serum levels of creatine kinase, though typically normal, may be mildly elevated. Autopsy studies suggest that variation among muscles is common. Muscle biopsy, including electron microscopy, is essential. In samples lacking specific structural markers, the various subtypes of CM exhibit common features. Fatty replacement of muscle in CM may occur with age. Muscle fibrosis is exceptional in CM but may be observed in central core disease and in severe infantile nemaline myopathy

CENTRONUCLEAR MYOPATHIES

Migration of reactive sarcolemmal nuclei away from the sarcolemma occurs in muscle regeneration and is a nonspecific alteration in chronic neuromuscular diseases of all types. Location of the nucleus in the exact center of most muscle fibers is the hallmark of centronuclear congenital myopathy (Figure 27-17). Sex-linked recessive, and autosomal dominant or recessive inheritance patterns of centronuclear myopathy are well documented (72–75). The autosomal recessive form is the most common. Severely affected infants are reported mainly in kindreds exhibiting an X-linked recessive inheritance pattern. Untypeable myotubes resembling the fetal myotube stage of development are prevalent in affected infants, but in contrast to the normal myotube, the perinuclear clear zone may extend for only a short distance on either side of the central nucleus. The clear zone contains glycogen, sarcoplasmic reticulum, mitochondria, and associated enzymes but lacks myofibrils. Overexpression of vimentin and desmin occurs only in the X-linked form (3). Mutations in the MTM1 gene that codes for myotubularin cause the X-linked disease (76). The dominant form is linked to the DNM2 gene, and the recessive form is linked to the BIN1 gene. Persistent myotubes uncommonly may be found in

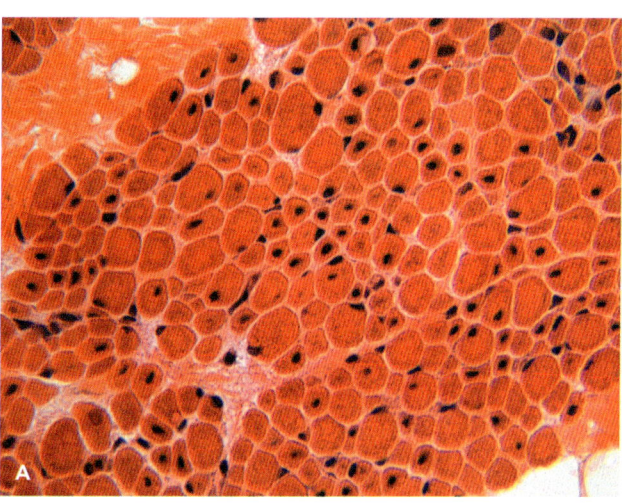
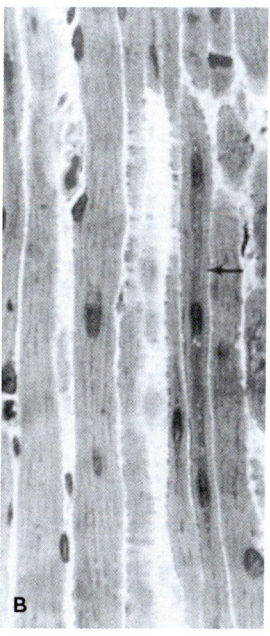

FIGURE 27-17 • **A:** Central nuclear and myotubular myopathy. Central nuclei are prominent and interstitium contains excess collagen. (Hematoxylin and eosin stain; original magnification ×300.) **B:** Central nuclear and myotubular myopathy. Myotubular configuration (*arrow*) is demonstrable in a variable percentage of fibers. (Methylene blue and azure II stain; original magnification ×800.)

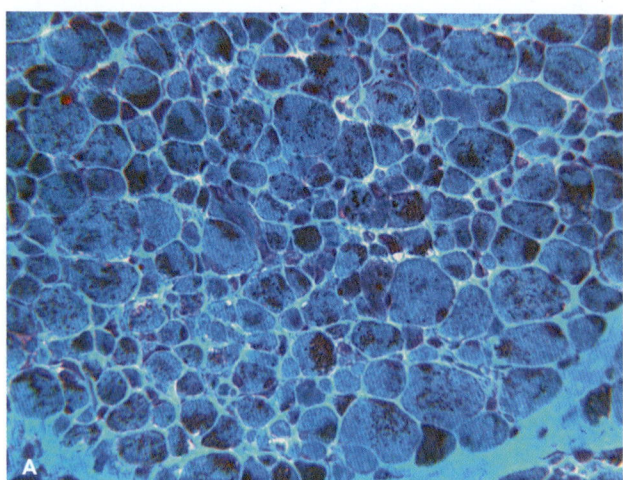
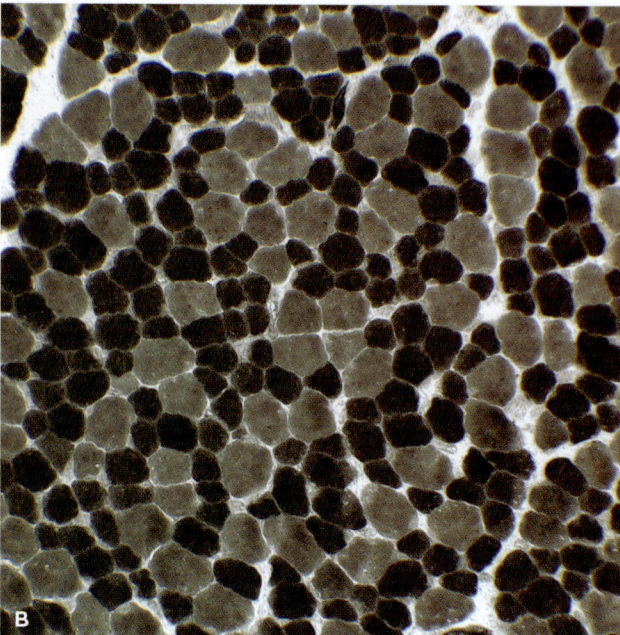

FIGURE 27-18 • **A:** Nemaline myopathy, infantile form. Dark-stained, rodlike granules tend to be most prevalent in smaller muscle fibers in symptomatic infants. (Trichrome stain; original magnification ×300.) **B:** Nemaline myopathy, infantile form. Type I fibers are smaller than type II fibers. Smallest fibers are untypeable. (Myosin ATPase stain with preincubation at pH 4.3; original magnification ×400.)

very young infants with other neuromuscular diseases such as myotonic dystrophy and type 1 spinal muscular atrophy.

Nemaline Myopathy

Nemaline (rod) myopathy (NM) is a distinctive and relatively common form of CM (77). Family data suggest two patterns of genetic expression: dominant with variable penetrance and autosomal recessive (78). Clinical subgroups include a rapidly fatal infantile form, a static or slowly progressive form with mild-to-moderate impairment, and a subclinical form in relatives. In most cases, the rods are readily observed in a cryostat section using a modification of the trichrome stain (Figure 27-18); rods are undetectable in sections stained with hematoxylin and eosin. Associated changes include type I fiber predominance and, in some instances, indistinct myosin ATPase fiber-typing reactions. Infants with nemaline myopathy usually have type I FSD.

Ultrastructural study of rods demonstrates discrete, electron-dense bodies with characteristic crystalline substructures (Figure 27-19). In some infants with severe CM, rods are difficult to detect by light microscopy, but rodlike Z-band changes are prevalent in electron micrographs. Rods contain multiple proteins including a-actinin (a Z-band protein) and actin and are contiguous with Z-bands, aggregated beneath the sarcolemma or in some patients, located within the nucleus (79). Molecular studies indicate that mutations in nebulin and skeletal muscle alpha-actin cause the majority of cases of autosomal recessive NM (80). Mutations in several other NM-associated genes such as tropomyosin and troponin are uncommon. Nebulin mutations associate only with autosomal recessive NM; in other respects, genotype–phenotype correlation is poor and not useful for prognosis.

Central Core Disease

Central core disease, the first defined form of CM, is usually detected in infancy or early childhood and may be mildly progressive (81). Dominant inheritance has been demonstrated, but many cases are sporadic. Severe involvement of

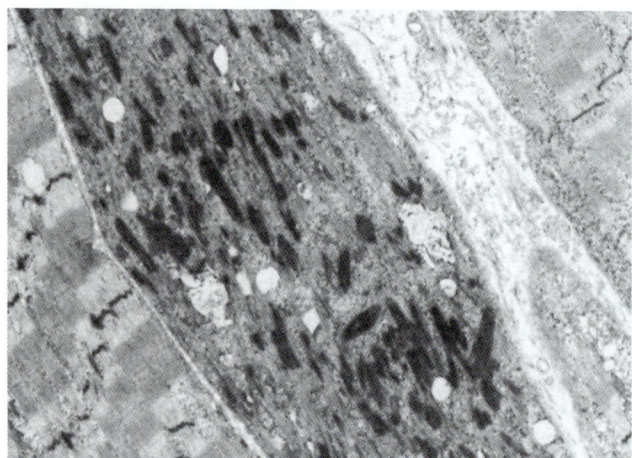

FIGURE 27-19 • Nemaline bodies are dense crystalline structures originating in the Z band. (Uranyl acetate and lead citrate stain; original magnification ×10,000.)

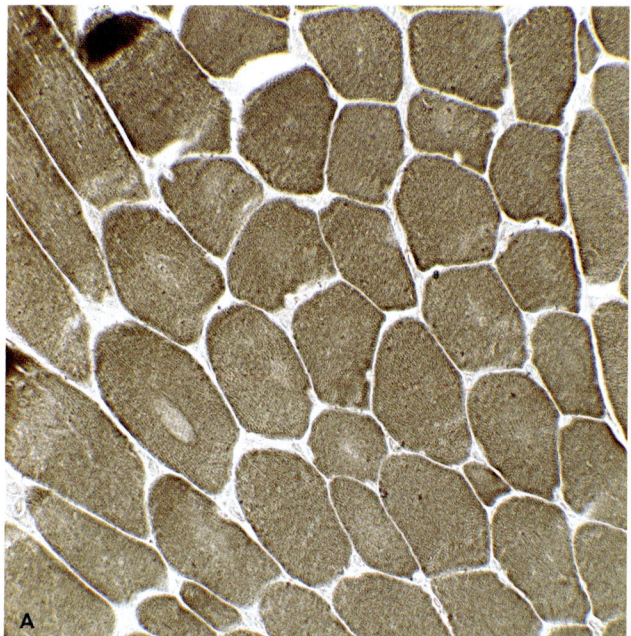
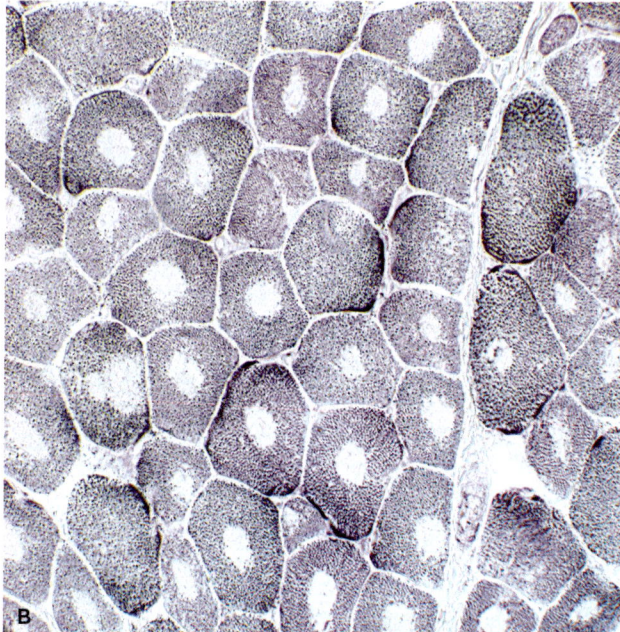

FIGURE 27-20 • **A:** Central core disease in the quadriceps muscle. A few unstructured cores show deficient myosin ATPase activity. (Myosin ATPase stain with preincubation at pH 4.6; original magnification ×400.) **B:** Central core disease with mitochondrial depletion corresponds to location of both unstructured and structured cores. (SDH reaction; original magnification ×400.)

the diaphragm is typical at autopsy. Cores have also been observed in the diaphragm in some patients with nemaline myopathy. Cores are well-demarcated (Figure 27-20), more or less centrally located, long contiguous zones usually found within the interior of type I muscle fibers. In cores, oxidative enzyme activity, mitochondria, lipid, glycogen, and phosphorylase activity are deficient. Myofibrils in the core area are intact (structured core) or are in disarray (unstructured core). Unstructured cores resemble target fibers, an acquired lesion commonly seen in disorders of chronic innervation, particularly in type I fibers. Variation in the prominence of cores within a single sample and poor differentiation of myofiber subtypes is common. Morphologically, atypical cases with incompletely developed cores, or with both cores and nemaline bodies, have been reported (82). Liability to malignant hyperthermia (MH) reaction associates with both central core disease and multiminicore disease; most patients with these forms of CM have mutations in the *RYR1* gene that codes for a calcium channel regulatory protein (83,84) located in the sarcoplasmic reticulum.

Multiminicore Disease

Minicore–multicore disease causes hypotonia that may be marked but most affected children ambulate. Axial weakness, scoliosis, and eventual respiratory insufficiency are the most common phenotype in older children (85). Minute foci of myofibrillar disorganization with local organelle depletion (Figure 27-21) resemble unstructured

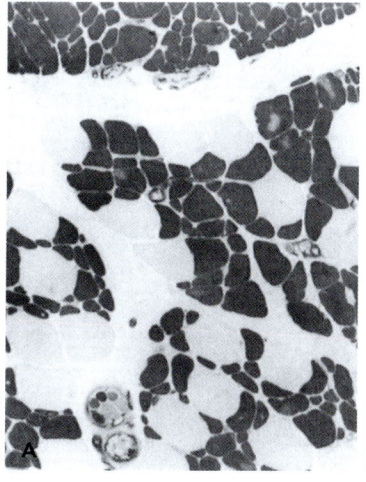
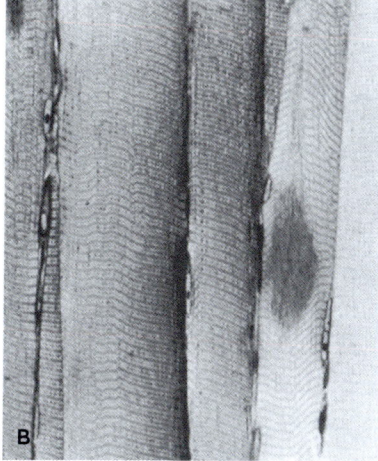

FIGURE 27-21 • **A:** Minicore–multicore disease. Limited cores in type I fibers display focally deficient myosin ATPase reaction. (Myosin ATPase stain with preincubation at pH 4.3; original magnification ×200.) **B:** Limited cores are focal zones of myofibrillar degeneration with loss of sarcomeres and deficient organelles. (Methylene blue and azure II stain; original magnification ×640.)

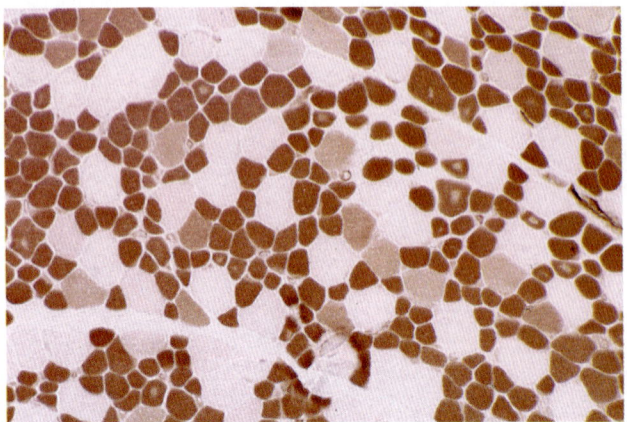

FIGURE 27-22 • Congenital myopathy with type I FSD. (Myosin ATPase stain with preincubation at pH 4.6; original magnification ×400.)

cores, except for their small dimensions. Distribution is less related than typical cores to the central region of muscle fibers. These lesions are demonstrable on frozen sections as random minute foci of reduced myosin ATPase and oxidative enzyme activity and in longitudinally oriented muscle fibers as foci of lost striations, a feature that is easily confirmed in plastic embedded tissue, and by electron microscopy.

Congenital Myopathy with Small Type I Fibers

Type I FSD (fiber size disproportion) is a common phenomenon in muscle specimens obtained during early infancy from hypotonic babies (86). Frequently associated with early-onset disorders of the nervous system and a component of many subtypes of CM, the clinical heterogeneity of patients with FSD has delayed acceptance of a CM characterized only by small size of type I fibers. In the absence of a structural marker, morphologic criteria less reliably distinguish primary myopathy with FSD from the more common secondary form. Nonetheless, CM with FSD typically has uniformly distributed excessive numbers of type I fibers, defined as greater than 60% of the fibers in a thigh muscle sample. This feature alone is unreliable because typically nonuniform numerical predominance may result from an acquired expansion of type I motor units caused by neuropathic injury. Despite these problems, after the age of 6 months, severe persistent FSD with uniformly small type 1 fibers, and numerical predominance, coupled with absence of clusters of type I fibers (Figure 27-22), identifies unequivocal cases of primary myopathy (46). Based upon analysis of kindreds with dominant and recessive familial patterns of FSD, CM with FSD appears to be a distinct entity with a relatively homogeneous clinical phenotype that includes normal intelligence, contractures, ophthalmoplegia, facial weakness, and some cases with early respiratory failure (87). Unlike most other forms of CM, clinical and morphologic improvement has been observed in some familial cases. A relationship of pure FSD to nemaline myopathy is suggested by cases of FSD with rods limited to a few fibers and mutations in skeletal muscle actin (88).

Other Congenital Myopathies

New subtypes of CM continue to be established, usually on the basis of clinical features, occasional familial occurrence, and a prevalent unusual structural abnormality in muscle fibers. Myofibrillary myopathy (MFM) is characterized by inclusions composed of protein aggregates that result from breakdown of Z-band–related proteins (89). Multiple genetically altered proteins have been identified in the inclusions of subtypes of MFM, such as myotilin, desmin, and alpha-B crystallin (90–92). Information about MFM in infants and children remains meager. Other examples of rare CM include reducing body myopathy (93), caused by mutation in the FLH1 gene, and cylindrical spiral myopathy, mutation unknown.

Less certain are putative myopathies characterized by fingerprint bodies, zebra bodies, tubular aggregates, trilaminar fibers, and cytoplasmic bodies. Cytoplasmic bodies are discrete eosinophilic dense masses of fine filaments found in a variety of acquired myopathic and denervating disorders of muscle, including infantile SMA (94) (Figure 27-23), but

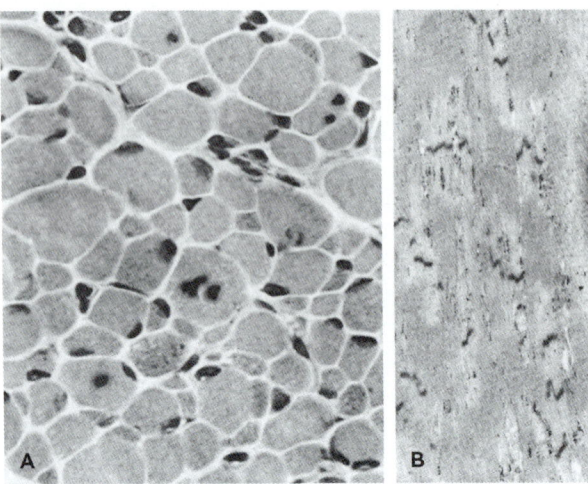

FIGURE 27-23 • **A:** Cytoplasmic bodies, dense purple-staining inclusions with a discernible halo, occur in infantile spinomuscular atrophy, as shown here, and in a rare congenital myopathy. (Trichrome stain; original magnification ×800.) **B:** Ultrastructure of cytoplasmic body shows granular center surrounded by disorganized filaments. (Uranyl acetate and lead citrate stain; original magnification ×6,000.)

they also seem to be a marker for an extremely rare, dominantly inherited CM (95). Fingerprint bodies have been described in myotonic dystrophy, oculopharyngeal dystrophy, and dermatomyositis. In some cases of clinically typical CM, muscle biopsy may show minimal changes that suggest a CM, but not a specific subtype, possibly because of sampling error. Excessive reliance on particular structural markers may lead to errors or misconceptions. Nemaline bodies may be acquired; target fibers, which resemble both cores and minicores, commonly develop in denervating disorders expression.

METABOLIC MYOPATHY

Lysosomal Storage Diseases

Skeletal muscle involvement is mild in most lysosomal enzyme deficiency diseases, and clinical manifestations are slight or absent. With the exception of type II glycogenosis, which features a vacuolar myopathy of variable severity (Figure 27-24), skeletal muscle biopsy is rarely used to define storage disease. However, if hypotonia or weakness prompts a muscle biopsy before a storage disease has been identified, morphologically specific types of lysosomal storage may be encountered (96). Usually, the storage vesicles are strongly positive for acid phosphatase, indicating the lysosomal nature of the disease. Infantile ceroid lipofuscinosis (Santavuori disease) is accompanied by dense homogeneously granular intramuscular inclusions, which are surprisingly similar to inclusions (see Figure 27-15D) that develop in the vitamin E deficiency–associated neuromyopathy complicating chronic cholestasis of infancy. Muscle fibers in the late infantile form (Jansky-Bielschowsky disease) may contain inclusions with curvilinear profiles.

In the mucopolysaccharidoses, endomysial fibroblasts may show typical acid phosphatase–positive vacuolar inclusions, but muscle fibers are usually normal. Characteristic inclusions of stored material occur in endothelium or smooth muscle cells in fucosidosis and Sandhoff disease. Storage inclusions occur in skeletal muscle fibers and vessel walls in Fabry disease and mannosidosis. Stored material accumulates in vascular endothelium and satellite cells but may not involve the muscle fibers of patients with I-cell disease and GM1 gangliosidosis (Figure 27-25A). In some of these rare conditions, too few patients have been studied to warrant conclusive statements. We have observed extensive intramuscular storage in one child with I-cell disease (Figure 27-25B; see Chapter 5).

Glycogen Storage Diseases

The glycogenoses include 13 metabolic disorders of glycogen metabolism in which tissue glycogen levels are excessive (except for disorders of terminal glycolysis), and availability for glycolysis is reduced (Table 27-5). Type I (liver) and type V (muscle) mainly affect single organs. In type II glycogenosis, lysosomal acid a-glucosidase activity is low or absent in all tissues including circulating leukocytes, and

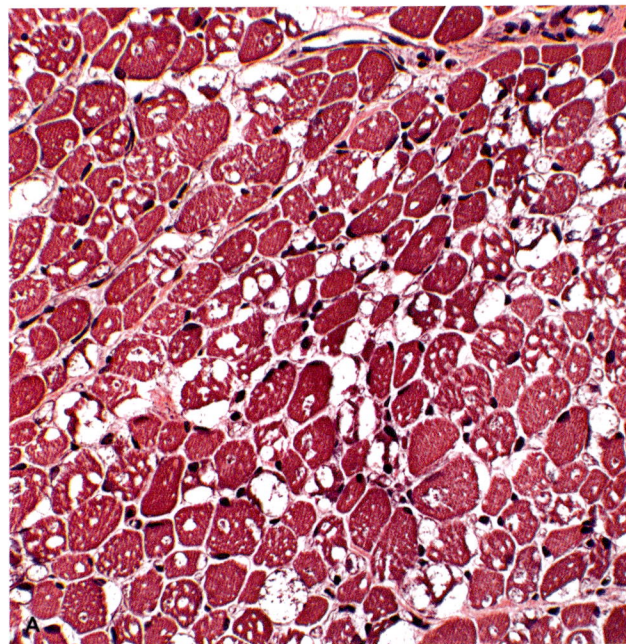
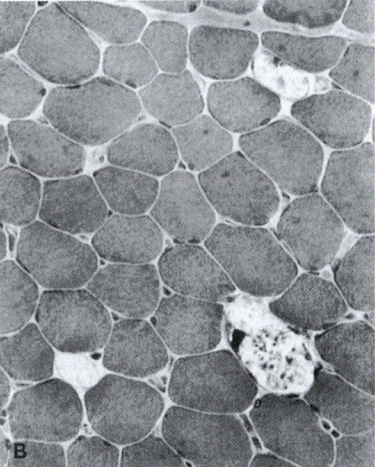

FIGURE 27-24 • **A:** Type IIa lysosomal glycogenosis features severe confluent vacuolar degeneration affecting all muscle fibers. (Hematoxylin and eosin stain; original magnification ×200.) **B:** Type IIb lysosomal glycogenosis features confluent vacuolar degeneration of isolated fibers. Ultrastructural lysosomal changes are more prevalent. (Trichrome stain; original magnifications ×600.)

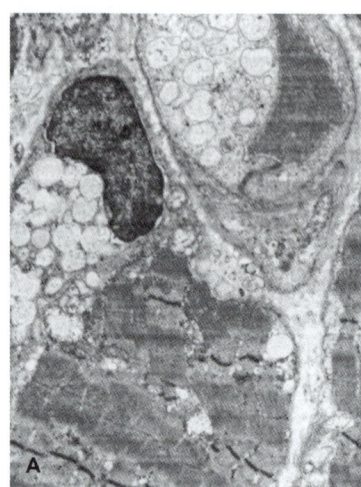 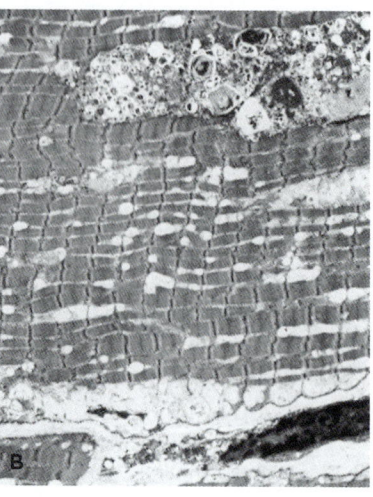

FIGURE 27-25 • **A:** Lysosomal inclusions containing amorphous material are located in endothelium and in muscle satellite cells of a patient with GM1 gangliosidosis. (Uranyl acetate and lead citrate stain; original magnification ×7,000.) **B:** Lysosomal inclusions containing polymorphous debris are present in skeletal muscle of this patient with I-cell disease. (Uranyl acetate and lead citrate stain; original magnification ×3,000.)

diagnosis is possible by electron microscopy of dermal or amnionic fibroblasts (97). Antenatal diagnosis is possible using a biochemical or morphologic approach. Because of multiple mutations, genetic analysis is only useful if an affected sibling has been previously analyzed. Early diagnosis of the infantile subtype is critically important now that both transgenic and recombinant enzyme replacement therapies have been shown to be effective if initiated in early infancy (98,99).

The precise mechanism responsible for hypotonia in type IIa glycogenosis is puzzling because nonlysosomal glycogen is abundant, and the glycolytic pathway is intact. Possible mechanisms include absolute loss, rather than simple displacement of myofibrils, increased work due to the mass of

TABLE 27-5 GLYCOGENOSES AND ASSOCIATED MUSCLE ABNORMALITIES

Type	Enzyme Defect	Tissues Affected	Muscle Morphology
I	Glucose-6-phosphatase	Liver	Normal muscle; secondary increase of lipid in type I fibers (rare)
IIA	Acid a-glucosidase	Generalized	Severe progressive vacuolar degeneration secondary to lysosomal storage of undegraded glycogen; sarcoplasmic glycogen increased
IIB	Acid a-glucosidase	Muscle, liver, heart	Variable (less severe) vacuolar degeneration secondary to lysosomal storage of undegraded glycogen
III	Debrancher enzyme	Liver, heart, muscle	Myopatic; excess intermyofibrillar and subsarcolemmal glycogen; rare vacuolar degeneration
IV	Brancher enzyme	Liver, muscle, heart	Abnormal polysaccharide (amylopectin)
V	Myophosphorylase	Muscle	Normal or myopathic; excess intermyofibrillar and subsarcolemmal glycogen
VI	Liver phosphorylase	Liver	Normal (no myopathy)
VII	Phosphofructokinase	Muscle	Normal or myopathic; similar to type V
VIII	Phosphorylase kinase: multiple subtypes	Liver, muscle, brain	Normal or myopathic; similar to type V
IX	Phosphorylase B kinase x-linked	Liver, muscle	Normal
X	Cyclic AMP-dependent phosphorylase kinase	Liver, muscle	Normal or myopathic
XI	Glut 2, liver transporter	Liver, kidney	Normal (no myopathy)
XII	Aldolase A	Muscle, anemia	?
Other	Phosphoglycerate kinase	Brain, muscle, anemia	Normal or myopathic
Other	Phosphoglycerate mutase	Systemic disease including muscle	Myopathy with tubular aggregates

accumulated glycogen, rupture of overdistended lysosomes with intramuscular proteolysis, and hypoinnervation secondary to glycogen storage in motor neurons.

Type II glycogenosis exists in less severe forms in older children or adults, who typically experience exercise intolerance associated with slowly progressive weakness. The deficiency of lysosomal glucosidase activity approximates that in the infantile form but residual activity may be somewhat greater. Skeletal muscle fibers show morphologic changes of variable severity and extent (see Figure 27-24B). Liver, heart, and leukocytes may contain only a few abnormal glycogen-laden lysosomes, despite low levels of acid a-glucosidase. Glycogen-filled lysosomes develop within a few weeks in cultured muscle or fibroblasts obtained from these patients and may also be seen in the resting fibroblasts. A biochemical test that identifies the infantile, childhood, and adult forms of type II glycogenosis is lacking. However, recent work suggests that subtyping may be based upon immunoassay of both enzyme protein and specific activity and lysosomal glycogen content of cultured fibroblasts (100). Approximately 100 mutations in the acid-a-glucosidase gene are known and have an unpredictable effect upon enzyme activity. Genotype–phenotype correlation is poor and does not explain the phenotype diversity in late-onset disease (101).

The pure myopathic phenotypes of type IV glycogenosis include fetal akinesia deformation sequence, congenital myopathy, and juvenile myopathy. Another phenotype, progressive liver failure due to hepatic fibrosis in infancy or early childhood, often occurs without clinical cardiomyopathy or skeletal muscle disease. A morphologically abnormal form of unbranched glycogen (amylopectin) accumulates in liver and variably in heart and skeletal muscle owing to deficiency of the brancher enzyme, which regulates the formation of normally branched glycogen molecules. This amylopectin stains blue-brown with Lugol iodine in frozen sections and has a characteristic granulofibrillar ultrastructure. Expression of the defect in type IV glycogenosis is extremely heterogeneous (see Chapter 15) (102).

The nonlysosomal glycogenoses that involve muscle feature accumulation of normal glycogen between myofibrils and in the subsarcolemmal region but glycogen accumulation may be absent in disorders of terminal glycolysis. In types III, V, VII, VIII, IX, and X, the periodic acid–Schiff (PAS) method applied to frozen or paraffin sections may demonstrate mild glycogen excess between myofibrils or beneath the sarcolemma, particularly in type 2 fibers (Figure 27-26A). Assessment of glycogen content by ultrastructural means (Figure 27-26B) can be misleading because aggregates may be artifactually produced by hypercontraction or enhanced by tangential sectioning. Direct measurement of glycogen and of glycolytic enzymes in muscle is reliable and should be considered if the history is suggestive of metabolic myopathy, glycogen excess is suspected, and/or focal myopathic features are otherwise unexplained. Histochemical methods are available for detecting the enzyme defect in type V and type VII glycogenosis. In both disorders, low-grade myopathy may be observed (Figure 27-26B). Segmental necrosis correlates with clinical myopathy or myoglobinuria precipitated by recent exercise.

Unusually, early presentation of myophosphorylase deficiency (type V glycogenosis) is reported in one case of fatal infantile hypotonia, and delayed motor development and proximal weakness occurred in an older child, simulating CM. An exceptionally severe presentation of phosphofructokinase deficiency is reported in a young child. Exercise intolerance and equivocal glycogen excess have been described in several other defects in terminal glycolysis, such as phosphoglycerate kinase and mutase deficiencies, conditions not previously classified with the glycogenoses.

Nonglycogen polysaccharide (polyglycan) storage diseases are poorly understood. First among these is Lafora disease, characterized by seizures, myoclonus, progressive dementia, and corpora amylacea–like deposits in neurons (Lafora bodies). Mutations in laforin, a unique phosphatase that contains a carbohydrate-binding module necessary for the maintenance of normal cellular glycogen, appear to cause Lafora disease (103). A puzzling cardioskeletal myopathy

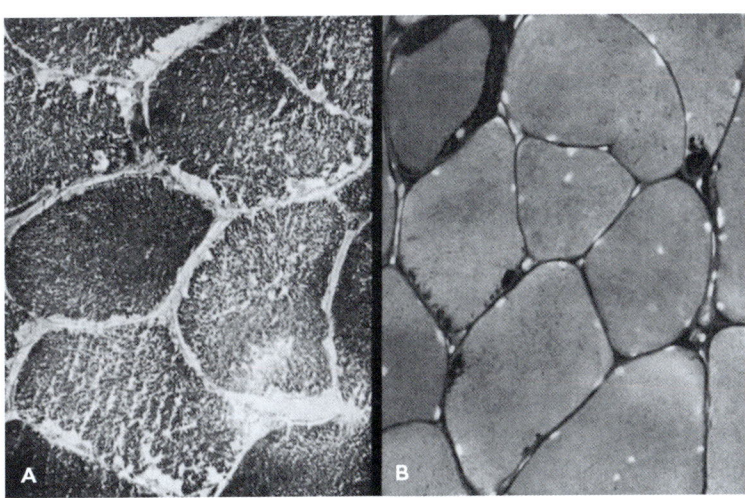

FIGURE 27-26 • **A:** Type V glycogenosis in a young adult. Coarse clumps of glycogen beneath sarcolemma and within fibers are excessive. (PAS stain, alcohol-fixed frozen section; original magnification ×400.) **B:** Type V glycogenosis. Low-grade changes include central nuclei and subsarcolemmal clearing at sites of glycogen accumulation. (Hematoxylin and eosin stain; original magnification ×400.)

TABLE 27-6	DISORDERS WITH TRIGLYCERIDE EXCESS IN MUSCLE

Shock carnitine transporter deficiency
Carnitine–acylcarnitine translocase deficiency
Carnitine palmitoyl transferase deficiency
Acyl-CoA dehydrogenase deficiency
- Long-, medium-, and short-chain
- Multiple (glutaric aciduria II)
3-Hydroxy-3-methylglutaryl-CoA synthase deficiency
Krebs cycle defects
- Fumarase deficiency
Electron transport system defects
Complex I, III, and IV

resembles type IV glycogenosis except for normal levels of brancher enzyme (104). In both conditions, PAS-positive, diastase-resistant, variably metachromatic, granulofibrillar material called polyglucosan accumulates in several tissues, including muscle. Ultrastructural study of muscle may help identify aggregates of material consistent with both conditions. However, typical well-formed Lafora bodies may be absent in skeletal muscle fibers in Lafora disease

Triglyceride Storage Diseases

Beta-oxidation of free fatty acids derived from circulating triglycerides is the major energy source for skeletal muscle fibers, both at rest and during prolonged exercise. In normal muscle fibers, a storage pool of minute neutral lipid droplets are evenly dispersed between myofibrils, more prominently in type I muscle fibers, signifying primary reliance on fatty acids for energy supply in these mitochondria-rich fibers. Muscle lipid content is probably a relatively labile feature, dependent on plasma fatty acid concentration, which may be altered in fasting states, starvation, or disease.

After entry into muscle, free fatty acids, conjugated with coenzyme A, are transported across the mitochondrial membrane by a biochemical shuttle involving carnitine acyltransferases. Transient increase of muscle neutral lipid occurs in many primary metabolic diseases, Reye syndrome, and probably in other clinical crises. Therefore, diagnostic specificity seems doubtful.

Many inborn errors that disrupt beta-oxidation of long, medium, and short chain lipids have been identified in the last two decades (Table 27-6) (105–108). Symptoms related to episodes of nonketotic hypoglycemia may begin in the neonatal period or later in life, typically fluctuate and may be precipitated in the form of a potentially lethal, metabolic crisis by a viral respiratory illness or low caloric intake (106,109,110). In older children, weakness and cramps may be precipitated by intense exercise, following which the serum level of creatine kinase rises, and myoglobinuria may appear (111).

Multiorgan triglyceride storage especially in heart, liver, kidney, and skeletal muscle suggest an inborn error in lipid oxidation and may be associated with recurrent episodes of acute encephalopathy resembling Reye syndrome, cardiac decompensation, or sudden death. A small subset of infants who die suddenly, and about 10% of cases of epidemic Reye syndrome, have been shown to have medium-chain acyl CoA dehydrogenase deficiency, a disorder that, during a crisis, promotes neutral lipid accumulation in the liver, myocardium, and in some instances, skeletal muscle (105,106). This is caused by a common point mutation in 80% of cases. The mechanism of sudden death in affected infants has not been established (see Chapters 5 and 15).

Specific metabolic defects that can lead to neutral lipid accumulation in muscle fibers (Figure 27-27A, B) include

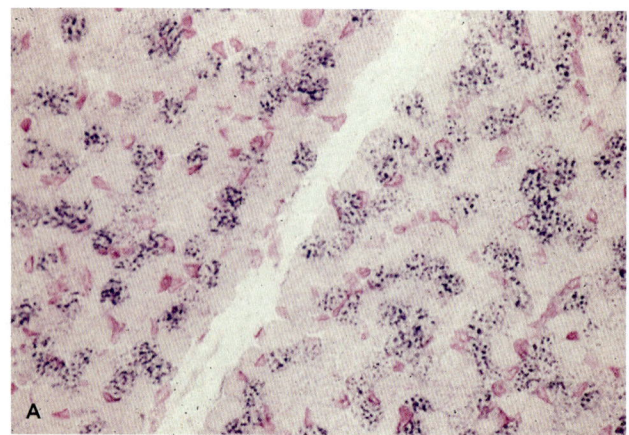
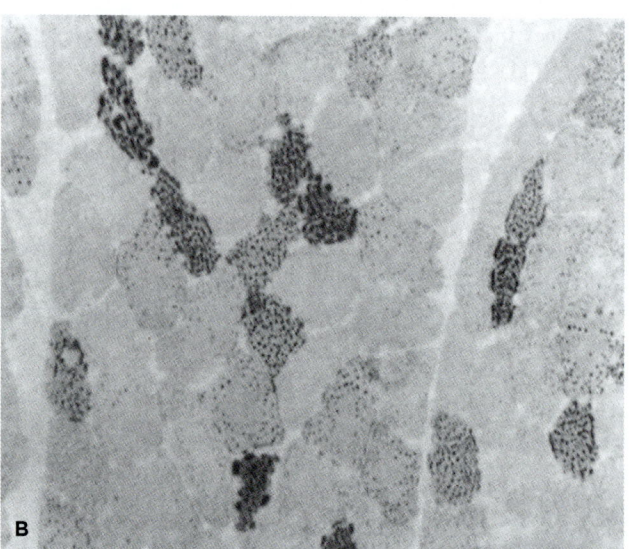

FIGURE 27-27 • **A:** Neutral lipid accumulation, mainly in type I fibers of a young adult with defect in lipid oxidation. (Sudan black stain; original magnification ×200.) **B:** Neutral lipid accumulation, mainly in type I fibers of an infant with lethal CPT II deficiency. (Sudan black stain; original magnification ×200.)

carnitine membrane transporter defect, carnitine palmitoyltransferase II deficiency, and defects in various components of the electron transport system (106,108). The pattern of acylcarnitine compounds excreted in urine has considerable diagnostic usefulness in disorders of lipid catabolism (107). Carnitine deficiency, based on the finding of low levels of carnitine in blood, usually is a secondary phenomenon caused by urinary loss of carnitine conjugated with organic acids resulting from defective lipid use. Carnitine transporter defect (112) is the basis for previously described cases of "primary" carnitine deficiency in which loss of carnitine in the urine is caused by failure of carnitine to transfer from blood to muscle after production in the liver. Among the listed disorders, muscle lipid accumulation is inconstant, and least likely to be seen in carnitine palmitoyltransferase II deficiency, an important cause of exercise-induced rhabdomyolysis in adults. In contrast, infants with this defect have prominent multiorgan lipid accumulation including intramuscular lipid droplets and lethal outcome (4). The phenotypic heterogeneity is explained by differing levels of residual enzyme activity and by extreme molecular genetic heterogeneity demonstrable in tissue and in fibroblast culture.

When a disorder of energy metabolism is suspected based on newborn screening, clinical history, or muscle biopsy findings, useful laboratory studies include determination of blood lactate, pyruvate, and carnitine levels; evaluation of a fasting urine sample for ketone bodies or acylcarnitine compounds; determination of unusual organic acids; measurement of tissue levels of carnitine transporter, carnitine, and carnitine palmityl transferase activity; and studies of fatty acid oxidation in fibroblast culture. Increasingly molecular studies are used to delineate these conditions.

Mitochondrial Myopathy

Mitochondrial diseases are a heterogeneous group of multisystemic disorders. Disorders of oxidative phosphorylation (OXPHOS) are caused by mitochondrial DNA (mtDNA) defects, mtRNA maintenance defect, or nuclear DNA (nDNA) defect (113). Disorders of mtDNA are often maternally inherited duplications or point mutations. Sporadic cases of OXPHOS defects result from postzygotic somatic mutation of the mitochondrial genome or autosomal recessive nuclear gene defects. Most primary mitochondrial disease is caused by a nuclear gene defect (114). The diagnosis of mitochondriopathy is based on clinical history, laboratory, genetic and biochemistry testing, and muscle biopsy findings (115). Major clinical presentations are unexplained multisystemic involvement, signs of clinical progression, or exacerbation with intercurrent illnesses and positive family history. Organs or tissues that are highly dependent on energy metabolism such as skeletal muscle, brain, heart, and peripheral nerve are most likely to be affected. Other organs such as the liver, kidney, eye, gastrointestinal tract, and pancreas may also be involved. Clinical and laboratory findings depend on the spectrum of organ involvement. In encephalomyopathy, a common combination, lactate and pyruvate levels may be elevated in both blood and spinal fluid. When skeletal muscle only is involved, unexplained weakness, lactic acidosis, episodic cramps, and rarely, myoglobinuria may occur. Measurement of activity of electron transport complexes in skeletal muscle samples plays a major role in the diagnosis of mitochondriopathy. Over 50 pathogenic point mutations and hundreds of large-scale deletions and duplications of mtDNA have been identified in a variety of mitochondriopathies (116,117). However, often in children who are suspected to have mitochondriopathy based upon currently accepted criteria, OXPHOS enzyme activity defects or pathogenic mutations are not identified (117).

Muscle biopsy is a primary investigative procedure in patients who are suspected to have a disorder of energy metabolism as a screening tool for morphologic features, which support the clinical suspicion and as a source of tissue for biochemical and molecular genetic study. By LM, muscle from patients with mitochondriopathies may appear normal, show nonspecific focal myopathic changes, or a few scattered diagnostic features such as "ragged-red" myofibers. Histochemical methods for succinic dehydrogenase (SDH) and cytochrome c oxidase (COX) demonstrate mitochondrial distribution and are a crude but useful measure of activity. Impaired lipid utilization is assessed with stains for neutral lipid. SDH is a component of complex II of the respiratory chain. COX is a component of complex IV of the respiratory chain that is coded for by both nuclear and mtDNA. Monoclonal antibodies to subunits of electron transport complexes can be used to differentiate deficiencies due to mtDNA or nDNA alone or in combination (118). This approach has not yet received wide use.

The most striking LM findings in mitochondriopathies are "ragged-red" myofibers (RRF); these are rare in infants but more common in older children. RRF contain large aggregates of SDH-reactive and COX-reactive or negative mitochondria between myofibrils and beneath the sarcolemma. RRF are best seen in cryostat sections stained with the modified trichrome method; ragged-blue fibers have hyperintense reaction product using the SDH method (Figure 27-28A, B). Small subsarcolemmal mitochondrial aggregates occur in up to 25% of myofibers in children and probably are of no consequence (Figure 27-29A). More than 2% of myofibers containing large subsarcolemmal mitochondrial aggregates based on the SDH reaction raises suspicion for mitochondriopathy (Figure 27-29B) (119). Neutral lipid storage is inconstant in mitochondrial myopathies. RRF often contain increased neutral lipid as well as clusters of pathologic mitochondria by EM. Muscle fibers in primary coenzyme Q_{10} deficiency, a rare encephalomyopathy, contain increased neutral lipid and aggregates of mitochondria that respond to replacement therapy (120). A general increase of lipid droplets in type 1 myofibers is more likely in disorders of lipid transport or oxidation than in disorders of electron transport.

Several different syndromes have been described in which activity of COX is reduced or absent in a few, most, or all

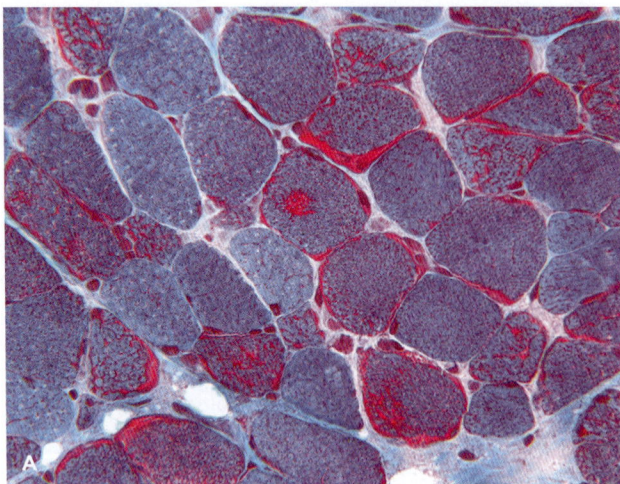
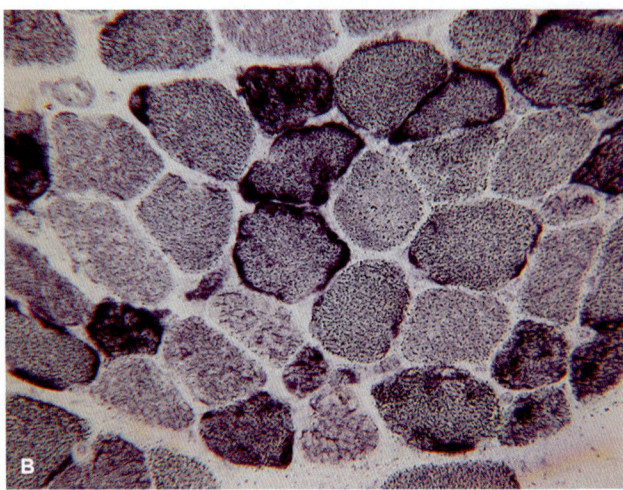

FIGURE 27-28 • **A:** Ragged red fibers in Kearns-Sayre syndrome contain coarse aggregates of pathologic mitochondria. (Modified Trichrome stain; original magnification ×200.)
B: Ragged blue fibers in Kearns-Sayre syndrome contain coarse aggregates of pathologic mitochondria. (SDH histochemistry; original magnification ×200.)

muscle fibers (116). All skeletal muscle fibers lack COX activity in lethal cytochrome oxidase deficiency of infancy (Figure 27-30) (121). In our experience, the mitochondria display subtle abnormalities only. A benign reversible form of this condition differs in histochemic characteristics (122). Isolated COX-negative fibers, common in adults with mitochondrial disease, are rarely seen in young children.

Electron microscopic (EM) examination of myofibers helps if unequivocally pathologic mitochondria are identified. Diagnostic changes include abnormal size or shape with paracrystalline inclusions, abnormal matrix density, and abnormal arrangements of cristae (Figure 27-31). Structurally abnormal mitochondria occur in both type I and type II fibers. Numerical excess, when extreme, is also helpful. Slight increase in apparent number, or variation in mitochondrial size, and mitochondrial budding and branching, or small aggregates are too subjective to be assigned a major role in support of that diagnosis (119).

Mitochondrial disorders with muscle involvement in infants or children include Kearns-Sayre syndrome (KSS); myoclonic epilepsy with ragged-red fibers (MERRF); mitochondrial encephalomyopathy, lactic acidosis, and stroke-like episodes (MELAS); Leigh syndrome (LS); fatal infantile mitochondrial myopathy with lactic acidosis and de Toni-Fanconi-Debre syndrome; infantile cytochrome oxidase deficiency (fatal and benign subtypes); and myoclonic epilepsy with weakness, short stature, and ataxia (123) (see Chapter 5).

KSS is usually sporadic with onset before age 20. Most patients have mtDNA deletions (124). Common clinical presentations include progressive external ophthalmoplegia, pigmentary retinopathy, and cardiomyopathy. Muscle samples contain scattered RRF and variable numbers of COX-negative fibers. Pathologic mitochondria are usually seen on EM. The disease is slowly progressive, and most patients die before the fourth decade.

The onset of MERRF may be in childhood or in adult life with variable disease progression. Patients typically present with myoclonic seizures, cerebellar ataxia, and mitochondrial myopathy with RRF. COX-negative fibers are also commonly seen. Biochemical studies may show defects in complex I, II, III, or IV. The discovery of a highly specific point mutation at nt 8344 (A8344G) in the tRNA-Lys gene of mtDNA facilitates the diagnosis of MERRF (122).

The onset of MELAS is usually before the age of 15 years. Common clinical presentations include seizures, hemianopia, and cortical blindness. Serum and CSF lactate is significantly increased. Muscle biopsy may show RRF or COX-negative fibers, but also may be normal. An interesting finding is mitochondrial accumulation in vascular smooth muscle detectable in the SDH reaction. Many patients have complex I deficiency. Demonstration of a point mutation at

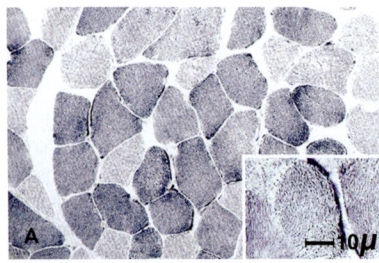
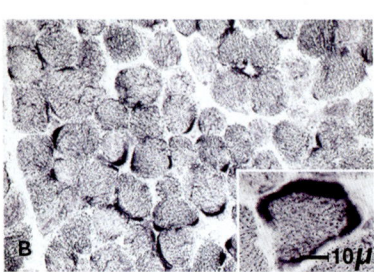

FIGURE 27-29 • **A:** Small subsarcolemmal mitochondrial aggregates but no intermyofibrillar aggregates are common in normal skeletal muscle fibers. (SDH histochemistry; original magnification ×200.) **B:** Greater than 2% subsarcolemmal mitochondrial aggregates larger than 4 μm in depth support a diagnosis of mitochondriopathy. (SDH histochemistry; original magnification ×200.)

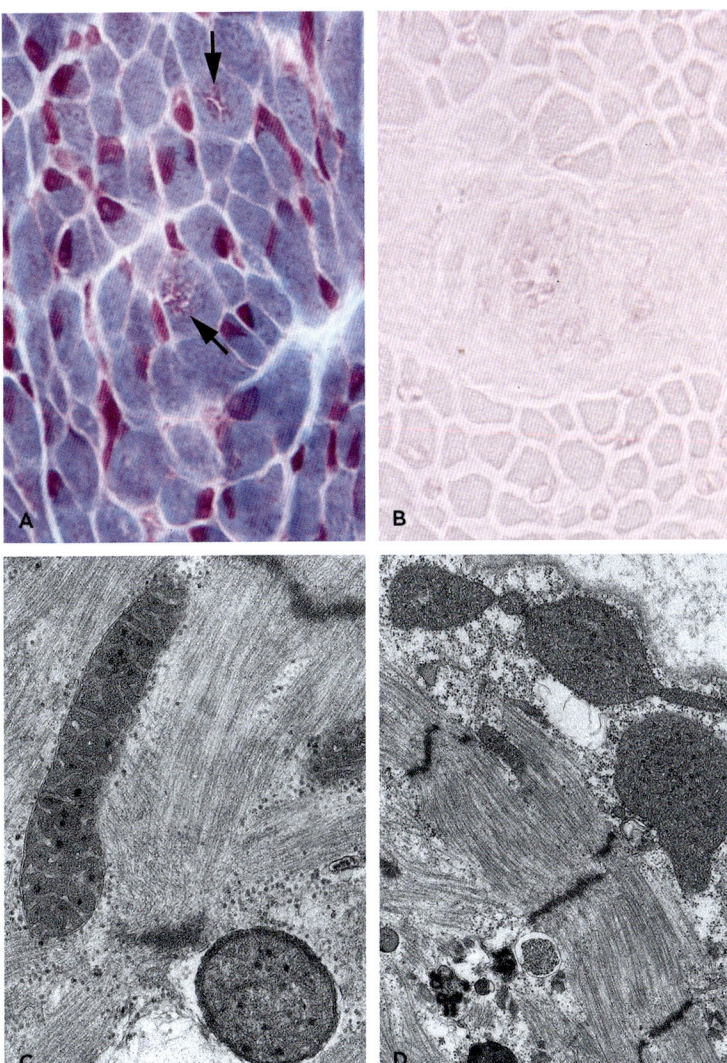

FIGURE 27-30 • **A:** Low-grade myopathic change with occasional near-ragged red fibers (*arrows*) in lethal infantile COX deficiency. (Hematoxylin and eosin stain; original magnification ×400.) **B:** Absent COX activity in muscle fibers and blood vessel. (Cytochrome oxidase histochemistry; original magnification ×400.) **C:** Pathologic mitochondria with dense matrix, excess matrix dense granules, dilatation of cristae, and fused outer membranes. (Uranyl acetate and lead citrate stain; original magnification ×15,000.) **D:** Pathologic mitochondria with prominent proliferation by budding. (Uranyl acetate and lead citrate stain; original magnification ×15,000.)

nt 3243 (A3243G) in the tRNALEU(UUR) gene of mtDNA is very helpful in the diagnosis (123).

Leigh syndrome presents in infants or young children with neuropathy, ataxia, and retinitis pigmentosa. Bilateral symmetric subacute necrotizing encephalomyelopathy is characteristic finding. Microscopy of muscle is normal in many cases, although myofibers that are COX negative or contain increased lipid are reported. RRF are consistently absent. Biochemical studies may show deficiencies in several of the electron transport complex complexes, the most common being complex IV. Although LS is usually inherited in autosomal recessive mode, sporadic, X-linked, and maternal modes of transmission also occur. Maternally inherited LS is associated with heteroplasmic point mutation of T8993G in the ATPase 6 gene of mtDNA. In these cases, genetic analysis of the muscle may be helpful (125).

The mtDNA depletion syndromes (MDSs) are autosomal recessive disorders with a decreased mitochondrial DNA copy number, which is due to mutations in eight different genes (*DGUOK, MPV17, POLG1, RRM2B, SUCLA2, SUCLG1, TK2,* and *PEO1*) (126). MDSs have a broad phenotypic spectrum.

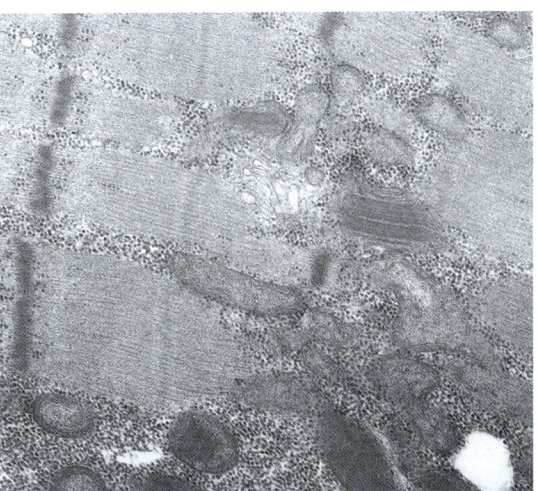

FIGURE 27-31 • Pathologic mitochondria in Kearns-Sayre syndrome exhibit two patterns. Some have central matrix clearing with margination of cristae at the periphery near the outer membrane. Others contain paracrystalline inclusions located in the inner crystal space. Typically, some mitochondria exhibit normal morphology. (Uranyl acetate and lead citrate stain; original magnification ×7500.)

Mutations in thymidine kinase 2 (TK2), a nDNA gene, have been associated with a myopathic form of MDS with onset in childhood. Microscopy demonstrates myopathic features with RRF, COX-deficient fibers, ultrastructural abnormalities in mitochondria, and in a few cases, progressive loss of muscle fibers, mimicking muscular dystrophy.

In current practice, many infants with unexplained hypotonia, seizures, developmental delay, sporadic elevation of blood lactate, and borderline abnormal brain imaging studies have a muscle biopsy to investigate for possible mitochondrial encephalomyopathy. The yield of diagnostic abnormality using a multimodal approach that includes light and electron microscopy, and measurement of electron transport activities is low (119). Better approaches for screening for disorders of energy metabolism are needed.

Other Metabolic Myopathies

Congenital lactic acidosis comprises a heterogeneous group of metabolic disorders characterized by generalized organ dysfunction, especially involving the brain, heart, skeletal muscle, and liver. The differential diagnosis includes defects in mitochondrial electron transport, especially in Complex I, mtDNA depletion of diverse genetic cause, organic acidemia of various types, deficiency of enzymes involved in gluconeogenesis, defects in the pyruvate dehydrogenase complex, and type I glycogenosis. Hypotonia with lactic acidosis often prompts a muscle biopsy. Muscle fibers may exhibit increased neutral lipid, abnormal accumulation of mitochondria, or both, but are often morphologically normal.

Myoadenylate deaminase activity in skeletal muscle in the general population is variable due to prevalent gene polymorphisms that result in functional proteins with reduced activity (127,128). Partially reduced enzyme activity due to polymorphisms is typically asymptomatic but is overrepresented in patients with muscular weakness or cramping after strenuous exercise in adults, and rarely, in children (129). Diagnosis is based on histochemical and/or biochemical assays, and mutation analysis. Molecular genetic confirmation is desirable because the histochemical and biochemical methods (130) may not distinguish secondary deficiency due to common polymorphisms, or from primary deficiency due to mutation. Myoadenylate deaminase deficiency has been reported in an infant with hypotonia and developmental delay and in a child whose symptoms resembled those in adults (131,132). The concept of synergistic heterozygosity proposes that combinations of polymorphisms or susceptibility alleles may result in triggerable myopathies as a result of partial defects in two or more enzyme activities such as myoadenylate deaminase, CPT II, or myophosphorylase (133).

EPISODIC MYOGLOBINURIA

Myoglobinuria may be caused by sepsis, myositis, malignant hyperthermia, severe transient electrolyte imbalance, drug reaction, or inherited metabolic disease (134). Repeated episodes precipitated by exercise or minor, usually febrile, viral illnesses signal the need for an investigation for an underlying metabolic disease or an unrecognized Becker dystrophinopathy (135,136). Major biochemical defects responsible for about half of the cases of episodic myoglobinuria, in approximate order of frequency, involve carnitine palmitoyltransferase II (CPT); myophosphorylase; phosphorylase kinase; b-oxidation lipolytic enzymes of several types, of which medium chain triglyceride acyl-CoA dehydrogenase is the most common; and phosphofructokinase. Other less frequent causes of recurrent myoglobinuria include phosphoglycerate kinase deficiency, myoadenylate deaminase deficiency, two types of muscle lactate dehydrogenase defect, lipoamide dehydrogenase deficiency, and most recently, as sophisticated molecular genetic tools are applied to this problem, defects in mitochondrial OXPHOS (137–140). Muscle biopsy is central to this formidable workup and requires that as much of the specimen as possible be frozen for biochemical and molecular studies. Several of the specific defects listed can be diagnosed on the basis of muscle morphology and histochemistry, and others, such as CPT II deficiency, can be determined in fibroblast culture.

MALIGNANT HYPERTHERMIA

MH is an intraoperative catastrophe characterized by acute rigidity and rapid temperature elevation associated with necrosis of muscle, gross pigmenturia due to myoglobin, and renal failure. Susceptibility to MH when exposed to halothane anesthetics or membrane depolarizers, such as succinylcholine, may be observed in persons with no antecedent myopathy having elective surgery or after recent trauma. The definition of susceptibility and anesthetic risk in children with a previous episode or family history of malignant hyperthermic reaction has relied on in vitro testing of strips of fresh muscle for susceptibility to contracture when exposed directly to halothane, caffeine, and/or ryanodine, a plant alkaloid. This method requires a special facility, and although the test is highly specific, it has a significant number of false-negative results (83). Noninvasive screening for common RYR1 mutations is a more practical method to detect susceptibility to MH (141) but sensitivity remains uncertain. Dantrolene, which inhibits calcium release from the sarcoplasmic reticulum, is effective in preventing or aborting malignant hyperthermic reactions. MH has been observed in patients with primary myopathies, especially central core disease and multimini core disease, but also in disorders of glycolysis, Duchenne muscular dystrophy (DMD), myotonic dystrophy, and congenital muscular dystrophy. Baseline alteration of creatine kinase levels, commonly found long after an attack, may be the only indication of underlying myopathy. The hazard of MH is magnified by the need for multiple orthopedic procedures engendered by the deformities that may develop in

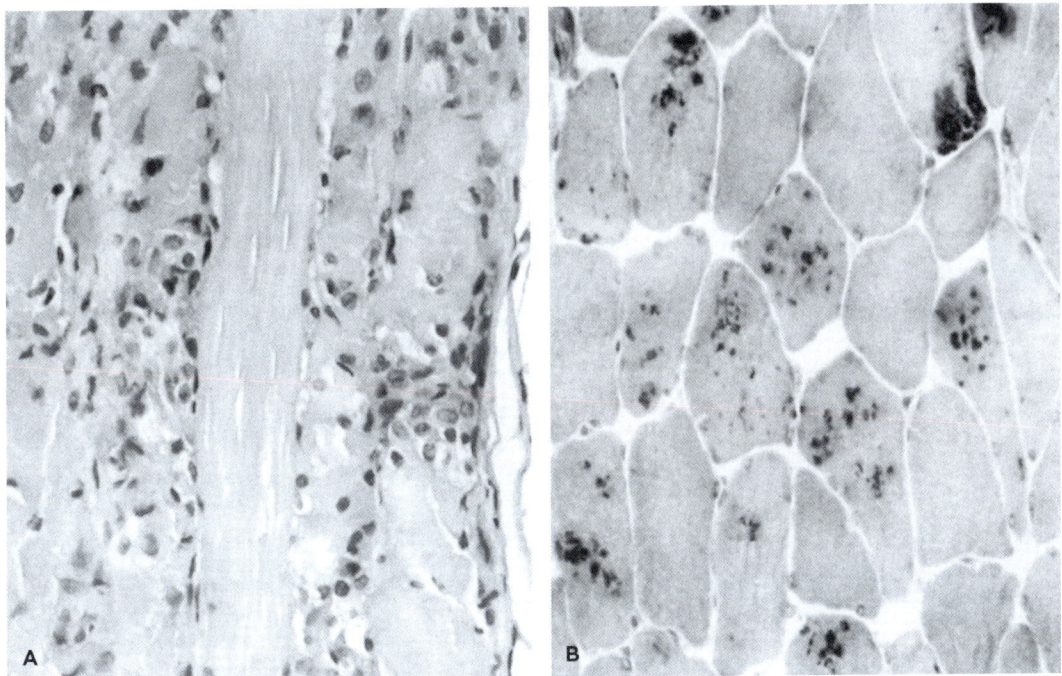

FIGURE 27-32 • **A:** Segmental necrosis of muscle fibers following massive ethanol binge, leading to myoglobinuria. (Hematoxylin and eosin stain; original magnification ×400.) **B:** Clumps of degenerating myofibrils in this teenage girl with ipecac-induced myopathy resemble cytoplasmic bodies. (Trichrome stain; original magnification ×400.)

children with neuromuscular disease. The lesion of MH, segmental muscle fiber necrosis (Figure 27-32A), is not specific and may be a final common pathway for any muscle injury (immune, drug, toxin, virus, extreme exercise) that triggers calcium-mediated proteolysis. This muscle lesion usually heals promptly with restoration of muscle fiber structure and no scarring.

SKELETAL MYOPATHY ASSOCIATED WITH CARDIOMYOPATHY

Patients with primary diseases of skeletal muscle sometimes exhibit cardiac dysfunction and may share similar molecular, anatomical, and clinical features. Cardiac involvement has been reported in many types of myopathies, including muscular dystrophies, particularly the dystrophinopathies (72,142). The genetic myofibrillinopathies, including desminopathies, are important cardioskeletal myopathies in adults and have been described in children (143). Metabolic diseases that may cause skeletal muscle and cardiac dysfunction include glycogenosis (types II-IV), disorders of b-oxidation, carnitine transporter defect, the infantile form of CPT II deficiency, and mitochondrial diseases. Mitochondrial encephalomyopathy and cardiomyopathy may be caused by complex I deficiency (144). Hypertrophic cardiomyopathy with unusually prominent left ventricular trabeculation occurs in Kearns-Sayre syndrome. Idiopathic cardiac hypertrophy, hypotonia, and RRF occur in a few patients with Leigh phenotype, a heterogeneous condition caused by at least six different biochemical defects. A maternally inherited myopathy and cardiomyopathy reported by Zeviani is due to a mtDNA defect (145). X-linked cardioskeletal myopathy, originally identified in infants by Neustein (146), includes several genetically distinct disorders, Barth syndrome, and Danon disease. Barth syndrome mainly affects older children and young adults and includes neutropenia and growth delay, morphologically abnormal mitochondria in heart and skeletal muscle, defects in OXPHOS, and deficiency of cardiolipin, a constituent of the inner mitochondrial membrane. A gene, TAZ, is linked, but the encoded proteins are not known. The best diagnostic test is quantitation of cardiolipin in platelets or cultured fibroblasts (147). Danon disease is a vacuolar cardioskeletal myopathy caused by deficiency of a lysosomal-associated membrane protein, LAMP-2 (148). Autophagic vacuoles are a hallmark of the associated myopathy (149) (Figure 27-33). Sengers syndrome is characterized by congenital cataracts, hypertrophic cardiomyopathy, hypotonia, and abnormal mitochondria in heart and skeletal muscle. Results of investigations of mitochondrial energetics in these rare conditions are inconsistent, suggesting that this

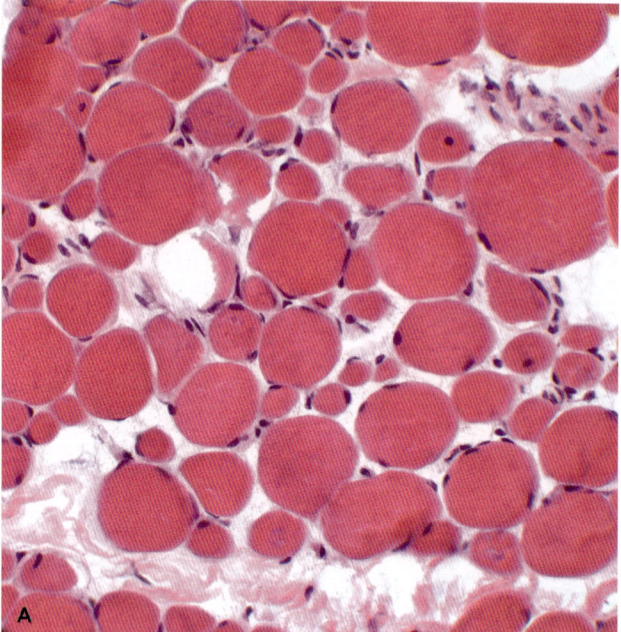
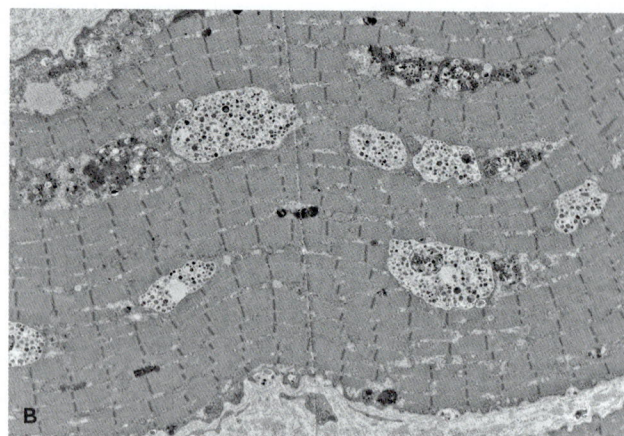
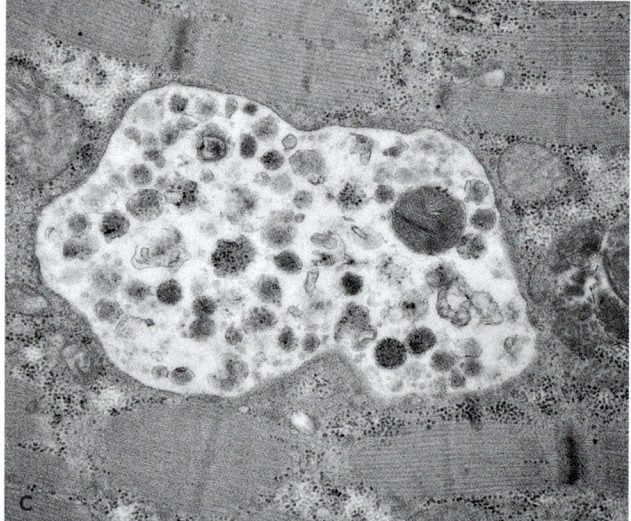

FIGURE 27-33 • **A:** A 34-month-old boy with Danon disease and maternal grandfather with vacuolar myopathy. Myofibers are variable in size; a minority contained vacuoles. (Hematoxylin and eosin stain; original magnification ×400). **B:** Numerous intermyofibrillar lysosomal inclusions (Uranyl acetate and lead citrate stain; original magnification ×4000). **C:** Complex lysosomal inclusions contain glycogen packets and degenerating mitochondria (Uranyl acetate and lead citrate stain; original magnification ×25,000).

phenotype may have multiple causes. Deficient activity of adenine nucleotide translocator is reported (150).

DRUG-INDUCED MYOPATHY

Examples of drug-induced muscle lesions include local acute or chronic myopathy at injection sites, acute or chronic proximal myopathy in myasthenic or polydermatomyositis-like disorders, myotonic syndromes, and malignant hyperthermia reactions. In the setting of critical care units, a number of different drugs (curare-like paralytic agents, corticosteroids, and aminoglycoside antibiotics), possibly augmented by the effects of sepsis, are associated with the development of acute myopathy or polyneuropathy, as discussed previously. Some drugs, such as alcohol, may produce several different clinical syndromes; most important in the pediatric age group are characteristic embryotoxicity and fetal myopathy (see Chapter 4) (151,152). Habitual use of Emetine or syrup of ipecac, usually observed in girls with eating disorders, may cause a significant proximal myopathy, clinically simulating dermatomyositis (153). Ipecac-induced myopathy features a distinctive form of myofibrillar degeneration, with coarse clumps of degenerated contractile elements (Figure 27-32B). Cimetidine and D-penicillamine both have been associated with the emergence of polymyositis, possibly by modulating T-cell–mediated reactions (154,155). Myopathy associated with chronic HIV infection resembles polymyositis. The myopathy associated with zidovudine therapy is a mitochondriopathy possibly being related to mtDNA depletion (156).

The range of morphologic reaction to injury of muscle fibers is limited. Reactions in metabolic myopathy, inflammatory myopathy, and drug-induced injury often overlap. Necrosis of muscle fiber segments, the basic lesion in all myoglobinuric muscle diseases, may be precipitated by anesthetic agents and after exposure to ethanol or heroin (Figure 27-32A). Low-grade, drug-induced myopathy often results in isolated basophilic muscle fibers, a manifestation of degeneration and regeneration cycles, without an inflammatory reaction. A common cause is electrolyte imbalance related to diuretic therapy. Overtly inflammatory drug-induced myopathies may be extremely difficult to distinguish from idiopathic inflammatory myopathy on the basis of histologic features. Clinical improvement after withdrawal of the suspect drug may prevent unnecessary muscle biopsy.

MUSCULAR DYSTROPHIES

Duchenne and Becker Dystrophinopathies

The muscular dystrophies are genetically determined diseases of skeletal muscle characterized by cumulative muscle fiber injury, progressive fibrosis, and loss of function. By far, the most common form is DMD, an X-linked disorder with an incidence of approximately 1 per 3,500 to 5,000 live born males (157). As many as two-third of the new cases of DMD are thought to be the result of new mutations in the dystrophin gene, either in the mother or in the affected boy (158).

Affected boys usually appear normal until about age 2 years, when clumsiness, proximal muscle weakness, and calf pseudohypertrophy prompt clinical investigation, which establishes the diagnosis. The serum creatine kinase level is usually very high at this stage, and electromyographic studies indicate widespread myopathy. Despite corticosteroid treatment and recent advances in experimental mutation-specific clinical trials (159), there is no cure for DMD. Most patients can no longer walk after the first decade, and few survive beyond the end of the second decade. Cardiac muscle involvement is a constant feature at autopsy and may cause clinical manifestations late in the course of the disease (see Chapter 13).

Becker muscular dystrophy (BMD) is a milder form of X-linked dystrophinopathy with a more protracted course and later onset of disease affecting 1 in 18,500 live born males. Despite milder skeletal muscle disease, patients with BMD are more likely to have clinical cardiomyopathy. An unusual presentation of the Becker form is recurrent myalgia with cramps but mild weakness (160), which is highly associated with the deletion of central and distal rod domains.

Both DMD and BMD are caused by intragenic deletions (in 60% to 65% of cases), duplications (in 5% to 10% of cases), or point mutations in the dystrophin gene. Specialized techniques have been developed to identify point mutations in families without deletions or duplications (161). Guidelines for molecular diagnosis have been recently published (162), but genetic definition for this disease is transforming rapidly. Dystrophin, absent in DMD and present in an altered form or reduced amounts in BMD, is spatially related to muscle sarcolemma. Currently, the use of all available techniques for DMD gene mutation screening permits a genetic definition in almost all cases. However, the great mutation heterogeneity largely complicates the genetic definition in dystrophinopathy. Furthermore, apparently easily interpretable mutations often have no predictable effect on phenotype, obviating the need for muscle biopsy.

Prenatal diagnosis for DMD/BMD is only done for male pregnancies. The familial mutation should be confirmed before the prenatal test. Polymorphic DNA sequences on the X chromosome, identified using restriction-enzyme digestion, are closely linked to expression of the DMD phenotype in families with one affected boy. This method remains useful for identifying carriers and affected fetuses when more specific methods are noninformative (163). Common deletions and duplications can be detected in chorionic villus samples and in amnion cells.

Muscle biopsy findings in DMD include random variation in muscle fiber size, with atrophic and isolated hypertrophic rounded, dense hypercontracted fibers with eosinophilic sarcoplasm; muscle fiber necrosis; fiber regeneration; and progressive increase in connective tissue and fat within and around muscle fascicles (Figure 27-34A, B). Inflammatory changes are typically minor, except during the active early phase of the disease when macrophages invade necrotic fibers. All muscle fiber subtypes are affected. None of the changes are specific, but the constellation is typical and diagnostic in most cases. Using specific antibodies to three dystrophin domains, DMD muscle lacks sarcolemmal labeling in the vast majority of myofibers (Figure 27-34A), except for rare revertant fibers. Muscle sections from BMD patients are characterized by subtle sarcolemmal labeling abnormalities (Figure 27-35B). BMD with an in-frame deletion may show strong sarcolemmal labeling of antibodies against the N- and C-termini but total absence of labeling using antibodies against the rod domain. These results may be further confirmed by western blots for quantitation and by more detailed characterization of mutations in the dystrophin gene.

Segmental necrosis of individual muscle fibers is the major feature in active DMD/BMD. A similar lesion in etiologically diverse skeletal muscle diseases is usually repaired without fibrosis, unlike DMD in which repeated breakdown of muscle fibers may exceed the capacity for repair. The prevalence of intact-appearing muscle fibers with highly stainable calcium content suggests that calcium-activated proteolysis may be exceptionally active in DMD (164).

Other Muscular Dystrophies

Other subtypes of muscular dystrophy that may be encountered in children are comparatively less common. Progressive muscle damage with fibrosis usually is less severe than in DMD. Classification, which is usually based on clinical information, is becoming more precise, as methods based on molecular genetics are developed. Myotonic dystrophy is notable because of myotonia, multiorgan involvement, dominant inheritance, and the devastating effect on some infants, but it is not a dystrophic disease in the morphologic sense (165). Genetically heterogeneous autosomal recessive forms of muscular dystrophy, some of which are clinically similar to DMD, may be responsible for some instances of the Duchenne phenotype in girls with a normal karyotype (166).

Limb-girdle muscular dystrophies (LGMD) are a heterogeneous group of genetic disorders characterized by

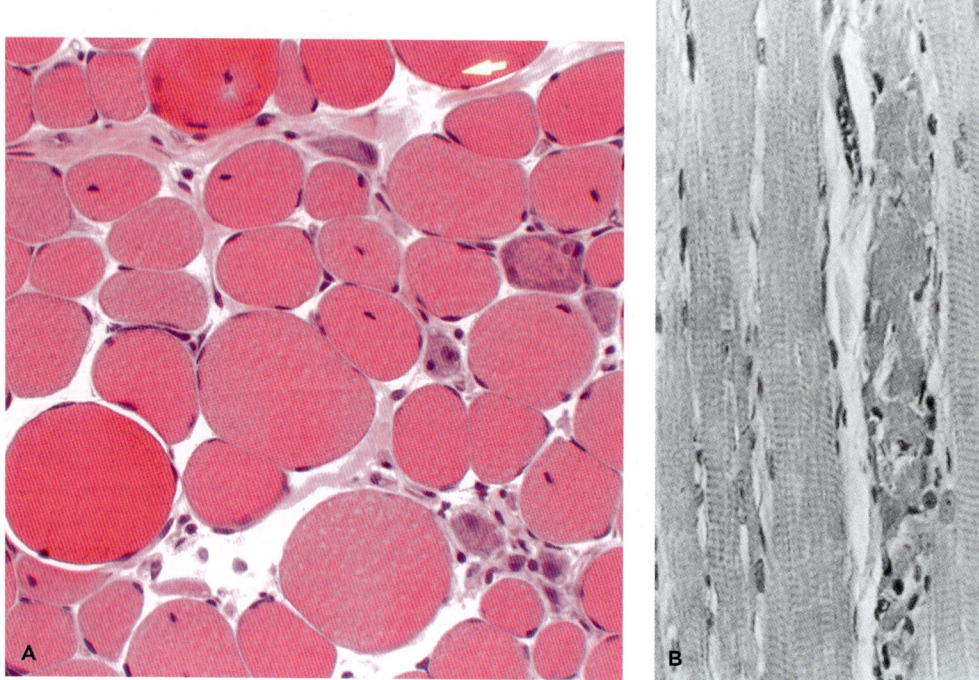

FIGURE 27-34 • **A:** Duchenne muscular dystrophy. Replacement fibrosis, focal active myopathy, and scattered, dense, rounded, hypercontracted fibers are typical. (Hematoxylin and eosin stain; original magnification ×400.) **B:** Duchenne muscular dystrophy. Segmental necrosis of isolated fibers is a consistent feature. (Hematoxylin and eosin stain; original magnification ×400.)

progressive muscle weakness with dystrophic muscle morphology caused by autosomal dominant or recessive gene mutations. Immunohistochemistry stains may demonstrate the absence of specific muscle proteins such as sarcoglycans, lamin A/C, caveolin 3, dysferlin, and dystroglycans. There has been rapid development in recognizing mutations in LGMD during the last decade. Most importantly, it was discovered that genes originally associated with other muscle diseases have also been linked to LGMD, and vice-versa (167).

The facioscapulohumeral form of muscular dystrophy often begins in childhood, and a rare severe infantile phenotype is described (168). Affected children may have

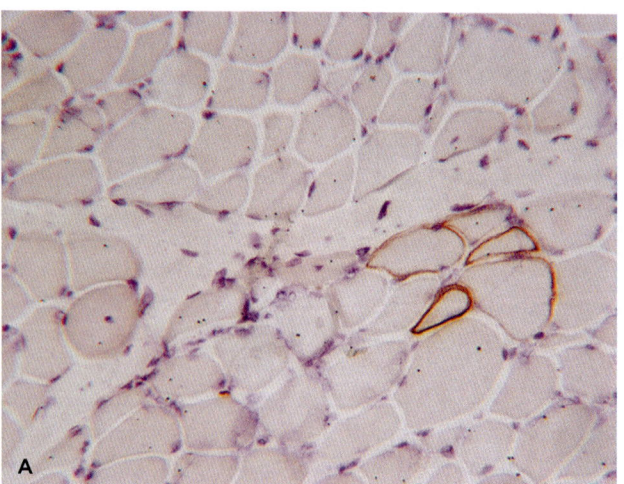
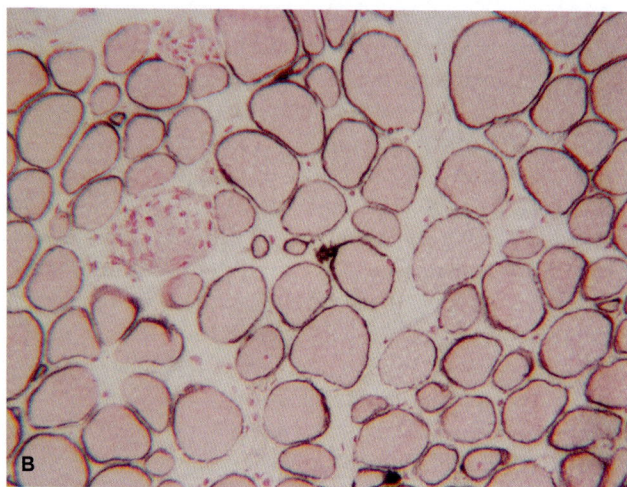

FIGURE 27-35 • **A:** In DMD, dystrophin is absent in the sarcolemma of 95% to 100% of myofibers. Rare positive myofibers may indicate partially successful transcription during muscle fiber regeneration. (Dystrophin immunostain; original magnification ×200.) **B:** In BMD, dystrophin is present in most muscle fibers, but the sarcolemmal pattern is often weak or interrupted. Dystrophin is absent in the necrotic muscle fiber. (Dystrophin immunostain; original magnification ×200.)

TABLE 27-7 CONGENITAL MUSCULAR DYSTROPHY

Congenital Muscular Dystrophy	Gene Defects	Organ/Tissue Involvement	Defects in IHC Stain
1. Abnormal extracellular matrix protein			
a. Congenital muscular dystrophy type I (MDC1A)	$LAMA_2$	Skeletal muscle, brain, and peripheral nerve	Merosin
b. Ullrich congenital muscular dystrophy (UCMD)	COL6A1, COL6A2, COL6A3	Skeletal muscle	Collagen VI
2. Abnormal membrane receptors for the extracellular matrix			
a. Fukuyama congenital muscular dystrophy (FCMD)	FUKUTIN	Skeletal muscle, brain, and heart	Glycosylated α-dystroglycan
b. Muscle-eye-brain disease	POMGnT1	Skeletal muscle, eye, and brain	Glycosylated α-dystroglycan and merosin
c. Walker-Warburg syndrome	POMT1, POMT2, FUKUTIN, FKRP	Skeletal muscle, eye, and brain	Glycosylated α-dystroglycan
d. Congenital muscular dystrophy type 1C (MDC1C)	FKRP	Skeletal muscle, heart, and brain	Glycosylated α-dystroglycan
e. Congenital muscular dystrophy type 1D (MDC1D)	LARGE	Skeletal muscle and brain	Glycosylated α-dystroglycan
3. Abnormal endoplasmic reticulum protein			
a. Rigid spine with muscular dystrophy type 1 (RSMD1)	SEPN1	Skeletal muscle and heart	None

neurodevelopmental delay and seizures. This dominantly inherited form of muscular dystrophy is recognized by careful attention to distribution of weakness and examination of relatives. Focal myositis is common, but the mechanism and the importance of inflammation are unclear. Deletion of tandem repeats at 4q35 is the basis for a reliable diagnostic test. The Emery-Dreifuss form of humeroperoneal muscular dystrophy is a rare disease recognizable in later childhood on the basis of an associated cardiac conduction disorder; both dominant and X-linked modes of inheritance are described. Defects in nuclear envelope proteins lamin A and emerin are demonstrable using immunostains (169).

CONGENITAL MUSCULAR DYSTROPHY

CMD is a heterogeneous group of disorders characterized by proximal muscle disease causing hypotonia, weakness, and a liability to contractures, which are often present at birth or develop soon thereafter (170). Affected infants are often floppy, and motor development is delayed. Involvement of the central nervous system is variable and helps define important subsets. This may take the form of gray matter migration defects or myelination disturbance. Elevations of the serum creatine kinase level vary. The clinical course of the disease ranges from severe, often with early demise, to mildly progressive with survival to adult life. Muscle fibrosis is often prominent and may be well developed at birth, but severe fibrosis in infants does not predict static versus progressive disease. Marked regional variations exist in incidence of different types of CMD, the highest being 0.46 per 10,000 live births in Japan making CMD one of the more common neuromuscular disorders. In recent years, great progress has been made in discerning the underlying molecular basis of congenital muscular dystrophies (171,172). The most recent classification of CMD is based on clinical presentation and immunohistologic, biochemical, and genetic defects (Table 27-7).

Muscle biopsy findings are generic in CMD and have no specificity for disease subtypes (Figures 27-36 to 27-38). The spectrum of pathologic features includes myofiber atrophy, hypertrophy with eosinophilic sarcoplasm, and the presence of scattered split, degenerative, necrotic, and regenerative myofibers. Fibrofatty replacement of myofibers is variable in amount and may be absent in the early stages of disease. Inflammation is limited to foci of fiber degeneration and is typically minor. Many of these features overlap with other forms of muscular dystrophy. Electron microscopy has no proven value in the diagnosis of CMD.

CMD with $α_2$-laminin deficiency (merosin-deficient CMD) includes almost 50% of the cases of CMD and is the basis for convenient subclassification based upon the merosin immunostain. These patients have mutations in the $α_2$ chain of laminin that lead to complete or partial deficiency of $α_2$ laminin (merosin) (173,174). Merosin is an extracellular

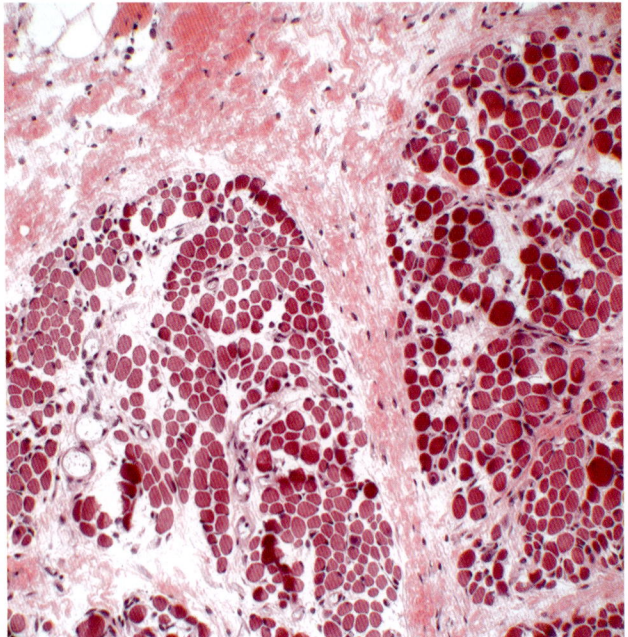

FIGURE 27-36 • Congenital muscular dystrophy shows extensive fibrosis but little evidence of active myopathy. This case was clinically static. (Hematoxylin and eosin stain; original magnification ×160.)

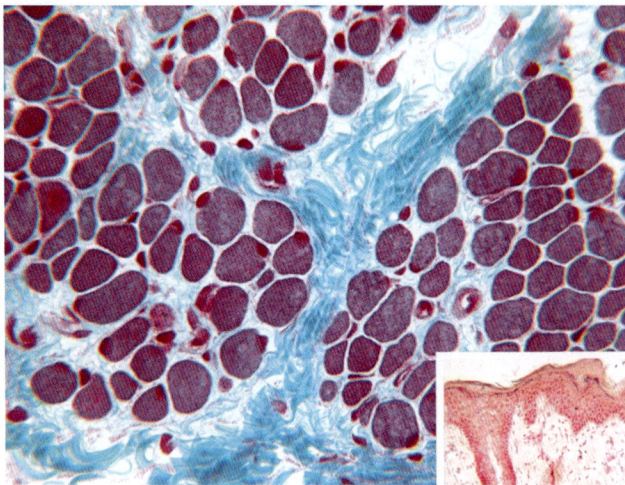

FIGURE 27-38 • Congenital muscular dystrophy with absent merosin in basement membranes of skeletal muscle fibers and skin (**inset**). (Merosin immunostain; original magnification ×200.)

matrix protein linked to the dystrophin-associated glycoproteins in basement membranes of muscle, peripheral nerves, trophoblast, and intracerebral blood vessels and glia limitans that form the blood brain barrier (175). Most patients with merosin deficiency (MDC1) learn to sit unsupported but are unable to walk. Progressive scoliosis is common. The majority have diffuse white matter abnormalities after 6 months of age. The internal capsule, corpus callosum, basal ganglia, thalami, and cerebellum are typically spared. Demyelinating motor neuropathy is common and sensory neuropathy may

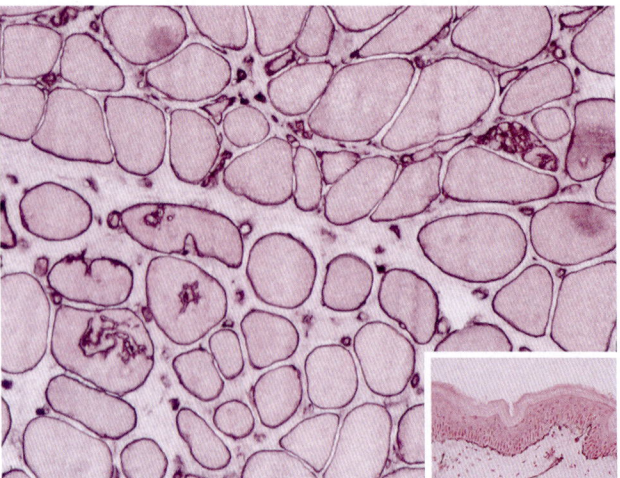

FIGURE 27-37 • Congenital muscular dystrophy with normal merosin in basement membranes of skeletal muscle fibers and skin (inset). Internalization of basement membrane in skeletal muscle fibers is a striking feature in some cases. (Merosin immunostain; original magnification ×200.)

develop in older children. Merosin status is determined on frozen sections of skeletal muscle, skin, or trophoblast (Figures 27-37 and 27-38) (175). Most, but not all, patients with merosin deficiency have demonstrable mutations; in some patients, the merosin deficiency may be secondary (176).

Ullrich congenital muscular dystrophy (UCMD) is probably the second most common CMD, with a likely autosomal recessive pattern of inheritance. Patients present in the neonatal period with muscle hypotonia, kyphosis of the spine, proximal joint contractures, hyperelasticity of the distal joints, and hip dislocation. Mutation in the COL6A gene leads to collagen VI deficiency in these patients. Collagen VI is a ubiquitous extracellular matrix protein that forms a microfibrillar network associated with basement membranes.

Although typical dystrophic features are seen in the muscle biopsies from most UCMD patients, pathologic findings may be limited to mild fiber size variation, myofibers containing central nuclei, and minimal endomysial fibrosis. The immunostain for collagen VI is an important diagnostic tool that can be applied to skin, where the protein can be detected in the papillary dermis and around hair follicles. In skeletal muscle, collagen VI is found in the epimysial, perimysial, and endomysial interstitium but is concentrated in particular in and adjacent to basement membrane of myofibers, blood vessels, and nerve twigs. In majority patients with UCMD, collagen VI is present in the interstitium but absent from the sarcolemma (177). Collagen VI stain may be falsely positive in patients with partial collagen VI deficiency, or falsely negative in patients with secondary downregulation of collagen VI. In both cases, genetic testing for COL6A may provide the definitive diagnosis. Mutations in the gene encoding collagen VI (COL6A) may also cause Bethlem myopathy (BM), which has similar but milder clinical features. BM is likely inherited as an autosomal dominant trait.

CMD with abnormal glycosylation of α-dystroglycan includes three severe forms of CMD that are associated with brain and/or eye involvement: Walker-Warburg syndrome (WWS), muscle-eye-brain (MEB) disease, and Fukuyama congenital muscular dystrophy (FCMD). Also included are congenital muscular dystrophy 1C (MDC1C), a milder form of LGMD2I, congenital muscular dystrophy 1D (MDC1D), and the myodystrophy mouse. All are caused by mutations that affect glycosyltransferases, and all share an abnormally glycosylated dystroglycan. Dystroglycan is an important component of the dystrophin–glycoprotein complex, and the glycosylation of α-dystroglycan is crucial for basement membrane function.

Muscle biopsies typically show low-grade myopathy with dystrophic features. Immunostain for a-dystroglycan is helpful in recognition of deficiency, but subclassification of this group of diseases is based on the clinical presentation and genetic testing.

WWS is the most severe disease in the category of muscular dystrophy–dystroglycanopathies (178). Patients present with severe early-onset hypotonia, profound developmental delay, type II lissencephaly, pontocerebellar hypoplasia, defective central myelination, and ocular dysgenesis. Death usually occurs in infancy. Marked dystrophic features plus a tendency to type I fiber predominance and size disproportion and persistence of type IIc fibers are present in muscle biopsies. The diagnosis depends on clinical, radiologic, and pathologic findings.

FCMD is particularly frequent in Japan but occurs in other ethnic groups and is characterized by dystrophic myopathy of early onset associated with central nervous system malformations, including cerebral and cerebellar microgyria, followed by the development of dilated cardiomyopathy (179). FCMD is caused by mutations of fukutin gene on chromosome 9q31 (180); evidence favors an autosomal recessive trait. Recognition depends on detection of appropriate central nervous system malformations, lack of sarcolemmal staining for α-dystroglycan, and genetic testing. Merosin expression may be reduced, but linkage studies indicate a different genomic locus in Fukuyama dystrophy than the one assigned to $α_2$ laminin.

MEB disease is an autosomal recessive disorder with a heterogeneous clinical spectrum. Characteristic clinical findings include early-onset hypotonia, congenital glaucoma, myopia, retinal hypoplasia, pachygyria, and cerebellar hypoplasia. The eye involvement is usually more severe than in FCMD. Mutation of POMGnT1, a gene encoding a glycotransferase, resulting in defective O-mannosyl glycan synthesis has been found in patients with MEB (181). Because POMGnT1 is a laminin-binding ligand of α-dystroglycan, muscle biopsies in these patients may lack sarcolemmal labeling with both α-dystroglycan and merosin antibodies.

MDC1C is caused by FKRP missense or null mutation. Broad variation in the clinical phenotype correlates with residual expression of α-dystroglycan. The severe form usually involves both muscle and brain, and LGMD2I represent the milder form with no brain involvement.

MDC1D is related to LARGE, an animal model of CMD with a loss of function mutation in the LARGE gene, encoding for a putative bifunctional glycosyltransferase. The human equivalent of the LARGE mutation was defined in a patient with muscular dystrophy, mental retardation, brain structural changes, and decreased muscle labeling for α-dystroglycan (182).

Included in the broad category of CMD are children with the rigid spine syndrome (RSMD1) (183). These are usually boys who have a fibrosing myopathy manifested as weakness in infancy; biopsy may show type I fiber numeric predominance or size disproportion. Upper spinal stiffness, scoliosis, and in some cases, cardiomyopathy develop in later childhood. The disease is caused by selenoprotein N gene mutation. There is substantial overlap of clinical manifestations and muscle abnormalities with other forms of muscular dystrophy and with CM. SPEN1 gene mutation has been reported in patients with multiminicore disease (184,185), which further complicates the diagnosis of RSMD1.

CMD may be considered when some other form of muscular dystrophy presents at an unusually early age. Another source of confusion may be the so-called congenital polymyositis (Figure 27-39), an incompletely defined condition that is distinguished from CMD mainly by foci of active "myositis" (186). This disorder has few clinical or morphologic features in common with childhood polydermatomyositis and is probably not an autoimmune disorder. Cerebral abnormalities in some of these infants suggest a nosologic relationship to CMD.

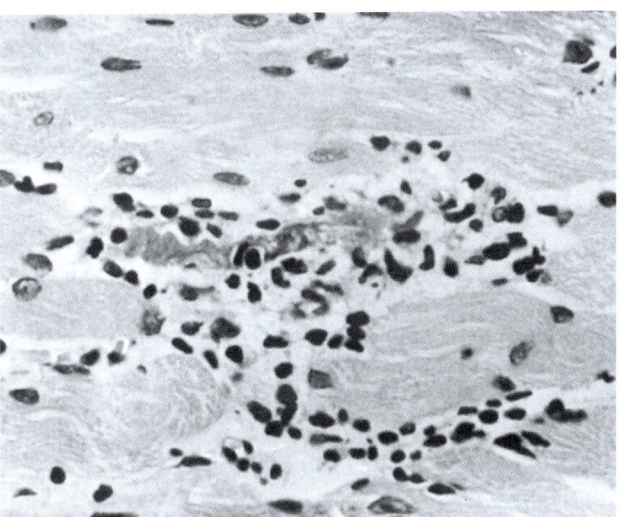

FIGURE 27-39 • Congenital "polymyositis" is indistinguishable from congenital muscular dystrophy except for occasional foci of necrotizing myositis. Contractures regressed and creatinine kinase normalized without therapy. (Hematoxylin and eosin stain; original magnification ×640.)

INFLAMMATORY MYOPATHY

Infectious Myositis

Acute, generalized myopathy may accompany acute bacterial or viral infections and may be severe enough to cause pigmenturia due to the release of myoglobin from damaged fibers. Local bacterial myositis may result by extension from cellulitis or acute necrotizing fasciitis, and it often follows trauma. A syndrome of "spontaneous" multifocal pyomyositis is prevalent in the tropics; most of these cases are due to Staphylococcus aureus sepsis (187).

Myalgia is a common component of the general malaise associated with flulike respiratory illnesses and may be exceptionally severe (188). Viruses most often implicated in acute myopathy include influenza virus and enteroviruses, particularly coxsackievirus and echovirus. Muscle biopsy in these cases has shown focal muscle fiber necrosis without inflammation or overt myositis. Virus has been recovered directly from muscle only rarely, and putative morphologic evidence for acute viral infection of muscle fibers is unconvincing. A cautionary note: muscle glycogen may be rearranged in a crystalline form, which resembles picornavirus particles in both antemortem and postmortem specimens (189,190). The serologic evidence that chronic inflammatory myopathy is associated with coxsackievirus type B is intriguing but inconclusive (191).

Local Myositis

Primary, noninfectious fasciitis arises in a variety of circumstances more common in adults than in children. Significant fasciitis is most likely to be encountered in full-thickness biopsy specimens in linear scleroderma, morphea, rheumatic fever, systemic sclerosis, or rheumatoid arthritis or in the syndrome of fasciitis with eosinophilia (192,193). Focal interstitial lymphocytic myositis is limited to the connective tissue framework of muscle contiguous with the involved fascia. Muscle fibers tend to be spared. Overlying fasciitis is surprisingly uncommon in juvenile dermatomyositis (JDM).

Macrophagic myofasciitis is a recently described histologically distinctive focal lesion incidentally encountered in muscle biopsies from adults and children performed to investigate muscle pain, fatigue and, often to rule out an underlying metabolic disorder as a cause of developmental delay (194). The macrophages contain cytoplasmic deposits of slate grey material that contain aluminum salts. Controversy exists over possible relationship to systemic disease, but the lesion is probably an innocuous local reaction to insoluble components of injected vaccines (195).

Local myositis, unrelated to fasciitis, infection, or overt trauma, is a self-limited, histologically florid, true myositis of undetermined cause (196). Changes seen in biopsy specimens from these tender lesions may resemble those of polymyositis.

IDIOPATHIC INFLAMMATORY MYOPATHY

Idiopathic inflammatory myopathy is a generic category that includes the childhood and adult forms of dermatomyositis, polymyositis as a component of systemic collagen–vascular disease, or in association with neoplasia (197). JDM and polymyositis are clinically and pathologically distinct diseases; the former is by far more common in children. Polymyositis also occurs in chronic HIV infection, certain drug reactions, and in chronic graft-versus-host disease.

JDM (juvenile dermatomyositis) is a clinically and morphologically distinct multisystem autoimmune disease (198,199) that is more common in girls usually with onset after the age of 5 years. Links to HLA-B8, and more recently, to HLA-DQA1, are reported (200). In a typical case, rash, insidious onset of fatigue, weight loss, and low-grade fever are accompanied by mucositis, arthralgia, myalgia, dysphonia, and dysphagia. Weakness, tenderness, and reduction in muscle mass most severely affect the proximal muscles. The skin lesion is a distinctive erythematous maculopapular rash involving the face and the extensor surfaces of the elbows, knees, and knuckles. The rash may be transient or subtle, but patients who never display it are rare. A few patients exhibit typical skin changes, but muscle involvement is delayed or never appears. Calcinosis cutis is common in chronic JDM, is usually not present initially, and has been linked to delay in diagnosis or therapy (201) (see Chapter 26).

Aids in establishing a diagnosis include elevated serum creatine kinase levels and electromyography, which usually reveals widespread signs of sarcolemmal membrane instability and nonuniform muscle fiber destruction. Noninvasive imaging methods help select a biopsy site and evaluate response to therapy (202). MRI evidence of involvement of subcutaneous fat may predict an aggressive chronic course (203). Tests for antinuclear antibodies, rheumatoid factor, and antimyoglobin are typically negative but may be transiently positive. A few patients eventually develop clinical and serologic features indicating another connective tissue disease, such as systemic lupus erythematosus or mixed connective tissue disease. Overlap occurs with some features of scleroderma (scleromyositis), but true systemic sclerosis is exceptionally rare in children.

Muscle biopsy is not necessary in typical cases but is useful in clinically uncertain cases and would find greater use if findings had predictive value for chronic disease, as has been suggested (204,205). Nondiagnostic muscle biopsy in a patient with inflammatory myopathy can result from nonuniform distribution of myositis, but subtle changes are easily overlooked. Efficiency is maximized by performing the muscle biopsy before starting therapy, sampling a muscle group that is clinically involved, and using immunostains to highlight subtle infiltration of inflammatory cells. Electron microscopy and direct immunofluorescence techniques increase detection of diagnostic microangiopathy. Selective expression on and beneath the sarcolemma of

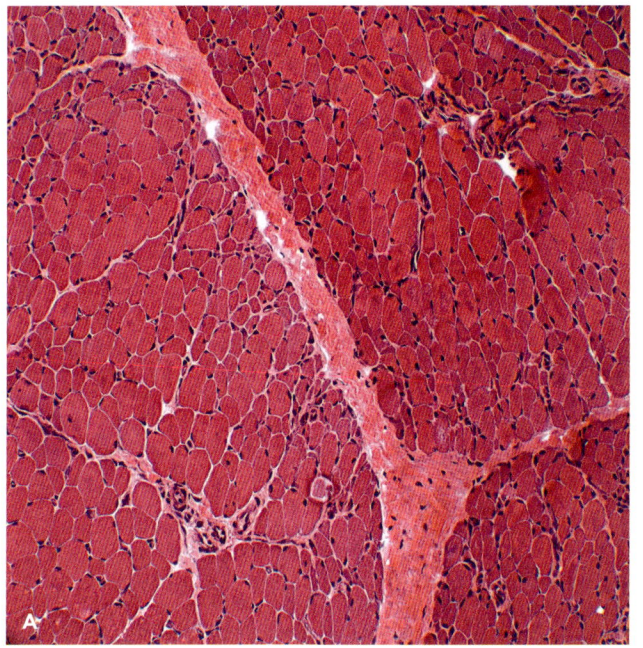
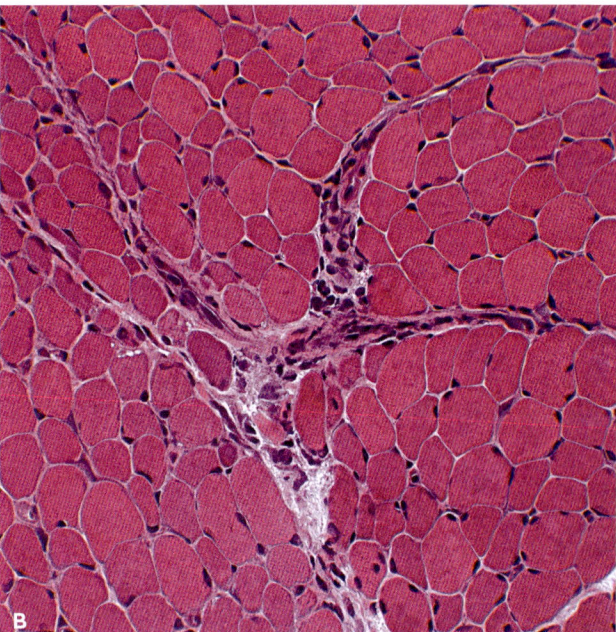
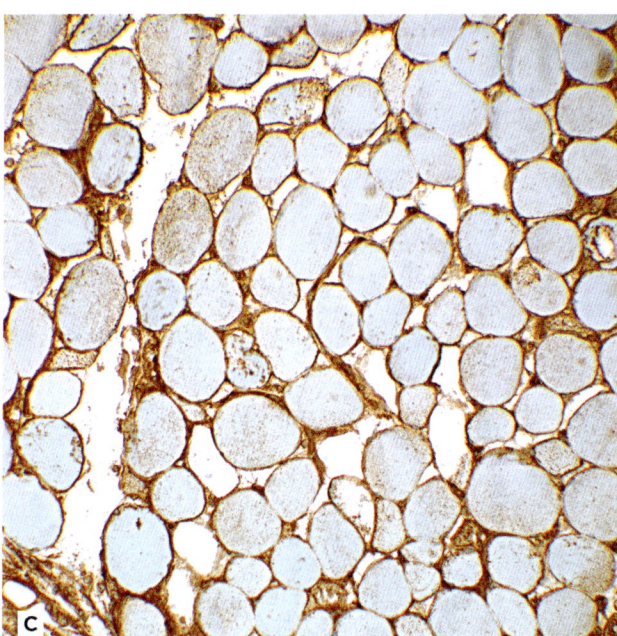

FIGURE 27-40 • **A:** Muscle in juvenile dermatomyositis (JDM) exhibiting selective fiber atrophy at the periphery of fascicles. (Hematoxylin and eosin stain; original magnification x200.) **B:** Mononuclear cell perivenulitis in JDM may coexist with true venulitis. CD68-positive macrophages, T cells, and less commonly B cells are demonstrable in this location. (Hematoxylin and eosin stain; original magnification x400.) **C:** Selective expression on and beneath the sarcolemma of class I histocompatibility antigens. (Class I histocompatibility antigen immunostain; original magnification x400.)

class II histocompatibility antigens in polymyositis (206) and class I histocompatibility antigens in JDM (207) (see Figure 27-41C) is extremely useful in muscle biopsy evaluation for inflammatory myopathy.

Histologic changes in new-onset JDM are highly variable and may be unexpectedly slight in patients who are profoundly weak. Myopathic/atrophic muscle fibers are usually more obvious at the periphery of muscle fascicles (Figure 27-40A). Necrosis may be absent or involve single fibers or small clusters of fibers with preservation of the sarcolemma. Infarcts are very uncommon. Perifascicular collagen fibers often are swollen and separated by interstitial fluid. Macrophages and lymphocytes aggregate around perimysial veins and may also infiltrate muscle fascicles (Figure 27-40B). In most cases, the small muscular arteries appear normal. However, the small arteries in muscle and subcutaneous fat may exhibit noninflammatory intimal cell swelling, degeneration, or lumen occlusion by cellular debris and fibrin, a thrombotic microangiopathy (Figure 27-41A.) The microangiopathy may cause ischemia that contributes to necrosis in skin, subcutaneous fat, and gastrointestinal tract (Figure 27-41B).

The microangiopathy is characterized by deposits of (Figure 27-41C and 27-42A) fibrin, IgM, Clq, C3, and C5 alone or as a component of C5-8 membrane attack complex (208). Virtually, all cases of active pretreatment JDM

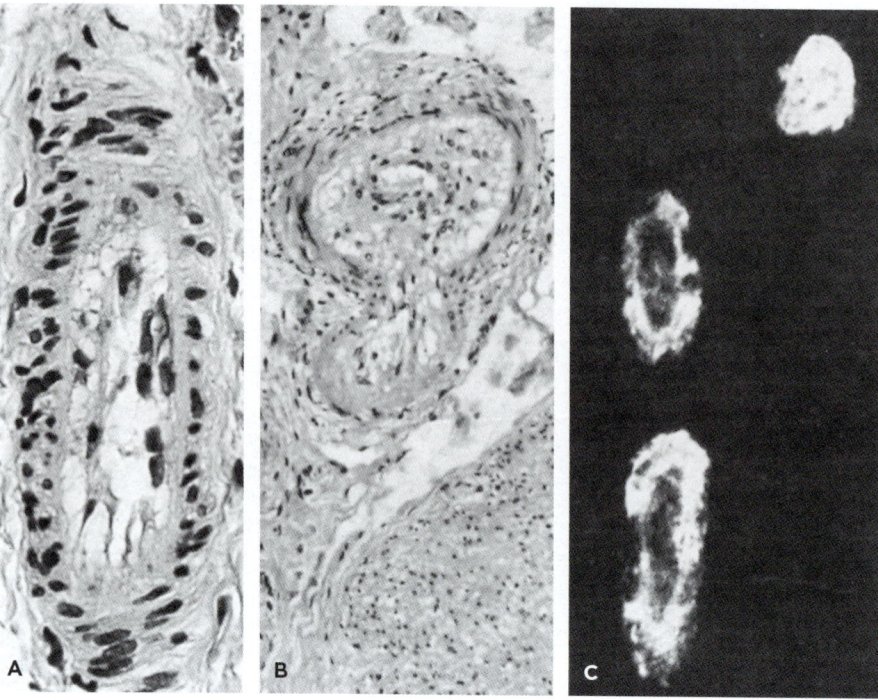

FIGURE 27-41 • **A:** Acute intimal arteriopathy in juvenile dermatomyositis (JDM). Endothelial cells are reactive. Prominent vacuolar changes usually reflect neutral lipid deposition. (Hematoxylin and eosin stain; original magnification ×800.) **B:** Chronic arteriopathy in JDM. Occlusive changes resulting from subintimal proliferation cause ischemic damage to the gut, skin, and muscle. (Hematoxylin and eosin stain; original magnification ×400.) **C:** JDM involvement displays positive direct fluorescence reaction in intramuscular arteries. (Anti-C3 stain; original magnification ×400.)

have ultrastructural evidence of endothelial cell alterations, including tubuloreticular inclusions, cytoplasmic swelling, and necrosis (Figure 27-42B, C). Similar inclusions also occur in lupus myositis and nephritis and occur in a variety of cell types, including circulating lymphocytes; it is possible that these inclusions result from complement-mediated cellular injury. The universal capillaropathy of JDM may resolve or permanent capillary obliteration may result (Figure 27-42D).

In contrast, polymyositis (inflammatory myopathy without rash), which is seen much more commonly in adults than in children, displays less prominent perivascular infiltrates, lacks a vasculopathy, and has a higher proportion of intrafascicular cytotoxic CD8 cells and macrophages locally reactive to isolated necrotic muscle fibers (Figure 27-43) (209). That finding is compatible with a cell-mediated cytotoxicity model.

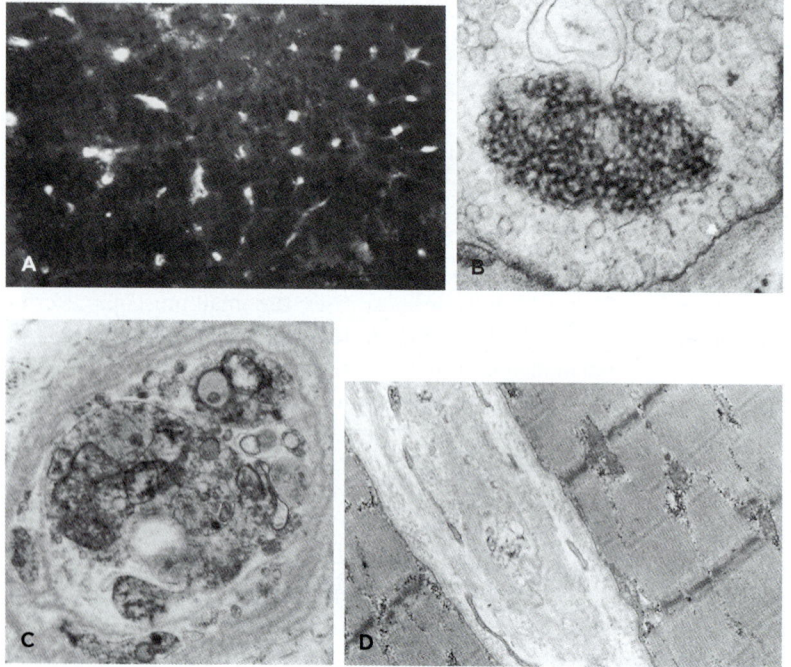

FIGURE 27-42 • **A:** Juvenile dermatomyositis (JDM) is apparent with positive direct immunofluorescence reaction in the intrafascicular muscle capillary bed. (Antifibrin stain; original magnification ×400.) **B:** JDM tubuloreticular inclusions are present in the endothelial cytoplasm. (Uranyl acetate and lead citrate stain; original magnification ×20,000.) **C:** In JDM, a capillary is occluded by cell debris and marked basement membrane redundancy. (Uranyl acetate and lead citrate stain; original magnification ×950.) **D:** Capillary obsolescence is present in chronic JDM. (Uranyl acetate and lead citrate stain; original magnification ×4,500.)

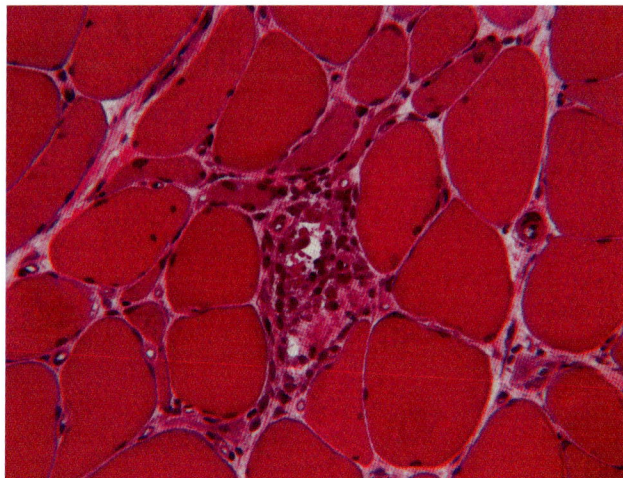

FIGURE 27-43 • Multifocal muscle fiber necrosis without histologic features of JDM in this child with arthritis/arthralgia, rheumatoid factor, antinuclear antibody, and no rash suggests polymyositis associated with a connective tissue disease. (Hematoxylin and eosin stain; original magnification ×200.)

Favorable outcome of JDM correlates directly with early treatment and is adversely influenced by the severity of the vasculopathy and prevalence of muscle fiber necrosis in pretreatment specimens (204,205). Cutaneous ulcers and gastrointestinal catastrophes, resulting from occlusive arteriopathy, are a common cause of morbidity and mortality. Many patients respond dramatically to therapy whereas others develop a chronic form of the disease.

References

1. Kablar B, Asakura A, Krastel K, et al. MyoD and Myf-5 define the specification of musculature of distinct embryonic origin. *Biochem Cell Biol* 1998;76:1079–1091.
2. Shi X, Garry DJ. Muscle stem cells in development, regeneration and disease. *Genes Dev* 2006;20:1692–1708.
3. Sarnat HB. Vimentin and desmin in maturing skeletal muscle and developmental myopathies. *Neurology* 1992;42:1616–1624.
4. Hug G, Bove K, Soukup S. Lethal neonatal multiorgan deficiency of carnitine palmitoyl transferase II. *N Engl J Med* 1991;325:1862–1864.
5. Vogler CA, Bove KE. Morphology of skeletal muscle in children. An assessment of normal growth and differentiation. *Arch Pathol Lab Med* 1985;109:238–242.
6. Brooke MH, Engel WK. The histographic analysis of human muscle biopsies with regard to fiber type: IV. Children's biopsies. *Neurology* 1969;19:591–605.
7. David TJ, Winter RM. Familial absence of the pectoralis major, serratus anterior and latissimus muscles. *J Med Genet* 1985;22:390–392.
8. Parker DL, Mitchell PR, Holmes GL. Poland-Mobius syndrome. *J Med Genet* 1981;18:317–320.
9. Bersu ET. Anatomical analysis of the developmental effects of aneuploidy in man: the Down syndrome. *Am J Med Genet* 1980;5:399–420.
10. Petterson JC, Colacino SC, Koltis GG, et al. A muscle phenotype characteristic of trisomy 13 based upon 8 subjects. *Pediatr Pathol* 1986;5:109(abst).
11. Ramirez-Castro JL, Bersu ET. Anatomical analysis of the developmental effects of aneuploidy in man—the trisomy 18 syndrome: II. Anomalies of the upper and lower limbs. *Am J Med Genet* 1978;2:285–306.
12. Manivel JC, Pettinato G, Reinberg Y, et al. Prune belly syndrome: clinicopathologic study of 29 cases. *Pediatr Pathol* 1989;9:691–711.
13. Goldstein JD, Reid LM. Pulmonary hypoplasia resulting from phrenic nerve agenesis and diaphragmatic amyoplasia. *J Pediatr* 1980;97:282–287.
14. Bove KE, Iannaccone ST. Atypical infantile spinomuscular atrophy presenting as acute diaphragmatic paralysis. *Pediatr Pathol* 1988;8:95–107.
15. Chudley AE, Barmada MA. Diaphragmatic elevation in neonatal myotonic dystrophy. *Am J Dis Child* 1979;133:1182–1185.
16. McWilliam RC, Gardner-Medwin D, Doyle D, et al. Diaphragmatic paralysis due to spinal muscular atrophy. *Arch Dis Child* 1985;60:145–149.
17. Hall JG. Analysis of Pena Shokeir phenotype. *Am J Med Genet* 1986;25:99–117.
18. Moessinger AC. Fetal akinesia deformation sequence. An animal model. *Pediatrics* 1983;72:857–863.
19. Witters I, Moerman P, Fryns JP. Fetal akinesia deformation sequence: a study of 30 consecutive in-utero diagnoses. *Am J Med Genet* 2002;15:23–28.
20. Reed SD, Hall JG, Riccardi VM, et al. Chromosomal abnormalities associated with congenital contractures (arthrogryposis). *Clin Genet* 1985;27:353–372.
21. Latta RJ, Graham CB, Aase JM, et al. Larsen's syndrome: a skeletal dysplasia with multiple joint dislocations and unusual facies. *J Pediatr* 1971;78:291–298.
22. Witt DR, Hayden MR, et al. Restrictive dermopathy: a newly recognized autosomal recessive skin dysplasia. *Am J Med Genet* 1986;24:631–648.
23. Muntoni F, Voit T. The congenital muscular dystrophies in 2004: a century of exciting progress. *Neuromuscul Disord* 2004;14:635–649.
24. Kho N, Czarnecki L, Kerrigan JF, et al. Pena-Shokier phenotype: case presentation and review. *J Child Neurol* 2002;17:397–399.
25. Hoganson G, Berlow S, Gilbert E, et al. Glutaric acidemia type II and flavin-dependent enzymes in morphogenesis. *Birth Defects Orig Artic Ser* 1987;23:65–74.
26. Miller ME, Higgenbottom MC, Smith DW. Short umbilical cord: its origin and relevance. *Pediatrics* 1981;67:618–621.
27. Banker BQ. Arthrogryposis multiplex congenita: spectrum of pathologic changes. *Hum Pathol* 1986;17:656–672.
28. Clarren SK, Hall JG. Neuropathologic findings in the spinal cords of 10 infants with arthrogryposis. *J Neurol Sci* 1983;58:89–102.
29. Kang PB, Lidov HG, David WS, et al. Diagnostic value of electromyography and muscle biopsy in arthrogryposis multiplex congenita. *Ann Neurol* 2003;54:790–795.
30. Agapitos M, Georgiou-Theodoropoulu M, Koutselinis A, et al. Arthrogryposis multiplex congenita, Pena-Shokier phenotype, with gastroschisis and agenesis of the leg. *Pediatr Pathol* 1988;8:409–413.
31. Lindhout D, Hageman G, et al. The Pena-Shokeir syndrome: report of nine Dutch cases. *Am J Med Genet* 1985;21:655–668.
32. Ouvrier RA, McLeod JG, Conchin TE. The hypertrophic forms of hereditary motor and sensory neuropathy. *Brain* 1987;110:121–148.
33. Moerman PH, Godderis P, Lauwerijns JM. Multiple ankyloses, facial anomalies and pulmonary hypoplasia associated with antenatal spinal muscular atrophy. *J Pediatr* 1983;103:238–241.
34. Choi BH, Ruess WR, Kim RC. Disturbances in neuronal migration and laminar cortical organization associated with multicystic encephalopathy in Pena-Shokier syndrome. *Acta Neuropathol* 1986;69:177–183.
35. Dimmick JE, Berry K, MacLeod PM, et al. Syndrome of ankylosis, facial anomalies and pulmonary hypoplasia: a pathologic analysis of one infant. In: Bergsma D, ed. *Embryology and Pathogenesis and Prenatal Diagnosis*, vol 13. New York: Alan R. Liss, 1977:133–137.
36. Dubowitz V, Brooke MH. *Muscle Biopsy: A Modern Approach*. London: WB Saunders, 1973:475.
37. Sarnat HB. *Muscle Pathology and Histochemistry*. Chicago, IL: American Society of Clinical Pathologists Press, 1983.
38. Cuisset JM, Maurage CA, Carpentier A, et al. Muscle biopsy in children: usefulness in 2012. *Rev Neurol (Paris)* 2013;169:632–639.
39. Gibreel WO, Selcen D, Zeiden MM, et al. Safety and yield of muscle biopsy in pediatric patients in the modern era. *J Pediatr Surg* 2014;49:1429–1432.

40. Johnson MA, Polgar J, Weightman D, et al. Data on the distribution of fiber types in thirty-six human muscles. *J Neurol Sci* 1973;18:111–129.
41. Lexell J, Downham D, Sjostrom M. Distribution of different fibre types in human skeletal muscles. A statistical and computational model for the study of fibre type grouping and early diagnosis of skeletal muscle fibre denervation and reinnervation. *J Neurol Sci* 1983;61:301–314.
42. Sallum AM, Varsani H, Holton JL, et al. Morphometric analysis of normal pediatric brachial and quadriceps muscle tissue. *Histol Histopathol* 2013;28:525–530.
43. Dastur DK, Daver SM, Manghani DK. Changes in muscle in human malnutrition with an emphasis on the fine structure in protein-calorie malnutrition. In: Zimmerman HM, ed. *Progress in Neuropathology*, vol 4. New York: Raven Press, 1979:29.
44. Robinson AJ, Clamann HP. Effects of glucocorticoids on motor units in cat hindlimb muscles. *Muscle Nerve* 1988;11:703–713.
45. Khan A, Sarnat HB, Spaetgens R. Congenital muscle fiber-type disproportion in a patient with congenital hypoventilation syndrome due to PHOX2B mutations. *J Child Neurol* 2008;23:829–831
46. Iannaccone ST, Bove KE, Vogler CA, et al. Type I fiber size disproportion. Morphometric data from 37 children with myopathic, neuropathic or idiopathic hypotonia. *Pediatr Pathol* 1987;7:395–419.
47. DeVito DC, DiMauro S. Mitochondrial defects of brain and muscle. *Biol Neonate* 1990;58(Suppl 1):54.
48. Castle ME, Reyman TA, Schneider M. Pathology of spastic muscle in cerebral palsy. *Clin Orthop Relat Res* 1979;142:223–232.
49. Schmitt HP, Volk B. The relationship between target targetoid and targetoid/core fibers in severe neurogenic muscular atrophy. *J Neurol* 1975;210:167–181.
50. Sladky JT, Rorke LB. Perinatal hypoxic/ischemic spinal cord injury. *Pediatr Pathol* 1986;6:87–101.
51. Monani UR, DeVivo DC. Neurodegeneration in spinomuscular atrophy: from disease phenotype and animal models to therapeutic strategies and beyond. *Future Neurol* 2014;9:49–65.
52. Tiziano FD, Melki J, Simard LR. Solving the puzzle of spinal muscular atrophy: what are the missing pieces? *Am J Med Genet A* 2013;161A:2836–2845.
53. Peeters K, Chamova T, Jordanova A. Clinical and genetic diversity of SMN1-negative proximal spinal muscular atrophies. *Brain* 2014;137(Pt 11):2879–2896.
54. Kaindl AM, Geunther UP, Rudnik-Schoneborn S, et al. Spinal muscular atrophy with respiratory distress type 1 (SMARD1). *J Child Neurol* 2008;23:199–204.
55. Dlamini N, Josifova DJ, Paine SM, et al. Clinical and neuropathological features of X-linked spinal muscular atrophy (SMAX2) associated with a novel mutation in the UBA1 gene. *Neuromuscul Disord* 2013;23:391–398.
56. Choi BO, Koo SK, Park MH, et al. Exome sequencing is an efficient tool for genetic screening of Charcot-Marie-Tooth disease, *Hum Mutat* 2012;33:1610–1615.
57. Baets J, De Jongh P, Timmerman V. Recent advances in Charcot-Marie-Tooth disease. *Curr Opin Neurol* 2014;27(5):532–540.
58. Charnas L, Trapp B, Griffin J. Congenital absence of peripheral myelin: abnormal Schwann cell development causes lethal arthrogryposis multiplex congenita. *Neurology* 1988;38:966–974.
59. Shorer Z, Philpot J, Muntoni F, et al. Demyelinating peripheral neuropathy in merosin-deficient congenital muscular dystrophy. *J Child Neurol* 1995;10:472–475.
60. Kararizou E, Karandreas N, Davaki P, et al. Polyneuropathies in teenagers: a clinicopathological study of 45 cases. *Neuromuscul Disord* 2006;16:304–307.
61. Sladky JT, Brown MJ, Berman PH. Chronic inflammatory demyelinating polyneuropathy of infancy: a corticosteroid responsive disorder. *Ann Neurol* 1986;20:76–81.
62. Sommer C, Koch S, Lammens M, et al. Macrophage clustering as a diagnostic marker in sural nerve biopsies of patients with CIDP. *Neurology* 2005;65:1924–1929.
63. Bouillot S, Martin-negrier ML, Vital A, et al. Peripheral neuropathy associated with mitochondrial disorders: 8 cases and review of the literature. *J Peripher Nerv Syst* 2002;7:213–220.
64. Landrieu P, Selva J, Alvarez F, et al. Peripheral nerve involvement in children with chronic cholestasis and vitamin E deficiency. A clinical, electrophysiological and morphological study. *Neuropediatrics* 1985;16:194–201.
65. Sokol R, Guggenheim M, et al. Improved neurologic function after long-term treatment of vitamin E deficiency in children with chronic cholestasis. *N Engl J Med* 1985;313:1580–1586.
66. Kinali M, Beeson D, Pitt MC, et al. Congenital myasthenic syndromes in childhood: diagnostic and management challenges. *J Neuroimmunol* 2008;201-202:6–12.
67. Kress JP, Hall JB. ICU-acquired weakness and recovery from critical illness. *N Engl J Med* 2014;370:1626–1635.
68. Rutledge ML, Hawkins EP, Langston C. Skeletal muscle growth failure induced in premature newborn infants by prolonged pancuronium treatment. *J Pediatr* 1986;109:883–886.
69. Sinha SK, Levene ML. Pancuronium bromide induced joint contractures in the newborn. *Arch Dis Child* 1984;59:7375.
70. North KN. Clinical approach to the diagnosis of congenital myopathies. *Semin Pediatr Neurol* 2011;18:216–220.
71. Nowak KJ, Ravenscroft G, Laing NG. Skeletal muscle alpha-actin diseases (actinopathies): pathology and mechanisms. *Acta Neuropathol* 2013;125:19–32.
72. Al-Rawaishid A, Vaisar J, Tein I, et al. Centronuclear myopathy and cardiomyopathy requiring transplant. *Brain Dev* 2003;25:62–66.
73. DeAngelis MS, Palmucci L, Leone M, et al. Centronuclear myopathy: clinical, morphological and genetic characters. A review of 288 cases. *J Neurol Sci* 1991;103:2–9.
74. Silver MM, Gilbert JJ, Stewart S, et al. Morphologic and morphometric analysis of muscle in X-linked myotubular myopathy. *Hum Pathol* 1986;7:1167–1178.
75. Romero NB. Centronuclear myopathies: a widening concept. *Neuromuscul Disord* 2010;20:223–228.
76. Pierson CR, Tomczak K, Agrawal P, et al. X-linked myotubular and centronuclear myopathies. *J Neuropathol Exp Neurol* 2005;64;555–564.
77. Wallgren-Pettersson C, Sewry CA, Nowak KJ et al. Nemaline myopathies. *Semin Pediatr Neurol* 2011;18:230–238.
78. Lehtokari VL, Pelin K, Sandbacka M, et al. Identification of 45 novel mutations in the nebulin gene associated with recessive nemaline myopathy. *Hum Mutat* 2006;27:946–956.
79. Hutchinson DO, Charlton A, Laing NG, et al. Autosomal dominant nemaline myopathy with intranuclear rods due to mutation of skeletal muscle ACTA1 gene: clinical and pathological variability within a kindred. *Neuromuscul Disord* 2006;16:113–121.
80. Agrawal PB, Greenleaf RS, Tomszak KK, et al. Nemaline myopathy with minicores caused by mutation of the CFL2 gene encoding the skeletal muscle actin-binding protein, cofilin2. *Am J Hum Genet* 2007;80:162–167.
81. Jungbluth H, Sewry CA, Muntoni F. Core myopathies. *Semin Pediatr Neurol* 2011;18:239–249.
82. Loke J, MacLennon DH. Malignant hyperthermia and central core disease: disorders of Ca2+ release channels. *Am J Med* 1998;104:470–486.
83. Robinson R, Carpenter D, Shaw MA, et al. Mutations in RYR1 in malignant hyperthermia and central core disease. *Hum Mutat* 2006;27:977–989.
84. Scacheri PC, Hoffman EP, Fratkin JD, et al. A novel ryanodine receptor gene mutation causing both cores and rods in congenital myopathy. *Neurology* 2000;12:1689–1696.
85. Jungbluth H, Sewry C, Brown SC, et al. Minicore myopathy in children: a clinical and histopathological study of 19 cases. *Neuromuscul Disord* 2000;10:264–273.
86. Clarke NF. Congenital fiber-type disproportion. *Semin Pediatr Neurol* 2011;18:264–271.
87. Clarke NF, North KN. Congenital fiber type disproportion—30 years on. *J Neuropathol Exp Neurol* 2003;62:977–989.

88. Laing NG, Clarke NF, Dye DE, et al. Actin mutations are one cause of congenital fiber type disproportion. *Ann Neurol* 2004;56:689–694.
89. Goebel HH, Blaschek A. Protein aggregation in congenital myopathies. *Semin Pediatr Neurol* 2011;18:272–276.
90. Selcen D, Ohno K, Engel AG. Myofibrillar myopathy: clinical morphologicaland genetic studies. *Brain* 2004;127:439–451.
91. Claeys KG, Fardeau M. Myofibrillar myopathies. *Handb Clin Neurol* 2013;113:1337–1342.
92. Forrest KM, Al-Sarraj S, Sewry C, et al. Infantile onset myofibrillar myopathy due to recessive CRYAB mutations. *Neuromuscul Disord* 2011;21;37–40.
93. Schessl J, Taratuto AL, Cewry C, et al. Clinical histological and genetic characterization of reducing body myopathy caused by mutations in FHL1. *Brain* 2009;132:452–464.
94. Buchino JJ, Bove KE, Iannaccone ST. Transient cytoplasmic bodies in muscle of three infants with Werdnig-Hoffmann disease. *Pediatr Pathol* 1990;10:563–573.
95. Patel H, Berry K, MacLeod P, et al. Cytoplasmic body myopathy: report on a family and review of the literature. *J Neurol Sci* 1983;60:281–292.
96. Carpenter S, Karpati G. Lysosomal storage in human skeletal muscle. *Hum Pathol* 1986;17:683–703.
97. DiMauro S, Costanza Lamperti. Muscle glycogenoses. *Muscle Nerve* 2001;24:984–999.
98. Raben N, Fukuda T, Gilbert AL, et al. Replacing acid alpha-glucosidase in Pompe disease: recombinant and transgenic enzymes are equipotent, but neither completely clears glycogen from type II muscle fibers. *Mol Ther* 2005;11:48–56.
99. Thurberg BL, Maloney CL, Vaccaro C, et al. Characterization of pre- and post-treatment pathology after enzyme replacement therapy for Pompe disease. *Lab Invest* 2006;86:1208–1220.
100. Umapathysivam K, Hopwood JJ, Meikle PJ. Correlation of alpha-glucosidase and glycogen content in skin fibroblasts with age of onset in Pompe disease. *Clin Chim Acta* 2005;361:191–198.
101. Palmer RE, Amartino HM, Niizawa G, et al. Pompe disease (glycogen storage disease type II) in Argentineans: clinical Manifestations and identification of 9 novel mutations. *Neuromuscul Disord* 2007;17:16–22.
102. Bruno C, van Diggelen OP, Cassandrini D, et al. Clinical and genetic heterogeneity of branching enzyme deficiency (glycogenosis type IV). *Neurology* 2004;63:1053–1058.
103. Worby CA, Gentry MS, Dixon JE. Laforin, a dual specificity phosphatase that dephosphorylates complex carbohydrates. *J Biol Chem* 2006;281:30412–30418.
104. Greene CM, Weldon DE, Ferrans VJ, et al. Juvenile polysaccharidosis with cardioskeletal myopathy. *Arch Pathol Lab Med* 1987;111:977–982.
105. Allison F, Bennett MJ, Variend S, et al. Acylcoenzyme A dehydrogenase deficiency in heart tissue from infants who die unexpectedly with fatty change in the liver. *Br Med J* 1988;296:11–12.
106. Roe CR, Millington DS, Maltby DA, et al. Recognition of medium-chain acyl-CoA dehydrogenase deficiency in asymptomatic siblings of children dying of sudden infant death or Reye-like syndromes. *J Pediatr* 1986;108:13–18.
107. Trumbull DM, Bartlett K, Stevens DL, et al. Short chain acyl-CoA dehydrogenase deficiency associated with lipid storage myopathy and secondary carnitine deficiency. *N Engl J Med* 1984;311:1232–1236.
108. Spiekerkoetter U. Mitochondrial fatty acid oxidation disorders: Clinical presentation of long-chain fatty oxidation defects before and after newborn screening. *J Inherit Metab Dis* 2010;33:527–532.
109. Bove KE. The metabolic crisis: a diagnostic challenge. *J Pediatr* 1997;131:181–182.
110. Chalmers RA, Stanley CA, English N, et al. Mitochondrial carnitine-acylcarnitine translocase deficiency presenting as sudden neonatal death. *J Pediatr* 1997;131:220.
111. Bank WJ, DiMauro S, Bonilla E, et al. A disorder of muscle lipid metabolism and myoglobinuria: absence of carnitine palmityl transferase. *N Engl J Med* 1975;292:443–449.
112. Longo N, Amat di San Fillipo C, Pasquali M. Disorders of carnitine transport and the carnitine cycle. *Am J Med Genet C Semin Med Genet* 2006;142:77–85.
113. DiMauro S, Schon EA, Carelli V, et al. The clinical maze of mitochondrial neurology. *Nat Rev Neurol* 2013;9(8):429–444.
114. Goldstein AC, Bhatia P, Vento JM. Mitochondrial disease in childhood: nuclear encoded. *Neurotherapeutics* 2013;10:212–226.
115. Bernier FP, Boneh A, Dennett X, et al. Diagnostic criteria for respiratory chain disorders in adults and children. *Neurology* 2002;59:1406–1411.
116. Darin N, Moslemi AR, Lebon S, et al. Genotypes and clinical phenotypes in children with cytochrome-c oxidase deficiency. *Neuropediatrics* 2003;34:311–317.
117. Shanske S, Wong LJ. Molecular analysis for mitochondrial DNA disorders. *Mitochondrion* 2004;4:403–415.
118. Hanson BJ, Capaldi RA, Marusich MF, et al. An immunohistochemical approach to detection of mitochondrial disorders. *J Histochem Cytochem* 2002;50:2181–1288.
119. Miles L, Bove KE, Wong B, et al. Investigation of children for mitochondriopathy confirms need for strict patient selection, improved morphological criteria, and better laboratory methods. *Hum Pathol* 2006;37:173–184.
120. Di Giovanni S, Mirabella M, Spinazzola A, et al. Coenzyme Q10 reverses pathological phenotype and reduces apoptosis in familial Co Q10 deficiency. *Neurology* 2001;57:515–518.
121. DiMauro S, Tanji K, Schon EA. The many clinical faces of cytochrome c oxidase deficiency. *Adv Exp Med Biol* 2012:748:341–357.
122. Finsterer J. Inherited mitochondrial disorders. *Adv Exp Med Biol* 2012:942:187–213.
123. Kaufmann P, Engelstad K, Wei Y, et al. Protean phenotypic features of the A3243G mitochondrial DNA mutation. *Arch Neurol* 2009;66:85–91.
124. Maceluch JA, Niedziela M. The clinical diagnosis and molecular genetics of kearns-sayre syndrome: a complex mitochondrial encephalomyopathy. *Pediatr Endocrinol Rev* 2006–2007;4:117–137.
125. Makino M, Horai S, Goto Y, et al. Mitochondrial DNA mutations in Leigh syndrome and their phylogenetic implications. *J Hum Genet* 2000;45(2):69–75.
126. Finsterer J, Ahting U. Mitochondrial depletion syndromes in children and adults. *Can J Neurol Sci* 2013;40(5):635–644.
127. Fishbein WN, Armbrustmacher VW, Griffin JL. Myoadenylate deaminase deficiency: a new disease of muscle. *Science* 1978;200:545–548.
128. Isackson PJ, Bujnicki H, Harding, CO, et al. Myoadenylate deaminase deficiency caused by alternate splicing due to a novel intronic mutation in the AMPD1 gene. *Mol Genet Metab* 2005;86:250–256.
129. Pantoja-Martinez J, Navarro Fernandez-Balbuena C, Gormaz-Moreno M, et al. Myoadenylate deaminase deficiency in a child with myalgias induced by physical exercise. *Rev Neurol* 2004;39:431–434.
130. Nagao H, Habara S, et al. AMP deaminase activity of skeletal muscle in neuromuscular disorders in childhood. Histochemical and biochemical studies. *Neuropediatrics* 1986;17:193–198.
131. Rossi LN, Cornelio F, et al. Myoadenylate deaminase deficiency in a 5-year-old boy with intermittent muscle pain. *Helv Paediatr Acta* 1984;39:89–93.
132. Shumate JB, Kaiser KK, Carroll JE, et al. Adenylate deaminase deficiency in a hypotonic infant. *J Pediatr* 1980;96:885–887.
133. Olpin SE, Afifi A, Clarke S, et al. Mutation and biochemical analysis in carnitine palmitoyltransferase type II (CPT II) deficiency. *J Inherit Metab Dis* 2003;26:543–557.
134. Melli G, Chaudhry V, Cornblath DR. Rhabdomyolysis: an evaluation of 475 hospitalized patients. *Medicine* 2005;84:377–385.
135. Tonin P, Lewis P, Servidei S, et al. Metabolic causes of myoglobinuria. *Ann Neurol* 1990;27:181–185.
136. Tsurui S, Sugie H, Ito M, et al. Clinical and biochemical analysis of 27 patients with myoglobinuria of unknown causes. *Clin Neurol (Japan)* 1995;35:24–28.
137. Elpeleg ON, Saada AB, Shaag A, et al. Lipoamide dehydrogenase deficiency: a new cause for recurrent myoglobinuria. *Muscle Nerve* 1997;20:238–240.
138. Kanno T, Maekawa M. Lactate dehydrogenase M-subunit deficiencies: clinical features, metabolic background, and genetic heterogeneities. *Muscle Nerve Suppl* 1995;3:S54–S60.

139. Keightley JA, Hoffbuhr KC, Burton MD, et al. A microdeletion in cytochrome c oxidase (COX) subunit III associated with COX deficiency and recurrent myoglobinuria. *Nat Genet* 1996;12:410–416.
140. Saunier P, Cretien D, Wood C, et al. Cytochrome c oxidase deficiency presenting as neonatal myoglobinuria. *Neuromuscul Disord* 1995;5:285–289.
141. Reuffert H, Olthoff D, Deutrich C, et al. Determination of a positive malignant hyperthermia (MH) disposition without the in vitro contraction test in families carrying the RYR1 Arg614Cys mutation. *Clin Genet* 2001;60:117–124.
142. Limongelli G, D'Alessandro R, Maddaloni V, et al. Skeletal muscle involvement in cardiomyopathies. *J Cardiovasc Med (Hagerstown)* 2013;14:837–861.
143. Selcen D. Myofibrillar myopathies. *Neuromuscul Disord* 2011;21:161–171.
144. Dhar R, Reardon W, McMahon CJ. Biventricular non-compaction hypertrophic cardiomyopathy in association with congenital complete heart block and type I mitochondrial complex deficiency. *Cardiol Young* 2014;15:1–3.
145. Zeviani M, Gellera C, Antozzi C, et al. Maternally-inherited myopathy and cardiomyopathy: association with mutation in mitochondrial DNA tRNA. *Lancet* 1991;338:143–147.
146. Neustein HB, Lurie PR, Dahms B, et al. An X-linked recessive cardiomyopathy with abnormal mitochondria. *Pediatrics* 1979;64:24–29.
147. Barth PG, Valianpour F, Bowen VM, et al. X-linked cardioskeletal myopathy and neutropenia (Barth Syndrome): an update. *Am J Med Genet* 2004;126:349–354.
148. Bertini E, Donati MA, Broda P, et al. Phenotypic heterogeneity in two unrelated Danon patients associated with LAMP-2 gene mutation. *Neuropediatrics* 2005;36:309–313.
149. Nishimo I. Autophagic vacuolar myopathy. *Semin Pediatr Neurol* 2006;13:90–95.
150. Morava E, Sengers R, Ter Laak H, et al. Congenital hypertrophic myopathy, cataract, mitochondrial myopathy and defective oxidative phosphorylation in two siblings with Senger-like syndrome. *Eur J Pediatr* 2004;163:467–471.
151. Adickes ED, Shuman RM. Fetal alcohol myopathy. *Pediatr Pathol* 1983;1:369–384.
152. Clarren SK, Smith DW. The fetal alcohol syndrome. *N Engl J Med* 1978;198:1063–1067.
153. Bennett HS, Spiro AJ, Pollack MA, et al. Ipecac-induced myopathy simulating dermatomyositis. *Neurology* 1982;32:91–94.
154. Carroll GJ, Will RK, Peter JB, et al. Penicillamine induced polymyositis and dermatomyositis. *J Rheumatol* 1987;14:995–101.
155. Watson AJ, Dalbow MH, et al. Immunologic studies in cimetidine induced nephropathy and polymyositis. *N Engl J Med* 1983;308:142–145.
156. Dalakas M, Illa I, Pezeshkpour GH, et al. Mitochondrial myopathy caused by long term zidovudine therapy. *N Engl J Med* 1990;332:1098–1105.
157. Emery AE. Population frequencies of inherited neuromuscular diseases-a world survey. *Neuromuscul Disord* 1991;1:19–29.
158. Dalkilic I, Kunkel LM. Muscular dystrophies: genes to pathogenesis. *Curr Opin Genet Dev* 2003;13;231–238.
159. Ferlini A, Neri M, Gualandi F. The medical genetics of dystrophinopathies: molecular genetic diagnosis and its impact on clinical practice. *Neuromuscul Disord* 2013;23:4–14.
160. Samaha FJ, Quinlan JG. Dystrophinopathies: clarification and complication. *J Child Neurol* 1996;11:13–20.
161. Flanigan KM, Dunn DM, von Niederhausern A, et al. Mutational spectrum of DMD mutations in dystrophinopathy patients: application of modern diagnostic techniques to a large cohort. *Hum Mutat* 2009;30:1657–1666.
162. Abbs S, Tuffery-Giraud S, Bakker E, et al. Best practice guidelines on molecular diagnostics in Duchenne/Becker muscular dystrophies. *Neuromuscul Disord* 2010;20:422–427.
163. Abbs S. Prenatal diagnosis of Duchenne and Becker muscular dystrophy. *Prenat Diagn* 1996;16:1187–1198.
164. Bodensteiner JB, Engel AG. Intracellular calcium accumulation in Duchenne dystrophy and other myopathies: a study of 567,000 muscle fibers in 114 biopsies. *Neurology* 1978;28:439–446.
165. Meola G, Cardani R. Myotonic dystrophies: an update on clinical aspects, genetic, pathology, and molecular pathomechanisms. *Biochim Biophys Acta* 2014.
166. Gardner-Medwin D, Johnston HM. Severe muscular dystrophy in girls. *J Neurol Sci* 1984;64:79–87.
167. Mitsuhashi S, Kang P. Update on the genetics of limb girdle muscular dystrophy. *Semin Pediatr Neurol* 2012;19:211–218.
168. Klinge L, Eagle M, Haggerty ID, et al. Severe phenotype in infantile facioscapulohumeral muscular dystrophy. *Neuromuscul Disord* 2006;16:553–558.
169. Ostlund C, Worman HJ. Nuclear envelope proteins and neuromuscular disease. *Muscle Nerve* 2003;27:393–406.
170. Kobayashi O, Hayashi Y, Arahata K, et al. Congenital muscular dystrophy: clinical and pathological study of 50 patients with the classical (Occidental) form. *Neurology* 1996;46:815–818.
171. Mendell JR, Boue DR, Martin PT. The congenital muscular dystrophies: recent advances and molecular insights. *Pediatr Dev Pathol* 2006;9:427–443.
172. Muntoni F, Voit T. The congenital muscular dystrophies in 2004: a century of exciting progress. *Neuromuscul Disord* 2004;14:635–649.
173. Philpot J, Pennock J, Cowan F, et al. Magnetic resonance imaging abnormalities in merosin-positive congenital muscular dystrophy. *Eur J Paediatr Neurol* 2000;4:109–114.
174. Villanova M, Malandrini A, Sabatelli P, et al. Localization of laminin alpha 2 chain in normal human central nervous system: an immunofluorescence and ultrastructural study. *Acta Neuropathol (Berl)* 1997;94:567–571.
175. Sewry CA, Philpot J, Sorokin LM, et al. Diagnosis of merosin (laminin-2) deficient congenital muscular dystrophy by skin biopsy. *Lancet* 1996;347:582–584.
176. Pegoraro E, Marks H, Garcia CA, et al. Laminin alpha2 muscular dystrophy: genotype/phenotype correlations of 22 patients. *Neurology* 1998;51:101–110.
177. Bonnemann CG. Collagen VI-related myopathies Ulrich congenital muscular dystrophy and Bethlem myopathy. *Hndb Clin Neurol* 2011;101:81–96.
178. Beltran-Valero de Bernabe D, Currier S, Steinbrecher A, et al. Mutations in the O-mannosyltransferase gene POMT1 give rise to the severe neuronal migration disorder Walker-Warburg syndrome. *Am J Hum Genet* 2002;71:1033–1043.
179. Fukuyama Y, Osawa M, Suzuki H. Congenital progressive muscular dystrophy of the Fukuyama type. Clinical, genetic and pathological considerations. *Brain Dev* 1981;3:1–29.
180. Toda T, Kobayashi K, Kondo-Lida E, et al. The Fukuyama congenital muscular dystrophy story. *Neuromuscul Disord* 2000;10:153–159.
181. Yoshida A, Kobayashi K, Manya H, et al. Muscular dystrophy and neuronal migration disorder caused by mutations in a glycosyltransferase, POMGnT1. *Dev Cell* 2001;1:717–724.
182. Longman C, Brockington M, Torelli S, et al. Mutations in the human LARGE gene cause MDC1D, a novel form of congenital muscular dystrophy with severe mental retardation and abnormal glycosylation of alpha-dystroglycan. *Hum Mol Genet* 2003;12:2853–2861.
183. Echenne B, Astruc J, et al. Congenital muscular dystrophy and rigid spine syndrome. *Neuropediatrics* 1983;14:97–101.
184. Ferreiro A, Quijano-Roy S, Pichereau C, et al. Mutations of the selenoprotein N gene, which is implicated in rigid spine muscular dystrophy, cause the classical phenotype of multiminicore disease: reassessing the nosology of early-onset myopathies. *Am J Hum Genet* 2002;71:739–749.
185. Claeys KG, Fardeau M. Myofibrillar myopathies. *Handbk Clin Neurol* 2013;113:1337–1342.
186. Shevell M, Rosenblatt B, Silver K, et al. Congenital inflammatory myopathy. *Neurology* 1990;40:111–114.
187. Shepherd JJ. Tropical myositis: is it an entity and what is its cause? *Lancet* 1983;2:1240–1242.
188. Bove KE, Partin JP, Farrell MK, et al. The morphology of myopathy associated with influenza B infection. *Pediatr Pathol* 1983;1:51–66.
189. Collins DN, Gilbert EF. Glycogen complexes in muscle in Reye's syndrome simulating virus-like particles. *Lab Invest* 1977;36:91–99.

190. Tang TT, Sedmak GV, Siegesmund KA, et al. Chronic myopathy associated with Coxsackie virus type A9. A combined electron microscopical and viral isolation study. *N Engl J Med* 1975;292:608–611.
191. Travers RL, Hughs GRV, Cambridge G, et al. Coxsackie B neutralisation titres in polymyositis/dermatomyositis [Letter]. *Lancet* 1977;1:1268.
192. Miller JJ. The fasciitis-morphea complex in children. *Am J Dis Child* 1992;146:733–736.
193. Simon DB, Ringel SP, Sufit RL. Clinical spectrum of fascial inflammation. *Muscle Nerve* 1982;5:525–537.
194. Lacson AG, D'Cruz CA, Gilbert-Barness E, et al. Aluminum phagocytosis in quadriceps muscle following vaccination in children: relationship to macrophagic myofasciitis. *Pediatr Dev Pathol* 2002 5:151–158.
195. Siegrist CA. Vaccine adjuvants and macrophagic myofasciitis. *Arch Pediatr* 2005;12:96–101.
196. Heffner RR, Armbrustmacher VW, Earle KM. Focal myositis. *Cancer* 1977;40:301–306.
197. Bohan A, Peter JB. Polymyositis and dermatomyositis (first of two parts). *N Engl J Med* 1975;292:344–347.
198. Bohan A, Peter JB. Polymyositis and dermatomyositis (second of two parts). *N Engl J Med* 1975;292:403–407.
199. Crowe WE, Bove KE, Levinson JE, et al. Clinical and pathogenetic implications of histopathology in childhood polydermatomyositis. *Arthritis Rheum* 1982;25:126–139.
200. Miller FW, Cooper RG, Vencvosky J, et al. Genome-wide association study of juvenile dermatomyositis reveals genetic overlap with other autoimmune disorders. *Arthritis Rheum* 2013;65:3239–3247.
201. Pachman LM, Hayford JR, Chung A, et al. Juvenile dermatomyositis at diagnosis: clinical characteristics in 79 children. *J Rheumatol* 1998;25:1198–1204.
202. Lofberg M, Liewendahl K, Lamminen A, et al. Antimyosin scintigraphy compared with magnetic resonance imaging in inflammatory myopathies. *Arch Neurol* 1998;55:987–993.
203. Ladd P, Emery K, Salisbury S, et al. Juvenile dermatomyositis: correlation of MRI at presentation with clinical outcome. *Am J Roentgenol* 2011;197:153–158.
204. Miles L, Bove KE, Lovell D, et al. The clinical course of juvenile dermatomyositis is predictable based on initial muscle biopsy: a retrospective study of 72 patients. *Arthritis Rheum* 2007;57:183–191.
205. Wargula JC, Lovell DJ, Passo MH, et al. What more can we learn from muscle histopathology in children with dermatomyositis/polymyositis? *Clin Exp Rheumatol* 2006;24:333–343.
206. Zuk JA, Fletcher A. Skeletal muscle expression of class II histocompatibility antigens (HLA-DR) in polymyositis and other muscle disorders with an inflammatory infiltrate. *J Clin Pathol* 1988;41:410–414.
207. Li CK, Varsani H, Holton JL, et al. MHC Class I overexpression on muscle in early juvenile dermatomyositis. *J Rheumatol* 2004;31:605–609.
208. Kissel JT, Mendell JR, Rammohan KW. Microvascular deposition of complement membrane attack complex in dermatomyositis. *N Engl J Med* 1986;314:329–334.
209. Emslie-Smith AM, Arahata K, Engel AG. Major histocompatibility complex class I antigen expression, immunolocalization of interferon subtypes and T-cell mediated cytotoxicity in myopathies. *Hum Pathol* 1989;20:224–231.

CHAPTER 28

Skeletal System

Louis P. Dehner, M.D., and Michael Kyriakos, M.D.

The complexity of the developing skeletal system was appreciated long before the advent of molecular biology. The molecular genetic understanding of skeletogenesis has continued to provide insights into the tightly regulated signaling pathways and transcription factors as highly conserved events throughout the vertebrate phyla (1–4). The morphologic events begin with the segregation of progenitor mesenchymal cells in the cranial portion of the neural crest (neuroectoderm) and mesoderm (craniofacial bone development, paraxial somite [axial skeleton], and lateral plate mesoderm [limb skeleton]). For instance, the neural crest cells have a central role in the development of bone and skeletal muscle in the head and neck (5). The blue print or patterning and migration are controlled by highly conserved transcriptional factors such as the HOX and PAX genes and their signaling pathways, which are integral to cell-to-cell communication and intracellular signaling. HOX genes are represented by 39 genes, which are critical for coordinated development of bone, tendons, and skeletal muscle in the axial and appendicular skeleton (6,7). Another set of developmental and patterning genes, PAX family, regulates the various pools of progenitor cells for various types of tissues, and the function of PAX1 is critical in the maintenance of a population of precursor mesenchymal cells for chondrogenesis (8). Mesenchymal cells after migration to their specific sites undergo the process of condensation whose end result is the formation of the 206 or so bones of the human skeleton. Once condensation has taken place, the next event is osteoblastic and chondrogenic differentiation, which is accompanied by a number of molecular events involved with lineage determination; SOX9 (SRY-box 9), a transcriptional factor gene, is critical in the differentiation of an osteochondral progenitor to a chondrocyte (9,10). Into this process of chondrogenesis and osteoblastogenesis, fibroblast growth factors and their high affinity receptors have critical roles in the activation of several transduction pathways (11). Goldring and associates (12) have pointed out that chondrogenesis is the earliest phase of skeletogenesis. Not only is SOX9 one of the earliest expressed genes in the condensation phase, but it is also necessary for the expression of COL2A1, which encodes the alpha-1 chain of type 2 collagen and other matrix proteins (13,14). The differentiation phase of chondrocytes occurs when two other members of the SOX family, SOX5 (SRY-box 5) and SOX6 (SRY-box 6), are expressed somewhat later than SOX9 (15,16). Extracellular matrix is synthesized with further chondrocytic differentiation to hypertrophic chondrocytes; these extracellular macromolecules include proteoglycans—aggrecan, decorin, biglycan, fibromodulin, and perlecan—in addition to collagens types II, IX, and XI (17). The next stage is the process of cartilage undergoing metamorphosis to bone (18). Just as SOX9 is critical in the development of chondroblasts, so the transcriptional factor, Runt-related 2 (Runx 2 or Cbfa-1) has a similar role in the differentiation of the osteoblast from the primordial osteochondral cell. The Runx 2 (Cbfa-1) is also involved in the development of the hypertrophic chondrocyte. In turn, there are several regulators of Runx 2 function.

The bones as the basic gross components of the skeleton develop by one of two processes, enchondral ossification in the formation of the appendicular and axial skeleton and membranous ossification in the formation of the craniofacial bones and portions of the clavicle (19–21). Membranous ossification is characterized by the direct differentiation of the common progenitor mesenchymal cell to an osteoblast even before the condensation stage; there is osteoid deposition with the formation of ossification centers that fuse into the platelike bone of the calvarium. The bone matrix proteins, osteocalcin/bone gla protein, collagen type 1, bone sialoprotein, and alkaline phosphatase, are induced by Runx 2 (Cbfa-1), which has been characterized as the "master regulator of osteoblast differentiation" despite the feat that Runx 2 does not induce osteoblastic differentiation alone, but interacts with TGF-β superfamily, bone morphogenic protein, and specific SMADs (22,23). Other important signaling molecules include Wnt/β-catenin and Hedgehog pathways (24,25).

Enchondral ossification requires the coordination of chondrocytes, osteoblasts, and osteoclasts. The osteoclast is a bone marrow–derived cell of the monocyte lineage, which is required for the process of bone remodeling. Following the stage of condensation (6 to 7 weeks of gestation), the formation of the cartilaginous anlage template (18 to 19 weeks of gestation) occurs in a proximal to distal fashion and in anterior before posterior structures. The primary center of ossification is found in the midshaft of the bone anlage in the vicinity of the hypertrophied or terminally differentiated chondrocytes (20,26,27). There is also vascular invasion as the hypertrophied chondrocytes express vascular endothelial growth factor. A periosteal bone collar is formed by mesenchymal cells that undergo osteoblastic differentiation to initiate the process of cortical bone formation. With the vascular invasion, hematopoietic precursors including preosteoclasts have gained access to the bone. Secondary centers of ossification are formed at the proximal and distal ends of the bone and are separated from the primary center by the growth plate where the epiphyseal cartilage proliferates, hypertrophies, and undergoes apoptosis (26,28). This latter process is in part under the control of the gene, Indian hedgehog. The invading front of ossification from the primary and secondary centers of ossification and the proliferating cartilage together account for bone growth.

We have not mentioned the roles of parathyroid hormone (PTH)-related peptide and its receptor, which is controlled by COL2A1 promoter and fibroblast growth factor receptor 3 (FGFR3) (28–30). The receptors are present on the cell membrane of the osteoblasts; the role of this receptor tyrosine kinase at the growth plate is an important one since activating mutations are involved in several types of skeletal dysplasia. The third basic cell type, the osteoclast, is a multinucleated cell of mononuclear phagocytic derivation whose function is bone matrix resorption through its resorptive organelle, the ruffled membrane (31). Defective function or differentiation of osteoclasts is the underlying pathogenesis of osteopetrosis (OP). Osteoblasts and osteoclasts interact through cytokines and growth factors, which serve to choreograph the initial modeling and remodeling of bone through autocrine, paracrine, and endocrine (parathormone) mechanisms (32). It has come to be appreciated that the osteoclast is more than a "bone-eater" but has a role in the regulation of hematopoiesis as well as immune response (33,34).

CONGENITAL AND DEVELOPMENTAL DISORDERS AND MALFORMATIONS

Skeletal anomalies consist of a broad range of anatomic defects, which may be an intrinsic abnormality in the development and growth of a single bone or is a generalized process affecting the entire skeleton as the manifestation of a mutated constitutional genetic determinant or an extrinsic teratogen (35–38). Examples of the former include the various chromosomal syndromes, heritable metabolic disorders, a multitude of congenital anomaly syndromes, and the numerous genetic skeletal disorders (GSDs) also known as skeletal dysplasias or osteochondrodysplasias. Several agents are well-documented or highly suspected teratogens affecting normal skeletal development (39–41) (Table 28-1). Some of the interpretive problems in the assessment of skeletal abnormalities as putatively teratogenic versus natural variations in skeletal development in humans are discussed thoughtfully elsewhere (42,43).

The estimated frequency of the various types of skeletal anomalies in children is derived from diverse sources including the experience of individual institutions, vital statistics, and registries (44,45). In one pediatric autopsy series that included children through 14 years of age, congenital anomalies and malformations were identified in 18% of cases; almost 20% of these were found in the skeletal system (46). Multiple organ anomalies were found in most of these children, and major musculoskeletal anomalies were documented at autopsy in 1.3% of previable fetuses and liveborn infants who died in the perinatal period with the exclusion of chromosomal syndromes (46). Major malformations of the limbs are found in approximately 2% of liveborn infants and minor limb abnormalities in another 5% to 7%. Overall, approximately 1:1000 neonates have some defective development of the limbs, most commonly limb reduction defects (LRDs) (44,46).

Among the three most common trisomy syndromes, trisomy 18 (Edwards syndrome) is characterized by overlapping fingers, radial aplasia, and other preaxial limb defects and less commonly rocker-bottom feet and equinovarus deformity, whereas trisomy 13 (Patau syndrome) has

TABLE 28-1 TERATOGEN AND SKELETAL ANOMALIES

Agent	Phenotype
Thalidomide	Phocomelia
Valproic acid and other antiepileptics	Limb reduction defects
	Polydactyly
Retinoids	"Lower limb defects"
Cyclophosphamide	Craniosynostosis
Warfarin	"Short limbs," stippled calcification of epiphyses of long bones, brachydactyly
Aminopterin	Craniosynostosis, oligodactyly, syndactyly, mesomelic shortening of forearms, talipes, equinovarus

postaxial polydactyly (47,48). Clinodactyly of the fifth finger with a hypoplastic middle phalanx is found in 50% to 60% of infants with trisomy 21 (49–51). Several other musculoskeletal abnormalities are found in the setting of trisomy 21 (52). Additional malformations of the axial skeleton in these three trisomic syndromes have been discussed elsewhere (52,53). Syndactyly and talipes equinovarus are the two most common limb anomalies in triploid fetuses (53).

Limb Reduction Defects

LRDs comprise one of the most common categories of congenital skeletal anomalies and is defined by the following anatomic categories: absence or hypoplasia of a phalanx, metacarpal, or metatarsal bone as a portion of any long bone with accompanying deformity; these anomalies are represented by the specific defects of amelia, aplasia to hypoplasia of individual long bones, oligodactyly, polydactyly, and syndactyly (Figure 28-1) (53,54). These developmental anomalies are seen as an isolated finding or as a component of a syndrome as one of several anomalies in other organ systems including the cardiovascular system, kidney, and intestinal tract. Approximately 70% to 75% of LRDs occur in the upper extremity, whereas 15% to 20% are detected in the lower extremity alone and both upper and lower in 10% of cases (55–58). The incidence of these defects is approximately 1:1000 to 2000 live births (59–61). LRDs are estimated to be present in 2% of perinatal autopsies and in less than 1% of stillborns (62). The genetic and developmental aspects of LRDs are discussed at length elsewhere (61,63,64).

The morphology of LRDs includes the following anatomic categories: terminal longitudinal defects (e.g., aplasia–hypoplasia of the radius with absence of the thumb), terminal transverse defects (loss of distal limb structure with preservation of proximal structure), intercalary defects (aplasia or hypoplasia of proximal limb structure), split hand–foot defects (loss of radial ray or central ray of hand or foot), and complex defects with multiple types of LRDs. The following distribution of 271 LRDs was reported in liveborn infants from the Congenital Malformation Registry: terminal longitudinal (25%), terminal transverse (35%), intercalary (10%), split hand–foot (26%), and multiple (4%) defects (65,66).

The etiopathogeneses of LRDs are divisible into the following categories: dominant—recessive inheritance (15% to 20% of cases), chromosomal abnormalities (5% to 10%), known syndromes, some with a multiorgan pattern of anomalies (5% to 10%), and teratogens (3% to 5%). The latter four categories are collectively thought to account for 30% to 35% of all LRDs, and another 30% to 35% of cases are ascribed to vascular disruption. A determination as to etiopathogenesis is inconclusive for almost one-third of cases. Among those LRDs associated with congenital anomalies (12% to 33% of cases), there are patterns or associations that repeat themselves (67). Seven specific anatomic categories of LRDs are defined in Table 28-2. The various LRDs have several associated major congenital anomalies, some of which are better known than others (61). Preaxial limb defects have the highest frequency (68); they are recognized in the VATER/VACTERL association, which acronymically refers to vertebra, anorectal atresia, congenital heart, tracheoesophageal fistula, renal and distal urinary tract, and limb anomalies (69–72). These may be a consequence of perturbations in the sonic hedgehog homologue gene (7q36) and its signaling pathway since a murine knockout produces a similar pattern of anomalies as seen clinically (73). Vertebral anomalies including vertebral fusion and butterfly vertebra as examples are present in approximately 25% of VACTERL cases, whereas limb defects are found in 10% of cases with the

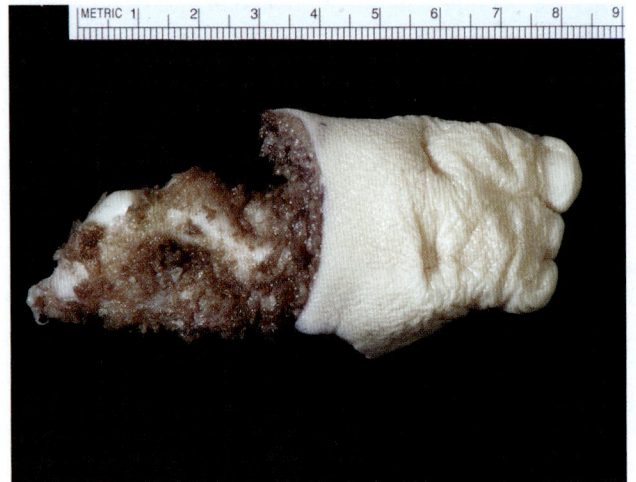
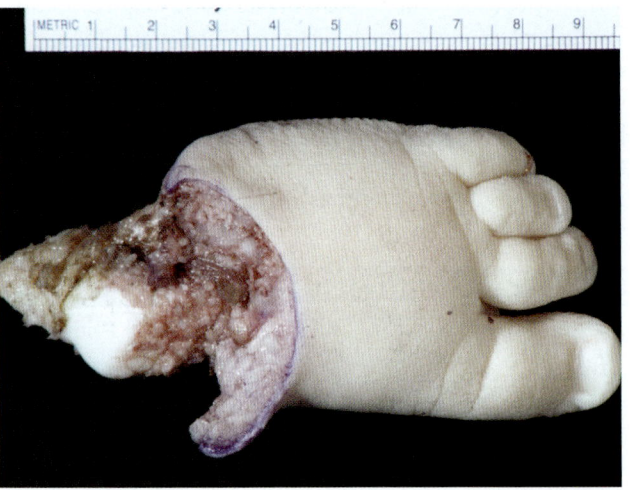

FIGURE 28-1 • Limb reduction defects. **A:** Symes amputation of the foot demonstrates absence of the fourth and fifth toes as an example of postaxial ray deficiency together with proximal syndactyly in a 9-month-old male. **B:** This amputation specimen of the foot from a 10-month-old female shows only four toes with absence of the fifth digit. The fibula was absent as well.

TABLE 28-2	ANATOMIC CATEGORIES OF LIMB DEFECTS
Type	Phenotype
Preaxial	Complete or partial absence of thumbs, first metacarpal and radius and/or absence of hallux, first metatarsal, and tibia
Transverse	Absence of distal metacarpal in phalanges with normal or deficient proximal structures
Postaxial	Complete or partial absence of fifth finger
Intercalary	Absence or hypoplasia of humerus or femur and remaining long bones as a single bone or multiple bones involvement, hands, and feet minimally involved
Split hand-foot	Defects in central ray including metacarpal-metatarsal with nearly normal lateral digits
Amelia	Complete or near complete limb absence
Mixed	Presence of multiple limb defects
Unspecified	Defects not included in previous definitions

preaxial absence of the radius and/or thumb and first metacarpal. A phenotype similar to VACTERL has been observed in the setting of Fanconi anemia (FA); the preaxial limb anomalies are more common in FA than in the VACTERL association (74). Tibial aplasia–hypoplasia, another preaxial defect, is very uncommon when it is compared to the radial aplasia in the VACTERL association (75).

Transverse limb defects with the loss of fingers and toes are associated with anorectal atresia, craniofacial anomalies, syndactyly, and genital defects. Absence of fingers and toes, cleft palate, and constriction band acrosyndactyly are anomalies associated with the *amniotic rupture sequence* (ARS) or *amniotic band syndrome* whose prevalence varies from 1: 1200 to 15,000 live births (76,77) but are commonly seen in stillbirths. Most cases of ARS are sporadic, but there is an apparent increased prevalence in type 4 Ehlers-Danlos syndrome and severe osteogenesis imperfecta (OI) (78). Similar distal limb defects are found in association with *ventral body wall defects*, which are commonly accompanied by a short umbilical cord (79). A vascular disruption has been proposed as a possible pathogenetic factor in both ARS and ventral body wall defect (80). Whether the tethered threads of amnion after the rupture of the amniotic sac are the entire explanation remains an unresolved issue.

Another preaxial limb defect, radial hypoplasia–aplasia, occurs in a number of syndromic settings, and it is estimated that as many as 50% to 80% of infants with absent radii have other anomalies as a component of a defined syndrome (81–85) (Table 28-3).

Lower limb deficiencies are less common than those in the upper extremities accounting for 20% to 40% of cases with or without defects in the upper extremity. Isolated deficiencies or defects of the lower extremity are uncommon, as illustrated by the fact that congenital deficiency of the tibia, or tibial hemimelia, is found in 1:1 million live births (86,87). Other anomalies are found in the same extremity, often other extremities and visceral organ systems in 70% to 80% of cases. Tibial hypoplasia/aplasia is found in almost 70% of cases of the VACTERL association (70). Congenital fibular deficiency in contrast to the rarity of congenital tibial deficiency is one of the most common lower extremity deficiencies (88). *Congenital radial–tibial deficiency* is defined by an absence or hypoplasia of the preaxial structures of the extremity including the thumb, first metacarpal, radius, hallux, first metatarsal, and tibia; this anomaly is associated with nonlimb abnormalities in 70% of cases (89). Among those are the Poland sequence and Holt-Oram syndrome (90). Isolated femoral or fibular deficiency is equally uncommon. Somewhat more frequent is ulnar–fibular deficiency, which

TABLE 28-3	SYNDROMIC ASSOCIATIONS WITH ABSENCE OF RADII

Tubulocytopenia—absent radius syndrome (HOXA11-IGKV3D-20 mutation on 7p15-p14)
Holt-Oram syndrome (TBX5 mutations on 12q24.1)
Fanconi anemia (FANCD1/BIRCA2 on 13q12.3, FANCN/PALB2 on 16p12.3 and FANCJ/BRIP1, TORCA2 mutations on 17q 22-24)
Renal hypoplasia—bilateral/radial ray aplasia
Hypothalamic hamartoblastoma syndrome
Multiple epiphyseal dysplasia (COL9A1 ON 6q12–q14, COL9A3 ON 20q13.3, COMP/TSP-5 on 5q31.2, MATS3 ON 1p33-p32)
Chromosome 22q11 deletion syndrome
Preaxial acrofacial dysostosis (Nager and de Reynier)
Trisomy 18
RAPADILINO syndrome (RECQ64 mutations on 8q24.3)
Baller-Gerold syndrome (craniosynostosis) (RECQ64 mutations on 8q24.3)

is typically manifested by postaxial ray deficiency in the hands and feet with defects of the ipsilateral ulna and fibula. In most cases, ulnar–fibular deficiency is an isolated defect without anomalies elsewhere (88).

Split hand–foot limb defect or malformation (SHFM) occurs as a sporadic (more common) or familial anomaly on the basis of a failure in the initiation and maintenance of the median apical ectodermal ridge (91,92). One case of SHFM is seen in 8500 to 25,000 newborns (93). Seven chromosomal foci have been identified in isolated cases (94). In the less common familial SHFM, both autosomal recessive and X-linked patterns of inheritance are documented (95). Duplication in 17p13.3 (BHLHA9) and mutations FGFR1 and WNT10B have been identified (96–98). In addition to the split hand malformation, polydactyly and syndactyly may be present. Congenital heart disease is found in almost 50% of those with an SHFM 5 mutation. Ectrodactyly, ectodermal dysplasia, and facial cleft syndrome are associated with a p63 (homologue of tumor suppressor gene, p53) mutation; p63 function is critical in the development of the limb bud and hair follicle (99).

Patellar aplasia (absence) and hypoplasia as a lower limb deficiency are found in a number of syndromes, which are discussed at length elsewhere (100,101). Some of these syndromes include neurofibromatosis type 1 (NF1), campomelic dysplasia (CD) with SOX9 (17q24.3) mutations, KAT6B-related disorders, and nail–patella syndrome (NPS) with LMX1B (9q 34.1) mutation, which has a downstream effect on collagen type 4 expression in the glomerular basement development (102). The so-called iliac horns are triangular-shaped outgrowths of the posterior ilium, which are diagnostic of NPS (see Chapter 17).

Amelia denotes incomplete or absent limb. This rare anomaly is seen in 0.15:10,000 live births and occurs with equal frequency in the upper and lower extremities (103,104). Amelia is associated with encephalocele, gastroschisis, omphalocele, anorectal atresia, trisomy 8, VACTERL association, and splenogonadal fusion. Severe lower limb defects are found in association with an omphalocele and diaphragmatic defect (105). A seemingly related or similar phenotypic association is the omphalocele–exstrophy–imperforate anus–spinal defects complex with severe lower limb defects.

Caudal Dysgenesis

CD or *caudal regression syndrome and sirenomelia* are pathogenetically related disorders of the caudal developmental field or axial mesodermal patterning (Figure 28-2) (106–108). Debate continues about the relationship between CD and sirenomelia (so-called mermaid syndrome) (109,110). Axial mesodermal dysplasia (oculo[facio]auriculovertebral spectrum and CD), CD, and sirenomelia are seen more commonly in infants of diabetic mothers to support the hypothesis of a diabetic embryopathy (111–114). However, there is no consensus whether the hyperglycemia itself is the teratogen. Limb deficiencies are another proposed manifestation of diabetic embryopathy. Dysgenesis or agenesis of the

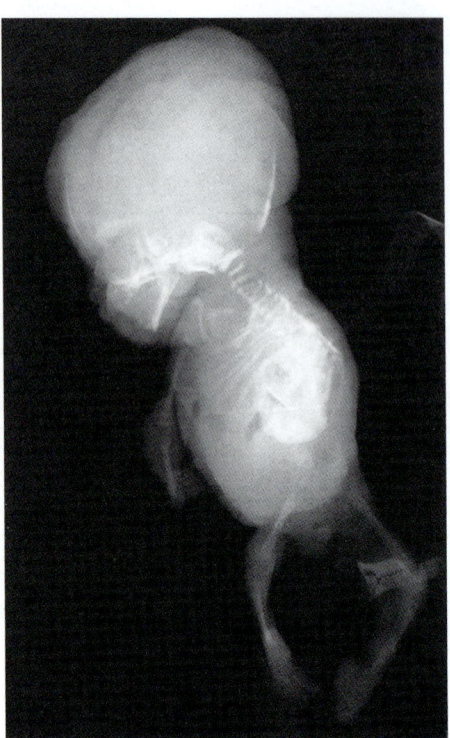

FIGURE 28-2 • Caudal dysgenesis (caudal regression syndrome). A constellation of findings is present including absence of the lumbosacral spine, hypoplastic and flattened pelvis, and absence of the pubis. Bilateral radial agenesis, one of the more common terminal longitudinal defects, is also present and the ribs are hypoplastic and deficient. Bilateral equinovarus deformities are also noted.

sacrum, renal agenesis, fused ectopic kidneys, ectopic ureters, müllerian duct agenesis or hypoplasia, agenesis of the bladder, cloacal exstrophy, cryptorchidism, anorectal atresia, penile–scrotal transposition, limb deficiencies, and fusion of a single dysmorphic lower limb are the range of anomalies in the genitourinary tract and lower extremities in sirenomelia (115). The estimated frequency of CD–sirenomelia is 1:7500 births. CD has been reported in i(18q), 18p-, and trisomy 18 syndromes, VACTERL association, and heterotaxy. Retinoic acid and synthetic retinoids have been shown to cause CD experimentally. Currarino syndrome is considered a variant of caudal regression by some; hemisacrum; anorectal malformation, usually stenosis or atresia; and presacral developmental cyst are the basic phenotypic features (116). The cyst has been interpreted as a cystic teratoma, but in some cases, it is not always clear as to the exact nature of the cyst. Hirschsprung disease and spinal dysraphia are other findings. Mutations in the homeobox gene H9 (HLXB9, MNX1 on 7q 36) have been detected in Currarino syndrome with a pattern of autosomal dominant (AD) transmission, but not in CD (116).

Anomalies of the axial skeleton include various abnormalities in the ribs, vertebra, and sacrum. Some of these are important in their own right, whereas others are associated with more severe anomalies, such as CD including the Currarino syndrome, anorectal malformations, and

VATER/VACTERL association (117). It has been reported that approximately 60% of those with congenital vertebral anomalies also have major or minor abnormalities in other organ systems.

Polydactyly and Syndactyly

Polydactyly is defined by the presence of six or more digits on the hand(s) or foot (feet) or both and is the obvious antithesis to the previously discussed LRDs. A defect in anterior–posterior patterning is considered the pathogenetic basis of polydactyly (118,119). Anatomically, similar designations to LRDs are applied to polydactyly: preaxial (lateral ray), postaxial (medial ray), and the rare central polydactyly. Polydactyly or duplication of the thumb (preaxial) is the most common example with an incidence of almost 1:100 live births. The overall prevalence is estimated to be 0.3 to 3.6:1000 live births (119). The duplicate digit is either partially formed or a severely hypoplastic structure with minimal features to suggest a digit but rather a small polyp (120). Histologically, the various fibrous, vascular, neural, and adipose tissues are not well organized; the peripheral nerve fibers may have traumatic neuroma-like appearance. Isolated preaxial polydactyly is more common in those of European descent, and isolated postaxial polydactyly occurs more frequently in those of African rather than European descent with incidences of 1:140–1300 live births, respectively (119). Postaxial polydactyly in a Caucasian infant has several syndromic associations (Table 28-4). Polydactyly can usually be observed by fetal ultrasonography at 14 to 16 weeks of gestation; one such study reported that 26 fetuses (0.15%) had polydactyly from a total of 17,760 examinations (121).

Preaxial and postaxial polydactyly have differing genetic mechanisms by which these malformations develop. In the case of preaxial polydactyly, point mutations in sonic hedgehog are expressed along the so-called zone of polarizing activity. Postaxial polydactyly has at least three different mutated genes: 7p13, 19p 13.2, and 13q21–32; there are also frameshift mutations in GL13 (122). The latter gene is a mediator of hedgehog signaling (123). Two types of postaxial polydactyly have two genophenotypic expressions: type A with a well-formed digit and a normal fifth digit and type B with a hypoplastic structure resembling a small papilloma or acrochordon. When these lesions autoamputate, a traumatic neuroma is a known sequel but is less common in those hypoplastic digits, which are surgically excised. There are in excess of 300 entities in syndromic and nonsyndromic settings with polydactyly as one phenotypic feature (118).

Syndactyly is defined by soft tissue fusion of fingers and toes with or without fusion of the small bones. Like the other anomalies in this section, syndactyly occurs as an isolated finding or as a manifestation of one of approximately 300 syndromes including acrocephalosyndactyly with its several types (Apert, Waardenburg, Pfeiffer, Summitt, and Saethre-Chotzen syndromes), Poland, Fraser, and F-syndrome (124). Syndactyly is also a well-documented feature of the amniotic band syndrome without any specific pattern of digital or

TABLE 28-4 SYNDROMIC ASSOCIATION WITH PREAXIAL AND POSTAXIAL POLYDACTYLY

Preaxial	Postaxial
Carpenter	Ellis van Creveld
Orofaciodigital II	Orofaciodigital III
Short rib—polydactyly II	Short-rib polydactyly I
Townes Brock	McKusick-Kaufmann
NF1	Smith-Lemli-Opitz
Diabetic embryopathy[a]	Bardet-Biedl[b]
Femoral-facial syndrome	Meckel-Gruber
Greig[b]	Jeune
Apert	Pallister-Hall[c]
Partial trisomy 4q	NF1
WAGR syndrome	Orofaciodigital IV[d]
14q(22) deletion	Deletion 22q11 (DiGeorge)[c]
Partial trisomy 1q	
Distal trisomy 10q	
Laurin-Sandrow	
Triphalangeal thumb polysyndactyly	
Amniotic band, cleft lip plate	
Trisomy 21	
VACTERL	

[a]Preaxial hallucal polydactyly.
[b]Pre- and postaxial polydactyly.
[c]Central polydactyly.
[d]Postaxial upper and preaxial lower extremities.

limb involvement. Polydactyly and syndactyly can also occur together with heterogeneous phenotypes.

Arthrogryposis

Arthrogryposis or congenital contracture is represented by two phenotypes: isolated or limited with single area involvement and multifocal with two or more joint contractures (125). Multiple congenital contractures are further classified into amyoplasia, distal arthrogryposis, and related syndromes (126,127). The latter category includes failure in forebrain development, chromosomal abnormalities, and motor neuron disorders like spinal muscular atrophy, congenital myopathies (myosinopathies), and heritable peripheral neuropathies (128). It has been estimated that more than 300 disorders are accompanied by multiple joint contractures and their arthrogryposis is not a specific diagnosis, but rather a phenotype (129). The contractures are often symmetrical in both upper and lower extremities in over 50% of cases (130) (Figure 28-3).

Fetal akinesia–hypokinesia deformation (FAD) sequence has an estimated prevalence of 1:12,000 to 19,000 live births, and it can be recognized after the first trimester (131,132). These infants have the so-called Pena-Shokeir phenotype

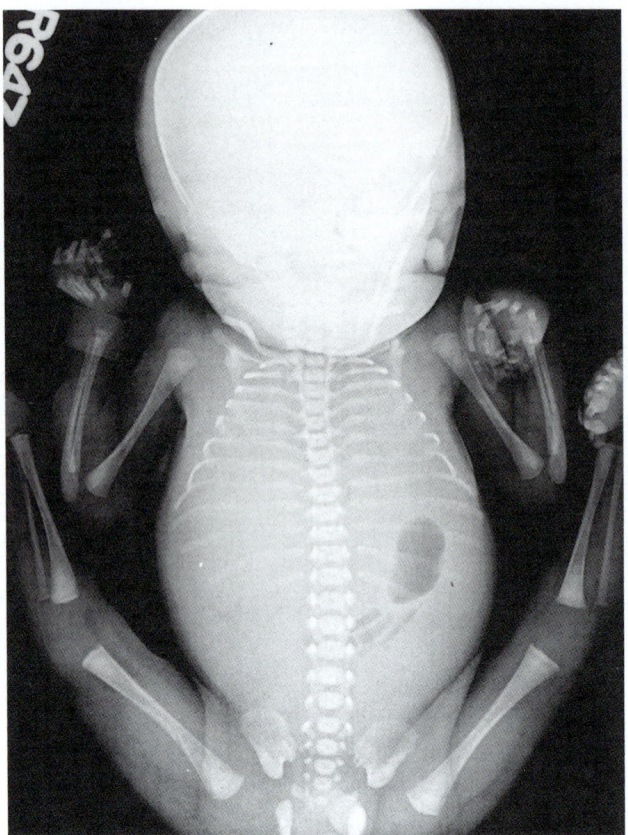 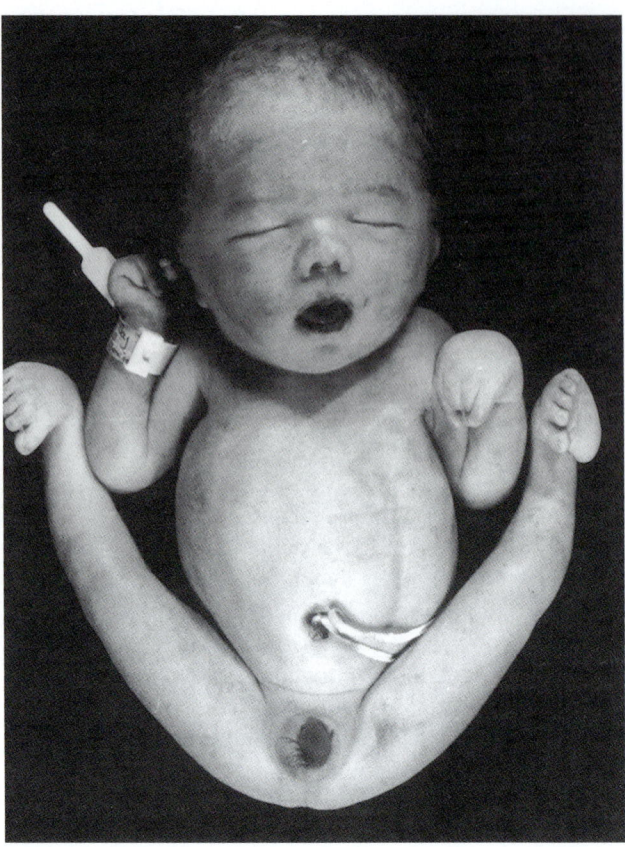

FIGURE 28-3 • Congenital arthrogryposis. **A:** Various deformities are present in these postmortem images. **B:** Severe contraction deformities are depicted in this postmortem image. Death occurred shortly after birth because of pulmonary hypoplasia.

with limb contractures (arthrogryposis), intrauterine growth restriction, an attenuated umbilical cord because of diminished fetal activity, secondary pulmonary hypoplasia, and craniofacial anomalies (133,134). The FAD sequence is itself a clinical phenotype with several specific genetic mutations including the Escobar syndrome (multiple pterygium syndrome) with multiple mutations involving the gamma subunit gene (CHRNG) of acetylcholine receptor (135,136).

Genetic Skeletal Disorders

GSD or skeletal dysplasias are the encompassing designation for the 40 groups of conditions that affect the normal development of bones and supporting tissues in terms of their shape and size and often with a reduction in normal stature (137). The number of recognized GSDs currently comprises some 456 conditions as of the 2010 revision of the Nosology and Classification of Genetic Skeletal Disorders (138). Among the 456 disorders, almost 70% are associated with mutations in 216 different genes. The 2010 revision was expanded to include 40 groups as defined by similar mutational and/or phenotypic characteristics (Table 28-5). These 40 groups are arranged in clusters: (a) groups 1 to 8 by common underlying gene or pathway defect; (b) groups 9 to 17 by specific bone structure or segment involvement by imaging studies; (c) groups 18 to 20 by macroscopic criteria and clinical features; (d) groups 21 to 25 and 28 by altered bone density, mineralization, stippling, or osteolysis; (e) group 27 by lysosomal disorders with skeletal manifestations; (f) group 29 by exostosis or enchondromas (ECs); (g) group 23 or OP group; (h) group 25 or OI group; (i) group 26 by hypophosphatemic rickets; (j) group 29 by disorganized skeletal development; (k) group 30 with overgrowth including skeleton; (l) group 31 by genetic inflammatory disorders involving bones and joints; and (m) groups 32 to 40 or dysostoses with abnormalities in individual bones or groups of bones (139).

The prevalence rate of the skeletal dysplasias is approximated at 2.4 to 34.5:10,000 stillbirths and live births, but among infants who died in the perinatal period, the frequency is higher at 9 to 10:1000 perinatal deaths (140–144). Several types of skeletal dysplasias are inconsistent with survival beyond the neonatal or early infancy period and are collectively referred to as lethal chondrodysplasias (145,146) (Table 28-6). The point prevalence at birth of the lethal chondrodysplasias was 15.4:100,000 births in one geographic region of Denmark (145,147). Whether the particular clinical observations had been obtained from prenatal diagnosis by ultrasonography or perinatal autopsies, thanatophoric dysplasia (TD) and OI type 2 are the most common lethal skeletal dysplasias, accounting for 50% to 65% of cases (148–150) (Table 28-7). Short-rib dysplasias (SRDs), achondrogenesis, and CD comprise the next most common lethal disorders (126,132). A somewhat different experience in the context of

TABLE 28-5	THE GROUPS OF GENETIC SKELETAL DISORDERS OF BONE: 2010 REVISION WITH PHENOTYPIC EXAMPLES

1. FGFR 3 chondrodysplasia group (e.g. thanatophoric dysplasia, types 1 and 2, TD type 2)
2. Type 2 collagen group (e.g., achondrogenesis type 2)
3. Type 11 collagen group (e.g., Stickler syndrome type 2)
4. Sulfation disorders group (e.g, achondrogenesis type1B)
5. Perlecan group (e.g., Schwartz-Jampel syndrome)
6. Aggrecan group (e.g., (spondylometaphyseal, Kimberly type))
7. Filamin group and related disorders (e.g., frontometaphyseal dysplasia)
8. TRPV4 group (e.g., metatropic dysplasia)
9. Short-ribs dysplasia (with or without polydactyly) group (e.g. chondroectodermal dysplasia)
10. Multiple epiphyseal dysplasia and pseudochondroplasia (e.g., pseudochondroplasia)
11. Metaphyseal dysplasia (e.g., metaphyseal dysplasia Schmid type)
12. Spondylometaphyseal dysplasia (e.g., spondyloenchondrodysplasia)
13. Spondyloepi (-meta) physeal dysplasias (e.g., immune-osseous dysplasia, Schimke)
14. Severe spondylodysplastic dysplasias (e.g., achondrogenesis type 1A)
15. Acromelic dysplasias (e.g., trichorhinophalangeal dysplasia types 1/3)
16. Acromesomelic dysplasias (e.g., acromesomelic dysplasia type Maroteaux)
17. Mesomelic and rhizo-mesomelic dysplasias (e.g., dyschondrosteosis, Leri-Weil)
18. Bent bone dysplasias (e.g., campomelic dysplasia)
19. Slender bone dysplasias (e.g., Kenny-Caffey dysplasia type 1)
20. Dysplasias with multiple joint dislocations (e.g., Desbuquois dysplasia)
21. Chondrodysplasia punctata group (e.g., Conradi-Hünermann type)
22. Neonatal osteosclerotic dysplasias (e.g., Caffey disease)
23. Increased bone density group (without modification of bone shape) (e.g., osteopetrosis, severe neonatal or infantile forms)
24. Increased bone density group with metaphyseal and/or diaphyseal involvement (e.g., craniometaphyseal dysplasia, autosomal dominant)
25. Osteogenesis imperfecta and decreased bone density group (e.g., OI type 1)
26. Defective mineralization group (e.g., hypophosphatasia, osteogenesis imperfecta, non-deforming, type 1, perinatal lethal and infantile forms)
27. Lysosomal storage diseases with skeletal involvement (dysostosis multiplex group) (e.g., mucopolysaccharidosis type 1H/1S)
28. Osteolysis group (e.g., progeria, Hutchinson-Gilford type)
29. Disorganized development of skeletal components group (e.g., multiple cartilaginous exostoses, types 1-3)
30. Overgrowth syndromes with skeletal involvement (e.g., Proteus syndrome)
31. Genetic inflammatory/rheumatoid-like osteoarthropathics (e.g., chronic recurrent multifocal osteomyelitis)
32. Cleidocranial dysplasia and isolated cranial ossification defects group (e.g., cleidocranial dysplasia)
33. Craniosynostosis syndrome (e.g., Pfeiffer syndrome [FGFR1-related]])
34. Dysostoses with predominant craniofacial involvement (e.g., mandibulo-facial dysostosis of Treacher-Collins)
35. Dysostosis with predominant vertebral with and without costal involvement (e.g., Currarino triad)
36. Patellar dysostoses (e.g., nail-patella syndrome)
37. Brachydactylies (with or without extraskeletal manifestations) (e.g., Albright hereditary osteodystrophy)
38. Limb hypoplasia-reduction defects group (e.g., Fanconi anemia)
39. Polydactyly-syndactyly-triphalangism group (e.g., Pallister-Hall syndrome)
40. Defects in joint formation and synostoses (e.g., radio-ulnar synostosis with amegakaryocytic thrombocytopenia)

Source: Adapted from Warman ML, Cormier-Daire V, Hall C, et al. Nosology and classification of genetic skeletal disorders: 2010 revision. *Am J Med Genet Part A* 2011;15:945–968.

TABLE 28-6 VARIOUS LETHAL SKELETAL DISORDERS AND SITES OF GENE MUTATION (IF KNOWN)

Disorder	Mutated Gene
TD	FGFR3
Achondroplasia (homozygous)	FGFR3
Achondrogenesis type 2	COL2
Kniest-like dysplasia	COL2
Platyspondylic dysplasia (Torrance type)	COL2
Achondrogenesis type 1B (Fracco type)	DTDST
Diastrophic dysplasia	DTDST
Dyssegmental dysplasia, Silverman-Handmaker type	HSPG2 (1p36.1-p34)
AO2	FLNB
Boomerang dysplasia	FLNB
Short rib polydactyly	
Type 1 (Saldino-Noonan)	DYNC2H1 (11q21–q22.1)
Type 2 (Majewski)	NEK1
Type 4 (Mohr-Majewski)	—
ATD	DYNC2H1 (11q21–q22.1)
Metaphyseal dysplasia, Jansen type	PTHRI
Metatrophic dysplasia, types 1 and 2	TRVP4
Achondrogenesis type 1A	TRIP11 (14q31–q32)
Spondylometaphyseal dysplasia, Sedaghatian type	—
Fibrochondrogenesis	COL11A1
Schneckenbecken dysplasia	SLC35DI
CD	SOX9
Rhizomelic CDP	
Type 1	PEX7 (6q23.3)
Type 2	6NPAT (1q42)
Type 3	AGPS (2q31.2)
Astley-Kendall dysplasia	—
Blomstrand dysplasia	PTHR1 (3p22-p21.1)
Osteosclerotic bone dysplasia (Raine syndrome)	FAM20C (7p22.3)
OI, type 2	CRTAP (3p22.3)
	LEPRE1 (1p34.1)
Spondylothoracic dysplasia (Jarcho-Levin syndrome)	DLL3(?), MESP2(?)
HP, perinatal lethal	ALP (1p36.12)
Desbuquois dysplasia	CANT1 19q25.3

International Skeletal Dysplasia Registry is based on referral cases with the following distribution: OI type 2 (20% of all cases), TD (11%), achondrogenesis type 2 (8%), CD (4%), and other specific disorders (36%) (157). Approximately 4.5% of cases were unclassified. In virtually all of the lethal GSDs, there is a severe narrowing or reduction in the volume of the thoracic cavity with restricted lung growth and resulting secondary pulmonary hypoplasia (158,159).

Postmortem examination in GSDs. Although it may seem obvious, radiographs with anterior–posterior and lateral views should be obtained as a prerequisite to the postmortem examination on any dysmorphic infant, including one with a suspected skeletal dysplasia (160). No conventional autopsy can hope to demonstrate the entire range of abnormalities in the skeletal system without a total body image (161,162). In fact, the GSDs were largely classified on the basis of their radiographic features, but molecular genetic and biochemical studies have served as the basis for classification in the majority of cases (138).

Acquisition of tissues, mainly soft tissues rich in fibroblasts, is recommended for standard metaphase cytogenetics. Although a few hours may have lapsed since death, it is still possible to obtain cellular growth, provided that the body has been placed in a temperature-controlled environment. Samples of cartilage at the costochondral junction or joint space can be snap frozen in liquid nitrogen. The utility of standardized sections from various specific sites for optimal pathologic examination has been discussed by Yang and associates (163).

Before the internal examination is performed, a careful documentation of the various standard measurements in the perinatal autopsy and photographs from the anterior, posterior, and lateral profiles should be obtained (164). Various sites, with particular emphasis on the regions of the growth plate, have been recommended for the sampling of membranous bone, including the ribs, vertebral bodies, proximal and distal humerus and/or femur, and cranium (163,165). The costochondral junctions of the fourth through sixth ribs are regarded by some as the optimal sites for identifying disturbances in the growth plate (166,167). Decalcified and undecalcified sections have complementary value. It is helpful to have microscopic sections available from the osteochondral junction of an age-matched infant without any known skeletal abnormalities for purposes of reference and orientation. A particularly useful review of the morphologic aspects of the growth plate has been provided by Brighton (26). Many of the histologic abnormalities in a GSD are semiquantitative, in addition to individual cellular alterations. The cellularity of the various zones of cartilage (resting, proliferating, and hypertrophic) and their organization into columns in the hypertrophic zone and the actual chondroosseous junction or zone of provisional ossification are the specific foci of histologic interest in this group of disorders. In some but not all disorders, the morphologic abnormalities are consistent from one case to another within a specific diagnostic entity. The discussion of chondrodysplasias by Gilbert-Barness with its high-quality images, which correlate the radiographic, gross, and microscopic features, is recommended (168).

The following discussion of GSDs is based on the various "groups" as defined in the 2010 revised classification (138). Selected groups are considered based upon their frequency and models of morphologic and molecular pathology.

TABLE 28-7	TYPES OF SKELETAL DYSPLASIAS BY PRENATAL DETECTION AND PERINATAL AUTOPSY						
	Schramm (148)	Bankova (143)	Stevenson (144)	Wood and Dimmick (160)	Lahmar-Bodfaroua (146)	Konstantinidou (148)	Total (%)
TD and other group 1	49	27	41	15	8	7	147 (31)
OI and other group 25	35	27	40	11	9	5	127 (27)
Achondrogenesis and other group 2	14	3	10	2	3	2	35 (7)
SRD and other group 9	26	9	5	3	3	5	51 (11)
CD and other group 18	8	1	6	1	—	4	20 (4)
CDP and other group 21	—	9	6	3	—	2	20 (4)
DD and other group 4	5	3	3	—	8	—	19 (4)
HP and other group 26	—	3	3	3	—	—	9 (2)
Metatrophic dysplasia and other group 8	—	—	—	1	—	—	1 (<1)
Severe spondylodysplastic dysplasias and other group 14	—	1	—	—	4	—	5 (1)
Other	—	24	39	2	—	16	81 (17)
Total	137	112	153	41	35	41	429

FGFR3 Chondrodysplasias (Group 1)

FGFR3 chondrodysplasia group is characterized by short limbs relative to a somewhat longer trunk. The individual entities in this group are achondroplasia (ACH), severe ACH with developmental delay and acanthosis nigricans (SADDAN), hypochondroplasia (HCP), hypochondrodysplasia-like dysplasia, and thanatophoric (TD) types 1 and 2 (169–171). Several mutations have been identified in the FGFR3 gene (4p16.3); the germ-line mutations in FGFR3 gene inhibit chondrocyte proliferation (172).

Achondroplasia, the most common type of chondrodysplasia, is a nonlethal disorder in the heterozygote (AD inheritance), with a birth prevalence of 1:10,000 to 30,000 live births (173). Most cases are sporadic, with greater than 80% of cases representing a new mutation. Approximately 50% of FGFR3 chondrodysplasias are examples of ACH (144). There is a gain of FGFR3 function, which at the growth plate has an arresting effect upon the chondrocytes with the development of rhizomelic shortening of the extremities. It has been reported that the mutation impairs endochondral bone growth by preventing SOX9 downregulation (174). Morphologically, the growth plate is regular with periosteal overgrowth.

Hypochondroplasia is also a nonlethal disorder with AD inheritance and a prevalence of 1.5:100,000 live births. The point mutations on the FGFR3 gene (p. ASN540 Lys) in 70% to 75% of cases differ from ACH (p.Glu 380 Arg); other mutations in the FGFR3 gene have been identified in HCP (175). The clinical and radiographic heterogeneity of HCP is substantial to serve as a challenge in the diagnosis. Compound carriers of the heterozygous mutations on the FGFR3 gene (G380R and N540K) appear to have a more morbid phenotype than those with either one or other point mutations (176). Like ACH, the growth plate is more or less normal appearing. The latter is not surprising in that there is considerable phenotypic overlap between ACH and HCP (176,177).

Thanatophoric dysplasia occurs in 1:20,000 to 60,000 births and is the most common type of lethal chondrodysplasia in most series based upon prenatal ultrasonography and/or autopsy (178–183). Like the other FGFR3 opathies, TD has AD inheritance. Two phenotypes of TD are recognized: type I with curved femora and missense point mutations, p.Arg 248 Lys and p.Tyr 373 Lys (90% of cases), and type II with straight femora and cloverleaf skull with the exclusive mutation, p. Lys 650 Glu (100% of cases) (176,178). Approximately 80% to 85% of TD cases are type I and the remainder are type II. In the ISDR with mutational analysis of the FGFR3 opathies, 65% of the cases were examples of TD types I and II, ACH (25%), and HCP (9%) (176).

Another phenotype of the FGFR3 opathies is severe achondrodysplasia with developmental delay and acanthosis nigricans (SADDAN) (184,185). In SADDAN, the point mutation is at codon 650 (p.Lys 650 Net) (184). Acanthosis nigricans and epidermal nevus are other expressions of FGFR3 mutations (186).

In population-based studies, both types of TD are almost as common as ACH (144). Type 1 TD is characterized by

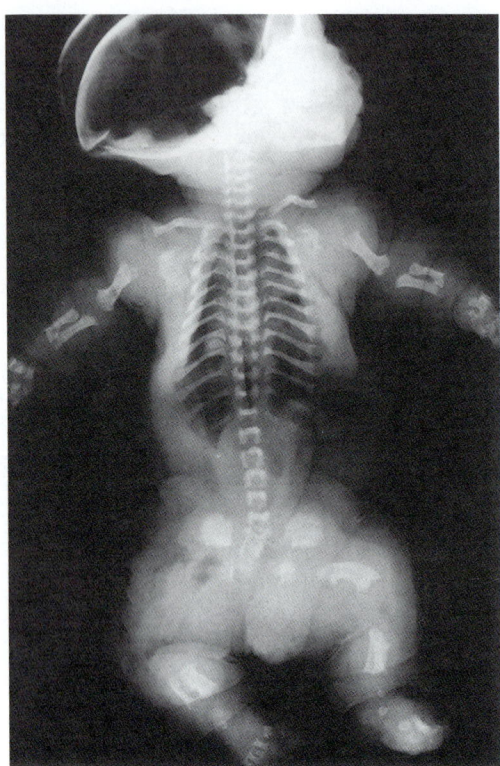
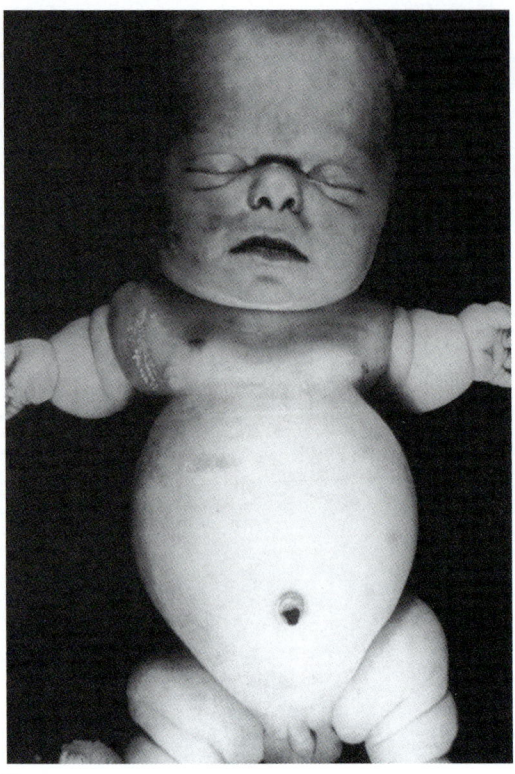

FIGURE 28-4 • Thanatophoric dysplasia type I. **A:** Radiograph shows flattened, U-shaped vertebrae; short, squared iliac bones with small sacrosciatic notches; shortened long bones with metaphyseal flaring; "French telephone receiver"–like left femur (right femur removed for special studies); and short ribs. **B:** The large head with frontal bossing, rhizomelic extremities, and narrow thorax are the characteristic external findings.

angulated or curved humeri and femora and craniosynostosis in 28% and mild cloverleaf skull in 3%, whereas type 2 is relatively straight femora, cloverleaf skull in 50%, and craniosynostosis in 90% (Figure 28-4) (178,179). Angulated femora are also present in CD and OI type II (178). Most infants die in the neonatal period of respiratory failure on the basis of severe secondary pulmonary hypoplasia as a consequence of the reduced volume of the thoracic cavity, which impedes normal lung growth (180,182). The lung/body weight ratio is low in contrast to the brain/body weight ratio (180). The chondroosseous junction of the growth plate is substantially reduced in width with disorderly columnation of the chondrocytes as a reflection of the impaired FGFR3 signaling; there is fibrosis in place of regular chondroid ossification (Figure 28-5) (181–183). Other findings include the flattening of ossification centers (platyspondyly). Another aspect of the pathologic findings in TD is the range of neuropathologic abnormalities, which include overgrowth of the temporal lobe, hyperconvolution, and neuronal heterotopia (187,188).

Osteogenesis Imperfecta and Decreased Bone Density Group

Group 25 (ISDS classification) or OI is represented by two general categories: the so-called collagenous types or COL1A1-/2-related disorders with AD inheritance (OI types I, II, III, and IV) and the noncollagenous types with autosomal recessive inheritance (Table 28-8) (189,190). It is estimated that 90% of all cases of OI have a defect in one of the type I collagen genes and the remainder are mutations in genes responsible for the synthesis of proteins that interact with collagen (190,191). With the failure of normal collagen type I synthesis by osteoblasts, the bones are less dense with the consequence

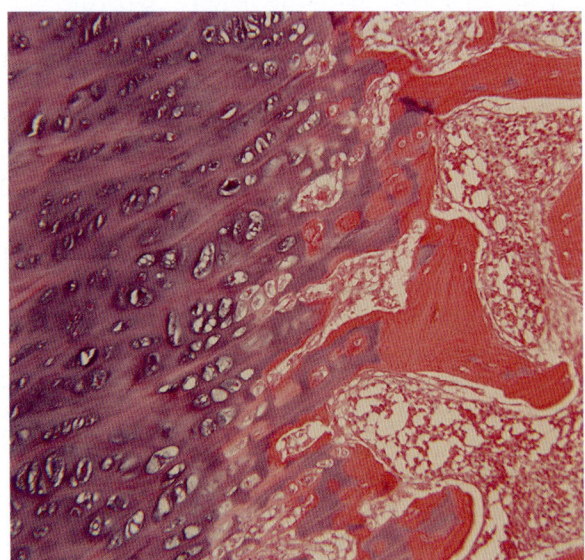

FIGURE 28-5 • Thanatophoric dysplasia type I. The chondroosseous function is reduced in width but retains some degree of organization though the chondrocyte columnation is modestly irregular.

TABLE 28-8 TYPES OF OSTEOGENESIS IMPERFECTA, INHERITANCE, MOLECULAR DEFECT, AND CLINICAL FEATURES

Gene	Inheritance	Phenotype (Sillence classification)	Specific characteristics
Type 1 Collagen Defects			
COL1A1	AD	Type I, II, III, and IV	Blue/gray/white sclerae, hypermobility, hearing loss, dentinogenesis imperfecta
COL1A2	AD	Type I, II, III, and IV	
Type 1 Collagen Processing and Maturation			
BMP1	AR		Increased bone mineral density, blue sclerae
Collagen Chaperone			
CRTAP	AR	Type II, III, and IV	
LEPRE1	AR	Type II and III	
PPIB	AR	Type II, III and IV	
SERPINH1	AR	Type II and III	Blue sclerae, dentinogenesis imperfecta (Dachshund model)
FKBP10	AR	Type III and IV	Congenital contractures of the limbs possible (Bruck syndrome type 1 and Kuskokwim syndrome)
PLOD2	AR	Type III	Pterigium, congenital contractures (Bruck syndrome type 2)
Bone Formation, Homeostasis and Regulation of Bone Density			
SERPINF1	AR	Type (III, IV) VI	Normal at birth, progressive course, poor response to bisphosphonate treatment
SP7	AR	Type III	Delayed dentition
LRP5 (WNT1 coreceptor)	AR	Type III and IV	Blind (osteoporosis–pseudoglioma syndrome)
WNT1	AR	Type III and IV	Progressive course, poor response to bisphosphonate treatment
TMEM38B	AR	Type III	
IFITM5	AR	Type V	Hypertrophic callus, metaphysical bands, interosseous membrane calcification
CREB3L1 (OASIS)	AR	Type III	Fractures in utero, IUGR, fractures, bone deformities, cardiac insufficiency
P4HB	AR	Cole-Carpenter syndrome OI-like	Craniofacial malformations, scoliosis, large epiphyses, deformity of upper and lower extremities, "popcorn epiphyses"
SEC24D	AR	Cole-Carpenter syndrome OI-like	Multiple pre- and postnatal fractures, craniofacial malformations
TAPT1 (transmembrane anterior–posterior transformation 1)	AR		
PLS3	AR	(I)	Osteoporosis with fractures

AD, autosomal dominant; AR, autosomal recessive; contributed through the kind efforts of Dr. Cecilia Giunta, April, 2015.

of structural fragility, which varies considerably in severity within the various types of OI (192,193). A severity index in a sense has been formulated and is based upon the type of OI (194). The incidence of OI including all types is estimated at 1:10,000 to 20,000 live births; one case of OI type II is encountered for every two to five cases of TD in the perinatal–neonatal period (195,196).

OI type II, known as the perinatal lethal type, is the manifestation of a new mutation in most cases and is characterized by severe osteopenia, blue sclera, short and bowed or angulated extremities, a diminutive thorax, and crumpled or collapsed long bones, especially the femora (Figure 28-6A, B) (195,197). The cranium is soft and intracranial hemorrhage is not uncommon. Shortened, deformed extremities are also features of

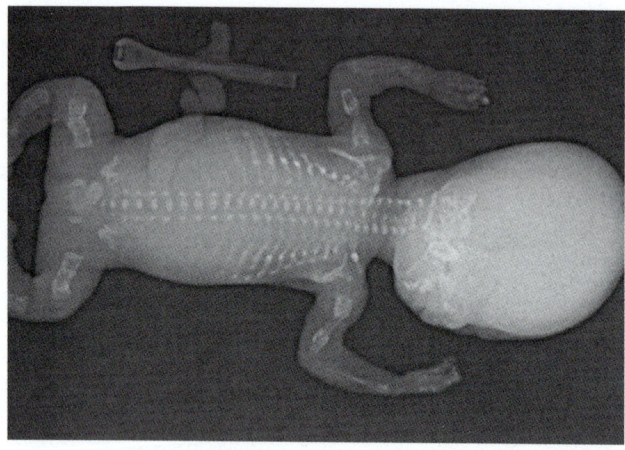 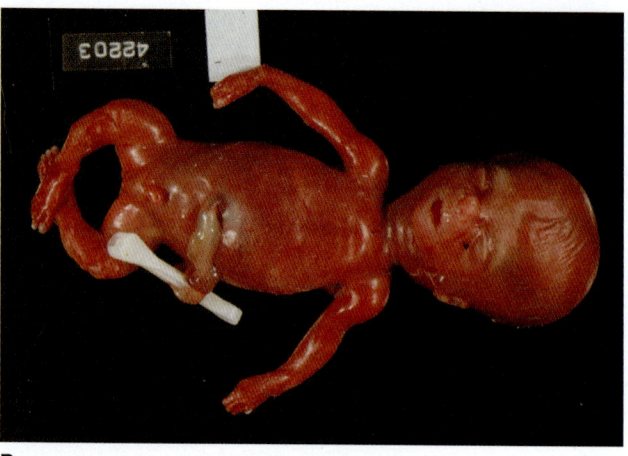

FIGURE 28-6 • Osteogenesis imperfecta, type II. **A:** This postmortem roentgenogram demonstrates poor ossification of the cranium and multiple fractures of the ribs, long bones, and pelvis and normal vertebra. **B:** Shortening of the femora secondary to fractures and marked curvature of the lower extremities are some of the more obvious external abnormalities. Note also the abnormal positioning of the upper extremities.

achondrogenesis types 1A and 2, TD, and hypophosphatasia (HP). A small thoracic cavity with its deformities results in severe pulmonary hypoplasia with smaller than normal weight of lungs for gestational age and structural abnormalities of the thoracic cage. The bones are shortened, with multiple fractures with minimal normal callus formation, and multinodular chondroid masses are present that resemble an endosteal cartilaginous neoplasm or EC (198). The cortex is quite attenuated, and the trabecular bone consists of delicate strands and is often disorganized, with an overall osteopenic appearance. The bone may appear hypercellular and the mosaic lines of osteoid seams are increased in number. The apparent hypercellularity is explained by a reduction in osteoid matrix secondary to defective type 1 collagen. The physis may be normal in many respects or may be disorganized (Figure 28-7A-D) (199,200). Chondrocyte columnation often appears normal, but osteoid forms directly on the cartilage without orderly endochondral ossification (201,202). These infants also exhibit neuropathologic changes, including perivenous microcalcifications and impaired neuroblastic–neuronal migration (203).

OI type III, unlike type II, is usually not lethal in the perinatal period, but its severe phenotype is characterized by fractures and deformities of the lower extremities; these complications are present at birth and continue throughout life with the development of severe kyphoscoliosis (194,204). In one series, 25% of infants and children with OI have type III (205). Lung infections with acute respiratory failure occur throughout the first decade of life because of the thoracic cage abnormalities (206,207). Marrow fibrosis and disorganized trabecular bone in OI type III can simulate fibrous dysplasia (FD). There are no specific histologic features to permit the differentiation of one type of OI from another (208). Immature woven bone is prominent, and lamellar bone is poorly formed.

OI type V, unlike OI types I to IV, is not defined by mutations in collagen type I, but rather by a mutation in IFITM5-like protein, which interferes with the collagen triple helix and bone mineralization (209–211). A moderate to severe phenotype and hyperplastic callus formation, especially in femoral fractures, can be mistaken for osteosarcoma (OS) (212). Pseudoarthrosis, aortic and mitral valvular insufficiency, and aortic dissection are other manifestations (213,214). Multiple fractures in the absence of a prior diagnosis of OI can be mistaken for child abuse (215). Rare examples of bone neoplasms and cysts have been reported in OI, including OS, chondrosarcoma (CS), ossifying fibroma (OF), and aneurysmal bone cyst (ABC) (216–218).

OI and its definition have been challenging with the recognition of the autosomal recessive forms of the disease accounting for 10% of cases (191,193,219,220). There are presently eight genes that have been identified. Clinically, the recessive forms of OI present with bone fragility. One of these, Bruck syndrome, is associated with joint contractures (221). The various recessive genes encode proteins, which are required for collagen transcriptional modification (220,222).

Defective Mineralization Group

Defective mineralization group (group 26) includes HP, an inborn error of metabolism associated with a deficiency of tissue nonspecific alkaline phosphatase with ALPL missense mutations in most cases (1p36.12) (223,224). The inheritance of the perinatal lethal and infantile forms of this disorder is AR with a prevalence of 1:100,000 births (223). Approximately 2% to 4% of lethal GSDs are examples of perinatal HP. There are six clinical forms of HP, and these reflect the heterogeneity of the missense mutations on the ALPL gene (225). There are some overlapping radiographic features among HP, OI types II and III, and achondrogenesis type 1A; however, these conditions can be differentiated from each other by radiographic analysis of the entire skeleton (139). The histopathologic findings at the physis

dysplasia (DD), and multiple epiphyseal dysplasia, recessiva (273). There is considerable phenotypic overlap between AO2 and DD (274). The pathologic features of DD and AO are similar: an attenuated growth plate, irregular clumping of chondrocytes in the resting zone, and foci of myxoid degeneration, not necessarily confined to the resting zone. One of the hallmark features is a dense rim of collagenous matrix around each lacuna (275,276). Giant chondrocytes may be found as well. ACG1B, in addition to severe micromelia with marked shortening of the femora and humeri, is characterized by minimal or absent ossification of the vertebral bodies and malformed tibiae and fibulae (Figure 28-13) (277).

Filamin Group and Related Disorders

Group 7 is defined by the presence of mutations in the FLNA gene (Xq28) that encodes filamin A and includes the following X-linked dominant dysplasias: frontometaphyseal dysplasia, Melnick-Needles osteodysplasia, and otopalatodigital syndromes types 1 and 2 (278). Mutations in FLNB gene (3p14.3) are both AD and AR and include the following: AO1, AO3, Larsen syndrome, spondylocarpotarsal syndrome, Piepkorn, and boomerang dysplasias (the latter two have been included with AO1) (138,279–281). The filamins are actin binding that stabilize the structure of actin and link them to the cell membrane (282). The filamin A–associated disorders are diverse from the skeletal dysplasia to periventricular nodular heterotopia to severe congenital lung disease with cysts and pulmonary vascular hypertensive changes (283–285). Otopalatodigital syndrome type 2 is a potentially lethal disorder with thoracic and pulmonary hypoplasia. Other defects include hypomineralized calvarium, poorly formed small bones of the hands and feet, septal and right ventricular outflow tract defects, omphalocele, and genitourinary tract anomalies. Boomerang dysplasia and AO1 are lethal disorders due to the small thorax and hypoplastic lungs (286,287). Multinucleated and giant chondrocytes may be seen in a focally hypocellular reserve or resting zone. Similar giant chondrocytes have been seen in Piepkorn dysplasia, which may be allelic to boomerang dysplasia (288). Near-complete

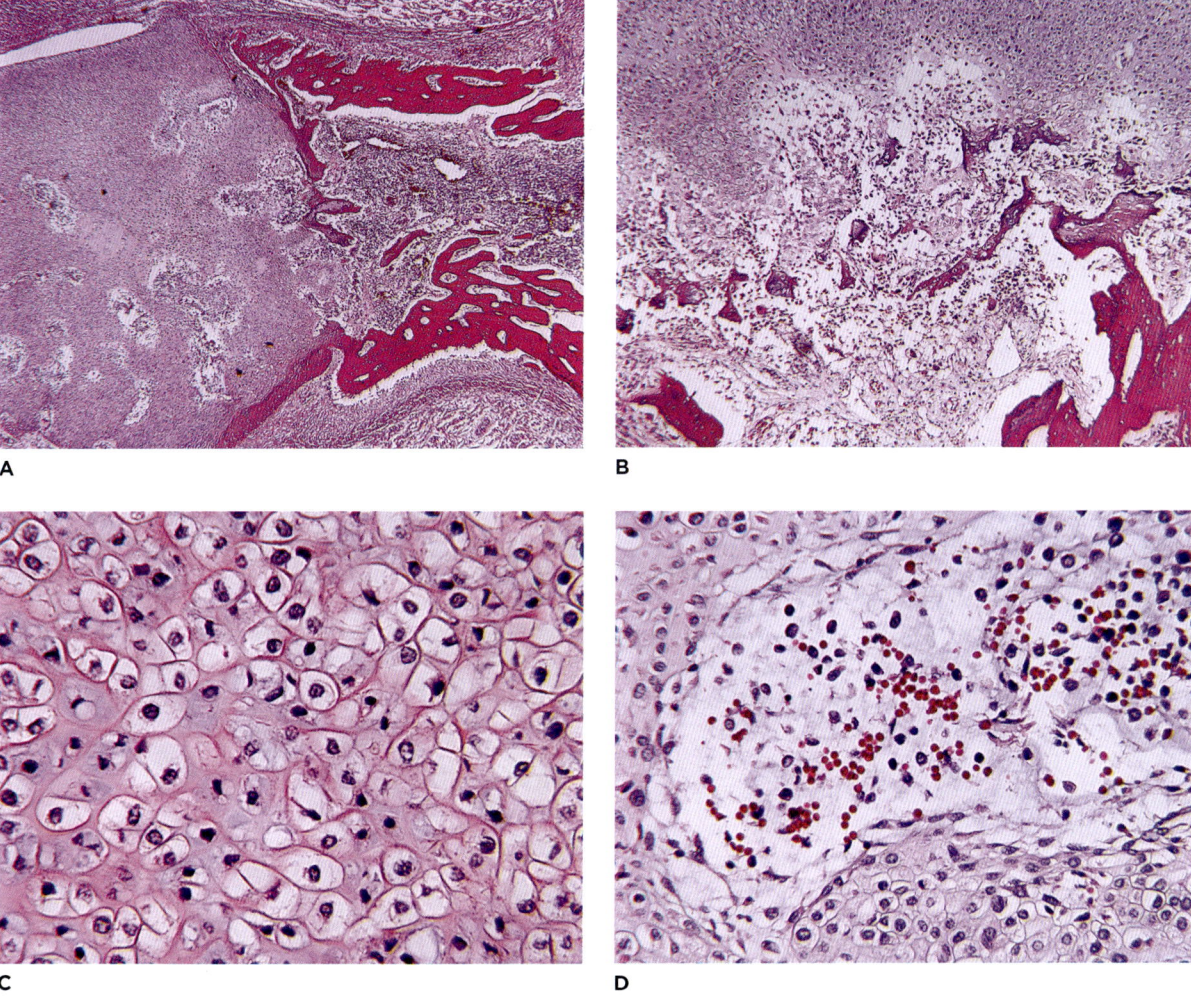

FIGURE 28-13 • Achondrogenesis type 1B. **A:** This field shows the epiphyseal cartilage and growth plate with obvious absence of any resemblance to a normal growth plate. **B:** The growth plate in another micromelic long bone shows a complete absence of any physeal organization. **C:** The zone of proliferating chondrocytes demonstrates an eosinophilic stroma in the background, which is collagen surrounding each cell. **D:** The multifocal cystic degeneration present in panel A is seen in this higher magnification field with hemorrhage and degenerating chondrocytes in the background. (Contributed by Bahig M. Shehata, MD, Atlanta, Georgia.)

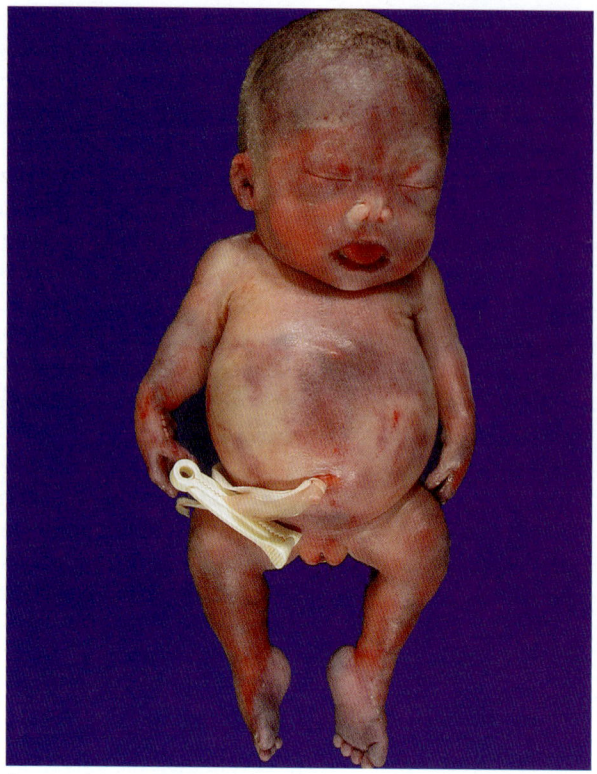

A

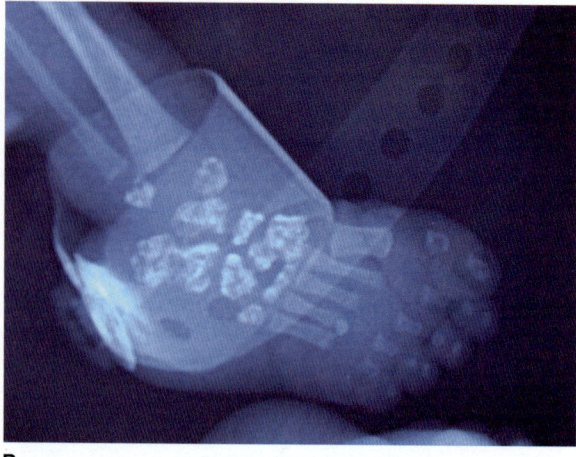

B

FIGURE 28-14 • Chondrodysplasia X-linked dominant (Conradi-Hünermann-Happle syndrome). **A:** The external examination reveals severe shortening of the upper and lower extremities with rhizomesoacromelic features. Note also the bilateral talipes equinovarus deformities. **B:** Multifocal stippled epiphyseal calcifications are the characteristic findings in CDP. This image of the foot shows the numerous calcifications in the epiphyses. (**Panel A** from Rakheja D, Read CP, Hull D et al. A severely affected female infant with X-linked dominant chondrodysplasia punctata: a case report and a brief review of the literature. *Pediatr Dev Pathol* 2007;10:142–148.)

absence of ossification and mineralization are seen in boomerang dysplasia. Marked disorganization in the columns of chondrocytes is the histologic features in boomerang dysplasia.

Chondrodysplasia Group

Chondrodysplasia (*CDP*) *group* (group 21) comprised 4% of GSDs in the Utah study (144). There are also acquired causes of CDP-like changes in children unrelated to the GSDs with similar punctate–stippled calcifications in the epiphyses and around the spine; examples are prenatal exposure to warfarin and neonatal lupus erythematosus (289). In terms of pathogenesis, CDP can be classified into inborn errors of cholesterol biosynthesis, peroxisomal biogenesis disorders, disruption of vitamin K metabolism, and chromosomal abnormalities (290,291). Rhizomelic CDP type I and Zellweger syndrome, both AR peroxisomal disorders, are lethal in most cases (292). Conradi-Hünermann-Happle (CHH) syndrome, with X-linked dominant inheritance (Xp11.23-p11.22), may be lethal in the affected neonate (Figure 28-14A, B) (293,294). One of the characteristic and accessible pathologic findings in CHH syndrome is lamellar orthokeratosis and dystrophic calcifications in keratotic plugs in a skin biopsy as the features of the linear ichthyosiform lesions (295). Rhizomelic CDP is represented by three AR disorders: peroxisomal CDP1 (PEX7 on 6q22-q24), CDP2 (DHAPAT on 1q42), and CDP3 (AGPS on 2q31) (296). The incidence is 1:100,000 live births. Severe shortening of proximal long bones (rhizomelia), cataracts, dysmorphic facies, and severe growth abnormalities are the various clinical features. Approximately 50% or more of children do not survive beyond the age of 6 years. The cause of death is usually respiratory in nature after multiple respiratory tract infections. Dystrophic calcifications in the region of an otherwise unremarkable growth plate and cystic myxoid degeneration in the subarticular cartilage are the principal histologic features in rhizomelic CDP (297). In other conditions, association with stippled calcifications, dystrophic calcifications, and degenerative changes in the chondroid matrix are the microscopic findings (Figure 28-15). OI-like features are present in the lethal Astley-Kendall syndrome as one of the overlap syndromes, which in this case is classified with the group 21 disorders (298).

Bent Bone Dysplasia

Bent bone dysplasias (*BBDs*) (group 18) are characterized by short limb dysplasia and bowing of the long bones of the lower extremity (299,300). However, the presence of "bent bones"

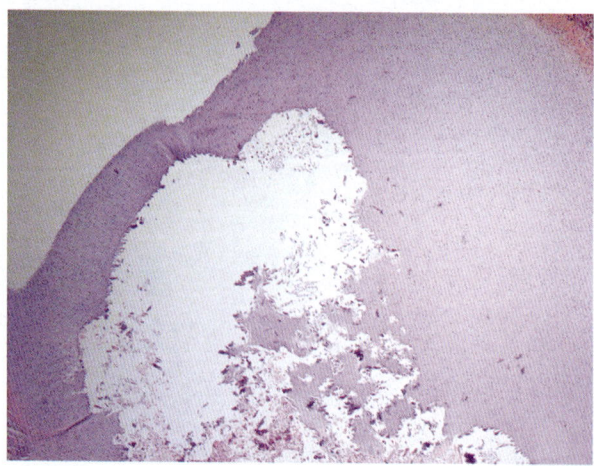

FIGURE 28-15 • Chondrodysplasia punctuate, X-linked dominant (Conradi-Hünermann-Happle syndrome). Dystrophic calcifications and cystic degeneration of the epiphysis are present. (Contributed by Charles Timmons, MD, Dallas, Texas.)

may be seen at birth in several other GSDs (138). The Utah study had six (4%) cases of BBD and five were examples of CD (144). CD has a reported incidence of 1:200,000 births and accounts for approximately 4% to 6% of all lethal skeletal dysplasias (301,302). Mutations in the SOX9 gene (17q24-q25) are the molecular genetic defect in this AD disorder (303). The role of SOX9 is multifold in development and in the context of this discussion—chondrogenesis with the activation of multiple cartilage-specific genes (304). Anterior bowing of the long bones of the lower extremities, hypoplastic thorax with secondary pulmonary hypoplasia, and craniofacial anomalies are the phenotypic abnormalities in addition to the characteristic sexual anomalies with so-called sex reversal; it is estimated that gonadal dysgenesis with male to female sex reversal is present in 75% of CD cases (305). Abnormalities of both müllerian and wolffian duct structures and incomplete ovarian or testicular development are other findings; gonadoblastoma may be seen in the dysgenetic testis (306,307). The physes of the long bones exhibit minimal histologic abnormalities; however, some alterations in the proliferative and hypertrophic zones of chondrocytes may be seen. In place of normal cortical bone, immature woven bone, osteoclastic activity, and vascularized intraosseous spaces are the microscopic features. Stuve-Wiedemann syndrome (SWS), another group 18 GSD, is a severe AR disorder with mutations in the LIFR gene (5p13.1) (308,309). Cortical thickening is present in bowed long bones with flared metaphyses and progressive decalcification. Dysautonomic hyperthermia, respiratory complications on the basis of aspiration pneumonitis, pulmonary artery hypertension, and cutaneous infections all contribute to death by 2 years of age (310,311). These children like those with CD have obstructive airway problems (312). BBD is also seen in FGFR2 mutation (313,314).

Neonatal Osteosclerotic Dysplasias

Neonatal osteosclerotic dysplasias (NOD) and increased bone density (IBD) group are designated as group 22 and group 23, respectively. Group 22 GSDs comprise five disorders including Caffey disease (infantile cortical hyperostosis), which is primarily an inflammatory and reactive condition arising in the diaphyseal region of long bones, but also in the mandible and clavicle in infants. There is fever and soft tissue swelling overlying the affected bone (315). The mandible is most commonly involved in 70% to 90% of cases (316). A mutation in the COL1A1 gene is present in the prenatal or infantile forms of Caffey disease but is uncommon in the later presenting form (317–319). Blomstrand dysplasia is an AR lethal neonatal disorder, which is characterized by generalized osteosclerosis and advanced skeletal maturation (320). Group 22 also includes desmosclerosis and Raine dysplasia. Inactivating recessive mutations in the PTH-related peptide type I receptor gene PTH PTH1 (3p22-21.1) are present in Blomstrand dysplasia (321,322). This same gene is mutated in Jansen chondrodysplasia. In addition to very short stature, the limbs are micromelic with accelerated ossification of virtually the entire skeleton. Like the other lethal skeletal dysplasias, the thorax is short and narrow. Early ossification of the epiphyseal center, a reduction in the epiphyseal cartilage, irregularity of the transformation zone, subperiosteal ossification, and cortical hyperostosis are some of the histologic findings.

Increased Bone Density: Osteopetrosis

IBD or OSP (group 23) is characterized by osseous hyperdensity without alteration in the shape of the bones. The basic defect occurs in the osteoclast in either development or function (323–325). Based upon the particular mutation, OSP is divided into the "osteoclast rich" whose mutations affect function and "osteoclast poor." The severe, neonatal forms with AR inheritance are seen in 1:250,000 births and are associated with several mutations (326–328). Loss-of-function mutations have been identified in five genes: TCIRG1 (11q13), CLCN7 (16p13), OSTM1(6q21), RANKL (TNFSF11, 13q14), and RANK (TNFRSF11A, 18q22.1) (325,329,330). Among these mutations in the AR OSP, the TCIRG1 mutation is detected in 50% to 60% and CLCN7 mutations account for 20% of cases and CLCN7 mutation in 20% to 25% of cases (324,325). Leukopenia and hepatosplenomegaly are the consequences of bony overgrowth of the marrow space with bone marrow failure, phthisic anemia, and organomegaly on the basis of extramedullary hematopoiesis. Early death may result from pathologic fractures, hydrocephalus, or anemia; the pathologic fractures are typically transverse breaks in the long bones. Without bone marrow or stem cell transplantation, survival beyond infancy is rare. Another expression of AR OSP is renal tubular acidosis (RTA) with cerebral calcifications; there are mutations in the carbonic anhydrase II gene (8q21.2). OSP–RTA is usually detected in the first 2 years of life with growth failure, mental retardation, visual and auditory deficiencies, pathologic fractures, and metabolic acidosis (325). Cerebral calcifications are detectable after 18 months of age. Cortical bone thickening is present in all forms of OSP, but in the most severe cases, the marrow cavity is obliterated and the corticomedullary demarcation is lost (Figure 28-16A to D). Osteosclerosis may be uniform or alternating, as seen in the vertebrae, where transverse striations of alternating lucent and dense bone formation with the so-called ruggerjersey spine. Lucency of the central portions of bones may convey the appearance of "bone within bone." Coxa vara and lateral bowing of the long bones are common findings, and rachitic features may be observed in infants. The microscopic hallmark is the persistence of calcified cartilage, surrounded by dense woven or lamellar bone of endochondral origin (Figure 28-17A, B) (331). The zone of proliferating cartilage is often extremely wide at sites of active endochondral ossification in infants, which reflects the failure in remodeling of mineralized cartilage and bone. Woven bone persists in the absence of lamellar bone formation. The number of osteoclasts in a bone biopsy may depend on the sampling or the osteoclast-rich or osteoclast-poor status of the particular type. Howship lacunae are often difficult to identify. Osteoblasts are generally present in normal numbers, but they often appear flattened and inactive. The marrow space is more or less obliterated by woven rather than lamellar bone, which is thought to account for the extreme fragility of the bone

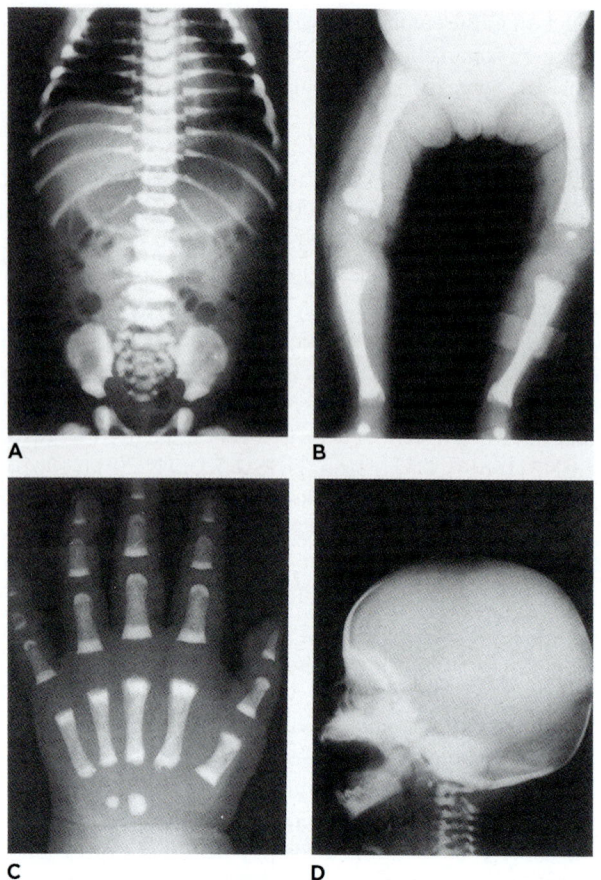

FIGURE 28-16 • Osteopetrosis, autosomal recessive lethal type. **A:** The images of the chest, abdomen, and pelvis demonstrate the generalized IBD. **B:** Sclerosis of the long bones of the lower extremities shows metaphyseal fragmentation, mild metaphyseal expansion, periosteal new bone formation, and an absence of the medullary canal. **C:** Sclerosis of the bones in the hand shows the most marked changes at the proximal ends of the phalanges and distal ends of the metacarpals. **D:** Lateral view of the skull demonstrates diffuse sclerosis, especially marked at the base. (Contributed by William H. McAlister, M.D., St. Louis, MO.)

despite its increased density. Ultrastructurally, the osteoclasts adjacent to the bone surface may lack the ruffled membrane that is necessary for bony resorption, which is impaired in all forms of OSP. AD OSP has mutations in CLCN7 and does not present until late childhood or adolescence with fractures, scoliosis, osteoarthropathy, and osteomyelitis of the mandible (325). The previous type of AD OSP with an LRP5 mutation is no longer regarded as a classic form of OSP (332).

Lysosomal Storage Disease

Lysosomal storage diseases (*LSDs*) with skeletal involvement or dysostosis multiplex group (group 27) comprise a family of heritable metabolic diseases with a defect in a specific acid hydrolase or enzyme activator whose functional and morphologic consequences are an accumulation or storage of the catabolic product at the blocked biochemical step. There are approximately 50 LSDs recognized, and the storage products include mucopolysaccharides, glycoproteins, amino acids, and lipids (333,334). Currently, 22 disorders with similar radiographic abnormalities are included in the ISDS classification (138). The incidence of LSDs is approximately 1:1500 to 8000 live births (335,336). Hypoplastic iliac bones with pseudoenlargement of the acetabula, pointed proximal metacarpals, defective development of the anterosuperior portions of the vertebral bodies at the thoracolumbar junctions, and widened ribs that taper near the vertebral margins are among the more consistent skeletal abnormalities among the LSDs with some differences among the specific types (Figure 28-18A to C) (337,338). The changes in the tubular bones, which are more pronounced in the upper extremities, include diaphyseal and metaphyseal expansion, delayed epiphyseal ossification, and osteopenia. Other changes include macrocrania, coxa valga, small carpal bones with V-shaped deformities of the distal radius and ulna, cardiomegaly, and hepatosplenomegaly. A consistent histologic finding in various parenchymal and mesenchymal cells, from hepatocytes to chondrocytes, is cellular enlargement, which

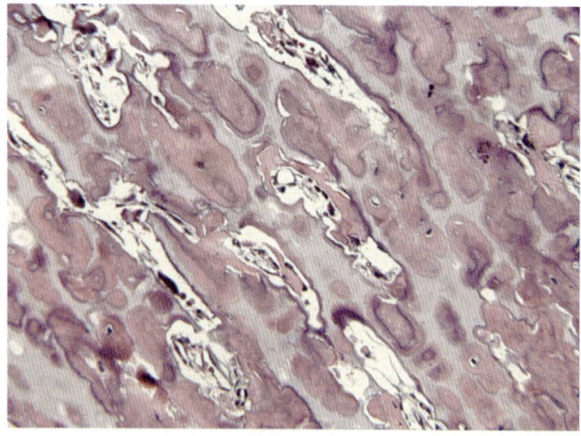 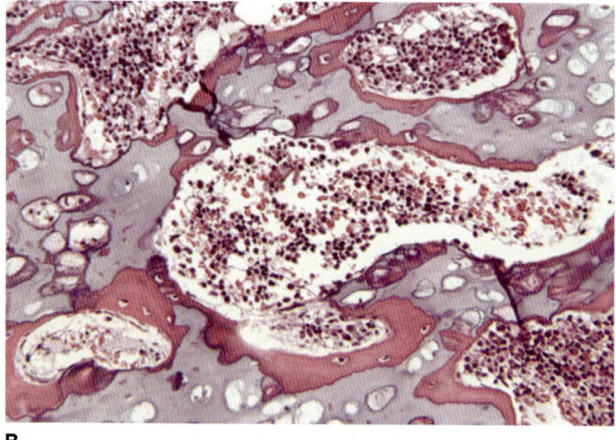

FIGURE 28-17 • Osteopetrosis, autosomal recessive type. **A:** The bone biopsy shows thickened trabeculae with retained central cores of cartilage. Note also the absence of bone marrow and hematopoiesis. **B:** A follow-up biopsy 2.5 years after a bone marrow transplant shows a reduction in the thickness of the trabeculae and the presence of hematopoiesis. A follow-up image at that time showed decreased bone density and an identifiable marrow. (From Tolar J, Teitelbaum SL, Orchard PJ. Mechanisms of Disease: Osteopetrosis. *N Engl J Med* 2004;351:2839–2849.)

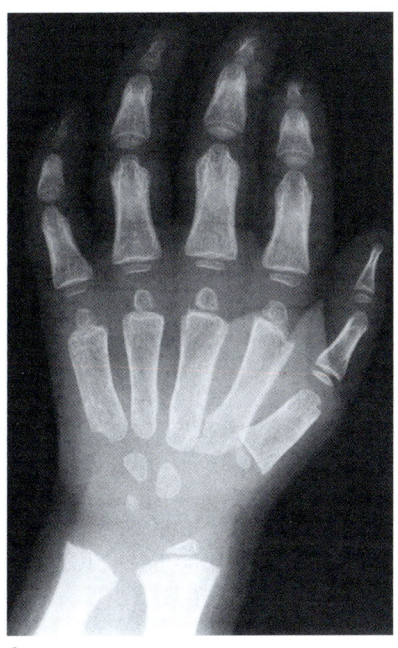
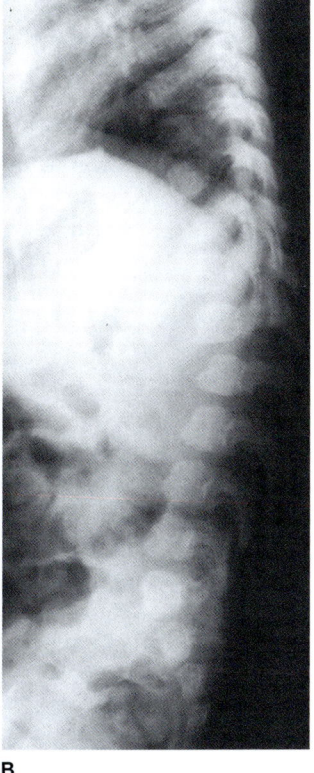
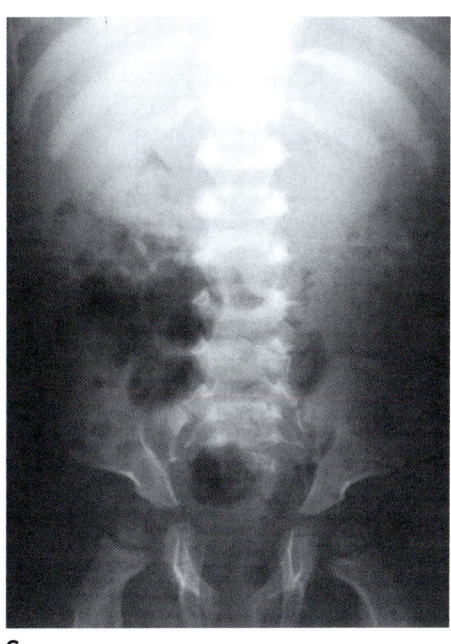

A B C

FIGURE 28-18 • Dysostosis multiplex congenita group. **A:** A 7-year-old boy with Hunter syndrome demonstrates proximal pointing of the metacarpals, widening of the proximal phalanges, tapering of the distal phalanges, and poor carpal bone development. **B:** A 9-month-old boy with Hurler syndrome shows the gibbous deformity of the spine and anterior beaking of the L2 vertebra. **C:** This 2-year-old boy with mucolipidosis has underdevelopment of the supra-acetabular portions of the iliac bones, coxa valga, and widening and tapering of the lower ribs near the spine. (Contributed by William H. McAlister, M.D., St. Louis, MO.)

reflects the presence of numerous membrane-bound vacuoles representing distended lysosomes that are clear or contain finely granular material (339–341) (see Chapter 5).

Mucopolysaccharidoses (*MPSs*) are the most familiar and common LSDs. There are seven distinct eponymic types of MPS with a total of 11 enzymatic defects (342,343). The overall incidence of the MPSs ranges from 1:100,000 to 600,000 live births with AR inheritance in all but MPS/H with X-linked recessive inheritance. A specific chromosomal defect has been identified in all of the MPSs. The natural history of the MPSs depends upon the severity of the CNS involvement and the development of cardiorespiratory complications (344–347). Shortened stature and progressive skeletal deformities are indicative of growth plate and bony abnormalities with subluxation of joints and progressive kyphoscoliosis, as in MPS type 7 (Sly syndrome). The growth plate is reduced in thickness and is disorganized in appearance. The prominence of enlarged, vacuolated chondrocytes varies somewhat among the types of MPS (Figure 28-19). Abrupt calcification of the cartilage without the formation of primary trabeculae is another feature of the growth plate in several of these disorders, including MPS type 1H (Hurler syndrome), MPS type IH/1S (Hurler-Scheie syndrome), and MPS type 4A (Morquio syndrome) (348). In addition to abnormalities in the axial and appendicular skeleton, histologic changes in the temporal bone have been correlated with deafness in MPS type 1H, type 1 IS (Scheie syndrome), MPS type 1H/1S, and MPS type 2 (Hunter syndrome).

Gaucher disease (GD), the most common LSD, occurs in 1:100,000 individuals in the general population, but 1:800 to 1000 Ashkenazi Jews (349). Type 1 GD accounts for 99% of cases, which becomes symptomatic in adolescence and early

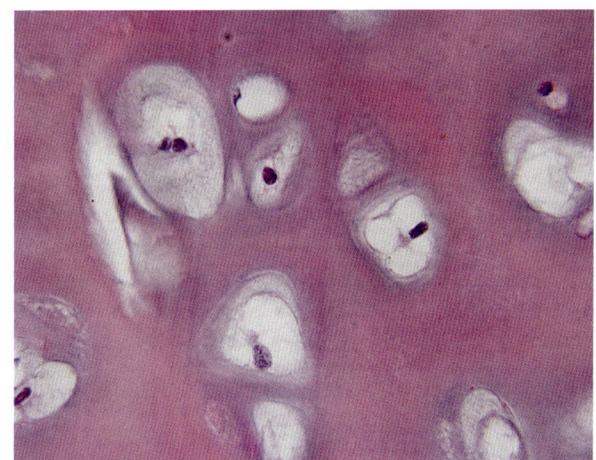

FIGURE 28-19 • Mucopolysaccharidosis, type 7 (Sly syndrome). The chondrocytes are distended with finely vacuolated cytoplasm.

adulthood. Bone changes in the distal femur and/or proximal tibia are present in 70% to 100% with type 1 GD (so-called adult) or type 3 (juvenile) GD (350–352). In addition to the Erlenmeyer flask–like deformities, osteopenia with pathologic fracture, bone infarcts, and osteomyelitis are the other skeletal complications. Macrophages with glucocerebrosides have a granular eosinophilic and fibrillary appearance.

Several other LSDs distinct from MPS also have dysostosis multiplex features, including mucolipidosis 2 (I-cell disease) and mucolipidosis 3 (pseudo-Hurler polydystrophy). Yet another category of metabolic disorders includes those in which glycoprotein degradation and structure are defective: fucosidosis, α-mannosidosis, β-mannosidosis, sialidosis, aspartylglycosaminuria, sialic acid storage disease, multiple sulfatase deficiency, and galactosialidosis (353–355). Carpal tunnel syndrome is a complication in both the MPSs and mucolipidoses secondary to the accumulation of material in swollen fibroblasts and the presence of foamy histiocytes (356).

Melorheostosis With and Without Osteopoikilosis, Pyknodysostosis, and Osteopathia Striata

Melorheostosis with and without osteopoikilosis, pyknodysostosis, and osteopathia striata is an example of a group 23 disorder (138). The estimated prevalence of melorheostosis is 1:1,000,000 individuals (357,358). The overwhelming majority of cases are sporadic in occurrence, but isolated examples have been reported in association with osteopoikilosis with mutations in the LEM domain containing 3 gene (12q14) (156). Mutations in this same gene are found in Buschke-Ollendorff syndrome. The diagnosis is rarely made in infancy, but 40% to 50% of cases are discovered before the age of 20 years (359). Any bone or bones may be affected; however, involvement is frequently unilateral, with one or more hyperostotic long bones, usually in the lower extremity, with so-called flowing hyperostosis (360). The fibrosing component in the contiguous soft tissues has fibromatosis-like or atypical decubitus fibroplasia-like histologic features, which result in contractures, a cause of substantial morbidity in this disorder (361). Fibrofatty and myositis ossificans-like lesions have also been observed. Unlike the marrow space in OP, the marrow space remains intact, but the cortex is thickened and dense, with a paucity of haversian canals. Mosaic lines may be prominent. Osteoclastic activity is inapparent, whereas osteoblasts are present, but not in appreciable numbers. Endochondral ossification extends well into the zone of articular cartilage. Osteopoikilosis is an AD disorder in which bone islands form at the ends of a bone and in the vicinity of the metaphysic. Histologically, the foci are identified as rounded expansions of hyperdense bone with some mosaic lines. Multiple dermal fibrous papules in association with osteopoikilosis are the features of Buschke-Ollendorff syndrome.

Metaphyseal Dysplasias

Metaphyseal dysplasias (*MPD*) (group 11) comprise a genetically heterogenous group of disorders, which are characterized by a failure in enchondral bone growth and remodeling of the end of the long bones with the development of Erlenmeyer flask–like deformity of the metaphysis with an increased diameter (362,363). The distal femur and proximal tibia are the most frequently affected sites. Similar deformities are seen in GD and other GSDs, which are not classified among the group 11 diseases. Shwachman-Diamond syndrome, one of the inherited bone marrow failure syndromes, in addition to FA, Diamond-Blackfan anemia, dyskeratosis congenita, and Kostmann severe congenital neutropenia, is an AR disorder with an incidence of 1:75,000 births; 90% of cases have mutations in the SBDS gene (7q11) (364,365). Metaphyseal dysplasia of the femoral head is present in 50% of cases, but abnormalities in ribs (shortened with flared ends) can result in a hypoplastic thorax with lethal consequences in the neonatal period (366). There is an apparent failure in the formation of the zone of hypertrophic cartilage; however, a case has been reported with features of spondylometaphyseal dysplasia in a neonate with a SBDS gene mutation in which the hypertrophic zone was hypercellular with minimal matrix extending into the metaphysis (367). Cartilage–hair hypoplasia (CHH, McKusick type) is one of four skeletal dysplasias with mutations in the RMRP gene (9p21-p13) (368,369). The incidence is 1:23,000 live births (370). In addition to short stature, these children have ectodermal dysplasia and T-cell immunodeficiency (371). Granulomatous inflammation of the skin may occur in infancy (372,373). Another type of MPD is the Schmid type with a mutation in COL10A1 gene (155,374).

Genetic Inflammatory Rheumatoid-Like Osteoarthropathies

Genetic inflammatory rheumatoid-like osteoarthropathies (*GIRLOs*) (group 31) include several autoinflammatory disorders with both AR inheritance and AD inheritance (138). The pathogenesis of these hereditary autoinflammatory disorders is an apparent disruption in the linkage of IL-1 function and the regulation of the innate immune response (375,376). Mutations in two IL-1–regulating genes, NLRP3 and IL1RN, are responsible for cryopyrin-associated periodic syndromes (CAPS) and deficiency of IL-1 receptor antagonist (DIRA). CAPS is a spectrum disorder whose earliest and severest manifestations are present in the neonatal-onset multisystem inflammatory disease (377,378). There is overgrowth in the region of the growth plate with exostosis-like features, defects in limb lengths, and contractures. A skin biopsy shows a neutrophilic infiltrate of an urticarial or neutrophilic dermatosis (pyoderma gangrenosum). In addition to growth retardation, there is diffuse osteopenia. Muckle-Wells syndrome is a less severe form of NOMID/CINCA spectrum (379). Chronic recurrent multifocal osteomyelitis (CRMO) and nonbacterial acute osteitis are associated with mutations in IL1RN or LPIN2 (Majeed syndrome) (380,381). Other mutations in CRMO include GALNTS and RAGS. The median age at diagnosis is 10 years ,and the presentation is the development of osteolytic bone lesions with the pathologic features of acute to subacute to chronic osteomyelitis; however, the lesions are sterile for microorganisms. Progressive pseudorheumatoid dysplasia develops in children between 3 and 6 years and has a mutation in the WISP3 gene (382). There are minimal signs of inflammation unlike the other disorders in this group. Growth abnormalities are present, and multiple large and small joints are involved with a particular early predilection for the hip joints where there is enlargement of the femoral heads.

Disorganized Development of Skeletal Component Group

Disorganized development of skeletal component group (group 29) constitutes several tumefactive lesions of bone, some of which are familiar to pathologists including polyostotic FD, multiple osteochondromas (OCs), or multiple hereditary exostoses, cherubism or multiple giant-cell reparative granulomas (GCRGs), and enchondromatosis with or without hemangiomas (138). These various tumor and tumorlike lesions are discussed in the subsequent section on neoplasms.

ACQUIRED DISORDERS

The major acquired disorders in children include infectious–inflammatory conditions involving bone or joint space, nutritional–metabolic conditions, and tumefactions of bone. Each of these three categories is related in the clinical differential diagnosis of a mass or swelling with or without pain and fever.

Metabolic and Nutritional Conditions

Vitamin deficiency disorders with notable clinical effects upon the skeletal system include vitamin C or ascorbic acid deficiency, which causes scurvy, and vitamin D deficiency, which causes rickets–osteomalacia. At one time in the past, both vitamin deficiencies were found with some frequency in infants.

Scurvy is characterized by a failure in the formation of the primary spongiosa of bone, where the earliest recognizable bone formation at the growth plate takes place. The inability to form extracellular collagenous matrix is secondary to the loss of hydroxylation of lysine and proline, which depends on vitamin C as a cofactor (383). Rather than bone formation, fibroblastic proliferation with extravasation of red cells occurs, reminiscent of nodular fasciitis. Subperiosteal hemorrhage and microfractures through the metaphyses are other findings. The medullary trabecular bone is markedly osteopenic; these radiographic changes are found predominantly in infancy and early childhood (384,385). The radiographic findings in the long tubular bones include diffuse demineralization; some sclerosis and irregularity in the provisional zone of calcification, in part secondary to microfractures; metaphyseal spurs; transverse metaphyseal bands of diminished bone density ("scurvy line") with peripheral fractures ("corner sign"); epiphyses with marked central rarefaction and relatively sclerotic margins (Wimberger sign); and periosteal new bone. Swelling of the knees is a presenting sign, and metaphyseal microfractures and dislocation may be falsely interpreted as evidence of child abuse. However, the presence of severe demineralization together with lateral metaphyseal spurs, and a dense irregular provisional zone of calcification makes differentiation relatively easy in most cases. Cupping of the epiphysis–metaphysis is a rare residual manifestation of infantile scurvy.

Rickets–osteomalacia is the consequence of deficient growth plate mineralization secondary to inadequate intake of calcium or a state of calciferol deficiency. There are numerous inherited and acquired disorders with rachitic and osteomalacic features (386–388). In congenital rickets secondary to maternal vitamin D deficiency, elements of hyperparathyroidism are noted in the fetus in response to maternal hypocalcemia. A substantial proportion of the childhood cases of rickets–osteomalacia in the developed countries of the world are secondary to hereditary defects in vitamin D activation or phosphate reabsorption by the renal tubules. However, rickets has been seen in recent years in the United States and Canada in infants breast-fed for a prolonged period without vitamin D supplementation (389,390). In some parts of the underdeveloped world, calcium malnutrition and/or vitamin D deficiency in children is a cause of rickets (391,392). Malabsorption syndromes, chronic hepatic disease, and infantile OP in children are complicated by rickets–osteomalacia. Linear sebaceous nevus syndrome, hemangiomatosis of bone, phosphaturic mesenchymal tumor (FGF23 mediated), nonossifying fibroma (NOF), osteoblastoma (OB), and OS are some of the causes of oncogenic hypophosphatemic rickets–osteomalacia (393,394). The radiographic appearance frequently differs according to the underlying disease. Infantile rickets is characterized by disruption of enchondral ossification and persistence and overgrowth of nonmineralized cartilage into the metaphysis (395). In undecalcified sections, the osteoid seams surrounding the bony trabeculae are widened and uncalcified. Myelofibrosis as a result of secondary hyperparathyroidism has been reported in an infant with vitamin D-deficient rickets (396). There has been discussion about the metaphyseal lesions of child abuse and their possible relationship to rickets since cartilaginous overgrowth is seen in both (397–399).

Hyperparathyroidism in the pediatric age population is usually secondary to chronic renal failure (400–402). Primary hyperparathyroidism is seen throughout the first two decades, even in the neonatal period, and is commonly associated with skeletal abnormalities and four gland hyperplasia (403,404). A classic but quite uncommon manifestation of hyperparathyroidism is the brown tumor, which has microscopic features very similar to GCRG. Both osteoclastic and osteoblastic activities, often with medullary fibrosis, in a bone biopsy should suggest the diagnosis of hyperparathyroidism (see Chapter 21).

Pseudohypoparathyroidism (PHP) is an inherited disorder, which is functionally characterized by peripheral resistance to PTH due to a mutation in the imprinted gene, GNAS (20q13.3) (405–407). There are two subtypes of PHP: type 1a with maternal inheritance and the Albright hereditary osteodystrophy (AOH) phenotype (short stature, brachydactyly, and extraskeletal osteomas in the dermis, subcutis, and skeletal muscles) and type 1b with paternal inheritance and AOH phenotype in the absence of the endocrinopathies (405). Progressive osseous heteroplasia (POH) is another of the GNAS-inactivating mutation disorders with heterotopic ossification in the skin with extension into the underlying soft tissues whose onset may be seen in infancy or in later childhood (407–409). There is an absence of the AOH phenotype; there is an overlap between PHP1b and POH in this respect. The formation of heterotopic bone resembles intramembrane bone with its direct development from mesenchymal-derived osteoblasts. A progressive osteodystrophy resembling that seen in PHP has been reported in mucolipidoses types I and II (410,411).

Primary hyperoxaluria 1 is an AR disorder with mutations in the alanine-glyoxylate aminotransferase (AGT) gene (2q37.3); AGT is responsible for the conversion of glyoxylate to glycine and in its absence glyoxylate is converted to oxalates, which accumulate in the kidney and other organs including the skeletal system (412). Dense and lucent metaphyseal bands that develop in the tubular (long) bones are characteristic findings (413–415). There is deposition of oxalate crystals in the medullary space and osteoblastic and osteoclastic activity in the trabecular bone, which reflects in part secondary hyperparathyroidism associated with chronic renal failure.

Tumor and Tumorlike Conditions

Neoplasms and other tumefactions of the skeletal system comprise a largely unique pathologic group of tumors, which are generally restricted to the first two decades of life but are also seen in young adults and tend to diminish in frequency beyond the age of 40 years (416). OC and OS account for 50% or more of all primary bone tumors in childhood, with OS accounting for 8% to 10% of all cases (417–419). Over 50% of all benign bone lesions in children are OCs, and almost 60% of all primary malignant neoplasms of bone in the same age group are OSs. The incidence of other primary skeletal lesions, including bone cysts and FD, tends to increase in incidence throughout the first two decades of life. In a review of the experience of biopsy-proven bone tumors in children from the Dutch Pathology Registry, the incidence per million children between 10 and 18 years of age rose from 3.9 in the first decade of life to a peak of 143 cases at 13 to 15 years of age (418). Primary bone tumors in the first 5 years of life are uncommon, but some examples include Langerhans cell histiocytosis (LCH), melanotic neuroectodermal tumor of infancy (MNTI), myofibroma, chest wall hamartoma, ABC, hemangioma, and Ewing sarcoma–primitive neuroectodermal tumor (EWS–PNET) (420,421). In fact, EWS–PNET of the bone is far more likely in a child less than 6 years old than OS (422). The most common malignant bone neoplasm in a child less than 6 years of age is metastatic neuroblastoma (NB).

There are few areas in anatomic and surgical pathology in which the formulation of the differential diagnosis is so fundamentally important to the ultimate interpretation. For the pathologist, challenges and potential pitfalls encountered along the way to the correct diagnosis include the generally infrequent nature of these tumors, and thus, a minimal or absent experience with many of them. The diminutive size of the biopsy specimens may be accompanied by artifacts, even to the point where the characteristic microscopic features of a specific entity may be muted or entirely absent in some cases. However, immunohistochemistry in a suspected malignant round-cell neoplasm may rescue a diagnosis even in the presence of substantial artifacts, which have compromised the morphology. A review of the skeletal imaging studies is also imperative when possible prior to formulating the final pathologic diagnosis.

In this section, our approach to the pathologic diagnosis focuses on the principal histologic features(s) in a biopsy or resection specimen. Although many lesions have mixed microscopic features, most skeletal tumors may be placed into one of three general morphologic categories: (a) osteoid and/or chondroid matrix-containing entities; (b) nonmatrix-associated lesions with a spindle cell stroma, with or without giant cells and with or without cyst formation; and (c) round-cell neoplasms with or without polymorphous features and an absence of apparent matrix production in most cases.

MATRIX-PRODUCING AND MATRIX-ASSOCIATED TUMORS

The overwhelming majority of benign and malignant neoplasms and tumorlike conditions arising in the skeletal system occurring in the first two decades of life are matrix-producing or matrix-associated tumors. Osteochondroma (OC), chondroblastoma (CB), chondromyxoid fibroma (CMF), and osteogenic lesions, osteoma, osteoid osteoma (OO), and OB account for 90% of all benign bone tumors in the first two decades, and 80% of these tumors are diagnosed in the second decade of life. Benign chondrogenic tumors alone comprise 60% to 70% of all benign bone tumors, and the overwhelming number of these are OCs (423). The number of OCs in our own files reflects the number of children who have had resections for multiple hereditary exostosis (MHE). Among primary malignant bone tumors in children, OS accounts for 60% to 70% of all cases; only 4% are CSs. OS accounts for 2% to 3% of all malignancies in the first two decades of life (424). Approximately 20% to 30% of cases are EWS–PNET, but this figure can vary depending upon the relative proportion of white and nonwhite children in a particular population as EWS–PNET is uncommon in nonwhite patients (425,426).

In addition to the more common osteogenic and chondrogenic neoplasms, others are somewhat ambiguous in terms of pathogenesis as in the case of aneurysmal and solitary bone cysts as "tumors of undefined neoplastic nature" and NOF as a fibrohistiocytic tumor (427). Some lesions such as FD and NOF are discovered incidentally, and their imaging characteristics are sufficiently diagnostic that the pathologist is less likely to encounter them as a biopsy or resection specimen unless some complication has occurred requiring surgical intervention such as a pathologic fracture.

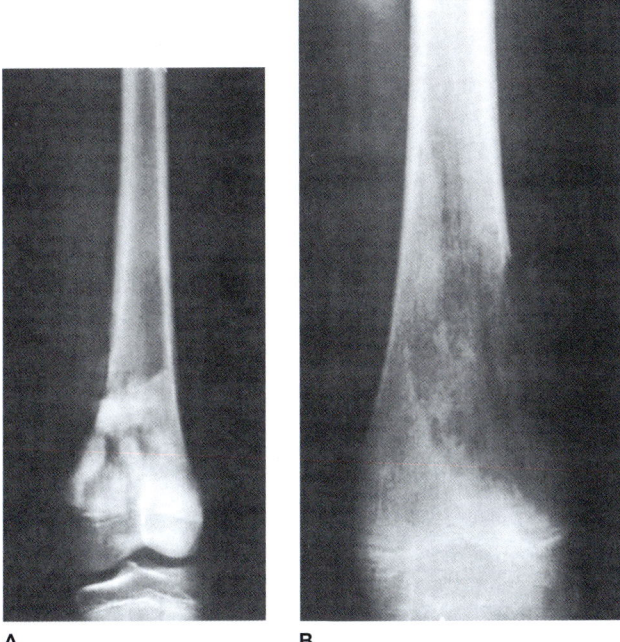

FIGURE 28-20 • Osteosarcomas in a 13-year-old girl and an 11-year-old girl show two patterns. **A:** Irregular, poorly defined, sclerotic lesion is seen in the distal femur. **B:** Purely osteolytic lesion in the distal femur may be associated with the telangiectatic variant of OS or fibroblastic OS with minimal ossification.

Osteosarcoma

OS should be considered in the presence of any long bone tumor in a patient between 10 and 25 years of age who has a radiologically poorly defined metaphyseal lesion, with a mixed lytic and sclerotic pattern of permeative growth, and cortical destruction (Figure 28-20A, B). The distal femur, proximal tibia, and proximal humerus account for 65% to 80% of all OSs. Although an associated soft tissue component may not be evident on routine imaging, magnetic resonance imaging (MRI) demonstrates that virtually all conventional OSs have extended into the soft tissue at the time of diagnosis (Figure 28-21A, B) (428,429). Less frequently, OS in children may present in the axial skeleton including the rib and head and neck region (430–432). A histologic diagnosis of OS depends upon the presence of osteoid or tumor bone being directly produced by malignant-appearing stromal cells. The so-called malignant osteoid has a fine, wispy, basophilic to eosinophilic histologic appearance; may be inapparent, especially in the telangiectatic form of OS; or presents as small extracellular deposits with or without obvious calcification or tumor bone formation; it is often seen as ribbon or lacelike strands around small groups or individual round to spindle-shaped cells (Figure 28-22A to D). It should be noted, however, that the diagnosis of osteoid is subjective in some cases and very much dependent upon individual experience, as nonspecific collagen and immature chondroid may mimic osteoid. The biopsy may show only a high-grade sarcoma composed of large round to epithelioid and/or spindle-shaped cells, without evident osteoid formation. Such lesions can be suspected as representing OS since few other malignancies of bone or soft tissues in children have this constellation of high-grade, pleomorphic features. Even in the total presence of highly atypical, if not overtly, malignant-appearing cartilage in the biopsy tissue, the tumor is more likely to represent a chondroblastic OS rather than a CS in a patient 20 years old or less. The suspicion of OS may be corroborated in most cases by a review of the pertinent imaging studies with a radiologist experienced in musculoskeletal disease. Infrequently, an innocuous image may belie the obvious presence of an OS in a biopsy specimen (433). On the other hand, a highly destructive, osteolytic lesion may

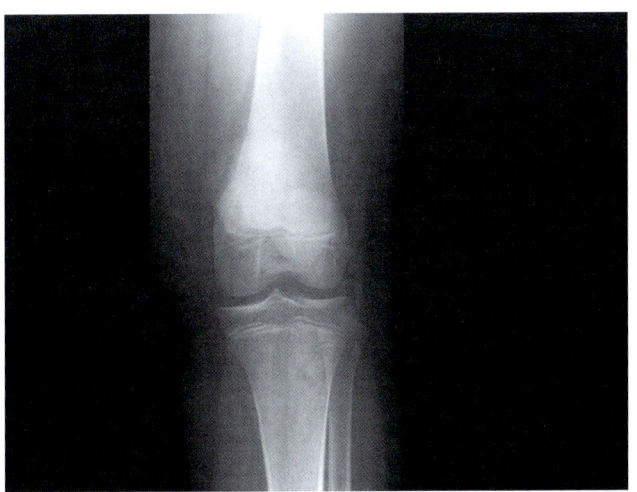
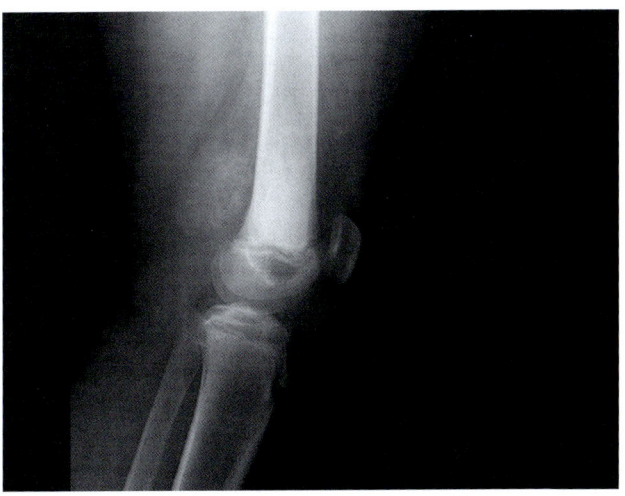

FIGURE 28-21 • Osteosarcoma in the distal femur of an 11-year-old girl. **A:** Anterior–posterior view of the distal femur shows medullary sclerosis. **B:** Lateral view demonstrates the sclerosis and suggestion of growth across the epiphyseal plate. There is a periosteal reaction with a prominent soft tissue mass.

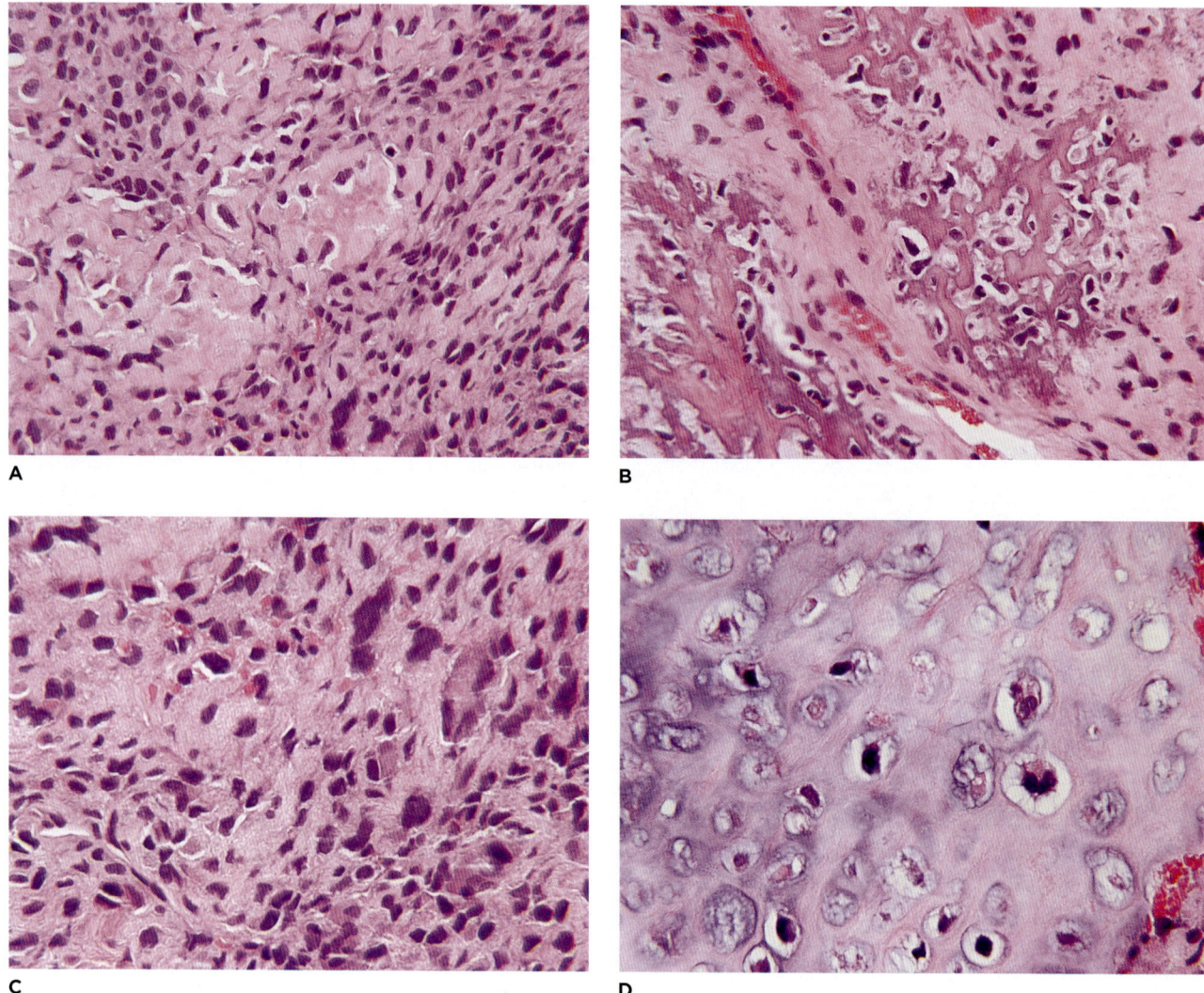

FIGURE 28-22 • Osteosarcoma in the distal femur of an 11-year-old girl. Several patterns are not unusual even in a relatively small biopsy. **A:** This microscopic field shows high-grade ovoid to spindle-shaped malignant cells with nuclear hyperchromatism. The appearance of the pink matrix may or may not qualify as osteoid. **B:** The presence of a lacelike pattern of formed calcified osteoid with associated malignant osteoblasts is seen in this field. **C:** Another field contains high-grade malignant mesenchymal cells with pale-staining matrix without clear osteoid formation. Tumor giant cells and atypical mitotic figures are also present. **D:** Another pattern in this tumor was the presence of malignant-appearing cartilage with high-grade features. The presence of malignant-appearing cartilage is a feature of OS, since conventional CS in children is typically low grade.

have imaging features more in keeping with EWS–PNET yet is an OS on biopsy. Although some EWS–PNETs may exhibit intraosseous foci resembling matrix formation due to the presence of necrotic bone on imaging studies, the presence of matrix in the adjacent soft tissue effectively rules out EWS–PNET as a diagnostic consideration.

OS of the "conventional" high-grade type comprises 65% to 80% of all cases (434). These tumors typically are intramedullary with expansile and infiltrative growth through the cortex into the soft tissues. A rare high-grade OS may also broadly originate from the surface of the bone and has a circumferential growth in 50% to 60% of cases; these latter tumors often arise from the diaphysis of the femur or tibia (435). High-grade conventional OS displays other features including patterns of pleomorphic sarcoma, sheets of osteoclast-like giant cells resembling giant-cell tumor (GCT), and/or nodules of malignant-appearing cartilage (434). Malignant osteoblasts with epithelioid features, some resembling rhabdoid cells, are present as either isolated foci or in a more diffuse pattern whose presence may be the source of a challenging differential diagnosis when osteoid is inapparent in which case epithelioid sarcoma, sclerosing epithelioid fibrosarcoma, myoepithelial tumor, and OB are among the other considerations (436–440). Additionally, unusual histologic patterns in conventional OS are those that have OB-like, CMF-like, CB-like, and malignant fibrous histiocytoma-like features (427). Anaplasia and mitotic figures, often atypical, are present to a greater or lesser degree in most conventional OSs. Dense osteoid formation, commonly in a sheetlike formation, rather than the more subtle intercellular ribbonlike eosinophilic matrix, may occur as appositional growth of "malignant bone" upon the surface of nonneoplastic residual cancellous bone; this feature is encountered more often in resection specimens than in a small biopsy that samples the periphery of the tumor.

"Nonconventional" OSs, representing 10% to 15% of cases, are represented by the following variants: telangiectatic, small-cell, periosteal, parosteal, and low-grade, central types (427,434). A predominantly telangiectatic OS may have the gross and low-power histologic features of an ABC, but on high-power view, anaplasia and pleomorphism of the cells within and lining the septa that form the walls of the ectatic blood-filled spaces are the diagnostic features. Pathologic fracture occurs in 40% to 50% of telangiectatic OSs at presentation, but does not have the dire prognostic implications that were once thought with improved management (441,442).

Small-cell OS accounts for only 1% to 2% of all OSs, and its histologic distinction from EWS–PNET of bone is based on the presence of osteoid among the relatively monotonous round to subtly spindle-shaped cells; there is also a degree of pleomorphism, mitotic activity, and cell size variation that also helps to differentiate a small-cell OS from a typical EWS–PNET (Figure 28-23A to C) (443). The tumor cells in small-cell OS are immunopositive for vimentin but nonreactive for cytokeratin and are focally reactive in some cases for CD99 and SATB2. Small-cell OS is not an EWSR1, FUS, or CIC–DUX4-associated neoplasm in at least one study (444).

Parosteal (juxtacortical) OS (3% to 4% of cases) is a markedly sclerotic tumor typically involving the distal posterior femur. A lobulated mass encircles the involved bone and may have a cartilaginous cap with OC-like features (445). This variant most commonly occurs in patients in the fourth to fifth decades of life. It is characterized by a spindle cell stroma containing bone that is frequently arrayed in parallel rows along the long axis of the lesion. The stromal cells may or may not show a mild degree of nuclear atypia (446). The bone varies from irregular metaplastic to mature bone lined by normal-appearing osteoblasts. The final diagnosis in those cases without overt cell atypia depends on its radiologic pattern of its broad attachment to the bone surface. Activating GNAS mutations, as seen in FD, have been found in parosteal OS as well as MDM2/CDK4 expression (447,448). Unlike conventional OS, surgical excision without chemotherapy is the usual treatment. Areas of dedifferentiation, with pleomorphic anaplastic change, may be present either at initial diagnosis or in recurrent lesions.

The tibial diaphysis is the characteristic site of the periosteal OS variant (1% to 2% of all cases) (Figure 28-24). This tumor is a high-grade chondroblastic form of OS. Its difference from a high-grade surface OS depends upon its characteristic speculated radiologic appearance (449). Like

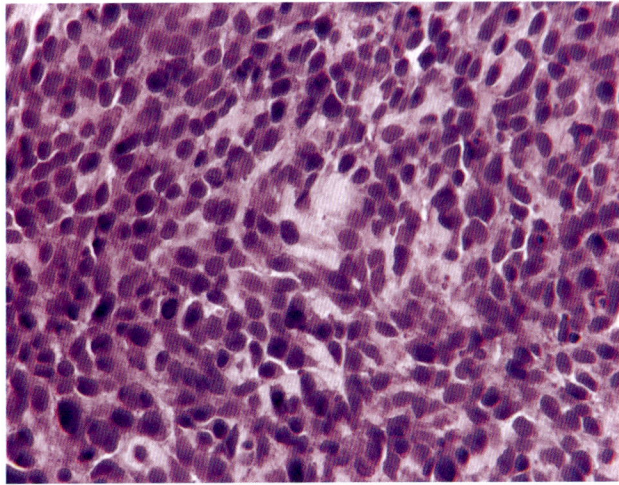

A

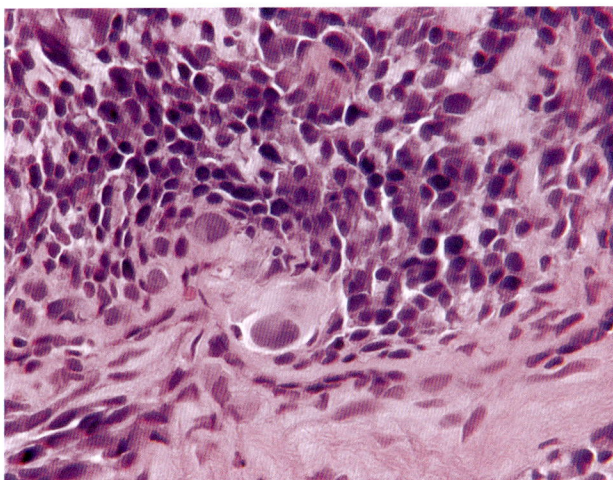

B

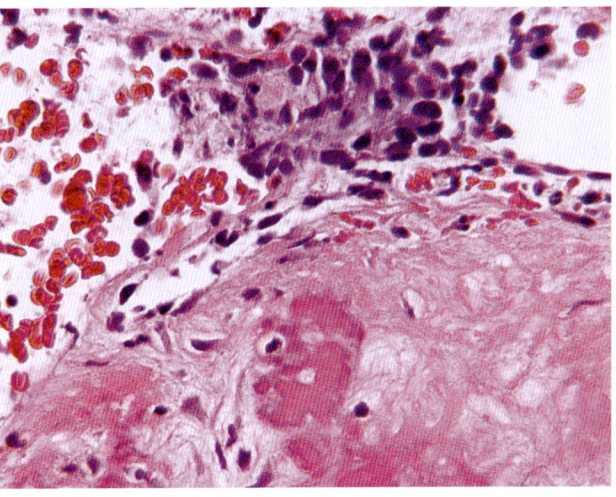

C

FIGURE 28-23 • Osteosarcoma in a 16-year-old boy. **A:** Sheets of malignant small round cells without apparent matrix are concerning for EWS–PNET. **B:** Larger pleomorphic cells among the round cells are unlikely findings in EWS–PNET and should initiate concern about an OS. **C:** Elsewhere, the focal presence of osteoid confirms the diagnosis of small-cell OS.

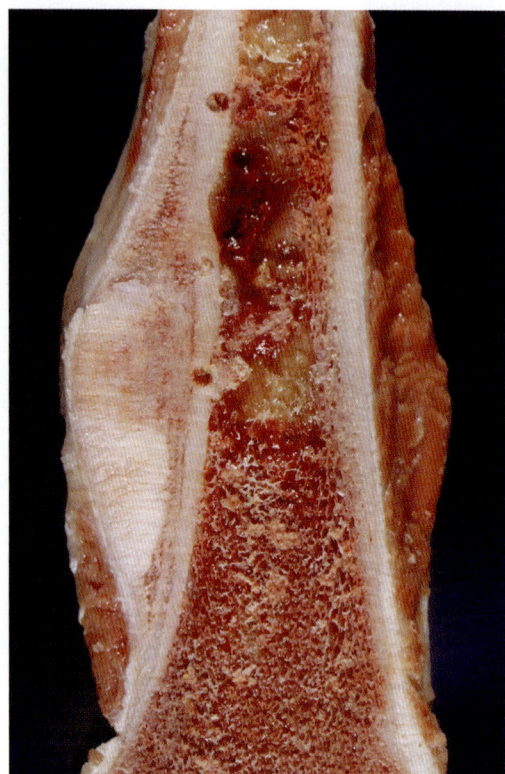

FIGURE 28-24 • Periosteal osteosarcoma. Note the presence of the mass with a prominent nodule of cartilage on the cortical surface.

parosteal OS, periosteal OS is associated with a more favorable prognosis than conventional type OS (Figure 28-25A to C) (449,450).

Low-grade central OS (1% or less of all cases) is a neoplasm with imaging and microscopic features that may in some cases be deceptively similar to those of FD, although in most cases, imaging studies are consistent with a malignant process (451–453). The spindle cell stroma and trabecular bone formation may also mimic FD, but in most cases, the stromal cell nuclear atypia and mitotic activity that is present are not encountered in FD. MDM2/CDK4 expression is reportedly helpful in differentiating low-grade central OS from FD (454). Activating mutation in GNAS is present in low-grade central OS (455). Intracortical or surface OS exists as individual reports of an otherwise conventional, high-grade neoplasm (456,457).

In most cases, contemporary management of conventional OS consists of a segmental surgical resection preceded by neoadjuvant chemotherapy. The gross appearance of the excised bone depends upon the proportions of fibrous, cartilaginous, and osseous tissue present and varies from soft fleshlike tumor to dense, sclerotic osseous areas. Cortical destruction with periosteal Codman triangles and soft tissue invasion are common features (Figure 28-26). Chemotherapy affects the microscopic appearance of the surgical specimen; those tumors with a "good response" to chemotherapy are defined as ablation of 90% or more of the cellular component of the tumor. There is an "empty" quality to the tumor area with minimal stromal cellularity and only acellular matrix

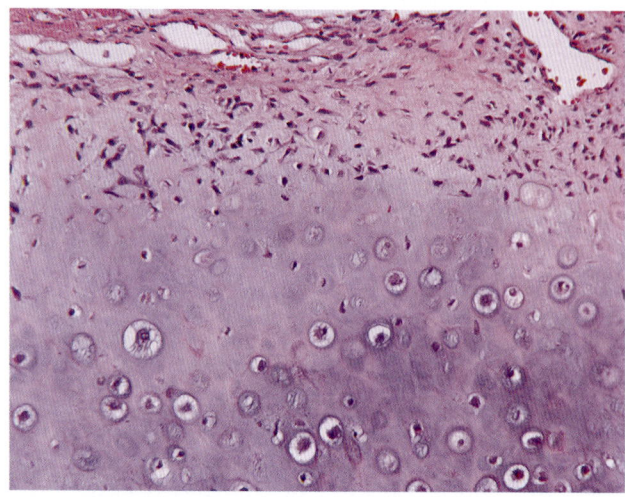

A

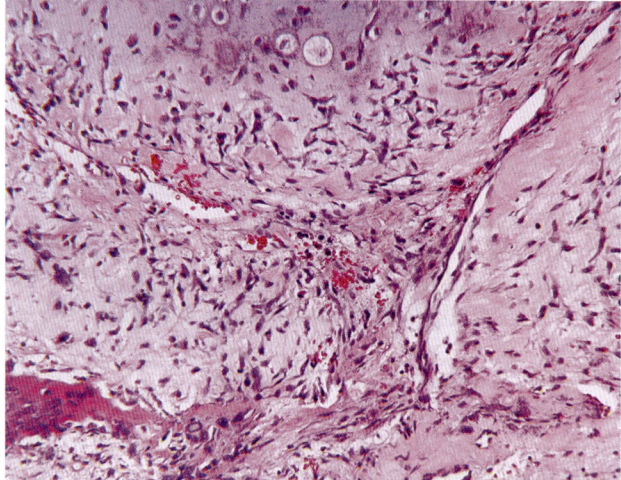

B

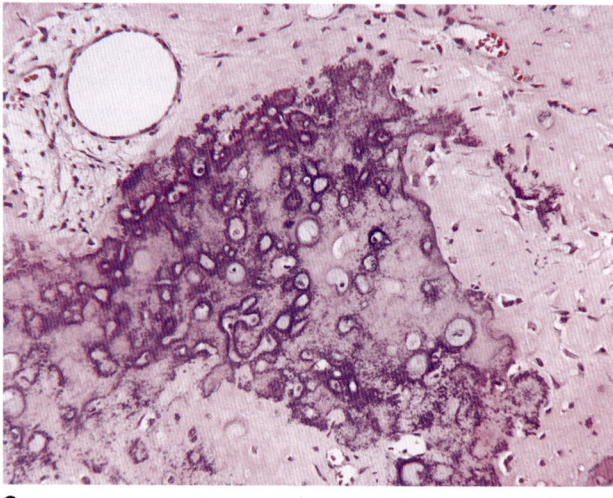

C

FIGURE 28-25 • Periosteal osteosarcoma. **A:** This field shows the periphery of the tumor with cartilage mimicking an OC in this tumor arising from the tibial diaphysis in a 13-year-old girl. **B:** Other areas in this tumor showed foci with spindle cell myxoid features. **C:** This focus shows the formation of calcified malignant osteoid with the basophilic features resembling cartilage.

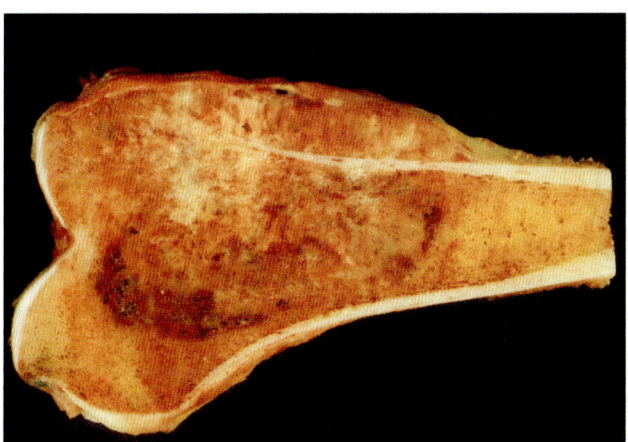

FIGURE 28-26 • Osteosarcoma of the distal femur in a 17-year-old boy. The mass in the region of the metaphysis measures 9.5 cm in greatest dimension and has a firm, densely sclerotic almost marbleized quality. Most OSs, like the present one, have been resected after chemotherapy. The College of American Pathologists' protocol for the examination of bone tumor specimens should be consulted for details (See *Arch Pathol Lab Med* 2010;134(4):e1–e7.)

evident (Figure 28-27A to D). If the tumor is soft, friable, and hemorrhagic and has a viable-appearing periosteal and soft tissue component, it can be surmised that the tumor did not respond favorably to chemotherapy. After fixation and photography of the bisected specimen, grid-oriented sections should be obtained for semiquantitative assessment of the effect of the chemotherapy on the tumor. Another important parameter of prognosis, which is optimally seen in the pretreatment images, is tumor size or volume (458,459). Children with "larger" OSs have a poorer outcome than those with smaller neoplasms (459).

Approximately 45% to 50% OSs are diagnosed before 20 years of age; however, only 5% of cases are recognized in the first decade of life and only rarely in children under age 5 years (460). By comparison, EWS–PNET is more likely in an infant or young child (461). Most OSs are sporadic, but there are several hereditary disorders with a predisposition for OS: Li-Fraumeni syndrome (TP53 on 17p13.1), RECQL4 gene (8q24.3) family syndrome (Rothmund-Thomson, Bloom, and Werner syndromes), and heritable retinoblastoma (RB) (RB1 on 13q14.2) (462–465). There may also be an increased risk for OS in association with Blackfan-Diamond anemia (466).

Microscopic foci of metastatic OS, most commonly involving the lung, and not visible on imaging studies, are present in 15% to 20% of cases at the time of initial clinical presentation. In addition, a subpopulation of patients may have overt metastatic lung deposits at presentation (467). These patients have an overall worse prognosis than the former. The metastases frequently show calcification. Another pattern of presentation is the presence of multifocal skeletal lesions of OS without pulmonary metastasis in 1% to 2% of cases; the incompletely resolved issue is whether this phenomenon constitutes multifocal synchronous primary tumors or is a unique pattern of metastases (468). The presence of a dominant mass in one of the sites has argued for the metastatic theory. Another problematic issue is the occurrence of skip metastases, which are detected in 2% to 7% of cases of conventional OS. A skip metastasis is defined as a separate, small focus of OS in the same site as the primary tumor but grossly proximal or distal to the main lesion. The overall prognosis of conventional OS in patients treated with combined surgical excisional and chemotherapy is now approximately 70% from its earlier 5-year survival of only 20% to 25% (469). However, there has been little if any improvement in this survival figure over the past decade.

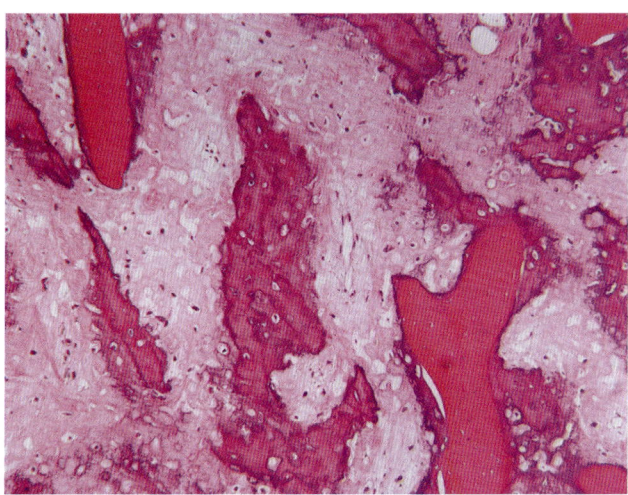
A

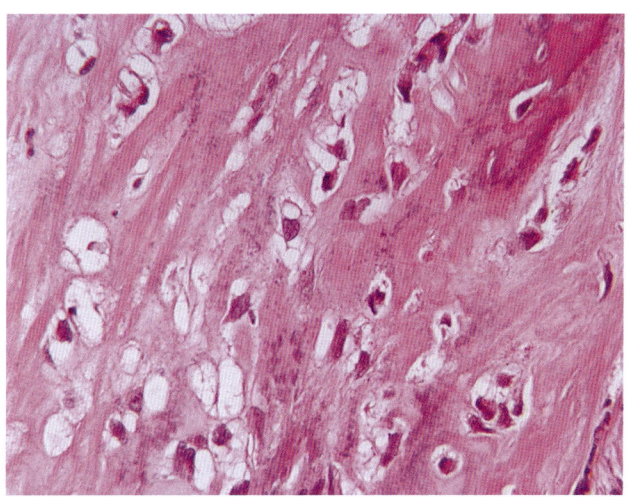
B

FIGURE 28-27 • Osteosarcoma in a postchemotherapy resection specimen in the distal femur of a 17-year-old boy. The sections require thorough decalcification especially in the case of an osteoblastic OS, and for that reason, the microscopic sections often have a pale eosinophilic quality. **A:** Acellular stroma containing trabeculae of tumor bone. **B:** Another focus is composed of "malignant"-appearing osteoid with atypical stromal cells.

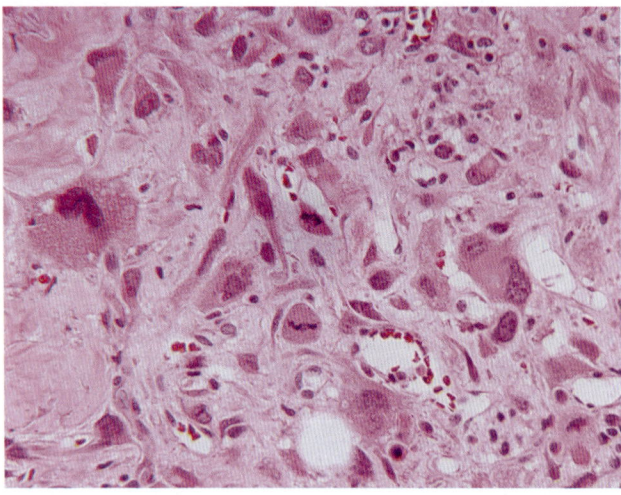 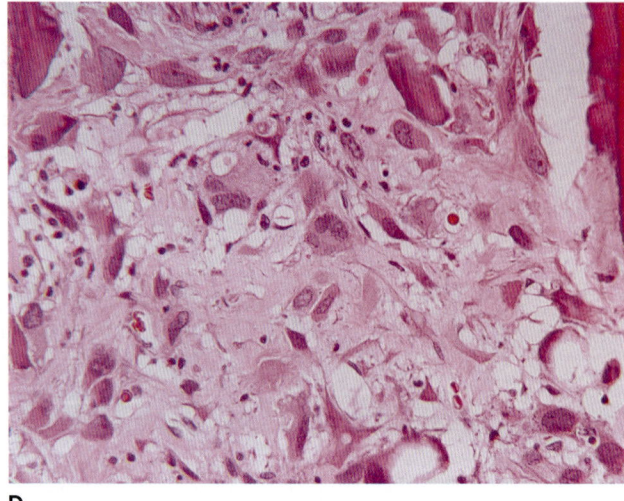

FIGURE 28-27 • (*continued*) **C:** A focus of bizarre-appearing tumor cells and mitoses is indicative of viable tumor. **D:** A comparison is made with the pretreatment biopsy tissue that demonstrates similar appearing tumor cells. There was less than 90% tumor ablation in this specimen and thus "a poor response."

Osteoid Osteoma and Osteoblastoma

These two neoplasms are regarded as closely related benign osteogenic neoplasms that account for approximately 8% to 20% of all bone tumors in children (470). From the perspective of bone biopsies in children, OO and OB accounted for 6% and 1.6%, respectively, of all biopsied bone lesions in children in one series (418). The microscopic similarities and examples of recurrent OO as larger, more locally aggressive OBs have served to support the hypothesis of a common histopathogenesis; however, there is no total agreement on this point (471–473). OO is the more common of the two tumors by a ratio of 4:1 overall, but in the first two decades, the ratio is 5:1–6:1, in favor of OO (474). The male to female ratio is 2:1–4:1 for both tumors. These lesions are seen most commonly in the second decade; however, OO is more likely than OB to present between the ages of 4 and 10 years; OB is known to occur infrequently in quite young children (475). The blood supply and unique innervation and production of prostaglandins in OO may be responsible for its characteristic occurrence of localized night pain relieved by salicylates; however, some patients with OB may also have a similar presentation (476,477).

The femur and tibia are sites of presentation of OO in 60% to 65% of cases, followed by the spine in 10% of cases (478,479). Less common sites include the mandible and small bones of the hands and feet and within a joint space (480). An intracortical area of radiolucency, the nidus, usually measuring 1 cm or less, and surrounded by dense sclerotic bone, is the typical roentgenographic appearance of OO, such that other imaging modalities, particularly computed tomography, may be required to identify the nidus. Because the nidus represents new bone and is encroached upon by the dense reactive cortical bone, it may eventually not be evident in routine images in 25% to 30% of cases (Figure 28-28). In the long bones, there is a preference for the corticodiaphyseal or metaphyseal location, but an OO may present in medullary as well as in subperiosteal sites; the sclerotic reactive bone that occurs with the intracortical lesions is lacking when OO occurs in these other locations. Rarely, OO may present as multicentric lesions (481).

In contrast to OO, OB presents in the femur or tibia in only 15% to 20% of cases, having a predilection for the axial skeleton in 60% to 65% of cases, with 5% to 8% of the tumors present in the craniofacial bones where the differential diagnosis

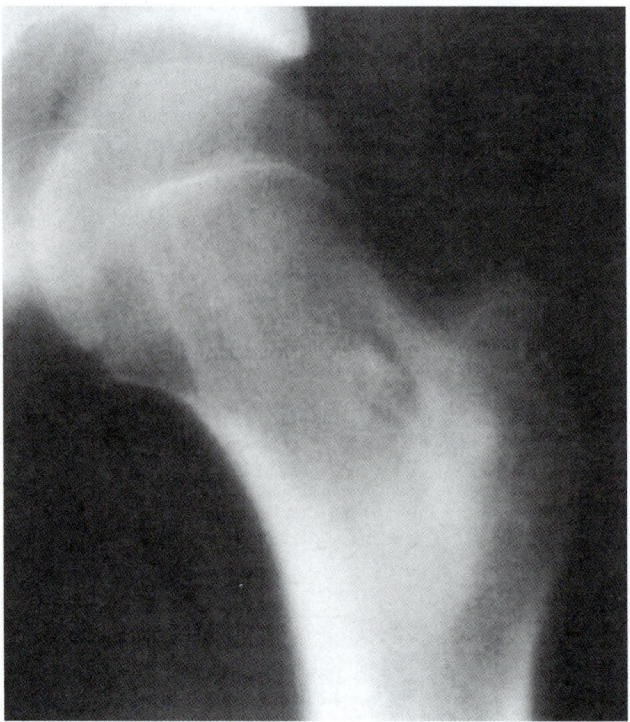

FIGURE 28-28 • Osteoid osteoma in the femoral neck of a 13-year-old boy. A central, lucent nidus surrounded by sclerotic bone is seen in this image.

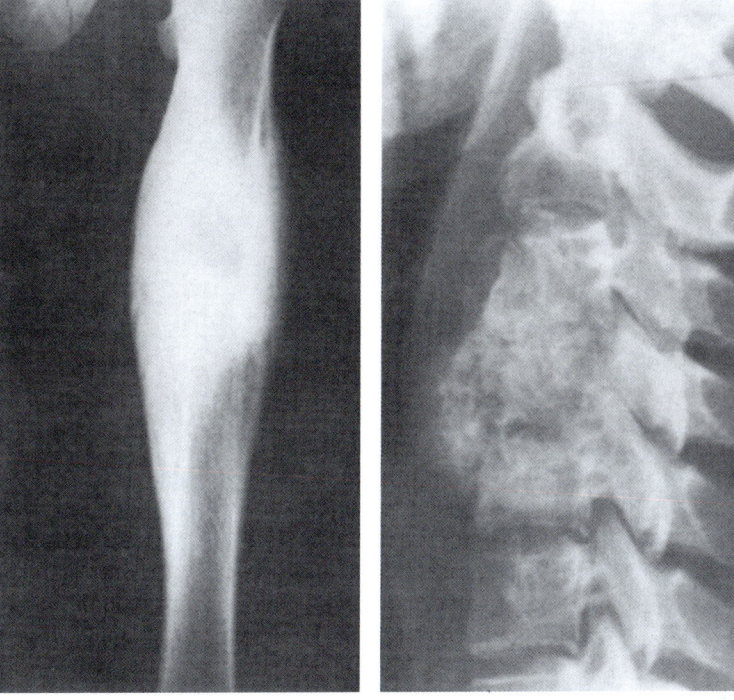

FIGURE 28-29 • Osteoblastoma generally has a benign radiologic appearance. Although most are well circumscribed, approximately 25% appear radiologically poorly marginated so that a malignant process is suspected. **A:** A femoral OB is shown with marked sclerosis. **B:** An Ob in the cervical vertebra is well circumscribed and composed of sclerotic and lucent areas.

includes juvenile-ossifying fibroma (482). The lumbosacral vertebra is the preferred site of presentation in the spine (483,484). A well-circumscribed, mixed sclerotic, and lucent or predominantly sclerotic lesion with cortical expansion is the frequent roentgenographic appearance of an OB although sclerosis is not as common as it is in OO (Figure 28-29) (485–487). Cortical destruction and apparent expansion beyond the bone account for an aggressive radiologic appearance that an OB may assume. There may even be extension into a contiguous vertebra. On MRI studies, increased signal intensity, interpreted as edema, is often noted both in the soft tissues surrounding the tumor and in the bone marrow proximal and distal to the lesion. This may convey the impression of a larger tumor than is the actual case. Rarely is an OB a multifocal tumor as an example of osteoblastomatosis (488).

In en bloc resection specimens, rarely encountered today, OO and the mass lesion of an OB often have a hemorrhagic appearance, and both are circumscribed and gritty with a surrounding zone of reactive-appearing sclerotic bone (Figure 28-30) (487,489). Although seemingly arbitrary, the principal distinction between OO and OB is the size of the nidus and does not include the size of any associated reactive bone. If the nidus is smaller than 2 cm, the lesion is designated as an OO, and if larger than 2 cm, an OB (490). The nidus of both lesions is composed of a well-vascularized stroma that contains an irregular network of variable calcified osteoid trabeculae and fully formed new bone lined by plump osteoblasts and some osteoclasts (Figure 28-31A, B). Although the fibrovascular stroma between trabeculae may contain scattered osteoblasts, it is not filled by these cells as often occurs in OS. The larger size and irregularly arranged osseous trabeculae of an OB may lead to concern about an OS (491). However, the fine, lacelike osteoid and relatively hypocellular vascularized stroma of OB does not display the degree of cellularity, mitotic activity, or anaplasia of an OS. OB also, unlike OS, does not show permeation at its interface with adjacent normal bone. The presence of plump epithelioid-like osteoblasts has been associated with so-called aggressive osteoblastoma, noted for an increased local recurrence rate, but these cells may also be focally present in OO, as well as in OBs that do not pursue a more aggressive clinical course. (Figure 28-32A to D) (492). A chondroid matrix has been described in a minority of OBs (493). OB-like OS and malignant transformation of OB exist as rarely reported

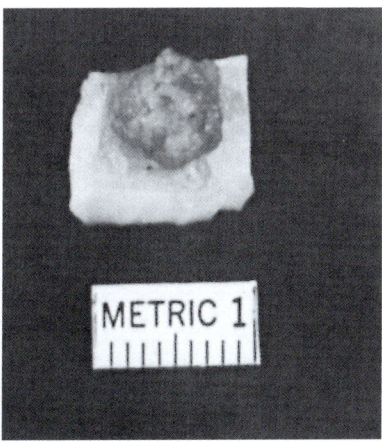

FIGURE 28-30 • Osteoid osteoma in this resection specimen shows an erythematous nidus surrounded by sclerotic bone. These tumors are frequently treated by radiofrequency and the specimen is fragmented, and the nidus is often in-apparent on gross and microscopic examination.

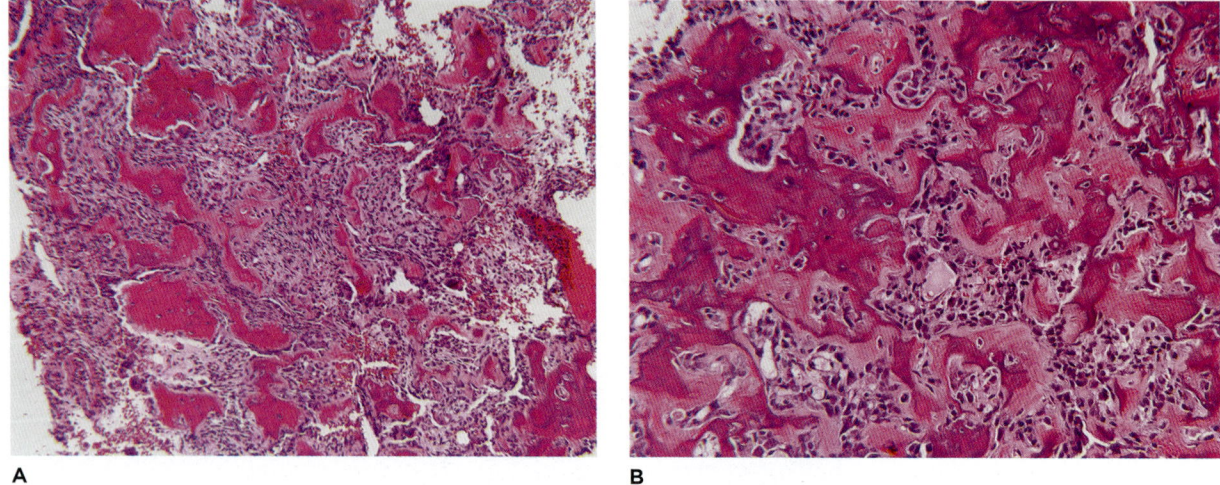

FIGURE 28-31 • Osteoid osteoma in the right proximal tibia of a 2-year-old boy. **A:** The nidus shows bone trabeculae that while varying in size and shape have an orderly appearance and a uniformly cellular stroma in the background. **B:** The nidus consists of a well-vascularized stroma, with new bone trabeculae rimmed by active, enlarged osteoblasts.

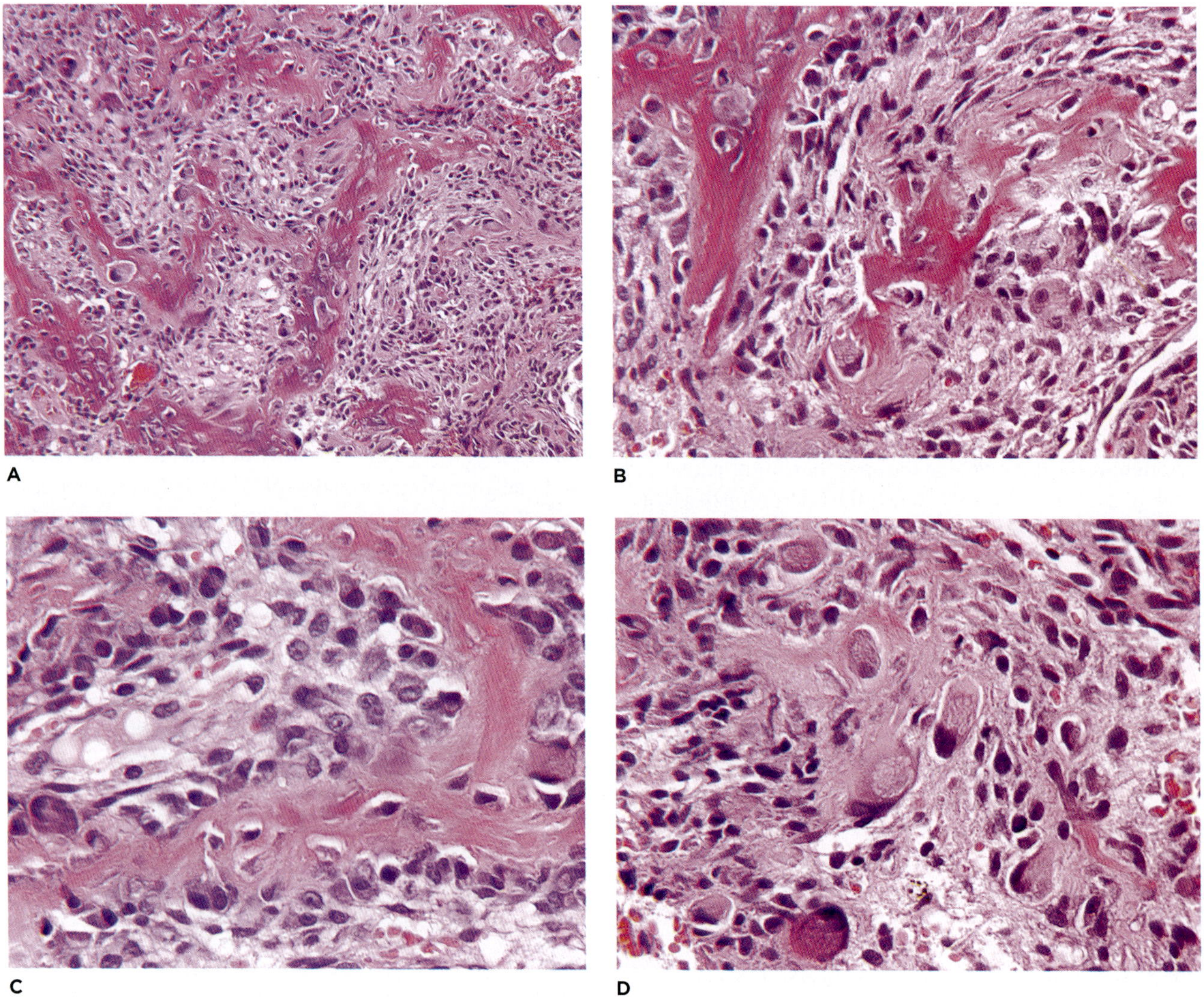

FIGURE 28-32 • Osteoblastoma presented in a 7-year-old boy. A 4-cm expansile medullary lesion was identified in the proximal femur. **A:** Nidus shows a mixed pattern of bony trabeculae with a regular pattern, accompanied by a vascular and cellular stroma. **B, C:** Features of the nidus are similar to those in OO. **D:** Some osteoblasts have a more abundant, pale eosinophilic cytoplasm and have an epithelioid appearance; similar cells are seen in OO.

entities (494). OOs are now only rarely encountered in an en bloc resection but more often as a specimen from radiofrequency ablation (495,496). These specimens consist of small bone fragments often without diagnostic features. Although ancillary studies do not have a large role in the diagnosis of OO and OB, the stroma is reportedly immunopositive for EMA and NSE and the nuclei for SATB2 and p63 (497–499).

Osteoma

Osteoma is a benign osseous lesion whose histologic features are those of dense compact or cancellous bone with or without an accompanying osteoblastic or vascular component similar to an OO or OB (473). There is almost exclusive involvement of craniofacial bones including the mandible and maxilla (500–502). The frontal sinus is the site of preference in some series, whereas in others, it is the mandible (503). Only 5% or so of osteomas are diagnosed before 20 years of age. However, an osteoma may be the initial clinical presentation of Gardner syndrome in which case there are commonly multiple osteomas and no history of intestinal polyps (503,504). Most osteomas are central, with an origin from the cancellous bone, and the remainder (peripheral osteoma) arises from the cortex (505). We have seen hybrid osseous tumors involving the paranasal sinuses with features of osteoma and FD (see Chapter 22).

Fibro-osseous Tumors

Ossifying fibroma (OF), osteofibrous dysplasia (OFD), and fibrous dysplasia (FD) are the other osseous matrix-associated lesions in children that have been collectively designated as "benign fibro-osseous lesions or tumors" and in the WHO classification are designated "tumors of undefined neoplastic nature" (427). At least one of these, FD, is not generally regarded as a true neoplasm, which may also be the case for OFD of the tibia and fibula whose pathologic features overlap with those of congenital pseudoarthrosis (CP) and adamantinoma (ADA). Because fibro-osseous lesions have a predilection for the facial and jaw bones, current classifications have tended to focus on maxillofacial fibro-osseous lesions, which include (a) FD; (b) OF, divisible into the three subtypes, conventional, juvenile trabecular, and juvenile psammomatoid; and (c) osseous dysplasia with four subtypes, periapical osseous dysplasia, focal osseous dysplasia, florid osseous dysplasia, and familial gigantiform cementoma (506–510). Osseous dysplasia is regarded as a hamartomatous lesion. The challenge of the benign fibro-osseous lesions of the craniofacial region is the thicket of diagnostic terms and the somewhat vague nature of the pathologic distinction between and among these lesions.

Juvenile-ossifying fibroma (JOF) includes two distinct histopathologic patterns with psammomatoid or trabecular features (511). In one series of benign fibro-osseous lesions of the jaws, 6% of cases were JOFs (512). A rapidly enlarging mass is present, whose radiologic features often depict a localized destructive process; this feature contrasts with the more indolent and diffuse ground-glass appearance of FD. Trabecular JOF is seen more often in the mandible and maxilla, whereas the psammomatoid JOF has a preference for the orbit and paranasal sinuses (Figure 28-33A, B) (513). A fibroblastic stroma, with islands of osteoid resembling cementicles or psammoma bodies (psammomatoid JOF), and a network of immature osteoid with prominent osteoblastic rimming merging with a spindle cell stroma, are the two basic histopathologic patterns. The small well-defined and smoothly contoured ossicles are distinct structures whose density can vary, with the result that the compact spindle cell stroma is more or less prominent in the background of the

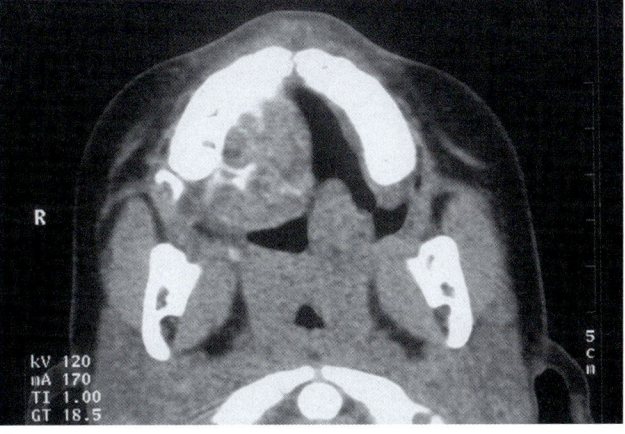
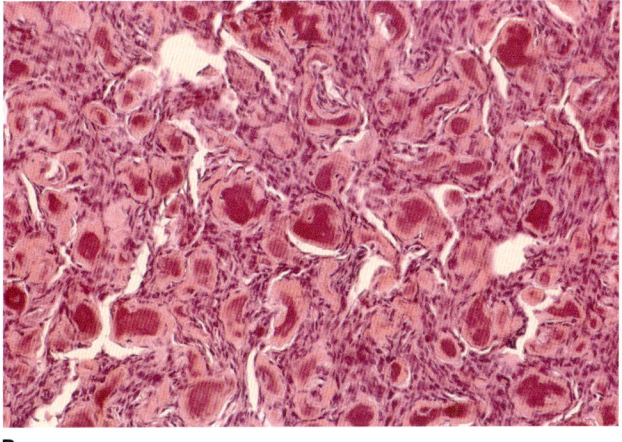

FIGURE 28-33 • Juvenile-ossifying fibroma, psammomatoid type. **A:** Computed tomogram shows a well-circumscribed mass present in the ethmoid sinus adjacent to the orbit. The lesion has a mixed radiolucent and radiodense appearance. **B:** The tumor is composed of relatively uniform calcified ossicles, which have been interpreted in the past as cementicles giving rise to the designation of cementifying fibroma. The spindle cell stroma may be inconspicuous, as in this microscopic field, or be predominant with only a few ossicles. (Contributed by Samir El-Mofty, DMD, PhD, St. Louis, MO.)

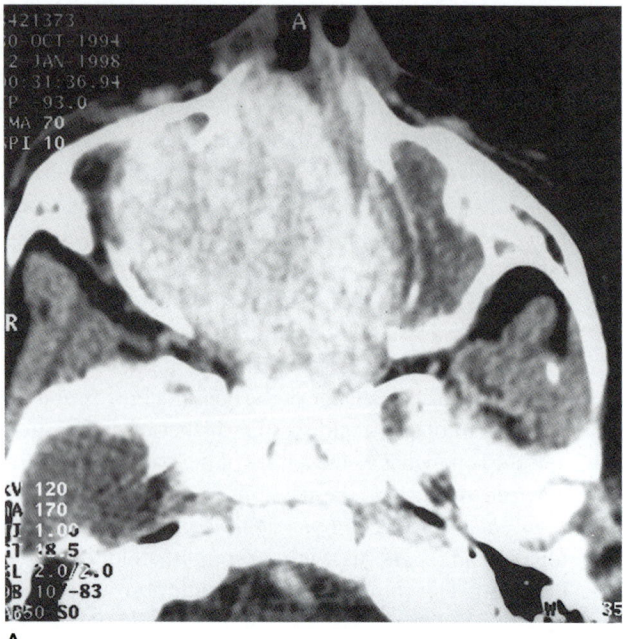 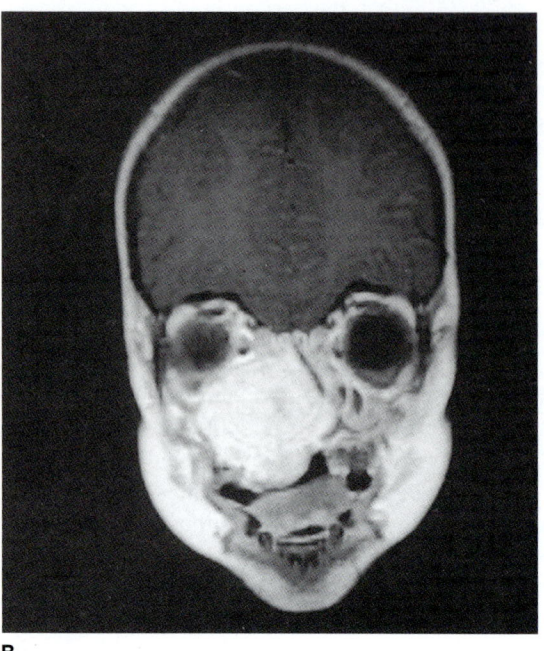

FIGURE 28-34 • Juvenile-ossifying fibroma, trabecular type. A 3-year-old boy had a rapidly enlarging mass filling the right maxillary sinus and depressing the palate inferiorly. **A:** Computed tomography shows the entire right maxilla and nasal cavity filled by a circumscribed, inhomogeneous mass. **B:** A frontal image shows the mass effect on the palate.

psammomatoid JOF. The latter tumor occurs in a broader age group than does trabecular JOF, which occurs in children less than 15 years of age and even in those younger than 5 years of age (Figure 28-34A, B) (513,514). The maxilla is more commonly involved than the mandible. A large, locally destructive mass is composed of a vascularized, reactive-appearing spindle cell stroma, with some resemblance to nodular fasciitis, and accompanying cellular osteoid-forming trabecular profiles in the background (Figure 28-35A, B). Both osteoblasts and osteoclasts are associated with the trabecular osteoid. The presence of immature woven bone may raise the possibility of FD except for the osteoblastic rimming. Scattered typical mitoses in the stroma should not be viewed with concern. Incomplete resection may be followed by rapid regrowth or persistence for a period of time (see Chapter 22).

Hyperparathyroidism–jaw tumor syndrome is an AD syndrome with mutations in the CDC73 (formerly HRPT2) gene (1q31.2), a tumor suppressor gene (515). In addition to

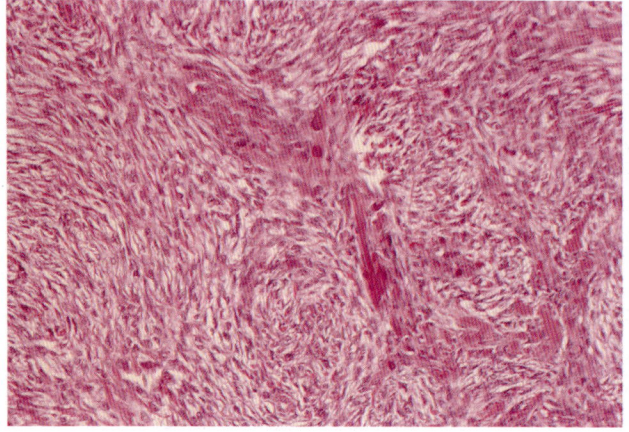 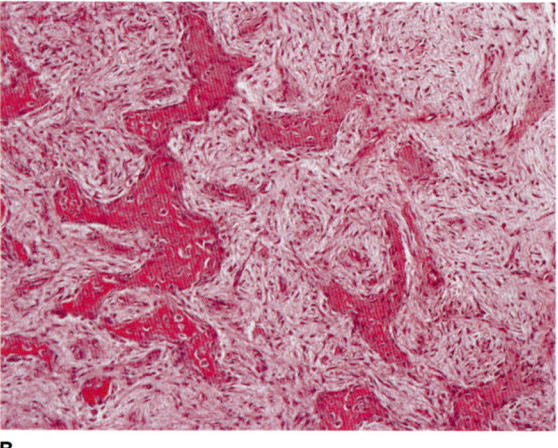

FIGURE 28-35 • Juvenile-ossifying fibroma, trabecular type. **A:** The lesion contains a spindle cell stroma, which with the hint of osteoid formation in the background has a resemblance to the center of myositis ossificans and without the osteoid formation to nodular fasciitis. Mitotic figures may be identified without difficulty, but are not atypical in form. **B:** Other foci are composed of immature woven bone, which is outlined in part by osteoblasts in a loose spindle cell stroma. Without the osteoblasts, there is a resemblance to FD. (Contributed by Samir El-Mofty, DMD, PhD, St. Louis, MO.)

mapped to 11p14.3-15.1 (GDD1/TMEM1GE gene); mutations have been reported in the ANO5 gene as well (519,520).

Osteofibrous dysplasia (OFD) is an uncommon lesion accounting for less than 1% of all bone tumors in children. It most commonly occurs as an expansile multiloculated radiolucent lesion with sclerotic margins in the diaphysis of the tibia and/or fibula in a child usually less than 10 years of age (Figure 28-36A, B) (521,522). OFD is only seen in the tibia or fibula and at times both simultaneously where it is a purely intracortical lesion. It most often involves the anterior cortex of the tibia as multiple lucent lesions with surrounding sclerosis, causing the characteristic anterior bowing of the bone (523). A pathologic fracture has been reported in the tibia of a neonate with OFD (524). Histologically, OFD has a loose spindle cell fibrous stroma, with or without a storiform pattern, in which are scattered irregularly sized trabeculae of woven bone similar to FD (525). This similarity led some to designate the lesion as intracortical FD; however, most trabeculae show peripheral osteoblastic rimming with the formation of lamellar bone, a pattern in sharp contrast to FD. A zonal pattern of maturation may be apparent, best seen in resection specimens, in which the central area of the lesion contains a few unrimmed trabeculae, with an increasing number of those with osteoblasts more peripherally located, with eventual interlocking of mature-appearing trabeculae and their fusion with the adjacent cortical bone (Figure 28-37A to D). Immunostains show the existence of cytokeratin-positive cells scattered within the fibrous stroma, usually in the form of single isolated cells, or in small nests of two to three cells. The lesions of OFD tend to stabilize at the time of puberty, and surgical therapy appears limited to correction of any existing bone deformity. In terms of the stromal component, there are also similarities to CP, which may be present together with OFD (526). The relationship of OFD to adamantinoma of bone is discussed later.

Fibrous dysplasia, the most common of the fibro-osseous lesions of bone in children, is seen in 6% to 10% of bone biopsies or curettage (418). Though discussed in terms of a bone tumor, FD is not considered a neoplasm in the strictest

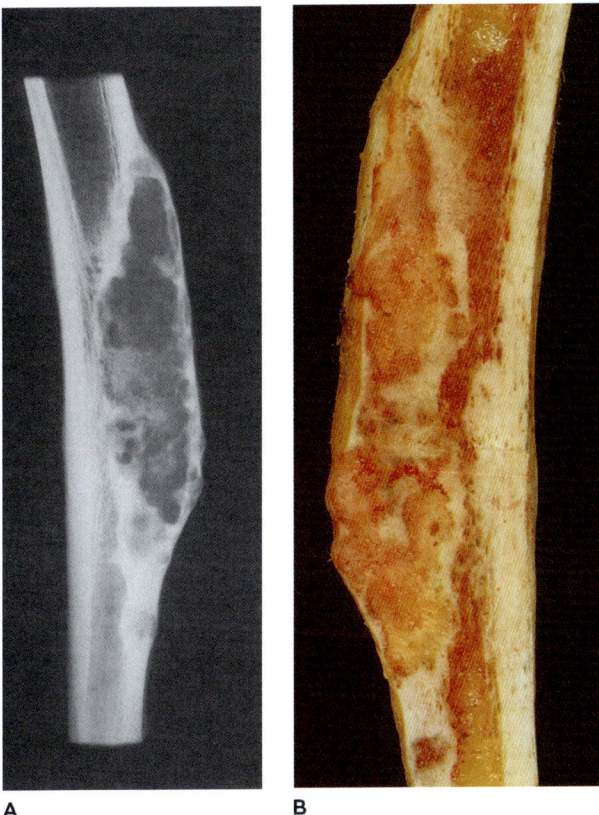

FIGURE 28-36 • Osteofibrous dysplasia of the tibia. **A:** This image of the resection specimen shows the cortical localization. **B:** The resected mass is composed of osseous and reddish stroma.

hyperparathyroidism, JOFs develop in the mandible or maxilla in approximately 30% of affected individuals and the tumors may be multiple (516). There is also an apparent increased risk for Wilms tumor and polycystic kidney disease (517). Another more generalized clinical setting in which psammomatoid JOF is reported is in gnathodiaphyseal dysplasia (GDD); this AD syndrome is also characterized by bone fragility and sclerosis and bowing of tubular bones (518). The GDD gene has been

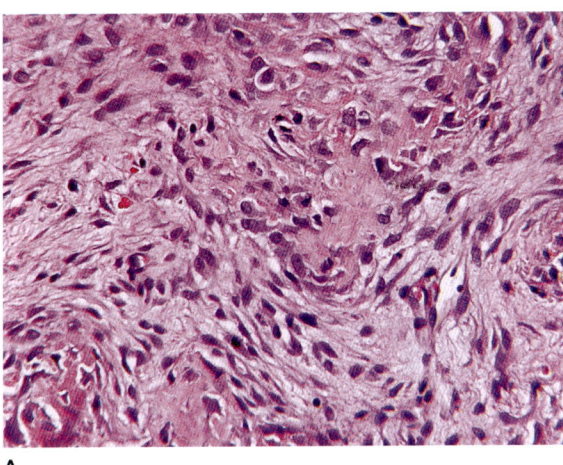
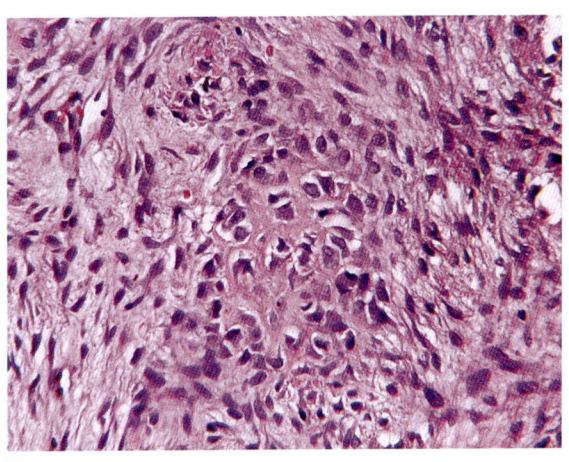

FIGURE 28-37 • Osteofibrous dysplasia of the tibia in a 4-year-old boy. **A:** Spindle stroma with only a hint of osteoid deposition. **B:** Adjacent focus shows early formation of bony trabeculae.

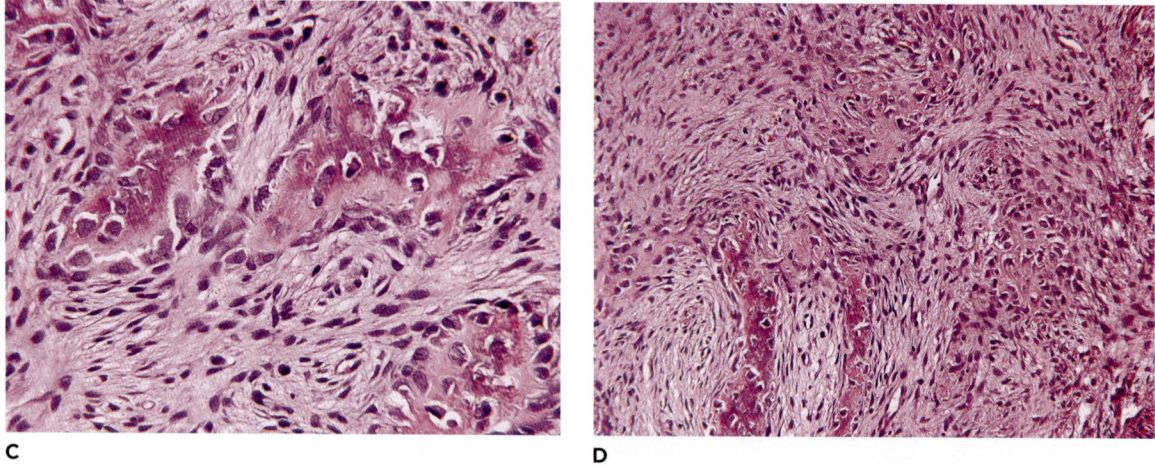

FIGURE 28-37 • (continued) **C:** This field shows bony trabeculae outlined by osteoblasts. **D:** This lower magnification field shows the pattern of spindle cells, osteoid formation, and bony trabeculae.

sense, but rather as a localized defect in normal bone formation and maturation, on the basis of an early embryonic postzygotic somatic activating mutations effecting the stimulatory alpha-subunit of G-protein on the GNAS gene (20q13.3); the protein product of this imprinted gene is an intermediate between receptor coupling and cyclic adenosine monophosphate (cAMP) generation. Increased levels of cAMP result in defective osteoblastic differentiation (527,528). Somatic mosaicism accounts for the highly variable expression in early development with differences in phenotype from solitary to multiple bone lesions and accompanying endocrinopathies including the McCune-Albright syndrome (MAS) (527). The latter explains the occurrence of monostotic and polyostotic bone lesions, with monostotic lesions in 70% to 80% of cases, and the remainder as polyostotic lesions with more than one lesion in either a single bone or involvement of multiple bones (529–531). Approximately 50% of cases of FD are diagnosed in the first two decades of life (532). The proximal femur, tibia, and ribs are the three most frequently involved individual bones. In the craniofacial region, monostotic lesions occur in the sphenoid bone, followed by the frontal bone; the maxilla and ethmoid are the common sites of involvement in children (Figure 28-38A, B) (533). Involvement of the proximal femur is one of the more

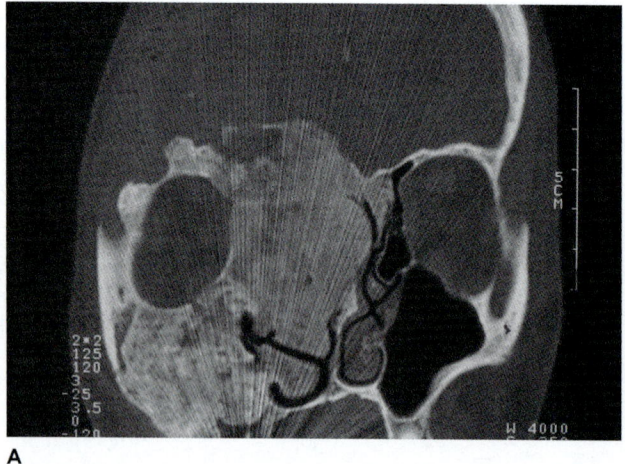

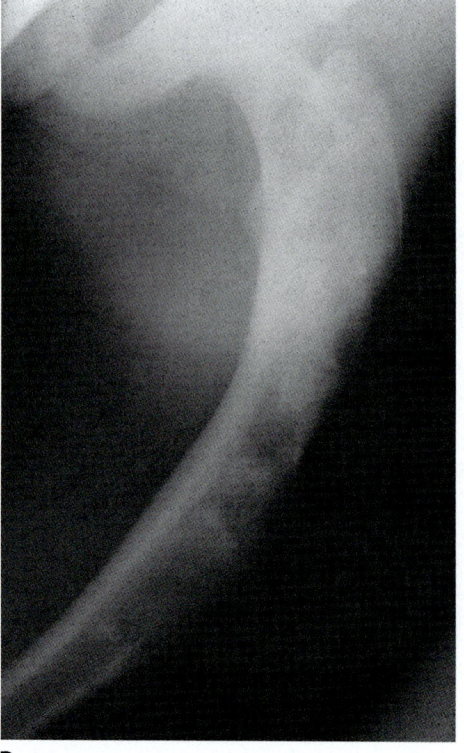

FIGURE 28-38 • Fibrous dysplasia. **A:** This image demonstrates a sizable mass involving the nasal–maxillary passages. **B:** The "shepherd crook" deformity of the femur is present in the polyostotic form of the disease.

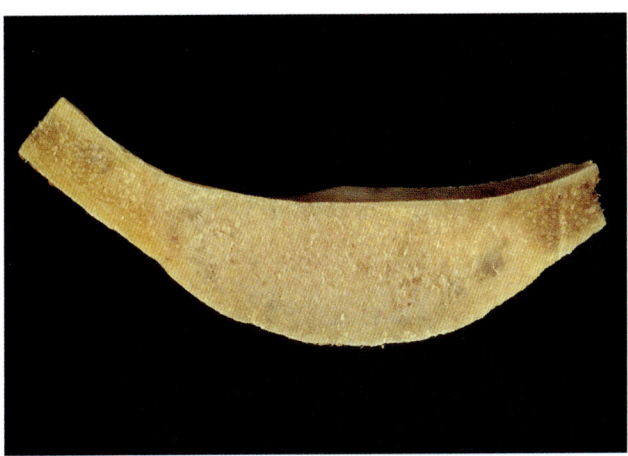

FIGURE 28-39 • Fibrous dysplasia. This lesion is presented in the calvarium and shows expansion of the inner and outer table of the skull.

common causes of pathologic fractures in children (534). The polyostotic presentation of FD may be recognized in the first decade of life with complications of severe bowing of weight-bearing long bones (so-called shepherd crook deformity in the proximal femur), and pathologic fractures (Figure 28-38B). Various endocrine disorders, with or without MAS, and the Mazabraud syndrome (FD with soft tissue myxoma) have been reported in association with FD (535,536). There is also an apparent association of FD with encephalocraniocutaneous lipomatosis (537).

The imaging features of FD in long bones are those of a demarcated, radiolucent, or dense lesion, within the medullary canal of the metaphysis or diaphysis (538). The gross appearance of the mass is that of an expansile lesion with a bony consistency (Figure 28-39). There is also the rare exophytic presentation (539). The so-called ground-glass radiologic appearance is correlated with the density of woven bone spicules relative to the amount of fibrous stroma (540). The islands of immature woven bone have different sizes and shapes, are devoid of osteoblasts, and are surrounded by a variably cellular fibrous stroma, which may have a storiform or diffuse nonspecific pattern (Figure 28-40A, B). The stromal cells are devoid of nuclear atypia or significant mitotic activity. There is an absence of differentiation to normal cancellous or trabecular bone. Exceptions to these features occur in FD of the craniofacial bones, where osteoblastic rimming of the bone trabeculae and lamellar transformation to mature bone may occur, which result in diagnostic uncertainty as to the specific type of fibro-osseous lesion (541). The distinction in these cases from OF depends in part upon the radiologic features, with FD having a diffuse, ill-defined interface with the adjacent uninvolved bone in contrast to OF that is well circumscribed and delimited from the adjacent bone.

Polarization microscopy discloses the mosaic pattern of woven bone in FD compared to normal lamellar bone (Figure 28-41). If an intramedullary FD-like lesion exhibits a sarcoma-like stroma and the imaging studies show aggressive features, a well-differentiated central OS is a strong possibility and most likely accounts for some reported putative examples of sarcomatous transformation in FD (542). However, some stromal cell atypia, in the absence of mitotic activity, may be observed and is thought to be "degenerative" in nature, much like the enlarged atypical cells seen in a schwannoma or leiomyoma (543). Solitary cystic change, as well as hemorrhage, is consistent with secondary ABC, and focal xanthomatous transformation of the stromal cells is another histologic finding. Cartilaginous metaplasia in FD is a recognized feature most often seen in polyostotic cases and is designated by some as "fibrocartilaginous dysplasia" (544). The spindle cell stroma of FD expresses periostin as a reflection of c-FOS activation (545). Fracture through FD, with subsequent callus formation, may cause concern for a serious pathologic process such as OS, but the absence of cellular pleomorphism and the nonaggressive radiologic

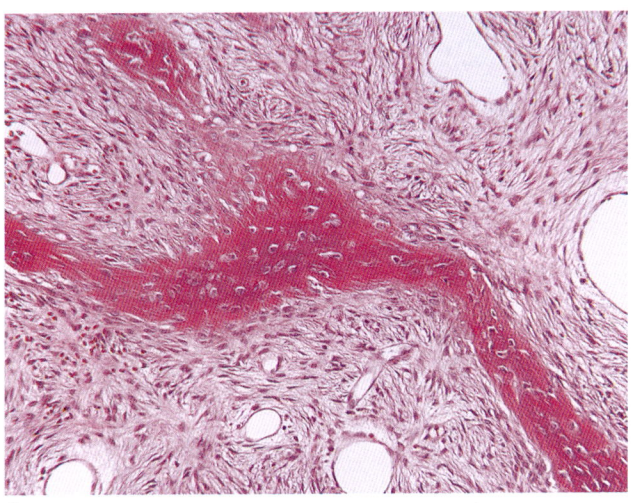
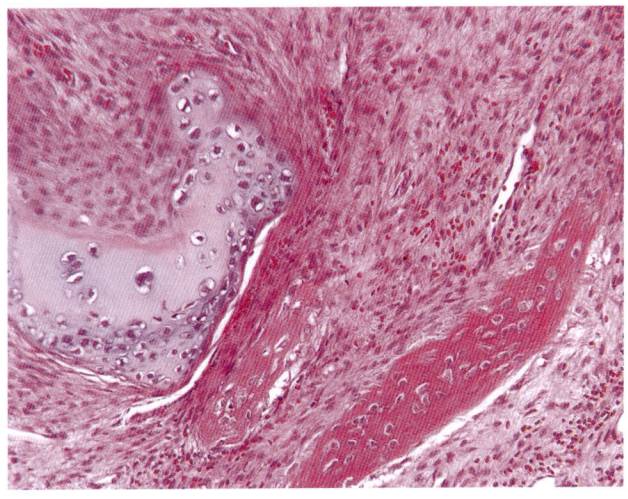

FIGURE 28-40 • Fibrous dysplasia in the femur of a 20-year-old male. **A:** Island of woven bone with irregular configuration is surrounded by a bland, loose spindle cell stroma. **B:** Islands of metaplastic cartilage may also be seen especially in polyostotic FD.

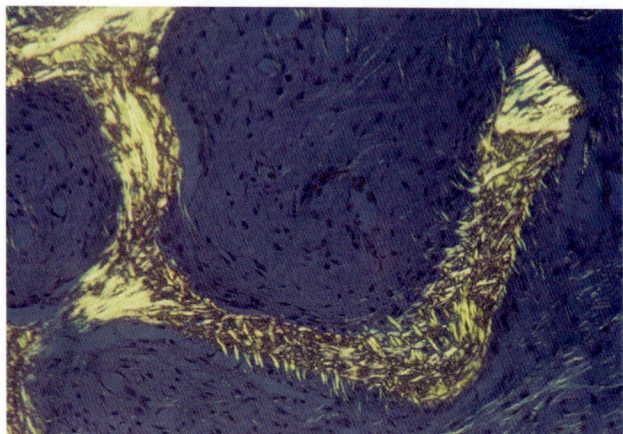

FIGURE 28-41 • Fibrous dysplasia. The characteristic pattern of woven bone is demonstrated by polarization microscopy.

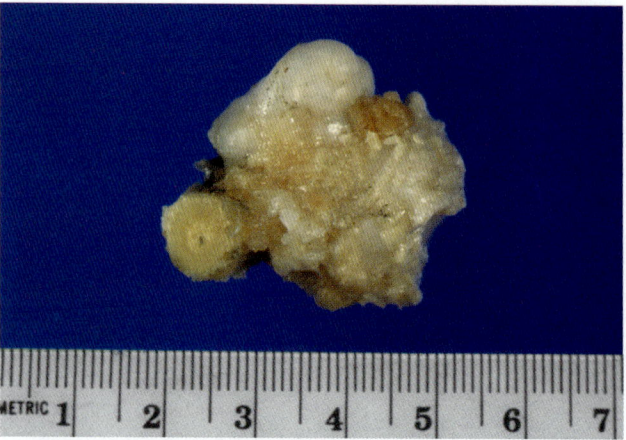

FIGURE 28-42 • Osteochondroma. This 3.5-cm mass with an irregular surface that is partially covered by a relatively thin cartilaginous cap arose from the proximal humerus of a 13-year-old male.

images serves to distinguish FD from OS. However, FD is known to present as a cortically destructive lesion on rare occasions (546).

Cartilaginous Tumors

Osteochondroma (OC) of the solitary type is the most common benign cartilaginous tumor, comprising 70% to 75% of cases, followed by EC (10% to 15% of all cases), CB (10%), and CMF (2% to 5%) (547,548). Approximately 40% to 50% of all bone tumors in children are OCs, and it has been estimated that 0.5% to 1% of all individuals before age 20 years may develop an OC. The average age at diagnosis ranges between 10 and 15 years, although OC may also be found in older adults, and there is an overall male predilection. Generally not included in a consideration of benign chondroid tumors are subungual exostosis, turret exostosis, focal fibrocartilaginous dysplasia, and bizarre parosteal osteochondromatous proliferation of the hands and feet (Nora lesion), all regarded as reactive pseudotumors (549–552).

OC in children is solitary in 85% to 90% of cases and multiple (MHE) in the remaining 10% to 15% (553). A painless mass arising in the distal femoral or proximal tibial metaphysis is the most common clinical presentation, with the proximal humerus the third most frequent site (Figure 28-42) (554). One of the more common benign tumors of the rib in a child is OC (555). However, OC is ubiquitous in its site distribution in the setting of MHE. The lesion, which may be pedunculated or sessile, has a translucent, bluish-tinted cartilaginous cap, which, in children, may be several centimeters thick. Radiologically, the medulla of the OC, be it pedunculated or sessile, is in direct continuity with the medulla of the underlying bone (Figure 28-43). When pedunculated, solitary, or multiple, the growth of the OC is away from the nearest joint.

Microscopically, the cartilaginous cap and underlying region of enchondral ossification recapitulate the histology of the epiphyseal growth plate (Figure 28-44A, B). Malignant change in solitary OC, most commonly to CS, occurs in less than 5% of cases (555). The differential diagnosis of OC includes dysplasia epiphysealis hemimelica (Trevor disease), which presents as an asymmetrical enlargement of the epiphysis of long bones (solitary or multiple) in children between 3 and 15 years of age (556–558). Islands of cartilage with enchondral ossification are the microscopic features.

Multiple hereditary exostosis (MHE) is an AD disorder characterized by the presence of two or more OCs. The incidence is 1:50,000 and is the most common inherited bone disorder (559). These lesions develop earlier, at 2 to 4 years of age on average, than do solitary OCs, and are more often

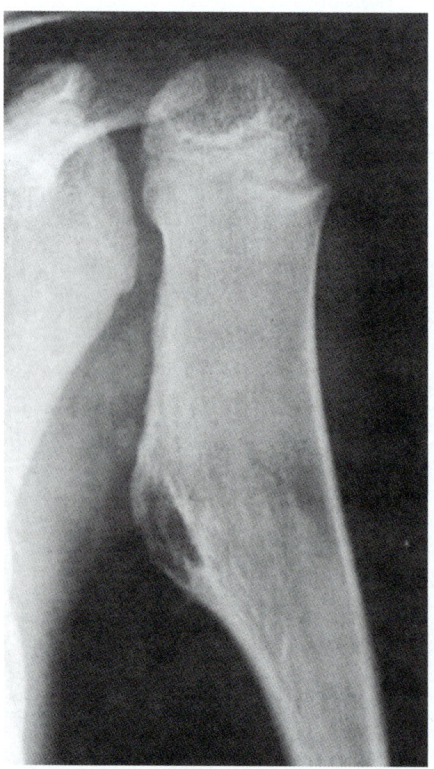

FIGURE 28-43 • Osteochondroma. This image shows a pedunculated lesion with the cortical and underlying medullary bone in continuity.

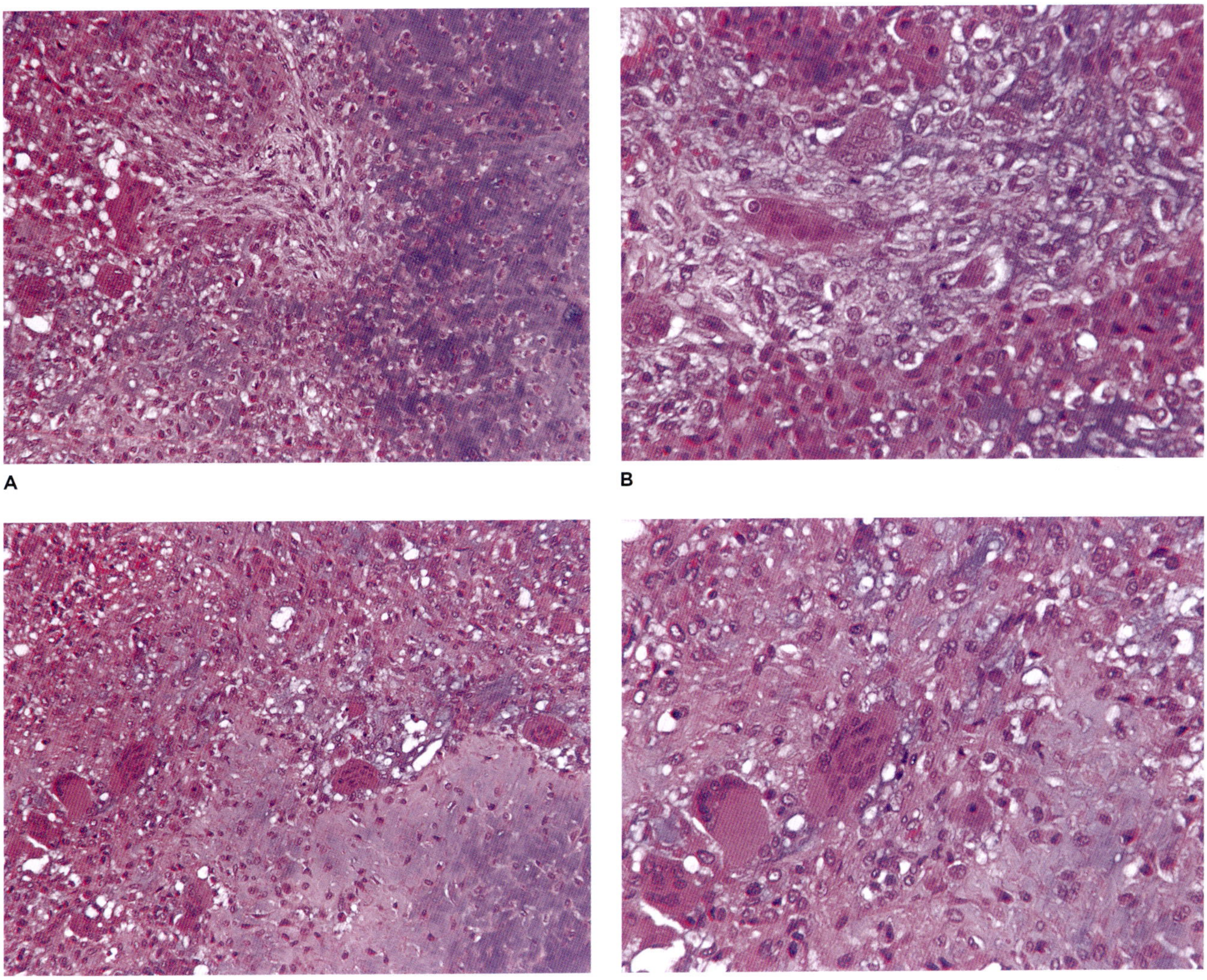

FIGURE 28-52 • Chondromyxoid fibroma. **A:** A chondroid focus is separated by a zone of cellular stroma and several osteoclast-like giant cells in this tumor of the proximal tibia of a 14-year-old female. **B:** A sheet of polygonal cells, resembling chondroblasts, is adjacent to stroma with osteoclast-like giant cells. **C:** Osteoclast-like giant cells are present at the periphery of a chondroid nodule. **D:** The three elements of this tumor are shown in this field: stroma, giant cells, and a portion of a chondroid nodule.

The component cells are stellate to spindle shaped with increased cellularity at the periphery of the lobules. Mild to moderate nuclear atypia may be present (Figure 28-52A to D) (587). At the confluence of the lobules, areas composed of chondroblasts and osteoclast-type giant cells may be present, simulating foci of CB. More mature chondroid areas may also occur with calcification. However, histologic calcifications are uncommonly present in CMFs in children. The nuclear atypia, especially when present in small biopsy specimens, may raise a suspicion of CS, but the benign-appearing imaging studies helps to distinguish CMF from CS. When possible, en bloc excision is preferable to curettage in order to decrease the local recurrence rate that varies from 10% to 20% (584,587). Malignant transformation is virtually nonexistent.

Chest wall hamartoma (mesenchymal hamartoma or chondromatous hamartoma of the chest wall) is a benign tumefaction of infancy, involving one or more ribs, presenting as a mass with or without respiratory symptoms (Figure 28-53) (588,589).

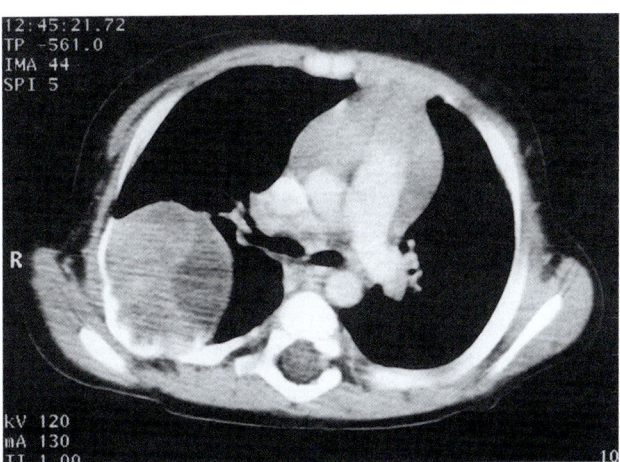

FIGURE 28-53 • Chest wall hamartoma in a 6-month-old male. This lesion arising in a rib projects into the thoracic space.

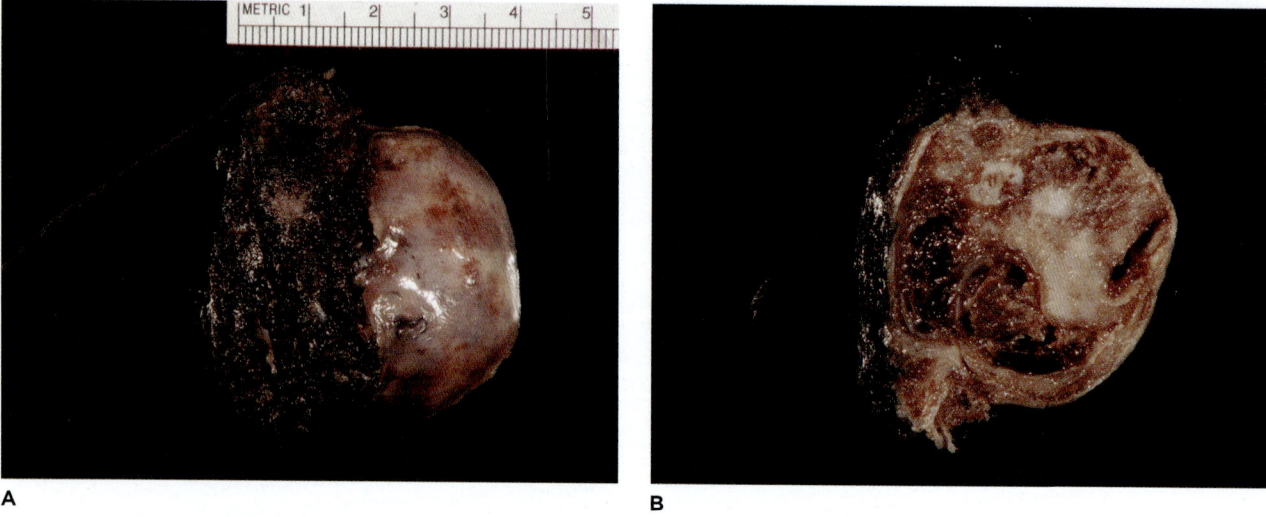

FIGURE 28-54 • Chest wall hamartoma in a 3-day-old boy who had two masses arising from, and involving, several ribs. **A:** The external surface of the mass has glistening appearance of cartilage. **B:** Cross section of the mass shows a varied appearance with cystic and solid cartilaginous foci with areas of hemorrhage.

The lesion consists of an expansile, intraosseous mass, measuring 3 to 5 cm in greatest dimension and usually having a hemorrhagic cystic to solid appearance (Figure 28-54A, B). Histologically, nodules of hypercellular hyaline cartilage, with foci of enchondral ossification that resemble growth plate tissue, are separated by a spindle cell stroma with or without osteoclast-type giant cells. Hemangioma-like areas, as well as ABC-like foci are common features (Figure 28-55A to D). The presence of woven bone imparts a similarity to FD. Local recurrence is uncommon but is seen in cases with incomplete resection. A seemingly comparable tumor, nasal chondromesenchymal hamartoma, is seen in the nasal–paranasal passages in infants or somewhat older children; this nasal tumor may be a manifestation of DICER1—pleuropulmonary blastoma tumor predisposition.

Chondrosarcoma (CS) comprises 5% or less of all primary malignant skeletal tumors in the first two decades of life, but approximately 25% of all such tumors when all age groups are included. Most CSs of bone in children are sporadically occurring neoplasms except for those cases of peripheral CS arising in the setting of MHE in 0.5% to 5% of cases or OD and MS. Both ECs and CMFs can mimic low-grade CS microscopically. Conventional or central CS in the child, as in the adult, tends to develop in the proximal long bones and the flat bones (590). The tumors are generally quite large and invade and destroy the cortex. CSs are histologically graded as well, moderate, or poorly differentiated or assigned a numerical grade of I to III. In children, as in adults, most CSs are well to moderately differentiated tumors (grades I to II)

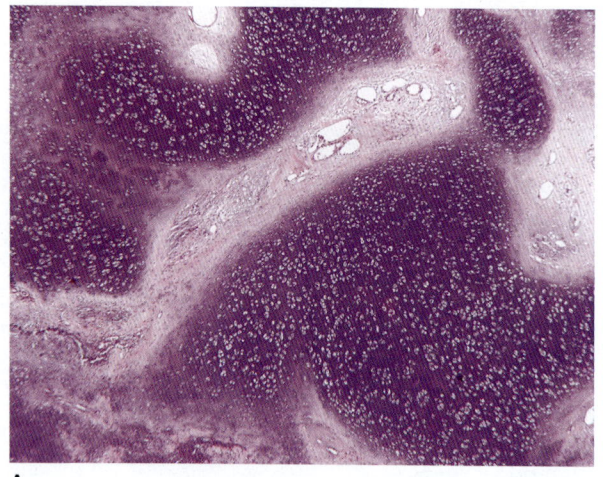
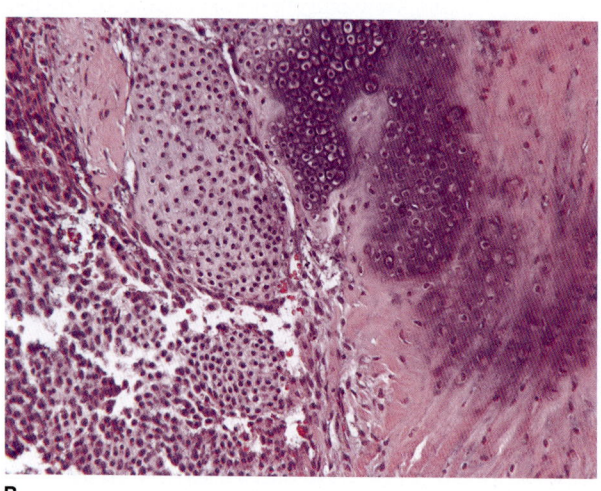

FIGURE 28-55 • Chest wall hamartoma. Several patterns are seen in these lesions. **A:** Nodules of well-differentiated cartilage comprise a substantial portion of the solid foci. **B:** Other areas have a bimorphic pattern of cartilage and polygonal cells with a resemblance to chondroblasts.

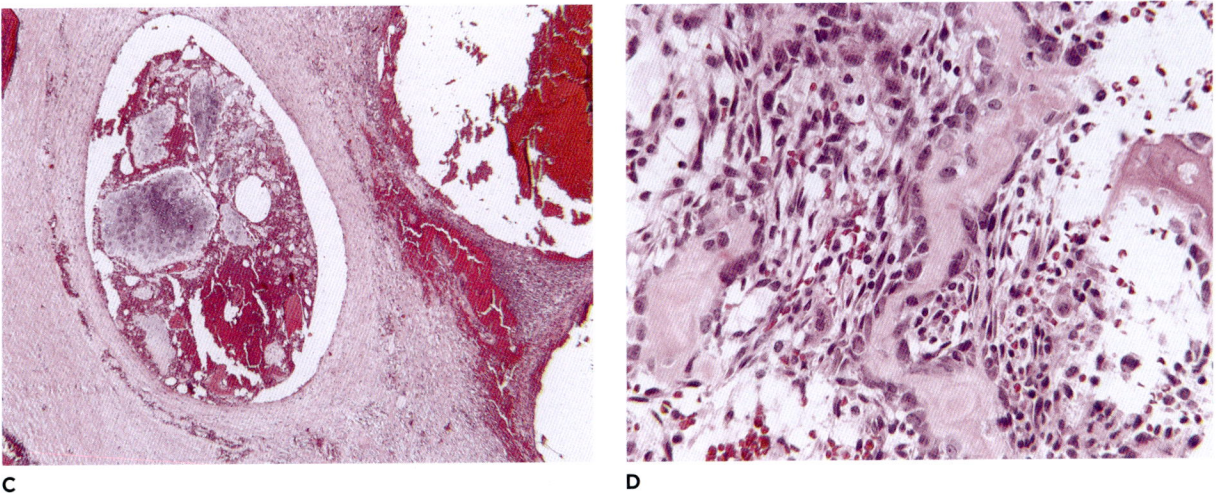

FIGURE 28-55 • (continued) C: Cystic and hemorrhagic foci have features of ABC. D: Another pattern is represented by bony trabeculae with osteoblastic rimming.

(Figure 28-56) (591). Three subtypes of CS are recognized in children: clear cell, mesenchymal, and myxoid; the latter two subtypes present as well in the soft tissues (591,592). Mesenchymal CS, though accounting for only 4% to 5% of all CSs, is the most common subtype in children with 25% to 30% presenting before 20 years of age (591). The head and neck (skull, mandible, maxilla, and meninges), ribs, and femur are the sites of predilection of mesenchymal CS (593). We have seen an example of myxoid CS in the phalanx of an adolescent girl whose tumor had a EWS breakapart translocation as occurs in extraosseous forms of this tumor (Figure 28-57A to D) (594). The pathologic features of mesenchymal and myxoid CS are discussed in the chapter on soft tissue lesions. A nonrandom translocation [t(1;5)(q42;q32)] has been reported in mesenchymal CS (595,596). Clear cell CS constitutes only 1% to 2% of all CSs. Unlike most conventional CSs, this tumor occurs in the second and third decades of life, with a predilection for the epiphysis of long bones, especially the proximal femur or humerus where it can be radiologically mistaken for CB or GCT (597). Histologically, lobules of hyaline cartilage are occupied by chondrocytes, many of which have an abundant clear cytoplasm. Small spicules of woven bone may be interspersed among the clear cells, as are osteoclast-type giant cells. The latter cells rarely occur in conventional CS. The presence of these giant cells around lobules of cartilage can be mistaken for CB or CMF. Clear cell CSs may express cytokeratin AE1/AE3 and SOX9 (598).

The diagnosis of CS in a child should be approached with caution and circumspection. When a biopsy from a bone neoplasm in a child has features of high-grade, malignant

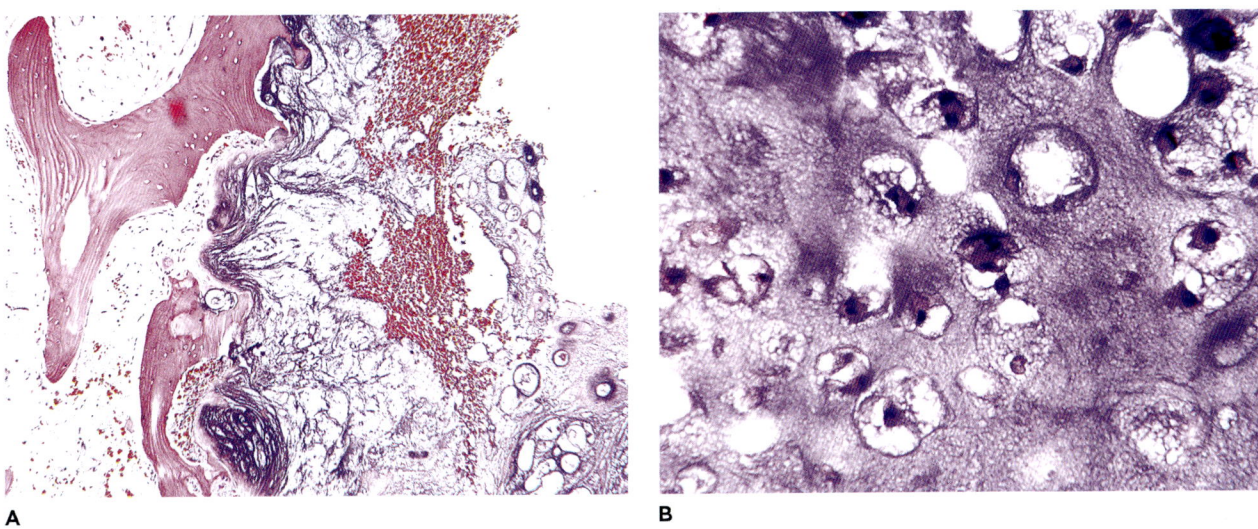

FIGURE 28-56 • Chondrosarcoma, conventional type. This tumor arose in the nasal cavity of a 16-year-old girl. A: The tumor is infiltrating through the bone. B: The tumor cells are enlarged with some nuclear atypism, but in the absence of any mitotic figures.

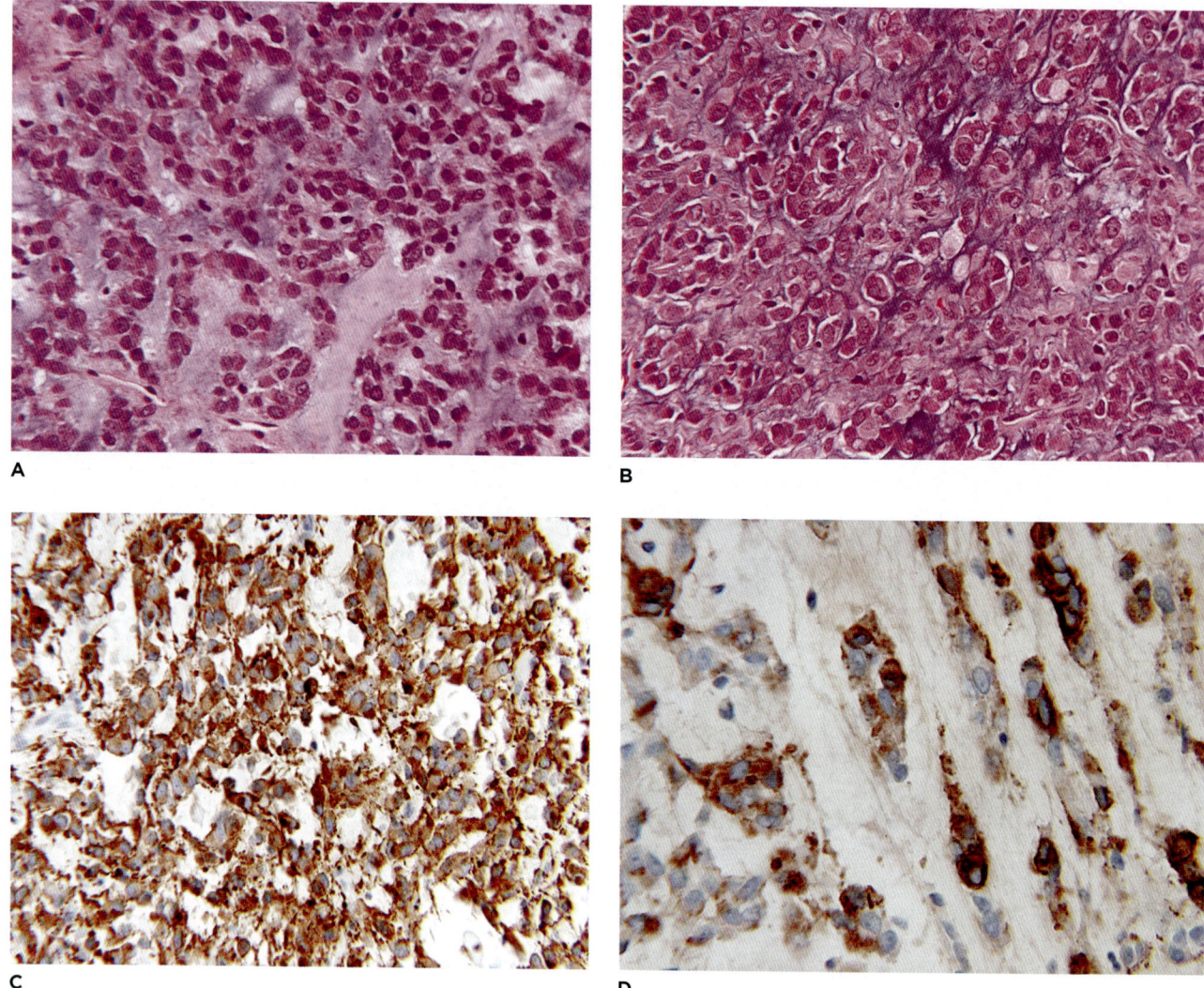

FIGURE 28-57 • Myxoid chondrosarcoma presented as an expansile osteolytic lesion in the middle phalanx of the right long finger in a 19-year-old woman. **A:** The tumor has a multi-lobular or nodular pattern composed of cords and strands of tumor cells in a myxoid stroma. **B:** The other pattern is one of solid sheets of relatively uniform epithelioid-appearing cells with wisps of extracellular mucoid material among the tumor cells. **C:** The tumor cells are diffusely positive for synaptophysin. **D:** These cells are also immunoreactive for chromogranin. One other feature of this particular intraosseous tumor was the presence of an EWS breakapart by FISH studies, an unusual finding in a myxoid CS of bone, being more commonly found in those arising in the soft tissue.

cartilage, it is more likely than not that the tumor is actually a chondroblastic OS since in children, conventional CS usually has low- to intermediate-grade features. The distinction between an EC and low-grade CS is an acknowledged difficult problem, even for those with considerable experience with skeletal tumors (599). Permeative growth between residual cancellous medullary bones, with entrapment of the bone, is a reasonably reliable feature associated with CS, as is invasion of cortical haversian systems. A review of the radiologic studies with a knowledgeable radiologist is often rewarding. The radiologic presence of aggressive features such as cortical disruption or a soft tissue component may be the only way to reach the correct diagnosis of CS, regardless of the age of the patient.

NONMATRIX-PRODUCING TUMORS AND CYSTS

Nonmatrix-producing lesions, with or without osteoclast-type giant cells, with or without cyst formation, include a variety of benign tumor or tumorlike conditions that in some cases may exhibit locally aggressive behavior. One pathologic subset comprises those lesions with osteoclast-type giant cells and an accompanying cellular stroma. In a wide variety of osseous lesions, osteoclast-like giant cells are a major or minor histologic component. Although these giant cells may reflect the true neoplastic element, they may also be, despite their abundance in some cases, only incidental to the actual pathologic process.

Giant-cell tumor (GCT) comprises only 1% to 2% of primary osseous neoplasms in children and adolescents, having a predilection for the skeletally mature with most patients between 30 and 50 years of age (418). The GCT is uncommon in those younger than age 20 years and very rare before age 10 years (600,601). An overall female preponderance of 1.5:1 is exaggerated in childhood, reflecting the earlier skeletal maturation of girls with fused physes, who are more prone to the development of GCTs (602). It should be kept in mind that most bone lesions with giant cells in children are unlikely to be GCTs, especially in those 10 years old or younger. The distal femur and proximal tibia together account for more than 50% of all cases, followed by the distal radius (Figure 28-58). The short tubular bones and vertebral bodies are uncommonly affected overall, but these sites are more often involved in children than in adults (603). Vertebral-based GCT above the sacrum is extremely uncommon. Multicentric GCTs, occurring in 1% of cases, have a particular predilection for the short tubular bones. When multiple GCTs are encountered, the possibility of hyperparathyroidism should be considered.

A metaphyseal, eccentric, osteolytic lesion that extends into the epiphysis to the subchondral bone and exhibiting expansion and cortical thinning is the characteristic radiologic appearance of GCT in tubular bones. In a skeletally immature patient, the tumor may be based in the metaphysis. Flat bones are uncommon sites, and in the absence of Paget disease, the craniofacial bones are not involved. Friable, reddish, and hemorrhagic tissue is the gross appearance of curetted fragments (Figure 28-59). A variably prominent and even inconspicuous oval to plump mononuclear spindle cell stroma accompanies numerous, usually evenly distributed sheetlike proliferation of osteoclastic-type giant cells (Figure 28-60). The giant cells are formed through fusion of mononuclear stromal cells that are of monocyte–macrophage derivation and exhibit osteoclastic differentiation. It is thought that a subset of the mononuclear stromal cells are the neoplastic element in GCT. The giant cells are relatively uniform in size and contain numerous overlapping nuclei that appear similar to the nuclei of the stromal cells. Any mitotic activity is confined to the stromal cells. Atypical pleomorphic nuclei in the stromal cells or atypical mitoses are not found in conventional GCT. The tumor has a well-vascularized background, and reactive bone may be observed at the tumor's advancing edge. Despite the usual view, focal bone formation may be found in GCT unrelated to any reactive repair process. Invasion of vascular spaces by giant cells should not be taken as evidence of aggressive behavior. Hemosiderin-laden macrophages reflect prior hemorrhage and ABC-like regions can occur. In some cases, the microscopic distinction between a GCT and an ABC (cystic and solid variants) is not always apparent as osteoclast-type giant cells may be abundant in ABC. Recourse to the radiologic imaging studies often helps reach the correct diagnosis in a skeletally immature patient. A xanthomatous and fibrohistiocytic pattern may either be seen focally or be so prominent as to obscure any evidence of the GCT. Such areas may resemble a benign fibrous histiocytoma or nonossifying fibroma and are thought to represent a lesion undergoing regression.

Depending upon the site of the GCT, curettage and en block resection are the therapies used. The former high rate of local recurrence (up to 50%) following curettage has been reduced to 5% to 10% by means of using greater operative

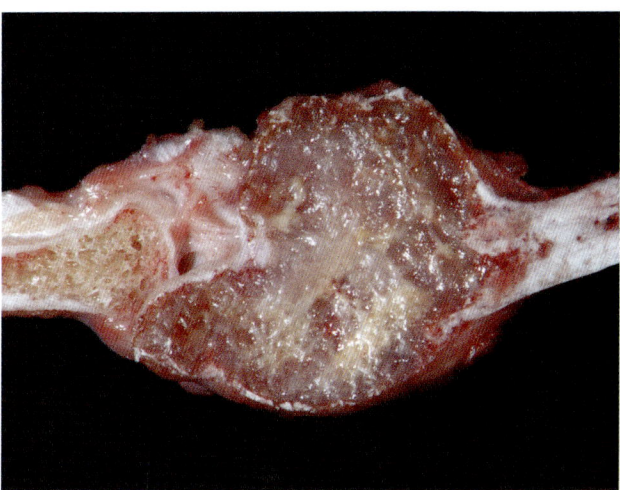

FIGURE 28-59 • Giant-cell tumor. This tumor presented in the right metacarpal bone of the right index finger of a 19-year-old male. An amputation was performed after an unsuccessful curettage. The tumor measured 4.2 cm in greatest dimension and extended beneath the articular cartilage. The brownish-tan, glistening tumor has destroyed the cortical bone.

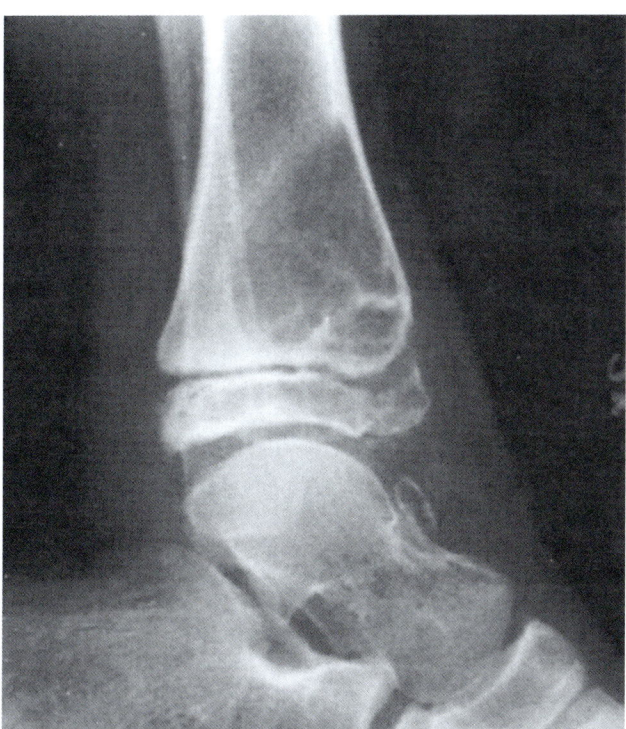

FIGURE 28-58 • Giant-cell tumor. This tumor arising in the distal tibia in an 8-year-old female is a lytic metaphyseal lesion that crosses the physis and lacks any bony sclerosis.

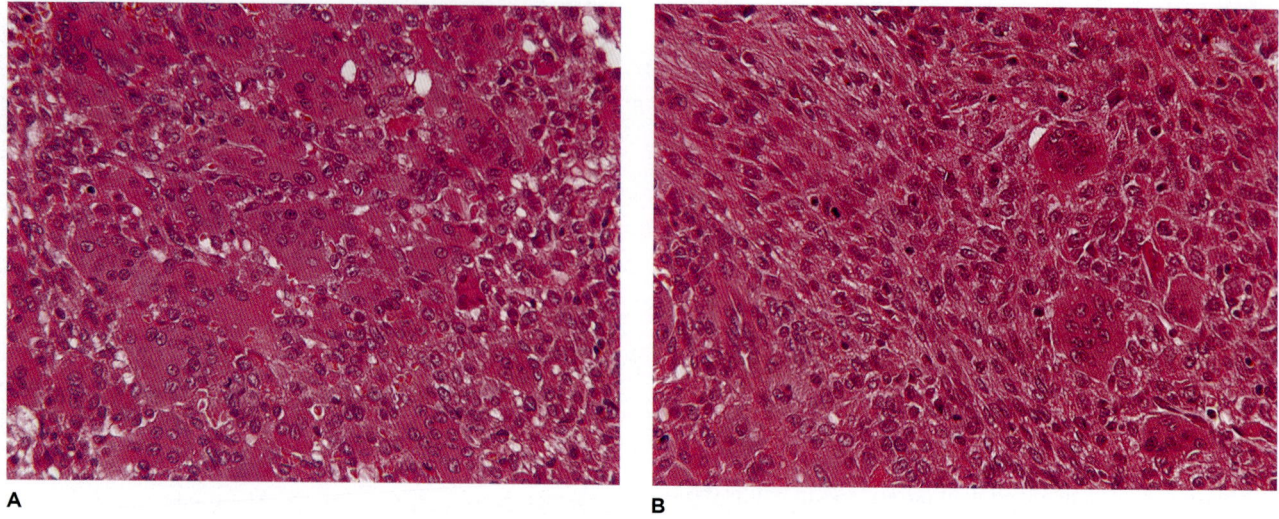

FIGURE 28-60 • Giant-cell tumor. This tumor arose in the distal tibia in a 17-year-old female. **A:** Area of tumor is composed of diffuse proliferation of relatively uniform osteoclast-like giant cells. **B:** Other fields have a less concentrated population of giant cells in a fibrous stromal background.

exposure, thorough curetting, and use of phenol solution. The stromal cells of GCT express RANK ligand (RANKL), a mediator of osteoclast formation and survival; osteoclasts express RANK (604). Denosumab, a human antibody that inhibits RANKL, and thus the osteolytic bone destruction caused by the osteoclasts in GCT, has been successfully used for unresectable and recurrent GCT and to reduce the size of some to make them operable (605). Secondary sarcomas in GCT may be in the form of fibrosarcoma, malignant fibrous histiocytoma, or OS. Primary malignant GCT is manifest by the presence of pleomorphic stromal cells with atypical mitoses intermixed with benign-appearing GCT. Pulmonary metastasis of GCT is a rare but known complication even in children (606).

Giant-cell reparative granuloma (GCRG) is a lesion that contains osteoclast-type giant cells and can be confused with true GCT, which commonly expresses p63 (607). Most GCRGs are diagnosed between the ages of 10 and 25 years, with 30% to 35% of cases recognized in the first two decades of life (608). Like GCT, there is a female predilection. Unlike GCT, the most common sites of involvement are the jaw bones (mandible more common than maxilla), orbit, paranasal sinuses, and temporal bone (608–610). Lesions similar to GCRG are also described in the short tubular bones of the hands and feet (611). The lesion described as solid ABC is regarded by some as a GCRG, but not by others (612). The lesions of cherubism represent GCRGs and not FD (613). Most lesions in the head and neck region are solitary, but multiquadrant lesions in jaw bones should raise the distinct likelihood of familial cherubism (SH3BP2 gene mutation on 4p16) (614–616). Another syndromic association is the Cohen-Gorlin syndrome (Noonan-like phenotype with GCRG-like lesions) (617). Likewise, GCRG and other giant-cell lesions of tendinous or synovial origin are found in NF1, Jaffe-Campanacci, and Noonan-NF1 syndromes (618).

A small apical lucency, to a large, destructive, multilocular, or unilocular lesion in the mandible or maxilla, is the range of radiographic features (Figure 28-61A, B). Friable, tan to red–brown tissue, with accompanying hemorrhage and cystic change, is the gross appearance of the curetted tissue, features that resemble GCT and ABC. Histologically, a predominantly fibrous and variably cellular background, containing interspersed aggregates of osteoclast-type giant cells, often around foci of stromal hemorrhage, is the typical feature (Figure 28-61B). The lack of a mononuclear stromal cell background population; the irregular distribution and focal aggregation of the giant cells, rather than their diffuse proliferation; and the prominent fibrous stroma serve to differentiate GCRG from GCT (619). However, especially in the short tubular bones of the hands and feet, the distinction from true GCT may be difficult, but the distinction is based in part on the patient's age, the location of the lesion in the bone, and its radiologic features. It has been reported that p63 expression in GCTs is not found in GCRG (620). Secondary ABC-like changes may be found in GCRG. Brown tumor of hyperparathyroidism is histologically indistinguishable from GCRG (621). Both LCH and juvenile xanthogranuloma (JXG) are considerations in the differential diagnosis. There are examples of an apparent nonhereditary presentation of GCRG in children without cherubism (622,623).

Osteoglophonic dysplasia (OGD) and *cherubism* are AD disorders in which abnormalities of the jaws have microscopic features resembling those of a GCRG and NOFs in long bones (30). Severe rhizomelic dysplasia and other craniofacial anomalies are present in OGD as well as mutations in FGFR1 (8p11.2-p11.1) (174,624). Cherubism ("familial FD") is generally not recognized clinically until the 2nd or 3rd year of life; it presents as fullness of the lower face secondary to symmetrical cystic lesions of the mandible and maxilla and less often of the floor and lateral wall of the

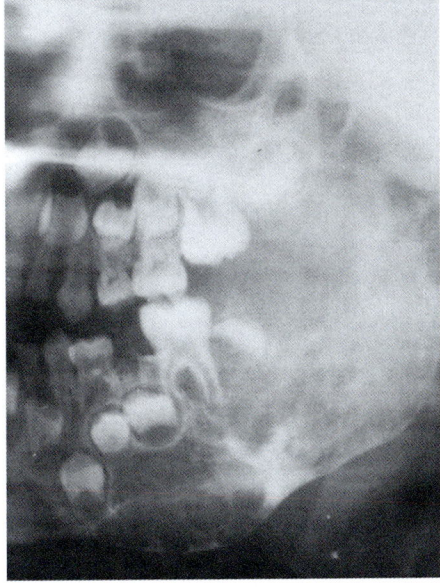
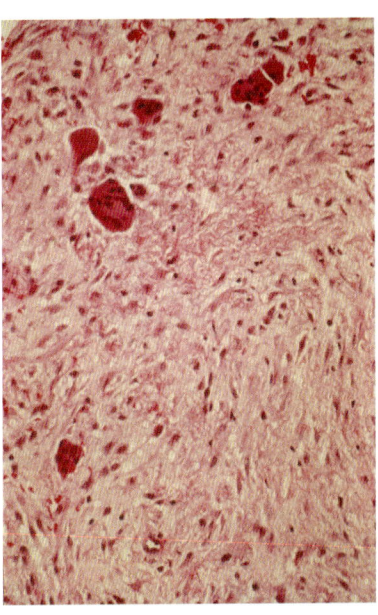

FIGURE 28-61 • Cherubism. **A:** A circumscribed multicystic lesion is present in the posterior mandible, but the same changes are found in the solitary GCRG. **B:** The histologic features of cherubism are also those of GCRG with scattered multinucleated giant cells in a loose to compact fibrous stroma with some similarities to nonossifying fibroma–fibrous histiocytoma of bone.

orbit (Figure 28-61). Some cases of cherubism are sporadic, while others are associated with Noonan and Ramon syndromes (gingival fibromatosis, juvenile rheumatoid arthritis (RA), seizure disorders, and a retinal pigmentary disorder). Microscopically, osteoclast-like giant cells are present within a fibrous spindle cell stroma in the cherubic lesion, without the features of a fibro-osseous lesion such as FD. The designation of cherubism as "familial FD" is a misnomer, as it relates to the typical histologic findings, although some affected families may also have fibro-osseous involvement of the jaws. The jaw lesions of cherubism resolve through adolescence and early adulthood, with loss of dentition, and the development of severe bony abnormalities.

Aneurysmal bone cyst (ABC) is predominantly a lesion of childhood, with a peak presentation in the second decade with a median age of 9 to 11 years and a male predilection (625,626). Approximately 10% to 15% of ABCs are diagnosed at or before 5 years of age. Overall, ABCs account for 5% to 8% of all bone "tumors" in children (418). The femur (20% to 25%), tibia (15% to 18%), spine (15% to 20%), humerus (8% to 10%), and fibula (5% to 6%) are the preferred sites, with localization to the metaphysis when in a long bone (627). However, any bone may be involved, even the soft tissues (628,629). Rarely, ABCs may present as multifocal lesions. The typical roentgenographic appearance is that of a lytic, "blown-out" eccentric lesion with a thin, expanded bony shell. Fluid–fluid levels, often present within the loculated spaces, are well shown on computed tomography (Figure 28-62A to C). Grossly, ABC has a cystic, hemorrhagic spongelike appearance that oozes blood upon

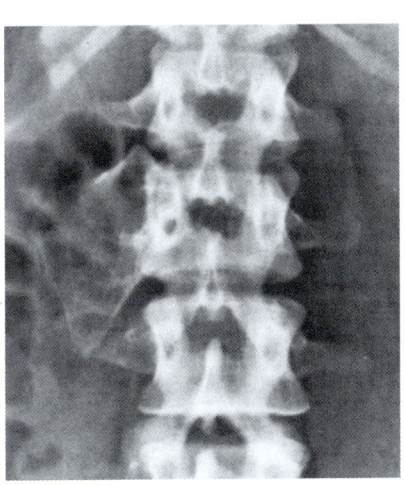
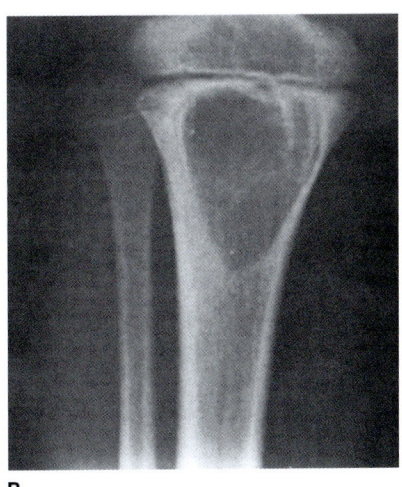
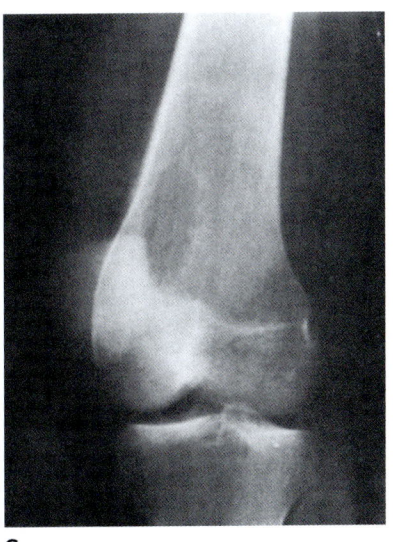

FIGURE 28-62 • Aneurysmal bone cyst. The appearance of an ABC varies from a well-circumscribed, benign lesion to a highly destructive one. **A:** The "blown-out" appearance of a vertebral lesion. **B:** A proximal tibial lesion crosses the open growth plate. **C:** A less well-defined distal femoral lesion with a periosteal reaction mimics an OS.

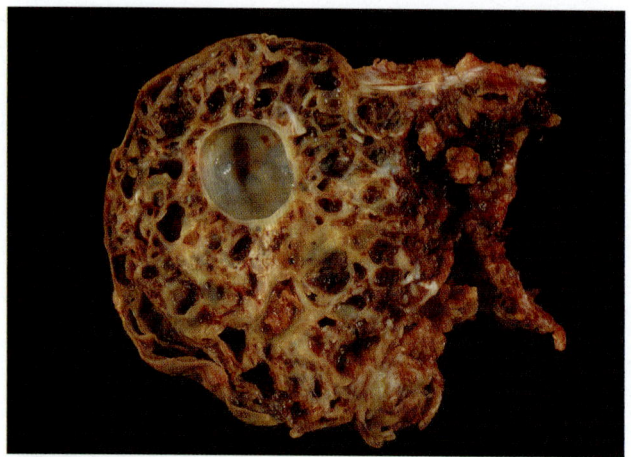

FIGURE 28-63 • Aneurysmal bone cyst. This resected intact lesion with its multicystic hemorrhagic appearance is the exception to the usual fragments of a bone curettage.

entering the lesion at operation (Figure 28-63). Friable hemorrhagic tissue fragments, often without intact cysts, are the nonspecific features of curetted tissue. Histologically, ABC shows multiple cavernous blood-filled spaces separated by fibrous septa that contain multinucleated osteoclast-type giant cells in a spindle background with or without seams of osteoid or bone (Figure 28-64A to D). The cells lack the pleomorphism and abnormal mitotic figures of a telangiectatic OS, which may mimic ABC at low-power histologic examination. A peculiar hematoxyphilic fibrochondroid material is frequently found in the walls and considered by some as virtually pathognomonic of ABC (Figure 28-64C,D). Although a vascular etiology is proposed for these lesions, the blood-filled cysts are not lined by endothelial cells. Similar aneurysmal cystic changes are seen in a wide variety of osseous lesions and the designation of ABC should be reserved for cases lacking the diagnostic features of another

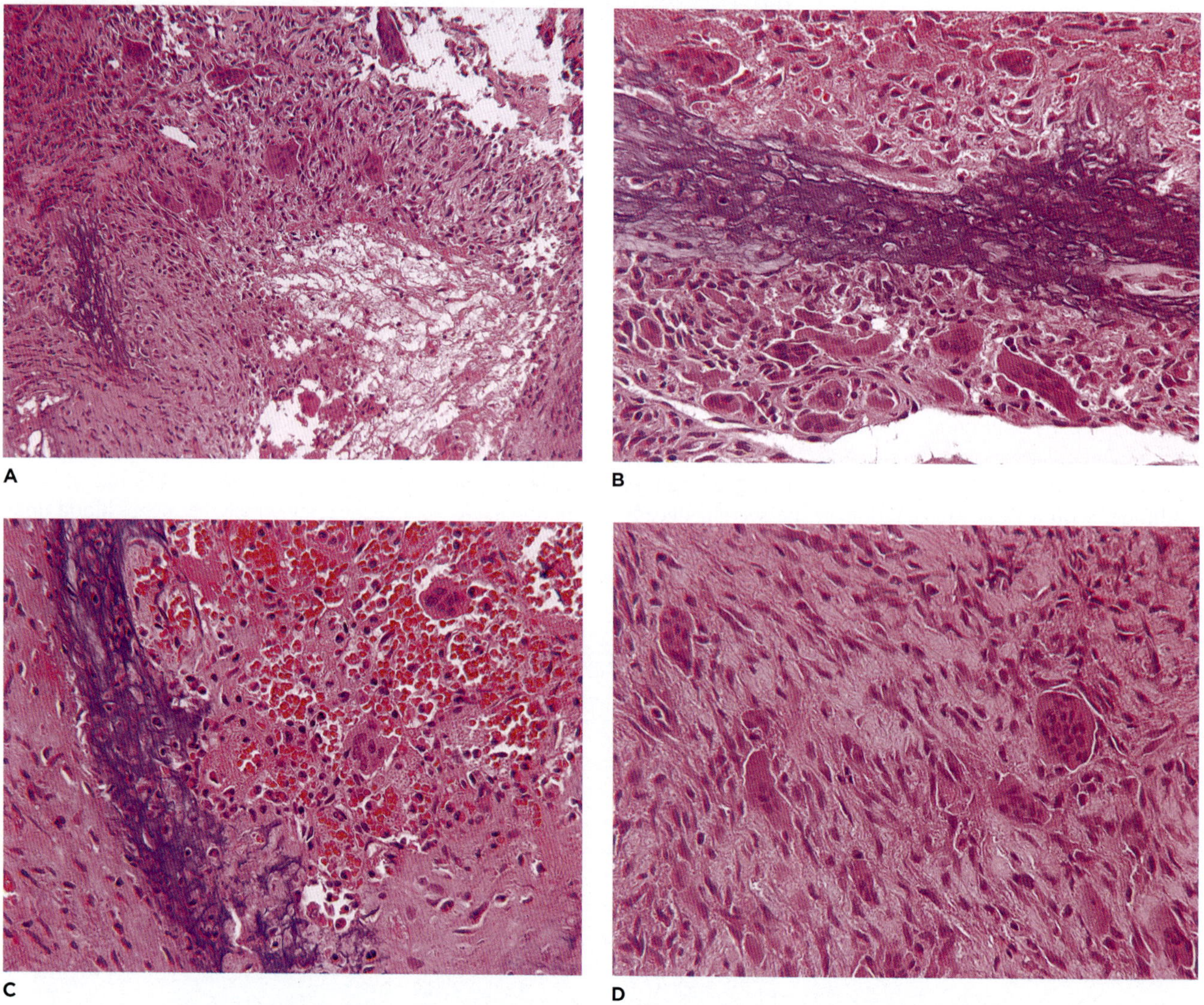

A

B

C

D

FIGURE 28-64 • Aneurysmal bone cyst. Several microscopic patterns are seen. **A:** Cystic spaces are filled with erythrocytes and fibrin and separated by variably thickened septa with multinucleated osteoclast-type giant cells and trabeculae of osteoid and bone. **B:** Septa often contain lacy fibrochondroid-like calcifications that are virtually diagnostic of ABC. **C:** This focus shows bone beneath the cyst lining with accompanying multinucleated giant cells. **D:** The thickened septa contain multinucleated giant cells and a reactive-appearing spindle cell stroma without appreciable atypia, which is not the case in the telangiectatic OS.

primary bone lesion (630). The local recurrence rate of ABC is 20% to 25% after curettage. Only rare cases of malignant change are reported (631). With the observation that primary ABC has a translocation involving the fusion partners, USP6 oncogene (17p13) and the CDH11 promoter, it is regarded as a related neoplastic process to nodular fasciitis (632). The so-called solid variant of ABC is considered by some as representing a GCRG (152).

Solitary–unicameral bone cyst (SUBC) occurs almost exclusively in children; 80% of cases present in the first decade and a half of life, and about two-thirds of all cases are found in adolescents; there is a male predilection (633). The proximal humerus and proximal femur are the most commonly affected bones; the talus, calcaneus, and ilium are less commonly involved (Figure 28-65) (634). The cyst is intramedullary, generally in the metaphysis at or near the physis; it frequently extends to the physis and may involve it, which has raised the possibility of a growth disturbance in its pathogenesis. As growth of the parent bone progresses, the physis moves away from the lesion. The latter grows in the long axis of the bone as a uniform expansion without the eccentric blown-out configuration of an ABC. Importantly, the cortex remains intact and soft tissue involvement does not occur; however, pathologic fracture is a common presenting clinical feature, especially in the cysts of the proximal humerus. Although typically unilocular, the cyst may radiologically appear to contain multiloculated cavities due to the presence of protruding bone ridges or trabeculations produced secondary to pressure scalloping of the cortical bone by the expanding cyst. An infrequent radiologic hallmark of SUBC is the "fallen fragment" sign, which occurs secondary to pathologic fracture whereby a small cortical bone fragment breaks free and falls by gravity to the bottom of the fluid-filled cyst. It is important to note that a totally lytic-appearing OS may rarely radiologically mimic an SUBC (635). Grossly, the cyst contains serous to serosanguineous fluid and is lined by a usually thin fibrous membrane, in contrast to the spongelike and abundantly hemorrhagic tissue of an ABC. There are no specific diagnostic microscopic features of SUBC. The cyst lining may be variable in amount but is usually scant and composed of a bland fibrous stroma in which osteoclast-type giant cells may be found and macrophages containing hemosiderin if a fracture has occurred (Figure 28-66A to C). In some cases, however, the lining may be thicker and have features indistinguishable from ABC. In such cases, the radiologic features, as well as the operative finding, are used to establish the diagnosis.

Eosinophilic fibrogranular deposits, incorrectly likened to odontogenic cementum, are a frequent finding; these deposits may undergo calcification and conversion to osteoid and new bone (Figure 28-66B, C) (636,637). Recurrence rates after steroid injections, or curettage with bone packing, range from 15% to 20%. EWS–PNET may present initially as a SUBC (638).

Other bone cysts occur in specific sites such as the mandible and maxilla where a variety of odontogenic-related lesions are recognized. Epidermoid cyst in the skull, or distal phalanx of the hand, histologically has a squamous lining and is filled with keratinous debris. So-called traumatic or hemorrhagic cysts are reported in the mandible or following a fracture especially in the region of the distal radius (639) (see Chapter 22).

Primary vascular neoplasms and other vascular lesions of bone in children comprise a small category of cases unlike their common occurrence in the skin and soft tissues. Several studies have examined vascular tumors in bone for the purpose of revising concepts about their pathogenesis as malformations or neoplasms (640,641). One of the larger series of pediatric vascular lesions of bone classified 44 of 77 (57%) as malformations of venous–lymphatic or arteriovenous types, with an equal number of cases in these two histogenetic categories (640). Some of the issues on the terminology of vascular lesions are discussed in the chapter on soft tissue tumors. Overall, it would appear that 5% to 10% of all "vascular tumors" of bone present in the first two decades. Craniofacial bones and vertebra are the most frequent sites for the occurrence of cavernous hemangiomas or venous malformations (Figure 28-67A to C). These lesions are uncommon in the long bones (642). Radiologically, most tumors are typically well-defined, lucent lesions. Uniform patent, thin-walled vascular spaces, with minimal stroma, are the basic

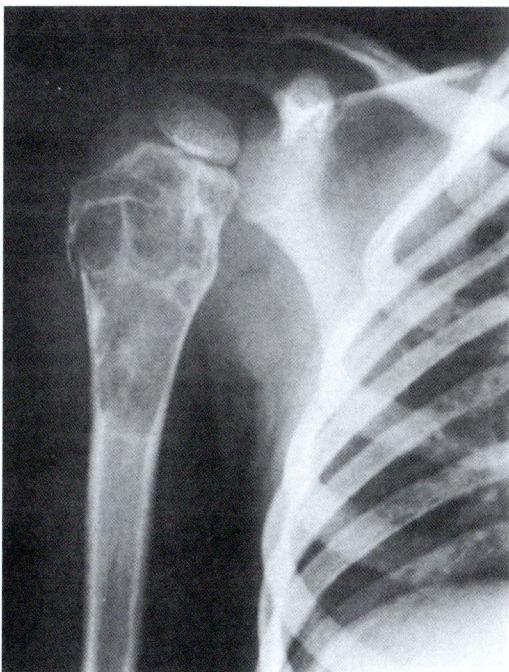

FIGURE 28-65 • Unicameral or simple bone cyst. A well-circumscribed, expansile medullary lytic lesion has a unilocular or septated appearance. Unlike ABC, the lesion lacks an eccentric blown-out appearance but expands the metaphysis uniformly.

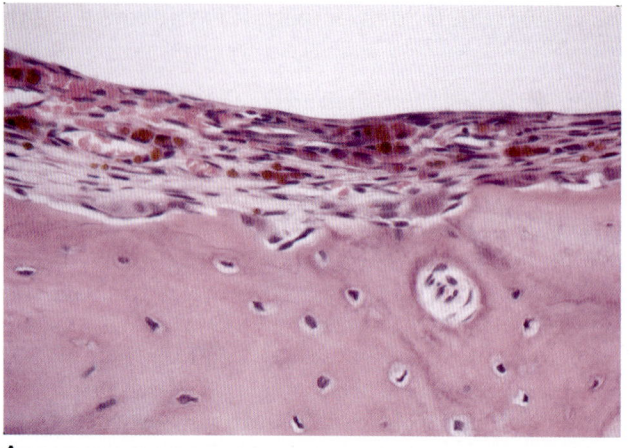
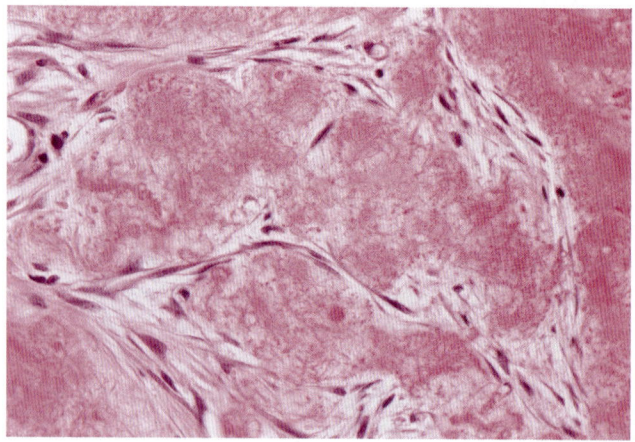
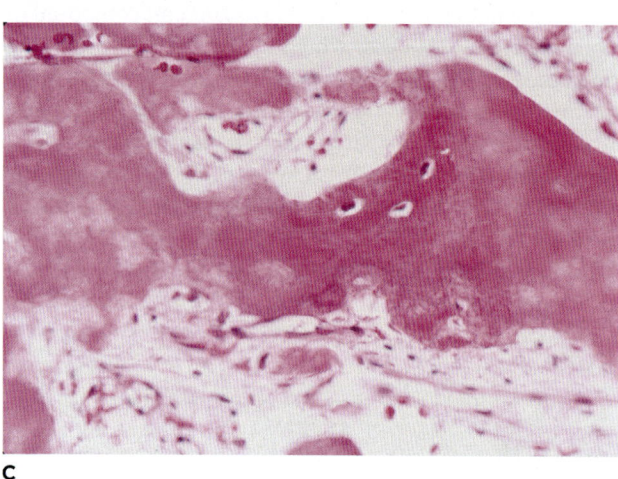

FIGURE 28-66 • Unicameral or simple bone cyst. **A:** The cyst lining often has a nondescript appearance. **B:** One of the characteristic findings is the pale eosinophilic fibrogranular material. **C:** This material can undergo transformation to osteoid.

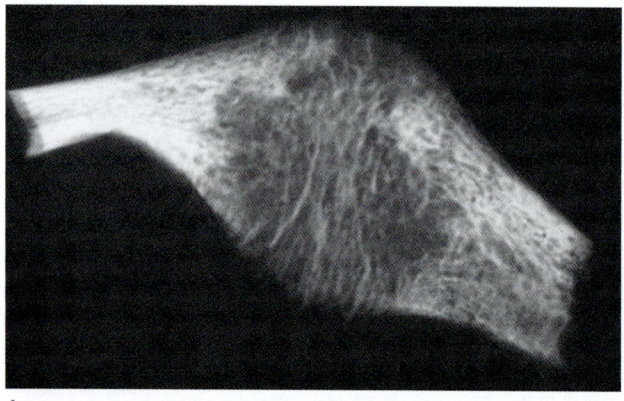
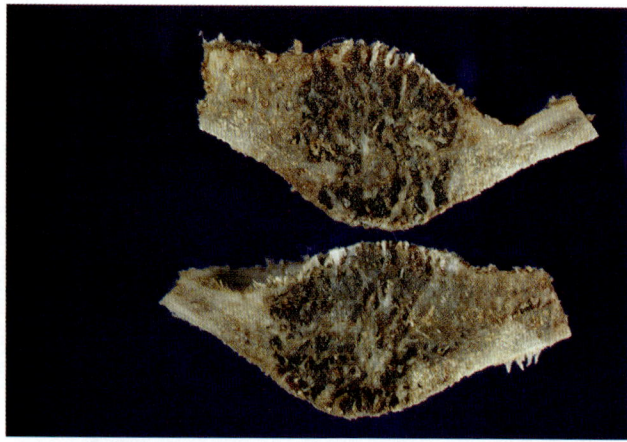
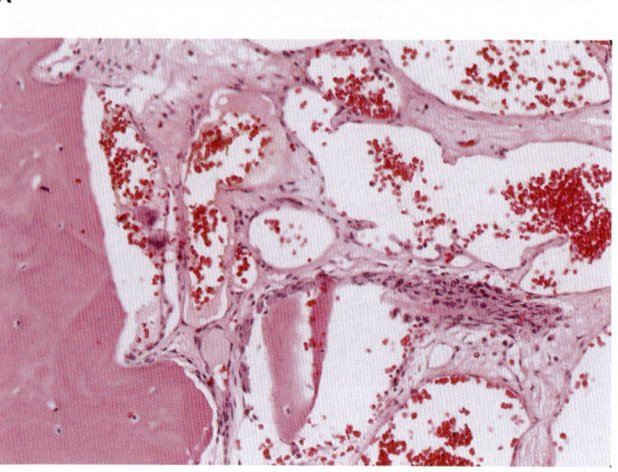

FIGURE 28-67 • Hemangioma. **A:** Thin skull-based lesion in a 9-year-old male. The specimen image shown presented an expansile lytic defect between the inner and outer table. **B:** The resection specimen has a porous, somewhat hemorrhagic appearance. **C:** Blood-filled vascular spaces are seen.

microscopic features (Figure 28-67C). The cavernous form of hemangioma is the most common in all bone sites (642). Organizing thrombi may be present in some vessels. Bone resorption and bone formation are found, respectively, in the vertebral and calvarial hemangiomas. These lesions are generally nonreactive for GLUT1 and D2-40. A less common vascular lesion is the epithelioid hemangioma (EH) whose histologic features are identical to its soft tissue counterpart. In one study, 10% of EHs occurred in individuals 20 years old or less and that these tumors occur in the long bones (643). Epithelioid hemangioendothelioma, kaposiform hemangioendothelioma, and angiosarcoma in aggregate are rare but documented in the bones of older children and adolescents (644–646).

Gorham-Stout disease (vanishing bone disease) is characterized by a proliferation of lymphatic spaces in bone that results in substantial loss of bone (osteolysis) in the axial and appendicular skeleton but with a predilection for the humerus, scapula, and pelvis (647–649). In some cases demonstrating a total loss of the involved bone, the process may extend beyond a joint space to involve adjacent bone. CD105 (endoglin) is expressed by the lymphatics in this disorder (650). Involvement of the pleura and/or thoracic duct may be accompanied by chylothorax. A more generalized form of the disease has been described with infiltration of soft tissues and even splenic involvement. There is a report of a 1-year-old male with a germ-line mutation in PTEN and concurrent progressive osteolysis (651).

FIBROUS SPINDLE CELL TUMORS

Nonossifying fibroma (NOF; benign fibrous histiocytoma of bone) is a relatively common incidental finding in skeletally immature individuals and is seen more often by the radiologist than the pathologist due to its very characteristic imaging features. It has been estimated that up to 40% of children have a small metaphyseal defect, presumably an NOF, which spontaneously disappears as it is incorporated into the growing bone (652,653). The distinction between a metaphyseal fibrous defect or fibrous cortical defect and NOF is the larger size of the NOF, which involves at least 50% of the bone width. In a pediatric bone tumor biopsy series, 3% of all cases were NOFs (418). Multifocal NOFs may be familial or associated with NF1, Jaffe-Campanacci syndrome, and osteoglophonic dysplasia with mutations in the FGFR1 gene (8p11.2-p11.1) (654). In the latter disorder, there are cystic lesions in the proximal femurs with NOF-like microscopic features. Like sporadic NOF, these lesions are subject to pathologic fracture.

Although the smaller lesions are usually asymptomatic, the larger NOF may cause pain with or without pathologic fracture in which case some have drawn a semantic distinction between NOF and benign fibrous histiocytoma or fibroxanthoma of bone (655,656). The distal femur and proximal tibia are the most common locations. This lesion is cortically based as an eccentric metaphyseal radiolucency in the

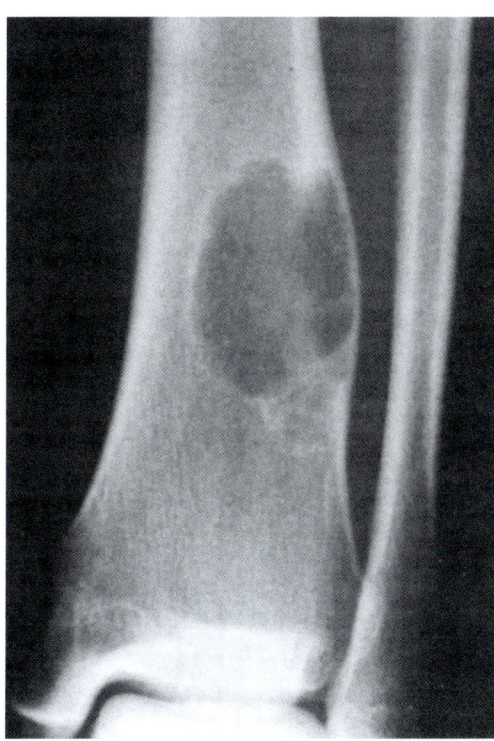

FIGURE 28-68 • Nonossifying fibroma or metaphyseal fibrous defect. An eccentric and well-circumscribed lesion with sclerotic borders is seen in this image. Lesions occupying 50% or more of the diameter of the bone may be complicated by a pathologic fracture.

long tubular bones with densely sclerotic scalloped borders (Figure 28-68) (657). In those very rare instances where the lesion has been treated by some sort of en bloc excision, rather than by thorough curettage, the lesion is grossly generally well demarcated and yellow to tan-brown, but aneurysmal cystic changes within may alter its appearance. The microscopic features are basically those of a bland, uniform spindle cell proliferation, frequently with storiform pattern, with a variable number of osteoclast-type giant cells. Small collections of giant cells may be localized in areas of interstitial hemorrhage (Figure 28-69A to D). Sheets or small aggregates of xanthoma cells tend to vary in frequency from one NOF to another. Hemorrhagic and cystic changes are present in some cases to the extent that the lesion resembles an ABC. Pathologic fracture through a NOF, with early callus formation, may distort much of the underlying features of the lesion.

Desmoplastic fibroma (DF) and myofibroma have their respective counterparts in the soft tissues in that DF is regarded as the intraosseous counterpart of desmoid-type fibromatosis, and myofibroma of bone can be either solitary or present in association with multifocal extraosseous myofibromas in an infant. Less than 1% of all bone tumors in children are DFs. In excess of 70% of all DFs present in the first three decades of life, with most cases diagnosed between 12 and 20 years of age, but are also seen as early as the first years of life (658,659). The mandible is the most common site of involvement (20% to 25% of cases), followed by the femur

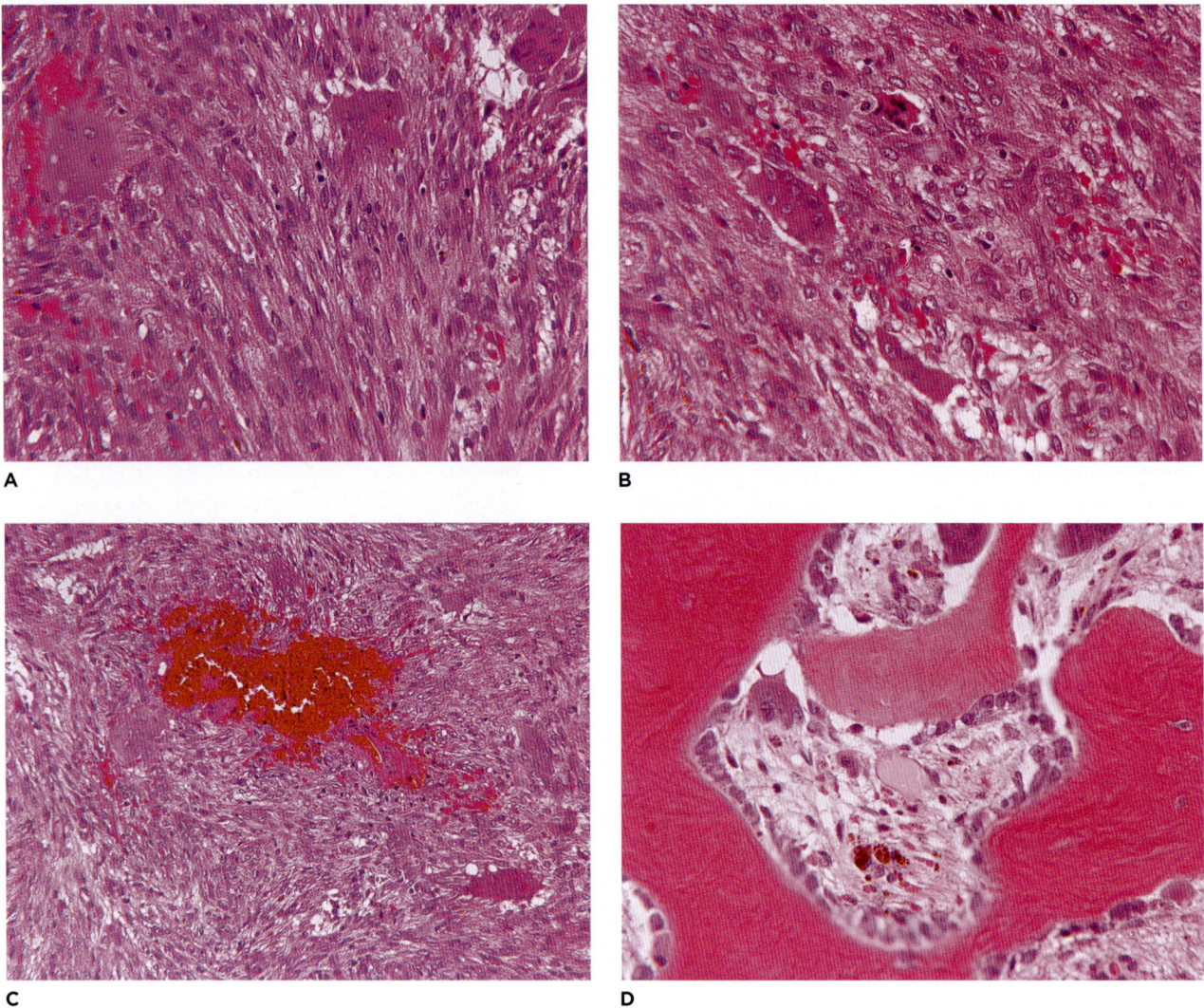

FIGURE 28-69 • Nonossifying fibroma. **A:** The basic microscopic features include multinucleated osteoclast-type giant cells in a bland spindle cell stroma with a storiform pattern. **B:** The multinucleated cells vary in number from one focus to another as well as in size and shape. **C:** Secondary changes include hemorrhage with or without features resembling an ABC. **D:** As these tumors expand into the cortex, there is often the presence of osteoblastic and osteoclastic activity as the bone is remodeled.

(12% to 15%), pelvic bones (10% to 13%), radius (10% to 12%), and tibia (8% to 10%) (660). In the mandible and maxilla, the tumor is located posteriorly in 20% to 80% of cases, while in the long bones, it is usually metaphyseal. A multiseptated radiolucency, or an ill-defined mass are the imaging features in the jaw and long bones. A juxtacortical mass, with erosion into the bone, is a less common presentation, but the latter most likely represents a soft tissue fibromatosis invading the bone. In 50% or more of cases, the tumor has extended into the adjacent soft tissues; this aggressive local growth accounts in part for the absence of a sclerotic border or an attenuated cortex. Histologically, DF is composed of spindle cells that are separated by a pale eosinophilic or more densely collagenized stroma. The nuclei are relatively uniform, and tapered, or plump appearing especially in foci with a fasciitis-like appearance. Nuclear pleomorphism and a more densely compacted cellularity with readily identifiable mitotic figures should be viewed with concern for myofibrosarcoma. Typical mitotic figures, in limited numbers, may be found in DF just as they may be present in a desmoid fibromatosis. The local recurrence rate following simple curettage is 30% to 40%, which is also similar to the recurrence of a desmoid fibromatosis in the soft tissues. It can be difficult in some cases to determine whether a fibromatosis in the head and neck region has arisen in bone as a DF or invaded into the bone from a soft tissue fibromatosis.

The differential diagnosis of DF in the mandible and maxilla is the *central odontogenic fibroma* (COF), which is not an insignificant distinction since the latter has a low recurrence rate in contrast to DF (661,662). COF has a female predilection and is more likely to occur in individuals over 20 years of age. The mandible and maxilla are equally involved with a multilocular or unilocular lesion in the absence of local extension into the surrounding soft tissues (663).

Histologically, the simple COF is a purely spindle cell proliferation with a myxoid stroma resembling a dental papilla.

Myofibroma of bone is one of the least common presentations for this tumor of childhood, with a male to female ratio of 2:1. Most examples are solitary lytic lesions, with sclerosis, and are found in the skull, orbit, or mandible, in an infant or young child (664–666). Less common is a presentation with cutaneous and soft tissue myofibromas and multiple skeletal lesions in an infant, and designated as congenital generalized myofibromatosis (667). Histologically, an infiltrative process expands and replaces the intraosseous space by nodules and bundles of bland-appearing spindle cells (Figure 28-70A to D). Some of the nodules have a juxtavascular orientation, whereas the spindle cells form interrupted bundles or fascicles. Bone lesions, like those in the soft tissue, have the capacity for spontaneous regression. Another fibroproliferative lesion presenting as a rapidly enlarging mass of the skull in an infant is *cranial fasciitis*. Its local growth may erode through the outer and inner table of the skull. Like the myofibroma, this lesion is composed of myofibroblasts, but its histologic features resemble nodular fasciitis (see Chapter 26).

Congenital pseudoarthrosis (CP, congenital tibial dysplasia) is a rare disorder of the tibia, but also reported in the fibula and rarer yet in the radius (668). The incidence is 1:190,000 live births. Approximately 1% of children with NF1 have CP, but 50% of those with CP have NF1 (669–671). Another rare association is with OFD of the tibia (672). There are varying degrees of severity noted radiologically, from slight angulation of the bone to cystification, and the most severe form of CP with tapered fragmented ends of bone merging into a fibrous mass-like area. The dense fibrous mass has a resemblance to an overly cellular desmoid fibromatosis. It has been

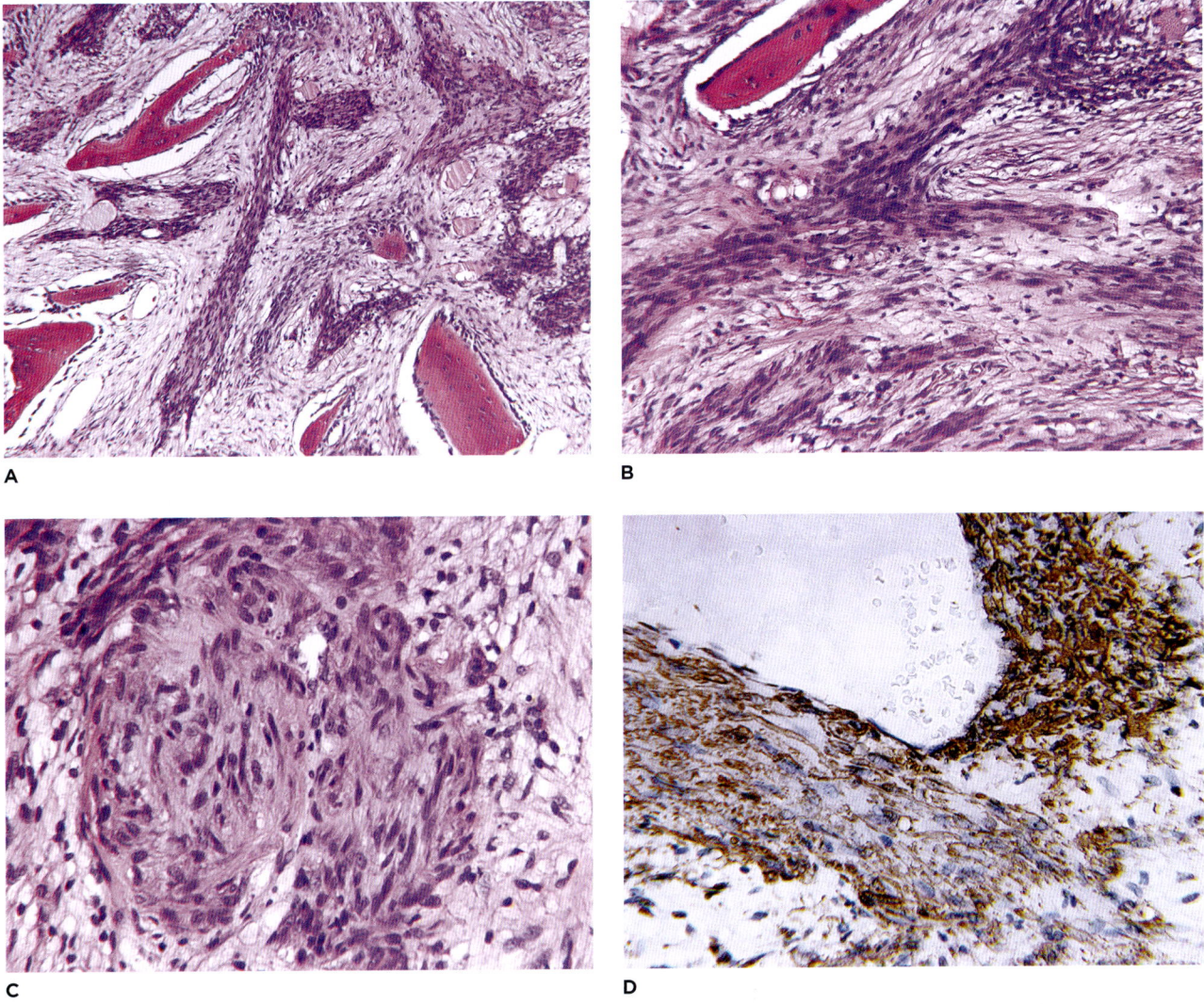

FIGURE 28-70 • Infantile myofibroma–myofibromatosis presented in the frontoparietal skull as an osteolytic focus in an 8-month-old boy. **A, B:** Biopsy tissue shows a spindle cell proliferation filling the intramedullary spaces and separating islands of bone. **C:** Nodules of loosely arranged spindle cells surround a small central vessel. This vasocentric pattern is characteristic of myofibroma. **D:** Immunohistochemical staining for smooth muscle actin yields a strongly positive reaction. (Contributed by Christine Reyes, MD, Washington, DC.)

claimed that schwannian elements are present among the fibroblasts, but the histologic features are not those of a neurofibroma. There are conflicting observations as to the nature of this stromal proliferation with the claim of a hamartomatous process in two cases of NF1-associated CP (673). Islands or spicules of woven bone, with accompanying osteoblasts, with maturation to lamellar bone, and a fibroblastic stroma containing cytokeratin-positive cells, are the features of an associated OFD.

Fibrosarcoma (FS) and *myofibrosarcoma* of bone in children are rare (674,675). Only 5% to 10% of all FSs of bone are diagnosed in the first two decades. Most FSs occur in the metaphysis of long bones; however, if a biopsy from a tumor with a FS-like pattern is seen in a child, the possibility of a fibroblastic OS should be suspected, with recourse to review of the radiologic images. Another fibrous tumor that has been described in the bone is inflammatory myofibroblastic tumor, which we have yet to see in our practice (153).

Adamantinoma (ADM), like OFD and CP, occurs predominantly in the tibia (85% to 90% of cases) especially in its anterior diaphysis (676). Involvement of the fibula, with or without a synchronous lesion in the tibia, is present in 5% to 10% of cases. This tumor accounts for 0.5% or less of bone tumors in children (154). As many as 25% to 30% are diagnosed in the second decade of life, with the infrequent example in a child less than 10 years of age.

ADM has been divided into two basic types, the classic form and a so-called "differentiated" or OFD-like ADM. The relationship between these lesions and OFD is controversial and still evolving. As with OFD, OFD-like ADM occurs exclusively as an intracortical lesion in the tibia and fibula, usually in patients younger than age 20 years. Radiologically, the lesion replicates those of OFD, including the anterior bowing of the tibia when it is involved. The histologic pattern is also similar to OFD with the exception that overt small islands of epithelial cells are visible in routine sections, unlike the individual cytokeratin-positive spindle cells in OFD. These epithelial nests are irregularly distributed in the stroma and never are a dominant component. As with OFD-like ADM, the classic form of ADM most often involves the tibia and fibula, but rare examples are reported in a variety of bones, and even within the soft tissues. The classic ADM is distinctly uncommon in children. The tumor also radiologically replicates that of OFD/OFD-like ADM, but in contrast, the classic form involves cortical as well as medullary bone and may show cortical destruction and soft tissue invasion. Histologically, ADM is dominated by large areas of epithelial cells with basaloid, squamoid, pseudoglandular, and spindle cell patterns (Figure 28-71). The epithelial component consists of large foci in contrast to the small, isolated areas in OFD-like ADM. Focally, and most commonly located at the periphery, areas similar to OFD may be found. OFD-like ADMs locally recur in 25% of cases, but have virtually no potential to metastasize, unlike classic ADM may spread to regional lymph nodes and lung in 15% or more of cases. Trisomies 7, 8, and 12 have been identified in ADMs (676). The relationship between OFD, OFD-like ADM, and ADM is controversial, with some proposing that OFD-like ADM is a regressing form of ADM, which eventually is indistinguishable from OFD, while others postulate that OFD and OFD-like ADM represents a continuum with OFD/OFD-like ADM being a precursor lesion to eventual classic ADM (677).

When biopsy tissue of a tibial diaphyseal lesion in a young patient shows the presence of nests of small cells in the stromal background, the neoplasm may represent an ADM-like EWS–PNET with its signature t(11;22) translocation (678).

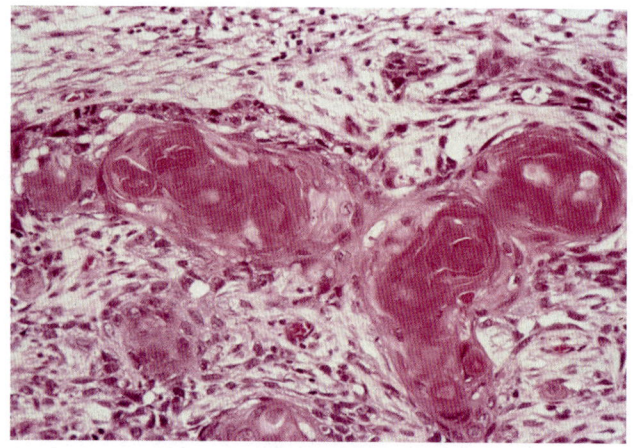
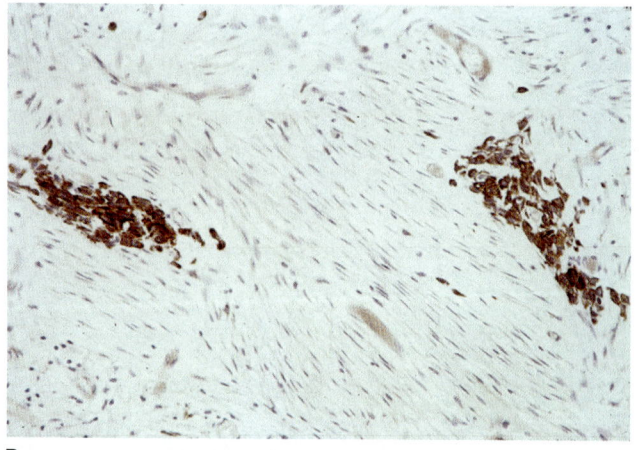

FIGURE 28-71 • Adamantinoma. Several histologic patterns are seen including tubular, basaloid, spindle cell, and squamous cell variants. In children and adolescents, OFD- and EWS-like variants are seen. **A:** Squamous variant has a resemblance to well-differentiated squamous cell carcinoma. **B:** Immunohistochemical stain for cytokeratin shows the presence of small positively staining small nests in a spindle cell background, representing the pattern of the differentiated or OFD-like ADM, which is the histologic type seen most often in children.

ROUND-CELL NEOPLASMS

Ewing sarcoma–primitive neuroectodermal tumor (EWS–PNET) is the second most common primary sarcoma of bone in children and adolescents but is third behind CS when all age groups are considered (424,426). It is estimated that there are approximately 250 newly diagnosed cases of osseous EWS–PNET per year in the United States and the incidence has changed little over the past 30 to 40 years, with the most recent figure of 0.128 case per 100,000 populations. There is a correlation between ethnic origin and the incidence of EWS–PNET with lower risks in those of African or Asian ancestry (679). There is one case of EWS–PNET of bone for every two to three cases of OS. Approximately 80% of cases of EWS–PNET present in the bone and the remained in a variety of extraosseous sites, including the soft tissues and kidney. Among 1,474 newly diagnosed primary bone tumors in children and adolescents to the age of 18 years, approximately 5% were EWS–PNET (418). Most patients are diagnosed between the ages of 10 and 25 years, but EWS–PNET in either bone or soft tissue may be seen in infancy and early childhood (680). The femur and tibia are the primary sites in 30% to 35% of cases, pelvic bones in 20% to 25%, axial spine and nonspine sites in 25% to 30%, and the head and neck in 2% to 3%. In the long bones, EWS–PNET has a preference for the diaphysis, where the tumor is a poorly marginated medullary lesion with permeative osseous destruction and cortical loss and a prominent periosteal, onionskin-like reaction representing new bone formation (Figure 28-72A, B). Rarely, the tumor may be located in the periosteum or as multifocal lesions (681). Histologic features of the reactive new bone may be initially unsettling, and worrisome for small-cell OS, until it is realized that the osteoblasts have an orderly arrangement around the islands of osteoid with an absence of anaplasia and atypical mitotic figures (Figure 28-73A). When EWS–PNET presents in the pelvis, the osteolytic focus in the pubis or ischium may be relatively inconspicuous compared to a sizable soft tissue component.

The diagnosis of EWS–PNET is facilitated to a considerable degree by the immunohistochemistry and molecular diagnostics since the basic cell morphology may be distorted by artifacts created at the time of biopsy and subsequent processing for microscopic examination. Because these tumors may be extensively hemorrhagic and necrotic, the biopsy tissue may be paucicellular. There are essentially no histopathologic differences between osseous and extraosseous EWS–PNET (see Chapter 26). There is a monolayer of nonoverlapping, small polygonal cells that have a distinct cell membrane, a uniform round to oval nucleus, with finely

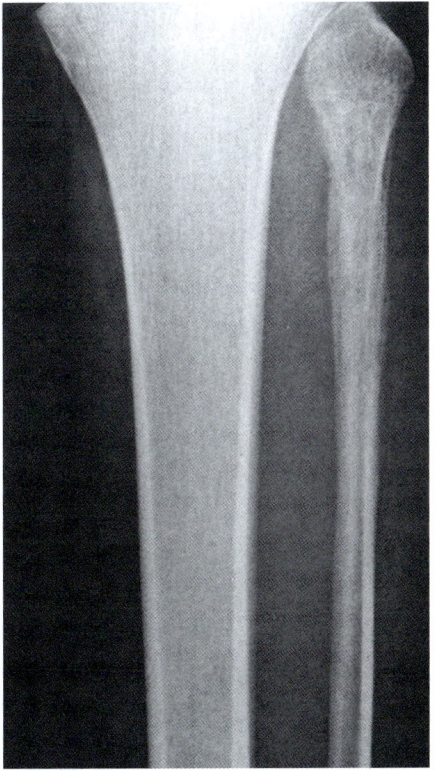
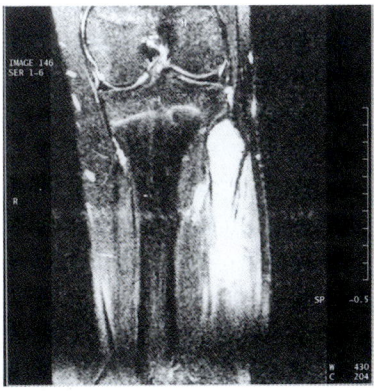

FIGURE 28-72 • Ewing sarcoma–primitive neuroectodermal tumor in the proximal fibula of a 16-year-old boy. **A:** Anterior–posterior roentgenogram shows a permeative, destructive-appearing medullary process with associated so-called onionskin periosteal reaction and a soft tissue mass in the space between the tibia and fibula. **B:** Magnetic resonance imaging study shows an intense signal in the proximal fibula and adjacent soft tissue.

dispersed chromatin, a small nucleolus, and a clear to finely vacuolated cytoplasm (Figure 28-73A to D). Mitotic figures are generally inconspicuous, but not in all cases. Indistinct cell borders, overlapping cells, nuclear hyperchromatism, scattered mitotic figures, and lobular–trabecular or rosette-like profiles are other features that may occur, the latter an indicator of neural differentiation. Any degree of anaplasia and substantial pleomorphism should be viewed with a question about the possibility of a small-cell OS, large-cell lymphoma, or metastatic alveolar rhabdomyosarcoma (ARMS) or one of the EWS-like sarcomas. Foci of necrosis, with or without a perithelial arrangement of tumor cells, and hemorrhage with a pseudovascular or peliosis-like appearance are other common microscopic features. Small contracted pyknotic or secondary cells (dark cells) may be seen among the better preserved tumor cells. If the biopsy tissue has been obtained from the soft tissue component, fibrous stroma with reactive features is often present and some of these nonneoplastic changes can obscure some of the diagnostic findings. The immunohistochemical and molecular genetic studies and their results are the same as those in the bone and soft tissue sites of EWS–PNET (Figure 28-74A to D) (682–685). Recently, small round-cell tumors histologically mimicking EWS–PNET have been

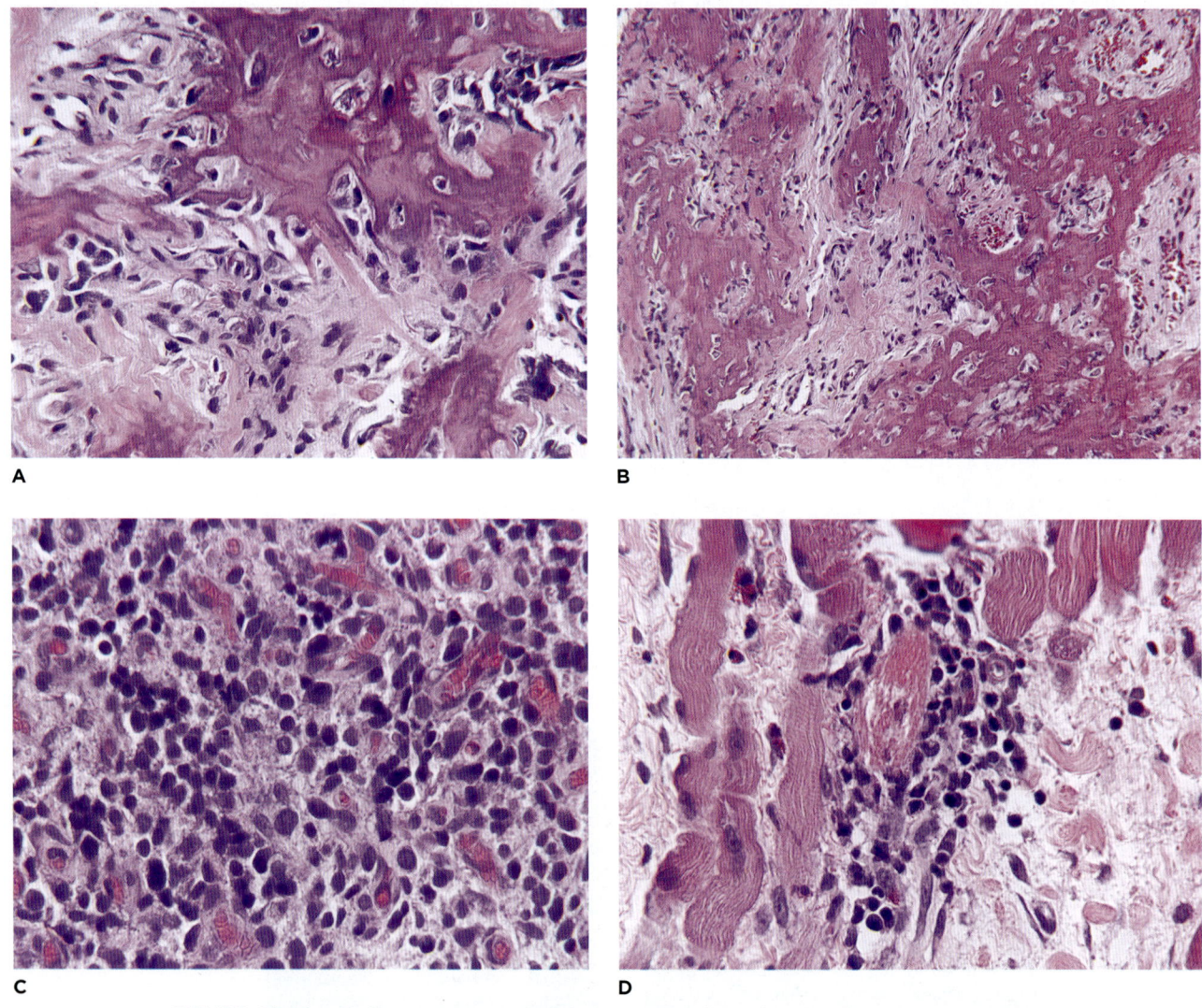

FIGURE 28-73 • Ewing sarcoma—primitive neuroectodermal tumor in a 3-year-old boy. **A:** Biopsy tissue shows extensive new bone formation with an accompanying population of osteoblasts and stromal cells with atypical features but in the absence of mitotic figures. **B:** Another field shows somewhat irregular sclerotic bone, which caused some concern about OS yet in the absence of anaplastic cells. **C:** A nodule in the adjacent soft tissues is composed of uniform hyperchromatic malignant round cells. **D:** Another focus consists of malignant round cells infiltrating skeletal muscle. The tumor cells were immunoreactive for vimentin, cytokeratin, and CD99. An EWS breakapart was demonstrated by FISH studies. (Contributed by D. Ashley Hill, MD, Washington, DC.)

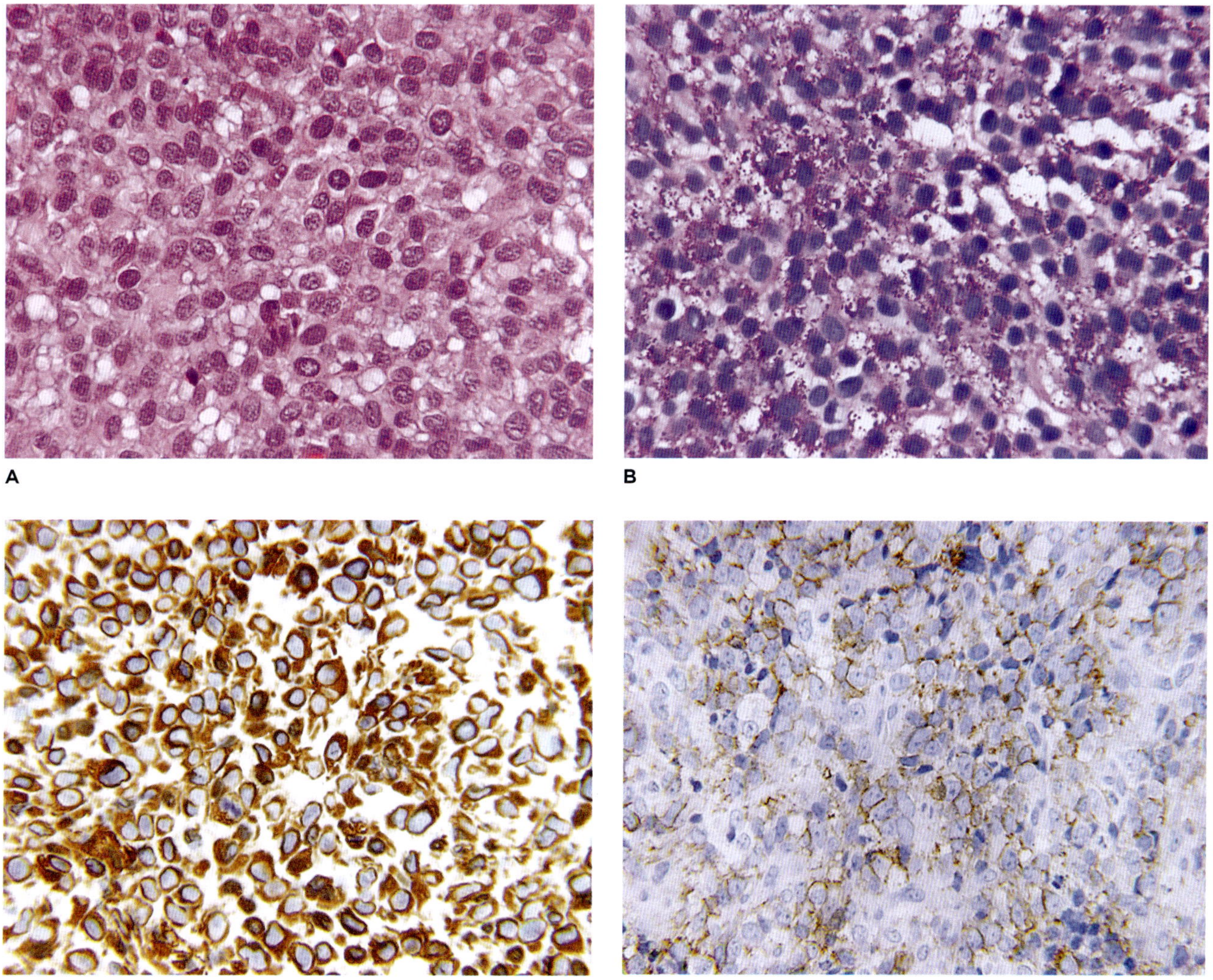

FIGURE 28-74 • Ewing sarcoma–primitive neuroectodermal tumor lends itself to several ancillary studies to confirm the suspected diagnosis. **A:** The tumor cells are uniform with clear to vacuolated cytoplasm due to the presence of cytoplasm confirmed by the glycogen. **B:** Periodic acid–Schiff stain that shows diffuse cytoplasmic positivity. **C:** The tumor cells demonstrate a diffuse cytoplasmic pattern of vimentin positivity by immunohistochemistry. **D:** Reactive CD99 immunostain shows diffuse membrane–cytoplasmic pattern with mosaic-like features.

described that demonstrate chromosomal translocations different from those in true EWS–PNETs (686–689).

The gross examination of the resected tumor follows neoadjuvant chemotherapy in virtually all cases, since initial primary resections is a treatment of the past. The gross features are variable, from a solid medullary focus of tumor to a hemorrhagic mass extending through the cortex into the subperiosteum of the diaphysis or beyond into the soft tissues (Figure 28-75). In some cases, the tumor may involve the medullary cavity along its length with associated cortical thickening (Figure 28-76). Though a substantial soft tissue component may have been present before chemotherapy, it is often reduced to a residual subcortical mass or may be totally absent. The presence of residual viable tumor postchemotherapy should be assessed in a fashion similar to OS. Blocks are obtained from grossly visible tumor and surrounding bone so as to provide a semiquantitative percentage of tumor

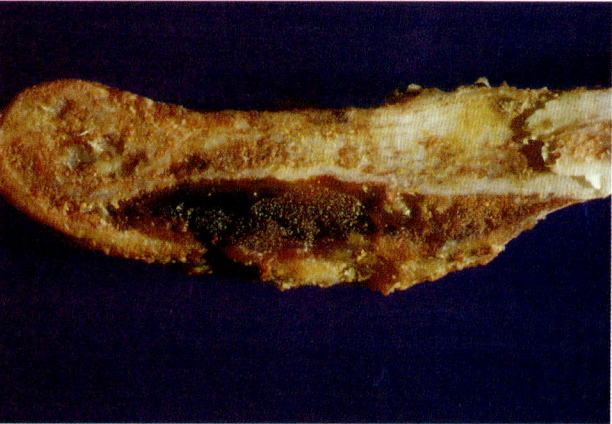

FIGURE 28-75 • Ewing sarcoma–primitive neuroectodermal tumor. The tumor in the clavicle has infiltrated through the cortex with the formation of a hemorrhagic mass elevating the periosteum.

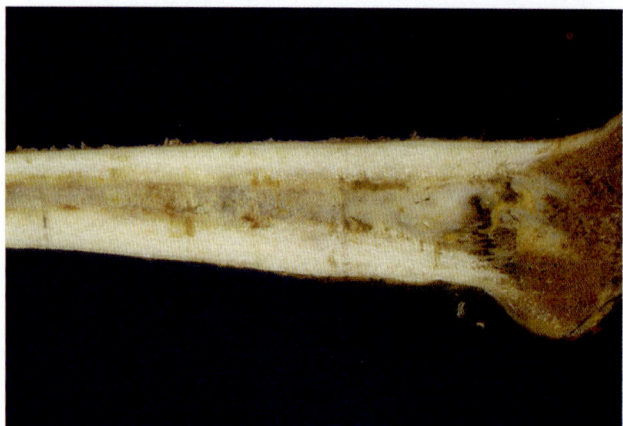

FIGURE 28-76 • Ewing sarcoma–primitive neuroectodermal tumor. Gray-white tumor has filled the medullary portion of bone and there is cortical thickening.

cell death, with an optimal ("good response") being tumor necrosis in the range of 90% or greater. Effectiveness of chemotherapy may also be judged by imaging studies of the soft tissue component (690). Fibrosis, hemorrhage, and cyst formation may be the only residual findings in the resected specimen. The prognostic determinants of outcome are location (axial, poor), size (8 cm or greater, poor), and complete surgical resection after chemotherapy, (favorable) (691–693). Those tumors arising in the appendicular skeleton have a more favorable outcome, and survival is no different between those with an osseous or extraosseous primary site (694). Patients with evidence of metastases at initial presentation have a poor prognosis, as do those who develop metastatic disease following initial therapy.

Melanotic neuroectodermal tumor of infancy (MNTI), most commonly presents in the bone (maxilla, mandible, or skull) but also may occur in nonosseous sites such as the brain and epididymis (695). About 90% or more of cases are diagnosed in children less than 1 year of age and located in the head and neck region (696). The tumor usually presents as an expansile mass in the maxilla (60% to 70% of MNTIs) with a nonulcerated mucosa. Radiologically, it is usually well circumscribed but often has infiltrative features histologically. Grossly, the tumor has a dense fibrous appearance and is variably pigmented from tan to an intense black. One of its notable microscopic features is a dense fibrous stroma containing small, angulated cell nests, some with a large-cell population with a central grouping of smaller hyperchromatic cells; the larger cells are epithelioid-appearing melanocyte-like cells, and the small cells are neuroblasts. The composition of the nests can vary from those composed almost exclusively of neuroblasts to nests of variably pigmented epithelioid cells. The neuroblasts are immunoreactive for chromogranin and synaptophysin, and the epithelioid cells express vimentin, cytokeratin AE1/AE3, HMB-45, and even desmin (Figure 28-77A to D) (697). Local recurrence develops postresection in 10% to 15% of cases, and 1% to 3% of tumors metastasize with morphologic features usually indistinguishable from classic neuroblastoma (CNB) (698) (see Chapter 22).

The differential diagnosis of MNTI is limited given the age and clinical presentation in the head and neck region of an infant. Metastatic NB is the most immediate consideration especially so when tissue contains crush artifact of the small cells without a readily recognizable population of melanin-containing cells. If the immunohistochemical

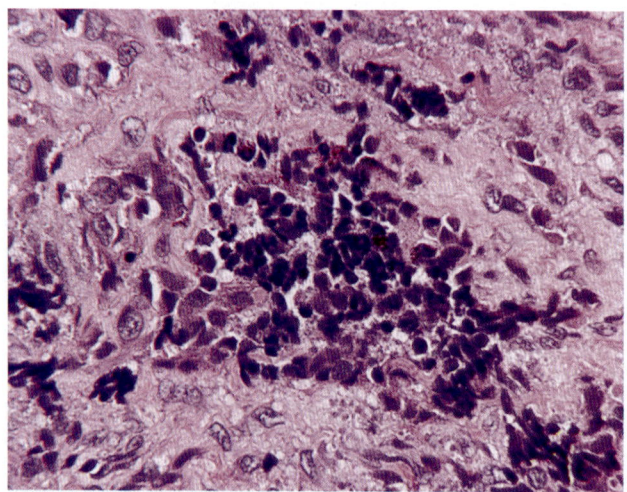
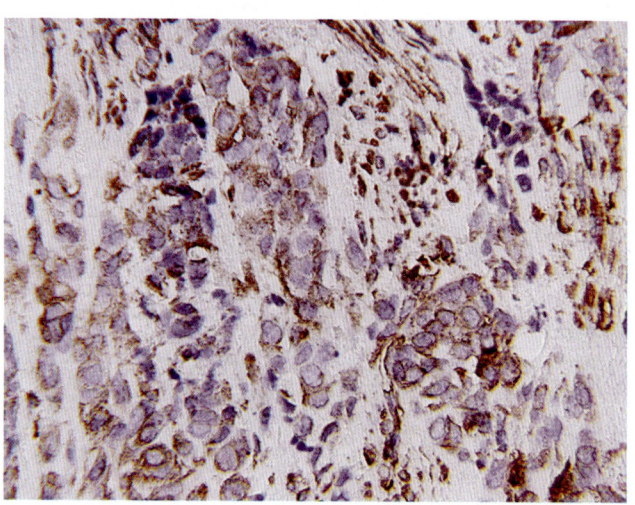

A

B

FIGURE 28-77 • Melanotic neuroectodermal tumor of infancy. **A:** The tumor presenting as a skull defect in a 10-week-old male is composed of multiple small nests of darkly staining cells within a dense fibrous background. Two populations of cells are shown, one population of larger, more epithelioid-appearing cells with finely pigmented cytoplasm and a second population of smaller more darkly staining cells representing neuroblasts. **B:** A vimentin immunostain shows the presence of staining of the larger rounded cells and some of the smaller cells. Cytokeratin was positive in scattered cells (not shown).

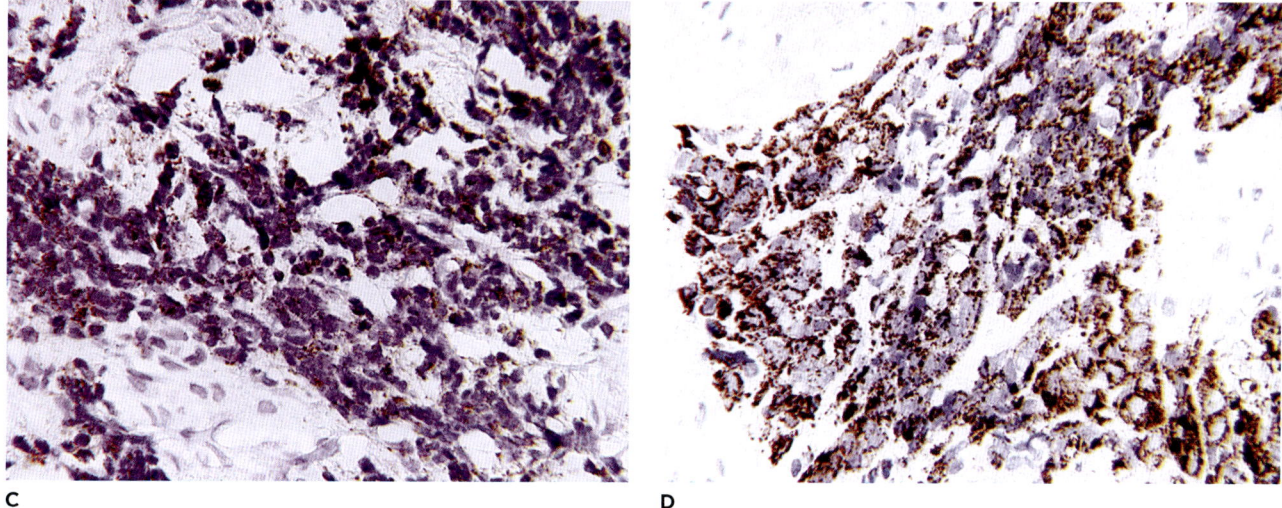

FIGURE 28-77 • (continued) C: Chromogranin immunostaining shows diffuse granular cytoplasmic positivity in the small neuroblastic cells. This tumor is also positive for neuron-specific enolase and chromogranin (not shown). D: HMB-45 immunostaining demonstrates diffuse cytoplasmic positivity in the larger epithelioid cells. This tumor also had a small population of cells staining for desmin (not shown). (Contributed by Deborah Perry, MD, Omaha, Nebraska.)

evaluation is restricted to "neural" markers, MNTI cannot be distinguished from CNB. Desmin and myogenin positivity in MNTI is another finding, which is not entirely surprising given the neural crest-like character of this tumor. Desmoplastic small round-cell tumor has been reported in the bone, and its histologic and some of its immunophenotypic features overlap with EWS–PNET and MNTI (699).

Primary lymphoma of bone constitutes only 1% or less of malignant skeletal neoplasms in the first two decades of life, but 5% to 10% of all lymphomas in children and adolescents present in the bone (700,701). In one review, approximately 10% of patients with lymphoma of bone were 20 years old or less (702). In most cases, children are diagnosed after the age of 10 years. An axial distribution of lesions, either solitary or multifocal, presents the differential diagnosis of LCH, EWS–PNET, metastatic NB, and osteomyelitis (Figure 28-78). Diffuse large B-cell (78%) and B-lymphoblastic lymphomas (12%) are the most common types in that order in a report by Chisholm et al. (Figure 28-79A, B) (703). A recent study has found a syndromic presentation of diffuse large B-cell lymphoma located in the proximal tibia of young patients and associated with sclerotic radiologic features and an excellent prognosis (704). Approximately 10% of anaplastic large-cell lymphomas (ALCL) are known to present in the bone with an axial skeletal and multifocal site distribution of lytic lesions (705,706). Children under 5 years of age may present with osseous lesions of ALCL in which case LCH or NB is often the favored clinical impression. Small biopsies can be problematic, especially in the presence of necrosis. An ALCL with its nested pattern in some cases may suggest a nonhematopoietic malignancy of possible metastatic nature. Lymphoblastic lymphoma is another potentially problematic diagnosis in the presence of CD99 positivity; however, ALCL in children is ALK and CD30 positive by immunohistochemistry (707). Hodgkin lymphoma rarely involves the skeletal system as a primary or secondary manifestation in children (708). Acute lymphoblastic leukemia in children is associated with multifocal osteolytic lesions in 20% to 25% of cases, which in most cases does not require a biopsy since the lesions have a

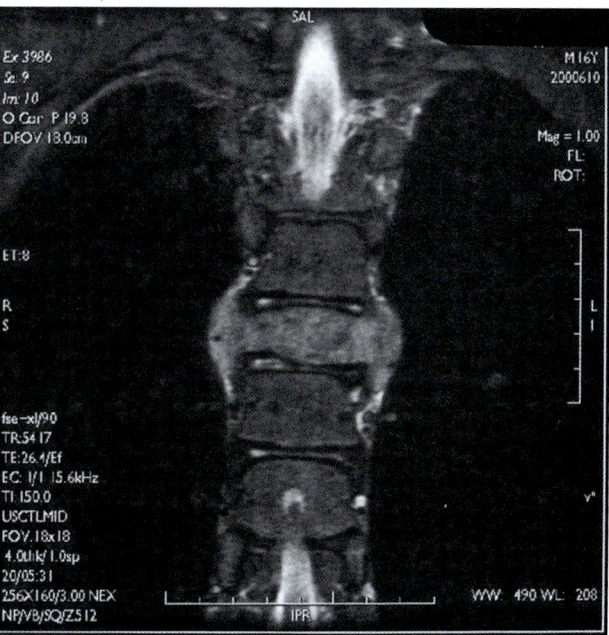

FIGURE 28-78 • Non-Hodgkin lymphoma with vertebral collapse presented with symptoms of spinal cord compression in a 17-year-old male. The collapsed vertebra (vertebra plana) raised the possibility of LCH.

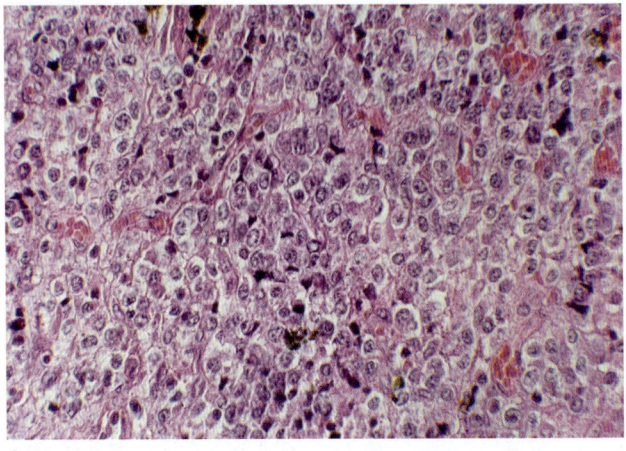 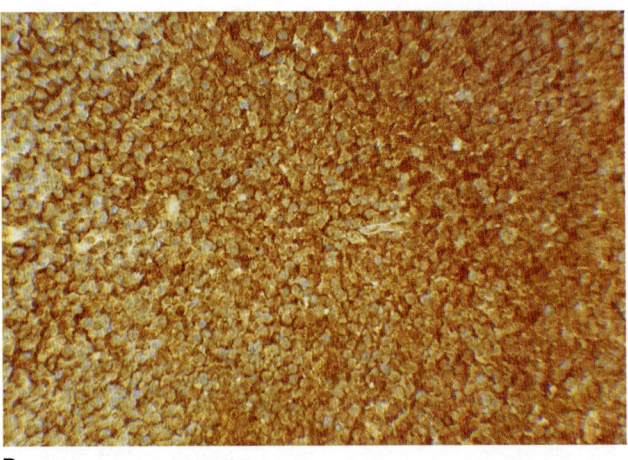

FIGURE 28-79 • Non-Hodgkin lymphoma. **A:** Biopsy tissue from the vertebra of a 17-year-old male shows the presence of uniform round cells with sharply defined cell borders and clear cytoplasm. Ewing sarcoma–primitive neuroectodermal tumor and a nonlymphomatous hematopoietic neoplasm were the other considerations in the differential diagnosis. **B:** Immunohistochemical positivity for CD20 establishes the diagnosis of large B-cell lymphoma.

characteristic appearance on imaging (709). Granulocytic sarcoma, as an extramedullary feature of acute myeloid leukemia, may present as a solitary osteolytic lesion in bone mimicking EWS–PNET or as multiple bone lesions in an infant to suggesting metastatic NB (710). There are a number of neoplastic and nonneoplastic manifestations of leukemia in children (711).

Multiple myeloma–plasma cell dyscrasia is the most common hematolymphoid malignancy to present in bone but occurs almost exclusively in adults usually older than age 40 years. Less than 1% of cases are diagnosed in individuals under 40 years of age. It is estimated that only 20 or so cases have been documented in children in the second decade of life (712,713).

Skeletal metastasis is well known and documented in the case of several childhood malignancies, exclusive of hematolymphoid neoplasms. Bone metastasis developed in 1.3% of children with a solid malignant neoplasm in a series from Denmark (714). Neuroblastoma is one of the more common solid malignancies of childhood to manifest skeletal metastasis either at the time of clinical presentation or during the clinical course, usually in setting of stage III disease. One or more osteolytic lesions are present in 75% to 80% of those who are found to have stage IV NB, mainly in children over 2 years of age at diagnosis. In an autopsy series of metastatic skeletal disease in children, 16 of 39 cases (41%) were NB (715). Clinically, it is important to differentiate between the metastasis to the bone marrow and a bone-destructive lesion in the setting of neuroblastoma to distinguish stage IVS from stage IV. The histologic features of metastatic NB are readily identifiable in most cases as nests or sheets of malignant small cells with a variably prominent fibrillary network of cytoplasmic processes. A ganglioneuromatous stroma may be seen in association with neuroblasts in some cases.

Metastatic retinoblastoma (RB) to bone is seen in 1% to 5% of those cases that have recurred, usually with involvement of the central nervous system. Malignant small cells, with minimal differentiation in the form of rosettes, are the basic microscopic features. Unlike NB, which may present with metastatic disease to the bone, this behavior is rare in RB. Metastatic RB to bone has a predilection for the mandible (716). Bone metastasis may present several years after the initial diagnosis (717,718).

Rhabdomyosarcoma (RMS) is the most common soft tissue sarcoma in childhood and is also the one with the highest frequency of bone metastases (719). Approximately 15% of children with RMS have metastatic tumor at the time of presentation, with the lung (47%), bone marrow (38%), bone (34%), and remote lymph nodes (26%) as the most common sites in descending order (720,721). In the presence of local invasion (T2), alveolar RMS is more likely to have bone metastasis (23%) than embryonal RMS (722).

Other sarcomas known to metastasize to bone include OS (multifocal), EWS–PNET (both osseous and extraosseous types), malignant rhabdoid tumor, alveolar soft part sarcoma, pleuropulmonary blastoma, and clear cell sarcoma of the kidney; Wilms tumor rarely metastasizes to bone.

Metastatic carcinoma to bone is rare in children. Nasopharyngeal carcinoma is the epithelial malignancy seen with some frequency in older children, with metastases to distant bone sites in 30% to 40% of cases (Figure 28-80A, B) (723). The translocation carcinoma [t(15;17)] of the respiratory tract in children (NUT-midline carcinoma), like carcinoma of the lung in adults, metastasizes to bone (724). Sialoblastoma, poorly differentiated carcinoma of the salivary gland, and adenocarcinoma of the colon are other examples of epithelial malignancies with metastatic potential to bone in children (725).

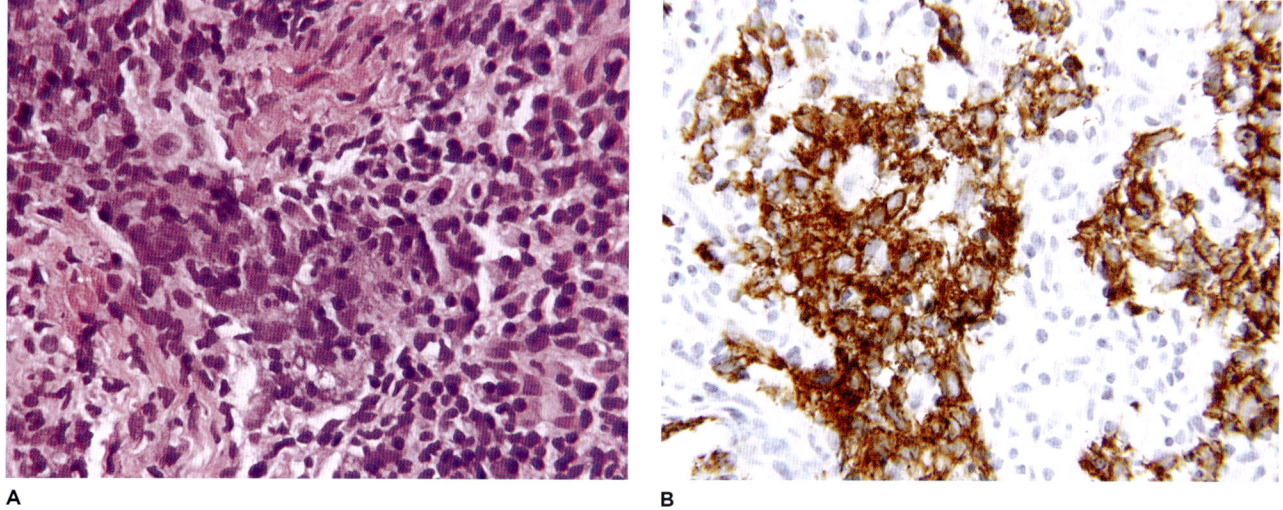

FIGURE 28-80 • Metastatic nasopharyngeal carcinoma. This lesion presented in the T12 vertebra in a 16-year-old male. **A:** A nest of malignant cells is accompanied by a dense lymphocytic infiltrate that is present in the primary and metastatic tumor in this disease, which is also known as lymphoepithelioma. **B:** Immunohistochemical stain for cytokeratin highlights the metastatic carcinoma in a dense background of lymphocytes.

HISTIOCYTIC DISORDERS

Histiocytic disorders with skeletal manifestations in children include LCH, JXG, and Rosai-Dorfman disease (RDD) (726). These rare disorders are not only important in their own regard, but their presentation as one or more predominantly osteolytic lesions is a diagnostic concern for infection or malignancy, especially metastatic disease.

Langerhans cell histiocytosis (LCH) is the most common of the histiocytic disorders with osseous lesion(s), which is often the only manifestation of the disease. It is now generally accepted that LCH in children is a clonal and therefore a neoplastic process (727). Monosystemic involvement is present in 75% to 80% of cases in children, with the skeletal system the most commonly affected single system in 60% to 80% of cases, followed by the skin, usually in a child with multisystemic disease (728–731). Approximately 60% of patients with osseous LCH have a single lesion, and the remainder is found to have two or more involved bones (732). It is estimated that 10% to 15% of children with bone lesion(s) have multisystem LCH. The average age at diagnosis of those with solitary or multiple bone lesions is 7 to 8 years, whereas those with multisystem LCH is usually 5 years old or younger, which also includes infants who have a more aggressive clinical course (733). There is validity to the statement that any bone may be involved, but there are preferred sites that include the skull, axial skeleton (vertebra, pelvic bones), and facial bones (orbit, mandible, and zygoma) (Figure 28-81) (Table 28-9). Facial bone involvement is often present in children with multisystem LCH. A sharply demarcated osteolytic focus, with a sclerotic margin, located in the diaphysis or metaphysis in a long bone or a similar lesion in a flat bone, is the appearance of a chronic lesion, whereas the early-stage LCH lesion is poorly marginated and has a more aggressive, if not malignant appearing, radiologic pattern, the latter suggestive of EWS–PNET or acute osteomyelitis (AO) (Figure 28-82) (732,733). A sizeable soft tissue component may accompany the latter features.

A biopsy, often accompanied by a request for frozen section consultation, usually consists of small fragments of otherwise nondescript tissue. When the clinical impression is LCH, touch imprints are useful to supplement the microscopic examination. Collections or aggregates of pale-staining, epithelioid-like mononuclear cells (Langerhans cells), with reniform nuclei and nuclear grooves, are found in association with a background that is variable in terms

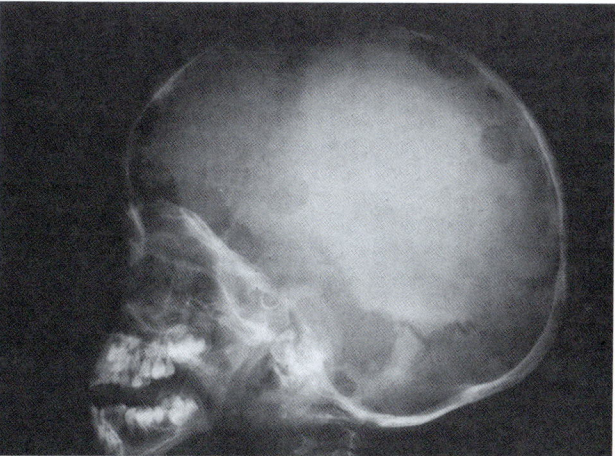

FIGURE 28-81 • Langerhans cell histiocytosis. The punched-out lesion in the skull of this child has a resemblance to multiple myeloma in an adult.

TABLE 28-9	LCH OF THE BONE (1989 TO 2009)		
Site	No. (%)	Age (Y) (Mean and Range)	Sex (M/F)
Skull	19 (19)	9 (1–19)	10/9
Temporal, mastoid, middle ear	16 (16)	6 (1–20)	9/7
Femur	15 (15)	8 (2–20)	11/4
Vertebra	12 (12)	6 (1–15)	8/4
Mandible (8) and maxilla (1)	9 (9)	5 (7 mo–13)	3/6
Pelvis (Ilium 6; ischium 1)	7 (7)	7 (1–15)	6/1
Humerus	6 (6)	6 (1–12)	5/1
Orbit	6 (6)	7 (5–11)	4/2
Rib	4 (6)	8 (1–20)	3/1
Radius(2); Ulna (1)	3 (3)	2 (2–3)	0/3
Scapula	3 (3)	7 (4–8)	1/2
Clavicle	1 (≤1)	11	0/1
Total	101 (~100)		60/41

From the files of the Lauren V. *Ackerman Laboratory of Surgical Pathology at Barnes-Jewish and St. Louis Children's Hospitals*. St. Louis, MO: Washington University Medical Center.

of other inflammatory cell types that may be present and necrosis in some cases (Figure 28-83A to D). In a site with an overlying mucous membrane that has undergone ulceration, neutrophils in association with a granulation tissue reaction may overwhelm and obscure the presence of Langerhans cells; these findings often accompany biopsy tissue from the middle ear or oral cavity with an underlying LCH in the mandible. Plasma cells are usually not prominent, but they can be seen especially in those lesions from the head and neck region in our experience. Extensive necrosis and/or collection of eosinophils, even with Charcot-Leyden crystals, can also obscure the underlying lesion, but the latter cells should suggest the possibility of an LCH as one attempts to correlate the histologic and imaging features. The diagnosis of LCH is corroborated by the presence of aggregates of CD1a-positive cells; Langerhans cells and multinucleated giant cells, including osteoclasts, are also often seen in the osseous lesions, and these cells are strongly reactive for CD68. S-100 protein also stains Langerhans cells, but it lacks specificity since the histiocytes in RDD and JXG are also immunoreactive for this marker. Despite the oft used name of "eosinophilic granuloma" to designate this lesion, eosinophils may be quite scarce or absent in some cases, and this does not distract from a diagnosis of LCH, which depends on the presence of CD1a Langerhans cells.

Rosai-Dorfman Disease (RDD) or sinus histiocytosis with lymphadenopathy is characterized by prominent bilateral cervical lymphadenopathy, but in as many as 35% to 40% of childhood cases, there are also extranodal sites of involvement or a single-site lesion is the only evidence of disease. Approximately 2% of cases have skeletal involvement with or without associated lymphadenopathy (734,735). Biopsy tissue from a bone lesion has polymorphic features, with a mixture of histiocytes, plasma cells, and lymphocytes whose features may be sufficiently nonspecific that chronic osteomyelitis is the initial impression, especially in a child without obvious disease elsewhere. Although the presence of epithelioid histiocytes may suggest LCH, lymphocytes and plasma cells are relatively uncommon in LCH, and CD1a immunohistochemical staining fails to demonstrate aggregates of positive Langerhans cells (Figure 28-84A, B). However,

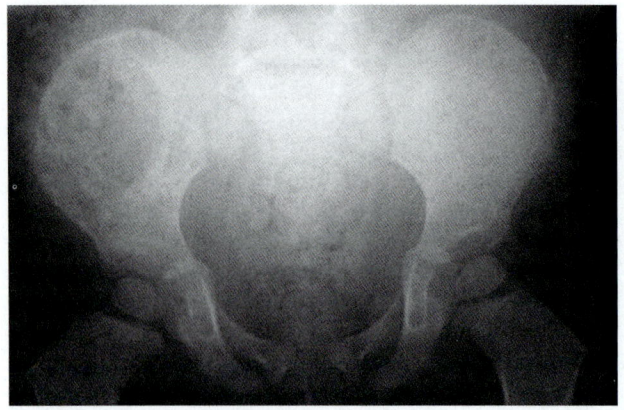
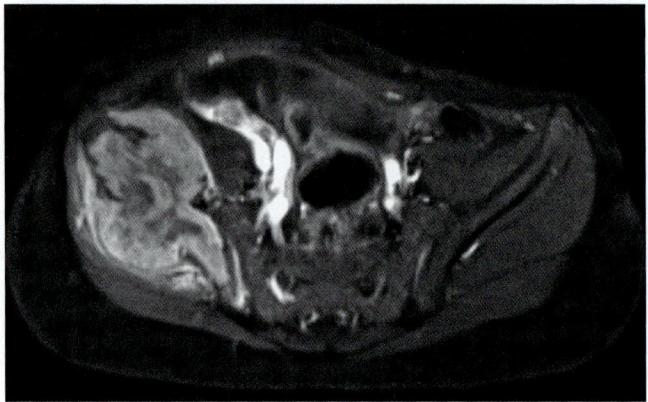

FIGURE 28-82 • Langerhans cell histiocytosis. An enlarging mass in the region of the hip of an 18-month-old male was worrisome for a malignant process. **A:** Imaging reveals the presence of a large, predominantly lytic, lesion involving the right ilium. **B:** MRI demonstrates the mass with a mixed signal, largely occupying and permeating the bone. This case illustrates that LCH can, during its active growth phase, produce an aggressive appearance. (Contributed by William McAlister, MD, St. Louis, MO.)

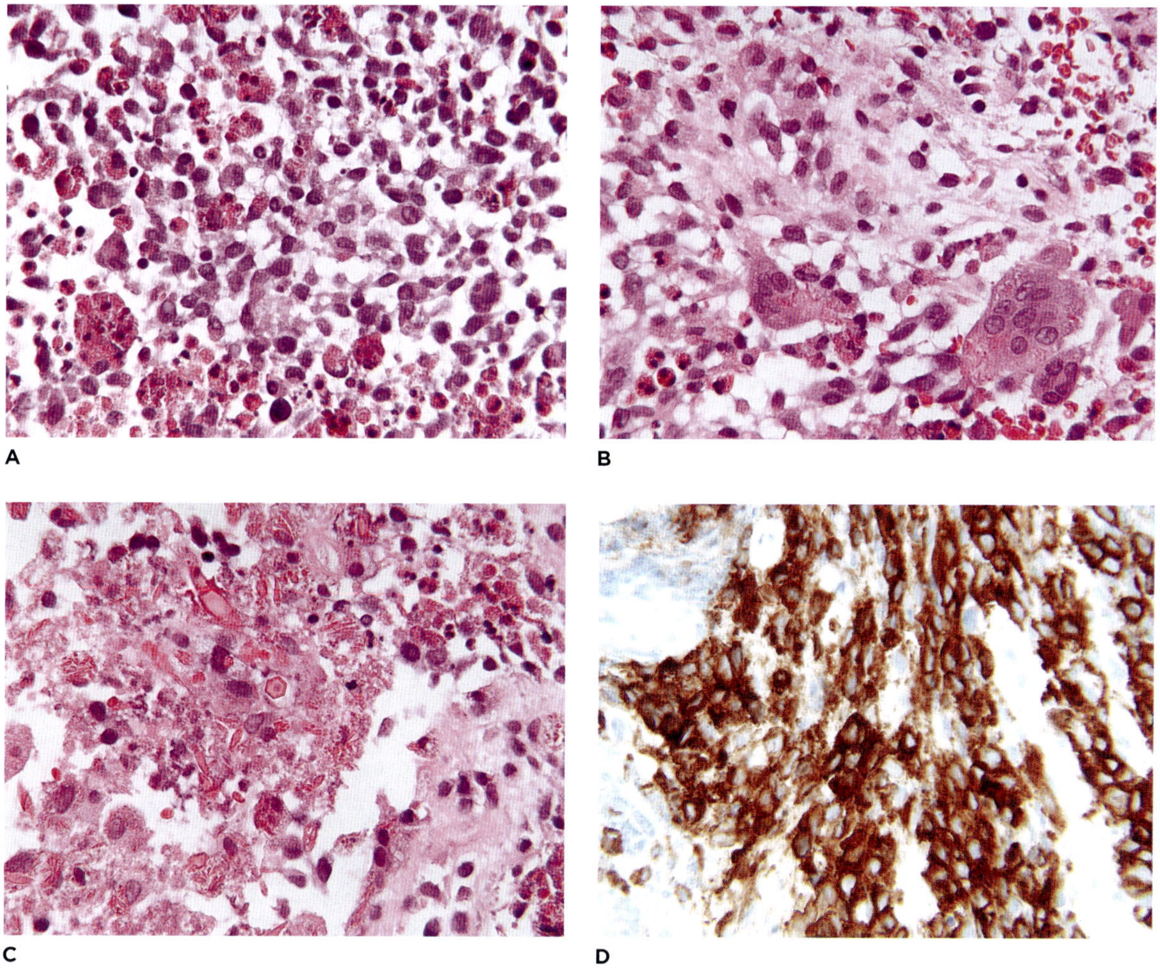

FIGURE 28-83 • Langerhans cell histiocytosis. **A:** Focus shows the presence of Langerhans cells (epithelioid histiocytes) comprising almost the entire lesion. **B:** Multinucleated giant cells may be found in LCH especially in the bone. In the background are Langerhans cells and scattered eosinophils. **C:** Numerous Charcot-Leyden crystals are present in this necrotic focus with degenerating eosinophils. **D:** CD1a immunostain shows reactivity in the Langerhans cells.

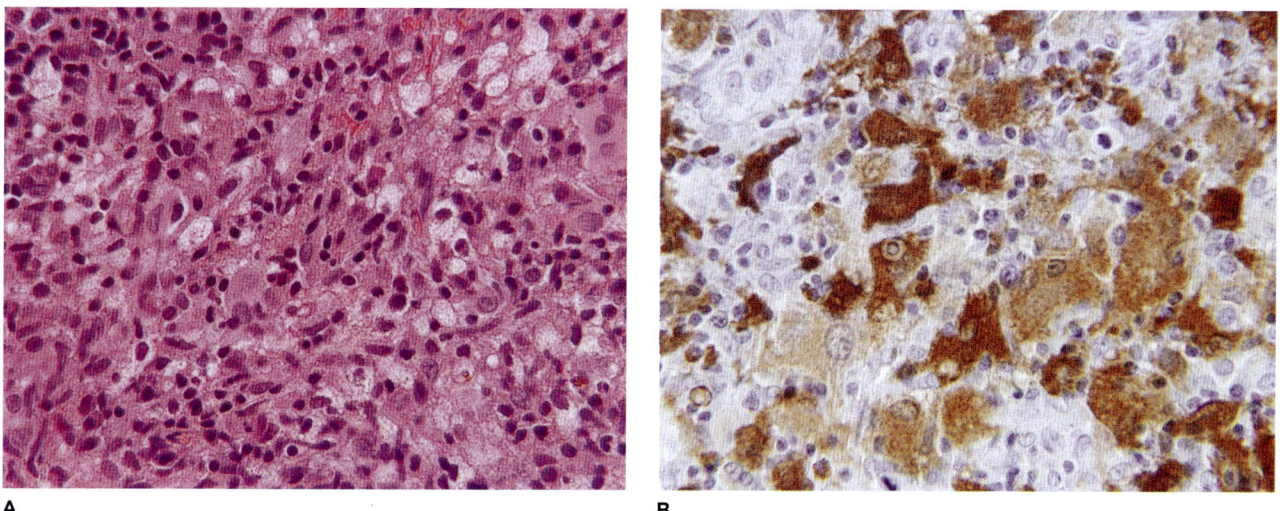

FIGURE 28-84 • Rosai-Dorfman disease. This solitary lesion presented a palpable scalp mass and a lytic defect in the left frontal bone of a 13-year-old male. **A:** Biopsy tissue shows a mixed inflammatory population consisting of histiocytes, plasma cells, and eosinophils. This histologic finding may easily be interpreted as LCH or chronic osteomyelitis. The finding of emperipolesis argues in favor of RDD. **B:** The histiocytes in RDD are typically S-100 positive but CD1a negative. The S-100 protein stain may highlight histiocytes with emperipolesis, which may not be readily apparent in the routine-stained sections. Plasma cells and large foamy histiocytes are features suggestive of the diagnosis of RDD in the appropriate clinical setting.

strong immunoreactivity for S-100 protein in group of histiocytes should suggest the possibility of RDD, and the presence of emperipolesis of lymphocytes, neutrophils, or plasma cells is the clue to the diagnosis of RDD; the engulfed cells may be surrounded by cytoplasmic halos. The histiocytes in RDD have abundant pale-staining cytoplasm and a central nucleus without the reniform contours of Langerhans cells. Eosinophils are not usually present in RDD.

Juvenile xanthogranuloma (JXG) is the least likely of the histiocytic disorders of childhood to have osseous manifestations (726). One of the difficulties in the diagnosis is the awareness that JXG may present as a solitary lesion in bone—involvement has been observed in the temporal bone and vertebra (736–739). The related entity of Erdheim-Chester disease (ECD), which occurs predominantly in adults, is characterized by bilateral sclerotic lesions in the metaphyses of long bones of the lower extremities but has been reported in the jaw bones and elsewhere in children (740–742). Microscopically, a mononuclear infiltrate, with or without xanthomatized histiocytes, and few, if any, Touton giant cells are the histologic features of JXG. Xanthomatized mononuclear and multinucleated cells, with or without features of Touton giant cells, and a more prominent fibrous component may convey a fibrohistiocytic appearance to JXG (736).

Xanthoma of bone may or may not represent a distinct clinicopathologic entity. The presence of xanthomatized histiocytes may represent an involuted LCH without residual Langerhans cells or the primary features of JXG or ECD. If these primary histiocytic disorders, or a chronic inflammatory process, have been excluded, then the default interpretation is xanthoma. Xanthoma cells may also be prominent in NOF, FD, and posttreatment EWS–PNET.

Chordoma is an uncommon axial-based osseous neoplasm whose histologic features and immunophenotype are similar to the embryonic notochord, yet this tumor is seen more often in adults than children with less than 5% of all cases appearing before 20 years of age (743). In children, chordoma is more likely to present in the basicranial and cervical regions of the spine (744–746). A soft, mucoid mass histologically composed of lobules of large, pale-staining cells and multivacuolated physaliferous cells are the classic features, but these tumors may also be poorly differentiated consisting of high-grade polygonal cells with a resemblance to rhabdoid cells (Figure 28-85) (747). Anaplastic chordoma has not only a rhabdoid appearance but also loss of SMARCI3I/INI1 expression (748,749). There is also a chondroid variant, usually found in basicranial lesions that may be histologically confused with CS. However, most chordomas coexpress vimentin and cytokeratin, as well as S-100 protein and epithelial membrane antigen, and most specifically are reactive for brachyury (750). Extraosseous chordoma has been reported in children (751).

INFECTION AND NONINFECTIOUS INFLAMMATORY CONDITIONS OF BONES AND JOINTS AND OSTEONECROSIS

The generic designation "osteomyelitis" is defined pathologically by the character of the inflammatory infiltrate: predominantly neutrophils in the acute phase; a mixture of

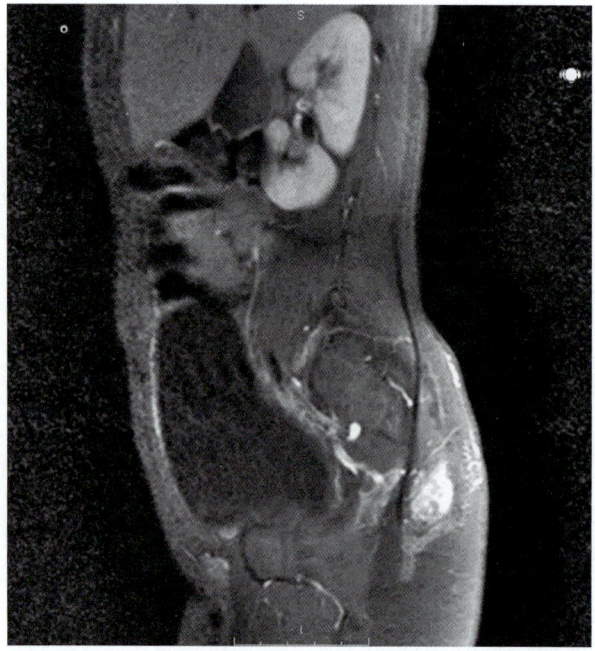
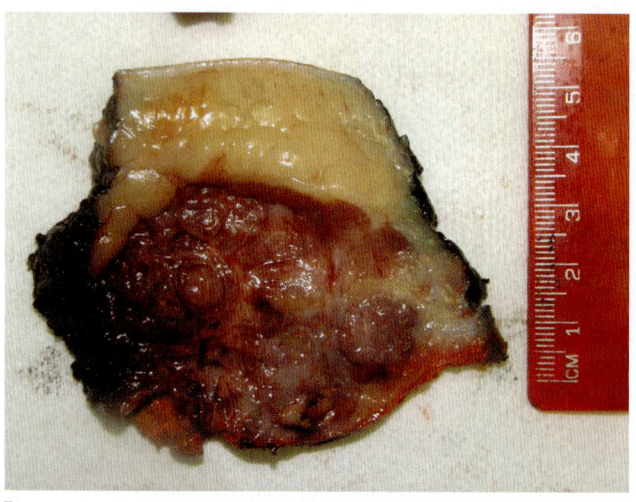

FIGURE 28-85 • Chordoma. The neoplasm presented as a mass in the gluteal region of a 3-year-old girl. **A:** This lateral image shows the sizable presacral mass, which presented in the gluteal region. **B:** The resected tumor was well circumscribed and has a gelatinous mucoid appearance.

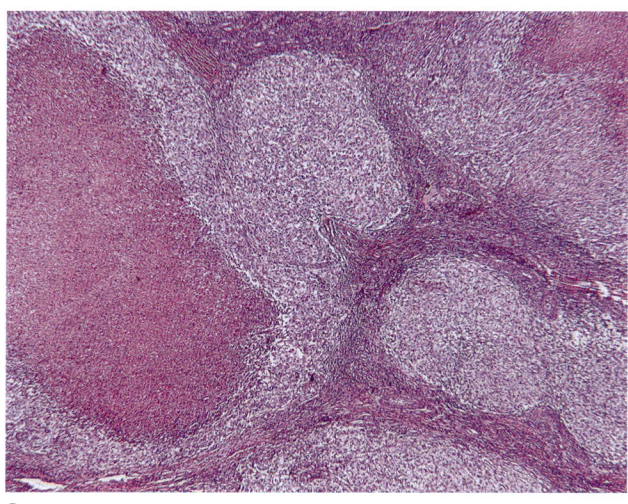 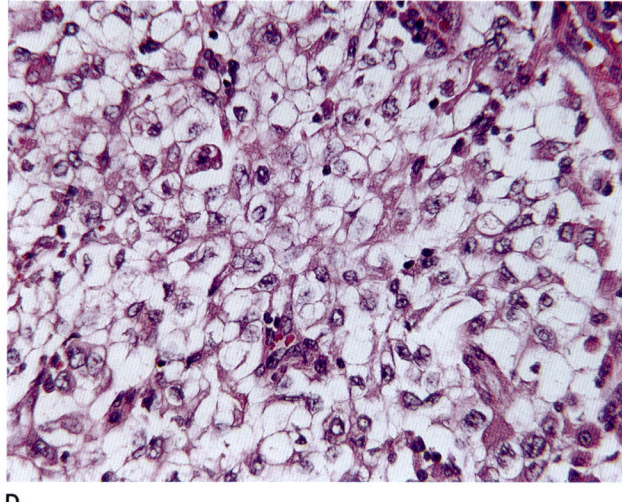

FIGURE 28-85 • (continued) C: The neoplasm was composed of well-circumscribed nests of uniform tumor cells. D: Higher magnification reveals the presence of epithelioid-appearing tumor cells with clear and vacuolated cytoplasm.

neutrophils, lymphocytes, and some plasma cells in the subacute phase; and lymphocytes, plasma cells, and histiocytes in the chronic phase (Figure 28-86A to C). Histiocytes and plasma cells are also features of RDD and a similar reaction may be seen in some cases of LCH. The composition of the inflammatory infiltrate does not necessarily correlate with the clinical duration in all cases. Necrotic bone fragments (sequestra) are identified in cases of AO in material from a vigorous curettage but is less often found in specimens from a drainage procedure. New bone formation on the surface of sequestra (involucra) is noted in the healing stage of osteomyelitis. Chronic osteomyelitis usually shows a filmy fibrous tissue replacement of the medullary space in which are scattered lymphocytes and plasma cells. Bone trabeculae may be seen undergoing lysis by osteoclasts despite the presence of osteocytes within the substance of the bone. The presence of inflammatory cells in a bone lesion does not imply that it is infectious in all cases. Often, a bone specimen from a presumptive case of osteomyelitis may only demonstrate the presence of reactive new bone formation and minimal evidence of inflammation.

Acute osteomyelitis (AO) in children is secondary to a bacterial infection in the overwhelming majority of cases, with 60% or more of cases caused by *Staphylococcus aureus* (*SA*) in both infants and older children; a variable proportion of methicillin-resistant *SA* (MRSA) and methicillin-sensitive strains are also found (752,753). There has been a considerable increase in the number of MRSA infections, but methicillin-susceptible SA accounts for 80% to 90% of cases with regional variation (752). Other bacterial agents of note are group-B streptococcus, *Streptococcus pneumoniae* and various gram-negative organisms including *Salmonella* in children with sickle cell disease (752). Approximately 40% to 50% of all cases of AO are diagnosed in the first two decades of life; children 5 years of age or younger are most frequently affected, and boys more often than girls (754). One gram-negative organism, *Kingella kingae*, has emerged as an important cause of AO and septic arthritis in children less than 36 months old (755). Most children in whom AO develops do not have a predisposing condition such as sickle cell disease or chronic granulomatous disease (CGD). A variety of organisms including *Serratia*, *Aspergillus*, *Candida*, and *Salmonella* are responsible for most cases of osteomyelitis in CGD, in addition to the other more common organisms (756–758). Many of these same pathogens are detected in children with primary or secondary immunodeficiency disorders. Tuberculous osteomyelitis has been on the increase in both developed and developing countries due to a host of epidemiologic factors. Skeletal involvement is present in 1% to 2% of all cases of tuberculosis but is seemingly higher in children (759). These infections are hematogenous in nature with a predilection for the anterior portion of the vertebral body. Joint space involvement may be present with epiphyseal lesions. Caseating granulomas are demonstrated on biopsy tissue in 50% or more of cases. Nontuberculous mycobacterial osteomyelitis is either due to puncture inoculation or as a consequence of immunosuppression or cystic fibrosis (760). Less than 1% of nontuberculous mycobacterial infections in children are associated with bone involvement alone. Though not an infection, *per se*, sarcoidosis with epithelioid granulomas may also rarely be seen in the small bones of the hands and feet in children with cystic fibrosis (761). *Bartonella henselae*, the causative organism in cat-scratch disease, is a reported cause of localized or multifocal osteomyelitis (762). Fungal osteomyelitis caused by *Candida* species may be seen in premature infants.

The femur and tibia are the most commonly involved bones in acute hematogenous osteomyelitis. Organisms typically are seeded at the junction of the epiphysis and metaphysis because of the unique pattern of vascular supply in this region. The infection and its inflammatory reaction are more likely to breach the attenuated cortex of an infant, with the subsequent development of pyomyositis. Permeative bone destruction is centered in the metaphysis with periosteal new bone formation. A large subperiosteal abscess is associated with the infrequent pathologic fracture in children with SA osteomyelitis (763). Subacute osteomyelitis, with formation of a so-called Brodie abscess, develops in the metaphyseal cortex at a site contiguous with the epicenter of AO, but it can be found throughout the skeletal system. Roentgenograms usually show a lytic area surrounded by osteosclerosis, which may resemble an OO or another neoplastic process.

Nonbacterial osteitis (NBO) or chronic recurrent multifocal osteomyelitis (CRMO) is a clinicopathologic entity that occurs in children and adults and is regarded as one entity in a family of autoinflammatory disorders as monogenic defect in innate immunity (764–766). Two autosomal recessive disorders with mutations of the IL1RN gene (2q14.2) and LPIN2 gene (18p11.31) are characterized by the onset of multisystem inflammation as early as infancy and congenital dyserythropoietic anemia in the latter (Majeed syndrome) (767,768). The multiple bone lesions may be symmetrical and widely distributed, but with a preference for the metaphysis of the long bones, pelvis, spine, clavicle, and mandible (Figure 28-87) (769). There is a female predilection and the mean age at diagnosis is 10 to 12 years (770).

The variable histologic changes in NBO include a predominantly neutrophilic or mixed type of inflammatory reaction and irregular bony trabeculae with prominent mosaic lines. The presence of acute inflammation is microscopically

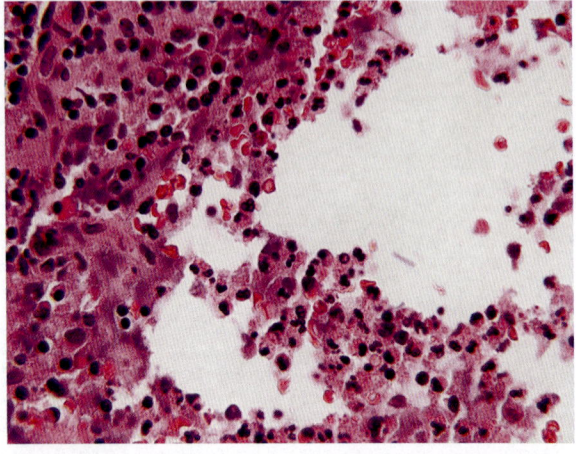

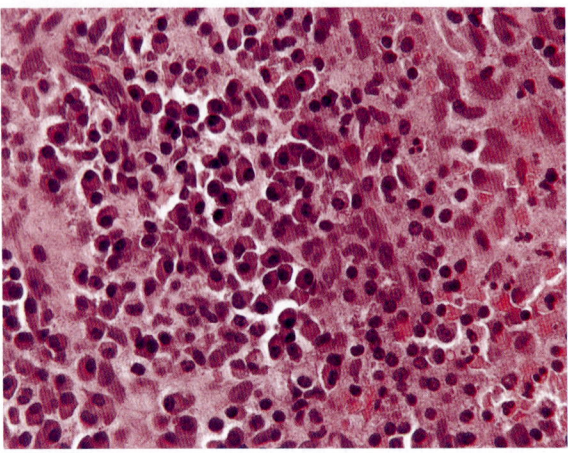

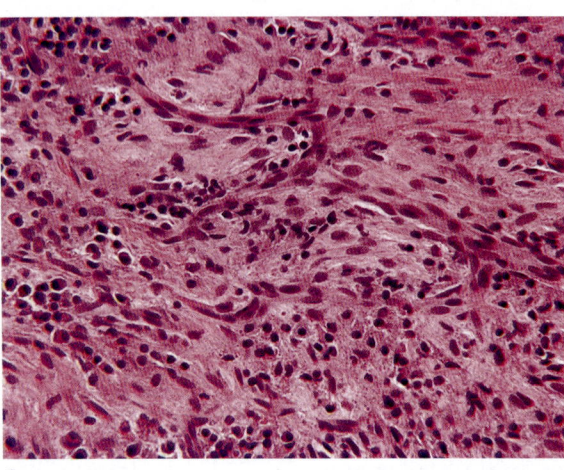

FIGURE 28-86 • Osteomyelitis in the mandible of a 13-year-old boy. By the time of surgical intervention in a case of osteomyelitis, the process is often characterized by a mixed population of inflammatory cells, since it has often been present for a period of time and under antibiotic treatment. **A:** The center of this lesion contains neutrophils, necrosis, and some hemorrhage. **B:** Plasma cells are either intermixed with macrophages or as monomorphous collections. **C:** Sheets of histiocytes with accompanying plasma cells are features of subacute to chronic osteomyelitis, but Rosai-Dorfman and NBO have similar features. There is essentially no difference in the histologic features of infection-associated osteomyelitis from NBO.

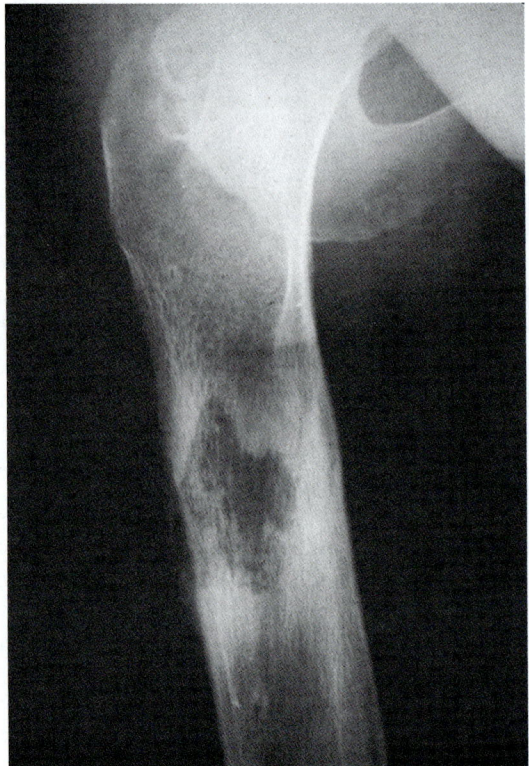

FIGURE 28-87 • Nonbacterial osteitis–chronic recurrent multifocal osteomyelitis. A lytic and sclerotic lesion is present in the metaphyseodiaphyseal region of the femur.

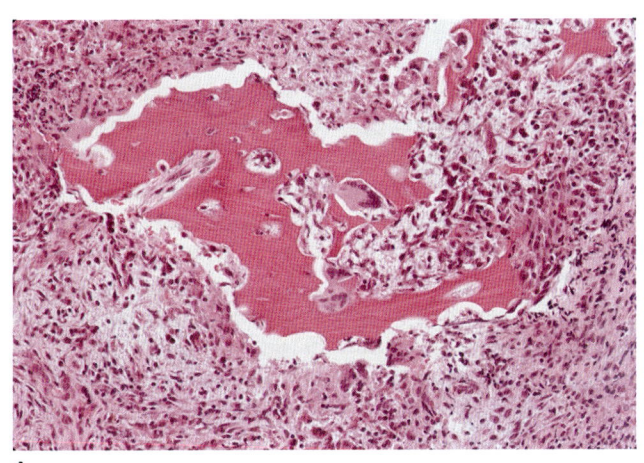
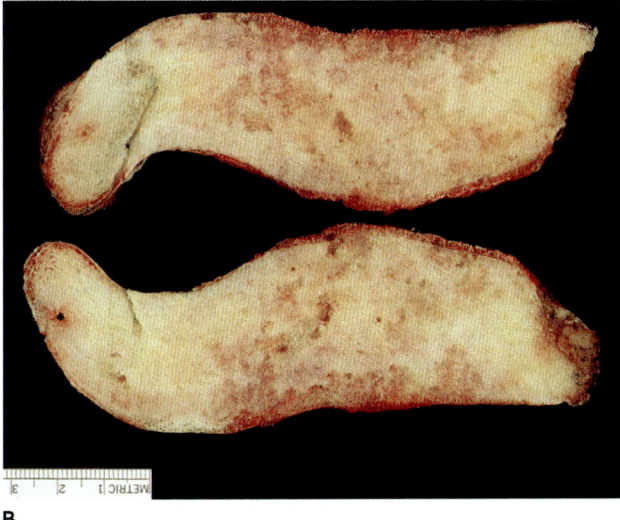

FIGURE 28-88 • Nonbacterial osteitis–chronic recurrent multifocal osteomyelitis. **A:** A mixed inflammatory reaction surrounds a bony fragment with osteoclastic activity. **B:** This resected portion of the clavicle shows dense sclerosis and medullary fibrosis.

indistinguishable from acute infectious osteomyelitis. Fibrosis of the marrow space and a modest degree of chronic inflammation with histiocytes and plasma cells are alternative histologic findings (Figure 28-88A, B) (771). In the long bones, a lytic area with larger areas of surrounding sclerosis is the usual radiographic finding. Expansion of the bone with sclerosis and small osteolytic areas is best seen in the clavicles and ribs. When the skin is involved, the histologic features are those of a neutrophilic dermatitis.

Infantile cortical hyperostosis (ICH, Caffey disease) has a familial or sporadic presentation, is manifested before 5 months of life, and has an incidence of 3 cases per 1000 infants less than 6 months of age. The familial form has an AD inheritance, with a missense mutation in the COL1A1 gene on chromosome 17q and is a related collagenopathy to OI and Ehlers-Danlos syndrome (772). The clinical course may wax and wane during the first 3 years of life. Soft tissue swellings, with accompanying inflammatory signs and constitutional symptoms, are the clinical manifestations. In sporadic ICH, the mandible is involved more often than in the familial form (773). ICH is now regarded as one of the GSDs. Involvement of single or multiple bones and bilateral symmetric involvement are the other patterns (774). Cortical thickening, without bone destruction, of the mandible, clavicle, and long tubular bones, often the ulna and ribs, is the characteristic alteration (Figure 28-89A, B). The ends of the

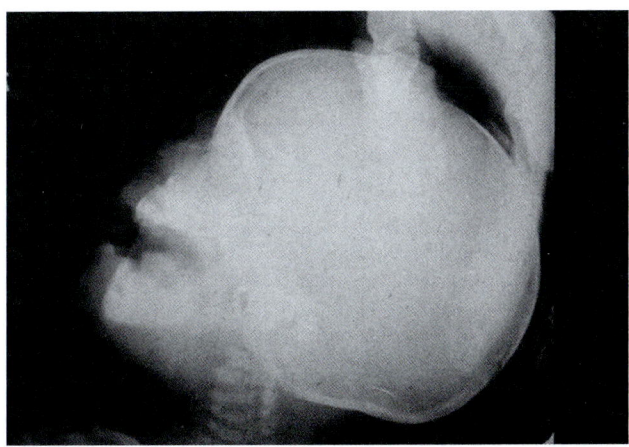
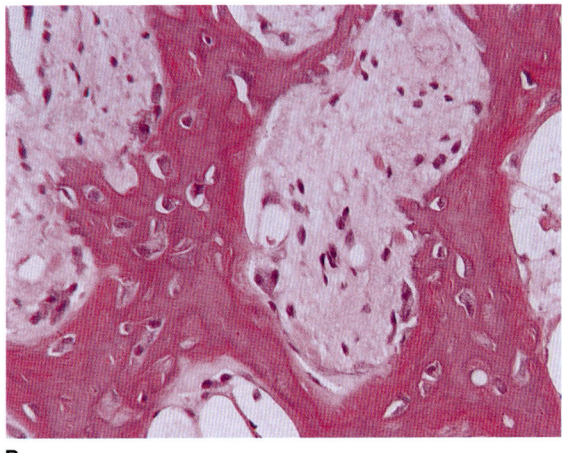

FIGURE 28-89 • Infantile cortical hyperostosis. This disorder presents in the first year of life but may be seen in toddlers. **A:** This image demonstrates the presence of a soft tissue mass in the region of the mandible whose cortical margins are indistinct because of subperiosteal new bone formation. **B:** Irregular bony trabeculae, with some osteoblastic activity, and fibrosis are some of the nonspecific histologic findings. The fibrous reaction with some accompanying inflammation is present in the advancing front into the adjacent soft tissues, which accounts for the soft tissue swelling. (Contributed by Samir El-Mofty, DMD, PhD, St.Louis, MO.)

bones are not involved. Reactive new bone formation with osteoblastic activity and a variably intense mixed inflammatory infiltrate with neutrophils are nonspecific findings that may suggest an acute to subacute osteomyelitis (775). The inflammation with edema and accompanying fibroplasia extends into the surrounding soft tissues. A self-limited clinical course is usual, although premature infants seem to fare less well than term infants. The diagnosis of ICH with or without nonimmune hydrops has been made prenatally (776).

Osteonecrosis (aseptic or avascular necrosis) is a known complication of chronic corticosteroid usage and hemoglobinopathy, particularly sickle cell disease. Children with acute lymphoblastic leukemia and non-Hodgkin lymphoma are especially at risk for osteonecrosis whereby the steroid therapy is thought to have an important role in the etiology of the necrosis (777–779). Other nontraumatic causes of ON in children include congenital hip dysplasia, slipped capital femoral epiphysis, and GD. Legg-Calve-Perthes (LCP) disease is defined by the presence of ON of the capital femoral epiphysis of the femoral head (780). The male to female ratio is 4 to 5:1, with a median age at diagnosis of 7 to 8 years, with a range of 3 to 12 years. Occlusion of vessels in the subchondral cortical bone in LCP may represent the complication of a primary thrombophilia such as protein C deficiency, factor V Leiden, and methylenetetrahydrofolate reductase C677T mutations (781,782).

Gaucher disease is associated with bone involvement in 70% to 100% of individuals with type 1 or type 3 disease (783,784). The ON in the femoral head is identical to that seen in LCP disease. Infarcts also occur in the head of the humerus, femoral condyle, and tibial plateau. Necrosis is first identified in the tissues of the medullary cavity with fat and coagulative necrosis of the hematopoietic elements. The cancellous bone acquires a pale, homogeneous appearance, and the osteocyte lacunae are empty. Often, the architecture of the bone is irregular due to past episodes of remodeling. In a study of femoral heads from those with GD, ON was present in 73% of cases, as well as the presence of Gaucher cells and osteoarthropathy (785).

Synovium

The joint space is at the junction of two contiguous bones held together by a joint capsule lined by a synovial membrane. Under normal circumstances, the synovial lining is inconspicuous, but in the presence of inflammation, regardless of the etiology, the synovial membrane and the underlying interstitial tissues are variably infiltrated by a range of inflammatory cells that reflect the nature of the etiology (infectious pathogens, metabolic abnormality, and autoimmunity) and the duration in some cases. Over a period of time, as the integrity of the synovial membrane is functionally compromised, there are degenerative changes in the adjacent articular cartilage. From our perspective, the synovial biopsy is an infrequent procedure in children to determine the nature of joint space pathology. It is usually restricted to those cases after clinical imaging and laboratory studies have failed to yield a diagnosis (786).

Acute synovitis is an infiltration of the synovial interstitium by neutrophils and is seen most frequently in the presence of a pyogenic infection of the joint space in septic arthritis. The latter is a complication of acute hematogenous osteomyelitis and occurs most frequently in the hip or knee joint. Kang and associates noted that the incidence is considerably lower in children in developed versus developing countries (1:100,000 versus 1:5000 to 20,000) (787). Lyme arthritis is associated with an acute inflammatory reaction, but persistent lyme arthritis, with the presence of lymphoid hyperplasia, histiocytes, and mast cells, resembles chronic idiopathic arthritis (788).

Chronic synovitis is characterized by an inflammatory reaction that is dominated by lymphocytes with a diffuse and/or nodular pattern with or without plasma cells, but accompanying clinical presentation may be relatively brief. There is hyperplasia of the synovial lining cells with or without a villous architecture. Mast cells are conspicuous in the background and whose presence can be demonstrated by a Leder stain. Fibrin deposition, lymphoid nodules, and plasma cells in appreciable numbers in the synovium have been associated with RA. The latter diagnostic entity, referenced in children as "juvenile RA," has been subsumed in the general category of juvenile idiopathic arthritis (JIA). The diagnosis relies on clinical criteria and is largely a diagnosis of exclusion (789,790). The pathogenesis is generally thought to be autoimmune or autoinflammatory in nature (791).

Hemophilic arthropathy is associated with chronic synovitis with proliferative features and a lymphocytic and histiocytic infiltrates, vascularized fibrosis, and striking hemosiderin deposition within the synovial lining cells as well as in the interstitium and within histiocytes (792). Hemarthrosis occurs when serum factor VIII or IX levels are below 1% of normal (793). The knee, ankle, and elbow joints are most prone to hemarthroses. There is progressive injury to the articular cartilage and bone, especially in the knee and ankle joints, in those with frequent episodes of hemarthroses. Since synovectomy is recommended in those children with progressive joint injury, these specimens are seen for pathologic examination. Another cause of nontraumatic hemarthrosis, especially of the knee and joint, is synovial hemangioma or hemangiomatosis (794).

Granulomatous synovitis may be observed in sarcoidosis in a child and also in AD-inherited disease, Blau syndrome, with its presentation of polyarthritis, uveitis, and an exanthematous skin rash; the mutation is in the CARD15/NOD2 (16q21) (795–797). The granulomas have sarcoid-like appearance. NOD2 mutations are also seen in Crohn disease.

Histiocytic synovitis or histiocytic infiltration of the synovium is seen in the camptodactyly, arthropathy, coxa vara, and pericarditis syndrome (798). The synovium contains CD68-positive multinucleated giant cells. Foamy histiocytes are found in the synovium in α-mannosidosis, which is accompanied by destructive joint disease and mental retardation in young individuals (799,800). Nontuberculous mycobacterial synovitis may have a diffuse histiocytic reaction rather than producing well-formed granulomas. A similar histiocytic synovial reaction, with destructive arthropathy, is present in multicentric reticulohistiocytosis and, although rare in childhood, is documented in several cases (801). There is mixture of mononuclear and multinuclear histiocytes.

Tumefactive lesions within and around the joints in children constitute a heterogeneous group of uncommon conditions. Some of these are intra-articular and are frequent in adults, such as synovial chondromatosis (802). Nodules of mature cartilage arise in the synovial membranes and/or free floating in the joint space of the knee, hip, and elbow. Rounded to faceted nodules vary from 1 mm to over 1 cm in diameter. A fibrous membrane surrounds the individual cartilaginous nodules, which are composed of haphazardly arranged or nested chondrocytes within a chondroid matrix. Some degree of cytologic atypia may exist in the chondrocytes, which does not have any importance in terms of prognosis. Another tumefaction is synovial lipomatosis (lipoma arborescens) presenting as a suprapatellar mass. Involvement of the synovial sheath of the tendon has been reported. This rare process is seen in children in a variety of joint spaces and bursa. The interstitial tissues of the synovium are largely replaced by lobules of mature adipose tissue. Nodular fasciitis, ganglion cyst, and synovial sarcoma have also been documented with intra-articular presentation (802,803). Pigmented villonodular synovitis is discussed in the chapter on soft tissue, together with GCT of tendon sheath, another periarticular soft tissue tumor. Ganglion cysts occur in children and represent 5% to 10% of all cases in all age groups. They are seen as early as infancy and throughout childhood. Most of these cysts are located in the wrist on the volar or dorsal aspect. There are a number of other sites of presentation, including the knee in the region of the anterior cruciate ligament, around the hip, spine, and adjacent to the spine. Rarely, ganglion cysts may be multifocal and referred to as "cystic ganglionosis" (804). Although referred to as "synovial," cysts in some cases arise in the tissues in and around tendons. Histologically, one or more rounded to elongated cysts with or without lining cells, and with or without pale mucoid material, are located within a dense fibrous background.

Osteoarthropathy (OAP) or degenerative joint disease is rarely encountered by the pathologist in a child. However, OAP is the consequence of any chronic inflammatory process or metabolic disorder with accompanying osteopenia, ON, and abnormal skeletal development with erosion and destruction of the articular cartilage. Some of these conditions include multiple epiphyseal dysplasia, PHP, Marfan syndrome, Ehlers-Danlos syndrome, cystic fibrosis, hemophiliac-associated hemarthrosis, chondrodysplasia punctata, dysostosis multiplex, ACH, and GD.

References

1. Kobayashi T, Kronenberg HM. Overview of skeletal development. *Methods Mol Biol* 2014;1130:3–12.
2. Murakami S, Akiyama H, De Crombrugghe B. The development of bone and cartilage. In: Epstein CJ, Erickson RP, Wynshaw-Boris A, eds. *Inborn Errors of Development: The Molecular Basis of Clinical Disorders of Morphogenesis*. New York: Oxford University Press, 2004:133–147.
3. Olsen BR, Reginato AM, Wang W. Bone development. *Annu Rev Cell Dev Biol* 2000;16:191–220.
4. Provot S, Schipani E, Wu J, et al. Development of the skeleton. In: Marcus R, Feldman D, Nelson DA, Rosen CJ, eds. *Osteoporosis*, 3rd ed. San Francisco, CA: Academic Press, 2008:241–269.
5. Le Douarin M, Dupin E. The neural crest in vertebrate evolution. *Curr Opin Genet Dev* 2012;22(4):381–389.
6. Pineault KM, Wellik DM. Hox genes and limb musculoskeletal development. *Curr Osteoporos Rep* 2014;12(4):420–427.
7. Soshnikova N. Hox genes regulation in vertebrates. *Dev Dyn* 2014;243(1):49–58.
8. Blake JA, Ziman MR. Pax genes: regulators of lineage specification and progenitor cell maintenance. *Development* 2014;141(4):737–751.
9. Oh CD, Lu Y, Liang S, et al. SOX9 regulates multiple genes in chondrocytes, including genes encoding ECM proteins, ECM modification enzymes, receptors, and transporters. *PLoS One* 2014;9(9):3107577.
10. Ono N, Ono W, Nagasawa T, et al. A subset of chondrogenic cells provides early mesenchymal progenitors in growing bones. *Nat Cell Biol* 2014;16(12):1157–1167.
11. Pierre JM. Fibroblast growth factor signaling controlling bone formation: an update. *Gene* 2012;498:1–4.
12. Goldring MB, Tsuchimochi K, Ijiri K. The control of chondrogenesis. *J Cell Biochem* 2006;97:33–44.
13. Bell DM, Leung KK, Wheatley SC, et al. SOX9 directly regulates the type-II collagen gene. *Nat Genet* 1997;16:174–178.
14. Leung VY, Gao B, Leung KK, et al. SOX9 governs differentiation stage-specific gene expression in growth plate chondrocytes via direct concomitant transactivation and repression. *PLoS Genet* 2011;7(11):e1002356.
15. Sarkar A, Hochedlinger K. The sox family of transcription factors: versatile regulators of stem and progenitor cell fate. *Cell Stem Cell* 2013;12(1):15–30.
16. Kamachi Y, Kondoh H. Sox proteins: regulators of cell fate specification and differentiation. *Development* 2013;140(20):4129–4144.
17. Malemud CJ. Matrix metalloproteinases: role in skeletal development and growth plate disorders. *Front Biosci* 2006;11:1702–1715.
18. Mackie EJ, Ahmed YA, Tatarczuch L, et al. Endochondral ossification: how cartilage is converted into bone in the developing skeleton. *Int J Biochem Cell Biol* 2008;40:46–62.
19. Chai Y, Maxson RE Jr. Recent advances in craniofacial morphogenesis. *Dev Dyn* 2006;235:2353–2375.
20. Cole WG. Structure of growth plate and bone matrix. In: Glorieux FH, ed. *Pediatric Bone. Biology & Diseases*. San Francisco, CA: Academic Press, 2003:1–41.
21. Karaplis AC. Embryonic development of bone and the molecular regulation of intramembranous and endochondral bone formation. In: Bilezikian JP, John P, Raisz G, Rodan GA, eds. *Principles of Bone Biology*, Vol. 1, 2nd ed. San Francisco, CA: Academic Press, 2002:33–58.
22. Fisher S, Franz-Odendaal T. Evolution of the bone gene regulatory network. *Curr Opin Genet Dev* 2012;22:390–397.
23. Okamoto M, Murai J, Yoshikawa H, et al. Bone morphogenetic proteins in bone stimulate osteoclasts and osteoblasts during bone development. *J Bone Miner Res* 2006;21:1022–1033.
24. Day TF, Yang Y. Wnt and hedgehog signaling pathways in bone development. *J Bone Joint Surg Am* 2008;90(suppl 1):19–24.
25. Liu F, Kohlmeier S, Wang CY. Wnt signaling and skeletal development. *Cell Signal* 2008;20:999–1009.
26. Brighton CT. Morphology and biochemistry of the growth plate. *Rheum Dis Clin North Am* 1987;13:75–100.
27. O'Rahilly R, Gardner E. The timing and sequence of events in the development of the limbs in the human embryo. *Anat Embryol (Berl)* 1975;148:1–23.
28. Burdan F, Szumilo J, Korobowicz A, et al. Morphology and physiology of the epiphyseal growth plate. *Folia Histochem Cytobiol* 2009;47:5–16.
29. Kronenberg HM. PTHrP and skeletal development. *Ann N Y Acad Sci* 2006;1068:1–13.

30. Wysolmerski JJ. Parathyroid hormone-related protein: an update. *J Clin Endocrinol Metab* 2012;97(9):2947–2956.
31. Novack DV, Teitelbaum SL. The osteoclast: friend or foe? *Annu Rev Pathol* 2008;3:457–484.
32. Aubin JE, Heersche JNM. Bone cell biology osteoblasts, osteocytes, and osteoclasts. In: Glorieux FH, ed. *Pediatric Bone. Biology and Diseases*. San Francisco, CA: Academic Press, 2002:43–76.
33. Charles JF, Aliprantis AO. Osteoclasts: more than 'bone eaters'. *Trends Mol Med* 2014;20:449–457.
34. Cappariello A, Maurizi A, Veeriah V, et al. The great beauty of the osteoclast. *Arch Biochem Biophys* 2014;558:70–78.
35. Nissim S. Development of the limbs. In: Epstein, CJ, Erickson RP, Wynshaw-Boris A, eds. *Inborn Errors of Development: The Molecular Basis of Clinical Disorders of Morphogenesis*. New York: Oxford University Press, 2004:148–167.
36. Rizzo R, Lammer EJ, Parano E, et al. Limb reduction defects in humans associated with prenatal isotretinoin exposure. *Teratology* 1991;44:599–604.
37. Fletcher I, Lambot-Juhan K, Teissier R, et al. Unexpected high frequency of skeletal dysplasia in idiopathic short stature and small for gestational age patients. *Eur J Endocrinol* 2014;170:677–684.
38. Zuniga A, Zeller R, Probst S. The molecular basis of human congenital limb malformations. *Wiley Interdiscip Rev Biol* 2012;1(6):803–822.
39. Barnicoat AJ, Seller MJ, Bennett CP. Fetus with features of Crane-Heise syndrome and aminopterin syndrome sine aminopterin (ASSAS). *Clin Dysmorphol* 1994;3:353–357.
40. Langer B, Haddad J, Gasser B, et al. Isolated fetal bilateral radial ray reduction associated with valproic acid usage. *Fetal Diagn Ther* 1994;9:155–158.
41. Milunsky A, Graef JW, Gaynor MF, Jr. Methotrexate-induced congenital malformations. *J Pediatr* 1968;72:790–795.
42. Daston GP, Seed J. Skeletal malformations and variations in developmental toxicity studies: interpretation issues for human risk assessment. *Birth Defects Res B Dev Reprod Toxicol* 2007;80:421–424.
43. Tyl RW, Chernoff N, Rogers JM. Altered axial skeletal development. *Birth Defects Res B Dev Reprod Toxicol* 2007;80:451–472.
44. Manouvrier-Hanu S, Holder-Espinasse M, Lyonnet S. Genetics of limb anomalies in humans. *Trends Genet* 1999;15:409–417.
45. Tretter AE, Saunders RC, Meyers CM, et al. Antenatal diagnosis of lethal skeletal dysplasias. *Am J Med Genet* 1998;75:518–522.
46. Mattos TC, Giugliani R, Haase HB. Congenital malformations detected in 731 autopsies of children aged 0 to 14 years. *Teratology* 1987;35:305–307.
47. Cereda A, Carey JC. The trisomy 18 syndrome. *Orphanet J Rare Dis* 2012;7:81.
48. Petry P, Polli JB, Mattos VF, et al. Clinical features and prognosis of a sample of patients with trisomy 13 (Patau syndrome) from Brazil. *Am J Med Genet A* 2013;161A(6):1278–1283.
49. Keeling JW, Hansen BF, Kjaer I. Pattern of malformations in the axial skeleton in human trisomy 21 fetuses. *Am J Med Genet* 1997;68:466–471.
50. Pfeiffer RA, Santelmann R. Limb anomalies in chromosomal aberrations. *Birth Defects Orig Artic Ser* 1977;13:319–337.
51. Stempfle N, Huten Y, Fredouille C, et al. Skeletal abnormalities in fetuses with Down's syndrome: a radiographic post-mortem study. *Pediatr Radiol* 1999;29:682–688.
52. Kamalakar A, Harris JR, McKelvey KD, et al. Aneuploidy and skeletal health. *Curr Osteoporos Rep* 2014;12:376–382.
53. Parker SE, Mai CT, Canfield MA, et al. Updated national birth prevalence estimates for selected birth defects in the United States, 2004–2006. *Birth Defects Res A Clin Mol Teratol* 2010;88:1008–1016.
54. Holder-Espinasse M, Devisme L, Thomas D, et al. Pre- and postnatal diagnosis of limb anomalies: a series of 107 cases. *Am J Med Genet A* 2004;124A:417–422.
55. Froster UG, Baird PA. Upper limb deficiencies and associated malformations: a population-based study. *Am J Med Genet* 1992;44:767–781.
56. Kozin SH. Upper-extremity congenital anomalies. *J Bone Joint Surg Am* 2003;85A:1564–1576.
57. McGuirk CK, Westgate MN, Holmes LB. Limb deficiencies in newborn infants. *Pediatrics* 2001;108:E64.
58. Stoll C, Wiesel A, Queisser-Luft A, et al. Evaluation of the prenatal diagnosis of limb reduction deficiencies. *Prenat Diagn* 2000;20:811–818.
59. Evans JA, Vitez M, Czeizel A. Congenital abnormalities associated with limb deficiency defects: a population study based on cases from the Hungarian Congenital Malformation Registry (1975-1984). *Am J Med Genet* 1994;49:52–66.
60. Kallen B. A prospective study of some aetiological factors in limb reduction defects in Sweden. *J Epidemiol Community Health* 1989;43:86–91.
61. Stoll C, Alembik Y, Dott B, et al. Risk factors in limb reduction defects. *Paediatr Perinat Epidemiol* 1992;6:323–338.
62. Goutas N, Simopoulou S, Petraki V, et al. Limb reduction defects—autopsy study. *Pediatr Pathol* 1993;13:29–35.
63. Gurrieri F, Kjaer KW, Sangiorgi E, et al. Limb anomalies: developmental and evolutionary aspects. *Am J Med Genet* 2002;115: 231–244.
64. Hill RE, Heaney SJ, Lettice LA. Sonic hedgehog: restricted expression and limb dysmorphologies. *J Anat* 2003;202:13–20.
65. Lin S, Marshall EG, Davidson GK, et al. Evaluation of congenital limb reduction defects in upstate New York. *Teratology* 1993;47:127–135.
66. Lin S, Marshall EG. Comparison of demographic and defect characteristics among different developmental stages of congenital limb reduction defects. *Paediatr Perinat Epidemiol* 1996;10:294–308.
67. Stoll C, Clementi M. Prenatal diagnosis of dysmorphic syndromes by routine fetal ultrasound examination across Europe. *Ultrasound Obstet Gynecol* 2003;21:543–551.
68. Rosano A, Botto LD, Olney RS, et al. Limb defects associated with major congenital anomalies: clinical and epidemiological study from the International Clearinghouse for Birth Defects Monitoring systems. *Am J Med Genet*, 2000,93:110–116.
69. Botto LD, Khoury MJ, Mastroiacovo P, et al. The spectrum of congenital anomalies of the VATER association: an international study. *Am J Med Genet* 1997;71:8–15.
70. Castori M, Rinaldi R, Cappellacci S, et al. Tibial developmental field defect is the most common lower limb malformation pattern in VACTERL association. *Am J Med Genet A* 2008;146A:1259–1266.
71. Shaw-Smith C. Oesophageal atresia, tracheo-oesophageal fistula, and the VACTERL association: review of genetics and epidemiology. *J Med Genet* 2006;43:545–554.
72. Solomon BD. VACTERL/VATER association. *Orphanet J Rare Dis* 2011;6:56.
73. Shaw-Smith C. Genetic factors in esophageal atresia, tracheo-esophageal fistula and the VACTERL association: roles for FOXF1 and the 16q24.1 FOX transcription factor gene cluster, and review of the literature. *Eur J Med Genet* 2010;53:6–13.
74. Alter BP, Rosenberg PS. VACTERL-H association and fanconi anemia. *Mol Syndromol* 2013;4:87–93.
75. Shafeghati Y, Kahrizi K, Najmabadi H, et al. Brachyphalangy, polydactyly and tibial aplasia/hypoplasia syndrome (OMIM 609945): case report and review of the literature. *Eur J Pediatr* 2010;169:1535–1539.
76. Bower C, Norwood F, Knowles S, et al. Amniotic band syndrome: a population-based study in two Australian states. *Paediatr Perinat Epidemiol* 1993;7:395–403.
77. Barros M, Gorgal G, Machado AP, et al. Revisiting amniotic band sequence: a wide spectrum of manifestations. *Fetal Diagn Ther* 2014;35:51–56.
78. Young ID, Lindenbaum RH, Thompson EM, et al. Amniotic bands in connective tissue disorders. *Arch Dis Child* 1985;60:1061–1063.
79. Hunter AG, Seaver LH, Stevenson RE. Limb-body wall defect. Is there a defensible hypothesis and can it explain all the associated anomalies? *Am J Med Genet A* 2011;155A:2045–2059.
80. Jamsheer A, Materna-Kiryluk A, Badura-Stronka M, et al. Comparative study of clinical characteristics of amniotic rupture sequence with and without body wall defect: further evidence for separation. *Birth Defects Res A Clin Mol Teratol* 2009;85:211–215.
81. Cox H, Viljoen D, Versfeld G, et al. Radial ray defects and associated anomalies. *Clin Genet* 1989;35:322–330.
82. Goldfarb CA, Wall L, Manske PR. Radial longitudinal deficiency: the incidence of associated medical and musculoskeletal conditions. *J Hand Surg Am* 2006;31:1176–1182.

83. Greenhalgh KL, Howell RT, Bottani A, et al. Thrombocytopenia-absent radius syndrome: a clinical genetic study. *J Med Genet* 2002;39:876–881.
84. Kaariainen H, Ryoppy S, Norio R. RAPADILINO syndrome with radial and patellar aplasia/hypoplasia as main manifestations. *Am J Med Genet* 1989;33:346–351.
85. Maschke SD, Seitz W, Lawton J. Radial longitudinal deficiency. *J Am Acad Orthop Surg* 2007;15:41–52.
86. Clinton R, Birch JG. Congenital tibial deficiency: a 37-year experience at 1 institution. *J Pediatr Orthop* 2015;35(4):385–390.
87. Fernandez-Palazzi F, Bendahan J, Rivas S. Congenital deficiency of the tibia: a report on 22 cases. *J Pediatr Orthop B* 1998;7:298–302.
88. Birch JG, Lincoln TL, Mack PW, et al. Congenital fibular deficiency: a review of thirty years' experience at one institution and a proposed classification system based on clinical deformity. *J Bone Joint Surg Am* 2011;93(12):1144–1451.
89. Czeizel AE, Vitéz M, Kodaj I, et al. A family study on isolated congenital radial and tibial deficiencies in Hungary, 1975–1984. *Clin Genet* 1993;44(1):32–36.
90. Pajkrt E, Cicero S, Griffin D, et al. Fetal forearm anomalies: prenatal diagnosis, associations and management strategy. *Prenat Diagn* 2012;32:1084–1093.
91. Basel D, Kilpatrick MW, Tsipouras P. The expanding panorama of split hand foot malformation. *Am J Med Genet A* 2006;140A:1359–1365.
92. Schwabe GC, Mundlos S. Genetics of congenital hand anomalies. *Handchir Mikrochir Plast Chir* 2004;36:85–97.
93. Gurrieri F, Everman DB. Clinical, genetic, and molecular aspects of split-hand/foot malformation: an update. *Am J Med Genet A* 2013;161A:2860–2872.
94. Sowińska-Seidler A, Socha M, Jamsheer A. Split-hand/foot malformation—molecular cause and implications in genetic counseling. *J Appl Genet* 2014;55:105–115.
95. Khan S, Basit S, Zimri FK, et al. A novel homozygous missense mutation in WNT10B in familial split-hand/foot malformation. *Clin Genet* 2012;82:48–55.
96. Petit F, Andrieux J, Demeer B, et al. Split-hand/foot malformation with long-bone deficiency and BHLHA9 duplication: two cases and expansion of the phenotype to radial agenesis. *Eur J Med Genet* 2013;56:88–92.
97. Nagata E, Kano H, Kato F, et al. Japanese founder duplications/triplications involving BHLHA9 are associated with split-hand/foot malformation with or without long bone deficiency and Gollop-Wolfgang complex. *Orphanet J Rare Dis* 2014;9(1):125.
98. Villanueva C, Jacobson-Dickman E, Xu C, et al. Congenital hypogonadotrophic hypogonadism with split hand/foot malformation: a clinical entity with a high frequency of FGFR1 mutations. *Genet Med* 2014; doi: 10.1038/gim. 2014;166.
99. Brunner HG, Hamel BC, Bokhoven HH. P63 gene mutations and human developmental syndromes. *Am J Med Genet* 2002;112:284–290.
100. Bongers EMHF, Gubler MC, Knoers NV. Nail-patella syndrome. Overview on clinical and molecular findings. *Pediatr Nephrol* 2002;17:703–712.
101. Bongers EMHF, van Kampen A, van Bokhoven H, et al. Human syndromes with congenital patellar anomalies and the underlying gene defects. *Clin Genet* 2005;68:302–319.
102. Campeau PM, Lu JT, Dawson BC, et al. The KAT6B-related disorders genitopatellar syndrome and Ohdo/SBBYS syndrome have distinct clinical features reflecting distinct molecular mechanisms. *Hum Mutat* 2012;33:1520–1525.
103. Froster-Iskenius UG, Baird PA. Amelia: incidence and associated defects in a large population. *Teratology* 1990;41:23–31.
104. Martinez-Frias ML, Bermejo E, Aparicio P, et al. Amelia: analysis of its epidemiological and clinical characteristics. *Am J Med Genet* 1997;73:189–193.
105. Syvänen J, Nietosvaara Y, Ritvanen A, et al. High risk for major non-limb anomalies associated with lower limb deficiency: a population-based study. *J Bone Joint Surg Am* 2014;96:1898–1904.
106. Adra A, Cordero D, Mejides A, et al. Caudal regression syndrome: etiopathogenesis, prenatal diagnosis, and perinatal management. *Obstet Gynecol Surv* 1994;49:508–516.
107. Bruce JH, Romaguera RL, Rodriguez MM, et al. Caudal dysplasia syndrome and sirenomelia: are they part of a spectrum? *Fetal Pediatr Pathol* 2009;28:109–131.
108. Stocker JT, Heifetz SA. Sirenomelia. A morphological study of 33 cases and review of the literature. *Perspect Pediatr Pathol* 1987;10:7–50.
109. Duesterhoeft SM, Ernst LM, Siebert JR, et al. Five cases of caudal regression with an aberrant abdominal umbilical artery: further support for a caudal regression-sirenomelia spectrum. *Am J Med Genet A* 2007;143A:3175–3184.
110. Valenzano M, Paoletti R, Rossi A, et al. Sirenomelia. Pathological features, antenatal ultrasonographic clues, and a review of current embryogenic theories. *Hum Reprod Update* 1999;5:82–86.
111. Allen VM, Armson BA, Wilson RD, et al. Teratogenicity associated with pre-existing and gestational diabetes. *J Obstet Gynaecol Can* 2007;29:927–944.
112. Eriksson UJ, Cederberg J, Wentzel P. Congenital malformations in offspring of diabetic mothers—animal and human studies. *Rev Endocr Metab Disord* 2003;4:79–93.
113. Castori M. Diabetic embryopathy: a developmental perspective from fertilization to adulthood. *Mol Syndromol* 2013;4:74–86.
114. Ramos-Arroyo MA, Rodriguez-Pinilla E, Cordero JF. Maternal diabetes: the risk for specific birth defects. *Eur J Epidemiol* 1992;8:503–508.
115. Chikkannaiah P, Mahadevan A, Gosavi M, et al. Sirenomelia with associated systemic anomalies: an autopsy pathologic illustration of a series of four cases. *Pathol Res Pract* 2014;210:444–449.
116. Crétolle C, Pelet A, Sanlaville D, et al. Spectrum of HLXB9 gene mutations in Currarino syndrome and genotype-phenotype correlation. *Hum Mutat* 2008;29:903–910.
117. Carli D, Garagnani L, Lando M, et al. VACTERL (vertebral defects, anal atresia, tracheoesophageal fistula with esophageal atresia, cardiac defects, renal and limb anomalies) association: disease spectrum in 25 patients ascertained for their upper limb involvement. *J Pediatr* 2014;164:458–462.
118. Biesecker LG. Polydactyly: how many disorders and how many genes? 2010 update. *Dev Dyn* 2011;240:931–942.
119. Malik S. Polydactyly: phenotypes, genetics and classification. *Clin Genet* 2014;85:203–212.
120. Leber GE, Gosain AK. Surgical excision of pedunculated supernumerary digits prevents traumatic amputation neuromas. *Pediatr Dermatol* 2003;20:108–112.
121. Zimmer EZ, Bronshtein M. Fetal polydactyly diagnosis during early pregnancy: clinical applications. *Am J Obstet Gynecol* 2000;183:755–758.
122. Verma PK, El-Harouni AA. Review of literatures: genes related to postaxial polydactyly. *Front Pediatr* 2015;3:8.
123. Quinn ME, Haaning A, Ware SM. Preaxial polydactyly caused by Gli3 haploinsufficiency is rescued by Zic3 loss of function in mice. *Hum Mol Genet* 2012;21:1888–1896.
124. Malik S. Syndactyly: phenotypes, genetics and current classification. *Eur J Hum Genet* 2012;20:817–824.
125. Bamshad M, Van Heest AE, Pleasure D. Arthrogryposis: a review and update. *J Bone Joint Surg Am* 2009;91 (Suppl 4):40–46.
126. Hall JG. Amyoplasia involving only the upper limbs or only involving the lower limbs with review of the relevant differential diagnoses. *Am J Med Genet A* 2014;164A:859–873.
127. Kalampokas E, Kalampokas T, Sofoudis C, et al. Diagnosing arthrogryposis multiplex congenital: a review. *ISRN Obstet Gynecol* 2012;2012:264918.
128. Tajsharghi H, Oldfors A. Myosinopathies: pathology and mechanisms. *Acta Neuropathol* 2013;125:3–18.
129. Rink BD. Arthrogryposis: a review and approach to prenatal diagnosis. *Obstet Gynecol Surv* 2011;66:369–377.
130. Hall JG, Aldinger KA, Tanaka KI. Amyoplasia revisited. *Am J Med Genet A* 2014;164A:700–730.
131. Moerman P, Fryns JP. The fetal akinesia deformation sequence. A fetopathological approach. *Genet Couns* 1990;1:25–33.
132. Haliloglu G, Topaloglu H. Arthrogryposis and fetal hypomobility syndrome. *Handb Clin Neurol* 2013;113:1311–1319.
133. Quinn CM, Wigglesworth JS, Heckmatt J. Lethal arthrogryposis multiplex congenita: a pathological study of 21 cases. *Histopathology* 1991;19:155–162.

134. Vuopala K, Leisti J, Herva R. Lethal arthrogryposis in Finland—a clinico-pathological study of 83 cases during thirteen years. *Neuropediatrics* 1994;25:308–315.
135. Michalk A, Stricker S, Becker J, et al. Acetylcholine receptor pathway mutations explain various fetal akinesia deformation sequence disorders. *Am J Hum Genet* 2008;82:464–476.
136. Chen CP. Prenatal diagnosis and genetic analysis of fetal akinesia deformation sequence and multiple pterygium syndrome associated with neuromuscular junction disorders: a review. *Taiwan J Obstet Gynecol* 2012;15:12–17.
137. Savarirayan R, Rimoin DL. The skeletal dysplasias. *Best Pract Res Clin Endocrinol Metab* 2002;16:547–560.
138. Warman ML, Cormier-Daire V, Hall C, et al. Nosology and classification of genetic skeletal disorders: 2010 revision. *Am J Med Genet* 2011;155A:943–968.
139. Spranger JW, Brill PW, Nishimura G, et al. *Bone Dysplasias. An Atlas of Genetic Disorders of Skeletal Development*, 3rd ed. New York: Oxford University Press, 2012.
140. Orioli IM, Castilla EE, Barbosa-Neto JG. The birth prevalence rates for the skeletal dysplasias. *J Med Genet* 1986;23:328–332.
141. Stoll C, Dott B, Roth MP, et al. Birth prevalence rates of skeletal dysplasias. *Clin Genet* 1989;35:88–92.
142. Al-Gazali LI, Bakir M, Hamid Z, et al. Birth prevalence and pattern of osteochondrodysplasias in an inbred high risk population. *Birth Defects Res A Clin Mol Teratol* 2003;67:125–132.
143. Barkova E, Mohan U, Chitayat D, et al. Fetal skeletal dysplasias in a tertiary care center: radiology, pathology and molecular analysis of 112 cases. *Clin Genet* 2015;87:330–337.
143a. Rasmussen SA, Bieber FR, Benacerraf BR, et al. Epidemiology of osteochondrodysplasias: changing trends due to advances in prenatal diagnosis. *Am J Med Genet* 1996;61:49–58.
144. Stevenson DA, Carey JC, Byrne JL. Analysis of skeletal dysplasia in the Utah population. *Am J Med Genet A* 2012;158A:1046–1054.
145. Cobben JM, Cornel MC, Dijkstra I, et al. Prevalence of lethal osteochondrodysplasias. *Am J Med Genet* 1990;36:377–378.
146. Lahmar-Boufaroua A, Yacoubi MT, Hmisssa S, et al. Lethal osteochondro-dysplasia: feto-pathological study of 32 cases. *Tunis Med* 2009;87:127–132.
147. Andersen PE Jr. Prevalence of lethal osteochondrodysplasias in Denmark. *Am J Med Genet* 1989;32:484–489.
148. Konstantinidou AE, Agrogiannis G, Sifakis S, et al. Genetic skeletal disorders of the fetus and infant: pathologic and molecular findings in a series of 41 cases. *Birth Defects Res A Clin Mol Teratol* 2009;85:811–821.
149. Schramm T, Gloning KP, Minderer S, et al. Prenatal sonographic diagnosis of skeletal dysplasias. *Ultrasound Obstet Gynecol* 2009;34:160–170.
150. Spranger J, Maroteaux P. The lethal osteochondrodysplasias. *Adv Hum Gent* 1990;19:1–103.
151. Pansuriya TC, Kroon HM, Bovée JV. Enchondromatosis: insights on the different subtypes. *Int J Clin Exp Pathol* 2010;3:557–569.
152. Ilaslan H, Sundaram M, Unni KK. Solid variant of aneurismal bone cysts in long tubular bones: giant cell reparative granuloma. *AJR Am J Roentgenol* 2003;180:1681–1687.
153. Inarejos Clemente EJ, Vilanova JC, Riaza Margin L, et al. A primary inflammatory myofibroblastic tumor of the scapula in a child: imaging findings. *Skeletal Radiol* 2015;44:733–777.
154. Moon NF. Adamantinoma of the appendicular skeleton in children. *Int Orthop* 1994;18:379–388.
155. Hasegawa K, Higuchi Y, Yamashita M, et al. Japanese familial case with metaphyseal dysplasia, Schmid type caused by the p.T555P mutation in the COL10A1 gene. *Clin Pediatr Endocrinol* 2015;24:33–36.
156. Nevin NC, Thomas PS, Davis RI, et al. Melorheostosis in a family with autosomal dominant osteopoikilosis. *Am J Med Genet* 1999;82:409–414.
157. Krakow D, Alanay Y, Rimoin LP, et al. Evaluation of prenatal-onset osteochondrodysplasias by ultrasonography: a retrospective and prospective analysis. *Am J Med Genet A* 2008;14A:1917–1924.
158. Aghabiklooei A, Goodarzi P, Kariminejad MH. Lung hypoplasia and its associated major congenital abnormalities in perinatal death: an autopsy study of 850 cases. *Indian J Pediatr* 2009;76:1137–1140.
159. Mogayzel PJ, Marcus CL. Skeletal dysplasias and their effect on the respiratory system. *Paediatr Respir Rev* 2001;2:365–371.
160. Wood B, Dimmick JE. Skeletal system. In: Dimmick JE, Kalousek DK, eds. *Developmental Pathology of the Embryo and Fetus*. Philadelphia, PA: JB Lippincott Co., 1992:662–706.
161. Borochowitz Z, Rimoin DL. The congenital chondroplasias. In: Reed GB, Claireaux AE, Cockburn F, eds. *Pathology, Imaging, Genetics and Management*, 2nd ed. London, UK: Chapman and Hall, 1995:787–802.
162. Parnell SE, Phillips GS. Neonatal skeletal dysplasias. *Pediatr Radiol* 2012;42(Suppl 1):S150–S157.
163. Yang SS, Kitchen E, Gilbert EF, et al. Histopathologic examination in osteochondrodysplasia. Time for standardization. *Arch Pathol Lab Med* 1986;110:10–12.
164. Offiah AC, Hall CM. Radiological diagnosis of the constitutional disorders of bone. As easy as A, B, C? *Pediatr Radiol* 2003;33:153–161.
165. Yang S. The skeletal system. In: Wigglesworth JS, Singer DB, eds. *Textbook of Fetal and Perinatal Pathology*, 2nd ed. Malden, MA: Blackwell Science, 1998:1039–1082.
166. Alman BA. Skeletal dysplasias and the growth plate. *Clin Genet* 2008;73:24–30.
167. Gilbert-Barness E, Opitz JM. Abnormal bone development: histopathology of skeletal dysplasias. *Birth Defects Orig Artic Ser* 1996;30:103–156.
168. Gilbert-Barness E. Osteochondrodysplasia—constitutional diseases of bone. In: *Potter's Pathology of the Fetus, Infant and Child*, 2nd ed. Philadelphia, PA: Mosby Elsevier, 2007:1836–1897.
169. Almeida MR, Campos-Xavier AB, Medeira A, et al. Clinical and molecular diagnosis of the skeletal dysplasias associated with mutations in the gene encoding Fibroblast Growth Factor Receptor 3 (FGFR3) in Portugal. *Clin Genet* 2009;75:150–156.
170. Bonaventure J, Rousseau F, Legeai-Mallet L, et al. Common mutations in the fibroblast growth factor receptor 3 (FGFR 3) gene account for achondroplasia, hypochondroplasia, and thanatophoric dwarfism. *Am J Med Genet* 1996;63:148–154.
171. Lemyre E, Azouz EM, Teebi AS, et al. Bone dysplasia series. Achondroplasia, hypochondroplasia and thanatophoric dysplasia: review and update. *Can Assoc Radiol J* 1999;50:185–197.
172. Krejci P. The paradox of FGFR3 signaling in skeletal dysplasia: why chondrocytes growth arrest while other cells over proliferate. *Mutat Res Rev Mutat Res* 2014;759:40–48.
173. Baujat G, Legeai-Mallet L, Finidori G, et al. Achondroplasia. *Best Pract Res Clin Rheumatol* 2008;22:3–18.
174. Zhou ZQ, Ota S, Deng C, et al. Mutant activated FGFR3 impairs endochondral bone growth by preventing SOX9 downregulation in differentiating chondrocytes. *Hum Mol Genet* 2015;24:1764–1773.
175. Prinster C, Carrera P, Del Maschio M, et al. Comparison of clinical-radiological and molecular findings in hypochondroplasia. *Am J Med Genet* 1998;75:109–112.
176. Xue Y, Sun A, Mekikian PB, et al. FGFR3 mutation frequency in 324 cases from the International Skeletal Dysplasia Registry. *Mol Genet Gen Med* 2014;2:497–503.
177. Bober M, Taylor M, Heinle R, et al. Achondroplasia-hypochondroplasia complex and abnormal pulmonary anatomy. *Am J Med Genet Part A* 2012;158A:2336–2341.
178. Alanay Y, Krakow D, Rimoin DL, et al. Angulated femurs and the skeletal dysplasias: experience of the International Skeletal Dysplasia Registry (1988–2006). *Am J Med Genet A* 2007;143A:1159–1168.
179. Karczeski B, Cutting GR. Thanatophoric dysplasia. In: Pagon RA, Adam MP, Ardinger HH, et al., eds. *GeneReviews®*[Internet]. Seattle, WA: University of Washington, Seattle, 1993–2014.
180. Vogt C, Blaas HG. Thanatophoric dysplasia: autopsy findings over a 25-year period. *Pediatr Dev Pathol* 2013;16:160–167.
181. Horton WA, Hood OJ, Machado MA, et al. Abnormal ossification in thanatophoric dysplasia. *Bone* 1988;9:53–61.

182. Weber M, Johannisson T, Thomsen M, et al. Thanatophoric dysplasia type I: new radiologic, morphologic, and histologic aspects toward the exact definition of the disorder. *J Pediatr Orthop B* 1998;7:1–9.
183. Wilcox WR, Tavormina PL, Krakow D, et al. Molecular, radiologic, and histopathologic correlations in thanatophoric dysplasia. *Am J Med Genet* 1998;78:274–281.
184. Farmakis SG, Shinawi M, Miller-Thomas M, et al. FGFR3-related condition: a skeletal dysplasia with similarities to thanatophoric dysplasia and SADDAN due to Lys650Met. *Skeletal Radiol* 2015;44:441–445.
185. Manickam K, Donoghue D, Meyer A, et al. Suppression of severe achondroplasia with developmental delay and acanthosis nigricans by the p.Thr651pro mutation. *Am J Med Genet Part A* 2014;164A:243–250.
186. Foldynova-Trantirkova S, Wilcox WR, Krejci P. Sixteen years and counting: the current understanding of fibroblast growth factor receptor 3 (FGFR3) signaling in skeletal dysplasias. *Hum Mutat* 2012;33:29–41.
187. Hevner RF. The cerebral cortex malformation in thanatophoric dysplasia: neuropathology and pathogenesis. *Acta Neuropathol* 2005;110:208–221.
188. Itoh K, Pooh R, Kanemura Y, et al. Brain malformation with loss of normal FGFR3 expression in thanatophoric dysplasia type I. *Neuropathology* 2013;33:663–666.
189. Steiner R, Adsit J, Basel D. COL1A1/2-related osteogenesis imperfecta. In: Pagon RA, Adam MP, Ardinger HH, et al., eds. *GeneReviews®*[Internet]. Seattle, WA: University of Washington, Seattle, 1993–2015.
190. Marini JC, Reich A, Smith SM. Osteogenesis imperfect due to mutations in non-collagenous genes: lessons in the biology of bone formation. *Curr Opin Pediatr* 2014;26:500–507.
191. Byers HP, Pyott SM. Recessively inherited forms of osteogenesis imperfecta. *Annu Rev Genet* 2012;46:475–497.
192. Rauch F, Lalic L, Roughley P, et al. Relationship between genotype and skeletal phenotype in children and adolescents with osteogenesis imperfecta. *J Bone Min Res* 2010;25:1367–1374.
193. Eyre DR, Weis MA. Bone collagen: new clues to its mineralization mechanism from recessive osteogenesis imperfecta. *Calcif Tissue Int* 2013;93:338–347.
194. Van Dijk FS, Sillence DO. Osteogenesis imperfect: clinical diagnosis, nomenclature and severity assessment. *Am J Med Genet Part A* 2014;164A:1470–1481.
195. Van Dijk FS, Cobben JM, Kariminejad A, et al. Osteogenesis imperfecta: a review with clinical examples. *Mol Syndromol* 2011;2:1–20.
196. Donnelly DE, McConnell V, Paterson A, et al. The prevalence of thanatophoric dysplasia and lethal osteogenesis imperfect type II in Northern Ireland—a complete population study. *Ulster Med J* 2010;79:114–118.
197. Cole WG, Dalgleish R. Perinatal lethal osteogenesis imperfecta. *J Med Genet* 1995;32:284–289.
198. Bullough PG, Davidson DD, Lorenzo JC. The morbid anatomy of the skeleton in osteogenesis imperfecta. *Clin Orthop Relat Res* 1981:42–57.
199. Cassella JP, Stamp TC, Ali SY. A morphological and ultrastructural study of bone in osteogenesis imperfecta. *Calcif Tissue Int* 1996;58:155–165.
200. Sanguinetti C, Greco F, De Palma L, et al. Morphological changes in growth-plate cartilage in osteogenesis imperfecta. *J Bone Joint Surg Br* 1990;72:475–479.
201. Marion MJ, Gannon FH, Fallon MD, et al. Skeletal dysplasia in perinatal lethal osteogenesis imperfecta. A complex disorder of endochondral and intramembranous ossification. *Clin Orthop Relat Res* 1993:327–337.
202. Stoss H. Pathologic anatomy of osteogenesis imperfecta. Light and electron microscopic studies of supportive tissue and skin. *Veroff Pathol* 1990;134:1–88.
203. Emery SC, Karpinski NC, Hansen L, et al. Abnormalities in central nervous system development in osteogenesis imperfecta type II. *Pediatr Dev Pathol* 1999;2:124–130.
204. Renaud A, Aucourt J, Weill J, et al. Radiographic features of osteogenesis imperfecta. *Insights Imaging* 2013;4:417–429.
205. Greeley CS, Donaruma-Kwoh M, Vettimattam M, et al. Fractures at diagnosis in infants and children with osteogenesis imperfecta. *J Pediatr Orthop* 2013;33:32–36.
206. Arcaro G, Braccioni F, Gallan F, et al. Noninvasive positive pressure ventilation in the management of acute respiratory failure due to osteogenesis imperfecta *J Clin Anesth* 2012;24:55–57.
207. Singer RB, Ogston SA, Paterson CR. Mortality in various types of osteogenesis imperfecta. *J Insur Med* 2001;33:216–220.
208. Sztrolovics R, Glorieux FH, Travers R, et al. Osteogenesis imperfecta: comparison of molecular defects with bone histological changes. *Bone* 1994;15:321–328.
209. Marini JC, Reich A, Smith SM. Osteogenesis imperfect due to mutations in non-collagenous genes: lessons in the biopsy of bone formation. *Curr Opin Pediatr* 2014;26:500–507.
210. Kim OH, Jin DK, Kosaki K, et al. Osteogenesis imperfecta type V: clinical and radiographic manifestations in mutation confirmed patients. *Am J Med Genet A* 2013;161A:1972–1979 .
211. Balasubramanian M, Parker M, Dalton A, et al. Genotype-phenotype study in type V osteogenesis imperfecta. *Clin Dysmorphol* 2013;22:93–101.
212. Cheung MS, Glorieux FH, Rauch F. Natural history of hyperplastic callus formation in osteogenesis imperfecta type V. *J Bone Miner Res* 2007;22:1181–1186.
213. McNeeley MF, Dontchos BN, Laflamme MA, et al. Aortic dissection in osteogenesis imperfecta: case report and review of the literature. *Emerg Radiol* 2012;19:553–556.
214. Lamanna A, Fayers T, Clarke S, et al. Valvular and aortic diseases in osteogenesis imperfecta. *Heart Lung Circ* 2013;22:801–810.
215. Tinkle BT, Wenstrup RJ. A genetic approach to fracture epidemiology in childhood. *Am J Med Genet C Semin Med Genet* 2005;139C:38–54.
216. Takahashi S, Okada K, Nagasawa H, et al. Osteosarcoma occurring in osteogenesis imperfecta. *Virchows Arch* 2004;444:454–458.
217. Mandziak DG, Clayer M. Chondrosarcoma in a patient with osteogenesis imperfecta. *ANZ J Surg* 2013;83:794–795.
218. Stig Jacobsen F. Aneurysmal bone cyst in a patient with osteogenesis imperfect. *J Pediatr Orthop B* 1997;6:225–227.
219. Rohbach M, Giunta C. Recessive osteogenesis imperfecta: clinical, radiological, and molecular findings. *Am J Med Genet C Semin Med Genet* 2012;160C:175–189.
220. Valadares ER, Carneiro TB, Santos PM, et al. What is new in genetics and osteogenesis imperfecta classification? *J Pediatr (Rio J)* 2014;90:536–541.
221. Schwarze U, Cundy T, Pyott SM, et al. Mutations in FKBP10, which result in Bruck syndrome and recessive forms of osteogenesis imperfecta, inhibit the hydroxylation of telopeptide lysines in bone collagen. *Hum Mol Genet* 2013;22:1–17.
222. Arnold WV, Fertala A. Skeletal diseases caused by mutations that affect collagen structure and function. *Int J Biochem Cell Biol* 2013;45:1556–1567.
223. Mornet E, Nunes ME. Hypophosphatasia. In: Pagon RA, Adam MP, Ardinger HH, et al., eds. *GeneReviews®*[Internet]. Seattle, WA: University of Washington, Seattle, 1993–2014.
224. Wenkert D, McAlister WH, Coburn SP, et al. Hypophosphatasia: nonlethal disease despite skeletal presentation in utero (17 new cases and literature review). *J Bone Min Res* 2011;26:2389–2398.
225. Reibel A, Maniere MC, Clauss F, et al. Orodental phenotype and genotype findings in all subtypes of hypophosphatasia. *Orphanet J Rare Dis* 2009;4:6.
226. Comstock JM, Putnam AR, Sangle N, et al. Recurrence of achondrogenesis type 2 in sibs: additional evidence for germline mosaicism. *Am J Med Genet Part A* 2010;152A:1822–1824.
227. Weisman, PS, Kashireddy PV, Ernst LM. Pathologic diagnosis of achondrogenesis type 2 in a fragmented fetus: case report and evidence-based differential diagnostic approach in the early midtrimester. *Pediatr Dev Pathol* 2014;17:10–20.
228. Wainwright H, Beighton P. Visceral manifestations of hypochondrogenesis. *Virchows Arch* 2008;453:203–207.
229. Wainwright H, Beighton P. Achondrogenesis type II with cutaneous hamartomata. *Clin Dysmorphol* 2008;17:207–209.
230. Baujat G, Le Merrer M. Ellis-van Creveld syndrome. *Orphanet J Rare Dis* 2007;2:27.

231. Sillence D, Kozlowski K, Bar-ziv J, et al. Perinatally lethal short rib-polydactyly syndromes. 1. Variability in known syndromes. *Pediatr Radiol* 1987;17:474–480.
232. Yang SS, Langer LO Jr, Cacciarelli A, et al. Three conditions in neonatal asphyxiating thoracic dysplasia (Jeune) and short rib-polydactyly syndrome spectrum: a clinicopathologic study. *Am J Med Genet Suppl* 1987;3:191–207.
233. Cavalcanti DP, Huber C, Le Quan Sang KH, et al. Mutation in IFT80 gene in a fetus with a phenotype of Verma-Naumoff provides molecular evidence for the Jeune-Verma-Naumoff dysplasia spectrum. *J Med Genet* 2011;48:88–92.
234. Baujat G, Huber C, El Hokayem J, et al. Asphysiating thoracic dysplasia: clinical and molecular review of 39 families. *J Med Genet* 2013;50:91–98.
235. Okiro P, Wainwright H, Spranger J, et al. Autopsy observations in lethal short-rib polydactyly syndromes. *Pediatr Dev Pathol* 2015;18:40–48.
236. Yuan S, Sun Z. Expanding Horizons: ciliary proteins reach beyond cilia. *Annu Rev Genet* 2013;47:353–376.
237. Huber C, Cormier-Daire V. Ciliary disorder of the skeleton. *Am J Med Genet Part C* 2012;160C:165–174.
238. Schmidts M. Clinical genetics and pathobiology of ciliary chondrodysplasias. *J Pediatr Genet* 2014;3:46–94.
239. Halbritter J, Bizet AA, Schmidts M, et al. Defects in the IFT-B component IFT172 cause Jeune and Mainzer-Saldino syndromes in humans. *Am J Hum Genet* 2013;93:915–925.
240. Hentze S, Sergi C, Troeger J, et al. Short-rib-polydactyly syndrome type Verma-Naumoff-Le Marec in a fetus with histological hallmarks of type Saldino-Noonan but lacking internal organ abnormalities. *Am J Med Genet* 1998;80:281–285.
241. Qureshi F, Jacques SM, Evans MI, et al. Skeletal histopathology in fetuses with chondroectodermal dysplasia (Ellis-van Creveld syndrome). *Am J Med Genet* 1993;45:471–476.
242. Yang SS, Lin CS, Al Saadi A, et al. Short rib-polydactyly syndrome, type 3 with chondrocytic inclusions: report of a case and review of the literature. *Am J Med Genet* 1980;7:205–213.
243. Erzen M, Stanescu R, Stanescu V, et al. Comparative histopathology of the growth cartilage in short-rib polydactyly syndromes type I and type III and in chondroectodermal dysplasia. *Ann Genet* 1988;31:144–150.
244. Copelovitch L, O'Brien MM, Guttenberg M, et al. Renal-hepatic-pancreatic dysplasia: a sibship with skeletal and central nervous system anomalies and NPHP3 mutation. *Am J Med Genet Part A* 2013; 161A:1743–1749.
245. Bendon RW. Ivemark's renal-hepatic-pancreatic dysplasia: analytic approach to a perinatal autopsy. *Pediatr Dev Pathol* 1999;2:94–100.
246. Brueton LA, Dillon MJ, Winter RM. Ellis-Van Creveld syndrome, Jeune syndrome, and renal-hepatic-pancreatic dysplasia: separate entities or disease spectrum? *J Med Genet* 1990;27:252–255.
247. Ruiz-Perez VL, Goodship JA. Ellis-van Creveld syndrome and Weyers acrodental dysostosis are caused by cilia-mediated diminished response to hedgehog ligands. *Am J Med Genet C Semin Med Genet* 2009;151C:341–351.
248. D'Asdia MC, Torrente I, Consoli F, et al. Novel and recurrent EVC and EVC2 mutations in Ellis-van Creveld syndrome and Weyers acrofacial dyostosis. *Eur J Med Genet* 2013;56:80–87.
249. Lin AE, Traum AZ, Sahai I, et al. Sensenbrenner syndrome (cranioectodermal dysplasia): clinical and molecular analyses of 39 patients including two new patients. *Am J Med Genet A* 2013;161A:2762–2776.
250. Grigelioniene G, Geiberger S, Papadogiannakis N, et al. The phenotype range of achondrogenesis 1A. *Am J Med Genet* 2013;161A:2554–2558.
251. Aigner T, Rau T, Niederhagen M, et al. Achondrogenesis type IA (Houston-Harris): a still-unresolved molecular phenotype. *Pediatr Dev Pathol* 2007;10:328–334.
252. Freeze HH. Achondrogenesis type 1A—from mouse to human. *N Engl J Med* 2010;362:266–267.
253. Smits P, Bolton AD, Funari V, et al. Lethal skeletal dysplasia in mice and humans lacking the golgin GMAP-210. *N Engl J Med* 2010;362:201–216.
254. Furuichi T, Kayserili H, Hiraoka S, et al. Identification of loss-of-function mutations of SLC35D1 in patients with Schneckenbecken dysplasia, but not with other severe spondylodysplastic dysplasias group diseases. *J Med Genet* 2009;46:562–568.
255. Mehawei C, Delahodde A, Legeai-Mallet L, et al. The impairment of MAGMAS function in human is responsible for a severe skeletal dysplasia. *PLoS Genet* 2014;10:e1004311.
256. Nikkels PG, Stigter RH, Knol IE, et al. Schneckenbecken dysplasia, radiology, and histology. *Pediatr Radiol* 2001;31:27–30.
257. Boerkoel CF, O'Neill S, Andre JL, et al. Manifestations and treatment of Schimke immuno-osseous dysplasia: 14 new cases and a review of the literature. *Eur J Pediatr* 2000;159:1–7.
258. Clewing JM, Antalfy BC, Lucke T, et al. Schimke immuno-osseous dysplasia: a clinicopathological correlation. *J Med Genet* 2007;44:122–130.
259. Hunter KB, Lücke T, Spranger J, et al. Schimke immunoosseous dysplasia: defining skeletal features. *Eur J Pediatr* 2010;169:801–811.
260. Morimoto M, Baradaran-Heravi A, Lücke T, et al. Schimke immunoosseous dysplasia. In: Pagon RA, Adam MP, Ardinger HH, et al., eds. *GeneReviews*®[Internet]. Seattle, WA: University of Washington, Seattle, 1993–2015.
261. Sarin S, Javidan A, Boivin F, et al. Insights into the renal pathogenesis in schimke immuno-osseous dysplasia: a renal histological characterization and expression analysis. *J Histochem Cytochem* 2015;63:32–44.
262. Elizondo LI, Cho KS, Zhang W, et al. Schimke immuno-osseous dysplasia: SMARCAL1 loss-of-function and phenotypic correlation. *J Med Genet* 2009;46:49–59.
263. Carroll C, Badu-Nkansah A, Hunley T, et al. Schimke immunoosseous dysplasia associated with undifferentiated carcinoma and a novel SMARCAL1 mutation in a child. *Pediatr Blood Cancer* 2013;60:88–90.
264. Baradaran-Heravi A, Raams A, Lubieniecka J, et al. SMARCAL1 deficiency predisposes to non-Hodgkin lymphoma and hypersensitivity to genotoxic agents in vivo. *Am J Med Genet* 2012;158A:2204–2213.
265. Morimoto M, Yu Z, Stenzel P, et al. Reduced elastogenesis: a clue to the arteriosclerosis and emphysematous changes in Schimke immuno-osseous dysplasia? *Orphanet J Rare Dis* 2012;7:70.
266. Schindler A, Sumner C, Hoover-Fong JE. TRPV4-associated disorders. In: Pagon RA, Adam MP, Ardinger HH, et al., eds. *GeneReviews*®[Internet]. Seattle, WA: University of Washington, Seattle, 1993–2014.
267. Unger S, Lausch E, Stanziel F, et al. Fetal akinesia in metatropic dysplasia: The combined phenotype of chondrodysplasia and neuropathy? *Am J Med Genet* 2011;155A:2860–2864.
268. Nishimura G, Lausch E, Savarirayan R, et al. TRPV4-associated skeletal dysplasias. *Am J Med Genet C Semin Med Genet* 2012;160C:190–204.
269. Hall BD. Lethality in Desbuquois dysplasia: three new cases. *Pediatr Radiol* 2001;31:43–47.
270. Kannu P, Aftimos S, Mayne V, et al. Metatropic dysplasia: clinical and radiographic findings in 11 patients demonstrating long-term natural history. *Am J Med Genet A* 2007;143A:2512–2522.
271. Cam N, Krakow D, Johnykutty S, et al. Dominant TRPV4 mutations in nonlethal and lethal metatropic dysplasia. *Am J Med Genet A* 2010;152A:1169–1177.
272. O'Sullivan MJ, McAllister WH, Ball RH, et al. Morphologic observations in a case of lethal variant (type I) metatropic dysplasia with atypical features: morphology of lethal metatropic dysplasia. *Pediatr Dev Pathol* 1998;1:405–412.
273. Dwyer E, Hyland H, Modaff P, et al. Genotype-Phenotype correlation in DTDST dysplasias: atelosteogenesis type II and diastropic dysplasia variant in one family. *Am J Med Gen Part A* 2010;152A:3043–3050.
274. Sillence D, Worthington S, Dixon J, et al. Atelosteogenesis syndromes: a review, with comments on their pathogenesis. *Pediatr Radiol* 1997;27:388–396.
275. Macias-Gomez NM, Megarbane A, Leal-Ugarte E, et al. Diastrophic dysplasia and atelosteogenesis type II as expression of compound heterozygosis: first report of a Mexican patient and genotype-phenotype correlation. *Am J Med Genet A* 2004;129A:190–192.
276. Maeda K, Miyamoto Y, Sawai H, et al. A compound heterozygote harboring novel and recurrent DTDST mutations with intermediate phenotype between atelosteogenesis type II and diastrophic dysplasia. *Am J Med Genet A* 2006;140:1143–1147.
277. Superti-Furga A. Achondrogenesis type 1B. *J Med Genet* 1996;33:957–961.

278. Robertson SP. Molecular pathology of filamin A: diverse phenotypes, many functions. *Clin Dysmorphol* 2004;13:123–131.
279. Bicknell LS, Morgan T, Bonafe L, et al. Mutations in FLNB cause boomerang dysplasia. *J Med Genet* 2005;42:e43.
280. Cordier AG, Mabille M, Delezoide AL, et al. Prenatal diagnosis of a rare skeletal dysplasia by ultrasound and scan tomography: atelosteogenesis III (AO III). Correlation with autopsy. *Prenat Diagn* 2008;28:975–977.
281. Lu J, Lian G, Lenkinski R, et al. Filamin B mutations cause chondrocyte defects in skeletal development. *Hum Mol Genet* 2007;16:1661–1675.
282. Zhou AX, Hartwig JH, Akyurek LM. Filamins in cell signaling, transcription and organ development. *Trends Cell Biol* 2010;20:113–123.
283. Masurel-Paulet A, Haan E, Thompson EM, et al. Lung disease associated with periventricular nodular heterotopia and an FLNA mutation. *Eur J Med Genet* 2011;54:25–28.
284. Robertson SP. Filamin A: phenotypic diversity. *Curr Opin Gen Dev* 2005;15:301–307.
285. Lord A, Shapiro AJ, Saint-Martin C, et al. Filamin A mutation may be associated with diffuse lung disease mimicking bronchopulmonary dysplasia in premature newborns. *Respir Care* 2014;59:e171–e177.
286. Bejjani BA, Oberg KC, Wilkins I, et al. Prenatal ultrasonographic description and postnatal pathological findings in atelosteogenesis type 1. *Am J Med Genet* 1998;79:392–395.
287. Hunter AG, Carpenter BF. Atelosteogenesis I and boomerang dysplasia: a question of nosology. *Clin Genet* 1991;39:471–480.
288. Canki-Klain N, Stanescu V, Stanescu R, et al. Lethal short limb dwarfism with dysmorphic face, omphalocele and severe ossification defect: Piepkorn syndrome or severe "boomerang dysplasia"? *Ann Genet* 1992;35:129–133.
289. Irving MD, Chitty LS, Mansour S, et al. Chondrodysplasia punctata: a clinical, diagnostic and radiological review. *Clin Dysmorphol* 2008;17:229–241.
290. Waterham HR, Ebberink MS. Genetics and molecular basis of human peroxisome biogenesis disorders. *Biochim Biophys Acta* 2012;1822:1430–1441.
291. Porter FD, Herman GE. Malformation syndromes caused by disorders of cholesterol synthesis. *J Lipid Res* 2011;52:6–34.
292. Braverman NE, D'Agostino MD, Maclean GE. Peroxisome biogenesis disorders: biological, clinical and pathophysiological perspectives. *Dev Disabil Res Rev* 2013;17:187–196.
293. Rakheja D, Read CP, Hull D, et al. A severely affected female infant with x-linked dominant chondrodysplasia punctata: a case report and a brief review of the literature. *Pediatr Dev Pathol* 2007;10:142–148.
294. Canueto J, Girós M, Ciria S, et al. Clinical, molecular and biochemical characterization of nine Spanish families with Conradi-Hünermann-Happle syndrome: new insights into X-linked dominant chondrodysplasia punctate with a comprehensive review of the literature. *Br J Dermatol* 2012;166:830–838.
295. Hoang MP, Carder KR, Pandya AG, et al. Ichthyosis and keratotic follicular plugs containing dystrophic calcification in newborns: distinctive histopathologic features of x-linked dominant chondrodysplasia punctata (Conradi-Hunermann-Happle syndrome). *Am J Dermatopathol* 2004;26:53–58.
296. White AL, Modaff P, Holland-Morris F, et al. Natural history of rhizomelic chondrodysplasia punctata. *Am J Med Genet A* 2003;118A:332–342.
297. Erzen M, Stanescu R, Stanescu V, et al. Comparative histopathology of the growth cartilage in short-rib polydactyly syndromes type I and type III and in chondroectodermal dysplasia. *Ann Genet* 1988;31:144–150.
298. Elcioglu N, Hall CM. A lethal skeletal dysplasia with features of chondrodysplasia punctata and osteogenesis imperfecta: an example of Astley-Kendall dysplasia. Further delineation of a rare genetic disorder. *J Med Genet* 1998;35:505–507.
299. Khoshhal K, Letts RM. Orthopaedic manifestations of campomelic dysplasia. *Clin Orthop Relat Res* 2002;401:65–74.
300. Lazjuk GI, Shved IA, Cherstvoy ED, et al. Campomelic syndrome: concepts of the bowing and shortening in the lower limbs. *Teratology* 1987;35:1–8.
301. Gimovsky M, Rosa E, Tolbert T, et al. Campomelic dysplasia: case report and review. *J Perinatol* 2008;28:71–73.
302. Mansour S, Hall CM, Pembrey ME, et al. A clinical and genetic study of campomelic dysplasia. *J Med Genet* 1995;32:415–420.
303. Wada Y, Nishimura G, Nagai T, et al. Mutation analysis of SOX9 and single copy number variant analysis of the upstream region in eight patients with campomelic dysplasia and acampomelic campomelic dysplasia. *Am J Med Genet A* 2009;149A:2882–2885.
304. Pritchett J, Athwal V, Roberts N, et al. Understanding the role of SOX9 in acquired diseases: lessons from development. *Trends Mol Med* 2011;17:166–174.
305. Chen SY, Lin SJ, Tsai LP, et al. Sex-reversed acampomelic campomelic dysplasia with a homozygous deletion mutation in SOX9 gene. *Urology* 2012;79:908–911.
306. Hong JR, Barber M, Scott CI, et al. 3-year-old phenotypic female with campomelic dysplasia and bilateral gonadoblastoma. *J Pediatr Surg* 1995;30:1735–1737.
307. Unger S, Scherer G, Superti-Furga A. Campomelic dysplasia. In: Pagon RA, Adam MP, Ardinger HH, et al. eds. *GeneReview*[Internet]. Seattle, WA: University of Washington, Seattle, 1993–2015.
308. Akawi NA, Ali BR, Al-Gazal L. Stüve-Wiedemann syndrome and related bent bone dysplasias. *Clin Genet* 2012;82:12–21.
309. Mikelonis D, Jorcyk CL, Tawara K, et al. Stüve-Wiedemann syndrome: LIFR and associated cytokines in clinical course and etiology. *Orphan J Rare Dis* 2014;9:34.
310. Yesil G, Lebre, AS, Santos SD, et al. Stüve-Wiedemann syndrome: is it underrecognized? *Am J Med Genet A* 2014;164A:2200–2205.
311. Raas-Rothschild A, Ergaz-Schaltiel Z, Bar-Ziv J, et al. Cardiovascular abnormalities associated with the Stüve-Wiedemann syndrome. *Am J Med Genet A* 2003;121A:156–158.
312. Nelson ME, Griffin GR, Innis JW, et al. Campomelic dysplasia: airway management in two patients and an update on clinical-molecular correlations in the head and neck. *Ann Otol Rhinol Laryngol* 2011;120:682–685.
313. Neben CL, Idoni B, Salva JE, et al. Bent bone dysplasia reveals nucleolar activity for FGFR2 in ribosomal DNA transcription. *Hum Mol Genet* 2014;23:5659–5671.
314. Collet C, Alessandri JL, Arnaud E, et al. Crouzon syndrome and Bent bone dysplasia associated with mutations at the same Tyr-381 residue in FGFR2 gene. *Clin Genet* 2014;85:598–599.
315. Shandilya R, Gadre KS, Sharma J, et al. Infantile cortical hyperostosis (caffey disease): a case report and review of the literature—where are we after 70 years? *J Oral Maxillofac Surg* 2013;71:1195–1201.
316. Nistala H, Mäkitie O, Jüppner H. Caffey disease: new perspectives on old questions. *Bone* 2014;60:246–251.
317. Kamoun-Goldrat A, Martinovic J, Saada J, et al. Prenatal cortical hyperostosis with COL1A1 gene mutation. *Am J Med Genet* 2008;146A:1820–1824.
318. Nemec SF, Rimoin DL, Lachman RS. Radiological aspects of prenatal-onset cortical hyperostosis [Caffey dysplasia]. *Eur J Radiol* 2012;81:e565–e572.
319. Navarre P, Pehlivanov I, Morin B. Recurrence of infantile cortical hyperostosis: a case report and review of the literature. *J Pediatr Orthop* 2013;33:e10–e17.
320. Oostra RJ, van der Harten JJ, Rijnders WP, et al. Blomstrand osteochondrodysplasia: three novel cases and histological evidence for heterogeneity. *Virchows Arch* 2000;436:28–35.
321. Duchatelet S, Ostergaard E, Cortes D, et al. Recessive mutations in PTHR1 cause contrasting skeletal dysplasias in Eiken and Blomstrand syndromes. *Hum Mol Genet* 2005;14:1–5.
322. Karaplis AC, He B, Nguyen MT, et al. Inactivating mutation in the human parathyroid hormone receptor type 1 gene in Blomstrand chondrodysplasia. *Endocrinology* 1998;139:5255–5258.
323. Segovia-Silvestre T, Neutzsky-Wulff AV, Sorensen MG, et al. Advances in osteoclast biology resulting in the study of osteopetrotic mutations. *Hum Genet* 2009;124:561–577.

324. Sobacchi C, Schultz A, Coxon FP, et al. Osteopetrosis: genetics, treatment and new insights into osteoclast function. *Nat Rev Endocrinol* 2013;9:522–536.
325. de Vernejoul MC, Schultz A, Kornak U. CLCN7-related osteopetrosis. In: Pagon RA, Adam MP, Ardinger HH, et al., eds. *GeneReviews*®[Internet]. Seattle, WA: University of Washington, Seattle, 1993–2014.
326. Stark Z, Savarirayan R. Osteopetrosis. *Orphanet J Rare Dis* 2009;4:5.
327. Villa A, Guerrini MM, Cassani B, et al. Infantile malignant, autosomal recessive osteopetrosis: the rich and the poor. *Calcif Tissue Int* 2009;84:1–12.
328. Mazzolari E, Forino C, Razza A, et al. A single-center experience in 20 patients with infantile malignant osteopetrosis. *Am J Hematol* 2009; 84:473–479.
329. Del Fattore A, Peruzzi B, Rucci N, et al. Clinical, genetic, and cellular analysis of 49 osteopetrotic patients: implications for diagnosis and treatment. *J Med Genet* 2006;43:315–325.
330. Waguespack SG, Hui SL, Dimeglio LA, et al. Autosomal dominant osteopetrosis: clinical severity and natural history of 94 subjects with a chloride channel 7 gene mutation. *J Clin Endocrinol Metab* 2007;92:771–778.
331. Helfrich MH, Aronson DC, Everts V, et al. Morphologic features of bone in human osteopetrosis. *Bone* 1991;12:411–419.
332. Bollerslev J, Henriksen K, Nielsen MF, et al. Autosomal dominant osteopetrosis revisited: lessons from recent studies. *Eur J Endocrinol* 2013;169:R39–R57.
333. Xing M, Parker EI, Moreno-De-Luca A, et al. Radiological and clinical characterization of the lysosomal storage disorders: non-lipid disorders. *Br J Radiol* 2014;87:20120467 (Correction Br J Radiol 2014; 87: 20149002).
334. Coutinho MF, Matos L, Alves S. From bedside to cell biology: a century of history on lysosomal dysfunction. *Gene* 2015;555:50–58.
335. Staretz-Chacham O, Lang TC, LaMarca ME, et al. Lysosomal storage disorders in the newborn. *Pediatrics* 2009;123:1191–1207.
336. Schultz ML, Tecedor L, Chang M, et al. Clarifying lysosomal storage diseases. *Trends Neurosci* 2011;34:401–410.
337. Aldenhoven M, Sakkers RJ, Boelens J, et al. Musculoskeletal manifestations of lysosomal storage disorders. *Ann Rheum Dis* 2009;68:1659–1665.
338. Pastores GM. Musculoskeletal complications encountered in the lysosomal storage disorders. *Best Pract Res Clin Rheumatol* 2008; 22:937–947.
339. Buchino JJ, Vogler C, Dimmick JE. Anatomical pathology and lysosomal storage diseases. In: Applegarth DA, Dimmick JE, Hall JG, eds. *Organelle Diseases*. London, UK: Chapman and Hall, 2007:117–142.
340. Dimmick JE. Pathology of peroxisomal disorders. In: Applegarth DA, Dimmick JE, Hall JG, eds. *Organelle Diseases*. London, UK: Chapman and Hall, 1997:211–232.
341. Silveri CP, Kaplan FS, Fallon MD, et al. Hurler syndrome with special reference to histologic abnormalities of the growth plate. *Clin Orthop Relat Res* 1991;(269):305–311.
342. Lacombe D, Germain DP. [Genetic aspects of mucopolysaccharidoses]. *Arch Pediatr* 2014;21(Suppl 1):S22–S26.
343. Muenzer J. Overview of the mucopolysaccharidoses. *Rheumatology (Oxford)* 2011;50(Suppl 5):v4–v12.
344. Vieira T, Schwartz I, Munoz V, et al. Mucopolysaccharidoses in Brazil: what happens from birth to biochemical diagnosis? *Am J Med Genet A* 2008;146A:1741–1747.
345. Braunlin EA, Harmatz PR, Scarpa M, et al. Cardiac disease in patients with mucopolysaccharidosis: presentation, diagnosis and management. *J Inherit Metab Dis* 2011;34:1183–1197.
346. Braunlin E, Orchard PJ, Whitley CB, et al. Unexpected coronary artery findings in mucopolysaccharidosis. Report of four cases and literature review. *Cardiovasc Pathol* 2014;23:145–151.
347. Muhlebach MS, Wooten W, Muenzer J. Respiratory manifestations in mucopolysaccharidoses. *Paediatr Res Rev* 2011;12:133–138.
348. McClure J, Smith PS, Sorby-Adams G, et al. The histological and ultrastructural features of the epiphyseal plate in Morquio type A syndrome (mucopolysaccharidosis type IVA). *Pathology* 1986;18:217–221.
349. Guggenbuhl P, Grosbois B, Chalés G. Gaucher disease. *Joint Bone Spine* 2008;75:116–124.
350. Elstein D, Abrahamov A, Dweck A, et al. Gaucher disease: pediatric concerns. *Paediatr Drugs* 2002;4:417–426.
351. Chen M, Wang J. Gaucher disease. Review of the literature. *Arch Pathol Lab Med* 2008;132:851–853.
352. Baris HN, Cohen IJ, Mistry PK. Gaucher disease: the metabolic defect, pathophysiology, phenotypes and natural history. *Pediatr Endocrinol Rev* 2014;12(Suppl 1):72–81.
353. Gerards AH, Winia WP, Westerga J, et al. Destructive joint disease in alpha-mannosidosis. A case report and review of the literature. *Clin Rheumatol* 2004;23:40–42.
354. Malm D, Nilssen O. Alpha-mannosidosis. *Orphanet J Rare Dis* 2008;3:21.
355. Stevenson DA, Steiner RD. Skeletal abnormalities in lysosomal storage diseases. *Pediatr Endocrinol Rev* 2013;10(Suppl 2):406–416.
356. Haddad FS, Jones DH, Vellodi A, et al. Carpal tunnel syndrome in the mucopolysaccharidoses and mucolipidoses. *J Bone Joint Surg Br* 1997;79:576–582.
357. Greenspan A, Azouz EM. Bone dysplasia series. Melorheostosis: review and update. *Can Assoc Radiol J* 1999;50:324–330.
358. Jain VK, Arya RK, Bharadwaj M, et al. Melorheostosis: clinicopathological features, diagnosis, and management. *Orthopedics* 2009;32:512.
359. Campbell CJ, Papademetriou T, Bonfiglio M. Melorheostosis. A report of the clinical, roentgenographic, and pathological findings in fourteen cases. *J Bone Joint Surg Am* 1968;50:1281–1304.
360. Ihde LL, Forrester DM, Gottsegen CJ, et al. Sclerosing bone dysplasias: review and differentiation from other causes of osteosclerosis. *Radiographics* 2011;31:1865–1882.
361. Ippolito V, Mirra JM, Motta C, et al. Case report 771: melorheostosis in association with desmoid tumor. *Skeletal Radiol* 1993;22:284–288.
362. Faden MA, Krakow D, Ezgu F, et al. The Erlenmeyer flask bone deformity in the skeletal dysplasias. *Am J Med Genet A* 2009;149A:1334–1345.
363. Verloes A, Lesenfants S, Barr M, et al. Fronto-otopalatodigital osteodysplasia: clinical evidence for a single entity encompassing Melnick-Needles syndrome, otopalatodigital syndrome types 1 and 2, and frontometaphyseal dysplasia. *Am J Med Genet* 2000;90:407–422.
364. Hashmi SK, Allen C, Klaassen R, et al. Comparative analysis of Shwachman-Diamond syndrome to other inherited bone marrow failure syndromes and genotype-phenotype correlation. *Clin Genet* 2011;79:448–458.
365. Chung NG, Kim M. Current insights into inherited bone marrow failure syndromes. *Korean J Pediatr* 2014;57:337–344.
366. McLennan TW, Steinbach HL. Schwachman's syndrome: the broad spectrum of bony abnormalities. *Radiology* 1974;112:167–173.
367. Nishimura G, Nakashima E, Hirose Y, et al. The Shwachman-Bodian-Diamond syndrome gene mutations cause a neonatal form of spondylometaphysial dysplasia (SMD) resembling SMD Sedaghatian type. *J Med Genet* 2007;44:e73.
368. Makitie O, Marttinen E, Kaitila I. Skeletal growth in cartilage-hair hypoplasia. A radiological study of 82 patients. *Pediatr Radiol* 1992;22:434–439.
369. Makitie O, Sulisalo T, de la Chapelle A, et al. Cartilage-hair hypoplasia. *J Med Genet* 1995;32:39–43.
370. Thiel CT, Rauch A. The molecular basis of the cartilage-hair hypoplasia-anauxetic dysplasia spectrum. *Best Pract Res Clin Endocrinol Metab* 2011;25:131–142.
371. Kwan A, Manning MA, Zollars LK, et al. Marked variability in the radiographic features of cartilage-hair hypoplasia: case report and review of the literature. *Am J Med Genet A* 2012;158A:2911–2916.
372. Crahes M, Saugier-Veber P, Patrier S, et al. Foetal presentation of cartilage hair hypoplasia with extensive granulomatous inflammation. *Eur J Med Genet* 2013;56:365–370.
373. McCann LJ, McPartland J, Barge D, et al. Phenotypic variations of cartilage hair hypoplasia: granulomatous skin inflammation and severe T cell immunodeficiency as initial clinical presentation in otherwise well child with short stature. *J Clin Immunol* 2014;34:42–48.
374. Park H, Hong S, Cho SI, et al. Case of mild Schmid-type metaphyseal chondrodysplasia with novel sequence variation involving an unusual mutational site of the COL10A1 gene. *Eur J Med Genet* 2015;58:175–179.

375. Jesus AA, Goldbach Mansky R. IL-1 blockade in autoinflammatory syndromes. *Annu Rev Med* 2014;65:223–244.
376. Rigante D, Vitale A, Lucherini OM, et al. The hereditary autoinflammatory disorders uncovered. *Autoimmun Rev* 2014;13:892–900.
377. Goldbach-Mansky R. Current status of understanding the pathogenesis and management of patients with NOMID/CINCA. *Curr Rheumatol Rep* 2011;13:123–131.
378. Federici S, Gattorno M. A practical approach to the diagnosis of autoinflammatory diseases in childhood. *Best Practice Res Clin Rheumatol* 2014;28:263–276.
379. Levy R, Gérard L, Keummerle-Deschner J, et al. Phenotypic and genotypic characteristics of cryopyrin-associated periodic syndrome: a series of 136 patients from the Eurofever Registry. *Ann Rheum Dis* 2014 Jul 18 [Epub ahead of print].
380. Costa-Reis P, Sullivan KE. Chronic recurrent multifocal osteomyelitis. *J Clin Immunol* 2013;33:1043–1056.
381. Hedrich CM, Hofmann SR, Pablik J, et al. Autoinflammatory bone disorders with special focus on chronic recurrent multifocal osteomyelitis (CRMO). *Pediatric Rheumatol Online J* 2013;11:47.
382. Garcia Segarra G, Mittaz L, Campos-Xavier AB, et al. The diagnostic challenge of progressive pseudorheumatoid dysplasia (PPRD): a review of clinical features, radiographic features, and WISP3 mutations in 63 affected individuals. *Am J Med Genet C Semin Med Genet* 2012;160C:217–219.
383. Pohanka M, Pejchal J, Snopkova S, et al. Ascorbic acid: an old player with a broad impact on body physiology including oxidative stress suppression and immunomodulation: a review. *Mini Rev Med Chem* 2012;12:35–43.
384. Pailhous S, Lamoureux S, Caietta E, et al. [Scurvy, an old disease still in the news: two case reports]. *Arch Pediatr* 2015;22:63–65.
385. Duggan CP, Westra SJ, Rosenberg AE. Case records of the Massachusetts General Hospital. Case 23-2007. A 9-year-old boy with bone pain, rash, and gingival hypertrophy. *N Eng J Med* 2007;357:392–400.
386. Elder CJ, Bishop NJ. Rickets. *Lancet* 2014;383:1665–1676.
387. Shore RM, Chesney RW. Rickets: part I. *Pediatr Radiol* 2013;43:140–151.
388. Shore RM, Chesney RW. Rickets: part II. *Pediatr Radiol* 2013;43:152–172.
389. Bhowmick SK, Johnson KR, Rettig KR. Rickets caused by vitamin D deficiency in breast-fed infants in the southern United States. *Am J Dis Child* 1991;145:127–130.
390. Marie PJ, Pettifor JM, Ross FP, et al. Histological osteomalacia due to dietary calcium deficiency in children. *N Engl J Med* 1982;307:584–588.
391. Holick MF. Resurrection of vitamin D deficiency and rickets. *J Clin Invest* 2006;116:2062–2072.
392. Iver P, Diamond F. Detecting disorders of vitamin D deficiency in children: an update. *Adv Pediatr* 2013;60:89–106.
393. Carey DE, Drezner MK, Hamdan JA, et al. Hypophosphatemic rickets/osteomalacia in linear sebaceous nevus syndrome: a variant of tumor-induced osteomalacia. *J Pediatr* 1986;109:994–1000.
394. Reyes-Mugica M, Arnsmeier SL, Backeljauw PF, et al. Phosphaturic mesenchymal tumor-induced rickets. *Pediatr Dev Pathol* 2000;3:61–69.
395. Oppenheimer SJ, Snodgrass GJ. Neonatal rickets. Histopathology and quantitative bone changes. *Arch Dis Child* 1980;55:945–949.
396. Teitelbaum SL. Pathological manifestations of osteomalacia and rickets. *Clin Endocrinol Metab* 1980;9:43–62.
397. Ayoub DM, Hyman C, Cohen M, et al. A critical review of the classic metaphyseal lesion: traumatic or metabolic? *AJR Am J Roentgenol* 2014;202:185–196.
398. Perez-Rossello JM, McDonald AG, Rosenberg AE, et al. Absence of rickets in infants with fatal abusive head trauma and classic metaphyseal lesions. *Radiology* 2015;275:141784.
399. Ogden JA, Ganey T, Light TR, et al. The pathology of acute chondro-osseous injury in the child. *Yale J Biol Med* 1993;66:219–233.
400. Schlosser K, Schmitt CP, Bartholomaeus JE, et al. Parathyroidectomy for renal hyperparathyroidism in children and adolescents. *World J Surg* 2008;32:801–806.
401. Wesseling-Perry K. Bone disease in pediatric chronic kidney disease. *Pediatr Nephrol* 2013;28:569–576.
402. Kemper MJ, van Husen M. Renal osteodystrophy in children: pathogenesis, diagnosis and treatment. *Curr Opin Pediatr* 2014;26:180–186.
403. Mallet E. Primary hyperparathyroidism in neonates and childhood. The French experience (1984–2004). *Horm Res* 2008;69:180–188.
404. Belcher R, Matrailer AM, Bodenner DL, et al. Characterization of hyperparathyroidism in youth and adolescents: a literature review. *Int J Pediatr Otorhinolaryngol* 2013;77:318–322.
405. Levine MA. An update on the clinical and molecular characteristics of pseudohypoparathyroidism. *Curr Opin Endocrinol Diabetes Obes* 2012;19:443–451.
406. Mantovani G, Elli FM, Spada A. GNAS epigenetic defects and pseudohypoparathyroidism: time for a new classification? *Horm Metab Res* 2012;44:716–723.
407. Adegbite NS, Xu M, Kaplan FS, et al. Diagnostic and mutational spectrum of progressive osseous heteroplasia (POH) and other forms of GNAS-based heterotopic ossification. *Am J Med Genet A* 2008;146A:1788–1796.
408. Schimmel RJ, Pasmans SG, Xu M, et al. GNAS-associated disorders of cutaneous ossification: two different clinical presentations. *Bone* 2009;46(3):868–872.
409. Pignolo RJ, Ramaswamy G, Fong JT, et al. Progressive osseous heteroplasia: diagnosis, treatment, and prognosis. *Appl Clin Genet* 2015;8:37–48.
410. David-Vizcarra G, Briody J, Ault J, et al. The natural history and osteodystrophy of mucolipidosis types II and III. *J Paediatr Child Health* 2010;46:316–322.
411. Unger S, Paul DA, Nino MC, et al. Mucolipidosis II presenting as severe neonatal hyperparathyroidism. *Eur J Pediatr* 2005;164:236–243.
412. Cochat P, Rumsby G. Primary hyperoxaluria. *N Engl J Med* 2013;369:649–658.
413. El Hage S, Ghanem I, Baradhi A, et al. Skeletal features of primary hyperoxaluria type 1, revisited. *J Child Orthop* 2008;2:205–210.
414. Orazi C, Picca S, Schingo PM, et al. Oxalosis in primary hyperoxaluria in infancy. Report of a case in a 3-month-old baby. Follow-up for 3 years and review of literature. *Skeletal Radiol* 2009;38:387–391.
415. Bacchetta J, Boivin G, Cochat P. Bone impairment in primary hyperoxaluria: a review. *Pediatr Nephrol* 2015; Jan 29 [Epub ahead of print].
416. Vlychou M, Athanasou NA. Radiological and pathological diagnosis of paediatric bone tumours and tumour-like lesions. *Pathology* 2008;40:196–216.
417. Stiller CA, Bielack SS, Jundt G, et al. Bone tumours in European children and adolescents, 1978–1997. Report from the Automated Childhood Cancer Information System project. *Eur J Cancer* 2006;42:2124–2135.
418. van den Berg H, Kroon HM, Slaar A, et al. Incidence of biopsy-proven bone tumors in children: a report based on the Dutch pathology registration "PALGA." *J Pediatr Orthop* 2008;28:29–35.
419. Mirabello L, Troisi RJ, Savage SA. Osteosarcoma incidence and survival rates from 1973 to 2004: data from the Surveillance, Epidemiology, and End Results Program. *Cancer* 2009;115:1531–1543.
420. Kozlowski K, Beluffi G, Cohen DH, et al. Primary bone tumours in infants. Short literature review and report of 10 cases. *Pediatr Radiol* 1985;15:359–367.
421. Maygarden SJ, Askin FB, Siegal GP, et al. Ewing sarcoma of bone in infants and toddlers. A clinicopathologic report from the Intergroup Ewing's Study. *Cancer* 1993;71:2109–2118.
422. De loris MA, Prete A, Cozza R, et al. Ewing sarcoma of the bone in children under 6 years of age. *PLoS One* 2013;8(1):e53223.
423. Estrada-Villasenor E, Delgado Cedillo EA, et al. Frequency of bone neoplasms in children. *Acta Ortop Mex* 2008;22:238–242.
424. Ottaviani G, Jaffe N. The epidemiology of osteosarcoma. *Cancer Treat Res* 2009;152:3–13.
425. Worch J, Matthay KK, Neuhaus J, et al. Ethnic and radical differences in patients with Ewing sarcoma. *Cancer* 2010;116:983–988.
426. Eyre R, Feltbower RG, Mubwandarikwa E, et al. Epidemiology of bone tumours in children and young adults. *Pediatr Blood Cancer* 2009;53:941–952.

427. Fletcher CDM, Bridge JA, Hogendoorn PCW, et al., eds. *WHO classification of Tumours, Soft Tissue and Bone*, 4th ed. Lyon, France: IARC Press, 2013.
428. Messerschmitt PJ, Garcia RM, Abdul-Karim FW, et al. Osteosarcoma. *J Am Acad Orthop Surg* 2009;17:515–527.
429. Picci P. Osteosarcoma (osteogenic sarcoma). *Orphanet J Rare Dis* 2007;2:6.
430. Daw NC, Mahmoud HH, Meyer WH, et al. Bone sarcomas of the head and neck in children: the St Jude Children's Research Hospital experience. *Cancer* 2000;88:2172–2180.
431. Gadwal SR, Gannon FH, Fanburg-Smith JC, et al. Primary osteosarcoma of the head and neck in pediatric patients: a clinicopathologic study of 22 cases with a review of the literature. *Cancer* 2001;91:598–605.
432. Huh WW, Holsinger FC, Levy A, et al. Osteosarcoma of the jaw in children and young adults. *Head Neck* 2012;34:981–984.
433. Ramo BA, Kyriakos M, McDonald DJ. Case reports; osteosarcoma without radiographic evidence of tumor. *Clin Orthopaedics Related Res* 2006;442:267–272.
434. Klein MJ, Siegal GP. Osteosarcoma. Anatomic and histologic variants. *Am J Clin Pathol* 2006;125:555–581.
435. Staals EL, Bacchini P, Bertoni F. High-grade surface osteosarcoma: a review of 25 cases from the Rizzoli Institute. *Cancer* 2008;112:1592–1599.
436. Wokcik JB, Bellizzi AM, Dal Cin P, et al. Primary sclerosing epithelioid fibrosarcoma of bone: analysis of a series. *Am J Surg Pathol* 2014;38:1538–1544.
437. Raoux D, Péoc'h M, Pedeutour F, et al. Primary epithelioid sarcoma of bone: report of a unique case, with immunohistochemical and fluorescent in situ hybridization confirmation of INI1 deletion. *Am J Surg Pathol* 2009;33:954–958.
438. Deyrub AT, Montag AG. Epithelioid and epithelial neoplasms of bone. *Arch Pathol Lab Med* 2007;131:205–216.
439. Franchi A, Palomba A, Roselli G, et al. Primary juxtacortical myoepithelioma/mixed tumor of the bone: a report of 3 cases with clinicopathologic, immunohistochemical, ultrastructural, and molecular characterization. *Hum Pathol* 2013;44:566–577.
440. Cozza R, Devito R, De loris MA, et al. Epithelioid osteosarcoma of the jaw. *Pediatr Blood Cancer* 2009;52:877–879.
441. Weiss A, Khoury JD, Hoffer FA, et al. Telangiectatic osteosarcoma: the St. Jude Children's Research Hospital's experience. *Cancer* 2007;109:1627–1637.
442. Salunke AA, Chen Y, Tan JH, et al. Does a pathological fracture affect the prognosis in patients with osteosarcoma of the extremities? A systematic review and meta-analysis. *Bone Joint J* 2014;96-B:1396–1403.
443. Nakajima H, Sim FH, Bond JR, et al. Small cell osteosarcoma of bone. Review of 72 cases. *Cancer* 1997;79:2095–2106.
444. Righi A, Gambarotti M, Longo S, et al. Small cell osteosarcoma: clinicopathologic, immunohistochemical, and molecular analysis of 36 cases. *Am J Surg Pathol* 2015;39(5):691–699.
445. Papathanassiou ZG, Alberghini M, Thiesse P, et al. Parosteal osteosarcoma mimicking osteochondroma: a radio-histologic approach on two cases. *Clin Sarcoma Res* 2011;1:2.
446. Hang JF, Chen PC. Parosteal osteosarcoma. *Arch Pathol Lab Med* 2014;138:694–699.
447. Righi A, Gambarotti M, Benini S, et al. MDM2 and CDK4 expression in periosteal osteosarcoma. *Hum Pathol* 2015;46:549–553.
448. Yoshida A, Ushiku T, Motoi T, et al. MDM2 and CDK4 immunohistochemical coexpression in high-grade osteosarcoma: correlation with a dedifferentiated subtype. *Am J Surg Pathol* 2012;36:423–431.
449. Cesari M, Alberghini M, Vanel D, et al. Periosteal osteosarcoma: a single-institution experience. *Cancer* 2011;117:1731–1735.
450. Grimer RJ, Bielack S, Flege S, et al. Periosteal osteosarcoma—a European review of outcome. *Eur J Cancer* 2005;41:2806–2811.
451. Choong PF, Pritchard DJ, Rock MG, et al. Low grade central osteogenic sarcoma. A long-term followup of 20 patients. *Clin Orthop Relat Res* 1996:(322):198–206.
452. Kurt AM, Unni KK, McLeod RA, et al. Low-grade intraosseous osteosarcoma. *Cancer* 1990;65:1418–1428.
453. Malhas AM, Sumathi VP, James SL, et al. Low-grade central osteosarcoma: a difficult condition to diagnose. *Sarcoma* 2012;2012:764796.
454. Dujardin F, Binh MB, Bouvier C, et al. MDM2 and CDK4 immunohistochemistry is a valuable tool in the differential diagnosis of low-grade osteosarcomas and other primary fibro-osseous lesions of the bone. *Mod Pathol* 2011;24:624–637.
455. Carter JM, Inwards CY, Jin L, et al. Activating GNAS mutations in parosteal osteosarcoma. *Am J Surg Pathol* 2014;38:402–409.
456. Blasius S, Link TM, Hillmann A, et al. Intracortical low grade osteosarcoma. A unique case and review of the literature on intracortical osteosarcoma. *Gen Diagn Pathol* 1996;141:273–278.
457. Kaste SC, Fuller CE, Saharia A, et al. Pediatric surface osteosarcoma: clinical, pathologic, and radiologic features. *Pediatr Blood Cancer* 2006;47:152–162.
458. Bieling P, Rehan N, Winkler P, et al. Tumor size and prognosis in aggressively treated osteosarcoma. *J Clin Oncol* 1996;14:848–858.
459. Lee JA, Kim MS, Kim DH, et al. Relative tumor burden predicts metastasis-free survival in pediatric osteosarcoma. *Pediatr Blood Cancer* 2008;50:195–200.
460. Rytting M, Pearson P, Raymond AK. Osteosarcoma in preadolescent patients. *Clin Orthop Relat Res* 2000;373:39–50.
461. van den Berg H, Dirksen U, Ranft A, et al. Ewing tumors in infants. *Pediatr Blood Cancer* 2008;50:761–764.
462. Ognjanovic S, Olivier M, Bergemann TL, et al. Sarcomas in TP53 germline mutation carriers: a review of the IARC TP53 database. *Cancer* 2012;118:1387–1396.
463. Larizza L, Roversi G, Volpi L. Rothmund-Thomson syndrome. *Orphanet J Rare Dis* 2010;5:2.
464. Siitonen HA, Sotkasiira J, Biervliet M, et al. The mutation spectrum in RECQL4 diseases. *Eur J Hum Genet* 2009;17:151–158.
465. Ottaviani G, Jaffe N. The etiology of osteosarcoma. *Cancer Treat Res* 2009;152:15–32.
466. Lipton JM, Federman N, Khabbaze Y, et al. Osteogenic sarcoma associated with Diamond-Blackfan anemia: a report from the Diamond-Blackfan Anemia Registry. *J Pediatr Hematol Oncol* 2001;23:39–44.
467. Kaste SC, Pratt CB, Cain AM, et al. Metastases detected at the time of diagnosis of primary pediatric extremity osteosarcoma at diagnosis? Imaging features. *Cancer* 1999;86:1602–1608.
468. Kunze B, Bürkle S, Kluba T. Multifocal osteosarcoma in childhood. *Chir Organi Mov* 2009;93:27–31.
469. Jaffe N. Historical perspective on the introduction and use of chemotherapy for the treatment of osteosarcoma. *Adv Exp Med Biol* 2014;804:1–30.
470. Frassica FJ, Waltrip RL, Sponseller PD, et al. Clinicopathologic features and treatment of osteoid osteoma and osteoblastoma in children and adolescents. *Orthop Clin North Am* 1996;27:559–574.
471. Bettelli G, Tigani D, Picci P. Recurring osteoblastoma initially presenting as a typical osteoid osteoma. Report of two cases. *Skeletal Radiol* 1991;20:1–4.
472. Morton KS, Quenville NF, Beauchamp CP. Aggressive osteoblastoma. A case previously reported as a recurrent osteoid osteoma. *J Bone Joint Surg Br* 1989;71:428–431.
473. Chotel F, Franck F, Solla F, et al. Osteoid osteoma transformation into osteoblastoma: fact or fiction? *Orthop Traumatol Surg Res* 2012;98(6 Suppl):S98–S104.
474. Greenspan A. Benign bone-forming lesions: osteoma, osteoid osteoma, and osteoblastoma. Clinical, imaging, pathologic, and differential considerations. *Skeletal Radiol* 1993;22:485–500.
475. Virayavanich W, Singh R, O'Donnell RJ, et al. Osteoid osteoma of the femur in a 7-month-old infant treated with radiofrequency ablation. *Skeletal Radiol* 2010;39:1145–1149.
476. de Chadarevian JP, Katsetos CD, Pascasio JM, et al. Histological study of osteoid osteoma's blood supply. *Pediatr Dev Pathol* 2007;10:358–368.
477. Boscainos PJ, Cousins GR, Kulshreshtha R, et al. Osteoid osteoma. *Orthopedics* 2013;36:792–800.
478. Klein MH, Shankman S. Osteoid osteoma: radiologic and pathologic correlation. *Skeletal Radiol* 1992;21:23–31.
479. Kransdorf MJ, Stull MA, Gilkey FW, et al. Osteoid osteoma. *Radiographics* 1991;11:671–696.

480. Farzan M, Ahangar P, Mazoochy H, et al. Osseous tumours of the hand: a review of 99 cases in 20 years. *Arch Bone Jt Surg* 2013;1:68–73.
481. Aynaci O, Turgutoglu O, Kerimoglu S, et al. Osteoid osteoma with a multicentric nidus: a case report and review of the literature. *Arch Orthop Trauma Surg* 2007;127:863–866.
482. Jones AC, Prihoda TJ, Kacher JE, et al. Osteoblastoma of the maxilla and mandible: a report of 24 cases, review of the literature, and discussion of its relationship to osteoid osteoma of the jaws. *Oral Surg Oral Med Oral Pathol Oral Radiol Endod* 2006;102:639–650.
483. Azouz EM, Kozlowski K, Marton D, et al. Osteoid osteoma and osteoblastoma of the spine in children. Report of 22 cases with brief literature review. *Pediatr Radiol* 1986;16:25–31.
484. Berry M, Mankin H, Gebhardt M, et al. Osteoblastoma: a 30-year study of 99 cases. *J Surg Oncol* 2008;98:179–183.
485. Trotta B, Fox MG. Benign osteoid-producing bone lesions: update on imaging and treatment. *Semin Musculoskelet Radiol* 2013;17:116–122.
486. Kroon HM, Schurmans J. Osteoblastoma: clinical and radiologic findings in 98 new cases. *Radiology* 1990;175:783–790.
487. Lucas DR, Unni KK, McLeod RA, et al. Osteoblastoma: clinicopathologic study of 306 cases. *Hum Pathol* 1994;25:117–134.
488. Kyriakos M, El-Khoury GY, McDonald DJ, et al. Osteoblastomatosis of bone. A benign, multifocal osteoblastic lesion, distinct from osteoid osteoma and osteoblastoma, radiologically simulating a vascular tumor. *Skeletal Radiol* 2007;36:237–247.
489. Green JT, Mills AM. Osteogenic tumors of bone. *Semin Diagn Pathol* 2014;31:21–29 [Epub ahead of print].
490. Papagelopoulos PJ, Galanis EC, Sim FH, et al. Clinicopathologic features, diagnosis, and treatment of osteoblastoma. *Orthopedics* 1999;22:244–247.
491. Oliveira CR, Mendonca BB, Camargo OP, et al. Classical osteoblastoma, atypical osteoblastoma, and osteosarcoma: a comparative study based on clinical, histological, and biological parameters. *Clinics (Sao Paulo)* 2007;62:167–174.
492. Angervall L, Persson S, Stenman G, et al. Large cell, epithelioid, telangiectatic osteoblastoma: a unique pseudosarcomatous variant of osteoblastoma. *Hum Pathol* 1999;30:1254–1259.
493. Bertoni F, Unni KK, Lucas DR, et al. Osteoblastoma with cartilaginous matrix. An unusual morphologic presentation in 18 cases. *Am J Surg Pathol* 1993;17:69–74.
494. Bertoni F, Bacchini P, Donati D, et al. Osteoblastoma-like osteosarcoma. The Rizzoli Institute experience. *Mod Pathol* 1993;6:707–716.
495. Atesok KI, Alman BA, Schemitsch EH, et al. Osteoid osteoma and osteoblastoma. *J Am Acad Orthop Surg* 2011;19:678–689.
496. Earhart J, Wellman D, Donaldson J, et al. Radiofrequency ablation in the treatment of osteoid osteoma: results and complications. *Pediatr Radiol* 2013;43:814–819.
497. Barlow E, Davies AM, Cool WP, et al. Osteoid osteoma and osteoblastoma: novel histological and immunohistochemical observations as evidence for a single entity. *J Clin Pathol* 2013;66:768–774.
498. Conner JR, Hornick JL. SATB2 is a novel maker of osteoblastic differentiation in bone and soft tissue tumours. *Histopathology* 2013;63:36–49.
499. Kallen ME, Sanders ME, Gonzalez AL, et al. Nuclear p63 expression in osteoblastic tumors. *Tumour Biol* 2012;33:1639–1644.
500. Kaplan I, Nicolaou Z, Hatuel D, et al. Solitary central osteoma of the jaws: a diagnostic dilemma. *Oral Surg Oral Med Pathol Oral Radiol Endod* 2008;106:e22–e29.
501. Herford AS, Stoffella E, Tandon R. Osteomas involving the facial skeleton: a report of 2 cases and review of the literature. *Oral Surg Oral Med Oral Pathol Oral Radiol* 2013;115:e1–e6.
502. Endo M, Tsukahara K, Nakamura K, et al. A case of giant osteoma in the middle turbinate of a child. *Jpn Clin Med* 2014;5:15–18.
503. McHugh JB, Mukherji SK, Lucas DR. Sino-orbital osteoma: a clinicopathologic study of 45 surgically treated cases with emphasis on tumors with osteoblastoma-like features. *Arch Pathol Lab Med* 2009;133:1587–1593.
504. Halawi AM, Maley JE, Robinson RA, et al. Craniofacial osteoma: clinical presentation and patterns of growth. *Am J Rhinol Allergy* 2013;27:128–133.
505. Sayan NB, Ucok C, Karasu HA, et al. Peripheral osteoma of the oral and maxillofacial region: a study of 35 new cases. *J Oral Maxillofac Surg* 2002;60:1299–1301.
506. El-Mofty SK. Fibro-osseous lesions of the craniofacial skeleton: an update. *Head Neck Pathol* 2014;8:432–444.
507. Brannon RB, Fowler CB. Benign fibro-osseous lesions: a review of current concepts. *Adv Anat Pathol* 2001;8:126–143.
508. Mehta D, Clifton N, McClelland L, et al. Paediatric fibro-osseous lesions of the nose and paranasal sinuses. *Int J Pediatr Otorhinolaryngol* 2006;70:193–199.
509. Regezi JA. Odontogenic cysts, odontogenic tumors, fibroosseous, and giant cell lesions of the jaws. *Mod Pathol* 2002;15:331–341.
510. Slootweg PJ. Lesions of the jaws. *Histopathology* 2009;54:401–418.
511. El-Mofty S. Psammomatoid and trabecular juvenile ossifying fibroma of the craniofacial skeleton: two distinct clinicopathologic entities. *Oral Surg Oral Med Oral Pathol Oral Radiol Endod* 2002;93:296–304.
512. Phattarataratip E, Pholjaroen C, Tiranon P. A Clinicopathologic analysis of 207 cases of benign fibro-osseous lesions of the jaws. *Int J Surg Pathol* 2013;22:326–333.
513. Wenig BM, Vinh TN, Smirniotopoulos JG, et al. Aggressive psammomatoid ossifying fibromas of the sinonasal region: a clinicopathologic study of a distinct group of fibro-osseous lesions. *Cancer* 1995;76:1155–1165.
514. Figueiredo LM, de Oliveira TF, Paraguassú GM, et al. Psammomatoid juvenile ossifying fibroma: case study and a review. *Oral Maxillofac Surg* 2014;18:87–93.
515. Jackson MA, Hu MI, Perrier ND, et al. CDC73-related disorders. In: Pagon RA, Adam MP, Ardinger HH, et al., eds. *GeneReviews® [Internet]*. Seattle, WA: University of Washington, Seattle, 1993–2014.
516. Wang TT, Zhang R, Wang L, et al. Two cases of multiple ossifying fibromas in the jaws. *Diagn Pathol* 2014;9:75.
517. Haven CJ, Wong FK, van Dam EW, et al. A genotypic and histopathological study of a large Dutch kindred with hyperparathyroidism-jaw tumor syndrome. *J Clin Endocrinol Metab* 2000;85:1449–1454.
518. Herman TE, Siegel MJ, Sargar K. Gnathodiaphyseal dysplasia. *J Perinatol* 2014;34:412–414.
519. Mizuta K, Tsutsumi S, Inoue H, et al. Molecular characterization of GDD1/TMEM16E, the gene product responsible for autosomal dominant gnathodiaphyseal dysplasia. *Biochem Biophys Res Commun* 2007;357:126–132.
520. Mclnerney-Leo AM, Duncan EL, Leo PJ, et al. COL1A1 C-propeptide cleavage site mutation causes high bone mass, bone fragility and jaw lesions: a new cause of gnathodiaphyseal dysplasia. *Clin Genet* 2015;88(1):49–55.
521. Nakashima Y, Yamamuro T, Fujiwara Y, et al. Osteofibrous dysplasia (ossifying fibroma of long bones). A study of 12 cases. *Cancer* 1983;52:909–914.
522. Park YK, Unni KK, McLeod RA, et al. Osteofibrous dysplasia: clinicopathologic study of 80 cases. *Hum Pathol* 1993;24:1339–1347.
523. Bethapudi S, Ritchie DA, Macduff E, et al. Imaging in osteofibrous dysplasia, osteofibrous dysplasia-like adamantinoma, and classic adamantinoma. *Clin Radiol* 2014;69:200–208.
524. Cetinkaya M, Özkan H, Köksal N, et al. Neonatal osteofibrous dysplasia associated with pathological tibia fracture: a case report and review of the literature. *J Pediatr Orthop B* 2012;21:183–186.
525. Khanna M, Delaney D, Tirabosco R, et al. Osteofibrous dysplasia, osteofibrous dysplasia-like adamantinoma and adamantinoma: correlation of radiological imaging features with surgical histology and assessment of the use of radiology in contributing to needle biopsy diagnosis. *Skeletal Radiol* 2008;37:1077–1084.
526. Teo HE, Peh WC, Akhilesh M, et al. Congenital osteofibrous dysplasia associated with pseudoarthrosis of the tibia and fibula. *Skeletal Radiol* 2007; 36(Suppl 1):S7–S14.
527. Boyce AM, Collins MT. Fibrous dysplasia/McCune-Albright syndrome. In: Pagon RA, Adam MP, Ardinger HH, et al., eds. *GeneReviews® [Internet]*. Seattle, WA: University of Washington, Seattle, 1993–2014.
528. Collins MT, Singer FR, Eugster E. McCune-Albright syndrome and the extraskeletal manifestations of fibrous dysplasia. *Orphanet J Rare Dis* 2012;7(Suppl 1):S4.

529. Riddle ND, Bui MM. Fibrous dysplasia. *Arch Pathol Lab Med* 2013;137:134–138.
530. DiCaprio MR, Enneking WF. Fibrous dysplasia. Pathophysiology, evaluation, and treatment. *J Bone Joint Surg Am* 2005;87A:1848–1864.
531. Parekh SG, Donthineni-Rao R, Ricchetti E, et al. Fibrous dysplasia. *J Am Acad Orthop Surg* 2004;12:305–313.
532. Ippolito E, Bray EW, Corsi A, et al. Natural history and treatment of fibrous dysplasia of bone: a multicenter clinicopathologic study promoted by the European Pediatric Orthopaedic Society. *J Pediatr Orthop B* 2003;12:155–177.
533. Fattah A, Khechoyan D, Phillips JH. et al. Paediatric craniofacial fibrous dysplasia: the Hospital for Sick Children experience and treatment philosophy. *J Plast Reconstr Aesthet Surg* 2013;66:1346–1355.
534. De Mattos CD, Binitie O, Dormans JP. Pathological fractures in children. *Bone Joint Res* 2012;1:272–280.
535. Lietman SA, Levine MA. Fibrous dysplasia. *Pediatr Endocrinol Rev* 2013;10(Suppl 2):389–396.
536. Munksgaard PS, Salkus G, Iyer VV, et al. Mazabraud's syndrome: case report and literature review. *Acta Radiol Short Rep* 2013;2(4):2047981613492532.
537. Delfino LN, Fariello G, Quattrocchi CC, et al. Encephalocraniocutaneous lipomatosis (ECCL): neuroradiological findings in three patients and a new association with fibrous dysplasia. *Am J Med Genet* 2011;155A:1690–1696.
538. Kransdorf MJ, Moser RP Jr, Gilkey FW. Fibrous dysplasia. *Radiographics* 1990;10:519–537.
539. Dorfman HD, Ishida T, Tsuneyoshi M. Exophytic variant of fibrous dysplasia (fibrous dysplasia protuberans). *Hum Pathol* 1994;25:1234–1237.
540. Jee WH, Choi KH, Choe BY, et al. Fibrous dysplasia: MR imaging characteristics with radiopathologic correlation. *AJR Am J Roentgenol* 1996;167:1523–1527.
541. Voytek TM, Ro JY, Edeiken J, et al. Fibrous dysplasia and cemento-ossifying fibroma. A histologic spectrum. *Am J Surg Pathol* 1995;19:775–781.
542. Qu N, Yao W, Cui X, et al. Malignant transformation in monostotic fibrous dysplasia: clinical features, imaging features, outcomes in 10 patients, and review. *Medicine (Baltimore)* 2015;94:e369.
543. Bertoni F, Fernando Arias L, Alberghini M, et al. Fibrous dysplasia with degenerative atypia: a benign lesion potentially mistaken for sarcoma. *Arch Pathol Lab Med* 2004;128:794–796.
544. Kyriakos M, McDonald DJ, Sundaram M. Fibrous dysplasia with cartilaginous differentiation ("fibrocartilaginous dysplasia"): a review, with an illustrative case followed for 18 years. *Skeletal Radiol* 2004;33:51–62.
545. Kashima TG, Nishiyama T, Shimazu K, et al. Periostin, a novel marker of intramembranous ossification, is expressed in fibrous dysplasia and in c-Fos-overexpressing bone lesions. *Hum Pathol* 2009;40:226–237.
546. Muthusamy S, Subhawong T, Conway SA, et al. Locally aggressive fibrous dysplasia mimicking malignancy: a report of four cases and review of the literature. *Clin Orthop Relat Res* 2015;473:742–750.
547. Romeo S, Hogendoorn PCW, Dei Tos AP. Benign cartilaginous tumors of bone: from morphology to somatic and germ-line genetics. *Adv Anat Pathol* 2009;16:307–315.
548. Vylchou M, Athanasou NA. Radiological and pathological diagnosis of paediatric bone tumours and tumour-like lesions. *Pathology* 2008;40:196–216.
549. Richardson RR. Variants of exostosis of the bone in children. *Semin Roentgenol* 2005;40:380–390.
550. Wick MR, McDermott MB, Swanson PE. Proliferative, reparative, and reactive benign bone lesions that may be confused diagnostically with true osseous neoplasms. *Semin Diagn Pathol* 2014;31:66–88.
551. Verhoeven N, De Smet L. Focal fibrocartilaginous dysplasia in the upper limb: case report and review of the literature. *Genet Couns* 2013;24:373–379.
552. Kumar A, Khan SA, Sampath Kumar V, et al. Bizarre parosteal osteochondromatous proliferation (Nora's lesion) of phalanx in a child. *BMJ Case Rep* 2014;2014. pii: bcr2013201714.
553. Qasem SA, DeYoung BR. Cartilage-forming tumors. *Semin Diagn Pathol* 2014;31:10–20.
554. Florez B, Mönckeberg J, Castillo G, et al. Solitary osteochondroma long-term follow-up. *J Pediatr Orthop B* 2008;17:91–94.
555. Kim S, Lee S, Arsenault DA, et al. Pediatric rib lesions: a 13-year experience. *J Pediatr Surg* 2008;43:1781–1785.
556. Bahk WJ, Lee HY, Kang YK. Dysplasia epiphysealis hemimelica: radiographic and magnetic resonance imaging features and clinical outcome of complete and incomplete resection. *Skeletal Radiol* 2010;39:85–90.
557. Glick R, Khaldi L, Ptaszynski K, et al. Dysplasia epiphysealis hemimelica (Trevor disease): a rare developmental disorder of bone mimicking osteochondroma of long bones. *Hum Pathol* 2007;38:1265–1272.
558. Baumfeld D, Pires R, Macedo B, et al. Trevor disease (hemimelic epiphyseal displasia): 12-year follow-up case report and literature review. *Ann Med Health Sci Res* 2014;4(Suppl 1):S9–S13.
559. Bovée JV. Multiple osteochondromas. *Orphanet J Rare Dis* 2008;3:3.
560. Jennes I, Pedrini E, Zuntini M, et al. Multiple osteochondromas: mutation update and description of the multiple osteochondromas mutation database (MOdb). *Hum Mutat* 2009;30:1620–1627.
561. Maas SM, Shaw AC, Bikker H, et al. Phenotype and genotype in 103 patients with tricho-rhino-phalangeal syndrome. *Eur J Med Genet* 2015;58(5):279–292. pii: S1769-7212(15)00059-2.
562. Sonne-Holm E, Wong C, Sone-Holm S. Multiple cartilaginous exostoses and development of chondrosarcoma—a systematic review. *Dan Med J* 2014;61:A4895.
563. Pierz KA, Womer RB, Dormans JP. Pediatric bone tumors: osteosarcoma, Ewing's sarcoma, and chondrosarcoma associated with multiple hereditary osteochondromatosis. *J Pediatr Orthop* 2001;21:412–418.
564. Pierz KA, Stieber JR, Kusumi K, et al. Hereditary multiple exostoses: one center's experience and review of etiology. *Clin Orthop Relat Res* 2002;(401):49–59.
565. Romeo S, Hogendoorn P, Dei Tos AP. Benign cartilaginous tumors of bone from morphology to somatic and germ-line genetics. *Adv Anat Pathol* 2009;16:307–315.
566. Bierry G, Kerr DA, Nielsen GP, et al. Enchondromas in children: imaging appearance with pathological correlation. *Skeletal Radiol* 2012;41:1223–1229.
567. Superti-Furga A, Spranger J, Nishimura G. Enchondromatosis revisited: new classification with molecular basis. *Am J Med Genet C Semin Med Genet* 2012;160C:154–164.
568. Verdegaal SH, Bovée JV, Pansuriya TC, et al. Incidence, predictive factors, and prognosis of chondrosarcoma in patients with Ollier disease and Maffucci syndrome: an international multicenter study of 161 patients. *Oncologist* 2011;16:1771–1779.
569. Fisher TJ, Williams N, Morris L, et al. Metachondromatosis: more than just multiple osteochondromas. *J Child Orthop* 2013;7:455–464.
570. Matsushima K, Matsuura K, Kayo M, et al. Periosteal chondroma of the rib possibly associated with hemothorax: a case report. *J Pediatr Surg* 2006;41:E31–E33.
571. Karabakhtsian R, Heller D, Hameed M, et al. Periosteal chondroma of the rib-report of a case and literature review. *J Pediatr Surg* 2005;40:1505–1507.
572. Rabarin F, Laulan J, Saint Cast Y, et al. Focal periosteal chondroma of the hand: a review of 24 cases. *Orthop Traumatol Surg Res* 2014;100:617–620.
573. Sailhan F, Chotel F, Parot R. Chondroblastoma of bone in a pediatric population. *J Bone Joint Surg Am* 2009;91A:2159–2168.
574. Maheshwari AV, Jelinek JS, Song AJ, et al. Metaphyseal and diaphyseal chondroblastomas. *Skeletal Radiol* 2011;40:1563–1573.
575. Demertzis JL, Kyriakos M, Connolly S, et al. Surface-based chondroblastoma of the tibia: a unique presentation. *Skeletal Radiol* 2015;44(7):1045–1050.
576. Cates JM, Rosenberg AE, O'Connell JX, et al. Chondroblastoma-like chondroma of soft tissue: an underrecognized variant and its differential diagnosis. *Am J Surg Pathol* 2001;25:661–666.
577. Raparia K, Lin JW, Donovan D, et al. Chondroblastoma-like chondroma of soft tissue: report of the first case in the base of skull. *Ann Diagn Pathol* 2013;17:298–301.
578. Tan H, Yan M, Yue B, et al. Chondroblastoma of the patella with aneurysmal bone cyst. *Orthopedics* 2014;37:e87–e91.

579. Aycan OF, Vanel D, Righi A, et al. Chondroblastoma-like osteosarcoma: a case report and review. *Skeletal Radiol* 2015;44(6):869–873.
580. De Mattos CB, Angsanuntsukh C, Arkader A, et al. Chondroblastoma and chondromyxoid fibroma. *J Am Acad Orthop Surg* 2013;21:225–233.
581. Kyriakos M, Land VJ, Penning HL, et al. Metastatic chondroblastoma. Report of a fatal case with a review of the literature on atypical, aggressive, and malignant chondroblastoma. *Cancer* 1985;55:1770–1789.
582. Behjati S, Tarpey PS, Presneau N, et al. Distinct H3F3A and H3F3B driver mutations define chondroblastoma and giant cell tumor of bone. *Nat Genet* 2013;45:1479–1482.
583. Engels C, Priemel M, Moller G, et al. Chondromyxoid fibroma. Morphological variations, site, incidence, radiologic criteria and differential diagnosis. *Pathologe* 1999;20:224–229.
584. Wilson AJ, Kyriakos M, Ackerman LV. Chondromyxoid fibroma: Radiographic appearance in 38 cases and in a review of the literature. *Radiology* 1991;179:513–518.
585. Marin C, Gallego C, Manjon P, et al. Juxtacortical chondromyxoid fibroma: imaging findings in three cases and a review of the literature. *Skeletal Radiol* 1997;26:642–649.
586. Meredith CC, Kepes JJ, Johnson P, et al. Chondromyxoid fibroma of the upper thoracic spine in a 7-year-old patient. A case report and review of the literature. *Pediatr Neurosurg* 2004;40:190–195.
587. Wu CT, Inwards CY, O'Laughlin S, et al. Chondromyxoid fibroma of bone: a clinicopathologic review of 278 cases. *Hum Pathol* 1998; 29:438–446.
588. Amstalden EMI, Carvalho RB, Pacheco EM, et al. Chondromatous hamartoma of the chest wall: description of 3 new cases and literature review. *Int J Surg Pathol* 2006;14:119–126.
589. Taweevisit M, Trinavarat P, Thorner PS. Aspiration cytology of mesenchymal hamartoma of the chest wall: a case report and literature review. *Diagn Cytopathol* 2014;42:890–894.
590. Mosier SM, Patel T, Strenge K, et al. Chondrosarcoma in childhood: the radiologic and clinical conundrum. *J Radiol Case Rep* 2012;6:32–42.
591. Huvos AG, Marcove RC. Chondrosarcoma in the young. A clinicopathologic analysis of 79 patients younger than 21 years of age. *Am J Surg Pathol* 1987;11:930–942.
592. Young CL, Sim FH, Unni KK, et al. Chondrosarcoma of bone in children. *Cancer* 1990;66:1641–1648.
593. Nakashima Y, Unni KK, Shives TC, et al. Mesenchymal chondrosarcoma of bone and soft tissue. A review of 111 cases. *Cancer* 1986;57:2444–2453.
594. Bumpass DB, Kyriakos M, Ribin DA, et al. Myxoid chondrosarcoma of the phalanx with an EWS translocation: a case report and review of the literature. *J Bone Joint Surg Am* 2011;93:e23(1–7).
595. Nyquist KB, Panagopoulos I, Thorsen J, et al. Whole-transcriptome sequencing identifies novel IRF2BP2-CDX1 fusion gene brought about by translocation t(1;5)(q42;q32) in mesenchymal chondrosarcoma. *PLoS One* 2012;7:e49705.
596. Panagopoulos I, Gorunova L, Bjerkehagen B, et al. Chromosome aberrations and HEY1-NCOA2 fusion gene in a mesenchymal chondrosarcoma. *Oncol Rep* 2014;32:40–44.
597. Collins MS, Koyama T, Swee RG, et al. Clear cell chondrosarcoma: radiographic, computed tomographic, and magnetic resonance findings in 34 patients with pathologic correlation. *Skeletal Radiol* 2003;32:687–694.
598. Matsuura S, Ishii T, Endo M, et al. Epithelial and cartilaginous differentiation in clear cell chondrosarcoma. *Hum Pathol* 2013;44:237–243.
599. The Skeletal Lesions Interobserver Correlation among Expert Diagnosticians (SLICED) Study Group. Reliability of histopathologic and radiologic grading of cartilaginous neoplasms in long bones. *J Bone Joint Surg Am* 2007;89:2113–2123.
600. McDonald DJ, Sim FH, McLeod RA, et al. Giant-cell tumor of bone. *J Bone Joint Surg Am* 1986;68:235–242.
601. Picci P, Manfrini M, Zucchi V, et al. Giant-cell tumor of bone in skeletally immature patients. *J Bone Joint Surg Am* 1983;65:486–490.
602. Hoeffel JC, Galloy MA, Grignon Y, et al. Giant cell tumor of bone in children and adolescents. *Rev Rhum Engl Ed* 1996;63:618–623.
603. Krajca-Radcliffe JB, Thomas JR, Nicholas RW. Giant-cell tumor of bone: a rare entity in the hands of children. *J Pediatr Orthop* 1994;14:776–780.
604. Federman N, Brien EW, Narasimhan V, et al. Giant cell tumor of bone in childhood: clinical aspects and novel therapeutic targets. *Paediatr Drugs* 2014;16:21–28.
605. Lucas DR. Giant cell tumor of bone. *Surg Pathol* 2012;5:183–200.
606. Jacopin S, Viehweger E, Glard Y, et al. Fatal lung metastasis secondary to index finger giant cell tumor in an 8-year-old child. *Orthop Traumatol Surg Res* 2010;96:310–313.
607. Hammas N, Laila C, Youssef AL, et al. Can p63 serve a biomarker for giant cell tumor of bone? A Moroccan experience. *Diagn Pathol* 2012;7:130.
608. de Lange J, van den Akker HP. Clinical and radiological features of central giant-cell lesions of the jaw. *Oral Surg Oral Med Oral Pathol Oral Radiol Endod* 2005;99:464–470.
609. de Lange J, van den Akker HP, van den Berg H. Central giant cell granuloma of the jaw: a review of the literature with emphasis on therapy options. *Oral Surg Oral Med Oral Pathol Oral Radiol Endod* 2007;104:603–615.
610. Murphey MD, Nomikos GC, Flemming DJ, et al. From the archives of AFIP. Imaging of giant cell tumor and giant cell reparative granuloma of bone: radiologic-pathologic correlation. *Radiographics* 2001; 21:1283–1309.
611. Wold LE, Dobyns JH, Swee RG, et al. Giant cell reaction (giant cell reparative granuloma) of the small bones of the hands and feet. *Am J Surg Pathol* 1986;10:491–496.
612. Agaram NP, LeLoarer FV, Zhang L, et al. USP6 gene rearrangements occur preferentially in giant cell reparative granulomas of the hands and feet but not in gnathic location. *Hum Pathol* 2014;45:1147–1152.
613. Yamaguchi T, Dorfman HD, Eisig S. Cherubism: clinicopathologic features. *Skeletal Radiol* 1999;28:350–353.
614. Reichenberger EJ, Levine MA, Olsen BR, et al. The role of SH3PB2 in the pathophysiology of cherubism. *Orphanet J Rare Dis* 2012; 7(Suppl 1):S5.
615. Papadaki ME, Lietman SA, Levine MA, et al. Cherubism: best clinical practice. *Orphanet J Rare Disc* 2012;7(Suppl 1):S6.
616. Prescott T, Redfors M, Rustad CF, et al. Characterization of a Norwegian cherubism cohort; molecular genetic findings, oral manifestations and quality of life. *Eur J Med Genet* 2013;56:131–137.
617. Beneteau C, Cavé H, Moncla A, et al. SOS1 and PTPN11 mutations in five cases of Noonan syndrome with multiple giant cell lesions. *Eur J Hum Genet* 2009;17:1216–1221.
618. Hachach-Haram N, Gerarchi P, Benyon SL, et al. Multidisciplinary surgical management of cherubism complicated by neurofibromatosis type 1. *J Craniofac Surg* 2011;22:2318–2322.
619. Auclair PL, Cuenin P, Kratochvil FJ, et al. A clinical and histomorphologic comparison of the central giant cell granuloma and the giant cell tumor. *Oral Surg Oral Med Oral Pathol* 1988;66:197–208.
620. Dickson BC, Li SQ, Wunder JS, et al. Giant cell tumor of bone express p63. *Mod Pathol* 2008;21:369–375.
621. Chowdhury S, Aggarwal A, Mittal N, et al. Brown tumor of hyperparathyroidism involving craniomaxillofacial region: a rare case report and literature review. *Minerva Stomatol* 2013;62:343–348.
622. Niranjan B, Shashikiran N, Singla S, et al. Non-hereditary cherubism. *J Oral Maxillofac Pathol* 2014;18:84–88.
623. Orhan E, Erol S, Deren O, et al. Idiopathic bilateral central giant cell reparative granuloma of jaws: a case report and literature review. *Int J Pediatr Otorhinolaryngol* 2010;74:547–552.
624. Azouz EM, Kozlowski K. Osteoglophonic dysplasia: appearance and progression of multiple nonossifying fibromata. *Pediatr Radiol* 1997;27:75–78.
625. Leithner A, Windhager R, Lang S, et al. Aneurysmal bone cyst. A population based epidemiologic study and literature review. *Clin Orthop Relat Res* 1999;(363):176–179.
626. Rapp TB, Ward JP, Alaia MJ. Aneurysmal bone cyst. *J Am Acad Orthop Surg* 2012;20:233–241.
627. Vergel De Dios AM, Bond JR, et al. Aneurysmal bone cyst. A clinicopathologic study of 238 cases. *Cancer* 1992;69:2921–2931.

628. Nielsen GP, Fletcher CD, Smith MA, et al. Soft tissue aneurysmal bone cyst: a clinicopathologic study of five cases. *Am J Surg Pathol* 2002;26:64–69.
629. Rodriguez-Peralto JL, Lopez-Barea F, Sanchez-Herrera S, et al. Primary aneurysmal cyst of soft tissues (extraosseous aneurysmal cyst). *Am J Surg Pathol* 1994;18:632–636.
630. Arora SS, Paul S, Arora S, et al. Secondary jaw aneurysmal bone cyst (JABC)—a possible misnomer? A review of literature on secondary JABCs, their pathogenesis and oncogenesis. *J Oral Pathol Med* 2014;43:647–651.
631. Kyriakos M, Hardy D. Malignant transformation of aneurysmal bone cyst, with an analysis of the literature. *Cancer* 1991;68:1770–1780.
632. Oliveira AM, Chou MM. USP6-induced neoplasms: the biologic spectrum of aneurysmal bone cyst and nodular fasciitis. *Hum Pathol* 2014;45:1–11.
633. Mascard E, Gomez-Brouchet A, Lambot K. Bone cysts: unicameral and aneurysmal bone cyst. *Orthop Traumatol Surg Res* 2015;101:S119–S127.
634. Amling M, Werner M, Posl M, et al. Solitary bone cysts. Morphologic variation, site, incidence and differential diagnosis. *Pathologe* 1996;17:63–67.
635. Mirra JM, Picci P, Gold RH. *Bone Tumors. Clinical, Radiologic, and Pathologic correlations*. Philadelphia, PA: Lee & Febiger, 1989:1250.
636. Amling M, Werner M, Posl M, et al. Calcifying solitary bone cyst: morphological aspects and differential diagnosis of sclerotic bone tumours. *Virchows Arch* 1995;426:235–242.
637. Amling M, Werner M, Pösi M, et al. Solitary bone cysts. Morphologic variation, site, incidence and differential diagnosis. *Pathologe* 1996;17:63–67.
638. Hammoud S, Frassica FJ, McCarthy EF. Ewing's sarcoma presenting as a solitary cyst. *Skeletal Radiol* 2006;35:533–535.
639. Huebner GR, Turlington EG. So-called traumatic (hemorrhagic) bone cysts of the jaws. Review of the literature and report of two unusual cases. *Oral Surg Oral Med Oral Pathol* 1971;31:354–365.
640. Bruder E, Perez-Atayde AR, Jundt G, et al. Vascular lesions of bone in children, adolescents, and young adults. A clinicopathologic reappraisal and application of the ISSVA classification. *Virchows Arch* 2009;454:161–179.
641. Wenger DE, Wold LE. Benign vascular lesions of bone: radiologic and pathologic features. *Skeletal Radiol* 2000;29:63–74.
642. Kaleem Z, Kyriakos M, Totty WG. Solitary skeletal hemangioma of the extremities. *Skeletal Radiol* 2000;29:502–513.
643. Nielsen GP, Srivastava A, Kattapuram S, et al. Epithelioid hemangioma of bone revisited. A study of 50 cases. *Am J Surg Pathol* 2009;33:270–277.
644. Nakaya T, Morita K, Kurata A, et al. Multifocal kaposiform hemangioendothelioma in multiple visceral organs: an autopsy of 9-day-old female baby. *Hum Pathol* 2014;45:1773–1777.
645. Palmerini E, Maki RG, Staals EL, et al. Primary angiosarcoma of bone: a retrospective analysis of 60 patients from 2 institutions. *Am J Clin Oncol* 2014;37:528–534.
646. Flucke U, Vogels RJ, de Saint Aubain Somerhausen N, et al. Epithelioid Hemangioendothelioma: clinicopathologic, immunohistochemical, and molecular genetic analysis of 39 cases. *Diagn Pathol* 2014;9:131.
647. Nikolaou VS, Chytas D, Korres D, et al. Vanishing bone disease (Gorham-Stout syndrome): a review of a rare entity. *World J Orthop* 2014; 5:694–698.
648. Dellinger MT, Garg N, Olsen BR. Viewpoints on vessels and vanishing bones in Gorham-Stout disease. *Bone* 2014;63:47–52.
649. Ruggieri P, Montalti M, Angelini A, et al. Gorham-Stout disease: the experience of the Rizzoli Institute review of the literature. *Skeletal Radiol* 2011;40:1391–1397.
650. Franchi A, Bertoni F, Bacchini P, et al. CD105/endoglin expression in Gorham disease of bone. *J Clin Pathol* 2009;62:163–167.
651. Hopman SM, Van Rijn RR, Eng C, et al. PTEN hamartoma tumor syndrome and Gorham-Stout phenomenon. *Am J Med Genet* 2012; 158A:1719–1723.
652. Betsy M, Kupersmith LM, Springfield DS. Metaphyseal fibrous defects. *J Am Acad Orthop Surg* 2004;12:89–95.
653. Caffey J. On fibrous defects in cortical walls of growing tubular bones: their radiologic appearance, structure, prevalence, natural course, and diagnostic significance. *Adv Pediatr* 1955;7:13–51.
654. Mankin HJ, Trahan CA, Fondren G, et al. Non-ossifying fibroma, fibrous cortical defect and Jaffe-Campanacci syndrome: a biologic and clinical review. *Chir Organi Mov* 2009;93:1–7.
655. Ceroni D, Dayer R, De Coulon G, et al. Benign fibrous histiocytoma of bone in a paediatric population: a report of 6 cases. *Musculoskelet Surg* 2011;95:107–114.
656. Moser RP Jr, Sweet DE, Haseman DB, et al. Multiple skeletal fibroxanthomas: radiologic-pathologic correlation of 72 cases. *Skeletal Radiol* 1987;16:353–359.
657. Jee WH, Choe BY, Kang HS, et al. Nonossifying fibroma: characteristics at MR imaging with pathologic correlation. *Radiology* 1998; 209:197–202.
658. Taconis WK, Schütte HE, van der Heul RO. Desmoplastic fibroma of bone: a report of 18 cases. *Skeletal Radiol* 1994;23:283–288.
659. Nedopil A, Raab P, Rudert M. Desmoplastic fibroma: a case report with three years of clinical and radiographic observation and review of the literature. *Open Orthop J* 2013;8:40–46.
660. Woods TR, Cohen DM, Islam MN, et al. Desmoplastic fibroma of the mandible: a series of three cases and review of literature. *Head Neck Pathol* 2015;9:196–204.
661. Hrichi R, Gargallo-Albiol J, Berini-Aytés L, et al. Central odontogenic fibroma: retrospective study of 8 clinical cases. *Med Oral Patol Oral Cir Bucal* 2012;17:e50–e55.
662. Lin HP, Chen HM, Vu CH, et al. Odontogenic fibroma: a clincopathological study of 15 cases. *J Formos Med Assoc* 2011;110.27–35.
663. Kaffe I, Buchner A. Radiologic features of central odontogenic fibroma. *Oral Surg Oral Med Oral Pathol* 1994;78:811–818.
664. Foss RD, Ellis GL. Myofibromas and myofibromatosis of the oral region: a clinicopathologic analysis of 79 cases. *Oral Surg Oral Med Oral Pathol Oral Radiol Endod* 2000;89:57–65.
665. Gibson SE, Prayson RA. Primary skull lesions in the pediatric population: a 25-year experience. *Arch Pathol Lab Med* 2007;131:761–766.
666. Yoon SH, Park SH. A study of 77 cases of surgically excised scalp and skull masses in pediatric patients. *Childs Nerv Syst* 2008;24:459–465.
667. Chan YF, Lau JH, Tong CY. Congenital generalized fibromatosis with predominant osseous involvement in a Chinese newborn. *J Pediatr Orthop* 1989;9:64–68.
668. Kameyama O, Ogawa R. Pseudarthrosis of the radius associated with neurofibromatosis: report of a case and review of the literature. *J Pediatr Orthop* 1990;10:128–131.
669. Hefti F, Bollini G, Dungl P, et al. Congenital pseudarthrosis of the tibia: history, etiology, classification, and epidemiologic data. *J Pediatr Orthop B* 2000;9:11–15.
670. Leskela HV, Kuorilehto T, Risteli J, et al. Congenital pseudarthrosis of neurofibromatosis type 1: impaired osteoblast differentiation and function and altered NF1 gene expression. *Bone* 2009;44:243–250.
671. Pannier S. Congenital pseudoarthrosis of the tibia. *Orthop Traumatol Surg Res* 2011;97:750–761.
672. Teo HE, Peh WC, Akhilesh M, et al. Congenital osteofibrous dysplasia associated with pseudoarthrosis of the tibia and fibula. *Skeletal Radiol* 2007;36(Suppl 1):S7–S14.
673. Mariaud-Schmidt RP, Rosales-Quintana S, Bitar E, et al. Hamartoma involving the pseudarthrosis site in patients with neurofibromatosis type 1. *Pediatr Dev Pathol* 2005;8:190–196.
674. Fisher C. Myofibrosarcoma. *Virchows Arch* 2004;445:215–223.
675. Kourelis K, Shnayder Y, Key V, et al. Mandibular myofibrosarcoma of childhood: surgical resection & reconstruction with fibula flap. *Braz J Otorhinolaryngol* 2011;77:404.
676. Camp MD, Tompkins RK, Spanier SS, et al. Best cases from the AFIP: adamantinoma of the tibia and fibula with cytogenetic analysis. *Radiographics* 2008;28:1215–1220.
677. Czerniak B, Rojas-Corona RR, Dorfman HD. Morphologic diversity of long bone adamantinoma. The concept of differentiated (regressing) adamantinoma and its relationship to osteofibrous dysplasia. *Cancer* 1989;64:2319–2334.

678. Kikuchi Y, Kishimoto T, Ota S, et al. Adamantinoma-like Ewing family tumor of soft tissue associated with the vagus nerve: a case report and review of the literature. *Am J Surg Pathol* 2013;37:772–779.
679. Worch J, Matthay KK, Neuhaus J, et al. Ethnic and racial differences in patients with Ewing sarcoma. *Cancer* 2010;116:983–988.
680. De Ioris MA, Prete A, Cozza R, et al. Ewing sarcoma of the bone in children under 6 years of age. *PLoS One* 2013;8:e53223.
681. Aymore IL Meohas W, Brito de Almeida AL, et al. Case report. Periosteal Ewing's sarcoma. Case report and literature review. *Clin Orthop Relat Res* 2005;434:265–272.
682. Puls F, Niblett AJ, Mangham DC. Molecular pathology of bone tumours: diagnostic implications. *Histopathology* 2014;64:461–476.
683. Li S, Siegal GP. Small cell tumors of bone. *Adv Anat Pathol* 2010;17:1–11.
684. Wei S, Siegal GP. Round cell tumors of bone: an update on recent molecular genetic advances. *Adv Anat Pathol* 2014;21:359–372.
685. Rekhi B, Vogel U, Basak R, et al. Clinicopathological and molecular spectrum of ewing sarcomas/PNETs, including validation of EWSR1 rearrangement by conventional and array FISH technique in certain cases. *Pathol Oncol Res* 2014;20:503–516.
686. Cohen-Gogo S, Cellier C, Coindre JM, et al. Ewing-like sarcomas with BCOR-CCNB3 fusion transcript: a clinical, radiological and pathological retrospective study from the Société Française des Cancers de L'Enfant. *Pediatr Blood Cancer* 2014;61:2191–2198.
687. Puls F, Niblett A, Marland G, et al. BCOR-CCNB3 (Ewing-like) sarcoma: a clinicopathologic analysis of 10 cases, in comparison with conventional Ewing sarcoma. *Am J Surg Pathol* 2014;38:1307–1318.
688. Specht K, Sung YS, Zhang L, et al. Distinct transcriptional signature and immunoprofile of CIC-DUX4 fusion-positive round cell tumors compared to EWSR1-rearranged Ewing sarcomas: further evidence toward distinct pathologic entities. *Genes Chromosomes Cancer* 2014;53:622–633.
689. Mariño-Enriquez A, Fletcher CD. Round cell sarcomas—biologically important refinements in subclassification. *Int J Biochem Cell Biol* 2014;53:493–504.
690. Lin PP, Jaffe N, Herzog CE, et al. Chemotherapy response is an important predictor of local recurrence in Ewing sarcoma. *Cancer* 2007;109:603–611.
691. Schrager J, Patzer RE, Mink PJ, et al. Survival outcomes of pediatric osteosarcoma and Ewing's sarcoma: a comparison of surgical type within the SEER database, 1988–2007. *J Registry Manag* 2011;38:153–161.
692. Duchman KR, Gao Y, Miller BJ. Prognostic factors for survival in patients with Ewing's sarcoma using the surveillance, epidemiology, and end results (SEER) program database. *Cancer Epidemiol* 2015;39:189–195.
693. Serlo J, Helenius I, Vettenranta K, et al. Surgically treated patients with axial and peripheral Ewing's sarcoma family of tumours: a population based study in Finland during 1990–2009. *Eur J Surg Oncol* 2015;41(7):893–898. pii: S0748-7983(15).
694. Pradhan A, Grimer RJ, Spooner D, et al. Oncological outcomes of patients with Ewing's sarcoma: is there a difference between skeletal and extra-skeletal Ewing's sarcoma? *J Bone Joint Surg Br* 2011;93:531–536.
695. Selim H, Shaheen S, Barakat K, et al. Melanotic neuroectodermal tumor of infancy: review of literature and case report. *J Pediatr Surg* 2008;43:E25–E29.
696. Kruse-Lösler B, Gaertner C, Bürger H, et al. Melanotic neuroectodermal tumor of infancy: systematic review of the literature and presentation of a case. *Oral Surg Oral Med Oral Pathol Oral Radiol Endod* 2006;102:204–216.
697. Pettinato G, Manivel JC, d'Amore ES, et al. Melanotic neuroectodermal tumor of infancy. A reexamination of a histogenetic problem based on immunohistochemical, flow cytometric, and ultrastructural study of 10 cases. *Am J Surg Pathol* 1991;15:233–245.
698. Derache AF, Rocourt N, Delattre C, et al. [Melanotic neuroectodermal tumors of infancy: current state of knowledge]. *Bull Cancer* 2014;101:626–636.
699. Küpeli S, Cağlar K, Birgen D, et al. Desmoplastic small round cell tumor of the mandible in a child with unusual plantar metastasis. *J Pediatr Hematol Oncol* 2010;32:e155–e157.
700. Furman WL, Fitch S, Hustu HO, et al. Primary lymphoma of bone in children. *J Clin Oncol* 1989;7:1275–1280.
701. Glotzbecker MP, Kersun LS, Choi JK, et al. Primary non-Hodgkin's lymphoma of bone in children. *J Bone Joint Surg Am* 2006;88:583–594.
702. Demircay E, Hornicek FJ Jr, Mankin HJ, et al. Malignant lymphoma of bone: a review of 119 patients. *Clin Orthop Relat Res* 2013;471:2684–2690.
703. Chisholm K, Ohgami RS, Tan B, et al. Primary lymphoma of bone in the pediatric population. *Society of Pediatric Pathology, Annual Meeting.* Boston, MA; March 21–22, 2015. [See abstracts online, Pediatr Dev Pathol 2015; 18(2)].
704. Subik MK, Herr MM, Hutchison RE, et al. A highly curable lymphoma occurs preferentially in the proximal tibia of young patients. *Mod Pathol* 2014;27:1430–1437.
705. Lowe EJ, Gross TG. Anaplastic large cell lymphoma in children and adolescents. *Pediatr Hematol Oncol* 2013;30:509–519.
706. Gajendra S, Sachdev R, Lipi L, et al. ALK positive anaplastic large cell lymphoma presenting as extensive bone involvement. *J Clin Diagn Res* 2015;9:XD04–XD05.
707. Kinnery MC, Higgins RA, Medina EA. Anaplastic large cell lymphoma: twenty-five years of discovery. *Arch Pathol Lab Med* 2011;135:19–43.
708. Singh P, Bakhshi S. Osseous involvement in pediatric Hodgkin's lymphoma. *Indian J Pediatr* 2010;77:565–566.
709. Shimonodan H, Nagayama J, Nagatoshi Y, et al. Acute lymphocytic leukemia in adolescence with multiple osteolytic lesions and hypercalcemia mediated by lymphoblast-producing parathyroid hormone-related peptide: a case report and review of the literature. *Pediatr Blood Cancer* 2005;45:333–339.
710. Athale UH, Kaste SC, Razzouk BI, et al. Skeletal manifestations of pediatric acute megakaryoblastic leukemia. *J Pediatr Hematol Oncol* 2002;24:561–565.
711. Mostoufi-Moab S, Halton J. Bone morbidity in childhood leukemia: epidemiology, mechanisms, diagnosis, and treatment. *Curr Osteoporos Rep* 2014;12:300–312.
712. Crusoe Ede Q, da Silva AM, Agareno J, et al. Multiple myeloma: a rare case in an 8-year-old child. *Clin Lymphoma Myeloma Leuk* 2015;15:e31–e33.
713. Garcia-Álvarez KG, Garibaldi-Covarrubias R, Flores-Márquez MR, et al. Plasma cell myeloma associated with Epstein-Barr virus infection in an 11-year-old girl. *Pediatr Dev Pathol* 2012;15:339–342.
714. Hernandez RK, Maegback ML, Liede A, et al. Bone metastases, skeletal-related events, and survival among children with cancer in Denmark. *J Pediatr Hematol Oncol* 2014;36:528–533.
715. Leeson MC, Makley JT, Carter JR. Metastatic skeletal disease in the pediatric population. *J Pediatr Orthop* 1985;5:261–267.
716. Ohba S, Tanizawa A, Yoshimura H, et al. A case of retinoblastoma metastasizing to the mandible and review of literature. *Cranio* 2015;Jan 28:2151090314y0000000032. [Epub ahead of print].
717. Cozza R, De Ioris MA, Ilari I, et al. Metastatic retinoblastoma: single institution experience over two decades. *Br J Ophthalmol* 2009;93:1163–1166.
718. George MK, Venkitaraman R, Chandra A, et al. Late solitary skeletal metastasis to the patella from retinoblastoma. *J Indian Med Assoc* 2008;106:313–314.
719. Yoshikawa H, Ueda T, Mori S, et al. Skeletal metastases from soft-tissue sarcomas. Incidence, patterns, and radiological features. *J Bone Joint Surg Br* 1997;79B:548–552.
720. Oberlin O, Rey A, Lyden E, et al. Prognostic factors in metastatic rhabdomyosarcomas: results of a pooled analysis from United States and European cooperative groups. *J Clin Oncol* 2008;26:2384–2389.
721. Shapeero LG, Couanet D, Vanel D, et al. Bone metastases as the presenting manifestation of rhabdomyosarcoma in childhood. *Skeletal Radiol* 1993;22:433–438.
722. Weiss AR, Lyden ER, Anderson JR, et al. Histologic and clinical characteristics can guide staging evaluations for children and adolescents with rhabdomyosaroma: a report from the Children's Oncology Group Soft Tissue Sarcoma Committee. *J Clin Oncol* 2013;31:3226–3232.

723. Caglar M, Ceylan E, Ozyar E. Frequency of skeletal metastases in nasopharyngeal carcinoma after initiation of therapy: should bone scans be used for follow-up? *Nucl Med Commun* 2003;24:1231–1236.
724. Puliyel MM, Mascarenhas L, Zhou S, et al. Nuclear protein in testis midline carcinoma misdiagnosed as adamantinoma. *J Clin Oncol* 2014;32:e57–e60.
725. Colangeli M, Calamelli C, Manfrini M, et al. Bone metastasis from colon carcinoma in an 11-year-old boy: radiological features and brief review of the literature. *Skeletal Radiol* 2015;44:743–748.
726. Zaveri J, La Q, Yarmish G, et al. More than just Langerhans cell histiocytosis: a radiologic review of histiocytic disorders. *Radiographics* 2014;34:2008–2024.
727. Badalian-Very G, Vergilio JA, Fleming M, et al. Pathogenesis of Langerhans cell histiocytosis. *Annu Rev Pathol* 2013;8:1–20.
728. Arkader A, Glotzbecker M, Hosalkar HS, et al. Primary musculoskeletal Langerhans cell histiocytosis in children: an analysis for a 3-decade period. *J Pediatr Orthop* 2009;29:201–207.
729. Imashuku S, Kinugawa N, Matsuzaki A, et al. Langerhans cell histiocytosis with multifocal bone lesions: comparative clinical features between single and multi-systems. *Int J Hematol* 2009;90:506–512.
730. Postini AM, Brach del Prever A, Pagana M, et al. Langerhans cell histiocytosis: 40 years' experience. *J Pediatr Hematol Oncol* 2012;34:353–358.
731. Postini AM, Andreacchio A, Boffano M, et al. Langerhans cell histiocytosis of bone in children: a long-term retrospective study. *J Pediatr Orthop B* 2012;21:457–462.
732. Kilpatrick SE, Wenger DE, Gilchrist GS, et al. Langerhans' cell histiocytosis (histiocytosis X) of bone. A clinicopathologic analysis of 263 pediatric and adult cases. *Cancer* 1995;76:2471–2484.
733. Khung S, Budzik JF, Amzallag-Bellenger E, et al. Skeletal involvement in Langerhans cell histiocytosis. *Insights Imaging* 2013;4:569–579.
734. Foucar E, Rosai J, Dorfman R. Sinus histiocytosis with massive lymphadenopathy (Rosai-Dorfman disease): review of the entity. *Semin Diagn Pathol* 1990;7:19–73.
735. Demicco EG, Rosenberg AE, Björnsson J, et al. Primary Rosai-Dorfman disease of bone: a clinicopathologic study of 15 cases. *Am J Surg Pathol* 2010;34:1324–1333.
736. Dehner LP. Juvenile xanthogranulomas in the first two decades of life: a clinicopathologic study of 174 cases with cutaneous and extracutaneous manifestations. *Am J Surg Pathol* 2003;27:579–593.
737. Janssen D, Harms D. Juvenile xanthogranuloma in childhood and adolescence: a clinicopathologic study of 129 patients from the Kiel Pediatric Tumor Registry. *Am J Surg Pathol* 2005;29(1):21–28.
738. Konar S, Pandey P, Yasha TC. Solitary juvenile xanthogranuloma in cervical spine: case report and review of the literature. *Turk Neurosurg* 2014;24:102–107.
739. Cornips EM, Cox KE, Creytens DH, et al. Solitary juvenile xanthogranuloma of the temporal muscle and bone penetrating the dura mater in a 2-month-old boy. *J Neurosurg Pediatr* 2009;4:588–591.
740. Tran TA, Fabre M, Pariente D, et al. Erdheim-Chester disease in childhood: a challenging diagnosis and treatment. *J Pediatr Hematol Oncol* 2009;31:782–786.
741. Song SY, Lee SW, Ryu KH, et al. Erdheim-Chester disease with multisystem involvement in a 4-year-old. *Pediatr Radiol* 2012;42:632–635.
742. Cives M, Simone V, Rizzo FM, et al. Erdheim-Chester disease: a systematic review. *Crit Rev Oncol Hematol* 2015;95(1):1-11. Pii: S1040-8428(15)00028-1.
743. Small NR, Gautschi OP, Radovanovic I, et al. Incidence and relative survival of chordomas. *Cancer* 2013;119:2029–2037.
744. Hock BL, Nielsen GP, Liebsch NJ, et al. Base of skull chordomas in children and adolescents: a clinicopathologic study of 73 cases. *Am J Surg Pathol* 2006;30:811–818.
745. Choi GH, Yang MS, Yoon DH, et al. Pediatric cervical chordoma: report of two cases and a review of the current literature. *Childs Nerv Syst* 2010;26:835–840.
746. Ridenour III RV, Ahrens WA, Folpe AL, et al. Clinical and histopathologic features of chordomas in children and young adults. *Pediatr Dev Pathol* 2010;13:9–17.
747. Renard C, Pissaloux D, Decouvelaere AV, et al. Non-rhabdoid pediatric SMARCB1-deficient tumors: overlap between chordomas and malignant rhabdoid tumors? *Cancer Genet* 2014;207:384–389.
748. Mobley BC, McKenney JK, Bangs CD, et al. Loss of SMARCB1/INI1 expression in poorly differentiated chordomas. *Acta Neuropathol* 2010;120:745–753.
749. Renard C, Pissaloux D, Decouvelaere AV, et al. Non-rhabdoid pediatric SMARCB1-deficient tumors: overlap between chordomas and malignant rhabdoid tumors? *Cancer Genet* 2014;207:384–389.
750. Sangoi AR, Karamchandani J, Lane B, et al. Specificity of brachyury in the distinction of chordoma from clear cell renal cell carcinoma and germ cell tumors: a study of 305 cases. *Mod Pathol* 2011;24:425–429.
751. Salazar Guilarte JX, Sancho Mestre M, Gras Albert JR. Extraosseous chordoma of nasopharynx in paediatric age. *Acta Otorrinolaringol Esp* 2012;63:321–323.
752. Krogstad P. Osteomyelitis. In: Cherry J, Demmler GJ, Kaplan SL, et al. *Feigin and Cherry's Textbook of Pediatric Infectious Diseases*, 7th ed. Philadelphia, PA: Saunders, 2013:711–727.
753. Peltola H, Pääkkömen M. Acute osteomyelitis in children. *N Engl J Med* 2014;370:352–370.
754. Offiah AC. Acute osteomyelitis, septic arthritis and discitis: differences between neonates and older children. *Eur J Radiol* 2006;60:221–232.
755. Yagupsky P. *Kingella kingae*: carriage, transmission, and disease. *Clin Microbiol Rev* 2015;28:54–79.
756. Soler-Palacin P, Margareto C, Llobet P, et al. Chronic granulomatous disease in pediatric patients: 25 years of experience. *Allergol Immunopathol (Madr)* 2007;35:83–89.
757. Winkelstein JA, Marino MC, Johnston RB Jr, et al. Chronic granulomatous disease. Report on a national registry of 368 patients. *Medicine (Baltimore)* 2000;79:155–169.
758. Leiding JW, Holland SM. Chronic granulomatous disease. In: Pagon RA, Adam MP, Ardinger HH, et al. eds. *GeneReviews© [Internet]*. Seattle, WA: University of Washington, Seattle, 1993–2012.
759. Teo HE, Peh WC. Skeletal tuberculosis in children. *Pediatr Radiol* 2004;34:853–860.
760. Blyth CC, Best EJ, Jones CA, et al. Nontuberculous mycobacterial infection in children. A prospective national study. *Pediatr Infect Dis J* 2009;28:801–805.
761. Bargagli E, Olivieri C, Penza F, et al. Rare localizations of bone sarcoidosis: two case reports and review of the literature. *Rheumatol Int* 2011;31:1503–1506.
762. Hajjaji N, Hocqueloux L, Kerdraon R, et al. Bone infection in cat-scratch disease: a review of the literature. *J Infect* 2007;54:417–421.
763. Belthur MV, Birchansky SB, Verdugo AA, et al. Pathologic fractures in children with acute *Staphylococcus aureus* osteomyelitis. *J Bone Joint Surg Am* 2012;94:34–42.
764. Kanazawa N. Rare hereditary autoinflammatory disorders: towards an understanding of critical in vivo inflammatory pathways. *J Dermatol Sci* 2012;66:183–189.
765. Moghaddas F, Masters SL. Monogenic autoinflammatory diseases: cytokinopathies. *Cytokine* 2015;74:237–246.
766. Sharma M, Ferguson PJ. Autoinflammatory bone disorders: update on immunologic abnormalities and clues about possible triggers. *Curr Opin Rheumatol* 2013;25:658–664.
767. Aksentijevich I, Masters SL, Ferguson PJ, et al. An autoinflammatory disease with deficiency of the interleukin-1-receptor antagonist. *N Engl J Med* 2009;360:2426–2437.
768. Ferguson PJ, Chen S, Taveh MK, et al. Homozygous mutations in LPIN2 are responsible for the syndrome of chronic recurrent multifocal osteomyelitis and congenital dyserythropoietic anaemia (Majeed syndrome). *J Med Genet* 2005;42:551–557.
769. Falip C, Alison M, Boutry N, et al. Chronic recurrent multifocal osteomyelitis (CRMO): a longitudinal case series review. *Pediatr Radiol* 2013;43:355–375.
770. Costa-Reis P, Sullivan KE. Chronic recurrent multifocal osteomyelitis. *J Clin Immunol* 2013;33:1043–1056.

771. Girschick HJ, Huppertz HI, Harmsen D, et al. Chronic recurrent multifocal osteomyelitis in children: diagnostic value of histopathology and microbial testing. *Hum Pathol* 1999;30:59–65.
772. Glorieux FH. Caffey disease: an unlikely collagenopathy. *J Clin Invest* 2005;115:1142–1144.
773. Kamoun-Goldrat A, le Merrer M. Infantile cortical hyperostosis (Caffey disease): a review. *J Oral Maxillofac Surg* 2008;66:2145–2150.
774. Suphapeetiporn K, Tongkobpetch S, Mahayosnond A, et al. Expanding the phenotypic spectrum of Caffey disease. *Clin Genet* 2007;71:280–284.
775. Pazzaglia UE, Byers PD, Beluffi G, et al. Pathology of infantile cortical hyperostosis (Caffey's disease). Report of a case. *J Bone Joint Surg Am* 1985;67:1417–1426.
776. Herman TE. Antenatal-onset infantile cortical hyperostosis and non-immune hydrops. *J Perinatol* 1996;16:137–139.
777. Lafforgue P. Pathophysiology and natural history of avascular necrosis of bone. *Joint Bone Spine* 2006;73:500–507.
778. Elmantaser M, Stewart G, Young D, et al. Skeletal morbidity in children receiving chemotherapy for acute lymphoblastic leukaemia. *Arch Dis Child* 2010;95:805–809.
779. Li X, Brazauskas R, Wang Z, et al. Avascular necrosis of bone after allogeneic hematopoietic cell transplantation in children and adolescents. *Biol Blood Marrow Transplant* 2014;20:587–592.
780. Gardner RO, Bradley CS, Howard A, et al. The incidence of avascular necrosis and the radiographic outcome following medial open reduction in children with developmental dysplasia of the hip: a systematic review. *Bone Joint J* 2014;96-B:279–286.
781. Kealey WD, Mayne EE, McDonald W, et al. The role of coagulation abnormalities in the development of Perthes' disease. *J Bone Joint Surg Br* 2000;82:744–746.
782. Kenet G, Ezra E, Wientroub S, et al. Perthes' disease and the search for genetic associations: collagen mutations, Gaucher's disease and thrombophilia. *J Bone Joint Surg Br* 2008;90:1507–1511.
783. Mignot C, Gelot A, Billette de Villemeur. Gaucher disease. In: Dulac O, Lassonde M, Sarnat HB, eds. *Handbook of Clinical Neurology*, Vol 113, 3rd series. Pediatric Neurology Part III. Elsevier BV, 2013:1709–1715.
784. van Dussen L, Lips P, van Essen HW, et al. Heterogeneous pattern of bone disease in adult type Gaucher disease: clinical and pathological correlates. *Blood Cells Mol Dis* 2014;53:118–123.
785. Lebel E, Elstein D, Peleg A, et al. Histologic findings of femoral heads from patients with Gaucher disease treated with enzyme replacement. *Am J Clin Pathol* 2013;140:91–96.
786. Gerlag D, Tak PP. Synovial biopsy. *Best Pract Res Clin Rheumatol* 2005;19:387–400.
787. Kang SN, Sanghera T, Mangwani J, et al. The management of septic arthritis in children: systematic review of the English language literature. *J Bone Joint Surg Br* 2009;91B:1127–1133.
788. Hendrickx G, De Boeck H, Goossens A, et al. Persistent synovitis in children with Lyme arthritis: two unusual cases. An immunogenetic approach. *Eur J Pediatr* 2004;163:646–650.
789. Eisenstein EM, Berkun Y. Diagnosis and classification of juvenile idiopathic arthritis. *J Autoimmunity* 2014;28–29:31–33.
790. Martini A. Systemic juvenile idiopathic arthritis. *Autoimmunity Rev* 2012;12:56–59.
791. Rigante D, Bosco A, Esposito S. The etiology of juvenile idiopathic arthritis. *Clin Rev Allergy Immunol* 2014 Nov 12 [Epub ahead of print].
792. Melchiorre D, Millia AF, Linari S, et al. RANK-RANKL-OPG in hemophilic arthropathy: from clinical and imaging diagnosis to histopathology. *J Rheumatol* 2012;39:1678–1686.
793. Jansen NW, Roosendaal G, Lafeber FP. Understanding haemophilic arthropathy: an exploration of current open issues. *Br J Haematol* 2008;143:632–640.
794. Demertzis J, Kyriakos M, Loomans R, et al. Synovial hemangioma of the hip joint in a pediatric patient. *Skeletal Radiol* 2014;433:107–113.
795. Borzutky A, Fried A, Chou J, et al. NOD2-associated diseases: bridging innate immunity and autoinflammation. *Clin Immunol* 2010;134:251–261.
796. Punzi L, Gava A, Galozzi P, et al. Miscellaneous non-inflammatory musculoskeletal conditions. Blau syndrome. *Best Pract Res Clin Rheumatol* 2011;25:703–714.
797. Janssen CE, Rose CD, De Hertogh G, et al. Morphologic and immunohistochemical characterization of granulomas in the nucleotide oligomerization domain 2-related disorders Blau syndrome and Crohn disease. *J Allergy Clin Immunol* 2012;129:1076–1084.
798. Shayan K, Ho M, Edwards V, et al. Synovial pathology in camptodactyly-arthropathy-coxa vara-pericarditis syndrome. *Pediatr Dev Pathol* 2005;8:26–33.
799. Borgwardt L, Lund AM, Dali CI. Alpha-mannosidosis—a review of genetic, clinical findings and options of treatment. *Pediatr Endocrinol Rev* 2014;12(Suppl 1):185–191.
800. Parker EI, Xing M, Moreno-dDe-Luca A, et al. Radiological and clinical characterization of the lysosomal storage disorders: non-lipid disorders. *Br J Radiol* 2014;87(1033):20130467.
801. Outland JD, Keiran SJ, Schikler KN, et al. Multicentric reticulohistiocytosis in a 14-year-old girl. *Pediatr Dermatol* 2002;19:527–531.
802. Hornick JL, Fletcher CD. Intraarticular nodular fasciitis—a rare lesion: clinicopathologic analysis of a series. *Am J Surg Pathol* 2006;30:237–241.
803. Friedman MV, Kyriakos M, Matava MJ. Intra-articular synovial sarcoma. Case report. *Skeletal Radiol* 2013;42:859–867.
804. Shinawi M, Hicks J, Guillerman RP, et al. Multiple ganglion cysts ('cystic ganglionosis'): an unusual presentation in a child. *Scand J Rheumatol* 2007;36:145–148.
805. Anninga JK, Gelderblom H, Fiocco M, et al. Chemotherapeutic adjuvant treatment for osteosarcoma: where do we stand? *Eur J Cancer* 2011;47:2431–2445.
806. Riminucci M, Liu B, Corsi A, et al. The histopathology of fibrous dysplasia of bone in patients with activating mutations of the Gs alpha gene: site-specific patterns and recurrent histological hallmarks. *J Pathol* 1999;187:249–258.
807. Farrow EG, Davis SI, Mooney SD, et al. Extended mutational analyses of FGFR1 in osteoglophonic dysplasia. *Am J Med Genet A* 2006;140:537–539.
808. Ko E, Mortimer E, Fraire AE. Extraarticular synovial chondromatosis: review of epidemiology, imaging studies, microscopy and pathogenesis, with a report of an additional case in a child. *Int J Surg Pathol* 2004;12:273–280.

List of Appendices

GROWTH AND DEVELOPMENT
1. Summary of Key Events During the Embryonic Period
2. Early Fetal Growth Characteristics
3. Late Fetal Growth Characteristics

ORGAN WEIGHTS AND BODY MEASUREMENTS
4. Expected Weights and SDs at Various Postmenstrual Gestational Ages
5. Expected Linear Measurements and SDs at Various Postmenstrual Gestational Ages
6. Gestational Age (GA) and Mean Organ Weights and Measurements with 1 Standard Deviation (SD)
7. Organ Weights for Fetuses from 24 to 44 Weeks of Menstrual Age
8. Female Birth Weight, Length, and HC Percentiles by GA
9. Male Birth Weight, Length, and HC Percentiles by GA
10. Means and Standard Deviations of Weights and Measurements of Stillborn Infants by Gestational Age
11. Means and Standard Deviations of Weights and Measurements of Stillborn Infants by Body Weight
12. Means and Standard Deviations of Weights and Measurements of Live-Born Infants by Gestational Age
13. Means and Standard Deviations of Weights and Measurements of Live-Born Infants by Body Weight
14. Selected Percentiles for Weight (in kg) from Age 1 to 12 Months (mo)
15. Selected Percentiles for Recumbent Length (in cm) from Age 1 to 12 Months (mo)
16. Infant Heart Weight Centiles (Boys)
17. Infant Heart Weight Centiles (Girls)
18. Infant Combined Lung Weight Centiles (Boys)
19. Infant Combined Lung Weight Centiles (Girls)
20. Infant Liver Weight Centiles (Boys)
21. Infant Liver Weight Centiles (Girls)
22. Infant Spleen Weight Centiles (Boys)
23. Infant Spleen Weight Centiles (Girls)
24. Infant Combined Kidney Weight Centiles (Boys)
25. Infant Combined Kidney Weight Centiles (Girls)
26. Infant Pancreas Weight Centiles (Boys)
27. Infant Pancreas Weight Centiles (Girls)
28. Infant Thymus Weight Centiles (Boys)
29. Infant Thymus Weight Centiles (Girls)
30. Infant Combined Adrenal Weight Centiles (Boys and Girls)
31. Head Circumference by Age in 0- to 18-Year-Old Boys (Per Centiles)
32. Head Circumference by Age in 0- to 18-Year-Old Girls (Per Centiles)
33. Organ Weights in Relation to Age and Body Length from Birth to 12 Years of Age
34. Average Weights of Organs According to Body Length from 31 to 170 cm
35. Brain Weights, Male and Female, from 1 Day to 19 Years of Age
36. Heart Weights, Male and Female, from 1 Day to 19 Years of Age
37. Lung Weights, Left and Right, Male and Female, from 1 Day to 19 Years of Age
38. Liver Weights, Male and Female, from 1 Day to 19 Years of Age
39. Spleen Weights, Male and Female, from 1 Day to 19 Years of Age
40. Kidney Weights, Left and Right, Male and Female, from 1 Day to 19 Years of Age
41. Penile Length by Menstrual Age
42. Penile Length by Age (0–22 Years; Percentiles)
43. Gyral Pattern of the Petal Brain
44. Gyral Pattern of the Perinatal Brain
45. Gestational Development of the Cerebral Hemispheres
46. Regional Development of the Cerebral Hemispheres

PLACENTA
47. Villous Characteristics
48. Growth Characteristics of Placenta and Fetus
49. Normative Values
50. Percentiles, Means, and Standard Deviations for Placental Weights by Gestational Age
51. Mean Weights and Percentiles for Twin Placentas
52. Mean Weights and Percentiles for Triplet Placentas

APPENDIX 1: Summary of Key Events During the Embryonic Period

Days	Somites	Length (mm)	Characteristic Features
14–15	0	0.2	Appearance of primitive streak
16–18	0	0.4	Notochordal process appears; hemopoietic cells in yolk sac
19–20	0	1.0–2.0	Intraembryonic mesoderm spread under cranial ectoderm; primitive streak continues; umbilical vessels and cranial neural folds beginning to form
20–21	1–4	2.0–3.0	Cranial neural folds elevated and deep neural groove established; embryo beginning to bend
22–23	5–12	3.0–3.5	Fusion of neural folds begins in cervical region; cranial and caudal neuropores open widely; visceral arches 1 and 2 present; heart tube beginning to fold
24–25	13–20	3.0–4.5	Cephalocaudal folding under way; cranial neuropore closing or closed; optic vesicles formed; otic placodes appear
26–27	21–29	3.5–5.0	Caudal neuropore closing or closed; upper limb buds appear; three pairs of visceral arches
28–30	30–35	4.0–6.0	Fourth visceral arch formed; hindlimb buds appear; otic vesicle and lens placode
31–35		7.0–10.0	Forelimbs paddle-shaped; nasal pits formed; embryo tightly C-shaped
36–42		9.0–14.0	Digital rays in hand and foot plates; brain vesicles prominent; external auricle forming from auricular hillocks; umbilical herniation initiated
43–49		13.0–22.0	Pigmentation of retina visible; digital rays separating; nipples and eyelids formed; maxillary swellings fuse with medial nasal swellings as upper lip forms; prominent umbilical herniation
50–56		21.0–31.0	Limbs long, bent at elbows and knees; fingers and toes free; face more human-like; tail disappears; umbilical herniation persists to end of 3rd month

From Sadler TW. *Langman's Medical Embryology*, 12th ed. Philadelphia, PA: Lippincott Williams & Wilkins, 2012, with permission.

APPENDIX 2: Early Fetal Growth Characteristics

Postovulation Age in Weeks (d)	Weight[a] (g)	CR Length[b] (mm)	CH Length[c] (mm)	Development
8 (56)	5	30	38	Eyes open; low-set ears; short neck; intestine in umbilical cord
9 (63)	6.5	40	52	Eyes closing or closed; head more rounded; external genitalia still not distinguishable as male or female
10 (70)	14	50	71	Intestine in abdomen; early fingernail development
11 (77)	26	62	84	
12 (84)	35	77	111	Sex distinguishable externally; well-defined neck
13 (91)	60	93	135	
14 (98)	85	107	156	Head erect; lower limbs well developed
15 (105)	100	118	175	
16 (112)	140	130	193	Ears stand out from head
17 (119)	210	141	209	
18 (126)	260	152	225	Vernix caseosa present; early toenail development
19 (133)	350	163	243	
20 (140)	385	174	260	Head and body hair (lanugo) visible
21 (147)	445	186	277	
22 (154)	590	197	294	Skin wrinkled and red
23 (161)	725	207	311	
24 (168)	820	216	325	Fingernails present; lean body

CH, crown–heel; CR, crown–rump.

[a]Adapted from Potter EL, Craig JM. *Pathology of the Fetus and Infant*, 3rd ed. Chicago, IL: Year Book, 1975, with permission. Weights beyond 21 weeks estimated from other sources.

[b]Adapted from Mall FP. Determination of the age of human embryos and fetuses. In: Keibel F, Mall FP, eds. *Manual of Human Embryology*. Philadelphia, PA: JB Lippincott Co., 1910.

[c]Adapted from Moore KL. *Before We Are Born. Basic Embryology and Birth Defects*, 3rd ed. Philadelphia, PA: WB Saunders, 1988, with permission.

APPENDIX 3: Late Fetal Growth Characteristics

Menstrual Age (wk)	Approximate CR Length (cm)	External Features
24	21	Skin wrinkled and red
26	23	Fingernails present; lean body
28	25	Eyes partially open; eyelashes present
30	27	Eyes open; good head of hair; skin slightly wrinkled
32	28	Toenails present; body filling out; testes descending
34	30	Fingernails reach fingertips; skin pink and smooth
38	34	Body usually plump; lanugo almost absent; toenails reach toe tips; flexed limbs; firm grasp
40	36	Prominent chest; breasts protrude; testes in scrotum or palpable in inguinal canals; fingernails extend beyond fingertips

CR, crown–rump.

From Moore KL. *The Developing Human*, 4th ed. Philadelphia, PA: WB Saunders, 1988, with permission.

APPENDIX 4: Expected Weights and SDs at Various Postmenstrual Gestational Ages[a]

Age (wk)	Body	Brain	Thymus	Lungs	Heart	Liver	Spleen	Adrenals	Pancreas	Kidneys
12	20.9 ± 6.6	3.20 ± 1.44	0.01 ± 0.01	0.50 ± 0.28	0.15 ± 0.02	1.01 ± 0.38	0.01 ± 0.01	0.10 ± 0.03	—	0.16 ± 0.04
13	31.2 ± 10.1	5.19 ± 1.95	0.03 ± 0.01	1.08 ± 0.45	0.20 ± 0.06	1.38 ± 0.57	0.01 ± 0.01	0.15 ± 0.05	—	0.22 ± 0.07
14	49.1 ± 14.5	8.14 ± 2.58	0.05 ± 0.02	1.79 ± 0.67	0.31 ± 0.11	2.18 ± 0.84	0.03 ± 0.02	0.23 ± 0.08	—	0.36 ± 0.13
15	74.7 ± 19.8	12.0 ± 3.3	0.09 ± 0.04	2.64 ± 0.92	0.50 ± 0.17	3.41 ± 1.18	0.05 ± 0.03	0.33 ± 0.12	—	0.59 ± 0.19
16	108 ± 26	16.9 ± 4.2	0.14 ± 0.06	3.61 ± 1.21	0.76 ± 0.24	5.06 ± 1.60	0.09 ± 0.05	0.47 ± 0.16	—	0.90 ± 0.28
17	149 ± 33	22.8 ± 5.2	0.20 ± 0.08	4.70 ± 1.55	1.10 ± 0.31	7.14 ± 2.10	0.15 ± 0.07	0.64 ± 0.22	—	1.30 ± 0.39
18	197 ± 42	29.7 ± 6.3	0.28 ± 0.12	5.92 ± 1.92	1.50 ± 0.40	9.65 ± 2.66	0.21 ± 0.10	0.84 ± 0.30	—	1.79 ± 0.51
19	255 ± 51	37.2 ± 7.6	0.41 ± 0.17	7.30 ± 2.34	1.88 ± 0.49	12.8 ± 3.3	0.30 ± 0.14	1.03 ± 0.34	—	2.36 ± 0.65
20	319 ± 61	45.7 ± 8.9	0.54 ± 0.23	8.84 ± 2.80	2.41 ± 0.59	16.5 ± 4.0	0.41 ± 0.18	1.29 ± 0.41	0.50 ± 0.14	3.00 ± 0.81
21	389 ± 72	54.6 ± 10.4	0.72 ± 0.29	10.4 ± 3.3	2.89 ± 0.71	19.9 ± 4.8	0.54 ± 0.22	1.51 ± 0.49	0.54 ± 0.21	3.63 ± 0.99
22	452 ± 84	63.7 ± 12.0	0.92 ± 0.37	12.0 ± 3.8	3.38 ± 0.82	22.7 ± 5.7	0.66 ± 0.28	1.73 ± 0.57	0.60 ± 0.26	4.23 ± 1.18
23	510 ± 97	72.3 ± 13.8	1.15 ± 0.46	13.5 ± 4.4	3.81 ± 0.96	24.3 ± 6.5	0.75 ± 0.32	1.88 ± 0.66	0.68 ± 0.31	4.77 ± 1.39
24	579 ± 115	82.8 ± 15.6	1.38 ± 0.58	15.0 ± 5.0	4.23 ± 1.12	26.4 ± 7.1	0.91 ± 0.36	2.00 ± 0.74	0.77 ± 0.34	5.65 ± 1.63
25	660 ± 134	93.4 ± 17.4	1.63 ± 0.71	16.8 ± 5.6	4.80 ± 1.31	29.4 ± 7.8	1.11 ± 0.44	2.16 ± 0.82	0.85 ± 0.36	6.55 ± 1.91
26	744 ± 163	105 ± 19	1.96 ± 0.86	18.7 ± 6.2	5.50 ± 1.57	33.2 ± 8.8	1.38 ± 0.55	2.36 ± 0.90	0.92 ± 0.38	7.46 ± 2.21
27	839 ± 199	118 ± 21	2.37 ± 1.02	20.6 ± 6.8	6.28 ± 1.84	37.8 ± 9.9	1.78 ± 0.71	2.58 ± 0.99	1.01 ± 0.38	8.53 ± 2.53
28	946 ± 239	135 ± 24	2.85 ± 1.22	22.7 ± 7.3	7.13 ± 2.11	42.6 ± 11.5	2.26 ± 0.96	2.83 ± 1.10	1.08 ± 0.37	9.75 ± 2.85
29	1064 ± 286	154 ± 26	3.44 ± 1.49	25.1 ± 7.9	7.95 ± 2.44	46.9 ± 13.3	2.73 ± 1.19	3.09 ± 1.21	1.14 ± 0.37	11.1 ± 3.2
30	1211 ± 330	173 ± 30	4.02 ± 1.85	27.4 ± 8.4	8.84 ± 2.71	51.3 ± 14.8	3.20 ± 1.36	3.36 ± 1.34	1.27 ± 0.39	12.5 ± 3.7
31	1351 ± 373	191 ± 33	4.52 ± 2.17	29.2 ± 8.8	9.83 ± 2.86	55.9 ± 15.8	3.74 ± 1.58	3.71 ± 1.42	1.46 ± 0.42	13.8 ± 4.0
32	1492 ± 406	206 ± 35	4.91 ± 2.43	31.2 ± 9.0	10.8 ± 3.0	61.2 ± 17.0	4.37 ± 1.87	4.07 ± 1.50	1.77 ± 0.47	15.0 ± 4.4
33	1650 ± 433	222 ± 36	5.40 ± 2.63	34.1 ± 9.4	11.9 ± 3.2	66.3 ± 18.8	5.06 ± 2.18	4.42 ± 1.56	1.95 ± 0.55	16.5 ± 4.9
34	1832 ± 457	242 ± 37	6.03 ± 2.84	37.5 ± 10.1	13.1 ± 3.5	72.8 ± 20.9	5.76 ± 2.51	4.77 ± 1.63	2.11 ± 0.63	18.0 ± 5.3
35	2040 ± 487	265 ± 39	6.87 ± 3.06	41.7 ± 11.0	14.5 ± 3.7	81.8 ± 22.3	6.47 ± 2.79	5.19 ± 1.92	2.36 ± 0.69	19.6 ± 5.7
36	2246 ± 511	292 ± 42	7.85 ± 3.22	45.1 ± 12.2	16.0 ± 4.0	92.8 ± 22.9	7.21 ± 3.07	5.74 ± 1.92	2.61 ± 0.77	21.3 ± 6.0
37	2424 ± 535	319 ± 44	8.95 ± 3.41	47.0 ± 13.2	17.6 ± 4.3	104 ± 23	8.11 ± 3.30	6.46 ± 2.10	2.84 ± 0.85	22.5 ± 6.4
38	2603 ± 559	340 ± 46	9.61 ± 3.60	48.4 ± 14.0	18.6 ± 4.5	116 ± 26	9.15 ± 3.53	7.01 ± 2.31	3.04 ± 0.94	23.9 ± 6.8
39	2787 ± 582	355 ± 49	9.98 ± 3.78	49.4 ± 14.8	19.4 ± 4.8	124 ± 29	9.83 ± 3.73	7.44 ± 2.55	3.33 ± 1.04	24.9 ± 7.1
40	2942 ± 603	368 ± 51	10.2 ± 3.9	50.8 ± 15.5	20.3 ± 5.0	130 ± 32	10.2 ± 3.9	7.75 ± 2.82	3.65 ± 1.15	25.7 ± 7.5
41	3098 ± 623	382 ± 53	10.2 ± 4.1	52.3 ± 16.1	21.3 ± 5.2	136 ± 36	10.5 ± 4.0	7.99 ± 3.11	4.01 ± 1.26	26.4 ± 7.8
42	3267 ± 641	395 ± 55	10.1 ± 4.3	54.0 ± 16.5	22.4 ± 5.3	141 ± 40	10.8 ± 4.0	8.14 ± 3.44	4.40 ± 1.39	27.0 ± 8.2
43	3444 ± 657	408 ± 57	9.83 ± 4.46	55.9 ± 16.8	23.6 ± 5.4	145 ± 45	10.9 ± 4.0	8.21 ± 3.79	—	27.6 ± 8.5
44	3633 ± 671	421 ± 59	9.44 ± 4.64	57.8 ± 16.9	24.8 ± 5.5	149 ± 50	11.1 ± 4.0	8.22 ± 4.17	—	28.3 ± 8.8

[a]Lungs, adrenals, and kidneys were weighed in pairs. Data are given as mean ± SD. Weights are given in grams.

From Archie JG, Collins JS, Lebel RR. Quantitative standards for fetal and neonatal autopsy. *Am J Clin Pathol* 2006;126(2):256–265, with permission.

APPENDIX 5: Expected Linear Measurements and SDs at Various Postmenstrual Gestational Ages[a]

Age (wk)	CHL	CRL	HC	BPD	OCD	ICD	PL	CC	IND	AC	HL	FL	SIL	LIL
12	93.0 ± 9.7	76.1 ± 6.7	67.7 ± 11.6	19.5 ± 3.5	14.0 ± 4.0	6.04 ± 1.55	—	—	14.1 ± 3.4	—	—	9.74 ± 1.11	194	20
13	114 ± 11	86.7 ± 78	82.1 ± 11.7	23.2 ± 3.6	16.7 ± 4.0	6.93 ± 1.56	2.80	76.7	16.3 ± 3.5	59.8	11.3	12.3 ± 1.1	282	39
14	134 ± 12	97.7 ± 8.8	96.2 ± 11.9	26.8 ± 3.6	19.3 ± 4.0	7.80 ± 1.57	3.09	86.1	18.5 ± 3.7	68.9	13.7	15.1 ± 1.1	370	58
15	154 ± 14	109 ± 10	110 ± 12	30.4 ± 3.7	21.9 ± 4.0	8.64 ± 1.58	3.39	95.4	20.7 ± 3.9	78.0	16.1	17.9 ± 1.1	458	77
16	174 ± 15	121 ± 11	123 ± 12	33.9 ± 3.8	24.4 ± 4.0	9.45 ± 1.59	3.68	105	22.9 ± 4.1	87.2	18.6	20.9 ± 1.2	547	96
17	193 ± 16	133 ± 11	136 ± 12	37.3 ± 3.8	26.8 ± 4.0	10.2 ± 1.6	3.98	114	25.0 ± 4.3	96.3	21.0	24.0 ± 1.2	635	115
18	212 ± 17	145 ± 12	149 ± 13	40.7 ± 3.9	29.2 ± 4.0	11.0 ± 1.6	4.27	124	27.2 ± 4.4	105	23.4	27.2 ± 1.4	723	134
19	230 ± 18	158 ± 13	161 ± 13	43.9 ± 4.0	31.5 ± 4.1	11.7 ± 1.6	4.57	133	29.4 ± 4.6	115	25.8	30.5 ± 1.5	811	152
20	247 ± 19	171 ± 14	173 ± 13	47.1 ± 4.1	33.8 ± 4.1	12.5 ± 1.6	4.86	142	31.6 ± 4.8	124	28.2	33.9 ± 1.7	900	171
21	264 ± 19	184 ± 14	185 ± 13	50.2 ± 4.1	35.9 ± 4.1	13.1 ± 1.7	5.16	152	33.8 ± 5.0	133	30.6	37.2 ± 1.9	988	190
22	278 ± 20	195 ± 15	196 ± 13	53.3 ± 4.2	38.1 ± 4.1	13.8 ± 1.7	5.45	161	36.0 ± 5.1	142	32.9	40.0 ± 2.1	1076	209
23	291 ± 20	204 ± 15	207 ± 14	56.2 ± 4.3	40.1 ± 4.1	14.4 ± 1.7	5.75	170	38.2 ± 5.3	151	35.3	41.7 ± 2.4	1164	228
24	303 ± 21	213 ± 16	218 ± 14	59.1 ± 4.3	42.1 ± 4.1	15.0 ± 1.7	6.04	180	40.4 ± 5.5	160	37.8	43.8 ± 2.6	1253	247
25	316 ± 22	223 ± 17	228 ± 14	61.9 ± 4.4	44.0 ± 4.1	15.6 ± 1.7	6.33	189	42.6 ± 5.7	169	40.4	46.0 ± 3.0	1341	266
26	328 ± 23	232 ± 18	238 ± 14	64.7 ± 4.5	45.9 ± 4.1	16.2 ± 1.7	6.63	199	44.8 ± 5.8	179	43.0	48.0 ± 3.5	—	—
27	340 ± 26	242 ± 19	248 ± 14	67.3 ± 4.5	47.7 ± 4.2	16.7 ± 1.7	—	208	47.0 ± 6.0	—	45.7	50.0 ± 3.9	—	—
28	351 ± 30	250 ± 21	257 ± 14	69.9 ± 4.6	49.4 ± 4.2	17.2 ± 1.7	—	217	49.2 ± 6.2	—	48.4	52.0 ± 4.3	—	—
29	362 ± 33	259 ± 24	266 ± 15	72.4 ± 4.7	51.1 ± 4.2	17.7 ± 1.7	—	227	51.4 ± 6.4	—	51.0	54.1 ± 4.9	—	—
30	374 ± 35	267 ± 27	275 ± 15	74.8 ± 4.8	52.7 ± 4.2	18.1 ± 1.8	—	236	53.5 ± 6.6	—	53.4	56.2 ± 5.4	—	—
31	386 ± 37	276 ± 30	283 ± 15	77.2 ± 4.8	54.2 ± 4.2	18.6 ± 1.8	—	245	55.7 ± 6.7	—	55.6	58.2 ± 6.0	—	—
32	397 ± 38	284 ± 32	291 ± 15	79.4 ± 4.9	55.7 ± 4.2	19.0 ± 1.8	—	255	57.9 ± 6.9	—	57.6 ± 2.1	60.4 ± 6.3	—	—
33	408 ± 40	292 ± 33	298 ± 15	81.6 ± 5.0	57.1 ± 4.2	19.3 ± 1.8	—	264	60.1 ± 7.1	—	59.2 ± 2.9	62.5 ± 6.4	—	—
34	419 ± 41	301 ± 33	306 ± 16	83.7 ± 5.0	58.5 ± 4.2	19.7 ± 1.8	—	274	62.3 ± 7.3	—	60.5 ± 4.1	64.7 ± 6.6	—	—
35	432 ± 43	310 ± 33	312 ± 16	85.8 ± 5.1	59.8 ± 4.2	20.0 ± 1.8	—	283	64.5 ± 7.4	—	61.9 ± 4.8	66.9 ± 6.7	—	—
36	444 ± 44	318 ± 33	319 ± 16	87.8 ± 5.2	61.0 ± 4.3	20.3 ± 1.8	—	292	66.7 ± 7.6	—	63.2 ± 5.1	69.2 ± 6.7	—	—
37	457 ± 44	327 ± 32	325 ± 16	89.6 ± 5.2	62.2 ± 4.3	20.6 ± 1.8	—	302	68.9 ± 7.8	—	64.4 ± 5.4	71.3 ± 6.7	—	—
38	470 ± 44	336 ± 32	331 ± 16	91.5 ± 5.3	63.3 ± 4.3	20.8 ± 1.9	—	311	71.1 ± 8.0	—	65.4 ± 5.5	73.4 ± 6.7	—	—
39	482 ± 44	344 ± 30	336 ± 17	93.2 ± 5.4	64.3 ± 4.3	21.0 ± 1.9	—	321	73.3 ± 8.1	—	66.3 ± 5.5	75.6 ± 6.7	—	—
40	493 ± 42	352 ± 29	342 ± 17	94.9 ± 5.5	65.3 ± 4.3	21.2 ± 1.9	—	330	75.5 ± 8.3	—	67.0 ± 5.3	77.8 ± 6.6	—	—
41	505 ± 41	360 ± 27	346 ± 17	96.4 ± 5.5	66.2 ± 4.3	21.4 ± 1.9	—	—	77.7 ± 8.5	—	67.6 ± 4.9	80.1 ± 6.4	—	—
42	516 ± 38	367 ± 25	351 ± 17	97.9 ± 5.6	67.0 ± 4.3	21.5 ± 1.9	—	—	79.9 ± 8.7	—	68.0 ± 4.2	82.5 ± 6.3	—	—

AC, abdominal circumference; BPD, biparietal diameter; CC, chest circumference; CHL, crown-heel length; CRL, crown-rump length; FL, foot length; HC, head circumference; HL, hand length; ICD, inner canthal distance; IND, internipple distance; LIL, large intestine length; OCD, outer canthal distance; PL, philtrum length; SIL, small intestine length.

[a] Data are given as mean or mean ± SD. Linear measurements are given in millimeters.

From Archie JG, Collins JS, Lebel RR. Quantitative standards for fetal and neonatal autopsy. *Am J Clin Pathol* 2006;126(2):256–265, with permission.

APPENDIX 6: Gestational Age (GA) and Mean Organ Weights and Measurements with 1 Standard Deviation (SD)

GA (wk)	Body Weight			Crown-Rump			Crown-Heel			Toe-Heel			Brain			Thymus		
	g	SD	n	cm	SD	n	cm	SD	n	cm	SD	n	g	SD	n	g	SD	n
12	21	±6.4	8	7.6	±0.6	10	9.3	±1.0	9	1.0	±0.1	11	3.5	±1.5	6	0.01		3
13	31	±10	21	8.7	±0.8	21	11.4	±1.0	16	1.2	±0.1	27	4.6	±1.7	11	0.03	±0.01	9
14	49	±16	18	9.8	±1.1	18	13.5	±1.5	17	1.5	±0.1	18	7.8	±4.1	12	0.05	±0.03	13
15	75	±22	49	10.9	±1.0	43	15.4	±1.4	40	1.8	±0.2	50	12.6	±3.4	31	0.09	±0.05	37
16	108	±25	36	12.0	±1.1	37	17.3	±1.5	36	2.1	±0.2	41	17.5	±3.7	23	0.14	±0.08	27
17	149	±32	50	13.2	±1.1	48	19.2	±1.6	47	2.4	±0.2	53	22.6	±4.7	34	0.18	±0.06	41
18	195	±44	44	14.3	±1.2	47	21.0	±1.6	44	2.7	±0.2	50	29.9	±7.5	40	0.27	±0.10	39
19	248	±46	52	15.4	±1.2	51	22.7	±1.4	44	3.0	±0.1	57	35.2	±6.6	43	0.39	±0.12	41
20	307	±47	66	16.5	±1.2	65	24.4	±1.8	64	3.3	±0.3	67	45.5	±7.2	54	0.53	±0.18	56
21	370	±60	38	17.7	±1.4	36	26.0	±2.1	35	3.6	±0.3	38	53.3	±8.8	33	0.70	±0.26	34
22	438	±74	50	18.8	±1.6	50	27.5	±2.1	50	3.9	±0.3	50	63.5	±10.5	45	0.91	±0.34	45
23	510	±77	39	19.9	±1.3	40	29.0	±1.8	40	4.2	±0.2	40	74.9	±13.5	34	1.14	±0.43	36
24	586	±74	29	21.0	±1.4	30	30.4	±1.4	30	4.4	±0.2	30	81.7	±14.8	28	1.41	±0.48	22
25	665	±104	24	22.1	±1.1	22	31.8	±1.8	24	4.6	±0.2	24	93.6	±12.2	23	1.70	±0.54	17
26	747	±110	13	23.3	±1.1	13	33.1	±1.6	13	4.8	±0.2	13	103.4	±12.9	12	2.04	±0.39	10

Modified from Hansen K, et al. Reference values for second trimester fetal and neonatal organ weights and measurements. *Pediatr Dev Pathol* 2003;6(2):160–167.

Heart			Lungs			Spleen			Liver			Kidneys			Adrenals		
g	SD	n	cm	SD	n	cm	SD	n	cm	SD	n	g	SD	n	g	SD	n
0.15	±0.02	5	0.5	±0.3	7	0.01		3	1.0	±0.4	7	0.16	±0.04	6	0.01	±0.04	6
0.2	±0.1	11	1.1	±0.4	12	0.01	±0.01	10	1.4	±0.5	14	0.21	±0.08	13	0.15	±0.04	11
0.3	±0.1	15	1.8	±0.7	16	0.03	±0.02	16	2.3	±1.1	15	0.35	±0.11	16	0.22	±0.11	15
0.5	±0.2	38	2.6	±0.9	37	0.06	±0.04	38	3.3	±1.2	37	0.61	±0.20	37	0.33	±0.11	38
0.8	±0.2	31	3.5	±1.3	33	0.09	±0.05	30	5.0	±1.4	30	0.97	±0.33	32	0.48	±0.19	33
1.1	±0.4	39	4.6	±1.5	40	0.14	±0.07	45	7.1	±1.9	39	1.33	±0.46	45	0.65	±0.22	44
1.5	±0.4	43	5.8	±2.2	40	0.19	±0.10	44	9.5	±2.5	38	1.75	±0.51	40	0.83	±0.31	43
1.9	±0.5	48	7.1	±2.0	45	0.27	±0.11	46	12.1	±3.2	47	2.28	±0.56	46	1.03	±0.34	47
2.3	±0.6	61	8.6	±2.6	55	0.36	±0.17	59	14.9	±3.8	56	2.89	±0.63	56	1.23	±0.38	61
2.8	±0.6	37	10.2	±3.0	38	0.47	±0.20	34	17.8	±4.1	37	3.46	±0.96	38	1.43	±0.45	37
3.3	±0.8	44	11.9	±3.5	43	0.60	±0.18	46	20.7	±4.3	6	4.20	±1.33	44	1.64	±0.48	45
3.8	±0.9	39	13.8	±3.8	31	0.73	±0.27	34	23.6	±6.8	36	5.01	±1.16	32	1.83	±0.50	36
4.4	±0.9	29	15.8	±5.3	26	0.89	±0.31	27	26.4	±5.9	24	5.66	±1.47	28	2.02	±0.57	25
5.0	±1.0	22	18.0	±5.3	18	1.05	±0.25	18	29.1	±4.7	18	6.52	±1.25	22	2.19	±0.54	21
5.6	±1.1	11	20.2	±5.4	10	1.24	±0.36	9	31.6	±6.3	11	7.50	±1.60	11	2.35	±0.63	10

APPENDIX 7: Organ Weights for Fetuses from 24 to 44 Weeks of Menstrual Age

Menstrual Age (wk)	Organ Weights (g)								No. of Cases
	Brain	Heart	Thymus	Lungs	Spleen	Liver	Kidneys	Adrenals	
24	92	4.9	2.7	17	1.7	32	6.4	2.9	108
	± 31	± 1.6	± 1.4	± 6	± 1.1	± 15	± 2.6	± 1.4	
26	111	6.4	3.0	18	2.2	39	7.9	3.4	143
	± 39	± 2.0	± 2.3	± 6	± 1.5	± 15	± 2.9	± 1.5	
28	139	7.6	3.8	23	2.6	46	10.4	3.7	139
	± 48	± 2.3	± 2.1	± 7	± 1.4	± 16	± 3.6	± 1.7	
30	166	9.3	4.6	28	3.4	53	12.3	4.2	148
	± 55	± 3.3	± 2.3	± 11	± 2.0	± 19	± 3.9	± 2.2	
32	209	11.0	5.5	34	4.1	65	14.5	4.3	150
	± 44	± 3.7	± 2.3	± 11	± 2.1	± 22	± 4.8	± 2.3	
34	246	13.4	7.5	40	5.2	74	17.7	5.5	104
	± 58	± 3.9	± 3.8	± 13	± 2.1	± 27	± 5.3	± 2.3	
36	288	15.1	8.1	46	6.7	87	21.6	6.4	87
	± 62	± 4.8	± 4.2	± 16	± 3.0	± 33	± 6.7	± 3.0	
38	349	18.5	9.7	53	8.8	111	23.8	8.4	102
	± 56	± 5.5	± 4.8	± 15	± 4.2	± 40	± 7.0	± 3.5	
40	362	20.4	9.5	56	10.0	130	25.6	8.6	220
	± 55	± 5.3	± 4.4	± 15	± 3.9	± 45	± 6.5	± 3.4	
42	405	21.9	10.4	56	10.2	139	25.8	9.1	112
	± 54	± 6.2	± 4.4	± 18	± 4.3	± 45	± 7.5	± 4.0	
44	417	25.8	10.3	60	11.2	149	28.4	9.3	42
	± 55	± 4.5	± 4.7	± 17	± 4.1	± 35	± 7.5	± 4.4	

Adapted from Gruenwald P, Minh HN. Evaluation of body and organ weights in perinatal pathology. I. Normal standards derived from autopsies. *Am J Clin Pathol* 1960;34:247, with permission.

APPENDIX 8: Female Birth Weight, Length, and HC Percentiles by GA

GA (wk)	Birth Size			Percentile						
	n	Mean	SD	3rd	10th	25th	50th	75th	90th	97th
Weight (g)										
23	133	587	80	NA[a]	477	528	584	639	687	NA[a]
24	438	649	89	464	524	585	651	715	772	828
25	603	738	121	511	584	657	737	816	885	953
26	773	822	143	558	645	732	827	921	1004	1085
27	966	934	168	615	719	822	936	1047	1147	1244
28	1187	1058	203	686	807	928	1061	1193	1310	1425
29	1254	1199	226	778	915	1052	1204	1354	1489	1621
30	1606	1376	246	902	1052	1204	1373	1542	1693	1842
31	2044	1548	271	1033	1196	1361	1546	1731	1897	2062
32	3007	1730	300	1177	1352	1530	1731	1933	2116	2297
33	4186	1960	328	1356	1545	1738	1956	2178	2379	2580
34	5936	2194	357	1523	1730	1944	2187	2434	2661	2888
35	5082	2420	440	1626	1869	2123	2413	2711	2985	3261
36	4690	2675	514	1745	2028	2324	2664	3015	3339	3667
37	4372	2946	551	1958	2260	2575	2937	3308	3651	3997
38	5755	3184	512	2235	2526	2829	3173	3525	3847	4172
39	5978	3342	489	2445	2724	3012	3338	3670	3973	4276
40	5529	3461	465	2581	2855	3136	3454	3776	4070	4363
41	1906	3546	477	2660	2933	3214	3530	3851	4142	4433

APPENDIX 8: Female Birth Weight, Length, and HC Percentiles by GA *(Continued)*

GA (wk)	n	Birth Size		Percentile						
		Mean	SD	3rd	10th	25th	50th	75th	90th	97th
Length (cm)										
23	133	29.9	1.8	NA[a]	27.7	28.7	29.9	31.0	31.9	NA[a]
24	438	31.0	1.7	27.5	28.7	29.8	31.1	32.3	33.3	34.3
25	603	32.3	2.0	28.3	29.7	31.0	32.3	33.6	34.8	35.9
26	773	33.4	2.2	29.2	30.7	32.1	33.6	35.1	36.3	37.4
27	966	35.0	2.3	30.2	31.9	33.4	35.0	36.6	37.9	39.1
28	1187	36.4	2.5	31.4	33.1	34.8	36.5	38.1	39.5	40.8
29	1254	37.8	2.7	32.8	34.6	36.3	38.0	39.7	41.2	42.5
30	1606	39.6	2.6	34.3	36.0	37.7	39.5	41.3	42.7	44.1
31	2044	40.9	2.6	35.7	37.5	39.2	41.0	42.7	44.1	45.5
32	3007	42.1	2.6	37.1	38.9	40.6	42.3	44.0	45.5	46.9
33	4186	43.7	2.6	38.6	40.3	41.9	43.7	45.4	46.9	48.3
34	5936	45.0	2.6	39.8	41.5	43.2	45.0	46.7	48.2	49.7
35	5082	46.0	2.7	40.9	42.6	44.3	46.2	48.0	49.5	51.0
36	4690	47.2	2.8	42.0	43.7	45.5	47.4	49.2	50.8	52.3
37	4372	48.4	2.8	43.2	44.9	46.6	48.5	50.3	51.9	53.4
38	5755	49.5	2.6	44.4	46.1	47.7	49.5	51.2	52.7	54.2
39	5978	50.1	2.5	45.3	46.9	48.5	50.2	51.9	53.3	54.7
40	5529	50.7	2.4	46.1	47.6	49.1	50.8	52.4	53.8	55.1
41	1906	51.3	2.4	46.7	48.2	49.7	51.3	52.8	54.2	55.5
HC (cm)										
23	133	20.8	1.2	NA[a]	19.5	20.1	20.9	21.6	22.2	NA[a]
24	438	21.7	1.1	19.6	20.3	21.0	21.8	22.5	23.2	23.8
25	603	22.7	1.2	20.4	21.1	21.9	22.7	23.4	24.1	24.8
26	773	23.5	1.2	21.2	22.0	22.7	23.6	24.4	25.1	25.9
27	966	24.5	1.3	21.9	22.8	23.6	24.5	25.4	26.2	27.0
28	1187	25.5	1.5	22.7	23.7	24.6	25.5	26.5	27.3	28.1
29	1254	26.5	1.5	23.6	24.6	25.5	26.5	27.5	28.4	29.2
30	1606	27.5	1.5	24.6	25.6	26.5	27.5	28.5	29.4	30.2
31	2044	28.4	1.5	25.5	26.5	27.4	28.4	29.4	30.3	31.1
32	3007	29.3	1.5	26.5	27.4	28.3	29.3	30.3	31.2	32.0
33	4186	30.2	1.5	27.3	28.3	29.2	30.2	31.2	32.1	33.0
34	5936	31.1	1.6	28.1	29.1	30.1	31.1	32.2	33.1	34.0
35	5082	31.9	1.6	28.8	29.8	30.8	31.9	33.0	34.0	34.9
36	4690	32.6	1.7	29.4	30.5	31.5	32.7	33.8	34.8	35.8
37	4372	33.3	1.7	30.1	31.1	32.2	33.3	34.4	35.4	36.3
38	5755	33.8	1.6	30.7	31.7	32.7	33.7	34.8	35.7	36.7
39	5978	34.0	1.5	31.1	32.0	33.0	34.0	35.1	36.0	36.9
40	5529	34.2	1.5	31.4	32.3	33.3	34.3	35.3	36.1	37.0
41	1906	34.5	1.5	31.7	32.6	33.5	34.5	35.5	36.3	37.1

[a]Not available because of small sample size.

From Olsen IE, et al. New intrauterine growth curves based on United States data. *Pediatrics* 2010;125(2): e214–e224, with permission. Adapted from Groveman SA. *New Preterm Infant Growth Curves Influence of Gender and Race on Birth Size [master's Thesis]*. Philadelphia, PA: Biotechnology and Bioscience, Drexel University, 2008.

APPENDIX 9: Male Birth Weight, Length, and HC Percentiles by GA

GA (wk)	n	Birth Size Mean	SD	Percentile 3rd	10th	25th	50th	75th	90th	97th
Weight (g)										
23	153	622	74	NA[a]	509	563	621	677	727	NA[a]
24	451	689	96	497	561	623	690	756	813	869
25	722	777	116	550	626	700	780	857	926	992
26	881	888	145	613	704	794	890	983	1065	1145
27	1030	1001	170	680	789	895	1009	1120	1218	1312
28	1281	1138	203	758	884	1007	1141	1271	1385	1496
29	1505	1277	218	845	988	1128	1280	1429	1560	1688
30	1992	1435	261	955	1114	1272	1443	1612	1761	1906
31	2460	1633	275	1093	1267	1441	1631	1818	1984	2147
32	3677	1823	306	1246	1433	1622	1829	2034	2218	2398
33	5014	2058	341	1422	1625	1830	2057	2284	2488	2688
34	7291	2288	364	1589	1810	2035	2285	2536	2763	2987
35	6952	2529	433	1728	1980	2238	2527	2819	3084	3348
36	7011	2798	498	1886	2170	2462	2792	3127	3432	3737
37	6692	3058	518	2103	2401	2708	3056	3411	3736	4060
38	8786	3319	527	2356	2652	2959	3306	3661	3986	4312
39	8324	3476	498	2545	2833	3131	3469	3813	4129	4446
40	7235	3582	493	2666	2950	3245	3579	3919	4232	4545
41	2538	3691	518	2755	3039	3333	3666	4007	4319	4633
Length (cm)										
23	153	30.5	1.6	NA[a]	28.0	29.1	30.3	31.4	32.4	NA[a]
24	451	31.5	1.8	27.9	29.1	30.3	31.5	32.8	33.9	34.9
25	722	32.7	2.1	28.8	30.2	31.5	32.9	34.2	35.4	36.5
26	881	34.2	2.2	29.9	31.3	32.8	34.3	35.7	37.0	38.2
27	1030	35.6	2.4	31.0	32.6	34.1	35.7	37.3	38.6	39.8
28	1281	37.2	2.5	32.2	33.9	35.5	37.2	38.8	40.2	41.5
29	1505	38.6	2.5	33.5	35.2	36.9	38.7	40.3	41.7	43.1
30	1992	39.9	2.8	34.8	36.6	38.3	40.1	41.8	43.2	44.6
31	2460	41.5	2.5	36.2	38.0	39.8	41.6	43.3	44.7	46.1
32	3677	42.8	2.7	37.7	39.5	41.2	43.0	44.7	46.1	47.5
33	5014	44.3	2.6	39.1	40.9	42.6	44.4	46.1	47.5	48.9
34	7291	45.6	2.6	40.4	42.2	43.9	45.7	47.4	48.9	50.3
35	6952	46.8	2.7	41.5	43.3	45.0	46.9	48.6	50.2	51.6
36	7011	48.0	2.8	42.7	44.5	46.2	48.1	49.9	51.5	53.0
37	6692	49.2	2.7	44.0	45.7	47.4	49.3	51.1	52.6	54.1
38	8786	50.2	2.7	45.2	46.8	48.5	50.2	52.0	53.5	55.0
39	8324	51.0	2.4	46.1	47.7	49.3	51.0	52.7	54.2	55.6
40	7235	51.6	2.4	46.9	48.4	49.9	51.6	53.2	54.7	56.1
41	2538	52.1	2.4	47.5	49.0	50.5	52.1	53.7	55.1	56.5
HC (cm)										
23	153	21.3	1.0	NA[a]	20.0	20.6	21.3	22.0	22.7	NA[a]
24[b]	451	22.2	1.1	20.1	20.8	21.5	22.2	23.0	23.6	24.3
25	722	23.1	1.1	20.9	21.7	22.4	23.2	23.9	24.6	25.3
26	881	24.1	1.3	21.8	22.5	23.3	24.2	25.0	25.7	26.4
27	1030	25.2	1.3	22.6	23.5	24.3	25.2	26.0	26.8	27.6
28	1281	26.1	1.4	23.5	24.3	25.2	26.1	27.1	27.9	28.6
29	1505	27.0	1.4	24.3	25.2	26.1	27.1	28.0	28.8	29.6
30	1992	27.9	1.5	25.1	26.1	27.0	28.0	29.0	29.8	30.6
31	2460	28.9	1.5	26.0	27.0	27.9	28.9	29.9	30.8	31.6
32	3677	29.8	1.5	26.9	27.8	28.8	29.9	30.9	31.8	32.6

APPENDIX 9: Male Birth Weight, Length, and HC Percentiles by GA *(Continued)*

GA (wk)	n	Birth Size Mean	SD	Percentile 3rd	10th	25th	50th	75th	90th	97th
33	5014	30.7	1.6	27.7	28.7	29.7	30.8	31.8	32.7	33.6
34	7291	31.6	1.6	28.5	29.5	30.5	31.6	32.7	33.6	34.6
35	6952	32.4	1.6	29.2	30.3	31.3	32.4	33.6	34.5	35.5
36	7011	33.2	1.7	29.9	31.0	32.1	33.2	34.3	35.3	36.3
37	6692	33.8	1.7	30.6	31.7	32.7	33.9	35.0	36.0	36.9
38	8786	34.4	1.7	31.2	32.2	33.2	34.4	35.5	36.4	37.3
39	8324	34.6	1.6	31.5	32.5	33.5	34.6	35.7	36.6	37.6
40	7235	34.8	1.5	31.8	32.8	33.8	34.8	35.9	36.8	37.7
41	2538	35.1	1.5	32.0	33.0	34.0	35.0	36.1	37.0	37.8

[a]Not available because of small sample size.
[b]Distribution skewed left.

From Olsen IE, et al. New intrauterine growth curves based on United States data. *Pediatrics* 2010;125(2):e214–e224, with permission. Adapted from Groveman SA. *New Preterm Infant Growth Curves Influence of Gender and Race on Birth Size [master's thesis]*. Philadelphia, PA: Biotechnology and Bioscience, Drexel University, 2008.

APPENDIX 10: Means and Standard Deviations of Weights and Measurements of Stillborn Infants by Gestational Age

Gestational Age (wk)	Body Weight (g)	Crown-Rump Length (cm)	Crown-Heel Length (cm)	Toe-Heel Length (cm)	Brain (g)	Thymus (g)
20	313	18	24.9	3.3	41	0.4
	± 139	± 2.0	± 2.3	± 0.6	± 24	± 0.3
21	353	18.9	26.2	3.5	48	0.5
	± 125	± 4.8	± 3.6	± 0.6	± 18	± 0.3
22	398	19.8	27.4	3.8	55	0.6
	± 117	± 9.6	± 2.5	± 0.4	± 15	± 0.4
23	450	20.6	28.7	4	64	0.8
	± 118	± 2.3	± 3.3	± 0.5	± 18	± 0.5
24	510	21.5	29.9	4.2	74	0.9
	± 179	± 3.1	± 4.3	± 0.8	± 25	± 0.7
25	581	22.3	31.1	4.4	85	1.1
	± 178	± 4.0	± 6.5	± 0.8	± 31	± 0.8
26	663	23.2	32.4	4.7	98	1.4
	± 227	± 4.1	± 5.3	± 0.9	± 37	± 1.4
27	758	24.1	33.6	4.9	112	1.7
	± 227	± 2.9	± 3.2	± 1.4	± 37	± 1.1
28	864	24.9	34.9	5.1	127	2
	± 247	± 2.2	± 5.6	± 1.2	± 39	± 2.1
29	984	25.8	36.1	5.3	143	2.4
	± 511	± 4.1	± 5.9	± 1.2	± 57	± 2.6
30	1115	26.6	37.3	5.6	160	2.8
	± 329	± 2.4	± 3.6	± 0.7	± 72	± 4.1
31	1259	27.5	38.6	5.8	178	3.2
	± 588	± 3.0	± 2.7	± 0.7	± 32	± 1.9
32	1413	28.4	39.8	6	196	3.7
	± 623	± 2.8	± 5.4	± 0.6	± 92	± 2.2
33	1578	29.2	41.1	6.2	216	4.3
	± 254	± 3.5	± 3.1	± 0.4	± 51	± 1.5
34	1750	30.1	42.3	6.5	236	4.8
	± 494	± 3.5	± 4.3	± 0.8	± 42	± 5.6
35	1930	30.9	43.5	6.7	256	5.4
	± 865	± 3.9	± 5.8	± 0.9	± 70	± 3.4
36	2114	31.8	44.8	6.9	277	6.1
	± 616	± 4.0	± 7.2	± 0.8	± 94	± 4.1
37	2300	32.7	46	7.2	297	6.7
	± 647	± 5.1	± 7.9	± 0.9	± 69	± 3.9
38	2485	33.5	47.3	7.4	317	7.4
	± 579	± 2.6	± 3.9	± 0.8	± 83	± 6.1
39	2667	34.4	48.5	7.6	337	8.1
	± 596	± 3.7	± 4.9	± 0.5	± 132	± 4.7
40	2842	35.2	49.7	7.8	355	8.9
	± 482	± 6.4	± 3.2	± 0.7	± 57	± 4.3
41	3006	36.1	51	8.1	373	9.6
	± 761	± 3.7	± 5.4	± 0.8	± 141	± 5.6
42	3156	36.9	52.2	8.3	389	10.4
	± 678	± 2.0	± 3.0	± 0.5	± 36	± 5.0

Compiled October 1, 1988, by CJ Sung and DB Singer with 1975–1984 data from Women and Infants' Hospital, Providence, Rhode Island.

Heart (g)	Lungs Combined (g)	Spleen (g)	Liver (g)	Kidneys Combined (g)	Adrenals Combined (g)	Pancreas (g)
2.4	7.1	0.3	17	2.7	1.3	0.5
± 1.0	± 3.0	± 1.0	± 9	± 2.9	± 0.6	± 0.1
2.6	7.9	0.4	18	3.1	1.4	0.5
± 0.9	± 3.8	± 0.6	± 7	± 1.3	± 0.7	± 0.4
2.8	8.7	0.5	19	3.5	1.4	0.6
± 0.9	± 3.1	± 0.4	± 10	± 0.8	± 0.6	± 0.5
3	9.5	0.7	21	4.1	1.5	0.7
± 1.4	± 5.7	± 0.5	± 7	± 1.7	± 0.8	± 0.3
3.3	10.5	0.9	22	4.6	1.5	0.7
± 1.8	± 5.6	± 0.7	± 8	± 2.4	± 0.8	± 0.3
3.7	11.6	1.2	24	5.3	1.6	0.8
± 1.3	± 4.9	± 0.4	± 35	± 2.4	± 0.8	± 0.7
4.2	12.9	1.5	26	6.1	1.7	0.8
± 2.2	± 8.7	± 1.1	± 16	± 3.6	± 0.9	± 0.7
4.8	14.4	1.9	29	7	1.9	0.9
± 3.6	± 9.7	± 1.0	± 24	± 3.1	± 1.5	± 0.3
5.4	16.1	2.3	32	7.9	2.1	1
± 2.6	± 7.0	± 1.1	± 32	± 2.5	± 1.6	± 0.3
6.2	18	2.7	36	9	2.4	1.1
± 2.4	± 13.6	± 2.0	± 23	± 4.5	± 1.2	± 1.2
7	20.1	3.1	40	10.1	2.7	1.2
± 2.8	± 8.6	± 1.5	± 22	± 6.0	± 1.3	± 0.2
8	22.5	3.6	46	11.3	3	1.4
± 3.1	± 10.1	± 4.0	± 38	± 4.1	± 1.8	± 1.4
9.1	25	4.2	52	12.6	3.5	1.6
± 4.1	± 10.7	± 2.4	± 32	± 8.0	± 1.8	± 0.6
10.2	27.8	4.7	58	13.9	3.9	1.8
± 2.0	± 5.8	± 2.3	± 17	± 3.5	± 1.4	± 0.8
11.4	30.7	5.3	66	15.3	4.4	2
± 3.2	± 15.2	± 2.5	± 22	± 5.1	± 1.3	± 0.5
12.6	33.7	5.9	74	16.7	4.9	2.3
± 5.3	± 14.3	± 6.8	± 46	± 7.1	± 1.9	± 0.7
13.9	36.7	6.5	82	18.1	5.4	2.6
± 5.8	± 16.8	± 2.9	± 36	± 6.3	± 2.4	± 2.6
15.1	39.8	7.2	91	19.4	5.8	2.9
± 9.9	± 11.1	± 6.3	± 57	± 9.7	± 6.2	± 3.1
16.4	42.9	7.8	100	20.8	6.3	3.2
± 4.4	± 15.7	± 5.9	± 44	± 6.0	± 2.1	± 1.6
17.5	45.8	8.5	109	22	6.7	3.5
± 3.9	± 15.2	± 4.5	± 53	± 5.8	± 5.3	± 1.9
18.6	48.6	9.2	118	23.1	7	3.9
±12.9	± 19.4	± 4.1	± 49	± 8.6	± 2.9	± 1.7
19.5	51.1	9.9	126	24.1	7.1	4.2
± 4.9	± 17.0	± 4.5	± 53	±10.5	± 3.0	
20.3	53.2	10.6	135	24.9	7.2	4.5
± 4.5	±10.1	± 3.7	± 54	± 8.1	± 2.9	± 2.3

APPENDIX 11: Means and Standard Deviations of Weights and Measurements of Stillborn Infants by Body Weight

Body Weight (g)	Gestational Age (wk)	Crown-Rump Length (cm)	Crown-Heel Length (cm)	Toe-Heel Length (cm)	Brain (g)	Thymus (g)
50-100	17	13.2	18.8	2.3	10	0.2
	± 3	± 0.4	± 1.1	± 0.3		
101-200	19	14.2	20.1	2.5	16	0.3
	± 3	± 1.0	± 1.3	± 0.2	± 1	± 0.3
201-300	21	16	22.7	3	33	0.4
	± 3	± 4.1	± 1.8	± 0.4	± 11	± 0.3
301-400	22	17.7	25.1	3.4	49	0.6
	± 2	± 1.3	± 2.1	± 0.4	± 12	± 0.5
401-500	24	19.3	27.3	3.8	65	0.9
	± 2	± 5.7	± 4.1	± 0.4	± 17	± 0.5
501-600	25	20.7	29.4	4.2	81	1.2
	± 2	± 2.2	± 2.1	0.3	± 19	± 0.5
601-700	26	22.1	31.3	4.6	96	1.5
	± 3	± 1.4	± 3.0	± 0.8	± 27	± 1.4
701-800	28	23.4	33.1	4.9	111	1.8
	± 3	± 2.0	± 3.9	± 0.5	± 29	± 0.8
801-900	29	24.5	34.7	5.2	126	2.1
	± 2	± 1.4	± 2.9	± 0.6	± 58	± 1.5
901-1000	30	25.6	36.2	5.5	140	2.4
	± 3	± 2.3	± 1.7	± 1.3	± 49	± 0.8
1001-1250	31	26.6	37.6	5.7	154	2.6
	± 3	± 1.7	± 3.7	± 0.7	± 37	± 1.7
1251-1500	33	28.7	40.6	6.3	188	3.4
	± 3	± 1.3	± 2.6	± 0.4	± 77	± 2.8
1501-1750	34	30.4	43	6.7	220	4.1
	± 3	± 5.6	± 5.6	± 0.4	± 67	± 2.9
1751-2000	36	31.8	44.8	7	249	4.9
	± 2	± 1.6	± 2.3	± 0.5	± 19	± 2.8
2001-2250	37	32.9	46.3	7.3	277	5.7
	± 3	± 1.9	± 2.8	± 0.6	± 69	± 2.8
2251-2500	38	33.7	47.5	7.4	302	6.5
	± 3	± 2.0	± 3.4	± 0.7	± 45	± 3.0
2501-2750	38	34.5	48.5	7.6	325	7.4
	± 3	± 3.2	± 2.6	± 0.5	± 89	± 4.6
2751-3000	39	35.1	49.5	7.7	345	8.4
	± 4	± 2.7	± 4.0	± 0.8	± 88	± 5.4
3001-3250	39	35.9	50.5	7.9	363	9.4
	± 2	± 2.2	± 3.5	± 0.6	± 111	± 4.3
3251-3500	39	36.7	51.7	8	379	10.5
	± 3	± 2.4	± 4.5	± 0.7	± 53	± 4.3
3501-3750	40	37.7	53.1	8.2	392	11.7
	± 2	± 2.4	± 3.1	± 0.4	± 85	6.0
3751-4000	40	39	54.9	8.5	403	13
	± 3	± 1.0	± 0.9	± 0.7	±124	± 1.0
4001-4500	41	40.6	57.1	8.9	411	14.4
	± 1	± 2.5	± 2.1	± 0.4	± 83	± 5.0

Compiled October 1, 1988, by CJ Sung and DB Singer with 1975–1984 data from Women and Infants' Hospital, Providence, Rhode Island.

Heart (g)	Lungs Combined (g)	Spleen (g)	Liver (g)	Kidneys Combined (g)	Adrenals Combined (g)	Pancreas (g)
0.9	3.9	0.1	6	1.4	0.1	0.1
± 1.4	± 1.2	± 0.1	± 4	± 0.3	± 0.4	
1.2	4.8	0.2	7	1.8	0.2	0.1
± 0.5	± 1.2	± 0.4	± 2	± 0.3	± 0.3	± 0.5
1.9	6.4	0.4	11	2.6	0.5	0.3
± 0.9	± 2.3	± 0.8	± 6	± 1.8	± 0.5	± 0.1
2.5	8	0.7	15	3.4	0.8	0.4
± 0.7	± 3.3	± 0.4	± 6	± 0.8	± 0.5	± 0.5
3.2	9.6	0.9	18	4.2	1.1	0.6
± 0.9	± 4.2	± 0.3	± 8	± 1.5	± 0.7	± 0.3
3.8	11.3	1.2	21	5.1	1.3	0.7
± 1.2	± 3.5	± 0.4	± 8	± 2.0	± 0.6	± 0.3
4.5	12.9	1.4	25	5.9	1.6	0.8
± 2.7	± 6.3	± 0.7	± 12	± 2.4	± 1.2	± 2.0
5.1	14.5	1.7	28	6.7	1.9	1
± 1.6	± 5.4	± 1.0	± 11	± 3.5	± 0.7	± 0.7
5.7	16.2	2	31	7.5	2.2	1.1
± 1.3	± 5.9	± 2.1	± 16	± 2.1	± 1.1	± 0.3
6.4	17.8	2.3	34	8.3	2.5	1.2
± 2.0	± 4.8	± 0.9	± 17	± 3.0	± 2.0	± 0.7
7	19.4	2.6	38	9.2	2.8	1.4
± 1.5	± 6.1	± 1.6	± 24	± 4.4	± 1.1	± 0.8
8.6	23.5	3.4	46	11.2	3.5	1.7
± 3.1	± 6.0	± 0.9	± 15	± 4.4	± 1.5	± 1.0
10.2	27.6	4.3	55	13.3	4.2	2
± 2.3	± 8.3	± 1.9	± 19	± 5.4	± 1.3	± 0.6
11.8	31.6	5.2	64	15.3	4.9	2.4
± 2.3	± 6.8	± 2.4	± 23	± 4.9	± 0.9	± 0.4
13.4	35.7	6.2	74	17.3	5.6	2.7
± 2.1	± 10.8	± 5.6	± 23	± 5.6	± 1.5	± 0.8
15	39.8	7.2	86	19.4	6.3	3.1
± 4.1	± 8.1	± 1.8	± 21	± 3.4	2.2	
16.7	43.9	8.3	98	21.4	7	3.4
± 11.9	± 9.6	± 3.3	± 31	± 5.4	± 2.2	± 2.3
18.3	47.9	9.4	113	23.5	7.7	3.7
± 3.7	± 15.2	± 3.7	± 28	± 6.2	± 2.8	± 0.1
19.9	52	10.6	129	25.5	8.4	4.1
± 8.3	± 15.6	± 4.4	± 43	± 7.9	± 2.7	± 1.3
21.5	56.1	11.8	147	27.6	9.1	4.4
± 3.5	± 13.6	± 6.4	± 30	± 7.8	± 5.0	
23.1	60.1	13.1	167	29.6	9.9	4.7
± 3.1	± 16.6	± 4.8	± 56	± 6.9	± 2.3	± 2.1
24.7	64.2	14.5	190	31.7	10.6	5.1
± 3.4	± 6.0	± 7.4	± 41	± 9.0	± 11.4	
26.3	68.3	15.9	216	33.7	11.3	5.4
± 4.1	± 7.3	± 4.9	± 32	± 6.5	± 1.3	

APPENDIX 12: Means and Standard Deviations of Weights and Measurements of Live-Born Infants by Gestational Age

Gestational Age (wk)	Body Weight (g)	Crown-Rump Length (cm)	Crown-Heel Length (cm)	Toe-Heel Length (cm)	Brain (g)	Thymus (g)
20	381	18.3	25.6	3.6	49	0.8
	± 104	± 2.2	± 2.2	± 0.7	± 15	± 2.3
21	426	19.1	26.7	3.8	57	1
	± 66	± 1.2	± 1.7	± 0.1	± 8	± 0.3
22	473	20	27.8	4	65	1.2
	± 63	± 1.3	± 1.6	± 0.4	± 13	± 0.3
23	524	20.8	28.9	4.2	74	1.4
	± 116	± 1.9	± 3.0	± 0.5	± 11	± 0.7
24	584	21.6	30	4.4	83	1.5
	± 92	± 1.4	± 1.7	± 0.3	± 15	± 0.7
25	655	22.5	31.1	4.6	94	1.8
	± 106	± 1.6	± 2.0	± 0.4	± 25	± 1.2
26	739	23.3	32.2	4.8	105	2
	± 181	± 1.9	± 2.4	± 0.7	± 21	± 1.1
27	836	24.2	33.4	5	118	2.3
	± 197	± 2.5	± 3.5	± 0.5	± 21	± 1.2
28	949	25	34.5	5.2	132	2.6
	± 190	± 1.7	± 2.3	± 0.6	± 29	± 1.5
29	1077	25.9	35.6	5.4	147	3
	± 449	± 2.8	± 4.4	± 0.8	± 49	± 1.9
30	1219	26.7	36.7	5.7	163	3.5
	± 431	± 3.3	± 4.2	± 0.7	± 38	± 2.6
31	1375	27.6	37.8	5.9	180	4
	± 281	± 3.8	± 3.1	± 0.7	± 34	± 3.4
32	1543	28.4	38.9	6.1	198	4.7
	± 519	± 9.5	± 5.7	± 1.1	± 48	± 3.6
33	1720	29.3	40	6.3	217	5.4
	± 580	± 3.3	± 3.5	± 0.7	± 49	± 3.2
34	1905	30.1	41.1	6.5	237	6.1
	± 625	± 4.3	± 4.0	± 0.6	± 53	± 3.8
35	2093	30.9	42.3	6.7	257	6.9
	± 309	± 2.0	± 2.9	± 0.4	± 45	± 4.5
36	2280	31.8	43.4	6.9	278	7.7
	± 615	± 3.9	± 5.9	± 1.1	± 96	± 5.0
37	2462	32.6	44.5	7.1	298	8.4
	± 821	± 5.0	± 7.0	± 1.2	± 70	± 5.6
38	2634	33.5	45.6	7.3	318	9
	± 534	± 3.2	± 5.1	± 0.8	± 106	± 2.8
39	2789	34.3	46.7	7.5	337	9.4
	± 520	± 1.9	± 4.4	± 0.5	± 91	± 2.5
40	2922	35.2	47.8	7.7	356	9.5
	± 450	± 2.8	± 4.2	± 0.8	± 79	± 5.0
41	3025	36	48.9	7.9	372	9.1
	± 600	± 3.1	± 5.4	± 0.8	± 65	± 4.8
42	391	36.9	50	8.1	387	8.1
	± 617	± 2.4	± 3.8	± 1.1	± 61	± 3.8

Compiled October 1, 1988, by CJ Sung and DB Singer with 1975–1984 data from Women and Infants' Hospital, Providence, Rhode Island.

Heart (g)	Lungs Combined (g)	Spleen (g)	Liver (g)	Kidneys Combined (g)	Adrenals Combined (g)	Pancreas (g)
2.8	11.5	0.7	22.4	3.7	1.8	0.5
± 1.0	± 2.9	± 0.3	± 8.0	± 1.3	± 1.0	± 0.5
3.2	12.9	0.7	24.1	4.2	2	0.5
± 0.4	± 2.8	± 0.2	± 4.2	± 0.7	± 0.5	
3.5	14.4	0.8	25.4	4.7	2	0.6
± 0.6	± 4.3	± 0.4	± 5.2	± 1.5	± 0.6	± 0.3
3.9	15.9	0.8	26.6	5.3	2.1	0.7
± 1.3	± 4.9	± 0.4	± 8.0	± 1.8	± 0.8	± 0.4
4.2	17.4	0.9	28	6	2.2	0.8
± 1.0	± 5.9	± 0.5	± 7.1	± 1.8	± 0.8	± 0.5
4.7	19	1.1	29.7	6.8	2.2	0.9
± 1.2	± 5.3	± 1.6	± 9.8	± 1.9	± 1.4	± 0.3
5.2	20.6	1.3	32.1	7.6	2.4	1
± 1.3	± 6.3	± 0.7	± 10.9	± 2.5	± 1.1	± 0.5
5.8	22.1	1.7	35.1	8.6	2.5	1.2
± 1.9	± 9.7	± 1.0	± 13.3	± 3.0	± 1.1	± 0.5
6.5	23.7	2.1	38.9	9.7	2.7	1.4
± 1.9	± 10.0	± 0.8	± 12.6	± 12.0	± 1.2	± 0.5
7.2	25.3	2.6	43.5	10.9	3	1.5
± 2.7	± 12.6	± 0.9	± 15.8	± 4.4	± 1.2	± 1.0
8.1	26.9	3.3	49.1	12.3	3.3	1.7
± 2.6	± 20.3	± 2.0	± 18.8	± 8.5	± 2.7	± 1.0
9	28.5	4	55.4	13.7	3.7	1.8
± 2.8	± 13.2	± 1.2	± 17.3	± 5.2	± 1.3	± 0.6
10.1	30.2	4.7	62.5	15.2	4.1	2
± 4.4	± 19.0	± 5.4	± 30.0	± 7.4	± 1.7	± 0.8
11.2	31.8	5.5	70.3	16.8	4.6	2.1
± 4.0	± 13.5	± 3.5	± 25.4	± 7.7	± 1.5	± 0.8
12.4	33.5	6.4	78.7	18.5	5.1	2.3
± 2.8	± 16.5	± 3.0	± 30.2	± 9.3	± 2.2	± 1.1
13.7	35.2	7.2	87.4	20.1	5.6	2.5
± 3.6	± 20.5	± 5.2	± 30.6	± 10.9	± 2.8	± 0.6
15	36.9	8.1	96.3	21.7	6.1	2.6
± 5.1	± 17.5	± 3.1	± 33.7	± 6.8	± 3.1	± 0.7
16.4	38.7	8.8	105.1	23.3	6.6	2.8
± 5.7	± 22.9	± 6.4	± 33.7	± 9.9	± 3.3	± 0.9
17.7	40.6	9.5	113.5	24.8	7.1	3
± 5.4	± 17.1	± 3.5	± 34.7	± 7.2	± 2.9	± 1.1
19.1	42.6	10.1	121.3	26.1	7.4	3.3
± 2.8	± 14.9	± 3.5	± 39.2	± 4.9	± 2.5	± 0.5
20.4	44.6	10.4	127.9	27.3	7.7	3.6
± 5.6	± 22.7	± 3.3	± 35.8	± 11.5	± 3.0	± 1.3
21.7	46.8	10.5	133.1	28.1	7.8	3.9
± 10.9	± 26.2	± 4.5	± 55.7	± 12.7	± 2.8	± 1.5
22.9	49.1	10.3	136.4	28.7	7.8	4.3
± 6.2	± 14.6	± 3.6	± 38.9	± 9.7	± 3.2	± 1.9

APPENDIX 13: Means and Standard Deviations of Weights and Measurements of Live-Born Infants by Body Weight

Body Weight (g)	Gestational Age (wk)	Crown-Rump Length (cm)	Crown-Heel Length (cm)	Toe-Heel Length (cm)	Brain (g)	Thymus (g)
100-200	20	15.3	21.7	2.8	20	0.2
	± 1	± 1.0	± 1.2	± 0.3	± 3	
201-300	21	16.9	23.7	3.2	36	0.4
	± 2	± 1.1	± 1.2	± 0.2	± 12	± 0.2
301-400	22	18.3	25.6	3.6	52	0.8
	± 2	± 1.1	± 1.4	± 0.4	± 9	± 0.3
401-500	23	19.6	27.4	4	68	1.1
	± 2	± 1.2	± 1.6	± 0.3	± 17	± 0.44
501-600	24	20.9	29.1	4.3	83	1.4
	± 3	± 1.2	± 2.0	± 0.5	± 25	± 1.0
601-700	25	22.1	30.7	4.6	98	1.8
	± 2	± 1.3	± 1.8	± 0.4	± 21	± 0.74
701-800	26	23.2	32.1	4.9	113	2.1
	± 2	± 1.2	± 2.0	± 0.4	± 24	± 1.2
801-900	27	24.2	33.5	5.1	127	2.5
	± 2	± 1.0	± 1.6	± 0.4	± 20	± 1.1
901-1000	28	25.2	34.8	5.4	141	2.8
	± 2	± 0.9	± 1.6	± 0.4	± 26	± 1.3
1001-1250	29	26.1	36	5.6	155	3.1
	± 2	± 1.6	± 2.1	± 0.4	± 2.2	± 1.4
1251-1500	31	28.1	38.6	6.1	188	4
	± 2	± 2.9	± 2.7	± 0.8	± 34	± 2.0
1501-1750	33	29.8	40.7	6.4	219	4.8
	± 3	± 1.9	± 2.7	± 0.6	± 47	± 4.1
1751-2000	34	31.2	42.5	6.7	249	5.6
	± 3	± 1.4	± 3.5	± 0.4	± 64	± 2.7
2001-2250	36	32.4	44	7	276	6.4
	± 3	± 2.1	± 12.8	± 0.5	± 69	± 3.3
2251-2500	37	33.4	45.3	7.2	301	7.2
	± 3	± 2.9	± 2.4	± 0.6	± 40	± 4.4
2501-2750	38	34.3	46.5	7.4	324	7.9
	± 3	± 2.5	± 3.9	± 0.7	± 1.3	± 4.3
2751-3000	39	35	47.5	7.5	345	8.7
	± 2	± 2.9	± 3.4	± 0.8	± 79	± 4.6
3001-3250	40	35.8	48.6	7.7	364	9.4
	± 3	± 1.9	± 3.1	± 0.7	± 87	± 5.4
3251-3500	40	36.5	49.7	7.9	381	10.1
	± 2	± 2.3	± 3.4	± 0.8	± 101	± 5.2
3501-3750	41	37.2	51	8.2	396	10
	± 1	± 1.6	± 4.0	± 0.6	± 32	± 2.6
3751-4000	41	38.1	52.5	8.5	409	11.5
	± 1	± 1.9	± 2.6	± 0.3	± 52	± 3.7
4001-4500	41	39.1	54.3	8.9	420	12.2
	± 1	± 1.0	± 1.5	± 0.4	± 33	± 2.7

Compiled October 1, 1988, by CJ Sung and DB Singer with 1975–1984 data from Women and Infants' Hospital, Providence, Rhode Island.

Heart (g)	Lungs Combined (g)	Spleen (g)	Liver (g)	Kidneys Combined (g)	Adrenals Combined (g)	Pancreas (g)
1.3	9.6	0.1	15	2.8	0.8	0.3
± 0.2	± 0.7		± 1	± 0.3	± 0.1	± 0.1
2	11.1	0.4	18	3.7	1.1	0.4
± 0.3	± 2.4	± 0.2	± 3	± 2.0	± 0.2	± 0.3
2.7	12.6	0.6	20	4.6	1.4	0.5
± 0.7	± 4.3	± 0.5	± 6	± 0.8	± 0.7	± 0.2
3.4	14.1	0.7	23	5.5	1.6	0.7
± 1.1	± 4.4	± 0.4	± 6	± 1.4	± 0.7	± 0.4
4.1	15.6	1.1	26	6.4	1.9	0.8
± 0.8	± 4.8	± 0.5	± 6	± 1.5	± 0.8	± 0.3
4.8	17.1	1.5	30	7.3	2.2	0.9
± 0.9	± 6.9	± 0.4	± 7	± 1.9	± 1.1	± 0.4
5.5	18.6	1.9	33	8.1	2.4	1
± 1.4	± 8.0	± 1.1	± 9	± 1.7	± 1.3	± 0.3
6.1	20.1	2.2	36	9	2.7	1.1
± 1.4	± 7.3	± 0.9	± 9	± 2.7	± 1.4	± 0.6
6.8	21.6	2.6	40	9.9	2.9	1.3
± 1.7	± 7.8	± 0.8	± 9	± 2.6	± 1.0	± 0.4
7.5	23.1	3	43	10.8	3.2	1.4
± 2.1	± 9.6	± 0.9	± 10	± 3.4	± 1.1	± 0.5
9.3	26.9	3.9	53	13	3.9	1.7
± 2.2	± 14.6	± 1.6	± 14	± 4.8	± 1.2	± 0.7
11	30.7	4.9	63	15.2	4.5	2
± 2.6	± 16.8	± 1.3	± 12	± 8.5	± 2.1	± 1.0
12.7	34.5	5.8	74	17.4	5.2	2.3
± 2.7	± 21.4	± 2.8	± 16	± 8.1	± 2.2	± 0.8
14.4	38.3	6.8	85	19.6	5.8	2.6
± 3.2	± 20	± 2.4	± 21	± 9.0	± 2.6	± 1.3
16.2	42.2	7.7	97	21.8	6.5	2.9
± 3.3	± 15.0	± 4.7	± 25	± 8.0	± 2.3	± 0.8
17.9	46.1	8.7	110	24	7.1	3.2
± 6.6	± 13.2	± 3.8	± 20	± 5.9	± 2.6	± 1.2
19.6	50	9.6	124	26.2	7.8	3.5
± 5.5	± 13.7	± 2.7	± 27	± 7.1	± 2.1	± 1.1
21.4	53.9	10.6	138	28.4	8.4	3.8
± 4.9	± 20.4	± 3.0	± 26	± 9.2	± 2.6	± 1.7
23.1	57.9	11.5	153	30.6	9.1	4.1
± 11.9	± 15.4	± 3.6	± 26	± 9.0	± 3.0	± 0.7
24.8	61.8	12.5	168	32.8	9.7	4.4
± 3.8	± 11.8	± 3.5	± 36	± 13.6	± 2.7	± 0.7
26.5	65.8	13.4	184	35	10.4	4.7
± 5.4	± 18.8	± 2.9	± 36	± 10.1	± 3.7	± 1.6
28.3	69.8	14.4	201	37.2	11.1	5
± 1.8	± 7.0	± 3.7	±40	± 17.4	± 2.8	

APPENDIX 14: Selected Percentiles for Weight (in kg) from Age 1 to 12 Months (mo)[a]

Age (mo)	1st	5th	10th	25th	50th	75th	90th	95th	99th	Value[b]
Boys[c]										
1	2.34	2.97	3.26	3.68	4.14	4.55	4.88	5.174	5.42	4.09 ± 0.66
2	3.78	4.33	4.58	5.00	5.48	5.81	6.17	6.29	6.75	5.41 ± 0.61
3	4.68	5.21	5.42	5.80	6.30	6.73	7.10	7.27	7.89	6.28 ± 0.65
4	5.39	5.85	6.01	6.45	6.96	7.44	7.83	8.06	8.77	6.95 ± 0.69
5	5.82	6.30	6.58	7.00	7.50	8.02	8.44	8.77	9.51	7.51 ± 0.73
6	6.20	6.72	7.00	7.45	7.95	8.51	8.98	9.27	10.12	7.99 ± 0.77
7	6.59	7.09	7.40	7.89	8.34	8.95	9.48	9.76	10.61	8.42 ± 0.80
8	7.03	7.46	7.74	8.25	8.71	9.36	9.91	10.19	11.04	8.81 ± 0.83
9	7.31	7.80	8.09	8.59	9.09	9.74	10.24	10.64	11.43	9.16 ± 0.87
10	7.53	8.11	8.39	8.92	9.42	10.07	10.60	11.04	11.83	9.49 ± 0.90
11	7.77	8.37	8.66	9.21	9.72	10.39	10.92	11.44	12.23	9.80 ± 0.93
12	8.02	8.59	8.91	9.48	10.01	10.70	11.23	11.82	12.58	10.09 ± 0.97
Girls[d]										
1	2.30	2.91	3.10	3.53	3.87	4.14	4.52	4.86	5.41	3.84 ± 0.56
2	3.66	3.96	4.15	4.63	4.95	5.30	5.73	5.89	6.42	4.96 ± 0.57
3	4.33	4.63	4.81	5.30	5.71	6.15	6.59	6.86	7.28	5.73 ± 0.65
4	4.82	5.17	5.39	5.86	6.34	6.84	7.25	7.56	7.98	6.35 ± 0.71
5	5.20	5.62	5.87	6.36	6.87	7.40	7.89	8.16	8.67	6.87 ± 0.76
6	5.56	5.96	6.28	6.77	7.31	7.90	8.46	8.63	9.26	7.33 ± 0.80
7	5.86	6.35	6.72	7.11	7.72	8.32	8.87	9.12	9.77	7.74 ± 0.83
8	6.15	6.69	7.01	7.48	8.10	8.71	9.27	9.52	10.24	8.12 ± 0.86
9	6.44	6.99	7.25	7.82	8.47	9.08	9.59	9.91	10.64	8.46 ± 0.88
10	6.72	7.28	7.57	8.15	8.79	9.43	9.95	10.22	11.02	8.79 ± 0.91
11	6.98	7.54	7.86	8.44	9.12	9.76	10.27	10.58	11.42	9.10 ± 0.93
12	7.22	7.81	8.11	8.71	9.42	10.07	10.60	10.91	11.80	9.39 ± 0.95

[a]From $f(x) = a + b(x)^{0.5} + c \log x$, where x is age in years and $f(x)$ is the weight (kg) at age x.
[b]$\bar{x}$ ± SD.
[c]$n = 265$.
[d]$n = 239$.

From Roche AF, Guo S, Moore WM. Weight and recumbent length from 1 to 12 mo of age: reference data for 1-mo increments. *Am J Clin Nutr* 1989;49(4):599–607, with permission.

APPENDIX 15: Selected Percentiles for Recumbent Length (in cm) from Age 1 to 12 Months (mo[a])

Age	1st	5th	10th	25th	50th	75th	90th	95th	99th	Value[b]
Boys[c]										
1	47.99	50.85	51.90	53.20	54.68	56.14	57.29	58.38	60.35	54.60 ± 2.38
2	52.78	55.44	56.02	57.04	57.51	59.98	61.05	62.02	63.61	58.50 ± 2.10
3	55.83	58.20	58.77	59.83	61.29	62.83	64.05	64.66	66.51	61.36 ± 2.07
4	58.10	60.33	61.13	62.29	63.64	65.22	66.60	67.16	68.95	63.73 ± 2.09
5	60.46	62.44	63.21	64.22	65.72	67.37	68.67	69.40	71.10	65.79 ± 2.12
6	62.35	64.03	65.06	66.07	67.53	69.19	70.44	71.30	73.05	67.63 ± 2.16
7	63.91	65.76	66.61	67.74	69.23	70.83	72.18	73.01	74.85	69.31 ± 2.21
8	65.25	67.22	68.10	69.37	70.86	72.30	73.62	74.70	76.57	70.66 ± 2.26
9	66.41	68.49	69.39	70.62	72.25	73.80	75.38	76.24	78.18	72.31 ± 2.31
10	67.41	69.76	70.70	72.14	73.64	75.19	76.85	77.63	79.69	73.68 ± 2.36
11	68.25	70.95	71.94	73.36	74.98	76.53	78.32	78.95	81.13	74.98 ± 2.42
12	69.05	72.14	73.18	74.61	76.22	77.88	79.60	80.49	82.49	76.21 ± 2.46
Girls[d]										
1	47.95	49.81	50.72	52.25	53.76	55.06	56.14	56.37	57.70	53.54 ± 2.11
2	51.23	53.63	54.26	55.69	57.06	58.46	59.49	60.08	61.39	57.01 ± 2.02
3	53.88	56.24	57.03	58.56	59.70	61.20	62.43	63.13	64.07	59.70 ± 2.05
4	56.17	58.42	59.35	60.72	61.65	63.42	64.68	65.56	66.39	61.97 ± 2.09
5	58.21	60.35	61.20	62.71	63.69	65.47	66.73	67.70	66.47	63.97 ± 2.13
6	60.08	62.10	62.89	64.53	65.61	67.31	68.56	69.69	70.47	65.79 ± 2.16
7	61.82	63.80	64.40	66.08	67.36	69.03	70.27	71.48	72.29	67.47 ± 2.19
8	63.44	65.41	65.93	67.59	68.95	70.49	71.83	73.11	73.98	69.03 ± 2.22
9	64.98	66.90	67.44	69.00	70.47	71.91	73.37	74.59	75.56	70.49 ± 2.25
10	66.36	68.22	68.77	70.28	71.84	73.36	74.82	75.98	77.05	71.88 ± 2.28
11	67.54	69.43	70.00	71.49	73.15	74.66	76.21	77.32	78.47	73.20 ± 2.32
12	68.77	70.61	71.22	72.76	74.42	75.95	77.49	78.57	79.81	74.46 ± 2.35

[a]From $f(x) = a + b(x)^{0.5} + c \log x$, where x is age in years and $f(x)$ is the weight (kg) at age x.
[b]$\bar{x}$ ± SD.
[c]n = 228.
[d]n = 202.
From Roche AF, Guo S, Moore WM. Weight and recumbent length from 1 to 12 mo of age: reference data for 1-mo increments. *Am J Clin Nutr* 1989;49(4):599–607, with permission.

APPENDIX 16: Infant Heart Weight Centiles (Boys)

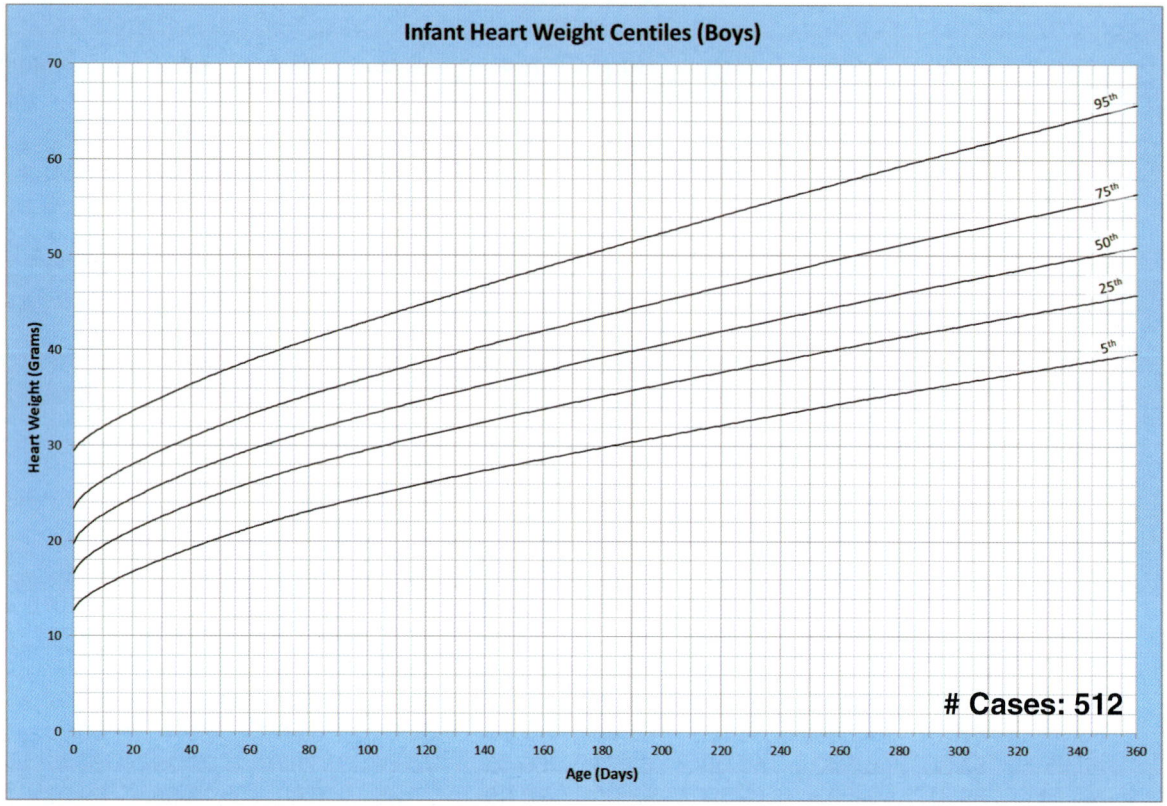

From Pryce JW, et al. Reference ranges for organ weights of infants at autopsy: results of >1,000 consecutive cases from a single centre. *BMC Clin Pathol* 2014;14:18, with permission.

APPENDIX 17: Infant Heart Weight Centiles (Girls)

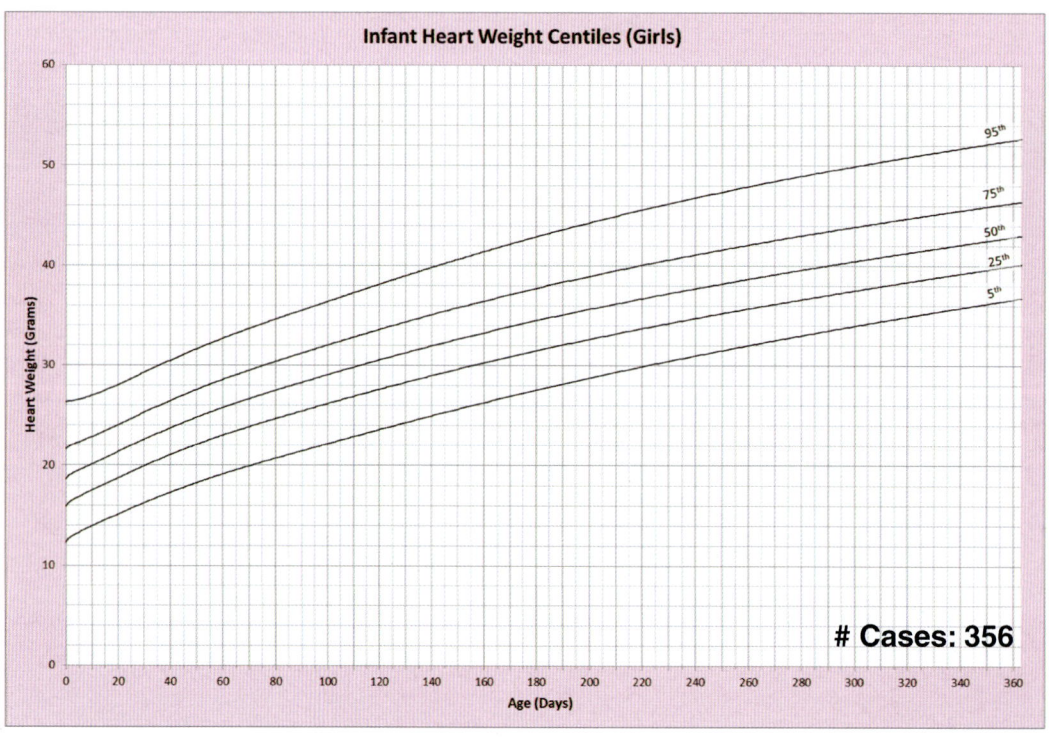

From Pryce JW, et al. Reference ranges for organ weights of infants at autopsy: results of >1,000 consecutive cases from a single centre. *BMC Clin Pathol* 2014;14:18, with permission.

APPENDIX 18: Infant Combined Lung Weight Centiles (Boys)

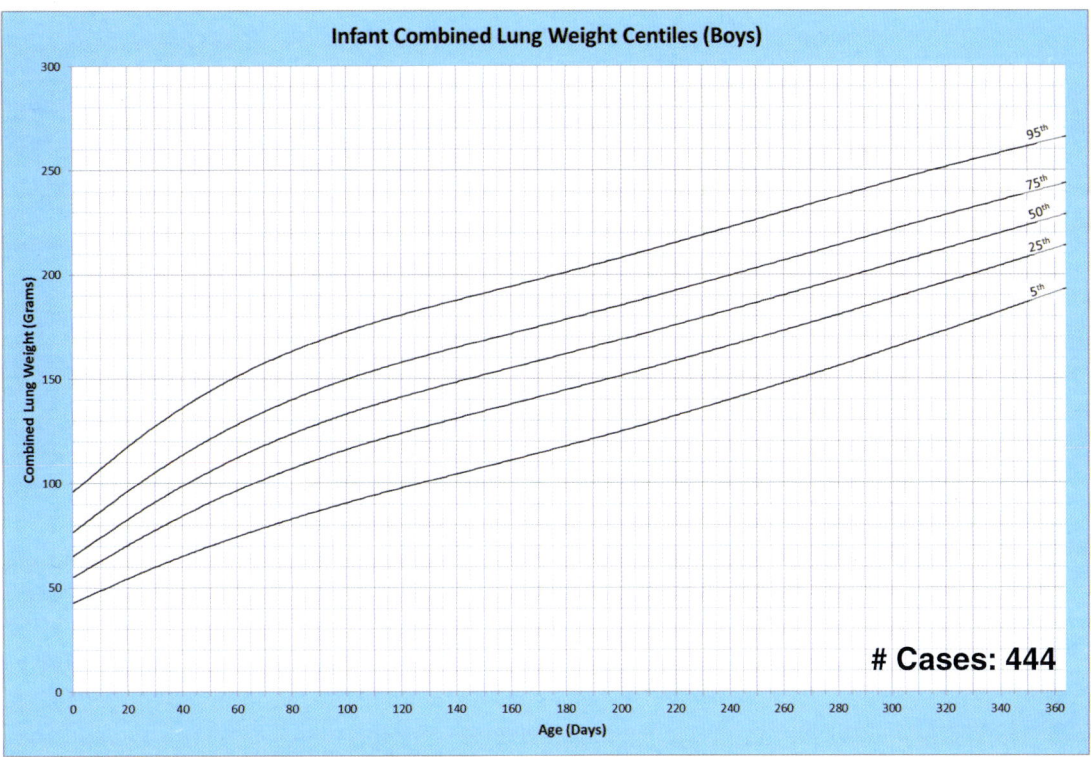

From Pryce JW, et al. Reference ranges for organ weights of infants at autopsy: results of >1,000 consecutive cases from a single centre. *BMC Clin Pathol* 2014;14:18, with permission.

APPENDIX 19: Infant Combined Lung Weight Centiles (Girls)

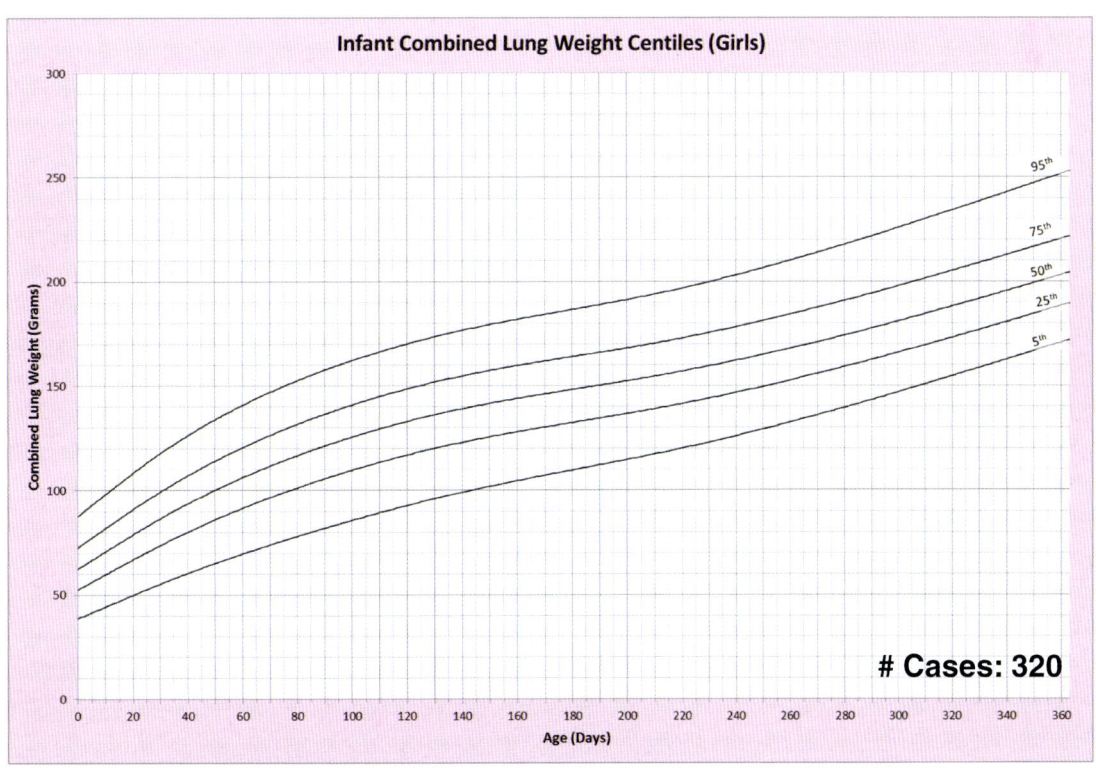

From Pryce JW, et al. Reference ranges for organ weights of infants at autopsy: results of >1,000 consecutive cases from a single centre. *BMC Clin Pathol* 2014;14:18, with permission.

APPENDIX 20: Infant Liver Weight Centiles (Boys)

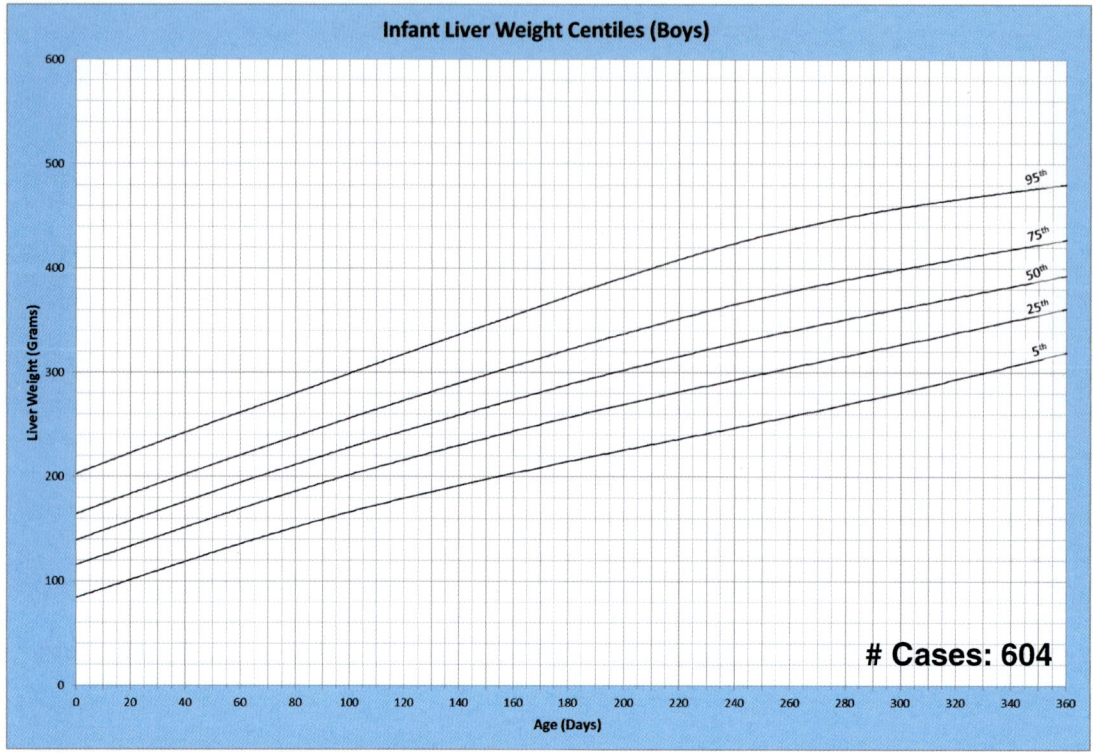

From Pryce JW, et al. Reference ranges for organ weights of infants at autopsy: results of >1,000 consecutive cases from a single centre. *BMC Clin Pathol* 2014;14:18, with permission.

APPENDIX 21: Infant Liver Weight Centiles (Girls)

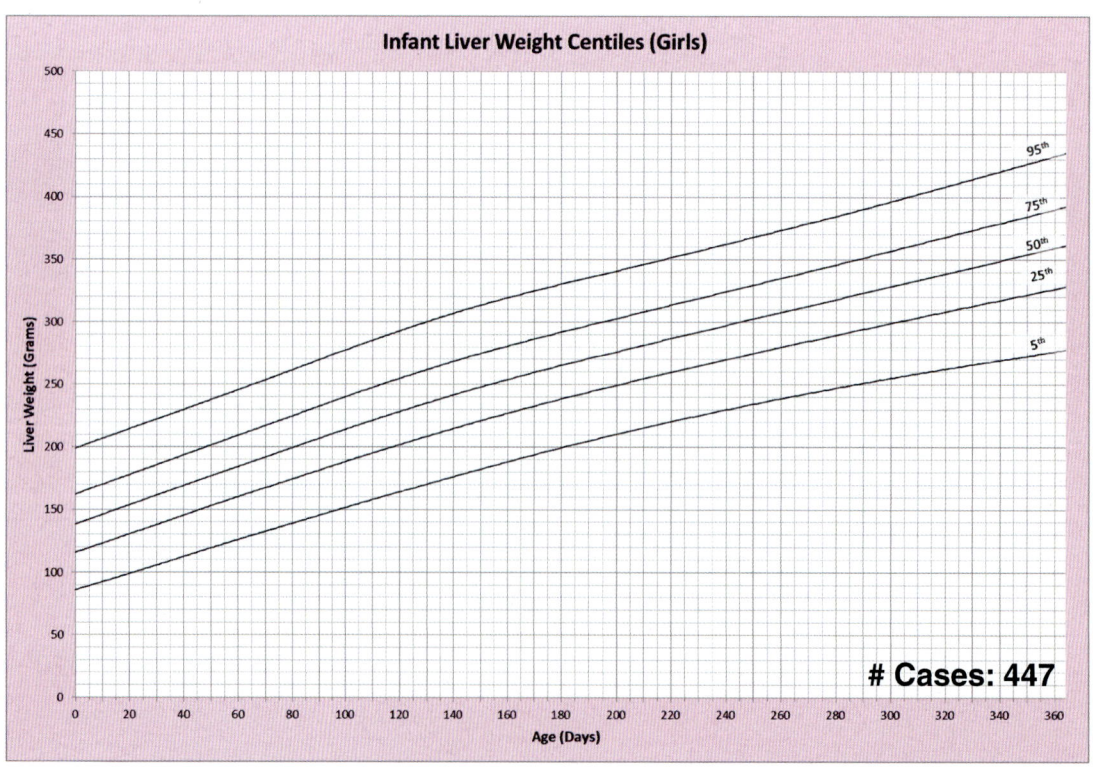

From Pryce JW, et al. Reference ranges for organ weights of infants at autopsy: results of >1,000 consecutive cases from a single centre. *BMC Clin Pathol* 2014;14:18, with permission.

APPENDIX 22: Infant Spleen Weight Centiles (Boys)

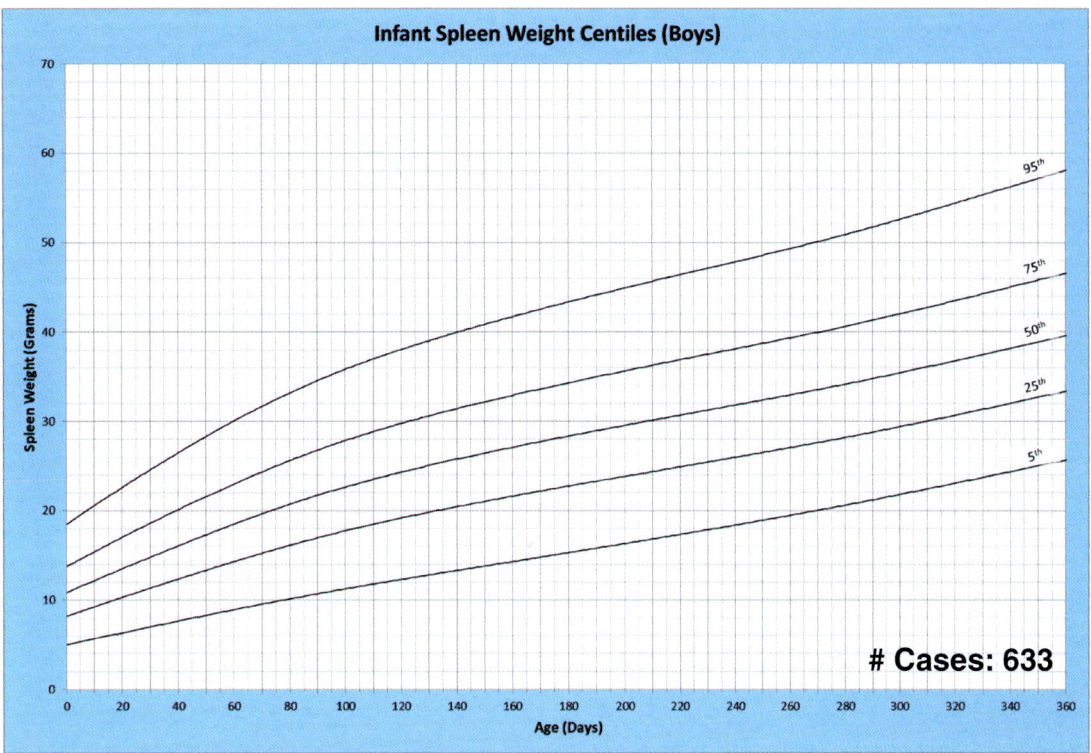

From Pryce, JW, et al. Reference ranges for organ weights of infants at autopsy: results of >1,000 consecutive cases from a single centre. *BMC Clin Pathol* 2014;14:18, with permission.

APPENDIX 23: Infant Spleen Weight Centiles (Girls)

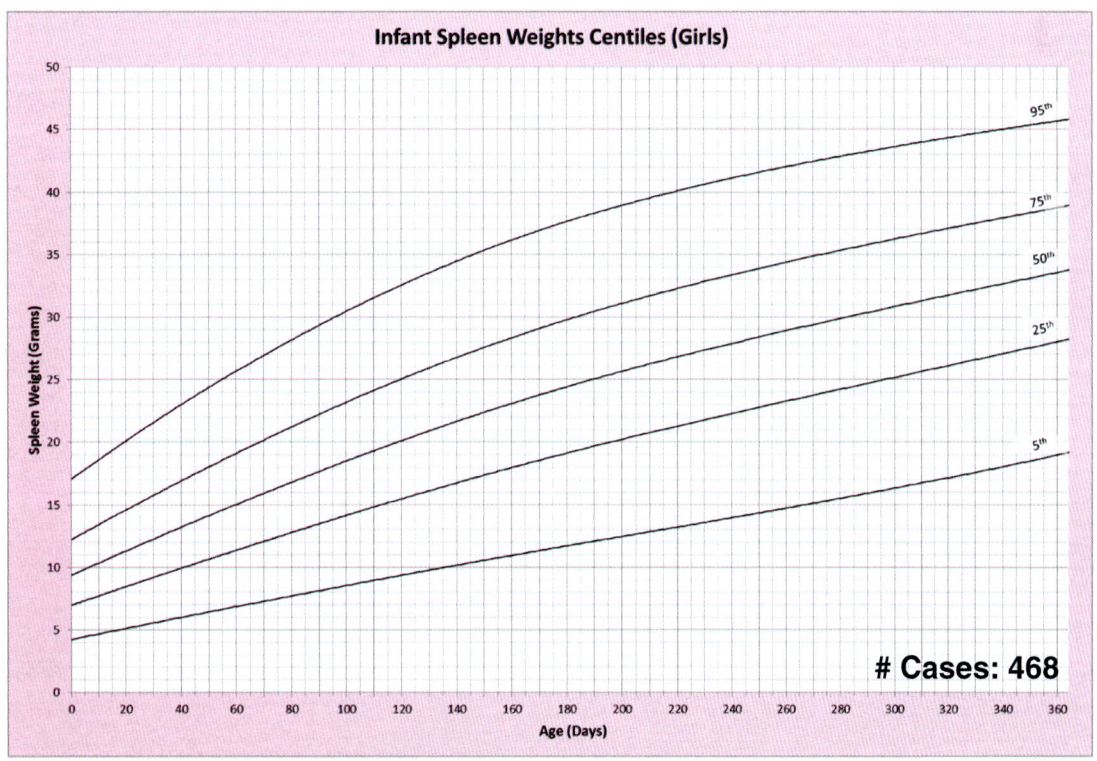

From Pryce JW, et al. Reference ranges for organ weights of infants at autopsy: results of >1,000 consecutive cases from a single centre. *BMC Clin Pathol* 2014;14:18, with permission.

APPENDIX 24: Infant Combined Kidney Weight Centiles (Boys)

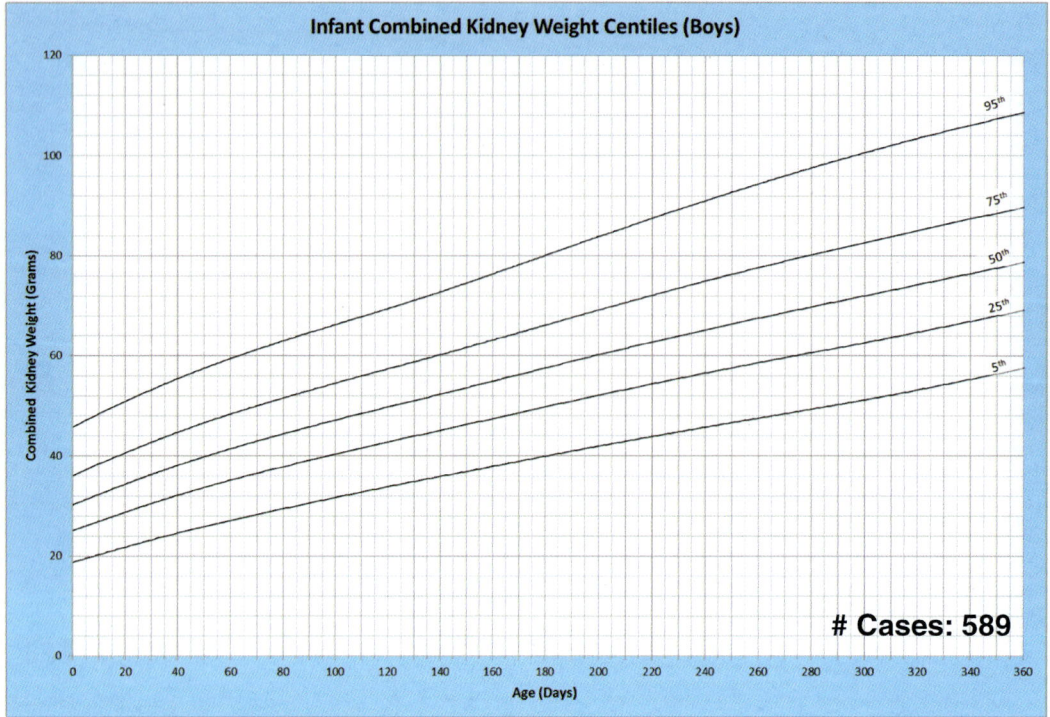

From Pryce JW, et al. Reference ranges for organ weights of infants at autopsy: results of >1,000 consecutive cases from a single centre. *BMC Clin Pathol* 2014;14:18, with permission.

APPENDIX 25: Infant Combined Kidney Weight Centiles (Girls)

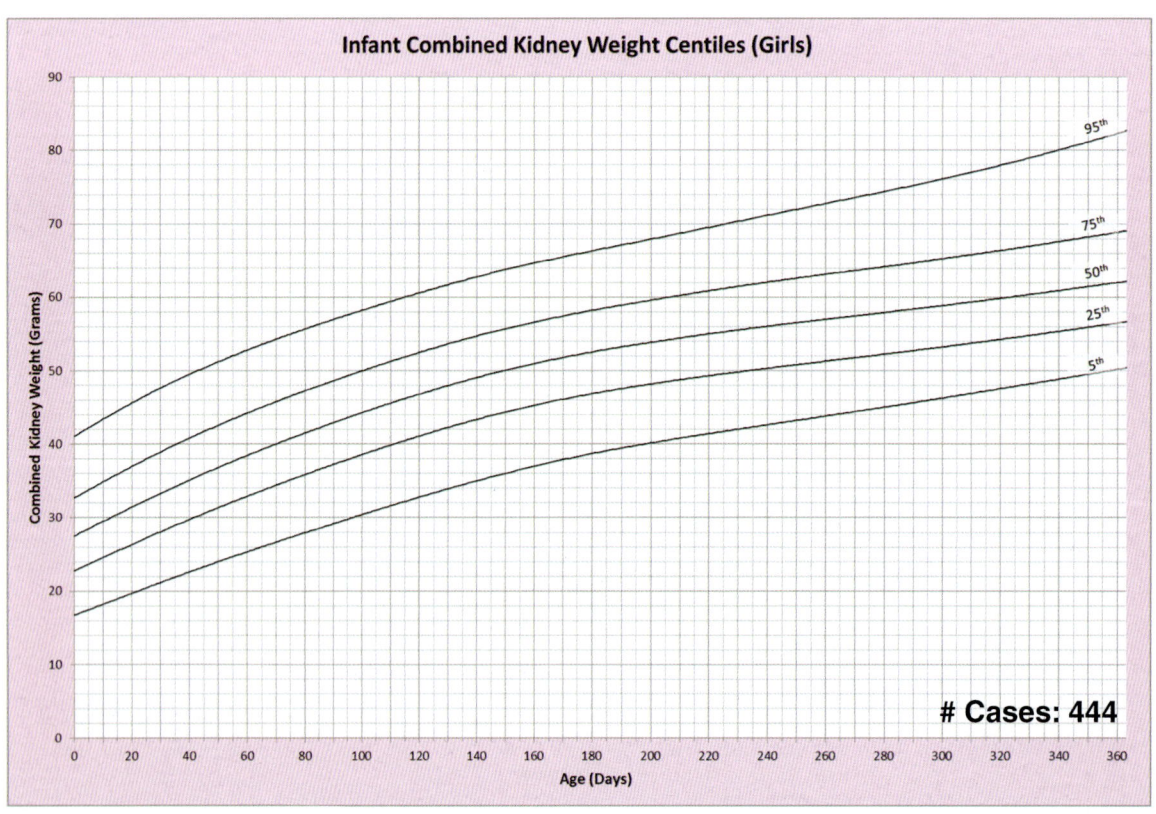

From Pryce JW, et al. Reference ranges for organ weights of infants at autopsy: results of >1,000 consecutive cases from a single centre. *BMC Clin Pathol* 2014;14:18, with permission.

APPENDIX 26: Infant Pancreas Weight Centiles (Boys)

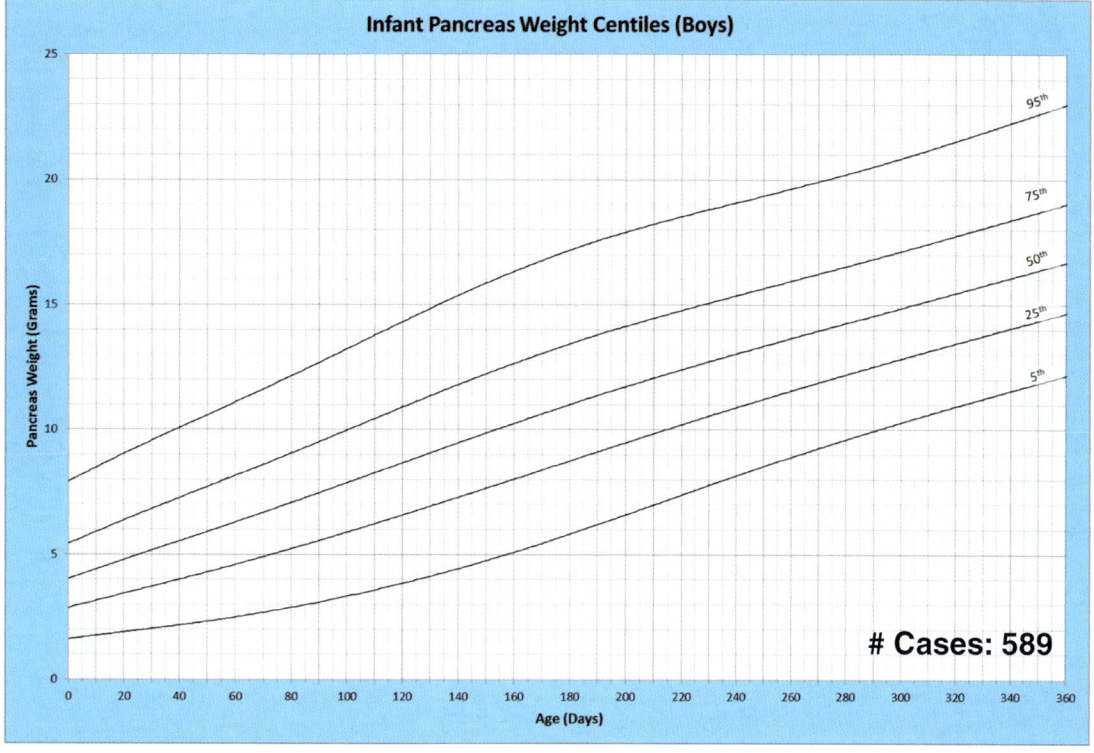

From Pryce JW, et al. Reference ranges for organ weights of infants at autopsy: results of >1,000 consecutive cases from a single centre. *BMC Clin Pathol* 2014;14:18, with permission.

APPENDIX 27: Infant Pancreas Weight Centiles (Girls)

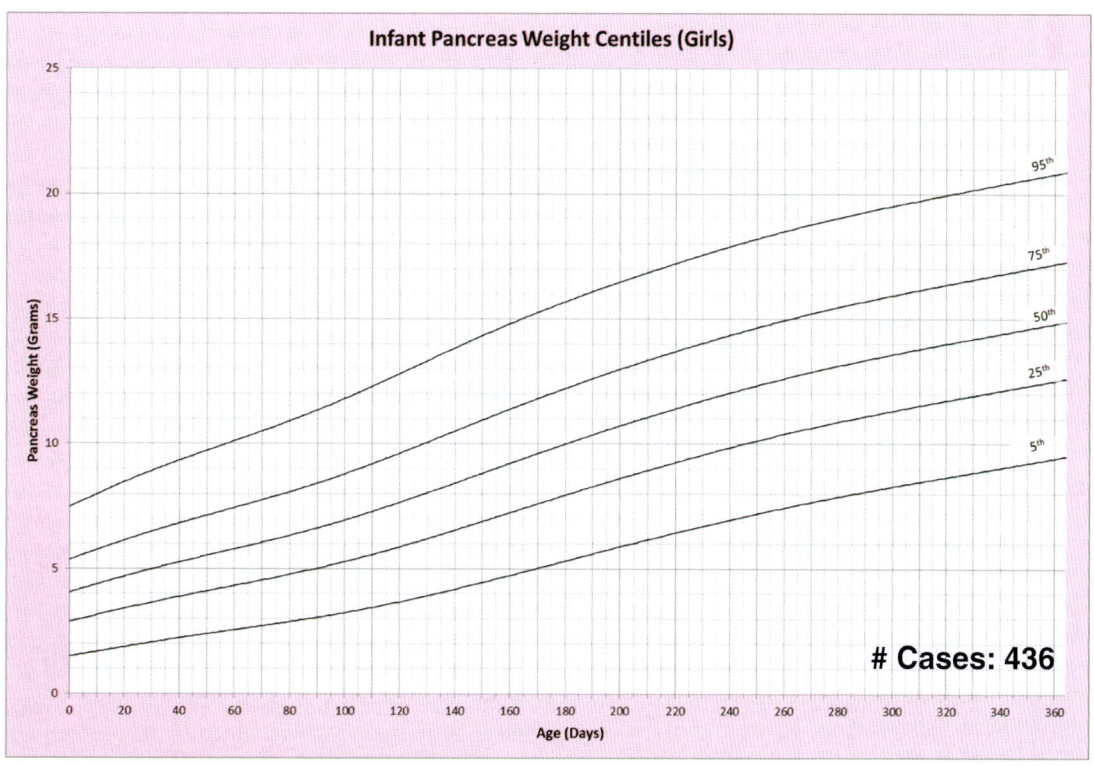

From Pryce JW, et al. Reference ranges for organ weights of infants at autopsy: results of >1,000 consecutive cases from a single centre. *BMC Clin Pathol* 2014;14:18, with permission.

APPENDIX 28: Infant Thymus Weight Centiles (Boys)

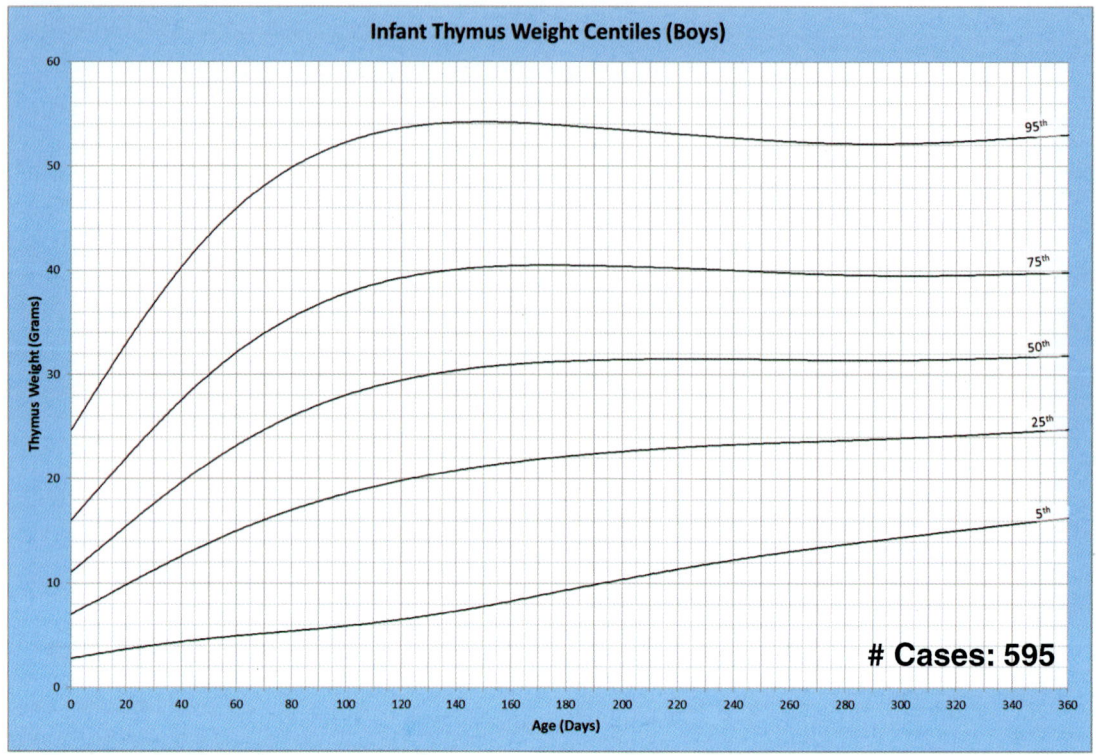

From Pryce JW, et al. Reference ranges for organ weights of infants at autopsy: results of >1,000 consecutive cases from a single centre. *BMC Clin Pathol* 2014;14:18, with permission.

APPENDIX 29: Infant Thymus Weight Centiles (Girls)

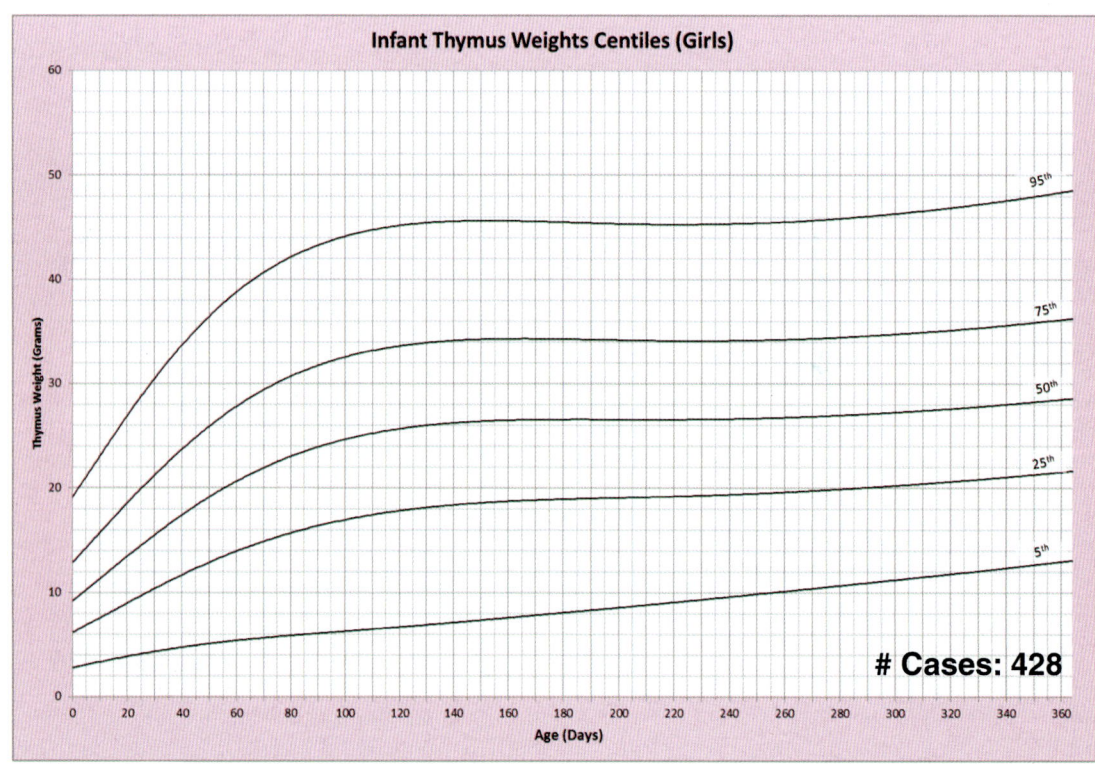

From Pryce JW, et al. Reference ranges for organ weights of infants at autopsy: results of >1,000 consecutive cases from a single centre. *BMC Clin Pathol* 2014;14:18, with permission.

APPENDIX 30: Infant Combined Adrenal Weight Centiles (Boys and Girls)

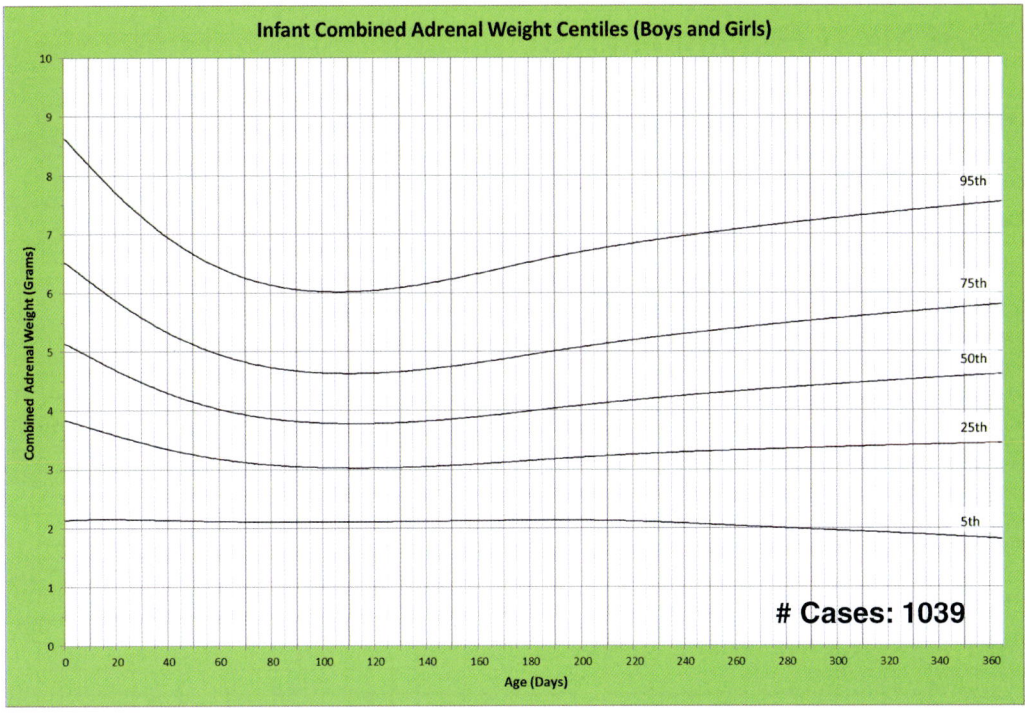

From Pryce JW, et al. Reference ranges for organ weights of infants at autopsy: results of >1,000 consecutive cases from a single centre. *BMC Clin Pathol* 2014;14:18, with permission.

APPENDIX 31: Head Circumference by Age in 0- to 18-Year-Old Boys (Per Centiles)

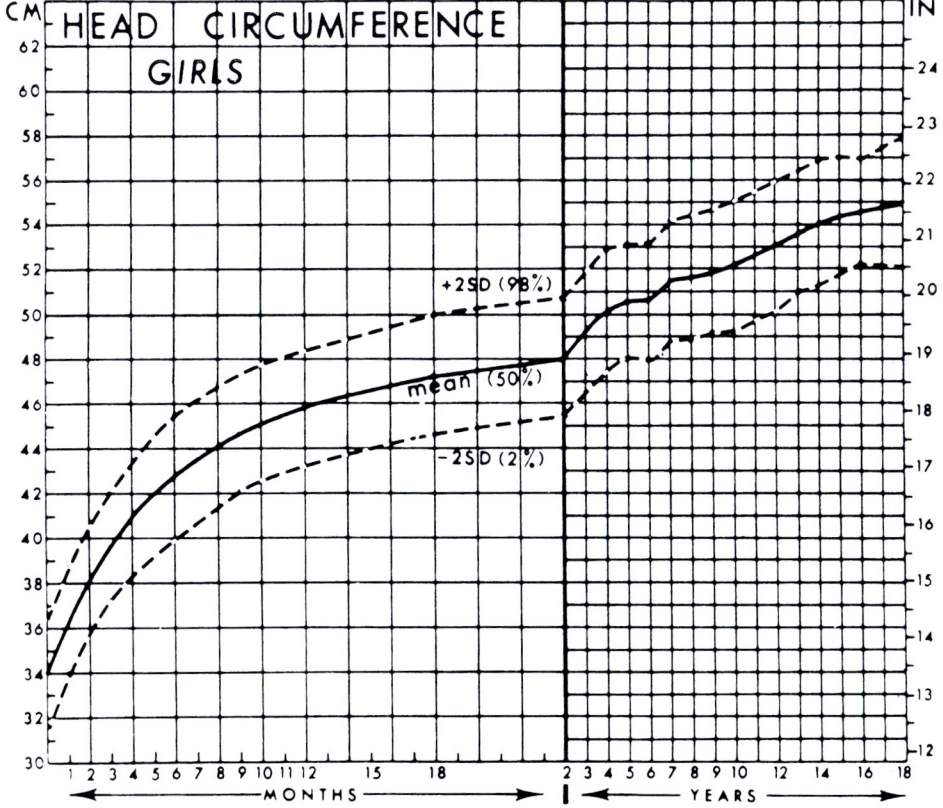

From Avery GB *Neonatology-Pathophysiology and Management of the Newborn*. Philadelphia, PA: JB Lippincott, 1975, with permission.

APPENDIX 32: Head Circumference by Age in 0- to 18-Year-Old Girls (Per Centiles)

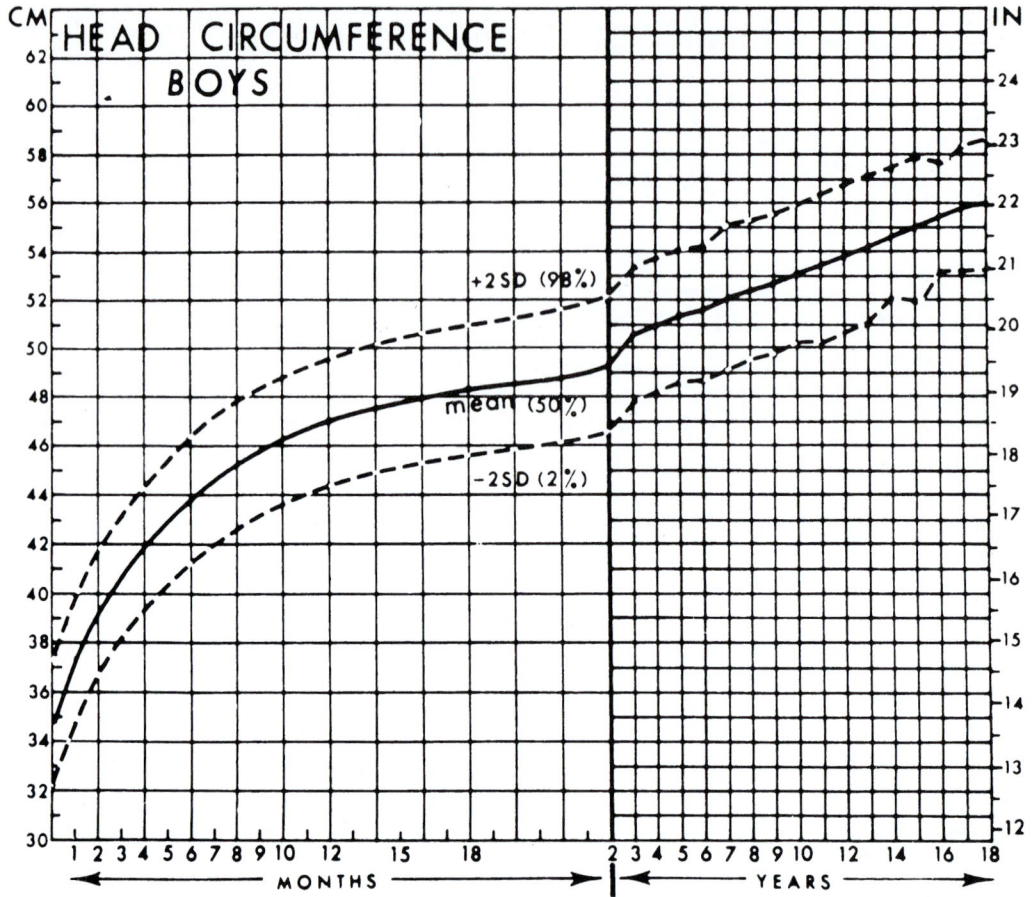

From Avery GB *Neonatology-Pathophysiology and Management of the Newborn.* Philadelphia, PA: JB Lippincott, 1975, with permission.

APPENDIX 33: Organ Weights in Relation to Age and Body Length from Birth to 12 Years of Age

Age	Body Length (cm)	Heart (g)	Lungs (g) Right	Lungs (g) Left	Spleen (g)	Liver (g)	Kidneys (g) Right	Kidneys (g) Left	Brain (g)
Birth to 3 d	49	17	21	18	8	78	13	14	335
3–7 d	49	18	24	22	9	96	14	14	358
1–3 wk	52	19	29	26	10	123	15	15	382
3–5 wk	52	20	31	27	12	127	16	16	413
5–7 wk	53	21	32	28	13	133	19	18	422
7–9 wk	55	23	32	29	13	136	19	18	489
9 wk–3 mo	56	23	35	30	14	140	20	19	516
4 mo	59	27	37	33	16	160	22	21	540
5 mo	61	29	38	35	16	188	25	25	644
6 mo	62	31	42	39	17	200	26	25	660
7 mo	65	34	49	41	19	227	30	30	691
8 mo	65	37	52	45	20	254	31	30	714
9 mo	67	37	53	47	20	260	31	30	750
10 mo	69	39	54	51	22	274	32	31	809
11 mo	70	40	59	53	25	277	34	33	852
12 mo	73	44	64	57	26	288	36	35	925
14 mo	74	45	66	60	26	304	36	35	944
16 mo	77	48	72	64	28	331	39	39	1010
18 mo	78	52	72	65	30	345	40	43	1042
20 mo	79	56	83	74	30	370	43	44	1050
22 mo	82	56	80	75	33	380	44	44	1059
24 mo	84	56	88	76	33	394	47	46	1064
3 y	88	59	89	77	37	413	48	49	1141
4 y	99	73	90	85	39	516	58	56	1191
5 y	106	85	107	104	47	596	65	64	1237
6 y	109	94	121	122	58	642	68	67	1243
7 y	113	100	130	123	66	680	69	70	1263
8 y	119	110	150	140	69	736	74	75	1273
9 y	129	115	174	152	73	756	82	83	1275
10 y	130	116	177	166	85	852	92	95	1290
11 y	135	122	201	190	87	909	94	95	1320
12 y	139	124			93	936	95	96	1351

From Coppelletta JM, Wolbach SB. Body length and organ weights of infants and children. *Am J Pathol* 1933;9:55, with permission.

APPENDIX 34: Average Weights of Organs According to Body Length from 31 to 170 cm

Crown-Heel (Standing) Length (cm)	Heart (g)	Lungs (g)		Spleen (g)	Liver (g)	Pancreas (g)	Adrenal (g)	Thymus (g)	Kidneys (g)	Brain (g)
		Right	Left							
31–35	4.5	23	16	5	51	2.1	4.2	3.2	15	220
35.1–39	5	27	19	7	66	3.0	4.3	4.1	18	250
39.1–41	6	29	21	8	78	3.1	4.3	4.5	20	280
41.1–44	7	30	23	9	88	3.4	4.4	4.9	21	290
44.1–47	8	33	27	11	100	4.0	4.5	5.5	26	320
47.1–49	11	37	29	11	118	4.2	4.6	6.1	30	365
49.1–52	12	40	31	12	128	5.0	4.7	7.5	32	410
52.1–55	16	44	37	15	155	6.0	4.8	9.0	38	470
55.1–58	20	48	39	16	180	7.0	5.0	10.4	42	520
58.1–62	23	54	43	19	212	8.6	5.3	11.8	50	615
62.1–65	30	58	48	24	235	10.0	5.4	12.2	52	665
65.1–70	42	69	57	29	288	13.0	5.6	13.5	62	770
70.1–75	51	80	65	35	330	16.2	5.9	14.5	72	860
75.1–80	54	90	75	42	378	20.0	6.2	15.5	82	990
80.1–85	63	103	86	49	442	23.0	6.4	16.5	90	1020
85.1–90	71	116	99	55	502	27.0	6.7	17.7	100	1100
90.1–95	74	131	111	62	550	30.0	7.0	18.7	112	1120
95.1–100	84	145	124	74	605	33.0	7.3	19.5	124	1165
100.1–105	94	160	138	85	652	35.0	7.5	20.2	136	1210
105.1–110	104	173	153	93	710	38.0	7.8	21.1	144	1250
110.1–115	123	186	166	101	770	41.0	8.0	22.0	155	1265
115.1–120	130	202	180	110	828	44.0	8.2	23.0	165	1305
121.1–125	140	220	195	120	885	46.0	8.6	23.4	175	1315
125.1–130	150	232	210	128	940	49.0	8.8	23.4	185	1345
130.1–135	165	250	225	138	992	51.0	9.1	22.5	196	1355
135.1–140	180	266	240	147	1050	54.0	9.4	21.5	207	1360
140.1–145	192	282	255	154	1110	57.0	9.7	20.5	219	1365
145.1–150	205	300	270	158	1170	59.0	10.1	19.6	231	1370
150.1–155	218	316	285	160	1220	62.0	10.5	18.8	243	1375
155.1–160	230	333	300	160	1275	65.0	10.8	17.7	258	1395
160.1–165	243	350	312	160	1310	67.0	11.0	17.0	270	1400
165.1–170	255	370	323	160	1350	71.0	11.1	15.5	283	1405

Data obtained from more than 30,000 pediatric autopsies.
From Stowens D. *Pediatric Pathology*. Baltimore, MD: Williams & Wilkins, 1959:3, with permission.

APPENDIX 35: Brain Weights, Male and Female, from 1 Day to 19 Years of Age

Age	Males			Females		
	n	Mean + Confidence Limits $p \geq 0.95$		n	Mean + Confidence Limits $p \geq 0.95$	
1 d	218	209.1　277.1　245.0		166	179.4　195.8　212.2	
2–30 d	63	348.8　383.3　417.8		30	388.7　436.6　484.5	
31–60 d	47	431.8　474.5　517.1		29	461.8　528.7　595.6	
61–90 d	43	543.7　595.3　647.0		26	451.4　503.1　554.8	
91–120 d	38	571.2　614.1　657.0		25	512.3　577.9　643.4	
121–150 d	17	587.8　665.2　742.7		25	504.7　571.9　639.1	
151–180 d	30	652.1　713.8　775.5		20	580.4　677.0　773.5	
1 y	25	738.2　851.4　964.6		22	655.1　786.8　918.4	
2 y	28	1083.1　1149.2　1215.3		15	1026.6　1090.3　1154.1	
3 y	29	1198.0　1257.4　1316.7		17	1112.4　1211.1　1309.8	
4 y	17	1217.1　1296.4　1375.8		14	1131.3　1204.2　1277.2	
5 y	17	1291.8　1363.5　1435.1		11	1167.1　1260.9　1354.6	
6 y	15	1329.5　1416.6　1503.8		15	1214.3　1263.0　1311.6	
7 y	7	1194.2　1381.4　1568.5		13	1079.3　1211.1　1342.9	
8 y	8	1252.8　1336.2　1419.6		6	1207.2　1295.8　1384.4	
9 y	12	1211.9　1370.0　1518.0		8	1111.8　1235.0　1358.1	
10 y	16	1177.4　1349.6　1521.9		10	1144.3　1299.0　1453.6	
11 y	8	1272.2　1390.6　1508.9		6	1146.8　1232.5　1318.1	
12 y	9	1081.1　1330.5　1579.9		4	1199.1　1337.5　1475.8	
13 y	9	1214.2　1370.5　1526.8		3	1045.3　1296.6　1547.9	
14 y	14	1414.7　1497.1　1579.5		9	1180.3　1292.7　1405.2	
15 y	13	1404.4　1446.1　1527.8		9	1255.2　1379.4　1503.6	
16 y	23	1292.7　1399.8　1506.9		5	1158.9　1266.0　1373.0	
17 y	19	1416.4　1466.3　1516.1		16	1209.0　1274.6　1340.3	
18 y	21	1391.3　1446.0　1500.7		13	1244.9　1291.5　1338.1	
19 y	27	1395.2　1446.6　1498.0		17	1217.1　1288.1　1359.1	

From Kayser K. *Height and Weight in Human Beings: Autopsy Report*. Munich: R. Oldenbourg, 1987, with permission.

APPENDIX 36: Heart Weights, Male and Female, from 1 Day to 19 Years of Age

	Males				Females		
		Mean + Confidence Limits $p \geq 0.95$				Mean + Confidence Limits $p \geq 0.95$	
Age	n				n		
1 d	348	12.1	13.2	14.4	312	11.2	12.4	13.5
2–30 d	87	20.8	25.4	30.0	63	18.0	20.4	22.8
31–60 d	76	21.9	26.4	30.9	49	19.1	29.9	40.8
61–90 d	62	24.7	27.4	30.1	57	21.9	26.1	30.4
91–120 d	58	24.2	30.4	36.6	37	21.1	29.9	38.8
121–150 d	53	26.1	28.3	30.5	36	23.8	28.2	32.7
151–180 d	33	31.5	38.0	44.4	33	30.1	39.2	48.2
1 y	48	38.5	48.5	58.5	42	39.8	43.1	46.3
2 y	49	62.2	66.4	70.7	31	50.3	55.0	59.7
3 y	52	70.4	75.7	80.9	36	60.0	64.9	69.7
4 y	26	73.8	83.3	92.9	22	69.5	77.5	85.6
5 y	40	86.8	94.9	102.9	20	72.1	85.2	98.3
6 y	26	101.1	115.9	130.8	38	90.3	96.9	103.6
7 y	21	95.4	106.6	117.8	18	92.2	107.0	121.7
8 y	30	117.2	131.7	146.1	20	102.4	126.0	149.5
9 y	22	116.4	131.1	145.7	20	118.0	135.3	152.6
10 y	28	139.1	158.5	177.9	12	97.3	117.0	136.6
11 y	18	146.8	170.2	193.7	9	117.3	155.0	192.6
12 y	25	159.4	178.6	197.7	15	135.5	170.4	205.3
13 y	19	173.0	195.6	218.2	15	158.2	177.0	195.7
14 y	27	189.4	213.1	236.8	19	179.1	207.8	236.5
15 y	24	204.3	232.3	260.3	30	172.8	190.3	207.7
16 y	39	239.7	258.8	277.9	17	199.8	229.1	258.3
17 y	56	261.8	278.4	295.1	37	210.5	230.1	249.7
18 y	62	262.7	279.4	296.0	34	216.5	235.1	253.7
19 y	54	271.6	294.9	318.2	36	212.1	231.0	249.8

From Kayser K. *Height and Weight in Human Beings: Autopsy Report*. Munich, Germany: R. Oldenbourg, 1987, with permission.

APPENDIX 37: Lung Weights, Left and Right, Male and Female, from 1 Day to 19 Years of Age

	Right Lung				Left Lung		
		Mean + Confidence Limits $p \geq 0.95$				Mean + Confidence Limits $p \geq 0.95$	
Age	n				n		
Males								
1 d	238	16.0	17.4	18.7	237	13.7	14.8	15.9
2–30 d	40	31.8	35.9	39.9	41	26.9	31.0	35.0
31–60 d	39	34.4	44.1	53.8	39	28.4	34.6	40.8
61–90 d	25	40.7	46.4	52.0	25	33.0	37.8	42.5
91–120 d	31	38.1	43.6	49.0	31	33.2	38.5	43.8
121–150 d	28	42.0	58.9	75.8	28	36.6	55.0	73.3
151–180 d	17	49.5	61.0	72.5	17	44.9	52.8	60.8
1 y	16	54.4	73.1	91.7	16	44.7	60.2	75.7
2 y	28	92.9	107.6	122.4	27	78.1	90.5	103.0
3 y	20	100.1	128.5	156.8	20	88.4	118.4	148.3

APPENDIX 37: Lung Weights, Left and Right, Male and Female, from 1 Day to 19 Years of Age (Continued)

Age	n	Right Lung Mean + Confidence Limits $p \geq 0.95$			n	Left Lung Mean + Confidence Limits $p \geq 0.95$		
4 y	12	90.9	150.5	210.0	12	86.1	125.0	163.8
5 y	14	125.8	160.6	195.3	14	106.8	141.5	176.1
6 y	13	120.5	159.3	198.2	13	108.6	141.4	174.2
7 y	12	174.6	203.1	231.7	12	160.7	189.6	218.5
8 y	9	155.8	187.7	219.7	9	154.8	187.2	219.5
9 y	8	162.5	253.7	344.9	8	129.6	228.1	326.5
10 y	17	202.2	250.4	298.6	17	179.0	213.2	247.5
11 y	7	238.6	270.8	303.0	7	177.9	257.2	336.6
12 y	15	263.5	349.6	435.7	15	212.3	286.0	359.6
13 y	9	272.3	375.5	478.7	9	244.8	328.8	412.8
14 y	12	285.1	375.8	466.5	12	287.9	361.2	434.5
15 y	15	347.9	448.0	548.0	15	309.8	420.0	530.1
16 y	15	316.9	406.6	496.3	15	291.8	365.6	439.4
17 y	18	450.7	527.5	604.3	18	411.3	487.7	564.2
18 y	10	370.0	460.0	549.9	10	323.1	403.2	483.2
19 y	18	498.3	593.8	689.3	17	435.7	497.0	558.3
Females								
1 d	200	14.5	15.8	17.1	203	12.3	13.5	14.7
2–30 d	29	23.4	39.6	55.7	29	20.1	34.3	48.5
31–60 d	31	32.7	37.9	43.0	32	29.2	34.5	39.7
61–90 d	27	36.1	40.8	45.5	27	30.9	35.2	39.5
91–120 d	17	35.2	43.5	51.8	17	31.6	39.8	48.0
121–150 d	19	34.8	44.2	53.6	19	30.6	38.2	45.7
151–180 d	17	40.9	48.4	56.0	17	37.1	43.8	50.4
1 y	13	38.3	54.9	71.5	13	32.5	49.9	67.3
2 y	13	88.5	116.4	144.4	13	83.1	103.0	122.9
3 y	13	107.9	121.9	135.9	13	86.5	104.3	122.0
4 y	10	111.3	132.4	153.4	10	100.1	115.7	131.2
5 y	6	106.1	156.1	206.1	6	101.9	142.0	182.0
6 y	20	151.0	178.7	206.4	20	140.5	169.7	198.9
7 y	10	145.0	211.0	276.9	10	124.4	159.8	195.1
8 y	14	156.3	232.7	309.1	14	155.9	204.2	252.6
9 y	9	165.3	212.2	259.0	9	136.4	175.5	214.6
10 y	5	82.8	251.0	419.1	5	65.0	218.0	370.9
11 y	6	214.6	247.5	280.3	6	196.7	232.5	268.2
12 y	6	121.0	205.0	288.9	6	110.4	182.5	254.5
13 y	12	286.3	345.8	405.2	12	253.1	297.0	340.9
14 y	7	178.1	263.5	348.9	7	151.0	237.1	323.1
15 y	11	299.9	363.1	426.3	11	237.4	282.7	327.9
16 y	6	233.2	464.1	695.0	6	193.8	430.8	667.7
17 y	14	360.3	475.0	589.6	14	305.2	391.4	477.6
18 y	8	287.6	415.0	542.3	8	227.2	326.2	425.2
19 y	13	327.7	456.1	584.5	13	290.7	377.3	463.9

From Kayser K. *Height and Weight in Human Beings: Autopsy Report*. Munich, Germany: R. Oldenbourg, 1987, with permission.

APPENDIX 38: Liver Weights, Male and Female, from 1 Day to 19 Years of Age

Age	Males n	Mean + Confidence Limits $p \geq 0.95$			Females n	Mean + Confidence Limits $p \geq 0.95$		
1 d	672	63.7	68.8	73.9	563	61.9	65.7	69.5
2–30 d	131	125.0	140.1	155.2	67	104.6	118.6	132.6
31–60 d	105	121.2	148.4	175.6	55	126.9	139.0	151.2
61–90 d	70	171.4	186.4	201.5	48	136.3	155.6	174.9
91–120 d	74	159.0	176.1	193.3	44	154.2	183.3	212.4
121–150 d	49	181.6	215.5	249.4	36	168.7	200.5	232.2
151–180 d	42	212.9	269.1	325.4	34	187.6	220.0	252.5
1 y	46	256.5	293.0	329.6	42	252.5	283.0	313.5
2 y	54	441.0	503.9	566.8	28	303.7	413.7	523.7
3 y	52	538.8	599.1	659.3	39	449.4	505.3	561.2
4 y	28	536.2	588.2	640.1	31	474.3	527.4	580.5
5 y	44	604.1	652.0	699.9	19	475.0	553.4	631.7
6 y	37	635.6	709.8	784.1	39	556.9	618.7	680.4
7 y	34	672.3	752.6	832.9	20	534.5	612.0	689.4
8 y	30	725.3	847.1	968.9	26	670.7	752.3	833.9
9 y	31	791.8	855.3	918.7	22	796.7	911.8	1026.8
10 y	28	861.3	956.9	1052.5	15	724.1	845.6	967.1
11 y	17	883.3	1060.2	1237.2	10	999.3	1095.0	1190.6
12 y	24	901.6	1075.2	1248.7	12	796.5	989.1	1181.7
13 y	21	1062.7	1201.4	1340.0	19	913.3	1050.2	1187.1
14 y	28	1095.3	1204.2	1313.2	11	1081.5	1194.5	1307.5
15 y	30	1246.8	1360.6	1474.5	28	1197.1	1307.6	1418.2
16 y	40	1506.4	1646.9	1787.4	16	1134.3	1347.5	1560.6
17 y	56	1485.8	1589.0	1692.2	36	1250.5	1398.4	1546.3
18 y	56	1609.7	1705.7	1801.6	26	1350.6	1504.4	1658.2
19 y	69	1563.0	1672.9	1782.8	36	1350.2	1456.3	1562.4

From Kayser K. *Height and Weight in Human Beings: Autopsy Report*. Munich, Germany: R. Oldenbourg, 1987, with permission.

APPENDIX 39: Spleen Weights, Male and Female, from 1 Day to 19 Years of Age

	Males				Females			
Age	n	Mean + Confidence Limits $p \geq 0.95$			n	Mean + Confidence Limits $p \geq 0.95$		
1 d	488	5.9	6.6	7.3	426	5.1	5.8	6.4
2–30 d	126	11.0	12.4	13.8	76	9.6	11.5	13.4
31–60 d	113	14.2	16.3	18.4	83	16.4	22.9	29.4
61–90 d	80	14.8	17.4	20.0	64	12.3	16.3	20.2
91–120 d	83	14.8	19.1	23.4	58	12.7	14.6	16.5
121–150 d	68	17.9	23.0	28.0	49	15.4	19.9	24.4
151–180 d	47	16.6	20.0	23.4	42	14.8	18.2	21.6
1 y	61	26.6	31.1	35.7	47	19.9	23.5	27.1
2 y	62	38.2	42.6	47.0	38	34.8	42.0	49.2
3 y	47	44.7	54.8	64.9	45	36.2	41.8	47.3
4 y	37	46.3	58.7	71.2	22	40.0	49.3	58.5
5 y	29	46.9	56.8	66.7	20	41.5	50.7	59.8
6 y	28	57.2	69.3	81.5	34	56.5	67.2	77.8
7 y	25	66.5	103.3	140.1	14	48.4	64.2	80.0
8 y	23	60.8	73.1	85.3	23	66.9	94.3	121.6
9 y	23	61.9	90.9	119.9	21	66.9	80.9	94.9
10 y	29	82.7	111.3	139.9	8	60.7	90.0	119.2
11 y	14	62.0	90.0	117.9	6	62.8	87.5	112.1
12 y	23	90.6	114.7	138.8	11	68.8	89.0	109.3
13 y	12	83.3	138.7	194.1	19	98.3	129.0	159.6
14 y	24	111.1	151.2	191.3	18	110.8	162.8	214.9
15 y	24	119.2	155.3	191.4	22	97.3	129.2	161.0
16 y	30	135.4	165.1	194.8	21	160.0	219.0	277.9
17 y	33	164.5	212.7	260.9	40	140.7	158.0	175.3
18 y	37	155.9	181.0	206.2	25	121.3	146.4	171.5
19 y	46	166.6	195.6	224.6	34	116.5	156.5	196.4

From Kayser K. *Height and Weight in Human Beings: Autopsy Report.* Munich, Germany: R. Oldenbourg, 1987, with permission.

APPENDIX 40: Kidney Weights, Left and Right, Male and Female, from 1 Day to 19 Years of Age

	Right Kidney				Left Kidney			
Age	n	Mean + Confidence Limits $p \geq 0.95$			n	Mean + Confidence Limits $p \geq 0.95$		
Males								
1 d	662	7.1	7.5	7.9	662	7.3	7.7	8.1
2–30 d	137	14.6	16.2	17.8	137	14.4	15.9	17.5
31–60 d	110	60.0	17.4	18.8	110	15.9	17.4	18.8
61–90 d	93	17.7	19.4	21.1	93	18.0	19.8	21.5
91–120 d	87	19.6	21.5	23.4	87	19.5	21.3	23.0
121–150 d	74	19.6	21.8	24.1	74	20.4	22.7	25.0
151–180 d	56	20.9	23.8	26.6	56	21.3	23.5	25.6
1 y	62	29.0	31.9	34.8	62	29.8	33.6	37.4
2 y	70	40.6	45.7	50.9	73	42.2	47.3	52.5

(Continued)

APPENDIX 40: Kidney Weights, Left and Right, Male and Female, from 1 Day to 19 Years of Age (Continued)

Age	n	Right Kidney Mean + Confidence Limits $p \geq 0.95$			n	Left Kidney Mean + Confidence Limits $p \geq 0.95$		
3 y	65	47.7	53.2	58.7	65	49.5	55.0	60.5
4 y	37	47.9	53.8	59.8	37	50.7	55.9	61.1
5 y	45	51.0	56.1	61.2	45	52.6	57.6	62.7
6 y	40	59.5	69.4	79.3	40	62.4	72.3	82.1
7 y	27	59.6	68.4	77.1	27	59.9	67.8	75.7
8 y	38	66.9	76.3	85.8	38	68.2	77.7	87.1
9 y	29	68.7	78.7	88.6	29	70.1	80.7	91.3
10 y	40	76.7	87.2	97.7	41	80.3	91.2	102.2
11 y	21	78.9	90.0	101.2	20	78.8	91.3	103.8
12 y	32	95.9	106.1	116.4	32	97.0	106.6	116.2
13 y	24	86.8	98.0	109.1	24	90.5	103.2	115.9
14 y	29	102.2	113.4	124.6	30	103.8	116.8	129.7
15 y	31	114.3	130.2	146.1	30	115.6	130.7	145.8
16 y	43	122.7	134.0	145.2	42	121.3	133.8	146.3
17 y	52	129.9	140.3	150.6	54	138.2	150.6	163.0
18 y	57	141.3	153.4	165.6	56	145.3	156.9	168.5
19 y	64	139.4	147.5	155.7	64	142.5	152.0	161.4
Females								
1 d	561	6.4	6.8	7.2	560	6.4	6.8	7.2
2–30 d	91	13.1	14.7	16.2	91	13.2	14.7	16.1
31–60 d	78	14.5	16.7	18.9	78	14.7	17.1	19.4
61–90 d	72	16.0	17.7	19.4	72	16.1	17.8	19.4
91–120 d	49	16.8	19.5	22.1	48	17.3	19.9	22.6
121–150 d	50	19.5	22.8	26.0	51	19.8	23.0	26.2
151–180 d	46	20.6	23.2	25.8	46	21.3	23.9	26.5
1 y	62	23.1	25.6	28.0	63	24.2	26.7	29.3
2 y	36	34.2	37.4	40.5	37	36.1	39.5	42.9
3 y	50	43.3	47.5	51.6	50	44.6	48.4	52.2
4 y	34	46.3	51.1	55.9	34	47.2	52.8	58.4
5 y	30	48.6	54.7	60.7	30	49.8	54.7	59.6
6 y	46	54.9	62.3	69.8	46	56.6	64.2	71.8
7 y	27	60.5	72.6	84.6	28	62.4	74.3	86.3
8 y	29	63.1	76.3	89.6	29	63.4	81.2	99.0
9 y	19	66.6	73.8	81.1	20	70.9	81.2	91.5
10 y	15	65.4	89.3	113.2	15	64.4	88.6	112.9
11 y	15	77.9	93.3	108.7	15	77.1	93.2	109.2
12 y	12	67.9	91.5	115.0	12	68.8	93.0	117.3
13 y	27	90.4	101.5	112.7	27	96.9	108.2	119.6
14 y	16	97.0	105.2	113.4	17	104.0	113.8	123.7
15 y	33	100.7	113.2	125.6	33	108.3	118.4	128.6
16 y	18	105.0	122.3	139.7	18	111.0	127.6	144.1
17 y	47	119.4	129.2	139.0	46	123.2	134.8	146.5
18 y	37	116.6	123.9	131.3	37	121.3	129.3	137.7
19 y	42	119.4	129.0	138.6	42	119.5	130.6	141.6

From Kayser K. *Height and Weight in Human Beings: Autopsy Report.* Munich, Germany: R. Oldenbourg, 1987, with permission.

APPENDIX 41: Penile Length by Menstrual Age

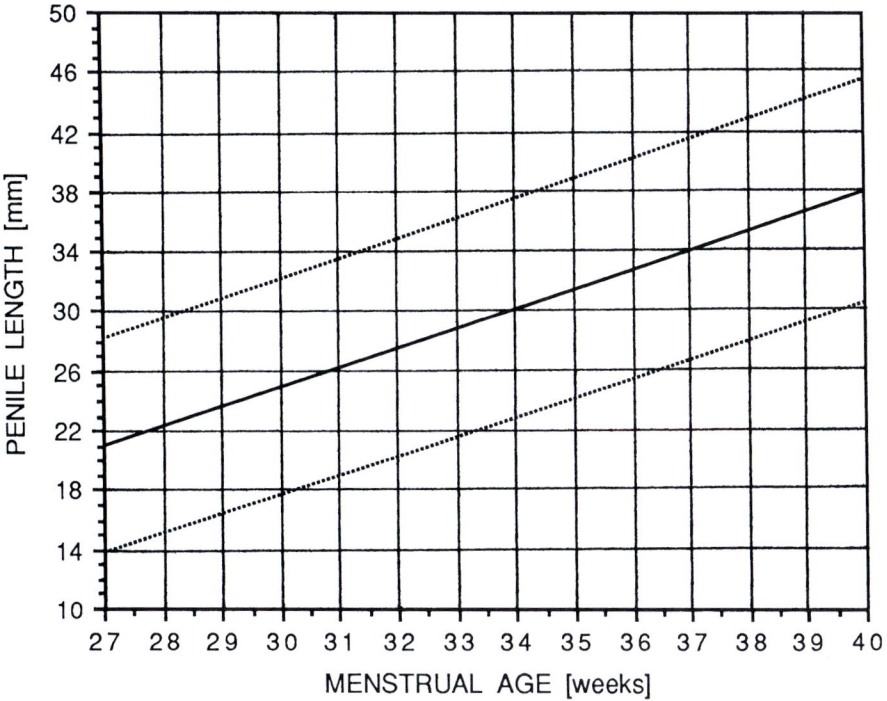

From Feldman KW, Smith DW. Fetal phallic growth and penile standards for newborn male infants. *J Pediatr* 1975;86:395, with permission.

APPENDIX 42: Penile Length by Age (0–22 Years; Percentiles)

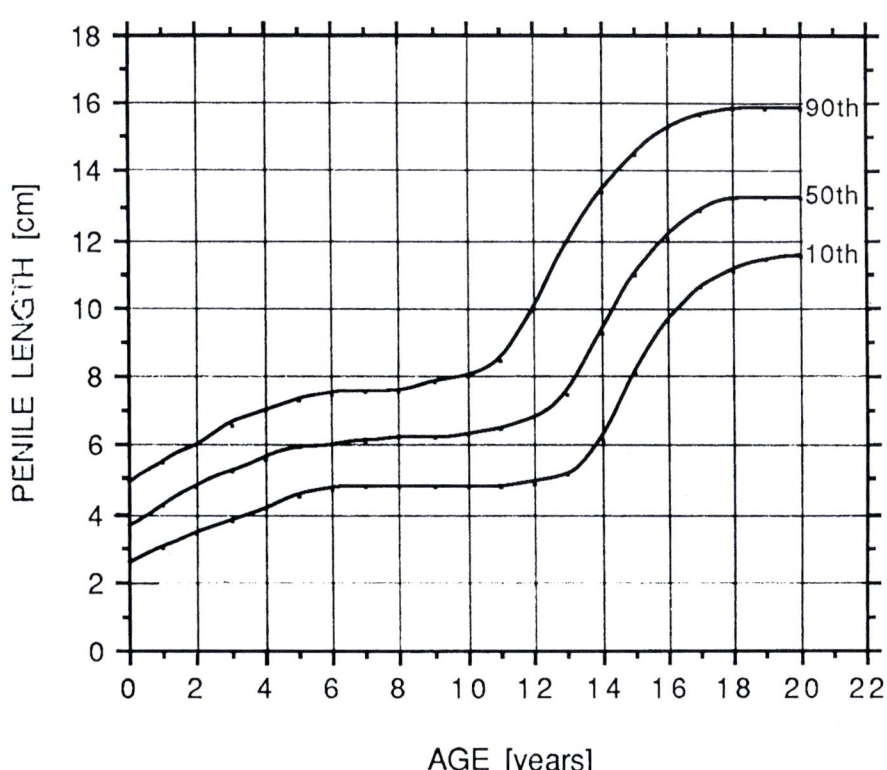

From Schonfield WA. Primary and secondary sexual characteristics: study of their development in males from birth through maturity, with biometric study of penis and testes. *Am J Dis Child* 1943;65:535, with permission.

APPENDIX 43: Gyral Pattern of the Petal Brain

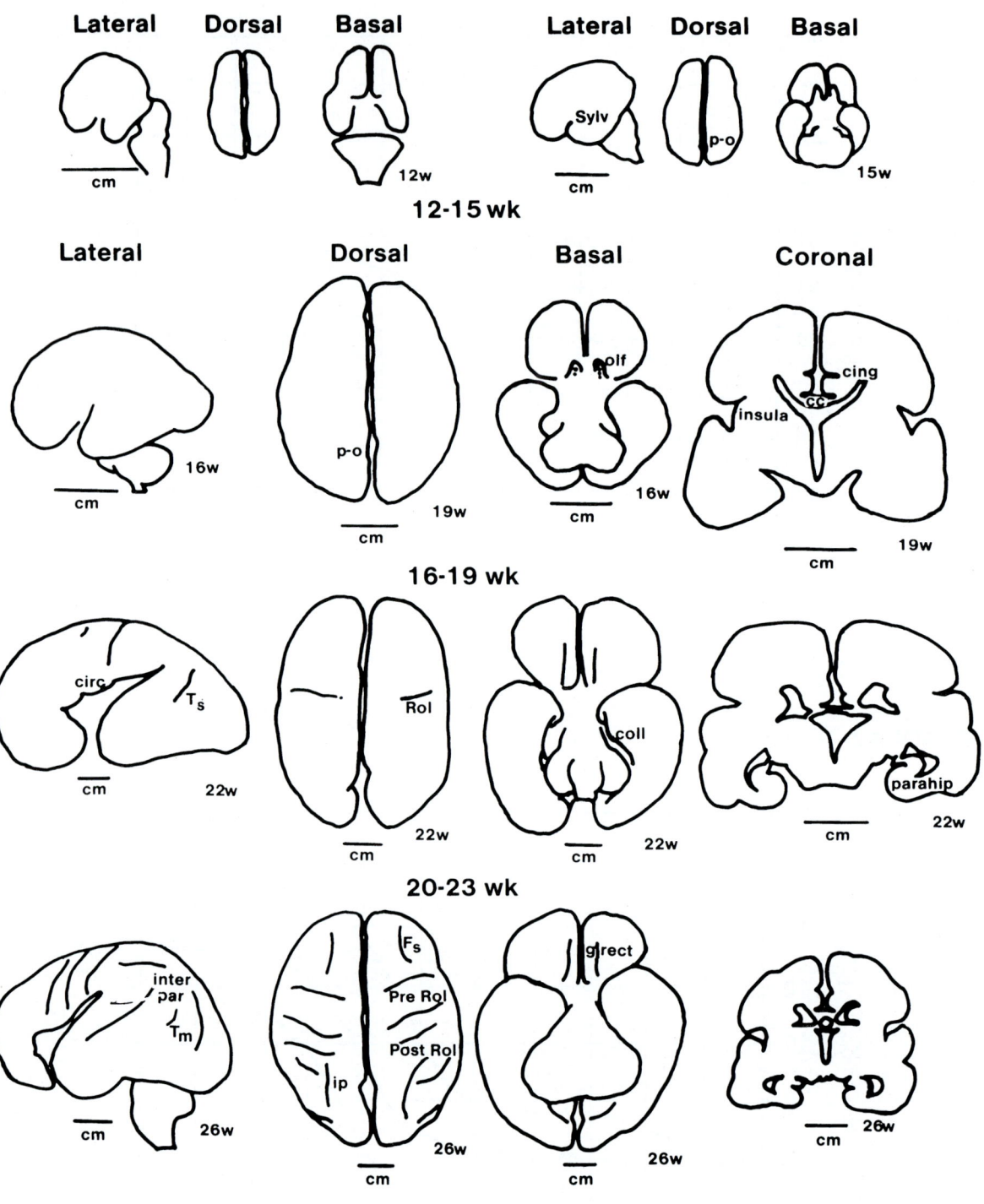

APPENDIX 44: Gyral Pattern of the Perinatal Brain

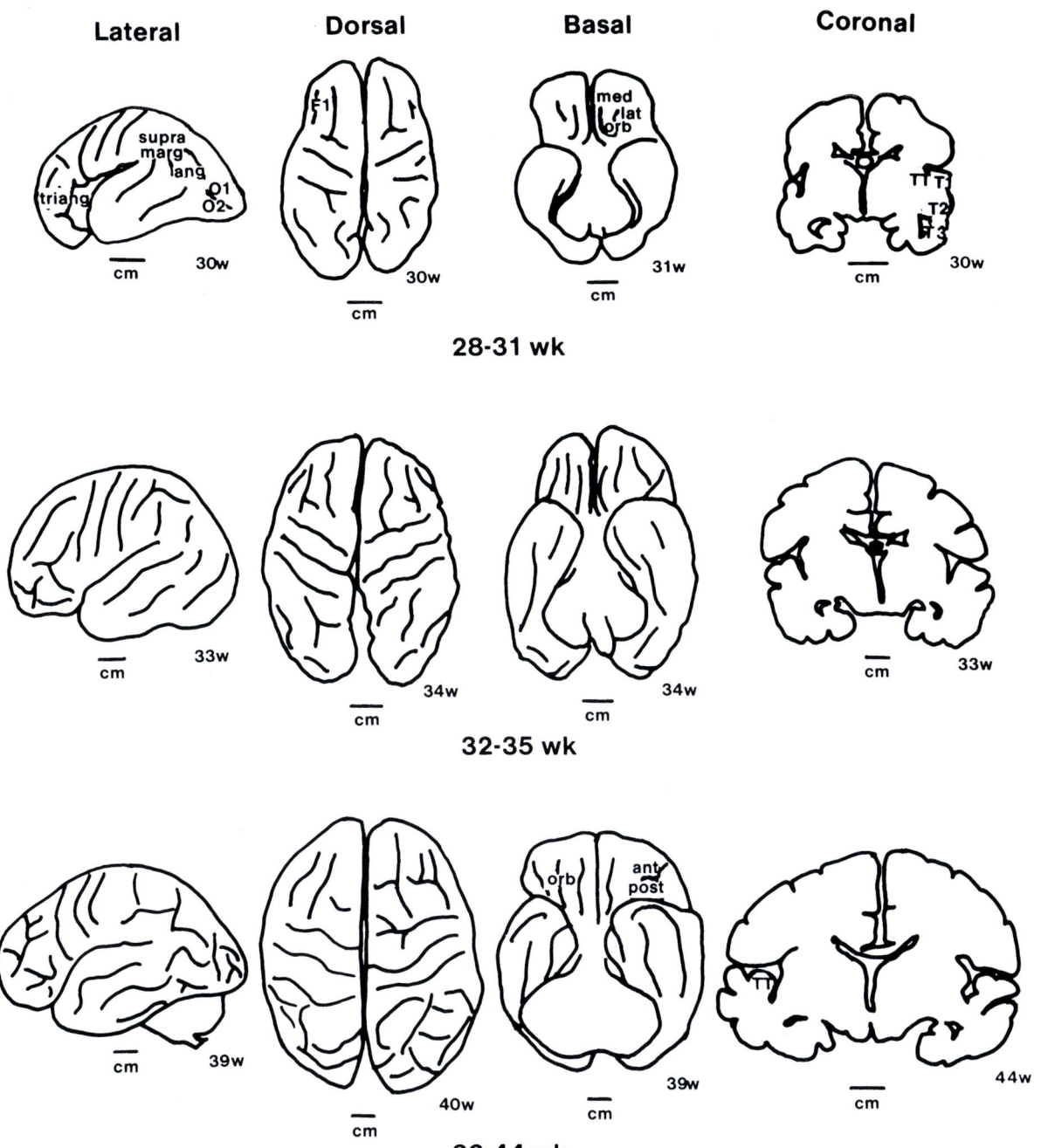

APPENDIX 45: Gestational Development of the Cerebral Hemispheres

Gestational Age (wk)	No. Examined	Sulci and Fissures	Gyri
10–15	6	Interhemispheric fissure, hippocampal sulcus, Sylvian fissure, transverse cerebral fissure, callosal sulcus	
16–19	13	Parietooccipital fissure, olfactory sulcus, circular sulcus, cingulate sulcus, calcarine fissure	Gyrus rectus, insula, cingulate gyrus
20–23	41	Rolandic sulcus, collateral sulcus, superior temporal sulcus	Parahippocampal gyrus, superior temporal gyrus
24–27	46	Prerolandic sulcus, middle temporal sulcus, postrolandic sulcus, interparietal sulcus, superior frontal sulcus, lateral occipital sulcus	Prerolandic gyrus, middle temporal gyrus, postrolandic gyrus, superior and inferior parietal lobules, superior and middle frontal gyri, superior and inferior occipital gyri, cuneus and lingual gyrus, fusiform gyrus
28–31	36	Inferior temporal sulcus, inferior frontal sulcus	Inferior temporal gyrus, triangular gyrus, medial and lateral orbital gyri, callosomarginal gyrus, transverse temporal gyrus, angular and supramarginal gyri, external occipitotemporal gyrus
32–35	29	Marginal sulcus; secondary superior, middle, and inferior frontal, superior and middle temporal, superior and inferior parietal, prerolandic and postrolandic, superior and inferior occipital sulci and gyri; insular gyri	Paracentral gyrus
36–39	31	Secondary transverse and inferior temporal and cingulate sulci and gyri, tertiary superior, middle, and inferior frontal and superior parietal sulci and gyri	Anterior and posterior orbital gyri
40–44	29	Secondary orbital, callosomarginal, and insular sulci and gyri, tertiary inferior temporal and superior and inferior occipital gyri and sulci	

From Gilles FH, Leviton A, Dooling EC. *The Developing Human Brain—Growth and Epidemiologic Neuropathology*. Boston, MA: John Wright, 1983, with permission.

APPENDIX 46: Regional Development of the Cerebral Hemispheres

Lobe	Fissures and Sulci	Gestational Age (wk)	Gyri	Gestational Age (wk)
Frontal	Interhemispheric fissure	10	Gyrus rectus	16
	Transverse cerebral fissure	10	Insula	18
	Hippocampal sulcus	10	Cingulate gyrus	18
	Callosal sulcus	14	Prerolandic gyrus	24
	Sylvian fissure	14	Superior frontal gyrus	25
	Olfactory sulcus	16	Middle frontal gyrus	27
	Circular sulcus	18	Triangular gyrus	28
	Cingulate sulcus	18	Medial and lateral orbital gyri	28
	Rolandic sulcus	20	Callosomarginal gyrus	28
	Prerolandic sulcus	24	Anterior and posterior orbital gyri	36
	Superior frontal sulcus	25		
	Inferior frontal sulcus	28		
Parietal	Interhemispheric fissure	10	Cingulate gyrus	18
	Transverse cerebral fissure	10	Postrolandic gyrus	25
	Sylvian fissure	14	Superior parietal lobule	26
	Parietooccipital fissure	16	Inferior parietal lobule	26
	Rolandic sulcus	20	Angular gyrus	28
	Postrolandic sulcus	25	Supramarginal gyrus	28
	Interparietal sulcus	26	Paracentral gyri	35
Temporal	Sylvian fissure	14	Superior temporal gyrus	23
	Superior temporal sulcus	23	Parahippocampal gyrus	23
	Collateral sulcus	23	Middle temporal gyrus	26
	Middle temporal sulcus	26	Fusiform gyrus	27
	Inferior temporal sulcus	30	Inferior temporal gyrus	30
			External occipitotemporal gyrus	30
			Transverse temporal gyrus	31
Occipital	Interhemispheric fissure	10	Superior occipital gyri	27
	Calcarine fissure	16	Inferior occipital gyri	27
	Parietooccipital sulcus	16	Cuneus	27
	Collateral sulcus	23	Lingual gyrus	27
	Lateral occipital sulcus	27	External occipitotemporal gyrus	30

From Gilles FH, Leviton A, Dooling EC. *The Developing Human Brain—Growth and Epidemiologic Neuropathology*. Boston, MA: John Wright, 1983, with permission.

APPENDIX 47: Villous Characteristics

Villous Type	When Present	When Maximum	% Volume at Term	Size	Characteristic Features
Mesenchymal villi	5-week term	0-8 weeks	<1%	120-250 μm (<8 wk) 60-100 μm (>8 wk)	Primitive stroma, thick trophoblastic cover, few vessels
Immature intermediate villi	8-week term	14-20 weeks	5%-10%	100-200 μm. May be up to 400 μm	Reticular stroma with fluid-filled stromal channels
Stem villi	12-week term	Term	20%-25%	150-300 μm	Fibrotic stroma, myofibroblastic perivascular sheath, large vessels
Mature intermediate villi	Third trimester	Third trimester	25%	80-150 μm	Cellular stroma with <50% capillaries
Terminal villi	Third trimester	Term	40%-50%	60 μm	>50% capillaries

From Baergen RN. *Manual of Pathology of the Human Placenta*, 2nd ed. New York: Springer, 2011, with permission.

APPENDIX 48: Growth Characteristics of Placenta and Fetus

Gestation (wk)	Placental Weight (g)	Expected Term Weight (%)	Fetal Weight (g)	Expected Term Weight (%)
24	195	41	680	21
26	220	47	880	27
28	280	58	1070	33
30	290	60	1330	41
32	320	68	1690	52
34	370	77	2090	62
36	420	87	2500	77
38	450	43	2960	91
41	480	100	3250	100
42	495	103	3410	105

From Wigglesworth JS, Singer DB. *Textbook of Fetal and Perinatal Pathology*, 2nd ed. Boston, MA: Blackwell Science, 1998, with permission.

APPENDIX 49: Normative Values

Pregnancy Week Postmenstrual	Crown-Rump Length (mm)	Foot Length (cm)	Embryonic/Fetal Weight (g)	Placental Weight (g)	Fetal/Placental Weight Ratio	Placental Thickness (cm)	Placental Diameter (cm)	Umbilical Cord Length (cm)
3								
4								0.2
5	2.5							0.4
6	5							0.7
7	9							1.2
8	14		1.1	6	0.18			2.0
9	20		2	8	0.25			3.3
10	26		5	13	0.38			5.5
11	33		11	19	0.58			9.2
12	40		17	26	0.65			12.6
13	48	1.2	23	32	0.72		5.0	15.8
14	56	1.7	30	41	0.73	1.0	5.6	18.8
15	65	1.9	40	50	0.80	1.1	6.2	21.5
16	75	2.2	60	60	1.00	1.2	6.9	24.0
17	88	2.5	90	70	1.29	1.2	7.5	26.4
18	99	2.8	130	80	1.63	1.3	8.1	28.7
19	112	2.9	180	101	1.78	1.4	8.7	30.9
20	125	3.3	250	112	2.23	1.5	9.4	33.0
21	137	3.6	320	126	2.54	1.5	10.0	35.0
22	150	3.9	400	144	2.78	1.6	10.6	36.9
23	163	4.2	480	162	2.96	1.7	11.2	38.7
24	176	4.5	560	180	3.11	1.8	11.9	40.4
25	188	4.7	650	198	3.28	1.8	12.5	42.0
26	200	5.0	750	216	3.47	1.9	13.1	43.5
27	213	5.3	870	234	3.72	1.9	13.7	45.0
28	226	5.5	1000	252	3.97	2.0	14.4	46.4
29	236	5.8	1130	270	4.19	2.0	15.0	47.7
30	250	6.0	1260	288	4.38	2.1	15.6	49.0
31	263	6.2	1400	306	4.58	2.1	16.2	50.2
32	276	6.5	1550	324	4.78	2.2	16.9	52.0
33	289	6.7	1700	342	4.97	2.2	17.5	53.0
34	302	6.9	1900	360	5.28	2.3	18.1	54.0
35	315	7.1	2100	378	5.56	2.3	18.7	54.9
36	328	7.4	2300	396	5.81	2.4	19.4	55.7
37	341	7.6	2500	414	6.04	2.4	20.0	56.5
38	354	7.8	2750	432	6.37	2.4	20.6	57.2
39	367	8.0	3000	451	6.65	2.5	21.3	57.9
40	380	8.1	3400	470	7.23	2.5	22.0	58.5

Portions of the table were modified from Kalousek et al. (1992).
From Baergen RN. *Manual of Pathology of the Human Placenta*, 2nd ed. New York: Springer, 2011, with permission.

APPENDIX 50: Percentiles, Means, and Standard Deviations for Placental Weights by Gestational Age

Gestational Age (wk)	N[a]	Mean	SD	Percentile								
				3	5	10	25	50	75	90	95	97
22	19	189	39		99	107	130	166	206	285	499	
23	16	100	41			127	168	188	208	262		
24	16	190	42			128	157	192	222	252		
25	26	197	70		105	128	153	184	216	299	400	
26	22	226	100		107	138	179	200	259	281	570	
27	22	240	77		119	130	166	242	310	332	381	
28	41	223	66	103	128	140	173	214	261	321	361	371
29	37	269	96	124	135	161	214	252	309	352	496	629
30	42	324	88	185	190	208	269	316	374	433	502	570
31	57	314	105	142	152	175	246	313	360	417	479	579
32	69	325	77	161	214	241	275	318	377	436	461	465
33	117	351	83	190	224	252	286	352	413	446	475	504
34	160	381	84	221	260	283	322	382	430	479	527	558
35	260	411	99	232	250	291	344	401	471	544	600	626
36	538	447	110	270	291	320	369	440	508	580	628	679
37	1103	467	107	303	324	349	390	452	531	607	660	692
38	2469	493	103	320	335	365	420	484	560	629	675	706
39	3932	500	103	330	350	379	426	490	564	635	683	713
40	4114	510	100	340	360	380	440	501	572	643	685	715
41	1982	524	100	358	379	403	452	515	583	655	705	738
42	321	532	99	370	388	412	460	525	592	658	700	771

SD, standard deviation.
[a]Number of placentas at each placental age.
From Kraus FT, Redline RW, Gersell DJ, et al. *Placental Pathology (Atlas of Nontumor Pathology)*, Vol. 3. Washington, DC: AFIP, 2004, with permission.

APPENDIX 51: Mean Weights and Percentiles for Twin Placentas

Gestational Age (wk)	90th Percentile	75th Percentile	Mean Twin Placental Weight (g)	25th Percentile	10th Percentile	Number of Cases
19	263	239	212	185	161	2
20	270	245	218	190	166	3
21	286	260	231	202	176	2
22	310	282	251	219	191	5
23	343	311	276	241	210	2
24	382	346	307	267	232	3
25	426	386	341	297	257	5
26	475	430	380	330	284	4
27	528	478	421	365	314	8
28	584	527	464	401	345	7
29	641	579	509	439	377	12
30	700	631	554	478	409	17
31	758	683	600	516	441	13
32	815	734	644	554	472	29
33	870	783	687	590	503	27
34	923	830	727	624	531	53
35	971	873	764	656	558	52
36	1014	912	798	684	582	66
37	1051	945	827	708	602	58
38	1082	972	850	728	619	54
39	1105	993	868	743	631	38
40	1118	1005	879	753	639	47
41	1123	1009	882	756	642	12

Both dichorionic and monochorionic placental weights were included.

From Pinar H, Sung CJ, Oyer CE, et al. Reference values for singleton and twin placental weights. *Pediatr Pathol Lab Med* 1996;16:904, with permission.

APPENDIX 52: Mean Weights and Percentiles for Triplet Placentas

Gestational Age (wk)	90th Percentile	Mean Triplet Placental Weight	10th Percentile	Cases (n)
20	285	253	226	3
21	320	284	257	2
22	345	319	289	2
23	400	361	331	3
24	445	406	371	5
25	498	456	408	6
26	558	509	444	6
27	630	564	480	4
28	697	621	516	5
29	772	679	553	6
30	849	738	591	10
31	925	797	631	15
32	1000	855	674	7
33	1072	911	719	14
34	1139	965	768	43
35	1200	1017	821	33
36	1253	1065	878	19
37	1297	1108	940	8
38	1330	1147	1007	5

From Pinar H, Singer D, et al. Triplet placentas: reference values for weights. *Pediatr Dev Pathol* 2002;5(5): 495–498, with permission.

Suggested Readings

Archie JG, Collins JS, Lebel RR. Quantitative standards for fetal and neonatal autopsy. *Am J Clin Pathol* 2006;126:256–265.

Baergen RN. *Manual of Pathology of the Human Placenta*, 2nd ed. Springer, 2011.

Gilbert-Barness E. Spicer DE, Steffensen TS, eds. *Handbook of Pediatric Autopsy Pathology*, 2nd ed. New York: Springer, 2014.

Hansen K, et al. Reference values for second trimester fetal and neonatal organ weights and measurements. *Pediatr Dev Pathol* 2003;6:160–167.

Jonathan SW. *Textbook of Fetal and Perinatal Pathology*, 2nd ed. In: Wigglesworth JS, Singer DB, eds. Blackwell Science, 1998.

Olsen IE, et al. New intrauterine growth curves based on United States data. *Pediatrics* 2010;125:e214–e224.

Pinar H, et al. Triplet placentas: reference values for weights. *Pediatr Dev Pathol* 2002;5:495–498.

Pryce JW, et al. Reference ranges for organ weights of infants at autopsy: results of >1,000 consecutive cases from a single centre. *BMC Clin Pathol* 2014;14:18.

Roche AF, Guo S, Moore WM. Weight and recumbent length from 1 to 12 mo of age: reference data for 1-mo increments. *Am J Clin Nutr* 1989;49:599–607.

Sadler TW. *Langman's Medical Embryology*, 13th ed. Philadelphia, PA: Lippincott Williams & Wilkins, 2015.

Stocker JT, Dehner LP, eds. *Pediatric Pathology*, 2nd ed. Philadelphia, PA: Lippincott Williams & Wilkins, 2001.

Index

Note: Page numbers followed by '*f*' indicate figures; those followed by '*t*' indicate tables.

A

Aagenaes syndrome. *See* Hereditary cholestasis with lymphedema
Abdominal muscle deficiency syndrome. *See* Prune belly syndrome
Aberrant right subclavian artery, 544
Abetalipoproteinemia, 617, 618*f*
Abruptio placenta, 347*f*
Abscesses, 706
Abusive head trauma, 279–282, 279*f*–282*f*
Acanthamoeba keratitis, 420, 420*f*
Accessory breast tissue, 928
Accessory diaphragm (AD), 513
Accidental blunt impact injuries, 278
Achondroplasia, 1307
Acid maltase deficiency, 675
Acinar cell carcinoma, 778–779, 779*f*, 1038–1039, 1039*f*
Acinar dysplasia, 466, 466*f*
Acne, 1238
Acquired immunodeficiency syndrome (AIDS), 775
Acrocephalosyndactyly syndrome, 120–122
Acrodermatitis enteropathica, 1222
ACTH-secreting adenomas, 954
Actinomycosis infections, 247
Acute allograft rejection, 293
Acute appendicitis, 644–645
Acute disease processes
  fetal hemorrhage, 348
  maternal arterial hemorrhages, 346
  umbilical cord accident, 347, 348*f*
Acute disseminated encephalomyelitis (ADEM), 399
Acute eosinophilic pneumonia (AEP), 491
Acute febrile neutrophilic dermatosis (Sweet syndrome), 1234
Acute interstitial pulmonary emphysema (AIPE), 482, 482*f*
Acute lung injury, 472–475
Acute lymphoblastic leukemia (ALL), 1092
  biologic basis, 1106*t*, 1107–1108, 1108*f*
  classification, 1105–1106
  clinical and laboratory features, 1108*t*
  incidence, 1105, 1109*t*
  morphologic basis, 1106, 1107*f*
  phenotypic basis, 1107, 1107*f*
Acute meningitis, 396, 397*f*
Acute monoblastic leukemia, 1117
Acute myelogenous leukemia (AML)
  biologic basis, 1109–1111, 1114–1115
  classification, 1108, 1109*t*
  incidence, 1108
  inv(16)(p13.1q22), 1111, 1115*f*
  monosomy 7, 1115
  morphologic diagnosis, 1108–1109, 1110*t*, 1111*f*
  myelodysplasia-related changes, 1115–1116, 1116*t*
  t(8;21)(q22;q22), 1109–1110
  t(9;11)(p22;q23), 1111, 1114
  t(15;17)(q22;q12), 1111, 1114*f*
  t(16;16)(p13.1;q22), 1111, 1115*f*
  WHO classification, 1109*t*, 1112*t*–1113*t*
Acute neuronal death, 351, 403
Acute nonspecific epididymitis, 919
Acute osteomyelitis (AO), 1365–1366
Acute pancreatitis, 775
Acute rheumatic carditis, 558*f*
Acute self-limited colitis, 629–630
Acute splenitis, 1079
Acute synovitis, 1368
Acute tubular necrosis (ATN), 834–835, 835*f*
Acyl-CoA oxidase deficiency, 181
Adamantinoma (ADM), 1354, 1354*f*
Adamantinomatous CPG, 391, 391*f*
Adenocarcinoma, 509, 509*f*
Adenohypophysis, 950, 953
Adenoid cystic carcinoma (ACC), 436, 438, 507–508
Adenomas, 930, 932, 932*f*
Adenomatoid odontogenic tumor (AOT), 1045–1046, 1047*f*
Adenomatoid tumor, 889, 921
Adenomatosis, 788
Adenomatous hyperplasia, 788
Adenomatous polyps and adenocarcinoma, 641–642, 642*f*
Adenomyoma, 764
Adenovirus, 491
Adipocytes, 959
Adipose tissue, exocrine acini, 771
Adrenal cortex, 980
Adrenal cortical tumor, 981*f*
Adrenal cysts, 991
Adrenal cytomegaly, 986–987, 987*f*
Adrenal fusion, 984
Adrenal glands
  acquired disorders
    adrenal cysts, 991
    adrenal hemorrhage, 991–992
    adrenocortical neoplasms, 992–995
    bacterial, fungal, parasitic, and viral infections, 991
    calcifications, 991
    neuroblastoma, 997–1011
  anatomy and physiology, 979–980
  congenital disorders of, 984
  cortex of, 979
  developmental disorders
    adrenal cytomegaly, 986–987
    adrenal fusion, 984
    adrenocortical hyperplasia, 991
    adrenocortical insufficiency, 991
    adrenoleukodystrophy, 986
    congenital adrenal hyperplasia, 989–991
    congenital adrenal hypoplasia, 987–989
    ectopic adrenal tissue, 984–985
    primary pigmented nodular adrenal disease, 991
    unilateral adrenal agenesis, 984
    Wolman disease, 985
  imaging, 980–983
  insufficiency, 988
  maldevelopment, 984*f*
  zonation, 979
Adrenal hemorrhage, 991
Adrenal medulla, 980
Adrenal medullary hyperplasia, 1011
Adrenocortical adenoma (AA), 992, 993*f*
Adrenocortical carcinoma (ACC), 992, 995, 997
Adrenocortical hyperplasia, 991
Adrenocortical insufficiency, 991
Adrenocortical neoplasms (ACNs), 994*f*
  bilateral, 992
  bimodal age distribution, 992
  cellular features, 995
  clinical outcome of, 995
  and Cushing syndrome, 993
  in genetic predisposition syndromes, 992
  mitotic activity, 995
  risk groups and staging, 996*t*, 997
Adrenogenital syndrome (AGS), 897
Adrenoleukodystrophy (ALD), 371*t*
Adult rhabdomyoma, 1180
Adult-type granulosa cell tumors (AGCTs), 887, 888*f*
α-dystroglycan glycosylation, 1289
Aeromonas, 613
Aganglionosis. *See* Hirschsprung disease (HSCR)
Agenesis
  agenesis of the corpus callosum (ACC), 360–362, 361*f*
  aplasia, parathyroids, 960
  common bile/hepatic duct, 669
  hypoplasia, parathyroids, 960
  of pituitary gland, 951
AGS. *See* Adrenogenital syndrome
Aicardi syndrome, 947
Alcohol embryopathy, 108–109, 109*t*
Alexander disease, 352, 371*t*
Allergic colitis (allergic proctocolitis), 636, 637*f*

1435

Allergic sinusitis, 1024, 1024f
Alloimmune gestational hepatitis, 688–689, 689f
Alobar holoprosencephaly, 360, 360f
Alpers disease, 606
Alpers-Huttenlocher syndrome, 374
Alpha-1-antitrypsin deficiency, 684–686
Alport syndrome, 827–829, 828f
Alveolar rhabdomyosarcoma (ARMS), 1185–1189, 1187f–1189f
Alveolar soft part sarcoma (ASPS), 1199, 1200f
Amblyopia, 410
Amelia, 1302
Ameloblastic fibroma (AF), 1045, 1045f
Ameloblastic fibro-odontoma, 1045, 1046f
Ameloblastic odontoma, 1045, 1046f
Ameloblastoma
    conventional, 1050–1051, 1050f
    extraosseous, 1051, 1051f
    therapeutic targets for, 1051
    unicystic, 1048–1050, 1049f
American Fertility Society classification, 870, 870f
AMH. See Antimüllerian hormone
Amino acid
    disorders, 373
    metabolic disorders, 677–678
Aminoacidopathies, 160–162
    homocystinuria, 161
    maple syrup urine disease, 162
    nonketotic hyperglycinemia, 161–162
    phenylketonuria, 160
    tyrosinemia type I, 160–161, 161f
    tyrosinemia type II, 161
Ammon horn sclerosis. See Mesial temporal sclerosis
Amniocentesis, 332
Amnion, 62
Amnionic sac, 326f
Amnion rupture disruption sequence, 111, 112f, 112t
Amniotic fluid infection, 342
    clinical correlation, 343
    fetomaternal hemorrhage, 345–346
    increased circulating fetal nucleated red blood cells, 345
    meconium-related changes, 343–345
    pathology, 342–343
Amylopectinosis, 164, 166, 675–676
Anal disorders
    acquired diseases, 648–649
    congenital abnormalities, 648, 648f
    perianal abscess and anal fistula, 649
Anal fistula, 649
Anaplastic astrocytoma, 384f
Anaplastic large cell lymphoma (ALCL), 1072–1073, 1073f
Andersen disease, 164, 166, 675–676
Anderson disease, 617
Androgen insensitivity syndrome, 900–901
Androgen receptor disorders, 900
Anembryonic gestation, 330
Anembryonic pregnancy, 330, 331f
Anemia, aplastic, 1101
Anencephaly, 357, 358f, 951
Aneuploidy
    definition, 81
    early spontaneous abortion, 61

    sex chromosome (See Sex chromosome aneuploidy)
Aneurysmal bone cyst (ABC), 1347–1349, 1347f–1348f
Angiocentric glioma, 386
Angiokeratomas, 878
Angiomatoid fibrous histiocytoma (AFH), 1163, 1164f
Angiomyolipomas, 851
Angiosarcoma (AS)
    breast, 941
    liver, 751–752, 751f–752f
    soft tissue, 1134, 1135f
    spleen, 1081
Annular pancreas, 764, 766f
Anogenital warts, 648–649
Anomalies. See also specific anomalies
    in pituitary gland, 951, 951t
    spleen, congenital
        accessory, 1077
        asplenia, 1077
        cysts, 1078
        hamartoma, 1077–1078
        polysplenia, 1077
        splenic fusion, 1077
Anomalous pulmonary venous connection, 528, 528f, 528t
Antenatal disruptive lesions, 365
Anterior basement membrane dystrophy. See Map-dot-fingerprint (MDF) dystrophy
Anterior chamber, 422
Anterior polar cataracts, 424
Anterior subcapsular cataract, 425f
Anthrax, 253, 254
Antibody-mediated rejection (AMR), 292
Antigen-processing cells, 414
Antigens, 26–30
    alpha-1-antitrypsin, 30
    cell cycle and apoptotic markers, 29–30
    cell surface, 27–28
    cytoskeleton, 26–27
    embryonal and cancer markers, 29
    hormones, 29
    limitations, 30
    pathogens, 28–29
    protooncogenes, 29
Antimüllerian hormone (AMH), 865, 868, 872, 894
Antiphospholipid antibody syndrome, 330
Antral web, 588
Antrochoanal polyps (AP), 1023, 1023f
Anus disorders, 648–649
Aortic arch
    interruption of, 544
    obstructive anomalies of, 543–545
Aortic arch-branching anomalies, 544
Aortic atresia, 542
Aortic outflow tract and valve malformations, 541
Aortic valvular stenosis, 541
Aortopulmonary septal defect, 535
Aortopulmonary window, 535–536
AOT. See Adenomatoid odontogenic tumor
AP. See Antrochoanal polyps
Apert syndrome, 120–121
Aplasia, 1256, 1258, 1258f
Aplasia cutis congenita, 1217

Aplastic anemia, 1101
Apocrine glands, 410
Apoptosis, signaling and activation, 141
Apoptotic neurons, 403
Appendiceal neuroendocrine (carcinoid) tumors, 647–648, 647f
Appendix
    acute appendicitis, 644–645
    anatomy and histology, 644
    appendiceal neuroendocrine (carcinoid) tumors, 647–648, 647f
    congenital and neuromuscular disorders, 644
    cystic fibrosis, 646–647, 647f
    interval appendectomy, 645
    mucosal melanosis, 646
    unusual infections, 645–646
Apple-peel variety, intestinal atresia, 596, 597f
Arachnoid cysts, 953
Area cerebrovasculosa, 357
Area medullovasculosa, 358
Arginase deficiency, 177
Argininemia, 177
Argininosuccinic aciduria, 177
Arrhythmia, 560t
Arrhythmogenic right ventricular dysplasia (ARVD), 546, 548
Arteriovenous malformations (AVMs), 405
Arthrogryposis, 1258–1260
    contractures, 1258–1260, 1259f
    pathogenetic classification, 1260t
    skeletal system, 1303
ASD. See Atrial septal defect
Ask-Upmark kidney, 805
Aspergillus, 615
Asphyxia, 268–270, 268f–226f
Asplenia, spleen, 1077
Assisted reproductive technologies (ARTs), 62
Asthma, 511–512, 512f
Astroblastomas, 386
Astrocytes, 351, 353
Astrocytosis, 351
Ataxia telangiectasia (AT), 390t, 795
Atherosclerosis, 568
Atopic dermatitis, 1225
Atresia
    bronchial, 454
    choanal, 447–448
    laryngeal stenosis and, 448
    and tracheoesophageal fistula, esophageal, 583–584
Atrial septal defect (ASD), 529, 529f
Atrial septum malformations, 529, 529t
Atrioventricular septum malformations, 531–532, 532f, 532t
Atrioventricular valves, 539
Atypical melanocytes, 416
Atypical teratoid rhabdoid tumor (ATRT), 378, 389–391, 391f
Autism, 376–377
Autoimmune enteropathy, 620, 621f
Autoimmune hepatitis, 704–706, 705f
Autoimmune lymphoproliferative syndrome (ALPS), 1065
Autopsy
    abdomen examination
        adrenals and kidneys, 13–14

bowel, 14–15, 14f
external, 5–6, 6f
internal, 7–8, 7f–8f
liver, 13, 14f
spleen, 13
blood culture, 8, 8f
body cavity, 10, 10f
brain, 15–16
calvarium, 15
cardiac-thoracic ratio, 9, 9f
central nervous system, 15, 15f
chest examination
external, 5, 5f
internal, 7–8, 7f–8f
of children with IEM, 186–187, 186t, 187t
crown-heel length measurement, 2, 3f
cytogenetics, 7, 9
ears, 3–4, 5f
external examination, 1–2, 3f
eyes, 3, 4f
face, 2–3, 3f
forensic pathology
algor mortis, 261
chemistry, 263–264
cultures, 264
decomposition, 262
livor mortis, 261, 262f
maceration, 262, 262f
metabolic analysis, 263
mummification, 262
odontology and anthropology, 264
photography, 263
putrefaction, 262
radiology, 263
rigor mortis, 261
scene investigation, 264–265, 265f
toxicology, 263
head measurement, 2, 3f
heart/lung, 11–13, 11f, 13f
instruments, 1, 2f, 2t
laboratory techniques, 6–7
lower extremities, 6, 6f
lung culture, 8
mouth, 4
nose, 3, 4f
organ removal, Rokitansky technique, 9
palms of the hands, 4
permit, 1
photography, 6
radiography, 6
remains, disposition, 17
respiratory system, 13
scalp, 15
standard, 1–2, 2f, 2t, 3f
testes/ovaries, 9
thymus, 8
upper extremities, 4
vertebral column/spinal cord, 10–11, 10f–11f
Autosomal dominant mutation, 118–120, 126–127
Autosomal dominant polycystic kidney disease, 812, 813f
Autosomal dominant transmission, 424
Autosomal monosomies, 87
Autosomal recessive mutation, 122–126, 122f, 125f

Autosomal recessive polycystic kidney disease, 809, 811–812, 811f, 812f
Autosomal trisomies, 82, 82t–85t, 86f–87f, 87, 88t
Avellino corneal dystrophy, 420
Axial mesodermal defects, 357, 359
Axial skeleton anomalies, 1302–1303
Axonal spheroids, 352, 355

B
Bacillary angiomatosis, 1079
Bacterial infections
in adrenal gland, 991
CNS
acute meningitis, 396, 397f
cerebral abscess, 397
chronic infection, 397–398
diarrhea
Aeromonas, 613
Campylobacter jejuni, 612
Clostridium difficile, 612–613
Escherichia coli, 611–612, 612f
Salmonella, 610–611
Shigella, 611
Vibrio cholerae, 611
Yersinia, 612
skin
ecthyma, 1230, 1230f
erysipelas, 1230, 1231
impetigo, 1229, 1229f
Staphylococcal scalded skin syndrome, 1229–1230, 1230f
toxic shock syndrome, 1230
spontaneous abortion, 65, 66
Balanitis xerotica obliterans (BXO), 921, 922
Balloon cells, 365, 365f
Band keratopathy, 421, 422f
Barrett esophagus, 585
Bartholin cysts, 876
Barth syndrome, 175
Bartonella henselae, 1079
Bartter syndrome, 840
Basal cell carcinoma, 413
Basal cell nevus syndrome, 413, 1243
Basal plate, 333, 334
Basket brain, 365
B-cell lymphoblastic lymphoma, 1070, 1071f
B-cell lymphomas, 1071–1072
Becker muscular dystrophy (BMD), 1285
Beckwith-Wiedemann syndrome (BWS), 114, 114f, 764, 768, 792, 793f, 955t, 986–987
Behçet disease, 875–876
Benign acquired medulloepitheliomas, 434
Benign cutaneous fibrous histiocytoma (BCFH), 1161, 1162f
Benign tumors
cardiac fibromas, 572
histiocytoid cardiomyopathy, 573
lower female genital tract
bacillary angiomatosis, 878
fibroepithelial polyp, 878
hidradenoma papilliferum, 878
Kaposi sarcoma, 878
müllerian/mesonephric papilloma, 878
prepubertal vulval fibroma, 878
malignant tumors, 574

myxomas, 572–573, 572t
rhabdomyomas, 571, 571f
teratomas, 572
Bent bone dysplasias, 1316–1317
Berger disease. *See* IgA nephropathy
Bergmann gliosis, 352
Beta-catenin mutations, 958
ß-catenin–mutated hepatocellular adenoma(bHCA), 722
Bilateral nodular hyperplasia, 990
Bilateral renal agenesis, 804
Bile acid metabolic disorders, 682–684
Biliary tract anomalies and disorders
agenesis, common bile/hepatic duct, 669
ciliated foregut cyst, 669
congenital bronchobiliary fistula (CBBF), 669
congenital dilatation, bile ducts, 669–670
embryonal rhabdomyosarcoma, 750–751, 750f
pancreatitis, 776
Biopsy
electron microscopic examination of specimens, 51–52, 52f
fine-needle aspiration as, 18–20
of lymph nodes
cytogenetic studies, 1058, 1060–1061, 1060t
immunophenotypic studies, 1058, 1059t–1060t
renal
electron microscopic examination of, 51–52, 52f
Birbeck granules, 53, 54f
Bladder, acquired lesions, 854–856
Bladder disorders
acquired lesions, 854–856
congenital lesions, 852
exstrophy, 852–853, 853f
megacystis–microcolon–intestinal hypoperistalsis syndrome, 854
tumors, 856–857
vesicoureteric reflux, 852
Blake pouch cyst, 367
Blastic plasmacytoid DC neoplasm (BPDCN), 1166
Blastocystis hominis, 614
Blood–brain barrier (BBB), 354
Blue nevi, 1245, 1245f, 1246
Blunt force injuries, 270–276, 270f–276f
Blunt impact injury, 273, 273f
Blunt trauma, 774
Bone marrow (BM)
biopsy, neuroblastoma, 1000
development, 1092
examination
aplastic anemia, 1011
benign erythroid disorders, 1011–1012, 1101f
constitutional hematologic disorders, 1099, 1099t, 1100t
indications, 1098t, 1099
inherited and congenital hematopoietic syndromes, granulocytes, 1102, 1102t
inherited bone marrow failure syndromes, 1099

Bone marrow (BM) (*Continued*)
    specialized techniques, 1098t
  features, 1093t
  hematologic profile, 1098–1099, 1098t
  hematopoiesis, 1093t
    lineages, 1094–1096, 1094f–1095f
    normal parameters, 1096, 1097t, 1098
  inherited immunodeficiency disorders
    B-cells and T-cells, 1103, 1104t
    hematogones, 1103, 1103f
    platelet and megakaryocytic disorders, 1103–1104
    specific disorders, 1103, 1104t
  neoplastic disorders
    acute leukemia, 1105
    acute lymphoblastic leukemia, 1105–1108
    acute myelogenous leukemia, 1108–1115
    chronic myeloproliferative disorders, 1116
    congenital leukemia, 1105–1108
    myelodysplastic/myeloproliferative neoplasm, 1115–1116, 1115f, 1116t
    myeloproliferative disorders, 1104
    t-AML/t-MDS, 1114–1115, 1115f
    transient abnormal myelopoiesis, 1104–1105, 1105f
  neoplastic histiocytic disorders
    complications, 1118–1119, 1118t
    dendritic cell–related disorders, 1117
    hematopoietic stem cell transplantation, 1118
    metastatic disorders, 1117–1118, 1117f
    neoplastic histiocytoses, 1116–1117, 1116f
  stem cells and progenitor cells, 1093–1094, 1094f
  structure, 1092–1093, 1093f
  transplantation, 142, 1118–1119
Boomerang dysplasia, 1315–1316, 1315f
Botulism, 240
Bowman membrane, 419, 420, 421, 422f
BPD. *See* Bronchopulmonary dysplasia
Brachmann–de Lange syndrome, 121–122, 122f
Brain
  edema, 354–355
  hydrocephalus, 354–355
  intracranial pressure, 354–355
  trauma
    birth, 355
    infancy and childhood, 355–356
    inflicted injury, 356
  tumors, 381t
Branched-chain ketoaciduria, 162
Branchial apparatus–associated anomalies, 968
Branching enzyme deficiency, 164, 166
Branchio-oto-renal syndrome, 119
Breast
  absence, 928
  adenomas, 930, 932, 932f
  adipose tissue, 927
  anatomy, 927
  carcinoma, 26
  congenital anomalies, 928
  cysts and ductal papillary lesions, 932–934
  displacement, 928
  earlier stages of, 927
  fibroadenomas, 929–930
  fibroepithelial neoplasms, 929–932
  fibrous tumors, 939–941, 940f
  forms subareolar nodule, 928f
  granular cell tumor, 938, 939f
  gynecomastia and juvenile macromastia, 934–935
  hematolymphoid neoplasms, 941–943
  lipomatous tumors, 939
  low- and high-grade malignant phyllodes tumor, 935–936, 936f, 937f
  mammary carcinoma, 936–937
  mesenchyme, 927
  metastatic neoplasms, 941–943
  myofibroblastic tumors, 939–941, 940f
  neurofibroma, 938
  pathologic processes, 929
  polythelia and supernumerary tissue, 928
  primary malignant neoplasms, 935–938
  rubbery fibrous/fibrofatty tissue, 935
  sarcomas, 941
  secretory carcinoma, 937, 938f
  soft tissue and secondary tumors, 938–943
  vascular lesions, 939
Brodie abscess, 1366
Bronchial atresia, 454
Bronchial isomerism syndromes, 454
Bronchiectasis, 485–487, 486f
Bronchiolitis obliterans (BO), 494
Bronchitis, plastic, 456–457
Bronchobiliary fistulae, 455
Bronchoesophageal fistulae, 455
Bronchogenic cyst, 455–456, 456f
Bronchomalacia, 454
Bronchopulmonary dysplasia (BPD), 475–478, 476f, 477f
Bronchus
  abnormal bronchial branching and origin, 454–455
  atresia, 454–457
  bronchobiliary and bronchoesophageal fistulae, 455
  bronchogenic cyst, 455–456, 456f
  bronchomalacia, 454
  isomerism syndromes, 454
  plastic bronchitis, 456–457
  tracheobronchomalacia, 454
Brucellosis, 240
Bruck syndrome, 1310
Budd-Chiari syndrome, 707–708, 708f
Bulbar conjunctiva, 414
Bullous diseases, 876
Bullous impetigo, 1229
Burkitt lymphoma, chromosome abnormalities, 31
Burns, 285, 285f–287f
BWS. *See* Beckwith-Wiedemann syndrome
BXO. *See* Balanitis xerotica obliterans

C

CAH. *See* Congenital adrenal hyperplasia
CAHP. *See* Congenital adrenal hypoplasia
Cajal-Retzius cells (CRCs), 362
Calcifications, adrenal glands, 992
Calcifying aponeurotic fibromatosis, 1152, 1152f
Calcifying epithelioma of Malherbe, 1242
Calcifying fibrous pseudotumor (CFP), 1153
Calcinosis cutis, 1240, 1240f
Calcium homeostasis, 959
Call-Exner bodies, 868, 868f
Campylobacter jejuni, 612
Canal of nuck, 876–877
Canavan disease, 371t
Cancer predisposition (neurocutaneous) syndromes, 390t, 396
Candida, 614
  esophagitis, 587
Caput succedaneum, 355
Carbamoyl phosphate synthetase I (CPS I) deficiency, 176–177
Carbohydrate metabolism abnormalities
  fructosemia, 673
  galactosemia, 162, 673
  glycogen storage diseases, 163–164, 163t, 165f–166f, 166, 673–677
  hereditary fructose intolerance, 162–163
Carcinoid tumor, 917
Carcinomas, 507
Cardiac fibromas, 572
Cardiac malformations
  monosomy X, 71
  trisomy 18, 70
  trisomy 21, 69–70
Cardiac situs, 526
Cardiomyopathy (CMP), 545–546
  dilated, 545, 546, 549–550, 549t
  hypertrophic, 545, 546, 547t–548t
  infant of diabetic mother, 559
  inflammatory, 551–552
  primary, 546–556
  restrictive, 550
  secondary, 554–556
  skeletal myopathy associated with, 1283–1284, 1284f
Cardiopulmonary resuscitation, 278
Carney complex, 955t
Carnitine deficiency, 169
Carnitine palmitoyltransferase (CPT) deficiency, 168, 169
Cartilaginous tumors
  chest wall hamartoma, 1341–1342, 1342f
  chondroblastoma, 1338–1339, 1339f–1340f
  chondroma, 1337–1338, 1338f
  chondromyxoid fibroma, 1339, 1340f–1341f, 1341–1342
  chondrosarcoma, 1342–1344, 1343f
  multiple hereditary exostosis, 1336–1337
  osteochondroma, 1336, 1336f–1337f
  periosteal chondroma, 1338
Castleman disease, 1063, 1063f
Cataractous lens, 426
Cat-scratch disease, 1066, 1066f
Caudal regression syndrome, 1302–1303, 1302f
Cavernous angiomas, 406
Cavernous transformation, portal vein, 707
CDGs. *See* Congenital disorders of glycosylation
CDH. *See* Congenital diaphragmatic hernia
CD10 immunohistochemistry, 876
CD34-positive spindle cell tumors, 1159, 1160
CDT. *See* Cystic dysplasia of the testis

Celiac disease, 620–623
Cell surface antigens, flow cytometry of, 27–28
Cemento-ossifying fibroma, 1031–1032, 1031f
Central giant cell granuloma, 1027–1028, 1028f
Central hypotonia, 1262–1263, 1264f
Central nervous system (CNS)
    autopsy, 15, 15f
    cystic lesions, 368
    cyst type, 368t
    infections, 396–402, 401t
    neuropathologic processes and principles, 351–353
    primitive neuroectodermal tumors, 389
    structural malformations
        agenesis of the corpus callosum, 360–362, 361f
        antenatal disruptive lesions, 365
        axial mesodermal defects, 357
        cell migration and specification disorders, 362
        cerebral heterotopia, 364
        Chiari and Dandy-Walker malformations, 366–368, 367f
        disorders of forebrain development, 359–360
        focal cortical dysplasia, 364–365
        hindbrain malformations, 366
        holoprosencephaly, 360–362, 360f
        lissencephaly, types I and II, 362–363, 363f
        malformations of cortical development, 364–365
        micrencephaly, 365
        microcephaly, 365
        neural tube defects, 357
        polymicrogyria, 363–364, 364f
        tail bud defects, 357
    sudden infant death syndrome, 356–357
    tumors, 396
        clinical considerations, 378
        IHC stains, 382t
        pathologic consideration, 378–382
        signs and symptoms, 381t
        stains, 382t
        WHO classification, 378, 378t–380t
    vascular disorders, 403–406
Central odontogenic fibroma (COF), 1352
Cerebral abscess, 397
Cerebral atrophy, 353
Cerebral blood flow (CBF), 354
Cerebral contusions, 356
Cerebral edema, 354
Cerebral hemispheres
    gestational development of, 1428t
    regional development of, 1429t
Cerebral heterotopia, 364
Cerebral palsy, 327
Cerebral perfusion pressure (CPP), 354
Cerebrohepatorenal syndrome, 181
Cerebro-oculo-facio-skeletal syndrome, 124–125
Cerebrospinal fluid (CSF), 354
    pleocytosis, 437
Cerulean cataract, 424
Cervical–thyroidal teratoma (CTT), 979

CFO. See Craniofacial osteomas
Chalazia, 411
Chalazion, 411, 412f
Chancroid, 875
Chaslin gliosis, 352
CHD. See Congenital heart disease
CHED. See Congenital hereditary endothelial dystrophy
Cherubism, 1346–1347, 1347f
Chest wall hamartoma, 1341–1342, 1342f
Chiari malformations, 366–368, 367f
Children's Hospital of Philadelphia (CHOP), 366
CHILD syndrome, 185–186
Chlamydial infections, 245–246, 246t
    Chlamydia pneumoniae, 491
    Chlamydia trachomatis, 415, 875
Choanal atresia, 447–448
Cholecystitis, 754–755, 754f, 755f
Cholelithiasis, 754–755, 754f, 755f
Cholera, 611
Cholestasis
    persistent intrahepatic (*See* Persistent intrahepatic cholestasis)
Cholestatic disorders, 659t. *See also* Liver
Cholesterol ester storage disease (CESD), 154–155, 155f
Chondroblastoma, 1338–1339, 1339f–1340f
Chondrodysplasia (CDP), 1316, 1316f
Chondroid neoplasms, 501
Chondroma, 1337–1338, 1338f
Chondromatous hamartoma, 502f
Chondromyxoid fibroma, 1339, 1340f–1341f, 1341–1342
Chondrosarcoma, 1342–1344, 1343f
Chordoma, 1364, 1364f
Chorioamnionitis, 342, 343f
    clinical correlation, 343
    fetomaternal hemorrhage, 345–346
    increased circulating fetal nucleated red blood cells, 345
    meconium-related changes, 343–345
    pathology, 342–343
Choriocarcinoma, 328, 329, 329f, 885, 885f, 912
Chorionic plate, 333
Chorionic villi, 62
Chorion leave, 334
Chorion sac, 111
Choroid plexus carcinoma (CPC), 395
Choroid plexus papilloma (CPP), 354, 395, 395f
Choroid plexus tumors (CPTs), 395–396, 395f
Christmas tree variety, intestinal atresia, 596, 597f
Chromaffin cells, 980
Chromosomal abnormalities
    acute lymphoblastic leukemia, 1107–1108
    constitutional
        aneuploidy, 81, 81t
        autosomal monosomies, 87
        autosomal trisomies, 82, 82t–85t, 86f–87f, 87, 88t
        chromosomal instability disorders, 95, 96, 96t, 97f
        confined placental mosaicism, 91–92, 91f

epigenetic chromosomal modifications, 96, 97
mitotic nondisjunction, 81–82
polyploidy, 92
polysomy, 88, 90, 91t
sex chromosome aneuploidies, 87
in spontaneous abortions, 81t
structural chromosomal abnormalities, 92, 93, 93f
submicroscopic abnormalities, 93
velocardiofacial/DiGeorge syndrome, 93, 94t, 95
cytogenetic techniques
    chromosomal microarray, 79, 81
    G-banding, 77, 79
    molecular analysis, 79
    indications, 79t
    online resources for, 79t
    translocations as, in solid tumors, 25f, 27f, 34
Chromosomal instability disorders, 95, 96, 96t, 97f
Chromosomally normal anembryonic pregnancies, 330
Chromosomal microarray, 79, 81, 381
Chronic bacterial infections, 397–398
Chronic bullous dermatosis of childhood. *See* Linear IgA bullous dermatosis
Chronic disease processes, 334
    chronic marginal abruption, 340–341
    fetal vascular malperfusion, 336–338
    maternal vascular malperfusion, 334–336
    perivillous fibrin/fibrinoid deposition, 341–342
    villitis of unknown etiology, 338–339
    villous stromal–vascular maldevelopment, 339–340
Chronic granulomatous disease, 1067
Chronic intermittent torsion, 905
Chronic leptomeningeal inflammation, 400
Chronic lung disease of infancy, 493
Chronic lung disease of prematurity (CLDP). *See* Bronchopulmonary dysplasia (BPD)
Chronic lymphocytic thyroiditis (CLT), 969–970
Chronic marginal abruption, 340–341, 341f
    clinical correlation, 341
    pathology, 341
Chronic maternal vascular malperfusion, 334
Chronic myeloproliferative disorders, 1116
Chronic pancreatitis, 775f, 777
Chronic progressive external ophthalmoplegia (CPEO), 174, 373
Chronic relapsing pancreatitis, 776
Chronic synovitis, 1368
Chronic villitis, 338f
Chylomicron retention (Anderson) disease, 617
Cilia, nasal, electron microscopic examination of, 56, 57f
Ciliated foregut cyst, 669
Cingulosynapsis, 361, 361f
Cirrhosis, 710–711, 711t, 712f
Citrobacter, 234
Citrullinemia type 1, 177
Clark dysplastic nevus, 1245f

Clear cell carcinoma of ovary, 891
Clear cell sarcoma (CCS), 1192–1193, 1194f
Clear cell sarcoma of the kidney (CCSK), 848–850
Cleft lip/palate, 64f, 71, 448
Clostridial infections, 240
Clostridium difficile, 612–613
CLT. *See* Chronic lymphocytic thyroiditis
CMP. *See* Cardiomyopathy (CMP)
CMV, 332, 332f, 398, 399
Coagulative necrosis, 402
Coarctation of the aorta, 543–544
Coats disease, 429
Cockayne syndrome, 123
Coenzyme Q_{10} (CoQ_{10}) deficiency, 175
Colitis
　acute self-limited colitis, 629–630
　allergic colitis (allergic proctocolitis), 636, 637f
　collagenous, 634
　Crohn disease, 632–633
　diversion, 635
　indeterminate, 633–634
　inflammatory bowel disease, 629
　lymphocytic, 634
　neonatal necrotizing enterocolitis, 635–636
　pseudomembranous, 634, 634f
　solitary rectal ulcer syndrome, 636–637
　spontaneous perforation, 636
　typhlitis (neutropenic enterocolitis), 635
　ulcerative colitis, 630–632
Collagenous colitis, 634
Collagen type III glomerulopathy, 825
Collagen vascular diseases
　lupus erythematosus, 26, 1238–1239, 1239f
　scleroderma, 1239, 1239f
Collision tumor, 958
Colloid goiter, 971
Colpocephaly, 361
Committee on Childhood Interstitial Lung Disease (ChILD), 492
Common-inlet ventricle, 539
Comparative genomic hybridization (CGH)
　early spontaneous abortion, 61
　first trimester spontaneous abortion, 62
Complete hydatidiform mole (CHM), 62, 66–67, 67f
Composite adrenal medullary neoplasms, 1011
Composite hemangioendothelioma (CHE), 1134
Conduction system abnormalities, 560–562
Condylomata lata, 875
Confined placental mosaicism, 91–92, 91f
Congenital abnormalities, 764
　abnormalities of unknown origin
　　nonimmune hydrops fetalis, 129–131, 129f, 130t
　　short-cord syndrome, 129
　acrocephalosyndactyly syndrome, 120–122
　　Apert syndrome, 120–121
　　Brachmann–de Lange syndrome, 121–122, 122f
　　Crouzon craniofacial dysostosis, 121
　　Noonan syndrome, 121
　　Pfeiffer syndrome, 121
　　Robinow syndrome, 121
　　Stickler syndrome, 121
　anal disorders, 648, 648f
　appendix, 644
　autosomal dominant conditions
　　branchio-oto-renal syndrome, 119
　　CHARGE syndrome, 118
　　Holt-Oram syndrome, 119
　　mandibulofacial dysostosis, 119
　　nail-patella syndrome, 118
　　Opitz-Frias syndrome, 119–120
　　oral-facial-digital syndrome type I, 118–119
　　Townes-Brocks syndrome, 119
　autosomal recessive conditions
　　Cockayne syndrome, 123
　　Dubowitz syndrome, 124
　　familial agnathia-holoprosencephaly, 125
　　hydrolethalus syndrome, 126
　　leprechaunism, 123
　　Meckel syndrome, 122–123, 122f
　　oral-facial-digital syndrome type II, 124
　　Pena-Shokeir phenotype type I, 124
　　Pena-Shokeir phenotype type II, 124–125
　　Robert syndrome, 125
　　Seckel syndrome, 123–124
　　Smith-Lemli-Opitz syndrome, 123
　　thrombocytopenia absent radius syndrome, 125–126
　biliary and hepatic ducts
　　agenesis, common bile/hepatic duct, 669
　　ciliated foregut cyst, 669
　　congenital bronchobiliary fistula (CBBF), 669
　　congenital dilatation, bile ducts, 669–670
　of breast, 928
　deformation, 105, 105f
　disruption, 105–113
　　amnion rupture disruption sequence, 111, 112f, 112t
　　chorion and yolk sac rupture sequence, 111
　　diabetes mellitus, 110, 110f, 111t
　　dysplastic disruptions, 113
　　hyperthermia, 113
　　infectious disruptions, 110–111
　　ionizing radiation, 105–106
　　ischemic and vascular disruptions, 111–113
　　metabolic disruptions, 110
　　phenylketonuria, 110
　　teratogenic disruptions, 106, 107t
　　twin reversed arterial perfusion, 113, 113f
　　twin-twin transfusion syndrome, 113
　esophagus disorders
　　esophageal atresia and tracheoesophageal fistula, 583–584
　　esophageal duplication, 582
　　esophageal stenosis, 584
　　heterotopic gastric mucosa (inlet patch), 581–582
　　neurenteric cyst (remnant) of the mediastinum, 583
　　persistent embryonic epithelium, 581
　etiology, 103
　heterogenous autosomal dominant and recessive dysplasias
　　chondrodysplasia, 126–127
　　osteochondrodysplasia, 126, 127
　intestinal epithelial differentiation, 617–620
　　congenital tufting enteropathy (CTE), 618, 619f
　　enteroendocrine cell dysgenesis (enteric anendocrinosis), 619–620
　　microvillus inclusion disease, 617–618, 619f
　kidney malformations
　　bilateral renal agenesis, 804
　　congenital mesoblastic nephroma, 847–848
　　hydronephrosis, 806–807
　　renal agenesis/hypoplasia, 804
　　renal duplication (duplex kidney), 806
　　renal ectopia, 802–803, 802t
　　renal fusion, 802t, 803–804, 803f
　　renal hypoplasia, 805
　　renal malformations, pediatric autopsies, 801, 802t
　　renal tubular dysgenesis, 805–806
　　renomegaly, 806
　　supernumerary kidney, 806
　　unilateral renal agenesis, 804–805
　liver, 655–656, 655f–656f
　malabsorption
　　congenital tufting enteropathy (CTE), 618, 619f
　　enteroendocrine cell dysgenesis (enteric anendocrinosis), 619–620
　　microvillus inclusion disease, 617–618, 619f
　metabolic dysplasia syndrome
　　Williams syndrome, 115
　　Zellweger syndrome, 115–116, 115t
　morphogenesis, 103–105, 105f
　MURCS association, 118
　nonmetabolic dysplasia syndrome
　　Beckwith-Wiedemann syndrome, 114, 114f
　　Perlman syndrome, 114–115
　Schisis association, 118
　sequence
　　prune belly sequence, 116–117, 117f
　　Robin sequence, 116
　skin (genodermatoses)
　　acrodermatitis enteropathica, 1222
　　aplasia cutis congenita, 1217
　　Darier disease, 1218, 1218f, 1219f
　　ectodermal dysplasias, 1219, 1220f, 1221f
　　epidermolysis bullosa, 1221–1222, 1221f
　　focal dermal hypoplasia, 1219, 1221
　　ichthyoses, 1217–1218, 1217f, 1218f
　　incontinentia pigmenti, 1222, 1222f
　　porokeratosis, 1218, 1219
　　restrictive dermopathy, 1219
　small and large intestine disorders
　　duplications, 596–598, 597f
　　gastroschisis, 594, 594f

intestinal atresia and stenosis, 595–596, 597f
malrotation, 582f, 594–595, 595f
Meckel diverticulum, 598–599, 599f
omphalocele, 594, 594f
vitelline (omphalomesenteric) duct anomalies, 598–599, 598f
sporadic abnormalities
Hallermann-Streiff syndrome, 128
hypomelanosis of Ito, 128–129
Klippel-Trenaunay-Weber vascular malformation, 128
Rubinstein-Taybi syndrome, 129
Sturge-Weber dysplasia, 128
stomach disorders
antral web, 588
duplication, 588
hypertrophic pyloric stenosis, 588
pancreatic heterotopia and pancreatic acinar metaplasia, 589
terminology of, 103–105
transport and enzymatic disorders, 616–617
ureter disorders, 851
VATER association, 117–118
X-linked mutations
Lesch-Nyhan syndrome, 127–128
Lowe syndrome, 127
Menkes syndrome, 127
Opitz-Kaveggia syndrome, 128
Pallister syndrome, 128
Congenital acinar dysplasia, 467f
Congenital adrenal hyperplasia (CAH), 980, 989–991, 990f
Congenital adrenal hypoplasia (CAHP), 987–989, 988f
Congenital alveolar capillary dysplasia, 472, 473f
Congenital bronchobiliary fistula (CBBF), 669
Congenital capillary alveolar dysplasia, 472t
Congenital cataracts, 424
Congenital diaphragmatic eventration (CDE), 513, 513f
Congenital diaphragmatic hernia (CDH), 512t, 513–514
Congenital dilatation, bile ducts, 669–670
Congenital disorders of glycosylation (CDG), 139, 182, 183t–184t, 184, 373
Congenital epulis of the newborn, 1027, 1027f
Congenital glaucoma, 423
Congenital heart defects, 525t
Congenital heart disease (CHD)
congenital malformations
aortic arch system, 542–545
cardiac situs, 526
classification, 526
coronary arteries, 545
dextrocardia, 526–527
etiology, 524
incidence, 524
pathophysiology, 525
septal malformations, 529–536
venous system, 527–529
ventricular inflow tracts, 536–539
ventricular outflow tracts, 539–545
hereditary and nonhereditary functional cardiovascular diseases

conduction system abnormalities, 560–562
endocardial diseases, 562–564
extracardiac vascular disease, 565–570
myocardial disease, 545–560
pericardial diseases, 564–565
tumors, 570–574, 571t, 574t
Congenital hemangioma (CH), 725, 1130–1131
Congenital hepatic fibrosis (CHF), 670–673, 672f
Congenital hereditary endothelial dystrophy (CHED), 420
Congenital hyperinsulinism, 787t
diazoxide-responsive, 791
Congenital hypothyroidism, 966–967, 967t
Congenital infantile fibrosarcoma (CIFS), 1156–1157, 1156f, 1156t, 1157f
Congenital infections
clinical correlation, 332
pathology, 332
Congenital lactic acidosis, 179–180, 1282
pyruvate carboxylase deficiency, 179, 180
pyruvate dehydrogenase deficiency, 179, 180f
Congenital laryngeal atresia, 448
Congenital lens opacities, 424
Congenital leukemia, 766f
Congenital lymphangiectasis, 895
Congenital medulloepitheliomas, 434
Congenital melanocytic nevi, 1243–1244, 1243f, 1244f
Congenital mesoblastic nephroma (CMN), 847–848
Congenital muscular dystrophy 1C (MDC1C), 1289
Congenital myopathies, 556
Congenital neuroblastoma, 917
Congenital nevus and malignant melanoma, 1244
Congenital ovarian cysts, 877
Congenital peribronchial myofibroblastic tumor (CPMT), 500, 501f
Congenital pseudoarthrosis (CP), 1353–1354
Congenital pulmonary airway malformation (CPAM), 466–472, 467f–472f
Congenital pulmonary lymphangiectasia (CPL), 459, 465–466, 466f
Congenital radial–tibial deficiency, 1301
Congenital spinal lipoma, 1167
Congenital surfactant deficiencies, 479t, 480f
Congenital syphilis, 766f
Congenital toxoplasmosis, 401
Congestion, spleen, 1078
Conjunctiva
biopsy, 418
developmental abnormalities, 415
inflammatory conditions, 415–416
melanocytic abnormalities, 416–418
melanoma of, 417
nevi, 416, 417f
pyogenic granuloma, 411
structure, 414, 414f
surgical procedures, 418
tissues of, 418
Conradi-Hunermann syndrome (CDPX2), 184–185

Constitutional hematologic disorders, 1099, 1099t, 1100t
Constitutional hematopoietic disorders
B-cells and T-cells, 1104t
granulocytes, 1102, 1102t
Contact dermatitis, 1225
Contact lens–like prosthesis, 439
Conus and truncus malformations, 533, 533t
Conventional ameloblastoma, 1050–1051, 1050f
Conventional cytogenetic analysis, 77, 79
Cori disease, 675
Cori-Forbes disease, 164
Cornea
degenerations, 421
developmental abnormalities, 419
dystrophic conditions, 420–421
structure, 418–419, 419f
surgical procedure, 422
Corneal dystrophies, 420
Corneal hydrops, 421f
Corneal stroma, 418
Coronary arteries malformations, 545
Coronary sinus ostium atresia, 527
Corpus callosum, 360–362, 361f
Cortical cysts, 814–815
Cortical dysplasia, 364
Corticotrophs, 950, 951
Cor triatriatum, 528–529
Cowden syndrome, 390t, 395, 955t
CPAM. See Congenital pulmonary airway malformation
CPP. See Choroid plexus papilloma
CPTs. See Choroid plexus tumors
C1q nephropathy, 820–821
Craniofacial osteomas (CFO), 1029–1030, 1029f
Craniopharyngioma (CPG), 391, 952, 953, 953f
Craniorachischisis, 357
CRCs. See Cajal-Retzius cells
Crescentic glomerulonephritis, 833–834
Creutzfeldt-Jakob disease (CJD), 374
Cribriform neuroepithelial tumors (CRINET), 391
Crigler-Najjar syndrome (CNS), 657–658
Crohn disease, 592, 632–633, 876
Crouzon craniofacial dysostosis, 121
Crown-heel length measurement, 2, 3f
CRP. See Craniopharyngioma
Cryopyrin-associated periodic syndromes (CAPS), 1320
Cryptorchidism, 895–896
Cryptorchid testis, 895, 896f
Sertoli cell nodule, 897f
Cryptosporidium, 613–614, 614f
Crystalline lens
developmental abnormalities, 423–424
dislocation, 426, 426f
structure, 423
surgical procedures, 426
CTT. See Cervical–thyroidal teratoma
Curettage, 1216
Cushing syndrome, 991
Cutaneous lesions, 410, 412
Cyst(s)
aneurysmal bone cyst, 1347–1349, 1347f–1348f

Cyst(s) (*Continued*)
  of breast, 932–934
  canal of nuck, 876–877
  epidermoid, 910–911, 910*f*, 1349
  of parathyroid, 961–962
  renal
    cortical, 814–815
    Meckel-Gruber syndrome, 816
    medullary cystic kidney disease, 814
    medullary sponge kidney, 813
    nephronophthisis, 813
    simple, 815
    tuberous sclerosis, 815, 815*f*
    Von Hippel-Lindau disease, 815–816
  solitary–unicameral bone cyst, 1349, 1349*f*–1350*f*
  spleen, 1078
Cystic dysplasia of the testis (CDT), 895
Cystic fibrosis, 486*f*, 772–773, 774*f*, 794, 1022
  appendix, 646–647, 647*f*
  gastrointestinal involvement, 600, 600*t*
  metabolic disorders, 686–687
  sinonasal polyp in, 1022, 1023*f*
Cystic fibrosis transmembrane conductance regulator (CFTR), 600, 600*t*
Cystic lesions
  CNS, 368
  female reproductive system
    Bartholin cysts, 876
    Gartner duct cysts, 876
    müllerian cysts, 876
    nonneoplastic ovarian cysts, 877–878
    peritoneal lined cysts, 876–877
    Skene duct cysts, 877
    vulvar mucous cysts, 876
Cystic teratomas, 880–881
Cystinosis, 156, 157
Cystitis, bladder and urethra
  cystica and glandularis, 855
  eosinophilic, 855
  granulomatous, 855
  hemorrhagic, 855–856
  interstitial, 855
  malakoplakia, 855
Cytogenetic studies, 33–35
  applications of, 24*f*, 27*f*, 35
  basis of methodology of, 33–35
  compared with other molecular methods, 22*t*
  limitations of, 35
Cytokeratin, 27
Cytomegalovirus (CMV), 69, 69*f*, 609–610, 610*f*
  clinical features, 205, 206*f*
  esophagitis, 587
  laboratory diagnosis, 207
  pancreatitis, 775*f*
  pathology, 205, 207
  prognosis and outcome, 207
  transmission, 201
Cytotoxic cerebral edema, 354

D

DAI. *See* Diffuse axonal injury
Dalen-Fuchs nodules, 438
Dandy-Walker malformation (DWM), 363, 366–368, 367*f*
Danlos syndrome, 276
Danon disease, 158, 554
Darier disease, 1218, 1218*f*, 1219*f*
Darier-White disease, 876
DAs. *See* Diffusely infiltrating astrocytomas
d-bifunctional protein deficiency, 182
Debranching enzyme disease, 675
Deep mycosis, 1233, 1234*f*
Defect in müllerian inhibiting system, 899–900
Defects in testosterone synthesis, 899
Degenerative-type atypia, 380–381
Delayed villous maturation, 339
Delta agent. *See* Hepatitis D virus (HDV)
Dendritic cell (DC) neoplasms, 1165
Dendritic melanocytes, 414
Denervation, fibers, 1265, 1266*f*, 1266*t*
Dense opacity, 415
Dentato-olivary dysplasia (DOD), 367
Dentigerous cyst, 1040–1042, 1041*f*
Denys-Drash syndrome, 904
Dermatofibroma (DF), 1161, 1161*f*
Dermatofibrosarcoma, 941, 942*f*
Dermatofibrosarcoma protuberans (DFSP), 1158–1159, 1159*f*, 1160*f*
Dermatomyofibroma, 1149, 1149*f*
Dermatopathic lymphadenopathy, 1068–1069, 1068*f*
Dermoid cyst, 436, 767, 953, 1241
Descemet stripping endothelial keratoplasty (DSEK), 422
Desmin, 26
Desmoid-type fibromatosis, 1149–1151, 1150*f*, 1151*f*
Desmoplastic fibroma (DF), 1032, 1032*f*, 1351–1353
Desmoplastic infantile ganglioglioma/desmoplastic infantile astrocytoma (DIG/DIA), 394
Desmoplastic nodular (DN), 387
Desmoplastic small round cell tumor (DSRCT), 920, 1191–1192, 1192*f*–1193*f*, 1192*t*
Developmental disorders
  adrenal glands
    adrenal cytomegaly, 986–987
    adrenal fusion, 984
    adrenocortical hyperplasia, 991
    adrenocortical insufficiency, 991
    adrenoleukodystrophy, 986
    congenital adrenal hyperplasia, 989–991
    congenital adrenal hypoplasia, 987–989
    ectopic adrenal tissue, 984–985
    primary pigmented nodular adrenal disease, 991
    unilateral adrenal agenesis, 984
    Wolman disease, 985
  conjunctiva, 415
  cornea, 419
  crystalline lens, 423–424
  parathyroid glands
    agenesis–hypoplasia, 960
    cyst, 961–962
    ectopic parathyroid, 960
    supernumerary parathyroid glands, 960
  pineal gland
    pineal agenesis, 947
    pineal cysts, 947–948
  pituitary gland
    agenesis of, 951
    anencephaly, 951
    anomalies in, 951, 951*t*
    ectopia, 951–952
    empty sella syndrome, 952
    hypopituitarism, 951
    mutations, 951, 952*t*
    nasopharyngeal teratomas, 952
    pituitary duplication, 952
    Rathke cleft cyst, 952
  thyroid gland
    branchial apparatus–associated anomalies, 968
    congenital hypothyroidism, 966–967, 967*t*
    dysgenesis, 965–967
    dysmorphism, 965
    ectopia, 967
    hemiagenesis, 967
    thyroglossal duct cyst, 967–968
Dextrocardia, 526
  ectopia cordis, 527
  juxtaposition of atrial appendages, 526–527
  situs ambiguus, 526
DFSP–giant cell fibroblastoma, 941
Diabetes mellitus, 110, 110*f*, 111*t*, 784–786
Diabetic nephropathy, 822–823, 823*f*
Diaphanous dysplasia, 70
Diaphragmatic hernia, 514*f*, 514*t*, 1258
Diarrhea
  bacterial
    Aeromonas, 613
    Campylobacter jejuni, 612
    Clostridium difficile, 612–613
    Escherichia coli, 611–612, 612*f*
    Salmonella, 610–611
    Shigella, 611
    Vibrio cholerae, 611
    Yersinia, 612
  viral
    cytomegalovirus, 609–610, 610*f*
    enteric adenovirus, 606*f*, 609
    herpes simplex virus, 610
    Norwalk virus, 609
    postenteritis enteropathy, 610
    rotaviruses, 609
Diazoxide-responsive congenital hyperinsulinism, 791
Diazoxide-unresponsive congenital hyperinsulinism, 787
Dientamoeba fragilis, 614
Dieterle stains, 875
Diffuse alveolar damage (DAD), 472
Diffuse axonal injury (DAI), 356
Diffuse hyperinsulinism, 787–788, 787*t*, 789*f*
Diffuse hyperplasia with clinical hyperthyroidis, 971
Diffuse intrinsic pontine glioma (DIPG), 383
Diffuse large B-cell lymphoma (DLBCL), 1071
Diffusely infiltrating astrocytomas (DAs), 383–384
Diffuse nesidioblastosis, 781
Diffuse placentitis, 332
Diffuse trophoblastic hyperplasia, 329
Diffuse-type giant cell tumor, 1161, 1163
Diffuse white matter gliosis, 404
DiGeorge anomaly, 1084

Dihydroepiandrosteindione sulfate, 980
Dilated cardiomyopathy (DCMP), 545, 546, 549–550, 549t
Diphenylhydantoin embryopathy, 110
Diphtheria infections, 232, 233
Diplopia, 412
Direct immunofluorescence (DIF), 30, 31f, 1216
Discretionary Advisory Committee on Heritable Disorders in Newborns and Children (DACHDNC), 136
Disorders of mitochondrial dysfunction, 139
Disorders of sex development (DSD), 897
   classification, 872t, 897, 898f
   clinical presentation, 872
   definition, 871
   etiologies, 871
   gonadal pathology in, 872–873
   tumors associated with gonadal dysgenesis, 873
Distal intestinal obstruction syndrome, 600
Distal villous immaturity, 339
Diversion, colitis, 635
DNT. See Dysembryoplastic neuroepithelial tumor
DOD. See Dentato-olivary dysplasia
DOLV. See Double-outlet left ventricle
Donlan syndrome, 772
Donohue syndrome, 794
Donovan bodies, 875
DORV. See Double-outlet right ventricle
Double-inlet ventricle, 538–539
Double-outlet left ventricle (DOLV), 534
Double-outlet right ventricle (DORV), 534
Drug-induced interstitial nephritis, 836
Drug-induced pancreatitis, 776
DSD. See Disorders of sex development
DSEK. See Descemet stripping endothelial keratoplasty
DSRCT. See Desmoplastic small round cell tumor
Dubin-Johnson syndrome, 657–658
Dubowitz syndrome, 124
Duchenne muscular dystrophy (DMD), 1285, 1286f
Ductal papillary lesions, breast, 932–934
Ductus arteriosus, 542–543
Duodenoduodenostomy, 764
Duplication
   esophageal, 582
   small and large intestine disorders, 596–598, 597f
   stomach, 588
   ureter disorders, 851–852
Dysembryoplastic neuroepithelial tumor (DNT), 386, 394, 394f
Dysgenesis, thyroid gland, 965–967
Dysgerminoma, 882–883, 883f
Dyshidrotic dermatitis, 1225
Dyshormonogenic goiter, 964, 964f
Dysmorphic neurons, 365, 393
Dysmorphic villi, 339
Dysmorphism, thyroid gland, 965
Dysmyelinating, 369
Dysostoses, 121
Dysplasia syndrome
   metabolic, 115, 115t
   nonmetabolic, 113–115, 114f
Dysplastic disruptions, 113

Dysplastic gangliocytoma of the cerebellum (DGCC), 395
Dystrophic conditions, cornea, 420–421

E
Eagle-Barrett syndrome. See Prune belly syndrome
Early pregnancy
   anembryonic pregnancy, 330, 331f
   congenital infections, 332
   development, 325–326, 326f
   gestational trophoblastic disease, 328–330
   miscarriage, 330, 331f, 332
   multiple, 326–328
Ebstein malformation, 536–537, 537f
Ectodermal dysplasias, 1219, 1220f, 1221f
Ectopia
   of adrenal tissue, 919f, 984–985
   cordis, 527
   lentis, 426, 426f
   of pancreas, 764, 767, 767f
   of parathyroid, 960
   of pituitary gland, 951–952
   of thyroid gland, 966f, 967
Eczematous dermatitis
   atopic dermatitis, 1225
   contact dermatitis, 1225
   dyshidrotic dermatitis, 1225
   nummular dermatitis, 1225
   spongiotic dermatitis, 1225–1226, 1227f
Edema, 328, 329
Edwards syndrome, 1299
Ehlers-Danlos syndrome, 568
Electron microscopy, 51–59
   in diagnosis
      of hematologic disorder, 56
      of peroxisomal disorders, 56, 56f
   economics of, 52
   in examination
      of autopsy specimens, 55, 55f
      of bowel biopsies, 58f, 59
      of cilia morphology, 56, 57f
      of fine-needle aspiration specimens, 55, 56f
      of frozen tissue, 55, 55f
   laboratory requirements for performing, 51–52
   specimen preparation for, 53
   suboptimal specimen processing and, 53, 54f
   surgical pathology specimens examined by, 51–52, 52f
   technique of, 52–59
   virus identification by, 56, 57f
Embryo
   cleft lip and coloboma, 64f
   encephaloceles, 64f
   growth-disorganized (See Growth-disorganized embryo)
   neural tube defects, 64–65
   normal development, 62–63, 63f
   triploid, 65, 65f
   trisomy 13, 120, 120f
Embryonal carcinoma (EC), 884–885, 885f, 911, 912f
Embryonal rhabdomyosarcoma (ERMS), 750–751, 750f, 879, 879f, 922, 923f, 1183–1185, 1184f–1186f, 1189f

Embryonal tumors, 387
   medulloblastomas, 387–389, 387f
   primitive neuroectodermal tumors, 389
Embryonal tumor with abundant neuropil and true rosettes (ETANTR), 389
Embryonic period events, 1388t
Emery-Dreifuss muscular dystrophy, 556
Empty sella syndrome (ESS), 952
Encephalitis, 398, 399f
Encephaloceles, 359, 359f
Encephalocraniocutaneous lipomatosis (ECCL), 1166
Encysted bradyzoites, 402
Endocardial diseases, 562
   infective, 562t, 563–564, 563t
   noninfective, 562–563, 562t
Endocardial fibroelastosis (EFE), 550
Endocardium and valves, 557
Endocrine aplasia, 783
Endocrine pancreas
   abnormalities, 783–792
   histogenesis, maturation, and morphology, 779–783, 781f, 782f
   syndromes/diseases, 792–795
   tumor in childhood, 795
   viral infections, 792
Endodermal sinus tumor (EST), 752, 753f–754f, 754, 879–880
   immature teratoma, 881, 882
   ovarian germ cell tumors, 883–884, 883f, 884f
Endometriosis, 877–878, 878f
Endometrium during childhood, 869
Endomyocardial biopsy and heart transplant, 559–560
End-organ defects, testis, 900–901
   androgen receptor disorders, 900
   disorder of peripheral testosterone metabolism, 901
   partial androgen insensitivity syndrome, 901
   testicular feminization, 900–901, 900f
Entamoeba histolytica, 252–253, 253f, 614, 615f
Enteric adenovirus, 606f, 609
Enterobacteriaceae infection, 230, 231f
Enterobius vermicularis (pinworm), 875
Enterococci, 229–230
Enteropathy, 776
Enteropeptidase, 771
Environmental lens opacities
   rubella cataract, 424, 425f
   toxic cataract, 425
   traumatic cataract, 425
Enzyme replacement therapy, 142
Eosinophilic cellulitis, 1234
Eosinophilic cystitis, 855
Eosinophilic esophagitis, 585–586, 587f, 587t
Eosinophilic gastroenteritis, 623–624
Eosinophilic granular bodies (EGBs), 352, 353f
Eosinophilic insulitis, 783f
Eosinophilic pneumonia, 491–492
Eosinophilic pustular folliculitis, 1238
Ependymoblastomas, 389
Ependymomas, 384–386
Epiblast, 325
Epidermal inclusion cyst, 1241, 1241f
Epidermal nevi, 1240–1241, 1241f
Epidermoid cyst, 910–911, 910f, 1349

Epidermolysis bullosa, 1221–1222, 1221f
Epididymal sarcoidosis, 920
Epididymis
　acquired abnormalities and lesions, 919–920
　adenomatoid tumor, 921
　congenital anomalies, 918–919
　developmental anomalies, 918–919
　papillary cystadenoma, 921
Epididymoorchitis, 905
Epidural hemorrhage, 356
Epigenetic chromosomal modifications, 96, 97
Epilepsy, 377
Episcleral osseous choristoma, 415
Epithelial growth factor receptor (EGFR), 1051
Epithelial membrane antigen (EMA), 385
Epithelial neoplasms
　female reproductive system, 889–891
　　ovary
　　　clear cell carcinoma, 891
　　　mucinous neoplasms, 890, 890f
　　　serous neoplasms, 889–890, 890f
　　　small cell carcinomas, 890–891
　respiratory tract, 504–506, 504t
Epithelioid cell nevus. See Spitz nevus
Epithelioid hemangioendothelioma (EHE), 502
Epithelioid hemangioma (EH), 1133, 1134f
Epithelioid sarcoma (ES), 1198–1199
Epithelioid trophoblastic tumor (ETT), 328–330, 329f
Epithelium-lined cysts, 767
Epstein-Barr virus (EBV), 220, 398
　infection, lymph nodes, 1063–1064, 1064f
　infectious mononucleosis, 221, 222f
　neoplasms, 221–223
Eruptive vellus hair cysts, 1241
Erysipelas, 1230, 1231
Erythema nodosum, 1236, 1236f
Erythroid disorders, benign, 1011–1012, 1101f
Erythropoiesis, 1095, 1095f
Escherichia coli, 611–612, 612f, 905, 922
Esophageal atresia (EA), 448, 451–453, 453f, 453t
　and tracheoesophageal fistula, 583–584
Esophageal cyst, 457
Esophageal duplication, 582
Esophageal stenosis, 584
Esophagitis, gastroesophageal reflux, 584–585, 584f, 584t
Esophagus disorders
　acquired diseases
　　Barrett esophagus, 585
　　Candida esophagitis, 587
　　cytomegalovirus esophagitis, 587
　　eosinophilic esophagitis, 585–586, 587f, 587t
　　esophagitis, gastroesophageal reflux, 584–585, 584f, 584t
　　herpes simplex esophagitis, 587, 588f
　　infectious esophagitis, 586
　congenital abnormalities
　　esophageal atresia and tracheoesophageal fistula, 583–584
　　esophageal duplication, 582

　　esophageal stenosis, 584
　　heterotopic gastric mucosa (inlet patch), 581–582
　　neurenteric cyst (remnant) of the mediastinum, 583
　　persistent embryonic epithelium, 581
ESS. *See* Empty sella syndrome
EST. *See* Endodermal sinus tumor
Esthesioneuroblastoma, 1034–1035, 1034f
ETT. *See* Epithelioid trophoblastic tumor
Ewing sarcoma, 494
Ewing sarcoma-like tumors, 1191, 1191f
Ewing sarcoma-primitive neuroectodermal tumor (EWS-PNET), 1189–1190, 1189t, 1190f, 1191f, 1356f–1357f
　diagnosis, 1355
　electron microscopic examination of, 55, 56f
　Gray–white tumor, 1358f
　gross examination, 1357
　immunohistochemical and molecular genetic studies, 1356
　incidence, 1355
　prognostic determinants, 1358
　proximal fibula, 1355f
Excisional biopsy, 1216
Exocrine acini, adipose tissue, 771
Exocrine atrophy, Shwachman-Diamond syndrome, 771, 772f
Exocrine pancreas
　abnormalities
　　cystic fibrosis, 772–773, 774f
　　exocrine acini by adipose tissue, 771
　　inspissation and pancreatic ducts changes, 773
　　isolated enzyme deficiencies, 771
　　Johanson-Blizzard syndrome, 772
　　neonatal hemochromatosis, 772
　　Pearson marrow–pancreas syndrome, 772
　　Shwachman-Diamond syndrome, 771, 772f
　functional development, 770–771
　pancreatitis in childhood, 773–776
　tumors, 777–779
　　acinar cell carcinoma, 778–779, 779f
　　pancreatic ductal adenocarcinoma, 779
　　pancreatoblastoma, 777, 778f
　　solid pseudopapillary neoplasm, 779
Exophthalmos, 412
Exstrophy, bladder, 852–853, 853f
Extracardiac vascular disease, 565–570
Extracorporeal membrane oxygenation (ECMO), 485, 485f
Extrahepatic biliary atresia (EHBA)
　biliary remnants classification, 663–664
　cholestasis, 661–662
　extrahepatic ducts, changes in, 662, 662f
　forms of, 659–660
　vs. neonatal hepatitis syndrome, 660t
Extramedullary hematopoiesis (EMH), 1080
Extraocular muscles, 418
Extraosseous ameloblastoma, 1051, 1051f

Extraskeletal myxoid chondrosarcoma (EMC), 1193, 1194
Extravaginal torsion, 905
Eye
　autopsy specimens of, 439–440
　structure, 413–414, 414f
Eyelid
　inflammatory abnormalities, 411–412
　neoplastic lesions, 412–413
　structure, 410, 411f
　surgical procedures, 412–413
　vascular abnormalities, 410–411

F

FA. *See* Fibroadenomas
Fabry disease, 555, 681
　sphingolipidoses, 142–144, 144f
Factitious disorder, 285–287
Familial adenomatous polyposis coli, 955t
Familial adenomatous polyposis syndrome, 1032
Familial agnathia-holoprosencephaly, 125
Familial and idiopathic pulmonary artery hypertension, 567
Familial exudative vitreoretinopathy, 427
Familial follicular thyroid carcinoma, 956t
Familial medullary thyroid carcinoma, 955t
Familial multinodular goiter with papillary thyroid carcinoma, 956t
Familial papillary carcinoma with oxyphilia, 956t
Familial papillary thyroid carcinoma with clear cell renal carcinoma, 956t
Familial paraganglioma–pheochromocytoma, 955t
Familial retinoblastoma syndrome, 390t
Fanconi-Bickel syndrome, 166
F-anisosplenia, 454
Farber disease, 149, 680–681
Fatty acid oxidation defects, 166–169, 555, 555t
　acyl-CoA dehydrogenase deficiencies, 167–168, 167t, 169f
　metabolic disorders, 694–695, 694f
　substrate transport defects, 168, 169
FCD. *See* Focal cortical dysplasia
FCMD. *See* Fukuyama congenital muscular dystrophy
Female external genitalia, 869–870
Female pseudohermaphroditism, 897
Female reproductive system
　anatomy and embryology
　　ductal system, 868–869
　　early gonadal development, 866, 866f
　　female external genitalia, 869–870
　　ovarian differentiation, 866–868, 867f, 868f
　　primordial germ cells, 865
　cystic lesions
　　Bartholin cysts, 876
　　Gartner duct cysts, 876
　　müllerian cysts, 876
　　nonneoplastic ovarian cysts, 877–878
　　peritoneal lined cysts, 876–877
　　Skene duct cysts, 877
　　vulvar mucous cysts, 876

disorders of sex development, 871
    classification, 872t
    gonadal pathology in, 872–873
    tumors associated with gonadal dysgenesis, 873
    neoplasms
        benign tumors, 878
        malignant tumors, 879–880
    nonneoplastic lesions
        chancroid, 875
        enterobius vermicularis, 875
        granuloma inguinale, 875
        infections, 874–875
        noninfectious inflammatory diseases, 875–876
    ovarian neoplasms
        epithelial neoplasms, 889–891
        germ cell tumors, 880–886
        sex cord–stromal tumors, 886–889
    structural abnormalities
        ductal system, 870–871
        external genitalia, 871
Ferritin, 1000
Fetal akinesia deformation sequence, 124
Fetal akinesia-hypokinesia deformation (FAD) sequence, 1303–1304
Fetal alcohol syndrome (FAS), 108
Fetal growth
    adrenal (combined) weight, 1415t
    from age 1 to 12 months
        recumbent length, 1407t
        weights, 1406t
    body length and organ weights, 1418t
    brain weight, 1419t
    characteristics
        early, 1389t
        late, 1389t
    expected linear measurements, 1391t
    expected weights, 1390t
    female
        adrenal (combined) weight, 1415t
        birth weight, 1394t–1395t
        HC percentiles, 1394t–1395t
        head circumference, 1416t
        heart weight, 1408t, 1420t
        kidney (combined) weight, 1412t, 1423t–1424t
        length, 1394t–1395t
        liver weight, 1410t, 1422t
        lung weight, 1409t, 1420t–1421t
        pancreas weight, 1413t
        spleen weight, 1411t, 1423t
        thymus weight, 1414t
    gyral pattern
        perinatal brain, 1427t
        petal brain, 1426t
    head circumference, 1415t, 1416t
    heart weight, 1408t, 1420t
    kidney (combined) weight, 1412t, 1423t–1424t
    liver weight, 1410t, 1422t
    lung weight, 1409t, 1420t–1421t
    male
        adrenal (combined) weight, 1415t
        birth weight, 1396t–1397t
        HC percentiles, 1396t–1397t
        head circumference, 1415t
        heart weight, 1408t, 1420t
        kidney (combined) weight, 1412t, 1423t–1424t
        length, 1396t–1397t
        liver weight, 1410t, 1422t
        lung weight, 1409t, 1420t–1421t
        pancreas weight, 1413t
        spleen weight, 1411t, 1423t
        thymus weight, 1414t
    organ weights
        from birth to 12 years of age, 1417t
        vs. body length from 31 to 170 cm, 1418t
        from 24 to 44 weeks of menstrual age, 1394t
    pancreas weight, 1413t
    penile length
        by age, 1425t
        by menstrual age, 1425t
    recumbent length, 1407t
    spleen weight, 1411t, 1423t
    thymus weight, 1414t
    weights
        from age 1 to 12 months, 1406t
        organ, 1394t
Fetal hemorrhage, 348
Fetal lung interstitial tumor (FLIT), 500, 500f
Fetal/neonatal deaths, 284–285
Fetal nucleated red blood cells, 345, 345f
Fetal rhabdomyoma, 1180, 1181f
Fetal surface. See Chorionic plate
Fetal thromboocclusive lesions, 337f
Fetal thrombotic vasculopathy (FTV), 336
Fetal vascular malperfusion, 336–337
    clinical correlation, 338
    pathology, 337–338
Fetal zone, 980
Fetomaternal hemorrhage (FMH), 345, 346f
    clinical correlation, 346
    pathology, 345–346
Fetoplacental vasculature, 333
Fibroadenomas (FA), 929–930
    benign phyllodes tumor, 931f
    cellular/juvenile type, 931f
    gelatinous cut surface, 930f
    hypercellular appearance, 931f
    with intracanalicular pattern, 929f
    intraductal papillary lesion, 931f
    papillary apocrine metaplasia, 931f
    with pericanalicular pattern, 930f
Fibroblastic and myofibroblastic tumors, soft tissue
    calcifying aponeurotic fibromatosis, 1152, 1152f
    calcifying fibrous pseudotumor, 1153
    CD34-positive spindle cell tumors, 1159, 1160
    of childhood, 1144
    congenital infantile fibrosarcoma, 1156–1157, 1156f, 1156t, 1157f
    dermatofibrosarcoma protuberans, 1158–1159, 1159f, 1160f
    dermatomyofibroma, 1149, 1149f
    desmoid-type fibromatosis, 1149–1151, 1150f, 1151f
    fibromatosis colli, 1153
    fibrosarcoma, 1155
    fibrous hamartoma of infancy, 1147–1148, 1148f
    gardner-nuchal fibroma, 1151
    inclusion body fibromatosis, 1148, 1148f, 1149
    infantile fibromatosis, 1146
    infantile myofibroma, 1144, 1144f–1145f
    infantile subcutaneous fibromatosis, 1146, 1147, 1147f
    inflammatory myofibroblastic tumor, 1153–1155, 1153t, 1154f
    juvenile hyaline fibromatosis, 1151–1152, 1151f
    juvenile nasopharyngeal angiofibroma, 1152, 1153
    low-grade fibromyxoid sarcoma, 1157–1158, 1157f–1158f
    low-grade myofibroblastic sarcoma, 1155
    myositis ossificans, 1141, 1143, 1143f
    myxoinflammatory fibroblastic sarcoma, 1155, 1155f
    nodular fasciitis, 1140, 1141t, 1142f
    palmar–plantar fibromatosis, 1151
    sclerosing epithelioid fibrosarcoma, 1158
    solitary fibrous, 1146, 1147f
Fibroepithelial neoplasms, breast, 929–932
Fibroepithelial polyp, 878, 922
Fibrohistiocytic tumors
    angiomatoid fibrous histiocytoma, 1163, 1164f
    benign cutaneous fibrous histiocytoma, 1161, 1162f
    blastic plasmacytoid DC neoplasm, 1166
    dendritic cell neoplasms, 1165
    dermatofibroma, 1161, 1161f
    diffuse-type giant cell tumor, 1161, 1163
    juvenile xanthogranuloma, 1165–1166, 1165f
    pigmented villonodular synovitis, 1161, 1163f
    plexiform fibrohistiocytic tumor, 1163, 1164f
    tenosynovial giant cell tumor, 1161, 1162f
    WHO classification of, 1160
Fibrolamellar HCC, 743–744, 743f
Fibroma, desmoplastic, 1032, 1032f
Fibromatosis colli, 1153
Fibromuscular dysplasia, 567
Fibrosarcoma (FS), 1155, 1354
Fibrosing colonopathy, 600
Fibrosis, 772, 953
Fibrous dysplasia, 1333–1336, 1334f–1336f
Fibrous hamartoma of infancy (FHI), 1147–1148, 1148f
Fibrous spindle cell tumors
    adamantinoma, 1354, 1354f
    central odontogenic fibroma, 1352
    congenital pseudoarthrosis, 1353–1354
    desmoplastic fibroma, 1351–1353
    fibrosarcoma, 1354
    myofibroma, 1353, 1353f
    myofibrosarcoma, 1354
    nonossifying fibroma, 1351, 1351f–1352f
Fibrous tumors, 939–941, 940f

Fine-needle aspiration (FNA), 18–20
    accuracy and sensitivity of, 20
    advantages, 18, 19t
    complications, 18
    control of patient for, 18–19
        papoose wrap, 19
    electron microscopic examination of, 55, 56f
    equipment for, 18, 19t
    indications, 18, 19t
    pitfalls in the diagnosis of lesions, 19–20
    technique of, 18, 19t
Fine-needle aspiration biopsy (FNAB), 968, 1216
First trimester spontaneous abortion, 62–67
    examination
        amnion, 62
        chorionic villi, 62
        complete hydatidiform mole, 66–67, 67f
        early pregnancy loss, 62
        embryo, normal development, 62–63, 63f
        growth-disorganized embryo, 63–64, 63f–64f
        GTN, 66
        histological findings, 65
        intervillositis, 65–66, 66f
        isolated/focal abnormalities, 63–65, 64f
        listeriosis, 65, 66, 66f
        partial hydatidiform mole, 66
        p57kip2 and p57 staining, 67
        placental tissues and decidua, 65–66
        products of conception, 62
        triploid embryo, 65, 65f, 66
        trisomy 13, 64–65, 65f
        trisomy 16, 61
        trisomy 22, 61
        viral and bacterial infections, 65, 66
    indication, cytogenetic analysis
        chromosome abnormality, 62
        IVF and ICSI, 62
        karyotype, 62
        morphological abnormalities, 62
Flexner-Wintersteiner rosettes, 431, 431f, 433
Floppy mitral valve (FMV), 538
Flow cytometry, 21–24, 1058
    applications of, 23–24
    basis of methodology in, 21–22
    method, 22–23
Fluorescein angiography, retinoblastoma, 430
Fluorescence *in situ* hybridization (FISH), 31–33, 32f, 33f, 381
    advantages, 31
    applications of, 31–33
    basis of methodology of, 31, 31f
Fluorescent-conjugated antibody technique, 875
FMH. *See* Fetomaternal hemorrhage
FNAB. *See* Fine-needle aspiration biopsy
Focal cortical dysplasia (FCD), 364–365, 377
Focal dermal hypoplasia, 1219, 1221
Focal hyperinsulinism, 787t, 788–791, 790f
Focal myositis (FM), 1180, 1181, 1182f

Focal nodular hyperplasia, liver
    age distribution, 713, 713f
    clinical features, 714–715
    gross appearance, 713f, 715
    histopathology, 714f, 715–716
    molecular pathology, 716
    pathogenesis, 713–714, 715t
    treatment, 715
Focal opacities, 429
Focal segmental glomerulosclerosis, 821
Follicular adenoma, 976–977
Follicular cyst, 877, 1040–1042, 1041f
Follicular hyperplasia
    lymph nodes
        Castleman disease, 1063, 1063f
        HIV-related adenopathy, 1061–1062, 1062f
        nonspecific reactive follicular hyperplasia, 1061
        progressive transformation of germinal centers, 1062, 1062f
        toxoplasmosis, 1062, 1062f
    spleen, 1081
Follicular neoplasms of thyroid, 976
Follicular thyroid carcinoma (FTC), 976–977, 976f
Folliculitis, skin, 1238
Folliculostellate cell, 950
Foramen ovale, premature closure of, 529
Forbes disease, 164, 675
Forebrain development disorders, 359–360
Forensic pathology
    autopsy
        algor mortis, 261
        chemistry, 263–264
        cultures, 264
        decomposition, 262
        livor mortis, 261, 262f
        maceration, 262, 262f
        metabolic analysis, 263
        mummification, 262
        odontology and anthropology, 264
        photography, 263
        putrefaction, 262
        radiology, 263
        rigor mortis, 261
        scene investigation, 264–265, 265f
        toxicology, 263
    cause of death, 260
    manner of death, 260
    medicolegal death, 260
    mimics
        abusive head trauma, 279–282, 279f–282f
        accidental blunt impact injuries, 278
        burns, 285, 285f–287f
        cardiopulmonary resuscitation, 278
        Danlos syndrome, 276
        factitious disorder, 285–287
        fetal/neonatal deaths, 284–285
        glutaric aciduria type I, 278
        gunshot wounds, 288–289
        impetigo contagiosa, 276, 277f
        Mongolian spots, 276, 277f
        neglect, 282–284, 283f
        osteogenesis imperfecta, 277
        rickets, 277–278

        shaken baby syndrome, 279–282, 279f–282f
        sharp force injuries, 287–288, 287f–288f
        staphylococcal scalded skin syndrome, 276
    polymerase chain reaction in, 47
    sudden death
        asphyxia, 268–270, 268f–226f
        blunt force injuries, 270–276, 270f–276f
        nonaccidental and accidental injuries, 270
        SIDS, 266–267
        SUID, 267–268, 267f
Fournier disease, 922
Fovea centralis, 428
Frasier syndrome, 904
Friedreich ataxia (FA), 375f, 556
Frozen tissue, electron microscopic examination of, 55, 55f
Fructosemia, 673
FTC. *See* Follicular thyroid carcinoma
FTV. *See* Fetal thrombotic vasculopathy
Fukuyama congenital muscular dystrophy (FCMD), 363, 1289
Fulminant hepatic failure, 701–702, 702f, 703f
Fungal infections
    in adrenal gland, 991
    aspergillosis, 249
    blastomycosis, 248
    candidiasis, 247, 247f
    CNS, 401
    Coccidioides immitis, 248, 249f
    Cryptococcus neoformans, 248, 249
    GI tract
        Aspergillus, 615
        Candida, 614
        Histoplasma capsulatum, 615
        zygomycosis, 615
    histoplasmosis, 248, 248f
    skin, 1233, 1233f, 1234f
    zygomycosis, 250

G

Galactocele, 932
Galactosemia, 162, 424, 673
Gallbladder disorders, 754–755, 754f, 755f
Gangliocytomas, 393, 958
Ganglioglioma (GG), 393–394, 393f
Ganglioneuroblastoma (GNB)
    intermixed subtype, 1002, 1002f, 1003, 1003f, 1006
    nodular, 1003–1004, 1004f
Ganglioneuroma, 1003, 1003f
Gangliosidoses, 554–555, 681
    sphingolipidoses, 144, 145
Gardner-nuchal fibroma, 1151
Gardner's syndrome, 955t, 1032
Gartner duct cysts, 876
Gas gangrene, 240
Gastritis, 589
Gastroenteritis and postenteritis enteropathy, 624–625
Gastroesophageal reflux disease (GERD), 584–585, 584f, 584t

Gastrointestinal stromal tumor (GIST), 592–593, 593f, 1179–1180
Gastrointestinal tract
  anal disorders
    acquired diseases, 648–649
    congenital abnormalities, 648, 648f
    perianal abscess and anal fistula, 649
  appendix
    acute appendicitis, 644–645
    anatomy and histology, 644
    appendiceal neuroendocrine (carcinoid) tumors, 647–648, 647f
    congenital and neuromuscular disorders, 644
    cystic fibrosis, 646–647, 647f
    interval appendectomy, 645
    mucosal melanosis, 646
    unusual infections, 645–646
  colitis
    acute self-limited colitis, 629–630
    allergic colitis (allergic proctocolitis), 636, 637f
    collagenous, 634
    Crohn disease, 632–633
    diversion, 635
    indeterminate, 633–634
    inflammatory bowel disease, 629
    lymphocytic, 634
    neonatal necrotizing enterocolitis, 635–636
    pseudomembranous, 634, 634f
    solitary rectal ulcer syndrome, 636–637
    spontaneous perforation, 636
    typhlitis (neutropenic enterocolitis), 635
    ulcerative colitis, 630–632
  embryology, 581, 582f, 583f
  esophagus disorders
    acquired diseases, 584–588
    congenital abnormalities, 581–584
  Hirschsprung disease, 600–604
    acquired diseases, 606–607
    chronic intestinal pseudo-obstruction, 604–606
  immunodeficiency, manifestations of
    graft versus host disease, 627–628
    Henoch-Schönlein purpura, 628–629, 629f
    pediatric HIV infection, 627
    primary immunodeficiencies, 626–627
  infections, 607t–608t
    bacterial diarrhea, 610–613
    fungal disease, 614–615
    protozoal infections, 613–614
    viral diarrhea, 609–610
  intestinal neoplasms, 638t
    adenomatous polyps and adenocarcinoma, 641–642, 642f
    juvenile polyps and juvenile polyposis syndrome, 637, 638f–640f, 639
    nonepithelial gastrointestinal tumors, 642–644
    Peutz-Jeghers polyposis syndrome, 640–641
    PTEN hamartoma tumor syndrome, 640

  malabsorption, 615–617
    autoimmune enteropathy, 620
    celiac disease (gluten-sensitive enteropathy (GSE)), 620–623
    congenital defects, intestinal epithelial differentiation, 617–620
    congenital transport and enzymatic disorders, 616–617
    eosinophilic gastroenteritis, 623–624
    gastroenteritis and postenteritis enteropathy, 624–625
    intestinal biopsy in children, 616
    intestinal lymphangiectasia, 624
    malnutrition, 625
    short bowel syndrome and bacterial overgrowth, 625
  small and large intestine disorders
    congenital abnormalities, 594–599
    gastrointestinal involvement, cystic fibrosis, 600
    meconium and meconium abnormalities, 599–600
  stomach disorders
    acquired diseases, 589–591
    congenital anomalies, 588–589
    Crohn disease, 592
    gastrointestinal stromal tumors, 592–593, 593f
    granulomatous gastritis, 591–592
    Ménétrier disease, 591
    peptic ulcer disease, 591
    polyps and tumors, 592, 594f
Gastroschisis, 594, 594f
Gastrospirillum hominis. See *Helicobacter heilmannii* gastritis
Gaucher disease (GD), 142, 143f, 682, 683f, 1079, 1319–1320, 1368
G-banding, 77, 79
GB virus C. See Hepatitis G virus (HGV)
Gene expression arrays, 47
Generalized arterial calcification of infancy (GACI), 567
Generalized glycogenosis, 675
Genetic diseases, lens opacities in, 424
Genetic skeletal disorders (GSD). See Skeletal dysplasia
Genital differentiation disorder, 897–900
Germ cell neoplasms, 510
Germ cell tumors (GCT), 392, 948. See also Mixed germ cell tumor (MGCT)
  ovaries
    dysgerminoma, 882–883, 883f
    gliomatosis peritonei, 882, 883f
    gonadoblastoma, 885–886, 885f, 886f
    hematologic malignancies associated with, 886
    histologic types of, 884–885
    immature teratoma, 881–882, 882f
    mature teratoma, 880–881, 881f
    serologic markers, 886, 886f
    yolk sac tumor, 883–884, 883f, 884f
  relative risk, 896
  staging, 907t
  XX male and XY female syndrome, 906
    embryonal carcinoma, 911, 912f
    epidermoid cyst, 910–911, 910f

    intratubular germ cell neoplasia, unclassified type, 911, 912f
    mixed germ cell tumor, 912–913
    seminoma, 911–912
    teratoma, 908–910, 909f
    yolk sac tumor, 907–908, 908f
Germinal matrix hemorrhage (GMH), 404, 405, 405f
Gestational age (GA) and mean organ weights, 1392t–1393t
Gestational sac, 326f
Gestational trophoblastic disease, 328–329, 330
Gestational trophoblastic neoplasia (GTN), 62, 66
Giant cell lesion of jaw, 1027–1028, 1028f
Giant-cell reparative granuloma (GCRG), 1346, 1347f
Giant-cell tumor (GCT), 1345–1346, 1345f–1346f
Giardia lamblia (Intestinalis), 613
Gingival granular cell tumor of infancy, 1027, 1027f
Glaucoma, 411, 422–423
  congenital, 423
  surgical treatment, 423
Glial fibrillary acid protein (GFAP), 26–27, 352, 431
Glial heterotopia, 1025
Gli 2 mutation, 951, 952t
Gli3 mutation, 952t
Gliomas, 948
  less common, 386–387
  pilocytic astrocytomas, 382–383
Gliomatosis peritonei, 882, 883f
Glioneuronal heterotopia, 1177
Glioneuronal tumors, 393–395
Gliosis, 351
Glomangioma, 1140, 1140f
Glomerular diseases
  causes, 816–817, 817f, 817t
  glomerulonephritis
    crescentic, 833–834
    membranoproliferative, 831–833, 832f
    postinfectious, 830–831, 831f
  with hematuria with/without proteinuria
    Alport syndrome, 827–829, 828f
    Henoch-Schönlein purpura nephritis, 827
    IgA nephropathy, 825–827
    loin pain hematuria syndrome, 830
    thin glomerular basement membrane disease, 829
  lupus nephritis, 833, 833f
  with proteinuria/nephrotic syndrome
    collagen type III glomerulopathy, 825
    complications, 820
    diabetic nephropathy, 822–823, 823f
    focal segmental glomerulosclerosis, 821
    incidence, 818
    membranous glomerulonephritis, 821–822, 822f
    minimal change disease, 820–821
    nail-patella syndrome, 825
    nephrotic syndrome, first year of life, 823–825, 824f
    Pierson syndrome, 825

Glomerulonephritis
    crescentic, 833–834
    membranoproliferative, 831–833, 832f
    postinfectious, 830–831, 831f
Glomus tumor, 1138
Glutamate dehydrogenase mutations, 791
Glutaric acidemia
    type I, 179
    type II, 168
Glutaric aciduria type I, 278
Gluten-sensitive enteropathy (GSE).
        See Celiac disease
Glycine encephalopathy, 161–162
Glycogen branching enzyme disease, 675–676
Glycogen storage diseases (GSD), 139,
        163–164, 163t, 165f–166f, 166, 554
    myopathy, 1275–1278, 1276t, 1277f
    type I, 674–675
    type II, 675
    type III, 675
    type IV, 675, 676f
    type IX, 676–677
    type VI, 676
    type VIII, 676
    type X, 676–677
    type XI, 676–677
Glycoprotein degradation disorders
    alpha-mannosidosis, 149
    aspartylglycosaminuria, 150
    beta-mannosidosis, 149
    fucosidosis, 149–150, 150f
    sialidosis, 150
GM2 gangliosidosis, 145
    activator protein deficiency, 145, 145f
    type 1, 145
    type 2, 145
GNB. See Ganglioneuroblastoma
Goblet cells, 414f
Goiter, simple/colloid, 971
Gonadal development, 866, 866f
Gonadal dysgenesis, 866, 872
    tumors associated with, 873
Gonadal neoplasms, 903
Gonadoblastoma
    feature, 885
    nodules of, 885f, 886f
    pathology, 873
    sex reversal, 916–917, 918f
    TSPY protein, 886
Gorham-Stout disease, 1351
Gorlin-Goltz syndromes, 413. See also basal
        cell nevus syndrome
Graft versus host disease (GVHD), 627–628
    skin, 1239–1240, 1240f
Granular cell tumor (GCT), 938, 939f,
        1176–1177, 1176f, 1177f, 1177t
Granular corneal dystrophy, 420
Granular ependymitis, 353
Granulation tissue reaction, 411
Granulocytes, hematopoietic syndromes,
        1102, 1102t
Granuloma
    annulare, 1235, 1235f
    inguinale, 875
    periapical cyst and, 1043–1044, 1043f
Granulomatous cystitis, 855
Granulomatous gastritis, 591–592

Granulomatous hepatitis, 707, 707t
Granulomatous hypophysitis, 953
Granulomatous inflammation, 427
Granulomatous synovitis, 1368
Granulopoiesis, 1094–1095, 1094f
Graves disease, 971–972, 972f
Growth-disorganized embryo, 62–63
    categories, 62–63
    cylindrical embryo, 63, 63f
    delayed organ development, 63, 64f
    incidence, 63
    intact empty sac, 63, 63f
    nodular embryo, 63, 63f
    ultrasound examination, 63–64
Growth hormone–secreting tumors, 954
Growth-promoting factors, 328
Gunshot wounds, 288–289
Gynecomastia, 934–935, 935f, 935t

H

Haemophilus ducreyi, 875
Haemophilus influenzae infection, 232, 232f
Hailey-Hailey disease, 876
Hallermann-Streiff syndrome, 128
Hallervorden-Spatz disease (HSD), 374, 375f
Halo nevus, 1245
Hamartoma, 941, 941f
    chest wall, 1341–1342, 1342f
    spleen, 1077–1078
Hand-Schüller-Christian disease, 436
HARP syndrome, 374
Hashimoto thyroiditis, 970
HCP. See Hydrocephalus
Headaches and pituitary adenoma, 954
Heart segments, 526t
Heart transplant pathology
    biopsy findings, 316, 317, 317f
    complications, 316
    infection, 316
    outcome, 317
    rejection, 314, 314t, 315f–317f
    surgical complications, 314
    volumes and indications, 314
Helicobacter heilmannii gastritis,
        590–591, 591f
Helicobacter pylori gastritis, 589–590, 590f
Hemangiomas, 411f, 725, 921, 1080–1081
Hematologic disorders
    constitutional, 1099, 1099t, 1100t
    neonate and infants, 1097t, 1098–1099
    ovarian germ cell tumors, 886
Hematolymphoid disorders, 503–504, 1004
Hematolymphoid neoplasms, 941–943
Hematopoiesis
    age-related physiologic variations, 1096,
        1097t, 1098
    constitutional disorders, 1099,
        1099t, 1100t
    erythropoiesis, 1095, 1095f
    features, 1093t
    granulopoiesis, 1094–1095, 1094f
    inherited and congenital, granulocytes,
        1102, 1102t
    lymphopoiesis, 1096
    malignancies
        flow cytometry in diagnosis of, 21–22
        polymerase chain reaction in diagnosis, 37

        megakaryocytopoiesis, 1094
        monopoiesis and dendritic cell
            development, 1095–1096
        natural killer cells development, 1095
    stem cells, 1093–1094, 1094f
Hematopoietic origin, tumors of, 917–918
Hematopoietic stem cell transplantation
        (HSCT)
    bone marrow, 1118
    pulmonary complications after, 321
Hematuria with/without proteinuria.
        See Glomerular diseases
Hemochromatosis, neonatal, 772, 773f
Hemophagocytic lymphohistiocytosis (HLH),
        1069
Hemophilic arthropathy, 1368
Hemorrhage, 355, 440, 440f
    adrenal cyst, 981f
    cystitis, 855–856
    epidural, 356
    and erosive gastritis, 589
    maternal arterial, 346
Henoch-Schönlein purpura, 628–629, 629f,
        920, 1237, 1238f
    nephritis, 827
Hepatic hemorrhage, 709
Hepatic steatosis and steatohepatitis, 692–694
Hepatic tumors, 712, 712t, 713t
Hepatitis A virus (HAV), 695–696, 696t
Hepatitis B virus (HBV), 697
Hepatitis C virus (HCV), 697
Hepatitis D virus (HDV), 697
Hepatitis E virus (HEV), 697–698
Hepatitis G virus (HGV), 698
Hepatobiliary morphogenesis, 654
Hepatoblastoma (HB), 494
    age distribution, 729, 730f
    clinical features, 731–732
    cytogenetic findings in, 739t
    fetal
        cholangioblastic HB, 737
        crowded fetal/fetal with mitoses HB,
            735–736
        embryonal HB, 736
        epithelial HB, 737
        macrotrabecular HB, 737
        mixed epithelial and mesenchymal
            HB, 737
        pleomorphic/anaplastic fetal/epithelial
            HB, 736
        small-cell undifferentiated HB,
            736–737
        teratoid HB, 737–738, 738f
        well-differentiated, 734f, 735
    gross appearance, 734–735, 734f
    histopathology, 735, 735t
    imaging, 731–732
    laboratory studies, 731–732
    molecular pathology, 738–740
    pathogenesis, 730–731
    prevalence, 729
    staging, 732–733, 732t
    treatment and outcomes, 733–734
Hepatocellular adenoma
    clinical features, 720
    gross pathology, 720
    histopathology, 719f, 720–721

Leukocoria, 429, 430f
Leukodystrophies, 369, 370f
Leydig cell
    deficiency, 899
    tumor, 913–914, 913f
Lhermitte-Duclos disease, 395
Lhx3 mutation, 951, 952t
Lhx4 mutation, 951, 952t
Lichen sclerosus, 876
Li-Fraumeni syndrome, 390t, 955t
Ligneous conjunctivitis, 416
Limbal dermoid, 415, 415f
Limb–body wall complex (LBWC), 73–74, 74f
Limb-girdle muscular dystrophies (LGMD), 1285–1286
Limb–mammary syndrome, 928
Limb reduction deficiency
    amelia, 1302
    anatomy, 1300 1301t
    caudal regression syndrome, 1302–1303, 1302f
    congenital radial–tibial deficiency, 1301
    etiopathogeneses, 1300
    lower limb deficiencies, 1301–1302, 1302f
    morphology, 1300
    patellar aplasia and hypoplasia, 1302
    sirenomelia, 1302
    split hand-foot limb defect, 1302
    transverse limb defects, 1301, 1301t
Limit dextrinosis, 675
Linear IgA bullous dermatosis, 1222–1223, 1223f
Lingual thyroid, 967, 968f
Lipid metabolism disorders, 184–186
    CHILD syndrome, 185–186
    Conradi-Hunermann syndrome, 184–185
    Smith-Lemli-Opitz syndrome, 184–185, 185f
Lipidoses, 154–155, 155f, 678, 679t
Lipid transport disorders, 617
Lipoblastoma (LPB), 1168, 1168f, 1168t, 1169f
Lipogranulomatous reaction, 411, 412
Lipomas, 1167–1168, 1167f
Lipomatosis, 772
Lipomatous lesion of heart, 1170
Lipomatous tumors, 116t, 939, 1166
Liposarcoma (LPS), 1169, 1170f, 1170t
Lissencephaly (LIS), types I and II, 362–363, 363f
Listeriosis
    first trimester abortion, 65–66, 66f
    infections, 234, 234f
    second trimester abortion, 68, 68f–69f
Littoral cell angiomas, spleen, 1081
Live-born infants, weights and measurements
    body weight, 1404t–1405t
    gestational age, 1402t–1403t
Liver
    abscesses, 706
    angiosarcoma, 751–752, 751f–752f
    biliary and hepatic ducts, anatomic anomalies and disorders, 669–670
    cirrhosis, 710–711, 711t, 712f
    congenital anomalies, 655–656, 655f–656f
    congenital hepatic fibrosis, 670–673
    development, 654
    embryonal rhabdomyosarcoma, biliary tract, 750–751, 750f
    endodermal sinus (yolk sac) tumor, 752, 753f–754f, 754
    extrahepatic biliary atresia, 659–664
    focal nodular hyperplasia
        age distribution, 713, 713f
        clinical features, 714–715
        gross appearance, 713f, 715
        histopathology, 714f, 715–716
        molecular pathology, 716
        pathogenesis, 713–714, 715t
        treatment, 715
    fulminant hepatic failure, 701–702, 702f, 703f
    gallbladder, 754–755, 754f, 755f
    granulomatous hepatitis, 707, 707t
    hepatic tumors, 712, 712t, 713t
    hepatoblastoma, 729–740
        (*See also* Hepatoblastoma)
    hepatocellular adenoma
        clinical features, 720
        gross pathology, 720
        histopathology, 719f, 720–721
        imaging features, 720
        laboratory features, 720
        molecular pathology, 721–722
        outcomes, 720
        pathogenesis, 719–720
        treatment, 720
    hepatocellular carcinoma, 740–744
    hereditary hyperbilirubinemias, 657–658
    histology, 654–655, 655f
    idiopathic neonatal hepatitis, 658–659
    lymphoma, 752, 753f–754f, 754
    malignant rhabdoid tumor, 752, 753f–754f, 754
    mesenchymal hamartoma
        clinical features, 722–723, 723f
        gross appearance, 724
        histopathology, 723f, 724
        imaging, 722–723, 723f
        laboratory studies, 722–723, 723f
        molecular pathology, 725
        outcomes, 724
        pathogenesis, 722
        treatment, 724
    metabolic disorders
        alpha-1-antitrypsin deficiency, 684–686
        amino acid, 677–678
        bile acid, 682–684
        carbohydrate, 673–677
        cystic fibrosis, 686–687
        fatty acid oxidation, defects, 694–695, 694f
        hepatic steatosis and steatohepatitis, 692–694
        iron storage disease, 687–689
        lysosomal storage, 678–682
        mitochondrial DNA depletion syndromes, 695
        porphyrias, 691
        Reye syndrome, 694
        urea cycle disorders, 691–692
        Wilson disease, 689–691
    nested stromal epithelial tumor, 748–749, 749f
    nodular regenerative hyperplasia
        clinical features, 717
        diagnosis, 717–718
        management, 717–718
        pathogenesis, 716–717, 717t
        pathology, 718–719
    parasitic diseases, 706–707
    persistent intrahepatic cholestasis, 664–669
    physiologic jaundice, 657, 658t
    primary sclerosing cholangitis and autoimmune hepatitis, 704–706
    teratoma, 729
    tissue triaging, 656–657, 657f
    total parenteral nutrition–related injury, 709–710
    transplant pathology
        acute cellular rejection, 300–301, 300f
        antibody-mediated rejection, 299–300
        biliary complications, 299
        in bone marrow transplantation, 304–305, 305f
        chronic rejection, 301–302, 301f
        complications, 298, 298t
        de novo and recurrent autoimmune hepatitis, 302, 302f
        hepatic artery thrombosis, 298, 299
        idiopathic posttransplantation chronic hepatitis, 303
        indications, 297t
        posttransplant opportunistic infections, 303–304, 304f
        preservation injury, 298, 299, 299f
        recurrent hepatitis C or B, 302–303
    undifferentiated embryonal sarcoma, 744–748
    vascular disorders
        Budd-Chiari syndrome, 707–708, 708f
        cavernous transformation, portal vein, 707
        hepatic hemorrhage, 709
        peliosis hepatis, 708–709, 709f
        venoocclusive disease, 708, 708f
    vascular tumors in children
        congenital hemangioma, 725
        hemangiomas, 725
        infantile hemangioma (IH), 725–729
    viral hepatitis
        hepatitis A, 695–696, 696t
        hepatitis B, 697
        hepatitis C, 697
        hepatitis D, 697
        hepatitis E, 697–698
        hepatitis G, 698
        pathology, 698–701, 698f–699f, 701t
Lobular capillary hemangioma–pyogenic granuloma, 1136, 1136f
Local myositis, 1290
Loeys-Dietz syndrome, 568
Loin pain hematuria syndrome, 830
Long-chain 3-hydroxyacyl-CoA dehydrogenase (LCHAD) deficiency, 168, 341
Long QT syndrome, 561t
Low- and high-grade malignant phyllodes tumor, 935–936, 936f, 937f
Lowe syndrome, 127
Low-grade fibromyxoid sarcoma (LGFS), 1155, 1157–1158, 1157f–1158f
LSDs. *See* Lysosomal storage diseases (LSDs)

Lumbosacral myelomeningocele, 358f
Lung disorders
    abnormal lobation, location, and shape, 457–458
    abscess, 487
    agenesis, 457
    alveolar proteinosis, 488
    aspiration, 483–484, 484f, 484t
    bronchiectasis, 485–487
    bronchiolitis obliterans, 494
    bronchopulmonary dysplasia, 475–478, 476f, 477f
    congenital alveolar capillary dysplasia, 472
    congenital pulmonary airway malformation, 466–472, 467f–472f
    congenital pulmonary lymphangiectasis, 465–466, 466f
    development, 444–447, 444t
        acinar or canalicular period, 444t, 445, 446f
        alveolar period, 444t, 447, 447f
        embryonic periods, 444, 444t, 445f
        pseudoglandular period, 444, 444t, 446f
        saccular period, 444t, 446, 447f
    diaphragm, 512–514
    eosinophilic pneumonia, 491–492
    extracorporeal membrane oxygenation, 485, 485f
    hemorrhage, 487
    hemosiderosis, 488–490
    herniation, 458
    hypoplasia, 462–464, 463f, 463t
    infantile (congenital) lobar emphysema (over inflation), 464–465, 464t, 465f
    infectious diseases
        adenovirus, 491
        human metapneumovirus, 491
        legionella pneumonia, 491
        pertussis, 491, 492f
        respiratory syncytial virus, 490–491, 490f
    interstitial lung diseases, 492–494
    interstitial pulmonary emphysema, 481–483
    peripheral cysts of, 472
    sequestration, 458–462
        extralobar, 458–459, 458f–459f
        intralobar, 460–462, 460f, 461f
        total, pulmonary hyperplasia, 460, 460f
    surfactant dysfunction disorders, 478
    transplant pathology
        acute rejection, 318–319, 319f
        airway anastomotic complications, 318
        antibody-mediated rejection, 318
        chronic rejection, 319–320, 320f
        infections, 320, 320f, 321f
        primary graft dysfunction, 318
        rejection, 318, 318t
        vascular complications, 318
        volumes and indications, 317–318
    tumors
        epithelial neoplasms, 504–506
        hematolymphoid and histiocytic disorders, 503–504
        metastatic disease, 494
        miscellaneous disorders, 510
        primary carcinomas, 507–510
        primary neoplasms, 494–503
        veno-occlusive disease, 488
Lung injury, transplant pathology, 321
Lupus nephritis, 833, 833f
Lyme disease
    clinical features, 238–239
    coinfections associated with, 239
    laboratory diagnosis, 239
    pathology, 239
    prognosis and outcomes, 239
    Tick-borne lymphadenopathy, 239
    transmission, 238
Lymphadenopathy
    clinical significance, in children, 1057–1058
    dermatopathic, 1068–1069, 1068f
    diagnostic approach, 1058, 1059t
    reactive, 1061, 1061t
    sinus histiocytosis, 1067–1068, 1067f–1068f
Lymphangioma, 437, 1080–1081
Lymphangiomatosis, 503
Lymphangiomyomatosis (LAM), 503
Lymphatic channels, 414
Lymphatic malformation, 770, 1137, 1138f
Lymph nodes
    anatomy, 1057, 1058f
    cytogenetic studies, 1058, 1060–1061, 1060t
    enlargement, 1069, 1070t
    follicular hyperplasia
        Castleman disease, 1063, 1063f
        HIV-related adenopathy, 1061–1062, 1062f
        nonspecific reactive follicular hyperplasia, 1061
        progressive transformation of germinal centers, 1062, 1062f
        toxoplasmosis, 1062, 1062f
    immunophenotypic studies, 1058, 1059t–1060t
    interfollicular granulomatous processes
        cat-scratch disease, 1066, 1066f
        chronic granulomatous disease, 1067
        with histiocytic proliferation (See Nongranulomatous proliferation)
        mycobacterial infections, 1066–1067
    interfollicular/paracortical reactions-immunoblastic
        autoimmune lymphoproliferative syndrome, 1065
        Epstein-Barr virus infection, 1063–1064, 1064f
        hypersensitivity-related lymphadenopathy, 1064
        juvenile rheumatoid arthritis, 1064
        Kawasaki disease, 1066
        Kikuchi-Fujimoto disease, 1065, 1065f
        non-EBV viral adenopathy, 1064
        systemic lupus erythematosus, 1065
    lymphadenopathy
        clinical significance, in children, 1057–1058
        diagnostic approach, 1058, 1059t
        reactive, 1061, 1061t
    malignant lymphadenopathy
        ALK-positive ALCL, 1072–1073, 1073f
        B-cell lymphoblastic lymphoma, 1070, 1071f
        B-cell lymphoma, 1071–1072
        Burkitt lymphoma, 1071, 1072t
        diffuse large B-cell lymphoma, 1071
        Hodgkin lymphoma, 1073–1075
        peripheral T-cell lymphomas, 1073
        T-cell lymphoblastic lymphoma, 1072
        tumors of monocyte/macrophage lineage, 1075
        WHO lymphoma classification, 1070t
    reactive, 1058f
    structure and function, 1057, 1058f
Lymphocyte-depleted Hodgkin lymphoma (LDHL), 1074
Lymphocyte–predominant Hodgkin lymphoma (LPHL), 1062
Lymphocytic colitis, 634
Lymphocytic hypophysitis, 953
Lymphocytic interstitial pneumonitis (LIP), 492, 503
Lymphoid hyperplasia, 1081–1082
Lymphoma
    anaplastic large cell, 1072–1073, 1073f
    B-cell, 1071–1072
    B-cell lymphoblastic, 1070, 1071f
    Burkitt, 1071, 1072t
    diffuse large B-cell lymphoma, 1071
    hematopoietic, 1251
    Hodgkin
        lymphocyte-depleted, 1074
        lymphocyte-rich classic, 1074
        mixed cellularity, 1074
        nodular lymphocyte–predominant, 1074–1075, 1075f
        nodular sclerosing, 1073, 1074, 1074f
    immunohistochemistry, 26
    liver, 752, 753f–754f, 754
    peripheral T-cell, 1073
    T-cell lymphoblastic, 1072
Lymphopoiesis, 1096
Lymphoproliferative disorders (LPDs), 503
Lysinuric protein intolerance (LPI), 177–178
Lysosomal storage diseases (LSDs), 139, 139t–140t, 368–369, 370t, 1318–1320, 1319f
    diagnosis, 141
    disorders of glycoprotein degradation, 149–150, 150f
    Fabry disease, 681
    Farber disease (Farber lipogranulomatosis), 680–681
    gangliosidoses, 681
    Gaucher disease, 1320
    glycogen storage disease, 150, 151f
    linked to defects in specific enzymes, 142–149, 143f–145f, 147f149f
    linked to nonenzymatic protein deficiencies, 155–157, 156f, 157f
    lipidoses, 154–155, 155f, 678, 679t
    metabolic disorders, 678–682
    metachromatic leukodystrophy, 680, 680f
    mucolipidoses, 678–679

mucopolysaccharidoses, 150–151, 152f–153f, 154, 154t, 681, 1319
myopathy, 158, 1275, 1275f–1276f
neuronal ceroid lipofuscinoses, 158, 159f, 159t
newborn screening, 136, 137–139, 137t, 138t
oligosaccharidoses (glycoproteinoses), 679–680
pathophysiology, 141
phenotype, 139–141
sphingolipidoses, 681–682, 682f, 683f
treatment, 142
X-linked vacuolar cardiomyopathy, 158

M

Maceration, second trimester abortion, 67, 70
MACIS (metastasis–age–completeness of resection–invasion–size) system, 976
Macroadenomas, 957
Macrodystrophia lipomatosa (MDL), 1167
Macrophagic myofasciitis, 1290
Macular corneal dystrophy, 420
Malabsorption, 615–617
    autoimmune enteropathy, 620, 621f
    causes, 615, 616t
    celiac disease (gluten-sensitive enteropathy (GSE)), 620–623
    congenital defects, intestinal epithelial differentiation
        congenital tufting enteropathy (CTE), 618, 619f
        enteroendocrine cell dysgenesis (enteric anendocrinosis), 619–620
        microvillus inclusion disease, 617–618, 619f
    congenital transport and enzymatic disorders, 616–617
    eosinophilic gastroenteritis, 623–624
    gastroenteritis and postenteritis enteropathy, 624–625
    intestinal biopsy in children, 616
    intestinal lymphangiectasia, 624
    lipid transport disorders, 617
    malnutrition, 625
    short bowel syndrome and bacterial overgrowth, 625
Malakoplakia, 855
Male pseudohermaphroditism, 898
Male reproductive system
    epididymis
        acquired abnormalities and lesions, 919–920
        congenital anomalies, 918–919
        developmental anomalies, 918–919
    paratesticular tissues
        acquired abnormalities and lesions, 919–920
        congenital anomalies, 918–919
        developmental anomalies, 918–919
        tumors of, 920–921
    spermatic cord
        acquired abnormalities and lesions, 919–920
        congenital anomalies, 918–919
        developmental anomalies, 918–919
    testis
        congenital anomalies, 894
        developmental anomalies, 894
        development and disorders, 894
        disorders of genital differentiation, 897–900
        disorders of sex development, 897
        disorders of sexual determination, 901–903
        end-organ defects, 900–901
    XX male and XY female syndrome
        acquired abnormalities and lesions, 904–906
        carcinoid tumor, 917
        defects in Wilms Tumor, 904
        germ cell tumors, 906–913
        gonadoblastoma, 916–917
        hematopoietic origin of tumors, 917–918
        neoplasms of testis, 906
        nephroblastoma, 917
        sex cord–stromal tumors, 913–196
Malformations of cortical development (MCD), 364–365
Malignant acquired medulloepitheliomas, 434
Malignant ectomesenchymoma, 1199, 1200f–1201f
Malignant histiocytosis, 1116–1117
Malignant hyperthermia (MH), 1282–1283, 1283f
Malignant lymphadenopathy
    ALK-positive ALCL, 1072–1073, 1073f
    B-cell lymphoblastic lymphoma, 1070, 1071f
    B-cell lymphoma, 1071–1072
    Burkitt lymphoma, 1071, 1072t
    diffuse large B-cell lymphoma, 1071
    Hodgkin lymphoma, 1073–1075
    lymph nodes, 1069, 1070t
    peripheral T-cell lymphomas, 1073
    T-cell lymphoblastic lymphoma, 1072
    tumors of monocyte/macrophage lineage, 1075
    WHO lymphoma classification, 1070t
Malignant mesothelioma, paratesticular region, 920
Malignant peripheral nerve sheath tumor, 1173–1175, 1174f–1175f
Malignant rhabdoid tumor (MRT), 752, 753f–754f, 754, 1196, 1197–1198, 1197t, 1198f
Malignant round cell neoplasm, 943, 943f
Malignant teratoma, 881
Malignant tumors, lower female genital tract
    rhabdomyosarcoma, 879
    yolk sac tumor, 879–880, 879f
Malnutrition, 625
Malrotation, small and large intestine disorders, 582f, 594–595, 595f
Mammary carcinoma, 936–937
Mandibulofacial dysostosis, 119
M-anisosplenia, 454
Map-dot-fingerprint (MDF) dystrophy, 420, 421f
Maple syrup urine disease (MSUD), 162
Marfan syndrome, 426, 568
Marginal sinus formation, 326

Massive choroidal invasion, 433
Massive ovarian edema, 878
Massive perivillous fibrin deposition/maternal floor infarction, 342f
Mass screening program, neuroblastoma, 1008–1011
Mast cell diseases, 1249, 1249f
Maternal arterial hemorrhages, 346
Maternal diabetes, 110, 110f, 111t
Maternal floor infarction/massive perivillous fibrin deposition (MFI/PVF), 341
Maternal vascular malperfusion, 334
    clinical correlation, 335–336
    pathology, 334–335, 335f–336f
matrix-producing and matrix-associated tumors, 1331–1336
Mature teratoma
    gross specimen of, 881f
    types, 880–881
Mayer-Rokitansky-Kuster-Hauser (MRKH) sequence, 871
McArdle disease, 166
McCune-Albright syndrome, 955t
MCD. See Malformations of cortical development
MCE. See Multicystic encephalopathy
MDF dystrophy. See Map-dot-fingerprint (MDF) dystrophy
Measles, 218–219, 400
    clinical features, 219, 220f
    pathology, 219, 220
    transmission, 219
Measles inclusion body encephalitis (MIBE), 400
MEC. See Mucoepidermoid carcinoma
Meckel diverticulum, 598–599, 599f
Meckel-Gruber syndrome, 359, 768–769, 816
Meckel syndrome, 122–123, 122f
Meconium and meconium abnormalities, 343, 344f
    clinical correlation, 345
    meconium ileus, 599
    meconium peritonitis, 599–600
    meconium plug, 600
    pathology, 344
Meconium aspiration syndrome (MAS), 484
Medium-chain acyl-CoA dehydrogenase deficiency (MCADD, MCAD), 168
Medullary cystic kidney disease, 814
Medullary sponge kidney, 813
Medullary thyroid carcinoma (MTC), 964–965, 974, 978f
    C-cell hyperplasia and, 977
    in children, 977
    immunohistochemical staining, 978
    MEN2 mutations, 966f
    pigmented variant, 977
    RET mutations, 972
    sporadic, 977
    syndromic, 979
    syndromic-associated, 977
    thyroidectomy, 978–979
Medulloblastomas, 387–389, 387f
Medulloblastoma with extensive nodularity (MBEN), 387
Medulloepithelioma, 427, 434

Megacystis-microcolon-intestinal hypoperistalsis syndrome (MMIHS), 605–606, 854
Megakaryocytic disorders, 1094, 1103–1104
Megalocornea, 419
Meibomian gland, 410, 411, 411f
Melanin granules, 428
Melanocyte-stimulating factor (MSH), 950
Melanocytic abnormalities, conjunctiva, 416–418
Melanocytic neoplasms
   malignant melanoma, 1246
   melanocytic nevi
      acquired melanocytic nevi, 1244
      blue nevi, 1245, 1245f, 1246
      Clark dysplastic nevus, 1245f
      congenital melanocytic nevi, 1243–1244, 1243f, 1244f
      congenital nevus and malignant melanoma, 1244
      halo nevus, 1245
      spitz nevus, 1244
Melanocytic nevi, 412
   acquired melanocytic nevi, 1244
   blue nevi, 1245, 1245f, 1246
   Clark dysplastic nevus, 1245f
   congenital melanocytic nevi, 1243–1244, 1243f, 1244f
   congenital nevus and malignant melanoma, 1244
   of conjunctiva, 416
   halo nevus, 1245
   spitz nevus, 1244
Melanocytosis, oculodermal, 413
Melanoma, conjunctiva, 417
Melanosis
   of conjunctiva, 416
   of episclera and scleral tissue, 416
   oculi, 417
Melanotic neuroectodermal tumor, 921
Melanotic neuroectodermal tumor of infancy (MNTI), 1033–1034, 1033f, 1358–1359, 1358f–1359f
Melanotic progonoma, 1033–1034, 1033f
Melatonin, 947
Melorheostosis, 1320
Membranoproliferative glomerulonephritis, 831–833, 832f
Membranous glomerulonephritis, 821–822, 822f
Ménétrier disease, 591
Meningioangiomatosis (MA), 406, 406f
Meningioma, optic nerve, 435
Meningitis, 355
Meningoceles, 359
Menkes disease, 568
Menkes syndrome, 127
MEN1 syndrome, 962
Mercury embryopathy, 108
Merosin, 1287–1288, 1288f
Mesenchymal chondrosarcoma (MCS), 1194–1195
Mesenchymal hamartoma
   clinical features, 722–723, 723f
   gross appearance, 724
   histopathology, 723f, 724
   imaging, 722–723, 723f
   laboratory studies, 722–723, 723f
   molecular pathology, 725

   outcomes, 724
   pathogenesis, 722
   treatment, 724
Mesenchymal neoplasms
   myofibroblastic/fibroblastic tumors
      congenital/infantile myofibromatosis, 1247, 1248f
      giant cell fibroblastoma, 1248, 1248f, 2149
      infantile digital fibromatosis, 1247, 1248, 1248f
   neurothekeoma, 1246–1247, 1247f
   vascular tumors, 1247
Mesenchyme, 927
Mesial temporal sclerosis (MTS), 377
Mesodermal stromal polyp, 878
Mesonephric duct, female embryo, 868, 869
Mesonephric papilloma, 878
Metabolic disorders
   acquired, 374
   alpha-1 antitrypsin deficiency, 684–686
   amino acid, 677–678, 678f
   bile acid, 682–684
   carbohydrate
      fructosemia, 673
      galactosemia, 673
      glycogen storage diseases, 673–677
   cystic fibrosis, 686–687
   fatty acid oxidation, defects, 694–695, 694f
   hepatic steatosis and steatohepatitis, 692–694
   iron storage disease
      alloimmune gestational hepatitis, 688–689, 689f
      secondary hemosiderosis, 687, 688f
   lysosomal storage
      Fabry disease, 681
      Farber disease (Farber lipogranulomatosis), 680–681
      gangliosidoses, 681
      lipidoses, 678, 679t
      metachromatic leukodystrophy, 680, 680f
      mucolipidoses, 678–679
      mucopolysaccharidoses, 681
      oligosaccharidoses (glycoproteinoses), 679–680
      sphingolipidoses, 681–682, 682f, 683f
   mitochondrial DNA depletion syndromes, 695
   porphyrias, 691
   Reye syndrome, 694
   urea cycle disorders, 691–692, 692f
   Wilson disease, 689–690, 690f–691f
Metabolic disruptions, 110
Metabolic dysplasia syndrome, 115, 115t
Metachromatic leukodystrophy (MLD), 371t, 680, 680f
   sphingolipidoses, 146, 148, 148f
Metanephric tumors, 851
Metaphyseal dysplasias, 1320
Metastasis, bone marrow, 1117–1118, 1117f
Metastatic disease, 494
Metastatic neoplasms, 941–943
Metastatic retinoblastoma (RB), 1360
2-Methylacyl-CoA racemase deficiency, 182
Methylmalonic acidemia, 179
MFI/PVF. *See* Maternal floor infarction/massive perivillous fibrin deposition

MGCT. *See* Mixed germ cell tumor
MGD. *See* Mixed gonadal dysgenesis
Micrencephaly, 365
Microarrays (gene chips), 47
Microbial infections, 415
Microcephaly, 365
Microcornea, 419
Microdysgenesis, 364
Microglia
   activated, 354f
   nodules of, 353
   perivascular, 353
   reactions of, 353
   resident, 353
Microphakia, 424
Microphthalmos, 419
Microvascular proliferation (MVP), 381
MIF. *See* Müllerian inhibiting factor
Mikulicz disease, SICCA syndrome, 1035–1036, 1036f
Minimal change disease (MCD), 820–821
Miscarriage, 330, 331f
   clinical correlation, 332
   pathology, 330, 332
Mitochondrial disorders, 169–170, 171t–174t, 174–175, 372–373, 372f
   age of onset, 170
   aspects, 170
   classification, 170, 174–175
   clinical presentations, 170
   diagnosis, 175
   genetics of, 170
   therapy of, 175
Mitochondrial DNA depletion syndrome, 175, 695
Mitochondrial electron transport chain disorders, 555–556
Mitochondrial encephalopathy with lactic acidosis and strokes (MELAS), 170, 372
Mitochondrial myopathy, 1279–1282, 1280f–1281f
Mitochondrial myopathy, epilepsy, lactic acidosis, and stroke like episodes (MELAS), 606
Mitochondrial myopathy, lactic acidosis, and "ragged red" muscle fibers (MELAR syndrome), 773
Mitochondrial neurogastrointestinal encephalomyopathy (MNGIE), 174–175, 606
Mitotic nondisjunction, 81–82
Mitral atresia, 538
Mitral stenosis, 537–538
Mitral valve malformations, 537–538, 537t
Mitral valve prolapse (MVP), 538
Mitral valve regurgitation (MVR), 538
Mixed germ cell tumor (MGCT), 912–913. *See also* Germ cell tumors (GCT)
Mixed glioneuronal tumors, 393–395
Mixed gonadal dysgenesis (MGD), 901–902, 902f
Moebius syndrome, 404
Mohr syndrome, 124
Molar pregnancies, 328, 328f, 330
Molecular diagnostic techniques
   antigens, 26–30
   cytogenetics as, 33–35
   flow cytometry as, 21–24
   future directions, 48
   gene expression arrays as, 47

Perlman syndrome, 114–115, 793, 794f
Peroxisomal biogenesis disorders, 181, 371
Peroxisomal disorders, 180–182, 369–371
  diagnosis of, by electron microscopy, 56
  peroxisomal biogenesis disorders, 181
  single peroxisomal enzyme deficiency, 181–182
Persistent embryonic epithelium, 581
Persistent hyperplastic primary vitreous (PHPV), 419
Persistent interstitial pulmonary emphysema (PIPE), 483, 483f
Persistent intrahepatic cholestasis
  Alagille syndrome, 664–665, 665t
  hereditary cholestasis with lymphedema, 669
  nonsyndromic paucity, intrahepatic ducts, 668–669
  progressive familial intrahepatic cholestasis, 665–668, 667f–668f
Persistent Müllerian duct syndrome (PMDS), 899–900
Persistent pulmonary hypertension of the newborn (PPHN), 566
Pertussis, 233, 491, 492f
Petechial hemorrhages, 355
Peters anomaly, 419
Peutz-Jeghers polyposis syndrome, 640–641
Peutz-Jeghers syndrome, 956t
Pfeiffer syndrome, 121
PGCs. See Primordial germ cells
PGD. See Pure gonadal dysgenesis
Phakomatous choristoma, 424
Phenylketonuria (PKU), 110, 160
PHEO. See Pheochromocytoma
Pheochromocytoma (PHEO), 982
  composite adrenal medullary neoplasms, 1011
  with hypertension, 983f
  malignancy prevalence, 1011
  mass screening program, 1008, 1009, 1009f
  principal histologic patterns in, 1010, 1010f
  serologic tests for, 995
Philadelphia chromosome, 35
Phosphatase and tensin homolog (PTEN) mutations, 384
PHOX2B, 1000
Phthisis, 439f
Phyllodes tumor (PT), 935–936, 936f, 937f
Physiologic gynecomastia, 934
Physiologic jaundice, 657, 658t
Pierson syndrome, 825
Pigmented epulis of infancy, 1033–1034, 1033f
Pigmented villonodular synovitis, 1161, 1163f
Pilocytic astrocytoma (PA), 352, 382–383, 383t
Pineal agenesis, 947
Pineal cysts, 947–948
Pineal gland
  acquired disorders
    neoplasms, 948
      pineal parenchymal tumors, 948
      pineoblastoma, 948, 949f
      pineocytoma, 948
    anatomy and physiology, 947

  computed tomography imaging, 947
  developmental disorders
    pineal agenesis, 947
    pineal cysts, 947–948
  hyperplasia, 947
  magnetic resonance imaging, 947
Pineal parenchymal tumors (PPTs), 392, 948. See also Pineal parenchymal tumors
Pineoblastoma, 392–393, 948, 949f
Pineoblastoma, pineocytoma, and PPT of intermediate grade (PPTIG), 392
Pineocytoma, 393f, 948
Pituitary adenoma (PA), 954–957, 957f
Pituitary apoplexy, 953, 954
Pituitary blastoma, 958
Pituitary duplication, 952
Pituitary dysfunction, 951
Pituitary gland
  acquired disorders, 952–958
    craniopharyngiomas, 953, 953f, 958
    granulomatous hypophysitis, 953
    heterotopia, 958
    inflammatory and infiltrative disorders, 952
    Langerhans cell histiocytosis, 958
    lymphocytic hypophysitis, 953
    nonneoplastic cysts, 953
    pituitary adenoma, 954–957, 957f
    pituitary blastoma, 958
    pituitary hyperplasia, 953–954
    salivary gland rest, 958
    vascular lesions, 953
    xanthogranulomatous inflammation, 953
  anatomy and physiology, 949–950
  developmental disorders
    agenesis of, 951
    anencephaly, 951
    anomalies in, 951, 951t
    ectopia, 951–952
    empty sella syndrome, 952
    hypopituitarism, 951
    mutations, 951, 952t
    nasopharyngeal teratomas, 952
    pituitary duplication, 952
    Rathke cleft cyst, 952
  imaging
    MR imaging, 950, 951
    T1-weighted images, 950, 951
Pituitary hyperplasia, 953–954
Pituitary stalk, 950, 958
Pituitary tumor apoplexy. See Pituitary apoplexy
PJOF. See Psammomatoid juvenile ossifying fibroma (PJOF)
Placenta
  aromatase deficiency in, 897
  chorangiomas in, 339
  diamnionic, dichorionic (DiDi), 327
  diamnionic, monochorionic (DiMo), 327
  early pregnancy
    anembryonic pregnancy, 330, 331f
    congenital infections, 332
    development, 325–326, 326f
    gestational trophoblastic disease, 328–330
    miscarriage, 330, 331f, 332

    multiple pregnancies, 326–328, 327f
  and fetus, growth characteristics, 1430t
  late pregnancy
    acute disease processes, 346–348
    anatomy, 333–334, 333f
    chronic disease processes, 334–342
    subacute disease processes, 342–346
  normative values, 1431t
  weights
    by gestational age, 1432t
    for triplets, 1434t
    for twins, 1433t
Placental site trophoblastic tumor (PSTT), 328–330, 329f
Plague, 254
Plastic bronchitis, 456–457
Platelet, 1103–1104
Pleocytosis, cerebrospinal fluid, 437
Pleomorphic adenoma (PA), 1036–1037, 1036f
Pleomorphic xanthoastrocytomas (PXA), 386
Pleuropulmonary blastoma (PPB), 494–497, 495f–498f
Plexiform fibrohistiocytic tumor (PFHT), 1163, 1164f
PMDS. See Persistent müllerian duct syndrome
PNET. See Primitive neuroectodermal tumors
Pneumonia, 491
Pneumopericardium, 481f
POF. See Peripheral ossifying fibroma
Poland syndrome, 928
Polar cataracts
  anterior, 424
  posterior, 424
Polycystic kidney disease
  autosomal dominant polycystic kidney disease, 812, 813f
  autosomal recessive polycystic kidney disease, 809, 811–812, 811f, 812f
Polycystic ovary syndrome (PCOS)
  diagnostic criteria for, 877
  etiology, 877
Polydactyly, skeletal system, 1303, 1303t
Polyendocrinopathy, 776
Polymerase chain reaction (PCR), 35–47
  applications, 37–47
    forensic identification, 47
    fusion gene transcripts detection, 38t–46t
    genetic testing for mutations, 47
    molecular microbiology, 37, 47
  basis of methodology of, 35–37, 36f
  compared with other molecular methods, 22t
  limitations, 47
  nested, 37
  vs. NGS, 47
  real-time, 28f, 37
  reverse transcriptase
    applications, 37
    basis of, 35, 36f
Polymerase gamma (POLG) gene, 374
Polymicrogyria, 363–364, 364f
Polymyositis, congenital, 1289, 1289f
Polyorchidism
  definition, 895
  histologic appearance, 895
Polyploidy, 92

Polyps, stomach, 592, 594f
Polysomy, 88, 90, 91t
Polysplenia syndrome, 454, 1077
Polythelia, 928
POMC. *See* Produce proopiomelanocortin
Pompe disease, 150, 554, 675
Pontomedullary rents, 356
Pontosubicular necrosis, 403
Porencephaly, 365
Porokeratosis, 1218, 1219
Porphyrias, metabolic disorders, 691
Postenteritis enteropathy, 610
Posterior fossa ependymoma, 385f
Posterior pituitary, 950, 953
   ectopia, 950
Posterior polar cataracts, 424
Posterior subcapsular cataract (PSC), 424, 425f
Postinfectious glomerulonephritis, 830–831, 831f
Postprocedure pregnancy loss, 74
Posttransplant lymphoproliferative disorder (PTLD), 321, 503
POU1F1 mutation, 951, 952t
PPNAD. *See* Primary pigmented nodular adrenal disease
Preeclampsia, 327
Pregnancy. *See* Early pregnancy; Late pregnancy
Premature delivery, 327
Prenatal diagnosis, cytogenetics in, 22t, 35
Prepubertal gynecomastia, 934, 935f
Prepubertal macroorchidism, 895
Prepubertal teratoma, 909, 909f
Prepubertal testicular tumors, 906, 912, 913, 915
Prepubertal vulval fibroma, 878
Preseptal cellulitis, 412
Primary acquired melanosis (PAM), 417
Primary aphakia, 424
Primary ciliary dyskinesia (PCD), 487
Primary CNS tumors, 378, 378t
Primary hyperoxaluria type 1, 1322
Primary immunodeficiency, 626–627, 1082
Primary lymphoma, 1359–1360
Primary pigmented nodular adrenal disease (PPNAD), 991
Primary pulmonary hypertension (PPH), 567
Primary sclerosing cholangitis (PSC), 704–706
Primary vascular neoplasms, 1349, 1351
Primary-villi, 326
Primitive neuroectodermal tumors (PNET), 389, 851
   family tumor, 1011
Primordial germ cells (PGCs), 865
Produce proopiomelanocortin (POMC), 950
Progestin, synthetic, fetal effects of, 108
Progressive familial intrahepatic cholestasis, 665–668, 667f–668f
Progressive multifocal leukoencephalopathy (PML), 353
Progressive neurodegeneration of childhood (PNDC), 374
Prolactinomas, 954
Propionic acidemia, 178–179
PROP1 mutation, 951, 952t
Proptosis, 412
Prostate
   acquired abnormalities and lesions, 922–923
   congenital anomalies, 922
   developmental anomalies, 922
Proteinuria/nephrotic syndrome. *See* Glomerular diseases
Proteus (PS) and proteus-like syndromes, 116
Protozoal infections, 252–253, 253f
   GI tract
      Blastocystis hominis, 614
      Cryptosporidium, 613–614, 614f
      Dientamoeba fragilis, 614
      Entamoeba histolytica, 614, 615f
      Giardia lamblia (Intestinalis), 613
Provisional cortex, 979–980
Prune belly syndrome, 116–117, 117f, 853–854, 854f
Psammomatoid juvenile ossifying fibroma (PJOF), 1030, 1031
PSC. *See* Posterior subcapsular cataract
Pseudocysts, 768
Pseudohermaphroditism, 897
Pseudohypoparathyroidism (PHP), 1321–1322
Pseudomembranous colitis, 240, 634, 634f
Pseudomonas aeruginosa infection, 233, 233f
Pseudoneonatal adrenoleukodystrophy, 181
Pseudosarcomatous tumor, 856
PSTT. *See* Placental site trophoblastic tumor
PTC. *See* Papillary thyroid carcinoma
PTEN-hamartoma syndromes (PTHS), 1166
PTEN hamartoma tumor syndrome, 640
PTX2 mutation, 952t
Pulmonary alveolar microlithiasis, 488
Pulmonary alveolar proteinosis (PAP), 488
Pulmonary arterial hypertension pathologic grading, 566t
Pulmonary artery stenosis, 540–541, 541t
Pulmonary atresia (PA)
   with ventricular septal defect, 540
   with VSD, 540
Pulmonary blastoma, 509
Pulmonary capillary hemangiomatosis (PCH), 502
Pulmonary hypertension, 565–567, 565t
   with obstructive left heart disease, 567
Pulmonary interstitial glycogenosis, 493–494, 493f
Pulmonary outflow tract and valve malformations, 539–540
Pulmonary stenosis with intact ventricular septum, 540
Pulmonary valve, absent, 540
Pulmonary vascular development, 566
Pulmonary vascular resistance (PVR), 525
Pulmonary vein atresia/stenosis, 528
Pulmonary veno-occlusive disease (PVOD), 488
Pulmonary venous anomalies, 527–529, 527t
Punch biopsy, 1216
Pure gonadal dysgenesis (PGD), 902
Pure red cell aplasia, 1101
PVL. *See* Periventricular leukomalacia
Pyknodysostosis, 1320
Pyloric stenosis (PS), 588
Pyoderma gangrenosum, 1235
Pyogenic granuloma, 411, 411f
Pyramidal cataract, 424
Pyramidal neurons, 351
Pyruvate carboxylase deficiency, 179, 180
Pyruvate dehydrogenase (PDH) deficiency, 179, 180f

R

Raccoon eyes, 998
Radiation disruption, 105–106
Radiation nephritis, 840
Ragged red fibers (RRF), 372
Rathke cleft cysts, 950, 952
   cystic dilatation of, 953
RDD. *See* Rosai-Dorfman disease
Reactive gliosis, 352f
Reddish lobulated mass, 411
Reflux esophagitis, 584–585, 584f, 584t
Refsum disease, 182
Renal agenesis/hypoplasia, 804
Renal artery stenosis, 839
Renal cell carcinoma, 850–851, 851f
Renal cortical necrosis, 839
Renal duplication (duplex kidney), 806
Renal dysplasia/cystic diseases, 807–809
   cortical cysts, 814–815
   cysts associated with syndromes
      Meckel-Gruber syndrome, 816
      tuberous sclerosis, 815, 815f
      Von Hippel-Lindau disease, 815–816
   medullary cysts
      medullary cystic kidney disease, 814
      medullary sponge kidney, 813
      nephronophthisis, 813
   polycystic kidney disease
      autosomal dominant polycystic kidney disease, 812, 813f
      autosomal recessive polycystic kidney disease, 809, 811–812, 811f, 812f
   renal dysplasia, 807–809
   simple cysts, 815
Renal ectopia, 802–803, 802t
Renal fusion, 802t, 803–804, 803f
Renal–hepatic–pancreatic dysplasia, 768
Renal hypoplasia, 805
Renal malformations, pediatric autopsies, 801, 802t
Renal neoplasms
   cystic variants, nephroblastic tumors
      cystic partially differentiated nephroblastoma, 845, 845f–846f
      nephroma, 845, 845f
   nephroblastoma (Wilms tumor)
      gross features, 842–843, 842f–843f
      microscopic features, 843–845, 843f–844f, 845t
      molecular and cellular biology, 841–842
      prevalence, 840–841
      staging, 845t
   nephrogenic rests and nephroblastomatosis, 846–847
Renal transplant pathology
   acute rejection, 307–310, 308t–310t
   allograft biopsies, 306
   chronic rejection, 310–311, 311f
   delayed graft function, 306–307
   hyperacute and accelerated acute rejection, 306–307
   immunosuppressive drug toxicity, 312, 313f
   polyomavirus nephropathy, 311–312, 312f

posttransplant lymphoproliferative disorders, 313–314
   recurrent disease, 313
Renal tubular dysgenesis, 805–806
Renal vein thrombosis, 839
Renomegaly, 806
Renovascular diseases
   Bartter syndrome, 840
   papillary necrosis, 839–840
   radiation nephritis, 840
   renal artery stenosis, 839
   renal cortical necrosis, 839
   renal involvement, systemic vasculitides, 838–839
   renal vein thrombosis, 839
   thrombotic microangiopathy syndrome, 837–838, 838f
Resident microglia, 353
Respiratory distress syndrome (RDS), 472–475
Respiratory papillomatosis, 1025–1027, 1026f
Respiratory syncytial virus (RSV), 490–491, 490f
Respiratory tract
   bronchus, 454–457
   diaphragm, 512–514
   lung (See Lung)
   nasopharynx, 447–450
   trachea, 450–453
Restrictive cardiomyopathy (RCMP), 550
Restrictive dermopathy, 1219
Rete mirabile, 361
Retiform hemangioendothelioma (RHE), 1134
Retina
   structure, 427, 427f
   tumors of, 428–434
Retinal anlage tumor, 1033–1034, 1033f
Retinal ischemia, 430
Retinal pigment epithelium (RPE), 427, 428
Retinoblastoma, 428–434, 429f–434f
Reverse transcriptase polymerase chain reaction (RT-PCR)
   applications, 37
   basis of, 35
Reye syndrome, 694
Rhabdoid tumor, 850, 850f
Rhabdomyoma, 571, 571f, 1180, 1180f
   dysplasia, 470
Rhabdomyosarcoma (RMS), 437, 494, 879, 879f, 906, 941–943, 1004, 1181, 1183, 1183t, 1360
   embryonal type, 922, 923f
   prostatic, 922–923
   renal, 856–857
Rheumatic fever (RF), 538, 557–559, 558t
Rheumatic heart disease, 557–559, 558t
Rheumatoid nodule, 1235–1236
Rhizomelic chondrodysplasia punctata
   type 1, 181
   type 2, 181
   type 3, 182
Richner-Hanhart syndrome, 161
Rickets, 277–278
Rickettsial infections, 243–244, 243t, 244f
Right-sided aortic arch, 544
Rigid-spine syndrome, 1289
RMS. See Rhabdomyosarcoma
Robertsonian translocation, 70

Robert syndrome, 125, 125f
Robinow syndrome, 121
Robin sequence, 116
Rocker bottom feet, 70
Rod cells, 353
Rokitansky technique, 9
Rosai-Dorfman disease (RDD), 958, 1067–1068, 1067f–1068f, 1251, 1362–1364, 1363f
Rosenthal fibers (RFs), 352, 353f
Rotaviruses, 609
Rotor syndrome, 657–658
Round-cell neoplasms
   EWS– PNET, 1355–1358, 1355f–1358f
   MNTI, 1358–1359, 1358f–1359f
   multiple myeloma–plasma cell dyscrasia, 1360
   non-Hodgkin lymphoma, 1359f–1360f
   primary lymphoma, 1359–1360
   skeletal metastasis, 1360
RPE. See Retinal pigment epithelium
RRF. See Ragged red fibers
Rubella, 424, 425f
   clinical features, 210
   laboratory diagnosis, 210
   pathology, 210
   prognosis and outcome, 210
   transmission, 209–210
Rubinstein-Taybi syndrome, 129
Rudimentary meningocele, 1177–1178, 1178f

S
Sacrococcygeal teratoma (SCT), 1201
Salivary gland rest, 958
Salmonella, 230–232, 905, 610–611
Sanger method, 47
Sarcoidosis, 418, 510–511, 511f, 1236
Sarcomas, 941
SC. See Secretory carcinoma
SCA. See Spinocerebellar atrophy
Scalp–ear–nipple syndrome, 928
Schiller-Duval bodies, 908
   yolk sac tumor, 883, 883f
Schisis, 118
Schizencephaly, 365
Schneckenbecken dysplasia, 1313f
Schwannian stroma-rich tumor, 1002
Schwannoma, 1172–1173, 1172f
Schwannomatosis, 1173
Sclera, 418
Sclerema neonatorum, 1236, 1237
Sclerosing epithelioid fibrosarcoma (SEF), 1158
Sclerosing stromal tumors, 888, 888f
SCT. See Sertoli cell tumor
SCTATs. See Sex cord tumors with annular tubules
Scurvy, 1321
SDH. See Subdural hemorrhage (SDH)
SDHB mutation, 1009, 1011
Sebaceous glands, 410
Seckel syndrome, 123–124
Secondary cardiomyopathies, 554–556
Secondary hemosiderosis, 687, 688f
Second trimester spontaneous abortion, 67–69
   ascending infection, 68
   CMV infection, 69, 69f
   cytogenetic studies, 68

hydrops fetalis, 72, 72f
internal and external examination, 68
limb–body wall complex, 73–74, 74f
listeriosis, 68, 68f–69f
maceration, 67, 70
monosomy X, 71, 71f
nonchromosomal factors, 67
postprocedure pregnancy loss, 74
syphilis, 69
triploidy, 71–72, 71f–72f
trisomy 13, 71, 71f
trisomy 18, 70, 70f
trisomy 21, 69–70, 70f
twinning, 72–73, 73f
umbilical cord compromise, 73, 73f
uterine anomalies, 68
Secretary's Advisory Committee on Heritable Disorders in Newborns and Children (SACHDNC), 136
Secretory carcinoma (SC), 937, 938f
SEER Program, 997
Semilobar HPE, 361
Seminal vesicle cysts, 918
Seminoma, germ cell tumors, 911–912
Sepsis, neonatal, 225–227, 226t
Septal malformations
   aortopulmonary window, 535–536
   atrial septum malformations, 529, 529t
   atrioventricular septum malformations, 531–532
   conus and truncus malformations, 533
   double-outlet ventricle, 534–535
   persistent truncus arteriosus, 535, 535f
   transposition of great vessels, 533–534
   ventricular septum malformations, 529–531
Serologic markers, 886, 886f
Serous neoplasms, ovary, 889–890, 890f
Serratia marcescens, 234
Sertoli cell tumor (SCT)
   in children, 914
   cryptorchid testis, 897f
   sex cord–stromal tumors, 914, 914f–915f
Sertoli-Leydig cell tumors, 889, 889f
^{99m}Tc Sestamibi, 960
Severe acute respiratory syndrome (SARS), 224
Severe combined immunodeficiency diseases (SCID), 1084–1085
Sex chromosome aneuploidy, 87
Sex cord–stromal tumors
   ovaries
      adenomatoid tumors, 889
      adult-type granulosa cell tumors, 887, 888f
      juvenile granulosa cell tumor, 886–887, 886f
      sclerosing stromal tumors, 888, 888f
      Sertoli cell tumors, 888
      Sertoli-Leydig cell tumors, 889, 889f
      sex cord tumors with annular tubules, 888, 888f
   XX male and XY female syndrome
      juvenile granulosa cell tumor, 915–196, 916f–917f
      Leydig cell tumor, 913–914, 913f
      Sertoli cell tumor, 914, 914f–915f
Sex cord tumors with annular tubules (SCTATs), 888, 888f

Sex reversal
    acquired abnormalities and lesions, 904–906
    carcinoid tumor, 917
    defects in Wilms tumor, 904
    germ cell tumors, 906
        embryonal carcinoma, 911, 912f
        epidermoid cyst, 910–911, 910f
        intratubular germ cell neoplasia, unclassified type, 911, 912f
        mixed germ cell tumor, 912–913
        seminoma, 911–912
        teratoma, 908–910, 909f
        yolk sac tumor, 907–908, 908f
    gonadoblastoma, 916–917
    hematopoietic origin of tumors, 917–918
    neoplasms of testis, 906
    nephroblastoma, 917
    sex cord–stromal tumors
        juvenile granulosa cell tumor, 915–196, 916f–917f
        Leydig cell tumor, 913–914, 913f
        Sertoli cell tumor, 914, 914f–915f
Sexual determination disorders, 901–903
Shaken baby syndrome, 279–282, 279f–282f, 356
Sharp force injuries, 287–288, 287f–288f
Shave biopsy, 1216
Sheehan syndrome, 953
Shigella, 611
Short bowel syndrome and bacterial overgrowth, 625
Short-chain acyl-CoA dehydrogenase deficiency (SCADD, SCAD), 167
Short-rib dysplasia (SRD), polydactyly, 1312–1313, 1312f
Shwachman-Diamond syndrome, 764, 771, 772f
Sialoblastoma, 1039–1040, 1040f
SIDS. *See* Sudden infant death syndrome
Simple goiter, 971
Single peroxisomal enzyme deficiency, 181–182
Single-photon emission computed tomography (SPECT), 960
Sinonasal inflammatory polyps, 1022–1023, 1023f
Sinonasal mycotic sinusitis, 1024–1025, 1024f
Sinus histiocytosis with massive lymphadenopathy (SHML), 1067–1068, 1067f–1068f
Sipple syndrome, 955t
Sirenomelia, 1302
Sjogren syndrome (SS) sialadenitis, 1035–1036, 1036f
Skeletal and smooth muscle neoplasms
    adult rhabdomyoma, 1180
    alveolar RMS, 1185–1189, 1187f–1189f
    in children, 1181, 1182f
    embryonal RMS, 1183–1185, 1184f–1186f, 1189f
    fetal rhabdomyoma, 1180, 1181f
    focal myositis, 1180, 1181, 1182f
    rhabdomyoma, 1180, 1180f
    rhabdomyosarcoma, 1181, 1183, 1183t
Skeletal dysplasia, 1299, 1305t
    achondroplasia, 1307
    bent bone dysplasias, 1316–1317
    bone density, 1317–1318, 1318f
    bone density group, 1308–1310
    Bruck syndrome, 1310
    chondrodysplasia group, 1316, 1316f
    defective mineralization group, 1310–1311
    FGFR3 chondrodysplasias, 1307–1308, 1308f
    filamin group, 1315–1316
    genetic inflammatory rheumatoid-like osteoarthropathies, 1320–1321
    hypochondroplasia, 1307
    lethal chondrodysplasias, 1304, 1306
    lysosomal storage diseases, 1318–1320, 1319f
    melorheostosis, osteopoikilosis, pyknodysostosis, and osteopathia striata, 1320
    metaphyseal dysplasias, 1320
    neonatal osteosclerotic dysplasias, 1317–1318, 1318f
    osteogenesis imperfecta, 1308–1310, 1309t, 1310f–1311f
    osteopetrosis, 1317–1318, 1318f
    perinatal lethal type, 1309–1310
    postmortem examination, 1306
    prevalence, 1304
    Schneckenbecken dysplasia, 1313f
    severe spondylodysplasias, 1313, 1313f
    skeletal component group, 1321
    spondyloepi(meta)physeal dysplasias, 1313
    SRD, polydactyly, 1312–1313, 1312f
    sulfation disorders, 1313, 1314f, 1315
    thanatophoric dysplasia, 1307, 1308f
    TRPV4-associated disorders, 1313, 1314f
    type 2 collagen group, 1311
    types, 1307t
Skeletal metastasis, 1360
Skeletal myopathy associated with cardiomyopathy, 1283–1284, 1284f
Skeletal system
    acquired disorders, 1321–1322
    congenital and developmental disorders and malformations
        arthrogryposis/congenital contracture, 1303
        axial skeleton anomalies, 1302–1303
        caudal dysgenesis, 1302–1303, 1302f
        FAD sequence, 1303–1304
        genetic skeletal disorders, 1304–1321
        limb reduction deficiency, 1300–1302
        polydactyly, 1303, 1303t
        skeletal dysplasias (*See* Skeletal dysplasia)
        syndactyly, 1303
        teratogen and anomalies, 1300–1302
    enchondral ossification, 1298–1299
    fibrous spindle cell tumors (*See* Fibrous spindle cell tumors)
    histiocytic disorders, 1361–1364, 1361f–1364f, 1362t
    infection and noninfectious inflammatory conditions
        acute osteomyelitis, 1365–1366
        Gaucher disease, 1368
        infantile cortical hyperostosis, 1367–1368, 1367f
        nonbacterial osteitis, 1366–1367, 1366f–1367f
        osteomyelitis, 1364–1365, 1366f
        osteonecrosis, 1368
    matrix-producing and matrix-associated tumors
        cartilaginous tumors (*See* Cartilaginous tumors)
        fibrous dysplasia, 1333–1336, 1334f–1336f
        hyperparathyroidism–jaw tumor syndrome, 1332–1333
        juvenile-ossifying fibroma, 1331–1332, 1331f–1332f
        osteofibrous dysplasia, 1333, 1333f
        osteoid osteoma and osteoblastoma, 1328–1329, 1328f–1330f, 1331
        osteoma, 1331
        osteosarcoma, 1323–1327, 1323f–1327f
    membranous ossification, 1298
    metabolic and nutritional conditions
        hyperparathyroidism, 1321
        primary hyperoxaluria type 1, 1322
        pseudohypoparathyroidism, 1321–1322
        rickets–osteomalacia, 1321
        scurvy, 1321
    nonmatrix-producing tumors and cysts, 1344
        aneurysmal bone cyst, 1347–1349, 1347f–1348f
        cherubism, 1346–1347, 1347f
        epidermoid cyst, 1349
        giant-cell reparative granuloma, 1346, 1347f
        giant-cell tumor, 1345–1346, 1345f–1346f
        Gorham-Stout disease, 1351
        osteoglophonic dysplasia, 1346–1347
        primary vascular neoplasms, 1349, 1351
        solitary–unicameral bone cyst, 1349, 1349f–1350f
    round-cell neoplasms
        EWS– PNET, 1355–1358, 1355f–1358f
        MNTI, 1358–1359, 1358f–1359f
        multiple myeloma–plasma cell dyscrasia, 1360
        non-Hodgkin lymphoma, 1359f–1360f
        primary lymphoma, 1359–1360
        skeletal metastasis, 1360
    synovium, 1368–1369
    tumor and tumorlike conditions, 1322
Skene duct cysts, 877
Skin
    adnexal tumors, 1242–1243, 1243f
    algorithmic approach, 1215t, 1217
    bacterial infections
        ecthyma, 1230, 1230f
        erysipelas, 1230, 1231
        impetigo, 1229, 1229f
        Staphylococcal scalded skin syndrome, 1229–1230, 1230f
        toxic shock syndrome, 1230
    biopsy
        electron microscopic examination of, 51, 52f
        techniques, 1216

carcinomas, 1243
congenital diseases (genodermatoses)
    acrodermatitis enteropathica, 1222
    aplasia cutis congenita, 1217
    Darier disease, 1218, 1218f, 1219f
    ectodermal dysplasias, 1219, 1220f, 1221f
    epidermolysis bullosa, 1221–1222, 1221f
    focal dermal hypoplasia, 1219, 1221
    ichthyoses, 1217–1218, 1217f, 1218f
    incontinentia pigmenti, 1222, 1222f
    porokeratosis, 1218, 1219
    restrictive dermopathy, 1219
dermoid cysts, 1241
eczematous dermatitis
    atopic dermatitis, 1225
    contact dermatitis, 1225
    dyshidrotic dermatitis, 1225
    nummular dermatitis, 1225
    spongiotic dermatitis, 1225–1226, 1227f
embryology, 1214, 1216f
epidermal inclusion cyst, 1241, 1241f
epidermal nevi, 1240–1241, 1241f
eruptive vellus hair cysts, 1241
folliculitis and perifolliculitis, 1238
fungal infections, 1233, 1233f, 1234f
graft versus host disease, 1239–1240, 1240f
hematopoietic, 1249, 1250, 1250f
    histiocytoses, 1249–1251, 1250f, 1251f
    leukemia and lymphoma, 1251
    mast cell diseases, 1249, 1249f
histology, 1214
infestations, 1233, 1234
leukocytoclastic vasculitis, 1237, 1238f
lymphocytic vasculitis, 1237, 1238
melanocytic neoplasms
    malignant melanoma, 1246
    melanocytic nevi, 1243–1246, 1243f–1246f
mesenchymal neoplasms
    myofibroblastic/fibroblastic tumors, 1247–1249, 1248f
    neurothekeoma, 1246–1247, 1247f
    vascular tumors, 1247
metabolic disorders, 1240, 1240f, 1241f
miscellaneous noninfectious vesiculopustular diseases, 1225
noninfectious acquired vesiculobullous diseases
    dermatitis herpetiformis, 1223, 1223f
    epidermolysis bullosa acquisita, 1224
    erythema multiforme, 1224, 1224f, 1225
    herpes gestationis, 1223
    linear IgA bullous dermatosis, 1222–1223, 1223f
    Stevens-Johnson syndrome, 1224, 1224f, 1225
    toxic epidermal necrolysis, 1224, 1224f, 1225
noninfectious granulomatous dermatoses
    granuloma annulare, 1235, 1235f
    necrobiosis lipoidica, 1235
    rheumatoid nodule, 1235–1236
    sarcoidosis, 1236
noninfectious inflammatory dermatoses
    acute febrile neutrophilic dermatosis, 1234
    eosinophilic cellulitis, 1234
    idiopathic palmoplantar hidradenitis, 1234
    neutrophilic eccrine hidradenitis, 1234
    pyoderma gangrenosum, 1235
noninfectious papulosquamous dermatoses
    lichen planus, 1226–1227, 1227f
    lichen sclerosus, 1228–1229, 1229f
    papular acrodermatitis of childhood, 1228
    pityriasis lichenoides, 1227–1228, 1228f
    pityriasis rosea, 1227
    pityriasis rubra pilaris, 1227, 1227f
    psoriasis vulgaris, 1226
    seborrheic dermatitis, 1226
panniculitis
    erythema nodosum, 1236, 1236f
    sclerema neonatorum, 1236, 1237
    subcutaneous fat necrosis, newborn, 1236, 1237f
routine processing, 1216
special processing, 1216–1217
steatocystoma multiplex, 1241, 1242f
systemic diseases, 1238–1239, 1239f
transient neonatal pustular melanosis, 1225
viral infections
    herpes viruses, 1232–1233, 1232f
    human papillomavirus, 1231, 1231f
    molluscum contagiosum, 1231, 1232f
Small and large intestine disorders
congenital abnormalities
    duplications, 596–598, 597f
    gastroschisis, 594, 594f
    intestinal atresia and stenosis, 595–596, 597f
    malrotation, 582f, 594–595, 595f
    Meckel diverticulum, 598–599, 599f
    omphalocele, 594, 594f
    vitelline (omphalomesenteric) duct anomalies, 598–599, 598f
cystic fibrosis, gastrointestinal involvement, 600, 600t
meconium and meconium abnormalities
    meconium ileus, 599
    meconium peritonitis, 599–600
    meconium plug, 600
Small cell carcinomas of ovary, 890–891
Smallpox, 253
Smith-Lemli-Opitz syndrome, 123, 184–185, 185f, 360
Soft tissue
congenital hemangioma, 131f, 1129–1131, 1130–1131, 1130f
fibroblast, 1140
fibroblastic and myofibroblastic tumors
    calcifying aponeurotic fibromatosis, 1152, 1152f
    calcifying fibrous pseudotumor, 1153
    CD34-positive spindle cell tumors, 1159, 1160
    of childhood, 1144
    congenital infantile fibrosarcoma, 1156–1157, 1156f, 1156t, 1157f
    dermatofibrosarcoma protuberans, 1158–1159, 1159f, 1160f
    dermatomyofibroma, 1149, 1149f
    desmoid-type fibromatosis, 1149–1151, 1150f, 1151f
    fibromatosis colli, 1153
    fibrosarcoma, 1155
    fibrous hamartoma of infancy, 1147–1148, 1148f
    gardner-nuchal fibroma, 1151
    inclusion body fibromatosis, 1148, 1148f, 1149
    infantile fibromatosis, 1146
    infantile myofibroma, 1144, 1144f–1145f
    infantile subcutaneous fibromatosis, 1146, 1147, 1147f
    inflammatory myofibroblastic tumor, 1153–1155, 1153t, 1154f
    juvenile hyaline fibromatosis, 1151–1152, 1151f
    juvenile nasopharyngeal angiofibroma, 1152, 1153
    low-grade fibromyxoid sarcoma, 1157–1158, 1157f–1158f
    low-grade myofibroblastic sarcoma, 1155
    myositis ossificans, 1141, 1143, 1143f
    myxoinflammatory fibroblastic sarcoma, 1155, 1155f
    nodular fasciitis, 1140, 1141t, 1142f
    palmar–plantar fibromatosis, 1151
    sclerosing epithelioid fibrosarcoma, 1158
    solitary fibrous, 1146, 1147f
fibrohistiocytic tumors
    angiomatoid fibrous histiocytoma, 1163, 1164f
    benign cutaneous fibrous histiocytoma, 1161, 1162f
    blastic plasmacytoid DC neoplasm, 1166
    dendritic cell neoplasms, 1165
    dermatofibroma, 1161, 1161f
    diffuse-type giant cell tumor, 1161, 1163
    juvenile xanthogranuloma, 1165–1166, 1165f
    pigmented villonodular synovitis, 1161, 1163f
    plexiform fibrohistiocytic tumor, 1163, 1164f
    tenosynovial giant cell tumor, 1161, 1162f
    WHO classification of, 1160
gastrointestinal stromal tumor, 1179–1180
infantile hemangiomas, 1129–1131, 1130f, 1131f
lipomatous hamartomas, 1166–1167
lipomatous tumors, 116t, 1166
neoplasms
    hibernoma, 1168
    lipoblastoma, 1168, 1168f, 1168t, 1169f
    lipomas, 1167–1168, 1167f
    lipomatous lesion of heart, 1170
    liposarcoma, 1169, 1170f, 1170t
neoplasms in children, 1125t–1126t

Soft tissue (*Continued*)
   peripheral nerve sheath tumors, 1170–1171
      glioneuronal heterotopia, 1177
      granular cell tumor, 1176–1177, 1176f, 1177f, 1177t
      malignant peripheral nerve sheath tumor, 1173–1175, 1174f–1175f
      nerve sheath myxoma, 1175–1176
      neurofibroma, 1171, 1171t, 1172f
      rudimentary meningocele, 1177–1178, 1178f
      schwannoma, 1172–1173, 1172f
      schwannomatosis, 1173
   perivascular epithelioid cell neoplasm (PEComa), 1178–1179, 1178f, 1179f
   sarcomas, 1127–1128
   sarcomas of uncertain histogenesis
      alveolar soft part sarcoma, 1199, 1200f
      clear cell sarcoma, 1192–1193, 1194f
      desmoplastic small round cell tumor, 1191–1192, 1192f–1193f, 1192t
      epithelioid sarcoma, 1198–1199
      Ewing sarcoma-like tumors, 1191, 1191f
      Ewing sarcoma-primitive neuroectodermal tumor, 1189–1190, 1189t, 1190f, 1191f
      extraskeletal myxoid chondrosarcoma, 1193, 1194
      malignant ectomesenchymoma, 1199, 1200f–1201f
      malignant rhabdoid tumor, 1196, 1197–1198, 1197t, 1198f
      mesenchymal chondrosarcoma, 1194–1195
      myoepithelial tumor, 1195
      NUT midline carcinomas, 1193
      sacrococcygeal teratoma, 1201
      synovial sarcoma, 1195–1196, 1195f, 1195t, 1196f
      undifferentiated sarcoma, 1189
   scar and keloid, 1140, 1140f
   skeletal and smooth muscle neoplasms
      adult rhabdomyoma, 1180
      alveolar rhabdomyosarcoma, 1185–1189, 1187f–1189f
      in children, 1181, 1182f
      embryonal rhabdomyosarcoma, 1183–1185, 1184f–1186f, 1189f
      fetal rhabdomyoma, 1180, 1181f
      focal myositis, 1180, 1181, 1182f
      rhabdomyoma, 1180, 1180f
      rhabdomyosarcoma, 1181, 1183, 1183t
   vascular malformations
      regional and diffuse syndromes associated with, 1136, 1137t
      glomangioma, 1140, 1140f
      glomus tumor, 1138
      lymphatic malformation, 1137, 1138f
      mixed venous and lymphatic malformation, 1137, 1138f
      morphologic features, 1137, 1137f
      PTEN hamartoma, 1138, 1139f
   vascular neoplasms
      angiosarcoma, 1134, 1135f
      composite hemangioendothelioma, 1134
      epithelioid hemangioma, 1133, 1134f
      kaposiform hemangioendothelioma, 1131, 1132f, 1133f
      kaposiform lymphangiomatosis, 1132–1133, 1133f, 1133t
      Kaposi sarcoma, 1136
      lobular capillary hemangioma–pyogenic granuloma, 1136, 1136f
      papillary intralymphatic angioendothelioma, 1134
      retiform hemangioendothelioma, 1134
      spindle cell hemangioma, 1134, 1135f
      tufted hemangioma, 1131
      vascular tumors, 1128–1129, 1129t
      verrucous hemangioma, 1131
Solid dermoid, 415f
Solid mature teratoma, 881
Solid pseudopapillary neoplasm, 779, 780f
Solitary fibrous tumor (SFT), 1146, 1147f
Solitary rectal ulcer syndrome, 636–637
Solitary–unicameral bone cyst (SUBC), 1349, 1349f–1350f
Somatotroph hyperplasia, 953
Somatotrophs, 950
Sonic hedgehog (Shh), 357, 388
   gene, 360
   signaling, 869
   signaling pathway, 951
Southern blotting, 37
SOX2 mutation, 951, 952t
SOX3 mutation, 951, 952t
Spermatic cord
   acquired abnormalities and lesions, 919–920
   congenital anomalies, 918–919
   cysts, 918
   developmental anomalies, 918–919
Sphingolipidoses, 681–682, 682f, 683f
   Fabry disease, 142–144, 144f
   Farber disease, 149
   gangliosidoses, 144, 145
   Gaucher disease, 142, 143f
   Krabbe disease, 148, 149f
   metachromatic leukodystrophy, 146, 148, 148f
   Niemann-Pick disease, 146, 147f
Spinal cord diseases, 1265–1266
Spinal muscular atrophy (SMA), 376, 376f
Spindle cell
   and epithelioid nevus, 413
   nevus (*See* Spitz nevus)
Spindle cell hemangioma (SCH), 1134, 1135f
Spinocerebellar atrophy (SCA), 375–376
Spitz nevus, 413, 1244
Spleen
   acquired abnormalities
      congestion, 1078
      extramedullary hematopoiesis, 1080
      follicular hyperplasia, 1081
      hemolytic anemia, 1078
      hereditary spherocytosis and elliptocytosis, 1078
      Hodgkin lymphoma, 1082
      immune thrombocytopenia, 1078
      inborn errors of metabolism, 1079–1080
      infection, 1079
      localized lymphoid hyperplasia, 1081–1082
      nonhematopoietic tumors, 1081
      non-Hodgkin lymphoma, 1082
      primary immunodeficiencies, 1082
      sickle cell anemia, 1078
      thalassemia syndromes, 1078
      vascular tumors, 1080–1081, 1081t
   congenital anomalies
      accessory, 1077
      asplenia, 1077
      cysts, 1078
      hamartoma, 1077–1078
      polysplenia, 1077
      splenic fusion, 1077
   embryology, 1075
   examination, 1076–1077, 1077t
   structure and function, 1075–1076, 1076f
   vascular tumors, 1080–1081
Split hand-foot limb defect, 1302
Spondylodysplasias, 1313, 1313f
Spongiotic dermatitis, 1225–1226, 1227f
Spontaneous abortion (SA), 81t
   causes, 60–62
   definition, 60
   early
      aneuploidy, 61
      CGH, 61
      chromosome abnormality, 61
      karyotype, 61
      maternal age, 61
      monosomy X, 61
      recurrent miscarriages, 61
      structural rearrangement, 61
      trisomy, 61
   first trimester
      examination, 62–67
      indication, 62
   incidence, 60
   pathologic examination, 60
   second trimester, 67–74
      hydrops fetalis, 72, 72f
      limb–body wall complex, 73–74, 74f
      monosomy X, 71, 71f
      postprocedure pregnancy loss, 74
      triploidy, 71–72, 72f
      trisomy 13, 71, 71f
      trisomy 18, 70, 70f
      trisomy 21, 69–70, 70f
      twinning, 72–73, 73f
      umbilical cord compromise, 73, 73f
Spontaneous perforation
   colitis, 636
   gastric, neonate, 589
Sporadic congenital abnormalities, 128–129
Squamous carcinoma, conjunctiva, 418
Squamous cell carcinoma (SCC), 508, 508f, 922
Squamous papillomatosis, laryngotracheal type, 1025–1027, 1026f
Staphylococcal infections, 227–228, 228f, 922, 1365
Staphylococcal scalded skin syndrome (SSSS), 276, 1229–1230, 1230f
Status marmoratus, 403
Stellate reticulum, 391
Stem cells, 1093–1094, 1094f
Stenosis, esophageal, 584
Steroidogenic acute regulatory protein (StAR), 980, 989

Sterol carrier protein X (SCPx) deficiency, 182
Stevens-Johnson syndrome, 876
Stickler syndrome, 121
Stillborn infants, weights and measurements
  body weight, 1400t–1401t
  gestational age, 1398t–1399t
Stomach disorders
  acquired diseases
    gastritis, 589
    Helicobacter heilmannii (*Gastrospirillum hominis*) gastritis, 590–591, 591f
    Helicobacter pylori gastritis, 589–590, 590f
    hemorrhagic and erosive gastritis, 589
    spontaneous gastric perforation, neonate, 589
  congenital anomalies
    antral web, 588
    duplication, 588
    hypertrophic pyloric stenosis, 588
    pancreatic heterotopia and pancreatic acinar metaplasia, 589
  Crohn disease, 592
  gastrointestinal stromal tumors, 592–593, 593f
  granulomatous gastritis, 591–592
  Ménétrier disease, 591
  peptic ulcer disease, 591
  polyps and tumors, 592, 594f
Storage histiocytosis (SH), 369
Streak gonads, 872, 872f, 873f
  disorders of sexual determination, 901
  hilar region of, 902
Streptococcal infections, 228–229, 229f
Structural chromosomal abnormalities, 92, 93, 93f
Sturge-Weber dysplasia, 128
Sty, 412
Subacute necrotizing encephalopathy, 373
Subacute sclerosing panencephalitis (SSPE), 400
Subarachnoid hemorrhage (SAH), 355
Subcutaneous fat necrosis, newborn, 1236, 1237f
Subdural hemorrhage (SDH), 355, 356
Subluxated lenses, 426
Submicroscopic abnormalities, 93
Substrate reduction therapy, 142
Subvalvular aortic stenosis, 541
Subvalvular stenosis, 540
Sudden infant death syndrome (SIDS), 266–267, 356–357, 791
Sudden unexplained infant death (SUID), 186, 267–268, 267f
Sulfation disorders (SDs), 1313, 1314f, 1315
Supernumerary breast tissue, 928
Supernumerary kidney, 806
Supernumerary nipples. *See* Polythelia
Supernumerary parathyroid glands, 960
Supratentorial primitive neuroectodermal tumor (sPNET), 389
Supravalvular aortic stenosis, 541
Supravalvular pullmonary artery stenosis, 540–541, 541t
Supraventricular tachycardias, 560
Surfactant dysfunction disorders, 478
Swiss cheese disease, 932
Sympathetic ophthalmia, 438, 439f

Syncytial trophoblasts stains, 329, 334
Syndactyly
  acrocephalosyndactyly syndrome, 120–122, 120t
  skeletal system, 1303
Synovial sarcoma (SS), 494, 1195–1196, 1195f, 1195t, 1196f
Synovium
  acute synovitis, 1368
  chronic synovitis, 1368
  granulomatous synovitis, 1368
  hemophilic arthropathy, 1368
  histiocytic synovitis, 1368–1369
  osteoarthropathy, 1369
  tumefactive lesions, 1369
Syphilis, 69, 332, 332f, 874–875
  clinical features, 234, 235f–236f, 236–237
  laboratory diagnosis, 237–238
  pathology, 237
  prognosis and outcome, 238
  transmission, 234
Syringoma, 1242
Systemic arterial disease, 567–570
  aneurysms, 567–568, 568t
  arteriopathy, 567
  atherosclerosis, 568
  vasculitis, 569
Systemic disease, 418
Systemic lupus erythematosus (SLE), 556–557, 1065
Systemic vasculitides, renal involvement, 838–839
Systemic venous anomalies, 527
Systemic viral infections
  adenoviral disease, 223–224
  enteroviral infections, 224
  HTLV infection, 224
  Mumps, 224, 225f

T
Tail bud defects, 357, 359
Takayasu arteritis, 570
TAPS. *See* Twin anemia polycythemia sequence
Tarsal conjunctiva, 411, 414
Tarsal plate, 410, 414
Tarui disease, 166
TBX19 mutation, 951
T-cell lymphoblastic lymphoma, 1072
TDC. *See* Thyroglossal duct cyst
Telangiectatic/inflammatory hepatocellular adenoma, 721–722
Tenosynovial giant cell tumor, 1161, 1162f
Teratocarcinoma teratoma, 881
Teratogenic disruptions, 106–110
  alcohol embryopathy, 108–109, 109t
  diphenylhydantoin embryopathy, 110
  fetal iodine deficiency, 107
  folic acid deficiency, 107
  isotretinoin embryopathy, 108
  mercury embryopathy, 108
  synthetic progestin embryopathy, 108
  thalidomide embryopathy, 106–107
  trimethadione syndrome, 107
  valproic acid embryopathy, 107–108
  warfarin embryopathy, 108

Teratogens
  critical periods in, 107t
  types, 106t
Teratoid medulloepithelioma, 434
Teratoma, 572
  definition, 880
  germ cell tumors, 908–910, 909f
  on gross examination, 909
  immature, 881–882, 882f
  liver, 729
  mature, 880–881, 881f
  in prepubertal testis, 909, 909f
Testicular adrenal rest tumors (TARTs), 990–991
Testicular feminization, 900–901, 900f
Testicular microliths, 905
Testicular regression syndrome (TRS), 898–899
Testicular torsion, 905f
  children, 906t
  extravaginal torsion, 905
  intravaginal torsion, 905
  pathology, 904
  types, 905
Testis
  congenital anomalies, 894
  developmental anomalies, 894
  development and disorders, 894
  disorders of genital differentiation, 897–900
  disorders of sex development, 897
  disorders of sexual determination, 901–903
  end-organ defects, 900–901
  microscopic changes, 905
  torsion of, 904
  vascular anomalies of, 895
Testosterone synthesis, defects in, 899
Tetanus, 240
Tetralogy of fallot (TOF), 539–540, 539f
TH. *See* True hermaphroditism
Thalidomide, 106, 107
Thanatophoric dysplasia, 1307
Thin glomerular basement membrane disease, 829
Third ventricle/suprasellar space tumors, 391–393
Thrombocytopenia absent radius (TAR) syndrome, 125–126
Thrombotic microangiopathy syndrome, 837–838, 838f
Thymic atrophy
  acquired hypoplasia, 1083
  DiGeorge anomaly, 1084
  SCID, 1084–1085
  thymic hypoplasia, 1083–1084
Thymic carcinomas, 1086
Thymic hypoplasia, 1083–1084
Thymus
  AIDS, 1085
  anatomy and histology, 1082–1083
  embryology, 1082
  lymphomas, 1086–1087, 1086f
  neoplastic proliferation, 1085–1086
  thymic atrophy, 1083–1085, 1083t–1084t
  thymic tumors, 1085
Thyroglossal duct cyst (TDC), 963–965, 965f, 967–968, 969f
Thyroidectomy, 978–979

Thyroid gland
    acquired disorders
        chronic lymphocytic thyroiditis, 969–970
        diffuse hyperplasia with clinical hyperthyroidism, 971
        Graves disease, 971–972
        hyperplasia, 970–971
    anatomy and physiology, 963–965
    C-cell, 964
    developmental disorders
        branchial apparatus–associated anomalies, 968
        congenital hypothyroidism, 966–967, 967t
        dysgenesis, 965–967
        dysmorphism, 965
        ectopia, 967
        hemiagenesis, 967
        thyroglossal duct cyst, 967–968
    heterotopias in, 968
    imaging, 965
    molecular pathology and cytogenetics, 973t–974t
    neoplasms, 972–979
    nodular enlargement, 969
    persistent diffuse, 969
Thyroid-stimulating hormone (TSH), 964
Thyrotrophs, 951
Thyrotropin-releasing hormone (TRH), 964
Tight cell–cell junctions formation, 325
Tiploidy, 770
Tissue triaging, 656–657, 657f
TJOF. See Trabecular juvenile ossifying fibroma (TJOF)
TOF. See Tetralogy of fallot
Topical steroids, 411
TORCH virus. See Toxoplasma, Other agents, Rubella virus, Cytomegalovirus, and Herpes simplex virus
Torsion of testis, 904
Total parenteral nutrition–related injury, 709–710
Townes-Brocks syndrome, 119
Toxic cataract, 425
Toxic injury, 906
Toxic shock syndrome, 1230
Toxoplasma, Other agents, Rubella virus, Cytomegalovirus, and Herpes simplex (TORCH) virus, 332
    infections, 332f
    titer test, 332
Toxoplasmosis, 250–252, 251f, 401, 402f
    acute, lymphadenopathy related to, 1062, 1062f
Tpit mutation, 952t
Trabecular juvenile ossifying fibroma (TJOF), 1030
Trachea
    agenesis, 450–451, 450t
    bronchus, 451
    esophageal atresia, 451–453, 453f, 453t
    stenosis, 451
    tracheobronchiomegaly, 451
    tracheoesophageal fistula, 451–453, 452f, 453f, 453t
    tracheomalacia, 451
Tracheal agenesis, 450–451, 450t

Tracheal bronchus, 451
Tracheal stenosis, 451
Tracheobronchiomegaly, 451
Tracheobronchomalacia, 454
Tracheoesophageal fistula (TEF), 451–453, 452f, 453f, 453t
Tracheomalacia, 451
Transient abnormal myelopoiesis (TAM), 1104–1105, 1105f
Transitional extravillous trophoblasts, 329
Transplant pathology
    bone marrow, 1118–1119
    heart
        biopsy findings, 316, 317, 317f
        complications, 316
        infection, 316
        outcome, 317
        rejection, 314, 314t, 315f–317f
        surgical complications, 314
        volumes and indications, 314
    immunology
        acute allograft rejection, 293
        allograft tolerance, 293–294
        antibody-mediated rejection, 292
        chronic allograft rejection, 293
    intestine
        acute rejection, 294–295, 295f
        chronic rejection, 295, 296
        complications of transplantation, 296, 296f
        gastrointestinal tract, 296–297
        graft *versus* host disease, 296–297
        hyperacute rejection, 294
        preservation injury, 294
    liver
        acute cellular rejection, 300–301, 300f
        antibody-mediated rejection, 299–300
        biliary complications, 299
        in bone marrow transplantation, 304–305, 305f
        chronic rejection, 301–302, 301f
        complications, 298, 298t
        de novo and recurrent autoimmune hepatitis, 302, 302f
        hepatic artery thrombosis, 298, 299
        idiopathic posttransplantation chronic hepatitis, 303
        indications, 297t
        posttransplant opportunistic infections, 303–304, 304f
        preservation injury, 298, 299, 299f
        recurrent hepatitis C or B, 302–303
    lung
        acute rejection, 318–319, 319f
        airway anastomotic complications, 318
        antibody-mediated rejection, 318
        chronic rejection, 319–320, 320f
        infections, 320, 320f, 321f
        primary graft dysfunction, 318
        rejection, 318, 318t
        vascular complications, 318
        volumes and indications, 317–318
    lung injury, 321
    pancreas, 306
    renal
        acute rejection, 307–310, 308t–310t
        allograft biopsies, 306
        chronic rejection, 310–311, 311f

        delayed graft function, 306–307
        hyperacute and accelerated acute rejection, 306–307
        immunosuppressive drug toxicity, 312, 313f
        polyomavirus nephropathy, 311–312, 312f
        posttransplant lymphoproliferative disorders, 313–314
        recurrent disease, 313
Transposition of great vessels, 533–534, 533f
Transverse limb defects, 1301, 1301t
Trauma
    nonaccidental, 440f
    orbital and ocular surgery after, 439
Traumatic cataract, 425
Traumatic pancreatitis, 774, 775f
TRH. See Thyrotropin-releasing hormone
Tricuspid atresia, 536, 536t
Tricuspid valve malformations
    Ebstein malformation, 536–537, 537f
    tricuspid atresia, 536
Trifunctional protein deficiency, 168
Triglyceride storage diseases, myopathy, 1278–1279, 1278f
Triple-risk model of SIDS, 357
Triploidy
    complete syndactyly, 71
    diandric triploid phenotype, 72, 72f
    digynic triploid phenotype, 72, 72f
    imprinting, 71
    second trimester abortion, 71–72, 72f
Trisomies, pancreatic pathology in, 770
Trisomy 13, 768
    congenital and developmental disorders, 1299–1300
    second trimester abortion, 71, 71f
Trisomy 18
    congenital and developmental disorders, 1299
    second trimester abortion, 70, 70f
Trisomy 21
    congenital and developmental disorders, 1300
    spontaneous abortion
        atrioventricular cardiac defect, 70
        hydrops fetalis, 69–70, 70f
        recurrence, 70
Trophoblast, 325, 326f
    coalesces, 334
    hyperplasia, 329
    tumors, 329f
    types, 328
TRS. See Testicular regression syndrome
True hermaphroditism (TH), 902–903
    causes of, 903
    gonadal tissues, 903
Truncus arteriosus, 535, 535f
    classification, 536t
TTTS. See Twin-to-twin transfusion syndrome
Tuberculosis, 240–241, 991
    clinical features, 241, 242f, 243
    laboratory diagnosis, 243
    pathology, 243
    transmission, 241
Tuberculous epididymitis, 920
Tuberous sclerosis (TS), 365, 815, 815f
Tubular adenoma, 930, 932, 932f

Tubular hypoplasia, 544
Tubulointerstitial diseases
    acute tubular necrosis, 834–835, 835f
    interstitial nephritis, 835–837
Tubulointerstitial nephritis. See Interstitial nephritis
Tufted hemangioma (TA), 1131
Tumefactive lesions, 1369
Tumors
    bladder, 856–857
    chromosome abnormalities associated with, 34
    cytogenetics associated with, 34–35
    electron microscopy in diagnosis of, 51, 52f
    immunohistochemistry, 25–26
    stomach, 592, 594f
Turcot syndrome, 390t
Turner-like mosaicism, 903
Turner syndrome, 903
    streak gonads, 872
Twin anemia polycythemia sequence (TAPS), 328
Twinning disruption, 113, 113f
Twin reversed arterial perfusion (TRAP), 73, 73f, 113, 113f, 327
Twins, 326
    dizygotic, 326
    monozygotic, 326, 327, 327f
Twin-to-twin transfusion syndrome (TTTS), 72–73, 73f, 113, 113f, 327–328
Type 1 diabetes mellitus, 784–785, 785f
Type 2 diabetes mellitus, 785
Typhlitis (neutropenic enterocolitis), 635
Tyrosinemia, 677–678, 678f, 766, 794
    type I, 160–161, 161f
    type II, 161

U
Ubiquinone deficiency, 175
UDT. See Undescended testis
Ulcerative colitis, 630–632
Ullrich congenital muscular dystrophy (UCMD), 1288
Umbilical cord (UC), 326
    accident, 347, 348f
    compromise, spontaneous abortion, 73, 73f
Undescended testis (UDT), 895–896
Undifferentiated embryonal sarcoma (UES)
    clinical features, 745–746
    gross appearance, 745f, 746
    histopathology, 745f, 747
    imaging, 745–746
    laboratory studies, 745–746
    molecular pathology, 747–748
    outcomes,–746
    pathogenesis, 744
    treatment, 746
Undifferentiated sarcoma (US), 1189
Unicystic ameloblastoma, 1048–1050, 1049f
Unilateral adrenal agenesis, 984
Unilateral renal agenesis, 804–805
Univentricular atrioventricular connection, 538, 538t
Upper rhombic lip, 366
Urachal remnants, 854, 854f
Urea cycle disorders, 691–692
Ureter disorders
    acquired lesions, 852
    agenesis, 851
    congenital malformations, 851
    duplication, 851–852
    ectopia, 852
    obstruction, 852, 852f
    ureterocele, 852
Ureterocele, 852
Urethral disorders
    acquired lesions, 854–856
    congenital lesions, 852
    fibroepithelial polyps of, 922
    tumors, 856–857
Uveal tract
    inflammation, 434
    structure, 427
    tumors of, 428–434

V
Vacuolization, 351
Vaginal plate, 869
Valproic acid embryopathy, 107–108
Vanillylmandelic acid (VMA), 1000, 1033, 1034
Varicella embryopathy, 400
Varicella infection, of lower genital tract, 874
Varicella zoster virus (VZV), 398, 399
    clinical features, 211–212, 211f
    laboratory diagnosis, 212
    pathology, 212
    prognosis and outcome, 212
    transmission, 211
Varicocele, 920
Vasa previa, 348
Vascular abnormalities
    CNS, 403–406
    eyelid, 410–411
    liver
        Budd-Chiari syndrome, 707–708, 708f
        cavernous transformation, portal vein, 707
        hepatic hemorrhage, 709
        peliosis hepatis, 708–709, 709f
        venoocclusive disease, 708, 708f
    testis, 895
Vascularized extraembryonic mesoderm, 326
Vascular lesions, 939, 953
Vascular malformations, soft tissue
    regional and diffuse syndromes associated with, 1136, 1137t
    glomangioma, 1140, 1140f
    glomus tumor, 1138
    lymphatic malformation, 1137, 1138f
    mixed venous and lymphatic malformation, 1137, 1138f
    morphologic features, 1137, 1137f
    PTEN hamartoma, 1138, 1139f
Vascular neoplasms, soft tissue
    angiosarcoma, 1134, 1135f
    composite hemangioendothelioma, 1134
    epithelioid hemangioma, 1133, 1134f
    kaposiform hemangioendothelioma, 1131, 1132f, 1133f
    kaposiform lymphangiomatosis, 1132–1133, 1133f, 1133t
    Kaposi sarcoma, 1136
    lobular capillary hemangioma–pyogenic granuloma, 1136, 1136f
    papillary intralymphatic angioendothelioma, 1134
    retiform hemangioendothelioma, 1134
    spindle cell hemangioma, 1134, 1135f
    tufted hemangioma, 1131
Vascular rings, 545
Vascular tumors, 501–503
    liver in children
        congenital hemangioma, 725
        hemangiomas, 725
        infantile hemangioma (IH), 725–729
    spleen
        angiosarcomas, 1081
        hemangiomas, 1080–1081
        immunophenotype, 1081t
        littoral cell angiomas, 1081
        lymphangiomas, 1080–1081
        myoid angioendothelioma, 1081
        peliosis, 1080–1081
Vasculitis, 569
    leukocytoclastic vasculitis, 1237, 1238f
    lymphocytic vasculitis, 1237, 1238
Vasculosyncytial membranes, 339
Vasopressin, 950
VATER association, 117–118
Vein of Galen aneurysms, 406
Velocardiofacial/DiGeorge syndrome, 93, 94t, 95
Venoocclusive disease, 708, 708f
Venous system malformations
    pulmonary venous anomalies, 527–529, 527t
    systemic venous anomalies, 527
Ventricular inflow tracts malformations, 536–539
Ventricular septal defect (VSD), 526, 529–531, 533
    pulmonary atresia with, 540
Ventricular septum malformations, 529–531, 530f, 530t, 531f, 531t
Ventricular tachycardia, 561
Verrucous hemangioma (VH), 1131
Very-long-chain acyl-CoA dehydrogenase deficiency (VLCADD, VLCAD), 168
Vesicoureteric reflux, bladder, 852
Vestibular glands, 870
Vibrio cholerae, 611
Villitis of unknown etiology, 338
    clinical correlation, 339
    pathology, 338–339
Villous capillary lesions, 339
Villous characteristics, 1430t
Villous choranigosis, 339
Villous fibrosis, 332f
Villous stromal–vascular lesions, 340
Villous stromal–vascular maldevelopment, 339
    clinical correlation, 339–340
    pathology, 339
Vimentin, 26
Viral diarrhea
    cytomegalovirus, 609–610, 610f
    enteric adenovirus, 606f, 609
    herpes simplex virus, 610
    Norwalk virus, 609
    postenteritis enteropathy, 610
    rotaviruses, 609
Viral encephalitis, 398
Viral hemorrhagic fevers, 223

Viral infections
    in adrenal gland, 991
    CNS, 398–401
    hepatitis
        hepatitis A, 695–696, 696t
        hepatitis B, 697
        hepatitis C, 697
        hepatitis D, 697
        hepatitis E, 697–698
        hepatitis G, 698
        pathology, 698–701, 698f–699f, 701t
    in neonates or infants, 201
    severe acute respiratory syndrome, 224
    skin
        herpes viruses, 1232–1233, 1232f
        human papillomavirus, 1231, 1231f
        molluscum contagiosum, 1231, 1232f
    spontaneous abortion, 65, 66
    systemic, 223–224 (See also Systemic viral infections)
Viral meningitis, 398
Viruses, identification of, by electron microscopy, 56, 57f
Visual field defects and pituitary adenoma, 954
Vitamin deficiency, 374, 1321–1322
Vitelline (omphalomesenteric) duct anomalies, 598–599, 598f
Vitrectomy, 426–427
Vitreous
    structure, 426
    surgical procedures, 426–427
von Gierke disease, 164, 674–675
von Hippel-Lindau (VHL) syndrome, 390t, 767, 768, 793, 815–816, 956t
Vulvar mucous cysts, 876

W

Wagenmann-Froboese syndrome, 956t
WAGR syndrome, 904
Walker-Warburg syndrome (WWS), 363, 1289
Warfarin, 108
Warthin-Starry silver stains, 875
Waterhouse-Friderichsen syndrome (WFS), 992, 992f
Well-differentiated fetal HB (WDFHB), 734f, 735
Well syndrome. See Eosinophilic cellulitis
Wermer syndrome, 955t
Werner syndrome, 956t
West Nile virus (WNV) infection, 224
WFS. See Waterhouse-Friderichsen syndrome
Williams-Campbell syndrome, 487
Williams syndrome, 115
Wilms tumor, 494. See also Nephroblastoma
    defects in, 904
Wilson disease, 689–691
Wolcott-Rallison syndrome, 793–794
Wolffian ducts, differentiation of, 894
Wolff-Parkinson-White (WPW) syndrome, 554
Wolman disease, 154–155, 155f, 678, 679t, 985–986, 985f

X

Xanthogranulomatous inflammation, 953
Xanthoma, 1364
Xeroderma pigmentosum, 413
X-linked adrenoleukodystrophy, 181, 986, 986f
X-linked mutations, 127–128
X-linked syndrome (IPEX), 776
X-linked vacuolar cardiomyopathy, 158
XX male and XY female syndrome
    acquired abnormalities and lesions, 904–906
    carcinoid tumor, 917
    defects in Wilms tumor, 904
    germ cell tumors, 906
        embryonal carcinoma, 911, 912f
        epidermoid cyst, 910–911, 910f
        intratubular germ cell neoplasia, unclassified type, 911, 912f
        mixed germ cell tumor, 912–913
        seminoma, 911–912
        teratoma, 908–910, 909f
        yolk sac tumor, 907–908, 908f
    gonadoblastoma, 916–917
    hematopoietic origin of tumors, 917–918
    neoplasms of testis, 906
    nephroblastoma, 917
    sex cord–stromal tumors
        juvenile granulosa cell tumor, 915–196, 916f–917f
        Leydig cell tumor, 913–914, 913f
        Sertoli cell tumor, 914, 914f–915f

Y

Yersinia, 612
Yolk sac rupture sequence, 111
Yolk sac tumor (YST), 510, 879–880, 879f
    germ cell tumors, 907–908, 908f
    ovarian germ cell tumors, 883–884, 883f, 884f
    Schiller-Duval bodies, 883, 883f

Z

Zellweger syndrome, 115–116, 115t, 181, 371
Zona reticularis, 980
Zonular apparatus, 426
Zonular congenital cataract, 424
Zonules, 423
Zygomycosis, 615